STANDARD EDITION

2011

ICD-9-CM

VOLUMES 1, 2, & 3

FOR HOSPITALS

STANDARD EDITION

2011

ICD-9-CM

VOLUMES 1, 2, & 3

FOR HOSPITALS

Carol J. Buck
MS, CPC, CPC-H, CCS-P

Program Director, Retired
Medical Secretary Programs
Northwest Technical College
East Grand Forks, Minnesota

SAUNDERS
ELSEVIER

AMA
AMERICAN
MEDICAL
ASSOCIATION

3251 Riverport Lane
St. Louis, Missouri 63043

2011 ICD-9-CM FOR HOSPITALS, VOLUMES 1, 2, & 3,
STANDARD EDITION

ISBN: 978-1-4377-1191-2

Notices

Knowledge and best practice in this field are constantly changing. As new research and experience broaden
our understanding, changes in research methods, professional practices, or medical treatment may become
necessary.

Practitioners and researchers must always rely on their own experience and knowledge in evaluating and
using any information, methods, compounds, or experiments described herein. In using such information
or methods they should be mindful of their own safety and the safety of others, including parties for whom
they have a professional responsibility.

With respect to any drug or pharmaceutical products identified, readers are advised to check the most
current information provided (i) on procedures featured or (ii) by the manufacturer of each product to be
administered, to verify the recommended dose or formula, the method and duration of administration, and
contraindications. It is the responsibility of practitioners, relying on their own experience and knowledge
of their patients, to make diagnoses, to determine dosages and the best treatment for each individual
patient, and to take all appropriate safety precautions.

To the fullest extent of the law, neither the Publisher nor the authors, contributors, or editors, assume
any liability for any injury and/or damage to persons or property as a matter of products liability,
negligence or otherwise, or from any use or operation of any methods, products, instructions, or ideas
contained in the material herein.

ISBN: 978-1-4377-1191-2

Publisher: Michael S. Ledbetter
Developmental Editor: Jenna Johnson
Publishing Services Manager: Pat Joiner-Myers

Printed in the United States of America

Last digit is the print number: 9 8 7 6 5 4 3 2 1

COLLABORATORS

Technical Collaborators:

Jacqueline Klitz Grass, MA, CPC
Coding Specialist
Grand Forks, North Dakota

Nancy Maguire, ACS, CRT, PCS, FCS, HCS-D, APC, AFC
Physician Consultant for Auditing and Education
Universal City, Texas

Technical Assistant:

Judith Neppel, RN, MS
Executive Director
Minnesota Rural Health Association
University of Minnesota, Crookston
Crookston, Minnesota

Hospital Reimbursement Specialist:

Lynn-Marie D. Wozniak, MS, RHIT
Product Manager
New York

Elsevier/MC Strategies Revenue Cycle, Coding and Compliance Staff

"Experts in providing e-learning on revenue cycle, coding and compliance."

Deborah Neville, RHIA, CCS-P
Director
Minnesota

Elizabeth Wheeler, RHIA, CCS-P
Product Manager
New York

Lynn-Marie D. Wozniak, MS, RHIT
Product Manager
New York

Therese M. Jorwic, MPH, RHIA, CCS, CCS-P, FAHIMA
Product Specialist
Illinois

Sandra L. Macica, MS, RHIA, CCS, ROCC
Product Specialist
New York

CONTENTS

2011 Inpatient Procedures will be posted on the companion website CodingUpdates.com when available.

Part VI contains 2010 MS-DRGs, Version 27.0, Appendixes A, B, D, and the Procedure Code Tables from Appendix E and are posted on the companion website CodingUpdates.com.

GUIDE TO USING THE 2011 ICD-9-CM FOR HOSPITALS, VOLUMES 1, 2, & 3, STANDARD EDITION

Medical coding has long been a part of the health care profession. Through the years medical coding systems have become more complex and extensive. Today, medical coding is an intricate and immense process that is present in every health care setting. The increased use of electronic submissions for health care services only increases the need for coders who understand the coding process.

2011 ICD-9-CM for Hospitals, Volumes 1, 2, & 3, Standard Edition was developed to help meet the needs of coding professionals at all levels by offering a comprehensive coding text at a reasonable price. This text combines the official coding guidelines and all three volumes of the ICD-9-CM in one book.

All material strictly adheres to the latest government versions available at the time of printing.

ILLUSTRATIONS AND ITEMS

The ICD-9-CM, Volume 1, Tabular List contains illustrations, pictures, and items to assist you in understanding difficult terminology, diseases/conditions, or coding in a specific category. Items are always printed in ▩▩▩▩ ink so the added material is not mistaken for official notations or instructions. ▩▩▩▩▩ ink is used for other annotations in the text. Your ideas on what other descriptions or illustrations should be in future editions of this text are always appreciated.

Annotated

Throughout the volumes, revisions, additions, and deleted codes or words are indicated by the following symbols:

- ◂▥▥ **Revised:** Revisions within the line or code from the previous edition are indicated by the arrow.

- ◂ **New:** Additions to the previous edition are indicated by the triangle.

- ~~deleted~~ **Deleted:** Deletions from the previous edition are struck through.

- ▩▩▩ **Omit code:** No code is to be assigned. The words *omit code* are highlighted in ▩▩▩ for easier reference.

ICD-9-CM, Volume 1, Tabular List Symbols

- ● **Unacceptable Principal Diagnosis:** These codes have a black dot before them and give additional information or describe the circumstances affecting the health care encounter but are unacceptable as principal diagnosis in the FY2010 *Definitions of Medicare Code Edits* (MCE) for inpatient admission.

- ● **Use Additional Digit(s):** The colored dot cautions that the code requires additional digit(s) to ensure the greatest specificity.

- OGCR **OGCR:** The *ICD-9-CM Official Guidelines for Coding and Reporting* symbol indicates the placement of a portion of a guideline as that guideline pertains to the code by which it is located. The complete OGCR are located in Part I.

  Coding Clinic identifies the year, quarter, and page number that presents information about an ICD-9-CM code in the American Hospital Association's *Coding Clinic for ICD-9-CM*.

- ▭ **Excludes:** Terms following the word "Excludes" are to be coded elsewhere and are highlighted in ▭ for easier reference.

Includes: This note appears immediately to further define or give examples of the content of codes and is highlighted in ▒▒▒ for easier reference.

Use additional: The words indicate an instructional note that another code may be needed and are highlighted in ▒▒▒ for easier reference.

Code first: The words indicate an instructional note that directs the coder to sequence the underlying condition before the manifestation. "Code first" is highlighted in ▒▒▒ for easier reference.

Omit code: No code is to be assigned. The words "omit code" are highlighted in ▒▒▒ for easier reference.

ICD-9-CM, Volume 3, Tabular List Symbols

● **Use Additional Digit(s):** The colored dot cautions that the code requires additional digit(s).

▭ **Excludes:** Terms following the word "Excludes" are to be coded elsewhere and are highlighted in ▭ for easier reference.

Includes: This note appears immediately under a code to further define or give examples of the content of codes and is highlighted in ▒▒▒ for easier reference.

Use additional: The words indicate an instructional note that another code may be needed, and they are highlighted in ▒▒▒ for easier reference.

Code also: This identifies synchronous procedures, which require reporting of individual components of a procedure.

Omit code: No code is to be assigned. The words are highlighted in ▒▒▒ for easier reference.

SYMBOLS AND CONVENTIONS

ICD-9-CM, Volumes 1, 2, & 3
Symbols Used to Identify New, Revised, or Deleted Material

Volume 1, Tabular List

237.70   **Neurofibromatosis, unspecified** ◄

Indicates **new** information or a new code.

V01.1   **Cholera** ◄▥

Indicates a **revision** within the line or code.

244.3   Other iatrogenic hypothyroidism
          Hypothyroidism resulting from:
              P-aminosalicylic acid [PAS]
              Phenylbutazone
              Resorcinol
              Iatrogenic hypothyroidism NOS
          Use additional E code to identify drug

Indicates **deleted** words/codes in the current edition.

Volume 2, Alphabetic Index

Tachypnea 786.06
    hysterical 300.11 ◄▥
    newborn (idiopathic) (transitory) 770.6 ◄

Congestion, congestive (chronic) (passive) ◄

Indicates a **revision** within the line or code.

Indicates **new** information or a new code.

Indicates a **deleted** entry in the current edition.

Volume 3, Procedures, Index

Biopsy
    peritoneum ◄▥
    closed 54.24 ◄

Lung (complete) (with mediastinal dissection) 32.5 32.59 ◄

Indicates a **revision** within the line or code.

Indicates **new** information or code.

Indicates a **deleted** entry in the current edition.

Volume 3, Procedures, Tabular List

00.19   **Disruption of blood brain barrier via infusion [BBBD]** ◄▥
              Infusion of substance to disrupt blood brain barrier ◄

00.74   **Hip replacement bearing surface, metal-on-polyethylene**

Indicates a **revision** within the line or code.

Indicates **new** information or a new code.

Indicates a **deleted** entry in the current edition.

Codes or index entries are for purposes of illustration only and may not be current.

Symbols for Volume 1, Tabular List

Use Additional Digit(s): The colored dot cautions you that the code requires additional digit(s) to ensure the greatest specificity.

→ ● **237.7   Neurofibromatosis**
            von Recklinghausen's disease

Unacceptable Principal Diagnosis: These codes have a black dot before them and give additional information or describe the circumstances affecting the health care encounter but are unacceptable as principal diagnosis in the FY2010 *Definitions of Medicare Code Edits* (MCE).

→ ● **284.2   Myelophthisis**

007.4   Cryptosporidiosis
          Coding Clinic: 1997, Q4, P30-31 ←

Indicates a Volume 1 reference in the American Hospital Association *Coding Clinic for ICD-9-CM.*

Codes or index entries are for purposes of illustration only and may not be current.

Conventions for Volume 1, Tabular List
2. NEOPLASMS (140–239)

Notes define terms or give coding instructions.

Notes

1. Content

   This chapter contains the following broad groups:

   140–195   Malignant neoplasms, stated or presumed to be primary, of specified sites, except of lymphatic and hematopoietic tissue

510   **Empyema**

Use additional code to identify infectious organism (041.0–041.9)

"Use additional" directs you to assign an additional code to give a more complete picture of the diagnosis.

Code first: The words indicate an instructional note that directs the coder to sequence the underlying condition (etiology) before the manifestation.

366.4   **Cataract associated with other disorders**

   366.41   *Diabetic cataract*

   Code first diabetes (249.5, 250.5)

A code with this note may be principal (first listed) if no causal condition is applicable or known.

428   **Heart failure**

Code, if applicable, heart failure due to hypertension first (402.0–402.9, with fifth-digit 1 or 404.0–404.9 with fifth-digit 1 or 3)

Terms following the word "Excludes" are to be coded elsewhere. The term "Excludes" means "Do Not Code Here."

150.2   **Abdominal esophagus**

   Excludes   *adenocarcinoma (151.0)*

   cardio-esophageal junction (151.0)

The "Includes" note appears to further define, or give example of, the contents of the code.

087   **Relapsing fever**

   Includes   recurrent fever

Codes or index entries are for purposes of illustration only and may not be current.

474   **Chronic disease of tonsils and adenoids**

"and" indicates a code that can be assigned if either of the conditions is present or if both of the conditions are present.

366.4   **Cataract associated with other disorders**

"with" indicates a code that can be used only if both conditions are present.

NEC means Not Elsewhere Classifiable and is to be used only when the information at hand specifies a condition but there is no more specific code for that condition.

244.8   **Other specified acquired hypothyroidism**
        Secondary hypothyroidism NEC

Bold type is used for all codes and titles.

159.0   **Intestinal tract, part unspecified**
        Intestine NOS

NOS means Not Otherwise Specified and is the equivalent of "unspecified."

426.89   **Other**
        Dissociation:
            atrioventricular [AV]

Brackets are used to enclose synonyms, alternative wording, or explanatory phrases.

158.8   **Specified parts of peritoneum**
        Cul-de-sac (of Douglas)
        Mesentery

Parentheses are used to enclose supplementary words that may be present or absent in the statement of a disease without affecting the code.

628.4   **Of cervical or vaginal origin**
        Infertility associated with:
            anomaly of cervical mucus
            congenital structural anomaly

A colon is used after an incomplete term that needs one or more of the modifiers that follow in order to make it assignable to a given category.

Codes or index entries are for purposes of illustration only and may not be current.

Conventions for Volume 2, Alphabetic Index

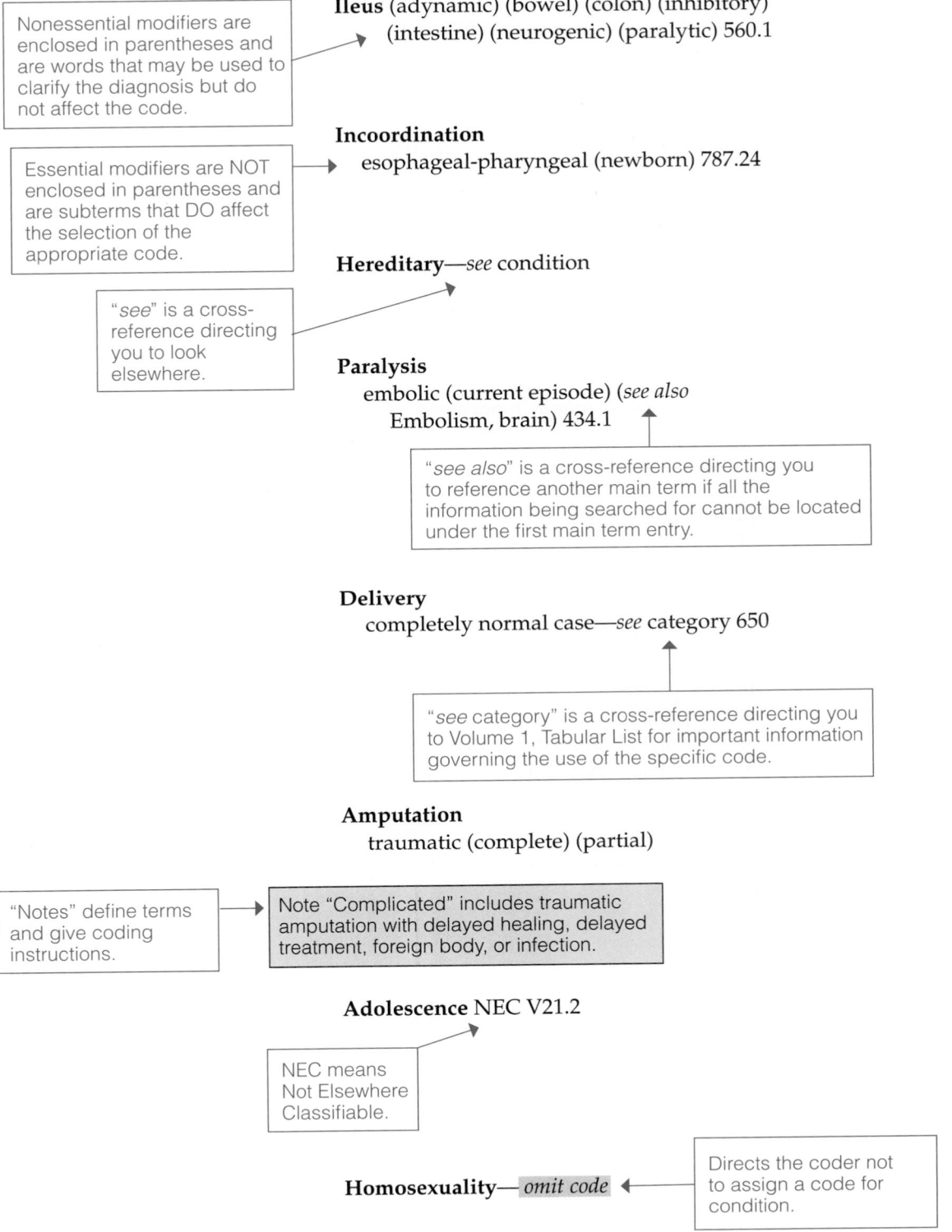

Ileus (adynamic) (bowel) (colon) (inhibitory) (intestine) (neurogenic) (paralytic) 560.1

Nonessential modifiers are enclosed in parentheses and are words that may be used to clarify the diagnosis but do not affect the code.

Incoordination
esophageal-pharyngeal (newborn) 787.24

Essential modifiers are NOT enclosed in parentheses and are subterms that DO affect the selection of the appropriate code.

Hereditary—*see* condition

"*see*" is a cross-reference directing you to look elsewhere.

Paralysis
embolic (current episode) (*see also* Embolism, brain) 434.1

"*see also*" is a cross-reference directing you to reference another main term if all the information being searched for cannot be located under the first main term entry.

Delivery
completely normal case—*see* category 650

"*see* category" is a cross-reference directing you to Volume 1, Tabular List for important information governing the use of the specific code.

Amputation
traumatic (complete) (partial)

"Notes" define terms and give coding instructions.

Note "Complicated" includes traumatic amputation with delayed healing, delayed treatment, foreign body, or infection.

Adolescence NEC V21.2

NEC means Not Elsewhere Classifiable.

Homosexuality—*omit code*

Directs the coder not to assign a code for condition.

Codes or index entries are for purposes of illustration only and may not be current.

Conventions for Volume 3, Procedures, Index

Arthrotomy 80.10

as operative approach—*omit code*

> "*omit code*" identifies procedures or services that are included in another larger procedure or service. For example, an incision that is part of the main surgical procedure is not coded separately.

Ileal

bladder

closed 57.87 *[45.51]*

> For some operative procedures it is necessary to record the individual components of the procedure. These procedures are termed **"synchronous procedures"** and are listed together in the Index. The codes are sequenced in the same order as displayed in the Index.

Operation

Thompson

cleft lip repair 27.54

correction of lymphedema 40.9

quadricepsplasty 83.86

> Eponyms are operations named for people and are listed in the Index both under the eponym and under the term "Operation."

Thompson

cleft lip repair 27.54

correction of lymphedema 40.9

quadricepsplasty 83.86

Volume 3, Index to Procedures, also contains "*see*," "*see also*," "*see* category," "essential modifiers," "nonessential modifiers," "notes," NEC, and NOS as in Volume 2, Alphabetic Index.

Codes or index entries are for purposes of illustration only and may not be current.

Symbols for Volume 3, Procedures, Tabular List

Use Additional Digit(s):
The colored dot cautions that the code requires additional digit(s) to ensure the greatest specificity.

● **31.9   Other operations on larynx and trachea**

00.0   Therapeutic ultrasound
▶ Coding Clinic: 2002, Q4, P90-91

Indicates a Volume 3 reference in the American Hospital Association *Coding Clinic for ICD-9-CM.*

Conventions for Volume 3, Procedures, Tabular List

The "Includes" note appears to further define, or give example of, the contents of the code.

88.4   Arteriography using contrast material ◀

Bold type is used for all codes and titles.

▶ **Includes** angiography of arteries
    arterial puncture for injection of contrast material
    radiography of arteries (by fluoroscopy)
    retrograde arteriography

Terms following the word "Excludes" are to be coded elsewhere. The term means "Do Not Code Here."

▶ **Excludes** *arteriography using:*
    radioisotopes or radionuclides (92.01–92.19)

For some operative procedures it is necessary to record the individual components of the procedure. These procedures are termed "synchronous procedures."

45.5   Isolation of intestinal segment

▶ Code also any synchronous:
    anastomosis other than end-to-end (45.90–45.94)
    enterostomy (46.10–46.39)

Codes or index entries are for purposes of illustration only and may not be current.

Symbols for Volume 3, Procedures, Tabular List

Use Additional Digit(s):
The colored dot cautions that the code requires additional digit(s) to ensure the greatest specificity.

● **31.9**   Other operations on larynx and trachea

Indicates a Volume 3 reference in the American Hospital Association *Coding Clinic for ICD-9-CM.*

00.0   **Therapeutic ultrasound**
Coding Clinic: 2002, Q4, P90-91

Conventions for Volume 3, Procedures, Tabular List

The "Includes" note appears to further define, or give example of, the contents of the code.

Bold type is used for all codes and titles.

88.4   **Arteriography using contrast material**
Includes angiography of arteries
arterial puncture for injection of contrast material
radiography of arteries (by fluoroscopy)
retrograde arteriography

Terms following the word "Excludes" are to be coded elsewhere. The term means "Do Not Code Here."

Excludes *arteriography using:*
radioisotopes or radionuclides (92.01–92.19)

For some operative procedures it is necessary to record the individual components of the procedure. These procedures are termed "synchronous procedures."

45.5   **Isolation of intestinal segment**
Code also any synchronous:
anastomosis other than end-to-end (45.90–45.94)
enterostomy (46.10–46.39)

Codes or index entries are for purposes of illustration only and may not be current.

GUIDE TO THE 2011 ICD-9-CM UPDATES

VOLUME 1 CHANGES EFFECTIVE OCTOBER 1, 2010

1. INFECTIOUS AND PARASITIC DISEASES (001-139)

Revise   **Excludes** *influenza (487.0-487.8, <u>488.01-488.19</u>)*

008 Intestinal infections due to other organisms

    008.8 Other organism, not elsewhere classified

Revise   **Excludes** *influenza with involvement of gastrointestinal tract (487.8, <u>488.09, 488.19</u>)*

189 Malignant neoplasm of kidney and other and unspecified urinary organs

Revise   **Excludes** *malignant carcinoid tumor of kidney (<u>209.24</u>)*

225 Benign neoplasm of brain and other parts of nervous system

Revise   **Excludes** *neurofibromatosis (237.7<u>0-237.79</u>)*

237 Neoplasm of uncertain behavior of endocrine glands and nervous system

    237.7 Neurofibromatosis

Delete   ~~von Recklinghausen's disease~~

New code   **237.73 Schwannomatosis**

New code   **237.79 Other neurofibromatosis**

244 Acquired hypothyroidism

    244.2 Iodine hypothyroidism

Add   **Excludes** *hypothyroidism resulting from administration of radioactive iodine (244.1)*

251 Other disorders of pancreatic internal secretion

    251.3 Postsurgical hypoinsulinemia

       Use additional code to identify (any associated):

Revise   acquired absence of pancreas (V88.11-V88.12)

275 Disorders of mineral metabolism

    275.0 Disorders of iron metabolism

Delete   ~~Bronzed diabetes~~

Delete   ~~Hemochromatosis~~

Delete   ~~Pigmentary cirrhosis (of liver)~~

New code   **275.01 Hereditary hemochromatosis**
       Bronzed diabetes
       Pigmentary cirrhosis (of liver)
       Primary (hereditary) hemochromatosis

New code   **275.02 Hemochromatosis due to repeated red blood cell transfusions**
       Iron overload due to repeated red blood cell transfusions
       Transfusion (red blood cell) associated hemochromatosis

New code   **275.03 Other hemochromatosis**
       Hemochromatosis NOS

New code   **275.09 Other disorders of iron metabolism**

276 Disorders of fluid, electrolyte, and acid-base balance

    276.6 Fluid overload

Delete   ~~Fluid retention~~

New code   **276.61 Transfusion associated circulatory overload**
       Fluid overload due to transfusion (blood) (blood components)
       TACO

New code   **276.69 Other fluid overload**
       Fluid retention

277 Other and unspecified disorders of metabolism

    277.7 Dysmetabolic syndrome X

       Use additional code for associated manifestation, such as:

Revise   obesity (278.00-278.03)

278 Overweight, obesity and other hyperalimentation

    278.0 Overweight and obesity

New code   **278.03 Obesity hypoventilation syndrome**
       Pickwickian syndrome

279 Disorders involving the immune mechanism

Add   Use additional code for associated manifestations

285 Other and unspecified anemias

    285.2 Anemia of chronic disease

      285.22 Anemia in neoplastic disease

Add   **Excludes** *aplastic anemia due to antineoplastic chemotherapy (284.89)*

287 Purpura and other hemorrhagic conditions

    287.4 Secondary thrombocytopenia

Delete   ~~Posttransfusion purpura~~

Delete   ~~Thrombocytopenia (due to):~~

Delete   ~~dilutional~~

Delete   ~~drugs~~

Delete   ~~extracorporeal circulation of blood~~

Delete   ~~massive blood transfusion~~

Delete   ~~platelet alloimmunization~~

New code   **287.41 Posttransfusion purpura**
       Posttransfusion purpura from whole blood (fresh) or blood products
       PTP

New code   **287.49 Other secondary thrombocytopenia**
       Thrombocytopenia (due to):
       dilutional
       drugs
       extracorporeal circulation of blood
       massive blood transfusion
       platelet alloimmunization
       secondary NOS

307 Special symptoms or syndromes, not elsewhere classified

Revise — **307.0** ~~Stuttering~~ Adult onset fluency disorder

Add — **Excludes** *childhood onset fluency disorder (315.35)*

Revise — *~~stuttering~~ (fluency disorder) due to late effect of cerebrovascular accident (438.14)*

Add — *fluency disorder in conditions classified elsewhere (784.52)*

307.7 Encopresis

Revise — **Excludes** *encopresis of unspecified cause (787.60-787.63)*

308 Acute reaction to stress

Add — **Includes** combat and operational stress reaction

315 Specific delays in development

315.3 Developmental speech or language disorder

New code — **315.35 Childhood onset fluency disorder**
Cluttering NOS
Stuttering NOS
Excludes *adult onset fluency disorder (307.0)*
fluency disorder due to late effect of cerebrovascular accident (438.14)
fluency disorder in conditions classified elsewhere (784.52)

315.39 Other

Delete — **Excludes** *~~stammering and stuttering (307.0)~~*

337 Disorders of the autonomic nervous system

337.3 Autonomic dysreflexia

Use additional code to identify the cause, such as:

Revise — fecal impaction (560.32)

345 Epilepsy and recurrent seizures

Delete — **Excludes** *~~progressive myoclonic epilepsy (333.2)~~*

360 Disorders of the globe

360.5 Retained (old) intraocular foreign body, magnetic

Add — Use additional code to identify foreign body (V90.11)

360.6 Retained (old) intraocular foreign body, nonmagnetic

Add — Use additional code to identify foreign body (V90.01-V90.10, V90.12, V90.2-V90.9)

365 Glaucoma

365.4 Glaucoma associated with congenital anomalies, dystrophies, and systemic syndromes

365.44 Glaucoma associated with systemic syndromes

Code first associated disease, as:
neurofibromatosis

Revise — (237.70-237.79)

374 Other disorder of eyelids

374.8 Other disorders of eyelid

374.86 Retained foreign body of eyelid

Add — Use additional code to identify foreign body (V90.01-V90.9)

376 Disorder of the orbit

376.6 Retained (old) foreign body following penetrating wound of orbit

Add — Use additional code to identify foreign body (V90.01-V90.9)

382 Suppurative and unspecified otitis media

382.0 Acute suppurative otitis media

382.02 Acute suppurative otitis media in diseases classified elsewhere

Code first underlying disease, as:
influenza (487.8, 488.09, 488.19)

Revise —

385 Other disorders of middle ear and mastoid

385.8 Other disorders of middle ear and mastoid

385.83 Retained foreign body of middle ear

Add — Use additional code to identify foreign body (V90.01-V90.9)

403 Hypertensive chronic kidney disease

Revise — any condition classifiable to 585 and 587 with any condition classifiable to 401

416 Chronic pulmonary heart disease

416.0 Primary pulmonary hypertension

Add — **Excludes** *pulmonary hypertension NOS (416.8)*

Add — *secondary pulmonary hypertension (416.8)*

416.8 Other chronic pulmonary heart diseases

Add — Pulmonary hypertension NOS

422 Acute myocarditis

422.0 Acute myocarditis in diseases classified elsewhere

Code first underlying disease, as:
myocarditis (acute):

Revise — influenzal (487.8, 488.09, 488.19)

428 Heart failure

428.0 Congestive heart failure, unspecified

Revise — **Excludes** *fluid overload NOS (276.69)*

438 Late effects of cerebrovascular disease

438.1 Speech and language deficits

438.14 Fluency disorder

Revise — Stuttering due to late effect of cerebrovascular accident

441 Aortic aneurysm and dissection

Add — **Excludes** *aortic ectasia (447.70-447.73)*

447 Other disorders of arteries and arterioles

447.7 Aortic ectasia

New sub — Ectasis aorta
Excludes *aortic aneurysm and dissection (441.00-441.9)*

New code — **447.70 Aortic ectasia, unspecified site**
New code — **447.71 Thoracic aortic ectasia**
New code — **447.72 Abdominal aortic ectasia**
New code — **447.73 Thoracoabdominal aortic ectasia**

453 Other venous embolism and thrombosis

453.5 Chronic venous embolism and thrombosis of deep vessels of lower extremity

453.51 Chronic venous embolism and thrombosis of deep vessels of proximal lower extremity

Add — Femoral
Add — Iliac
Add — Popliteal
Add — Thigh
Add — Upper leg NOS

	453.52 Chronic venous embolism and thrombosis of deep vessels of distal lower extremity
Add	Calf
Add	Lower leg NOS
Add	Peroneal
Add	Tibial
	453.6 Venous embolism and thrombosis of superficial vessels of lower extremity
Add	Use additional code, if applicable, for associated long-term (current) use of anticoagulants (V58.61)

ACUTE RESPIRATORY INFECTIONS (460-466)

Revise	**Excludes** *pneumonia and influenza (480.0-488.19)*

462 Acute pharyngitis

	Excludes *that specified as (due to):*
Revise	*influenza (487.1, 488.02, 488.12)*

464 Acute laryngitis and tracheitis

Revise	**Excludes** *that associated with influenza (487.1, 488.02, 488.12)*

464.0 Acute laryngitis

Revise	**Excludes** *influenzal laryngitis (487.1, 488.02, 488.12)*

465 Acute upper respiratory infections of multiple or unspecified sites

Revise	**Excludes** *upper respiratory infection due to: influenza (487.1, 488.02, 488.12)*

480 Viral pneumonia

480.8 Pneumonia due to other virus not elsewhere classified

Delete	**Excludes** ~~*influenza with pneumonia, any form (487.0)*~~

484 Pneumonia in infectious diseases classified elsewhere

Delete	**Excludes** ~~*influenza with pneumonia, any form (487.0)*~~

486 Pneumonia, organism unspecified

Delete	**Excludes** ~~*influenza with pneumonia, any form (487.0)*~~

487 Influenza

Revise	**Excludes** *influenza due to novel 2009 H1N1 [swine] influenza virus (488.11-488.19)*
Revise	*influenza due to identified avian influenza virus (488.01-488.09)*
Revise	*influenza due to identified novel H1N1 influenza virus (488.11-488.19)*

487.1 With other respiratory manifestations

Add	Influenza NEC

488 Influenza due to certain identified influenza viruses

488.0 Influenza due to identified avian influenza virus

New code	**488.01 Influenza due to identified avian influenza virus with pneumonia**
	Avian influenzal:
	bronchopneumonia
	pneumonia
	Influenza due to identified avian influenza virus with pneumonia, any form
	Use additional code to identify the type of pneumonia (480.0-480.9, 481, 482.0-482.9, 483.0-483.8, 485)

New code	**488.02 Influenza due to identified avian influenza virus with other respiratory manifestations**
	Avian influenzal:
	laryngitis
	pharyngitis
	respiratory infection (acute) (upper)
	Identified avian influenza NOS
New code	**488.09 Influenza due to identified avian influenza virus with other manifestations**
	Avian influenza with involvement of gastrointestinal tract
	Encephalopathy due to identified avian influenza
	Excludes *"intestinal flu" [viral gastroenteritis] (008.8)*

488.1 Influenza due to identified novel H1N1 influenza virus

New code	**488.11 Influenza due to identified novel H1N1 influenza virus with pneumonia**
	Influenza due to identified novel H1N1 with pneumonia, any form
	Novel H1N1 influenzal:
	bronchopneumonia
	pneumonia
	Use additional code to identify the type of pneumonia (480.0-480.9, 481, 482.0-482.9, 483.0-483.8, 485)
New code	**488.12 Influenza due to identified novel H1N1 influenza virus with other respiratory manifestations**
	Novel H1N1 influenza NOS
	Novel H1N1 influenzal:
	laryngitis
	pharyngitis
	respiratory infection (acute) (upper)
New code	**488.19 Influenza due to identified novel H1N1 influenza virus with other manifestations**
	Encephalopathy due to identified novel H1N1 influenza
	Novel H1N1 influenza with involvement of gastrointestinal tract
	Excludes *"intestinal flu" [viral gastroenteritis] (008.8)*

514 Pulmonary congestion and hypostasis

Revise	**Excludes** *hypostatic pneumonia due to or specified as a specific type of pneumonia - code to the type of pneumonia (480.0-480.9, 481, 482.0-482.9, 483.0-483.8, 485, 486, 487.0, 488.01, 488.11)*

516 Other alveolar and parietoalveolar pneumonopathy

516.1 Idiopathic pulmonary hemosiderosis

Revise	*Code first underlying disease (275.01-275.09)*
Add	**Excludes** *acute idiopathic pulmonary hemorrhage in infants [AIPHI] (786.31)*

552 Other hernia of abdominal cavity, with obstruction, but without mention of gangrene

    552.8 Hernia of other specified sites, with obstruction

Delete | Excludes | ~~hernia due to adhesion with obstruction (560.81)~~

560 Intestinal obstruction without mention of hernia

    560.3 Impaction of intestine

New code   560.32 Fecal impaction

         | Excludes | *constipation (564.00-564.09)* *incomplete defecation (787.61)*

    560.39 Other

Delete   ~~Fecal impaction~~

564 Functional digestive disorders, not elsewhere classified

    564.0 Constipation

Add | Excludes | *fecal impaction (560.32)*
Add   *incomplete defecation (787.61)*

569 Other disorders of intestine

    569.4 Other specified disorders of rectum and anus

        569.43 Anal sphincter tear (healed) (old)

Revise   Use additional code for any associated fecal incontinence (787.60-787.63)

        569.49 Other

Add   Use additional code for associated fecal incontinence (787.60-787.63)

Delete | Excludes | ~~incontinence of sphincter ani (787.6)~~

572 Liver abscess and sequelae of chronic liver disease

    572.3 Portal hypertension

Add   Use additional code for any associated complications, such as: portal hypertensive gastropathy (537.89)

583 Nephritis and nephropathy, not specified as acute or chronic

    583.6 With lesion of renal cortical necrosis

Revise   Nephropathy NOS with (renal) cortical necrosis

618 Genital prolapse

    618.0 Prolapse of vaginal walls without mention of uterine prolapse

        618.04 Rectocele

Add   Use additional code for associated fecal incontinence (787.60-787.63)

621 Disorders of uterus, not elsewhere classified

    621.4 Hematometra

Revise | Excludes | *that in congenital anomaly (752.2-752.39)*

626 Disorders of menstruation and other abnormal bleeding from female genital tract

Add | Excludes | *precocious puberty (259.1)*

629 Other disorders of female genital organs

    629.8 Other specified disorders of female genital organs

Revise   629.81 ~~Habitual aborter~~ Recurrent pregnancy loss without current pregnancy

Revise | Excludes | ~~habitual aborter~~ *recurrent pregnancy loss with current pregnancy (646.3)*

646 Other complications of pregnancy, not elsewhere classified

Revise   646.3 ~~Habitual aborter~~ Recurrent pregnancy loss

649 Other conditions or status of the mother complicating pregnancy, childbirth, or the puerperium

    649.1 Obesity complicating pregnancy, childbirth, or the puerperium

Revise   Use additional code to identify the obesity (278.00-278.03)

651 Multiple gestation

Add   Use additional code to specify placenta status (V91.00-V91.99)

664 Trauma to perineum and vulva during delivery

    664.8 Other specified trauma to perineum and vulva

Add   Periurethral trauma

665 Other obstetrical trauma

    665.5 Other injury to pelvic organs

Add | Excludes | *periurethral trauma (664.8)*

670 Major puerperal infection

    670.2 Puerperal sepsis

Add   Use additional code to identify severe sepsis (995.92) and any associated acute organ dysfunction, if applicable

671 Venous complications in pregnancy and the puerperium

    671.2 Superficial thrombophlebitis

Add   Use additional code to identify the superficial thrombophlebitis (453.6, 453.71, 453.81)

709 Other disorders of skin and subcutaneous tissue

    709.4 Foreign body granuloma of skin and subcutaneous tissue

Add   Use additional code to identify foreign body (V90.01-V90.9)

713 Arthropathy associated with other disorders classified elsewhere

    713.0 Arthropathy associated with other endocrine and metabolic disorders

Revise   *Code first* underlying disease, as: hemochromatosis (275.01-275.09)

721 Spondylosis and allied disorders

    721.4 Thoracic or lumbar spondylosis with myelopathy

        721.42 Lumbar region

Delete   ~~Spondylogenic compression of lumbar spinal cord~~

724 Other and unspecified disorders of *back*

    724.0 *Spinal* stenosis, *other than cervical*

Revise   **724.02 Lumbar region, without neurogenic claudication**

Add   Lumbar region NOS

New code   **724.03 Lumbar region, with neurogenic claudication**

728 Disorders of muscle, ligament, and fascia

    728.8 Other disorders of muscle, ligament, and fascia

        728.82 Foreign body granuloma of muscle

Add   Use additional code to identify foreign body (V90.01-V90.9)

729 Other disorders of soft tissues

    729.6 Residual foreign body in soft tissue

Add   Use additional code to identify foreign body (V90.01-V90.9)

737 Curvature of spine

    737.4 Curvature of spine associated with other conditions

        Code first *associated condition, as:*

Revise   neurofibromatosis (237.70-237.79)

742 Other congenital anomalies of nervous system

    742.8 Other specified anomalies of nervous system

Revise   Excludes *neurofibromatosis (237.70-237.79)*

748 Congenital anomalies of respiratory system

    748.1 Other anomalies of nose

        Congenital:

Revise   perforation of wall of nasal sinus

751 Other congenital anomalies of digestive system

    751.2 Atresia and stenosis of large intestine, rectum, and anal canal

        Absence:

Revise   large intestine, congenital

    751.3 Hirschsprung's disease and other congenital functional disorders of colon

Revise   Macrocolon

752 Congenital anomalies of genital organs

    752.3 Other anomalies of uterus

Delete   Absence, congenital, of uterus

Delete   Agenesis of uterus

Delete   Aplasia of uterus

Delete   Bicornuate uterus

Delete   Uterus unicornis

Delete   Uterus with only one functioning horn

New code   **752.31 Agenesis of uterus**

           Congenital absence of uterus

New code   **752.32 Hypoplasia of uterus**

New code   **752.33 Unicornuate uterus**

           Unicornate uterus with or without a separate uterine horn

           Uterus with only one functioning horn

New code   **752.34 Bicornuate uterus**

           Bicornuate uterus, complete or partial

New code   **752.35 Septate uterus**

           Septate uterus, complete or partial

New code   **752.36 Arcuate uterus**

New code   **752.39 Other anomalies of uterus**

           Aplasia of uterus NOS

           Müllerian anomaly of the uterus, NEC

           Excludes *anomaly of uterus due to exposure to diethylstilbestrol [DES] in utero (760.76)*

                didelphic uterus (752.2)

                doubling of uterus (752.2)

    752.4 Anomalies of cervix, vagina, and external female genitalia

New code   **752.43 Cervical agenesis**

           Cervical hypoplasia

New code   **752.44 Cervical duplication**

New code   **752.45 Vaginal agenesis**

           Agenesis of vagina, total or partial

New code   **752.46 Transverse vaginal septum**

New code   **752.47 Longitudinal vaginal septum**

           Longitudinal vaginal septum with or without obstruction

        752.49 Other anomalies of cervix, vagina, and external female genitalia

Revise   Absence of cervix, clitoris, vagina, or vulva

Revise   Agenesis of cervix, clitoris, vagina, or vulva

Add   Anomalies of cervix, NEC

Add   Anomalies of hymen, NEC

Add   Müllerian anomalies of the cervix and vagina, NEC

753 Congenital anomalies of urinary system

    753.4 Other specified anomalies of ureter

Revise   Deviation of ureter

759 Other and unspecified congenital anomalies

    759.6 Other hamartoses, NEC

Revise   Excludes *neurofibromatosis (237.70-237.79)*

763 Fetus or newborn affected by other complications of labor and delivery

    763.5 Maternal anesthesia and analgesia

Revise   Reactions and intoxications from maternal opiates and tranquilizers during labor and delivery

771 Infections specific to the perinatal period

    771.8 Other infections specific to the perinatal period

Revise   Use additional code to identify organism or specific infection (041.00-041.9)

780 General symptoms

    780.3 Convulsions

New code   **780.33 Post traumatic seizures**

           Excludes *post traumatic epilepsy (345.00-345.91)*

    780.6 Fever and other physiologic disturbances of temperature regulation

        780.62 Postprocedural fever

Add   Excludes *posttransfusion fever (780.66)*

New code   **780.66 Febrile nonhemolytic transfusion reaction**

           FNHTR

           Posttransfusion fever

781 Symptoms involving nervous and musculoskeletal systems

Revise   **781.8 Neurologic neglect syndrome**

Add   **Excludes**   *visuospatial deficit (799.53)*

782 Symptoms involving skin and other integumentary tissue

     782.3 Edema

Revise   **Excludes**   *fluid retention (276.69)*

784 Symptoms involving head and neck

     784.5 Other speech disturbance

Revise   **Excludes**   *stammering and stuttering (315.35)*
Delete   *that of nonorganic origin (307.0, 307.9)*

New code   **784.52 Fluency disorder in conditions classified elsewhere**
Stuttering in conditions classified elsewhere

Code first underlying disease or condition, such as:
Parkinson's disease (332.0)

Excludes   *adult onset fluency disorder (307.0)*
childhood onset fluency disorder (315.35)
fluency disorder due to late effect of cerebrovascular accident (438.14)

     784.8 Hemorrhage from throat

Revise   **Excludes**   *hemoptysis (786.30-786.39)*

     784.9 Other symptoms involving head and neck

New code   **784.92 Jaw pain**
Mandibular pain
Maxilla pain

Excludes   *temporomandibular joint arthralgia (524.62)*

786 Symptoms involving respiratory system and other chest symptoms

     786.2 Cough

Excludes   *cough:*
Revise   *with hemorrhage (786.39)*

     786.3 Hemoptysis

Delete   ~~Cough with hemorrhage~~
Delete   ~~Pulmonary hemorrhage NOS~~
Delete   **Excludes**   *pulmonary hemorrhage of newborn (770.3)*

New code   **786.30 Hemoptysis, unspecified**
Pulmonary hemorrhage NOS

New code   **786.31 Acute idiopathic pulmonary hemorrhage in infants [AIPHI]**
Acute idiopathic pulmonary hemorrhage in infant over 28 days old

Excludes   *pulmonary hemorrhage of newborn under 28 days old (770.3)*
von Willebrand's disease (286.4)

New code   **786.39 Other hemoptysis**
Cough with hemorrhage

787 Symptoms involving digestive system

     787.6 Incontinence of feces

New code   **787.60 Full incontinence of feces**
Fecal incontinence NOS

New code   **787.61 Incomplete defecation**

Excludes   *constipation (564.00-564.09)*
fecal impaction (560.32)

New code   **787.62 Fecal smearing**
Fecal soiling

New code   **787.63 Fecal urgency**

796 Other nonspecific abnormal findings

     796.0 Nonspecific abnormal toxicological findings

Add   Use additional code for retained foreign body, if applicable, (V90.01-V90.9)

799 Other ill-defined and unknown causes of morbidity and mortality

New sub   **799.5 Signs and symptoms involving cognition**

Excludes   *amnesia (780.93)*
amnestic syndrome (294.0)
attention deficit disorder (314.00-314.01)
late effects of cerebrovascular disease (438)
memory loss (780.93)
mild cognitive impairment, so stated (331.83)
specific problems in developmental delay (315.00-315.9)
transient global amnesia (437.7)
visuospatial neglect 781.8

New code   **799.51 Attention or concentration deficit**
New code   **799.52 Cognitive communication deficit**
New code   **799.53 Visuospatial deficit**
New code   **799.54 Psychomotor deficit**
New code   **799.55 Frontal lobe and executive function deficit**
New code   **799.59 Other signs and symptoms involving cognition**

     799.8 Other ill-defined conditions

     799.82 Apparent life threatening event in infant

Add   *Code first* confirmed diagnosis, if known

Revise   Use additional code(s) for associated signs and symptoms if no confirmed diagnosis established, or if signs and symptoms are not associated routinely with confirmed diagnosis, or provide additional information for cause of ALTE

Delete   **Excludes**   *signs and symptoms associated with a confirmed diagnosis code to confirmed diagnosis*

17. INJURY AND POISONING (800-999)

Add — Use additional code for retained foreign body, if applicable, V90.01-V90.9)

836 Dislocation of knee

836.5 Other dislocation of knee, closed

836.51 Anterior dislocation of tibia, proximal end

Revise — Posterior dislocation of femur, distal end, closed

836.52 Posterior dislocation of tibia, proximal end

Revise — Anterior dislocation of femur, distal end, closed

836.6 Other dislocation of knee, open

836.61 Anterior dislocation of tibia, proximal end

Add — Posterior dislocation of femur, distal end, open

836.62 Posterior dislocation of tibia, proximal end

Add — Anterior dislocation of femur, distal end, open

SPRAINS AND STRAINS OF JOINTS AND ADJACENT MUSCLES (840-848)

Revise — **Includes** avulsion of joint capsule, ligament, muscle, tendon

Revise — hemarthrosis of joint capsule, ligament, muscle, tendon

Revise — laceration of joint capsule, ligament, muscle, tendon

Revise — rupture of joint capsule, ligament, muscle, tendon

Revise — sprain of joint capsule, ligament, muscle, tendon

Revise — strain of joint capsule, ligament, muscle, tendon

Revise — tear of joint capsule, ligament, muscle, tendon

970 Poisoning by central nervous system stimulants

970.8 Other specified central nervous system stimulants

New code — **970.81 Cocaine**
Crack

New code — **970.89 Other central nervous system stimulants**

TOXIC EFFECTS OF SUBSTANCES CHIEFLY NONMEDICINAL AS TO SOURCE (980-989)

Add — Use additional code to identify:

Add — personal history of retained foreign body fully removed (V15.53)

Add — retained foreign body status, if applicable (V90.01-V90.9)

992 Effects of heat and light

992.0 Heat stroke and sunstroke

Add — Use additional code(s) to identify any associated complication of heat stroke, such as:

Add — alterations of consciousness (780.01-780.09)

Add — systemic inflammatory response syndrome (995.93-995.94)

995 Certain adverse effects not elsewhere classified

Revise — **995.2 Other and unspecified adverse effect of drug, medicinal and biological substance (due) to correct medicinal substance properly administered**

Delete — Adverse effect to correct medicinal substance properly administered

Delete — Allergic reaction to correct medicinal substance properly administered

Delete — Hypersensitivity to correct medicinal substance properly administered

Delete — Idiosyncrasy due to correct medicinal substance properly administered

Delete — Drug:
Delete — hypersensitivity NOS
Delete — reaction NOS

995.20 Unspecified adverse effect of unspecified drug, medicinal and biological substance

Add — Unspecified adverse effect of unspecified medicinal substance properly administered

995.27 Other drug allergy

Add — Allergic reaction NEC (due) to correct medical substance properly administered

Add — Hypersensitivity (due) to correct medical substance properly administered

995.29 Unspecified adverse effect of other drug, medicinal and biological substance

Add — Unspecified adverse effect of medicinal substance NEC properly administered

995.9 Systemic inflammatory response syndrome (SIRS)

995.94 Systemic inflammatory response syndrome due to non- infectious process with acute organ dysfunction

Code first underlying conditions, such as:

Add — heat stroke (992.0)

998 Other complications of procedures, not elsewhere classified

Add — **Excludes** fluid overload due to transfusion (blood) (276.61)
TACO (276.61)
transfusion associated circulatory overload (276.61)

999 Complications of medical care, not elsewhere classified

Revise — **999.6 ABO incompatibility reaction due to transfusion of blood or blood products**

Delete — Incompatible blood transfusion
Delete — Reaction to blood group incompatibility in infusion or transfusion

New code — **999.60 ABO incompatibility reaction, unspecified**
ABO incompatible blood transfusion NOS
Reaction to ABO incompatibility from transfusion NOS

New code   **999.61 ABO incompatibility with hemolytic transfusion reaction not specified as acute or delayed**
ABO incompatibility with hemolytic transfusion reaction at unspecified time after transfusion
Hemolytic transfusion reaction (HTR) due to ABO incompatibility

New code   **999.62 ABO incompatibility with acute hemolytictransfusion reaction**
ABO incompatibility with hemolytic transfusion reaction less than 24 hoursafter transfusion
Acute hemolytic transfusion reaction (AHTR) due to ABO incompatibility

New code   **999.63 ABO incompatibility with delayed hemolytic transfusion reaction**
ABO incompatibility with hemolytic transfusion reaction 24 hours or more after transfusion
Delayed hemolytic transfusion reaction (DHTR) due to ABO incompatibility

New code   **999.69 Other ABO incompatibility reaction**
Delayed serologic transfusion reaction (DSTR) from ABO incompatibility
Other ABO incompatible blood transfusion
Other reaction to ABO incompatibility from transfusion

Revise   **999.7 Rh and other non-ABO incompatibility reaction due to transfusion of blood or blood products**

Delete   ~~Reactions due to Rh factor in infusion or transfusion~~

New code   **999.70 Rh incompatibility reaction, unspecified**
Reaction due to Rh factor in transfusion NOS
Rh incompatible blood transfusion NOS
Unspecified reaction due to incompatibility related to Rh antigens (C) (c) (D) (E) (e)
Unspecified reaction to Rh incompatibility

New code   **999.71 Rh incompatibility with hemolytic transfusion reaction not specified as acute or delayed**
Hemolytic transfusion reaction (HTR) due to Rh incompatibility
HTR due to incompatibility related to Rh antigens (C) (c) (D) (E) (e), not specified as acute or delayed
Rh incompatibility with hemolytic transfusion reaction at unspecified time after transfusion

New code   **999.72 Rh incompatibility with acute hemolytic transfusion reaction**
Acute hemolytic transfusion reaction (AHTR) due to Rh incompatibility
AHTR due to incompatibility related to Rh antigens (C) (c) (D) (E) (e)
Rh incompatibility with hemolytic transfusion reaction less than 24 hours after transfusion

New code   **999.73 Rh incompatibility with delayed hemolytic transfusion reaction**
Delayed hemolytic transfusion reaction (DHTR) due to Rh incompatibility
DHTR due to incompatibility related to Rh antigens (C) (c) (D) (E) (e)
Rh incompatibility with hemolytic transfusion reaction 24 hours or more after transfusion

New code   **999.74 Other Rh incompatibility reaction**
Delayed serologic transfusion reaction (DSTR) from Rh incompatibility
Other reaction due to incompatibility related to Rh antigens (C) (c) (D) (E) (e)
Other reaction to Rh incompatible bloodtransfusion

New code   **999.75 Non-ABO incompatibility reaction, unspecified**
Non-ABO incompatible blood transfusion NOS
Reaction to non-ABO antigen incompatibility from transfusion NOS
Unspecified reaction due to incompatibility related to minor antigens (Duffy) (Kell) (Kidd) (Lewis) (M) (N) (P) (S)

New code   **999.76 Non-ABO incompatibility with hemolytic transfusion reaction not specified as acute or delayed**
Hemolytic transfusion reaction (HTR) due to non-ABO incompatibility
HTR from incompatibility related to minor antigens (Duffy) (Kell) (Kidd) (Lewis) (M) (N) (P) (S)
Non-ABO incompatibility with hemolytic transfusion reaction at unspecified timeafter transfusion

New code   **999.77 Non-ABO incompatibility with acute hemolytic transfusion reaction**
Acute hemolytic transfusion reaction (AHTR) due to non-ABO incompatibility
AHTR from incompatibility related to minor antigens (Duffy) (Kell) (Kidd) (Lewis) (M) (N) (P) (S)
Non-ABO incompatibility with hemolytic transfusion reaction less than 24 hours after transfusion

New code   **999.78 Non-ABO incompatibility with delayed hemolytic transfusion reaction**
Delayed hemolytic transfusion reaction (DHTR) due to non-ABO incompatibility
DHTR from incompatibility related to minor antigens (Duffy) (Kell) (Kidd) (Lewis) (M) (N) (P) (S)
Non-ABO incompatibility with hemolytic transfusion reaction 24 hours or more after transfusion

New code   **999.79 Other non-ABO incompatibility reaction**
Delayed serologic transfusion reaction (DSTR) from non-ABO incompatibility
Other non-ABO incompatible blood transfusion
Other reaction due to incompatibility related to minor antigens (Duffy) (Kell) (Kidd) (Lewis) (M) (N) (P) (S)
Other reaction to non-ABO incompatibility from transfusion

Revise   **999.8 Other and unspecified infusion and transfusion reaction**

Add   **Excludes** *ABO incompatibility reactions (999.60-999.69)*
Add   *febrile nonhemolytic transfusion reaction (FNHTR) (780.66)*
Add   *hemochromatosis due to repeated red blood cell transfusions (275.02)*
Add   *non-ABO incompatibility reactions (999.70-999.79)*
Add   *posttransfusion purpura (287.41)*
Add   *Rh incompatibility reactions (999.70-999.74)*
Add   *transfusion associated circulatory overload (TACO) (276.61)*

New code   **999.80 Transfusion reaction, unspecified**
Incompatible blood transfusion NOS
Reaction to blood group incompatibility in infusion or transfusion NOS

New code   **999.83 Hemolytic transfusion reaction, incompatibility unspecified**
Hemolytic transfusion reaction (HTR) with antigen incompatibility unspecified, not specified as acute or delayed
HTR with incompatibility unspecified at unspecified time after transfusion

New code   **999.84 Acute hemolytic transfusion reaction, incompatibility unspecified**
Acute hemolytic transfusion reaction (AHTR) with antigen incompatibility unspecified
AHTR, incompatibility unspecified

New code   **999.85 Delayed hemolytic transfusion reaction, incompatibility unspecified**
Delayed hemolytic transfusion reaction (DHTR) with antigen incompatibility unspecified
DHTR, incompatibility unspecified

    999.89 Other transfusion reaction
Delete   ~~Transfusion reaction NOS~~
Add   Delayed serologic transfusion reaction (DSTR), incompatibility unspecified

Revise section heading   **SUPPLEMENTARY CLASSIFICATION OF FACTORS INFLUENCING HEALTH STATUS AND CONTACT WITH HEALTH SERVICES (V01-V90)**

Revise   **V07 Need for isolation and other prophylactic or treatment measures**

Add   **Excludes** *long-term (current) (prophylactic) use of certain specific drugs (V58.61-V58.69)*

Revise   **V07.5 ~~Prophylactic u~~Use of agents affecting estrogen receptors and estrogen levels**

Revise   **V07.51 ~~Prophylactic u~~Use of selective estrogen receptor modulators (SERMs)**
Revise   ~~Prophylactic u~~Use of:

Revise   **V07.52 ~~Prophylactic u~~Use of aromatase inhibitors**
Revise   ~~Prophylactic u~~Use of:

Revise   **V07.59 ~~Prophylactic u~~Use of other agents affecting estrogen receptors and estrogen levels**
Revise   ~~Prophylactic u~~Use of:

Revise   **V07.8 Other specified prophylactic or treatment measure**

Revise   **V07.9 Unspecified prophylactic or treatment measure**

    V10 Personal history of malignant neoplasm

    V10.5 Urinary organs

Add   **Excludes** *personal history of malignant carcinoid tumor (V10.91)*
Add   *personal history of malignant neuroendocrine tumor (V10.91)*

    V11 Personal history of mental disorder

New code   **V11.4 Combat and operational stress reaction**

    V13 Personal history of other diseases

    V13.2 Other genital system and obstetric disorders

Revise   **Excludes** *~~habitual aborter~~ recurrent pregnancy loss (646.3)*

New code   **V13.23 Personal history of vaginal dysplasia**
Personal history of conditions classifiable to 623.0

    Excludes *personal history of malignant neoplasm of vagina (V10.44)*

New code	**V13.24**	**Personal history of vulvar dysplasia**

Personal history of conditions classifiable to 624.01-624.02

> **Excludes** *personal history of malignant neoplasm of vulva (V10.44)*

Revise	**V13.6**	**Congenital (corrected) malformations**
Revise	**V13.61**	**Personal history of (corrected) hHypospadias**
New code	**V13.62**	**Personal history of other (corrected) congenital malformations of genitourinary system**
New code	**V13.63**	**Personal history of (corrected) congenital malformations of nervous system**
New code	**V13.64**	**Personal history of (corrected) congenital malformations of eye, ear, face and neck**

Corrected cleft lip and palate

New code	**V13.65**	**Personal history of (corrected) congenital malformations of heart and circulatory system**
New code	**V13.66**	**Personal history of (corrected) congenital malformations of respiratory system**
New code	**V13.67**	**Personal history of (corrected) congenital malformations of digestive system**
New code	**V13.68**	**Personal history of (corrected) congenital malformations of integument, limbs, and musculoskeletal systems**
Revise	**V13.69**	**Personal history of other (corrected) congenital malformations**

	V15	**Other personal history presenting hazards to health**
	V15.5	**Injury**
New code	**V15.53**	**Personal history of retained foreign body fully removed**
	V15.8	**Other specified personal history presenting hazards to health**
	V15.89	**Other**

Revise		

> **Excludes** *contact with and (suspected) exposure to otherpotentially other potentially hazardous substances (V87.39)*

	V23	**Supervision of high-risk pregnancy**
	V23.2	**Pregnancy with history of abortion**

Revise		

> **Excludes** *habitual aborter recurrent pregnancy loss:*

	V25	**Encounter for contraceptive management**
Revise	**V25.1**	**Encounter for insertion or removal of intrauterine contraceptive device**

Add		

> **Excludes** *encounter for routine checking of intrauterine contraceptive device (V25.42)*

New code	**V25.11**	**Encounter for insertion of intrauterine contraceptive device**

New code	**V25.12**	**Encounter for removal of intrauterine contraceptive device**
New code	**V25.13**	**Encounter for removal and reinsertion of intrauterine contraceptive device**

Encounter for replacement of intrauterine contraceptive device

	V25.4	**Surveillance of previously prescribed contraceptive methods**
Delete		

> **Excludes** *presence of intrauterine contraceptive device as incidental finding (V45.5)*

	V25.42	**Intrauterine contraceptive device**
Revise		Checking, reinsertion, or removal of intrauterine device

Add		

> **Excludes** *insertion or removal of intrauterine contraceptive device (V25.11-V25.13)*

Add		

> *presence of intrauterine contraceptive device as incidental finding (V45.5)*

	V26	**Procreative management**
	V26.3	**Genetic counseling and testing**
	V26.32	**Other genetic testing of female**
Revise		Use additional code to identify habitual aborter recurrent pregnancy loss (629.81, 646.3)
Revise	**V26.35**	**Encounter for testing of male partner of habitual aborter female with recurrent pregnancy loss**

	V45	**Other postprocedural states**
	V45.0	**Cardiac device in situ**
	V45.01	**Cardiac pacemaker**
Add		

> **Excludes** *cardiac defibrillator with synchronous cardiac pacemaker (V45.02)*

	V45.02	**Automatic implantable cardiac defibrillator**
Add		With synchronous cardiac pacemaker

	V45.5	**Presence of contraceptive device**
Delete		

> **Excludes** *checking, reinsertion, or removal of device (V25.42)*
> *complication from device (996.32)*
> *insertion of device (V25.1)*

	V45.51	**Intrauterine contraceptive device**
Add		

> **Excludes** *checking of device (V25.42)*

Add		

> *complication from device (996.32)*

Add		

> *insertion and removal of device (V25.11-V25.13)*

	V45.7	Acquired absence of organ
		V45.79 Other acquired absence of organ
Add			Excludes	acquired absence of pancreas (V88.11-V88.12)

V46 Other dependence on machines and devices

V46.3 Wheelchair dependence

Revise — *Code first cause of dependence, such as:* obesity (278.00-278.03)

V49 Other conditions influencing health status

V49.8 Other specified conditions influencing health status

New code — V49.86 Do not resuscitate status

New code — V49.87 Physical restraints status

Add — Excludes *restraint due to a procedure – omit code*

V53 Fitting and adjustment of other device

V53.3 Cardiac device

V53.31 Cardiac pacemaker

Add — Excludes *automatic implantable cardiac defibrillator with synchronous cardiac pacemaker (V53.32)*

V53.32 Automatic implantable cardiac defibrillator

Add — With synchronous cardiac pacemaker

V55 Attention to artificial openings

Revise — Excludes *complications of external stoma (519.00-519.09, 569.60-569.69, 997.4, 997.5)*

V58 Encounter for other and unspecified procedures and aftercare

V58.6 Long-term (current) drug use

Add — Long-term (current) prophylactic drug use

Revise — Excludes *prophylactic use of agents affecting estrogen receptors and estrogen levels (V07.51-V07.59)*

V62 Other psychosocial circumstances

V62.8 Other psychological or physical stress, not elsewhere classified

New code — V62.85 Homicidal ideation

V76 Special screening for malignant neoplasms

V76.5 Intestine

V76.51 Colon

Add — Screening colonoscopy NOS

V85 Body mass index (BMI)

V85.4 Body Mass Index 40 and over, adult

New code — V85.41 Body Mass Index 40.0-44.9, adult

New code — V85.42 Body Mass Index 45.0-49.9, adult

New code — V85.43 Body Mass Index 50.0-59.9, adult

New code — V85.44 Body Mass Index 60.0-69.9, adult

New code — V85.45 Body Mass Index 70 and over, adult

V87 Other specified personal exposures and history presenting hazards to health

V87.3 Contact with and (suspected) exposure to other potentially hazardous substances

Add — Excludes *personal history of retained foreign body fully removed (V15.53)*

V88 Acquired absence of other organs and tissue

New sub — V88.1 Acquired absence of pancreas

Use additional code to identify any associated:
insulin use (V58.67)
secondary diabetes mellitus (249.00-249.91)

New code — V88.11 Acquired total absence of pancreas
Acquired absence of pancreas NOS

New code — V88.12 Acquired partial absence of pancreas

New section — **RETAINED FOREIGN BODY (V90)**

New category — **V90 Retained foreign body**
Embedded fragment (status)
Embedded splinter (status)
Retained foreign body status

Excludes *artificial joint prosthesis status (V43.60-V43.69)*
foreign body accidentally left during a procedure (998.4)
foreign body entering through orifice (930.0-939.9)
in situ cardiac devices (V45.00-V45.09)
organ or tissue replaced by other means (V43.0-V43.89)
organ or tissue replaced by transplant (V42.0-V42.9)
personal history of retained foreign body removed (V15.53)
superficial foreign body (splinter) (categories 910-917 and 919 with 4th character 6 or 7, 918.0)

New sub — V90.0 Retained radioactive fragment

New code — V90.01 Retained depleted uranium fragments

New code — V90.09 Other retained radioactive fragments
Other retained depleted isotope fragments
Retained nontherapeutic radioactive fragments

New sub — V90.1 Retained metal fragments

Excludes *retained radioactive metal fragments (V90.01-V90.09)*

New code — V90.10 Retained metal fragments, unspecified
Retained metal fragment NOS

New code — V90.11 Retained magnetic metal fragments

New code — V90.12 Retained nonmagnetic metal fragments

New code — V90.2 Retained plastic fragments
Acrylics fragments
Diethylhexylphthalates fragments
Isocyanate fragments

New sub	**V90.3**	**Retained organic fragments**
New code	**V90.31**	**Retained animal quills or spines**
New code	**V90.32**	**Retained tooth**
New code	**V90.33**	**Retained wood fragments**
New code	**V90.39**	**Other retained organic fragments**
New sub	**V90.8**	**Other specified retained foreign body**
New code	**V90.81**	**Retained glass fragments**
New code	**V90.83**	**Retained stone or crystalline fragments**
		Retained concrete or cement fragments
New code	**V90.89**	**Other specified retained foreign body**
New code	**V90.9**	**Retained foreign body, unspecified material**

MULTIPLE GESTATION PLACENTA STATUS (V91)

New section

New category	**V91**	**Multiple gestation placenta status**
		Code first multiple gestation (651.0-651.9)
New sub	**V91.0**	**Twin gestation placenta status**
New code	**V91.00**	**Twin gestation, unspecified number of placenta, unspecified number of amniotic sacs**
New code	**V91.01**	**Twin gestation, monochorionic/monoamniotic (one placenta, one amniotic sac)**
New code	**V91.02**	**Twin gestation, monochorionic/diamniotic (one placenta, two amniotic sacs)**
New code	**V91.03**	**Twin gestation, dichorionic/diamniotic (two placentae, two amniotic sacs)**
New code	**V91.09**	**Twin gestation, unable to determine number of placenta and number of amniotic sacs**
New sub	**V91.1**	**Triplet gestation placenta status**
New code	**V91.10**	**Triplet gestation, unspecified number of placenta and unspecified number of amniotic sacs**
New code	**V91.11**	**Triplet gestation, with two or more monochorionic fetuses**
New code	**V91.12**	**Triplet gestation, with two or more monoamniotic fetuses**
New code	**V91.19**	**Triplet gestation, unable to determine number of placenta and number of amniotic sacs**
New sub	**V91.2**	**Quadruplet gestation placenta status**
New code	**V91.20**	**Quadruplet gestation, unspecified number of placenta and unspecified number of amniotic sacs**
New code	**V91.21**	**Quadruplet gestation, with two or more monochorionic fetuses**
New code	**V91.22**	**Quadruplet gestation, with two or more monoamniotic fetuses**
New code	**V91.29**	**Quadruplet gestation, unable to determine number of placenta and number of amniotic sacs**

New sub	**V91.9**	**Other specified multiple gestation placenta status**
		Placenta status for multiple gestations greater than quadruplets
New code	**V91.90**	**Other specified multiple gestation, unspecified number of placenta and unspecified number of amniotic sacs**
New code	**V91.91**	**Other specified multiple gestation, with two or more monochorionic fetuses**
New code	**V91.92**	**Other specified multiple gestation, with two or more monoamniotic fetuses**
New code	**V91.99**	**Other specified multiple gestation, unable to determine number of placenta and number of amniotic sacs**
	E000	**External cause status**
New code	**E000.2**	**Volunteer activity**
		Excludes *activity of child or other family member assisting in compensated work of other family member (E000.8)*
	E000.8	**Other external cause status**
Add		Activity of child or other family member assisting in compensated work of other family member
Delete		~~Volunteer activity~~
	E017	**Activities involving roller coasters and other types of external motion**
Revise	**E017.0**	Roller coaster riding

TRANSPORT ACCIDENTS (E800-E848)

Definitions and examples related to transport accidents

(q) pedestrian conveyance is any human powered device by which a pedestrian may move other than by walking or by which a walking person may move another pedestrian.

Add		**Includes** motorized mobility scooter
Revise		wheelchair (electric)

Revise   **PLACE OF OCCURRENCE (E849)**

	E865	**Accidental poisoning from poisonous foodstuffs and poisonous plants**
Revise		**Excludes** *anaphylactic shock due to adverse food reaction (995.60-995.69)*
	E884	**Other fall from one level to another**
	E884.3	**Fall from wheelchair**
Add		Fall from motorized mobility scooter
Add		Fall from motorized wheelchair
	E885	**Fall on same level from slipping, tripping, or stumbling**
	E885.0	**Fall from (nonmotorized) scooter**
Add		**Excludes** *fall from motorized mobility scooter (E884.3)*

VOLUME 3 CHANGES EFFECTIVE OCTOBER 1, 2010

Tabular

Revise code title — **00.55 Insertion of drug-eluting ~~peripheral vessel~~ stent(s) of other peripheral vessel(s)**

Add exclusion term — *Excludes insertion of drug-eluting stent(s) of superficial femoral artery (00.60)*

Revise exclusion term — *~~that for aneurysm repair~~ that for other endovascular procedure (39.71-39.79)*

New code — **00.60 Insertion of drug-eluting stent(s) of superficial femoral artery**
  Code also any:
    angioplasty or atherectomy of other non-coronary vessel(s) (39.50)
    non-drug-eluting peripheral stents (39.90)
    number of vascular stents inserted (00.45-00.48)
    number of vessels treated (00.40-00.43)
    procedure on vessel bifurcation (00.44)
  Excludes insertion of drug-eluting stent(s) of other peripheral vessel (00.55)
  that for other endovascular procedure (39.71-39.79)

New code — **01.20 Cranial implantation or replacement of neurostimulator pulse generator**
  Code also any associated lead implantation (02.93)
  Excludes implantation or replacement of subcutaneous neurostimulator pulse generator (86.94-86.98)

New code — **01.29 Removal of cranial neurostimulator pulse generator**

01.59 Other excision or destruction of lesion or tissue of brain
Add inclusion term — Amygdalohippocampectomy

02.93 Implantation or replacement of intracranial neurostimulator lead(s)
Revise code also note — **Code also** any:
Add code also note — insertion of cranial implantation or replacement of neurostimulator pulse generator (01.20)
Revise code also note — insertion of subcutaneous neurostimulator pulse generator (86.94-86.98)

04.92 Implantation or replacement of peripheral neurostimulator lead(s)
Add exclusion term — *Excludes implantation or replacement of carotid sinus stimulation lead(s) (39.82)*

---

07 Operations on other endocrine glands
  Excludes operations on:
Revise exclusion term — *aortic and carotid bodies (39.81-39.89)*

New code — **17.71 Non-coronary intra-operative fluorescence vascular angiography [IFVA]**
    Intraoperative laser arteriogram
    SPY arteriogram
    SPY arteriography
  Excludes intra-operative coronary fluorescence vascular angiography (88.59)

32.26 Other and unspecified ablation of lung lesion or tissue
Add exclusion term — *Excludes bronchoscopic bronchial thermoplasty, ablation of smooth airway muscle (32.27)*

New code — **32.27 Bronchoscopic bronchial thermoplasty, ablation of airway smooth muscle**

33.24 Closed [endoscopic] biopsy of bronchus
Revise inclusion term — Transbronchoscopic needle aspiration [TBNA] of bronchus
Add exclusion term — *Excludes mini-bronchoalveolar lavage [mini-BAL] (33.29)*

33.27 Closed endoscopic biopsy of lung
Add inclusion term — Transbronchoscopic needle aspiration [TBNA] of lung

33.29 Other diagnostic procedures on lung and bronchus
Add exclusion term — *Excludes bronchoalveolar lavage [BAL] (33.24)*

33.73 Endoscopic insertion or replacement of bronchial valve(s), multiple lobes
Add inclusion term — Endobronchial airflow redirection valve
Add inclusion term — Intrabronchial airflow redirection valve

35.24 Other replacement of mitral valve
Add exclusion term — *Excludes percutaneous repair with implant or leaflet clip (35.97)*

Revise code title — **35.96 Percutaneous balloon valvuloplasty**
Delete inclusion term — ~~Percutaneous balloon valvuloplasty~~
Add inclusion term — Balloon dilation of valve
Add exclusion term — *Excludes mitral valve repair with implant (35.97)*

New code   35.97 **Percutaneous mitral valve repair with implant**
Endovascular mitral valve repair
Implantation of mitral valve leaflet clip
Transcatheter mitral valve repair

Code also any transesophageal echocardiography [TEE] (88.72)

Excludes *percutaneous balloon valvuloplasty (35.96)*

37.3 **Pericardiectomy and excision of lesion of heart**

Revise code also note
Code also cardiopulmonary bypass [extracorporeal circulation] [heart-lung machine], if performed (39.61)

37.33 **Excision or destruction of other lesion or tissue of heart, open approach**

Revise inclusion term
Ablation or incision of heart tissue (cryoablation) (electrocautery) (laser) (microwave) (radiofrequency) (resection) (ultrasound), open chest approach

Delete inclusion term
~~Modified maze procedure, transthoracic approach~~

Add inclusion term
That by median sternotomy

Add inclusion term
That by thoracotomy without use of thoracoscope

Excludes *ablation, excision, or destruction of lesion or tissue of heart:*

Add exclusion term
thoracoscopic approach (37.37)

Revise code title
37.34 **Excision or destruction of other lesion or tissue of heart, ~~other~~ endovascular approach**

Revise inclusion term
Ablation of heart tissue (cryoablation) (electrocautery) (laser) (microwave) (radiofrequency) (~~resection~~) (ultrasound), via peripherally inserted catheter

Revise inclusion term
Modified maze procedure, ~~endovascular~~ percutaneous approach

Add exclusion term
Excludes *ablation, excision or destruction of lesion of tissue of heart:*
open approach (37.33)
thoracoscopic approach (37.37)

New code   37.37 **Excision or destruction of other lesion or tissue of heart, thoracoscopic approach**
Ablation or incision of heart tissue (cryoablation) (electrocautery) (laser) (microwave) (radiofrequency) (resection) (ultrasound), via thoracoscope
Modified maze procedure, thoracoscopic approach
That via thoracoscopically-assisted approach (without thoracotomy) (with port access) (with sub-xiphoid incision)

Excludes *ablation, excision or destruction of lesion or tissue of heart:*
open approach (37.33)
endovascular approach (37.34)
thoracoscopic excision or destruction of left atrial appendage [LAA] (37.36)

37.62 **Insertion of temporary non-implantable extracorporeal circulatory assist device**

Delete inclusion term
~~Acute circulatory support device~~

Delete inclusion term
~~Short-term circulatory support (up to six hours)~~

38.93 **Venous catheterization, not elsewhere classified**

Add exclusion term
Excludes *that with guidance (electrocardiogram) (fluoroscopy) (ultrasound) (38.97)*

New code   38.97 **Central venous catheter placement with guidance**
Includes guidance by:
electrocardiogram
fluoroscopy
ultrasound

New category   39.8 **Operations on carotid body, carotid sinus and other vascular bodies**

Delete inclusion term
~~Chemodectomy~~

Delete inclusion term
~~Denervation of:~~

Delete inclusion term
~~aortic body~~

Delete inclusion term
~~carotid body~~

Delete inclusion term
~~Electronic stimulator~~

Delete inclusion term
~~Glomectomy, carotid~~

Delete inclusion term
~~Implantation or replacement of carotid sinus baroreflex activation device~~

Delete excludes term
Excludes *replacement of carotid sinus lead(s) only (04.92)*

New code | **39.81** | **Implantation or replacement of carotid sinus stimulation device, total system**
Carotid sinus baroreflex activation device
Implantation of carotid sinus stimulator and lead(s)

Includes carotid explorations

Excludes *implantation or replacement of carotid sinus stimulation lead(s) only (39.82)*
implantation or replacement of carotid sinus stimulation pulse generator only (39.83)

New code | **39.82** | **Implantation or replacement of carotid sinus stimulation lead(s) only**

Excludes *implantation or replacement of carotid sinus stimulation device, total system (39.81)*

New code | **39.83** | **Implantation or replacement of carotid sinus stimulation pulse generator only**

Excludes *implantation or replacement of carotid sinus stimulation device, total system (39.81)*

New code | **39.84** | **Revision of carotid sinus stimulation lead(s) only**
Repair of electrode [removal with re-insertion]
Repositioning of lead(s) [electrode]

New code | **39.85** | **Revision of carotid sinus stimulation pulse generator**
Debridement and reforming pocket (skin and subcutaneous tissue)
Relocation of pocket [creation of new pocket]
Repositioning of pulse generator
Revision of carotid sinus stimulation pulse generator pocket

New code | **39.86** | **Removal of carotid sinus stimulation device, total system**

New code | **39.87** | **Removal of carotid sinus stimulation lead(s) only**

New code | **39.88** | **Removal of carotid sinus stimulation pulse generator only**

New code | **39.89** | **Other operations on carotid body, carotid sinus and other vascular bodies**
Chemodectomy
Denervation of:
aortic body
carotid body
Glomectomy, carotid

Excludes *excision of glomus jugulare (20.51)*

40.11 | **Biopsy of lymphatic structure**

Add inclusion term
Transbronchoscopic needle aspiration [TBNA] of lymph node

53.59 | **Repair of other hernia of anterior abdominal wall**

Add inclusion term
That by laparoscopic approach

78.5 | **Internal fixation of bone without fracture reduction**

Add exclusion term
Excludes *insertion of sternal fixation device with rigid plates (84.94)*

81.0 | **Spinal fusion**

Add note
Note: Spinal fusion is classified by the anatomic portion (column) fused and the technique (approach) used to perform the fusion.

For the anterior column, the body (corpus) of adjacent vertebrae are fused (interbody fusion). The anterior column can be fused using an anterior, lateral, or posterior technique.

For the posterior column, posterior structures of adjacent vertebrae are fused (pedicle, lamina, facet, transverse process, or "gutter" fusion). A posterior column fusion can be performed using a posterior, posterolateral, or lateral transverse technique.

Revise code title | **81.02** | **Other cervical fusion of the, anterior column, anterior technique**

Revise inclusion term
Arthrodesis of C2 level or below: anterior (interbody ~~technique~~) fusion

Revise code title | **81.03** | **Other cervical fusion of the, posterior column, posterior technique**

Revise inclusion term
Arthrodesis of C2 level or below:, posterolateral technique

Delete inclusion term
~~posterior (interbody) technique~~

Delete inclusion term
~~posterolateral technique~~

Revise code title | **81.04** | **Dorsal and dorsolumbar fusion of the, anterior column, anterior technique**
Arthrodesis of thoracic or thoracolumbar region:

Revise inclusion term
anterior (interbody ~~technique~~) fusion

Add inclusion term
Extracavitary technique

Revise code title | **81.05** | **Dorsal and dorsolumbar fusion of the, posterior column, posterior technique**
Arthrodesis of thoracic or

Revise inclusion term
thoracolumbar regionn:, posterolateral technique

Delete inclusion term
~~posterior (interbody) technique~~

Delete inclusion term
~~posterolateral technique~~

Revise code title	81.06	**Lumbar and lumbosacral fusion of the, anterior column, anterior technique**
		Arthrodesis of lumbar or lumbosacral region:
Revise inclusion term		anterior (interbody ~~technique~~) fusion
Add inclusion term		retroperitoneal
Add inclusion term		transperitoneal
Add inclusion term		Direct lateral interbody fusion [DLIF]
Add inclusion term		Extreme lateral interbody fusion [XLIF]
Revise code title	81.07	**Lumbar and lumbosacral fusion of the, posterior column, posterior ~~or lateral transverse process~~ technique**
Add inclusion term		Facet fusion
Add inclusion term		Posterolateral technique
Add inclusion term		Transverse process technique
Revise code title	81.08	**Lumbar and lumbosacral fusion of the, anterior column, posterior technique**
		Arthrodesis of lumbar or lumbosacral region:,
Revise inclusion term		posterior (interbody) ~~technique~~ fusion
Delete inclusion term		~~posterolateral technique~~
Add inclusion term		Axial lumbar interbody fusion [AxiaLIF]
	81.3	**Refusion of spine**
Add note		Note: Spine fusion is classified by the anatomic portion (column) fused and the technique (approach) used to perform the fusion.
		For the anterior column, the body (corpus) of adjacent vertebrae are fused (interbody fusion). The anterior column can be fused using an anterior, lateral, or posterior technique.
		For the posterior column, posterior structures of adjacent vertebrae are fused (pedicle, lamina, facet, transverse process, or "gutter" fusion). A posterior column fusion can be performed using a posterior, posterolateral, or lateral transverse technique.
Revise code title	81.32	**Refusion of other cervical spine, anterior column, anterior technique**
		Arthrodesis of C2 level or below: anterior (interbody ~~technique~~) fusion
Revise inclusion term		

Revise code title	81.33	**Refusion of other cervical spine, posterior column, posterior technique**
		Arthrodesis of C2 level or below:, posterolateral technique
Revise inclusion term		
Delete inclusion term		~~Posterior (interbody) technique~~
Delete inclusion term		~~Posterolateral technique~~
Revise code title	81.34	**Refusion of dorsal and dorsolumbar spine, anterior column, anterior technique**
		Arthrodesis of thoracic or thoracolumbar region: anterior (interbody ~~technique~~) fusion
Revise inclusion term		
Add inclusion term		Extracavitary technique
Revise code title	81.35	**Refusion of dorsal and dorsolumbar spine, posterior column, posterior technique**
		Arthrodesis of thoracic or thoracolumbar region:, posterolateral technique
Revise inclusion term		
Delete inclusion term		~~posterior (interbody) technique~~
Delete inclusion term		~~posterolateral technique~~
Revise code title	81.36	**Refusion of lumbar and lumbosacral spine, anterior column, anterior technique**
		Arthrodesis of lumbar or lumbosacral region: anterior (interbody ~~technique~~) fusion
Revise inclusion term		
Add inclusion term		retroperitoneal
Add inclusion term		transperitoneal
Add inclusion term		Direct lateral interbody fusion [DLIF]
Add inclusion term		Extreme lateral interbody fusion [XLIF]
Revise code title	81.37	**Refusion of lumbar and lumbosacral spine, posterior column, posterior ~~or lateral transverse process~~ technique**
		Facet fusion
Add inclusion term		Posterolateral technique
Add inclusion term		Transverse process technique
Add inclusion term		

Revise
code title

81.38 Refusion of lumbar and lumbosacral spine, anterior column, posterior technique

Revise
inclusion
term

> Arthrodesis of lumbar or lumbosacral region:,

Revise
inclusion
term

> posterior (interbody) technique fusion

Delete
inclusion
term

> posterolateral technique

Add
inclusion
term

> Axial lumbar interbody fusion [AxiaLIF]

Revise
code title

81.80 Other Ttotal shoulder replacement

Add
exclusion
term

> | Excludes | *reverse total shoulder replacement (81.88)*

81.83 Other repair of shoulder

> Revision of arthroplasty of shoulder

Delete
inclusion
term

New code

81.88 Reverse total shoulder replacement

> Reverse ball-and-socket of the shoulder

> | Excludes | *conversion of prior (failed) total shoulder replacement (arthroplasty) to reverse total shoulder replacement (81.97)*

81.97 Revision of joint replacement of upper extremity

Add
inclusion
term

> Revision of arthroplasty of shoulder

Revise
code title

83.21 Open Bbiopsy of soft tissue

Revise
exclusion
term

> | Excludes | *closed biopsy of skin and subcutaneous tissue (86.11)*

New code

84.94 Insertion of sternal fixation device with rigid plates

> | Excludes | *insertion of sternal fixation device for internalfixation of fracture (79.39) internal fixation of bone without fracture reduction (78.59)*

85.51 Unilateral injection into breast for augmentation

Add
exclusion
term

> | Excludes | *injection of fat graft of breast (85.55)*

85.52 Bilateral injection into breast for augmentation

Add
exclusion
term

> | Excludes | *injection of fat graft of breast (85.55)*

New code

85.55 Fat graft to breast

> | Includes | extraction of fat for autologous graft Autologous fat transplantation or transfer Fat graft to breast NOS Fat graft to breast with or without use of enriched graft Micro-fat grafting

> | Excludes | *that with reconstruction of breast (85.70-85.79)*

85.92 Injection of therapeutic agent into breast

Revise
exclusion
term

> | Excludes | *that for augmentation of breast (85.51-85.52, 85.55)*

Revise
code title

86.11 Closed Bbiopsy of skin and subcutaneous tissue

86.83 Size reduction plastic operation

Add
exclusion
term

> | Excludes | *liposuction to harvest fat graft (86.90)*

New code

86.87 Fat graft of skin and subcutaneous tissue

> | Includes | extraction of fat for autologous graft Autologous fat transplantation or transfer Fat graft NOS Fat graft of skin and subcutaneous tissue with orwithout use of enriched graft Micro-fat grafting

> | Excludes | *fat graft to breast (85.55)*

New code

86.90 Extraction of fat for graft or banking

> Harvest of fat for extraction of cells for future use Liposuction to harvest fat graft

> | Excludes | *that with graft at same operative episode (85.55, 86.87)*

86.94 Insertion or replacement of single array neurostimulator pulse generator, not specified as rechargeable

Add
exclusion
term

> | Excludes | *cranial implantation or replacement of neurostimulator pulse generator (01.20)*

86.95 Insertion or replacement of dual array neurostimulator pulse generator, not specified as rechargeable

Add
exclusion
term

> | Excludes | *cranial implantation or replacement of neurostimulator pulse generator (01.20)*

Add exclusion term

86.96   Insertion or replacement of other neurostimulator pulse generator

> **Excludes** *cranial implantation or replacement of neurostimulator pulse generator (01.20)*

86.97   Insertion or replacement of single array rechargeable neurostimulator pulse generator

Add exclusion term

> **Excludes** *cranial implantation or replacement of neurostimulator pulse generator (01.20)*

Add exclusion term

86.98   Insertion or replacement of dual array rechargeable neurostimulator pulse generator

> **Excludes** *cranial implantation or replacement of neurostimulator pulse generator (01.20)*

Revise code title

88.59   Intra-operative <u>coronary</u> fluorescence vascular angiography

Revise code title

Add inclusion term

99.14   Injection or infusion of ~~gamma globulin~~ immunoglobulin

> <u>Injection or infusion of gamma globulin</u>

PART I

Introduction

ICD-9-CM BACKGROUND

The International Classification of Diseases, 9th Revision, Clinical Modification (ICD-9-CM) is based on the official version of the World Health Organization's 9th Revision, International Classification of Diseases (ICD-9). ICD-9 is designed for the classification of morbidity and mortality information for statistical purposes, and for the indexing of hospital records by disease and operations, for data storage and retrieval. The historical background of the International Classification of Diseases may be found in the Introduction to ICD-9 (Manual of the International Classification of Diseases, Injuries, and Causes of Death, World Health Organization, Geneva, Switzerland, 1977).

ICD-9-CM is a clinical modification of the World Health Organization's International Classification of Diseases, 9th Revision (ICD-9). The term "clinical" is used to emphasize the modification's intent: to serve as a useful tool in the area of classification of morbidity data for indexing of medical records, medical care review, and ambulatory and other medical care programs, as well as for basic health statistics. To describe the clinical picture of the patient, the codes must be more precise than those needed only for statistical groupings and trend analysis.

COORDINATION AND MAINTENANCE COMMITTEE

Annual modifications are made to the ICD-9-CM through the ICD-9-CM Coordination and Maintenance Committee (C&M). The Committee

is made up of representatives from two Federal Government agencies, the National Center for Health Statistics and the Health Care Financing Administration. The Committee holds meetings twice a year which are open to the public. Modification proposals submitted to the Committee for consideration are presented at the meetings for public discussion. Those modification proposals which are approved are incorporated into the official government version of the ICD-9-CM and become effective for use October 1 of the year following their presentation. The C&M also prepares updates for use April 1 of each year. To date, no April 1 updates have been released.

CHARACTERISTICS OF ICD-9-CM

ICD-9-CM far exceeds its predecessors in the number of codes provided. The disease classification has been expanded to include health-related conditions and to provide greater specificity at the fifth-digit level of detail. These fifth digits are not optional; they are intended for use in recording the information substantiated in the clinical record.

Volume I of ICD-9-CM contains five appendices:

Appendix A	Morphology of Neoplasms
Appendix B	Glossary of Mental Disorders (Deleted in 2004)
Appendix C	Classification of Drugs by American Hospital Formulary Service List Number and Their ICD-9-CM Equivalents
Appendix D	Classification of Industrial Accidents According to Agency
Appendix E	List of Three-Digit Categories

These appendices are included as a reference to the user in order to provide further information about the patient's clinical picture, to further define a diagnostic statement, to aid in classifying new drugs, or to reference three-digit categories.

Volume 2 of ICD-9-CM contains many diagnostic terms which do not appear in Volume 1 since the index includes most diagnostic terms currently in use.

The Disease Classification

ICD-9-CM is totally compatible with its parent system, ICD-9, thus meeting the need for comparability of morbidity and mortality statistics at the international level. A few fourth-digit codes were created in existing three-digit rubrics only when the necessary detail could not be accommodated by the use of a fifth-digit subclassification. To ensure that each rubric of ICD-9-CM collapses back to its ICD-9 counterpart, the following specifications governed the ICD-9-CM disease classification:

Specifications for the Tabular List

1. Three-digit rubrics and their contents are unchanged from ICD-9.
2. The sequence of three-digit rubrics is unchanged from ICD-9.
3. Unsubdivided three-digit rubrics are subdivided where necessary to:
   a) Add clinical detail
   b) Isolate terms for clinical accuracy
4. The modification in ICD-9-CM is accomplished by the addition of a fifth digit to existing ICD-9 rubrics.
5. The optional dual classification in ICD-9 is modified.
   a) Duplicate rubrics are deleted:
      1) Four-digit manifestation categories duplicating etiology entries.
      2) Manifestation inclusion terms duplicating etiology entries.
   b) Manifestations of diseases are identified, to the extent possible, by creating five-digit codes in the etiology rubrics.
   c) When the manifestation of a disease cannot be included in the etiology rubrics, provision for its identification is made by retaining the ICD-9 rubrics used for classifying manifestations of disease.
6. The format of ICD-9-CM is revised from that used in ICD-9.
   a) American spelling of medical terms is used.
   b) Inclusion terms are indented beneath the titles of codes.
   c) Codes not to be used for principal tabulation of disease are printed with the notation, "Code first underlying disease."

Specifications for the Alphabetic Index

1. Format of the Alphabetic Index follows the format of ICD-9.
2. When two codes are required to indicate etiology and manifestation, the manifestation code appears in brackets, e.g., diabetic cataract 250.5X [366.41]. The etiology code is always sequenced first followed by the manifestation code.

The following guidelines were the most current at the time of publication. Check the website at http://codingupdates.com for the latest updates to the Guidelines.

ICD-9-CM OFFICIAL GUIDELINES FOR CODING AND REPORTING

Effective October 1, 2009
Narrative changes appear in bold text
Items underlined have been moved within the guidelines since October 1, 2008
The guidelines include the updated V Code Table

The Centers for Medicare and Medicaid Services (CMS) and the National Center for Health Statistics (NCHS), two departments within the U.S. Federal Government's Department of Health and Human Services (DHHS) provide the following guidelines for coding and reporting using the International Classification of Diseases, 9th Revision, Clinical Modification (ICD-9-CM). These guidelines should be used as a companion document to the official version of the ICD-9-CM as published on CD-ROM by the U.S. Government Printing Office (GPO).

These guidelines have been approved by the four organizations that make up the Cooperating Parties for the ICD-9-CM: the American Hospital Association (AHA), the American Health Information Management Association (AHIMA), CMS, and NCHS. These guidelines are included on the official government version of the ICD-9-CM, and also appear in "Coding Clinic for ICD-9-CM" published by the AHA.

These guidelines are a set of rules that have been developed to accompany and complement the official conventions and instructions provided within the ICD-9-CM itself. **The instructions and conventions of the classification take precedence over guidelines.** These guidelines are based on the coding and sequencing instructions in Volumes I, II and III of ICD-9-CM, but provide additional instruction. Adherence to these guidelines when assigning ICD-9-CM diagnosis and procedure codes is required under the Health Insurance Portability and Accountability Act (HIPAA). The diagnosis codes (Volumes 1-2) have been adopted under HIPAA for all healthcare settings. Volume 3 procedure codes have been adopted for inpatient procedures reported by hospitals. A joint effort between the healthcare provider and the coder is essential to achieve complete and accurate documentation, code assignment, and reporting of diagnoses and procedures. These guidelines have been developed to assist both the healthcare provider and the coder in identifying those diagnoses and procedures that are to be reported. The importance of consistent, complete documentation in the medical record cannot be overemphasized. Without such documentation accurate coding cannot be achieved. The entire record should be reviewed to determine the specific reason for the encounter and the conditions treated.

The term encounter is used for all settings, including hospital admissions. In the context of these guidelines, the term provider is used throughout the guidelines to mean physician or any qualified health care practitioner who is legally accountable for establishing the patient's diagnosis. Only this set of guidelines, approved by the Cooperating Parties, is official.

The guidelines are organized into sections. Section I includes the structure and conventions of the classification and general guidelines that apply to the entire classification, and chapter-specific guidelines that correspond to the chapters as they are arranged in the classification. Section II includes guidelines for selection of principal diagnosis for non-outpatient settings. Section III includes guidelines for reporting additional diagnoses in non-outpatient settings. Section IV is for outpatient coding and reporting.

ICD-9-CM Official Guidelines for Coding and Reporting

Section I. Conventions, general coding guidelines and chapter specific guidelines

A. Conventions for the ICD-9-CM
   1. Format:
   2. Abbreviations
      a. Index abbreviations
      b. Tabular abbreviations
   3. Punctuation
   4. Includes and Excludes Notes and Inclusion terms
   5. Other and Unspecified codes
      a. "Other" codes
      b. "Unspecified" codes
   6. Etiology/manifestation convention ("code first", "use additional code" and "in diseases classified elsewhere" notes)
   7. "And"
   8. "With"
   9. "See" and "See Also"

B. General Coding Guidelines
   1. Use of Both Alphabetic Index and Tabular List
   2. Locate each term in the Alphabetic Index
   3. Level of Detail in Coding
   4. Code or codes from 001.0 through V89.**09**
   5. Selection of codes 001.0 through 999.9
   6. Signs and symptoms
   7. Conditions that are an integral part of a disease process
   8. Conditions that are not an integral part of a disease process
   9. Multiple coding for a single condition
   10. Acute and Chronic Conditions
   11. Combination Code
   12. Late Effects
   13. Impending or Threatened Condition
   14. Reporting Same Diagnosis Code More than Once
   15. Admissions/Encounters for Rehabilitation
   16. Documentation for BMI and Pressure Ulcer Stages
   17. **Syndromes**

C. Chapter-Specific Coding Guidelines
   1. Chapter 1: Infectious and Parasitic Diseases (001-139)
      a. Human Immunodeficiency Virus (HIV) Infections
      b. Septicemia, Systemic Inflammatory Response Syndrome (SIRS), Sepsis, Severe Sepsis, and Septic Shock
      c. Methicillin Resistant *Staphylococcus aureus* (MRSA) Conditions
   2. Chapter 2: Neoplasms (140-239)
      a. Treatment directed at the malignancy
      b. Treatment of secondary site
      c. Coding and sequencing of complications
      d. Primary malignancy previously excised
      e. Admissions/Encounters involving chemotherapy, immunotherapy and radiation therapy
      f. Admission/encounter to determine extent of malignancy
      g. Symptoms, signs, and ill-defined conditions listed in Chapter 16 associated with neoplasms
      h. Admission/encounter for pain control/management
      i. Malignant neoplasm associated with transplanted organ

GUIDELINES

f. Undetermined Cause
g. Late Effects of External Cause Guidelines
h. Misadventures and Complications of Care Guidelines
i. Terrorism Guidelines
j. Activity Code Guidelines
k. **External cause status**

Section II. Selection of Principal Diagnosis

A. Codes for symptoms, signs, and ill-defined conditions
B. Two or more interrelated conditions, each potentially meeting the definition for principal diagnosis
C. Two or more diagnoses that equally meet the definition for principal diagnosis
D. Two or more comparative or contrasting conditions
E. A symptom(s) followed by contrasting/comparative diagnoses
F. Original treatment plan not carried out
G. Complications of surgery and other medical care
H. Uncertain Diagnosis
I. Admission from Observation Unit
   1. Admission Following Medical Observation
   2. Admission Following Post-Operative Observation
J. Admission from Outpatient Surgery

Section III. Reporting Additional Diagnoses

A. Previous conditions
B. Abnormal findings
C. Uncertain Diagnosis

Section IV. Diagnostic Coding and Reporting Guidelines for Outpatient Services

A. Selection of first-listed condition
   1. Outpatient Surgery
   2. Observation Stay
B. Codes from 001.0 through V89
C. Accurate reporting of ICD-9-CM diagnosis codes
D. Selection of codes 001.0 through 999.9
E. Codes that describe symptoms and signs
F. Encounters for circumstances other than a disease or injury
G. Level of Detail in Coding
   1. ICD-9-CM codes with 3, 4, or 5 digits
   2. Use of full number of digits required for a code

H. ICD-9-CM code for the diagnosis, condition, problem, or other reason for encounter/visit
I. Uncertain diagnosis
J. Chronic diseases
K. Code all documented conditions that coexist
L. Patients receiving diagnostic services only
M. Patients receiving therapeutic services only
N. Patients receiving preoperative evaluations only
O. Ambulatory surgery
P. Routine outpatient prenatal visits

Appendix I: Present on Admission Reporting Guidelines

Section I. Conventions, general coding guidelines and chapter specific guidelines

The conventions, general guidelines and chapter-specific guidelines are applicable to all health care settings unless otherwise indicated. **The conventions and instructions of the classification take precedence over guidelines.**

A. **Conventions for the ICD-9-CM**

The conventions for the ICD-9-CM are the general rules for use of the classification independent of the guidelines. These conventions are incorporated within the index and tabular of the ICD-9-CM as instructional notes. The conventions are as follows:

1. **Format:**
   The ICD-9-CM uses an indented format for ease in reference

2. **Abbreviations**
   a. **Index abbreviations**
      NEC "Not elsewhere classifiable" This abbreviation in the index represents "other specified" when a specific code is not available for a condition the index directs the coder to the "other specified" code in the tabular.

   b. **Tabular abbreviations**
      NEC "Not elsewhere classifiable" This abbreviation in the tabular represents "other specified". When a specific code is not available for a condition the tabular includes an NEC entry under a code to identify the code as the "other specified" code. (*See Section I.A.5.a. "Other" codes*).
      NOS "Not otherwise specified" This abbreviation is the equivalent of unspecified. (*See Section I.A.5.b., "Unspecified" codes*)

5

3. **Punctuation**

[ ] Brackets are used in the tabular list to enclose synonyms, alternative wording or explanatory phrases. Brackets are used in the index to identify manifestation codes. *(See Section I.A.6. "Etiology/manifestations")*

( ) Parentheses are used in both the index and tabular to enclose supplementary words that may be present or absent in the statement of a disease or procedure without affecting the code number to which it is assigned. The terms within the parentheses are referred to as nonessential modifiers.

: Colons are used in the Tabular list after an incomplete term which needs one or more of the modifiers following the colon to make it assignable to a given category.

4. **Includes and Excludes Notes and Inclusion terms**

Includes: This note appears immediately under a three-digit code title to further define, or give examples of, the content of the category.

Excludes: An excludes note under a code indicates that the terms excluded from the code are to be coded elsewhere. In some cases the codes for the excluded terms should not be used in conjunction with the code from which it is excluded. An example of this is a congenital condition excluded from an acquired form of the same condition. The congenital and acquired codes should not be used together. In other cases, the excluded terms may be used together with an excluded code. An example of this is when fractures of different bones are coded to different codes. Both codes may be used together if both types of fractures are present.

Inclusion terms: List of terms is included under certain four and five digit codes. These terms are the conditions for which that code number is to be used. The terms may be synonyms of the code title, or, in the case of "other specified" codes, the terms are a list of the various conditions assigned to that code. The inclusion terms are not necessarily exhaustive. Additional terms found only in the index may also be assigned to a code.

5. **Other and Unspecified codes**

a. **"Other" codes**

Codes titled "other" or "other specified" (usually a code with a 4th digit 8 or fifth-digit 9 for diagnosis codes) are for use when the information in the medical record provides detail for which a specific code does not exist. Index entries with NEC in the line designate "other" codes in the tabular. These index entries represent specific disease entities for which no specific code exists so the term is included within an "other" code.

b. **"Unspecified" codes**

Codes (usually a code with a 4th digit 9 or 5th digit 0 for diagnosis codes) titled "unspecified" are for use when the information in the medical record is insufficient to assign a more specific code.

6. **Etiology/manifestation convention ("code first", "use additional code" and "in diseases classified elsewhere" notes)**

Certain conditions have both an underlying etiology and multiple body system manifestations due to the underlying etiology. For such conditions, the ICD-9-CM has a coding convention that requires the underlying condition be sequenced first followed by the manifestation. Wherever such a combination exists, there is a "use additional code" note at the etiology code, and a "code first" note at the manifestation code. These instructional notes indicate the proper sequencing order of the codes, etiology followed by manifestation.

In most cases the manifestation codes will have in the code title, "in diseases classified elsewhere." Codes with this title are a component of the etiology/manifestation convention. The code title indicates that it is a manifestation code. "In diseases classified elsewhere" codes are never permitted to be used as first listed or principal diagnosis codes. They must be used in conjunction with an underlying condition code and they must be listed following the underlying condition.

There are manifestation codes that do not have "in diseases classified elsewhere" in the title. For such codes a "use additional code" note will still be present and the rules for sequencing apply.

In addition to the notes in the tabular, these conditions also have a specific index entry structure. In the index both conditions are listed together with the etiology code first followed by the manifestation codes in brackets. The code in brackets is always to be sequenced second.

The most commonly used etiology/manifestation combinations are the codes for Diabetes mellitus, category 250. For each code under category 250 there is a use additional code note for the manifestation that is specific for that particular diabetic manifestation. Should a patient have more than one manifestation of diabetes, more than one code from category 250 may be used with as many manifestation codes as are needed to fully describe the patient's complete diabetic condition. The category 250 diabetes codes should be sequenced first, followed by the manifestation codes.

"Code first" and "Use additional code" notes are also used as sequencing rules in the classification for certain codes that are not part of an etiology/manifestation combination.

See - Section I.B.9. "Multiple coding for a single condition".

7. "And"

The word "and" should be interpreted to mean either "and" or "or" when it appears in a title.

8. "With"

The word "with" in the alphabetic index is sequenced immediately following the main term, not in alphabetical order.

9. "See" and "See Also"

The "see" instruction following a main term in the index indicates that another term should be referenced. It is necessary to go to the main term referenced with the "see" note to locate the correct code.

A "see also" instruction following a main term in the index instructs that there is another main term that may also be referenced that may provide additional index entries that may be useful. It is not necessary to follow the "see also" note when the original main term provides the necessary code.

B. General Coding Guidelines

1. Use of Both Alphabetic Index and Tabular List

Use both the Alphabetic Index and the Tabular List when locating and assigning a code. Reliance on only the Alphabetic Index or the Tabular List leads to errors in code assignments and less specificity in code selection.

2. Locate each term in the Alphabetic Index

Locate each term in the Alphabetic Index and verify the code selected in the Tabular List. Read and be guided by instructional notations that appear in both the Alphabetic Index and the Tabular List.

3. Level of Detail in Coding

Diagnosis and procedure codes are to be used at their highest number of digits available.

ICD-9-CM diagnosis codes are composed of codes with 3, 4, or 5 digits. Codes with three digits are included in ICD-9-CM as the heading of a category of codes that may be further subdivided by the use of fourth and/or fifth digits, which provide greater detail.

A three-digit code is to be used only if it is not further subdivided. Where fourth-digit subcategories and/or fifth-digit subclassifications are provided, they must be assigned. A code is invalid if it has not been coded to the full number of digits required for that code. For example, Acute myocardial infarction, code 410, has fourth digits that describe the location of the infarction (e.g., 410.2, Of inferolateral wall), and fifth digits that identify the episode of care. It would be incorrect to report a code in category 410 without a fourth and fifth digit.

ICD-9-CM Volume 3 procedure codes are composed of codes with either 3 or 4 digits. Codes with two digits are included in ICD-9-CM as the heading of a category of codes that may be further subdivided by the use of third and/or fourth digits, which provide greater detail.

4. Code or codes from 001.0 through V89.09

The appropriate code or codes from 001.0 through V89.09 must be used to identify diagnoses, symptoms, conditions, problems, complaints or other reason(s) for the encounter/visit.

5. Selection of codes 001.0 through 999.9

The selection of codes 001.0 through 999.9 will frequently be used to describe the reason for the admission/encounter. These codes are from the section of ICD-9-CM for the classification of diseases and injuries (e.g., infectious and parasitic diseases; neoplasms; symptoms, signs, and ill-defined conditions, etc.).

6. Signs and symptoms

Codes that describe symptoms and signs, as opposed to diagnoses, are acceptable for reporting purposes when a related definitive diagnosis has not been established (confirmed) by the provider. Chapter 16 of ICD-9-CM, Symptoms, Signs, and Ill-defined conditions (codes 780.0 - 799.9) contain many, but not all codes for symptoms.

7. Conditions that are an integral part of a disease process

Signs and symptoms that are associated routinely with a disease process should not be assigned as additional codes, unless otherwise instructed by the classification.

8. **Conditions that are not an integral part of a disease process**

Additional signs and symptoms that may not be associated routinely with a disease process should be coded when present.

9. **Multiple coding for a single condition**

In addition to the etiology/manifestation convention that requires two codes to fully describe a single condition that affects multiple body systems, there are other single conditions that also require more than one code. "Use additional code" notes are found in the tabular at codes that are not part of an etiology/manifestation pair where a secondary code is useful to fully describe a condition. The sequencing rule is the same as the etiology/manifestation pair - , "use additional code" indicates that a secondary code should be added.

For example, for infections that are not included in chapter 1, a secondary code from category 041, Bacterial infection in conditions classified elsewhere and of unspecified site, may be required to identify the bacterial organism causing the infection. A "use additional code" note will normally be found at the infectious disease code, indicating a need for the organism code to be added as a secondary code.

"Code first" notes are also under certain codes that are not specifically manifestation codes but may be due to an underlying cause. When a "code first" note is present and an underlying condition is present the underlying condition should be sequenced first.

"Code, if applicable, any causal condition first", notes indicate that this code may be assigned as a principal diagnosis when the causal condition is unknown or not applicable. If a causal condition is known, then the code for that condition should be sequenced as the principal or first-listed diagnosis.

Multiple codes may be needed for late effects, complication codes and obstetric codes to more fully describe a condition. See the specific guidelines for these conditions for further instruction.

10. **Acute and Chronic Conditions**

If the same condition is described as both acute (subacute) and chronic, and separate subentries exist in the Alphabetic Index at the same indentation level, code both and sequence the acute (subacute) code first.

11. **Combination Code**

A combination code is a single code used to classify:
Two diagnoses, or

A diagnosis with an associated secondary process (manifestation)
A diagnosis with an associated complication

Combination codes are identified by referring to subterm entries in the Alphabetic Index and by reading the inclusion and exclusion notes in the Tabular List.

Assign only the combination code when that code fully identifies the diagnostic conditions involved or when the Alphabetic Index so directs. Multiple coding should not be used when the classification provides a combination code that clearly identifies all of the elements documented in the diagnosis. When the combination code lacks necessary specificity in describing the manifestation or complication, an additional code should be used as a secondary code.

12. **Late Effects**

A late effect is the residual effect (condition produced) after the acute phase of an illness or injury has terminated. There is no time limit on when a late effect code can be used. The residual may be apparent early, such as in cerebrovascular accident cases, or it may occur months or years later, such as that due to a previous injury. Coding of late effects generally requires two codes sequenced in the following order: The condition or nature of the late effect is sequenced first. The late effect code is sequenced second.

An exception to the above guidelines are those instances where the code for late effect is followed by a manifestation code identified in the Tabular List and title, or the late effect code has been expanded (at the fourth and fifth-digit levels) to include the manifestation(s). The code for the acute phase of an illness or injury that led to the late effect is never used with a code for the late effect.

13. **Impending or Threatened Condition**

Code any condition described at the time of discharge as "impending" or "threatened" as follows:

If it did occur, code as confirmed diagnosis.

If it did not occur, reference the Alphabetic Index to determine if the condition has a subentry term for "impending" or "threatened" and also reference main term entries for "Impending" and for "Threatened."

If the subterms are listed, assign the given code.

If the subterms are not listed, code the existing underlying condition(s) and not the condition described as impending or threatened.

14. Reporting Same Diagnosis Code More than Once

Each unique ICD-9-CM diagnosis code may be reported only once for an encounter. This applies to bilateral conditions or two different conditions classified to the same ICD-9-CM diagnosis code.

15. Admissions/Encounters for Rehabilitation

When the purpose for the admission/encounter is rehabilitation, sequence the appropriate V code from category V57, Care involving use of rehabilitation procedures, as the principal/first-listed diagnosis. The code for the condition for which the service is being performed should be reported as an additional diagnosis.

Only one code from category V57 is required. Code V57.89, Other specified rehabilitation procedures, should be assigned if more than one type of rehabilitation is performed during a single encounter. A procedure code should be reported to identify each type of rehabilitation therapy actually performed.

16. Documentation for BMI and Pressure Ulcer Stages

For the Body Mass Index (BMI) and pressure ulcer stage codes, code assignment may be based on medical record documentation from clinicians who are not the patient's provider (i.e., physician or other qualified healthcare practitioner legally accountable for establishing the patient's diagnosis), since this information is typically documented by other clinicians involved in the care of the patient (e.g., a dietitian often documents the BMI and nurses often documents the pressure ulcer stages). However, the associated diagnosis (such as overweight, obesity, or pressure ulcer) must be documented by the patient's provider. If there is conflicting medical record documentation, either from the same clinician or different clinicians, the patient's attending provider should be queried for clarification.

The BMI and pressure ulcer stage codes should only be reported as secondary diagnoses. As with all other secondary diagnosis codes, the BMI and pressure ulcer stage codes should only be assigned when they meet the definition of a reportable additional diagnosis (see Section III, Reporting Additional Diagnoses).

17. Syndromes

Follow the Alphabetic Index guidance when coding syndromes. In the absence of index guidance, assign codes for the documented manifestations of the syndrome.

C. Chapter-Specific Coding Guidelines

In addition to general coding guidelines, there are guidelines for specific diagnoses and/or conditions in the classification. Unless otherwise indicated, these guidelines apply to all health care settings. Please refer to Section II for guidelines on the selection of principal diagnosis.

1. Chapter 1: Infectious and Parasitic Diseases (001-139)

a. Human Immunodeficiency Virus (HIV) Infections

1) Code only confirmed cases

Code only confirmed cases of HIV infection/illness. This is an exception to the hospital inpatient guideline Section II, H.

In this context, "confirmation" does not require documentation of positive serology or culture for HIV; the provider's diagnostic statement that the patient is HIV positive, or has an HIV-related illness is sufficient.

2) Selection and sequencing of HIV codes

(a) Patient admitted for HIV-related condition

If a patient is admitted for an HIV-related condition, the principal diagnosis should be 042, followed by additional diagnosis codes for all reported HIV-related conditions.

(b) Patient with HIV disease admitted for unrelated condition

If a patient with HIV disease is admitted for an unrelated condition (such as a traumatic injury), the code for the unrelated condition (e.g., the nature of injury code) should be the principal diagnosis. Other diagnoses would be 042 followed by additional diagnosis codes for all reported HIV-related conditions.

(c) Whether the patient is newly diagnosed

Whether the patient is newly diagnosed or has had previous admissions/encounters for HIV conditions is irrelevant to the sequencing decision.

(d) Asymptomatic human immunodeficiency virus

V08 Asymptomatic human immunodeficiency virus [HIV]

infection, is to be applied when the patient without any documentation of symptoms is listed as being "HIV positive," "known HIV," "HIV test positive," or similar terminology. Do not use this code if the term "AIDS" is used or if the patient is treated for any HIV-related illness or is described as having any condition(s) resulting from his/her HIV positive status; use 042 in these cases.

(e) Patients with inconclusive HIV serology

Patients with inconclusive HIV serology, but no definitive diagnosis or manifestations of the illness, may be assigned code 795.71, Inconclusive serologic test for Human Immunodeficiency Virus [HIV].

(f) Previously diagnosed HIV-related illness

Patients with any known prior diagnosis of an HIV-related illness should be coded to 042. Once a patient has developed an HIV-related illness, the patient should always be assigned code 042 on every subsequent admission/encounter. Patients previously diagnosed with any HIV illness (042) should never be assigned to 795.71 or V08.

(g) HIV Infection in Pregnancy, Childbirth and the Puerperium

During pregnancy, childbirth or the puerperium, a patient admitted (or presenting for a health care encounter) because of an HIV-related illness should receive a principal diagnosis code of 647.6X, Other specified infectious and parasitic diseases in the mother classifiable elsewhere, but complicating the pregnancy, childbirth or the puerperium, followed by 042 and the code(s) for the HIV-related illness(es). Codes from Chapter 15 always take sequencing priority.

Patients with asymptomatic HIV infection status admitted (or presenting for a health care encounter) during pregnancy, childbirth, or the puerperium should receive codes of 647.6X and V08.

(h) Encounters for testing for HIV

If a patient is being seen to determine his/her HIV status, use code V73.89, Screening for other specified viral disease. Use code V69.8, Other problems related to lifestyle, as a secondary code if an asymptomatic patient is in a known high risk group for HIV. Should a patient with signs or symptoms or illness, or a confirmed HIV related diagnosis be tested for HIV, code the signs and symptoms or the diagnosis. An additional counseling code V65.44 may be used if counseling is provided during the encounter for the test.

When a patient returns to be informed of his/her HIV test results use code V65.44, HIV counseling, if the results of the test are negative.

If the results are positive but the patient is asymptomatic use code V08, Asymptomatic HIV infection. If the results are positive and the patient is symptomatic use code 042, HIV infection, with codes for the HIV related symptoms or diagnosis. The HIV counseling code may also be used if counseling is provided for patients with positive test results.

b. Septicemia, Systemic Inflammatory Response Syndrome (SIRS), Sepsis, Severe Sepsis, and Septic Shock

1) SIRS, Septicemia, and Sepsis

(a) The terms *septicemia* and *sepsis* are often used interchangeably by providers, however they are not considered synonymous terms. The following descriptions are provided for reference but do not preclude querying the provider for clarification about terms used in the documentation:

(i)   Septicemia generally refers to a systemic disease associated with the presence of pathological microorganisms or toxins in the blood, which can include bacteria, viruses, fungi or other organisms.

(ii)   Systemic inflammatory response syndrome (SIRS) generally refers to the systemic response to infection, trauma/burns, or other insult (such as cancer) with symptoms including fever, tachycardia, tachypnea, and leukocytosis.

   (iii) Sepsis generally refers to SIRS due to infection.

   (iv) Severe sepsis generally refers to sepsis with associated acute organ dysfunction.

(b) The Coding of SIRS, sepsis and severe sepsis

The coding of SIRS, sepsis and severe sepsis requires a minimum of 2 codes: a code for the underlying cause (such as infection or trauma) and a code from subcategory 995.9 Systemic inflammatory response syndrome (SIRS).

   (i) The code for the underlying cause (such as infection or trauma) must be sequenced before the code from subcategory 995.9 Systemic inflammatory response syndrome (SIRS).

   (ii) Sepsis and severe sepsis require a code for the systemic infection (038.xx, 112.5, etc.) and either code 995.91, Sepsis, or 995.92, Severe sepsis. If the causal organism is not documented, assign code 038.9, Unspecified septicemia.

   (iii) Severe sepsis requires additional code(s) for the associated acute organ dysfunction(s).

   (iv) If a patient has sepsis with multiple organ dysfunctions, follow the instructions for coding severe sepsis.

   (v) Either the term sepsis or SIRS must be documented to assign a code from subcategory 995.9.

      See Section I.C.17.g), Injury and poisoning, for information regarding systemic inflammatory response syndrome (SIRS) due to trauma/burns and other non-infectious processes.

(c) Due to the complex nature of sepsis and severe sepsis, some cases may require querying the provider prior to assignment of the codes.

2) Sequencing sepsis and severe sepsis

(a) Sepsis and severe sepsis as principal diagnosis

If sepsis or severe sepsis is present on admission, and meets the definition of principal diagnosis, the systemic infection code (e.g., 038.xx, 112.5, etc) should be assigned as the principal diagnosis, followed by code 995.91, Sepsis, or 995.92, Severe sepsis, as required by the sequencing rules in the Tabular List. Codes from subcategory 995.9 can never be assigned as a principal diagnosis. A code should also be assigned for any localized infection, if present.

If the sepsis or severe sepsis is due to a postprocedural infection, see Section I.C.1.b.10 for guidelines related to sepsis due to postprocedural infection.

(b) Sepsis and severe sepsis as secondary diagnoses

When sepsis or severe sepsis develops during the encounter (it was not present on admission), the systemic infection code and code 995.91 or 995.92 should be assigned as secondary diagnoses.

(c) Documentation unclear as to whether sepsis or severe sepsis is present on admission

Sepsis or severe sepsis may be present on admission but the diagnosis may not be confirmed until sometime after admission. If the documentation is not clear whether the sepsis or severe sepsis was present on admission, the provider should be queried.

3) Sepsis/SIRS with Localized Infection

If the reason for admission is both sepsis, severe sepsis, or SIRS and a localized infection, such as pneumonia or cellulitis, a code for the systemic infection (038.xx, 112.5, etc) should be assigned first, then code 995.91 or 995.92, followed by the code for the localized infection. If the patient is admitted with a localized infection, such as pneumonia, and sepsis/SIRS doesn't develop until after admission, see guideline I.C.1.b.2.b).

If the localized infection is postprocedural, *see Section I.C.1.b.10 for guidelines related to sepsis due to postprocedural infection.*

Note: The term urosepsis is a nonspecific term. If that is the only term documented then only code 599.0 should be assigned based on the default for the term in the ICD-9-CM index, in addition to the code for the causal organism if known.

4) **Bacterial Sepsis and Septicemia**

In most cases, it will be a code from category 038, Septicemia, that will be used in conjunction with a code from subcategory 995.9 such as the following:

(a) **Streptococcal sepsis**

If the documentation in the record states streptococcal sepsis, codes 038.0, Streptococcal septicemia, and code 995.91 should be used, in that sequence.

(b) **Streptococcal septicemia**

If the documentation states streptococcal septicemia, only code 038.0 should be assigned, however, the provider should be queried whether the patient has sepsis, an infection with SIRS.

5) **Acute organ dysfunction that is not clearly associated with the sepsis**

If a patient has sepsis and an acute organ dysfunction, but the medical record documentation indicates that the acute organ dysfunction is related to a medical condition other than the sepsis, do not assign code 995.92, Severe sepsis. An acute organ dysfunction must be associated with the sepsis in order to assign the severe sepsis code. If the documentation is not clear as to whether an acute organ dysfunction is related to the sepsis or another medical condition, query the provider.

6) **Septic shock**

(a) **Sequencing of septic shock**

Septic shock generally refers to circulatory failure associated with severe sepsis, and, therefore, it represents a type of acute organ dysfunction.

For all cases of septic shock, the code for the systemic infection should be sequenced first, followed by codes 995.92 and 785.52. Any additional codes for other acute organ dysfunctions should also be assigned. As noted in the sequencing instructions in the Tabular List, the code for septic shock cannot be assigned as a principal diagnosis.

(b) **Septic Shock without documentation of severe sepsis**

Septic shock indicates the presence of severe sepsis.

Code 995.92, Severe sepsis, must be assigned with code 785.52, Septic shock, even if the term severe sepsis is not documented in the record. The "use additional code" note and the "code first" note in the tabular support this guideline.

7) **Sepsis and septic shock complicating abortion and pregnancy**

Sepsis and septic shock complicating abortion, ectopic pregnancy, and molar pregnancy are classified to category codes in Chapter 11 (630-639).

See section I.C.11.i.7 for information on the coding of puerperal sepsis.

8) **Negative or inconclusive blood cultures**

Negative or inconclusive blood cultures do not preclude a diagnosis of septicemia or sepsis in patients with clinical evidence of the condition, however, the provider should be queried.

9) **Newborn sepsis**

See Section I.C.15.j for information on the coding of newborn sepsis.

10) **Sepsis due to a Postprocedural Infection**

(a) **Documentation of causal relationship**

As with all postprocedural complications, code assignment is based on the provider's documentation of the relationship between the infection and the procedure.

(b) **Sepsis due to postprocedural infection**

In cases of postprocedural sepsis, the complication code, such as code 998.59, Other postoperative infection, or 674.3x, Other complications of obstetrical surgical wounds should be coded first followed by the appropriate sepsis codes (systemic infection code and either code 995.91or

995.92). An additional code(s) for any acute organ dysfunction should also be assigned for cases of severe sepsis.

11) External cause of injury codes with SIRS

Refer to Section I.C.19.a.7 for instruction on the use of external cause of injury codes with codes for SIRS resulting from trauma.

12) Sepsis and Severe Sepsis Associated with Non-infectious Process

In some cases, a non-infectious process, such as trauma, may lead to an infection which can result in sepsis or severe sepsis. If sepsis or severe sepsis is documented as associated with a non-infectious condition, such as a burn or serious injury, and this condition meets the definition for principal diagnosis, the code for the non-infectious condition should be sequenced first, followed by the code for the systemic infection and either code 995.91, Sepsis, or 995.92, Severe sepsis. Additional codes for any associated acute organ dysfunction(s) should also be assigned for cases of severe sepsis. If the sepsis or severe sepsis meets the definition of principal diagnosis, the systemic infection and sepsis codes should be sequenced before the non-infectious condition. When both the associated non-infectious condition and the sepsis or severe sepsis meet the definition of principal diagnosis, either may be assigned as principal diagnosis.

See Section I.C.1.b.2.a for guidelines pertaining to sepsis or severe sepsis as the principal diagnosis.

Only one code from subcategory 995.9 should be assigned. Therefore, when a non-infectious condition leads to an infection resulting in sepsis or severe sepsis, assign either code 995.91 or 995.92. Do not additionally assign code 995.93, Systemic inflammatory response syndrome due to non-infectious process without acute organ dysfunction, or 995.94, Systemic inflammatory response syndrome with acute organ dysfunction.

See Section I.C.17.g for information on the coding of SIRS due to trauma/burns or other non-infectious disease processes.

c. Methicillin Resistant *Staphylococcus aureus* (MRSA) Conditions

1) Selection and sequencing of MRSA codes

(a) Combination codes for MRSA infection

When a patient is diagnosed with an infection that is due to methicillin resistant *Staphylococcus aureus* (MRSA), and that infection has a combination code that includes the causal organism (e.g., septicemia, pneumonia) assign the appropriate code for the condition (e.g., code 038.12, Methicillin resistant Staphylococcus aureus septicemia or code 482.42, Methicillin resistant pneumonia due to Staphylococcus aureus). Do not assign code 041.12, Methicillin resistant Staphylococcus aureus, as an additional code because the code includes the type of infection and the MRSA organism. Do not assign a code from subcategory V09.0, Infection with microorganisms resistant to penicillins, as an additional diagnosis.

See Section C.1.b.1 for instructions on coding and sequencing of septicemia.

(b) Other codes for MRSA infection

When there is documentation of a current infection (e.g., wound infection, stitch abscess, urinary tract infection) due to MRSA, and that infection does not have a combination code that includes the causal organism, select the appropriate code to identify the condition along with code 041.12, Methicillin resistant Staphylococcus aureus, for the MRSA infection. Do not assign a code from subcategory V09.0, Infection with microorganisms resistant to penicillins.

(c) Methicillin susceptible Staphylococcus aureus (MSSA) and MRSA colonization

The condition or state of being colonized or carrying MSSA or MRSA is called colonization or carriage, while an individual person is described as being colonized or being a carrier. Colonization means that MSSA or MSRA is present on or in the body without necessarily causing illness. A positive MRSA colonization test might be documented by the provider as "MRSA screen positive" or "MRSA nasal swab positive".

Assign code V02.54, Carrier or suspected carrier, Methicillin resistant Staphylococcus aureus, for patients documented as having MRSA colonization. Assign code V02.53, Carrier or suspected carrier, Methicillin susceptible Staphylococcus aureus, for patient documented as having MSSA colonization. Colonization is not necessarily indicative of a disease process or as the cause of a specific condition the patient may have unless documented as such by the provider.

Code V02.59, Other specified bacterial diseases, should be assigned for other types of staphylococcal colonization (e.g., *S. epidermidis, S. saprophyticus*). Code V02.59 should not be assigned for colonization with any type of *Staphylococcus aureus* (MRSA, MSSA).

(d) MRSA colonization and infection

If a patient is documented as having both MRSA colonization and infection during a hospital admission, code V02.54, Carrier or suspected carrier, Methicillin resistant *Staphylococcus aureus*, and a code for the MRSA infection may both be assigned.

2. **Chapter 2: Neoplasms (140-239)**

General guidelines

Chapter 2 of the ICD-9-CM contains the codes for most benign and all malignant neoplasms. Certain benign neoplasms, such as prostatic adenomas, may be found in the specific body system chapters. To properly code a neoplasm it is necessary to determine from the record if the neoplasm is benign, in-situ, malignant, or of uncertain histologic behavior. If malignant, any secondary (metastatic) sites should also be determined.

The neoplasm table in the Alphabetic Index should be referenced first. However, if the histological term is documented, that term should be referenced first, rather than going immediately to the Neoplasm Table, in order to determine which column in the Neoplasm Table is appropriate. For example, if the documentation indicates "adenoma," refer to the term in the Alphabetic Index to review the entries under this term and the instructional note to "see also neoplasm, by site, benign." The table provides the proper code based on the type of neoplasm and the site. It is important to select the proper column in the table that corresponds to the type of neoplasm. The tabular should then be referenced to verify that the correct code has been selected from the table and that a more specific site code does not exist.

See Section I. C. 18.d.4. for information regarding V codes for genetic susceptibility to cancer.

a. **Treatment directed at the malignancy**

If the treatment is directed at the malignancy, designate the malignancy as the principal diagnosis.

The only exception to this guideline is if a patient admission/encounter is solely for the administration of chemotherapy, immunotherapy or radiation therapy, assign the appropriate V58.x code as the first-listed or principal diagnosis, and the diagnosis or problem for which the service is being performed as a secondary diagnosis.

b. **Treatment of secondary site**

When a patient is admitted because of a primary neoplasm with metastasis and treatment is directed toward the secondary site only, the secondary neoplasm is designated as the principal diagnosis even though the primary malignancy is still present.

c. **Coding and sequencing of complications**

Coding and sequencing of complications associated with the malignancies or with the therapy thereof are subject to the following guidelines:

1) **Anemia associated with malignancy**

When admission/encounter is for management of an anemia associated with the malignancy, and the treatment is only for anemia, the appropriate anemia code (such as code 285.22, Anemia in neoplastic disease) is designated as the principal diagnosis and is followed by the appropriate code(s) for the malignancy.

Code 285.22 may also be used as a secondary code if the patient suffers from anemia and is being treated for the malignancy.

Code 285.22, Anemia in neoplastic disease, and code 285.3, Antineoplastic chemotherapy induced anemia, may both be assigned if anemia in neoplastic disease and anemia due to antineoplastic chemotherapy are both documented.

2) **Anemia associated with chemotherapy, immunotherapy and radiation therapy**

When the admission/encounter is for management of an anemia associated with chemotherapy, immunotherapy or radiotherapy and the only treatment is for the anemia, the anemia is sequenced first. The appropriate neoplasm code should be assigned as an additional code.

3) **Management of dehydration due to the malignancy**

When the admission/encounter is for management of dehydration due to the malignancy or the therapy, or a combination of both, and only the dehydration is being treated (intravenous rehydration), the dehydration is sequenced first, followed by the code(s) for the malignancy.

4) **Treatment of a complication resulting from a surgical procedure**

When the admission/encounter is for treatment of a complication resulting from a surgical procedure, designate the complication as the principal or first-listed diagnosis if treatment is directed at resolving the complication.

d. **Primary malignancy previously excised**

When a primary malignancy has been previously excised or eradicated from its site and there is no further treatment directed to that site and there is no evidence of any existing primary malignancy, a code from category V10, Personal history of malignant neoplasm, should be used to indicate the former site of the malignancy. Any mention of extension, invasion, or metastasis to another site is coded as a secondary malignant neoplasm to that site. The secondary site may be the principal or first-listed with the V10 code used as a secondary code.

e. **Admissions/Encounters involving chemotherapy, immunotherapy and radiation therapy**

1) **Episode of care involves surgical removal of neoplasm**

When an episode of care involves the surgical removal of a neoplasm, primary or secondary site, followed by adjunct chemotherapy or radiation treatment during the same episode of care, the neoplasm code should be assigned as principal or first-listed diagnosis, using codes in the 140-198 series or where appropriate in the 200-203 series.

2) **Patient admission/encounter solely for administration of chemotherapy, immunotherapy and radiation therapy**

If a patient admission/encounter is solely for the administration of chemotherapy, immunotherapy or radiation therapy assign code V58.0, Encounter for radiation therapy, or V58.11, Encounter for antineoplastic chemotherapy, or V58.12, Encounter for antineoplastic immunotherapy as the first-listed or principal diagnosis. If a patient receives more than one of these therapies during the same admission more than one of these codes may be assigned, in any sequence.

The malignancy for which the therapy is being administered should be assigned as a secondary diagnosis.

3) **Patient admitted for radiotherapy/ chemotherapy and immunotherapy and develops complications**

When a patient is admitted for the purpose of radiotherapy, immunotherapy or chemotherapy and develops complications such as uncontrolled nausea and vomiting or dehydration, the principal or first-listed diagnosis is V58.0, Encounter for radiotherapy, or V58.11, Encounter for antineoplastic chemotherapy, or V58.12, Encounter for antineoplastic immunotherapy followed by any codes for the complications.

f. **Admission/encounter to determine extent of malignancy**

When the reason for admission/encounter is to determine the extent of the malignancy, or for a procedure such as paracentesis or thoracentesis, the primary malignancy or appropriate metastatic site is designated as the principal or first-listed diagnosis, even though chemotherapy or radiotherapy is administered.

g. **Symptoms, signs, and ill-defined conditions listed in Chapter 16 associated with neoplasms**

Symptoms, signs, and ill-defined conditions listed in Chapter 16 characteristic of, or associated with, an existing primary or secondary site malignancy cannot be used to replace the malignancy as principal or first-listed diagnosis, regardless of the number of admissions or encounters for treatment and care of the neoplasm.

h. **Admission/encounter for pain control/ management**

See Section I.C.6.a.5 for information on coding admission/encounter for pain control/ management.

i. **Malignant neoplasm associated with transplanted organ**

A malignant neoplasm of a transplanted organ should be coded as a transplant complication. Assign first the appropriate code from subcategory 996.8, Complications of transplanted organ, followed by code 199.2, Malignant neoplasm associated with transplanted organ. Use an additional code for the specific malignancy.

3. **Chapter 3: Endocrine, Nutritional, and Metabolic Diseases and Immunity Disorders (240-279)**

a. **Diabetes mellitus**

Codes under category 250, Diabetes mellitus, identify complications/ manifestations associated with diabetes mellitus. A fifth-digit is required for all category 250 codes to identify the type of diabetes mellitus and whether the diabetes is controlled or uncontrolled.

See I.C.3.a.7 for secondary diabetes

1) **Fifth-digits for category 250:**

The following are the fifth-digits for the codes under category 250:

0   type II or unspecified type, not stated as uncontrolled

1   type I, [juvenile type], not stated as uncontrolled

2   type II or unspecified type, uncontrolled

3   type I, [juvenile type], uncontrolled

The age of a patient is not the sole determining factor, though most type I diabetics develop the condition before reaching puberty. For this reason type I diabetes mellitus is also referred to as juvenile diabetes.

2) **Type of diabetes mellitus not documented**

If the type of diabetes mellitus is not documented in the medical record the default is type II.

3) **Diabetes mellitus and the use of insulin**

All type I diabetics must use insulin to replace what their bodies do not produce. However, the use of insulin does not mean that a patient is a type I diabetic. Some patients with type II diabetes mellitus are unable to control their blood sugar through diet and oral medication alone and do require insulin. If the documentation in a medical record does not indicate the type of diabetes but does indicate that the patient uses insulin, the appropriate fifth-digit for type II must be used. For type II patients who routinely use insulin, code V58.67, Long-term (current) use of insulin, should also be assigned to indicate that the patient uses insulin. Code V58.67 should not be assigned if insulin is given temporarily to bring a type II patient's blood sugar under control during an encounter.

4) **Assigning and sequencing diabetes codes and associated conditions**

When assigning codes for diabetes and its associated conditions, the code(s) from category 250 must be sequenced before the codes for the associated conditions. The diabetes codes and the secondary codes that correspond to them are paired codes that follow the etiology/manifestation convention of the classification *(See Section I.A.6., Etiology/manifestation convention)*. Assign as many codes from category 250 as needed to identify all of the associated conditions that the patient has. The corresponding secondary codes are listed under each of the diabetes codes.

(a) **Diabetic retinopathy/diabetic macular edema**

Diabetic macular edema, code 362.07, is only present with diabetic retinopathy. Another code from subcategory 362.0, Diabetic retinopathy, must be used with code 362.07. Codes under subcategory 362.0 are diabetes manifestation codes, so they must be used following the appropriate diabetes code.

5) **Diabetes mellitus in pregnancy and gestational diabetes**

(a) For diabetes mellitus complicating pregnancy, see Section I.C.11.f., Diabetes mellitus in pregnancy.

(b) For gestational diabetes, see Section I.C.11, g., Gestational diabetes.

6) Insulin pump malfunction

(a) Underdose of insulin due insulin pump failure

An underdose of insulin due to an insulin pump failure should be assigned 996.57, Mechanical complication due to insulin pump, as the principal or first listed code, followed by the appropriate diabetes mellitus code based on documentation.

(b) Overdose of insulin due to insulin pump failure

The principal or first listed code for an encounter due to an insulin pump malfunction resulting in an overdose of insulin, should also be 996.57, Mechanical complication due to insulin pump, followed by code 962.3, Poisoning by insulins and antidiabetic agents, and the appropriate diabetes mellitus code based on documentation.

7) Secondary Diabetes Mellitus

Codes under category 249, Secondary diabetes mellitus, identify complications/manifestations associated with secondary diabetes mellitus. Secondary diabetes is always caused by another condition or event (e.g., cystic fibrosis, malignant neoplasm of pancreas, pancreatectomy, adverse effect of drug, or poisoning).

(a) Fifth-digits for category 249:

A fifth-digit is required for all category 249 codes to identify whether the diabetes is controlled or uncontrolled.

(b) Secondary diabetes mellitus and the use of insulin

For patients who routinely use insulin, code V58.67, Long-term (current) use of insulin, should also be assigned. Code V58.67 should not be assigned if insulin is given temporarily to bring a patient's blood sugar under control during an encounter.

(c) Assigning and sequencing secondary diabetes codes and associated conditions

When assigning codes for secondary diabetes and its associated conditions (e.g. renal manifestations), the code(s) from category 249 must be sequenced before the codes for the associated conditions. The secondary diabetes codes and the diabetic manifestation codes that correspond to them are paired codes that follow the etiology/manifestation convention of the classification. Assign as many codes from category 249 as needed to identify all of the associated conditions that the patient has. The corresponding codes for the associated conditions are listed under each of the secondary diabetes codes. For example, secondary diabetes with diabetic nephrosis is assigned to code 249.40, followed by 581.81.

(d) Assigning and sequencing secondary diabetes codes and its causes

The sequencing of the secondary diabetes codes in relationship to codes for the cause of the diabetes is based on the reason for the encounter, applicable ICD-9-CM sequencing conventions, and chapter-specific guidelines.

If a patient is seen for treatment of the secondary diabetes or one of its associated conditions, a code from category 249 is sequenced as the principal or first-listed diagnosis, with the cause of the secondary diabetes (e.g. cystic fibrosis) sequenced as an additional diagnosis.

If, however, the patient is seen for the treatment of the condition causing the secondary diabetes (e.g., malignant neoplasm of pancreas), the code for the cause of the secondary diabetes should be sequenced as the principal or first-listed diagnosis followed by a code from category 249.

(i) Secondary diabetes mellitus due to pancreatectomy

For postpancreatectomy diabetes mellitus (lack of insulin due to the surgical removal of all or part of the pancreas), assign code 251.3, Postsurgical hypoinsulinemia. **Assign a code from subcategory 249 and code V45.79, Other acquired absence of organ, as additional codes.** Code also any diabetic manifestations (e.g. diabetic nephrosis 581.81).

(ii) Secondary diabetes due to drugs

Secondary diabetes may be caused by an adverse effect of correctly administered medications, poisoning or late effect of poisoning.

See section I.C.17.e for coding of adverse effects and poisoning, and section I.C.19 for E code reporting.

4. Chapter 4: Diseases of Blood and Blood Forming Organs (280-289)

a. Anemia of chronic disease

Subcategory 285.2, Anemia in chronic illness, has codes for anemia in chronic kidney disease, code 285.21; anemia in neoplastic disease, code 285.22; and anemia in other chronic illness, code 285.29. These codes can be used as the principal/first listed code if the reason for the encounter is to treat the anemia. They may also be used as secondary codes if treatment of the anemia is a component of an encounter, but not the primary reason for the encounter. When using a code from subcategory 285 it is also necessary to use the code for the chronic condition causing the anemia.

1) Anemia in chronic kidney disease

When assigning code 285.21, Anemia in chronic kidney disease, it is also necessary to assign a code from category 585, Chronic kidney disease, to indicate the stage of chronic kidney disease.

See I.C.10.a. Chronic kidney disease (CKD).

2) Anemia in neoplastic disease

When assigning code 285.22, Anemia in neoplastic disease, it is also necessary to assign the neoplasm code that is responsible for the anemia. Code 285.22 is for use for anemia that is due to the malignancy, not for anemia due to antineoplastic chemotherapy drugs. **Assign code 285.3 for anemia due to antineoplastic chemotherapy.**

See I.C.2.c.1 Anemia associated with malignancy.

See I.C.2.c.2 Anemia associated with chemotherapy, immunotherapy and radiation therapy.

See I.C.17.e.1. Adverse effects.

5. Chapter 5: Mental Disorders (290-319)

Reserved for future guideline expansion

6. Chapter 6: Diseases of Nervous System and Sense Organs (320-389)

a. Pain - Category 338

1) General coding information

Codes in category 338 may be used in conjunction with codes from other categories and chapters to provide more detail about acute or chronic pain and neoplasm-related pain, unless otherwise indicated below.

If the pain is not specified as acute or chronic, do not assign codes from category 338, except for post-thoracotomy pain, postoperative pain, neoplasm related pain, or central pain syndrome.

A code from subcategories 338.1 and 338.2 should not be assigned if the underlying (definitive) diagnosis is known, unless the reason for the encounter is pain control/management and not management of the underlying condition.

(a) Category 338 Codes as Principal or First-Listed Diagnosis

Category 338 codes are acceptable as principal diagnosis or the first-listed code:

- When pain control or pain management is the reason for the admission/encounter (e.g., a patient with displaced intervertebral disc, nerve impingement and severe back pain presents for injection of steroid into the spinal canal). The underlying cause of the pain should be reported as an additional diagnosis, if known.

- When an admission or encounter is for a procedure aimed at treating the underlying condition (e.g., spinal fusion, kyphoplasty), a code for the underlying condition (e.g., vertebral fracture, spinal stenosis) should be assigned as the principal diagnosis. No code from category 338 should be assigned.

- When a patient is admitted for the insertion of a neurostimulator for pain control, assign the appropriate pain code as the principal or first listed diagnosis. When an admission or encounter is for a procedure aimed at treating the underlying condition and a neurostimulator is inserted for pain control during the same admission/encounter, a code for the underlying condition should be assigned as the principal diagnosis and the appropriate pain code should be assigned as a secondary diagnosis.

(b) Use of Category 338 Codes in Conjunction with Site Specific Pain Codes

(i) Assigning Category 338 Codes and Site-Specific Pain Codes

Codes from category 338 may be used in conjunction with codes that identify the site of pain (including codes from chapter 16) if the category 338 code provides additional information. For example, if the code describes the site of the pain, but does not fully describe whether the pain is acute or chronic, then both codes should be assigned.

(ii) Sequencing of Category 338 Codes with Site-Specific Pain Codes

The sequencing of category 338 codes with site-specific pain codes (including chapter 16 codes), is dependent on the circumstances of the encounter/admission as follows:

- If the encounter is for pain control or pain management, assign the code from category 338 followed by the code identifying the specific site of pain (e.g., encounter for pain management for acute neck pain from trauma is assigned code 338.11, Acute pain due to trauma, followed by code 723.1, Cervicalgia, to identify the site of pain).

- If the encounter is for any other reason except pain control or pain management, and a related definitive diagnosis has not been established (confirmed) by the provider, assign the code for the specific site of pain first, followed by the appropriate code from category 338.

2) Pain due to devices, implants and grafts

Pain associated with devices, implants or grafts left in a surgical site (for example painful hip prosthesis) is assigned to the appropriate code(s) found in Chapter 17, Injury and Poisoning. Use additional code(s) from category 338 to identify acute or chronic pain due to presence of the device, implant or graft (338.18-338.19 or 338.28-338.29).

3) Postoperative Pain

Post-thoracotomy pain and other postoperative pain are classified to subcategories 338.1 and 338.2, depending on whether the pain is acute or chronic. The default for post-thoracotomy and other postoperative pain not specified as acute or chronic is the code for the acute form.

Routine or expected postoperative pain immediately after surgery should not be coded.

(a) Postoperative pain not associated with specific postoperative complication

Postoperative pain not associated with a specific postoperative complication is assigned to the appropriate postoperative pain code in category 338.

(b) Postoperative pain associated with specific postoperative complication

Postoperative pain associated with a specific postoperative complication (such as painful wire sutures) is assigned to the appropriate code(s) found in Chapter 17, Injury and Poisoning. If appropriate, use additional code(s) from category 338 to identify acute or chronic pain (338.18 or 338.28). If pain control/management is the reason for the encounter, a code from category 338 should be assigned as the principal or first-listed diagnosis in accordance with *Section I.C.6.a.1.a above*.

(c) Postoperative pain as principal or first-listed diagnosis

Postoperative pain may be reported as the principal or first-listed diagnosis when the stated reason for the admission/encounter is documented as postoperative pain control/management.

(d) Postoperative pain as secondary diagnosis

Postoperative pain may be reported as a secondary diagnosis code when a patient presents for outpatient surgery and develops an unusual or inordinate amount of postoperative pain.

The provider's documentation should be used to guide the coding of postoperative pain, as well as *Section III. Reporting Additional Diagnoses* and *Section IV. Diagnostic Coding and Reporting in the Outpatient Setting.*

See Section II.I.2 for information on sequencing of diagnoses for patients admitted to hospital inpatient care following post-operative observation.

See Section II.J for information on sequencing of diagnoses for patients admitted to hospital inpatient care from outpatient surgery.

See Section IV.A.2 for information on sequencing of diagnoses for patients admitted for observation.

4) Chronic pain

Chronic pain is classified to subcategory 338.2. There is no time frame defining when pain becomes chronic pain. The provider's documentation should be used to guide use of these codes.

5) Neoplasm Related Pain

Code 338.3 is assigned to pain documented as being related, associated or due to cancer, primary or secondary malignancy, or tumor. This code is assigned regardless of whether the pain is acute or chronic.

This code may be assigned as the principal or first-listed code when the stated reason for the admission/encounter is documented as pain control/pain management. The underlying neoplasm should be reported as an additional diagnosis.

When the reason for the admission/encounter is management of the neoplasm and the pain associated with the neoplasm is also documented, code 338.3 may be assigned as an additional diagnosis.

See Section I.C.2 for instructions on the sequencing of neoplasms for all other stated reasons for the admission/encounter (except for pain control/pain management).

6) Chronic pain syndrome

This condition is different than the term "chronic pain," and therefore this code should only be used when the provider has specifically documented this condition.

7. Chapter 7: Diseases of Circulatory System (390-459)

a. Hypertension
Hypertension Table

The Hypertension Table, found under the main term, "Hypertension", in the Alphabetic Index, contains a complete listing of all conditions due to or associated with hypertension and classifies them according to malignant, benign, and unspecified.

1) Hypertension, Essential, or NOS

Assign hypertension (arterial) (essential) (primary) (systemic) (NOS) to category code 401 with the appropriate fourth digit to indicate malignant (.0), benign (.1), or unspecified (.9). Do not use either .0 malignant or .1 benign unless medical record documentation supports such a designation.

2) Hypertension with Heart Disease

Heart conditions (425.8, 429.0-429.3, 429.8, 429.9) are assigned to a code from category 402 when a causal relationship is stated (due to hypertension) or implied (hypertensive). Use an additional code from category 428 to identify the type of heart failure in those patients with heart failure. More than one code from category 428 may be assigned if the patient has systolic or diastolic failure and congestive heart failure.

The same heart conditions (425.8, 429.0-429.3, 429.8, 429.9) with hypertension, but without a stated causal relationship, are coded separately. Sequence according to the circumstances of the admission/encounter.

3) Hypertensive Chronic Kidney Disease

Assign codes from category 403, Hypertensive chronic kidney disease, when conditions classified to category 585 are present. Unlike hypertension with heart disease, ICD-9-CM presumes a cause-and-effect relationship and classifies chronic kidney disease (CKD) with hypertension as hypertensive chronic kidney disease.

Fifth digits for category 403 should be assigned as follows:

- 0 with CKD stage I through stage IV, or unspecified.
- 1 with CKD stage V or end stage renal disease.

The appropriate code from category 585, Chronic kidney disease, should be used as a secondary code with a code from category 403 to identify the stage of chronic kidney disease.

See Section I.C.10.a for information on the coding of chronic kidney disease.

4) Hypertensive Heart and Chronic Kidney Disease

Assign codes from combination category 404, Hypertensive heart and chronic kidney disease, when both hypertensive kidney disease and hypertensive heart disease are stated in the diagnosis. Assume a relationship between the hypertension and the chronic kidney disease, whether or not the condition is so designated. Assign an additional code from category 428, to identify the type of heart failure. More than one code from category 428 may be assigned if the patient has systolic or diastolic failure and congestive heart failure.

Fifth digits for category 404 should be assigned as follows:

- 0 without heart failure and with chronic kidney disease (CKD) stage I through stage IV, or unspecified
- 1 with heart failure and with CKD stage I through stage IV, or unspecified
- 2 without heart failure and with CKD stage V or end stage renal disease
- 3 with heart failure and with CKD stage V or end stage renal disease

The appropriate code from category 585, Chronic kidney disease, should be used as a secondary code with a code from category 404 to identify the stage of kidney disease.

See Section I.C.10.a for information on the coding of chronic kidney disease.

5) Hypertensive Cerebrovascular Disease

First assign codes from 430-438, Cerebrovascular disease, then the appropriate hypertension code from categories 401-405.

6) Hypertensive Retinopathy

Two codes are necessary to identify the condition. First assign the code from subcategory 362.11, Hypertensive retinopathy, then the appropriate code from categories 401-405 to indicate the type of hypertension.

7) Hypertension, Secondary

Two codes are required: one to identify the underlying etiology and one from category 405 to identify the hypertension. Sequencing of codes is determined by the reason for admission/encounter.

8) Hypertension, Transient

Assign code 796.2, Elevated blood pressure reading without diagnosis of hypertension, unless patient has an established diagnosis of hypertension. Assign code 642.3x for transient hypertension of pregnancy.

9) Hypertension, Controlled

Assign appropriate code from categories 401-405. This diagnostic statement usually refers to an existing state of hypertension under control by therapy.

10) Hypertension, Uncontrolled

Uncontrolled hypertension may refer to untreated hypertension or hypertension not responding to current therapeutic regimen. In either case, assign the appropriate code from categories 401-405 to designate the stage and type of hypertension. Code to the type of hypertension.

11) Elevated Blood Pressure

For a statement of elevated blood pressure without further specificity, assign code 796.2, Elevated blood pressure reading without diagnosis of hypertension, rather than a code from category 401.

b. **Cerebral infarction/stroke/cerebrovascular accident (CVA)**

The terms stroke and CVA are often used interchangeably to refer to a cerebral infarction. The terms stroke, CVA, and cerebral infarction NOS are all indexed to the default code 434.91, Cerebral artery occlusion, unspecified, with infarction. Code 436, Acute, but ill-defined, cerebrovascular disease, should not be used when the documentation states stroke or CVA.

See Section I.C.18.d.3 for information on coding status post administration of tPA in a different facility within the last 24 hours.

c. **Postoperative cerebrovascular accident**

A cerebrovascular hemorrhage or infarction that occurs as a result of medical intervention is coded to 997.02, Iatrogenic cerebrovascular infarction or hemorrhage. Medical record documentation should clearly specify the cause- and-effect relationship between the medical intervention and the cerebrovascular accident in order to assign this code. A secondary code from the code range 430-432 or from a code from subcategories 433 or 434 with a fifth digit of "1" should also be used to identify the type of hemorrhage or infarct.

This guideline conforms to the use additional code note instruction at category 997. Code 436, Acute, but ill-defined, cerebrovascular disease, should not be used as a secondary code with code 997.02.

d. **Late Effects of Cerebrovascular Disease**

1) **Category 438, Late Effects of Cerebrovascular disease**

Category 438 is used to indicate conditions classifiable to categories 430-437 as the causes of late effects (neurologic deficits), themselves classified elsewhere. These "late effects" include neurologic deficits that persist after initial onset of conditions classifiable to 430-437. The neurologic deficits caused by cerebrovascular disease may be present from the onset or may arise at any time after the onset of the condition classifiable to 430-437.

2) **Codes from category 438 with codes from 430-437**

Codes from category 438 may be assigned on a health care record with codes from 430-437, if the patient has a current cerebrovascular accident (CVA) and deficits from an old CVA.

3) **Code V12.54**

Assign code V12.54, Transient ischemic attack (TIA), and cerebral infarction without residual deficits (and not a code from category 438) as an additional code for history of cerebrovascular disease when no neurologic deficits are present.

e. **Acute myocardial infarction (AMI)**

1) **ST elevation myocardial infarction (STEMI) and non ST elevation myocardial infarction (NSTEMI)**

The ICD-9-CM codes for acute myocardial infarction (AMI) identify the site, such as anterolateral wall or true posterior wall. Subcategories 410.0-410.6 and 410.8 are used for ST elevation myocardial infarction (STEMI). Subcategory 410.7, Subendocardial infarction, is used for non ST elevation myocardial infarction (NSTEMI) and nontransmural MIs.

2) **Acute myocardial infarction, unspecified**

Subcategory 410.9 is the default for the unspecified term acute myocardial infarction. If only STEMI or transmural MI without the site is documented, query the provider as to the site, or assign a code from subcategory 410.9.

3) **AMI documented as nontransmural or subendocardial but site provided**

If an AMI is documented as nontransmural or subendocardial, but the site is provided, it is still coded as a subendocardial AMI. If NSTEMI evolves to STEMI, assign the STEMI code. If STEMI converts to NSTEMI due to thrombolytic therapy, it is still coded as STEMI.

See Section I.C.18.d.3 for information on coding status post administration of tPA in a different facility within the last 24 hours.

8. **Chapter 8: Diseases of Respiratory System (460-519)**

See I.C.17.f. for ventilator-associated pneumonia.

a. **Chronic Obstructive Pulmonary Disease [COPD] and Asthma**

1) **Conditions that comprise COPD and Asthma**

The conditions that comprise COPD are obstructive chronic bronchitis, subcategory 491.2, and emphysema, category 492. All asthma codes are under category 493, Asthma. Code

496, Chronic airway obstruction, not elsewhere classified, is a nonspecific code that should only be used when the documentation in a medical record does not specify the type of COPD being treated.

2) Acute exacerbation of chronic obstructive bronchitis and asthma

The codes for chronic obstructive bronchitis and asthma distinguish between uncomplicated cases and those in acute exacerbation. An acute exacerbation is a worsening or a decompensation of a chronic condition. An acute exacerbation is not equivalent to an infection superimposed on a chronic condition, though an exacerbation may be triggered by an infection.

3) Overlapping nature of the conditions that comprise COPD and asthma

Due to the overlapping nature of the conditions that make up COPD and asthma, there are many variations in the way these conditions are documented. Code selection must be based on the terms as documented. When selecting the correct code for the documented type of COPD and asthma, it is essential to first review the index, and then verify the code in the tabular list. There are many instructional notes under the different COPD subcategories and codes. It is important that all such notes be reviewed to assure correct code assignment.

4) Acute exacerbation of asthma and status asthmaticus

An acute exacerbation of asthma is an increased severity of the asthma symptoms, such as wheezing and shortness of breath. Status asthmaticus refers to a patient's failure to respond to therapy administered during an asthmatic episode and is a life threatening complication that requires emergency care. If status asthmaticus is documented by the provider with any type of COPD or with acute bronchitis, the status asthmaticus should be sequenced first. It supersedes any type of COPD including that with acute exacerbation or acute bronchitis. It is inappropriate to assign an asthma code with 5th digit 2, with acute exacerbation, together with an asthma code with 5th digit 1, with status

asthmatics. Only the 5th digit 1 should be assigned.

b. Chronic Obstructive Pulmonary Disease [COPD] and Bronchitis

1) Acute bronchitis with COPD

Acute bronchitis, code 466.0, is due to an infectious organism. When acute bronchitis is documented with COPD, code 491.22, Obstructive chronic bronchitis with acute bronchitis, should be assigned. It is not necessary to also assign code 466.0. If a medical record documents acute bronchitis with COPD with acute exacerbation, only code 491.22 should be assigned. The acute bronchitis included in code 491.22 supersedes the acute exacerbation. If a medical record documents COPD with acute exacerbation without mention of acute bronchitis, only code 491.21 should be assigned.

c. Acute Respiratory Failure

1) Acute respiratory failure as principal diagnosis

Code 518.81, Acute respiratory failure, may be assigned as a principal diagnosis when it is the condition established after study to be chiefly responsible for occasioning the admission to the hospital, and the selection is supported by the Alphabetic Index and Tabular List. However, chapter-specific coding guidelines (such as obstetrics, poisoning, HIV, newborn) that provide sequencing direction take precedence.

2) Acute respiratory failure as secondary diagnosis

Respiratory failure may be listed as a secondary diagnosis if it occurs after admission, or if it is present on admission, but does not meet the definition of principal diagnosis.

3) Sequencing of acute respiratory failure and another acute condition

When a patient is admitted with respiratory failure and another acute condition, (e.g., myocardial infarction, cerebrovascular accident, aspiration pneumonia), the principal diagnosis will not be the same in every situation. This applies whether the other acute condition is a respiratory or nonrespiratory condition. Selection of the principal diagnosis will be dependent on the circumstances of admission. If both the respiratory failure and the other acute condition are equally responsible for occasioning the admission to the hospital, and there are no chapter-specific sequencing rules, the guideline regarding two or more diagnoses that equally meet the definition for principal diagnosis *(Section II, C.)* may be applied in these situations.

If the documentation is not clear as to whether acute respiratory failure and another condition are equally responsible for occasioning the admission, query the provider for clarification.

d. **Influenza due to** *certain* **identified avian influenza** *viruses*

Code only confirmed cases of avian influenza **(code 488.0, Influenza due to indentified avian influenza virus) or novel H1N1 influenza virus (H1N1 or swine flu, code 488.1)**. This is an exception to the hospital inpatient guideline Section II, H. (Uncertain Diagnosis).

In this context, "confirmation" does not require documentation of positive laboratory testing specific for avian **or novel H1N1** influenza. However, coding should be based on the provider's diagnostic statement that the patient has avian **or novel H1N1 (H1N1 or swine flu)** influenza.

If the provider records "suspected or possible or probable avian **or novel H1N1** influenza **(H1N1 or swine flu)**," the appropriate influenza code from category 487 should be assigned. **A code from category** 488, Influenza due to **certain** identified avian influenza virus**es**, should not be assigned.

9. **Chapter 9: Diseases of Digestive System (520-579)**

Reserved for future guideline expansion

10. **Chapter 10: Diseases of Genitourinary System (580-629)**

a. **Chronic kidney disease**

1) **Stages of chronic kidney disease (CKD)**

The ICD-9-CM classifies CKD based on severity. The severity of CKD is designated by stages I-V. Stage II, code 585.2, equates to mild CKD; stage III, code 585.3, equates to moderate CKD; and stage IV, code 585.4, equates to severe CKD. Code 585.6, End stage renal disease (ESRD), is assigned when the provider has documented end-stage-renal disease (ESRD).

If both a stage of CKD and ESRD are documented, assign code 585.6 only.

2) **Chronic kidney disease and kidney transplant status**

Patients who have undergone kidney transplant may still have some form of CKD, because the kidney transplant may not fully restore kidney function. Therefore, the presence of CKD alone does not constitute a transplant complication. Assign the appropriate 585 code for the patient's stage of CKD and code V42.0. If a transplant complication such as failure or rejection is documented, see section I.C.17.f.2.b for information on coding complications of a kidney transplant. If the documentation is unclear as to whether the patient has a complication of the transplant, query the provider.

3) **Chronic kidney disease with other conditions**

Patients with CKD may also suffer from other serious conditions, most commonly diabetes mellitus and hypertension. The sequencing of the CKD code in relationship to codes for other contributing conditions is based on the conventions in the tabular list.

See I.C.3.a.4 for sequencing instructions for diabetes.

See I.C.4.a.1 for anemia in CKD.

See I.C.7.a.3 for hypertensive chronic kidney disease.

See I.C.17.f.2.b, Kidney transplant complications, for instructions on coding of documented rejection or failure.

11. **Chapter 11: Complications of Pregnancy, Childbirth, and the Puerperium (630-679)**

a. **General Rules for Obstetric Cases**

1) **Codes from chapter 11 and sequencing priority**

Obstetric cases require codes from chapter 11, codes in the range 630-679, Complications of Pregnancy, Childbirth, and the Puerperium. Chapter 11 codes have sequencing priority over codes from other chapters. Additional codes from other chapters may be used in conjunction with chapter 11 codes to further specify conditions. Should the provider document that the pregnancy is incidental to the encounter, then code V22.2 should be used in place of any chapter 11 codes. It is the provider's responsibility to state that the condition being treated is not affecting the pregnancy.

2) Chapter 11 codes used only on the maternal record

Chapter 11 codes are to be used only on the maternal record, never on the record of the newborn.

3) Chapter 11 fifth-digits

Categories 640-648, 651-676 have required fifth-digits, which indicate whether the encounter is antepartum, postpartum and whether a delivery has also occurred.

4) Fifth-digits, appropriate for each code

The fifth-digits, which are appropriate for each code number, are listed in brackets under each code. The fifth-digits on each code should all be consistent with each other. That is, should a delivery occur all of the fifth-digits should indicate the delivery.

b. Selection of OB Principal or First-listed Diagnosis

1) Routine outpatient prenatal visits

For routine outpatient prenatal visits when no complications are present codes V22.0, Supervision of normal first pregnancy, and V22.1, Supervision of other normal pregnancy, should be used as the first-listed diagnoses. These codes should not be used in conjunction with chapter 11 codes.

2) Prenatal outpatient visits for high-risk patients

For **routine** prenatal outpatient visits for patients with high-risk pregnancies, a code from category V23, Supervision of high-risk pregnancy, should be used as the first-listed diagnosis. Secondary chapter 11 codes may be used in conjunction with these codes if appropriate.

3) Episodes when no delivery occurs

In episodes when no delivery occurs, the principal diagnosis should correspond to the principal complication of the pregnancy, which necessitated the encounter. Should more than one complication exist, all of which are treated or monitored, any of the complications codes may be sequenced first.

4) When a delivery occurs

When a delivery occurs, the principal diagnosis should correspond to the main circumstances or complication of the delivery. In cases of cesarean delivery, the selection of the principal diagnosis **should be the condition established after study that was responsible for the patient's admission. If the patient was admitted with a condition that resulted in the performance of a cesarean procedure, that condition should be selected as the principal diagnosis. If the** reason for **the** admission/encounter was unrelated to the condition resulting in the cesarean delivery, **the condition related to the reason for the admission/encounter should be selected as the principal diagnosis, even if a cesarean was performed.**

5) Outcome of delivery

An outcome of delivery code, V27.0-V27.9, should be included on every maternal record when a delivery has occurred. These codes are not to be used on subsequent records or on the newborn record.

c. Fetal Conditions Affecting the Management of the Mother

1) Codes from category 655

Known or suspected fetal abnormality affecting management of the mother, and category 656, Other fetal and placental problems affecting the management of the mother, are assigned only when the fetal condition is actually responsible for modifying the management of the mother, i.e., by requiring diagnostic studies, additional observation, special care, or termination of pregnancy. The fact that the fetal condition exists does not justify assigning a code from this series to the mother's record.

See I.C.18.d. for suspected maternal and fetal conditions not found

2) In utero surgery

In cases when surgery is performed on the fetus, a diagnosis code from category 655, Known or suspected fetal abnormalities affecting management of the mother, should be assigned identifying the fetal condition. Procedure code 75.36, Correction of fetal defect, should be assigned on the hospital inpatient record.

No code from Chapter 15, the perinatal codes, should be used on the mother's record to identify fetal conditions. Surgery performed in utero on a fetus is still to be coded as an obstetric encounter.

d. **HIV Infection in Pregnancy, Childbirth and the Puerperium**

During pregnancy, childbirth or the puerperium, a patient admitted because of an HIV-related illness should receive a principal diagnosis of 647.6X, Other specified infectious and parasitic diseases in the mother classifiable elsewhere, but complicating the pregnancy, childbirth or the puerperium, followed by 042 and the code(s) for the HIV-related illness(es).

Patients with asymptomatic HIV infection status admitted during pregnancy, childbirth, or the puerperium should receive codes of 647.6X and V08.

e. **Current Conditions Complicating Pregnancy**

Assign a code from subcategory 648.x for patients that have current conditions when the condition affects the management of the pregnancy, childbirth, or the puerperium. Use additional secondary codes from other chapters to identify the conditions, as appropriate.

f. **Diabetes mellitus in pregnancy**

Diabetes mellitus is a significant complicating factor in pregnancy. Pregnant women who are diabetic should be assigned code 648.0x, Diabetes mellitus complicating pregnancy, and a secondary code from category 250, Diabetes mellitus, or category 249, Secondary diabetes to identify the type of diabetes.

Code V58.67, Long-term (current) use of insulin, should also be assigned if the diabetes mellitus is being treated with insulin.

g. **Gestational diabetes**

Gestational diabetes can occur during the second and third trimester of pregnancy in women who were not diabetic prior to pregnancy. Gestational diabetes can cause complications in the pregnancy similar to those of pre-existing diabetes mellitus. It also puts the woman at greater risk of developing diabetes after the pregnancy. Gestational diabetes is coded to 648.8x, Abnormal glucose tolerance. Codes 648.0x and 648.8x should never be used together on the same record.

Code V58.67, Long-term (current) use of insulin, should also be assigned if the gestational diabetes is being treated with insulin.

h. **Normal Delivery, Code 650**

1) **Normal delivery**

Code 650 is for use in cases when a woman is admitted for a full-term normal delivery and delivers a single, healthy infant without any complications antepartum, during the delivery, or postpartum during the delivery episode. Code 650 is always a principal diagnosis. It is not to be used if any other code from chapter 11 is needed to describe a current complication of the antenatal, delivery, or perinatal period. Additional codes from other chapters may be used with code 650 if they are not related to or are in any way complicating the pregnancy.

2) **Normal delivery with resolved antepartum complication**

Code 650 may be used if the patient had a complication at some point during her pregnancy, but the complication is not present at the time of the admission for delivery.

3) **V27.0, Single liveborn, outcome of delivery**

V27.0, Single liveborn, is the only outcome of delivery code appropriate for use with 650.

i. **The Postpartum and Peripartum Periods**

1) **Postpartum and peripartum periods**

The postpartum period begins immediately after delivery and continues for six weeks following delivery. The peripartum period is defined as the last month of pregnancy to five months postpartum.

2) **Postpartum complication**

A postpartum complication is any complication occurring within the six-week period.

3) **Pregnancy-related complications after 6 week period**

Chapter 11 codes may also be used to describe pregnancy-related complications after the six-week period should the provider document that a condition is pregnancy related.

4) **Postpartum complications occurring during the same admission as delivery**

Postpartum complications that occur during the same admission as the delivery are identified with a fifth digit of "2." Subsequent admissions/encounters for postpartum complications should be identified with a fifth digit of "4."

5) Admission for routine postpartum care following delivery outside hospital

When the mother delivers outside the hospital prior to admission and is admitted for routine postpartum care and no complications are noted, code V24.0, Postpartum care and examination immediately after delivery, should be assigned as the principal diagnosis.

6) Admission following delivery outside hospital with postpartum conditions

A delivery diagnosis code should not be used for a woman who has delivered prior to admission to the hospital. Any postpartum conditions and/or postpartum procedures should be coded.

7) Puerperal sepsis

Code 670.2x, Puerperal sepsis, should be assigned with a secondary code to identify the causal organism (e.g., for a bacterial infection, assign a code from category 041, Bacterial infections in conditions classified elsewhere and of unspecified site). A code from category 038, Septicemia, should not be used for puerperal sepsis. Do not assign code 995.91, Sepsis, as code 670.2x describes the sepsis. If applicable, use additional codes to identify severe sepsis (995.92) and any associated acute organ dysfunction.

j. Code 677, Late effect of complication of pregnancy

1) Code 677

Code 677, Late effect of complication of pregnancy, childbirth, and the puerperium is for use in those cases when an initial complication of a pregnancy develops a sequelae requiring care or treatment at a future date.

2) After the initial postpartum period

This code may be used at any time after the initial postpartum period.

3) Sequencing of Code 677

This code, like all late effect codes, is to be sequenced following the code describing the sequelae of the complication.

k. Abortions

1) Fifth-digits required for abortion categories

Fifth-digits are required for abortion categories 634-637. **Fifth digit assignment is based on the status of the patient at the beginning (or start) of the encounter.** Fifth-digit 1, incomplete, indicates that all of the products of conception have not been expelled from the uterus. Fifth-digit 2, complete, indicates that all products of conception have been expelled from the uterus.

2) Code from categories 640-648 and 651-659

A code from categories 640-648 and 651-659 may be used as additional codes with an abortion code to indicate the complication leading to the abortion.

Fifth digit 3 is assigned with codes from these categories when used with an abortion code because the other fifth digits will not apply. Codes from the 660-669 series are not to be used for complications of abortion.

3) Code 639 for complications

Code 639 is to be used for all complications following abortion. Code 639 cannot be assigned with codes from categories 634-638.

4) Abortion with Liveborn Fetus

When an attempted termination of pregnancy results in a liveborn fetus assign code 644.21, Early onset of delivery, with an appropriate code from category V27, Outcome of Delivery. The procedure code for the attempted termination of pregnancy should also be assigned.

5) Retained Products of Conception following an abortion

Subsequent admissions for retained products of conception following a spontaneous or legally induced abortion are assigned the appropriate code from category 634, Spontaneous abortion, or 635 Legally induced abortion, with a fifth digit of "1" (incomplete). This advice is appropriate even when the patient was discharged previously with a discharge diagnosis of complete abortion.

12. **Chapter 12: Diseases Skin and Subcutaneous Tissue (680-709)**

a. **Pressure ulcer stage codes**

1) **Pressure ulcer stages**

Two codes are needed to completely describe a pressure ulcer: A code from subcategory 707.0, Pressure ulcer, to identify the site of the pressure ulcer and a code from subcategory 707.2, Pressure ulcer stages.

The codes in subcategory 707.2, Pressure ulcer stages, are to be used as an additional diagnosis with a code(s) from subcategory 707.0, Pressure Ulcer. Codes from 707.2, Pressure ulcer stages, may not be assigned as a principal or first-listed diagnosis. The pressure ulcer stage codes should only be used with pressure ulcers and not with other types of ulcers (e.g., stasis ulcer).

The ICD-9-CM classifies pressure ulcer stages based on severity, which is designated by stages I-IV and unstageable.

2) **Unstageable pressure ulcers**

Assignment of code 707.25, Pressure ulcer, unstageable, should be based on the clinical documentation. Code 707.25 is used for pressure ulcers whose stage cannot be clinically determined (e.g., the ulcer is covered by eschar or has been treated with a skin or muscle graft) and pressure ulcers that are documented as deep tissue injury but not documented as due to trauma. This code should not be confused with code 707.20, Pressure ulcer, stage unspecified. Code 707.20 should be assigned when there is no documentation regarding the stage of the pressure ulcer.

3) **Documented pressure ulcer stage**

Assignment of the pressure ulcer stage code should be guided by clinical documentation of the stage or documentation of the terms found in the index. For clinical terms describing the stage that are not found in the index, and there is no documentation of the stage, the provider should be queried.

4) **Bilateral pressure ulcers with same stage**

When a patient has bilateral pressure ulcers (e.g., both buttocks) and both pressure ulcers are documented as being the same stage, only the code for the site and one code for the stage should be reported.

5) **Bilateral pressure ulcers with different stages**

When a patient has bilateral pressure ulcers at the same site (e.g., both buttocks) and each pressure ulcer is documented as being at a different stage, assign one code for the site and the appropriate codes for the pressure ulcer stage.

6) **Multiple pressure ulcers of different sites and stages**

When a patient has multiple pressure ulcers at different sites (e.g., buttock, heel, shoulder) and each pressure ulcer is documented as being at different stages (e.g., stage 3 and stage 4), assign the appropriate codes for each different site and a code for each different pressure ulcer stage.

7) **Patients admitted with pressure ulcers documented as healed**

No code is assigned if the documentation states that the pressure ulcer is completely healed.

8) **Patients admitted with pressure ulcers documented as healing**

Pressure ulcers described as healing should be assigned the appropriate pressure ulcer stage code based on the documentation in the medical record. If the documentation does not provide information about the stage of the healing pressure ulcer, assign code 707.20, Pressure ulcer stage, unspecified.

If the documentation is unclear as to whether the patient has a current (new) pressure ulcer or if the patient is being treated for a healing pressure ulcer, query the provider.

9) **Patient admitted with pressure ulcer evolving into another stage during the admission**

If a patient is admitted with a pressure ulcer at one stage and it progresses to a higher stage, assign the code for highest stage reported for that site.

13. **Chapter 13: Diseases of Musculoskeletal and Connective Tissue (710-739)**

a. **Coding of Pathologic Fractures**

1) **Acute Fractures vs. Aftercare**

Pathologic fractures are reported using subcategory 733.1, when the fracture is newly diagnosed. Subcategory 733.1 may be used while the patient is receiving active treatment for the fracture. Examples of active treatment are: surgical treatment, emergency department encounter, evaluation and treatment by a new physician.

Fractures are coded using the aftercare codes (subcategories V54.0, V54.2, V54.8 or V54.9) for encounters after the patient has completed active treatment of the fracture and is receiving routine care for the fracture during the healing or recovery phase. Examples of fracture aftercare are: cast change or removal, removal of external or internal fixation device, medication adjustment, and follow up visits following fracture treatment.

Care for complications of surgical treatment for fracture repairs during the healing or recovery phase should be coded with the appropriate complication codes.

Care of complications of fractures, such as malunion and nonunion, should be reported with the appropriate codes.

See Section I. C. 17.b for information on the coding of traumatic fractures.

14. **Chapter 14: Congenital Anomalies (740-759)**

   a. **Codes in categories 740-759, Congenital Anomalies**

   Assign an appropriate code(s) from categories 740-759, Congenital Anomalies, when an anomaly is documented. A congenital anomaly may be the principal/first listed diagnosis on a record or a secondary diagnosis.

   When a congenital anomaly does not have a unique code assignment, assign additional code(s) for any manifestations that may be present.

   When the code assignment specifically identifies the congenital anomaly, manifestations that are an inherent component of the anomaly should not be coded separately. Additional codes should be assigned for manifestations that are not an inherent component.

   Codes from Chapter 14 may be used throughout the life of the patient. If a congenital anomaly has been corrected, a personal history code should be used to identify the history of the anomaly. Although present at birth, a congenital anomaly may not be identified until later in life. Whenever the condition is diagnosed by the physician, it is appropriate to assign a code from codes 740-759.

For the birth admission, the appropriate code from category V30, Liveborn infants, according to type of birth should be sequenced as the principal diagnosis, followed by any congenital anomaly codes, 740-759.

15. **Chapter 15: Newborn (Perinatal) Guidelines (760-779)**

   For coding and reporting purposes the perinatal period is defined as before birth through the 28th day following birth. The following guidelines are provided for reporting purposes. Hospitals may record other diagnoses as needed for internal data use.

   a. **General Perinatal Rules**

      1) **Chapter 15 Codes**

         They are <u>never</u> for use on the maternal record. Codes from Chapter 11, the obstetric chapter, are never permitted on the newborn record. Chapter 15 code may be used throughout the life of the patient if the condition is still present.

      2) **Sequencing of perinatal codes**

         Generally, codes from Chapter 15 should be sequenced as the principal/first-listed diagnosis on the newborn record, with the exception of the appropriate V30 code for the birth episode, followed by codes from any other chapter that provide additional detail. The "use additional code" note at the beginning of the chapter supports this guideline. If the index does not provide a specific code for a perinatal condition, assign code 779.89, Other specified conditions originating in the perinatal period, followed by the code from another chapter that specifies the condition. Codes for signs and symptoms may be assigned when a definitive diagnosis has not been established.

      3) **Birth process or community acquired conditions**

         If a newborn has a condition that may be either due to the birth process or community acquired and the documentation does not indicate which it is, the default is due to the birth process and the code from Chapter 15 should be used. If the condition is community-acquired, a code from Chapter 15 should not be assigned.

4) Code all clinically significant conditions

All clinically significant conditions noted on routine newborn examination should be coded. A condition is clinically significant if it requires:

- clinical evaluation; or
- therapeutic treatment; or
- diagnostic procedures; or
- extended length of hospital stay; or
- increased nursing care and/or monitoring; or
- has implications for future health care needs

Note: The perinatal guidelines listed above are the same as the general coding guidelines for "additional diagnoses", except for the final point regarding implications for future health care needs. Codes should be assigned for conditions that have been specified by the provider as having implications for future health care needs. Codes from the perinatal chapter should not be assigned unless the provider has established a definitive diagnosis.

b. Use of codes V30-V39

When coding the birth of an infant, assign a code from categories V30-V39, according to the type of birth. A code from this series is assigned as a principal diagnosis, and assigned only once to a newborn at the time of birth.

c. Newborn transfers

If the newborn is transferred to another institution, the V30 series is not used at the receiving hospital.

d. Use of category V29

1) Assigning a code from category V29

Assign a code from category V29, Observation and evaluation of newborns and infants for suspected conditions not found, to identify those instances when a healthy newborn is evaluated for a suspected condition that is determined after study not to be present. Do not use a code from category V29 when the patient has identified signs or symptoms of a suspected problem; in such cases, code the sign or symptom.

A code from category V29 may also be assigned as a principal code for readmissions or encounters when the V30 code no longer applies. Codes from category V29 are for use only for healthy newborns and infants for which no condition after study is found to be present.

2) V29 code on a birth record

A V29 code is to be used as a secondary code after the V30, Outcome of delivery, code.

e. Use of other V codes on perinatal records

V codes other than V30 and V29 may be assigned on a perinatal or newborn record code. The codes may be used as a principal or first-listed diagnosis for specific types of encounters or for readmissions or encounters when the V30 code no longer applies.

See Section I.C.18 for information regarding the assignment of V codes.

f. Maternal Causes of Perinatal Morbidity

Codes from categories 760-763, Maternal causes of perinatal morbidity and mortality, are assigned only when the maternal condition has actually affected the fetus or newborn. The fact that the mother has an associated medical condition or experiences some complication of pregnancy, labor or delivery does not justify the routine assignment of codes from these categories to the newborn record.

g. Congenital Anomalies in Newborns

For the birth admission, the appropriate code from category V30, Liveborn infants according to type of birth, should be used, followed by any congenital anomaly codes, categories 740-759. Use additional secondary codes from other chapters to specify conditions associated with the anomaly, if applicable.

Also, see Section I.C.14 for information on the coding of congenital anomalies.

h. Coding Additional Perinatal Diagnoses

1) Assigning codes for conditions that require treatment

Assign codes for conditions that require treatment or further investigation, prolong the length of stay, or require resource utilization.

2) Codes for conditions specified as having implications for future health care needs

Assign codes for conditions that have been specified by the provider as having implications for future health care needs.

Note: This guideline should not be used for adult patients.

3) Codes for newborn conditions originating in the perinatal period

Assign a code for newborn conditions originating in the perinatal period (categories 760-779), as well as complications arising during the current episode of care classified in other chapters, only if the diagnoses have been documented by the responsible provider at the time of transfer or discharge as having affected the fetus or newborn.

i. Prematurity and Fetal Growth Retardation

Providers utilize different criteria in determining prematurity. A code for prematurity should not be assigned unless it is documented. The 5th digit assignment for codes from category 764 and subcategories 765.0 and 765.1 should be based on the recorded birth weight and estimated gestational age.

A code from subcategory 765.2, Weeks of gestation, should be assigned as an additional code with category 764 and codes from 765.0 and 765.1 to specify weeks of gestation as documented by the provider in the record.

j. Newborn sepsis

Code 771.81, Septicemia [sepsis] of newborn, should be assigned with a secondary code from category 041, Bacterial infections in conditions classified elsewhere and of unspecified site, to identify the organism. A code from category 038, Septicemia, should not be used on a newborn record. Do not assign code 995.91, Sepsis, as code 771.81 describes the sepsis. If applicable, use additional codes to identify severe sepsis (995.92) and any associated acute organ dysfunction.

16. Chapter 16: Signs, Symptoms and Ill-Defined Conditions (780-799)

Reserved for future guideline expansion

17. Chapter 17: Injury and Poisoning (800-999)

a. Coding of Injuries

When coding injuries, assign separate codes for each injury unless a combination code is provided, in which case the combination code is assigned. Multiple injury codes are provided in ICD-9-CM, but should not be assigned unless information for a more specific code is not available. These **traumatic injury** codes are not to be used for normal, healing surgical wounds or to identify complications of surgical wounds.

The code for the most serious injury, as determined by the provider and the focus of treatment, is sequenced first.

1) Superficial injuries

Superficial injuries such as abrasions or contusions are not coded when associated with more severe injuries of the same site.

2) Primary injury with damage to nerves/blood vessels

When a primary injury results in minor damage to peripheral nerves or blood vessels, the primary injury is sequenced first with additional code(s) from categories 950-957, Injury to nerves and spinal cord, and/or 900-904, Injury to blood vessels. When the primary injury is to the blood vessels or nerves, that injury should be sequenced first.

b. Coding of Traumatic Fractures

The principles of multiple coding of injuries should be followed in coding fractures. Fractures of specified sites are coded individually by site in accordance with both the provisions within categories 800-829 and the level of detail furnished by medical record content. Combination categories for multiple fractures are provided for use when there is insufficient detail in the medical record (such as trauma cases transferred to another hospital), when the reporting form limits the number of codes that can be used in reporting pertinent clinical data, or when there is insufficient specificity at the fourth-digit or fifth-digit level. More specific guidelines are as follows:

1) Acute Fractures vs. Aftercare

Traumatic fractures are coded using the acute fracture codes (800-829) while the patient is receiving active treatment for the fracture. Examples of active treatment are: surgical treatment, emergency department encounter, and evaluation and treatment by a new physician.

Fractures are coded using the aftercare codes (subcategories V54.0, V54.1, V54.8, or V54.9) for encounters after the patient has completed active treatment of the fracture and is receiving routine care for the fracture during the healing or recovery phase. Examples of fracture aftercare are: cast change or removal, removal of external or internal fixation device, medication adjustment, and follow up visits following fracture treatment.

Care for complications of surgical treatment for fracture repairs during the healing or recovery phase should be coded with the appropriate complication codes.

Care of complications of fractures, such as malunion and nonunion, should be reported with the appropriate codes.

Pathologic fractures are not coded in the 800-829 range, but instead are assigned to subcategory 733.1. *See Section I.C.13.a for additional information.*

2) Multiple fractures of same limb

Multiple fractures of same limb classifiable to the same three-digit or four-digit category are coded to that category.

3) Multiple unilateral or bilateral fractures of same bone

Multiple unilateral or bilateral fractures of same bone(s) but classified to different fourth-digit subdivisions (bone part) within the same three-digit category are coded individually by site.

4) Multiple fracture categories 819 and 828

Multiple fracture categories 819 and 828 classify bilateral fractures of both upper limbs (819) and both lower limbs (828), but without any detail at the fourth-digit level other than open and closed type of fractures.

5) Multiple fractures sequencing

Multiple fractures are sequenced in accordance with the severity of the fracture. The provider should be asked to list the fracture diagnoses in the order of severity.

c. Coding of Burns

Current burns (940-948) are classified by depth, extent and by agent (E code). Burns are classified by depth as first degree (erythema), second degree (blistering), and third degree (full-thickness involvement).

1) Sequencing of burn and related condition codes

Sequence first the code that reflects the highest degree of burn when more than one burn is present.

a. When the reason for the admission or encounter is for treatment of external multiple burns, sequence first the code that reflects the burn of the highest degree.

b. When a patient has both internal and external burns, the circumstances of admission govern the selection of the principal diagnosis or first-listed diagnosis.

c. When a patient is admitted for burn injuries and other related conditions such as smoke inhalation and/or respiratory failure, the circumstances of admission govern the selection of the principal or first-listed diagnosis.

2) Burns of the same local site

Classify burns of the same local site (three-digit category level, 940-947) but of different degrees to the subcategory identifying the highest degree recorded in the diagnosis.

3) Non-healing burns

Non-healing burns are coded as acute burns.

Necrosis of burned skin should be coded as a non-healed burn.

4) Code 958.3, Posttraumatic wound infection

Assign code 958.3, Posttraumatic wound infection, not elsewhere classified, as an additional code for any documented infected burn site.

5) Assign separate codes for each burn site

When coding burns, assign separate codes for each burn site. Category 946 Burns of Multiple specified sites, should only be used if the location of the burns are not documented. Category 949, Burn, unspecified, is extremely vague and should rarely be used.

6) Assign codes from category 948, Burns

Burns classified according to extent of body surface involved, when the site of the burn is not specified or when there is a need for additional data. It is advisable to use category 948 as additional coding when needed to provide data for evaluating burn mortality, such as that needed by burn units. It is also advisable to use category 948 as an additional code for reporting purposes when there is mention of a third-degree burn involving 20 percent or more of the body surface.

In assigning a code from category 948:

Fourth-digit codes are used to identify the percentage of total body surface involved in a burn (all degree).

Fifth-digits are assigned to identify the percentage of body surface involved in third-degree burn.

Fifth-digit zero (0) is assigned when less than 10 percent or when no body surface is involved in a third-degree burn.

Category 948 is based on the classic "rule of nines" in estimating body surface involved: head and neck are assigned nine percent, each arm nine percent, each leg 18 percent, the anterior trunk 18 percent, posterior trunk 18 percent, and genitalia one percent. Providers may change these percentage assignments where necessary to accommodate infants and children who have proportionately larger heads than adults and patients who have large buttocks, thighs, or abdomen that involve burns.

7) Encounters for treatment of late effects of burns

Encounters for the treatment of the late effects of burns (i.e., scars or joint contractures) should be coded to the residual condition (sequelae) followed by the appropriate late effect code (906.5-906.9). A late effect E code may also be used, if desired.

8) Sequelae with a late effect code and current burn

When appropriate, both a sequelae with a late effect code, and a current burn code may be assigned on the same record (when both a current burn and sequelae of an old burn exist).

d. Coding of Debridement of Wound, Infection, or Burn

Excisional debridement involves surgical removal or cutting away, as opposed to a mechanical (brushing, scrubbing, washing) debridement.

For coding purposes, excisional debridement is assigned to code 86.22.

Nonexcisional debridement is assigned to code 86.28.

e. Adverse Effects, Poisoning and Toxic Effects

The properties of certain drugs, medicinal and biological substances or combinations of such substances, may cause toxic reactions. The occurrence of drug toxicity is classified in ICD-9-CM as follows:

1) Adverse Effect

When the drug was correctly prescribed and properly administered, code the reaction plus the appropriate code from the E930-E949 series. Codes from the E930-E949 series must be used to identify the causative substance for an adverse effect of drug, medicinal and biological substances, correctly prescribed and properly administered. The effect, such as tachycardia, delirium, gastrointestinal hemorrhaging, vomiting, hypokalemia, hepatitis, renal failure, or respiratory failure, is coded and followed by the appropriate code from the E930-E949 series.

Adverse effects of therapeutic substances correctly prescribed and properly administered (toxicity, synergistic reaction, side effect, and idiosyncratic reaction) may be due to (1) differences among patients, such as age, sex, disease, and genetic factors, and (2) drug-related factors, such as type of drug, route of administration, duration of therapy, dosage, and bioavailability.

2) Poisoning

(a) Error was made in drug prescription

Errors made in drug prescription or in the administration of the drug by provider, nurse, patient, or other person, use the appropriate poisoning code from the 960-979 series.

(b) Overdose of a drug intentionally taken

If an overdose of a drug was intentionally taken or administered and resulted in drug toxicity, it would be coded as a poisoning (960-979 series).

33

(c) **Nonprescribed drug taken with correctly prescribed and properly administered drug**

If a nonprescribed drug or medicinal agent was taken in combination with a correctly prescribed and properly administered drug, any drug toxicity or other reaction resulting from the interaction of the two drugs would be classified as a poisoning.

(d) **Interaction of drug(s) and alcohol**

When a reaction results from the interaction of a drug(s) and alcohol, this would be classified as poisoning.

(e) **Sequencing of poisoning**

When coding a poisoning or reaction to the improper use of a medication (e.g., wrong dose, wrong substance, wrong route of administration) the poisoning code is sequenced first, followed by a code for the manifestation. If there is also a diagnosis of drug abuse or dependence to the substance, the abuse or dependence is coded as an additional code.

See Section I.C.3.a.6.b. if poisoning is the result of insulin pump malfunctions and Section I.C.19 for general use of E-codes.

3) **Toxic Effects**

(a) **Toxic effect codes**

When a harmful substance is ingested or comes in contact with a person, this is classified as a toxic effect. The toxic effect codes are in categories 980-989.

(b) **Sequencing toxic effect codes**

A toxic effect code should be sequenced first, followed by the code(s) that identify the result of the toxic effect.

(c) **External cause codes for toxic effects**

An external cause code from categories E860-E869 for accidental exposure, codes E950.6 or E950.7 for intentional self-harm, category E962 for assault, or categories E980-E982, for undetermined, should also be assigned to indicate intent.

f. **Complications of care**

1) **Complications of care**

(a) **Documentation of complications of care**

As with all procedural or postprocedural complications, code assignment is based on the provider's documentation of the relationship between the condition and the procedure.

2) **Transplant complications**

(a) **Transplant complications other than kidney**

Codes under subcategory 996.8, Complications of transplanted organ, are for use for both complications and rejection of transplanted organs. A transplant complication code is only assigned if the complication affects the function of the transplanted organ. Two codes are required to fully describe a transplant complication, the appropriate code from subcategory 996.8 and a secondary code that identifies the complication.

Pre-existing conditions or conditions that develop after the transplant are not coded as complications unless they affect the function of the transplanted organs.

See I.C.18.d.3) for transplant organ removal status

See I.C.2.i for malignant neoplasm associated with transplanted organ.

(b) **Chronic kidney disease and kidney transplant complications**

Patients who have undergone kidney transplant may still have some form of chronic kidney disease (CKD) because the kidney transplant may not fully restore kidney function. Code 996.81 should be assigned for documented complications of a kidney transplant, such as transplant failure or rejection or other transplant complication. Code 996.81 should not be assigned for post kidney transplant patients who have chronic kidney (CKD) unless a transplant complication such as transplant failure or rejection is documented. If the documentation is unclear as to whether the patient has a complication of the transplant, query the provider.

For patients with CKD following a kidney transplant, but who do not have a complication such as failure or rejection, *see section I.C.10. a.2, Chronic kidney disease and kidney transplant status.*

3) Ventilator associated pneumonia

(a) Documentation of Ventilator associated Pneumonia

As with all procedural or postprocedural complications, code assignment is based on the provider's documentation of the relationship between the condition and the procedure.

Code 997.31, Ventilator associated pneumonia, should be assigned only when the provider has documented ventilator associated pneumonia (VAP). An additional code to identify the organism (e.g., Pseudomonas aeruginosa, code 041.7) should also be assigned. Do not assign an additional code from categories 480-484 to identify the type of pneumonia.

Code 997.31 should not be assigned for cases where the patient has pneumonia and is on a mechanical ventilator but the provider has not specifically stated that the pneumonia is ventilator-associated pneumonia.

If the documentation is unclear as to whether the patient has a pneumonia that is a complication attributable to the mechanical ventilator, query the provider.

(b) Patient admitted with pneumonia and develops VAP

A patient may be admitted with one type of pneumonia (e.g., code 481, Pneumococcal pneumonia) and subsequently develop VAP. In this instance, the principal diagnosis would be the appropriate code from categories 480-484 for the pneumonia diagnosed at the time of admission. Code 997.31, Ventilator associated pneumonia, would be assigned as an additional diagnosis when the provider has also documented the presence of ventilator associated pneumonia.

g. SIRS due to Non-infectious Process

The systemic inflammatory response syndrome (SIRS) can develop as a result of certain non-infectious disease processes, such as trauma, malignant neoplasm, or pancreatitis. When SIRS is documented with a noninfectious condition, and no subsequent infection is documented, the code for the underlying condition, such as an injury, should be assigned, followed by code 995.93, Systemic inflammatory response syndrome due to noninfectious process without acute organ dysfunction, or 995.94, Systemic inflammatory response syndrome due to non-infectious process with acute organ dysfunction. If an acute organ dysfunction is documented, the appropriate code(s) for the associated acute organ dysfunction(s) should be assigned in addition to code 995.94. If acute organ dysfunction is documented, but it cannot be determined if the acute organ dysfunction is associated with SIRS or due to another condition (e.g., directly due to the trauma), the provider should be queried.

When the non-infectious condition has led to an infection that results in SIRS, *see Section I.C.1.b.12 for the guideline for sepsis and severe sepsis associated with a non-infectious process.*

18. Classification of Factors Influencing Health Status and Contact with Health Service (Supplemental V01-V89)

Note: The chapter specific guidelines provide additional information about the use of V codes for specified encounters.

a. Introduction

ICD-9-CM provides codes to deal with encounters for circumstances other than a disease or injury. The Supplementary Classification of Factors Influencing Health Status and Contact with Health Services (V01.0 - V89.09) is provided to deal with occasions when circumstances other than a disease or injury (codes 001-999) are recorded as a diagnosis or problem.

There are four primary circumstances for the use of V codes:

1) A person who is not currently sick encounters the health services for some specific reason, such as to act as an organ donor, to receive prophylactic care, such as inoculations or health screenings, or to receive counseling on health related issues.

2) A person with a resolving disease or injury, or a chronic, long-term condition requiring continuous care, encounters the health care system for specific aftercare of that disease or injury (e.g., dialysis for renal disease; chemotherapy for malignancy; cast change). A diagnosis/symptom code should be used whenever a current, acute, diagnosis is being treated or a sign or symptom is being studied.

3) Circumstances or problems influence a person's health status but are not in themselves a current illness or injury.

4) Newborns, to indicate birth status

b. **V codes use in any healthcare setting**

V codes are for use in any healthcare setting. V codes may be used as either a first listed (principal diagnosis code in the inpatient setting) or secondary code, depending on the circumstances of the encounter. Certain V codes may only be used as first listed, others only as secondary codes.

See Section I.C.18.e, **V Codes That May Only be Principal/First-Listed Diagnosis.**

c. **V Codes indicate a reason for an encounter**

They are not procedure codes. A corresponding procedure code must accompany a V code to describe the procedure performed.

d. **Categories of V Codes**

1) **Contact/Exposure**

Category V01 indicates contact with or exposure to communicable diseases. These codes are for patients who do not show any sign or symptom of a disease but have been exposed to it by close personal contact with an infected individual or are in an area where a disease is epidemic. These codes may be used as a first listed code to explain an encounter for testing, or, more commonly, as a secondary code to identify a potential risk.

2) **Inoculations and vaccinations**

Categories V03-V06 are for encounters for inoculations and vaccinations. They indicate that a patient is being seen to receive a prophylactic inoculation against a disease. The injection itself must be represented by the appropriate procedure code. A code from V03-V06 may be used as a secondary code if the inoculation is given as a routine part of preventive health care, such as a well-baby visit.

3) **Status**

Status codes indicate that a patient is either a carrier of a disease or has the sequelae or residual of a past disease or condition. This includes such things as the presence of prosthetic or mechanical devices resulting from past treatment. A status code is informative, because the status may affect the course of treatment and its outcome. A status code is distinct from a history code. The history code indicates that the patient no longer has the condition.

A status code should not be used with a diagnosis code from one of the body system chapters, if the diagnosis code includes the information provided by the status code. For example, code V42.1, Heart transplant status, should not be used with code 996.83, Complications of transplanted heart. The status code does not provide additional information. The complication code indicates that the patient is a heart transplant patient.

The status V codes/categories are:

V02   Carrier or suspected carrier of infectious diseases

Carrier status indicates that a person harbors the specific organisms of a disease without manifest symptoms and is capable of transmitting the infection.

V07.5X   Prophylactic use of agents affecting estrogen receptors and estrogen level

This code indicates when a patient is receiving a drug that affects estrogen receptors and estrogen levels for prevention of cancer.

V08   Asymptomatic HIV infection status

This code indicates that a patient has tested positive for HIV but has manifested no signs or symptoms of the disease.

V09   Infection with drug-resistant microorganisms

This category indicates that a patient has an infection that is resistant to drug treatment. Sequence the infection code first.

V21   Constitutional states in development

V22.2   Pregnant state, incidental

This code is a secondary code only for use when the pregnancy is in no way complicating the reason for visit. Otherwise, a code from the obstetric chapter is required.

V26.5x   Sterilization status

V42   Organ or tissue replaced by transplant

V43   Organ or tissue replaced by other means

V44   Artificial opening status

V45   Other postsurgical states

Assign code V45.87, Transplant organ removal status, to indicate that a transplanted organ has been previously removed. This code should not be assigned for the encounter in which the transplanted organ is removed. The complication necessitating removal of the transplant organ should be assigned for that encounter.

See section I.C17.f.2. for information on the coding of organ transplant complications.

Assign code V45.88, Status post administration of tPA (rtPA) in a different facility within the last 24 hours prior to admission to the current facility, as a secondary diagnosis when a patient is received by transfer into a facility and documentation indicates they were administered tissue plasminogen activator (tPA) within the last 24 hours prior to admission to the current facility.

This guideline applies even if the patient is still receiving the tPA at the time they are received into the current facility.

The appropriate code for the condition for which the tPA was administered (such as cerebrovascular disease or myocardial infarction) should be assigned first.

Code V45.88 is only applicable to the receiving facility record and not to the transferring facility record.

V46   Other dependence on machines

V49.6   Upper limb amputation status

V49.7   Lower limb amputation status

Note: Categories V42-V46, and subcategories V49.6, V49.7 are for use only if there are no complications or malfunctions of the organ or tissue replaced, the amputation site or the equipment on which the patient is dependent.

V49.81   Postmenopausal status

V49.82   Dental sealant status

V49.83   Awaiting organ transplant status

V58.6x   Long-term (current) drug use

Codes from this subcategory indicate a patient's continuous use of a prescribed drug (including such things as aspirin therapy) for the long-term treatment of a condition or for prophylactic use. It is not for use for patients who have addictions to drugs. This subcategory is not for use of medications for detoxification or maintenance programs to prevent withdrawal symptoms in patients with drug dependence (e.g., methadone maintenance for opiate dependence). Assign the appropriate code for the drug dependence instead.

Assign a code from subcategory V58.6, Long-term (current) drug use, if the patient is receiving a medication for an extended period as a prophylactic measure (such as for the prevention of deep vein thrombosis) or as treatment of a chronic condition (such as arthritis) or a disease requiring a lengthy course of treatment (such as cancer). Do not assign a code from subcategory V58.6 for medication being administered for a brief period of time to treat an acute illness or injury (such as a course of antibiotics to treat acute bronchitis).

V83   Genetic carrier status

Genetic carrier status indicates that a person carries a gene, associated with a particular disease, which may be passed to offspring who may develop that disease. The person does not have the disease and is not at risk of developing the disease.

V84   Genetic susceptibility status

Genetic susceptibility indicates that a person has a gene that increases the risk of that person developing the disease.

Codes from category V84, Genetic susceptibility to disease, should not be used as principal or first-listed codes. If the patient has the condition to which he/she is susceptible, and that condition is the reason for the encounter, the code for the current condition should be sequenced first. If the patient is being seen for follow-up after completed treatment for this condition, and the condition no longer exists, a follow-up code should be sequenced first, followed by the appropriate personal history and genetic susceptibility codes. If the purpose of the encounter is genetic counseling associated with procreative management, a code from subcategory V26.3, Genetic counseling and testing, should be assigned as the first-listed code, followed by a code from category V84. Additional codes should be assigned for any applicable family or personal history.

See Section I.C. 18.d.14 for information on prophylactic organ removal due to a genetic susceptibility.

V85   Body Mass Index (BMI)

V86   Estrogen receptor status

V88   Acquired absence of other organs and tissue

4) **History (of)**

There are two types of history V codes, personal and family. Personal history codes explain a patient's past medical condition that no longer exists and is not receiving any treatment, but that has the potential for recurrence, and therefore may require continued monitoring. The exceptions to this general rule are category V14, Personal history of allergy to medicinal agents, and subcategory V15.0, Allergy, other than to medicinal agents. A person who has had an allergic episode to a substance or food in the past should always be considered allergic to the substance.

Family history codes are for use when a patient has a family member(s) who has had a particular disease that causes the patient to be at higher risk of also contracting the disease.

Personal history codes may be used in conjunction with follow-up codes and family history codes may be used in conjunction with screening codes to explain the need for a test or procedure. History codes are also acceptable on any medical record regardless of the reason for visit. A history of an illness, even if no longer present, is important information that may alter the type of treatment ordered.

The history V code categories are:

V10   Personal history of malignant neoplasm

V12   Personal history of certain other diseases

V13   Personal history of other diseases

Except: V13.4, Personal history of arthritis, and V13.6, Personal history of congenital malformations. These conditions are life-long so are not true history codes.

V14   Personal history of allergy to medicinal agents

V15   Other personal history presenting hazards to health

Except: V15.7, Personal history of contraception.

V16   Family history of malignant neoplasm

V17 Family history of certain chronic disabling diseases

V18 Family history of certain other specific diseases

V19 Family history of other conditions

V87 Other specified personal exposures and history presenting hazards to health

5) Screening

Screening is the testing for disease or disease precursors in seemingly well individuals so that early detection and treatment can be provided for those who test positive for the disease. Screenings that are recommended for many subgroups in a population include: routine mammograms for women over 40, a fecal occult blood test for everyone over 50, an amniocentesis to rule out a fetal anomaly for pregnant women over 35, because the incidence of breast cancer and colon cancer in these subgroups is higher than in the general population, as is the incidence of Down's syndrome in older mothers.

The testing of a person to rule out or confirm a suspected diagnosis because the patient has some sign or symptom is a diagnostic examination, not a screening. In these cases, the sign or symptom is used to explain the reason for the test.

A screening code may be a first listed code if the reason for the visit is specifically the screening exam. It may also be used as an additional code if the screening is done during an office visit for other health problems. A screening code is not necessary if the screening is inherent to a routine examination, such as a pap smear done during a routine pelvic examination.

Should a condition be discovered during the screening then the code for the condition may be assigned as an additional diagnosis.

The V code indicates that a screening exam is planned. A procedure code is required to confirm that the screening was performed.

The screening V code categories:

V28 Antenatal screening

V73-V82 Special screening examinations

6) Observation

There are three observation V code categories. They are for use in very limited circumstances when a person is being observed for a suspected condition that is ruled out. The observation codes are not for use if an injury or illness or any signs or symptoms related to the suspected condition are present. In such cases the diagnosis/symptom code is used with the corresponding E code to identify any external cause.

The observation codes are to be used as principal diagnosis only. The only exception to this is when the principal diagnosis is required to be a code from the V30, Live born infant, category. Then the V29 observation code is sequenced after the V30 code. Additional codes may be used in addition to the observation code but only if they are unrelated to the suspected condition being observed.

Codes from subcategory V89.0, Suspected maternal and fetal conditions not found, may either be used as a first listed or as an additional code assignment depending on the case. They are for use in very limited circumstances on a maternal record when an encounter is for a suspected maternal or fetal condition that is ruled out during that encounter (for example, a maternal or fetal condition may be suspected due to an abnormal test result). These codes should not be used when the condition is confirmed. In those cases, the confirmed condition should be coded. In addition, these codes are not for use if an illness or any signs or symptoms related to the suspected condition or problem are present. In such cases the diagnosis/symptom code is used.

Additional codes may be used in addition to the code from subcategory V89.0, but only if they are unrelated to the suspected condition being evaluated.

Codes from subcategory V89.0 may not be used for encounters for antenatal screening of mother. *See Section I.C.18.d., Screening).*

For encounters for suspected fetal condition that are inconclusive following testing and evaluation, assign the appropriate code from category 655, 656, 657 or 658.

The observation V code categories:

V29   Observation and evaluation of newborns for suspected condition not found

For the birth encounter, a code from category V30 should be sequenced before the V29 code.

V71   Observation and evaluation for suspected condition not found

V89   Suspected maternal and fetal conditions not found

7) Aftercare

Aftercare visit codes cover situations when the initial treatment of a disease or injury has been performed and the patient requires continued care during the healing or recovery phase, or for the long-term consequences of the disease. The aftercare V code should not be used if treatment is directed at a current, acute disease or injury. The diagnosis code is to be used in these cases. Exceptions to this rule are codes V58.0, Radiotherapy, and codes from subcategory V58.1, Encounter for chemotherapy and immunotherapy for neoplastic conditions. These codes are to be first listed, followed by the diagnosis code when a patient's encounter is solely to receive radiation therapy or chemotherapy for the treatment of a neoplasm. Should a patient receive both chemotherapy and radiation therapy during the same encounter code V58.0 and V58.1 may be used together on a record with either one being sequenced first.

The aftercare codes are generally first listed to explain the specific reason for the encounter. An aftercare code may be used as an additional code when some type of aftercare is provided in addition to the reason for admission and no diagnosis code is applicable. An example of this would be the closure of a colostomy during an encounter for treatment of another condition.

Aftercare codes should be used in conjunction with any other aftercare codes or other diagnosis codes to provide better detail on the specifics of an aftercare encounter visit, unless otherwise directed by the classification. The sequencing of multiple aftercare codes is discretionary.

Certain aftercare V code categories need a secondary diagnosis code to describe the resolving condition or sequelae, for others, the condition is inherent in the code title.

Additional V code aftercare category terms include fitting and adjustment, and attention to artificial openings.

Status V codes may be used with aftercare V codes to indicate the nature of the aftercare. For example code V45.81, Aortocoronary bypass status, may be used with code V58.73, Aftercare following surgery of the circulatory system, NEC, to indicate the surgery for which the aftercare is being performed. Also, a transplant status code may be used following code V58.44, Aftercare following organ transplant, to identify the organ transplanted. A status code should not be used when the aftercare code indicates the type of status, such as using V55.0, Attention to tracheostomy with V44.0, Tracheostomy status.

See Section I. B.16 Admissions/Encounter for Rehabilitation

The aftercare V category/codes:

V51.0   Encounter for breast reconstruction following mastectomy

V52   Fitting and adjustment of prosthetic device and implant

V53   Fitting and adjustment of other device

V54   Other orthopedic aftercare

V55   Attention to artificial openings

V56   Encounter for dialysis and dialysis catheter care

V57   Care involving the use of rehabilitation procedures

V58.0   Radiotherapy

V58.11   Encounter for antineoplastic chemotherapy

V58.12   Encounter for antineoplastic immunotherapy

V58.3x   Attention to dressings and sutures

V58.41   Encounter for planned post-operative wound closure

V58.42   Aftercare, surgery, neoplasm

V58.43   Aftercare, surgery, trauma

V58.44   Aftercare involving organ transplant

V58.49   Other specified aftercare following surgery

V58.7x   Aftercare following surgery

V58.81   Fitting and adjustment of vascular catheter

V58.82   Fitting and adjustment of non-vascular catheter

V58.83   Monitoring therapeutic drug

V58.89   Other specified aftercare

8) Follow-up

The follow-up codes are used to explain continuing surveillance following completed treatment of a disease, condition, or injury. They imply that the condition has been fully treated and no longer exists. They should not be confused with aftercare codes that explain current treatment for a healing condition or its sequelae. Follow-up codes may be used in conjunction with history codes to provide the full picture of the healed condition and its treatment. The follow-up code is sequenced first, followed by the history code.

A follow-up code may be used to explain repeated visits. Should a condition be found to have recurred on the follow-up visit, then the diagnosis code should be used in place of the follow-up code.

The follow-up V code categories:

V24   Postpartum care and evaluation

V67   Follow-up examination

9) Donor

Category V59 is the donor codes. They are used for living individuals who are donating blood or other body tissue. These codes are only for individuals donating for others, not for self donations. They are not for use to identify cadaveric donations.

10) Counseling

Counseling V codes are used when a patient or family member receives assistance in the aftermath of an illness or injury, or when support is required in coping with family or social problems. They are not necessary for use in conjunction with a diagnosis code when the counseling component of care is considered integral to standard treatment.

The counseling V categories/codes:

V25.0   General counseling and advice for contraceptive management

V26.3   Genetic counseling

V26.4   General counseling and advice for procreative management

V61.**X**   Other family circumstances

V65.1   Person consulted on behalf of another person

V65.3   Dietary surveillance and counseling

V65.4   Other counseling, not elsewhere classified

11) Obstetrics and related conditions

See Section I.C.11., the Obstetrics guidelines for further instruction on the use of these codes.

V codes for pregnancy are for use in those circumstances when none of the problems or complications included in the codes from the Obstetrics chapter exist (a routine prenatal visit or postpartum care). Codes V22.0, Supervision of normal first pregnancy, and V22.1, Supervision of other normal pregnancy, are always first listed and are not to be used with any other code from the OB chapter.

The outcome of delivery, category V27, should be included on all maternal delivery records. It is always a secondary code.

V codes for family planning (contraceptive) or procreative management and counseling should be included on an obstetric record either during the pregnancy or the postpartum stage, if applicable.

Obstetrics and related conditions V code categories:

V22   Normal pregnancy

V23   Supervision of high-risk pregnancy

Except: V23.2, Pregnancy with history of abortion. Code 646.3, Habitual aborter, from the OB chapter is required to indicate a history of abortion during a pregnancy.

V24   Postpartum care and evaluation

V25 Encounter for contraceptive management

Except V25.0x

(See Section I.C.18.d.11, Counseling)

V26 Procreative management

Except V26.5x, Sterilization status, V26.3 and V26.4

(See Section I.C.18.d.11., Counseling)

V27 Outcome of delivery

V28 Antenatal screening

(See Section I.C.18.d.6., Screening)

12) Newborn, infant and child

See Section I.C.15, the Newborn guidelines for further instruction on the use of these codes.

Newborn V code categories:

V20 Health supervision of infant or child

V29 Observation and evaluation of newborns for suspected condition not found

(See Section I.C.18.d.7, Observation)

V30-V39 Liveborn infant according to type of birth

13) Routine and administrative examinations

The V codes allow for the description of encounters for routine examinations, such as, a general check-up, or examinations for administrative purposes, such as a pre-employment physical. The codes are not to be used if the examination is for diagnosis of a suspected condition or for treatment purposes. In such cases the diagnosis code is used. During a routine exam, should a diagnosis or condition be discovered, it should be coded as an additional code. Pre-existing and chronic conditions and history codes may also be included as additional codes as long as the examination is for administrative purposes and not focused on any particular condition.

Pre-operative examination **and pre-procedural laboratory examination** V codes are for use only in those situations when a patient is being cleared for **a procedure or** surgery and no treatment is given.

The V codes categories/code for routine and administrative examinations:

V20.2 Routine infant or child health check

Any injections given should have a corresponding procedure code.

V70 General medical examination

V72 Special investigations and examinations

Codes V72.5 and V72.6**2** may be used if the reason for the patient encounter is for routine laboratory/radiology testing in the absence of any signs, symptoms, or associated diagnosis. If routine testing is performed during the same encounter as a test to evaluate a sign, symptom, or diagnosis, it is appropriate to assign both the V code and the code describing the reason for the non-routine test.

14) Miscellaneous V codes

The miscellaneous V codes capture a number of other health care encounters that do not fall into one of the other categories. Certain of these codes identify the reason for the encounter, others are for use as additional codes that provide useful information on circumstances that may affect a patient's care and treatment.

Prophylactic Organ Removal

For encounters specifically for prophylactic removal of breasts, ovaries, or another organ due to a genetic susceptibility to cancer or a family history of cancer, the principal or first listed code should be a code from subcategory V50.4, Prophylactic organ removal, followed by the appropriate genetic susceptibility code and the appropriate family history code.

If the patient has a malignancy of one site and is having prophylactic removal at another site to prevent either a new primary malignancy or metastatic disease, a code for the malignancy should also be assigned in addition to a code from subcategory V50.4. A V50.4 code should not be assigned if the patient is having organ removal for treatment of a malignancy, such as the removal of the testes for the treatment of prostate cancer.

Miscellaneous V code categories/codes:

V07	Need for isolation and other prophylactic measures
	Except V07.5, Prophylactic use of agents affecting estrogen receptors and estrogen levels
V50	Elective surgery for purposes other than remedying health states
V58.5	Orthodontics
V60	Housing, household, and economic circumstances
V62	Other psychosocial circumstances
V63	Unavailability of other medical facilities for care
V64	Persons encountering health services for specific procedures, not carried out
V66	Convalescence and Palliative Care
V68	Encounters for administrative purposes
V69	Problems related to lifestyle
V85	Body Mass Index

15) Nonspecific V codes

Certain V codes are so non-specific, or potentially redundant with other codes in the classification, that there can be little justification for their use in the inpatient setting. Their use in the outpatient setting should be limited to those instances when there is no further documentation to permit more precise coding. Otherwise, any sign or symptom or any other reason for visit that is captured in another code should be used.

Nonspecific V code categories/codes:

V11	Personal history of mental disorder
	A code from the mental disorders chapter, with an in remission fifth-digit, should be used.
V13.4	Personal history of arthritis
V13.6	Personal history of congenital malformations
V15.7	Personal history of contraception
V23.2	Pregnancy with history of abortion
V40	Mental and behavioral problems
V41	Problems with special senses and other special functions
V47	Other problems with internal organs
V48	Problems with head, neck, and trunk
V49	Problems with limbs and other problems

Exceptions:

	V49.6	Upper limb amputation status
	V49.7	Lower limb amputation status
	V49.81	Postmenopausal status
	V49.82	Dental sealant status
	V49.83	Awaiting organ transplant status
V51.8	Other aftercare involving the use of plastic surgery	
V58.2	Blood transfusion, without reported diagnosis	
V58.9	Unspecified aftercare	

See Section IV.K. and Section IV.L. of the Outpatient guidelines.

e. **V Codes That May Only be Principal/First-Listed Diagnosis**

The list of V codes/categories below may only be reported as the principal/first-listed diagnosis, except when there are multiple encounters on the same day and the medical records for the encounters are combined or when there is more than one V code that meets the definition of principal diagnosis (e.g., a patient is admitted to home healthcare for both aftercare and rehabilitation and they equally meet the definition of principal diagnosis). These codes should not be reported if they do not meet the definition of principal or first-listed diagnosis.

See Section II and Section IV.A for information on selection of principal and first-listed diagnosis.

See Section II.C for information on two or more diagnoses that equally meet the definition for principal diagnosis.

V20.X	Health supervision of infant or child
V22.0	Supervision of normal first pregnancy
V22.1	Supervision of other normal pregnancy
V24.X	Postpartum care and examination
V26.81	Encounter for assisted reproductive fertility procedure cycle
V26.82	**Encounter for fertility preservation procedure**
V30.X	Single liveborn
V31.X	Twin, mate liveborn
V32.X	Twin, mate stillborn
V33.X	Twin, unspecified
V34.X	Other multiple, mates all liveborn
V35.X	Other multiple, mates all stillborn
V36.X	Other multiple, mates live- and stillborn
V37.X	Other multiple, unspecified
V39.X	Unspecified
V46.12	Encounter for respirator dependence during power failure
V46.13	Encounter for weaning from respirator [ventilator]
V51.0	Encounter for breast reconstruction following mastectomy
V56.0	Extracorporeal dialysis
V57.X	Care involving use of rehabilitation procedures
V58.0	Radiotherapy
V58.11	Encounter for antineoplastic chemotherapy
V58.12	Encounter for antineoplastic immunotherapy
V59.X	Donors
V66.0	Convalescence and palliative care following surgery
V66.1	Convalescence and palliative care following radiotherapy
V66.2	Convalescence and palliative care following chemotherapy
V66.3	Convalescence and palliative care following psychotherapy and other treatment for mental disorder
V66.4	Convalescence and palliative care following treatment of fracture
V66.5	Convalescence and palliative care following other treatment
V66.6	Convalescence and palliative care following combined treatment
V66.9	Unspecified convalescence
V68.X	Encounters for administrative purposes
V70.0	Routine general medical examination at a health care facility
V70.1	General psychiatric examination, requested by the authority
V70.2	General psychiatric examination, other and unspecified
V70.3	Other medical examination for administrative purposes
V70.4	Examination for medicolegal reasons
V70.5	Health examination of defined subpopulations
V70.6	Health examination in population surveys
V70.8	Other specified general medical examinations
V70.9	Unspecified general medical examination
V71.X	Observation and evaluation for suspected conditions not found

19. **Supplemental Classification of External Causes of Injury and Poisoning (E-codes, E800-E999)**

Introduction: These guidelines are provided for those who are currently collecting E codes in order that there will be standardization in the process. If your institution plans to begin collecting E codes, these guidelines are to be applied. The use of E codes is supplemental to the application of ICD-9-CM diagnosis codes.

External causes of injury and poisoning codes (**categories E000 and E800-E999**) are intended to provide data for injury research and evaluation of injury prevention strategies. **Activity codes (categories E001-E030) are intended to be used to describe the activity of a person seeking care for injuries as well as other health conditions, when the injury or other health condition resulted from an activity or the activity contributed to a condition.** E codes capture how the injury, **poisoning, or adverse effect** happened (cause), the intent (unintentional or accidental; or intentional, such as suicide or assault), **the person's status (e.g. civilian, military), the associated activity** and the place where the event occurred.

Some major categories of E codes include:

transport accidents

poisoning and adverse effects of drugs, medicinal substances and biologicals

accidental falls

accidents caused by fire and flames

accidents due to natural and environmental factors

late effects of accidents, assaults or self injury

assaults or purposely inflicted injury

suicide or self inflicted injury

These guidelines apply for the coding and collection of E codes from records in hospitals, outpatient clinics, emergency departments, other ambulatory care settings and provider offices, and nonacute care settings, except when other specific guidelines apply.

a. **General E Code Coding Guidelines**

1) **Used with any code in the range of 001-V89**

An E code **from categories E800-E999** may be used with any code in the range of 001-V89, which indicates an injury, poisoning, or adverse effect due to an external cause.

An activity E code (categories E001-E030) may be used with any code in the range of 001-V89 that indicates an injury, or other health condition that resulted from an activity, or the activity contributed to a condition.

2) **Assign the appropriate E code for all initial treatments**

Assign the appropriate E code for the initial encounter of an injury, poisoning, or adverse effect of drugs, not for subsequent treatment.

External cause of injury codes (E-codes) may be assigned while the acute fracture codes are still applicable.

See Section I.C.17.b.1 for coding of acute fractures.

3) **Use the full range of E codes**

Use the full range of E codes (**E800–E999**) to completely describe the cause, the intent and the place of occurrence, if applicable, for all injuries, poisonings, and adverse effects of drugs.

See a.1.), j.), and k.) in this section for information on the use of status and activity E codes.

4) **Assign as many E codes as necessary**

Assign as many E codes as necessary to fully explain each cause. If only one E code can be recorded, assign the E code most related to the principal diagnosis.

5) **The selection of the appropriate E code**

The selection of the appropriate E code is guided by the Index to External Causes, which is located after the alphabetical index to diseases and by Inclusion and Exclusion notes in the Tabular List.

6) **E code can never be a principal diagnosis**

An E code can never be a principal (first listed) diagnosis.

7) **External cause code(s) with systemic inflammatory response syndrome (SIRS)**

An external cause code is not appropriate with a code from subcategory 995.9, unless the patient also has **another condition for which an E code would be appropriate (such as** an injury, poisoning, or adverse effect of drugs.

8) **Multiple Cause E Code Coding Guidelines**

More than one E-code is required to fully describe the external cause of an illness, injury or poisoning. The assignment of E-codes should be sequenced in the following priority:

If two or more events cause separate injuries, an E code should be assigned for each cause. The first listed E code will be selected in the following order:

E codes for child and adult abuse take priority over all other E codes.

See Section I.C.19.e., Child and Adult abuse guidelines.

E codes for terrorism events take priority over all other E codes except child and adult abuse.

E codes for cataclysmic events take priority over all other E codes except child and adult abuse and terrorism.

E codes for transport accidents take priority over all other E codes except cataclysmic events, child and adult abuse and terrorism.

Activity and external cause status codes are assigned following all causal (intent) E codes.

The first-listed E code should correspond to the cause of the most serious diagnosis due to an assault, accident, or self-harm, following the order of hierarchy listed above.

9) **If the reporting format limits the number of E codes**

If the reporting format limits the number of E codes that can be used in reporting clinical data, report the code for the cause/intent most related to the principal diagnosis. If the format permits capture of additional E codes, the cause/intent, including medical misadventures, of the additional events should be reported rather than the codes for place, activity or external status.

b. **Place of Occurrence Guideline**

Use an additional code from category E849 to indicate the Place of Occurrence for injuries and poisonings. The Place of Occurrence describes the place where the event occurred and not the patient's activity at the time of the event.

Do not use E849.9 if the place of occurrence is not stated.

c. **Adverse Effects of Drugs, Medicinal and Biological Substances Guidelines**

1) **Do not code directly from the Table of Drugs**

Do not code directly from the Table of Drugs and Chemicals. Always refer back to the Tabular List.

2) **Use as many codes as necessary to describe**

Use as many codes as necessary to describe completely all drugs, medicinal or biological substances.

If the reporting format limits the number of E codes, and there are different fourth digit codes in the same three digit category, use the code for "Other specified" of that category of drugs, medicinal or biological substances. If there is no "Other specified" code in that category, use the appropriate "Unspecified" code in that category.

If the reporting format limits the number of E codes, and the codes are in different three digit categories, assign the appropriate E code for other multiple drugs and medicinal substances.

3) **If the same E code would describe the causative agent**

If the same E code would describe the causative agent for more than one adverse reaction, assign the code only once.

4) **If two or more drugs, medicinal or biological substances**

If two or more drugs, medicinal or biological substances are reported, code each individually unless the combination code is listed in the Table of Drugs and Chemicals. In that case, assign the E code for the combination.

5) **When a reaction results from the interaction of a drug(s)**

When a reaction results from the interaction of a drug(s) and alcohol, use poisoning codes and E codes for both.

6) **Codes from the E930-E949 series**

Codes from the E930-E949 series must be used to identify the causative substance for an adverse effect of drug, medicinal and biological substances, correctly prescribed and properly administered. The effect, such as tachycardia, delirium, gastrointestinal hemorrhaging, vomiting, hypokalemia, hepatitis, renal failure, or respiratory failure, is coded and followed by the appropriate code from the E930-E949 series.

d. **Child and Adult Abuse Guideline**

   1) **Intentional injury**

      When the cause of an injury or neglect is intentional child or adult abuse, the first listed E code should be assigned from categories E960-E968, Homicide and injury purposely inflicted by other persons, (except category E967). An E code from category E967, Child and adult battering and other maltreatment, should be added as an additional code to identify the perpetrator, if known.

   2) **Accidental intent**

      In cases of neglect when the intent is determined to be accidental E code E904.0, Abandonment or neglect of infant and helpless person, should be the first listed E code.

e. **Unknown or Suspected Intent Guideline**

   1) **If the intent (accident, self-harm, assault) of the cause of an injury or poisoning is unknown**

      If the intent (accident, self-harm, assault) of the cause of an injury or poisoning is unknown or unspecified, code the intent as undetermined E980-E989.

   2) **If the intent (accident, self-harm, assault) of the cause of an injury or poisoning is questionable**

      If the intent (accident, self-harm, assault) of the cause of an injury or poisoning is questionable, probable or suspected, code the intent as undetermined E980-E989.

f. **Undetermined Cause**

   When the intent of an injury or poisoning is known, but the cause is unknown, use codes: E928.9, Unspecified accident, E958.9, Suicide and self-inflicted injury by unspecified means, and E968.9, Assault by unspecified means.

   These E codes should rarely be used, as the documentation in the medical record, in both the inpatient outpatient and other settings, should normally provide sufficient detail to determine the cause of the injury.

g. **Late Effects of External Cause Guidelines**

   1) **Late effect E codes**

      Late effect E codes exist for injuries and poisonings but not for adverse effects of drugs, misadventures and surgical complications.

   2) **Late effect E codes (E929, E959, E969, E977, E989, or E999.1)**

      A late effect E code (E929, E959, E969, E977, E989, or E999.1) should be used with any report of a late effect or sequela resulting from a previous injury or poisoning (905-909).

   3) **Late effect E code with a related current injury**

      A late effect E code should never be used with a related current nature of injury code.

   4) **Use of late effect E codes for subsequent visits**

      Use a late effect E code for subsequent visits when a late effect of the initial injury or poisoning is being treated. There is no late effect E code for adverse effects of drugs.

      Do not use a late effect E code for subsequent visits for follow-up care (e.g., to assess healing, to receive rehabilitative therapy) of the injury or poisoning when no late effect of the injury has been documented.

h. **Misadventures and Complications of Care Guidelines**

   1) **Code range E870-E876**

      Assign a code in the range of E870-E876 if misadventures are stated by the provider. **When applying the E code guidelines pertaining to sequencing, these E codes are considered causal codes.**

   2) **Code range E878-E879**

      Assign a code in the range of E878-E879 if the provider attributes an abnormal reaction or later complication to a surgical or medical procedure, but does not mention misadventure at the time of the procedure as the cause of the reaction.

i. Terrorism Guidelines

1) **Cause of injury identified by the Federal Government (FBI) as terrorism**

When the cause of an injury is identified by the Federal Government (FBI) as terrorism, the first-listed E-code should be a code from category E979, Terrorism. The definition of terrorism employed by the FBI is found at the inclusion note at E979. The terrorism E-code is the only E-code that should be assigned. Additional E codes from the assault categories should not be assigned.

2) **Cause of an injury is suspected to be the result of terrorism**

When the cause of an injury is suspected to be the result of terrorism a code from category E979 should not be assigned. Assign a code in the range of E codes based circumstances on the documentation of intent and mechanism.

3) **Code E979.9, Terrorism, secondary effects**

Assign code E979.9, Terrorism, secondary effects, for conditions occurring subsequent to the terrorist event. This code should not be assigned for conditions that are due to the initial terrorist act.

4) **Statistical tabulation of terrorism codes**

For statistical purposes these codes will be tabulated within the category for assault, expanding the current category from E960-E969 to include E979 and E999.1.

j. Activity Code Guidelines

Assign a code from category E001-E030 to describe the activity that caused or contributed to the injury or other health condition.

Unlike other E codes, activity E codes may be assigned to indicate a health condition (not just injuries) resulted from an activity, or the activity contributed to the condition.

The activity codes are not applicable to poisonings, adverse effects, misadventures or late effects.

k. External cause status

A code from category E000, External cause status, should be assigned whenever any other E code is assigned for an encounter, including an Activity E code, except for the events noted below. Assign a code from category E000, External cause status, to indicate the work status of the person at the time the event occurred. The status code indicates whether the event occurred during military activity, whether a non-military person was at work, whether an individual including a student or volunteer was involved in a non-work activity at the time of the causal event.

A code from E000, External cause status, should be assigned, when applicable, with other external cause codes, such as transport accidents and falls. The external cause status codes are not applicable to poisonings, adverse effects, misadventures or late effects.

Do not assign a code from category E000 if no other E codes (cause, activity) are applicable for the encounter.

Do not assign code E000.9, Unspecified external cause status, if the status is not stated.

Section II. Selection of Principal Diagnosis

The circumstances of inpatient admission always govern the selection of principal diagnosis. The principal diagnosis is defined in the Uniform Hospital Discharge Data Set (UHDDS) as "that condition established after study to be chiefly responsible for occasioning the admission of the patient to the hospital for care."

The UHDDS definitions are used by hospitals to report inpatient data elements in a standardized manner. These data elements and their definitions can be found in the July 31, 1985, Federal Register (Vol. 50, No, 147), pp. 31038-40.

Since that time the application of the UHDDS definitions has been expanded to include all non-outpatient settings (acute care, short term, long term care and psychiatric hospitals; home health agencies; rehab facilities; nursing homes, etc).

In determining principal diagnosis the coding conventions in the ICD-9-CM, Volumes I and II take precedence over these official coding guidelines.

(See Section I.A., Conventions for the ICD-9-CM)

The importance of consistent, complete documentation in the medical record cannot be overemphasized. Without such documentation the application of all coding guidelines is a difficult, if not impossible, task.

A. **Codes for symptoms, signs, and ill-defined conditions**

Codes for symptoms, signs, and ill-defined conditions from Chapter 16 are not to be used as principal diagnosis when a related definitive diagnosis has been established.

B. **Two or more interrelated conditions, each potentially meeting the definition for principal diagnosis.**

When there are two or more interrelated conditions (such as diseases in the same ICD-9-CM chapter or manifestations characteristically associated with a certain disease) potentially meeting the definition of principal diagnosis, either condition may be sequenced first, unless the circumstances of the admission, the therapy provided, the Tabular List, or the Alphabetic Index indicate otherwise.

C. **Two or more diagnoses that equally meet the definition for principal diagnosis**

In the unusual instance when two or more diagnoses equally meet the criteria for principal diagnosis as determined by the circumstances of admission, diagnostic workup and/or therapy provided, and the Alphabetic Index, Tabular List, or another coding guidelines does not provide sequencing direction, any one of the diagnoses may be sequenced first.

D. **Two or more comparative or contrasting conditions.**

In those rare instances when two or more contrasting or comparative diagnoses are documented as "either/or" (or similar terminology), they are coded as if the diagnoses were confirmed and the diagnoses are sequenced according to the circumstances of the admission. If no further determination can be made as to which diagnosis should be principal, either diagnosis may be sequenced first.

E. **A symptom(s) followed by contrasting/ comparative diagnoses**

When a symptom(s) is followed by contrasting/ comparative diagnoses, the symptom code is sequenced first. All the contrasting/comparative diagnoses should be coded as additional diagnoses.

F. **Original treatment plan not carried out**

Sequence as the principal diagnosis the condition, which after study occasioned the admission to the hospital, even though treatment may not have been carried out due to unforeseen circumstances.

G. **Complications of surgery and other medical care**

When the admission is for treatment of a complication resulting from surgery or other medical care, the complication code is sequenced as the principal diagnosis. If the complication is classified to the 996-999 series and the code lacks the necessary specificity in describing the complication, an additional code for the specific complication should be assigned.

H. **Uncertain Diagnosis**

If the diagnosis documented at the time of discharge is qualified as "probable", "suspected", "likely", "questionable", "possible", or "still to be ruled out", or other similar terms indicating uncertainty, code the condition as if it existed or was established. The bases for these guidelines are the diagnostic workup, arrangements for further workup or observation, and initial therapeutic approach that correspond most closely with the established diagnosis.

Note: This guideline is applicable only to inpatient admissions to short-term, acute, long-term care and psychiatric hospitals.

I. **Admission from Observation Unit**

1. **Admission Following Medical Observation**

When a patient is admitted to an observation unit for a medical condition, which either worsens or does not improve, and is subsequently admitted as an inpatient of the same hospital for this same medical condition, the principal diagnosis would be the medical condition which led to the hospital admission.

2. **Admission Following Post-Operative Observation**

When a patient is admitted to an observation unit to monitor a condition (or complication) that develops following outpatient surgery, and then is subsequently admitted as an inpatient of the same hospital, hospitals should apply the Uniform Hospital Discharge Data Set (UHDDS) definition of principal diagnosis as "that condition established after study to be chiefly responsible for occasioning the admission of the patient to the hospital for care."

J. Admission from Outpatient Surgery

When a patient receives surgery in the hospital's outpatient surgery department and is subsequently admitted for continuing inpatient care at the same hospital, the following guidelines should be followed in selecting the principal diagnosis for the inpatient admission:

- If the reason for the inpatient admission is a complication, assign the complication as the principal diagnosis.

- If no complication, or other condition, is documented as the reason for the inpatient admission, assign the reason for the outpatient surgery as the principal diagnosis.

- If the reason for the inpatient admission is another condition unrelated to the surgery, assign the unrelated condition as the principal diagnosis.

Section III. Reporting Additional Diagnoses

GENERAL RULES FOR OTHER (ADDITIONAL) DIAGNOSES

For reporting purposes the definition for "other diagnoses" is interpreted as additional conditions that affect patient care in terms of requiring:

clinical evaluation; or
therapeutic treatment; or
diagnostic procedures; or
extended length of hospital stay; or
increased nursing care and/or monitoring.

The UHDDS item #11-b defines Other Diagnoses as "all conditions that coexist at the time of admission, that develop subsequently, or that affect the treatment received and/or the length of stay. Diagnoses that relate to an earlier episode which have no bearing on the current hospital stay are to be excluded." UHDDS definitions apply to inpatients in acute care, short-term, long term care and psychiatric hospital setting. The UHDDS definitions are used by acute care short-term hospitals to report inpatient data elements in a standardized manner. These data elements and their definitions can be found in the July 31, 1985, Federal Register (Vol. 50, No, 147), pp. 31038-40.

Since that time the application of the UHDDS definitions has been expanded to include all non-outpatient settings (acute care, short term, long term care and psychiatric hospitals; home health agencies; rehab facilities; nursing homes, etc).

The following guidelines are to be applied in designating "other diagnoses" when neither the Alphabetic Index nor the Tabular List in ICD-9-CM provide direction. The listing of the diagnoses in the patient record is the responsibility of the attending provider.

A. Previous conditions

If the provider has included a diagnosis in the final diagnostic statement, such as the discharge summary or the face sheet, it should ordinarily be coded. Some providers include in the diagnostic statement resolved conditions or diagnoses and status-post procedures from previous admission that have no bearing on the current stay. Such conditions are not to be reported and are coded only if required by hospital policy.

However, history codes (V10-V19) may be used as secondary codes if the historical condition or family history has an impact on current care or influences treatment.

B. Abnormal findings

Abnormal findings (laboratory, x-ray, pathologic, and other diagnostic results) are not coded and reported unless the provider indicates their clinical significance. If the findings are outside the normal range and the attending provider has ordered other tests to evaluate the condition or prescribed treatment, it is appropriate to ask the provider whether the abnormal finding should be added.

Please note: This differs from the coding practices in the outpatient setting for coding encounters for diagnostic tests that have been interpreted by a provider.

C. Uncertain Diagnosis

If the diagnosis documented at the time of discharge is qualified as "probable", "suspected", "likely", "questionable", "possible", or "still to be ruled out" or other similar terms indicating uncertainty, code the condition as if it existed or was established. The bases for these guidelines are the diagnostic workup, arrangements for further workup or observation, and initial therapeutic approach that correspond most closely with the established diagnosis.

Note: This guideline is applicable only to inpatient admissions to short-term, acute, long-term care and psychiatric hospitals.

Section IV. Diagnostic Coding and Reporting Guidelines for Outpatient Services

These coding guidelines for outpatient diagnoses have been approved for use by hospitals/providers in coding and reporting hospital-based outpatient services and provider-based office visits.

Information about the use of certain abbreviations, punctuation, symbols, and other conventions used in the ICD-9-CM Tabular List (code numbers and titles), can be found in Section IA of these guidelines, under "Conventions Used in the Tabular List." Information about the correct sequence to use in finding a code is also described in Section I.

The terms encounter and visit are often used interchangeably in describing outpatient service contacts and, therefore, appear together in these guidelines without distinguishing one from the other.

Though the conventions and general guidelines apply to all settings, coding guidelines for outpatient and provider reporting of diagnoses will vary in a number of instances from those for inpatient diagnoses, recognizing that:

The Uniform Hospital Discharge Data Set (UHDDS) definition of principal diagnosis applies only to inpatients in acute, short-term, long-term care and psychiatric hospitals.

Coding guidelines for inconclusive diagnoses (probable, suspected, rule out, etc.) were developed for inpatient reporting and do not apply to outpatients.

A. Selection of first-listed condition

In the outpatient setting, the term first-listed diagnosis is used in lieu of principal diagnosis.

In determining the first-listed diagnosis the coding conventions of ICD-9-CM, as well as the general and disease specific guidelines take precedence over the outpatient guidelines.

Diagnoses often are not established at the time of the initial encounter/visit. It may take two or more visits before the diagnosis is confirmed.

The most critical rule involves beginning the search for the correct code assignment through the Alphabetic Index. Never begin searching initially in the Tabular List as this will lead to coding errors.

1. Outpatient Surgery

When a patient presents for outpatient surgery, code the reason for the surgery as the first-listed diagnosis (reason for the encounter), even if the surgery is not performed due to a contraindication.

2. Observation Stay

When a patient is admitted for observation for a medical condition, assign a code for the medical condition as the first-listed diagnosis.

When a patient presents for outpatient surgery and develops complications requiring admission to observation, code the reason for the surgery as the first reported diagnosis (reason for the encounter), followed by codes for the complications as secondary diagnoses.

B. Codes from 001.0 through V89

The appropriate code or codes from 001.0 through **V89** must be used to identify diagnoses, symptoms, conditions, problems, complaints, or other reason(s) for the encounter/visit.

C. Accurate reporting of ICD-9-CM diagnosis codes

For accurate reporting of ICD-9-CM diagnosis codes, the documentation should describe the patient's condition, using terminology which includes specific diagnoses as well as symptoms, problems, or reasons for the encounter. There are ICD-9-CM codes to describe all of these.

D. Selection of codes 001.0 through 999.9

The selection of codes 001.0 through 999.9 will frequently be used to describe the reason for the encounter. These codes are from the section of ICD-9-CM for the classification of diseases and injuries (e.g. infectious and parasitic diseases; neoplasms; symptoms, signs, and ill-defined conditions, etc.).

E. Codes that describe symptoms and signs

Codes that describe symptoms and signs, as opposed to diagnoses, are acceptable for reporting purposes when a diagnosis has not been established (confirmed) by the provider. Chapter 16 of ICD-9-CM, Symptoms, Signs, and Ill-defined conditions (codes 780.0 - 799.9) contain many, but not all codes for symptoms.

F. Encounters for circumstances other than a disease or injury

ICD-9-CM provides codes to deal with encounters for circumstances other than a disease or injury. The Supplementary Classification of factors Influencing Health Status and Contact with Health Services (V01.0- **V89**) is provided to deal with occasions when circumstances other than a disease or injury are recorded as diagnosis or problems. *See Section I.C. 18 for information on V-codes.*

G. Level of Detail in Coding

1. ICD-9-CM codes with 3, 4, or 5 digits

ICD-9-CM is composed of codes with either 3, 4, or 5 digits. Codes with three digits are included in ICD-9-CM as the heading of a category of codes that may be further subdivided by the use of fourth and/or fifth digits, which provide greater specificity.

2. **Use of full number of digits required for a code**

A three-digit code is to be used only if it is not further subdivided. Where fourth-digit subcategories and/or fifth-digit subclassifications are provided, they must be assigned. A code is invalid if it has not been coded to the full number of digits required for that code.

See also discussion under Section I.b.3., General Coding Guidelines, Level of Detail in Coding.

H. ICD-9-CM code for the diagnosis, condition, problem, or other reason for encounter/visit

List first the ICD-9-CM code for the diagnosis, condition, problem, or other reason for encounter/visit shown in the medical record to be chiefly responsible for the services provided. List additional codes that describe any coexisting conditions. In some cases the first-listed diagnosis may be a symptom when a diagnosis has not been established (confirmed) by the physician.

I. Uncertain diagnosis

Do not code diagnoses documented as "probable", "suspected," "questionable," "rule out," or "working diagnosis" or other similar terms indicating uncertainty. Rather, code the condition(s) to the highest degree of certainty for that encounter/visit, such as symptoms, signs, abnormal test results, or other reason for the visit.

Please note: This differs from the coding practices used by short-term, acute care, long-term care and psychiatric hospitals.

J. Chronic diseases

Chronic diseases treated on an ongoing basis may be coded and reported as many times as the patient receives treatment and care for the condition(s)

K. Code all documented conditions that coexist

Code all documented conditions that coexist at the time of the encounter/visit, and require or affect patient care treatment or management. Do not code conditions that were previously treated and no longer exist. However, history codes (V10-V19) may be used as secondary codes if the historical condition or family history has an impact on current care or influences treatment.

L. Patients receiving diagnostic services only

For patients receiving diagnostic services only during an encounter/visit, sequence first the diagnosis, condition, problem, or other reason for encounter/visit shown in the medical record to be chiefly responsible for the outpatient services provided during the encounter/visit. Codes for other diagnoses (e.g., chronic conditions) may be sequenced as additional diagnoses.

For encounters for routine laboratory/radiology testing in the absence of any signs, symptoms, or associated diagnosis, assign V72.5 and **a code from subcategory** V72.6. If routine testing is performed during the same encounter as a test to evaluate a sign, symptom, or diagnosis, it is appropriate to assign both the V code and the code describing the reason for the non-routine test.

For outpatient encounters for diagnostic tests that have been interpreted by a physician, and the final report is available at the time of coding, code any confirmed or definitive diagnosis(es) documented in the interpretation. Do not code related signs and symptoms as additional diagnoses.

Please note: This differs from the coding practice in the hospital inpatient setting regarding abnormal findings on test results.

M. Patients receiving therapeutic services only

For patients receiving therapeutic services only during an encounter/visit, sequence first the diagnosis, condition, problem, or other reason for encounter/visit shown in the medical record to be chiefly responsible for the outpatient services provided during the encounter/visit. Codes for other diagnoses (e.g., chronic conditions) may be sequenced as additional diagnoses.

The only exception to this rule is that when the primary reason for the admission/encounter is chemotherapy, radiation therapy, or rehabilitation, the appropriate V code for the service is listed first, and the diagnosis or problem for which the service is being performed listed second.

N. Patients receiving preoperative evaluations only

For patients receiving preoperative evaluations only, sequence first a code from category V72.8, Other specified examinations, to describe the pre-op consultations. Assign a code for the condition to describe the reason for the surgery as an additional diagnosis. Code also any findings related to the pre-op evaluation.

O. Ambulatory surgery

For ambulatory surgery, code the diagnosis for which the surgery was performed. If the postoperative diagnosis is known to be different from the preoperative diagnosis at the time the diagnosis is confirmed, select the postoperative diagnosis for coding, since it is the most definitive.

P. Routine outpatient prenatal visits

For routine outpatient prenatal visits when no complications are present, codes V22.0, Supervision of normal first pregnancy, or V22.1, Supervision of other normal pregnancy, should be used as the principal diagnosis. These codes should not be used in conjunction with chapter 11 codes.

Appendix I Present on Admission Reporting Guidelines

Introduction

These guidelines are to be used as a supplement to the *ICD-9-CM Official Guidelines for Coding and Reporting* to facilitate the assignment of the Present on Admission (POA) indicator for each diagnosis and external cause of injury code reported on claim forms (UB-04 and 837 Institutional).

These guidelines are not intended to replace any guidelines in the main body of the *ICD-9-CM Official Guidelines for Coding and Reporting.* The POA guidelines are not intended to provide guidance on when a condition should be coded, but rather, how to apply the POA indicator to the final set of diagnosis codes that have been assigned in accordance with Sections I, II, and III of the official coding guidelines. Subsequent to the assignment of the ICD-9-CM codes, the POA indicator should then be assigned to those conditions that have been coded.

As stated in the Introduction to the ICD-9-CM Official Guidelines for Coding and Reporting, a joint effort between the healthcare provider and the coder is essential to achieve complete and accurate documentation, code assignment, and reporting of diagnoses and procedures. The importance of consistent, complete documentation in the medical record cannot be overemphasized. Medical record documentation from any provider involved in the care and treatment of the patient may be used to support the determination of whether a condition was present on admission or not. In the context of the official coding guidelines, the term "provider" means a physician or any qualified healthcare practitioner who is legally accountable for establishing the patient's diagnosis.

These guidelines are not a substitute for the provider's clinical judgment as to the determination of whether a condition was/was not present on admission. The provider should be queried regarding issues related to the linking of signs/symptoms, timing of test results, and the timing of findings.

General Reporting Requirements

All claims involving inpatient admissions to general acute care hospitals or other facilities that are subject to a law or regulation mandating collection of present on admission information.

Present on admission is defined as present at the time the order for inpatient admission occurs — conditions that develop during an outpatient encounter, including emergency department, observation, or outpatient surgery, are considered as present on admission.

POA indicator is assigned to principal and secondary diagnoses (as defined in Section II of the Official Guidelines for Coding and Reporting) and the external cause of injury codes.

Issues related to inconsistent, missing, conflicting or unclear documentation must still be resolved by the provider.

If a condition would not be coded and reported based on UHDDS definitions and current official coding guidelines, then the POA indicator would not be reported.

Reporting Options

Y - Yes

N - No

U - Unknown

W – Clinically undetermined

Unreported/Not used (or "1" for Medicare usage) – (Exempt from POA reporting)

For more specific instructions on Medicare POA indicator reporting options, refer to http://www.cms.hhs.gov/HospitalAcqCond/02_ Statute_Regulations _Program_Instructions. asp#TopOfPage

Reporting Definitions

Y = present at the time of inpatient admission

N = not present at the time of inpatient admission

U = documentation is insufficient to determine if condition is present on admission

W = provider is unable to clinically determine whether condition was present on admission or not

Timeframe for POA Identification and Documentation

There is no required timeframe as to when a provider (per the definition of "provider" used in these guidelines) must identify or document a condition to be present on admission. In some clinical situations, it may not be possible for a provider to make a definitive diagnosis (or a condition may not be recognized or reported by the patient) for a period of time after admission. In some cases it may be several days before the provider arrives at a definitive diagnosis. This does not mean that the condition was not present on admission. Determination of whether the condition was present on admission or not will be based on the applicable POA guideline as identified in this document, or on the provider's best clinical judgment.

If at the time of code assignment the documentation is unclear as to whether a condition was present on admission or not, it is appropriate to query the provider for clarification.

Assigning the POA Indicator

Condition is on the "Exempt from Reporting" list

Leave the "present on admission" field blank if the condition is on the list of ICD-9-CM codes for which this field is not applicable. This is the only circumstance in which the field may be left blank.

POA Explicitly Documented

Assign Y for any condition the provider explicitly documents as being present on admission.

Assign N for any condition the provider explicitly documents as not present at the time of admission.

Conditions diagnosed prior to inpatient admission

Assign "Y" for conditions that were diagnosed prior to admission (example: hypertension, diabetes mellitus, asthma)

Conditions diagnosed during the admission but clearly present before admission

Assign "Y" for conditions diagnosed during the admission that were clearly present but not diagnosed until after admission occurred.

Diagnoses subsequently confirmed after admission are considered present on admission if at the time of admission they are documented as suspected, possible, rule out, differential diagnosis, or constitute an underlying cause of a symptom that is present at the time of admission.

Condition develops during outpatient encounter prior to inpatient admission

Assign Y for any condition that develops during an outpatient encounter prior to a written order for inpatient admission.

Documentation does not indicate whether condition was present on admission

Assign "U" when the medical record documentation is unclear as to whether the condition was present on admission. "U" should not be routinely assigned and used only in very limited circumstances. Coders are encouraged to query the providers when the documentation is unclear.

Documentation states that it cannot be determined whether the condition was or was not present on admission

Assign "W" when the medical record documentation indicates that it cannot be clinically determined whether or not the condition was present on admission.

Chronic condition with acute exacerbation during the admission

If the code is a combination code that identifies both the chronic condition and the acute exacerbation, see POA guidelines pertaining to combination codes.

If the combination code only identifies the chronic condition and not the acute exacerbation (e.g., acute exacerbation of CHF), assign "Y."

Conditions documented as possible, probable, suspected, or rule out at the time of discharge

If the final diagnosis contains a possible, probable, suspected, or rule out diagnosis, and this diagnosis was **based on signs, symptoms, or clinical findings** suspected at the time of inpatient admission, assign "Y."

If the final diagnosis contains a possible, probable, suspected, or rule out diagnosis, and this diagnosis was based on **signs,** symptoms or clinical findings that were not present on admission, assign "N".

Conditions documented as impending or threatened at the time of discharge

If the final diagnosis contains an impending or threatened diagnosis, and this diagnosis is based on symptoms or clinical findings that were present on admission, assign "Y".

If the final diagnosis contains an impending or threatened diagnosis, and this diagnosis is based on symptoms or clinical findings that were not present on admission, assign "N".

Acute and Chronic Conditions

Assign "Y" for acute conditions that are present at time of admission and N for acute conditions that are not present at time of admission.

Assign "Y" for chronic conditions, even though the condition may not be diagnosed until after admission.

If a single code identifies both an acute and chronic condition, see the POA guidelines for combination codes.

Combination Codes

Assign "N" if any part of the combination code was not present on admission (e.g., obstructive chronic bronchitis with acute exacerbation and the exacerbation was not present on admission; gastric ulcer that does not start bleeding until after admission; asthma patient develops status asthmaticus after admission)

Assign "Y" if all parts of the combination code were present on admission (e.g., patient with diabetic nephropathy is admitted with uncontrolled diabetes)

If the final diagnosis includes comparative or contrasting diagnoses, and both were present, or suspected, at the time of admission, assign "Y".

For infection codes that include the causal organism, assign "Y" if the infection (or signs of the infection) was present on admission, even though the culture results may not be known until after admission (e.g., patient is admitted with pneumonia and the provider documents pseudomonas as the causal organism a few days later).

Same Diagnosis Code for Two or More Conditions

When the same ICD-9-CM diagnosis code applies to two or more conditions during the same encounter (e.g. bilateral condition, or two separate conditions classified to the same ICD-9-CM diagnosis code):

Assign "Y" if all conditions represented by the single ICD-9-CM code were present on admission (e.g. bilateral fracture of the same bone, same site, and both fractures were present on admission)

Assign "N" if any of the conditions represented by the single ICD-9-CM code was not present on admission (e.g. dehydration with hyponatremia is assigned to code 276.1, but only one of these conditions was present on admission).

Obstetrical conditions

Whether or not the patient delivers during the current hospitalization does not affect assignment of the POA indicator. The determining factor for POA assignment is whether the pregnancy complication or obstetrical condition described by the code was present at the time of admission or not.

If the pregnancy complication or obstetrical condition was present on admission (e.g., patient admitted in preterm labor), assign "Y".

If the pregnancy complication or obstetrical condition was not present on admission (e.g., 2nd degree laceration during delivery, postpartum hemorrhage that occurred during current hospitalization, fetal distress develops after admission), assign "N".

If the obstetrical code includes more than one diagnosis and any of the diagnoses identified by the code were not present on admission assign "N".

> (e.g., Code 642.7, Pre-eclampsia or eclampsia superimposed on pre-existing hypertension).

If the obstetrical code includes information that is not a diagnosis, do not consider that information in the POA determination.

> (e.g. Code 652.1x, Breech or other malpresentation successfully converted to cephalic presentation should be reported as present on admission if the fetus was breech on admission but was converted to cephalic presentation after admission (since the conversion to cephalic presentation does not represent a diagnosis, the fact that the conversion occurred after admission has no bearing on the POA determination).

Perinatal conditions

Newborns are not considered to be admitted until after birth. Therefore, any condition present at birth or that developed in utero is considered present at admission and should be assigned "Y". This includes conditions that occur during delivery (e.g., injury during delivery, meconium aspiration, exposure to streptococcus B in the vaginal canal).

Congenital conditions and anomalies

Assign "Y" for congenital conditions and anomalies. Congenital conditions are always considered present on admission.

External cause of injury codes

Assign "Y" for any E code representing an external cause of injury or poisoning that occurred prior to inpatient admission (e.g., patient fell out of bed at home, patient fell out of bed in emergency room prior to admission)

Assign "N" for any E code representing an external cause of injury or poisoning that occurred during inpatient hospitalization (e.g., patient fell out of hospital bed during hospital stay, patient experienced an adverse reaction to a medication administered after inpatient admission)

Categories and Codes Exempt from Diagnosis Present on Admission Requirement

Effective Date: October 1, 2008

Note: "Diagnosis present on admission" for these code categories are exempt because they represent circumstances regarding the healthcare encounter or factors influencing health status that do not represent a current disease or injury or are always present on admission

137-139, Late effects of infectious and parasitic diseases

268.1, Rickets, late effect

326, Late effects of intracranial abscess or pyogenic infection

412, Old myocardial infarction

438, Late effects of cerebrovascular disease

650, Normal delivery

660.7, Failed forceps or vacuum extractor, unspecified

677, Late effect of complication of pregnancy, childbirth, and the puerperium

905-909, Late effects of injuries, poisonings, toxic effects, and other external causes

V02, Carrier or suspected carrier of infectious diseases

V03, Need for prophylactic vaccination and inoculation against bacterial diseases

V04, Need for prophylactic vaccination and inoculation against certain viral diseases

V05, Need for other prophylactic vaccination and inoculation against single diseases

V06, Need for prophylactic vaccination and inoculation against combinations of diseases

V07, Need for isolation and other prophylactic measures

V10, Personal history of malignant neoplasm

V11, Personal history of mental disorder

V12, Personal history of certain other diseases

V13, Personal history of other diseases

V14, Personal history of allergy to medicinal agents

V15.01-V15.09, Other personal history, Allergy, other than to medicinal agents

V15.1, Other personal history, Surgery to heart and great vessels

V15.2, Other personal history, Surgery to other major organs

V15.3, Other personal history, Irradiation

V15.4, Other personal history, Psychological trauma

V15.5, Other personal history, Injury

V15.6, Other personal history, Poisoning

V15.7, Other personal history, Contraception

V15.80, Other personal history, History of failed moderate sedation

V15.81, Other personal history, Noncompliance with medical treatment

V15.82, Other personal history, History of tobacco use

V15.83, Other personal history, Underimmunization status

V15.84, Other personal history, Contact with and (suspected) exposure to asbestos

V15.85, Other personal history, Contact with and (suspected) exposure to potentially hazardous body fluids

V15.86, Other personal history, Contact with and (suspected) exposure to lead

V15.88, Other personal history, History of fall

V15.89, Other personal history, Other

V15.9 Unspecified personal history presenting hazards to health

V16, Family history of malignant neoplasm

V17, Family history of certain chronic disabling diseases

V18, Family history of certain other specific conditions

V19, Family history of other conditions

V20, Health supervision of infant or child

V21, Constitutional states in development

V22, Normal pregnancy

V23, Supervision of high-risk pregnancy

V24, Postpartum care and examination

V25, Encounter for contraceptive management

V26, Procreative management

V27, Outcome of delivery

V28, Antenatal screening

V29, Observation and evaluation of newborns for suspected condition not found

V30-V39, Liveborn infants according to type of birth

V42, Organ or tissue replaced by transplant

V43, Organ or tissue replaced by other means

V44, Artificial opening status

V45, Other postprocedural states

V46, Other dependence on machines

V49.60-V49.77, Upper and lower limb amputation status

V49.81-V49.84, Other specified conditions influencing health status

V50, Elective surgery for purposes other than remedying health states

V51, Aftercare involving the use of plastic surgery

V52, Fitting and adjustment of prosthetic device and implant

V53, Fitting and adjustment of other device

V54, Other orthopedic aftercare

V55, Attention to artificial openings

V56, Encounter for dialysis and dialysis catheter care

V57, Care involving use of rehabilitation procedures

V58, Encounter for other and unspecified procedures and aftercare

V59, Donors

V60, Housing, household, and economic circumstances

V61, Other family circumstances

V62, Other psychosocial circumstances

V64, Persons encountering health services for specific procedures, not carried out

V65, Other persons seeking consultation

V66, Convalescence and palliative care

V67, Follow-up examination

V68, Encounters for administrative purposes

V69, Problems related to lifestyle

V70, General medical examination

V71, Observation and evaluation for suspected condition not found

V72, Special investigations and examinations

V73, Special screening examination for viral and chlamydial diseases

V74, Special screening examination for bacterial and spirochetal diseases

V75, Special screening examination for other infectious diseases

V76, Special screening for malignant neoplasms

V77, Special screening for endocrine, nutritional, metabolic, and immunity disorders

V78, Special screening for disorders of blood and blood-forming organs

V79, Special screening for mental disorders and developmental handicaps

V80, Special screening for neurological, eye, and ear diseases

V81, Special screening for cardiovascular, respiratory, and genitourinary diseases

V82, Special screening for other conditions

V83, Genetic carrier status

V84, Genetic susceptibility to disease

V85, Body Mass Index

V86, Estrogen receptor status

V87.32, Contact with and (suspected) exposure to algae bloom

V87.4, Personal history of drug therapy

V88, Acquired absence of cervix and uterus

V89, Suspected maternal and fetal conditions not found

E000, External cause status

E001-E030, Activity

E800-E807, Railway accidents

E810-E819, Motor vehicle traffic accidents

E820-E825, Motor vehicle nontraffic accidents

E826-E829, Other road vehicle accidents

E830-E838, Water transport accidents

E840-E845, Air and space transport accidents

E846-E848, Vehicle accidents not elsewhere classifiable

E849.0-E849.6, Place of occurrence

E849.8-E849.9, Place of occurrence

E883.1, Accidental fall into well

E883.2, Accidental fall into storm drain or manhole

E884.0, Fall from playground equipment

E884.1, Fall from cliff

E885.0, Fall from (nonmotorized) scooter

E885.1, Fall from roller skates

E885.2, Fall from skateboard

E885.3, Fall from skis

E885.4, Fall from snowboard

E886.0, Fall on same level from collision, pushing, or shoving, by or with other person, In sports

E890.0-E890.9, Conflagration in private dwelling

E893.0, Accident caused by ignition of clothing, from controlled fire in private dwelling

E893.2, Accident caused by ignition of clothing, from controlled fire not in building or structure

E894, Ignition of highly inflammable material

E895, Accident caused by controlled fire in private dwelling

E897, Accident caused by controlled fire not in building or structure

E898.0-E898.1, Accident caused by other specified fire and flames

E917.0, Striking against or struck accidentally by objects or persons, in sports without subsequent fall

E917.1, Striking against or struck accidentally by objects or persons, caused by a crowd, by collective fear or panic without subsequent fall

E917.2, Striking against or struck accidentally by objects or persons, in running water without subsequent fall

E917.5, Striking against or struck accidentally by objects or persons, object in sports with subsequent fall

E917.6, Striking against or struck accidentally by objects or persons, caused by a crowd, by collective fear or panic with subsequent fall

E919.0-E919.1, Accidents caused by machinery

E919.3-E919.9, Accidents caused by machinery

E921.0-E921.9, Accident caused by explosion of pressure vessel

E922.0-E922.9, Accident caused by firearm and air gun missile

E924.1, Caustic and corrosive substances

E926.2, Visible and ultraviolet light sources

E928.0-E928.8, Other and unspecified environmental and accidental causes

E929.0-E929.9, Late effects of accidental injury

E959, Late effects of self-inflicted injury

E970-E978, Legal intervention

E979, Terrorism

E981.0-E981.8, Poisoning by gases in domestic use, undetermined whether accidentally or purposely inflicted

E982.0-E982.9, Poisoning by other gases, undetermined whether accidentally or purposely inflicted

E985.0-E985.7, Injury by firearms, air guns and explosives, undetermined whether accidentally or purposely inflicted

E987.0, Falling from high place, undetermined whether accidentally or purposely inflicted, residential premises

E987.2, Falling from high place, undetermined whether accidentally or purposely inflicted, natural sites

E989, Late effects of injury, undetermined whether accidentally or purposely inflicted

E990-E999, Injury resulting from operations of war

POA Examples

The POA examples have been removed from the guidelines.

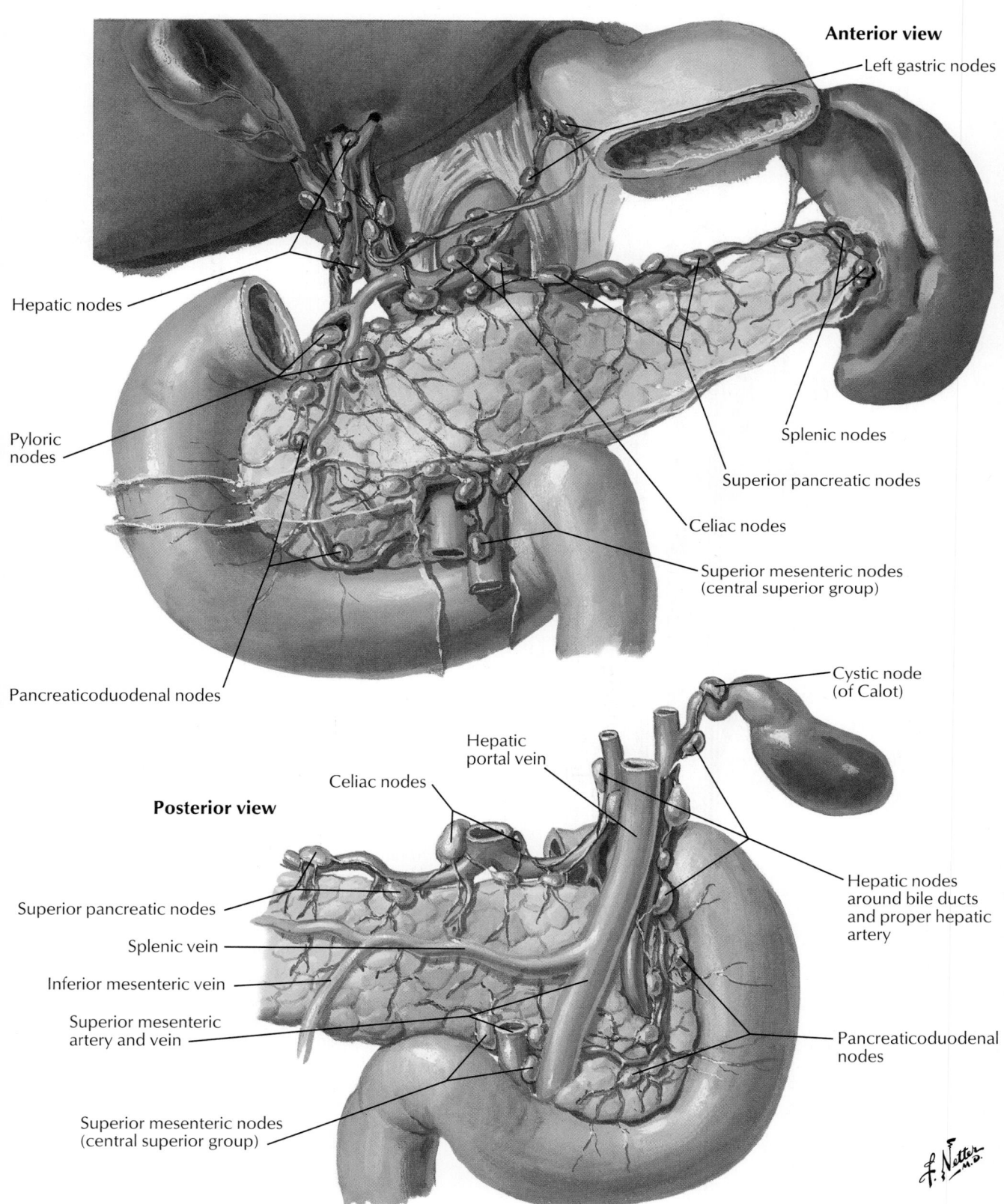

Left gastric nodes

Hepatic nodes

Pyloric
nodes

Pancreaticoduodenal nodes

Splenic nodes

Superior pancreatic nodes

Celiac nodes

Superior mesenteric nodes
(central superior group)

Cystic node
(of Calot)

Hepatic
portal vein

Celiac nodes

Posterior view

Hepatic nodes
around bile ducts
and proper hepatic
artery

Superior pancreatic nodes

Splenic vein

Inferior mesenteric vein

Superior mesenteric
artery and vein

Pancreaticoduodenal
nodes

Superior mesenteric nodes
(central superior group)

NETTER ANATOMY PLATE

Plate 315 Lymph Vessels and Nodes of Pancreas. (Netter: Atlas of Human Anatomy, 4 ed, 2006, Saunders.)

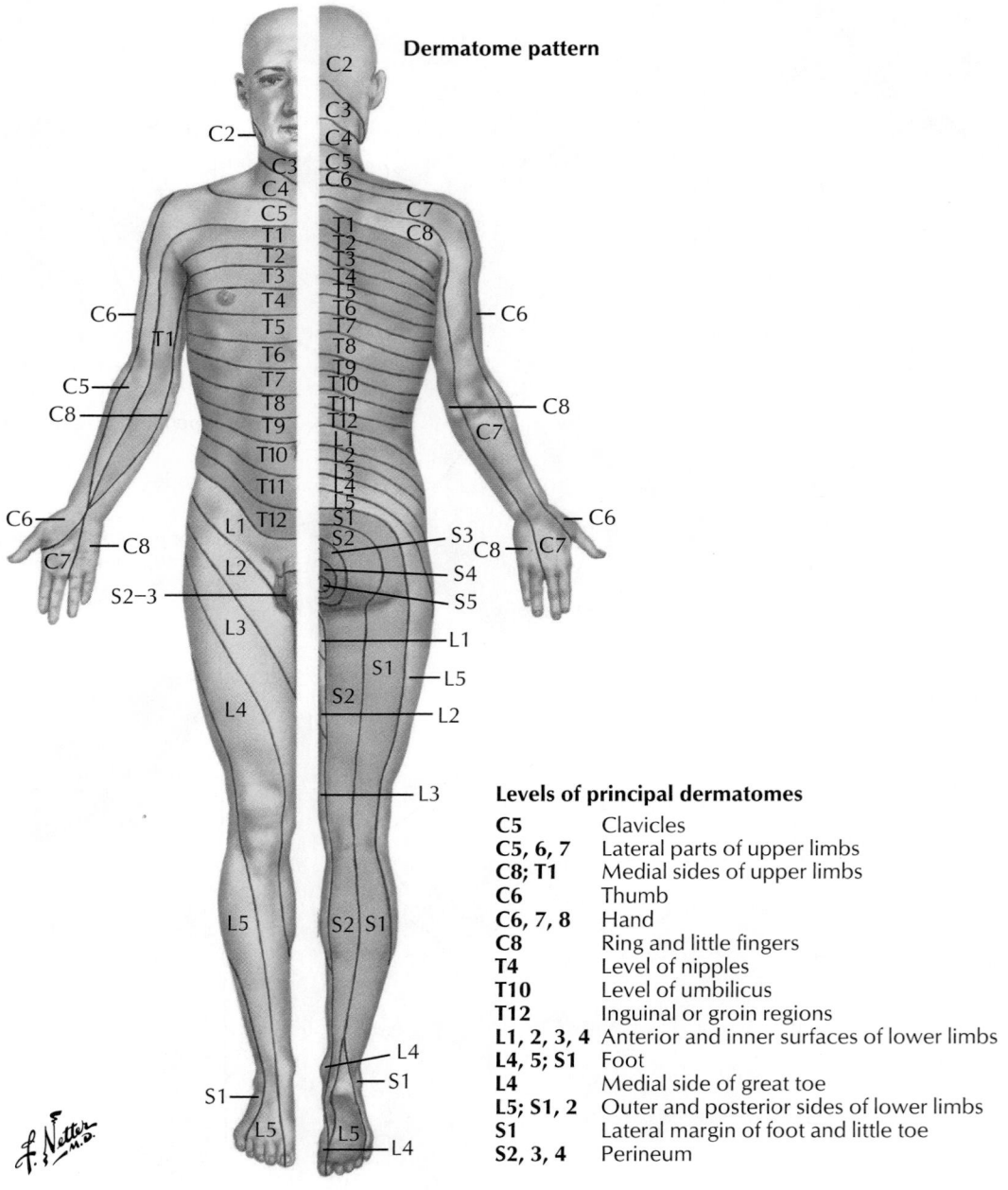

Dermatome pattern

Levels of principal dermatomes

C5	Clavicles
C5, 6, 7	Lateral parts of upper limbs
C8; T1	Medial sides of upper limbs
C6	Thumb
C6, 7, 8	Hand
C8	Ring and little fingers
T4	Level of nipples
T10	Level of umbilicus
T12	Inguinal or groin regions
L1, 2, 3, 4	Anterior and inner surfaces of lower limbs
L4, 5; S1	Foot
L4	Medial side of great toe
L5; S1, 2	Outer and posterior sides of lower limbs
S1	Lateral margin of foot and little toe
S2, 3, 4	Perineum

Plate 164   Dermatomes. (Netter: Atlas of Human Anatomy, 4 ed, 2006, Saunders.)

Female: frontal section

- Peritoneum
- Body of bladder
- Fundus of bladder
- Interureteric crest
- Left ureteric orifice
- Trigone of bladder
- Neck of bladder
- Paravesical endopelvic fascia and vesical venous plexus
- Vesical fascia
- Tendinous arch of levator ani muscle
- Obturator internus muscle
- Levator ani muscle
- Tendinous arch of pelvic fascia
- Urethra
- Sphincter urethrae muscle
- Perineal membrane
- Inferior pubic ramus
- Crus of clitoris and ischiocavernosus muscle
- Bulb of vestibule and bulbospongiosus muscle
- Deep perineal (investing or Gallaudet's) fascia
- Superficial perineal (Colles') fascia

Round ligament of uterus

Vagina

Male: frontal section

- Peritoneum
- Body of bladder
- Fundus of bladder
- Ductus (vas) deferens
- Interureteric crest
- Right ureteric orifice
- Trigone of bladder
- Neck of bladder
- Paravesical endopelvic fascia and vesical venous plexus
- Tendinous arch of levator ani muscle
- Uvula of bladder
- Obturator internus muscle
- Levator ani muscle
- Capsule of prostate
- Prostate and prostatic urethra
- Seminal colliculus
- Bulbourethral (Cowper's) gland
- Perineal membrane and sphincter urethrae muscle
- Bulbous portion of spongy urethra
- Corpus spongiosum and bulbospongiosus muscle
- Deep perineal (investing or Gallaudet's) fascia

- Internal urethral sphincter
- Tendinous arch of pelvic fascia
- Anterior recess of ischio-anal fossa
- Inferior pubic ramus
- Crus of penis and ischiocavernosus muscle
- Superficial perineal (Colles') fascia

Plate 366 Urinary Bladder: Female and Male. (Netter: Atlas of Human Anatomy, 4 ed, 2006, Saunders.)

Sites of ectopic implantation

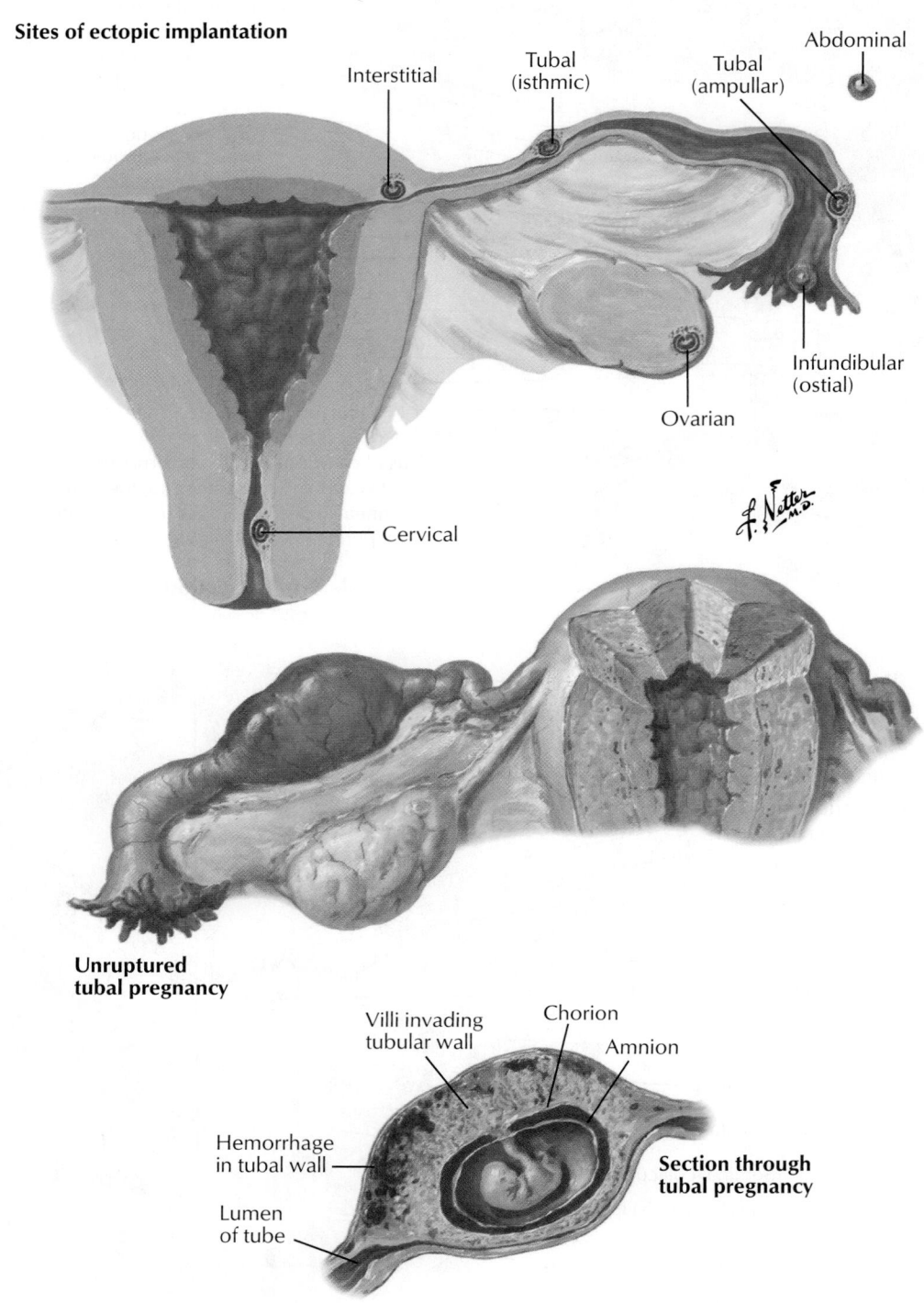

Interstitial

Tubal (isthmic)

Tubal (ampullar)

Abdominal

Infundibular (ostial)

Ovarian

Cervical

Unruptured tubal pregnancy

Villi invading tubular wall

Chorion

Amnion

Hemorrhage in tubal wall

Lumen of tube

Section through tubal pregnancy

Plate 375   Ectopic Pregnancy. (Netter: Atlas of Human Anatomy, 4 ed, 2006, Saunders.)

Superficial inguinal ring

External spermatic fascia

Cremaster muscle and fascia

Septum of scrotum (formed by dartos fascia)

Superficial (dartos) fascia of scrotum

Skin of scrotum

Skin of penis

Superficial fascia of penis (Colles' fascia)

Deep (Buck's) fascia of penis

Testicular artery

Ductus deferens

Artery to ductus deferens

Genital branch of genitofemoral nerve

Pampiniform (venous) plexus

Epididymis

Appendix of epididymis

Appendix of testis

Testis (covered by visceral layer of tunica vaginalis)

Parietal layer of tunica vaginalis

Superficial (dartos) fascia of scrotum

External spermatic fascia

Cremaster muscle and fascia

Internal spermatic fascia

Parietal layer of tunica vaginalis

Epididymis

Testis (covered by visceral layer of tunica vaginalis)

Skin of scrotum

Plate 387   Scrotum and Contents. (Netter: Atlas of Human Anatomy, 4 ed, 2006, Saunders.)

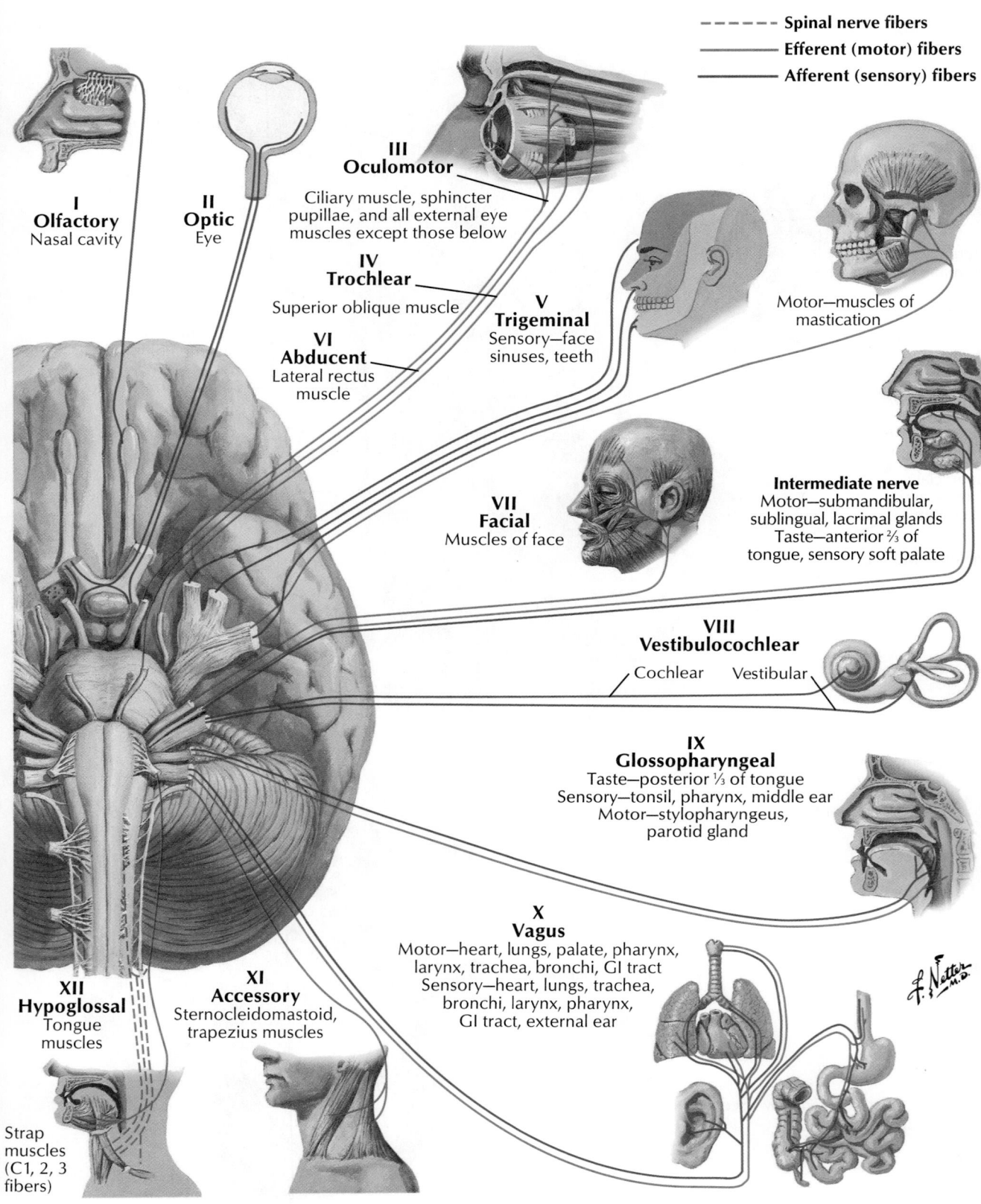

- - - - - Spinal nerve fibers
———— Efferent (motor) fibers
———— Afferent (sensory) fibers

I
Olfactory
Nasal cavity

II
Optic
Eye

III
Oculomotor
Ciliary muscle, sphincter pupillae, and all external eye muscles except those below

IV
Trochlear
Superior oblique muscle

VI
Abducent
Lateral rectus muscle

V
Trigeminal
Sensory—face sinuses, teeth

Motor—muscles of mastication

VII
Facial
Muscles of face

Intermediate nerve
Motor—submandibular, sublingual, lacrimal glands
Taste—anterior ⅔ of tongue, sensory soft palate

VIII
Vestibulocochlear
Cochlear   Vestibular

IX
Glossopharyngeal
Taste—posterior ⅓ of tongue
Sensory—tonsil, pharynx, middle ear
Motor—stylopharyngeus, parotid gland

X
Vagus
Motor—heart, lungs, palate, pharynx, larynx, trachea, bronchi, GI tract
Sensory—heart, lungs, trachea, bronchi, larynx, pharynx, GI tract, external ear

XII
Hypoglossal
Tongue muscles

Strap muscles (C1, 2, 3 fibers)

XI
Accessory
Sternocleidomastoid, trapezius muscles

Plate 118   Cranial Nerves (Motor and Sensory Distribution): Schema. (Netter: Atlas of Human Anatomy, 4 ed, 2006, Saunders.)

Superior view

Supratrochlear nerve

Medial rectus muscle

Superior oblique muscle

Infratrochlear nerve

Nasociliary nerve

Trochlear nerve (IV)

Common tendinous ring

Ophthalmic nerve (V₁)

Optic nerve (II)

Internal carotid artery
and nerve plexus

Oculomotor nerve (III)

Trochlear nerve (IV)

Abducent nerve (VI)

Tentorium cerebelli

Medial branch } Supraorbital nerve
Lateral branch

Levator palpebrae superioris muscle

Superior rectus muscle

Lacrimal gland

Lacrimal nerve

Lateral rectus muscle

Frontal nerve

Maxillary nerve (V₂)

Meningeal branch
of maxillary nerve

Mandibular nerve (V₃)

Lesser petrosal nerve

Meningeal branch
of mandibular nerve

Greater petrosal nerve

Trigeminal (semilunar) ganglion

Tentorial (meningeal)
branch of ophthalmic nerve

Superior view:
levator palpebrae superioris,
superior rectus, and superior
oblique muscles partially
cut away

Supratrochlear nerve *(cut)*

Supraorbital nerve branches *(cut)*

Infratrochlear nerve

Anterior ethmoidal nerve

Optic nerve (II)

Posterior ethmoidal nerve

Superior branch of
oculomotor nerve (III) *(cut)*

Nasociliary nerve

Internal carotid plexus

Trochlear nerve (IV) *(cut)*

Oculomotor nerve (III)

Abducent nerve (VI)

Long ciliary nerves

Short ciliary nerves

Lacrimal nerve

Ciliary ganglion

Parasympathetic root of ciliary
ganglion (from inferior branch
of oculomotor nerve)

Sympathetic root of ciliary
ganglion (from internal
carotid plexus)

Sensory root of ciliary ganglion
(from nasociliary nerve)

Branches to inferior
and medial rectus muscles

Abducent nerve (VI)

Inferior branch of
oculomotor nerve (III)

Lacrimal nerve

Frontal nerve *(cut)*

Ophthalmic nerve (V₁)

f. Netter M.D.

NETTER ANATOMY PLATE

Plate 86 Nerves of Orbit. (Netter: Atlas of Human Anatomy, 4 ed, 2006, Saunders.)

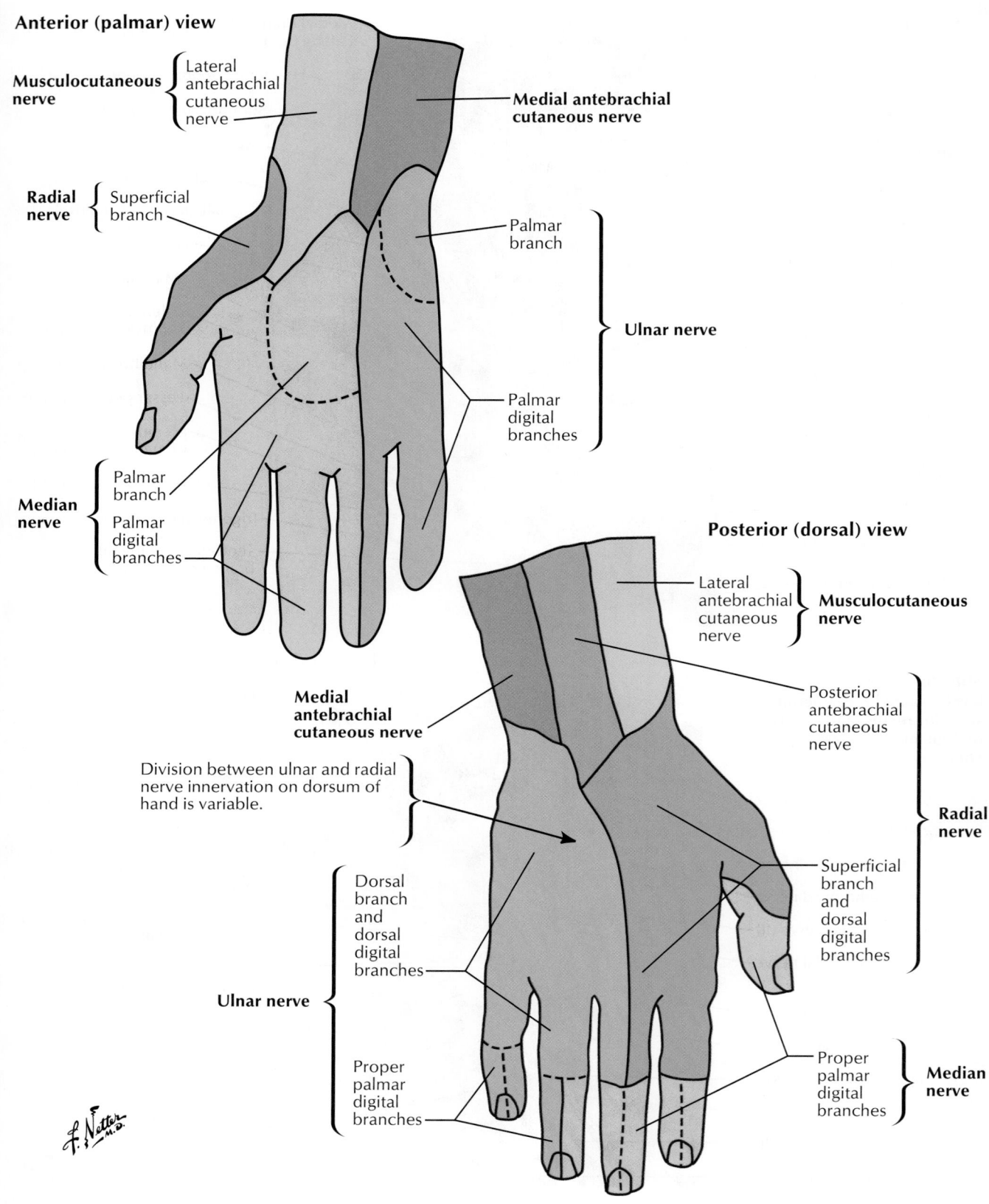

Anterior (palmar) view

Musculocutaneous nerve — Lateral antebrachial cutaneous nerve

Medial antebrachial cutaneous nerve

Radial nerve — Superficial branch

Palmar branch

Ulnar nerve

Palmar digital branches

Palmar branch

Median nerve

Palmar digital branches

Posterior (dorsal) view

Lateral antebrachial cutaneous nerve — **Musculocutaneous nerve**

Posterior antebrachial cutaneous nerve

Medial antebrachial cutaneous nerve

Division between ulnar and radial nerve innervation on dorsum of hand is variable.

Radial nerve

Superficial branch and dorsal digital branches

Dorsal branch and dorsal digital branches

Ulnar nerve

Proper palmar digital branches

Proper palmar digital branches — **Median nerve**

Plate 472 Cutaneous Innervation of Wrist and Hand. (Netter: Atlas of Human Anatomy, 4 ed, 2006, Saunders.)

Anterior view

Deltoid muscle

Coracobrachialis muscle

Biceps brachii muscle { Short head (*cut*)
Long head (*cut*)

Musculocutaneous nerve

Brachialis muscle

Biceps brachii muscle (*cut*) and tendon

Lateral antebrachial cutaneous nerve (from musculocutaneous nerve)

Radial nerve { Deep branch
Superficial branch

Supinator muscle

Brachioradialis muscle

Radial artery

Pronator teres muscle (*partially cut*)

Median nerve

Flexor pollicis longus muscle

Flexor carpi radialis tendon (*cut*)

Flexor retinaculum (transverse carpal ligament)

Superficial branch of radial nerve

Recurrent (motor) branch of median nerve to thenar muscles

Common palmar digital branches of median nerve

Proper palmar digital branches of median nerve

Intercostobrachial nerve

Medial brachial cutaneous nerve

Radial nerve

Ulnar nerve

Medial antebrachial cutaneous nerve

Median nerve

Brachial artery

Bicipital aponeurosis

Humeral head (*cut*)
Ulnar head } Pronator teres muscle

Flexor carpi radialis muscle (*cut*)

Humeroulnar head
Radial head } Flexor digitorum superficialis muscle (*cut*)

Flexor digitorum profundus muscle

Flexor carpi ulnaris muscle

Ulnar artery and nerve

Dorsal branch of ulnar nerve

Flexor digitorum superficialis tendons (*cut*)

Deep palmar branch of ulnar artery and deep branch of ulnar nerve

Superficial branch of ulnar nerve

Superficial palmar arch (*cut*)

Common palmar digital branch of ulnar nerve

Communicating branch of median nerve with ulnar nerve

Proper palmar digital branches of ulnar nerve

f. Netter
M.D.

NETTER ANATOMY PLATE

Plate 473 Arteries and Nerves of Upper Limb. (Netter: Atlas of Human Anatomy, 4 ed, 2006, Saunders.)

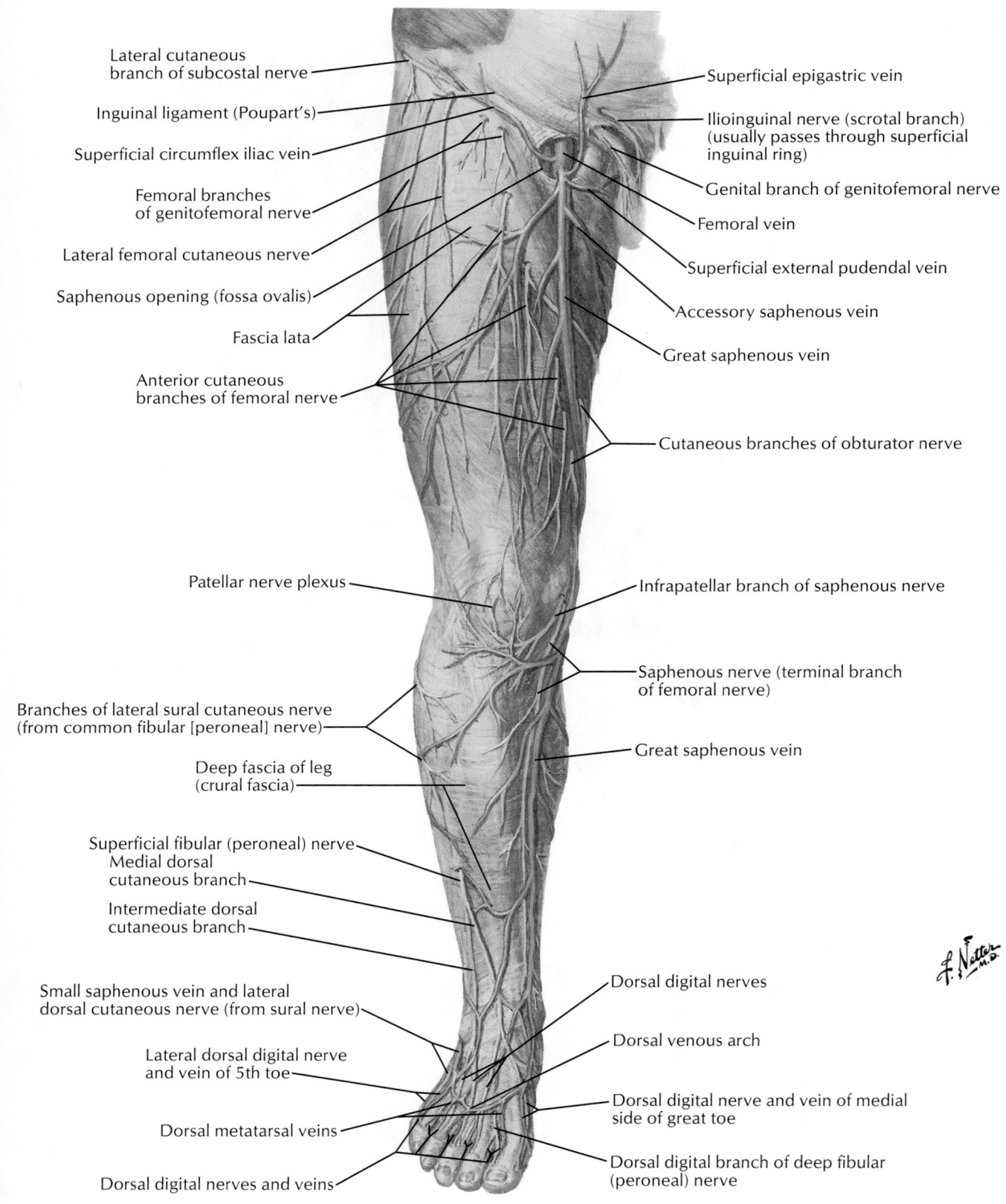

Lateral cutaneous branch of subcostal nerve

Inguinal ligament (Poupart's)

Superficial circumflex iliac vein

Femoral branches of genitofemoral nerve

Lateral femoral cutaneous nerve

Saphenous opening (fossa ovalis)

Fascia lata

Anterior cutaneous branches of femoral nerve

Patellar nerve plexus

Branches of lateral sural cutaneous nerve (from common fibular [peroneal] nerve)

Deep fascia of leg (crural fascia)

Superficial fibular (peroneal) nerve
Medial dorsal cutaneous branch

Intermediate dorsal cutaneous branch

Small saphenous vein and lateral dorsal cutaneous nerve (from sural nerve)

Lateral dorsal digital nerve and vein of 5th toe

Dorsal metatarsal veins

Dorsal digital nerves and veins

Superficial epigastric vein

Ilioinguinal nerve (scrotal branch) (usually passes through superficial inguinal ring)

Genital branch of genitofemoral nerve

Femoral vein

Superficial external pudendal vein

Accessory saphenous vein

Great saphenous vein

Cutaneous branches of obturator nerve

Infrapatellar branch of saphenous nerve

Saphenous nerve (terminal branch of femoral nerve)

Great saphenous vein

Dorsal digital nerves

Dorsal venous arch

Dorsal digital nerve and vein of medial side of great toe

Dorsal digital branch of deep fibular (peroneal) nerve

F. Netter M.D.

Plate 544   Superficial Nerves and Veins of Lower Limb: Anterior View. (Netter: Atlas of Human Anatomy, 4 ed, 2006, Saunders.)

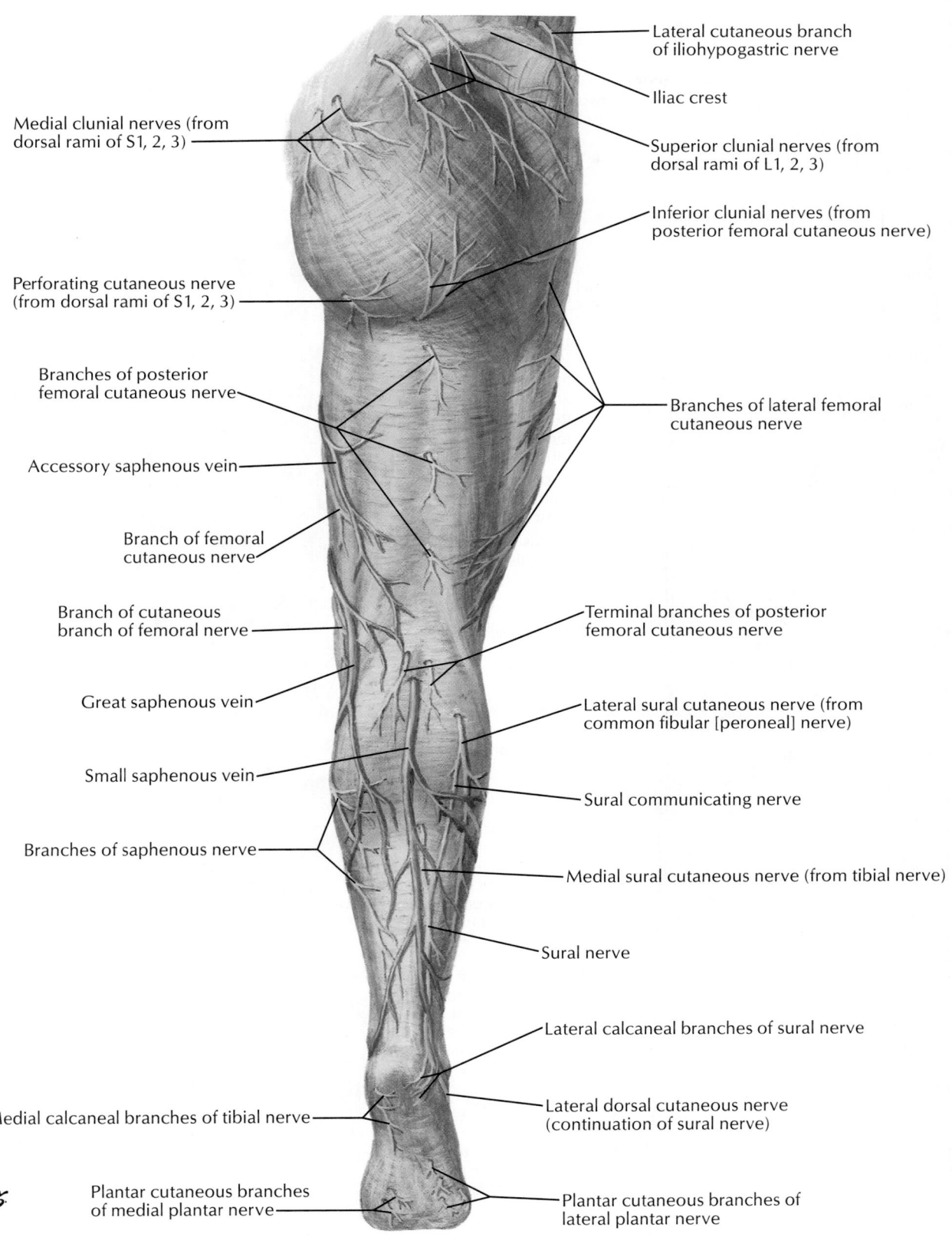

Lateral cutaneous branch of iliohypogastric nerve

Iliac crest

Superior clunial nerves (from dorsal rami of L1, 2, 3)

Inferior clunial nerves (from posterior femoral cutaneous nerve)

Branches of lateral femoral cutaneous nerve

Terminal branches of posterior femoral cutaneous nerve

Lateral sural cutaneous nerve (from common fibular [peroneal] nerve)

Sural communicating nerve

Medial sural cutaneous nerve (from tibial nerve)

Sural nerve

Lateral calcaneal branches of sural nerve

Lateral dorsal cutaneous nerve (continuation of sural nerve)

Plantar cutaneous branches of lateral plantar nerve

Medial clunial nerves (from dorsal rami of S1, 2, 3)

Perforating cutaneous nerve (from dorsal rami of S1, 2, 3)

Branches of posterior femoral cutaneous nerve

Accessory saphenous vein

Branch of femoral cutaneous nerve

Branch of cutaneous branch of femoral nerve

Great saphenous vein

Small saphenous vein

Branches of saphenous nerve

Medial calcaneal branches of tibial nerve

Plantar cutaneous branches of medial plantar nerve

Plate 545 Superficial Nerves and Veins of Lower Limb: Posterior View. (Netter: Atlas of Human Anatomy, 4 ed, 2006, Saunders.)

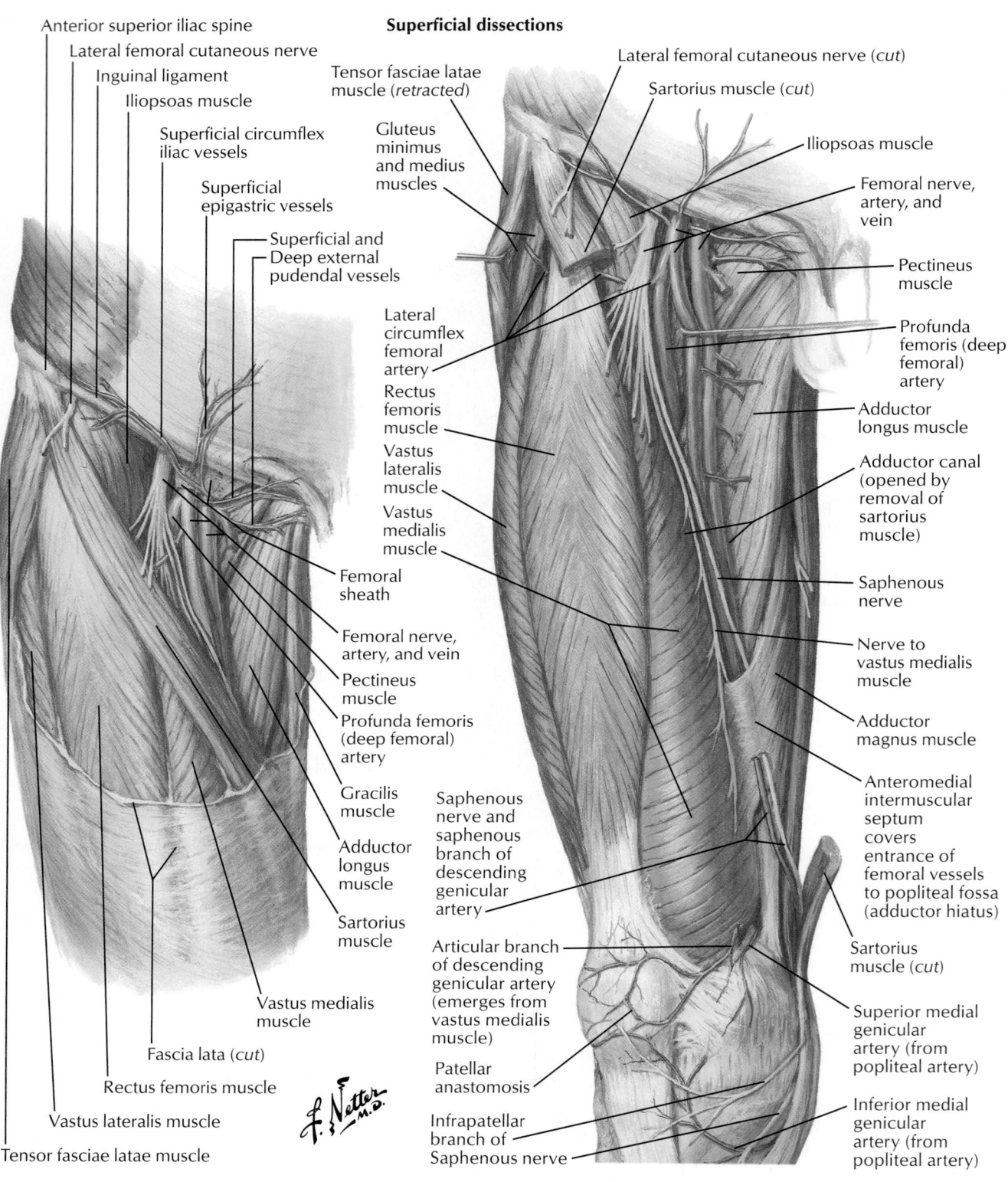

Superficial dissections

Anterior superior iliac spine

Lateral femoral cutaneous nerve

Inguinal ligament

Iliopsoas muscle

Superficial circumflex iliac vessels

Superficial epigastric vessels

Superficial and Deep external pudendal vessels

Tensor fasciae latae muscle (*retracted*)

Gluteus minimus and medius muscles

Lateral circumflex femoral artery

Rectus femoris muscle

Vastus lateralis muscle

Vastus medialis muscle

Femoral sheath

Femoral nerve, artery, and vein

Pectineus muscle

Profunda femoris (deep femoral) artery

Gracilis muscle

Adductor longus muscle

Sartorius muscle

Saphenous nerve and saphenous branch of descending genicular artery

Articular branch of descending genicular artery (emerges from vastus medialis muscle)

Patellar anastomosis

Infrapatellar branch of Saphenous nerve

Vastus medialis muscle

Fascia lata (*cut*)

Rectus femoris muscle

Vastus lateralis muscle

Tensor fasciae latae muscle

Lateral femoral cutaneous nerve (*cut*)

Sartorius muscle (*cut*)

Iliopsoas muscle

Femoral nerve, artery, and vein

Pectineus muscle

Profunda femoris (deep femoral) artery

Adductor longus muscle

Adductor canal (opened by removal of sartorius muscle)

Saphenous nerve

Nerve to vastus medialis muscle

Adductor magnus muscle

Anteromedial intermuscular septum covers entrance of femoral vessels to popliteal fossa (adductor hiatus)

Sartorius muscle (*cut*)

Superior medial genicular artery (from popliteal artery)

Inferior medial genicular artery (from popliteal artery)

F. Netter M.D.

Plate 500 Arteries and Nerves of Thigh: Anterior View. (Netter: Atlas of Human Anatomy, 4 ed, 2006, Saunders.)

Deep dissection

Deep circumflex iliac artery

Lateral femoral cutaneous nerve

Sartorius muscle (cut)

Iliopsoas muscle

Tensor fasciae latae muscle (retracted)

Gluteus medius and minimus muscles

Femoral nerve

Rectus femoris muscle (cut)

Ascending, transverse and descending branches of Lateral circumflex femoral artery

Medial circumflex femoral artery

Pectineus muscle (cut)

Profunda femoris (deep femoral) artery

Perforating branches

Adductor longus muscle (cut)

Vastus lateralis muscle

Vastus intermedius muscle

Rectus femoris muscle (cut)

Saphenous nerve

Anteromedial intermuscular septum (opened)

Vastus medialis muscle

Quadriceps femoris tendon

Patella and patellar anastomosis

Medial patellar retinaculum

Patellar ligament

External iliac artery and vein

Inguinal ligament (Poupart's)

Femoral artery and vein (cut)

Pectineus muscle (cut)

Obturator canal

Obturator externus muscle

Adductor longus muscle (cut)

Anterior branch and Posterior branch of obturator nerve

Quadratus femoris muscle

Adductor brevis muscle

Branches of posterior branch of obturator nerve

Adductor magnus muscle

Gracilis muscle

Cutaneous branch of obturator nerve

Femoral artery and vein (cut)

Descending genicular artery
Articular branch
Saphenous branch

Adductor hiatus

Sartorius muscle (cut)

Adductor magnus tendon

Adductor tubercle on medial epicondyle of femur

Superior medial genicular artery (from popliteal artery)

Infrapatellar branch of Saphenous nerve

Inferior medial genicular artery (from popliteal artery)

NETTER ANATOMY PLATE

Plate 501   Arteries and Nerves of Thigh: Anterior View. (Netter: Atlas of Human Anatomy, 4 ed, 2006, Saunders.)

Deep dissection

Superior clunial nerves

Gluteus maximus muscle (*cut*)

Medial clunial nerves

Inferior gluteal artery and nerve

Pudendal nerve

Nerve to obturator internus (and superior gemellus)

Posterior femoral cutaneous nerve

Sacrotuberous ligament

Ischial tuberosity

Inferior clunial nerves (*cut*)

Adductor magnus muscle

Gracilis muscle

Sciatic nerve

Muscular branches of sciatic nerve

Semitendinosus muscle (*retracted*)

Semimembranosus muscle

Sciatic nerve

Articular branch

Adductor hiatus

Popliteal vein and artery

Superior medial genicular artery

Medial epicondyle of femur

Tibial nerve

Gastrocnemius muscle (medial head)

Medial sural cutaneous nerve

Small saphenous vein

Iliac crest

Gluteal aponeurosis and gluteus medius muscle (*cut*)

Superior gluteal artery and nerve

Gluteus minimus muscle

Tensor fasciae latae muscle

Piriformis muscle

Gluteus medius muscle (*cut*)

Superior gemellus muscle

Greater trochanter of femur

Obturator internus muscle

Inferior gemellus muscle

Gluteus maximus muscle (*cut*)

Quadratus femoris muscle

Medial circumflex femoral artery

Vastus lateralis muscle and iliotibial tract

Adductor minimus part of adductor magnus muscle

1st perforating artery (from profunda femoris artery)

Adductor magnus muscle

2nd and 3rd perforating arteries (from profunda femoris artery)

4th perforating artery (from profunda femoris artery)

Long head (*retracted*) ⎱ Biceps femoris
Short head   ⎰ muscle

Superior lateral genicular artery

Common fibular (peroneal) nerve

Plantaris muscle

Gastrocnemius muscle (lateral head)

Lateral sural cutaneous nerve

Plate 502 Arteries and Nerves of Thigh: Posterior View. (Netter: Atlas of Human Anatomy, 4 ed, 2006, Saunders.)

Horizontal section

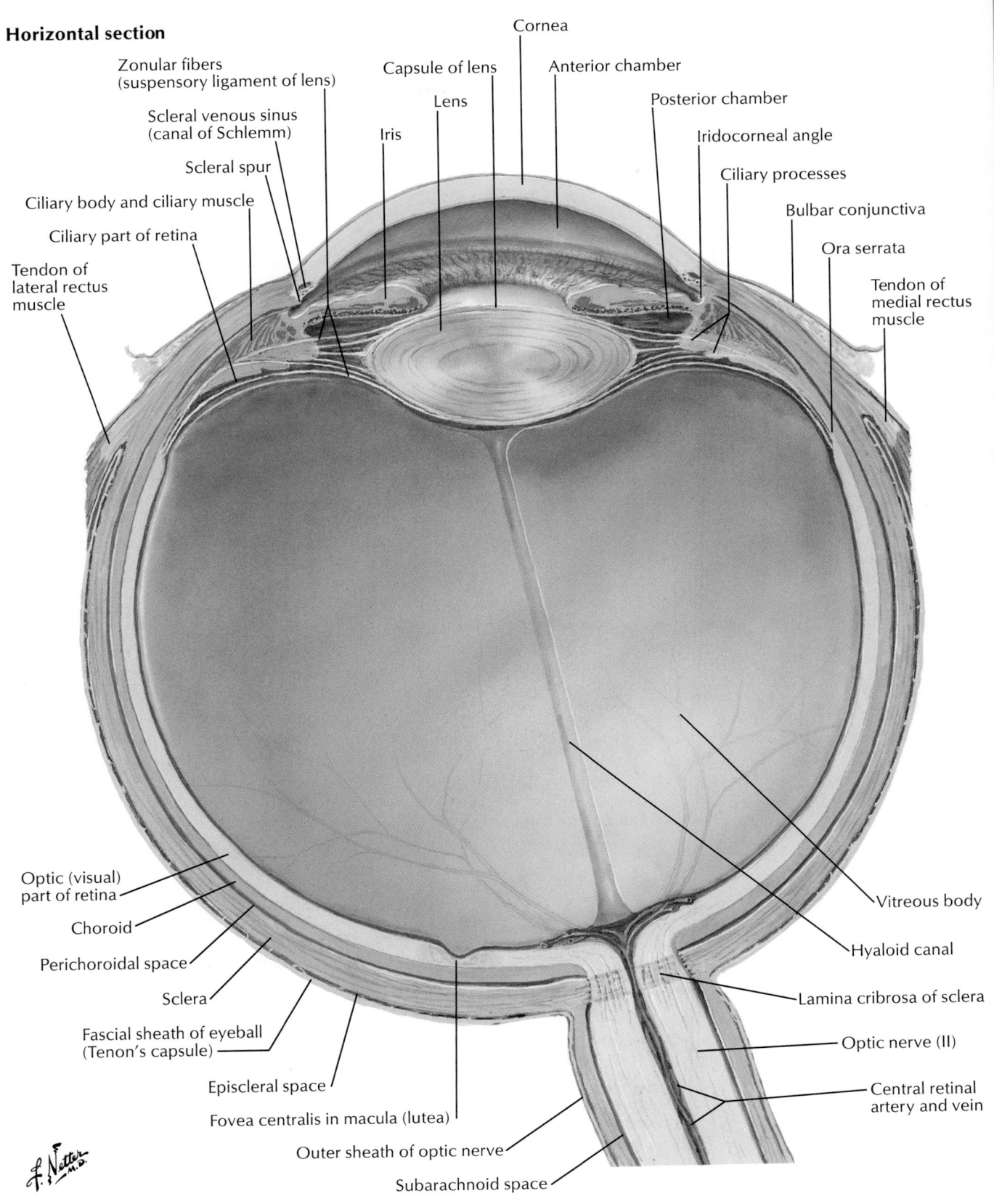

Zonular fibers (suspensory ligament of lens)

Scleral venous sinus (canal of Schlemm)

Scleral spur

Ciliary body and ciliary muscle

Ciliary part of retina

Tendon of lateral rectus muscle

Capsule of lens

Lens

Iris

Cornea

Anterior chamber

Posterior chamber

Iridocorneal angle

Ciliary processes

Bulbar conjunctiva

Ora serrata

Tendon of medial rectus muscle

Optic (visual) part of retina

Choroid

Perichoroidal space

Sclera

Fascial sheath of eyeball (Tenon's capsule)

Episcleral space

Fovea centralis in macula (lutea)

Outer sheath of optic nerve

Subarachnoid space

Vitreous body

Hyaloid canal

Lamina cribrosa of sclera

Optic nerve (II)

Central retinal artery and vein

NETTER ANATOMY PLATE

Plate 87   Eyeball. (Netter: Atlas of Human Anatomy, 4 ed, 2006, Saunders.)

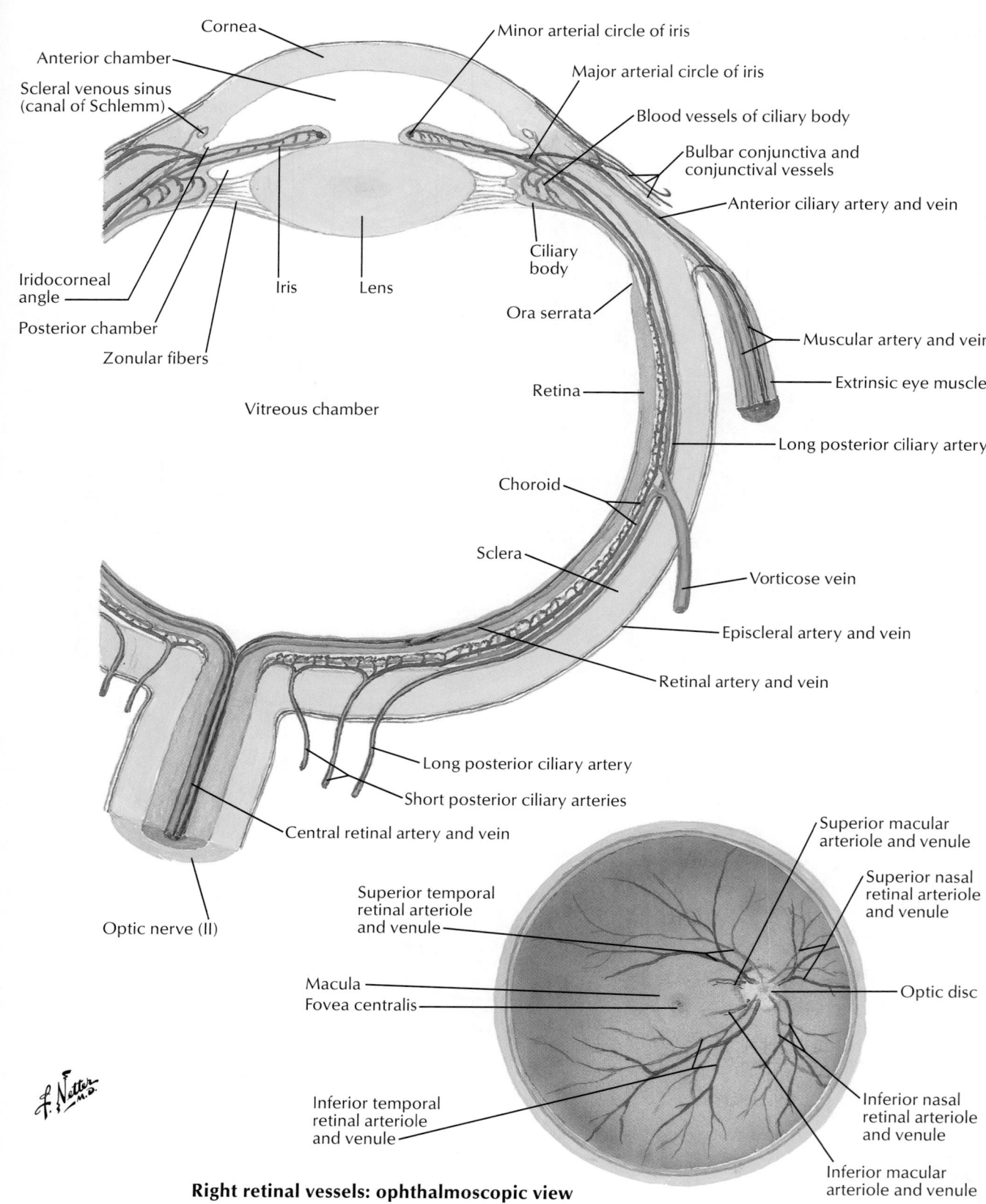

Cornea

Minor arterial circle of iris

Anterior chamber

Major arterial circle of iris

Scleral venous sinus
(canal of Schlemm)

Blood vessels of ciliary body

Bulbar conjunctiva and
conjunctival vessels

Anterior ciliary artery and vein

Iridocorneal
angle

Iris

Lens

Ciliary
body

Posterior chamber

Ora serrata

Muscular artery and vein

Zonular fibers

Extrinsic eye muscle

Retina

Vitreous chamber

Long posterior ciliary artery

Choroid

Sclera

Vorticose vein

Episcleral artery and vein

Retinal artery and vein

Long posterior ciliary artery

Short posterior ciliary arteries

Central retinal artery and vein

Optic nerve (II)

Superior macular
arteriole and venule

Superior temporal
retinal arteriole
and venule

Superior nasal
retinal arteriole
and venule

Macula

Optic disc

Fovea centralis

Inferior temporal
retinal arteriole
and venule

Inferior nasal
retinal arteriole
and venule

Inferior macular
arteriole and venule

Right retinal vessels: ophthalmoscopic view

Plate 90 Intrinsic Arteries and Veins of Eye. (Netter: Atlas of Human Anatomy, 4 ed, 2006, Saunders.)

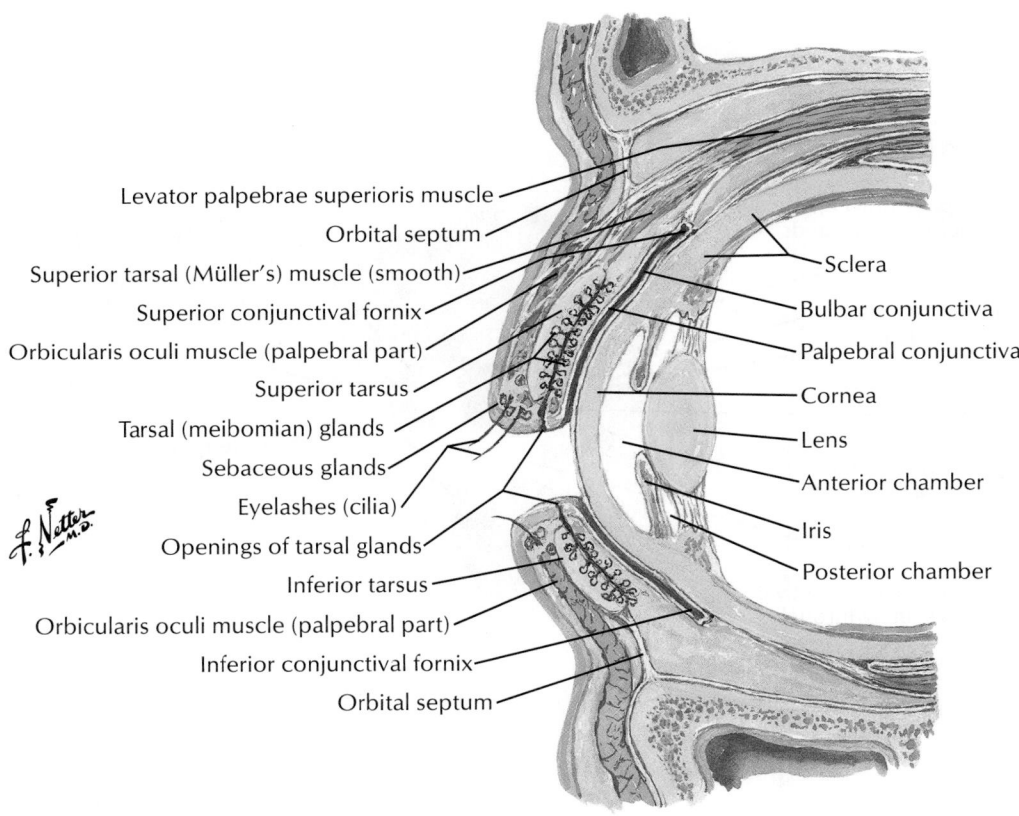

Levator palpebrae superioris muscle

Orbital septum

Superior tarsal (Müller's) muscle (smooth)

Superior conjunctival fornix

Orbicularis oculi muscle (palpebral part)

Superior tarsus

Tarsal (meibomian) glands

Sebaceous glands

Eyelashes (cilia)

Openings of tarsal glands

Inferior tarsus

Orbicularis oculi muscle (palpebral part)

Inferior conjunctival fornix

Orbital septum

Sclera

Bulbar conjunctiva

Palpebral conjunctiva

Cornea

Lens

Anterior chamber

Iris

Posterior chamber

Plate 81, Middle   Eyelid. (Netter: Atlas of Human Anatomy, 4 ed, 2006, Saunders.)

Superior palpebral conjunctiva:
tarsal (meibomian) glands
shining through

Seen through { Pupil
cornea { Iris

Corneoscleral junction
(corneal limbus)

Bulbar conjunctiva
over sclera

Inferior conjunctival fornix

Inferior palpebral conjunctiva:
tarsal glands shining through

Superior lacrimal papilla and
punctum

Plica semilunaris

Lacrimal caruncle in
lacrimal lake (lacus lacrimalis)

Inferior lacrimal papilla and
punctum

Plate 81, Upper   Eyelid. (Netter: Atlas of Human Anatomy, 4 ed, 2006, Saunders.)

Orbital part of
lacrimal gland

Palpebral part of
lacrimal gland

Excretory ducts of
lacrimal gland

Plica semilunaris

Lacrimal caruncle

Inferior lacrimal papilla and punctum

Superior lacrimal papilla and punctum

Lacrimal canaliculi

Lacrimal sac

Nasolacrimal duct

Opening of
nasolacrimal duct

Frontal bone (cut away)

Orbital part of
lacrimal gland

Palpebral part of
lacrimal gland

Excretory ducts of
lacrimal gland

Plica semilunaris
and lacrimal lake

Lacrimal caruncle

Inferior lacrimal papilla and punctum

Opening of nasolacrimal duct

Superior lacrimal papilla and punctum

Lacrimal canaliculi

Lacrimal sac

Nasolacrimal duct

Middle nasal
concha

Nasal cavity

Inferior nasal
concha (cut)

Inferior nasal meatus

Plate 82   Lacrimal Apparatus. (Netter: Atlas of Human Anatomy, 4 ed, 2006, Saunders.)

Frontal section

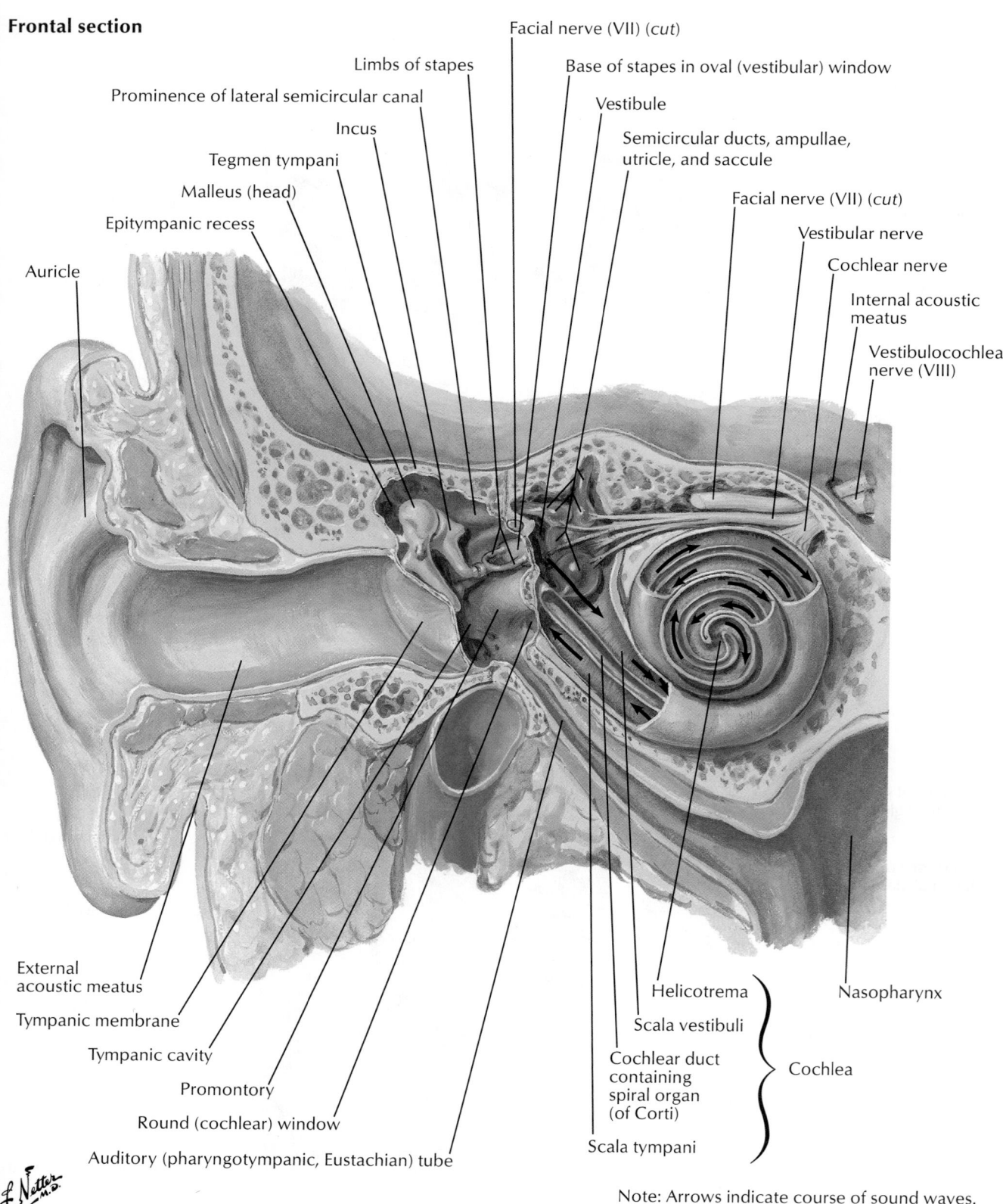

Facial nerve (VII) (*cut*)

Limbs of stapes

Base of stapes in oval (vestibular) window

Prominence of lateral semicircular canal

Vestibule

Incus

Semicircular ducts, ampullae, utricle, and saccule

Tegmen tympani

Malleus (head)

Facial nerve (VII) (*cut*)

Epitympanic recess

Vestibular nerve

Auricle

Cochlear nerve

Internal acoustic meatus

Vestibulocochlear nerve (VIII)

External acoustic meatus

Tympanic membrane

Tympanic cavity

Promontory

Round (cochlear) window

Auditory (pharyngotympanic, Eustachian) tube

Helicotrema

Scala vestibuli

Nasopharynx

Cochlear duct containing spiral organ (of Corti)

Cochlea

Scala tympani

Note: Arrows indicate course of sound waves.

NETTER ANATOMY PLATE

Plate 92 Pathway of Sound Reception. (Netter: Atlas of Human Anatomy, 4 ed, 2006, Saunders.)

Medial wall of tympanic cavity: lateral view

Prominence of lateral semicircular canal

Prominence of facial canal

Geniculum (geniculate ganglion) of facial nerve

Greater petrosal nerve

Mastoid antrum

Base of stapes in fossa of oval (vestibular) window

Limbs of stapes

Pyramidal eminence

Chorda tympani nerve (*cut*)

Mastoid cells

Tendon of stapedius muscle

Fossa of round (cochlear) window

Facial nerve (VII) in stylomastoid foramen

Jugular fossa

Tympanic cells

Tensor tympani muscle (*tendon cut*)

Auditory (pharyngotympanic, Eustachian) tube

Levator veli palatini muscle

Promontory with tympanic nerve (of Jacobson) and plexus under mucosa

Internal carotid artery

Plate 94 Tympanic Cavity. (Netter: Atlas of Human Anatomy, 4 ed, 2006, Saunders.)

Dissected right bony labyrinth (otic capsule): membranous labyrinth removed

Posterior
Lateral
Anterior } Semicircular canals

Elliptical recess
Cochlear recess
Spherical recess } Vestibule (note perforations for nerve fibers)

Helicotrema

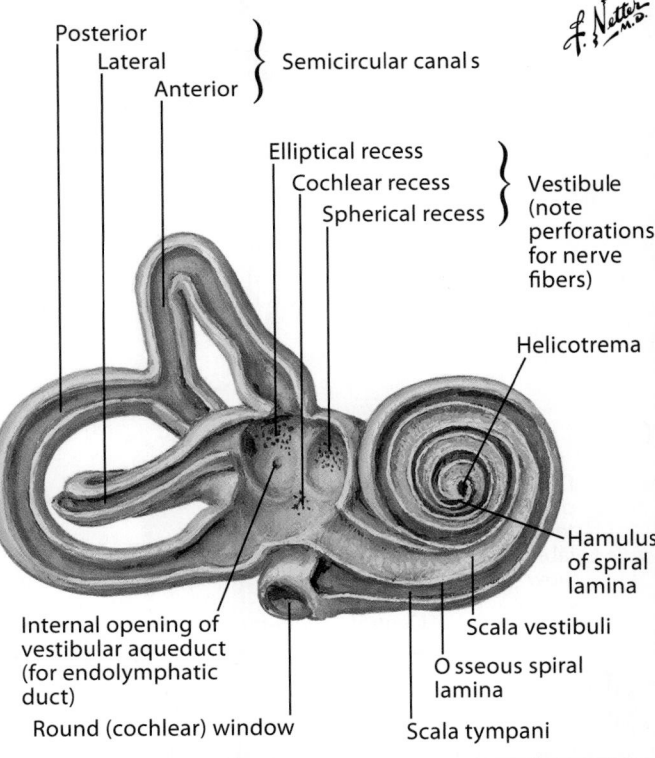

Internal opening of vestibular aqueduct (for endolymphatic duct)

Round (cochlear) window

Hamulus of spiral lamina

Scala vestibuli

Osseous spiral lamina

Scala tympani

Plate 95 Bony Membranous Labyrinth. (Netter: Atlas of Human Anatomy, 4 ed, 2006, Saunders.)

Otoscopic view of right tympanic membrane

Pars flaccida

Posterior mallear fold

Lateral process of malleus

Anterior mallear fold

Long limb of incus

Handle of malleus

Umbo

Cone of light

Tympanic

Pars tensa

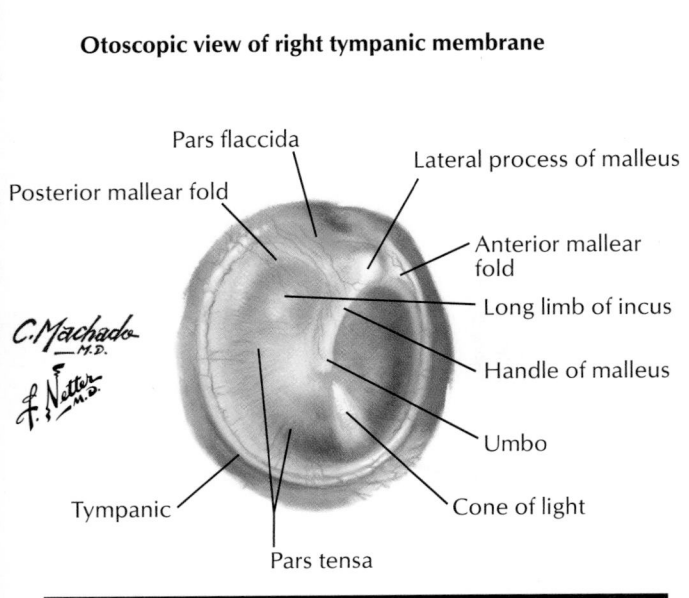

Plate 93 Tympanic Cavity. (Netter: Atlas of Human Anatomy, 4 ed, 2006, Saunders.)

NETTER ANATOMY PLATE

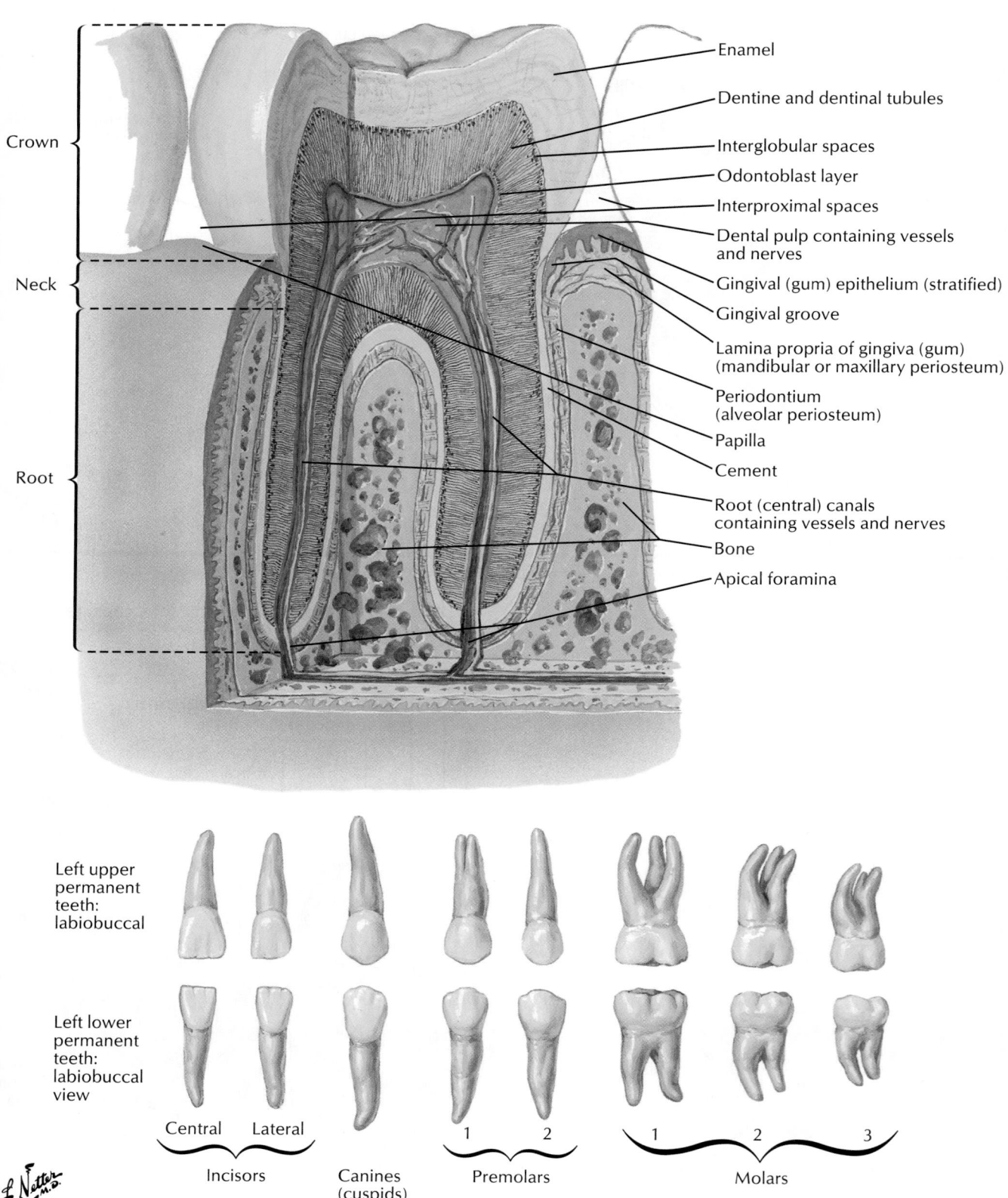

Crown

Neck

Root

Enamel

Dentine and dentinal tubules

Interglobular spaces

Odontoblast layer

Interproximal spaces

Dental pulp containing vessels and nerves

Gingival (gum) epithelium (stratified)

Gingival groove

Lamina propria of gingiva (gum) (mandibular or maxillary periosteum)

Periodontium (alveolar periosteum)

Papilla

Cement

Root (central) canals containing vessels and nerves

Bone

Apical foramina

Left upper permanent teeth: labiobuccal

Left lower permanent teeth: labiobuccal view

Central   Lateral

Incisors

Canines (cuspids)

1   2

Premolars

1   2   3

Molars

Plate 57   Teeth. (Netter: Atlas of Human Anatomy, 4 ed, 2006, Saunders.)

Tongue

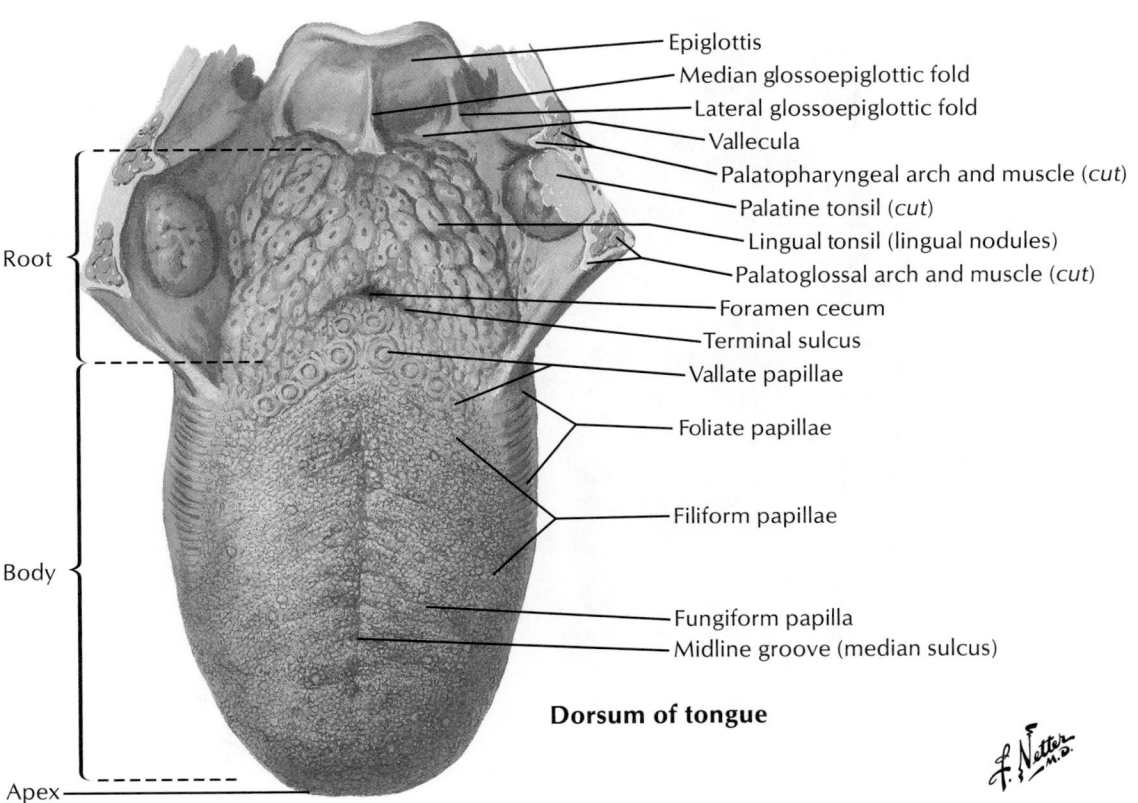

Epiglottis

Median glossoepiglottic fold

Lateral glossoepiglottic fold

Vallecula

Palatopharyngeal arch and muscle (*cut*)

Palatine tonsil (*cut*)

Lingual tonsil (lingual nodules)

Palatoglossal arch and muscle (*cut*)

Foramen cecum

Terminal sulcus

Vallate papillae

Foliate papillae

Filiform papillae

Fungiform papilla

Midline groove (median sulcus)

Root

Body

Apex

Dorsum of tongue

Plate 58   Tongue. (Netter: Atlas of Human Anatomy, 4 ed, 2006, Saunders.)

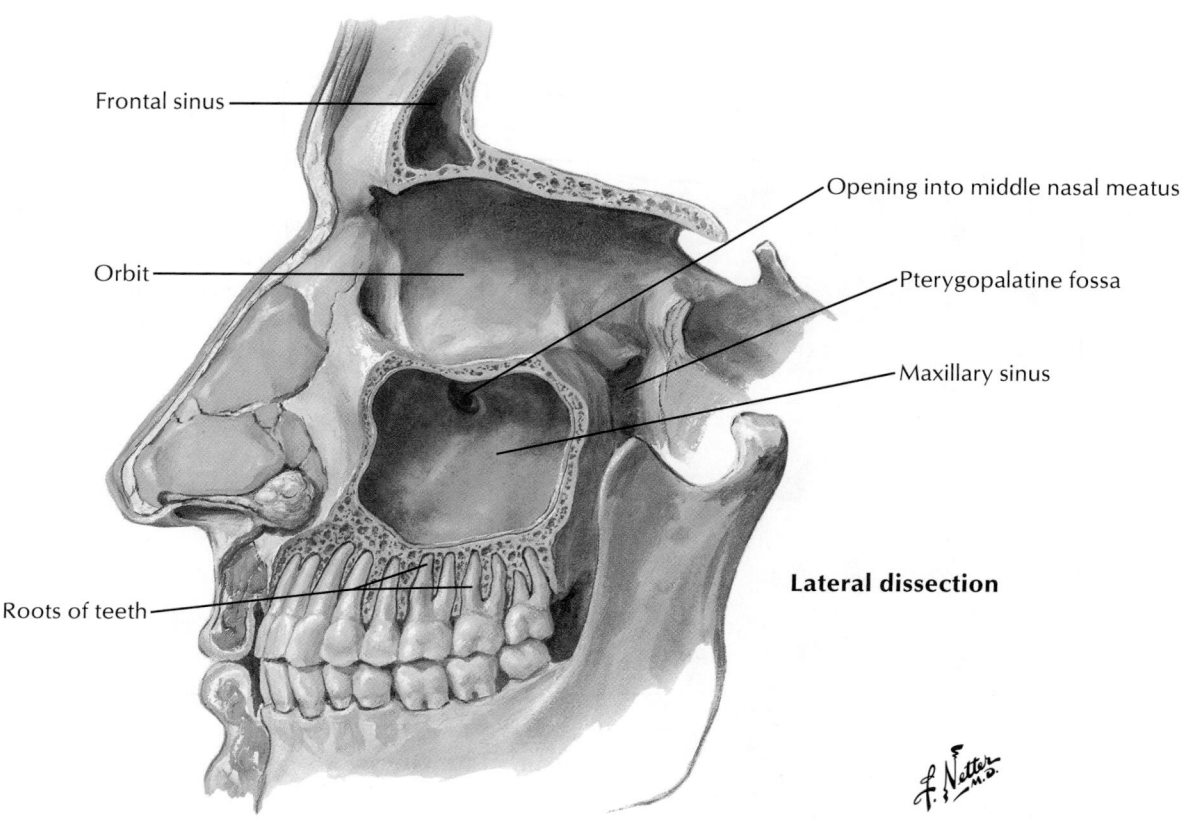

Frontal sinus

Orbit

Opening into middle nasal meatus

Pterygopalatine fossa

Maxillary sinus

Roots of teeth

Lateral dissection

Plate 49   Paranasal Sinuses. (Netter: Atlas of Human Anatomy, 4 ed, 2006, Saunders.)

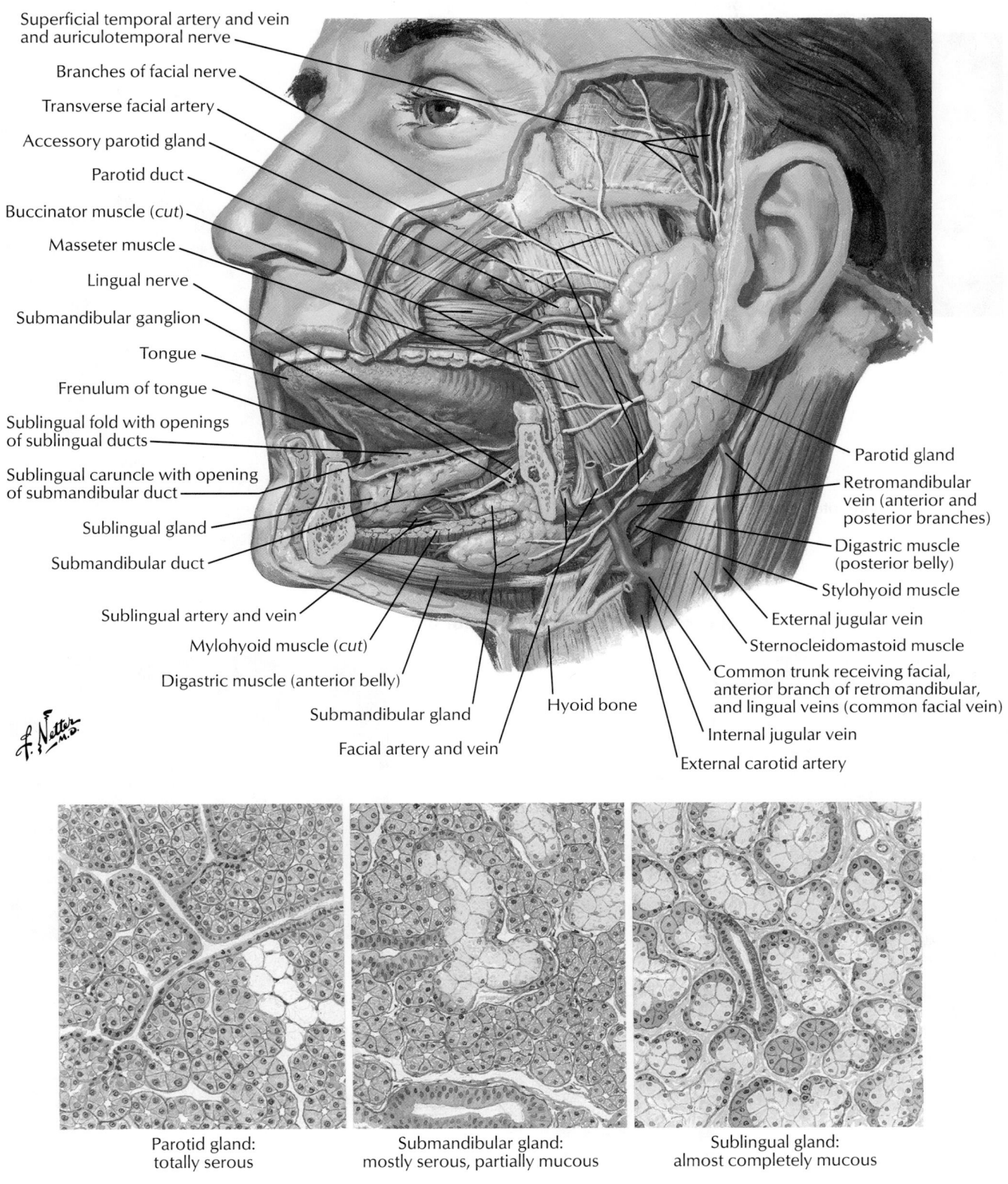

Superficial temporal artery and vein and auriculotemporal nerve

Branches of facial nerve

Transverse facial artery

Accessory parotid gland

Parotid duct

Buccinator muscle (*cut*)

Masseter muscle

Lingual nerve

Submandibular ganglion

Tongue

Frenulum of tongue

Sublingual fold with openings of sublingual ducts

Sublingual caruncle with opening of submandibular duct

Sublingual gland

Submandibular duct

Sublingual artery and vein

Mylohyoid muscle (*cut*)

Digastric muscle (anterior belly)

Submandibular gland

Facial artery and vein

Hyoid bone

Parotid gland

Retromandibular vein (anterior and posterior branches)

Digastric muscle (posterior belly)

Stylohyoid muscle

External jugular vein

Sternocleidomastoid muscle

Common trunk receiving facial, anterior branch of retromandibular, and lingual veins (common facial vein)

Internal jugular vein

External carotid artery

Parotid gland: totally serous

Submandibular gland: mostly serous, partially mucous

Sublingual gland: almost completely mucous

Plate 61 Salivary Glands. (Netter: Atlas of Human Anatomy, 4 ed, 2006, Saunders.)

Right coronary artery: left anterior oblique view

Arteriogram

Sinuatrial (SA) nodal branch

Right coronary artery

Atrioventricular (AV) nodal branch

Branches to back of left ventricle

Right marginal branch

Posterior interventricular branch (posterior descending artery)

Right coronary artery: right anterior oblique view

Sinuatrial (SA) nodal branch

Conus (arteriosus) branch

Right coronary artery

Right marginal branch

Arteriogram

Atrioventricular (AV) nodal branch

Right posterolateral branches (to back of left ventricle)

Posterior interventricular branch (posterior descending artery)

Plate 218   Coronary Arteries: Arteriographic Views. (Netter: Atlas of Human Anatomy, 4 ed, 2006, Saunders.)

Left coronary artery: left anterior oblique view

Left coronary artery

Circumflex branch

Arteriogram

Anterior interventricular branch (left anterior descending)

Diagonal branches of anterior interventricular branch

Atrioventricular branch of circumflex branch

Left (obtuse) marginal branch

Posterolateral branches

(Perforating) interventricular septal branches

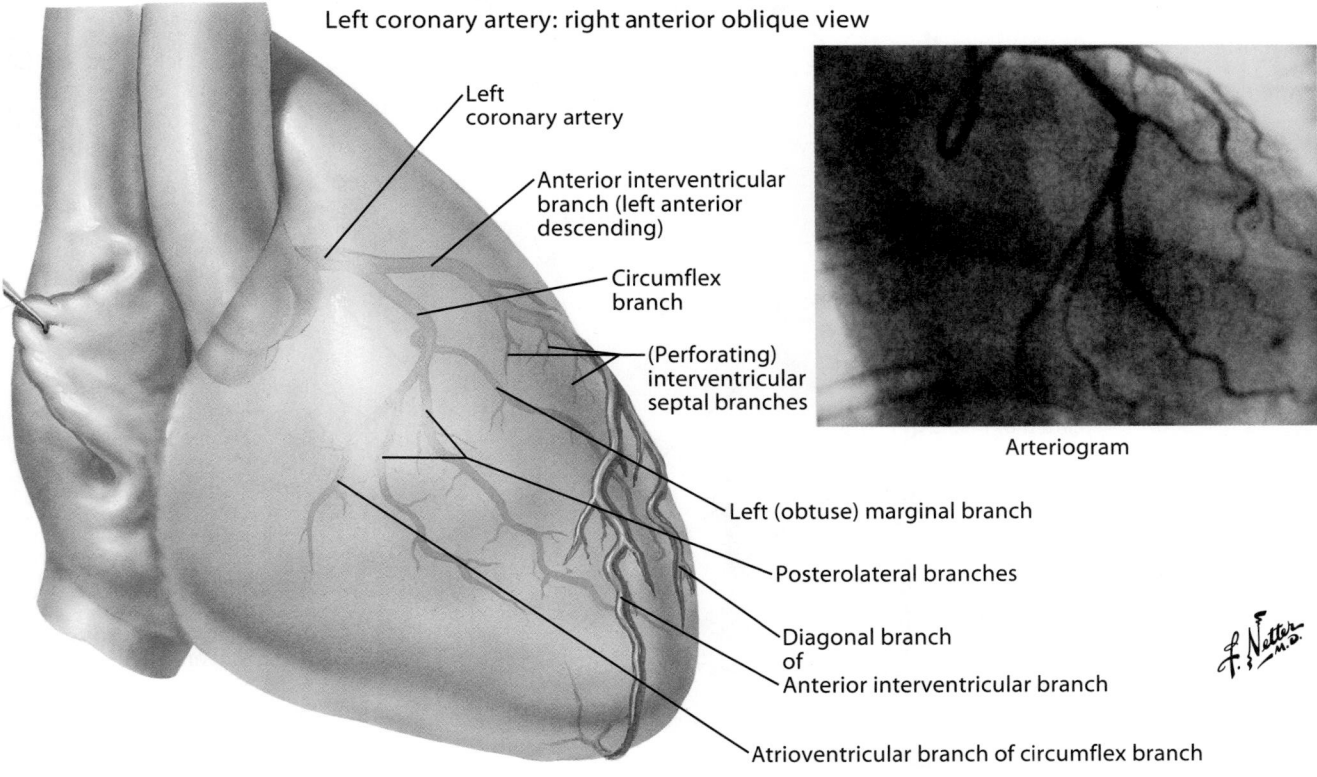

Left coronary artery: right anterior oblique view

Left coronary artery

Anterior interventricular branch (left anterior descending)

Circumflex branch

(Perforating) interventricular septal branches

Arteriogram

Left (obtuse) marginal branch

Posterolateral branches

Diagonal branch of Anterior interventricular branch

Atrioventricular branch of circumflex branch

Plate 219 Coronary Arteries: Arteriographic Views. (Netter: Atlas of Human Anatomy, 4 ed, 2006, Saunders.)

Corpus callosum

Anterolateral central (lenticulostriate) arteries

Lateral frontobasal (orbitofrontal) artery

Prefrontal artery

Precentral (pre-Rolandic) and central (Rolandic) sulcal arteries

Anterior parietal (postcentral sulcal) artery

Posterior parietal artery

Branch to angular gyrus

Temporal branches (anterior, middle, and posterior)

Middle cerebral artery and branches (deep in lateral cerebral [Sylvian] sulcus)

Anterior communicating artery

Posterior communicating artery

Anterior inferior cerebellar artery (AICA)

Posterior spinal artery

Paracentral artery

Medial frontal branches

Pericallosal artery

Callosomarginal artery

Polar frontal artery

Anterior cerebral arteries

Medial frontobasal (orbitofrontal) artery

Distal medial striate artery (recurrent artery of Heubner)

Internal carotid artery

Anterior choroidal artery

Posterior cerebral artery

Superior cerebellar artery

Basilar and pontine arteries

Labyrinthine (internal acoustic) artery

Vertebral artery

Posterior inferior cerebellar artery (PICA)

Anterior spinal artery

Corpus striatum (caudate and lentiform nuclei)

Anterolateral central (lenticulostriate) arteries

Insula (island of Reil)

Limen of insula

Precentral (pre-Rolandic), central (Rolandic) sulcal, and parietal arteries

Lateral cerebral (Sylvian) sulcus

Temporal branches of middle cerebral artery

Temporal lobe

Middle cerebral artery

Internal carotid artery

Falx cerebri

Callosomarginal arteries and Pericallosal arteries (branches of anterior cerebral arteries)

Trunk of corpus callosum

Internal capsule

Septum pellucidum

Rostrum of corpus callosum

Anterior cerebral arteries

Distal medial striate artery (recurrent artery of Heubner)

Anterior communicating artery

Optic chiasm

Plate 141 Arteries of Brain: Frontal View and Section. (Netter: Atlas of Human Anatomy, 4 ed, 2006, Saunders.)

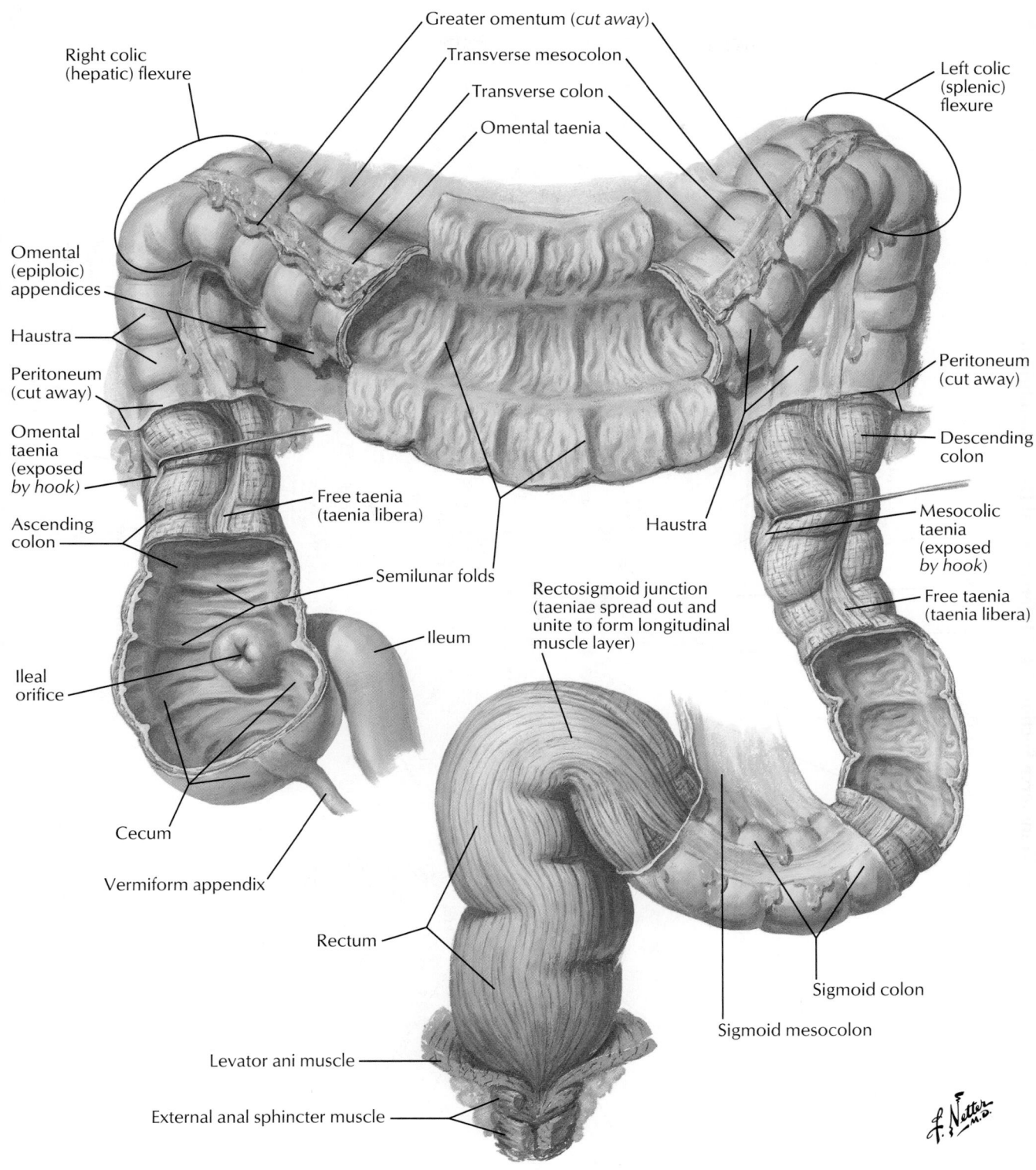

Right colic (hepatic) flexure

Greater omentum (*cut away*)

Transverse mesocolon

Transverse colon

Omental taenia

Left colic (splenic) flexure

Omental (epiploic) appendices

Haustra

Peritoneum (cut away)

Omental taenia (exposed *by hook*)

Ascending colon

Ileal orifice

Cecum

Vermiform appendix

Free taenia (taenia libera)

Semilunar folds

Ileum

Peritoneum (cut away)

Descending colon

Haustra

Mesocolic taenia (exposed *by hook*)

Free taenia (taenia libera)

Rectosigmoid junction (taeniae spread out and unite to form longitudinal muscle layer)

Rectum

Sigmoid colon

Sigmoid mesocolon

Levator ani muscle

External anal sphincter muscle

NETTER ANATOMY PLATE

Plate 284 Mucosa and Musculature of Large Intestine. (Netter: Atlas of Human Anatomy, 4 ed, 2006, Saunders.)

Transverse Section: T3–4 Intervertebral Disc, Manubrium

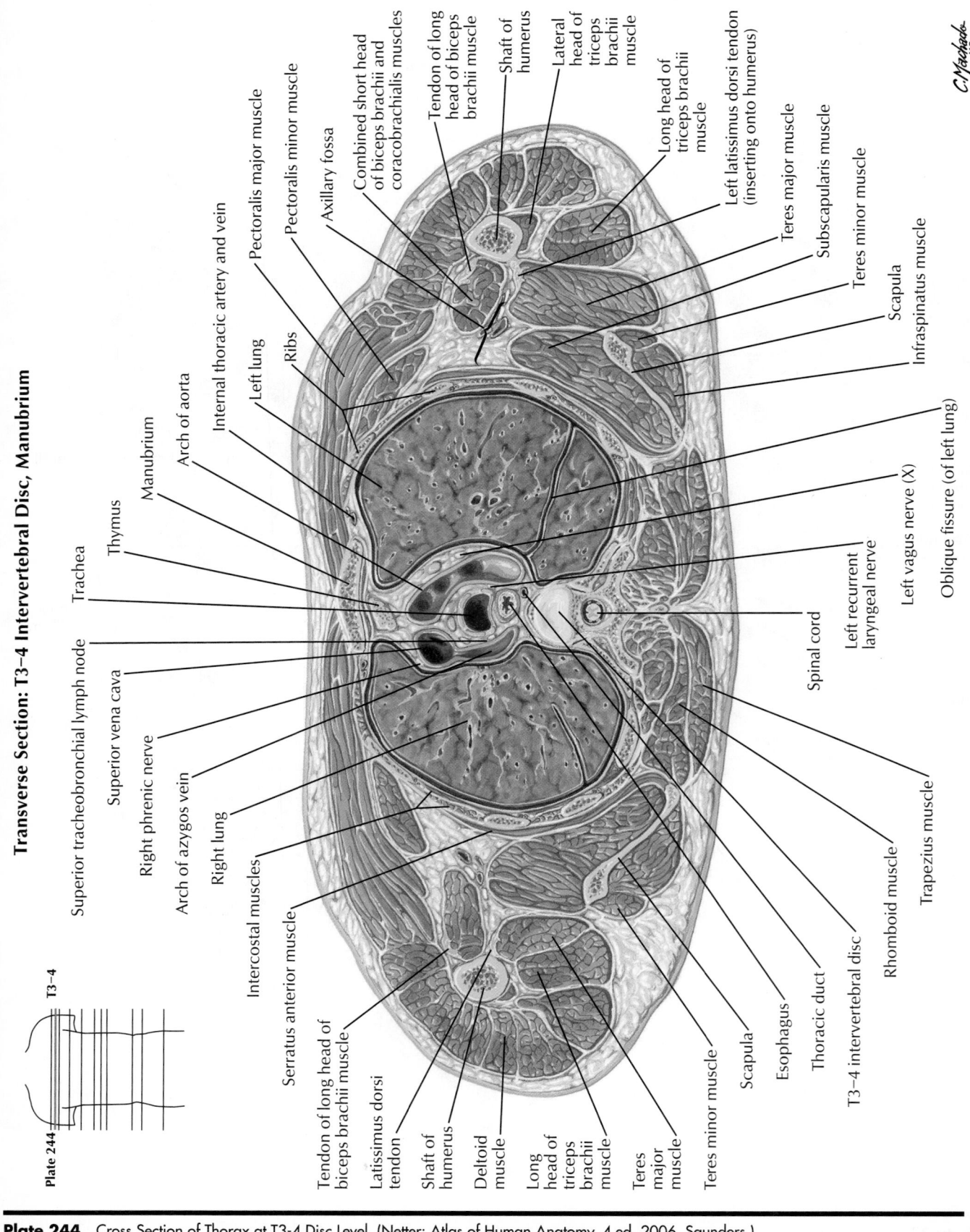

Superior tracheobronchial lymph node
Trachea
Thymus
Manubrium
Arch of aorta
Internal thoracic artery and vein
Left lung
Ribs
Pectoralis minor muscle
Pectoralis major muscle
Axillary fossa
Combined short head of biceps brachii and coracobrachialis muscles
Tendon of long head of biceps brachii muscle
Shaft of humerus
Lateral head of triceps brachii muscle
Long head of triceps brachii muscle
Left latissimus dorsi tendon (inserting onto humerus)
Teres major muscle
Subscapularis muscle
Teres minor muscle
Scapula
Infraspinatus muscle

Superior vena cava
Right phrenic nerve
Arch of azygos vein
Right lung

Oblique fissure (of left lung)
Left vagus nerve (X)
Left recurrent laryngeal nerve
Spinal cord

Intercostal muscles
Serratus anterior muscle
Tendon of long head of biceps brachii muscle
Latissimus dorsi tendon
Shaft of humerus
Deltoid muscle
Long head of triceps brachii muscle
Teres major muscle
Teres minor muscle
Scapula
Esophagus
Thoracic duct
T3–4 intervertebral disc
Rhomboid muscle
Trapezius muscle

Plate 244 Cross Section of Thorax at T3-4 Disc Level. (Netter: Atlas of Human Anatomy, 4 ed, 2006, Saunders.)

Plate 244

T3–4

Right knee in extension: posterior view

Posterior cruciate ligament

Anterior cruciate ligament

Posterior meniscofemoral ligament

Lateral condyle of femur (articular surface)

Popliteus tendon

Fibular collateral ligament

Lateral meniscus

Head of fibula

Adductor tubercle on medial epicondyle of femur

Medial condyle of femur (articular surface)

Medial meniscus

Tibial collateral ligament

Medial condyle of tibia

Plate 509   Knee: Cruciate and Collateral Ligaments. (Netter: Atlas of Human Anatomy, 4 ed, 2006, Saunders.)

Paramedian (sagittal) dissection

Ureter

Uterine (fallopian) tube

Ovary

Ligament of ovary

Round ligament of uterus

Broad ligament (cut)

Superior pubic ramus (cut)

Inferior pubic ramus (cut)

Ischiocavernosus muscle

Body of clitoris

Labia minora

Labium majus

Rectouterine pouch (of Douglas)

Peritoneum (cut edge)

Vesicouterine pouch

Rectum

Ureter

Urinary bladder

Vagina

Pelvic diaphragm (levator ani muscle)

Deep transverse perineal muscle (cut)

External anal sphincter muscle

Median (sagittal) section

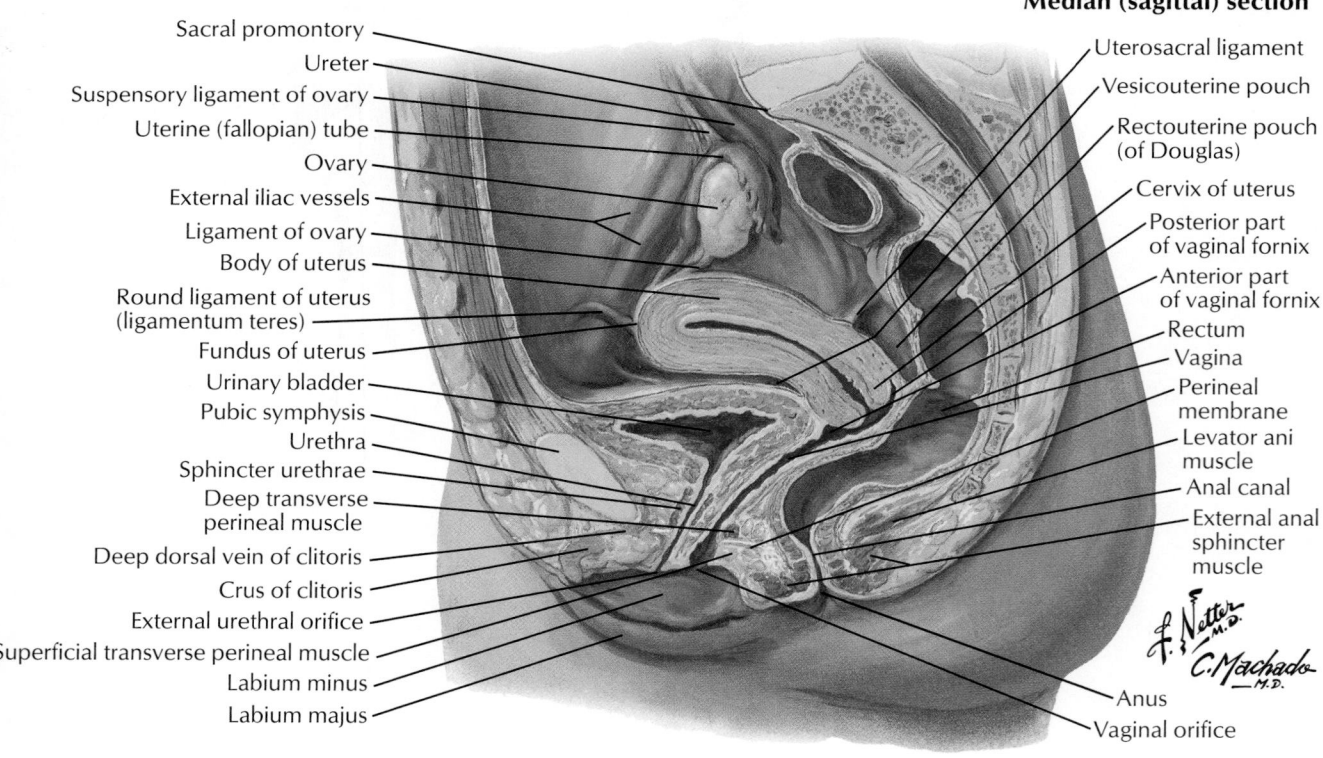

Sacral promontory

Ureter

Suspensory ligament of ovary

Uterine (fallopian) tube

Ovary

External iliac vessels

Ligament of ovary

Body of uterus

Round ligament of uterus (ligamentum teres)

Fundus of uterus

Urinary bladder

Pubic symphysis

Urethra

Sphincter urethrae

Deep transverse perineal muscle

Deep dorsal vein of clitoris

Crus of clitoris

External urethral orifice

Superficial transverse perineal muscle

Labium minus

Labium majus

Uterosacral ligament

Vesicouterine pouch

Rectouterine pouch (of Douglas)

Cervix of uterus

Posterior part of vaginal fornix

Anterior part of vaginal fornix

Rectum

Vagina

Perineal membrane

Levator ani muscle

Anal canal

External anal sphincter muscle

Anus

Vaginal orifice

Plate 360 Pelvic Viscera and Perineum: Female. (Netter: Atlas of Human Anatomy, 4 ed, 2006, Saunders.)

PART II

Alphabetic Index
Volume 2

A

AAT (alpha-1 antitrypsin) deficiency 273.4
AAV (disease) (illness) (infection) - *see*
Human immunodeficiency virus
(disease) (illness) (infection)
Abactio - *see* Abortion, induced
Abactus venter - *see* Abortion, induced
Abarognosis 781.99
Abasia (-astasia) 307.9
    atactica 781.3
    choreic 781.3
    hysterical 300.11
    paroxysmal trepidant 781.3
    spastic 781.3
    trembling 781.3
    trepidans 781.3
Abderhalden-Kaufmann-Lignac
    syndrome (cystinosis) 270.0
Abdomen, abdominal - *see also* condition
    accordion 306.4
    acute 789.0●
    angina 557.1
    burst 868.00
    convulsive equivalent (*see also*
        Epilepsy) 345.5●
    heart 746.87
    muscle deficiency syndrome 756.79
    obstipum 756.79
Abdominalgia 789.0●
    periodic 277.31
Abduction contracture, hip or other
    joint - *see* Contraction, joint
Abercrombie's syndrome (amyloid
    degeneration) 277.39
Aberrant (congenital) - *see also*
    Malposition, congenital
    adrenal gland 759.1
    blood vessel NEC 747.60
        arteriovenous NEC 747.60
        cerebrovascular 747.81
        gastrointestinal 747.61
        lower limb 747.64
        renal 747.62
        spinal 747.82
        upper limb 747.63
    breast 757.6
    endocrine gland NEC 759.2
    gastrointestinal vessel (peripheral) 747.61
    hepatic duct 751.69
    lower limb vessel (peripheral) 747.64
    pancreas 751.7
    parathyroid gland 759.2
    peripheral vascular vessel NEC 747.60
    pituitary gland (pharyngeal) 759.2
    renal blood vessel 747.62
    sebaceous glands, mucous membrane,
        mouth 750.26
    spinal vessel 747.82
    spleen 759.0
    testis (descent) 752.51
    thymus gland 759.2
    thyroid gland 759.2
    upper limb vessel (peripheral) 747.63
Aberratio
    lactis 757.6
    testis 752.51
Aberration - *see also* Anomaly
    chromosome - *see* Anomaly,
        chromosome(s)
    distantial 368.9
    mental (*see also* Disorder, mental,
        nonpsychotic) 300.9

Abetalipoproteinemia 272.5
Abionarce 780.79
Abiotrophy 799.89
Ablatio
    placentae - *see* Placenta, ablatio
    retinae (*see also* Detachment, retina)
        361.9
Ablation
    pituitary (gland) (with hypofunction)
        253.7
    placenta - *see* Placenta, ablatio
    uterus 621.8
Ablepharia, ablepharon, ablephary
    743.62
Ablepsia - *see* Blindness
Ablepsy - *see* Blindness
Ablutomania 300.3
Abnormal, abnormality, abnormalities -
    see also Anomaly
    acid-base balance 276.4
        fetus or newborn - *see* Distress, fetal
    adaptation curve, dark 368.63
    alveolar ridge 525.9
    amnion 658.9●
        affecting fetus or newborn 762.9
    anatomical relationship NEC 759.9
    apertures, congenital, diaphragm
        756.6
    auditory perception NEC 388.40
    autosomes NEC 758.5
        13 758.1
        18 758.2
        21 or 22 758.0
        D_1 758.1
        E_3 758.2
        G 758.0
    ballistocardiogram 794.39
    basal metabolic rate (BMR) 794.7
    biosynthesis, testicular androgen
        257.2
    blood level (of)
        cobalt 790.6
        copper 790.6
        iron 790.6
        lead 790.6
        lithium 790.6
        magnesium 790.6
        mineral 790.6
        zinc 790.6
    blood pressure
        elevated (without diagnosis of
            hypertension) 796.2
        low (*see also* Hypotension) 458.9
            reading (incidental) (isolated)
                (nonspecific) 796.3
    blood sugar 790.29
    bowel sounds 787.5
    breathing behavior - *see* Respiration
    caloric test 794.19
    cervix (acquired) NEC 622.9
        congenital 752.40
        in pregnancy or childbirth 654.6●
            causing obstructed labor 660.2●
                affecting fetus or newborn
                    763.1
    chemistry, blood NEC 790.6
    chest sounds 786.7
    chorion 658.9●
        affecting fetus or newborn 762.9
    chromosomal NEC 758.89
        analysis, nonspecific result 795.2
        autosomes (*see also* Abnormal,
            autosomes NEC) 758.5

Abnormal, abnormality, abnormalities
    (*Continued*)
    chromosomal NEC (*Continued*)
        fetal, (suspected) affecting
            management of pregnancy
            655.1●
        sex 758.81
    clinical findings NEC 796.4
    communication - *see* Fistula
    configuration of pupils 379.49
    coronary
        artery 746.85
        vein 746.9
    cortisol-binding globulin 255.8
    course, Eustachian tube 744.24
    creatinine clearance 794.4
    dentofacial NEC 524.9
        functional 524.50
        specified type NEC 524.89
    development, developmental NEC
        759.9
        bone 756.9
        central nervous system 742.9
    direction, teeth 524.30
    dynia (*see also* Defect, coagulation)
        286.9
    Ebstein 746.2
    echocardiogram 793.2
    echoencephalogram 794.01
    echogram NEC - *see* Findings,
        abnormal, structure
    electrocardiogram (ECG) (EKG) 794.31
    electroencephalogram (EEG) 794.02
    electromyogram (EMG) 794.17
        ocular 794.14
    electro-oculogram (EOG) 794.12
    electroretinogram (ERG) 794.11
    erythrocytes 289.9
        congenital, with perinatal jaundice
            282.9 [774.0]
    eustachian valve 746.9
    excitability under minor stress 301.9
    fat distribution 782.9
    feces 787.7
    fetal heart rate - *see* Distress, fetal
    fetus NEC
        affecting management of
            pregnancy - *see* Pregnancy,
            management affected by, fetal
        causing disproportion 653.7●
            affecting fetus or newborn 763.1
            causing obstructed labor 660.1●
                affecting fetus or newborn
                    763.1
    findings without manifest disease - *see*
        Findings, abnormal
    fluid
        amniotic 792.3
        cerebrospinal 792.0
        peritoneal 792.9
        pleural 792.9
        synovial 792.9
        vaginal 792.9
    forces of labor NEC 661.9●
        affecting fetus or newborn 763.7
    form, teeth 520.2
    function studies
        auditory 794.15
        bladder 794.9
        brain 794.00
        cardiovascular 794.30
        endocrine NEC 794.6
        kidney 794.4

◀ New ◀||| Revised ~~deleted~~ Deleted ● Use Additional Digit(s) ▨ Omit code

Abnormal, abnormality, abnormalities
  (Continued)
  function studies (Continued)
    liver 794.8
    nervous system
      central 794.00
      peripheral 794.19
    oculomotor 794.14
    pancreas 794.9
    placenta 794.9
    pulmonary 794.2
    retina 794.11
    special senses 794.19
    spleen 794.9
    thyroid 794.5
    vestibular 794.16
  gait 781.2
    hysterical 300.11
  gastrin secretion 251.5
  globulin
    cortisol-binding 255.8
    thyroid-binding 246.8
  glucagon secretion 251.4
  glucose 790.29
    in pregnancy, childbirth, or
        puerperium 648.8●
      fetus or newborn 775.0
    non-fasting 790.29
  gravitational (G) forces or states 994.9
  hair NEC 704.2
  hard tissue formation in pulp 522.3
  head movement 781.0
  heart
    rate
      fetus, affecting liveborn infant
        before the onset of labor 763.81
        during labor 763.82
        unspecified as to time of onset
            763.83
      intrauterine
        before the onset of labor 763.81
        during labor 763.82
        unspecified as to time of onset
            763.83
      newborn
        before the onset of labor 763.81
        during labor 763.82
        unspecified as to time of onset
            763.83
    shadow 793.2
    sounds NEC 785.3
  hemoglobin (see also Disease,
      hemoglobin) 282.7
    trait - see Trait, hemoglobin,
        abnormal
  hemorrhage, uterus - see Hemorrhage,
      uterus
  histology NEC 795.4
  increase in
    appetite 783.6
    development 783.9
  involuntary movement 781.0
  jaw closure 524.51
  karyotype 795.2
  knee jerk 796.1
  labor NEC 661.9●
    affecting fetus or newborn 763.7
  laboratory findings - see Findings,
      abnormal
  length, organ or site, congenital - see
      Distortion
  liver function test 790.6
  loss of height 781.91
  loss of weight 783.21

Abnormal, abnormality, abnormalities
  (Continued)
  lung shadow 793.1
  mammogram 793.80
    calcification 793.89
    calculus 793.89
    microcalcification 793.81
  Mantoux test 795.5
  membranes (fetal)
    affecting fetus or newborn 762.9
    complicating pregnancy 658.8●
  menstruation - see Menstruation
  metabolism (see also condition) 783.9
  movement 781.0
    disorder NEC 333.90
      sleep related, unspecified 780.58
      specified NEC 333.99
    head 781.0
    involuntary 781.0
    specified type NEC 333.99
  muscle contraction, localized 728.85
  myoglobin (Aberdeen) (Annapolis)
      289.9
  narrowness, eyelid 743.62
  optokinetic response 379.57
  organs or tissues of pelvis NEC
    in pregnancy or childbirth 654.9●
      affecting fetus or newborn
          763.89
      causing obstructed labor 660.2●
        affecting fetus or newborn
            763.1
  origin - see Malposition, congenital
  palmar creases 757.2
  Papanicolaou (smear)
    anus 796.70
      with
        atypical squamous cells
          cannot exclude high grade
              squamous
              intraepithelial lesion
              (ASC-H) 796.72
          of undetermined
              significance (ASC-US)
              796.71
        cytologic evidence of
            malignancy 796.76
        high grade squamous
            intraepithelial lesion
            (HGSIL) 796.74
        low grade squamous
            intraepithelial lesion
            (LGSIL) 796.73
      glandular 796.70
      specified finding NEC 796.79
    cervix 795.00
      with
        atypical squamous cells
          cannot exclude high grade
              squamous
              intraepithelial lesion
              (ASC-H) 795.02
          of undetermined
              significance (ASC-US)
              795.01
        cytologic evidence of
            malignancy 795.06
        high grade squamous
            intraepithelial lesion
            (HGSIL) 795.04
        low grade squamous
            intraepithelial lesion
            (LGSIL) 795.03
      nonspecific finding NEC 795.09

Abnormal, abnormality, abnormalities
  (Continued)
  Papanicolaou (smear) (Continued)
    other site 796.9
    vagina 795.10
      with
        atypical squamous cells
          cannot exclude high grade
              squamous
              intraepithelial lesion
              (ASC-H) 795.12
          of undetermined
              significance (ASC-US)
              795.11
        cytologic evidence of
            malignancy 795.16
        high grade squamous
            intraepithelial lesion
            (HGSIL)795.14
        low grade squamous
            intraepithelial lesion
            (LGSIL) 795.13
      glandular 795.10
      specified finding NEC 795.19
  parturition
    affecting fetus or newborn 763.9
    mother - see Delivery, complicated
  pelvis (bony) - see Deformity, pelvis
  percussion, chest 786.7
  periods (grossly) (see also
      Menstruation) 626.9
  phonocardiogram 794.39
  placenta - see Placenta, abnormal
  plantar reflex 796.1
  plasma protein - see Deficiency, plasma,
      protein
  pleural folds 748.8
  position - see also Malposition
    gravid uterus 654.4●
      causing obstructed labor 660.2●
        affecting fetus or newborn
            763.1
  posture NEC 781.92
  presentation (fetus) - see Presentation,
      fetus, abnormal
  product of conception NEC 631
  puberty - see Puberty
  pulmonary
    artery 747.3
    function, newborn 770.89
    test results 794.2
    ventilation, newborn 770.89
      hyperventilation 786.01
  pulsations in neck 785.1
  pupil reflexes 379.40
  quality of milk 676.8●
  radiological examination 793.99
    abdomen NEC 793.6
    biliary tract 793.3
    breast 793.89
      mammogram NOS 793.80
      mammographic
        calcification 793.89
        calculus 793.89
        microcalcification 793.81
    gastrointestinal tract 793.4
    genitourinary organs 793.5
    head 793.0
    image test inconclusive due to
        excess body fat 793.91
    intrathoracic organ NEC 793.2
    lung (field) 793.1
    musculoskeletal system 793.7
    retroperitoneum 793.6

Abnormal, abnormality, abnormalities
   (Continued)
   radiological examination *(Continued)*
      skin and subcutaneous tissue 793.99
      skull 793.0
   red blood cells 790.09
      morphology 790.09
      volume 790.09
   reflex NEC 796.1
   renal function test 794.4
   respiration signs - *see* Respiration
   response to nerve stimulation 794.10
   retinal correspondence 368.34
   rhythm, heart - *see also* Arrhythmia
      fetus - *see* Distress, fetal
   saliva 792.4
   scan
      brain 794.09
      kidney 794.4
      liver 794.8
      lung 794.2
      thyroid 794.5
   secretion
      gastrin 251.5
      glucagon 251.4
   semen 792.2
   serum level (of)
      acid phosphatase 790.5
      alkaline phosphatase 790.5
      amylase 790.5
      enzymes NEC 790.5
      lipase 790.5
   shape
      cornea 743.41
      gallbladder 751.69
      gravid uterus 654.4●
         affecting fetus or newborn 763.89
         causing obstructed labor 660.2●
            affecting fetus or newborn 763.1
      head (*see also* Anomaly, skull) 756.0
      organ or site, congenital NEC - *see*
         Distortion
   sinus venosus 747.40
   size
      fetus, complicating delivery 653.5●
         causing obstructed labor 660.1●
      gallbladder 751.69
      head (*see also* Anomaly, skull) 756.0
      organ or site, congenital NEC - *see*
         Distortion
      teeth 520.2
   skin and appendages, congenital NEC
      757.9
   soft parts of pelvis - *see* Abnormal,
      organs or tissues of pelvis
   spermatozoa 792.2
   sputum (amount) (color) (excessive)
      (odor) (purulent) 786.4
   stool NEC 787.7
      bloody 578.1
         occult 792.1
      bulky 787.7
      color (dark) (light) 792.1
      content (fat) (mucus) (pus) 792.1
      occult blood 792.1
   synchondrosis 756.9
   test results without manifest disease -
      see Findings, abnormal
   thebesian valve 746.9
   thermography - *see* Findings, abnormal,
      structure
   threshold, cones or rods (eye) 368.63
   thyroid-binding globulin 246.8
   thyroid product 246.8
   toxicology (findings) NEC 796.0
   tracheal cartilage (congenital) 748.3

Abnormal, abnormality, abnormalities
   (Continued)
   transport protein 273.8
   ultrasound results - *see* Findings,
      abnormal, structure
   umbilical cord
      affecting fetus or newborn 762.6
      complicating delivery 663.9●
      specified NEC 663.8●
   union
      cricoid cartilage and thyroid
         cartilage 748.3
      larynx and trachea 748.3
      thyroid cartilage and hyoid bone
         748.3
   urination NEC 788.69
      psychogenic 306.53
      stream
         intermittent 788.61
         slowing 788.62
         splitting 788.61
         weak 788.62
      urgency 788.63
   urine (constituents) NEC 791.9
   uterine hemorrhage (*see also*
      Hemorrhage, uterus) 626.9
      climacteric 627.0
      postmenopausal 627.1
   vagina (acquired) (congenital)
      in pregnancy or childbirth 654.7●
         affecting fetus or newborn 763.89
         causing obstructed labor 660.2●
            affecting fetus or newborn
               763.1
   vascular sounds 785.9
   vectorcardiogram 794.39
   visually evoked potential (VEP)
      794.13
   vulva (acquired) (congenital)
      in pregnancy or childbirth 654.8●
         affecting fetus or newborn 763.89
         causing obstructed labor 660.2●
            affecting fetus or newborn 763.1
   weight
      gain 783.1
         of pregnancy 646.1●
            with hypertension - *see*
               Toxemia, of pregnancy
      loss 783.21
   x-ray examination - *see* Abnormal,
      radiological examination
Abnormally formed uterus - *see* Anomaly,
   uterus
Abnormity (any organ or part) - *see*
   Anomaly
ABO
   hemolytic disease 773.1
   incompatibility (due to transfusion of
      blood or blood products) ~~reaction~~
      ~~999.6~~ ◀▥
      with hemolytic transfusion reaction
         (HTR) (not specified as acute
         or delayed) 999.61 ◀
      24 hours or more after
         transfusion 999.63 ◀
      acute 999.62 ◀
      delayed 999.63 ◀
      less than 24 hours after
         transfusion 999.62 ◀
      unspecified time after transfusion
         999.61 ◀
   reaction 999.60 ◀
      specified NEC 999.69 ◀
Abocclusion 524.20
Abolition, language 784.69

Aborter, habitual or recurrent NEC
   without current pregnancy 629.81
   current abortion (*see also* Abortion,
      spontaneous) 634.9●
      affecting fetus or newborn 761.8
   observation in current pregnancy
      646.3●
Abortion (complete) (incomplete)
   (inevitable) (with retained products
   of conception) 637.9●

Note: Use the following fifth-digit
subclassification with categories 634-637:

0   unspecified
1   incomplete
2   complete

---

   with
      complication(s) (any) following
         previous abortion - *see*
         category 639
      damage to pelvic organ (laceration)
         (rupture) (tear) 637.2●
      embolism (air) (amniotic fluid)
         (blood clot) (pulmonary)
         (pyemic) (septic) (soap) 637.6●
      genital tract and pelvic infection
         637.0●
      hemorrhage, delayed or excessive
         637.1●
      metabolic disorder 637.4●
      renal failure (acute) 637.3●
      sepsis (genital tract) (pelvic organ)
         637.0●
         urinary tract 637.7●
      shock (postoperative) (septic)
         637.5●
      specified complication NEC 637.7●
      toxemia 637.3●
      unspecified complication(s) 637.8●
      urinary tract infection 637.7●
   accidental - *see* Abortion, spontaneous
   artificial - *see* Abortion, induced
   attempted (failed) - *see* Abortion, failed
   criminal - *see* Abortion, illegal
   early - *see* Abortion, spontaneous
   elective - *see* Abortion, legal
   failed (legal) 638.9
      with
         damage to pelvic organ
            (laceration) (rupture) (tear)
            638.2
         embolism (air) (amniotic fluid)
            (blood clot) (pulmonary)
            (pyemic) (septic) (soap)
            638.6
         genital tract and pelvic infection
            638.0
         hemorrhage, delayed or excessive
            638.1
         metabolic disorder 638.4
         renal failure (acute) 638.3
         sepsis (genital tract) (pelvic
            organ) 638.0
            urinary tract 638.7
         shock (postoperative) (septic)
            638.5
         specified complication NEC 638.7
         toxemia 638.3
         unspecified complication(s) 638.8
         urinary tract infection 638.7
   fetal indication - *see* Abortion, legal
   fetus 779.6
   following threatened abortion - *see*
      Abortion, by type

◀ New   ◀▥ Revised   ~~deleted~~ Deleted   ● Use Additional Digit(s)   ▥ Omit code

Abortion (*Continued*)
habitual or recurrent (care during
pregnancy) 646.3 ●
with current abortion (*see also*
Abortion, spontaneous) 634.9 ●
affecting fetus or newborn 761.8
without current pregnancy 629.81
homicidal - *see* Abortion, illegal
illegal 636.9 ●
with
damage to pelvic organ
(laceration) (rupture)
(tear) 636.2 ●
embolism (air) (amniotic fluid)
(blood clot) (pulmonary)
(pyemic) (septic) (soap)
636.6 ●
genital tract and pelvic infection
636.0 ●
hemorrhage, delayed or excessive
636.1 ●
metabolic disorder 636.4 ●
renal failure 636.3 ●
sepsis (genital tract) (pelvic
organ) 636.0 ●
urinary tract 636.7 ●
shock (postoperative) (septic)
636.5 ●
specified complication NEC
636.7 ●
toxemia 636.3 ●
unspecified complication(s)
636.8 ●
urinary tract infection 636.7 ●
fetus 779.6
induced 637.9 ●
illegal - *see* Abortion, illegal
legal indications - *see* Abortion, legal
medical indications - *see* Abortion,
legal
therapeutic - *see* Abortion, legal
late - *see* Abortion, spontaneous
legal (legal indication) (medical
indication) (under medical
supervision) 635.9 ●
with
damage to pelvic organ
(laceration) (rupture)
(tear) 635.2 ●
embolism (air) (amniotic fluid)
(blood clot) (pulmonary)
(pyemic) (septic) (soap)
635.6 ●
genital tract and pelvic infection
635.0 ●
hemorrhage, delayed or excessive
635.1 ●
metabolic disorder 635.4 ●
renal failure (acute) 635.3 ●
sepsis (genital tract) (pelvic
organ) 635.0 ●
urinary tract 635.7 ●
shock (postoperative) (septic)
635.5 ●
specified complication NEC
635.7 ●
toxemia 635.3 ●
unspecified complication(s)
635.8 ●
urinary tract infection 635.7 ●
fetus 779.6
medical indication - *see* Abortion, legal
mental hygiene problem - *see* Abortion,
legal
missed 632

Abortion (*Continued*)
operative - *see* Abortion, legal
psychiatric indication - *see* Abortion,
legal
recurrent - *see* Abortion, spontaneous
self-induced - *see* Abortion, illegal
septic - *see* Abortion, by type, with sepsis
spontaneous 634.9 ●
with
damage to pelvic organ
(laceration) (rupture)
(tear) 634.2 ●
embolism (air) (amniotic fluid)
(blood clot) (pulmonary)
(pyemic) (septic) (soap)
634.6 ●
genital tract and pelvic infection
634.0 ●
hemorrhage, delayed or excessive
634.1 ●
metabolic disorder 634.4 ●
renal failure 634.3 ●
sepsis (genital tract) (pelvic
organ) 634.0 ●
urinary tract 634.7 ●
shock (postoperative) (septic)
634.5 ●
specified complication NEC
634.7 ●
toxemia 634.3 ●
unspecified complication(s)
634.8 ●
urinary tract infection 634.7 ●
fetus 761.8
threatened 640.0 ●
affecting fetus or newborn 762.1
surgical - *see* Abortion, legal
therapeutic - *see* Abortion, legal
threatened 640.0 ●
affecting fetus or newborn 762.1
tubal - *see* Pregnancy, tubal
voluntary - *see* Abortion, legal
Abortus fever 023.9
Aboulomania 301.6
Abrachia 755.20
Abrachiatism 755.20
Abrachiocephalia 759.89
Abrachiocephalus 759.89
Abrami's disease (acquired hemolytic
jaundice) 283.9
Abramov-Fiedler myocarditis (acute
isolated myocarditis) 422.91
Abrasion - *see also* Injury, superficial, by
site
cornea 918.1
dental 521.20
extending into
dentine 521.22
pulp 521.23
generalized 521.25
limited to enamel 521.21
localized 521.24
teeth, tooth (dentifrice) (habitual) (hard
tissues) (occupational) (ritual)
(traditional) (wedge defect) (*see*
also Abrasion, dental) 521.20
Abrikossov's tumor (M9580/0) - *see also*
Neoplasm, connective tissue, benign
malignant (M9580/3) - *see* Neoplasm,
connective tissue, malignant
Abrism 988.8
Abruption, placenta - *see* Placenta,
abruptio
Abruptio placentae - *see* Placenta,
abruptio

Abscess (acute) (chronic) (infectional)
(lymphangitic) (metastatic)
(multiple) (pyogenic) (septic) (with
lymphangitis) (*see also* Cellulitis)
682.9
abdomen, abdominal
cavity 567.22
wall 682.2
abdominopelvic 567.22
accessory sinus (chronic) (*see also*
Sinusitis) 473.9
adrenal (capsule) (gland) 255.8
alveolar 522.5
with sinus 522.7
amebic 006.3
bladder 006.8
brain (with liver or lung abscess)
006.5
liver (without mention of brain or
lung abscess) 006.3
with
brain abscess (and lung
abscess) 006.5
lung abscess 006.4
lung (with liver abscess) 006.4
with brain abscess 006.5
seminal vesicle 006.8
specified site NEC 006.8
spleen 006.8
anaerobic 040.0
ankle 682.6
anorectal 566
antecubital space 682.3
antrum (chronic) (Highmore)
(*see also* Sinusitis, maxillary)
473.0
anus 566
apical (tooth) 522.5
with sinus (alveolar) 522.7
appendix 540.1
areola (acute) (chronic) (nonpuerperal)
611.0
puerperal, postpartum 675.1 ●
arm (any part, above wrist) 682.3
artery (wall) 447.2
atheromatous 447.2
auditory canal (external) 380.10
auricle (ear) (staphylococcal)
(streptococcal) 380.10
axilla, axillary (region) 682.3
lymph gland or node 683
back (any part) 682.2
Bartholin's gland 616.3
with
abortion - *see* Abortion, by type,
with sepsis
ectopic pregnancy (*see also*
categories 633.0-633.9)
639.0
molar pregnancy (*see also*
categories 630-632)
639.0
complicating pregnancy or
puerperium 646.6 ●
following
abortion 639.0
ectopic or molar pregnancy
639.0
bartholinian 616.3
Bezold's 383.01
bile, biliary, duct or tract (*see also*
Cholecystitis) 576.8
bilharziasis 120.1
bladder (wall) 595.89
amebic 006.8

A

Abscess *(Continued)*
  bone (subperiosteal) *(see also*
      Osteomyelitis)* 730.0●
    accessory sinus (chronic) *(see also*
        Sinusitis)* 473.9
    acute 730.0●
    chronic or old 730.1●
    jaw (lower) (upper) 526.4
    mastoid - *see* Mastoiditis, acute
    petrous *(see also* Petrositis)
        383.20
    spinal (tuberculous) *(see also*
        Tuberculosis)* 015.0●
        [730.88]
      nontuberculous 730.08
  bowel 569.5
  brain (any part) 324.0
    amebic (with liver or lung abscess)
        006.5
    cystic 324.0
    late effect - *see* category 326
    otogenic 324.0
    tuberculous *(see also* Tuberculosis)
        013.3●
  breast (acute) (chronic) (nonpuerperal)
        611.0
    newborn 771.5
    puerperal, postpartum 675.1●
    tuberculous *(see also* Tuberculosis)
        017.9●
  broad ligament (chronic) *(see also*
        Disease, pelvis, inflammatory)*
        614.4
    acute 614.3
  Brodie's (chronic) (localized) *(see also*
        Osteomyelitis)* 730.1●
  bronchus 519.19
  buccal cavity 528.3
  bulbourethral gland 597.0
  bursa 727.89
    pharyngeal 478.29
  buttock 682.5
  canaliculus, breast 611.0
  canthus 372.20
  cartilage 733.99
  cecum 569.5
    with appendicitis 540.1
  cerebellum, cerebellar 324.0
    late effect - *see* category 326
  cerebral (embolic) 324.0
    late effect - *see* category 326
  cervical (neck region) 682.1
    lymph gland or node 683
    stump *(see also* Cervicitis)* 616.0
  cervix (stump) (uteri) *(see also*
        Cervicitis)* 616.0
  cheek, external 682.0
    inner 528.3
  chest 510.9
    with fistula 510.0
    wall 682.2
  chin 682.0
  choroid 363.00
  ciliary body 364.3
  circumtonsillar 475
  cold (tuberculous) - *see also*
        Tuberculosis, abscess
    articular - *see* Tuberculosis, joint
  colon (wall) 569.5
  colostomy or enterostomy 569.61
  conjunctiva 372.00
  connective tissue NEC 682.9
  cornea 370.55
    with ulcer 370.00

Abscess *(Continued)*
  corpus
    cavernosum 607.2
    luteum *(see also* Salpingo-oophoritis)
        614.2
  Cowper's gland 597.0
  cranium 324.0
  cul-de-sac (Douglas') (posterior) *(see*
        also Disease, pelvis,
        inflammatory)* 614.4
    acute 614.3
  dental 522.5
    with sinus (alveolar) 522.7
  dentoalveolar 522.5
    with sinus (alveolar) 522.7
  diaphragm, diaphragmatic 567.22
  digit NEC 681.9
  Douglas' cul-de-sac or pouch *(see also*
        Disease, pelvis, inflammatory)*
        614.4
    acute 614.3
  Dubois' 090.5
  ductless gland 259.8
  ear
    acute 382.00
    external 380.10
    inner 386.30
    middle - *see* Otitis media
  elbow 682.3
  endamebic - *see* Abscess, amebic
  entamebic - *see* Abscess, amebic
  enterostomy 569.61
  epididymis 604.0
  epidural 324.9
    brain 324.0
    late effect - *see* category 326
    spinal cord 324.1
  epiglottis 478.79
  epiploon, epiploic 567.22
  erysipelatous *(see also* Erysipelas)* 035
  esophagostomy 530.86
  esophagus 530.19
  ethmoid (bone) (chronic) (sinus) *(see*
        also Sinusitis, ethmoidal)* 473.2
  external auditory canal 380.10
  extradural 324.9
    brain 324.0
    late effect - *see* category 326
    spinal cord 324.1
  extraperitoneal - *see* Abscess,
        peritoneum
  eye 360.00
  eyelid 373.13
  face (any part, except eye) 682.0
  fallopian tube *(see also* Salpingo-
        oophoritis)* 614.2
  fascia 728.89
  fauces 478.29
  fecal 569.5
  femoral (region) 682.6
  filaria, filarial *(see also* Infestation,
        filarial)* 125.9
  finger (any) (intrathecal) (periosteal)
        (subcutaneous) (subcuticular)
        681.00
  fistulous NEC 682.9
  flank 682.2
  foot (except toe) 682.7
  forearm 682.3
  forehead 682.0
  frontal (sinus) (chronic) *(see also*
        Sinusitis, frontal)* 473.1
  gallbladder *(see also* Cholecystitis,
        acute)* 575.0

Abscess *(Continued)*
  gastric 535.0●
  genital organ or tract NEC
    female 616.9
      with
        abortion - *see* Abortion, by
            type, with sepsis
        ectopic pregnancy *(see also*
            categories 633.0-633.9)*
            639.0
        molar pregnancy *(see also*
            categories 630-632)*
            639.0
      following
        abortion 639.0
        ectopic or molar pregnancy
            639.0
      puerperal, postpartum,
            childbirth 670.8●
    male 608.4
  genitourinary system, tuberculous *(see*
        also Tuberculosis)* 016.9●
  gingival 523.30
  gland, glandular (lymph) (acute) NEC
        683
  glottis 478.79
  gluteal (region) 682.5
  gonorrheal NEC *(see also* Gonococcus)*
        098.0
  groin 682.2
  gum 523.30
  hand (except finger or thumb) 682.4
  head (except face) 682.8
  heart 429.89
  heel 682.7
  helminthic *(see also* Infestation, by
        specific parasite)* 128.9
  hepatic 572.0
    amebic *(see also* Abscess, liver,
        amebic)* 006.3
    duct 576.8
  hip 682.6
    tuberculous (active) *(see also*
        Tuberculosis)* 015.1●
  ileocecal 540.1
  ileostomy (bud) 569.61
  iliac (region) 682.2
    fossa 540.1
  iliopsoas 567.31
    tuberculous *(see also* Tuberculosis)
        015.0● *[730.88]*
  infraclavicular (fossa) 682.3
  inguinal (region) 682.2
    lymph gland or node 683
  intersphincteric (anus) 566
  intestine, intestinal 569.5
    rectal 566
  intra-abdominal *(see also* Abscess,
        peritoneum)* 567.22
    postoperative 998.59
  intracranial 324.0
    late effect - *see* category 326
  intramammary - *see* Abscess, breast
  intramastoid *(see also* Mastoiditis,
        acute)* 383.00
  intraorbital 376.01
  intraperitoneal 567.22
  intraspinal 324.1
    late effect - *see* category 326
  intratonsillar 475
  iris 364.3
  ischiorectal 566
  jaw (bone) (lower) (upper) 526.4
    skin 682.0

◀ New   ◀▥ Revised   ~~deleted~~ Deleted   ● Use Additional Digit(s)   ▢ Omit code

Abscess *(Continued)*
  joint *(see also* Arthritis, pyogenic)
    711.0●
    vertebral (tuberculous) *(see also*
      Tuberculosis) 015.0● *[730.88]*
      nontuberculous 724.8
  kidney 590.2
    with
      abortion - *see* Abortion, by type,
        with urinary tract infection
      calculus 592.0
      ectopic pregnancy *(see also*
        categories 633.0-633.9)
        639.8
      molar pregnancy *(see also*
        categories 630-632) 639.8
      complicating pregnancy or
        puerperium 646.6●
        affecting fetus or newborn
          760.1
    following
      abortion 639.8
      ectopic or molar pregnancy
        639.8
  knee 682.6
    joint 711.06
    tuberculous (active) *(see also*
      Tuberculosis) 015.2●
  labium (majus) (minus) 616.4
    complicating pregnancy, childbirth,
      or puerperium 646.6●
  lacrimal (passages) (sac) *(see also*
    Dacryocystitis) 375.30
    caruncle 375.30
    gland *(see also* Dacryoadenitis)
      375.00
  lacunar 597.0
  larynx 478.79
  lateral (alveolar) 522.5
    with sinus 522.7
  leg, except foot 682.6
  lens 360.00
  lid 373.13
  lingual 529.0
    tonsil 475
  lip 528.5
  Littre's gland 597.0
  liver 572.0
    amebic 006.3
      with
        brain abscess (and lung
          abscess) 006.5
        lung abscess 006.4
      due to Entamoeba histolytica 006.3
    dysenteric *(see also* Abscess, liver,
      amebic) 006.3
    pyogenic 572.0
    tropical *(see also* Abscess, liver,
      amebic) 006.3
  loin (region) 682.2
  lumbar (tuberculous) *(see also*
    Tuberculosis) 015.0● *[730.88]*
    nontuberculous 682.2
  lung (miliary) (putrid) 513.0
    amebic (with liver abscess) 006.4
      with brain abscess 006.5
  lymph, lymphatic, gland or node
    (acute) 683
    any site, except mesenteric 683
    mesentery 289.2
  lymphangitic, acute - *see* Cellulitis
  malar 526.4
  mammary gland - *see* Abscess, breast
  marginal (anus) 566

Abscess *(Continued)*
  mastoid (process) *(see also* Mastoiditis,
    acute) 383.00
    subperiosteal 383.01
  maxilla, maxillary 526.4
    molar (tooth) 522.5
      with sinus 522.7
    premolar 522.5
    sinus (chronic) *(see also* Sinusitis,
      maxillary) 473.0
  mediastinum 513.1
  meibomian gland 373.12
  meninges *(see also* Meningitis) 320.9
  mesentery, mesenteric 567.22
  mesosalpinx *(see also* Salpingo-
    oophoritis) 614.2
  milk 675.1●
  Monro's (psoriasis) 696.1
  mons pubis 682.2
  mouth (floor) 528.3
  multiple sites NEC 682.9
  mural 682.2
  muscle 728.89
    psoas 567.31
  myocardium 422.92
  nabothian (follicle) *(see also* Cervicitis)
    616.0
  nail (chronic) (with lymphangitis) 681.9
    finger 681.02
    toe 681.11
  nasal (fossa) (septum) 478.19
    sinus (chronic) *(see also* Sinusitis)
      473.9
  nasopharyngeal 478.29
  nates 682.5
  navel 682.2
    newborn NEC 771.4
  neck (region) 682.1
    lymph gland or node 683
  nephritic *(see also* Abscess, kidney)
    590.2
  nipple 611.0
    puerperal, postpartum 675.0●
  nose (septum) 478.19
    external 682.0
  omentum 567.22
  operative wound 998.59
  orbit, orbital 376.01
  ossifluent - *see* Abscess, bone
  ovary, ovarian (corpus luteum) *(see also*
    Salpingo-oophoritis) 614.2
  oviduct *(see also* Salpingo-oophoritis)
    614.2
  palate (soft) 528.3
    hard 526.4
  palmar (space) 682.4
  pancreas (duct) 577.0
  paradontal 523.30
  parafrenal 607.2
  parametric, parametrium (chronic) *(see*
    also Disease, pelvis,
    inflammatory) 614.4
    acute 614.3
  paranephric 590.2
  parapancreatic 577.0
  parapharyngeal 478.22
  pararectal 566
  parasinus *(see also* Sinusitis) 473.9
  parauterine *(see also* Disease, pelvis,
    inflammatory) 614.4
    acute 614.3
  paravaginal *(see also* Vaginitis) 616.10
  parietal region 682.8
  parodontal 523.30

Abscess *(Continued)*
  parotid (duct) (gland) 527.3
    region 528.3
  parumbilical 682.2
    newborn 771.4
  pectoral (region) 682.2
  pelvirectal 567.22
  pelvis, pelvic
    female (chronic) *(see also* Disease,
      pelvis, inflammatory) 614.4
      acute 614.3
    male, peritoneal (cellular tissue) - *see*
      Abscess, peritoneum
    tuberculous *(see also* Tuberculosis)
      016.9●
  penis 607.2
    gonococcal (acute) 098.0
      chronic or duration of 2 months
        or over 098.2
  perianal 566
  periapical 522.5
    with sinus (alveolar) 522.7
  periappendiceal 540.1
  pericecal 540.1
  pericardial 420.99
  pericemental 523.30
  pericholecystic *(see also* Cholecystitis,
    acute) 575.0
  pericoronal 523.30
  peridental 523.30
  perigastric 535.0●
  perimetric *(see also* Disease, pelvis,
    inflammatory) 614.4
    acute 614.3
  perinephric, perinephritic *(see also*
    Abscess, kidney) 590.2
  perineum, perineal (superficial) 682.2
    deep (with urethral involvement)
      597.0
    urethra 597.0
  periodontal (parietal) 523.31
    apical 522.5
  periosteum, periosteal *(see also*
    Periostitis) 730.3●
    with osteomyelitis *(see also*
      Osteomyelitis) 730.2●
      acute or subacute 730.0●
      chronic or old 730.1●
  peripleuritic 510.9
    with fistula 510.0
  periproctic 566
  periprostatic 601.2
  perirectal (staphylococcal) 566
  perirenal (tissue) *(see also* Abscess,
    kidney) 590.2
  perisinuous (nose) *(see also* Sinusitis)
    473.9
  peritoneum, peritoneal (perforated)
    (ruptured) 567.22
    with
      abortion - *see* Abortion, by type,
        with sepsis
      appendicitis 540.1
      ectopic pregnancy *(see also*
        categories 633.0-633.9)
        639.0
      molar pregnancy *(see also*
        categories 630-632) 639.0
    following
      abortion 639.0
      ectopic or molar pregnancy 639.0
    pelvic, female *(see also* Disease,
      pelvis, inflammatory) 614.4
      acute 614.3

Abscess *(Continued)*
  umbilicus NEC 682.2
    newborn 771.4
  upper arm 682.3
  upper respiratory 478.9
  urachus 682.2
  urethra (gland) 597.0
  urinary 597.0
  uterus, uterine (wall) *(see also* Endometritis) 615.9
    ligament *(see also* Disease, pelvis, inflammatory) 614.4
      acute 614.3
    neck *(see also* Cervicitis) 616.0
  uvula 528.3
  vagina (wall) *(see also* Vaginitis) 616.10
  vaginorectal *(see also* Vaginitis) 616.10
  vas deferens 608.4
  vermiform appendix 540.1
  vertebra (column) (tuberculous) *(see also* Tuberculosis) 015.0● *[730.88]*
    nontuberculous 730.0●
  vesical 595.89
  vesicouterine pouch *(see also* Disease, pelvis, inflammatory) 614.4
  vitreous (humor) (pneumococcal) 360.04
  vocal cord 478.5
  von Bezold's 383.01
  vulva 616.4
    complicating pregnancy, childbirth, or puerperium 646.6●
  vulvovaginal gland *(see also* Vaginitis) 616.3
  web-space 682.4
  wrist 682.4
Absence (organ or part) (complete or partial)
  acoustic nerve 742.8
  adrenal (gland) (congenital) 759.1
    acquired V45.79
  albumin (blood) 273.8
  alimentary tract (complete) (congenital) (partial) 751.8
    lower 751.5
    upper 750.8
  alpha-fucosidase 271.8
  alveolar process (acquired) 525.8
    congenital 750.26
  anus, anal (canal) (congenital) 751.2
  aorta (congenital) 747.22
  aortic valve (congenital) 746.89
  appendix, congenital 751.2
  arm (acquired) V49.60
    above elbow V49.66
    below elbow V49.65
    congenital *(see also* Deformity, reduction, upper limb) 755.20
      lower - *see* Absence, forearm, congenital
      upper (complete) (partial) (with absence of distal elements, incomplete) 755.24
        with
          complete absence of distal elements 755.21
          forearm (incomplete) 755.23
  artery (congenital) (peripheral) NEC *(see also* Anomaly, peripheral vascular system) 747.60
    brain 747.81
    cerebral 747.81
    coronary 746.85

Absence *(Continued)*
  artery NEC *(Continued)*
    pulmonary 747.3
    umbilical 747.5
  atrial septum 745.69
  auditory canal (congenital) (external) 744.01
  auricle (ear) (with stenosis or atresia of auditory canal), congenital 744.01
  bile, biliary duct (common) or passage (congenital) 751.61
  bladder (acquired) V45.74
    congenital 753.8
  bone (congenital) NEC 756.9
    marrow 284.9
      acquired (secondary) 284.89
      congenital 284.09
      hereditary 284.09
      idiopathic 284.9
    skull 756.0
  bowel sounds 787.5
  brain 740.0
    specified part 742.2
  breast(s) (acquired) V45.71
    congenital 757.6
  broad ligament (congenital) 752.19
  bronchus (congenital) 748.3
  calvarium, calvaria (skull) 756.0
  canaliculus lacrimalis, congenital 743.65
  carpal(s) (congenital) (complete) (partial) (with absence of distal elements, incomplete) *(see also* Deformity, reduction, upper limb) 755.28
    with complete absence of distal elements 755.21
  cartilage 756.9
  caudal spine 756.13
  cecum (acquired) (postoperative) (posttraumatic) V45.72
    congenital 751.2
  cementum 520.4
  cerebellum (congenital) (vermis) 742.2
  cervix (acquired) (uteri) V88.01
    with remaining uterus V88.03
    and uterus V88.01
    congenital 752.43 ◀▥
  chin, congenital 744.89
  cilia (congenital) 743.63
    acquired 374.89
  circulatory system, part NEC 747.89
  clavicle 755.51
  clitoris (congenital) 752.49
  coccyx, congenital 756.13
  cold sense *(see also* Disturbance, sensation) 782.0
  colon (acquired) (postoperative) V45.72
    congenital 751.2
  congenital
    lumen - *see* Atresia
    organ or site NEC - *see* Agenesis
    septum - *see* Imperfect, closure
  corpus callosum (congenital) 742.2
  cricoid cartilage 748.3
  diaphragm (congenital) (with hernia) 756.6
    with obstruction 756.6
  digestive organ(s) or tract, congenital (complete) (partial) 751.8
    acquired V45.79
    lower 751.5
    upper 750.8

Absence *(Continued)*
  ductus arteriosus 747.89
  duodenum (acquired) (postoperative) V45.72
    congenital 751.1
  ear, congenital 744.09
    acquired V45.79
    auricle 744.01
    external 744.01
    inner 744.05
    lobe, lobule 744.21
    middle, except ossicles 744.03
      ossicles 744.04
    ossicles 744.04
  ejaculatory duct (congenital) 752.89
  endocrine gland NEC (congenital) 759.2
  epididymis (congenital) 752.89
    acquired V45.77
  epiglottis, congenital 748.3
  epileptic (atonic) (typical) *(see also* Epilepsy) 345.0●
  erythrocyte 284.9
  erythropoiesis 284.9
    congenital 284.01
  esophagus (congenital) 750.3
  eustachian tube (congenital) 744.24
  extremity (acquired)
    congenital *(see also* Deformity, reduction) 755.4
    lower V49.70
    upper V49.60
  extrinsic muscle, eye 743.69
  eye (acquired) V45.78
    adnexa (congenital) 743.69
    congenital 743.00
    muscle (congenital) 743.69
  eyelid (fold), congenital 743.62
    acquired 374.89
  face
    bones NEC 756.0
    specified part NEC 744.89
  fallopian tube(s) (acquired) V45.77
    congenital 752.19
  femur, congenital (complete) (partial) (with absence of distal elements, incomplete) *(see also* Deformity, reduction, lower limb) 755.34
    with
      complete absence of distal elements 755.31
      tibia and fibula (incomplete) 755.33
  fibrin 790.92
  fibrinogen (congenital) 286.3
    acquired 286.6
  fibula, congenital (complete) (partial) (with absence of distal elements, incomplete) *(see also* Deformity, reduction, lower limb) 755.37
    with
      complete absence of distal elements 755.31
      tibia 755.35
        with
          complete absence of distal elements 755.31
          femur (incomplete) 755.33
            with complete absence of distal elements 755.31

Absence (*Continued*)
finger (acquired) V49.62
    congenital (complete) (partial) (*see also* Deformity, reduction, upper limb) 755.29
      meaning all fingers (complete) (partial) 755.21
      transverse 755.21
fissures of lungs (congenital) 748.5
foot (acquired) V49.73
    congenital (complete) 755.31
forearm (acquired) V49.65
    congenital (complete) (partial) (with absence of distal elements, incomplete) (*see also* Deformity, reduction, upper limb) 755.25
      with
        complete absence of distal elements (hand and fingers) 755.21
        humerus (incomplete) 755.23
fovea centralis 743.55
fucosidase 271.8
gallbladder (acquired) V45.79
    congenital 751.69
gamma globulin (blood) 279.00
genital organs
    acquired V45.77
    congenital
      female 752.89
        external 752.49
        internal NEC 752.89
      male 752.89
        penis 752.69
genitourinary organs, congenital NEC 752.89
glottis 748.3
gonadal, congenital NEC 758.6
hair (congenital) 757.4
    acquired - *see* Alopecia
hand (acquired) V49.63
    congenital (complete) (*see also* Deformity, reduction, upper limb) 755.21
heart (congenital) 759.89
    acquired - *see* Status, organ replacement
heat sense (*see also* Disturbance, sensation) 782.0
humerus, congenital (complete) (partial) (with absence of distal elements, incomplete) (*see also* Deformity, reduction, upper limb) 755.24
    with
      complete absence of distal elements 755.21
      radius and ulna (incomplete) 755.23
hymen (congenital) 752.49
ileum (acquired) (postoperative) (posttraumatic) V45.72
    congenital 751.1
immunoglobulin, isolated NEC 279.03
    IgA 279.01
    IgG 279.03
    IgM 279.02
incus (acquired) 385.24
    congenital 744.04
internal ear (congenital) 744.05
intestine (acquired) (small) V45.72
    congenital 751.1
      large 751.2

Absence (*Continued*)
intestine (*Continued*)
    large V45.72
      congenital 751.2
iris (congenital) 743.45
jaw - *see* Absence, mandible
jejunum (acquired) V45.72
    congenital 751.1
joint, congenital NEC 755.8
kidney(s) (acquired) V45.73
    congenital 753.0
labium (congenital) (majus) (minus) 752.49
labyrinth, membranous 744.05
lacrimal apparatus (congenital) 743.65
larynx (congenital) 748.3
leg (acquired) V49.70
    above knee V49.76
    below knee V49.75
    congenital (partial) (unilateral) (*see also* Deformity, reduction, lower limb) 755.31
      lower (complete) (partial) (with absence of distal elements, incomplete) 755.35
        with
          complete absence of distal elements (foot and toes) 755.31
        thigh (incomplete) 755.33
          with complete absence of distal elements 755.31
      upper - *see* Absence, femur
lens (congenital) 743.35
    acquired 379.31
ligament, broad (congenital) 752.19
limb (acquired)
    congenital (complete) (partial) (*see also* Deformity, reduction) 755.4
      lower 755.30
        complete 755.31
        incomplete 755.32
        longitudinal - *see* Deficiency, lower limb, longitudinal
        transverse 755.31
      upper 755.20
        complete 755.21
        incomplete 755.22
        longitudinal - *see* Deficiency, upper limb, longitudinal
        transverse 755.21
    lower NEC V49.70
    upper NEC V49.60
lip 750.26
liver (congenital) (lobe) 751.69
lumbar (congenital) (vertebra) 756.13
    isthmus 756.11
    pars articularis 756.11
lumen - *see* Atresia
lung (bilateral) (congenital) (fissure) (lobe) (unilateral) 748.5
    acquired (any part) V45.76
mandible (congenital) 524.09
maxilla (congenital) 524.09
menstruation 626.0
metacarpal(s), congenital (complete) (partial) (with absence of distal elements, incomplete) (*see also* Deformity, reduction, upper limb) 755.28
    with all fingers, complete 755.21

Absence (*Continued*)
metatarsal(s), congenital (complete) (partial) (with absence of distal elements, incomplete) (*see also* Deformity, reduction, lower limb) 755.38
    with complete absence of distal elements 755.31
muscle (congenital) (pectoral) 756.81
    ocular 743.69
musculoskeletal system (congenital) NEC 756.9
nail(s) (congenital) 757.5
neck, part 744.89
nerve 742.8
nervous system, part NEC 742.8
neutrophil 288.00
nipple (congenital) 757.6
    acquired V45.71
nose (congenital) 748.1
    acquired 738.0
nuclear 742.8
ocular muscle (congenital) 743.69
organ
    of Corti (congenital) 744.05
    or site
      acquired V45.79
      congenital NEC 759.89
osseous meatus (ear) 744.03
ovary (acquired) V45.77
    congenital 752.0
oviduct (acquired) V45.77
    congenital 752.19
pancreas (congenital) 751.7
    acquired (postoperative) (posttraumatic) V88.11 ◀▥
      partial V88.12 ◀
      total V88.11 ◀
parathyroid gland (congenital) 759.2
parotid gland(s) (congenital) 750.21
patella, congenital 755.64
pelvic girdle (congenital) 755.69
penis (congenital) 752.69
    acquired V45.77
pericardium (congenital) 746.89
perineal body (congenital) 756.81
phalange(s), congenital 755.4
    lower limb (complete) (intercalary) (partial) (terminal) (*see also* Deformity, reduction, lower limb) 755.39
      meaning all toes (complete) (partial) 755.31
      transverse 755.31
    upper limb (complete) (intercalary) (partial) (terminal) (*see also* Deformity, reduction, upper limb) 755.29
      meaning all digits (complete) (partial) 755.21
      transverse 755.21
pituitary gland (congenital) 759.2
postoperative - *see* Absence, by site, acquired
prostate (congenital) 752.89
    acquired V45.77
pulmonary
    artery 747.3
    trunk 747.3
    valve (congenital) 746.01
    vein 747.49
punctum lacrimale (congenital) 743.65

Absence *(Continued)*
  radius, congenital (complete) (partial)
      (with absence of distal elements,
      incomplete) 755.26
    with
      complete absence of distal
          elements 755.21
      ulna 755.25
        with
          complete absence of distal
              elements 755.21
          humerus (incomplete) 755.23
  ray, congenital 755.4
    lower limb (complete) (partial) *(see
        also* Deformity, reduction,
        lower limb) 755.38
      meaning all rays 755.31
      transverse 755.31
    upper limb (complete) (partial) *(see
        also* Deformity, reduction,
        upper limb) 755.28
      meaning all rays 755.21
      transverse 755.21
  rectum (congenital) 751.2
    acquired V45.79
  red cell 284.9
    acquired (secondary) 284.81
    congenital 284.01
    hereditary 284.01
    idiopathic 284.9
  respiratory organ (congenital) NEC
      748.9
  rib (acquired) 738.3
    congenital 756.3
  roof of orbit (congenital) 742.0
  round ligament (congenital) 752.89
  sacrum, congenital 756.13
  salivary gland(s) (congenital) 750.21
  scapula 755.59
  scrotum, congenital 752.89
  seminal tract or duct (congenital)
      752.89
    acquired V45.77
  septum (congenital) - *see also* Imperfect,
      closure, septum
    atrial 745.69
      and ventricular 745.7
    between aorta and pulmonary
        artery 745.0
    ventricular 745.3
      and atrial 745.7
  sex chromosomes 758.81
  shoulder girdle, congenital (complete)
      (partial) 755.59
  skin (congenital) 757.39
  skull bone 756.0
    with
      anencephalus 740.0
      encephalocele 742.0
      hydrocephalus 742.3
        with spina bifida *(see also*
            Spina bifida) 741.0●
      microcephalus 742.1
  spermatic cord (congenital) 752.89
  spinal cord 742.59
  spine, congenital 756.13
  spleen (congenital) 759.0
    acquired V45.79
  sternum, congenital 756.3
  stomach (acquired) (partial)
      (postoperative) V45.75
    with postgastric surgery syndrome
        564.2
    congenital 750.7

Absence *(Continued)*
  submaxillary gland(s) (congenital)
      750.21
  superior vena cava (congenital)
      747.49
  tarsal(s), congenital (complete)
      (partial) (with absence of distal
      elements, incomplete) *(see also*
      Deformity, reduction, lower
      limb) 755.38
  teeth, tooth (congenital) 520.0
    with abnormal spacing 524.30
    acquired 525.10
      with malocclusion 524.30
      due to
        caries 525.13
        extraction 525.10
        periodontal disease 525.12
        trauma 525.11
  tendon (congenital) 756.81
  testis (congenital) 752.89
    acquired V45.77
  thigh (acquired) 736.89
  thumb (acquired) V49.61
    congenital 755.29
  thymus gland (congenital) 759.2
  thyroid (gland) (surgical) 246.8
    with hypothyroidism 244.0
    cartilage, congenital 748.3
    congenital 243
  tibia, congenital (complete) (partial)
      (with absence of distal elements,
      incomplete) *(see also* Deformity,
      reduction, lower limb) 755.36
    with
      complete absence of distal
          elements 755.31
      fibula 755.35
        with
          complete absence of distal
              elements 755.31
          femur (incomplete)
              755.33
            with complete absence
                of distal elements
                755.31
  toe (acquired) V49.72
    congenital (complete) (partial)
        755.39
      meaning all toes 755.31
      transverse 755.31
    great V49.71
  tongue (congenital) 750.11
  tooth, teeth (congenital) 520.0
    with abnormal spacing 524.30
    acquired 525.10
      with malocclusion 524.30
      due to
        caries 525.13
        extraction 525.10
        periodontal disease 525.12
        trauma 525.11
  trachea (cartilage) (congenital) (rings)
      748.3
  transverse aortic arch (congenital)
      747.21
  tricuspid valve 746.1
  ulna, congenital (complete) (partial)
      (with absence of distal elements,
      incomplete) *(see also* Deformity,
      reduction, upper limb) 755.27
    with
      complete absence of distal
          elements 755.21

Absence *(Continued)*
  ulna, congenital *(Continued)*
    with *(Continued)*
      radius 755.25
        with
          complete absence of distal
              elements 755.21
          humerus (incomplete)
              755.23
  umbilical artery (congenital) 747.5
  ureter (congenital) 753.4
    acquired V45.74
  urethra, congenital 753.8
    acquired V45.74
  urinary system, part NEC, congenital
      753.8
    acquired V45.74
  uterus (acquired) V88.01
    with remaining cervical stump
        V88.02
    and cervix V88.01
    congenital 752.31 ◀▥
  uvula (congenital) 750.26
  vagina, congenital 752.45 ◀▥
    acquired V45.77
  vas deferens (congenital) 752.89
    acquired V45.77
  vein (congenital) (peripheral) NEC *(see
      also* Anomaly, peripheral vascular
      system) 747.60
    brain 747.81
    great 747.49
    portal 747.49
    pulmonary 747.49
  vena cava (congenital) (inferior)
      (superior) 747.49
  ventral horn cell 742.59
  ventricular septum 745.3
  vermis of cerebellum 742.2
  vertebra, congenital 756.13
  vulva, congenital 752.49
Absentia epileptica *(see also* Epilepsy)
    345.0●
Absinthemia *(see also* Dependence)
    304.6●
Absinthism *(see also* Dependence)
    304.6●
Absorbent system disease 459.89
Absorption
  alcohol, through placenta or breast
      milk 760.71
  antibiotics, through placenta or breast
      milk 760.74
  anticonvulsants, through placenta or
      breast milk 760.77
  antifungals, through placenta or breast
      milk 760.74
  anti-infective, through placenta or
      breast milk 760.74
  antimetabolics, through placenta or
      breast milk 760.78
  chemical NEC 989.9
    specified chemical or substance - *see*
        Table of Drugs and Chemicals
    through placenta or breast milk
        (fetus or newborn) 760.70
      alcohol 760.71
      anticonvulsants 760.77
      antifungals 760.74
      anti-infective agents 760.74
      antimetabolics 760.78
      cocaine 760.75
      "crack" 760.75
      diethylstilbestrol [DES] 760.76

Absorption (*Continued*)
  chemical NEC (*Continued*)
    through placenta or breast milk
      (*Continued*)
      hallucinogenic agents 760.73
      medicinal agents NEC 760.79
      narcotics 760.72
      obstetric anesthetic or analgesic
        drug 763.5
      specified agent NEC 760.79
      suspected, affecting
        management of
        pregnancy 655.5●
  cocaine, through placenta or breast
    milk 760.75
  drug NEC (*see also* Reaction, drug)
    through placenta or breast milk
      (fetus or newborn) 760.70
      alcohol 760.71
      anticonvulsants 760.77
      antifungals 760.74
      anti-infective agents 760.74
      antimetabolics 760.78
      cocaine 760.75
      "crack" 760.75
      diethylstilbestrol (DES) 760.76
      hallucinogenic agents 760.73
      medicinal agents NEC 760.79
      narcotics 760.72
      obstetric anesthetic or analgesic
        drug 763.5
      specified agent NEC 760.79
      suspected, affecting
        management of
        pregnancy 655.5●
  fat, disturbance 579.8
  hallucinogenic agents, through
    placenta or breast milk 760.73
  immune sera, through placenta or
    breast milk 760.79
  lactose defect 271.3
  medicinal agents NEC, through
    placenta or breast milk 760.79
  narcotics, through placenta or breast
    milk 760.72
  noxious substance - *see* Absorption,
    chemical
  protein, disturbance 579.8
  pus or septic, general - *see* Septicemia
  quinine, through placenta or breast
    milk 760.74
  toxic substance - *see* Absorption,
    chemical
  uremic - *see* Uremia
Abstinence symptoms or syndrome
  alcohol 291.81
  drug 292.0
  neonatal 779.5
Abt-Letterer-Siwe syndrome (acute
  histiocytosis X) (M9722/3)
  202.5●
Abulia 799.89
Abulomania 301.6
Abuse
  adult 995.80
    emotional 995.82
    multiple forms 995.85
    neglect (nutritional) 995.84
    physical 995.81
    psychological 995.82
    sexual 995.83
  alcohol (*see also* Alcoholism) 305.0●
    dependent 303.9●
    nondependent 305.0●

Abuse (*Continued*)
  child 995.50
    counseling
      perpetrator
        non-parent V62.83
        parent V61.22
      victim V61.21
    emotional 995.51
    multiple forms 995.59
    neglect (nutritional) 995.52
    physical 995.54
      shaken infant syndrome 995.55
    psychological 995.51
    sexual 995.53
  drugs, nondependent 305.9●

> Note: Use the following fifth-digit
> subclassification with the following
> codes: 305.0, 305.2-305.9:
>
> 0   unspecified
> 1   continuous
> 2   episodic
> 3   in remission

    amphetamine type 305.7●
    antidepressants 305.8●
    anxiolytic 305.4●
    barbiturates 305.4●
    caffeine 305.9●
    cannabis 305.2●
    cocaine type 305.6●
    hallucinogens 305.3●
    hashish 305.2●
    hypnotic 305.4●
    inhalant 305.9●
    LSD 305.3●
    marijuana 305.2●
    mixed 305.9●
    morphine type 305.5●
    opioid type 305.5●
    phencyclidine (PCP) 305.9●
    sedative 305.4●
    specified NEC 305.9●
    tranquilizers 305.4●
  spouse 995.80
  tobacco 305.1
Acalcerosis 275.40
Acalcicosis 275.40
Acalculia 784.69
  developmental 315.1
Acanthocheilonemiasis 125.4
Acanthocytosis 272.5
Acanthokeratodermia 701.1
Acantholysis 701.8
  bullosa 757.39
Acanthoma (benign) (M8070/0) - *see also*
  Neoplasm, by site, benign
  malignant (M8070/3) - *see* Neoplasm,
    by site, malignant
Acanthosis (acquired) (nigricans) 701.2
  adult 701.2
  benign (congenital) 757.39
  congenital 757.39
  glycogenic
    esophagus 530.89
  juvenile 701.2
  tongue 529.8
Acanthrocytosis 272.5
Acapnia 276.3
Acarbia 276.2
Acardia 759.89
Acardiacus amorphus 759.89
Acardiotrophia 429.1
Acardius 759.89

Acariasis 133.9
  sarcoptic 133.0
Acaridiasis 133.9
Acarinosis 133.9
Acariosis 133.9
Acarodermatitis 133.9
  urticarioides 133.9
Acarophobia 300.29
Acatalasemia 277.89
Acatalasia 277.89
Acatamathesia 784.69
Acataphasia 784.59
Acathisia 781.0
  due to drugs 333.99
Acceleration, accelerated
  atrioventricular conduction 426.7
  idioventricular rhythm 427.89
Accessory (congenital)
  adrenal gland 759.1
  anus 751.5
  appendix 751.5
  atrioventricular conduction 426.7
  auditory ossicles 744.04
  auricle (ear) 744.1
  autosome(s) NEC 758.5
    21 or 22 758.0
  biliary duct or passage 751.69
  bladder 753.8
  blood vessels (peripheral) (congenital)
    NEC (*see also* Anomaly,
    peripheral vascular system)
    747.60
    cerebral 747.81
    coronary 746.85
  bone NEC 756.9
    foot 755.67
  breast tissue, axilla 757.6
  carpal bones 755.56
  cecum 751.5
  cervix 752.44 ◀▥
  chromosome(s) NEC 758.5
    13-15 758.1
    16-18 758.2
    21 or 22 758.0
    autosome(s) NEC 758.5
    D_1 758.1
    E_3 758.2
    G 758.0
    sex 758.81
  coronary artery 746.85
  cusp(s), heart valve NEC 746.89
    pulmonary 746.09
  cystic duct 751.69
  digits 755.00
  ear (auricle) (lobe) 744.1
  endocrine gland NEC 759.2
  external os 752.44 ◀▥
  eyelid 743.62
  eye muscle 743.69
  face bone(s) 756.0
  fallopian tube (fimbria) (ostium)
    752.19
  fingers 755.01
  foreskin 605
  frontonasal process 756.0
  gallbladder 751.69
  genital organ(s)
    female 752.89
      external 752.49
      internal NEC 752.89
    male NEC 752.89
      penis 752.69
  genitourinary organs NEC 752.89

◀ New   ◀▥ Revised   ~~deleted~~ Deleted   ● Use Additional Digit(s)   ▥ Omit code

Accessory *(Continued)*
heart 746.89
valve NEC 746.89
pulmonary 746.09
hepatic ducts 751.69
hymen 752.49
intestine (large) (small) 751.5
kidney 753.3
lacrimal canal 743.65
leaflet, heart valve NEC 746.89
pulmonary 746.09
ligament, broad 752.19
liver (duct) 751.69
lobule (ear) 744.1
lung (lobe) 748.69
muscle 756.82
navicular of carpus 755.56
nervous system, part NEC 742.8
nipple 757.6
nose 748.1
organ or site NEC - *see* Anomaly,
specified type NEC
ovary 752.0
oviduct 752.19
pancreas 751.7
parathyroid gland 759.2
parotid gland (and duct) 750.22
pituitary gland 759.2
placental lobe - *see* Placenta, abnormal
preauricular appendage 744.1
prepuce 605
renal arteries (multiple) 747.62
rib 756.3
cervical 756.2
roots (teeth) 520.2
salivary gland 750.22
sesamoids 755.8
sinus - *see* Condition
skin tags 757.39
spleen 759.0
sternum 756.3
submaxillary gland 750.22
tarsal bones 755.67
teeth, tooth 520.1
causing crowding 524.31
tendon 756.89
thumb 755.01
thymus gland 759.2
thyroid gland 759.2
toes 755.02
tongue 750.13
tragus 744.1
ureter 753.4
urethra 753.8
urinary organ or tract NEC 753.8
uterus 752.2
vagina 752.49
valve, heart NEC 746.89
pulmonary 746.09
vertebra 756.19
vocal cords 748.3
vulva 752.49
Accident, accidental - *see also* condition
birth NEC 767.9
cardiovascular (*see also* Disease,
cardiovascular) 429.2
cerebral (*see also* Disease,
cerebrovascular, acute) 434.91
cerebrovascular (current) (CVA) (*see
also* Disease, cerebrovascular,
acute) 434.91
aborted 434.91
embolic 434.11
healed or old V12.54

Accident, accidental *(Continued)*
cerebrovascular *(Continued)*
hemorrhagic - *see* Hemorrhage,
brain
impending 435.9
ischemic 434.91
late effect - *see* Late effect(s) (of)
cerebrovascular disease
postoperative 997.02
thrombotic 434.01
coronary (*see also* Infarct, myocardium)
410.9●
craniovascular (*see also* Disease,
cerebrovascular, acute) 436
during pregnancy, to mother, affecting
fetus or newborn 760.5
heart, cardiac (*see also* Infarct,
myocardium) 410.9●
intrauterine 779.89
vascular - *see* Disease, cerebrovascular,
acute
Accommodation
disorder of 367.51
drug-induced 367.89
toxic 367.89
insufficiency of 367.4
paralysis of 367.51
hysterical 300.11
spasm of 367.53
Accouchement - *see* Delivery
Accreta placenta (without hemorrhage)
667.0●
with hemorrhage 666.0●
Accretio cordis (nonrheumatic) 423.1
Accretions on teeth 523.6
Accumulation secretion, prostate 602.8
Acephalia, acephalism, acephaly 740.0
Acephalic 740.0
Acephalobrachia 759.89
Acephalocardia 759.89
Acephalocardius 759.89
Acephalochiria 759.89
Acephalochirus 759.89
Acephalogaster 759.89
Acephalostomus 759.89
Acephalothorax 759.89
Acephalus 740.0
Acetonemia 790.6
diabetic 250.1●
due to secondary diabetes 249.1●
Acetonglycosuria 982.8
Acetonuria 791.6
Achalasia 530.0
cardia 530.0
digestive organs congenital NEC 751.8
esophagus 530.0
pelvirectal 751.3
psychogenic 306.4
pylorus 750.5
sphincteral NEC 564.89
Achard-Thiers syndrome (adrenogenital)
255.2
Ache(s) - *see* Pain
Acheilia 750.26
Acheiria 755.21
Achilloborsitis 726.71
Achillodynia 726.71
Achlorhydria, achlorhydric 536.0
anemia 280.9
diarrhea 536.0
neurogenic 536.0
postvagotomy 564.2
psychogenic 306.4
secondary to vagotomy 564.2

Achloroblepsia 368.52
Achloropsia 368.52
Acholia 575.8
Acholuric jaundice (familial)
(splenomegalic) (*see also*
Spherocytosis) 282.0
acquired 283.9
Achondroplasia 756.4
Achrestic anemia 281.8
Achroacytosis, lacrimal gland 375.00
tuberculous (*see also* Tuberculosis)
017.3●
Achroma, cutis 709.00
Achromate (congenital) 368.54
Achromatopia 368.54
Achromatopsia (congenital) 368.54
Achromia
congenital 270.2
parasitica 111.0
unguium 703.8
Achylia
gastrica 536.8
neurogenic 536.3
psychogenic 306.4
pancreatica 577.1
Achylosis 536.8
Acid
burn - *see also* Burn, by site
from swallowing acid - *see* Burn,
internal organs
deficiency
amide nicotinic 265.2
amino 270.9
ascorbic 267
folic 266.2
nicotinic (amide) 265.2
pantothenic 266.2
intoxication 276.2
peptic disease 536.8
stomach 536.8
psychogenic 306.4
Acidemia 276.2
arginosuccinic 270.6
fetal
affecting management of pregnancy
656.3●
before onset of labor, in liveborn
infant 768.2
during labor and delivery, in
liveborn infant 768.3
intrauterine 656.3●
unspecified as to time of onset, in
liveborn infant 768.4
newborn 775.81
pipecolic 270.7
Acidity, gastric (high) (low) 536.8
psychogenic 306.4
Acidocytopenia 288.59
Acidocytosis 288.3
Acidopenia 288.59
Acidosis 276.2
diabetic 250.1●
due to secondary diabetes
249.1●
fetal, affecting management of
pregnancy 656.8●
fetal, affecting newborn 775.81
kidney tubular 588.89
lactic 276.2
metabolic NEC 276.2
with respiratory acidosis 276.4
of newborn 775.81
late, of newborn 775.7
newborn 775.81

Acidosis *(Continued)*
  renal
    hyperchloremic 588.89
    tubular (distal) (proximal) 588.89
  respiratory 276.2
    complicated by
      metabolic acidosis 276.4
        of newborn 775.81
      metabolic alkalosis 276.4
Aciduria 791.9
  arginosuccinic 270.6
  beta-aminoisobutyric (BAIB) 277.2
  glutaric
    type I 270.7
    type II (type IIA, IIB, IIC) 277.85
    type III 277.86
  glycolic 271.8
  methylmalonic 270.3
    with glycinemia 270.7
  organic 270.9
  orotic (congenital) (hereditary)
    (pyrimidine deficiency) 281.4
Acladiosis 111.8
  skin 111.8
Aclasis
  diaphyseal 756.4
  tarsoepiphyseal 756.59
Acleistocardia 745.5
Aclusion 524.4
Acmesthesia 782.0
Acne (pustular) (vulgaris) 706.1
  agminata (*see also* Tuberculosis) 017.0●
  artificialis 706.1
  atrophica 706.0
  cachecticorum (Hebra) 706.1
  conglobata 706.1
  conjunctiva 706.1
  cystic 706.1
  decalvans 704.09
  erythematosa 695.3
  eyelid 706.1
  frontalis 706.0
  indurata 706.1
  keloid 706.1
  lupoid 706.0
  necrotic, necrotica 706.0
    miliaris 704.8
  neonatal 706.1
  nodular 706.1
  occupational 706.1
  papulosa 706.1
  rodens 706.0
  rosacea 695.3
  scorbutica 267
  scrofulosorum (Bazin) (*see also*
    Tuberculosis) 017.0●
  summer 692.72
  tropical 706.1
  varioliformis 706.0
Acneiform drug eruptions 692.3
Acnitis (primary) (*see also* Tuberculosis)
    017.0●
Acomia 704.00
Acontractile bladder 344.61
Aconuresis (*see also* Incontinence) 788.30
Acosta's disease 993.2
Acousma 780.1
Acoustic - *see* condition
Acousticophobia 300.29
Acquired - *see* condition
Acquired immune deficiency
    syndrome - *see* Human
    immunodeficiency virus (disease)
    (illness) (infection)

Acquired immunodeficiency
    syndrome - *see* Human
    immunodeficiency virus (disease)
    (illness) (infection)
Acragnosis 781.99
Acrania 740.0
Acroagnosis 781.99
Acroasphyxia, chronic 443.89
Acrobrachycephaly 756.0
Acrobystiolith 608.89
Acrobystitis 607.2
Acrocephalopolysyndactyly 755.55
Acrocephalosyndactyly 755.55
Acrocephaly 756.0
Acrochondrohyperplasia 759.82
Acrocyanosis 443.89
  newborn 770.83
    meaning transient blue hands and
      feet - *omit code*
Acrodermatitis 686.8
  atrophicans (chronica) 701.8
  continua (Hallopeau) 696.1
  enteropathica 686.8
  Hallopeau's 696.1
  perstans 696.1
  pustulosa continua 696.1
  recalcitrant pustular 696.1
Acrodynia 985.0
Acrodysplasia 755.55
Acrohyperhidrosis (*see also*
    Hyperhidrosis) 780.8
Acrokeratosis verruciformis 757.39
Acromastitis 611.0
Acromegaly, acromegalia (skin) 253.0
Acromelalgia 443.82
Acromicria, acromikria 756.59
Acronyx 703.0
Acropachy, thyroid (*see also*
    Thyrotoxicosis) 242.9●
Acropachyderma 757.39
Acroparesthesia 443.89
  simple (Schultz's type) 443.89
  vasomotor (Nothnagel's type) 443.89
Acropathy thyroid (*see also*
    Thyrotoxicosis) 242.9●
Acrophobia 300.29
Acroposthitis 607.2
Acroscleriasis (*see also* Scleroderma) 710.1
Acroscleroderma (*see also* Scleroderma)
    710.1
Acrosclerosis (*see also* Scleroderma)
    710.1
Acrosphacelus 785.4
Acrosphenosyndactylia 755.55
Acrospiroma, eccrine (M8402/0) - *see*
    Neoplasm, skin, benign
Acrostealgia 732.9
Acrosyndactyly (*see also* Syndactylism)
    755.10
Acrotrophodynia 991.4
Actinic - *see also* condition
  cheilitis (due to sun) 692.72
    chronic NEC 692.74
    due to radiation, except from sun
      692.82
  conjunctivitis 370.24
  dermatitis (due to sun) (*see also*
    Dermatitis, actinic) 692.70
  due to
    roentgen rays or radioactive
      substance 692.82
    ultraviolet radiation, except from
      sun 692.82
    sun NEC 692.70

Actinic *(Continued)*
  elastosis solare 692.74
  granuloma 692.73
  keratitis 370.24
  ophthalmia 370.24
  reticuloid 692.73
Actinobacillosis, general 027.8
Actinobacillus
  lignieresii 027.8
  mallei 024
  muris 026.1
Actinocutitis NEC (*see also* Dermatitis,
    actinic) 692.70
Actinodermatitis NEC (*see also*
    Dermatitis, actinic) 692.70
Actinomyces
  israelii (infection) - *see*
    Actinomycosis
  muris-ratti (infection) 026.1
Actinomycosis, actinomycotic 039.9
  with
    pneumonia 039.1
  abdominal 039.2
  cervicofacial 039.3
  cutaneous 039.0
  pulmonary 039.1
  specified site NEC 039.8
  thoracic 039.1
Actinoneuritis 357.89
Action, heart
  disorder 427.9
    postoperative 997.1
  irregular 427.9
    postoperative 997.1
    psychogenic 306.2
Active - *see* condition
Activity decrease, functional 780.99
Acute - *see also* condition
  abdomen NEC 789.0●
  gallbladder (*see also* Cholecystitis,
    acute) 575.0
Acyanoblepsia 368.53
Acyanopsia 368.53
Acystia 753.8
Acystinervia - *see* Neurogenic, bladder
Acystineuria - *see* Neurogenic, bladder
Adactylia, adactyly (congenital) 755.4
  lower limb (complete) (intercalary)
    (partial) (terminal) (*see also*
    Deformity, reduction, lower limb)
    755.39
    meaning all digits (complete)
      (partial) 755.31
    transverse (complete) (partial)
      755.31
  upper limb (complete) (intercalary)
    (partial) (terminal) (*see also*
    Deformity, reduction, upper limb)
    755.29
    meaning all digits (complete)
      (partial) 755.21
    transverse (complete) (partial)
      755.21
Adair-Dighton syndrome (brittle bones
    and blue sclera, deafness) 756.51
Adamantinoblastoma (M9310/0) - *see*
    Ameloblastoma
Adamantinoma (M9310/0) - *see*
    Ameloblastoma
Adamantoblastoma (M9310/0) - *see*
    Ameloblastoma
Adams-Stokes (-Morgagni) disease or
    syndrome (syncope with heart
    block) 426.9

◀ New   ◀▥ Revised   ~~deleted~~ Deleted   ● Use Additional Digit(s)   ▨ Omit code

Adaptation reaction (*see also* Reaction, adjustment) 309.9

Addiction - *see also* Dependence
  absinthe 304.6●
  alcoholic (ethyl) (methyl) (wood) 303.9●
    complicating pregnancy, childbirth, or puerperium 648.4●
      affecting fetus or newborn 760.71
      suspected damage to fetus affecting management of pregnancy 655.4●
  drug (*see also* Dependence) 304.9●
  ethyl alcohol 303.9●
  heroin 304.0●
  hospital 301.51
  methyl alcohol 303.9●
  methylated spirit 303.9●
  morphine (-like substances) 304.0●
  nicotine 305.1
  opium 304.0●
  tobacco 305.1
  wine 303.9●

Addison's
  anemia (pernicious) 281.0
  disease (bronze) (primary adrenal insufficiency) 255.41
    tuberculous (*see also* Tuberculosis) 017.6●
  keloid (morphea) 701.0
  melanoderma (adrenal cortical hypofunction) 255.41

Addison-Biermer anemia (pernicious) 281.0

Addison-Gull disease - *see* Xanthoma

Addisonian crisis or melanosis (acute adrenocortical insufficiency) 255.41

Additional - *see also* Accessory
  chromosome(s) 758.5
    13-15 758.1
    16-18 758.2
    21 758.0
    autosome(s) NEC 758.5
    sex 758.81

Adduction contracture, hip or other joint - *see* Contraction, joint

ADEM (acute disseminated encephalomyelitis) (postinfectious) 136.9 [323.61]
  infectious 136.9 [323.61]
  noninfectious 323.81

Adenasthenia gastrica 536.0

Aden fever 061

Adenitis (*see also* Lymphadenitis) 289.3
  acute, unspecified site 683
    epidemic infectious 075
  axillary 289.3
    acute 683
    chronic or subacute 289.1
  Bartholin's gland 616.89
  bulbourethral gland (*see also* Urethritis) 597.89
  cervical 289.3
    acute 683
    chronic or subacute 289.1
  chancroid (Ducrey's bacillus) 099.0
  chronic (any lymph node, except mesenteric) 289.1
    mesenteric 289.2
  Cowper's gland (*see also* Urethritis) 597.89
  epidemic, acute 075
  gangrenous 683
  gonorrheal NEC 098.89

Adenitis (*Continued*)
  groin 289.3
    acute 683
    chronic or subacute 289.1
  infectious 075
  inguinal (region) 289.3
    acute 683
    chronic or subacute 289.1
  lymph gland or node, except mesenteric 289.3
    acute 683
    chronic or subacute 289.1
    mesenteric (acute) (chronic) (nonspecific) (subacute) 289.2
  mesenteric (acute) (chronic) (nonspecific) (subacute) 289.2
  due to Pasteurella multocida (P. septica) 027.2
  parotid gland (suppurative) 527.2
  phlegmonous 683
  salivary duct or gland (any) (recurring) (suppurative) 527.2
  scrofulous (*see also* Tuberculosis) 017.2●
  septic 289.3
  Skene's duct or gland (*see also* Urethritis) 597.89
  strumous, tuberculous (*see also* Tuberculosis) 017.2●
  subacute, unspecified site 289.1
  sublingual gland (suppurative) 527.2
  submandibular gland (suppurative) 527.2
  submaxillary gland (suppurative) 527.2
  suppurative 683
  tuberculous - *see* Tuberculosis, lymph gland
  urethral gland (*see also* Urethritis) 597.89
  venereal NEC 099.8
  Wharton's duct (suppurative) 527.2

Adenoacanthoma (M8570/3) - *see* Neoplasm, by site, malignant

Adenoameloblastoma (M9300/0) 213.1
  upper jaw (bone) 213.0

Adenocarcinoma (M8140/3) - *see also* Neoplasm, by site, malignant

> Note: The list of adjectival modifiers below is not exhaustive. A description of adenocarcinoma that does not appear in this list should be coded in the same manner as carcinoma with that description. Thus, "mixed acidophil-basophil adenocarcinoma," should be coded in the same manner as "mixed acidophil-basophil carcinoma," which appears in the list under "Carcinoma."
>
> Except where otherwise indicated, the morphological varieties of adenocarcinoma in the list below should be coded by site as for "Neoplasm, malignant."

  with
    apocrine metaplasia (M8573/3)
    cartilaginous (and osseous) metaplasia (M8571/3)
    osseous (and cartilaginous) metaplasia (M8571/3)
    spindle cell metaplasia (M8572/3)
    squamous metaplasia (M8570/3)

Adenocarcinoma (*Continued*)
  acidophil (M8280/3)
    specified site - *see* Neoplasm, by site, malignant
    unspecified site 194.3
  acinar (M8550/3)
  acinic cell (M8550/3)
  adrenal cortical (M8370/3) 194.0
  alveolar (M8251/3)
    and
      epidermoid carcinoma, mixed (M8560/3)
      squamous cell carcinoma, mixed (M8560/3)
  apocrine (M8401/3)
    breast - *see* Neoplasm, breast, malignant
    specified site NEC - *see* Neoplasm, skin, malignant
    unspecified site 173.9
  basophil (M8300/3)
    specified site - *see* Neoplasm, by site, malignant
    unspecified site 194.3
  bile duct type (M8160/3)
    liver 155.1
    specified site NEC - *see* Neoplasm, by site, malignant
    unspecified site 155.1
  bronchiolar (M8250/3) - *see* Neoplasm, lung, malignant
  ceruminous (M8420/3) 173.2
  chromophobe (M8270/3)
    specified site - *see* Neoplasm, by site, malignant
    unspecified site 194.3
  clear cell (mesonephroid type) (M8310/3)
  colloid (M8480/3)
  cylindroid type (M8200/3)
  diffuse type (M8145/3)
    specified site - *see* Neoplasm, by site, malignant
    unspecified site 151.9
  duct (infiltrating) (M8500/3)
    with Paget's disease (M8541/3) - *see* Neoplasm, breast, malignant
    specified site - *see* Neoplasm, by site, malignant
    unspecified site 174.9
  embryonal (M9070/3)
  endometrioid (M8380/3) - *see* Neoplasm, by site, malignant
  eosinophil (M8280/3)
    specified site - *see* Neoplasm, by site, malignant
    unspecified site 194.3
  follicular (M8330/3)
    and papillary (M8340/3) 193
    moderately differentiated type (M8332/3) 193
    pure follicle type (M8331/3) 193
    specified site - *see* Neoplasm, by site, malignant
    trabecular type (M8332/3) 193
    unspecified type 193
    well differentiated type (M8331/3) 193
  gelatinous (M8480/3)
  granular cell (M8320/3)
  Hürthle cell (M8290/3) 193
  in
    adenomatous
      polyp (M8210/3)
      polyposis coli (M8220/3) 153.9

Adenocarcinoma *(Continued)*
  in *(Continued)*
    polypoid adenoma (M8210/3)
    tubular adenoma (M8210/3)
    villous adenoma (M8261/3)
  infiltrating duct (M8500/3)
    with Paget's disease (M8541/3) -
      see Neoplasm, breast,
      malignant
    specified site - *see* Neoplasm, by site,
      malignant
    unspecified site 174.9
  inflammatory (M8530/3)
    specified site - *see* Neoplasm, by site,
      malignant
    unspecified site 174.9
  in situ (M8140/2) - *see* Neoplasm, by
    site, in situ
  intestinal type (M8144/3)
    specified site - *see* Neoplasm, by site,
      malignant
    unspecified site 151.9
  intraductal (noninfiltrating)
    (M8500/2)
    papillary (M8503/2)
      specified site - *see* Neoplasm, by
        site, in situ
      unspecified site 233.0
    specified site - *see* Neoplasm, by site,
      in situ
    unspecified site 233.0
  islet cell (M8150/3)
    and exocrine, mixed (M8154/3)
      specified site - *see* Neoplasm, by
        site, malignant
      unspecified site 157.9
    pancreas 157.4
    specified site NEC - *see* Neoplasm,
      by site, malignant
    unspecified site 157.4
  lobular (M8520/3)
    specified site - *see* Neoplasm, by site,
      malignant
    unspecified site 174.9
  medullary (M8510/3)
  mesonephric (M9110/3)
  mixed cell (M8323/3)
  mucinous (M8480/3)
  mucin-producing (M8481/3)
  mucoid (M8480/3) - *see also* Neoplasm,
    by site, malignant
    cell (M8300/3)
      specified site - *see* Neoplasm, by
        site, malignant
      unspecified site 194.3
  nonencapsulated sclerosing (M8350/3)
    193
  oncocytic (M8290/3)
  oxyphilic (M8290/3)
  papillary (M8260/3)
    and follicular (M8340/3) 193
    intraductal (noninfiltrating)
      (M8503/2)
    specified site - *see* Neoplasm, by
      site, in situ
    unspecified site 233.0
  serous (M8460/3)
    specified site - *see* Neoplasm, by
      site, malignant
    unspecified site 183.0
  papillocystic (M8450/3)
    specified site - *see* Neoplasm, by site,
      malignant
    unspecified site 183.0

Adenocarcinoma *(Continued)*
  pseudomucinous (M8470/3)
    specified site - *see* Neoplasm, by site,
      malignant
    unspecified site 183.0
  renal cell (M8312/3) 189.0
  sebaceous (M8410/3)
  serous (M8441/3) - *see also* Neoplasm,
    by site, malignant
    papillary
      specified site - *see* Neoplasm, by
        site, malignant
      unspecified site 183.0
  signet ring cell (M8490/3)
  superficial spreading (M8143/3)
  sweat gland (M8400/3) - *see* Neoplasm,
    skin, malignant
  trabecular (M8190/3)
  tubular (M8211/3)
  villous (M8262/3)
  water-clear cell (M8322/3) 194.1
Adenofibroma (M9013/0)
  clear cell (M8313/0) - *see* Neoplasm, by
    site, benign
  endometrioid (M8381/0) 220
    borderline malignancy (M8381/1)
      236.2
    malignant (M8381/3) 183.0
  mucinous (M9015/0)
    specified site - *see* Neoplasm, by site,
      benign
    unspecified site 220
  prostate 600.20
    with
      other lower urinary tract
        symptoms (LUTS) 600.21
      urinary
        obstruction 600.21
        retention 600.21
  serous (M9014/0)
    specified site - *see* Neoplasm, by site,
      benign
    unspecified site 220
  specified site - *see* Neoplasm, by site,
    benign
  unspecified site 220
Adenofibrosis
  breast 610.2
  endometrioid 617.0
Adenoiditis 474.01
  acute 463
  chronic 474.01
    with chronic tonsillitis 474.02
Adenoids (congenital) (of nasal fossa) 474.9
  hypertrophy 474.12
  vegetations 474.2
Adenolipomatosis (symmetrical) 272.8
Adenolymphoma (M8561/0)
  specified site - *see* Neoplasm, by site,
    benign
  unspecified 210.2
Adenoma (sessile) (M8140/0) - *see also*
  Neoplasm, by site, benign

> Note: Except where otherwise indicated, the morphological varieties of adenoma in the list below should be coded by site as for "Neoplasm, benign."

  acidophil (M8280/0)
    specified site - *see* Neoplasm, by site,
      benign
    unspecified site 227.3

Adenoma *(Continued)*
  acinar (cell) (M8550/0)
  acinic cell (M8550/0)
  adrenal (cortex) (cortical) (functioning)
    (M8370/0) 227.0
    clear cell type (M8373/0) 227.0
    compact cell type (M8371/0) 227.0
    glomerulosa cell type (M8374/0)
      227.0
    heavily pigmented variant
      (M8372/0) 227.0
    mixed cell type (M8375/0) 227.0
  alpha cell (M8152/0)
    pancreas 211.7
    specified site NEC - *see* Neoplasm,
      by site, benign
    unspecified site 211.7
  alveolar (M8251/0)
  apocrine (M8401/0)
    breast 217
    specified site NEC - *see* Neoplasm,
      skin, benign
    unspecified site 216.9
  basal cell (M8147/0)
  basophil (M8300/0)
    specified site - *see* Neoplasm, by site,
      benign
    unspecified site 227.3
  beta cell (M8151/0)
    pancreas 211.7
    specified site NEC - *see* Neoplasm,
      by site, benign
    unspecified site 211.7
  bile duct (M8160/0) 211.5
  black (M8372/0) 227.0
  bronchial (M8140/1) 235.7
    carcinoid type (M8240/3) - *see*
      Neoplasm, lung, malignant
    cylindroid type (M8200/3) - *see*
      Neoplasm, lung, malignant
  ceruminous (M8420/0) 216.2
  chief cell (M8321/0) 227.1
  chromophobe (M8270/0)
    specified site - *see* Neoplasm, by site,
      benign
    unspecified site 227.3
  clear cell (M8310/0)
  colloid (M8334/0)
    specified site - *see* Neoplasm, by site,
      benign
    unspecified site 226
  cylindroid type, bronchus (M8200/3) -
    see Neoplasm, lung, malignant
  duct (M8503/0)
  embryonal (M8191/0)
  endocrine, multiple (M8360/1)
    single specified site - *see* Neoplasm,
      by site, uncertain behavior
    two or more specified sites 237.4
    unspecified site 237.4
  endometrioid (M8380/0) - *see also*
    Neoplasm, by site, benign
    borderline malignancy (M8380/1) -
      see Neoplasm, by site,
      uncertain behavior
  eosinophil (M8280/0)
    specified site - *see* Neoplasm, by site,
      benign
    unspecified site 227.3
  fetal (M8333/0)
    specified site - *see* Neoplasm, by site,
      benign
    unspecified site 226

◀ New   ◀▥ Revised   ~~deleted~~ Deleted   ● Use Additional Digit(s)   ▥ Omit code

Adenoma *(Continued)*
  follicular (M8330/0)
    specified site - *see* Neoplasm, by site,
      benign
    unspecified site 226
  hepatocellular (M8170/0) 211.5
  Hürthle cell (M8290/0) 226
  intracystic papillary (M8504/0)
  islet cell (functioning) (M8150/0)
    pancreas 211.7
    specified site NEC - *see* Neoplasm,
      by site, benign
    unspecified site 211.7
  liver cell (M8170/0) 211.5
  macrofollicular (M8334/0)
    specified site NEC - *see* Neoplasm,
      by site, benign
    unspecified site 226
  malignant, malignum (M8140/3) - *see*
    Neoplasm, by site, malignant
  mesonephric (M9110/0)
  microfollicular (M8333/0)
    specified site - *see* Neoplasm, by site,
      benign
    unspecified site 226
  mixed cell (M8323/0)
  monomorphic (M8146/0)
  mucinous (M8480/0)
  mucoid cell (M8300/0)
    specified site - *see* Neoplasm, by site,
      benign
    unspecified site 227.3
  multiple endocrine (M8360/1)
    single specified site - *see* Neoplasm,
      by site, uncertain behavior
    two or more specified sites 237.4
    unspecified site 237.4
  nipple (M8506/0) 217
  oncocytic (M8290/0)
  oxyphilic (M8290/0)
  papillary (M8260/0) - *see also*
    Neoplasm, by site, benign
    intracystic (M8504/0)
  papillotubular (M8263/0)
  Pick's tubular (M8640/0)
    specified site - *see* Neoplasm, by site,
      benign
    unspecified site
      female 220
      male 222.0
  pleomorphic (M8940/0)
  polypoid (M8210/0)
  prostate (benign) 600.20
    with
      other lower urinary tract
        symptoms (LUTS)
        600.21
      urinary
        obstruction 600.21
        retention 600.21
  rete cell 222.0
  sebaceous, sebaceum (gland) (senile)
    (M8410/0) - *see also* Neoplasm,
    skin, benign
    disseminata 759.5
  Sertoli cell (M8640/0)
    specified site - *see* Neoplasm, by site,
      benign
    unspecified site
      female 220
      male 222.0
  skin appendage (M8390/0) - *see*
    Neoplasm, skin, benign
  sudoriferous gland (M8400/0) - *see*
    Neoplasm, skin, benign

Adenoma *(Continued)*
  sweat gland or duct (M8400/0) - *see*
    Neoplasm, skin, benign
  testicular (M8640/0)
    specified site - *see* Neoplasm, by site,
      benign
    unspecified site
      female 220
      male 222.0
  thyroid 226
  trabecular (M8190/0)
  tubular (M8211/0) - *see also* Neoplasm,
    by site, benign
    papillary (M8460/3)
    Pick's (M8640/0)
      specified site - *see* Neoplasm, by
        site, benign
      unspecified site
        female 220
        male 222.0
  tubulovillous (M8263/0)
  villoglandular (M8263/0)
  villous (M8261/1) - *see* Neoplasm, by
    site, uncertain behavior
  water-clear cell (M8322/0) 227.1
  wolffian duct (M9110/0)
Adenomatosis (M8220/0)
  endocrine (multiple) (M8360/1)
    single specified site - *see* Neoplasm,
      by site, uncertain behavior
    two or more specified sites 237.4
    unspecified site 237.4
  erosive of nipple (M8506/0) 217
  pluriendocrine - *see* Adenomatosis,
    endocrine
  pulmonary (M8250/1) 235.7
    malignant (M8250/3) - *see*
      Neoplasm, lung, malignant
  specified site - *see* Neoplasm, by site,
    benign
  unspecified site 211.3
Adenomatous
  cyst, thyroid (gland) - *see* Goiter,
    nodular
  goiter (nontoxic) (*see also* Goiter,
    nodular) 241.9
    toxic or with hyperthyroidism
      242.3●
Adenomyoma (M8932/0) - *see also*
  Neoplasm, by site, benign
  prostate 600.20
    with
      other lower urinary tract
        symptoms (LUTS) 600.21
      urinary
        obstruction 600.21
        retention 600.21
Adenomyometritis 617.0
Adenomyosis (uterus) (internal) 617.0
Adenopathy (lymph gland) 785.6
  inguinal 785.6
  mediastinal 785.6
  mesentery 785.6
  syphilitic (secondary) 091.4
  tracheobronchial 785.6
    tuberculous (*see also* Tuberculosis)
      012.1●
      primary, progressive 010.8●
  tuberculous (*see also* Tuberculosis,
    lymph gland) 017.2●
    tracheobronchial 012.1●
      primary, progressive 010.8●
Adenopharyngitis 462
Adenophlegmon 683

Adenosalpingitis 614.1
Adenosarcoma (M8960/3) 189.0
Adenosclerosis 289.3
Adenosis
  breast (sclerosing) 610.2
  vagina, congenital 752.49
Adentia (complete) (partial) (*see also*
  Absence, teeth) 520.0
Adherent
  labium (minus) 624.4
  pericardium (nonrheumatic) 423.1
    rheumatic 393
  placenta 667.0●
    with hemorrhage 666.0●
  prepuce 605
  scar (skin) NEC 709.2
  tendon in scar 709.2
Adhesion(s), adhesive (postinfectional)
  (postoperative)
  abdominal (wall) (*see also* Adhesions,
    peritoneum) 568.0
  amnion to fetus 658.8●
    affecting fetus or newborn 762.8
  appendix 543.9
  arachnoiditis - *see* Meningitis
  auditory tube (Eustachian) 381.89
  bands - *see* Adhesions,
    peritoneum
    cervix 622.3
    uterus 621.5
  bile duct (any) 576.8
  bladder (sphincter) 596.8
  bowel (*see also* Adhesions, peritoneum)
    568.0
  cardiac 423.1
    rheumatic 398.99
  cecum (*see also* Adhesions, peritoneum)
    568.0
  cervicovaginal 622.3
    congenital 752.49
    postpartal 674.8●
      old 622.3
  cervix 622.3
  clitoris 624.4
  colon (*see also* Adhesions, peritoneum)
    568.0
  common duct 576.8
  congenital - *see also* Anomaly, specified
    type NEC
    fingers (*see also* Syndactylism,
      fingers) 755.11
    labium (majus) (minus) 752.49
    omental, anomalous 751.4
    ovary 752.0
    peritoneal 751.4
    toes (*see also* Syndactylism, toes)
      755.13
    tongue (to gum or roof of mouth)
      750.12
  conjunctiva (acquired) (localized)
    372.62
    congenital 743.63
    extensive 372.63
  cornea - *see* Opacity, cornea
  cystic duct 575.8
  diaphragm (*see also* Adhesions,
    peritoneum) 568.0
  due to foreign body - *see* Foreign body
  duodenum (*see also* Adhesions,
    peritoneum) 568.0
    with obstruction 537.3
  ear, middle - *see* Adhesions, middle ear
  epididymis 608.89
  epidural - *see* Adhesions, meninges

Adhesion(s) (*Continued*)
　epiglottis 478.79
　Eustachian tube 381.89
　eyelid 374.46
　　postoperative 997.99
　　　surgically created V45.69
　gallbladder (*see also* Disease,
　　gallbladder) 575.8
　globe 360.89
　heart 423.1
　　rheumatic 398.99
　ileocecal (coil) (*see also* Adhesions,
　　peritoneum) 568.0
　ileum (*see also* Adhesions, peritoneum)
　　568.0
　intestine (postoperative) (*see also*
　　Adhesions, peritoneum) 568.0
　　with obstruction 560.81
　　　with hernia - *see also* Hernia, by
　　　　site, with obstruction
　　　　　gangrenous - *see* Hernia, by
　　　　　　site, with gangrene
　intra-abdominal (*see also* Adhesions,
　　peritoneum) 568.0
　iris 364.70
　　to corneal graft 996.79
　joint (*see also* Ankylosis) 718.5●
　kidney 593.89
　labium (majus) (minus), congenital
　　752.49
　liver 572.8
　lung 511.0
　mediastinum 519.3
　meninges 349.2
　　cerebral (any) 349.2
　　　congenital 742.4
　　congenital 742.8
　　spinal (any) 349.2
　　　congenital 742.59
　　tuberculous (cerebral) (spinal) (*see
　　　also* Tuberculosis, meninges)
　　　013.0●
　mesenteric (*see also* Adhesions,
　　peritoneum) 568.0
　middle ear (fibrous) 385.10
　　drum head 385.19
　　　to
　　　　incus 385.11
　　　　promontorium 385.13
　　　　stapes 385.12
　　　specified NEC 385.19
　nasal (septum) (to turbinates)
　　478.19
　nerve NEC 355.9
　　spinal 355.9
　　　root 724.9
　　　　cervical NEC 723.4
　　　　lumbar NEC 724.4
　　　　lumbosacral 724.4
　　　　thoracic 724.4
　ocular muscle 378.60
　omentum (*see also* Adhesions,
　　peritoneum) 568.0
　organ or site, congenital NEC -
　　see Anomaly, specified type
　　NEC
　ovary 614.6
　　congenital (to cecum, kidney, or
　　　omentum) 752.0
　parauterine 614.6
　parovarian 614.6
　pelvic (peritoneal)
　　female (postoperative)
　　　(postinfection) 614.6

Adhesion(s) (*Continued*)
　pelvic (*Continued*)
　　male (postoperative) (postinfection)
　　　(*see also* Adhesions,
　　　peritoneum) 568.0
　　postpartal (old) 614.6
　　tuberculous (*see also* Tuberculosis)
　　　016.9●
　penis to scrotum (congenital) 752.69
　periappendiceal (*see also* Adhesions,
　　peritoneum) 568.0
　pericardium (nonrheumatic) 423.1
　　rheumatic 393
　　tuberculous (*see also* Tuberculosis)
　　　017.9● [420.0]
　pericholecystic 575.8
　perigastric (*see also* Adhesions,
　　peritoneum) 568.0
　periovarian 614.6
　periprostatic 602.8
　perirectal (*see also* Adhesions,
　　peritoneum) 568.0
　perirenal 593.89
　peritoneum, peritoneal (fibrous)
　　(postoperative) 568.0
　　with obstruction (intestinal) 560.81
　　　with hernia - *see also* Hernia, by
　　　　site, with obstruction
　　　　　gangrenous - *see* Hernia, by
　　　　　　site, with gangrene
　　　duodenum 537.3
　　congenital 751.4
　　female (postoperative)
　　　(postinfective) 614.6
　　pelvic, female 614.6
　　pelvic, male 568.0
　　postpartal, pelvic 614.6
　　to uterus 614.6
　peritubal 614.6
　periureteral 593.89
　periuterine 621.5
　perivesical 596.8
　perivesicular (seminal vesicle) 608.89
　pleura, pleuritic 511.0
　　tuberculous (*see also* Tuberculosis,
　　　pleura) 012.0●
　pleuropericardial 511.0
　postoperative (gastrointestinal tract)
　　(*see also* Adhesions, peritoneum)
　　eyelid 997.99
　　　surgically created V45.69
　　pelvic, female 614.9
　　pelvic, male 568.0
　　urethra 598.2
　postpartal, old 624.4
　preputial, prepuce 605
　pulmonary 511.0
　pylorus (*see also* Adhesions,
　　peritoneum) 568.0
　Rosenmüller's fossa 478.29
　sciatic nerve 355.0
　seminal vesicle 608.89
　shoulder (joint) 726.0
　sigmoid flexure (*see also* Adhesions,
　　peritoneum) 568.0
　spermatic cord (acquired) 608.89
　　congenital 752.89
　spinal canal 349.2
　　nerve 355.9
　　　root 724.9
　　　　cervical NEC 723.4
　　　　lumbar NEC 724.4
　　　　lumbosacral 724.4
　　　　thoracic 724.4

Adhesion(s) (*Continued*)
　stomach (*see also* Adhesions,
　　peritoneum) 568.0
　subscapular 726.2
　tendonitis 726.90
　　shoulder 726.0
　testicle 608.89
　tongue (congenital) (to gum or roof of
　　mouth) 750.12
　　acquired 529.8
　trachea 519.19
　tubo-ovarian 614.6
　tunica vaginalis 608.89
　ureter 593.89
　uterus 621.5
　　to abdominal wall 614.6
　　　in pregnancy or childbirth 654.4●
　　　　affecting fetus or newborn
　　　　　763.89
　vagina (chronic) (postoperative)
　　(postradiation) 623.2
　vaginitis (congenital) 752.49
　vesical 596.8
　vitreous 379.29
Adie (-Holmes) syndrome (tonic pupillary
　reaction) 379.46
Adiponecrosis neonatorum 778.1
Adiposa dolorosa 272.8
Adiposalgia 272.8
Adiposis
　cerebralis 253.8
　dolorosa 272.8
　tuberosa simplex 272.8
Adiposity 278.02
　heart (*see also* Degeneration,
　　myocardial) 429.1
　localized 278.1
Adiposogenital dystrophy 253.8
Adjustment
　prosthesis or other device - *see* Fitting
　　of
　reaction - *see* Reaction, adjustment
Administration, prophylactic
　antibiotics, long-term V58.62 ◄▥
　　short-term use - *omit code* ◄
　antitoxin, any V07.2
　antivenin V07.2
　chemotherapeutic agent NEC V07.39
　chemotherapy NEC V07.39
　diphtheria antitoxin V07.2
　fluoride V07.31
　gamma globulin V07.2
　immune sera (gamma globulin) V07.2
　passive immunization agent V07.2
　RhoGAM V07.2
Admission (encounter)
　as organ donor - *see* Donor
　by mistake V68.9
　for
　　adequacy testing (for)
　　　hemodialysis V56.31
　　　peritoneal dialysis V56.32
　　adjustment (of)
　　　artificial
　　　　arm (complete) (partial) V52.0
　　　　eye V52.2
　　　　leg (complete) (partial) V52.1
　　　brain neuropacemaker V53.02
　　　breast
　　　　implant V52.4
　　　　　exchange (different
　　　　　　material) (different
　　　　　　size) V52.4
　　　　prosthesis V52.4

◄ New　◄▥ Revised　~~deleted~~ Deleted　● Use Additional Digit(s)　▨ Omit code

Admission *(Continued)*
  for *(Continued)*
    adjustment (of) *(Continued)*
      cardiac device V53.39
        defibrillator, automatic
          implantable (with
          synchronous cardiac
          pacemaker) V53.32 ◀▥
        pacemaker V53.31
          carotid sinus V53.39
      catheter
        non-vascular V58.82
        vascular V58.81
      cerebral ventricle (communicating)
        shunt V53.01
      colostomy belt V55.3
      contact lenses V53.1
      cystostomy device V53.6
      dental prosthesis V52.3
      device, unspecified type V53.90
        abdominal V53.59
        cardiac V53.39
          defibrillator, automatic
            implantable (with
            synchronous cardiac
            pacemaker) V53.32 ◀▥
          pacemaker V53.31
        carotid sinus V53.39
        cerebral ventricle
          (communicating)
          shunt V53.01
        gastrointestinal NEC V53.59
        insulin pump V53.91
        intestinal V53.50
        ~~intrauterine contraceptive V25.1~~
        nervous system V53.09
        orthodontic V53.4
        other device V53.99
        prosthetic V52.9
          breast V52.4
          dental V52.3
          eye V52.2
          specified type NEC V52.8
        special senses V53.09
        substitution
          auditory V53.09
          nervous system V53.09
          visual V53.09
        urinary V53.6
      dialysis catheter
        extracorporeal V56.1
        peritoneal V56.2
      diaphragm (contraceptive) V25.02
      gastric lap band V53.51
      gastrointestinal appliance and
        device NEC V53.59
      growth rod V54.02
      hearing aid V53.2
      ileostomy device V55.2
      intestinal appliance and device
        V53.50
      ~~intrauterine contraceptive device~~
        ~~V25.1~~
      neuropacemaker (brain)
        (peripheral nerve) (spinal
        cord) V53.02
      orthodontic device V53.4
      orthopedic (device) V53.7
        brace V53.7
        cast V53.7
        shoes V53.7
      pacemaker
        brain V53.02
        cardiac V53.31
        carotid sinus V53.39
        peripheral nerve V53.02
        spinal cord V53.02

Admission *(Continued)*
  for *(Continued)*
    adjustment (of) *(Continued)*
      prosthesis V52.9
        arm (complete) (partial) V52.0
        breast V52.4
        dental V52.3
        eye V52.2
        leg (complete) (partial) V52.1
        specified type NEC V52.8
      spectacles V53.1
      wheelchair V53.8
    adoption referral or proceedings
      V68.89
    aftercare (*see also* Aftercare) V58.9
      cardiac pacemaker V53.31
      chemotherapy (oral) (intravenous)
        V58.11
      dialysis
        extracorporeal (renal) V56.0
        peritoneal V56.8
        renal V56.0
      fracture (*see also* Aftercare,
        fracture) V54.9
      medical NEC V58.89
      organ transplant V58.44
      orthopedic V54.9
        specified care NEC V54.89
      pacemaker device
        brain V53.02
        cardiac V53.31
        carotid sinus V53.39
        nervous system V53.02
        spinal cord V53.02
      postoperative NEC V58.49
        wound closure, planned V58.41
      postpartum
        immediately after delivery
          V24.0
        routine follow-up V24.2
      postradiation V58.0
      radiation therapy V58.0
      removal of
        non-vascular catheter V58.82
        vascular catheter V58.81
      specified NEC V58.89
      surgical NEC V58.49
        wound closure, planned V58.41
    antineoplastic
      chemotherapy (oral) (intravenous)
        V58.11
      immunotherapy V58.12
    artificial insemination V26.1
    assisted reproductive fertility
        procedure cycle V26.81
    attention to artificial opening (of)
      V55.9
      artificial vagina V55.7
      colostomy V55.3
      cystostomy V55.5
      enterostomy V55.4
      gastrostomy V55.1
      ileostomy V55.2
      jejunostomy V55.4
      nephrostomy V55.6
      specified site NEC V55.8
        intestinal tract V55.4
        urinary tract V55.6
      tracheostomy V55.0
      ureterostomy V55.6
      urethrostomy V55.6
    battery replacement
      cardiac pacemaker V53.31
    blood typing V72.86
      Rh typing V72.86

Admission *(Continued)*
  for *(Continued)*
    boarding V65.0
    breast
      augmentation or reduction V50.1
      implant exchange (different
        material) (different size)
        V52.4
      reconstruction following
        mastectomy V51.0
      removal
        prophylactic V50.41
        tissue expander without
          synchronous insertion of
          permanent implant V52.4
    change of
      cardiac pacemaker (battery) 53.31
      carotid sinus pacemaker V53.39
      catheter in artificial opening - *see*
        Attention to, artificial,
        opening
      drains V58.49
      dressing
        wound V58.30
          nonsurgical V58.30
          surgical V58.31
      fixation device
        external V54.89
        internal V54.01
      Kirschner wire V54.89
      neuropacemaker device (brain)
        (peripheral nerve) (spinal
        cord) V53.02
      nonsurgical wound dressing
        V58.30
      pacemaker device
        brain V53.02
        cardiac V53.31
        carotid sinus V53.39
        nervous system V53.02
      plaster cast V54.89
      splint, external V54.89
      Steinmann pin V54.89
      surgical wound dressing V58.31
      traction device V54.89
      wound packing V58.30
        nonsurgical V58.30
        surgical V58.31
    checkup only V70.0
    chemotherapy, (oral) (intravenous)
      antineoplastic V58.11
    circumcision, ritual or routine (in
      absence of medical indication)
      V50.2
    clinical research investigation
      (control) (normal comparison)
      (participant) V70.7
    closure of artificial opening - *see*
      Attention to, artificial, opening
    contraceptive
      counseling V25.09
        emergency V25.03
        postcoital V25.03
      management V25.9
        specified type NEC V25.8
    convalescence following V66.9
      chemotherapy V66.2
      psychotherapy V66.3
      radiotherapy V66.1
      surgery V66.0
      treatment (for) V66.5
        combined V66.6
        fracture V66.4
        mental disorder NEC V66.3
        specified condition NEC V66.5

A

Admission (*Continued*)
  for (*Continued*)
    cosmetic surgery NEC V50.1
      breast reconstruction following
          mastectomy V51.0
      following healed injury or
          operation V51.8
    counseling (*see also* Counseling)
        V65.40
      without complaint or sickness
          V65.49
      contraceptive management
          V25.09
        emergency V25.03
        postcoital V25.03
      dietary V65.3
      exercise V65.41
      fertility preservation (prior to
          cancer therapy) (prior to
          surgical removal of gonads)
          V26.42
      for
        nonattending third party
            V65.19
        pediatric
          pre-adoption visit for
              adoptive parent(s)
              V65.11
          pre-birth visit for
              expectant parent(s)
              V65.11
        victim of abuse
          child V61.21
          partner or spouse V61.11
      genetic V26.33
      gonorrhea V65.45
      HIV V65.44
      human immunodeficiency virus
          V65.44
      injury prevention V65.43
      insulin pump training V65.46
      natural family planning
          procreative V26.41
          to avoid pregnancy V25.04
      procreative management
          V26.49
        using natural family planning
            V26.41
      sexually transmitted disease NEC
          V65.45
        HIV V65.44
      specified reason NEC V65.49
      substance use and abuse
          V65.42
      syphilis V65.45
      victim of abuse
          child V61.21
          partner or spouse V61.11
    desensitization to allergens V07.1
    dialysis V56.0
      catheter
        fitting and adjustment
            extracorporeal V56.1
            peritoneal V56.2
        removal or replacement
            extracorporeal V56.1
            peritoneal V56.2
      extracorporeal (renal) V56.0
      peritoneal V56.8
      renal V56.0
    dietary surveillance and counseling
        V65.3
    drug monitoring, therapeutic
        V58.83
    ear piercing V50.3

Admission (*Continued*)
  for (*Continued*)
    elective surgery
      breast
        augmentation or reduction
            V50.1
        reconstruction following
            mastectomy V51.0
        removal, prophylactic V50.41
      circumcision, ritual or routine (in
          absence of medical
          indication) V50.2
      cosmetic NEC V50.1
        breast reconstruction following
            mastectomy V51.0
        following healed injury or
            operation V51.8
      ear piercing V50.3
      face-lift V50.1
      hair transplant V50.0
      plastic
        breast reconstruction following
            mastectomy V51.0
        cosmetic NEC V50.1
        following healed injury or
            operation V51.8
      prophylactic organ removal V50.49
        breast V50.41
        ovary V50.42
      repair of scarred tissue (following
          healed injury or operation)
          V51.8
      specified type NEC V50.8
    end-of-life care V66.7
    examination (*see also* Examination)
        V70.9
      administrative purpose NEC V70.3
      adoption V70.3
      allergy V72.7
      antibody response V72.61
      at health care facility V70.0
      athletic team V70.3
      camp V70.3
      cardiovascular, preoperative
          V72.81
      clinical research investigation
          (control) (participant) V70.7
      dental V72.2
      developmental testing (child)
          (infant) V20.2
      donor (potential) V70.8
      driver's license V70.3
      ear V72.19
      employment V70.5
      eye V72.0
      follow-up (routine) - *see*
          Examination, follow-up
      for admission to
          old age home V70.3
          school V70.3
      general V70.9
          specified reason NEC V70.8
      gynecological V72.31
      health supervision
          child (over 28 days old) V20.2
          infant (over 28 days old) V20.2
          newborn
            8 to 28 days old V20.32
            under 8 days old V20.31
      hearing V72.19
          following failed hearing
              screening V72.11
      immigration V70.3
      infant
          8 to 28 days old V20.32
          over 28 days old, routine V20.2
          under 8 days old V20.31

Admission (*Continued*)
  for (*Continued*)
    examination (*Continued*)
      insurance certification V70.3
      laboratory V72.60
          ordered as part of a routine
              general medical
              examination V72.62
      pre-operative V72.63
      pre-procedural V72.63
      specified NEC V72.69
      marriage license V70.3
      medical (general) (*see also*
          Examination, medical) V70.9
      medicolegal reasons V70.4
      naturalization V70.3
      pelvic (annual) (periodic) V72.31
      postpartum checkup V24.2
      pregnancy (possible)
          (unconfirmed) V72.40
          negative result V72.41
          positive result V72.42
      preoperative V72.84
          cardiovascular V72.81
          respiratory V72.82
          specified NEC V72.83
      preprocedural V72.84
          cardiovascular V72.81
          general physical V72.83
          respiratory V72.82
          specified NEC V72.83
      prior to chemotherapy V72.83
      prison V70.3
      psychiatric (general) V70.2
          requested by authority V70.1
      radiological NEC V72.5
      respiratory, preoperative V72.82
      school V70.3
      screening - *see* Screening
      skin hypersensitivity V72.7
      specified type NEC V72.85
      sport competition V70.3
      vision V72.0
      well baby and child care V20.2
    exercise therapy V57.1
    face-lift, cosmetic reason V50.1
    fertility preservation (prior to cancer
        therapy) (prior to surgical
        removal of gonads) V26.82
    fitting (of)
      artificial
        arm (complete) (partial) V52.0
        eye V52.2
        leg (complete) (partial) V52.1
      biliary drainage tube V58.82
      brain neuropacemaker V53.02
      breast V52.4
        implant V52.4
        prosthesis V52.4
      cardiac pacemaker V53.31
      catheter
        non-vascular V58.82
        vascular V58.81
      cerebral ventricle (communicating)
          shunt V53.01
      chest tube V58.82
      colostomy belt V55.2
      contact lenses V53.1
      cystostomy device V53.6
      dental prosthesis V52.3
      device, unspecified type V53.90
        abdominal V53.59
        cerebral ventricle
            (communicating)
            shunt V53.01
        gastrointestinal NEC V53.59
        insulin pump V53.91

◀ New   ◀▥ Revised   ~~deleted~~ Deleted   ● Use Additional Digit(s)   ▨ Omit code

Admission *(Continued)*
  for *(Continued)*
    fitting *(Continued)*
      device, unspecified type
        (Continued)
        intestinal V53.50
        intrauterine contraceptive
          V25.1 ◀▥
          insertion V25.11 ◀
          removal V25.12 ◀
            and reinsertion V25.13 ◀
          replacement V25.13 ◀
        nervous system V53.09
        orthodontic V53.4
        other device V53.99
        prosthetic V52.9
          breast V52.4
          dental V52.3
          eye V52.2
        special senses V53.09
        substitution
          auditory V53.09
          nervous system V53.09
          visual V53.09
      diaphragm (contraceptive) V25.02
      fistula (sinus tract) drainage tube
        V58.82
      gastric lap band V53.51
      gastrointestinal appliance and
        device NEC V53.59
      growth rod V54.02
      hearing aid V53.2
      ileostomy device V55.2
      intestinal appliance and device
        V53.50
      intrauterine contraceptive device
        V25.1 ◀▥
        insertion V25.11 ◀
        removal V25.12 ◀
          and reinsertion V25.13 ◀
        replacement V25.13 ◀
      neuropacemaker (brain)
        (peripheral nerve) (spinal
        cord) V53.02
      orthodontic device V53.4
      orthopedic (device) V53.7
        brace V53.7
        cast V53.7
        shoes V53.7
      pacemaker
        brain V53.02
        cardiac V53.31
        carotid sinus V53.39
        spinal cord V53.02
      pleural drainage tube V58.82
      portacath V58.81
      prosthesis V52.9
        arm (complete) (partial) V52.0
        breast V52.4
        dental V52.3
        eye V52.2
        leg (complete) (partial) V52.1
        specified type NEC V52.8
      spectacles V53.1
      wheelchair V53.8
    follow-up examination (routine)
      (following) V67.9
      cancer chemotherapy V67.2
      chemotherapy V67.2
      high-risk medication NEC V67.51
      injury NEC V67.59
      psychiatric V67.3
      psychotherapy V67.3
      radiotherapy V67.1
      specified surgery NEC V67.09
      surgery V67.00
        vaginal pap smear V67.01

Admission *(Continued)*
  for *(Continued)*
    follow-up examination *(Continued)*
      treatment (for) V67.9
        combined V67.6
        fracture V67.4
        involving high-risk medication
          NEC V67.51
        mental disorder V67.3
        specified NEC V67.59
    hair transplant, for cosmetic reason
      V50.0
    health advice, education, or
      instruction V65.4
    hearing conservation and treatment
      V72.12
    hormone replacement therapy
      (postmenopausal) V07.4
    hospice care V66.7
    immunizations (childhood)
      appropriate for age V20.2
    immunotherapy, antineoplastic V58.12
    insertion (of)
      intrauterine contraceptive device
        V25.11 ◀
      subdermal implantable
        contraceptive V25.5
    insulin pump titration V53.91
    insulin pump training V65.46
    intrauterine device
      insertion V25.11 ◀▥
      management V25.42
      removal V25.12 ◀
        and reinsertion V25.13 ◀
      replacement V25.13 ◀
    investigation to determine further
      disposition V63.8
    in vitro fertilization cycle V26.81
    isolation V07.0
    issue of
      disability examination certificate
        V68.01
      medical certificate NEC V68.09
      repeat prescription NEC V68.1
        contraceptive device NEC
          V25.49
    kidney dialysis V56.0
    lengthening of growth rod V54.02
    mental health evaluation V70.2
      requested by authority V70.1
    natural family planning counseling
      and advice
      procreative V26.41
      to avoid pregnancy V25.04
    nonmedical reason NEC V68.89
    nursing care evaluation V63.8
    observation (without need for
      further medical care) *(see also*
      Observation) V71.9
      accident V71.4
      alleged rape or seduction V71.5
      criminal assault V71.6
      following accident V71.4
        at work V71.3
      foreign body ingestion V71.89
      growth and development
        variations, childhood V21.0
      inflicted injury NEC V71.6
      ingestion of deleterious agent or
        foreign body V71.89
      injury V71.6
      malignant neoplasm V71.1
      mental disorder V71.09
      newborn - *see* Observation,
        suspected, condition,
        newborn

Admission *(Continued)*
  for *(Continued)*
    observation *(Continued)*
      rape V71.5
      specified NEC V71.89
        disorder V71.9
          abuse V71.81
          accident V71.4
            at work V71.3
          benign neoplasm V71.89
          cardiovascular V71.7
          exposure
            anthrax V71.82
            biological agent NEC
              V71.83
            SARS V71.83
          heart V71.7
          inflicted injury NEC V71.6
          malignant neoplasm V71.1
          mental NEC V71.09
          neglect V71.81
          specified condition NEC
            V71.89
          tuberculosis V71.2
        maternal and fetal problem not
          found
          amniotic cavity and
            membrane V89.01
          cervical shortening V89.05
          fetal anomaly V89.03
          fetal growth V89.04
          oligohydramnios V89.01
          other specified NEC V89.09
          placenta V89.02
          polyhydramnios V89.01
      tuberculosis V71.2
    occupational therapy V57.21
    organ transplant, donor - *see* Donor
    ovary, ovarian removal, prophylactic
      V50.42
    palliative care V66.7
    Papanicolaou smear
      cervix V76.2
        for suspected malignant
          neoplasm V76.2
        no disease found V71.1
        routine, as part of
          gynecological
          examination V72.31
        to confirm findings of recent
          normal smear following
          initial abnormal smear
          V72.32
      vaginal V76.47
        following hysterectomy for
          malignant condition
          V67.01
    passage of sounds or bougie in
      artificial opening - *see*
      Attention to, artificial, opening
    paternity testing V70.4
    peritoneal dialysis V56.32
    physical therapy NEC V57.1
    plastic surgery
      breast reconstruction following
        mastectomy V51.0
      cosmetic NEC V50.1
      following healed injury or
        operation V51.8
    postmenopausal hormone
      replacement therapy V07.4
    postpartum observation
      immediately after delivery V24.0
      routine follow-up V24.2
    poststerilization (for restoration)
      V26.0

Admission *(Continued)*
  for *(Continued)*
    procreative management V26.9
      assisted reproductive fertility
        procedure cycle V26.81
      in vitro fertilization cycle V26.81
      specified type NEC V26.89
    prophylactic
      administration of
        antibiotics, long-term V58.62 ◀▥
          short-term use - *omit code* ◀
        antitoxin, any V07.2
        antivenin V07.2
        chemotherapeutic agent NEC
          V07.39
        chemotherapy NEC V07.39
        diphtheria antitoxin V07.2
        fluoride V07.31
        gamma globulin V07.2
        immune sera (gamma
          globulin) V07.2
        RhoGAM V07.2
        tetanus antitoxin V07.2
      breathing exercises V57.0
      chemotherapy NEC V07.39
        fluoride V07.31
      measure V07.9
        specified type NEC V07.8
      organ removal V50.49
        breast V50.41
        ovary V50.42
    psychiatric examination (general)
      V70.2
      requested by authority V70.1
    radiation management V58.0
    radiotherapy V58.0
    reconstruction following
      mastectomy V51.0
    reforming of artificial opening -
      see Attention to, artificial,
      opening
    rehabilitation V57.9
      multiple types V57.89
      occupational V57.21
      orthoptic V57.4
      orthotic V57.81
      physical NEC V57.1
      specified type NEC V57.89
      speech (-language) V57.3
      vocational V57.22
    removal of
      breast tissue expander without
        synchronous insertion of
        permanent implant V52.4
      cardiac pacemaker V53.31
      cast (plaster) V54.89
      catheter from artificial opening -
        see Attention to, artificial,
        opening
      cerebral ventricle (communicating)
        shunt V53.01
      cystostomy catheter V55.5
      device
        cerebral ventricle
          (communicating)
          shunt V53.01
        fixation
          external V54.89
          internal V54.01
        intrauterine contraceptive
          V25.12 ◀▥
        traction, external V54.89
      drains V58.49
      dressing
        wound V58.30
          nonsurgical V58.30
          surgical V58.31

Admission *(Continued)*
  for *(Continued)*
    removal of *(Continued)*
      fixation device
        external V54.89
        internal V54.01
      intrauterine contraceptive device
        V25.12 ◀▥
      Kirschner wire V54.89
      neuropacemaker (brain)
        (peripheral nerve) (spinal
        cord) V53.02
      nonsurgical wound dressing
        V58.30
      orthopedic fixation device
        external V54.89
        internal V54.01
      pacemaker device
        brain V53.02
        cardiac V53.31
        carotid sinus V53.39
        nervous system V53.02
      plaster cast V54.89
      plate (fracture) V54.01
      rod V54.01
      screw (fracture) V54.01
      splint, traction V54.89
      staples V58.32
      Steinmann pin V54.89
      subdermal implantable
        contraceptive V25.43
      surgical wound dressing V58.31
      sutures V58.32
      traction device, external V54.89
      ureteral stent V53.6
      wound packing V58.30
        nonsurgical V58.30
        surgical V58.31
    repair of scarred tissue (following
      healed injury or operation)
      V51.8
    replacement of intrauterine
      contraceptive device V25.13 ◀
    reprogramming of cardiac
      pacemaker V53.31
    respirator [ventilator] dependence
      during
        mechanical failure V46.14
        power failure V46.12
      for weaning V46.13
    restoration of organ continuity
      (poststerilization) (tuboplasty)
      (vasoplasty) V26.0
    Rh typing V72.86
    routine infant and child vision and
      hearing testing V20.2
    sensitivity test - *see also* Test, skin
      allergy NEC V72.7
      bacterial disease NEC V74.9
      Dick V74.8
      Kveim V82.89
      Mantoux V74.1
      mycotic infection NEC V75.4
      parasitic disease NEC V75.8
      Schick V74.3
      Schultz-Charlton V74.8
    social service (agency) referral or
      evaluation V63.8
    speech (-language) therapy V57.3
    sterilization V25.2
    suspected disorder (ruled out)
      (without need for further
      care) - *see* Observation
    terminal care V66.7
    tests only - *see* Test
    therapeutic drug monitoring
      V58.83

Admission *(Continued)*
  for *(Continued)*
    therapy
      blood transfusion, without
        reported diagnosis V58.2
      breathing exercises V57.0
      chemotherapy, antineoplastic
        V58.11
        prophylactic NEC V07.39
          fluoride V07.31
      dialysis (intermittent) (treatment)
        extracorporeal V56.0
        peritoneal V56.8
        renal V56.0
        specified type NEC V56.8
      exercise (remedial) NEC V57.1
        breathing V57.0
      immunotherapy, antineoplastic
        V58.12
      long-term (current) (prophylactic)
        drug use NEC V58.69 ◀▥
        antibiotics V58.62
          short-term use - *omit code* ◀
        anticoagulants V58.61
        anti-inflammatories, non-
          steroidal (NSAID)
          V58.64
        antiplatelets V58.63
        antithrombotics V58.63
        aspirin V58.66
        high-risk medications NEC
          V58.69
        insulin V58.67
        methadone V58.69
        opiate analgesic V58.69
        steroids V58.65
      occupational V57.21
      orthoptic V57.4
      physical NEC V57.1
      radiation V58.0
      speech (-language) V57.3
      vocational V57.22
    toilet or cleaning
      of artificial opening - *see* Attention
        to, artificial, opening
      of non-vascular catheter V58.82
      of vascular catheter V58.81
    treatment ◀
      measure V07.9 ◀
        specified type NEC V07.8 ◀
    tubal ligation V25.2
    tuboplasty for previous sterilization
      V26.0
    ultrasound, routine fetal V28.3
    vaccination, prophylactic (against)
      arthropod-borne virus, viral NEC
        V05.1
        disease NEC V05.1
        encephalitis V05.0
      Bacille Calmette Guérin (BCG)
        V03.2
      BCG V03.2
      chickenpox V05.4
      cholera alone V03.0
        with typhoid-paratyphoid
          (cholera + TAB) V06.0
      common cold V04.7
      dengue V05.1
      diphtheria alone V03.5
      diphtheria-tetanus-pertussis
        (DTP) (DTaP) V06.1
        with
          poliomyelitis (DTP polio)
          V06.3
          typhoid-paratyphoid
          (DTP + TAB) V06.2
      diphtheria-tetanus [Td] [DT]
        without pertussis V06.5

Admission *(Continued)*
  for *(Continued)*
    vaccination, prophylactic *(Continued)*
      disease (single) NEC V05.9
        bacterial NEC V03.9
          specified type NEC V03.89
        combinations NEC V06.9
          specified type NEC V06.8
        specified type NEC V05.8
        viral NEC V04.89
      encephalitis, viral, arthropod-
        borne V05.0
      Hemophilus influenzae, type B
        [Hib] V03.81
      hepatitis, viral V05.3
      human papillomavirus (HPV)
        V04.89
      immune sera (gamma globulin)
        V07.2
      influenza V04.81
        with
          Streptococcus pneumoniae
            [pneumococcus] V06.6
      Leishmaniasis V05.2
      measles alone V04.2
      measles-mumps-rubella (MMR)
        V06.4
      mumps alone V04.6
        with measles and rubella
          (MMR) V06.4
      not done because of
        contraindication V64.09
      pertussis alone V03.6
      plague V03.3
      pneumonia V03.82
      poliomyelitis V04.0
        with diphtheria-tetanus-
          pertussis (DTP polio)
          V06.3
      rabies V04.5
      respiratory syncytial virus (RSV)
        V04.82
      rubella alone V04.3
        with measles and mumps
          (MMR) V06.4
      smallpox V04.1
      specified type NEC V05.8
      Streptococcus pneumoniae
        [pneumococcus] V03.82
        with
          influenza V06.6
      tetanus toxoid alone V03.7
        with diphtheria [Td] [DT] V06.5
          and pertussis (DTP) (DTaP)
          V06.1
      tuberculosis (BCG) V03.2
      tularemia V03.4
      typhoid alone V03.1
        with diphtheria-tetanus-
          pertussis (TAB + DTP)
          V06.2
      typhoid-paratyphoid alone (TAB)
        V03.1
      typhus V05.8
      varicella (chicken pox) V05.4
      viral encephalitis, arthropod-
        borne V05.0
      viral hepatitis V05.3
      yellow fever V04.4
    vasectomy V25.2
    vasoplasty for previous sterilization
      V26.0
    vision examination V72.0
    vocational therapy V57.22
    waiting period for admission to
      other facility V63.2
    undergoing social agency
      investigation V63.8

Admission *(Continued)*
  for *(Continued)*
    well baby and child care V20.2
    x-ray of chest
      for suspected tuberculosis V71.2
      routine V72.5
Adnexitis (suppurative) *(see also* Salpingo-
  oophoritis) 614.2
Adolescence NEC V21.2
Adoption
  agency referral V68.89
  examination V70.3
  held for V68.89
Adrenal gland - *see* condition
Adrenalism 255.9
  tuberculous *(see also* Tuberculosis)
    017.6●
Adrenalitis, adrenitis 255.8
  meningococcal hemorrhagic 036.3
Adrenarche, precocious 259.1
Adrenocortical syndrome 255.2
Adrenogenital syndrome (acquired)
  (congenital) 255.2
  iatrogenic, fetus or newborn 760.79
Adrenoleukodystrophy 277.86
  neonatal 277.86
  x-linked 277.86
Adrenomyeloneuropathy 277.86
Adventitious bursa - *see* Bursitis
Adynamia (episodica) (hereditary)
  (periodic) 359.3
Adynamic
  ileus or intestine *(see also* Ileus) 560.1
  ureter 753.22
Aeration lung, imperfect, newborn 770.5
Aerobullosis 993.3
Aerocele - *see* Embolism, air
Aerodermectasia
  subcutaneous (traumatic) 958.7
    surgical 998.81
  surgical 998.81
Aerodontalgia 993.2
Aeroembolism 993.3
Aerogenes capsulatus infection *(see also*
  Gangrene, gas) 040.0
Aero-otitis media 993.0
Aerophagy, aerophagia 306.4
  psychogenic 306.4
Aerosinusitis 993.1
Aerotitis 993.0
Affection, affections - *see also* Disease
  sacroiliac (joint), old 724.6
  shoulder region NEC 726.2
Afibrinogenemia 286.3
  acquired 286.6
  congenital 286.3
  postpartum 666.3●
African
  sleeping sickness 086.5
  tick fever 087.1
  trypanosomiasis 086.5
    Gambian 086.3
    Rhodesian 086.4
Aftercare V58.9
  amputation stump V54.89
  artificial openings - *see* Attention to,
    artificial, opening
  blood transfusion without reported
    diagnosis V58.2
  breathing exercise V57.0
  cardiac device V53.39
    defibrillator, automatic implantable
      (with synchronous cardiac
      pacemaker) V53.32 ◀▥
    pacemaker V53.31
      carotid sinus V53.39
  carotid sinus pacemaker V53.39

Aftercare *(Continued)*
  cerebral ventricle (communicating)
    shunt V53.01
  chemotherapy (oral) (intravenous)
    session (adjunctive)
    (maintenance) V58.11
  defibrillator, automatic implantable
    cardiac (with synchronous
    cardiac pacemaker) V53.32 ◀▥
  exercise (remedial) (therapeutic) V57.1
    breathing V57.0
  extracorporeal dialysis (intermittent)
    (treatment) V56.0
  following surgery NEC V58.49
    for
      injury V58.43
      neoplasm V58.42
      organ transplant V58.44
      trauma V58.43
    joint replacement V54.81
    of
      circulatory system V58.73
      digestive system V58.75
      genital organs V58.76
      genitourinary system V58.76
      musculoskeletal system V58.78
      nervous system V58.72
      oral cavity V58.75
      respiratory system V58.74
      sense organs V58.71
      skin V58.77
      subcutaneous tissue V58.77
      teeth V58.75
      urinary system V58.76
    spinal - *see* Aftercare, following
      surgery, of, specified body
      system
    wound closure, planned V58.41
  fracture V54.9
    healing V54.89
      pathologic
        ankle V54.29
        arm V54.20
          lower V54.22
          upper V54.21
        finger V54.29
        foot V54.29
        hand V54.29
        hip V54.23
        leg V54.24
          lower V54.26
          upper V54.25
        pelvis V54.29
        specified site NEC V54.29
        toe(s) V54.29
        vertebrae V54.27
        wrist V54.29
      traumatic
        ankle V54.19
        arm V54.10
          lower V54.12
          upper V54.11
        finger V54.19
        foot V54.19
        hand V54.19
        hip V54.13
        leg V54.14
          lower V54.16
          upper V54.15
        pelvis V54.19
        specified site NEC V54.19
        toe(s) V54.19
        vertebrae V54.17
        wrist V54.19
    removal of
      external fixation device V54.89
      internal fixation device V54.01
    specified care NEC V54.89

Aftercare (Continued)
gait training V57.1
    for use of artificial limb(s) V57.81
internal fixation device V54.09
involving
    dialysis (intermittent) (treatment)
        extracorporeal V56.0
        peritoneal V56.8
        renal V56.0
    gait training V57.1
        for use of artificial limb(s) V57.81
    growth rod
        adjustment V54.02
        lengthening V54.02
    internal fixation device V54.09
    orthoptic training V57.4
    orthotic training V57.81
    radiotherapy session V58.0
    removal of
        drains V58.49
        dressings
            wound V58.30
                nonsurgical V58.30
                surgical V58.31
        fixation device
            external V54.89
            internal V54.01
        fracture plate V54.01
        nonsurgical wound dressing
            V58.30
        pins V54.01
        plaster cast V54.89
        rods V54.01
        screws V54.01
        staples V58.32
        surgical wound dressings V58.31
        sutures V58.32
        traction device, external V54.89
        wound packing V58.30
            nonsurgical V58.30
            surgical V58.31
neuropacemaker (brain) (peripheral
    nerve) (spinal cord) V53.02
occupational therapy V57.21
orthodontic V58.5
orthopedic V54.9
    change of external fixation or
        traction device V54.89
    following joint replacement V54.81
    internal fixation device V54.09
    removal of fixation device
        external V54.89
        internal V54.01
    specified care NEC V54.89
orthoptic training V57.4
orthotic training V57.81
pacemaker
    brain V53.02
    cardiac V53.31
    carotid sinus V53.39
    peripheral nerve V53.02
    spinal cord V53.02
peritoneal dialysis (intermittent)
    (treatment) V56.8
physical therapy NEC V57.1
    breathing exercises V57.0
radiotherapy session V58.0
rehabilitation procedure V57.9
    breathing exercises V57.0
    multiple types V57.89
    occupational V57.21
    orthoptic V57.4
    orthotic V57.81
    physical therapy NEC V57.1
    remedial exercises V57.1
    specified type NEC V57.89

Aftercare (Continued)
rehabilitation procedure (Continued)
    speech (-language) V57.3
    therapeutic exercises V57.1
    vocational V57.22
renal dialysis (intermittent) (treatment)
    V56.0
specified type NEC V58.89
    removal of non-vascular catheter
        V58.82
    removal of vascular catheter V58.81
speech (-language) therapy V57.3
stump, amputation V54.89
vocational rehabilitation V57.22
After-cataract 366.50
obscuring vision 366.53
specified type, not obscuring vision
    366.52
Agalactia 676.4●
Agammaglobulinemia 279.00
with lymphopenia 279.2
acquired (primary) (secondary)
    279.06
Bruton's X-linked 279.04
infantile sex-linked (Bruton's)
    (congenital) 279.04
Swiss-type 279.2
Aganglionosis (bowel) (colon) 751.3
Age (old) (see also Senile) 797
Agenesis - see also Absence, by site,
    congenital
acoustic nerve 742.8
adrenal (gland) 759.1
alimentary tract (complete) (partial)
    NEC 751.8
    lower 751.2
    upper 750.8
anus, anal (canal) 751.2
aorta 747.22
appendix 751.2
arm (complete) (partial) (see also
    Deformity, reduction, upper limb)
    755.20
artery (peripheral) NEC (see also
    Anomaly, peripheral vascular
    system) 747.60
    brain 747.81
    coronary 746.85
    pulmonary 747.3
    umbilical 747.5
auditory (canal) (external) 744.01
auricle (ear) 744.01
bile, biliary duct or passage 751.61
bone NEC 756.9
brain 740.0
    specified part 742.2
breast 757.6
bronchus 748.3
canaliculus lacrimalis 743.65
carpus NEC (see also Deformity,
    reduction, upper limb) 755.28
cartilage 756.9
cecum 751.2
cerebellum 742.2
cervix 752.43 ◀▥
chin 744.89
cilia 743.63
circulatory system, part NEC 747.89
clavicle 755.51
clitoris 752.49
coccyx 756.13
colon 751.2
corpus callosum 742.2
cricoid cartilage 748.3
diaphragm (with hernia) 756.6

Agenesis (Continued)
digestive organ(s) or tract (complete)
    (partial) NEC 751.8
    lower 751.2
    upper 750.8
ductus arteriosus 747.89
duodenum 751.1
ear NEC 744.09
    auricle 744.01
    lobe 744.21
ejaculatory duct 752.89
endocrine (gland) NEC 759.2
epiglottis 748.3
esophagus 750.3
Eustachian tube 744.24
extrinsic muscle, eye 743.69
eye 743.00
    adnexa 743.69
eyelid (fold) 743.62
face
    bones NEC 756.0
    specified part NEC 744.89
fallopian tube 752.19
femur NEC (see also Absence, femur,
    congenital) 755.34
fibula NEC (see also Absence, fibula,
    congenital) 755.37
finger NEC (see also Absence, finger,
    congenital) 755.29
foot (complete) (see also Deformity,
    reduction, lower limb) 755.31
gallbladder 751.69
gastric 750.8
genitalia, genital (organ)
    female 752.89
        external 752.49
        internal NEC 752.89
    male 752.89
        penis 752.69
glottis 748.3
gonadal 758.6
hair 757.4
hand (complete) (see also Deformity,
    reduction, upper limb) 755.21
heart 746.89
    valve NEC 746.89
        aortic 746.89
        mitral 746.89
        pulmonary 746.01
hepatic 751.69
humerus NEC (see also Absence,
    humerus, congenital) 755.24
hymen 752.49
ileum 751.1
incus 744.04
intestine (small) 751.1
    large 751.2
iris (dilator fibers) 743.45
jaw 524.09
jejunum 751.1
kidney(s) (partial) (unilateral) 753.0
labium (majus) (minus) 752.49
labyrinth, membranous 744.05
lacrimal apparatus (congenital) 743.65
larynx 748.3
leg NEC (see also Deformity, reduction,
    lower limb) 755.30
lens 743.35
limb (complete) (partial) (see also
    Deformity, reduction) 755.4
    lower NEC 755.30
    upper 755.20
lip 750.26
liver 751.69
lung (bilateral) (fissures) (lobe)
    (unilateral) 748.5

◀ New   ◀▥ Revised   ~~deleted~~ Deleted   ● Use Additional Digit(s)   ▨ Omit code

Agenesis *(Continued)*
  mandible 524.09
  maxilla 524.09
  metacarpus NEC 755.28
  metatarsus NEC 755.38
  muscle (any) 756.81
  musculoskeletal system NEC 756.9
  nail(s) 757.5
  neck, part 744.89
  nerve 742.8
  nervous system, part NEC 742.8
  nipple 757.6
  nose 748.1
  nuclear 742.8
  organ
      of Corti 744.05
      or site not listed - *see* Anomaly,
          specified type NEC
  osseous meatus (ear) 744.03
  ovary 752.0
  oviduct 752.19
  pancreas 751.7
  parathyroid (gland) 759.2
  patella 755.64
  pelvic girdle (complete) (partial) 755.69
  penis 752.69
  pericardium 746.89
  perineal body 756.81
  pituitary (gland) 759.2
  prostate 752.89
  pulmonary
      artery 747.3
      trunk 747.3
      vein 747.49
  punctum lacrimale 743.65
  radioulnar NEC (*see also* Absence,
      forearm, congenital) 755.25
  radius NEC (*see also* Absence, radius,
      congenital) 755.26
  rectum 751.2
  renal 753.0
  respiratory organ NEC 748.9
  rib 756.3
  roof of orbit 742.0
  round ligament 752.89
  sacrum 756.13
  salivary gland 750.21
  scapula 755.59
  scrotum 752.89
  seminal duct or tract 752.89
  septum
      atrial 745.69
      between aorta and pulmonary
          artery 745.0
      ventricular 745.3
  shoulder girdle (complete) (partial)
      755.59
  skull (bone) 756.0
      with
          anencephalus 740.0
          encephalocele 742.0
          hydrocephalus 742.3
              with spina bifida (*see also*
                  Spina bifida) 741.0●
          microcephalus 742.1
  spermatic cord 752.89
  spinal cord 742.59
  spine 756.13
      lumbar 756.13
          isthmus 756.11
          pars articularis 756.11
  spleen 759.0
  sternum 756.3
  stomach 750.7
  tarsus NEC 755.38

Agenesis *(Continued)*
  tendon 756.81
  testicular 752.89
  testis 752.89
  thymus (gland) 759.2
  thyroid (gland) 243
      cartilage 748.3
  tibia NEC (*see also* Absence, tibia,
      congenital) 755.36
  tibiofibular NEC 755.35
  toe (complete) (partial) (*see also*
      Absence, toe, congenital) 755.39
  tongue 750.11
  trachea (cartilage) 748.3
  ulna NEC (*see also* Absence, ulna,
      congenital) 755.27
  ureter 753.4
  urethra 753.8
  urinary tract NEC 753.8
  uterus 752.31 ◄▦
  uvula 750.26
  vagina (total) (partial) 752.45 ◄▦
  vas deferens 752.89
  vein(s) (peripheral) NEC (*see also*
      Anomaly, peripheral vascular
      system) 747.60
      brain 747.81
      great 747.49
      portal 747.49
      pulmonary 747.49
  vena cava (inferior) (superior) 747.49
  vermis of cerebellum 742.2
  vertebra 756.13
      lumbar 756.13
          isthmus 756.11
          pars articularis 756.11
  vulva 752.49
Ageusia (*see also* Disturbance, sensation)
  781.1
Aggressiveness 301.3
Aggressive outburst (*see also* Disturbance,
  conduct) 312.0●
  in children or adolescents 313.9
Aging skin 701.8
Agitated - *see* condition
Agitation 307.9
  catatonic (*see also* Schizophrenia) 295.2●
Aglossia (congenital) 750.11
Aglycogenosis 271.0
Agnail (finger) (with lymphangitis) 681.02
Agnosia (body image) (tactile) 784.69
  verbal 784.69
      auditory 784.69
          secondary to organic lesion 784.69
      developmental 315.8
      secondary to organic lesion 784.69
  visual 368.16
      object 368.16
Agoraphobia 300.22
  with panic disorder 300.21
Agrammatism 784.69
Agranulocytopenia (*see also*
  Agranulocytosis) 288.09
Agranulocytosis (*see also* Neutropenia)
  288.09
  chronic 288.09
  cyclical 288.02
  due to infection 288.04
  genetic 288.01
  infantile 288.01
  periodic 288.02
  pernicious 288.09
Agraphia (absolute) 784.69
  with alexia 784.61
  developmental 315.39
Agrypnia (*see also* Insomnia) 780.52

Ague (*see also* Malaria) 084.6
  brass-founders' 985.8
  dumb 084.6
  tertian 084.1
Agyria 742.2
AHTR (acute hemolytic transfusion
  reaction) - *see* Complications,
  transfusion ◄
Ahumada-del Castillo syndrome
  (nonpuerperal galactorrhea and
  amenorrhea) 253.1
AIDS 042
AIDS-associated retrovirus (disease)
  (illness) 042
  infection - *see* Human
      immunodeficiency virus,
      infection
AIDS-associated virus (disease) (illness)
  042
  infection - *see* Human
      immunodeficiency virus,
      infection
AIDS-like disease (illness) (syndrome) 042
AIDS-related complex 042
AIDS-related conditions 042
AIDS-related virus (disease) (illness) 042
  infection - *see* Human
      immunodeficiency virus,
      infection
AIDS virus (disease) (illness) 042
  infection - *see* Human
      immunodeficiency virus,
      infection
Ailment, heart - *see* Disease, heart
Ailurophobia 300.29
AIN I (anal intraepithelial neoplasia I)
  (histologically confirmed) 569.44 ◄▦
AIN II (anal intraepithelial neoplasia II)
  (histologically confirmed) 569.44 ◄▦
AIN III (anal intraepithelial neoplasia III)
  230.6 ◄▦
  anal canal 230.5
Ainhum (disease) 136.0
AIPHI (acute idiopathic pulmonary
  hemorrhage in infants (over 28 days
  old) 786.31 ◄
Air
  anterior mediastinum 518.1
  compressed, disease 993.3
  embolism (any site) (artery) (cerebral)
      958.0
      with
          abortion - *see* Abortion, by type,
              with embolism
          ectopic pregnancy (*see also*
              categories 633.0-633.9) 639.6
          molar pregnancy (*see also*
              categories 630-632) 639.6
      due to implanted device - *see*
          Complications, due to
          (presence of) any device,
          implant, or graft classified to
          996.0-996.5 NEC
      following
          abortion 639.6
          ectopic or molar pregnancy 639.6
          infusion, perfusion, or
              transfusion 999.1
      in pregnancy, childbirth, or
          puerperium 673.0●
      traumatic 958.0
  hunger 786.09
      psychogenic 306.1
  leak (lung) (pulmonary) (thorax) 512.8
      iatrogenic 512.1
      postoperative 512.1

Air *(Continued)*
 rarefied, effects of - *see* Effect, adverse,
  high altitude
 sickness 994.6
Airplane sickness 994.6
Akathisia, acathisia 781.0
 due to drugs 333.99
 neuroleptic-induced acute 333.99
Akinesia algeria 352.6
Akiyami 100.89
Akureyri disease (epidemic
  neuromyasthenia) 049.8
Alacrima (congenital) 743.65
Alactasia (hereditary) 271.3
Alagille syndrome 759.89
Alalia 784.3
 developmental 315.31
  receptive-expressive 315.32
 secondary to organic lesion 784.3
Alaninemia 270.8
Alastrim 050.1
Albarrán's disease (colibacilluria) 791.9
Albers-Schönberg's disease (marble
  bones) 756.52
Albert's disease 726.71
Albinism, albino (choroid) (cutaneous)
  (eye) (generalized) (isolated) (ocular)
  (oculocutaneous) (partial) 270.2
Albinismus 270.2
Albright (-Martin) (-Bantam) disease
  (pseudohypoparathyroidism) 275.49
Albright (-McCune) (-Sternberg)
  syndrome (osteitis fibrosa
  disseminata) 756.59
Albuminous - *see* Condition
Albuminuria, albuminuric (acute)
  (chronic) (subacute) 791.0
 Bence-Jones 791.0
 cardiac 785.9
 complicating pregnancy, childbirth, or
  puerperium 646.2●
  with hypertension - *see* Toxemia, of
   pregnancy
  affecting fetus or newborn 760.1
 cyclic 593.6
 gestational 646.2●
 gravidarum 646.2●
  with hypertension - *see* Toxemia, of
   pregnancy
  affecting fetus or newborn 760.1
 heart 785.9
 idiopathic 593.6
 orthostatic 593.6
 postural 593.6
 pre-eclamptic (mild) 642.4●
  affecting fetus or newborn 760.0
  severe 642.5●
   affecting fetus or newborn 760.0
 recurrent physiologic 593.6
 scarlatinal 034.1
Albumosuria 791.0
 Bence-Jones 791.0
 myelopathic (M9730/3) 203.0●
Alcaptonuria 270.2
Alcohol, alcoholic
 abstinence 291.81
 acute intoxication 305.0●
  with dependence 303.0●
 addiction (*see also* Alcoholism) 303.9●
  maternal
   with suspected fetal damage
    affecting management of
    pregnancy 655.4●
   affecting fetus or newborn 760.71
 amnestic disorder, persisting 291.1

Alcohol, alcoholic *(Continued)*
 anxiety 291.89
 brain syndrome, chronic 291.2
 cardiopathy 425.5
 chronic (*see also* Alcoholism) 303.9●
 cirrhosis (liver) 571.2
 delirium 291.0
  acute 291.0
  chronic 291.1
  tremens 291.0
  withdrawal 291.0
 dementia NEC 291.2
 deterioration 291.2
 drunkenness (simple) 305.0●
 hallucinosis (acute) 291.3
 induced
  circadian rhythm sleep disorder
   291.82
  hypersomnia 291.82
  insomnia 291.82
  mental disorder 291.9
   anxiety 291.89
   mood 291.89
   sexual 291.89
   sleep 291.82
   specified type 291.89
  parasomnia 291.82
  persisting
   amnestic disorder 291.1
   dementia 291.2
  psychotic disorder
   with
    delusions 291.5
    hallucinations 291.3
  sleep disorder 291.82
 insanity 291.9
 intoxication (acute) 305.0●
  with dependence 303.0●
  pathological 291.4
 jealousy 291.5
 Korsakoff's, Korsakov's, Korsakow's
  291.1
 liver NEC 571.3
  acute 571.1
  chronic 571.2
 mania (acute) (chronic) 291.9
 mood 291.89
 paranoia 291.5
 paranoid (type) psychosis 291.5
 pellagra 265.2
 poisoning, accidental (acute) NEC 980.9
  specified type of alcohol - *see* Table
   of Drugs and Chemicals
 psychosis (*see also* Psychosis, alcoholic)
  291.9
  Korsakoff's, Korsakov's, Korsakow's
   291.1
  polyneuritic 291.1
   with
    delusions 291.5
    hallucinations 291.3
 related disorder 291.9
 withdrawal symptoms, syndrome NEC
  291.81
  delirium 291.0
  hallucinosis 291.3
Alcoholism 303.9●

Note: Use the following fifth-digit
subclassification with category 303:

0 unspecified
1 continuous
2 episodic
3 in remission

Alcoholism *(Continued)*
 with psychosis (*see also* Psychosis,
  alcoholic) 291.9
 acute 303.0●
 chronic 303.9●
  with psychosis 291.9
 complicating pregnancy, childbirth, or
  puerperium 648.4●
  affecting fetus or newborn 760.71
 history V11.3
 Korsakoff's, Korsakov's, Korsakow's
  291.1
 suspected damage to fetus affecting
  management of pregnancy
  655.4●
Alder's anomaly or syndrome
  (leukocyte granulation anomaly)
  288.2
Alder-Reilly anomaly (leukocyte
  granulation) 288.2
Aldosteronism (primary) 255.10
 congenital 255.10
 familial type I 255.11
 glucocorticoid-remediable 255.11
 secondary 255.14
Aldosteronoma (M8370/1) 237.2
Aldrich (-Wiskott) syndrome (eczema-
  thrombocytopenia) 279.12
Aleppo boil 085.1
Aleukemic - *see* condition
Aleukia
 congenital 288.09
 hemorrhagica 284.9
  acquired (secondary) 284.89
  congenital 284.09
  idiopathic 284.9
 splenica 289.4
Alexia (congenital) (developmental)
  315.01
 secondary to organic lesion 784.61
Algoneurodystrophy 733.7
Algophobia 300.29
Alibert's disease (mycosis fungoides)
  (M9700/3) 202.1●
Alibert-Bazin disease (M9700/3) 202.1●
Alice in Wonderland syndrome 293.89
Alienation, mental (*see also* Psychosis)
  298.9
Alkalemia 276.3
Alkalosis 276.3
 metabolic 276.3
  with respiratory acidosis 276.4
 respiratory 276.3
Alkaptonuria 270.2
Allen-Masters syndrome 620.6
Allergic bronchopulmonary aspergillosis
  518.6
Allergy, allergic (reaction) 995.3
 air-borne substance (*see also* Fever, hay)
  477.9
  specified allergen NEC 477.8
 alveolitis (extrinsic) 495.9
  due to
   Aspergillus clavatus 495.4
   cryptostroma corticale 495.6
   organisms (fungal, thermophilic
    actinomycete, other)
    growing in ventilation
    (air conditioning systems)
    495.7
  specified type NEC 495.8
 anaphylactic shock 995.0 ◀
  due to food - *see* Anaphylactic shock,
   due to, food
 angioneurotic edema 995.1

◀ New   ◀ Revised   ~~deleted~~ Deleted   ● Use Additional Digit(s)   Omit code

Allergy, allergic *(Continued)*
  animal (cat) (dog) (epidermal) 477.8
    dander 477.2
    hair 477.2
  arthritis *(see also* Arthritis, allergic)
      716.2●
  asthma - *see* Asthma
  bee sting (anaphylactic shock) 989.5
  biological - *see* Allergy, drug
  bronchial asthma - *see* Asthma
  conjunctivitis (eczematous) 372.14
  dander, animal (cat) (dog) 477.2
  dandruff 477.8
  dermatitis (venenata) - *see* Dermatitis
  diathesis V15.09
  drug, medicinal substance, and
      biological (any) (correct medicinal
      substance properly administered)
      (external) (internal) 995.27
    wrong substance given or taken
        NEC 977.9
      specified drug or substance - *see*
          Table of Drugs and
          Chemicals
  dust (house) (stock) 477.8
  eczema - *see* Eczema
  endophthalmitis 360.19
  epidermal (animal) 477.8
  existing dental restorative material
      525.66
  feathers 477.8
  food (any) (ingested) 693.1
    atopic 691.8
    in contact with skin 692.5
  gastritis 535.4●
  gastroenteritis 558.3
  gastrointestinal 558.3
  grain 477.0
  grass (pollen) 477.0
    asthma *(see also* Asthma) 493.0●
    hay fever 477.0
  hair, animal (cat) (dog) 477.2
  hay fever (grass) (pollen) (ragweed)
      (tree) *(see also* Fever, hay) 477.9
  history (of) V15.09
    to
        arachnid bite V15.06
        eggs V15.03
        food additives V15.05
        insect bite V15.06
        latex V15.07
        milk products V15.02
        nuts V15.05
          peanuts V15.01
        radiographic dye V15.08
        seafood V15.04
        specified food NEC V15.05
        spider bite V15.06
  horse serum - *see* Allergy, serum
  inhalant 477.9
    dust 477.8
    pollen 477.0
    specified allergen other than pollen
        477.8
  kapok 477.8
  medicine - *see* Allergy, drug
  migraine 339.00
  milk protein 558.3
  pannus 370.62
  pneumonia 518.3
  pollen (any) (hay fever) 477.0
    asthma *(see also* Asthma) 493.0●
  primrose 477.0
  primula 477.0
  purpura 287.0

Allergy, allergic *(Continued)*
  ragweed (pollen) (Senecio jacobae)
      477.0
    asthma *(see also* Asthma) 493.0●
    hay fever 477.0
  respiratory *(see also* Allergy, inhalant)
      477.9
    due to
        drug - *see* Allergy, drug
        food - *see* Allergy, food
  rhinitis *(see also* Fever, hay) 477.9
    due to food 477.1
  rose 477.0
  Senecio jacobae 477.0
  serum (prophylactic) (therapeutic)
      999.5
    anaphylactic shock 999.4
  shock (anaphylactic) (due to adverse
      effect of correct medicinal
      substance properly administered)
      995.0
    food - *see* Anaphylactic shock, due
        to, food
    from serum or immunization 999.5
      anaphylactic 999.4
  sinusitis *(see also* Fever, hay) 477.9
  skin reaction 692.9
    specified substance - *see* Dermatitis,
        due to
  tree (any) (hay fever) (pollen) 477.0
    asthma *(see also* Asthma) 493.0●
  upper respiratory *(see also* Fever, hay)
      477.9
  urethritis 597.89
  urticaria 708.0
  vaccine - *see* Allergy, serum
Allescheriosis 117.6
Alligator skin disease (ichthyosis
      congenita) 757.1
    acquired 701.1
Allocheiria, allochiria *(see also*
      Disturbance, sensation) 782.0
Almeida's disease (Brazilian
      blastomycosis) 116.1
Alopecia (atrophicans) (pregnancy)
      (premature) (senile) 704.00
    adnata 757.4
    areata 704.01
    celsi 704.01
    cicatrisata 704.09
    circumscripta 704.01
    congenital, congenitalis 757.4
    disseminata 704.01
    effluvium (telogen) 704.02
    febrile 704.09
    generalisata 704.09
    hereditaria 704.09
    marginalis 704.01
    mucinosa 704.09
    postinfectional 704.09
    seborrheica 704.09
    specific 091.82
    syphilitic (secondary) 091.82
    telogen effluvium 704.02
    totalis 704.09
    toxica 704.09
    universalis 704.09
    x-ray 704.09
Alpers' disease 330.8
Alpha-lipoproteinemia 272.4
Alpha thalassemia 282.49
Alphos 696.1
Alpine sickness 993.2
Alport's syndrome (hereditary hematuria-
      nephropathy-deafness) 759.89

ALPS (autoimmune lymphoproliferative
      syndrome) 279.41
ALTE (apparent life threatening event)
      in newborn and infant 799.82
Alteration (of), altered
    awareness 780.09
      transient 780.02
    consciousness 780.09
      persistent vegetative state 780.03
      transient 780.02
    mental status 780.97
      amnesia (retrograde) 780.93
      memory loss 780.93
Alternaria (infection) 118
Alternating - *see* condition
Altitude, high (effects) - *see* Effect,
      adverse, high altitude
Aluminosis (of lung) 503
Alvarez syndrome (transient cerebral
      ischemia) 435.9
Alveolar capillary block syndrome 516.3
Alveolitis
    allergic (extrinsic) 495.9
      due to organisms (fungal,
          thermophilic actinomycete,
          other) growing in ventilation
          (air conditioning systems) 495.7
      specified type NEC 495.8
    due to
        Aspergillus clavatus 495.4
        Cryptostroma corticale 495.6
    fibrosing (chronic) (cryptogenic) (lung)
        516.3
      idiopathic 516.3
      rheumatoid 714.81
    jaw 526.5
    sicca dolorosa 526.5
Alveolus, alveolar - *see* condition
Alymphocytosis (pure) 279.2
Alymphoplasia, thymic 279.2
Alzheimer's
    dementia (senile)
      with behavioral disturbance 331.0
          [294.11]
      without behavioral disturbance
          331.0 *[294.10]*
    disease or sclerosis 331.0
      with dementia - *see* Alzheimer's,
          dementia
Amastia *(see also* Absence, breast) 611.89
Amaurosis (acquired) (congenital) *(see
      also* Blindness) 369.00
    fugax 362.34
    hysterical 300.11
    Leber's (congenital) 362.76
    tobacco 377.34
    uremic - *see* Uremia
Amaurotic familial idiocy (infantile)
      (juvenile) (late) 330.1
Ambisexual 752.7
Amblyopia (acquired) (congenital)
      (partial) 368.00
    color 368.59
      acquired 368.55
    deprivation 368.02
    ex anopsia 368.00
    hysterical 300.11
    nocturnal 368.60
      vitamin A deficiency 264.5
    refractive 368.03
    strabismic 368.01
    suppression 368.01
    tobacco 377.34
    toxic NEC 377.34
    uremic - *see* Uremia

A

Ameba, amebic (histolytica) - *see also*
   Amebiasis
   abscess 006.3
      bladder 006.8
      brain (with liver and lung abscess)
         006.5
      liver 006.3
         with
            brain abscess (and lung
               abscess) 006.5
            lung abscess 006.4
         lung (with liver abscess) 006.4
            with brain abscess 006.5
      seminal vesicle 006.8
      spleen 006.8
   carrier (suspected of) V02.2
   meningoencephalitis
      due to Naegleria (gruberi) 136.29
      primary 136.29
Amebiasis NEC 006.9
   with
      brain abscess (with liver or lung
         abscess) 006.5
      liver abscess (without mention of
         brain or lung abscess) 006.3
      lung abscess (with liver abscess)
         006.4
         with brain abscess 006.5
   acute 006.0
   bladder 006.8
   chronic 006.1
   cutaneous 006.6
   cutis 006.6
   due to organism other than Entamoeba
      histolytica 007.8
   hepatic (*see also* Abscess, liver, amebic)
      006.3
   nondysenteric 006.2
   seminal vesicle 006.8
   specified
      organism NEC 007.8
      site NEC 006.8
Ameboma 006.8
Amelia 755.4
   lower limb 755.31
   upper limb 755.21
Ameloblastoma (M9310/0) 213.1
   jaw (bone) (lower) 213.1
      upper 213.0
   long bones (M9261/3) - *see* Neoplasm,
      bone, malignant
   malignant (M9310/3) 170.1
      jaw (bone) (lower) 170.1
         upper 170.0
   mandible 213.1
   tibial (M9261/3) 170.7
Amelogenesis imperfecta 520.5
   nonhereditaria (segmentalis) 520.4
Amenorrhea (primary) (secondary) 626.0
   due to ovarian dysfunction 256.8
   hyperhormonal 256.8
Amentia (*see also* Retardation, mental) 319
   Meynert's (nonalcoholic) 294.0
      alcoholic 291.1
   nevoid 759.6
American
   leishmaniasis 085.5
   mountain tick fever 066.1
   trypanosomiasis - *see* Trypanosomiasis,
      American
Ametropia (*see also* Disorder,
      accommodation) 367.9
Amianthosis 501
Amimia 784.69

Amino acid
   deficiency 270.9
      anemia 281.4
   metabolic disorder (*see also* Disorder,
      amino acid) 270.9
Aminoaciduria 270.9
   imidazole 270.5
Amnesia (retrograde) 780.93
   auditory 784.69
      developmental 315.31
      secondary to organic lesion 784.69
   dissociative 300.12
   hysterical or dissociative type 300.12
   psychogenic 300.12
   transient global 437.7
Amnestic (confabulatory) syndrome 294.0
   alcohol-induced persisting 291.1
   drug-induced persisting 292.83
   posttraumatic 294.0
Amniocentesis screening (for) V28.2
   alphafetoprotein level, raised V28.1
   chromosomal anomalies V28.0
Amnion, amniotic - *see also* condition
   nodosum 658.8●
Amnionitis (complicating pregnancy)
      658.4●
   affecting fetus or newborn 762.7
Amoral trends 301.7
Amotio retinae (*see also* Detachment,
      retina) 361.9
Ampulla
   lower esophagus 530.89
   phrenic 530.89
Amputation
   any part of fetus, to facilitate delivery
      763.89
   cervix (supravaginal) (uteri) 622.8
      in pregnancy or childbirth 654.6●
         affecting fetus or newborn
            763.89
   clitoris - *see* Wound, open, clitoris
   congenital
      lower limb 755.31
      upper limb 755.21
   neuroma (traumatic) - *see also* Injury,
      nerve, by site
   surgical complication (late) 997.61
   penis - *see* Amputation, traumatic,
      penis
   status (without complication) - *see*
      Absence, by site, acquired
   stump (surgical) (posttraumatic)
      abnormal, painful, or with
         complication (late) 997.60
      healed or old NEC - *see also* Absence,
         by site, acquired
         lower V49.70
         upper V49.60
   traumatic (complete) (partial)

> Note: "Complicated" includes
> traumatic amputation with delayed
> healing, delayed treatment, foreign
> body, or infection.

      arm 887.4
         at or above elbow 887.2
            complicated 887.3
         below elbow 887.0
            complicated 887.1
         both (bilateral) (any level(s))
            887.6
            complicated 887.7
         complicated 887.5

Amputation (*Continued*)
   traumatic (*Continued*)
      finger(s) (one or both hands) 886.0
         with thumb(s) 885.0
            complicated 885.1
         complicated 886.1
      foot (except toe(s) only) 896.0
         and other leg 897.6
            complicated 897.7
         both (bilateral) 896.2
            complicated 896.3
         complicated 896.1
      toe(s) only (one or both feet) 895.0
         complicated 895.1
      genital organ(s) (external) NEC
         878.8
         complicated 878.9
      hand (except finger(s) only) 887.0
         and other arm 887.6
            complicated 887.7
         both (bilateral) 887.6
            complicated 887.7
         complicated 887.1
      finger(s) (one or both hands)
         886.0
         with thumb(s) 885.0
            complicated 885.1
         complicated 886.1
      thumb(s) (with fingers of either
         hand) 885.0
         complicated 885.1
      head 874.9
      late effect - *see* Late, effects (of),
         amputation
      leg 897.4
         and other foot 897.6
            complicated 897.7
         at or above knee 897.2
            complicated 897.3
         below knee 897.0
            complicated 897.1
         both (bilateral) 897.6
            complicated 897.7
         complicated 897.5
      lower limb(s) except toe(s) - *see*
         Amputation, traumatic, leg
      nose - *see* Wound, open, nose
      penis 878.0
         complicated 878.1
      sites other than limbs - *see* Wound,
         open, by site
      thumb(s) (with finger(s) of either
         hand) 885.0
         complicated 885.1
      toe(s) (one or both feet) 895.0
         complicated 895.1
      upper limb(s) - *see* Amputation,
         traumatic, arm
Amputee (bilateral) (old) - *see also*
      Absence, by site, acquired V49.70
Amusia 784.69
   developmental 315.39
   secondary to organic lesion 784.69
Amyelencephalus 740.0
Amyelia 742.59
Amygdalitis - *see* Tonsillitis
Amygdalolith 474.8
Amyloid disease or degeneration 277.30
   heart 277.39 [425.7]
Amyloidosis (familial) (general)
      (generalized) (genetic) (primary)
      277.30
   with lung involvement 277.39 [517.8]
   cardiac, hereditary 277.39

◀ New   ◀‖‖ Revised   ~~deleted~~ Deleted   ● Use Additional Digit(s)   ▨ Omit code

Amyloidosis (Continued)
  heart 277.39 [425.7]
  nephropathic 277.39 [583.81]
  neuropathic (Portuguese) (Swiss)
    277.39 [357.4]
  pulmonary 277.39 [517.8]
  secondary 277.39
  systemic, inherited 277.39
Amylopectinosis (brancher enzyme
    deficiency) 271.0
Amylophagia 307.52
Amyoplasia, congenita 756.89
Amyotonia 728.2
  congenita 358.8
Amyotrophia, amyotrophy, amyotrophic
    728.2
  congenita 756.89
  diabetic 250.6● [353.5]
    due to secondary diabetes 249.6●
      [353.5]
  lateral sclerosis (syndrome)
    335.20
  neuralgic 353.5
  sclerosis (lateral) 335.20
  spinal progressive 335.21
Anacidity, gastric 536.0
  psychogenic 306.4
Anaerosis of newborn 770.88
Analbuminemia 273.8
Analgesia (see also Anesthesia) 782.0
Analphalipoproteinemia 272.5
Anaphylactic shock or reaction (correct
    substance properly administered)
    995.0
  due to
    food 995.60
      additives 995.66
      crustaceans 995.62
      eggs 995.68
      fish 995.65
      fruits 995.63
      milk products 995.67
      nuts (tree) 995.64
      peanuts 995.61
      seeds 995.64
      specified NEC 995.69
      tree nuts 995.64
      vegetables 995.63
    immunization 999.4
    overdose or wrong substance given
      or taken 977.9
      specified drug - see Table of
        Drugs and Chemicals
    serum 999.4
  following sting(s) 989.5
  purpura 287.0
  serum 999.4
Anaphylactoid shock or reaction - see
    Anaphylactic shock
Anaphylaxis - see Anaphylactic shock
Anaplasia, cervix 622.10
Anarthria 784.51
Anarthritic rheumatoid disease
    446.5
Anasarca 782.3
  cardiac (see also Failure, heart)
    428.0
  fetus or newborn 778.0
  lung 514
  nutritional 262
  pulmonary 514
  renal (see also Nephrosis) 581.9
Anaspadias 752.62

Anastomosis
  aneurysmal - see Aneurysm
  arteriovenous, congenital NEC (see also
    Anomaly, arteriovenous) 747.60
  ruptured, of brain (see also
      Hemorrhage, subarachnoid)
      430
  intestinal 569.89
    complicated NEC 997.4
      involving urinary tract 997.5
  retinal and choroidal vessels 743.58
    acquired 362.17
Anatomical narrow angle (glaucoma)
    365.02
Ancylostoma (infection) (infestation)
    126.9
  americanus 126.1
  braziliense 126.2
  caninum 126.8
  ceylanicum 126.3
  duodenale 126.0
  Necator americanus 126.1
Ancylostomiasis (intestinal) 126.9
  ancylostoma
    americanus 126.1
    caninum 126.8
    ceylanicum 126.3
    duodenale 126.0
  braziliense 126.2
  Necator americanus 126.1
Anders' disease or syndrome (adiposis
    tuberosa simplex) 272.8
Andersen's glycogen storage disease
    271.0
Anderson's disease 272.7
Andes disease 993.2
Andrews' disease (bacterid) 686.8
Androblastoma (M8630/1)
  benign (M8630/0)
    specified site - see Neoplasm, by site,
      benign
    unspecified site
      female 220
      male 222.0
  malignant (M8630/3)
    specified site - see Neoplasm, by site,
      malignant
    unspecified site
      female 183.0
      male 186.9
  specified site - see Neoplasm, by site,
    uncertain behavior
  tubular (M8640/0)
    with lipid storage (M8641/0)
      specified site - see Neoplasm, by
        site, benign
      unspecified site
        female 220
        male 222.0
    specified site - see Neoplasm, by site,
      benign
    unspecified site
      female 220
      male 222.0
  unspecified site
    female 236.2
    male 236.4
Android pelvis 755.69
  with disproportion (fetopelvic) 653.3●
    affecting fetus or newborn 763.1
    causing obstructed labor 660.1●
      affecting fetus or newborn 763.1
Anectasis, pulmonary (newborn or fetus)
    770.5

Anemia 285.9
  with
    disorder of
      anaerobic glycolysis 282.3
      pentose phosphate pathway 282.2
    koilonychia 280.9
  6-phosphogluconic dehydrogenase
    deficiency 282.2
  achlorhydric 280.9
  achrestic 281.8
  Addison's (pernicious) 281.0
  Addison-Biermer (pernicious) 281.0
  agranulocytic 288.09
  amino acid deficiency 281.4
  antineoplastic chemotherapy induced
    285.3
  aplastic 284.9
    acquired (secondary) 284.89
    congenital 284.01
    constitutional 284.01
    due to
      antineoplastic chemotherapy
        284.89
      chronic systemic disease 284.89
      drugs 284.89
      infection 284.89
      radiation 284.89
    idiopathic 284.9
    myxedema 244.9
    of or complicating pregnancy 648.2●
    red cell (acquired) (adult) (with
      thymoma) 284.81
      congenital 284.01
      pure 284.01
    specified type NEC 284.89
    toxic (paralytic) 284.89
  aregenerative 284.9
    congenital 284.01
  asiderotic 280.9
  atypical (primary) 285.9
  autohemolysis of Selwyn and Dacie
    (type I) 282.2
  autoimmune hemolytic 283.0
  Baghdad Spring 282.2
  Balantidium coli 007.0
  Biermer's (pernicious) 281.0
  blood loss (chronic) 280.0
    acute 285.1
  bothriocephalus 123.4
  brickmakers' (see also Ancylostomiasis)
    126.9
  cerebral 437.8
  childhood 282.9
  chlorotic 280.9
  chronica congenita aregenerativa
    284.01
  chronic simple 281.9
  combined system disease NEC 281.0
    [336.2]
    due to dietary deficiency 281.1 [336.2]
  complicating pregnancy or childbirth
    648.2●
  congenital (following fetal blood loss)
    776.5
    aplastic 284.01
    due to isoimmunization NEC 773.2
    Heinz-body 282.7
    hereditary hemolytic NEC 282.9
    nonspherocytic
      type I 282.2
      type II 282.3
    pernicious 281.0
    spherocytic (see also Spherocytosis)
      282.0

Anemia (Continued)
  Cooley's (erythroblastic) 282.49
  crescent - see Disease, sickle-cell
  cytogenic 281.0
  Dacie's (nonspherocytic)
    type I 282.2
    type II 282.3
  Davidson's (refractory) 284.9
  deficiency 281.9
    2, 3 diphosphoglycurate mutase
        282.3
    2, 3 PG 282.3
    6-PGD 282.2
    6-phosphogluronic dehydrogenase
        282.2
    amino acid 281.4
    combined B₁₂ and folate 281.3
    enzyme, drug-induced (hemolytic)
        282.2
    erythrocytic glutathione 282.2
    folate 281.2
      dietary 281.2
      drug-induced 281.2
    folic acid 281.2
      dietary 281.2
      drug-induced 281.2
    G-6-PD 282.2
    GGS-R 282.2
    glucose-6-phosphate dehydrogenase
        (G-6-PD) 282.2
    glucose-phosphate isomerase 282.3
    glutathione peroxidase 282.2
    glutathione reductase 282.2
    glyceraldehyde phosphate
        dehydrogenase 282.3
    GPI 282.3
    G SH 282.2
    hexokinase 282.3
    iron (Fe) 280.9
      specified NEC 280.8
    nutritional 281.9
      with
        poor iron absorption 280.9
        specified deficiency NEC 281.8
      due to inadequate dietary iron
          intake 280.1
      specified type NEC 281.8
    of or complicating pregnancy 648.2 ●
    pentose phosphate pathway 282.2
    PFK 282.3
    phosphofructo-aldolase 282.3
    phosphofructokinase 282.3
    phosphoglycerate kinase 282.3
    PK 282.3
    protein 281.4
    pyruvate kinase (PK) 282.3
    TPI 282.3
    triosephosphate isomerase 282.3
    vitamin B₁₂ NEC 281.1
      dietary 281.1
      pernicious 281.0
  Diamond-Blackfan (congenital
      hypoplastic) 284.01
  dibothriocephalus 123.4
  dimorphic 281.9
  diphasic 281.8
  diphtheritic 032.89
  Diphyllobothrium 123.4
  drepanocytic (see also Disease, sickle-
      cell) 282.60
  due to
    antineoplastic chemotherapy 285.3
    blood loss (chronic) 280.0
      acute 285.1

Anemia (Continued)
  due to (Continued)
    chemotherapy, antineoplastic 285.3
    defect of Embden-Meyerhof
        pathway glycolysis 282.3
    disorder of glutathione metabolism
        282.2
    drug - see Anemia, by type (see also
        Table of Drugs and Chemicals)
      chemotherapy, antineoplastic
          285.3
    fetal blood loss 776.5
    fish tapeworm (D. latum) infestation
        123.4
    glutathione metabolism disorder
        282.2
    hemorrhage (chronic) 280.0
      acute 285.1
    hexose monophosphate (HMP)
        shunt deficiency 282.2
    impaired absorption 280.9
    loss of blood (chronic) 280.0
      acute 285.1
    myxedema 244.9
    Necator americanus 126.1
    prematurity 776.6
    selective vitamin B₁₂ malabsorption
        with proteinuria 281.1
  Dyke-Young type (secondary)
      (symptomatic) 283.9
  dyserythropoietic (congenital) (types I,
      II, III) 285.8
  dyshemopoietic (congenital) 285.8
  Egypt (see also Ancylostomiasis) 126.9
  elliptocytosis (see also Elliptocytosis)
      282.1
  enzyme deficiency, drug-induced 282.2
  epidemic (see also Ancylostomiasis)
      126.9
  EPO resistant 285.21
  erythroblastic
    familial 282.49
    fetus or newborn (see also Disease,
        hemolytic) 773.2
      late 773.5
  erythrocytic glutathione deficiency 282.2
  erythropoietin-resistant (EPO resistant
      anemia) 285.21
  essential 285.9
  Faber's (achlorhydric anemia) 280.9
  factitious (self-induced bloodletting)
      280.0
  familial erythroblastic (microcytic)
      282.49
  Fanconi's (congenital pancytopenia)
      284.09
  favism 282.2
  fetal 678.0 ●
    following blood loss, affecting
        newborn 776.5
  fetus or newborn
    due to
      ABO
        antibodies 773.1
        incompatibility, maternal/fetal
            773.1
        isoimmunization 773.1
      Rh
        antibodies 773.0
        incompatibility, maternal/fetal
            773.0
        isoimmunization 773.0
    following fetal blood loss 776.5
  fish tapeworm (D. latum) infestation
      123.4

Anemia (Continued)
  folate (folic acid) deficiency 281.2
    dietary 281.2
    drug-induced 281.2
  folate malabsorption, congenital 281.2
  folic acid deficiency 281.2
    dietary 281.2
    drug-induced 281.2
  G-6-PD 282.2
  general 285.9
  glucose-6-phosphate dehydrogenase
      deficiency 282.2
  glutathione-reductase deficiency 282.2
  goat's milk 281.2
  granulocytic 288.09
  Heinz-body, congenital 282.7
  hemoglobin deficiency 285.9
  hemolytic 283.9
    acquired 283.9
      with hemoglobinuria NEC 283.2
      autoimmune (cold type)
          (idiopathic) (primary)
          (secondary) (symptomatic)
          (warm type) 283.0
      due to
        cold reactive antibodies 283.0
        drug exposure 283.0
        warm reactive antibodies 283.0
      fragmentation 283.19
      idiopathic (chronic) 283.9
      infectious 283.19
        autoimmune 283.0
      non-autoimmune 283.10
      toxic 283.19
      traumatic cardiac 283.19
    acute 283.9
      due to enzyme deficiency NEC
          282.3
      fetus or newborn (see also Disease,
          hemolytic) 773.2
        late 773.5
      Lederer's (acquired infectious
          hemolytic anemia) 283.19
    autoimmune (acquired) 283.0
    chronic 282.9
      idiopathic 283.9
    cold type (secondary) (symptomatic)
        283.0
    congenital (spherocytic) (see also
        Spherocytosis) 282.0
      nonspherocytic - see Anemia,
          hemolytic, nonspherocytic,
          congenital
    drug-induced 283.0
      enzyme deficiency 282.2
    due to
      cardiac conditions 283.19
      drugs 283.0
      enzyme deficiency NEC 282.3
        drug-induced 282.2
      presence of shunt or other
          internal prosthetic device
          283.19
      thrombotic thrombocytopenic
          purpura 446.6
    elliptocytotic (see also Elliptocytosis)
        282.1
    familial 282.9
    hereditary 282.9
      due to enzyme deficiency NEC
          282.3
      specified NEC 282.8
    idiopathic (chronic) 283.9
    infectious (acquired) 283.19

◄ New   ◄▥ Revised   ~~deleted~~ Deleted   ● Use Additional Digit(s)   ▨ Omit code

Anemia *(Continued)*
  hemolytic *(Continued)*
    mechanical 283.19
    microangiopathic 283.19
    nonautoimmune 283.10
    nonspherocytic
      congenital or hereditary NEC 282.3
        glucose-6-phosphate dehydrogenase deficiency 282.2
        pyruvate kinase (PK) deficiency 282.3
        type I 282.2
        type II 282.3
      type I 282.2
      type II 282.3
      of or complicating pregnancy 648.2●
    resulting from presence of shunt or other internal prosthetic device 283.19
    secondary 283.19
      autoimmune 283.0
    sickle-cell - *see* Disease, sickle-cell
    Stransky-Regala type (Hb-E) *(see also* Disease, hemoglobin) 282.7
    symptomatic 283.19
      autoimmune 283.0
    toxic (acquired) 283.19
    uremic (adult) (child) 283.11
    warm type (secondary) (symptomatic) 283.0
  hemorrhagic (chronic) 280.0
    acute 285.1
  HEMPAS 285.8
  hereditary erythroblast multinuclearity-positive acidified serum test 285.8
  Herrick's (hemoglobin S disease) 282.61
  hexokinase deficiency 282.3
  high A_2 282.49
  hookworm *(see also* Ancylostomiasis) 126.9
  hypochromic (idiopathic) (microcytic) (normoblastic) 280.9
    with iron loading 285.0
    due to blood loss (chronic) 280.0
      acute 285.1
    familial sex linked 285.0
    pyridoxine-responsive 285.0
  hypoplasia, red blood cells 284.81
    congenital or familial 284.01
  hypoplastic (idiopathic) 284.9
    congenital 284.01
    familial 284.01
    of childhood 284.09
  idiopathic 285.9
    hemolytic, chronic 283.9
  in (due to) (with)
    chronic illness NEC 285.29
    chronic kidney disease 285.21
    end-stage renal disease 285.21
    neoplastic disease 285.22
  infantile 285.9
  infective, infectional 285.9
  intertropical *(see also* Ancylostomiasis) 126.9
  iron (Fe) deficiency 280.9
    due to blood loss (chronic) 280.0
      acute 285.1
    of or complicating pregnancy 648.2●
    specified NEC 280.8

Anemia *(Continued)*
  Jaksch's (pseudoleukemia infantum) 285.8
  Joseph-Diamond-Blackfan (congenital hypoplastic) 284.01
  labyrinth 386.50
  Lederer's (acquired infectious hemolytic anemia) 283.19
  leptocytosis (hereditary) 282.49
  leukoerythroblastic 284.2
  macrocytic 281.9
    nutritional 281.2
    of or complicating pregnancy 648.2●
    tropical 281.2
  malabsorption (familial), selective B_{12} with proteinuria 281.1
  malarial *(see also* Malaria) 084.6
  malignant (progressive) 281.0
  malnutrition 281.9
  marsh *(see also* Malaria) 084.6
  Mediterranean (with hemoglobinopathy) 282.49
  megaloblastic 281.9
    combined B_{12} and folate deficiency 281.3
    nutritional (of infancy) 281.2
    of infancy 281.2
    of or complicating pregnancy 648.2●
    refractory 281.3
    specified NEC 281.3
  megalocytic 281.9
  microangiopathic hemolytic 283.19
  microcytic (hypochromic) 280.9
    due to blood loss (chronic) 280.0
      acute 285.1
    familial 282.49
    hypochromic 280.9
  microdrepanocytosis 282.49
  miners' *(see also* Ancylostomiasis) 126.9
  myelopathic 285.8
  myelophthisic (normocytic) 284.2
  newborn *(see also* Disease, hemolytic) 773.2
    due to isoimmunization *(see also* Disease, hemolytic) 773.2
    late, due to isoimmunization 773.5
    posthemorrhagic 776.5
  nonregenerative 284.9
  nonspherocytic hemolytic - *see* Anemia, hemolytic, nonspherocytic
  normocytic (infectional) (not due to blood loss) 285.9
    due to blood loss (chronic) 280.0
      acute 285.1
    myelophthisic 284.2
  nutritional (deficiency) 281.9
    with
      poor iron absorption 280.9
      specified deficiency NEC 281.8
    due to inadequate dietary iron intake 280.1
    megaloblastic (of infancy) 281.2
  of childhood 282.9
  of chronic
    disease NEC 285.29
    illness NEC 285.29
  of or complicating pregnancy 648.2●
    affecting fetus or newborn 760.8
  of prematurity 776.6
  orotic aciduric (congenital) (hereditary) 281.4
  osteosclerotic 289.89
  ovalocytosis (hereditary) *(see also* Elliptocytosis) 282.1

Anemia *(Continued)*
  paludal *(see also* Malaria) 084.6
  pentose phosphate pathway deficiency 282.2
  pernicious (combined system disease) (congenital) (dorsolateral spinal degeneration) (juvenile) (myelopathy) (neuropathy) (posterior sclerosis) (primary) (progressive) (spleen) 281.0
    of or complicating pregnancy 648.2●
  pleochromic 285.9
    of sprue 281.8
  portal 285.8
  posthemorrhagic (chronic) 280.0
    acute 285.1
    newborn 776.5
  postoperative
    due to (acute) blood loss 285.1
      chronic blood loss 280.0
    other 285.9
  postpartum 648.2●
  pressure 285.9
  primary 285.9
  profound 285.9
  progressive 285.9
    malignant 281.0
    pernicious 281.0
  protein-deficiency 281.4
  pseudoleukemica infantum 285.8
  puerperal 648.2●
  pure red cell 284.81
    congenital 284.01
  pyridoxine-responsive (hypochromic) 285.0
  pyruvate kinase (PK) deficiency 282.3
  refractoria sideroblastica 238.72
  refractory (primary) 238.72
    with
      excess
        blasts-1 (RAEB-1) 238.72
        blasts-2 (RAEB-2) 238.73
      hemochromatosis 238.72
      ringed sideroblasts (RARS) 238.72
    due to
      drug 285.0
      myelodysplastic syndrome 238.72
      toxin 285.0
    hereditary 285.0
    idiopathic 238.72
    megaloblastic 281.3
    sideroblastic 238.72
      hereditary 285.0
    sideropenic 280.9
  Rietti-Greppi-Micheli (thalassemia minor) 282.49
  scorbutic 281.8
  secondary (to) 285.9
    blood loss (chronic) 280.0
      acute 285.1
    hemorrhage 280.0
      acute 285.1
    inadequate dietary iron intake 280.1
  semiplastic 284.9
  septic 285.9
  sickle-cell *(see also* Disease, sickle-cell) 282.60
  sideroachrestic 285.0

A

◀ New   ⁐ Revised   ~~deleted~~ Deleted   ● Use Additional Digit(s)   ▨ Omit code

Anemia (Continued)
  sideroblastic (acquired) (any type)
    (congenital) (drug-induced) (due
    to disease) (hereditary) (primary)
    (secondary) (sex-linked
    hypochromic) (vitamin B_6
    responsive) 285.0
    refractory 238.72
      congenital 285.0
      drug-induced 285.0
      hereditary 285.0
      sex-linked hypochromic 285.0
      vitamin B_6-responsive 285.0
  sideropenic 280.9
    due to blood loss (chronic) 280.0
      acute 285.1
  simple chronic 281.9
  specified type NEC 285.8
  spherocytic (hereditary) (see also
    Spherocytosis) 282.0
  splenic 285.8
    familial (Gaucher's) 272.7
  splenomegalic 285.8
  stomatocytosis 282.8
  syphilitic 095.8
  target cell (oval) 282.49
  thalassemia 282.49
  thrombocytopenic (see also
    Thrombocytopenia) 287.5
  toxic 284.89
  triosephosphate isomerase deficiency
    282.3
  tropical, macrocytic 281.2
  tuberculous (see also Tuberculosis)
    017.9 ●
  Vegan's 281.1
  vitamin
    B_6-responsive 285.0
    B_{12} deficiency (dietary) 281.1
      pernicious 281.0
  von Jaksch's (pseudoleukemia
    infantum) 285.8
  Witts' (achlorhydric anemia) 280.9
  Zuelzer (-Ogden) (nutritional
    megaloblastic anemia) 281.2
Anencephalus, anencephaly 740.0
  fetal, affecting management of
    pregnancy 655.0 ●
Anergasia (see also Psychosis, organic)
  294.9
  senile 290.0
Anesthesia, anesthetic 782.0
  complication or reaction NEC 995.22
    due to
      correct substance properly
        administered 995.22
      overdose or wrong substance
        given 968.4
        specified anesthetic - see Table
          of Drugs and Chemicals
  cornea 371.81
  death from
    correct substance properly
      administered 995.4
    during delivery 668.9 ●
    overdose or wrong substance given
      968.4
      specified anesthetic - see Table of
        Drugs and Chemicals
  eye 371.81
  functional 300.11
  hyperesthetic, thalamic 338.0
  hysterical 300.11
  local skin lesion 782.0

Anesthesia, anesthetic (Continued)
  olfactory 781.1
  sexual (psychogenic) 302.72
  shock
    due to
      correct substance properly
        administered 995.4
      overdose or wrong substance
        given 968.4
        specified anesthetic - see Table
          of Drugs and Chemicals
  skin 782.0
  tactile 782.0
  testicular 608.9
  thermal 782.0
Anetoderma (maculosum) 701.3
Aneuploidy NEC 758.5
Aneurin deficiency 265.1
Aneurysm (anastomotic) (artery)
  (cirsoid) (diffuse) (false) (fusiform)
  (multiple) (ruptured) (saccular)
  (varicose) 442.9
  abdominal (aorta) 441.4
    ruptured 441.3
    syphilitic 093.0
  aorta, aortic (nonsyphilitic) 441.9
    abdominal 441.4
      dissecting 441.02
      ruptured 441.3
      syphilitic 093.0
    arch 441.2
      ruptured 441.1
    arteriosclerotic NEC 441.9
      ruptured 441.5
    ascending 441.2
      ruptured 441.1
    congenital 747.29
    descending 441.9
      abdominal 441.4
        ruptured 441.3
      ruptured 441.5
      thoracic 441.2
        ruptured 441.1
    dissecting 441.00
      abdominal 441.02
      thoracic 441.01
      thoracoabdominal 441.03
    due to coarctation (aorta) 747.10
    ruptured 441.5
    sinus, right 747.29
    syphilitic 093.0
    thoracoabdominal 441.7
      ruptured 441.6
    thorax, thoracic (arch)
      (nonsyphilitic) 441.2
      dissecting 441.01
      ruptured 441.1
      syphilitic 093.0
    transverse 441.2
      ruptured 441.1
    valve (heart) (see also Endocarditis,
      aortic) 424.1
  arteriosclerotic NEC 442.9
    cerebral 437.3
      ruptured (see also Hemorrhage,
        subarachnoid) 430
  arteriovenous (congenital)
    (peripheral) NEC (see also
    Anomaly, arteriovenous) 747.60
    acquired NEC 447.0
      brain 437.3
        ruptured (see also Hemorrhage,
          subarachnoid) 430

Aneurysm (Continued)
  arteriovenous (Continued)
    acquired NEC (Continued)
      coronary 414.11
      pulmonary 417.0
    brain (cerebral) 747.81
      ruptured (see also Hemorrhage,
        subarachnoid) 430
    coronary 746.85
    pulmonary 747.3
    retina 743.58
    specified site NEC 747.89
      acquired 447.0
    traumatic (see also Injury, blood
      vessel, by site) 904.9
  basal - see Aneurysm, brain
  berry (congenital) (ruptured)
    (see also Hemorrhage,
    subarachnoid) 430
  brain 437.3
    arteriosclerotic 437.3
      ruptured (see also Hemorrhage,
        subarachnoid) 430
    arteriovenous 747.81
      acquired 437.3
        ruptured (see also Hemorrhage,
          subarachnoid) 430
      ruptured (see also Hemorrhage,
        subarachnoid) 430
    berry (congenital) (ruptured) (see
      also Hemorrhage,
      subarachnoid) 430
    congenital 747.81
      ruptured (see also Hemorrhage,
        subarachnoid) 430
    meninges 437.3
      ruptured (see also Hemorrhage,
        subarachnoid) 430
    miliary (congenital) (ruptured) (see
      also Hemorrhage,
      subarachnoid) 430
    mycotic 421.0
      ruptured (see also Hemorrhage,
        subarachnoid) 430
    nonruptured 437.3
    ruptured (see also Hemorrhage,
      subarachnoid) 430
    syphilitic 094.87
    syphilitic (hemorrhage) 094.87
    traumatic - see Injury, intracranial
  cardiac (false) (see also Aneurysm,
    heart) 414.10
  carotid artery (common) (external)
    442.81
    internal (intracranial portion) 437.3
      extracranial portion 442.81
      ruptured into brain (see also
        Hemorrhage, subarachnoid)
        430
    syphilitic 093.89
      intracranial 094.87
  cavernous sinus (see also Aneurysm,
    brain) 437.3
    arteriovenous 747.81
      ruptured (see also Hemorrhage,
        subarachnoid) 430
    congenital 747.81
      ruptured (see also Hemorrhage,
        subarachnoid) 430
  celiac 442.84
  central nervous system, syphilitic
    094.89
  cerebral - see Aneurysm, brain
  chest - see Aneurysm, thorax

◀ New   ⇐ Revised   ~~deleted~~ Deleted   ● Use Additional Digit(s)   ▢ Omit code

Aneurysm *(Continued)*
  circle of Willis *(see also* Aneurysm,
    brain) 437.3
    congenital 747.81
      ruptured *(see also* Hemorrhage,
        subarachnoid) 430
    ruptured *(see also* Hemorrhage,
      subarachnoid) 430
  common iliac artery 442.2
  congenital (peripheral) NEC 747.60
    brain 747.81
      ruptured *(see also* Hemorrhage,
        subarachnoid) 430
    cerebral - *see* Aneurysm, brain,
      congenital
    coronary 746.85
    gastrointestinal 747.61
    lower limb 747.64
    pulmonary 747.3
    renal 747.62
    retina 743.58
    specified site NEC 747.89
    spinal 747.82
    upper limb 747.63
  conjunctiva 372.74
  conus arteriosus *(see also* Aneurysm,
    heart) 414.10
  coronary (arteriosclerotic) (artery)
    (vein) *(see also* Aneurysm, heart)
    414.11
    arteriovenous 746.85
    congenital 746.85
    syphilitic 093.89
  cylindrical 441.9
    ruptured 441.5
    syphilitic 093.9
  dissecting 442.9
    aorta 441.00
      abdominal 441.02
      thoracic 441.01
      thoracoabdominal 441.03
    syphilitic 093.9
  ductus arteriosus 747.0
  embolic - *see* Embolism, artery
  endocardial, infective (any valve) 421.0
  femoral 442.3
  gastroduodenal 442.84
  gastroepiploic 442.84
  heart (chronic or with a stated duration
    of over 8 weeks) (infectional)
    (wall) 414.10
    acute or with a stated duration of 8
      weeks or less *(see also* Infarct,
      myocardium) 410.9●
    congenital 746.89
    valve - *see* Endocarditis
  hepatic 442.84
  iliac (common) 442.2
  infective (any valve) 421.0
  innominate (nonsyphilitic) 442.89
    syphilitic 093.89
  interauricular septum *(see also*
    Aneurysm, heart) 414.10
  interventricular septum *(see also*
    Aneurysm, heart) 414.10
  intracranial - *see* Aneurysm, brain
  intrathoracic (nonsyphilitic) 441.2
    ruptured 441.1
    syphilitic 093.0
  jugular vein (acute) 453.89 ◀▥
    chronic 453.76 ◀
  lower extremity 442.3
  lung (pulmonary artery) 417.1
  malignant 093.9

Aneurysm *(Continued)*
  mediastinal (nonsyphilitic) 442.89
    syphilitic 093.89
  miliary (congenital) (ruptured) *(see also*
    Hemorrhage, subarachnoid) 430
  mitral (heart) (valve) 424.0
  mural (arteriovenous) (heart) *(see also*
    Aneurysm, heart) 414.10
  mycotic, any site 421.0
    without endocarditis - *see*
      Aneurysm, by site
    ruptured, brain *(see also*
      Hemorrhage, subarachnoid)
      430
  myocardium *(see also* Aneurysm, heart)
    414.10
  neck 442.81
  pancreaticoduodenal 442.84
  patent ductus arteriosus 747.0
  peripheral NEC 442.89
    congenital NEC *(see also* Aneurysm,
      congenital) 747.60
  popliteal 442.3
  pulmonary 417.1
    arteriovenous 747.3
      acquired 417.0
    syphilitic 093.89
    valve (heart) *(see also* Endocarditis,
      pulmonary) 424.3
  racemose 442.9
    congenital (peripheral) NEC 747.60
  radial 442.0
  Rasmussen's *(see also* Tuberculosis)
    011.2●
  renal 442.1
  retinal (acquired) 362.17
    congenital 743.58
    diabetic 250.5● *[362.01]*
      due to secondary diabetes 249.5●
        [362.01]
  sinus, aortic (of Valsalva) 747.29
  specified site NEC 442.89
  spinal (cord) 442.89
    congenital 747.82
    syphilitic (hemorrhage) 094.89
  spleen, splenic 442.83
  subclavian 442.82
    syphilitic 093.89
  superior mesenteric 442.84
  syphilitic 093.9
    aorta 093.0
    central nervous system 094.89
    congenital 090.5
    spine, spinal 094.89
  thoracoabdominal 441.7
    ruptured 441.6
  thorax, thoracic (arch) (nonsyphilitic)
    441.2
    dissecting 441.01
    ruptured 441.1
    syphilitic 093.0
  traumatic (complication) (early) - *see*
    Injury, blood vessel, by site
  tricuspid (heart) (valve) - *see*
    Endocarditis, tricuspid
  ulnar 442.0
  upper extremity 442.0
  valve, valvular - *see* Endocarditis
  venous 456.8
    congenital NEC *(see also* Aneurysm,
      congenital) 747.60
  ventricle (arteriovenous) *(see also*
    Aneurysm, heart) 414.10
  visceral artery NEC 442.84

Angiectasis 459.89
Angiectopia 459.9
Angiitis 447.6
  allergic granulomatous 446.4
  hypersensitivity 446.20
    Goodpasture's syndrome 446.21
    specified NEC 446.29
  necrotizing 446.0
  Wegener's (necrotizing respiratory
    granulomatosis) 446.4
Angina (attack) (cardiac) (chest) (effort)
  (heart) (pectoris) (syndrome)
  (vasomotor) 413.9
  abdominal 557.1
  accelerated 411.1
  agranulocytic 288.03
  aphthous 074.0
  catarrhal 462
  crescendo 411.1
  croupous 464.4
  cruris 443.9
    due to atherosclerosis NEC *(see also*
      Arteriosclerosis, extremities)
      440.20
  decubitus 413.0
  diphtheritic (membranous) 032.0
  equivalent 413.9
  erysipelatous 034.0
  erythematous 462
  exudative, chronic 476.0
  faucium 478.29
  gangrenous 462
    diphtheritic 032.0
  infectious 462
  initial 411.1
  intestinal 557.1
  ludovici 528.3
  Ludwig's 528.3
  malignant 462
    diphtheritic 032.0
  membranous 464.4
    diphtheritic 032.0
  mesenteric 557.1
  monocytic 075
  nocturnal 413.0
  phlegmonous 475
    diphtheritic 032.0
  preinfarctional 411.1
  Prinzmetal's 413.1
  progressive 411.1
  pseudomembranous 101
  psychogenic 306.2
  pultaceous, diphtheritic 032.0
  scarlatinal 034.1
  septic 034.0
  simple 462
  stable NEC 413.9
  staphylococcal 462
  streptococcal 034.0
  stridulous, diphtheritic 032.3
  syphilitic 093.9
    congenital 090.5
  tonsil 475
  trachealis 464.4
  unstable 411.1
  variant 413.1
  Vincent's 101
Angioblastoma (M9161/1) - *see*
  Neoplasm, connective tissue,
  uncertain behavior
Angiocholecystitis *(see also* Cholecystitis,
  acute) 575.0
Angiocholitis *(see also* Cholecystitis,
  acute) 576.1

Angiodysgensis spinalis 336.1
Angiodysplasia (intestinalis) (intestine) 569.84
  with hemorrhage 569.85
  duodenum 537.82
    with hemorrhage 537.83
  stomach 537.82
    with hemorrhage 537.83
Angioedema (allergic) (any site) (with urticaria) 995.1
  hereditary 277.6
Angioendothelioma (M9130/1) - see also Neoplasm, by site, uncertain behavior
  benign (M9130/0) (see also Hemangioma, by site) 228.00
  bone (M9260/3) - see Neoplasm, bone, malignant
  Ewing's (M9260/3) - see Neoplasm, bone, malignant
  nervous system (M9130/0) 228.09
Angiofibroma (M9160/0) - see also Neoplasm, by site, benign
  juvenile (M9160/0) 210.7
    specified site - see Neoplasm, by site, benign
    unspecified site 210.7
Angiohemophilia (A) (B) 286.4
Angioid streaks (choroid) (retina) 363.43
Angiokeratoma (M9141/0) - see also Neoplasm, skin, benign
  corporis diffusum 272.7
Angiokeratosis
  diffuse 272.7
Angioleiomyoma (M8894/0) - see Neoplasm, connective tissue, benign
Angioleucitis 683
Angiolipoma (M8861/0) (see also Lipoma, by site) 214.9
  infiltrating (M8861/1) - see Neoplasm, connective tissue, uncertain behavior
Angioma (M9120/0) (see also Hemangioma, by site) 228.00
  capillary 448.1
  hemorrhagicum hereditaria 448.0
  malignant (M9120/3) - see Neoplasm, connective tissue, malignant
  pigmentosum et atrophicum 757.33
  placenta - see Placenta, abnormal
  plexiform (M9131/0) - see Hemangioma, by site
  senile 448.1
  serpiginosum 709.1
  spider 448.1
  stellate 448.1
Angiomatosis 757.32
  bacillary 083.8
  corporis diffusum universale 272.7
  cutaneocerebral 759.6
  encephalocutaneous 759.6
  encephalofacial 759.6
  encephalotrigeminal 759.6
  hemorrhagic familial 448.0
  hereditary familial 448.0
  heredofamilial 448.0
  meningo-oculofacial 759.6
  multiple sites 228.09
  neuro-oculocutaneous 759.6
  retina (Hippel's disease) 759.6
  retinocerebellosa 759.6
  retinocerebral 759.6
  systemic 228.09

Angiomyolipoma (M8860/0)
  specified site - see Neoplasm, connective tissue, benign
  unspecified site 223.0
Angiomyoliposarcoma (M8860/3) - see Neoplasm, connective tissue, malignant
Angiomyoma (M8894/0) - see Neoplasm, connective tissue, benign
Angiomyosarcoma (M8894/3) - see Neoplasm, connective tissue, malignant
Angioneurosis 306.2
Angioneurotic edema (allergic) (any site) (with urticaria) 995.1
  hereditary 277.6
Angiopathia, angiopathy 459.9
  diabetic (peripheral) 250.7● [443.81]
    due to secondary diabetes 249.7● [443.81]
  peripheral 443.9
    diabetic 250.7● [443.81]
      due to secondary diabetes 249.7● [443.81]
    specified type NEC 443.89
  retinae syphilitica 093.89
  retinalis (juvenilis) 362.18
    background 362.10
    diabetic 250.5● [362.01]
      due to secondary diabetes 249.5● [362.01]
    proliferative 362.29
    tuberculous (see also Tuberculosis) 017.3● [362.18]
Angiosarcoma (M9120/3) - see Neoplasm, connective tissue, malignant
Angiosclerosis - see Arteriosclerosis
Angioscotoma, enlarged 368.42
Angiospasm 443.9
  brachial plexus 353.0
  cerebral 435.9
  cervical plexus 353.2
  nerve
    arm 354.9
      axillary 353.0
      median 354.1
      ulnar 354.2
    autonomic (see also Neuropathy, peripheral, autonomic) 337.9
    axillary 353.0
    leg 355.8
      plantar 355.6
    lower extremity - see Angiospasm, nerve, leg
    median 354.1
    peripheral NEC 355.9
    spinal NEC 355.9
    sympathetic (see also Neuropathy, peripheral, autonomic) 337.9
    ulnar 354.2
    upper extremity - see Angiospasm, nerve, arm
  peripheral NEC 443.9
  traumatic 443.9
    foot 443.9
    leg 443.9
  vessel 443.9
Angiospastic disease or edema 443.9
Angle's
  class I 524.21
  class II 524.22
  class III 524.23
Anguillulosis 127.2

Angulation
  cecum (see also Obstruction, intestine) 560.9
  coccyx (acquired) 738.6
    congenital 756.19
  femur (acquired) 736.39
    congenital 755.69
  intestine (large) (small) (see also Obstruction, intestine) 560.9
  sacrum (acquired) 738.5
    congenital 756.19
  sigmoid (flexure) (see also Obstruction, intestine) 560.9
  spine (see also Curvature, spine) 737.9
  tibia (acquired) 736.89
    congenital 755.69
  ureter 593.3
  wrist (acquired) 736.09
    congenital 755.59
Angulus infectiosus 686.8
Anhedonia 780.99
Anhidrosis (lid) (neurogenic) (thermogenic) 705.0
Anhydration 276.51
  with
    hypernatremia 276.0
    hyponatremia 276.1
Anhydremia 276.52
  with
    hypernatremia 276.0
    hyponatremia 276.1
Anidrosis 705.0
Aniridia (congenital) 743.45
Anisakiasis (infection) (infestation) 127.1
Anisakis larva infestation 127.1
Aniseikonia 367.32
Anisocoria (pupil) 379.41
  congenital 743.46
Anisocytosis 790.09
Anisometropia (congenital) 367.31
Ankle - see condition
Ankyloblepharon (acquired) (eyelid) 374.46
  filiforme (adnatum) (congenital) 743.62
  total 743.62
Ankylodactly (see also Syndactylism) 755.10
Ankyloglossia 750.0
Ankylosis (fibrous) (osseous) 718.50
  ankle 718.57
  any joint, produced by surgical fusion V45.4
  cricoarytenoid (cartilage) (joint) (larynx) 478.79
  dental 521.6
  ear ossicle NEC 385.22
    malleus 385.21
  elbow 718.52
  finger 718.54
  hip 718.55
  incostapedial joint (infectional) 385.22
  joint, produced by surgical fusion NEC V45.4
  knee 718.56
  lumbosacral (joint) 724.6
  malleus 385.21
  multiple sites 718.59
  postoperative (status) V45.4
  sacroiliac (joint) 724.6
  shoulder 718.51
  specified site NEC 718.58
  spine NEC 724.9
  surgical V45.4
  teeth, tooth (hard tissues) 521.6

◀ New   ◀▥ Revised   deleted Deleted   ● Use Additional Digit(s)   Omit code

Ankylosis *(Continued)*
  temporomandibular joint 524.61
  wrist 718.53
Ankylostoma - *see* Ancylostoma
Ankylostomiasis (intestinal) - *see*
    Ancylostomiasis
Ankylurethria *(see also* Stricture, urethra)
    598.9
Annular - *see also* condition
  detachment, cervix 622.8
  organ or site, congenital NEC - *see*
    Distortion
  pancreas (congenital) 751.7
Anodontia (complete) (partial) (vera) 520.0
  with abnormal spacing 524.30
  acquired 525.10
    causing malocclusion 524.30
    due to
      caries 525.13
      extraction 525.10
      periodontal disease 525.12
      trauma 525.11
Anomaly, anomalous (congenital)
    (unspecified type) 759.9
  abdomen 759.9
  abdominal wall 756.70
  acoustic nerve 742.9
  adrenal (gland) 759.1
  Alder (-Reilly) (leukocyte granulation)
      288.2
  alimentary tract 751.9
    lower 751.5
    specified type NEC 751.8
    upper (any part, except tongue)
        750.9
      tongue 750.10
        specified type NEC 750.19
  alveolar 524.70
    ridge (process) 525.8
    specified NEC 524.79
  ankle (joint) 755.69
  anus, anal (canal) 751.5
  aorta, aortic 747.20
    arch 747.21
    coarctation (postductal) (preductal)
        747.10
    cusp or valve NEC 746.9
    septum 745.0
    specified type NEC 747.29
  aorticopulmonary septum 745.0
  apertures, diaphragm 756.6
  appendix 751.5
  aqueduct of Sylvius 742.3
    with spina bifida *(see also* Spina
        bifida) 741.0●
  arm 755.50
    reduction *(see also* Deformity,
        reduction, upper limb) 755.20
  arteriovenous (congenital) (peripheral)
        NEC 747.60
    brain 747.81
    cerebral 747.81
    coronary 746.85
    gastrointestinal 747.61
      acquired - *see* Angiodysplasia
    lower limb 747.64
    renal 747.62
    specified site NEC 747.69
    spinal 747.82
    upper limb 747.63
  artery *(see also* Anomaly, peripheral
      vascular system) NEC 747.60
    brain 747.81
    cerebral 747.81

Anomaly, anomalous *(Continued)*
  artery NEC *(Continued)*
    coronary 746.85
    eye 743.9
    pulmonary 747.3
    renal 747.62
    retina 743.9
    umbilical 747.5
  arytenoepiglottic folds 748.3
  atrial
    bands 746.9
    folds 746.9
    septa 745.5
  atrioventricular
    canal 745.69
    common 745.69
    conduction 426.7
    excitation 426.7
    septum 745.4
  atrium - *see* Anomaly, atrial
  auditory canal 744.3
    specified type NEC 744.29
      with hearing impairment 744.02
  auricle
    ear 744.3
      causing impairment of hearing
          744.02
    heart 746.9
      septum 745.5
  autosomes, autosomal NEC 758.5
  Axenfeld's 743.44
  back 759.9
  band
    atrial 746.9
    heart 746.9
    ventricular 746.9
  Bartholin's duct 750.9
  biliary duct or passage 751.60
    atresia 751.61
  bladder (neck) (sphincter) (trigone) 753.9
    specified type NEC 753.8
  blood vessel 747.9
    artery - *see* Anomaly, artery
    peripheral vascular - *see* Anomaly,
        peripheral vascular system
    vein - *see* Anomaly, vein
  bone NEC 756.9
    ankle 755.69
    arm 755.50
    chest 756.3
    cranium 756.0
    face 756.0
    finger 755.50
    foot 755.67
    forearm 755.50
    frontal 756.0
    head 756.0
    hip 755.63
    leg 755.60
    lumbosacral 756.10
    nose 748.1
    pelvic girdle 755.60
    rachitic 756.4
    rib 756.3
    shoulder girdle 755.50
    skull 756.0
      with
        anencephalus 740.0
        encephalocele 742.0
        hydrocephalus 742.3
          with spina bifida *(see also*
              Spina bifida) 741.0●
        microcephalus 742.1
    toe 755.66

Anomaly, anomalous *(Continued)*
  brain 742.9
    multiple 742.4
    reduction 742.2
    specified type NEC 742.4
    vessel 747.81
  branchial cleft NEC 744.49
    cyst 744.42
    fistula 744.41
    persistent 744.41
    sinus (external) (internal) 744.41
  breast 757.6
  broad ligament 752.10
    specified type NEC 752.19
  bronchus 748.3
  bulbar septum 745.0
  bulbus cordis 745.9
    persistent (in left ventricle) 745.8
  bursa 756.9
  canal of Nuck 752.9
  canthus 743.9
  capillary NEC *(see also* Anomaly,
      peripheral vascular system)
      747.60
  cardiac 746.9
    septal closure 745.9
      acquired 429.71
    valve NEC 746.9
      pulmonary 746.00
      specified type NEC 746.89
  cardiovascular system 746.9
    complicating pregnancy, childbirth,
        or puerperium 648.5●
  carpus 755.50
  cartilage, trachea 748.3
  cartilaginous 756.9
  caruncle, lacrimal, lachrymal 743.9
  cascade stomach 750.7
  cauda equina 742.59
  cecum 751.5
  cerebral - *see also* Anomaly, brain
      vessels 747.81
  cerebrovascular system 747.81
  cervix (uterus) 752.40
    with doubling of vagina and uterus
        752.2
    in pregnancy or childbirth 654.6●
      affecting fetus or newborn 763.89
      causing obstructed labor 660.2●
        affecting fetus or newborn
            763.1
  Chédiak-Higashi (-Steinbrinck)
      (congenital gigantism of
      peroxidase granules) 288.2
  cheek 744.9
  chest (wall) 756.3
  chin 744.9
    specified type NEC 744.89
  chordae tendineae 746.9
  choroid 743.9
    plexus 742.9
  chromosomes, chromosomal 758.9
    13 (13-15) 758.1
    18 (16-18) 758.2
    21 or 22 758.0
    autosomes NEC *(see also* Abnormal,
        autosomes) 758.5
    deletion 758.39
    Christchurch 758.39
    D_1 758.1
    E_3 758.2
    G 758.0
    mitochondrial 758.9

Anomaly, anomalous *(Continued)*
  chromosomes, chromosomal
    (Continued)
    mosaics 758.89
    sex 758.81
      complement, XO 758.6
      complement, XXX 758.81
      complement, XXY 758.7
      complement, XYY 758.81
      gonadal dysgenesis 758.6
      Klinefelter's 758.7
      Turner's 758.6
    trisomy 21 758.0
  cilia 743.9
  circulatory system 747.9
    specified type NEC 747.89
  clavicle 755.51
  clitoris 752.40
  coccyx 756.10
  colon 751.5
  common duct 751.60
  communication
    coronary artery 746.85
    left ventricle with right atrium
      745.4
  concha (ear) 744.3
  connection
    renal vessels with kidney 747.62
    total pulmonary venous 747.41
  connective tissue 756.9
    specified type NEC 756.89
  cornea 743.9
    shape 743.41
    size 743.41
    specified type NEC 743.49
  coronary
    artery 746.85
    vein 746.89
  cranium - *see* Anomaly, skull
  cricoid cartilage 748.3
  cushion, endocardial 745.60
    specified type NEC 745.69
  cystic duct 751.60
  dental arch 524.20
    specified NEC 524.29
  dental arch relationship 524.20
    angle's class I 524.21
    angle's class II 524.22
    angle's class III 524.23
    articulation
      anterior 524.27
      posterior 524.27
      reverse 524.27
    disto-occlusion 524.22
      division I 524.22
      division II 524.22
    excessive horizontal overlap 524.26
    interarch distance (excessive)
      (inadequate) 524.28
    mesio-occlusion 524.23
    neutro-occlusion 524.21
    open
      anterior occlusal relationship
        524.24
      posterior occlusal relationship
        524.25
    specified NEC 524.29
  dentition 520.6
  dentofacial NEC 524.9
    functional 524.50
    specified type NEC 524.89
  dermatoglyphic 757.2
  Descemet's membrane 743.9
    specified type NEC 743.49

Anomaly, anomalous *(Continued)*
  development
    cervix 752.40
    vagina 752.40
    vulva 752.40
  diaphragm, diaphragmatic (apertures)
    NEC 756.6
  digestive organ(s) or system 751.9
    lower 751.5
    specified type NEC 751.8
    upper 750.9
  distribution, coronary artery 746.85
  ductus
    arteriosus 747.0
    Botalli 747.0
  duodenum 751.5
  dura 742.9
    brain 742.4
    spinal cord 742.59
  ear 744.3
    causing impairment of hearing
      744.00
      specified type NEC 744.09
    external 744.3
      causing impairment of hearing
        744.02
      specified type NEC 744.29
    inner (causing impairment of
      hearing) 744.05
    middle, except ossicles (causing
      impairment of hearing) 744.03
      ossicles 744.04
    ossicles 744.04
    prominent auricle 744.29
    specified type NEC 744.29
      with hearing impairment 744.09
  Ebstein's (heart) 746.2
    tricuspid valve 746.2
  ectodermal 757.9
  Eisenmenger's (ventricular septal
    defect) 745.4
  ejaculatory duct 752.9
    specified type NEC 752.89
  elbow (joint) 755.50
  endocardial cushion 745.60
    specified type NEC 745.69
  endocrine gland NEC 759.2
  epididymis 752.9
  epiglottis 748.3
  esophagus 750.9
    specified type NEC 750.4
  Eustachian tube 744.3
    specified type NEC 744.24
  eye (any part) 743.9
    adnexa 743.9
      specified type NEC 743.69
    anophthalmos 743.00
    anterior
      chamber and related structures
        743.9
        angle 743.9
          specified type NEC 743.44
        specified type NEC 743.44
      segment 743.9
        combined 743.48
        multiple 743.48
        specified type NEC 743.49
    cataract (*see also* Cataract) 743.30
    glaucoma (*see also* Buphthalmia)
      743.20
    lid 743.9
      specified type NEC 743.63
    microphthalmos (*see also*
      Microphthalmos) 743.10

Anomaly, anomalous *(Continued)*
  eye *(Continued)*
    posterior segment 743.9
      specified type NEC 743.59
      vascular 743.58
      vitreous 743.9
        specified type NEC 743.51
    ptosis (eyelid) 743.61
    retina 743.9
      specified type NEC 743.59
    sclera 743.9
      specified type NEC 743.47
    specified type NEC 743.8
  eyebrow 744.89
  eyelid 743.9
    specified type NEC 743.63
  face (any part) 744.9
    bone(s) 756.0
    specified type NEC 744.89
  fallopian tube 752.10
    specified type NEC 752.19
  fascia 756.9
    specified type NEC 756.89
  femur 755.60
  fibula 755.60
  finger 755.50
    supernumerary 755.01
    webbed (*see also* Syndactylism,
      fingers) 755.11
  fixation, intestine 751.4
  flexion (joint) 755.9
    hip or thigh (*see also* Dislocation,
      hip, congenital) 754.30
  folds, heart 746.9
  foot 755.67
  foramen
    Botalli 745.5
    ovale 745.5
  forearm 755.50
  forehead (*see also* Anomaly, skull)
    756.0
  form, teeth 520.2
  fovea centralis 743.9
  frontal bone (*see also* Anomaly, skull)
    756.0
  gallbladder 751.60
  Gartner's duct 752.41
  gastrointestinal tract 751.9
    specified type NEC 751.8
    vessel 747.61
  genitalia, genital organ(s) or system
    female 752.9
      external 752.40
        specified type NEC 752.49
      internal NEC 752.9
    male (external and internal) 752.9
      epispadias 752.62
      hidden penis 752.65
      hydrocele, congenital 778.6
      hypospadias 752.61
      micropenis 752.64
      testis, undescended 752.51
        retractile 752.52
    specified type NEC 752.89
  genitourinary NEC 752.9
  Gerbode 745.4
  globe (eye) 743.9
  glottis 748.3
  granulation or granulocyte, genetic
    288.2
    constitutional 288.2
    leukocyte 288.2
  gum 750.9
  gyri 742.9

◀ New   ◀ɪɪɪ Revised   ~~deleted~~ Deleted   ● Use Additional Digit(s)   Omit code

Anomaly, anomalous (Continued)
hair 757.9
   specified type NEC 757.4
hand 755.50
hard tissue formation in pulp 522.3
head (see also Anomaly, skull) 756.0
heart 746.9
   auricle 746.9
   bands 746.9
   fibroelastosis cordis 425.3
   folds 746.9
   malposition 746.87
   maternal, affecting fetus or newborn 760.3
   obstructive NEC 746.84
   patent ductus arteriosus (Botalli) 747.0
   septum 745.9
      acquired 429.71
      aortic 745.0
      aorticopulmonary 745.0
      atrial 745.5
      auricular 745.5
      between aorta and pulmonary artery 745.0
      endocardial cushion type 745.60
         specified type NEC 745.69
      interatrial 745.5
      interventricular 745.4
         with pulmonary stenosis or atresia, dextraposition of aorta, and hypertrophy of right ventricle 745.2
         acquired 429.71
      specified type NEC 745.8
      ventricular 745.4
         with pulmonary stenosis or atresia, dextraposition of aorta, and hypertrophy of right ventricle 745.2
         acquired 429.71
   specified type NEC 746.89
   tetralogy of Fallot 745.2
   valve NEC 746.9
      aortic 746.9
         atresia 746.89
         bicuspid valve 746.4
         insufficiency 746.4
         specified type NEC 746.89
         stenosis 746.3
            subaortic 746.81
            supravalvular 747.22
      mitral 746.9
         atresia 746.89
         insufficiency 746.6
         specified type NEC 746.89
         stenosis 746.5
      pulmonary 746.00
         atresia 746.01
         insufficiency 746.09
         stenosis 746.02
            infundibular 746.83
            subvalvular 746.83
      tricuspid 746.9
         atresia 746.1
         stenosis 746.1
   ventricle 746.9
heel 755.67
Hegglin's 288.2
hemianencephaly 740.0
hemicephaly 740.0
hemicrania 740.0
hepatic duct 751.60
hip (joint) 755.63

Anomaly, anomalous (Continued)
hourglass
   bladder 753.8
   gallbladder 751.69
   stomach 750.7
humerus 755.50
hymen 752.40
hypersegmentation of neutrophils, hereditary 288.2
hypophyseal 759.2
ileocecal (coil) (valve) 751.5
ileum (intestine) 751.5
ilium 755.60
integument 757.9
   specified type NEC 757.8
interarch distance (excessive) (inadequate) 524.28
intervertebral cartilage or disc 756.10
intestine (large) (small) 751.5
   fixational type 751.4
iris 743.9
   specified type NEC 743.46
ischium 755.60
jaw NEC 524.9
   closure 524.51
   size (major) NEC 524.00
   specified type NEC 524.89
jaw-cranial base relationship 524.10
   specified NEC 524.19
jejunum 751.5
joint 755.9
   hip
      dislocation (see also Dislocation, hip, congenital) 754.30
      predislocation (see also Subluxation, congenital, hip) 754.32
      preluxation (see also Subluxation, congenital, hip) 754.32
      subluxation (see also Subluxation, congenital, hip) 754.32
   lumbosacral 756.10
      spondylolisthesis 756.12
      spondylosis 756.11
   multiple arthrogryposis 754.89
   sacroiliac 755.69
Jordan's 288.2
kidney(s) (calyx) (pelvis) 753.9
   vessel 747.62
Klippel-Feil (brevicollis) 756.16
knee (joint) 755.64
labium (majus) (minus) 752.40
labyrinth, membranous (causing impairment of hearing) 744.05
lacrimal
   apparatus, duct or passage 743.9
      specified type NEC 743.65
   gland 743.9
      specified type NEC 743.64
Langdon Down (mongolism) 758.0
larynx, laryngeal (muscle) 748.3
   web, webbed 748.2
leg (lower) (upper) 755.60
   reduction NEC (see also Deformity, reduction, lower limb) 755.30
lens 743.9
   shape 743.36
   specified type NEC 743.39
leukocytes, genetic 288.2
   granulation (constitutional) 288.2
lid (fold) 743.9
ligament 756.9
   broad 752.10
   round 752.9

Anomaly, anomalous (Continued)
limb, except reduction deformity 755.8
   lower 755.60
      reduction deformity (see also Deformity, reduction, lower limb) 755.30
      specified type NEC 755.69
   upper 755.50
      reduction deformity (see also Deformity, reduction, upper limb) 755.20
      specified type NEC 755.59
lip 750.9
   harelip (see also Cleft, lip) 749.10
   specified type NEC 750.26
liver (duct) 751.60
   atresia 751.69
lower extremity 755.60
   vessel 747.64
lumbosacral (joint) (region) 756.10
lung (fissure) (lobe) NEC 748.60
   agenesis 748.5
   specified type NEC 748.69
lymphatic system 759.9
Madelung's (radius) 755.54
mandible 524.9
   size NEC 524.00
maxilla 524.90
   size NEC 524.00
May (-Hegglin) 288.2
meatus urinarius 753.9
   specified type NEC 753.8
meningeal bands or folds, constriction of 742.8
meninges 742.9
   brain 742.4
   spinal 742.59
meningocele (see also Spina bifida) 741.9 ●
   acquired 349.2
mesentery 751.9
metacarpus 755.50
metatarsus 755.67
middle ear, except ossicles (causing impairment of hearing) 744.03
   ossicles 744.04
mitral (leaflets) (valve) 746.9
   atresia 746.89
   insufficiency 746.6
   specified type NEC 746.89
   stenosis 746.5
mouth 750.9
   specified type NEC 750.26
multiple NEC 759.7
   specified type NEC 759.89
muscle 756.9
   eye 743.9
      specified type NEC 743.69
   specified type NEC 756.89
musculoskeletal system, except limbs 756.9
   specified type NEC 756.9
nail 757.9
   specified type NEC 757.5
narrowness, eyelid 743.62
nasal sinus or septum 748.1
neck (any part) 744.9
   specified type NEC 744.89
nerve 742.9
   acoustic 742.9
      specified type NEC 742.8
   optic 742.9
      specified type NEC 742.8
   specified type NEC 742.8

Anomaly, anomalous *(Continued)*
- nervous system NEC 742.9
  - brain 742.9
    - specified type NEC 742.4
  - specified type NEC 742.8
- neurological 742.9
- nipple 757.6
- nonteratogenic NEC 754.89
- nose, nasal (bone) (cartilage) (septum) (sinus) 748.1
- ocular muscle 743.9
- omphalomesenteric duct 751.0
- opening, pulmonary veins 747.49
- optic
  - disc 743.9
    - specified type NEC 743.57
  - nerve 742.9
- opticociliary vessels 743.9
- orbit (eye) 743.9
  - specified type NEC 743.66
- organ
  - of Corti (causing impairment of hearing) 744.05
  - or site 759.9
    - specified type NEC 759.89
- origin
  - both great arteries from same ventricle 745.11
  - coronary artery 746.85
  - innominate artery 747.69
  - left coronary artery from pulmonary artery 746.85
  - pulmonary artery 747.3
  - renal vessels 747.62
  - subclavian artery (left) (right) 747.21
- osseous meatus (ear) 744.03
- ovary 752.0
- oviduct 752.10
- palate (hard) (soft) 750.9
  - cleft (*see also* Cleft, palate) 749.00
- pancreas (duct) 751.7
- papillary muscles 746.9
- parathyroid gland 759.2
- paraurethral ducts 753.9
- parotid (gland) 750.9
- patella 755.64
- Pelger-Huët (hereditary hyposegmentation) 288.2
- pelvic girdle 755.60
  - specified type NEC 755.69
- pelvis (bony) 755.60
  - complicating delivery 653.0●
  - rachitic 268.1
    - fetal 756.4
- penis (glans) 752.69
- pericardium 746.89
- peripheral vascular system NEC 747.60
  - gastrointestinal 747.61
  - lower limb 747.64
  - renal 747.62
  - specified site NEC 747.69
  - spinal 747.82
  - upper limb 747.63
- Peter's 743.44
- pharynx 750.9
  - branchial cleft 744.41
  - specified type NEC 750.29
- Pierre Robin 756.0
- pigmentation 709.00
  - congenital 757.33
  - specified NEC 709.09
- pituitary (gland) 759.2
- pleural folds 748.8

Anomaly, anomalous *(Continued)*
- portal vein 747.40
- position tooth, teeth 524.30
  - crowding 524.31
  - displacement 524.30
    - horizontal 524.33
    - vertical 524.34
  - distance
    - interocclusal
      - excessive 524.37
      - insufficient 524.36
  - excessive spacing 524.32
  - rotation 524.35
  - specified NEC 524.39
- preauricular sinus 744.46
- prepuce 752.9
- prostate 752.9
- pulmonary 748.60
  - artery 747.3
  - circulation 747.3
  - specified type NEC 748.69
  - valve 746.00
    - atresia 746.01
    - insufficiency 746.09
    - specified type NEC 746.09
    - stenosis 746.02
      - infundibular 746.83
      - subvalvular 746.83
  - vein 747.40
  - venous
    - connection 747.49
      - partial 747.42
      - total 747.41
    - return 747.49
      - partial 747.42
      - total (TAPVR) (complete) (subdiaphragmatic) (supradiaphragmatic) 747.41
- pupil 743.9
- pylorus 750.9
  - hypertrophy 750.5
  - stenosis 750.5
- rachitic, fetal 756.4
- radius 755.50
- rectovaginal (septum) 752.40
- rectum 751.5
- refraction 367.9
- renal 753.9
  - vessel 747.62
- respiratory system 748.9
  - specified type NEC 748.8
- rib 756.3
  - cervical 756.2
- Rieger's 743.44
- rings, trachea 748.3
- rotation - *see also* Malrotation
  - hip or thigh (*see also* Subluxation, congenital, hip) 754.32
- round ligament 752.9
- sacroiliac (joint) 755.69
- sacrum 756.10
- saddle
  - back 754.2
  - nose 754.0
    - syphilitic 090.5
- salivary gland or duct 750.9
  - specified type NEC 750.26
- scapula 755.50
- sclera 743.9
  - specified type NEC 743.47
- scrotum 752.9
- sebaceous gland 757.9

Anomaly, anomalous *(Continued)*
- seminal duct or tract 752.9
- sense organs 742.9
  - specified type NEC 742.8
- septum
  - heart - *see* Anomaly, heart, septum
  - nasal 748.1
- sex chromosomes NEC (*see also* Anomaly, chromosomes) 758.81
- shoulder (girdle) (joint) 755.50
  - specified type NEC 755.59
- sigmoid (flexure) 751.5
- sinus of Valsalva 747.29
- site NEC 759.9
- skeleton generalized NEC 756.50
- skin (appendage) 757.9
  - specified type NEC 757.39
- skull (bone) 756.0
  - with
    - anencephalus 740.0
    - encephalocele 742.0
    - hydrocephalus 742.3
      - with spina bifida (*see also* Spina bifida) 741.0●
    - microcephalus 742.1
- specified type NEC
  - adrenal (gland) 759.1
  - alimentary tract (complete) (partial) 751.8
    - lower 751.5
    - upper 750.8
  - ankle 755.69
  - anus, anal (canal) 751.5
  - aorta, aortic 747.29
    - arch 747.21
  - appendix 751.5
  - arm 755.59
  - artery (peripheral) NEC (*see also* Anomaly, peripheral vascular system) 747.60
    - brain 747.81
    - coronary 746.85
    - eye 743.58
    - pulmonary 747.3
    - retinal 743.58
    - umbilical 747.5
  - auditory canal 744.29
    - causing impairment of hearing 744.02
  - bile duct or passage 751.69
  - bladder 753.8
    - neck 753.8
  - bone(s) 756.9
    - arm 755.59
    - face 756.0
    - leg 755.69
    - pelvic girdle 755.69
    - shoulder girdle 755.59
    - skull 756.0
      - with
        - anencephalus 740.0
        - encephalocele 742.0
        - hydrocephalus 742.3
          - with spina bifida (*see also* Spina bifida) 741.0●
        - microcephalus 742.1
  - brain 742.4
  - breast 757.6
  - broad ligament 752.19
  - bronchus 748.3
  - canal of Nuck 752.89

◀ New   ◀║║ Revised   ~~deleted~~ Deleted   ● Use Additional Digit(s)   ▨ Omit code

Anomaly, anomalous *(Continued)*
  specified type NEC *(Continued)*
    cardiac septal closure 745.8
    carpus 755.59
    cartilaginous 756.9
    cecum 751.5
    cervix 752.49
    chest (wall) 756.3
    chin 744.89
    ciliary body 743.46
    circulatory system 747.89
    clavicle 755.51
    clitoris 752.49
    coccyx 756.19
    colon 751.5
    common duct 751.69
    connective tissue 756.89
    cricoid cartilage 748.3
    cystic duct 751.69
    diaphragm 756.6
    digestive organ(s) or tract 751.8
      lower 751.5
      upper 750.8
    duodenum 751.5
    ear 744.29
      auricle 744.29
        causing impairment of
            hearing 744.02
        causing impairment of hearing
            744.09
      inner (causing impairment of
          hearing) 744.05
      middle, except ossicles 744.03
        ossicles 744.04
    ejaculatory duct 752.89
    endocrine 759.2
    epiglottis 748.3
    esophagus 750.4
    eustachian tube 744.24
    eye 743.8
      lid 743.63
      muscle 743.69
    face 744.89
      bone(s) 756.0
    fallopian tube 752.19
    fascia 756.89
    femur 755.69
    fibula 755.69
    finger 755.59
    foot 755.67
    fovea centralis 743.55
    gallbladder 751.69
    Gartner's duct 752.89
    gastrointestinal tract 751.8
    genitalia, genital organ(s)
      female 752.89
        external 752.49
        internal NEC 752.89
      male 752.89
        penis 752.69
        scrotal transposition 752.81
    genitourinary tract NEC 752.89
    glottis 748.3
    hair 757.4
    hand 755.59
    heart 746.89
      valve NEC 746.89
        pulmonary 746.09
    hepatic duct 751.69
    hydatid of Morgagni 752.89
    hymen 752.49
    integument 757.8
    intestine (large) (small) 751.5
      fixational type 751.4

Anomaly, anomalous *(Continued)*
  specified type NEC *(Continued)*
    iris 743.46
    jejunum 751.5
    joint 755.8
    kidney 753.3
    knee 755.64
    labium (majus) (minus) 752.49
    labyrinth, membranous 744.05
    larynx 748.3
    leg 755.69
    lens 743.39
    limb, except reduction deformity
        755.8
      lower 755.69
        reduction deformity *(see also*
            Deformity, reduction,
            lower limb) 755.30
      upper 755.59
        reduction deformity *(see also*
            Deformity, reduction,
            upper limb) 755.20
    lip 750.26
    liver 751.69
    lung (fissure) (lobe) 748.69
    meatus urinarius 753.8
    metacarpus 755.59
    mouth 750.26
    Müllerian ◄
      cervix 752.49 ◄
      uterus 752.39 ◄
      vagina 752.49 ◄
    muscle 756.89
      eye 743.69
    musculoskeletal system, except
        limbs 756.9
    nail 757.5
    neck 744.89
    nerve 742.8
      acoustic 742.8
      optic 742.8
    nervous system 742.8
    nipple 757.6
    nose 748.1
    organ NEC 759.89
      of Corti 744.05
    osseous meatus (ear) 744.03
    ovary 752.0
    oviduct 752.19
    pancreas 751.7
    parathyroid 759.2
    patella 755.64
    pelvic girdle 755.69
    penis 752.69
    pericardium 746.89
    peripheral vascular system NEC
        (see also Anomaly, peripheral
        vascular system) 747.60
    pharynx 750.29
    pituitary 759.2
    prostate 752.89
    radius 755.59
    rectum 751.5
    respiratory system 748.8
    rib 756.3
    round ligament 752.89
    sacrum 756.19
    salivary duct or gland 750.26
    scapula 755.59
    sclera 743.47
    scrotum 752.89
      transposition 752.81
    seminal duct or tract 752.89
    shoulder girdle 755.59
    site NEC 759.89

Anomaly, anomalous *(Continued)*
  specified type NEC *(Continued)*
    skin 757.39
    skull (bone(s)) 756.0
      with
        anencephalus 740.0
        encephalocele 742.0
        hydrocephalus 742.3
          with spina bifida *(see also*
              Spina bifida) 741.0●
        microcephalus 742.1
    specified organ or site NEC 759.89
    spermatic cord 752.89
    spinal cord 742.59
    spine 756.19
    spleen 759.0
    sternum 756.3
    stomach 750.7
    tarsus 755.67
    tendon 756.89
    testis 752.89
    thorax (wall) 756.3
    thymus 759.2
    thyroid (gland) 759.2
      cartilage 748.3
    tibia 755.69
    toe 755.66
    tongue 750.19
    trachea (cartilage) 748.3
    ulna 755.59
    urachus 753.7
    ureter 753.4
      obstructive 753.29
    urethra 753.8
      obstructive 753.6
    urinary tract 753.8
    uterus (Müllerian) 752.39 ◄▥
    uvula 750.26
    vagina 752.49
    vascular NEC *(see also* Anomaly,
        peripheral vascular system)
        747.60
      brain 747.81
    vas deferens 752.89
    vein(s) (peripheral) NEC *(see also*
        Anomaly, peripheral vascular
        system) 747.60
      brain 747.81
      great 747.49
      portal 747.49
      pulmonary 747.49
    vena cava (inferior) (superior) 747.49
    vertebra 756.19
    vulva 752.49
  spermatic cord 752.9
  spine, spinal 756.10
    column 756.10
    cord 742.9
      meningocele *(see also* Spina
          bifida) 741.9●
      specified type NEC 742.59
      spina bifida *(see also* Spina bifida)
          741.9●
      vessel 747.82
    meninges 742.59
    nerve root 742.9
  spleen 759.0
  Sprengel's 755.52
  sternum 756.3
  stomach 750.9
    specified type NEC 750.7
  submaxillary gland 750.9
  superior vena cava 747.40
  talipes - *see* Talipes

Anomaly, anomalous (*Continued*)
  tarsus 755.67
    with complete absence of distal
      elements 755.31
  teeth, tooth NEC 520.9
    position 524.30
      crowding 524.31
      displacement 524.30
        horizontal 524.33
        vertical 524.34
      distance
        interocclusal
          excessive 524.37
          insufficient 524.36
      excessive spacing 524.32
      rotation 524.35
      specified NEC 524.39
      spacing 524.30
  tendon 756.9
    specified type NEC 756.89
  termination
    coronary artery 746.85
  testis 752.9
  thebesian valve 746.9
  thigh 755.60
    flexion (*see also* Subluxation,
      congenital, hip) 754.32
  thorax (wall) 756.3
  throat 750.9
  thumb 755.50
    supernumerary 755.01
  thymus gland 759.2
  thyroid (gland) 759.2
    cartilage 748.3
  tibia 755.60
    saber 090.5
  toe 755.66
    supernumerary 755.02
    webbed (*see also* Syndactylism,
      toes) 755.13
  tongue 750.10
    specified type NEC 750.19
  trachea, tracheal 748.3
    cartilage 748.3
    rings 748.3
  tragus 744.3
  transverse aortic arch 747.21
  trichromata 368.59
  trichromatopsia 368.59
  tricuspid (leaflet) (valve) 746.9
    atresia 746.1
    Ebstein's 746.2
    specified type NEC 746.89
    stenosis 746.1
  trunk 759.9
  Uhl's (hypoplasia of myocardium,
    right ventricle) 746.84
  ulna 755.50
  umbilicus 759.9
    artery 747.5
  union, trachea with larynx 748.3
  unspecified site 759.9
  upper extremity 755.50
    vessel 747.63
  urachus 753.7
    specified type NEC 753.7
  ureter 753.9
    obstructive 753.20
    specified type NEC 753.4
      obstructive 753.29
  urethra (valve) 753.9
    obstructive 753.6
    specified type NEC 753.8

Anomaly, anomalous (*Continued*)
  urinary tract or system (any part,
    except urachus) 753.9
    specified type NEC 753.8
    urachus 753.7
  uterus 752.39 ◀▥
    with only one functioning horn
      752.33 ◀▥
    in pregnancy or childbirth 654.0●
      affecting fetus or newborn 763.89
      causing obstructed labor 660.2●
        affecting fetus or newborn
          763.1
  uvula 750.9
  vagina 752.40
  valleculae 748.3
  valve (heart) NEC 746.9
    formation, ureter 753.29
    pulmonary 746.00
    specified type NEC 746.89
  vascular NEC (*see also* Anomaly,
    peripheral vascular system)
    747.60
    ring 747.21
  vas deferens 752.9
  vein(s) (peripheral) NEC (*see also*
    Anomaly, peripheral vascular
    system) 747.60
    brain 747.81
    cerebral 747.81
    coronary 746.89
    great 747.40
      specified type NEC 747.49
    portal 747.40
    pulmonary 747.40
    retina 743.9
  vena cava (inferior) (superior) 747.40
  venous - *see* Anomaly, vein
  venous return (pulmonary) 747.49
    partial 747.42
    total 747.41
  ventricle, ventricular (heart) 746.9
    bands 746.9
    folds 746.9
    septa 745.4
  vertebra 756.10
  vesicourethral orifice 753.9
  vessels NEC (*see also* Anomaly,
    peripheral vascular system)
    747.60
    optic papilla 743.9
  vitelline duct 751.0
  vitreous humor 743.9
    specified type NEC 743.51
  vulva 752.40
  wrist (joint) 755.50
Anomia 784.69
Anonychia 757.5
  acquired 703.8
Anophthalmos, anophthalmus (clinical)
  (congenital) (globe) 743.00
  acquired V45.78
Anopsia (altitudinal) (quadrant) 368.46
Anorchia 752.89
Anorchism, anorchidism 752.89
Anorexia 783.0
  hysterical 300.11
  nervosa 307.1
Anosmia (*see also* Disturbance, sensation)
  781.1
  hysterical 300.11
  postinfectional 478.9
  psychogenic 306.7
  traumatic 951.8

Anosognosia 780.99
Anosphrasia 781.1
Anosteoplasia 756.50
Anotia 744.09
Anovulatory cycle 628.0
Anoxemia 799.02
  newborn 770.88
Anoxia 799.02
  altitude 993.2
  cerebral 348.1
    with
      abortion - *see* Abortion, by type,
        with specified complication
        NEC
      ectopic pregnancy (*see also*
        categories 633.0-633.9) 639.8
      molar pregnancy (*see also*
        categories 630-632) 639.8
    complicating
      delivery (cesarean) (instrumental)
        669.4●
      ectopic or molar pregnancy 639.8
      obstetric anesthesia or sedation
        668.2●
    during or resulting from a
      procedure 997.01
    following
      abortion 639.8
      ectopic or molar pregnancy
        639.8
    newborn (*see also* Distress, fetal,
      liveborn infant) 770.88
  due to drowning 994.1
  fetal, affecting newborn 770.88
  heart - *see* Insufficiency, coronary
  high altitude 993.2
  intrauterine
    fetal death (before onset of labor)
      768.0
      during labor 768.1
    liveborn infant - *see* Distress, fetal,
      liveborn infant
  myocardial - *see* Insufficiency, coronary
  newborn 768.9
    mild or moderate 768.6
    severe 768.5
  pathological 799.02
Anteflexion - *see* Anteversion
Antenatal
  care, normal pregnancy V22.1
    first V22.0
  sampling
    chorionic villus V28.89
  screening of mother (for) V28.9
    based on amniocentesis NEC V28.2
      chromosomal anomalies V28.0
      raised alphafetoprotein levels
        V28.1
    chromosomal anomalies V28.0
    fetal growth retardation using
      ultrasonics V28.4
    genomic V28.89
    isoimmunization V28.5
    malformations using ultrasonics
      V28.3
    proteomic V28.89
    raised alphafetoprotein levels in
      amniotic fluid V28.1
    risk
      pre-term labor V28.82
    specified condition NEC V28.89
    Streptococcus B V28.6
  survey
    fetal anatomic V28.81

Antenatal (Continued)
  testing
    nuchal translucency V28.89
Antepartum - see condition
Anterior - see also condition
  spinal artery compression syndrome
      721.1
Antero-occlusion 524.24
Anteversion
  cervix - see Anteversion, uterus
  femur (neck), congenital 755.63
  uterus, uterine (cervix) (postinfectional)
      (postpartal, old) 621.6
    congenital 752.39 ◀▥
    in pregnancy or childbirth 654.4●
      affecting fetus or newborn 763.89
      causing obstructed labor 660.2●
        affecting fetus or newborn 763.1
Anthracosilicosis (occupational) 500
Anthracosis (lung) (occupational) 500
  lingua 529.3
Anthrax 022.9
  with pneumonia 022.1 [484.5]
  colitis 022.2
  cutaneous 022.0
  gastrointestinal 022.2
  intestinal 022.2
  pulmonary 022.1
  respiratory 022.1
  septicemia 022.3
  specified manifestation NEC 022.8
Anthropoid pelvis 755.69
  with disproportion (fetopelvic) 653.2●
    affecting fetus or newborn 763.1
    causing obstructed labor 660.1●
      affecting fetus or newborn 763.1
Anthropophobia 300.29
Antibioma, breast 611.0
Antibodies
  maternal (blood group) (see also
      Incompatibility) 656.2●
    anti-D, cord blood 656.1●
      fetus or newborn 773.0
Antibody deficiency syndrome
  agammaglobulinemic 279.00
  congenital 279.04
  hypogammaglobulinemic 279.00
Anticoagulant, intrinsic, circulating,
    causing hemorrhagic disorder (see
    also Circulating anticoagulants) 286.5
Antimongolism syndrome 758.39
Antimonial cholera 985.4
Antisocial personality 301.7
Antithrombinemia (see also Circulating
    anticoagulants) 286.5
Antithromboplastinemia (see also
    Circulating anticoagulants) 286.5
Antithromboplastinogenemia (see also
    Circulating anticoagulants) 286.5
Antitoxin complication or reaction - see
    Complications, vaccination
Anton (-Babinski) syndrome
    (hemiasomatognosia) 307.9
Antritis (chronic) 473.0
  maxilla 473.0
    acute 461.0
  stomach 535.4●
Antrum, antral - see condition
Anuria 788.5
  with
    abortion - see Abortion, by type,
        with renal failure
    ectopic pregnancy (see also
        categories 633.0-633.9) 639.3

Anuria (Continued)
  with (Continued)
    molar pregnancy (see also categories
        630-632) 639.3
    calculus (impacted) (recurrent) 592.9
      kidney 592.0
      ureter 592.1
    congenital 753.3
    due to a procedure 997.5
    following
      abortion 639.3
      ectopic or molar pregnancy 639.3
    newborn 753.3
    postrenal 593.4
    puerperal, postpartum, childbirth
        669.3●
    specified as due to a procedure 997.5
    sulfonamide
      correct substance properly
          administered 788.5
      overdose or wrong substance given
          or taken 961.0
    traumatic (following crushing) 958.5
Anus, anal - see also condition
  high risk human papillomavirus (HPV)
      DNA test positive 796.75
  low risk human papillomavirus (HPV)
      DNA test positive 796.79
Anusitis 569.49
Anxiety (neurosis) (reaction) (state) 300.00
  alcohol-induced 291.89
  depression 300.4
  drug-induced 292.89
  due to or associated with physical
      condition 293.84
  generalized 300.02
  hysteria 300.20
  in
    acute stress reaction 308.0
    transient adjustment reaction
        309.24
  panic type 300.01
  separation, abnormal 309.21
  syndrome (organic) (transient) 293.84
Aorta, aortic - see condition
Aortectasia 441.9 (see also Ectasia, aortic)
    447.70 ◀▥
  with aneurysm 441.9 ◀
Aortitis (nonsyphilitic) 447.6
  arteriosclerotic 440.0
  calcific 447.6
  Döhle-Heller 093.1
  luetic 093.1
  rheumatic (see also Endocarditis, acute,
      rheumatic) 391.1
  rheumatoid - see Arthritis, rheumatoid
  specific 093.1
  syphilitic 093.1
    congenital 090.5
Apathetic 799.25
  thyroid storm (see also Thyrotoxicosis)
      242.9●
Apathy 799.25
Apepsia 536.8
  achlorhydric 536.0
  psychogenic 306.4
Aperistalsis, esophagus 530.0
Apert's syndrome
    (acrocephalosyndactyly) 755.55
Apert-Gallais syndrome (adrenogenital)
    255.2
Apertognathia 524.20
Aphagia 787.20
  psychogenic 307.1

Aphakia (acquired) (bilateral)
    (postoperative) (unilateral) 379.31
  congenital 743.35
Aphalangia (congenital) 755.4
  lower limb (complete) (intercalary)
      (partial) (terminal) 755.39
    meaning all digits (complete)
        (partial) 755.31
    transverse 755.31
  upper limb (complete) (intercalary)
      (partial) (terminal) 755.29
    meaning all digits (complete)
        (partial) 755.21
    transverse 755.21
Aphasia (amnestic) (ataxic) (auditory)
    (Broca's) (choreatic) (classic)
    (expressive) (global) (ideational)
    (ideokinetic) (ideomotor) (jargon)
    (motor) (nominal) (receptive)
    (semantic) (sensory) (syntactic)
    (verbal) (visual) (Wernicke's) 784.3
  developmental 315.31
  syphilis, tertiary 094.89
  uremic - see Uremia
Aphemia 784.3
  uremic - see Uremia
Aphonia 784.41
  clericorum 784.49
  hysterical 300.11
  organic 784.41
  psychogenic 306.1
Aphthae, aphthous - see also condition
  Bednar's 528.2
  cachectic 529.0
  epizootic 078.4
  fever 078.4
  oral 528.2
  stomatitis 528.2
  thrush 112.0
  ulcer (oral) (recurrent) 528.2
    genital organ(s) NEC
      female 616.50
      male 608.89
    larynx 478.79
Apical - see condition
Apical ballooning syndrome 429.83
Aplasia - see also Agenesis
  alveolar process (acquired) 525.8
    congenital 750.26
  aorta (congenital) 747.22
  aortic valve (congenital) 746.89
  axialis extracorticalis (congenital) 330.0
  bone marrow (myeloid) 284.9
    acquired (secondary) 284.89
    congenital 284.01
    idiopathic 284.9
  brain 740.0
    specified part 742.2
  breast 757.6
  bronchus 748.3
  cementum 520.4
  cerebellar 742.2
  congenital (pure) red cell 284.01
  corpus callosum 742.2
  erythrocyte 284.81
    congenital 284.01
  extracortical axial 330.0
  eye (congenital) 743.00
  fovea centralis (congenital) 743.55
  germinal (cell) 606.0
  iris 743.45
  labyrinth, membranous 744.05
  limb (congenital) 755.4
    lower NEC 755.30
    upper NEC 755.20

Aplasia *(Continued)*
   lung (bilateral) (congenital) (unilateral)
      748.5
   nervous system NEC 742.8
   nuclear 742.8
   ovary 752.0
   Pelizaeus-Merzbacher 330.0
   prostate (congenital) 752.89
   red cell (with thymoma) (adult) 284.81
      acquired (secondary) 284.81
      congenital 284.01
      hereditary 284.01
      of infants 284.01
      primary 284.01
      pure 284.01
   round ligament (congenital) 752.89
   salivary gland 750.21
   skin (congenital) 757.39
   spinal cord 742.59
   spleen 759.0
   testis (congenital) 752.89
   thymic, with immunodeficiency 279.2
   thyroid 243
   uterus 752.39 ◀▥
   ventral horn cell 742.59
Apleuria 756.3
Apnea, apneic (spells) 786.03
   newborn, neonatorum 770.81
      essential 770.81
      obstructive 770.82
      primary 770.81
      sleep 770.81
      specified NEC 770.82
   psychogenic 306.1
   sleep 780.57
      with
         hypersomnia, unspecified 780.53
         hyposomnia, unspecified 780.51
         insomnia, unspecified 780.51
         sleep disturbance 780.57
      central, in conditions classified
         elsewhere 327.27
      obstructive (adult) (pediatric)
         327.23
      organic 327.20
         other 327.29
      primary central 327.21
Apneumatosis newborn 770.4
Apodia 755.31
Apophysitis (bone) *(see also*
      Osteochondrosis) 732.9
   calcaneus 732.5
   juvenile 732.6
Apoplectiform convulsions *(see also*
      Disease, cerebrovascular, acute) 436
Apoplexia, apoplexy, apoplectic *(see also*
      Disease, cerebrovascular, acute) 436
   abdominal 569.89
   adrenal 036.3
   attack 436
   basilar *(see also* Disease,
      cerebrovascular, acute) 436
   brain *(see also* Disease, cerebrovascular,
      acute) 436
   bulbar *(see also* Disease,
      cerebrovascular, acute) 436
   capillary *(see also* Disease,
      cerebrovascular, acute) 436
   cardiac *(see also* Infarct, myocardium)
      410.9●
   cerebral *(see also* Disease,
      cerebrovascular, acute) 436
   chorea *(see also* Disease,
      cerebrovascular, acute) 436

Apoplexia, apoplexy, apoplectic
   (Continued)
   congestive *(see also* Disease,
      cerebrovascular, acute) 436
      newborn 767.4
   embolic *(see also* Embolism, brain)
      434.1●
   fetus 767.0
   fit *(see also* Disease, cerebrovascular,
      acute) 436
   healed or old V12.54
   heart (auricle) (ventricle) *(see also*
      Infarct, myocardium) 410.9●
   heat 992.0
   hemiplegia *(see also* Disease,
      cerebrovascular, acute) 436
   hemorrhagic (stroke) *(see also*
      Hemorrhage, brain) 432.9
   ingravescent *(see also* Disease,
      cerebrovascular, acute) 436
   late effect - *see* Late effect(s) (of)
      cerebrovascular disease
   lung - *see* Embolism, pulmonary
   meninges, hemorrhagic *(see also*
      Hemorrhage, subarachnoid) 430
   neonatorum 767.0
   newborn 767.0
   pancreatitis 577.0
   placenta 641.2●
   progressive *(see also* Disease,
      cerebrovascular, acute) 436
   pulmonary (artery) (vein) - *see*
      Embolism, pulmonary
   sanguineous *(see also* Disease,
      cerebrovascular, acute) 436
   seizure *(see also* Disease,
      cerebrovascular, acute) 436
   serous *(see also* Disease,
      cerebrovascular, acute) 436
   spleen 289.59
   stroke *(see also* Disease, cerebrovascular,
      acute) 436
   thrombotic *(see also* Thrombosis, brain)
      434.0●
   uremic - *see* Uremia
   uteroplacental 641.2●
Appendage
   fallopian tube (cyst of Morgagni) 752.11
   intestine (epiploic) 751.5
   preauricular 744.1
   testicular (organ of Morgagni) 752.89
Appendicitis 541
   with
      perforation, peritonitis
         (generalized), or rupture 540.0
         with peritoneal abscess 540.1
      peritoneal abscess 540.1
   acute (catarrhal) (fulminating)
      (gangrenous) (inflammatory)
      (obstructive) (retrocecal)
      (suppurative) 540.9
      with
         perforation, peritonitis, or
          rupture 540.0
          with peritoneal abscess 540.1
         peritoneal abscess 540.1
   amebic 006.8
   chronic (recurrent) 542
   exacerbation - *see* Appendicitis, acute
   fulminating - *see* Appendicitis, acute
   gangrenous - *see* Appendicitis, acute
   healed (obliterative) 542
   interval 542
   neurogenic 542

Appendicitis *(Continued)*
   obstructive 542
   pneumococcal 541
   recurrent 542
   relapsing 542
   retrocecal 541
   subacute (adhesive) 542
   subsiding 542
   suppurative - *see* Appendicitis, acute
   tuberculous *(see also* Tuberculosis)
      014.8●
Appendiclausis 543.9
Appendicolithiasis 543.9
Appendicopathia oxyurica 127.4
Appendix, appendicular - *see also* condition
   Morgagni (male) 752.89
      fallopian tube 752.11
Appetite
   depraved 307.52
   excessive 783.6
      psychogenic 307.51
   lack or loss *(see also* Anorexia) 783.0
      nonorganic origin 307.59
   perverted 307.52
      hysterical 300.11
Apprehension, apprehensiveness
   (abnormal) (state) 300.00
   specified type NEC 300.09
Approximal wear 521.10
Apraxia (classic) (ideational) (ideokinetic)
   (ideomotor) (motor) 784.69
   oculomotor, congenital 379.51
   verbal 784.69
Aptyalism 527.7
Aqueous misdirection 365.83
Arabicum elephantiasis *(see also*
   Infestation, filarial) 125.9
Arachnidism 989.5
Arachnitis - *see* Meningitis
Arachnodactyly 759.82
Arachnoidism 989.5
Arachnoiditis (acute) (adhesive) (basic)
   (brain) (cerebrospinal) (chiasmal)
   (chronic) (spinal) *(see also*
   Meningitis) 322.9
   meningococcal (chronic) 036.0
   syphilitic 094.2
   tuberculous *(see also* Tuberculosis,
      meninges) 013.0●
Araneism 989.5
Arboencephalitis, Australian 062.4
Arborization block (heart) 426.6
Arbor virus, arbovirus (infection) NEC
   066.9
ARC 042
Arches - *see* condition
Arcuate uterus 752.36 ◀
Arcuatus uterus 752.36 ◀▥
Arcus (cornea)
   juvenilis 743.43
      interfering with vision 743.42
   senilis 371.41
Arc-welders' lung 503
Arc-welders' syndrome (photokeratitis)
   370.24
Areflexia 796.1
Areola - *see* condition
Argentaffinoma (M8241/1) - *see also*
   Neoplasm, by site, uncertain
   behavior
   benign (M8241/0) - *see* Neoplasm, by
      site, benign
   malignant (M8241/3) - *see* Neoplasm,
      by site, malignant
   syndrome 259.2

◀ New   ◀▥ Revised   ~~deleted~~ Deleted   ● Use Additional Digit(s)   ▦ Omit code

Argentinian hemorrhagic fever 078.7
Arginosuccinicaciduria 270.6
Argonz-Del Castillo syndrome
    (nonpuerperal galactorrhea and
    amenorrhea) 253.1
Argyll-Robertson phenomenon, pupil, or
    syndrome (syphilitic) 094.89
  atypical 379.45
  nonluetic 379.45
  nonsyphilitic 379.45
  reversed 379.45
Argyria, argyriasis NEC 985.8
  conjunctiva 372.55
  cornea 371.16
  from drug or medicinal agent
    correct substance properly
      administered 709.09
    overdose or wrong substance given
      or taken 961.2
Arhinencephaly 742.2
Arias-Stella phenomenon 621.30
Ariboflavinosis 266.0
Arizona enteritis 008.1
Arm - see condition
Armenian disease 277.31
Arnold-Chiari obstruction or syndrome
    (see also Spina bifida) 741.0●
  type I 348.4
  type II (see also Spina bifida) 741.0●
  type III 742.0
  type IV 742.2
Arousals
  confusional 327.41
Arrest, arrested
  active phase of labor 661.1●
    affecting fetus or newborn 763.7
  any plane in pelvis
    complicating delivery 660.1●
      affecting fetus or newborn 763.1
  bone marrow (see also Anemia, aplastic)
    284.9
  cardiac 427.5
    with
      abortion - see Abortion, by type,
        with specified complication
        NEC
      ectopic pregnancy (see also
        categories 633.0-633.9) 639.8
      molar pregnancy (see also
        categories 630-632) 639.8
    complicating
      anesthesia
        correct substance properly
          administered 427.5
        obstetric 668.1●
        overdose or wrong substance
          given 968.4
        specified anesthetic - see
          Table of Drugs and
          Chemicals
      delivery (cesarean) (instrumental)
        669.4●
    ectopic or molar pregnancy 639.8
    surgery (nontherapeutic)
      (therapeutic) 997.1
    fetus or newborn 779.85
    following
      abortion 639.8
      ectopic or molar pregnancy 639.8
    personal history, successfully
      rescucitated V12.53
    postoperative (immediate) 997.1
      long-term effect of cardiac
        surgery 429.4

Arrest, arrested (Continued)
  cardiorespiratory (see also Arrest,
    cardiac) 427.5
  deep transverse 660.3●
    affecting fetus or newborn 763.1
  development or growth
    bone 733.91
    child 783.40
    fetus 764.9●
      affecting management of
        pregnancy 656.5●
    tracheal rings 748.3
  epiphyseal 733.91
  granulopoiesis 288.09
  heart - see Arrest, cardiac
  respiratory 799.1
    newborn 770.87
  sinus 426.6
  transverse (deep) 660.3●
    affecting fetus or newborn 763.1
Arrhenoblastoma (M8630/1)
  benign (M8630/0)
    specified site - see Neoplasm, by site,
      benign
    unspecified site
      female 220
      male 222.0
  malignant (M8630/3)
    specified site - see Neoplasm, by site,
      malignant
    unspecified site
      female 183.0
      male 186.9
  specified site - see Neoplasm, by site,
    uncertain behavior
  unspecified site
    female 236.2
    male 236.4
Arrhinencephaly 742.2
  due to
    trisomy 13 (13-15) 758.1
    trisomy 18 (16-18) 758.2
Arrhythmia (auricle) (cardiac) (cordis)
    (gallop rhythm) (juvenile) (nodal)
    (reflex) (sinus) (supraventricular)
    (transitory) (ventricle) 427.9
  bigeminal rhythm 427.89
  block 426.9
  bradycardia 427.89
  contractions, premature 427.60
  coronary sinus 427.89
  ectopic 427.89
  extrasystolic 427.60
  postoperative 997.1
  psychogenic 306.2
  vagal 780.2
Arrillaga-Ayerza syndrome (pulmonary
    artery sclerosis with pulmonary
    hypertension) 416.0
Arsenical
  dermatitis 692.4
  keratosis 692.4
  pigmentation 985.1
    from drug or medicinal agent
      correct substance properly
        administered 709.09
      overdose or wrong substance
        given or taken 961.1
Arsenism 985.1
  from drug or medicinal agent
    correct substance properly
      administered 692.4
    overdose or wrong substance given
      or taken 961.1

Arterial - see condition
Arteriectasis 447.8
Arteriofibrosis - see Arteriosclerosis
Arteriolar sclerosis - see Arteriosclerosis
Arteriolith - see Arteriosclerosis
Arteriolitis 447.6
  necrotizing, kidney 447.5
  renal - see Hypertension, kidney
Arteriolosclerosis - see Arteriosclerosis
Arterionephrosclerosis (see also
    Hypertension, kidney) 403.90
Arteriopathy 447.9
Arteriosclerosis, arteriosclerotic (artery)
    (deformans) (diffuse) (disease)
    (endarteritis) (general) (obliterans)
    (obliterative) (occlusive) (senile)
    (with calcification) 440.9
  with
    gangrene 440.24
    psychosis (see also Psychosis,
      arteriosclerotic) 290.40
    ulceration 440.23
  aorta 440.0
  arteries of extremities - see
    Arteriosclerosis, extremities
  basilar (artery) (see also Occlusion,
    artery, basilar) 433.0●
  brain 437.0
  bypass graft
    coronary artery 414.05
      autologous artery
        (gastroepiploic) (internal
        mammary) 414.04
      autologous vein 414.02
      nonautologous biological 414.03
      of transplanted heart 414.07
    extremity 440.30
      autologous vein 440.31
      nonautologous biological 440.32
  cardiac - see Arteriosclerosis, coronary
  cardiopathy - see Arteriosclerosis,
    coronary
  cardiorenal (see also Hypertension,
    cardiorenal) 404.90
  cardiovascular (see also Disease,
    cardiovascular) 429.2
  carotid (artery) (common) (internal)
    (see also Occlusion, artery, carotid)
    433.1●
  central nervous system 437.0
  cerebral 437.0
    late effect - see Late effect(s) (of)
      cerebrovascular disease
  cerebrospinal 437.0
  cerebrovascular 437.0
  coronary (artery) 414.00
    due to lipid rich plaque 414.3
    graft - see Arteriosclerosis, bypass
      graft
    native artery 414.01
      of transplanted heart 414.06
  extremities (native artery) NEC 440.20
    bypass graft 440.30
      autologous vein 440.31
      nonautologous biological 440.32
    claudication (intermittent) 440.21
    and
      gangrene 440.24
      rest pain 440.22
      and
        gangrene 440.24
        ulceration 440.23
          and gangrene 440.24
      ulceration 440.23
        and gangrene 440.24

Arteriosclerosis, arteriosclerotic (Continued)
 extremities NEC (Continued)
  gangrene 440.24
  rest pain 440.22
  and
    gangrene 440.24
    ulceration 440.23
     and gangrene 440.24
  specified site NEC 440.29
  ulceration 440.23
   and gangrene 440.24
 heart (disease) - see also
   Arteriosclerosis, coronary
  valve 424.99
   aortic 424.1
   mitral 424.0
   pulmonary 424.3
   tricuspid 424.2
 iliac 440.8 ◄
 kidney (see also Hypertension, kidney)
   403.90
 labyrinth, labyrinthine 388.00
 medial NEC (see also Arteriosclerosis,
   extremities) 440.20
 mesentery (artery) 557.1
 Mönckeberg's (see also Arteriosclerosis,
   extremities) 440.20
 myocarditis 429.0
 nephrosclerosis (see also Hypertension,
   kidney) 403.90
 peripheral (of extremities) - see
   Arteriosclerosis, extremities
 precerebral 433.9●
  specified artery NEC 433.8●
 pulmonary (idiopathic) 416.0
 renal (see also Hypertension, kidney)
   403.90
  arterioles (see also Hypertension,
    kidney) 403.90
  artery 440.1
 retinal (vascular) 440.8 [362.13]
 specified artery NEC 440.8
  with gangrene 440.8 [785.4]
 spinal (cord) 437.0
 vertebral (artery) (see also Occlusion,
   artery, vertebral) 433.2●
Arteriospasm 443.9
Arteriovenous - see condition
Arteritis 447.6
 allergic (see also Angiitis,
   hypersensitivity) 446.20
 aorta (nonsyphilitic) 447.6
  syphilitic 093.1
 aortic arch 446.7
 brachiocephalica 446.7
 brain 437.4
  syphilitic 094.89
 branchial 446.7
 cerebral 437.4
  late effect - see Late effect(s) (of)
    cerebrovascular disease
  syphilitic 094.89
 coronary (artery) - see also
   Arteriosclerosis, coronary
  rheumatic 391.9
   chronic 398.99
  syphilitic 093.89
 cranial (left) (right) 446.5
 deformans - see Arteriosclerosis
 giant cell 446.5
 necrosing or necrotizing 446.0
 nodosa 446.0
 obliterans - see also Arteriosclerosis
  subclaviocarotica 446.7

Arteritis (Continued)
 pulmonary 417.8
 retina 362.18
 rheumatic - see Fever, rheumatic
 senile - see Arteriosclerosis
 suppurative 447.2
 syphilitic (general) 093.89
  brain 094.89
  coronary 093.89
  spinal 094.89
 temporal 446.5
 young female, syndrome 446.7
Artery, arterial - see condition
Arthralgia (see also Pain, joint) 719.4●
 allergic (see also Pain, joint) 719.4●
 in caisson disease 993.3
 psychogenic 307.89
 rubella 056.71
 Salmonella 003.23
 temporomandibular joint 524.62
Arthritis, arthritic (acute) (chronic)
  (subacute) 716.9●
 meaning Osteoarthritis - see
   Osteoarthrosis

> Note: Use the following fifth-digit
> subclassification with categories
> 711-712, 715-716:
>
> 0   site unspecified
> 1   shoulder region
> 2   upper arm
> 3   forearm
> 4   hand
> 5   pelvic region and thigh
> 6   lower leg
> 7   ankle and foot
> 8   other specified sites
> 9   multiple sites

 allergic 716.2●
 ankylosing (crippling) (spine) 720.0
   [713.2]
  sites other than spine 716.9●
 atrophic 714.0
  spine 720.9
 back (see also Arthritis, spine) 721.90
 Bechterew's (ankylosing spondylitis)
   720.0
 blennorrhagic 098.50 [711.6]●
 cervical, cervicodorsal (see also
   Spondylosis, cervical) 721.0
 Charcôt's 094.0 [713.5]
  diabetic 250.6● [713.5]
   due to secondary diabetes 249.6●
     [713.5]
  syringomyelic 336.0 [713.5]
  tabetic 094.0 [713.5]
 chylous (see also Filariasis) 125.9
   [711.7]●
 climacteric NEC 716.3●
 coccyx 721.8
 cricoarytenoid 478.79
 crystal (-induced) - see Arthritis, due to
   crystals
 deformans (see also Osteoarthrosis)
   715.9●
  spine 721.90
   with myelopathy 721.91
 degenerative (see also Osteoarthrosis)
   715.9●
  idiopathic 715.09
  polyarticular 715.09
  spine 721.90
   with myelopathy 721.91

Arthritis, arthritic (Continued)
 dermatoarthritis, lipoid 272.8 [713.0]
 due to or associated with
  acromegaly 253.0 [713.0]
  actinomycosis 039.8 [711.4]●
  amyloidosis 277.39 [713.7]
  bacterial disease NEC 040.89
    [711.4]●
  Behçet's syndrome 136.1 [711.2]●
  blastomycosis 116.0 [711.6]●
  brucellosis (see also Brucellosis) 023.9
    [711.4]●
  caisson disease 993.3
  coccidioidomycosis 114.3 [711.6]●
  coliform (Escherichia coli) 711.0●
  colitis, ulcerative (see also Colitis,
    ulcerative) 556.9 [713.1]
  cowpox 051.01 [711.5]●
  crystals (see also Gout)
   dicalcium phosphate 275.49
     [712.1]●
   pyrophosphate 275.49 [712.2]●
   specified NEC 275.49 [712.8]●
  dermatoarthritis, lipoid 272.8 [713.0]
  dermatological disorder NEC 709.9
    [713.3]
  diabetes 250.6● [713.5]
   due to secondary diabetes 249.6●
     [713.5]
  diphtheria 032.89 [711.4]●
  dracontiasis 125.7 [711.7]●
  dysentery 009.0 [711.3]●
  endocrine disorder NEC 259.9
    [713.0]
  enteritis NEC 009.1 [711.3]●
   infectious (see also Enteritis,
     infectious) 009.0 [711.3]●
    specified organism NEC 008.8
      [711.3]●
   regional (see also Enteritis,
     regional) 555.9 [713.1]
   specified organism NEC 008.8
     [711.3]●
  epiphyseal slip, nontraumatic (old)
    716.8●
  erysipelas 035 [711.4]●
  erythema
   epidemic 026.1
   multiforme 695.10 [713.3]
   nodosum 695.2 [713.3]
  Escherichia coli 711.0●
  filariasis NEC 125.9 [711.7]●
  gastrointestinal condition NEC 569.9
    [713.1]
  glanders 024 [711.4]●
  Gonococcus 098.50
  gout 274.00
  H. influenzae 711.0●
  helminthiasis NEC 128.9 [711.7]●
  hematological disorder NEC 289.9
    [713.2]
  hemochromatosis 275.03 [713.0] ◄▥
  hemoglobinopathy NEC (see also
    Disease, hemoglobin) 282.7
    [713.2]
  hemophilia (see also Hemophilia)
    286.0 [713.2]
  Hemophilus influenzae (H.
    influenzae) 711.0●
  Henoch (-Schönlein) purpura 287.0
    [713.6]
  histoplasmosis NEC (see also
    Histoplasmosis) 115.99
    [711.6]●

◄ New   ◄▥ Revised   ~~deleted~~ Deleted   ● Use Additional Digit(s)   ▥ Omit code

Arthritis, arthritic (Continued)
  due to or associated with (Continued)
    human parvovirus 079.83
      [711.5]●
    hyperparathyroidism 252.00
      [713.0]
    hypersensitivity reaction NEC
      995.3 [713.6]
    hypogammaglobulinemia (see also
      Hypogammaglobulinemia)
      279.00 [713.0]
    hypothyroidism NEC 244.9
      [713.0]
    infection (see also Arthritis,
      infectious) 711.9●
    infectious disease NEC 136.9
      [711.8]●
    leprosy (see also Leprosy) 030.9
      [711.4]●
    leukemia NEC (M9800/3) 208.9●
      [713.2]
    lipoid dermatoarthritis 272.8
      [713.0]
    Lyme disease 088.81 [711.8]●
    Mediterranean fever, familial 277.31
      [713.7]
    meningococcal infection 036.82
    metabolic disorder NEC 277.9
      [713.0]
    multiple myelomatosis (M9730/3)
      203.0● [713.2]
    mumps 072.79 [711.5]●
    mycobacteria 031.8 [711.4]●
    mycosis NEC 117.9 [711.6]●
    neurological disorder NEC 349.9
      [713.5]
    ochronosis 270.2 [713.0]
    O'Nyong Nyong 066.3 [711.5]●
    parasitic disease NEC 136.9
      [711.8]●
    paratyphoid fever (see also Fever,
      paratyphoid) 002.9 [711.3]●
    parvovirus B19 079.83 [711.5]●
    Pneumococcus 711.0●
    poliomyelitis (see also Poliomyelitis)
      045.9● [711.5]●
    Pseudomonas 711.0●
    psoriasis 696.0
    pyogenic organism (E. coli) (H.
      influenzae) (Pseudomonas)
      (Streptococcus) 711.0●
    rat-bite fever 026.1 [711.4]●
    regional enteritis (see also Enteritis,
      regional) 555.9 [713.1]
    Reiter's disease 099.3 [711.1]●
    respiratory disorder NEC 519.9
      [713.4]
    reticulosis, malignant (M9720/3)
      202.3● [713.2]
    rubella 056.71
    salmonellosis 003.23
    sarcoidosis 135 [713.7]
    serum sickness 999.5 [713.6]
    Staphylococcus 711.0●
    Streptococcus 711.0●
    syphilis (see also Syphilis) 094.0
      [711.4]●
    syringomyelia 336.0 [713.5]
    thalassemia 282.49 [713.2]
    tuberculosis (see also Tuberculosis,
      arthritis) 015.9● [711.4]●
    typhoid fever 002.0 [711.3]●
    ulcerative colitis (see also Colitis,
      ulcerative) 556.9 [713.1]

Arthritis, arthritic (Continued)
  due to or associated with (Continued)
    urethritis
      nongonococcal (see also Urethritis,
        nongonococcal) 099.40
        [711.1]●
      nonspecific (see also Urethritis,
        nongonococcal) 099.40
        [711.1]●
      Reiter's 099.3 [711.1]●
    viral disease NEC 079.99 [711.5]●
  erythema epidemic 026.1
  gonococcal 098.50
  gouty 274.00
    acute 274.01
  hypertrophic (see also Osteoarthrosis)
    715.9●
    spine 721.90
      with myelopathy 721.91
  idiopathic, blennorrheal 099.3
  in caisson disease 993.3 [713.8]
  infectious or infective (acute) (chronic)
    (subacute) NEC 711.9●
    nonpyogenic 711.9●
    spine 720.9
  inflammatory NEC 714.9
  juvenile rheumatoid (chronic)
    (polyarticular) 714.30
    acute 714.31
    monoarticular 714.33
    pauciarticular 714.32
  lumbar (see also Spondylosis, lumbar)
    721.3
  meningococcal 036.82
  menopausal NEC 716.3●
  migratory - see Fever, rheumatic
  neuropathic (Charcôt's) 094.0 [713.5]
    diabetic 250.6● [713.5]
      due to secondary diabetes 249.6●
        [713.5]
    nonsyphilitic NEC 349.9 [713.5]
    syringomyelic 336.0 [713.5]
    tabetic 094.0 [713.5]
  nodosa (see also Osteoarthrosis) 715.9●
    spine 721.90
      with myelopathy 721.91
  nonpyogenic NEC 716.9●
    spine 721.90
      with myelopathy 721.91
  ochronotic 270.2 [713.0]
  palindromic (see also Rheumatism,
    palindromic) 719.3●
  pneumococcal 711.0●
  postdysenteric 009.0 [711.3]●
  postrheumatic, chronic (Jaccoud's)
    714.4
  primary progressive 714.0
    spine 720.9
  proliferative 714.0
    spine 720.0
  psoriatic 696.0
  purulent 711.0●
  pyogenic or pyemic 711.0●
  rheumatic 714.0
    acute or subacute - see Fever,
      rheumatic
    chronic 714.0
    spine 720.9
  rheumatoid (nodular) 714.0
    with
      splenoadenomegaly and
        leukopenia 714.1
      visceral or systemic involvement
        714.2

Arthritis, arthritic (Continued)
  rheumatoid (Continued)
    aortitis 714.89
    carditis 714.2
    heart disease 714.2
    juvenile (chronic) (polyarticular)
      714.30
      acute 714.31
      monoarticular 714.33
      pauciarticular 714.32
    spine 720.0
    rubella 056.71
    sacral, sacroiliac, sacrococcygeal (see
      also Spondylosis, sacral) 721.3
    scorbutic 267
    senile or senescent (see also
      Osteoarthrosis) 715.9●
      spine 721.90
        with myelopathy 721.91
    septic 711.0●
    serum (nontherapeutic) (therapeutic)
      999.5 [713.6]
    specified form NEC 716.8●
    spine 721.90
      with myelopathy 721.91
      atrophic 720.9
      degenerative 721.90
        with myelopathy 721.91
      hypertrophic (with deformity) 721.90
        with myelopathy 721.91
      infectious or infective NEC 720.9
      Marie-Strümpell 720.0
      nonpyogenic 721.90
        with myelopathy 721.91
      pyogenic 720.9
      rheumatoid 720.0
      traumatic (old) 721.7
      tuberculous (see also Tuberculosis)
        015.0● [720.81]
    staphylococcal 711.0●
    streptococcal 711.0●
    suppurative 711.0●
    syphilitic 094.0 [713.5]
      congenital 090.49 [713.5]
    syphilitica deformans (Charcôt) 094.0
      [713.5]
    temporomandibular joint 524.69
    thoracic (see also Spondylosis, thoracic)
      721.2
    toxic of menopause 716.3●
    transient 716.4●
    traumatic (chronic) (old) (post) 716.1●
      current injury - see nature of injury
    tuberculous (see also Tuberculosis,
      arthritis) 015.9● [711.4]●
    urethritica 099.3 [711.1]●
    urica, uratic 274.00
    venereal 099.3 [711.1]●
    vertebral (see also Arthritis, spine)
      721.90
    villous 716.8●
    von Bechterew's 720.0
Arthrocele (see also Effusion, joint) 719.0●
Arthrochondritis - see Arthritis
Arthrodesis status V45.4
Arthrodynia (see also Pain, joint) 719.4●
  psychogenic 307.89
Arthrodysplasia 755.9
Arthrofibrosis, joint (see also Ankylosis)
  718.5●
Arthrogryposis 728.3
  multiplex, congenita 754.89
Arthrokatadysis 715.35
Arthrolithiasis 274.00

Arthro-onychodysplasia 756.89
Arthro-osteo-onychodysplasia 756.89
Arthropathy (see also Arthritis) 716.9●

> Note: Use the following fifth-digit subclassification with categories 711-712, 716:
>
> 0 site unspecified
> 1 shoulder region
> 2 upper arm
> 3 forearm
> 4 hand
> 5 pelvic region and thigh
> 6 lower leg
> 7 ankle and foot
> 8 other specified sites
> 9 multiple sites

Behçet's 136.1 [711.2]●
Charcôt's 094.0 [713.5]
    diabetic 250.6● [713.5]
        due to secondary diabetes 249.6● [713.5]
    syringomyelic 336.0 [713.5]
    tabetic 094.0 [713.5]
crystal (-induced) - see Arthritis, due to crystals
gouty 274.00
    acute 274.01
    chronic (without mention of tophus (tophi)) 274.02
        with tophus (tophi) 274.03
neurogenic, neuropathic (Charcôt's) (tabetic) 094.0 [713.5]
    diabetic 250.6● [713.5]
        due to secondary diabetes 249.6● [713.5]
    nonsyphilitic NEC 349.9 [713.5]
    syringomyelic 336.0 [713.5]
postdysenteric NEC 009.0 [711.3]●
postrheumatic, chronic (Jaccoud's) 714.4
psoriatic 696.0
pulmonary 731.2
specified NEC 716.8●
syringomyelia 336.0 [713.5]
tabes dorsalis 094.0 [713.5]
tabetic 094.0 [713.5]
transient 716.4●
traumatic 716.1●
uric acid 274.00
Arthrophyte (see also Loose, body, joint) 718.1●
Arthrophytis 719.80
    ankle 719.87
    elbow 719.82
    foot 719.87
    hand 719.84
    hip 719.85
    knee 719.86
    multiple sites 719.89
    pelvic region 719.85
    shoulder (region) 719.81
    specified site NEC 719.88
    wrist 719.83
Arthropyosis (see also Arthritis, pyogenic) 711.0●
Arthroscopic surgical procedure converted to open procedure V64.43
Arthrosis (deformans) (degenerative) (see also Osteoarthrosis) 715.9●
    Charcôt's 094.0 [713.5]
    polyarticular 715.09
    spine (see also Spondylosis) 721.90

Arthus phenomenon 995.21
    due to
        correct substance properly administered 995.21
        overdose or wrong substance given or taken 977.9
        specified drug - see Table of Drugs and Chemicals
    serum 999.5
Articular - see also condition
    disc disorder (reducing or non-reducing) 524.63
    spondylolisthesis 756.12
Articulation
    anterior 524.27
    posterior 524.27
    reverse 524.27
Artificial
    device (prosthetic) - see Fitting, device
    insemination V26.1
    menopause (states) (symptoms) (syndrome) 627.4
    opening status (functioning) (without complication) V44.9
        anus (colostomy) V44.3
        colostomy V44.3
        cystostomy V44.50
            appendico-vesicostomy V44.52
            cutaneous-vesicostomy V44.51
            specified type NEC V44.59
        enterostomy V44.4
        gastrostomy V44.1
        ileostomy V44.2
        intestinal tract NEC V44.4
        jejunostomy V44.4
        nephrostomy V44.6
        specified site NEC V44.8
    tracheostomy V44.0
    ureterostomy V44.6
    urethrostomy V44.6
    urinary tract NEC V44.6
    vagina V44.7
    vagina status V44.7
ARV (disease) (illness) (infection) - see Human immunodeficiency virus (disease) (illness) (infection)
Arytenoid - see condition
Asbestosis (occupational) 501
Asboe-Hansen's disease (incontinentia pigmenti) 757.33
Ascariasis (intestinal) (lung) 127.0
Ascaridiasis 127.0
Ascaridosis 127.0
Ascaris 127.0
    lumbricoides (infestation) 127.0
    pneumonia 127.0
Ascending - see condition
Aschoff's bodies (see also Myocarditis, rheumatic) 398.0
Ascites 789.59
    abdominal NEC 789.59
    cancerous (M8000/6) 789.51
    cardiac 428.0
    chylous (nonfilarial) 457.8
        filarial (see also Infestation, filarial) 125.9
    congenital 778.0
    due to S. japonicum 120.2
    fetal, causing fetopelvic disproportion 653.7●
    heart 428.0
    joint (see also Effusion, joint) 719.0●
    malignant (M8000/6) 789.51
    pseudochylous 789.59

Ascites (Continued)
    syphilitic 095.2
    tuberculous (see also Tuberculosis) 014.0●
Ascorbic acid (vitamin C) deficiency (scurvy) 267
ASC-H (atypical squamous cells cannot exclude high grade squamous intraepithelial lesion)
    anus 796.72
    cervix 795.02
    vagina 795.12
ASC-US (atypical squamous cells of undetermined significance)
    anus 796.71
    cervix 795.01
    vagina 795.11
ASCVD (arteriosclerotic cardiovascular disease) 429.2
Aseptic - see condition
Asherman's syndrome 621.5
Asialia 527.7
Asiatic cholera (see also Cholera) 001.9
Asocial personality or trends 301.7
Asomatognosia 781.8
Aspergillosis 117.3
    with pneumonia 117.3 [484.6]
    allergic bronchopulmonary 518.6
    nonsyphilitic NEC 117.3
Aspergillus (flavus) (fumigatus) (infection) (terreus) 117.3
Aspermatogenesis 606.0
Aspermia (testis) 606.0
Asphyxia, asphyxiation (by) 799.01
    antenatal - see Distress, fetal
    bedclothes 994.7
    birth (see also Asphyxia, newborn) 768.9
    bunny bag 994.7
    carbon monoxide 986
    caul (see also Asphyxia, newborn) 768.9
    cave-in 994.7
        crushing - see Injury, internal, intrathoracic organs
    constriction 994.7
    crushing - see Injury, internal, intrathoracic organs
    drowning 994.1
    fetal, affecting newborn 768.9
    food or foreign body (in larynx) 933.1
        bronchioles 934.8
        bronchus (main) 934.1
        lung 934.8
        nasopharynx 933.0
        nose, nasal passages 932
        pharynx 933.0
        respiratory tract 934.9
            specified part NEC 934.8
        throat 933.0
        trachea 934.0
    gas, fumes, or vapor NEC 987.9
        specified - see Table of Drugs and Chemicals
    gravitational changes 994.7
    hanging 994.7
    inhalation - see Inhalation
    intrauterine
        fetal death (before onset of labor) 768.0
            during labor 768.1
        liveborn infant - see Distress, fetal, liveborn infant
    local 443.0

◀ New   ◀▦ Revised   ~~deleted~~ Deleted   ● Use Additional Digit(s)   ▨ Omit code

Asphyxia, asphyxiation (Continued)
  mechanical 994.7
    during birth (see also Distress, fetal)
      768.9
    mucus 933.1
      bronchus (main) 934.1
      larynx 933.1
      lung 934.8
      nasal passages 932
      newborn 770.18
      pharynx 933.0
      respiratory tract 934.9
        specified part NEC 934.8
      throat 933.0
      trachea 934.0
      vaginal (fetus or newborn) 770.18
    newborn 768.9
      with neurologic involvement 768.5
      blue 768.6
      livida 768.6
      mild or moderate 768.6
      pallida 768.5
      severe 768.5
      white 768.5
    pathological 799.01
    plastic bag 994.7
    postnatal (see also Asphyxia, newborn)
      768.9
      mechanical 994.7
    pressure 994.7
    reticularis 782.61
    strangulation 994.7
    submersion 994.1
    traumatic NEC - see Injury, internal,
      intrathoracic organs
    vomiting, vomitus - see Asphyxia, food
      or foreign body
Aspiration
  acid pulmonary (syndrome) 997.39
    obstetric 668.0●
  amniotic fluid 770.13
    with respiratory symptoms 770.14
  bronchitis 507.0
  clear amniotic fluid 770.13
    with
      pneumonia 770.14
      pneumonitis 770.14
      respiratory symptoms 770.14
  contents of birth canal 770.17
    with respiratory symptoms 770.18
  fetal 770.10
    blood 770.15
      with
        pneumonia 770.16
        pneumonitis 770.16
      pneumonitis 770.18
  food, foreign body, or gasoline (with
    asphyxiation) - see Asphyxia,
    food or foreign body
  meconium 770.11
    with
      pneumonia 770.12
      pneumonitis 770.12
      respiratory symptoms 770.12
    below vocal cords 770.11
      with respiratory symptoms
        770.12
  mucus 933.1
    into
      bronchus (main) 934.1
      lung 934.8
      respiratory tract 934.9
        specified part NEC 934.8
      trachea 934.0

Aspiration (Continued)
  mucus (Continued)
    newborn 770.17
      vaginal (fetus or newborn) 770.17
    newborn 770.10
      with respiratory symptoms 770.18
      blood 770.15
        with
          pneumonia 770.16
          pneumonitis 770.16
          respiratory symptoms
            770.16
    pneumonia 507.0
      fetus or newborn 770.18
        meconium 770.12
    pneumonitis 507.0
      fetus or newborn 770.18
        meconium 770.12
      obstetric 668.0●
    postnatal stomach contents 770.85
      with
        pneumonia 770.86
        pneumonitis 770.86
        respiratory symptoms 770.86
    syndrome of newborn (massive)
      770.18
      meconium 770.12
    vernix caseosa 770.17
Asplenia 759.0
  with mesocardia 746.87
Assam fever 085.0
Assimilation, pelvis
  with disproportion 653.2●
    affecting fetus or newborn 763.1
    causing obstructed labor 660.1●
      affecting fetus or newborn
        763.1
Assmann's focus (see also Tuberculosis)
  011.0●
Astasia (-abasia) 307.9
  hysterical 300.11
Asteatosis 706.8
  cutis 706.8
Astereognosis 780.99
Asterixis 781.3
  in liver disease 572.8
Asteroid hyalitis 379.22
Asthenia, asthenic 780.79
  cardiac (see also Failure, heart) 428.9
    psychogenic 306.2
  cardiovascular (see also Failure, heart)
    428.9
    psychogenic 306.2
  heart (see also Failure, heart) 428.9
    psychogenic 306.2
  hysterical 300.11
  myocardial (see also Failure, heart)
    428.9
    psychogenic 306.2
  nervous 300.5
  neurocirculatory 306.2
  neurotic 300.5
  psychogenic 300.5
  psychoneurotic 300.5
  psychophysiologic 300.5
  reaction, psychoneurotic 300.5
  senile 797
  Stiller's 780.79
  tropical anhidrotic 705.1
Asthenopia 368.13
  accommodative 367.4
  hysterical (muscular) 300.11
  psychogenic 306.7
Asthenospermia 792.2

Asthma, asthmatic (bronchial) (catarrh)
  (spasmodic) 493.9●

Note: The following fifth digit
subclassification is for use with codes
493.0-493.2, 493.9:

0   unspecified
1   with status asthmaticus
2   with (acute) exacerbation

  with
    chronic obstructive pulmonary
      disease (COPD) 493.2●
    hay fever 493.0●
    rhinitis, allergic 493.0●
  allergic 493.9●
    stated cause (external allergen)
      493.0●
  atopic 493.0●
  cardiac (see also Failure, ventricular,
    left) 428.1
  cardiobronchial (see also Failure,
    ventricular, left) 428.1
  cardiorenal (see also Hypertension,
    cardiorenal) 404.90
  childhood 493.0●
  Colliers' 500
  cough variant 493.82
  croup 493.9●
  detergent 507.8
  due to
    detergent 507.8
    inhalation of fumes 506.3
    internal immunological process
      493.0●
  endogenous (intrinsic) 493.1●
  eosinophilic 518.3
  exercise induced bronchospasm 493.81
  exogenous (cosmetics) (dander or dust)
    (drugs) (dust) (feathers) (food)
    (hay) (platinum) (pollen) 493.0●
  extrinsic 493.0●
  grinders' 502
  hay 493.0●
  heart (see also Failure, ventricular, left)
    428.1
  IgE 493.0●
  infective 493.1●
  intrinsic 493.1●
  Kopp's 254.8
  late-onset 493.1●
  meat-wrappers' 506.9
  Millar's (laryngismus stridulus) 478.75
  millstone makers' 502
  miners' 500
  Monday morning 504
  New Orleans (epidemic) 493.0●
  platinum 493.0●
  pneumoconiotic (occupational) NEC 505
  potters' 502
  psychogenic 316 [493.9]●
  pulmonary eosinophilic 518.3
  red cedar 495.8
  Rostan's (see also Failure, ventricular,
    left) 428.1
  sandblasters' 502
  sequoiosis 495.8
  stonemasons' 502
  thymic 254.8
  tuberculous (see also Tuberculosis,
    pulmonary) 011.9●
  Wichmann's (laryngismus stridulus)
    478.75
  wood 495.8

A

Astigmatism (compound) (congenital) 367.20
   irregular 367.22
   regular 367.21
Astroblastoma (M9430/3)
   nose 748.1
   specified site - see Neoplasm, by site, malignant
   unspecified site 191.9
Astrocytoma (cystic) (M9400/3)
   anaplastic type (M9401/3)
      specified site - see Neoplasm, by site, malignant
      unspecified site 191.9
   fibrillary (M9420/3)
      specified site - see Neoplasm, by site, malignant
      unspecified site 191.9
   fibrous (M9420/3)
      specified site - see Neoplasm, by site, malignant
      unspecified site 191.9
   gemistocytic (M9411/3)
      specified site - see Neoplasm, by site, malignant
      unspecified site 191.9
   juvenile (M9421/3)
      specified site - see Neoplasm, by site, malignant
      unspecified site 191.9
   nose 748.1
   pilocytic (M9421/3)
      specified site - see Neoplasm, by site, malignant
      unspecified site 191.9
   piloid (M9421/3)
      specified site - see Neoplasm, by site, malignant
      unspecified site 191.9
   protoplasmic (M9410/3)
      specified site - see Neoplasm, by site, malignant
      unspecified site 191.9
   specified site - see Neoplasm, by site, malignant
   subependymal (M9383/1) 237.5
      giant cell (M9384/1) 237.5
   unspecified site 191.9
Astroglioma (M9400/3)
   nose 748.1
   specified site - see Neoplasm, by site, malignant
   unspecified site 191.9
Asymbolia 784.60
Asymmetrical breathing 786.09
Asymmetry - see also Distortion
   breast, between native and reconstructed 612.1
   chest 786.9
   face 754.0
   jaw NEC 524.12
      maxillary 524.11
   pelvis with disproportion 653.0●
      affecting fetus or newborn 763.1
      causing obstructed labor 660.1●
         affecting fetus or newborn 763.1
Synergia 781.3
Asynergy 781.3
   ventricular 429.89
Asystole (heart) (see also Arrest, cardiac) 427.5
At risk for falling V15.88

Ataxia, ataxy, ataxic 781.3
   acute 781.3
   brain 331.89
   cerebellar 334.3
      hereditary (Marie's) 334.2
      in
         alcoholism 303.9● [334.4]
         myxedema (see also Myxedema) 244.9 [334.4]
         neoplastic disease NEC 239.9 [334.4]
   cerebral 331.89
   family, familial 334.2
      cerebral (Marie's) 334.2
      spinal (Friedreich's) 334.0
   Friedreich's (heredofamilial) (spinal) 334.0
   frontal lobe 781.3
   gait 781.2
      hysterical 300.11
   general 781.3
   hereditary NEC 334.2
      cerebellar 334.2
      spastic 334.1
      spinal 334.0
   heredofamilial (Marie's) 334.2
   hysterical 300.11
   locomotor (progressive) 094.0
      diabetic 250.6● [337.1]
         due to secondary diabetes 249.6● [337.1]
   Marie's (cerebellar) (heredofamilial) 334.2
   nonorganic origin 307.9
   partial 094.0
   postchickenpox 052.7
   progressive locomotor 094.0
   psychogenic 307.9
   Sanger-Brown's 334.2
   spastic 094.0
      hereditary 334.1
      syphilitic 094.0
   spinal
      hereditary 334.0
      progressive locomotor 094.0
   telangiectasia 334.8
Ataxia-telangiectasia 334.8
Atelectasis (absorption collapse) (complete) (compression) (massive) (partial) (postinfective) (pressure collapse) (pulmonary) (relaxation) 518.0
   newborn (congenital) (partial) 770.5
      primary 770.4
   primary 770.4
   tuberculous (see also Tuberculosis, pulmonary) 011.9●
Ateleiosis, ateliosis 253.3
Atelia - see Distortion
Ateliosis 253.3
Atelocardia 746.9
Atelomyelia 742.59
Athelia 757.6
Atheroembolism
   extremity
      lower 445.02
      upper 445.01
   kidney 445.81
   specified site NEC 445.89
Atheroma, atheromatous (see also Arteriosclerosis) 440.9
   aorta, aortic 440.0
      valve (see also Endocarditis, aortic) 424.1

Atheroma, atheromatous (Continued)
   artery - see Arteriosclerosis
   basilar (artery) (see also Occlusion, artery, basilar) 433.0●
   carotid (artery) (common) (internal) (see also Occlusion, artery, carotid) 433.1●
   cerebral (arteries) 437.0
   coronary (artery) - see Arteriosclerosis, coronary
   degeneration - see Arteriosclerosis
   heart, cardiac - see Arteriosclerosis, coronary
   mitral (valve) 424.0
   myocardium, myocardial - see Arteriosclerosis, coronary
   pulmonary valve (heart) (see also Endocarditis, pulmonary) 424.3
   skin 706.2
   tricuspid (heart) (valve) 424.2
   valve, valvular - see Endocarditis
   vertebral (artery) (see also Occlusion, artery, vertebral) 433.2●
Atheromatosis - see also Arteriosclerosis
   arterial, congenital 272.8
Atherosclerosis - see Arteriosclerosis
Athetosis (acquired) 781.0
   bilateral 333.79
   congenital (bilateral) 333.6
   double 333.71
   unilateral 781.0
Athlete's
   foot 110.4
   heart 429.3
Athletic team examination V70.3
Athrepsia 261
Athyrea (acquired) (see also Hypothyroidism) 244.9
   congenital 243
Athyreosis (congenital) 243
   acquired - see Hypothyroidism
Athyroidism (acquired) (see also Hypothyroidism) 244.9
   congenital 243
Atmospheric pyrexia 992.0
Atonia, atony, atonic
   abdominal wall 728.2
   bladder (sphincter) 596.4
      neurogenic NEC 596.54
         with cauda equina syndrome 344.61
   capillary 448.9
   cecum 564.89
      psychogenic 306.4
   colon 564.89
      psychogenic 306.4
   congenital 779.89
   dyspepsia 536.3
      psychogenic 306.4
   intestine 564.89
      psychogenic 306.4
   stomach 536.3
      neurotic or psychogenic 306.4
      psychogenic 306.4
   uterus 661.2●
      with hemorrhage (postpartum) 666.1●
         affecting fetus or newborn 763.7
      without hemorrhage
         intrapartum 661.2●
         postpartum 669.8●
   vesical 596.4
Atopy NEC V15.09
Atransferrinemia, congenital 273.8

◄ New   ◄|||| Revised   ~~deleted~~ Deleted   ● Use Additional Digit(s)   ▒ Omit code

Atresia, atretic (congenital) 759.89
  alimentary organ or tract NEC
       751.8
    lower 751.2
    upper 750.8
  ani, anus, anal (canal) 751.2
  aorta 747.22
    with hypoplasia of ascending aorta
         and defective development of
         left ventricle (with mitral valve
         atresia) 746.7
    arch 747.11
    ring 747.21
  aortic (orifice) (valve) 746.89
    arch 747.11
  aqueduct of Sylvius 742.3
    with spina bifida (see also Spina
         bifida) 741.0●
  artery NEC (see also Atresia, blood
       vessel) 747.60
    cerebral 747.81
    coronary 746.85
    eye 743.58
    pulmonary 747.3
    umbilical 747.5
  auditory canal (external) 744.02
  bile, biliary duct (common) or passage
       751.61
    acquired (see also Obstruction,
         biliary) 576.2
  bladder (neck) 753.6
  blood vessel (peripheral) NEC
       747.60
    cerebral 747.81
    gastrointestinal 747.61
    lower limb 747.64
    pulmonary artery 747.3
    renal 747.62
    spinal 747.82
    upper limb 747.63
  bronchus 748.3
  canal, ear 744.02
  cardiac
    valve 746.89
       aortic 746.89
       mitral 746.89
       pulmonary 746.01
       tricuspid 746.1
  cecum 751.2
  cervix (acquired) 622.4
    congenital 752.43 ◄▥
    in pregnancy or childbirth 654.6●
       affecting fetus or newborn
            763.89
       causing obstructed labor 660.2●
         affecting fetus or newborn
              763.1
  choana 748.0
  colon 751.2
  cystic duct 751.61
    acquired 575.8
       with obstruction (see also
            Obstruction, gallbladder)
            575.2
  digestive organs NEC 751.8
  duodenum 751.1
  ear canal 744.02
  ejaculatory duct 752.89
  epiglottis 748.3
  esophagus 750.3
  Eustachian tube 744.24
  fallopian tube (acquired) 628.2
    congenital 752.19
  follicular cyst 620.0

Atresia, atretic (Continued)
  foramen of
    Luschka 742.3
       with spina bifida (see also Spina
            bifida) 741.0●
    Magendie 742.3
       with spina bifida (see also Spina
            bifida) 741.0●
  gallbladder 751.69
  genital organ
    external
       female 752.49
       male NEC 752.89
         penis 752.69
    internal
       female 752.89
       male 752.89
  glottis 748.3
  gullet 750.3
  heart
    valve NEC 746.89
       aortic 746.89
       mitral 746.89
       pulmonary 746.01
       tricuspid 746.1
  hymen 752.42
    acquired 623.3
    postinfective 623.3
  ileum 751.1
  intestine (small) 751.1
    large 751.2
  iris, filtration angle (see also
       Buphthalmia) 743.20
  jejunum 751.1
  kidney 753.3
  lacrimal, apparatus 743.65
    acquired - see Stenosis, lacrimal
  larynx 748.3
  ligament, broad 752.19
  lung 748.5
  meatus urinarius 753.6
  mitral valve 746.89
    with atresia or hypoplasia of aortic
         orifice or valve, with
         hypoplasia of ascending aorta
         and defective development of
         left ventricle 746.7
  nares (anterior) (posterior) 748.0
  nasolacrimal duct 743.65
  nasopharynx 748.8
  nose, nostril 748.0
    acquired 738.0
  organ or site NEC - see Anomaly,
       specified type NEC
  osseous meatus (ear) 744.03
  oviduct (acquired) 628.2
    congenital 752.19
  parotid duct 750.23
    acquired 527.8
  pulmonary (artery) 747.3
    valve 746.01
    vein 747.49
  pulmonic 746.01
  pupil 743.46
  rectum 751.2
  salivary duct or gland 750.23
    acquired 527.8
  sublingual duct 750.23
    acquired 527.8
  submaxillary duct or gland 750.23
    acquired 527.8
  trachea 748.3
  tricuspid valve 746.1
  ureter 753.29

Atresia, atretic (Continued)
  ureteropelvic junction 753.21
  ureterovesical orifice 753.22
  urethra (valvular) 753.6
  urinary tract NEC 753.29
  uterus 752.31 ◄▥
    acquired 621.8
  vagina (acquired) 623.2
    congenital (total) (partial) 752.45 ◄▥
    postgonococcal (old) 098.2
    postinfectional 623.2
    senile 623.2
  vascular NEC (see also Atresia, blood
       vessel) 747.60
    cerebral 747.81
  vas deferens 752.89
  vein NEC (see also Atresia, blood
       vessel) 747.60
    cardiac 746.89
    great 747.49
    portal 747.49
    pulmonary 747.49
  vena cava (inferior) (superior) 747.49
  vesicourethral orifice 753.6
  vulva 752.49
    acquired 624.8
Atrichia, atrichosis 704.00
  congenital (universal) 757.4
Atrioventricularis commune 745.69
Atrophia - see also Atrophy
  alba 709.09
  cutis 701.8
    idiopathica progressiva 701.8
    senilis 701.8
  dermatological, diffuse (idiopathic)
       701.8
  flava hepatis (acuta) (subacuta) (see also
       Necrosis, liver) 570
  gyrata of choroid and retina (central)
       363.54
    generalized 363.57
  senilis 797
    dermatological 701.8
  unguium 703.8
    congenita 757.5
Atrophoderma, atrophodermia 701.9
  diffusum (idiopathic) 701.8
  maculatum 701.3
    et striatum 701.3
       due to syphilis 095.8
    syphilitic 091.3
  neuriticum 701.8
  pigmentosum 757.33
  reticulatum symmetricum faciei 701.8
  senile 701.8
  symmetrical 701.8
  vermiculata 701.8
Atrophy, atrophic
  adrenal (autoimmune) (capsule)
       (cortex) (gland) 255.41
    with hypofunction 255.41
  alveolar process or ridge (edentulous)
       525.20
    mandible 525.20
       minimal 525.21
       moderate 525.22
       severe 525.23
    maxilla 525.20
       minimal 525.24
       moderate 525.25
       severe 525.26
  appendix 543.9
  Aran-Duchenne muscular 335.21
  arm 728.2

A

Atrophy, atrophic *(Continued)*
arteriosclerotic - *see* Arteriosclerosis
arthritis 714.0
   spine 720.9
bile duct (any) 576.8
bladder 596.8
blanche (of Milian) 701.3
bone (senile) 733.99
   due to
      disuse 733.7
      infection 733.99
      tabes dorsalis (neurogenic) 094.0
   posttraumatic 733.99
brain (cortex) (progressive) 331.9
   with dementia 290.10
   Alzheimer's 331.0
      with dementia - *see* Alzheimer's, dementia
   circumscribed (Pick's) 331.11
      with dementia
         with behavioral disturbance 331.11 [294.11]
         without behavioral disturbance 331.11 [294.10]
   congenital 742.4
   hereditary 331.9
   senile 331.2
breast 611.4
   puerperal, postpartum 676.3●
buccal cavity 528.9
cardiac (brown) (senile) (*see also* Degeneration, myocardial) 429.1
cartilage (infectional) (joint) 733.99
cast, plaster of Paris 728.2
cerebellar - *see* Atrophy, brain
cerebral - *see* Atrophy, brain
cervix (endometrium) (mucosa) (myometrium) (senile) (uteri) 622.8
   menopausal 627.8
Charcôt-Marie-Tooth 356.1
choroid 363.40
   diffuse secondary 363.42
   hereditary (*see also* Dystrophy, choroid) 363.50
      gyrate
         central 363.54
         diffuse 363.57
         generalized 363.57
   senile 363.41
ciliary body 364.57
colloid, degenerative 701.3
conjunctiva (senile) 372.89
corpus cavernosum 607.89
cortical (*see also* Atrophy, brain) 331.9
Cruveilhier's 335.21
cystic duct 576.8
dacryosialadenopathy 710.2
degenerative
   colloid 701.3
   senile 701.3
Déjérine-Thomas 333.0
diffuse idiopathic, dermatological 701.8
disuse
   bone 733.7
   muscle 728.2
   pelvic muscles and anal sphincter 618.83
Duchenne-Aran 335.21
ear 388.9

Atrophy, atrophic *(Continued)*
edentulous alveolar ridge 525.20
   mandible 525.20
      minimal 525.21
      moderate 525.22
      severe 525.23
   maxilla 525.20
      minimal 525.24
      moderate 525.25
      severe 525.26
emphysema, lung 492.8
endometrium (senile) 621.8
   cervix 622.8
enteric 569.89
epididymis 608.3
eyeball, cause unknown 360.41
eyelid (senile) 374.50
facial (skin) 701.9
facioscapulohumeral (Landouzy-Déjérine) 359.1
fallopian tube (senile), acquired 620.3
fatty, thymus (gland) 254.8
gallbladder 575.8
gastric 537.89
gastritis (chronic) 535.1●
gastrointestinal 569.89
genital organ, male 608.89
glandular 289.3
globe (phthisis bulbi) 360.41
gum (*see also* Recession, gingival) 523.20
hair 704.2
heart (brown) (senile) (*see also* Degeneration, myocardial) 429.1
hemifacial 754.0
   Romberg 349.89
hydronephrosis 591
infantile 261
   paralysis, acute (*see also* Poliomyelitis, with paralysis) 045.1●
intestine 569.89
iris (generalized) (postinfectional) (sector shaped) 364.59
   essential 364.51
   progressive 364.51
   sphincter 364.54
kidney (senile) (*see also* Sclerosis, renal) 587
   with hypertension (*see also* Hypertension, kidney) 403.90
   congenital 753.0
   hydronephrotic 591
   infantile 753.0
lacrimal apparatus (primary) 375.13
   secondary 375.14
Landouzy-Déjérine 359.1
laryngitis, infection 476.0
larynx 478.79
Leber's optic 377.16
lip 528.5
liver (acute) (subacute) (*see also* Necrosis, liver) 570
   chronic (yellow) 571.8
   yellow (congenital) 570
      with
         abortion - *see* Abortion, by type, with specified complication NEC
         ectopic pregnancy (*see also* categories 633.0-633.9) 639.8
         molar pregnancy (*see also* categories 630-632) 639.8

Atrophy, atrophic *(Continued)*
liver *(Continued)*
   yellow *(Continued)*
      chronic 571.8
      complicating pregnancy 646.7●
      following
         abortion 639.8
         ectopic or molar pregnancy 639.8
      from injection, inoculation or transfusion (onset within 8 months after administration) - *see* Hepatitis, viral
      healed 571.5
      obstetric 646.7●
      postabortal 639.8
      postimmunization - *see* Hepatitis, viral
      posttransfusion - *see* Hepatitis, viral
      puerperal, postpartum 674.8●
lung (senile) 518.89
   congenital 748.69
macular (dermatological) 701.3
   syphilitic, skin 091.3
      striated 095.8
muscle, muscular 728.2
   disuse 728.2
   Duchenne-Aran 335.21
   extremity (lower) (upper) 728.2
   familial spinal 335.11
   general 728.2
   idiopathic 728.2
   infantile spinal 335.0
   myelopathic (progressive) 335.10
   myotonic 359.21
   neuritic 356.1
   neuropathic (peroneal) (progressive) 356.1
   peroneal 356.1
   primary (idiopathic) 728.2
   progressive (familial) (hereditary) (pure) 335.21
      adult (spinal) 335.19
      infantile (spinal) 335.0
      juvenile (spinal) 335.11
      spinal 335.10
         adult 335.19
         hereditary or familial 335.11
         infantile 335.0
   pseudohypertrophic 359.1
   spinal (progressive) 335.10
      adult 335.19
      Aran-Duchenne 335.21
      familial 335.11
      hereditary 335.11
      infantile 335.0
      juvenile 335.11
   syphilitic 095.6
myocardium (*see also* Degeneration, myocardial) 429.1
myometrium (senile) 621.8
   cervix 622.8
myotatic 728.2
myotonia 359.21
nail 703.8
   congenital 757.5
nasopharynx 472.2
nerve - *see also* Disorder, nerve
   abducens 378.54
   accessory 352.4
   acoustic or auditory 388.5

◀ New   ◀║║ Revised   ~~deleted~~ Deleted   ● Use Additional Digit(s)   ▬ Omit code

Atrophy, atrophic (Continued)
nerve (Continued)
cranial 352.9
first (olfactory) 352.0
second (optic) (see also Atrophy,
optic nerve) 377.10
third (oculomotor) (partial)
378.51
total 378.52
fourth (trochlear) 378.53
fifth (trigeminal) 350.8
sixth (abducens) 378.54
seventh (facial) 351.8
eighth (auditory) 388.5
ninth (glossopharyngeal) 352.2
tenth (pneumogastric) (vagus)
352.3
eleventh (accessory) 352.4
twelfth (hypoglossal) 352.5
facial 351.8
glossopharyngeal 352.2
hypoglossal 352.5
oculomotor (partial) 378.51
total 378.52
olfactory 352.0
peripheral 355.9
pneumogastric 352.3
trigeminal 350.8
trochlear 378.53
vagus (pneumogastric) 352.3
nervous system, congenital 742.8
neuritic (see also Disorder, nerve) 355.9
neurogenic NEC 355.9
bone
tabetic 094.0
nutritional 261
old age 797
olivopontocerebellar 333.0
optic nerve (ascending) (descending)
(infectional) (nonfamilial)
(papillomacular bundle)
(postretinal) (secondary NEC)
(simple) 377.10
associated with retinal dystrophy
377.13
dominant hereditary 377.16
glaucomatous 377.14
hereditary (dominant) (Leber's)
377.16
Leber's (hereditary) 377.16
partial 377.15
postinflammatory 377.12
primary 377.11
syphilitic 094.84
congenital 090.49
tabes dorsalis 094.0
orbit 376.45
ovary (senile), acquired 620.3
oviduct (senile), acquired 620.3
palsy, diffuse 335.20
pancreas (duct) (senile) 577.8
papillary muscle 429.81
paralysis 355.9
parotid gland 527.0
patches skin 701.3
senile 701.8
penis 607.89
pharyngitis 472.1
pharynx 478.29
pluriglandular 258.8
polyarthritis 714.0
prostate 602.2
pseudohypertrophic 359.1
renal (see also Sclerosis, renal) 587

Atrophy, atrophic (Continued)
reticulata 701.8
retina (see also Degeneration, retina)
362.60
hereditary (see also Dystrophy,
retina) 362.70
rhinitis 472.0
salivary duct or gland 527.0
scar NEC 709.2
sclerosis, lobar (of brain) 331.0
with dementia
with behavioral disturbance 331.0
[294.11]
without behavioral disturbance
331.0 [294.10]
scrotum 608.89
seminal vesicle 608.89
senile 797
degenerative, of skin 701.3
skin (patches) (senile) 701.8
spermatic cord 608.89
spinal (cord) 336.8
acute 336.8
muscular (chronic) 335.10
adult 335.19
familial 335.11
juvenile 335.10
paralysis 335.10
acute (see also Poliomyelitis, with
paralysis) 045.1 ●
spine (column) 733.99
spleen (senile) 289.59
spots (skin) 701.3
senile 701.8
stomach 537.89
striate and macular 701.3
syphilitic 095.8
subcutaneous 701.9
due to injection 999.9
sublingual gland 527.0
submaxillary gland 527.0
Sudeck's 733.7
suprarenal (autoimmune) (capsule)
(gland) 255.41
with hypofunction 255.41
tarso-orbital fascia, congenital 743.66
testis 608.3
thenar, partial 354.0
throat 478.29
thymus (fat) 254.8
thyroid (gland) 246.8
with
cretinism 243
myxedema 244.9
congenital 243
tongue (senile) 529.8
papillae 529.4
smooth 529.4
trachea 519.19
tunica vaginalis 608.89
turbinate 733.99
tympanic membrane (nonflaccid)
384.82
flaccid 384.81
ulcer (see also Ulcer, skin) 707.9
upper respiratory tract 478.9
uterus, uterine (acquired) (senile) 621.8
cervix 622.8
due to radiation (intended effect) 621.8
vagina (senile) 627.3
vascular 459.89
vas deferens 608.89
vertebra (senile) 733.99
vulva (primary) (senile) 624.1

Atrophy, atrophic (Continued)
Werdnig-Hoffmann 335.0
yellow (acute) (congenital) (liver)
(subacute) (see also Necrosis,
liver) 570
chronic 571.8
resulting from administration of
blood, plasma, serum, or other
biological substance (within 8
months of administration) - see
Hepatitis, viral
Attack
akinetic (see also Epilepsy) 345.0 ●
angina - see Angina
apoplectic (see also Disease,
cerebrovascular, acute) 436
benign shuddering 333.93
bilious - see Vomiting
cataleptic 300.11
cerebral (see also Disease,
cerebrovascular, acute) 436
coronary (see also Infarct, myocardium)
410.9 ●
cyanotic, newborn 770.83
epileptic (see also Epilepsy) 345.9 ●
epileptiform 780.39
heart (see also Infarct, myocardium)
410.9 ●
hemiplegia (see also Disease,
cerebrovascular, acute) 436
hysterical 300.11
jacksonian (see also Epilepsy) 345.5 ●
myocardium, myocardial (see also
Infarct, myocardium) 410.9 ●
myoclonic (see also Epilepsy) 345.1 ●
panic 300.01
paralysis (see also Disease,
cerebrovascular, acute) 436
paroxysmal 780.39
psychomotor (see also Epilepsy) 345.4 ●
salaam (see also Epilepsy) 345.6 ●
schizophreniform (see also
Schizophrenia) 295.4 ●
sensory and motor 780.39
syncope 780.2
toxic, cerebral 780.39
transient ischemic (TIA) 435.9
unconsciousness 780.2
hysterical 300.11
vasomotor 780.2
vasovagal (idiopathic) (paroxysmal)
780.2
Attention to
artificial
opening (of) V55.9
digestive tract NEC V55.4
specified site NEC V55.8
urinary tract NEC V55.6
vagina V55.7
colostomy V55.3
cystostomy V55.5
dressing
wound V58.30
nonsurgical V58.30
surgical V58.31
gastrostomy V55.1
ileostomy V55.2
jejunostomy V55.4
nephrostomy V55.6
surgical dressings V58.31
sutures V58.32
tracheostomy V55.0
ureterostomy V55.6
urethrostomy V55.6

Attrition
gum (*see also* Recession, gingival) 523.20
teeth (hard tissues) 521.10
excessive 521.10
extending into
dentine 521.12
pulp 521.13
generalized 521.15
limited to enamel 521.11
localized 521.14
Atypical - *see also* condition
cells
endocervical 795.00
endometrial 795.00
glandular
anus 796.70
cervical 795.00
vaginal 795.10
distribution, vessel (congenital) (peripheral) NEC 747.60
endometrium 621.9
kidney 593.89
Atypism, cervix 622.10
Audible tinnitus (*see also* Tinnitus) 388.30
Auditory - *see* condition
Audry's syndrome (acropachyderma) 757.39
Aujeszky's disease 078.89
Aura
jacksonian (*see also* Epilepsy) 345.5●
persistent migraine 346.5●
with cerebral infarction 346.6●
without cerebral infarction 346.5●
Aurantiasis, cutis 278.3
Auricle, auricular - *see* condition
Auriculotemporal syndrome 350.8
Australian
Q fever 083.0
X disease 062.4
Autism, autistic (child) (infantile) 299.0●
Autodigestion 799.89
Autoerythrocyte sensitization 287.2
Autographism 708.3
Autoimmune
cold sensitivity 283.0
disease NEC 279.49
hemolytic anemia 283.0
lymphoproliferative syndrome (ALPS) 279.41
thyroiditis 245.2
Autoinfection, septic - *see* Septicemia
Autointoxication 799.89
Automatism 348.89
epileptic (*see also* Epilepsy) 345.4●
paroxysmal, idiopathic (*see also* Epilepsy) 345.4●

Autonomic, autonomous
bladder 596.54
neurogenic 596.54
with cauda equina 344.61
dysreflexia 337.3
faciocephalalgia (*see also* Neuropathy, peripheral, autonomic) 337.9
hysterical seizure 300.11
imbalance (*see also* Neuropathy, peripheral, autonomic 337.9
Autophony 388.40
Autosensitivity, erythrocyte 287.2
Autotopagnosia 780.99
Autotoxemia 799.89
Autumn - *see* condition
Avellis' syndrome 344.89
Aviators
disease or sickness (*see also* Effect, adverse, high altitude) 993.2
ear 993.0
effort syndrome 306.2
Avitaminosis (multiple NEC) (*see also* Deficiency, vitamin) 269.2
A 264.9
B 266.9
with
beriberi 265.0
pellagra 265.2
B$_1$ 265.1
B$_2$ 266.0
B$_6$ 266.1
B$_{12}$ 266.2
C (with scurvy) 267
D 268.9
with
osteomalacia 268.2
rickets 268.0
E 269.1
G 266.0
H 269.1
K 269.0
multiple 269.2
nicotinic acid 265.2
P 269.1
Avulsion (traumatic) 879.8
blood vessel - *see* Injury, blood vessel, by site
cartilage - *see also* Dislocation, by site
knee, current (*see also* Tear, meniscus) 836.2
symphyseal (inner), complicating delivery 665.6●
complicated 879.9
diaphragm - *see* Injury, internal, diaphragm

Avulsion (*Continued*)
ear - *see* Wound, open, ear
epiphysis of bone - *see* Fracture, by site
external site other than limb - *see* Wound, open, by site
eye 871.3
fingernail - *see* Wound, open, finger
fracture - *see* Fracture, by site
genital organs, external - *see* Wound, open, genital organs
head (intracranial) NEC - *see also* Injury, intracranial, with open intracranial wound
complete 874.9
external site NEC 873.8
complicated 873.9
internal organ or site - *see* Injury, internal, by site
joint - *see also* Dislocation, by site
capsule - *see* Sprain, by site
ligament - *see* Sprain, by site
limb - *see also* Amputation, traumatic, by site
skin and subcutaneous tissue - *see* Wound, open, by site
muscle - *see* Sprain, by site
nerve (root) - *see* Injury, nerve, by site
scalp - *see* Wound, open, scalp
skin and subcutaneous tissue - *see* Wound, open, by site
symphyseal cartilage (inner), complicating delivery 665.6●
tendon - *see also* Sprain, by site
with open wound - *see* Wound, open, by site
toenail - *see* Wound, open, toe(s)
tooth 873.63
complicated 873.73
Awaiting organ transplant status V49.83
Awareness of heart beat 785.1
Axe grinders' disease 502
Axenfeld's anomaly or syndrome 743.44
Axilla, axillary - *see also* condition
breast 757.6
Axonotmesis - *see* Injury, nerve, by site
Ayala's disease 756.89
Ayerza's disease or syndrome (pulmonary artery sclerosis with pulmonary hypertension) 416.0
Azoospermia 606.0
Azorean disease (of the nervous system) 334.8
Azotemia 790.6
meaning uremia (*see also* Uremia) 586
Aztec ear 744.29
Azygos lobe, lung (fissure) 748.69

◀ New ◀ Revised ~~deleted~~ Deleted ● Use Additional Digit(s) ▨ Omit code

B

Baader's syndrome (erythema multiforme exudativum) 695.19
Baastrup's syndrome 721.5
Babesiasis 088.82
Babesiosis 088.82
Babington's disease (familial hemorrhagic telangiectasia) 448.0
Babinski's syndrome (cardiovascular syphilis) 093.89
Babinski-Fröhlich syndrome (adiposogenital dystrophy) 253.8
Babinski-Nageotte syndrome 344.89
Bacillary - see condition
Bacilluria 791.9
  asymptomatic, in pregnancy or puerperium 646.5●
  tuberculous (see also Tuberculosis) 016.9●
Bacillus - see also Infection, bacillus
  abortus infection 023.1
  anthracis infection 022.9
  coli
    infection 041.4
      generalized 038.42
      intestinal 008.00
      pyemia 038.42
      septicemia 038.42
  Flexner's 004.1
  fusiformis infestation 101
  mallei infection 024
  Shiga's 004.0
  suipestifer infection (see also Infection, Salmonella) 003.9
Back - see condition
Backache (postural) 724.5
  psychogenic 307.89
  sacroiliac 724.6
Backflow (pyelovenous) (see also Disease, renal) 593.9
Backknee (see also Genu, recurvatum) 736.5
Bacteremia 790.7
  newborn 771.83
Bacteria
  in blood (see also Bacteremia) 790.7
  in urine (see also Bacteriuria) 791.9
Bacterial - see condition
Bactericholia (see also Cholecystitis, acute) 575.0
Bacterid, bacteride (Andrews' pustular) 686.8
Bacteriuria, bacteruria 791.9
  with
    urinary tract infection 599.0
  asymptomatic 791.9
    in pregnancy or puerperium 646.5●
      affecting fetus or newborn 760.1
Bad
  breath 784.99
  heart - see Disease, heart
  trip (see also Abuse, drugs, nondependent) 305.3●
Baehr-Schiffrin disease (thrombotic thrombocytopenic purpura) 446.6
Baelz's disease (cheilitis glandularis apostematosa) 528.5
Baerensprung's disease (eczema marginatum) 110.3
Bagassosis (occupational) 495.1
Baghdad boil 085.1
Bagratuni's syndrome (temporal arteritis) 446.5

Baker's
  cyst (knee) 727.51
    tuberculous (see also Tuberculosis) 015.2●
  itch 692.89
Bakwin-Krida syndrome (craniometa-physeal dysplasia) 756.89
Balanitis (circinata) (gangraenosa) (infectious) (vulgaris) 607.1
  amebic 006.8
  candidal 112.2
  chlamydial 099.53
  due to Ducrey's bacillus 099.0
  erosiva circinata et gangraenosa 607.1
  gangrenous 607.1
  gonococcal (acute) 098.0
    chronic or duration of 2 months or over 098.2
  nongonococcal 607.1
  phagedenic 607.1
  venereal NEC 099.8
  xerotica obliterans 607.81
Balanoposthitis 607.1
  chlamydial 099.53
  gonococcal (acute) 098.0
    chronic or duration of 2 months or over 098.2
  ulcerative NEC 099.8
Balanorrhagia - see Balanitis
Balantidiasis 007.0
Balantidiosis 007.0
Balbuties, balbutio (see also Disorder, fluency) 315.35 ◀||||
Bald
  patches on scalp 704.00
  tongue 529.4
Baldness (see also Alopecia) 704.00
Balfour's disease (chloroma) 205.3●
Balint's syndrome (psychic paralysis of visual fixation) 368.16
Balkan grippe 083.0
Ball
  food 938
  hair 938
Ballantyne (-Runge) syndrome (postmaturity) 766.22
Balloon disease (see also Effect, adverse, high altitude) 993.2
Ballooning posterior leaflet syndrome 424.0
Baló's disease or concentric sclerosis 341.1
Bamberger's disease (hypertrophic pulmonary osteoarthropathy) 731.2
Bamberger-Marie disease (hypertrophic pulmonary osteoarthropathy) 731.2
Bamboo spine 720.0
Bancroft's filariasis 125.0
Band(s)
  adhesive (see also Adhesions, peritoneum) 568.0
  amniotic 658.8●
    affecting fetus or newborn 762.8
  anomalous or congenital - see also Anomaly, specified type NEC
    atrial 746.9
    heart 746.9
    intestine 751.4
    omentum 751.4
    ventricular 746.9
  cervix 622.3
  gallbladder (congenital) 751.69
  intestinal (adhesive) (see also Adhesions, peritoneum) 568.0
    congenital 751.4

Band(s) (Continued)
  obstructive (see also Obstruction, intestine) 560.81
  periappendiceal (congenital) 751.4
  peritoneal (adhesive) (see also Adhesions, peritoneum) 568.0
    with intestinal obstruction 560.81
    congenital 751.4
  uterus 621.5
  vagina 623.2
Bandemia (without diagnosis of specific infection) 288.66
Bandl's ring (contraction)
  complicating delivery 661.4●
  affecting fetus or newborn 763.7
Bang's disease (Brucella abortus) 023.1
Bangkok hemorrhagic fever 065.4
Bannister's disease 995.1
Bantam-Albright-Martin disease (pseudohypoparathyroidism) 275.49
Banti's disease or syndrome (with cirrhosis) (with portal hypertension) - see Cirrhosis, liver
Bar
  calcaneocuboid 755.67
  calcaneonavicular 755.67
  cubonavicular 755.67
  prostate 600.90
    with
      other lower urinary tract symptoms (LUTS) 600.91
      urinary
        obstruction 600.91
        retention 600.91
  talocalcaneal 755.67
Baragnosis 780.99
Barasheh, barashek 266.2
Barcoo disease or rot (see also Ulcer, skin) 707.9
Bard-Pic syndrome (carcinoma, head of pancreas) 157.0
Bärensprung's disease (eczema marginatum) 110.3
Baritosis 503
Barium lung disease 503
Barlow's syndrome (meaning mitral valve prolapse) 424.0
Barlow (-Möller) disease or syndrome (meaning infantile scurvy) 267
Barodontalgia 993.2
Baron Münchausen syndrome 301.51
Barosinusitis 993.1
Barotitis 993.0
Barotrauma 993.2
  odontalgia 993.2
  otitic 993.0
  sinus 993.1
Barraquer's disease or syndrome (progressive lipodystrophy) 272.6
Barré-Guillain syndrome 357.0
Barré-Liéou syndrome (posterior cervical sympathetic) 723.2
Barrel chest 738.3
Barrett's esophagus 530.85
Barrett's syndrome or ulcer (chronic peptic ulcer of esophagus) 530.85
Bársony-Polgár syndrome (corkscrew esophagus) 530.5
Bársony-Teschendorf syndrome (corkscrew esophagus) 530.5
Barth syndrome 759.89
Bartholin's
  adenitis (see also Bartholinitis) 616.89
  gland - see condition

Bartholinitis (suppurating) 616.89
  gonococcal (acute) 098.0
    chronic or duration of 2 months or
      over 098.2
Bartonellosis 088.0
Bartter's syndrome (secondary
    hyperaldosteronism with
    juxtaglomerular hyperplasia)
    255.13
Basal - see condition
Basan's (hidrotic) ectodermal dysplasia
    757.31
Baseball finger 842.13
Basedow's disease or syndrome
    (exophthalmic goiter) 242.0●
Basic - see condition
Basilar - see condition
Bason's (hidrotic) ectodermal dysplasia
    757.31
Basopenia 288.59
Basophilia 288.65
Basophilism (corticoadrenal) (Cushing's)
    (pituitary) (thymic) 255.0
Bassen-Kornzweig syndrome
    (abetalipoproteinemia) 272.5
Bat ear 744.29
Bateman's
  disease 078.0
  purpura (senile) 287.2
Bathing cramp 994.1
Bathophobia 300.23
Batten's disease, retina 330.1 [362.71]
Batten-Mayou disease 330.1 [362.71]
Batten-Steinert syndrome 359.21
Battered
  adult (syndrome) 995.81
  baby or child (syndrome) 995.54
  spouse (syndrome) 995.81
Battey mycobacterium infection 031.0
Battledore placenta - see Placenta,
    abnormal
Battle exhaustion (see also Reaction,
    stress, acute) 308.9
Baumgarten-Cruveilhier (cirrhosis)
    disease, or syndrome 571.5
Bauxite
  fibrosis (of lung) 503
  workers' disease 503
Bayle's disease (dementia paralytica)
    094.1
Bazin's disease (primary) (see also
    Tuberculosis) 017.1●
Beach ear 380.12
Beaded hair (congenital) 757.4
Beals syndrome 759.82
Beard's disease (neurasthenia) 300.5
Bearn-Kunkel (-Slater) syndrome (lupoid
    hepatitis) 571.49
Beat
  elbow 727.2
  hand 727.2
  knee 727.2
Beats
  ectopic 427.60
  escaped, heart 427.60
    postoperative 997.1
  premature (nodal) 427.60
    atrial 427.61
    auricular 427.61
    postoperative 997.1
    specified type NEC 427.69
    supraventricular 427.61
    ventricular 427.69

Beau's
  disease or syndrome (see also
    Degeneration, myocardial) 429.1
  lines (transverse furrows on
    fingernails) 703.8
Bechterew's disease (ankylosing
    spondylitis) 720.0
Bechterew-Strümpell-Marie syndrome
    (ankylosing spondylitis) 720.0
Beck's syndrome (anterior spinal artery
    occlusion) 433.8●
Becker's
  disease
    idiopathic mural endomyocardial
      disease 425.2
    myotonia congenita, recessive form
      359.22
  dystrophy 359.22
Beckwith (-Wiedemann) syndrome
    759.89
Bedbugs bite(s) - see Injury, superficial,
    by site
Bedclothes, asphyxiation or suffocation
    by 994.7
Bed confinement status V49.84
Bednar's aphthae 528.2
Bedsore (see also Ulcer, pressure)
    707.00
  with gangrene 707.00 [785.4]
Bedwetting (see also Enuresis) 788.36
Beer-drinkers' heart (disease) 425.5
Bee sting (with allergic or anaphylactic
    shock) 989.5
Begbie's disease (exophthalmic goiter)
    242.0●
Behavior disorder, disturbance - see also
    Disturbance, conduct
  antisocial, without manifest psychiatric
    disorder
    adolescent V71.02
    adult V71.01
    child V71.02
  dyssocial, without manifest psychiatric
    disorder
    adolescent V71.02
    adult V71.01
    child V71.02
  high-risk- see problem
Behçet's syndrome 136.1
Behr's disease 362.50
Beigel's disease or morbus (white piedra)
    111.2
Bejel 104.0
Bekhterev's disease (ankylosing
    spondylitis) 720.0
Bekhterev-Strümpell-Marie syndrome
    (ankylosing spondylitis) 720.0
Belching (see also Eructation) 787.3
Bell's
  disease (see also Psychosis, affective)
    296.0●
  mania (see also Psychosis, affective)
    296.0●
  palsy, paralysis 351.0
    infant 767.5
    newborn 767.5
    syphilitic 094.89
  spasm 351.0
Bence-Jones albuminuria,
    albuminosuria, or proteinuria
    791.0
Bends 993.3
Benedikt's syndrome (paralysis)
    344.89

Benign - see also condition
  cellular changes, cervix 795.09
  prostate
    hyperplasia 600.20
      with
        other lower urinary tract
          symptoms (LUTS)
          600.21
        urinary
          obstruction 600.21
          retention 600.21
    neoplasm 222.2
Bennett's
  disease (leukemia) 208.9●
  fracture (closed) 815.01
    open 815.11
Benson's disease 379.22
Bent
  back (hysterical) 300.11
  nose 738.0
    congenital 754.0
Bereavement V62.82
  as adjustment reaction 309.0
Berger's paresthesia (lower limb)
    782.0
Bergeron's disease (hysteroepilepsy)
    300.11
Beriberi (acute) (atrophic) (chronic)
    (dry) (subacute) (wet) 265.0
  with polyneuropathy 265.0 [357.4]
  heart (disease) 265.0 [425.7]
  leprosy 030.1
  neuritis 265.0 [357.4]
Berlin's disease or edema (traumatic)
    921.3
Berloque dermatitis 692.72
Bernard-Horner syndrome (see also
    Neuropathy, peripheral, autonomic)
    337.9
Bernard-Sergent syndrome (acute
    adrenocortical insufficiency)
    255.41
Bernard-Soulier disease or
    thrombopathy 287.1
Bernhardt's disease or paresthesia
    355.1
Bernhardt-Roth disease or syndrome
    (parasthesia) 355.1
Bernheim's syndrome (see also Failure,
    heart) 428.0
Bertielliasis 123.8
Bertolotti's syndrome (sacralization of
    fifth lumbar vertebra) 756.15
Berylliosis (acute) (chronic) (lung)
    (occupational) 503
Besnier's
  lupus pernio 135
  prurigo (atopic dermatitis) (infantile
    eczema) 691.8
Besnier-Boeck disease or sarcoid
    135
Besnier-Boeck-Schaumann disease
    (sarcoidosis) 135
Best's disease 362.76
Bestiality 302.1
Beta-adrenergic hyperdynamic
    circulatory state 429.82
Beta-aminoisobutyric aciduria 277.2
Beta-mercaptolactate-cysteine
    disulfiduria 270.0
Beta thalassemia (major) (minor) (mixed)
    282.49
Beurmann's disease (sporotrichosis)
    117.1

◄ New   ◄‖‖ Revised   ~~deleted~~ Deleted   ● Use Additional Digit(s)   ▒ Omit code

Bezoar 938
  intestine 936
  stomach 935.2
Bezold's abscess (*see also* Mastoiditis)
  383.01
Bianchi's syndrome (aphasia-apraxia-
  alexia) 784.69
Bicornuate or bicornis uterus (complete)
  (partial) 752.34 ◄▥
  in pregnancy or childbirth 654.0●
    with obstructed labor 660.2●
      affecting fetus or newborn 763.1
    affecting fetus or newborn 763.89
Bicuspid aortic valve 746.4
Biedl-Bardet syndrome 759.89
Bielschowsky's disease 330.1
Bielschowsky-Jansky
  amaurotic familial idiocy 330.1
  disease 330.1
Biemond's syndrome (obesity, polydactyly,
  and mental retardation) 759.89
Biermer's anemia or disease (pernicious
  anemia) 281.0
Biett's disease 695.4
Bifid (congenital) - *see also* Imperfect,
  closure
  apex, heart 746.89
  clitoris 752.49
  epiglottis 748.3
  kidney 753.3
  nose 748.1
  patella 755.64
  scrotum 752.89
  toe 755.66
  tongue 750.13
  ureter 753.4 ◄▥
  uterus 752.34 ◄▥
  uvula 749.02
    with cleft lip (*see also* Cleft, palate,
      with cleft lip) 749.20
Biforis uterus (suprasimplex) 752.34 ◄▥
Bifurcation (congenital) - *see also*
    Imperfect, closure
  gallbladder 751.69
  kidney pelvis 753.3
  renal pelvis 753.3
  rib 756.3
  tongue 750.13
  trachea 748.3
  ureter 753.4
  urethra 753.8
  uvula 749.02
    with cleft lip (*see also* Cleft, palate,
      with cleft lip) 749.20
  vertebra 756.19
Bigeminal pulse 427.89
Bigeminy 427.89
Big spleen syndrome 289.4
Bilateral - *see* condition
Bile duct - *see* condition
Bile pigments in urine 791.4
Bilharziasis (*see also* Schistosomiasis) 120.9
  chyluria 120.0
  cutaneous 120.3
  galacturia 120.0
  hematochyluria 120.0
  intestinal 120.1
  lipemia 120.9
  lipuria 120.0
  Oriental 120.2
  piarhemia 120.9
  pulmonary 120.2
  tropical hematuria 120.0
  vesical 120.0

Biliary - *see* condition
Bilious (attack) - *see also* Vomiting
  fever, hemoglobinuric 084.8
Bilirubinuria 791.4
Biliuria 791.4
Billroth's disease
  meningocele (*see also* Spina bifida)
    741.9●
Bilobate placenta - *see* Placenta, abnormal
Bilocular
  heart 745.7
  stomach 536.8
Bing-Horton syndrome (histamine
  cephalgia) 339.00
Binswanger's disease or dementia
  290.12
Biörck (-Thorson) syndrome (malignant
  carcinoid) 259.2
Biparta, bipartite - *see also* Imperfect,
  closure
  carpal scaphoid 755.59
  patella 755.64
  placenta - *see* Placenta, abnormal
  vagina 752.49
Bird
  face 756.0
  fanciers' lung or disease 495.2
  flu (*see also* Influenza, avian) 488.02 ◄▥
Bird's disease (oxaluria) 271.8
Birth
  abnormal fetus or newborn 763.9
  accident, fetus or newborn - *see* Birth,
    injury
  complications in mother - *see* Delivery,
    complicated
  compression during NEC 767.9
  defect - *see* Anomaly
  delayed, fetus 763.9
  difficult NEC, affecting fetus or
    newborn 763.9
  dry, affecting fetus or newborn 761.1
  forced, NEC, affecting fetus or
    newborn 763.89
  forceps, affecting fetus or newborn
    763.2
  hematoma of sternomastoid 767.8
  immature 765.1●
    extremely 765.0●
  inattention, after or at 995.52
  induced, affecting fetus or newborn
    763.89
  infant - *see* Newborn
  injury NEC 767.9
    adrenal gland 767.8
    basal ganglia 767.0
    brachial plexus (paralysis) 767.6
    brain (compression) (pressure)
      767.0
    cerebellum 767.0
    cerebral hemorrhage 767.0
    conjunctiva 767.8
    eye 767.8
    fracture
      bone, any except clavicle or spine
        767.3
      clavicle 767.2
      femur 767.3
      humerus 767.3
      long bone 767.3
      radius and ulna 767.3
      skeleton NEC 767.3
      skull 767.3
      spine 767.4
      tibia and fibula 767.3

Birth (*Continued*)
  injury NEC (*Continued*)
    hematoma 767.8
      liver (subcapsular) 767.8
      mastoid 767.8
      skull 767.19
      sternomastoid 767.8
      testes 767.8
      vulva 767.8
    intracranial (edema) 767.0
    laceration
      brain 767.0
      by scalpel 767.8
      peripheral nerve 767.7
    liver 767.8
    meninges
      brain 767.0
      spinal cord 767.4
    nerves (cranial, peripheral) 767.7
      brachial plexus 767.6
      facial 767.5
    paralysis 767.7
      brachial plexus 767.6
      Erb (-Duchenne) 767.6
      facial nerve 767.5
      Klumpke (-Déjérine) 767.6
      radial nerve 767.6
      spinal (cord) (hemorrhage)
        (laceration) (rupture) 767.4
    rupture
      intracranial 767.0
      liver 767.8
      spinal cord 767.4
      spleen 767.8
      viscera 767.8
    scalp 767.19
    scalpel wound 767.8
    skeleton NEC 767.3
    specified NEC 767.8
    spinal cord 767.4
    spleen 767.8
    subdural hemorrhage 767.0
    tentorial, tear 767.0
    testes 767.8
    vulva 767.8
  instrumental, NEC, affecting fetus or
    newborn 763.2
  lack of care, after or at 995.52
  multiple
    affected by maternal complications
      of pregnancy 761.5
    healthy liveborn - *see* Newborn,
      multiple
  neglect, after or at 995.52
  newborn - *see* Newborn
  palsy or paralysis NEC 767.7
  precipitate, fetus or newborn 763.6
  premature (infant) 765.1●
  prolonged, affecting fetus or newborn
    763.9
  retarded, fetus or newborn 763.9
  shock, newborn 779.89
  strangulation or suffocation
    due to aspiration of clear amniotic
      fluid 770.13
      with respiratory symptoms
        770.14
    mechanical 767.8
  trauma NEC 767.9
  triplet
    affected by maternal complications
      of pregnancy 761.5
    healthy liveborn - *see* Newborn,
      multiple

Birth *(Continued)*
  twin
    affected by maternal complications
      of pregnancy 761.5
    healthy liveborn - *see* Newborn, twin
  ventouse, affecting fetus or newborn
    763.3
Birthmark 757.32
Birt-Hogg-Dube syndrome 759.89
Bisalbuminemia 273.8
Biskra button 085.1
Bite(s)
  with intact skin surface - *see* Contusion
  animal - *see* Wound, open, by site
    intact skin surface - *see* Contusion
  bedbug - *see* Injury, superficial, by site
  centipede 989.5
  chigger 133.8
  fire ant 989.5
  flea - *see* Injury, superficial, by site
  human (open wound) - *see also* Wound,
    open, by site
    intact skin surface - *see* Contusion
  insect
    nonvenomous - *see* Injury,
      superficial, by site
    venomous 989.5
  mad dog (death from) 071
  open
    anterior 524.24
    posterior 524.25
  poisonous 989.5
  red bug 133.8
  reptile 989.5
    nonvenomous - *see* Wound, open, by
      site
  snake 989.5
    nonvenomous - *see* Wound, open, by
      site
  spider (venomous) 989.5
    nonvenomous - *see* Injury,
      superficial, by site
  venomous 989.5
Biting
  cheek or lip 528.9
  nail 307.9
Black
  death 020.9
  eye NEC 921.0
  hairy tongue 529.3
  heel 924.20
  lung disease 500
  palm 923.20
Blackfan-Diamond anemia or syndrome
  (congenital hypoplastic anemia)
  284.01
Blackhead 706.1
Blackout 780.2
Blackwater fever 084.8
Bladder - *see* condition
Blast
  blindness 921.3
  concussion - *see* Blast, injury
  injury 869.0
    with open wound into cavity 869.1
    abdomen or thorax - *see* Injury,
      internal, by site
    brain (*see also* Concussion, brain)
      850.9
      with skull fracture - *see* Fracture,
        skull
    ear (acoustic nerve trauma) 951.5
      with perforation, tympanic
        membrane - *see* Wound,
        open, ear, drum

Blast *(Continued)*
  injury *(Continued)*
    lung (*see also* Injury, internal, lung)
      861.20
    otitic (explosive) 388.11
Blastomycosis, blastomycotic (chronic)
  (cutaneous) (disseminated) (lung)
  (pulmonary) (systemic) 116.0
  Brazilian 116.1
  European 117.5
  keloidal 116.2
  North American 116.0
  primary pulmonary 116.0
  South American 116.1
Bleb(s) 709.8
  emphysematous (bullous) (diffuse)
    (lung) (ruptured) (solitary) 492.0
  filtering, eye (postglaucoma) (status)
    V45.69
    with complication 997.99
    postcataract extraction
      (complication) 997.99
  lung (ruptured) 492.0
    congenital 770.5
  subpleural (emphysematous) 492.0
Bleeder (familial) (hereditary) (*see also*
  Defect, coagulation) 286.9
  nonfamilial 286.9
Bleeding (*see also* Hemorrhage) 459.0
  anal 569.3
  anovulatory 628.0
  atonic, following delivery 666.1●
  capillary 448.9
  due to subinvolution 621.1
    puerperal 666.2●
  ear 388.69
  excessive, associated with menopausal
    onset 627.0
  familial (*see also* Defect, coagulation)
    286.9
  following intercourse 626.7
  gastrointestinal 578.9
  gums 523.8
  hemorrhoids - *see* Hemorrhoids,
    bleeding
  intermenstrual
    irregular 626.6
    regular 626.5
  intraoperative 998.11
  irregular NEC 626.4
  menopausal 627.0
  mouth 528.9
  nipple 611.79
  nose 784.7
  ovulation 626.5
  postclimacteric 627.1
  postcoital 626.7
  postmenopausal 627.1
    following induced menopause 627.4
  postoperative 998.11
  preclimacteric 627.0
  puberty 626.3
    excessive, with onset of menstrual
      periods 626.3
  rectum, rectal 569.3
  tendencies (*see also* Defect, coagulation)
    286.9
  throat 784.8
  umbilical stump 772.3
  umbilicus 789.9
  unrelated to menstrual cycle 626.6
  uterus, uterine 626.9
    climacteric 627.0
    dysfunctional 626.8

Bleeding *(Continued)*
  uterus, uterine *(Continued)*
    functional 626.8
    unrelated to menstrual cycle
      626.6
  vagina, vaginal 623.8
    functional 626.8
  vicarious 625.8
Blennorrhagia, blennorrhagic - *see*
  Blennorrhea
Blennorrhea (acute) 098.0
  adultorum 098.40
  alveolaris 523.40
  chronic or duration of 2 months or over
    098.2
  gonococcal (neonatorum) 098.40
  inclusion (neonatal) (newborn) 771.6
  neonatorum 098.40
Blepharelosis (*see also* Entropion) 374.00
Blepharitis (eyelid) 373.00
  angularis 373.01
  ciliaris 373.00
    with ulcer 373.01
  marginal 373.00
    with ulcer 373.01
  scrofulous (*see also* Tuberculosis)
    017.3● *[373.00]*
  squamous 373.02
  ulcerative 373.01
Blepharochalasis 374.34
  congenital 743.62
Blepharoclonus 333.81
Blepharoconjunctivitis (*see also*
  Conjunctivitis) 372.20
  angular 372.21
  contact 372.22
Blepharophimosis (eyelid) 374.46
  congenital 743.62
Blepharoplegia 374.89
Blepharoptosis 374.30
  congenital 743.61
Blepharopyorrhea 098.49
Blepharospasm 333.81
  due to drugs 333.85
Blessig's cyst 362.62
Blighted ovum 631
Blind
  bronchus (congenital) 748.3
  eye - *see also* Blindness
    hypertensive 360.42
    hypotensive 360.41
  loop syndrome (postoperative) 579.2
  sac, fallopian tube (congenital) 752.19
  spot, enlarged 368.42
  tract or tube (congenital) NEC - *see*
    Atresia
Blindness (acquired) (congenital) (both
  eyes) 369.00
  with deafness V49.85
  blast 921.3
    with nerve injury - *see* Injury, nerve,
      optic
  Bright's - *see* Uremia
  color (congenital) 368.59
    acquired 368.55
    blue 368.53
    green 368.52
    red 368.51
    total 368.54
  concussion 950.9
  cortical 377.75
  day 368.10
    acquired 368.10
    congenital 368.10

◀ New   ◀||| Revised   ~~deleted~~ Deleted   ● Use Additional Digit(s)   ▓ Omit code

Blindness *(Continued)*
  day *(Continued)*
    hereditary 368.10
    specified type NEC 368.10
  due to
    injury NEC 950.9
    refractive error - *see* Error, refractive
  eclipse (total) 363.31
  emotional 300.11
  face 368.16
  hysterical 300.11
  legal (both eyes) (USA definition) 369.4
    with impairment of better (less
      impaired) eye
      near-total 369.02
        with
          lesser eye impairment 369.02
            near-total 369.04
            total 369.03
      profound 369.05
        with
          lesser eye impairment 369.05
            near-total 369.07
            profound 369.08
            total 369.06
      severe 369.21
        with
          lesser eye impairment
            369.21
            blind 369.11
            near-total 369.13
            profound 369.14
            severe 369.22
            total 369.12
      total
        with lesser eye impairment
          total 369.01
  mind 784.69
  moderate
    both eyes 369.25
      with impairment of lesser eye
        (specified as)
        blind, not further specified
          369.15
        low vision, not further
          specified 369.23
        near-total 369.17
        profound 369.18
        severe 369.24
        total 369.16
    one eye 369.74
      with vision of other eye (specified
        as)
        near-normal 369.75
        normal 369.76
  near-total
    both eyes 369.04
      with impairment of lesser eye
        (specified as)
        blind, not further specified
          369.02
        total 369.03
    one eye 369.64
      with vision of other eye (specified
        as)
        near-normal 369.65
        normal 369.66
  night 368.60
    acquired 368.62
    congenital (Japanese) 368.61
    hereditary 368.61
    specified type NEC 368.69
    vitamin A deficiency 264.5
  nocturnal - *see* Blindness, night

Blindness *(Continued)*
  one eye 369.60
    with low vision of other eye 369.10
  profound
    both eyes 369.08
      with impairment of lesser eye
        (specified as)
        blind, not further specified
          369.05
        near-total 369.07
        total 369.06
    one eye 369.67
      with vision of other eye (specified
        as)
        near-normal 369.68
        normal 369.69
  psychic 784.69
  severe
    both eyes 369.22
      with impairment of lesser eye
        (specified as)
        blind, not further specified
          369.11
        low vision, not further
          specified 369.21
        near-total 369.13
        profound 369.14
        total 369.12
    one eye 369.71
      with vision of other eye (specified
        as)
        near-normal 369.72
        normal 369.73
  snow 370.24
  sun 363.31
  temporary 368.12
  total
    both eyes 369.01
    one eye 369.61
      with vision of other eye (specified
        as)
        near-normal 369.62
        normal 369.63
  transient 368.12
  traumatic NEC 950.9
  word (developmental) 315.01
    acquired 784.61
    secondary to organic lesion 784.61
Blister - *see also* Injury, superficial,
  by site
  beetle dermatitis 692.89
  due to burn - *see* Burn, by site, second
    degree
  fever 054.9
  fracture - *omit code* ◄
  multiple, skin, nontraumatic 709.8
Bloating 787.3
Bloch-Siemens syndrome (incontinentia
  pigmenti) 757.33
Bloch-Stauffer dyshormonal dermatosis
  757.33
Bloch-Sulzberger disease or syndrome
  (incontinentia pigmenti)
  (melanoblastosis) 757.33
Block
  alveolar capillary 516.3
  arborization (heart) 426.6
  arrhythmic 426.9
  atrioventricular (AV) (incomplete)
    (partial) 426.10
    with
      2:1 atrioventricular response
        block 426.13
      atrioventricular dissociation 426.0

Block *(Continued)*
  atrioventricular *(Continued)*
    first degree (incomplete) 426.11
    second degree (Mobitz type I)
      426.13
      Mobitz (type II) 426.12
    third degree 426.0
    complete 426.0
      congenital 746.86
    congenital 746.86
    Mobitz (incomplete)
      type I (Wenckebach's) 426.13
      type II 426.12
    partial 426.13
  auriculoventricular (*see also* Block,
    atrioventricular) 426.10
    complete 426.0
      congenital 746.86
    congenital 746.86
  bifascicular (cardiac) 426.53
  bundle branch (complete) (false)
    (incomplete) 426.50
    bilateral 426.53
    left (complete) (main stem) 426.3
      with right bundle branch block
        426.53
      anterior fascicular 426.2
        with
          posterior fascicular block
            426.3
          right bundle branch block
            426.52
      hemiblock 426.2
      incomplete 426.2
        with right bundle branch block
          426.53
      posterior fascicular 426.2
        with
          anterior fascicular block
            426.3
          right bundle branch block
            426.51
    right 426.4
      with
        left bundle branch block
          (incomplete) (main stem)
          426.53
        left fascicular block 426.53
          anterior 426.52
          posterior 426.51
    Wilson's type 426.4
  cardiac 426.9
  conduction 426.9
    complete 426.0
  Eustachian tube (*see also* Obstruction,
    Eustachian tube) 381.60
  fascicular (left anterior) (left posterior)
    426.2
  foramen Magendie (acquired) 331.3
    congenital 742.3
      with spina bifida (*see also* Spina
        bifida) 741.0●
  heart 426.9
    first degree (atrioventricular) 426.11
    second degree (atrioventricular)
      426.13
    third degree (atrioventricular) 426.0
    bundle branch (complete) (false)
      (incomplete) 426.50
      bilateral 426.53
      left (*see also* Block, bundle branch,
        left) 426.3
      right (*see also* Block, bundle
        branch, right) 426.4

Block *(Continued)*
  heart *(Continued)*
    complete (atrioventricular) 426.0
    congenital 746.86
    incomplete 426.13
    intra-atrial 426.6
    intraventricular NEC 426.6
    sinoatrial 426.6
    specified type NEC 426.6
  hepatic vein 453.0
  intraventricular (diffuse) (myofibrillar) 426.6
    bundle branch (complete) (false) (incomplete) 426.50
      bilateral 426.53
      left *(see also* Block, bundle branch, left) 426.3
      right *(see also* Block, bundle branch, right) 426.4
  kidney *(see also* Disease, renal) 593.9
    postcystoscopic 997.5
  myocardial *(see also* Block, heart) 426.9
  nodal 426.10
  optic nerve 377.49
  organ or site (congenital) NEC - *see* Atresia
  parietal 426.6
  peri-infarction 426.6
  portal (vein) 452
  sinoatrial 426.6
  sinoauricular 426.6
  spinal cord 336.9
  trifascicular 426.54
  tubal 628.2
  vein NEC 453.9
Blocq's disease or syndrome (astasia-abasia) 307.9
Blood
  constituents, abnormal NEC 790.6
  disease 289.9
    specified NEC 289.89
  donor V59.01
    other blood components V59.09
    stem cells V59.02
    whole blood V59.01
  dyscrasia 289.9
    with
      abortion - *see* Abortion, by type, with hemorrhage, delayed or excessive
      ectopic pregnancy *(see also* categories 633.0–633.9) 639.1
      molar pregnancy *(see also* categories 630–632) 639.1
    following
      abortion 639.1
      ectopic or molar pregnancy 639.1
    newborn NEC 776.9
    puerperal, postpartum 666.3●
  flukes NEC *(see also* Infestation, Schistosoma) 120.9
  in
    feces *(see also* Melena) 578.1
      occult 792.1
    urine *(see also* Hematuria) 599.70
  mole 631
  occult 792.1
  poisoning *(see also* Septicemia) 038.9
  pressure
    decreased, due to shock following injury 958.4
    fluctuating 796.4

Blood *(Continued)*
  pressure *(Continued)*
    high *(see also* Hypertension) 401.9
      incidental reading (isolated) (nonspecific), without diagnosis of hypertension 796.2
    low *(see also* Hypotension) 458.9
      incidental reading (isolated) (nonspecific), without diagnosis of hypotension 796.3
  spitting *(see also* Hemoptysis) 786.30 ◀▥
  staining cornea 371.12
  transfusion
    without reported diagnosis V58.2
    donor V59.01
      stem cells V59.02
    reaction or complication - *see* Complications, transfusion
  tumor - *see* Hematoma
  vessel rupture - *see* Hemorrhage
  vomiting *(see also* Hematemesis) 578.0
Blood-forming organ disease 289.9
Bloodgood's disease 610.1
Bloodshot eye 379.93
Bloom (-Machacek) (-Torre) syndrome 757.39
Blotch, palpebral 372.55
Blount's disease (tibia vara) 732.4
Blount-Barber syndrome (tibia vara) 732.4
Blue
  baby 746.9
  bloater 491.20
    with
      acute bronchitis 491.22
      exacerbation (acute) 491.21
  diaper syndrome 270.0
  disease 746.9
  dome cyst 610.0
  drum syndrome 381.02
  sclera 743.47
    with fragility of bone and deafness 756.51
  toe syndrome 445.02
Blueness *(see also* Cyanosis) 782.5
Blurring, visual 368.8
Blushing (abnormal) (excessive) 782.62
BMI (body mass index)
  adult
    25.0–25.9 V85.21
    26.0–26.9 V85.22
    27.0–27.9 V85.23
    28.0–28.9 V85.24
    29.0–29.9 V85.25
    30.0–30.9 V85.30
    31.0–31.9 V85.31
    32.0–32.9 V85.32
    33.0–33.9 V85.33
    34.0–34.9 V85.34
    35.0–35.9 V85.35
    36.0–36.9 V85.36
    37.0–37.9 V85.37
    38.0–38.9 V85.38
    39.0–39.9 V85.39
    40.0–44.9 ~~and over~~ V85.41 ◀▥
    45.0-49.9 V85.42 ◀
    50.0-59.9 V85.43 ◀
    60.0-69.9 V85.44 ◀
    70 and over V85.45 ◀
    between 19–24 V85.1
    less than 19 V85.0

BMI *(Continued)*
  pediatric
    5th percentile to less than 85th percentile for age V85.52
    85th percentile to less than 95th percentile for age V85.53
    greater than or equal to 95th percentile for age V85.54
    less than 5th percentile for age V85.51
Boarder, hospital V65.0
  infant V65.0
Bockhart's impetigo (superficial folliculitis) 704.8
Bodechtel-Guttmann disease (subacute sclerosing panencephalitis) 046.2
Boder-Sedgwick syndrome (ataxia-telangiectasia) 334.8
Body, bodies
  Aschoff *(see also* Myocarditis, rheumatic) 398.0
  asteroid, vitreous 379.22
  choroid, colloid (degenerative) 362.57
    hereditary 362.77
  cytoid (retina) 362.82
  drusen (retina) *(see also* Drusen) 362.57
    optic disc 377.21
  fibrin, pleura 511.0
  foreign - *see* Foreign body
  Hassall-Henle 371.41
  loose
    joint *(see also* Loose, body, joint) 718.1●
      knee 717.6
    knee 717.6
    sheath, tendon 727.82
  Mallory's 034.1
  mass index (BMI)
    adult
      25.0–25.9 V85.21
      26.0–26.9 V85.22
      27.0–27.9 V85.23
      28.0–28.9 V85.24
      29.0–29.9 V85.25
      30.0–30.9 V85.30
      31.0–31.9 V85.31
      32.0–32.9 V85.32
      33.0–33.9 V85.33
      34.0–34.9 V85.34
      35.0–35.9 V85.35
      36.0–36.9 V85.36
      37.0–37.9 V85.37
      38.0–38.9 V85.38
      39.0–39.9 V85.39
      40.0-44.9 ~~and over~~ V85.41 ◀▥
      45.0-49.9 V85.42 ◀
      50.0-59.9 V85.43 ◀
      60.0-69.9 V85.44 ◀
      70 and over V85.45 ◀
      between 19–24 V85.1
      less than 19 V85.0
    pediatric
      5th percentile to less than 85th percentile for age V85.52
      85th percentile to less than 95th percentile for age V85.53
      greater than or equal to 95th percentile for age V85.54
      less than 5th percentile for age V85.51
  Mooser 081.0
  Negri 071
  rice (joint) *(see also* Loose, body, joint) 718.1●
    knee 717.6
  rocking 307.3

◀ New   ◀▥ Revised   ~~deleted~~ Deleted   ● Use Additional Digit(s)   ▦ Omit code

Boeck's
   disease (sarcoidosis) 135
   lupoid (miliary) 135
   sarcoid 135
Boerhaave's syndrome (spontaneous
      esophageal rupture) 530.4
Boggy
   cervix 622.8
   uterus 621.8
Boil (see also Carbuncle) 680.9
   abdominal wall 680.2
   Aleppo 085.1
   ankle 680.6
   anus 680.5
   arm (any part, above wrist) 680.3
   auditory canal, external 680.0
   axilla 680.3
   back (any part) 680.2
   Baghdad 085.1
   breast 680.2
   buttock 680.5
   chest wall 680.2
   corpus cavernosum 607.2
   Delhi 085.1
   ear (any part) 680.0
   eyelid 373.13
   face (any part, except eye) 680.0
   finger (any) 680.4
   flank 680.2
   foot (any part) 680.7
   forearm 680.3
   Gafsa 085.1
   genital organ, male 608.4
   gluteal (region) 680.5
   groin 680.2
   hand (any part) 680.4
   head (any part, except face) 680.8
   heel 680.7
   hip 680.6
   knee 680.6
   labia 616.4
   lacrimal (see also Dacryocystitis) 375.30
      gland (see also Dacryoadenitis) 375.00
      passages (duct) (sac) (see also
         Dacryocystitis) 375.30
   leg, any part, except foot 680.6
   multiple sites 680.9
   natal 085.1
   neck 680.1
   nose (external) (septum) 680.0
   orbit, orbital 376.01
   partes posteriores 680.5
   pectoral region 680.2
   penis 607.2
   perineum 680.2
   pinna 680.0
   scalp (any part) 680.8
   scrotum 608.4
   seminal vesicle 608.0
   shoulder 680.3
   skin NEC 680.9
   specified site NEC 680.8
   spermatic cord 608.4
   temple (region) 680.0
   testis 608.4
   thigh 680.6
   thumb 680.4
   toe (any) 680.7
   tropical 085.1
   trunk 680.2
   tunica vaginalis 608.4
   umbilicus 680.2
   upper arm 680.3
   vas deferens 608.4

Boil (Continued)
   vulva 616.4
   wrist 680.4
Bold hives (see also Urticaria) 708.9
Bolivian hemorrhagic fever 078.7
Bombé, iris 364.74
Bomford-Rhoads anemia (refractory)
      238.72
Bone - see condition
Bonnevie-Ullrich syndrome 758.6
Bonnier's syndrome 386.19
Bonvale Dam fever 780.79
Bony block of joint 718.80
   ankle 718.87
   elbow 718.82
   foot 718.87
   hand 718.84
   hip 718.85
   knee 718.86
   multiple sites 718.89
   pelvic region 718.85
   shoulder (region) 718.81
   specified site NEC 718.88
   wrist 718.83
BOOP (bronchiolitis obliterans organized
      pneumonia) 516.8
Borderline
   intellectual functioning V62.89
   osteopenia 733.90
   pelvis 653.1●
      with obstruction during labor 660.1●
         affecting fetus or newborn 763.1
   psychosis (see also Schizophrenia)
      295.5●
      of childhood (see also Psychosis,
         childhood) 299.8●
   schizophrenia (see also Schizophrenia)
      295.5●
Borna disease 062.9
Bornholm disease (epidemic
      pleurodynia) 074.1
Borrelia vincentii (mouth) (pharynx)
      (tonsils) 101
Bostock's catarrh (see also Fever, hay) 477.9
Boston exanthem 048
Botalli, ductus (patent) (persistent) 747.0
Bothriocephalus latus infestation 123.4
Botulism 005.1
   food poisoning 005.1
   infant 040.41
   non-foodborne 040.42
   wound 040.42
Bouba (see also Yaws) 102.9
Bouffée délirante 298.3
Bouillaud's disease or syndrome
      (rheumatic heart disease) 391.9
Bourneville's disease (tuberous sclerosis)
      759.5
Boutonneuse fever 082.1
Boutonniere
   deformity (finger) 736.21
   hand (intrinsic) 736.21
Bouveret (-Hoffmann) disease or
      syndrome (paroxysmal tachycardia)
      427.2
Bovine heart - see Hypertrophy, cardiac
Bowel - see condition
Bowen's
   dermatosis (precancerous) (M8081/2) -
      see Neoplasm, skin, in situ
   disease (M8081/2) - see Neoplasm,
      skin, in situ
   epithelioma (M8081/2) - see Neoplasm,
      skin, in situ

Bowen's (Continued)
   type
      epidermoid carcinoma in situ
         (M8081/2) - see Neoplasm,
         skin, in situ
      intraepidermal squamous cell
         carcinoma (M8081/2) - see
         Neoplasm, skin, in situ
Bowing
   femur 736.89
      congenital 754.42
   fibula 736.89
      congenital 754.43
   forearm 736.09
      away from midline (cubitus valgus)
         736.01
      toward midline (cubitus varus) 736.02
   leg(s), long bones, congenital 754.44
   radius 736.09
      away from midline (cubitus valgus)
         736.01
      toward midline (cubitus varus) 736.02
   tibia 736.89
      congenital 754.43
Bowleg(s) 736.42
   congenital 754.44
   rachitic 268.1
Boyd's dysentery 004.2
Brachial - see condition
Brachman-de Lange syndrome
      (Amsterdam dwarf, mental
      retardation, and brachycephaly)
      759.89
Brachycardia 427.89
Brachycephaly 756.0
Brachymorphism and ectopia lentis 759.89
Bradley's disease (epidemic vomiting)
      078.82
Bradycardia 427.89
   chronic (sinus) 427.81
   newborn 779.81
   nodal 427.89
   postoperative 997.1
   reflex 337.09
   sinoatrial 427.89
      with paroxysmal tachyarrhythmia
         or tachycardia 427.81
      chronic 427.81
   sinus 427.89
      with paroxysmal tachyarrhythmia
         or tachycardia 427.81
      chronic 427.81
      persistent 427.81
      severe 427.81
   tachycardia syndrome 427.81
   vagal 427.89
Bradykinesia 781.0
Bradypnea 786.09
Brailsford's disease 732.3
   radial head 732.3
   tarsal scaphoid 732.5
Brailsford-Morquio disease or syndrome
      (mucopolysaccharidosis IV) 277.5
Brain - see also condition
   death 348.89
   syndrome (acute) (chronic)
      (nonpsychotic) (organic) (with
      neurotic reaction) (with
      behavioral reaction) (see also
      Syndrome, brain) 310.9
      with
         presenile brain disease 290.10
         psychosis, psychotic reaction (see
            also Psychosis, organic) 294.9

Brain *(Continued)*
  syndrome *(Continued)*
    congenital (*see also* Retardation,
      mental) 319
Branched-chain amino-acid disease 270.3
Branchial - *see* condition
Brandt's syndrome (acrodermatitis
  enteropathica) 686.8
Brash (water) 787.1
Brass-founders' ague 985.8
Bravais-Jacksonian epilepsy (*see also*
  Epilepsy) 345.5●
Braxton Hicks contractions 644.1●
Braziers' disease 985.8
Brazilian
  blastomycosis 116.1
  leishmaniasis 085.5
BRBPR (bright red blood per rectum)
  569.3
Break
  cardiorenal - *see* Hypertension,
    cardiorenal
  retina (*see also* Defect, retina) 361.30
Breakbone fever 061
Breakdown
  device, implant, or graft - *see*
    Complications, mechanical
  nervous (*see also* Disorder, mental,
    nonpsychotic) 300.9
  perineum 674.2●
Breast - *see also* condition
  buds 259.1
    in newborn 779.89
  dense 793.82
  nodule 793.89
Breast feeding difficulties 676.8●
Breath
  foul 784.99
  holder, child 312.81
  holding spells 786.9
  shortness 786.05
Breathing
  asymmetrical 786.09
  bronchial 786.09
  exercises V57.0
  labored 786.09
  mouth 784.99
    causing malocclusion 524.59
  periodic 786.09
    high altitude 327.22
  tic 307.20
Breathlessness 786.09
Breda's disease (*see also* Yaws) 102.9
Breech
  delivery, affecting fetus or newborn
    763.0
  extraction, affecting fetus or newborn
    763.0
  presentation (buttocks) (complete)
    (frank) 652.2●
    with successful version 652.1●
    before labor, affecting fetus or
      newborn 761.7
    during labor, affecting fetus or
      newborn 763.0
Breisky's disease (kraurosis vulvae) 624.09
Brennemann's syndrome (acute
  mesenteric lymphadenitis) 289.2
Brenner's
  tumor (benign) (M9000/0) 220
    borderline malignancy (M9000/1)
      236.2
    malignant (M9000/3) 183.0
    proliferating (M9000/1) 236.2

Bretonneau's disease (diphtheritic
  malignant angina) 032.0
Breus' mole 631
Brevicollis 756.16
Bricklayers' itch 692.89
Brickmakers' anemia 126.9
Bridge
  myocardial 746.85
Bright red blood per rectum (BRBPR) 569.3
Bright's
  blindness - *see* Uremia
  disease (*see also* Nephritis) 583.9
    arteriosclerotic (*see also*
      Hypertension, kidney) 403.90
Brill's disease (recrudescent typhus) 081.1
  flea-borne 081.0
  louse-borne 081.1
Brill-Symmers disease (follicular
  lymphoma) (M9690/3) 202.0●
Brill-Zinsser disease (recrudescent
  typhus) 081.1
Brinton's disease (linitis plastica)
  (M8142/3) 151.9
Brion-Kayser disease (*see also* Fever,
  paratyphoid) 002.9
Briquet's disorder or syndrome 300.81
Brissaud's
  infantilism (infantile myxedema) 244.9
  motor-verbal tic 307.23
Brissaud-Meige syndrome (infantile
  myxedema) 244.9
Brittle
  bones (congenital) 756.51
  nails 703.8
    congenital 757.5
Broad - *see also* condition
  beta disease 272.2
  ligament laceration syndrome 620.6
Brock's syndrome (atelectasis due to
  enlarged lymph nodes) 518.0
Brocq's disease 691.8
  atopic (diffuse) neurodermatitis 691.8
  lichen simplex chronicus 698.3
  parakeratosis psoriasiformis 696.2
  parapsoriasis 696.2
Brocq-Duhring disease (dermatitis
  herpetiformis) 694.0
Brodie's
  abscess (localized) (chronic) (*see also*
    Osteomyelitis) 730.1●
  disease (joint) (*see also* Osteomyelitis)
    730.1●
Broken
  arches 734
    congenital 755.67
  back - *see* Fracture, vertebra, by site
  bone - *see* Fracture, by site
  compensation - *see* Disease, heart
  heart syndrome 429.83
  implant or internal device - *see* listing
    under Complications, mechanical
  neck - *see* Fracture, vertebra, cervical
  nose 802.0
    open 802.1
  tooth, teeth 873.63
    complicated 873.73
Bromhidrosis 705.89
Bromidism, bromism
  acute 967.3
    correct substance properly
      administered 349.82
    overdose or wrong substance given
      or taken 967.3
  chronic (*see also* Dependence) 304.1●

Bromidrosiphobia 300.23
Bromidrosis 705.89
Bronchi, bronchial - *see* condition
Bronchiectasis (cylindrical) (diffuse)
  (fusiform) (localized) (moniliform)
  (postinfectious) (recurrent)
  (saccular) 494.0
  with acute exacerbation 494.1
  congenital 748.61
  tuberculosis (*see also* Tuberculosis)
    011.5●
Bronchiolectasis - *see* Bronchiectasis
Bronchiolitis (acute) (infectious)
  (subacute) 466.19
  with
    bronchospasm or obstruction 466.19
    influenza, flu, or grippe (*see also*
      Influenza) 487.1 ◄▥
  catarrhal (acute) (subacute) 466.19
  chemical 506.0
    chronic 506.4
  chronic (obliterative) 491.8
  due to external agent - *see* Bronchitis,
    acute, due to
  fibrosa obliterans 491.8
  influenzal (*see also* Influenza) 487.1 ◄▥
  obliterans 491.8
    with organizing pneumonia (BOOP)
      516.8
    status post lung transplant 996.84
  obliterative (chronic) (diffuse)
    (subacute) 491.8
    due to fumes or vapors 506.4
  respiratory syncytial virus 466.11
  vesicular - *see* Pneumonia, broncho-
Bronchitis (diffuse) (hypostatic) (infectious)
  (inflammatory) (simple) 490
  with
    emphysema - *see* Emphysema
    influenza, flu, or grippe (*see also*
      Influenza) 487.1 ◄▥
    obstruction airway, chronic 491.20
      with
        acute bronchitis 491.22
        exacerbation (acute) 491.21
    tracheitis 490
      acute or subacute 466.0
        with bronchospasm or
          obstruction 466.0
      chronic 491.8
  acute or subacute 466.0
    with
      bronchiectasis 494.1
      bronchospasm 466.0
      obstruction 466.0
      tracheitis 466.0
    chemical (due to fumes or vapors)
      506.0
    due to
      fumes or vapors 506.0
      radiation 508.8
  allergic (acute) (*see also* Asthma) 493.9●
  arachidic 934.1
  aspiration 507.0
    due to fumes or vapors 506.0
  asthmatic (acute) 493.90
    with
      acute exacerbation 493.92
      status asthmaticus 493.91
    chronic 493.2●
  capillary 466.19
    with bronchospasm or obstruction
      466.19
    chronic 491.8

◄ New   ◄▥ Revised   ~~deleted~~ Deleted   ● Use Additional Digit(s)   ▨ Omit code

Bronchitis (*Continued*)
caseous (*see also* Tuberculosis) 011.3●
Castellani's 104.8
catarrhal 490
  acute - *see* Bronchitis, acute
  chronic 491.0
chemical (acute) (subacute) 506.0
  chronic 506.4
  due to fumes or vapors (acute)
     (subacute) 506.0
    chronic 506.4
chronic 491.9
  with
    tracheitis (chronic) 491.8
  asthmatic 493.2●
  catarrhal 491.0
  chemical (due to fumes and vapors)
    506.4
  due to
    fumes or vapors (chemical)
      (inhalation) 506.4
    radiation 508.8
    tobacco smoking 491.0
  mucopurulent 491.1
  obstructive 491.20
    with
      acute bronchitis 491.22
      exacerbation (acute) 491.21
  purulent 491.1
  simple 491.0
  specified type NEC 491.8
croupous 466.0
  with bronchospasm or obstruction
    466.0
  due to fumes or vapors 506.0
emphysematous 491.20
  with
    acute bronchitis 491.22
    exacerbation (acute) 491.21
exudative 466.0
fetid (chronic) (recurrent) 491.1
fibrinous, acute or subacute 466.0
  with bronchospasm or obstruction
    466.0
grippal (*see also* Influenza) 487.1 ◀▥
influenzal (*see also* Influenza) 487.1 ◀▥
membranous, acute or subacute 466.0
  with bronchospasm or obstruction
    466.0
moulders' 502
mucopurulent (chronic) (recurrent)
  491.1
  acute or subacute 466.0
obliterans 491.8
obstructive (chronic) 491.20
  with
    acute bronchitis 491.22
    exacerbation (acute) 491.21
pituitous 491.1
plastic (inflammatory) 466.0
pneumococcal, acute or subacute 466.0
  with bronchospasm or obstruction
    466.0
pseudomembranous 466.0
purulent (chronic) (recurrent) 491.1
  acute or subacute 466.0
    with bronchospasm or
      obstruction 466.0
putrid 491.1
scrofulous (*see also* Tuberculosis) 011.3●
senile 491.9
septic, acute or subacute 466.0
  with bronchospasm or obstruction
    466.0

Bronchitis (*Continued*)
smokers' 491.0
spirochetal 104.8
suffocative, acute or subacute 466.0
summer (*see also* Asthma) 493.9●
suppurative (chronic) 491.1
  acute or subacute 466.0
tuberculous (*see also* Tuberculosis)
  011.3●
ulcerative 491.8
  Vincent's 101
Vincent's 101
viral, acute or subacute 466.0
Bronchoalveolitis 485
Bronchoaspergillosis 117.3
Bronchocele
meaning
  dilatation of bronchus 519.19
  goiter 240.9
Bronchogenic carcinoma 162.9
Bronchohemisporosis 117.9
Broncholithiasis 518.89
tuberculous (*see also* Tuberculosis)
  011.3●
Bronchomalacia 748.3
Bronchomoniliasis 112.89
Bronchomycosis 112.89
Bronchonocardiosis 039.1
Bronchopleuropneumonia - *see*
  Pneumonia, broncho-
Bronchopneumonia - *see* Pneumonia,
  broncho-
Bronchopneumonitis - *see* Pneumonia,
  broncho-
Bronchopulmonary - *see* condition
Bronchopulmonitis - *see* Pneumonia,
  broncho-
Bronchorrhagia 786.30 ◀▥
newborn 770.3
tuberculous (*see also* Tuberculosis)
  011.3●
Bronchorrhea (chronic) (purulent)
  491.0
acute 466.0
Bronchospasm 519.11
with
  asthma - *see* Asthma
  bronchiolitis, acute 466.19
    due to respiratory syncytial
      virus 466.11
  bronchitis - *see* Bronchitis
  chronic obstructive pulmonary
    disease (COPD) 496
  emphysema - *see* Emphysema
  due to external agent - *see*
      Condition, respiratory,
      acute, due to
  acute 519.11
  exercise induced 493.81
Bronchospirochetosis 104.8
Bronchostenosis 519.19
Bronchus - *see* condition
Bronze, bronzed
diabetes 275.01 ◀▥
disease (Addison's) (skin) 255.41
  tuberculous (*see also* Tuberculosis)
    017.6●
Brooke's disease or tumor (M8100/0) -
  see Neoplasm, skin, benign
Brown's tendon sheath syndrome
  378.61
Brown enamel of teeth (hereditary)
  520.5

Brown-Séquard's paralysis (syndrome)
  344.89
Brow presentation complicating delivery
  652.4●
Brucella, brucellosis (infection) 023.9
abortus 023.1
canis 023.3
dermatitis, skin 023.9
melitensis 023.0
mixed 023.8
suis 023.2
Bruck's disease 733.99
Bruck-de Lange disease or syndrome
  (Amsterdam dwarf, mental
  retardation, and brachycephaly)
  759.89
Brugada syndrome 746.89
Brug's filariasis 125.1
Brugsch's syndrome (acropachyderma)
  757.39
Bruhl's disease (splenic anemia with
  fever) 285.8
Bruise (skin surface intact) - *see also*
  Contusion
with
  fracture - *see* Fracture, by site
  open wound - *see* Wound, open, by
    site
  internal organ (abdomen, chest, or
    pelvis) - *see* Injury, internal, by
    site
  umbilical cord 663.6●
    affecting fetus or newborn 762.6
Bruit 785.9
arterial (abdominal) (carotid) 785.9
supraclavicular 785.9
Brushburn - *see* Injury, superficial, by
  site
Bruton's X-linked agammaglobulinemia
  279.04
Bruxism 306.8
sleep related 327.53
Bubbly lung syndrome 770.7
Bubo 289.3
blennorrhagic 098.89
chancroidal 099.0
climatic 099.1
due to Hemophilus ducreyi 099.0
gonococcal 098.89
indolent NEC 099.8
inguinal NEC 099.8
  chancroidal 099.0
  climatic 099.1
  due to H. ducreyi 099.0
scrofulous (*see also* Tuberculosis)
  017.2●
soft chancre 099.0
suppurating 683
syphilitic 091.0
  congenital 090.0
tropical 099.1
venereal NEC 099.8
virulent 099.0
Bubonic plague 020.0
Bubonocele - *see* Hernia, inguinal
Buccal - *see* condition
Buchanan's disease (juvenile
  osteochondrosis of iliac crest)
  732.1
Buchem's syndrome (hyperostosis
  corticalis) 733.3
Buchman's disease (osteochondrosis,
  juvenile) 732.1

Bucket handle fracture (semilunar cartilage) (*see also* Tear, meniscus) 836.2

Budd-Chiari syndrome (hepatic vein thrombosis) 453.0

Budgerigar-fanciers' disease or lung 495.2

Büdinger-Ludloff-Läwen disease 717.89

Buds
breast 259.1
in newborn 779.89

Buerger's disease (thromboangiitis obliterans) 443.1

Bulbar - *see* condition

Bulbus cordis 745.9
persistent (in left ventricle) 745.8

Bulging fontanels (congenital) 756.0

Bulimia 783.6
nervosa 307.51
nonorganic origin 307.51

Bulky uterus 621.2

Bulla(e) 709.8
lung (emphysematous) (solitary) 492.0

Bullet wound - *see also* Wound, open, by site
fracture - *see* Fracture, by site, open
internal organ (abdomen, chest, or pelvis) - *see* Injury, internal, by site, with open wound
intracranial - *see* Laceration, brain, with open wound

Bullis fever 082.8

Bullying (*see also* Disturbance, conduct) 312.0●

Bundle
branch block (complete) (false) (incomplete) 426.50
bilateral 426.53
left (*see also* Block, bundle branch, left) 426.3
hemiblock 426.2
right (*see also* Block, bundle branch, right) 426.4
of His - *see* condition
of Kent syndrome (anomalous atrioventricular excitation) 426.7

Bungpagga 040.81

Bunion 727.1

Bunionette 727.1

Bunyamwera fever 066.3

Buphthalmia, buphthalmos (congenital) 743.20
associated with
keratoglobus, congenital 743.22
megalocornea 743.22
ocular anomalies NEC 743.22
isolated 743.21
simple 743.21

Bürger-Grütz disease or syndrome (essential familial hyperlipemia) 272.3

Buried roots 525.3

Burke's syndrome 577.8

Burkitt's
tumor (M9750/3) 200.2●
type malignant, lymphoma, lymphoblastic, or undifferentiated (M9750/3) 200.2●

Burn (acid) (cathode ray) (caustic) (chemical) (electric heating appliance) (electricity) (fire) (flame) (hot liquid or object) (irradiation) (lime) (radiation) (steam) (thermal) (x-ray) 949.0

Note: Use the following fifth-digit subclassification with category 948 to indicate the percent of body surface with third degree burn:

0   less than 10 percent or unspecified
1   10–19 percent
2   20–29 percent
3   30–39 percent
4   40–49 percent
5   50–59 percent
6   60–69 percent
7   70–79 percent
8   80–89 percent
9   90 percent or more of body surface

with
blisters - *see* Burn, by site, second degree
erythema - *see* Burn, by site, first degree
skin loss (epidermal) - *see also* Burn, by site, second degree
full thickness - *see also* Burn, by site, third degree
with necrosis of underlying tissues - *see* Burn, by site, third degree, deep
first degree - *see* Burn, by site, first degree
second degree - *see* Burn, by site, second degree
third degree - *see also* Burn, by site, third degree
deep - *see* Burn, by site, third degree, deep
abdomen, abdominal (muscle) (wall) 942.03
with
trunk - *see* Burn, trunk, multiple sites
first degree 942.13
second degree 942.23
third degree 942.33
deep 942.43
with loss of body part 942.53
ankle 945.03
with
lower limb(s) - *see* Burn, leg, multiple sites
first degree 945.13
second degree 945.23
third degree 945.33
deep 945.43
with loss of body part 945.53
anus - *see* Burn, trunk, specified site NEC
arm(s) 943.00
first degree 943.10
second degree 943.20
third degree 943.30
deep 943.40
with loss of body part 943.50
lower - *see* Burn, forearm(s)

Burn (*Continued*)
arm(s) (*Continued*)
multiple sites, except hand(s) or wrist(s) 943.09
first degree 943.19
second degree 943.29
third degree 943.39
deep 943.49
with loss of body part 943.59
upper 943.03
first degree 943.13
second degree 943.23
third degree 943.33
deep 943.43
with loss of body part 943.53
auditory canal (external) - *see* Burn, ear
auricle (ear) - *see* Burn, ear
axilla 943.04
with
upper limb(s), except hand(s) or wrist(s) - *see* Burn, arm(s), multiple sites
first degree 943.14
second degree 943.24
third degree 943.34
deep 943.44
with loss of body part 943.54
back 942.04
with
trunk - *see* Burn, trunk, multiple sites
first degree 942.14
second degree 942.24
third degree 942.34
deep 942.44
with loss of body part 942.54
biceps
brachii - *see* Burn, arm(s), upper
femoris - *see* Burn, thigh
breast(s) 942.01
with
trunk - *see* Burn, trunk, multiple sites
first degree 942.11
second degree 942.21
third degree 942.31
deep 942.41
with loss of body part 942.51
brow - *see* Burn, forehead
buttock(s) - *see* Burn, back
canthus (eye) 940.1
chemical 940.0
cervix (uteri) 947.4
cheek (cutaneous) 941.07
with
face or head - *see* Burn, head, multiple sites
first degree 941.17
second degree 941.27
third degree 941.37
deep 941.47
with loss of body part 941.57
chest wall (anterior) 942.02
with
trunk - *see* Burn, trunk, multiple sites
first degree 942.12
second degree 942.22
third degree 942.32
deep 942.42
with loss of body part 942.52

◄ New   ◄▮▮ Revised   ~~deleted~~ Deleted   ● Use Additional Digit(s)   ▓▓ Omit code

Burn (Continued)
  chin 941.04
    with
      face or head - see Burn, head,
        multiple sites
      first degree 941.14
      second degree 941.24
      third degree 941.34
        deep 941.44
          with loss of body part 941.54
  clitoris - see Burn, genitourinary
    organs, external
  colon 947.3
  conjunctiva (and cornea) 940.4
    chemical
      acid 940.3
      alkaline 940.2
  cornea (and conjunctiva) 940.4
    chemical
      acid 940.3
      alkaline 940.2
  costal region - see Burn, chest wall
  due to ingested chemical agent - see
    Burn, internal organs
  ear (auricle) (canal) (drum) (external)
    941.01
    with
      face or head - see Burn, head,
        multiple sites
      first degree 941.11
      second degree 941.21
      third degree 941.31
        deep 941.41
          with loss of a body part 941.51
  elbow 943.02
    with
      hand(s) and wrist(s) - see Burn,
        multiple specified sites
      upper limb(s), except hand(s) or
        wrist(s) - see also Burn,
        arm(s), multiple sites
      first degree 943.12
      second degree 943.22
      third degree 943.32
        deep 943.42
          with loss of body part 943.52
  electricity, electric current - see Burn, by
    site
  entire body - see Burn, multiple,
    specified sites
  epididymis - see Burn, genitourinary
    organs, external
  epigastric region - see Burn, abdomen
  epiglottis 947.1
  esophagus 947.2
  extent (percent of body surface)
    less than 10 percent 948.0●
    10–19 percent 948.1●
    20–29 percent 948.2●
    30–39 percent 948.3●
    40–49 percent 948.4●
    50–59 percent 948.5●
    60–69 percent 948.6●
    70–79 percent 948.7●
    80–89 percent 948.8●
    90 percent or more 948.9●
  extremity
    lower - see Burn, leg
    upper - see Burn, arm(s)
  eye(s) (and adnexa) (only) 940.9
    with
      face, head, or neck 941.02
        first degree 941.12
        second degree 941.22

Burn (Continued)
  eye(s) (Continued)
    with (Continued)
      face, head, or neck (Continued)
        third degree 941.32
          deep 941.42
            with loss of body part
              941.52
      other sites (classifiable to more
        than one category in 940–
        945) - see Burn, multiple,
        specified sites
      resulting rupture and destruction
        of eyeball 940.5
      specified part - see Burn, by site
  eyeball - see also Burn, eye
    with resulting rupture and
      destruction of eyeball 940.5
  eyelid(s) 940.1
    chemical 940.0
  face - see Burn, head
  finger (nail) (subungual) 944.01
    with
      hand(s) - see Burn, hand(s),
        multiple sites
      other sites - see Burn, multiple,
        specified sites
      thumb 944.04
        first degree 944.14
        second degree 944.24
        third degree 944.34
          deep 944.44
            with loss of body part
              944.54
      first degree 944.11
      second degree 944.21
      third degree 944.31
        deep 944.41
          with loss of body part 944.51
    multiple (digits) 944.03
      with thumb - see Burn, finger,
        with thumb
      first degree 944.13
      second degree 944.23
      third degree 944.33
        deep 944.43
          with loss of body part
            944.53
  flank - see Burn, abdomen
  foot 945.02
    with
      lower limb(s) - see Burn, leg,
        multiple sites
      first degree 945.12
      second degree 945.22
      third degree 945.32
        deep 945.42
          with loss of body part 945.52
  forearm(s) 943.01
    with
      upper limb(s), except hand(s) or
        wrist(s) - see Burn, arm(s),
        multiple sites
      first degree 943.11
      second degree 943.21
      third degree 943.31
        deep 943.41
          with loss of body part 943.51
  forehead 941.07
    with
      face or head - see Burn, head,
        multiple sites
      first degree 941.17
      second degree 941.27

Burn (Continued)
  forehead (Continued)
    third degree 941.37
      deep 941.47
        with loss of body part 941.57
  fourth degree - see Burn, by site, third
    degree, deep
  friction - see Injury, superficial, by site
  from swallowing caustic or corrosive
    substance NEC - see Burn,
    internal organs
  full thickness - see Burn, by site, third
    degree
  gastrointestinal tract 947.3
  genitourinary organs
    external 942.05
      with
        trunk - see Burn, trunk,
          multiple sites
        first degree 942.15
        second degree 942.25
        third degree 942.35
          deep 942.45
            with loss of body part
              942.55
    internal 947.8
  globe (eye) - see Burn, eyeball
  groin - see Burn, abdomen
  gum 947.0
  hand(s) (phalanges) (and wrist) 944.00
    first degree 944.10
    second degree 944.20
    third degree 944.30
      deep 944.40
        with loss of body part 944.50
    back (dorsal surface) 944.06
      first degree 944.16
      second degree 944.26
      third degree 944.36
        deep 944.46
          with loss of body part
            944.56
    multiple sites 944.08
      first degree 944.18
      second degree 944.28
      third degree 944.38
        deep 944.48
          with loss of body part
            944.58
  head (and face) 941.00
    eye(s) only 940.9
      specified part - see Burn, by site
    first degree 941.10
    second degree 941.20
    third degree 941.30
      deep 941.40
        with loss of body part 941.50
    multiple sites 941.09
      with eyes - see Burn, eyes, with
        face, head, or neck
      first degree 941.19
      second degree 941.29
      third degree 941.39
        deep 941.49
          with loss of body part
            941.59
  heel - see Burn, foot
  hip - see Burn, trunk, specified site
    NEC
  iliac region - see Burn, trunk, specified
    site NEC
  infected 958.3
  inhalation (see also Burn, internal
    organs) 947.9

Burn *(Continued)*
  internal organs 947.9
    from caustic or corrosive substance
        (swallowing) NEC 947.9
    specified NEC *(see also* Burn, by site)
        947.8
  interscapular region - *see* Burn, back
  intestine (large) (small) 947.3
  iris - *see* Burn, eyeball
  knee 945.05
    with
        lower limb(s) - *see* Burn, leg,
            multiple sites
    first degree 945.15
    second degree 945.25
    third degree 945.35
        deep 945.45
            with loss of body part 945.55
  labium (majus) (minus) - *see* Burn,
      genitourinary organs, external
  lacrimal apparatus, duct, gland, or sac
      940.1
    chemical 940.0
  larynx 947.1
  late effect - *see* Late, effects (of), burn
  leg 945.00
    first degree 945.10
    second degree 945.20
    third degree 945.30
        deep 945.40
            with loss of body part
                945.50
    lower 945.04
        with other part(s) of lower
            limb(s) - *see* Burn, leg,
            multiple sites
        first degree 945.14
        second degree 945.24
        third degree 945.34
            deep 945.44
                with loss of body part
                    945.54
    multiple sites 945.09
        first degree 945.19
        second degree 945.29
        third degree 945.39
            deep 945.49
                with loss of body part
                    945.59
    upper - *see* Burn, thigh
  lightning - *see* Burn, by site
  limb(s)
    lower (including foot or toe(s)) -
        see Burn, leg
    upper (except wrist and hand) -
        see Burn, arm(s)
  lip(s) 941.03
    with
        face or head - *see* Burn, head,
            multiple sites
    first degree 941.13
    second degree 941.23
    third degree 941.33
        deep 941.43
            with loss of body part
                941.53
  lumbar region - *see* Burn, back
  lung 947.1
  malar region - *see* Burn, cheek
  mastoid region - *see* Burn, scalp
  membrane, tympanic - *see* Burn, ear
  midthoracic region - *see* Burn, chest
      wall
  mouth 947.0

Burn *(Continued)*
  multiple *(see also* Burn, unspecified)
      949.0
    specified sites classifiable to more
        than one category in 940–945
        946.0
    first degree 946.1
    second degree 946.2
    third degree 946.3
        deep 946.4
            with loss of body part
                946.5
  muscle, abdominal - *see* Burn,
      abdomen
  nasal (septum) - *see* Burn, nose
  neck 941.08
    with
        face or head - *see* Burn, head,
            multiple sites
    first degree 941.18
    second degree 941.28
    third degree 941.38
        deep 941.48
            with loss of body part 941.58
  nose (septum) 941.05
    with
        face or head - *see* Burn, head,
            multiple sites
    first degree 941.15
    second degree 941.25
    third degree 941.35
        deep 941.45
            with loss of body part 941.55
  occipital region - *see* Burn, scalp
  orbit region 940.1
    chemical 940.0
  oronasopharynx 947.0
  palate 947.0
  palm(s) 944.05
    with
        hand(s) and wrist(s) - *see* Burn,
            hand(s), multiple sites
    first degree 944.15
    second degree 944.25
    third degree 944.35
        deep 944.45
            with loss of a body part 944.55
  parietal region - *see* Burn, scalp
  penis - *see* Burn, genitourinary organs,
      external
  perineum - *see* Burn, genitourinary
      organs, external
  periocular area 940.1
    chemical 940.0
  pharynx 947.0
  pleura 947.1
  popliteal space - *see* Burn, knee
  prepuce - *see* Burn, genitourinary
      organs, external
  pubic region - *see* Burn, genitourinary
      organs, external
  pudenda - *see* Burn, genitourinary
      organs, external
  rectum 947.3
  sac, lacrimal 940.1
    chemical 940.0
  sacral region - *see* Burn, back
  salivary (ducts) (glands) 947.0
  scalp 941.06
    with
        face or neck - *see* Burn, head,
            multiple sites
    first degree 941.16
    second degree 941.26

Burn *(Continued)*
  scalp *(Continued)*
    third degree 941.36
        deep 941.46
            with loss of body part
                941.56
  scapular region 943.06
    with
        upper limb(s), except hand(s) or
            wrist(s) - *see* Burn, arm(s),
            multiple sites
    first degree 943.16
    second degree 943.26
    third degree 943.36
        deep 943.46
            with loss of body part 943.56
  sclera - *see* Burn, eyeball
  scrotum - *see* Burn, genitourinary
      organs, external
  septum, nasal - *see* Burn, nose
  shoulder(s) 943.05
    with
        hand(s) and wrist(s) - *see* Burn,
            multiple, specified sites
        upper limb(s), except hand(s) or
            wrist(s) - *see* Burn, arm(s),
            multiple sites
    first degree 943.15
    second degree 943.25
    third degree 943.35
        deep 943.45
            with loss of body part 943.55
  skin NEC *(see also* Burn, unspecified)
      949.0
  skull - *see* Burn, head
  small intestine 947.3
  sternal region - *see* Burn, chest wall
  stomach 947.3
  subconjunctival - *see* Burn, conjunctiva
  subcutaneous - *see* Burn, by site, third
      degree
  submaxillary region - *see* Burn, head
  submental region - *see* Burn, chin
  sun - *see* Sunburn
  supraclavicular fossa - *see* Burn, neck
  supraorbital - *see* Burn, forehead
  temple - *see* Burn, scalp
  temporal region - *see* Burn, scalp
  testicle - *see* Burn, genitourinary
      organs, external
  testis - *see* Burn, genitourinary organs,
      external
  thigh 945.06
    with
        lower limb(s) - *see* Burn, leg,
            multiple sites
    first degree 945.16
    second degree 945.26
    third degree 945.36
        deep 945.46
            with loss of body part 945.56
  thorax (external) - *see* Burn, chest wall
  throat 947.0
  thumb(s) (nail) (subungual) 944.02
    with
        finger(s) - *see* Burn, finger, with
            other sites, thumb
        hand(s) and wrist(s) - *see* Burn,
            hand(s), multiple sites
    first degree 944.12
    second degree 944.22
    third degree 944.32
        deep 944.42
            with loss of body part 944.52

◀ New   ◀▥ Revised   ~~deleted~~ Deleted   ● Use Additional Digit(s)   ▨ Omit code

Burn (Continued)
toe (nail) (subungual) 945.01
with
lower limb(s) - see Burn, leg,
multiple sites
first degree 945.11
second degree 945.21
third degree 945.31
deep 945.41
with loss of body part 945.51
tongue 947.0
tonsil 947.0
trachea 947.1
trunk 942.00
first degree 942.10
second degree 942.20
third degree 942.30
deep 942.40
with loss of body part 942.50
multiple sites 942.09
first degree 942.19
second degree 942.29
third degree 942.39
deep 942.49
with loss of body part
942.59
specified site NEC 942.09
first degree 942.19
second degree 942.29
third degree 942.39
deep 942.49
with loss of body part
942.59
tunica vaginalis - see Burn,
genitourinary organs, external
tympanic membrane - see Burn, ear
tympanum - see Burn, ear
ultraviolet 692.82
unspecified site (multiple) 949.0
with extent of body surface involved
specified
less than 10 percent 948.0 ●
10–19 percent 948.1 ●
20–29 percent 948.2 ●
30–39 percent 948.3 ●
40–49 percent 948.4 ●
50–59 percent 948.5 ●
60–69 percent 948.6 ●
70–79 percent 948.7 ●
80–89 percent 948.8 ●
90 percent or more 948.9 ●

Burn (Continued)
unspecified site (Continued)
first degree 949.1
second degree 949.2
third degree 949.3
deep 949.4
with loss of body part 949.5
uterus 947.4
uvula 947.0
vagina 947.4
vulva - see Burn, genitourinary organs,
external
wrist(s) 944.07
with
hand(s) - see Burn, hand(s),
multiple sites
first degree 944.17
second degree 944.27
third degree 944.37
deep 944.47
with loss of body part
944.57
Burnett's syndrome (milk-alkali)
275.42
Burnier's syndrome (hypophyseal
dwarfism) 253.3
Burning
feet syndrome 266.2
sensation (see also Disturbance,
sensation) 782.0
tongue 529.6
Burns' disease (osteochondrosis, lower
ulna) 732.3
Bursa - see also condition
pharynx 478.29
Bursitis NEC 727.3
Achilles tendon 726.71
adhesive 726.90
shoulder 726.0
ankle 726.79
buttock 726.5
calcaneal 726.79
collateral ligament
fibular 726.63
tibial 726.62
Duplay's 726.2
elbow 726.33
finger 726.8
foot 726.79
gonococcal 098.52
hand 726.4

Bursitis NEC (Continued)
hip 726.5
infrapatellar 726.69
ischiogluteal 726.5
knee 726.60
occupational NEC 727.2
olecranon 726.33
pes anserinus 726.61
pharyngeal 478.29
popliteal 727.51
prepatellar 726.65
radiohumeral 727.3
scapulohumeral 726.19
adhesive 726.0
shoulder 726.10
adhesive 726.0
subacromial 726.19
adhesive 726.0
subcoracoid 726.19
subdeltoid 726.19
adhesive 726.0
subpatellar 726.69
syphilitic 095.7
Thornwaldt's, Tornwaldt's
(pharyngeal) 478.29
toe 726.79
trochanteric area 726.5
wrist 726.4
Burst stitches or sutures (complication of
surgery) (external) (see also
Dehiscence) 998.32
internal 998.31
Buruli ulcer 031.1
Bury's disease (erythema elevatum
diutinum) 695.89
Buschke's disease or scleredema
(adultorum) 710.1
Busquet's disease (osteoperiostitis) (see
also Osteomyelitis) 730.1 ●
Busse-Buschke disease (cryptococcosis)
117.5
Buttock - see condition
Button
Biskra 085.1
Delhi 085.1
oriental 085.1
Buttonhole hand (intrinsic) 736.21
Bwamba fever (encephalitis) 066.3
Byssinosis (occupational) 504
Bywaters' syndrome 958.5

C

Cacergasia 300.9
Cachexia 799.4
   cancerous - *see also* Neoplasm, by site,
     malignant 799.4
   cardiac - *see* Disease, heart
   dehydration 276.51
     with
       hypernatremia 276.0
       hyponatremia 276.1
   due to malnutrition 799.4
   exophthalmic 242.0●
   heart - *see* Disease, heart
   hypophyseal 253.2
   hypopituitary 253.2
   lead 984.9
     specified type of lead - *see* Table of
      Drugs and Chemicals
   malaria 084.9
   malignant *see also* Neoplasm, by site,
     malignant 799.4
   marsh 084.9
   nervous 300.5
   old age 797
   pachydermic - *see* Hypothyroidism
   paludal 084.9
   pituitary (postpartum) 253.2
   renal (*see also* Disease, renal) 593.9
   saturnine 984.9
     specified type of lead - *see* Table of
      Drugs and Chemicals
   senile 797
   Simmonds' (pituitary cachexia) 253.2
   splenica 289.59
   strumipriva (*see also* Hypothyroidism)
     244.9
   tuberculous NEC (*see also* Tuberculosis)
     011.9●
Café au lait spots 709.09
Caffey's disease or syndrome (infantile
   cortical hyperostosis) 756.59
Caisson disease 993.3
Caked breast (puerperal, postpartum)
   676.2●
Cake kidney 753.3
Calabar swelling 125.2
Calcaneal spur 726.73
Calcaneoapophysitis 732.5
Calcaneonavicular bar 755.67
Calcareous - *see* condition
Calcicosis (occupational) 502
Calciferol (vitamin D) deficiency 268.9
   with
     osteomalacia 268.2
     rickets (*see also* Rickets) 268.0
Calcification
   adrenal (capsule) (gland) 255.41
     tuberculous (*see also* Tuberculosis)
      017.6●
   aorta 440.0
   artery (annular) - *see* Arteriosclerosis
   auricle (ear) 380.89
   bladder 596.8
     due to S. hematobium 120.0
   brain (cortex) - *see* Calcification,
     cerebral
   bronchus 519.19
   bursa 727.82
   cardiac (*see also* Degeneration,
     myocardial) 429.1
   cartilage (postinfectional) 733.99
   cerebral (cortex) 348.89
     artery 437.0

Calcification (*Continued*)
   cervix (uteri) 622.8
   choroid plexus 349.2
   conjunctiva 372.54
   corpora cavernosa (penis) 607.89
   cortex (brain) - *see* Calcification,
     cerebral
   dental pulp (nodular) 522.2
   dentinal papilla 520.4
   disc, intervertebral 722.90
     cervical, cervicothoracic 722.91
     lumbar, lumbosacral 722.93
     thoracic, thoracolumbar 722.92
   fallopian tube 620.8
   falx cerebri - *see* Calcification, cerebral
   fascia 728.89
   gallbladder 575.8
   general 275.40
   heart (*see also* Degeneration,
     myocardial) 429.1
     valve - *see* Endocarditis
   intervertebral cartilage or disc
     (postinfectional) 722.90
     cervical, cervicothoracic 722.91
     lumbar, lumbosacral 722.93
     thoracic, thoracolumbar 722.92
   intracranial - *see* Calcification, cerebral
   intraspinal ligament 728.89
   joint 719.80
     ankle 719.87
     elbow 719.82
     foot 719.87
     hand 719.84
     hip 719.85
     knee 719.86
     multiple sites 719.89
     pelvic region 719.85
     shoulder (region) 719.81
     specified site NEC 719.88
     wrist 719.83
   kidney 593.89
     tuberculous (*see also* Tuberculosis)
      016.0●
   larynx (senile) 478.79
   lens 366.8
   ligament 728.89
     intraspinal 728.89
     knee (medial collateral) 717.89
   lung 518.89
     active 518.89
     postinfectional 518.89
     tuberculous (*see also* Tuberculosis,
      pulmonary) 011.9●
   lymph gland or node (postinfectional)
     289.3
     tuberculous (*see also* Tuberculosis,
      lymph gland) 017.2●
   mammographic 793.89
   massive (paraplegic) 728.10
   medial (*see also* Arteriosclerosis,
     extremities) 440.20
   meninges (cerebral) 349.2
   metastatic 275.40
   Mönckeberg's - *see* Arteriosclerosis
   muscle 728.10
     heterotopic, postoperative 728.13
   myocardium, myocardial (*see also*
     Degeneration, myocardial) 429.1
   ovary 620.8
   pancreas 577.8
   penis 607.89
   periarticular 728.89
   pericardium (*see also* Pericarditis) 423.8
   pineal gland 259.8

Calcification (*Continued*)
   pleura 511.0
     postinfectional 518.89
     tuberculous (*see also* Tuberculosis,
      pleura) 012.0●
   pulp (dental) (nodular) 522.2
   renal 593.89
   Rider's bone 733.99
   sclera 379.16
   semilunar cartilage 717.89
   spleen 289.59
   subcutaneous 709.3
   suprarenal (capsule) (gland) 255.41
   tendon (sheath) 727.82
     with bursitis, synovitis or
      tenosynovitis 727.82
   trachea 519.19
   ureter 593.89
   uterus 621.8
   vitreous 379.29
Calcified - *see also* Calcification
   hematoma NEC 959.9
Calcinosis (generalized) (interstitial)
   (tumoral) (universalis) 275.49
   circumscripta 709.3
   cutis 709.3
   intervertebralis 275.49 [722.90]
   Raynaud's phenomenon
     sclerodactylytelangiectasis
     (CRST) 710.1
Calciphylaxis (*see also* Calcification, by
   site) 275.49
Calcium
   blood
     high (*see also* Hypercalcemia) 275.42
     low (*see also* Hypocalcemia) 275.41
   deposits - *see also* Calcification, by site
     in bursa 727.82
     in tendon (sheath) 727.82
      with bursitis, synovitis or
       tenosynovitis 727.82
   salts or soaps in vitreous 379.22
Calciuria 791.9
Calculi - *see* Calculus
Calculosis, intrahepatic - *see*
   Choledocholithiasis
Calculus, calculi, calculous 592.9
   ampulla of Vater - *see*
     Choledocholithiasis
   anuria (impacted) (recurrent) 592.0
   appendix 543.9
   bile duct (any) - *see* Choledocholithiasis
   biliary - *see* Cholelithiasis
   bilirubin, multiple - *see* Cholelithiasis
   bladder (encysted) (impacted)
     (urinary) 594.1
     diverticulum 594.0
   bronchus 518.89
   calyx (kidney) (renal) 592.0
     congenital 753.3
   cholesterol (pure) (solitary) - *see*
     Cholelithiasis
   common duct (bile) - *see*
     Choledocholithiasis
   conjunctiva 372.54
   cystic 594.1
     duct - *see* Cholelithiasis
   dental 523.6
     subgingival 523.6
     supragingival 523.6
   epididymis 608.89
   gallbladder - *see also* Cholelithiasis
     congenital 751.69
   hepatic (duct) - *see* Choledocholithiasis

◀ New   ◀▥ Revised   ~~deleted~~ Deleted   ● Use Additional Digit(s)   ▦ Omit code

Calculus, calculi, calculous (*Continued*)
  intestine (impaction) (obstruction) 560.39
  kidney (impacted) (multiple) (pelvis)
      (recurrent) (staghorn) 592.0
    congenital 753.3
  lacrimal (passages) 375.57
  liver (impacted) - *see* Choledocholithiasis
  lung 518.89
  mammographic 793.89
  nephritic (impacted) (recurrent) 592.0
  nose 478.19
  pancreas (duct) 577.8
  parotid gland 527.5
  pelvis, encysted 592.0
  prostate 602.0
  pulmonary 518.89
  renal (impacted) (recurrent) 592.0
    congenital 753.3
  salivary (duct) (gland) 527.5
  seminal vesicle 608.89
  staghorn 592.0
  Stensen's duct 527.5
  sublingual duct or gland 527.5
    congenital 750.26
  submaxillary duct, gland, or region 527.5
  suburethral 594.8
  tonsil 474.8
  tooth, teeth 523.6
  tunica vaginalis 608.89
  ureter (impacted) (recurrent) 592.1
  urethra (impacted) 594.2
  urinary (duct) (impacted) (passage)
      (tract) 592.9
    lower tract NEC 594.9
      specified site 594.8
  vagina 623.8
  vesical (impacted) 594.1
  Wharton's duct 527.5
Caliectasis 593.89
California
  disease 114.0
  encephalitis 062.5
Caligo cornea 371.03
Callositas, callosity (infected) 700
Callus (infected) 700
  bone 726.91
  excessive, following fracture - *see also*
      Late, effect (of), fracture
Calvé (-Perthes) disease (osteochondrosis,
    femoral capital) 732.1
Calvities (*see also* Alopecia) 704.00
Cameroon fever (*see also* Malaria) 084.6
Camptocormia 300.11
Camptodactyly (congenital) 755.59
Camurati-Engelmann disease
    (diaphyseal sclerosis) 756.59
Canal - *see* condition
Canaliculitis (lacrimal) (acute) 375.31
  Actinomyces 039.8
  chronic 375.41
Canavan's disease 330.0
Cancer (M8000/3) - *see also* Neoplasm, by
    site, malignant

Note: The term "cancer" when modified by an adjective or adjectival phrase indicating a morphological type should be coded in the same manner as "carcinoma" with that adjective or phrase. Thus, "squamous-cell cancer" should be coded in the same manner as "squamous-cell carcinoma," which appears in the list under "Carcinoma."

Cancer (*Continued*)
  bile duct type (M8160/3), liver 155.1
  hepatocellular (M8170/3) 155.0
Cancerous (M8000/3) - *see* Neoplasm, by
    site, malignant
Cancerphobia 300.29
Cancrum oris 528.1
Candidiasis, candidal 112.9
  with pneumonia 112.4
  balanitis 112.2
  congenital 771.7
  disseminated 112.5
  endocarditis 112.81
  esophagus 112.84
  intertrigo 112.3
  intestine 112.85
  lung 112.4
  meningitis 112.83
  mouth 112.0
  nails 112.3
  neonatal 771.7
  onychia 112.3
  otitis externa 112.82
  otomycosis 112.82
  paronychia 112.3
  perionyxis 112.3
  pneumonia 112.4
  pneumonitis 112.4
  skin 112.3
  specified site NEC 112.89
  systemic 112.5
  urogenital site NEC 112.2
  vagina 112.1
  vulva 112.1
  vulvovaginitis 112.1
Candidiosis - *see* Candidiasis
Candiru infection or infestation 136.8
Canities (premature) 704.3
  congenital 757.4
Canker (mouth) (sore) 528.2
  rash 034.1
Cannabinosis 504
Canton fever 081.9
Cap
  cradle 690.11
Capillariasis 127.5
Capillary - *see* condition
Caplan's syndrome 714.81
Caplan-Colinet syndrome 714.81
Capsule - *see* condition
Capsulitis (joint) 726.90
  adhesive (shoulder) 726.0
  hip 726.5
  knee 726.60
  labyrinthine 387.8
  thyroid 245.9
  wrist 726.4
Caput
  crepitus 756.0
  medusae 456.8
  succedaneum 767.19
Carapata disease 087.1
Carate - *see* Pinta
Carbohydrate-deficient glycoprotein
    syndrome (CDGS) 271.8
Carboxyhemoglobinemia 986
Carbuncle 680.9
  abdominal wall 680.2
  ankle 680.6
  anus 680.5
  arm (any part, above wrist) 680.3
  auditory canal, external 680.0
  axilla 680.3
  back (any part) 680.2

Carbuncle (*Continued*)
  breast 680.2
  buttock 680.5
  chest wall 680.2
  corpus cavernosum 607.2
  ear (any part) (external) 680.0
  eyelid 373.13
  face (any part, except eye) 680.0
  finger (any) 680.4
  flank 680.2
  foot (any part) 680.7
  forearm 680.3
  genital organ (male) 608.4
  gluteal (region) 680.5
  groin 680.2
  hand (any part) 680.4
  head (any part, except face) 680.8
  heel 680.7
  hip 680.6
  kidney (*see also* Abscess, kidney)
      590.2
  knee 680.6
  labia 616.4
  lacrimal
    gland (*see also* Dacryoadenitis)
        375.00
    passages (duct) (sac) (*see also*
        Dacryocystitis) 375.30
  leg, any part except foot 680.6
  lower extremity, any part except foot
      680.6
  malignant 022.0
  multiple sites 680.9
  neck 680.1
  nose (external) (septum) 680.0
  orbit, orbital 376.01
  partes posteriores 680.5
  pectoral region 680.2
  penis 607.2
  perineum 680.2
  pinna 680.0
  scalp (any part) 680.8
  scrotum 608.4
  seminal vesicle 608.0
  shoulder 680.3
  skin NEC 680.9
  specified site NEC 680.8
  spermatic cord 608.4
  temple (region) 680.0
  testis 608.4
  thigh 680.6
  thumb 680.4
  toe (any) 680.7
  trunk 680.2
  tunica vaginalis 608.4
  umbilicus 680.2
  upper arm 680.3
  urethra 597.0
  vas deferens 608.4
  vulva 616.4
  wrist 680.4
Carbunculus (*see also* Carbuncle) 680.9
Carcinoid (tumor) (M8240/1) - *see* Tumor,
    carcinoid
Carcinoidosis 259.2
Carcinoma (M8010/3) - *see also* Neoplasm,
    by site, malignant

Note: Except where otherwise indicated, the morphological varieties of carcinoma in the list below should be coded by site as for "Neoplasm, malignant."

Carcinoma (Continued)
  with
    apocrine metaplasia (M8573/3)
    cartilaginous (and osseous)
        metaplasia (M8571/3)
    osseous (and cartilaginous)
        metaplasia (M8571/3)
    productive fibrosis (M8141/3)
    spindle cell metaplasia (M8572/3)
    squamous metaplasia (M8570/3)
  acidophil (M8280/3)
    specified site - see Neoplasm, by site,
        malignant
    unspecified site 194.3
  acidophil-basophil, mixed
      (M8281/3)
    specified site - see Neoplasm,
        by site, malignant
    unspecified site 194.3
  acinar (cell) (M8550/3)
  acinic cell (M8550/3)
  adenocystic (M8200/3)
  adenoid
    cystic (M8200/3)
    squamous cell (M8075/3)
  adenosquamous (M8560/3)
  adnexal (skin) (M8390/3) - see
      Neoplasm, skin, malignant
  adrenal cortical (M8370/3) 194.0
  alveolar (M8251/3)
    cell (M8250/3) - see Neoplasm, lung,
        malignant
  anaplastic type (M8021/3)
  apocrine (M8401/3)
    breast - see Neoplasm, breast,
        malignant
    specified site NEC - see Neoplasm,
        skin, malignant
    unspecified site 173.9
  basal cell (pigmented) (M8090/3) -
      see also Neoplasm, skin,
        malignant
    fibro-epithelial type (M8093/3) -
        see Neoplasm, skin,
        malignant
    morphea type (M8092/3) - see
        Neoplasm, skin, malignant
    multicentric (M8091/3) - see
        Neoplasm, skin, malignant
  basaloid (M8123/3)
  basal-squamous cell, mixed
      (M8094/3) - see Neoplasm, skin,
        malignant
  basophil (M8300/3)
    specified site - see Neoplasm, by site,
        malignant
    unspecified site 194.3
  basophil-acidophil, mixed (M8281/3)
    specified site - see Neoplasm, by site,
        malignant
    unspecified site 194.3
  basosquamous (M8094/3) - see
      Neoplasm, skin, malignant
  bile duct type (M8160/3)
    and hepatocellular, mixed
        (M8180/3) 155.0
    liver 155.1
    specified site NEC - see Neoplasm,
        by site, malignant
    unspecified site 155.1
  branchial or branchiogenic 146.8

Carcinoma (Continued)
  bronchial or bronchogenic - see
      Neoplasm, lung, malignant
  bronchiolar (terminal) (M8250/3) -
      see Neoplasm, lung,
        malignant
  bronchiolo-alveolar (M8250/3) -
      see Neoplasm, lung, malignant
  bronchogenic (epidermoid) 162.9
  C cell (M8510/3)
    specified site - see Neoplasm, by site,
        malignant
    unspecified site 193
  ceruminous (M8420/3) 173.2
  chorionic (M9100/3)
    specified site - see Neoplasm, by site,
        malignant
    unspecified site
      female 181
      male 186.9
  chromophobe (M8270/3)
    specified site - see Neoplasm, by site,
        malignant
    unspecified site 194.3
  clear cell (mesonephroid type)
      (M8310/3)
  cloacogenic (M8124/3)
    specified site - see Neoplasm, by site,
        malignant
    unspecified site 154.8
  colloid (M8480/3)
  cribriform (M8201/3)
  cylindroid type (M8200/3)
  diffuse type (M8145/3)
    specified site - see Neoplasm, by site,
        malignant
    unspecified site 151.9
  duct (cell) (M8500/3)
    with Paget's disease (M8541/3) -
        see Neoplasm, breast,
        malignant
    infiltrating (M8500/3)
      specified site - see Neoplasm, by
          site, malignant
      unspecified site 174.9
  ductal (M8500/3)
  ductular, infiltrating (M8521/3)
  embryonal (M9070/3)
    and teratoma, mixed (M9081/3)
    combined with choriocarcinoma
        (M9101/3) - see Neoplasm, by
        site, malignant
    infantile type (M9071/3)
    liver 155.0
    polyembryonal type (M9072/3)
  endometrioid (M8380/3)
  eosinophil (M8280/3)
    specified site - see Neoplasm, by site,
        malignant
    unspecified site 194.3
  epidermoid (M8070/3) - see also
      Carcinoma, squamous cell
    and adenocarcinoma, mixed
        (M8560/3)
    in situ, Bowen's type (M8081/2) - see
        Neoplasm, skin, in situ
    intradermal - see Neoplasm, skin, in
        situ
  fibroepithelial type basal cell
      (M8093/3) - see Neoplasm,
        skin, malignant

Carcinoma (Continued)
  follicular (M8330/3)
    and papillary (mixed) (M8340/3) 193
    moderately differentiated type
        (M8332/3) 193
    pure follicle type (M8331/3) 193
    specified site - see Neoplasm, by site,
        malignant
    trabecular type (M8332/3) 193
    unspecified site 193
    well differentiated type (M8331/3)
        193
  gelatinous (M8480/3)
  giant cell (M8031/3)
    and spindle cell (M8030/3)
  granular cell (M8320/3)
  granulosa cell (M8620/3) 183.0
  hepatic cell (M8170/3) 155.0
  hepatocellular (M8170/3) 155.0
    and bile duct, mixed (M8180/3)
        155.0
  hepatocholangiolitic (M8180/3) 155.0
  Hürthle cell (thyroid) 193
  hypernephroid (M8311/3)
  in
    adenomatous
      polyp (M8210/3)
      polyposis coli (M8220/3) 153.9
    pleomorphic adenoma (M8940/3)
    polypoid adenoma (M8210/3)
    situ (M8010/3) - see Carcinoma, in
        situ
    tubular adenoma (M8210/3)
    villous adenoma (M8261/3)
  infiltrating duct (M8500/3)
    with Paget's disease (M8541/3) - see
        Neoplasm, breast, malignant
    specified site - see Neoplasm, by site,
        malignant
    unspecified site 174.9
  inflammatory (M8530/3)
    specified site - see Neoplasm, by site,
        malignant
    unspecified site 174.9
  in situ (M8010/2) - see also Neoplasm,
      by site, in situ
    epidermoid (M8070/2) - see also
        Neoplasm, by site, in situ
      with questionable stromal
          invasion (M8076/2)
        specified site - see Neoplasm,
            by site, in situ
        unspecified site 233.1
      Bowen's type (M8081/2) - see
          Neoplasm, skin, in situ
    intraductal (M8500/2)
      specified site - see Neoplasm, by
          site, in situ
      unspecified site 233.0
    lobular (M8520/2)
      specified site - see Neoplasm, by
          site, in situ
      unspecified site 233.0
    papillary (M8050/2) - see Neoplasm,
        by site, in situ
    squamous cell (M8070/2) - see also
        Neoplasm, by site, in situ
      with questionable stromal
          invasion (M8076/2)
        specified site - see Neoplasm,
            by site, in situ
        unspecified site 233.1

◀ New   ◀▥ Revised   ~~deleted~~ Deleted   ● Use Additional Digit(s)   ▨ Omit code

Carcinoma (Continued)
  in situ (Continued)
    transitional cell (M8120/2) - see
      Neoplasm, by site, in situ
  intestinal type (M8144/3)
    specified site - see Neoplasm, by site,
      malignant
    unspecified site 151.9
  intraductal (noninfiltrating)
      (M8500/2)
    papillary (M8503/2)
      specified site - see Neoplasm, by
        site, in situ
      unspecified site 233.0
    specified site - see Neoplasm, by site,
      in situ
    unspecified site 233.0
  intraepidermal (M8070/2) - see also
      Neoplasm, skin, in situ
    squamous cell, Bowen's type
      (M8081/2) - see Neoplasm,
      skin, in situ
  intraepithelial (M8010/2) - see also
      Neoplasm, by site, in situ
    squamous cell (M8072/2) - see
      Neoplasm, by site, in situ
  intraosseous (M9270/3) 170.1
    upper jaw (bone) 170.0
  islet cell (M8150/3)
    and exocrine, mixed (M8154/3)
      specified site - see Neoplasm, by
        site, malignant
      unspecified site 157.9
    pancreas 157.4
    specified site NEC - see Neoplasm,
      by site, malignant
    unspecified site 157.4
  juvenile, breast (M8502/3) -
    see Neoplasm, breast,
    malignant
  Kulchitsky's cell (carcinoid tumor of
    intestine) 259.2
  large cell (M8012/3)
    squamous cell, non-keratinizing
      type (M8072/3)
  Leydig cell (testis) (M8650/3)
    specified site - see Neoplasm, by site,
      malignant
    unspecified site 186.9
      female 183.0
      male 186.9
  liver cell (M8170/3) 155.0
  lobular (infiltrating) (M8520/3)
    noninfiltrating (M8520/3)
      specified site - see Neoplasm, by
        site, in situ
      unspecified site 233.0
    specified site - see Neoplasm, by site,
      malignant
    unspecified site 174.9
  lymphoepithelial (M8082/3)
  medullary (M8510/3)
    with
      amyloid stroma (M8511/3)
        specified site - see Neoplasm,
          by site, malignant
        unspecified site 193
      lymphoid stroma (M8512/3)
        specified site - see Neoplasm,
          by site, malignant
        unspecified site 174.9

Carcinoma (Continued)
  medullary (Continued)
    Merkel cell 209.36
      buttock 209.36
      ear 209.31
      eyelid, including canthus 209.31
      face 209.31
      genitals 209.36
      lip 209.31
      lower limb 209.34
      neck 209.32
      nodal presentation 209.75
      scalp 209.32
      secondary (any site) 209.75
      specified site NEC 209.36
      trunk 209.35
      unknown primary site 209.75
      upper limb 209.33
      visceral metastatic presentation
        209.75
  mesometanephric (M9110/3)
  mesonephric (M9110/3)
  metastatic (M8010/6) - see Metastasis,
    cancer
  metatypical (M8095/3) - see Neoplasm,
    skin, malignant
  morphea type basal cell (M8092/3) - see
    Neoplasm, skin, malignant
  mucinous (M8480/3)
  mucin-producing (M8481/3)
  mucin-secreting (M8481/3)
  mucoepidermoid (M8430/3)
  mucoid (M8480/3)
    cell (M8300/3)
      specified site - see Neoplasm, by
        site, malignant
      unspecified site 194.3
  mucous (M8480/3)
  neuroendocrine
    high grade (M8240/3) 209.30
    malignant poorly differentiated
      (M8240/3) 209.30
  nonencapsulated sclerosing (M8350/3)
    193
  noninfiltrating
    intracystic (M8504/2) - see
      Neoplasm, by site, in situ
    intraductal (M8500/2)
      papillary (M8503/2)
        specified site - see Neoplasm,
          by site, in situ
        unspecified site 233.0
      specified site - see Neoplasm, by
        site, in situ
      unspecified site 233.0
    lobular (M8520/2)
      specified site - see Neoplasm, by
        site, in situ
      unspecified site 233.0
  oat cell (M8042/3)
    specified site - see Neoplasm, by site,
      malignant
    unspecified site 162.9
  odontogenic (M9270/3) 170.1
    upper jaw (bone) 170.0
  onocytic (M8290/3)
  oxyphilic (M8290/3)
  papillary (M8050/3)
    and follicular (mixed) (M8340/3)
      193
    epidermoid (M8052/3)

Carcinoma (Continued)
  papillary (Continued)
    intraductal (noninfiltrating)
      (M8503/2)
      specified site - see Neoplasm, by
        site, in situ
      unspecified site 233.0
    serous (M8460/3)
      specified site - see Neoplasm, by
        site, malignant
      surface (M8461/3)
        specified site - see Neoplasm,
          by site, malignant
        unspecified site 183.0
      unspecified site 183.0
    squamous cell (M8052/3)
    transitional cell (M8130/3)
  papillocystic (M8450/3)
    specified site - see Neoplasm, by site,
      malignant
    unspecified site 183.0
  parafollicular cell (M8510/3)
    specified site - see Neoplasm, by site,
      malignant
    unspecified site 193
  pleomorphic (M8022/3)
  polygonal cell (M8034/3)
  prickle cell (M8070/3)
  pseudoglandular, squamous cell
    (M8075/3)
  pseudomucinous (M8470/3)
    specified site - see Neoplasm, by site,
      malignant
    unspecified site 183.0
  pseudosarcomatous (M8033/3)
  regaud type (M8082/3) - see
    Neoplasm, nasopharynx,
    malignant
  renal cell (M8312/3) 189.0
  reserve cell (M8041/3)
  round cell (M8041/3)
  Schmincke (M8082/3) - see
    Neoplasm, nasopharynx,
    malignant
  Schneiderian (M8121/3)
    specified site - see Neoplasm, by site,
      malignant
    unspecified site 160.0
  scirrhous (M8141/3)
  sebaceous (M8410/3) - see Neoplasm,
    skin, malignant
  secondary (M8010/6) - see Neoplasm,
    by site, malignant, secondary
  secretory, breast (M8502/3) - see
    Neoplasm, breast, malignant
  serous (M8441/3)
    papillary (M8460/3)
      specified site - see Neoplasm, by
        site, malignant
      unspecified site 183.0
    surface, papillary (M8461/3)
      specified site - see Neoplasm, by
        site, malignant
      unspecified site 183.0
  Sertoli cell (M8640/3)
    specified site - see Neoplasm, by site,
      malignant
    unspecified site 186.9
  signet ring cell (M8490/3)
    metastatic (M8490/6) - see
      Neoplasm, by site,
      secondary
  simplex (M8231/3)

Carcinoma *(Continued)*
  skin appendage (M8390/3) - *see*
    Neoplasm, skin, malignant
  small cell (M8041/3)
    fusiform cell type (M8043/3)
    squamous cell, nonkeratinizing type
      (M8073/3)
  solid (M8230/3)
    with amyloid stroma (M8511/3)
      specified site - *see* Neoplasm, by
        site, malignant
      unspecified site 193
  spheroidal cell (M8035/3)
  spindle cell (M8032/3)
    and giant cell (M8030/3)
  spinous cell (M8070/3)
  squamous (cell) (M8070/3)
    adenoid type (M8075/3)
    and adenocarcinoma, mixed
      (M8560/3)
    intraepidermal, Bowen's type - *see*
      Neoplasm, skin, in situ
    keratinizing type (large cell)
      (M8071/3)
    large cell, nonkeratinizing type
      (M8072/3)
    microinvasive (M8076/3)
      specified site - *see* Neoplasm, by
        site, malignant
      unspecified site 180.9
    nonkeratinizing type (M8072/3)
    papillary (M8052/3)
    pseudoglandular (M8075/3)
    small cell, nonkeratinizing type
      (M8073/3)
    spindle cell type (M8074/3)
    verrucous (M8051/3)
  superficial spreading (M8143/3)
  sweat gland (M8400/3) - *see* Neoplasm,
    skin, malignant
  theca cell (M8600/3) 183.0
  thymic (M8580/3) 164.0
  trabecular (M8190/3)
  transitional (cell) (M8120/3)
    papillary (M8130/3)
    spindle cell type (M8122/3)
  tubular (M8211/3)
  undifferentiated type (M8020/3)
  urothelial (M8120/3)
  ventriculi 151.9
  verrucous (epidermoid) (squamous
    cell) (M8051/3)
  villous (M8262/3)
  water-clear cell (M8322/3) 194.1
  wolffian duct (M9110/3)
Carcinomaphobia 300.29
Carcinomatosis
  peritonei (M8010/6) 197.6
  specified site NEC (M8010/3) - *see*
    Neoplasm, by site, malignant
  unspecified site (M8010/6) 199.0
Carcinosarcoma (M8980/3) - *see also*
  Neoplasm, by site, malignant
  embryonal type (M8981/3) - *see*
    Neoplasm, by site, malignant
Cardia, cardial - *see* condition
Cardiac - *see also* condition
  death - *see* Disease, heart
  device
    defibrillator, automatic implantable
      (with synchronous cardiac
      pacemaker) V45.02 ◀▥
    in situ NEC V45.00
    pacemaker
      cardiac
        fitting or adjustment V53.31
        in situ V45.01

Cardiac *(Continued)*
  device *(Continued)*
    carotid sinus
      fitting or adjustment V53.39
      in situ V45.09
    pacemaker - *see* Cardiac, device,
      pacemaker
    tamponade 423.3
Cardialgia (*see also* Pain, precordial)
  786.51
Cardiectasis - *see* Hypertrophy, cardiac
Cardiochalasia 530.81
Cardiomalacia (*see also* Degeneration,
  myocardial) 429.1
Cardiomegalia glycogenica diffusa 271.0
Cardiomegaly (*see also* Hypertrophy,
  cardiac) 429.3
  congenital 746.89
  glycogen 271.0
  hypertensive (*see also* Hypertension,
    heart) 402.90
  idiopathic 425.4
Cardiomyoliposis (*see also* Degeneration,
  myocardial) 429.1
Cardiomyopathy (congestive) (constrictive)
  (familial) (infiltrative) (obstructive)
  (restrictive) (sporadic) 425.4
  alcoholic 425.5
  amyloid 277.39 [425.7]
  beriberi 265.0 [425.7]
  cobalt-beer 425.5
  congenital 425.3
  due to
    amyloidosis 277.39 [425.7]
    beriberi 265.0 [425.7]
    cardiac glycogenosis 271.0 [425.7]
    Chagas' disease 086.0
    Friedreich's ataxia 334.0 [425.8]
    hypertension - *see* Hypertension,
      with, heart involvement
    mucopolysaccharidosis 277.5 [425.7]
    myotonia atrophica 359.21 [425.8]
    progressive muscular dystrophy
      359.1 [425.8]
    sarcoidosis 135 [425.8]
  glycogen storage 271.0 [425.7]
  hypertensive - *see* Hypertension, with,
    heart involvement
  hypertrophic
    nonobstructive 425.4
    obstructive 425.1
      congenital 746.84
  idiopathic (concentric) 425.4
  in
    Chagas' disease 086.0
    sarcoidosis 135 [425.8]
  ischemic 414.8
  metabolic NEC 277.9 [425.7]
    amyloid 277.39 [425.7]
    thyrotoxic (*see also* Thyrotoxicosis)
      242.9● [425.7]
    thyrotoxicosis (*see also*
      Thyrotoxicosis) 242.9● [425.7]
  newborn 425.4
    congenital 425.3
  nutritional 269.9 [425.7]
    beriberi 265.0 [425.7]
  obscure of Africa 425.2
  peripartum 674.5●
  postpartum 674.5●
  primary 425.4
  secondary 425.9
  stress induced 429.83
  takotsubo 429.83
  thyrotoxic (*see also* Thyrotoxicosis)
    242.9● [425.7]

Cardiomyopathy *(Continued)*
  toxic NEC 425.9
  tuberculous (*see also* Tuberculosis)
    017.9● [425.8]
Cardionephritis - *see* Hypertension,
  cardiorenal
Cardionephropathy - *see* Hypertension,
  cardiorenal
Cardionephrosis - *see* Hypertension,
  cardiorenal
Cardioneurosis 306.2
Cardiopathia nigra 416.0
Cardiopathy (*see also* Disease, heart)
  429.9
  hypertensive (*see also* Hypertension,
    heart) 402.90
  idiopathic 425.4
  mucopolysaccharidosis 277.5 [425.7]
Cardiopericarditis (*see also* Pericarditis)
  423.9
Cardiophobia 300.29
Cardioptosis 746.87
Cardiorenal - *see* condition
Cardiorrhexis (*see also* Infarct,
  myocardium) 410.9●
Cardiosclerosis - *see* Arteriosclerosis,
  coronary
Cardiosis - *see* Disease, heart
Cardiospasm (esophagus) (reflex)
  (stomach) 530.0
  congenital 750.7
Cardiostenosis - *see* Disease, heart
Cardiosymphysis 423.1
Cardiothyrotoxicosis - *see*
  Hyperthyroidism
Cardiovascular - *see* condition
Carditis (acute) (bacterial) (chronic)
  (subacute) 429.89
  Coxsackie 074.20
  hypertensive (*see also* Hypertension,
    heart) 402.90
  meningococcal 036.40
  rheumatic - *see* Disease, heart,
    rheumatic
  rheumatoid 714.2
Care (of)
  child (routine) V20.1
  convalescent following V66.9
    chemotherapy V66.2
    medical NEC V66.5
    psychotherapy V66.3
    radiotherapy V66.1
    surgery V66.0
    surgical NEC V66.0
    treatment (for) V66.5
      combined V66.6
      fracture V66.4
      mental disorder NEC V66.3
      specified type NEC V66.5
  end-of-life V66.7
  family member (handicapped) (sick)
    creating problem for family V61.49
    provided away from home for
      holiday relief V60.5
    unavailable, due to
      absence (person rendering care)
        (sufferer) V60.4
      inability (any reason) of person
        rendering care V60.4
  holiday relief V60.5
  hospice V66.7
  lack of (at or after birth) (infant) (child)
    995.52
    adult 995.84
  lactation of mother V24.1
  palliative V66.7

◀ New   ◀▥ Revised   ~~deleted~~ Deleted   ● Use Additional Digit(s)   ▤ Omit code

Care *(Continued)*
  postpartum
    immediately after delivery V24.0
    routine follow-up V24.2
  prenatal V22.1
    first pregnancy V22.0
    high-risk pregnancy V23.9
      specified problem NEC V23.89
  terminal V66.7
  unavailable, due to
    absence of person rendering care
      V60.4
    inability (any reason) of person
      rendering care V60.4
  well baby V20.1
Caries (bone) *(see also* Tuberculosis, bone)
  015.9● *[730.8]*●
  arrested 521.04
  cementum 521.03
  cerebrospinal (tuberculous) 015.0●
    [730.88]
  dental (acute) (chronic) (incipient)
    (infected) 521.00
    with pulp exposure 521.03
    extending to
      dentine 521.02
      pulp 521.03
    other specified NEC 521.09
    pit and fissure 521.06
    primary
      pit and fissure origin 521.06
      root surface 521.08
      smooth surface origin 521.07
    root surface 521.08
    smooth surface 521.07
  dentin (acute) (chronic) 521.02
  enamel (acute) (chronic) (incipient)
    521.01
  external meatus 380.89
  hip *(see also* Tuberculosis) 015.1● *[730.85]*
  initial 521.01
  knee 015.2● *[730.86]*
  labyrinth 386.8
  limb NEC 015.7● *[730.88]*
  mastoid (chronic) (process) 383.1
  middle ear 385.89
  nose 015.7● *[730.88]*
  orbit 015.7● *[730.88]*
  ossicle 385.24
  petrous bone 383.20
  sacrum (tuberculous) 015.0● *[730.88]*
  spine, spinal (column) (tuberculous)
    015.0● *[730.88]*
  syphilitic 095.5
    congenital 090.0 *[730.8]*●
  teeth (internal) 521.00
    initial 521.01
  vertebra (column) (tuberculous) 015.0●
    [730.88]
Carini's syndrome (ichthyosis congenita)
  757.1
Carious teeth 521.00
Carneous mole 631
Carnosinemia 270.5
Carotid body or sinus syndrome 337.01
Carotidynia 337.01
Carotinemia (dietary) 278.3
Carotinosis (cutis) (skin) 278.3
Carpal tunnel syndrome 354.0
Carpenter's syndrome 759.89
Carpopedal spasm *(see also* Tetany) 781.7
Carpoptosis 736.05
Carrier (suspected) of
  amebiasis V02.2
  bacterial disease (meningococcal,
    staphylococcal) NEC V02.59

Carrier *(Continued)*
  cholera V02.0
  cystic fibrosis gene V83.81
  defective gene V83.89
  diphtheria V02.4
  dysentery (bacillary) V02.3
    amebic V02.2
  Endamoeba histolytica V02.2
  gastrointestinal pathogens NEC V02.3
  genetic defect V83.89
  gonorrhea V02.7
  group B streptococcus V02.51
  HAA (hepatitis Australian-antigen)
    V02.61
  hemophilia A (asymptomatic) V83.01
    symptomatic V83.02
  hepatitis V02.60
    Australian-antigen (HAA) V02.61
    B V02.61
    C V02.62
    specified type NEC V02.69
    serum V02.61
    viral V02.60
  infective organism NEC V02.9
  malaria V02.9
  paratyphoid V02.3
  Salmonella V02.3
    typhosa V02.1
  serum hepatitis V02.61
  Shigella V02.3
  Staphylococcus NEC V02.59
    methicillin
      resistant Staphylococcus aureus
        V02.54
      susceptible Staphylococcus
        aureus V02.53
  Streptococcus NEC V02.52
    group B V02.51
  typhoid V02.1
  venereal disease NEC V02.8
Carrión's disease (Bartonellosis) 088.0
Car sickness 994.6
Carter's
  relapsing fever (Asiatic) 087.0
Cartilage - *see* condition
Caruncle (inflamed)
  abscess, lacrimal *(see also*
    Dacryocystitis) 375.30
  conjunctiva 372.00
    acute 372.00
  eyelid 373.00
  labium (majus) (minus) 616.89
  lacrimal 375.30
  urethra (benign) 599.3
  vagina (wall) 616.89
Cascade stomach 537.6
Caseation lymphatic gland *(see also*
  Tuberculosis) 017.2●
Caseous
  bronchitis - *see* Tuberculosis,
    pulmonary
  meningitis 013.0●
  pneumonia - *see* Tuberculosis,
    pulmonary
Cassidy (-Scholte) syndrome (malignant
  carcinoid) 259.2
Castellani's bronchitis 104.8
Castleman's tumor or lymphoma
  (mediastinal lymph node
  hyperplasia) 785.6
Castration, traumatic 878.2
  complicated 878.3
Casts in urine 791.7
Cat's ear 744.29
Catalepsy 300.11
  catatonic (acute) *(see also*
    Schizophrenia) 295.2●

Catalepsy *(Continued)*
  hysterical 300.11
  schizophrenic *(see also* Schizophrenia)
    295.2●
Cataphasia *(see also* Disorder, fluency)
  315.35 ◀▥
Cataplexy (idiopathic) *see also* Narcolepsy
Cataract (anterior cortical) (anterior polar)
  (black) (capsular) (central) (cortical)
  (hypermature) (immature)
  (incipient) (mature) 366.9
  anterior
    and posterior axial embryonal
      743.33
    pyramidal 743.31
    subcapsular polar
      infantile, juvenile, or presenile
        366.01
      senile 366.13
  associated with
    calcinosis 275.40 *[366.42]*
    craniofacial dysostosis 756.0 *[366.44]*
    galactosemia 271.1 *[366.44]*
    hypoparathyroidism 252.1 *[366.42]*
    myotonic disorders 359.21 *[366.43]*
    neovascularization 366.33
  blue dot 743.39
  cerulean 743.39
  complicated NEC 366.30
  congenital 743.30
    capsular or subcapsular 743.31
    cortical 743.32
    nuclear 743.33
    specified type NEC 743.39
    total or subtotal 743.34
    zonular 743.32
  coronary (congenital) 743.39
    acquired 366.12
  cupuliform 366.14
  diabetic 250.5● *[366.41]*
    due to secondary diabetes 249.5●
      [366.41]
  drug-induced 366.45
  due to
    chalcosis 360.24 *[366.34]*
    chronic choroiditis *(see also*
      Choroiditis) 363.20 *[366.32]*
    degenerative myopia 360.21 *[366.34]*
    glaucoma *(see also* Glaucoma) 365.9
      [366.31]
    infection, intraocular NEC 366.32
    inflammatory ocular disorder NEC
      366.32
    iridocyclitis, chronic 364.10 *[366.33]*
    pigmentary retinal dystrophy 362.74
      [366.34]
    radiation 366.46
  electric 366.46
  glassblowers' 366.46
  heat ray 366.46
  heterochromic 366.33
  in eye disease NEC 366.30
  infantile *(see also* Cataract, juvenile)
    366.00
  intumescent 366.12
  irradiational 366.46
  juvenile 366.00
    anterior subcapsular polar 366.01
    combined forms 366.09
    cortical 366.03
    lamellar 366.03
    nuclear 366.04
    posterior subcapsular polar 366.02
    specified NEC 366.09
    zonular 366.03

Cataract *(Continued)*
  lamellar 743.32
    infantile juvenile, or presenile 366.03
  morgagnian 366.18
  myotonic 359.21 *[366.43]*
  myxedema 244.9 *[366.44]*
    nuclear 366.16
  posterior, polar (capsular) 743.31
    infantile, juvenile, or presenile 366.02
    senile 366.14
  presenile *(see also* Cataract, juvenile) 366.00
  punctate
    acquired 366.12
    congenital 743.39
  secondary (membrane) 366.50
    obscuring vision 366.53
    specified type, not obscuring vision 366.52
  senile 366.10
    anterior subcapsular polar 366.13
    combined forms 366.19
    cortical 366.15
    hypermature 366.18
    immature 366.12
    incipient 366.12
    mature 366.17
    nuclear 366.16
    posterior subcapsular polar 366.14
    specified NEC 366.19
    total or subtotal 366.17
  snowflake 250.5● *[366.41]*
    due to secondary diabetes 249.5● *[366.41]*
  specified NEC 366.8
  subtotal (senile) 366.17
    congenital 743.34
  sunflower 360.24 *[366.34]*
  tetanic NEC 252.1 *[366.42]*
  total (mature) (senile) 366.17
    congenital 743.34
    localized 366.21
    traumatic 366.22
  toxic 366.45
  traumatic 366.20
    partially resolved 366.23
    total 366.22
  zonular (perinuclear) 743.32
    infantile, juvenile, or presenile 366.03
Cataracta 366.10
  brunescens 366.16
  cerulea 743.39
  complicata 366.30
  congenita 743.30
  coralliformis 743.39
  coronaria (congenital) 743.39
    acquired 366.12
  diabetic 250.5● *[366.41]*
    due to secondary diabetes 249.5● *[366.41]*
  floriformis 360.24 *[366.34]*
  membranacea
    accreta 366.50
    congenita 743.39
  nigra 366.16
Catarrh, catarrhal (inflammation) *(see also* condition) 460
  acute 460
  asthma, asthmatic *(see also* Asthma) 493.9●
  Bostock's *(see also* Fever, hay) 477.9
  bowel - *see* Enteritis

Catarrh, catarrhal *(Continued)*
  bronchial 490
    acute 466.0
    chronic 491.0
    subacute 466.0
  cervix, cervical (canal) (uteri) - *see* Cervicitis
  chest *(see also* Bronchitis) 490
  chronic 472.0
  congestion 472.0
  conjunctivitis 372.03
  due to syphilis 095.9
    congenital 090.0
  enteric - *see* Enteritis
  epidemic *(see also* Influenza) 487.1 ◀▥
  Eustachian 381.50
  eye (acute) (vernal) 372.03
  fauces *(see also* Pharyngitis) 462
  febrile 460
  fibrinous acute 466.0
  gastroenteric - *see* Enteritis
  gastrointestinal - *see* Enteritis
  gingivitis 523.00
  hay *(see also* Fever, hay) 477.9
  infectious 460
  intestinal - *see* Enteritis
  larynx *(see also* Laryngitis, chronic) 476.0
  liver 070.1
    with hepatic coma 070.0
  lung *(see also* Bronchitis) 490
    acute 466.0
    chronic 491.0
  middle ear (chronic) - *see* Otitis media, chronic
  mouth 528.00
  nasal (chronic) *(see also* Rhinitis) 472.0
    acute 460
  nasobronchial 472.2
  nasopharyngeal (chronic) 472.2
    acute 460
  nose - *see* Catarrh, nasal
  ophthalmia 372.03
  pneumococcal, acute 466.0
  pulmonary *(see also* Bronchitis) 490
    acute 466.0
    chronic 491.0
  spring (eye) 372.13
  suffocating *(see also* Asthma) 493.9●
  summer (hay) *(see also* Fever, hay) 477.9
  throat 472.1
  tracheitis 464.10
    with obstruction 464.11
  tubotympanal 381.4
    acute *(see also* Otitis media, acute, nonsuppurative) 381.00
    chronic 381.10
  vasomotor *(see also* Fever, hay) 477.9
  vesical (bladder) - *see* Cystitis
Catarrhus aestivus *(see also* Fever, hay) 477.9
Catastrophe, cerebral *(see also* Disease, cerebrovascular, acute) 436
Catatonia, catatonic (acute) 781.99
  with
    affective psychosis - *see* Psychosis, affective
  agitation 295.2●
  dementia (praecox) 295.2●
  due to or associated with physical condition 293.89
  excitation 295.2●

Catatonia, catatonic *(Continued)*
  excited type 295.2●
  in conditions classified elsewhere 293.89
  schizophrenia 295.2●
  stupor 295.2●
Cat-scratch - *see also* Injury, superficial disease or fever 078.3
Cauda equina - *see also* condition
  syndrome 344.60
Cauliflower ear 738.7
Caul over face 768.9
Causalgia 355.9
  lower limb 355.71
  upper limb 354.4
Cause
  external, general effects NEC 994.9
  not stated 799.9
  unknown 799.9
Caustic burn - *see also* Burn, by site
  from swallowing caustic or corrosive substance - *see* Burn, internal organs
Cavare's disease (familial periodic paralysis) 359.3
Cave-in, injury
  crushing (severe) *(see also* Crush, by site) 869.1
  suffocation 994.7
Cavernitis (penis) 607.2
  lymph vessel - *see* Lymphangioma
Cavernositis 607.2
Cavernous - *see* condition
Cavitation of lung *(see also* Tuberculosis) 011.2●
  nontuberculous 518.89
  primary, progressive 010.8●
Cavity
  lung - *see* Cavitation of lung
  optic papilla 743.57
  pulmonary - *see* Cavitation of lung
  teeth 521.00
  vitreous (humor) 379.21
Cavovarus foot, congenital 754.59
Cavus foot (congenital) 754.71
  acquired 736.73
Cazenave's
  disease (pemphigus) NEC 694.4
  lupus (erythematosus) 695.4
CDGS (carbohydrate-deficient glycoprotein syndrome) 271.8
Cecitis - *see* Appendicitis
Cecocele - *see* Hernia
Cecum - *see* condition
Celiac
  artery compression syndrome 447.4
  disease 579.0
  infantilism 579.0
Cell, cellular - *see also* condition
  anterior chamber (eye) (positive aqueous ray) 364.04
Cellulitis (diffuse) (with lymphangitis) *(see also* Abscess) 682.9
  abdominal wall 682.2
  anaerobic *(see also* Gas gangrene) 040.0
  ankle 682.6
  anus 566
  areola 611.0
  arm (any part, above wrist) 682.3
  auditory canal (external) 380.10
  axilla 682.3
  back (any part) 682.2
  breast 611.0
    postpartum 675.1●

Cellulitis (Continued)
broad ligament (see also Disease, pelvis, inflammatory) 614.4
 acute 614.3
buttock 682.5
cervical (neck region) 682.1
cervix (uteri) (see also Cervicitis) 616.0
cheek, external 682.0
 internal 528.3
chest wall 682.2
chronic NEC 682.9
colostomy 569.61
corpus cavernosum 607.2
digit 681.9
Douglas' cul-de-sac or pouch (chronic) (see also Disease, pelvis, inflammatory) 614.4
 acute 614.3
drainage site (following operation) 998.59
ear, external 380.10
enterostomy 569.61
erysipelar (see also Erysipelas) 035
esophagostomy 530.86
eyelid 373.13
face (any part, except eye) 682.0
finger (intrathecal) (periosteal) (subcutaneous) (subcuticular) 681.00
flank 682.2
foot (except toe) 682.7
forearm 682.3
gangrenous (see also Gangrene) 785.4
genital organ NEC
 female - see Abscess, genital organ, female
 male 608.4
glottis 478.71
gluteal (region) 682.5
gonococcal NEC 098.0
groin 682.2
hand (except finger or thumb) 682.4
head (except face) NEC 682.8
heel 682.7
hip 682.6
jaw (region) 682.0
knee 682.6
labium (majus) (minus) (see also Vulvitis) 616.10
larynx 478.71
leg, except foot 682.6
lip 528.5
mammary gland 611.0
mouth (floor) 528.3
multiple sites NEC 682.9
nasopharynx 478.21
navel 682.2
 newborn NEC 771.4
neck (region) 682.1
nipple 611.0
nose 478.19
 external 682.0
orbit, orbital 376.01
palate (soft) 528.3
pectoral (region) 682.2
pelvis, pelvic
 with
 abortion - see Abortion, by type, with sepsis
 ectopic pregnancy (see also categories 633.0–633.9) 639.0
 molar pregnancy (see also categories 630–632) 639.0

Cellulitis (Continued)
pelvis, pelvic (Continued)
 female (see also Disease, pelvis, inflammatory) 614.4
 acute 614.3
 following
 abortion 639.0
 ectopic or molar pregnancy 639.0
 male 567.21
 puerperal, postpartum, childbirth 670.8●
penis 607.2
perineal, perineum 682.2
perirectal 566
peritonsillar 475
periurethral 597.0
periuterine (see also Disease, pelvis, inflammatory) 614.4
 acute 614.3
pharynx 478.21
phlegmonous NEC 682.9
rectum 566
retromammary 611.0
retroperitoneal (see also Peritonitis) 567.38
round ligament (see also Disease, pelvis, inflammatory) 614.4
 acute 614.3
scalp (any part) 682.8
 dissecting 704.8
scrotum 608.4
seminal vesicle 608.0
septic NEC 682.9
shoulder 682.3
specified sites NEC 682.8
spermatic cord 608.4
submandibular (region) (space) (triangle) 682.0
 gland 527.3
submaxillary 528.3
 gland 527.3
submental (pyogenic) 682.0
 gland 527.3
suppurative NEC 682.9
testis 608.4
thigh 682.6
thumb (intrathecal) (periosteal) (subcutaneous) (subcuticular) 681.00
toe (intrathecal) (periosteal) (subcutaneous) (subcuticular) 681.10
tonsil 475
trunk 682.2
tuberculous (primary) (see also Tuberculosis) 017.0●
tunica vaginalis 608.4
umbilical 682.2
 newborn NEC 771.4
vaccinal 999.39
vagina - see Vaginitis
vas deferens 608.4
vocal cords 478.5
vulva (see also Vulvitis) 616.10
wrist 682.4
Cementoblastoma, benign (M9273/0) 213.1
 upper jaw (bone) 213.0
Cementoma (M9273/0) 213.1
 gigantiform (M9276/0) 213.1
 upper jaw (bone) 213.0
 upper jaw (bone) 213.0
Cementoperiostitis 523.40
 acute 523.33
 apical 523.40

Cephalgia, cephalagia (see also Headache) 784.0
 histamine 339.00
 nonorganic origin 307.81
 other trigeminal autonomic (TACS) 339.09
 psychogenic 307.81
 tension 307.81
Cephalhematocele, cephalematocele
 due to birth injury 767.19
 fetus or newborn 767.19
 traumatic (see also Contusion, head) 920
Cephalhematoma, cephalematoma (calcified)
 due to birth injury 767.19
 fetus or newborn 767.19
 traumatic (see also Contusion, head) 920
Cephalic - see condition
Cephalitis - see Encephalitis
Cephalocele 742.0
Cephaloma - see Neoplasm, by site, malignant
Cephalomenia 625.8
Cephalopelvic - see condition
Cercomoniasis 007.3
Cerebellitis - see Encephalitis
Cerebellum (cerebellar) - see condition
Cerebral - see condition
Cerebritis - see Encephalitis
Cerebrohepatorenal syndrome 759.89
Cerebromacular degeneration 330.1
Cerebromalacia (see also Softening, brain) 348.89 ◄▥
 due to cerebrovascular accident 438.89 ◄
Cerebrosidosis 272.7
Cerebrospasticity - see Palsy, cerebral
Cerebrospinal - see condition
Cerebrum - see condition
Ceroid storage disease 272.7
Cerumen (accumulation) (impacted) 380.4
Cervical - see also condition
 auricle 744.43
 high risk human papillomavirus (HPV) DNA test positive 795.05
 intraepithelial glandular neoplasia 233.1
 low risk human papillomavirus (HPV) DNA test positive 795.09
 rib 756.2
 shortening - see Short, cervical
Cervicalgia 723.1
Cervicitis (acute) (chronic) (nonvenereal) (subacute) (with erosion or ectropion) 616.0
 with
 abortion - see Abortion, by type, with sepsis
 ectopic pregnancy (see also categories 633.0-633.9) 639.0
 molar pregnancy (see also categories 630-632) 639.0
 ulceration 616.0
 chlamydial 099.53
 complicating pregnancy or puerperium 646.6●
 affecting fetus or newborn 760.8
 following
 abortion 639.0
 ectopic or molar pregnancy 639.0
 gonococcal (acute) 098.15
 chronic or duration of 2 months or more 098.35
 senile (atrophic) 616.0
 syphilitic 095.8

Cervicitis *(Continued)*
  trichomonal 131.09
  tuberculous *(see also* Tuberculosis)
    016.7●
Cervicoaural fistula 744.49
Cervicocolpitis (emphysematosa) *(see also*
    Cervicitis) 616.0
Cervix - *see* condition
Cesarean delivery, operation or section
    NEC 669.7●
  affecting fetus or newborn 763.4
  post mortem, affecting fetus or
    newborn 761.6
  previous, affecting management of
    pregnancy 654.2●
Céstan's syndrome 344.89
Céstan-Chenais paralysis 344.89
Céstan-Raymond syndrome 433.8●
Cestode infestation NEC 123.9
  specified type NEC 123.8
Cestodiasis 123.9
CGF (congenital generalized fibromatosis)
    759.89
Chabert's disease 022.9
Chacaleh 266.2
Chafing 709.8
Chagas' disease *(see also* Trypanosomiasis,
    American) 086.2
  with heart involvement 086.0
Chagres fever 084.0
Chalasia (cardiac sphincter) 530.81
Chalazion 373.2
Chalazoderma 757.39
Chalcosis 360.24
  cornea 371.15
  crystalline lens 360.24 *[366.34]*
  retina 360.24
Chalicosis (occupational) (pulmonum) 502
Chancre (any genital site) (hard)
    (indurated) (infecting) (primary)
    (recurrent) 091.0
  congenital 090.0
  conjunctiva 091.2
  Ducrey's 099.0
  extragenital 091.2
  eyelid 091.2
  Hunterian 091.0
  lip (syphilis) 091.2
  mixed 099.8
  nipple 091.2
  Nisbet's 099.0
  of
    carate 103.0
    pinta 103.0
    yaws 102.0
  palate, soft 091.2
  phagedenic 099.0
  Ricord's 091.0
  Rollet's (syphilitic) 091.0
  seronegative 091.0
  seropositive 091.0
  simple 099.0
  soft 099.0
    bubo 099.0
  urethra 091.0
  yaws 102.0
Chancriform syndrome 114.1
Chancroid 099.0
  anus 099.0
  penis (Ducrey's bacillus) 099.0
  perineum 099.0
  rectum 099.0
  scrotum 099.0
  urethra 099.0
  vulva 099.0

Chandipura fever 066.8
Chandler's disease (osteochondritis
    dissecans, hip) 732.7
Change(s) (of) - *see also* Removal of
  arteriosclerotic - *see* Arteriosclerosis
  battery
    cardiac pacemaker V53.31
  bone 733.90
    diabetic 250.8● *[731.8]*
      due to secondary diabetes 249.8●
        [731.8]
    in disease, unknown cause 733.90
  bowel habits 787.99
  cardiorenal (vascular) *(see also*
      Hypertension, cardiorenal) 404.90
  cardiovascular - *see* Disease,
      cardiovascular
  circulatory 459.9
  cognitive or personality change of
      other type, nonpsychotic 310.1
  color, teeth, tooth
    during formation 520.8
    extrinsic 523.6
    intrinsic posteruptive 521.7
  contraceptive device V25.42
  cornea, corneal
    degenerative NEC 371.40
    membrane NEC 371.30
    senile 371.41
  coronary *(see also* Ischemia, heart) 414.9
  degenerative
    chamber angle (anterior) (iris) 364.56
    ciliary body 364.57
    spine or vertebra *(see also*
        Spondylosis) 721.90
  dental pulp, regressive 522.2
  drains V58.49
  dressing
    wound V58.30
      nonsurgical V58.30
      surgical V58.31
  fixation device V54.89
    external V54.89
    internal V54.01
  heart - *see also* Disease, heart
  hip joint 718.95
  hyperplastic larynx 478.79
  hypertrophic
    nasal sinus *(see also* Sinusitis) 473.9
    turbinate, nasal 478.0
    upper respiratory tract 478.9
  inflammatory - *see* Inflammation
  joint *(see also* Derangement, joint) 718.90
    sacroiliac 724.6
  Kirschner wire V54.89
  knee 717.9
  macular, congenital 743.55
  malignant (M----/3) - *see also*
      Neoplasm, by site, malignant

> Note: For malignant change
> occurring in a neoplasm, use the
> appropriate M code with behavior
> digit/3 e.g., malignant change
> in uterine fibroid-M8890/3. For
> malignant change occurring in a
> nonneoplastic condition (e.g., gastric
> ulcer) use the M code M8000/3.

  mental (status) NEC 780.97
    due to or associated with physical
        condition - *see* Syndrome, brain
  myocardium, myocardial - *see*
      Degeneration, myocardial
  of life *(see also* Menopause) 627.2

Change(s) *(Continued)*
  pacemaker battery (cardiac) V53.31
  peripheral nerve 355.9
  personality (nonpsychotic) NEC 310.1
  plaster cast V54.89
  refractive, transient 367.81
  regressive, dental pulp 522.2
  retina 362.9
    myopic (degenerative) (malignant)
        360.21
    vascular appearance 362.13
  sacroiliac joint 724.6
  scleral 379.19
    degenerative 379.16
  senile *(see also* Senility) 797
  sensory *(see also* Disturbance,
      sensation) 782.0
  skin texture 782.8
  spinal cord 336.9
  splint, external V54.89
  subdermal implantable contraceptive
      V25.5
  suture V58.32
  traction device V54.89
  trophic 355.9
    arm NEC 354.9
    leg NEC 355.8
    lower extremity NEC 355.8
    upper extremity NEC 354.9
  vascular 459.9
  vasomotor 443.9
  voice 784.49
    psychogenic 306.1
  wound packing V58.30
    nonsurgical V58.30
    surgical V58.31
Changing sleep-work schedule, affecting
    sleep 327.36
Changuinola fever 066.0
Chapping skin 709.8
Character
  depressive 301.12
Charcôt's
  arthropathy 094.0 *[713.5]*
  cirrhosis - *see* Cirrhosis, biliary
  disease 094.0
    spinal cord 094.0
  fever (biliary) (hepatic) (intermittent) -
      see Choledocholithiasis
  joint (disease) 094.0 *[713.5]*
    diabetic 250.6● *[713.5]*
      due to secondary diabetes 249.6●
        [713.5]
    syringomyelic 336.0 *[713.5]*
  syndrome (intermittent claudication)
      443.9
    due to atherosclerosis 440.21
Charcôt-Marie-Tooth disease, paralysis,
    or syndrome 356.1
CHARGE association (syndrome) 759.89
Charleyhorse (quadriceps) 843.8
  muscle, except quadriceps - *see* Sprain,
      by site
Charlouis' disease *(see also* Yaws) 102.9
Chauffeur's fracture - *see* Fracture, ulna,
    lower end
Cheadle (-Möller) (-Barlow) disease or
    syndrome (infantile scurvy) 267
Checking (of)
  contraceptive device (intrauterine)
      V25.42
  device
    fixation V54.89
      external V54.89
      internal V54.09
    traction V54.89

◀ New   ◀▥ Revised   ~~deleted~~ Deleted   ● Use Additional Digit(s)   ▨ Omit code

Checking (Continued)
Kirschner wire V54.89
plaster cast V54.89
splint, external V54.89
Checkup
following treatment - see Examination
health V70.0
infant (over 28 days old) (not sick)
V20.2
newborn, routine
8 to 28 days old V20.32
over 28 days old, routine V20.2
under 8 days old V20.31
weight V20.32
pregnancy (normal) V22.1
first V22.0
high-risk pregnancy V23.9
specified problem NEC V23.89
Chédiak-Higashi (-Steinbrinck) anomaly,
disease, or syndrome (congenital
gigantism of peroxidase granules)
288.2
Cheek - see also condition
biting 528.9
Cheese itch 133.8
Cheese washers' lung 495.8
Cheilitis 528.5
actinic (due to sun) 692.72
chronic NEC 692.74
due to radiation, except from sun
692.82
due to radiation, except from sun
692.82
acute 528.5
angular 528.5
catarrhal 528.5
chronic 528.5
exfoliative 528.5
gangrenous 528.5
glandularis apostematosa 528.5
granulomatosa 351.8
infectional 528.5
membranous 528.5
Miescher's 351.8
suppurative 528.5
ulcerative 528.5
vesicular 528.5
Cheilodynia 528.5
Cheilopalatoschisis (see also Cleft, palate,
with cleft lip) 749.20
Cheilophagia 528.9
Cheiloschisis (see also Cleft, lip) 749.10
Cheilosis 528.5
with pellagra 265.2
angular 528.5
due to
dietary deficiency 266.0
vitamin deficiency 266.0
Cheiromegaly 729.89
Cheiropompholyx 705.81
Cheloid (see also Keloid) 701.4
Chemical burn - see also Burn, by site
from swallowing chemical - see Burn,
internal organs
Chemodectoma (M8693/1) - see
Paraganglioma, nonchromaffin
Chemoprophylaxis NEC V07.39
Chemosis, conjunctiva 372.73
Chemotherapy
convalescence V66.2
encounter (for) (oral) (intravenous)
V58.11
maintenance (oral) (intravenous)
V58.11

Chemotherapy (Continued)
prophylactic NEC V07.39
fluoride V07.31
Cherubism 526.89
Chest - see condition
Cheyne-Stokes respiration (periodic)
786.04
Chiari's
disease or syndrome (hepatic vein
thrombosis) 453.0
malformation
type I 348.4
type II (see also Spina bifida) 741.0●
type III 742.0
type IV 742.2
network 746.89
Chiari-Frommel syndrome 676.6●
Chicago disease (North American
blastomycosis) 116.0
Chickenpox (see also Varicella) 052.9
exposure to V01.71
vaccination and inoculation
(prophylactic) V05.4
Chiclero ulcer 085.4
Chiggers 133.8
Chignon 111.2
fetus or newborn (from vacuum
extraction) 767.19
Chigoe disease 134.1
Chikungunya fever 066.3
Chilaiditi's syndrome (subphrenic
displacement, colon) 751.4
Chilblains 991.5
lupus 991.5
Child
behavior causing concern V61.20
adopted child V61.24
biological child V61.23
foster child V61.25
Childbed fever 670.8●
Childbirth - see also Delivery
puerperal complications - see Puerperal
Childhood, period of rapid growth V21.0
Chill(s) 780.64
with fever 780.60
without fever 780.64
congestive 780.99
in malarial regions 084.6
septic - see Septicemia
urethral 599.84
Chilomastigiasis 007.8
Chin - see condition
Chinese dysentery 004.9
Chiropractic dislocation (see also Lesion,
nonallopathic, by site) 739.9
Chitral fever 066.0
Chlamydia, chlamydial - see condition
Chloasma 709.09
cachecticorum 709.09
eyelid 374.52
congenital 757.33
hyperthyroid 242.0●
gravidarum 646.8●
idiopathic 709.09
skin 709.09
symptomatic 709.09
Chloroma (M9930/3) 205.3●
Chlorosis 280.9
Egyptian (see also Ancylostomiasis) 126.9
miners' (see also Ancylostomiasis) 126.9
Chlorotic anemia 280.9
Chocolate cyst (ovary) 617.1
Choked
disk or disc - see Papilledema
on food, phlegm, or vomitus NEC (see
also Asphyxia, food) 933.1

Choked (Continued)
phlegm 933.1
while vomiting NEC (see also Asphyxia,
food) 933.1
Chokes (resulting from bends) 993.3
Choking sensation 784.99
Cholangiectasis (see also Disease,
gallbladder) 575.8
Cholangiocarcinoma (M8160/3)
and hepatocellular carcinoma,
combined (M8180/3) 155.0
liver 155.1
specified site NEC - see Neoplasm, by
site, malignant
unspecified site 155.1
Cholangiohepatitis 575.8
due to fluke infestation 121.1
Cholangiohepatoma (M8180/3) 155.0
Cholangiolitis (acute) (chronic)
(extrahepatic) (gangrenous) 576.1
intrahepatic 575.8
paratyphoidal (see also Fever,
paratyphoid) 002.9
typhoidal 002.0
Cholangioma (M8160/0) 211.5
malignant - see Cholangiocarcinoma
Cholangitis (acute) (ascending)
(catarrhal) (chronic) (infective)
(malignant) (primary) (recurrent)
(sclerosing) (secondary) (stenosing)
(suppurative) 576.1
chronic nonsuppurative destructive
571.6
nonsuppurative destructive (chronic)
571.6
Cholecystdocholithiasis - see
Choledocholithiasis
Cholecystitis 575.10
with
calculus, stones in
bile duct (common) (hepatic) -
see Choledocholithiasis
gallbladder - see Cholelithiasis
acute 575.0
acute and chronic 575.12
chronic 575.11
emphysematous (acute) (see also
Cholecystitis, acute) 575.0
gangrenous (see also Cholecystitis,
acute) 575.0
paratyphoidal, current (see also Fever,
paratyphoid) 002.9
suppurative (see also Cholecystitis,
acute) 575.0
typhoidal 002.0
Choledochitis (suppurative) 576.1
Choledocholith - see Choledocholithiasis
Choledocholithiasis 574.5●

Note: Use the following fifth-digit
subclassification with category 574:

0   without mention of obstruction
1   with obstruction

with
cholecystitis 574.4●
acute 574.3●
chronic 574.4●
cholelithiasis 574.9●
with
cholecystitis 574.7●
acute 574.6●
and chronic 574.8●
chronic 574.7●

Cholelithiasis (impacted) (multiple) 574.2●

Note: Use the following fifth-digit subclassification with category 574:

0   without mention of obstruction
1   with obstruction

with
cholecystitis 574.1●
acute 574.0●
chronic 574.1●
choledocholithiasis 574.9●
with
cholecystitis 574.7●
acute 574.6●
and chronic 574.8●
chronic cholecystitis 574.7●
Cholemia (*see also* Jaundice) 782.4
familial 277.4
Gilbert's (familial nonhemolytic) 277.4
Cholemic gallstone - *see* Cholelithiasis
Choleperitoneum, choleperitonitis (*see also* Disease, gallbladder) 567.81
Cholera (algid) (Asiatic) (asphyctic) (epidemic) (gravis) (Indian) (malignant) (morbus) (pestilential) (spasmodic) 001.9
antimonial 985.4
carrier (suspected) of V02.0
classical 001.0
contact V01.0
due to
Vibrio
cholerae (Inaba, Ogawa, Hikojima serotypes) 001.0
el Tor 001.1
el Tor 001.1
exposure to V01.0
vaccination, prophylactic (against) V03.0
Cholerine (*see also* Cholera) 001.9
Cholestasis 576.8
due to total parenteral nutrition (TPN) 573.8
Cholesteatoma (ear) 385.30
attic (primary) 385.31
diffuse 385.35
external ear (canal) 380.21
marginal (middle ear) 385.32
with involvement of mastoid cavity 385.33
secondary (with middle ear involvement) 385.33
mastoid cavity 385.30
middle ear (secondary) 385.32
with involvement of mastoid cavity 385.33
postmastoidectomy cavity (recurrent) 383.32
primary 385.31
recurrent, postmastoidectomy cavity 383.32
secondary (middle ear) 385.32
with involvement of mastoid cavity 385.33
Cholesteatosis (middle ear) (*see also* Cholesteatoma) 385.30
diffuse 385.35
Cholesteremia 272.0
Cholesterin
granuloma, middle ear 385.82
in vitreous 379.22

Cholesterol
deposit
retina 362.82
vitreous 379.22
elevated (high) 272.0
with elevated (high) triglycerides 272.2
imbibition of gallbladder (*see also* Disease, gallbladder) 575.6
Cholesterolemia 272.0
essential 272.0
familial 272.0
hereditary 272.0
Cholesterosis, cholesterolosis (gallbladder) 575.6
with
cholecystitis - *see* Cholecystitis
cholelithiasis - *see* Cholelithiasis
middle ear (*see also* Cholesteatoma) 385.30
Cholocolic fistula (*see also* Fistula, gallbladder) 575.5
Choluria 791.4
Chondritis (purulent) 733.99
auricle 380.03
costal 733.6
Tietze's 733.6
patella, posttraumatic 717.7
pinna 380.03
posttraumatica patellae 717.7
tuberculous (active) (*see also* Tuberculosis) 015.9●
intervertebral 015.0● [730.88]
Chondroangiopathia calcarea seu punctate 756.59
Chondroblastoma (M9230/0) - *see also* Neoplasm, bone, benign
malignant (M9230/3) - *see* Neoplasm, bone, malignant
Chondrocalcinosis (articular) (crystal deposition) (dihydrate) (*see also* Arthritis, due to, crystals) 275.49 [712.3]●
due to
calcium pyrophosphate 275.49 [712.2]●
dicalcium phosphate crystals 275.49 [712.1]●
pyrophosphate crystals 275.49 [712.2]●
Chondrodermatitis nodularis helicis 380.00
Chondrodysplasia 756.4
angiomatose 756.4
calcificans congenita 756.59
epiphysialis punctata 756.59
hereditary deforming 756.4
rhizomelic punctata 277.86
Chondrodystrophia (fetalis) 756.4
calcarea 756.4
calcificans congenita 756.59
fetalis hypoplastica 756.59
hypoplastica calcinosa 756.59
punctata 756.59
tarda 277.5
Chondrodystrophy (familial) (hypoplastic) 756.4
myotonic (congenital) 359.23
Chondroectodermal dysplasia 756.55
Chondrolysis 733.99
Chondroma (M9220/0) - *see also* Neoplasm, cartilage, benign
juxtacortical (M9221/0) - *see* Neoplasm, bone, benign

Chondroma (*Continued*)
periosteal (M9221/0) - *see* Neoplasm, bone, benign
Chondromalacia 733.92
epiglottis (congenital) 748.3
generalized 733.92
knee 717.7
larynx (congenital) 748.3
localized, except patella 733.92
patella, patellae 717.7
systemic 733.92
tibial plateau 733.92
trachea (congenital) 748.3
Chondromatosis (M9220/1) - *see* Neoplasm, cartilage, uncertain behavior
Chondromyxosarcoma (M9220/3) - *see* Neoplasm, cartilage, malignant
Chondro-osteodysplasia (Morquio-Brailsford type) 277.5
Chondro-osteodystrophy 277.5
Chondro-osteoma (M9210/0) - *see* Neoplasm, bone, benign
Chondropathia tuberosa 733.6
Chondrosarcoma (M9220/3) - *see also* Neoplasm, cartilage, malignant
juxtacortical (M9221/3) - *see* Neoplasm, bone, malignant
mesenchymal (M9240/3) - *see* Neoplasm, connective tissue, malignant
Chordae tendineae rupture (chronic) 429.5
Chordee (nonvenereal) 607.89
congenital 752.63
gonococcal 098.2
Chorditis (fibrinous) (nodosa) (tuberosa) 478.5
Chordoma (M9370/3) - *see* Neoplasm, by site, malignant
Chorea (gravis) (minor) (spasmodic) 333.5
with
heart involvement - *see* Chorea with rheumatic heart disease
rheumatic heart disease (chronic, inactive, or quiescent) (conditions classifiable to 393–398) - *see*- rheumatic heart condition involved,
active or acute (conditions classifiable to 391) 392.0
acute - *see* Chorea, Sydenham's
apoplectic (*see also* Disease, cerebrovascular, acute) 436
chronic 333.4
electric 049.8
gravidarum - *see* Eclampsia, pregnancy
habit 307.22
hereditary 333.4
Huntington's 333.4
posthemiplegic 344.89
pregnancy - *see* Eclampsia, pregnancy
progressive 333.4
chronic 333.4
hereditary 333.4
rheumatic (chronic) 392.9
with heart disease or involvement - *see* Chorea, with rheumatic heart disease
senile 333.5
Sydenham's 392.9
with heart involvement - *see* Chorea, with rheumatic heart disease
nonrheumatic 333.5
variabilis 307.23

Choreoathetosis (paroxysmal) 333.5
Chorioadenoma (destruens) (M9100/1) 236.1
Chorioamnionitis 658.4●
    affecting fetus or newborn 762.7
Chorioangioma (M9120/0) 219.8
Choriocarcinoma (M9100/3)
    combined with
        embryonal carcinoma (M9101/3) -
            see Neoplasm, by site,
            malignant
        teratoma (M9101/3) - see Neoplasm,
            by site, malignant
    specified site - see Neoplasm, by site,
        malignant
    unspecified site
        female 181
        male 186.9
Chorioencephalitis, lymphocytic (acute)
    (serous) 049.0
Chorioepithelioma (M9100/3) - see
    Choriocarcinoma
Choriomeningitis (acute) (benign)
    (lymphocytic) (serous) 049.0
Chorionepithelioma (M9100/3) - see
    Choriocarcinoma
Chorionitis (see also Scleroderma)
    710.1
Chorioretinitis 363.20
    disseminated 363.10
        generalized 363.13
        in
            neurosyphilis 094.83
            secondary syphilis 091.51
        peripheral 363.12
        posterior pole 363.11
        tuberculous (see also Tuberculosis)
            017.3● [363.13]
    due to
        histoplasmosis (see also
            Histoplasmosis) 115.92
        toxoplasmosis (acquired) 130.2
            congenital (active) 771.2
    focal 363.00
        juxtapapillary 363.01
        peripheral 363.04
        posterior pole NEC 363.03
    juxtapapillaris, juxtapapillary 363.01
    progressive myopia (degeneration)
        360.21
    syphilitic (secondary) 091.51
        congenital (early) 090.0 [363.13]
            late 090.5 [363.13]
        late 095.8 [363.13]
    tuberculous (see also Tuberculosis)
        017.3● [363.13]
Choristoma - see Neoplasm, by site,
    benign
Choroid - see condition
Choroideremia, choroidermia (initial
    stage) (late stage) (partial or total
    atrophy) 363.55
Choroiditis (see also Chorioretinitis)
    363.20
    leprous 030.9 [363.13]
    senile guttate 363.41
    sympathetic 360.11
    syphilitic (secondary) 091.51
        congenital (early) 090.0 [363.13]
            late 090.5 [363.13]
        late 095.8 [363.13]
    Tay's 363.41
    tuberculous (see also Tuberculosis)
        017.3 ● [363.13]

Choroidopathy NEC 363.9
    degenerative (see also Degeneration,
        choroid) 363.40
    hereditary (see also Dystrophy, choroid)
        363.50
    specified type NEC 363.8
Choroidoretinitis - see Chorioretinitis
Choroidosis, central serous 362.41
Choroidretinopathy, serous 362.41
Christian's syndrome (chronic
    histiocytosis X) 277.89
Christian-Weber disease (nodular
    nonsuppurative panniculitis) 729.30
Christmas disease 286.1
Chromaffinoma (M8700/0) - see also
    Neoplasm, by site, benign
    malignant (M8700/3) - see Neoplasm,
        by site, malignant
Chromatopsia 368.59
Chromhidrosis, chromidrosis 705.89
Chromoblastomycosis 117.2
Chromomycosis 117.2
Chromophytosis 111.0
Chromotrichomycosis 111.8
Chronic - see condition
Churg-Strauss syndrome 446.4
Chyle cyst, mesentery 457.8
Chylocele (nonfilarial) 457.8
    filarial (see also Infestation, filarial)
        125.9
    tunica vaginalis (nonfilarial) 608.84
        filarial (see also Infestation, filarial)
            125.9
Chylomicronemia (fasting) (with
    hyperprebetalipoproteinemia)
    272.3
Chylopericardium (acute) 420.90
Chylothorax (nonfilarial) 457.8
    filarial (see also Infestation, filarial)
        125.9
Chylous
    ascites 457.8
    cyst of peritoneum 457.8
    hydrocele 603.9
    hydrothorax (nonfilarial) 457.8
        filarial (see also Infestation, filarial)
            125.9
Chyluria 791.1
    bilharziasis 120.0
    due to
        Brugia (malayi) 125.1
        Wuchereria (bancrofti) 125.0
            malayi 125.1
    filarial (see also Infestation, filarial)
        125.9
    filariasis (see also Infestation, filarial)
        125.9
    nonfilarial 791.1
Cicatricial (deformity) - see Cicatrix
Cicatrix (adherent) (contracted) (painful)
    (vicious) 709.2
    adenoid 474.8
    alveolar process 525.8
    anus 569.49
    auricle 380.89
    bile duct (see also Disease, biliary)
        576.8
    bladder 596.8
    bone 733.99
    brain 348.89
    cervix (postoperative) (postpartal)
        622.3
        in pregnancy or childbirth 654.6●
            causing obstructed labor 660.2●

Cicatrix (Continued)
    chorioretinal 363.30
        disseminated 363.35
        macular 363.32
        peripheral 363.34
        posterior pole NEC 363.33
    choroid - see Cicatrix, chorioretinal
    common duct (see also Disease, biliary)
        576.8
    congenital 757.39
    conjunctiva 372.64
    cornea 371.00
        tuberculous (see also Tuberculosis)
            017.3● [371.05]
    duodenum (bulb) 537.3
    esophagus 530.3
    eyelid 374.46
        with
            ectropion - see Ectropion
            entropion - see Entropion
    hypopharynx 478.29
    knee, semilunar cartilage 717.5
    lacrimal
        canaliculi 375.53
        duct
            acquired 375.56
            neonatal 375.55
        punctum 375.52
        sac 375.54
    larynx 478.79
    limbus (cystoid) 372.64
    lung 518.89
    macular 363.32
        disseminated 363.35
        peripheral 363.34
    middle ear 385.89
    mouth 528.9
    muscle 728.89
    nasolacrimal duct
        acquired 375.56
        neonatal 375.55
    nasopharynx 478.29
    palate (soft) 528.9
    penis 607.89
    prostate 602.8
    rectum 569.49
    retina 363.30
        disseminated 363.35
        macular 363.32
        peripheral 363.34
        posterior pole NEC 363.33
    semilunar cartilage - see Derangement,
        meniscus
    seminal vesicle 608.89
    skin 709.2
        infected 686.8
        postinfectional 709.2
        tuberculous (see also Tuberculosis)
            017.0●
    specified site NEC 709.2
    throat 478.29
    tongue 529.8
    tonsil (and adenoid) 474.8
    trachea 478.9
    tuberculous NEC (see also Tuberculosis)
        011.9●
    ureter 593.89
    urethra 599.84
    uterus 621.8
    vagina 623.4
        in pregnancy or childbirth 654.7●
            causing obstructed labor 660.2●
    vocal cord 478.5
    wrist, constricting (annular) 709.2

CIDP (chronic inflammatory demyelinating polyneuropathy) 357.81
CIN I (cervical intraepithelial neoplasia I) 622.11 ◄▥
CIN II (cervical intraepithelial neoplasia II) 622.12 ◄▥
CIN III (cervical intraepithelial neoplasia III) 233.1 ◄▥
Cinchonism
  correct substance properly administered 386.9
  overdose or wrong substance given or taken 961.4
Circine herpes 110.5
Circle of Willis - see condition
Circular - see also condition
  hymen 752.49
Circulating, intrinsic anticoagulants causing hemorrhagic disorder 286.5
  following childbirth 666.3●
  postpartum 666.3●
Circulation
  collateral (venous), any site 459.89
  defective 459.9
    congenital 747.9
    lower extremity 459.89
  embryonic 747.9
  failure 799.89
    fetus or newborn 779.89
    peripheral 785.59
  fetal, persistent 747.83
  heart, incomplete 747.9
Circulatory system - see condition
Circulus senilis 371.41
Circumcision
  in absence of medical indication V50.2
  ritual V50.2
  routine V50.2
Circumscribed - see condition
Circumvallata placenta - see Placenta, abnormal
Cirrhosis, cirrhotic 571.5
  with alcoholism 571.2
  alcoholic (liver) 571.2
  atrophic (of liver) - see Cirrhosis, portal
  Baumgarten-Cruveilhier 571.5
  biliary (cholangiolitic) (cholangitic) (cholestatic) (extrahepatic) (hypertrophic) (intrahepatic) (nonobstructive) (obstructive) (pericholangiolitic) (posthepatic) (primary) (secondary) (xanthomatous) 571.6
    due to
      clonorchiasis 121.1
      flukes 121.3
  brain 331.9
  capsular - see Cirrhosis, portal
  cardiac 571.5
    alcoholic 571.2
  central (liver) - see Cirrhosis, liver
  Charcôt's 571.6
  cholangiolitic - see Cirrhosis, biliary
  cholangitic - see Cirrhosis, biliary
  cholestatic - see Cirrhosis, biliary
  clitoris (hypertrophic) 624.2
  coarsely nodular 571.5
  congestive (liver) - see Cirrhosis, cardiac
  Cruveilhier-Baumgarten 571.5
  cryptogenic (of liver) 571.5
    alcoholic 571.2
  dietary (see also Cirrhosis, portal) 571.5

Cirrhosis, cirrhotic (Continued)
  due to
    bronzed diabetes 275.01 ◄▥
    congestive hepatomegaly - see Cirrhosis, cardiac
    cystic fibrosis 277.00
    hemochromatosis (see also Hemochromatosis) 275.03 ◄▥
    hepatolenticular degeneration 275.1
    passive congestion (chronic) - see Cirrhosis, cardiac
    Wilson's disease 275.1
    xanthomatosis 272.2
  extrahepatic (obstructive) - see Cirrhosis, biliary
  fatty 571.8
    alcoholic 571.0
  florid 571.2
  Glisson's - see Cirrhosis, portal
  Hanot's (hypertrophic) - see Cirrhosis, biliary
  hepatic - see Cirrhosis, liver
  hepatolienal - see Cirrhosis, liver
  hobnail - see Cirrhosis, portal
  hypertrophic - see also Cirrhosis, liver
    biliary - see Cirrhosis, biliary
    Hanot's - see Cirrhosis, biliary
  infectious NEC - see Cirrhosis, portal
  insular - see Cirrhosis, portal
  intrahepatic (obstructive) (primary) (secondary) - see Cirrhosis, biliary
  juvenile (see also Cirrhosis, portal) 571.5
  kidney (see also Sclerosis, renal) 587
  Laennec's (of liver) 571.2
    nonalcoholic 571.5
  liver (chronic) (hepatolienal) (hypertrophic) (nodular) (splenomegalic) (unilobar) 571.5
    with alcoholism 571.2
    alcoholic 571.2
    congenital (due to failure of obliteration of umbilical vein) 777.8
    cryptogenic 571.5
      alcoholic 571.2
    fatty 571.8
      alcoholic 571.0
    macronodular 571.5
      alcoholic 571.2
    micronodular 571.5
      alcoholic 571.2
    nodular, diffuse 571.5
      alcoholic 571.2
    pigmentary 275.01 ◄▥
    portal 571.5
      alcoholic 571.2
    postnecrotic 571.5
      alcoholic 571.2
    syphilitic 095.3
  lung (chronic) (see also Fibrosis, lung) 515
  macronodular (of liver) 571.5
    alcoholic 571.2
  malarial 084.9
  metabolic NEC 571.5
  micronodular (of liver) 571.5
    alcoholic 571.2
  monolobular - see Cirrhosis, portal
  multilobular - see Cirrhosis, portal
  nephritis (see also Sclerosis, renal) 587
  nodular - see Cirrhosis, liver
  nutritional (fatty) 571.5
  obstructive (biliary) (extrahepatic) (intrahepatic) - see Cirrhosis, biliary

Cirrhosis, cirrhotic (Continued)
  ovarian 620.8
  paludal 084.9
  pancreas (duct) 577.8
  pericholangiolitic - see Cirrhosis, biliary
  periportal - see Cirrhosis, portal
  pigment, pigmentary (of liver) 275.01 ◄▥
  portal (of liver) 571.5
    alcoholic 571.2
  posthepatitic (see also Cirrhosis, postnecrotic) 571.5
  postnecrotic (of liver) 571.5
    alcoholic 571.2
  primary (intrahepatic) - see Cirrhosis, biliary
  pulmonary (see also Fibrosis, lung) 515
  renal (see also Sclerosis, renal) 587
  septal (see also Cirrhosis, postnecrotic) 571.5
  spleen 289.51
  splenomegalic (of liver) - see Cirrhosis, liver
  stasis (liver) - see Cirrhosis, liver
  stomach 535.4●
  Todd's (see also Cirrhosis, biliary) 571.6
  toxic (nodular) - see Cirrhosis, postnecrotic
  trabecular - see Cirrhosis, postnecrotic
  unilobar - see Cirrhosis, liver
  vascular (of liver) - see Cirrhosis, liver
  xanthomatous (biliary) (see also Cirrhosis, biliary) 571.6
    due to xanthomatosis (familial) (metabolic) (primary) 272.2
Cistern, subarachnoid 793.0
Citrullinemia 270.6
Citrullinuria 270.6
Ciuffini-Pancoast tumor (M8010/3) (carcinoma, pulmonary apex) 162.3
Civatte's disease or poikiloderma 709.09
CJD (Creutzfeldt-Jakob disease) 046.19
  variant (vCJD) 046.11
Clam diggers' itch 120.3
Clap - see Gonorrhea
Clark's paralysis 343.9
Clarke-Hadfield syndrome (pancreatic infantilism) 577.8
Clastothrix 704.2
Claude's syndrome 352.6
Claude Bernard-Horner syndrome (see also Neuropathy, peripheral, autonomic) 337.9
Claudication, intermittent 443.9
  cerebral (artery) (see also Ischemia, cerebral, transient) 435.9
  due to atherosclerosis 440.21
  spinal cord (arteriosclerotic) 435.1
    syphilitic 094.89
  spinalis 435.1
  venous (axillary) 453.89
Claudicatio venosa intermittens 453.89
Claustrophobia 300.29
Clavus (infected) 700
Clawfoot (congenital) 754.71
  acquired 736.74
Clawhand (acquired) 736.06
  congenital 755.59
Clawtoe (congenital) 754.71
  acquired 735.5
Clay eating 307.52
Clay shovelers' fracture - see Fracture, vertebra, cervical
Cleansing of artificial opening (see also Attention to artificial opening) V55.9

◄ New   ◄▥ Revised   d̶e̶l̶e̶t̶e̶d̶ Deleted   ● Use Additional Digit(s)   ▥ Omit code

Cleft (congenital) - *see also* Imperfect, closure
  alveolar process 525.8
  branchial (persistent) 744.41
    cyst 744.42
  clitoris 752.49
  cricoid cartilage, posterior 748.3
  facial (*see also* Cleft, lip) 749.10
  lip 749.10
    with cleft palate 749.20
      bilateral (lip and palate) 749.24
        with unilateral lip or palate 749.25
        complete 749.23
        incomplete 749.24
      unilateral (lip and palate) 749.22
        with bilateral lip or palate 749.25
        complete 749.21
        incomplete 749.22
    bilateral 749.14
      with cleft palate, unilateral 749.25
      complete 749.13
      incomplete 749.14
    unilateral 749.12
      with cleft palate, bilateral 749.25
      complete 749.11
      incomplete 749.12
  nose 748.1
  palate 749.00
    with cleft lip 749.20
      bilateral (lip and palate) 749.24
        with unilateral lip or palate 749.25
        complete 749.23
        incomplete 749.24
      unilateral (lip and palate) 749.22
        with bilateral lip or palate 749.25
        complete 749.21
        incomplete 749.22
    bilateral 749.04
      with cleft lip, unilateral 749.25
      complete 749.03
      incomplete 749.04
    unilateral 749.02
      with cleft lip, bilateral 749.25
      complete 749.01
      incomplete 749.02
  penis 752.69
  posterior, cricoid cartilage 748.3
  scrotum 752.89
  sternum (congenital) 756.3
  thyroid cartilage (congenital) 748.3
  tongue 750.13
  uvula 749.02
    with cleft lip (*see also* Cleft, lip, with cleft palate) 749.20
  water 366.12
Cleft hand (congenital) 755.58
Cleidocranial dysostosis 755.59
Cleidotomy, fetal 763.89
Cleptomania 312.32
Clérambault's syndrome 297.8
  erotomania 302.89
Clergyman's sore throat 784.49
Click, clicking
  systolic syndrome 785.2
Clifford's syndrome (postmaturity) 766.22
Climacteric (*see also* Menopause) 627.2
  arthritis NEC (*see also* Arthritis, climacteric) 716.3●

Climacteric (*Continued*)
  depression (*see also* Psychosis, affective) 296.2●
  disease 627.2
    recurrent episode 296.3●
    single episode 296.2●
  female (symptoms) 627.2
  male (symptoms) (syndrome) 608.89
  melancholia (*see also* Psychosis, affective) 296.2●
    recurrent episode 296.3●
    single episode 296.2●
  paranoid state 297.2
  paraphrenia 297.2
  polyarthritis NEC 716.39
    male 608.89
  symptoms (female) 627.2
Clinical research investigation (control) (participant) V70.7
Clinodactyly 755.59
Clitoris - *see* condition
Cloaca, persistent 751.5
Clonorchiasis 121.1
Clonorchiosis 121.1
Clonorchis infection, liver 121.1
Clonus 781.0
Closed bite 524.20
Closed surgical procedure converted to open procedure
  arthroscopic V64.43
  laparoscopic V64.41
  thoracoscopic V64.42
Closure
  artificial opening (*see also* Attention to artificial opening) V55.9
  congenital, nose 748.0
  cranial sutures, premature 756.0
  defective or imperfect NEC - *see* Imperfect, closure
  fistula, delayed - *see* Fistula
  fontanelle, delayed 756.0
  foramen ovale, imperfect 745.5
  hymen 623.3
  interauricular septum, defective 745.5
  interventricular septum, defective 745.4
  lacrimal duct 375.56
    congenital 743.65
    neonatal 375.55
  nose (congenital) 748.0
    acquired 738.0
  vagina 623.2
  valve - *see* Endocarditis
  vulva 624.8
Clot (blood)
  artery (obstruction) (occlusion) (*see also* Embolism) 444.9
  atrial appendage 429.89
  bladder 596.7
  brain (extradural or intradural) (*see also* Thrombosis, brain) 434.0●
    late effect - *see* Late effect(s) (of) cerebrovascular disease
  circulation 444.9
  heart (*see also* Infarct, myocardium) 410.9●
    without myocardial infarction 429.89
  vein (*see also* Thrombosis) 453.9
Clotting defect NEC (*see also* Defect, coagulation) 286.9
Clouded state 780.09
  epileptic (*see also* Epilepsy) 345.9●
  paroxysmal (idiopathic) (*see also* Epilepsy) 345.9●

Clouding
  corneal graft 996.51
Cloudy
  antrum, antra 473.0
  dialysis effluent 792.5
Clouston's (hidrotic) ectodermal dysplasia 757.31
Clubbing of fingers 781.5
Clubfinger 736.29
  acquired 736.29
  congenital 754.89
Clubfoot (congenital) 754.70
  acquired 736.71
  equinovarus 754.51
  paralytic 736.71
Club hand (congenital) 754.89
  acquired 736.07
Clubnail (acquired) 703.8
  congenital 757.5
Clump kidney 753.3
Clumsiness 781.3
  syndrome 315.4
Cluttering (*see also* Disorder, fluency) 315.35 ◀▥
Clutton's joints 090.5
Coagulation, intravascular (diffuse) (disseminated) (*see also* Fibrinolysis) 286.6
  newborn 776.2
Coagulopathy (*see also* Defect, coagulation) 286.9
  consumption 286.6
  intravascular (disseminated) NEC 286.6
  newborn 776.2
Coalition
  calcaneoscaphoid 755.67
  calcaneus 755.67
  tarsal 755.67
Coal miners'
  elbow 727.2
  lung 500
Coal workers' lung or pneumoconiosis 500
Coarctation
  aorta (postductal) (preductal) 747.10
  pulmonary artery 747.3
Coated tongue 529.3
Coats' disease 362.12
Cocainism (*see also* Dependence) 304.2●
Coccidioidal granuloma 114.3
Coccidioidomycosis 114.9
  with pneumonia 114.0
  cutaneous (primary) 114.1
  disseminated 114.3
  extrapulmonary (primary) 114.1
  lung 114.5
    acute 114.0
    chronic 114.4
    primary 114.0
  meninges 114.2
  primary (pulmonary) 114.0
    acute 114.0
  prostate 114.3
  pulmonary 114.5
    acute 114.0
    chronic 114.4
    primary 114.0
  specified site NEC 114.3
Coccidioidosis 114.9
  lung 114.5
    acute 114.0
    chronic 114.4
    primary 114.0
  meninges 114.2

Coccidiosis (colitis) (diarrhea) (dysentery) 007.2
Cocciuria 791.9
Coccus in urine 791.9
Coccydynia 724.79
Coccygodynia 724.79
Coccyx - *see* condition
Cochin-China
   diarrhea 579.1
      anguilluliasis 127.2
      ulcer 085.1
Cock's peculiar tumor 706.2
Cockayne's disease or syndrome
      (microcephaly and dwarfism) 759.89
Cockayne-Weber syndrome
      (epidermolysis bullosa) 757.39
Cocked-up toe 735.2
Codman's tumor (benign
      chondroblastoma) (M9230/0) - *see*
      Neoplasm, bone, benign
Coenurosis 123.8
Coffee workers' lung 495.8
Cogan's syndrome 370.52
   congenital oculomotor apraxia 379.51
   nonsyphilitic interstitial keratitis 370.52
Coiling, umbilical cord - *see*
      Complications, umbilical cord
Coitus, painful (female) 625.0
   male 608.89
   psychogenic 302.76
Cold 460
   with influenza, flu, or grippe (*see also*
      Influenza) 487.1 ◀▥
   abscess - *see also* Tuberculosis, abscess
      articular - *see* Tuberculosis, joint
   agglutinin
      disease (chronic) or syndrome 283.0
      hemoglobinuria 283.0
         paroxysmal (cold) (nocturnal)
          283.2
   allergic (*see also* Fever, hay) 477.9
   bronchus or chest - *see* Bronchitis
      with grippe or influenza (*see also*
         Influenza) 487.1 ◀▥
   common (head) 460
      vaccination, prophylactic (against)
         V04.7
   deep 464.10
   effects of 991.9
      specified effect NEC 991.8
   excessive 991.9
      specified effect NEC 991.8
   exhaustion from 991.8
   exposure to 991.9
      specified effect NEC 991.8
   grippy (*see also* Influenza) 487.1 ◀▥
   head 460
   injury syndrome (newborn) 778.2
   intolerance 780.99
   on lung - *see* Bronchitis
   rose 477.0
   sensitivity, autoimmune 283.0
   virus 460
Coldsore (*see also* Herpes, simplex) 054.9
Colibacillosis 041.4
   generalized 038.42
Colibacilluria 791.9
Colic (recurrent) 789.7
   abdomen 789.7
      psychogenic 307.89
   appendicular 543.9
   appendix 543.9
   bile duct - *see* Choledocholithiasis
   biliary - *see* Cholelithiasis
   bilious - *see* Cholelithiasis

Colic (*Continued*)
   common duct - *see* Choledocholithiasis
   Devonshire NEC 984.9
      specified type of lead - *see* Table of
         Drugs and Chemicals
   flatulent 787.3
   gallbladder or gallstone - *see*
      Cholelithiasis
   gastric 536.8
   hepatic (duct) - *see* Choledocholithiasis
   hysterical 300.11
   in
      adult 789.0
      child over 12 months old 789.0
      infant 789.7
   infantile 789.7
   intestinal 789.7
   kidney 788.0
   lead NEC 984.9
      specified type of lead - *see* Table of
         Drugs and Chemicals
   liver (duct) - *see* Choledocholithiasis
   mucous 564.9
      psychogenic 316 [564.9]
   nephritic 788.0
   Painter's NEC 984.9
   pancreas 577.8
   psychogenic 306.4
   renal 788.0
   saturnine NEC 984.9
      specified type of lead - *see* Table of
         Drugs and Chemicals
   spasmodic 789.7
   ureter 788.0
   urethral 599.84
      due to calculus 594.2
   uterus 625.8
      menstrual 625.3
   vermicular 543.9
   virus 460
   worm NEC 128.9
Colicystitis (*see also* Cystitis) 595.9
Colitis (acute) (catarrhal) (croupous)
      (cystica superficialis) (exudative)
      (hemorrhagic) (noninfectious)
      (phlegmonous) (presumed
      noninfectious) 558.9
   adaptive 564.9
   allergic 558.3
   amebic (*see also* Amebiasis) 006.9
      nondysenteric 006.2
   anthrax 022.2
   bacillary (*see also* Infection, Shigella)
      004.9
   balantidial 007.0
   chronic 558.9
      ulcerative (*see also* Colitis, ulcerative)
         556.9
   coccidial 007.2
   dietetic 558.9
   due to radiation 558.1
   eosinophilic 558.42
   functional 558.9
   gangrenous 009.0
   giardial 007.1
   granulomatous 555.1
   gravis (*see also* Colitis, ulcerative) 556.9
   infectious (*see also* Enteritis, due to,
      specific organism) 009.0
      presumed 009.1
   ischemic 557.9
      acute 557.0
      chronic 557.1
      due to mesenteric artery
         insufficiency 557.1

Colitis (*Continued*)
   membranous 564.9
      psychogenic 316 [564.9]
   mucous 564.9
      psychogenic 316 [564.9]
   necrotic 009.0
   polyposa (*see also* Colitis, ulcerative)
      556.9
   protozoal NEC 007.9
   pseudomembranous 008.45
   pseudomucinous 564.9
   regional 555.1
   segmental 555.1
   septic (*see also* Enteritis, due to, specific
      organism) 009.0
   spastic 564.9
      psychogenic 316 [564.9]
   Staphylococcus 008.41
      food 005.0
   thromboulcerative 557.0
   toxic 558.2
   transmural 555.1
   trichomonal 007.3
   tuberculous (ulcerative) 014.8●
   ulcerative (chronic) (idiopathic)
      (nonspecific) 556.9
      entero- 556.0
      fulminant 557.0
      ileo- 556.1
      left-sided 556.5
      procto- 556.2
      proctosigmoid 556.3
      psychogenic 316 [556]
      specified NEC 556.8
      universal 556.6
Collagen disease NEC 710.9
   nonvascular 710.9
   vascular (allergic) (*see also* Angiitis,
      hypersensitivity) 446.20
Collagenosis (*see also* Collagen disease)
      710.9
   cardiovascular 425.4
   mediastinal 519.3
Collapse 780.2
   adrenal 255.8
   cardiorenal (*see also* Hypertension,
      cardiorenal) 404.90
   cardiorespiratory 785.51
      fetus or newborn 779.85
   cardiovascular (*see also* Disease, heart)
      785.51
      fetus or newborn 779.85
   circulatory (peripheral) 785.59
      with
         abortion - *see* Abortion, by type,
           with shock
         ectopic pregnancy (*see also*
           categories 633.0–633.9) 639.5
         molar pregnancy (*see also*
           categories 630–632) 639.5
      during or after labor and delivery
         669.1●
      fetus or newborn 779.85
      following
         abortion 639.5
         ectopic or molar pregnancy 639.5
   during or after labor and delivery
      669.1●
      fetus or newborn 779.89
   external ear canal 380.50
      secondary to
         inflammation 380.53
         surgery 380.52
         trauma 380.51
   general 780.2

◀ New   ◀▥ Revised   ~~deleted~~ Deleted   ● Use Additional Digit(s)   ▨ Omit code

Collapse (Continued)
   heart - see Disease, heart
   heat 992.1
   hysterical 300.11
   labyrinth, membranous (congenital)
      744.05
   lung (massive) (see also Atelectasis) 518.0
      pressure, during labor 668.0●
   myocardial - see Disease, heart
   nervous (see also Disorder, mental,
      nonpsychotic) 300.9
   neurocirculatory 306.2
   nose 738.0
   postoperative (cardiovascular) 998.0
   pulmonary (see also Atelectasis) 518.0
      fetus or newborn 770.5
         partial 770.5
         primary 770.4
   thorax 512.8
      iatrogenic 512.1
      postoperative 512.1
   trachea 519.19
   valvular - see Endocarditis
   vascular (peripheral) 785.59
      with
         abortion - see Abortion, by type,
            with shock
         ectopic pregnancy (see also
            categories 633.0–633.9) 639.5
         molar pregnancy (see also
            categories 630–632) 639.5
         cerebral (see also Disease,
            cerebrovascular, acute) 436
         during or after labor and delivery
            669.1●
         fetus or newborn 779.89
         following
            abortion 639.5
            ectopic or molar pregnancy 639.5
      vasomotor 785.59
      vertebra 733.13
Collateral - see also condition
   circulation (venous) 459.89
   dilation, veins 459.89
Colles' fracture (closed) (reversed)
   (separation) 813.41
   open 813.51
Collet's syndrome 352.6
Collet-Sicard syndrome 352.6
Colliculitis urethralis (see also Urethritis)
   597.89
Colliers'
   asthma 500
   lung 500
   phthisis (see also Tuberculosis) 011.4●
Collodion baby (ichthyosis congenita)
   757.1
Colloid milium 709.3
Coloboma NEC 743.49
   choroid 743.59
   fundus 743.52
   iris 743.46
   lens 743.36
   lids 743.62
   optic disc (congenital) 743.57
      acquired 377.23
   retina 743.56
   sclera 743.47
Coloenteritis - see Enteritis
Colon - see condition
Colonization
   MRSA (methicillin resistant
      Staphylococcus aureus) V02.54
   MSSA (methicillin susceptible
      Staphylococcus aureus) V02.53

Coloptosis 569.89
Color
   amblyopia NEC 368.59
      acquired 368.55
   blindness NEC (congenital) 368.59
      acquired 368.55
Colostomy
   attention to V55.3
   fitting or adjustment V55.3
   malfunctioning 569.62
   status V44.3
Colpitis (see also Vaginitis) 616.10
Colpocele 618.6
Colpocystitis (see also Vaginitis) 616.10
Colporrhexis 665.4●
Colpospasm 625.1
Column, spinal, vertebral - see condition
Coma 780.01
   apoplectic (see also Disease,
      cerebrovascular, acute) 436
   diabetic (with ketoacidosis) 250.3●
      due to secondary diabetes 249.3●
      hyperosmolar 250.2●
         due to secondary diabetes
            249.2●
   eclamptic (see also Eclampsia) 780.39
   epileptic 345.3
   hepatic 572.2
   hyperglycemic 250.2●
      due to secondary diabetes 249.2●
   hyperosmolar (diabetic) (nonketotic)
      250.2●
      due to secondary diabetes 249.2●
   hypoglycemic 251.0
      diabetic 250.3●
         due to secondary diabetes
            249.3●
   insulin 250.3●
      due to secondary diabetes 249.3●
      hyperosmolar 250.2●
         due to secondary diabetes
            249.2●
      nondiabetic 251.0
      organic hyperinsulinism 251.0
   Kussmaul's (diabetic) 250.3●
      due to secondary diabetes 249.3●
   liver 572.2
   newborn 779.2
   prediabetic 250.2●
      due to secondary diabetes 249.2●
   uremic - see Uremia
Combat fatigue (see also Reaction, stress,
   acute) 308.9
Combined - see condition
Comedo 706.1
Comedocarcinoma (M8501/3) - see also
   Neoplasm, breast, malignant
   noninfiltrating (M8501/2)
      specified site - see Neoplasm, by site,
         in situ
      unspecified site 233.0
Comedomastitis 610.4
Comedones 706.1
   lanugo 757.4
Comma bacillus, carrier (suspected) of
   V02.3
Comminuted fracture - see Fracture, by
   site
Common
   aortopulmonary trunk 745.0
   atrioventricular canal (defect) 745.69
   atrium 745.69
   cold (head) 460
      vaccination, prophylactic (against)
         V04.7

Common (Continued)
   truncus (arteriosus) 745.0
   ventricle 745.3
Commotio (current)
   cerebri (see also Concussion, brain) 850.9
      with skull fracture - see Fracture,
         skull, by site
   retinae 921.3
   spinalis - see Injury, spinal, by site
Commotion (current)
   brain (without skull fracture) (see also
      Concussion, brain) 850.9
      with skull fracture - see Fracture,
         skull, by site
   spinal cord - see Injury, spinal, by site
Communication
   abnormal - see also Fistula
      between
         base of aorta and pulmonary
            artery 745.0
         left ventricle and right atrium
            745.4
         pericardial sac and pleural sac
            748.8
         pulmonary artery and pulmonary
            vein 747.3
         congenital, between uterus and
            anterior abdominal wall
            752.39 ◀▥
            bladder 752.39 ◀▥
            intestine 752.39 ◀▥
            rectum 752.39 ◀▥
      left ventricular-right atrial 745.4
      pulmonary artery-pulmonary vein 747.3
Compartment syndrome - see Syndrome,
   compartment
Compensation
   broken - see Failure, heart
   failure - see Failure, heart
   neurosis, psychoneurosis 300.11
Complaint - see also Disease
   bowel, functional 564.9
      psychogenic 306.4
   intestine, functional 564.9
      psychogenic 306.4
   kidney (see also Disease, renal) 593.9
   liver 573.9
   miners' 500
Complete - see condition
Complex
   cardiorenal (see also Hypertension,
      cardiorenal) 404.90
   castration 300.9
   Costen's 524.60
   ego-dystonic homosexuality 302.0
   Eisenmenger's (ventricular septal
      defect) 745.4
   homosexual, ego-dystonic 302.0
   hypersexual 302.89
   inferiority 301.9
   jumped process
      spine - see Dislocation, vertebra
   primary, tuberculosis (see also
      Tuberculosis) 010.0●
   regional pain syndrome 355.9
      type I 337.20
         lower limb 337.22
         specified site NEC 337.29
         upper limb 337.21
      type II
         lower limb 355.71
         upper limb 354.4
   Taussig-Bing (transposition, aorta and
      overriding pulmonary artery)
      745.11

Complications
- abortion NEC - *see* categories 634–639
- accidental puncture or laceration during a procedure 998.2
- amniocentesis, fetal 679.1●
- amputation stump (late) (surgical) 997.60
  - traumatic - *see* Amputation, traumatic
- anastomosis (and bypass) - *see also* Complications, due to (presence of) any device, implant, or graft classified to 996.0–996.5 NEC
  - hemorrhage NEC 998.11
  - intestinal (internal) NEC 997.4
    - involving urinary tract 997.5
  - mechanical - *see* Complications, mechanical, graft
  - urinary tract (involving intestinal tract) 997.5
- anesthesia, anesthetic NEC (*see also* Anesthesia, complication) 995.22
  - in labor and delivery 668.9●
    - affecting fetus or newborn 763.5
    - cardiac 668.1●
    - central nervous system 668.2●
    - pulmonary 668.0●
    - specified type NEC 668.8●
- aortocoronary (bypass) graft 996.03
  - atherosclerosis - *see* Arteriosclerosis, coronary
  - embolism 996.72
  - occlusion NEC 996.72
  - thrombus 996.72
- arthroplasty (*see also* Complications, prosthetic joint) 996.49
- artificial opening
  - cecostomy 569.60
  - colostomy 569.60
  - cystostomy 997.5
  - enterostomy 569.60
  - esophagostomy 530.87
    - infection 530.86
    - mechanical 530.87
  - gastrostomy 536.40
  - ileostomy 569.60
  - jejunostomy 569.60
  - nephrostomy 997.5
  - tracheostomy 519.00
  - ureterostomy 997.5
  - urethrostomy 997.5
- bariatric surgery 997.4
- bile duct implant (prosthetic) NEC 996.79
  - infection or inflammation 996.69
  - mechanical 996.59
- bleeding (intraoperative) (postoperative) 998.11
- blood vessel graft 996.1
  - aortocoronary 996.03
    - atherosclerosis - *see* Arteriosclerosis, coronary
    - embolism 996.72
    - occlusion NEC 996.72
    - thrombus 996.72
  - atherosclerosis - *see* Arteriosclerosis, extremities
  - embolism 996.74
  - occlusion NEC 996.74
  - thrombus 996.74
- bone growth stimulator NEC 996.78
  - infection or inflammation 996.67
- bone marrow transplant 996.85

Complications (*Continued*)
- breast implant (prosthetic) NEC 996.79
  - infection or inflammation 996.69
  - mechanical 996.54
- bypass - *see also* Complications, anastomosis
  - aortocoronary 996.03
    - atherosclerosis - *see* Arteriosclerosis, coronary
    - embolism 996.72
    - occlusion NEC 996.72
    - thrombus 996.72
  - carotid artery 996.1
    - atherosclerosis - *see* Arteriosclerosis, coronary
    - embolism 996.74
    - occlusion NEC 996.74
    - thrombus 996.74
- cardiac (*see also* Disease, heart) 429.9
  - device, implant, or graft NEC 996.72
    - infection or inflammation 996.61
    - long-term effect 429.4
    - mechanical (*see also* Complications, mechanical, by type) 996.00
    - valve prosthesis 996.71
      - infection or inflammation 996.61
  - postoperative NEC 997.1
    - long-term effect 429.4
- cardiorenal (*see also* Hypertension, cardiorenal) 404.90
- carotid artery bypass graft 996.1
  - atherosclerosis - *see* Arteriosclerosis, coronary
  - embolism 996.74
  - occlusion NEC 996.74
  - thrombus 996.74
- cataract fragments in eye 998.82
- catheter device NEC - *see also* Complications, due to (presence of) any device, implant, or graft classified to 996.0-996.5 NEC
  - mechanical - *see* Complications, mechanical, catheter
- cecostomy 569.60
- cesarean section wound 674.3●
- chemotherapy (antineoplastic) 995.29
- chin implant (prosthetic) NEC 996.79
  - infection or inflammation 996.69
  - mechanical 996.59
- colostomy (enterostomy) 569.60
  - specified type NEC 569.69
- contraceptive device, intrauterine NEC 996.76
  - infection 996.65
  - inflammation 996.65
  - mechanical 996.32
- cord (umbilical) - *see* Complications, umbilical cord
- cornea
  - due to
    - contact lens 371.82
- coronary (artery) bypass (graft) NEC 996.03
  - atherosclerosis - *see* Arteriosclerosis, coronary
  - embolism 996.72
  - infection or inflammation 996.61
  - mechanical 996.03
  - occlusion NEC 996.72
  - specified type NEC 996.72
  - thrombus 996.72

Complications (*Continued*)
- cystostomy 997.5
- delivery 669.9●
  - procedure (instrumental) (manual) (surgical) 669.4●
  - specified type NEC 669.8●
- dialysis (hemodialysis) (peritoneal) (renal) NEC 999.9
  - catheter NEC - *see also* Complications, due to (presence of) any device, implant, or graft classified to 996.0–996.5 NEC
    - infection or inflammation 996.62
      - peritoneal 996.68
    - mechanical 996.1
      - peritoneal 996.56
- drug NEC 995.29
- due to (presence of) any device, implant, or graft classified to 996.0–996.5 NEC
  - with infection or inflammation - *see* Complications, infection or inflammation, due to (presence of) any device, implant, or graft classified to 996.0–996.5 NEC
  - arterial NEC 996.74
    - coronary NEC 996.03
      - atherosclerosis - *see* Arteriosclerosis, coronary
      - embolism 996.72
      - occlusion NEC 996.72
      - specified type NEC 996.72
      - thrombus 996.72
    - renal dialysis 996.73
  - arteriovenous fistula or shunt NEC 996.74
  - bone growth stimulator 996.78
  - breast NEC 996.79
  - cardiac NEC 996.72
    - defibrillator 996.72
    - pacemaker 996.72
    - valve prosthesis 996.71
  - catheter NEC 996.79
    - spinal 996.75
    - urinary, indwelling 996.76
    - vascular NEC 996.74
      - renal dialysis 996.73
    - ventricular shunt 996.75
  - coronary (artery) bypass (graft) NEC 996.03
    - atherosclerosis - *see* Arteriosclerosis, coronary
    - embolism 996.72
    - occlusion NEC 996.72
    - thrombus 996.72
  - electrodes
    - brain 996.75
    - heart 996.72
  - esophagostomy 530.87
  - gastrointestinal NEC 996.79
  - genitourinary NEC 996.76
  - heart valve prosthesis NEC 996.71
  - infusion pump 996.74
  - insulin pump 996.57
  - internal
    - joint prosthesis 996.77
    - orthopedic NEC 996.78
    - specified type NEC 996.79
  - intrauterine contraceptive device NEC 996.76

◀ New ◀▥ Revised ~~deleted~~ Deleted ● Use Additional Digit(s) ▦ Omit code

Complications *(Continued)*
due to any device, implant, or graft
classified to 996.0–996.5 NEC
(Continued)
joint prosthesis, internal NEC 996.77
mechanical - *see* Complications,
mechanical
nervous system NEC 996.75
ocular lens NEC 996.79
orbital NEC 996.79
orthopedic NEC 996.78
joint, internal 996.77
renal dialysis 996.73
specified type NEC 996.79
urinary catheter, indwelling 996.76
vascular NEC 996.74
ventricular shunt 996.75
during dialysis NEC 999.9
ectopic or molar pregnancy NEC 639.9
electroshock therapy NEC 999.9
enterostomy 569.60
specified type NEC 569.69
esophagostomy 530.87
infection 530.86
mechanical 530.87
external (fixation) device with internal
component(s) NEC 996.78
infection or inflammation 996.67
mechanical 996.49
extracorporeal circulation NEC 999.9
eye implant (prosthetic) NEC 996.79
infection or inflammation 996.69
mechanical
ocular lens 996.53
orbital globe 996.59
fetal, from amniocentesis 679.1●
gastrointestinal, postoperative NEC
(see also Complications, surgical
procedures) 997.4
gastrostomy 536.40
specified type NEC 536.49
genitourinary device, implant or graft
NEC 996.76
infection or inflammation 996.65
urinary catheter, indwelling 996.64
mechanical *(see also* Complications,
mechanical, by type) 996.30
specified NEC 996.39
graft (bypass) (patch) - *see also*
Complications, due to (presence
of) any device, implant, or graft
classified to 996.0–996.5 NEC
bone marrow 996.85
corneal NEC 996.79
infection or inflammation 996.69
rejection or reaction 996.51
retroprosthetic membrane
996.51 ◀
mechanical - *see* Complications,
mechanical, graft
organ (immune or nonimmune
cause) (partial) (total) 996.80
bone marrow 996.85
heart 996.83
intestines 996.87
kidney 996.81
liver 996.82
lung 996.84
pancreas 996.86
specified NEC 996.89
skin NEC 996.79
infection or inflammation 996.69
rejection 996.52
artificial 996.55
decellularized allodermis 996.55

Complications *(Continued)*
heart - *see also* Disease, heart transplant
(immune or nonimmune cause)
996.83
hematoma (intraoperative)
(postoperative) 998.12
hemorrhage (intraoperative)
(postoperative) 998.11
hyperalimentation therapy NEC 999.9
immunization (procedure) - *see*
Complications, vaccination
implant - *see also* Complications, due to
(presence of) any device, implant,
or graft classified to 996.0–996.5
NEC
dental placement, hemorrhagic
525.71
mechanical, - *see* Complications,
mechanical, implant
infection and inflammation
due to (presence of) any device,
implant or graft classified to
996.0–996.5 NEC 996.60
arterial NEC 996.62
coronary 996.61
renal dialysis 996.62
arteriovenous fistula or shunt
996.62
artificial heart 996.61
bone growth stimulator 996.67
breast 996.69
cardiac 996.61
catheter NEC 996.69
central venous 999.31
Hickman 999.31
peripherally inserted central
(PICC) 999.31
peritoneal 996.68
portacath (port-a-cath) 999.31
spinal 996.63
triple lumen 999.31
umbilical venous 999.31
urinary, indwelling 996.64
vascular (arterial) (dialysis)
(peripheral venous) NEC
996.62
ventricular shunt 996.63
central venous catheter 999.31
coronary artery bypass 996.61
electrodes
brain 996.63
heart 996.61
gastrointestinal NEC 996.69
genitourinary NEC 996.65
indwelling urinary catheter
996.64
heart assist device 996.61
heart valve 996.61
Hickman catheter 999.31
infusion pump 996.62
insulin pump 996.69
intrauterine contraceptive device
996.65
joint prosthesis, internal 996.66
ocular lens 996.69
orbital (implant) 996.69
orthopedic NEC 996.67
joint, internal 996.66
peripherally inserted central
catheter (PICC) 999.31
portacath (port-a-cath) 999.31
specified type NEC 996.69
triple lumen catheter 999.31
umbilical venous catheter 999.31

Complications *(Continued)*
infection and inflammation *(Continued)*
due to any device *(Continued)*
urinary catheter, indwelling 996.64
ventricular shunt 996.63
infusion (procedure) 999.88
blood - *see* Complications,
transfusion
infection NEC 999.39
sepsis NEC 999.39
inhalation therapy NEC 999.9
injection (procedure) 999.9
drug reaction *(see also* Reaction,
drug) 995.27
infection NEC 999.39
sepsis NEC 999.39
serum (prophylactic) (therapeutic) -
see Complications, vaccination
vaccine (any) - *see* Complications,
vaccination
inoculation (any) - *see* Complications,
vaccination
insulin pump 996.57
internal device (catheter) (electronic)
(fixation) (prosthetic) - *see also*
Complications, due to (presence
of) any device, implant, or graft
classified to 996.0–996.5 NEC
mechanical - *see* Complications,
mechanical
intestinal pouch, specified NEC
569.79
intestinal transplant (immune or
nonimmune cause) 996.87
intraoperative bleeding or hemorrhage
998.11
intrauterine contraceptive device *(see
also* Complications, contraceptive
device) 996.76
with fetal damage affecting
management of pregnancy
655.8●
infection or inflammation 996.65
in utero procedure
fetal 679.1●
maternal 679.0●
jejunostomy 569.60
kidney transplant (immune or
nonimmune cause) 996.81
labor 669.9●
specified condition NEC 669.8●
liver transplant (immune or
nonimmune cause) 996.82
lumbar puncture 349.0
mechanical
anastomosis - *see* Complications,
mechanical, graft
artificial heart 996.09
bypass - *see* Complications,
mechanical, graft
catheter NEC 996.59
cardiac 996.09
cystostomy 996.39
dialysis (hemodialysis) 996.1
peritoneal 996.56
during a procedure 998.2
urethral, indwelling 996.31
colostomy 569.62
device NEC 996.59
balloon (counterpulsation),
intra-aortic 996.1
cardiac 996.00
automatic implantable
defibrillator 996.04
long-term effect 429.4
specified NEC 996.09

Complications (Continued)
mechanical (Continued)
device NEC (Continued)
contraceptive, intrauterine 996.32
counterpulsation, intra-aortic 996.1
fixation, external, with internal components 996.49
fixation, internal (nail, rod, plate) 996.40
genitourinary 996.30
specified NEC 996.39
insulin pump 996.57
nervous system 996.2
orthopedic, internal 996.40
prosthetic joint (see also Complications, mechanical, device, orthopedic, prosthetic, joint) 996.47
prosthetic NEC 996.59
joint 996.47
articular bearing surface wear 996.46
aseptic loosening 996.41
breakage 996.43
dislocation 996.42
failure 996.47
fracture 996.43
around prosthetic 996.44
peri-prosthetic 996.44
instability 996.42
loosening 996.41
peri-prosthetic osteolysis 996.45
subluxation 996.42
wear 996.46
umbrella, vena cava 996.1
vascular 996.1
dorsal column stimulator 996.2
electrode NEC 996.59
brain 996.2
cardiac 996.01
spinal column 996.2
enterostomy 569.62
esophagostomy 530.87
fistula, arteriovenous, surgically created 996.1
gastrostomy 536.42
graft NEC 996.52
aortic (bifurcation) 996.1
aortocoronary bypass 996.03
blood vessel NEC 996.1
bone 996.49
cardiac 996.00
carotid artery bypass 996.1
cartilage 996.49
corneal 996.51
coronary bypass 996.03
decellularized allodermis 996.55
genitourinary 996.30
specified NEC 996.39
muscle 996.49
nervous system 996.2
organ (immune or nonimmune cause) 996.80
heart 996.83
intestines 996.87
kidney 996.81
liver 996.82
lung 996.84
pancreas 996.86
specified NEC 996.89

Complications (Continued)
mechanical (Continued)
graft NEC (Continued)
orthopedic, internal 996.49
peripheral nerve 996.2
prosthetic NEC 996.59
skin 996.52
artificial 996.55
specified NEC 996.59
tendon 996.49
tissue NEC 996.52
tooth 996.59
ureter, without mention of resection 996.39
vascular 996.1
heart valve prosthesis 996.02
long-term effect 429.4
implant NEC 996.59
cardiac 996.00
automatic implantable defibrillator 996.04
long-term effect 429.4
specified NEC 996.09
electrode NEC 996.59
brain 996.2
cardiac 996.01
spinal column 996.2
genitourinary 996.30
nervous system 996.2
orthopedic, internal 996.49
prosthetic NEC 996.59
in
bile duct 996.59
breast 996.54
chin 996.59
eye
ocular lens 996.53
orbital globe 996.59
vascular 996.1
insulin pump 996.57
nonabsorbable surgical material 996.59
pacemaker NEC 996.59
brain 996.2
cardiac 996.01
nerve (phrenic) 996.2
patch - see Complications, mechanical, graft
prosthesis NEC 996.59
bile duct 996.59
breast 996.54
chin 996.59
ocular lens 996.53
reconstruction, vas deferens 996.39
reimplant NEC 996.59
extremity (see also Complications, reattached, extremity) 996.90
organ (see also Complications, transplant, organ, by site) 996.80
repair - see Complications, mechanical, graft
respirator [ventilator] V46.14
shunt NEC 996.59
arteriovenous, surgically created 996.1
ventricular (communicating) 996.2
stent NEC 996.59
tracheostomy 519.02
vas deferens reconstruction 996.39
ventilator [respirator] V46.14

Complications (Continued)
medical care NEC 999.9
cardiac NEC 997.1
gastrointestinal NEC 997.4
nervous system NEC 997.00
peripheral vascular NEC 997.2
respiratory NEC 997.39
urinary NEC 997.5
vascular
mesenteric artery 997.71
other vessels 997.79
peripheral vessels 997.2
renal artery 997.72
nephrostomy 997.5
nervous system
device, implant, or graft NEC 349.1
mechanical 996.2
postoperative NEC 997.00
obstetric 669.9●
procedure (instrumental) (manual) (surgical) 669.4●
specified NEC 669.8●
surgical wound 674.3●
ocular lens implant NEC 996.79
infection or inflammation 996.69
mechanical 996.53
organ transplant - see Complications, transplant, organ, by site
orthopedic device, implant, or graft
internal (fixation) (nail) (plate) (rod) NEC 996.78
infection or inflammation 996.67
joint prosthesis 996.77
infection or inflammation 996.66
mechanical 996.40
pacemaker (cardiac) 996.72
infection or inflammation 996.61
mechanical 996.01
pancreas transplant (immune or nonimmune cause) 996.86
perfusion NEC 999.9
perineal repair (obstetrical) 674.3●
disruption 674.2●
pessary (uterus) (vagina) - see Complications, contraceptive device
phototherapy 990
postcystoscopic 997.5
postmastoidectomy NEC 383.30
postoperative - see Complications, surgical procedures
pregnancy NEC 646.9●
affecting fetus or newborn 761.9
prosthetic device, internal - see also Complications, due to (presence of) any device, implant or graft classified to 996.0–996.5 NEC
mechanical NEC (see also Complications, mechanical) 996.59
puerperium NEC (see also Puerperal) 674.9●
puncture, spinal 349.0
pyelogram 997.5
radiation 990
radiotherapy 990
reattached
body part, except extremity 996.99
extremity (infection) (rejection) 996.90
arm(s) 996.94
digit(s) (hand) 996.93
foot 996.95
finger(s) 996.93
foot 996.95

Complications (*Continued*)
  reattached (*Continued*)
    extremity (*Continued*)
      forearm 996.91
      hand 996.92
      leg 996.96
      lower NEC 996.96
      toe(s) 996.95
      upper NEC 996.94
    reimplant NEC - *see also* Complications,
      due to (presence of) any device,
      implant, or graft classified to
      996.0–996.5 NEC
      bone marrow 996.85
      extremity (*see also* Complications,
        reattached, extremity) 996.90
        due to infection 996.90
      mechanical - *see* Complications,
        mechanical, reimplant
      organ (immune or nonimmune
        cause) (partial) (total) (*see also*
        Complications, transplant,
        organ, by site) 996.80
  renal allograft 996.81
  renal dialysis - *see* Complications,
    dialysis
  respirator [ventilator], mechanical
    V46.14
  respiratory 519.9
    device, implant or graft NEC
      996.79
      infection or inflammation 996.69
      mechanical 996.59
    distress syndrome, adult, following
      trauma or surgery 518.5
    insufficiency, acute, postoperative
      518.5
    postoperative NEC 997.39
    therapy NEC 999.9
  sedation during labor and delivery
    668.9●
    affecting fetus or newborn 763.5
    cardiac 668.1●
    central nervous system 668.2●
    pulmonary 668.0●
    specified type NEC 668.8●
  seroma (intraoperative) (postoperative)
    (noninfected) 998.13
    infected 998.51
  shunt - *see also* Complications, due to
    (presence of) any device, implant,
    or graft classified to 996.0–996.5
    NEC
    mechanical - *see* Complications,
      mechanical, shunt
  specified body system NEC
    device, implant, or graft - *see*
      Complications, due to
      (presence of) any device,
      implant, or graft classified to
      996.0–996.5 NEC
    postoperative NEC 997.99
  spinal puncture or tap 349.0
  stoma, external
    gastrointestinal tract
      colostomy 569.60
      enterostomy 569.60
      esophagostomy 530.87
        infection 530.86
        mechanical 530.87
      gastrostomy 536.40
    urinary tract 997.5
  stomach banding 997.4
  stomach stapling 997.4

Complications (*Continued*)
  surgical procedures 998.9
    accidental puncture or laceration
      998.2
    amputation stump (late) 997.60
    anastomosis - *see* Complications,
      anastomosis
    burst stitches or sutures (external)
      (*see also* Dehiscence) 998.32
      internal 998.31
    cardiac 997.1
      long-term effect following cardiac
        surgery 429.4
    catheter device - *see* Complications,
      catheter device
    cataract fragments in eye 998.82
    cecostomy malfunction 569.62
    colostomy malfunction 569.62
    cystostomy malfunction 997.5
    dehiscence (of incision) (external)
      (*see also* Dehiscence) 998.32
      internal 998.31
    dialysis NEC (*see also* Complications,
      dialysis) 999.9
    disruption (*see also* Dehiscence)
      anastomosis (internal) - *see*
        Complications, mechanical,
        graft
      internal suture (line) 998.31
      wound (external) 998.32
        internal 998.31
    dumping syndrome
      (postgastrectomy) 564.2
    elephantiasis or lymphedema 997.99
      postmastectomy 457.0
    emphysema (surgical) 998.81
    enterostomy malfunction 569.62
    esophagostomy malfunction 530.87
    evisceration 998.32
    fistula (persistent postoperative) 998.6
    foreign body inadvertently left in
      wound (sponge) (suture)
      (swab) 998.4
    from nonabsorbable surgical material
      (Dacron) (mesh) (permanent
      suture) (reinforcing) (Teflon) -
      see Complications due to
      (presence of) any device,
      implant, or graft classified to
      996.0–996.5 NEC
    gastrointestinal NEC 997.4
    gastrostomy malfunction 536.42
    hematoma 998.12
    hemorrhage 998.11
    ileostomy malfunction 569.62
    internal prosthetic device NEC (*see*
      also Complications, internal
      device) 996.70
      hemolytic anemia 283.19
      infection or inflammation 996.60
      malfunction - *see* Complications,
        mechanical
      mechanical complication - *see*
        Complications, mechanical
      thrombus 996.70
    jejunostomy malfunction 569.62
    nervous system NEC 997.00
    obstruction, internal anastomosis -
      see Complications, mechanical,
      graft
    other body system NEC 997.99
    peripheral vascular NEC 997.2
    postcardiotomy syndrome 429.4
    postcholecystectomy syndrome 576.0

Complications (*Continued*)
  surgical procedures (*Continued*)
    postcommissurotomy syndrome
      429.4
    postgastrectomy dumping
      syndrome 564.2
    postmastectomy lymphedema
      syndrome 457.0
    postmastoidectomy 383.30
      cholesteatoma, recurrent 383.32
      cyst, mucosal 383.31
      granulation 383.33
      inflammation, chronic 383.33
    postvagotomy syndrome 564.2
    postvalvulotomy syndrome 429.4
    reattached extremity (infection)
      (rejection) (*see also*
      Complications, reattached,
      extremity) 996.90
    respiratory NEC 997.39
    seroma 998.13
    shock (endotoxic) (hypovolemic)
      (septic) 998.0
    shunt, prosthetic (thrombus) - *see also*
      Complications, due to (presence
      of) any device, implant, or graft
      classified to 996.0–996.5 NEC
      hemolytic anemia 283.19
    specified complication NEC 998.89
    stitch abscess 998.59
    transplant - *see* Complications, graft
    ureterostomy malfunction 997.5
    urethrostomy malfunction 997.5
    urinary NEC 997.5
    vascular
      mesenteric artery 997.71
      other vessels 997.79
      peripheral vessels 997.2
      renal artery 997.72
    wound infection 998.59
  therapeutic misadventure NEC 999.9
    surgical treatment 998.9
  tracheostomy 519.00
  transfusion (blood) (lymphocytes)
    (plasma) ~~NEC~~ 999.80 ◀▦
    acute lung injury (TRALI) 518.7
    atrophy, liver, yellow, subacute
      (within 8 months of
      administration) - *see* Hepatitis,
      viral
    bone marrow 996.85
    embolism
      air 999.1
      thrombus 999.2
    febrile nonhemolytic reaction
      (FNHTR) 780.66 ◀
    hemolysis NEC 999.89
      bone marrow 996.85
    hemolytic reaction, incompatibility
      unspecified 999.83 ◀
      acute 999.84 ◀
      delayed 999.85 ◀
    hepatitis (serum) (type B) (within 8
      months after administration) -
      see Hepatitis, viral
    incompatibility reaction
      ABO 999.60 ◀▦
        with hemolytic transfusion
          reaction (HTR) (not
          specified as acute or
          delayed) 999.61 ◀
          acute 999.62 ◀
          delayed 999.63 ◀
          specified type NEC 999.69 ◀

Complications *(Continued)*
  transfusion *(Continued)*
    incompatibility reaction *(Continued)*
      minor blood group 999.89
      non-ABO (minor antigens) (Duffy)
        (Kell) (Kidd) (Lewis) (M) (N)
        (P) (S) 999.75 ◄
        with hemolytic transfusion
          reaction (HTR) (not
          specified as acute or
          delayed) 999.76 ◄
          acute 999.77 ◄
          delayed 999.78 ◄
          specified type NEC 999.79 ◄
      Rh antigen (C) (c) (D) (E) (e)
        (factor) 999.70 ◄▦
        with hemolytic transfusion
          reaction (HTR) (not
          specified as acute or
          delayed) 999.71 ◄
          acute 999.72 ◄
          delayed 999.73 ◄
          specified type NEC 999.74 ◄
    infection 999.39
    jaundice (serum) (within 8 months
      after administration) - *see*
      Hepatitis, viral
    sepsis 999.39
    specified reaction NEC 999.89 ◄
    shock or reaction NEC 999.89
      bone marrow 996.85
    subacute yellow atrophy of liver
      (within 8 months after
      administration) - *see* Hepatitis,
      viral
    thromboembolism 999.2
  transplant NEC - *see also* Complications,
    due to (presence of) any device,
    implant, or graft classified to
    996.0–996.5 NEC
    bone marrow 996.85
    organ (immune or nonimmune
      cause) (partial) (total) 996.80
      bone marrow 996.85
      heart 996.83
      intestines 996.87
      kidney 996.81
      liver 996.82
      lung 996.84
      pancreas 996.86
      specified NEC 996.89
  trauma NEC (early) 958.8
  ultrasound therapy NEC 999.9
  umbilical cord
    affecting fetus or newborn 762.6
    complicating delivery 663.9●
      affecting fetus or newborn 762.6
      specified type NEC 663.8●
  urethral catheter NEC 996.76
    infection or inflammation 996.64
    mechanical 996.31
  urinary, postoperative NEC 997.5
  vaccination 999.9
    anaphylaxis NEC 999.4
    cellulitis 999.39
    encephalitis or encephalomyelitis
      323.51
    hepatitis (serum) (type B) (within 8
      months after administration) -
      see Hepatitis, viral
    infection (general) (local) NEC 999.39
    jaundice (serum) (within 8 months
      after administration) - *see*
      Hepatitis, viral
    meningitis 997.09 *[321.8]*

Complications *(Continued)*
  vaccination *(Continued)*
    myelitis 323.52
    protein sickness 999.5
    reaction (allergic) 999.5
      Herxheimer's 995.0
      serum 999.5
    sepsis 999.39
    serum intoxication, sickness, rash, or
      other serum reaction NEC 999.5
    shock (allergic) (anaphylactic) 999.4
    subacute yellow atrophy of liver
      (within 8 months after
      administration) - *see* Hepatitis,
      viral
    vaccinia (generalized) 999.0
      localized 999.39
  vascular
    device, implant, or graft NEC 996.74
      infection or inflammation 996.62
      mechanical NEC 996.1
        cardiac (*see also* Complications,
          mechanical, by type)
          996.00
    following infusion, perfusion, or
      transfusion 999.2
    postoperative NEC 997.2
      mesenteric artery 997.71
      other vessels 997.79
      peripheral vessels 997.2
      renal artery 997.72
  ventilation therapy NEC 999.9
  ventilator [respirator], mechanical
    V46.14
Compound presentation, complicating
  delivery 652.8●
  causing obstructed labor 660.0●
Compressed air disease 993.3
Compression
  with injury - *see* specific injury
  arm NEC 354.9
  artery 447.1
    celiac, syndrome 447.4
  brachial plexus 353.0
  brain (stem) 348.4
    due to
      contusion, brain - *see* Contusion,
        brain
      injury NEC - *see also* Hemorrhage,
        brain, traumatic
      birth - *see* Birth, injury, brain
      laceration, brain - *see* Laceration,
        brain
    osteopathic 739.0
  bronchus 519.19
  by cicatrix - *see* Cicatrix
  cardiac 423.9
  cauda equina 344.60
    with neurogenic bladder 344.61
  celiac (artery) (axis) 447.4
  cerebral - *see* Compression, brain
  cervical plexus 353.2
  cord (umbilical) - *see* Compression,
    umbilical cord
  cranial nerve 352.9
    second 377.49
    third (partial) 378.51
      total 378.52
    fourth 378.53
    fifth 350.8
    sixth 378.54
    seventh 351.8
  divers' squeeze 993.3
  duodenum (external) (*see also*
    Obstruction, duodenum) 537.3

Compression *(Continued)*
  during birth 767.9
  esophagus 530.3
    congenital, external 750.3
  Eustachian tube 381.63
  facies (congenital) 754.0
  fracture - *see* Fracture, by site
  heart - *see* Disease, heart
  intestine (*see also* Obstruction, intestine)
    560.9
    with hernia - *see* Hernia, by site,
      with obstruction
  laryngeal nerve, recurrent 478.79
  leg NEC 355.8
  lower extremity NEC 355.8
  lumbosacral plexus 353.1
  lung 518.89
  lymphatic vessel 457.1
  medulla - *see* Compression, brain
  nerve NEC - *see also* Disorder, nerve
    arm NEC 354.9
    autonomic nervous system (*see also*
      Neuropathy, peripheral,
      autonomic) 337.9
    axillary 353.0
    cranial NEC 352.9
    due to displacement of
      intervertebral disc 722.2
      with myelopathy 722.70
      cervical 722.0
        with myelopathy 722.71
      lumbar, lumbosacral 722.10
        with myelopathy 722.73
      thoracic, thoracolumbar 722.11
        with myelopathy 722.72
    iliohypogastric 355.79
    ilioinguinal 355.79
    leg NEC 355.8
    lower extremity NEC 355.8
    median (in carpal tunnel) 354.0
    obturator 355.79
    optic 377.49
    plantar 355.6
    posterior tibial (in tarsal tunnel) 355.5
    root (by scar tissue) NEC 724.9
      cervical NEC 723.4
      lumbar NEC 724.4
      lumbosacral 724.4
      thoracic 724.4
    saphenous 355.79
    sciatic (acute) 355.0
    sympathetic 337.9
    traumatic - *see* Injury, nerve
    ulnar 354.2
    upper extremity NEC 354.9
  peripheral - *see* Compression, nerve
  spinal (cord) (old or nontraumatic)
    336.9
    by displacement of intervertebral
      disc - *see* Displacement,
      intervertebral disc
    nerve
      root NEC 724.9
        postoperative 722.80
          cervical region 722.81
          lumbar region 722.83
          thoracic region 722.82
          traumatic - *see* Injury, nerve,
            spinal
        traumatic - *see* Injury, nerve,
          spinal
    spondylogenic 721.91
      cervical 721.1
      lumbar, lumbosacral 721.42
      thoracic 721.41

Compression (*Continued*)
  spinal (*Continued*)
    traumatic - *see also* Injury, spinal, by
      site
      with fracture, vertebra - *see*
        Fracture, vertebra, by site,
        with spinal cord injury
    spondylogenic - *see* Compression,
      spinal cord, spondylogenic
  subcostal nerve (syndrome) 354.8
  sympathetic nerve NEC 337.9
  syndrome 958.5
  thorax 512.8
    iatrogenic 512.1
    postoperative 512.1
  trachea 519.19
    congenital 748.3
  ulnar nerve (by scar tissue) 354.2
  umbilical cord
    affecting fetus or newborn 762.5
      cord prolapsed 762.4
    complicating delivery 663.2●
      cord around neck 663.1●
      cord prolapsed 663.0●
  upper extremity NEC 354.9
  ureter 593.3
  urethra - *see* Stricture, urethra
  vein 459.2
  vena cava (inferior) (superior) 459.2
  vertebral NEC - *see* Compression,
    spinal (cord)
Compulsion, compulsive
  eating 307.51
  neurosis (obsessive) 300.3
  personality 301.4
  states (mixed) 300.3
  swearing 300.3
    in Gilles de la Tourette's syndrome
      307.23
  tics and spasms 307.22
  water drinking NEC (syndrome) 307.9
Concato's disease (pericardial
  polyserositis) 423.2
  peritoneal 568.82
  pleural - *see* Pleurisy
Concavity, chest wall 738.3
Concealed
  hemorrhage NEC 459.0
  penis 752.65
Concentric fading 368.12
Concern (normal) about sick person in
  family V61.49
Concrescence (teeth) 520.2
Concretio cordis 423.1
  rheumatic 393
Concretion - *see also* Calculus
  appendicular 543.9
  canaliculus 375.57
  clitoris 624.8
  conjunctiva 372.54
  eyelid 374.56
  intestine (impaction) (obstruction) 560.39
  lacrimal (passages) 375.57
  prepuce (male) 605
    female (clitoris) 624.8
  salivary gland (any) 527.5
  seminal vesicle 608.89
  stomach 537.89
  tonsil 474.8
Concussion (current) 850.9
  with
    loss of consciousness 850.5
      brief (less than one hour)
        30 minutes or less 850.11
        31–59 minutes 850.12
      moderate (1–24 hours) 850.2

Concussion (*Continued*)
  with (*Continued*)
    loss of consciousness (*Continued*)
      prolonged (more than 24 hours)
        (with complete recovery)
        (with return to pre-existing
        conscious level) 850.3
        without return to pre-existing
        conscious level 850.4
      mental confusion or disorientation
        (without loss of consciousness)
        850.0
      with loss of consciousness - *see*
        Concussion, with, loss of
        consciousness
    without loss of consciousness 850.0
  blast (air) (hydraulic) (immersion)
    (underwater) 869.0
    with open wound into cavity 869.1
    abdomen or thorax - *see* Injury,
      internal, by site
    brain - *see* Concussion, brain
    ear (acoustic nerve trauma) 951.5
      with perforation, tympanic
        membrane - *see* Wound,
        open, ear drum
    thorax - *see* Injury, internal,
      intrathoracic organs NEC
  brain or cerebral (without skull
    fracture) 850.9
    with
      loss of consciousness 850.5
        brief (less than one hour)
          30 minutes or less 850.11
          31–59 minutes 850.12
        moderate (1–24 hours) 850.2
        prolonged (more than 24
          hours) (with complete
          recovery) (with return to
          pre-existing conscious
          level) 850.3
        without return to pre-
          existing conscious
          level 850.4
      mental confusion or
        disorientation (without loss
        of consciousness) 850.0
      with loss of consciousness - *see*
        Concussion, brain, with,
        loss of consciousness
      skull fracture - *see* Fracture, skull,
        by site
    without loss of consciousness 850.0
  cauda equina 952.4
  cerebral - *see* Concussion, brain
  conus medullaris (spine) 952.4
  hydraulic - *see* Concussion, blast
  internal organs - *see* Injury, internal, by
    site
  labyrinth - *see* Injury, intracranial
  ocular 921.3
  osseous labyrinth - *see* Injury, intracranial
  spinal (cord) - *see also* Injury, spinal, by
    site
    due to
      broken
        back - *see* Fracture, vertebra,
          by site, with spinal cord
          injury
        neck - *see* Fracture, vertebra,
          cervical, with spinal cord
          injury
      fracture, fracture dislocation, or
        compression fracture of
        spine or vertebra - *see*
        Fracture, vertebra, by site,
        with spinal cord injury

Concussion (*Continued*)
  syndrome 310.2
  underwater blast - *see* Concussion, blast
Condition - *see also* Disease
  fetal hematologic 678.0●
  psychiatric 298.9
  respiratory NEC 519.9
    acute or subacute NEC 519.9
      due to
        external agent 508.9
          specified type NEC 508.8
          fumes or vapors (chemical)
          (inhalation) 506.3
          radiation 508.0
    chronic NEC 519.9
      due to
        external agent 508.9
          specified type NEC 508.8
          fumes or vapors (chemical)
          (inhalation) 506.4
          radiation 508.1
    due to
      external agent 508.9
        specified type NEC 508.8
      fumes or vapors (chemical)
        inhalation 506.9
Conduct disturbance (*see also*
  Disturbance, conduct) 312.9
  adjustment reaction 309.3
  hyperkinetic 314.2
Condyloma NEC 078.11
  acuminatum 078.11
  gonorrheal 098.0
  latum 091.3
  syphilitic 091.3
    congenital 090.0
  venereal, syphilitic 091.3
Confinement - *see* Delivery
Conflagration - *see also* Burn, by site
  asphyxia (by inhalation of smoke,
    gases, fumes, or vapors) 987.9
    specified agent - *see* Table of Drugs
      and Chemicals
Conflict
  family V61.9
    specified circumstance NEC V61.8
  interpersonal NEC V62.81
  marital V61.10
    involving
      divorce V61.03
      estrangement V61.09
  parent (guardian)-child V61.20
    adopted child V61.24
    biological child V61.23
    foster child V61.25
  partner V61.10
Confluent - *see* condition
Confusion, confused (mental) (state) (*see*
  also State, confusional) 298.9
  acute 293.0
  epileptic 293.0
  postoperative 293.9
  psychogenic 298.2
  reactive (from emotional stress,
    psychological trauma) 298.2
  subacute 293.1
Confusional arousals 327.41
Congelation 991.9
Congenital - *see also* condition
  aortic septum 747.29
  generalized fibromatosis (CGF) 759.89
  intrinsic factor deficiency 281.0
  malformation - *see* Anomaly
Congestion, congestive
  asphyxia, newborn 768.9
  bladder 596.8
  bowel 569.89

Congestion, congestive (*Continued*)
- brain (*see also* Disease, cerebrovascular NEC) 437.8
  - malarial 084.9
- breast 611.79
- bronchi 519.19
- bronchial tube 519.19
- catarrhal 472.0
- cerebral - *see* Congestion, brain
- cerebrospinal - *see* Congestion, brain
- chest 786.9
- chill 780.99
  - malarial (*see also* Malaria) 084.6
- circulatory NEC 459.9
- conjunctiva 372.71
- due to disturbance of circulation 459.9
- duodenum 537.3
- enteritis - *see* Enteritis
- eye 372.71
- fibrosis syndrome (pelvic) 625.5
- gastroenteritis - *see* Enteritis
- general 799.89
- glottis 476.0
- heart (*see also* Failure, heart) 428.0
- hepatic 573.0
- hypostatic (lung) 514
- intestine 569.89
- intracranial - *see* Congestion, brain
- kidney 593.89
- labyrinth 386.50
- larynx 476.0
- liver 573.0
- lung 786.9
  - active or acute (*see also* Pneumonia) 486
    - congenital 770.0
  - chronic 514
  - hypostatic 514
  - idiopathic, acute 518.5
  - passive 514
- malaria, malarial (brain) (fever) (*see also* Malaria) 084.6
- medulla - *see* Congestion, brain
- nasal 478.19
- nose 478.19
- orbit, orbital 376.33
  - inflammatory (chronic) 376.10
    - acute 376.00
- ovary 620.8
- pancreas 577.8
- pelvic, female 625.5
- pleural 511.0
- prostate (active) 602.1
- pulmonary - *see* Congestion, lung
- renal 593.89
- retina 362.89
- seminal vesicle 608.89
- spinal cord 336.1
- spleen 289.51
  - chronic 289.51
- stomach 537.89
- trachea 464.11
- urethra 599.84
- uterus 625.5
  - with subinvolution 621.1
- viscera 799.89

Congestive - *see* Congestion

Conical
- cervix 622.6
- cornea 371.60
- teeth 520.2

Conjoined twins 759.4
- causing disproportion (fetopelvic) 678.1●
- fetal 678.1●

Conjugal maladjustment V61.10
- involving
  - divorce V61.03
  - estrangement V61.09

Conjunctiva - *see* condition

Conjunctivitis (exposure) (infectious) (nondiphtheritic) (pneumococcal) (pustular) (staphylococcal) (streptococcal) NEC 372.30
- actinic 370.24
- acute 372.00
  - atopic 372.05
  - chemical 372.06
  - contagious 372.03
  - follicular 372.02
  - hemorrhagic (viral) 077.4
  - toxic 372.06
- adenoviral (acute) 077.3
- allergic (chronic) 372.14
  - with hay fever 372.05
- anaphylactic 372.05
- angular 372.03
- Apollo (viral) 077.4
- atopic 372.05
- blennorrhagic (neonatorum) 098.40
- catarrhal 372.03
- chemical 372.06
  - allergic 372.05
  - meaning corrosion - *see* Burn, conjunctiva
- chlamydial 077.98
  - due to
    - Chlamydia trachomatis - *see* Trachoma
    - paratrachoma 077.0
- chronic 372.10
  - allergic 372.14
  - follicular 372.12
  - simple 372.11
  - specified type NEC 372.14
  - vernal 372.13
- diphtheritic 032.81
- due to
  - dust 372.05
  - enterovirus type 70 077.4
  - erythema multiforme 695.10 [372.33]
  - filariasis (*see also* Filariasis) 125.9 [372.15]
  - mucocutaneous
    - disease NEC 372.33
    - leishmaniasis 085.5 [372.15]
  - Reiter's disease 099.3 [372.33]
  - syphilis 095.8 [372.10]
  - toxoplasmosis (acquired) 130.1
    - congenital (active) 771.2
  - trachoma - *see* Trachoma
- dust 372.05
- eczematous 370.31
- epidemic 077.1
  - hemorrhagic 077.4
- follicular (acute) 372.02
  - adenoviral (acute) 077.3
  - chronic 372.12
- glare 370.24
- gonococcal (neonatorum) 098.40
- granular (trachomatous) 076.1
  - late effect 139.1
- hemorrhagic (acute) (epidemic) 077.4
- herpetic (simplex) 054.43
  - zoster 053.21
- inclusion 077.0
- infantile 771.6
- influenzal 372.03
- Koch-Weeks 372.03
- light 372.05
- medicamentosa 372.05

Conjunctivitis (*Continued*)
- membranous 372.04
- meningococcic 036.89
- Morax-Axenfeld 372.02
- mucopurulent NEC 372.03
- neonatal 771.6
  - gonococcal 098.40
- Newcastle's 077.8
- nodosa 360.14
- of Beal 077.3
- parasitic 372.15
  - filariasis (*see also* Filariasis) 125.9 [372.15]
  - mucocutaneous leishmaniasis 085.5 [372.15]
- Parinaud's 372.02
- petrificans 372.39
- phlyctenular 370.31
- pseudomembranous 372.04
  - diphtheritic 032.81
- purulent 372.03
- Reiter's 099.3 [372.33]
- rosacea 695.3 [372.31]
- serous 372.01
  - viral 077.99
- simple chronic 372.11
- specified NEC 372.39
- sunlamp 372.04
- swimming pool 077.0
- toxic 372.06
- trachomatous (follicular) 076.1
  - acute 076.0
  - late effect 139.1
- traumatic NEC 372.39
- tuberculous (*see also* Tuberculosis) 017.3● [370.31]
- tularemic 021.3
- tularensis 021.3
- vernal 372.13
  - limbar 372.13 [370.32]
- viral 077.99
  - acute hemorrhagic 077.4
  - specified NEC 077.8

Conjunctivochalasis 372.81

Conjunctoblepharitis - *see* Conjunctivitis

Conn (-Louis) syndrome (primary aldosteronism) 255.12

Connective tissue - *see* condition

Conradi (-Hünermann) syndrome or disease (chondrodysplasia calcificans congenita) 756.59

Consanguinity V19.7

Consecutive - *see* condition

Consolidated lung (base) - *see* Pneumonia, lobar

Constipation 564.00
- atonic 564.09
- drug induced
  - correct substance properly administered 564.09
  - overdose or wrong substance given or taken 977.9
    - specified drug - *see* Table of Drugs and Chemicals
- neurogenic 564.09
- other specified NEC 564.09
- outlet dysfunction 564.02
- psychogenic 306.4
- simple 564.00
- slow transit 564.01
- spastic 564.09

Constitutional - *see also* condition
- arterial hypotension (*see also* Hypotension) 458.9
- obesity 278.00
  - morbid 278.01

◀ New   ◀ Revised   ~~deleted~~ Deleted   ● Use Additional Digit(s)   Omit code

Constitutional (*Continued*)
psychopathic state 301.9
short stature in childhood 783.43
state, developmental V21.9
specified development NEC V21.8
substandard 301.6
Constitutionally substandard 301.6
Constriction
anomalous, meningeal bands or folds
742.8
aortic arch (congenital) 747.10
asphyxiation or suffocation by 994.7
bronchus 519.19
canal, ear (*see also* Stricture, ear canal,
acquired) 380.50
duodenum 537.3
gallbladder (*see also* Obstruction,
gallbladder) 575.2
congenital 751.69
intestine (*see also* Obstruction, intestine)
560.9
larynx 478.74
congenital 748.3
meningeal bands or folds, anomalous
742.8
organ or site, congenital NEC - *see*
Atresia
prepuce (congenital) 605
pylorus 537.0
adult hypertrophic 537.0
congenital or infantile 750.5
newborn 750.5
ring (uterus) 661.4●
affecting fetus or newborn 763.7
spastic - *see also* Spasm
ureter 593.3
urethra - *see* Stricture, urethra
stomach 537.89
ureter 593.3
urethra - *see* Stricture, urethra
visual field (functional) (peripheral)
368.45
Constrictive - *see* condition
Consultation V65.9
medical - *see also* Counseling, medical
specified reason NEC V65.8
without complaint or sickness V65.9
feared complaint unfounded V65.5
specified reason NEC V65.8
Consumption - *see* Tuberculosis
Contact
with
AIDS virus V01.79
anthrax V01.81
asbestos V15.84
cholera V01.0
communicable disease V01.9
specified type NEC V01.89
viral NEC V01.79
Escherichia coli (E. coli) V01.83
German measles V01.4
gonorrhea V01.6
HIV V01.79
human immunodeficiency virus
V01.79
lead V15.86
meningococcus V01.84
parasitic disease NEC V01.89
poliomyelitis V01.2
potentially hazardous body fluids
V15.85
rabies V01.5
rubella V01.4
SARS-associated coronavirus V01.82
smallpox V01.3
syphilis V01.6
tuberculosis V01.1

Contact (*Continued*)
with (*Continued*)
varicella V01.71
venereal disease V01.6
viral disease NEC V01.79
dermatitis - *see* Dermatitis
Contamination, food (*see also* Poisoning,
food) 005.9
Contraception, contraceptive
advice NEC V25.09
family planning V25.09
fitting of diaphragm V25.02
prescribing or use of
oral contraceptive agent V25.01
specified agent NEC V25.02
counseling NEC V25.09
emergency V25.03
family planning V25.09
fitting of diaphragm V25.02
prescribing or use of
oral contraceptive agent V25.01
emergency V25.03
postcoital V25.03
specified agent NEC V25.02
device (in situ) V45.59
causing menorrhagia 996.76
checking V25.42
complications 996.32
insertion V25.11 ◀▥
intrauterine V45.51
reinsertion V25.13 ◀▥
removal V25.12 ◀▥
and reinsertion V25.13 ◀
replacement V25.13 ◀
subdermal V45.52
fitting of diaphragm V25.02
insertion
intrauterine contraceptive device
V25.11 ◀▥
subdermal implantable V25.5
maintenance V25.40
examination V25.40
intrauterine device V25.42
oral contraceptive V25.41
specified method NEC V25.49
subdermal implantable V25.43
intrauterine device V25.42
oral contraceptive V25.41
specified method NEC V25.49
subdermal implantable V25.43
management NEC V25.49
prescription
oral contraceptive agent V25.01
emergency V25.03
postcoital V25.03
repeat V25.41
specified agent NEC V25.02
repeat V25.49
sterilization V25.2
surveillance V25.40
intrauterine device V25.42
oral contraceptive agent V25.41
specified method NEC V25.49
subdermal implantable V25.43
Contraction, contracture, contracted
Achilles tendon (*see also* Short, tendon,
Achilles) 727.81
anus 564.89
axilla 729.90
bile duct (*see also* Disease, biliary) 576.8
bladder 596.8
neck or sphincter 596.0
bowel (*see also* Obstruction, intestine)
560.9
Braxton Hicks 644.1●
breast implant, capsular 611.83
bronchus 519.19

Contraction, contracture, contracted
(*Continued*)
burn (old) - *see* Cicatrix
capsular, of breast implant 611.83
cecum (*see also* Obstruction, intestine)
560.9
cervix (*see also* Stricture, cervix) 622.4
congenital 752.49
cicatricial - *see* Cicatrix
colon (*see also* Obstruction, intestine)
560.9
conjunctiva, trachomatous, active 076.1
late effect 139.1
Dupuytren's 728.6
eyelid 374.41
eye socket (after enucleation) 372.64
face 729.90
fascia (lata) (postural) 728.89
Dupuytren's 728.6
palmar 728.6
plantar 728.71
finger NEC 736.29
congenital 755.59
joint (*see also* Contraction, joint)
718.44
flaccid, paralytic
joint (*see also* Contraction, joint)
718.4●
muscle 728.85
ocular 378.50
gallbladder (*see also* Obstruction,
gallbladder) 575.2
hamstring 728.89
tendon 727.81
heart valve - *see* Endocarditis
Hicks' 644.1●
hip (*see also* Contraction, joint) 718.4●
hourglass
bladder 596.8
congenital 753.8
gallbladder (*see also* Obstruction,
gallbladder) 575.2
congenital 751.69
stomach 536.8
congenital 750.7
psychogenic 306.4
uterus 661.4●
affecting fetus or newborn 763.7
hysterical 300.11
infantile (*see also* Epilepsy) 345.6●
internal os (*see also* Stricture, cervix) 622.4
intestine (*see also* Obstruction, intestine)
560.9
joint (abduction) (acquired) (adduction)
(flexion) (rotation) 718.40
ankle 718.47
congenital NEC 755.8
generalized or multiple 754.89
lower limb joints 754.89
hip (*see also* Subluxation,
congenital, hip) 754.32
lower limb (including pelvic
girdle) not involving hip
754.89
upper limb (including shoulder
girdle) 755.59
elbow 718.42
foot 718.47
hand 718.44
hip 718.45
hysterical 300.11
knee 718.46
multiple sites 718.49
pelvic region 718.45
shoulder (region) 718.41
specified site NEC 718.48
wrist 718.43

Contraction, contracture, contracted
(*Continued*)
kidney (granular) (secondary) (*see also*
Sclerosis, renal) 587
congenital 753.3
hydronephritic 591
pyelonephritic (*see also* Pyelitis,
chronic) 590.00
tuberculous (*see also* Tuberculosis)
016.0●
ligament 728.89
congenital 756.89
liver - *see* Cirrhosis, liver
muscle (postinfectional) (postural)
NEC 728.85
congenital 756.89
sternocleidomastoid 754.1
extraocular 378.60
eye (extrinsic) (*see also* Strabismus)
378.9
paralytic (*see also* Strabismus,
paralytic) 378.50
flaccid 728.85
hysterical 300.11
ischemic (Volkmann's) 958.6
paralytic 728.85
posttraumatic 958.6
psychogenic 306.0
specified as conversion reaction
300.11
myotonic 728.85
neck (*see also* Torticollis) 723.5
congenital 754.1
psychogenic 306.0
ocular muscle (*see also* Strabismus)
378.9
paralytic (*see also* Strabismus,
paralytic) 378.50
organ or site, congenital NEC - *see*
Atresia
outlet (pelvis) - *see* Contraction, pelvis
palmar fascia 728.6
paralytic
joint (*see also* Contraction, joint)
718.4●
muscle 728.85
ocular (*see also* Strabismus,
paralytic) 378.50
pelvis (acquired) (general) 738.6
affecting fetus or newborn 763.1
complicating delivery 653.1●
causing obstructed labor
660.1●
generally contracted 653.1●
causing obstructed labor
660.1●
inlet 653.2●
causing obstructed labor
660.1●
midpelvic 653.8●
causing obstructed labor
660.1●
midplane 653.8●
causing obstructed labor
660.1●
outlet 653.3●
causing obstructed labor
660.1●
plantar fascia 728.71
premature
atrial 427.61
auricular 427.61
auriculoventricular 427.61
heart (junctional) (nodal) 427.60

Contraction, contracture, contracted
(*Continued*)
premature (*Continued*)
supraventricular 427.61
ventricular 427.69
prostate 602.8
pylorus (*see also* Pylorospasm) 537.81
rectosigmoid (*see also* Obstruction,
intestine) 560.9
rectum, rectal (sphincter) 564.89
psychogenic 306.4
ring (Bandl's) 661.4●
affecting fetus or newborn 763.7
scar - *see* Cicatrix
sigmoid (*see also* Obstruction, intestine)
560.9
socket, eye 372.64
spine (*see also* Curvature, spine) 737.9
stomach 536.8
hourglass 536.8
congenital 750.7
psychogenic 306.4
psychogenic 306.4
tendon (sheath) (*see also* Short, tendon)
727.81
toe 735.8
ureterovesical orifice (postinfectional)
593.3
urethra 599.84
uterus 621.8
abnormal 661.9●
affecting fetus or newborn 763.7
clonic, hourglass or tetanic 661.4●
affecting fetus or newborn 763.7
dyscoordinate 661.4●
affecting fetus or newborn 763.7
hourglass 661.4●
affecting fetus or newborn 763.7
hypotonic NEC 661.2●
affecting fetus or newborn 763.7
incoordinate 661.4●
affecting fetus or newborn 763.7
inefficient or poor 661.2●
affecting fetus or newborn 763.7
irregular 661.2●
affecting fetus or newborn 763.7
tetanic 661.4●
affecting fetus or newborn 763.7
vagina (outlet) 623.2
vesical 596.8
neck or urethral orifice 596.0
visual field, generalized 368.45
Volkmann's (ischemic) 958.6
Contusion (skin surface intact) 924.9
with
crush injury - *see* Crush
dislocation - *see* Dislocation, by site
fracture - *see* Fracture, by site
internal injury - *see also* Injury,
internal, by site
heart - *see* Contusion, cardiac
kidney - *see* Contusion, kidney
liver - *see* Contusion, liver
lung - *see* Contusion, lung
spleen - *see* Contusion, spleen
intracranial injury - *see* Injury,
intracranial
nerve injury - *see* Injury, nerve
open wound - *see* Wound, open, by
site
abdomen, abdominal (muscle) (wall)
922.2
organ(s) NEC 868.00
adnexa, eye NEC 921.9

Contusion (*Continued*)
ankle 924.21
with other parts of foot 924.20
arm 923.9
lower (with elbow) 923.10
upper 923.03
with shoulder or axillary region
923.09
auditory canal (external) (meatus) (and
other part(s) of neck, scalp, or
face, except eye) 920
auricle, ear (and other part(s) of neck,
scalp, or face except eye) 920
axilla 923.02
with shoulder or upper arm 923.09
back 922.31
bone NEC 924.9
brain (cerebral) (membrane) (with
hemorrhage) 851.8●

> Note: Use the following fifth-digit
> subclassification with categories
> 851–854:
>
> 0   unspecified state of
>   consciousness
> 1   with no loss of consciousness
> 2   with brief [less than one hour]
>   loss of consciousness
> 3   with moderate [1-24 hours] loss
>   of consciousness
> 4   with prolonged [more than 24
>   hours] loss of consciousness
>   and return to pre-existing
>   conscious level
> 5   with prolonged [more than 24
>   hours] loss of
>   consciousness, without
>   return to pre-existing
>   conscious level
>
> Use fifth-digit 5 to designate when a
> patient is unconscious and dies before
> regaining consciousness, regardless of
> the duration of the loss of consciousness
>
> 6   with loss of consciousness of
>   unspecified duration
> 9   with concussion, unspecified

with
open intracranial wound 851.9●
skull fracture - *see* Fracture, skull,
by site
cerebellum 851.4●
with open intracranial wound
851.5●
cortex 851.0●
with open intracranial wound
851.1●
occipital lobe 851.4●
with open intracranial wound
851.5●
stem 851.4●
with open intracranial wound
851.5●
breast 922.0
brow (and other part(s) of neck, scalp,
or face, except eye) 920
buttock 922.32
canthus 921.1
cardiac 861.01
with open wound into thorax 861.11
cauda equina (spine) 952.4
cerebellum - *see* Contusion, brain,
cerebellum

◀ New   ◀∥∥ Revised   ~~deleted~~ Deleted   ● Use Additional Digit(s)   ▬ Omit code

Contusion (*Continued*)
cerebral - *see* Contusion, brain
cheek(s) (and other part(s) of neck, scalp, or face, except eye) 920
chest (wall) 922.1
chin (and other part(s) of neck, scalp, or face, except eye) 920
clitoris 922.4
conjunctiva 921.1
conus medullaris (spine) 952.4
cornea 921.3
corpus cavernosum 922.4
cortex (brain) (cerebral) - *see* Contusion, brain, cortex
costal region 922.1
ear (and other part(s) of neck, scalp, or face except eye) 920
elbow 923.11
   with forearm 923.10
epididymis 922.4
epigastric region 922.2
eye NEC 921.9
eyeball 921.3
eyelid(s) (and periocular area) 921.1
face (and neck, or scalp, any part, except eye) 920
femoral triangle 922.2
fetus or newborn 772.6
finger(s) (nail) (subungual) 923.3
flank 922.2
foot (with ankle) (excluding toe(s)) 924.20
forearm (and elbow) 923.10
forehead (and other part(s) of neck, scalp, or face, except eye) 920
genital organs, external 922.4
globe (eye) 921.3
groin 922.2
gum(s) (and other part(s) of neck, scalp, or face, except eye) 920
hand(s) (except fingers alone) 923.20
head (any part, except eye) (and face) (and neck) 920
heart - *see* Contusion, cardiac
heel 924.20
hip 924.01
   with thigh 924.00
iliac region 922.2
inguinal region 922.2
internal organs (abdomen, chest, or pelvis) NEC - *see* Injury, internal, by site
interscapular region 922.33
iris (eye) 921.3
kidney 866.01
   with open wound into cavity 866.11
knee 924.11
   with lower leg 924.10
labium (majus) (minus) 922.4
lacrimal apparatus, gland, or sac 921.1
larynx (and other part(s) of neck, scalp, or face, except eye) 920
late effect - *see* Late, effects (of), contusion
leg 924.5
   lower (with knee) 924.10
lens 921.3
lingual (and other part(s) of neck, scalp, or face, except eye) 920
lip(s) (and other part(s) of neck, scalp, or face, except eye) 920

Contusion (*Continued*)
liver 864.01
   with
      laceration - *see* Laceration, liver
      open wound into cavity 864.11
lower extremity 924.5
   multiple sites 924.4
lumbar region 922.31
lung 861.21
   with open wound into thorax 861.31
malar region (and other part(s) of neck, scalp, or face, except eye) 920
mandibular joint (and other part(s) of neck, scalp, or face, except eye) 920
mastoid region (and other part(s) of neck, scalp, or face, except eye) 920
membrane, brain - *see* Contusion, brain
midthoracic region 922.1
mouth (and other part(s) of neck, scalp, or face, except eye) 920
multiple sites (not classifiable to same three-digit category) 924.8
   lower limb 924.4
   trunk 922.8
   upper limb 923.8
muscle NEC 924.9
myocardium - *see* Contusion, cardiac
nasal (septum) (and other part(s) of neck, scalp, or face, except eye) 920
neck (and scalp, or face, any part, except eye) 920
nerve - *see* Injury, nerve, by site
nose (and other part(s) of neck, scalp, or face, except eye) 920
occipital region (scalp) (and neck or face, except eye) 920
   lobe - *see* Contusion, brain, occipital lobe
orbit (region) (tissues) 921.2
palate (soft) (and other part(s) of neck, scalp, or face, except eye) 920
parietal region (scalp) (and neck, or face, except eye) 920
   lobe - *see* Contusion, brain
penis 922.4
pericardium - *see* Contusion, cardiac
perineum 922.4
periocular area 921.1
pharynx (and other part(s) of neck, scalp, or face, except eye) 920
popliteal space (*see also* Contusion, knee) 924.11
prepuce 922.4
pubic region 922.4
pudenda 922.4
pulmonary - *see* Contusion, lung
quadriceps femoralis 924.00
rib cage 922.1
sacral region 922.32
salivary ducts or glands (and other part(s) of neck, scalp, or face, except eye) 920
scalp (and neck, or face, any part, except eye) 920
scapular region 923.01
   with shoulder or upper arm 923.09
sclera (eye) 921.3
scrotum 922.4
shoulder 923.00
   with upper arm or axillar regions 923.09

Contusion (*Continued*)
skin NEC 924.9
skull 920
spermatic cord 922.4
spinal cord - *see also* Injury, spinal, by site
   cauda equina 952.4
   conus medullaris 952.4
spleen 865.01
   with open wound into cavity 865.11
sternal region 922.1
stomach - *see* Injury, internal, stomach
subconjunctival 921.1
subcutaneous NEC 924.9
submaxillary region (and other part(s) of neck, scalp, or face, except eye) 920
submental region (and other part(s) of neck, scalp, or face, except eye) 920
subperiosteal NEC 924.9
supraclavicular fossa (and other part(s) of neck, scalp, or face, except eye) 920
supraorbital (and other part(s) of neck, scalp, or face, except eye) 920
temple (region) (and other part(s) of neck, scalp, or face, except eye) 920
testis 922.4
thigh (and hip) 924.00
thorax 922.1
   organ - *see* Injury, internal, intrathoracic
throat (and other part(s) of neck, scalp, or face, except eye) 920
thumb(s) (nail) (subungual) 923.3
toe(s) (nail) (subungual) 924.3
tongue (and other part(s) of neck, scalp, or face, except eye) 920
trunk 922.9
   multiple sites 922.8
   specified site - *see* Contusion, by site
tunica vaginalis 922.4
tympanum (membrane) (and other part(s) of neck, scalp, or face, except eye) 920
upper extremity 923.9
   multiple sites 923.8
uvula (and other part(s) of neck, scalp, or face, except eye) 920
vagina 922.4
vocal cord(s) (and other part(s) of neck, scalp, or face, except eye) 920
vulva 922.4
wrist 923.21
   with hand(s), except finger(s) alone 923.20
Conus (any type) (congenital) 743.57
acquired 371.60
medullaris syndrome 336.8
Convalescence (following) V66.9
chemotherapy V66.2
medical NEC V66.5
psychotherapy V66.3
radiotherapy V66.1
surgery NEC V66.0
treatment (for) NEC V66.5
   combined V66.6
   fracture V66.4
   mental disorder NEC V66.3
   specified disorder NEC V66.5

Conversion
  closed surgical procedure to open
      procedure
    arthroscopic V64.43
    laparoscopic V64.41
    thoracoscopic V64.42
  hysteria, hysterical, any type 300.11
  neurosis, any 300.11
  reaction, any 300.11
Converter, tuberculosis (test reaction)
  795.5
Convulsions (idiopathic) 780.39
  apoplectiform (*see also* Disease,
    cerebrovascular, acute) 436
  brain 780.39
  cerebral 780.39
  cerebrospinal 780.39
  due to trauma NEC - *see* Injury,
    intracranial
  eclamptic (*see also* Eclampsia) 780.39
  epileptic (*see also* Epilepsy) 345.9●
  epileptiform (*see also* Seizure,
    epileptiform) 780.39
  epileptoid (*see also* Seizure,
    epileptiform) 780.39
  ether
    anesthetic
      correct substance properly
        administered 780.39
      overdose or wrong substance
        given 968.2
    other specified type - *see* Table of
      Drugs and Chemicals
  febrile (simple) 780.31
    complex 780.32
  generalized 780.39
  hysterical 300.11
  infantile 780.39
    epilepsy - *see* Epilepsy
  internal 780.39
  jacksonian (*see also* Epilepsy) 345.5●
  myoclonic 333.2
  newborn 779.0
  paretic 094.1
  pregnancy (nephritic) (uremic) - *see*
    Eclampsia, pregnancy
  psychomotor (*see also* Epilepsy)
    345.4●
  puerperal, postpartum - *see* Eclampsia,
    pregnancy
  recurrent 780.39
    epileptic - *see* Epilepsy
  reflex 781.0
  repetitive 780.39
    epileptic - *see* Epilepsy
  salaam (*see also* Epilepsy) 345.6●
  scarlatinal 034.1
  spasmodic 780.39
  tetanus, tetanic (*see also* Tetanus) 037
  thymic 254.8
  uncinate 780.39
  uremic 586
Convulsive - *see also* Convulsions
  disorder or state 780.39
    epileptic - *see* Epilepsy
  equivalent, abdominal (*see also*
    Epilepsy) 345.5●
Cooke-Apert-Gallais syndrome
  (adrenogenital) 255.2
Cooley's anemia (erythroblastic) 282.49
Coolie itch 126.9
Cooper's
  disease 610.1
  hernia - *see* Hernia, Cooper's

Coordination disturbance 781.3
Copper wire arteries, retina 362.13
Copra itch 133.8
Coprolith 560.39
Coprophilia 302.89
Coproporphyria, hereditary 277.1
Coprostasis 560.39
  with hernia - *see also* Hernia, by site,
    with obstruction
    gangrenous - *see* Hernia, by site,
      with gangrene
Cor
  biloculare 745.7
  bovinum - *see* Hypertrophy, cardiac
  bovis - *see* Hypertrophy, cardiac
  pulmonale (chronic) 416.9
    acute 415.0
  triatriatum, triatrium 746.82
  triloculare 745.8
    biatriatum 745.3
    biventriculare 745.69
Corbus' disease 607.1
Cord - *see also* condition
  around neck (tightly) (with
    compression)
    affecting fetus or newborn 762.5
    complicating delivery 663.1●
      without compression 663.3●
        affecting fetus or newborn
          762.6
  bladder NEC 344.61
    tabetic 094.0
  prolapse
    affecting fetus or newborn 762.4
    complicating delivery 663.0●
Cord's angiopathy (*see also* Tuberculosis)
  017.3● *[362.18]*
Cordis ectopia 746.87
Corditis (spermatic) 608.4
Corectopia 743.46
Cori type glycogen storage disease - *see*
  Disease, glycogen storage
Cork-handlers' disease or lung 495.3
Corkscrew esophagus 530.5
Corlett's pyosis (impetigo) 684
Corn (infected) 700
Cornea - *see also* condition
  donor V59.5
  guttata (dystrophy) 371.57
  plana 743.41
Cornelia de Lange's syndrome
  (Amsterdam dwarf, mental
  retardation, and brachycephaly)
  759.89
Cornual gestation or pregnancy - *see*
  Pregnancy, cornual
Cornu cutaneum 702.8
Coronary (artery) - *see also* condition
  arising from aorta or pulmonary trunk
    746.85
Corpora - *see also* condition
  amylacea (prostate) 602.8
  cavernosa - *see* condition
Corpulence (*see also* Obesity)
Corpus - *see* condition
Corrigan's disease - *see* Insufficiency,
  aortic
Corrosive burn - *see* Burn, by site
Corsican fever (*see also* Malaria) 084.6
Cortical - *see also* condition
  blindness 377.75
  necrosis, kidney (bilateral) 583.6
Corticoadrenal - *see* condition
Corticosexual syndrome 255.2

Coryza (acute) 460
  with grippe or influenza (*see also*
    Influenza) 487.1 ◀▥
  syphilitic 095.8
    congenital (chronic) 090.0
Costen's syndrome or complex 524.60
Costiveness (*see also* Constipation) 564.00
Costochondritis 733.6
Cotard's syndrome (paranoia) 297.1
Cot death 798.0
Cotia virus 059.8
Cotungo's disease 724.3
Cough 786.2
  with hemorrhage (*see also* Hemoptysis)
    786.39 ◀▥
  affected 786.2
  bronchial 786.2
    with grippe or influenza (*see also*
      Influenza) 487.1 ◀▥
  chronic 786.2
  epidemic 786.2
  functional 306.1
  hemorrhagic 786.39 ◀▥
  hysterical 300.11
  laryngeal, spasmodic 786.2
  nervous 786.2
  psychogenic 306.1
  smokers' 491.0
  tea tasters' 112.89
Counseling NEC V65.40
  without complaint or sickness V65.49
  abuse victim NEC V62.89
    child V61.21
    partner V61.11
    spouse V61.11
  child abuse, maltreatment, or neglect
    V61.21
  contraceptive NEC V25.09
    device (intrauterine) V25.02
    maintenance V25.40
      intrauterine contraceptive device
        V25.42
      oral contraceptive (pill) V25.41
      specified type NEC V25.49
      subdermal implantable V25.43
    management NEC V25.9
    oral contraceptive (pill) V25.01
      emergency V25.03
      postcoital V25.03
    prescription NEC V25.02
      oral contraceptive (pill) V25.01
        emergency V25.03
        postcoital V25.03
        repeat prescription V25.41
      repeat prescription V25.40
    subdermal implantable V25.43
    surveillance NEC V25.40
  dietary V65.3
  exercise V65.41
  expectant parent(s)
    pediatric pre-adoption visit V65.11
    pediatric pre-birth visit V65.11
  explanation of
    investigation finding NEC V65.49
    medication NEC V65.49
  family planning V25.09
    natural
      procreative V26.41
      to avoid pregnancy V25.04
  for nonattending third party V65.19
  genetic V26.33
  gonorrhea V65.45
  health (advice) (education)
    (instruction) NEC V65.49

◀ New   ◀▥ Revised   ~~deleted~~ Deleted   ● Use Additional Digit(s)   ▨ Omit code

Counseling NEC (Continued)
  HIV V65.44
  human immunodeficiency virus V65.44
  injury prevention V65.43
  insulin pump training V65.46
  marital V61.10
  medical (for) V65.9
    boarding school resident V60.6
    condition not demonstrated V65.5
    feared complaint and no disease
        found V65.5
    institutional resident V60.6
    on behalf of another V65.19
    person living alone V60.3
  natural family planning
    procreative V26.41
    to avoid pregnancy V25.04
  parent (guardian)-child conflict V61.20
    adopted child V61.24
    biological child V61.23
    foster child V61.25
    specified problem NEC V61.29
  partner abuse
    perpetrator V61.12
    victim V61.11
  pediatric
    pre-adoption visit for adoptive
        parent(s) V65.11
    pre-birth visit for expectant parents
        V65.11
  perpetrator of
    child abuse V62.83
      parental V61.22
    partner abuse V61.12
    spouse abuse V61.12
  procreative V65.49
  sex NEC V65.49
    transmitted disease NEC V65.45
      HIV V65.44
  specified reason NEC V65.49
  spousal abuse
    perpetrator V61.12
    victim V61.11
  substance use and abuse V65.42
  syphilis V65.45
  victim (of)
    abuse NEC V62.89
    child abuse V61.21
    partner abuse V61.11
    spousal abuse V61.11
Coupled rhythm 427.89
Couvelaire uterus (complicating
    delivery) - see Placenta, separation
Cowper's gland - see condition
Cowperitis (see also Urethritis) 597.89
  gonorrheal (acute) 098.0
    chronic or duration of 2 months or
        over 098.2
Cowpox (abortive) 051.01
  due to vaccination 999.0
  eyelid 051.01 [373.5]
    postvaccination 999.0 [373.5]
Coxa
  plana 732.1
  valga (acquired) 736.31
    congenital 755.61
    late effect of rickets 268.1
  vara (acquired) 736.32
    congenital 755.62
    late effect of rickets 268.1
Coxae malum senilis 715.25
Coxalgia (nontuberculous) 719.45
  tuberculous (see also Tuberculosis)
    015.1 ● [730.85]

Coxalgic pelvis 736.30
Coxitis 716.65
Coxsackie (infection) (virus) 079.2
  central nervous system NEC 048
  endocarditis 074.22
  enteritis 008.67
  meningitis (aseptic) 047.0
  myocarditis 074.23
  pericarditis 074.21
  pharyngitis 074.0
  pleurodynia 074.1
  specific disease NEC 074.8
Crabs, meaning pubic lice 132.2
Crack baby 760.75
Cracked
  nipple 611.2
    puerperal, postpartum 676.1 ●
  tooth 521.81
Cradle cap 690.11
Craft neurosis 300.89
Craigiasis 007.8
Cramp(s) 729.82
  abdominal 789.0 ●
  bathing 994.1
  colic 789.7
    infantile 789.7
    psychogenic 306.4
  due to immersion 994.1
  extremity (lower) (upper) NEC 729.82
  fireman 992.2
  heat 992.2
  hysterical 300.11
  immersion 994.1
  intestinal 789.0 ●
    psychogenic 306.4
  linotypist's 300.89
    organic 333.84
  muscle (extremity) (general) 729.82
    due to immersion 994.1
    hysterical 300.11
  occupational (hand) 300.89
    organic 333.84
  psychogenic 307.89
  salt depletion 276.1
  sleep related leg 327.52
  stoker 992.2
  stomach 789.0 ●
  telegraphers' 300.89
    organic 333.84
  typists' 300.89
    organic 333.84
  uterus 625.8
    menstrual 625.3
  writers' 333.84
    organic 333.84
    psychogenic 300.89
Cranial - see condition
Cranioclasis, fetal 763.89
Craniocleidodysostosis 755.59
Craniofenestria (skull) 756.0
Craniolacunia (skull) 756.0
Craniopagus 759.4
Craniopathy, metabolic 733.3
Craniopharyngeal - see condition
Craniopharyngioma (M9350/1) 237.0
Craniorachischisis (totalis) 740.1
Cranioschisis 756.0
Craniostenosis 756.0
Craniosynostosis 756.0
Craniotabes (cause unknown) 733.3
  rachitic 268.1
  syphilitic 090.5
Craniotomy, fetal 763.89
Cranium - see condition
Craw-craw 125.3

CRBSI (catheter-related bloodstream
    infection) 999.31
Creaking joint 719.60
  ankle 719.67
  elbow 719.62
  foot 719.67
  hand 719.64
  hip 719.65
  knee 719.66
  multiple sites 719.69
  pelvic region 719.65
  shoulder (region) 719.61
  specified site NEC 719.68
  wrist 719.63
Creeping
  eruption 126.9
  palsy 335.21
  paralysis 335.21
Crenated tongue 529.8
Creotoxism 005.9
Crepitus
  caput 756.0
  joint 719.60
    ankle 719.67
    elbow 719.62
    foot 719.67
    hand 719.64
    hip 719.65
    knee 719.66
    multiple sites 719.69
    pelvic region 719.65
    shoulder (region) 719.61
    specified site NEC 719.68
    wrist 719.63
Crescent or conus choroid, congenital
    743.57
Cretin, cretinism (athyrotic) (congenital)
    (endemic) (metabolic) (nongoitrous)
    (sporadic) 243
  goitrous (sporadic) 246.1
  pelvis (dwarf type) (male type) 243
    with disproportion (fetopelvic)
        653.1 ●
      affecting fetus or newborn
          763.1
      causing obstructed labor 660.1 ●
        affecting fetus or newborn
            763.1
  pituitary 253.3
Cretinoid degeneration 243
Creutzfeldt-Jakob disease (CJD)
    (syndrome) 046.19
  with dementia
    with behavioral disturbance 046.19
        [294.11]
    without behavioral disturbance
        046.19 [294.10]
  familial 046.19
  iatrogenic 046.19
  specified NEC 046.19
  sporadic 046.19
  variant (vCJD) 046.11
    with dementia
      with behavioral disturbance
          046.11 [294.11]
      without behavioral disturbance
          046.11 [294.10]
Crib death 798.0
Cribriform hymen 752.49
Cri-du-chat syndrome 758.31
Crigler-Najjar disease or syndrome
    (congenital hyperbilirubinemia)
    277.4
Crimean hemorrhagic fever 065.0
Criminalism 301.7

Crisis
abdomen 789.0●
addisonian (acute adrenocortical
insufficiency) 255.41
adrenal (cortical) 255.41
asthmatic - *see* Asthma
brain, cerebral (*see also* Disease,
cerebrovascular, acute) 436
celiac 579.0
Dietl's 593.4
emotional NEC 309.29
acute reaction to stress 308.0
adjustment reaction 309.9
specific to childhood or adolescence
313.9
gastric (tabetic) 094.0
glaucomatocyclitic 364.22
heart (*see also* Failure, heart) 428.9
hypertensive - *see* Hypertension
nitritoid
correct substance properly
administered 458.29
overdose or wrong substance given
or taken 961.1
oculogyric 378.87
psychogenic 306.7
Pel's 094.0
psychosexual identity 302.6
rectum 094.0
renal 593.81
sickle cell 282.62
stomach (tabetic) 094.0
tabetic 094.0
thyroid (*see also* Thyrotoxicosis) 242.9●
thyrotoxic (*see also* Thyrotoxicosis)
242.9●
vascular - *see* Disease, cerebrovascular,
acute
Crocq's disease (acrocyanosis) 443.89
Crohn's disease (*see also* Enteritis,
regional) 555.9
Cronkhite-Canada syndrome 211.3
Crooked septum, nasal 470
Cross
birth (of fetus) complicating delivery
652.3●
with successful version 652.1●
causing obstructed labor 660.0●
bite, anterior or posterior 524.27
eye (*see also* Esotropia) 378.00
Crossed ectopia of kidney 753.3
Crossfoot 754.50
Croup, croupous (acute) (angina)
(catarrhal) (infective)
(inflammatory) (laryngeal)
(membranous) (nondiphtheritic)
(pseudomembranous) 464.4
asthmatic (*see also* Asthma) 493.9●
bronchial 466.0
diphtheritic (membranous) 032.3
false 478.75
spasmodic 478.75
diphtheritic 032.3
stridulous 478.75
diphtheritic 032.3
Crouzon's disease (craniofacial
dysostosis) 756.0
Crowding, teeth 524.31
CRST syndrome (cutaneous systemic
sclerosis) 710.1
Cruchet's disease (encephalitis lethargica)
049.8
Cruelty in children (*see also* Disturbance,
conduct) 312.9

Crural ulcer (*see also* Ulcer, lower
extremity) 707.10
Crush, crushed, crushing (injury) 929.9
abdomen 926.19
internal - *see* Injury, internal,
abdomen
ankle 928.21
with other parts of foot 928.20
arm 927.9
lower (and elbow) 927.10
upper 927.03
with shoulder or axillary region
927.09
axilla 927.02
with shoulder or upper arm 927.09
back 926.11
breast 926.19
buttock 926.12
cheek 925.1
chest - *see* Injury, internal, chest
ear 925.1
elbow 927.11
with forearm 927.10
face 925.1
finger(s) 927.3
with hand(s) 927.20
and wrist(s) 927.21
flank 926.19
foot, excluding toe(s) alone (with
ankle) 928.20
forearm (and elbow) 927.10
genitalia, external (female) (male) 926.0
internal - *see* Injury, internal, genital
organ NEC
hand, except finger(s) alone (and wrist)
927.20
head - *see* Fracture, skull, by site
heel 928.20
hip 928.01
with thigh 928.00
internal organ (abdomen, chest, or
pelvis) - *see* Injury, internal, by
site
knee 928.11
with leg, lower 928.10
labium (majus) (minus) 926.0
larynx 925.2
late effect - *see* Late, effects (of), crushing
leg 928.9
lower 928.10
and knee 928.11
upper 928.00
limb
lower 928.9
multiple sites 928.8
upper 927.9
multiple sites 927.8
multiple sites NEC 929.0
neck 925.2
nerve - *see* Injury, nerve, by site
nose 802.0
open 802.1
penis 926.0
pharynx 925.2
scalp 925.1
scapular region 927.01
with shoulder or upper arm 927.09
scrotum 926.0
shoulder 927.00
with upper arm or axillary region
927.09
skull or cranium - *see* Fracture, skull, by
site
spinal cord - *see* Injury, spinal, by site

Crush, crushed, crushing (*Continued*)
syndrome (complication of trauma)
958.5
testis 926.0
thigh (with hip) 928.00
throat 925.2
thumb(s) (and fingers) 927.3
toe(s) 928.3
with foot 928.20
and ankle 928.21
tonsil 925.2
trunk 926.9
chest - *see* Injury, internal,
intrathoracic organs NEC
internal organ - *see* Injury, internal,
by site
multiple sites 926.8
specified site NEC 926.19
vulva 926.0
wrist 927.21
with hand(s), except fingers alone
927.20
Crusta lactea 690.11
Crusts 782.8
Crutch paralysis 953.4
Cruveilhier's disease 335.21
**Cruveilhier-Baumgarten cirrhosis,
disease, or syndrome** 571.5
Cruz-Chagas disease (*see also*
Trypanosomiasis) 086.2
Crying
constant, continuous
adolescent 780.95
adult 780.95
baby 780.92
child 780.95
infant 780.92
newborn 780.92
excessive
adolescent 780.95
adult 780.95
baby 780.92
child 780.95
infant 780.92
newborn 780.92
Cryofibrinogenemia 273.2
Cryoglobulinemia (mixed) 273.2
Crypt (anal) (rectal) 569.49
Cryptitis (anal) (rectal) 569.49
Cryptococcosis (European) (pulmonary)
(systemic) 117.5
Cryptococcus 117.5
epidermicus 117.5
neoformans, infection by 117.5
Cryptopapillitis (anus) 569.49
Cryptophthalmos (eyelid) 743.06
**Cryptorchid, cryptorchism,
cryptorchidism** 752.51
Cryptosporidiosis 007.4
hepatobiliary 136.8
respiratory 136.8
Cryptotia 744.29
Crystallopathy
calcium pyrophosphate (*see also*
Arthritis) 275.49 [712.2]●
dicalcium phosphate (*see also* Arthritis)
275.49 [712.1]●
gouty 274.00
pyrophosphate NEC (*see also* Arthritis)
275.49 [712.2]●
uric acid 274.00
Crystalluria 791.9
Csillag's disease (lichen sclerosus et
atrophicus) 701.0
Cuban itch 050.1

◀ New　◀▥ Revised　~~deleted~~ Deleted　● Use Additional Digit(s)　▨ Omit code

Cubitus
  valgus (acquired) 736.01
    congenital 755.59
    late effect of rickets 268.1
  varus (acquired) 736.02
    congenital 755.59
    late effect of rickets 268.1
Cultural deprivation V62.4
Cupping of optic disc 377.14
Curling's ulcer - *see* Ulcer, duodenum
Curling esophagus 530.5
Curschmann (-Batten) (-Steinert) disease
  or syndrome 359.21
Curvature
  organ or site, congenital NEC - *see*
    Distortion
  penis (lateral) 752.69
  Pott's (spinal) (*see also* Tuberculosis)
    015.0● *[737.43]*
  radius, idiopathic, progressive
    (congenital) 755.54
  spine (acquired) (angular) (idiopathic)
    (incorrect) (postural) 737.9
    congenital 754.2
    due to or associated with
      Charcôt-Marie-Tooth disease
        356.1 *[737.40]*
      mucopolysaccharidosis 277.5
        [737.40]
      neurofibromatosis 237.71 *[737.40]*
      osteitis
        deformans 731.0 *[737.40]*
        fibrosa cystica 252.01 *[737.40]*
      osteoporosis (*see also*
        Osteoporosis) 733.00
        [737.40]
      poliomyelitis (*see also*
        Poliomyelitis) 138 *[737.40]*
      tuberculosis (Pott's curvature) (*see*
        also Tuberculosis) 015.0●
        [737.43]
    kyphoscoliotic (*see also*
      Kyphoscoliosis) 737.30
    kyphotic (*see also* Kyphosis) 737.10
    late effect of rickets 268.1 *[737.40]*
    Pott's 015.0● *[737.40]*
    scoliotic (*see also* Scoliosis) 737.30
    specified NEC 737.8
    tuberculous 015.0● *[737.40]*
Cushing's
  basophilism, disease, or syndrome
    (iatrogenic) (idiopathic) (pituitary
    basophilism) (pituitary
    dependent) 255.0
  ulcer - *see* Ulcer, peptic
Cushingoid due to steroid therapy
  correct substance properly
    administered 255.0
  overdose or wrong substance given or
    taken 962.0
Cut (external) - *see* Wound, open, by site
Cutaneous - *see also* condition
  hemorrhage 782.7
  horn (cheek) (eyelid) (mouth) 702.8
  larva migrans 126.9
Cutis - *see also* condition
  hyperelastic 756.83
    acquired 701.8
  laxa 756.83
    senilis 701.8
  marmorata 782.61
  osteosis 709.3
  pendula 756.83
    acquired 701.8

Cutis (*Continued*)
  rhomboidalis nuchae 701.8
  verticis gyrata 757.39
    acquired 701.8
Cyanopathy, newborn 770.83
Cyanosis 782.5
  autotoxic 289.7
  common atrioventricular canal
    745.69
  congenital 770.83
  conjunctiva 372.71
  due to
    endocardial cushion defect
      745.60
    nonclosure, foramen botalli 745.5
    patent foramen botalli 745.5
    persistent foramen ovale 745.5
  enterogenous 289.7
  fetus or newborn 770.83
  ostium primum defect 745.61
  paroxysmal digital 443.0
  retina, retinal 362.10
Cycle
  anovulatory 628.0
  menstrual, irregular 626.4
Cyclencephaly 759.89
Cyclical vomiting 536.2
  associated with migraine 346.2●
  psychogenic 306.4
Cyclitic membrane 364.74
Cyclitis (*see also* Iridocyclitis) 364.3
  acute 364.00
    primary 364.01
    recurrent 364.02
  chronic 364.10
    in
      sarcoidosis 135 *[364.11]*
      tuberculosis (*see also* Tuberculosis)
        017.3● *[364.11]*
  Fuchs' heterochromic 364.21
  granulomatous 364.10
  lens induced 364.23
  nongranulomatous 364.00
  posterior 363.21
  primary 364.01
  recurrent 364.02
  secondary (noninfectious) 364.04
    infectious 364.03
  subacute 364.00
    primary 364.01
    recurrent 364.02
Cyclokeratitis - *see* Keratitis
Cyclophoria 378.44
Cyclopia, cyclops 759.89
Cycloplegia 367.51
Cyclospasm 367.53
Cyclosporiasis 007.5
Cyclothymia 301.13
Cyclothymic personality 301.13
Cyclotropia 378.33
Cyesis - *see* Pregnancy
Cylindroma (M8200/3) - *see also*
  Neoplasm, by site, malignant
  eccrine dermal (M8200/0) - *see*
    Neoplasm, skin, benign
  skin (M8200/0) - *see* Neoplasm, skin,
    benign
Cylindruria 791.7
Cyllosoma 759.89
Cynanche
  diphtheritic 032.3
  tonsillaris 475
Cynorexia 783.6
Cyphosis - *see* Kyphosis

Cyprus fever (*see also* Brucellosis) 023.9
Cyriax's syndrome (slipping rib) 733.99
Cyst (mucus) (retention) (serous) (simple)

> Note: In general, cysts are not
> neoplastic and are classified to the
> appropriate category for disease of
> the specified anatomical site. This
> generalization does not apply to certain
> types of cysts which are neoplastic in
> nature, for example, dermoid, nor does
> it apply to cysts of certain structures,
> for example, branchial cleft, which are
> classified as developmental anomalies.
>
> The following listing includes some
> of the most frequently reported sites
> of cysts as well as qualifiers which
> indicate the type of cyst. The latter
> qualifiers usually are not repeated
> under the anatomical sites. Since the
> code assignment for a given site may
> vary depending upon the type of cyst,
> the coder should refer to the listings
> under the specified type of cyst before
> consideration is given to the site.

  accessory, fallopian tube 752.11
  adenoid (infected) 474.8
  adrenal gland 255.8
    congenital 759.1
  air, lung 518.89
  allantoic 753.7
  alveolar process (jaw bone) 526.2
  amnion, amniotic 658.8●
  anterior chamber (eye) 364.60
    exudative 364.62
    implantation (surgical) (traumatic)
      364.61
    parasitic 360.13
  anterior nasopalatine 526.1
  antrum 478.19
  anus 569.49
  apical (periodontal) (tooth) 522.8
  appendix 543.9
  arachnoid, brain 348.0
  arytenoid 478.79
  auricle 706.2
  Baker's (knee) 727.51
    tuberculous (*see also* Tuberculosis)
      015.2●
  Bartholin's gland or duct 616.2
  bile duct (*see also* Disease, biliary)
    576.8
  bladder (multiple) (trigone) 596.8
  Blessig's 362.62
  blood, endocardial (*see also*
    Endocarditis) 424.90
  blue dome 610.0
  bone (local) 733.20
    aneurysmal 733.22
    jaw 526.2
      developmental (odontogenic)
        526.0
      fissural 526.1
      latent 526.89
    solitary 733.21
    unicameral 733.21
  brain 348.0
    congenital 742.4
    hydatid (*see also* Echinococcus)
      122.9
    third ventricle (colloid) 742.4
  branchial (cleft) 744.42
  branchiogenic 744.42

Cyst (Continued)
    breast (benign) (blue dome)
        (pedunculated) (solitary)
        (traumatic) 610.0
        involution 610.4
        sebaceous 610.8
    broad ligament (benign) 620.8
        embryonic 752.11
    bronchogenic (mediastinal)
        (sequestration) 518.89
        congenital 748.4
    buccal 528.4
    bulbourethral gland (Cowper's) 599.89
    bursa, bursal 727.49
        pharyngeal 478.26
    calcifying odontogenic (M9301/0) 213.1
        upper jaw (bone) 213.0
    canal of Nuck (acquired) (serous) 629.1
        congenital 752.41
    canthus 372.75
    carcinomatous (M8010/3) - see
        Neoplasm, by site, malignant
    cartilage (joint) - see Derangement, joint
    cauda equina 336.8
    cavum septi pellucidi NEC 348.0
    celomic (pericardium) 746.89
    cerebellopontine (angle) - see Cyst,
        brain
    cerebellum - see Cyst, brain
    cerebral - see Cyst, brain
    cervical lateral 744.42
    cervix 622.8
        embryonal 752.41
        nabothian (gland) 616.0
    chamber, anterior (eye) 364.60
        exudative 364.62
        implantation (surgical) (traumatic)
            364.61
        parasitic 360.13
    chiasmal, optic NEC (see also Lesion,
        chiasmal) 377.54
    chocolate (ovary) 617.1
    choledochal (congenital) 751.69
        acquired 576.8
    choledochus 751.69
    chorion 658.8 ●
    choroid plexus 348.0
    chyle, mesentery 457.8
    ciliary body 364.60
        exudative 364.64
        implantation 364.61
        primary 364.63
    clitoris 624.8
    coccyx (see also Cyst, bone) 733.20
    colloid
        third ventricle (brain) 742.4
        thyroid gland - see Goiter
    colon 569.89
    common (bile) duct (see also Disease,
        biliary) 576.8
    congenital NEC 759.89
        adrenal glands 759.1
        epiglottis 748.3
        esophagus 750.4
        fallopian tube 752.11
        kidney 753.10
            multiple 753.19
            single 753.11
        larynx 748.3
        liver 751.62
        lung 748.4
        mediastinum 748.8
        ovary 752.0
        oviduct 752.11

Cyst (Continued)
    congenital NEC (Continued)
        pancreas 751.7
        periurethral (tissue) 753.8
        prepuce NEC 752.69
            penis 752.69
        sublingual 750.26
        submaxillary gland 750.26
        thymus (gland) 759.2
        tongue 750.19
        ureterovesical orifice 753.4
        vulva 752.41
    conjunctiva 372.75
    cornea 371.23
    corpora quadrigemina 348.0
    corpus
        albicans (ovary) 620.2
        luteum (ruptured) 620.1
    Cowper's gland (benign) (infected)
        599.89
    cranial meninges 348.0
    craniobuccal pouch 253.8
    craniopharyngeal pouch 253.8
    cystic duct (see also Disease,
        gallbladder) 575.8
    Cysticercus (any site) 123.1
    Dandy-Walker 742.3
        with spina bifida (see also Spina
            bifida) 741.0 ●
    dental 522.8
        developmental 526.0
        eruption 526.0
        lateral periodontal 526.0
        primordial (keratocyst) 526.0
        root 522.8
    dentigerous 526.0
        mandible 526.0
        maxilla 526.0
    dermoid (M9084/0) - see also
        Neoplasm, by site, benign
        with malignant transformation
            (M9084/3) 183.0
        implantation
            external area or site (skin) NEC
                709.8
            iris 364.61
            skin 709.8
            vagina 623.8
            vulva 624.8
        mouth 528.4
        oral soft tissue 528.4
        sacrococcygeal 685.1
            with abscess 685.0
    developmental of ovary, ovarian
        752.0
    dura (cerebral) 348.0
        spinal 349.2
    ear (external) 706.2
    echinococcal (see also Echinococcus)
        122.9
    embryonal
        cervix uteri 752.41
        genitalia, female external 752.41
        uterus 752.39 ◄
        vagina 752.41
    endometrial 621.8
        ectopic 617.9
    endometrium (uterus) 621.8
        ectopic - see Endometriosis
    enteric 751.5
    enterogenous 751.5
    epidermal (inclusion) (see also Cyst,
        skin) 706.2

Cyst (Continued)
    epidermoid (inclusion) (see also Cyst,
        skin) 706.2
        mouth 528.4
        not of skin - see Cyst, by site
        oral soft tissue 528.4
    epididymis 608.89
    epiglottis 478.79
    epiphysis cerebri 259.8
    epithelial (inclusion) (see also Cyst,
        skin) 706.2
    epoophoron 752.11
    eruption 526.0
    esophagus 530.89
    ethmoid sinus 478.19
    eye (retention) 379.8
        congenital 743.03
        posterior segment, congenital 743.54
    eyebrow 706.2
    eyelid (sebaceous) 374.84
        infected 373.13
        sweat glands or ducts 374.84
    falciform ligament (inflammatory)
        573.8
    fallopian tube 620.8
        congenital 752.11
    female genital organs NEC 629.89
    fimbrial (congenital) 752.11
    fissural (oral region) 526.1
    follicle (atretic) (graafian) (ovarian)
        620.0
        nabothian (gland) 616.0
    follicular (atretic) (ovarian) 620.0
        dentigerous 526.0
    frontal sinus 478.19
    gallbladder or duct 575.8
    ganglion 727.43
    Gartner's duct 752.41
    gas, of mesentery 568.89
    gingiva 523.8
    gland of moll 374.84
    globulomaxillary 526.1
    graafian follicle 620.0
    granulosal lutein 620.2
    hemangiomatous (M9121/0) (see also
        Hemangioma) 228.00
    hydatid (see also Echinococcus) 122.9
        fallopian tube (Morgagni) 752.11
        liver NEC 122.8
        lung NEC 122.9
        Morgagni 752.89
            fallopian tube 752.11
        specified site NEC 122.9
    hymen 623.8
        embryonal 752.41
    hypopharynx 478.26
    hypophysis, hypophyseal (duct)
        (recurrent) 253.8
        cerebri 253.8
    implantation (dermoid)
        anterior chamber (eye) 364.61
        external area or site (skin) NEC
            709.8
        iris 364.61
        vagina 623.8
        vulva 624.8
    incisor, incisive canal 526.1
    inclusion (epidermal) (epithelial)
        (epidermoid) (mucous)
        (squamous) (see also Cyst, skin)
        706.2
        not of skin - see Neoplasm, by site,
            benign
    intestine (large) (small) 569.89

◄ New   ◄▥ Revised   ~~deleted~~ Deleted   ● Use Additional Digit(s)   ▨ Omit code

Cyst (Continued)
  intracranial - see Cyst, brain
  intraligamentous 728.89
    knee 717.89
  intrasellar 253.8
  iris (idiopathic) 364.60
    exudative 364.62
    implantation (surgical) (traumatic)
      364.61
    miotic pupillary 364.55
    parasitic 360.13
  Iwanoff's 362.62
  jaw (bone) (aneurysmal)
      (extravasation) (hemorrhagic)
      (traumatic) 526.2
    developmental (odontogenic) 526.0
    fissural 526.1
  keratin 706.2
  kidney (congenital) 753.10
    acquired 593.2
    calyceal (see also Hydronephrosis)
      591
    multiple 753.19
    pyelogenic (see also Hydronephrosis)
      591
    simple 593.2
    single 753.11
    solitary (not congenital) 593.2
  labium (majus) (minus) 624.8
    sebaceous 624.8
  lacrimal
    apparatus 375.43
    gland or sac 375.12
  larynx 478.79
  lens 379.39
    congenital 743.39
  lip (gland) 528.5
  liver 573.8
    congenital 751.62
    hydatid (see also Echinococcus) 122.8
      granulosis 122.0
      multilocularis 122.5
  lung 518.89
    congenital 748.4
    giant bullous 492.0
  lutein 620.1
  lymphangiomatous (M9173/0) 228.1
  lymphoepithelial
    mouth 528.4
    oral soft tissue 528.4
  macula 362.54
  malignant (M8000/3) - see Neoplasm,
    by site, malignant
  mammary gland (sweat gland) (see also
    Cyst, breast) 610.0
  mandible 526.2
    dentigerous 526.0
    radicular 522.8
  maxilla 526.2
    dentigerous 526.0
    radicular 522.8
  median
    anterior maxillary 526.1
    palatal 526.1
  mediastinum (congenital) 748.8
  meibomian (gland) (retention) 373.2
    infected 373.12
  membrane, brain 348.0
  meninges (cerebral) 348.0
    spinal 349.2
  meniscus knee 717.5
  mesentery, mesenteric (gas) 568.89
    chyle 457.8
    gas 568.89

Cyst (Continued)
  mesonephric duct 752.89
  mesothelial
    peritoneum 568.89
    pleura (peritoneal) 568.89
  milk 611.5
  miotic pupillary (iris) 364.55
  Morgagni (hydatid) 752.89
    fallopian tube 752.11
  mouth 528.4
  Müllerian duct 752.89
    appendix testis 608.89
    cervix (embryonal) 752.41
    fallopian tube 752.11
    prostatic utricle 599.89
    vagina (embryonal) 752.41
  multilocular (ovary) (M8000/1)
    239.5
  myometrium 621.8
  nabothian (follicle) (ruptured) 616.0
  nasal sinus 478.19
  nasoalveolar 528.4
  nasolabial 528.4
  nasopalatine (duct) 526.1
    anterior 526.1
  nasopharynx 478.26
  neoplastic (M8000/1) - see also
      Neoplasm, by site, unspecified
      nature
    benign (M8000/0) - see Neoplasm,
        by site, benign
      uterus 621.8
  nervous system - see Cyst, brain
  neuroenteric 742.59
  neuroepithelial ventricle 348.0
  nipple 610.0
  nose 478.19
    skin of 706.2
  odontogenic, developmental 526.0
  omentum (lesser) 568.89
    congenital 751.8
  oral soft tissue (dermoid) (epidermoid)
    (lymphoepithelial) 528.4
  ora serrata 361.19
  orbit 376.81
  ovary, ovarian (twisted) 620.2
    adherent 620.2
    chocolate 617.1
    corpus
      albicans 620.2
      luteum 620.1
    dermoid (M9084/0) 220
    developmental 752.0
    due to failure of involution NEC
      620.2
    endometrial 617.1
    follicular (atretic) (graafian)
      (hemorrhagic) 620.0
    hemorrhagic 620.2
    in pregnancy or childbirth 654.4●
      affecting fetus or newborn 763.89
      causing obstructed labor 660.2●
        affecting fetus or newborn
          763.1
    multilocular (M8000/1) 239.5
    pseudomucinous (M8470/0) 220
    retention 620.2
    serous 620.2
    theca lutein 620.2
    tuberculous (see also Tuberculosis)
      016.6●
    unspecified 620.2
  oviduct 620.8
  palatal papilla (jaw) 526.1

Cyst (Continued)
  palate 526.1
    fissural 526.1
      median (fissural) 526.1
  palatine, of papilla 526.1
  pancreas, pancreatic 577.2
    congenital 751.7
    false 577.2
    hemorrhagic 577.2
    true 577.2
  paralabral
    hip 718.85
    shoulder 840.7
  paramesonephric duct - see Cyst,
    Müllerian duct
  paranephric 593.2
  paraovarian 752.11
  paraphysis, cerebri 742.4
  parasitic NEC 136.9
  parathyroid (gland) 252.8
  paratubal (fallopian) 620.8
  paraurethral duct 599.89
  paroophoron 752.11
  parotid gland 527.6
    mucous extravasation or retention
      527.6
  parovarian 752.11
  pars planus 364.60
    exudative 364.64
    primary 364.63
  pelvis, female
    in pregnancy or childbirth 654.4●
      affecting fetus or newborn 763.89
      causing obstructed labor 660.2●
        affecting fetus or newborn
          763.1
  penis (sebaceous) 607.89
  periapical 522.8
  pericardial (congenital) 746.89
    acquired (secondary) 423.8
  pericoronal 526.0
  perineural (Tarlov's) 355.9
  periodontal 522.8
    lateral 526.0
  peripancreatic 577.2
  peripelvic (lymphatic) 593.2
  peritoneum 568.89
    chylous 457.8
  pharynx (wall) 478.26
  pilonidal (infected) (rectum) 685.1
    with abscess 685.0
    malignant (M9084/3) 173.5
  pituitary (duct) (gland) 253.8
  placenta (amniotic) - see Placenta,
    abnormal
  pleura 519.8
  popliteal 727.51
  porencephalic 742.4
    acquired 348.0
  postanal (infected) 685.1
    with abscess 685.0
  posterior segment of eye, congenital
    743.54
  postmastoidectomy cavity 383.31
  preauricular 744.47
  prepuce 607.89
    congenital 752.69
  primordial (jaw) 526.0
  prostate 600.3
  pseudomucinous (ovary) (M8470/0) 220
  pudenda (sweat glands) 624.8
  pupillary, miotic 364.55
    sebaceous 624.8
  radicular (residual) 522.8

Cyst (Continued)
  radiculodental 522.8
  ranular 527.6
  Rathke's pouch 253.8
  rectum (epithelium) (mucous) 569.49
  renal - see Cyst, kidney
  residual (radicular) 522.8
  retention (ovary) 620.2
  retina 361.19
    macular 362.54
    parasitic 360.13
    primary 361.13
    secondary 361.14
  retroperitoneal 568.89
  sacrococcygeal (dermoid) 685.1
    with abscess 685.0
  salivary gland or duct 527.6
    mucous extravasation or retention
      527.6
  Sampson's 617.1
  sclera 379.19
  scrotum (sebaceous) 706.2
    sweat glands 706.2
  sebaceous (duct) (gland) 706.2
    breast 610.8
    eyelid 374.84
    genital organ NEC
      female 629.89
      male 608.89
    scrotum 706.2
  semilunar cartilage (knee) (multiple)
    717.5
  seminal vesicle 608.89
  serous (ovary) 620.2
  sinus (antral) (ethmoidal) (frontal)
    (maxillary) (nasal) (sphenoidal)
    478.19
  Skene's gland 599.89
  skin (epidermal) (epidermoid,
    inclusion) (epithelial) (inclusion)
    (retention) (sebaceous) 706.2
    breast 610.8
    eyelid 374.84
    genital organ NEC
      female 629.89
      male 608.89
    neoplastic 216.3
    scrotum 706.2
    sweat gland or duct 705.89
  solitary
    bone 733.21
    kidney 593.2
  spermatic cord 608.89
  sphenoid sinus 478.19
  spinal meninges 349.2
  spine (see also Cyst, bone) 733.20
  spleen NEC 289.59
    congenital 759.0
    hydatid (see also Echinococcus) 122.9
  spring water (pericardium) 746.89
  subarachnoid 348.0
    intrasellar 793.0
  subdural (cerebral) 348.0
    spinal cord 349.2
  sublingual gland 527.6
    mucous extravasation or retention
      527.6
  submaxillary gland 527.6
    mucous extravasation or retention
      527.6
  suburethral 599.89
  suprarenal gland 255.8
  suprasellar - see Cyst, brain
  sweat gland or duct 705.89

Cyst (Continued)
  sympathetic nervous system 337.9
  synovial 727.40
    popliteal space 727.51
  Tarlov's 355.9
  tarsal 373.2
  tendon (sheath) 727.42
  testis 608.89
  theca-lutein (ovary) 620.2
  Thornwaldt's, Tornwaldt's 478.26
  thymus (gland) 254.8
  thyroglossal (duct) (infected)
    (persistent) 759.2
  thyroid (gland) 246.2
    adenomatous - see Goiter, nodular
    colloid (see also Goiter) 240.9
  thyrolingual duct (infected) (persistent)
    759.2
  tongue (mucous) 529.8
  tonsil 474.8
  tooth (dental root) 522.8
  tubo-ovarian 620.8
    inflammatory 614.1
  tunica vaginalis 608.89
  turbinate (nose) (see also Cyst, bone)
    733.20
  Tyson's gland (benign) (infected)
    607.89
  umbilicus 759.89
  urachus 753.7
  ureter 593.89
  ureterovesical orifice 593.89
    congenital 753.4
  urethra 599.84
  urethral gland (Cowper's) 599.89
  uterine
    ligament 620.8
      embryonic 752.11
    tube 620.8
  uterus (body) (corpus) (recurrent) 621.8
    embryonal 752.39 ◀▥
  utricle (ear) 386.8
    prostatic 599.89
  utriculus masculinus 599.89
  vagina, vaginal (squamous cell) (wall)
    623.8
    embryonal 752.41
    implantation 623.8
    inclusion 623.8
  vallecula, vallecular 478.79
  ventricle, neuroepithelial 348.0
  verumontanum 599.89
  vesical (orifice) 596.8
  vitreous humor 379.29
  vulva (sweat glands) 624.8
    congenital 752.41
    implantation 624.8
    inclusion 624.8
    sebaceous gland 624.8
  vulvovaginal gland 624.8
  wolffian 752.89
Cystadenocarcinoma (M8440/3) - see also
    Neoplasm, by site, malignant
  bile duct type (M8161/3) 155.1
  endometrioid (M8380/3) - see
    Neoplasm, by site, malignant
  mucinous (M8470/3)
    papillary (M8471/3)
      specified site - see Neoplasm, by
        site, malignant
      unspecified site 183.0
    specified site - see Neoplasm, by site,
      malignant
    unspecified site 183.0

Cystadenocarcinoma (Continued)
  papillary (M8450/3)
    mucinous (M8471/3)
      specified site - see Neoplasm, by
        site, malignant
      unspecified site 183.0
    pseudomucinous (M8471/3)
      specified site - see Neoplasm, by
        site, malignant
      unspecified site 183.0
    serous (M8460/3)
      specified site - see Neoplasm, by
        site, malignant
      unspecified site 183.0
    specified site - see Neoplasm, by site,
      malignant
    unspecified 183.0
  pseudomucinous (M8470/3)
    papillary (M8471/3)
      specified site - see Neoplasm, by
        site, malignant
      unspecified site 183.0
    specified site - see Neoplasm, by site,
      malignant
    unspecified site 183.0
  serous (M8441/3)
    papillary (M8460/3)
      specified site - see Neoplasm, by
        site, malignant
      unspecified site 183.0
    specified site - see Neoplasm, by site,
      malignant
    unspecified site 183.0
Cystadenofibroma (M9013/0)
  clear cell (M8313/0) - see Neoplasm, by
    site, benign
  endometrioid (M8381/0) 220
    borderline malignancy (M8381/1)
      236.2
    malignant (M8381/3) 183.0
  mucinous (M9015/0)
    specified site - see Neoplasm, by site,
      benign
    unspecified site 220
  serous (M9014/0)
    specified site - see Neoplasm, by site,
      benign
    unspecified site 220
  specified site - see Neoplasm, by site,
    benign
  unspecified site 220
Cystadenoma (M8440/0) - see also
    Neoplasm, by site, benign
  bile duct (M8161/0) 211.5
  endometrioid (M8380/0) - see also
    Neoplasm, by site, benign
    borderline malignancy (M8380/1) -
      see Neoplasm, by site,
      uncertain behavior
  malignant (M8440/3) - see Neoplasm,
    by site, malignant
  mucinous (M8470/0)
    borderline malignancy
      (M8470/1)
      specified site - see Neoplasm,
        uncertain behavior
      unspecified site 236.2
    papillary (M8471/0)
      borderline malignancy
        (M8471/1)
        specified site - see Neoplasm,
          by site, uncertain
          behavior
      unspecified site 236.2

Cystadenoma *(Continued)*
  mucinous *(Continued)*
    papillary *(Continued)*
      specified site - *see* Neoplasm, by
        site, benign
      unspecified site 220
    specified site - *see* Neoplasm, by site,
      benign
    unspecified site 220
  papillary (M8450/0)
    borderline malignancy (M8450/1)
      specified site - *see* Neoplasm, by
        site, uncertain behavior
      unspecified site 236.2
    lymphomatosum (M8561/0) 210.2
    mucinous (M8471/0)
      borderline malignancy (M8471/1)
        specified site - *see* Neoplasm, by
          site, uncertain behavior
        unspecified site 236.2
      specified site - *see* Neoplasm, by
        site, benign
      unspecified site 220
    pseudomucinous (M8471/0)
      borderline malignancy (M8471/1)
        specified site - *see* Neoplasm,
          by site uncertain
          behavior
        unspecified site 236.2
      specified site - *see* Neoplasm, by
        site, benign
      unspecified site 220
  serous (M8460/0)
    borderline malignancy (M8460/1)
      specified site - *see* Neoplasm,
        by site, uncertain
        behavior
      unspecified site 236.2
    specified site - *see* Neoplasm, by
      site, benign
    unspecified site 220
    specified site - *see* Neoplasm, by site,
      benign
    unspecified site 220
  pseudomucinous (M8470/0)
    borderline malignancy (M8470/1)
      specified site - *see* Neoplasm, by
        site uncertain behavior
      unspecified site 236.2
    papillary (M8471/0)
      borderline malignancy (M8471/1)
        specified site - *see* Neoplasm,
          by site uncertain
          behavior
        unspecified site 236.2
      specified site - *see* Neoplasm, by
        site, benign
      unspecified site 220
    specified site - *see* Neoplasm, by site,
      benign
    unspecified site 220
  serous (M8441/0)
    borderline malignancy (M8441/1)
      specified site - *see* Neoplasm, by
        site, uncertain behavior
      unspecified site 236.2
    papillary (M8460/0)
      borderline malignancy (M8460/1)
        specified site - *see* Neoplasm,
          by site, uncertain
          behavior
        unspecified site 236.2
      specified site - *see* Neoplasm, by
        site, benign
      unspecified site 220

Cystadenoma *(Continued)*
  serous *(Continued)*
    specified site - *see* Neoplasm, by site,
      benign
    unspecified site 220
  thyroid 226
Cystathioninemia 270.4
Cystathioninuria 270.4
Cystic - *see also* condition
  breast, chronic 610.1
  corpora lutea 620.1
  degeneration, congenital
    brain 742.4
    kidney (*see also* Cystic, disease,
      kidney) 753.10
  disease
    breast, chronic 610.1
    kidney, congenital 753.10
      medullary 753.16
      multiple 753.19
      polycystic - *see* Polycystic, kidney
      single 753.11
      specified NEC 753.19
    liver, congenital 751.62
    lung 518.89
      congenital 748.4
    pancreas, congenital 751.7
    semilunar cartilage 717.5
  duct - *see* condition
  eyeball, congenital 743.03
  fibrosis (pancreas) 277.00
    with
      manifestations
        gastrointestinal 277.03
        pulmonary 277.02
        specified NEC 277.09
      meconium ileus 277.01
      pulmonary exacerbation 277.02
  hygroma (M9173/0) 228.1
  kidney, congenital 753.10
    medullary 753.16
    multiple 753.19
    polycystic - *see* Polycystic, kidney
    single 753.11
    specified NEC 753.19
  liver, congenital 751.62
  lung 518.89
    congenital 748.4
  mass - *see* Cyst
  mastitis, chronic 610.1
  ovary 620.2
  pancreas, congenital 751.7
Cysticerciasis 123.1
Cysticercosis (mammary) (subretinal)
  123.1
Cysticercus 123.1
  cellulosae infestation 123.1
Cystinosis (malignant) 270.0
Cystinuria 270.0
Cystitis (bacillary) (colli) (diffuse)
    (exudative) (hemorrhagic)
    (purulent) (recurrent) (septic)
    (suppurative) (ulcerative) 595.9
  with
    abortion - *see* Abortion, by type,
      with urinary tract infection
    ectopic pregnancy (*see also*
      categories 633.0–633.9) 639.8
    fibrosis 595.1
    leukoplakia 595.1
    malakoplakia 595.1
    metaplasia 595.1
    molar pregnancy (*see also* categories
      630–632) 639.8

Cystitis *(Continued)*
  actinomycotic 039.8 *[595.4]*
  acute 595.0
    of trigone 595.3
  allergic 595.89
  amebic 006.8 *[595.4]*
  bilharzial 120.9 *[595.4]*
  blennorrhagic (acute) 098.11
    chronic or duration of 2 months or
      more 098.31
  bullous 595.89
  calculous 594.1
  chlamydial 099.53
  chronic 595.2
    interstitial 595.1
    of trigone 595.3
  complicating pregnancy, childbirth, or
    puerperium 646.6●
    affecting fetus or newborn 760.1
  cystic(a) 595.81
  diphtheritic 032.84
  echinococcal
    glanulosus 122.3 *[595.4]*
    multilocularis 122.6 *[595.4]*
  emphysematous 595.89
  encysted 595.81
  follicular 595.3
  following
    abortion 639.8
    ectopic or molar pregnancy 639.8
  gangrenous 595.89
  glandularis 595.89
  gonococcal (acute) 098.11
    chronic or duration of 2 months or
      more 098.31
  incrusted 595.89
  interstitial 595.1
  irradiation 595.82
  irritation 595.89
  malignant 595.89
  monilial 112.2
  of trigone 595.3
  panmural 595.1
  polyposa 595.89
  prostatic 601.3
  radiation 595.82
  Reiter's (abacterial) 099.3
  specified NEC 595.89
  subacute 595.2
  submucous 595.1
  syphilitic 095.8
  trichomoniasis 131.09
  tuberculous (*see also* Tuberculosis)
    016.1●
  ulcerative 595.1
Cystocele
  female (without uterine prolapse)
    618.01
    with uterine prolapse 618.4
      complete 618.3
      incomplete 618.2
    lateral 618.02
    midline 618.01
    paravaginal 618.02
  in pregnancy or childbirth 654.4●
    affecting fetus or newborn 763.89
    causing obstructed labor 660.2●
      affecting fetus or newborn 763.1
  male 596.8
Cystoid
  cicatrix limbus 372.64
  degeneration macula 362.53
Cystolithiasis 594.1

◀ New   ◀║ Revised   ~~deleted~~ Deleted   ● Use Additional Digit(s)   Omit code

Cystoma (M8440/0) - *see also* Neoplasm, by site, benign
  endometrial, ovary 617.1
  mucinous (M8470/0)
    specified site - *see* Neoplasm, by site, benign
    unspecified site 220
  serous (M8441/0)
    specified site - *see* Neoplasm, by site, benign
    unspecified site 220
  simple (ovary) 620.2
Cystoplegia 596.53
Cystoptosis 596.8
Cystopyelitis (*see also* Pyelitis) 590.80
Cystorrhagia 596.8

Cystosarcoma phyllodes (M9020/1) 238.3
  benign (M9020/0) 217
  malignant (M9020/3) - *see* Neoplasm, breast, malignant
Cystostomy status V44.50
  with complication 997.5
  appendico-vesicostomy V44.52
  cutaneous-vesicostomy V44.51
  specified type NEC V44.59
Cystourethritis (*see also* Urethritis) 597.89
Cystourethrocele (*see also* Cystocele)
  female (without uterine prolapse) 618.09
    with uterine prolapse 618.4
      complete 618.3
      incomplete 618.2
  male 596.8

Cytomegalic inclusion disease 078.5
  congenital 771.1
Cytomycosis, reticuloendothelial (*see also* Histoplasmosis, American) 115.00
Cytopenia 289.9
  refractory
    with
      multilineage dysplasia (RCMD) 238.72
      and ringed sideroblasts (RCMD-RS) 238.72

◄ New   ◄▥ Revised   ~~deleted~~ Deleted   ● Use Additional Digit(s)   ▥ Omit code

D

Daae (-Finsen) disease (epidemic pleurodynia) 074.1
Dabney's grip 074.1
Da Costa's syndrome (neurocirculatory asthenia) 306.2
Dacryoadenitis, dacryadenitis 375.00
  acute 375.01
  chronic 375.02
Dacryocystitis 375.30
  acute 375.32
  chronic 375.42
  neonatal 771.6
  phlegmonous 375.33
  syphilitic 095.8
    congenital 090.0
  trachomatous, active 076.1
    late effect 139.1
  tuberculous (see also Tuberculosis) 017.3●
Dacryocystoblenorrhea 375.42
Dacryocystocele 375.43
Dacryolith, dacryolithiasis 375.57
Dacryoma 375.43
Dacryopericystitis (acute) (subacute) 375.32
  chronic 375.42
Dacryops 375.11
Dacryosialadenopathy, atrophic 710.2
Dacryostenosis 375.56
  congenital 743.65
Dactylitis
  bone (see also Osteomyelitis) 730.2●
  sickle-cell 282.62
    Hb-C 282.64
    Hb-SS 282.62
    specified NEC 282.69
  syphilitic 095.5
  tuberculous (see also Tuberculosis) 015.5●
Dactylolysis spontanea 136.0
Dactylosymphysis (see also Syndactylism) 755.10
Damage
  arteriosclerotic - see Arteriosclerosis
  brain 348.9
    anoxic, hypoxic 348.1
      during or resulting from a procedure 997.01
      ischemic, in newborn 768.70
        mild 768.71
        moderate 768.72
        severe 768.73
    child NEC 343.9
    due to birth injury 767.0
    minimal (child) (see also Hyperkinesia) 314.9
    newborn 767.0
  cardiac - see also Disease, heart
  cardiorenal (vascular) (see also Hypertension, cardiorenal) 404.90
  central nervous system - see Damage, brain
  cerebral NEC - see Damage, brain
  coccyx, complicating delivery 665.6●
  coronary (see also Ischemia, heart) 414.9
  eye, birth injury 767.8
  heart - see also Disease, heart
    valve - see Endocarditis
  hypothalamus NEC 348.9
  liver 571.9
    alcoholic 571.3
  medication 995.20
  myocardium (see also Degeneration, myocardial) 429.1
  pelvic

Damage (Continued)
  pelvic (Continued)
    joint or ligament, during delivery 665.6●
    organ NEC
      with
        abortion - see Abortion, by type, with damage to pelvic organs
        ectopic pregnancy (see also categories 633.0–633.9) 639.2
        molar pregnancy (see also categories 630–632) 639.2
      during delivery 665.5●
      following
        abortion 639.2
        ectopic or molar pregnancy 639.2
  renal (see also Disease, renal) 593.9
  skin, solar 692.79
    acute 692.72
    chronic 692.74
  subendocardium, subendocardial (see also Degeneration, myocardial) 429.1
  vascular 459.9
Dameshek's syndrome (erythroblastic anemia) 282.49
Dana-Putnam syndrome (subacute combined sclerosis with pernicious anemia) 281.0 [336.2]
Danbolt (-Closs) syndrome (acrodermatitis enteropathica) 686.8
Dandruff 690.18
Dandy fever 061
Dandy-Walker deformity or syndrome (atresia, foramen of Magendie) 742.3
  with spina bifida (see also Spina bifida) 741.0●
Dangle foot 736.79
Danielssen's disease (anesthetic leprosy) 030.1
Danlos' syndrome 756.83
Darier's disease (congenital) (keratosis follicularis) 757.39
  due to vitamin A deficiency 264.8
  meaning erythema annulare centrifugum 695.0
Darier-Roussy sarcoid 135
Dark area on retina 239.81
Darling's
  disease (see also Histoplasmosis, American) 115.00
  histoplasmosis (see also Histoplasmosis, American) 115.00
Dartre 054.9
Darwin's tubercle 744.29
Davidson's anemia (refractory) 284.9
Davies' disease 425.0
Davies-Colley syndrome (slipping rib) 733.99
Dawson's encephalitis 046.2
Day blindness (see also Blindness, day) 368.60
Dead
  fetus
    retained (in utero) 656.4●
      early pregnancy (death before 22 completed weeks' gestation) 632
      late (death after 22 completed weeks' gestation) 656.4●
  syndrome 641.3●

Dead (Continued)
  labyrinth 386.50
  ovum, retained 631
Deaf and dumb NEC 389.7
Deaf mutism (acquired) (congenital) NEC 389.7
  endemic 243
  hysterical 300.11
  syphilitic, congenital 090.0
Deafness (acquired) (complete) (congenital) (hereditary) (middle ear) (partial) 389.9
  with
    blindness V49.85
    blue sclera and fragility of bone 756.51
  auditory fatigue 389.9
  aviation 993.0
    nerve injury 951.5
  boilermakers' 951.5
  central 389.14
    with conductive hearing loss 389.20
      bilateral 389.22
      unilateral 389.21
  conductive (air) 389.00
    with sensorineural hearing loss 389.20
      bilateral 389.22
      unilateral 389.21
    bilateral 389.06
    combined types 389.08
    external ear 389.01
    inner ear 389.04
    middle ear 389.03
    multiple types 389.08
    tympanic membrane 389.02
    unilateral 389.05
  emotional (complete) 300.11
  functional (complete) 300.11
  high frequency 389.8
  hysterical (complete) 300.11
  injury 951.5
  low frequency 389.8
  mental 784.69
  mixed conductive and sensorineural 389.20
    bilateral 389.22
    unilateral 389.21
  nerve
    with conductive hearing loss 389.20
      bilateral 389.22
      unilateral 389.21
    bilateral 389.12
    unilateral 389.13
  neural
    with conductive hearing loss 389.20
      bilateral 389.22
      unilateral 389.21
    bilateral 389.12
    unilateral 389.13
  noise-induced 388.12
    nerve injury 951.5
  nonspeaking 389.7
  perceptive 389.10
    with conductive hearing loss 389.20
      bilateral 389.22
      unilateral 389.21
    central 389.14
    neural
      bilateral 389.12
      unilateral 389.13

Deafness *(Continued)*
 perceptive *(Continued)*
  sensorineural 389.10
   asymmetrical 389.16
   bilateral 389.18
   unilateral 389.15
  sensory
   bilateral 389.11
   unilateral 389.17
 psychogenic (complete) 306.7
 sensorineural *(see also* Deafness, perceptive) 389.10
  asymmetrical 389.16
  bilateral 389.18
  unilateral 389.15
 sensory
  with conductive hearing loss 389.20
   bilateral 389.22
   unilateral 389.21
  bilateral 389.11
  unilateral 389.17
 specified type NEC 389.8
 sudden NEC 388.2
 syphilitic 094.89
 transient ischemic 388.02
 transmission - *see* Deafness, conductive
 traumatic 951.5
 word (secondary to organic lesion) 784.69
  developmental 315.31
Death
 after delivery (cause not stated) (sudden) 674.9●
 anesthetic
  due to
   correct substance properly administered 995.4
   overdose or wrong substance given 968.4
    specified anesthetic - *see* Table of Drugs and Chemicals
  during delivery 668.9●
 brain 348.89
 cardiac (sudden) (SCD) - *code to* underlying condition
  family history of V17.41
  personal history of, successfully resuscitated V12.53
 cause unknown 798.2
 cot (infant) 798.0
 crib (infant) 798.0
 fetus, fetal (cause not stated) (intrauterine) 779.9
  early, with retention (before 22 completed weeks' gestation) 632
  from asphyxia or anoxia (before labor) 768.0
   during labor 768.1
  late, affecting management of pregnancy (after 22 completed weeks' gestation) 656.4●
 from pregnancy NEC 646.9●
 instantaneous 798.1
 intrauterine *(see also* Death, fetus) 779.9
  complicating pregnancy 656.4●
 maternal, affecting fetus or newborn 761.6
 neonatal NEC 779.9
 sudden (cause unknown) 798.1
  cardiac (SCD)
   family history of V17.41
   personal history of, successfully resuscitated V12.53

Death *(Continued)*
 sudden *(Continued)*
  during delivery 669.9●
   under anesthesia NEC 668.9●
  infant, syndrome (SIDS) 798.0
  puerperal, during puerperium 674.9●
  unattended (cause unknown) 798.9
  under anesthesia NEC
   due to
    correct substance properly administered 995.4
    overdose or wrong substance given 968.4
     specified anesthetic - *see* Table of Drugs and Chemicals
   during delivery 668.9●
  violent 798.1
de Beurmann-Gougerot disease (sporotrichosis) 117.1
Debility (general) (infantile) (postinfectional) 799.3
 with nutritional difficulty 269.9
 congenital or neonatal NEC 779.9
 nervous 300.5
 old age 797
 senile 797
Débove's disease (splenomegaly) 789.2
Decalcification
 bone *(see also* Osteoporosis) 733.00
 teeth 521.89
Decapitation 874.9
 fetal (to facilitate delivery) 763.89
Decapsulation, kidney 593.89
Decay
 dental 521.00
 senile 797
 tooth, teeth 521.00
Decensus, uterus - *see* Prolapse, uterus
Deciduitis (acute)
 with
  abortion - *see* Abortion, by type, with sepsis
  ectopic pregnancy *(see also* categories 633.0–633.9) 639.0
  molar pregnancy *(see also* categories 630–632) 639.0
 affecting fetus or newborn 760.8
 following
  abortion 639.0
  ectopic or molar pregnancy 639.0
 in pregnancy 646.6●
 puerperal, postpartum 670.1●
Deciduoma malignum (M9100/3) 181
Deciduous tooth (retained) 520.6
Decline (general) *(see also* Debility) 799.3
Decompensation
 cardiac (acute) (chronic) *(see also* Disease, heart) 429.9
  failure - *see* Failure, heart
 cardiorenal *(see also* Hypertension, cardiorenal) 404.90
 cardiovascular *(see also* Disease, cardiovascular) 429.2
 heart *(see also* Disease, heart) 429.9
  failure - *see* Failure, heart
 hepatic 572.2
 myocardial (acute) (chronic) *(see also* Disease, heart) 429.9
  failure - *see* Failure, heart
 respiratory 519.9
Decompression sickness 993.3

Decrease, decreased
 blood
  platelets *(see also* Thrombocytopenia) 287.5
  pressure 796.3
   due to shock following injury 958.4
    operation 998.0
  white cell count 288.50
   specified NEC 288.59
 cardiac reserve - *see* Disease, heart
 estrogen 256.39
  postablative 256.2
 fetal movements 655.7●
 fragility of erythrocytes 289.89
 function
  adrenal (cortex) 255.41
   medulla 255.5
  ovary in hypopituitarism 253.4
  parenchyma of pancreas 577.8
  pituitary (gland) (lobe) (anterior) 253.2
   posterior (lobe) 253.8
 functional activity 780.99
 glucose 790.29
 haptoglobin (serum) NEC 273.8
 leukocytes 288.50
 libido 799.81
 lymphocytes 288.51
 platelets *(see also* Thrombocytopenia) 287.5
 pulse pressure 785.9
 respiration due to shock following injury 958.4
 sexual desire 799.81
 tear secretion NEC 375.15
 tolerance
  fat 579.8
  salt and water 276.9
 vision NEC 369.9
 white blood cell count 288.50
Decubital gangrene *(see also* Ulcer, pressure) 707.00 [785.4]
Decubiti *(see also* Ulcer, pressure) 707.00
Decubitus (ulcer) *(see also* Ulcer, pressure) 707.00
 with gangrene 707.00 [785.4]
 ankle 707.06
 back
  lower 707.03
  upper 707.02
 buttock 707.05
 coccyx 707.03
 elbow 707.01
 head 707.09
 heel 707.07
 hip 707.04
 other site 707.09
 sacrum 707.03
 shoulder blades 707.02
Deepening acetabulum 718.85
Defect, defective 759.9
 3-beta-hydroxysteroid dehydrogenase 255.2
 11-hydroxylase 255.2
 21-hydroxylase 255.2
 abdominal wall, congenital 756.70
 aorticopulmonary septum 745.0
 aortic septal 745.0
 atrial septal (ostium secundum type) 745.5
  acquired 429.71
  ostium primum type 745.61
  sinus venosus 745.8

Defect, defective *(Continued)*
  atrioventricular
    canal 745.69
    septum 745.4
      acquired 429.71
  atrium secundum 745.5
    acquired 429.71
  auricular septal 745.5
    acquired 429.71
  bilirubin excretion 277.4
  biosynthesis, testicular androgen 257.2
  bridge 525.60
  bulbar septum 745.0
  butanol-insoluble iodide 246.1
  chromosome - *see* Anomaly, chromosome
  circulation (acquired) 459.9
    congenital 747.9
    newborn 747.9
  clotting NEC (*see also* Defect, coagulation) 286.9
  coagulation (factor) (*see also* Deficiency, coagulation factor) 286.9
    with
      abortion - *see* Abortion, by type, with hemorrhage
      ectopic pregnancy (*see also* categories 634–638) 639.1
      molar pregnancy (*see also* categories 630–632) 639.1
    acquired (any) 286.7
    antepartum or intrapartum 641.3●
      affecting fetus or newborn 762.1
    causing hemorrhage of pregnancy or delivery 641.3●
    complicating pregnancy, childbirth, or puerperium 649.3●
    due to
      liver disease 286.7
      vitamin K deficiency 286.7
    newborn, transient 776.3
    postpartum 666.3●
    specified type NEC 286.9
  conduction (heart) 426.9
    bone (*see also* Deafness, conductive) 389.00
  congenital, organ or site NEC - *see also* Anomaly
    circulation 747.9
    Descemet's membrane 743.9
      specified type NEC 743.49
    diaphragm 756.6
    ectodermal 757.9
    esophagus 750.9
    pulmonic cusps - *see* Anomaly, heart valve
    respiratory system 748.9
      specified type NEC 748.8
  crown 525.60
  cushion endocardial 745.60
  dental restoration 525.60
  dentin (hereditary) 520.5
  Descemet's membrane (congenital) 743.9
    acquired 371.30
    specific type NEC 743.49
  deutan 368.52

Defect, defective *(Continued)*
  developmental - *see also* Anomaly, by site
    cauda equina 742.59
    left ventricle 746.9
      with atresia or hypoplasia of aortic orifice or valve, with hypoplasia of ascending aorta 746.7
      in hypoplastic left heart syndrome 746.7
    testis 752.9
    vessel 747.9
  diaphragm
    with elevation, eventration, or hernia - *see* Hernia, diaphragm
    congenital 756.6
      with elevation, eventration, or hernia 756.6
      gross (with elevation, eventration, or hernia) 756.6
  ectodermal, congenital 757.9
  Eisenmenger's (ventricular septal defect) 745.4
  endocardial cushion 745.60
    specified type NEC 745.69
  esophagus, congenital 750.9
  extensor retinaculum 728.9
  fibrin polymerization (*see also* Defect, coagulation) 286.3
  filling
    biliary tract 793.3
    bladder 793.5
    dental 525.60
    gallbladder 793.3
    kidney 793.5
    stomach 793.4
    ureter 793.5
  fossa ovalis 745.5
  gene, carrier (suspected) of V83.89
  Gerbode 745.4
  glaucomatous, without elevated tension 365.89
  Hageman (factor) (*see also* Defect, coagulation) 286.3
  hearing (*see also* Deafness) 389.9
  high grade 317
  homogentisic acid 270.2
  interatrial septal 745.5
    acquired 429.71
  interauricular septal 745.5
    acquired 429.71
  interventricular septal 745.4
    with pulmonary stenosis or atresia, dextraposition of aorta, and hypertrophy of right ventricle 745.2
    acquired 429.71
    in tetralogy of Fallot 745.2
  iodide trapping 246.1
  iodotyrosine dehalogenase 246.1
  kynureninase 270.2
  learning, specific 315.2
  major osseous 731.3
  mental (*see also* Retardation, mental) 319
  osseous, major 731.3
  osteochondral NEC 738.8
  ostium
    primum 745.61
    secundum 745.5
  pericardium 746.89
  peroxidase-binding 246.1
  placental blood supply - *see* Placenta, insufficiency
  platelet (qualitative) 287.1
    constitutional 286.4

Defect, defective *(Continued)*
  postural, spine 737.9
  protan 368.51
  pulmonic cusps, congenital 746.00
  renal pelvis 753.9
    obstructive 753.29
    specified type NEC 753.3
  respiratory system, congenital 748.9
    specified type NEC 748.8
  retina, retinal 361.30
    with detachment (*see also* Detachment, retina, with retinal defect) 361.00
    multiple 361.33
      with detachment 361.02
    nerve fiber bundle 362.85
    single 361.30
      with detachment 361.01
  septal (closure) (heart) NEC 745.9
    acquired 429.71
    atrial 745.5
    specified type NEC 745.8
  speech NEC 784.59
    developmental 315.39
    late effect of cerebrovascular disease - *see* Late effect(s) (of) cerebrovascular disease, speech and language deficit
    secondary to organic lesion 784.59
  Taussig-Bing (transposition, aorta and overriding pulmonary artery) 745.11
  teeth, wedge 521.20
  thyroid hormone synthesis 246.1
  tritan 368.53
  ureter 753.9
    obstructive 753.29
  vascular (acquired) (local) 459.9
    congenital (peripheral) NEC 747.60
      gastrointestinal 747.61
      lower limb 747.64
      renal 747.62
      specified NEC 747.69
      spinal 747.82
      upper limb 747.63
  ventricular septal 745.4
    with pulmonary stenosis or atresia, dextraposition of aorta, and hypertrophy of right ventricle 745.2
    acquired 429.71
    atrioventricular canal type 745.69
    between infundibulum and anterior portion 745.4
    in tetralogy of Fallot 745.2
    isolated anterior 745.4
  vision NEC 369.9
  visual field 368.40
    arcuate 368.43
    heteronymous, bilateral 368.47
    homonymous, bilateral 368.46
    localized NEC 368.44
    nasal step 368.44
    peripheral 368.44
    sector 368.43
  voice and resonance 784.40
  wedge, teeth (abrasion) 521.20
Defeminization syndrome 255.2
Deferentitis 608.4
  gonorrheal (acute) 098.14
    chronic or duration of 2 months or over 098.34
Defibrination syndrome (*see also* Fibrinolysis) 286.6

Deficiency, deficient
- 3-beta-hydroxysteroid dehydrogenase 255.2
- 6-phosphogluconic dehydrogenase (anemia) 282.2
- 11-beta-hydroxylase 255.2
- 17-alpha-hydroxylase 255.2
- 18-hydroxysteroid dehydrogenase 255.2
- 20-alpha-hydroxylase 255.2
- 21-hydroxylase 255.2
- AAT (alpha-1 antitrypsin) 273.4
- abdominal muscle syndrome 756.79
- accelerator globulin (Ac G) (blood) (*see also* Defect, coagulation) 286.3
- AC globulin (congenital) (*see also* Defect, coagulation) 286.3
    - acquired 286.7
- activating factor (blood) (*see also* Defect, coagulation) 286.3
- adenohypophyseal 253.2
- adenosine deaminase 277.2
- aldolase (hereditary) 271.2
- alpha-1-antitrypsin 273.4
- alpha-1-trypsin inhibitor 273.4
- alpha-fucosidase 271.8
- alpha-lipoprotein 272.5
- alpha-mannosidase 271.8
- amino acid 270.9
- anemia - *see* Anemia, deficiency
- aneurin 265.1
    - with beriberi 265.0
- antibody NEC 279.00
- antidiuretic hormone 253.5
- antihemophilic
    - factor (A) 286.0
        - B 286.1
        - C 286.2
    - globulin (AHG) NEC 286.0
- antithrombin III 289.81
- antitrypsin 273.4
- argininosuccinate synthetase or lyase 270.6
- ascorbic acid (with scurvy) 267
- autoprothrombin
    - I (*see also* Defect, coagulation) 286.3
    - II 286.1
    - C (*see also* Defect, coagulation) 286.3
- bile salt 579.8
- biotin 266.2
- biotinidase 277.6
- bradykinase-1 277.6
- brancher enzyme (amylopectinosis) 271.0
- calciferol 268.9
    - with
        - osteomalacia 268.2
        - rickets (*see also* Rickets) 268.0
- calcium 275.40
    - dietary 269.3
- calorie, severe 261
- carbamyl phosphate synthetase 270.6
- cardiac (*see also* Insufficiency, myocardial) 428.0
- carnitine 277.81
    - due to
        - hemodialysis 277.83
        - inborn errors of metabolism 277.82
        - valproic acid therapy 277.83
    - iatrogenic 277.83
    - palmitoyltransferase (CPT1, CPT2) 277.85

Deficiency, deficient (*Continued*)
- carnitine (*Continued*)
    - palmityl transferase (CPT1, CPT2) 277.85
    - primary 277.81
    - secondary 277.84
- carotene 264.9
- Carr factor (*see also* Defect, coagulation) 286.9
- central nervous system 349.9
- ceruloplasmin 275.1
- cevitamic acid (with scurvy) 267
- choline 266.2
- Christmas factor 286.1
- chromium 269.3
- citrin 269.1
- clotting (blood) (*see also* Defect, coagulation) 286.9
- coagulation factor NEC 286.9
    - with
        - abortion - *see* Abortion, by type, with hemorrhage
        - ectopic pregnancy (*see also* categories 634–638) 639.1
        - molar pregnancy (*see also* categories 630–632) 639.1
    - acquired (any) 286.7
    - antepartum or intrapartum 641.3●
        - affecting fetus or newborn 762.1
    - complicating pregnancy, childbirth, or puerperium 649.3●
    - due to
        - liver disease 286.7
        - vitamin K deficiency 286.7
    - newborn, transient 776.3
    - postpartum 666.3●
    - specified type NEC 286.3
- color vision (congenital) 368.59
    - acquired 368.55
- combined glucocorticoid and mineralocorticoid 255.41
- combined, two or more coagulation factors (*see also* Defect, coagulation) 286.9
- complement factor NEC 279.8
- contact factor (*see also* Defect, coagulation) 286.3
- copper NEC 275.1
- corticoadrenal 255.41
- craniofacial axis 756.0
- cyanocobalamin (vitamin B_{12}) 266.2
- debrancher enzyme (limit dextrinosis) 271.0
- desmolase 255.2
- diet 269.9
- dihydrofolate reductase 281.2
- dihydropteridine reductase 270.1
- dihydropyrimidine dehydrogenase (DPD) 277.6 ◀
- disaccharidase (intestinal) 271.3
- disease NEC 269.9
- ear(s) V48.8
- edema 262
- endocrine 259.9
- enzymes, circulating NEC (*see also* Deficiency, by specific enzyme) 277.6
- ergosterol 268.9
    - with
        - osteomalacia 268.2
        - rickets (*see also* Rickets) 268.0
- erythrocytic glutathione (anemia) 282.2
- eyelid(s) V48.8

Deficiency, deficient (*Continued*)
- factor (*see also* Defect, coagulation) 286.9
    - I (congenital) (fibrinogen) 286.3
        - antepartum or intrapartum 641.3●
            - affecting fetus or newborn 762.1
        - newborn, transient 776.3
        - postpartum 666.3●
    - II (congenital) (prothrombin) 286.3
    - V (congenital) (labile) 286.3
    - VII (congenital) (stable) 286.3
    - VIII (congenital) (functional) 286.0
        - with
            - functional defect 286.0
            - vascular defect 286.4
    - IX (Christmas) (congenital) (functional) 286.1
    - X (congenital) (Stuart-Prower) 286.3
    - XI (congenital) (plasma thromboplastin antecedent) 286.2
    - XII (congenital) (Hageman) 286.3
    - XIII (congenital) (fibrin stabilizing) 286.3
    - Hageman 286.3
    - multiple (congenital) 286.9
        - acquired 286.7
- fibrinase (*see also* Defect, coagulation) 286.3
- fibrinogen (congenital) (*see also* Defect, coagulation) 286.3
    - acquired 286.6
- fibrin-stabilizing factor (congenital) (*see also* Defect, coagulation) 286.3
    - acquired 286.7
- finger - *see* Absence, finger
- fletcher factor (*see also* Defect, coagulation) 286.9
- fluorine 269.3
- folate, anemia 281.2
- folic acid (vitamin B_C) 266.2
    - anemia 281.2
- follicle-stimulating hormone (FSH) 253.4
- fructokinase 271.2
- fructose-1, 6-diphosphate 271.2
- fructose-1-phosphate aldolase 271.2
- FSH (follicle-stimulating hormone) 253.4
- fucosidase 271.8
- galactokinase 271.1
- galactose-1-phosphate uridyl transferase 271.1
- gamma globulin in blood 279.00
- glass factor (*see also* Defect, coagulation) 286.3
- glucocorticoid 255.41
- glucose-6-phosphatase 271.0
- glucose-6-phosphate dehydrogenase anemia 282.2
- glucuronyl transferase 277.4
- glutathione-reductase (anemia) 282.2
- glycogen synthetase 271.0
- growth hormone 253.3
- Hageman factor (congenital) (*see also* Defect, coagulation) 286.3
- head V48.0
- hemoglobin (*see also* Anemia) 285.9
- hepatophosphorylase 271.0
- hexose monophosphate (HMP) shunt 282.2
- HGH (human growth hormone) 253.3

Deficiency, deficient (*Continued*)
HG-PRT 277.2
homogentisic acid oxidase 270.2
hormone - *see also* Deficiency, by
　　specific hormone
　　anterior pituitary (isolated) (partial)
　　　NEC 253.4
　　　growth (human) 253.3
　　follicle-stimulating 253.4
　　growth (human) (isolated) 253.3
　　human growth 253.3
　　interstitial cell-stimulating 253.4
　　luteinizing 253.4
　　melanocyte-stimulating 253.4
　　testicular 257.2
human growth hormone 253.3
humoral 279.00
　　with
　　　hyper-IgM 279.05
　　　　autosomal recessive 279.05
　　　　X-linked 279.05
　　　increased IgM 279.05
　　　congenital hypogammaglobulinemia
　　　　279.04
　　　non-sex-linked 279.06
　　　selective immunoglobulin NEC
　　　　279.03
　　　　IgA 279.01
　　　　IgG 279.03
　　　　IgM 279.02
　　　　　increased 279.05
　　　specified NEC 279.09
hydroxylase 255.2
hypoxanthine-guanine
　　phosphoribosyltransferase
　　(HG-PRT) 277.2
ICSH (interstitial cell-stimulating
　　hormone) 253.4
immunity NEC 279.3
　　cell-mediated 279.10
　　　with
　　　　hyperimmunoglobulinemia
　　　　　279.2
　　　　thrombocytopenia and eczema
　　　　　279.12
　　　specified NEC 279.19
　　combined (severe) 279.2
　　　syndrome 279.2
　　common variable 279.06
　　humoral NEC 279.00
　　IgA (secretory) 279.01
　　IgG 279.03
　　IgM 279.02
immunoglobulin, selective NEC 279.03
　　IgA 279.01
　　IgG 279.03
　　IgM 279.02
inositol (B complex) 266.2
interferon 279.49
internal organ V47.0
interstitial cell-stimulating hormone
　　(ICSH) 253.4
intrinsic factor (Castle's) (congenital)
　　281.0
intrinsic (urethral) sphincter (ISD)
　　599.82
invertase 271.3
iodine 269.3
iron, anemia 280.9
labile factor (congenital) (*see also*
　　Defect, coagulation) 286.3
　　acquired 286.7
lacrimal fluid (acquired) 375.15
　　congenital 743.64

Deficiency, deficient (*Continued*)
lactase 271.3
Laki-Lorand factor (*see also* Defect,
　　coagulation) 286.3
lecithin-cholesterol acyltranferase
　　272.5
LH (luteinizing hormone) 253.4
limb V49.0
　　lower V49.0
　　　congenital (*see also* Deficiency,
　　　　lower limb, congenital)
　　　　755.30
　　upper V49.0
　　　congenital (*see also* Deficiency,
　　　　upper limb, congenital)
　　　　755.20
lipocaic 577.8
lipoid (high-density) 272.5
lipoprotein (familial) (high-density)
　　272.5
liver phosphorylase 271.0
long chain 3-hydroxyacyl CoA
　　dehydrogenase (LCHAD) 277.85
long chain/very long chain acyl CoA
　　dehydrogenase (LCAD, VLCAD)
　　277.85
lower limb V49.0
　　congenital 755.30
　　　with complete absence of distal
　　　　elements 755.31
　　　longitudinal (complete) (partial)
　　　　(with distal deficiencies,
　　　　incomplete) 755.32
　　　with complete absence of
　　　　distal elements 755.31
　　　combined femoral, tibial,
　　　　fibular (incomplete)
　　　　755.33
　　　femoral 755.34
　　　fibular 755.37
　　　metatarsal(s) 755.38
　　　phalange(s) 755.39
　　　　meaning all digits 755.31
　　　tarsal(s) 755.38
　　　tibia 755.36
　　　tibiofibular 755.35
　　　transverse 755.31
luteinizing hormone (LH) 253.4
lysosomal alpha-1, 4 glucosidase
　　271.0
magnesium 275.2
mannosidase 271.8
medium chain acyl CoA
　　dehydrogenase (MCAD) 277.85
melanocyte-stimulating hormone
　　(MSH) 253.4
menadione (vitamin K) 269.0
　　newborn 776.0
mental (familial) (hereditary) (*see also*
　　Retardation, mental) 319
methylenetetrahydrofolate reductase
　　(MTHFR) 270.4
mineral NEC 269.3
mineralocorticoid 255.42
molybdenum 269.3
moral 301.7
multiple, syndrome 260
myocardial (*see also* Insufficiency,
　　myocardial) 428.0
myophosphorylase 271.0
NADH (DPNH)-methemoglobin-
　　reductase (congenital) 289.7
NADH diaphorase or reductase
　　(congenital) 289.7

Deficiency, deficient (*Continued*)
neck V48.1
niacin (amide) (-tryptophan) 265.2
nicotinamide 265.2
nicotinic acid (amide) 265.2
nose V48.8
number of teeth (*see also* Anodontia)
　　520.0
nutrition, nutritional 269.9
　　specified NEC 269.8
ornithine transcarbamylase 270.6
ovarian 256.39
oxygen (*see also* Anoxia) 799.02
pantothenic acid 266.2
parathyroid (gland) 252.1
phenylalanine hydroxylase 270.1
phosphoenolpyruvate carboxykinase
　　271.8
phosphofructokinase 271.2
phosphoglucomutase 271.0
phosphohexosisomerase 271.0
phosphomannomutase 271.8
phosphomannose isomerase 271.8
phosphomannosyl mutase 271.8
phosphorylase kinase, liver 271.0
pituitary (anterior) 253.2
　　posterior 253.5
placenta - *see* Placenta, insufficiency
plasma
　　cell 279.00
　　protein (paraproteinemia)
　　　(pyroglobulinemia) 273.8
　　　gamma globulin 279.00
　　thromboplastin
　　　antecedent (PTA) 286.2
　　　component (PTC) 286.1
platelet NEC 287.1
　　constitutional 286.4
polyglandular 258.9
potassium (K) 276.8
proaccelerin (congenital) (*see also*
　　Defect, congenital) 286.3
　　acquired 286.7
proconvertin factor (congenital) (*see
　　also* Defect, coagulation) 286.3
　　acquired 286.7
prolactin 253.4
protein 260
　　anemia 281.4
　　C 289.81
　　plasma - *see* Deficiency, plasma,
　　　protein
　　S 289.81
prothrombin (congenital) (*see also*
　　Defect, coagulation) 286.3
　　acquired 286.7
Prower factor (*see also* Defect,
　　coagulation) 286.3
PRT 277.2
pseudocholinesterase 289.89
psychobiological 301.6
PTA 286.2
PTC 286.1
purine nucleoside phosphorylase 277.2
pyracin (alpha) (beta) 266.1
pyridoxal 266.1
pyridoxamine 266.1
pyridoxine (derivatives) 266.1
pyruvate carboxylase 271.8
pyruvate dehydrogenase 271.8
pyruvate kinase (PK) 282.3
riboflavin (vitamin B_2) 266.0
saccadic eye movements 379.57
salivation 527.7

Deficiency, deficient *(Continued)*
salt 276.1
secretion
  ovary 256.39
  salivary gland (any) 527.7
  urine 788.5
selenium 269.3
serum
  antitrypsin, familial 273.4
  protein (congenital) 273.8
short chain acyl CoA dehydrogenase
  (SCAD) 277.85
short stature homeobox gene (SHOX)
  with
    dyschondrosteosis 756.89
    short stature (idiopathic) 783.43
    Turner's syndrome 758.6
smooth pursuit movements (eye) 379.58
sodium (Na) 276.1
SPCA (*see also* Defect, coagulation) 286.3
specified NEC 269.8
stable factor (congenital) (*see also*
  Defect, coagulation) 286.3
  acquired 286.7
Stuart (-Prower) factor (*see also* Defect,
  coagulation) 286.3
sucrase 271.3
sucrase-isomaltase 271.3
sulfite oxidase 270.0
syndrome, multiple 260
thiamine, thiaminic (chloride) 265.1
thrombokinase (*see also* Defect,
  coagulation) 286.3
  newborn 776.0
thrombopoieten 287.39
thymolymphatic 279.2
thyroid (gland) 244.9
tocopherol 269.1
toe - *see* Absence, toe
tooth bud (*see also* Anodontia) 520.0
trunk V48.1
UDPG-glycogen transferase 271.0
upper limb V49.0
  congenital 755.20
    with complete absence of distal
      elements 755.21
    longitudinal (complete) (partial)
      (with distal deficiencies,
      incomplete) 755.22
      carpal(s) 755.28
      combined humeral, radial,
        ulnar (incomplete) 755.23
      humeral 755.24
      metacarpal(s) 755.28
      phalange(s) 755.29
        meaning all digits 755.21
      radial 755.26
      radioulnar 755.25
      ulnar 755.27
    transverse (complete) (partial)
      755.21
vascular 459.9
vasopressin 253.5
viosterol (*see also* Deficiency, calciferol)
  268.9
vitamin (multiple) NEC 269.2
  A 264.9
    with
      Bitôt's spot 264.1
      corneal 264.2
        with corneal ulceration
          264.3
      keratomalacia 264.4
      keratosis, follicular 264.8
      night blindness 264.5

Deficiency, deficient *(Continued)*
vitamin *(Continued)*
  A *(Continued)*
    with *(Continued)*
      scar of cornea, xerophthalmic
        264.6
      specified manifestation NEC
        264.8
      ocular 264.7
    xeroderma 264.8
    xerophthalmia 264.7
    xerosis
      conjunctival 264.0
        with Bitôt's spot 264.1
      corneal 264.2
        with corneal ulceration
          264.3
  B (complex) NEC 266.9
    with
      beriberi 265.0
      pellagra 265.2
    specified type NEC 266.2
  B_1 NEC 265.1
    beriberi 265.0
  B_2 266.0
  B_6 266.1
  B_{12} 266.2
  B_C (folic acid) 266.2
  C (ascorbic acid) (with scurvy) 267
  D (calciferol) (ergosterol) 268.9
    with
      osteomalacia 268.2
      rickets (*see also* Rickets) 268.0
  E 269.1
  folic acid 266.2
  G 266.0
  H 266.2
  K 269.0
    of newborn 776.0
  nicotinic acid 265.2
  P 269.1
  PP 265.2
  specified NEC 269.1
  zinc 269.3
Deficient - *see also* Deficiency
blink reflex 374.45
craniofacial axis 756.0
number of teeth (*see also* Anodontia) 520.0
secretion of urine 788.5
Deficit
attention 799.51 ◄
cognitive communication 799.52 ◄
concentration 799.51 ◄
executive function 799.55 ◄
frontal lobe 799.55 ◄
neurologic NEC 781.99
  due to
    cerebrovascular lesion (*see also*
      Disease, cerebrovascular,
      acute) 436
      late effect - *see* Late effect(s) (of)
        cerebrovascular disease
    transient ischemic attack 435.9
  ischemic
    reversible (RIND) 434.91
      history of (personal) V12.54
    prolonged (PRIND) 434.91
      history of (personal) V12.54
oxygen 799.02
psychomotor 799.54 ◄
visuospatial 799.53 ◄
Deflection
radius 736.09
septum (acquired) (nasal) (nose) 470
spine - *see* Curvature, spine
turbinate (nose) 470

Defluvium
capillorum (*see also* Alopecia) 704.00
ciliorum 374.55
unguium 703.8
Deformity 738.9
abdomen, congenital 759.9
abdominal wall
  acquired 738.8
  congenital 756.70
  muscle deficiency syndrome
    756.79
acquired (unspecified site) 738.9
  specified site NEC 738.8
adrenal gland (congenital) 759.1
alimentary tract, congenital 751.9
  lower 751.5
  specified type NEC 751.8
  upper (any part, except tongue)
    750.9
    specified type NEC 750.8
    tongue 750.10
      specified type NEC 750.19
ankle (joint) (acquired) 736.70
  abduction 718.47
  congenital 755.69
  contraction 718.47
  specified NEC 736.79
anus (congenital) 751.5
  acquired 569.49
aorta (congenital) 747.20
  acquired 447.8
  arch 747.21
    acquired 447.8
  coarctation 747.10
aortic
  arch 747.21
    acquired 447.8
  cusp or valve (congenital) 746.9
    acquired (*see also* Endocarditis,
      aortic) 424.1
  ring 747.21
appendix 751.5
arm (acquired) 736.89
  congenital 755.50
arteriovenous (congenital) (peripheral)
  NEC 747.60
  gastrointestinal 747.61
  lower limb 747.64
  renal 747.62
  specified NEC 747.69
  spinal 747.82
  upper limb 747.63
artery (congenital) (peripheral) NEC
  (*see also* Deformity, vascular)
  747.60
  acquired 447.8
  cerebral 747.81
  coronary (congenital) 746.85
    acquired (*see also* Ischemia, heart)
      414.9
  retinal 743.9
  umbilical 747.5
atrial septal (congenital) (heart)
  745.5
auditory canal (congenital) (external)
  (*see also* Deformity, ear) 744.3
  acquired 380.50
auricle
  ear (congenital) (*see also* Deformity,
    ear) 744.3
    acquired 380.32
  heart (congenital) 746.9
back (acquired) - *see* Deformity,
  spine
Bartholin's duct (congenital) 750.9

◄ New   ◄⊪ Revised   ~~deleted~~ Deleted   ● Use Additional Digit(s)   ▨ Omit code

Deformity (*Continued*)
bile duct (congenital) 751.60
  acquired 576.8
    with calculus, choledocholithiasis,
      or stones - *see*
      Choledocholithiasis
biliary duct or passage (congenital)
  751.60
  acquired 576.8
    with calculus, choledocholithiasis,
      or stones - *see*
      Choledocholithiasis
bladder (neck) (sphincter) (trigone)
  (acquired) 596.8
  congenital 753.9
bone (acquired) NEC 738.9
  congenital 756.9
  turbinate 738.0
boutonniere (finger) 736.21
brain (congenital) 742.9
  acquired 348.89
  multiple 742.4
  reduction 742.2
  vessel (congenital) 747.81
breast (acquired) 611.89
  congenital 757.6
  reconstructed 612.0
bronchus (congenital) 748.3
  acquired 519.19
bursa, congenital 756.9
canal of Nuck 752.9
canthus (congenital) 743.9
  acquired 374.89
capillary (acquired) 448.9
  congenital NEC (*see also* Deformity,
    vascular) 747.60
cardiac - *see* Deformity, heart
cardiovascular system (congenital)
  746.9
caruncle, lacrimal (congenital)
  743.9
  acquired 375.69
cascade, stomach 537.6
cecum (congenital) 751.5
  acquired 569.89
cerebral (congenital) 742.9
  acquired 348.89
cervix (congenital) (uterus) 622.8
  congenital 752.40
cheek (acquired) 738.19
  congenital 744.9
chest (wall) (acquired) 738.3
  congenital 754.89
  late effect of rickets 268.1
chin (acquired) 738.19
  congenital 744.9
choroid (congenital) 743.9
  acquired 363.8
  plexus (congenital) 742.9
    acquired 349.2
cicatricial - *see* Cicatrix
cilia (congenital) 743.9
  acquired 374.89
circulatory system (congenital)
  747.9
clavicle (acquired) 738.8
  congenital 755.51
clitoris (congenital) 752.40
  acquired 624.8
clubfoot - *see* Clubfoot
coccyx (acquired) 738.6
  congenital 756.10
colon (congenital) 751.5
  acquired 569.89

Deformity (*Continued*)
concha (ear) (congenital) (*see also*
  Deformity, ear) 744.3
  acquired 380.32
congenital, organ or site not listed (*see*
  also Anomaly) 759.9
cornea (congenital) 743.9
  acquired 371.70
coronary artery (congenital) 746.85
  acquired (*see also* Ischemia, heart)
    414.9
cranium (acquired) 738.19
  congenital (*see also* Deformity, skull,
    congenital) 756.0
cricoid cartilage (congenital) 748.3
  acquired 478.79
cystic duct (congenital) 751.60
  acquired 575.8
Dandy-Walker 742.3
  with spina bifida (*see also* Spina
    bifida) 741.0●
diaphragm (congenital) 756.6
  acquired 738.8
digestive organ(s) or system
  (congenital) NEC 751.9
  specified type NEC 751.8
ductus arteriosus 747.0
duodenal bulb 537.89
duodenum (congenital) 751.5
  acquired 537.89
dura (congenital) 742.9
  brain 742.4
    acquired 349.2
  spinal 742.59
    acquired 349.2
ear (congenital) 744.3
  acquired 380.32
  auricle 744.3
    causing impairment of hearing
      744.02
  causing impairment of hearing
    744.00
  external 744.3
    causing impairment of hearing
      744.02
  internal 744.05
  lobule 744.3
  middle 744.03
    ossicles 744.04
  ossicles 744.04
ectodermal (congenital) NEC 757.9
  specified type NEC 757.8
ejaculatory duct (congenital) 752.9
  acquired 608.89
elbow (joint) (acquired) 736.00
  congenital 755.50
  contraction 718.42
endocrine gland NEC 759.2
epididymis (congenital) 752.9
  acquired 608.89
  torsion 608.24
epiglottis (congenital) 748.3
  acquired 478.79
esophagus (congenital) 750.9
  acquired 530.89
Eustachian tube (congenital) NEC
  744.3
  specified type NEC 744.24
extremity (acquired) 736.9
  congenital, except reduction
    deformity 755.9
    lower 755.60
    upper 755.50
  reduction - *see* Deformity, reduction

Deformity (*Continued*)
eye (congenital) 743.9
  acquired 379.8
  muscle 743.9
eyebrow (congenital) 744.89
eyelid (congenital) 743.9
  acquired 374.89
  specified type NEC 743.62
face (acquired) 738.19
  congenital (any part) 744.9
    due to intrauterine malposition
      and pressure 754.0
fallopian tube (congenital) 752.10
  acquired 620.8
femur (acquired) 736.89
  congenital 755.60
fetal
  with fetopelvic disproportion
    653.7●
    affecting fetus or newborn 763.1
    causing obstructed labor 660.1●
    affecting fetus or newborn 763.1
  known or suspected, affecting
    management of pregnancy
    655.9●
finger (acquired) 736.20
  boutonniere type 736.21
  congenital 755.50
  flexion contracture 718.44
  swan neck 736.22
flexion (joint) (acquired) 736.9
  congenital NEC 755.9
  hip or thigh (acquired) 736.39
    congenital (*see also* Subluxation,
      congenital, hip) 754.32
foot (acquired) 736.70
  cavovarus 736.75
    congenital 754.59
  congenital NEC 754.70
    specified type NEC 754.79
  valgus (acquired) 736.79
    congenital 754.60
      specified type NEC 754.69
  varus (acquired) 736.79
    congenital 754.50
      specified type NEC 754.59
forearm (acquired) 736.00
  congenital 755.50
forehead (acquired) 738.19
  congenital (*see also* Deformity, skull,
    congenital) 756.0
frontal bone (acquired) 738.19
  congenital (*see also* Deformity, skull,
    congenital) 756.0
gallbladder (congenital) 751.60
  acquired 575.8
gastrointestinal tract (congenital) NEC
  751.9
  acquired 569.89
  specified type NEC 751.8
genitalia, genital organ(s) or system
  NEC
  congenital 752.9
  female (congenital) 752.9
    acquired 629.89
    external 752.40
    internal 752.9
  male (congenital) 752.9
    acquired 608.89
globe (eye) (congenital) 743.9
  acquired 360.89
gum (congenital) 750.9
  acquired 523.9
gunstock 736.02

Deformity (*Continued*)
  hand (acquired) 736.00
    claw 736.06
    congenital 755.50
    minus (and plus) (intrinsic) 736.09
    pill roller (intrinsic) 736.09
    plus (and minus) (intrinsic) 736.09
    swan neck (intrinsic) 736.09
  head (acquired) 738.10
    congenital (*see also* Deformity, skull,
        congenital) 756.0
    specified NEC 738.19
  heart (congenital) 746.9
    auricle (congenital) 746.9
    septum 745.9
      auricular 745.5
      specified type NEC 745.8
      ventricular 745.4
    valve (congenital) NEC 746.9
      acquired - *see* Endocarditis
      pulmonary (congenital) 746.00
      specified type NEC 746.89
    ventricle (congenital) 746.9
  heel (acquired) 736.76
    congenital 755.67
  hepatic duct (congenital) 751.60
    acquired 576.8
      with calculus, choledocholithiasis,
          or stones - *see*
          Choledocholithiasis
  hip (joint) (acquired) 736.30
    congenital NEC 755.63
    flexion 718.45
      congenital (*see also* Subluxation,
          congenital, hip) 754.32
  hourglass - *see* Contraction, hourglass
  humerus (acquired) 736.89
    congenital 755.50
  hymen (congenital) 752.40
  hypophyseal (congenital) 759.2
  ileocecal (coil) (valve) (congenital)
      751.5
    acquired 569.89
  ileum (intestine) (congenital) 751.5
    acquired 569.89
  ilium (acquired) 738.6
    congenital 755.60
  integument (congenital) 757.9
  intervertebral cartilage or disc
      (acquired) - *see also* Displacement,
      intervertebral disc
    congenital 756.10
  intestine (large) (small) (congenital)
      751.5
    acquired 569.89
  iris (acquired) 364.75
    congenital 743.9
    prolapse 364.89
  ischium (acquired) 738.6
    congenital 755.60
  jaw (acquired) (congenital) NEC 524.9
    due to intrauterine malposition and
        pressure 754.0
  joint (acquired) NEC 738.8
    congenital 755.9
    contraction (abduction) (adduction)
        (extension) (flexion) - *see*
        Contraction, joint
  kidney(s) (calyx) (pelvis) (congenital)
      753.9
    acquired 593.89
    vessel 747.62
      acquired 459.9
  Klippel-Feil (brevicollis) 756.16

Deformity (*Continued*)
  knee (acquired) NEC 736.6
    congenital 755.64
  labium (majus) (minus) (congenital)
      752.40
    acquired 624.8
  lacrimal apparatus or duct (congenital)
      743.9
    acquired 375.69
  larynx (muscle) (congenital)
      748.3
    acquired 478.79
    web (glottic) (subglottic) 748.2
  leg (lower) (upper) (acquired) NEC
      736.89
    congenital 755.60
      reduction - *see* Deformity,
          reduction, lower limb
  lens (congenital) 743.9
    acquired 379.39
  lid (fold) (congenital) 743.9
    acquired 374.89
  ligament (acquired) 728.9
    congenital 756.9
  limb (acquired) 736.9
    congenital, except reduction
        deformity 755.9
      lower 755.60
        reduction (*see also*
            Deformity, reduction,
            lower limb) 755.30
      upper 755.50
        reduction (*see also*
            Deformity, reduction,
            lower limb) 755.20
    specified NEC 736.89
  lip (congenital) NEC 750.9
    acquired 528.5
    specified type NEC 750.26
  liver (congenital) 751.60
    acquired 573.8
    duct (congenital) 751.60
      acquired 576.8
        with calculus,
            choledocholithiasis,
            or stones - *see*
            Choledocholithiasis
  lower extremity - *see* Deformity, leg
  lumbosacral (joint) (region)
      (congenital) 756.10
    acquired 738.5
  lung (congenital) 748.60
    acquired 518.89
    specified type NEC 748.69
  lymphatic system, congenital
      759.9
  Madelung's (radius) 755.54
  maxilla (acquired) (congenital)
      524.9
  meninges or membrane (congenital)
      742.9
    brain 742.4
      acquired 349.2
    spinal (cord) 742.59
      acquired 349.2
  mesentery (congenital) 751.9
    acquired 568.89
  metacarpus (acquired) 736.00
    congenital 755.50
  metatarsus (acquired) 736.70
    congenital 754.70
  middle ear, except ossicles (congenital)
      744.03
    ossicles 744.04

Deformity (*Continued*)
  mitral (leaflets) (valve) (congenital)
      746.9
    acquired - *see* Endocarditis, mitral
    Ebstein's 746.89
    parachute 746.5
    specified type NEC 746.89
    stenosis, congenital 746.5
  mouth (acquired) 528.9
    congenital NEC 750.9
      specified type NEC 750.26
  multiple, congenital NEC 759.7
    specified type NEC 759.89
  muscle (acquired) 728.9
    congenital 756.9
      specified type NEC 756.89
      sternocleidomastoid (due to
          intrauterine malposition
          and pressure) 754.1
  musculoskeletal system, congenital
      NEC 756.9
    specified type NEC 756.9
  nail (acquired) 703.9
    congenital 757.9
  nasal - *see* Deformity, nose
  neck (acquired) NEC 738.2
    congenital (any part) 744.9
      sternocleidomastoid 754.1
  nervous system (congenital) 742.9
  nipple (congenital) 757.6
    acquired 611.89
  nose, nasal (cartilage) (acquired) 738.0
    bone (turbinate) 738.0
    congenital 748.1
      bent 754.0
      squashed 754.0
    saddle 738.0
      syphilitic 090.5
    septum 470
      congenital 748.1
    sinus (wall) (congenital) 748.1
      acquired 738.0
    syphilitic (congenital) 090.5
      late 095.8
  ocular muscle (congenital) 743.9
    acquired 378.60
  opticociliary vessels (congenital) 743.9
  orbit (congenital) (eye) 743.9
    acquired NEC 376.40
      associated with craniofacial
          deformities 376.44
      due to
        bone disease 376.43
        surgery 376.47
        trauma 376.47
  organ of Corti (congenital) 744.05
  ovary (congenital) 752.0
    acquired 620.8
  oviduct (congenital) 752.10
    acquired 620.8
  palate (congenital) 750.9
    acquired 526.89
    cleft (congenital) (*see also* Cleft,
        palate) 749.00
    hard, acquired 526.89
    soft, acquired 528.9
  pancreas (congenital) 751.7
    acquired 577.8
  parachute, mitral valve 746.5
  parathyroid (gland) 759.2
  parotid (gland) (congenital) 750.9
    acquired 527.8
  patella (acquired) 736.6
    congenital 755.64

◀ New   ◀▥ Revised   ~~deleted~~ Deleted   ● Use Additional Digit(s)   ▨ Omit code

Deformity (*Continued*)
  pelvis, pelvic (acquired) (bony) 738.6
    with disproportion (fetopelvic)
        653.0●
      affecting fetus or newborn 763.1
      causing obstructed labor 660.1●
        affecting fetus or newborn
            763.1
    congenital 755.60
    rachitic (late effect) 268.1
  penis (glans) (congenital) 752.9
    acquired 607.89
  pericardium (congenital) 746.9
    acquired - *see* Pericarditis
  pharynx (congenital) 750.9
    acquired 478.29
  Pierre Robin (congenital) 756.0
  pinna (acquired) 380.32
    congenital 744.3
  pituitary (congenital) 759.2
  pleural folds (congenital) 748.8
  portal vein (congenital) 747.40
  posture - *see* Curvature, spine
  prepuce (congenital) 752.9
    acquired 607.89
  prostate (congenital) 752.9
    acquired 602.8
  pulmonary valve - *see* Endocarditis,
      pulmonary
  pupil (congenital) 743.9
    acquired 364.75
  pylorus (congenital) 750.9
    acquired 537.89
  rachitic (acquired), healed or old 268.1
  radius (acquired) 736.00
    congenital 755.50
      reduction - *see* Deformity,
          reduction, upper limb
  rectovaginal septum (congenital)
      752.40
    acquired 623.8
  rectum (congenital) 751.5
    acquired 569.49
  reduction (extremity) (limb) 755.4
    brain 742.2
    lower limb 755.30
      with complete absence of distal
          elements 755.31
      longitudinal (complete) (partial)
          (with distal deficiencies,
          incomplete) 755.32
        with complete absence of
            distal elements 755.31
        combined femoral, tibial,
            fibular (incomplete)
            755.33
        femoral 755.34
        fibular 755.37
        metatarsal(s) 755.38
        phalange(s) 755.39
          meaning all digits 755.31
        tarsal(s) 755.38
        tibia 755.36
        tibiofibular 755.35
      transverse 755.31
    upper limb 755.20
      with complete absence of distal
          elements 755.21
      longitudinal (complete) (partial)
          (with distal deficiencies,
          incomplete) 755.22
        with complete absence of
            distal elements 755.21
        carpal(s) 755.28

Deformity (*Continued*)
  reduction (*Continued*)
    upper limb (*Continued*)
      longitudinal (*Continued*)
        combined humeral, radial,
            ulnar (incomplete) 755.23
        humeral 755.24
        metacarpal(s) 755.28
        phalange(s) 755.29
          meaning all digits 755.21
        radial 755.26
        radioulnar 755.25
        ulnar 755.27
      transverse (complete) (partial)
          755.21
  renal - *see* Deformity, kidney
  respiratory system (congenital) 748.9
    specified type NEC 748.8
  rib (acquired) 738.3
    congenital 756.3
    cervical 756.2
  rotation (joint) (acquired) 736.9
    congenital 755.9
    hip or thigh 736.39
      congenital (*see also* Subluxation,
          congenital, hip) 754.32
  sacroiliac joint (congenital) 755.69
    acquired 738.5
  sacrum (acquired) 738.5
    congenital 756.10
  saddle
    back 737.8
    nose 738.0
      syphilitic 090.5
  salivary gland or duct (congenital)
      750.9
    acquired 527.8
  scapula (acquired) 736.89
    congenital 755.50
  scrotum (congenital) 752.9
    acquired 608.89
  sebaceous gland, acquired 706.8
  seminal tract or duct (congenital)
      752.9
    acquired 608.89
  septum (nasal) (acquired) 470
    congenital 748.1
  shoulder (joint) (acquired) 736.89
    congenital 755.50
      specified type NEC 755.59
    contraction 718.41
  sigmoid (flexure) (congenital) 751.5
    acquired 569.89
  sinus of Valsalva 747.29
  skin (congenital) 757.9
    acquired NEC 709.8
  skull (acquired) 738.19
    congenital 756.0
      with
        anencephalus 740.0
        encephalocele 742.0
        hydrocephalus 742.3
          with spina bifida (*see also*
              Spina bifida) 741.0●
        microcephalus 742.1
      due to intrauterine malposition
          and pressure 754.0
  soft parts, organs or tissues (of pelvis)
      in pregnancy or childbirth NEC
      654.9●
      affecting fetus or newborn 763.89
      causing obstructed labor 660.2●
        affecting fetus or newborn
            763.1

Deformity (*Continued*)
  spermatic cord (congenital) 752.9
    acquired 608.89
      torsion 608.22
        extravaginal 608.21
        intravaginal 608.22
  spinal
    column - *see* Deformity, spine
    cord (congenital) 742.9
      acquired 336.8
      vessel (congenital) 747.82
    nerve root (congenital) 742.9
      acquired 724.9
  spine (acquired) NEC 738.5
    congenital 756.10
      due to intrauterine malposition
          and pressure 754.2
    kyphoscoliotic (*see also*
        Kyphoscoliosis) 737.30
    kyphotic (*see also* Kyphosis) 737.10
    lordotic (*see also* Lordosis) 737.20
    rachitic 268.1
    scoliotic (*see also* Scoliosis) 737.30
  spleen
    acquired 289.59
    congenital 759.0
  Sprengel's (congenital) 755.52
  sternum (acquired) 738.3
    congenital 756.3
  stomach (congenital) 750.9
    acquired 537.89
  submaxillary gland (congenital) 750.9
    acquired 527.8
  swan neck (acquired)
    finger 736.22
    hand 736.09
  talipes - *see* Talipes
  teeth, tooth NEC 520.9
  testis (congenital) 752.9
    acquired 608.89
      torsion 608.20
  thigh (acquired) 736.89
    congenital 755.60
  thorax (acquired) (wall) 738.3
    congenital 754.89
    late effect of rickets 268.1
  thumb (acquired) 736.20
    congenital 755.50
  thymus (tissue) (congenital) 759.2
  thyroid (gland) (congenital) 759.2
    cartilage 748.3
      acquired 478.79
  tibia (acquired) 736.89
    congenital 755.60
    saber 090.5
  toe (acquired) 735.9
    congenital 755.66
    specified NEC 735.8
  tongue (congenital) 750.10
    acquired 529.8
  tooth, teeth NEC 520.9
  trachea (rings) (congenital) 748.3
    acquired 519.19
  transverse aortic arch (congenital)
      747.21
  tricuspid (leaflets) (valve) (congenital)
      746.9
    acquired - *see* Endocarditis, tricuspid
    atresia or stenosis 746.1
    specified type NEC 746.89
  trunk (acquired) 738.3
    congenital 759.9
  ulna (acquired) 736.00
    congenital 755.50

Deformity *(Continued)*
   upper extremity - *see* Deformity,
      arm
   urachus (congenital) 753.7
   ureter (opening) (congenital) 753.9
      acquired 593.89
   urethra (valve) (congenital) 753.9
      acquired 599.84
   urinary tract or system (congenital)
      753.9
      urachus 753.7
   uterus (congenital) 752.39 ◄▥
      acquired 621.8
   uvula (congenital) 750.9
      acquired 528.9
   vagina (congenital) 752.40
      acquired 623.8
   valve, valvular (heart) (congenital)
      746.9
      acquired - *see* Endocarditis
      pulmonary 746.00
      specified type NEC 746.89
   vascular (congenital) (peripheral) NEC
      747.60
      acquired 459.9
      gastrointestinal 747.61
      lower limb 747.64
      renal 747.62
      specified site NEC 747.69
      spinal 747.82
      upper limb 747.63
   vas deferens (congenital) 752.9
      acquired 608.89
   vein (congenital) NEC (*see also*
      Deformity, vascular) 747.60
      brain 747.81
      coronary 746.9
      great 747.40
   vena cava (inferior) (superior)
      (congenital) 747.40
   vertebra - *see* Deformity, spine
   vesicourethral orifice (acquired)
      596.8
      congenital NEC 753.9
        specified type NEC 753.8
   vessels of optic papilla (congenital)
      743.9
   visual field (contraction) 368.45
   vitreous humor (congenital) 743.9
      acquired 379.29
   vulva (congenital) 752.40
      acquired 624.8
   wrist (joint) (acquired) 736.00
      congenital 755.50
      contraction 718.43
      valgus 736.03
        congenital 755.59
      varus 736.04
        congenital 755.59

Degeneration, degenerative
   adrenal (capsule) (gland) 255.8
      with hypofunction 255.41
      fatty 255.8
      hyaline 255.8
      infectional 255.8
      lardaceous 277.39
   amyloid (any site) (general) 277.39
   anterior cornua, spinal cord 336.8
   anterior labral 840.8
   aorta, aortic 440.0
      fatty 447.8
      valve (heart) (*see also* Endocarditis,
        aortic) 424.1
   arteriovascular - *see* Arteriosclerosis

Degeneration, degenerative *(Continued)*
   artery, arterial (atheromatous)
      (calcareous) - *see also*
        Arteriosclerosis
      amyloid 277.39
      lardaceous 277.39
      medial NEC (*see also*
        Arteriosclerosis, extremities)
        440.20
   articular cartilage NEC (*see also*
      Disorder, cartilage, articular)
      718.0●
      elbow 718.02
      knee 717.5
      patella 717.7
      shoulder 718.01
      spine (*see also* Spondylosis)
        721.90
   atheromatous - *see* Arteriosclerosis
   bacony (any site) 277.39
   basal nuclei or ganglia NEC 333.0
   bone 733.90
   brachial plexus 353.0
   brain (cortical) (progressive) 331.9
      arteriosclerotic 437.0
      childhood 330.9
        specified type NEC 330.8
      congenital 742.4
      cystic 348.0
        congenital 742.4
      familial NEC 331.89
      grey matter 330.8
      heredofamilial NEC 331.89
      in
        alcoholism 303.9● [331.7]
        beriberi 265.0 [331.7]
        cerebrovascular disease 437.9
          [331.7]
        congenital hydrocephalus 742.3
          [331.7]
          with spina bifida (*see also*
            Spina bifida) 741.0●
            [331.7]
        Babry's disease 272.7 [330.2]
        Gaucher's disease 272.7 [330.2]
        Hunter's disease or syndrome
          277.5 [330.3]
        lipidosis
          cerebral 330.1
          generalized 272.7 [330.2]
        mucopolysaccharidosis 277.5
          [330.3]
        myxedema (*see also* Myxedema)
          244.9 [331.7]
        neoplastic disease NEC
          (M8000/1) 239.9 [331.7]
        Niemann-Pick disease 272.7
          [330.2]
        sphingolipidosis 272.7 [330.2]
        vitamin B$_{12}$ deficiency 266.2
          [331.7]
      motor centers 331.89
      senile 331.2
      specified type NEC 331.89
   breast - *see* Disease, breast
   Bruch's membrane 363.40
   bundle of His 426.50
      left 426.3
      right 426.4
   calcareous NEC 275.49
   capillaries 448.9
      amyloid 277.39
      fatty 448.9
      lardaceous 277.39

Degeneration, degenerative *(Continued)*
   cardiac (brown) (calcareous) (fatty)
      (fibrous) (hyaline) (mural)
      (muscular) (pigmentary) (senile)
      (with arteriosclerosis) (*see also*
      Degeneration, myocardial) 429.1
      valve, valvular - *see* Endocarditis
   cardiorenal (*see also* Hypertension,
      cardiorenal) 404.90
   cardiovascular (*see also* Disease,
      cardiovascular) 429.2
      renal (*see also* Hypertension,
        cardiorenal) 404.90
   cartilage (joint) - *see* Derangement, joint
   cerebellar NEC 334.9
      primary (hereditary) (sporadic)
        334.2
   cerebral - *see* Degeneration, brain
   cerebromacular 330.1
   cerebrovascular 437.1
      due to hypertension 437.2
      late effect - *see* Late effect(s) (of)
        cerebrovascular disease
   cervical plexus 353.2
   cervix 622.8
      due to radiation (intended effect)
        622.8
        adverse effect or misadventure
          622.8
   changes, spine or vertebra (*see also*
      Spondylosis) 721.90
   chitinous 277.39
   chorioretinal 363.40
      congenital 743.53
      hereditary 363.50
   choroid (colloid) (drusen) 363.40
      hereditary 363.50
      senile 363.41
        diffuse secondary 363.42
   cochlear 386.8
   collateral ligament (knee) (medial)
      717.82
      lateral 717.81
   combined (spinal cord) (subacute)
      266.2 [336.2]
      with anemia (pernicious) 281.0
        [336.2]
        due to dietary deficiency 281.1
          [336.2]
      due to vitamin B$_{12}$ deficiency anemia
        (dietary) 281.1 [336.2]
   conjunctiva 372.50
      amyloid 277.39 [372.50]
   cornea 371.40
      calcerous 371.44
      familial (hereditary) (*see also*
        Dystrophy, cornea) 371.50
        macular 371.55
        reticular 371.54
      hyaline (of old scars) 371.41
      marginal (Terrien's) 371.48
      mosaic (shagreen) 371.41
      nodular 371.46
      peripheral 371.48
      senile 371.41
   cortical (cerebellar) (parenchymatous)
      334.2
      alcoholic 303.9● [334.4]
      diffuse, due to arteriopathy 437.0
   corticostriatal-spinal 334.8
   cretinoid 243
   cruciate ligament (knee) (posterior)
      717.84
      anterior 717.83

◄ New   ◄▥ Revised   ~~deleted~~ Deleted   ● Use Additional Digit(s)   ▨ Omit code

Degeneration, degenerative (*Continued*)
  cutis 709.3
    amyloid 277.39
  dental pulp 522.2
  disc disease - *see* Degeneration,
      intervertebral disc
  dorsolateral (spinal cord) - *see*
      Degeneration, combined
  endocardial 424.90
  extrapyramidal NEC 333.90
  eye NEC 360.40
    macular (*see also* Degeneration,
        macula) 362.50
      congenital 362.75
      hereditary 362.76
  fatty (diffuse) (general) 272.8
    liver 571.8
      alcoholic 571.0
    localized site - *see* Degeneration, by
        site, fatty
    placenta - *see* Placenta, abnormal
  globe (eye) NEC 360.40
    macular - *see* Degeneration,
        macula
  grey matter 330.8
  heart (brown) (calcareous) (fatty)
      (fibrous) (hyaline) (mural)
      (muscular) (pigmentary) (senile)
      (with arteriosclerosis) (*see also*
      Degeneration, myocardial)
      429.1
    amyloid 277.39 [425.7]
    atheromatous - *see* Arteriosclerosis,
        coronary
    gouty 274.82
    hypertensive (*see also* Hypertension,
        heart) 402.90
    ischemic 414.9
    valve, valvular - *see* Endocarditis
  hepatolenticular (Wilson's) 275.1
  hepatorenal 572.4
  heredofamilial
    brain NEC 331.89
    spinal cord NEC 336.8
  hyaline (diffuse) (generalized) 728.9
    localized - *see also* Degeneration, by
        site
      cornea 371.41
      keratitis 371.41
  hypertensive vascular - *see*
      Hypertension
  infrapatellar fat pad 729.31
  internal semilunar cartilage 717.3
  intervertebral disc 722.6
    with myelopathy 722.70
    cervical, cervicothoracic 722.4
      with myelopathy 722.71
    lumbar, lumbosacral 722.52
      with myelopathy 722.73
    thoracic, thoracolumbar 722.51
      with myelopathy 722.72
  intestine 569.89
    amyloid 277.39
    lardaceous 277.39
  iris (generalized) (*see also* Atrophy, iris)
      364.59
    pigmentary 364.53
    pupillary margin 364.54
  ischemic - *see* Ischemia
  joint disease (*see also* Osteoarthrosis)
      715.9 ●
    multiple sites 715.09
    spine (*see also* Spondylosis)
        721.90

Degeneration, degenerative (*Continued*)
  kidney (*see also* Sclerosis, renal) 587
    amyloid 277.39 [583.81]
    cyst, cystic (multiple) (solitary) 593.2
      congenital (*see also* Cystic,
          disease, kidney) 753.10
    fatty 593.89
    fibrocystic (congenital) 753.19
    lardaceous 277.39 [583.81]
    polycystic (congenital) 753.12
      adult type (APKD) 753.13
      autosomal dominant 753.13
      autosomal recessive 753.14
      childhood type (CPKD) 753.14
      infantile type 753.14
    waxy 277.39 [583.81]
  Kuhnt-Junius (retina) 362.52
  labyrinth, osseous 386.8
  lacrimal passages, cystic 375.12
  lardaceous (any site) 277.39
  lateral column (posterior), spinal cord
      (*see also* Degeneration, combined)
      266.2 [336.2]
  lattice 362.63
  lens 366.9
    infantile, juvenile, or presenile
        366.00
    senile 366.10
  lenticular (familial) (progressive)
      (Wilson's) (with cirrhosis of liver)
      275.1
    striate artery 437.0
  lethal ball, prosthetic heart valve 996.02
  ligament
    collateral (knee) (medial) 717.82
      lateral 717.81
    cruciate (knee) (posterior) 717.84
      anterior 717.83
  liver (diffuse) 572.8
    amyloid 277.39
    congenital (cystic) 751.62
    cystic 572.8
      congenital 751.62
    fatty 571.8
      alcoholic 571.0
    hypertrophic 572.8
    lardaceous 277.39
    parenchymatous, acute or subacute
        (*see also* Necrosis, liver) 570
    pigmentary 572.8
    toxic (acute) 573.8
    waxy 277.39
  lung 518.89
  lymph gland 289.3
    hyaline 289.3
    lardaceous 277.39
  macula (acquired) (senile) 362.50
    atrophic 362.51
    Best's 362.76
    congenital 362.75
    cystic 362.54
    cystoid 362.53
    disciform 362.52
    dry 362.51
    exudative 362.52
    familial pseudoinflammatory
        362.77
    hereditary 362.76
    hole 362.54
    juvenile (Stargardt's) 362.75
    nonexudative 362.51
    pseudohole 362.54
    wet 362.52
  medullary - *see* Degeneration, brain

Degeneration, degenerative (*Continued*)
  membranous labyrinth, congenital
      (causing impairment of hearing)
      744.05
  meniscus - *see* Derangement, joint
  microcystoid 362.62
  mitral - *see* Insufficiency, mitral
  Mönckeberg's (*see also* Arteriosclerosis,
      extremities) 440.20
  moral 301.7
  motor centers, senile 331.2
  mural (*see also* Degeneration,
      myocardial) 429.1
    heart, cardiac (*see also* Degeneration,
        myocardial) 429.1
    myocardium, myocardial (*see also*
        Degeneration, myocardial)
        429.1
  muscle 728.9
    fatty 728.9
    fibrous 728.9
    heart (*see also* Degeneration,
        myocardial) 429.1
    hyaline 728.9
  muscular progressive 728.2
  myelin, central nervous system NEC
      341.9
  myocardium, myocardial (brown)
      (calcareous) (fatty) (fibrous)
      (hyaline) (mural) (muscular)
      (pigmentary) (senile) (with
      arteriosclerosis) 429.1
    with rheumatic fever (conditions
        classifiable to 390) 398.0
      active, acute, or subacute 391.2
        with chorea 392.0
      inactive or quiescent (with
          chorea) 398.0
    amyloid 277.39 [425.7]
    congenital 746.89
    fetus or newborn 779.89
    gouty 274.82
    hypertensive (*see also* Hypertension,
        heart) 402.90
    ischemic 414.8
    rheumatic (*see also* Degeneration,
        myocardium, with rheumatic
        fever) 398.0
    syphilitic 093.82
  nasal sinus (mucosa) (*see also* Sinusitis)
      473.9
    frontal 473.1
    maxillary 473.0
  nerve - *see* Disorder, nerve
  nervous system 349.89
    amyloid 277.39 [357.4]
    autonomic (*see also* Neuropathy,
        peripheral, autonomic) 337.9
    fatty 349.89
    peripheral autonomic NEC (*see also*
        Neuropathy, peripheral,
        autonomic) 337.9
  nipple 611.9
  nose 478.19
  oculoacousticocerebral, congenital
      (progressive) 743.8
  olivopontocerebellar (familial)
      (hereditary) 333.0
  osseous labyrinth 386.8
  ovary 620.8
    cystic 620.2
    microcystic 620.2
  pallidal, pigmentary (progressive)
      333.0

Degeneration, degenerative *(Continued)*
  pancreas 577.8
    tuberculous *(see also* Tuberculosis)
      017.9●
  papillary muscle 429.81
  paving stone 362.61
  penis 607.89
  peritoneum 568.89
  pigmentary (diffuse) (general)
    localized - *see* Degeneration, by site
    pallidal (progressive) 333.0
    secondary 362.65
  pineal gland 259.8
  pituitary (gland) 253.8
  placenta (fatty) (fibrinoid) (fibroid) -
    see Placenta, abnormal
  popliteal fat pad 729.31
  posterolateral (spinal cord) *(see also*
    Degeneration, combined) 266.2
    [336.2]
  pulmonary valve (heart) *(see also*
    Endocarditis, pulmonary) 424.3
  pulp (tooth) 522.2
  pupillary margin 364.54
  renal *(see also* Sclerosis, renal) 587
    fibrocystic 753.19
    polycystic 753.12
      adult type (APKD) 753.13
      autosomal dominant 753.13
      autosomal recessive 753.14
      childhood type (CPKD) 753.14
      infantile type 753.14
  reticuloendothelial system 289.89
  retina (peripheral) 362.60
    with retinal defect *(see also*
      Detachment, retina, with
      retinal defect) 361.00
    cystic (senile) 362.50
    cystoid 362.53
    hereditary *(see also* Dystrophy,
      retina) 362.70
      cerebroretinal 362.71
      congenital 362.75
      juvenile (Stargardt's) 362.75
      macula 362.76
    Kuhnt-Junius 362.52
    lattice 362.63
    macular *(see also* Degeneration,
      macula) 362.50
    microcystoid 362.62
    palisade 362.63
    paving stone 362.61
    pigmentary (primary) 362.74
      secondary 362.65
    posterior pole *(see also* Degeneration,
      macula) 362.50
    secondary 362.66
    senile 362.60
      cystic 362.53
      reticular 362.64
  saccule, congenital (causing
    impairment of hearing) 744.05
  sacculocochlear 386.8
  senile 797
    brain 331.2
    cardiac, heart, or myocardium *(see*
      also Degeneration, myocardial)
      429.1
    motor centers 331.2
    reticule 362.64
    retina, cystic 362.50
    vascular - *see* Arteriosclerosis
  silicone rubber poppet (prosthetic
    valve) 996.02

Degeneration, degenerative *(Continued)*
  sinus (cystic) *(see also* Sinusitis)
    473.9
    polypoid 471.1
  skin 709.3
    amyloid 277.39
    colloid 709.3
  spinal (cord) 336.8
    amyloid 277.39
    column 733.90
    combined (subacute) *(see also*
      Degeneration, combined)
      266.2 *[336.2]*
      with anemia (pernicious) 281.0
        [336.2]
    dorsolateral *(see also* Degeneration,
      combined) 266.2 *[336.2]*
    familial NEC 336.8
    fatty 336.8
    funicular *(see also* Degeneration,
      combined) 266.2 *[336.2]*
    heredofamilial NEC 336.8
    posterolateral *(see also* Degeneration,
      combined) 266.2 *[336.2]*
    subacute combined - *see*
      Degeneration, combined
    tuberculous *(see also* Tuberculosis)
      013.8●
  spine 733.90
  spleen 289.59
    amyloid 277.39
    lardaceous 277.39
  stomach 537.89
    lardaceous 277.39
  strionigral 333.0
  sudoriparous (cystic) 705.89
  suprarenal (capsule) (gland) 255.8
    with hypofunction 255.41
  sweat gland 705.89
  synovial membrane (pulpy) 727.9
  tapetoretinal 362.74
    adult or presenile form 362.50
  testis (postinfectional) 608.89
  thymus (gland) 254.8
    fatty 254.8
    lardaceous 277.39
  thyroid (gland) 246.8
  tricuspid (heart) (valve) - *see*
    Endocarditis, tricuspid
  tuberculous NEC *(see also* Tuberculosis)
    011.9●
  turbinate 733.90
  uterus 621.8
    cystic 621.8
  vascular (senile) - *see also*
    Arteriosclerosis
    hypertensive - *see* Hypertension
  vitreoretinal (primary) 362.73
    secondary 362.66
  vitreous humor (with infiltration) 379.21
  wallerian NEC - *see* Disorder, nerve
  waxy (any site) 277.39
  Wilson's hepatolenticular 275.1
Deglutition
  paralysis 784.99
    hysterical 300.11
  pneumonia 507.0
Degos' disease or syndrome 447.8
Degradation disorder, branched-chain
  amino-acid 270.3
Dehiscence
  anastomosis - *see* Complications,
    anastomosis
  cesarean wound 674.1●

Dehiscence *(Continued)*
  closure of
    cornea 998.32
    fascia, superficial or muscular 998.31
    internal organ 998.31
    mucosa 998.32
    muscle or muscle flap 998.31
    ribs or rib cage 998.31
    skin 998.32
    skull or craniotomy 998.31
    sternum or sternotomy 998.31
    subcutaneous tissue 998.32
    tendon or ligament 998.31
    traumatic laceration (external)
      (internal) 998.33
  episiotomy 674.2●
  operation wound 998.32
    deep 998.31
    external 998.32
    internal 998.31
    superficial 998.32
  perineal wound (postpartum) 674.2●
  postoperative 998.32
    abdomen 998.32
      internal 998.31
    internal 998.31
  traumatic injury wound repair 998.33
  uterine wound 674.1●
Dehydration (cachexia) 276.51
  with
    hypernatremia 276.0
    hyponatremia 276.1
  newborn 775.5
Deiters' nucleus syndrome 386.19
Déjérine's disease 356.0
Déjérine-Klumpke paralysis 767.6
Déjérine-Roussy syndrome 338.0
Déjérine-Sottas disease or neuropathy
  (hypertrophic) 356.0
Déjérine-Thomas atrophy or syndrome
  333.0
de Lange's syndrome (Amsterdam dwarf,
  mental retardation, and
  brachycephaly) 759.89
Delay, delayed
  adaptation, cones or rods 368.63
  any plane in pelvis
    affecting fetus or newborn 763.1
    complicating delivery 660.1●
  birth or delivery NEC 662.1●
    affecting fetus or newborn 763.9
    second twin, triplet, or multiple
      mate 662.3●
  closure - *see also* Fistula
    cranial suture 756.0
    fontanel 756.0
  coagulation NEC 790.92
  conduction (cardiac) (ventricular) 426.9
  delivery NEC 662.1●
    second twin, triplet, etc. 662.3●
      affecting fetus or newborn 763.89
  development
    in childhood 783.40
      physiological 783.40
    intellectual NEC 315.9
    learning NEC 315.2
    reading 315.00
    sexual 259.0
    speech 315.39
      and language due to hearing loss
        315.34
      associated with hyperkinesis
        314.1
    spelling 315.09

Delay, delayed (*Continued*)
gastric emptying 536.8
menarche 256.39
  due to pituitary hypofunction
    253.4
menstruation (cause unknown)
    626.8
milestone in childhood 783.42
motility - *see* Hypomotility
passage of meconium (newborn)
    777.1
primary respiration 768.9
puberty 259.0
separation of umbilical cord 779.83
sexual maturation, female 259.0
vaccination V64.00
Del Castillo's syndrome (germinal
    aplasia) 606.0
Deleage's disease 359.89
Deletion syndrome
  5p 758.31
  22q11.2 758.32
  autosomal NEC 758.39
  constitutional 5q deletion 758.39
Delhi (boil) (button) (sore) 085.1
Delinquency (juvenile) 312.9
  group (*see also* Disturbance, conduct)
    312.2●
  neurotic 312.4
Delirium, delirious 780.09
  acute (psychotic) 780.09 ◀▥
    due to conditions classified
      elsewhere 293.0 ◀
  alcoholic 291.0
    acute 291.0
    chronic 291.1
  alcoholicum 291.0
  chronic (*see also* Psychosis) 293.89
    due to or associated with physical
      condition - *see* Psychosis,
      organic
  drug-induced 292.81
  due to conditions classified elsewhere
    293.0
  eclamptic (*see also* Eclampsia) 780.39
  exhaustion (*see also* Reaction, stress,
    acute) 308.9
  hysterical 300.11
  in
    presenile dementia 290.11
    senile dementia 290.3
  induced by drug 292.81
  manic, maniacal (acute) (*see also*
    Psychosis, affective) 296.0●
    recurrent episode 296.1●
    single episode 296.0●
  puerperal 293.9
  senile 290.3
  subacute (psychotic) 293.1
  thyroid (*see also* Thyrotoxicosis) 242.9●
  traumatic - *see also* Injury,
    intracranial
    with
      lesion, spinal cord - *see* Injury,
        spinal, by site
      shock, spinal - *see* Injury, spinal,
        by site
  tremens (impending) 291.0
  uremic - *see* Uremia
  withdrawal
    alcoholic (acute) 291.0
      chronic 291.1
    drug 292.0

Delivery

Note: Use the following fifth-digit
subclassification with categories
640–649, 651–676:

  0 unspecified as to episode of care
  1 delivered, with or without
       mention of antepartum
       condition
  2 delivered, with mention of
       postpartum complication
  3 antepartum condition or
       complication
  4 postpartum condition or
       complication

breech (assisted) (buttocks) (complete)
    (frank) (spontaneous) 652.2●
  affecting fetus or newborn 763.0
  extraction NEC 669.6●
cesarean (for) 669.7●
  abnormal
    cervix 654.6●
    pelvic organs of tissues 654.9●
    pelvis (bony) (major) NEC 653.0●
    presentation or position 652.9●
      in multiple gestation 652.6●
    size, fetus 653.5●
    soft parts (of pelvis) 654.9●
    uterus, congenital 654.0●
    vagina 654.7●
    vulva 654.8●
  abruptio placentae 641.2●
  acromion presentation 652.8●
  affecting fetus or newborn 763.4
  anteversion, cervix or uterus 654.4●
  atony, uterus 661.2●
    with hemorrhage 666.1●
  bicornis or bicornuate uterus 654.0●
  breech presentation (buttocks)
    (complete) (frank) 652.2●
  brow presentation 652.4●
  cephalopelvic disproportion
    (normally formed fetus)
    653.4●
  chin presentation 652.4●
  cicatrix of cervix 654.6●
  contracted pelvis (general) 653.1●
    inlet 653.2●
    outlet 653.3●
  cord presentation or prolapse 663.0●
  cystocele 654.4●
  deformity (acquired) (congenital)
    pelvic organs or tissues NEC
      654.9●
    pelvis (bony) NEC 653.0●
  displacement, uterus NEC 654.4●
  disproportion NEC 653.9●
  distress
    fetal 656.8●
    maternal 669.0●
  eclampsia 642.6●
  face presentation 652.4●
  failed
    forceps 660.7●
    trial of labor NEC 660.6●
    vacuum extraction 660.7●
    ventouse 660.7●
  fetal deformity 653.7●
  fetal-maternal hemorrhage 656.0●
  fetus, fetal
    distress 656.8●
    prematurity 656.8●
  fibroid (tumor) (uterus) 654.1●

Delivery (*Continued*)
cesarean (*Continued*)
  footling 652.8●
    with successful version 652.1●
  hemorrhage (antepartum)
    (intrapartum) NEC 641.9●
  hydrocephalic fetus 653.6●
  incarceration of uterus 654.3●
  incoordinate uterine action 661.4●
  inertia, uterus 661.2●
    primary 661.0●
    secondary 661.1●
  lateroversion, uterus or cervix
    654.4●
  mal lie 652.9●
  malposition
    fetus 652.9●
      in multiple gestation 652.6●
    pelvic organs or tissues NEC
      654.9●
    uterus NEC or cervix 654.4●
  malpresentation NEC 652.9●
    in multiple gestation 652.6●
  maternal
    diabetes mellitus (conditions
      classifiable to 249 and 250)
      648.0●
    heart disease NEC 648.6●
  meconium in liquor 656.8●
    staining only 792.3
  oblique presentation 652.3●
  oversize fetus 653.5●
  pelvic tumor NEC 654.9●
  placental insufficiency 656.5●
  placenta previa 641.0●
    with hemorrhage 641.1●
  poor dilation, cervix 661.0●
  pre-eclampsia 642.4●
    severe 642.5●
  previous
    cesarean delivery, section
      654.2●
    surgery (to)
      cervix 654.6●
      gynecological NEC 654.9●
      rectum 654.8●
      uterus NEC 654.9●
        previous cesarean delivery,
          section 654.2●
      vagina 654.7●
  prolapse
    arm or hand 652.7●
    uterus 654.4●
  prolonged labor 662.1●
  rectocele 654.4●
  retroversion, uterus or cervix
    654.3●
  rigid
    cervix 654.6●
    pelvic floor 654.4●
    perineum 654.8●
    vagina 654.7●
    vulva 654.8●
  sacculation, pregnant uterus 654.4●
  scar(s)
    cervix 654.6●
    cesarean delivery, section 654.2●
    uterus NEC 654.9●
      due to previous cesarean
        delivery, section 654.2●
  Shirodkar suture in situ 654.5●
  shoulder presentation 652.8●
  stenosis or stricture, cervix 654.6●
  transverse presentation or lie 652.3●

Delivery (Continued)
  cesarean (Continued)
    tumor, pelvic organs or tissues NEC
        654.4●
    umbilical cord presentation or
        prolapse 663.0●
  completely normal case - see category
      650
  complicated (by) NEC 669.9●
    abdominal tumor, fetal 653.7●
      causing obstructed labor 660.1●
    abnormal, abnormality of
      cervix 654.6●
        causing obstructed labor
            660.2●
      forces of labor 661.9●
      formation of uterus 654.0●
      pelvic organs or tissues 654.9●
        causing obstructed labor
            660.2●
      pelvis (bony) (major) NEC 653.0●
        causing obstructed labor
            660.1●
      presentation or position NEC
          652.9●
        causing obstructed labor
            660.0●
      size, fetus 653.5●
        causing obstructed labor
            660.1●
      soft parts (of pelvis) 654.9●
        causing obstructed labor
            660.2●
      uterine contractions NEC 661.9●
      uterus (formation) 654.0●
        causing obstructed labor
            660.2●
      vagina 654.7●
        causing obstructed labor
            660.2●
    abnormally formed uterus (any
        type) (congenital) 654.0●
      causing obstructed labor 660.2●
    acromion presentation 652.8●
      causing obstructed labor 660.0●
    adherent placenta 667.0●
      with hemorrhage 666.0●
    adhesions, uterus (to abdominal
        wall) 654.4●
    advanced maternal age NEC
        659.6●
      multigravida 659.6●
      primigravida 659.5●
    air embolism 673.0●
    amnionitis 658.4●
    amniotic fluid embolism 673.1●
    anesthetic death 668.9●
    annular detachment, cervix 665.3●
    antepartum hemorrhage - see
        Delivery, complicated,
        hemorrhage
    anteversion, cervix or uterus 654.4●
      causing obstructed labor 660.2●
    apoplexy 674.0●
      placenta 641.2●
    arrested active phase 661.1●
    asymmetrical pelvis bone 653.0●
      causing obstructed labor 660.1●
    atony, uterus with hemorrhage
        (hypotonic) (inertia) 666.1●
      hypertonic 661.4●
    Bandl's ring 661.4●
    Battledore placenta - see Placenta,
        abnormal

Delivery (Continued)
  complicated (by) NEC (Continued)
    bicornis or bicornuate uterus
        654.0●
      causing obstructed labor 660.2●
    birth injury to mother NEC 665.9●
    bleeding (see also Delivery,
        complicated, hemorrhage)
        641.9●
    breech presentation (assisted)
        (buttocks) (complete) (frank)
        (spontaneous) 652.2●
      with successful version 652.1●
    brow presentation 652.4●
    cephalopelvic disproportion
        (normally formed fetus)
        653.4●
      causing obstructed labor 660.1●
    cerebral hemorrhage 674.0●
    cervical dystocia 661.2●
    chin presentation 652.4●
      causing obstructed labor 660.0●
    cicatrix
      cervix 654.6●
        causing obstructed labor
            660.2●
      vagina 654.7●
        causing obstructed labor
            660.2●
    coagulation defect 649.3●
    colporrhexis 665.4●
      with perineal laceration 664.0●
    compound presentation 652.8●
      causing obstructed labor 660.0●
    compression of cord (umbilical)
        663.2●
      around neck 663.1●
      cord prolapsed 663.0●
    contraction, contracted pelvis
        653.1●
      causing obstructed labor 660.1●
      general 653.1●
        causing obstructed labor
            660.1●
      inlet 653.2●
        causing obstructed labor
            660.1●
      midpelvic 653.8●
        causing obstructed labor
            660.1●
      midplane 653.8●
        causing obstructed labor
            660.1●
      outlet 653.3●
        causing obstructed labor
            660.1●
    contraction ring 661.4●
    cord (umbilical) 663.9●
      around neck, tightly or with
          compression 663.1●
        without compression 663.3●
      bruising 663.6●
      complication NEC 663.9●
        specified type NEC 663.8●
      compression NEC 663.2●
      entanglement NEC 663.3●
        with compression 663.2●
      forelying 663.0●
      hematoma 663.6●
      marginal attachment 663.8●
      presentation 663.0●
      prolapse (complete) (occult)
          (partial) 663.0●
      short 663.4●

Delivery (Continued)
  complicated (by) NEC (Continued)
    cord (Continued)
      specified complication NEC
          663.8●
      thrombosis (vessels) 663.6●
      vascular lesion 663.6●
      velamentous insertion 663.8●
    Couvelaire uterus 641.2●
    cretin pelvis (dwarf type) (male
        type) 653.1●
      causing obstructed labor 660.1●
    crossbirth 652.3●
      with successful version 652.1●
      causing obstructed labor 660.0●
    cyst (Gartner's duct) 654.7●
    cystocele 654.4●
      causing obstructed labor 660.2●
    death of fetus (near term) 656.4●
      early (before 22 completed weeks'
          gestation) 632
    deformity (acquired) (congenital)
      fetus 653.7●
        causing obstructed labor
            660.1●
      pelvic organs or tissues NEC
          654.9●
        causing obstructed labor
            660.2●
      pelvis (bony) NEC 653.0●
        causing obstructed labor
            660.1●
    delay, delayed
      delivery in multiple pregnancy
          662.3●
      due to locked mates 660.5●
      following rupture of membranes
          (spontaneous) 658.2●
        artificial 658.3●
    depressed fetal heart tones 659.7●
    diastasis recti 665.8●
    dilatation
      bladder 654.4●
        causing obstructed labor
            660.2●
      cervix, incomplete, poor or slow
          661.0●
    diseased placenta 656.7●
    displacement uterus NEC 654.4●
      causing obstructed labor 660.2●
    disproportion NEC 653.9●
      causing obstructed labor 660.1●
    disruptio uteri - see Delivery,
        complicated, rupture, uterus
    distress
      fetal 656.8●
      maternal 669.0●
    double uterus (congenital) 654.0●
      causing obstructed labor
          660.2●
    dropsy amnion 657●
    dysfunction, uterus 661.9●
      hypertonic 661.4●
      hypotonic 661.2●
        primary 661.0●
        secondary 661.1●
      incoordinate 661.4●
    dystocia
      cervical 661.2●
      fetal - see Delivery, complicated,
          abnormal, presentation
      maternal - see Delivery,
          complicated, prolonged
          labor

◀ New   ◀╫ Revised   deleted Deleted   ● Use Additional Digit(s)   ▨ Omit code

Delivery *(Continued)*
  complicated (by) NEC *(Continued)*
    dystocia *(Continued)*
      pelvic - *see* Delivery, complicated, contraction pelvis
      positional 652.8●
      shoulder girdle 660.4●
    eclampsia 642.6●
    ectopic kidney 654.4●
      causing obstructed labor 660.2●
    edema, cervix 654.6●
      causing obstructed labor 660.2●
    effusion, amniotic fluid 658.1●
    elderly multigravida 659.6●
    elderly primigravida 659.5●
    embolism (pulmonary) 673.2●
      air 673.0●
      amniotic fluid 673.1●
      blood-clot 673.2●
      cerebral 674.0●
      fat 673.8●
      pyemic 673.3●
      septic 673.3●
    entanglement, umbilical cord 663.3●
      with compression 663.2●
      around neck (with compression) 663.1●
    eversion, cervix or uterus 665.2●
    excessive
      fetal growth 653.5●
        causing obstructed labor 660.1●
      size of fetus 653.5●
        causing obstructed labor 660.1●
    face presentation 652.4●
      causing obstructed labor 660.0●
      to pubes 660.3●
    failure, fetal head to enter pelvic brim 652.5●
      causing obstructed labor 660.0●
    female genital mutilation 660.8●
    fetal
      acid-base balance 656.8●
      death (near term) NEC 656.4●
        early (before 22 completed weeks' gestation) 632
      deformity 653.7●
        causing obstructed labor 660.1●
      distress 656.8●
      heart rate or rhythm 659.7●
      reduction of multiple fetuses reduced to single fetus 651.7●
    fetopelvic disproportion 653.4●
      causing obstructed labor 660.1●
    fever during labor 659.2●
    fibroid (tumor) (uterus) 654.1●
      causing obstructed labor 660.2●
    fibromyomata 654.1●
      causing obstructed labor 660.2●
    forelying umbilical cord 663.0●
    fracture of coccyx 665.6●
    hematoma 664.5●
      broad ligament 665.7●
      ischial spine 665.7●
      pelvic 665.7●
      perineum 664.5●
      soft tissues 665.7●
      subdural 674.0●
      umbilical cord 663.6●
      vagina 665.7●
      vulva or perineum 664.5●

Delivery *(Continued)*
  complicated (by) NEC *(Continued)*
    hemorrhage (uterine) (antepartum) (intrapartum) (pregnancy) 641.9●
      accidental 641.2●
      associated with
        afibrinogenemia 641.3●
        coagulation defect 641.3●
          hyperfibrinolysis 641.3●
          hypofibrinogenemia 641.3●
      cerebral 674.0●
      due to
        low-lying placenta 641.1●
        placenta previa 641.1●
        premature separation of placenta (normally implanted) 641.2●
        retained placenta 666.0●
        trauma 641.8●
        uterine leiomyoma 641.8●
      marginal sinus rupture 641.2●
      placenta NEC 641.9●
      postpartum (atonic) (immediate) (within 24 hours) 666.1●
        with retained or trapped placenta 666.0●
        delayed 666.2●
        secondary 666.2●
        third stage 666.0●
    hourglass contraction, uterus 661.4●
    hydramnios 657●
    hydrocephalic fetus 653.6●
      causing obstructed labor 660.1●
    hydrops fetalis 653.7●
      causing obstructed labor 660.1●
    hypertension - *see* Hypertension, complicating pregnancy
    hypertonic uterine dysfunction 661.4●
    hypotonic uterine dysfunction 661.2●
    impacted shoulders 660.4●
    incarceration, uterus 654.3●
      causing obstructed labor 660.2●
    incomplete dilation (cervix) 661.0●
    incoordinate uterus 661.4●
    indication NEC 659.9●
      specified type NEC 659.8●
    inertia, uterus 661.2●
      hypertonic 661.4●
      hypotonic 661.2●
      primary 661.0●
      secondary 661.1●
    infantile
      genitalia 654.4●
        causing obstructed labor 660.2●
      uterus (os) 654.4●
        causing obstructed labor 660.2●
    injury (to mother) NEC 665.9●
    intrauterine fetal death (near term) NEC 656.4●
      early (before 22 completed weeks' gestation) 632
    inversion, uterus 665.2●
    kidney, ectopic 654.4●
      causing obstructed labor 660.2●
    knot (true), umbilical cord 663.2●
    labor, premature (before 37 completed weeks' gestation) 644.2●

Delivery *(Continued)*
  complicated (by) NEC *(Continued)*
    laceration 664.9●
      anus (sphincter) (healed) (old) 654.8●
        with mucosa 664.3●
        not associated with third-degree perineal laceration 664.6●
      bladder (urinary) 665.5●
      bowel 665.5●
      central 664.4●
      cervix (uteri) 665.3●
      fourchette 664.0●
      hymen 664.0●
      labia (majora) (minora) 664.0●
      pelvic
        floor 664.1●
        organ NEC 665.5●
      perineum, perineal 664.4●
        first degree 664.0●
        second degree 664.1●
        third degree 664.2●
        fourth degree 664.3●
        central 664.4●
        extensive NEC 664.4●
        muscles 664.1●
        skin 664.0●
        slight 664.0●
      peritoneum (pelvic) 665.5● ◀▥
      periurethral tissue 664.8●
      rectovaginal (septum) (without perineal laceration) 665.4●
        with perineum 664.2●
          with anal or rectal mucosa 664.3●
      skin (perineum) 664.0●
      specified site or type NEC 664.8●
      sphincter ani (healed) (old) 654.8●
        with mucosa 664.3●
        not associated with third-degree perineal laceration 664.6●
      urethra 665.5●
      uterus 665.1●
        before labor 665.0●
      vagina, vaginal (deep) (high) (sulcus) (wall) (without perineal laceration) 665.4●
        with perineum 664.0●
        muscles, with perineum 664.1●
      vulva 664.0●
    lateroversion, uterus or cervix 654.4●
      causing obstructed labor 660.2●
    locked mates 660.5●
    low implantation of placenta - *see* Delivery, complicated, placenta, previa
    mal lie 652.9●
    malposition
      fetus NEC 652.9●
        causing obstructed labor 660.0●
      pelvic organs or tissues NEC 654.9●
        causing obstructed labor 660.2●
    placenta 641.1●
      without hemorrhage 641.0●

Delivery (Continued)
  complicated (by) NEC (Continued)
    malposition (Continued)
      uterus NEC or cervix 654.4●
        causing obstructed labor
          660.2●
    malpresentation 652.9●
      causing obstructed labor 660.0●
    marginal sinus (bleeding) (rupture)
      641.2●
    maternal hypotension syndrome
      669.2●
    meconium in liquor 656.8●
    membranes, retained - see Delivery,
      complicated, placenta,
      retained
    mentum presentation 652.4●
      causing obstructed labor 660.0●
    metrorrhagia (myopathia) - see
      Delivery, complicated,
      hemorrhage
    metrorrhexis - see Delivery,
      complicated, rupture, uterus
    multiparity (grand) 659.4●
    myelomeningocele, fetus 653.7●
      causing obstructed labor 660.1●
    Nägele's pelvis 653.0●
      causing obstructed labor 660.1●
    nonengagement, fetal head 652.5●
      causing obstructed labor 660.0●
    oblique presentation 652.3●
      causing obstructed labor
        660.0●
    obstetric
      shock 669.1●
      trauma NEC 665.9●
    obstructed labor 660.9●
      due to
        abnormality of pelvic organs
          or tissues (conditions
          classifiable to 654.0–
          654.9) 660.2●
        deep transverse arrest 660.3●
        impacted shoulders 660.4●
        locked twins 660.5●
        malposition and
          malpresentation of fetus
          (conditions classifiable to
          652.0–652.9) 660.0●
        persistent occipitoposterior
          660.3●
        shoulder dystocia 660.4●
    occult prolapse of umbilical cord
      663.0●
    oversize fetus 653.5●
      causing obstructed labor 660.1●
    pathological retraction ring, uterus
      661.4●
    pelvic
      arrest (deep) (high) (of fetal head)
        (transverse) 660.3●
      deformity (bone) - see also
        Deformity, pelvis, with
        disproportion
      soft tissue 654.9●
        causing obstructed labor
          660.2●
      tumor NEC 654.9●
        causing obstructed labor
          660.2●
    penetration, pregnant uterus by
      instrument 665.1●
    perforation - see Delivery,
      complicated, laceration

Delivery (Continued)
  complicated (by) NEC (Continued)
    persistent
      hymen 654.8●
        causing obstructed labor
          660.2●
      occipitoposterior 660.3●
    placenta, placental
      ablatio 641.2●
      abnormality 656.7●
        with hemorrhage 641.2●
      abruptio 641.2●
      accreta 667.0●
        with hemorrhage 666.0●
      adherent (without hemorrhage)
        667.0●
        with hemorrhage 666.0●
      apoplexy 641.2●
      Battledore - see Placenta,
        abnormal
      detachment (premature)
        641.2●
      disease 656.7●
      hemorrhage NEC 641.9●
      increta (without hemorrhage)
        667.0●
        with hemorrhage 666.0●
      low (implantation) 641.1●
        without hemorrhage 641.0●
      malformation 656.7●
        with hemorrhage 641.2●
      malposition 641.1●
        without hemorrhage 641.0●
      marginal sinus rupture 641.2●
      percreta 667.0●
        with hemorrhage 666.0●
      premature separation 641.2●
      previa (central) (lateral)
        (marginal) (partial) 641.1●
        without hemorrhage 641.0●
      retained (with hemorrhage)
        666.0●
        without hemorrhage 667.0●
      rupture of marginal sinus 641.2●
      separation (premature) 641.2●
      trapped 666.0●
        without hemorrhage 667.0●
      vicious insertion 641.1●
    polyhydramnios 657●
    polyp, cervix 654.6●
      causing obstructed labor 660.2●
    precipitate labor 661.3●
    premature
      labor (before 37 completed
        weeks' gestation) 644.2●
      rupture, membranes 658.1●
        delayed delivery following
          658.2●
    presenting umbilical cord 663.0●
    previous
      cesarean delivery, section 654.2●
      surgery
        cervix 654.6●
          causing obstructed labor
            660.2●
        gynecological NEC 654.9●
          causing obstructed labor
            660.2●
        perineum 654.8●
        rectum 654.8●
        uterus NEC 654.9●
          due to previous cesarean
            delivery, section
            654.2●

Delivery (Continued)
  complicated (by) NEC (Continued)
    previous (Continued)
      surgery (Continued)
        vagina 654.7●
          causing obstructed labor
            660.2●
        vulva 654.8●
    primary uterine inertia 661.0●
    primipara, elderly or old 659.5●
    prolapse
      arm or hand 652.7●
        causing obstructed labor
          660.0●
      cord (umbilical) 663.0●
      fetal extremity 652.8●
      foot or leg 652.8●
        causing obstructed labor
          660.0●
      umbilical cord (complete) (occult)
        (partial) 663.0●
      uterus 654.4●
        causing obstructed labor
          660.2●
    prolonged labor 662.1●
      first stage 662.0●
      second stage 662.2●
      active phase 661.2●
      due to
        cervical dystocia 661.2●
        contraction ring 661.4●
        tetanic uterus 661.4●
        uterine inertia 661.2●
          primary 661.0●
          secondary 661.1●
      latent phase 661.0●
    pyrexia during labor 659.2●
    rachitic pelvis 653.2●
      causing obstructed labor 660.1●
    rectocele 654.4●
      causing obstructed labor 660.2●
    retained membranes or portions of
      placenta 666.2●
      without hemorrhage 667.1●
    retarded (prolonged) birth 662.1●
    retention secundines (with
      hemorrhage) 666.2●
      without hemorrhage 667.1●
    retroversion, uterus or cervix
      654.3●
      causing obstructed labor 660.2●
    rigid
      cervix 654.6●
        causing obstructed labor
          660.2●
      pelvic floor 654.4●
        causing obstructed labor
          660.2●
      perineum or vulva 654.8●
        causing obstructed labor
          660.2●
      vagina 654.7●
        causing obstructed labor
          660.2●
    Robert's pelvis 653.0●
      causing obstructed labor
        660.1●
    rupture - see also Delivery,
      complicated, laceration
      bladder (urinary) 665.5●
      cervix 665.3●
      marginal sinus 641.2●
      membranes, premature 658.1●
      pelvic organ NEC 665.5●

◀ New   ◀▥ Revised   deleted Deleted   ● Use Additional Digit(s)   Omit code

Delivery (Continued)
    complicated (by) NEC (Continued)
        rupture (Continued)
            perineum (without mention of
                other laceration) - see
                Delivery, complicated,
                laceration, perineum
            peritoneum (pelvic) 665.5● ◀▥
            urethra 665.5●
            uterus (during labor) 665.1●
                before labor 665.0●
        sacculation, pregnant uterus 654.4●
        sacral teratomas, fetal 653.7●
            causing obstructed labor 660.1●
        scar(s)
            cervix 654.6●
                causing obstructed labor
                    660.2●
            cesarean delivery, section
                654.2●
                causing obstructed labor
                    660.2●
            perineum 654.8●
                causing obstructed labor
                    660.2●
            uterus NEC 654.9●
                causing obstructed labor
                    660.2●
                due to previous cesarean
                    delivery, section 654.2●
            vagina 654.7●
                causing obstructed labor
                    660.2●
            vulva 654.8●
                causing obstructed labor
                    660.2●
        scoliotic pelvis 653.0●
            causing obstructed labor 660.1●
        secondary uterine inertia 661.1●
        secundines, retained - see Delivery,
            complicated, placenta,
            retained
        separation
            placenta (premature) 641.2●
            pubic bone 665.6●
            symphysis pubis 665.6●
        septate vagina 654.7●
            causing obstructed labor 660.2●
        shock (birth) (obstetric) (puerperal)
            669.1●
        short cord syndrome 663.4●
        shoulder
            girdle dystocia 660.4●
            presentation 652.8●
                causing obstructed labor
                    660.0●
        Siamese twins 678.1●
        slow slope active phase 661.2●
        spasm
            cervix 661.4●
            uterus 661.4●
        spondylolisthesis, pelvis 653.3●
            causing obstructed labor 660.1●
        spondylolysis (lumbosacral) 653.3●
            causing obstructed labor 660.1●
        spondylosis 653.0●
            causing obstructed labor 660.1●
        stenosis or stricture
            cervix 654.6●
                causing obstructed labor
                    660.2●
            vagina 654.7●
                causing obstructed labor
                    660.2●

Delivery (Continued)
    complicated (by) NEC (Continued)
        sudden death, unknown cause
            669.9●
        tear (pelvic organ) (see also Delivery,
            complicated, laceration)
            664.9●
            anal sphincter (healed) (old)
                654.8●
                not associated with third-
                    degree perineal
                    laceration 664.6●
        teratomas, sacral, fetal 653.7●
            causing obstructed labor 660.1●
        tetanic uterus 661.4●
        tipping pelvis 653.0●
            causing obstructed labor 660.1●
        transverse
            arrest (deep) 660.3●
            presentation or lie 652.3●
                with successful version
                    652.1●
                causing obstructed labor
                    660.0●
        trauma (obstetrical) NEC 665.9●
            periurethral 664.8 ◀
        tumor
            abdominal, fetal 653.7●
                causing obstructed labor
                    660.1●
            pelvic organs or tissues NEC
                654.9●
                causing obstructed labor
                    660.2●
        umbilical cord (see also Delivery,
            complicated, cord) 663.9●
            around neck tightly, or with
                compression 663.1●
            entanglement NEC 663.3●
                with compression 663.2●
            prolapse (complete) (occult)
                (partial) 663.0●
        unstable lie 652.0●
            causing obstructed labor
                660.0●
        uterine
            inertia (see also Delivery,
                complicated, inertia,
                uterus) 661.2●
            spasm 661.4●
        vasa previa 663.5●
        velamentous insertion of cord
            663.8●
        young maternal age 659.8●
    delayed NEC 662.1●
        following rupture of membranes
            (spontaneous) 658.2●
            artificial 658.3●
        second twin, triplet, etc. 662.3●
    difficult NEC 669.9●
        previous, affecting management of
            pregnancy or childbirth V23.49
        specified type NEC 669.8●
    early onset (spontaneous) 644.2●
    footling 652.8●
        with successful version 652.1●
    forceps NEC 669.5●
        affecting fetus or newborn 763.2
    missed (at or near term) 656.4●
    multiple gestation NEC 651.9●
        with fetal loss and retention of one
            or more fetus(es) 651.6●
        following (elective) fetal reduction
            651.7●

Delivery (Continued)
    multiple gestation NEC (Continued)
        specified type NEC 651.8●
            with fetal loss and retention of
                one or more fetus(es)
                651.6●
            following (elective) fetal
                reduction 651.7●
    nonviable infant 656.4●
    normal - see category 650
    precipitate 661.3●
        affecting fetus or newborn 763.6
    premature NEC (before 37 completed
        weeks' gestation) 644.2●
        previous, affecting management of
            pregnancy V23.41
    quadruplet NEC 651.2●
        with fetal loss and retention of one
            or more fetus(es) 651.5●
        following (elective) fetal reduction
            651.7●
    quintuplet NEC 651.8●
        with fetal loss and retention of one
            or more fetus(es) 651.6●
        following (elective) fetal reduction
            651.7●
    sextuplet NEC 651.8●
        with fetal loss and retention of one
            or more fetus(es) 651.6●
        following (elective) fetal reduction
            651.7●
    specified complication NEC
        669.8●
    stillbirth (near term) NEC 656.4●
        early (before 22 completed weeks'
            gestation) 632
    term pregnancy (live birth) NEC - see
        category 650
        stillbirth NEC 656.4●
    threatened premature 644.2●
    triplets NEC 651.1●
        with fetal loss and retention of one
            or more fetus(es) 651.4●
        delayed delivery (one or more
            mates) 662.3●
        following (elective) fetal reduction
            651.7●
        locked mates 660.5●
    twins NEC 651.0●
        with fetal loss and retention of one
            fetus 651.3●
        delayed delivery (one or more
            mates) 662.3●
        following (elective) fetal reduction
            651.7●
        locked mates 660.5●
    uncomplicated - see category 650
    vacuum extractor NEC 669.5●
        affecting fetus or newborn
            763.3
    ventouse NEC 669.5●
        affecting fetus or newborn
            763.3
Dellen, cornea 371.41
Delusions (paranoid) 297.9
    grandiose 297.1
    parasitosis 300.29
    systematized 297.1
Dementia 294.8
    alcohol-induced persisting (see
        also Psychosis, alcoholic)
        291.2
    Alzheimer's - see Alzheimer's,
        dementia

Dementia (Continued)
  arteriosclerotic (simple type)
      (uncomplicated) 290.40
    with
      acute confusional state 290.41
      delirium 290.41
      delusions 290.42
      depressed mood 290.43
    depressed type 290.43
    paranoid type 290.42
  Binswanger's 290.12
  catatonic (acute) (see also
      Schizophrenia) 295.2●
  congenital (see also Retardation, mental)
      319
  degenerative 290.9
    presenile-onset - see Dementia,
        presenile
    senile-onset - see Dementia, senile
  developmental (see also Schizophrenia)
      295.9●
  dialysis 294.8
    transient 293.9
  drug-induced persisting (see also
      Psychosis, drug) 292.82
  due to or associated with condition(s)
      classified elsewhere
    Alzheimer's
      with behavioral disturbance 331.0
          [294.11]
      without behavioral disturbance
          331.0 [294.10]
    cerebral lipidoses
      with behavioral disturbance 330.1
          [294.11]
      without behavioral disturbance
          330.1 [294.10]
    epilepsy
      with behavioral disturbance
          345.9● [294.11]
      without behavioral disturbance
          345.9● [294.10]
    hepatolenticular degeneration
      with behavioral disturbance 275.1
          [294.11]
      without behavioral disturbance
          275.1 [294.10]
    HIV
      with behavioral disturbance 042
          [294.11]
      without behavioral disturbance
          042 [294.10]
    Huntington's chorea
      with behavioral disturbance 333.4
          [294.11]
      without behavioral disturbance
          333.4 [294.10]
    Jakob-Creutzfeldt disease (CJD)
      with behavioral disturbance
          046.19 [294.11]
      without behavioral disturbance
          046.19 [294.10]
      variant (vCJD) 046.11
        with dementia
          with behavioral disturbance
              046.11 [294.11]
          without behavioral
              disturbance 046.11
              [294.10]
    Lewy bodies
      with behavioral disturbance
          331.82 [294.11]
      without behavioral disturbance
          331.82 [294.10]

Dementia (Continued)
  due to or associated with condition(s)
      classified elsewhere (Continued)
    multiple sclerosis
      with behavioral disturbance 340
          [294.11]
      without behavioral disturbance
          340 [294.10]
    neurosyphilis
      with behavioral disturbance 094.9
          [294.11]
      without behavioral disturbance
          094.9 [294.10]
    Parkinsonism
      with behavioral disturbance
          331.82 [294.11]
      without behavioral disturbance
          331.82 [294.10]
    Pelizaeus-Merzbacher disease
      with behavioral disturbance 333.0
          [294.11]
      without behavioral disturbance
          333.0 [294.10]
    Pick's disease
      with behavioral disturbance
          331.11 [294.11]
      without behavioral disturbance
          331.11 [294.10]
    polyarteritis nodosa
      with behavioral disturbance 446.0
          [294.11]
      without behavioral disturbance
          446.0 [294.10]
    syphilis
      with behavioral disturbance 094.1
          [294.11]
      without behavioral disturbance
          094.1 [294.10]
    Wilson's disease
      with behavioral disturbance 275.1
          [294.11]
      without behavioral disturbance
          275.1 [294.10]
  frontal 331.19
    with behavioral disturbance 331.19
        [294.11]
    without behavioral disturbance
        331.19 [294.10]
  frontotemporal 331.19
    with behavioral disturbance 331.19
        [294.11]
    without behavioral disturbance
        331.19 [294.10]
  hebephrenic (acute) 295.1●
  Heller's (infantile psychosis) (see also
      Psychosis, childhood) 299.1●
  idiopathic 290.9
    presenile-onset - see Dementia,
        presenile
    senile-onset - see Dementia, senile
  in
    arteriosclerotic brain disease 290.40
    senility 290.0
  induced by drug 292.82
  infantile, infantilia (see also Psychosis,
      childhood) 299.0●
  Lewy body 331.82
    with behavioral disturbance 331.82
        [294.11]
    without behavioral disturbance
        331.82 [294.10]
  multi-infarct (cerebrovascular) (see also
      Dementia, arteriosclerotic) 290.40
  old age 290.0

Dementia (Continued)
  paralytica, paralytic 094.1
    juvenilis 090.40
    syphilitic 094.1
      congenital 090.40
    tabetic form 094.1
  paranoid (see also Schizophrenia)
      295.3●
  paraphrenic (see also Schizophrenia)
      295.3●
  paretic 094.1
  praecox (see also Schizophrenia) 295.9●
  presenile 290.10
    with
      acute confusional state 290.11
      delirium 290.11
      delusional features 290.12
      depressive features 290.13
    depressed type 290.13
    paranoid type 290.12
    simple type 290.10
    uncomplicated 290.10
  primary (acute) (see also Schizophrenia)
      295.0●
  progressive, syphilitic 094.1
  puerperal - see Psychosis, puerperal
  schizophrenic (see also Schizophrenia)
      295.9●
  senile 290.0
    with
      acute confusional state 290.3
      delirium 290.3
      delusional features 290.20
      depressive features 290.21
    depressed type 290.21
    exhaustion 290.0
    paranoid type 290.20
  simple type (acute) (see also
      Schizophrenia) 295.0●
  simplex (acute) (see also Schizophrenia)
      295.0●
  syphilitic 094.1
  uremic - see Uremia
  vascular 290.40
    with
      delirium 290.41
      delusions 290.42
      depressed mood 290.43
Demerol dependence (see also
    Dependence) 304.0●
Demineralization, ankle (see also
    Osteoporosis) 733.00
Demodex folliculorum (infestation) 133.8
Demoralization 799.25
de Morgan's spots (senile angiomas) 448.1
Demyelinating
  polyneuritis, chronic inflammatory
      357.81
Demyelination, demyelinization
  central nervous system 341.9
    specified NEC 341.8
  corpus callosum (central) 341.8
  global 340
Dengue (fever) 061
  sandfly 061
  vaccination, prophylactic (against)
      V05.1
  virus hemorrhagic fever 065.4
Dens
  evaginatus 520.2
  in dente 520.2
  invaginatus 520.2
Dense
  breast(s) - omit code

◀ New   ◀▥ Revised   ~~deleted~~ Deleted   ● Use Additional Digit(s)   ▨ Omit code

Density
  increased, bone (disseminated) (generalized) (spotted) 733.99
  lung (nodular) 518.89
Dental - *see also* condition
  examination only V72.2
Dentia praecox 520.6
Denticles (in pulp) 522.2
Dentigerous cyst 526.0
Dentin
  irregular (in pulp) 522.3
  opalescent 520.5
  secondary (in pulp) 522.3
  sensitive 521.89
Dentinogenesis imperfecta 520.5
Dentinoma (M9271/0) 213.1
  upper jaw (bone) 213.0
Dentition 520.7
  abnormal 520.6
  anomaly 520.6
  delayed 520.6
  difficult 520.7
  disorder of 520.6
  precocious 520.6
  retarded 520.6
Denture sore (mouth) 528.9
Dependence

> Note: Use the following fifth-digit subclassification with category 304:
>
> 0 unspecified
> 1 continuous
> 2 episodic
> 3 in remission

  with
    withdrawal symptoms
      alcohol 291.81
      drug 292.0
  14-hydroxy-dihydromorphinone 304.0●
  absinthe 304.6●
  acemorphan 304.0●
  acetanilid(e) 304.6●
  acetophenetidin 304.6●
  acetorphine 304.0●
  acetyldihydrocodeine 304.0●
  acetyldihydrocodeinone 304.0●
  Adalin 304.1●
  Afghanistan black 304.3●
  agrypnal 304.1●
  alcohol, alcoholic (ethyl) (methyl) (wood) 303.9●
    maternal, with suspected fetal damage affecting management of pregnancy 655.4●
  allobarbitone 304.1●
  allonal 304.1●
  allylisopropylacetylurea 304.1●
  alphaprodine (hydrochloride) 304.0●
  Alurate 304.1●
  Alvodine 304.0●
  amethocaine 304.6●
  amidone 304.0●
  amidopyrine 304.6●
  aminopyrine 304.6●
  amobarbital 304.1●
  amphetamine(s) (type) (drugs classifiable to 969.72) 304.4●
  amylene hydrate 304.6●
  amylobarbitone 304.1●
  amylocaine 304.6●
  Amytal (sodium) 304.1●

Dependence (*Continued*)
  analgesic (drug) NEC 304.6●
    synthetic with morphine-like effect 304.0●
  anesthetic (agent) (drug) (gas) (general) (local) NEC 304.6●
  Angel dust 304.6●
  anileridine 304.0●
  antipyrine 304.6●
  anxiolytic 304.1●
  aprobarbital 304.1●
  aprobarbitone 304.1●
  atropine 304.6●
  Avertin (bromide) 304.6●
  barbenyl 304.1●
  barbital(s) 304.1●
  barbitone 304.1●
  barbiturate(s) (compounds) (drugs classifiable to 967.0) 304.1●
  barbituric acid (and compounds) 304.1●
  benzedrine 304.4●
  benzylmorphine 304.0●
  Beta-chlor 304.1●
  bhang 304.3●
  blue velvet 304.0●
  Brevital 304.1●
  bromal (hydrate) 304.1●
  bromide(s) NEC 304.1●
  bromine compounds NEC 304.1●
  bromisovalum 304.1●
  bromoform 304.1●
  Bromo-seltzer 304.1●
  bromural 304.1●
  butabarbital (sodium) 304.1●
  butabarpal 304.1●
  butallylonal 304.1●
  butethal 304.1●
  buthalitone (sodium) 304.1●
  Butisol 304.1●
  butobarbitone 304.1●
  butyl chloral (hydrate) 304.1●
  caffeine 304.4●
  cannabis (indica) (sativa) (resin) (derivatives) (type) 304.3●
  carbamazepine 304.6●
  Carbrital 304.1●
  carbromal 304.1●
  carisoprodol 304.6●
  Catha (edulis) 304.4●
  chloral (betaine) (hydrate) 304.1●
  chloralamide 304.1●
  chloralformamide 304.1●
  chloralose 304.1●
  chlordiazepoxide 304.1●
  Chloretone 304.1●
  chlorobutanol 304.1●
  chlorodyne 304.1●
  chloroform 304.6●
  Cliradon 304.0●
  coca (leaf) and derivatives 304.2●
  cocaine 304.2●
    hydrochloride 304.2●
    salt (any) 304.2●
  codeine 304.0●
  combination of drugs (excluding morphine or opioid type drug) NEC 304.8●
    morphine or opioid type drug with any other drug 304.7●
  croton-chloral 304.1●
  cyclobarbital 304.1●
  cyclobarbitone 304.1●
  dagga 304.3●

Dependence (*Continued*)
  Delvinal 304.1●
  Demerol 304.0●
  desocodeine 304.0●
  desomorphine 304.0●
  desoxyephedrine 304.4●
  DET 304.5●
  dexamphetamine 304.4●
  dexedrine 304.4●
  dextromethorphan 304.0●
  dextromoramide 304.0●
  dextronorpseudoephedrine 304.4●
  dextrorphan 304.0●
  diacetylmorphine 304.0●
  Dial 304.1●
  diallylbarbituric acid 304.1●
  diamorphine 304.0●
  diazepam 304.1●
  dibucaine 304.6●
  dichloroethane 304.6●
  diethyl barbituric acid 304.1●
  diethylsulfone-diethylmethane 304.1●
  difencloxazine 304.0●
  dihydrocodeine 304.0●
  dihydrocodeinone 304.0●
  dihydrohydroxycodeinone 304.0●
  dihydroisocodeine 304.0●
  dihydromorphine 304.0●
  dihydromorphinone 304.0●
  dihydroxcodeinone 304.0●
  Dilaudid 304.0●
  dimenhydrinate 304.6●
  dimethylmeperidine 304.0●
  dimethyltriptamine 304.5●
  Dionin 304.0●
  diphenoxylate 304.6●
  dipipanone 304.0●
  d-lysergic acid diethylamide 304.5●
  DMT 304.5●
  Dolophine 304.0●
  DOM 304.2●
  doriden 304.1●
  dormiral 304.1●
  Dormison 304.1●
  Dromoran 304.0●
  drug NEC 304.9●
    analgesic NEC 304.6●
    combination (excluding morphine or opioid type drug) NEC 304.8●
      morphine or opioid type drug with any other drug 304.7●
    complicating pregnancy, childbirth, or puerperium 648.3●
      affecting fetus or newborn 779.5
    hallucinogenic 304.5●
    hypnotic NEC 304.1●
    narcotic NEC 304.9●
    psychostimulant NEC 304.4●
    sedative 304.1●
    soporific NEC 304.1●
    specified type NEC 304.6●
    suspected damage to fetus affecting management of pregnancy 655.5●
    synthetic, with morphine-like effect 304.0●
    tranquilizing 304.1●
  duboisine 304.6●
  ectylurea 304.1●
  Endocaine 304.6●
  Equanil 304.1●
  Eskabarb 304.1●
  ethchlorvynol 304.1●

Dependence (*Continued*)

ether (ethyl) (liquid) (vapor) (vinyl) 304.6●
ethidene 304.6●
ethinamate 304.1●
ethoheptazine 304.6●
ethyl
    alcohol 303.9●
    bromide 304.6●
    carbamate 304.6●
    chloride 304.6●
    morphine 304.0●
ethylene (gas) 304.6●
    dichloride 304.6●
ethylidene chloride 304.6●
etilfen 304.1●
etorphine 304.0●
etoval 304.1●
eucodal 304.0●
euneryl 304.1●
Evipal 304.1●
Evipan 304.1●
fentanyl 304.0●
ganja 304.3●
gardenal 304.1●
gardenpanyl 304.1●
gelsemine 304.6●
Gelsemium 304.6●
Gemonil 304.1●
glucochloral 304.1●
glue (airplane) (sniffing) 304.6●
glutethimide 304.1●
hallucinogenics 304.5●
hashish 304.3●
headache powder NEC 304.6●
Heavenly Blue 304.5●
hedonal 304.1●
hemp 304.3●
heptabarbital 304.1●
Heptalgin 304.0●
heptobarbitone 304.1●
heroin 304.0●
    salt (any) 304.0●
hexethal (sodium) 304.1●
hexobarbital 304.1●
Hycodan 304.0●
hydrocodone 304.0●
hydromorphinol 304.0●
hydromorphinone 304.0●
hydromorphone 304.0●
hydroxycodeine 304.0●
hypnotic NEC 304.1●
Indian hemp 304.3●
inhalant 304.6●
intranarcon 304.1●
Kemithal 304.1●
ketobemidone 304.0●
khat 304.4●
kif 304.3●
Lactuca (virosa) extract 304.1●
lactucarium 304.1●
laudanum 304.0●
Lebanese red 304.3●
Leritine 304.0●
lettuce opium 304.1●
Levanil 304.1●
Levo-Dromoran 304.0●
levo-iso-methadone 304.0●
levorphanol 304.0●
Librium 304.1●
Lomotil 304.6●
Lotusate 304.1●
LSD (-25) (and derivatives) 304.5●
Luminal 304.1●

Dependence (*Continued*)

lysergic acid 304.5●
    amide 304.5●
maconha 304.3●
magic mushroom 304.5●
marihuana 304.3●
MDA (methylene dioxyamphetamine) 304.4●
Mebaral 304.1●
Medinal 304.1●
Medomin 304.1●
megahallucinogenics 304.5●
meperidine 304.0●
mephobarbital 304.1●
meprobamate 304.1●
mescaline 304.5●
methadone 304.0●
methamphetamine(s) 304.4●
methaqualone 304.1●
metharbital 304.1●
methitural 304.1●
methobarbitone 304.1●
methohexital 304.1●
methopholine 304.6●
methyl●
    alcohol 303.9●
    bromide 304.6●
    morphine 304.0●
    sulfonal 304.1●
methylated spirit 303.9●
methylbutinol 304.6●
methyldihydromorphinone 304.0●
methylene●
    chloride 304.6●
    dichloride 304.6●
    dioxyamphetamine (MDA) 304.4●
methylparafynol 304.1●
methylphenidate 304.4●
methyprylone 304.1●
metopon 304.0●
Miltown 304.1●
morning glory seeds 304.5●
morphinan(s) 304.0●
morphine (sulfate) (sulfite) (type) (drugs classifiable to 965.00–965.09) 304.0●
morphine or opioid type drug (drugs classifiable to 965.00–965.09) with any other drug 304.7●
morphinol(s) 304.0●
morphinon 304.0●
morpholinylethylmorphine 304.0●
mylomide 304.1●
myristicin 304.5●
narcotic (drug) NEC 304.9●
nealbarbital 304.1●
nealbarbitone 304.1●
Nembutal 304.1●
Neonal 304.1●
Neraval 304.1●
Neravan 304.1●
neurobarb 304.1●
nicotine 305.1
Nisentil 304.0●
nitrous oxide 304.6●
Noctec 304.1●
Noludar 304.1●
nonbarbiturate sedatives and tranquilizers with similar effect 304.1●
noptil 304.1●
normorphine 304.0●
noscapine 304.0●
Novocaine 304.6●
Numorphan 304.0●

Dependence (*Continued*)

nunol 304.1●
Nupercaine 304.6●
Oblivon 304.1●
on
    aspirator V46.0
    hemodialysis V45.11
    hyperbaric chamber V46.8
    iron lung V46.11
    machine (enabling) V46.9
        specified type NEC V46.8
    peritoneal dialysis V45.11
    Possum (patient-operated-selector-mechanism) V46.8
    renal dialysis machine V45.11
    respirator [ventilator] V46.11
        encounter
            during
                power failure V46.12
                mechanical failure V46.14
            for weaning V46.13
    supplemental oxygen V46.2
    wheelchair V46.3
opiate 304.0●
opioids 304.0●
opioid type drug 304.0●
    with any other drug 304.7●
opium (alkaloids) (derivatives) (tincture) 304.0●
ortal 304.1●
oxazepam 304.1●
oxycodone 304.0●
oxymorphone 304.0●
Palfium 304.0●
Panadol 304.6●
pantopium 304.0●
pantopon 304.0●
papaverine 304.0●
paracetamol 304.6●
paracodin 304.0●
paraldehyde 304.1●
paregoric 304.0●
Parzone 304.0●
PCP (phencyclidine) 304.6●
Pearly Gates 304.5●
pentazocine 304.0●
pentobarbital 304.1●
pentobarbitone (sodium) 304.1●
Pentothal 304.1●
Percaine 304.6●
Percodan 304.0●
Perichlor 304.1●
Pernocton 304.1●
Pernoston 304.1●
peronine 304.0●
pethidine (hydrochloride) 304.0●
petrichloral 304.1●
peyote 304.5●
Phanodorn 304.1●
phenacetin 304.6●
phenadoxone 304.0●
phenaglycodol 304.1●
phenazocine 304.0●
phencyclidine 304.6●
phenmetrazine 304.4●
phenobal 304.1●
phenobarbital 304.1●
phenobarbitone 304.1●
phenomorphan 304.0●
phenonyl 304.1●
phenoperidine 304.0●
pholcodine 304.0●
piminodine 304.0●
Pipadone 304.0●
Pitkin's solution 304.6●

◀ New   ◀▥ Revised   ~~deleted~~ Deleted   ● Use Additional Digit(s)   ▨ Omit code

Dependence (Continued)
Placidyl 304.1 ●
polysubstance 304.8 ●
Pontocaine 304.6 ●
pot 304.3 ●
potassium bromide 304.1 ●
Preludin 304.4 ●
Prinadol 304.0 ●
probarbital 304.1 ●
procaine 304.6 ●
propanal 304.1 ●
propoxyphene 304.6 ●
psilocibin 304.5 ●
psilocin 304.5 ●
psilocybin 304.5 ●
psilocyline 304.5 ●
psilocyn 304.5 ●
psychedelic agents 304.5 ●
psychostimulant NEC 304.4 ●
psychotomimetic agents 304.5 ●
pyrahexyl 304.3 ●
Pyramidon 304.6 ●
quinalbarbitone 304.1 ●
racemoramide 304.0 ●
racemorphan 304.0 ●
Rela 304.6 ●
scopolamine 304.6 ●
secobarbital 304.1 ●
seconal 304.1 ●
sedative NEC 304.1 ●
 nonbarbiturate with barbiturate
  effect 304.1 ●
Sedormid 304.1 ●
sernyl 304.1 ●
sodium bromide 304.1 ●
Soma 304.6 ●
Somnal 304.1 ●
Somnos 304.1 ●
Soneryl 304.1 ●
soporific (drug) NEC 304.1 ●
specified drug NEC 304.6 ●
speed 304.4 ●
spinocaine 304.6 ●
stovaine 304.6 ●
STP 304.5 ●
stramonium 304.6 ●
Sulfonal 304.1 ●
sulfonethylmethane 304.1 ●
sulfonmethane 304.1 ●
Surital 304.1 ●
synthetic drug with morphine-like
  effect 304.0 ●
talbutal 304.1 ●
tetracaine 304.6 ●
tetrahydrocannabinol 304.3 ●
tetronal 304.1 ●
THC 304.3 ●
thebacon 304.0 ●
thebaine 304.0 ●
thiamil 304.1 ●
thiamylal 304.1 ●
thiopental 304.1 ●
tobacco 305.1
toluene, toluol 304.6 ●
tranquilizer NEC 304.1 ●
 nonbarbiturate with barbiturate
  effect 304.1 ●
tribromacetaldehyde 304.6 ●
tribromethanol 304.6 ●
tribromomethane 304.6 ●
trichloroethanol 304.6 ●
trichoroethyl phosphate 304.1 ●
triclofos 304.1 ●
Trional 304.1 ●
Tuinal 304.1 ●

Dependence (Continued)
Turkish green 304.3 ●
urethan(e) 304.6 ●
Valium 304.1 ●
Valmid 304.1 ●
veganin 304.0 ●
veramon 304.1 ●
Veronal 304.1 ●
versidyne 304.6 ●
vinbarbital 304.1 ●
vinbarbitone 304.1 ●
vinyl bitone 304.1 ●
vitamin B₆ 266.1
wine 303.9 ●
Zactane 304.6 ●
Dependency
passive 301.6
reactions 301.6
Depersonalization (episode, in neurotic
 state) (neurotic) (syndrome) 300.6
Depletion
carbohydrates 271.9
complement factor 279.8
extracellular fluid 276.52
plasma 276.52
potassium 276.8
 nephropathy 588.89
salt or sodium 276.1
 causing heat exhaustion or
  prostration 992.4
 nephropathy 593.9
volume 276.50
 extracellular fluid 276.52
 plasma 276.52
Deployment (military)
personal history of V62.22
returned from V62.22
status V62.21
Deposit
argentous, cornea 371.16
bone, in Boeck's sarcoid 135
calcareous, calcium - see Calcification
cholesterol
 retina 362.82
 skin 709.3
 vitreous (humor) 379.22
conjunctival 372.56
cornea, corneal NEC 371.10
 argentous 371.16
 in
  cystinosis 270.0 [371.15]
  mucopolysaccharidosis 277.5
   [371.15]
crystalline, vitreous (humor) 379.22
hemosiderin, in old scars of cornea
 371.11
metallic, in lens 366.45
skin 709.3
teeth, tooth (betel) (black) (green)
 (materia alba) (orange) (soft)
 (tobacco) 523.6
urate, in kidney (see also Disease, renal)
 593.9
Depraved appetite 307.52
Depression 311
acute (see also Psychosis, affective)
 296.2 ●
 recurrent episode 296.3 ●
 single episode 296.2 ●
agitated (see also Psychosis, affective)
 296.2 ●
 recurrent episode 296.3 ●
 single episode 296.2 ●
anaclitic 309.21
anxiety 300.4

Depression (Continued)
arches 734
 congenital 754.61
autogenous (see also Psychosis,
  affective) 296.2 ●
 recurrent episode 296.3 ●
 single episode 296.2 ●
basal metabolic rate (BMR) 794.7
bone marrow 289.9
central nervous system 799.1
 newborn 779.2
cerebral 331.9
 newborn 779.2
cerebrovascular 437.8
 newborn 779.2
chest wall 738.3
endogenous (see also Psychosis,
  affective) 296.2 ●
 recurrent episode 296.3 ●
 single episode 296.2 ●
functional activity 780.99
hysterical 300.11
involutional, climacteric, or
  menopausal (see also Psychosis,
  affective) 296.2 ●
 recurrent episode 296.3 ●
 single episode 296.2 ●
major 296.2 ◄
 recurrent episode 296.3 ◄
 single episode 296.2 ◄
manic (see also Psychosis, affective)
 296.80
medullary 348.89
 newborn 779.2
mental 300.4
metatarsal heads - see Depression,
 arches
metatarsus - see Depression, arches
monopolar (see also Psychosis,
  affective) 296.2 ●
 recurrent episode 296.3 ●
 single episode 296.2 ●
nervous 300.4
neurotic 300.4
nose 738.0
postpartum 648.4 ●
psychogenic 300.4
 reactive 298.0
psychoneurotic 300.4
psychotic (see also Psychosis, affective)
 296.2 ●
 reactive 298.0
 recurrent episode 296.3 ●
 single episode 296.2 ●
reactive 300.4
 neurotic 300.4
 psychogenic 298.0
 psychoneurotic 300.4
 psychotic 298.0
recurrent 296.3 ●
respiratory center 348.89
 newborn 770.89
scapula 736.89
senile 290.21
situational (acute) (brief) 309.0
 prolonged 309.1
skull 754.0
sternum 738.3
visual field 368.40
Depressive reaction - see also Reaction,
 depressive
acute (transient) 309.0
 with anxiety 309.28
prolonged 309.1
situational (acute) 309.0
 prolonged 309.1

Deprivation
  cultural V62.4
  emotional V62.89
    affecting
      adult 995.82
      infant or child 995.51
  food 994.2
    specific substance NEC 269.8
  protein (familial) (kwashiorkor)
    260
  sleep V69.4
  social V62.4
    affecting
      adult 995.82
      infant or child 995.51
  symptoms, syndrome
    alcohol 291.81
    drug 292.0
  vitamins (*see also* Deficiency, vitamin)
    269.2
  water 994.3
de Quervain's
  disease (tendon sheath) 727.04
  syndrome 259.51
  thyroiditis (subacute granulomatous
    thyroiditis) 245.1
Derangement
  ankle (internal) 718.97
    current injury (*see also* Dislocation,
      ankle) 837.0
    recurrent 718.37
  cartilage (articular) NEC (*see also*
    Disorder, cartilage, articular)
    718.0●
    knee 717.9
      recurrent 718.36
    recurrent 718.3●
  collateral ligament (knee) (medial)
    (tibial) 717.82
    current injury 844.1
      lateral (fibular) 844.0
    lateral (fibular) 717.81
      current injury 844.0
  cruciate ligament (knee) (posterior)
    717.84
    anterior 717.83
      current injury 844.2
    current injury 844.2
  elbow (internal) 718.92
    current injury (*see also* Dislocation,
      elbow) 832.00
    recurrent 718.32
  gastrointestinal 536.9
  heart - *see* Disease, heart
  hip (joint) (internal) (old) 718.95
    current injury (*see also* Dislocation,
      hip) 835.00
    recurrent 718.35
  intervertebral disc - *see* Displacement,
    intervertebral disc
  joint (internal) 718.90
    ankle 718.97
    current injury - *see also* Dislocation,
      by site
      knee, meniscus or cartilage
        (*see also* Tear, meniscus)
        836.2
    elbow 718.92
    foot 718.97
    hand 718.94
    hip 718.95
    knee 717.9
    multiple sites 718.99
    pelvic region 718.95

Derangement (*Continued*)
  joint (*Continued*)
    recurrent 718.30
      ankle 718.37
      elbow 718.32
      foot 718.37
      hand 718.34
      hip 718.35
      knee 718.36
      multiple sites 718.39
      pelvic region 718.35
      shoulder (region) 718.31
      specified site NEC 718.38
      temporomandibular (old) 524.69
      wrist 718.33
    shoulder (region) 718.91
    specified site NEC 718.98
    spine NEC 724.9
    temporomandibular 524.69
    wrist 718.93
  knee (cartilage) (internal) 717.9
    current injury (*see also* Tear,
      meniscus) 836.2
    ligament 717.89
      capsular 717.85
      collateral - *see* Derangement,
        collateral ligament
      cruciate - *see* Derangement,
        cruciate ligament
      specified NEC 717.85
    recurrent 718.36
  low back NEC 724.9
  meniscus NEC (knee) 717.5
    current injury (*see also* Tear,
      meniscus) 836.2
    lateral 717.40
      anterior horn 717.42
      posterior horn 717.43
      specified NEC 717.49
    medial 717.3
      anterior horn 717.1
      posterior horn 717.2
    recurrent 718.3●
    site other than knee - *see* Disorder,
      cartilage, articular
  mental (*see also* Psychosis) 298.9
  rotator cuff (recurrent) (tear) 726.10
    current 840.4
  sacroiliac (old) 724.6
    current - *see* Dislocation, sacroiliac
  semilunar cartilage (knee) 717.5
    current injury 836.2
      lateral 836.1
      medial 836.0
    recurrent 718.3●
  shoulder (internal) 718.91
    current injury (*see also* Dislocation,
      shoulder) 831.00
    recurrent 718.31
  spine (recurrent) NEC 724.9
    current - *see* Dislocation, spine
  temporomandibular (internal) (joint)
    (old) 524.69
    current - *see* Dislocation, jaw
Dercum's disease or syndrome (adiposis
  dolorosa) 272.8
Derealization (neurotic) 300.6
Dermal - *see* condition
Dermaphytid - *see* Dermatophytosis
Dermatergosis - *see* Dermatitis
Dermatitis (allergic) (contact)
  (occupational) (venenata) 692.9
  ab igne 692.82
  acneiform 692.9

Dermatitis (*Continued*)
  actinic (due to sun) 692.70
    acute 692.72
    chronic NEC 692.74
    other than from sun NEC 692.82
  ambustionis
    due to
      burn or scald - *see* Burn, by site
      sunburn (*see also* Sunburn)
        692.71
  amebic 006.6
  ammonia 691.0
  anaphylactoid NEC 692.9
  arsenical 692.4
  artefacta 698.4
    psychogenic 316 [698.4]
  asthmatic 691.8
  atopic (allergic) (intrinsic) 691.8
    psychogenic 316 [691.8]
  atrophicans 701.8
    diffusa 701.8
    maculosa 701.3
  autoimmune progesterone 279.49
  berlock, berloque 692.72
  blastomycetic 116.0
  blister beetle 692.89
  Brucella NEC 023.9
  bullosa 694.9
    striata pratensis 692.6
  bullous 694.9
    mucosynechial, atrophic 694.60
      with ocular involvement 694.61
    seasonal 694.8
  calorica
    due to
      burn or scald - *see* Burn, by site
      cold 692.89
      sunburn (*see also* Sunburn) 692.71
  caterpillar 692.89
  cercarial 120.3
  combustionis
    due to
      burn or scald - *see* Burn, by
        site
      sunburn (*see also* Sunburn)
        692.71
  congelationis 991.5
  contusiformis 695.2
  diabetic 250.8●
  diaper 691.0
  diphtheritica 032.85
  due to
    acetone 692.2
    acids 692.4
    adhesive plaster 692.4
    alcohol (skin contact) (substances
      classifiable to 980.0–980.9)
      692.4
      taken internally 693.8
    alkalis 692.4
    allergy NEC 692.9
    ammonia (household) (liquid)
      692.4
    animal
      dander (cat) (dog) 692.84
      hair (cat) (dog) 692.84
    arnica 692.3
    arsenic 692.4
      taken internally 693.8
    blister beetle 692.89
    cantharides 692.3
    carbon disulphide 692.2
    caterpillar 692.89
    caustics 692.4

◄ New   ◄▥ Revised   ~~deleted~~ Deleted   ● Use Additional Digit(s)   ▨ Omit code

Dermatitis *(Continued)*
due to *(Continued)*
cereal (ingested) 693.1
contact with skin 692.5
chemical(s) NEC 692.4
internal 693.8
irritant NEC 692.4
taken internally 693.8
chlorocompounds 692.2
coffee (ingested) 693.1
contact with skin 692.5
cold weather 692.89
cosmetics 692.81
cyclohexanes 692.2
dander, animal (cat) (dog)
692.84
deodorant 692.81
detergents 692.0
dichromate 692.4
drugs and medicinals (correct
substance properly
administered) (internal use)
693.0
external (in contact with skin)
692.3
wrong substance given or
taken 976.9
specified substance - *see*
Table of Drugs and
Chemicals
wrong substance given or taken
977.9
specified substance - *see*
Table of Drugs and
Chemicals
dyes 692.89
hair 692.89
epidermophytosis - *see*
Dermatophytosis
esters 692.2
external irritant NEC 692.9
specified agent NEC 692.89
eye shadow 692.81
fish (ingested) 693.1
contact with skin 692.5
flour (ingested) 693.1
contact with skin 692.5
food (ingested) 693.1
in contact with skin 692.5
fruit (ingested) 693.1
contact with skin 692.5
fungicides 692.3
furs 692.84
glycols 692.2
greases NEC 692.1
hair, animal (cat) (dog) 692.84
hair dyes 692.89
hot
objects and materials - *see* Burn,
by site
weather or places 692.89
hydrocarbons 692.2
infrared rays, except from sun
692.82
solar NEC *(see also* Dermatitis,
due to, sun) 692.70
ingested substance 693.9
drugs and medicinals *(see
also* Dermatitis, due to,
drugs and medicinals)
693.0
food 693.1
specified substance NEC
693.8

Dermatitis *(Continued)*
due to *(Continued)*
ingestion or injection of
chemical 693.8
drug (correct substance properly
administered) 693.0
wrong substance given or
taken 977.9
specified substance - *see*
Table of Drugs and
Chemicals
insecticides 692.4
internal agent 693.9
drugs and medicinals *(see also*
Dermatitis, due to, drugs
and medicinals) 693.0
food (ingested) 693.1
in contact with skin 692.5
specified agent NEC 693.8
iodine 692.3
iodoform 692.3
irradiation 692.82
jewelry 692.83
keratolytics 692.3
ketones 692.2
lacquer tree (Rhus verniciflua)
692.6
light (sun) NEC *(see also* Dermatitis,
due to, sun) 692.70
other 692.82
low temperature 692.89
mascara 692.81
meat (ingested) 693.1
contact with skin 692.5
mercury, mercurials 692.3
metals 692.83
milk (ingested) 693.1
contact with skin 692.5
Neomycin 692.3
nylon 692.4
oils NEC 692.1
paint solvent 692.2
pediculocides 692.3
petroleum products (substances
classifiable to 981) 692.4
phenol 692.3
photosensitiveness, photosensitivity
(sun) 692.72
other light 692.82
plants NEC 692.6
plasters, medicated (any) 692.3
plastic 692.4
poison
ivy (Rhus toxicodendron) 692.6
oak (Rhus diversiloba) 692.6
plant or vine 692.6
sumac (Rhus venenata) 692.6
vine (Rhus radicans) 692.6
preservatives 692.89
primrose (primula) 692.6
primula 692.6
radiation 692.82
sun NEC *(see also* Dermatitis,
due to, sun) 692.70
tanning bed 692.82
radioactive substance 692.82
radium 692.82
ragweed (Senecio jacobae) 692.6
Rhus (diversiloba) (radicans)
(toxicodendron) (venenata)
(verniciflua) 692.6
rubber 692.4
scabicides 692.3
Senecio jacobae 692.6

Dermatitis *(Continued)*
due to *(Continued)*
solar radiation - *see* Dermatitis, due
to, sun
solvents (any) (substances
classifiable to 982.0–982.8)
692.2
chlorocompound group 692.2
cyclohexane group 692.2
ester group 692.2
glycol group 692.2
hydrocarbon group 692.2
ketone group 692.2
paint 692.2
specified agent NEC 692.89
sun 692.70
acute 692.72
chronic NEC 692.74
specified NEC 692.79
sunburn *(see also* Sunburn) 692.71
sunshine NEC *(see also* Dermatitis,
due to, sun) 692.70
tanning bed 692.82
tetrachlorethylene 692.2
toluene 692.2
topical medications 692.3
turpentine 692.2
ultraviolet rays, except from sun
692.82
sun NEC *(see also* Dermatitis, due
to, sun) 692.70
vaccine or vaccination (correct
substance properly
administered) 693.0
wrong substance given or taken
bacterial vaccine 978.8
specified - *see* Table
of Drugs and
Chemicals
other vaccines NEC 979.9
specified - *see* Table of
Drugs and
Chemicals
varicose veins *(see also* Varicose,
vein, inflamed or infected)
454.1
x-rays 692.82
dyshydrotic 705.81
dysmenorrheica 625.8
eczematoid NEC 692.9
infectious 690.8
eczematous NEC 692.9
epidemica 695.89
erysipelatosa 695.81
escharotica - *see* Burn, by site
exfoliativa, exfoliative 695.89
generalized 695.89
infantum 695.81
neonatorum 695.81
eyelid 373.31
allergic 373.32
contact 373.32
eczematous 373.31
herpes (zoster) 053.20
simplex 054.41
infective 373.5
due to
actinomycosis 039.3 *[373.5]*
herpes
simplex 054.41
zoster 053.20
impetigo 684 *[373.5]*
leprosy *(see also* Leprosy) 030.0
[373.4]

Dermatitis *(Continued)*
  eyelid *(Continued)*
    infective *(Continued)*
      due to *(Continued)*
        lupus vulgaris (tuberculous)
          (see also Tuberculosis)
          017.0 ● [373.4]
        mycotic dermatitis *(see also*
          Dermatomycosis) 111.9
          [373.5]
        vaccinia 051.02 [373.5]
          postvaccination 999.0
            [373.5]
        yaws *(see also* Yaws) 102.9 [373.4]
  facta, factitia 698.4
    psychogenic 316 [698.4]
  ficta 698.4
    psychogenic 316 [698.4]
  flexural 691.8
  follicularis 704.8
  friction 709.8
  fungus 111.9
    specified type NEC 111.8
  gangrenosa, gangrenous (infantum)
    (see also Gangrene) 785.4
  gestationis 646.8●
  gonococcal 098.89
  gouty 274.89
  harvest mite 133.8
  heat 692.89
  herpetiformis (bullous) (erythematous)
    (pustular) (vesicular) 694.0
    juvenile 694.2
    senile 694.5
  hiemalis 692.89
  hypostatic, hypostatica 454.1
    with ulcer 454.2
  impetiginous 684
  infantile (acute) (chronic)
    (intertriginous) (intrinsic)
    (seborrheic) 690.12
  infectiosa eczematoides 690.8
  infectious (staphylococcal)
    (streptococcal) 686.9
    eczematoid 690.8
  infective eczematoid 690.8
  Jacquet's (diaper dermatitis) 691.0
  leptus 133.8
  lichenified NEC 692.9
  lichenoid, chronic 701.0
  lichenoides purpurica pigmentosa
    709.1
  meadow 692.6
  medicamentosa (correct substance
    properly administered) (internal
    use) *(see also* Dermatitis, due to,
    drugs or medicinals) 693.0
    due to contact with skin 692.3
  mite 133.8
  multiformis 694.0
    juvenile 694.2
    senile 694.5
  napkin 691.0
  neuro 698.3
  neurotica 694.0
  nummular NEC 692.9
  osteatosis, osteatotic 706.8
  papillaris capillitii 706.1
  pellagrous 265.2
  perioral 695.3
  perstans 696.1
  photosensitivity (sun) 692.72
    other light 692.82
  pigmented purpuric lichenoid 709.1

Dermatitis *(Continued)*
  polymorpha dolorosa 694.0
  primary irritant 692.9
  pruriginosa 694.0
  pruritic NEC 692.9
  psoriasiform nodularis 696.2
  psychogenic 316
  purulent 686.00
  pustular contagious 051.2
  pyococcal 686.00
  pyocyaneus 686.09
  pyogenica 686.00
  radiation 692.82
  repens 696.1
  Ritter's (exfoliativa) 695.81
  Schamberg's (progressive pigmentary
    dermatosis) 709.09
  schistosome 120.3
  seasonal bullous 694.8
  seborrheic 690.10
    infantile 690.12
  sensitization NEC 692.9
  septic *(see also* Septicemia) 686.00
    gonococcal 098.89
  solar, solare NEC *(see also* Dermatitis,
    due to, sun) 692.70
  stasis 454.1
    due to
      postphlebitic syndrome 459.12
        with ulcer 459.13
      varicose veins - *see* Varicose
    ulcerated or with ulcer (varicose)
      454.2
  sunburn *(see also* Sunburn) 692.71
  suppurative 686.00
  traumatic NEC 709.8
  trophoneurotica 694.0
  ultraviolet, except from sun 692.82
    due to sun NEC *(see also* Dermatitis,
      due to, sun) 692.70
  varicose 454.1
    with ulcer 454.2
  vegetans 686.8
  verrucosa 117.2
  xerotic 706.8
Dermatoarthritis, lipoid 272.8 [713.0]
Dermatochalasia, dermatochalasis 374.87
Dermatofibroma (lenticulare) (M8832/0) -
  see also Neoplasm, skin, benign
  protuberans (M8832/1) - *see* Neoplasm,
    skin, uncertain behavior
Dermatofibrosarcoma (protuberans)
  (M8832/3) - *see* Neoplasm, skin,
  malignant
Dermatographia 708.3
Dermatolysis (congenital) (exfoliativa)
  757.39
  acquired 701.8
  eyelids 374.34
  palpebrarum 374.34
  senile 701.8
Dermatomegaly NEC 701.8
Dermatomucomyositis 710.3
Dermatomycosis 111.9
  furfuracea 111.0
  specified type NEC 111.8
Dermatomyositis (acute) (chronic) 710.3
Dermatoneuritis of children 985.0
Dermatophiliasis 134.1
Dermatophytide - *see* Dermatophytosis
Dermatophytosis (Epidermophyton)
  (infection) (microsporum) (tinea)
  (Trichophyton) 110.9
  beard 110.0

Dermatophytosis *(Continued)*
  body 110.5
  deep seated 110.6
  fingernails 110.1
  foot 110.4
  groin 110.3
  hand 110.2
  nail 110.1
  perianal (area) 110.3
  scalp 110.0
  scrotal 110.8
  specified site NEC 110.8
  toenails 110.1
  vulva 110.8
Dermatopolyneuritis 985.0
Dermatorrhexis 756.83
  acquired 701.8
Dermatosclerosis *(see also* Scleroderma)
  710.1
  localized 701.0
Dermatosis 709.9
  Andrews' 686.8
  atopic 691.8
  Bowen's (M8081/2) - *see* Neoplasm,
    skin, in situ
  bullous 694.9
    specified type NEC 694.8
  erythematosquamous 690.8
  exfoliativa 695.89
  factitial 698.4
  gonococcal 098.89
  herpetiformis 694.0
    juvenile 694.2
    senile 694.5
  hysterical 300.11
  linear IgA 694.8
  menstrual NEC 709.8
  neutrophilic, acute febrile 695.89
  occupational *(see also* Dermatitis)
    692.9
  papulosa nigra 709.8
  pigmentary NEC 709.00
    progressive 709.09
    Schamberg's 709.09
    Siemens-Bloch 757.33
  progressive pigmentary 709.09
  psychogenic 316
  pustular subcorneal 694.1
  Schamberg's (progressive pigmentary)
    709.09
  senile NEC 709.3
  specified NEC 702.8
  Unna's (seborrheic dermatitis) 690.10
Dermographia 708.3
Dermographism 708.3
Dermoid (cyst) (M9084/0) - *see also*
  Neoplasm, by site, benign
  with malignant transformation
    (M9084/3) 183.0
Dermopathy
  infiltrative, with thyrotoxicosis
    242.0●
  nephrogenic fibrosing 701.8
  senile NEC 709.3
Dermophytosis - *see* Dermatophytosis
Descemet's membrane - *see* condition
Descemetocele 371.72
Descending - *see* condition
Descensus uteri (complete) (incomplete)
  (partial) (without vaginal wall
  prolapse) 618.1
  with mention of vaginal wall prolapse -
    see Prolapse, uterovaginal
Desensitization to allergens V07.1

Desert
  rheumatism 114.0
  sore (see also Ulcer, skin) 707.9
Desertion (child) (newborn) 995.52
  adult 995.84
Desmoid (extra-abdominal) (tumor)
  (M8821/1) - see also Neoplasm,
  connective tissue, uncertain
  behavior
  abdominal (M8822/1) - see Neoplasm,
    connective tissue, uncertain
    behavior
Despondency 300.4
Desquamative dermatitis NEC 695.89
Destruction
  articular facet (see also Derangement,
    joint) 718.9●
    vertebra 724.9
  bone 733.90
    syphilitic 095.5
  joint (see also Derangement, joint)
    718.9●
    sacroiliac 724.6
  kidney 593.89
  live fetus to facilitate birth NEC 763.89
  ossicles (ear) 385.24
  rectal sphincter 569.49
  septum (nasal) 478.19
  tuberculous NEC (see also Tuberculosis)
    011.9●
  tympanic membrane 384.82
  tympanum 385.89
  vertebral disc - see Degeneration,
    intervertebral disc
Destructiveness (see also Disturbance,
  conduct) 312.9
  adjustment reaction 309.3
Detachment
  cartilage - see also Sprain, by site
    knee - see Tear, meniscus
  cervix, annular 622.8
    complicating delivery 665.3●
  choroid (old) (postinfectional)
    (simple) (spontaneous)
    363.70
    hemorrhagic 363.72
    serous 363.71
  knee, medial meniscus (old) 717.3
    current injury 836.0
  ligament - see Sprain, by site
  placenta (premature) - see Placenta,
    separation
  retina (recent) 361.9
    with retinal defect
      (rhegmatogenous) 361.00
      giant tear 361.03
      multiple 361.02
      partial
        with
          giant tear 361.03
          multiple defects 361.02
          retinal dialysis (juvenile)
            361.04
          single defect 361.01
      retinal dialysis (juvenile)
        361.04
      single 361.01
      subtotal 361.05
      total 361.05
    delimited (old) (partial) 361.06
    old
      delimited 361.06
      partial 361.06
      total or subtotal 361.07

Detachment (Continued)
  retina (Continued)
    pigment epithelium (RPE) (serous)
      362.42
      exudative 362.42
      hemorrhagic 362.43
    rhegmatogenous (see also
      Detachment, retina, with retinal
      defect) 361.00
    serous (without retinal defect)
      361.2
    specified type NEC 361.89
    traction (with vitreoretinal
      organization) 361.81
    vitreous humor 379.21
Detergent asthma 507.8
Deterioration
  epileptic
    with behavioral disturbance 345.9●
      [294.11]
    without behavioral disturbance
      345.9● [294.10]
  heart, cardiac (see also Degeneration,
    myocardial) 429.1
  mental (see also Psychosis) 298.9
  myocardium, myocardial (see also
    Degeneration, myocardial)
    429.1
  senile (simple) 797
    transplanted organ - see
      Complications, transplant,
      organ, by site
de Toni-Fanconi syndrome (cystinosis)
  270.0
Deuteranomaly 368.52
Deuteranopia (anomalous trichromat)
  (complete) (incomplete) 368.52
Deutschländer's disease - see Fracture,
  foot
Development
  abnormal, bone 756.9
  arrested 783.40
    bone 733.91
    child 783.40
    due to malnutrition (protein-calorie)
      263.2
    fetus or newborn 764.9●
    tracheal rings (congenital) 748.3
  defective, congenital - see also Anomaly
    cauda equina 742.59
    left ventricle 746.9
      with atresia or hypoplasia of
        aortic orifice or valve with
        hypoplasia of ascending
        aorta 746.7
      in hypoplastic left heart
        syndrome 746.7
  delayed (see also Delay, development)
    783.40
    arithmetical skills 315.1
    language (skills) 315.31
      and speech due to hearing loss
        315.34
      expressive 315.31
      mixed receptive-expressive
        315.32
    learning skill, specified NEC 315.2
    mixed skills 315.5
    motor coordination 315.4
    reading 315.00
    specified
      learning skill NEC 315.2
      type NEC, except learning
        315.8

Development (Continued)
  delayed (Continued)
    speech 315.39
      and language due to hearing loss
        315.34
      associated with hyperkinesia
        314.1
      phonological 315.39
    spelling 315.09
    written expression 315.2
  imperfect, congenital - see also Anomaly
    heart 746.9
    lungs 748.60
  improper (fetus or newborn) 764.9●
  incomplete (fetus or newborn) 764.9●
    affecting management of pregnancy
      656.5●
    bronchial tree 748.3
    organ or site not listed - see
      Hypoplasia
    respiratory system 748.9
  sexual, precocious NEC 259.1
  tardy, mental (see also Retardation,
    mental) 319
Developmental - see condition
Devergie's disease (pityriasis rubra
  pilaris) 696.4
Deviation
  conjugate (eye) 378.87
    palsy 378.81
    spasm, spastic 378.82
  esophagus 530.89
  eye, skew 378.87
  mandible, opening and closing 524.53
  midline (jaw) (teeth) 524.29
    specified site NEC - see Malposition
  occlusal plane 524.76
  organ or site, congenital NEC - see
    Malposition, congenital
  septum (acquired) (nasal) 470
    congenital 754.0
  sexual 302.9
    bestiality 302.1
    coprophilia 302.89
    ego-dystonic
      homosexuality 302.0
      lesbianism 302.0
    erotomania 302.89
      Clérambault's 297.8
    exhibitionism (sexual) 302.4
    fetishism 302.81
      transvestic 302.3
    frotteurism 302.89
    homosexuality, ego-dystonic 302.0
      pedophilic 302.2
    lesbianism, ego-dystonic 302.0
    masochism 302.83
    narcissism 302.89
    necrophilia 302.89
    nymphomania 302.89
    pederosis 302.2
    pedophilia 302.2
    sadism 302.84
    sadomasochism 302.84
    satyriasis 302.89
    specified type NEC 302.89
    transvestic fetishism 302.3
    transvestism 302.3
    voyeurism 302.82
    zoophilia (erotica) 302.1
  teeth, midline 524.29
  trachea 519.19
  ureter (congenital) 753.4
Devic's disease 341.0

Device
  cerebral ventricle (communicating) in
    situ V45.2
  contraceptive - *see* Contraceptive,
    device
  drainage, cerebrospinal fluid V45.2
Devil's
  grip 074.1
  pinches (purpura simplex) 287.2
Devitalized tooth 522.9
Devonshire colic 984.9
  specified type of lead - *see* Table of
    Drugs and Chemicals
Dextraposition, aorta 747.21
  with ventricular septal defect,
    pulmonary stenosis or atresia,
    and hypertrophy of right
    ventricle 745.2
  in tetralogy of Fallot 745.2
Dextratransposition, aorta 745.11
Dextrinosis, limit (debrancher enzyme
    deficiency) 271.0
Dextrocardia (corrected) (false) (isolated)
    (secondary) (true) 746.87
  with
    complete transposition of viscera
      759.3
    situs inversus 759.3
Dextroversion, kidney (left) 753.3
Dhobie itch 110.3
DHTR (delayed hemolytic transfusion
    reaction) - *see* Complications,
    transfusion ◄
Diabetes, diabetic (brittle) (congenital)
    (familial) (mellitus) (severe)
    (slight) (without complication)
    250.0●

> Note: Use the following fifth-digit
> subclassification with category 250:
>
> 0   type II or unspecified type, not
>   stated as uncontrolled
>
>   Fifth-digit 0 is for use for type II
>   patients, even if the patient
>   requires insulin
>
> 1   type I [juvenile type], not stated
>   as uncontrolled
>
> 2   type II or unspecified type,
>   uncontrolled
>
>   Fifth-digit 2 is for use for type II
>   patients, even if the patient
>   requires insulin
>
> 3   type I [juvenile type],
>   uncontrolled

  with
    coma (with ketoacidosis) 250.3●
      due to secondary diabetes 249.3●
      hyperosmolar (nonketotic) 250.2●
        due to secondary diabetes 249.2●
    complication NEC 250.9●
      due to secondary diabetes 249.9●
      specified NEC 250.8●
        due to secondary diabetes
          249.8●
    gangrene 250.7● *[785.4]*
      due to secondary diabetes
        249.7● *[785.4]*
    hyperglycemia - *code to* Diabetes, by
      type, with 5th digit for not
      stated as uncontrolled

Diabetes, diabetic *(Continued)*
  with *(Continued)*
    hyperosmolarity 250.2●
      due to secondary diabetes 249.2●
    ketosis, ketoacidosis 250.1●
      due to secondary diabetes 249.1●
    loss of protective sensation (LOPS) -
      see Diabetes, neuropathy ◄
    osteomyelitis 250.8● *[731.8]*
      due to secondary diabetes 249.8●
        [731.8]
    specified manifestations NEC 250.8●
      due to secondary diabetes 249.8●
  acetonemia 250.1●
    due to secondary diabetes 249.1●
  acidosis 250.1●
    due to secondary diabetes 249.1●
  amyotrophy 250.6● *[353.5]*
    due to secondary diabetes 249.6●
      [353.5]
  angiopathy, peripheral 250.7● *[443.81]*
    due to secondary diabetes 249.7●
      [443.81]
  asymptomatic 790.29
  autonomic neuropathy (peripheral)
    250.6● *[337.1]*
    due to secondary diabetes 249.6●
      [337.1]
  bone change 250.8● *[731.8]*
    due to secondary diabetes 249.8●
      [731.8]
  bronze, bronzed 275.01 ◄▥
  cataract 250.5● *[366.41]*
    due to secondary diabetes 249.5●
      [366.41]
  chemical induced - *see* Diabetes,
    secondary
    complicating pregnancy, childbirth,
      or puerperium 648.0●
  coma (with ketoacidosis) 250.3●
    due to secondary diabetes 249.3●
    hyperglycemic 250.3●
      due to secondary diabetes 249.3●
    hyperosmolar (nonketotic) 250.2●
      due to secondary diabetes 249.2●
    hypoglycemic 250.3●
      due to secondary diabetes 249.3●
    insulin 250.3●
      due to secondary diabetes 249.3●
  complicating pregnancy, childbirth, or
    puerperium (maternal)
    (conditions classifiable to 249 and
    250) 648.0●
    affecting fetus or newborn 775.0
  complication NEC 250.9●
    due to secondary diabetes 249.9●
    specified NEC 250.8●
      due to secondary diabetes 249.8●
  dorsal sclerosis 250.6● *[340]*
    due to secondary diabetes 249.6●
      [340]
  drug-induced - *see also* Diabetes,
    secondary
    overdose or wrong substance given
      or taken - *see* Table of Drugs
      and Chemicals
  due to
    cystic fibrosis - *see* Diabetes,
      secondary
    infection - *see* Diabetes, secondary
  dwarfism-obesity syndrome 258.1
  gangrene 250.7● *[785.4]*
    due to secondary diabetes 249.7●
      [785.4]
  gastroparesis 250.6● *[536.3]*
    due to secondary diabetes 249.6●
      [536.3]

Diabetes, diabetic *(Continued)*
  gestational 648.8●
    complicating pregnancy, childbirth,
      or puerperium 648.8●
  glaucoma 250.5● *[365.44]*
    due to secondary diabetes 249.5●
      [365.44]
  glomerulosclerosis (intercapillary)
    250.4● *[581.81]*
    due to secondary diabetes 249.4●
      [581.81]
  glycogenosis, secondary 250.8● *[259.8]*
    due to secondary diabetes 249.8●
      [259.8]
  hemochromatosis (*see also*
    Hemochromatosis) 275.03 ◄▥
  hyperosmolar coma 250.2●
    due to secondary diabetes 249.2●
  hyperosmolarity 250.2●
    due to secondary diabetes 249.2●
  hypertension-nephrosis syndrome
    250.4● *[581.81]*
    due to secondary diabetes 249.4●
      [581.81]
  hypoglycemia 250.8●
    due to secondary diabetes 249.8●
  hypoglycemic shock 250.8●
    due to secondary diabetes 249.8●
  inadequately controlled - *code to*
    Diabetes, by type, with 5th digit
    for not stated as uncontrolled
  insipidus 253.5
    nephrogenic 588.1
    pituitary 253.5
    vasopression-resistant 588.1
  intercapillary glomerulosclerosis
    250.4● *[581.81]*
    due to secondary diabetes 249.4●
      [581.81]
  iritis 250.5● *[364.42]*
    due to secondary diabetes 249.5●
      [364.42]
  ketosis, ketoacidosis 250.1●
    due to secondary diabetes 249.1●
  Kimmelstiel (-Wilson) disease or
    syndrome (intercapillary
    glomerulosclerosis) 250.4●
    [581.81]
    due to secondary diabetes 249.4●
      [581.81]
  Lancereaux's (diabetes mellitus with
    marked emaciation) 250.8● *[261]*
    due to secondary diabetes 249.8●
      [261]
  latent (chemical) - *see* Diabetes,
    secondary
    complicating pregnancy, childbirth,
      or puerperium 648.0●
  lipoidosis 250.8● *[272.7]*
    due to secondary diabetes 249.8●
      [272.7]
  macular edema 250.5● *[362.07]*
    due to secondary diabetes 249.5●
      [362.07]
  maternal
    with manifest disease in the infant
      775.1
    affecting fetus or newborn 775.0
  microaneurysms, retinal 250.5●
    [362.01]
    due to secondary diabetes 249.5●
      [362.01]
  mononeuropathy 250.6● *[355.9]*
    due to secondary diabetes 249.6●
      [355.9]
  neonatal, transient 775.1

Diabetes, diabetic (*Continued*)
nephropathy 250.4● [583.81]
  due to secondary diabetes 249.4●
    [583.81]
nephrosis (syndrome) 250.4●
  [581.81]
  due to secondary diabetes 249.4●
    [583.81]
neuralgia 250.6● [357.2]
  due to secondary diabetes 249.6●
    [357.2]
neuritis 250.6● [357.2]
  due to secondary diabetes 249.6●
    [357.2]
neurogenic arthropathy 250.6●
  [713.5]
  due to secondary diabetes 249.6●
    [713.5]
neuropathy 250.6● [357.2]
  autonomic (peripheral) 250.6
    [337.1]
    due to secondary diabetes
      249.6 [337.1]
  due to secondary diabetes 249.6●
    [357.2]
nonclinical 790.29
osteomyelitis 250.8● [731.8]
  due to secondary diabetes 249.8●
    [731.8]
out of control - *code to* Diabetes, by type,
  with 5th digit for uncontrolled
peripheral autonomic neuropathy
  250.6● [337.1]
  due to secondary diabetes 249.6●
    [337.1]
phosphate 275.3
polyneuropathy 250.6● [357.2]
  due to secondary diabetes 249.6●
    [357.2]
poorly controlled - *code to* Diabetes, by
  type, with 5th digit for not stated
  as uncontrolled
renal (true) 271.4
retinal
  edema 250.5● [362.07]
    due to secondary diabetes 249.5●
      [362.07]
  hemorrhage 250.5● [362.01]
    due to secondary diabetes 249.5●
      [362.01]
  microaneurysms 250.5● [362.01]
    due to secondary diabetes 249.5●
      [362.01]
  retinitis 250.5● [362.01]
    due to secondary diabetes 249.5●
      [362.01]
  retinopathy 250.5● [362.01]
    due to secondary diabetes 249.5●
      [362.01]
    background 250.5● [362.01]
      due to secondary diabetes 249.5●
        [362.01]
    nonproliferative 250.5● [362.03]
      due to secondary diabetes 249.5●
        [362.03]
      mild 250.5● [362.04]
        due to secondary diabetes
          249.5● [362.04]
      moderate 250.5● [362.05]
        due to secondary diabetes
          249.5● [362.05]
      severe 250.5● [362.06]
        due to secondary diabetes
          249.5● [362.06]

Diabetes, diabetic (*Continued*)
retinopathy (*Continued*)
  proliferative 250.5● [362.02]
    due to secondary diabetes 249.5●
      [362.02]
secondary (chemical-induced) (due to
  chronic condition) (due to
  infection) (drug-induced)
  249.0●
  with
    coma (with ketoacidosis)
      249.3●
      hyperosmolar (nonketotic)
        249.2●
    complication NEC 249.9●
      specified NEC 249.8●
    gangrene 249.7● [785.4]
    hyperosmolarity 249.2●
    ketosis, ketoacidosis 249.1●
    osteomyelitis 249.8● [731.8]
    specified manifestations NEC
      249.8●
  acetonemia 249.1●
  acidosis 249.1●
  amyotrophy 249.6 ● [353.5]
  angiopathy, peripheral 249.7●
    [443.81]
  autonomic neuropathy (peripheral)
    249.6● [337.1]
  bone change 249.8● [731.8]
  cataract 249.5● [366.41]
  coma (with ketoacidosis) 249.3●
    hyperglycemic 249.3●
    hyperosmolar (nonketotic)
      249.2●
    hypoglycemic 249.3●
    insulin 249.3●
  complicating pregnancy, childbirth,
    or puerperium (maternal)
    648.0●
    affecting fetus or newborn
      775.0
  complication NEC 249.9●
    specified NEC 249.8●
  dorsal sclerosis 249.6● [340]
  due to overdose or wrong
    substance given or taken -
    see Table of Drugs and
    Chemicals
  gangrene 249.7● [785.4]
  gastroparesis 249.6● [536.3]
  glaucoma 249.5● [365.44]
  glomerulosclerosis (intercapillary)
    249.4● [581.81]
  glycogenosis, secondary 249.8●
    [259.8]
  hyperosmolar coma 249.2●
  hyperosmolarity 249.2●
  hypertension-nephrosis syndrome
    249.4● [581.81]
  hypoglycemia 249.8●
  hypoglycemic shock 249.8●
  intercapillary glomerulosclerosis
    249.4● [581.81]
  iritis 249.5● [364.42]
  ketosis, ketoacidosis 249.1●
  Kimmelstiel (-Wilson) disease or
    syndrome (intercapillary
    glomerulosclerosis) 249.4●
    [581.81]
  Lancereaux's (diabetes mellitus
    with marked emaciation)
    249.8● [261]
  lipoidosis 249.8● [272.7]
  macular edema 249.5● [362.07]

Diabetes, diabetic (*Continued*)
secondary (*Continued*)
  maternal
    with manifest disease in the
      infant 775.1
    affecting fetus or newborn 775.0
  microaneurysms, retinal 249.5●
    [362.01]
  mononeuropathy 249.6● [355.9]
  nephropathy 249.4● [583.81]
  nephrosis (syndrome) 249.4● [581.81]
  neuralgia 249.6● [357.2]
  neuritis 249.6● [357.2]
  neurogenic arthropathy 249.6●
    [713.5]
  neuropathy 249.6● [357.2]
    autonomic (peripheral) 249.6
      [337.1]
  osteomyelitis 249.8● [731.8]
  peripheral autonomic neuropathy
    249.6● [337.1]
  polyneuropathy 249.6● [357.2]
  retinal
    edema 249.5● [362.07]
    hemorrhage 249.5● [362.01]
    microaneurysms 249.5● [362.01]
  retinitis 249.5● [362.01]
  retinopathy 249.5● [362.01]
    background 249.5● [362.01]
    nonproliferative 249.5● [362.03]
      mild 249.5● [362.04]
      moderate 249.5● [362.05]
      severe 249.5● [362.06]
    proliferative 249.5● [362.02]
  ulcer (skin) 249.8● [707.9]
    lower extremity 249.8● [707.10]
      ankle 249.8● [707.13]
      calf 249.8● [707.12]
      foot 249.8● [707.15]
      heel 249.8● [707.14]
      knee 249.8● [707.19]
      specified site NEC 249.8●
        [707.19]
      thigh 249.8● [707.11]
      toes 249.8● [707.15]
    specified site NEC 249.8● [707.8]
  xanthoma 249.8● [272.2]
steroid induced - *see also* Diabetes,
  secondary
  overdose or wrong substance given
    or taken 962.0
stress 790.29
subclinical 790.29
subliminal 790.29
sugar 250.0●
ulcer (skin) 250.8● [707.9]
  due to secondary diabetes 249.8●
    [707.9]
  lower extremity 250.8● [707.10]
    due to secondary diabetes 249.8●
      [707.10]
    ankle 250.8● [707.13]
      due to secondary diabetes
        249.8● [707.13]
    calf 250.8● [707.12]
      due to secondary diabetes
        249.8● [707.12]
    foot 250.8● [707.15]
      due to secondary diabetes
        249.8● [707.15]
    heel 250.8● [707.14]
      due to secondary diabetes
        249.8● [707.14]
    knee 250.8● [707.19]
      due to secondary diabetes
        249.8● [707.19]

Diabetes, diabetic (Continued)
  ulcer (Continued)
    lower extremity (Continued)
      specified site NEC 250.8● [707.19]
        due to secondary diabetes 249.8● [707.19]
      thigh 250.8● [707.11]
        due to secondary diabetes 249.8● [707.11]
      toes 250.8● [707.15]
        due to secondary diabetes 249.8● [707.15]
    specified site NEC 250.8● [707.8]
      due to secondary diabetes 249.8● [707.8]
  xanthoma 250.8● [272.2]
    due to secondary diabetes 249.8● [272.2]
Diacyclothrombopathia 287.1
Diagnosis deferred 799.9
Dialysis (intermittent) (treatment)
  anterior retinal (juvenile) (with detachment) 361.04
  extracorporeal V56.0
  hemodialysis V56.0
    status only V45.11
  peritoneal V56.8
    status only V45.11
  renal V56.0
    status only V45.11
  specified type NEC V56.8
Diamond-Blackfan anemia or syndrome (congenital hypoplastic anemia) 284.01
Diamond-Gardener syndrome (autoerythrocyte sensitization) 287.2
Diaper rash 691.0
Diaphoresis (excessive) NEC (see also Hyperhidrosis) 780.8
Diaphragm - see condition
Diaphragmalgia 786.52
Diaphragmitis 519.4
Diaphyseal aclasis 756.4
Diaphysitis 733.99
Diarrhea, diarrheal (acute) (autumn) (bilious) (bloody) (catarrhal) (choleraic) (chronic) (gravis) (green) (infantile) (lienteric) (noninfectious) (presumed noninfectious) (putrefactive) (secondary) (sporadic) (summer) (symptomatic) (thermic) 787.91
  achlorhydric 536.0
  allergic 558.3
  amebic (see also Amebiasis) 006.9
    with abscess - see Abscess, amebic
    acute 006.0
    chronic 006.1
    nondysenteric 006.2
  bacillary - see Dysentery, bacillary
  bacterial NEC 008.5
  balantidial 007.0
  bile salt-induced 579.8
  cachectic NEC 787.91
  chilomastix 007.8
  choleriformis 001.1
  coccidial 007.2
  Cochin-China 579.1
    anguilluliasis 127.2
    psilosis 579.1
  Dientamoeba 007.8
  dietetic 787.91

Diarrhea, diarrheal (Continued)
  due to
    achylia gastrica 536.8
    Aerobacter aerogenes 008.2
    Bacillus coli - see Enteritis, E. coli
    bacteria NEC 008.5
    bile salts 579.8
    Capillaria
      hepatica 128.8
      philippinensis 127.5
    Clostridium perfringens (C) (F) 008.46
    Enterobacter aerogenes 008.2
    enterococci 008.49
    Escherichia coli - see Enteritis, E. coli
    Giardia lamblia 007.1
    Heterophyes heterophyes 121.6
    irritating foods 787.91
    Metagonimus yokogawai 121.5
    Necator americanus 126.1
    Paracolobactrum arizonae 008.1
    Paracolon bacillus NEC 008.47
      Arizona 008.1
    Proteus (bacillus) (mirabilis) (Morganii) 008.3
    Pseudomonas aeruginosa 008.42
    S. japonicum 120.2
    specified organism NEC 008.8
      bacterial 008.49
      viral NEC 008.69
    Staphylococcus 008.41
    Streptococcus 008.49
      anaerobic 008.46
    Strongyloides stercoralis 127.2
    Trichuris trichiuria 127.3
    virus NEC (see also Enteritis, viral) 008.69
  dysenteric 009.2
    due to specified organism NEC 008.8
  dyspeptic 787.91
  endemic 009.3
    due to specified organism NEC 008.8
  epidemic 009.2
    due to specified organism NEC 008.8
  fermentative 787.91
  flagellate 007.9
  Flexner's (ulcerative) 004.1
  functional 564.5
    following gastrointestinal surgery 564.4
    psychogenic 306.4
  giardial 007.1
  Giardia lamblia 007.1
  hill 579.1
  hyperperistalsis (nervous) 306.4
  infectious 009.2
    due to specified organism NEC 008.8
    presumed 009.3
  inflammatory 787.91
    due to specified organism NEC 008.8
  malarial (see also Malaria) 084.6
  mite 133.8
  mycotic 117.9
  nervous 306.4
  neurogenic 564.5
  parenteral NEC 009.2
  postgastrectomy 564.4
  postvagotomy 564.4
  prostaglandin induced 579.8

Diarrhea, diarrheal (Continued)
  protozoal NEC 007.9
  psychogenic 306.4
  septic 009.2
    due to specified organism NEC 008.8
  specified organism NEC 008.8
    bacterial 008.49
    viral NEC 008.69
  Staphylococcus 008.41
  Streptococcus 008.49
    anaerobic 008.46
  toxic 558.2
  travelers' 009.2
    due to specified organism NEC 008.8
  trichomonal 007.3
  tropical 579.1
  tuberculous 014.8●
  ulcerative (chronic) (see also Colitis, ulcerative) 556.9
  viral (see also Enteritis, viral) 008.8
  zymotic NEC 009.2
Diastasis
  cranial bones 733.99
    congenital 756.0
  joint (traumatic) - see Dislocation, by site
  muscle 728.84
    congenital 756.89
  recti (abdomen) 728.84
    complicating delivery 665.8●
    congenital 756.79
Diastema, teeth, tooth 524.30
Diastematomyelia 742.51
Diataxia, cerebral, infantile 343.0
Diathesis
  allergic V15.09
  bleeding (familial) 287.9
  cystine (familial) 270.0
  gouty 274.9
  hemorrhagic (familial) 287.9
    newborn NEC 776.0
  oxalic 271.8
  scrofulous (see also Tuberculosis) 017.2●
  spasmophilic (see also Tetany) 781.7
  ulcer 536.9
  uric acid 274.9
Diaz's disease or osteochondrosis 732.5
Dibothriocephaliasis 123.4
  larval 123.5
Dibothriocephalus (infection) (infestation) (latus) 123.4
  larval 123.5
Dicephalus 759.4
Dichotomy, teeth 520.2
Dichromat, dichromata (congenital) 368.59
Dichromatopsia (congenital) 368.59
Dichuchwa 104.0
Dicroceliasis 121.8
Didelphys, didelphic (see also Double uterus) 752.2
Didymitis (see also Epididymitis) 604.90
Died - see also Death
  without
    medical attention (cause unknown) 798.9
  sign of disease 798.2
Dientamoeba diarrhea 007.8
Dietary
  inadequacy or deficiency 269.9
  surveillance and counseling V65.3

◀ New   ◀◀◀ Revised   ~~deleted~~ Deleted   ● Use Additional Digit(s)   ▇ Omit code

Dietl's crisis 593.4
Dieulafoy lesion (hemorrhagic)
    of
        duodenum 537.84
        esophagus 530.82
        intestine 569.86
        stomach 537.84
Difficult
    birth, affecting fetus or newborn 763.9
    delivery NEC 669.9●
Difficulty
    feeding 783.3
        adult 783.3
        breast 676.8●
        child 783.3
        elderly 783.3
        infant 783.3
        newborn 779.31
        nonorganic (infant) NEC 307.59
    mechanical, gastroduodenal stoma
        537.89
    reading 315.00
    specific, spelling 315.09
    swallowing (see also Dysphagia) 787.20
    walking 719.7
Diffuse - see condition
Diffused ganglion 727.42
Di George's syndrome (thymic
    hypoplasia) 279.11
Digestive - see condition
Di Guglielmo's disease or syndrome
    (M9841/3) 207.0●
Dihydropyrimidine dehydrogenase
    disease (DPD) 277.6 ◄
Diktyoma (M9051/3) - see Neoplasm, by
    site, malignant
Dilaceration, tooth 520.4
Dilatation
    anus 564.89
        venule - see Hemorrhoids
    aorta (focal) (general) (see also
        Aneurysm, aorta) 441.9 (see also
        Ectasia, aortic) 447.70 ◄||||
        with aneurysm 441.9 ◄
        congenital 747.29
        infectional 093.0
        ruptured 441.5
        syphilitic 093.0
    appendix (cystic) 543.9
    artery 447.8
    bile duct (common) (cystic)
        (congenital) 751.69
        acquired 576.8
    bladder (sphincter) 596.8
        congenital 753.8
        in pregnancy or childbirth 654.4●
            causing obstructed labor 660.2●
                affecting fetus or newborn
                    763.1
    blood vessel 459.89
    bronchus, bronchi 494.0
        with acute exacerbation 494.1
    calyx (due to obstruction) 593.89
    capillaries 448.9
    cardiac (acute) (chronic) (see also
        Hypertrophy, cardiac) 429.3
        congenital 746.89
            valve NEC 746.89
                pulmonary 746.09
        hypertensive (see also Hypertension,
            heart) 402.90
    cavum septi pellucidi 742.4
    cecum 564.89
        psychogenic 306.4

Dilatation (Continued)
    cervix (uteri) - see also Incompetency,
        cervix
        incomplete, poor, slow
            affecting fetus or newborn 763.7
            complicating delivery 661.0●
                affecting fetus or newborn
                    763.7
    colon 564.7
        congenital 751.3
        due to mechanical obstruction
            560.89
        psychogenic 306.4
    common bile duct (congenital) 751.69
        acquired 576.8
            with calculus,
                choledocholithiasis, or
                stones - see
                Choledocholithiasis
    cystic duct 751.69
        acquired (any bile duct) 575.8
    duct, mammary 610.4
    duodenum 564.89
    esophagus 530.89
        congenital 750.4
        due to
            achalasia 530.0
            cardiospasm 530.0
    Eustachian tube, congenital 744.24
    fontanel 756.0
    gallbladder 575.8
        congenital 751.69
    gastric 536.8
        acute 536.1
        psychogenic 306.4
    heart (acute) (chronic) (see also
        Hypertrophy, cardiac) 429.3
        congenital 746.89
        hypertensive (see also Hypertension,
            heart) 402.90
        valve - see also Endocarditis
            congenital 746.89
    ileum 564.89
        psychogenic 306.4
    inguinal rings - see Hernia, inguinal
    jejunum 564.89
        psychogenic 306.4
    kidney (calyx) (collecting structures)
        (cystic) (parenchyma) (pelvis)
        593.89
    lacrimal passages 375.69
    lymphatic vessel 457.1
    mammary duct 610.4
    Meckel's diverticulum (congenital)
        751.0
    meningeal vessels, congenital 742.8
    myocardium (acute) (chronic) (see also
        Hypertrophy, cardiac) 429.3
    organ or site, congenital NEC - see
        Distortion
    pancreatic duct 577.8
    pelvis, kidney 593.89
    pericardium - see Pericarditis
    pharynx 478.29
    prostate 602.8
    pulmonary
        artery (idiopathic) 417.8
            congenital 747.3
        valve, congenital 746.09
    pupil 379.43
    rectum 564.89
    renal 593.89
    saccule vestibularis, congenital 744.05
    salivary gland (duct) 527.8

Dilatation (Continued)
    sphincter ani 564.89
    stomach 536.8
        acute 536.1
        psychogenic 306.4
    submaxillary duct 527.8
    trachea, congenital 748.3
    ureter (idiopathic) 593.89
        congenital 753.20
        due to obstruction 593.5
    urethra (acquired) 599.84
    vasomotor 443.9
    vein 459.89
    ventricular, ventricle (acute) (chronic)
        (see also Hypertrophy, cardiac)
        429.3
        cerebral, congenital 742.4
        hypertensive (see also Hypertension,
            heart) 402.90
    venule 459.89
        anus - see Hemorrhoids
    vesical orifice 596.8
Dilated, dilation - see Dilatation
Diminished
    hearing (acuity) (see also Deafness)
        389.9
    pulse pressure 785.9
    vision NEC 369.9
    vital capacity 794.2
Diminuta taenia 123.6
Diminution, sense or sensation (cold)
    (heat) (tactile) (vibratory) (see also
    Disturbance, sensation) 782.0
Dimitri-Sturge-Weber disease
    (encephalocutaneous angiomatosis)
    759.6
Dimple
    parasacral 685.1
        with abscess 685.0
    pilonidal 685.1
        with abscess 685.0
    postanal 685.1
        with abscess 685.0
Dioctophyma renale (infection)
    (infestation) 128.8
Dipetalonemiasis 125.4
Diphallus 752.69
Diphtheria, diphtheritic (gangrenous)
    (hemorrhagic) 032.9
    carrier (suspected) of V02.4
    cutaneous 032.85
    cystitis 032.84
    faucial 032.0
    infection of wound 032.85
    inoculation (anti) (not sick) V03.5
    laryngeal 032.3
    myocarditis 032.82
    nasal anterior 032.2
    nasopharyngeal 032.1
    neurological complication 032.89
    peritonitis 032.83
    specified site NEC 032.89
Diphyllobothriasis (intestine) 123.4
    larval 123.5
Diplacusis 388.41
Diplegia (upper limbs) 344.2
    brain or cerebral 437.8
    congenital 343.0
    facial 351.0
        congenital 352.6
    infantile or congenital (cerebral)
        (spastic) (spinal) 343.0
    lower limbs 344.1
    syphilitic, congenital 090.49

Diplococcus, diplococcal - *see* condition
Diplomyelia 742.59
Diplopia 368.2
  refractive 368.15
Dipsomania (*see also* Alcoholism) 303.9●
  with psychosis (*see also* Psychosis, alcoholic) 291.9
Dipylidiasis 123.8
  intestine 123.8
Direction, teeth, abnormal 524.30
Dirt-eating child 307.52
Disability
  heart - *see* Disease, heart
  learning NEC 315.2
  special spelling 315.09
Disarticulation (*see also* Derangement, joint) 718.9●
  meaning
    amputation
      status - *see* Absence, by site
      traumatic - *see* Amputation, traumatic
    dislocation, traumatic or congenital - *see* Dislocation
Disaster, cerebrovascular (*see also* Disease, cerebrovascular, acute) 436
Discharge
  anal NEC 787.99
  breast (female) (male) 611.79
  conjunctiva 372.89
  continued locomotor idiopathic (*see also* Epilepsy) 345.5●
  diencephalic autonomic idiopathic (*see also* Epilepsy) 345.5●
  ear 388.60
    blood 388.69
    cerebrospinal fluid 388.61
  excessive urine 788.42
  eye 379.93
  nasal 478.19
  nipple 611.79
  patterned motor idiopathic (*see also* Epilepsy) 345.5●
  penile 788.7
  postnasal - *see* Sinusitis
  sinus, from mediastinum 510.0
  umbilicus 789.9
  urethral 788.7
    bloody 599.84
  vaginal 623.5
Discitis 722.90
  cervical, cervicothoracic 722.91
  lumbar, lumbosacral 722.93
  thoracic, thoracolumbar 722.92
Discogenic syndrome - *see* Displacement, intervertebral disc
Discoid
  kidney 753.3
  meniscus, congenital 717.5
  semilunar cartilage 717.5
Discoloration
  mouth 528.9
  nails 703.8
  teeth 521.7
    due to
      drugs 521.7
      metals (copper) (silver) 521.7
      pulpal bleeding 521.7
    during formation 520.8
    extrinsic 523.6
    intrinsic posteruptive 521.7
Discomfort
  chest 786.59
  visual 368.13

Discomycosis - *see* Actinomycosis
Discontinuity, ossicles, ossicular chain 385.23
Discrepancy
  centric occlusion
    maximum intercuspation 524.55
    of teeth 524.55
  leg length (acquired) 736.81
    congenital 755.30
  uterine size-date 649.6●
Discrimination
  political V62.4
  racial V62.4
  religious V62.4
  sex V62.4
Disease, diseased - *see also* Syndrome
  Abrami's (acquired hemolytic jaundice) 283.9
  absorbent system 459.89
  accumulation - *see* Thesaurismosis
  acid-peptic 536.8
  Acosta's 993.2
  Adams-Stokes (-Morgagni) (syncope with heart block) 426.9
  Addison's (bronze) (primary adrenal insufficiency) 255.41
    anemia (pernicious) 281.0
    tuberculous (*see also* Tuberculosis) 017.6●
  Addison-Gull - *see* Xanthoma
  adenoids (and tonsils) (chronic) 474.9
  adrenal (gland) (capsule) (cortex) 255.9
    hyperfunction 255.3
    hypofunction 255.41
    specified type NEC 255.8
  ainhum (dactylolysis spontanea) 136.0
  akamushi (scrub typhus) 081.2
  Akureyri (epidemic neuromyasthenia) 049.8
  Albarrán's (colibacilluria) 791.9
  Albers-Schönberg's (marble bones) 756.52
  Albert's 726.71
  Albright (-Martin) (-Bantam) 275.49
  Alibert's (mycosis fungoides) (M9700/3) 202.1●
  Alibert-Bazin (M9700/3) 202.1●
  alimentary canal 569.9
  alligator skin (ichthyosis congenita) 757.1
    acquired 701.1
  Almeida's (Brazilian blastomycosis) 116.1
  Alpers' 330.8
  alpine 993.2
  altitude 993.2
  alveoli, teeth 525.9
  Alzheimer's - *see* Alzheimer's
  amyloid (any site) 277.30
  anarthritic rheumatoid 446.5
  Anders' (adiposis tuberosa simplex) 272.8
  Andersen's (glycogenosis IV) 271.0
  Anderson's (angiokeratoma corporis diffusum) 272.7
  Andes 993.2
  Andrews' (bacterid) 686.8
  angiopastic, angiospasmodic 443.9
    cerebral 435.9
      with transient neurologic deficit 435.9
    vein 459.89

Disease, diseased (*Continued*)
  anterior
    chamber 364.9
    horn cell 335.9
      specified type NEC 335.8
  antral (chronic) 473.0
    acute 461.0
  anus NEC 569.49
  aorta (nonsyphilitic) 447.9
    syphilitic NEC 093.89
  aortic (heart) (valve) (*see also* Endocarditis, aortic) 424.1
  apollo 077.4
  aponeurosis 726.90
  appendix 543.9
  aqueous (chamber) 364.9
  arc-welders' lung 503
  Armenian 277.31
  Arnold-Chiari (*see also* Spina bifida) 741.0●
  arterial 447.9
    occlusive (*see also* Occlusion, by site) 444.22
      with embolus or thrombus - *see* Occlusion, by site
      due to stricture or stenosis 447.1
    specified type NEC 447.8
  arteriocardiorenal (*see also* Hypertension, cardiorenal) 404.90
  arteriolar (generalized) (obliterative) 447.90
    specified type NEC 447.8
  arteriorenal - *see* Hypertension, kidney
  arteriosclerotic - *see also* Arteriosclerosis
    cardiovascular 429.2
    coronary - *see* Arteriosclerosis, coronary
    heart - *see* Arteriosclerosis, coronary
    vascular - *see* Arteriosclerosis
  artery 447.9
    cerebral 437.9
    coronary - *see* Arteriosclerosis, coronary
    specified type NEC 447.8
  arthropod-borne NEC 088.9
    specified type NEC 088.89
  Asboe-Hansen's (incontinentia pigmenti) 757.33
  atticoantral, chronic (with posterior or superior marginal perforation of ear drum) 382.2
  auditory canal, ear 380.9
  Aujeszky's 078.89
  auricle, ear NEC 380.30
  Australian X 062.4
  autoimmune NEC 279.49
    hemolytic (cold type) (warm type) 283.0
    parathyroid 252.1
    thyroid 245.2
  aviators' (*see also* Effect, adverse, high altitude) 993.2
  ax(e)-grinders' 502
  Ayala's 756.89
  Ayerza's (pulmonary artery sclerosis with pulmonary hypertension) 416.0
  Azorean (of the nervous system) 334.8
  Babington's (familial hemorrhagic telangiectasia) 448.0
  back bone NEC 733.90
  bacterial NEC 040.89
    zoonotic NEC 027.9
      specified type NEC 027.8

◀ New   ◀▥ Revised   ~~deleted~~ Deleted   ● Use Additional Digit(s)   ▦ Omit code

Disease, diseased *(Continued)*
  Baehr-Schiffrin (thrombotic
    thrombocytopenic purpura)
    446.6
  Baelz's (cheilitis glandularis
    apostematosa) 528.5
  Baerensprung's (eczema marginatum)
    110.3
  Balfour's (chloroma) 205.3●
  balloon *(see also* Effect, adverse, high
    altitude) 993.2
  Baló's 341.1
  Bamberger (-Marie) (hypertrophic
    pulmonary osteoarthropathy)
    731.2
  Bang's (Brucella abortus) 023.1
  Bannister's 995.1
  Banti's (with cirrhosis) (with portal
    hypertension) - *see* Cirrhosis, liver
  Barcoo *(see also* Ulcer, skin) 707.9
  barium lung 503
  Barlow (-Möller) (infantile scurvy) 267
  barometer makers' 985.0
  Barraquer (-Simons) (progressive
    lipodystrophy) 272.6
  basal ganglia 333.90
    degenerative NEC 333.0
    specified NEC 333.89
  Basedow's (exophthalmic goiter)
    242.0●
  basement membrane NEC 583.89
    with
      pulmonary hemorrhage
        (Goodpasture's syndrome)
        446.21 *[583.81]*
  Bateman's 078.0
    purpura (senile) 287.2
  Batten's 330.1 *[362.71]*
  Batten-Mayou (retina) 330.1 *[362.71]*
  Batten-Steinert 359.21
  Battey 031.0
  Baumgarten-Cruveilhier (cirrhosis of
    liver) 571.5
  bauxite-workers' 503
  Bayle's (dementia paralytica) 094.1
  Bazin's (primary) *(see also* Tuberculosis)
    017.1●
  Beard's (neurasthenia) 300.5
  Beau's *(see also* Degeneration,
    myocardial) 429.1
  Bechterew's (ankylosing spondylitis)
    720.0
  Becker's
    idiopathic mural endomyocardial
      disease 425.2
    myotonia congenita, recessive form
      359.22
  Begbie's (exophthalmic goiter) 242.0●
  Behr's 362.50
  Beigel's (white piedra) 111.2
  Bekhterev's (ankylosing spondylitis)
    720.0
  Bell's *(see also* Psychosis, affective)
    296.0●
  Bennett's (leukemia) 208.9●
  Benson's 379.22
  Bergeron's (hysteroepilepsy) 300.11
  Berlin's 921.3
  Bernard-Soulier (thrombopathy) 287.1
  Bernhardt (-Roth) 355.1
  beryllium 503
  Besnier-Boeck (-Schaumann)
    (sarcoidosis) 135
  Best's 362.76

Disease, diseased *(Continued)*
  Beurmann's (sporotrichosis) 117.1
  Bielschowsky (-Jansky) 330.1
  Biermer's (pernicious anemia) 281.0
  Biett's (discoid lupus erythematosus)
    695.4
  bile duct *(see also* Disease, biliary) 576.9
  biliary (duct) (tract) 576.9
    with calculus, choledocholithiasis,
      or stones - *see*
      Choledocholithiasis
  Billroth's (meningocele) *(see also* Spina
    bifida) 741.9●
  Binswanger's 290.12
  Bird's (oxaluria) 271.8
  bird fanciers' 495.2
  black lung 500
  bladder 596.9
    specified NEC 596.8
  bleeder's 286.0
  Bloch-Sulzberger (incontinentia
    pigmenti) 757.33
  Blocq's (astasia-abasia) 307.9
  blood (-forming organs) 289.9
    specified NEC 289.89
    vessel 459.9
  Bloodgood's 610.1
  Blount's (tibia vara) 732.4
  blue 746.9
  Bodechtel-Guttmann (subacute
    sclerosing panencephalitis) 046.2
  Boeck's (sarcoidosis) 135
  bone 733.90
    fibrocystic NEC 733.29
      jaw 526.2
    marrow 289.9
    Paget's (osteitis deformans) 731.0
    specified type NEC 733.99
    von Recklinghausen's (osteitis
      fibrosa cystica) 252.01
  Bonfils' - *see* Disease, Hodgkin's
  Borna 062.9
  Bornholm (epidemic pleurodynia)
    074.1
  Bostock's *(see also* Fever, hay) 477.9
  Bouchard's (myopathic dilatation of
    the stomach) 536.1
  Bouillaud's (rheumatic heart disease)
    391.9
  Bourneville (-Brissaud) (tuberous
    sclerosis) 759.5
  Bouveret (-Hoffmann) (paroxysmal
    tachycardia) 427.2
  bowel 569.9
    functional 564.9
      psychogenic 306.4
  Bowen's (M8081/2) - *see* Neoplasm,
    skin, in situ
  Bozzolo's (multiple myeloma)
    (M9730/3) 203.0●
  Bradley's (epidemic vomiting)
    078.82
  Brailsford's 732.3
    radius, head 732.3
    tarsal, scaphoid 732.5
  Brailsford-Morquio
    (mucopolysaccharidosis IV)
    277.5
  brain 348.9
    Alzheimer's 331.0
      with dementia - *see* Alzheimer's,
        dementia
    arterial, artery 437.9
    arteriosclerotic 437.0

Disease, diseased *(Continued)*
  brain *(Continued)*
    congenital 742.9
    degenerative - *see* Degeneration,
      brain
    inflammatory - *see also* Encephalitis
      late effect - *see* category 326
    organic 348.9
      arteriosclerotic 437.0
    parasitic NEC 123.9
    Pick's 331.11
      with dementia
        with behavioral disturbance
          331.11 *[294.11]*
        without behavioral
          disturbance 331.11
          [294.10]
    senile 331.2
  braziers' 985.8
  breast 611.9
    cystic (chronic) 610.1
    fibrocystic 610.1
    inflammatory 611.0
    Paget's (M8540/3) 174.0
    puerperal, postpartum NEC 676.3●
    specified NEC 611.89
  Breda's *(see also* Yaws) 102.9
  Breisky's (kraurosis vulvae) 624.09
  Bretonneau's (diphtheritic malignant
    angina) 032.0
  Bright's *(see also* Nephritis) 583.9
    arteriosclerotic *(see also*
      Hypertension, kidney) 403.90
  Brill's (recrudescent typhus) 081.1
    flea-borne 081.0
    louse-borne 081.1
  Brill-Symmers (follicular lymphoma)
    (M9690/3) 202.0●
  Brill-Zinsser (recrudescent typhus)
    081.1
  Brinton's (leather bottle stomach)
    (M8142/3) 151.9
  Brion-Kayser *(see also* Fever,
    paratyphoid) 002.9
  broad
    beta 272.2
    ligament, noninflammatory 620.9
      specified NEC 620.8
  Brocq's 691.8
    meaning
      atopic (diffuse) neurodermatitis
        691.8
      dermatitis herpetiformis 694.0
      lichen simplex chronicus 698.3
      parapsoriasis 696.2
      prurigo 698.2
  Brocq-Duhring (dermatitis
    herpetiformis) 694.0
  Brodie's (joint) *(see also* Osteomyelitis)
    730.1●
  bronchi 519.19
  bronchopulmonary 519.19
  bronze (Addison's) 255.41
    tuberculous *(see also* Tuberculosis)
      017.6●
  Brown-Séquard 344.89
  Bruck's 733.99
  Bruck-de Lange (Amsterdam dwarf,
    mental retardation, and
    brachycephaly) 759.89
  Bruhl's (splenic anemia with fever)
    285.8
  Bruton's (X-linked
    agammaglobulinemia) 279.04

Disease, diseased *(Continued)*
  buccal cavity 528.9
  Buchanan's (juvenile osteochondrosis, iliac crest) 732.1
  Buchman's (osteochondrosis juvenile) 732.1
  Budgerigar-Fanciers' 495.2
  Budinger-Ludloff-Läwen 717.89
  Büerger's (thromboangiitis obliterans) 443.1
  Burger-Grütz (essential familial hyperlipemia) 272.3
  Burns' (lower ulna) 732.3
  bursa 727.9
  Bury's (erythema elevatum diutinum) 695.89
  Buschke's 710.1
  Busquet's *(see also* Osteomyelitis) 730.1●
  Busse-Buschke (cryptococcosis) 117.5
  C₂ *(see also* Alcoholism) 303.9●
  Caffey's (infantile cortical hyperostosis) 756.59
  caisson 993.3
  calculous 592.9
  California 114.0
  Calvé (-Perthes) (osteochondrosis, femoral capital) 732.1
  Camurati-Engelmann (diaphyseal sclerosis) 756.59
  Canavan's 330.0
  capillaries 448.9
  Carapata 087.1
  cardiac - *see* Disease, heart
  cardiopulmonary, chronic 416.9
  cardiorenal (arteriosclerotic) (hepatic) (hypertensive) (vascular) *(see also* Hypertension, cardiorenal) 404.90
  cardiovascular (arteriosclerotic) 429.2
    congenital 746.9
    hypertensive *(see also* Hypertension, heart) 402.90
      benign 402.10
      malignant 402.00
    renal *(see also* Hypertension, cardiorenal) 404.90
    syphilitic (asymptomatic) 093.9
  carotid gland 259.8
  Carrión's (Bartonellosis) 088.0
  cartilage NEC 733.90
    specified NEC 733.99
  Castellani's 104.8
  cat-scratch 078.3
  Cavare's (familial periodic paralysis) 359.3
  Cazenave's (pemphigus) 694.4
  cecum 569.9
  celiac (adult) 579.0
    infantile 579.0
  cellular tissue NEC 709.9
  central core 359.0
  cerebellar, cerebellum - *see* Disease, brain
  cerebral *(see also* Disease, brain) 348.9
    arterial, artery 437.9
    degenerative - *see* Degeneration, brain
  cerebrospinal 349.9
  cerebrovascular NEC 437.9
    acute 436
      embolic - *see* Embolism, brain
      late effect - *see* Late effect(s) (of) cerebrovascular disease

Disease, diseased *(Continued)*
  cerebrovascular NEC *(Continued)*
    acute *(Continued)*
      puerperal, postpartum, childbirth 674.0●
      thrombotic - *see* Thrombosis, brain
    arteriosclerotic 437.0
    embolic - *see* Embolism, brain
    ischemic, generalized NEC 437.1
    late effect - *see* Late effect(s) (of) cerebrovascular disease
    occlusive 437.1
    puerperal, postpartum, childbirth 674.0●
    specified type NEC 437.8
    thrombotic - *see* Thrombosis, brain
  ceroid storage 272.7
  cervix (uteri)
    inflammatory 616.0
    noninflammatory 622.9
      specified NEC 622.8
  Chabert's 022.9
  Chagas' *(see also* Trypanosomiasis, American) 086.2
  Chandler's (osteochondritis dissecans, hip) 732.7
  Charcôt's (joint) 094.0 *[713.5]*
    spinal cord 094.0
  Charcôt-Marie-Tooth 356.1
  Charlouis' *(see also* Yaws) 102.9
  Cheadle (-Möller) (-Barlow) (infantile scurvy) 267
  Chédiak-Steinbrinck (-Higashi) (congenital gigantism of peroxidase granules) 288.2
  cheek, inner 528.9
  chest 519.9
  Chiari's (hepatic vein thrombosis) 453.0
  Chicago (North American blastomycosis) 116.0
  chignon (white piedra) 111.2
  chigoe, chigo (jigger) 134.1
  childhood granulomatous 288.1
  Chinese liver fluke 121.1
  chlamydial NEC 078.88
  cholecystic *(see also* Disease, gallbladder) 575.9
  choroid 363.9
    degenerative *(see also* Degeneration, choroid) 363.40
    hereditary *(see also* Dystrophy, choroid) 363.50
    specified type NEC 363.8
  Christian's (chronic histiocytosis X) 277.89
  Christian-Weber (nodular nonsuppurative panniculitis) 729.30
  Christmas 286.1
  ciliary body 364.9
    specified NEC 364.89
  circulatory (system) NEC 459.9
    chronic, maternal, affecting fetus or newborn 760.3
    specified NEC 459.89
    syphilitic 093.9
      congenital 090.5
  Civatte's (poikiloderma) 709.09
  climacteric 627.2
    male 608.89
  coagulation factor deficiency (congenital) *(see also* Defect, coagulation) 286.9

Disease, diseased *(Continued)*
  Coats' 362.12
  coccidioidal pulmonary 114.5
    acute 114.0
    chronic 114.4
    primary 114.0
    residual 114.4
  Cockayne's (microcephaly and dwarfism) 759.89
  Cogan's 370.52
  cold
    agglutinin 283.0
      or hemoglobinuria 283.0
        paroxysmal (cold) (nocturnal) 283.2
    hemagglutinin (chronic) 283.0
  collagen NEC 710.9
    nonvascular 710.9
    specified NEC 710.8
    vascular (allergic) *(see also* Angiitis, hypersensitivity) 446.20
  colon 569.9
    functional 564.9
      congenital 751.3
    ischemic 557.0
  combined system (of spinal cord) 266.2 *[336.2]*
    with anemia (pernicious) 281.0 *[336.2]*
  compressed air 993.3
  Concato's (pericardial polyserositis) 423.2
    peritoneal 568.82
    pleural - *see* Pleurisy
  congenital NEC 799.89
  conjunctiva 372.9
    chlamydial 077.98
      specified NEC 077.8
    specified type NEC 372.89
    viral 077.99
      specified NEC 077.8
  connective tissue, diffuse *(see also* Disease, collagen) 710.9
  Conor and Bruch's (boutonneuse fever) 082.1
  Conradi (-Hünermann) 756.59
  Cooley's (erythroblastic anemia) 282.49
  Cooper's 610.1
  Corbus' 607.1
  cork-handlers' 495.3
  cornea *(see also* Keratopathy) 371.9
  coronary *(see also* Ischemia, heart) 414.9
    congenital 746.85
    ostial, syphilitic 093.20
      aortic 093.22
      mitral 093.21
      pulmonary 093.24
      tricuspid 093.23
  Corrigan's - *see* Insufficiency, aortic
  Cotugno's 724.3
  Coxsackie (virus) NEC 074.8
  cranial nerve NEC 352.9
  Creutzfeldt-Jakob (CJD) 046.19
    with dementia
      with behavioral disturbance 046.19 *[294.11]*
      without behavioral disturbance 046.19 *[294.10]*
    familial 046.19
    iatrogenic 046.19
    specified NEC 046.19
    sporadic 046.19

◀ New   ◀◀◀ Revised   ~~deleted~~ Deleted   ● Use Additional Digit(s)   ▨ Omit code

Disease, diseased (*Continued*)
Creutzfeldt-Jakob (*Continued*)
variant (vCJD) 046.11
with dementia
with behavioral disturbance
046.11 [294.11]
without behavioral
disturbance 046.11
[294.10]
Crigler-Najjar (congenital
hyperbilirubinemia) 277.4
Crocq's (acrocyanosis) 443.89
Crohn's (intestine) (*see also* Enteritis,
regional) 555.9
Crouzon's (craniofacial dysostosis)
756.0
Cruchet's (encephalitis lethargica)
049.8
Cruveilhier's 335.21
Cruz-Chagas (*see also*
Trypanosomiasis,
American) 086.2
crystal deposition (*see also* Arthritis,
due to, crystals) 712.9●
Csillag's (lichen sclerosus et
atrophicus) 701.0
Curschmann's 359.21
Cushing's (pituitary basophilism)
255.0
cystic
breast (chronic) 610.1
kidney, congenital (*see also* Cystic,
disease, kidney) 753.10
liver, congenital 751.62
lung 518.89
congenital 748.4
pancreas 577.2
congenital 751.7
renal, congenital (*see also* Cystic,
disease, kidney) 753.10
semilunar cartilage 717.5
cysticercus 123.1
cystine storage (with renal sclerosis)
270.0
cytomegalic inclusion (generalized)
078.5
with
pneumonia 078.5 [484.1]
congenital 771.1
Daae (-Finsen) (epidemic pleurodynia)
074.1
dancing 297.8
Danielssen's (anesthetic leprosy)
030.1
Darier's (congenital) (keratosis
follicularis) 757.39
erythema annulare centrifugum
695.0
vitamin A deficiency 264.8
Darling's (histoplasmosis) (*see also*
Histoplasmosis, American)
115.00
Davies' 425.0
de Beurmann-Gougerot
(sporotrichosis) 117.1
Débove's (splenomegaly) 789.2
deer fly (*see also* Tularemia) 021.9
deficiency 269.9
degenerative - *see also* Degeneration
disc - *see* Degeneration,
intervertebral disc
Degos' 447.8
Déjérine (-Sottas) 356.0
Déleage's 359.89

Disease, diseased (*Continued*)
demyelinating, demyelinizating (brain
stem) (central nervous system)
341.9
multiple sclerosis 340
specified NEC 341.8
de Quervain's (tendon sheath) 727.04
thyroid (subacute granulomatous
thyroiditis) 245.1
Dercum's (adiposis dolorosa) 272.8
Deutschländer's - *see* Fracture, foot
Devergie's (pityriasis rubra pilaris)
696.4
Devic's 341.0
diaphorase deficiency 289.7
diaphragm 519.4
diarrheal, infectious 009.2
diatomaceous earth 502
Diaz's (osteochondrosis astragalus)
732.5
digestive system 569.9
Di Guglielmo's (erythemic myelosis)
(M9841/3) 207.0●
Dimitri-Sturge-Weber
(encephalocutaneous
angiomatosis) 759.6
disc, degenerative - *see* Degeneration,
intervertebral disc
discogenic (*see also* Disease,
intervertebral disc) 722.90
diverticular - *see* Diverticula
Down's (mongolism) 758.0
Dubini's (electric chorea) 049.8
Dubois' (thymus gland) 090.5
Duchenne's 094.0
locomotor ataxia 094.0
muscular dystrophy 359.1
paralysis 335.22
pseudohypertrophy, muscles 359.1
Duchenne-Griesinger 359.1
ductless glands 259.9
Duhring's (dermatitis herpetiformis)
694.0
Dukes (-Filatov) 057.8
duodenum NEC 537.9
specified NEC 537.89
Duplay's 726.2
Dupré's (meningism) 781.6
Dupuytren's (muscle contracture) 728.6
Durand-Nicolas-Favre (climatic bubo)
099.1
Duroziez's (congenital mitral stenosis)
746.5
Dutton's (trypanosomiasis) 086.9
Eales' 362.18
ear (chronic) (inner) NEC 388.9
middle 385.9
adhesive (*see also* Adhesions,
middle ear) 385.10
specified NEC 385.89
Eberth's (typhoid fever) 002.0
Ebstein's
heart 746.2
meaning diabetes 250.4● [581.81]
due to secondary diabetes 249.4●
[581.81]
Echinococcus (*see also* Echinococcus)
122.9
ECHO virus NEC 078.89
Economo's (encephalitis lethargica)
049.8
Eddowes' (brittle bones and blue
sclera) 756.51
Edsall's 992.2

Disease, diseased (*Continued*)
Eichstedt's (pityriasis versicolor) 111.0
Ellis-van Creveld (chondroectodermal
dysplasia) 756.55
endocardium - *see* Endocarditis
endocrine glands or system NEC 259.9
specified NEC 259.8
endomyocardial, idiopathic mural 425.2
Engel-von Recklinghausen (osteitis
fibrosa cystica) 252.01
Engelmann's (diaphyseal sclerosis)
756.59
English (rickets) 268.0
Engman's (infectious eczematoid
dermatitis) 690.8
enteroviral, enterovirus NEC 078.89
central nervous system NEC 048
epidemic NEC 136.9
epididymis 608.9
epigastric, functional 536.9
psychogenic 306.4
Erb (-Landouzy) 359.1
Erb-Goldflam 358.00
Erdheim-Chester (ECD) 277.89
Erichsen's (railway spine) 300.16
esophagus 530.9
functional 530.5
psychogenic 306.4
Eulenburg's (congenital paramyotonia)
359.29
Eustachian tube 381.9
Evans' (thrombocytopenic purpura)
287.32
external auditory canal 380.9
extrapyramidal NEC 333.90
eye 379.90
anterior chamber 364.9
inflammatory NEC 364.3
muscle 378.9
eyeball 360.9
eyelid 374.9
eyeworm of Africa 125.2
Fabry's (angiokeratoma corporis
diffusum) 272.7
facial nerve (seventh) 351.9
newborn 767.5
Fahr-Volhard (malignant
nephrosclerosis) 403.00
fallopian tube, noninflammatory 620.9
specified NEC 620.8
familial periodic 277.31
paralysis 359.3
Fanconi's (congenital pancytopenia)
284.09
Farber's (disseminated
lipogranulomatosis) 272.8
fascia 728.9
inflammatory 728.9
Fauchard's (periodontitis) 523.40
Favre-Durand-Nicolas (climatic bubo)
099.1
Favre-Racouchot (elastoidosis cutanea
nodularis) 701.8
Fede's 529.0
Feer's 985.0
Felix's (juvenile osteochondrosis, hip)
732.1
Fenwick's (gastric atrophy) 537.89
Fernels' (aortic aneurysm) 441.9
fibrocaseous, of lung (*see also*
Tuberculosis, pulmonary) 011.9●
fibrocystic - *see also* Fibrocystic, disease
newborn 277.01
Fiedler's (leptospiral jaundice) 100.0

Disease, diseased (*Continued*)
fifth 057.0
Filatoff's (infectious mononucleosis) 075
Filatov's (infectious mononucleosis) 075
file-cutters' 984.9
   specified type of lead - *see* Table of Drugs and Chemicals
filterable virus NEC 078.89
fish skin 757.1
   acquired 701.1
Flajani (-Basedow) (exophthalmic goiter) 242.0●
Flatau-Schilder 341.1
flax-dressers' 504
Fleischner's 732.3
flint 502
fluke - *see* Infestation, fluke
Følling's (phenylketonuria) 270.1
foot and mouth 078.4
foot process 581.3
Forbes' (glycogenosis III) 271.0
Fordyce's (ectopic sebaceous glands) (mouth) 750.26
Fordyce-Fox (apocrine miliaria) 705.82
Fothergill's
   meaning scarlatina anginosa 034.1
   neuralgia (*see also* Neuralgia, trigeminal) 350.1
Fournier's 608.83
fourth 057.8
Fox (-Fordyce) (apocrine miliaria) 705.82
Francis' (*see also* Tularemia) 021.9
Franklin's (heavy chain) 273.2
Frei's (climatic bubo) 099.1
Freiberg's (flattening metatarsal) 732.5
Friedländer's (endarteritis obliterans) - *see* Arteriosclerosis
Friedreich's
   combined systemic or ataxia 334.0
   facial hemihypertrophy 756.0
   myoclonia 333.2
Fröhlich's (adiposogenital dystrophy) 253.8
Frommel's 676.6●
frontal sinus (chronic) 473.1
   acute 461.1
Fuller's earth 502
fungus, fungous NEC 117.9
Gaisböck's (polycythemia hypertonica) 289.0
gallbladder 575.9
   congenital 751.60
Gamna's (siderotic splenomegaly) 289.51
Gamstorp's (adynamia episodica hereditaria) 359.3
Gandy-Nanta (siderotic splenomegaly) 289.51
Gannister (occupational) 502
Garré's (*see also* Osteomyelitis) 730.1●
gastric (*see also* Disease, stomach) 537.9
gastroesophageal reflux (GERD) 530.81
gastrointestinal (tract) 569.9
   amyloid 277.39
   functional 536.9
      psychogenic 306.4
Gaucher's (adult) (cerebroside lipidosis) (infantile) 272.7
Gayet's (superior hemorrhagic polioencephalitis) 265.1

Disease, diseased (*Continued*)
Gee (-Herter) (-Heubner) (-Thaysen) (nontropical sprue) 579.0
generalized neoplastic (M8000/6) 199.0
genital organs NEC
   female 629.9
      specified NEC 629.89
   male 608.9
Gerhardt's (erythromelalgia) 443.82
Gerlier's (epidemic vertigo) 078.81
Gibert's (pityriasis rosea) 696.3
Gibney's (perispondylitis) 720.9
Gierke's (glycogenosis I) 271.0
Gilbert's (familial nonhemolytic jaundice) 277.4
Gilchrist's (North American blastomycosis) 116.0
Gilford (-Hutchinson) (progeria) 259.8
Gilles de la Tourette's (motor-verbal tic) 307.23
Giovannini's 117.9
gland (lymph) 289.9
Glanzmann's (hereditary hemorrhagic thrombasthenia) 287.1
glassblowers' 527.1
Glénard's (enteroptosis) 569.89
Glisson's (*see also* Rickets) 268.0
glomerular
   membranous, idiopathic 581.1
   minimal change 581.3
glycogen storage (Andersen's) (Cori types 1-7) (Forbes') (McArdle-Schmid-Pearson) (Pompe's) (types I-VII) 271.0
   cardiac 271.0 [425.7]
   generalized 271.0
   glucose-6-phosphatase deficiency 271.0
   heart 271.0 [425.7]
   hepatorenal 271.0
   liver and kidneys 271.0
   myocardium 271.0 [425.7]
   von Gierke's (glycogenosis I) 271.0
Goldflam-Erb 358.00
Goldscheider's (epidermolysis bullosa) 757.39
Goldstein's (familial hemorrhagic telangiectasia) 448.0
gonococcal NEC 098.0
Goodall's (epidemic vomiting) 078.82
Gordon's (exudative enteropathy) 579.8
Gougerot's (trisymptomatic) 709.1
Gougerot-Carteaud (confluent reticulate papillomatosis) 701.8
Gougerot-Hailey-Hailey (benign familial chronic pemphigus) 757.39
graft-versus-host 279.50
   acute 279.51
      on chronic 279.53
   chronic 279.52
grain-handlers' 495.8
Grancher's (splenopneumonia) - *see* Pneumonia
granulomatous (childhood) (chronic) 288.1
graphite lung 503
Graves' (exophthalmic goiter) 242.0●
Greenfield's 330.0
green monkey 078.89
Griesinger's (*see also* Ancylostomiasis) 126.9

Disease, diseased (*Continued*)
grinders' 502
Grisel's 723.5
Gruby's (tinea tonsurans) 110.0
Guertin's (electric chorea) 049.8
Guillain-Barré 357.0
Guinon's (motor-verbal tic) 307.23
Gull's (thyroid atrophy with myxedema) 244.8
Gull and Sutton's - *see* Hypertension, kidney
gum NEC 523.9
Günther's (congenital erythropoietic porphyria) 277.1
gynecological 629.9
   specified NEC 629.89
H 270.0
Haas' 732.3
Habermann's (acute parapsoriasis varioliformis) 696.2
Haff 985.1
Hageman (congenital factor XII deficiency) (*see also* Defect, congenital) 286.3
Haglund's (osteochondrosis os tibiale externum) 732.5
Hagner's (hypertrophic pulmonary osteoarthropathy) 731.2
Hailey-Hailey (benign familial chronic pemphigus) 757.39
hair (follicles) NEC 704.9
   specified type NEC 704.8
Hallervorden-Spatz 333.0
Hallopeau's (lichen sclerosus et atrophicus) 701.0
Hamman's (spontaneous mediastinal emphysema) 518.1
hand, foot, and mouth 074.3
Hand-Schüller-Christian (chronic histiocytosis X) 277.89
Hanot's - *see* Cirrhosis, biliary
Hansen's (leprosy) 030.9
   benign form 030.1
   malignant form 030.0
Harada's 363.22
Harley's (intermittent hemoglobinuria) 283.2
Hart's (pellagra-cerebellar ataxia-renal aminoaciduria) 270.0
Hartnup (pellagra-cerebellar ataxia-renal aminoaciduria) 270.0
Hashimoto's (struma lymphomatosa) 245.2
Hb - *see* Disease, hemoglobin
heart (organic) 429.9
   with
      acute pulmonary edema (*see also* Failure, ventricular, left) 428.1
      hypertensive 402.91
         with renal failure 404.92
         benign 402.11
            with renal failure 404.12
         malignant 402.01
            with renal failure 404.02
      kidney disease - *see* Hypertension, cardiorenal
      rheumatic fever (conditions classifiable to 390)
         active 391.9
            with chorea 392.0
         inactive or quiescent (with chorea) 398.90

◀ New   ◀▥ Revised   ~~deleted~~ Deleted   ● Use Additional Digit(s)   ▨ Omit code

Disease, diseased *(Continued)*
  heart *(Continued)*
    amyloid 277.39 *[425.7]*
    aortic (valve) *(see also* Endocarditis,
      aortic) 424.1
    arteriosclerotic or sclerotic (minimal)
      (senile) - *see* Arteriosclerosis,
      coronary
    artery, arterial - *see* Arteriosclerosis,
      coronary
    atherosclerotic - *see* Arteriosclerosis,
      coronary
    beer drinkers' 425.5
    beriberi 265.0 *[425.7]*
    black 416.0
    congenital NEC 746.9
      cyanotic 746.9
      maternal, affecting fetus or
        newborn 760.3
      specified type NEC 746.89
    congestive *(see also* Failure, heart)
      428.0
    coronary 414.9
    cryptogenic 429.9
    due to
      amyloidosis 277.39 *[425.7]*
      beriberi 265.0 *[425.7]*
      cardiac glycogenosis 271.0 *[425.7]*
      Friedreich's ataxia 334.0 *[425.8]*
      gout 274.82
      mucopolysaccharidosis 277.5
        [425.7]
      myotonia atrophica 359.21 *[425.8]*
      progressive muscular dystrophy
        359.1 *[425.8]*
      sarcoidosis 135 *[425.8]*
    fetal 746.9
      inflammatory 746.89
    fibroid *(see also* Myocarditis) 429.0
    functional 427.9
      postoperative 997.1
      psychogenic 306.2
    glycogen storage 271.0 *[425.7]*
    gonococcal NEC 098.85
    gouty 274.82
    hypertensive *(see also* Hypertension,
      heart) 402.90
      benign 402.10
      malignant 402.00
    hyperthyroid *(see also*
      Hyperthyroidism) 242.9●
      [425.7]
    incompletely diagnosed - *see*
      Disease, heart
    ischemic (chronic) *(see also* Ischemia,
      heart) 414.9
      acute *(see also* Infarct,
        myocardium) 410.9●
        without myocardial infarction
          411.89
          with coronary (artery)
            occlusion 411.81
      asymptomatic 412
      diagnosed on ECG or other
        special investigation but
        currently presenting no
        symptoms 412
    kyphoscoliotic 416.1
    mitral *(see also* Endocarditis, mitral)
      394.9
    muscular *(see also* Degeneration,
      myocardial) 429.1
    postpartum 674.8●
    psychogenic (functional) 306.2

Disease, diseased *(Continued)*
  heart *(Continued)*
    pulmonary (chronic) 416.9
      acute 415.0
      specified NEC 416.8
    rheumatic (chronic) (inactive) (old)
      (quiescent) (with chorea)
      398.90
      active or acute 391.9
        with chorea (active)
          (rheumatic)
          (Sydenham's) 392.0
        specified type NEC 391.8
      maternal, affecting fetus or
        newborn 760.3
    rheumatoid - *see* Arthritis,
      rheumatoid
    sclerotic - *see* Arteriosclerosis,
      coronary
    senile *(see also* Myocarditis) 429.0
    specified type NEC 429.89
    syphilitic 093.89
      aortic 093.1
        aneurysm 093.0
      asymptomatic 093.89
      congenital 090.5
    thyroid (gland) *(see also*
      Hyperthyroidism) 242.9●
      [425.7]
    thyrotoxic *(see also* Thyrotoxicosis)
      242.9● *[425.7]*
    tuberculous *(see also* Tuberculosis)
      017.9● *[425.8]*
    valve, valvular (obstructive)
      (regurgitant) - *see also*
      Endocarditis
      congenital NEC *(see also* Anomaly,
        heart, valve) 746.9
      pulmonary 746.00
      specified type NEC 746.89
    vascular - *see* Disease,
      cardiovascular
  heavy-chain (gamma G) 273.2
  Heberden's 715.04
  Hebra's
    dermatitis exfoliativa 695.89
    erythema multiforme exudativum
      695.19
    pityriasis
      maculata et circinata 696.3
      rubra 695.89
      pilaris 696.4
    prurigo 698.2
  Heerfordt's (uveoparotitis) 135
  Heidenhain's 290.10
    with dementia 290.10
  Heilmeyer-Schöner (M9842/3)
    207.1●
  Heine-Medin *(see also* Poliomyelitis)
    045.9●
  Heller's *(see also* Psychosis, childhood)
    299.1●
  Heller-Döhle (syphilitic aortitis) 093.1
  hematopoietic organs 289.9
  hemoglobin (Hb) 282.7
    with thalassemia 282.49
    abnormal (mixed) NEC 282.7
      with thalassemia 282.49
    AS genotype 282.5
    Bart's 282.49
    C (Hb-C) 282.7
      with other abnormal hemoglobin
        NEC 282.7
      elliptocytosis 282.7

Disease, diseased *(Continued)*
  hemoglobin (Hb) *(Continued)*
    C (Hb-C) *(Continued)*
      Hb-S (without crisis) 282.63
        with
          crisis 282.64
          vaso-occlusive pain 282.64
      sickle-cell (without crisis) 282.63
        with
          crisis 282.64
          vaso-occlusive pain 282.64
      thalassemia 282.49
    constant spring 282.7
    D (Hb-D) 282.7
      with other abnormal hemoglobin
        NEC 282.7
      Hb-S (without crisis) 282.68
        with crisis 282.69
      sickle-cell (without crisis) 282.68
        with crisis 282.69
      thalassemia 282.49
    E (Hb-E) 282.7
      with other abnormal hemoglobin
        NEC 282.7
      Hb-S (without crisis) 282.68
        with crisis 282.69
      sickle-cell (without crisis) 282.68
        with crisis 282.69
      thalassemia 282.49
    elliptocytosis 282.7
    F (Hb-F) 282.7
    G (Hb-G) 282.7
    H (Hb-H) 282.49
    hereditary persistence, fetal (HPFH)
      ("Swiss variety") 282.7
    high fetal gene 282.7
    I thalassemia 282.49
    M 289.7
    S - *see also* Disease, sickle-cell, Hb-S
      thalassemia (without crisis)
        282.41
        with
          crisis 282.42
          vaso-occlusive pain 282.42
    spherocytosis 282.7
    unstable, hemolytic 282.7
    Zurich (Hb-Zurich) 282.7
  hemolytic (fetus) (newborn) 773.2
    autoimmune (cold type) (warm
      type) 283.0
    due to or with
      incompatibility
        ABO (blood group) 773.1
        blood (group) (Duffy) (Kell)
          (Kidd) (Lewis) (M) (S)
          NEC 773.2
        Rh (blood group) (factor) 773.0
          Rh negative mother 773.0
    unstable hemoglobin 282.7
  hemorrhagic 287.9
    newborn 776.0
  Henoch (-Schönlein) (purpura nervosa)
    287.0
  hepatic - *see* Disease, liver
  hepatolenticular 275.1
  heredodegenerative NEC
    brain 331.89
    spinal cord 336.8
  Hers' (glycogenosis VI) 271.0
  Herter (-Gee) (-Heubner) (nontropical
    sprue) 579.0
  Herxheimer's (diffuse idiopathic
    cutaneous atrophy) 701.8
  Heubner's 094.89

Disease, diseased (Continued)

Heubner-Herter (nontropical sprue) 579.0

high fetal gene or hemoglobin thalassemia 282.49

Hildenbrand's (typhus) 081.9

hip (joint) NEC 719.95
  congenital 755.63
  suppurative 711.05
  tuberculous (see also Tuberculosis) 015.1● [730.85]

Hippel's (retinocerebral angiomatosis) 759.6

Hirschfeld's (acute diabetes mellitus) (see also Diabetes) 250.0●
  due to secondary diabetes 249.0●

Hirschsprung's (congenital megacolon) 751.3

His (-Werner) (trench fever) 083.1

HIV 042

Hodgkin's (M9650/3) 201.9●

> **Note:** Use the following fifth-digit subclassification with category 201:
> 0 unspecified site
> 1 lymph nodes of head, face, and neck
> 2 intrathoracic lymph nodes
> 3 intra-abdominal lymph nodes
> 4 lymph nodes of axilla and upper limb
> 5 lymph nodes of inguinal region and lower limb
> 6 intrapelvic lymph nodes
> 7 spleen
> 8 lymph nodes of multiple sites

  lymphocytic
    depletion (M9653/3) 201.7●
      diffuse fibrosis (M9654/3) 201.7●
      reticular type (M9655/3) 201.7●
      predominance (M9651/3) 201.4●
  lymphocytic-histiocytic predominance (M9651/3) 201.4●
  mixed cellularity (M9652/3) 201.6●
  nodular sclerosis (M9656/3) 201.5●
    cellular phase (M9657/3) 201.5●

Hodgson's 441.9
  ruptured 441.5

Hoffa (-Kastert) (liposynovitis prepatellaris) 272.8

Holla (see also Spherocytosis) 282.0

homozygous-Hb-S 282.61

hoof and mouth 078.4

hookworm (see also Ancylostomiasis) 126.9

Horton's (temporal arteritis) 446.5

host-versus-graft (immune or nonimmune cause) 279.50

HPFH (hereditary persistence of fetal hemoglobin) ("Swiss variety") 282.7

Huchard's (continued arterial hypertension) 401.9

Huguier's (uterine fibroma) 218.9

human immunodeficiency (virus) 042

hunger 251.1

Disease, diseased (Continued)

Hunt's
  dyssynergia cerebellaris myoclonica 334.2
  herpetic geniculate ganglionitis 053.11

Huntington's 333.4

Huppert's (multiple myeloma) (M9730/3) 203.0●

Hurler's (mucopolysaccharidosis I) 277.5

Hutchinson's, meaning
  angioma serpiginosum 709.1
  cheiropompholyx 705.81
  prurigo estivalis 692.72

Hutchinson-Boeck (sarcoidosis) 135

Hutchinson-Gilford (progeria) 259.8

hyaline (diffuse) (generalized) 728.9
  membrane (lung) (newborn) 769

hydatid (see also Echinococcus) 122.9

Hyde's (prurigo nodularis) 698.3

hyperkinetic (see also Hyperkinesia) 314.9
  heart 429.82

hypertensive (see also Hypertension) 401.9

hypophysis 253.9
  hyperfunction 253.1
  hypofunction 253.2

Iceland (epidemic neuromyasthenia) 049.8

I cell 272.7

ill-defined 799.89

immunologic NEC 279.9

immunoproliferative 203.8●

inclusion 078.5
  salivary gland 078.5

infancy, early NEC 779.9

infective NEC 136.9

inguinal gland 289.9

internal semilunar cartilage, cystic 717.5

intervertebral disc 722.90
  with myelopathy 722.70
  cervical, cervicothoracic 722.91
    with myelopathy 722.71
  lumbar, lumbosacral 722.93
    with myelopathy 722.73
  thoracic, thoracolumbar 722.92
    with myelopathy 722.72

intestine 569.9
  functional 564.9
    congenital 751.3
    psychogenic 306.4
  lardaceous 277.39
  organic 569.9
  protozoal NEC 007.9

iris 364.9
  specified NEC 364.89

iron
  metabolism (see also Hemochromatosis) 275.03 ◀
  storage (see also Hemochromatosis) 275.03 ◀

Isambert's (see also Tuberculosis, larynx) 012.3●

Iselin's (osteochondrosis, fifth metatarsal) 732.5

island (scrub typhus) 081.2

itai-itai 985.5

Jadassohn's (maculopapular erythroderma) 696.2

Jadassohn-Pellizari's (anetoderma) 701.3

Disease, diseased (Continued)

Jakob-Creutzfeldt (CJD) 046.19
  with dementia
    with behavioral disturbance 046.19 [294.11]
    without behavioral disturbance 046.19 [294.10]
  familial 046.19
  iatrogenic 046.19
  specified NEC 046.19
  sporadic 046.19
  variant (vCJD) 046.11
    with dementia
      with behavioral disturbance 046.11 [294.11]
      without behavioral disturbance 046.11 [294.10]

Jaksch (-Luzet) (pseudoleukemia infantum) 285.8

Janet's 300.89

Jansky-Bielschowsky 330.1

jaw NEC 526.9
  fibrocystic 526.2

Jensen's 363.05

Jeune's (asphyxiating thoracic dystrophy) 756.4

Jigger 134.1

Johnson-Stevens (erythema multiforme exudativum) 695.13

joint NEC 719.9●
  ankle 719.97
  Charcôt 094.0 [713.5]
  degenerative (see also Osteoarthrosis) 715.9●
    multiple 715.09
    spine (see also Spondylosis) 721.90
  elbow 719.92
  foot 719.97
  hand 719.94
  hip 719.95
  hypertrophic (chronic) (degenerative) (see also Osteoarthrosis) 715.9●
    spine (see also Spondylosis) 721.90
  knee 719.96
  Luschka 721.90
  multiple sites 719.99
  pelvic region 719.95
  sacroiliac 724.6
  shoulder (region) 719.91
  specified site NEC 719.98
  spine NEC 724.9
    pseudarthrosis following fusion 733.82
    sacroiliac 724.6
  wrist 719.93

Jourdain's (acute gingivitis) 523.00

Jüngling's (sarcoidosis) 135

Kahler (-Bozzolo) (multiple myeloma) (M9730/3) 203.0●

Kalischer's 759.6

Kaposi's 757.33
  lichen ruber 697.8
    acuminatus 696.4
    moniliformis 697.8
  xeroderma pigmentosum 757.33

Kaschin-Beck (endemic polyarthritis) 716.00
  ankle 716.07
  arm 716.02
    lower (and wrist) 716.03
    upper (and elbow) 716.02
  foot (and ankle) 716.07

Disease, diseased *(Continued)*
  Kaschin-Beck *(Continued)*
    forearm (and wrist) 716.03
    hand 716.04
    leg 716.06
      lower 716.06
      upper 716.05
    multiple sites 716.09
    pelvic region (hip) (thigh) 716.05
    shoulder region 716.01
    specified site NEC 716.08
  Katayama 120.2
  Kawasaki 446.1
  Kedani (scrub typhus) 081.2
  kidney (functional) (pelvis) *(see also*
    Disease, renal) 593.9
    chronic 585.9
      requiring chronic dialysis 585.6
      stage
        I 585.1
        II (mild) 585.2
        III (moderate) 585.3
        IV (severe) 585.4
        V 585.5
    cystic (congenital) 753.10
      multiple 753.19
      single 753.11
      specified NEC 753.19
    fibrocystic (congenital) 753.19
    in gout 274.10
    polycystic (congenital) 753.12
      adult type (APKD) 753.13
      autosomal dominant 753.13
      autosomal recessive 753.14
      childhood type (CPKD) 753.14
      infantile type 753.14
  Kienböck's (carpal lunate) (wrist) 732.3
  Kimmelstiel (-Wilson) (intercapillary
    glomerulosclerosis) 250.4 ●
    [581.81]
    due to secondary diabetes 249.4 ●
    [581.81]
  Kinnier Wilson's (hepatolenticular
    degeneration) 275.1
  kissing 075
  Kleb's *(see also* Nephritis) 583.9
  Klinger's 446.4
  Klippel's 723.8
  Klippel-Feil (brevicollis) 756.16
  Knight's 911.1
  Köbner's (epidermolysis bullosa)
    757.39
  Koenig-Wichmann (pemphigus) 694.4
  Köhler's
    first (osteoarthrosis juvenilis) 732.5
    second (Freiberg's infraction,
      metatarsal head) 732.5
    patellar 732.4
    tarsal navicular (bone)
      (osteoarthrosis juvenilis) 732.5
  Köhler-Freiberg (infraction, metatarsal
    head) 732.5
  Köhler-Mouchet (osteoarthrosis
    juvenilis) 732.5
  Köhler-Pellegrini-Stieda (calcification,
    knee joint) 726.62
  Kok 759.89
  König's (osteochondritis dissecans)
    732.7
  Korsakoff's (nonalcoholic) 294.0
    alcoholic 291.1
  Kostmann's (infantile genetic
    agranulocytosis) 288.01
  Krabbe's 330.0

Disease, diseased *(Continued)*
  Kraepelin-Morel *(see also*
    Schizophrenia) 295.9 ●
  Kraft-Weber-Dimitri 759.6
  Kufs' 330.1
  Kugelberg-Welander 335.11
  Kuhnt-Junius 362.52
  Kümmell's (-Verneuil) (spondylitis)
    721.7
  Kundrat's (lymphosarcoma) 200.1 ●
  kuru 046.0
  Kussmaul (-Meier) (polyarteritis
    nodosa) 446.0
  Kyasanur Forest 065.2
  Kyrle's (hyperkeratosis follicularis in
    cutem penetrans) 701.1
  labia
    inflammatory 616.10
    noninflammatory 624.9
      specified NEC 624.8
  labyrinth, ear 386.8
  lacrimal system (apparatus) (passages)
    375.9
    gland 375.00
    specified NEC 375.89
  Lafora's 333.2
  Lagleyze-von Hippel (retinocerebral
    angiomatosis) 759.6
  Lancereaux-Mathieu (leptospiral
    jaundice) 100.0
  Landry's 357.0
  Lane's 569.89
  lardaceous (any site) 277.39
  Larrey-Weil (leptospiral jaundice)
    100.0
  Larsen (-Johansson) (juvenile
    osteopathia patellae) 732.4
  larynx 478.70
  Lasègue's (persecution mania) 297.9
  Leber's 377.16
  Lederer's (acquired infectious
    hemolytic anemia) 283.19
  Legg's (capital femoral
    osteochondrosis) 732.1
  Legg-Calvé-Perthes (capital femoral
    osteochondrosis) 732.1
  Legg-Calvé-Waldenström (femoral
    capital osteochondrosis) 732.1
  Legg-Perthes (femoral capital
    osteochrondosis) 732.1
  Legionnaires' 482.84
  Leigh's 330.8
  Leiner's (exfoliative dermatitis)
    695.89
  Leloir's (lupus erythematosus) 695.4
  Lenegre's 426.0
  lens (eye) 379.39
  Leriche's (osteoporosis, posttraumatic)
    733.7
  Letterer-Siwe (acute histiocytosis X)
    (M9722/3) 202.5 ●
  Lev's (acquired complete heart block)
    426.0
  Lewandowski's *(see also* Tuberculosis)
    017.0 ●
  Lewandowski-Lutz
    (epidermodysplasia
    verruciformis) 078.19
  Lewy body 331.82
    with dementia
      with behavioral disturbance
        331.82 *[294.11]*
      without behavioral disturbance
        331.82 *[294.10]*

Disease, diseased *(Continued)*
  Leyden's (periodic vomiting) 536.2
  Libman-Sacks (verrucous endocarditis)
    710.0 *[424.91]*
  Lichtheim's (subacute combined
    sclerosis with pernicious anemia)
    281.0 *[336.2]*
  ligament 728.9
  light chain 203.0 ●
  Lightwood's (renal tubular acidosis)
    588.89
  Lignac's (cystinosis) 270.0
  Lindau's (retinocerebral angiomatosis)
    759.6
  Lindau-von Hippel (angiomatosis
    retinocerebellosa) 759.6
  lip NEC 528.5
  lipidosis 272.7
  lipoid storage NEC 272.7
  Lipschütz's 616.50
  Little's - *see* Palsy, cerebral
  liver 573.9
    alcoholic 571.3
      acute 571.1
      chronic 571.3
    chronic 571.9
      alcoholic 571.3
    cystic, congenital 751.62
    drug-induced 573.3
    due to
      chemicals 573.3
      fluorinated agents 573.3
      hypersensitivity drugs 573.3
      isoniazids 573.3
    end stage NEC 572.8
      due to hepatitis - *see* Hepatitis
    fibrocystic (congenital) 751.62
    glycogen storage 271.0
    organic 573.9
    polycystic (congenital) 751.62
  Lobo's (keloid blastomycosis) 116.2
  Lobstein's (brittle bones and blue
    sclera) 756.51
  locomotor system 334.9
  Lorain's (pituitary dwarfism) 253.3
  Lou Gehrig's 335.20
  Lucas-Championnière (fibrinous
    bronchitis) 466.0
  Ludwig's (submaxillary cellulitis)
    528.3
  luetic - *see* Syphilis
  lumbosacral region 724.6
  lung NEC 518.89
    black 500
    congenital 748.60
    cystic 518.89
      congenital 748.4
    fibroid (chronic) *(see also* Fibrosis,
      lung) 515
    fluke 121.2
      oriental 121.2
    in
      amyloidosis 277.39 *[517.8]*
      polymyositis 710.4 *[517.8]*
      sarcoidosis 135 *[517.8]*
      Sjögren's syndrome 710.2
        [517.8]
      syphilis 095.1
      systemic lupus erythematosus
        710.0 *[517.8]*
      systemic sclerosis 710.1 *[517.2]*
    interstitial (chronic) 515
      acute 136.3
    nonspecific, chronic 496

Disease, diseased *(Continued)*
  lung NEC *(Continued)*
    obstructive (chronic) (COPD) 496
      with
        acute
          bronchitis 491.22
          exacerbation NEC 491.21
        alveolitis, allergic *(see also*
          Alveolitis, allergic) 495.9
        asthma (chronic) (obstructive)
          493.2●
        bronchiectasis 494.0
          with acute exacerbation
            494.1
        bronchitis (chronic) 491.20
          with
            acute bronchitis 491.22
            exacerbation (acute)
              491.21
        decompensated 491.21
          with exacerbation 491.21
        emphysema NEC 492.8
      diffuse (with fibrosis) 496
    polycystic 518.89
      asthma (chronic) (obstructive)
        493.2●
      congenital 748.4
    purulent (cavitary) 513.0
    restrictive 518.89
    rheumatoid 714.81
      diffuse interstitial 714.81
    specified NEC 518.89
  Lutembacher's (atrial septal defect
    with mitral stenosis) 745.5
  Lutz-Miescher (elastosis perforans
    serpiginosa) 701.1
  Lutz-Splendore-de Almeida (Brazilian
    blastomycosis) 116.1
  Lyell's (toxic epidermal necrolysis)
    695.15
    due to drug
      correct substance properly
        administered 695.15
      overdose or wrong substance
        given or taken 977.9
      specific drug - *see* Table of
        Drugs and Chemicals
  Lyme 088.81
  lymphatic (gland) (system) 289.9
    channel (noninfective) 457.9
    vessel (noninfective) 457.9
      specified NEC 457.8
  lymphoproliferative (chronic)
    (M9970/1) 238.79
  Machado-Joseph 334.8
  Madelung's (lipomatosis) 272.8
  Madura (actinomycotic) 039.9
    mycotic 117.4
  Magitot's 526.4
  Majocchi's (purpura annularis
    telangiectodes) 709.1
  malarial *(see also* Malaria) 084.6
  Malassez's (cystic) 608.89
  Malibu 919.8
    infected 919.9
  malignant (M8000/3) - *see also*
    Neoplasm, by site, malignant
    previous, affecting management of
      pregnancy V23.89
  Manson's 120.1
  maple bark 495.6
  maple syrup (urine) 270.3
  Marburg (virus) 078.89
  Marchiafava (-Bignami) 341.8

Disease, diseased *(Continued)*
  Marfan's 090.49
    congenital syphilis 090.49
    meaning Marfan's syndrome 759.82
  Marie-Bamberger (hypertrophic
    pulmonary osteoarthropathy)
    (secondary) 731.2
    primary or idiopathic
      (acropachyderma) 757.39
    pulmonary (hypertrophic
      osteoarthropathy) 731.2
  Marie-Strümpell (ankylosing
    spondylitis) 720.0
  Marion's (bladder neck obstruction) 596.0
  Marsh's (exophthalmic goiter) 242.0●
  Martin's 715.27
  mast cell 757.33
    systemic (M9741/3) 202.6●
  mastoid *(see also* Mastoiditis) 383.9
    process 385.9
  maternal, unrelated to pregnancy NEC,
    affecting fetus or newborn 760.9
  Mathieu's (leptospiral jaundice) 100.0
  Mauclaire's 732.3
  Mauriac's (erythema nodosum
    syphiliticum) 091.3
  Maxcy's 081.0
  McArdle (-Schmid-Pearson)
    (glycogenosis V) 271.0
  mediastinum NEC 519.3
  Medin's *(see also* Poliomyelitis) 045.9●
  Mediterranean (with
    hemoglobinopathy) 282.49
  medullary center (idiopathic)
    (respiratory) 348.89
  Meige's (chronic hereditary edema)
    757.0
  Meleda 757.39
  Ménétrier's (hypertrophic gastritis)
    535.2●
  Ménière's (active) 386.00
    cochlear 386.02
    cochleovestibular 386.01
    inactive 386.04
    in remission 386.04
    vestibular 386.03
  meningeal - *see* Meningitis
  mental *(see also* Psychosis) 298.9
  Merzbacher-Pelizaeus 330.0
  mesenchymal 710.9
  mesenteric embolic 557.0
  metabolic NEC 277.9
  metal polishers' 502
  metastatic - *see* Metastasis
  Mibelli's 757.39
  microdrepanocytic 282.49
  microvascular - *code to* condition
  microvillus inclusion (MVD) 751.5 ◀
  Miescher's 709.3
  Mikulicz's (dryness of mouth, absent
    or decreased lacrimation) 527.1
  Milkman (-Looser) (osteomalacia with
    pseudofractures) 268.2
  Miller's (osteomalacia) 268.2
  Mills' 335.29
  Milroy's (chronic hereditary edema)
    757.0
  Minamata 985.0
  Minor's 336.1
  Minot's (hemorrhagic disease,
    newborn) 776.0
  Minot-von Willebrand-Jürgens
    (angiohemophilia) 286.4
  Mitchell's (erythromelalgia) 443.82

Disease, diseased *(Continued)*
  mitral - *see* Endocarditis, mitral
  Mljet (mal de Meleda) 757.39
  Möbius', Moebius' 346.2●
  Möeller's 267
  Möller (-Barlow) (infantile scurvy)
    267
  Mönckeberg's *(see also* Arteriosclerosis,
    extremities) 440.20
  Mondor's (thrombophlebitis of breast)
    451.89
  Monge's 993.2
  Morel-Kraepelin *(see also*
    Schizophrenia) 295.9●
  Morgagni's (syndrome) (hyperostosis
    frontalis interna) 733.3
  Morgagni-Adams-Stokes (syncope
    with heart block) 426.9
  Morquio (-Brailsford) (-Ullrich)
    (mucopolysaccharidosis IV) 277.5
  Morton's (with metatarsalgia) 355.6
  Morvan's 336.0
  motor neuron (bulbar) (mixed type)
    335.20
  Mouchet's (juvenile osteochondrosis,
    foot) 732.5
  mouth 528.9
  Moyamoya 437.5
  Mucha's (acute parapsoriasis
    varioliformis) 696.2
  mu-chain 273.2
  mucolipidosis (I) (II) (III) 272.7
  Münchmeyer's (exostosis luxurians)
    728.11
  Murri's (intermittent hemoglobinuria)
    283.2
  muscle 359.9
    inflammatory 728.9
    ocular 378.9
  musculoskeletal system 729.90
  mushroom workers' 495.5
  Myà's (congenital dilation, colon) 751.3
  mycotic 117.9
  myeloproliferative (chronic) (M9960/1)
    238.79
  myocardium, myocardial *(see also*
    Degeneration, myocardial) 429.1
    hypertensive *(see also* Hypertension,
      heart) 402.90
    primary (idiopathic) 425.4
  myoneural 358.9
  Naegeli's 287.1
  nail 703.9
    specified type NEC 703.8
  Nairobi sheep 066.1
  nasal 478.19
    cavity NEC 478.19
    sinus (chronic) - *see* Sinusitis
  navel (newborn) NEC 779.89
    delayed separation of umbilical cord
      779.83
  nemaline body 359.0
  neoplastic, generalized (M8000/6)
    199.0
  nerve - *see* Disorder, nerve
  nervous system (central) 349.9
    autonomic, peripheral *(see also*
      Neuropathy, peripheral,
      autonomic) 337.9
    congenital 742.9
    inflammatory - *see* Encephalitis
    parasympathetic *(see also*
      Neuropathy, peripheral,
      autonomic) 337.9

◀ New   ◀▥ Revised   ~~deleted~~ Deleted   ● Use Additional Digit(s)   ▨ Omit code

Disease, diseased *(Continued)*
  nervous system *(Continued)*
    peripheral NEC 355.9
    prion NEC 046.79
    specified NEC 349.89
    sympathetic *(see also* Neuropathy,
        peripheral, autonomic) 337.9
    vegetative *(see also* Neuropathy,
        peripheral, autonomic) 337.9
  Nettleship's (urticaria pigmentosa)
      757.33
  Neumann's (pemphigus vegetans)
      694.4
  neurologic (central) NEC *(see also*
      Disease, nervous system) 349.9
    peripheral NEC 355.9
  neuromuscular system NEC 358.9
  Newcastle 077.8
  Nicolas (-Durand) -Favre (climatic
      bubo) 099.1
  Niemann-Pick (lipid histiocytosis)
      272.7
  nipple 611.9
    Paget's (M8540/3) 174.0
  Nishimoto (-Takeuchi) 437.5
  nonarthropod-borne NEC 078.89
    central nervous system NEC 049.9
    enterovirus NEC 078.89
  nonautoimmune hemolytic NEC 283.10
  Nonne-Milroy-Meige (chronic
      hereditary edema) 757.0
  Norrie's (congenital progressive
      oculoacousticocerebral
      degeneration) 743.8
  nose 478.19
  nucleus pulposus - *see* Disease,
      intervertebral disc
  nutritional 269.9
    maternal, affecting fetus or newborn
        760.4
  oasthouse, urine 270.2
  obliterative vascular 447.1
  Odelberg's (juvenile osteochondrosis)
      732.1
  Oguchi's (retina) 368.61
  Ohara's *(see also* Tularemia) 021.9
  Ollier's (chondrodysplasia) 756.4
  Opitz's (congestive splenomegaly)
      289.51
  Oppenheim's 358.8
  Oppenheim-Urbach (necrobiosis
      lipoidica diabeticorum) 250.8●
      [709.3]
    due to secondary diabetes 249.8●
        [709.3]
  optic nerve NEC 377.49
  orbit 376.9
    specified NEC 376.89
  Oriental liver fluke 121.1
  Oriental lung fluke 121.2
  Ormond's 593.4
  Osgood's tibia (tubercle) 732.4
  Osgood-Schlatter 732.4
  Osler (-Vaquez) (polycythemia vera)
      (M9950/1) 238.4
  Osler-Rendu (familial hemorrhagic
      telangiectasia) 448.0
  osteofibrocystic 252.01
  Otto's 715.35
  outer ear 380.9
  ovary (noninflammatory) NEC 620.9
    cystic 620.2
    polycystic 256.4
    specified NEC 620.8

Disease, diseased *(Continued)*
  Owren's (congenital) *(see also* Defect,
      coagulation) 286.3
  Paas' 756.59
  Paget's (osteitis deformans) 731.0
    with infiltrating duct carcinoma of
        the breast (M8541/3) - *see*
        Neoplasm, breast, malignant
    bone 731.0
      osteosarcoma in (M9184/3) - *see*
          Neoplasm, bone, malignant
    breast (M8540/3) 174.0
    extramammary (M8542/3) - *see also*
        Neoplasm, skin, malignant
      anus 154.3
      skin 173.5
    malignant (M8540/3)
      breast 174.0
      specified site NEC (M8542/3) -
          see Neoplasm, skin,
          malignant
      unspecified site 174.0
    mammary (M8540/3) 174.0
    nipple (M8540/3) 174.0
  palate (soft) 528.9
  Paltauf-Sternberg 201.9●
  pancreas 577.9
    cystic 577.2
      congenital 751.7
    fibrocystic 277.00
  Panner's 732.3
    capitellum humeri 732.3
    head of humerus 732.3
    tarsal navicular (bone)
        (osteochondrosis) 732.5
  panvalvular - *see* Endocarditis, mitral
  parametrium 629.9
  parasitic NEC 136.9
    cerebral NEC 123.9
    intestinal NEC 129
    mouth 112.0
    skin NEC 134.9
    specified type - *see* Infestation
    tongue 112.0
  parathyroid (gland) 252.9
    specified NEC 252.8
  Parkinson's 332.0
  parodontal 523.9
  Parrot's (syphilitic osteochondritis)
      090.0
  Parry's (exophthalmic goiter) 242.0●
  Parson's (exophthalmic goiter)
      242.0●
  Pavy's 593.6
  Paxton's (white piedra) 111.2
  Payr's (splenic flexure syndrome)
      569.89
  pearl-workers' (chronic osteomyelitis)
      (see also Osteomyelitis) 730.1●
  Pel-Ebstein - *see* Disease, Hodgkin's
  Pelizaeus-Merzbacher 330.0
    with dementia
      with behavioral disturbance 330.0
          [294.11]
      without behavioral disturbance
          330.0 *[294.10]*
  Pellegrini-Stieda (calcification, knee
      joint) 726.62
  pelvis, pelvic
    female NEC 629.9
      specified NEC 629.89
    gonococcal (acute) 098.19
      chronic or duration of 2 months
          or over 098.39

Disease, diseased *(Continued)*
  pelvis, pelvic *(Continued)*
    infection *(see also* Disease, pelvis,
        inflammatory) 614.9
    inflammatory (female) (PID) 614.9
      with
        abortion - *see* Abortion, by
            type, with sepsis
        ectopic pregnancy *(see also*
            categories 633.0–633.9)
            639.0
        molar pregnancy *(see also*
            categories 630–632) 639.0
      acute 614.3
      chronic 614.4
      complicating pregnancy 646.6●
        affecting fetus or newborn
            760.8
      following
        abortion 639.0
        ectopic or molar pregnancy
            639.0
      peritonitis (acute) 614.5
        chronic NEC 614.7
      puerperal, postpartum, childbirth
          670.8●
      specified NEC 614.8
    organ, female NEC 629.9
      specified NEC 629.89
    peritoneum, female NEC 629.9
      specified NEC 629.89
  penis 607.9
    inflammatory 607.2
  peptic NEC 536.9
    acid 536.8
  periapical tissues NEC 522.9
  pericardium 423.9
    specified type NEC 423.8
  perineum
    female
      inflammatory 616.9
        specified NEC 616.89
      noninflammatory 624.9
        specified NEC 624.8
    male (inflammatory) 682.2
  periodic (familial) (Reimann's) NEC
      277.31
    paralysis 359.3
  periodontal NEC 523.9
    specified NEC 523.8
  periosteum 733.90
  peripheral
    arterial 443.9
    autonomic nervous system *(see also*
        Neuropathy, autonomic) 337.9
    nerve NEC *(see also* Neuropathy)
        356.9
      multiple - *see* Polyneuropathy
    vascular 443.9
      specified type NEC 443.89
  peritoneum 568.9
    pelvic, female 629.9
      specified NEC 629.89
  Perrin-Ferraton (snapping hip) 719.65
  persistent mucosal (middle ear) (with
      posterior or superior marginal
      perforation of ear drum) 382.2
  Perthes' (capital femoral
      osteochondrosis) 732.1
  Petit's *(see also* Hernia, lumbar) 553.8
  Peutz-Jeghers 759.6
  Peyronie's 607.85
  Pfeiffer's (infectious mononucleosis)
      075

Disease, diseased (Continued)
  pharynx 478.20
  Phocas' 610.1
  photochromogenic (acid-fast bacilli)
    (pulmonary) 031.0
    nonpulmonary 031.9
  Pick's
    brain 331.11
      with dementia
        with behavioral disturbance
          331.11 [294.11]
        without behavioral
          disturbance 331.11
          [294.10]
    cerebral atrophy 331.11
      with dementia
        with behavioral disturbance
          331.11 [294.11]
        without behavioral
          disturbance 331.11
          [294.10]
    lipid histiocytosis 272.7
    liver (pericardial pseudocirrhosis of
      liver) 423.2
    pericardium (pericardial
      pseudocirrhosis of liver) 423.2
    polyserositis (pericardial
      pseudocirrhosis of liver)
      423.2
  Pierson's (osteochondrosis) 732.1
  pigeon fanciers' or breeders' 495.2
  pineal gland 259.8
  pink 985.0
  Pinkus' (lichen nitidus) 697.1
  pinworm 127.4
  pituitary (gland) 253.9
    hyperfunction 253.1
    hypofunction 253.2
  pituitary snuff-takers' 495.8
  placenta
    affecting fetus or newborn 762.2
    complicating pregnancy or
      childbirth 656.7●
  pleura (cavity) (see also Pleurisy)
    511.0
  Plummer's (toxic nodular goiter)
    242.3●
  pneumatic
    drill 994.9
    hammer 994.9
  policeman's 729.2
  Pollitzer's (hidradenitis suppurativa)
    705.83
  polycystic (congenital) 759.89
    kidney or renal 753.12
      adult type (APKD) 753.13
      autosomal dominant 753.13
      autosomal recessive 753.14
      childhood type (CPKD) 753.14
      infantile type 753.14
    liver or hepatic 751.62
    lung or pulmonary 518.89
      congenital 748.4
    ovary, ovaries 256.4
    spleen 759.0
  Pompe's (glycogenosis II) 271.0
  Poncet's (tuberculous rheumatism) (see
    also Tuberculosis) 015.9●
  Posada-Wernicke 114.9
  Potain's (pulmonary edema) 514
  Pott's (see also Tuberculosis) 015.0 ●
    [730.88]
    osteomyelitis 015.0 ● [730.88]
    paraplegia 015.0 ● [730.88]

Disease, diseased (Continued)
  Pott's (Continued)
    spinal curvature 015.0● [737.43]
    spondylitis 015.0● [720.81]
  Potter's 753.0
  Poulet's 714.2
  pregnancy NEC (see also Pregnancy)
    646.9●
  Preiser's (osteoporosis) 733.09
  Pringle's (tuberous sclerosis) 759.5
  Profichet's 729.90
  prostate 602.9
    specified type NEC 602.8
  protozoal NEC 136.8
    intestine, intestinal NEC 007.9
  pseudo-Hurler's (mucolipidosis III)
    272.7
  psychiatric (see also Psychosis) 298.9
  psychotic (see also Psychosis) 298.9
  Puente's (simple glandular cheilitis)
    528.5
  puerperal NEC (see also Puerperal)
    674.9●
  pulmonary - see also Disease, lung
    amyloid 277.39 [517.8]
    artery 417.9
    circulation, circulatory 417.9
      specified NEC 417.8
    diffuse obstructive (chronic) 496
      with
        acute bronchitis 491.22
        asthma (chronic) (obstructive)
          493.2●
        exacerbation NEC (acute)
          491.21
    heart (chronic) 416.9
      specified NEC 416.8
    hypertensive (vascular) 416.0
      cardiovascular 416.0
    obstructive diffuse (chronic) 496
      with
        acute bronchitis 491.22
        asthma (chronic) (obstructive)
          493.2●
        bronchitis (chronic) 491.20
          with
            exacerbation (acute)
              491.21
            acute 491.22
        exacerbation NEC (acute)
          491.21
      decompensated 491.21
        with exacerbation 491.21
    valve (see also Endocarditis,
      pulmonary) 424.3
  pulp (dental) NEC 522.9
  pulseless 446.7
  Putnam's (subacute combined sclerosis
    with pernicious anemia) 281.0
    [336.2]
  Pyle (-Cohn) (craniometaphyseal
    dysplasia) 756.89
  pyramidal tract 333.90
  Quervain's
    tendon sheath 727.04
    thyroid (subacute granulomatous
      thyroiditis) 245.1
  Quincke's - see Edema,
    angioneurotic
  Quinquaud (acne decalvans)
    704.09
  rag sorters' 022.1
  Raynaud's (paroxysmal digital
    cyanosis) 443.0

Disease, diseased (Continued)
  reactive airway - see Asthma
  Recklinghausen's (M9540/1) 237.71
    bone (osteitis fibrosa cystica) 252.01
  Recklinghausen-Applebaum
    (hemochromatosis) (see also
    Hemochromatosis) 275.03 ◀▥
  Reclus' (cystic) 610.1
  rectum NEC 569.49
  Refsum's (heredopathia atactica
    polyneuritiformis) 356.3
  Reichmann's (gastrosuccorrhea) 536.8
  Reimann's (periodic) 277.31
  Reiter's 099.3
  renal (functional) (pelvis) (see also
    Disease, kidney) 593.9
    with
      edema (see also Nephrosis) 581.9
      exudative nephritis 583.89
      lesion of interstitial nephritis 583.89
      stated generalized cause - see
        Nephritis
    acute 593.9
    basement membrane NEC 583.89
      with
        pulmonary hemorrhage
          (Goodpasture's
          syndrome) 446.21
          [583.81]
    chronic (see also Disease, kidney,
      chronic) 585.9
    complicating pregnancy or
      puerperium NEC 646.2●
      with hypertension - see Toxemia,
        of pregnancy
      affecting fetus or newborn 760.1
    cystic, congenital (see also Cystic,
      disease, kidney) 753.10
    diabetic 250.4● [583.81]
      due to secondary diabetes 249.4●
        [581.81]
    due to
      amyloidosis 277.39 [583.81]
      diabetes mellitus 250.4 ●
        [583.81]
        due to secondary diabetes
          249.4 ● [581.81]
      systemic lupus erythematosis
        710.0 [583.81]
    end-stage 585.6
    exudative 583.89
    fibrocystic (congenital) 753.19
    gonococcal 098.19 [583.81]
    gouty 274.10
    hypertensive (see also Hypertension,
      kidney) 403.90
    immune complex NEC 583.89
    interstitial (diffuse) (focal) 583.89
    lupus 710.0 [583.81]
    maternal, affecting fetus or newborn
      760.1
      hypertensive 760.0
    phosphate-losing (tubular) 588.0
    polycystic (congenital) 753.12
      adult type (APKD) 753.13
      autosomal dominant 753.13
      autosomal recessive 753.14
      childhood type (CPKD) 753.14
      infantile type 753.14
    specified lesion or cause NEC (see
      also Glomerulonephritis)
      583.89
    subacute 581.9
    syphilitic 095.4

◀ New   ◀▥ Revised   ~~deleted~~ Deleted   ● Use Additional Digit(s)   ▨ Omit code

Disease, diseased *(Continued)*
  renal *(Continued)*
    tuberculous *(see also* Tuberculosis)
      016.0● *[583.81]*
    tubular *(see also* Nephrosis, tubular)
      584.5
  Rendu-Osler-Weber (familial
      hemorrhagic telangiectasia) 448.0
  renovascular (arteriosclerotic) *(see also*
      Hypertension, kidney) 403.90
  respiratory (tract) 519.9
    acute or subacute (upper) NEC
      465.9
      due to fumes or vapors 506.3
      multiple sites NEC 465.8
      noninfectious 478.9
      streptococcal 034.0
    chronic 519.9
      arising in the perinatal period
        770.7
      due to fumes or vapors 506.4
    due to
      aspiration of liquids or solids
        508.9
      external agents NEC 508.9
        specified NEC 508.8
      fumes or vapors 506.9
        acute or subacute NEC 506.3
        chronic 506.4
    fetus or newborn NEC 770.9
    obstructive 496
    specified type NEC 519.8
    upper (acute) (infectious) NEC
      465.9
      multiple sites NEC 465.8
      noninfectious NEC 478.9
      streptococcal 034.0
  retina, retinal NEC 362.9
    Batten's or Batten-Mayou 330.1
      [362.71]
    degeneration 362.89
    vascular lesion 362.17
  rheumatic *(see also* Arthritis) 716.8●
    heart - *see* Disease, heart, rheumatic
  rheumatoid (heart) - *see* Arthritis,
      rheumatoid
  rickettsial NEC 083.9
    specified type NEC 083.8
  Riedel's (ligneous thyroiditis) 245.3
  Riga (-Fede) (cachectic aphthae) 529.0
  Riggs' (compound periodontitis)
      523.40
  Ritter's 695.81
  Rivalta's (cervicofacial actinomycosis)
      039.3
  Robles' (onchocerciasis) 125.3 *[360.13]*
  Roger's (congenital interventricular
      septal defect) 745.4
  Rokitansky's *(see also* Necrosis, liver)
      570
  Romberg's 349.89
  Rosenthal's (factor XI deficiency) 286.2
  Rossbach's (hyperchlorhydria) 536.8
    psychogenic 306.4
  Roth (-Bernhardt) 355.1
  Runeberg's (progressive pernicious
      anemia) 281.0
  Rust's (tuberculous spondylitis) *(see
      also* Tuberculosis) 015.0 ● *[720.81]*
  Rustitskii's (multiple myeloma)
      (M9730/3) 203.0●
  Ruysch's (Hirschsprung's disease) 751.3
  Sachs (-Tay) 330.1
  sacroiliac NEC 724.6

Disease, diseased *(Continued)*
  salivary gland or duct NEC 527.9
    inclusion 078.5
      streptococcal 034.0
    virus 078.5
  Sander's (paranoia) 297.1
  Sandhoff's 330.1
  sandworm 126.9
  Savill's (epidemic exfoliative
      dermatitis) 695.89
  Schamberg's (progressive pigmentary
      dermatosis) 709.09
  Schaumann's (sarcoidosis) 135
  Schenck's (sporotrichosis) 117.1
  Scheuermann's (osteochondrosis) 732.0
  Schilder (-Flatau) 341.1
  Schimmelbusch's 610.1
  Schlatter's tibia (tubercle) 732.4
  Schlatter-Osgood 732.4
  Schmorl's 722.30
    cervical 722.39
    lumbar, lumbosacral 722.32
    specified region NEC 722.39
    thoracic, thoracolumbar 722.31
  Scholz's 330.0
  Schönlein (-Henoch) (purpura
      rheumatica) 287.0
  Schottmüller's *(see also* Fever,
      paratyphoid) 002.9
  Schüller-Christian (chronic
      histiocytosis X) 277.89
  Schultz's (agranulocytosis) 288.09
  Schwalbe-Ziehen-Oppenheimer 333.6
  Schwartz-Jampel 359.23
  Schweninger-Buzzi (macular atrophy)
      701.3
  sclera 379.19
  scrofulous *(see also* Tuberculosis)
      017.2●
  scrotum 608.9
  sebaceous glands NEC 706.9
  Secretan's (posttraumatic edema) 782.3
  semilunar cartilage, cystic 717.5
  seminal vesicle 608.9
  Senear-Usher (pemphigus
      erythematosus) 694.4
  serum NEC 999.5
  Sever's (osteochondrosis calcaneum)
      732.5
  sexually transmitted - *see* Disease,
      venereal
  Sézary's (reticulosis) (M9701/3)
      202.2●
  Shaver's (bauxite pneumoconiosis)
      503
  Sheehan's (postpartum pituitary
      necrosis) 253.2
  shimamushi (scrub typhus) 081.2
  shipyard 077.1
  sickle-cell 282.60
    with
      crisis 282.62
      Hb-S disease 282.61
      other abnormal hemoglobin
        (Hb-D) (Hb-E) (Hb-G)
        (Hb-J) (Hb-K) (Hb-O)
        (Hb-P) (high fetal gene)
        (without crisis) 282.68
        with crisis 282.69
    elliptocytosis 282.60
    Hb-C (without crisis) 282.63
      with
        crisis 282.64
        vaso-occlusive pain 282.64

Disease, diseased *(Continued)*
  sickle-cell *(Continued)*
    Hb-S 282.61
      with
        crisis 282.62
        Hb-C (without crisis) 282.63
          with
            crisis 282.64
            vaso-occlusive pain
              282.64
        other abnormal hemoglobin
          (Hb-D) (Hb-E) (Hb-G)
          (Hb-J) (Hb-K) (Hb-O)
          (Hb-P) (high fetal gene)
          (without crisis) 282.68
          with crisis 282.69
    spherocytosis 282.60
    thalassemia (without crisis) 282.41
      with
        crisis 282.42
        vaso-occlusive pain 282.42
  Siegal-Cattan-Mamou (periodic) 277.31
  silo fillers' 506.9
  Simian B 054.3
  Simmonds' (pituitary cachexia) 253.2
  Simons' (progressive lipodystrophy)
      272.6
  Sinding-Larsen (juvenile osteopathia
      patellae) 732.4
  sinus - *see also* Sinusitis
    brain 437.9
    specified NEC 478.19
  Sirkari's 085.0
  sixth *(see also* Exanthem subitum)
      058.10
  Sjögren (-Gougerot) 710.2
    with lung involvement 710.2 *[517.8]*
  Skevas-Zerfus 989.5
  skin NEC 709.9
    due to metabolic disorder 277.9
    specified type NEC 709.8
  sleeping *(see also* Narcolepsy) 347.00
    meaning sleeping sickness *(see also*
        Trypanosomiasis) 086.5
  small vessel 443.9
  Smith-Strang (oasthouse urine) 270.2
  Sneddon-Wilkinson (subcorneal
      pustular dermatosis) 694.1
  South African creeping 133.8
  Spencer's (epidemic vomiting) 078.82
  Spielmeyer-Stock 330.1
  Spielmeyer-Vogt 330.1
  spine, spinal 733.90
    combined system *(see also*
        Degeneration, combined) 266.2
        [336.2]
      with pernicious anemia 281.0
          [336.2]
    cord NEC 336.9
      congenital 742.9
    demyelinating NEC 341.8
    joint *(see also* Disease, joint, spine)
        724.9
    tuberculous 015.0● *[730.8]*●
  spinocerebellar 334.9
    specified NEC 334.8
  spleen (organic) (postinfectional)
      289.50
    amyloid 277.39
    lardaceous 277.39
    polycystic 759.0
    specified NEC 289.59
  sponge divers' 989.5
  Stanton's (melioidosis) 025

Disease, diseased *(Continued)*
  Stargardt's 362.75
  Startle 759.89
  Steinert's 359.21
  Sternberg's - *see* Disease, Hodgkin's
  Stevens-Johnson (erythema multiforme
      exudativum) 695.13
  Sticker's (erythema infectiosum) 057.0
  Stieda's (calcification, knee joint) 726.62
  Still's (juvenile rheumatoid arthritis)
      714.30
    adult onset 714.2
  Stiller's (asthenia) 780.79
  Stokes' (exophthalmic goiter) 242.0●
  Stokes-Adams (syncope with heart
      block) 426.9
  Stokvis (-Talma) (enterogenous
      cyanosis) 289.7
  stomach NEC (organic) 537.9
    functional 536.9
      psychogenic 306.4
    lardaceous 277.39
  stonemasons' 502
  storage
    glycogen (*see also* Disease, glycogen
        storage) 271.0
    lipid 272.7
    mucopolysaccharide 277.5
  striatopallidal system 333.90
    specified NEC 333.89
  Strümpell-Marie (ankylosing
      spondylitis) 720.0
  Stuart's (congenital factor X deficiency)
      (*see also* Defect, coagulation) 286.3
  Stuart-Prower (congenital factor X
      deficiency) (*see also* Defect,
      coagulation) 286.3
  Sturge (-Weber) (-Dimitri)
      (encephalocutaneous
      angiomatosis) 759.6
  Stuttgart 100.89
  Sudeck's 733.7
  supporting structures of teeth NEC
      525.9
  suprarenal (gland) (capsule) 255.9
    hyperfunction 255.3
    hypofunction 255.41
  Sutton's 709.09
  Sutton and Gull's - *see* Hypertension,
      kidney
  sweat glands NEC 705.9
    specified type NEC 705.89
  sweating 078.2
  Sweeley-Klionsky 272.4
  Swift (-Feer) 985.0
  swimming pool (bacillus) 031.1
  swineherd's 100.89
  Sylvest's (epidemic pleurodynia) 074.1
  Symmers (follicular lymphoma)
      (M9690/3) 202.0●
  sympathetic nervous system (*see also*
      Neuropathy, peripheral,
      autonomic) 337.9
  synovium 727.9
  syphilitic - *see* Syphilis
  systemic tissue mast cell (M9741/3)
      202.6●
  Taenzer's 757.4
  Takayasu's (pulseless) 446.7
  Talma's 728.85
  Tangier (familial high-density
      lipoprotein deficiency) 272.5
  Tarral-Besnier (pityriasis rubra pilaris)
      696.4

Disease, diseased *(Continued)*
  Tay-Sachs 330.1
  Taylor's 701.8
  tear duct 375.69
  teeth, tooth 525.9
    hard tissues 521.9
      specified NEC 521.89
    pulp NEC 522.9
  tendon 727.9
    inflammatory NEC 727.9
  terminal vessel 443.9
  testis 608.9
  Thaysen-Gee (nontropical sprue) 579.0
  Thomsen's 359.22
  Thomson's (congenital poikiloderma)
      757.33
  Thornwaldt's, Tornwaldt's (pharyngeal
      bursitis) 478.29
  throat 478.20
    septic 034.0
  thromboembolic (*see also* Embolism)
      444.9
  thymus (gland) 254.9
    specified NEC 254.8
  thyroid (gland) NEC 246.9
    heart (*see also* Hyperthyroidism)
        242.9 ● [*425.7*]
    lardaceous 277.39
    specified NEC 246.8
  Tietze's 733.6
  Tommaselli's
    correct substance properly
        administered 599.70
    overdose or wrong substance given
        or taken 961.4
  tongue 529.9
  tonsils, tonsillar (and adenoids)
      (chronic) 474.9
    specified NEC 474.8
  tooth, teeth 525.9
    hard tissues 521.9
      specified NEC 521.89
    pulp NEC 522.9
  Tornwaldt's (pharyngeal bursitis)
      478.29
  Tourette's 307.23
  trachea 519.19
  tricuspid - *see* Endocarditis, tricuspid
  triglyceride-storage, type I, II, III
      272.7
  triple vessel - *see* Arteriosclerosis,
      coronary
  trisymptomatic, Gougerot's 709.1
  trophoblastic (*see also* Hydatidiform
      mole) 630
    previous, affecting management of
        pregnancy V23.1
  tsutsugamushi (scrub typhus) 081.2
  tube (fallopian), noninflammatory
      620.9
    specified NEC 620.8
  tuberculous NEC (*see also* Tuberculosis)
      011.9●
  tubo-ovarian
    inflammatory (*see also* Salpingo-
        oophoritis) 614.2
    noninflammatory 620.9
      specified NEC 620.8
  tubotympanic, chronic (with anterior
      perforation of ear drum) 382.1
  tympanum 385.9
  Uhl's 746.84
  umbilicus (newborn) NEC 779.89
    delayed separation 779.83

Disease, diseased *(Continued)*
  Underwood's (sclerema neonatorum)
      778.1
  undiagnosed 799.9
  Unna's (seborrheic dermatitis) 690.18
  unstable hemoglobin hemolytic
      282.7
  Unverricht (-Lundborg) 345.1●
  Urbach-Oppenheim (necrobiosis
      lipoidica diabeticorum) 250.8●
      [*709.3*]
    due to secondary diabetes 249.8●
      [*709.3*]
  Urbach-Wiethe (lipoid proteinosis)
      272.8
  ureter 593.9
  urethra 599.9
    specified type NEC 599.84
  urinary (tract) 599.9
    bladder 596.9
      specified NEC 596.8
    maternal, affecting fetus or newborn
        760.1
  Usher-Senear (pemphigus
      erythematosus) 694.4
  uterus (organic) 621.9
    infective (*see also* Endometritis) 615.9
    inflammatory (*see also* Endometritis)
        615.9
    noninflammatory 621.9
      specified type NEC 621.8
  uveal tract
    anterior 364.9
    posterior 363.9
  vagabonds' 132.1
  vagina, vaginal
    inflammatory 616.10
    noninflammatory 623.9
      specified NEC 623.8
  Valsuani's (progressive pernicious
      anemia, puerperal) 648.2●
    complicating pregnancy or
        puerperium 648.2●
  valve, valvular - *see also* Endocarditis
    congenital NEC (*see also* Anomaly,
        heart, valve) 746.9
      pulmonary 746.00
      specified type NEC 746.89
  van Bogaert-Nijssen (-Peiffer) 330.0
  van Creveld-von Gierke (glycogenosis
      I) 271.0
  van den Bergh's (enterogenous
      cyanosis) 289.7
  van Neck's (juvenile osteochondrosis)
      732.1
  Vaquez (-Osler) (polycythemia vera)
      (M9950/1) 238.4
  vascular 459.9
    arteriosclerotic - *see* Arteriosclerosis
    hypertensive - *see* Hypertension
    obliterative 447.1
      peripheral 443.9
    occlusive 459.9
    peripheral (occlusive) 443.9
      in (due to) (with) diabetes
          mellitus 250.7● [*443.81*]
      in (due to) (with) secondary
          diabetes 249.7●
          [*443.81*]
      specified type NEC 443.89
  vas deferens 608.9
  vasomotor 443.9
  vasospastic 443.9
  vein 459.9

◄ New   ◄▥ Revised   ~~deleted~~ Deleted   ● Use Additional Digit(s)   ▨ Omit code

Disease, diseased *(Continued)*
  venereal 099.9
    chlamydial NEC 099.50
      anus 099.52
      bladder 099.53
      cervix 099.53
      epididymis 099.54
      genitourinary NEC 099.55
        lower 099.53
        specified NEC 099.54
      pelvic inflammatory disease
        099.54
      perihepatic 099.56
      peritoneum 099.56
      pharynx 099.51
      rectum 099.52
      specified site NEC 099.59
      testis 099.54
      vagina 099.53
      vulva 099.53
    fifth 099.1
    sixth 099.1
    complicating pregnancy, childbirth,
      or puerperium 647.2●
    specified nature or type NEC
      099.8
      chlamydial - *see* Disease,
        venereal, chlamydial
  Verneuil's (syphilitic bursitis) 095.7
  Verse's (calcinosis intervertebralis)
    275.49 *[722.90]*
  vertebra, vertebral NEC 733.90
    disc - *see* Disease, Intervertebral disc
  vibration NEC 994.9
  Vidal's (lichen simplex chronicus) 698.3
  Vincent's (trench mouth) 101
  Virchow's 733.99
  virus (filterable) NEC 078.89
    arbovirus NEC 066.9
    arthropod-borne NEC 066.9
    central nervous system NEC
      049.9
      specified type NEC 049.8
    complicating pregnancy, childbirth,
      or puerperium 647.6●
    contact (with) V01.79
      varicella V01.71
    exposure to V01.79
      varicella V01.71
    Marburg 078.89
    maternal
      with fetal damage affecting
        management of pregnancy
        655.3●
    nonarthropod-borne NEC 078.89
      central nervous system NEC
        049.9
        specified NEC 049.8
    vaccination, prophylactic (against)
      V04.89
  vitreous 379.29
  vocal cords NEC 478.5
  Vogt's (Cecile) 333.71
  Vogt-Spielmeyer 330.1
  Volhard-Fahr (malignant
    nephrosclerosis) 403.00
  Volkmann's
    acquired 958.6
  von Bechterew's (ankylosing
    spondylitis) 720.0
  von Economo's (encephalitis
    lethargica) 049.8
  von Eulenburg's (congenital
    paramyotonia) 359.29

Disease, diseased *(Continued)*
  von Gierke's (glycogenosis I) 271.0
  von Graefe's 378.72
  von Hippel's (retinocerebral
    angiomatosis) 759.6
  von Hippel-Lindau (angiomatosis
    retinocerebellosa) 759.6
  von Jaksch's (pseudoleukemia
    infantum) 285.8
  von Recklinghausen's (M9540/1)
    237.71
    bone (osteitis fibrosa cystica) 252.01
  von Recklinghausen-Applebaum
    (hemochromatosis) *(see also*
      Hemochromatosis) 275.03 ←▥
  von Willebrand (-Jürgens)
    (angiohemophilia) 286.4
  von Zambusch's (lichen sclerosus et
    atrophicus) 701.0
  Voorhoeve's (dyschondroplasia) 756.4
  Vrolik's (osteogenesis imperfecta)
    756.51
  vulva
    inflammatory 616.10
    noninflammatory 624.9
      specified NEC 624.8
  Wagner's (colloid milium) 709.3
  Waldenström's (osteochondrosis
    capital femoral) 732.1
  Wallgren's (obstruction of splenic vein
    with collateral circulation) 459.89
  Wardrop's (with lymphangitis) 681.9
    finger 681.02
    toe 681.11
  Wassilieff's (leptospiral jaundice) 100.0
  wasting NEC 799.4
    due to malnutrition 261
    paralysis 335.21
  Waterhouse-Friderichsen 036.3
  waxy (any site) 277.39
  Weber-Christian (nodular
    nonsuppurative panniculitis)
    729.30
  Wegner's (syphilitic osteochondritis)
    090.0
  Weil's (leptospiral jaundice) 100.0
    of lung 100.0
  Weir Mitchell's (erythromelalgia)
    443.82
  Werdnig-Hoffmann 335.0
  Werlhof's *(see also* Purpura,
    thrombocytopenic) 287.39
  Wermer's 258.01
  Werner's (progeria adultorum) 259.8
  Werner-His (trench fever) 083.1
  Werner-Schultz (agranulocytosis) 288.09
  Wernicke's (superior hemorrhagic
    polioencephalitis) 265.1
  Wernicke-Posadas 114.9
  Whipple's (intestinal lipodystrophy)
    040.2
  whipworm 127.3
  white
    blood cell 288.9
      specified NEC 288.8
    spot 701.0
  White's (congenital) (keratosis
    follicularis) 757.39
  Whitmore's (melioidosis) 025
  Widal-Abrami (acquired hemolytic
    jaundice) 283.9
  Wilkie's 557.1
  Wilkinson-Sneddon (subcorneal
    pustular dermatosis) 694.1

Disease, diseased *(Continued)*
  Willis' (diabetes mellitus) *(see also*
    Diabetes) 250.0●
    due to secondary diabetes 249.0●
  Wilson's (hepatolenticular
    degeneration) 275.1
  Wilson-Brocq (dermatitis exfoliativa)
    695.89
  winter vomiting 078.82
  Wise's 696.2
  Wohlfart-Kugelberg-Welander 335.11
  Woillez's (acute idiopathic pulmonary
    congestion) 518.5
  Wolman's (primary familial
    xanthomatosis) 272.7
  wool-sorters' 022.1
  Zagari's (xerostomia) 527.7
  Zahorsky's (exanthem subitum) 058.10
  Ziehen-Oppenheim 333.6
  zoonotic, bacterial NEC 027.9
    specified type NEC 027.8
Disfigurement (due to scar) 709.2
  head V48.6
  limb V49.4
  neck V48.7
  trunk V48.7
Disgerminoma - *see* Dysgerminoma
Disinsertion, retina 361.04
Disintegration, complete, of the body
  799.89
  traumatic 869.1
Disk kidney 753.3
Dislocatable hip, congenital *(see also*
  Dislocation, hip, congenital) 754.30
Dislocation (articulation) (closed)
    (displacement) (simple) (subluxation)
    839.8

Note:

"Closed" includes simple, complete,
partial, uncomplicated, and
unspecified dislocation.

"Open" includes dislocation specified
as infected or compound and
dislocation with foreign body.

"Chronic," "habitual," "old," or
"recurrent" dislocations should be
coded as indicated under the entry
"Dislocation, recurrent"; and
"pathological" as indicated under the
entry "Dislocation, pathological."

For late effect of dislocation *see* Late,
effect, dislocation.

---

  with fracture - *see* Fracture, by site
  acromioclavicular (joint) (closed)
    831.04
    open 831.14
  anatomical site (closed)
    specified NEC 839.69
      open 839.79
    unspecified or ill-defined 839.8
      open 839.9
  ankle (scaphoid bone) (closed) 837.0
    open 837.1
  arm (closed) 839.8
    open 839.9
  astragalus (closed) 837.0
    open 837.1
  atlanto-axial (closed) 839.01
    open 839.11

Dislocation *(Continued)*
  atlas (closed) 839.01
    open 839.11
  axis (closed) 839.02
    open 839.12
  back (closed) 839.8
    open 839.9
  Bell-Daly 723.8
  breast bone (closed) 839.61
    open 839.71
  capsule, joint - *see* Dislocation, by site
  carpal (bone) - *see* Dislocation, wrist
  carpometacarpal (joint) (closed) 833.04
    open 833.14
  cartilage (joint) - *see also* Dislocation, by
      site
    knee - *see* Tear, meniscus
  cervical, cervicodorsal, or
      cervicothoracic (spine)
      (vertebra) - *see* Dislocation,
      vertebra, cervical
  chiropractic (*see also* Lesion,
      nonallopathic) 739.9
  chondrocostal - *see* Dislocation,
      costochondral
  chronic - *see* Dislocation, recurrent
  clavicle (closed) 831.04
    open 831.14
  coccyx (closed) 839.41
    open 839.51
  collar bone (closed) 831.04
    open 831.14
  compound (open) NEC 839.9
  congenital NEC 755.8
    hip (*see also* Dislocation, hip,
        congenital) 754.30
    lens 743.37
    rib 756.3
    sacroiliac 755.69
    spine NEC 756.19
    vertebra 756.19
  coracoid (closed) 831.09
    open 831.19
  costal cartilage (closed) 839.69
    open 839.79
  costochondral (closed) 839.69
    open 839.79
  cricoarytenoid articulation (closed)
      839.69
    open 839.79
  cricothyroid (cartilage) articulation
      (closed) 839.69
    open 839.79
  dorsal vertebra (closed) 839.21
    open 839.31
  ear ossicle 385.23
  elbow (closed) 832.00
    anterior (closed) 832.01
      open 832.11
    congenital 754.89
    divergent (closed) 832.09
      open 832.19
    lateral (closed) 832.04
      open 832.14
    medial (closed) 832.03
      open 832.13
    open 832.10
    posterior (closed) 832.02
      open 832.12
    recurrent 718.32
    specified type NEC 832.09
      open 832.19
  eye 360.81
    lateral 376.36

Dislocation *(Continued)*
  eyeball 360.81
    lateral 376.36
  femur
    distal end (closed) 836.50
      anterior 836.52
        open 836.62
      lateral 836.54
        open 836.64
      medial 836.53
        open 836.63
      open 836.60
      posterior 836.51
        open 836.61
    proximal end (closed) 835.00
      anterior (pubic) 835.03
        open 835.13
      obturator 835.02
        open 835.12
      open 835.10
      posterior 835.01
        open 835.11
  fibula
    distal end (closed) 837.0
      open 837.1
    proximal end (closed) 836.59
      open 836.69
  finger(s) (phalanx) (thumb) (closed)
      834.00
    interphalangeal (joint) 834.02
      open 834.12
    metacarpal (bone), distal end
        834.01
      open 834.11
    metacarpophalangeal (joint) 834.01
      open 834.11
    open 834.10
    recurrent 718.34
  foot (closed) 838.00
    open 838.10
    recurrent 718.37
  forearm (closed) 839.8
    open 839.9
  fracture - *see* Fracture, by site
  glenoid (closed) 831.09
    open 831.19
  habitual - *see* Dislocation, recurrent
  hand (closed) 839.8
    open 839.9
  hip (closed) 835.00
    anterior 835.03
      obturator 835.02
        open 835.12
      open 835.13
    congenital (unilateral) 754.30
      with subluxation of other hip
          754.35
      bilateral 754.31
    developmental 718.75
    open 835.10
    posterior 835.01
      open 835.11
    recurrent 718.35
  humerus (closed) 831.00
    distal end (*see also* Dislocation,
        elbow) 832.00
    open 831.10
    proximal end (closed) 831.00
      anterior (subclavicular)
          (subcoracoid) (subglenoid)
          (closed) 831.01
        open 831.11
      inferior (closed) 831.03
        open 831.13

Dislocation *(Continued)*
  humerus *(Continued)*
    proximal end *(Continued)*
      open 831.10
      posterior (closed) 831.02
        open 831.12
  implant - *see* Complications,
      mechanical
  incus 385.23
  infracoracoid (closed) 831.01
    open 831.11
  innominate (pubic junction) (sacral
      junction) (closed) 839.69
    acetabulum (*see also* Dislocation,
        hip) 835.00
    open 839.79
  interphalangeal (joint)
    finger or hand (closed) 834.02
      open 834.12
    foot or toe (closed) 838.06
      open 838.16
  jaw (cartilage) (meniscus) (closed)
      830.0
    open 830.1
    recurrent 524.69
  joint NEC (closed) 839.8
    developmental 718.7●
    open 839.9
    pathological - *see* Dislocation,
        pathological
    recurrent - *see* Dislocation,
        recurrent
  knee (closed) 836.50
    anterior 836.51
      open 836.61
    congenital (with genu recurvatum)
        754.41
    habitual 718.36
    lateral 836.54
      open 836.64
    medial 836.53
      open 836.63
    old 718.36
    open 836.60
    posterior 836.52
      open 836.62
    recurrent 718.36
    rotatory 836.59
      open 836.69
  lacrimal gland 375.16
  leg (closed) 839.8
    open 839.9
  lens (crystalline) (complete) (partial)
      379.32
    anterior 379.33
    congenital 743.37
    ocular implant 996.53
    posterior 379.34
    traumatic 921.3
  ligament - *see* Dislocation, by site
  lumbar (vertebrae) (closed) 839.20
    open 839.30
  lumbosacral (vertebrae) (closed)
      839.20
    congenital 756.19
    open 839.30
  mandible (closed) 830.0
    open 830.1
  maxilla (inferior) (closed) 830.0
    open 830.1
  meniscus (knee) - *see also* Tear,
      meniscus
    other sites - *see* Dislocation, by
        site

◄ New   ◄▥ Revised   ~~deleted~~ Deleted   ● Use Additional Digit(s)   ▨ Omit code

Dislocation *(Continued)*
  metacarpal (bone)
    distal end (closed) 834.01
      open 834.11
    proximal end (closed) 833.05
      open 833.15
  metacarpophalangeal (joint) (closed)
    834.01
    open 834.11
  metatarsal (bone) (closed) 838.04
    open 838.14
  metatarsophalangeal (joint) (closed)
    838.05
    open 838.15
  midcarpal (joint) (closed) 833.03
    open 833.13
  midtarsal (joint) (closed) 838.02
    open 838.12
  Monteggia's - *see* Dislocation, hip
  multiple locations (except fingers only
    or toes only) (closed) 839.8
    open 839.9
  navicular (bone) foot (closed) 837.0
    open 837.1
  neck (*see also* Dislocation, vertebra,
    cervical) 839.00
  Nélaton's - *see* Dislocation, ankle
  nontraumatic (joint) - *see* Dislocation,
    pathological
  nose (closed) 839.69
    open 839.79
  not recurrent, not current injury - *see*
    Dislocation, pathological
  occiput from atlas (closed) 839.01
    open 839.11
  old - *see* Dislocation, recurrent
  open (compound) NEC 839.9
  ossicle, ear 385.23
  paralytic (flaccid) (spastic) - *see*
    Dislocation, pathological
  patella (closed) 836.3
    congenital 755.64
    open 836.4
  pathological NEC 718.20
    ankle 718.27
    elbow 718.22
    foot 718.27
    hand 718.24
    hip 718.25
    knee 718.26
    lumbosacral joint 724.6
    multiple sites 718.29
    pelvic region 718.25
    sacroiliac 724.6
    shoulder (region) 718.21
    specified site NEC 718.28
    spine 724.8
      sacroiliac 724.6
    wrist 718.23
  pelvis (closed) 839.69
    acetabulum (*see also* Dislocation,
      hip) 835.00
    open 839.79
  phalanx
    foot or toe (closed) 838.09
      open 838.19
    hand or finger (*see also* Dislocation,
      finger) 834.00
  postpoliomyelitic - *see* Dislocation,
    pathological
  prosthesis, internal - *see* Complications,
    mechanical
  radiocarpal (joint) (closed) 833.02
    open 833.12

Dislocation *(Continued)*
  radioulnar (joint)
    distal end (closed) 833.01
      open 833.11
    proximal end (*see also* Dislocation,
      elbow) 832.00
  radius
    distal end (closed) 833.00
      open 833.10
    proximal end (closed) 832.01
      open 832.11
  recurrent (*see also* Derangement, joint,
    recurrent) 718.3●
    elbow 718.32
    hip 718.35
    joint NEC 718.38
    knee 718.36
    lumbosacral (joint) 724.6
    patella 718.36
    sacroiliac 724.6
    shoulder 718.31
    temporomandibular 524.69
  rib (cartilage) (closed) 839.69
    congenital 756.3
    open 839.79
  sacrococcygeal (closed) 839.42
    open 839.52
  sacroiliac (joint) (ligament) (closed)
    839.42
    congenital 755.69
    open 839.52
    recurrent 724.6
  sacrum (closed) 839.42
    open 839.52
  scaphoid (bone)
    ankle or foot (closed) 837.0
      open 837.1
    wrist (closed) (*see also* Dislocation,
      wrist) 833.00
      open 833.10
  scapula (closed) 831.09
    open 831.19
  semilunar cartilage, knee - *see* Tear,
    meniscus
  septal cartilage (nose) (closed) 839.69
    open 839.79
  septum (nasal) (old) 470
  sesamoid bone - *see* Dislocation, by site
  shoulder (blade) (ligament) (closed)
    831.00
    anterior (subclavicular) (subcoracoid)
      (subglenoid) (closed) 831.01
      open 831.11
    chronic 718.31
    inferior 831.03
      open 831.13
    open 831.10
    posterior (closed) 831.02
      open 831.12
    recurrent 718.31
  skull - *see* Injury, intracranial
  Smith's - *see* Dislocation, foot
  spine (articular process) (*see also*
    Dislocation, vertebra) (closed)
    839.40
    atlanto-axial (closed) 839.01
      open 839.11
      recurrent 723.8
    cervical, cervicodorsal,
      cervicothoracic (closed) (*see*
      also Dislocation, vertebrae,
      cervical) 839.00
      open 839.10
      recurrent 723.8

Dislocation *(Continued)*
  spine *(Continued)*
    coccyx 839.41
      open 839.51
    congenital 756.19
    due to birth trauma 767.4
    open 839.50
    recurrent 724.9
    sacroiliac 839.42
      recurrent 724.6
    sacrum (sacrococcygeal) (sacroiliac)
      839.42
      open 839.52
  spontaneous - *see* Dislocation,
    pathological
  sternoclavicular (joint) (closed)
    839.61
    open 839.71
  sternum (closed) 839.61
    open 839.71
  subastragalar - *see* Dislocation, foot
  subglenoid (closed) 831.01
    open 831.11
  symphysis
    jaw (closed) 830.0
      open 830.1
    mandibular (closed) 830.0
      open 830.1
    pubis (closed) 839.69
      open 839.79
  tarsal (bone) (joint) 838.01
    open 838.11
  tarsometatarsal (joint) 838.03
    open 838.13
  temporomandibular (joint) (closed)
    830.0
    open 830.1
    recurrent 524.69
  thigh
    distal end (*see also* Dislocation,
      femur, distal end) 836.50
    proximal end (*see also* Dislocation,
      hip) 835.00
  thoracic (vertebrae) (closed) 839.21
    open 839.31
  thumb(s) (*see also* Dislocation, finger)
    834.00
  thyroid cartilage (closed) 839.69
    open 839.79
  tibia
    distal end (closed) 837.0
      open 837.1
    proximal end (closed) 836.50
      anterior 836.51
        open 836.61
      lateral 836.54
        open 836.64
      medial 836.53
        open 836.63
      open 836.60
      posterior 836.52
        open 836.62
      rotatory 836.59
        open 836.69
  tibiofibular
    distal (closed) 837.0
      open 837.1
    superior (closed) 836.59
      open 836.69
  toe(s) (closed) 838.09
    open 838.19
  trachea (closed) 839.69
    open 839.79

◀ New   ◀⁞ Revised   ~~deleted~~ Deleted   ● Use Additional Digit(s)   ▨ Omit code

Dislocation *(Continued)*
  ulna
    distal end (closed) 833.09
      open 833.19
    proximal end - *see* Dislocation,
      elbow
    vertebra (articular process) (body)
      (closed) (traumatic) 839.40
      cervical, cervicodorsal or
        cervicothoracic (closed) 839.00
        first (atlas) 839.01
          open 839.11
        second (axis) 839.02
          open 839.12
        third 839.03
          open 839.13
        fourth 839.04
          open 839.14
        fifth 839.05
          open 839.15
        sixth 839.06
          open 839.16
        seventh 839.07
          open 839.17
        congenital 756.19
        multiple sites 839.08
          open 839.18
        open 839.10
      congenital 756.19
      dorsal 839.21
        open 839.31
        recurrent 724.9
      lumbar, lumbosacral 839.20
        open 839.30
      non-traumatic - *see* Displacement,
        intervertebral disc
      open NEC 839.50
      recurrent 724.9
      specified region NEC 839.49
        open 839.59
      thoracic 839.21
        open 839.31
  wrist (carpal bone) (scaphoid)
    (semilunar) (closed) 833.00
    carpometacarpal (joint) 833.04
      open 833.14
    metacarpal bone, proximal end
      833.05
      open 833.15
    midcarpal (joint) 833.03
      open 833.13
    open 833.10
    radiocarpal (joint) 833.02
      open 833.12
    radioulnar (joint) 833.01
      open 833.11
    recurrent 718.33
    specified site NEC 833.09
      open 833.19
  xiphoid cartilage (closed) 839.61
    open 839.71
Dislodgement
  artificial skin graft 996.55
  decellularized allodermis graft
    996.55
Disobedience, hostile (covert) (overt)
  (*see also* Disturbance, conduct)
  312.0●
Disorder - *see also* Disease
  academic underachievement,
    childhood and adolescence 313.83
  accommodation 367.51
    drug-induced 367.89
    toxic 367.89

Disorder *(Continued)*
  adjustment (*see also* Reaction,
    adjustment) 309.9
    with
      anxiety 309.24
      anxiety and depressed mood
        309.28
      depressed mood 309.0
      disturbance of conduct 309.3
      disturbance of emotions and
        conduct 309.4
  adrenal (capsule) (cortex) (gland) 255.9
    specified type NEC 255.8
  adrenogenital 255.2
  affective (*see also* Psychosis, affective)
    296.90
    atypical 296.81
  aggressive, unsocialized (*see also*
    Disturbance, conduct) 312.0●
  alcohol, alcoholic (*see also* Alcohol)
    291.9
  allergic - *see* Allergy
  amino acid (metabolic) (*see also*
    Disturbance, metabolism, amino
    acid) 270.9
    albinism 270.2
    alkaptonuria 270.2
    argininosuccinicaciduria 270.6
    beta-amino-isobutyricaciduria 277.2
    cystathioninuria 270.4
    cystinosis 270.0
    cystinuria 270.0
    glycinuria 270.0
    homocystinuria 270.4
    imidazole 270.5
    maple syrup (urine) disease 270.3
    neonatal, transitory 775.89
    oasthouse urine disease 270.2
    ochronosis 270.2
    phenylketonuria 270.1
    phenylpyruvic oligophrenia 270.1
    purine NEC 277.2
    pyrimidine NEC 277.2
    renal transport NEC 270.0
    specified type NEC 270.8
    transport NEC 270.0
      renal 270.0
    xanthinuria 277.2
  amnestic (*see also* Amnestic syndrome)
    294.8
    alcohol-induced persisting 291.1
    drug-induced persisting 292.83
    in conditions classified elsewhere
      294.0
  anaerobic glycolysis with anemia 282.3
  anxiety (*see also* Anxiety) 300.00
    due to or associated with physical
      condition 293.84
  arteriole 447.9
    specified type NEC 447.8
  artery 447.9
    specified type NEC 447.8
  articulation - *see* Disorder, joint
  Asperger's 299.8●
  attachment of infancy or early
    childhood 313.89
  attention deficit 314.00
    with hyperactivity 314.01
    predominantly
    combined hyperactive/inattentive
      314.01
      hyperactive/impulsive 314.01
      inattentive 314.00
    residual type 314.8

Disorder *(Continued)*
  auditory processing disorder 388.45
    acquired 388.45
    developmental 315.32
  autistic 299.0●
  autoimmune NEC 279.49
    hemolytic (cold type) (warm type)
      283.0
    parathyroid 252.1
    thyroid 245.2
  avoidant, childhood or adolescence
    313.21
  balance
    acid-base 276.9
      mixed (with hypercapnia)
        276.4
    electrolyte 276.9
    fluid 276.9
  behavior NEC (*see also* Disturbance,
    conduct) 312.9
    disruptive 312.9
  bilirubin excretion 277.4
  bipolar (affective) (alternating)
    296.80

Note: Use the following fifth-digit subclassification with categories 296.0–296.6:
0 unspecified
1 mild
2 moderate
3 severe, without mention of psychotic behavior
4 severe, specified as with psychotic behavior
5 in partial or unspecified remission
6 in full remission

    atypical 296.7
    specified type NEC 296.89
    type I 296.7
      most recent episode (or current)
        depressed 296.5●
        hypomanic 296.4●
        manic 296.4●
        mixed 296.6●
        unspecified 296.7
      single manic episode 296.0●
    type II (recurrent major depressive
      episodes with hypomania)
      296.89
  bladder 596.9
    functional NEC 596.59
    specified NEC 596.8
  bleeding 286.9
  bone NEC 733.90
    specified NEC 733.99
  brachial plexus 353.0
  branched-chain amino-acid
    degradation 270.3
  breast 611.9
    puerperal, postpartum 676.3●
    specified NEC 611.89
  Briquet's 300.81
  bursa 727.9
    shoulder region 726.10
  carbohydrate metabolism, congenital
    271.9
  cardiac, functional 427.9
    postoperative 997.1
    psychogenic 306.2
  cardiovascular, psychogenic 306.2

◀ New   ◀▥ Revised   ~~deleted~~ Deleted   ● Use Additional Digit(s)   ▨ Omit code

Disorder (Continued)
cartilage NEC 733.90
  articular 718.00
    ankle 718.07
    elbow 718.02
    foot 718.07
    hand 718.04
    hip 718.05
    knee 717.9
    multiple sites 718.09
    pelvic region 718.05
    shoulder region 718.01
    specified
      site NEC 718.08
      type NEC 733.99
    wrist 718.03
catatonic - see Catatonia
central auditory processing 315.32
  acquired 388.45
  developmental 315.32
cervical region NEC 723.9
cervical root (nerve) NEC 353.2
character NEC (see also Disorder,
    personality) 301.9
ciliary body 364.9
  specified NEC 364.89
coagulation (factor) (see also Defect,
    coagulation) 286.9
  factor VIII (congenital) (functional)
    286.0
  factor IX (congenital) (functional)
    286.1
  neonatal, transitory 776.3
coccyx 724.70
  specified NEC 724.79
cognitive 294.9
colon 569.9
  functional 564.9
    congenital 751.3
communication 307.9
conduct (see also Disturbance, conduct)
    312.9
  adjustment reaction 309.3
  adolescent onset type 312.82
  childhood onset type 312.81
  compulsive 312.30
    specified type NEC 312.39
  hyperkinetic 314.2
  onset unspecified 312.89
  socialized (type) 312.20
    aggressive 312.23
    unaggressive 312.21
  specified NEC 312.89
conduction, heart 426.9
  specified NEC 426.89
conflict
  sexual orientation 302.0
congenital
  glycosylation (CDG) 271.8
convulsive (secondary) (see also
    Convulsions) 780.39
  due to injury at birth 767.0
  idiopathic 780.39
coordination 781.3
cornea NEC 371.89
  due to contact lens 371.82
corticosteroid metabolism NEC
    255.2
cranial nerve - see Disorder, nerve,
    cranial
cyclothymic 301.13
degradation, branched-chain amino
    acid 270.3
delusional 297.1

Disorder (Continued)
dentition 520.6
depersonalization 300.6
depressive NEC 311
  atypical 296.82
  major (see also Psychosis, affective)
    296.2●
    recurrent episode 296.3●
    single episode 296.2●
development, specific 315.9
  associated with hyperkinesia
    314.1
  coordination 315.4
  language 315.31
    and speech due to hearing loss
    315.34
  learning 315.2
    arithmetical 315.1
    reading 315.00
  mixed 315.5
  motor coordination 315.4
  specified type NEC 315.8
  speech 315.39
    and language due to hearing loss
    315.34
diaphragm 519.4
digestive 536.9
  fetus or newborn 777.9
    specified NEC 777.8
  psychogenic 306.4
disintegrative childhood 299.1●
dissociative 300.15
  identity 300.14
  nocturnal 307.47
drug-related 292.9
dysmorphic body 300.7
dysthymic 300.4
ear 388.9
  degenerative NEC 388.00
  external 380.9
    specified 380.89
  pinna 380.30
  specified type NEC 388.8
  vascular NEC 388.00
eating NEC 307.50
electrolyte NEC 276.9
  with
    abortion - see Abortion, by type,
      with metabolic disorder
    ectopic pregnancy (see also
      categories 633.0–633.9)
      639.4
    molar pregnancy (see also
      categories 630–632) 639.4
  acidosis 276.2
    metabolic 276.2
    respiratory 276.2
  alkalosis 276.3
    metabolic 276.3
    respiratory 276.3
  following
    abortion 639.4
    ectopic or molar pregnancy
      639.4
  neonatal, transitory NEC 775.5
emancipation as adjustment reaction
    309.22
emotional (see also Disorder, mental,
    nonpsychotic) V40.9
endocrine 259.9
  specified type NEC 259.8
esophagus 530.9
  functional 530.5
  psychogenic 306.4

Disorder (Continued)
explosive
  intermittent 312.34
  isolated 312.35
expressive language 315.31
eye 379.90
  globe - see Disorder, globe
  ill-defined NEC 379.99
  limited duction NEC 378.63
  specified NEC 379.8
eyelid 374.9
  degenerative 374.50
  sensory 374.44
  specified type NEC 374.89
  vascular 374.85
factitious (with combined
    psychological and physical
    signs and symptoms) (with
    predominantly physical signs
    and symptoms) 300.19
  with predominantly psychological
    signs and symptoms 300.16
factor, coagulation (see also Defect,
    coagulation) 286.9
  VIII (congenital) (functional) 286.0
  IX (congenital) (functional) 286.1
fascia 728.9
fatty acid oxidation 277.85
feeding - see Feeding
female sexual arousal 302.72
fluency 315.35 ◀
  adult onset 307.0 ◀
  childhood onset 315.35 ◀
  due to late effect of cerebrovascular
    accident 438.14 ◀
  in conditions classified elsewhere
    784.52 ◀
fluid NEC 276.9
gastric (functional) 536.9
  motility 536.8
  psychogenic 306.4
  secretion 536.8
gastrointestinal (functional) NEC 536.9
  newborn (neonatal) 777.9
    specified NEC 777.8
  psychogenic 306.4
gender (child) 302.6
  adult 302.85
gender identity (childhood) 302.6
  adolescents 302.85
  adults (-life) 302.85
genitourinary system, psychogenic
    306.50
globe 360.9
  degenerative 360.20
    specified NEC 360.29
  specified type NEC 360.89
hearing - see also Deafness
  conductive type (air) (see also
    Deafness, conductive) 389.00
  mixed conductive and
    sensorineural 389.20
    bilateral 389.22
    unilateral 389.21
  nerve
    bilateral 389.12
    unilateral 389.13
  perceptive (see also Deafness,
    perceptive) 389.10
  sensorineural type NEC (see also
    Deafness, sensorineural) 389.10
heart action 427.9
  postoperative 997.1
hematological, transient neonatal 776.9
  specified type NEC 776.8
hematopoietic organs 289.9

Disorder (*Continued*)
  hemorrhagic NEC 287.9
    due to intrinsic circulating
      anticoagulants 286.5
    specified type NEC 287.8
  hemostasis (*see also* Defect, coagulation)
    286.9
  homosexual conflict 302.0
  hypomanic (chronic) 301.11
  identity
    childhood and adolescence 313.82
      gender 302.6
  immune mechanism (immunity) 279.9
    single complement (C₁–C₉) 279.8
    specified type NEC 279.8
  impulse control (*see also* Disturbance,
    conduct, compulsive) 312.30
  infant sialic acid storage 271.8
  integument, fetus or newborn 778.9
    specified type NEC 778.8
  interactional psychotic (childhood) (*see
    also* Psychosis, childhood) 299.1●
  intermittent explosive 312.34
  intervertebral disc 722.90
    cervical, cervicothoracic 722.91
    lumbar, lumbosacral 722.93
    thoracic, thoracolumbar 722.92
  intestinal 569.9
    functional NEC 564.9
      congenital 751.3
      postoperative 564.4
    psychogenic 306.4
  introverted, of childhood and
    adolescence 313.22
  involuntary emotional expression
    (IEED) 310.8
  iris 364.9
    specified NEC 364.89
  iron, metabolism 275.09 ◀▥
    specified type NEC 275.09 ◀
  isolated explosive 312.35
  joint NEC 719.90
    ankle 719.97
    elbow 719.92
    foot 719.97
    hand 719.94
    hip 719.95
    knee 719.96
    multiple sites 719.99
    pelvic region 719.95
    psychogenic 306.0
    shoulder (region) 719.91
    specified site NEC 719.98
    temporomandibular 524.60
      sounds on opening or closing
        524.64
      specified NEC 524.69
    wrist 719.93
  kidney 593.9
    functional 588.9
      specified NEC 588.89
  labyrinth, labyrinthine 386.9
    specified type NEC 386.8
  lactation 676.9●
  language (developmental) (expressive)
    315.31
    mixed receptive-expressive 315.32
  learning 315.9
  ligament 728.9
  ligamentous attachments, peripheral -
    see also Enthesopathy
    spine 720.1
  limb NEC 729.90
    psychogenic 306.0

Disorder (*Continued*)
  lipid
    metabolism, congenital 272.9
    storage 272.7
  lipoprotein deficiency (familial) 272.5
  low back NEC 724.9
    psychogenic 306.0
  lumbosacral
    plexus 353.1
    root (nerve) NEC 353.4
  lymphoproliferative (chronic) NEC
    (M9970/1) 238.79
    post-transplant (PTLD) 238.77
  major depressive (*see also* Psychosis,
    affective) 296.2●
    recurrent episode 296.3●
    single episode 296.2●
  male erectile 607.84
    nonorganic origin 302.72
  manic (*see also* Psychosis, affective)
    296.0●
    atypical 296.81
  mathematics 315.1
  meniscus NEC (*see also* Disorder,
    cartilage, articular) 718.0●
  menopausal 627.9
    specified NEC 627.8
  menstrual 626.9
    psychogenic 306.52
    specified NEC 626.8
  mental (nonpsychotic) 300.9
    affecting management of pregnancy,
      childbirth, or puerperium
      648.4●
    drug-induced 292.9
      hallucinogen persisting
        perception 292.89
      specified type NEC 292.89
    due to or associated with
      alcoholism 291.9
      drug consumption NEC 292.9
        specified type NEC 292.89
      physical condition NEC 293.9
    induced by drug 292.9
      specified type NEC 292.89
    neurotic (*see also* Neurosis) 300.9
    of infancy, childhood or adolescence
      313.9
    persistent
      other
        due to conditions classified
          elsewhere 294.8
      unspecified
        due to conditions classified
          elsewhere 294.9
    presenile 310.1
      psychotic NEC 290.10
    previous, affecting management of
      pregnancy V23.89
    psychoneurotic (*see also* Neurosis)
      300.9
    psychotic (*see also* Psychosis) 298.9
      brief 298.8
      senile 290.20
    specific, following organic brain
      damage 310.9
      cognitive or personality change
        of other type 310.1
      frontal lobe syndrome 310.0
      postconcussional syndrome 310.2
      specified type NEC 310.8
    transient
      in conditions classified elsewhere
        293.9

Disorder (*Continued*)
  metabolism NEC 277.9
    with
      abortion - *see* Abortion, by type,
        with metabolic disorder
      ectopic pregnancy (*see also*
        categories 633.0–633.9)
        639.4
      molar pregnancy (*see also*
        categories 630–632) 639.4
    alkaptonuria 270.2
    amino acid (*see also* Disorder, amino
      acid) 270.9
      specified type NEC 270.8
    ammonia 270.6
    arginine 270.6
    argininosuccinic acid 270.6
    basal 794.7
    bilirubin 277.4
    calcium 275.40
    carbohydrate 271.9
      specified type NEC 271.8
    cholesterol 272.9
    citrulline 270.6
    copper 275.1
    corticosteroid 255.2
    cystine storage 270.0
    cystinuria 270.0
    fat 272.9
      fatty acid oxidation 277.85
    following
      abortion 639.4
      ectopic or molar pregnancy 639.4
    fructosemia 271.2
    fructosuria 271.2
    fucosidosis 271.8
    galactose-1-phosphate uridyl
      transferase 271.1
    glutamine 270.7
    glycine 270.7
    glycogen storage NEC 271.0
      hepatorenal 271.0
    hemochromatosis (*see also*
      Hemochromatosis) 275.03 ◀▥
    in labor and delivery 669.0●
    iron 275.09 ◀▥
    lactose 271.3
    lipid 272.9
      specified type NEC 272.8
      storage 272.7
    lipoprotein - *see also* Hyperlipemia
      deficiency (familial) 272.5
    lysine 270.7
    magnesium 275.2
    mannosidosis 271.8
    mineral 275.9
      specified type NEC 275.8
      mitochondrial 277.87
    mucopolysaccharide 277.5
    nitrogen 270.9
    ornithine 270.6
    oxalosis 271.8
    pentosuria 271.8
    phenylketonuria 270.1
    phosphate 275.3
    phosphorus 275.3
    plasma protein 273.9
      specified type NEC 273.8
    porphyrin 277.1
    purine 277.2
    pyrimidine 277.2
    serine 270.7
    sodium 276.9
    specified type NEC 277.89

◀ New   ◀▥ Revised   ~~deleted~~ Deleted   ● Use Additional Digit(s)   ▥ Omit code

Disorder (*Continued*)
  metabolism NEC (*Continued*)
    steroid 255.2
    threonine 270.7
    urea cycle 270.6
    xylose 271.8
  micturition NEC 788.69
    psychogenic 306.53
  misery and unhappiness, of childhood
    and adolescence 313.1
  mitochondrial metabolism 277.87
  mitral valve 424.0
  mood (*see also* Disorder, bipolar) 296.90
    episodic 296.90
      specified NEC 296.99
    in conditions classified elsewhere
      293.83
  motor tic 307.20
    chronic 307.22
    transient (childhood) 307.21
  movement NEC 333.90
    hysterical 300.11
    medication-induced 333.90
    periodic limb 327.51
    sleep related unspecified 780.58
      other organic 327.59
    specified type NEC 333.99
    stereotypic 307.3
  mucopolysaccharide 277.5
  muscle 728.9
    psychogenic 306.0
    specified type NEC 728.3
  muscular attachments, peripheral - *see*
    also Enthesopathy
    spine 720.1
  musculoskeletal system NEC 729.90
    psychogenic 306.0
  myeloproliferative (chronic) NEC
    (M9960/1) 238.79
  myoneural 358.9
    due to lead 358.2
    specified type NEC 358.8
    toxic 358.2
  myotonic 359.29
  neck region NEC 723.9
  nerve 349.9
    abducens NEC 378.54
    accessory 352.4
    acoustic 388.5
    auditory 388.5
    auriculotemporal 350.8
    axillary 353.0
    cerebral - *see* Disorder, nerve, cranial
    cranial 352.9
      first 352.0
      second 377.49
      third
        partial 378.51
        total 378.52
      fourth 378.53
      fifth 350.9
      sixth 378.54
      seventh NEC 351.9
      eighth 388.5
      ninth 352.2
      tenth 352.3
      eleventh 352.4
      twelfth 352.5
      multiple 352.6
    entrapment - *see* Neuropathy,
      entrapment
    facial 351.9
      specified NEC 351.8
    femoral 355.2

Disorder (*Continued*)
  nerve (*Continued*)
    glossopharyngeal NEC 352.2
    hypoglossal 352.5
    iliohypogastric 355.79
    ilioinguinal 355.79
    intercostal 353.8
    lateral
      cutaneous of thigh 355.1
      popliteal 355.3
    lower limb NEC 355.8
    medial, popliteal 355.4
    median NEC 354.1
    obturator 355.79
    oculomotor
      partial 378.51
      total 378.52
    olfactory 352.0
    optic 377.49
      hypoplasia 377.43
      ischemic 377.41
      nutritional 377.33
      toxic 377.34
    peroneal 355.3
    phrenic 354.8
    plantar 355.6
    pneumogastric 352.3
    posterior tibial 355.5
    radial 354.3
    recurrent laryngeal 352.3
    root 353.9
      specified NEC 353.8
    saphenous 355.79
    sciatic NEC 355.0
    specified NEC 355.9
      lower limb 355.79
      upper limb 354.8
    spinal 355.9
    sympathetic NEC 337.9
    trigeminal 350.9
      specified NEC 350.8
    trochlear 378.53
    ulnar 354.2
    upper limb NEC 354.9
    vagus 352.3
  nervous system NEC 349.9
    autonomic (peripheral) (*see also*
      Neuropathy, peripheral,
      autonomic) 337.9
    cranial 352.9
    parasympathetic (*see also*
      Neuropathy, peripheral,
      autonomic) 337.9
    specified type NEC 349.89
    sympathetic (*see also* Neuropathy,
      peripheral, autonomic) 337.9
    vegetative (*see also* Neuropathy,
      peripheral, autonomic) 337.9
  neurohypophysis NEC 253.6
  neurological NEC 781.99
    peripheral NEC 355.9
  neuromuscular NEC 358.9
    hereditary NEC 359.1
    specified NEC 358.8
    toxic 358.2
  neurotic 300.9
    specified type NEC 300.89
  neutrophil, polymorphonuclear
    (functional) 288.1
  nightmare 307.47
  night terror 307.46
  obsessive-compulsive 300.3
  oppositional defiant, childhood and
    adolescence 313.81

Disorder (*Continued*)
  optic
    chiasm 377.54
      associated with
        inflammatory disorders 377.54
        neoplasm NEC 377.52
          pituitary 377.51
        pituitary disorders 377.51
        vascular disorders 377.53
    nerve 377.49
    radiations 377.63
    tracts 377.63
  orbit 376.9
    specified NEC 376.89
  orgasmic
    female 302.73
    male 302.74
  overanxious, of childhood and
    adolescence 313.0
  oxidation, fatty acid 277.85
  pancreas, internal secretion (other than
    diabetes mellitus) 251.9
    specified type NEC 251.8
  panic 300.01
    with agoraphobia 300.21
  papillary muscle NEC 429.81
  paranoid 297.9
    induced 297.3
    shared 297.3
  parathyroid 252.9
    specified type NEC 252.8
  paroxysmal, mixed 780.39
  pentose phosphate pathway with
    anemia 282.2
  periodic limb movement 327.51
  peroxisomal 277.86
  personality 301.9
    affective 301.10
    aggressive 301.3
    amoral 301.7
    anancastic, anankastic 301.4
    antisocial 301.7
    asocial 301.7
    asthenic 301.6
    avoidant 301.82
    borderline 301.83
    compulsive 301.4
    cyclothymic 301.13
    dependent-passive 301.6
    dyssocial 301.7
    emotional instability 301.59
    epileptoid 301.3
    explosive 301.3
    following organic brain damage
      310.1
    histrionic 301.50
    hyperthymic 301.11
    hypomanic (chronic) 301.11
    hypothymic 301.12
    hysterical 301.50
    immature 301.89
    inadequate 301.6
    introverted 301.21
    labile 301.59
    moral deficiency 301.7
    narcissistic 301.81
    obsessional 301.4
    obsessive-compulsive 301.4
    overconscientious 301.4
    paranoid 301.0
    passive (-dependent) 301.6
    passive-aggressive 301.84
    pathological NEC 301.9
    pseudosocial 301.7

Disorder *(Continued)*
  personality *(Continued)*
    psychopathic 301.9
    schizoid 301.20
      introverted 301.21
      schizotypal 301.22
    schizotypal 301.22
    seductive 301.59
    type A 301.4
    unstable 301.59
  pervasive developmental 299.9●
    childhood-onset 299.8●
    specified NEC 299.8●
  phonological 315.39
  pigmentation, choroid (congenital)
      743.53
  pinna 380.30
    specified type NEC 380.39
  pituitary, thalamic 253.9
    anterior NEC 253.4
    iatrogenic 253.7
    postablative 253.7
    specified NEC 253.8
  pityriasis-like NEC 696.8
  platelets (blood) 287.1
  polymorphonuclear neutrophils
      (functional) 288.1
  porphyrin metabolism 277.1
  postmenopausal 627.9
    specified type NEC 627.8
  post-transplant lymphoproliferative
      (PTLD) 238.77
  post-traumatic stress (PTSD) 309.81
  posttraumatic stress 309.81
    acute 309.81
    brief 309.81
    chronic 309.81
  premenstrual dysphoric (PMDD)
      625.4
  psoriatic-like NEC 696.8
  psychic, with diseases classified
      elsewhere 316
  psychogenic NEC *(see also* condition)
      300.9
    allergic NEC
      respiratory 306.1
    anxiety 300.00
      atypical 300.00
      generalized 300.02
    appetite 307.59
    articulation, joint 306.0
    asthenic 300.5
    blood 306.8
    cardiovascular (system) 306.2
    compulsive 300.3
    cutaneous 306.3
    depressive 300.4
    digestive (system) 306.4
    dysmenorrheic 306.52
    dyspneic 306.1
    eczematous 306.3
    endocrine (system) 306.6
    eye 306.7
    feeding 307.59
    functional NEC 306.9
    gastric 306.4
    gastrointestinal (system) 306.4
    genitourinary (system) 306.50
    heart (function) (rhythm) 306.2
    hemic 306.8
    hyperventilatory 306.1
    hypochondriacal 300.7
    hysterical 300.10
    intestinal 306.4

Disorder *(Continued)*
  psychogenic NEC *(Continued)*
    joint 306.0
    learning 315.2
    limb 306.0
    lymphatic (system) 306.8
    menstrual 306.52
    micturition 306.53
    monoplegic NEC 306.0
    motor 307.9
    muscle 306.0
    musculoskeletal 306.0
    neurocirculatory 306.2
    obsessive 300.3
    occupational 300.89
    organ or part of body NEC 306.9
    organs of special sense 306.7
    paralytic NEC 306.0
    phobic 300.20
    physical NEC 306.9
    pruritic 306.3
    rectal 306.4
    respiratory (system) 306.1
    rheumatic 306.0
    sexual (function) 302.70
      specified type NEC 302.79
    sexual orientation conflict 302.0
    skin (allergic) (eczematous)
        (pruritic) 306.3
    sleep 307.40
      initiation or maintenance 307.41
        persistent 307.42
        transient 307.41
      movement 780.58
      sleep terror 307.46
      specified type NEC 307.49
    specified part of body NEC 306.8
    stomach 306.4
  psychomotor NEC 307.9
    hysterical 300.11
  psychoneurotic *(see also* Neurosis) 300.9
    mixed NEC 300.89
  psychophysiologic *(see also* Disorder,
      psychosomatic) 306.9
  psychosexual identity (childhood)
      302.6
    adult-life 302.85
  psychosomatic NEC 306.9
    allergic NEC
      respiratory 306.1
    articulation, joint 306.0
    cardiovascular (system) 306.2
    cutaneous 306.3
    digestive (system) 306.4
    dysmenorrheic 306.52
    dyspneic 306.1
    endocrine (system) 306.6
    eye 306.7
    gastric 306.4
    gastrointestinal (system) 306.4
    genitourinary (system) 306.50
    heart (functional) (rhythm) 306.2
    hyperventilatory 306.1
    intestinal 306.4
    joint 306.0
    limb 306.0
    lymphatic (system) 306.8
    menstrual 306.52
    micturition 306.53
    monoplegic NEC 306.0
    muscle 306.0
    musculoskeletal 306.0
    neurocirculatory 306.2
    organs of special sense 306.7

Disorder *(Continued)*
  psychosomatic NEC *(Continued)*
    paralytic NEC 306.0
    pruritic 306.3
    rectal 306.4
    respiratory (system) 306.1
    rheumatic 306.0
    sexual (function) 302.70
      specified type NEC 302.79
    skin 306.3
    specified part of body NEC 306.8
    stomach 306.4
  psychotic *(see also* Psychosis) 298.9
    brief 298.8
  purine metabolism NEC 277.2
  pyrimidine metabolism NEC 277.2
  reactive attachment of infancy or early
      childhood 313.89
  reading, developmental 315.00
  reflex 796.1
  REM sleep behavior 327.42
  renal function, impaired 588.9
    specified type NEC 588.89
  renal transport NEC 588.89
  respiration, respiratory NEC 519.9
    due to
      aspiration of liquids or solids
          508.9
      inhalation of fumes or vapors
          506.9
    psychogenic 306.1
  retina 362.9
    specified type NEC 362.89
  rumination 307.53
  sacroiliac joint NEC 724.6
  sacrum 724.6
  schizo-affective *(see also* Schizophrenia)
      295.7●
  schizoid, childhood or adolescence
      313.22
  schizophreniform 295.4●
  schizotypal personality 301.22
  secretion, thyrocalcitonin 246.0
  seizure 345.9●
    recurrent 345.9●
      epileptic - *see* Epilepsy
  semantic pragmatic 315.39
    with autism 299.0●
  sense of smell 781.1
    psychogenic 306.7
  separation anxiety 309.21
  sexual *(see also* Deviation, sexual) 302.9
    aversion 302.79
    desire, hypoactive 302.71
    function, psychogenic 302.70
  shyness, of childhood and adolescence
      313.21
  single complement $(C_1–C_9)$ 279.8
  skin NEC 709.9
    fetus or newborn 778.9
      specified type 778.8
    psychogenic (allergic) (eczematous)
        (pruritic) 306.3
    specified type NEC 709.8
    vascular 709.1
  sleep 780.50
    with apnea - *see* Apnea, sleep
    alcohol induced 291.82
    arousal 307.46
      confusional 327.41
    circadian rhythm 327.30
      advanced sleep phase type 327.32
      alcohol induced 291.82
      delayed sleep phase type 327.31

◀ New   ◀▥ Revised   ~~deleted~~ Deleted   ● Use Additional Digit(s)   ▨ Omit code

Disorder *(Continued)*
  sleep *(Continued)*
    circadian rhythm *(Continued)*
      drug induced 292.85
      free running type 327.34
      in conditions classified elsewhere 327.37
      irregular sleep-wake type 327.33
      jet lag type 327.35
      other 327.39
      shift work type 327.36
    drug induced 292.85
    initiation or maintenance *(see also* Insomnia) 780.52
      nonorganic origin (transient) 307.41
        persistent 307.42
    nonorganic origin 307.40
      specified type NEC 307.49
    organic specified type NEC 327.8
    periodic limb movement 327.51
    specified NEC 780.59
    wake
      cycle - *see* Disorder, sleep, circadian rhythm
      schedule - *see* Disorder, sleep, circadian rhythm
  social, of childhood and adolescence 313.22
  soft tissue 729.90
    specified type NEC 729.99
  somatization 300.81
  somatoform (atypical) (undifferentiated) 300.82
    severe 300.81
    specified type NEC 300.89
  speech NEC 784.59
    nonorganic origin 307.9
  spine NEC 724.9
    ligamentous or muscular attachments, peripheral 720.1
  steroid metabolism NEC 255.2
  stomach (functional) *(see also* Disorder, gastric) 536.9
    psychogenic 306.4
  storage, iron 275.09 ◀▥
  stress *(see also* Reaction, stress, acute) 308.3
    posttraumatic
      acute 309.81
      brief 309.81
      chronic (motor or vocal) 309.81
  substitution 300.11
  suspected - *see* Observation
  synovium 727.9
  temperature regulation, fetus or newborn 778.4
  temporomandibular joint NEC 524.60
    sounds on opening or closing 524.64
    specified NEC 524.69
  tendon 727.9
    shoulder region 726.10
  thoracic root (nerve) NEC 353.3
  thyrocalcitonin secretion 246.0
  thyroid (gland) NEC 246.9
    specified type NEC 246.8
  tic 307.20
    chronic (motor or vocal) 307.22
    motor-verbal 307.23
    organic origin 333.1
    transient (of childhood) 307.21

Disorder *(Continued)*
  tooth NEC 525.9
    development NEC 520.9
      specified type NEC 520.8
    eruption 520.6
    specified type NEC 525.8
  Tourette's 307.23
  transport, carbohydrate 271.9
    specified type NEC 271.8
  tubular, phosphate-losing 588.0
  tympanic membrane 384.9
  unaggressive, unsocialized *(see also* Disturbance, conduct) 312.1●
  undersocialized, unsocialized *(see also* Disturbance, conduct)
    aggressive (type) 312.0●
    unaggressive (type) 312.1●
  vision, visual NEC 368.9
    binocular NEC 368.30
    cortex 377.73
      associated with
        inflammatory disorders 377.73
        neoplasms 377.71
        vascular disorders 377.72
    pathway NEC 377.63
      associated with
        inflammatory disorders 377.63
        neoplasms 377.61
        vascular disorders 377.62
  vocal tic
    chronic 307.22
  wakefulness *(see also* Hypersomnia) 780.54
    nonorganic origin (transient) 307.43
      persistent 307.44
  written expression 315.2
Disorganized globe 360.29
Displacement, displaced

> Note: For acquired displacement of bones, cartilage, joints, tendons, due to injury, *see also* Dislocation.
>
> Displacements at ages under one year should be considered congenital, provided there is no indication the condition was acquired after birth.

  acquired traumatic of bone, cartilage, joint, tendon NEC (without fracture) *(see also* Dislocation) 839.8
    with fracture - *see* Fracture, by site
  adrenal gland (congenital) 759.1
  alveolus and teeth, vertical 524.75
  appendix, retrocecal (congenital) 751.5
  auricle (congenital) 744.29
  bladder (acquired) 596.8
    congenital 753.8
  brachial plexus (congenital) 742.8
  brain stem, caudal 742.4
  canaliculus lacrimalis 743.65
  cardia, through esophageal hiatus 750.6
  cerebellum, caudal 742.4
  cervix - *see* Displacement, uterus
  colon (congenital) 751.4
  device, implant, or graft - *see* Complications, mechanical
  epithelium
    columnar of cervix 622.10
    cuboidal, beyond limits of external os (uterus) 752.49
  esophageal mucosa into cardia of stomach, congenital 750.4

Displacement, displaced *(Continued)*
  esophagus (acquired) 530.89
    congenital 750.4
  eyeball (acquired) (old) 376.36
    congenital 743.8
    current injury 871.3
    lateral 376.36
  fallopian tube (acquired) 620.4
    congenital 752.19
    opening (congenital) 752.19
  gallbladder (congenital) 751.69
  gastric mucosa 750.7
    into
      duodenum 750.7
      esophagus 750.7
      Meckel's diverticulum, congenital 750.7
  globe (acquired) (lateral) (old) 376.36
    current injury 871.3
  graft
    artificial skin graft 996.55
    decellularized allodermis graft 996.55
  heart (congenital) 746.87
    acquired 429.89
  hymen (congenital) (upward) 752.49
  internal prosthesis NEC - *see* Complications, mechanical
  intervertebral disc (with neuritis, radiculitis, sciatica, or other pain) 722.2
    with myelopathy 722.70
    cervical, cervicodorsal, cervicothoracic 722.0
      with myelopathy 722.71
      due to major trauma - *see* Dislocation, vertebra, cervical
    due to trauma - *see* Dislocation, vertebra
    lumbar, lumbosacral 722.10
      with myelopathy 722.73
      due to major trauma - *see* Dislocation, vertebra, lumbar
    thoracic, thoracolumbar 722.11
      with myelopathy 722.72
      due to major trauma - *see* Dislocation, vertebra, thoracic
  intrauterine device 996.32
  kidney (acquired) 593.0
    congenital 753.3
  lacrimal apparatus or duct (congenital) 743.65
  macula (congenital) 743.55
  Meckel's diverticulum (congenital) 751.0
  nail (congenital) 757.5
    acquired 703.8
  opening of Wharton's duct in mouth 750.26
  organ or site, congenital NEC - *see* Malposition, congenital
  ovary (acquired) 620.4
    congenital 752.0
    free in peritoneal cavity (congenital) 752.0
    into hernial sac 620.4
  oviduct (acquired) 620.4
    congenital 752.19
  parathyroid (gland) 252.8
  parotid gland (congenital) 750.26
  punctum lacrimale (congenital) 743.65

◀ New   ◀▥ Revised   ~~deleted~~ Deleted   ● Use Additional Digit(s)   ▥ Omit code

Displacement, displaced (Continued)
 sacroiliac (congenital) (joint) 755.69
  current injury - see Dislocation,
   sacroiliac
  old 724.6
 spine (congenital) 756.19
 spleen, congenital 759.0
 stomach (congenital) 750.7
  acquired 537.89
 subglenoid (closed) 831.01
 sublingual duct (congenital) 750.26
 teeth, tooth 524.30
  horizontal 524.33
  vertical 524.34
 tongue (congenital) (downward)
  750.19
 trachea (congenital) 748.3
 ureter or ureteric opening or orifice
  (congenital) 753.4
 uterine opening of oviducts or
  fallopian tubes 752.19
 uterus, uterine (see also Malposition,
  uterus) 621.6
  congenital 752.39 ◄▓
 ventricular septum 746.89
  with rudimentary ventricle 746.89
 xyphoid bone (process) 738.3
Disproportion 653.9●
 affecting fetus or newborn 763.1
 breast, reconstructed 612.1
  between native and reconstructed
   612.1
 caused by
  conjoined twins 678.1●
  contraction, pelvis (general) 653.1●
   inlet 653.2●
   midpelvic 653.8●
   midplane 653.8●
   outlet 653.3●
  fetal
   ascites 653.7●
   hydrocephalus 653.6●
   hydrops 653.7●
   meningomyelocele 653.7●
   sacral teratoma 653.7●
   tumor 653.7●
  hydrocephalic fetus 653.6●
  pelvis, pelvic, abnormality (bony)
   NEC 653.0●
  unusually large fetus 653.5●
 causing obstructed labor 660.1●
 cephalopelvic, normally formed fetus
  653.4●
  causing obstructed labor 660.1●
 fetal NEC 653.5●
  causing obstructed labor 660.1●
 fetopelvic, normally formed fetus
  653.4●
  causing obstructed labor 660.1●
 mixed maternal and fetal origin,
  normally, formed fetus 653.4●
 pelvis, pelvic (bony) NEC 653.1●
  causing obstructed labor 660.1●
 specified type NEC 653.8●
Disruption
 cesarean wound 674.1●
 family V61.09
  due to
   child in
    care of non-parental family
     member V61.06
    foster care V61.06
    welfare custody V61.05
   death of family member V61.07
   divorce V61.03

Disruption (Continued)
 family (Continued)
  due to (Continued)
   estrangement V61.09
    parent-child V61.04
   extended absence of family
    member NEC V61.08
   family member
    on military deployment V61.01
    return from military
     deployment V61.02
   legal separation V61.03
 gastrointestinal anastomosis 997.4
 ligament(s) - see also Sprain
  knee
   current injury - see Dislocation,
    knee
   old 717.89
    capsular 717.85
    collateral (medial) 717.82
     lateral 717.81
    cruciate (posterior) 717.84
     anterior 717.83
    specified site NEC 717.85
 marital V61.10
  involving
   divorce V61.03
   estrangement V61.09
 operation wound (external) (see also
  Dehiscence) 998.32
  internal 998.31
 organ transplant, anastomosis site - see
  Complications, transplant, organ,
  by site
 ossicles, ossicular chain 385.23
  traumatic - see Fracture, skull, base
 parenchyma
  liver (hepatic) - see Laceration, liver,
   major
  spleen - see Laceration, spleen,
   parenchyma, massive
 phase-shift, of 24 hour sleep-wake
  cycle, unspecified 780.55
  nonorganic origin 307.45
 sleep-wake cycle (24 hour), unspecified
  780.55
  circadian rhythm 327.33
  nonorganic origin 307.45
 suture line (external) (see also
  Dehiscence) 998.32
  internal 998.31
 wound 998.30
  cesarean operation 674.1●
  episiotomy 674.2●
  operation (surgical) 998.32
   cesarean 674.1●
   internal 998.31
  perineal (obstetric) 674.2●
  uterine 674.1●
Disruptio uteri - see also Rupture, uterus
 complicating delivery - see Delivery,
  complicated, rupture, uterus
Dissatisfaction with
 employment V62.29
 school environment V62.3
Dissecting - see condition
Dissection
 aorta 441.00
  abdominal 441.02
  thoracic 441.01
  thoracoabdominal 441.03
 artery, arterial
  carotid 443.21
  coronary 414.12
  iliac 443.22

Dissection (Continued)
 artery, arterial (Continued)
  renal 443.23
  specified NEC 443.29
  vertebral 443.24
  vascular 459.9
  wound - see Wound, open, by site
Disseminated - see condition
Dissociated personality NEC 300.15
Dissociation
 auriculoventricular or atrioventricular
  (any degree) (AV) 426.89
  with heart block 426.0
 interference 426.89
 isorhythmic 426.89
 rhythm
  atrioventricular (AV) 426.89
  interference 426.89
Dissociative
 identity disorder 300.14
 reaction NEC 300.15
Dissolution, vertebra (see also
 Osteoporosis) 733.00
Distention
 abdomen (gaseous) 787.3
 bladder 596.8
 cecum 569.89
 colon 569.89
 gallbladder 575.8
 gaseous (abdomen) 787.3
 intestine 569.89
 kidney 593.89
 liver 573.9
 seminal vesicle 608.89
 stomach 536.8
  acute 536.1
  psychogenic 306.4
 ureter 593.5
 uterus 621.8
Distichia, distichiasis (eyelid) 743.63
Distoma hepaticum infestation 121.3
Distomiasis 121.9
 bile passages 121.3
  due to Clonorchis sinensis 121.1
 hemic 120.9
 hepatic (liver) 121.3
  due to Clonorchis sinensis
   (clonorchiasis) 121.1
 intestinal 121.4
 liver 121.3
  due to Clonorchis sinensis 121.1
 lung 121.2
 pulmonary 121.2
Distomolar (fourth molar) 520.1
 causing crowding 524.31
Disto-occlusion (division I) (division II)
 524.22
Distortion (congenital)
 adrenal (gland) 759.1
 ankle (joint) 755.69
 anus 751.5
 aorta 747.29
 appendix 751.5
 arm 755.59
 artery (peripheral) NEC (see also
  Distortion, peripheral vascular
  system) 747.60
  cerebral 747.81
  coronary 746.85
  pulmonary 747.3
  retinal 743.58
  umbilical 747.5
 auditory canal 744.29
  causing impairment of hearing
   744.02

Distortion (Continued)
  bile duct or passage 751.69
  bladder 753.8
  brain 742.4
  bronchus 748.3
  cecum 751.5
  cervix (uteri) 752.49
  chest (wall) 756.3
  clavicle 755.51
  clitoris 752.49
  coccyx 756.19
  colon 751.5
  common duct 751.69
  cornea 743.41
  cricoid cartilage 748.3
  cystic duct 751.69
  duodenum 751.5
  ear 744.29
    auricle 744.29
      causing impairment of hearing
        744.02
      causing impairment of hearing
        744.09
    external 744.29
      causing impairment of hearing
        744.02
    inner 744.05
    middle, except ossicles 744.03
      ossicles 744.04
    ossicles 744.04
  endocrine (gland) NEC 759.2
  epiglottis 748.3
  Eustachian tube 744.24
  eye 743.8
    adnexa 743.69
  face bone(s) 756.0
  fallopian tube 752.19
  femur 755.69
  fibula 755.69
  finger(s) 755.59
  foot 755.67
  gallbladder 751.69
  genitalia, genital organ(s)
    female 752.89
      external 752.49
      internal NEC 752.89
    male 752.89
      penis 752.69
  glottis 748.3
  gyri 742.4
  hand bone(s) 755.59
  heart (auricle) (ventricle) 746.89
    valve (cusp) 746.89
  hepatic duct 751.69
  humerus 755.59
  hymen 752.49
  ileum 751.5
  intestine (large) (small) 751.5
    with anomalous adhesions, fixation
      or malrotation 751.4
  jaw NEC 524.89
  jejunum 751.5
  kidney 753.3
  knee (joint) 755.64
  labium (majus) (minus) 752.49
  larynx 748.3
  leg 755.69
  lens 743.36
  liver 751.69
  lumbar spine 756.19
    with disproportion (fetopelvic)
      653.0●
      affecting fetus or newborn
        763.1
      causing obstructed labor 660.1●

Distortion (Continued)
  lumbosacral (joint) (region) 756.19
  lung (fissures) (lobe) 748.69
  nerve 742.8
  nose 748.1
  organ
    of Corti 744.05
    of site not listed - see Anomaly,
      specified type NEC
  ossicles, ear 744.04
  ovary 752.0
  oviduct 752.19
  pancreas 751.7
  parathyroid (gland) 759.2
  patella 755.64
  peripheral vascular system NEC
    747.60
    gastrointestinal 747.61
    lower limb 747.64
    renal 747.62
    spinal 747.82
    upper limb 747.63
  pituitary (gland) 759.2
  radius 755.59
  rectum 751.5
  rib 756.3
  sacroiliac joint 755.69
  sacrum 756.19
  scapula 755.59
  shoulder girdle 755.59
  site not listed - see Anomaly, specified
    type NEC
  skull bone(s) 756.0
    with
      anencephalus 740.0
      encephalocele 742.0
      hydrocephalus 742.3
        with spina bifida (see also
          Spina bifida) 741.0●
      microcephalus 742.1
  spinal cord 742.59
  spine 756.19
  spleen 759.0
  sternum 756.3
  thorax (wall) 756.3
  thymus (gland) 759.2
  thyroid (gland) 759.2
    cartilage 748.3
  tibia 755.69
  toe(s) 755.66
  tongue 750.19
  trachea (cartilage) 748.3
  ulna 755.59
  ureter 753.4
    causing obstruction 753.20
  urethra 753.8
    causing obstruction 753.6
  uterus 752.39 ◄▦
  vagina 752.49
  vein (peripheral) NEC (see also
    Distortion, peripheral vascular
    system) 747.60
    great 747.49
    portal 747.49
    pulmonary 747.49
  vena cava (inferior) (superior)
    747.49
  vertebra 756.19
  visual NEC 368.15
    shape or size 368.14
  vulva 752.49
  wrist (bones) (joint) 755.59
Distress
  abdomen 789.0●
  colon 564.9

Distress (Continued)
  emotional V40.9
  epigastric 789.0●
  fetal (syndrome) 768.4
    affecting management of
      pregnancy or childbirth
      656.8●
    liveborn infant 768.4
      first noted
        before onset of labor 768.2
        during labor and delivery
          768.3
    stillborn infant (death before onset
      of labor) 768.0
      death during labor 768.1
  gastrointestinal (functional) 536.9
    psychogenic 306.4
  intestinal (functional) NEC 564.9
    psychogenic 306.4
  intrauterine - see Distress, fetal
  leg 729.5
  maternal 669.0●
  mental V40.9
  respiratory 786.09
    acute (adult) 518.82
    adult syndrome (following
      shock, surgery, or trauma)
      518.5
      specified NEC 518.82
    fetus or newborn 770.89
    syndrome (idiopathic) (newborn)
      769
  stomach 536.9
    psychogenic 306.4
Distribution vessel, atypical NEC
    747.60
  coronary artery 746.85
  spinal 747.82
Districhiasis 704.2
Disturbance - see also Disease
  absorption NEC 579.9
    calcium 269.3
    carbohydrate 579.8
    fat 579.8
    protein 579.8
    specified type NEC 579.8
    vitamin (see also Deficiency,
      vitamin) 269.2
  acid-base equilibrium 276.9
  activity and attention, simple, with
    hyperkinesis 314.01
  amino acid (metabolic) (see also
    Disorder, amino acid) 270.9
    imidazole 270.5
    maple syrup (urine) disease
      270.3
    transport 270.0
  assimilation, food 579.9
  attention, simple 314.00
    with hyperactivity 314.01
  auditory, nerve, except deafness
    388.5
  behavior (see also Disturbance, conduct)
    312.9
  blood clotting (hypoproteinemia)
    (mechanism) (see also Defect,
    coagulation) 286.9
  central nervous system NEC
    349.9
  cerebral nerve NEC 352.9
  circulatory 459.9
  conduct 312.9
    adjustment reaction 309.3
    adolescent onset type 312.82

Disturbance *(Continued)*
  conduct *(Continued)*
    childhood onset type 312.81

> Note: Use the following fifth-digit
> subclassification with categories
> 312.0–312.2:
>
> 0   unspecified
> 1   mild
> 2   moderate
> 3   severe

    compulsive 312.30
      intermittent explosive disorder
        312.34
      isolated explosive disorder 312.35
      kleptomania 312.32
      pathological gambling 312.31
      pyromania 312.33
    hyperkinetic 314.2
    intermittent explosive 312.34
    isolated explosive 312.35
    mixed with emotions 312.4
    socialized (type) 312.20
      aggressive 312.23
      unaggressive 312.21
    specified type NEC 312.89
    undersocialized, unsocialized
      aggressive (type) 312.0●
      unaggressive (type) 312.1●
  coordination 781.3
  cranial nerve NEC 352.9
  deep sensibility - *see* Disturbance,
    sensation
  digestive 536.9
    psychogenic 306.4
  electrolyte - *see* Imbalance, electrolyte
  emotions specific to childhood or
    adolescence 313.9
    with
      academic underachievement
        313.83
      anxiety and fearfulness 313.0
      elective mutism 313.23
      identity disorder 313.82
      jealousy 313.3
      misery and unhappiness 313.1
      oppositional defiant disorder
        313.81
      overanxiousness 313.0
      sensitivity 313.21
      shyness 313.21
      social withdrawal 313.22
      withdrawal reaction 313.22
    involving relationship problems
      313.3
    mixed 313.89
    specified type NEC 313.89
  endocrine (gland) 259.9
    neonatal, transitory 775.9
      specified NEC 775.89
  equilibrium 780.4
  feeding (elderly) (infant) 783.3
    newborn 779.31
    nonorganic origin NEC 307.59
    psychogenic NEC 307.59
  fructose metabolism 271.2
  gait 781.2
    hysterical 300.11
  gastric (functional) 536.9
    motility 536.8
    psychogenic 306.4
    secretion 536.8

Disturbance *(Continued)*
  gastrointestinal (functional) 536.9
    psychogenic 306.4
  habit, child 307.9
  hearing, except deafness 388.40
  heart, functional (conditions
      classifiable to 426, 427, 428)
    due to presence of (cardiac)
        prosthesis 429.4
    postoperative (immediate) 997.1
      long-term effect of cardiac
        surgery 429.4
    psychogenic 306.2
  hormone 259.9
  innervation uterus, sympathetic,
      parasympathetic 621.8
  keratinization NEC
    gingiva 523.10
    lip 528.5
    oral (mucosa) (soft tissue) 528.79
      residual ridge mucosa
        excessive 528.72
        minimal 528.71
    tongue 528.79
  labyrinth, labyrinthine (vestibule) 386.9
  learning, specific NEC 315.2
  memory *(see also* Amnesia) 780.93
    mild, following organic brain
      damage 310.8
  mental *(see also* Disorder, mental) 300.9
    associated with diseases classified
      elsewhere 316
  metabolism (acquired) (congenital) *(see
      also* Disorder, metabolism) 277.9
    with
      abortion - *see* Abortion, by type,
        with metabolic disorder
      ectopic pregnancy *(see also*
        categories 633.0–633.9)
        639.4
      molar pregnancy *(see also*
        categories 630–632) 639.4
    amino acid *(see also* Disorder, amino
        acid) 270.9
      aromatic NEC 270.2
      branched-chain 270.3
      specified type NEC 270.8
      straight-chain NEC 270.7
      sulfur-bearing 270.4
      transport 270.0
    ammonia 270.6
    arginine 270.6
    argininosuccinic acid 270.6
    carbohydrate NEC 271.9
    cholesterol 272.9
    citrulline 270.6
    cystathionine 270.4
    fat 272.9
    following
      abortion 639.4
      ectopic or molar pregnancy
        639.4
    general 277.9
      carbohydrate 271.9
      iron 275.09 ◀▥
      phosphate 275.3
      sodium 276.9
    glutamine 270.7
    glycine 270.7
    histidine 270.5
    homocystine 270.4
    in labor or delivery 669.0●
    iron 275.09 ◀▥
    isoleucine 270.3

Disturbance *(Continued)*
  metabolism *(Continued)*
    leucine 270.3
    lipoid 272.9
      specified type NEC 272.8
    lysine 270.7
    methionine 270.4
    neonatal, transitory 775.9
      specified type NEC 775.89
    nitrogen 788.99
    ornithine 270.6
    phosphate 275.3
    phosphatides 272.7
    serine 270.7
    sodium NEC 276.9
    threonine 270.7
    tryptophan 270.2
    tyrosine 270.2
    urea cycle 270.6
    valine 270.3
  motor 796.1
  nervous functional 799.21
  neuromuscular mechanism (eye) due
    to syphilis 094.84
  nutritional 269.9
    nail 703.8
  ocular motion 378.87
    psychogenic 306.7
  oculogyric 378.87
    psychogenic 306.7
  oculomotor NEC 378.87
    psychogenic 306.7
  olfactory nerve 781.1
  optic nerve NEC 377.49
  oral epithelium, including tongue
    528.79
    residual ridge mucosa
      excessive 528.72
      minimal 528.71
  personality (pattern) (trait) *(see also*
      Disorder, personality) 301.9
    following organic brain damage
      310.1
  polyglandular 258.9
  psychomotor 307.9
  pupillary 379.49
  reflex 796.1
  rhythm, heart 427.9
    postoperative (immediate) 997.1
      long-term effect of cardiac
        surgery 429.4
    psychogenic 306.2
  salivary secretion 527.7
  sensation (cold) (heat) (localization)
      (tactile discrimination
      localization) (texture) (vibratory)
      NEC 782.0
    hysterical 300.11
    skin 782.0
    smell 781.1
    taste 781.1
  sensory *(see also* Disturbance,
      sensation) 782.0
    innervation 782.0
  situational (transient) *(see also* Reaction,
      adjustment) 309.9
    acute 308.3
  sleep 780.50
    with apnea - *see* Apnea, sleep
    initiation or maintenance *(see also*
      Insomnia) 780.52
      nonorganic origin 307.41
    nonorganic origin 307.40
      specified type NEC 307.49

◀ New   ◀▥ Revised   ~~deleted~~ Deleted   ● Use Additional Digit(s)   ▨ Omit code

Disturbance *(Continued)*
  sleep *(Continued)*
    specified NEC 780.59
      nonorganic origin 307.49
      wakefulness *(see also* Hypersomnia)
        780.54
      nonorganic origin 307.43
  sociopathic 301.7
  speech NEC 784.59
    developmental 315.39
      associated with hyperkinesis
        314.1
    secondary to organic lesion 784.59
  stomach (functional) *(see also*
    Disturbance, gastric) 536.9
  sympathetic (nerve) *(see also*
    Neuropathy, peripheral,
    autonomic) 337.9
  temperature sense 782.0
    hysterical 300.11
  tooth
    eruption 520.6
    formation 520.4
    structure, hereditary NEC 520.5
  touch *(see also* Disturbance, sensation)
    782.0
  vascular 459.9
    arteriosclerotic - *see* Arteriosclerosis
  vasomotor 443.9
  vasospastic 443.9
  vestibular labyrinth 386.9
  vision, visual NEC 368.9
    psychophysical 368.16
    specified NEC 368.8
    subjective 368.10
  voice and resonance 784.40
  wakefulness (initiation or
    maintenance) *(see also*
    Hypersomnia) 780.54
    nonorganic origin 307.43
Disulfiduria, beta-mercaptolactate-
  cysteine 270.0
Disuse atrophy, bone 733.7
Ditthomska syndrome 307.81
Diuresis 788.42
Divers'
  palsy or paralysis 993.3
  squeeze 993.3
Diverticula, diverticulosis, diverticulum
    (acute) (multiple) (perforated)
    (ruptured) 562.10
  with diverticulitis 562.11
  aorta (Kommerell's) 747.21
  appendix (noninflammatory) 543.9
  bladder (acquired) (sphincter) 596.3
    congenital 753.8
  broad ligament 620.8
  bronchus (congenital) 748.3
    acquired 494.0
      with acute exacerbation 494.1
  calyx, calyceal (kidney) 593.89
  cardia (stomach) 537.1
  cecum 562.10
    with
      diverticulitis 562.11
        with hemorrhage 562.13
      hemorrhage 562.12
    congenital 751.5
  colon (acquired) 562.10
    with
      diverticulitis 562.11
        with hemorrhage 562.13
      hemorrhage 562.12
    congenital 751.5

Diverticula, diverticulosis,
    diverticulum *(Continued)*
  duodenum 562.00
    with
      diverticulitis 562.01
        with hemorrhage 562.03
      hemorrhage 562.02
    congenital 751.5
  epiphrenic (esophagus) 530.6
  esophagus (congenital) 750.4
    acquired 530.6
    epiphrenic 530.6
    pulsion 530.6
    traction 530.6
    Zenker's 530.6
  Eustachian tube 381.89
  fallopian tube 620.8
  gallbladder (congenital) 751.69
  gastric 537.1
  heart (congenital) 746.89
  ileum 562.00
    with
      diverticulitis 562.01
        with hemorrhage 562.03
      hemorrhage 562.03
  intestine (large) 562.10
    with
      diverticulitis 562.11
        with hemorrhage 562.13
      hemorrhage 562.12
    congenital 751.5
    small 562.00
      with
        diverticulitis 562.01
          with hemorrhage 562.03
        hemorrhage 562.02
      congenital 751.5
  jejunum 562.00
    with
      diverticulitis 562.01
        with hemorrhage 562.03
      hemorrhage 562.02
  kidney (calyx) (pelvis) 593.89
    with calculus 592.0
  Kommerell's 747.21
  laryngeal ventricle (congenital)
    748.3
  Meckel's (displaced) (hypertrophic)
    751.0
  midthoracic 530.6
  organ or site, congenital NEC - *see*
    Distortion
  pericardium (congenital) (cyst)
    746.89
    acquired (true) 423.8
  pharyngoesophageal (pulsion)
    530.6
  pharynx (congenital) 750.27
  pulsion (esophagus) 530.6
  rectosigmoid 562.10
    with
      diverticulitis 562.11
        with hemorrhage 562.13
      hemorrhage 562.12
    congenital 751.5
  rectum 562.10
    with
      diverticulitis 562.11
        with hemorrhage 562.13
      hemorrhage 562.12
  renal (calyces) (pelvis) 593.89
    with calculus 592.0
  Rokitansky's 530.6
  seminal vesicle 608.0

Diverticula, diverticulosis,
    diverticulum *(Continued)*
  sigmoid 562.10
    with
      diverticulitis 562.11
        with hemorrhage 562.13
      hemorrhage 562.12
    congenital 751.5
  small intestine 562.00
    with
      diverticulitis 562.01
        with hemorrhage 562.03
      hemorrhage 562.02
  stomach (cardia) (juxtacardia)
    (juxtapyloric) (acquired) 537.1
    congenital 750.7
  subdiaphragmatic 530.6
  trachea (congenital) 748.3
    acquired 519.19
  traction (esophagus) 530.6
  ureter (acquired) 593.89
    congenital 753.4
  ureterovesical orifice 593.89
  urethra (acquired) 599.2
    congenital 753.8
  ventricle, left (congenital) 746.89
  vesical (urinary) 596.3
    congenital 753.8
  Zenker's (esophagus) 530.6
Diverticulitis (acute) *(see also* Diverticula)
    562.11
  with hemorrhage 562.13
  bladder (urinary) 596.3
  cecum (perforated) 562.11
    with hemorrhage 562.13
  colon (perforated) 562.11
    with hemorrhage 562.13
  duodenum 562.01
    with hemorrhage 562.03
  esophagus 530.6
  ileum (perforated) 562.01
    with hemorrhage 562.03
  intestine (large) (perforated) 562.11
    with hemorrhage 562.13
    small 562.01
      with hemorrhage 562.03
  jejunum (perforated) 562.01
    with hemorrhage 562.03
  Meckel's (perforated) 751.0
  pharyngoesophageal 530.6
  rectosigmoid (perforated) 562.11
    with hemorrhage 562.13
  rectum 562.11
    with hemorrhage 562.13
  sigmoid (old) (perforated) 562.11
    with hemorrhage 562.13
  small intestine (perforated) 562.01
    with hemorrhage 562.03
  vesical (urinary) 596.3
Diverticulosis - *see* Diverticula
Division
  cervix uteri 622.8
    external os into two openings by
      frenum 752.44 ◀▥
    external (cervical) into two openings
      by frenum 752.44 ◀▥
  glans penis 752.69
  hymen 752.49
  labia minora (congenital) 752.49
  ligament (partial or complete)
    (current) - *see also* Sprain, by
    site
    with open wound - *see* Wound,
      open, by site

Division *(Continued)*
    muscle (partial or complete) (current) -
        see also Sprain, by site
            with open wound - *see* Wound,
                open, by site
    nerve - *see* Injury, nerve, by site
    penis glans 752.69
    spinal cord - *see* Injury, spinal, by site
    vein 459.9
            traumatic - *see* Injury, vascular, by
                site
Divorce V61.03
Dix-Hallpike neurolabyrinthitis
    386.12
Dizziness 780.4
    hysterical 300.11
    psychogenic 306.9
Doan-Wiseman syndrome (primary
    splenic neutropenia) 289.53
Dog bite - *see* Wound, open, by site
Döhle-Heller aortitis 093.1
Döhle body-panmyelopathic syndrome
    288.2
Dolichocephaly, dolichocephalus
    754.0
Dolichocolon 751.5
Dolichostenomelia 759.82
Donohue's syndrome (leprechaunism)
    259.8
Donor
    blood V59.01
        other blood components V59.09
        stem cells V59.02
        whole blood V59.01
    bone V59.2
        marrow V59.3
    cornea V59.5
    egg (oocyte) (ovum) V59.70
        over age 35 V59.73
            anonymous recipient V59.73
            designated recipient V59.74
        under age 35 V59.71
            anonymous recipient V59.71
            designated recipient V59.72
    heart V59.8
    kidney V59.4
    liver V59.6
    lung V59.8
    lymphocyte V59.8
    organ V59.9
        specified NEC V59.8
    potential, examination of V70.8
    skin V59.1
    specified organ or tissue NEC V59.8
    sperm V59.8
    stem cells V59.02
    tissue V59.9
        specified type NEC V59.8
Donovanosis (granuloma venereum)
    099.2
DOPS (diffuse obstructive pulmonary
    syndrome) 496
Double
    albumin 273.8
    aortic arch 747.21
    auditory canal 744.29
    auricle (heart) 746.82
    bladder 753.8
    external (cervical) os 752.44 ◄▥
    kidney with double pelvis (renal)
        753.3
    larynx 748.3
    meatus urinarius 753.8
    organ or site NEC - *see* Accessory

Double *(Continued)*
    orifice
        heart valve NEC 746.89
            pulmonary 746.09
    outlet, right ventricle 745.11
    pelvis (renal) with double ureter 753.4
    penis 752.69
    tongue 750.13
    ureter (one or both sides) 753.4
        with double pelvis (renal) 753.4
    urethra 753.8
    urinary meatus 753.8
    uterus (any degree) 752.2
        with doubling of cervix and vagina
            752.2
        in pregnancy or childbirth 654.0●
            affecting fetus or newborn 763.89
    vagina 752.47 ◄▥
        with doubling of cervix and uterus
            752.2
    vision 368.2
    vocal cords 748.3
    vulva 752.49
    whammy (syndrome) 360.81
Douglas' pouch, cul-de-sac - *see* condition
Down's disease or syndrome
    (mongolism) 758.0
Down-growth, epithelial (anterior
    chamber) 364.61
DPD (dihydropyrimidine dehydrogenase
    deficiency) 277.6 ◄
Dracontiasis 125.7
Dracunculiasis 125.7
Dracunculosis 125.7
Drainage
    abscess (spontaneous) - *see* Abscess
    anomalous pulmonary veins to hepatic
        veins or right atrium 747.41
    stump (amputation) (surgical) 997.62
    suprapubic, bladder 596.8
Dream state, hysterical 300.13
Drepanocytic anemia (*see also* Disease,
    sickle cell) 282.60
Dresbach's syndrome (elliptocytosis)
    282.1
Dreschlera (infection) 118
    hawaiiensis 117.8
Dressler's syndrome (postmyocardial
    infarction) 411.0
Dribbling (post-void) 788.35
Drift, ulnar 736.09
Drinking (alcohol) - *see also* Alcoholism
    excessive, to excess NEC (*see also* Abuse,
        drugs, nondependent) 305.0●
        bouts, periodic 305.0●
        continual 303.9●
        episodic 305.0●
        habitual 303.9●
        periodic 305.0●
Drip, postnasal (chronic) 784.91
    due to:
        allergic rhinitis - *see* Rhinitis, allergic
        common cold 460
        gastroesophageal reflux - *see* Reflux,
            gastroesophageal
        nasopharyngitis - *see*
            Nasopharyngitis
        other known condition - *code to*
            condition
        sinusitis - *see* Sinusitis
Drivers' license examination V70.3
Droop
    Cooper's 611.81
    facial 781.94

Drop
    finger 736.29
    foot 736.79
    hematocrit (precipitous) 790.01
    hemoglobin 790.01
    toe 735.8
    wrist 736.05
Dropped
    dead 798.1
    heart beats 426.6
Dropsy, dropsical (*see also* Edema) 782.3
    abdomen 789.59
    amnion (*see also* Hydramnios) 657●
    brain - *see* Hydrocephalus
    cardiac (*see also* Failure, heart) 428.0
    cardiorenal (*see also* Hypertension,
        cardiorenal) 404.90
    chest 511.9
    fetus or newborn 778.0
        due to isoimmunization 773.3
    gangrenous (*see also* Gangrene) 785.4
    heart (*see also* Failure, heart) 428.0
    hepatic - *see* Cirrhosis, liver
    infantile - *see* Hydrops, fetalis
    kidney (*see also* Nephrosis) 581.9
    liver - *see* Cirrhosis, liver
    lung 514
    malarial (*see also* Malaria) 084.9
    neonatorum - *see* Hydrops, fetalis
    nephritic 581.9
    newborn - *see* Hydrops, fetalis
    nutritional 269.9
    ovary 620.8
    pericardium (*see also* Pericarditis) 423.9
    renal (*see also* Nephrosis) 581.9
    uremic - *see* Uremia
Drowned, drowning (near) 994.1
    lung 518.5
Drowsiness 780.09
Drug - *see also* condition
    addiction (*see also* Dependence)
        304.9●
    adverse effect NEC, correct substance
        properly administered 995.20 ◄▥
    allergy 995.27
    dependence (*see also* Dependence)
        304.9●
    habit (*see also* Dependence) 304.9●
    hypersensitivity 995.27
    induced
        circadian rhythm sleep disorder
            292.85
        hypersomnia 292.85
        insomnia 292.85
        mental disorder 292.9
            anxiety 292.89
            mood 292.84
            sexual 292.89
            sleep 292.85
            specified type 292.89
        parasomnia 292.85
        persisting
            amnestic disorder 292.83
            dementia 292.82
        psychotic disorder
            with
                delusions 292.11
                hallucinations 292.12
        sleep disorder 292.85
    intoxication 292.89
    overdose - *see* Table of Drugs and
        Chemicals
    poisoning - *see* Table of Drugs and
        Chemicals

◄ New   ◄▥ Revised   ~~deleted~~ Deleted   ● Use Additional Digit(s)   ▥ Omit code

Drug (Continued)
  therapy (maintenance) status NEC
    chemotherapy, antineoplastic
      V58.11
    immunotherapy, antineoplastic
      V58.12
    long-term (current) (prophylactic)
      use V58.69 ◀▥
      antibiotics V58.62
      anticoagulants V58.61
      anti-inflammatories, non-
        steroidal (NSAID) V58.64
      antiplatelets V58.63
      antithrombotics V58.63
      aspirin V58.66
      high-risk medications NEC V58.69
      insulin V58.67
      methadone V58.69
      opiate analgesic V58.69
      steroids V58.65
  wrong substance given or taken in
    error - see Table of Drugs and
    Chemicals
Drunkenness (see also Abuse, drugs,
  nondependent) 305.0●
  acute in alcoholism (see also
    Alcoholism) 303.0●
  chronic (see also Alcoholism) 303.9●
  pathologic 291.4
  simple (acute) 305.0●
    in alcoholism 303.0●
  sleep 307.47
Drusen
  optic disc or papilla 377.21
  retina (colloid) (hyaloid degeneration)
    362.57
    hereditary 362.77
Drusenfieber 075
Dry, dryness - see also condition
  eye 375.15
    syndrome 375.15
  larynx 478.79
  mouth 527.7
  nose 478.19
  skin syndrome 701.1
  socket (teeth) 526.5
  throat 478.29
DSAP (disseminated superficial actinic
  porokeratosis) 692.75
DSTR (delayed serologic transfusion
  reaction) ◀
  due to or resulting from ◀
    incompatibility ◀
      ABO 999.69 ◀
      non-ABO antigen (minor) (Duffy)
        (Kell) (Kidd) (Lewis) (M)
        (N) (P) (S) 999.79 ◀
      Rh antigen (C) (c) (D) (E) (e)
        999.74 ◀
Duane's retraction syndrome 378.71
Duane-Stilling-Türk syndrome (ocular
  retraction syndrome) 378.71
Dubin-Johnson disease or syndrome 277.4
Dubini's disease (electric chorea) 049.8
Dubois' abscess or disease 090.5
Duchenne's
  disease 094.0
    locomotor ataxia 094.0
    muscular dystrophy 359.1
    pseudohypertrophy, muscles 359.1
  paralysis 335.22
  syndrome 335.22
Duchenne-Aran myelopathic, muscular
  atrophy (nonprogressive)
  (progressive) 335.21
Duchenne-Griesinger disease 359.1

Ducrey's
  bacillus 099.0
  chancre 099.0
  disease (chancroid) 099.0
Duct, ductus - see condition
Duengero 061
Duhring's disease (dermatitis
  herpetiformis) 694.0
Dukes (-Filatov) disease 057.8
Dullness
  cardiac (decreased) (increased) 785.3
Dumb ague (see also Malaria) 084.6
Dumbness (see also Aphasia) 784.3
Dumdum fever 085.0
Dumping syndrome (postgastrectomy)
  564.2
  nonsurgical 536.8
Duodenitis (nonspecific) (peptic) 535.60
  with hemorrhage 535.61
  due to
    strongyloides stercoralis 127.2
Duodenocholangitis 575.8
Duodenum, duodenal - see condition
Duplay's disease, periarthritis, or
  syndrome 726.2
Duplex - see also Accessory
  kidney 753.3
  placenta - see Placenta, abnormal
  uterus 752.2
Duplication - see also Accessory
  anus 751.5
  aortic arch 747.21
  appendix 751.5
  biliary duct (any) 751.69
  bladder 753.8
  cecum 751.5
    and appendix 751.5
  cervical, cervix 752.44 ◀
  clitoris 752.49
  cystic duct 751.69
  digestive organs 751.8
  duodenum 751.5
  esophagus 750.4
  fallopian tube 752.19
  frontonasal process 756.0
  gallbladder 751.69
  ileum 751.5
  intestine (large) (small) 751.5
  jejunum 751.5
  kidney 753.3
  liver 751.69
  nose 748.1
  pancreas 751.7
  penis 752.69
  respiratory organs NEC 748.9
  salivary duct 750.22
  spinal cord (incomplete) 742.51
  stomach 750.7
  ureter 753.4
  vagina 752.47 ◀▥
  vas deferens 752.89
  vocal cords 748.3
Dupré's disease or syndrome
  (meningism) 781.6
Dupuytren's
  contraction 728.6
  disease (muscle contracture) 728.6
  fracture (closed) 824.4
    ankle (closed) 824.4
      open 824.5
    fibula (closed) 824.4
      open 824.5
    open 824.5
    radius (closed) 813.42
      open 813.52
  muscle contracture 728.6

Durand-Nicolas-Favre disease (climatic
  bubo) 099.1
Durotomy, incidental (inadvertent) (see
  also Tear, dural) 349.31
Duroziez's disease (congenital mitral
  stenosis) 746.5
Dust
  conjunctivitis 372.05
  reticulation (occupational) 504
Dutton's
  disease (trypanosomiasis) 086.9
  relapsing fever (West African) 087.1
Dwarf, dwarfism 259.4
  with infantilism (hypophyseal) 253.3
  achondroplastic 756.4
  Amsterdam 759.89
  bird-headed 759.89
  congenital 259.4
  constitutional 259.4
  hypophyseal 253.3
  infantile 259.4
  Levi type 253.3
  Lorain-Levi (pituitary) 253.3
  Lorain type (pituitary) 253.3
  metatropic 756.4
  nephrotic-glycosuric, with
    hypophosphatemic rickets 270.0
  nutritional 263.2
  ovarian 758.6
  pancreatic 577.8
  pituitary 253.3
  polydystrophic 277.5
  primordial 253.3
  psychosocial 259.4
  renal 588.0
    with hypertension - see
      Hypertension, kidney
  Russell's (uterine dwarfism and
    craniofacial dysostosis) 759.89
Dyke-Young anemia or syndrome
  (acquired macrocytic hemolytic
  anemia) (secondary) (symptomatic)
  283.9
Dynia abnormality (see also Defect,
  coagulation) 286.9
Dysacousis 388.40
Dysadrenocortism 255.9
  hyperfunction 255.3
  hypofunction 255.41
Dysarthria 784.51
  due to late effect of cerebrovascular
    disease (see also Late effect(s) (of)
    cerebrovascular disease) 438.13
Dysautonomia (see also Neuropathy,
  peripheral, autonomic) 337.9
  familial 742.8
Dysbarism 993.3
Dysbasia 719.7
  angiosclerotica intermittens 443.9
    due to atherosclerosis 440.21
  hysterical 300.11
  lordotica (progressiva) 333.6
  nonorganic origin 307.9
  psychogenic 307.9
Dysbetalipoproteinemia (familial) 272.2
Dyscalculia 315.1
Dyschezia (see also Constipation) 564.00
Dyschondroplasia (with hemangiomata)
  756.4
  Voorhoeve's 756.4
Dyschondrosteosis 756.59
Dyschromia 709.00
Dyscollagenosis 710.9
Dyscoria 743.41
Dyscraniopyophalangy 759.89

Dyscrasia
blood 289.9
with antepartum hemorrhage
641.3●
hemorrhage, subungual 287.8
newborn NEC 776.9
puerperal, postpartum 666.3●
ovary 256.8
plasma cell 273.9
pluriglandular 258.9
polyglandular 258.9
Dysdiadochokinesia 781.3
Dysectasia, vesical neck 596.8
Dysendocrinism 259.9
Dysentery, dysenteric (bilious)
(catarrhal) (diarrhea) (epidemic)
(gangrenous) (hemorrhagic)
(infectious) (sporadic) (tropical)
(ulcerative) 009.0
abscess, liver (see also Abscess, amebic)
006.3
amebic (see also Amebiasis) 006.9
with abscess - see Abscess, amebic
acute 006.0
carrier (suspected) of V02.2
chronic 006.1
arthritis (see also Arthritis, due to,
dysentery) 009.0 [711.3]●
bacillary 004.9 [711.3]●
asylum 004.9
bacillary 004.9
arthritis 004.9 [711.3]●
Boyd 004.2
Flexner 004.1
Schmitz (-Stutzer) 004.0
Shiga 004.0
Shigella 004.9
group A 004.0
group B 004.1
group C 004.2
group D 004.3
specified type NEC 004.8
Sonne 004.3
specified type NEC 004.8
bacterium 004.9
balantidial 007.0
Balantidium coli 007.0
Boyd's 004.2
Chilomastix 007.8
Chinese 004.9
choleriform 001.1
coccidial 007.2
Dientamoeba fragilis 007.8
due to specified organism NEC - see
Enteritis, due to, by organism
Embadomonas 007.8
Endolimax nana - see Dysentery, amebic
Entamoba, entamebic - see Dysentery,
amebic
Flexner's 004.1
Flexner-Boyd 004.2
giardial 007.1
Giardia lamblia 007.1
Hiss-Russell 004.1
lamblia 007.1
leishmanial 085.0
malarial (see also Malaria) 084.6
metazoal 127.9
Monilia 112.89
protozoal NEC 007.9
Russell's 004.8
salmonella 003.0
schistosomal 120.1
Schmitz (-Stutzer) 004.0

Dysentery, dysenteric (Continued)
Shiga 004.0
Shigella NEC (see also Dysentery,
bacillary) 004.9
boydii 004.2
dysenteriae 004.0
Schmitz 004.0
Shiga 004.0
flexneri 004.1
group A 004.0
group B 004.1
group C 004.2
group D 004.3
Schmitz 004.0
Shiga 004.0
Sonnei 004.3
Sonne 004.3
strongyloidiasis 127.2
trichomonal 007.3
tuberculous (see also Tuberculosis)
014.8●
viral (see also Enteritis, viral) 008.8
Dysequilibrium 780.4
Dysesthesia 782.0
hysterical 300.11
Dysfibrinogenemia (congenital) (see also
Defect, coagulation) 286.3
Dysfunction
adrenal (cortical) 255.9
hyperfunction 255.3
hypofunction 255.41
associated with sleep stages or arousal
from sleep 780.56
nonorganic origin 307.47
bladder NEC 596.59
bleeding, uterus 626.8
brain, minimal (see also Hyperkinesia)
314.9
cerebral 348.30
colon 564.9
psychogenic 306.4
colostomy or enterostomy 569.62
cystic duct 575.8
diastolic 429.9
with heart failure - see Failure, heart
due to
cardiomyopathy - see
Cardiomyopathy
hypertension - see Hypertension,
heart
endocrine NEC 259.9
endometrium 621.8
enteric stoma 569.62
enterostomy 569.62
erectile 607.84
nonorganic origin 302.72
esophagostomy 530.87
Eustachian tube 381.81
gallbladder 575.8
gastrointestinal 536.9
gland, glandular NEC 259.9
heart 427.9
postoperative (immediate) 997.1
long-term effect of cardiac
surgery 429.4
hemoglobin 289.89
hepatic 573.9
hepatocellular NEC 573.9
hypophysis 253.9
hyperfunction 253.1
hypofunction 253.2
posterior lobe 253.6
hypofunction 253.5
kidney (see also Disease, renal) 593.9

Dysfunction (Continued)
labyrinthine 386.50
specified NEC 386.58
liver 573.9
constitutional 277.4
minimal brain (child) (see also
Hyperkinesia) 314.9
ovary, ovarian 256.9
hyperfunction 256.1
estrogen 256.0
hypofunction 256.39
postablative 256.2
postablative 256.2
specified NEC 256.8
papillary muscle 429.81
with myocardial infarction 410.8●
parathyroid 252.8
hyperfunction 252.00
hypofunction 252.1
pineal gland 259.8
pituitary (gland) 253.9
hyperfunction 253.1
hypofunction 253.2
posterior 253.6
hypofunction 253.5
placental - see Placenta, insufficiency
platelets (blood) 287.1
polyglandular 258.9
specified NEC 258.8
psychosexual 302.70
with
dyspareunia (functional)
(psychogenic) 302.76
frigidity 302.72
impotence 302.72
inhibition
orgasm
female 302.73
male 302.74
sexual
desire 302.71
excitement 302.72
premature ejaculation 302.75
sexual aversion 302.79
specified disorder NEC 302.79
vaginismus 306.51
pylorus 537.9
rectum 564.9
psychogenic 306.4
segmental (see also Dysfunction,
somatic) 739.9
senile 797
sexual 302.70
sinoatrial node 427.81
somatic 739.9
abdomen 739.9
acromioclavicular 739.7
cervical 739.1
cervicothoracic 739.1
costochondral 739.8
costovertebral 739.8
extremities
lower 739.6
upper 739.7
head 739.0
hip 739.5
lumbar, lumbosacral 739.3
occipitocervical 739.0
pelvic 739.5
pubic 739.5
rib cage 739.8
sacral 739.4
sacrococcygeal 739.4
sacroiliac 739.4

◀ New ◀ Revised ~~deleted~~ Deleted ● Use Additional Digit(s) Omit code

Dysfunction *(Continued)*
  somatic *(Continued)*
    specified site NEC 739.9
    sternochondral 739.8
    sternoclavicular 739.7
    temporomandibular 739.0
    thoracic, thoracolumbar 739.2
  stomach 536.9
    psychogenic 306.4
  suprarenal 255.9
    hyperfunction 255.3
    hypofunction 255.41
  symbolic NEC 784.60
    specified type NEC 784.69
  systolic 429.9
    with heart failure - *see* Failure,
        heart
  temporomandibular (joint) (joint-pain-
      syndrome) NEC 524.60
    sounds on opening or closing
        524.64
    specified NEC 524.69
  testicular 257.9
    hyperfunction 257.0
    hypofunction 257.2
    specified type NEC 257.8
  thymus 254.9
  thyroid 246.9
    complicating pregnancy, childbirth,
        or puerperium 648.1●
    hyperfunction - *see* Hyperthyroidism
    hypofunction - *see* Hypothyroidism
  uterus, complicating delivery 661.9●
    affecting fetus or newborn 763.7
    hypertonic 661.4●
    hypotonic 661.2●
      primary 661.0●
      secondary 661.1●
  velopharyngeal (acquired) 528.9
    congenital 750.29
  ventricular 429.9
    with congestive heart failure *(see also*
        Failure, heart) 428.0
    due to
      cardiomyopathy - *see*
          Cardiomyopathy
      hypertension - *see* Hypertension,
          heart
    left, reversible following sudden
        emotional stress 429.83
  vesicourethral NEC 596.59
  vestibular 386.50
    specified type NEC 386.58
Dysgammaglobulinemia 279.06
Dysgenesis
  gonadal (due to chromosomal
      anomaly) 758.6
    pure 752.7
  kidney(s) 753.0
  ovarian 758.6
  renal 753.0
  reticular 279.2
  seminiferous tubules 758.6
  tidal platelet 287.31
Dysgerminoma (M9060/3)
  specified site - *see* Neoplasm, by site,
      malignant
  unspecified site
    female 183.0
    male 186.9
Dysgeusia 781.1
Dysgraphia 781.3
Dyshidrosis 705.81
Dysidrosis 705.81

Dysinsulinism 251.8
Dyskaryotic cervical smear 795.09
Dyskeratosis *(see also* Keratosis) 701.1
  bullosa hereditaria 757.39
  cervix 622.10
  congenital 757.39
  follicularis 757.39
    vitamin A deficiency 264.8
  gingiva 523.8
  oral soft tissue NEC 528.79
  tongue 528.79
  uterus NEC 621.8
Dyskinesia 781.3
  biliary 575.8
  esophagus 530.5
  hysterical 300.11
  intestinal 564.89
  neuroleptic-induced tardive 333.85
  nonorganic origin 307.9
  orofacial 333.82
    due to drugs 333.85
  psychogenic 307.9
  subacute, due to drugs 333.85
  tardive (oral) 333.85
Dyslalia 784.59
  developmental 315.39
Dyslexia 784.61
  developmental 315.02
  secondary to organic lesion 784.61
Dyslipidemia 272.4
Dysmaturity *(see also* Immaturity)
      765.1●
  lung 770.4
  pulmonary 770.4
Dysmenorrhea (essential) (exfoliative)
      (functional) (intrinsic)
      (membranous) (primary)
      (secondary) 625.3
  psychogenic 306.52
Dysmetabolic syndrome X 277.7
Dysmetria 781.3
Dysmorodystrophia mesodermalis
      congenita 759.82
Dysnomia 784.3
Dysorexia 783.0
  hysterical 300.11
Dysostosis
  cleidocranial, cleidocranialis 755.59
  craniofacial 756.0
  Fairbank's (idiopathic familial
      generalized osteophytosis)
      756.50
  mandibularis 756.0
  mandibulofacial, incomplete 756.0
  multiplex 277.5
  orodigitofacial 759.89
Dyspareunia (female) 625.0
  male 608.89
  psychogenic 302.76
Dyspepsia (allergic) (congenital)
      (fermentative) (flatulent)
      (functional) (gastric)
      (gastrointestinal) (neurogenic)
      (occupational) (reflex) 536.8
  acid 536.8
  atonic 536.3
    psychogenic 306.4
  diarrhea 787.91
    psychogenic 306.4
  intestinal 564.89
    psychogenic 306.4
  nervous 306.4
  neurotic 306.4
  psychogenic 306.4

Dysphagia 787.20
  cervical 787.29
  functional 300.11
  hysterical 300.11
  nervous 300.11
  neurogenic 787.29
  oral phase 787.21
  oropharyngeal phase 787.22
  pharyngeal phase 787.23
  pharyngoesophageal phase 787.24
  psychogenic 306.4
  sideropenic 280.8
  spastica 530.5
  specified NEC 787.29
Dysphagocytosis, congenital 288.1
Dysphasia 784.59
Dysphonia 784.42
  clericorum 784.49
  functional 300.11
  hysterical 300.11
  psychogenic 306.1
  spastica 478.79
Dyspigmentation - *see also* Pigmentation
  eyelid (acquired) 374.52
Dyspituitarism 253.9
  hyperfunction 253.1
  hypofunction 253.2
  posterior lobe 253.6
Dysplasia - *see also* Anomaly
  anus 569.44
    intraepithelial neoplasia I (AIN I)
        (histologically confirmed)
        569.44 ◀▥
    intraepithelial neoplasia II (AIN II)
        (histologically confirmed)
        569.44 ◀▥
    intraepithelial neoplasia III (AIN III)
        230.6 ◀▥
    anal canal 230.5
    mild (histologically confirmed)
        569.44
    moderate (histologically confirmed)
        569.44
    severe 230.6
    anal canal 230.5
  artery
    fibromuscular NEC 447.8
      carotid 447.8
      renal 447.3
  bladder 596.8
  bone (fibrous) NEC 733.29
    diaphyseal, progressive 756.59
    jaw 526.89
    monostotic 733.29
    polyostotic 756.54
    solitary 733.29
  brain 742.9
  bronchopulmonary, fetus or newborn
      770.7
  cervix (uteri) 622.10
    cervical intraepithelial neoplasia I
        (CIN I) 622.11 ◀▥
    cervical intraepithelial neoplasia II
        (CIN II) 622.12 ◀▥
    cervical intraepithelial neoplasia III
        (CIN III) 233.1 ◀▥
    CIN I 622.11
    CIN II 622.12
    CIN III 233.1
    mild 622.11
    moderate 622.12
    severe 233.1
  chondroectodermal 756.55
  chondromatose 756.4

Dysplasia (*Continued*)
  colon 211.3
  craniocarpotarsal 759.89
  craniometaphyseal 756.89
  dentinal 520.5
  diaphyseal, progressive 756.59
  ectodermal (anhidrotic) (Bason)
        (Clouston's) (congenital)
        (Feinmesser) (hereditary)
        (hidrotic) (Marshall)
        (Robinson's) 757.31
  epiphysealis 756.9
      multiplex 756.56
      punctata 756.59
  epiphysis 756.9
      multiple 756.56
  epithelial
      epiglottis 478.79
      uterine cervix 622.10
  erythroid NEC 289.89
  eye (*see also* Microphthalmos)
        743.10
  familial metaphyseal 756.89
  fibromuscular, artery NEC 447.8
      carotid 447.8
      renal 447.3
  fibrous
      bone NEC 733.29
      diaphyseal, progressive 756.59
      jaw 526.89
      monostotic 733.29
      polyostotic 756.54
      solitary 733.29
  high grade, focal - *see* Neoplasm, by
        site, benign
  hip (congenital) 755.63
      with dislocation (*see also* Dislocation,
          hip, congenital) 754.30
  hypohidrotic ectodermal 757.31
  joint 755.8
  kidney 753.15
  leg 755.69
  linguofacialis 759.89
  lung 748.5
  macular 743.55
  mammary (benign) (gland) 610.9
      cystic 610.1
      specified type NEC 610.8
  metaphyseal 756.9
      familial 756.89
  monostotic fibrous 733.29
  muscle 756.89
  myeloid NEC 289.89
  nervous system (general) 742.9
  neuroectodermal 759.6
  oculoauriculovertebral 756.0
  oculodentodigital 759.89
  olfactogenital 253.4
  osteo-onycho-arthro (hereditary) 756.89
  periosteum 733.99
  polyostotic fibrous 756.54
  progressive diaphyseal 756.59
  prostate 602.3
      intraepithelial neoplasia I
          [PIN I] 602.3
      intraepithelial neoplasia II
          [PIN II] 602.3
      intraepithelial neoplasia III
          [PIN III] 233.4
  renal 753.15
  renofacialis 753.0
  retinal NEC 743.56
  retrolental (*see also* Retinopathy of
        prematurity) 362.21

Dysplasia (*Continued*)
  skin 709.8
  spinal cord 742.9
  thymic, with immunodeficiency
        279.2
  vagina 623.0
      mild 623.0
      moderate 623.0
      severe 233.31
  vocal cord 478.5
  vulva 624.8
      intraepithelial neoplasia I (VIN I)
          624.01 ◀▥
      intraepithelial neoplasia II (VIN II)
          624.02 ◀▥
      intraepithelial neoplasia III (VIN III)
          233.32 ◀▥
      mild 624.01
      moderate 624.02
      severe 233.32
      VIN I 624.01
      VIN II 624.02
      VIN III 233.32
Dyspnea (nocturnal) (paroxysmal) 786.09
  asthmatic (bronchial) (*see also* Asthma)
        493.9●
      with bronchitis (*see also* Asthma)
          493.9●
      chronic 493.2●
  cardiac (*see also* Failure, ventricular,
        left) 428.1
  cardiac (*see also* Failure, ventricular,
        left) 428.1
  functional 300.11
  hyperventilation 786.01
  hysterical 300.11
  Monday morning 504
  newborn 770.89
  psychogenic 306.1
  uremic - *see* Uremia
Dyspraxia 781.3
  syndrome 315.4
Dysproteinemia 273.8
  transient with copper deficiency
        281.4
Dysprothrombinemia (constitutional)
        (*see also* Defect, coagulation) 286.3
Dysreflexia, autonomic 337.3
Dysrhythmia
  cardiac 427.9
      postoperative (immediate) 997.1
          long-term effect of cardiac
              surgery 429.4
      specified type NEC 427.89
  cerebral or cortical 348.30
Dyssecretosis, mucoserous 710.2
Dyssocial reaction, without manifest
        psychiatric disorder
  adolescent V71.02
  adult V71.01
  child V71.02
Dyssomnia NEC 780.56
  nonorganic origin 307.47
Dyssplenism 289.4
Dyssynergia
  biliary (*see also* Disease, biliary)
        576.8
  cerebellaris myoclonica 334.2
  detrusor sphincter (bladder) 596.55
  ventricular 429.89
Dystasia, hereditary areflexic 334.3
Dysthymia 300.4
Dysthymic disorder 300.4
Dysthyroidism 246.9

Dystocia 660.9●
  affecting fetus or newborn 763.1
  cervical 661.2●
      affecting fetus or newborn 763.7
  contraction ring 661.4●
      affecting fetus or newborn 763.7
  fetal 660.9●
      abnormal size 653.5●
      affecting fetus or newborn 763.1
      deformity 653.7●
  maternal 660.9●
      affecting fetus or newborn 763.1
  positional 660.0●
      affecting fetus or newborn 763.1
  shoulder (girdle) 660.4●
      affecting fetus or newborn 763.1
  uterine NEC 661.4●
      affecting fetus or newborn 763.7
Dystonia
  acute
      due to drugs 333.72
          neuroleptic-induced acute 333.72
  deformans progressiva 333.6
  lenticularis 333.6
  musculorum deformans 333.6
  torsion (idiopathic) 333.6
      acquired 333.79
      fragments (of) 333.89
      genetic 333.6
      symptomatic 333.79
Dystonic
  movements 781.0
Dystopia kidney 753.3
Dystrophy, dystrophia 783.9
  adiposogenital 253.8
  asphyxiating thoracic 756.4
  Becker's type 359.22
  brevicollis 756.16
  Bruch's membrane 362.77
  cervical (sympathetic) NEC 337.09
  chondro-osseus with punctate
        epiphyseal dysplasia 756.59
  choroid (hereditary) 363.50
      central (areolar) (partial) 363.53
          total (gyrate) 363.54
      circinate 363.53
      circumpapillary (partial) 363.51
          total 363.52
      diffuse
          partial 363.56
          total 363.57
      generalized
          partial 363.56
          total 363.57
      gyrate
          central 363.54
          generalized 363.57
      helicoid 363.52
      peripapillary - *see* Dystrophy,
            choroid, circumpapillary
      serpiginous 363.54
  cornea (hereditary) 371.50
      anterior NEC 371.52
      Cogan's 371.52
      combined 371.57
      crystalline 371.56
      endothelial (Fuchs') 371.57
      epithelial 371.50
          juvenile 371.51
          microscopic cystic 371.52
      granular 371.53
      lattice 371.54
      macular 371.55
      marginal (Terrien's) 371.48

◀ New   ◀▥ Revised   ~~deleted~~ Deleted   ● Use Additional Digit(s)   ▥ Omit code

Dystrophy, dystrophia *(Continued)*
  cornea *(Continued)*
    Meesman's 371.51
    microscopic cystic (epithelial)
      371.52
    nodular, Salzmann's 371.46
    polymorphous 371.58
    posterior NEC 371.58
    ring-like 371.52
    Salzmann's nodular 371.46
    stromal NEC 371.56
  dermatochondrocorneal 371.50
  Duchenne's 359.1
  due to malnutrition 263.9
  Erb's 359.1
  familial
    hyperplastic periosteal 756.59
    osseous 277.5
  foveal 362.77
  Fuchs', cornea 371.57
  Gowers' muscular 359.1
  hair 704.2
  hereditary, progressive muscular
    359.1
  hypogenital, with diabetic tendency
    759.81
  Landouzy-Déjérine 359.1
  Leyden-Möbius 359.1
  mesodermalis congenita 759.82
  muscular 359.1
    congenital (hereditary) 359.0
      myotonic 359.22
    distal 359.1
    Duchenne's 359.1
    Erb's 359.1
    fascioscapulohumeral 359.1
    Gowers' 359.1
    hereditary (progressive) 359.1

Dystrophy, dystrophia *(Continued)*
  muscular *(Continued)*
    Landouzy-Déjérine 359.1
    limb-girdle 359.1
    myotonic 359.21
    progressive (hereditary) 359.1
      Charcôt-Marie-Tooth 356.1
    pseudohypertrophic (infantile)
      359.1
  myocardium, myocardial *(see also*
    Degeneration, myocardial)
    429.1
  myotonic 359.21
  myotonica 359.21
  nail 703.8
    congenital 757.5
  neurovascular (traumatic) *(see also*
    Neuropathy, peripheral,
    autonomic) 337.9
  nutritional 263.9
  ocular 359.1
  oculocerebrorenal 270.8
  oculopharyngeal 359.1
  ovarian 620.8
  papillary (and pigmentary) 701.1
  pelvicrural atrophic 359.1
  pigmentary *(see also* Acanthosis)
    701.2
  pituitary (gland) 253.8
  polyglandular 258.8
  posttraumatic sympathetic - *see*
    Dystrophy, symphatic
  progressive ophthalmoplegic 359.1
  reflex neuromuscular - *see* Dystrophy,
    sympathetic
  retina, retinal (hereditary) 362.70
    albipunctate 362.74
    Bruch's membrane 362.77

Dystrophy, dystrophia *(Continued)*
  retina, retinal *(Continued)*
    cone, progressive 362.75
    hyaline 362.77
    in
      Bassen-Kornzweig syndrome
        272.5 *[362.72]*
      cerebroretinal lipidosis 330.1
        [362.71]
      Refsum's disease 356.3 *[362.72]*
      systemic lipidosis 272.7 *[362.71]*
    juvenile (Stargardt's) 362.75
    pigmentary 362.74
    pigment epithelium 362.76
    progressive cone (-rod) 362.75
    pseudoinflammatory foveal
      362.77
    rod, progressive 362.75
    sensory 362.75
    vitelliform 362.76
  Salzmann's nodular 371.46
  scapuloperoneal 359.1
  skin NEC 709.9
  sympathetic (posttraumatic) (reflex)
    337.20
    lower limb 337.22
    specified site NEC 337.29
    upper limb 337.21
  tapetoretinal NEC 362.74
  thoracic asphyxiating 756.4
  unguium 703.8
    congenital 757.5
  vitreoretinal (primary) 362.73
    secondary 362.66
  vulva 624.09
Dysuria 788.1
  psychogenic 306.53

E

Eagle-Barrett syndrome 756.71
Eales' disease (syndrome) 362.18
Ear - *see also* condition
  ache 388.70
    otogenic 388.71
    referred 388.72
  lop 744.29
  piercing V50.3
  swimmers' acute 380.12
  tank 380.12
  tropical 111.8 *[380.15]*
  wax 380.4
Earache 388.70
  otogenic 388.71
  referred 388.72
Early satiety 780.94
Eaton-Lambert syndrome (*see also*
  Neoplasm, by site, malignant)
  199.1 *[358.1]*
Eberth's disease (typhoid fever) 002.0
Ebstein's
  anomaly or syndrome (downward
    displacement, tricuspid valve
    into right ventricle) 746.2
  disease (diabetes) 250.4● *[581.81]*
    due to secondary diabetes 249.4●
      [581.81]
Eccentro-osteochondrodysplasia
  277.5
Ecchondroma (M9210/0) - *see* Neoplasm,
  bone, benign
Ecchondrosis (M9210/1) 238.0
Ecchordosis physaliphora 756.0
Ecchymosis (multiple) 459.89
  conjunctiva 372.72
  eye (traumatic) 921.0
  eyelids (traumatic) 921.1
  newborn 772.6
  spontaneous 782.7
  traumatic - *see* Contusion
ECD (Erdheim-Chester disease)
  277.89
Echinococciasis - *see* Echinococcus
Echinococcosis - *see* Echinococcus
Echinococcus (infection) 122.9
  granulosus 122.4
    liver 122.0
    lung 122.1
    orbit 122.3 *[376.13]*
    specified site NEC 122.3
    thyroid 122.2
  liver NEC 122.8
    granulosus 122.0
    multilocularis 122.5
  lung NEC 122.9
    granulosus 122.1
    multilocularis 122.6
  multilocularis 122.7
    liver 122.5
    specified site NEC 122.6
  orbit 122.9 *[376.13]*
    granulosus 122.3 *[376.13]*
    multilocularis 122.6 *[376.13]*
  specified site NEC 122.9
    granulosus 122.3
    multilocularis 122.6 *[376.13]*
  thyroid NEC 122.9
    granulosus 122.2
    multilocularis 122.6
Echinorhynchiasis 127.7
Echinostomiasis 121.8
Echolalia 784.69
ECHO virus infection NEC 079.1

Eclampsia, eclamptic (coma)
  (convulsions) (delirium) 780.39
  female, child-bearing age NEC - *see*
    Eclampsia, pregnancy
  gravidarum - *see* Eclampsia, pregnancy
  male 780.39
  not associated with pregnancy or
    childbirth 780.39
  pregnancy, childbirth, or puerperium
    642.6●
    with pre-existing hypertension
      642.7●
    affecting fetus or newborn 760.0
  uremic 586
Eclipse blindness (total) 363.31
Economic circumstance affecting care
  V60.9
  specified type NEC V60.89
Economo's disease (encephalitis
  lethargica) 049.8
Ectasia, ectasis
  annuloaortic 424.1 ◀
  aorta (see also Aneurysm, aorta) 441.9
    (*see also* Ectasia, aortic) 447.70 ◀▥
    with aneurysm 441.9 ◀
    ruptured 441.5
  aortic 447.70 ◀
    with aneurysm 441.9 ◀
    abdominal 447.72 ◀
    thoracic 447.71 ◀
    thoracoabdominal 447.73 ◀
  breast 610.4
  capillary 448.9
  cornea (marginal) (postinfectional) 371.71
  duct (mammary) 610.4
  gastric antral vascular (GAVE) 537.82
    with hemorrhage 537.83
    without hemorrhage 537.82
  kidney 593.89
  mammary duct (gland) 610.4
  papillary 448.9
  renal 593.89
  salivary gland (duct) 527.8
  scar, cornea 371.71
  sclera 379.11
Ecthyma 686.8
  contagiosum 051.2
  gangrenosum 686.09
  infectiosum 051.2
Ectocardia 746.87
Ectodermal dysplasia, congenital 757.31
Ectodermosis erosiva pluriorificialis 695.19
Ectopic, ectopia (congenital) 759.89
  abdominal viscera 751.8
    due to defect in anterior abdominal
      wall 756.79
  ACTH syndrome 255.0
  adrenal gland 759.1
  anus 751.5
  auricular beats 427.61
  beats 427.60
  bladder 753.5
  bone and cartilage in lung 748.69
  brain 742.4
  breast tissue 757.6
  cardiac 746.87
  cerebral 742.4
  cordis 746.87
  endometrium 617.9
  gallbladder 751.69
  gastric mucosa 750.7
  gestation - *see* Pregnancy, ectopic
  heart 746.87
  hormone secretion NEC 259.3
  hyperparathyroidism 259.3

Ectopic, ectopia (*Continued*)
  kidney (crossed) (intrathoracic) (pelvis)
    753.3
    in pregnancy or childbirth 654.4●
      causing obstructed labor 660.2●
  lens 743.37
  lentis 743.37
  mole - *see* Pregnancy, ectopic
  organ or site NEC - *see* Malposition,
    congenital
  ovary 752.0
  pancreas, pancreatic tissue 751.7
  pregnancy - *see* Pregnancy, ectopic
  pupil 364.75
  renal 753.3
  sebaceous glands of mouth 750.26
  secretion
    ACTH 255.0
    adrenal hormone 259.3
    adrenalin 259.3
    adrenocorticotropin 255.0
    antidiuretic hormone (ADH) 259.3
    epinephrine 259.3
    hormone NEC 259.3
    norepinephrine 259.3
    pituitary (posterior) 259.3
  spleen 759.0
  testis 752.51
  thyroid 759.2
  ureter 753.4
  ventricular beats 427.69
  vesicae 753.5
Ectrodactyly 755.4
  finger (*see also* Absence, finger,
    congenital) 755.29
  toe (*see also* Absence, toe, congenital)
    755.39
Ectromelia 755.4
  lower limb 755.30
  upper limb 755.20
Ectropion 374.10
  anus 569.49
  cervix 622.0
    with mention of cervicitis 616.0
  cicatricial 374.14
  congenital 743.62
  eyelid 374.10
    cicatricial 374.14
    congenital 743.62
    mechanical 374.12
    paralytic 374.12
    senile 374.11
    spastic 374.13
  iris (pigment epithelium) 364.54
  lip (congenital) 750.26
    acquired 528.5
  mechanical 374.12
  paralytic 374.12
  rectum 569.49
  senile 374.11
  spastic 374.13
  urethra 599.84
  uvea 364.54
Eczema (acute) (allergic) (chronic)
  (erythematous) (fissum)
  (occupational) (rubrum) (squamous)
  692.9
  asteatotic 706.8
  atopic 691.8
  contact NEC 692.9
  dermatitis NEC 692.9
  due to specified cause - *see* Dermatitis,
    due to
  dyshidrotic 705.81
  external ear 380.22

◀ New   ◀▥ Revised   ~~deleted~~ Deleted   ● Use Additional Digit(s)   ▨ Omit code

Eczema *(Continued)*
flexural 691.8
gouty 274.89
herpeticum 054.0
hypertrophicum 701.8
hypostatic - *see* Varicose, vein
impetiginous 684
infantile (acute) (chronic) (due to any
substance) (intertriginous)
(seborrheic) 690.12
intertriginous NEC 692.9
infantile 690.12
intrinsic 691.8
lichenified NEC 692.9
marginatum 110.3
nummular 692.9
pustular 686.8
seborrheic 690.18
infantile 690.12
solare 692.72
stasis (lower extremity) 454.1
ulcerated 454.2
vaccination, vaccinatum 999.0
varicose (lower extremity) - *see*
Varicose, vein
verrucosum callosum 698.3
Eczematoid, exudative 691.8
Eddowes' syndrome (brittle bones and
blue sclera) 756.51
Edema, edematous 782.3
with nephritis (*see also* Nephrosis)
581.9
allergic 995.1
angioneurotic (allergic) (any site)
(with urticaria) 995.1
hereditary 277.6
angiospastic 443.9
Berlin's (traumatic) 921.3
brain (cytotoxic) (vasogenic) 348.5 ◀▥
due to birth injury 767.8
fetus or newborn 767.8
cardiac (*see also* Failure, heart) 428.0
cardiovascular (*see also* Failure, heart)
428.0
cerebral - *see* Edema, brain
cerebrospinal vessel - *see* Edema,
brain
cervix (acute) (uteri) 622.8
puerperal, postpartum 674.8●
chronic hereditary 757.0
circumscribed, acute 995.1
hereditary 277.6
complicating pregnancy (gestational)
646.1●
with hypertension - *see* Toxemia, of
pregnancy
conjunctiva 372.73
connective tissue 782.3
cornea 371.20
due to contact lenses 371.24
idiopathic 371.21
secondary 371.22
cystoid macular 362.53
due to
lymphatic obstruction - *see* Edema,
lymphatic
salt retention 276.0
epiglottis - *see* Edema, glottis
essential, acute 995.1
hereditary 277.6
extremities, lower - *see* Edema, legs
eyelid NEC 374.82
familial, hereditary (legs) 757.0
famine 262
fetus or newborn 778.5

Edema, edematous *(Continued)*
genital organs
female 629.89
male 608.86
gestational 646.1●
with hypertension - *see* Toxemia, of
pregnancy
glottis, glottic, glottides (obstructive)
(passive) 478.6
allergic 995.1
hereditary 277.6
due to external agent - *see*
Condition, respiratory, acute,
due to specified agent
heart (*see also* Failure, heart) 428.0
newborn 779.89
heat 992.7
hereditary (legs) 757.0
inanition 262
infectious 782.3
intracranial 348.5
due to injury at birth 767.8
iris 364.89
joint (*see also* Effusion, joint) 719.0●
larynx (*see also* Edema, glottis) 478.6
legs 782.3
due to venous obstruction 459.2
hereditary 757.0
localized 782.3
due to venous obstruction 459.2
lower extremity 459.2
lower extremities - *see* Edema, legs
lung 514
acute 518.4
with heart disease or failure (*see*
also Failure, ventricular, left)
428.1
congestive 428.0
chemical (due to fumes or
vapors) 506.1
due to
external agent(s) NEC 508.9
specified NEC 508.8
fumes and vapors (chemical)
(inhalation) 506.1
radiation 508.0
chemical (acute) 506.1
chronic 506.4
chronic 514
chemical (due to fumes or
vapors) 506.4
due to
external agent(s) NEC 508.9
specified NEC 508.8
fumes or vapors (chemical)
(inhalation) 506.4
radiation 508.1
due to
external agent 508.9
specified NEC 508.8
high altitude 993.2
near drowning 994.1
postoperative 518.4
terminal 514
lymphatic 457.1
due to mastectomy operation 457.0
macula 362.83
cystoid 362.53
diabetic 250.5● [362.07]
due to secondary diabetes 249.5●
[362.07]
malignant (*see also* Gangrene, gas) 040.0
Milroy's 757.0
nasopharynx 478.25
neonatorum 778.5

Edema, edematous *(Continued)*
nutritional (newborn) 262
with dyspigmentation, skin and hair
260
optic disc or nerve - *see* Papilledema
orbit 376.33
circulatory 459.89
palate (soft) (hard) 528.9
pancreas 577.8
penis 607.83
periodic 995.1
hereditary 277.6
pharynx 478.25
pitting 782.3
pulmonary - *see* Edema, lung
Quincke's 995.1
hereditary 277.6
renal (*see also* Nephrosis) 581.9
retina (localized) (macular) (peripheral)
362.83
cystoid 362.53
diabetic 250.5● [362.07]
due to secondary diabetes 249.5●
[362.07]
salt 276.0
scrotum 608.86
seminal vesicle 608.86
spermatic cord 608.86
spinal cord 336.1
starvation 262
stasis - *see also* Hypertension, venous
459.30
subconjunctival 372.73
subglottic (*see also* Edema, glottis)
478.6
supraglottic (*see also* Edema, glottis)
478.6
testis 608.86
toxic NEC 782.3
traumatic NEC 782.3
tunica vaginalis 608.86
vas deferens 608.86
vocal cord - *see* Edema, glottis
vulva (acute) 624.8
Edentia (complete) (partial) (*see also*
Absence, tooth) 520.0
acquired (*see also* Edentulism) 525.40
due to
caries 525.13
extraction 525.10
periodontal disease 525.12
specified NEC 525.19
trauma 525.11
causing malocclusion 524.30
congenital (deficiency of tooth buds)
520.0
Edentulism 525.40
complete 525.40
class I 525.41
class II 525.42
class III 525.43
class IV 525.44
partial 525.50
class I 525.51
class II 525.52
class III 525.53
class IV 525.54
Edsall's disease 992.2
Educational handicap V62.3
Edwards' syndrome 758.2
Effect, adverse NEC
abnormal gravitational (G) forces or
states 994.9
air pressure - *see* Effect, adverse,
atmospheric pressure

Effect, adverse NEC (*Continued*)
altitude (high) - *see* Effect, adverse, high altitude
anesthetic
  in labor and delivery NEC 668.9●
    affecting fetus or newborn 763.5
antitoxin - *see* Complications, vaccination
atmospheric pressure 993.9
  due to explosion 993.4
  high 993.3
  low - *see* Effect, adverse, high altitude
  specified effect NEC 993.8
biological, correct substance properly administered (*see also* Effect, adverse, drug) 995.20
blood (derivatives) (serum) (transfusion) - *see* Complications, transfusion
chemical substance NEC 989.9
  specified - *see* Table of Drugs and Chemicals
cobalt, radioactive (*see also* Effect, adverse, radioactive substance) 990
cold (temperature) (weather) 991.9
  chilblains 991.5
  frostbite - *see* Frostbite
  specified effect NEC 991.8
drugs and medicinals 995.20
  correct substance properly administered 995.20
  overdose or wrong substance given or taken 977.9
  specified drug - *see* Table of Drugs and Chemicals
electric current (shock) 994.8
  burn - *see* Burn, by site
electricity (electrocution) (shock) 994.8
  burn - *see* Burn, by site
exertion (excessive) 994.5
exposure 994.9
  exhaustion 994.4
external cause NEC 994.9
fallout (radioactive) NEC 990
fluoroscopy NEC 990
foodstuffs
  allergic reaction (*see also* Allergy, food) 693.1
    anaphylactic shock due to food NEC 995.60
  noxious 988.9
    specified type NEC (*see also* Poisoning, by name of noxious foodstuff) 988.8
gases, fumes, or vapors - *see* Table of Drugs and Chemicals
glue (airplane) sniffing 304.6●
heat - *see* Heat
high altitude NEC 993.2
  anoxia 993.2
  on
    ears 993.0
    sinuses 993.1
  polycythemia 289.0
hot weather - *see* Heat
hunger 994.2
immersion, foot 991.4
immunization - *see* Complications, vaccination
immunological agents - *see* Complications, vaccination
implantation (removable) of isotope or radium NEC 990

Effect, adverse NEC (*Continued*)
infrared (radiation) (rays) NEC 990
  burn - *see* Burn, by site
  dermatitis or eczema 692.82
infusion - *see* Complications, infusion
ingestion or injection of isotope (therapeutic) NEC 990
irradiation NEC (*see also* Effect, adverse, radiation) 990
isotope (radioactive) NEC 990
lack of care (child) (infant) (newborn) 995.52
  adult 995.84
lightning 994.0
  burn - *see* Burn, by site
Lirugin - *see* Complications, vaccination
medicinal substance, correct, properly administered (*see also* Effect, adverse, drugs) 995.20
mesothorium NEC 990
motion 994.6
noise, inner ear 388.10
other drug, medicinal and biological substance 995.29
overheated places - *see* Heat
polonium NEC 990
psychosocial, of work environment V62.1
radiation (diagnostic) (fallout) (infrared) (natural source) (therapeutic) (tracer) (ultraviolet) (x-ray) NEC 990
  with pulmonary manifestations
    acute 508.0
    chronic 508.1
  dermatitis or eczema 692.82
    due to sun NEC (*see also* Dermatitis, due to, sun) 692.70
  fibrosis of lungs 508.1
  maternal with suspected damage to fetus affecting management of pregnancy 655.6●
  pneumonitis 508.0
radioactive substance NEC 990
  dermatitis or eczema 692.82
radioactivity NEC 990
radiotherapy NEC 990
  dermatitis or eczema 692.82
radium NEC 990
reduced temperature 991.9
  frostbite - *see* Frostbite
  immersion, foot (hand) 991.4
  specified effect NEC 991.8
roentgenography NEC 990
roentgenoscopy NEC 990
roentgen rays NEC 990
serum (prophylactic) (therapeutic) NEC 999.5
specified NEC 995.89
  external cause NEC 994.9
strangulation 994.7
submersion 994.1
teletherapy NEC 990
thirst 994.3
transfusion - *see* Complications, transfusion
ultraviolet (radiation) (rays) NEC 990
  burn - *see also* Burn, by site
    from sun (*see also* Sunburn) 692.71
  dermatitis or eczema 692.82
    due to sun NEC (*see also* Dermatitis, due to, sun) 692.70

Effect, adverse NEC (*Continued*)
uranium NEC 990
vaccine (any) - *see* Complications, vaccination
weightlessness 994.9
whole blood - *see also* Complications, transfusion
  overdose or wrong substance given (*see also* Table of Drugs and Chemicals) 964.7
working environment V62.1
x-rays NEC 990
  dermatitis or eczema 692.82
Effect, remote
of cancer - *see* condition
Effects, late - *see* Late, effect (of)
Effluvium, telogen 704.02
Effort
intolerance 306.2
syndrome (aviators) (psychogenic) 306.2
Effusion
amniotic fluid (*see also* Rupture, membranes, premature) 658.1●
brain (serous) 348.5
bronchial (*see also* Bronchitis) 490
cerebral 348.5
cerebrospinal (*see also* Meningitis) 322.9
  vessel 348.5
chest - *see* Effusion, pleura
intracranial 348.5
joint 719.00
  ankle 719.07
  elbow 719.02
  foot 719.07
  hand 719.04
  hip 719.05
  knee 719.06
  multiple sites 719.09
  pelvic region 719.05
  shoulder (region) 719.01
  specified site NEC 719.08
  wrist 719.03
meninges (*see also* Meningitis) 322.9
pericardium, pericardial (*see also* Pericarditis) 423.9
  acute 420.90
peritoneal (chronic) 568.82
pleura, pleurisy, pleuritic, pleuropericardial 511.9
  bacterial, nontuberculous 511.1
  fetus or newborn 511.9
  malignant 511.81
  nontuberculous 511.9
    bacterial 511.1
  pneumococcal 511.1
  staphylococcal 511.1
  streptococcal 511.1
  traumatic 862.29
    with open wound 862.39
  tuberculous (*see also* Tuberculosis, pleura) 012.0●
    primary progressive 010.1●
pulmonary - *see* Effusion, pleura
spinal (*see also* Meningitis) 322.9
thorax, thoracic - *see* Effusion, pleura
Egg (oocyte) (ovum)
donor V59.70
  over age 35 V59.73
    anonymous recipient V59.73
    designated recipient V59.74
  under age 35 V59.71
    anonymous recipient V59.71
    designated recipient V59.72
Eggshell nails 703.8
congenital 757.5

◄ New   ◄▦ Revised   ~~deleted~~ Deleted   ● Use Additional Digit(s)   ▦ Omit code

Ego-dystonic
  homosexuality 302.0
  lesbianism 302.0
  sexual orientation 302.0
Egyptian splenomegaly 120.1
Ehlers-Danlos syndrome 756.83
Ehrlichiosis 082.40
  chaffeensis 082.41
  specified type NEC 082.49
Eichstedt's disease (pityriasis versicolor)
  111.0
EIN (endometrial intraepithelial
  neoplasia) 621.35
Eisenmenger's complex or syndrome
  (ventricular septal defect) 745.4
Ejaculation, semen
  painful 608.89
    psychogenic 306.59
  premature 302.75
  retrograde 608.87
Ekbom syndrome (restless legs) 333.94
Ekman's syndrome (brittle bones and
  blue sclera) 756.51
Elastic skin 756.83
  acquired 701.8
Elastofibroma (M8820/0) - see Neoplasm,
  connective tissue, benign
Elastoidosis
  cutanea nodularis 701.8
  cutis cystica et comedonica 701.8
Elastoma 757.39
  juvenile 757.39
  Miescher's (elastosis perforans
    serpiginosa) 701.1
Elastomyofibrosis 425.3
Elastosis 701.8
  atrophicans 701.8
  perforans serpiginosa 701.1
  reactive perforating 701.1
  senilis 701.8
  solar (actinic) 692.74
Elbow - see condition
Electric
  current, electricity, effects (concussion)
    (fatal) (nonfatal) (shock) 994.8
    burn - see Burn, by site
  feet (foot) syndrome 266.2
  shock from electroshock gun (taser)
    994.8
Electrocution 994.8
Electrolyte imbalance 276.9
  with
    abortion - see Abortion, by type,
      with metabolic disorder
    ectopic pregnancy (see also
      categories 633.0–633.9) 639.4
    hyperemesis gravidarum (before 22
      completed weeks' gestation)
      643.1●
    molar pregnancy (see also categories
      630–632) 639.4
  following
    abortion 639.4
    ectopic or molar pregnancy 639.4
Elephant man syndrome 237.71
Elephantiasis (nonfilarial) 457.1
  arabicum (see also Infestation, filarial)
    125.9
  congenita hereditaria 757.0
  congenital (any site) 757.0
  due to
    Brugia (malayi) 125.1
    mastectomy operation 457.0
    Wuchereria (bancrofti) 125.0
      malayi 125.1

Elephantiasis (Continued)
  eyelid 374.83
  filarial (see also Infestation, filarial)
    125.9
  filariensis (see also Infestation, filarial)
    125.9
  gingival 523.8
  glandular 457.1
  graecorum 030.9
  lymphangiectatic 457.1
  lymphatic vessel 457.1
    due to mastectomy operation 457.0
  neuromatosa 237.71
  postmastectomy 457.0
  scrotum 457.1
  streptococcal 457.1
  surgical 997.99
    postmastectomy 457.0
  telangiectodes 457.1
  vulva (nonfilarial) 624.8
Elevated - see Elevation
  findings on laboratory examination -
    see Findings, abnormal, without
    diagnosis (examination)
    (laboratory test)
  GFR (glomerular filtration rate) -
    see Findings, abnormal, without
    diagnosis (examination)
    (laboratory test)
Elevation
  17-ketosteroids 791.9
  acid phosphatase 790.5
  alkaline phosphatase 790.5
  amylase 790.5
  antibody titers 795.79
  basal metabolic rate (BMR) 794.7
  blood pressure (see also Hypertension)
    401.9
    reading (incidental) (isolated)
      (nonspecific), no diagnosis of
      hypertension 796.2
  blood sugar 790.29
  body temperature (of unknown origin)
    (see also Pyrexia) 780.60
  C-reactive protein (CRP) 790.95
  cancer antigen 125 [CA 125] 795.82
  carcinoembryonic antigen [CEA]
    795.81
  cholesterol 272.0
    with high triglycerides 272.2
  conjugate, eye 378.81
  CRP (C-reactive protein) 790.95
  diaphragm, congenital 756.6
  GFR (glomerular filtration rate) - see
    Findings, abnormal, without
    diagnosis (examination)
    (laboratory test)
  glucose
    fasting 790.21
    tolerance test 790.22
  immunoglobulin level 795.79
  indolacetic acid 791.9
  lactic acid dehydrogenase (LDH) level
    790.4
  leukocytes 288.60
  lipase 790.5
  lipoprotein a level 272.8
  liver function test (LFT) 790.6
    alkaline phosphatase 790.5
    aminotransferase 790.4
    bilirubin 782.4
    hepatic enzyme NEC 790.5
    lactate dehydrogenase 790.4
  lymphocytes 288.61
  prostate specific antigen (PSA)
    790.93

Elevation (Continued)
  renin 790.99
    in hypertension (see also
      Hypertension, renovascular)
      405.91
  Rh titer (see also Complications,
    transfusion) 999.70 ◀▥
  scapula, congenital 755.52
  sedimentation rate 790.1
  SGOT 790.4
  SGPT 790.4
  transaminase 790.4
  triglycerides 272.1
    with high cholesterol 272.2
  vanillylmandelic acid 791.9
  venous pressure 459.89
  VMA 791.9
  white blood cell count 288.60
    specified NEC 288.69
Elliptocytosis (congenital) (hereditary)
  282.1
  Hb-C (disease) 282.7
  hemoglobin disease 282.7
  sickle-cell (disease) 282.60
    trait 282.5
Ellis-van Creveld disease or syndrome
  (chondroectodermal dysplasia) 756.55
Ellison-Zollinger syndrome
  (gastric hypersecretion with pancreatic
    islet cell tumor) 251.5
Elongation, elongated (congenital) - see
  also Distortion
  bone 756.9
  cervix (uteri) 752.49
    acquired 622.6
    hypertrophic 622.6
  colon 751.5
  common bile duct 751.69
  cystic duct 751.69
  frenulum, penis 752.69
  labia minora, acquired 624.8
  ligamentum patellae 756.89
  petiolus (epiglottidis) 748.3
  styloid bone (process) 733.99
  tooth, teeth 520.2
  uvula 750.26
    acquired 528.9
Elschnig bodies or pearls 366.51
El Tor cholera 001.1
Emaciation (due to malnutrition) 261
Emancipation disorder 309.22
Embadomoniasis 007.8
Embarrassment heart, cardiac - see
  Disease, heart
Embedded tooth, teeth 520.6 ◀▥
  fragment (status) - see Foreign body,
    retained ◀
  root only 525.3
  splinter (status) - see Foreign body,
    retained ◀
  tooth, teeth 520.6 ◀
Embolic - see condition
Embolism 444.9
  with
    abortion - see Abortion, by type,
      with embolism
    ectopic pregnancy (see also
      categories 633.0–633.9) 639.6
    molar pregnancy (see also categories
      630–632) 639.6
  air (any site) 958.0
    with
      abortion - see Abortion, by type,
        with embolism
      ectopic pregnancy (see also
        categories 633.0–633.9) 639.6

m

Embolism *(Continued)*
  air *(Continued)*
    with *(Continued)*
      molar pregnancy *(see also*
        categories 630–632) 639.6
      due to implanted device - *see*
        Complications, due to (presence
        of) any device, implant, or graft
        classified to 996.0–996.5 NEC
      following
        abortion 639.6
        ectopic or molar pregnancy 639.6
      infusion, perfusion, or
        transfusion 999.1
      in pregnancy, childbirth, or
        puerperium 673.0●
      traumatic 958.0
  amniotic fluid (pulmonary) 673.1●
    with
      abortion - *see* Abortion, by type,
        with embolism
      ectopic pregnancy *(see also*
        categories 633.0–633.9) 639.6
      molar pregnancy *(see also*
        categories 630–632) 639.6
    following
      abortion 639.6
      ectopic or molar pregnancy 639.6
  aorta, aortic 444.1
    abdominal 444.0
    bifurcation 444.0
    saddle 444.0
    thoracic 444.1
  artery 444.9
    auditory, internal 433.8●
    basilar *(see also* Occlusion, artery,
      basilar) 433.0●
    bladder 444.89
    carotid (common) (internal) *(see also*
      Occlusion, artery, carotid)
      433.1●
    cerebellar (anterior inferior)
      (posterior inferior) (superior)
      433.8●
    cerebral *(see also* Embolism, brain)
      434.1●
    choroidal (anterior) 433.8●
    communicating posterior 433.8●
    coronary *(see also* Infarct,
      myocardium) 410.9●
      without myocardial infarction
        411.81
    extremity 444.22
      lower 444.22
      upper 444.21
    hypophyseal 433.8●
    mesenteric (with gangrene) 557.0
    ophthalmic *(see also* Occlusion,
      retina) 362.30
    peripheral 444.22
    pontine 433.8●
    precerebral NEC - *see* Occlusion,
      artery, precerebral
    pulmonary - *see* Embolism, pulmonary
    pyemic 449
      pulmonary 415.12
    renal 593.81
    retinal *(see also* Occlusion, retina)
      362.30
    septic 449
      pulmonary 415.12
    specified site NEC 444.89
    vertebral *(see also* Occlusion, artery,
      vertebral) 433.2●
  auditory, internal 433.8●
  basilar (artery) *(see also* Occlusion,
    artery, basilar) 433.0●

Embolism *(Continued)*
  birth, mother - *see* Embolism,
    obstetrical
  blood-clot
    with
      abortion - *see* Abortion, by type,
        with embolism
      ectopic pregnancy *(see also*
        categories 633.0–633.9) 639.6
      molar pregnancy *(see also*
        categories 630–632) 639.6
    following
      abortion 639.6
      ectopic or molar pregnancy 639.6
    in pregnancy, childbirth, or
      puerperium 673.2●
  brain 434.1●
    with
      abortion - *see* Abortion, by type,
        with embolism
      ectopic pregnancy *(see also*
        categories 633.0–633.9)
        639.6
      molar pregnancy *(see also*
        categories 630–632) 639.6
    following
      abortion 639.6
      ectopic or molar pregnancy 639.6
    late effect - *see* Late effect(s) (of)
      cerebrovascular disease
    puerperal, postpartum, childbirth
      674.0●
  capillary 448.9
  cardiac *(see also* Infarct, myocardium)
    410.9●
  carotid (artery) (common) (internal)
    (see also Occlusion, artery, carotid)
    433.1●
  cavernous sinus (venous) - *see*
    Embolism, intracranial venous
    sinus
  cerebral *(see also* Embolism, brain)
    434.1●
  cholesterol - *see* Atheroembolism
  choroidal (anterior) (artery) 433.8●
  coronary (artery or vein) (systemic) *(see
    also* Infarct, myocardium) 410.9●
    without myocardial infarction 411.81
  due to (presence of) any device,
    implant, or graft classifiable to
    996.0–996.5 - *see* Complications,
    due to (presence of) any device,
    implant, or graft classified to
    996.0–996.5 NEC
  encephalomalacia *(see also* Embolism,
    brain) 434.1●
  extremities 444.22
    lower 444.22
    upper 444.21
  eye 362.30
  fat (cerebral) (pulmonary) (systemic)
    958.1
    with
      abortion - *see* Abortion, by type,
        with embolism
      ectopic pregnancy *(see also*
        categories 633.0–633.9) 639.6
      molar pregnancy *(see also*
        categories 630–632) 639.6
    complicating delivery or
      puerperium 673.8●
    following
      abortion 639.6
      ectopic or molar pregnancy
        639.6
    in pregnancy, childbirth, or the
      puerperium 673.8●

Embolism *(Continued)*
  femoral (artery) 444.22
    vein 453.6
      deep 453.41
  following
    abortion 639.6
    ectopic or molar pregnancy
      639.6
    infusion, perfusion, or transfusion
      air 999.1
      thrombus 999.2
  heart (fatty) *(see also* Infarct,
    myocardium) 410.9●
  hepatic (vein) 453.0
  iliac (artery) 444.81
  iliofemoral 444.81
  in pregnancy, childbirth, or
    puerperium (pulmonary) - *see*
    Embolism, obstetrical
  intestine (artery) (vein) (with gangrene)
    557.0
  intracranial *(see also* Embolism, brain)
    434.1●
    venous sinus (any) 325
      late effect - *see* category 326
      nonpyogenic 437.6
        in pregnancy or puerperium
          671.5●
  kidney (artery) 593.81
  lateral sinus (venous) - *see*
    Embolism, intracranial venous
    sinus
  longitudinal sinus (venous) - *see*
    Embolism, intracranial venous
    sinus
  lower extremity 444.22
  lung (massive) - *see* Embolism,
    pulmonary
  meninges *(see also* Embolism, brain)
    434.1●
  mesenteric (artery) (with gangrene)
    557.0
  multiple NEC 444.9
  obstetrical (pulmonary) 673.2●
    air 673.0●
    amniotic fluid (pulmonary) 673.1●
    blood-clot 673.2●
    cardiac 674.8●
    fat 673.8●
    heart 674.8●
    pyemic 673.3●
    septic 673.3●
    specified NEC 674.8●
  ophthalmic *(see also* Occlusion, retina)
    362.30
  paradoxical NEC 444.9
  penis 607.82
  peripheral arteries NEC 444.22
    lower 444.22
    upper 444.21
  pituitary 253.8
  popliteal (artery) 444.22
  portal (vein) 452
  postoperative NEC 997.2
    cerebral 997.02
    mesenteric artery 997.71
    other vessels 997.79
    peripheral vascular 997.2
    pulmonary 415.11
      septic 415.11
    renal artery 997.72
  precerebral artery *(see also*
    Occlusion, artery, precerebral)
    433.9●
  puerperal - *see* Embolism,
    obstetrical

Embolism (Continued)
pulmonary (acute) (artery) (vein)
415.19
with
abortion - see Abortion, by type,
with embolism
ectopic pregnancy (see also
categories 633.0–633.9) 639.6
molar pregnancy (see also
categories 630–632) 639.6
chronic 416.2
following
abortion 639.6
ectopic or molar pregnancy 639.6
healed or old V12.51
iatrogenic 415.11
in pregnancy, childbirth, or
puerperium - see Embolism,
obstetrical
personal history of V12.51
postoperative 415.11
septic 415.12
pyemic (multiple) (see also Septicemia)
415.12
with
abortion - see Abortion, by type,
with embolism
ectopic pregnancy (see also
categories 633.0–633.9) 639.6
molar pregnancy (see also
categories 630–632) 639.6
Aerobacter aerogenes 415.12
enteric gram-negative bacilli 415.12
Enterobacter aerogenes 415.12
Escherichia coli 415.12
following
abortion 639.6
ectopic or molar pregnancy 639.6
Hemophilus influenzae 415.12
pneumococcal 415.12
Proteus vulgaris 415.12
Pseudomonas (aeruginosa) 415.12
puerperal, postpartum, childbirth
(any organism) 673.3 ●
Serratia 415.12
specified organism NEC 415.12
staphylococcal 415.12
aureus 415.12
specified organism NEC 415.12
streptococcal 415.12
renal (artery) 593.81
vein 453.3
retina, retinal (see also Occlusion, retina)
362.30
saddle (aorta) 444.0
septic 415.12
arterial 449
septicemic - see Embolism, pyemic
sinus - see Embolism, intracranial
venous sinus
soap
with
abortion - see Abortion, by type,
with embolism
ectopic pregnancy (see also
categories 633.0–633.9) 639.6
molar pregnancy (see also
categories 630–632) 639.6
following
abortion 639.6
ectopic or molar pregnancy 639.6
spinal cord (nonpyogenic) 336.1
in pregnancy or puerperium 671.5 ●
pyogenic origin 324.1
late effect - see category 326
spleen, splenic (artery) 444.89

Embolism (Continued)
thrombus (thromboembolism)
following infusion, perfusion, or
transfusion 999.2
upper extremity 444.21
vein 453.9
with inflammation or phlebitis - see
Thrombophlebitis
antecubital (acute) 453.81 ◄
acute 453.81
chronic 453.71
axillary (acute) 453.84 ◄
acute 453.84
chronic 453.74
basilic (acute) 453.81 ◄
acute 453.81
chronic 453.71
brachial (acute) 453.82 ◄
acute 453.82
chronic 453.72
brachiocephalic (acute) (innominate)
453.87 ◄
acute 453.87
chronic 453.77
cephalic (acute) 453.81 ◄
acute 453.81
chronic 453.71
cerebral (see also Embolism, brain)
434.1 ●
coronary (see also Infarct,
myocardium) 410.9 ●
without myocardial infarction
411.81
hepatic 453.0
internal jugular (acute) 453.86 ◄
acute 453.86
chronic 453.76
lower extremity (superficial)
453.6
deep 453.40
acute 453.40
calf 453.42
distal (lower leg) 453.42
femoral 453.41
iliac 453.41
lower leg 453.42
peroneal 453.42
popliteal 453.41
proximal (upper leg)
453.41
thigh 453.41
tibial 453.42
chronic 453.50
calf 453.52
distal (lower leg) 453.52
femoral 453.51
iliac 453.51
lower leg 453.52
peroneal 453.52
popliteal 453.51
proximal (upper leg)
453.51
thigh 453.51
tibial 453.52
saphenous (greater) (lesser)
453.6
superficial 453.6
mesenteric (with gangrene)
557.0
portal 452
pulmonary - see Embolism,
pulmonary
radial (acute) 453.82 ◄
acute 453.82
chronic 453.72
renal 453.3

Embolism (Continued)
vein (Continued)
saphenous (greater) (lesser) 453.6
specified NEC (acute) 453.89
with inflammation or phlebitis -
see Thrombophlebitis
chronic 453.79
subclavian (acute) 453.85 ◄
acute 453.85
chronic 453.75
superior vena cava (acute)
453.87 ◄
acute 453.87
chronic 453.77
thoracic (acute) 453.87 ◄
acute 453.87
chronic 453.77
ulnar (acute) 453.82 ◄
acute 453.82
chronic 453.72
upper extremity 453.83
acute 453.83
deep 453.82
superficial 453.81
chronic 453.73
deep 453.72
superficial 453.71
vena cava
inferior 453.2 ◄
superior (acute) 453.87 ◄
acute 453.87
chronic 453.77
vessels of brain (see also Embolism,
brain) 434.1 ●
Embolization - see Embolism
Embolus - see Embolism
Embryoma (M9080/1) - see also
Neoplasm, by site, uncertain
behavior
benign (M9080/0) - see Neoplasm, by
site, benign
kidney (M8960/3) 189.0
liver (M8970/3) 155.0
malignant (M9080/3) - see also
Neoplasm, by site, malignant
kidney (M8960/3) 189.0
liver (M8970/3) 155.0
testis (M9070/3) 186.9
undescended 186.0
testis (M9070/3) 186.9
undescended 186.0
Embryonic
circulation 747.9
heart 747.9
vas deferens 752.89
Embryopathia NEC 759.9
Embryotomy, fetal 763.89
Embryotoxon 743.43
interfering with vision 743.42
Emesis - see also Vomiting
bilious 787.04
gravidarum - see Hyperemesis,
gravidarum
Emissions, nocturnal (semen) 608.89
Emotional
crisis - see Crisis, emotional
disorder (see also Disorder, mental)
300.9
instability (excessive) 301.3
lability 799.24
overlay - see Reaction, adjustment
upset 300.9
Emotionality, pathological 301.3
Emotogenic disease (see also Disorder,
psychogenic) 306.9

Emphysema (atrophic) (centriacinar)
(centrilobular) (chronic) (diffuse)
(essential) (hypertrophic)
(interlobular) (lung) (obstructive)
(panlobular) (paracicatricial)
(paracinar) (postural) (pulmonary)
(senile) (subpleural) (traction)
(unilateral) (unilobular) (vesicular)
492.8
with bronchitis
chronic 491.20
with
acute bronchitis 491.22
exacerbation (acute) 491.21
bullous (giant) 492.0
cellular tissue 958.7
surgical 998.81
compensatory 518.2
congenital 770.2
conjunctiva 372.89
connective tissue 958.7
surgical 998.81
due to fumes or vapors 506.4
eye 376.89
eyelid 374.85
surgical 998.81
traumatic 958.7
fetus or newborn (interstitial)
(mediastinal) (unilobular) 770.2
heart 416.9
interstitial 518.1
congenital 770.2
fetus or newborn 770.2
laminated tissue 958.7
surgical 998.81
mediastinal 518.1
fetus or newborn 770.2
newborn (interstitial) (mediastinal)
(unilobular) 770.2
obstructive diffuse with fibrosis 492.8
orbit 376.89
subcutaneous 958.7
due to trauma 958.7
nontraumatic 518.1
surgical 998.81
surgical 998.81
thymus (gland) (congenital)254.8
traumatic 958.7
tuberculous (see also Tuberculosis,
pulmonary) 011.9●
Employment examination (certification)
V70.5
Empty sella (turcica) syndrome 253.8
Empyema (chest) (diaphragmatic)
(double) (encapsulated) (general)
(interlobar) (lung) (medial)
(necessitatis) (perforating chest wall)
(pleura) (pneumococcal) (residual)
(sacculated) (streptococcal)
(supradiaphragmatic) 510.9
with fistula 510.0
accessory sinus (chronic) (see also
Sinusitis) 473.9
acute 510.9
with fistula 510.0
antrum (chronic) (see also Sinusitis,
maxillary) 473.0
brain (any part) (see also Abscess, brain)
324.0
ethmoidal (sinus) (chronic) (see also
Sinusitis, ethmoidal) 473.2
extradural (see also Abscess, extradural)
324.9
frontal (sinus) (chronic) (see also
Sinusitis, frontal) 473.1
gallbladder (see also Cholecystitis,
acute) 575.0

Empyema (Continued)
mastoid (process) (acute) (see also
Mastoiditis, acute) 383.00
maxilla, maxillary 526.4
sinus (chronic) (see also Sinusitis,
maxillary) 473.0
nasal sinus (chronic) (see also Sinusitis)
473.9
sinus (accessory) (nasal) (see also
Sinusitis) 473.9
sphenoidal (chronic) (sinus) (see also
Sinusitis, sphenoidal) 473.3
subarachnoid (see also Abscess,
extradural) 324.9
subdural (see also Abscess, extradural)
324.9
tuberculous (see also Tuberculosis,
pleura) 012.0●
ureter (see also Ureteritis) 593.89
ventricular (see also Abscess, brain) 324.0
Enameloma 520.2
Encephalitis (bacterial) (chronic)
(hemorrhagic) (idiopathic)
(nonepidemic) (spurious) (subacute)
323.9
acute - see also Encephalitis, viral
disseminated (postinfectious) NEC
136.9 [323.61]
postimmunization or
postvaccination 323.51
inclusional 049.8
inclusion body 049.8
necrotizing 049.8
arboviral, arbovirus NEC 064
arthropod-borne (see also Encephalitis,
viral, arthropod-borne) 064
Australian X 062.4
Bwamba fever 066.3
California (virus) 062.5
Central European 063.2
Czechoslovakian 063.2
Dawson's (inclusion body) 046.2
diffuse sclerosing 046.2
due to
actinomycosis 039.8 [323.41]
cat-scratch disease 078.3 [323.01]
human herpesvirus 6 058.21
human herpesvirus 7 058.29
human herpesvirus NEC 058.29
infection classified elsewhere 136.9
[323.41]
infectious mononucleosis 075
[323.01]
malaria (see also Malaria) 084.6 [323.2]
Negishi virus 064
ornithosis 073.7 [323.01]
prophylactic inoculation against
smallpox 323.51
rickettsiosis (see also Rickettsiosis)
083.9 [323.1]
rubella 056.01
toxoplasmosis (acquired) 130.0
congenital (active) 771.2 [323.41]
typhus (fever) (see also Typhus) 081.9
[323.1]
vaccination (smallpox) 323.51
Eastern equine 062.2
endemic 049.8
epidemic 049.8
equine (acute) (infectious) (viral) 062.9
eastern 062.2
Venezuelan 066.2
western 062.1
Far Eastern 063.0
following vaccination or other
immunization procedure 323.51
herpes 054.3

Encephalitis (Continued)
human herpesvirus 6 058.21
human herpesvirus 7 058.29
human herpesvirus NEC 058.29
Ilheus (virus) 062.8
inclusion body 046.2
infectious (acute) (virus) NEC 049.8
influenzal (see also Influenza) 487.8
[323.41] ◀▥
lethargic 049.8
Japanese (B type) 062.0
La Crosse 062.5
Langat 063.8
late effect - see Late, effect, encephalitis
lead 984.9 [323.71]
lethargic (acute) (infectious)
(influenzal) 049.8
lethargica 049.8
louping ill 063.1
lupus 710.0 [323.81]
lymphatica 049.0
Mengo 049.8
meningococcal 036.1
mumps 072.2
Murray Valley 062.4
myoclonic 049.8
Negishi virus 064
otitic NEC 382.4 [323.41]
parasitic NEC 123.9 [323.41]
periaxialis (concentrica) (diffusa) 341.1
postchickenpox 052.0
postexanthematous NEC 057.9 [323.62]
postimmunization 323.51
postinfectious NEC 136.9 [323.62]
postmeasles 055.0
posttraumatic 323.81
postvaccinal (smallpox) 323.51
postvaricella 052.0
postviral NEC 079.99 [323.62]
postexanthematous 057.9 [323.62]
specified NEC 057.8 [323.62]
Powassan 063.8
progressive subcortical (Binswanger's)
290.12
Rasmussen 323.81
Rio Bravo 049.8
rubella 056.01
Russian
autumnal 062.0
spring-summer type (taiga) 063.0
saturnine 984.9 [323.71]
Semliki Forest 062.8
serous 048
slow-acting virus NEC 046.8
specified cause NEC 323.81
St. Louis type 062.3
subacute sclerosing 046.2
subcorticalis chronica 290.12
summer 062.0
suppurative 324.0
syphilitic 094.81
congenital 090.41
tick-borne 063.9
torula, torular 117.5 [323.41]
toxic NEC 989.9 [323.71]
toxoplasmic (acquired) 130.0
congenital (active) 771.2 [323.41]
trichinosis 124 [323.41]
Trypanosomiasis (see also
Trypanosomiasis) 086.9 [323.2]
tuberculous (see also Tuberculosis)
013.6●
type B (Japanese) 062.0
type C 062.3
van Bogaert's 046.2
Venezuelan 066.2
Vienna type 049.8

◀ New ◀▥ Revised ~~deleted~~ Deleted ● Use Additional Digit(s) ▦ Omit code

Encephalitis (*Continued*)
  viral, virus 049.9
    arthropod-borne NEC 064
      mosquito-borne 062.9
        Australian X disease 062.4
        California virus 062.5
        Eastern equine 062.2
        Ilheus virus 062.8
        Japanese (B type) 062.0
        Murray Valley 062.4
        specified type NEC 062.8
        St. Louis 062.3
        type B 062.0
        type C 062.3
        Western equine 062.1
      tick-borne 063.9
        biundulant 063.2
        Central European 063.2
        Czechoslovakian 063.2
        diphasic meningoencephalitis
          063.2
        Far Eastern 063.0
        Langat 063.8
        louping ill 063.1
        Powassan 063.8
        Russian spring-summer (taiga)
          063.0
        specified type NEC 063.8
        vector unknown 064
      slow acting NEC 046.8
      specified type NEC 049.8
      vaccination, prophylactic (against)
        V05.0
    von Economo's 049.8
    Western equine 062.1
    West Nile type 066.41
Encephalocele 742.0
  orbit 376.81
Encephalocystocele 742.0
Encephalomalacia (brain) (cerebellar)
    (cerebral) (cerebrospinal) (*see also*
    Softening, brain) 348.89 ◄▥
  due to
    hemorrhage (*see also* Hemorrhage,
      brain) 431
    recurrent spasm of artery 435.9
  embolic (cerebral) (*see also* Embolism,
    brain) 434.1●
  subcorticalis chronicus arteriosclerotica
    290.12
  thrombotic (*see also* Thrombosis, brain)
    434.0●
Encephalomeningitis - *see*
  Meningoencephalitis
Encephalomeningocele 742.0
Encephalomeningomyelitis - *see*
  Meningoencephalitis
Encephalomeningopathy (*see also*
  Meningoencephalitis) 349.9
Encephalomyelitis (chronic)
    (granulomatous) (myalgic, benign)
    (*see also* Encephalitis) 323.9
  abortive disseminated 049.8
  acute disseminated (ADEM)
    (postinfectious) 136.9
    [323.61]
    infectious 136.9 [323.61]
    noninfectious 323.81
    postimmunization 323.51
  due to
    cat-scratch disease 078.3 [323.01]
    infectious mononucleosis 075
      [323.01]
    ornithosis 073.7 [323.01]
    vaccination (any) 323.51

Encephalomyelitis (*Continued*)
  equine (acute) (infectious) 062.9
    eastern 062.2
    Venezuelan 066.2
    western 062.1
  funicularis infectiosa 049.8
  late effect - *see* Late, effect, encephalitis
  Munch-Peterson's 049.8
  postchickenpox 052.0
  postimmunization 323.51
  postmeasles 055.0
  postvaccinal (smallpox) 323.51
  rubella 056.01
  specified cause NEC 323.81
  syphilitic 094.81
  West Nile 066.41
Encephalomyelocele 742.0
Encephalomyelomeningitis - *see*
  Meningoencephalitis
Encephalomyeloneuropathy 349.9
Encephalomyelopathy 349.9
  subacute necrotizing (infantile) 330.8
Encephalomyeloradiculitis (acute) 357.0
Encephalomyeloradiculoneuritis (acute)
  357.0
Encephalomyeloradiculopathy 349.9
Encephalomyocarditis 074.23
Encephalopathia hyperbilirubinemica,
  newborn 774.7
  due to isoimmunization (conditions
    classifiable to 773.0–773.2) 773.4
Encephalopathy (acute) 348.30
  alcoholic 291.2
  anoxic - *see* Damage, brain, anoxic
  arteriosclerotic 437.0
    late effect - *see* Late effect(s) (of)
      cerebrovascular disease
  bilirubin, newborn 774.7
    due to isoimmunization 773.4
  congenital 742.9
  demyelinating (callosal) 341.8
  due to
    birth injury (intracranial) 767.8
    dialysis 294.8
      transient 293.9
    drugs - (*see also* Table of Drugs and
      Chemicals) 348.39
    hyperinsulinism - *see*
      Hyperinsulinism
    influenza (virus) (*see also* Influenza)
      487.8 ◄▥
      identified ◄
        avian 488.09 ◄
        novel H1N1 488.19 ◄
    lack of vitamin (*see also* Deficiency,
      vitamin) 269.2
    nicotinic acid deficiency 291.2
    serum (nontherapeutic)
      (therapeutic) 999.5
    syphilis 094.81
    trauma (postconcussional) 310.2
      current (*see also* Concussion,
        brain) 850.9
        with skull fracture - *see*
          Fracture, skull, by site,
          with intracranial injury
    vaccination 323.51
  hepatic 572.2
  hyperbilirubinemic, newborn 774.7
    due to isoimmunization (conditions
      classifiable to 773.0–773.2) 773.4
  hypertensive 437.2
  hypoglycemic 251.2
  hypoxic - *see also* Damage, brain, anoxic
    ischemic (HIE) 768.70
      mild 768.71
      moderate 768.72
      severe 768.73

Encephalopathy (*Continued*)
  infantile cystic necrotizing (congenital)
    341.8
  lead 984.9 [323.71]
  leukopolio 330.0
  metabolic (*see also* Delirium) 348.31
    toxic 349.82
  necrotizing
    hemorrhagic (acute) 323.61
    subacute 330.8
  other specified type NEC 348.39
  pellagrous 265.2
  portal-systemic 572.2
  postcontusional 310.2
  posttraumatic 310.2
  saturnine 984.9 [323.71]
  septic 348.31
  spongiform, subacute (viral) 046.19
  subacute
    necrotizing 330.8
    spongiform 046.19
    viral, spongiform 046.19
  subcortical progressive (Schilder) 341.1
    chronic (Binswanger's) 290.12
  toxic 349.82
    metabolic 349.82
  traumatic (postconcussional) 310.2
    current (*see also* Concussion, brain)
      850.9
      with skull fracture - *see* Fracture,
        skull, by site, with
        intracranial injury
  vitamin B deficiency NEC 266.9
  Wernicke's (superior hemorrhagic
    polioencephalitis) 265.1
Encephalorrhagia (*see also* Hemorrhage,
    brain) 432.9
  healed or old V12.54
  late effect - *see* Late effect(s) (of)
    cerebrovascular disease
Encephalosis, posttraumatic 310.2
Enchondroma (M9220/0) - *see also*
  Neoplasm, bone, benign
  multiple, congenital 756.4
Enchondromatosis (cartilaginous)
  (congenital) (multiple) 756.4
Enchondroses, multiple (cartilaginous)
  (congenital) 756.4
Encopresis (*see also* Incontinence, feces)
  787.60 ◄▥
  nonorganic origin 307.7
Encounter for - *see also* Admission for
  administrative purpose only V68.9
    referral of patient without exami-
      nation or treatment V68.81
    specified purpose NEC V68.89
  chemotherapy, (oral) (intravenous),
    antineoplastic V58.11
  dialysis
    extracorporeal (renal) V56.0
    peritoneal V56.8
  disability examination V68.01
  end-of-life care V66.7
  hospice care V66.7
  immunizations (childhood)
    appropriate for age V20.2
  immunotherapy, antineoplastic V58.12
  palliative care V66.7
  paternity testing V70.4
  radiotherapy V58.0
  respirator [ventilator] dependence
    during
      mechanical failure V46.14
      power failure V46.12
    for weaning V46.13
  routine infant and child vision and
    hearing testing V20.2
  school examination V70.3
    following surgery V67.09

◄ New   ◄▥ Revised   ~~deleted~~ Deleted   ● Use Additional Digit(s)   ▨ Omit code   **227**

Encounter for *(Continued)*
  screening mammogram NEC V76.12
    for high-risk patient V76.11
  terminal care V66.7
  weaning from respirator [ventilator]
    V46.13
Encystment - *see* Cyst
End-of-life care V66.7
Endamebiasis - *see* Amebiasis
Endamoeba - *see* Amebiasis
Endarteritis (bacterial, subacute)
    (infective) (septic) 447.6
  brain, cerebral or cerebrospinal 437.4
    late effect - *see* Late effect(s) (of)
      cerebrovascular disease
  coronary (artery) - *see* Arteriosclerosis,
    coronary
  deformans - *see* Arteriosclerosis
  embolic (*see also* Embolism) 444.9
  obliterans - *see also* Arteriosclerosis
    pulmonary 417.8
  pulmonary 417.8
  retina 362.18
  senile - *see* Arteriosclerosis
  syphilitic 093.89
    brain or cerebral 094.89
    congenital 090.5
    spinal 094.89
  tuberculous (*see also* Tuberculosis)
    017.9●
Endemic - *see* condition
Endocarditis (chronic) (indeterminate)
    (interstitial) (marantic) (nonbacterial
    thrombotic) (residual) (sclerotic)
    (sclerous) (senile) (valvular) 424.90
  with
    rheumatic fever (conditions
      classifiable to 390)
      active - *see* Endocarditis, acute,
        rheumatic
      inactive or quiescent (with
        chorea) 397.9
  acute or subacute 421.9
    rheumatic (aortic) (mitral)
      (pulmonary) (tricuspid) 391.1
      with chorea (acute) (rheumatic)
        (Sydenham's) 392.0
  aortic (heart) (nonrheumatic) (valve)
    424.1
    with
      mitral (valve) disease 396.9
        active or acute 391.1
          with chorea (acute)
            (rheumatic)
            (Sydenham's) 392.0
        bacterial 421.0
      rheumatic fever (conditions
        classifiable to 390)
        active - *see* Endocarditis, acute,
          rheumatic
        inactive or quiescent (with
          chorea) 395.9
          with mitral disease 396.9
    acute or subacute 421.9
    arteriosclerotic 424.1
    congenital 746.89
    hypertensive 424.1
    rheumatic (chronic) (inactive) 395.9
      with mitral (valve) disease 396.9
        active or acute 391.1
          with chorea (acute)
            (rheumatic)
            (Sydenham's) 392.0
        active or acute 391.1
          with chorea (acute)
            (rheumatic)
            (Sydenham's) 392.0

Endocarditis *(Continued)*
  aortic *(Continued)*
    specified cause, except rheumatic
      424.1
    syphilitic 093.22
  arteriosclerotic or due to
    arteriosclerosis 424.99
  atypical verrucous (Libman-Sacks)
    710.0 *[424.91]*
  bacterial (acute) (any valve) (chronic)
    (subacute) 421.0
  blastomycotic 116.0 *[421.1]*
  candidal 112.81
  congenital 425.3
  constrictive 421.0
  Coxsackie 074.22
  due to
    blastomycosis 116.0 *[421.1]*
    candidiasis 112.81
    Coxsackie (virus) 074.22
    disseminated lupus erythematosus
      710.0 *[424.91]*
    histoplasmosis (*see also*
      Histoplasmosis) 115.94
    hypertension (benign) 424.99
    moniliasis 112.81
    prosthetic cardiac valve 996.61
    Q fever 083.0 *[421.1]*
    serratia marcescens 421.0
    typhoid (fever) 002.0 *[421.1]*
  fetal 425.3
  gonococcal 098.84
  hypertensive 424.99
  infectious or infective (acute) (any
    valve) (chronic) (subacute)
    421.0
  lenta (acute) (any valve) (chronic)
    (subacute) 421.0
  Libman-Sacks 710.0 *[424.91]*
  Loeffler's (parietal fibroplastic)
    421.0
  malignant (acute) (any valve) (chronic)
    (subacute) 421.0
  meningococcal 036.42
  mitral (chronic) (double) (fibroid)
    (heart) (inactive) (valve) (with
    chorea) 394.9
    with
      aortic (valve) disease 396.9
        active or acute 391.1
          with chorea (acute)
            (rheumatic)
            (Sydenham's) 392.0
      rheumatic fever (conditions
        classifiable to 390)
        active - *see* Endocarditis,
          acute, rheumatic
        inactive or quiescent (with
          chorea) 394.9
          with aortic valve disease
            396.9
    active or acute 391.1
      with chorea (acute) (rheumatic)
        (Sydenham's) 392.0
    bacterial 421.0
    arteriosclerotic 424.0
    congenital 746.89
    hypertensive 424.0
    nonrheumatic 424.0
      acute or subacute 421.9
    syphilitic 093.21
  monilial 112.81
  mycotic (acute) (any valve) (chronic)
    (subacute) 421.0
  pneumococcic (acute) (any valve)
    (chronic) (subacute)
    421.0

Endocarditis *(Continued)*
  pulmonary (chronic) (heart) (valve) 424.3
    with
      rheumatic fever (conditions
        classifiable to 390)
        active - *see* Endocarditis, acute,
          rheumatic
        inactive or quiescent (with
          chorea) 397.1
    acute or subacute 421.9
      rheumatic 391.1
        with chorea (acute)
          (rheumatic)
          (Sydenham's) 392.0
    arteriosclerotic or due to
      arteriosclerosis 424.3
    congenital 746.09
    hypertensive or due to hypertension
      (benign) 424.3
    rheumatic (chronic) (inactive) (with
      chorea) 397.1
      active or acute 391.1
        with chorea (acute)
          (rheumatic)
          (Sydenham's) 392.0
    syphilitic 093.24
  purulent (acute) (any valve) (chronic)
    (subacute) 421.0
  rheumatic (chronic) (inactive) (with
    chorea) 397.9
    active or acute (aortic) (mitral)
      (pulmonary) (tricuspid) 391.1
      with chorea (acute) (rheumatic)
        (Sydenham's) 392.0
  septic (acute) (any valve) (chronic)
    (subacute) 421.0
  specified cause, except rheumatic
    424.99
  streptococcal (acute) (any valve)
    (chronic) (subacute) 421.0
  subacute - *see* Endocarditis, acute
  suppurative (any valve) (acute)
    (chronic) (subacute) 421.0
  syphilitic NEC 093.20
  toxic (*see also* Endocarditis, acute) 421.9
  tricuspid (chronic) (heart) (inactive)
    (rheumatic) (valve) (with chorea)
    397.0
    with
      rheumatic fever (conditions
        classifiable to 390)
        active - *see* Endocarditis, acute,
          rheumatic
        inactive or quiescent (with
          chorea) 397.0
    active or acute 391.1
      with chorea (acute) (rheumatic)
        (Sydenham's) 392.0
    arteriosclerotic 424.2
    congenital 746.89
    hypertensive 424.2
    nonrheumatic 424.2
      acute or subacute 421.9
    specified cause, except rheumatic
      424.2
    syphilitic 093.23
  tuberculous (*see also* Tuberculosis)
    017.9● *[424.91]*
  typhoid 002.0 *[421.1]*
  ulcerative (acute) (any valve) (chronic)
    (subacute) 421.0
  vegetative (acute) (any valve) (chronic)
    (subacute) 421.0
  verrucous (acute) (any valve) (chronic)
    (subacute) NEC 710.0 *[424.91]*
    nonbacterial 710.0 *[424.91]*
    nonrheumatic 710.0 *[424.91]*

◀ New   ◀▥ Revised   ~~deleted~~ Deleted   ● Use Additional Digit(s)   ▥ Omit code

Endocardium, endocardial - *see also*
  condition
  cushion defect 745.60
    specified type NEC 745.69
Endocervicitis (*see also* Cervicitis) 616.0
  due to
    intrauterine (contraceptive) device
      996.65
    gonorrheal (acute) 098.15
      chronic or duration of 2 months or
        over 098.35
  hyperplastic 616.0
  syphilitic 095.8
  trichomonal 131.09
  tuberculous (*see also* Tuberculosis) 016.7●
Endocrine - *see* condition
Endocrinopathy, pluriglandular 258.9
Endodontitis 522.0
Endomastoiditis (*see also* Mastoiditis)
  383.9
Endometrioma 617.9
Endometriosis 617.9
  appendix 617.5
  bladder 617.8
  bowel 617.5
  broad ligament 617.3
  cervix 617.0
  colon 617.5
  cul-de-sac (Douglas') 617.3
  exocervix 617.0
  fallopian tube 617.2
  female genital organ NEC 617.8
  gallbladder 617.8
  in scar of skin 617.6
  internal 617.0
  intestine 617.5
  lung 617.8
  myometrium 617.0
  ovary 617.1
  parametrium 617.3
  pelvic peritoneum 617.3
  peritoneal (pelvic) 617.3
  rectovaginal septum 617.4
  rectum 617.5
  round ligament 617.3
  skin 617.6
  specified site NEC 617.8
  stromal (M8931/1) 236.0
  umbilicus 617.8
  uterus 617.0
    internal 617.0
  vagina 617.4
  vulva 617.8
Endometritis (nonspecific) (purulent)
    (septic) (suppurative) 615.9
  with
    abortion - *see* Abortion, by type,
      with sepsis
    ectopic pregnancy (*see also*
      categories 633.0-633.9) 639.0
    molar pregnancy (*see also* categories
      630-632) 639.0
  acute 615.0
  blennorrhagic 098.16
    acute 098.16
    chronic or duration of 2 months or
      over 098.36
  cervix, cervical (*see also* Cervicitis) 616.0
    hyperplastic 616.0
  chronic 615.1
  complicating pregnancy 670.1●
    affecting fetus or newborn 760.8
    septic 670.2●
  decidual 615.9
  following
    abortion 639.0
    ectopic or molar pregnancy 639.0

Endometritis (*Continued*)
  gonorrheal (acute) 098.16
    chronic or duration of 2 months or
      over 098.36
  hyperplastic (*see also* Hyperplasia,
    endometrium) 621.30
    cervix 616.0
  polypoid - *see* Endometritis,
    hyperplastic
  puerperal, postpartum, childbirth
    670.1●
    septic 670.2●
  senile (atrophic) 615.9
  subacute 615.0
  tuberculous (*see also* Tuberculosis)
    016.7●
Endometrium - *see* condition
Endomyocardiopathy, South African
  425.2
Endomyocarditis - *see* Endocarditis
Endomyofibrosis 425.0
Endomyometritis (*see also* Endometritis)
  615.9
Endopericarditis - *see* Endocarditis
Endoperineuritis - *see* Disorder, nerve
Endophlebitis (*see also* Phlebitis) 451.9
  leg 451.2
    deep (vessels) 451.19
    superficial (vessels) 451.0
  portal (vein) 572.1
  retina 362.18
  specified site NEC 451.89
  syphilitic 093.89
Endophthalmia (*see also* Endophthalmitis)
  360.00
  gonorrheal 098.42
Endophthalmitis (globe) (infective)
    (metastatic) (purulent) (subacute)
    360.00
  acute 360.01
  bleb associated 379.63
  chronic 360.03
  parasitic 360.13
  phacoanaphylactic 360.19
  specified type NEC 360.19
  sympathetic 360.11
Endosalpingioma (M9111/1) 236.2
Endosalpingiosis 629.89
Endosteitis - *see* Osteomyelitis
Endothelioma, bone (M9260/3) - *see*
  Neoplasm, bone, malignant
Endotheliosis 287.8
  hemorrhagic infectional 287.8
Endotoxemia - *code to* condition
Endotoxic shock 785.52
Endotrachelitis (*see also* Cervicitis) 616.0
Enema rash 692.89
Engel-von Recklinghausen disease or
  syndrome (osteitis fibrosa cystica)
  252.01
Engelmann's disease (diaphyseal
  sclerosis) 756.59
English disease (*see also* Rickets) 268.0
Engman's disease (infectious eczematoid
  dermatitis) 690.8
Engorgement
  breast 611.79
    newborn 778.7
    puerperal, postpartum 676.2●
  liver 573.9
  lung 514
  pulmonary 514
  retina, venous 362.37
  stomach 536.8
  venous, retina 362.37
Enlargement, enlarged - *see also*
  Hypertrophy

Enlargement, enlarged (*Continued*)
  abdomen 789.3●
  adenoids 474.12
    and tonsils 474.10
  alveolar process or ridge 525.8
  apertures of diaphragm (congenital)
    756.6
  blind spot, visual field 368.42
  gingival 523.8
  heart, cardiac (*see also* Hypertrophy,
    cardiac) 429.3
  lacrimal gland, chronic 375.03
  liver (*see also* Hypertrophy, liver) 789.1
  lymph gland or node 785.6
  orbit 376.46
  organ or site, congenital NEC - *see*
    Anomaly, specified type NEC
  parathyroid (gland) 252.01
  pituitary fossa 793.0
  prostate (simple) (soft) 600.00
    with
      other lower urinary tract
        symptoms (LUTS) 600.01
      urinary
        obstruction 600.01
        retention 600.01
  sella turcica 793.0
  spleen (*see also* Splenomegaly) 789.2
    congenital 759.0
  thymus (congenital) (gland) 254.0
  thyroid (gland) (*see also* Goiter) 240.9
  tongue 529.8
  tonsils 474.11
    and adenoids 474.10
  uterus 621.2
Enophthalmos 376.50
  due to
    atrophy of orbital tissue 376.51
    surgery 376.52
    trauma 376.52
Enostosis 526.89
Entamebiasis - *see* Amebiasis
Entamebic - *see* Amebiasis
Entanglement, umbilical cord(s)
    663.3●
  with compression 663.2●
  affecting fetus or newborn 762.5
  around neck with compression 663.1●
  twins in monoamniotic sac 663.2●
Enteralgia 789.0●
Enteric - *see* condition
Enteritis (acute) (catarrhal) (choleraic)
    (chronic) (congestive) (diarrheal)
    (exudative) (follicular)
    (hemorrhagic) (infantile) (lienteric)
    (noninfectious) (perforative)
    (phlegmonous) (presumed
    noninfectious)
    (pseudomembranous) 558.9
  adaptive 564.9
  aertrycke infection 003.0
  allergic 558.3
  amebic (*see also* Amebiasis) 006.9
    with abscess - *see* Abscess, amebic
    acute 006.0
      with abscess - *see* Abscess, amebic
      nondysenteric 006.2
    chronic 006.1
      with abscess - *see* Abscess, amebic
      nondysenteric 006.2
    nondysenteric 006.2
  anaerobic (cocci) (gram-negative)
    (gram-positive) (mixed) NEC
    008.46
  bacillary NEC 004.9
  bacterial NEC 008.5
    specified NEC 008.49

Enteritis *(Continued)*
  Bacteroides (fragilis)
        (melaninogeniscus) (oralis) 008.46
  Butyrivibrio (fibriosolvens) 008.46
  Campylobacter 008.43
  Candida 112.85
  Chilomastix 007.8
  choleriformis 001.1
  chronic 558.9
    ulcerative *(see also* Colitis, ulcerative)
        556.9
  cicatrizing (chronic) 555.0
  Clostridium
    botulinum 005.1
    difficile 008.45
    haemolyticum 008.46
    novyi 008.46
    perfringens (C) (F) 008.46
    specified type NEC 008.46
  coccidial 007.2
  dietetic 558.9
  due to
    achylia gastrica 536.8
    adenovirus 008.62
    Aerobacter aerogenes 008.2
    anaerobes *(see also* Enteritis,
        anaerobic) 008.46
    Arizona (bacillus) 008.1
    astrovirus 008.66
    Bacillus coli - *see* Enteritis, E. coli
    bacteria NEC 008.5
      specified NEC 008.49
    Bacteroides *(see also* Enteritis,
        Bacteroides) 008.46
    Butyrivibrio (fibriosolvens)
        008.46
    calicivirus 008.65
    Campylobacter 008.43
    Clostridium - *see* Enteritis,
        Clostridium
    Cockle agent 008.64
    Coxsackie (virus) 008.67
    Ditchling agent 008.64
    ECHO virus 008.67
    Enterobacter aerogenes 008.2
    enterococci 008.49
    enterovirus NEC 008.67
    Escherichia coli - *see* Enteritis, E. coli
    Eubacterium 008.46
    Fusobacterium (nucleatum) 008.46
    gram-negative bacteria NEC 008.47
      anaerobic NEC 008.46
    Hawaii agent 008.63
    irritating foods 558.9
    Klebsiella aerogenes 008.47
    Marin County agent 008.66
    Montgomery County agent 008.63
    norovirus 008.63
    Norwalk-like agent 008.63
    Norwalk virus 008.63
    Otofuke agent 008.63
    Paracolobactrum arizonae 008.1
    paracolon bacillus NEC 008.47
        Arizona 008.1
    Paramatta agent 008.64
    Peptococcus 008.46
    Peptostreptococcus 008.46
    Proprionibacterium 008.46
    Proteus (bacillus) (mirabilis)
        (morganii) 008.3
    Pseudomonas aeruginosa 008.42
    Rotavirus 008.61
    Sapporo agent 008.63
    small round virus (SRV) NEC
        008.64
      featureless NEC 008.63
      structured NEC 008.63

Enteritis *(Continued)*
  due to *(Continued)*
    Snow Mountain (SM) agent 008.63
    specified
      bacteria NEC 008.49
      organism, nonbacterial NEC 008.8
      virus NEC 008.69
    Staphylococcus 008.41
    Streptococcus 008.49
      anaerobic 008.46
    Taunton agent 008.63
    Torovirus 008.69
    Treponema 008.46
    Veillonella 008.46
    virus 008.8
      specified type NEC 008.69
    Wollan (W) agent 008.64
    Yersinia enterocolitica 008.44
  dysentery - *see* Dysentery
  E. coli 008.00
    enterohemorrhagic 008.04
    enteroinvasive 008.03
    enteropathogenic 008.01
    enterotoxigenic 008.02
    specified type NEC 008.09
  El Tor 001.1
  embadomonial 007.8
  eosinophilic 558.41
  epidemic 009.0
  Eubacterium 008.46
  fermentative 558.9
  fulminant 557.0
  Fusobacterium (nucleatum) 008.46
  gangrenous *(see also* Enteritis, due to,
        by organism) 009.0
  giardial 007.1
  gram-negative bacteria NEC 008.47
    anaerobic NEC 008.46
  infectious NEC *(see also* Enteritis, due
        to, by organism) 009.0
    presumed 009.1
  influenzal *(see also* Influenza) 487.8 ◀▥
  ischemic 557.9
    acute 557.0
    chronic 557.1
    due to mesenteric artery
        insufficiency 557.1
  membranous 564.9
  mucous 564.9
  myxomembranous 564.9
  necrotic *(see also* Enteritis, due to, by
        organism) 009.0
  necroticans 005.2
  necrotizing of fetus or newborn *(see also*
        Enterocolitis, necrotizing,
        newborn) 777.50
  neurogenic 564.9
  newborn 777.8
    necrotizing *(see also* Enterocolitis,
        necrotizing, newborn)
        777.50
  parasitic NEC 129
  paratyphoid (fever) *(see also* Fever,
        paratyphoid) 002.9
  Peptococcus 008.46
  Peptostreptococcus 008.46
  Proprionibacterium 008.46
  protozoal NEC 007.9
  radiation 558.1
  regional (of) 555.9
    intestine
      large (bowel, colon, or rectum)
        555.1
        with small intestine 555.2
      small (duodenum, ileum, or
        jejunum) 555.0
        with large intestine 555.2

Enteritis *(Continued)*
  Salmonella infection 003.0
  salmonellosis 003.0
  segmental *(see also* Enteritis, regional)
        555.9
  septic *(see also* Enteritis, due to, by
        organism) 009.0
  Shigella 004.9
  simple 558.9
  spasmodic 564.9
  spastic 564.9
  staphylococcal 008.41
    due to food 005.0
  streptococcal 008.49
    anaerobic 008.46
  toxic 558.2
  Treponema (denticola) (macrodentium)
        008.46
  trichomonal 007.3
  tuberculous *(see also* Tuberculosis) 014.8●
  typhosa 002.0
  ulcerative (chronic) *(see also* Colitis,
        ulcerative) 556.9
  Veillonella 008.46
  viral 008.8
    adenovirus 008.62
    enterovirus 008.67
    specified virus NEC 008.69
  Yersinia enterocolitica 008.44
  zymotic 009.0
Enteroarticular syndrome 099.3
Enterobiasis 127.4
Enterobius vermicularis 127.4
Enterocele *(see also* Hernia) 553.9
  pelvis, pelvic (acquired) (congenital)
        618.6
  vagina, vaginal (acquired) (congenital)
        618.6
Enterocolitis - *see also* Enteritis
  fetus or newborn *(see also* Enterocolitis,
        necrotizing, newborn) 777.8
    necrotizing 777.50
  fulminant 557.0
  granulomatous 555.2
  hemorrhagic (acute) 557.0
    chronic 557.1
  necrotizing (acute) (membranous) 557.0
    newborn 777.50
      with
        perforation 777.53
        pneumatosis without
            perforation 777.52
        pneumatosis and perforation
            777.53
        without pneumatosis, without
            perforation 777.51
      stage I 777.51
      stage II 777.52
      stage III 777.53
  primary necrotizing *(see also*
        Enterocolitis, necrotizing,
        newborn) 777.50
  pseudomembranous 008.45
    newborn 008.45
  radiation 558.1
    newborn *(see also* Enterocolitis,
        necrotizing, newborn) 777.50
  ulcerative 556.0
Enterocystoma 751.5
Enterogastritis - *see* Enteritis
Enterogenous cyanosis 289.7
Enterolith, enterolithiasis (impaction)
        560.39
  with hernia - *see also* Hernia, by site,
        with obstruction
    gangrenous - *see* Hernia, by site,
        with gangrene

◀ New   ◀▥ Revised   ~~deleted~~ Deleted   ● Use Additional Digit(s)   ▨ Omit code

Enteropathy 569.9
  exudative (of Gordon) 579.8
  gluten 579.0
  hemorrhagic, terminal 557.0
  protein-losing 579.8
Enteroperitonitis (see also Peritonitis)
    567.9
Enteroptosis 569.89
Enterorrhagia 578.9
Enterospasm 564.9
  psychogenic 306.4
Enterostenosis (see also Obstruction,
    intestine) 560.9
Enterostomy status V44.4
  with complication 569.60
Enthesopathy 726.90
  ankle and tarsus 726.70
  elbow region 726.30
    specified NEC 726.39
  hip 726.5
  knee 726.60
  peripheral NEC 726.8
  shoulder region 726.10
    adhesive 726.0
  spinal 720.1
  wrist and carpus 726.4
Entrance, air into vein - see Embolism,
    air
Entrapment, nerve - see Neuropathy,
    entrapment
Entropion (eyelid) 374.00
  cicatricial 374.04
  congenital 743.62
  late effect of trachoma (healed)
      139.1
  mechanical 374.02
  paralytic 374.02
  senile 374.01
  spastic 374.03
Enucleation of eye (current) (traumatic)
    871.3
Enuresis 788.30
  habit disturbance 307.6
  nocturnal 788.36
    psychogenic 307.6
  nonorganic origin 307.6
  psychogenic 307.6
Enzymopathy 277.9
Eosinopenia 288.59
Eosinophilia 288.3
  allergic 288.3
  hereditary 288.3
  idiopathic 288.3
  infiltrative 518.3
  Loeffler's 518.3
  myalgia syndrome 710.5
  pulmonary (tropical) 518.3
  secondary 288.3
  tropical 518.3
Eosinophilic - see also condition
  fasciitis 728.89
  granuloma (bone) 277.89
  infiltration lung 518.3
Ependymitis (acute) (cerebral) (chronic)
    (granular) (see also Meningitis)
    322.9
Ependymoblastoma (M9392/3)
  specified site - see Neoplasm, by site,
    malignant
  unspecified site 191.9
Ependymoma (epithelial) (malignant)
    (M9391/3)
  anaplastic type (M9392/3)
    specified site - see Neoplasm, by site,
      malignant
    unspecified site 191.9

Ependymoma (Continued)
  benign (M9391/0)
    specified site - see Neoplasm, by site,
      benign
    unspecified site 225.0
  myxopapillary (M9394/1) 237.5
  papillary (M9393/1) 237.5
    specified site - see Neoplasm, by site,
      malignant
    unspecified site 191.9
Ependymopathy 349.2
  spinal cord 349.2
Ephelides, ephelis 709.09
Ephemeral fever (see also Pyrexia)
    780.60
Epiblepharon (congenital) 743.62
Epicanthus, epicanthic fold (congenital)
    (eyelid) 743.63
Epicondylitis (elbow) (lateral) 726.32
  medial 726.31
Epicystitis (see also Cystitis) 595.9
Epidemic - see condition
Epidermidalization, cervix - see condition
Epidermidization, cervix - see condition
Epidermis, epidermal - see condition
Epidermization, cervix - see condition
Epidermodysplasia verruciformis
    078.19
Epidermoid
  cholesteatoma - see Cholesteatoma
  inclusion (see also Cyst, skin) 706.2
Epidermolysis
  acuta (combustiformis) (toxica)
      695.15
  bullosa 757.39
  necroticans combustiformis 695.15
    due to drug
      correct substance properly
        administered 695.15
      overdose or wrong substance
        given or taken 977.9
      specified drug - see Table of
        Drugs and Chemicals
Epidermophytid - see Dermatophytosis
Epidermophytosis (infected) - see
    Dermatophytosis
Epidermosis, ear (middle) (see also
    Cholesteatoma) 385.30
Epididymis - see condition
Epididymitis (nonvenereal) 604.90
  with abscess 604.0
  acute 604.99
  blennorrhagic (acute) 098.0
    chronic or duration of 2 months or
      over 098.2
  caseous (see also Tuberculosis) 016.4●
  chlamydial 099.54
  diphtheritic 032.89 [604.91]
  filarial 125.9 [604.91]
  gonococcal (acute) 098.0
    chronic or duration of 2 months or
      over 098.2
  recurrent 604.99
  residual 604.99
  syphilitic 095.8 [604.91]
  tuberculous (see also Tuberculosis)
      016.4●
Epididymo-orchitis (see also Epididymitis)
    604.90
  with abscess 604.0
  chlamydial 099.54
  gonococcal (acute) 098.13
    chronic or duration of 2 months or
      over 098.33
Epidural - see condition
Epigastritis (see also Gastritis) 535.5●
Epigastrium, epigastric - see condition

Epigastrocele (see also Hernia, epigastric)
    553.29
Epiglottiditis (acute) 464.30
  with obstruction 464.31
  chronic 476.1
  viral 464.30
    with obstruction 464.31
Epiglottis - see condition
Epiglottitis (acute) 464.30
  with obstruction 464.31
  chronic 476.1
  viral 464.30
    with obstruction 464.31
Epignathus 759.4
Epilepsia
  partialis continua (see also Epilepsy)
      345.7●
  procursiva (see also Epilepsy)
      345.8●
Epilepsy, epileptic (idiopathic)
    345.9●

Note: Use the following fifth-digit
subclassifications with categories 345.0,
345.1, 345.4–345.9

  0   without mention of intractable
       epilepsy
  1   with intractable epilepsy
       pharmacoresistant
          (pharmacologically
          resistant)
       poorly controlled
       refractory (medically)
       treatment resistant

  abdominal 345.5●
  absence (attack) 345.0●
  akinetic 345.0●
    psychomotor 345.4●
  automatism 345.4●
  autonomic diencephalic 345.5●
  brain 345.9●
  Bravais-Jacksonian 345.5●
  cerebral 345.9●
  climacteric 345.9●
  clonic 345.1●
  clouded state 345.9●
  coma 345.3●
  communicating 345.4●
  complicating pregnancy, childbirth, or
      the puerperium 649.4●
  congenital 345.9●
  convulsions 345.9●
  cortical (focal) (motor) 345.5●
  cursive (running) 345.8●
  cysticercosis 123.1
  deterioration
    with behavioral disturbance 345.9●
      [294.11]
    without behavioral disturbance
      345.9● [294.10]
  due to syphilis 094.89
  equivalent 345.5●
  fit 345.9●
  focal (motor) 345.5●
  gelastic 345.8●
  generalized 345.9●
    convulsive 345.1●
    flexion 345.1●
    nonconvulsive 345.0●
  grand mal (idiopathic) 345.1●
  Jacksonian (motor) (sensory) 345.5●
  Kojevnikoff's, Kojevnikov's,
      Kojewnikoff's 345.7●
  laryngeal 786.2
  limbic system 345.4●

Epilepsy, epileptic *(Continued)*
  localization related (focal) (partial) and
     epileptic syndromes
    with
      complex partial seizures 345.4●
      simple partial seizures 345.5●
  major (motor) 345.1●
  minor 345.0●
  mixed (type) 345.9●
  motor partial 345.5●
  musicogenic 345.1●
  myoclonus, myoclonic 345.1●
    progressive (familial) 345.1●
  nonconvulsive, generalized
    345.0●
  parasitic NEC 123.9
  partial (focalized) 345.5●
    with
      impairment of consciousness
        345.4●
      memory and ideational
        disturbances 345.4●
      without impairment of
        consciousness 345.5●
    abdominal type 345.5●
    motor type 345.5●
    psychomotor type 345.4●
    psychosensory type 345.4●
    secondarily generalized
      345.4●
    sensory type 345.5●
    somatomotor type 345.5●
    somatosensory type 345.5●
    temporal lobe type 345.4●
    visceral type 345.5●
    visual type 345.5●
  peripheral 345.9●
  petit mal 345.0●
  photokinetic 345.8●
  progressive myoclonic (familial)
    345.1●
  psychic equivalent 345.5●
  psychomotor 345.4●
  psychosensory 345.4●
  reflex 345.1●
  seizure 345.9●
  senile 345.9●
  sensory-induced 345.5●
  sleep *(see also* Narcolepsy) 347.00
  somatomotor type 345.5●
  somatosensory 345.5●
  specified type NEC 345.8●
  status (grand mal) 345.3
    focal motor 345.7●
    petit mal 345.2●
    psychomotor 345.7●
    temporal lobe 345.7●
  symptomatic 345.9●
  temporal lobe 345.4●
  tonic (-clonic) 345.1●
  traumatic (injury unspecified)
    907.0
    injury specified - *see* Late, effect (of)
      specified injury
  twilight 293.0
  uncinate (gyrus) 345.4●
  Unverricht (-Lundborg) (familial
    myoclonic) 345.1●
  visceral 345.5●
  visual 345.5●
Epileptiform
  convulsions 780.39
  seizure 780.39
Epiloia 759.5
Epimenorrhea 626.2
Epipharyngitis *(see also* Nasopharyngitis)
  460

Epiphora 375.20
  due to
    excess lacrimation 375.21
    insufficient drainage 375.22
Epiphyseal arrest 733.91
  femoral head 732.2
Epiphyseolysis, epiphysiolysis *(see also*
  Osteochondrosis) 732.9
Epiphysitis *(see also* Osteochondrosis)
  732.9
  juvenile 732.6
  marginal (Scheuermann's) 732.0
  os calcis 732.5
  syphilitic (congenital) 090.0
  vertebral (Scheuermann's) 732.0
Epiplocele *(see also* Hernia)553.9
Epiploitis *(see also* Peritonitis) 567.9
Epiplosarcomphalocele *(see also* Hernia,
  umbilicus) 553.1
Episcleritis 379.00
  gouty 274.89 *[379.09]*
  nodular 379.02
  periodica fugax 379.01
    angioneurotic - *see* Edema,
      angioneurotic
  specified NEC 379.09
  staphylococcal 379.00
  suppurative 379.00
  syphilitic 095.0
  tuberculous *(see also* Tuberculosis)
    017.3● *[379.09]*
Episode
  brain *(see also* Disease, cerebrovascular,
    acute) 436
  cerebral *(see also* Disease,
    cerebrovascular, acute) 436
  depersonalization (in neurotic
    state) 300.6
  hyporesponsive 780.09
  psychotic *(see also* Psychosis) 298.9
    organic, transient 293.9
  schizophrenic (acute) NEC *(see also*
    Schizophrenia) 295.4●
Epispadias
  female 753.8
  male 752.62
Episplenitis 289.59
Epistaxis (multiple) 784.7
  hereditary 448.0
  vicarious menstruation 625.8
Epithelioma (malignant) (M8011/3) - *see*
  also Neoplasm, by site, malignant
  adenoides cysticum (M8100/0) - *see*
    Neoplasm, skin, benign
  basal cell (M8090/3) - *see* Neoplasm,
    skin, malignant
  benign (M8011/0) - *see* Neoplasm, by
    site, benign
  Bowen's (M8081/2) - *see* Neoplasm,
    skin, in situ
  calcifying (benign) (Malherbe's)
    (M8110/0) - *see* Neoplasm, skin,
    benign
  external site - *see* Neoplasm, skin,
    malignant
  intraepidermal, Jadassohn (M8096/0) -
    see Neoplasm, skin, benign
  squamous cell (M8070/3) - *see*
    Neoplasm, by site, malignant
Epitheliopathy
  pigment, retina 363.15
  posterior multifocal placoid (acute)
    363.15
Epithelium, epithelial - *see* condition
Epituberculosis (allergic) (with
  atelectasis) *(see also* Tuberculosis)
  010.8●

Eponychia 757.5
Epstein's
  nephrosis or syndrome *(see also*
    Nephrosis) 581.9
  pearl (mouth) 528.4
Epstein-Barr infection (viral) 075
  chronic 780.79 *[139.8]*
Epulis (giant cell) (gingiva) 523.8
Equinia 024
Equinovarus (congenital) 754.51
  acquired 736.71
Equivalent
  angina 413.9
  convulsive (abdominal) *(see also*
    Epilepsy) 345.5●
  epileptic (psychic) *(see also* Epilepsy)
    345.5●
Erb's
  disease 359.1
  palsy, paralysis (birth) (brachial)
    (newborn) 767.6
    spinal (spastic) syphilitic 094.89
  pseudohypertrophic muscular
    dystrophy 359.1
Erb (-Duchenne) paralysis (birth injury)
  (newborn) 767.6
Erb-Goldflam disease or syndrome
  358.00
Erdheim-Chester disease (ECD) 277.89
Erdheim's syndrome (acromegalic
  macrospondylitis) 253.0
Erection, painful (persistent) 607.3
Ergosterol deficiency (vitamin D) 268.9
  with
    osteomalacia 268.2
    rickets *(see also* Rickets) 268.0
Ergotism (ergotized grain) 988.2
  from ergot used as drug (migraine
    therapy)
    correct substance properly
      administered 349.82
    overdose or wrong substance given
      or taken 975.0
Erichsen's disease (railway spine) 300.16
Erlacher-Blount syndrome (tibia vara)
  732.4
Erosio interdigitalis blastomycetica 112.3
Erosion
  arteriosclerotic plaque - *see*
    Arteriosclerosis, by site
  artery NEC 447.2
    without rupture 447.8
  bone 733.99
  bronchus 519.19
  cartilage (joint) 733.99
  cervix (uteri) (acquired) (chronic)
    (congenital) 622.0
    with mention of cervicitis 616.0
  cornea (recurrent) *(see also* Keratitis)
    371.42
    traumatic 918.1
  dental (idiopathic) (occupational)
    521.30
    extending into
      dentine 521.32
      pulp 521.33
    generalized 521.35
    limited to enamel 521.31
    localized 521.34
  duodenum, postpyloric - *see* Ulcer,
    duodenum
  esophagus 530.89
  gastric 535.4●
  intestine 569.89
  lymphatic vessel 457.8
  pylorus, pyloric (ulcer) 535.4●
  sclera 379.16

Erosion (Continued)
spine, aneurysmal 094.89
spleen 289.59 ●
stomach 535.4 ●
teeth (idiopathic) (occupational) (see also Erosion, dental) 521.30
due to
medicine 521.30
persistent vomiting 521.30
urethra 599.84
uterus 621.8
vertebra 733.99
Erotomania 302.89
Clerambault's 297.8
Error
in diet 269.9
refractive 367.9
astigmatism (see also Astigmatism) 367.20
drug-induced 367.89
hypermetropia 367.0
hyperopia 367.0
myopia 367.1
presbyopia 367.4
toxic 367.89
Eructation 787.3
nervous 306.4
psychogenic 306.4
Eruption
creeping 126.9
drug - see Dermatitis, due to, drug
Hutchinson, summer 692.72
Kaposi's varicelliform 054.0
napkin (psoriasiform) 691.0
polymorphous
light (sun) 692.72
other source 692.82
psoriasiform, napkin 691.0
recalcitrant pustular 694.8
ringed 695.89
skin (see also Dermatitis) 782.1
creeping (meaning hookworm) 126.9
due to
chemical(s) NEC 692.4
internal use 693.8
drug - see Dermatitis, due to, drug
prophylactic inoculation or vaccination against disease - see Dermatitis, due to, vaccine
smallpox vaccination NEC - see Dermatitis, due to, vaccine
erysipeloid 027.1
feigned 698.4
Hutchinson, summer 692.72
Kaposi's, varicelliform 054.0
vaccinia 999.0
lichenoid, axilla 698.3
polymorphous, due to light 692.72
toxic NEC 695.0
vesicular 709.8
teeth, tooth
accelerated 520.6
delayed 520.6
difficult 520.6
disturbance of 520.6
in abnormal sequence 520.6
incomplete 520.6
late 520.6
natal 520.6
neonatal 520.6
obstructed 520.6
partial 520.6
persistent primary 520.6
premature 520.6
prenatal 520.6
vesicular 709.8

Erysipelas (gangrenous) (infantile) (newborn) (phlegmonous) (suppurative) 035
external ear 035 [380.13]
puerperal, postpartum, childbirth 670.8 ●
Erysipelatoid (Rosenbach's) 027.1
Erysipeloid (Rosenbach's) 027.1
Erythema, erythematous (generalized) 695.9
ab igne - see Burn, by site, first degree
annulare (centrifugum) (rheumaticum) 695.0
arthriticum epidemicum 026.1
brucellum (see also Brucellosis) 023.9
bullosum 695.19
caloricum - see Burn, by site, first degree
chronicum migrans 088.81
circinatum 695.19
diaper 691.0
due to
chemical (contact) NEC 692.4
internal 693.8
drug (internal use) 693.0
contact 692.3
elevatum diutinum 695.89
endemic 265.2
epidemic, arthritic 026.1
figuratum perstans 695.0
gluteal 691.0
gyratum (perstans) (repens) 695.19
heat - see Burn, by site, first degree
ichthyosiforme congenitum 757.1
induratum (primary) (scrofulosorum) (see also Tuberculosis) 017.1 ●
nontuberculous 695.2
infantum febrile 057.8
infectional NEC 695.9
infectiosum 057.0
inflammation NEC 695.9
intertrigo 695.89
iris 695.10
lupus (discoid) (localized) (see also Lupus, erythematosus) 695.4
marginatum 695.0
rheumaticum - see Fever, rheumatic
medicamentosum - see Dermatitis, due to, drug
migrans 529.1
chronicum 088.81
multiforme 695.10
bullosum 695.19
conjunctiva 695.19
exudativum (Hebra) 695.19
major 695.12
minor 695.11
pemphigoides 694.5
napkin 691.0
neonatorum 778.8
nodosum 695.2
tuberculous (see also Tuberculosis) 017.1 ●
nummular, nummulare 695.19
palmar 695.0
palmaris hereditarium 695.0
pernio 991.5
perstans solare 692.72
rash, newborn 778.8
scarlatiniform (exfoliative) (recurrent) 695.0
simplex marginatum 057.8
solare (see also Sunburn) 692.71
streptogenes 696.5
toxic, toxicum NEC 695.0
newborn 778.8

Erythema, erythematous (Continued)
tuberculous (primary) (see also Tuberculosis) 017.0 ●
venenatum 695.0
Erythematosus - see condition
Erythematous - see condition
Erythermalgia (primary) 443.82
Erythralgia 443.82
Erythrasma 039.0
Erythredema 985.0
polyneuritica 985.0
polyneuropathy 985.0
Erythremia (acute) (M9841/3) 207.0 ●
chronic (M9842/3) 207.1 ●
secondary 289.0
Erythroblastopenia (acquired) 284.89
congenital 284.01
Erythroblastophthisis 284.01
Erythroblastosis (fetalis) (newborn) 773.2
due to
ABO
antibodies 773.1
incompatibility, maternal/fetal 773.1
isoimmunization 773.1
Rh
antibodies 773.0
incompatibility, maternal/fetal 773.0
isoimmunization 773.0
Erythrocyanosis (crurum) 443.89
Erythrocythemia - see Erythremia
Erythrocytopenia 285.9
Erythrocytosis (megalosplenic)
familial 289.6
oval, hereditary (see also Elliptocytosis) 282.1
secondary 289.0
stress 289.0
Erythroderma (see also Erythema) 695.9
desquamativa (in infants) 695.89
exfoliative 695.89
ichthyosiform, congenital 757.1
infantum 695.89
maculopapular 696.2
neonatorum 778.8
psoriaticum 696.1
secondary 695.9
Erythrodysesthesia, palmar plantar (PPE) 693.0
Erythrogenesis imperfecta 284.09
Erythroleukemia (M9840/3) 207.0 ●
Erythromelalgia 443.82
Erythromelia 701.8
Erythropenia 285.9
Erythrophagocytosis 289.9
Erythrophobia 300.23
Erythroplakia
oral mucosa 528.79
tongue 528.79
Erythroplasia (Queyrat) (M8080/2)
specified site - see Neoplasm, skin, in situ
unspecified site 233.5
Erythropoiesis, idiopathic ineffective 285.0
Escaped beats, heart 427.60
postoperative 997.1
Esoenteritis - see Enteritis
Esophagalgia 530.89
Esophagectasis 530.89
due to cardiospasm 530.0
Esophagismus 530.5
Esophagitis (alkaline) (chemical) (chronic) (infectional) (necrotic) (peptic) (postoperative) (regurgitant) 530.10

Esophagitis *(Continued)*
  acute 530.12
  candidal 112.84
  eosinophilic 530.13
  reflux 530.11
  specified NEC 530.19
  tuberculous *(see also* Tuberculosis)
    017.8●
  ulcerative 530.19
Esophagocele 530.6
Esophagodynia 530.89
Esophagomalacia 530.89
Esophagoptosis 530.89
Esophagospasm 530.5
Esophagostenosis 530.3
Esophagostomiasis 127.7
Esophagostomy
  complication 530.87
    infection 530.86
    malfunctioning 530.87
    mechanical 530.87
Esophagotracheal *- see* condition
Esophagus *- see* condition
Esophoria 378.41
  convergence, excess 378.84
  divergence, insufficiency 378.85
Esotropia (nonaccommodative) 378.00
  accommodative 378.35
  alternating 378.05
    with
      A pattern 378.06
      specified noncomitancy NEC
        378.08
      V pattern 378.07
      X pattern 378.08
      Y pattern 378.08
    intermittent 378.22
  intermittent 378.20
    alternating 378.22
    monocular 378.21
  monocular 378.01
    with
      A pattern 378.02
      specified noncomitancy NEC
        378.04
      V pattern 378.03
      X pattern 378.04
      Y pattern 378.04
    intermittent 378.21
Espundia 085.5
Essential *- see* condition
Esterapenia 289.89
Esthesioneuroblastoma (M9522/3) 160.0
Esthesioneurocytoma (M9521/3) 160.0
Esthesioneuroepithelioma (M9523/3)
  160.0
Esthiomene 099.1
Estivo-autumnal
  fever 084.0
  malaria 084.0
Estrangement V61.09
Estriasis 134.0
Ethanolaminuria 270.8
Ethanolism *(see also* Alcoholism) 303.9●
Ether dependence, dependency *(see also*
  Dependence) 304.6●
Etherism *(see also* Dependence) 304.6●
Ethmoid, ethmoidal *- see* condition
Ethmoiditis (chronic) (nonpurulent)
  (purulent) *(see also* Sinusitis,
  ethmoidal) 473.2
  influenzal *(see also* Influenza) 487.1 ◀▥
  Woakes' 471.1
Ethylism *(see also* Alcoholism) 303.9●

Eulenburg's disease (congenital
  paramyotonia) 359.29
Eunuchism 257.2
Eunuchoidism 257.2
  hypogonadotropic 257.2
European blastomycosis 117.5
Eustachian *- see* condition
Euthyroid sick syndrome 790.94
Euthyroidism 244.9
Evaluation
  fetal lung maturity 659.8●
  for suspected condition *(see also*
    Observation) V71.9
    abuse V71.81
    exposure
      anthrax V71.82
      biologic agent NEC V71.83
      SARS V71.83
    neglect V71.81
    newborn *- see* Observation,
      suspected, condition, newborn
    specified condition NEC V71.89
  mental health V70.2
  requested by authority V70.1
  nursing care V63.8
  social service V63.8
Evans' syndrome (thrombocytopenic
  purpura) 287.32
Event, apparent life threatening in
  newborn and infant (ALTE) 799.82
Eventration
  colon into chest *- see* Hernia,
    diaphragm
  diaphragm (congenital) 756.6
Eversion
  bladder 596.8
  cervix (uteri) 622.0
    with mention of cervicitis 616.0
  foot NEC 736.79
    congenital 755.67
  lacrimal punctum 375.51
  punctum lacrimale (postinfectional)
    (senile) 375.51
  ureter (meatus) 593.89
  urethra (meatus) 599.84
  uterus 618.1
    complicating delivery 665.2●
      affecting fetus or newborn 763.89
    puerperal, postpartum 674.8●
Evidence
  of malignancy
    cytologic
      without histologic confirmation
        anus 796.76
        cervix 795.06
        vagina 795.16
Evisceration
  birth injury 767.8
  bowel (congenital) *- see* Hernia, ventral
  congenital *(see also* Hernia, ventral)
    553.29
  operative wound 998.32
  traumatic NEC 869.1
    eye 871.3
Evulsion *- see* Avulsion
Ewing's
  angioendothelioma (M9260/3) *- see*
    Neoplasm, bone, malignant
  sarcoma (M9260/3) *- see* Neoplasm,
    bone, malignant
  tumor (M9260/3) *- see* Neoplasm, bone,
    malignant
Exaggerated lumbosacral angle (with
  impinging spine) 756.12

Examination (general) (routine) (of) (for)
  V70.9
  allergy V72.7
  annual V70.0
  cardiovascular preoperative V72.81
  cervical Papanicolaou smear V76.2
    as a part of routine gynecological
      examination V72.31
    to confirm findings of recent normal
      smear following initial
      abnormal smear V72.32
  child care (routine) V20.2
  clinical research investigation (normal
    control patient) (participant)
    V70.7
  dental V72.2
  developmental testing (child) (infant)
    V20.2
  donor (potential) V70.8
  ear V72.19
  eye V72.0
  following
    accident (motor vehicle) V71.4
    alleged rape or seduction (victim or
      culprit) V71.5
    inflicted injury (victim or culprit)
      NEC V71.6
    rape or seduction, alleged (victim or
      culprit) V71.5
    treatment (for) V67.9
      combined V67.6
      fracture V67.4
      involving high-risk medication
        NEC V67.51
      mental disorder V67.3
      specified condition NEC V67.59
  follow-up (routine) (following) V67.9
    cancer chemotherapy V67.2
    chemotherapy V67.2
    disease NEC V67.59
    high-risk medication NEC V67.51
    injury NEC V67.59
    population survey V70.6
    postpartum V24.2
    psychiatric V67.3
    psychotherapy V67.3
    radiotherapy V67.1
    specified surgery NEC V67.09
    surgery V67.00
      vaginal pap smear V67.01
  gynecological V72.31
    for contraceptive maintenance V25.40
      intrauterine device V25.42
      pill V25.41
      specified method NEC V25.49
  health (of)
    armed forces personnel V70.5
    checkup V70.0
    child, routine V20.2
    defined subpopulation NEC V70.5
    inhabitants of institutions V70.5
    occupational V70.5
    pre-employment screening V70.5
    preschool children V70.5
      for admission to school V70.3
    prisoners V70.5
      for entrance into prison V70.3
    prostitutes V70.5
    refugees V70.5
    school children V70.5
    students V70.5
  hearing V72.19
    following failed hearing screening
      V72.11

◀ New   ◀▥ Revised   ~~deleted~~ Deleted   ● Use Additional Digit(s)   ▨ Omit code

Examination *(Continued)*
  infant
    8 to 28 days old V20.32
    over 28 days old, routine V20.2
    under 8 days old V20.31
  laboratory V72.60
    ordered as part of a routine general
      medical examination V72.62
    pre-operative V72.63
    pre-procedural V72.63
    specified NEC V72.69
  lactating mother V24.1
  medical (for) (of) V70.9
    administrative purpose NEC
      V70.3
    admission to
      old age home V70.3
      prison V70.3
      school V70.3
    adoption V70.3
    armed forces personnel V70.5
    at health care facility V70.0
    camp V70.3
    child, routine V20.2
    clinical research (control) (normal
      comparison) (participant)
      V70.7
    defined subpopulation NEC V70.5
    donor (potential) V70.8
    driving license V70.3
    general V70.9
      routine V70.0
      specified reason NEC V70.8
    immigration V70.3
    inhabitants of institutions V70.5
    insurance certification V70.3
    marriage V70.3
    medicolegal reasons V70.4
    naturalization V70.3
    occupational V70.5
    population survey V70.6
    pre-employment V70.5
    preschool children V70.5
      for admission to school V70.3
    prison V70.3
    prisoners V70.5
      for entrance into prison V70.3
    prostitutes V70.5
    refugees V70.5
    school children V70.5
    specified reason NEC V70.8
    sport competition V70.3
    students V70.5
  medicolegal reason V70.4
  pelvic (annual) (periodic) V72.31
  periodic (annual) (routine) V70.0
  postpartum
    immediately after delivery V24.0
    routine follow-up V24.2
  pregnancy (unconfirmed) (possible)
    V72.40
    negative result V72.41
    positive result V72.42
  prenatal V22.1
    first pregnancy V22.0
    high-risk pregnancy V23.9
      specified problem NEC V23.89
  preoperative V72.84
    cardiovascular V72.81
    respiratory V72.82
    specified NEC V72.83
  preprocedural V72.84
    cardiovascular V72.81
    general physical V72.83
    respiratory V72.82
    specified NEC V72.83

Examination *(Continued)*
  prior to chemotherapy V72.83
  psychiatric V70.2
    follow-up not needing further care
      V67.3
    requested by authority V70.1
  radiological NEC V72.5
  respiratory preoperative V72.82
  screening - *see* Screening
  sensitization V72.7
  skin V72.7
    hypersensitivity V72.7
  special V72.9
  specified type or reason NEC V72.85
    preoperative V72.83
      specified NEC V72.83
  teeth V72.2
  vaginal Papanicolaou smear V76.47
    following hysterectomy for
      malignant condition V67.01
  victim or culprit following
    alleged rape or seduction V71.5
    inflicted injury NEC V71.6
  vision V72.0
  well baby V20.2
Exanthem, exanthema *(see also* Rash) 782.1
  Boston 048
  epidemic, with meningitis 048
  lichenoid psoriasiform 696.2
  subitum 058.10
    due to
      human herpesvirus 6 058.11
      human herpesvirus 7 058.12
  viral, virus NEC 057.9
    specified type NEC 057.8
Excess, excessive, excessively
  alcohol level in blood 790.3
  carbohydrate tissue, localized 278.1
  carotene (dietary) 278.3
  cold 991.9
    specified effect NEC 991.8
  convergence 378.84
  crying 780.95
    of
      adolescent 780.95
      adult 780.95
      baby 780.92
      child 780.95
      infant (baby) 780.92
      newborn 780.92
  development, breast 611.1
  diaphoresis *(see also* Hyperhidrosis)
    780.8
  distance, interarch 524.28
  divergence 378.85
  drinking (alcohol) NEC *(see also*
    Abuse, drugs, nondependent)
    305.0●
    continual *(see also* Alcoholism)
      303.9●
    habitual *(see also* Alcoholism) 303.9●
  eating 783.6
  eyelid fold (congenital) 743.62
  fat 278.02
    in heart *(see also* Degeneration,
      myocardial) 429.1
    tissue, localized 278.1
  foreskin 605
  gas 787.3
  gastrin 251.5
  glucagon 251.4
  heat *(see also* Heat) 992.9
  horizontal
    overjet 524.26
    overlap 524.26
  interarch distance 524.28

Excess, excessive, excessively *(Continued)*
  intermaxillary vertical dimension
    524.37
  interocclusal distance of teeth 524.37
  large
    colon 564.7
      congenital 751.3
    fetus or infant 766.0
      with obstructed labor 660.1●
        affecting management of
          pregnancy 656.6●
      causing disproportion 653.5●
    newborn (weight of 4500 grams or
      more) 766.0
    organ or site, congenital NEC - *see*
      Anomaly, specified type NEC
  lid fold (congenital) 743.62
  long
    colon 751.5
    organ or site, congenital NEC - *see*
      Anomaly, specified type NEC
    umbilical cord (entangled)
      affecting fetus or newborn 762.5
      in pregnancy or childbirth 663.3●
        with compression 663.2●
  menstruation 626.2
  number of teeth 520.1
    causing crowding 524.31
  nutrients (dietary) NEC 783.6
  potassium (K) 276.7
  salivation *(see also* Ptyalism) 527.7
  secretion - *see also* Hypersecretion
    milk 676.6●
    sputum 786.4
    sweat *(see also* Hyperhidrosis)
      780.8
  short
    organ or site, congenital NEC - *see*
      Anomaly, specified type NEC
    umbilical cord
      affecting fetus or newborn 762.6
      in pregnancy or childbirth
        663.4●
  skin NEC 701.9
    eyelid 743.62
      acquired 374.30
  sodium (Na) 276.0
  spacing of teeth 524.32
  sputum 786.4
  sweating *(see also* Hyperhidrosis)
    780.8
  tearing (ducts) (eye) *(see also* Epiphora)
    375.20
  thirst 783.5
    due to deprivation of water 994.3
  tissue in reconstructed breast 612.0
  tuberosity 524.07
  vitamin
    A (dietary) 278.2
      administered as drug (chronic)
        (prolonged excessive
        intake) 278.2
      reaction to sudden overdose
        963.5
    D (dietary) 278.4
      administered as drug (chronic)
        (prolonged excessive
        intake) 278.4
      reaction to sudden overdose
        963.5
  weight 278.02
    gain 783.1
      of pregnancy 646.1●
    loss 783.21
Excitability, abnormal, under minor
  stress 309.29

Excitation
  catatonic (*see also* Schizophrenia)
      295.2●
  psychogenic 298.1
  reactive (from emotional stress,
      psychological trauma) 298.1
Excitement
  manic (*see also* Psychosis, affective)
      296.0●
      recurrent episode 296.1●
      single episode 296.0●
  mental, reactive (from emotional stress,
      psychological trauma) 298.1
  state, reactive (from emotional stress,
      psychological trauma) 298.1
Excluded pupils 364.76
Excoriation (traumatic) (*see also* Injury,
      superficial, by site) 919.8
  neurotic 698.4
Excyclophoria 378.44
Excyclotropia 378.33
Exencephalus, exencephaly 742.0
Exercise
  breathing V57.0
  remedial NEC V57.1
  therapeutic NEC V57.1
Exfoliation
  skin
      due to erythematous condition
          695.50
          involving (percent of body
              surface)
              less than 10 percent 695.50
              10-19 percent 695.51
              20-29 percent 695.52
              30-39 percent 695.53
              40-49 percent 695.54
              50-59 percent 695.55
              60-69 percent 695.56
              70-79 percent 695.57
              80-89 percent 695.58
              90 percent or more 695.59
  teeth
      due to systemic causes 525.0
Exfoliative - *see also* condition
  dermatitis 695.89
Exhaustion, exhaustive (physical NEC)
      780.79
  battle (*see also* Reaction, stress, acute)
      308.9
  cardiac (*see also* Failure, heart) 428.9
  delirium (*see also* Reaction, stress,
      acute) 308.9
  due to
      cold 991.8
      excessive exertion 994.5
      exposure 994.4
      overexertion 994.5
  fetus or newborn 779.89
  heart (*see also* Failure, heart) 428.9
  heat 992.5
      due to
          salt depletion 992.4
          water depletion 992.3
  manic (*see also* Psychosis, affective)
      296.0●
      recurrent episode 296.1●
      single episode 296.0●
  maternal, complicating delivery 669.8●
      affecting fetus or newborn 763.89
  mental 300.5
  myocardium, myocardial (*see also*
      Failure, heart) 428.9
  nervous 300.5

Exhaustion, exhaustive (*Continued*)
  old age 797
  postinfectional NEC 780.79
  psychogenic 300.5
  psychosis (*see also* Reaction, stress,
      acute) 308.9
  senile 797
      dementia 290.0
Exhibitionism (sexual) 302.4
Exomphalos 756.72
Exophoria 378.42
  convergence, insufficiency 378.83
  divergence, excess 378.85
Exophthalmic
  cachexia 242.0●
  goiter 242.0●
  ophthalmoplegia 242.0● [376.22]
Exophthalmos 376.30
  congenital 743.66
  constant 376.31
  endocrine NEC 259.9 [376.22]
  hyperthyroidism 242.0● [376.21]
  intermittent NEC 376.34
  malignant 242.0● [376.21]
  pulsating 376.35
      endocrine NEC 259.9 [376.22]
  thyrotoxic 242.0● [376.21]
Exostosis 726.91
  cartilaginous (M9210/0) - *see*
      Neoplasm, bone, benign
  congenital 756.4
  ear canal, external 380.81
  gonococcal 098.89
  hip 726.5
  intracranial 733.3
  jaw (bone) 526.81
  luxurians 728.11
  multiple (cancellous) (congenital)
      (hereditary) 756.4
  nasal bones 726.91
  orbit, orbital 376.42
  osteocartilaginous (M9210/0) - *see*
      Neoplasm, bone, benign
  spine 721.8
      with spondylosis - *see*
          Spondylosis
  syphilitic 095.5
  wrist 726.4
Exotropia 378.10
  alternating 378.15
      with
          A pattern 378.16
          specified noncomitancy NEC
              378.18
          V pattern 378.17
          X pattern 378.18
          Y pattern 378.18
      intermittent 378.24
  intermittent 378.20
      alternating 378.24
      monocular 378.23
  monocular 378.11
      with
          A pattern 378.12
          specified noncomitancy NEC
              378.14
          V pattern 378.13
          X pattern 378.14
          Y pattern 378.14
      intermittent 378.23
Explanation of
  investigation finding V65.4
  medication V65.4

Exposure (suspected) 994.9
  algae bloom V87.32
  cold 991.9
      specified effect NEC 991.8
  effects of 994.9
  exhaustion due to 994.4
  to
      AIDS virus V01.79
      anthrax V01.81
      aromatic
          amines V87.11
          dyes V87.19
      arsenic V87.01
      asbestos V15.84
      benzene V87.12
      body fluids (hazardous) V15.85
      cholera V01.0
      chromium compounds V87.09
      communicable disease V01.9
          specified type NEC V01.89
      dyes V87.2
          aromatic V87.19
      Escherichia coli (E. coli) V01.83
      German measles V01.4
      gonorrhea V01.6
      hazardous
          aromatic compounds NEC
              V87.19
          body fluids V15.85
          chemicals NEC V87.2
          metals V87.09
          substances V87.39
      HIV V01.79
      human immunodeficiency virus
          V01.79
      lead V15.86
      meningococcus V01.84
      mold V87.31
      nickel dust V87.09
      parasitic disease V01.89
      poliomyelitis V01.2
      polycyclic aromatic hydrocarbons
          V87.19
      potentially hazardous body fluids
          V15.85
      rabies V01.5
      rubella V01.4
      SARS-associated coronavirus V01.82
      smallpox V01.3
      syphilis V01.6
      tuberculosis V01.1
      varicella V01.71
      venereal disease V01.6
      viral disease NEC V01.79
          varicella V01.71
Exsanguination, fetal 772.0
Exstrophy
  abdominal content 751.8
  bladder (urinary) 753.5
Extensive - *see* condition
Extra - *see also* Accessory
  rib 756.3
      cervical 756.2
Extraction
  with hook 763.89
  breech NEC 669.6●
      affecting fetus or newborn 763.0
  cataract postsurgical V45.61
  manual NEC 669.8●
      affecting fetus or newborn 763.89
Extrasystole 427.60
  atrial 427.61
  postoperative 997.1
  ventricular 427.69

◄ New   ◄IIII Revised   ~~deleted~~ Deleted   ● Use Additional Digit(s)   ▨ Omit code

Extrauterine gestation or pregnancy - *see*
 Pregnancy, ectopic
Extravasation
 blood 459.0
  lower extremity 459.0
 chemotherapy, vesicant 999.81
 chyle into mesentery 457.8
 pelvicalyceal 593.4
 pyelosinus 593.4
 urine 788.8
  from ureter 788.8
 vesicant
  agent NEC 999.82
  chemotherapy 999.81
Extremity - *see* condition

Extrophy - *see* Exstrophy
Extroversion
 bladder 753.5
 uterus 618.1
  complicating delivery 665.2●
   affecting fetus or newborn
    763.89
  postpartal (old) 618.1
Extruded tooth 524.34
Extrusion
 alveolus and teeth 524.75
 breast implant (prosthetic) 996.54
 device, implant, or graft - *see*
  Complications, mechanical
 eye implant (ball) (globe) 996.59

Extrusion (*Continued*)
 intervertebral disc - *see* Displacement,
  intervertebral disc
 lacrimal gland 375.43
 mesh (reinforcing) 996.59
 ocular lens implant 996.53
 prosthetic device NEC - *see*
  Complications, mechanical
 vitreous 379.26
Exudate, pleura - *see* Effusion, pleura
Exudates, retina 362.82
Exudative - *see* condition
Eye, eyeball, eyelid - *see* condition
Eyestrain 368.13
Eyeworm disease of Africa 125.2

F

Faber's anemia or syndrome
(achlorhydric anemia) 280.9
Fabry's disease (angiokeratoma corporis
diffusum) 272.7
Face, facial - see condition
Facet of cornea 371.44
Faciocephalalgia, autonomic (see also
Neuropathy, peripheral, autonomic)
337.9
Facioscapulohumeral myopathy 359.1
Factitious disorder, illness - see Illness,
factitious
Factor
deficiency - see Deficiency, factor
psychic, associated with diseases
classified elsewhere 316
risk-see problem
Fahr-Volhard disease (malignant
nephrosclerosis) 403.00
Failure, failed
adenohypophyseal 253.2
attempted abortion (legal) (see also
Abortion, failed) 638.9
bone marrow (anemia) 284.9
acquired (secondary) 284.89
congenital 284.09
idiopathic 284.9
cardiac (see also Failure, heart) 428.9
newborn 779.89
cardiorenal (chronic) 428.9
hypertensive (see also Hypertension,
cardiorenal) 404.93
cardiorespiratory 799.1
specified during or due to a
procedure 997.1
long-term effect of cardiac
surgery 429.4
cardiovascular (chronic) 428.9
cerebrovascular 437.8
cervical dilatation in labor 661.0●
affecting fetus or newborn 763.7
circulation, circulatory 799.89
fetus or newborn 779.89
peripheral 785.50
compensation - see Disease, heart
congestive (see also Failure, heart) 428.0
conscious sedation, during
procedure 995.24
coronary (see also Insufficiency,
coronary) 411.89
dental implant 525.79
due to
infection 525.71
lack of attached gingiva
525.72
occlusal trauma (caused by poor
prosthetic design) 525.72
parafunctional habits 525.72
periodontal infection
(periimplantitis) 525.72
poor oral hygiene 525.72
unintentional loading 525.71
endosseous NEC 525.79
mechanical 525.73
osseointegration 525.71
due to
complications of systemic
disease 525.71
poor bone quality 525.71
premature loading 525.71
iatrogenic 525.71
prior to intentional prosthetic
loading 525.71

Failure, failed (Continued)
dental implant (Continued)
post-osseointegration
biological 525.72
iatrogenic 525.72
due to complications of systemic
disease 525.72
mechanical 525.73
pre-integration 525.71
pre-osseointegration 525.71
dental prosthesis causing loss of dental
implant 525.73
dental restoration
marginal integrity 525.61
periodontal anatomical integrity
525.65
descent of head (at term) 652.5●
affecting fetus or newborn 763.1
in labor 660.0●
affecting fetus or newborn
763.1
device, implant, or graft - see
Complications, mechanical
engagement of head NEC 652.5●
in labor 660.0●
extrarenal 788.99
fetal head to enter pelvic brim
652.5●
affecting fetus or newborn 763.1
in labor 660.0●
affecting fetus or newborn 763.1
forceps NEC 660.7●
affecting fetus or newborn 763.1
fusion (joint) (spinal) 996.49
growth in childhood 783.43
heart (acute) (sudden) 428.9
with
abortion - see Abortion, by type,
with specified complication
NEC
acute pulmonary edema (see also
Failure, ventricular, left)
428.1
with congestion (see also
Failure, heart) 428.0
decompensation (see also Failure,
heart) 428.0
dilation - see Disease, heart
ectopic pregnancy (see also
categories 633.0–633.9)
639.8
molar pregnancy (see also
categories 630–632) 639.8
arteriosclerotic 440.9
combined left-right sided 428.0
combined systolic and diastolic
428.40
acute 428.41
acute on chronic 428.43
chronic 428.42
compensated (see also Failure, heart)
428.0
complicating
abortion - see Abortion, by type,
with specified complication
NEC
delivery (cesarean) (instrumental)
669.4●
ectopic pregnancy (see also
categories 633.0–633.9) 639.8
molar pregnancy (see also
categories 630–632) 639.8
obstetric anesthesia or sedation
668.1●
surgery 997.1

Failure, failed (Continued)
heart (Continued)
congestive (compensated)
(decompensated) (see also
Failure, heart) 428.0
with rheumatic fever (conditions
classifiable to 390)
active 391.8
inactive or quiescent (with
chorea) 398.91
fetus or newborn 779.89
hypertensive (see also
Hypertension, heart)
402.91
with renal disease (see also
Hypertension,
cardiorenal) 404.91
with renal failure 404.93
benign 402.11
malignant 402.01
rheumatic (chronic) (inactive)
(with chorea) 398.91
active or acute 391.8
with chorea (Sydenham's)
392.0
decompensated (see also Failure,
heart) 428.0
degenerative (see also Degeneration,
myocardial) 429.1
diastolic 428.30
acute 428.31
acute on chronic 428.33
chronic 428.32
due to presence of (cardiac)
prosthesis 429.4
fetus or newborn 779.89
following
abortion 639.8
cardiac surgery 429.4
ectopic or molar pregnancy
639.8
high output NEC 428.9
hypertensive (see also Hypertension,
heart) 402.91
with renal disease (see also
Hypertension, cardiorenal)
404.91
with renal failure 404.93
benign 402.11
malignant 402.01
left (ventricular) (see also Failure,
ventricular, left) 428.1
with right-sided failure (see also
Failure, heart) 428.0
low output (syndrome) NEC
428.9
organic - see Disease, heart
postoperative (immediate) 997.1
long term effect of cardiac
surgery 429.4
rheumatic (chronic) (congestive)
(inactive) 398.91
right (secondary to left heart failure,
conditions classifiable to 428.1)
(ventricular) (see also Failure,
heart) 428.0
senile 797
specified during or due to a
procedure 997.1
long-term effect of cardiac
surgery 429.4
systolic 428.20
acute 428.21
acute on chronic 428.23
chronic 428.22

◀ New   ◀▥ Revised   ~~deleted~~ Deleted   ● Use Additional Digit(s)   ▨ Omit code

Failure, failed (Continued)
  heart (Continued)
    thyrotoxic (see also Thyrotoxicosis)
      242.9● [425.7]
    valvular - see Endocarditis
  hepatic 572.8
    acute 570
    due to a procedure 997.4
  hepatorenal 572.4
  hypertensive heart (see also
      Hypertension, heart) 402.91
    benign 402.11
    malignant 402.01
  induction (of labor) 659.1●
    abortion (legal) (see also Abortion,
        failed) 638.9
    affecting fetus or newborn 763.89
    by oxytocic drugs 659.1●
    instrumental 659.0●
    mechanical 659.0●
    medical 659.1●
    surgical 659.0●
  initial alveolar expansion, newborn
      770.4
  involution, thymus (gland) 254.8
  kidney - see Failure, renal
  lactation 676.4●
  Leydig's cell, adult 257.2
  liver 572.8
    acute 570
  medullary 799.89
  mitral - see Endocarditis, mitral
  moderate sedation, during
      procedure 995.24
  myocardium, myocardial (see also
      Failure, heart) 428.9
    chronic (see also Failure, heart)
        428.0
    congestive (see also Failure, heart)
        428.0
  ovarian (primary) 256.39
    iatrogenic 256.2
    postablative 256.2
    postirradiation 256.2
    postsurgical 256.2
  ovulation 628.0
  prerenal 788.99
  renal (kidney) 586
    with
      abortion - see Abortion, by type,
          with renal failure
      ectopic pregnancy (see also
          categories 633.0–633.9) 639.3
      edema (see also Nephrosis) 581.9
      hypertension (see also
          Hypertension, kidney)
          403.91
      hypertensive heart disease
          (conditions classifiable to
          402) 404.92
        with heart failure 404.93
        benign 404.12
          with heart failure 404.13
        malignant 404.02
          with heart failure 404.03
      molar pregnancy (see also
          categories 630–632) 639.3
      tubular necrosis (acute) 584.5
    acute 584.9
      with lesion of
        necrosis
          cortical (renal) 584.6
          medullary (renal)
              (papillary) 584.7
          tubular 584.5
        specified pathology NEC
            584.8

Failure, failed (Continued)
  renal (Continued)
    chronic 585.9
      hypertensive or with
          hypertension (see also
          Hypertension, kidney)
          403.91
      due to a procedure 997.5
      following
        abortion 639.3
        crushing 958.5
        ectopic or molar pregnancy
            639.3
        labor and delivery (acute)
            669.3●
      hypertensive (see also Hypertension,
          kidney) 403.91
      puerperal, postpartum 669.3●
    respiration, respiratory 518.81
      acute 518.81
      acute and chronic 518.84
      center 348.89
        newborn 770.84
      chronic 518.83
      due to trauma, surgery or shock
          518.5
      newborn 770.84
    rotation
      cecum 751.4
      colon 751.4
      intestine 751.4
      kidney 753.3
    sedation, during procedure
      conscious 995.24
      moderate 995.24
    segmentation - see also Fusion
      fingers (see also Syndactylism,
          fingers) 755.11
      toes (see also Syndactylism, toes)
          755.13
    seminiferous tubule, adult 257.2
    senile (general) 797
      with psychosis 290.20
    testis, primary (seminal) 257.2
    to progress 661.2●
    to thrive
      adult 783.7
      child 783.41
      newborn 779.34
    transplant 996.80
      bone marrow 996.85
      organ (immune or nonimmune
          cause) 996.80
        bone marrow 996.85
        heart 996.83
        intestines 996.87
        kidney 996.81
        liver 996.82
        lung 996.84
        pancreas 996.86
        specified NEC 996.89
      skin 996.52
        artificial 996.55
        decellularized allodermis
            996.55
        temporary allograft or pigskin
            graft - *omit code*
    trial of labor NEC 660.6●
      affecting fetus or newborn 763.1
    tubal ligation 998.89
    urinary 586
    vacuum extraction
      abortion - see Abortion, failed
      delivery NEC 660.7●
        affecting fetus or newborn
            763.1
    vasectomy 998.89

Failure, failed (Continued)
  ventouse NEC 660.7●
    affecting fetus or newborn 763.1
  ventricular (see also Failure, heart) 428.9
    left 428.1
      with rheumatic fever (conditions
          classifiable to 390)
        active 391.8
          with chorea 392.0
        inactive or quiescent (with
            chorea) 398.91
      hypertensive (see also
          Hypertension, heart)
          402.91
        benign 402.11
        malignant 402.01
      rheumatic (chronic) (inactive)
          (with chorea) 398.91
        active or acute 391.8
          with chorea 392.0
    right (see also Failure, heart) 428.0
  vital centers, fetus or newborn
      779.89
  weight gain in childhood 783.41
Fainting (fit) (spell) 780.2
Falciform hymen 752.49
**Fall, maternal, affecting fetus or
    newborn** 760.5
Fallen arches 734
Falling, any organ or part - see Prolapse
Fallopian
  insufflation
    fertility testing V26.21
    following sterilization reversal
        V26.22
  tube - see condition
Fallot's
  pentalogy 745.2
  tetrad or tetralogy 745.2
  triad or trilogy 746.09
Fallout, radioactive (adverse effect) NEC
    990
False - see also condition
  bundle branch block 426.50
  bursa 727.89
  croup 478.75
  joint 733.82
  labor (pains) 644.1●
  opening, urinary, male 752.69
  passage, urethra (prostatic) 599.4
  positive
    serological test for syphilis 795.6
    Wassermann reaction 795.6
  pregnancy 300.11
Family, familial - see also condition
  affected by
    family member
      currently on deployment
          (military) V61.01
      returned from deployment
          (military) (current or past
          conflict) V61.02
  disruption (see also Disruption, family)
      V61.09
  estrangement V61.09
  hemophagocytic
    lymphohistiocytosis 288.4
    reticulosis 288.4
  Li-Fraumeni (syndrome) V84.01
  planning advice V25.09
    natural
      procreative V26.41
      to avoid pregnancy V25.04
  problem V61.9
    specified circumstance NEC
        V61.8
  retinoblastoma (syndrome) 190.5

Famine 994.2
  edema 262
Fanconi's anemia (congenital
      pancytopenia) 284.09
Fanconi (-de Toni) (-Debré) syndrome
      (cystinosis) 270.0
Farber (-Uzman) syndrome or disease
      (disseminated lipogranulomatosis)
      272.8
Farcin 024
Farcy 024
Farmers'
  lung 495.0
  skin 692.74
Farsightedness 367.0
Fascia - see condition
Fasciculation 781.0
Fasciculitis optica 377.32
Fasciitis 729.4
  eosinophilic 728.89
  necrotizing 728.86
  nodular 728.79
  perirenal 593.4
  plantar 728.71
  pseudosarcomatous 728.79
  traumatic (old) NEC 728.79
    current - see Sprain, by site
Fasciola hepatica infestation 121.3
Fascioliasis 121.3
Fasciolopsiasis (small intestine) 121.4
Fasciolopsis (small intestine) 121.4
Fast pulse 785.0
Fat
  embolism (cerebral) (pulmonary)
        (systemic) 958.1
    with
      abortion - see Abortion, by type,
            with embolism
      ectopic pregnancy (see also
            categories 633.0–633.9) 639.6
      molar pregnancy (see also
            categories 630–632) 639.6
      complicating delivery or
            puerperium 673.8●
    following
      abortion 639.6
      ectopic or molar pregnancy
            639.6
    in pregnancy, childbirth, or the
          puerperium 673.8●
  excessive 278.02
    in heart (see also Degeneration,
          myocardial) 429.1
  general 278.02
  hernia, herniation 729.30
    eyelid 374.34
    knee 729.31
    orbit 374.34
    retro-orbital 374.34
    retropatellar 729.31
    specified site NEC 729.39
  indigestion 579.8
  in stool 792.1
  localized (pad) 278.1
    heart (see also Degeneration,
          myocardial) 429.1
    knee 729.31
    retropatellar 729.31
  necrosis - see also Fatty, degeneration
    breast (aseptic) (segmental) 611.3
    mesentery 567.82
    omentum 567.82
    peritoneum 567.82
  pad 278.1

Fatal familial insomnia (FFI) 046.72
Fatal syncope 798.1
Fatigue 780.79
  auditory deafness (see also Deafness)
        389.9
  chronic, syndrome 780.71
  combat (see also Reaction, stress, acute)
        308.9
  during pregnancy 646.8●
  general 780.79
    psychogenic 300.5
  heat (transient) 992.6
  muscle 729.89
  myocardium (see also Failure, heart)
        428.9
  nervous 300.5
  neurosis 300.5
  operational 300.89
  postural 729.89
  posture 729.89
  psychogenic (general) 300.5
  senile 797
  syndrome NEC 300.5
    chronic 780.71
  undue 780.79
  voice 784.49
Fatness 278.02
Fatty - see also condition
  apron 278.1
  degeneration (diffuse) (general) NEC
        272.8
    localized - see Degeneration, by site,
          fatty
    placenta - see Placenta, abnormal
  heart (enlarged) (see also Degeneration,
        myocardial) 429.1
  infiltration (diffuse) (general) (see also
        Degeneration, by site, fatty) 272.8
    heart (enlarged) (see also
          Degeneration, myocardial)
          429.1
  liver 571.8
    alcoholic 571.0
  necrosis - see Degeneration, fatty
  phanerosis 272.8
Fauces - see condition
Fauchard's disease (periodontitis) 523.40
Faucitis 478.29
Faulty - see also condition
  position of teeth 524.30
Favism (anemia) 282.2
Favre-Racouchot disease (elastoidosis
      cutanea nodularis) 701.8
Favus 110.9
  beard 110.0
  capitis 110.0
  corporis 110.5
  eyelid 110.8
  foot 110.4
  hand 110.2
  scalp 110.0
  specified site NEC 110.8
Fear, fearfulness (complex) (reaction)
      300.20
  child 313.0
  of
    animals 300.29
    closed spaces 300.29
    crowds 300.29
    eating in public 300.23
    heights 300.29
    open spaces 300.22
      with panic attacks 300.21
    public speaking 300.23

Fear, fearfulness (Continued)
  of (Continued)
    streets 300.22
      with panic attacks 300.21
    travel 300.22
      with panic attacks 300.21
    washing in public 300.23
  transient 308.0
Feared complaint unfounded V65.5
Febricula (continued) (simple) (see also
      Pyrexia) 780.60
Febrile (see also Pyrexia) 780.60
  convulsion (simple) 780.31
    complex 780.32
  nonhemolytic transfusion reaction
        (FNHTR) 780.66 ◄
  seizure (simple) 780.31
    atypical 780.32
    complex 780.32
    complicated 780.32
Febris (see also Fever) 780.60
  aestiva (see also Fever, hay) 477.9
  flava (see also Fever, yellow) 060.9
  melitensis 023.0
  pestis (see also Plague) 020.9
  puerperalis 672●
  recurrens (see also Fever, relapsing)
        087.9
    pediculo vestimenti 087.0
  rubra 034.1
  typhoidea 002.0
  typhosa 002.0
Fecal - see condition
Fecalith (impaction) 560.32 ◄▥
  with hernia - see also Hernia, by site,
        with obstruction
    gangrenous - see Hernia, by site,
          with gangrene
  appendix 543.9
  congenital 777.1
Fede's disease 529.0
Feeble-minded 317
Feeble rapid pulse due to shock
      following injury 958.4
Feeding
  faulty (elderly) (infant) 783.3
    newborn 779.31
  formula check V20.2
  improper (elderly) (infant) 783.3
    newborn 779.31
  problem (elderly) (infant) 783.3
    newborn 779.31
  nonorganic origin 307.59
Feeling of foreign body in throat 784.99
Feer's disease 985.0
Feet - see condition
Feigned illness V65.2
Feil-Klippel syndrome (brevicollis) 756.16
Feinmesser's (hidrotic) ectodermal
      dysplasia 757.31
Felix's disease (juvenile osteochondrosis,
      hip) 732.1
Felon (any digit) (with lymphangitis) 681.01
  herpetic 054.6
Felty's syndrome (rheumatoid arthritis
      with splenomegaly and leukopenia)
      714.1
Feminism in boys 302.6
Feminization, testicular 259.51
  with pseudohermaphroditism, male
        259.51
Femoral hernia - see Hernia, femoral
Femora vara 736.32
Femur, femoral - see condition

◄ New   ◄▥ Revised   ~~deleted~~ Deleted   ● Use Additional Digit(s)   ▥ Omit code

Fenestrata placenta - *see* Placenta, abnormal
Fenestration, fenestrated - *see also*
    Imperfect, closure
  aorta-pulmonary 745.0
  aorticopulmonary 745.0
  aortopulmonary 745.0
  cusps, heart valve NEC 746.89
    pulmonary 746.09
  hymen 752.49
  pulmonic cusps 746.09
Fenwick's disease 537.89
Fermentation (gastric) (gastrointestinal)
    (stomach) 536.8
  intestine 564.89
    psychogenic 306.4
  psychogenic 306.4
Fernell's disease (aortic aneurysm) 441.9
Fertile eunuch syndrome 257.2
Fertility, meaning multiparity - *see*
    Multiparity
Fetal
  alcohol syndrome 760.71
  anemia 678.0●
  thrombocytopenia 678.0●
  twin to twin transfusion 678.0●
Fetalis uterus 752.39 ◀▥
Fetid
  breath 784.99
  sweat 705.89
Fetishism 302.81
  transvestic 302.3
Fetomaternal hemorrhage
  affecting management of pregnancy
    656.0●
  fetus or newborn 772.0
Fetus, fetal - *see also* condition
  papyraceous 779.89
  type lung tissue 770.4
Fever 780.60
  with chills 780.60
    in malarial regions (*see also* Malaria)
      084.6
  abortus NEC 023.9
  aden 061
  African tick-borne 087.1
  American
    mountain tick 066.1
    spotted 082.0
  and ague (*see also* Malaria) 084.6
  aphthous 078.4
  arbovirus hemorrhagic 065.9
  Assam 085.0
  Australian A or Q 083.0
  Bangkok hemorrhagic 065.4
  biliary, Charcôt's intermittent - *see*
    Choledocholithiasis
  bilious, hemoglobinuric 084.8
  blackwater 084.8
  blister 054.9
  Bonvale Dam 780.79
  boutonneuse 082.1
  brain 323.9
    late effect - *see* category 326
  breakbone 061
  Bullis 082.8
  Bunyamwera 066.3
  Burdwan 085.0
  Bwamba (encephalitis) 066.3
  Cameroon (*see also* Malaria) 084.6
  Canton 081.9
  catarrhal (acute) 460
    chronic 472.0
  cat-scratch 078.3
  cerebral 323.9
    late effect - *see* category 326

Fever *(Continued)*
  cerebrospinal (meningococcal) (*see also*
    Meningitis, cerebrospinal) 036.0
  Chagres 084.0
  Chandipura 066.8
  changuinola 066.0
  Charcôt's (biliary) (hepatic)
    (intermittent) *see*
    Choledocholithiasis
  Chikungunya (viral) 066.3
    hemorrhagic 065.4
  childbed 670.8●
  Chitral 066.0
  Colombo (*see also* Fever, paratyphoid)
    002.9
  Colorado tick (virus) 066.1
  congestive
    malarial (*see also* Malaria) 084.6
    remittent (*see also* Malaria) 084.6
  Congo virus 065.0
  continued 780.60
    malarial 084.0
  Corsican (*see also* Malaria) 084.6
  Crimean hemorrhagic 065.0
  Cyprus (*see also* Brucellosis) 023.9
  dandy 061
  deer fly (*see also* Tularemia) 021.9
  dehydration, newborn 778.4
  dengue (virus) 061
    hemorrhagic 065.4
  desert 114.0
  due to heat 992.0
  Dumdum 085.0
  enteric 002.0
  ephemeral (of unknown origin) (*see also*
    Pyrexia) 780.60
  epidemic, hemorrhagic of the Far East
    065.0
  erysipelatous (*see also* Erysipelas) 035
  estivo-autumnal (malarial) 084.0
  etiocholanolone 277.31
  famine - *see also* Fever, relapsing
    meaning typhus - *see* Typhus
  Far Eastern hemorrhagic 065.0
  five day 083.1
  Fort Bragg 100.89
  gastroenteric 002.0
  gastromalarial (*see also* Malaria) 084.6
  Gibraltar (*see also* Brucellosis) 023.9
  glandular 075
  Guama (viral) 066.3
  Haverhill 026.1
  hay (allergic) (with rhinitis) 477.9
    with
      asthma (bronchial) (*see also*
        Asthma) 493.0●
    due to
      dander, animal (cat) (dog) 477.2
      dust 477.8
      fowl 477.8
      hair, animal (cat) (dog) 477.2
      pollen, any plant or tree 477.0
      specified allergen other than
        pollen 477.8
  heat (effects) 992.0
  hematuric, bilious 084.8
  hemoglobinuric (malarial) 084.8
    bilious 084.8
  hemorrhagic (arthropod-borne) NEC
    065.9
    with renal syndrome 078.6
    arenaviral 078.7
    Argentine 078.7
    Bangkok 065.4

Fever *(Continued)*
  hemorrhagic NEC *(Continued)*
    Bolivian 078.7
    Central Asian 065.0
    chikungunya 065.4
    Crimean 065.0
    dengue (virus) 065.4
    Ebola 065.8
    epidemic 078.6
      of Far East 065.0
    Far Eastern 065.0
    Junin virus 078.7
    Korean 078.6
    Kyasanur forest 065.2
    Machupo virus 078.7
    mite-borne NEC 065.8
    mosquito-borne 065.4
    Omsk 065.1
    Philippine 065.4
    Russian (Yaroslav) 078.6
    Singapore 065.4
    Southeast Asia 065.4
    Thailand 065.4
    tick-borne NEC 065.3
  hepatic (*see also* Cholecystitis) 575.8
    intermittent (Charcôt's) - *see*
      Choledocholithiasis
  herpetic (*see also* Herpes) 054.9
  hyalomma tick 065.0
  icterohemorrhagic 100.0
  inanition 780.60
    newborn 778.4
  in conditions classified elsewhere
    780.61
  infective NEC 136.9
  intermittent (bilious) (*see also* Malaria)
    084.6
    hepatic (Charcôt) - *see*
      Choledocholithiasis
    of unknown origin (*see also* Pyrexia)
      780.60
    pernicious 084.0
  iodide
    correct substance properly
      administered 780.60
    overdose or wrong substance given
      or taken 975.5
  Japanese river 081.2
  jungle yellow 060.0
  Junin virus, hemorrhagic 078.7
  Katayama 120.2
  Kedani 081.2
  Kenya 082.1
  Korean hemorrhagic 078.6
  Lassa 078.89
  Lone Star 082.8
  lung - *see* Pneumonia
  Machupo virus, hemorrhagic 078.7
  malaria, malarial (*see also* Malaria)
    084.6
  Malta (*see also* Brucellosis) 023.9
  Marseilles 082.1
  marsh (*see also* Malaria) 084.6
  Mayaro (viral) 066.3
  Mediterranean (*see also* Brucellosis)
    023.9
    familial 277.31
    tick 082.1
  meningeal - *see* Meningitis
  metal fumes NEC 985.8
  Meuse 083.1
  Mexican - *see* Typhus, Mexican
  Mianeh 087.1
  miasmatic (*see also* Malaria) 084.6

Fever (*Continued*)
  miliary 078.2
  milk, female 672●
  mill 504
  mite-borne hemorrhagic 065.8
  Monday 504
  mosquito-borne NEC 066.3
    hemorrhagic NEC 065.4
  mountain 066.1
    meaning
      Rocky Mountain spotted 082.0
      undulant fever (*see also*
        Brucellosis) 023.9
    tick (American) 066.1
  Mucambo (viral) 066.3
  mud 100.89
  Neapolitan (*see also* Brucellosis) 023.9
  neutropenic 288.00
  newborn (environmentally-induced)
    778.4
  nine-mile 083.0
  nonexanthematous tick 066.1
  North Asian tick-borne typhus 082.2
  Omsk hemorrhagic 065.1
  O'nyong nyong (viral) 066.3
  Oropouche (viral) 066.3
  Oroya 088.0
  paludal (*see also* Malaria) 084.6
  Panama 084.0
  pappataci 066.0
  paratyphoid 002.9
    A 002.1
    B (Schottmüller's) 002.2
    C (Hirschfeld) 002.3
  parrot 073.9
  periodic 277.31
  pernicious, acute 084.0
  persistent (of unknown origin) (*see also*
    Pyrexia) 780.60
  petechial 036.0
  pharyngoconjunctival 077.2
    adenoviral type 3 077.2
  Philippine hemorrhagic 065.4
  phlebotomus 066.0
  Piry 066.8
  Pixuna (viral) 066.3
  Plasmodium ovale 084.3
  pleural (*see also* Pleurisy) 511.0
  pneumonic - *see* Pneumonia
  polymer fume 987.8
  postimmunization 780.63
  postoperative 780.62
    due to infection 998.59
  posttransfusion 780.66 ◀
  postvaccination 780.63
  pretibial 100.89
  puerperal, postpartum 672●
  putrid - *see* Septicemia
  pyemic - *see* Septicemia
  Q 083.0
    with pneumonia 083.0 *[484.8]*
  quadrilateral 083.0
  quartan (malaria) 084.2
  Queensland (coastal) 083.0
    seven-day 100.89
  Quintan (A) 083.1
  quotidian 084.0
  rabbit (*see also* Tularemia) 021.9
  rat-bite 026.9
    due to
      Spirillum minor or minus 026.0
      Spirochaeta morsus muris 026.0
      Streptobacillus moniliformis 026.1
  recurrent - *see* Fever, relapsing

Fever (*Continued*)
  relapsing 087.9
    Carter's (Asiatic) 087.0
    Dutton's (West African) 087.1
    Koch's 087.9
    louse-borne (epidemic) 087.0
    Novy's (American) 087.1
    Obermeyer's (European) 087.0
    spirillum NEC 087.9
    tick-borne (endemic) 087.1
  remittent (bilious) (congestive) (gastric)
    (*see also* Malaria) 084.6
  rheumatic (active) (acute) (chronic)
    (subacute) 390
    with heart involvement 391.9
      carditis 391.9
      endocarditis (aortic) (mitral)
        (pulmonary) (tricuspid)
        391.1
      multiple sites 391.8
      myocarditis 391.2
      pancarditis, acute 391.8
      pericarditis 391.0
      specified type NEC 391.8
      valvulitis 391.1
    inactive or quiescent with
      cardiac hypertrophy 398.99
      carditis 398.90
      endocarditis 397.9
        aortic (valve) 395.9
          with mitral (valve) disease
            396.9
        mitral (valve) 394.9
          with aortic (valve) disease
            396.9
        pulmonary (valve) 397.1
        tricuspid (valve) 397.0
      heart conditions (classifiable to
        429.3, 429.6, 429.9) 398.99
      failure (congestive) (conditions
        classifiable to 428.0,
        428.9) 398.91
      left ventricular failure
        (conditions classifiable
        to 428.1) 398.91
      myocardial degeneration
        (conditions classifiable to
        429.1) 398.0
      myocarditis (conditions
        classifiable to 429.0) 398.0
      pancarditis 398.99
      pericarditis 393
  Rift Valley (viral) 066.3
  Rocky Mountain spotted 082.0
  rose 477.0
  Ross river (viral) 066.3
  Russian hemorrhagic 078.6
  sandfly 066.0
  San Joaquin (valley) 114.0
  Sao Paulo 082.0
  scarlet 034.1
  septic - *see* Septicemia
  seven-day 061
    Japan 100.89
    Queensland 100.89
  shin bone 083.1
  Singapore hemorrhagic 065.4
  solar 061
  sore 054.9
  South African tick-bite 087.1
  Southeast Asia hemorrhagic 065.4
  spinal - *see* Meningitis
  spirillary 026.0
  splenic (*see also* Anthrax) 022.9

Fever (*Continued*)
  spotted (Rocky Mountain) 082.0
    American 082.0
    Brazilian 082.0
    Colombian 082.0
    meaning
      cerebrospinal meningitis 036.0
      typhus 082.9
  spring 309.23
  steroid
    correct substance properly
      administered 780.60
    overdose or wrong substance given
      or taken 962.0
  streptobacillary 026.1
  subtertian 084.0
  Sumatran mite 081.2
  sun 061
  swamp 100.89
  sweating 078.2
  swine 003.8
  sylvatic yellow 060.0
  Tahyna 062.5
  tertian - *see* Malaria, tertian
  Thailand hemorrhagic 065.4
  thermic 992.0
  three day 066.0
    with Coxsackie exanthem 074.8
  tick
    American mountain 066.1
    Colorado 066.1
    Kemerovo 066.1
    Mediterranean 082.1
    mountain 066.1
    nonexanthematous 066.1
    Quaranfil 066.1
  tick-bite NEC 066.1
  tick-borne NEC 066.1
    hemorrhagic NEC 065.3
  transitory of newborn 778.4
  trench 083.1
  tsutsugamushi 081.2
  typhogastric 002.0
  typhoid (abortive) (ambulant) (any
    site) (hemorrhagic) (infection)
    (intermittent) (malignant)
    (rheumatic) 002.0
  typhomalarial (*see also* Malaria) 084.6
  typhus - *see* Typhus
  undulant (*see also* Brucellosis) 023.9
  unknown origin (*see also* Pyrexia)
    780.60
  uremic - *see* Uremia
  uveoparotid 135
  valley (Coccidioidomycosis) 114.0
  Venezuelan equine 066.2
  Volhynian 083.1
  Wesselsbron (viral) 066.3
  West
    African 084.8
    Nile (viral) 066.40
      with
        cranial nerve disorders
          066.42
        encephalitis 066.41
        optic neuritis 066.42
        other complications 066.49
        other neurologic manifestations
          066.42
        polyradiculitis 066.42
  Whitmore's 025
  Wolhynian 083.1
  worm 128.9
  Yaroslav hemorrhagic 078.6

◀ New   ◀▥ Revised   ~~deleted~~ Deleted   ● Use Additional Digit(s)   ▨ Omit code

Fever (*Continued*)
  yellow 060.9
    jungle 060.0
    sylvatic 060.0
    urban 060.1
    vaccination, prophylactic (against)
      V04.4
  Zika (viral) 066.3
Fibrillation
  atrial (established) (paroxysmal) 427.31
  auricular (atrial) (established) 427.31
  cardiac (ventricular) 427.41
  coronary (*see also* Infarct, myocardium)
    410.9●
  heart (ventricular) 427.41
  muscular 728.9
  postoperative 997.1
  ventricular 427.41
Fibrin
  ball or bodies, pleural (sac) 511.0
  chamber, anterior (eye) (gelatinous
    exudate) 364.04
Fibrinogenolysis (hemorrhagic) - *see*
    Fibrinolysis
Fibrinogenopenia (congenital) (hereditary)
    (*see also* Defect, coagulation) 286.3
  acquired 286.6
Fibrinolysis (acquired) (hemorrhagic)
    (pathologic) 286.6
  with
    abortion - *see* Abortion, by type, with
      hemorrhage, delayed or
      excessive
    ectopic pregnancy (*see also*
      categories 633.0–633.9) 639.1
    molar pregnancy (*see also* categories
      630–632) 639.1
  antepartum or intrapartum 641.3●
    affecting fetus or newborn 762.1
  following
    abortion 639.1
    ectopic or molar pregnancy 639.1
  newborn, transient 776.2
  postpartum 666.3●
Fibrinopenia (hereditary) (*see also* Defect,
    coagulation) 286.3
  acquired 286.6
Fibrinopurulent - *see* condition
Fibrinous - *see* condition
Fibroadenoma (M9010/0)
  cellular intracanalicular (M9020/0) 217
  giant (intracanalicular) (M9020/0) 217
  intracanalicular (M9011/0)
    cellular (M9020/0) 217
    giant (M9020/0) 217
    specified site - *see* Neoplasm, by site,
      benign
    unspecified site 217
  juvenile (M9030/0) 217
  pericanicular (M9012/0)
    specified site - *see* Neoplasm, by site,
      benign
    unspecified site 217
  phyllodes (M9020/0) 217
  prostate 600.20
    with
      other lower urinary tract
        symptoms (LUTS) 600.21
      urinary
        obstruction 600.21
        retention 600.21
  specified site - *see* Neoplasm, by site,
    benign
  unspecified site 217

Fibroadenosis, breast (chronic) (cystic)
    (diffuse) (periodic) (segmental) 610.2
Fibroangioma (M9160/0) - *see also*
    Neoplasm, by site, benign
  juvenile (M9160/0)
    specified site - *see* Neoplasm, by site,
      benign
    unspecified site 210.7
Fibrocellulitis progressiva ossificans
    728.11
Fibrochondrosarcoma (M9220/3) - *see*
    Neoplasm, cartilage, malignant
Fibrocystic
  disease 277.00
    bone NEC 733.29
    breast 610.1
    jaw 526.2
    kidney (congenital) 753.19
    liver 751.62
    lung 518.89
      congenital 748.4
    pancreas 277.00
  kidney (congenital) 753.19
Fibrodysplasia ossificans multiplex
    (progressiva) 728.11
Fibroelastosis (cordis) (endocardial)
    (endomyocardial) 425.3
Fibroid (tumor) (M8890/0) - *see also*
    Neoplasm, connective tissue, benign
  disease, lung (chronic) (*see also* Fibrosis,
    lung) 515
  heart (disease) (*see also* Myocarditis)
    429.0
  induration, lung (chronic) (*see also*
    Fibrosis, lung) 515
  in pregnancy or childbirth 654.1●
    affecting fetus or newborn 763.89
    causing obstructed labor 660.2●
      affecting fetus or newborn
        763.1
  liver - *see* Cirrhosis, liver
  lung (*see also* Fibrosis, lung) 515
  pneumonia (chronic) (*see also* Fibrosis,
    lung) 515
  uterus (M8890/0) (*see also* Leiomyoma,
    uterus) 218.9
Fibrolipoma (M8851/0) (*see also* Lipoma,
    by site) 214.9
Fibroliposarcoma (M8850/3) - *see*
    Neoplasm, connective tissue,
    malignant
Fibroma (M8810/0) - *see also* Neoplasm,
    connective tissue, benign
  ameloblastic (M9330/0) 213.1
    upper jaw (bone) 213.0
  bone (nonossifying) 733.99
    ossifying (M9262/0) - *see* Neoplasm,
      bone, benign
  cementifying (M9274/0) - *see*
    Neoplasm, bone, benign
  chondromyxoid (M9241/0) - *see*
    Neoplasm, bone, benign
  desmoplastic (M8823/1) - *see*
    Neoplasm, connective tissue,
    uncertain behavior
  facial (M8813/0) - *see* Neoplasm,
    connective tissue, benign
  invasive (M8821/1) - *see* Neoplasm,
    connective tissue, uncertain
    behavior
  molle (M8851/0) (*see also* Lipoma, by
    site) 214.9
  myxoid (M8811/0) - *see* Neoplasm,
    connective tissue, benign

Fibroma (*Continued*)
  nasopharynx, nasopharyngeal
    (juvenile) (M9160/0) 210.7
  nonosteogenic (nonossifying) - *see*
    Dysplasia, fibrous
  odontogenic (M9321/0) 213.1
    upper jaw (bone) 213.0
  ossifying (M9262/0) - *see* Neoplasm,
    bone, benign
  periosteal (M8812/0) - *see* Neoplasm,
    bone, benign
  prostate 600.20
    with
      other lower urinary tract
        symptoms (LUTS) 600.21
      urinary
        obstruction 600.21
        retention 600.21
  soft (M8851/0) (*see also* Lipoma, by
    site) 214.9
Fibromatosis 728.79
  abdominal (M8822/1) - *see* Neoplasm,
    connective tissue, uncertain
    behavior
  aggressive (M8821/1) - *see* Neoplasm,
    connective tissue, uncertain
    behavior
  congenital generalized (CGF) 759.89
  Dupuytren's 728.6
  gingival 523.8
  plantar fascia 728.71
  proliferative 728.79
  pseudosarcomatous (proliferative)
    (subcutaneous) 728.79
  subcutaneous pseudosarcomatous
    (proliferative) 728.79
Fibromyalgia 729.1
Fibromyoma (M8890/0) - *see also*
    Neoplasm, connective tissue, benign
  uterus (corpus) (*see also* Leiomyoma,
    uterus) 218.9
    in pregnancy or childbirth 654.1●
      affecting fetus or newborn 763.89
      causing obstructed labor 660.2●
        affecting fetus or newborn
          763.1
Fibromyositis (*see also* Myositis) 729.1
  scapulohumeral 726.2
Fibromyxolipoma (M8852/0) (*see also*
    Lipoma, by site) 214.9
Fibromyxoma (M8811/0) - *see* Neoplasm,
    connective tissue, benign
Fibromyxosarcoma (M8811/3) - *see*
    Neoplasm, connective tissue,
    malignant
Fibro-odontoma, ameloblastic (M9290/0)
    213.1
  upper jaw (bone) 213.0
Fibro-osteoma (M9262/0) - *see* Neoplasm,
    bone, benign
Fibroplasia, retrolental (*see also*
    Retinopathy of prematurity) 362.21
Fibropurulent - *see* condition
Fibrosarcoma (M8810/3) - *see also*
    Neoplasm, connective tissue,
    malignant
  ameloblastic (M9330/3) 170.1
    upper jaw (bone) 170.0
  congenital (M8814/3) - *see* Neoplasm,
    connective tissue, malignant
  fascial (M8813/3) - *see* Neoplasm,
    connective tissue, malignant
  infantile (M8814/3) - *see* Neoplasm,
    connective tissue, malignant

Fibrosarcoma *(Continued)*
  odontogenic (M9330/3) 170.1
    upper jaw (bone) 170.0
  periosteal (M8812/3) - *see* Neoplasm,
    bone, malignant
Fibrosclerosis
  breast 610.3
  corpora cavernosa (penis) 607.89
  familial multifocal NEC 710.8
  multifocal (idiopathic) NEC 710.8
  penis (corpora cavernosa) 607.89
Fibrosis, fibrotic
  adrenal (gland) 255.8
  alveolar (diffuse) 516.3
  amnion 658.8●
  anal papillae 569.49
  anus 569.49
  appendix, appendiceal,
    noninflammatory 543.9
  arteriocapillary - *see* Arteriosclerosis
  bauxite (of lung) 503
  biliary 576.8
    due to Clonorchis sinensis 121.1
  bladder 596.8
    interstitial 595.1
    localized submucosal 595.1
    panmural 595.1
  bone, diffuse 756.59
  breast 610.3
  capillary - *see also* Arteriosclerosis
    lung (chronic) (*see also* Fibrosis,
      lung) 515
  cardiac (*see also* Myocarditis) 429.0
  cervix 622.8
  chorion 658.8●
  corpus cavernosum 607.89
  cystic (of pancreas) 277.00
    with
      manifestations
        gastrointestinal 277.03
        pulmonary 277.02
        specified NEC 277.09
      meconium ileus 277.01
      pulmonary exacerbation 277.02
  due to (presence of) any device,
    implant, or graft - *see*
    Complications, due to
    (presence of) any device, implant,
    or graft classified to 996.0–996.5
    NEC
  ejaculatory duct 608.89
  endocardium (*see also* Endocarditis)
    424.90
  endomyocardial (African) 425.0
  epididymis 608.89
  eye muscle 378.62
  graphite (of lung) 503
  heart (*see also* Myocarditis) 429.0
  hepatic - *see also* Cirrhosis, liver
    due to Clonorchis sinensis 121.1
  hepatolienal - *see* Cirrhosis, liver
  hepatosplenic - *see* Cirrhosis, liver
  infrapatellar fat pad 729.31
  interstitial pulmonary, newborn
    770.7
  intrascrotal 608.89
  kidney (*see also* Sclerosis, renal) 587
  liver - *see* Cirrhosis, liver
  lung (atrophic) (capillary) (chronic)
    (confluent) (massive)
    (perialveolar) (peribronchial)
    515
    with
      anthracosilicosis (occupational)
        500

Fibrosis, fibrotic *(Continued)*
  lung *(Continued)*
    with *(Continued)*
      anthracosis (occupational) 500
      asbestosis (occupational) 501
      bagassosis (occupational) 495.1
      bauxite 503
      berylliosis (occupational) 503
      byssinosis (occupational) 504
      calcicosis (occupational) 502
      chalicosis (occupational) 502
      dust reticulation (occupational)
        504
      farmers' lung 495.0
      gannister disease (occupational)
        502
      graphite 503
      pneumonoconiosis (occupational)
        505
      pneumosiderosis (occupational)
        503
      siderosis (occupational) 503
      silicosis (occupational) 502
      tuberculosis (*see also* Tuberculosis)
        011.4●
    diffuse (idiopathic) (interstitial)
      516.3
    due to
      bauxite 503
      fumes or vapors (chemical)
        (inhalation) 506.4
      graphite 503
    following radiation 508.1
    postinflammatory 515
    silicotic (massive) (occupational)
      502
    tuberculous (*see also* Tuberculosis)
      011.4●
  lymphatic gland 289.3
  median bar 600.90
    with
      other lower urinary tract
        symptoms (LUTS) 600.91
      urinary
        obstruction 600.91
        retention 600.91
  mediastinum (idiopathic) 519.3
  meninges 349.2
  muscle NEC 728.2
    iatrogenic (from injection) 999.9
  myocardium, myocardial (*see also*
    Myocarditis) 429.0
  oral submucous 528.8
  ovary 620.8
  oviduct 620.8
  pancreas 577.8
    cystic 277.00
      with
        manifestations
          gastrointestinal 277.03
          pulmonary 277.02
          specified NEC 277.09
        meconium ileus 277.01
        pulmonary exacerbation
          277.02
  penis 607.89
  periappendiceal 543.9
  periarticular (*see also* Ankylosis)
    718.5●
  pericardium 423.1
  perineum, in pregnancy or childbirth
    654.8●
    affecting fetus or newborn 763.89
    causing obstructed labor 660.2●
      affecting fetus or newborn 763.1

Fibrosis, fibrotic *(Continued)*
  perineural NEC 355.9
    foot 355.6
  periureteral 593.89
  placenta - *see* Placenta, abnormal
  pleura 511.0
  popliteal fat pad 729.31
  preretinal 362.56
  prostate (chronic) 600.90
    with
      other lower urinary tract
        symptoms (LUTS) 600.91
      urinary
        obstruction 600.91
        retention 600.91
  pulmonary (chronic) (*see also* Fibrosis,
    lung) 515
    alveolar capillary block 516.3
    interstitial
      diffuse (idiopathic) 516.3
      newborn 770.7
  radiation - *see* Effect, adverse, radiation
  rectal sphincter 569.49
  retroperitoneal, idiopathic 593.4
  sclerosing mesenteric (idiopathic)
    567.82
  scrotum 608.89
  seminal vesicle 608.89
  senile 797
  skin NEC 709.2
  spermatic cord 608.89
  spleen 289.59
    bilharzial (*see also* Schistosomiasis)
      120.9
  subepidermal nodular (M8832/0) - *see*
    Neoplasm, skin, benign
  submucous NEC 709.2
    oral 528.8
    tongue 528.8
  syncytium - *see* Placenta, abnormal
  testis 608.89
    chronic, due to syphilis 095.8
  thymus (gland) 254.8
  tunica vaginalis 608.89
  ureter 593.89
  urethra 599.84
  uterus (nonneoplastic) 621.8
    bilharzial (*see also* Schistosomiasis)
      120.9
    neoplastic (*see also* Leiomyoma,
      uterus) 218.9
  vagina 623.8
  valve, heart (*see also* Endocarditis)
    424.90
  vas deferens 608.89
  vein 459.89
    lower extremities 459.89
  vesical 595.1
Fibrositis (periarticular) (rheumatoid)
  729.0
  humeroscapular region 726.2
  nodular, chronic
    Jaccoud's 714.4
    rheumatoid 714.4
  ossificans 728.11
  scapulohumeral 726.2
Fibrothorax 511.0
Fibrotic - *see* Fibrosis
Fibrous - *see* condition
Fibroxanthoma (M8831/0) - *see also*
  Neoplasm, connective tissue,
  benign
  atypical (M8831/1) - *see* Neoplasm,
    connective tissue, uncertain
    behavior

Fibroxanthoma *(Continued)*
  malignant (M8831/3) - *see* Neoplasm,
    connective tissue, malignant
Fibroxanthosarcoma (M8831/3) - *see*
    Neoplasm, connective tissue,
    malignant
Fiedler's
  disease (leptospiral jaundice) 100.0
  myocarditis or syndrome (acute
    isolated myocarditis) 422.91
Fiessinger-Leroy (-Reiter) syndrome 099.3
Fiessinger-Rendu syndrome (erythema
    muliforme exudativum) 695.19
Fifth disease (eruptive) 057.0
  venereal 099.1
Filaria, filarial - *see* Infestation, filarial
Filariasis (*see also* Infestation, filarial) 125.9
  bancroftian 125.0
  Brug's 125.1
  due to
    bancrofti 125.0
    Brugia (Wuchereria) (malayi) 125.1
    Loa loa 125.2
    malayi 125.1
    organism NEC 125.6
    Wuchereria (bancrofti) 125.0
      malayi 125.1
  Malayan 125.1
  ozzardi 125.5
  specified type NEC 125.6
Filatoff's, Filatov's, Filatow's disease
    (infectious mononucleosis) 075
File-cutters' disease 984.9
  specified type of lead - *see* Table of
    Drugs and Chemicals
Filling defect
  biliary tract 793.3
  bladder 793.5
  duodenum 793.4
  gallbladder 793.3
  gastrointestinal tract 793.4
  intestine 793.4
  kidney 793.5
  stomach 793.4
  ureter 793.5
Filtering bleb, eye (postglaucoma)
    (status) V45.69
  with complication or rupture 997.99
  postcataract extraction (complication)
    997.99
Fimbrial cyst (congenital) 752.11
Fimbriated hymen 752.49
Financial problem affecting care V60.2
Findings, (abnormal), without diagnosis
    (examination) (laboratory
    test) 796.4
  17-ketosteroids, elevated 791.9
  acetonuria 791.6
  acid phosphatase 790.5
  albumin-globulin ratio 790.99
  albuminuria 791.0
  alcohol in blood 790.3
  alkaline phosphatase 790.5
  amniotic fluid 792.3
  amylase 790.5
  antenatal screening 796.5
  anisocytosis 790.09
  anthrax, positive 795.31
  antibody titers, elevated 795.79
  anticardiolipin antibody 795.79
  antigen-antibody reaction 795.79
  antiphospholipid antibody 795.79
  bacteriuria 791.9
  ballistocardiogram 794.39
  bile in urine 791.4
  bilirubin 277.4

Findings *(Continued)*
  bleeding time (prolonged) 790.92
  blood culture, positive 790.7
  blood gas level (arterial) 790.91
  blood sugar level 790.29
    high 790.29
      fasting glucose 790.21
      glucose tolerance test 790.22
    low 251.2
  C-reactive protein (CRP) 790.95
  calcium 275.40
  cancer antigen 125 [CA 125] 795.82
  carbonate 276.9
  carcinoembryonic antigen [CEA] 795.81
  casts, urine 791.7
  catecholamines 791.9
  cells, urine 791.7
  cerebrospinal fluid (color) (content)
    (pressure) 792.0
  cervical
    high risk human papillomavirus
      (HPV) DNA test positive
      795.05
    low risk human papillomavirus
      (HPV) DNA test positive
      795.09
    non-atypical endometrial cells
      795.09 ◄
  chloride 276.9
  cholesterol 272.9
    high 272.0
      with high triglycerides 272.2
  chromosome analysis 795.2
  chyluria 791.1
  circulation time 794.39
  cloudy dialysis effluent 792.5
  cloudy urine 791.9
  coagulation study 790.92
  cobalt, blood 790.6
  color of urine (unusual) NEC 791.9
  copper, blood 790.6
  creatinine clearance 794.4
  crystals, urine 791.9
  culture, positive NEC 795.39
    blood 790.7
    HIV V08
    human immunodeficiency virus V08
    nose 795.39
      Staphylococcus - *see* Carrier
        (suspected) of,
        Staphylococcus
    skin lesion NEC 795.39
    spinal fluid 792.0
    sputum 795.39
    stool 792.1
    throat 795.39
    urine 791.9
    viral
      human immunodeficiency V08
    wound 795.39
  cytology specified site NEC 796.9
  echocardiogram 793.2
  echoencephalogram 794.01
  echogram NEC - *see* Findings,
    abnormal, structure
  electrocardiogram (ECG) (EKG)
    794.31
  electroencephalogram (EEG) 794.02
  electrolyte level, urinary 791.9
  electromyogram (EMG) 794.17
    ocular 794.14
  electro-oculogram (EOG) 794.12
  electroretinogram (ERG) 794.11
  enzymes, serum NEC 790.5
  fibrinogen titer coagulation study 790.92
  filling defect - *see* Filling defect

Findings *(Continued)*
  function study NEC 794.9
    auditory 794.15
    bladder 794.9
    brain 794.00
    cardiac 794.30
    endocrine NEC 794.6
      thyroid 794.5
    kidney 794.4
    liver 794.8
    nervous system
      central 794.00
      peripheral 794.19
    oculomotor 794.14
    pancreas 794.9
    placenta 794.9
    pulmonary 794.2
    retina 794.11
    special senses 794.19
    spleen 794.9
    vestibular 794.16
  gallbladder, nonvisualization 793.3
  glucose 790.29
    elevated
      fasting 790.21
      tolerance test 790.22
  glycosuria 791.5
  heart
    shadow 793.2
    sounds 785.3
  hematinuria 791.2
  hematocrit
    drop (precipitous) 790.01
    elevated 282.7
    low 285.9
  hematologic NEC 790.99
  hematuria 599.70
  hemoglobin
    drop 790.01
    elevated 282.7
    low 285.9
  hemoglobinuria 791.2
  histological NEC 795.4
  hormones 259.9
  immunoglobulins, elevated 795.79
  indolacetic acid, elevated 791.9
  iron 790.6
  karyotype 795.2
  ketonuria 791.6
  lactic acid dehydrogenase
    (LDH) 790.4
  lead 790.6
  lipase 790.5
  lipids NEC 272.9
  lithium, blood 790.6
  liver function test 790.6
  lung field (coin lesion) (shadow)
    793.1
  magnesium, blood 790.6
  mammogram 793.80
    calcification 793.89
    calculus 793.89
    dense breasts 793.82
    inconclusive 793.82
      due to dense breasts 793.82
    microcalcification 793.81
  mediastinal shift 793.2
  melanin, urine 791.9
  microbiologic NEC 795.39
  mineral, blood NEC 790.6
  myoglobinuria 791.3
  nasal swab, anthrax 795.31
  neonatal screening 796.6
  nitrogen derivatives, blood 790.6
  nonvisualization of gallbladder 793.3
  nose culture, positive 795.39

Findings *(Continued)*
odor of urine (unusual) NEC 791.9
oxygen saturation 790.91
Papanicolaou (smear) 796.9
  anus 796.70
    with
      atypical squamous cells
        cannot exclude high
          grade squamous
          intraepithelial
          lesion (ASC-H) 796.72
        of undetermined
          significance
          (ASC-US) 796.71
      cytologic evidence of
        malignancy 796.76
      high grade squamous
        intraepithelial lesion
        (HGSIL) 796.74
      low grade squamous
        intraepithelial lesion
        (LGSIL) 796.73
  glandular 796.70
  specified finding NEC 796.79
  cervix 795.00
    with
      atypical squamous cells
        cannot exclude high grade
          squamous
          intraepithelial lesion
          (ASC-H) 795.02
        of undetermined significance
          (ASC-US) 795.01
      cytologic evidence of
        malignancy 795.06
      high grade squamous
        intraepithelial lesion
        (HGSIL) 795.04
      low grade squamous
        intraepithelial lesion
        (LGSIL) 795.03
      non-atypical endometrial cells
        795.09 ◀
    dyskaryotic 795.09
    non-atypical endometrial cells
      795.09 ◀
    nonspecific finding NEC 795.09
  other site 796.9
  vagina 795.10
    with
      atypical squamous cells
        cannot exclude high grade
          squamous
          intraepithelial lesion
          (ASC-H) 795.12
        of undetermined significance
          (ASC-US) 795.11
      cytologic evidence of
        malignancy 795.16
      high grade squamous
        intraepithelial lesion
        (HGSIL) 795.14
      low grade squamous
        intraepithelial lesion
        (LGSIL) 795.13
  glandular 795.10
  specified NEC 795.19
peritoneal fluid 792.9
phonocardiogram 794.39
phosphorus 275.3
pleural fluid 792.9
pneumoencephalogram 793.0
PO$_2$-oxygen ratio 790.91
poikilocytosis 790.09

Findings *(Continued)*
potassium
  deficiency 276.8
  excess 276.7
PPD 795.5
prostate specific antigen (PSA)
  790.93
protein, serum NEC 790.99
proteinuria 791.0
prothrombin time (prolonged) (partial)
  (PT) (PTT) 790.92
pyuria 791.9
radiologic (x-ray) 793.99
  abdomen 793.6
  biliary tract 793.3
  breast 793.89
    abnormal mammogram NOS
      793.80
    mammographic
      calcification 793.89
      calculus 793.89
      microcalcification 793.81
  gastrointestinal tract 793.4
  genitourinary organs 793.5
  head 793.0
  image test inconclusive due to
    excess body fat 793.91
  intrathoracic organs NEC 793.2
  lung 793.1
  musculoskeletal 793.7
  placenta 793.99
  retroperitoneum 793.6
  skin 793.99
  skull 793.0
  subcutaneous tissue 793.99
red blood cell 790.09
  count 790.09
  morphology 790.09
  sickling 790.09
  volume 790.09
saliva 792.4
scan NEC 794.9
  bladder 794.9
  bone 794.9
  brain 794.09
  kidney 794.4
  liver 794.8
  lung 794.2
  pancreas 794.9
  placental 794.9
  spleen 794.9
  thyroid 794.5
sedimentation rate, elevated 790.1
semen 792.2
serological (for)
  human immunodeficiency virus
    (HIV)
    inconclusive 795.71
    positive V08
  syphilis - *see* Findings, serology for
    syphilis
serology for syphilis
  false positive 795.6
  positive 097.1
    false 795.6
    follow-up of latent syphilis - *see*
      Syphilis, latent
    only finding - *see* Syphilis, latent
serum 790.99
  blood NEC 790.99
  enzymes NEC 790.5
  proteins 790.99
SGOT 790.4
SGPT 790.4

Findings *(Continued)*
sickling of red blood cells 790.09
skin test, positive 795.79
  tuberculin (without active
    tuberculosis) 795.5
sodium 790.6
  deficiency 276.1
  excess 276.0
specified NEC 796.9
spermatozoa 792.2
spinal fluid 792.0
  culture, positive 792.0
sputum culture, positive 795.39
  for acid-fast bacilli 795.39
stool NEC 792.1
  bloody 578.1
    occult 792.1
  color 792.1
  culture, positive 792.1
  occult blood 792.1
stress test 794.39
structure, body (echogram)
  (thermogram) (ultrasound) (x-ray)
  NEC 793.99
  abdomen 793.6
  breast 793.89
    abnormal mammogram 793.80
    mammographic
      calcification 793.89
      calculus 793.89
      microcalcification 793.81
  gastrointestinal tract 793.4
  genitourinary organs 793.5
  head 793.0
    echogram (ultrasound) 794.01
  intrathoracic organs NEC 793.2
  lung 793.1
  musculoskeletal 793.7
  placenta 793.99
  retroperitoneum 793.6
  skin 793.99
  subcutaneous tissue NEC 793.99
synovial fluid 792.9
thermogram - *see* Findings, abnormal,
  structure
throat culture, positive 795.39
thyroid (function) 794.5
  metabolism (rate) 794.5
  scan 794.5
  uptake 794.5
total proteins 790.99
toxicology (drugs) (heavy metals) 796.0
transaminase (level) 790.4
triglycerides 272.9
  high 272.1
    with high cholesterol 272.2
tuberculin skin test (without active
  tuberculosis) 795.5
tumor markers NEC 795.89
ultrasound - *see also* Findings,
  abnormal, structure
  cardiogram 793.2
uric acid, blood 790.6
urine, urinary constituents 791.9
  acetone 791.6
  albumin 791.0
  bacteria 791.9
  bile 791.4
  blood 599.70
  casts or cells 791.7
  chyle 791.1
  culture, positive 791.9
  glucose 791.5
  hemoglobin 791.2

◀ New   ◀▥ Revised   ~~deleted~~ Deleted   ● Use Additional Digit(s)   ▥ Omit code

Findings (*Continued*)
  urine, urinary constituents (*Continued*)
    ketone 791.6
    protein 791.0
    pus 791.9
    sugar 791.5
  vaginal
    fluid 792.9
    high risk human papillomavirus
        (HPV) DNA test positive
        795.15
    low risk human papillomavirus
        (HPV) DNA test positive
        795.19
  vanillylmandelic acid, elevated
      791.9
  vectorcardiogram (VCG) 794.39
  ventriculogram (cerebral) 793.0
  VMA, elevated 791.9
  Wassermann reaction
    false positive 795.6
    positive 097.1
      follow-up of latent syphilis - *see*
          Syphilis, latent
      only finding - *see* Syphilis, latent
  white blood cell 288.9
    count 288.9
      elevated 288.60
      low 288.50
    differential 288.9
    morphology 288.9
  wound culture 795.39
  xerography 793.89
  zinc, blood 790.6
Finger - *see* condition
Finnish type nephrosis (congenital)
    759.89
Fire, St. Anthony's (*see also* Erysipelas) 035
Fish
  hook stomach 537.89
  meal workers' lung 495.8
Fisher's syndrome 357.0
Fissure, fissured
  abdominal wall (congenital) 756.79
  anus, anal 565.0
    congenital 751.5
  buccal cavity 528.9
  clitoris (congenital) 752.49
  ear, lobule (congenital) 744.29
  epiglottis (congenital) 748.3
  larynx 478.79
    congenital 748.3
  lip 528.5
    congenital (*see also* Cleft, lip) 749.10
  nipple 611.2
    puerperal, postpartum 676.1●
  palate (congenital) (*see also* Cleft,
      palate) 749.00
  postanal 565.0
  rectum 565.0
  skin 709.8
    streptococcal 686.9
  spine (congenital) (*see also* Spina bifida)
      741.9●
  sternum (congenital) 756.3
  tongue (acquired) 529.5
    congenital 750.13
Fistula (sinus) 686.9
  abdomen (wall) 569.81
    bladder 596.2
    intestine 569.81
    ureter 593.82
    uterus 619.2
  abdominorectal 569.81
  abdominosigmoidal 569.81

Fistula (*Continued*)
  abdominothoracic 510.0
  abdominouterine 619.2
    congenital 752.39 ◀▥
  abdominovesical 596.2
  accessory sinuses (*see also* Sinusitis)
      473.9
  actinomycotic - *see* Actinomycosis
  alveolar
    antrum (*see also* Sinusitis, maxillary)
        473.0
    process 522.7
  anorectal 565.1
  antrobuccal (*see also* Sinusitis,
      maxillary) 473.0
  antrum (*see also* Sinusitis, maxillary)
      473.0
  anus, anal (infectional) (recurrent)
      565.1
    congenital 751.5
    tuberculous (*see also* Tuberculosis)
        014.8●
  aortic sinus 747.29
  aortoduodenal 447.2
  appendix, appendicular 543.9
  arteriovenous (acquired) 447.0
    brain 437.3
      congenital 747.81
        ruptured (*see also*
            Hemorrhage,
            subarachnoid) 430
      ruptured (*see also* Hemorrhage,
          subarachnoid) 430
    cerebral 437.3
      congenital 747.81
    congenital (peripheral) 747.60
      brain - *see* Fistula,
          arteriovenous,
            brain, congenital
      coronary 746.85
      gastrointestinal 747.61
      lower limb 747.64
      pulmonary 747.3
      renal 747.62
      specified site NEC 747.69
      upper limb 747.63
    coronary 414.19
      congenital 746.85
    heart 414.19
    pulmonary (vessels) 417.0
      congenital 747.3
    surgically created (for dialysis)
        V45.11
      complication NEC 996.73
        atherosclerosis - *see*
            Arteriosclerosis,
            extremities
        embolism 996.74
        infection or inflammation
            996.62
        mechanical 996.1
        occlusion NEC 996.74
        thrombus 996.74
    traumatic - *see* Injury, blood vessel,
        by site
  artery 447.2
  aural 383.81
    congenital 744.49
  auricle 383.81
    congenital 744.49
  Bartholin's gland 619.8
  bile duct (*see also* Fistula, biliary)
      576.4
  biliary (duct) (tract) 576.4
    congenital 751.69

Fistula (*Continued*)
  bladder (neck) (sphincter) 596.2
    into seminal vesicle 596.2
  bone 733.99
  brain 348.89
    arteriovenous - *see* Fistula,
        arteriovenous, brain
  branchial (cleft) 744.41
  branchiogenous 744.41
  breast 611.0
    puerperal, postpartum 675.1●
  bronchial 510.0
  bronchocutaneous,
      bronchomediastinal,
      bronchopleural,
      bronchopleuromediastinal
      (infective) 510.0
    tuberculous (*see also* Tuberculosis)
        011.3●
  bronchoesophageal 530.84
    congenital 750.3
  buccal cavity (infective) 528.3
  canal, ear 380.89
  carotid-cavernous
    congenital 747.81
      with hemorrhage 430
    traumatic 900.82
      with hemorrhage (*see also*
          Hemorrhage, brain,
          traumatic) 853.0●
    late effect 908.3
  cecosigmoidal 569.81
  cecum 569.81
  cerebrospinal (fluid) 349.81
  cervical, lateral (congenital)
      744.41
  cervicoaural (congenital) 744.49
  cervicosigmoidal 619.1
  cervicovesical 619.0
  cervix 619.8
  chest (wall) 510.0
  cholecystocolic (*see also* Fistula,
      gallbladder) 575.5
  cholecystocolonic (*see also* Fistula,
      gallbladder) 575.5
  cholecystoduodenal (*see also* Fistula,
      gallbladder) 575.5
  cholecystoenteric (*see also* Fistula,
      gallbladder) 575.5
  cholecystogastric (*see also* Fistula,
      gallbladder) 575.5
  cholecystointestinal (*see also* Fistula,
      gallbladder) 575.5
  choledochoduodenal 576.4
  cholocolic (*see also* Fistula, gallbladder)
      575.5
  coccyx 685.1
    with abscess 685.0
  colon 569.81
  colostomy 569.69
  colovaginal (acquired) 619.1
  common duct (bile duct) 576.4
  congenital, NEC - *see* Anomaly,
      specified type NEC
  cornea, causing hypotony
      360.32
  coronary, arteriovenous 414.19
    congenital 746.85
  costal region 510.0
  cul-de-sac, Douglas' 619.8
  cutaneous 686.9
  cystic duct (*see also* Fistula, gallbladder)
      575.5
    congenital 751.69
  dental 522.7

Fistula *(Continued)*
  diaphragm 510.0
    bronchovisceral 510.0
    pleuroperitoneal 510.0
    pulmonoperitoneal 510.0
  duodenum 537.4
  ear (canal) (external) 380.89
  enterocolic 569.81
  enterocutaneous 569.81
  enteroenteric 569.81
  entero-uterine 619.1
    congenital 752.39 ◄▥
  enterovaginal 619.1
    congenital 752.49
  enterovesical 596.1
  epididymis 608.89
    tuberculous *(see also* Tuberculosis)
      016.4●
  esophagobronchial 530.89
    congenital 750.3
  esophagocutaneous 530.89
  esophagopleurocutaneous 530.89
  esophagotracheal 530.84
    congenital 750.3
  esophagus 530.89
    congenital 750.4
  ethmoid *(see also* Sinusitis, ethmoidal)
    473.2
  eyeball (cornea) (sclera) 360.32
  eyelid 373.11
  fallopian tube (external) 619.2
  fecal 569.81
    congenital 751.5
  from periapical lesion 522.7
  frontal sinus *(see also* Sinusitis, frontal)
    473.1
  gallbladder 575.5
    with calculus, cholelithiasis, stones
      (see also Cholelithiasis) 574.2●
    congenital 751.69
  gastric 537.4
  gastrocolic 537.4
    congenital 750.7
    tuberculous *(see also* Tuberculosis)
      014.8●
  gastroenterocolic 537.4
  gastroesophageal 537.4
  gastrojejunal 537.4
  gastrojejunocolic 537.4
  genital
    organs
      female 619.9
        specified site NEC 619.8
      male 608.89
    tract-skin (female) 619.2
  hepatopleural 510.0
  hepatopulmonary 510.0
  horseshoe 565.1
  ileorectal 569.81
  ileosigmoidal 569.81
  ileostomy 569.69
  ileovesical 596.1
  ileum 569.81
  in ano 565.1
    tuberculous *(see also* Tuberculosis)
      014.8●
  inner ear *(see also* Fistula, labyrinth)
    386.40
  intestine 569.81
  intestinocolonic (abdominal) 569.81
  intestinoureteral 593.82
  intestinouterine 619.1
  intestinovaginal 619.1
    congenital 752.49
  intestinovesical 596.1

Fistula *(Continued)*
  involving female genital tract 619.9
    digestive-genital 619.1
    genital tract-skin 619.2
    specified site NEC 619.8
    urinary-genital 619.0
  ischiorectal (fossa) 566
  jejunostomy 569.69
  jejunum 569.81
  joint 719.80
    ankle 719.87
    elbow 719.82
    foot 719.87
    hand 719.84
    hip 719.85
    knee 719.86
    multiple sites 719.89
    pelvic region 719.85
    shoulder (region) 719.81
    specified site NEC 719.88
    tuberculous - *see* Tuberculosis, joint
    wrist 719.83
  kidney 593.89
  labium (majus) (minus) 619.8
  labyrinth, labyrinthine NEC 386.40
    combined sites 386.48
    multiple sites 386.48
    oval window 386.42
    round window 386.41
    semicircular canal 386.43
  lacrimal, lachrymal (duct) (gland) (sac)
    375.61
  lacrimonasal duct 375.61
  laryngotracheal 748.3
  larynx 478.79
  lip 528.5
    congenital 750.25
  lumbar, tuberculous *(see also*
    Tuberculosis) 015.0● *[730.8]*●
  lung 510.0
  lymphatic (node) (vessel) 457.8
  mamillary 611.0
  mammary (gland) 611.0
    puerperal, postpartum 675.1●
  mastoid (process) (region) 383.1
  maxillary *(see also* Sinusitis, maxillary)
    473.0
  mediastinal 510.0
  mediastinobronchial 510.0
  mediastinocutaneous 510.0
  middle ear 385.89
  mouth 528.3
  nasal 478.19
    sinus *(see also* Sinusitis) 473.9
  nasopharynx 478.29
  nipple - *see* Fistula, breast
  nose 478.19
  oral (cutaneous) 528.3
    maxillary *(see also* Sinusitis,
      maxillary) 473.0
    nasal (with cleft palate) *(see also*
      Cleft, palate) 749.00
  orbit, orbital 376.10
  oro-antral *(see also* Sinusitis, maxillary)
    473.0
  oval window (internal ear) 386.42
  oviduct (external) 619.2
  palate (hard) 526.89
    soft 528.9
  pancreatic 577.8
  pancreaticoduodenal 577.8
  parotid (gland) 527.4
    region 528.3
  pelvoabdominointestinal 569.81
  penis 607.89

Fistula *(Continued)*
  perianal 565.1
  pericardium (pleura) (sac) *(see also*
    Pericarditis) 423.8
  pericecal 569.81
  perineal - *see* Fistula, perineum
  perineorectal 569.81
  perineosigmoidal 569.81
  perineo-urethroscrotal 608.89
  perineum, perineal (with urethral
    involvement) NEC 599.1
    tuberculous *(see also* Tuberculosis)
      017.9●
    ureter 593.82
  perirectal 565.1
    tuberculous *(see also* Tuberculosis)
      014.8●
  peritoneum *(see also* Peritonitis) 567.22
  periurethral 599.1
  pharyngo-esophageal 478.29
  pharynx 478.29
    branchial cleft (congenital) 744.41
  pilonidal (infected) (rectum) 685.1
    with abscess 685.0
  pleura, pleural, pleurocutaneous,
    pleuroperitoneal 510.0
    stomach 510.0
    tuberculous *(see also* Tuberculosis)
      012.0●
  pleuropericardial 423.8
  postauricular 383.81
  postoperative, persistent 998.6
  preauricular (congenital) 744.46
  prostate 602.8
  pulmonary 510.0
    arteriovenous 417.0
      congenital 747.3
    tuberculous *(see also* Tuberculosis,
      pulmonary) 011.9●
  pulmonoperitoneal 510.0
  rectolabial 619.1
  rectosigmoid (intercommunicating)
    569.81
  rectoureteral 593.82
  rectourethral 599.1
    congenital 753.8
  rectouterine 619.1
    congenital 752.39 ◄▥
  rectovaginal 619.1
    congenital 752.49
    old, postpartal 619.1
    tuberculous *(see also* Tuberculosis)
      014.8●
  rectovesical 596.1
    congenital 753.8
  rectovesicovaginal 619.1
  rectovulvar 619.1
    congenital 752.49
  rectum (to skin) 565.1
    tuberculous *(see also* Tuberculosis)
      014.8●
  renal 593.89
  retroauricular 383.81
  round window (internal ear) 386.41
  salivary duct or gland 527.4
    congenital 750.24
  sclera 360.32
  scrotum (urinary) 608.89
    tuberculous *(see also* Tuberculosis)
      016.5●
  semicircular canals (internal ear) 386.43
  sigmoid 569.81
    vesicoabdominal 596.1
  sigmoidovaginal 619.1
    congenital 752.49

◄ New   ◄▥ Revised   ~~deleted~~ Deleted   ● Use Additional Digit(s)   ▨ Omit code

Fistula *(Continued)*
  skin 686.9
    ureter 593.82
    vagina 619.2
  sphenoidal sinus *(see also* Sinusitis,
     sphenoidal) 473.3
  splenocolic 289.59
  stercoral 569.81
  stomach 537.4
  sublingual gland 527.4
    congenital 750.24
  submaxillary
    gland 527.4
      congenital 750.24
    region 528.3
  thoracic 510.0
    duct 457.8
  thoracicoabdominal 510.0
  thoracicogastric 510.0
  thoracicointestinal 510.0
  thoracoabdominal 510.0
  thoracogastric 510.0
  thorax 510.0
  thyroglossal duct 759.2
  thyroid 246.8
  trachea (congenital) (external)
    (internal) 748.3
  tracheoesophageal 530.84
    congenital 750.3
    following tracheostomy 519.09
  traumatic
    arteriovenous *(see also* Injury, blood
     vessel, by site) 904.9
    brain - *see* Injury, intracranial
  tuberculous - *see* Tuberculosis, by site
  typhoid 002.0
  umbilical 759.89
  umbilico-urinary 753.8
  urachal, urachus 753.7
  ureter (persistent) 593.82
  ureteroabdominal 593.82
  ureterocervical 593.82
  ureterorectal 593.82
  ureterosigmoido-abdominal 593.82
  ureterovaginal 619.0
  ureterovesical 596.2
  urethra 599.1
    congenital 753.8
    tuberculous *(see also* Tuberculosis)
     016.3●
  urethroperineal 599.1
  urethroperineovesical 596.2
  urethrorectal 599.1
    congenital 753.8
  urethroscrotal 608.89
  urethrovaginal 619.0
  urethrovesical 596.2
  urethrovesicovaginal 619.0
  urinary (persistent) (recurrent) 599.1
  uteroabdominal (anterior wall)
    619.2
    congenital 752.39 ◄▥
  uteroenteric 619.1
  uterofecal 619.1
  uterointestinal 619.1
    congenital 752.39 ◄▥
  uterorectal 619.1
    congenital 752.39 ◄▥
  uteroureteric 619.0
  uterovaginal 619.8
  uterovesical 619.0
    congenital 752.39 ◄▥
  uterus 619.8
  vagina (wall) 619.8
    postpartal, old 619.8

Fistula *(Continued)*
  vaginocutaneous (postpartal) 619.2
  vaginoileal (acquired) 619.1
  vaginoperineal 619.2
  vesical NEC 596.2
  vesicoabdominal 596.2
  vesicocervicovaginal 619.0
  vesicocolic 596.1
  vesicocutaneous 596.2
  vesicoenteric 596.1
  vesicointestinal 596.1
  vesicometrorectal 619.1
  vesicoperineal 596.2
  vesicorectal 596.1
    congenital 753.8
  vesicosigmoidal 596.1
  vesicosigmoidovaginal 619.1
  vesicoureteral 596.2
  vesicoureterovaginal 619.0
  vesicourethral 596.2
  vesicourethrorectal 596.1
  vesicouterine 619.0
    congenital 752.39 ◄▥
  vesicovaginal 619.0
  vulvorectal 619.1
    congenital 752.49
Fit 780.39
  apoplectic *(see also* Disease,
    cerebrovascular, acute) 436
    late effect - *see* Late effect(s) (of)
     cerebrovascular disease
  epileptic *(see also* Epilepsy) 345.9●
  fainting 780.2
  hysterical 300.11
  newborn 779.0
Fitting (of)
  artificial
    arm (complete) (partial) V52.0
    breast V52.4
     implant exchange (different
      material) (different size)
      V52.4
    eye(s) V52.2
    leg(s) (complete) (partial) V52.1
  brain neuropacemaker V53.02
  cardiac pacemaker V53.31
  carotid sinus pacemaker V53.39
  cerebral ventricle (communicating)
    shunt V53.01
  colostomy belt V55.3
  contact lenses V53.1
  cystostomy device V53.6
  defibrillator, automatic implantable
    cardiac (with synchronous
     cardiac pacemaker) V53.32 ◄▥
  dentures V52.3
  device, unspecified type V53.90
    abdominal V53.59
    cardiac
     defibrillator, automatic
      implantable (with
      synchronous cardiac
      pacemaker) V53.32 ◄▥
     pacemaker V53.31
     specified NEC V53.39
    cerebral ventricle (communicating)
     shunt V53.01
    gastrointestinal NEC V53.59
    insulin pump V53.91
    intestinal V53.50
    intrauterine contraceptive V25.1 ◄▥
     insertion V25.11 ◄
     removal V25.12 ◄
      and reinsertion V25.13 ◄
     replacement V25.13 ◄
    nervous system V53.09

Fitting *(Continued)*
  device, unspecified type *(Continued)*
    orthodontic V53.4
    orthoptic V53.1
    other device V53.99
    prosthetic V52.9
     breast V52.4
     dental V52.3
     eye V52.2
     specified type NEC V52.8
    special senses V53.09
    substitution
     auditory V53.09
     nervous system V53.09
     visual V53.09
    urinary V53.6
  diaphragm (contraceptive) V25.02
  gastric lap band V53.51
  gastrointestinal appliance and device
    NEC V53.59
  glasses (reading) V53.1
  growth rod V54.02
  hearing aid V53.2
  ileostomy device V55.2
  intestinal appliance and device V53.50
  intrauterine contraceptive device
    V25.1 ◄▥
    insertion V25.11 ◄
    removal V25.12 ◄
     and reinsertion V25.13 ◄
    replacement V25.13 ◄
  neuropacemaker (brain) (peripheral
    nerve) (spinal cord) V53.02
  orthodontic device V53.4
  orthopedic (device) V53.7
    brace V53.7
    cast V53.7
    corset V53.7
    shoes V53.7
  pacemaker (cardiac) V53.31
    brain V53.02
    carotid sinus V53.39
    peripheral nerve V53.02
    spinal cord V53.02
  prosthesis V52.9
    arm (complete) (partial) V52.0
    breast V52.4
     implant exchange (different
      material) (different size)
      V52.4
    dental V52.3
    eye V52.2
    leg (complete) (partial) V52.1
    specified type NEC V52.8
  spectacles V53.1
  wheelchair V53.8
Fitz's syndrome (acute hemorrhagic
  pancreatitis) 577.0
Fitz-Hugh and Curtis syndrome 098.86
  due to
    Chlamydia trachomatis 099.56
    Neisseria gonorrhoeae (gonococcal
     peritonitis) 098.86
Fixation
  joint - *see* Ankylosis
  larynx 478.79
  pupil 364.76
  stapes 385.22
    deafness *(see also* Deafness,
     conductive) 389.04
  uterus (acquired) - *see* Malposition,
    uterus
  vocal cord 478.5
Flaccid - *see also* condition
  foot 736.79
  forearm 736.09
  palate, congenital 750.26

Flail
- chest 807.4
  - newborn 767.3
- joint (paralytic) 718.80
  - ankle 718.87
  - elbow 718.82
  - foot 718.87
  - hand 718.84
  - hip 718.85
  - knee 718.86
  - multiple sites 718.89
  - pelvic region 718.85
  - shoulder (region) 718.81
  - specified site NEC 718.88
  - wrist 718.83

Flajani (-Basedow) syndrome or disease (exophthalmic goiter) 242.0●

Flap, liver 572.8

Flare, anterior chamber (aqueous) (eye) 364.04

Flashback phenomena (drug) (hallucinogenic) 292.89

Flat
- chamber (anterior) (eye) 360.34
- chest, congenital 754.89
- electroencephalogram (EEG) 348.89
- foot (acquired) (fixed type) (painful) (postural) (spastic) 734
  - congenital 754.61
    - rocker bottom 754.61
    - vertical talus 754.61
  - rachitic 268.1
  - rocker bottom (congenital) 754.61
  - vertical talus, congenital 754.61
- organ or site, congenital NEC - *see* Anomaly, specified type NEC
- pelvis 738.6
  - with disproportion (fetopelvic) 653.2●
    - affecting fetus or newborn 763.1
    - causing obstructed labor 660.1●
      - affecting fetus or newborn 763.1
  - congenital 755.69

Flatau-Schilder disease 341.1

Flattening
- head, femur 736.39
- hip 736.39
- lip (congenital) 744.89
- nose (congenital) 754.0
  - acquired 738.0

Flatulence 787.3

Flatus 787.3
- vaginalis 629.89

Flax dressers' disease 504

Flea bite - *see* Injury, superficial, by site

Fleischer (-Kayser) ring (corneal pigmentation) 275.1 [371.14]

Fleischner's disease 732.3

Fleshy mole 631

Flexibilitas cerea (*see also* Catalepsy) 300.11

Flexion
- cervix - *see* Flexion, uterus
- contracture, joint (*see also* Contraction, joint) 718.4●
- deformity, joint (*see also* Contraction, joint) 736.9
  - hip, congenital (*see also* Subluxation, congenital, hip) 754.32
- uterus (*see also* Malposition, uterus) 621.6

Flexner's
- bacillus 004.1
- diarrhea (ulcerative) 004.1
- dysentery 004.1

Flexner-Boyd dysentery 004.2

Flexure - *see* condition

Floater, vitreous 379.24

Floating
- cartilage (joint) (*see also* Disorder, cartilage, articular) 718.0●
  - knee 717.6
- gallbladder (congenital) 751.69
- kidney 593.0
  - congenital 753.3
- liver (congenital) 751.69
- rib 756.3
- spleen 289.59

Flooding 626.2

Floor - *see* condition

Floppy
- infant NEC 781.99
- iris syndrome 364.81
- valve syndrome (mitral) 424.0

Flu - *see also* Influenza
- bird (*see also* Influenza, avian) 488.02 ◄▦
- gastric NEC 008.8
- swine (*see also* Influenza, novel H1N1) 488.12 ◄▦

Fluctuating blood pressure 796.4

Fluid
- abdomen 789.59
- chest (*see also* Pleurisy, with effusion) 511.9
- heart (*see also* Failure, heart) 428.0
- joint (*see also* Effusion, joint) 719.0●
- loss (acute) 276.50
  - with
    - hypernatremia 276.0
    - hyponatremia 276.1
- lung - *see also* Edema, lung
  - encysted 511.89
- peritoneal cavity 789.59
  - malignant 789.51
- pleural cavity (*see also* Pleurisy, with effusion) 511.9
- retention 276.69 ◄▦

Flukes NEC (*see also* Infestation, fluke) 121.9
- blood NEC (*see also* Infestation, Schistosoma) 120.9
- liver 121.3

Fluor (albus) (vaginalis) 623.5
- trichomonal (Trichomonas vaginalis) 131.00

Fluorosis (dental) (chronic) 520.3

Flushing 782.62
- menopausal 627.2

Flush syndrome 259.2

Flutter
- atrial or auricular 427.32
- heart (ventricular) 427.42
  - atrial 427.32
- impure 427.32
- postoperative 997.1
- ventricular 427.42

Flux (bloody) (serosanguineous) 009.0

FNHTR (febrile nonhemolytic transfusion reaction) 780.66 ◄

Focal - *see* condition

Fochier's abscess - *see* Abscess, by site

Focus, Assmann's (*see also* Tuberculosis) 011.0●

Fogo selvagem 694.4

Foix-Alajouanine syndrome 336.1

Folds, anomalous - *see also* Anomaly, specified type NEC
- Bowman's membrane 371.31
- Descemet's membrane 371.32
- epicanthic 743.63
- heart 746.89
- posterior segment of eye, congenital 743.54

Folie a deux 297.3

Follicle
- cervix (nabothian) (ruptured) 616.0
- graafian, ruptured, with hemorrhage 620.0
- nabothian 616.0

Folliclis (primary) (*see also* Tuberculosis) 017.0●

Follicular - *see also* condition
- cyst (atretic) 620.0

Folliculitis 704.8
- abscedens et suffodiens 704.8
- decalvans 704.09
- gonorrheal (acute) 098.0
  - chronic or duration of 2 months or more 098.2
- keloid, keloidalis 706.1
- pustular 704.8
- ulerythematosa reticulata 701.8

Folliculosis, conjunctival 372.02

Følling's disease (phenylketonuria) 270.1

Follow-up (examination) (routine) (following) V67.9
- cancer chemotherapy V67.2
- chemotherapy V67.2
- fracture V67.4
- high-risk medication V67.51
- injury NEC V67.59
- postpartum
  - immediately after delivery V24.0
  - routine V24.2
- psychiatric V67.3
- psychotherapy V67.3
- radiotherapy V67.1
- specified condition NEC V67.59
- specified surgery NEC V67.09
- surgery V67.00
  - vaginal pap smear V67.01
- treatment V67.9
  - combined NEC V67.6
  - fracture V67.4
  - involving high-risk medication NEC V67.51
  - mental disorder V67.3
  - specified NEC V67.59

Fong's syndrome (hereditary osteoonychodysplasia) 756.89

Food
- allergy 693.1
- anaphylactic shock - *see* Anaphylactic shock, due to food
- asphyxia (from aspiration or inhalation) (*see also* Asphyxia, food) 933.1
- choked on (*see also* Asphyxia, food) 933.1
- deprivation 994.2
  - specified kind of food NEC 269.8
- intoxication (*see also* Poisoning, food) 005.9
- lack of 994.2
- poisoning (*see also* Poisoning, food) 005.9
- refusal or rejection NEC 307.59
- strangulation or suffocation (*see also* Asphyxia, food) 933.1
- toxemia (*see also* Poisoning, food) 005.9

Foot - *see also* condition
- and mouth disease 078.4
- process disease 581.3

Foramen ovale (nonclosure) (patent) (persistent) 745.5

Forbes' (glycogen storage) disease 271.0

Forbes-Albright syndrome (nonpuerperal amenorrhea and lactation associated with pituitary tumor) 253.1

◄ New   ◄▦ Revised   ~~deleted~~ Deleted   ● Use Additional Digit(s)   ▦ Omit code

Forced birth or delivery NEC 669.8●
  affecting fetus or newborn NEC 763.89
Forceps
  delivery NEC 669.5●
    affecting fetus or newborn 763.2
Fordyce's disease (ectopic sebaceous
    glands) (mouth) 750.26
Fordyce-Fox disease (apocrine miliaria)
    705.82
Forearm - *see* condition
Foreign body

> Note: For foreign body with open
> wound or other injury, see Wound,
> open, or the type of injury specified.

  accidentally left during a procedure
    998.4
  anterior chamber (eye) 871.6
    magnetic 871.5
      retained or old 360.51
    retained or old 360.61
  ciliary body (eye) 871.6
    magnetic 871.5
      retained or old 360.52
    retained or old 360.62
  entering through orifice (current) (old)
    accessory sinus 932
    air passage (upper) 933.0
      lower 934.8
    alimentary canal 938
    alveolar process 935.0
    antrum (Highmore) 932
    anus 937
    appendix 936
    asphyxia due to (*see also* Asphyxia,
        food) 933.1
    auditory canal 931
    auricle 931
    bladder 939.0
    bronchioles 934.8
    bronchus (main) 934.1
    buccal cavity 935.0
    canthus (inner) 930.1
    cecum 936
    cervix (canal) uterine 939.1
    coil, ileocecal 936
    colon 936
    conjunctiva 930.1
    conjunctival sac 930.1
    cornea 930.0
    digestive organ or tract NEC 938
    duodenum 936
    ear (external) 931
    esophagus 935.1
    eye (external) 930.9
      combined sites 930.8
      intraocular - *see* Foreign body, by
          site
      specified site NEC 930.8
    eyeball 930.8
      intraocular - *see* Foreign body,
          intraocular
    eyelid 930.1
      retained or old 374.86
    frontal sinus 932
    gastrointestinal tract 938
    genitourinary tract 939.9
    globe 930.8
      penetrating 871.6
        magnetic 871.5
          retained or old 360.50
        retained or old 360.60
    gum 935.0

Foreign body (*Continued*)
  entering through orifice (*Continued*)
    Highmore's antrum 932
    hypopharynx 933.0
    ileocecal coil 936
    ileum 936
    inspiration (of) 933.1
    intestine (large) (small) 936
    lacrimal apparatus, duct, gland, or
        sac 930.2
    larynx 933.1
    lung 934.8
    maxillary sinus 932
    mouth 935.0
    nasal sinus 932
    nasopharynx 933.0
    nose (passage) 932
    nostril 932
    oral cavity 935.0
    palate 935.0
    penis 939.3
    pharynx 933.0
    pyriform sinus 933.0
    rectosigmoid 937
      junction 937
    rectum 937
    respiratory tract 934.9
      specified part NEC 934.8
    sclera 930.1
    sinus 932
      accessory 932
      frontal 932
      maxillary 932
      nasal 932
      pyriform 933.0
    small intestine 936
    stomach (hairball) 935.2
    suffocation by (*see also* Asphyxia,
        food) 933.1
    swallowed 938
      tongue 933.0
    tear ducts or glands 930.2
    throat 933.0
    tongue 935.0
      swallowed 933.0
    tonsil, tonsillar 933.0
      fossa 933.0
    trachea 934.0
    ureter 939.0
    urethra 939.0
    uterus (any part) 939.1
    vagina 939.2
    vulva 939.2
    wind pipe 934.0
  feeling of, in throat 784.99
  granuloma (old) 728.82
    bone 733.99
    in operative wound (inadvertently
        left) 998.4
      due to surgical material
          intentionally left - *see*
          Complications, due to
          (presence of) any device,
          implant, or graft classified
          to 996.0–996.5 NEC
    muscle 728.82
    skin 709.4
    soft tissue NEC 709.4
    subcutaneous tissue 709.4
  in
    bone (residual) 733.99
    open wound - *see* Wound, open, by
        site complicated
    soft tissue (residual) 729.6

Foreign body (*Continued*)
  inadvertently left in operation
      wound (causing adhesions,
      obstruction, or perforation)
      998.4
  ingestion, ingested NEC 938
  inhalation or inspiration (*see also*
      Asphyxia, food) 933.1
  internal organ, not entering
      through an orifice - *see* Injury,
      internal, by site, with open
      wound
  intraocular (nonmagnetic) 871.6
    combined sites 871.6
      magnetic 871.5
        retained or old 360.59
      retained or old 360.69
    magnetic 871.5
      retained or old 360.50
    retained or old 360.60
    specified site NEC 871.6
      magnetic 871.5
        retained or old 360.59
      retained or old 360.69
  iris (nonmagnetic) 871.6
    magnetic 871.5
      retained or old 360.52
    retained or old 360.62
  lens (nonmagnetic) 871.6
    magnetic 871.5
      retained or old 360.53
    retained or old 360.63
  lid, eye 930.1
  ocular muscle 870.4
    retained or old 376.6
  old or residual
    bone 733.99
    eyelid 374.86
    middle ear 385.83
    muscle 729.6
      ocular 376.6
    retrobulbar 376.6
    skin 729.6
      with granuloma 709.4
    soft tissue 729.6
      with granuloma 709.4
    subcutaneous tissue 729.6
      with granuloma 709.4
  operation wound, left accidentally 998.4
  orbit 870.4
    retained or old 376.6
  posterior wall, eye 871.6
    magnetic 871.5
      retained or old 360.55
    retained or old 360.65
  respiratory tree 934.9
    specified site NEC 934.8
  retained (old) (nonmagnetic) (in)
      V90.9 ◀▥
    anterior chamber (eye) 360.61
      magnetic 360.51
    ciliary body 360.62
      magnetic 360.52
    eyelid 374.86
    fragment(s) ◀
      acrylics V90.2 ◀
      animal quills V90.31 ◀
      animal spines V90.31 ◀
      cement V90.83 ◀
      concrete V90.83 ◀
      crystalline V90.83 ◀
      depleted ◀
        isotope V90.09 ◀
        uranium V90.01 ◀

Foreign body (Continued)
  retained (Continued)
    fragment(s) (Continued)
      diethylhexylphthalates V90.2 ◄
      glass V90.81 ◄
      isocyanate V90.2 ◄
      metal V90.10 ◄
        magnetic V90.11 ◄
        nonmagnetic V90.12 ◄
      organic NEC V90.39 ◄
      plastic V90.2 ◄
      radioactive ◄
        nontherapeutic V90.09 ◄
        specified NEC V90.09 ◄
      stone V90.83 ◄
      tooth V90.32 ◄
      wood V90.33 ◄
    globe 360.60
      magnetic 360.50
    intraocular 360.60
      magnetic 360.50
      specified site NEC 360.69
        magnetic 360.59
    iris 360.62
      magnetic 360.52
    lens 360.63
      magnetic 360.53
    muscle 729.6
    orbit 376.6
    posterior wall of globe 360.65
      magnetic 360.55
    retina 360.65
      magnetic 360.55
    retrobulbar 376.6
    skin 729.6
      with granuloma 709.4
    soft tissue 729.6
      with granuloma 709.4
    specified NEC V90.89 ◄
    subcutaneous tissue 729.6
      with granuloma 709.4
    vitreous 360.64
      magnetic 360.54
  retina 871.6
    magnetic 871.5
      retained or old 360.55
    retained or old 360.65
  superficial, without major open wound
      (see also Injury, superficial, by site)
      919.6
  swallowed NEC 938
  throat, feeling of 784.99
  vitreous (humor) 871.6
    magnetic 871.5
      retained or old 360.54
    retained or old 360.64
Forking, aqueduct of Sylvius 742.3
  with spina bifida (see also
      Spina bifida) 741.0●
Formation
  bone in scar tissue (skin) 709.3
  connective tissue in vitreous 379.25
  Elschnig pearls (postcataract
      extraction) 366.51
  hyaline in cornea 371.49
  sequestrum in bone (due to infection)
      (see also Osteomyelitis) 730.1●
  valve
    colon, congenital 751.5
    ureter (congenital) 753.29
Formication 782.0
Fort Bragg fever 100.89
Fossa - see also condition
  pyriform - see condition
Foster care (status) V60.81
Foster-Kennedy syndrome 377.04

Fothergill's
  disease, meaning scarlatina anginosa
      034.1
  neuralgia (see also Neuralgia,
      trigeminal) 350.1
Foul breath 784.99
Found dead (cause unknown) 798.9
Foundling V20.0
Fournier's disease (idiopathic gangrene)
      608.83
Fourth
  cranial nerve - see condition
  disease 057.8
  molar 520.1
Foville's syndrome 344.89
Fox's
  disease (apocrine miliaria) 705.82
  impetigo (contagiosa) 684
Fox-Fordyce disease (apocrine miliaria)
      705.82
Fracture (abduction) (adduction) (avulsion)
      (compression) (crush) (dislocation)
      (oblique) (separation) (closed) 829.0

Note: For fracture of any of the
following sites with fracture of other
bones - see Fracture, multiple.

"Closed" includes the following
descriptions of fractures, with or
without delayed healing, unless they
are specified as open or compound:

  comminuted
  depressed
  elevated
  fissured
  greenstick
  impacted
  linear
  simple
  slipped epiphysis
  spiral
  unspecified

"Open" includes the following
descriptions of fractures, with or
without delayed healing:

  compound
  infected
  missile
  puncture
  with foreign body

For late effect of fracture, see Late,
effect, fracture, by site.

---

  with
      internal injuries in same region
          (conditions classifiable to
          860–869) - see also Injury,
          internal, by site
      pelvic region - see Fracture,
          pelvis
  acetabulum (with visceral injury)
      (closed) 808.0
    open 808.1
  acromion (process) (closed) 811.01
    open 811.11
  alveolus (closed) 802.8
    open 802.9
  ankle (malleolus) (closed) 824.8
    bimalleolar (Dupuytren's) (Pott's)
        824.4
      open 824.5
    bone 825.21
      open 825.31

Fracture (Continued)
  ankle (Continued)
    lateral malleolus only (fibular) 824.2
      open 824.3
    medial malleolus only (tibial) 824.0
      open 824.1
    open 824.9
    pathologic 733.16
    talus 825.21
      open 825.31
    trimalleolar 824.6
      open 824.7
  antrum - see Fracture, skull, base
  arm (closed) 818.0
    and leg(s) (any bones) 828.0
      open 828.1
    both (any bones) (with rib(s)) (with
        sternum) 819.0
      open 819.1
    lower 813.80
      open 813.90
    open 818.1
    upper - see Fracture, humerus
  astragalus (closed) 825.21
    open 825.31
  atlas - see Fracture, vertebra, cervical,
      first
  axis - see Fracture, vertebra, cervical,
      second
  back - see Fracture, vertebra, by site
  Barton's - see Fracture, radius, lower end
  basal (skull) - see Fracture, skull, base
  Bennett's (closed) 815.01
    open 815.11
  bimalleolar (closed) 824.4
    open 824.5
  bone (closed) NEC 829.0
    birth injury NEC 767.3
    open 829.1
    pathological NEC (see also Fracture,
        pathologic) 733.10
    stress NEC (see also Fracture, stress)
        733.95
  boot top - see Fracture, fibula
  boxers' - see Fracture, metacarpal bone(s)
  breast bone - see Fracture, sternum
  buckle - see Fracture, torus
  bucket handle (semilunar cartilage) -
      see Tear, meniscus
  burst - see Fracture, traumatic, by site
  bursting - see Fracture, phalanx, hand,
      distal
  calcaneus (closed) 825.0
    open 825.1
  capitate (bone) (closed) 814.07
    open 814.17
  capitellum (humerus) (closed) 812.49
    open 812.59
  carpal bone(s) (wrist NEC) (closed)
      814.00
    open 814.10
    specified site NEC 814.09
      open 814.19
  cartilage, knee (semilunar) - see Tear,
      meniscus
  cervical - see Fracture, vertebra, cervical
  chauffeur's - see Fracture, ulna, lower end
  chisel - see Fracture, radius, upper end
  chronic - see Fracture, pathologic
  clavicle (interligamentous part)
      (closed) 810.00
    acromial end 810.03
      open 810.13
    due to birth trauma 767.2
    open 810.10

◄ New   ◄▌ Revised   ~~deleted~~ Deleted   ● Use Additional Digit(s)   � Omit code

Fracture *(Continued)*
  clavicle *(Continued)*
    shaft (middle third) 810.02
      open 810.12
    sternal end 810.01
      open 810.11
  clayshovelers' - *see* Fracture, vertebra,
      cervical
  coccyx - *see also* Fracture, vertebra,
      coccyx
    complicating delivery 665.6●
  collar bone - *see* Fracture, clavicle
  Colles' (reversed) (closed) 813.41
    open 813.51
  comminuted - *see* Fracture, by site
  compression - *see also* Fracture, by site
    nontraumatic - *see* Fracture,
        pathologic
  congenital 756.9
  coracoid process (closed) 811.02
    open 811.12
  coronoid process (ulna) (closed) 813.02
    mandible (closed) 802.23
      open 802.33
    open 813.12
  corpus cavernosum penis 959.13
  costochondral junction - *see* Fracture, rib
  costosternal junction - *see* Fracture, rib
  cranium - *see* Fracture, skull, by site
  cricoid cartilage (closed) 807.5
    open 807.6
  cuboid (ankle) (closed) 825.23
    open 825.33
  cuneiform
    foot (closed) 825.24
      open 825.34
    wrist (closed) 814.03
      open 814.13
  dental implant 525.73
  dental restorative material
    with loss of material 525.64
    without loss of material 525.63
  due to
    birth injury - *see* Birth injury, fracture
    gunshot - *see* Fracture, by site, open
    neoplasm - *see* Fracture, pathologic
    osteoporosis - *see* Fracture,
        pathologic
  Dupuytren's (ankle) (fibula) (closed)
      824.4
    open 824.5
    radius 813.42
      open 813.52
  Duverney's - *see* Fracture, ilium
  elbow - *see also* Fracture, humerus,
      lower end
    olecranon (process) (closed) 813.01
      open 813.11
    supracondylar (closed) 812.41
      open 812.51
  ethmoid (bone) (sinus) - *see* Fracture,
      skull, base
  face bone(s) (closed) NEC 802.8
    with
      other bone(s) - *see* Fracture,
          multiple, skull
      skull - *see also* Fracture, skull
        involving other bones - *see*
            Fracture, multiple, skull
    open 802.9
  fatigue - *see* Fracture, march
  femur, femoral (closed) 821.00
    cervicotrochanteric 820.03
      open 820.13
    condyles, epicondyles 821.21
      open 821.31

Fracture *(Continued)*
  femur, femoral *(Continued)*
    distal end - *see* Fracture, femur,
        lower end
    epiphysis (separation)
      capital 820.01
        open 820.11
      head 820.01
        open 820.11
      lower 821.22
        open 821.32
      trochanteric 820.01
        open 820.11
      upper 820.01
        open 820.11
    head 820.09
      open 820.19
    lower end or extremity (distal end)
        (closed) 821.20
      condyles, epicondyles 821.21
        open 821.31
      epiphysis (separation) 821.22
        open 821.32
      multiple sites 821.29
        open 821.39
      open 821.30
      specified site NEC 821.29
        open 821.39
      supracondylar 821.23
        open 821.33
      T-shaped 821.21
        open 821.31
    neck (closed) 820.8
      base (cervicotrochanteric) 820.03
        open 820.13
      extracapsular 820.20
        open 820.30
      intertrochanteric (section) 820.21
        open 820.31
      intracapsular 820.00
        open 820.10
      intratrochanteric 820.21
        open 820.31
      midcervical 820.02
        open 820.12
      open 820.9
      pathologic 733.14
        specified part NEC 733.15
      specified site NEC 820.09
        open 820.19
      transcervical 820.02
        open 820.12
      transtrochanteric 820.20
        open 820.30
    open 821.10
    pathologic 733.14
      specified part NEC 733.15
    peritrochanteric (section) 820.20
      open 820.30
    shaft (lower third) (middle third)
        (upper third) 821.01
      open 821.11
    subcapital 820.09
      open 820.19
    subtrochanteric (region) (section)
        820.22
      open 820.32
    supracondylar 821.23
      open 821.33
    transepiphyseal 820.01
      open 820.11
    trochanter (greater) (lesser) (*see also*
        Fracture, femur, neck, by site)
        820.20
      open 820.30

Fracture *(Continued)*
  femur, femoral *(Continued)*
    T-shaped, into knee joint 821.21
      open 821.31
    upper end 820.8
      open 820.9
  fibula (closed) 823.81
    with tibia 823.82
      open 823.92
    distal end 824.8
      open 824.9
    epiphysis
      lower 824.8
        open 824.9
      upper - *see* Fracture, fibula, upper
          end
    head - *see* Fracture, fibula, upper end
    involving ankle 824.2
      open 824.3
    lower end or extremity 824.8
      open 824.9
    malleolus (external) (lateral) 824.2
      open 824.3
    open NEC 823.91
    pathologic 733.16
    proximal end - *see* Fracture, fibula,
        upper end
    shaft 823.21
      with tibia 823.22
        open 823.32
      open 823.31
    stress 733.93
    torus 823.41
      with tibia 823.42
    upper end or extremity (epiphysis)
        (head) (proximal end) (styloid)
        823.01
      with tibia 823.02
        open 823.12
      open 823.11
  finger(s), of one hand (closed) (*see also*
      Fracture, phalanx, hand) 816.00
    with
      metacarpal bone(s), of same hand
          817.0
        open 817.1
      thumb of same hand 816.03
        open 816.13
    open 816.10
  foot, except toe(s) alone (closed) 825.20
    open 825.30
  forearm (closed) NEC 813.80
    lower end (distal end) (lower
        epiphysis) 813.40
      open 813.50
    open 813.90
    shaft 813.20
      open 813.30
    upper end (proximal end) (upper
        epiphysis) 813.00
      open 813.10
  fossa, anterior, middle, or posterior -
      see Fracture, skull, base
  frontal (bone) - *see also* Fracture, skull,
      vault
    sinus - *see* Fracture, skull, base
  Galeazzi's - *see* Fracture, radius, lower
      end
  glenoid (cavity) (fossa) (scapula)
      (closed) 811.03
    open 811.13
  Gosselin's - *see* Fracture, ankle
  greenstick - *see* Fracture, by site
  grenade-throwers' - *see* Fracture,
      humerus, shaft

Fracture (*Continued*)
  gutter - *see* Fracture, skull, vault
  hamate (closed) 814.08
    open 814.18
  hand, one (closed) 815.00
    carpals 814.00
      open 814.10
      specified site NEC 814.09
        open 814.19
    metacarpals 815.00
      open 815.10
    multiple, bones of one hand 817.0
      open 817.1
    open 815.10
    phalanges (*see also* Fracture,
      phalanx, hand) 816.00
      open 816.10
  healing
    aftercare (*see also* Aftercare, fracture)
      V54.89
    change of cast V54.89
    complications - *see* condition
    convalescence V66.4
    removal of
      cast V54.89
      fixation device
        external V54.89
        internal V54.01
  heel bone (closed) 825.0
    open 825.1
  Hill-Sachs 812.09
  hip (closed) (*see also* Fracture, femur,
    neck) 820.8
    open 820.9
    pathologic 733.14
  humerus (closed) 812.20
    anatomical neck 812.02
      open 812.12
    articular process (*see also* Fracture
      humerus, condyle(s)) 812.44
      open 812.54
    capitellum 812.49
      open 812.59
    condyle(s) 812.44
      lateral (external) 812.42
        open 812.52
      medial (internal epicondyle)
        812.43
        open 812.53
      open 812.54
    distal end - *see* Fracture, humerus,
      lower end
    epiphysis
      lower (*see also* Fracture, humerus,
        condyle(s)) 812.44
        open 812.54
      upper 812.09
        open 812.19
    external condyle 812.42
      open 812.52
    great tuberosity 812.03
      open 812.13
    head 812.09
      open 812.19
    internal epicondyle 812.43
      open 812.53
    lesser tuberosity 812.09
      open 812.19
    lower end or extremity (distal end)
      (*see also* Fracture, humerus, by
      site) 812.40
      multiple sites NEC 812.49
        open 812.59
      open 812.50
      specified site NEC 812.49
        open 812.59

Fracture (*Continued*)
  humerus (*Continued*)
    neck 812.01
      open 812.11
    open 812.30
    pathologic 733.11
    proximal end - *see* Fracture,
      humerus, upper end
    shaft 812.21
      open 812.31
    supracondylar 812.41
      open 812.51
    surgical neck 812.01
      open 812.11
    trochlea 812.49
      open 812.59
    T-shaped 812.44
      open 812.54
    tuberosity - *see* Fracture, humerus,
      upper end
    upper end or extremity (proximal
      end) (*see also* Fracture,
      humerus, by site) 812.00
      open 812.10
      specified site NEC 812.09
        open 812.19
  hyoid bone (closed) 807.5
    open 807.6
  hyperextension - *see* Fracture, radius,
    lower end
  ilium (with visceral injury) (closed)
    808.41
    open 808.51
  impaction, impacted - *see* Fracture, by
    site
  incus - *see* Fracture, skull, base
  innominate bone (with visceral injury)
    (closed) 808.49
    open 808.59
  instep, of one foot (closed) 825.20
    with toe(s) of same foot 827.0
      open 827.1
    open 825.30
  insufficiency - *see* Fracture, pathologic,
    by site
  internal
    ear - *see* Fracture, skull, base
    semilunar cartilage, knee - *see* Tear,
      meniscus, medial
  intertrochanteric - *see* Fracture, femur,
    neck, intertrochanteric
  ischium (with visceral injury) (closed)
    808.42
    open 808.52
  jaw (bone) (lower) (closed) (*see also*
    Fracture, mandible) 802.20
    angle 802.25
      open 802.35
    open 802.30
    upper - *see* Fracture, maxilla
  knee
    cap (closed) 822.0
      open 822.1
    cartilage (semilunar) - *see* Tear,
      meniscus
  labyrinth (osseous) - *see* Fracture, skull,
    base
  larynx (closed) 807.5
    open 807.6
  late effect - *see* Late, effects (of),
    fracture
  Le Fort's - *see* Fracture, maxilla
  leg (closed) 827.0
    with rib(s) or sternum 828.0
      open 828.1

Fracture (*Continued*)
  leg (*Continued*)
    both (any bones) 828.0
      open 828.1
    lower - *see* Fracture, tibia
    open 827.1
    upper - *see* Fracture, femur
  limb
    lower (multiple) (closed) NEC 827.0
      open 827.1
    upper (multiple) (closed) NEC
      818.0
      open 818.1
  long bones, due to birth trauma - *see*
    Birth injury, fracture
  lumbar - *see* Fracture, vertebra, lumbar
  lunate bone (closed) 814.02
    open 814.12
  malar bone (closed) 802.4
    open 802.5
  Malgaigne's (closed) 808.43
    open 808.53
  malleolus (closed) 824.8
    bimalleolar 824.4
      open 824.5
    lateral 824.2
      and medial - *see also* Fracture,
        malleolus, bimalleolar
        with lip of tibia - *see*
          Fracture, malleolus,
          trimalleolar
      open 824.3
    medial (closed) 824.0
      and lateral - *see also* Fracture,
        malleolus, bimalleolar
        with lip of tibia - *see*
          Fracture, malleolus,
          trimalleolar
      open 824.1
    open 824.9
    trimalleolar (closed) 824.6
      open 824.7
  malleus - *see* Fracture, skull, base
  malunion 733.81
  mandible (closed) 802.20
    angle 802.25
      open 802.35
    body 802.28
      alveolar border 802.27
        open 802.37
      open 802.38
      symphysis 802.26
        open 802.36
    condylar process 802.21
      open 802.31
    coronoid process 802.23
      open 802.33
    multiple sites 802.29
      open 802.39
    open 802.30
    ramus NEC 802.24
      open 802.34
    subcondylar 802.22
      open 802.32
  manubrium - *see* Fracture, sternum
  march 733.95
    fibula 733.93
    metatarsals 733.94
    tibia 733.93
  maxilla, maxillary (superior) (upper
    jaw) (closed) 802.4
    inferior - *see* Fracture, mandible
    open 802.5
  meniscus, knee - *see* Tear, meniscus

◀ New   ◀▥ Revised   ~~deleted~~ Deleted   ● Use Additional Digit(s)   ▨ Omit code

Fracture *(Continued)*
   metacarpus, metacarpal (bone(s)), of
      one hand (closed) 815.00
     with phalanx, phalanges, hand
       (finger(s)) (thumb) of same
       hand 817.0
       open 817.1
     base 815.02
      first metacarpal 815.01
       open 815.11
      open 815.12
      thumb 815.01
       open 815.11
     multiple sites 815.09
      open 815.19
     neck 815.04
      open 815.14
     open 815.10
     shaft 815.03
      open 815.13
   metatarsus, metatarsal (bone(s)), of one
      foot (closed) 825.25
     with tarsal bone(s) 825.29
      open 825.39
     open 825.35
   Monteggia's (closed) 813.03
     open 813.13
   Moore's - *see* Fracture, radius, lower
     end
   multangular bone (closed)
     larger 814.05
      open 814.15
     smaller 814.06
      open 814.16
   multiple (closed) 829.0

> Note: Multiple fractures of sites
> classifiable to the same three- or
> four-digit category are coded to that
> category, except for sites classifiable
> to 810–818 or 820–827 in different
> limbs.
>
> Multiple fractures of sites classifiable to
> different fourth-digit subdivisions
> within the same three-digit category
> should be dealt with according to
> coding rules.
>
> Multiple fractures of sites classifiable to
> different three-digit categories
> (identifiable from the listing under
> "Fracture"), and of sites classifiable to
> 810–818 or 820–827 in different limbs
> should be coded according to the
> following list, which should be referred
> to in the following priority order: skull
> or face bones, pelvis or vertebral
> column, legs, arms.

   arm (multiple bones in same arm
      except in hand alone) (sites
      classifiable to 810–817 with
      sites classifiable to a different
      three-digit category in
      810–817 in same arm) (closed)
      818.0
     open 818.1
   arms, both or arm(s) with rib(s) or
      sternum (sites classifiable to
      810–818 with sites classifiable
      to same range of categories in
      other limb or to 807) (closed)
      819.0
     open 819.1

Fracture *(Continued)*
   multiple *(Continued)*
     bones of trunk NEC (closed) 809.0
      open 809.1
     hand, metacarpal bone(s) with
      phalanx or phalanges of same
      hand (sites classifiable to 815
      with sites classifiable to 816 in
      same hand) (closed) 817.0
      open 817.1
     leg (multiple bones in same leg)
      (sites classifiable to 820–826
      with sites classifiable to a
      different three-digit category
      in that range in same leg)
      (closed) 827.0
      open 827.1
     legs, both or leg(s) with arm(s),
      rib(s), or sternum (sites
      classifiable to 820–827 with
      sites classifiable to same range
      of categories in other leg or to
      807 or 810–819) (closed) 828.0
      open 828.1
     open 829.1
     pelvis with other bones except skull
      or face bones (sites classifiable
      to 808 with sites classifiable to
      805–807 or 810–829) (closed)
      809.0
      open 809.1
     skull, specified or unspecified bones,
      or face bone(s) with any other
      bone(s) (sites classifiable to
      800–803 with sites classifiable
      to 805–829) (closed) 804.0 ●

> Note: Use the following fifth-digit
> subclassification with categories 800,
> 801, 803, and 804:
>
> 0 unspecified state of
>   consciousness
> 1 with no loss of consciousness
> 2 with brief [less than one hour]
>   loss of consciousness
> 3 with moderate [1–24 hours] loss
>   of consciousness
> 4 with prolonged [more than 24
>   hours] loss of
>   consciousness and return
>   to pre-existing conscious
>   level
> 5 with prolonged [more than 24
>   hours] loss of
>   consciousness, without
>   return to pre-existing
>   conscious level
>
> Use fifth-digit 5 to designate when a
> patient is unconscious and dies before
> regaining consciousness, regardless of
> the duration of the loss of
> consciousness
>
> 6 with loss of consciousness of
>   unspecified duration
> 9 with concussion, unspecified

     with
      contusion, cerebral 804.1 ●
      epidural hemorrhage 804.2 ●
      extradural hemorrhage 804.2 ●
      hemorrhage (intracranial) NEC
       804.3 ●
      intracranial injury NEC 804.4 ●
      laceration, cerebral 804.1 ●

Fracture *(Continued)*
   multiple *(Continued)*
     with *(Continued)*
      subarachnoid hemorrhage 804.2 ●
      subdural hemorrhage 804.2 ●
     open 804.5 ●
      with
       contusion, cerebral 804.6 ●
       epidural hemorrhage 804.7 ●
       extradural hemorrhage 804.7 ●
       hemorrhage (intracranial)
        NEC 804.8 ●
       intracranial injury NEC 804.9 ●
       laceration, cerebral 804.6 ●
       subarachnoid hemorrhage
        804.7 ●
       subdural hemorrhage 804.7 ●
   vertebral column with other bones,
      except skull or face bones (sites
      classifiable to 805 or 806 with
      sites classifiable to 807–808 or
      810–829) (closed) 809.0
     open 809.1
   nasal (bone(s)) (closed) 802.0
     open 802.1
     sinus - *see* Fracture, skull, base
   navicular
     carpal (wrist) (closed) 814.01
      open 814.11
     tarsal (ankle) (closed) 825.22
      open 825.32
   neck - *see* Fracture, vertebra, cervical
   neural arch - *see* Fracture, vertebra, by
     site
   nonunion 733.82
   nose, nasal, (bone) (septum) (closed)
     802.0
     open 802.1
   occiput - *see* Fracture, skull, base
   odontoid process - *see* Fracture,
     vertebra, cervical
   olecranon (process) (ulna) (closed)
     813.01
     open 813.11
   open 829.1
   orbit, orbital (bone) (region) (closed)
     802.8
     floor (blow-out) 802.6
      open 802.7
     open 802.9
     roof - *see* Fracture, skull, base
     specified part NEC 802.8
      open 802.9
   os
     calcis (closed) 825.0
      open 825.1
     magnum (closed) 814.07
      open 814.17
     pubis (with visceral injury) (closed)
      808.2
      open 808.3
     triquetrum (closed) 814.03
      open 814.13
   osseous
     auditory meatus - *see* Fracture, skull,
      base
     labyrinth - *see* Fracture, skull, base
   ossicles, auditory (incus) (malleus)
     (stapes) - *see* Fracture, skull, base
   osteoporotic - *see* Fracture, pathologic
   palate (closed) 802.8
     open 802.9
   paratrooper - *see* Fracture, tibia, lower
     end

Fracture (*Continued*)
  parietal bone - *see* Fracture, skull, vault
  parry - *see* Fracture, Monteggia's
  patella (closed) 822.0
    open 822.1
  pathologic (cause unknown) 733.10
    ankle 733.16
    femur (neck) 733.14
      specified NEC 733.15
    fibula 733.16
    hip 733.14
    humerus 733.11
    radius (distal) 733.12
    specified site NEC 733.19
    tibia 733.16
    ulna 733.12
    vertebrae (collapse) 733.13
    wrist 733.12
  pedicle (of vertebral arch) - *see*
    Fracture, vertebra, by site
  pelvis, pelvic (bone(s)) (with visceral
    injury) (closed) 808.8
    multiple ~~(with disruption of pelvic~~
      ~~circle)~~ with disruption of
      pelvic circle 808.43 ◀▥
      open 808.53
    open 808.9
    rim (closed) 808.49
      open 808.59
  peritrochanteric (closed) 820.20
    open 820.30
  phalanx, phalanges, of one
    foot (closed) 826.0
      with bone(s) of same lower limb
        827.0
        open 827.1
      open 826.1
    hand (closed) 816.00
      with metacarpal bone(s) of same
        hand 817.0
        open 817.1
      distal 816.02
        open 816.12
      middle 816.01
        open 816.11
      multiple sites NEC 816.03
        open 816.13
      open 816.10
      proximal 816.01
        open 816.11
  pisiform (closed) 814.04
    open 814.14
  pond - *see* Fracture, skull, vault
  Pott's (closed) 824.4
    open 824.5
  prosthetic device, internal - *see*
    Complications, mechanical
  pubis (with visceral injury) (closed)
    808.2
    open 808.3
  Quervain's (closed) 814.01
    open 814.11
  radius (alone) (closed) 813.81
    with ulna NEC 813.83
      open 813.93
    distal end - *see* Fracture, radius,
      lower end
    epiphysis
      lower - *see* Fracture, radius, lower
        end
      upper - *see* Fracture, radius,
        upper end
    head - *see* Fracture, radius, upper
      end

Fracture (*Continued*)
  radius (*Continued*)
    lower end or extremity (distal end)
      (lower epiphysis) 813.42
      with ulna (lower end) 813.44
        open 813.54
      open 813.52
      torus 813.45
        with ulna 813.47
    neck - *see* Fracture, radius, upper
      end
    open NEC 813.91
    pathologic 733.12
    proximal end - *see* Fracture, radius,
      upper end
    shaft (closed) 813.21
      with ulna (shaft) 813.23
        open 813.33
      open 813.31
    upper end 813.07
      with ulna (upper end) 813.08
        open 813.18
      epiphysis 813.05
        open 813.15
      head 813.05
        open 813.15
      multiple sites 813.07
        open 813.17
      neck 813.06
        open 813.16
      open 813.17
      specified site NEC 813.07
        open 813.17
  ramus
    inferior or superior (with visceral
      injury) (closed) 808.2
      open 808.3
    ischium - *see* Fracture, ischium
    mandible 802.24
      open 802.34
  rib(s) (closed) 807.0●

Note: Use the following fifth-digit
subclassification with categories
807.0–807.1:

  0   rib(s), unspecified
  1   one rib
  2   two ribs
  3   three ribs
  4   four ribs
  5   five ribs
  6   six ribs
  7   seven ribs
  8   eight or more ribs
  9   multiple ribs, unspecified

    with flail chest (open) 807.4
      open 807.1●
  root, tooth 873.63
    complicated 873.73
  sacrum - *see* Fracture, vertebra, sacrum
  scaphoid
    ankle (closed) 825.22
      open 825.32
    wrist (closed) 814.01
      open 814.11
  scapula (closed) 811.00
    acromial, acromion (process) 811.01
      open 811.11
    body 811.09
      open 811.19
    coracoid process 811.02
      open 811.12

Fracture (*Continued*)
  scapula (*Continued*)
    glenoid (cavity) (fossa) 811.03
      open 811.13
    neck 811.03
      open 811.13
    open 811.10
  semilunar
    bone, wrist (closed) 814.02
      open 814.12
    cartilage (interior) (knee) - *see* Tear,
      meniscus
  sesamoid bone - *see* Fracture, by site
  Shepherd's (closed) 825.21
    open 825.31
  shoulder - *see also* Fracture, humerus,
    upper end
    blade - *see* Fracture, scapula
  silverfork - *see* Fracture, radius, lower
    end
  sinus (ethmoid) (frontal) (maxillary)
    (nasal) (sphenoidal) - *see* Fracture,
    skull, base
  Skillern's - *see* Fracture, radius, shaft
  skull (multiple NEC) (with face bones)
    (closed) 803.0●

Note: Use the following fifth-digit
subclassification with categories 800,
801, 803, and 804:

  0   unspecified state of
        consciousness
  1   with no loss of consciousness
  2   with brief [less than one hour]
        loss of consciousness
  3   with moderate [1-24 hours] loss
        of consciousness
  4   with prolonged [more than 24
        hours] loss of
        consciousness and return
        to pre-existing conscious
        level
  5   with prolonged [more than 24
        hours] loss of
        consciousness, without
        return to pre-existing
        conscious level

Use fifth-digit 5 to designate when a
patient is unconscious and dies before
regaining consciousness, regardless of
the duration of the loss of consciousness

  6   with loss of consciousness of
        unspecified duration
  9   with concussion, unspecified

    with
      contusion, cerebral 803.1●
      epidural hemorrhage 803.2●
      extradural hemorrhage 803.2●
      hemorrhage (intracranial) NEC
        803.3●
      intracranial injury NEC 803.4●
      laceration, cerebral 803.1●
      other bones - *see* Fracture,
        multiple, skull
      subarachnoid hemorrhage 803.2●
      subdural hemorrhage 803.2●
    base (antrum) (ethmoid bone) (fossa)
      (internal ear) (nasal sinus)
      (occiput) (sphenoid) (temporal
      bone) (closed) 801.0●
      with
        contusion, cerebral 801.1●
        epidural hemorrhage 801.2●

◀ New   ◀▥ Revised   ~~deleted~~ Deleted   ● Use Additional Digit(s)   ▥ Omit code

Fracture *(Continued)*
skull *(Continued)*
base *(Continued)*
with *(Continued)*
extradural hemorrhage 801.2●
hemorrhage (intracranial)
NEC 801.3●
intracranial injury NEC 801.4●
laceration, cerebral 801.1●
subarachnoid hemorrhage
801.2●
subdural hemorrhage 801.2●
open 801.5●
with
contusion, cerebral 801.6●
epidural hemorrhage
801.7●
extradural hemorrhage
801.7●
hemorrhage (intracranial)
NEC 801.8●
intracranial injury NEC
801.9●
laceration, cerebral 801.6●
subarachnoid hemorrhage
801.7●
subdural hemorrhage
801.7●
birth injury 767.3
face bones - *see* Fracture, face bones
open 803.5●
with
contusion, cerebral 803.6●
epidural hemorrhage 803.7●
extradural hemorrhage 803.7●
hemorrhage (intracranial)
NEC 803.8●
intracranial injury NEC 803.9●
laceration, cerebral 803.6●
subarachnoid hemorrhage
803.7●
subdural hemorrhage 803.7●
vault (frontal bone) (parietal bone)
(vertex) (closed) 800.0●
with
contusion, cerebral 800.1●
epidural hemorrhage 800.2●
extradural hemorrhage 800.2●
hemorrhage (intracranial)
NEC 800.3●
intracranial injury NEC
800.4●
laceration, cerebral 800.1●
subarachnoid hemorrhage
800.2●
subdural hemorrhage
800.2●
open 800.5●
with
contusion, cerebral
800.6●
epidural hemorrhage
800.7●
extradural hemorrhage
800.7●
hemorrhage (intracranial)
NEC 800.8●
intracranial injury NEC
800.9●
laceration, cerebral 800.6●
subarachnoid hemorrhage
800.7●
subdural hemorrhage
800.7●

Fracture *(Continued)*
Smith's 813.41
open 813.51
sphenoid (bone) (sinus) - *see* Fracture,
skull, base
spine - *see also* Fracture, vertebra,
by site due to birth trauma
767.4
spinous process - *see* Fracture,
vertebra, by site
spontaneous - *see* Fracture, pathologic
sprinters' - *see* Fracture, ilium
stapes - *see* Fracture, skull, base
stave - *see also* Fracture, metacarpus,
metacarpal bone(s)
spine - *see* Fracture, tibia, upper
end
sternum (closed) 807.2
with flail chest (open) 807.4
open 807.3
Stieda's - *see* Fracture, femur, lower
end
stress 733.95
fibula 733.93
metatarsals 733.94
specified site NEC 733.95
tibia 733.93
styloid process
metacarpal (closed) 815.02
open 815.12
radius - *see* Fracture, radius, lower
end
temporal bone - *see* Fracture, skull,
base
ulna - *see* Fracture, ulna, lower
end
supracondylar, elbow 812.41
open 812.51
symphysis pubis (with visceral injury)
(closed) 808.2
open 808.3
talus (ankle bone) (closed) 825.21
open 825.31
tarsus, tarsal bone(s) (with
metatarsus) of one foot
(closed) NEC 825.29
open 825.39
temporal bone (styloid) - *see* Fracture,
skull, base
tendon - *see* Sprain, by site
thigh - *see* Fracture, femur, shaft
thumb (and finger(s)) of one hand
(closed) (*see also* Fracture,
phalanx, hand) 816.00
with metacarpal bone(s) of same
hand 817.0
open 817.1
metacarpal(s) - *see* Fracture,
metacarpus
open 816.10
thyroid cartilage (closed) 807.5
open 807.6
tibia (closed) 823.80
with fibula 823.82
open 823.92
condyles - *see* Fracture, tibia, upper
end
distal end 824.8
open 824.9
epiphysis
lower 824.8
open 824.9
upper - *see* Fracture, tibia, upper
end

Fracture *(Continued)*
tibia *(Continued)*
head (involving knee joint) - *see*
Fracture, tibia, upper end
intercondyloid eminence - *see*
Fracture, tibia, upper end
involving ankle 824.0
open 824.1
lower end or extremity (anterior
lip) (posterior lip) 824.8
open 824.9
malleolus (internal) (medial) 824.0
open 824.1
open NEC 823.90
pathologic 733.16
proximal end - *see* Fracture, tibia,
upper end
shaft 823.20
with fibula 823.22
open 823.32
open 823.30
spine - *see* Fracture, tibia, upper end
stress 733.93
torus 823.40
with fibula 823.42
tuberosity - *see* Fracture, tibia, upper
end
upper end or extremity (condyle)
(epiphysis) (head) (spine)
(proximal end) (tuberosity)
823.00
with fibula 823.02
open 823.12
open 823.10
toe(s), of one foot (closed) 826.0
with bone(s) of same lower limb
827.0
open 827.1
open 826.1
tooth (root) 873.63
complicated 873.73
torus
fibula 823.41
with tibia 823.42
humerus 812.49
radius (alone) 813.45
with ulna 813.47
tibia 823.40
with fibula 823.42
ulna (alone) 813.46
with radius 813.47
trachea (closed) 807.5
open 807.6
transverse process - *see* Fracture,
vertebra, by site
trapezium (closed) 814.05
open 814.15
trapezoid bone (closed) 814.06
open 814.16
trimalleolar (closed) 824.6
open 824.7
triquetral (bone) (closed) 814.03
open 814.13
trochanter (greater) (lesser) (closed)
(*see also* Fracture, femur, neck,
by site) 820.20
open 820.30
trunk (bones) (closed) 809.0
open 809.1
tuberosity (external) - *see* Fracture,
by site
ulna (alone) (closed) 813.82
with radius NEC 813.83
open 813.93

Fracture *(Continued)*
  ulna *(Continued)*
    coronoid process (closed) 813.02
      open 813.12
    distal end - *see* Fracture, ulna, lower
        end
    epiphysis
      lower - *see* Fracture, ulna, lower
          end
      upper - *see* Fracture, ulna, upper,
          end
    head - *see* Fracture, ulna, lower
        end
    lower end (distal end) (head)
        (lower epiphysis) (styloid
        process) 813.43
      with radius (lower end) 813.44
        open 813.54
      open 813.53
    olecranon process (closed) 813.01
      open 813.11
    open NEC 813.92
    pathologic 733.12
    proximal end - *see* Fracture, ulna,
        upper end
    shaft 813.22
      with radius (shaft) 813.23
        open 813.33
      open 813.32
    styloid process - *see* Fracture, ulna,
        lower end
    torus 813.46
      with radius 813.47
    transverse - *see* Fracture, ulna, by
        site
    upper end (epiphysis) 813.04
      with radius (upper end)
          813.08
        open 813.18
      multiple sites 813.04
        open 813.14
      open 813.14
      specified site NEC 813.04
        open 813.14
  unciform (closed) 814.08
    open 814.18
  vertebra, vertebral (back) (body)
      (column) (neural arch) (pedicle)
      (spine) (spinous process)
      (transverse process) (closed)
      805.8
    with
      hematomyelia - *see* Fracture,
          vertebra, by site, with
          spinal cord injury
      injury to
        cauda equina - *see* Fracture,
            vertebra, sacrum, with
            spinal cord injury
        nerve - *see* Fracture, vertebra,
            by site, with spinal cord
            injury
      paralysis - *see* Fracture, vertebra,
          by site, with spinal cord
          injury
      paraplegia - *see* Fracture,
          vertebra, by site, with
          spinal cord injury
      quadriplegia - *see* Fracture,
          vertebra, by site, with
          spinal cord injury
      spinal concussion - *see* Fracture,
          vertebra, by site, with
          spinal cord injury

Fracture *(Continued)*
  vertebra, vertebral *(Continued)*
    with *(Continued)*
      spinal cord injury (closed) NEC
          806.8

Note: Use the following fifth-digit
subclassification with categories
806.0–806.3:

C_1–C_4 or unspecified level and D_1–D_6
(T_1–T_6) or unspecified level with:

0   unspecified spinal cord injury
1   complete lesion of cord
2   anterior cord syndrome
3   central cord syndrome
4   specified injury NEC

level and D_1–D_{12} level with:

5   unspecified spinal cord injury
6   complete lesion of cord
7   anterior cord syndrome
8   central cord syndrome
9   specified injury NEC

      cervical 806.0●
        open 806.1●
      chronic 733.13
      dorsal, dorsolumbar 806.2●
        open 806.3●
      open 806.9
      thoracic, thoracolumbar
          806.2●
        open 806.3●
    atlanto-axial - *see* Fracture,
        vertebra, cervical
    cervical (hangman) (teardrop)
        (closed) 805.00
      with spinal cord injury -
          see Fracture, vertebra,
          with spinal cord injury,
          cervical
      first (atlas) 805.01
        open 805.11
      second (axis) 805.02
        open 805.12
      third 805.03
        open 805.13
      fourth 805.04
        open 805.14
      fifth 805.05
        open 805.15
      sixth 805.06
        open 805.16
      seventh 805.07
        open 805.17
      multiple sites 805.08
        open 805.18
      open 805.10
    coccyx (closed) 805.6
      with spinal cord injury (closed)
          806.60
        cauda equina injury 806.62
          complete lesion 806.61
            open 806.71
          open 806.72
        open 806.70
          specified type NEC
              806.69
        open 806.79
      open 805.7
    collapsed 733.13
    compression, not due to trauma
        733.13

Fracture *(Continued)*
  dorsal (closed) 805.2
    with spinal cord injury - *see* Fracture,
        vertebra, with spinal cord
        injury, dorsal
    open 805.3
  dorsolumbar (closed) 805.2
    with spinal cord injury - *see* Fracture,
        vertebra, with spinal cord
        injury, dorsal
    open 805.3
  due to osteoporosis 733.13
  fetus or newborn 767.4
  lumbar (closed) 805.4
    with spinal cord injury (closed)
        806.4
      open 806.5
    open 805.5
  nontraumatic 733.13
  open NEC 805.9
  pathologic (any site) 733.13
  sacrum (closed) 805.6
    with spinal cord injury 806.60
      cauda equina injury 806.62
        complete lesion 806.61
          open 806.71
        open 806.72
      open 806.70
      specified type NEC 806.69
        open 806.79
    open 805.7
  site unspecified (closed) 805.8
    with spinal cord injury (closed)
        806.8
      open 806.9
    open 805.9
  stress (any site) 733.95
  thoracic (closed) 805.2
    with spinal cord injury - *see* Fracture,
        vertebra, with spinal cord
        injury, thoracic
    open 805.3
  vertex - *see* Fracture, skull, vault
  vomer (bone) 802.0
    open 802.1
  Wagstaffe's - *see* Fracture, ankle
  wrist (closed) 814.00
    open 814.10
    pathologic 733.12
  xiphoid (process) - *see* Fracture,
      sternum
  zygoma (zygomatic arch) (closed) 802.4
    open 802.5
Fragile X syndrome 759.83
Fragilitas
  crinium 704.2
  hair 704.2
  ossium 756.51
    with blue sclera 756.51
  unguium 703.8
    congenital 757.5
Fragility
  bone 756.51
    with deafness and blue sclera
        756.51
  capillary (hereditary) 287.8
  hair 704.2
  nails 703.8
Fragmentation - *see* Fracture, by site
Frailty 797
Frambesia, frambesial (tropica) (*see also*
    Yaws) 102.9
  initial lesion or ulcer 102.0
  primary 102.0

◀ New   ◀▥ Revised   ~~deleted~~ Deleted   ● Use Additional Digit(s)   ▨ Omit code

Frambeside
  gummatous 102.4
  of early yaws 102.2
Frambesioma 102.1
Franceschetti's syndrome
    (mandibulofacial dysostosis)
    756.0
Francis' disease (*see also* Tularemia)
    021.9
Frank's essential thrombocytopenia (*see
    also* Purpura, thrombocytopenic)
    287.39
Franklin's disease (heavy chain) 273.2
Fraser's syndrome 759.89
Freckle 709.09
  malignant melanoma in (M8742/3) - *see*
    Melanoma
  melanotic (of Hutchinson) (M8742/2) -
    see Neoplasm, skin, in situ
  retinal 239.81
Freeman-Sheldon syndrome 759.89
Freezing 991.9
  specified effect NEC 991.8
Frei's disease (climatic bubo) 099.1
Freiberg's
  disease (osteochondrosis, second
    metatarsal) 732.5
  infraction of metatarsal head 732.5
  osteochondrosis 732.5
Fremitus, friction, cardiac 785.3
Frenulum linguae 750.0
Frenum
  external os 752.44 ◀▥
  tongue 750.0
Frequency (urinary) NEC 788.41
  micturition 788.41
  nocturnal 788.43
  polyuria 788.42
  psychogenic 306.53
Frey's syndrome (auriculotemporal
    syndrome) 705.22
Friction
  burn (*see also* Injury, superficial, by site)
    919.0
  fremitus, cardiac 785.3
  precordial 785.3
  sounds, chest 786.7
Friderichsen-Waterhouse syndrome or
    disease 036.3
Friedländer's
  B (bacillus) NEC (*see also* condition)
    041.3
    sepsis or septicemia 038.49
  disease (endarteritis obliterans) - *see*
    Arteriosclerosis
Friedreich's
  ataxia 334.0
  combined systemic disease 334.0
  disease 333.2
    combined systemic 334.0
  myoclonia 333.2
  sclerosis (spinal cord) 334.0
Friedrich-Erb-Arnold syndrome
    (acropachyderma) 757.39
Frigidity 302.72
  psychic or psychogenic 302.72
Fröhlich's disease or syndrome
    (adiposogenital dystrophy) 253.8
Froin's syndrome 336.8
Frommel's disease 676.6●
Frommel-Chiari syndrome 676.6●
Frontal - *see also* condition
  lobe syndrome 310.0

Frostbite 991.3
  face 991.0
  foot 991.2
  hand 991.1
  specified site NEC 991.3
Frotteurism 302.89
Frozen 991.9
  pelvis 620.8
  shoulder 726.0
Fructosemia 271.2
Fructosuria (benign) (essential) 271.2
Fuchs'
  black spot (myopic) 360.21
  corneal dystrophy (endothelial)
    371.57
  heterochromic cyclitis 364.21
Fucosidosis 271.8
Fugue 780.99
  dissociative 300.13
  hysterical (dissociative) 300.13
  reaction to exceptional stress (transient)
    308.1
Fukuhara syndrome 277.87
Fuller Albright's syndrome (osteitis
    fibrosa disseminata) 756.59
Fuller's earth disease 502
Fulminant, fulminating - *see* condition
Functional - *see* condition
Functioning
  borderline intellectual V62.89
Fundus - *see also* condition
  flavimaculatus 362.76
Fungemia 117.9
Fungus, fungous
  cerebral 348.89
  disease NEC 117.9
  infection - *see* Infection, fungus
  testis (*see also* Tuberculosis) 016.5●
    [608.81]
Funiculitis (acute) 608.4
  chronic 608.4
  endemic 608.4
  gonococcal (acute) 098.14
    chronic or duration of 2 months or
      over 098.34
  tuberculous (*see also* Tuberculosis)
    016.5●
FUO (*see also* Pyrexia) 780.60
Funnel
  breast (acquired) 738.3
    congenital 754.81
    late effect of rickets 268.1
  chest (acquired) 738.3
    congenital 754.81
    late effect of rickets 268.1
  pelvis (acquired) 738.6
    with disproportion (fetopelvic)
      653.3●
      affecting fetus or newborn
        763.1
      causing obstructed labor
        660.1●
        affecting fetus or newborn
          763.1
    congenital 755.69
    tuberculous (*see also* Tuberculosis)
      016.9●
Furfur 690.18
  microsporon 111.0
Furor, paroxysmal (idiopathic) (*see also*
    Epilepsy) 345.8●
Furriers' lung 495.8
Furrowed tongue 529.5
  congenital 750.13

Furrowing nail(s) (transverse) 703.8
  congenital 757.5
Furuncle 680.9
  abdominal wall 680.2
  ankle 680.6
  anus 680.5
  arm (any part, above wrist) 680.3
  auditory canal, external 680.0
  axilla 680.3
  back (any part) 680.2
  breast 680.2
  buttock 680.5
  chest wall 680.2
  corpus cavernosum 607.2
  ear (any part) 680.0
  eyelid 373.13
  face (any part, except eye) 680.0
  finger (any) 680.4
  flank 680.2
  foot (any part) 680.7
  forearm 680.3
  gluteal (region) 680.5
  groin 680.2
  hand (any part) 680.4
  head (any part, except face) 680.8
  heel 680.7
  hip 680.6
  kidney (*see also* Abscess, kidney) 590.2
  knee 680.6
  labium (majus) (minus) 616.4
  lacrimal
    gland (*see also* Dacryoadenitis)
      375.00
    passages (duct) (sac) (*see also*
      Dacryocystitis) 375.30
  leg, any part except foot 680.6
  malignant 022.0
  multiple sites 680.9
  neck 680.1
  nose (external) (septum) 680.0
  orbit 376.01
  partes posteriores 680.5
  pectoral region 680.2
  penis 607.2
  perineum 680.2
  pinna 680.0
  scalp (any part) 680.8
  scrotum 608.4
  seminal vesicle 608.0
  shoulder 680.3
  skin NEC 680.9
  specified site NEC 680.8
  spermatic cord 608.4
  temple (region) 680.0
  testis 604.90
  thigh 680.6
  thumb 680.4
  toe (any) 680.7
  trunk 680.2
  tunica vaginalis 608.4
  umbilicus 680.2
  upper arm 680.3
  vas deferens 608.4
  vulva 616.4
  wrist 680.4
Furunculosis (*see also* Furuncle) 680.9
  external auditory meatus 680.0 [380.13]
Fusarium (infection) 118
Fusion, fused (congenital)
  anal (with urogenital canal) 751.5
  aorta and pulmonary artery 745.0
  astragaloscaphoid 755.67
  atria 745.5
  atrium and ventricle 745.69

Fusion, fused (Continued)
  auditory canal 744.02
  auricles, heart 745.5
  binocular, with defective stereopsis
      368.33
  bone 756.9
  cervical spine - see Fusion, spine
  choanal 748.0
  commissure, mitral valve 746.5
  cranial sutures, premature 756.0
  cusps, heart valve NEC 746.89
      mitral 746.5
      tricuspid 746.89
  ear ossicles 744.04
  fingers (see also Syndactylism, fingers)
      755.11
  hymen 752.42
  hymeno-urethral 599.89
      causing obstructed labor 660.1 ●
          affecting fetus or newborn
              763.1
  joint (acquired) - see also Ankylosis
      congenital 755.8
  kidneys (incomplete) 753.3

Fusion, fused (Continued)
  labium (majus) (minus) 752.49
  larynx and trachea 748.3
  limb 755.8
      lower 755.69
      upper 755.59
  lobe, lung 748.5
  lumbosacral (acquired) 724.6
      congenital 756.15
      surgical V45.4
  nares (anterior) (posterior) 748.0
  nose, nasal 748.0
  nostril(s) 748.0
  organ or site NEC - see Anomaly,
      specified type NEC
  ossicles 756.9
      auditory 744.04
  pulmonary valve segment 746.02
  pulmonic cusps 746.02
  ribs 756.3
  sacroiliac (acquired) (joint) 724.6
      congenital 755.69
      surgical V45.4
  skull, imperfect 756.0

Fusion, fused (Continued)
  spine (acquired) 724.9
      arthrodesis status V45.4
      congenital (vertebra) 756.15
      postoperative status V45.4
  sublingual duct with submaxillary duct
      at opening in mouth 750.26
  talonavicular (bar) 755.67
  teeth, tooth 520.2
  testes 752.89
  toes (see also Syndactylism, toes) 755.13
  trachea and esophagus 750.3
  twins 759.4
  urethral-hymenal 599.89
  vagina 752.49
  valve cusps - see Fusion, cusps, heart
      valve
  ventricles, heart 745.4
  vertebra (arch) - see Fusion, spine
  vulva 752.49
Fusospirillosis (mouth) (tongue) (tonsil)
      101
Fussy infant (baby) 780.91

◀ New   ◀▥ Revised   deleted Deleted   ● Use Additional Digit(s)   ▨ Omit code

G

Gafsa boil 085.1
Gain, weight (abnormal) (excessive) (see also Weight, gain) 783.1
Gaisböck's disease or syndrome (polycythemia hypertonica) 289.0
Gait
  abnormality 781.2
    hysterical 300.11
  ataxic 781.2
    hysterical 300.11
  disturbance 781.2
    hysterical 300.11
  paralytic 781.2
  scissor 781.2
  spastic 781.2
  staggering 781.2
    hysterical 300.11
Galactocele (breast) (infected) 611.5
  puerperal, postpartum 676.8●
Galactophoritis 611.0
  puerperal, postpartum 675.2●
Galactorrhea 676.6●
  not associated with childbirth 611.6
Galactosemia (classic) (congenital) 271.1
Galactosuria 271.1
Galacturia 791.1
  bilharziasis 120.0
Galen's vein - see condition
Gallbladder - see also condition
  acute (see also Disease, gallbladder) 575.0
Gall duct - see condition
Gallop rhythm 427.89
Gallstone (cholemic) (colic) (impacted) - see also Cholelithiasis
  causing intestinal obstruction 560.31
Gambling, pathological 312.31
Gammaloidosis 277.39
Gammopathy 273.9
  macroglobulinemia 273.3
  monoclonal (benign) (essential) (idiopathic) (with lymphoplasmacytic dyscrasia) 273.1
Gamna's disease (siderotic splenomegaly) 289.51
Gampsodactylia (congenital) 754.71
Gamstorp's disease (adynamia episodica hereditaria) 359.3
Gandy-Nanta disease (siderotic splenomegaly) 289.51
Gang activity, without manifest psychiatric disorder V71.09
  adolescent V71.02
  adult V71.01
  child V71.02
Gangliocytoma (M9490/0) - see Neoplasm, connective tissue, benign
Ganglioglioma (M9505/1) - see Neoplasm, by site, uncertain behavior
Ganglion 727.43
  joint 727.41
  of yaws (early) (late) 102.6
  periosteal (see also Periostitis) 730.3●
  tendon sheath (compound) (diffuse) 727.42
  tuberculous (see also Tuberculosis) 015.9●
Ganglioneuroblastoma (M9490/3) - see Neoplasm, connective tissue, malignant

Ganglioneuroma (M9490/0) - see also Neoplasm, connective tissue, benign
  malignant (M9490/3) - see Neoplasm, connective tissue, malignant
Ganglioneuromatosis (M9491/0) - see Neoplasm, connective tissue, benign
Ganglionitis
  fifth nerve (see also Neuralgia, trigeminal) 350.1
  gasserian 350.1
  geniculate 351.1
    herpetic 053.11
    newborn 767.5
  herpes zoster 053.11
  herpetic geniculate (Hunt's syndrome) 053.11
Gangliosidosis 330.1
Gangosa 102.5
Gangrene, gangrenous (anemia) (artery) (cellulitis) (dermatitis) (dry) (infective) (moist) (pemphigus) (septic) (skin) (stasis) (ulcer) 785.4
  with
    arteriosclerosis (native artery) 440.24
      bypass graft 440.30
        autologous vein 440.31
        nonautologous biological 440.32
    diabetes (mellitus) 250.7● [785.4]
      due to secondary diabetes 249.7● [785.4]
  abdomen (wall) 785.4
  adenitis 683
  alveolar 526.5
  angina 462
    diphtheritic 032.0
  anus 569.49
  appendices epiploicae - see Gangrene, mesentery
  appendix - see Appendicitis, acute
  arteriosclerotic - see Arteriosclerosis, with, gangrene
  auricle 785.4
  Bacillus welchii (see also Gangrene, gas) 040.0
  bile duct (see also Cholangitis) 576.8
  bladder 595.89
  bowel - see Gangrene, intestine
  cecum - see Gangrene, intestine
  Clostridium perfringens or welchii (see also Gangrene, gas) 040.0
  colon - see Gangrene, intestine
  connective tissue 785.4
  cornea 371.40
  corpora cavernosa (infective) 607.2
    noninfective 607.89
  cutaneous, spreading 785.4
  decubital (see also Ulcer, pressure) 707.00 [785.4]
  diabetic (any site) 250.7● [785.4]
    due to secondary diabetes 249.7● [785.4]
  dropsical 785.4
  emphysematous (see also Gangrene, gas) 040.0
  epidemic (ergotized grain) 988.2
  epididymis (infectional) (see also Epididymitis) 604.99
  erysipelas (see also Erysipelas) 035
  extremity (lower) (upper) 785.4
  gallbladder or duct (see also Cholecystitis, acute) 575.0

Gangrene, gangrenous (Continued)
  gas (bacillus) 040.0
    with
      abortion - see Abortion, by type, with sepsis
      ectopic pregnancy (see also categories 633.0–633.9) 639.0
      molar pregnancy (see also categories 630–632) 639.0
    following
      abortion 639.0
      ectopic or molar pregnancy 639.0
    puerperal, postpartum, childbirth 670.8●
  glossitis 529.0
  gum 523.8
  hernia - see Hernia, by site, with gangrene
  hospital noma 528.1
  intestine, intestinal (acute) (hemorrhagic) (massive) 557.0
    with
      hernia - see Hernia, by site, with gangrene
      mesenteric embolism or infarction 557.0
      obstruction (see also Obstruction, intestine) 560.9
  laryngitis 464.00
    with obstruction 464.01
  liver 573.8
  lung 513.0
    spirochetal 104.8
  lymphangitis 457.2
  Meleney's (cutaneous) 686.09
  mesentery 557.0
    with
      embolism or infarction 557.0
      intestinal obstruction (see also Obstruction, intestine) 560.9
  mouth 528.1
  noma 528.1
  orchitis 604.90
  ovary (see also Salpingo-oophoritis) 614.2
  pancreas 577.0
  penis (infectional) 607.2
    noninfective 607.89
  perineum 785.4
  pharynx 462
    septic 034.0
  pneumonia 513.0
  Pott's 440.24
  presenile 443.1
  pulmonary 513.0
  pulp, tooth 522.1
  quinsy 475
  Raynaud's (symmetric gangrene) 443.0 [785.4]
  rectum 569.49
  retropharyngeal 478.24
  rupture - see Hernia, by site, with gangrene
  scrotum 608.4
    noninfective 608.83
  senile 440.24
  sore throat 462
  spermatic cord 608.4
    noninfective 608.89
  spine 785.4
  spirochetal NEC 104.8
  spreading cutaneous 785.4
  stomach 537.89
  stomatitis 528.1

Gangrene, gangrenous (*Continued*)
  symmetrical 443.0 [785.4]
  testis (infectional) (*see also* Orchitis)
    604.99
    noninfective 608.89
  throat 462
    diphtheritic 032.0
  thyroid (gland) 246.8
  tonsillitis (acute) 463
  tooth (pulp) 522.1
  tuberculous NEC (*see also* Tuberculosis)
    011.9●
  tunica vaginalis 608.4
    noninfective 608.89
  umbilicus 785.4
  uterus (*see also* Endometritis) 615.9
  uvulitis 528.3
  vas deferens 608.4
    noninfective 608.89
  vulva (*see also* Vulvitis) 616.10
Gannister disease (occupational) 502
  with tuberculosis - *see* Tuberculosis,
    pulmonary
Ganser's syndrome, hysterical 300.16
Gardner-Diamond syndrome
  (autoerythrocyte sensitization) 287.2
Gargoylism 277.5
Garré's
  disease (*see also* Osteomyelitis) 730.1●
  osteitis (sclerosing) (*see also*
    Osteomyelitis) 730.1●
  osteomyelitis (*see also* Osteomyelitis)
    730.1●
Garrod's pads, knuckle 728.79
Gartner's duct
  cyst 752.41
  persistent 752.41
Gas 787.3
  asphyxia, asphyxiation, inhalation,
    poisoning, suffocation NEC 987.9
    specified gas - *see* Table of Drugs
      and Chemicals
  bacillus gangrene or infection - *see* Gas,
    gangrene
  cyst, mesentery 568.89
  excessive 787.3
  gangrene 040.0
    with
      abortion - *see* Abortion, by type,
        with sepsis
      ectopic pregnancy (*see also*
        categories 633.0–633.9) 639.0
      molar pregnancy (*see also*
        categories 630–632) 639.0
    following
      abortion 639.0
      ectopic or molar pregnancy
        639.0
    puerperal, postpartum,
      childbirth 670.8●
  on stomach 787.3
  pains 787.3
Gastradenitis 535.0●
Gastralgia 536.8
  psychogenic 307.89
Gastrectasis, gastrectasia 536.1
  psychogenic 306.4
Gastric - *see* condition
Gastrinoma (M8153/1)
  malignant (M8153/3)
    pancreas 157.4
    specified site NEC - *see* Neoplasm,
      by site, malignant
    unspecified site 157.4

Gastrinoma (*Continued*)
  specified site - *see* Neoplasm, by site,
    uncertain behavior
  unspecified site 235.5
Gastritis 535.5●

> Note: Use the following fifth-digit
> subclassification for category 535:
> 0   without mention of hemorrhage
> 1   with hemorrhage

  acute 535.0●
  alcoholic 535.3●
  allergic 535.4●
  antral 535.4●
  atrophic 535.1●
  atrophic-hyperplastic 535.1●
  bile-induced 535.4●
  catarrhal 535.0●
  chronic (atrophic) 535.1●
  cirrhotic 535.4●
  corrosive (acute) 535.4●
  dietetic 535.4●
  due to diet deficiency 269.9 [535.4]●
  eosinophilic 535.7●
  erosive 535.4●
  follicular 535.4●
    chronic 535.1●
  giant hypertrophic 535.2●
  glandular 535.4●
    chronic 535.1●
  hypertrophic (mucosa) 535.2●
    chronic giant 211.1
  irritant 535.4●
  nervous 306.4
  phlegmonous 535.0●
  psychogenic 306.4
  sclerotic 535.4●
  spastic 536.8
  subacute 535.0●
  superficial 535.4●
  suppurative 535.0●
  toxic 535.4●
  tuberculous (*see also* Tuberculosis)
    017.9●
Gastrocarcinoma (M8010/3) 151.9
Gastrocolic - *see* condition
Gastrocolitis - *see* Enteritis
Gastrodisciasis 121.8
Gastroduodenitis (*see also* Gastritis)
  535.5●
  catarrhal 535.0●
  infectional 535.0●
  virus, viral 008.8
    specified type NEC 008.69
Gastrodynia 536.8
Gastroenteritis (acute) (catarrhal)
  (congestive) (hemorrhagic)
  (noninfectious) (*see also* Enteritis)
  558.9
  aertrycke infection 003.0
  allergic 558.3
  chronic 558.9
    ulcerative (*see also* Colitis, ulcerative)
      556.9
  dietetic 558.9
  due to
    antineoplastic chemotherapy 558.9
    food poisoning (*see also* Poisoning,
      food) 005.9
    radiation 558.1
  eosinophilic 558.41
  epidemic 009.0

Gastroenteritis (*Continued*)
  functional 558.9
  infectious (*see also* Enteritis, due to, by
    organism) 009.0
    presumed 009.1
  salmonella 003.0
  septic (*see also* Enteritis, due to, by
    organism) 009.0
  toxic 558.2
  tuberculous (*see also* Tuberculosis)
    014.8●
  ulcerative (*see also* Colitis, ulcerative)
    556.9
  viral NEC 008.8
    specified type NEC 008.69
  zymotic 009.0
Gastroenterocolitis - *see* Enteritis
Gastroenteropathy, protein-losing 579.8
Gastroenteroptosis 569.89
Gastroesophageal laceration-hemorrhage
  syndrome 530.7
Gastroesophagitis 530.19
Gastrohepatitis (*see also* Gastritis) 535.5●
Gastrointestinal - *see* condition
Gastrojejunal - *see* condition
Gastrojejunitis (*see also* Gastritis) 535.5●
Gastrojejunocolic - *see* condition
Gastroliths 537.89
Gastromalacia 537.89
Gastroparalysis 536.3
  diabetic 250.6● [536.3]
    due to secondary diabetes 249.6●
      [536.3]
Gastroparesis 536.3
  diabetic 250.6● [536.3]
    due to secondary diabetes 249.6●
      [536.3]
Gastropathy 537.9
  congestive portal 537.89
  erythematous 535.5●
  exudative 579.8
  portal hypertensive 537.89
Gastroptosis 537.5
Gastrorrhagia 578.0
Gastrorrhea 536.8
  psychogenic 306.4
Gastroschisis (congenital) 756.73
  acquired 569.89
Gastrospasm (neurogenic) (reflex) 536.8
  neurotic 306.4
  psychogenic 306.4
Gastrostaxis 578.0
Gastrostenosis 537.89
Gastrostomy
  attention to V55.1
  complication 536.40
    specified type 536.49
  infection 536.41
  malfunctioning 536.42
  status V44.1
Gastrosuccorrhea (continuous)
  (intermittent) 536.8
  neurotic 306.4
  psychogenic 306.4
Gaucher's
  disease (adult) (cerebroside lipidosis)
    (infantile) 272.7
  hepatomegaly 272.7
  splenomegaly (cerebroside lipidosis)
    272.7
GAVE (gastric antral vascular ectasia)
  537.82
  with hemorrhage 537.83
  without hemorrhage 537.82

◄ New   ◄▥ Revised   ~~deleted~~ Deleted   ● Use Additional Digit(s)   ▓ Omit code

Gayet's disease (superior hemorrhagic polioencephalitis) 265.1
Gayet-Wernicke's syndrome (superior hemorrhagic polioencephalitis) 265.1
Gee (-Herter) (-Heubner) (-Thaysen) disease or syndrome (nontropical sprue) 579.0
Gélineau's syndrome (see also Narcolepsy) 347.00
Gemination, teeth 520.2
Gemistocytoma (M9411/3)
    specified site - see Neoplasm, by site, malignant
    unspecified site 191.9
General, generalized - see condition
Genetic
    susceptibility to
        MEN (multiple endocrine neoplasia) V84.81
        neoplasia
            multiple endocrine (MEN) V84.81 ◀▥
        neoplasm
            malignant, of
                breast V84.01
                endometrium V84.04
                other V84.09
                ovary V84.02
                prostate V84.03
        specified disease NEC V84.89
Genital - see condition
    warts 078.11
Genito-anorectal syndrome 099.1
Genitourinary system - see condition
Genu
    congenital 755.64
    extrorsum (acquired) 736.42
        congenital 755.64
        late effects of rickets 268.1
    introrsum (acquired) 736.41
        congenital 755.64
        late effects of rickets 268.1
    rachitic (old) 268.1
    recurvatum (acquired) 736.5
        congenital 754.40
            with dislocation of knee 754.41
        late effects of rickets 268.1
    valgum (acquired) (knock-knee) 736.41
        congenital 755.64
        late effects of rickets 268.1
    varum (acquired) (bowleg) 736.42
        congenital 755.64
        late effect of rickets 268.1
Geographic tongue 529.1
Geophagia 307.52
Geotrichosis 117.9
    intestine 117.9
    lung 117.9
    mouth 117.9
Gephyrophobia 300.29
Gerbode defect 745.4
GERD (gastroesophageal reflux disease) 530.81
Gerhardt's
    disease (erythromelalgia) 443.82
    syndrome (vocal cord paralysis) 478.30
Gerlier's disease (epidemic vertigo) 078.81
German measles 056.9
    exposure to V01.4
Germinoblastoma (diffuse) (M9614/3) 202.8●
    follicular (M9692/3) 202.0●
Germinoma (M9064/3) - see Neoplasm, by site, malignant
Gerontoxon 371.41

Gerstmann-Sträussler-Scheinker syndrome (GSS) 046.71
Gerstmann's syndrome (finger agnosia) 784.69
Gestation (period) - see also Pregnancy
    ectopic NEC (see also Pregnancy, ectopic) 633.90
        with intrauterine pregnancy 633.91
    multiple ◀
        placenta status ◀
            quadruplet ◀
                two or more monoamniotic fetuses V91.22 ◀
                two or more monochorionic fetuses V91.21 ◀
                unable to determine number of placenta and number of amniotic sacs V91.29 ◀
                unspecified number of placenta and unspecified number of amniotic sacs V91.20 ◀
            specified (greater than quadruplets) NEC ◀
                two or more monoamniotic fetuses V91.92 ◀
                two or more monochorionic fetuses V91.91 ◀
                unable to determine number of placenta and number of amniotic sacs V91.99 ◀
                unspecified number of placenta and unspecified number of amniotic sacs V91.90 ◀
            triplet ◀
                two or more monoamniotic fetuses V91.12 ◀
                two or more monochorionic fetuses V91.11 ◀
                unable to determine number of placenta and number of amniotic sacs V91.19 ◀
                unspecified number of placenta, unspecified number of amniotic sacs V91.10 ◀
            twin ◀
                dichorionic/diamniotic (two placentae, two amniotic sacs) V91.03 ◀
                monochorionic/diamniotic (one placenta, two amniotic sacs) V91.02 ◀
                monochorionic/monoamniotic (one placenta, one amniotic sac) V91.01 ◀
                unable to determine number of placenta and number of amniotic sacs V91.09 ◀
                unspecified number of placenta, unspecified number of amniotic sacs V91.00 ◀
Gestational proteinuria 646.2●
    with hypertension - see Toxemia, of pregnancy
Ghon tubercle primary infection (see also Tuberculosis) 010.0●
Ghost
    teeth 520.4
    vessels, cornea 370.64

Ghoul hand 102.3
Gianotti Crosti syndrome 057.8
    due to known virus - see Infection, virus
    due to unknown virus 057.8
Giant
    cell
        epulis 523.8
        peripheral (gingiva) 523.8
        tumor, tendon sheath 727.02
    colon (congenital) 751.3
    esophagus (congenital) 750.4
    kidney 753.3
    urticaria 995.1
        hereditary 277.6
Giardia lamblia infestation 007.1
Giardiasis 007.1
Gibert's disease (pityriasis rosea) 696.3
Gibraltar fever - see Brucellosis
Giddiness 780.4
    hysterical 300.11
    psychogenic 306.9
Gierke's disease (glycogenosis I) 271.0
Gigantism (cerebral) (hypophyseal) (pituitary) 253.0
Gilbert's disease or cholemia (familial nonhemolytic jaundice) 277.4
Gilchrist's disease (North American blastomycosis) 116.0
Gilford (-Hutchinson) disease or syndrome (progeria) 259.8
Gilles de la Tourette's disease (motor-verbal tic) 307.23
Gillespie's syndrome (dysplasia oculodentodigitalis) 759.89
Gingivitis 523.10
    acute 523.00
        necrotizing 101
        non-plaque induced 523.01
        plaque induced 523.00
    catarrhal 523.00
    chronic 523.10
        non-plaque induced 523.11
    desquamative 523.10
    expulsiva 523.40
    hyperplastic 523.10
    marginal, simple 523.10
    necrotizing, acute 101
    non-plaque induced 523.11
    pellagrous 265.2
    plaque induced 523.10
    ulcerative 523.10
        acute necrotizing 101
    Vincent's 101
Gingivoglossitis 529.0
Gingivopericementitis 523.40
Gingivosis 523.10
Gingivostomatitis 523.10
    herpetic 054.2
Giovannini's disease 117.9
GISA (glycopeptide intermediate staphylococcus aureus) V09.8
Gland, glandular - see condition
Glanders 024
Glanzmann (-Naegeli) disease or thrombasthenia 287.1
Glassblowers' disease 527.1
Glaucoma (capsular) (inflammatory) (noninflammatory) (primary) 365.9
    with increased episcleral venous pressure 365.82
    absolute 360.42
    acute 365.22
        narrow angle 365.22
        secondary 365.60

◀ New ◀▥ Revised ~~deleted~~ Deleted ● Use Additional Digit(s) ▨ Omit code

Glomerulonephritis (Continued)
due to or associated with
amyloidosis 277.39 [583.81]
with nephrotic syndrome 277.39 [581.81]
chronic 277.39 [582.81]
diabetes mellitus 250.4 ● [583.81]
due to secondary diabetes 249.4 ● [581.81]
with nephrotic syndrome 250.4 ● [581.81]
due to secondary diabetes 249.4 ● [581.81]
diphtheria 032.89 [580.81]
gonococcal infection (acute) 098.19 [583.81]
chronic or duration of 2 months or over 098.39 [583.81]
infectious hepatitis 070.9 [580.81]
malaria (with nephrotic syndrome) 084.9 [581.81]
mumps 072.79 [580.81]
polyarteritis (nodosa) (with nephrotic syndrome) 446.0 [581.81]
specified pathology NEC 583.89
acute 580.89
chronic 582.89
streptotrichosis 039.8 [583.81]
subacute bacterial endocarditis 421.0 [580.81]
syphilis (late) 095.4
congenital 090.5 [583.81]
early 091.69 [583.81]
systemic lupus erythematosus 710.0 [583.81]
with nephrotic syndrome 710.0 [581.81]
chronic 710.0 [582.81]
tuberculosis (see also Tuberculosis) 016.0 ● [583.81]
typhoid fever 002.0 [580.81]
extracapillary with epithelial crescents 583.4
acute 580.4
chronic 582.4
exudative 583.89
acute 580.89
chronic 582.89
focal (see also Nephritis) 583.9
embolic 580.4
granular 582.89
granulomatous 582.89
hydremic (see also Nephrosis) 581.9
hypocomplementemic persistent 583.2
with nephrotic syndrome 581.2
chronic 582.2
immune complex NEC 583.89
infective (see also Pyelitis) 590.80
interstitial (diffuse) (focal) 583.89
with nephrotic syndrome 581.89
acute 580.89
chronic 582.89
latent or quiescent 582.9
lobular 583.2
with nephrotic syndrome 581.2
chronic 582.2
membranoproliferative 583.2
with nephrotic syndrome 581.2
chronic 582.2
membranous 583.1
with nephrotic syndrome 581.1
and proliferative (mixed) 583.2
with nephrotic syndrome 581.2
chronic 582.2
chronic 582.1
sclerosing 582.1
with nephrotic syndrome 581.1

Glomerulonephritis (Continued)
mesangiocapillary 583.2
with nephrotic syndrome 581.2
chronic 582.2
minimal change 581.3
mixed membranous and proliferative 583.2
with nephrotic syndrome 581.2
chronic 582.2
necrotizing 583.4
acute 580.4
chronic 582.4
nephrotic (see also Nephrosis) 581.9
old - see Glomerulonephritis, chronic
parenchymatous 581.89
poststreptococcal 580.0
proliferative (diffuse) 583.0
with nephrotic syndrome 581.0
acute 580.0
chronic 582.0
purulent (see also Pyelitis) 590.80
quiescent - see Nephritis, chronic
rapidly progressive 583.4
acute 580.4
chronic 582.4
sclerosing membranous (chronic) 582.1
with nephrotic syndrome 581.1
septic (see also Pyelitis) 590.80
specified pathology or lesion NEC 583.89
with nephrotic syndrome 581.89
acute 580.89
chronic 582.89
suppurative (acute) (disseminated) (see also Pyelitis) 590.80
toxic - see Nephritis, acute
tubal, tubular - see Nephrosis, tubular
type II (Ellis) - see Nephrosis
vascular - see Hypertension, kidney
Glomerulosclerosis (see also Sclerosis, renal) 587
focal 582.1
with nephrotic syndrome 581.1
intercapillary (nodular) (with diabetes) 250.4 ● [581.81]
due to secondary diabetes 249.4 ● [581.81]
Glossagra 529.6
Glossalgia 529.6
Glossitis 529.0
areata exfoliativa 529.1
atrophic 529.4
benign migratory 529.1
gangrenous 529.0
Hunter's 529.4
median rhomboid 529.2
Moeller's 529.4
pellagrous 265.2
Glossocele 529.8
Glossodynia 529.6
exfoliativa 529.4
Glossoncus 529.8
Glossophytia 529.3
Glossoplegia 529.8
Glossoptosis 529.8
Glossopyrosis 529.6
Glossotrichia 529.3
Glossy skin 701.9
Glottis - see condition
Glottitis - see Glossitis
Glucagonoma (M8152/0)
malignant (M8152/3)
pancreas 157.4
specified site NEC - see Neoplasm, by site, malignant
unspecified site 157.4
pancreas 211.7

Glucagonoma (Continued)
specified site NEC - see Neoplasm, by site, benign
unspecified site 211.7
Glucoglycinuria 270.7
Glue ear syndrome 381.20
Glue sniffing (airplane glue) (see also Dependence) 304.6 ●
Glycinemia (with methylmalonic acidemia) 270.7
Glycinuria (renal) (with ketosis) 270.0
Glycogen
infiltration (see also Disease, glycogen storage) 271.0
storage disease (see also Disease, glycogen storage) 271.0
Glycogenosis (see also Disease, glycogen storage) 271.0
cardiac 271.0 [425.7]
Cori, types I-VII 271.0
diabetic, secondary 250.8 ● [259.8]
due to secondary diabetes 249.8 ● [259.8]
diffuse (with hepatic cirrhosis) 271.0
generalized 271.0
glucose-6-phosphatase deficiency 271.0
hepatophosphorylase deficiency 271.0
hepatorenal 271.0
myophosphorylase deficiency 271.0
Glycopenia 251.2
Glycopeptide
intermediate staphylococcus aureus (GISA) V09.8
resistant
enterococcus V09.8
staphylococcus aureus (GRSA) V09.8
Glycoprolinuria 270.8
Glycosuria 791.5
renal 271.4
Gnathostoma (spinigerum) (infection) (infestation) 128.1
wandering swellings from 128.1
Gnathostomiasis 128.1
Goiter (adolescent) (colloid) (diffuse) (dipping) (due to iodine deficiency) (endemic) (euthyroid) (heart) (hyperplastic) (internal) (intrathoracic) (juvenile) (mixed type) (nonendemic) (parenchymatous) (plunging) (sporadic) (subclavicular) (substernal) 240.9
with
hyperthyroidism (recurrent) (see also Goiter, toxic) 242.0 ●
thyrotoxicosis (see also Goiter, toxic) 242.0 ●
adenomatous (see also Goiter, nodular) 241.9
cancerous (M8000/3) 193
complicating pregnancy, childbirth, or puerperium 648.1 ●
congenital 246.1
cystic (see also Goiter, nodular) 241.9
due to enzyme defect in synthesis of thyroid hormone (butane-insoluble iodine) (coupling) (deiodinase) (iodide trapping or organification) (iodotyrosine dehalogenase) (peroxidase) 246.1
dyshormonogenic 246.1
exophthalmic (see also Goiter, toxic) 242.0 ●
familial (with deaf-mutism) 243
fibrous 245.3
lingual 759.2
lymphadenoid 245.2

Goiter (*Continued*)
  malignant (M8000/3) 193
  multinodular (nontoxic) 241.1
    toxic or with hyperthyroidism (*see also* Goiter, toxic) 242.2●
  nodular (nontoxic) 241.9
    with
      hyperthyroidism (*see also* Goiter, toxic) 242.3●
      thyrotoxicosis (*see also* Goiter, toxic) 242.3●
    endemic 241.9
    exophthalmic (diffuse) (*see also* Goiter, toxic) 242.0●
    multinodular (nontoxic) 241.1
    sporadic 241.9
    toxic (*see also* Goiter, toxic) 242.3●
    uninodular (nontoxic) 241.0
  nontoxic (nodular) 241.9
    multinodular 241.1
    uninodular 241.0
  pulsating (*see also* Goiter, toxic) 242.0●
  simple 240.0
  toxic 242.0●

> Note: Use the following fifth-digit subclassification with category 242:
>
> 0   without mention of thyrotoxic crisis or storm
> 1   with mention of thyrotoxic crisis or storm

    adenomatous 242.3●
      multinodular 242.2●
      uninodular 242.1●
    multinodular 242.2●
    nodular 242.3●
      multinodular 242.2●
      uninodular 242.1●
    uninodular 242.1●
  uninodular (nontoxic) 241.0
    toxic or with hyperthyroidism (*see also* Goiter, toxic) 242.1●
Goldberg (-Maxwell) (-Morris) syndrome (testicular feminization) 259.51
Goldblatt's
  hypertension 440.1
  kidney 440.1
Goldenhar's syndrome (oculoauriculovertebral dysplasia) 756.0
Goldflam-Erb disease or syndrome 358.00
Goldscheider's disease (epidermolysis bullosa) 757.39
Goldstein's disease (familial hemorrhagic telangiectasia) 448.0
Golfer's elbow 726.32
Goltz-Gorlin syndrome (dermal hypoplasia) 757.39
Gonadoblastoma (M9073/1)
  specified site - *see* Neoplasm, by site uncertain behavior
  unspecified site
    female 236.2
    male 236.4
Gonecystitis (*see also* Vesiculitis) 608.0
Gongylonemiasis 125.6
  mouth 125.6
Goniosynechiae 364.73
Gonococcemia 098.89
Gonococcus, gonococcal (disease) (infection) (*see also* condition) 098.0
  anus 098.7
  bursa 098.52

Gonococcus, gonococcal (*Continued*)
  chronic NEC 098.2
  complicating pregnancy, childbirth, or puerperium 647.1●
    affecting fetus or newborn 760.2
  conjunctiva, conjunctivitis (neonatorum) 098.40
  dermatosis 098.89
  endocardium 098.84
  epididymo-orchitis 098.13
    chronic or duration of 2 months or over 098.33
  eye (newborn) 098.40
  fallopian tube (chronic) 098.37
    acute 098.17
  genitourinary (acute) (organ) (system) (tract) (*see also* Gonorrhea) 098.0
    lower 098.0
      chronic 098.2
    upper 098.10
      chronic 098.30
  heart NEC 098.85
  joint 098.50
  keratoderma 098.81
  keratosis (blennorrhagica) 098.81
  lymphatic (gland) (node) 098.89
  meninges 098.82
  orchitis (acute) 098.13
    chronic or duration of 2 months or over 098.33
  pelvis (acute) 098.19
    chronic or duration of 2 months or over 098.39
  pericarditis 098.83
  peritonitis 098.86
  pharyngitis 098.6
  pharynx 098.6
  proctitis 098.7
  pyosalpinx (chronic) 098.37
    acute 098.17
  rectum 098.7
  septicemia 098.89
  skin 098.89
  specified site NEC 098.89
  synovitis 098.51
  tendon sheath 098.51
  throat 098.6
  urethra (acute) 098.0
    chronic or duration of 2 months or over 098.2
  vulva (acute) 098.0
    chronic or duration of 2 months or over 098.2
Gonocytoma (M9073/1)
  specified site - *see* Neoplasm, by site, uncertain behavior
  unspecified site
    female 236.2
    male 236.4
Gonorrhea 098.0
  acute 098.0
  Bartholin's gland (acute) 098.0
    chronic or duration of 2 months or over 098.2
  bladder (acute) 098.11
    chronic or duration of 2 months or over 098.31
  carrier (suspected of) V02.7
  cervix (acute) 098.15
    chronic or duration of 2 months or over 098.35
  chronic 098.2
  complicating pregnancy, childbirth, or puerperium 647.1●
    affecting fetus or newborn 760.2

Gonorrhea (*Continued*)
  conjunctiva, conjunctivitis (neonatorum) 098.40
  contact V01.6
  Cowper's gland (acute) 098.0
    chronic or duration of 2 months or over 098.2
  duration of 2 months or over 098.2
  exposure to V01.6
  fallopian tube (chronic) 098.37
    acute 098.17
  genitourinary (acute) (organ) (system) (tract) 098.0
    chronic 098.2
    duration of 2 months or over 098.2
  kidney (acute) 098.19
    chronic or duration of 2 months or over 098.39
  ovary (acute) 098.19
    chronic or duration of 2 months or over 098.39
  pelvis (acute) 098.19
    chronic or duration of 2 months or over 098.39
  penis (acute) 098.0
    chronic or duration of 2 months or over 098.2
  prostate (acute) 098.12
    chronic or duration of 2 months or over 098.32
  seminal vesicle (acute) 098.14
    chronic or duration of 2 months or over 098.34
  specified site NEC - *see* Gonococcus
  spermatic cord (acute) 098.14
    chronic or duration of 2 months or over 098.34
  urethra (acute) 098.0
    chronic or duration of 2 months or over 098.2
  vagina (acute) 098.0
    chronic or duration of 2 months or over 098.2
  vas deferens (acute) 098.14
    chronic or duration of 2 months or over 098.34
  vulva (acute) 098.0
    chronic or duration of 2 months or over 098.2
Goodpasture's syndrome (pneumorenal) 446.21
Good's syndrome 279.06
Gopalan's syndrome (burning feet) 266.2
Gordon's disease (exudative enteropathy) 579.8
Gorlin-Chaudhry-Moss syndrome 759.89
Gougerot's syndrome (trisymptomatic) 709.1
Gougerot-Blum syndrome (pigmented purpuric lichenoid dermatitis) 709.1
Gougerot-Carteaud disease or syndrome (confluent reticulate papillomatosis) 701.8
Gougerot-Hailey-Hailey disease (benign familial chronic pemphigus) 757.39
Gougerot (-Houwer)-Sjögren syndrome (keratoconjunctivitis sicca) 710.2
Gouley's syndrome (constrictive pericarditis) 423.2
Goundou 102.6
Gout, gouty 274.9
  with
    specified manifestations NEC 274.89
    tophi (tophus) 274.03

Gout, gouty *(Continued)*
  acute 274.01
  arthritis 274.00
    acute 274.01
  arthropathy 274.00
    acute 274.01
    chronic (without mention of tophus (tophi)) 274.02
      with tophus (tophi) 274.03
  attack 274.01
  chronic 274.02
    tophaceous 274.03
  degeneration, heart 274.82
  diathesis 274.9
  eczema 274.89
  episcleritis 274.89 *[379.09]*
  external ear (tophus) 274.81
  flare 274.01
  glomerulonephritis 274.10
  iritis 274.89 *[364.11]*
  joint 274.00
  kidney 274.10
  lead 984.9
    specified type of lead - *see* Table of Drugs and Chemicals
  nephritis 274.10
  neuritis 274.89 *[357.4]*
  phlebitis 274.89 *[451.9]*
  rheumatic 714.0
  saturnine 984.9
    specified type of lead - *see* Table of Drugs and Chemicals
  spondylitis 274.00
  synovitis 274.00
  syphilitic 095.8
  tophi 274.03
    ear 274.81
    heart 274.82
    specified site NEC 274.82
Gowers'
  muscular dystrophy 359.1
  syndrome (vasovagal attack) 780.2
Gowers-Paton-Kennedy syndrome 377.04
Gradenigo's syndrome 383.02
Graft-versus-host disease 279.50
  due to organ transplant NEC - *see* Complications, transplant, organ
Graham Steell's murmur (pulmonic regurgitation) (*see also* Endocarditis, pulmonary) 424.3
Grain-handlers' disease or lung 495.8
Grain mite (itch) 133.8
Grand
  mal (idiopathic) (*see also* Epilepsy) 345.1●
    hysteria of Charcôt 300.11
    nonrecurrent or isolated 780.39
  multipara
    affecting management of labor and delivery 659.4●
    status only (not pregnant) V61.5
Granite workers' lung 502
Granular - *see also* condition
  inflammation, pharynx 472.1
  kidney (contracting) (*see also* Sclerosis, renal) 587
  liver - *see* Cirrhosis, liver
  nephritis - *see* Nephritis
Granulation tissue, abnormal - *see also* Granuloma
  abnormal or excessive 701.5
  postmastoidectomy cavity 383.33
  postoperative 701.5
  skin 701.5

Granulocytopenia, granulocytopenic (primary) 288.00
  malignant 288.09
Granuloma NEC 686.1
  abdomen (wall) 568.89
    skin (pyogenicum) 686.1
      from residual foreign body 709.4
  annulare 695.89
  anus 569.49
  apical 522.6
  appendix 543.9
  aural 380.23
  beryllium (skin) 709.4
    lung 503
  bone (*see also* Osteomyelitis) 730.1●
    eosinophilic 277.89
    from residual foreign body 733.99
  canaliculus lacrimalis 375.81
  cerebral 348.89
  cholesterin, middle ear 385.82
  coccidioidal (progressive) 114.3
    lung 114.4
    meninges 114.2
    primary (lung) 114.0
  colon 569.89
  conjunctiva 372.61
  dental 522.6
  ear, middle (cholesterin) 385.82
    with otitis media - *see* Otitis media
  eosinophilic 277.89
    bone 277.89
    lung 277.89
    oral mucosa 528.9
  exuberant 701.5
  eyelid 374.89
  facial
    lethal midline 446.3
    malignant 446.3
  faciale 701.8
  fissuratum (gum) 523.8
  foot NEC 686.1
  foreign body (in soft tissue) NEC 728.82
    bone 733.99
    in operative wound 998.4
    muscle 728.82
    skin 709.4
    subcutaneous tissue 709.4
  fungoides 202.1●
  gangraenescens 446.3
  giant cell (central) (jaw) (reparative) 526.3
    gingiva 523.8
    peripheral (gingiva) 523.8
  gland (lymph) 289.3
  Hodgkin's (M9661/3) 201.1●
  ileum 569.89
  infectious NEC 136.9
  inguinale (Donovan) 099.2
    venereal 099.2
  intestine 569.89
  iridocyclitis 364.10
  iris 364.10
  jaw (bone) 526.3
    reparative giant cell 526.3
  kidney (*see also* Infection, kidney) 590.9
  lacrimal sac 375.81
  larynx 478.79
  lethal midline 446.3
  lipid 277.89
  lipoid 277.89
  liver 572.8
  lung (infectious) (*see also* Fibrosis, lung) 515
    coccidioidal 114.4
    eosinophilic 277.89

Granuloma NEC *(Continued)*
  lymph gland 289.3
  Majocchi's 110.6
  malignant, face 446.3
  mandible 526.3
  mediastinum 519.3
  midline 446.3
  monilial 112.3
  muscle 728.82
    from residual foreign body 728.82
  nasal sinus (*see also* Sinusitis) 473.9
  operation wound 998.59
    foreign body 998.4
    stitch (external) 998.89
      internal wound 998.89
    talc 998.7
  oral mucosa, eosinophilic or pyogenic 528.9
  orbit, orbital 376.11
  paracoccidioidal 116.1
  penis, venereal 099.2
  periapical 522.6
  peritoneum 568.89
    due to ova of helminths NEC (*see also* Helminthiasis) 128.9
  postmastoidectomy cavity 383.33
  postoperative - *see* Granuloma, operation wound
  prostate 601.8
  pudendi (ulcerating) 099.2
  pudendorum (ulcerative) 099.2
  pulp, internal (tooth) 521.49
  pyogenic, pyogenicum (skin) 686.1
    maxillary alveolar ridge 522.6
    oral mucosa 528.9
  rectum 569.49
  reticulohistiocytic 277.89
  rubrum nasi 705.89
  sarcoid 135
  Schistosoma 120.9
  septic (skin) 686.1
  silica (skin) 709.4
  sinus (accessory) (infectional) (nasal) (*see also* Sinusitis) 473.9
  skin (pyogenicum) 686.1
    from foreign body or material 709.4
  sperm 608.89
  spine
    syphilitic (epidural) 094.89
    tuberculous (*see also* Tuberculosis) 015.0● *[730.88]*
  stitch (postoperative) 998.89
    internal wound 998.89
  suppurative (skin) 686.1
  suture (postoperative) 998.89
    internal wound 998.89
  swimming pool 031.1
  talc 728.82
    in operation wound 998.7
  telangiectaticum (skin) 686.1
  tracheostomy 519.09
  trichophyticum 110.6
  tropicum 102.4
  umbilicus 686.1
    newborn 771.4
  urethra 599.84
  uveitis 364.10
  vagina 099.2
  venereum 099.2
  vocal cords 478.5
  Wegener's (necrotizing respiratory granulomatosis) 446.4

Granulomatosis NEC 686.1
  disciformis chronica et progressiva 709.3
  infantiseptica 771.2
  lipoid 277.89
  lipophagic, intestinal 040.2
  miliary 027.0
  necrotizing, respiratory 446.4
  progressive, septic 288.1
  Wegener's (necrotizing respiratory)
    446.4
Granulomatous tissue - *see* Granuloma
Granulosis rubra nasi 705.89
Graphite fibrosis (of lung) 503
Graphospasm 300.89
  organic 333.84
Grating scapula 733.99
Gravel (urinary) (*see also* Calculus) 592.9
Graves' disease (exophthalmic goiter) (*see also* Goiter, toxic) 242.0●
Gravis - *see* condition
Grawitz's tumor (hypernephroma)
  (M8312/3) 189.0
Grayness, hair (premature) 704.3
  congenital 757.4
Gray or grey syndrome
    (chloramphenicol) (newborn)
    779.4
Greenfield's disease 330.0
Green sickness 280.9
Greenstick fracture - *see* Fracture,
  by site
Greig's syndrome (hypertelorism) 756.0
Grief 309.0
Griesinger's disease (*see also*
  Ancylostomiasis) 126.9
Grinders'
  asthma 502
  lung 502
  phthisis (*see also* Tuberculosis) 011.4●
Grinding, teeth 306.8
Grip
  Dabney's 074.1
  devil's 074.1
Grippe, grippal - *see also* Influenza
  Balkan 083.0
  intestinal (*see also* Influenza) 487.8 ◀▥
  summer 074.8
Grippy cold (*see also* Influenza) 487.1 ◀▥
Grisel's disease 723.5
Groin - *see* condition
Grooved
  nails (transverse) 703.8
  tongue 529.5
    congenital 750.13
Ground itch 126.9
Growing pains, children 781.99

Growth (fungoid) (neoplastic) (new)
  (M8000/1) - *see also* Neoplasm, by
  site, unspecified nature
  adenoid (vegetative) 474.12
  benign (M8000/0) - *see* Neoplasm, by
    site, benign
  fetal, poor 764.9●
    affecting management of pregnancy
      656.5●
  malignant (M8000/3) - *see* Neoplasm,
    by site, malignant
  rapid, childhood V21.0
  secondary (M8000/6) - *see* Neoplasm,
    by site, malignant, secondary
GRSA (glycopeptide resistant
  staphylococcus aureus) V09.8
Gruber's hernia - *see* Hernia, Gruber's
Gruby's disease (tinea tonsurans) 110.0
GSS (Gerstmann-Sträussler-Scheinker
  syndrome) 046.71
G-trisomy 758.0
Guama fever 066.3
Gubler (-Millard) paralysis or syndrome
  344.89
Guérin-Stern syndrome (arthrogryposis
  multiplex congenita) 754.89
Guertin's disease (electric chorea) 049.8
Guillain-Barré disease or syndrome 357.0
Guinea worms (infection) (infestation)
  125.7
Guinon's disease (motor-verbal tic)
  307.23
Gull's disease (thyroid atrophy with
  myxedema) 244.8
Gull and Sutton's disease - *see*
  Hypertension, kidney
Gum - *see* condition
Gumboil 522.7
Gumma (syphilitic) 095.9
  artery 093.89
    cerebral or spinal 094.89
  bone 095.5
    of yaws (late) 102.6
  brain 094.89
  cauda equina 094.89
  central nervous system NEC 094.9
  ciliary body 095.8 [364.11]
  congenital 090.5
    testis 090.5
  eyelid 095.8 [373.5]
  heart 093.89
  intracranial 094.89
  iris 095.8 [364.11]
  kidney 095.4
  larynx 095.8
  leptomeninges 094.2

Gumma (*Continued*)
  liver 095.3
  meninges 094.2
  myocardium 093.82
  nasopharynx 095.8
  neurosyphilitic 094.9
  nose 095.8
  orbit 095.8
  palate (soft) 095.8
  penis 095.8
  pericardium 093.81
  pharynx 095.8
  pituitary 095.8
  scrofulous (*see also* Tuberculosis) 017.0●
  skin 095.8
  specified site NEC 095.8
  spinal cord 094.89
  tongue 095.8
  tonsil 095.8
  trachea 095.8
  tuberculous (*see also* Tuberculosis)
    017.0●
  ulcerative due to yaws 102.4
  ureter 095.8
  yaws 102.4
    bone 102.6
Gunn's syndrome (jaw-winking
  syndrome) 742.8
Gunshot wound - *see also* Wound, open,
  by site
  fracture - *see* Fracture, by site, open
  internal organs (abdomen, chest, or
    pelvis) - *see* Injury, internal, by
    site, with open wound
  intracranial - *see* Laceration, brain,
    with open intracranial wound
Günther's disease or syndrome
  (congenital erythropoietic
  porphyria) 277.1
Gustatory hallucination 780.1
Gynandrism 752.7
Gynandroblastoma (M8632/1)
  specified site - *see* Neoplasm, by site,
    uncertain behavior
  unspecified site
    female 236.2
    male 236.4
Gynandromorphism 752.7
Gynatresia (congenital) 752.49
Gynecoid pelvis, male 738.6
Gynecological examination V72.31
  for contraceptive maintenance
    V25.40
Gynecomastia 611.1
Gynephobia 300.29
Gyrate scalp 757.39

H

Haas' disease (osteochondrosis head of humerus) 732.3
Habermann's disease (acute parapsoriasis varioliformis) 696.2
Habit, habituation
  chorea 307.22
  disturbance, child 307.9
  drug (*see also* Dependence) 304.9 ●
  laxative (*see also* Abuse, drugs, nondependent) 305.9 ●
  spasm 307.20
    chronic 307.22
    transient (of childhood) 307.21
  tic 307.20
    chronic 307.22
    transient (of childhood) 307.21
  use of
    nonprescribed drugs (*see also* Abuse, drugs, nondependent) 305.9 ●
    patent medicines (*see also* Abuse, drugs, nondependent) 305.9 ●
  vomiting 536.2
Hadfield-Clarke syndrome (pancreatic infantilism) 577.8
Haff disease 985.1
Hag teeth, tooth 524.39
Hageman factor defect, deficiency, or disease (*see also* Defect, coagulation) 286.3
Haglund's disease (osteochondrosis os tibiale externum) 732.5
Haglund-Läwen-Fründ syndrome 717.89
Hagner's disease (hypertrophic pulmonary osteoarthropathy) 731.2
Hailey-Hailey disease (benign familial chronic pemphigus) 757.39
Hair - *see also* condition
  plucking 307.9
Hairball in stomach 935.2
Hairy black tongue 529.3
Half vertebra 756.14
Halitosis 784.99
Hallermann-Streiff syndrome 756.0
Hallervorden-Spatz disease or syndrome 333.0
Hallopeau's
  acrodermatitis (continua) 696.1
  disease (lichen sclerosis et atrophicus) 701.0
Hallucination (auditory) (gustatory) (olfactory) (tactile) 780.1
  alcohol-induced 291.3
  drug-induced 292.12
  visual 368.16
Hallucinosis 298.9
  alcohol-induced (acute) 291.3
  drug-induced 292.12
Hallus - *see* Hallux
Hallux 735.9
  limitus 735.8
  malleus (acquired) 735.3
  rigidus (acquired) 735.2
    congenital 755.66
    late effects of rickets 268.1
  valgus (acquired) 735.0
    congenital 755.66
  varus (acquired) 735.1
    congenital 755.66
Halo, visual 368.15
Hamartoblastoma 759.6

Hamartoma 759.6
  epithelial (gingival), odontogenic, central, or peripheral (M9321/0) 213.1
    upper jaw (bone) 213.0
  vascular 757.32
Hamartosis, hamartoses NEC 759.6
Hamman's disease or syndrome (spontaneous mediastinal emphysema) 518.1
Hamman-Rich syndrome (diffuse interstitial pulmonary fibrosis) 516.3
Hammer toe (acquired) 735.4
  congenital 755.66
  late effects of rickets 268.1
Hand - *see* condition
Hand-Schüller-Christian disease or syndrome (chronic histiocytosis x) 277.89
Hand-foot syndrome 693.0
Hanging (asphyxia) (strangulation) (suffocation) 994.7
Hangnail (finger) (with lymphangitis) 681.02
Hangover (alcohol) (*see also* Abuse, drugs, nondependent) 305.0 ●
Hanot's cirrhosis or disease - *see* Cirrhosis, biliary
Hanot-Chauffard (-Troisier) syndrome (bronze diabetes) 275.01 ◀▥
Hansen's disease (leprosy) 030.9
  benign form 030.1
  malignant form 030.0
Harada's disease or syndrome 363.22
Hard chancre 091.0
Hard firm prostate 600.10
  with
    urinary
      obstruction 600.11
      retention 600.11
Hardening
  artery - *see* Arteriosclerosis
  brain 348.89
  liver 571.8
Hare's syndrome (M8010/3) (carcinoma, pulmonary apex) 162.3
Harelip (*see also* Cleft, lip) 749.10
Harkavy's syndrome 446.0
Harlequin (fetus) 757.1
  color change syndrome 779.89
Harley's disease (intermittent hemoglobinuria) 283.2
Harris'
  lines 733.91
  syndrome (organic hyperinsulinism) 251.1
Hart's disease or syndrome (pellagra-cerebellar ataxia-renal aminoaciduria) 270.0
Hartmann's pouch (abnormal sacculation of gallbladder neck) 575.8
  of intestine V44.3
    attention to V55.3
Hartnup disease (pellagra-cerebellar ataxia-renal aminoaciduria) 270.0
Harvester lung 495.0
Hashimoto's disease or struma (struma lymphomatosa) 245.2
Hassall-Henle bodies (corneal warts) 371.41
Haut mal (*see also* Epilepsy) 345.1 ●
Haverhill fever 026.1
Hawaiian wood rose dependence 304.5 ●
Hawkins' keloid 701.4

Hay
  asthma (*see also* Asthma) 493.0 ●
  fever (allergic) (with rhinitis) 477.9
    with asthma (bronchial) (*see also* Asthma) 493.0 ●
    allergic, due to grass, pollen, ragweed, or tree 477.0
    conjunctivitis 372.05
    due to
      dander, animal (cat) (dog) 477.2
      dust 477.8
      fowl 477.8
      hair, animal (cat) (dog) 477.2
      pollen 477.0
      specified allergen other than pollen 477.8
Hayem-Faber syndrome (achlorhydric anemia) 280.9
Hayem-Widal syndrome (acquired hemolytic jaundice) 283.9
Haygarth's nodosities 715.04
Hazard-Crile tumor (M8350/3) 193
Hb (abnormal)
  disease - *see* Disease, hemoglobin
  trait - *see* Trait
H disease 270.0
Head - *see also* condition
  banging 307.3
Headache 784.0
  allergic 339.00
  associated with sexual activity 339.82
  cluster 339.00
    chronic 339.02
    episodic 339.01
  daily
    chronic 784.0
    new persistent (NPDH) 339.42
  drug induced 339.3
  due to
    loss, spinal fluid 349.0
    lumbar puncture 349.0
    saddle block 349.0
  emotional 307.81
  histamine 339.00
  hypnic 339.81
  lumbar puncture 349.0
  medication overuse 339.3
  menopausal 627.2
  menstrual 346.4 ●
  migraine 346.9 ●
  nasal septum 784.0
  nonorganic origin 307.81
  orgasmic 339.82
  postspinal 349.0
  post-traumatic 339.20
    acute 339.21
    chronic 339.22
  premenstrual 346.4 ●
  preorgasmic 339.82
  primary
    cough 339.83
    exertional 339.84
    stabbing 339.85
    thunderclap 339.43
  psychogenic 307.81
  psychophysiologic 307.81
  rebound 339.3
  short lasting unilateral neuralgiform with conjunctival injection and tearing (SUNCT) 339.05
  sick 346.9 ●

Headache *(Continued)*
  spinal 349.0
    complicating labor and delivery 668.8●
    postpartum 668.8●
  spinal fluid loss 349.0
  syndrome
    cluster 339.00
    complicated NEC 339.44
    periodic in child or adolescent 346.2●
    specified NEC 339.89
  tension 307.81
    type 339.10
      chronic 339.12
      episodic 339.11
  vascular 784.0
    migraine type 346.9●
  vasomotor 346.9●
Health
  advice V65.4
  audit V70.0
  checkup V70.0
  education V65.4
  hazard *(see also* History of) V15.9
    falling V15.88
    specified cause NEC V15.89
  instruction V65.4
  services provided because (of)
    boarding school residence V60.6
    holiday relief for person providing home care V60.5
    inadequate
      housing V60.1
      resources V60.2
    lack of housing V60.0
    no care available in home V60.4
    person living alone V60.3
    poverty V60.3
    residence in institution V60.6
    specified cause NEC V60.89
    vacation relief for person providing home care V60.5
Healthy
  donor *(see also* Donor) V59.9
  infant or child
    accompanying sick mother V65.0
    receiving care V20.1
  person
    accompanying sick relative V65.0
    admitted for sterilization V25.2
    receiving prophylactic inoculation or vaccination *(see also* Vaccination, prophylactic) V05.9
Hearing
  conservation and treatment V72.12
  examination V72.19
    following failed hearing screening V72.11
Heart - *see* condition
Heartburn 787.1
  psychogenic 306.4
Heat (effects) 992.9
  apoplexy 992.0
  burn - *see also* Burn, by site
    from sun *(see also* Sunburn) 692.71
  collapse 992.1
  cramps 992.2
  dermatitis or eczema 692.89
  edema 992.7
  erythema - *see* Burn, by site
  excessive 992.9
    specified effect NEC 992.8

Heat *(Continued)*
  exhaustion 992.5
    anhydrotic 992.3
    due to
      salt (and water) depletion 992.4
      water depletion 992.3
  fatigue (transient) 992.6
  fever 992.0
  hyperpyrexia 992.0
  prickly 705.1
  prostration - *see* Heat, exhaustion
  pyrexia 992.0
  rash 705.1
  specified effect NEC 992.8
  stroke 992.0
  sunburn *(see also* Sunburn) 692.71
  syncope 992.1
Heavy-chain disease 273.2
Heavy-for-dates (fetus or infant) 766.1
  4500 grams or more 766.0
  exceptionally 766.0
Hebephrenia, hebephrenic (acute) *(see also* Schizophrenia) 295.1●
  dementia (praecox) *(see also* Schizophrenia) 295.1●
  schizophrenia *(see also* Schizophrenia) 295.1●
Heberden's
  disease or nodes 715.04
  syndrome (angina pectoris) 413.9
Hebra's disease
  dermatitis exfoliativa 695.89
  erythema multiforme exudativum 695.19
  pityriasis 695.89
    maculata et circinata 696.3
    rubra 695.89
      pilaris 696.4
  prurigo 698.2
Hebra, nose 040.1
Hedinger's syndrome (malignant carcinoid) 259.2
Heel - *see* condition
Heerfordt's disease or syndrome (uveoparotitis) 135
Hegglin's anomaly or syndrome 288.2
Heidenhain's disease 290.10
  with dementia 290.10
Heilmeyer-Schoner disease (M9842/3) 207.1●
Heine-Medin disease *(see also* Poliomyelitis) 045.9●
Heinz-body anemia, congenital 282.7
Heller's disease or syndrome (infantile psychosis) *(see also* Psychosis, childhood) 299.1●
H.E.L.L.P. 642.5●
Helminthiasis *(see also* Infestation, by specific parasite) 128.9
  Ancylostoma *(see also* Ancylostoma) 126.9
  intestinal 127.9
    mixed types (types classifiable to more than one of the categories 120.0–127.7) 127.8
    specified type 127.7
  mixed types (intestinal) (types classifiable to more than one of the categories 120.0–127.7) 127.8
  Necator americanus 126.1
  specified type NEC 128.8
  Trichinella 124

Heloma 700
Hemangioblastoma (M9161/1) - *see also* Neoplasm, connective tissue, uncertain behavior
  malignant (M9161/3) - *see* Neoplasm, connective tissue, malignant
Hemangioblastomatosis, cerebelloretinal 759.6
Hemangioendothelioma (M9130/1) - *see also* Neoplasm, by site, uncertain behavior
  benign (M9130/0) 228.00
  bone (diffuse) (M9130/3) - *see* Neoplasm, bone, malignant
  malignant (M9130/3) - *see* Neoplasm, connective tissue, malignant
  nervous system (M9130/0) 228.09
Hemangioendotheliosarcoma (M9130/3) - *see* Neoplasm, connective tissue, malignant
Hemangiofibroma (M9160/0) - *see* Neoplasm, by site, benign
Hemangiolipoma (M8861/0) - *see* Lipoma
Hemangioma (M9120/0) 228.00
  arteriovenous (M9123/0) - *see* Hemangioma, by site
  brain 228.02
  capillary (M9131/0) - *see* Hemangioma, by site
  cavernous (M9121/0) - *see* Hemangioma, by site
  central nervous system NEC 228.09
  choroid 228.09
  heart 228.09
  infantile (M9131/0) - *see* Hemangioma, by site
  intra-abdominal structures 228.04
  intracranial structures 228.02
  intramuscular (M9132/0) - *see* Hemangioma, by site
  iris 228.09
  juvenile (M9131/0) - *see* Hemangioma, by site
  malignant (M9120/3) - *see* Neoplasm, connective tissue, malignant
  meninges 228.09
    brain 228.02
    spinal cord 228.09
  peritoneum 228.04
  placenta - *see* Placenta, abnormal
  plexiform (M9131/0) - *see* Hemangioma, by site
  racemose (M9123/0) - *see* Hemangioma, by site
  retina 228.03
  retroperitoneal tissue 228.04
  sclerosing (M8832/0) - *see* Neoplasm, skin, benign
  simplex (M9131/0) - *see* Hemangioma, by site
  skin and subcutaneous tissue 228.01
  specified site NEC 228.09
  spinal cord 228.09
  venous (M9122/0) - *see* Hemangioma, by site
  verrucous keratotic (M9142/0) - *see* Hemangioma, by site
Hemangiomatosis (systemic) 757.32
  involving single site - *see* Hemangioma

◀ New   ◀▥ Revised   ~~deleted~~ Deleted   ● Use Additional Digit(s)   ▨ Omit code

Hemangiopericytoma (M9150/1) - *see also*
　　Neoplasm, connective tissue,
　　uncertain behavior
　　benign (M9150/0) - *see* Neoplasm,
　　　connective tissue, benign
　　malignant (M9150/3) - *see* Neoplasm,
　　　connective tissue, malignant
Hemangiosarcoma (M9120/3) - *see*
　　Neoplasm, connective tissue,
　　malignant
Hemarthrosis (nontraumatic) 719.10
　　ankle 719.17
　　elbow 719.12
　　foot 719.17
　　hand 719.14
　　hip 719.15
　　knee 719.16
　　multiple sites 719.19
　　pelvic region 719.15
　　shoulder (region) 719.11
　　specified site NEC 719.18
　　traumatic - *see* Sprain, by site
　　wrist 719.13
Hematemesis 578.0
　　with ulcer - *see* Ulcer, by site, with
　　　hemorrhage
　　due to S. japonicum 120.2
　　Goldstein's (familial hemorrhagic
　　　telangiectasia) 448.0
　　newborn 772.4
　　　due to swallowed maternal blood
　　　　777.3
Hematidrosis 705.89
Hematinuria (*see also* Hemoglobinuria)
　　791.2
　　malarial 084.8
　　paroxysmal 283.2
Hematite miners' lung 503
Hematobilia 576.8
Hematocele (congenital) (diffuse)
　　(idiopathic) 608.83
　　broad ligament 620.7
　　canal of Nuck 629.0
　　cord, male 608.83
　　fallopian tube 620.8
　　female NEC 629.0
　　ischiorectal 569.89
　　male NEC 608.83
　　ovary 629.0
　　pelvis, pelvic
　　　female 629.0
　　　　with ectopic pregnancy (*see also*
　　　　　Pregnancy, ectopic) 633.90
　　　　　with intrauterine pregnancy
　　　　　　633.91
　　　male 608.83
　　periuterine 629.0
　　retrouterine 629.0
　　scrotum 608.83
　　spermatic cord (diffuse) 608.83
　　testis 608.84
　　traumatic - *see* Injury, internal, pelvis
　　tunica vaginalis 608.83
　　uterine ligament 629.0
　　uterus 621.4
　　vagina 623.6
　　vulva 624.5
Hematocephalus 742.4
Hematochezia (*see also* Melena) 578.1
Hematochyluria (*see also* Infestation,
　　filarial) 125.9
Hematocolpos 626.8
Hematocornea 371.12
Hematogenous - *see* condition

Hematoma (skin surface intact)
　　(traumatic) - *see also* Contusion

> Note: Hematomas are coded
> according to origin and the nature and
> site of the hematoma or the
> accompanying injury. Hematomas of
> unspecified origin are coded as injuries
> of the sites involved, except:
>
> (a) hematomas of genital organs
> 　　which are coded as
> 　　diseases of the organ
> 　　involved unless they
> 　　complicate pregnancy or
> 　　delivery
> (b) hematomas of the eye which are
> 　　coded as diseases of the eye.
>
> For late effect of hematoma classifiable
> to 920–924 *see* Late, effect, contusion.

　　with
　　　crush injury - *see* Crush
　　　fracture - *see* Fracture, by site
　　　injury of internal organs - *see also*
　　　　Injury, internal, by site
　　　　kidney - *see* Hematoma, kidney,
　　　　　traumatic
　　　　liver - *see* Hematoma, liver,
　　　　　traumatic
　　　　spleen - *see* Hematoma, spleen
　　　nerve injury - *see* Injury, nerve
　　　open wound - *see* Wound, open, by
　　　　site
　　　skin surface intact - *see* Contusion
　　abdomen (wall) - *see* Contusion,
　　　abdomen
　　amnion 658.8●
　　aorta, dissecting 441.00
　　　abdominal 441.02
　　　thoracic 441.01
　　　thoracoabdominal 441.03
　　arterial (complicating trauma) 904.9
　　　specified site - *see* Injury, blood
　　　　vessel, by site
　　auricle (ear) 380.31
　　birth injury 767.8
　　　skull 767.19
　　brain (traumatic) 853.0●

> Note: Use the following fifth-digit
> subclassification with categories 851–854:
>
> 0　unspecified state of
> 　　consciousness
> 1　with no loss of consciousness
> 2　with brief [less than one hour]
> 　　loss of consciousness
> 3　with moderate [1–24 hours] loss
> 　　of consciousness
> 4　with prolonged [more than 24
> 　　hours] loss of consciousness
> 　　and return to pre-existing
> 　　conscious level
> 5　with prolonged [more than 24
> 　　hours] loss of
> 　　consciousness, without
> 　　return to pre-existing
> 　　conscious level
>
> Use fifth-digit 5 to designate when a
> patient is unconscious and dies before
> regaining consciousness, regardless of
> the duration of the loss of consciousness
>
> 6　with loss of consciousness of
> 　　unspecified duration
> 9　with concussion, unspecified

Hematoma (Continued)
　　brain (Continued)
　　　with
　　　　cerebral
　　　　　contusion - *see* Contusion,
　　　　　　brain
　　　　　laceration - *see* Laceration,
　　　　　　brain
　　　　open intracranial wound
　　　　　853.1●
　　　　skull fracture - *see* Fracture,
　　　　　skull, by site
　　　extradural or epidural 852.4●
　　　　with open intracranial wound
　　　　　852.5●
　　　　fetus or newborn 767.0
　　　　nontraumatic 432.0
　　　fetus or newborn NEC 767.0
　　　nontraumatic (*see also* Hemorrhage,
　　　　brain) 431
　　　　epidural or extradural 432.0
　　　　newborn NEC 772.8
　　　　subarachnoid, arachnoid, or
　　　　　meningeal (*see also*
　　　　　Hemorrhage, subarachnoid)
　　　　　430
　　　　subdural (*see also* Hemorrhage,
　　　　　subdural) 432.1
　　　subarachnoid, arachnoid, or
　　　　meningeal 852.0●
　　　　with open intracranial wound
　　　　　852.1●
　　　　fetus or newborn 772.2
　　　　nontraumatic (*see also*
　　　　　Hemorrhage,
　　　　　subarachnoid) 430
　　　subdural 852.2●
　　　　with open intracranial wound
　　　　　852.3●
　　　　fetus or newborn (localized)
　　　　　767.0
　　　　nontraumatic (*see also*
　　　　　Hemorrhage, subdural)
　　　　　432.1
　　breast (nontraumatic) 611.89
　　broad ligament (nontraumatic)
　　　620.7
　　　complicating delivery 665.7●
　　　traumatic - *see* Injury, internal,
　　　　broad ligament
　　calcified NEC 959.9
　　capitis 920
　　　due to birth injury 767.19
　　　newborn 767.19
　　cerebral - *see* Hematoma, brain
　　cesarean section wound 674.3●
　　chorion - *see* Placenta, abnormal
　　complicating delivery (perineum)
　　　(vulva) 664.5●
　　　pelvic 665.7●
　　　vagina 665.7●
　　corpus
　　　cavernosum (nontraumatic)
　　　　607.82
　　　luteum (nontraumatic) (ruptured)
　　　　620.1
　　dura (mater) - *see* Hematoma, brain,
　　　subdural
　　epididymis (nontraumatic) 608.83
　　epidural (traumatic) - *see also*
　　　Hematoma, brain, extradural
　　　spinal - *see* Injury, spinal, by site
　　episiotomy 674.3●
　　external ear 380.31

Hematoma (*Continued*)
  extradural - *see also* Hematoma, brain, extradural
    fetus or newborn 767.0
    nontraumatic 432.0
      fetus or newborn 767.0
  fallopian tube 620.8
  genital organ (nontraumatic)
    female NEC 629.89
    male NEC 608.83
    traumatic (external site) 922.4
      internal - *see* Injury, internal, genital organ
  graafian follicle (ruptured) 620.0
  internal organs (abdomen, chest, or pelvis) - *see also* Injury, internal, by site
    kidney - *see* Hematoma, kidney, traumatic
    liver - *see* Hematoma, liver, traumatic
    spleen - *see* Hematoma, spleen
  intracranial - *see* Hematoma, brain
  kidney, cystic 593.81
    traumatic 866.01
      with open wound into cavity 866.11
  labia (nontraumatic) 624.5
  lingual (and other parts of neck, scalp, or face, except eye) 920
  liver (subcapsular) 573.8
    birth injury 767.8
    fetus or newborn 767.8
    traumatic NEC 864.01
      with
        laceration - *see* Laceration, liver
        open wound into cavity 864.11
  mediastinum - *see* Injury, internal, mediastinum
  meninges, meningeal (brain) - *see also* Hematoma, brain, subarachnoid
    spinal - *see* Injury, spinal, by site
  mesosalpinx (nontraumatic) 620.8
    traumatic - *see* Injury, internal, pelvis
  muscle (traumatic) - *see* Contusion, by site
    nontraumatic 729.92
  nasal (septum) (and other part(s) of neck, scalp, or face, except eye) 920
  obstetrical surgical wound 674.3●
  orbit, orbital (nontraumatic) 376.32
    traumatic 921.2
  ovary (corpus luteum) (nontraumatic) 620.1
    traumatic - *see* Injury, internal, ovary
  pelvis (female) (nontraumatic) 629.89
    complicating delivery 665.7●
    male 608.83
    traumatic - *see also* Injury, internal, pelvis
      specified organ NEC (*see also* Injury, internal, pelvis) 867.6
  penis (nontraumatic) 607.82
  pericranial (and neck, or face any part, except eye) 920
    due to injury at birth 767.19
  perineal wound (obstetrical) 674.3●
    complicating delivery 664.5●
  perirenal, cystic 593.81
  pinna 380.31

Hematoma (*Continued*)
  placenta - *see* Placenta, abnormal
  postoperative 998.12
  retroperitoneal (nontraumatic) 568.81
    traumatic - *see* Injury, internal, retroperitoneum
  retropubic, male 568.81
  scalp (and neck, or face any part, except eye) 920
    fetus or newborn 767.19
  scrotum (nontraumatic) 608.83
    traumatic 922.4
  seminal vesicle (nontraumatic) 608.83
    traumatic - *see* Injury, internal, seminal, vesicle
  soft tissue, nontraumatic 729.92
  spermatic cord - *see also* Injury, internal, spermatic cord
    nontraumatic 608.83
  spinal (cord) (meninges) - *see also* Injury, spinal, by site
    fetus or newborn 767.4
    nontraumatic 336.1
  spleen 865.01
    with
      laceration - *see* Laceration, spleen
      open wound into cavity 865.11
  sternocleidomastoid, birth injury 767.8
  sternomastoid, birth injury 767.8
  subarachnoid - *see also* Hematoma, brain, subarachnoid
    fetus or newborn 772.2
    nontraumatic (*see also* Hemorrhage, subarachnoid) 430
      newborn 772.2
  subdural - *see also* Hematoma, brain, subdural
    fetus or newborn (localized) 767.0
    nontraumatic (*see also* Hemorrhage, subdural) 432.1
  subperiosteal (syndrome) 267
    traumatic - *see* Hematoma, by site
  superficial, fetus or newborn 772.6
  syncytium - *see* Placenta, abnormal
  testis (nontraumatic) 608.83
    birth injury 767.8
    traumatic 922.4
  tunica vaginalis (nontraumatic) 608.83
  umbilical cord 663.6●
    affecting fetus or newborn 762.6
  uterine ligament (nontraumatic) 620.7
    traumatic - *see* Injury, internal, pelvis
  uterus 621.4
    traumatic - *see* Injury, internal, pelvis
  vagina (nontraumatic) (ruptured) 623.6
    complicating delivery 665.7●
    traumatic 922.4
  vas deferens (nontraumatic) 608.83
    traumatic - *see* Injury, internal, vas deferens
  vitreous 379.23
  vocal cord 920
  vulva (nontraumatic) 624.5
    complicating delivery 664.5●
    fetus or newborn 767.8
    traumatic 922.4
Hematometra 621.4
Hematomyelia 336.1
  with fracture of vertebra (*see also* Fracture, vertebra, by site, with spinal cord injury) 806.8
  fetus or newborn 767.4
Hematomyelitis 323.9
  late effect - *see* category 326

Hematoperitoneum (*see also* Hemoperitoneum) 568.81
Hematopneumothorax (*see also* Hemothorax) 511.89
Hematopoiesis, cyclic 288.02
Hematoporphyria (acquired) (congenital) 277.1
Hematoporphyrinuria (acquired) (congenital) 277.1
Hematorachis, hematorrhachis 336.1
  fetus or newborn 767.4
Hematosalpinx 620.8
  with
    ectopic pregnancy (*see also* categories 633.0–633.9) 639.2
    molar pregnancy (*see also* categories 630–632) 639.2
  infectional (*see also* Salpingo-oophoritis) 614.2
Hematospermia 608.82
Hematothorax (*see also* Hemothorax) 511.89
Hematotympanum 381.03
Hematuria (benign) (essential) (idiopathic) 599.70
  due to S. hematobium 120.0
  endemic 120.0
  gross 599.71
  intermittent 599.70
  malarial 084.8
  microscopic 599.72
  paroxysmal 599.70
  sulfonamide
    correct substance properly administered 599.70
    overdose or wrong substance given or taken 961.0
  tropical (bilharziasis) 120.0
  tuberculous (*see also* Tuberculosis) 016.9●
Hematuric bilious fever 084.8
Hemeralopia 368.10
Hemiabiotrophy 799.89
Hemi-akinesia 781.8
Hemianalgesia (*see also* Disturbance, sensation) 782.0
Hemianencephaly 740.0
Hemianesthesia (*see also* Disturbance, sensation) 782.0
Hemianopia, hemianopsia (altitudinal) (homonymous) 368.46
  binasal 368.47
  bitemporal 368.47
  heteronymous 368.47
  syphilitic 095.8
Hemiasomatognosia 307.9
Hemiathetosis 781.0
Hemiatrophy 799.89
  cerebellar 334.8
  face 349.89
    progressive 349.89
  fascia 728.9
  leg 728.2
  tongue 529.8
Hemiballism (us) 333.5
Hemiblock (cardiac) (heart) (left) 426.2
Hemicardia 746.89
Hemicephalus, hemicephaly 740.0
Hemichorea 333.5
Hemicrania 346.9●
  congenital malformation 740.0
  continua 339.41
  paroxysmal 339.03
    chronic 339.04
    episodic 339.03

◀ New ◀◀◀ Revised ~~deleted~~ Deleted ● Use Additional Digit(s) ▬ Omit code

Hemidystrophy - *see* Hemiatrophy
Hemiectromelia 755.4
Hemihypalgesia (*see also* Disturbance, sensation) 782.0
Hemihypertrophy (congenital) 759.89
cranial 756.0
Hemihypesthesia (*see also* Disturbance, sensation) 782.0
Hemi-inattention 781.8
Hemimelia 755.4
lower limb 755.30
paraxial (complete) (incomplete) (intercalary) (terminal) 755.32
fibula 755.37
tibia 755.36
transverse (complete) (partial) 755.31
upper limb 755.20
paraxial (complete) (incomplete) (intercalary) (terminal) 755.22
radial 755.26
ulnar 755.27
transverse (complete) (partial) 755.21
Hemiparalysis (*see also* Hemiplegia) 342.9●
Hemiparesis (*see also* Hemiplegia) 342.9●
Hemiparesthesia (*see also* Disturbance, sensation) 782.0
Hemiplegia 342.9●
acute (*see also* Disease, cerebrovascular, acute) 436
alternans facialis 344.89
apoplectic (*see also* Disease, cerebrovascular, acute) 436
late effect or residual
affecting
dominant side 438.21
nondominant side 438.22
unspecified side 438.20
arteriosclerotic 437.0
late effect or residual
affecting
dominant side 438.21
nondominant side 438.22
unspecified side 438.20
ascending (spinal) NEC 344.89
attack (*see also* Disease, cerebrovascular, acute) 436
brain, cerebral (current episode) 437.8
congenital 343.1
cerebral - *see* Hemiplegia, brain
congenital (cerebral) (spastic) (spinal) 343.1
conversion neurosis (hysterical) 300.11
cortical - *see* Hemiplegia, brain
due to
arteriosclerosis 437.0
late effect or residual
affecting
dominant side 438.21
nondominant side 438.22
unspecified side 438.20
cerebrovascular lesion (*see also* Disease, cerebrovascular, acute) 436
late effect
affecting
dominant side 438.21
nondominant side 438.22
unspecified side 438.20

Hemiplegia (*Continued*)
embolic (current) (*see also* Embolism, brain) 434.1●
late effect
affecting
dominant side 438.21
nondominant side 438.22
unspecified side 438.20
flaccid 342.0●
hypertensive (current episode) 437.8
infantile (postnatal) 343.4
late effect
birth injury, intracranial or spinal 343.4
cerebrovascular lesion - *see* Late effect(s) (of) cerebrovascular disease
viral encephalitis 139.0
middle alternating NEC 344.89
newborn NEC 767.0
seizure (current episode) (*see also* Disease, cerebrovascular, acute) 436
spastic 342.1●
congenital or infantile 343.1
specified NEC 342.8●
thrombotic (current) (*see also* Thrombosis, brain) 434.0●
late effect - *see* Late effect(s) (of) cerebrovascular disease
Hemisection, spinal cord - *see* Fracture, vertebra, by site, with spinal cord injury
Hemispasm 781.0
facial 781.0
Hemispatial neglect 781.8
Hemisporosis 117.9
Hemitremor 781.0
Hemivertebra 756.14
Hemobilia 576.8
Hemocholecyst 575.8
Hemochromatosis (acquired) ~~(diabetic)~~ ~~(hereditary)~~ (liver) (myocardium) ~~(primary idiopathic)~~ (secondary) 275.03 ◄▥
with refractory anemia 238.72
diabetic 275.01 ◄
due to repeated red blood cell transfusions 275.02 ◄
hereditary 275.01 ◄
primary idiopathic 275.01 ◄
specified NEC 275.03 ◄
transfusion associated (red blood cell) 275.02 ◄
Hemodialysis V56.0
Hemoglobin - *see also* condition
abnormal (disease) - *see* Disease, hemoglobin
AS genotype 282.5
fetal, hereditary persistence 282.7
high-oxygen-affinity 289.0
low NEC 285.9
S (Hb-S), heterozygous 282.5
Hemoglobinemia 283.2
due to blood transfusion NEC 999.89
bone marrow 996.85
paroxysmal 283.2
Hemoglobinopathy (mixed) (*see also* Disease, hemoglobin) 282.7
with thalassemia 282.49
sickle-cell 282.60
with thalassemia (without crisis) 282.41
with
crisis 282.42
vaso-occlusive pain 282.42

Hemoglobinuria, hemoglobinuric 791.2
with anemia, hemolytic, acquired (chronic) NEC 283.2
cold (agglutinin) (paroxysmal) (with Raynaud's syndrome) 283.2
due to
exertion 283.2
hemolysis (from external causes) NEC 283.2
exercise 283.2
fever (malaria) 084.8
infantile 791.2
intermittent 283.2
malarial 084.8
march 283.2
nocturnal (paroxysmal) 283.2
paroxysmal (cold) (nocturnal) 283.2
Hemolymphangioma (M9175/0) 228.1
Hemolysis
fetal - *see* Jaundice, fetus or newborn
intravascular (disseminated) NEC 286.6
with
abortion - *see* Abortion, by type, with hemorrhage, delayed or excessive
ectopic pregnancy (*see also* categories 633.0–633.9) 639.1
hemorrhage of pregnancy 641.3●
affecting fetus or newborn 762.1
molar pregnancy (*see also* categories 630–632) 639.1
acute 283.2
following
abortion 639.1
ectopic or molar pregnancy 639.1
neonatal - *see* Jaundice, fetus or newborn
transfusion NEC 999.89
bone marrow 996.85
Hemolytic - *see also* condition
anemia - *see* Anemia, hemolytic
uremic syndrome 283.11
Hemometra 621.4
Hemopericardium (with effusion) 423.0
newborn 772.8
traumatic (*see also* Hemothorax, traumatic) 860.2
with open wound into thorax 860.3
Hemoperitoneum 568.81
infectional (*see also* Peritonitis) 567.29
traumatic - *see* Injury, internal, peritoneum
Hemophagocytic syndrome 288.4
infection-associated 288.4
Hemophilia (familial) (hereditary) 286.0
A 286.0
carrier (asymptomatic) V83.01
symptomatic V83.02
acquired 286.5
B (Leyden) 286.1
C 286.2
calcipriva (*see also* Fibrinolysis) 286.7
classical 286.0
nonfamilial 286.7
secondary 286.5
vascular 286.4
Hemophilus influenzae NEC 041.5
arachnoiditis (basic) (brain) (spinal) 320.0
late effect - *see* category 326
bronchopneumonia 482.2
cerebral ventriculitis 320.0
late effect - *see* category 326

◄ New   ◄▥ Revised   ~~deleted~~ Deleted   ● Use Additional Digit(s)   ▨ Omit code

Hemophilus influenzae NEC *(Continued)*
cerebrospinal inflammation 320.0
late effect - *see* category 326
infection NEC 041.5
leptomeningitis 320.0
late effect - *see* category 326
meningitis (cerebral) (cerebrospinal)
(spinal) 320.0
late effect - *see* category 326
meningomyelitis 320.0
late effect - *see* category 326
pachymeningitis (adhesive) (fibrous)
(hemorrhagic) (hypertrophic)
(spinal) 320.0
late effect - *see* category 326
pneumonia (broncho-) 482.2
Hemophthalmos 360.43
Hemopneumothorax *(see also*
Hemothorax) 511.89
traumatic 860.4
with open wound into thorax 860.5
Hemoptysis 786.30 ◀▥
due to Paragonimus (westermani) 121.2
newborn 770.3
specified NEC 786.39 ◀
tuberculous (*see also* Tuberculosis,
pulmonary) 011.9●
Hemorrhage, hemorrhagic
(nontraumatic) 459.0
abdomen 459.0
accidental (antepartum) 641.2●
affecting fetus or newborn 762.1
adenoid 474.8
adrenal (capsule) (gland) (medulla)
255.41
newborn 772.5
after labor - *see* Hemorrhage,
postpartum
alveolar
lung, newborn 770.3
process 525.8
alveolus 525.8
amputation stump (surgical) 998.11
secondary, delayed 997.69
anemia (chronic) 280.0
acute 285.1
antepartum - *see* Hemorrhage,
pregnancy
anus (sphincter) 569.3
apoplexy (stroke) 432.9
arachnoid - *see* Hemorrhage,
subarachnoid
artery NEC 459.0
brain (*see also* Hemorrhage, brain) 431
middle meningeal - *see* Hemorrhage,
subarachnoid
basilar (ganglion) (*see also* Hemorrhage,
brain) 431
bladder 596.8
blood dyscrasia 289.9
bowel 578.9
newborn 772.4
brain (miliary) (nontraumatic) 431
with
birth injury 767.0
arachnoid - *see* Hemorrhage,
subarachnoid
due to
birth injury 767.0
rupture of aneurysm (congenital)
(*see also* Hemorrhage,
subarachnoid) 430
mycotic 431
syphilis 094.89

Hemorrhage, hemorrhagic *(Continued)*
brain *(Continued)*
epidural or extradural - *see*
Hemorrhage, extradural
fetus or newborn (anoxic) (hypoxic)
(due to birth trauma)
(nontraumatic) 767.0
intraventricular 772.10
grade I 772.11
grade II 772.12
grade III 772.13
grade IV 772.14
iatrogenic 997.02
postoperative 997.02
puerperal, postpartum, childbirth
674.0●
stem 431
subarachnoid, arachnoid, or
meningeal - *see* Hemorrhage,
subarachnoid
subdural - *see* Hemorrhage,
subdural
traumatic NEC 853.0●

Note: Use the following fifth-digit
subclassification with categories 851–854:

0 unspecified state of
consciousness
1 with no loss of consciousness
2 with brief [less than one hour]
loss of consciousness
3 with moderate [1–24 hours] loss
of consciousness
4 with prolonged [more than 24
hours] loss of
consciousness and return
to pre-existing conscious
level
5 with prolonged [more than 24
hours] loss of
consciousness, without
return to pre-existing
conscious level

Use fifth-digit 5 to designate when a
patient is unconscious and dies before
regaining consciousness, regardless of
the duration of the loss of consciousness

6 with loss of consciousness of
unspecified duration
9 with concussion, unspecified

with
cerebral
contusion - *see* Contusion,
brain
laceration - *see* Laceration,
brain
open intracranial wound
853.1●
skull fracture - *see* Fracture,
skull, by site
extradural or epidural 852.4●
with open intracranial wound
852.5●
subarachnoid 852.0●
with open intracranial wound
852.1●
subdural 852.2●
with open intracranial wound
852.3●
breast 611.79
bronchial tube - *see* Hemorrhage, lung
bronchopulmonary - *see* Hemorrhage,
lung

Hemorrhage, hemorrhagic *(Continued)*
bronchus (cause unknown) (*see also*
Hemorrhage, lung) 786.30 ◀▥
bulbar (*see also* Hemorrhage, brain) 431
bursa 727.89
capillary 448.9
primary 287.8
capsular - *see* Hemorrhage, brain
cardiovascular 429.89
cecum 578.9
cephalic (*see also* Hemorrhage, brain)
431
cerebellar (*see also* Hemorrhage, brain)
431
cerebellum (*see also* Hemorrhage, brain)
431
cerebral (*see also* Hemorrhage, brain)
431
fetus or newborn (anoxic)
(traumatic) 767.0
cerebromeningeal (*see also*
Hemorrhage, brain) 431
cerebrospinal (*see also* Hemorrhage,
brain) 431
cerebrovascular accident - *see*
Hemorrhage, brain
cerebrum (*see also* Hemorrhage, brain)
431
cervix (stump) (uteri) 622.8
cesarean section wound 674.3●
chamber, anterior (eye) 364.41
childbirth - *see* Hemorrhage,
complicating, delivery
choroid 363.61
expulsive 363.62
ciliary body 364.41
cochlea 386.8
colon - *see* Hemorrhage, intestine
complicating
delivery 641.9●
affecting fetus or newborn 762.1
associated with
afibrinogenemia 641.3●
affecting fetus or newborn
763.89
coagulation defect 641.3●
affecting fetus or newborn
763.89
hyperfibrinolysis 641.3●
affecting fetus or newborn
763.89
hypofibrinogenemia 641.3●
affecting fetus or newborn
763.89
due to
low-lying placenta 641.1●
affecting fetus or newborn
762.0
placenta previa 641.1●
affecting fetus or newborn
762.0
premature separation of
placenta 641.2●
affecting fetus or newborn
762.1
retained
placenta 666.0●
secundines 666.2●
trauma 641.8●
affecting fetus or newborn
763.89
uterine leiomyoma 641.8●
affecting fetus or newborn
763.89

◀ New ◀▥ Revised deleted Deleted ● Use Additional Digit(s) Omit code

Hemorrhage, hemorrhagic *(Continued)*
  complication(s)
    of dental implant placement 525.71
    surgical procedure 998.11
  concealed NEC 459.0
  congenital 772.9
  conjunctiva 372.72
    newborn 772.8
  cord, newborn 772.0
    slipped ligature 772.3
    stump 772.3
  corpus luteum (ruptured) 620.1
  cortical (*see also* Hemorrhage, brain)
      431
  cranial 432.9
  cutaneous 782.7
    newborn 772.6
  cyst, pancreas 577.2
  cystitis - *see* Cystitis
  delayed
    with
      abortion - *see* Abortion, by type,
          with hemorrhage, delayed
          or excessive
      ectopic pregnancy (*see also*
          categories 633.0–633.9) 639.1
      molar pregnancy (*see also*
          categories 630–632) 639.1
    following
      abortion 639.1
      ectopic or molar pregnancy
          639.1
    postpartum 666.2●
  diathesis (familial) 287.9
    newborn 776.0
  disease 287.9
    newborn 776.0
    specified type NEC 287.8
  disorder 287.9
    due to intrinsic circulating
        anticoagulants 286.5
    specified type NEC 287.8
  due to
    any device, implant, or graft
        (presence of) classifiable to
        996.0–996.5 - *see*
        Complications, due to
        (presence of) any device,
        implant, or graft classified to
        996.0–996.5 NEC
    intrinsic circulating anticoagulant
        286.5
  duodenum, duodenal 537.89
    ulcer - *see* Ulcer, duodenum, with
        hemorrhage
  dura mater - *see* Hemorrhage, subdural
  endotracheal - *see* Hemorrhage, lung
  epicranial subaponeurotic (massive)
      767.11
  epidural - *see* Hemorrhage, extradural
  episiotomy 674.3●
  esophagus 530.82
    varix (*see also* Varix, esophagus,
        bleeding) 456.0
  excessive
    with
      abortion - *see* Abortion, by type,
          with hemorrhage, delayed
          or excessive
      ectopic pregnancy (*see also*
          categories 633.0–633.9)
          639.1
      molar pregnancy (*see also*
          categories 630–632) 639.1

Hemorrhage, hemorrhagic *(Continued)*
  excessive *(Continued)*
    following
      abortion 639.1
      ectopic or molar pregnancy 639.1
  external 459.0
  extradural (traumatic) - *see also*
        Hemorrhage, brain, traumatic,
        extradural
    birth injury 767.0
    fetus or newborn (anoxic)
        (traumatic) 767.0
    nontraumatic 432.0
  eye 360.43
    chamber (anterior) (aqueous) 364.41
    fundus 362.81
  eyelid 374.81
  fallopian tube 620.8
  fetomaternal 772.0
    affecting management of pregnancy
        or puerperium 656.0●
  fetus, fetal, affecting newborn 772.0
    from
      cut end of co-twin's cord 772.0
      placenta 772.0
      ruptured cord 772.0
      vasa previa 772.0
    into
      co-twin 772.0
      mother's circulation 772.0
        affecting management of
            pregnancy or
            puerperium 656.0●
  fever (*see also* Fever, hemorrhagic) 065.9
    with renal syndrome 078.6
    arthropod-borne NEC 065.9
    Bangkok 065.4
    Crimean 065.0
    dengue virus 065.4
    epidemic 078.6
    Junin virus 078.7
    Korean 078.6
    Machupo virus 078.7
    mite-borne 065.8
    mosquito-borne 065.4
    Philippine 065.4
    Russian (Yaroslav) 078.6
    Singapore 065.4
    Southeast Asia 065.4
    Thailand 065.4
    tick-borne NEC 065.3
  fibrinogenolysis (*see also* Fibrinolysis)
      286.6
  fibrinolytic (acquired) (*see also*
      Fibrinolysis) 286.6
  fontanel 767.19
  from tracheostomy stoma 519.09
  fundus, eye 362.81
  funis
    affecting fetus or newborn 772.0
    complicating delivery 663.8●
  gastric (*see also* Hemorrhage, stomach)
      578.9
  gastroenteric 578.9
    newborn 772.4
  gastrointestinal (tract) 578.9
    newborn 772.4
  genitourinary (tract) NEC 599.89
  gingiva 523.8
  globe 360.43
  gravidarum - *see* Hemorrhage,
      pregnancy
  gum 523.8
  heart 429.89

Hemorrhage, hemorrhagic *(Continued)*
  hypopharyngeal (throat) 784.8
  intermenstrual 626.6
    irregular 626.6
    regular 626.5
  internal (organs) 459.0
    capsule (*see also* Hemorrhage brain)
        431
    ear 386.8
    newborn 772.8
  intestine 578.9
    congenital 772.4
    newborn 772.4
  into
    bladder wall 596.7
    bursa 727.89
    corpus luysii (*see also* Hemorrhage,
        brain) 431
  intra-abdominal 459.0
    during or following surgery 998.11
  intra-alveolar, newborn (lung) 770.3
  intracerebral (*see also* Hemorrhage,
      brain) 431
  intracranial NEC 432.9
    puerperal, postpartum, childbirth
        674.0●
    traumatic - *see* Hemorrhage, brain,
        traumatic
  intramedullary NEC 336.1
  intraocular 360.43
  intraoperative 998.11
  intrapartum - *see* Hemorrhage,
      complicating, delivery
  intrapelvic
    female 629.89
    male 459.0
  intraperitoneal 459.0
  intrapontine (*see also* Hemorrhage,
      brain) 431
  intrauterine 621.4
    complicating delivery - *see*
        Hemorrhage, complicating,
        delivery
    in pregnancy or childbirth - *see*
        Hemorrhage, pregnancy
    postpartum (*see also* Hemorrhage,
        postpartum) 666.1●
  intraventricular (*see also* Hemorrhage,
      brain) 431
    fetus or newborn (anoxic)
        (traumatic) 772.10
      grade I 772.11
      grade II 772.12
      grade III 772.13
      grade IV 772.14
  intravesical 596.7
  iris (postinfectional)
      (postinflammatory) (toxic) 364.41
  joint (nontraumatic) 719.10
    ankle 719.17
    elbow 719.12
    foot 719.17
    forearm 719.13
    hand 719.14
    hip 719.15
    knee 719.16
    lower leg 719.16
    multiple sites 719.19
    pelvic region 719.15
    shoulder (region) 719.11
    specified site NEC 719.18
    thigh 719.15
    upper arm 719.12
    wrist 719.13

Hemorrhage, hemorrhagic (*Continued*)
kidney 593.81
knee (joint) 719.16
labyrinth 386.8
leg NEC 459.0
lenticular striate artery (*see also*
    Hemorrhage, brain) 431
ligature, vessel 998.11
liver 573.8
lower extremity NEC 459.0
lung 786.30 ◄▦
    newborn 770.3
    tuberculous (*see also* Tuberculosis,
        pulmonary) 011.9●
malaria 084.8
marginal sinus 641.2●
massive subaponeurotic, birth injury
    767.11
maternal, affecting fetus or newborn
    762.1
mediastinum 786.30 ◄▦
medulla (*see also* Hemorrhage, brain)
    431
membrane (brain) (*see also*
    Hemorrhage, subarachnoid)
    430
    spinal cord - *see* Hemorrhage,
        spinal cord
meninges, meningeal (brain) (middle)
    (*see also* Hemorrhage,
    subarachnoid) 430
    spinal cord - *see* Hemorrhage, spinal
        cord
mesentery 568.81
metritis 626.8
midbrain (*see also* Hemorrhage, brain)
    431
mole 631
mouth 528.9
mucous membrane NEC 459.0
    newborn 772.8
muscle 728.89
nail (subungual) 703.8
nasal turbinate 784.7
    newborn 772.8
nasopharynx 478.29
navel, newborn 772.3
newborn 772.9
    adrenal 772.5
    alveolar (lung) 770.3
    brain (anoxic) (hypoxic) (due to
        birth trauma) 767.0
    cerebral (anoxic) (hypoxic) (due to
        birth trauma) 767.0
    conjunctiva 772.8
    cutaneous 772.6
    diathesis 776.0
    due to vitamin K deficiency
        776.0
    epicranial subaponeurotic
        (massive) 767.11
    gastrointestinal 772.4
    internal (organs) 772.8
    intestines 772.4
    intra-alveolar (lung) 770.3
    intracranial (from any perinatal
        cause) 767.0
    intraventricular (from any perinatal
        cause) 772.10
        grade I 772.11
        grade II 772.12
        grade III 772.13
        grade IV 772.14
    lung 770.3

Hemorrhage, hemorrhagic (*Continued*)
newborn (*Continued*)
    pulmonary (massive) 770.3
    spinal cord, traumatic 767.4
    stomach 772.4
    subaponeurotic (massive) 767.11
    subarachnoid (from any perinatal
        cause) 772.2
    subconjunctival 772.8
    subgaleal 767.11
    umbilicus 772.0
        slipped ligature 772.3
        vasa previa 772.0
nipple 611.79
nose 784.7
    newborn 772.8
obstetrical surgical wound 674.3●
omentum 568.89
    newborn 772.4
optic nerve (sheath) 377.42
orbit 376.32
ovary 620.1
oviduct 620.8
pancreas 577.8
parathyroid (gland) (spontaneous)
    252.8
parturition - *see* Hemorrhage,
    complicating, delivery
penis 607.82
pericardium, pericarditis 423.0
perineal wound (obstetrical) 674.3●
peritoneum, peritoneal 459.0
peritonsillar tissue 474.8
    after operation on tonsils 998.11
    due to infection 475
petechial 782.7
pituitary (gland) 253.8
placenta NEC 641.9●
    affecting fetus or newborn 762.1
    from surgical or instrumental
        damage 641.8●
    affecting fetus or newborn
        762.1
    previa 641.1●
        affecting fetus or newborn
            762.0
pleura - *see* Hemorrhage, lung
polioencephalitis, superior 265.1
polymyositis - *see* Polymyositis
pons (*see also* Hemorrhage, brain) 431
pontine (*see also* Hemorrhage, brain)
    431
popliteal 459.0
postcoital 626.7
postextraction (dental) 998.11
postmenopausal 627.1
postnasal 784.7
postoperative 998.11
postpartum (atonic) (following
    delivery of placenta) 666.1●
    delayed or secondary (after 24
        hours) 666.2●
    retained placenta 666.0●
    third stage 666.0●
pregnancy (concealed) 641.9●
    accidental 641.2●
        affecting fetus or newborn
            762.1
    affecting fetus or newborn
        762.1
    before 22 completed weeks'
        gestation 640.9●
    affecting fetus or newborn
        762.1

Hemorrhage, hemorrhagic (*Continued*)
pregnancy (*Continued*)
    due to
        abruptio placenta 641.2●
            affecting fetus or newborn
                762.1
        afibrinogenemia or other
            coagulation defect
            (conditions classifiable to
            286.0–286.9) 641.3●
            affecting fetus or newborn
                762.1
        coagulation defect 641.3●
            affecting fetus or newborn
                762.1
        hyperfibrinolysis 641.3●
            affecting fetus or newborn
                762.1
        hypofibrinogenemia 641.3●
            affecting fetus or newborn
                762.1
        leiomyoma, uterus 641.8●
            affecting fetus or newborn
                762.1
        low-lying placenta 641.1●
            affecting fetus or newborn
                762.1
        marginal sinus (rupture)
            641.2●
            affecting fetus or newborn
                762.1
        placenta previa 641.1●
            affecting fetus or newborn
                762.0
        premature separation of placenta
            (normally implanted)
            641.2●
            affecting fetus or newborn
                762.1
        threatened abortion 640.0●
            affecting fetus or newborn
                762.1
        trauma 641.8●
            affecting fetus or newborn
                762.1
    early (before 22 completed weeks'
        gestation) 640.9●
    affecting fetus or newborn 762.1
    previous, affecting management of
        pregnancy or childbirth V23.49
    unavoidable - *see* Hemorrhage,
        pregnancy, due to placenta
        previa
prepartum (mother) - *see* Hemorrhage,
    pregnancy
preretinal, cause unspecified 362.81
prostate 602.1
puerperal (*see also* Hemorrhage,
    postpartum) 666.1●
pulmonary (*see also* Hemorrhage, lung)
    786.30 ◄▦
    acute idiopathic in infants (AIPHI)
        (over 28 days old) 786.31 ◄
    newborn (massive) 770.3
    renal syndrome 446.21
purpura (primary) (*see also* Purpura,
    thrombocytopenic) 287.39
rectum (sphincter) 569.3
recurring, following initial hemorrhage
    at time of injury 958.2
renal 593.81
    pulmonary syndrome 446.21
respiratory tract (*see also* Hemorrhage,
    lung) 786.30 ◄▦

◄ New   ◄▦ Revised   ~~deleted~~ Deleted   ● Use Additional Digit(s)   ▦ Omit code

Hemorrhage, hemorrhagic *(Continued)*
  retina, retinal (deep) (superficial)
      (vessels) 362.81
    diabetic 250.5● *[362.01]*
      due to secondary diabetes 249.5●
          [362.01]
    due to birth injury 772.8
  retrobulbar 376.89
  retroperitoneal 459.0
  retroplacental (*see also* Placenta,
      separation) 641.2●
  scalp 459.0
    due to injury at birth 767.19
  scrotum 608.83
  secondary (nontraumatic) 459.0
    following initial hemorrhage at time
        of injury 958.2
  seminal vesicle 608.83
  skin 782.7
    newborn 772.6
  spermatic cord 608.83
  spinal (cord) 336.1
    aneurysm (ruptured) 336.1
      syphilitic 094.89
    due to birth injury 767.4
    fetus or newborn 767.4
  spleen 289.59
  spontaneous NEC 459.0
    petechial 782.7
  stomach 578.9
    newborn 772.4
    ulcer - *see* Ulcer, stomach, with
        hemorrhage
  subaponeurotic, newborn 767.11
    massive (birth injury) 767.11
  subarachnoid (nontraumatic) 430
    fetus or newborn (anoxic)
        (traumatic) 772.2
    puerperal, postpartum, childbirth
        674.0●
    traumatic - *see* Hemorrhage, brain,
        traumatic, subarachnoid
  subconjunctival 372.72
    due to birth injury 772.8
    newborn 772.8
  subcortical (*see also* Hemorrhage, brain)
      431
  subcutaneous 782.7
  subdiaphragmatic 459.0
  subdural (nontraumatic) 432.1
    due to birth injury 767.0
    fetus or newborn (anoxic) (hypoxic)
        (due to birth trauma) 767.0
    puerperal, postpartum, childbirth
        674.0●
    spinal 336.1
    traumatic - *see* Hemorrhage, brain,
        traumatic, subdural
  subgaleal 767.11
  subhyaloid 362.81
  subperiosteal 733.99
  subretinal 362.81
  subtentorial (*see also* Hemorrhage,
      subdural) 432.1
  subungual 703.8
    due to blood dyscrasia 287.8
  suprarenal (capsule) (gland) 255.41
    fetus or newborn 772.5
  tentorium (traumatic) - *see also*
      Hemorrhage, brain, traumatic
    fetus or newborn 767.0
    nontraumatic - *see* Hemorrhage,
        subdural
  testis 608.83

Hemorrhage, hemorrhagic *(Continued)*
  thigh 459.0
  third stage 666.0●
  thorax - *see* Hemorrhage, lung
  throat 784.8
  thrombocythemia 238.71
  thymus (gland) 254.8
  thyroid (gland) 246.3
    cyst 246.3
  tongue 529.8
  tonsil 474.8
    postoperative 998.11
  tooth socket (postextraction) 998.11
  trachea - *see* Hemorrhage, lung
  traumatic - *see also* nature of injury
    brain - *see* Hemorrhage, brain,
        traumatic
    recurring or secondary (following
        initial hemorrhage at time of
        injury) 958.2
  tuberculous NEC (*see also* Tuberculosis,
      pulmonary) 011.9●
  tunica vaginalis 608.83
  ulcer - *see* Ulcer, by site, with
      hemorrhage
  umbilicus, umbilical cord 772.0
    after birth, newborn 772.3
    complicating delivery 663.8●
      affecting fetus or newborn
          772.0
    slipped ligature 772.3
    stump 772.3
  unavoidable (due to placenta previa)
      641.1●
    affecting fetus or newborn
        762.0
  upper extremity 459.0
  urethra (idiopathic) 599.84
  uterus, uterine (abnormal) 626.9
    climacteric 627.0
    complicating delivery - *see*
        Hemorrhage, complicating,
        delivery
    due to
      intrauterine contraceptive device
          996.76
      perforating uterus 996.32
    functional or dysfunctional
        626.8
    in pregnancy - *see* Hemorrhage,
        pregnancy
    intermenstrual 626.6
      irregular 626.6
      regular 626.5
    postmenopausal 627.1
    postpartum (*see also* Hemorrhage,
        postpartum) 666.1●
    prepubertal 626.8
    pubertal 626.3
    puerperal (immediate) 666.1●
  vagina 623.8
  vasa previa 663.5●
    affecting fetus or newborn
        772.0
  vas deferens 608.83
  ventricular (*see also* Hemorrhage,
      brain) 431
  vesical 596.8
  viscera 459.0
    newborn 772.8
  vitreous (humor) (intraocular)
      379.23
  vocal cord 478.5
  vulva 624.8

Hemorrhoids (anus) (rectum) (without
    complication) 455.6
  bleeding, prolapsed, strangulated, or
      ulcerated NEC 455.8
    external 455.5
    internal 455.2
  complicated NEC 455.8
  complicating pregnancy and
      puerperium 671.8●
  external 455.3
    with complication NEC 455.5
      bleeding, prolapsed, strangulated,
          or ulcerated 455.5
    thrombosed 455.4
  internal 455.0
    with complication NEC 455.2
      bleeding, prolapsed, strangulated,
          or ulcerated 455.2
    thrombosed 455.1
  residual skin tag 455.9
  sentinel pile 455.9
  thrombosed NEC 455.7
    external 455.4
    internal 455.1
Hemosalpinx 620.8
Hemosiderosis 275.09 ◀▥
  dietary 275.09 ◀▥
  pulmonary (idiopathic) 275.09 *[516.1]* ◀▥
  transfusion NEC 275.02 ◀▥
    bone marrow 996.85
Hemospermia 608.82
Hemothorax 511.89
  bacterial, nontuberculous 511.1
  newborn 772.8
  nontuberculous 511.89
    bacterial 511.1
  pneumococcal 511.1
  postoperative 998.11
  staphylococcal 511.1
  streptococcal 511.1
  traumatic 860.2
    with
      open wound into thorax 860.3
      pneumothorax 860.4
        with open wound into thorax
            860.5
  tuberculous (*see also* Tuberculosis,
      pleura) 012.0●
Hemotympanum 385.89
Hench-Rosenberg syndrome
    (palindromic arthritis) (*see also*
    Rheumatism, palindromic)
    719.3●
Henle's warts 371.41
Henoch (-Schönlein)
  disease or syndrome (allergic purpura)
      287.0
  purpura (allergic) 287.0
Henpue, henpuye 102.6
Heparin-induced thrombocytopenia
    (HIT) 289.84
Heparitinuria 277.5
Hepar lobatum 095.3
Hepatalgia 573.8
Hepatic - *see also* condition
  flexure syndrome 569.89
Hepatitis 573.3
  acute (*see also* Necrosis, liver) 570
    alcoholic 571.1
    infective 070.1
      with hepatic coma 070.0
  alcoholic 571.1
  amebic - *see* Abscess, liver, amebic
  anicteric (acute) - *see* Hepatitis, viral

Hepatitis (Continued)
  antigen-associated (HAA) - see
      Hepatitis, viral, type B
  Australian antigen (positive) - see
      Hepatitis, viral, type B
  autoimmune 571.42
  catarrhal (acute) 070.1
    with hepatic coma 070.0
    chronic 571.40
    newborn 070.1
      with hepatic coma 070.0
  chemical 573.3
  cholangiolitic 573.8
  cholestatic 573.8
  chronic 571.40
    active 571.49
      viral - see Hepatitis, viral
    aggressive 571.49
    persistent 571.41
    viral - see Hepatitis, viral
  cytomegalic inclusion virus 078.5 [573.1]
  diffuse 573.3
  "dirty needle" - see Hepatitis, viral
  drug-induced 573.3
  due to
    Coxsackie 074.8 [573.1]
    cytomegalic inclusion virus 078.5
        [573.1]
    infectious mononucleosis 075 [573.1]
    malaria 084.9 [573.2]
    mumps 072.71
    secondary syphilis 091.62
    toxoplasmosis (acquired) 130.5
      congenital (active) 771.2
  epidemic - see Hepatitis, viral, type A
  fetus or newborn 774.4
  fibrous (chronic) 571.49
    acute 570
  from injection, inoculation, or
      transfusion (blood) (other
      substance) (plasma) (serum)
      (onset within 8 months after
      administration) - see Hepatitis,
      viral
  fulminant (viral) (see also Hepatitis,
      viral) 070.9
    with hepatic coma 070.6
    type A 070.1
      with hepatic coma 070.0
    type B - see Hepatitis, viral, type B
  giant cell (neonatal) 774.4
  hemorrhagic 573.8
  history of
    B V12.09
    C V12.09
  homologous serum - see Hepatitis, viral
  hypertrophic (chronic) 571.49
    acute 570
  infectious, infective (acute) (chronic)
      (subacute) 070.1
    with hepatic coma 070.0
  inoculation - see Hepatitis, viral
  interstitial (chronic) 571.49
    acute 570
  lupoid 571.49
  malarial 084.9 [573.2]
  malignant (see also Necrosis, liver) 570
  neonatal (toxic) 774.4
  newborn 774.4
  parenchymatous (acute) (see also
      Necrosis, liver) 570
  peliosis 573.3
  persistent, chronic 571.41
  plasma cell 571.49

Hepatitis (Continued)
  postimmunization - see Hepatitis, viral
  postnecrotic 571.49
  posttransfusion - see Hepatitis, viral
  recurrent 571.49
  septic 573.3
  serum - see Hepatitis, viral
    carrier (suspected of) V02.61
  subacute (see also Necrosis, liver) 570
  suppurative (diffuse) 572.0
  syphilitic (late) 095.3
    congenital (early) 090.0 [573.2]
      late 090.5 [573.2]
    secondary 091.62
  toxic (noninfectious) 573.3
    fetus or newborn 774.4
  tuberculous (see also Tuberculosis)
      017.9●
  viral (acute) (anicteric) (cholangiolitic)
      (cholestatic) (chronic) (subacute)
      070.9
    with hepatic coma 070.6
    AU-SH type virus - see Hepatitis,
        viral, type B
    Australian antigen - see Hepatitis,
        viral, type B
    B-antigen - see Hepatitis, viral, type B
    Coxsackie 074.8 [573.1]
    cytomegalic inclusion 078.5 [573.1]
    IH (virus) - see Hepatitis, viral, type A
    infectious hepatitis virus - see
        Hepatitis, viral, type A
    serum hepatitis virus - see Hepatitis,
        viral, type B
    SH - see Hepatitis, viral, type B
    specified type NEC 070.59
      with hepatic coma 070.49
    type A 070.1
      with hepatic coma 070.0
    type B (acute) 070.30
      with
        hepatic coma 070.20
      carrier status V02.61
      chronic 070.32
        with
          hepatic coma 070.22
            with hepatitis delta
                070.23
          hepatitis delta 070.33
            with hepatic coma 070.23
            with hepatitis delta 070.21
          hepatitis delta 070.31
            with hepatic coma 070.21
    type C
      acute 070.51
        with hepatic coma 070.41
      carrier status V02.62
      chronic 070.54
        with hepatic coma 070.44
        in remission 070.54
      unspecified 070.70
        with hepatic coma 070.71
    type delta (with hepatitis B carrier
        state) 070.52
      with
        active hepatitis B disease - see
            Hepatitis, viral, type B
        hepatic coma 070.42
    type E 070.53
      with hepatic coma 070.43
    vaccination and inoculation
        (prophylactic) V05.3
  Waldenström's (lupoid hepatitis)
      571.49

Hepatization, lung (acute) - see also
    Pneumonia, lobar
  chronic (see also Fibrosis, lung) 515
Hepatoblastoma (M8970/3) 155.0
Hepatocarcinoma (M8170/3) 155.0
Hepatocholangiocarcinoma (M8180/3)
    155.0
Hepatocholangioma, benign (M8180/0)
    211.5
Hepatocholangitis 573.8
Hepatocystitis (see also Cholecystitis)
    575.10
Hepatodystrophy 570
Hepatolenticular degeneration 275.1
Hepatolithiasis - see Choledocholithiasis
Hepatoma (malignant) (M8170/3) 155.0
  benign (M8170/0) 211.5
  congenital (M8970/3) 155.0
  embryonal (M8970/3) 155.0
Hepatomegalia glycogenica diffusa 271.0
Hepatomegaly (see also Hypertrophy,
    liver) 789.1
  congenital 751.69
    syphilitic 090.0
  due to Clonorchis sinensis 121.1
  Gaucher's 272.7
  syphilitic (congenital) 090.0
Hepatoptosis 573.8
Hepatorrhexis 573.8
Hepatosis, toxic 573.8
Hepatosplenomegaly 571.8
  due to S. japonicum 120.2
  hyperlipemic (Bürger-Grutz type)
      272.3
Herald patch 696.3
Hereditary - see condition
Heredodegeneration 330.9
  macular 362.70
Heredopathia atactica polyneuritiformis
    356.3
Heredosyphilis (see also Syphilis,
    congenital) 090.9
Hermaphroditism (true) 752.7
  with specified chromosomal anomaly -
      see Anomaly, chromosomes, sex
Hernia, hernial (acquired) (recurrent)
    553.9
  with
    gangrene (obstructed) NEC 551.9
    obstruction NEC 552.9
      and gangrene 551.9
  abdomen (wall) - see Hernia, ventral
  abdominal, specified site NEC 553.8
    with
      gangrene (obstructed) 551.8
      obstruction 552.8
        and gangrene 551.8
  appendix 553.8
    with
      gangrene (obstructed) 551.8
      obstruction 552.8
        and gangrene 551.8
  bilateral (inguinal) - see Hernia,
      inguinal
  bladder (sphincter)
    congenital (female) (male) 756.71
    female (see also Cystocele, female)
        618.01
    male 596.8
  brain 348.4
    congenital 742.0
  broad ligament 553.8
  cartilage, vertebral - see Displacement,
      intervertebral disc

◄ New   ◄▥ Revised   ~~deleted~~ Deleted   ● Use Additional Digit(s)   ▨ Omit code

Hernia, hernial (*Continued*)
cerebral 348.4
  congenital 742.0
  endaural 742.0
ciliary body 364.89
  traumatic 871.1
colic 553.9
  with
    gangrene (obstructed) 551.9
    obstruction 552.9
      and gangrene 551.9
colon 553.9
  with
    gangrene (obstructed) 551.9
    obstruction 552.9
      and gangrene 551.9
colostomy (stoma) 569.69
Cooper's (retroperitoneal) 553.8
  with
    gangrene (obstructed) 551.8
    obstruction 552.8
      and gangrene 551.8
crural - *see* Hernia, femoral
diaphragm, diaphragmatic 553.3
  with
    gangrene (obstructed) 551.3
    obstruction 552.3
      and gangrene 551.3
  congenital 756.6
  due to gross defect of diaphragm
    756.6
  traumatic 862.0
    with open wound into cavity
      862.1
direct (inguinal) - *see* Hernia, inguinal
disc, intervertebral - *see* Displacement,
  intervertebral disc
diverticulum, intestine 553.9
  with
    gangrene (obstructed) 551.9
    obstruction 552.9
      and gangrene 551.9
double (inguinal) - *see* Hernia,
  inguinal
due to adhesion with obstruction
  552.9 ◀▥
duodenojejunal 553.8
  with
    gangrene (obstructed) 551.8
    obstruction 552.8
      and gangrene 551.8
en glissade - *see* Hernia, inguinal
enterostomy (stoma) 569.69
epigastric 553.29
  with
    gangrene (obstruction) 551.29
    obstruction 552.29
      and gangrene 551.29
  recurrent 553.21
    with
      gangrene (obstructed)
        551.21
      obstruction 552.21
        and gangrene 551.21
esophageal hiatus (sliding) 553.3
  with
    gangrene (obstructed) 551.3
    obstruction 552.3
      and gangrene 551.3
  congenital 750.6
external (inguinal) - *see* Hernia,
  inguinal
fallopian tube 620.4
fascia 728.89

Hernia, hernial (*Continued*)
fat 729.30
  eyelid 374.34
  orbital 374.34
  pad 729.30
    eye, eyelid 374.34
    knee 729.31
    orbit 374.34
    popliteal (space) 729.31
    specified site NEC 729.39
femoral (unilateral) 553.00
  with
    gangrene (obstructed) 551.00
    obstruction 552.00
      with gangrene 551.00
  bilateral 553.02
    gangrenous (obstructed)
      551.02
    obstructed 552.02
      with gangrene 551.02
    recurrent 553.03
      gangrenous (obstructed)
        551.03
      obstructed 552.03
        with gangrene 551.03
  recurrent (unilateral) 553.01
    bilateral 553.03
      gangrenous (obstructed)
        551.03
      obstructed 552.03
        with gangrene 551.03
    gangrenous (obstructed)
      551.01
    obstructed 552.01
      with gangrene 551.01
foramen
  Bochdalek 553.3
    with
      gangrene (obstructed) 551.3
      obstruction 552.3
        and gangrene 551.3
    congenital 756.6
  magnum 348.4
  Morgagni, Morgagnian 553.3
    with
      gangrene 551.3
      obstruction 552.3
        and gangrene 551.3
    congenital 756.6
funicular (umbilical) 553.1
  with
    gangrene (obstructed) 551.1
    obstruction 552.1
      and gangrene 551.1
  spermatic cord - *see* Hernia, inguinal
gangrenous - *see* Hernia, by site, with
  gangrene
gastrointestinal tract 553.9
  with
    gangrene (obstructed) 551.9
    obstruction 552.9
      and gangrene 551.9
gluteal - *see* Hernia, femoral
Gruber's (internal mesogastric)
  553.8
  with
    gangrene (obstructed) 551.8
    obstruction 552.8
      and gangrene 551.8
Hesselbach's 553.8
  with
    gangrene (obstructed) 551.8
    obstruction 552.8
      and gangrene 551.8

Hernia, hernial (*Continued*)
hiatal (esophageal) (sliding) 553.3
  with
    gangrene (obstructed) 551.3
    obstruction 552.3
      and gangrene 551.3
  congenital 750.6
incarcerated (*see also* Hernia, by site,
  with obstruction) 552.9
  gangrenous (*see also* Hernia, by site,
    with gangrene) 551.9
incisional 553.21
  with
    gangrene (obstructed) 551.21
    obstruction 552.21
      and gangrene 551.21
  lumbar - *see* Hernia, lumbar
  recurrent 553.21
    with
      gangrene (obstructed) 551.21
      obstruction 552.21
        and gangrene 551.21
indirect (inguinal) - *see* Hernia, inguinal
infantile - *see* Hernia, inguinal
infrapatellar fat pad 729.31
inguinal (direct) (double) (encysted)
  (external) (funicular) (indirect)
  (infantile) (internal) (interstitial)
  (oblique) (scrotal) (sliding)
  550.9●

> Note: Use the following fifth-digit
> subclassification with category 550:
>
> 0   unilateral or unspecified (not
>   specified as recurrent)
> 1   unilateral or unspecified,
>   recurrent
> 2   bilateral (not specified as
>   recurrent)
> 3   bilateral, recurrent

  with
    gangrene (obstructed) 550.0●
    obstruction 550.1●
      and gangrene 550.0●
internal 553.8
  with
    gangrene (obstructed) 551.8
    obstruction 552.8
      and gangrene 551.8
  inguinal - *see* Hernia, inguinal
interstitial 553.9
  with
    gangrene (obstructed) 551.9
    obstruction 552.9
      and gangrene 551.9
  inguinal - *see* Hernia, inguinal
intervertebral cartilage or disc - *see*
  Displacement, intervertebral disc
intestine, intestinal 553.9
  with
    gangrene (obstructed) 551.9
    obstruction 552.9
      and gangrene 551.9
intra-abdominal 553.9
  with
    gangrene (obstructed) 551.9
    obstruction 552.9
      and gangrene 551.9
intraparietal 553.9
  with
    gangrene (obstructed) 551.9
    obstruction 552.9
      and gangrene 551.9

Hernia, hernial (*Continued*)
  iris 364.89
    traumatic 871.1
  irreducible (*see also* Hernia, by site,
      with obstruction) 552.9
    gangrenous (with obstruction) (*see
      also* Hernia, by site, with
      gangrene) 551.9
  ischiatic 553.8
    with
      gangrene (obstructed) 551.8
      obstruction 552.8
        and gangrene 551.8
  ischiorectal 553.8
    with
      gangrene (obstructed) 551.8
      obstruction 552.8
        and gangrene 551.8
  lens 379.32
    traumatic 871.1
  linea
    alba - *see* Hernia, epigastric
    semilunaris - *see* Hernia,
      spigelian
  Littre's (diverticular) 553.9
    with
      gangrene (obstructed) 551.9
      obstruction 552.9
        and gangrene 551.9
  lumbar 553.8
    with
      gangrene (obstructed) 551.8
      obstruction 552.8
        and gangrene 551.8
    intervertebral disc 722.10
  lung (subcutaneous) 518.89
    congenital 748.69
  mediastinum 519.3
  mesenteric (internal) 553.8
    with
      gangrene (obstructed) 551.8
      obstruction 552.8
        and gangrene 551.8
  mesocolon 553.8
    with
      gangrene (obstructed) 551.8
      obstruction 552.8
        and gangrene 551.8
  muscle (sheath) 728.89
  nucleus pulposus - *see* Displacement,
      intervertebral disc
  oblique (inguinal) - *see* Hernia,
      inguinal
  obstructive (*see also* Hernia, by site,
      with obstruction) 552.9
    gangrenous (with obstruction)
      (*see also* Hernia, by site,
      with gangrene) 551.9
  obturator 553.8
    with
      gangrene (obstructed)
        551.8
      obstruction 552.8
        and gangrene 551.8
  omental 553.8
    with
      gangrene (obstructed)
        551.8
      obstruction 552.8
        and gangrene 551.8
  orbital fat (pad) 374.34
  ovary 620.4
  oviduct 620.4
  paracolostomy (stoma) 569.69

Hernia, hernial (*Continued*)
  paraduodenal 553.8
    with
      gangrene (obstructed) 551.8
      obstruction 552.8
        and gangrene 551.8
  paraesophageal 553.3
    with
      gangrene (obstructed) 551.3
      obstruction 552.3
        and gangrene 551.3
    congenital 750.6
  parahiatal 553.3
    with
      gangrene (obstructed) 551.3
      obstruction 552.3
        and gangrene 551.3
  paraumbilical 553.1
    with
      gangrene (obstructed) 551.1
      obstruction 552.1
        and gangrene 551.1
  parietal 553.9
    with
      gangrene (obstructed) 551.9
      obstruction 552.9
        and gangrene 551.9
  perineal 553.8
    with
      gangrene (obstructed) 551.8
      obstruction 552.8
        and gangrene 551.8
  peritoneal sac, lesser 553.8
    with
      gangrene (obstructed) 551.8
      obstruction 552.8
        and gangrene 551.8
  popliteal fat pad 729.31
  postoperative 553.21
    with
      gangrene (obstructed) 551.21
      obstruction 552.21
        and gangrene 551.21
  pregnant uterus 654.4●
  prevesical 596.8
  properitoneal 553.8
    with
      gangrene (obstructed) 551.8
      obstruction 552.8
        and gangrene 551.8
  pudendal 553.8
    with
      gangrene (obstructed) 551.8
      obstruction 552.8
        and gangrene 551.8
  rectovaginal 618.6
  retroperitoneal 553.8
    with
      gangrene (obstructed)
        551.8
      obstruction 552.8
        and gangrene 551.8
  Richter's (parietal) 553.9
    with
      gangrene (obstructed)
        551.9
      obstruction 552.9
        and gangrene 551.9
  Rieux's, Riex's (retrocecal) 553.8
    with
      gangrene (obstructed)
        551.8
      obstruction 552.8
        and gangrene 551.8

Hernia, hernial (*Continued*)
  sciatic 553.8
    with
      gangrene (obstructed) 551.8
      obstruction 552.8
        and gangrene 551.8
  scrotum, scrotal - *see* Hernia, inguinal
  sliding (inguinal) - *see also* Hernia,
      inguinal
    hiatus - *see* Hernia, hiatal
  spigelian 553.29
    with
      gangrene (obstructed) 551.29
      obstruction 552.29
        and gangrene 551.29
  spinal (*see also* Spina bifida) 741.9●
    with hydrocephalus 741.0●
  strangulated (*see also* Hernia, by site,
      with obstruction) 552.9
    gangrenous (with obstruction) (*see
      also* Hernia, by site, with
      gangrene) 551.9
  supraumbilicus (linea alba) - *see*
      Hernia, epigastric
  tendon 727.9
  testis (nontraumatic) 550.9●
    meaning
      scrotal hernia 550.9●
      symptomatic late syphilis 095.8
  Treitz's (fossa) 553.8
    with
      gangrene (obstructed) 551.8
      obstruction 552.8
        and gangrene 551.8
  tunica
    albuginea 608.89
    vaginalis 752.89
  umbilicus, umbilical 553.1
    with
      gangrene (obstructed) 551.1
      obstruction 552.1
        and gangrene 551.1
  ureter 593.89
    with obstruction 593.4
  uterus 621.8
    pregnant 654.4●
  vaginal (posterior) 618.6
  Velpeau's (femoral) (*see also* Hernia,
      femoral) 553.00
  ventral 553.20
    with
      gangrene (obstructed) 551.20
      obstruction 552.20
        and gangrene 551.20
    incisional 553.21
    recurrent 553.21
      with
        gangrene (obstructed) 551.21
        obstruction 552.21
          and gangrene 551.21
  vesical
    congenital (female) (male) 756.71
    female (*see also* Cystocele, female)
      618.01
    male 596.8
  vitreous (into anterior chamber)
      379.21
    traumatic 871.1
Herniation - *see also* Hernia
  brain (stem) 348.4
  cerebral 348.4
  gastric mucosa (into duodenal bulb)
      537.89
  mediastinum 519.3

◄ New   ◄◖ Revised   ~~deleted~~ Deleted   ● Use Additional Digit(s)   ▒ Omit code

Herniation *(Continued)*
  nucleus pulposus - *see* Displacement,
    intervertebral disc
Herpangina 074.0
Herpes, herpetic 054.9
  auricularis (zoster) 053.71
    simplex 054.73
  blepharitis (zoster) 053.20
    simplex 054.41
  circinate 110.5
  circinatus 110.5
    bullous 694.5
  conjunctiva (simplex) 054.43
    zoster 053.21
  cornea (simplex) 054.43
    disciform (simplex) 054.43
    zoster 053.21
  encephalitis 054.3
  eye (zoster) 053.29
    simplex 054.40
  eyelid (zoster) 053.20
    simplex 054.41
  febrilis 054.9
  fever 054.9
  geniculate ganglionitis 053.11
  genital, genitalis 054.10
    specified site NEC 054.19
  gestationis 646.8●
  gingivostomatitis 054.2
  iridocyclitis (simplex) 054.44
    zoster 053.22
  iris (any site) 695.10
  iritis (simplex) 054.44
  keratitis (simplex) 054.43
    dendritic 054.42
    disciform 054.43
    interstitial 054.43
      zoster 053.21
  keratoconjunctivitis (simplex) 054.43
    zoster 053.21
  labialis 054.9
    meningococcal 036.89
  lip 054.9
  meningitis (simplex) 054.72
    zoster 053.0
  ophthalmicus (zoster) 053.20
    simplex 054.40
  otitis externa (zoster) 053.71
    simplex 054.73
  penis 054.13
  perianal 054.10
  pharyngitis 054.79
  progenitalis 054.10
  scrotum 054.19
  septicemia 054.5
  simplex 054.9
    complicated 054.8
      ophthalmic 054.40
        specified NEC 054.49
      specified NEC 054.79
    congenital 771.2
    external ear 054.73
    keratitis 054.43
      dendritic 054.42
    meningitis 054.72
    myelitis 054.74
    neuritis 054.79
    specified complication NEC 054.79
      ophthalmic 054.49
    visceral 054.71
  stomatitis 054.2
  tonsurans 110.0
    maculosus (of Hebra) 696.3
  visceral 054.71
  vulva 054.12

Herpes, herpetic *(Continued)*
  vulvovaginitis 054.11
  whitlow 054.6
  zoster 053.9
    auricularis 053.71
    complicated 053.8
      specified NEC 053.79
    conjunctiva 053.21
    cornea 053.21
    ear 053.71
    eye 053.29
    geniculate 053.11
    keratitis 053.21
      interstitial 053.21
    myelitis 053.14
    neuritis 053.10
    ophthalmicus(a) 053.20
    oticus 053.71
    otitis externa 053.71
    specified complication NEC 053.79
    specified site NEC 053.9
  zosteriform, intermediate type 053.9
Herrick's
  anemia (hemoglobin S disease) 282.61
  syndrome (hemoglobin S disease)
    282.61
Hers' disease (glycogenosis VI) 271.0
Herter's infantilism (nontropical sprue)
  579.0
Herter (-Gee) disease or syndrome
  (nontropical sprue) 579.0
Herxheimer's disease (diffuse idiopathic
  cutaneous atrophy) 701.8
Herxheimer's reaction 995.0
Hesitancy, urinary 788.64
Hesselbach's hernia - *see* Hernia,
  Hesselbach's
Heterochromia (congenital) 743.46
  acquired 364.53
  cataract 366.33
  cyclitis 364.21
  hair 704.3
  iritis 364.21
  retained metallic foreign body 360.62
    magnetic 360.52
  uveitis 364.21
Heterophoria 378.40
  alternating 378.45
  vertical 378.43
Heterophyes, small intestine 121.6
Heterophyiasis 121.6
Heteropsia 368.8
Heterotopia, heterotopic - *see also*
  Malposition, congenital
  cerebralis 742.4
  pancreas, pancreatic 751.7
  spinalis 742.59
Heterotropia 378.30
  intermittent 378.20
    vertical 378.31
  vertical (constant) (intermittent) 378.31
Heubner's disease 094.89
Heubner-Herter disease or syndrome
  (nontropical sprue) 579.0
Hexadactylism 755.00
Heyd's syndrome (hepatorenal) 572.4
HGSIL (high grade squamous
  intraepithelial lesion) (cytologic
  finding) (Pap smear finding)
  anus 796.74
  cervix 795.04
    biopsy finding - *code to* CIN II or
      CIN III
  vagina 795.14
Hibernoma (M8880/0) - *see* Lipoma

Hiccough 786.8
  epidemic 078.89
  psychogenic 306.1
Hiccup (*see also* Hiccough) 786.8
Hicks (-Braxton) contractures 644.1●
Hidden penis 752.65
Hidradenitis (axillaris) (suppurative)
  705.83
Hidradenoma (nodular) (M8400/0) -
  see also Neoplasm, skin, benign
  clear cell (M8402/0) - *see* Neoplasm,
    skin, benign
  papillary (M8405/0) - *see* Neoplasm,
    skin, benign
Hidrocystoma (M8404/0) - *see* Neoplasm,
  skin, benign
HIE (hypoxic-ischemic encephalopathy)
  768.70
  mild 768.71
  moderate 768.72
  severe 768.73
High
  A$_2$ anemia 282.49
  altitude effects 993.2
    anoxia 993.2
    on
      ears 993.0
      sinuses 993.1
    polycythemia 289.0
  arch
    foot 755.67
    palate 750.26
  artery (arterial) tension (*see also*
    Hypertension) 401.9
    without diagnosis of hypertension
      796.2
  basal metabolic rate (BMR) 794.7
  blood pressure (*see also* Hypertension)
    401.9
    incidental reading (isolated)
      (nonspecific), no diagnosis of
      hypertension 796.2
  cholesterol 272.0
    with high triglycerides 272.2
  compliance bladder 596.4
  diaphragm (congenital) 756.6
  frequency deafness (congenital)
    (regional) 389.8
  head at term 652.5●
    affecting fetus or newborn 763.1
  output failure (cardiac) (*see also* Failure,
    heart) 428.9
  oxygen-affinity hemoglobin 289.0
  palate 750.26
  risk
    behavior -*see* problem
    family situation V61.9
      specified circumstance NEC V61.8
    human papillomavirus (HPV) DNA
      test positive
      anal 796.75
      cervical 795.05
      vaginal 795.15
    individual NEC V62.89
    infant NEC V20.1
    patient taking drugs (prescribed)
      V67.51
      nonprescribed (*see also* Abuse,
        drugs, nondependent)
        305.9●
    pregnancy V23.9
      inadequate prenatal care V23.7
      specified problem NEC V23.89
  temperature (of unknown origin) (*see
    also* Pyrexia) 780.60

High (Continued)
thoracic rib 756.3
triglycerides 272.1
with high cholesterol 272.2
Hildenbrand's disease (typhus) 081.9
Hilger's syndrome 337.09
Hill diarrhea 579.1
Hilliard's lupus (see also Tuberculosis) 017.0●
Hilum - see condition
Hip - see condition
Hippel's disease (retinocerebral angiomatosis) 759.6
Hippus 379.49
Hirschfeld's disease (acute diabetes mellitus) (see also Diabetes) 250.0●
due to secondary diabetes 249.0●
Hirschsprung's disease or megacolon (congenital) 751.3
Hirsuties (see also Hypertrichosis) 704.1
Hirsutism (see also Hypertrichosis) 704.1
Hirudiniasis (external) (internal) 134.2
His-Werner disease (trench fever) 083.1
Hiss-Russell dysentery 004.1
Histamine cephalgia 339.00
Histidinemia 270.5
Histidinuria 270.5
Histiocytic syndromes 288.4
Histiocytoma (M8832/0) - see also Neoplasm, skin, benign
fibrous (M8830/0) - see also Neoplasm, skin, benign
atypical (M8830/1) - see Neoplasm, connective tissue, uncertain behavior
malignant (M8830/3) - see Neoplasm, connective tissue, malignant
Histiocytosis (acute) (chronic) (subacute) 277.89
acute differentiated progressive (M9722/3) 202.5●
cholesterol 277.89
essential 277.89
lipid, lipoid (essential) 272.7
lipochrome (familial) 288.1
malignant (M9720/3) 202.3●
non-Langerhans cell 277.89
polyostotic sclerosing 277.89
X (chronic) 277.89
acute (progressive) (M9722/3) 202.5●
Histoplasmosis 115.90
with
endocarditis 115.94
meningitis 115.91
pericarditis 115.93
pneumonia 115.95
retinitis 115.92
specified manifestation NEC 115.99
African (due to Histoplasma duboisii) 115.10
with
endocarditis 115.14
meningitis 115.11
pericarditis 115.13
pneumonia 115.15
retinitis 115.12
specified manifestation NEC 115.19

Histoplasmosis (Continued)
American (due to Histoplasma capsulatum) 115.00
with
endocarditis 115.04
meningitis 115.01
pericarditis 115.03
pneumonia 115.05
retinitis 115.02
specified manifestation NEC 115.09
Darling's - see Histoplasmosis, American
large form (see also Histoplasmosis, African) 115.10
lung 115.05
small form (see also Histoplasmosis, American) 115.00
History (personal) of
abuse
emotional V15.42
neglect V15.42
physical V15.41
sexual V15.41
affective psychosis V11.1
alcoholism V11.3
specified as drinking problem (see also Abuse, drugs, nondependent) 305.0●
allergy (to) V15.09 ◀▦
analgesic agent NEC V14.6
anesthetic NEC V14.4
antibiotic agent NEC V14.1
penicillin V14.0
anti-infective agent NEC V14.3
arachnid bite V15.06
diathesis V15.09
drug V14.9
specified type NEC V14.8
eggs V15.03
food additives V15.05
insect bite V15.06
latex V15.07
medicinal agents V14.9
specified type NEC V14.8
milk products V15.02
narcotic agent NEC V14.5
nuts V15.05
peanuts V15.01
penicillin V14.0
radiographic dye V15.08
seafood V15.04
serum V14.7
specified food NEC V15.05
specified nonmedicinal agents NEC V15.09
spider bite V15.06
sulfa V14.2
sulfonamides V14.2
therapeutic agent NEC V15.09
vaccine V14.7
anaphylactic shock V15.09 ◀
anemia V12.3
arrest, sudden cardiac V12.53
arthritis V13.4
attack, transient ischemic (TIA) V12.54
benign neoplasm of brain V12.41
blood disease V12.3
calculi, urinary V13.01
cardiovascular disease V12.50
myocardial infarction 412
chemotherapy, antineoplastic V87.41
child abuse V15.41
cigarette smoking V15.82
circulatory system disease V12.50
myocardial infarction 412
cleft lip and palate, corrected V13.64 ◀

History (Continued)
combat and operational stress reaction V11.4 ◀
congenital malformation (corrected)
~~V13.69~~ ◀▦
circulatory system V13.65 ◀
digestive system V13.67 ◀
ear V13.64 ◀
eye V13.64 ◀
face V13.64 ◀
genitourinary system V13.62 ◀
heart V13.65 ◀
integument V13.68 ◀
limbs V13.68 ◀
musculoskeletal V13.68 ◀
neck V13.64 ◀
nervous system V13.63 ◀
respiratory system V13.66 ◀
specified type NEC V13.69 ◀
contraception V15.7
death, sudden, successfully resuscitated V12.53
deficit
prolonged reversible ischemic neurologic (PRIND) V12.54
reversible ischemic neurologic (RIND) V12.54
diathesis, allergic V15.09
digestive system disease V12.70
peptic ulcer V12.71
polyps, colonic V12.72
specified NEC V12.79
disease (of) V13.9
blood V12.3
blood-forming organs V12.3
cardiovascular system V12.50
circulatory system V12.50
specified NEC V12.59
digestive system V12.70
peptic ulcer V12.71
polyps, colonic V12.72
specified NEC V12.79
infectious V12.00
malaria V12.03
methicillin resistant Staphylococcus aureus (MRSA) V12.04
MRSA (methicillin resistant Staphylococcus aureus) V12.04
poliomyelitis V12.02
specified NEC V12.09
tuberculosis V12.01
parasitic V12.00
specified NEC V12.09
respiratory system V12.60
pneumonia V12.61
specified NEC V12.69
skin V13.3
specified site NEC V13.8
subcutaneous tissue V13.3
trophoblastic V13.1
affecting management of pregnancy V23.1
disorder (of) V13.9
endocrine V12.2
genital system V13.29
hematological V12.3
immunity V12.2
mental V11.9
affective type V11.1
manic-depressive V11.1
neurosis V11.2
schizophrenia V11.0
specified type NEC V11.8
metabolic V12.2

◀ New   ◀▦ Revised   ~~deleted~~ Deleted   ● Use Additional Digit(s)   ▦ Omit code

History *(Continued)*
  disorder *(Continued)*
    musculoskeletal NEC V13.59
    nervous system V12.40
      specified type NEC V12.49
    obstetric V13.29
      affecting management of current
          pregnancy V23.49
          pre-term labor V23.41
      pre-term labor V13.21
    sense organs V12.40
      specified type NEC V12.49
    specified site NEC V13.8
    urinary system V13.00
      calculi V13.01
      infection V13.02
      nephrotic syndrome V13.03
      specified NEC V13.09
  drug use
    nonprescribed *(see also* Abuse,
        drugs, nondependent) 305.9●
    patent *(see also* Abuse, drugs,
        nondependent) 305.9●
  dysplasia
    cervical (conditions classifiable to
        622.10–622.12) V13.22
    vaginal (conditions classifiable to
        623.0) V13.23 ◀
    vulvar (conditions classifiable to
        624.01-624.02) V13.24 ◀
  effect NEC of external cause V15.89
  embolism (pulmonary) V12.51
  emotional abuse V15.42
  encephalitis V12.42
  endocrine disorder V12.2
  estrogen therapy V87.43
  extracorporeal membrane oxygenation
    (ECMO) V15.87
  failed
    conscious sedation V15.80
    moderate sedation V15.80
  falling V15.88
  family
    allergy V19.6
    anemia V18.2
    arteriosclerosis V17.49
    arthritis V17.7
    asthma V17.5
    blindness V19.0
    blood disorder NEC V18.3
    cardiovascular disease V17.49
    carrier, genetic disease V18.9
    cerebrovascular disease V17.1
    chronic respiratory condition NEC
      V17.6
    colonic polyps V18.51
    congenital anomalies V19.5
    consanguinity V19.7
    coronary artery disease V17.3
    cystic fibrosis V18.19
    deafness V19.2
    diabetes mellitus V18.0
    digestive disorders V18.59
    disease or disorder (of)
      allergic V19.6
      blood NEC V18.3
      cardiovascular NEC V17.49
      cerebrovascular V17.1
      colonic polyps V18.51
      coronary artery V17.3
      death, sudden cardiac (SCD)
        V17.41
      digestive V18.59
      ear NEC V19.3
      endocrine V18.19
        multiple neoplasia (MEN)
          syndrome V18.11 ◀▦

History *(Continued)*
  family *(Continued)*
    disease or disorder *(Continued)*
      eye NEC V19.1
      genitourinary NEC V18.7
      hypertensive V17.49
      infectious V18.8
      ischemic heart V17.3
      kidney V18.69
        polycystic V18.61
      mental V17.0
      metabolic V18.19
      musculoskeletal NEC V17.89
        osteoporosis V17.81
      neurological NEC V17.2
      parasitic V18.8
      psychiatric condition V17.0
      skin condition V19.4
    ear disorder NEC V19.3
    endocrine disease V18.19
      multiple neoplasia (MEN)
        syndrome V18.11 ◀▦
    epilepsy V17.2
    eye disorder NEC V19.1
    genetic disease carrier V18.9
    genitourinary disease NEC V18.7
    glomerulonephritis V18.69
    gout V18.19
    hay fever V17.6
    hearing loss V19.2
    hematopoietic neoplasia V16.7
    Hodgkin's disease V16.7
    Huntington's chorea V17.2
    hydrocephalus V19.5
    hypertension V17.49
    infarction, myocardial V17.3
    infectious disease V18.8
    ischemic heart disease V17.3
    kidney disease V18.69
      polycystic V18.61
    leukemia V16.6
    lymphatic malignant neoplasia
      NEC V16.7
    malignant neoplasm (of) NEC V16.9
      anorectal V16.0
      anus V16.0
      appendix V16.0
      bladder V16.52
      bone V16.8
      brain V16.8
      breast V16.3
        male V16.8
      bronchus V16.1
      cecum V16.0
      cervix V16.49
      colon V16.0
      duodenum V16.0
      esophagus V16.0
      eye V16.8
      gallbladder V16.0
      gastrointestinal tract V16.0
      genital organs V16.40
      hemopoietic NEC V16.7
      ileum V16.0
      ilium V16.8
      intestine V16.0
      intrathoracic organs NEC V16.2
      kidney V16.51
      larynx V16.2
      liver V16.0
      lung V16.1
      lymphatic NEC V16.7
      ovary V16.41
      oviduct V16.41
      pancreas V16.0
      penis V16.49
      prostate V16.42

History *(Continued)*
  family *(Continued)*
    malignant neoplasm *(Continued)*
      rectum V16.0
      respiratory organs NEC V16.2
      skin V16.8
      specified site NEC V16.8
      stomach V16.0
      testis V16.43
      trachea V16.1
      ureter V16.59
      urethra V16.59
      urinary organs V16.59
      uterus V16.49
      vagina V16.49
      vulva V16.49
    MEN (multiple endocrine neoplasia
      syndrome) V18.11
    mental retardation V18.4
    metabolic disease NEC V18.19
    mongolism V19.5
    multiple
      endocrine neoplasia (MEN)
        syndrome V18.11 ◀▦
      myeloma V16.7
    musculoskeletal disease NEC V17.89
      osteoporosis V17.81
    myocardial infarction V17.3
    nephritis V18.69
    nephrosis V18.69
      osteoporosis V17.81
    parasitic disease V18.8
    polycystic kidney disease V18.61
    psychiatric disorder V17.0
    psychosis V17.0
    retardation, mental V18.4
    retinitis pigmentosa V19.1
    schizophrenia V17.0
    skin conditions V19.4
    specified condition NEC V19.8
    stroke (cerebrovascular) V17.1
    sudden cardiac death (SCD) V17.41
    visual loss V19.0
  foreign body fully removed V15.53 ◀
  fracture, healed
    pathologic V13.51
    stress V13.52
    traumatic V15.51
  genital system disorder V13.29
    pre-term labor V13.21
  health hazard V15.9
    falling V15.88
    specified cause NEC V15.89
  hepatitis
    B V12.09
    C V12.09
  Hodgkin's disease V10.72
  hypospadias (corrected) V13.61 ◀▦
  immunity disorder V12.2
  immunosuppression therapy V87.46
  infarction, cerebral, without residual
    deficits V12.54
  infection
    central nervous system V12.42
    urinary (tract) V13.02
  infectious disease V12.00
    malaria V12.03
    methicillin resistant Staphylococcus
      aureus (MRSA) V12.04
    MRSA (methicillin resistant
      Staphylococcus aureus)
      V12.04 poliomyelitis V12.02
    specified NEC V12.09
    tuberculosis V12.01
  injury NEC V15.59
    traumatic brain V15.52
  insufficient prenatal care V23.7

History *(Continued)*
  in utero procedure
      during pregnancy V15.21
        while a fetus V15.22
  irradiation V15.3
  leukemia V10.60
      lymphoid V10.61
      monocytic V10.63
      myeloid V10.62
      specified type NEC V10.69
  little or no prenatal care V23.7
  low birth weight *(see also* Status, low
        birth weight) V21.30
  lymphosarcoma V10.71
  malaria V12.03
  malignant carcinoid tumor V10.91
  malignant neoplasm (of) V10.90
      accessory sinus V10.22
      adrenal V10.88
      anus V10.06
      bile duct V10.09
      bladder V10.51
      bone V10.81
      brain V10.85
      breast V10.3
      bronchus V10.11
      cervix uteri V10.41
      colon V10.05
      connective tissue NEC V10.89
      corpus uteri V10.42
      digestive system V10.00
        specified part NEC V10.09
      duodenum V10.09
      endocrine gland NEC V10.88
      epididymis V10.48
      esophagus V10.03
      eye V10.84
      fallopian tube V10.44
      female genital organ V10.40
        specified site NEC V10.44
      gallbladder V10.09
      gastrointestinal tract V10.00
      gum V10.02
      hematopoietic NEC V10.79
      hypopharynx V10.02
      ileum V10.09
      intrathoracic organs NEC V10.20
      jejunum V10.09
      kidney V10.52
      large intestine V10.05
      larynx V10.21
      lip V10.02
      liver V10.07
      lung V10.11
      lymphatic NEC V10.79
      lymph glands or nodes NEC V10.79
      male genital organ V10.45
        specified site NEC V10.49
      mediastinum V10.29
      melanoma (of skin) V10.82
      middle ear V10.22
      mouth V10.02
        specified part NEC V10.02
      nasal cavities V10.22
      nasopharynx V10.02
      nervous system NEC V10.86
      nose V10.22
      oropharynx V10.02
      ovary V10.43
      pancreas V10.09
      parathyroid V10.88
      penis V10.49
      pharynx V10.02
      pineal V10.88
      pituitary V10.88
      placenta V10.44
      pleura V10.29

History *(Continued)*
  malignant neoplasm *(Continued)*
      prostate V10.46
      rectosigmoid junction V10.06
      rectum V10.06
      renal pelvis V10.53
      respiratory organs NEC V10.20
      salivary gland V10.02
      skin V10.83
        melanoma V10.82
      small intestine NEC V10.09
      soft tissue NEC V10.89
      specified site NEC V10.89
      stomach V10.04
      testis V10.47
      thymus V10.29
      thyroid V10.87
      tongue V10.01
      trachea V10.12
      ureter V10.59
      urethra V10.59
      urinary organ V10.50
      uterine adnexa V10.44
      uterus V10.42
      vagina V10.44
      vulva V10.44
  malignant neuroendocrine tumor V10.91
  manic-depressive psychosis V11.1
  meningitis V12.42
  mental disorder V11.9
      affective type V11.1
      manic-depressive V11.1
      neurosis V11.2
      schizophrenia V11.0
      specified type NEC V11.8
  Merkel cell carcinoma V10.91
  metabolic disorder V12.2
  methicillin resistant Staphylococcus
        aureus (MRSA) V12.04
  MRSA (methicillin resistant
        Staphylococcus aureus) V12.04
  musculoskeletal disorder NEC V13.59
  myocardial infarction 412
  neglect (emotional) V15.42
  nephrotic syndrome V13.03
  nervous system disorder V12.40
      specified type NEC V12.49
  neurosis V11.2
  noncompliance with medical treatment
        V15.81
  nutritional deficiency V12.1
  obstetric disorder V13.29
      affecting management of current
            pregnancy V23.49
        pre-term labor V23.41
      pre-term labor V13.21
  parasitic disease V12.00
      specified NEC V12.09
  perinatal problems V13.7
      low birth weight *(see also* Status,
            low birth weight) V21.30
  physical abuse V15.41
  poisoning V15.6
  poliomyelitis V12.02
  polyps, colonic V12.72
  poor obstetric V13.29
      affecting management of current
            pregnancy V23.49
        pre-term labor V23.41
      pre-term labor V13.21
  prolonged reversible ischemic
        neurologic deficit (PRIND)
        V12.54
  psychiatric disorder V11.9
      affective type V11.1
      manic-depressive V11.1
      neurosis V11.2

History *(Continued)*
  psychiatric disorder *(Continued)*
      schizophrenia V11.0
      specified type NEC V11.8
  psychological trauma V15.49
      emotional abuse V15.42
      neglect V15.42
      physical abuse V15.41
      rape V15.41
  psychoneurosis V11.2
  radiation therapy V15.3
  rape V15.41
  respiratory system disease
        V12.60
      pneumonia V12.61
      specified NEC V12.69
  reticulosarcoma V10.71
  return from military deployment
        V62.22
  reversible ischemic neurologic deficit
        (RIND) V12.54
  schizophrenia V11.0
  skin disease V13.3
  smoking (tobacco) V15.82
  steroid therapy V87.45
      inhaled V87.44
      systemic V87.45
  stroke without residual deficits
        V12.54
  subcutaneous tissue disease V13.3
  sudden
      cardiac
        arrest V12.53
        death (successfully resuscitated)
            V12.53
  surgery to
      great vessels V15.1
      heart V15.1
      in utero
        during pregnancy V15.21
        while a fetus V15.22
      organs NEC V15.29
  syndrome, nephrotic V13.03
  therapy
      antineoplastic drug V87.41
      drug NEC V87.49
      estrogen V87.43
      immunosuppression V87.46
      monoclonal drug V87.42
      steroid V87.45
        inhaled V87.44
        systemic V87.45
  thrombophlebitis V12.52
  thrombosis V12.51
  tobacco use V15.82
  trophoblastic disease V13.1
      affecting management of pregnancy
            V23.1
  tuberculosis V12.01
  ulcer, peptic V12.71
  urinary system disorder V13.00
      calculi V13.01
      infection V13.02
      nephrotic syndrome V13.03
      specified NEC V13.09
HIT (heparin-induced thrombocytopenia)
        289.84
HIV infection (disease) (illness) - *see*
        Human immunodeficiency virus
        (disease) (illness) (infection)
Hives (bold) *(see also* Urticaria)
        708.9
Hoarseness 784.42
Hobnail liver - *see* Cirrhosis, portal
Hobo, hoboism V60.0

◀ New   ◀▥ Revised   ~~deleted~~ Deleted   ● Use Additional Digit(s)   ▨ Omit code

Hodgkin's
  disease (M9650/3) 201.9●
    lymphocytic
      depletion (M9653/3) 201.7●
        diffuse fibrosis (M9654/3)
          201.7●
        reticular type (M9655/3)
          201.7●
      predominance (M9651/3)
        201.4●
    lymphocytic-histiocytic
      predominance (M9651/3)
        201.4●
    mixed cellularity (M9652/3) 201.6●
    nodular sclerosis (M9656/3) 201.5●
      cellular phase (M9657/3) 201.5●
  granuloma (M9661/3) 201.1●
  lymphogranulomatosis (M9650/3)
    201.9●
  lymphoma (M9650/3) 201.9●
  lymphosarcoma (M9650/3) 201.9●
  paragranuloma (M9660/3) 201.0●
  sarcoma (M9662/3) 201.2●
Hodgson's disease (aneurysmal dilatation
    of aorta) 441.9
  ruptured 441.5
Hodi-potsy 111.0
Hoffa (-Kastert) disease or syndrome
    (liposynovitis prepatellaris) 272.8
Hoffmann's syndrome 244.9 [359.5]
Hoffmann-Bouveret syndrome
    (paroxysmal tachycardia) 427.2
Hole
  macula 362.54
  optic disc, crater-like 377.22
  retina (macula) 362.54
    round 361.31
      with detachment 361.01
Holla disease (see also Spherocytosis) 282.0
Holländer-Simons syndrome
    (progressive lipodystrophy) 272.6
Hollow foot (congenital) 754.71
  acquired 736.73
Holmes' syndrome (visual disorientation)
    368.16
Holoprosencephaly 742.2
  due to
    trisomy 13 758.1
    trisomy 18 758.2
Holthouse's hernia - see Hernia, inguinal
Homesickness 309.89
Homicidal ideation V62.85 ◀
Homocystinemia 270.4
Homocystinuria 270.4
Homologous serum jaundice
    (prophylactic) (therapeutic) - see
    Hepatitis, viral
Homosexuality - omit code
  ego-dystonic 302.0
  pedophilic 302.2
  problems with 302.0
Homozygous Hb-S disease 282.61
Honeycomb lung 518.89
  congenital 748.4
Hong Kong ear 117.3
HOOD (hereditary osteo-
    onychodysplasia) 756.89
Hooded
  clitoris 752.49
  penis 752.69
Hookworm (anemia) (disease)
    (infestation) - see Ancylostomiasis
Hoppe-Goldflam syndrome 358.00
Hordeolum (external) (eyelid) 373.11
  internal 373.12

Horn
  cutaneous 702.8
    cheek 702.8
    eyelid 702.8
    penis 702.8
  iliac 756.89
  nail 703.8
    congenital 757.5
  papillary 700
Horner's
  syndrome (see also Neuropathy,
    peripheral, autonomic) 337.9
    traumatic 954.0
  teeth 520.4
Horseshoe kidney (congenital) 753.3
Horton's
  disease (temporal arteritis) 446.5
  headache or neuralgia 339.00
Hospice care V66.7
Hospitalism (in children) NEC 309.83
Hourglass contraction, contracture
  bladder 596.8
  gallbladder 575.2
    congenital 751.69
  stomach 536.8
    congenital 750.7
    psychogenic 306.4
  uterus 661.4●
    affecting fetus or newborn 763.7
Household circumstance affecting care
    V60.9
  specified type NEC V60.89
Housemaid's knee 727.2
Housing circumstance affecting care V60.9
  specified type NEC V60.89
HTR (hemolytic transfusion reaction) ◀
  due to or resulting from ◀
    incompatibility ◀
      ABO 999.61 ◀
        acute 999.62 ◀
        delayed 999.63 ◀
      non-ABO antigen (minor) (Duffy)
        (Kell) (Kidd) (Lewis) (M) (N)
        (P) (S) 999.76 ◀
        acute 999.77 ◀
        delayed 999.78 ◀
      Rh antigen (C) (c) (D) (E) (e)
        999.71 ◀
        acute 999.72 ◀
        delayed 999.73 ◀
Huchard's disease (continued arterial
    hypertension) 401.9
Hudson-Stähli lines 371.11
Huguier's disease (uterine fibroma) 218.9
Hum, venous - omit code
Human bite (open wound) - (see also
    Wound, open, by site)
  intact skin surface - see Contusion
Human immunodeficiency virus
    (disease) (illness) 042
  infection V08
    with symptoms, symptomatic 042
Human immunodeficiency virus-2
    infection 079.53
Human immunovirus (disease) (illness)
    (infection) - see Human
    immunodeficiency virus (disease)
    (illness) (infection)
Human papillomavirus 079.4
  high risk, DNA test positive
    anal 796.75
    cervical 795.05
    vaginal 795.15
  low risk, DNA test positive
    anal 796.79
    cervical 795.09
    vaginal 795.19

Human parvovirus 079.83
Human T-cell lymphotrophic virus I
    infection 079.51
Human T-cell lymphotrophic virus II
    infection 079.52
Human T-cell lymphotropic virus-III
    (disease) (illness) (infection) - see
    Human immunodeficiency virus
    (disease) (illness) (infection)
HTLV-I infection 079.51
HTLV-II infection 079.52
HTLV-III (disease) (illness) (infection) -
    see Human immunodeficiency
    virus (disease) (illness) (infection)
HTLV-III/LAV (disease) (illness)
    (infection) - see Human
    immunodeficiency virus (disease)
    (illness) (infection)
Humpback (acquired) 737.9
  congenital 756.19
Hunchback (acquired) 737.9
  congenital 756.19
Hunger 994.2
  air, psychogenic 306.1
  disease 251.1
Hungry bone syndrome 275.5
Hunner's ulcer (see also Cystitis) 595.1
Hunt's
  neuralgia 053.11
  syndrome (herpetic geniculate
    ganglionitis) 053.11
    dyssynergia cerebellaris myoclonica
      334.2
Hunter's glossitis 529.4
Hunter (-Hurler) syndrome
    (mucopolysaccharidosis II) 277.5
Hunterian chancre 091.0
Huntington's
  chorea 333.4
  disease 333.4
Huppert's disease (multiple myeloma)
    (M9730/3) 203.0●
Hurler (-Hunter) disease or syndrome
    (mucopolysaccharidosis II) 277.5
Hürthle cell
  adenocarcinoma (M8290/3) 193
  adenoma (M8290/0) 226
  carcinoma (M8290/3) 193
  tumor (M8290/0) 226
Hutchinson's
  disease meaning
    angioma serpiginosum 709.1
    cheiropompholyx 705.81
    prurigo estivalis 692.72
    summer eruption, or summer
      prurigo 692.72
  incisors 090.5
  melanotic freckle (M8742/2) - see also
    Neoplasm, skin, in situ
    malignant melanoma in (M8742/3) -
      see Melanoma
  teeth or incisors (congenital syphilis)
    090.5
Hutchinson-Boeck disease or syndrome
    (sarcoidosis) 135
Hutchinson-Gilford disease or syndrome
    (progeria) 259.8
Hyaline
  degeneration (diffuse) (generalized)
    728.9
    localized - see Degeneration, by site
  membrane (disease) (lung) (newborn)
    769
Hyalinosis cutis et mucosae 272.8
Hyalin plaque, sclera, senile 379.16

Hyalitis (asteroid) 379.22
  syphilitic 095.8
Hydatid
  cyst or tumor - *see also* Echinococcus
    fallopian tube 752.11
  mole - *see* Hydatidiform mole
  Morgagni (congenital) 752.89
    fallopian tube 752.11
Hydatidiform mole (benign)
    (complicating pregnancy)
    (delivered) (undelivered) 630
  invasive (M9100/1) 236.1
  malignant (M9100/1) 236.1
  previous, affecting management of
    pregnancy V23.1
Hydatidosis - *see* Echinococcus
Hyde's disease (prurigo nodularis) 698.3
Hydradenitis 705.83
Hydradenoma (M8400/0) - *see*
    Hidradenoma
Hydralazine lupus or syndrome
  correct substance properly
    administered 695.4
  overdose or wrong substance given or
    taken 972.6
Hydramnios 657●
  affecting fetus or newborn 761.3
Hydrancephaly 742.3
  with spina bifida (*see also* Spina bifida)
    741.0●
Hydranencephaly 742.3
  with spina bifida (*see also* Spina bifida)
    741.0●
Hydrargyrism NEC 985.0
Hydrarthrosis (*see also* Effusion, joint)
    719.0●
  gonococcal 098.50
  intermittent (*see also* Rheumatism,
    palindromic) 719.3●
  of yaws (early) (late) 102.6
  syphilitic 095.8
    congenital 090.5
Hydremia 285.9
Hydrencephalocele (congenital) 742.0
Hydrencephalomeningocele (congenital)
    742.0
Hydroa 694.0
  aestivale 692.72
  gestationis 646.8●
  herpetiformis 694.0
  pruriginosa 694.0
  vacciniforme 692.72
Hydroadenitis 705.83
Hydrocalycosis (*see also* Hydronephrosis)
    591
  congenital 753.29
Hydrocalyx (*see also* Hydronephrosis) 591
Hydrocele (calcified) (chylous)
    (idiopathic) (infantile) (inguinal
    canal) (recurrent) (senile) (spermatic
    cord) (testis) (tunica vaginalis) 603.9
  canal of Nuck (female) 629.1
    male 603.9
  congenital 778.6
  encysted 603.0
    congenital 778.6
  female NEC 629.89
  infected 603.1
  round ligament 629.89
  specified type NEC 603.8
    congenital 778.6
  spinalis (*see also* Spina bifida) 741.9●
  vulva 624.8
Hydrocephalic fetus
  affecting management or pregnancy
    655.0●

Hydrocephalic fetus (*Continued*)
  causing disproportion 653.6●
    with obstructed labor 660.1●
      affecting fetus or newborn 763.1
Hydrocephalus (acquired) (external)
    (internal) (malignant)
    (noncommunicating) (obstructive)
    (recurrent) 331.4
  aqueduct of Sylvius stricture 742.3
    with spina bifida (*see also* Spina
      bifida) 741.0●
  chronic 742.3
    with spina bifida (*see also* Spina
      bifida) 741.0●
  communicating 331.3
  congenital (external) (internal) 742.3
    with spina bifida (*see also* Spina
      bifida) 741.0●
  due to
    stricture of aqueduct of Sylvius 742.3
      with spina bifida (*see also* Spina
        bifida) 741.0●
    toxoplasmosis (congenital) 771.2
  fetal affecting management of
    pregnancy 655.0●
  foramen Magendie block (acquired) 331.3
    congenital 742.3
      with spina bifida (*see also* Spina
        bifida) 741.0●
  newborn 742.3
    with spina bifida (*see also* Spina
      bifida) 741.0●
  normal pressure 331.5
    idiopathic (INPH) 331.5
    secondary 331.3
  otitic 348.2
  syphilitic, congenital 090.49
  tuberculous (*see also* Tuberculosis)
    013.8●
Hydrocolpos (congenital) 623.8
Hydrocystoma (M8404/0) - *see* Neoplasm,
    skin, benign
Hydroencephalocele (congenital) 742.0
Hydroencephalomeningocele
    (congenital) 742.0
Hydrohematopneumothorax (*see also*
    Hemothorax) 511.89
Hydromeningitis - *see* Meningitis
Hydromeningocele (spinal) (*see also* Spina
    bifida) 741.9●
  cranial 742.0
Hydrometra 621.8
Hydrometrocolpos 623.8
Hydromicrocephaly 742.1
Hydromphalus (congenital) (since birth)
    757.39
Hydromyelia 742.53
Hydromyelocele (*see also* Spina bifida)
    741.9●
Hydronephrosis 591
  atrophic 591
  congenital 753.29
  due to S. hematobium 120.0
  early 591
  functionless (infected) 591
  infected 591
  intermittent 591
  primary 591
  secondary 591
  tuberculous (*see also* Tuberculosis)
    016.0●
Hydropericarditis (*see also* Pericarditis)
    423.9
Hydropericardium (*see also* Pericarditis)
    423.9

Hydroperitoneum 789.59
Hydrophobia 071
Hydrophthalmos (*see also* Buphthalmia)
    743.20
Hydropneumohemothorax (*see also*
    Hemothorax) 511.89
Hydropneumopericarditis (*see also*
    Pericarditis) 423.9
Hydropneumopericardium (*see also*
    Pericarditis) 423.9
Hydropneumothorax 511.89
  nontuberculous 511.89
    bacterial 511.1
  pneumococcal 511.1
  staphylococcal 511.1
  streptococcal 511.1
  traumatic 860.0
    with open wound into thorax 860.1
  tuberculous (*see also* Tuberculosis,
    pleura) 012.0●
Hydrops 782.3
  abdominis 789.59
  amnii (complicating pregnancy) (*see
    also* Hydramnios) 657●
  articulorum intermittens (*see also*
    Rheumatism, palindromic)
    719.3●
  cardiac (*see also* Failure, heart) 428.0
  congenital - *see* Hydrops, fetalis
  endolymphatic (*see also* Disease,
    Ménière's) 386.00
  fetal(is) or newborn 778.0
    due to isoimmunization 773.3
    not due to isoimmunization 778.0
  gallbladder 575.3
  idiopathic (fetus or newborn) 778.0
  joint (*see also* Effusion, joint) 719.0●
  labyrinth (*see also* Disease, Ménière's)
    386.00
  meningeal NEC 331.4
  nutritional 262
  pericardium - *see* Pericarditis
  pleura (*see also* Hydrothorax) 511.89
  renal (*see also* Nephrosis) 581.9
  spermatic cord (*see also* Hydrocele) 603.9
Hydropyonephrosis (*see also* Pyelitis)
    590.80
  chronic 590.00
Hydrorachis 742.53
Hydrorrhea (nasal) 478.19
  gravidarum 658.1●
  pregnancy 658.1●
Hydrosadenitis 705.83
Hydrosalpinx (fallopian tube)
    (follicularis) 614.1
Hydrothorax (double) (pleural) 511.89
  chylous (nonfilarial) 457.8
    filaria (*see also* Infestation, filarial)
      125.9
  nontuberculous 511.89
    bacterial 511.1
  pneumococcal 511.1
  staphylococcal 511.1
  streptococcal 511.1
  traumatic 862.29
    with open wound into thorax 862.39
  tuberculous (*see also* Tuberculosis,
    pleura) 012.0●
Hydroureter 593.5
  congenital 753.22
Hydroureteronephrosis (*see also*
    Hydronephrosis) 591
Hydrourethra 599.84
Hydroxykynureninuria 270.2
Hydroxyprolinemia 270.8
Hydroxyprolinuria 270.8

Hygroma (congenital) (cystic) (M9173/0) 228.1
  prepatellar 727.3
  subdural - *see* Hematoma, subdural
Hymen - *see* condition
Hymenolepiasis (diminuta) (infection) (infestation) (nana) 123.6
Hymenolepsis (diminuta) (infection) (infestation) (nana) 123.6
Hypalgesia (*see also* Disturbance, sensation) 782.0
Hyperabduction syndrome 447.8
Hyperacidity, gastric 536.8
  psychogenic 306.4
Hyperactive, hyperactivity 314.01
  basal cell, uterine cervix 622.10
  bladder 596.51
  bowel (syndrome) 564.9
    sounds 787.5
  cervix epithelial (basal) 622.10
  child 314.01
  colon 564.9
  gastrointestinal 536.8
    psychogenic 306.4
  intestine 564.9
  labyrinth (unilateral) 386.51
    with loss of labyrinthine reactivity 386.58
    bilateral 386.52
  nasal mucous membrane 478.19
  stomach 536.8
  thyroid (gland) (*see also* Thyrotoxicosis) 242.9●
Hyperacusis 388.42
Hyperadrenalism (cortical) 255.3
  medullary 255.6
Hyperadrenocorticism 255.3
  congenital 255.2
  iatrogenic
    correct substance properly administered 255.3
    overdose or wrong substance given or taken 962.0
Hyperaffectivity 301.11
Hyperaldosteronism (atypical) (hyperplastic) (normoaldosteronal) (nor-motensive) (primary) 255.10
  secondary 255.14
Hyperalgesia (*see also* Disturbance, sensation) 782.0
Hyperalimentation 783.6
  carotene 278.3
  specified NEC 278.8
  vitamin A 278.2
  vitamin D 278.4
Hyperaminoaciduria 270.9
  arginine 270.6
  citrulline 270.6
  cystine 270.0
  glycine 270.0
  lysine 270.7
  ornithine 270.6
  renal (types I, II, III) 270.0
Hyperammonemia (congenital) 270.6
Hyperamnesia 780.99
Hyperamylasemia 790.5
Hyperaphia 782.0
Hyperazotemia 791.9
Hyperbetalipoproteinemia (acquired) (essential) (familial) (hereditary) (primary) (secondary) 272.0
  with prebetalipoproteinemia 272.2
Hyperbilirubinemia 782.4
  congenital 277.4
  constitutional 277.4
  neonatal (transient) (*see also* Jaundice, fetus or newborn) 774.6
  of prematurity 774.2

Hyperbilirubinemica encephalopathia, newborn 774.7
  due to isoimmunization 773.4
Hypercalcemia, hypercalcemic (idiopathic) 275.42
  nephropathy 588.89
Hypercalcinuria 275.40
Hypercapnia 786.09
  with mixed acid-based disorder 276.4
  fetal, affecting newborn 770.89
Hypercarotinemia 278.3
Hypercementosis 521.5
Hyperchloremia 276.9
Hyperchlorhydria 536.8
  neurotic 306.4
  psychogenic 306.4
Hypercholesterinemia - *see* Hypercholesterolemia
Hypercholesterolemia 272.0
  with hyperglyceridemia, endogenous 272.2
  essential 272.0
  familial 272.0
  hereditary 272.0
  primary 272.0
  pure 272.0
Hypercholesterolosis 272.0
Hyperchylia gastrica 536.8
  psychogenic 306.4
Hyperchylomicronemia (familial) (with hyperbetalipoproteinemia) 272.3
Hypercoagulation syndrome (primary) 289.81
  secondary 289.82
Hypercorticosteronism
  correct substance properly administered 255.3
  overdose or wrong substance given or taken 962.0
Hypercortisonism
  correct substance properly administered 255.3
  overdose or wrong substance given or taken 962.0
Hyperdynamic beta-adrenergic state or syndrome (circulatory) 429.82
Hyperekplexia 759.89
Hyperelectrolytemia 276.9
Hyperemesis 536.2
  arising during pregnancy - *see* Hyperemesis, gravidarum
  gravidarum (mild) (before 22 completed weeks' gestation) 643.0●
    with
      carbohydrate depletion 643.1●
      dehydration 643.1●
      electrolyte imbalance 643.1●
      metabolic disturbance 643.1●
    affecting fetus or newborn 761.8
    severe (with metabolic disturbance) 643.1●
  psychogenic 306.4
Hyperemia (acute) 780.99
  anal mucosa 569.49
  bladder 596.7
  cerebral 437.8
  conjunctiva 372.71
  ear, internal, acute 386.30
  enteric 564.89
  eye 372.71
  eyelid (active) (passive) 374.82
  intestine 564.89
  iris 364.41
  kidney 593.81

Hyperemia (*Continued*)
  labyrinth 386.30
  liver (active) (passive) 573.8
  lung 514
  ovary 620.8
  passive 780.99
  pulmonary 514
  renal 593.81
  retina 362.89
  spleen 289.59
  stomach 537.89
Hyperesthesia (body surface) (*see also* Disturbance, sensation) 782.0
  larynx (reflex) 478.79
    hysterical 300.11
  pharynx (reflex) 478.29
Hyperestrinism 256.0
Hyperestrogenism 256.0
Hyperestrogenosis 256.0
Hyperexplexia 759.89
Hyperextension, joint 718.80
  ankle 718.87
  elbow 718.82
  foot 718.87
  hand 718.84
  hip 718.85
  knee 718.86
  multiple sites 718.89
  pelvic region 718.85
  shoulder (region) 718.81
  specified site NEC 718.88
  wrist 718.83
Hyperfibrinolysis - *see* Fibrinolysis
Hyperfolliculinism 256.0
Hyperfructosemia 271.2
Hyperfunction
  adrenal (cortex) 255.3
    androgenic, acquired benign 255.3
    medulla 255.6
    virilism 255.2
  corticoadrenal NEC 255.3
  labyrinth - *see* Hyperactive, labyrinth
  medulloadrenal 255.6
  ovary 256.1
    estrogen 256.0
  pancreas 577.8
  parathyroid (gland) 252.00
  pituitary (anterior) (gland) (lobe) 253.1
  testicular 257.0
Hypergammaglobulinemia 289.89
  monoclonal, benign (BMH) 273.1
  polyclonal 273.0
  Waldenström's 273.0
Hyperglobulinemia 273.8
Hyperglycemia 790.29
  maternal
    affecting fetus or newborn 775.0
    manifest diabetes in infant 775.1
  postpancreatectomy (complete) (partial) 251.3
Hyperglyceridemia 272.1
  endogenous 272.1
  essential 272.1
  familial 272.1
  hereditary 272.1
  mixed 272.3
  pure 272.1
Hyperglycinemia 270.7
Hypergonadism
  ovarian 256.1
  testicular (infantile) (primary) 257.0
Hyperheparinemia (*see also* Circulating anticoagulants) 286.5
Hyperhidrosis, hyperidrosis 705.21
  axilla 705.21
  face 705.21

Hyperhidrosis, hyperidrosis *(Continued)*
  focal (localized) 705.21
    primary 705.21
      axilla 705.21
      face 705.21
      palms 705.21
      soles 705.21
    secondary 705.22
      axilla 705.22
      face 705.22
      palms 705.22
      soles 705.22
  generalized 780.8
  palms 705.21
  psychogenic 306.3
  secondary 780.8
  soles 705.21
Hyperhistidinemia 270.5
Hyperinsulinism (ectopic) (functional)
    (organic) NEC 251.1
  iatrogenic 251.0
  reactive 251.2
  spontaneous 251.2
  therapeutic misadventure (from
      administration of insulin) 962.3
Hyperiodemia 276.9
Hyperirritability (cerebral), in newborn
    779.1
Hyperkalemia 276.7
Hyperkeratosis *(see also* Keratosis) 701.1
  cervix 622.2
  congenital 757.39
  cornea 371.89
  due to yaws (early) (late) (palmar or
      plantar) 102.3
  eccentrica 757.39
  figurata centrifuga atrophica 757.39
  follicularis 757.39
    in cutem penetrans 701.1
  limbic (cornea) 371.89
  palmoplantaris climacterica 701.1
  pinta (carate) 103.1
  senile (with pruritus) 702.0
  tongue 528.79
  universalis congenita 757.1
  vagina 623.1
  vocal cord 478.5
  vulva 624.09
Hyperkinesia, hyperkinetic (disease)
    (reaction) (syndrome) 314.9
  with
    attention deficit - *see* Disorder,
        attention deficit
    conduct disorder 314.2
    developmental delay 314.1
    simple disturbance of activity and
        attention 314.01
    specified manifestation NEC 314.8
  heart (disease) 429.82
  of childhood or adolescence NEC 314.9
Hyperlacrimation *(see also* Epiphora)
    375.20
Hyperlipemia *(see also* Hyperlipidemia)
    272.4
Hyperlipidemia 272.4
  carbohydrate-induced 272.1
  combined 272.2
  endogenous 272.1
  exogenous 272.3
  fat-induced 272.3
  group
    A 272.0
    B 272.1
    C 272.2
    D 272.3
  mixed 272.2
  specified type NEC 272.4

Hyperlipidosis 272.7
  hereditary 272.7
Hyperlipoproteinemia (acquired)
    (essential) (familial) (hereditary)
    (primary) (secondary) 272.4
  Fredrickson type
    I 272.3
    IIA 272.0
    IIB 272.2
    III 272.2
    IV 272.1
    V 272.3
  low-density-lipoid-type (LDL) 272.0
  very-low-density-lipoid-type [VLDL]
    272.1
Hyperlucent lung, unilateral 492.8
Hyperluteinization 256.1
Hyperlysinemia 270.7
Hypermagnesemia 275.2
  neonatal 775.5
Hypermaturity (fetus or newborn)
  post-term infant 766.21
  prolonged gestation infant 766.22
Hypermenorrhea 626.2
Hypermetabolism 794.7
Hypermethioninemia 270.4
Hypermetropia (congenital) 367.0
Hypermobility
  cecum 564.9
  coccyx 724.71
  colon 564.9
    psychogenic 306.4
  ileum 564.89
  joint (acquired) 718.80
    ankle 718.87
    elbow 718.82
    foot 718.87
    hand 718.84
    hip 718.85
    knee 718.86
    multiple sites 718.89
    pelvic region 718.85
    shoulder (region) 718.81
    specified site NEC 718.88
    wrist 718.83
  kidney, congenital 753.3
  meniscus (knee) 717.5
  scapula 718.81
  stomach 536.8
    psychogenic 306.4
  syndrome 728.5
  testis, congenital 752.52
  urethral 599.81
Hypermotility
  gastrointestinal 536.8
  intestine 564.9
    psychogenic 306.4
  stomach 536.8
Hypernasality 784.43
Hypernatremia 276.0
  with water depletion 276.0
Hypernephroma (M8312/3) 189.0
Hyperopia 367.0
Hyperorexia 783.6
Hyperornithinemia 270.6
Hyperosmia *(see also* Disturbance,
    sensation) 781.1
Hyperosmolality 276.0
Hyperosteogenesis 733.99
Hyperostosis 733.99
  calvarial 733.3
  cortical 733.3
    infantile 756.59
  frontal, internal of skull 733.3

Hyperostosis *(Continued)*
  interna frontalis 733.3
  monomelic 733.99
  skull 733.3
    congenital 756.0
  vertebral 721.8
    with spondylosis - *see* Spondylosis
    ankylosing 721.6
Hyperovarianism 256.1
Hyperovarism, hyperovaria 256.1
Hyperoxaluria (primary) 271.8
Hyperoxia 987.8
Hyperparathyroidism 252.00
  ectopic 259.3
  other 252.08
  primary 252.01
  secondary (of renal origin) 588.81
    non-renal 252.02
  tertiary 252.08
Hyperpathia *(see also* Disturbance,
    sensation) 782.0
  psychogenic 307.80
Hyperperistalsis 787.4
  psychogenic 306.4
Hyperpermeability, capillary 448.9
Hyperphagia 783.6
Hyperphenylalaninemia 270.1
Hyperphoria 378.40
  alternating 378.45
Hyperphosphatemia 275.3
Hyperpiesia *(see also* Hypertension) 401.9
Hyperpiesis *(see also* Hypertension) 401.9
Hyperpigmentation - *see* Pigmentation
Hyperpinealism 259.8
Hyperpipecolatemia 270.7
Hyperpituitarism 253.1
Hyperplasia, hyperplastic
  adenoids (lymphoid tissue) 474.12
    and tonsils 474.10
  adrenal (capsule) (cortex) (gland) 255.8
    with
      sexual precocity (male) 255.2
      virilism, adrenal 255.2
      virilization (female) 255.2
    congenital 255.2
    due to excess ACTH (ectopic)
        (pituitary) 255.0
    medulla 255.8
  alpha cells (pancreatic)
    with
      gastrin excess 251.5
      glucagon excess 251.4
  appendix (lymphoid) 543.0
  artery, fibromuscular NEC 447.8
    carotid 447.8
    renal 447.3
  bone 733.99
    marrow 289.9
  breast *(see also* Hypertrophy, breast)
      611.1
    ductal 610.8
      atypical 610.8
  carotid artery 447.8
  cementation, cementum (teeth) (tooth)
      521.5
  cervical gland 785.6
  cervix (uteri) 622.10
    basal cell 622.10
    congenital 752.49
    endometrium 622.10
    polypoid 622.10
  chin 524.05
  clitoris, congenital 752.49
  dentin 521.5
  endocervicitis 616.0

◀ New   ◀▦ Revised   ~~deleted~~ Deleted   ● Use Additional Digit(s)   ▨ Omit code

Hyperplasia, hyperplastic *(Continued)*
  endometrium, endometrial
      (adenomatous) (atypical) (cystic)
      (glandular) (polypoid) (uterus)
      621.30
    with atypia 621.33
    without atypia
      complex 621.32
      simple 621.31
    benign 621.34
  cervix 622.10
  epithelial 709.8
    focal, oral, including tongue 528.79
    mouth (focal) 528.79
    nipple 611.89
    skin 709.8
    tongue (focal) 528.79
    vaginal wall 623.0
  erythroid 289.9
  fascialis ossificans (progressiva) 728.11
  fibromuscular, artery NEC 447.8
    carotid 447.8
    renal 447.3
  genital
    female 629.89
    male 608.89
  gingiva 523.8
  glandularis
    cystica uteri 621.30
    endometrium (uterus) 621.30
    interstitialis uteri 621.30
  granulocytic 288.69
  gum 523.8
  hymen, congenital 752.49
  islands of Langerhans 251.1
  islet cell (pancreatic) 251.9
    alpha cells
      with excess
        gastrin 251.5
        glucagon 251.4
    beta cells 251.1
  juxtaglomerular (complex) (kidney)
      593.89
  kidney (congenital) 753.3
  liver (congenital) 751.69
  lymph node (gland) 785.6
  lymphoid (diffuse) (nodular) 785.6
    appendix 543.0
    intestine 569.89
  mandibular 524.02
    alveolar 524.72
    unilateral condylar 526.89
  Marchand multiple nodular (liver) -
      see Cirrhosis, postnecrotic
  maxillary 524.01
    alveolar 524.71
  medulla, adrenal 255.8
  myometrium, myometrial 621.2
  nose (lymphoid) (polypoid) 478.19
  oral soft tissue (inflammatory)
      (irritative) (mucosa) NEC 528.9
    gingiva 523.8
    tongue 529.8
  organ or site, congenital NEC - *see*
      Anomaly, specified type NEC
  ovary 620.8
  palate, papillary 528.9
  pancreatic islet cells 251.9
    alpha
      with excess
        gastrin 251.5
        glucagon 251.4
    beta 251.1
  parathyroid (gland) 252.01
  persistent, vitreous (primary) 743.51

Hyperplasia, hyperplastic *(Continued)*
  pharynx (lymphoid) 478.29
  prostate 600.90
    with
      other lower urinary tract
          symptoms (LUTS) 600.91
      urinary
          obstruction 600.91
          retention 600.91
    adenofibromatous 600.20
      with
        other lower urinary tract
            symptoms (LUTS)
            600.21
        urinary
            obstruction 600.21
            retention 600.21
    nodular 600.10
      with
        urinary
            obstruction 600.11
            retention 600.11
  renal artery (fibromuscular) 447.3
  reticuloendothelial (cell) 289.9
  salivary gland (any) 527.1
  Schimmelbusch's 610.1
  suprarenal (capsule) (gland) 255.8
  thymus (gland) (persistent) 254.0
  thyroid (*see also* Goiter) 240.9
    primary 242.0●
    secondary 242.2●
  tonsil (lymphoid tissue) 474.11
    and adenoids 474.10
  urethrovaginal 599.89
  uterus, uterine (myometrium) 621.2
    endometrium (*see also* Hyperplasia,
        endometrium) 621.30
  vitreous (humor), primary persistent
      743.51
  vulva 624.3
  zygoma 738.11
Hyperpnea (*see also* Hyperventilation)
    786.01
Hyperpotassemia 276.7
Hyperprebetalipoproteinemia 272.1
  with chylomicronemia 272.3
  familial 272.1
Hyperprolactinemia 253.1
Hyperprolinemia 270.8
Hyperproteinemia 273.8
Hyperprothrombinemia 289.89
Hyperpselaphesia 782.0
Hyperpyrexia 780.60
  heat (effects of) 992.0
  malarial (*see also* Malaria) 084.6
  malignant, due to anesthetic 995.86
  rheumatic - *see* Fever, rheumatic
  unknown origin (*see also* Pyrexia)
      780.60
Hyperreactor, vascular 780.2
Hyperreflexia 796.1
  bladder, autonomic 596.54
    with cauda equina 344.61
  detrusor 344.61
Hypersalivation (*see also* Ptyalism)
    527.7
Hypersarcosinemia 270.8
Hypersecretion
  ACTH 255.3
  androgens (ovarian) 256.1
  calcitonin 246.0
  corticoadrenal 255.3
  cortisol 255.0
  estrogen 256.0
  gastric 536.8
    psychogenic 306.4

Hypersecretion *(Continued)*
  gastrin 251.5
  glucagon 251.4
  hormone
    ACTH 255.3
    anterior pituitary 253.1
    growth NEC 253.0
    ovarian androgen 256.1
    testicular 257.0
    thyroid stimulating 242.8●
  insulin - *see* Hyperinsulinism
  lacrimal glands (*see also* Epiphora) 375.20
  medulloadrenal 255.6
  milk 676.6●
  ovarian androgens 256.1
  pituitary (anterior) 253.1
  salivary gland (any) 527.7
  testicular hormones 257.0
  thyrocalcitonin 246.0
  upper respiratory 478.9
Hypersegmentation, hereditary 288.2
  eosinophils 288.2
  neutrophil nuclei 288.2
Hypersensitive, hypersensitiveness,
    hypersensitivity - *see also* Allergy
  angiitis 446.20
    specified NEC 446.29
  carotid sinus 337.01
  colon 564.9
    psychogenic 306.4
  DNA (deoxyribonucleic acid) NEC 287.2
  drug (*see also* Allergy, drug) 995.27
  due to correct medical substance
      properly administered 995.27 ◄
  esophagus 530.89
  insect bites - *see* Injury, superficial, by site
  labyrinth 386.58
  pain (*see also* Disturbance, sensation)
      782.0
  pneumonitis NEC 495.9
  reaction (*see also* Allergy) 995.3
    upper respiratory tract NEC 478.8
  stomach (allergic) (nonallergic) 536.8
    psychogenic 306.4
Hypersomatotropism (classic) 253.0
Hypersomnia, unspecified 780.54
  with sleep apnea, unspecified 780.53
  alcohol induced 291.82
  drug induced 292.85
  due to
    medical condition classified
        elsewhere 327.14
    mental disorder 327.15
  idiopathic
    with long sleep time 327.11
    without long sleep time 327.12
  menstrual related 327.13
  nonorganic origin 307.43
    persistent (primary) 307.44
    transient 307.43
  organic 327.10
    other 327.19
  primary 307.44
  recurrent 327.13
Hypersplenia 289.4
Hypersplenism 289.4
Hypersteatosis 706.3
Hyperstimulation, ovarian 256.1
Hypersuprarenalism 255.3
Hypersusceptibility - *see* Allergy
Hyper-TBG-nemia 246.8
Hypertelorism 756.0
  orbit, orbital 376.41
Hypertension, hypertensive - *see* table
    on pages 290–293

OGCR Section I.C.7.a.1
Assign hypertension (arterial) (essential) (systemic) (NOS) to category code 401 with appropriate fourth digit to indicate malignant (.0), benign (.1), or unspecified (.9). Do not use either .0 malignant or .1 benign unless medical record documentation supports such a designation.

	Malignant	Benign	Unspecified
Hypertension, hypertensive (arterial) (arteriolar) (crisis) (degeneration) (disease) (essential) (fluctuating) (idiopathic) (intermittent) (labile) (low renin) (orthostatic) (paroxysmal) (primary) (systemic) (uncontrolled) (vascular)	**401.0**	**401.1**	**401.9**
with			
chronic kidney disease	—	—	—
stage I through stage IV, or unspecified	**403.00**	**403.10**	**403.90**
stage V or end stage renal disease	**403.01**	**403.11**	**403.91**
heart involvement (conditions classifiable to 429.0–429.3, 429.8, 429.9 due to hypertension) (*see also* Hypertension, heart)	**402.00**	**402.10**	**402.90**
with kidney involvement - *see* Hypertension, cardiorenal			
renal (kidney) involvement ~~(only conditions classifiable to 585)~~ (only conditions classifiable to 585, 587) (excludes conditions classifiable to 584) (*see also* Hypertension, kidney)	**403.00**	**403.10**	**403.90** ◀
with heart involvement - *see* Hypertension, cardiorenal failure (and sclerosis) (*see also* Hypertension, kidney)	**403.01**	**403.11**	**403.91**
sclerosis without failure (*see also* Hypertension, kidney)	**403.00**	**403.10**	**403.90**
accelerated (*see also* Hypertension, by type, malignant)	**401.0**	—	—
antepartum - *see* Hypertension, complicating pregnancy, childbirth, or the puerperium			
cardiorenal (disease)	**404.00**	**404.10**	**404.90**
with			
chronic kidney disease	—	—	—
stage I through stage IV, or unspecified	**404.00**	**404.10**	**404.90**
and heart failure	**404.01**	**404.11**	**404.91**
stage V or end stage renal disease	**404.02**	**404.12**	**404.92**
and heart failure	**404.03**	**404.13**	**404.93**
heart failure	**404.01**	**404.11**	**404.91**
and chronic kidney disease	**404.01**	**404.11**	**404.91**
stage I through stage IV or unspecified	**404.01**	**404.11**	**404.91**
stage V or end stage renal disease	**404.03**	**404.13**	**404.93**
cardiovascular disease (arteriosclerotic) (sclerotic)	**402.00**	**402.10**	**402.90**
with			
heart failure	**402.01**	**402.11**	**402.91**
renal involvement (conditions classifiable to 403) (*see also* Hypertension, cardiorenal)	**404.00**	**404.10**	**404.90**
cardiovascular renal (disease) (sclerosis) (*see also* Hypertension, cardiorenal)	**404.00**	**404.10**	**404.90**
cerebrovascular disease NEC	**437.2**	**437.2**	**437.2**
complicating pregnancy, childbirth, or the puerperium	**642.2**●	**642.0**●	**642.9**●
with			
albuminuria (and edema) (mild)	—	—	**642.4**●
severe	—	—	**642.5**●
chronic kidney disease	**642.2**●	**642.2**●	**642.2**●
and heart disease	**642.2**●	**642.2**●	**642.2**●
edema (mild)	—	—	**642.4**●
severe	—	—	**642.5**●
heart disease	**642.2**●	**642.2**●	**642.2**●
and chronic kidney disease	**642.2**●	**642.2**●	**642.2**●
renal disease	**642.2**●	**642.2**●	**642.2**●
and heart disease	**642.2**●	**642.2**●	**642.2**●

◀ New　◀▥ Revised　~~deleted~~ Deleted　● Use Additional Digit(s)　▨ Omit code

	Malignant	Benign	Unspecified
Hypertension, hypertensive *(Continued)*			
complicating pregnancy, childbirth, or the puerperium *(Continued)*			
chronic	642.2●	642.0●	642.0●
with pre-eclampsia or eclampsia	642.7●	642.7●	642.7●
fetus or newborn	760.0	760.0	760.0
essential	—	642.0●	642.0●
with pre-eclampsia or eclampsia	—	642.7●	642.7●
fetus or newborn	760.0	760.0	760.0
fetus or newborn	760.0	760.0	760.0
gestational	—	—	642.3●
pre-existing	642.2●	642.0●	642.0●
with pre-eclampsia or eclampsia	642.7●	642.7●	642.7●
fetus or newborn	760.0	760.0	760.0
secondary to renal disease	642.1●	642.1●	642.1●
with pre-eclampsia or eclampsia	642.7●	642.7●	642.7●
fetus or newborn	760.0	760.0	760.0
transient	—	—	642.3●
due to			
aldosteronism, primary	405.09	405.19	405.99
brain tumor	405.09	405.19	405.99
bulbar poliomyelitis	405.09	405.19	405.99
calculus			
kidney	405.09	405.19	405.99
ureter	405.09	405.19	405.99
coarctation, aorta	405.09	405.19	405.99
Cushing's disease	405.09	405.19	405.99
glomerulosclerosis (*see also* Hypertension, kidney)	403.00	403.10	403.90
periarteritis nodosa	405.09	405.19	405.99
pheochromocytoma	405.09	405.19	405.99
polycystic kidney(s)	405.09	405.19	405.99
polycythemia	405.09	405.19	405.99
porphyria	405.09	405.19	405.99
pyelonephritis	405.09	405.19	405.99
renal (artery)			
aneurysm	405.01	405.11	405.91
anomaly	405.01	405.11	405.91
embolism	405.01	405.11	405.91
fibromuscular hyperplasia	405.01	405.11	405.91
occlusion	405.01	405.11	405.91
stenosis	405.01	405.11	405.91
thrombosis	405.01	405.11	405.91
encephalopathy	437.2	437.2	437.2
gestational (transient) NEC	—	—	642.3●
Goldblatt's	440.1	440.1	440.1

◀ New   ◀‖‖ Revised   ~~deleted~~ Deleted   ● Use Additional Digit(s)   ▨ Omit code

	Malignant	Benign	Unspecified
Hypertension, hypertensive *(Continued)*			
heart (disease) (conditions classifiable to 429.0–429.3, 429.8, 429.9 due to hypertension)	402.00	402.10	402.90
with			
heart failure	402.01	402.11	402.91
hypertensive kidney disease (conditions classifiable to 403) (*see also* Hypertension, cardiorenal)	404.00	404.10	404.90
renal sclerosis (*see also* Hypertension, cardiorenal)	404.00	404.10	404.90
intracranial, benign	—	348.2	—
intraocular	—	—	365.04
kidney	403.00	403.10	403.90
with			
chronic kidney disease	—	—	—
stage I through stage IV, or unspecified	403.00	403.10	403.90
stage V or end stage renal disease	403.01	403.11	403.91
heart involvement (conditions classifiable to 429.0–429.3, 429.8, 429.9 due to hypertension) (*see also* Hypertension, cardiorenal)	404.00	404.10	404.90
hypertensive heart (disease) (conditions classifiable to 402) (*see also* Hypertension, cardiorenal)	404.00	404.10	404.90
lesser circulation	—	—	416.0
necrotizing	401.0	—	—
pancreatic duct - *code to* underlying condition			
with			
chronic pancreatitis	—	—	577.11
ocular			365.04
portal (due to chronic liver disease)	—	—	572.3
postoperative			997.91
psychogenic	—	—	306.2
puerperal, postpartum - *see* Hypertension, complicating pregnancy, childbirth, or the puerperium			
pulmonary (artery) (secondary)	—	—	416.8
with cor pulmonale (chronic)	—	—	416.8
acute	—	—	415.0
idiopathic	—	—	416.0
primary	—	—	416.0
of newborn	—	—	747.83
secondary	—	—	416.8
renal (disease) (*see also* Hypertension, kidney)	403.00	403.10	403.90
renovascular NEC	405.01	405.11	405.91

◀ New   ◀▦ Revised   ~~deleted~~ Deleted   ● Use Additional Digit(s)   ▨ Omit code

	Malignant	Benign	Unspecified
Hypertension, hypertensive *(Continued)*			
secondary NEC	405.09	405.19	405.99
due to			
aldosteronism, primary	405.09	405.19	405.99
brain tumor	405.09	405.19	405.99
bulbar poliomyelitis	405.09	405.19	405.99
calculus			
kidney	405.09	405.19	405.99
ureter	405.09	405.19	405.99
coarctation, aorta	405.09	405.19	405.99
Cushing's disease	405.09	405.19	405.99
glomerulosclerosis (*see also* Hypertension, kidney)	403.00	403.10	403.90
periarteritis nodosa	405.09	405.19	405.99
pheochromocytoma	405.09	405.19	405.99
polycystic kidney(s)	405.09	405.19	405.99
polycythemia	405.09	405.19	405.99
porphyria	405.09	405.19	405.99
pyelonephritis	405.09	405.19	405.99
renal (artery)			
aneurysm	405.01	405.11	405.91
anomaly	405.01	405.11	405.91
embolism	405.01	405.11	405.91
fibromuscular hyperplasia	405.01	405.11	405.91
occlusion	405.01	405.11	405.91
stenosis	405.01	405.11	405.91
thrombosis	405.01	405.11	405.91
transient	—	—	796.2
of pregnancy	—	—	642.3●
venous, chronic (asymptomatic) (idiopathic)	—	—	459.30
with			
complication, NEC	—	—	459.39
inflammation	—	—	459.32
with ulcer	—	—	459.33
ulcer	—	—	459.31
with inflammation	—	—	459.33
due to			
deep vein thrombosis (*see also* Syndrome, postphlebitic)	—	—	459.10

Hypertensive urgency - *see*
　　Hypertension ◀
Hyperthecosis, ovary 256.8
Hyperthermia (of unknown origin) (*see also* Pyrexia) 780.60
　　malignant (due to anesthesia) 995.86
　　newborn 778.4
Hyperthymergasia (*see also* Psychosis, affective) 296.0●
　　reactive (from emotional stress, psychological trauma) 298.1
　　recurrent episode 296.1●
　　single episode 296.0●
Hyperthymism 254.8
Hyperthyroid (recurrent) - *see* Hyperthyroidism
Hyperthyroidism (latent) (preadult) (recurrent) (without goiter) 242.9●

Note:　Use the following fifth-digit subclassification with category 242:

0　without mention of thyrotoxic crisis or storm
1　with mention of thyrotoxic crisis or storm

---

　　with
　　　　goiter (diffuse) 242.0●
　　　　　　adenomatous 242.3●
　　　　　　　　multinodular 242.2●
　　　　　　　　uninodular 242.1●
　　　　　　nodular 242.3●
　　　　　　　　multinodular 242.2●
　　　　　　　　uninodular 242.1●
　　　　　　thyroid nodule 242.1●
　　complicating pregnancy, childbirth, or puerperium 648.1●
　　neonatal (transient) 775.3
Hypertonia - *see* Hypertonicity
Hypertonicity
　　bladder 596.51
　　fetus or newborn 779.89
　　gastrointestinal (tract) 536.8
　　infancy 779.89
　　　　due to electrolyte imbalance 779.89
　　muscle 728.85
　　stomach 536.8
　　　　psychogenic 306.4
　　uterus, uterine (contractions) 661.4●
　　　　affecting fetus or newborn 763.7
Hypertony - *see* Hypertonicity
Hypertransaminemia 790.4
Hypertrichosis 704.1
　　congenital 757.4
　　eyelid 374.54
　　lanuginosa 757.4
　　　　acquired 704.1
Hypertriglyceridemia, essential 272.1
Hypertrophy, hypertrophic
　　adenoids (infectional) 474.12
　　　　and tonsils (faucial) (infective) (lingual) (lymphoid) 474.10
　　adrenal 255.8
　　alveolar process or ridge 525.8
　　anal papillae 569.49
　　apocrine gland 705.82
　　artery NEC 447.8
　　　　carotid 447.8
　　　　congenital (peripheral) NEC 747.60
　　　　　　gastrointestinal 747.61
　　　　　　lower limb 747.64
　　　　　　renal 747.62
　　　　　　specified NEC 747.69
　　　　　　spinal 747.82
　　　　　　upper limb 747.63
　　　　renal 447.3

Hypertrophy, hypertrophic (*Continued*)
　　arthritis (chronic) (*see also* Osteoarthrosis) 715.9●
　　　　spine (*see also* Spondylosis) 721.90
　　arytenoid 478.79
　　asymmetrical (heart) 429.9
　　auricular - *see* Hypertrophy, cardiac
　　Bartholin's gland 624.8
　　bile duct 576.8
　　bladder (sphincter) (trigone) 596.8
　　blind spot, visual field 368.42
　　bone 733.99
　　brain 348.89
　　breast 611.1
　　　　cystic 610.1
　　　　fetus or newborn 778.7
　　　　fibrocystic 610.1
　　　　massive pubertal 611.1
　　　　puerperal, postpartum 676.3●
　　　　senile (parenchymatous) 611.1
　　cardiac (chronic) (idiopathic) 429.3
　　　　with
　　　　　　rheumatic fever (conditions classifiable to 390)
　　　　　　　　active 391.8
　　　　　　　　　　with chorea 392.0
　　　　　　　　inactive or quiescent (with chorea) 398.99
　　　　congenital NEC 746.89
　　　　fatty (*see also* Degeneration, myocardial) 429.1
　　　　hypertensive (*see also* Hypertension, heart) 402.90
　　　　rheumatic (with chorea) 398.99
　　　　　　active or acute 391.8
　　　　　　　　with chorea 392.0
　　　　valve (*see also* Endocarditis) 424.90
　　　　　　congenital NEC 746.89
　　cartilage 733.99
　　cecum 569.89
　　cervix (uteri) 622.6
　　　　congenital 752.49
　　　　elongation 622.6
　　clitoris (cirrhotic) 624.2
　　　　congenital 752.49
　　colon 569.89
　　　　congenital 751.3
　　conjunctiva, lymphoid 372.73
　　cornea 371.89
　　corpora cavernosa 607.89
　　duodenum 537.89
　　endometrium (uterus) (*see also* Hyperplasia, endometrium) 621.30
　　　　cervix 622.6
　　epididymis 608.89
　　esophageal hiatus (congenital) 756.6
　　　　with hernia - *see* Hernia, diaphragm
　　eyelid 374.30
　　falx, skull 733.99
　　fat pad 729.30
　　　　infrapatellar 729.31
　　　　knee 729.31
　　　　orbital 374.34
　　　　popliteal 729.31
　　　　prepatellar 729.31
　　　　retropatellar 729.31
　　　　specified site NEC 729.39
　　foot (congenital) 755.67
　　frenum, frenulum (tongue) 529.8
　　　　linguae 529.8
　　　　lip 528.5
　　gallbladder or cystic duct 575.8

Hypertrophy, hypertrophic (*Continued*)
　　gastric mucosa 535.2●
　　gingiva 523.8
　　gland, glandular (general) NEC 785.6
　　gum (mucous membrane) 523.8
　　heart (idiopathic) - *see also* Hypertrophy, cardiac
　　　　valve - *see also* Endocarditis
　　　　congenital NEC 746.89
　　hemifacial 754.0
　　hepatic - *see* Hypertrophy, liver
　　hiatus (esophageal) 756.6
　　hilus gland 785.6
　　hymen, congenital 752.49
　　ileum 569.89
　　infrapatellar fat pad 729.31
　　intestine 569.89
　　jejunum 569.89
　　kidney (compensatory) 593.1
　　　　congenital 753.3
　　labial frenulum 528.5
　　labium (majus) (minus) 624.3
　　lacrimal gland, chronic 375.03
　　ligament 728.9
　　　　spinal 724.8
　　linguae frenulum 529.8
　　lingual tonsil (infectional) 474.11
　　lip (frenum) 528.5
　　　　congenital 744.81
　　liver 789.1
　　　　acute 573.8
　　　　cirrhotic - *see* Cirrhosis, liver
　　　　congenital 751.69
　　　　fatty - *see* Fatty, liver
　　lymph gland 785.6
　　　　tuberculous - *see* Tuberculosis, lymph gland
　　mammary gland - *see* Hypertrophy, breast
　　maxillary frenulum 528.5
　　Meckel's diverticulum (congenital) 751.0
　　medial meniscus, acquired 717.3
　　median bar 600.90
　　　　with
　　　　　　other lower urinary tract symptoms (LUTS) 600.91
　　　　　　urinary
　　　　　　　　obstruction 600.91
　　　　　　　　retention 600.91
　　mediastinum 519.3
　　meibomian gland 373.2
　　meniscus, knee, congenital 755.64
　　metatarsal head 733.99
　　metatarsus 733.99
　　mouth 528.9
　　mucous membrane
　　　　alveolar process 523.8
　　　　nose 478.19
　　　　turbinate (nasal) 478.0
　　muscle 728.9
　　muscular coat, artery NEC 447.8
　　　　carotid 447.8
　　　　renal 447.3
　　myocardium (*see also* Hypertrophy, cardiac) 429.3
　　　　idiopathic 425.4
　　myometrium 621.2
　　nail 703.8
　　　　congenital 757.5
　　nasal 478.19
　　　　alae 478.19
　　　　bone 738.0
　　　　cartilage 478.19

　　◀ New　◀▥ Revised　~~deleted~~ Deleted　● Use Additional Digit(s)　▨ Omit code

Hypertrophy, hypertrophic (*Continued*)
  nasal (*Continued*)
    mucous membrane (septum) 478.19
    sinus (*see also* Sinusitis) 473.9
    turbinate 478.0
  nasopharynx, lymphoid (infectional) (tissue) (wall) 478.29
  neck, uterus 622.6
  nipple 611.1
  normal aperture diaphragm (congenital) 756.6
  nose (*see also* Hypertrophy, nasal) 478.19
  orbit 376.46
  organ or site, congenital NEC - *see* Anomaly, specified type NEC
  osteoarthropathy (pulmonary) 731.2
  ovary 620.8
  palate (hard) 526.89
    soft 528.9
  pancreas (congenital) 751.7
  papillae
    anal 569.49
    tongue 529.3
  parathyroid (gland) 252.01
  parotid gland 527.1
  penis 607.89
  phallus 607.89
    female (clitoris) 624.2
  pharyngeal tonsil 474.12
  pharyngitis 472.1
  pharynx 478.29
    lymphoid (infectional) (tissue) (wall) 478.29
  pituitary (fossa) (gland) 253.8
  popliteal fat pad 729.31
  preauricular (lymph) gland (Hampstead) 785.6
  prepuce (congenital) 605
    female 624.2
  prostate (asymptomatic) (early) (recurrent) 600.90
    with
      other lower urinary tract symptoms (LUTS) 600.91
      urinary
        obstruction 600.91
        retention 600.91
    adenofibromatous 600.20
      with
        other lower urinary tract symptoms (LUTS) 600.21
        urinary
          obstruction 600.21
          retention 600.21
    benign 600.00
      with
        other lower urinary tract symptoms (LUTS) 600.01
        urinary
          obstruction 600.01
          retention 600.01
    congenital 752.89
  pseudoedematous hypodermal 757.0
  pseudomuscular 359.1
  pylorus (muscle) (sphincter) 537.0
    congenital 750.5
    infantile 750.5
  rectal sphincter 569.49
  rectum 569.49
  renal 593.1

Hypertrophy, hypertrophic (*Continued*)
  rhinitis (turbinate) 472.0
  salivary duct or gland 527.1
    congenital 750.26
  scaphoid (tarsal) 733.99
  scar 701.4
  scrotum 608.89
  sella turcica 253.8
  seminal vesicle 608.89
  sigmoid 569.89
  skin condition NEC 701.9
  spermatic cord 608.89
  spinal ligament 724.8
  spleen - *see* Splenomegaly
  spondylitis (spine) (*see also* Spondylosis) 721.90
  stomach 537.89
  subaortic stenosis (idiopathic) 425.1
  sublingual gland 527.1
    congenital 750.26
  submaxillary gland 527.1
  suprarenal (gland) 255.8
  tendon 727.9
  testis 608.89
    congenital 752.89
  thymic, thymus (congenital) (gland) 254.0
  thyroid (gland) (*see also* Goiter) 240.9
    primary 242.0●
    secondary 242.2●
  toe (congenital) 755.65
    acquired 735.8
  tongue 529.8
    congenital 750.15
    frenum 529.8
    papillae (foliate) 529.3
  tonsil (faucial) (infective) (lingual) (lymphoid) 474.11
    with
      adenoiditis 474.01
      tonsillitis 474.00
        and adenoiditis 474.02
      and adenoids 474.10
  tunica vaginalis 608.89
  turbinate (mucous membrane) 478.0
  ureter 593.89
  urethra 599.84
  uterus 621.2
    puerperal, postpartum 674.8●
  uvula 528.9
  vagina 623.8
  vas deferens 608.89
  vein 459.89
  ventricle, ventricular (heart) (left) (right) - *see also* Hypertrophy, cardiac
    congenital 746.89
    due to hypertension (left) (right) (*see also* Hypertension, heart) 402.90
      benign 402.10
      malignant 402.00
    right with ventricular septal defect, pulmonary stenosis or atresia, and dextraposition of aorta 745.2
  verumontanum 599.89
  vesical 596.8
  vocal cord 478.5
  vulva 624.3
    stasis (nonfilarial) 624.3
Hypertropia (intermittent) (periodic) 378.31
Hypertyrosinemia 270.2

Hyperuricemia 790.6
Hypervalinemia 270.3
Hyperventilation (tetany) 786.01
  hysterical 300.11
  psychogenic 306.1
  syndrome 306.1
Hyperviscidosis 277.00
Hyperviscosity (of serum) (syndrome) NEC 273.3
  polycythemic 289.0
  sclerocythemic 282.8
Hypervitaminosis (dietary) NEC 278.8
  A (dietary) 278.2
  D (dietary) 278.4
  from excessive administration or use of vitamin preparations (chronic) 278.8
    reaction to sudden overdose 963.5
    vitamin A 278.2
      reaction to sudden overdose 963.5
    vitamin D 278.4
      reaction to sudden overdose 963.5
    vitamin K
      correct substance properly administered 278.8
      overdose or wrong substance given or taken 964.3
Hypervolemia 276.69 ◀▥
Hypesthesia (*see also* Disturbance, sensation) 782.0
  cornea 371.81
Hyphema (anterior chamber) (ciliary body) (iris) 364.41
  traumatic 921.3
Hyphemia - *see* Hyphema
Hypoacidity, gastric 536.8
  psychogenic 306.4
Hypoactive labyrinth (function) - *see* Hypofunction, labyrinth
Hypoadrenalism 255.41
  tuberculous (*see also* Tuberculosis) 017.6●
Hypoadrenocorticism 255.41
  pituitary 253.4
Hypoalbuminemia 273.8
Hypoaldosteronism 255.42
Hypoalphalipoproteinemia 272.5
Hypobarism 993.2
Hypobaropathy 993.2
Hypobetalipoproteinemia (familial) 272.5
Hypocalcemia 275.41
  cow's milk 775.4
  dietary 269.3
  neonatal 775.4
  phosphate-loading 775.4
Hypocalcification, teeth 520.4
Hypochloremia 276.9
Hypochlorhydria 536.8
  neurotic 306.4
  psychogenic 306.4
Hypocholesteremia 272.5
Hypochondria (reaction) 300.7
Hypochondriac 300.7
Hypochondriasis 300.7
Hypochromasia blood cells 280.9
Hypochromic anemia 280.9
  due to blood loss (chronic) 280.0
    acute 285.1
  microcytic 280.9
Hypocoagulability (*see also* Defect, coagulation) 286.9
Hypocomplementemia 279.8
Hypocythemia (progressive) 284.9
Hypodontia (*see also* Anodontia) 520.0

Hypoeosinophilia 288.59
Hypoesthesia (*see also* Disturbance, sensation) 782.0
    cornea 371.81
    tactile 782.0
Hypoestrinism 256.39
Hypoestrogenism 256.39
Hypoferremia 280.9
    due to blood loss (chronic) 280.0
Hypofertility
    female 628.9
    male 606.1
Hypofibrinogenemia 286.3
    acquired 286.6
    congenital 286.3
Hypofunction
    adrenal (gland) 255.41
        cortex 255.41
        medulla 255.5
        specified NEC 255.5
    cerebral 331.9
    corticoadrenal NEC 255.41
    intestinal 564.89
    labyrinth (unilateral) 386.53
        with loss of labyrinthine reactivity 386.55
        bilateral 386.54
            with loss of labyrinthine reactivity 386.56
    Leydig cell 257.2
    ovary 256.39
        postablative 256.2
    pituitary (anterior) (gland) (lobe) 253.2
        posterior 253.5
    testicular 257.2
        iatrogenic 257.1
        postablative 257.1
        postirradiation 257.1
        postsurgical 257.1
Hypogammaglobulinemia 279.00
    acquired primary 279.06
    non-sex-linked, congenital 279.06
    sporadic 279.06
    transient of infancy 279.09
Hypogenitalism (congenital) (female) (male) 752.89
    penis 752.69
Hypoglycemia (spontaneous) 251.2
    coma 251.0
        diabetic 250.3 ●
            due to secondary diabetes 249.3 ●
        diabetic 250.8 ●
            due to secondary diabetes 249.8 ●
        due to insulin 251.0
            therapeutic misadventure 962.3
    familial (idiopathic) 251.2
    following gastrointestinal surgery 579.3
    infantile (idiopathic) 251.2
    in infant of diabetic mother 775.0
    leucine-induced 270.3
    neonatal 775.6
    reactive 251.2
    specified NEC 251.1
Hypoglycemic shock 251.0
    diabetic 250.8 ●
        due to secondary diabetes 249.8 ●
    due to insulin 251.0
    functional (syndrome) 251.1

Hypogonadism
    female 256.39
    gonadotrophic (isolated) 253.4
    hypogonadotropic (isolated) (with anosmia) 253.4
    isolated 253.4
    male 257.2
        hereditary familial (Reifenstein's syndrome) 259.52
    ovarian (primary) 256.39
    pituitary (secondary) 253.4
    testicular (primary) (secondary) 257.2
Hypohidrosis 705.0
Hypohidrotic ectodermal dysplasia 757.31
Hypoidrosis 705.0
Hypoinsulinemia, postsurgical 251.3
    postpancreatectomy (complete) (partial) 251.3
Hypokalemia 276.8
Hypokinesia 780.99
Hypoleukia splenica 289.4
Hypoleukocytosis 288.50
Hypolipidemia 272.5
Hypolipoproteinemia 272.5
Hypomagnesemia 275.2
    neonatal 775.4
Hypomania, hypomanic reaction (*see also* Psychosis, affective) 296.0 ●
    recurrent episode 296.1 ●
    single episode 296.0 ●
Hypomastia (congenital) 611.82
Hypomenorrhea 626.1
Hypometabolism 783.9
Hypomotility
    gastrointestinal tract 536.8
        psychogenic 306.4
    intestine 564.89
        psychogenic 306.4
    stomach 536.8
        psychogenic 306.4
Hyponasality 784.44
Hyponatremia 276.1
Hypo-ovarianism 256.39
Hypo-ovarism 256.39
Hypoparathyroidism (idiopathic) (surgically induced) 252.1
    neonatal 775.4
Hypoperfusion (in) ◀
    newborn 779.89 ◀
Hypopharyngitis 462
Hypophoria 378.40
Hypophosphatasia 275.3
Hypophosphatemia (acquired) (congenital) (familial) 275.3
    renal 275.3
Hypophyseal, hypophysis - *see also* condition
    dwarfism 253.3
    gigantism 253.0
    syndrome 253.8
Hypophyseothalamic syndrome 253.8
Hypopiesis - *see* Hypotension
Hypopigmentation 709.00
    eyelid 374.53
Hypopinealism 259.8
Hypopituitarism (juvenile) (syndrome) 253.2
    due to
        hormone therapy 253.7
        hypophysectomy 253.7
        radiotherapy 253.7
    postablative 253.7
    postpartum hemorrhage 253.2

Hypoplasia, hypoplasis 759.89
    adrenal (gland) 759.1
    alimentary tract 751.8
        lower 751.2
        upper 750.8
    anus, anal (canal) 751.2
    aorta 747.22
    aortic
        arch (tubular) 747.10
            orifice or valve with hypoplasia of ascending aorta and defective development of left ventricle (with mitral valve atresia) 746.7
    appendix 751.2
    areola 757.6
    arm (*see also* Absence, arm, congenital) 755.20
    artery (congenital) (peripheral) 747.60
        brain 747.81
        cerebral 747.81
        coronary 746.85
        gastrointestinal 747.61
        lower limb 747.64
        pulmonary 747.3
        renal 747.62
        retinal 743.58
        specified NEC 747.69
        spinal 747.82
        umbilical 747.5
        upper limb 747.63
    auditory canal 744.29
        causing impairment of hearing 744.02
    biliary duct (common) or passage 751.61
    bladder 753.8
    bone NEC 756.9
        face 756.0
        malar 756.0
        mandible 524.04
            alveolar 524.74
        marrow 284.9
            acquired (secondary) 284.89
            congenital 284.09
            idiopathic 284.9
        maxilla 524.03
            alveolar 524.73
        skull (*see also* Hypoplasia, skull) 756.0
    brain 742.1
        gyri 742.2
        specified part 742.2
    breast (areola) 611.82
    bronchus (tree) 748.3
    cardiac 746.89
        valve - *see* Hypoplasia, heart, valve
        vein 746.89
    carpus (*see also* Absence, carpal, congenital) 755.28
    cartilaginous 756.9
    cecum 751.2
    cementum 520.4
        hereditary 520.5
    cephalic 742.1
    cerebellum 742.2
    cervix (uteri) 752.43 ◀▥
    chin 524.06
    clavicle 755.51
    coccyx 756.19
    colon 751.2
    corpus callosum 742.2
    cricoid cartilage 748.3
    dermal, focal (Goltz) 757.39

Hypoplasia, hypoplasis *(Continued)*
digestive organ(s) or tract NEC 751.8
  lower 751.2
  upper 750.8
ear 744.29
  auricle 744.23
  lobe 744.29
  middle, except ossicles 744.03
    ossicles 744.04
  ossicles 744.04
enamel of teeth (neonatal) (postnatal)
    (prenatal) 520.4
  hereditary 520.5
endocrine (gland) NEC 759.2
endometrium 621.8
epididymis 752.89
epiglottis 748.3
erythroid, congenital 284.01
erythropoietic, chronic acquired 284.81
esophagus 750.3
Eustachian tube 744.24
eye (*see also* Microphthalmos) 743.10
  lid 743.62
face 744.89
  bone(s) 756.0
fallopian tube 752.19
femur (*see also* Absence, femur,
    congenital) 755.34
fibula (*see also* Absence, fibula,
    congenital) 755.37
finger (*see also* Absence, finger,
    congenital) 755.29
focal dermal 757.39
foot 755.31
gallbladder 751.69
genitalia, genital organ(s)
  female 752.89
    external 752.49
    internal NEC 752.89
  in adiposogenital dystrophy 253.8
  male 752.89
    penis 752.69
glottis 748.3
hair 757.4
hand 755.21
heart 746.89
  left (complex) (syndrome) 746.7
  valve NEC 746.89
    pulmonary 746.01
humerus (*see also* Absence, humerus,
    congenital) 755.24
hymen 752.49
intestine (small) 751.1
  large 751.2
iris 743.46
jaw 524.09
kidney(s) 753.0
labium (majus) (minus) 752.49
labyrinth, membranous 744.05
lacrimal duct (apparatus) 743.65
larynx 748.3
leg (*see also* Absence, limb, congenital,
    lower) 755.30
limb 755.4
  lower (*see also* Absence, limb,
    congenital, lower) 755.30
  upper (*see also* Absence, limb,
    congenital, upper) 755.20
liver 751.69
lung (lobe) 748.5
mammary (areolar) 611.82
mandibular 524.04
  alveolar 524.74
  unilateral condylar 526.89

Hypoplasia, hypoplasis *(Continued)*
maxillary 524.03
  alveolar 524.73
medullary 284.9
megakaryocytic 287.30
metacarpus (*see also* Absence,
    metacarpal, congenital) 755.28
metatarsus (*see also* Absence,
    metatarsal, congenital) 755.38
muscle 756.89
  eye 743.69
myocardium (congenital) (Uhl's
    anomaly) 746.84
nail(s) 757.5
nasolacrimal duct 743.65
nervous system NEC 742.8
neural 742.8
nose, nasal 748.1
ophthalmic (*see also* Microphthalmos)
    743.10
optic nerve 377.43
organ
  of Corti 744.05
  or site NEC - *see* Anomaly, by site
osseous meatus (ear) 744.03
ovary 752.0
oviduct 752.19
pancreas 751.7
parathyroid (gland) 759.2
parotid gland 750.26
patella 755.64
pelvis, pelvic girdle 755.69
penis 752.69
peripheral vascular system (congenital)
    NEC 747.60
  gastrointestinal 747.61
  lower limb 747.64
  renal 747.62
  specified NEC 747.69
  spinal 747.82
  upper limb 747.63
pituitary (gland) 759.2
pulmonary 748.5
  arteriovenous 747.3
  artery 747.3
  valve 746.01
punctum lacrimale 743.65
radioulnar (*see also* Absence, radius,
    congenital, with ulna) 755.25
radius (*see also* Absence, radius,
    congenital) 755.26
rectum 751.2
respiratory system NEC 748.9
rib 756.3
sacrum 756.19
scapula 755.59
shoulder girdle 755.59
skin 757.39
skull (bone) 756.0
  with
    anencephalus 740.0
    encephalocele 742.0
    hydrocephalus 742.3
      with spina bifida (*see also*
        Spina bifida) 741.0 ●
    microcephalus 742.1
spinal (cord) (ventral horn cell) 742.59
  vessel 747.82
spine 756.19
spleen 759.0
sternum 756.3
tarsus (*see also* Absence, tarsal,
    congenital) 755.38
testis, testicle 752.89

Hypoplasia, hypoplasis *(Continued)*
thymus (gland) 279.11
thyroid (gland) 243
  cartilage 748.3
tibiofibular (*see also* Absence, tibia,
    congenital, with fibula) 755.35
toe (*see also* Absence, toe, congenital)
    755.39
tongue 750.16
trachea (cartilage) (rings) 748.3
Turner's (tooth) 520.4
ulna (*see also* Absence, ulna, congenital)
    755.27
umbilical artery 747.5
ureter 753.29
uterus 752.32 ◀▥
vagina 752.45 ◀▥
vascular (peripheral) NEC (*see also*
    Hypoplasia, peripheral vascular
    system) 747.60
  brain 747.81
vein(s) (peripheral) NEC (*see also*
    Hypoplasia, peripheral vascular
    system) 747.60
  brain 747.81
  cardiac 746.89
  great 747.49
  portal 747.49
  pulmonary 747.49
  vena cava (inferior) (superior) 747.49
vertebra 756.19
vulva 752.49
zonule (ciliary) 743.39
zygoma 738.12
Hypopotassemia 276.8
Hypoproaccelerinemia (*see also* Defect,
    coagulation) 286.3
Hypoproconvertinemia (congenital) (*see
    also* Defect, coagulation) 286.3
Hypoproteinemia (essential)
    (hypermetabolic) (idiopathic) 273.8
Hypoproteinosis 260
Hypoprothrombinemia (congenital)
    (hereditary) (idiopathic) (*see also*
    Defect, coagulation) 286.3
  acquired 286.7
  newborn 776.3
Hypopselaphesia 782.0
Hypopyon (anterior chamber) (eye)
    364.05
  iritis 364.05
  ulcer (cornea) 370.04
Hypopyrexia 780.99
Hyporeflex 796.1
Hyporeninemia, extreme 790.99
  in primary aldosteronism 255.10
Hyporesponsive episode 780.09
Hyposecretion
  ACTH 253.4
  ovary 256.39
    postablative 256.2
  salivary gland (any) 527.7
Hyposegmentation of neutrophils,
    hereditary 288.2
Hyposiderinemia 280.9
Hyposmolality 276.1
  syndrome 276.1
Hyposomatotropism 253.3
Hyposomnia, unspecified (*see also*
    Insomnia) 780.52
  with sleep apnea, unspecified 780.51
Hypospadias (male) 752.61
  female 753.8
Hypospermatogenesis 606.1

Hyposphagma 372.72
Hyposplenism 289.59
Hypostasis, pulmonary 514
Hypostatic - *see* condition
Hyposthenuria 593.89
Hyposuprarenalism 255.41
Hypo-TBG-nemia 246.8
Hypotension (arterial) (constitutional)
    458.9
  chronic 458.1
  iatrogenic 458.29
  maternal, syndrome (following labor
      and delivery) 669.2●
  of hemodialysis 458.21
  orthostatic (chronic) 458.0
    dysautonomic-dyskinetic syndrome
      333.0
  permanent idiopathic 458.1
  postoperative 458.29
  postural 458.0
  specified type NEC 458.8
  transient 796.3
Hypothermia (accidental) 991.6
  anesthetic 995.89
  associated with low environmental
    temperature 991.6
  newborn NEC 778.3
  not associated with low environmental
    temperature 780.65
Hypothymergasia (*see also* Psychosis,
    affective) 296.2●
  recurrent episode 296.3●
  single episode 296.2●
Hypothyroidism (acquired) 244.9
  complicating pregnancy, childbirth, or
    puerperium 648.1●
  congenital 243
  due to
    ablation 244.1
      radioactive iodine 244.1
      surgical 244.0
    iodine (administration) (ingestion)
      244.2
      radioactive 244.1
    irradiation therapy 244.1

Hypothyroidism (*Continued*)
  due to (*Continued*)
    p-aminosalicylic acid (PAS) 244.3
    phenylbutazone 244.3
    resorcinol 244.3
    specified cause NEC 244.8
    surgery 244.0
  goitrous (sporadic) 246.1
  iatrogenic NEC 244.3
  iodine 244.2
  pituitary 244.8
  postablative NEC 244.1
  postsurgical 244.0
  primary 244.9
  secondary NEC 244.8
  specified cause NEC 244.8
  sporadic goitrous 246.1
Hypotonia, hypotonicity, hypotony
    781.3
  benign congenital 358.8
  bladder 596.4
  congenital 779.89
    benign 358.8
  eye 360.30
    due to
      fistula 360.32
        ocular disorder NEC 360.33
      following loss of aqueous or
        vitreous 360.33
      primary 360.31
  infantile muscular (benign) 359.0
  muscle 728.9
  uterus, uterine (contractions) - *see*
    Inertia, uterus
Hypotrichosis 704.09
  congenital 757.4
  lid (congenital) 757.4
    acquired 374.55
  postinfectional NEC 704.09
Hypotropia 378.32
Hypoventilation 786.09
  congenital central alveolar syndrome
    327.25
  idiopathic sleep related nonobstructive
    alveolar 327.24

Hypoventilation (*Continued*)
  obesity 278.03 ◀
  sleep related, in conditions classifiable
    elsewhere 327.26
Hypovitaminosis (*see also* Deficiency,
    vitamin) 269.2
Hypovolemia 276.52
  surgical shock 998.0
  traumatic (shock) 958.4
Hypoxemia (*see also* Anoxia) 799.02
  sleep related, in conditions classifiable
    elsewhere 327.26
Hypoxia (*see also* Anoxia) 799.02
  cerebral 348.1
    during or resulting from a
      procedure 997.01
    newborn 770.88
      mild or moderate 768.6
      severe 768.5
  fetal, affecting newborn 770.88
  intrauterine - *see* Distress, fetal
  myocardial (*see also* Insufficiency,
    coronary) 411.89
    arteriosclerotic - *see* Arteriosclerosis,
      coronary
  newborn 770.88
  sleep related 327.24
Hypoxic-ischemic encephalopathy
    (HIE) 768.70
  mild 768.71
  moderate 768.72
  severe 768.73
Hypsarrhythmia (*see also* Epilepsy)
    345.6●
Hysteralgia, pregnant uterus 646.8●
Hysteria, hysterical 300.10
  anxiety 300.20
  Charcôt's gland 300.11
  conversion (any manifestation)
    300.11
  dissociative type NEC 300.15
  psychosis, acute 298.1
Hysteroepilepsy 300.11
Hysterotomy, affecting fetus or newborn
    763.89

◀ New   ◀⫶ Revised   ~~deleted~~ Deleted   ● Use Additional Digit(s)   Omit code

I

Iatrogenic syndrome of excess cortisol 255.0
IBM (inclusion body myositis) 359.71
Iceland disease (epidemic neuromyasthenia) 049.8
Ichthyosis (congenita) 757.1
    acquired 701.1
    fetalis gravior 757.1
    follicularis 757.1
    hystrix 757.39
    lamellar 757.1
    lingual 528.6
    palmaris and plantaris 757.39
    simplex 757.1
    vera 757.1
    vulgaris 757.1
Ichthyotoxism 988.0
    bacterial (see also Poisoning, food) 005.9
Icteroanemia, hemolytic (acquired) 283.9
    congenital (see also Spherocytosis) 282.0
Icterus (see also Jaundice) 782.4
    catarrhal - see Icterus, infectious
    conjunctiva 782.4
        newborn 774.6
    epidemic - see Icterus, infectious
    febrilis - see Icterus, infectious
    fetus or newborn - see Jaundice, fetus or newborn
    gravis (see also Necrosis, liver) 570
        complicating pregnancy 646.7●
            affecting fetus or newborn 760.8
        fetus or newborn NEC 773.0
        obstetrical 646.7●
            affecting fetus or newborn 760.8
    hematogenous (acquired) 283.9
    hemolytic (acquired) 283.9
        congenital (see also Spherocytosis) 282.0
    hemorrhagic (acute) 100.0
        leptospiral 100.0
        newborn 776.0
        spirochetal 100.0
    infectious 070.1
        with hepatic coma 070.0
        leptospiral 100.0
        spirochetal 100.0
    intermittens juvenilis 277.4
    malignant (see also Necrosis, liver) 570
    neonatorum (see also Jaundice, fetus or newborn) 774.6
    pernicious (see also Necrosis, liver) 570
    spirochetal 100.0
Ictus solaris, solis 992.0
Id reaction (due to bacteria) 692.89
Ideation
    homicidal V62.85 ◄
    suicidal V62.84
Identity disorder 313.82
    dissociative 300.14
    gender role (child) 302.6
        adult 302.85
    psychosexual (child) 302.6
        adult 302.85
Idioglossia 307.9
Idiopathic - see condition
Idiosyncrasy (see also Allergy) 995.3
    drug, medicinal substance, and biological - see Allergy, drug
Idiot, idiocy (congenital) 318.2
    amaurotic (Bielschowsky) (-Jansky) (family) (infantile (late)) (juvenile (late)) (Vogt-Spielmeyer) 330.1
    microcephalic 742.1
    Mongolian 758.0
    oxycephalic 756.0

IEED (involuntary emotional expression disorder) 310.8
IFIS (intraoperative floppy iris syndrome) 364.81
IgE asthma 493.0●
Ileitis (chronic) (see also Enteritis) 558.9
    infectious 009.0
    noninfectious 558.9
    regional (ulcerative) 555.0
        with large intestine 555.2
    segmental 555.0
        with large intestine 555.2
    terminal (ulcerative) 555.0
        with large intestine 555.2
Ileocolitis (see also Enteritis) 558.9
    infectious 009.0
    regional 555.2
    ulcerative 556.1
Ileostomy status V44.2
    with complication 569.60
Ileotyphus 002.0
Ileum - see condition
Ileus (adynamic) (bowel) (colon) (inhibitory) (intestine) (neurogenic) (paralytic) 560.1
    arteriomesenteric duodenal 537.2
    due to gallstone (in intestine) 560.31
    duodenal, chronic 537.2
    following gastrointestinal surgery 997.4
    gallstone 560.31
    mechanical (see also Obstruction, intestine) 560.9
    meconium 777.1
        due to cystic fibrosis 277.01
    myxedema 564.89
    postoperative 997.4
    transitory, newborn 777.4
Iliac - see condition
Iliotibial band friction syndrome 728.89
Ill, louping 063.1
Illegitimacy V61.6
Illness - see also Disease
    factitious 300.19
        with
            combined psychological and physical signs and symptoms 300.19
            physical symptoms 300.19
            predominantly
                physical signs and symptoms 300.19
                psychological symptoms 300.16
        chronic (with physical symptoms) 301.51
    heart - see Disease, heart
    manic-depressive (see also Psychosis, affective) 296.80
    mental (see also Disorder, mental) 300.9
Imbalance 781.2
    autonomic (see also Neuropathy, peripheral, autonomic) 337.9
    electrolyte 276.9
        with
            abortion - see Abortion, by type, with metabolic disorder
            ectopic pregnancy (see also categories 633.0–633.9) 639.4
            hyperemesis gravidarum (before 22 completed weeks' gestation) 643.1●
            molar pregnancy (see also categories 630–632) 639.4

Imbalance (Continued)
    electrolyte (Continued)
        following
            abortion 639.4
            ectopic or molar pregnancy 639.4
            neonatal, transitory NEC 775.5
        endocrine 259.9
        eye muscle NEC 378.9
            heterophoria - see Heterophoria
        glomerulotubular NEC 593.89
        hormone 259.9
        hysterical (see also Hysteria) 300.10
        labyrinth NEC 386.50
        posture 729.90
        sympathetic (see also Neuropathy, peripheral, autonomic) 337.9
Imbecile, imbecility 318.0
    moral 301.7
    old age 290.9
    senile 290.9
    specified IQ - see IQ
    unspecified IQ 318.0
Imbedding, intrauterine device 996.32
Imbibition, cholesterol (gallbladder) 575.6
Imerslund (-Gräsbeck) syndrome (anemia due to familial selective vitamin B_{12} malabsorption) 281.1
Iminoacidopathy 270.8
Iminoglycinuria, familial 270.8
Immature - see also Immaturity
    personality 301.89
Immaturity 765.1●
    extreme 765.0●
    fetus or infant light-for-dates - see Light-for-dates
    lung, fetus or newborn 770.4
    organ or site NEC - see Hypoplasia
    pulmonary, fetus or newborn 770.4
    reaction 301.89
    sexual (female) (male) 259.0
Immersion 994.1
    foot 991.4
    hand 991.4
Immobile, immobility
    complete
        due to severe physical disability or frality 780.72
    intestine 564.89
    joint - see Ankylosis
    syndrome (paraplegic) 728.3
Immunization
    ABO
        affecting management of pregnancy 656.2●
        fetus or newborn 773.1
    complication - see Complications, vaccination
    Rh factor
        affecting management of pregnancy 656.1●
        fetus or newborn 773.0
        from transfusion (see also Complications, transfusion) 999.70 ◄▥
Immunodeficiency 279.3
    with
        adenosine-deaminase deficiency 279.2
        defect, predominant
            B-cell 279.00
            T-cell 279.10
        hyperimmunoglobulinemia 279.2
        lymphopenia, hereditary 279.2
        thrombocytopenia and eczema 279.12

Immunodeficiency *(Continued)*
  with *(Continued)*
    thymic
      aplasia 279.2
      dysplasia 279.2
    autosomal recessive, Swiss-type
      279.2
    common variable 279.06
    severe combined (SCID) 279.2
    to Rh factor
      affecting management of pregnancy
        656.1 ●
      fetus or newborn 773.0
    X-linked, with increased IgM 279.05
Immunotherapy, prophylactic V07.2
  antineoplastic V58.12
Impaction, impacted
  bowel, colon, rectum 560.30
    with hernia - *see also* Hernia, by site,
      with, obstruction
        gangrenous - *see* Hernia, by site,
          with gangrene
    by
      calculus 560.39
      gallstone 560.31
      fecal 560.32 ◀▥
    specified type NEC 560.39
  calculus - *see* Calculus
  cerumen (ear) (external) 380.4
  cuspid 520.6
  dental 520.6
  fecal, feces 560.32 ◀▥
    with hernia - *see also* Hernia, by site,
      with obstruction
        gangrenous - *see* Hernia, by site,
          with gangrene
  fracture - *see* Fracture, by site
  gallbladder - *see* Cholelithiasis
  gallstone(s) - *see* Cholelithiasis
    in intestine (any part) 560.31
  intestine(s) 560.30
    with hernia - *see also* Hernia, by site,
      with obstruction
        gangrenous - *see* Hernia, by site,
          with gangrene
    by
      calculus 560.39
      gallstone 560.31
      fecal 560.32 ◀▥
    specified type NEC 560.39
  intrauterine device (IUD) 996.32
  molar 520.6
  shoulder 660.4 ●
    affecting fetus or newborn 763.1
  tooth, teeth 520.6
  turbinate 733.99
Impaired, impairment (function)
  arm V49.1
    movement, involving
      musculoskeletal system V49.1
      nervous system V49.2
  auditory discrimination 388.43
  back V48.3
  body (entire) V49.89
  cognitive, mild, so stated 331.83
  combined visual hearing V49.85
  dual sensory V49.85
  glucose
    fasting 790.21
    tolerance test (oral) 790.22
  hearing (*see also* Deafness) 389.9
    combined with visual impairment
      V49.85
  heart - *see* Disease, heart

Impaired, impairment *(Continued)*
  kidney (*see also* Disease, renal)
    593.9
    disorder resulting from 588.9
      specified NEC 588.89
  leg V49.1
    movement, involving
      musculoskeletal system
        V49.1
      nervous system V49.2
  limb V49.1
    movement, involving
      musculoskeletal system
        V49.1
      nervous system V49.2
  liver 573.8
  mastication 524.9
  mild cognitive, so stated 331.83
  mobility
    ear ossicles NEC 385.22
    incostapedial joint 385.22
    malleus 385.21
  myocardium, myocardial (*see also*
    Insufficiency, myocardial)
    428.0
  neuromusculoskeletal NEC V49.89
    back V48.3
    head V48.2
    limb V49.2
    neck V48.3
    spine V48.3
    trunk V48.3
  rectal sphincter 787.99
  renal (*see also* Disease, renal) 593.9
    disorder resulting from 588.9
      specified NEC 588.89
  spine V48.3
  vision NEC 369.9
    both eyes NEC 369.3
    combined with hearing impairment
      V49.85
    moderate 369.74
      both eyes 369.25
        with impairment of lesser eye
          (specified as)
          blind, not further specified
            369.15
          low vision, not further
            specified 369.23
          near-total 369.17
          profound 369.18
          severe 369.24
          total 369.16
      one eye 369.74
        with vision of other eye
          (specified as)
          near-normal 369.75
          normal 369.76
    near-total 369.64
      both eyes 369.04
        with impairment of lesser eye
          (specified as)
          blind, not further specified
            369.02
          total 369.03
      one eye 369.64
        with vision of other eye
          (specified as)
          near-normal 369.65
          normal 369.66
    one eye 369.60
      with low vision of other eye
        369.10

Impaired, impairment *(Continued)*
  vision NEC *(Continued)*
    profound 369.67
      both eyes 369.08
        with impairment of lesser eye
          (specified as)
          blind, not further specified
            369.05
          near-total 369.07
          total 369.06
      one eye 369.67
        with vision of other eye
          (specified as)
          near-normal 369.68
          normal 369.69
    severe 369.71
      both eyes 369.22
        with impairment of lesser eye
          (specified as)
          blind, not further specified
            369.11
        low vision, not further
          specified 369.21
        near-total 369.13
        profound 369.14
        total 369.12
    one eye 369.71
      with vision of other eye
        (specified as)
        near-normal 369.72
        normal 369.73
    total
      both eyes 369.01
      one eye 369.61
        with vision of other eye
        (specified as)
        near-normal 369.62
        normal 369.63
Impaludism - *see* Malaria
Impediment, speech NEC 784.59
  psychogenic 307.9
  secondary to organic lesion 784.59
Impending
  cerebrovascular accident or attack 435.9
  coronary syndrome 411.1
  delirium tremens 291.0
  myocardial infarction 411.1
Imperception, auditory (acquired)
  (congenital) 389.9
Imperfect
  aeration, lung (newborn) 770.5
  closure (congenital)
    alimentary tract NEC 751.8
      lower 751.5
      upper 750.8
    atrioventricular ostium 745.69
    atrium (secundum) 745.5
      primum 745.61
    branchial cleft or sinus 744.41
    choroid 743.59
    cricoid cartilage 748.3
    cusps, heart valve NEC 746.89
      pulmonary 746.09
    ductus
      arteriosus 747.0
      Botalli 747.0
    ear drum 744.29
      causing impairment of hearing
        744.03
    endocardial cushion 745.60
    epiglottis 748.3
    esophagus with communication to
      bronchus or trachea 750.3
    Eustachian valve 746.89

Imperfect *(Continued)*
  closure *(Continued)*
    eyelid 743.62
    face, facial *(see also* Cleft, lip) 749.10
    foramen
      Botalli 745.5
      ovale 745.5
    genitalia, genital organ(s) or system
      female 752.89
        external 752.49
        internal NEC 752.89
          uterus 752.39 ◀▥
      male 752.89
        penis 752.69
    glottis 748.3
    heart valve (cusps) NEC 746.89
    interatrial ostium or septum 745.5
    interauricular ostium or septum 745.5
    interventricular ostium or septum 745.4
    iris 743.46
    kidney 753.3
    larynx 748.3
    lens 743.36
    lip *(see also* Cleft, lip) 749.10
    nasal septum or sinus 748.1
    nose 748.1
    omphalomesenteric duct 751.0
    optic nerve entry 743.57
    organ or site NEC - *see* Anomaly, specified type, by site
    ostium
      interatrial 745.5
      interauricular 745.5
      interventricular 745.4
    palate *(see also* Cleft, palate) 749.00
    preauricular sinus 744.46
    retina 743.56
    roof of orbit 742.0
    sclera 743.47
    septum
      aortic 745.0
      aorticopulmonary 745.0
      atrial (secundum) 745.5
        primum 745.61
      between aorta and pulmonary artery 745.0
      heart 745.9
      interatrial (secundum) 745.5
        primum 745.61
      interauricular (secundum) 745.5
        primum 745.61
      interventricular 745.4
        with pulmonary stenosis or atresia, dextraposition of aorta, and hypertrophy of right ventricle 745.2
        in tetralogy of Fallot 745.2
      nasal 748.1
      ventricular 745.4
        with pulmonary stenosis or atresia, dextraposition of aorta, and hypertrophy of right ventricle 745.2
        in tetralogy of Fallot 745.2
    skull 756.0
      with
        anencephalus 740.0
        encephalocele 742.0
        hydrocephalus 742.3
          with spina bifida *(see also* Spina bifida) 741.0●
        microcephalus 742.1

Imperfect *(Continued)*
  closure *(Continued)*
    spine (with meningocele) *(see also* Spina bifida) 741.90
    thyroid cartilage 748.3
    trachea 748.3
    tympanic membrane 744.29
      causing impairment of hearing 744.03
    uterus (with communication to bladder, intestine, or rectum) 752.39 ◀▥
      with cleft lip *(see also* Cleft, palate, with cleft lip) 749.20
    uvula 749.02
    vitelline duct 751.0
  development - *see* Anomaly, by site
  erection 607.84
  fusion - *see* Imperfect, closure
  inflation lung (newborn) 770.5
  intestinal canal 751.5
  poise 729.90
  rotation - *see* Malrotation
  septum, ventricular 745.4
Imperfectly descended testis 752.51
Imperforate (congenital) - *see also* Atresia
  anus 751.2
  bile duct 751.61
  cervix (uteri) 752.49
  esophagus 750.3
  hymen 752.42
  intestine (small) 751.1
    large 751.2
  jejunum 751.1
  pharynx 750.29
  rectum 751.2
  salivary duct 750.23
  urethra 753.6
  urinary meatus 753.6
  vagina 752.49
Impervious (congenital) - *see also* Atresia
  anus 751.2
  bile duct 751.61
  esophagus 750.3
  intestine (small) 751.1
    large 751.5
  rectum 751.2
  urethra 753.6
Impetiginization of other dermatoses 684
Impetigo (any organism) (any site) (bullous) (circinate) (contagiosa) (neonatorum) (simplex) 684
  Bockhart's (superficial folliculitis) 704.8
  external ear 684 *[380.13]*
  eyelid 684 *[373.5]*
  Fox's (contagiosa) 684
  furfuracea 696.5
  herpetiformis 694.3
    nonobstetrical 694.3
  staphylococcal infection 684
  ulcerative 686.8
  vulgaris 684
Impingement, soft tissue between teeth 524.89
  anterior 524.81
  posterior 524.82
Implant, endometrial 617.9
Implantation
  anomalous - *see also* Anomaly, specified type, by site
    ureter 753.4

Implantation *(Continued)*
  cyst
    external area or site (skin) NEC 709.8
    iris 364.61
    vagina 623.8
    vulva 624.8
  dermoid (cyst)
    external area or site (skin) NEC 709.8
    iris 364.61
    vagina 623.8
    vulva 624.8
  placenta, low or marginal - *see* Placenta previa
Impotence (sexual) 607.84
  organic origin NEC 607.84
  psychogenic 302.72
Impoverished blood 285.9
Impression, basilar 756.0
Imprisonment V62.5
Improper
  development, infant 764.9●
Improperly tied umbilical cord (causing hemorrhage) 772.3
Impulses, obsessional 300.3
Impulsive 799.23
  neurosis 300.3
Impulsiveness 799.23
Inaction, kidney *(see also* Disease, renal) 593.9
Inactive - *see* condition
Inadequate, inadequacy
  aesthetics of dental restoration 525.67
  biologic 301.6
  cardiac and renal - *see* Hypertension, cardiorenal
  constitutional 301.6
  development
    child 783.40
    fetus 764.9●
      affecting management of pregnancy 656.5●
    genitalia
      after puberty NEC 259.0
      congenital - *see* Hypoplasia, genitalia
    lungs 748.5
    organ or site NEC - *see* Hypoplasia, by site
  dietary 269.9
  distance, interarch 524.28
  education V62.3
  environment
    economic problem V60.2
    household condition NEC V60.1
    poverty V60.2
    unemployment V62.0
  functional 301.6
  household care, due to
    family member
      handicapped or ill V60.4
      temporarily away from home V60.4
      on vacation V60.5
    technical defects in home V60.1
    temporary absence from home of person rendering care V60.4
  housing (heating) (space) V60.1
  interarch distance 524.28
  material resources V60.2
  mental *(see also* Retardation, mental) 319
  nervous system 799.29
  personality 301.6

Inadequate, inadequacy *(Continued)*
 prenatal care in current pregnancy V23.7
 pulmonary
  function 786.09
   newborn 770.89
  ventilation, newborn 770.89
 respiration 786.09
  newborn 770.89
 sample
  cytology
   anal 796.78
   cervical 795.08
   vaginal 795.18
 social 301.6
Inanition 263.9
 with edema 262
 due to
  deprivation of food 994.2
  malnutrition 263.9
 fever 780.60
Inappropriate secretion
 ACTH 255.0
 antidiuretic hormone (ADH) (excessive) 253.6
  deficiency 253.5
 ectopic hormone NEC 259.3
 pituitary (posterior) 253.6
Inattention after or at birth 995.52
Inborn errors of metabolism - *see* Disorder, metabolism
Incarceration, incarcerated
 bubonocele - *see also* Hernia, inguinal, with obstruction
  gangrenous - *see* Hernia, inguinal, with gangrene
 colon (by hernia) - *see also* Hernia, by site with obstruction
  gangrenous - *see* Hernia, by site, with gangrene
 enterocele 552.9
  gangrenous 551.9
 epigastrocele 552.29
  gangrenous 551.29
 epiplocele 552.9
  gangrenous 551.9
 exomphalos 552.1
  gangrenous 551.1
 fallopian tube 620.8
 hernia - *see also* Hernia, by site, with obstruction
  gangrenous - *see* Hernia, by site, with gangrene
 iris, in wound 871.1
 lens, in wound 871.1
 merocele (*see also* Hernia, femoral, with obstruction) 552.00
 omentum (by hernia) - *see also* Hernia, by site, with obstruction
  gangrenous - *see* Hernia, by site, with gangrene
 omphalocele 756.72
 rupture (meaning hernia) (*see also* Hernia, by site, with obstruction) 552.9
  gangrenous (*see also* Hernia, by site, with gangrene) 551.9
 sarcoepiplocele 552.9
  gangrenous 551.9
 sarcoepiplomphalocele 552.1
  with gangrene 551.1
 uterus 621.8
  gravid 654.3●
   causing obstructed labor 660.2●
    affecting fetus or newborn 763.1

Incident, cerebrovascular (*see also* Disease, cerebrovascular, acute) 436
Incineration (entire body) (from fire, conflagration, electricity, or lightning) - *see* Burn, multiple, specified sites
Incised wound
 external - *see* Wound, open, by site
 internal organs (abdomen, chest, or pelvis) - *see* Injury, internal, by site, with open wound
Incision, incisional
 hernia - *see* Hernia, incisional
 surgical, complication - *see* Complications, surgical procedures
 traumatic
  external - *see* Wound, open, by site
  internal organs (abdomen, chest, or pelvis) - *see* Injury, internal, by site, with open wound
Inclusion
 azurophilic leukocytic 288.2
 blennorrhea (neonatal) (newborn) 771.6
 cyst - *see* Cyst, skin
 gallbladder in liver (congenital) 751.69
Incompatibility
 ABO
  affecting management of pregnancy 656.2●
  fetus or newborn 773.1
  infusion or transfusion reaction (*see also* Complications, transfusion) 999.60 ◀▥
 blood (group) (Duffy) (E) (K(ell)) (Kidd) (Lewis) (M) (N) (P) (S) NEC
  affecting management of pregnancy 656.2●
  fetus or newborn 773.2
  infusion or transfusion reaction (*see also* Complications, transfusion) 999.75 ◀▥
 contour of existing restoration of tooth with oral health 525.65
 marital V61.10
  involving
   divorce V61.03
   estrangement V61.09
 non-ABO (*see also* Complications, transfusion) 999.75 ◀
 Rh (antigen) (C) (c) (D) (E) (e) (blood group) (factor) ◀▥
  affecting management of pregnancy 656.1●
  fetus or newborn 773.0
  infusion or transfusion reaction (*see also* Complications, transfusion) 999.70 ◀▥
 Rhesus - *see* Incompatibility, Rh
Incompetency, incompetence, incompetent
 annular
  aortic (valve) (*see also* Insufficiency, aortic) 424.1
  mitral (valve) - (*see also* Insufficiency, mitral) 424.0
  pulmonary valve (heart) (*see also* Endocarditis, pulmonary) 424.3
 aortic (valve) (*see also* Insufficiency, aortic) 424.1
  syphilitic 093.22
 cardiac (orifice) 530.0
  valve - *see* Endocarditis
 cervix, cervical (os) 622.5
  in pregnancy 654.5●
   affecting fetus or newborn 761.0

Incompetency, incompetence, incompetent *(Continued)*
 chronotropic 426.89
  with
   autonomic dysfunction 337.9
   ischemic heart disease 414.9
   left ventricular dysfunction 429.89
   sinus node dysfunction 427.81
 esophagogastric (junction) (sphincter) 530.0
 heart valve, congenital 746.89
 mitral (valve) - *see* Insufficiency, mitral
 papillary muscle (heart) 429.81
 pelvic fundus
  pubocervical tissue 618.81
  rectovaginal tissue 618.82
 pulmonary valve (heart) (*see also* Endocarditis, pulmonary) 424.3
  congenital 746.09
 tricuspid (annular) (rheumatic) (valve) (*see also* Endocarditis, tricuspid) 397.0
 valvular - *see* Endocarditis
 vein, venous (saphenous) (varicose) (*see also* Varicose, vein) 454.9
 velopharyngeal (closure)
  acquired 528.9
  congenital 750.29
Incomplete - *see also* condition
 bladder emptying 788.21
 defecation 787.61 ◀
 expansion lungs (newborn) 770.5
 gestation (liveborn) - *see* Immaturity
 rotation - *see* Malrotation
Inconclusive
 image test due to excess body fat 793.91
 mammogram, mammography 793.82
  due to dense breasts 793.82
Incontinence 788.30
 without sensory awareness 788.34
 anal sphincter 787.60 ◀▥
 continuous leakage 788.37
 feces, fecal 787.60 ◀▥
  due to hysteria 300.11
  nonorganic origin 307.7
 hysterical 300.11
 mixed (male) (female) (urge and stress) 788.33
 overflow 788.38
 paradoxical 788.39
 rectal 787.60 ◀▥
 specified NEC 788.39
 stress (female) 625.6
  male NEC 788.32
 urethral sphincter 599.84
 urge 788.31
  and stress (male) (female) 788.33
 urine 788.30
  active 788.30
  due to
   cognitive impairment 788.91
   severe physical disability 788.91
   immobility 788.91
  functional 788.91
  male 788.30
   stress 788.32
    and urge 788.33
  neurogenic 788.39
  nonorganic origin 307.6
  stress (female) 625.6
   male NEC 788.32
  urge 788.31
   and stress 788.33
Incontinentia pigmenti 757.33

Incoordinate
uterus (action) (contractions) 661.4●
affecting fetus or newborn 763.7
Incoordination
esophageal-pharyngeal (newborn) 787.24
muscular 781.3
papillary muscle 429.81
Increase, increased
abnormal, in development 783.9
androgens (ovarian) 256.1
anticoagulants (antithrombin) (anti-VIIIa) (anti-IXa) (anti-Xa) (anti-XIa) 286.5
postpartum 666.3●
cold sense (see also Disturbance, sensation) 782.0
estrogen 256.0
function
adrenal (cortex) 255.3
medulla 255.6
pituitary (anterior) (gland) (lobe) 253.1
posterior 253.6
heat sense (see also Disturbance, sensation) 782.0
intracranial pressure 781.99
injury at birth 767.8
light reflex of retina 362.13
permeability, capillary 448.9
pressure
intracranial 781.99
injury at birth 767.8
intraocular 365.00
pulsations 785.9
pulse pressure 785.9
sphericity, lens 743.36
splenic activity 289.4
venous pressure 459.89
portal 572.3
Incrustation, cornea, lead, or zinc 930.0
Incyclophoria 378.44
Incyclotropia 378.33
Indeterminate sex 752.7
India rubber skin 756.83
Indicanuria 270.2
Indigestion (bilious) (functional) 536.8
acid 536.8
catarrhal 536.8
due to decomposed food NEC 005.9
fat 579.8
nervous 306.4
psychogenic 306.4
Indirect - see condition
Indolent bubo NEC 099.8
Induced
abortion - see Abortion, induced
birth, affecting fetus or newborn 763.89
delivery - see Delivery
labor - see Delivery
Induration, indurated
brain 348.89
breast (fibrous) 611.79
puerperal, postpartum 676.3●
broad ligament 620.8
chancre 091.0
anus 091.1
congenital 090.0
extragenital NEC 091.2
corpora cavernosa (penis) (plastic) 607.89
liver (chronic) 573.8
acute 573.8

Induration, indurated (Continued)
lung (black) (brown) (chronic) (fibroid) (see also Fibrosis, lung) 515
essential brown 275.09 [516.1] ◀▥
penile 607.89
phlebitic - see Phlebitis
skin 782.8
stomach 537.89
Induratio penis plastica 607.89
Industrial - see condition
Inebriety (see also Abuse, drugs, nondependent) 305.0●
Inefficiency
kidney (see also Disease, renal) 593.9
thyroid (acquired) (gland) 244.9
Inelasticity, skin 782.8
Inequality, leg (acquired) (length) 736.81
congenital 755.30
Inertia
bladder 596.4
neurogenic 596.54
with cauda equina syndrome 344.61
stomach 536.8
psychogenic 306.4
uterus, uterine 661.2●
affecting fetus or newborn 763.7
primary 661.0●
secondary 661.1●
vesical 596.4
neurogenic 596.54
with cauda equina 344.61
Infant - see also condition
excessive crying of 780.92
fussy (baby) 780.91
held for adoption V68.89
newborn - see Newborn
post-term (gestation period over 40 completed weeks to 42 completed weeks) 766.21
prolonged gestation of (period over 42 completed weeks) 766.22
syndrome of diabetic mother 775.0
"Infant Hercules" syndrome 255.2
Infantile - see also condition
genitalia, genitals 259.0
in pregnancy or childbirth NEC 654.4●
affecting fetus or newborn 763.89
causing obstructed labor 660.2●
affecting fetus or newborn 763.1
heart 746.9
kidney 753.3
lack of care 995.52
macula degeneration 362.75
melanodontia 521.05
os, uterus (see also Infantile, genitalia) 259.0
pelvis 738.6
with disproportion (fetopelvic) 653.1●
affecting fetus or newborn 763.1
causing obstructed labor 660.1●
affecting fetus or newborn 763.1
penis 259.0
testis 257.2
uterus (see also Infantile, genitalia)259.0
vulva 752.49
Infantilism 259.9
with dwarfism (hypophyseal) 253.3
Brissaud's (infantile myxedema) 244.9
celiac 579.0

Infantilism (Continued)
Herter's (nontropical sprue) 579.0
hypophyseal 253.3
hypothalamic (with obesity) 253.8
idiopathic 259.9
intestinal 579.0
pancreatic 577.8
pituitary 253.3
renal 588.0
sexual (with obesity) 259.0
Infants, healthy liveborn - see Newborn
Infarct, infarction
adrenal (capsule) (gland) 255.41
amnion 658.8●
anterior (with contiguous portion of intraventricular septum) NEC (see also Infarct, myocardium) 410.1●
appendices epiploicae 557.0
bowel 557.0
brain (stem) 434.91
embolic (see also Embolism, brain) 434.11
healed or old without residuals V12.54
iatrogenic 997.02
lacunar 434.91
late effect - see Late effect(s) (of) cerebrovascular disease
postoperative 997.02
puerperal, postpartum, childbirth 674.0●
thrombotic (see also Thrombosis, brain) 434.01
breast 611.89
Brewer's (kidney) 593.81
cardiac (see also Infarct, myocardium) 410.9●
cerebellar (see also Infarct, brain) 434.91
embolic (see also Embolism, brain) 434.11
cerebral (see also Infarct, brain) 434.91
aborted 434.91
embolic (see also Embolism, brain) 434.11
thrombotic (see also Infarct, brain) 434.01
chorion 658.8●
colon (acute) (agnogenic) (embolic) (hemorrhagic) (nonocclusive) (nonthrombotic) (occlusive) (segmental) (thrombotic) (with gangrene) 557.0
coronary artery (see also Infarct, myocardium) 410.9●
cortical 434.91
embolic (see also Embolism) 444.9
fallopian tube 620.8
gallbladder 575.8
heart (see also Infarct, myocardium) 410.9●
hepatic 573.4
hypophysis (anterior lobe) 253.8
impending (myocardium) 411.1
intestine (acute) (agnogenic) (embolic) (hemorrhagic) (nonocclusive) (nonthrombotic) (occlusive) (thrombotic) (with gangrene) 557.0
kidney 593.81
lacunar 434.91
liver 573.4

Infarct, infarction (*Continued*)
  lung (embolic) (thrombotic) 415.19
    with
      abortion - *see* Abortion, by type,
        with, embolism
      ectopic pregnancy (*see also*
        categories 633.0–633.9) 639.6
      molar pregnancy (*see also*
        categories 630–632) 639.6
    following
      abortion 639.6
      ectopic or molar pregnancy 639.6
    iatrogenic 415.11
    in pregnancy, childbirth, or
      puerperium - *see* Embolism,
      obstetrical
    postoperative 415.11
    septic 415.12
  lymph node or vessel 457.8
  medullary (brain) - *see* Infarct, brain
  meibomian gland (eyelid) 374.85
  mesentery, mesenteric (embolic)
    (thrombotic) (with gangrene)
    557.0
  midbrain - *see* Infarct, brain
  myocardium, myocardial (acute or
    with a stated duration of 8 weeks
    or less) (with hypertension)
    410.9●

Note: Use the following fifth-digit
subclassification with category 410:

  0   episode unspecified
  1   initial episode
  2   subsequent episode without
         recurrence

---

    with symptoms after 8 weeks from
      date of infarction 414.8
    anterior (wall) (with contiguous
      portion of intraventricular
      septum) NEC 410.1●
    anteroapical (with contiguous
      portion of intraventricular
      septum) 410.1●
    anterolateral (wall) 410.0●
    anteroseptal (with contiguous
      portion of intraventricular
      septum) 410.1●
    apical-lateral 410.5●
    atrial 410.8●
    basal-lateral 410.5●
    chronic (with symptoms after 8
      weeks from date of infarction)
      414.8
    diagnosed on ECG, but presenting
      no symptoms 412
    diaphragmatic wall (with
      contiguous portion of
      intraventricular septum)
      410.4●
    healed or old, currently presenting
      no symptoms 412
    high lateral 410.5●
    impending 411.1
    inferior (wall) (with contiguous
      portion of intraventricular
      septum) 410.4●
    inferolateral (wall) 410.2●
    inferoposterior wall 410.3●
    intraoperative 997.1
    lateral wall 410.5●
    non-Q wave 410.7●

Infarct, infarction (*Continued*)
  myocardium, myocardial (*Continued*)
    non-ST elevation (NSTEMI) 410.7●
    nontransmural 410.7●
    papillary muscle 410.8●
    past (diagnosed on ECG or other
      special investigation, but
      currently presenting no
      symptoms) 412
      with symptoms NEC 414.8
    posterior (strictly) (true) (wall)
      410.6●
    posterobasal 410.6●
    posteroinferior 410.3●
    posterolateral 410.5●
    postprocedural 997.1
    previous, currently presenting no
      symptoms 412
    Q wave (*see also* Infarct,
      myocardium, by site) 410.9●
    septal 410.8●
    specified site NEC 410.8●
    ST elevation (STEMI) 410.9●
      anterior (wall) 410.1●
      anterolateral (wall) 410.0●
      inferior (wall) 410.4●
      inferolateral (wall) 410.2●
      inferoposterior wall 410.3●
      lateral wall 410.5●
      posterior (strictly) (true) (wall)
        410.6●
      specified site NEC 410.8●
    subendocardial 410.7●
    syphilitic 093.82
  non-ST elevation myocardial infarction
    (NSTEMI) 410.7●
  nontransmural 410.7●
  omentum 557.0
  ovary 620.8
  pancreas 577.8
  papillary muscle (*see also* Infarct,
    myocardium) 410.8●
  parathyroid gland 252.8
  pituitary (gland) 253.8
  placenta (complicating pregnancy)
    656.7●
    affecting fetus or newborn 762.2
  pontine - *see* Infarct, brain
  posterior NEC (*see also* Infarct,
    myocardium) 410.6●
  prostate 602.8
  pulmonary (artery) (hemorrhagic)
    (vein) 415.19
    with
      abortion - *see* Abortion, by type,
        with embolism
      ectopic pregnancy (*see also*
        categories 633.0–633.9)
        639.6
      molar pregnancy (*see also*
        categories 630–632) 639.6
    following
      abortion 639.6
      ectopic or molar pregnancy 639.6
    iatrogenic 415.11
    in pregnancy, childbirth, or
      puerperium - *see* Embolism,
      obstetrical
    postoperative 415.11
    septic 415.12
  renal 593.81
    embolic or thrombotic 593.81
  retina, retinal 362.84
    with occlusion - *see* Occlusion, retina

Infarct, infarction (*Continued*)
  spinal (acute) (cord) (embolic)
    (nonembolic) 336.1
  spleen 289.59
    embolic or thrombotic 444.89
  subchorionic - *see* Infarct, placenta
  subendocardial (*see also* Infarct,
    myocardium) 410.7●
  suprarenal (capsule) (gland) 255.41
  syncytium - *see* Infarct, placenta
  testis 608.83
  thrombotic (*see also* Thrombosis)
    453.9
    artery, arterial - *see* Embolism
  thyroid (gland) 246.3
  ventricle (heart) (*see also* Infarct,
    myocardium) 410.9●
Infecting - *see* condition
Infection, infected, infective
    (opportunistic) 136.9
  with lymphangitis - *see* Lymphangitis
  abortion - *see* Abortion, by type, with,
    sepsis
  abscess (skin) - *see* Abscess, by site
  Absidia 117.7
  acanthamoeba 136.21
  Acanthocheilonema (perstans) 125.4
    streptocerca 125.6
  accessory sinus (chronic) (*see also*
    Sinusitis) 473.9
  Achorion - *see* Dermatophytosis
  Acremonium falciforme 117.4
  acromioclavicular (joint) 711.91
  Actinobacillus
    lignieresii 027.8
    mallei 024
    muris 026.1
  Actinomadura - *see* Actinomycosis
  Actinomyces (israelii) - *see also*
    Actinomycosis
    muris-ratti 026.1
  Actinomycetales (Actinomadura)
    (Actinomyces) (Nocardia)
    (Streptomyces) - *see*
    Actinomycosis
  actinomycotic NEC (*see also*
    Actinomycosis) 039.9
  adenoid (chronic) 474.01
    acute 463
    and tonsil (chronic) 474.02
      acute or subacute 463
  adenovirus NEC 079.0
    in diseases classified elsewhere - *see*
      category 079
    unspecified nature or site 079.0
  Aerobacter aerogenes NEC 041.85
    enteritis 008.2
  Aerogenes capsulatus (*see also*
    Gangrene, gas) 040.0
  aertrycke (*see also* Infection,
    Salmonella) 003.9
  Ajellomyces dermatitidis 116.0
  alimentary canal NEC (*see also*
    Enteritis, due to, by organism)
    009.0
  Allescheria boydii 117.6
  Alternaria 118
  alveolus, alveolar (process) (pulpal
    origin) 522.4
  ameba, amebic (histolytica) (*see also*
    Amebiasis) 006.9
    acute 006.0
    chronic 006.1
    free-living 136.29

Infection, infected, infective *(Continued)*
  ameba, amebic *(Continued)*
    hartmanni 007.8
    specified
      site NEC 006.8
      type NEC 007.8
  amniotic fluid or cavity 658.4 ●
    affecting fetus or newborn 762.7
  anaerobes (cocci) (gram-negative)
    (gram-positive) (mixed) NEC
    041.84
  anal canal 569.49
  Ancylostoma braziliense 126.2
  Angiostrongylus cantonensis 128.8
  anisakiasis 127.1
  Anisakis larva 127.1
  anthrax *(see also* Anthrax) 022.9
  antrum (chronic) *(see also* Sinusitis,
    maxillary) 473.0
  anus (papillae) (sphincter) 569.49
  arbor virus NEC 066.9
  arbovirus NEC 066.9
  argentophil-rod 027.0
  Ascaris lumbricoides 127.0
  ascomycetes 117.4
  Aspergillus (flavus) (fumigatus)
    (terreus) 117.3
  atypical
    acid-fast (bacilli) *(see also*
      Mycobacterium, atypical)
      031.9
    mycobacteria *(see also*
      Mycobacterium, atypical)
      031.9
  auditory meatus (circumscribed)
    (diffuse) (external) *(see also* Otitis,
    externa) 380.10
  auricle (ear) *(see also* Otitis, externa)
    380.10
  axillary gland 683
  Babesiasis 088.82
  Babesiosis 088.82
  Bacillus NEC 041.89
    abortus 023.1
    anthracis *(see also* Anthrax) 022.9
    cereus (food poisoning) 005.89
    coli - *see* Infection, Escherichia coli
    coliform NEC 041.85
    Ducrey's (any location) 099.0
    Flexner's 004.1
    Friedländer's NEC 041.3
    fusiformis 101
    gas (gangrene) *(see also* Gangrene,
      gas) 040.0
    mallei 024
    melitensis 023.0
    paratyphoid, paratyphosus 002.9
      A 002.1
      B 002.2
      C 002.3
    Schmorl's 040.3
    Shiga 004.0
    suipestifer *(see also* Infection,
      Salmonella) 003.9
    swimming pool 031.1
    typhosa 002.0
    welchii *(see also* Gangrene, gas)
      040.0
    Whitmore's 025
  bacterial NEC 041.9
    specified NEC 041.89
      anaerobic NEC 041.84
      gram-negative NEC 041.85
        anaerobic NEC 041.84

Infection, infected, infective *(Continued)*
  Bacterium
    paratyphosum 002.9
      A 002.1
      B 002.2
      C 002.3
    typhosum 002.9
  Bacteroides (fragilis) (melaninogenicus)
    (oralis) NEC 041.82
  Balantidium coli 007.0
  Bartholin's gland 616.89
  Basidiobolus 117.7
  Bedsonia 079.98
    specified NEC 079.88
  bile duct 576.1
  bladder *(see also* Cystitis) 595.9
  Blastomyces, blastomycotic 116.0
    brasiliensis 116.1
    dermatitidis 116.0
    European 117.5
    loboi 116.2
    North American 116.0
    South American 116.1
  bleb
    postprocedural 379.60
      stage 1 379.61
      stage 2 379.62
      stage 3 379.63
  blood stream - *see also* Septicemia
    catheter-related (CRBSI) 999.31
  bone 730.9 ●
    specified - *see* Osteomyelitis
  Bordetella 033.9
    bronchiseptica 033.8
    parapertussis 033.1
    pertussis 033.0
  Borrelia
    bergdorfi 088.81
    vincentii (mouth) (pharynx) (tonsil)
      101
  bovine stomatitis 059.11
  brain *(see also* Encephalitis) 323.9
    late effect - *see* category 326
    membranes - *(see also* Meningitis)
      322.9
    septic 324.0
      late effect - *see* category 326
      meninges *(see also* Meningitis)
        320.9
  branchial cyst 744.42
  breast 611.0
    puerperal, postpartum 675.2 ●
      with nipple 675.9 ●
        specified type NEC 675.8 ●
      nonpurulent 675.2 ●
      purulent 675.1 ●
  bronchus *(see also* Bronchitis) 490
    fungus NEC 117.9
  Brucella 023.9
    abortus 023.1
    canis 023.3
    melitensis 023.0
    mixed 023.8
    suis 023.2
  Brugia (Wuchereria) malayi 125.1
  bursa - *see* Bursitis
  buttocks (skin) 686.9
  Candida (albicans) (tropicalis) *(see also*
    Candidiasis) 112.9
    congenital 771.7
  Candiru 136.8
  Capillaria
    hepatica 128.8
    philippinensis 127.5

Infection, infected, infective *(Continued)*
  cartilage 733.99
  cat liver fluke 121.0
  catheter-related bloodstream (CRBSI)
    999.31
  cellulitis - *see* Cellulitis, by site
  Cephalosporum falciforme 117.4
  Cercomonas hominis (intestinal) 007.3
  cerebrospinal *(see also* Meningitis) 322.9
    late effect - *see* category 326
  cervical gland 683
  cervix *(see also* Cervicitis) 616.0
  cesarean section wound 674.3 ●
  Chilomastix (intestinal) 007.8
  Chlamydia 079.98
    specified NEC 079.88
  Cholera *(see also* Cholera) 001.9
  chorionic plate 658.8 ●
  Cladosporium
    bantianum 117.8
    carrionii 117.2
    mansoni 111.1
    trichoides 117.8
    wernecki 111.1
  Clonorchis (sinensis) (liver) 121.1
  Clostridium (haemolyticum) (novyi)
    NEC 041.84
    botulinum 005.1
    histolyticum *(see also* Gangrene, gas)
      040.0
    oedematiens *(see also* Gangrene, gas)
      040.0
    perfringens 041.83
      due to food 005.2
    septicum *(see also* Gangrene, gas)
      040.0
    sordellii *(see also* Gangrene, gas)
      040.0
    welchii *(see also* Gangrene, gas)
      040.0
      due to food 005.2
  Coccidioides (immitis) *(see also*
    Coccidioidomycosis) 114.9
  coccus NEC 041.89
  colon *(see also* Enteritis, due to, by
    organism) 009.0
    bacillus - *see* Infection, Escherichia
      coli
  colostomy or enterostomy 569.61
  common duct 576.1
  complicating pregnancy, childbirth, or
    puerperium NEC 647.9 ●
    affecting fetus or newborn 760.2
  Condiobolus 117.7
  congenital NEC 771.89
    Candida albicans 771.7
    chronic 771.2
    Cytomegalovirus 771.1
    hepatitis, viral 771.2
    herpes simplex 771.2
    listeriosis 771.2
    malaria 771.2
    poliomyelitis 771.2
    rubella 771.0
    toxoplasmosis 771.2
    tuberculosis 771.2
    urinary (tract) 771.82
    vaccinia 771.2
  coronavirus 079.89
    SARS-associated 079.82
  corpus luteum *(see also* Salpingo-
    oophoritis) 614.2
  Corynebacterium diphtheriae - *see*
    Diphtheria

Infection, infected, infective (*Continued*)
cotia virus 059.8
Coxsackie (*see also* Coxsackie) 079.2
    endocardium 074.22
    heart NEC 074.20
    in diseases classified elsewhere - *see*
        category 079
    meninges 047.0
    myocardium 074.23
    pericardium 074.21
    pharynx 074.0
    specified disease NEC 074.8
    unspecified nature or site 079.2
Cryptococcus neoformans 117.5
Cryptosporidia 007.4
Cunninghamella 117.7
cyst - *see* Cyst
Cysticercus cellulosae 123.1
cytomegalovirus 078.5
    congenital 771.1
dental (pulpal origin) 522.4
deuteromycetes 117.4
Dicrocoelium dendriticum 121.8
Dipetalonema (perstans) 125.4
    streptocerca 125.6
diphtherial - *see* Diphtheria
Diphyllobothrium (adult) (latum)
        (pacificum) 123.4
    larval 123.5
Diplogonoporus (grandis) 123.8
Dipylidium (caninum) 123.8
Dirofilaria 125.6
dog tapeworm 123.8
Dracunculus medinensis 125.7
Dreschlera 118
    hawaiiensis 117.8
Ducrey's bacillus (any site) 099.0
due to or resulting from
    central venous catheter 999.31
    device, implant, or graft (any)
        (presence of) - *see*
        Complications, infection and
        inflammation, due to (presence
        of) any device, implant, or
        graft classified to 996.0–996.5
        NEC
    injection, inoculation, infusion,
        transfusion, or vaccination
        (prophylactic) (therapeutic)
        999.39
    injury NEC - *see* Wound, open, by
        site, complicated
    surgery 998.59
duodenum 535.6●
ear - *see also* Otitis
    external (*see also* Otitis, externa)
        380.10
    inner (*see also* Labyrinthitis) 386.30
    middle - *see* Otitis, media
Eaton's agent NEC 041.81
Eberthella typhosa 002.0
Ebola 078.89
echinococcosis 122.9
Echinococcus (*see also* Echinococcus)
    122.9
Echinostoma 121.8
ECHO virus 079.1
    in diseases classified elsewhere - *see*
        category 079
    unspecified nature or site 079.1
Ehrlichiosis 082.40
    chaffeensis 082.41
    specified type NEC 082.49
Endamoeba - *see* Infection, ameba

Infection, infected, infective (*Continued*)
endocardium (*see also* Endocarditis)
    421.0
endocervix (*see also* Cervicitis) 616.0
Entamoeba - *see* Infection, ameba
enteric (*see also* Enteritis, due to, by
    organism) 009.0
Enterobacter aerogenes NEC 041.85
Enterobacter sakazakii 041.85
Enterobius vermicularis 127.4
enterococcus NEC 041.04
enterovirus NEC 079.89
    central nervous system NEC 048
    enteritis 008.67
    meningitis 047.9
Entomophthora 117.7
Epidermophyton - *see* Dermatophytosis
epidermophytosis - *see*
    Dermatophytosis
episiotomy 674.3●
Epstein-Barr virus 075
    chronic 780.79 [139.8]
erysipeloid 027.1
Erysipelothrix (insidiosa)
    (rhusiopathiae) 027.1
erythema infectiosum 057.0
Escherichia coli NEC 041.4
    enteritis - *see* Enteritis, E. coli
    generalized 038.42
    intestinal - *see* Enteritis, E. coli
esophagostomy 530.86
ethmoidal (chronic) (sinus) (*see also*
    Sinusitis, ethmoidal) 473.2
Eubacterium 041.84
Eustachian tube (ear) 381.50
    acute 381.51
    chronic 381.52
exanthema subitum (*see also* Exanthem
    subitum) 058.10
external auditory canal (meatus) (*see*
    also Otitis, externa) 380.10
eye NEC 360.00
eyelid 373.9
    specified NEC 373.8
fallopian tube (*see also* Salpingo-
    oophoritis) 614.2
fascia 728.89
Fasciola
    gigantica 121.3
    hepatica 121.3
Fasciolopsis (buski) 121.4
fetus (intra-amniotic) - *see* Infection,
    congenital
filarial - *see* Infestation, filarial
finger (skin) 686.9
    abscess (with lymphangitis) 681.00
        pulp 681.01
    cellulitis (with lymphangitis)
        681.00
    distal closed space (with
        lymphangitis) 681.00
    nail 681.02
        fungus 110.1
fish tapeworm 123.4
    larval 123.5
flagellate, intestinal 007.9
fluke - *see* Infestation, fluke
focal
    teeth (pulpal origin) 522.4
    tonsils 474.00
        and adenoids 474.02
Fonsecaea
    compactum 117.2
    pedrosoi 117.2

Infection, infected, infective (*Continued*)
food (*see also* Poisoning, food) 005.9
foot (skin) 686.9
    fungus 110.4
Francisella tularensis (*see also*
    Tularemia) 021.9
frontal sinus (chronic) (*see also* Sinusitis,
    frontal) 473.1
fungus NEC 117.9
    beard 110.0
    body 110.5
    dermatiacious NEC 117.8
    foot 110.4
    groin 110.3
    hand 110.2
    nail 110.1
    pathogenic to compromised host
        only 118
    perianal (area) 110.3
    scalp 110.0
    scrotum 110.8
    skin 111.9
        foot 110.4
        hand 110.2
    toenails 110.1
    trachea 117.9
Fusarium 118
Fusobacterium 041.84
gallbladder (*see also* Cholecystitis,
    acute) 575.0
Gardnerella vaginalis 041.89
gas bacillus (*see also* Gas, gangrene)
    040.0
gastric (*see also* Gastritis) 535.5●
Gastrodiscoides hominis 121.8
gastroenteric (*see also* Enteritis, due to,
    by organism) 009.0
gastrointestinal (*see also* Enteritis, due
    to, by organism) 009.0
gastrostomy 536.41
generalized NEC (*see also* Septicemia)
    038.9
genital organ or tract NEC
    female 614.9
        with
            abortion - *see* Abortion, by
                type, with sepsis
            ectopic pregnancy (*see also*
                categories 633.0–633.9)
                639.0
            molar pregnancy (*see also*
                categories 630–632)
                639.0
        complicating pregnancy 646.6●
            affecting fetus or newborn
                760.8
        following
            abortion 639.0
            ectopic or molar pregnancy
                639.0
        puerperal, postpartum, childbirth
            670.8●
        minor or localized 646.6●
            affecting fetus or newborn
                760.8
    male 608.4
genitourinary tract NEC 599.0
Ghon tubercle, primary (*see also*
    Tuberculosis) 010.0●
Giardia lamblia 007.1
gingival (chronic) 523.10
    acute 523.00
    Vincent's 101
glanders 024

◀ New   ◀‖‖ Revised   ~~deleted~~ Deleted   ● Use Additional Digit(s)   ▨ Omit code

Infection, infected, infective *(Continued)*
  Glenosporopsis amazonica 116.2
  Gnathostoma spinigerum 128.1
  Gongylonema 125.6
  gonococcal NEC *(see also* Gonococcus)
    098.0
  gram-negative bacilli NEC 041.85
    anaerobic 041.84
  guinea worm 125.7
  gum *(see also* Infection, gingival) 523.10
  Hantavirus 079.81
  heart 429.89
  Helicobacter pylori [H. pylori]
    041.86
  helminths NEC 128.9
    intestinal 127.9
      mixed (types classifiable to more
        than one category in 120.0–
        127.7) 127.8
      specified type NEC 127.7
    specified type NEC 128.8
  Hemophilus influenzae NEC 041.5
    generalized 038.41
  Herpes (simplex) *(see also* Herpes,
    simplex) 054.9
    congenital 771.2
    zoster *(see also* Herpes, zoster) 053.9
      eye NEC 053.29
  Heterophyes heterophyes 121.6
  Histoplasma *(see also* Histoplasmosis)
    115.90
    capsulatum *(see also* Histoplasmosis,
      American) 115.00
    duboisii *(see also* Histoplasmosis,
      African) 115.10
  HIV V08
    with symptoms, symptomatic 042
  hookworm *(see also* Ancylostomiasis)
    126.9
  human herpesvirus 6 058.81
  human herpesvirus 7 058.82
  human herpesvirus 8 058.89
  human herpesvirus NEC 058.89
  human immunodeficiency virus V08
    with symptoms, symptomatic 042
  human papillomavirus 079.4
  hydrocele 603.1
  hydronephrosis 591
  Hymenolepis 123.6
  hypopharynx 478.29
  inguinal glands 683
    due to soft chancre 099.0
  intestine, intestinal *(see also* Enteritis,
    due to, by organism) 009.0
  intrauterine *(see also* Endometritis)
    615.9
    complicating delivery 646.6●
  isospora belli or hominis 007.2
  Japanese B encephalitis 062.0
  jaw (bone) (acute) (chronic) (lower)
    (subacute) (upper) 526.4
  joint - *see* Arthritis, infectious or
    infective
  Kaposi's sarcoma-associated
    herpesvirus 058.89
  kidney (cortex) (hematogenous) 590.9
    with
      abortion - *see* Abortion, by type,
        with urinary tract infection
      calculus 592.0
      ectopic pregnancy *(see also*
        categories 633.0–633.9) 639.8
      molar pregnancy *(see also*
        categories 630–632) 639.8

Infection, infected, infective *(Continued)*
  kidney *(Continued)*
    complicating pregnancy or
      puerperium 646.6●
      affecting fetus or newborn 760.1
    following
      abortion 639.8
      ectopic or molar pregnancy 639.8
    pelvis and ureter 590.3
  Klebsiella pneumoniae NEC 041.3
  knee (skin) NEC 686.9
    joint - *see* Arthritis, infectious
  Koch's *(see also* Tuberculosis,
    pulmonary) 011.9●
  labia (majora) (minora) *(see also*
    Vulvitis) 616.10
  lacrimal
    gland *(see also* Dacryoadenitis)
      375.00
    passages (duct) (sac) *(see also*
      Dacryocystitis) 375.30
  larynx NEC 478.79
  leg (skin) NEC 686.9
  Leishmania *(see also* Leishmaniasis)
    085.9
    braziliensis 085.5
    donovani 085.0
    Ethiopica 085.3
    furunculosa 085.1
    infantum 085.0
    Mexicana 085.4
    tropica (minor) 085.1
      major 085.2
  Leptosphaeria senegalensis 117.4
  Leptospira *(see also* Leptospirosis)
    100.9
    australis 100.89
    bataviae 100.89
    pyrogenes 100.89
    specified type NEC 100.89
  leptospirochetal NEC *(see also*
    Leptospirosis) 100.9
  Leptothrix - *see* Actinomycosis
  Listeria monocytogenes (listeriosis)
    027.0
    congenital 771.2
  liver fluke - *see* Infestation, fluke,
    liver
  Loa loa 125.2
    eyelid 125.2 *[373.6]*
  Loboa loboi 116.2
  local, skin (staphylococcal)
    (streptococcal) NEC 686.9
    abscess - *see* Abscess, by site
    cellulitis - *see* Cellulitis, by site
    ulcer *(see also* Ulcer, skin) 707.9
  Loefflerella
    mallei 024
    whitmori 025
  lung 518.89
    atypical Mycobacterium 031.0
      tuberculous *(see also*
        Tuberculosis,
        pulmonary) 011.9●
    basilar 518.89
    chronic 518.89
    fungus NEC 117.9
    spirochetal 104.8
    virus - *see* Pneumonia, virus
  lymph gland (axillary) (cervical)
    (inguinal) 683
    mesenteric 289.2
  lymphoid tissue, base of tongue or
    posterior pharynx, NEC 474.00

Infection, infected, infective *(Continued)*
  Madurella
    grisea 117.4
    mycetomii 117.4
  major
    with
      abortion - *see* Abortion, by type,
        with sepsis
      ectopic pregnancy *(see also*
        categories 633.0–633.9) 639.0
      molar pregnancy *(see also*
        categories 630–632) 639.0
    following
      abortion 639.0
      ectopic or molar pregnancy
        639.0
    puerperal, postpartum,
      childbirth 670.0●
  malarial - *see* Malaria
  Malassezia furfur 111.0
  Malleomyces
    mallei 024
    pseudomallei 025
  mammary gland 611.0
    puerperal, postpartum 675.2●
  Mansonella (ozzardi) 125.5
  mastoid (suppurative) - *see*
    Mastoiditis
  maxilla, maxillary 526.4
    sinus (chronic) *(see also* Sinusitis,
      maxillary) 473.0
  mediastinum 519.2
  medina 125.7
  meibomian
    cyst 373.12
    gland 373.12
  melioidosis 025
  meninges *(see also* Meningitis) 320.9
  meningococcal *(see also* condition)
    036.9
    brain 036.1
    cerebrospinal 036.0
    endocardium 036.42
    generalized 036.2
    meninges 036.0
    meningococcemia 036.2
    specified site NEC 036.89
  mesenteric lymph nodes or glands
    NEC 289.2
  Metagonimus 121.5
  metatarsophalangeal 711.97
  methicillin
    resistant Staphylococcus aureus
      (MRSA) 041.12
    susceptible Staphylococcus aureus
      (MSSA) 041.11
  microorganism resistant to drugs - *see*
    Resistance (to), drugs by
    microorganisms
  Microsporidia 136.8
  microsporum, microsporic - *see*
    Dermatophytosis
  mima polymorpha NEC 041.85
  mixed flora NEC 041.89
  Monilia *(see also* Candidiasis) 112.9
    neonatal 771.7
  monkeypox 059.01
  Monosporium apiospermum 117.6
  mouth (focus) NEC 528.9
    parasitic 136.9
  MRSA (methicillin resistant
    Staphylococcus aureus) 041.12
  MSSA (methicillin susceptible
    Staphylococcus aureus) 041.11

Infection, infected, infective (*Continued*)
Mucor 117.7
muscle NEC 728.89
mycelium NEC 117.9
mycetoma
  actinomycotic NEC (*see also*
      Actinomycosis) 039.9
  mycotic NEC 117.4
Mycobacterium, mycobacterial (*see also*
    Mycobacterium) 031.9
Mycoplasma NEC 041.81
mycotic NEC 117.9
  pathogenic to compromised host
      only 118
  skin NEC 111.9
  systemic 117.9
myocardium NEC 422.90
nail (chronic) (with lymphangitis)
    681.9
  finger 681.02
    fungus 110.1
  ingrowing 703.0
  toe 681.11
    fungus 110.1
nasal sinus (chronic (*see also* Sinusitis)
    473.9
nasopharynx (chronic) 478.29
  acute 460
navel 686.9
  newborn 771.4
Neisserian - *see* Gonococcus
Neotestudina rosatii 117.4
newborn, generalized 771.89
nipple 611.0
  puerperal, postpartum 675.0●
    with breast 675.9●
      specified type NEC 675.8●
Nocardia - *see* Actinomycosis
nose 478.19
nostril 478.19
obstetrical surgical wound 674.3●
Oesophagostomum (apiostomum)
    127.7
Oestrus ovis 134.0
Oidium albicans (*see also* Candidiasis)
    112.9
Onchocerca (volvulus) 125.3
  eye 125.3 [360.13]
  eyelid 125.3 [373.6]
operation wound 998.59
Opisthorchis (felineus) (tenuicollis)
    (viverrini) 121.0
orbit 376.00
  chronic 376.10
orthopoxvirus 059.00
  specified NEC 059.09
ovary (*see also* Salpingo-oophoritis)
    614.2
Oxyuris vermicularis 127.4
pancreas 577.0
Paracoccidioides brasiliensis 116.1
Paragonimus (westermani) 121.2
parainfluenza virus 079.89
parameningococcus NEC 036.9
  with meningitis 036.0
parapoxvirus 059.10
  specified NEC 059.19
parasitic NEC 136.9
paratyphoid 002.9
  type A 002.1
  type B 002.2
  type C 002.3
paraurethral ducts 597.89
parotid gland 527.2

Infection, infected, infective (*Continued*)
Pasteurella NEC 027.2
  multocida (cat-bite) (dog-bite)
      027.2
  pestis (*see also* Plague) 020.9
  pseudotuberculosis 027.2
  septica (cat-bite) (dog-bite) 027.2
  tularensis (*see also* Tularemia) 021.9
pelvic, female (*see also* Disease, pelvis,
    inflammatory) 614.9
penis (glans) (retention) NEC 607.2
  herpetic 054.13
Peptococcus 041.84
Peptostreptococcus 041.84
periapical (pulpal origin) 522.4
peridental 523.30
perineal wound (obstetrical) 674.3●
periodontal 523.31
periorbital 376.00
  chronic 376.10
perirectal 569.49
perirenal (*see also* Infection, kidney)
    590.9
peritoneal (*see also* Peritonitis) 567.9
periureteral 593.89
periurethral 597.89
Petriellidium boydii 117.6
pharynx 478.29
  Coxsackie virus 074.0
  phlegmonous 462
  posterior, lymphoid 474.00
Phialophora
  gougerotii 117.8
  jeanselmei 117.8
  verrucosa 117.2
Piedraia hortai 111.3
pinna, acute 380.11
pinta 103.9
  intermediate 103.1
  late 103.2
  mixed 103.3
  primary 103.0
pinworm 127.4
pityrosporum furfur 111.0
pleuropneumonia-like organisms NEC
    (PPLO) 041.81
pneumococcal NEC 041.2
  generalized (purulent) 038.2
Pneumococcus NEC 041.2
postoperative wound 998.59
posttraumatic NEC 958.3
postvaccinal 999.39
poxvirus 059.9
  specified NEC 059.8
prepuce NEC 607.1
Proprionibacterium 041.84
prostate (capsule) (*see also* Prostatitis)
    601.9
Proteus (mirabilis) (morganii)
    (vulgaris) NEC 041.6
  enteritis 008.3
protozoal NEC 136.8
  intestinal NEC 007.9
Pseudomonas NEC 041.7
  mallei 024
  pneumonia 482.1
  pseudomallei 025
psittacosis 073.9
puerperal, postpartum (major) 670.0●
  minor 646.6●
pulmonary - *see* Infection, lung
purulent - *see* Abscess
putrid, generalized - *see* Septicemia
pyemic - *see* Septicemia

Infection, infected, infective (*Continued*)
Pyrenochaeta romeroi 117.4
Q fever 083.0
rabies 071
rectum (sphincter) 569.49
renal (*see also* Infection, kidney) 590.9
  pelvis and ureter 590.3
resistant to drugs - *see* Resistance (to),
    drugs by microorganisms
respiratory 519.8
  chronic 519.8
  influenzal (acute) (upper) (*see also*
      Influenza) 487.1 ◀▦
  lung 518.89
  rhinovirus 460
  syncytial virus 079.6
  upper (acute) (infectious) NEC 465.9
    with flu, grippe, or influenza (*see
        also* Influenza) 487.1 ◀▦
    influenzal (*see also* Influenza)
        487.1 ◀▦
    multiple sites NEC 465.8
    streptococcal 034.0
    viral NEC 465.9
respiratory syncytial virus (RSV)
    079.6
resulting from presence of shunt or
    other internal prosthetic device -
    see Complications, infection and
    inflammation, due to (presence
    of) any device, implant, or graft
    classified to 996.0–996.5 NEC
retroperitoneal 567.39
retrovirus 079.50
  human immunodeficiency virus
      type 2 (HIV 2) 079.53 ◀▦
  human T-cell lymphotrophic virus
      type I (HTLV-I) 079.51 ◀▦
  human T-cell lymphotrophic virus
      type II (HTLV-II) 079.52 ◀▦
  specified NEC 079.59
Rhinocladium 117.1
Rhinosporidium (seeberi) 117.0
rhinovirus
  in diseases classified elsewhere - *see*
      category 079
  unspecified nature or site 079.3
Rhizopus 117.7
rickettsial 083.9
rickettsialpox 083.2
rubella (*see also* Rubella) 056.9
  congenital 771.0
Saccharomyces (*see also* Candidiasis)
    112.9
Saksenaea 117.7
salivary duct or gland (any) 527.2
Salmonella (aertrycke) (callinarum)
    (choleraesuis) (enteritidis)
    (suipestifer) (typhimurium) 003.9
  with
    arthritis 003.23
    gastroenteritis 003.0
    localized infection 003.20
      specified type NEC 003.29
    meningitis 003.21
    osteomyelitis 003.24
    pneumonia 003.22
    septicemia 003.1
    specified manifestation NEC
        003.8
  due to food (poisoning) (any
      serotype) (*see also* Poisoning,
      food, due to, Salmonella)
  hirschfeldii 002.3

◀ New   ◀▦ Revised   ~~deleted~~ Deleted   ● Use Additional Digit(s)   ▦ Omit code

Infection, infected, infective *(Continued)*
Salmonella *(Continued)*
  localized 003.20
    specified type NEC 003.29
  paratyphi 002.9
    A 002.1
    B 002.2
    C 002.3
  schottmuelleri 002.2
  specified type NEC 003.8
  typhi 002.0
  typhosa 002.0
saprophytic 136.8
Sarcocystis, lindemanni 136.5
SARS-associated coronavirus 079.82
scabies 133.0
Schistosoma - *see* Infestation,
    Schistosoma
Schmorl's bacillus 040.3
scratch or other superficial injury - *see*
    Injury, superficial, by site
scrotum (acute) NEC 608.4
sealpox 059.12
secondary, burn or open wound
    (dislocation) (fracture) 958.3
seminal vesicle (*see also* Vesiculitis)
    608.0
septic
  generalized - *see* Septicemia
  localized, skin (*see also* Abscess)
    682.9
septicemic - *see* Septicemia
seroma 998.51
Serratia (marcescens) 041.85
  generalized 038.44
sheep liver fluke 121.3
Shigella 004.9
  boydii 004.2
  dysenteriae 004.0
  Flexneri 004.1
  group
    A 004.0
    B 004.1
    C 004.2
    D 004.3
  Schmitz (-Stutzer) 004.0
  Schmitzii 004.0
  Shiga 004.0
  Sonnei 004.3
  specified type NEC 004.8
Sin Nombre virus 079.81
sinus (*see also* Sinusitis) 473.9
  pilonidal 685.1
    with abscess 685.0
  skin NEC 686.9
Skene's duct or gland (*see also*
    Urethritis) 597.89
skin (local) (staphylococcal)
    (streptococcal) NEC 686.9
  abscess - *see* Abscess, by site
  cellulitis - *see* Cellulitis, by site
  due to fungus 111.9
    specified type NEC 111.8
  mycotic 111.9
    specified type NEC 111.8
  ulcer (*see also* Ulcer, skin) 707.9
slow virus 046.9
  specified condition NEC 046.8
Sparganum (mansoni) (proliferum)
    123.5
spermatic cord NEC 608.4
sphenoidal (chronic) (sinus) (*see also*
    Sinusitis, sphenoidal) 473.3
Spherophorus necrophorus 040.3

Infection, infected, infective *(Continued)*
spinal cord NEC (*see also* Encephalitis)
    323.9
  abscess 324.1
    late effect - *see* category 326
  late effect - *see* category 326
  meninges - *see* Meningitis
  streptococcal 320.2
Spirillum
  minus or minor 026.0
  morsus muris 026.0
  obermeieri 087.0
spirochetal NEC 104.9
  lung 104.8
  specified nature or site NEC
    104.8
spleen 289.59
Sporothrix schenckii 117.1
Sporotrichum (schenckii) 117.1
Sporozoa 136.8
staphylococcal NEC 041.10
  aureus 041.11
    methicillin
      resistant (MRSA) 041.12
      susceptible MSSA) 041.11
  food poisoning 005.0
  generalized (purulent) 038.10
    aureus 038.11
      methicillin
        resistant 038.12
        susceptible 038.11
    specified organism NEC 038.19
  pneumonia 482.40
    aureus 482.41
      methicillin
        resistant (MRSA) 482.42
        susceptible (MSSA)
          482.41
    MRSA (methicillin resistant
      staphylococcus aureus)
      482.42
    MSSA (methicillin susceptible
      staphylococcus aureus)
      482.41
    specified type NEC 482.49
  septicemia 038.10
    aureus 038.11
      methicillin
        resistant (MRSA) 038.12
        susceptible (MSSA) 038.11
    MRSA (methicillin resistant
      staphylococcus aureus)
      038.12
    MSSA (methicillin susceptible
      staphylococcus aureus)
      038.11
    specified organism NEC 038.19
  specified NEC 041.19
steatoma 706.2
Stellantchasmus falcatus 121.6
Streptobacillus moniliformis 026.1
streptococcal NEC 041.00
  generalized (purulent) 038.0
  group
    A 041.01
    B 041.02
    C 041.03
    D [enterococcus] 041.04
    G 041.05
  pneumonia - *see* Pneumonia,
    streptococcal
  septicemia 038.0
  sore throat 034.0
  specified NEC 041.09

Infection, infected, infective *(Continued)*
Streptomyces - *see* Actinomycosis
streptotrichosis - *see* Actinomycosis
Strongyloides (stercoralis) 127.2
stump (amputation) (posttraumatic)
    (surgical) 997.62
  traumatic - *see* Amputation,
    traumatic, by site, complicated
subcutaneous tissue, local NEC 686.9
submaxillary region 528.9
suipestifer (*see also* Infection,
    Salmonella) 003.9
swimming pool bacillus 031.1
syphilitic - *see* Syphilis
systemic - *see* Septicemia
Taenia - *see* Infestation, Taenia
Taeniarhynchus saginatus 123.2
tanapox 059.21
tapeworm - *see* Infestation, tapeworm
tendon (sheath) 727.89
Ternidens diminutus 127.7
testis (*see also* Orchitis) 604.90
thigh (skin) 686.9
threadworm 127.4
throat 478.29
  pneumococcal 462
  staphylococcal 462
  streptococcal 034.0
  viral NEC (*see also* Pharyngitis) 462
thumb (skin) 686.9
  abscess (with lymphangitis)
    681.00
    pulp 681.01
  cellulitis (with lymphangitis)
    681.00
  nail 681.02
thyroglossal duct 529.8
toe (skin) 686.9
  abscess (with lymphangitis)
    681.10
  cellulitis (with lymphangitis)
    681.10
  nail 681.11
    fungus 110.1
tongue NEC 529.0
  parasitic 112.0
tonsil (faucial) (lingual) (pharyngeal)
    474.00
  acute or subacute 463
  and adenoid 474.02
  tag 474.00
tooth, teeth 522.4
  periapical (pulpal origin) 522.4
  peridental 523.30
  periodontal 523.31
  pulp 522.0
  socket 526.5
TORCH - *see* Infection, congenital
    NEC
  without active infection 760.2
Torula histolytica 117.5
Toxocara (cani) (cati) (felis) 128.0
Toxoplasma gondii (*see also*
    Toxoplasmosis) 130.9
trachea, chronic 491.8
  fungus 117.9
traumatic NEC 958.3
trematode NEC 121.9
trench fever 083.1
Treponema
  denticola 041.84
  macrodenticum 041.84
  pallidum (*see also* Syphilis) 097.9
Trichinella (spiralis) 124

Infection, infected, infective (Continued)
Trichomonas 131.9
  bladder 131.09
  cervix 131.09
  hominis 007.3
  intestine 007.3
  prostate 131.03
  specified site NEC 131.8
  urethra 131.02
  urogenitalis 131.00
  vagina 131.01
  vulva 131.01
Trichophyton, trichophytid - see
  Dermatophytosis
Trichosporon (beigelii) cutaneum 111.2
Trichostrongylus 127.6
Trichuris (trichiura) 127.3
Trombicula (irritans) 133.8
Trypanosoma (see also
  Trypanosomiasis) 086.9
  cruzi 086.2
tubal (see also Salpingo-oophoritis)
  614.2
tuberculous NEC (see also Tuberculosis)
  011.9●
tubo-ovarian (see also Salpingo-
  oophoritis) 614.2
tunica vaginalis 608.4
tympanic membrane - see Myringitis
typhoid (abortive) (ambulant)
  (bacillus) 002.0
typhus 081.9
  flea-borne (endemic) 081.0
  louse-borne (epidemic) 080
  mite-borne 081.2
  recrudescent 081.1
  tick-borne 082.9
    African 082.1
    North Asian 082.2
umbilicus (septic) 686.9
  newborn NEC 771.4
ureter 593.89
urethra (see also Urethritis) 597.80
urinary (tract) NEC 599.0
  with
    abortion - see Abortion, by type,
      with urinary tract infection
    ectopic pregnancy (see also
      categories 633.0–633.9) 639.8
    molar pregnancy (see also
      categories 630–632) 639.8
  candidal 112.2
  complicating pregnancy, childbirth,
    or puerperium 646.6●
    affecting fetus or newborn 760.1
    asymptomatic 646.5●
      affecting fetus or newborn
        760.1
  diplococcal (acute) 098.0
    chronic 098.2
  due to Trichomonas (vaginalis)
    131.00
  following
    abortion 639.8
    ectopic or molar pregnancy 639.8
  gonococcal (acute) 098.0
    chronic or duration of 2 months
      or over 098.2
  newborn 771.82
  trichomonal 131.00
  tuberculous (see also Tuberculosis)
    016.3●
uterus, uterine (see also Endometritis)
  615.9

Infection, infected, infective (Continued)
utriculus masculinus NEC 597.89
vaccination 999.39
vagina (granulation tissue) (wall) (see
  also Vaginitis) 616.10
varicella 052.9
varicose veins - see Varicose, veins
variola 050.9
  major 050.0
  minor 050.1
vas deferens NEC 608.4
Veillonella 041.84
verumontanum 597.89
vesical (see also Cystitis) 595.9
Vibrio
  cholerae 001.0
    El Tor 001.1
  parahaemolyticus (food poisoning)
    005.4
  vulnificus 041.85
Vincent's (gums) (mouth) (tonsil) 101
virus, viral 079.99
  adenovirus
    in diseases classified elsewhere -
      see category 079
    unspecified nature or site 079.0
  central nervous system NEC 049.9
    enterovirus 048
      meningitis 047.9
        specified type NEC 047.8
    slow virus 046.9
      specified condition NEC 046.8
  chest 519.8
  conjunctivitis 077.99
    specified type NEC 077.89
  coronavirus 079.89
    SARS-associated 079.82
  Coxsackie (see also Infection,
    Coxsackie) 079.2
  Ebola 065.8
  ECHO
    in diseases classified elsewhere -
      see category 079
    unspecified nature or site 079.1
  encephalitis 049.9
    arthropod-borne NEC 064
    tick-borne 063.9
      specified type NEC 063.8
  enteritis NEC (see also Enteritis,
    viral) 008.8
  exanthem NEC 057.9
  Hantavirus 079.81
  human papilloma 079.4
  in diseases classified elsewhere - see
    category 079
  intestine (see also Enteritis, viral)
    008.8
  lung - see Pneumonia, viral
  respiratory syncytial (RSV) 079.6
  Retrovirus 079.50
  rhinovirus
    in diseases classified elsewhere -
      see category 079
    unspecified nature or site 079.3
  salivary gland disease 078.5
  slow 046.9
    specified condition NEC 046.8
  specified type NEC 079.89
    in diseases classified elsewhere -
      see category 079
  unspecified nature or site 079.99
  warts 078.10
    specified NEC 078.19
  yaba monkey tumor 059.22

Infection, infected, infective (Continued)
vulva (see also Vulvitis) 616.10
whipworm 127.3
Whitmore's bacillus 025
wound (local) (posttraumatic) NEC
  958.3
  with
    dislocation - see Dislocation, by
      site, open
    fracture - see Fracture, by site,
      open
    open wound - see Wound, open,
      by site, complicated
  postoperative 998.59
  surgical 998.59
Wuchereria 125.0
  bancrofti 125.0
  malayi 125.1
yaba monkey tumor virus 059.22
yatapoxvirus 059.20
yaws - see Yaws
yeast (see also Candidiasis) 112.9
yellow fever (see also Fever, yellow)
  060.9
Yersinia pestis (see also Plague) 020.9
Zeis' gland 373.12
zoonotic bacterial NEC 027.9
Zopfia senegalensis 117.4
Infective, infectious - see condition
Inferiority complex 301.9
  constitutional psychopathic 301.9
Infertility
  female 628.9
    age related 628.8
    associated with
      adhesions, peritubal 614.6 [628.2]
      anomaly
        cervical mucus 628.4
        congenital
          cervix 628.4
          fallopian tube 628.2
          uterus 628.3
          vagina 628.4
      anovulation 628.0
      dysmucorrhea 628.4
      endometritis, tuberculous (see also
        Tuberculosis) 016.7● [628.3]
      Stein-Leventhal syndrome 256.4
        [628.0]
    due to
      adiposogenital dystrophy 253.8
        [628.1]
      anterior pituitary disorder NEC
        253.4 [628.1]
        hyperfunction 253.1 [628.1]
      cervical anomaly 628.4
      fallopian tube anomaly 628.2
      ovarian failure 256.39 [628.0]
      Stein-Leventhal syndrome 256.4
        [628.0]
      uterine anomaly 628.3
      vaginal anomaly 628.4
    nonimplantation 628.3
    origin
      cervical 628.4
      pituitary-hypothalamus NEC
        253.8 [628.1]
        anterior pituitary NEC 253.4
          [628.1]
          hyperfunction NEC 253.1
            [628.1]
        dwarfism 253.3 [628.1]
        panhypopituitarism 253.2
          [628.1]

◀ New   ◀▥ Revised   deleted Deleted   ● Use Additional Digit(s)   ▨ Omit code

Infertility (*Continued*)
  female (*Continued*)
    origin (*Continued*)
      specified NEC 628.8
      tubal (block) (occlusion)
          (stenosis) 628.2
        adhesions 614.6 *[628.2]*
      uterine 628.3
      vaginal 628.4
    previous, requiring supervision of
        pregnancy V23.0
  male 606.9
    absolute 606.0
    due to
      azoospermia 606.0
      drug therapy 606.8
      extratesticular cause NEC
          606.8
      germinal cell
        aplasia 606.0
        desquamation 606.1
      hypospermatogenesis 606.1
      infection 606.8
      obstruction, afferent ducts 606.8
      oligospermia 606.1
      radiation 606.8
      spermatogenic arrest (complete)
          606.0
        incomplete 606.1
      systemic disease 606.8
Infestation 134.9
  Acanthocheilonema (perstans)
      125.4
    streptocerca 125.6
  Acariasis 133.9
    demodex folliculorum 133.8
    sarcoptes scabiei 133.0
    trombiculae 133.8
  Agamofilaria streptocerca 125.6
  Ancylostoma, Ankylostoma 126.9
    americanum 126.1
    braziliense 126.2
    canium 126.8
    ceylanicum 126.3
    duodenale 126.0
    new world 126.1
    old world 126.0
  Angiostrongylus cantonensis 128.8
  anisakiasis 127.1
  Anisakis larva 127.1
  arthropod NEC 134.1
  Ascaris lumbricoides 127.0
  Bacillus fusiformis 101
  Balantidium coli 007.0
  beef tapeworm 123.2
  Bothriocephalus (latus) 123.4
    larval 123.5
  broad tapeworm 123.4
    larval 123.5
  Brugia malayi 125.1
  Candiru 136.8
  Capillaria
    hepatica 128.8
    philippinensis 127.5
  cat liver fluke 121.0
  Cercomonas hominis (intestinal)
      007.3
  cestodes 123.9
    specified type NEC 123.8
  chigger 133.8
  chigoe 134.1
  Chilomastix 007.8
  Clonorchis (sinensis) (liver) 121.1
  coccidia 007.2

Infestation (*Continued*)
  complicating pregnancy, childbirth, or
      puerperium 647.9●
    affecting fetus or newborn 760.8
  Cysticercus cellulosae 123.1
  Demodex folliculorum 133.8
  Dermatobia (hominis) 134.0
  Dibothriocephalus (latus) 123.4
    larval 123.5
  Dicrocoelium dendriticum 121.8
  Diphyllobothrium (adult) (intestinal)
      (latum) (pacificum) 123.4
    larval 123.5
  Diplogonoporus (grandis) 123.8
  Dipylidium (caninum) 123.8
  Distoma hepaticum 121.3
  dog tapeworm 123.8
  Dracunculus medinensis 125.7
  dragon worm 125.7
  dwarf tapeworm 123.6
  Echinococcus (*see also* Echinococcus)
      122.9
  Echinostoma ilocanum 121.8
  Embadomonas 007.8
  Endamoeba (histolytica) - *see* Infection,
      ameba
  Entamoeba (histolytica) - *see* Infection,
      ameba
  Enterobius vermicularis 127.4
  Epidermophyton - *see*
      Dermatophytosis
  eyeworm 125.2
  Fasciola
    gigantica 121.3
    hepatica 121.3
  Fasciolopsis (buski) (small intestine)
      121.4
  filarial 125.9
    due to
      acanthocheilonema (perstans)
          125.4
        streptocerca 125.6
      Brugia (Wuchereria) malayi
          125.1
      Dracunculus medinensis 125.7
      guinea worms 125.7
      Mansonella (ozzardi) 125.5
      Onchocerca volvulus 125.3
        eye 125.3 *[360.13]*
        eyelid 125.3 *[373.6]*
      Wuchereria (bancrofti) 125.0
        malayi 125.1
    specified type NEC 125.6
  fish tapeworm 123.4
    larval 123.5
  fluke 121.9
    blood NEC (*see also* Schistosomiasis)
        120.9
    cat liver 121.0
    intestinal (giant) 121.4
    liver (sheep) 121.3
      cat 121.0
      Chinese 121.1
      clonorchiasis 121.1
      fascioliasis 121.3
      Oriental 121.1
    lung (oriental) 121.2
    sheep liver 121.3
  fly larva 134.0
  Gasterophilus (intestinalis) 134.0
  Gastrodiscoides hominis 121.8
  Giardia lamblia 007.1
  Gnathostoma (spinigerum) 128.1
  Gongylonema 125.6

Infestation (*Continued*)
  guinea worm 125.7
  helminth NEC 128.9
    intestinal 127.9
      mixed (types classifiable to more
          than one category in 120.0–
          127.7) 127.8
      specified type NEC 127.7
    specified type NEC 128.8
  Heterophyes heterophyes (small
      intestine) 121.6
  hookworm (*see also* Infestation,
      ancylostoma) 126.9
  Hymenolepis (diminuta) (nana) 123.6
  intestinal NEC 129
  leeches (aquatic) (land) 134.2
  Leishmania - *see* Leishmaniasis
  lice (*see also* Infestation, pediculus)
      132.9
  Linguatulidae, linguatula (pentastoma)
      (serrata) 134.1
  Loa loa 125.2
    eyelid 125.2 *[373.6]*
  louse (*see also* Infestation, pediculus)
      132.9
    body 132.1
    head 132.0
    pubic 132.2
  maggots 134.0
  Mansonella (ozzardi) 125.5
  medina 125.7
  Metagonimus yokogawai (small
      intestine) 121.5
  Microfilaria streptocerca 125.3
    eye 125.3 *[360.13]*
    eyelid 125.3 *[373.6]*
  Microsporon furfur 111.0
  microsporum - *see* Dermatophytosis
  mites 133.9
    scabic 133.0
    specified type NEC 133.8
  Monilia (albicans) (*see also* Candidiasis)
      112.9
    vagina 112.1
    vulva 112.1
  mouth 112.0
  Necator americanus 126.1
  nematode (intestinal) 127.9
    Ancylostoma (*see also* Ancylostoma)
        126.9
    Ascaris lumbricoides 127.0
    conjunctiva NEC 128.9
    Dioctophyma 128.8
    Enterobius vermicularis 127.4
    Gnathostoma spinigerum 128.1
    Oesophagostomum (apiostomum)
        127.7
    Physaloptera 127.4
    specified type NEC 127.7
    Strongyloides stercoralis 127.2
    Ternidens diminutus 127.7
    Trichinella spiralis 124
    Trichostrongylus 127.6
    Trichuris (trichiuria) 127.3
  Oesophagostomum (apiostomum)
      127.7
  Oestrus ovis 134.0
  Onchocerca (volvulus) 125.3
    eye 125.3 *[360.13]*
    eyelid 125.3 *[373.6]*
  Opisthorchis (felineus) (tenuicollis)
      (viverrini) 121.0
  Oxyuris vermicularis 127.4
  Paragonimus (westermani) 121.2

Infestation (*Continued*)
  parasite, parasitic NEC 136.9
    eyelid 134.9 *[373.6]*
    intestinal 129
    mouth 112.0
    orbit 376.13
    skin 134.9
    tongue 112.0
  pediculus 132.9
    capitis (humanus) (any site) 132.0
    corporis (humanus) (any site) 132.1
    eyelid 132.0 *[373.6]*
    mixed (classifiable to more than
      one category in 132.0–132.2)
      132.3
    pubis (any site) 132.2
  phthirus (pubis) (any site) 132.2
    with any infestation classifiable to
      132.0 and 132.1 132.3
  pinworm 127.4
  pork tapeworm (adult) 123.0
  protozoal NEC 136.8
  pubic louse 132.2
  rat tapeworm 123.6
  red bug 133.8
  roundworm (large) NEC 127.0
  sand flea 134.1
  saprophytic NEC 136.8
  Sarcoptes scabiei 133.0
  scabies 133.0
  Schistosoma 120.9
    bovis 120.8
    cercariae 120.3
    hematobium 120.0
    intercalatum 120.8
    japonicum 120.2
    mansoni 120.1
    mattheii 120.8
    specified
      site - *see* Schistosomiasis
      type NEC 120.8
    spindale 120.8
  screw worms 134.0
  skin NEC 134.9
  Sparganum (mansoni) (proliferum)
    123.5
    larval 123.5
  specified type NEC 134.8
  Spirometra larvae 123.5
  Sporozoa NEC 136.8
  Stellantchasmus falcatus 121.6
  Strongyloides 127.2
  Strongylus (gibsoni) 127.7
  Taenia 123.3
    diminuta 123.6
    Echinococcus (*see also* Echinococcus)
      122.9
    mediocanellata 123.2
    nana 123.6
    saginata (mediocanellata) 123.2
    solium (intestinal form) 123.0
      larval form 123.1
  Taeniarhynchus saginatus 123.2
  tapeworm 123.9
    beef 123.2
    broad 123.4
      larval 123.5
    dog 123.8
    dwarf 123.6
    fish 123.4
      larval 123.5
    pork 123.0
    rat 123.6
  Ternidens diminutus 127.7

Infestation (*Continued*)
  Tetranychus molestissimus 133.8
  threadworm 127.4
  tongue 112.0
  Toxocara (cani) (cati) (felis) 128.0
  trematode(s) NEC 121.9
  Trichina spiralis 124
  Trichinella spiralis 124
  Trichocephalus 127.3
  Trichomonas 131.9
    bladder 131.09
    cervix 131.09
    intestine 007.3
    prostate 131.03
    specified site NEC 131.8
    urethra (female) (male) 131.02
    urogenital 131.00
    vagina 131.01
    vulva 131.01
  Trichophyton - *see* Dermatophytosis
  Trichostrongylus instabilis 127.6
  Trichuris (trichiuria) 127.3
  Trombicula (irritans) 133.8
  Trypanosoma - *see* Trypanosomiasis
  Tunga penetrans 134.1
  Uncinaria americana 126.1
  whipworm 127.3
  worms NEC 128.9
    intestinal 127.9
  Wuchereria 125.0
    bancrofti 125.0
    malayi 125.1
Infiltrate, infiltration
  with an iron compound 275.09 ◀▥
  amyloid (any site) (generalized)
    277.39
  calcareous (muscle) NEC 275.49
    localized - *see* Degeneration, by
      site
  calcium salt (muscle) 275.49
  chemotherapy, vesicant 999.81
  corneal (*see also* Edema, cornea)
    371.20
  eyelid 373.9
  fatty (diffuse) (generalized) 272.8
    localized - *see* Degeneration, by site,
      fatty
  glycogen, glycogenic (*see also* Disease,
    glycogen storage) 271.0
  heart, cardiac
    fatty (*see also* Degeneration,
      myocardial) 429.1
    glycogenic 271.0 *[425.7]*
  inflammatory in vitreous 379.29
  kidney (*see also* Disease, renal) 593.9
  leukemic (M9800/3) - *see* Leukemia
  liver 573.8
    fatty - *see* Fatty, liver
    glycogen (*see also* Disease, glycogen
      storage) 271.0
  lung (*see also* Infiltrate, pulmonary)
    518.3
    eosinophilic 518.3
    x-ray finding only 793.1
  lymphatic (*see also* Leukemia,
    lymphatic) 204.9●
    gland, pigmentary 289.3
  muscle, fatty 728.9
  myelogenous (*see also* Leukemia,
    myeloid) 205.9●
  myocardium, myocardial
    fatty (*see also* Degeneration,
      myocardial) 429.1
    glycogenic 271.0 *[425.7]*

Infiltrate, infiltration (*Continued*)
  pulmonary 518.3
    with
      eosinophilia 518.3
      pneumonia - *see* Pneumonia, by
        type
    x-ray finding only 793.1
  Ranke's primary (*see also* Tuberculosis)
    010.0●
  skin, lymphocytic (benign) 709.8
  thymus (gland) (fatty) 254.8
  urine 788.8
  vesicant
    agent NEC 999.82
    chemotherapy 999.81
  vitreous humor 379.29
Infirmity 799.89
  senile 797
Inflammation, inflamed, inflammatory
  (with exudation)
  abducens (nerve) 378.54
  accessory sinus (chronic) (*see also*
    Sinusitis) 473.9
  adrenal (gland) 255.8
  alimentary canal - *see* Enteritis
  alveoli (teeth) 526.5
    scorbutic 267
  amnion - *see* Amnionitis
  anal canal 569.49
  antrum (chronic) (*see also* Sinusitis,
    maxillary) 473.0
  anus 569.49
  appendix (*see also* Appendicitis) 541
  arachnoid - *see* Meningitis
  areola 611.0
    puerperal, postpartum 675.0●
  areolar tissue NEC 686.9
  artery - *see* Arteritis
  auditory meatus (external) (*see also*
    Otitis, externa) 380.10
  Bartholin's gland 616.89
  bile duct or passage 576.1
  bladder (*see also* Cystitis) 595.9
  bleb
    postprocedural 379.60
      stage 1 379.61
      stage 2 379.62
      stage 3 379.63
  bone - *see* Osteomyelitis
  bowel (*see also* Enteritis) 558.9
  brain (*see also* Encephalitis) 323.9
    late effect - *see* category 326
    membrane - *see* Meningitis
  breast 611.0
    puerperal, postpartum 675.2●
  broad ligament (*see also* Disease, pelvis,
    inflammatory) 614.4
    acute 614.3
  bronchus - *see* Bronchitis
  bursa - *see* Bursitis
  capsule
    liver 573.3
    spleen 289.59
  catarrhal (*see also* Catarrh) 460
    vagina 616.10
  cecum (*see also* Appendicitis) 541
  cerebral (*see also* Encephalitis) 323.9
    late effect - *see* category 326
    membrane - *see* Meningitis
  cerebrospinal (*see also* Meningitis) 322.9
    late effect - *see* category 326
    meningococcal 036.0
    tuberculous (*see also* Tuberculosis)
      013.6●

    ◀ New   ◀▥ Revised   ~~deleted~~ Deleted   ● Use Additional Digit(s)   ▨ Omit code

Inflammation, inflamed, inflammatory
(*Continued*)
cervix (uteri) (*see also* Cervicitis) 616.0
chest 519.9
choroid NEC (*see also* Choroiditis)
363.20
cicatrix (tissue) - *see* Cicatrix
colon (*see also* Enteritis) 558.9
granulomatous 555.1
newborn 558.9
connective tissue (diffuse) NEC 728.9
cornea (*see also* Keratitis) 370.9
with ulcer (*see also* Ulcer, cornea)
370.00
corpora cavernosa (penis) 607.2
cranial nerve - *see* Disorder, nerve,
cranial
diarrhea - *see* Diarrhea
disc (intervertebral) (space) 722.90
cervical, cervicothoracic 722.91
lumbar, lumbosacral 722.93
thoracic, thoracolumbar 722.92
Douglas' cul-de-sac or pouch (chronic)
(*see also* Disease, pelvis,
inflammatory) 614.4
acute 614.3
due to (presence of) any device,
implant, or graft classifiable to
996.0–996.5 - *see* Complications,
infection and inflammation, due
to (presence of) any device,
implant, or graft classified to
996.0–996.5 NEC
duodenum 535.6●
dura mater - *see* Meningitis
ear - *see also* Otitis
external (*see also* Otitis, externa)
380.10
inner (*see also* Labyrinthitis) 386.30
middle - *see* Otitis media
esophagus 530.10
ethmoidal (chronic) (sinus) (*see also*
Sinusitis, ethmoidal) 473.2
Eustachian tube (catarrhal) 381.50
acute 381.51
chronic 381.52
extrarectal 569.49
eye 379.99
eyelid 373.9
specified NEC 373.8
fallopian tube (*see also* Salpingo-
oophoritis) 614.2
fascia 728.9
fetal membranes (acute) 658.4●
affecting fetus or newborn 762.7
follicular, pharynx 472.1
frontal (chronic) (sinus) (*see also*
Sinusitis, frontal) 473.1
gallbladder (*see also* Cholecystitis,
acute) 575.0
gall duct (*see also* Cholecystitis) 575.10
gastrointestinal (*see also* Enteritis)
558.9
genital organ (diffuse) (internal)
female 614.9
with
abortion - *see* Abortion, by
type, with sepsis
ectopic pregnancy (*see also*
categories 633.0–633.9)
639.0
molar pregnancy (*see also*
categories 630–632)
639.0

Inflammation, inflamed, inflammatory
(*Continued*)
genital organ (*Continued*)
female (*Continued*)
complicating pregnancy,
childbirth, or puerperium
646.6●
affecting fetus or newborn
760.8
following
abortion 639.0
ectopic or molar pregnancy
639.0
male 608.4
gland (lymph) (*see also* Lymphadenitis)
289.3
glottis (*see also* Laryngitis) 464.00
with obstruction 464.01
granular, pharynx 472.1
gum 523.10
heart (*see also* Carditis) 429.89
hepatic duct 576.8
hernial sac - *see* Hernia, by site
ileum (*see also* Enteritis) 558.9
terminal or regional 555.0
with large intestine 555.2
intervertebral disc 722.90
cervical, cervicothoracic 722.91
lumbar, lumbosacral 722.93
thoracic, thoracolumbar 722.92
intestine (*see also* Enteritis) 558.9
jaw (acute) (bone) (chronic) (lower)
(suppurative) (upper) 526.4
jejunum - *see* Enteritis
joint NEC (*see also* Arthritis) 716.9●
sacroiliac 720.2
kidney (*see also* Nephritis) 583.9
knee (joint) 716.66
tuberculous (active) (*see also*
Tuberculosis) 015.2●
labium (majus) (minus) (*see also*
Vulvitis) 616.10
lacrimal
gland (*see also* Dacryoadenitis)
375.00
passages (duct) (sac) (*see also*
Dacryocystitis) 375.30
larynx (*see also* Laryngitis) 464.00
with obstruction 464.01
diphtheritic 032.3
leg NEC 686.9
lip 528.5
liver (capsule) (*see also* Hepatitis) 573.3
acute 570
chronic 571.40
suppurative 572.0
lung (acute) (*see also* Pneumonia) 486
chronic (interstitial) 518.89
lymphatic vessel (*see also*
Lymphangitis) 457.2
lymph node or gland (*see also*
Lymphadenitis) 289.3
mammary gland 611.0
puerperal, postpartum 675.2●
maxilla, maxillary 526.4
sinus (chronic) (*see also* Sinusitis,
maxillary) 473.0
membranes of brain or spinal cord - *see*
Meningitis
meninges - *see* Meningitis
mouth 528.00
muscle 728.9
myocardium (*see also* Myocarditis)
429.0

Inflammation, inflamed, inflammatory
(*Continued*)
nasal sinus (chronic) (*see also* Sinusitis)
473.9
nasopharynx - *see* Nasopharyngitis
navel 686.9
newborn NEC 771.4
nerve NEC 729.2
nipple 611.0
puerperal, postpartum 675.0●
nose 478.19
suppurative 472.0
oculomotor nerve 378.51
optic nerve 377.30
orbit (chronic) 376.10
acute 376.00
chronic 376.10
ovary (*see also* Salpingo-oophoritis)
614.2
oviduct (*see also* Salpingo-oophoritis)
614.2
pancreas - *see* Pancreatitis
parametrium (chronic) (*see also* Disease,
pelvis, inflammatory) 614.4
acute 614.3
parotid region 686.9
gland 527.2
pelvis, female (*see also* Disease, pelvis,
inflammatory) 614.9
penis (corpora cavernosa) 607.2
perianal 569.49
pericardium (*see also* Pericarditis) 423.9
perineum (female) (male) 686.9
perirectal 569.49
peritoneum (*see also* Peritonitis) 567.9
periuterine (*see also* Disease, pelvis,
inflammatory) 614.9
perivesical (*see also* Cystitis) 595.9
petrous bone (*see also* Petrositis) 383.20
pharynx (*see also* Pharyngitis) 462
follicular 472.1
granular 472.1
pia mater - *see* Meningitis
pleura - *see* Pleurisy
postmastoidectomy cavity 383.30
chronic 383.33
pouch, internal ileoanal 569.71
prostate (*see also* Prostatitis) 601.9
rectosigmoid - *see* Rectosigmoiditis
rectum (*see also* Proctitis) 569.49
respiratory, upper (*see also* Infection,
respiratory, upper) 465.9
chronic, due to external agent - *see*
Condition, respiratory, chronic,
due to, external agent
due to
fumes or vapors (chemical)
(inhalation) 506.2
radiation 508.1
retina (*see also* Retinitis) 363.20
retrocecal (*see also* Appendicitis) 541
retroperitoneal (*see also* Peritonitis) 567.9
salivary duct or gland (any)
(suppurative) 527.2
scorbutic, alveoli, teeth 267
scrotum 608.4
sigmoid - *see* Enteritis
sinus (*see also* Sinusitis) 473.9
Skene's duct or gland (*see also*
Urethritis) 597.89
skin 686.9
spermatic cord 608.4
sphenoidal (sinus) (*see also* Sinusitis,
sphenoidal) 473.3

Inflammation, inflamed, inflammatory
(Continued)
spinal
cord (see also Encephalitis) 323.9
late effect - see category 326
membrane - see Meningitis
nerve - see Disorder, nerve
spine (see also Spondylitis) 720.9
spleen (capsule) 289.59
stomach - see Gastritis
stricture, rectum 569.49
subcutaneous tissue NEC 686.9
suprarenal (gland) 255.8
synovial (fringe) (membrane) - see
Bursitis
tendon (sheath) NEC 726.90
testis (see also Orchitis) 604.90
thigh 686.9
throat (see also Sore throat) 462
thymus (gland) 254.8
thyroid (gland) (see also Thyroiditis)
245.9
tongue 529.0
tonsil - see Tonsillitis
trachea - see Tracheitis
trochlear nerve 378.53
tubal (see also Salpingo-oophoritis) 614.2
tuberculous NEC (see also Tuberculosis)
011.9●
tubo-ovarian (see also Salpingo-
oophoritis) 614.2
tunica vaginalis 608.4
tympanic membrane - see Myringitis
umbilicus, umbilical 686.9
newborn NEC 771.4
uterine ligament (see also Disease,
pelvis, inflammatory) 614.4
acute 614.3
uterus (catarrhal) (see also Endometritis)
615.9
uveal tract (anterior) (see also
Iridocyclitis) 364.3
posterior - see Chorioretinitis
sympathetic 360.11
vagina (see also Vaginitis) 616.10
vas deferens 608.4
vein (see also Phlebitis) 451.9
thrombotic 451.9
cerebral (see also Thrombosis,
brain) 434.0●
leg 451.2
deep (vessels) NEC 451.19
superficial (vessels) 451.0
lower extremity 451.2
deep (vessels) NEC 451.19
superficial (vessels) 451.0
vocal cord 478.5
vulva (see also Vulvitis) 616.10
Inflation, lung imperfect (newborn)
770.5
Influenza, influenzal 487.1
with
bronchitis 487.1
bronchopneumonia 487.0
cold (any type) 487.1
digestive manifestations 487.8
hemoptysis 487.1
involvement of
gastrointestinal tract 487.8
nervous system 487.8
laryngitis 487.1
manifestations NEC 487.8
respiratory 487.1
pneumonia 487.0
pharyngitis 487.1
pneumonia (any form classifiable to
480–483, 485–486) 487.0

Influenza, influenzal (Continued)
with (Continued)
respiratory manifestations NEC 487.1
sinusitis 487.1
sore throat 487.1
tonsillitis 487.1
tracheitis 487.1
upper respiratory infection (acute)
487.1
A/H5N1 (see also Influenza, avian)
488.02 ◀▥
abdominal 487.8
Asian 487.1
avian 488.02 ◀▥
with involvement of gastrointestinal
tract 488.09 ◀
bronchopneumonia 488.01 ◀
laryngitis 488.02 ◀
manifestations NEC 488.09 ◀
respiratory 488.02 ◀
pharyngitis 488.02 ◀
pneumonia (any form classifiable to
480-483, 485-486) 488.01 ◀
respiratory infection (acute) (upper)
488.02 ◀
bronchial 487.1
bronchopneumonia 487.0
catarrhal 487.1
due to identified
avian influenza virus 488.02 ◀▥
with ◀
manifestations NEC 488.09 ◀
respiratory 488.02 ◀
pneumonia (any form
classifiable to 480-483,
485-486) 488.01 ◀
novel H1N1 influenza virus
488.12 ◀▥
with ◀
manifestations NEC 488.19 ◀
respiratory 488.12 ◀
pneumonia 488.11 ◀
epidemic 487.1
gastric 487.8
intestinal 487.8
laryngitis 487.1
maternal affecting fetus or newborn 760.2
manifest influenza in infant 771.2
novel (2009) H1N1 488.12 ◀▥
with involvement of gastrointestinal
tract 488.19 ◀
bronchopneumonia 488.11 ◀
laryngitis 488.12 ◀
manifestations NEC 488.19 ◀
respiratory 488.12 ◀
pharyngitis 488.12 ◀
pneumonia (any form classifiable to
480-483, 485-486) 488.11 ◀
respiratory infection (acute) (upper)
488.12 ◀
novel A/H1N1 (see also Influenza,
novel H1N1) 488.12 ◀▥
pharyngitis 487.1
pneumonia (any form) 487.0
respiratory (upper) 487.1
specified NEC 487.1
stomach 487.8
vaccination, prophylactic (against)
V04.81
Influenza-like disease (see also Influenza)
487.1 ◀▥
Infraction, Freiberg's (metatarsal head)
732.5
Infraeruption, teeth 524.34
**Infusion complication, misadventure, or
reaction** - see Complication, infusion

Ingestion
chemical - see Table of Drugs and
Chemicals
drug or medicinal substance
overdose or wrong substance given
or taken 977.9
specified drug - see Table of
Drugs and Chemicals
foreign body NEC (see also Foreign
body) 938
Ingrowing
hair 704.8
nail (finger) (toe) (infected) 703.0
Inguinal - see also condition
testis 752.51
Inhalation
carbon monoxide 986
flame
mouth 947.0
lung 947.1
food or foreign body (see also Asphyxia,
food or foreign body) 933.1
gas, fumes, or vapor (noxious) 987.9
specified agent - see Table of Drugs
and Chemicals
liquid or vomitus (see also Asphyxia,
food or foreign body) 933.1
lower respiratory tract NEC 934.9
meconium (fetus or newborn) 770.11
with respiratory symptoms 770.12
mucus (see also Asphyxia, mucus) 933.1
oil (causing suffocation) (see also
Asphyxia, food or foreign body)
933.1
pneumonia - see Pneumonia, aspiration
smoke 987.9
steam 987.9
stomach contents or secretions (see also
Asphyxia, food or foreign body)
933.1
in labor and delivery 668.0●
Inhibition, inhibited
academic as adjustment reaction 309.23
orgasm
female 302.73
male 302.74
sexual
desire 302.71
excitement 302.72
work as adjustment reaction 309.23
Inhibitor, systemic lupus erythematosus
(presence of) 286.5
Iniencephalus, iniencephaly 740.2
Injected eye 372.74
Injury 959.9

Note: For abrasion, insect bite
(nonvenomous), blister, or scratch, see
Injury, superficial.

For laceration, traumatic rupture, tear,
or penetrating wound of internal
organs, such as heart, lung, liver,
kidney, pelvic organs, whether or not
accompanied by open wound in the
same region, see Injury, internal.

For nerve injury, see Injury, nerve.

For late effect of injuries classifiable to
850–854, 860–869, 900–919, 950–959, see
Late, effect, injury, by type.

abdomen, abdominal (viscera) - see also
Injury, internal, abdomen
muscle or wall 959.12

◀ New   ◀▥ Revised   ~~deleted~~ Deleted   ● Use Additional Digit(s)   ▨ Omit code

Injury (Continued)
  acoustic, resulting in deafness 951.5
  adenoid 959.09
  adrenal (gland) - see Injury, internal, adrenal
  alveolar (process) 959.09
  ankle (and foot) (and knee) (and leg, except thigh) 959.7
  anterior chamber, eye 921.3
  anus 959.19
  aorta (thoracic) 901.0
    abdominal 902.0
  appendix - see Injury, internal, appendix
  arm, upper (and shoulder) 959.2
  artery (complicating trauma) (see also Injury, blood vessel, by site) 904.9
    cerebral or meningeal (see also Hemorrhage, brain, traumatic, subarachnoid) 852.0 ●
  auditory canal (external) (meatus) 959.09
  auricle, auris, ear 959.09
  axilla 959.2
  back 959.19
  bile duct - see Injury, internal, bile duct
  birth - see also Birth, injury
    canal NEC, complicating delivery 665.9 ●
  bladder (sphincter) - see Injury, internal, bladder
  blast (air) (hydraulic) (immersion) (underwater) NEC 869.0
    with open wound into cavity NEC 869.1
    abdomen or thorax - see Injury, internal, by site
    brain - see Concussion, brain
    ear (acoustic nerve trauma) 951.5
      with perforation of tympanic membrane - see Wound, open, ear, drum
  blood vessel NEC 904.9
    abdomen 902.9
      multiple 902.87
      specified NEC 902.89
    aorta (thoracic) 901.0
      abdominal 902.0
    arm NEC 903.9
    axillary 903.00
      artery 903.1
      vein 903.02
    azygos vein 901.89
    basilic vein 903.1
    brachial (artery) (vein) 903.1
    bronchial 901.89
    carotid artery 900.00
      common 900.01
      external 900.02
      internal 900.03
    celiac artery 902.20
      specified branch NEC 902.24
    cephalic vein (arm) 903.1
    colica dextra 902.26
    cystic
      artery 902.24
      vein 902.39
    deep plantar 904.6
    digital (artery) (vein) 903.5
    due to accidental puncture or laceration during procedure 998.2
    extremity
      lower 904.8
        multiple 904.7
        specified NEC 904.7
      upper 903.9
        multiple 903.8
        specified NEC 903.8

Injury (Continued)
  blood vessel (Continued)
    femoral
      artery (superficial) 904.1
        above profunda origin 904.0
        common 904.0
      vein 904.2
    gastric
      artery 902.21
      vein 902.39
    head 900.9
      intracranial - see Injury, intracranial
      multiple 900.82
      specified NEC 900.89
    hemiazygos vein 901.89
    hepatic
      artery 902.22
      vein 902.11
    hypogastric 902.59
      artery 902.51
      vein 902.52
    ileocolic
      artery 902.26
      vein 902.31
    iliac 902.50
      artery 902.53
      specified branch NEC 902.59
      vein 902.54
    innominate
      artery 901.1
      vein 901.3
    intercostal (artery) (vein) 901.81
    jugular vein (external) 900.81
      internal 900.1
    leg NEC 904.8
    mammary (artery) (vein) 901.82
    mesenteric
      artery 902.20
        inferior 902.27
        specified branch NEC 902.29
        superior (trunk) 902.25
          branches, primary 902.26
      vein 902.39
        inferior 902.32
        superior (and primary subdivisions) 902.31
    neck 900.9
      multiple 900.82
      specified NEC 900.89
    ovarian 902.89
      artery 902.81
      vein 902.82
    palmar artery 903.4
    pelvis 902.9
      multiple 902.87
      specified NEC 902.89
    plantar (deep) (artery) (vein) 904.6
    popliteal 904.40
      artery 904.41
      vein 904.42
    portal 902.33
    pulmonary 901.40
      artery 901.41
      vein 901.42
    radial (artery) (vein) 903.2
    renal 902.40
      artery 902.41
      specified NEC 902.49
      vein 902.42
    saphenous
      artery 904.7
      vein (greater) (lesser) 904.3
    splenic
      artery 902.23
      vein 902.34

Injury (Continued)
  blood vessel (Continued)
    subclavian
      artery 901.1
      vein 901.3
    suprarenal 902.49
    thoracic 901.9
      multiple 901.83
      specified NEC 901.89
    tibial 904.50
      artery 904.50
        anterior 904.51
        posterior 904.53
      vein 904.50
        anterior 904.52
        posterior 904.54
    ulnar (artery) (vein) 903.3
    uterine 902.59
      artery 902.55
      vein 902.56
    vena cava
      inferior 902.10
        specified branches NEC 902.19
      superior 901.2
  brachial plexus 953.4
    newborn 767.6
  brain (traumatic) NEC (see also Injury, intracranial) 854.0 ●
    due to fracture of skull - see Fracture, skull, by site
  breast 959.19
  broad ligament - see Injury, internal, broad ligament
  bronchus, bronchi - see Injury, internal, bronchus
  brow 959.09
  buttock 959.19
  canthus, eye 921.1
  cathode ray 990
  cauda equina 952.4
    with fracture, vertebra - see Fracture, vertebra, sacrum
  cavernous sinus (see also Injury, intracranial) 854.0 ●
  cecum - see Injury, internal, cecum
  celiac ganglion or plexus 954.1
  cerebellum (see also Injury, intracranial) 854.0 ●
  cervix (uteri) - see Injury, internal, cervix
  cheek 959.09
  chest - see Injury, internal, chest
    wall 959.11
  childbirth - see also Birth, injury
    maternal NEC 665.9 ●
  chin 959.09
  choroid (eye) 921.3
  clitoris 959.14
  coccyx 959.19
    complicating delivery 665.6 ●
  colon - see Injury, internal, colon
  common duct - see Injury, internal, common duct
  conjunctiva 921.1
    superficial 918.2
  cord
    spermatic - see Injury, internal, spermatic cord
    spinal - see Injury, spinal, by site
  cornea 921.3
    abrasion 918.1
    due to contact lens 371.82
    penetrating - see Injury, eyeball, penetrating
    superficial 918.1
    due to contact lens 371.82

Injury (Continued)
   cortex (cerebral) (see also Injury,
      intracranial) 854.0●
     visual 950.3
   costal region 959.11
   costochondral 959.11
   cranial
     bones - see Fracture, skull, by site
     cavity (see also Injury, intracranial)
      854.0●
     nerve - see Injury, nerve, cranial
   crushing - see Crush
   cutaneous sensory nerve
     lower limb 956.4
     upper limb 955.5
   deep tissue - see Contusion, by site
     meaning pressure ulcer 707.25
   delivery - see also Birth, injury
     maternal NEC 665.9●
   Descemet's membrane - see Injury,
     eyeball, penetrating
   diaphragm - see Injury, internal,
     diaphragm
   diffuse axonal - see Injury, intracranial
   duodenum - see Injury, internal,
     duodenum
   ear (auricle) (canal) (drum) (external)
     959.09
   elbow (and forearm) (and wrist)
     959.3
   epididymis 959.14
   epigastric region 959.12
   epiglottis 959.09
   epiphyseal, current - see Fracture, by
     site
   esophagus - see Injury, internal,
     esophagus
   Eustachian tube 959.09
   extremity (lower) (upper) NEC 959.8
   eye 921.9
     penetrating eyeball - see Injury,
      eyeball, penetrating
     superficial 918.9
   eyeball 921.3
     penetrating 871.7
      with
        partial loss (of intraocular
          tissue) 871.2
        prolapse or exposure (of
          intraocular tissue) 871.1
      without prolapse 871.0
      foreign body (nonmagnetic)
        871.6
        magnetic 871.5
     superficial 918.9
   eyebrow 959.09
   eyelid(s) 921.1
     laceration - see Laceration, eyelid
     superficial 918.0
   face (and neck) 959.09
   fallopian tube - see Injury, internal,
     fallopian tube
   fingers(s) (nail) 959.5
   flank 959.19
   foot (and ankle) (and knee) (and leg,
     except thigh) 959.7
   forceps NEC 767.9
     scalp 767.19
   forearm (and elbow) (and wrist) 959.3
   forehead 959.09
   gallbladder - see Injury, internal,
     gallbladder
   gasserian ganglion 951.2
   gastrointestinal tract - see Injury,
     internal, gastrointestinal tract

Injury (Continued)
   genital organ(s)
     with
      abortion - see Abortion, by type,
        with, damage to pelvic
        organs
      ectopic pregnancy (see also
        categories 633.0–633.9) 639.2
      molar pregnancy (see also
        categories 630–632) 639.2
     external 959.14
     fracture of corpus cavernosum penis
      959.13
     following
      abortion 639.2
      ectopic or molar pregnancy 639.2
     internal - see Injury, internal, genital
      organs
     obstetrical trauma NEC 665.9●
      affecting fetus or newborn 763.89
   gland
     lacrimal 921.1
      laceration 870.8
     parathyroid 959.09
     salivary 959.09
     thyroid 959.09
   globe (eye) (see also Injury, eyeball) 921.3
   grease gun - see Wound, open, by site,
     complicated
   groin 959.19
   gum 959.09
   hand(s) (except fingers) 959.4
   head NEC 959.01
     with
      loss of consciousness 850.5
      skull fracture - see Fracture, skull,
        by site
   heart - see Injury, internal, heart
   heel 959.7
   hip (and thigh) 959.6
   hymen 959.14
   hyperextension (cervical) (vertebra) 847.0
   ileum - see Injury, internal, ileum
   iliac region 959.19
   infrared rays NEC 990
   instrumental (during surgery) 998.2
     birth injury - see Birth, injury
     nonsurgical (see also Injury, by site)
      959.9
     obstetrical 665.9●
      affecting fetus or newborn 763.89
      bladder 665.5●
      cervix 665.3●
      high vaginal 665.4●
      perineal NEC 664.9●
      urethra 665.5●
      uterus 665.5●
   internal 869.0

Note: For injury of internal organ(s)
by foreign body entering through a
natural orifice (e.g., inhaled, ingested,
or swallowed)-see Foreign body,
entering through orifice.

For internal injury of any of the
following sites with internal injury of
any other of the sites-see Injury,
internal, multiple.

---

     with
      fracture
        pelvis - see Fracture, pelvis
        specified site, except pelvis -
          see Injury, internal, by
          site
      open wound into cavity 869.1

Injury (Continued)
   internal (Continued)
     abdomen, abdominal (viscera) NEC
      868.00
      with
        fracture, pelvis - see Fracture,
          pelvis
        open wound into cavity
          868.10
      specified site NEC 868.09
        with open wound into cavity
          868.19
     adrenal (gland) 868.01
      with open wound into cavity
        868.11
     aorta (thoracic) 901.0
      abdominal 902.0
     appendix 863.85
      with open wound into cavity
        863.95
     bile duct 868.02
      with open wound into cavity
        868.12
     bladder (sphincter) 867.0
      with
        abortion - see Abortion, by
          type, with, damage to
          pelvic organs
        ectopic pregnancy (see also
          categories 633.0–633.9)
          639.2
        molar pregnancy (see also
          categories 630–632) 639.2
        open wound into cavity 867.1
      following
        abortion 639.2
        ectopic or molar pregnancy
          639.2
      obstetrical trauma 665.5●
        affecting fetus or newborn
          763.89
     blood vessel - see Injury, blood
      vessel, by site
     broad ligament 867.6
      with open wound into cavity
        867.7
     bronchus, bronchi 862.21
      with open wound into cavity
        862.31
     cecum 863.89
      with open wound into cavity
        863.99
     cervix (uteri) 867.4
      with
        abortion - see Abortion, by
          type, with damage to
          pelvic organs
        ectopic pregnancy (see also
          categories 633.0–633.9)
          639.2
        molar pregnancy (see also
          categories 630–632)
          639.2
        open wound into cavity 867.5
      following
        abortion 639.2
        ectopic or molar pregnancy
          639.2
      obstetrical trauma 665.3●
        affecting fetus or newborn
          763.89
     chest (see also Injury, internal,
      intrathoracic organs) 862.8
      with open wound into cavity
        862.9

◀ New   ◀||||| Revised   ~~deleted~~ Deleted   ● Use Additional Digit(s)   Omit code

Injury (Continued)
  internal (Continued)
    colon 863.40
      with
        open wound into cavity 863.50
        rectum 863.46
          with open wound into
            cavity 863.56
      ascending (right) 863.41
        with open wound into cavity
          863.51
      descending (left) 863.43
        with open wound into cavity
          863.53
      multiple sites 863.46
        with open wound into cavity
          863.56
      sigmoid 863.44
        with open wound into cavity
          863.54
      specified site NEC 863.49
        with open wound into cavity
          863.59
      transverse 863.42
        with open wound into cavity
          863.52
    common duct 868.02
      with open wound into cavity
        868.12
    complicating delivery 665.9●
      affecting fetus or newborn 763.89
    diaphragm 862.0
      with open wound into cavity
        862.1
    duodenum 863.21
      with open wound into cavity
        863.31
    esophagus (intrathoracic) 862.22
      with open wound into cavity
        862.32
      cervical region 874.4
        complicated 874.5
    fallopian tube 867.6
      with open wound into cavity 867.7
    gallbladder 868.02
      with open wound into cavity
        868.12
    gastrointestinal tract NEC 863.80
      with open wound into cavity
        863.90
    genital organ NEC 867.6
      with open wound into cavity 867.7
    heart 861.00
      with open wound into thorax
        861.10
    ileum 863.29
      with open wound into cavity 863.39
    intestine NEC 863.89
      with open wound into cavity
        863.99
      large NEC 863.40
        with open wound into cavity
          863.50
      small NEC 863.20
        with open wound into cavity
          863.30
    intra-abdominal (organ) 868.00
      with open wound into cavity
        868.10
      multiple sites 868.09
        with open wound into cavity
          868.19
      specified site NEC 868.09
        with open wound into cavity
          868.19

Injury (Continued)
  internal (Continued)
    intrathoracic organs (multiple) 862.8
      with open wound into cavity 862.9
      diaphragm (only) - see Injury,
        internal, diaphragm
      heart (only) - see Injury, internal,
        heart
      lung (only) - see Injury, internal,
        lung
      specified site NEC 862.29
        with open wound into cavity
          862.39
    intrauterine (see also Injury, internal,
      uterus) 867.4
      with open wound into cavity
        867.5
    jejunum 863.29
      with open wound into cavity
        863.39
    kidney (subcapsular) 866.00
      with
        disruption of parenchyma
          (complete) 866.03
          with open wound into
            cavity 866.13
        hematoma (without rupture of
          capsule) 866.01
          with open wound into
            cavity 866.11
        laceration 866.02
          with open wound into
            cavity 866.12
        open wound into cavity
          866.10
    liver 864.00
      with
        contusion 864.01
          with open wound into
            cavity 864.11
        hematoma 864.01
          with open wound into
            cavity 864.11
        laceration 864.05
          with open wound into
            cavity 864.15
        major (disruption of hepatic
          parenchyma) 864.04
          with open wound into
            cavity 864.14
        minor (capsule only)
          864.02
          with open wound into
            cavity 864.12
        moderate (involving
          parenchyma) 864.03
          with open wound into
            cavity 864.13
        multiple 864.04
        stellate 864.04
          with open wound into
            cavity 864.14
        open wound into cavity
          864.10
    lung 861.20
      with open wound into thorax
        861.30
      hemopneumothorax - see
        Hemopneumothorax,
        traumatic
      hemothorax - see Hemothorax,
        traumatic
      pneumohemothorax - see
        Pneumohemothorax,
        traumatic

Injury (Continued)
  internal (Continued)
    lung (Continued)
      pneumothorax - see
        Pneumothorax,
        traumatic
      transfusion related, acute
        (TRALI) 518.7
    mediastinum 862.29
      with open wound into cavity
        862.39
    mesentery 863.89
      with open wound into cavity
        863.99
    mesosalpinx 867.6
      with open wound into cavity
        867.7
    multiple 869.0

> Note: Multiple internal injuries of
> sites classifiable to the same three- or
> four-digit category should be classified
> to that category.
>
> Multiple injuries classifiable to
> different fourth-digit subdivisions of
> 861.-(heart and lung injuries) should
> be dealt with according to coding
> rules.

      internal 869.0
        with open wound into cavity
          869.1
      intra-abdominal organ (sites
        classifiable to 863–868)
        with
          intrathoracic organ(s) (sites
            classifiable to 861–862)
            869.0
            with open wound into
              cavity 869.1
          other intra-abdominal
            organ(s) (sites
            classifiable to
            863–868, except
            where classifiable
            to the same three-
            digit category)
            868.09
            with open wound into
              cavity 868.19
      intrathoracic organ (sites
        classifiable to 861–862)
        with
          intra-abdominal organ(s)
            (sites classifiable to
            863–868) 869.0
            with open wound into
              cavity 869.1
          other intrathoracic organs(s)
            (sites classifiable to
            861–862, except where
            classifiable to the same
            three-digit category)
            862.8
            with open wound into cavity
              862.9
    myocardium - see Injury, internal,
      heart
    ovary 867.6
      with open wound into cavity
        867.7
    pancreas (multiple sites) 863.84
      with open wound into cavity
        863.94

Injury (Continued)
  internal (Continued)
    pancreas (Continued)
      body 863.82
        with open wound into cavity
          863.92
      head 863.81
        with open wound into cavity
          863.91
      tail 863.83
      with open wound into cavity
        863.93
    pelvis, pelvic (organs) (viscera) 867.8
      with
        fracture, pelvis - see Fracture,
          pelvis
        open wound into cavity 867.9
      specified site NEC 867.6
        with open wound into cavity
          867.7
    peritoneum 868.03
      with open wound into cavity
        868.13
    pleura 862.29
      with open wound into cavity
        862.39
    prostate 867.6
      with open wound into cavity
        867.7
    rectum 863.45
      with
        colon 863.46
          with open wound into
            cavity 863.56
        open wound into cavity
          863.55
    retroperitoneum 868.04
      with open wound into cavity
        868.14
    round ligament 867.6
      with open wound into cavity
        867.7
    seminal vesicle 867.6
      with open wound into cavity
        867.7
    spermatic cord 867.6
      with open wound into cavity
        867.7
    scrotal - see Wound, open,
      spermatic cord
    spleen 865.00
      with
        disruption of parenchyma
          (massive) 865.04
          with open wound into
            cavity 865.14
        hematoma (without rupture of
          capsule) 865.01
          with open wound into
            cavity 865.11
        open wound into cavity 865.10
        tear, capsular 865.02
          with open wound into
            cavity 865.12
          extending into parenchyma
            865.03
            with open wound into
              cavity 865.13
    stomach 863.0
      with open wound into cavity
        863.1
    suprarenal gland (multiple) 868.01
      with open wound into cavity
        868.11

Injury (Continued)
  internal (Continued)
    thorax, thoracic (cavity) (organs)
      (multiple) (see also Injury,
      internal, intrathoracic organs)
      862.8
      with open wound into cavity
        862.9
    thymus (gland) 862.29
      with open wound into cavity
        862.39
    trachea (intrathoracic) 862.29
      with open wound into cavity
        862.39
      cervical region (see also Wound,
        open, trachea) 874.02
    ureter 867.2
      with open wound into cavity
        867.3
    urethra (sphincter) 867.0
      with
        abortion - see Abortion, by
          type, with, damage to
          pelvic organs
        ectopic pregnancy (see also
          categories 633.0–633.9)
          639.2
        molar pregnancy (see also
          categories 630–632)
          639.2
        open wound into cavity 867.1
      following
        abortion 639.2
        ectopic or molar pregnancy
          639.2
      obstetrical trauma 665.5●
        affecting fetus or newborn
          763.89
    uterus 867.4
      with
        abortion - see Abortion, by
          type, with, damage to
          pelvic organs
        ectopic pregnancy (see also
          categories 633.0–633.9)
          639.2
        molar pregnancy (see also
          categories 630–632)
          639.2
        open wound into cavity 867.5
      following
        abortion 639.2
        ectopic or molar pregnancy
          639.2
      obstetrical trauma NEC 665.5●
        affecting fetus or newborn
          763.89
    vas deferens 867.6
      with open wound into cavity
        867.7
    vesical (sphincter) 867.0
      with open wound into cavity
        867.1
    viscera (abdominal) (see also Injury,
      internal, multiple) 868.00
      with
        fracture, pelvis - see Fracture,
          pelvis
        open wound into cavity 868.10
      thoracic NEC (see also Injury,
        internal, intrathoracic
        organs) 862.8
        with open wound into cavity
          862.9

Injury (Continued)
  interscapular region 959.19
  intervertebral disc 959.19
  intestine - see Injury, internal, intestine
  intra-abdominal (organs) NEC - see
    Injury, internal, intra-abdominal
  intracranial (traumatic) 854.0●

> Note: Use the following fifth-digit
> subclassification with categories 851–854:
>
> 0   unspecified state of
>   consciousness
> 1   with no loss of consciousness
> 2   with brief [less than one hour]
>   loss of consciousness
> 3   with moderate [1–24 hours] loss
>   of consciousness
> 4   with prolonged [more than 24
>   hours] loss of
>   consciousness and return
>   to pre-existing conscious
>   level
> 5   with prolonged [more than 24
>   hours] loss of
>   consciousness, without
>   return to pre-existing
>   conscious level
>
> Use fifth-digit 5 to designate when a
> patient is unconscious and dies before
> regaining consciousness, regardless of
> the duration of the loss of consciousness
>
> 6   with loss of consciousness of
>   unspecified duration
> 9   with concussion, unspecified

    with
      open intracranial wound
        854.1●
      skull fracture - see Fracture,
        skull, by site
    contusion 851.8●
      with open intracranial wound
        851.9●
      brain stem 851.4●
        with open intracranial wound
          851.5●
      cerebellum 851.4●
        with open intracranial wound
          851.5●
      cortex (cerebral) 851.0●
        with open intracranial wound
          851.2●
      hematoma - see Injury,
        intracranial, hemorrhage
      hemorrhage 853.0●
        with
          laceration - see Injury,
            intracranial,
            laceration
          open intracranial wound
            853.1●
        extradural 852.4●
          with open intracranial
            wound 852.5●
        subarachnoid 852.0●
          with open intracranial
            wound 852.1●
        subdural 852.2●
          with open intracranial
            wound 852.3●
      laceration 851.8●
        with open intracranial wound
          851.9●

◀ New   ⇚ Revised   ~~deleted~~ Deleted   ● Use Additional Digit(s)   ▮ Omit code

Injury *(Continued)*
  intracranial *(Continued)*
    contusion *(Continued)*
      laceration *(Continued)*
        brain stem 851.6●
          with open intracranial
            wound 851.7●
        cerebellum 851.6●
          with open intracranial
            wound 851.7●
        cortex (cerebral) 851.2●
          with open intracranial
            wound 851.3●
  intraocular - *see* Injury, eyeball, penetrating
  intrathoracic organs (multiple) - *see* Injury, internal, intrathoracic organs
  intrauterine - *see* Injury, internal, intrauterine
  iris 921.3
    penetrating - *see* Injury, eyeball, penetrating
  jaw 959.09
  jejunum - *see* Injury, internal, jejunum
  joint NEC 959.9
    old or residual 718.80
      ankle 718.87
      elbow 718.82
      foot 718.87
      hand 718.84
      hip 718.85
      knee 718.86
      multiple sites 718.89
      pelvic region 718.85
      shoulder (region) 718.81
      specified site NEC 718.88
      wrist 718.83
  kidney - *see* Injury, internal, kidney
    acute (nontraumatic) 584.9
  knee (and ankle) (and foot) (and leg, except thigh) 959.7
  labium (majus) (minus) 959.14
  labyrinth, ear 959.09
  lacrimal apparatus, gland, or sac 921.1
    laceration 870.8
  larynx 959.09
  late effect - *see* Late, effects (of), injury
  leg, except thigh (and ankle) (and foot) (and knee) 959.7
    upper or thigh 959.6
  lens, eye 921.3
    penetrating - *see* Injury, eyeball, penetrating
  lid, eye - *see* Injury, eyelid
  lip 959.09
  liver - *see* Injury, internal, liver
  lobe, parietal - *see* Injury, intracranial
  lumbar (region) 959.19
    plexus 953.5
  lumbosacral (region) 959.19
    plexus 953.5
  lung - *see* Injury, internal, lung
  malar region 959.09
  mastoid region 959.09
  maternal, during pregnancy, affecting fetus or newborn 760.5
  maxilla 959.09
  mediastinum - *see* Injury, internal, mediastinum
  membrane
    brain (*see also* Injury, intracranial) 854.0●
    tympanic 959.09

Injury *(Continued)*
  meningeal artery - *see* Hemorrhage, brain, traumatic, subarachnoid
  meninges (cerebral) - *see* Injury, intracranial
  mesenteric
    artery - *see* Injury, blood vessel, mesenteric, artery
    plexus, inferior 954.1
    vein - *see* Injury, blood vessel, mesenteric, vein
  mesentery - *see* Injury, internal, mesentery
  mesosalpinx - *see* Injury, internal, mesosalpinx
  middle ear 959.09
  midthoracic region 959.11
  mouth 959.09
  multiple (sites not classifiable to the same four-digit category in 959.0–959.7) 959.8
    internal 869.0
      with open wound into cavity 869.1
  musculocutaneous nerve 955.4
  nail
    finger 959.5
    toe 959.7
  nasal (septum) (sinus) 959.09
  nasopharynx 959.09
  neck (and face) 959.09
  nerve 957.9
    abducens 951.3
    abducent 951.3
    accessory 951.6
    acoustic 951.5
    ankle and foot 956.9
    anterior crural, femoral 956.1
    arm (*see also* Injury, nerve, upper limb) 955.9
    auditory 951.5
    axillary 955.0
    brachial plexus 953.4
    cervical sympathetic 954.0
    cranial 951.9
      first or olfactory 951.8
      second or optic 950.0
      third or oculomotor 951.0
      fourth or trochlear 951.1
      fifth or trigeminal 951.2
      sixth or abducens 951.3
      seventh or facial 951.4
      eighth, acoustic, or auditory 951.5
      ninth or glossopharyngeal 951.8
      tenth, pneumogastric, or vagus 951.8
      eleventh or accessory 951.6
      twelfth or hypoglossal 951.7
      newborn 767.7
    cutaneous sensory
      lower limb 956.4
      upper limb 955.5
    digital (finger) 955.6
      toe 956.5
    facial 951.4
      newborn 767.5
    femoral 956.1
    finger 955.9
    foot and ankle 956.9
    forearm 955.9
    glossopharyngeal 951.8
    hand and wrist 955.9
    head and neck, superficial 957.0

Injury *(Continued)*
  nerve *(Continued)*
    hypoglossal 951.7
    involving several parts of body 957.8
    leg (*see also* Injury, nerve, lower limb) 956.9
    lower limb 956.9
      multiple 956.8
      specified site NEC 956.5
    lumbar plexus 953.5
    lumbosacral plexus 953.5
    median 955.1
      forearm 955.1
      wrist and hand 955.1
    multiple (in several parts of body) (sites not classifiable to the same three-digit category) 957.8
    musculocutaneous 955.4
    musculospiral 955.3
      upper arm 955.3
    oculomotor 951.0
    olfactory 951.8
    optic 950.0
    pelvic girdle 956.9
      multiple sites 956.8
      specified site NEC 956.5
    peripheral 957.9
      multiple (in several regions) (sites not classifiable to the same three-digit category) 957.8
      specified site NEC 957.1
    peroneal 956.3
      ankle and foot 956.3
      lower leg 956.3
    plantar 956.5
    plexus 957.9
      celiac 954.1
      mesenteric, inferior 954.1
      spinal 953.9
        brachial 953.4
        lumbosacral 953.5
        multiple sites 953.8
      sympathetic NEC 954.1
    pneumogastric 951.8
    radial 955.3
      wrist and hand 955.3
    sacral plexus 953.5
    sciatic 956.0
      thigh 956.0
    shoulder girdle 955.9
      multiple 955.8
      specified site NEC 955.7
    specified site NEC 957.1
    spinal 953.9
      plexus - *see* Injury, nerve, plexus, spinal
      root 953.9
        cervical 953.0
        dorsal 953.1
        lumbar 953.2
        multiple sites 953.8
        sacral 953.3
    splanchnic 954.1
    sympathetic NEC 954.1
      cervical 954.0
    thigh 956.9
    tibial 956.5
      ankle and foot 956.2
      lower leg 956.5
      posterior 956.2
    toe 956.9

Injury (Continued)
  nerve (Continued)
    trigeminal 951.2
    trochlear 951.1
    trunk, excluding shoulder and
      pelvic girdles 954.9
      specified site NEC 954.8
      sympathetic NEC 954.1
    ulnar 955.2
      forearm 955.2
      wrist (and hand) 955.2
    upper limb 955.9
      multiple 955.8
      specified site NEC 955.7
    vagus 951.8
    wrist and hand 955.9
  nervous system, diffuse 957.8
  nose (septum) 959.09
  obstetrical NEC 665.9●
    affecting fetus or newborn 763.89
  occipital (region) (scalp) 959.09
    lobe (see also Injury, intracranial)
      854.0●
  optic 950.9
    chiasm 950.1
    cortex 950.3
    nerve 950.0
    pathways 950.2
  orbit, orbital (region) 921.2
    penetrating 870.3
      with foreign body 870.4
  ovary - see Injury, internal, ovary
  paint-gun - see Wound, open, by site,
    complicated
  palate (soft) 959.09
  pancreas - see Injury, internal, pancreas
  parathyroid (gland) 959.09
  parietal (region) (scalp) 959.09
    lobe - see Injury, intracranial
  pelvic
    floor 959.19
      complicating delivery 664.1●
        affecting fetus or newborn
          763.89
    joint or ligament, complicating
      delivery 665.6●
      affecting fetus or newborn
        763.89
    organs - see also Injury, internal,
      pelvis
      with
        abortion - see Abortion, by
          type, with damage to
          pelvic organs
        ectopic pregnancy (see also
          categories 633.0–633.9)
          639.2
        molar pregnancy (see also
          categories 633.0–633.9)
          639.2
      following
        abortion 639.2
        ectopic or molar pregnancy
          639.2
      obstetrical trauma 665.5●
        affecting fetus or newborn
          763.89
  pelvis 959.19
  penis 959.14
    fracture of corpus cavernosum
      959.13
  perineum 959.14
  peritoneum - see Injury, internal,
    peritoneum

Injury (Continued)
  periurethral tissue
    with
      abortion - see Abortion, by type,
        with damage to pelvic
        organs
      ectopic pregnancy (see also
        categories 633.0–633.9) 639.2
      molar pregnancy (see also
        categories 630–632) 639.2
    complicating delivery 664.8● ◀▥
      affecting fetus or newborn 763.89
    following
      abortion 639.2
      ectopic or molar pregnancy
        639.2
  phalanges
    foot 959.7
    hand 959.5
  pharynx 959.09
  pleura - see Injury, internal, pleura
  popliteal space 959.7
  post-cardiac surgery (syndrome)
    429.4
  prepuce 959.14
  prostate - see Injury, internal, prostate
  pubic region 959.19
  pudenda 959.14
  radiation NEC 990
  radioactive substance or radium NEC
    990
  rectovaginal septum 959.14
  rectum - see Injury, internal, rectum
  retina 921.3
    penetrating - see Injury, eyeball,
      penetrating
  retroperitoneal - see Injury, internal,
    retroperitoneum
  roentgen rays NEC 990
  round ligament - see Injury, internal,
    round ligament
  sacral (region) 959.19
    plexus 953.5
  sacroiliac ligament NEC 959.19
  sacrum 959.19
  salivary ducts or glands 959.09
  scalp 959.09
    due to birth trauma 767.19
    fetus or newborn 767.19
  scapular region 959.2
  sclera 921.3
    penetrating - see Injury, eyeball,
      penetrating
    superficial 918.2
  scrotum 959.14
  seminal vesicle - see Injury, internal,
    seminal vesicle
  shoulder (and upper arm) 959.2
  sinus
    cavernous (see also Injury,
      intracranial) 854.0●
    nasal 959.09
  skeleton NEC, birth injury 767.3
  skin NEC 959.9
  skull - see Fracture, skull, by site
  soft tissue (of external sites) (severe) -
    see Wound, open, by site
  specified site NEC 959.8
  spermatic cord - see Injury, internal,
    spermatic cord
  spinal (cord) 952.9
    with fracture, vertebra - see Fracture,
      vertebra, by site, with spinal
      cord injury

Injury (Continued)
  spinal (Continued)
    cervical (C_1–C_4) 952.00
      with
        anterior cord syndrome 952.02
        central cord syndrome 952.03
        complete lesion of cord 952.01
        incomplete lesion NEC 952.04
        posterior cord syndrome
          952.04
      C_5–C_7 level 952.05
        with
          anterior cord syndrome
            952.07
          central cord syndrome
            952.08
          complete lesion of cord
            952.06
          incomplete lesion NEC
            952.09
          posterior cord syndrome
            952.09
        specified type NEC 952.09
      specified type NEC 952.04
    dorsal (D_1–D_6) (T_1–T_6) (thoracic)
      952.10
      with
        anterior cord syndrome
          952.12
        central cord syndrome
          952.13
        complete lesion of cord
          952.11
        incomplete lesion NEC
          952.14
        posterior cord syndrome
          952.14
    D_7–D_{12} level (T_7–T_{12}) 952.15
      with
        anterior cord syndrome
          952.17
        central cord syndrome
          952.18
        complete lesion of cord
          952.16
        incomplete lesion NEC
          952.19
        posterior cord syndrome
          952.19
      specified type NEC 952.19
    specified type NEC 952.14
    lumbar 952.2
    multiple sites 952.8
    nerve (root) NEC - see Injury, nerve,
      spinal, root
    plexus 953.9
      brachial 953.4
      lumbosacral 953.5
      multiple sites 953.8
    sacral 952.3
    thoracic (see also Injury, spinal,
      dorsal) 952.10
  spleen - see Injury, internal, spleen
  stellate ganglion 954.1
  sternal region 959.11
  stomach - see Injury, internal, stomach
  subconjunctival 921.1
  subcutaneous 959.9
  subdural - see Injury, intracranial
  submaxillary region 959.09
  submental region 959.09
  subungual
    fingers 959.5
    toes 959.7

◀ New   ◀▥ Revised   deleted Deleted   ● Use Additional Digit(s)   ▥ Omit code

Injury (Continued)
  superficial 919

Note: Use the following fourth-digit subdivisions with categories 910–919:

.0 abrasion or friction burn without mention of infection
.1 abrasion or friction burn, infected
.2 blister without mention of infection
.3 blister, infected
.4 insect bite, nonvenomous, without mention of infection
.5 insect bite, nonvenomous, infected
.6 superficial foreign body (splinter) without major open wound and without mention of infection
.7 superficial foreign body (splinter) without major open wound, infected
.8 other and unspecified superficial injury without mention of infection
.9 other and unspecified superficial injury, infected

For late effects of superficial injury, see category 906.2.

abdomen, abdominal (muscle) (wall) (and other part(s) of trunk) 911
ankle (and hip, knee, leg, or thigh) 916
anus (and other part(s) of trunk) 911
arm 913
  upper (and shoulder) 912
auditory canal (external) (meatus) (and other part(s) of face, neck, or scalp, except eye) 910
axilla (and upper arm) 912
back (and other part(s) of trunk) 911
breast (and other part(s) of trunk) 911
brow (and other part(s) of face, neck, or scalp, except eye) 910
buttock (and other part(s) of trunk) 911
canthus, eye 918.0
cheek(s) (and other part(s) of face, neck, or scalp, except eye) 910
chest wall (and other part(s) of trunk) 911
chin (and other part(s) of face, neck, or scalp, except eye) 910
clitoris (and other part(s) of trunk) 911
conjunctiva 918.2
cornea 918.1
  due to contact lens 371.82
costal region (and other part(s) of trunk) 911
ear(s) (auricle) (canal) (drum) (external) (and other part(s) of face, neck, or scalp, except eye) 910
elbow (and forearm) (and wrist) 913

Injury (Continued)
  superficial (Continued)
    epididymis (and other part(s) of trunk) 911
    epigastric region (and other part(s) of trunk) 911
    epiglottis (and other part(s) of face, neck, or scalp, except eye) 910
    eye(s) (and adnexa) NEC 918.9
    eyelid(s) (and periocular area) 918.0
    face (any part(s), except eye) (and neck or scalp) 910
    finger(s) (nail) (any) 915
    flank (and other part(s) of trunk) 911
    foot (phalanges) (and toe(s)) 917
    forearm (and elbow) (and wrist) 913
    forehead (and other part(s) of face, neck, or scalp, except eye) 910
    globe (eye) 918.9
    groin (and other part(s) of trunk) 911
    gum(s) (and other part(s) of face, neck, or scalp, except eye) 910
    hand(s) (except fingers alone) 914
    head (and other part(s) of face, neck, or scalp, except eye) 910
    heel (and foot or toe) 917
    hip (and ankle, knee, leg, or thigh) 916
    iliac region (and other part(s) of trunk) 911
    interscapular region (and other part(s) of trunk) 911
    iris 918.9
    knee (and ankle, hip, leg, or thigh) 916
    labium (majus) (minus) (and other part(s) of trunk) 911
    lacrimal (apparatus) (gland) (sac) 918.0
    leg (lower) (upper) (and ankle, hip, knee, or thigh) 916
    lip(s) (and other part(s) of face, neck, or scalp, except eye) 910
    lower extremity (except foot) 916
    lumbar region (and other part(s) of trunk) 911
    malar region (and other part(s) of face, neck, or scalp, except eye) 910
    mastoid region (and other part(s) of face, neck, or scalp, except eye) 910
    midthoracic region (and other part(s) of trunk) 911
    mouth (and other part(s) of face, neck, or scalp, except eye) 910
    multiple sites (not classifiable to the same three-digit category) 919
    nasal (septum) (and other part(s) of face, neck, or scalp, except eye) 910
    neck (and face or scalp, any part(s), except eye) 910
    nose (septum) (and other part(s) of face, neck, or scalp, except eye) 910
    occipital region (and other part(s) of face, neck, or scalp, except eye) 910
    orbital region 918.0
    palate (soft) (and other part(s) of face, neck, or scalp, except eye) 910

Injury (Continued)
  superficial (Continued)
    parietal region (and other part(s) of face, neck, or scalp, except eye) 910
    penis (and other part(s) of trunk) 911
    perineum (and other part(s) of trunk) 911
    periocular area 918.0
    pharynx (and other part(s) of face, neck, or scalp, except eye) 910
    popliteal space (and ankle, hip, leg, or thigh) 916
    prepuce (and other part(s) of trunk) 911
    pubic region (and other part(s) of trunk) 911
    pudenda (and other part(s) of trunk) 911
    sacral region (and other part(s) of trunk) 911
    salivary (ducts) (glands) (and other part(s) of face, neck, or scalp, except eye) 910
    scalp (and other part(s) of face or neck, except eye) 910
    scapular region (and upper arm) 912
    sclera 918.2
    scrotum (and other part(s) of trunk) 911
    shoulder (and upper arm) 912
    skin NEC 919
    specified site(s) NEC 919
    sternal region (and other part(s) of trunk) 911
    subconjunctival 918.2
    subcutaneous NEC 919
    submaxillary region (and other part(s) of face, neck, or scalp, except eye) 910
    submental region (and other part(s) of face, neck, or scalp, except eye) 910
    supraclavicular fossa (and other part(s) of face, neck, or scalp, except eye) 910
    supraorbital 918.0
    temple (and other part(s) of face, neck, or scalp, except eye) 910
    temporal region (and other part(s) of face, neck, or scalp, except eye) 910
    testis (and other part(s) of trunk) 911
    thigh (and ankle, hip, knee, or leg) 916
    thorax, thoracic (external) (and other part(s) of trunk) 911
    throat (and other part(s) of face, neck, or scalp, except eye) 910
    thumb(s) (nail) 915
    toe(s) (nail) (subungual) (and foot) 917
    tongue (and other part(s) of face, neck, or scalp, except eye) 910
    tooth, teeth (see also Abrasion, dental) 521.20
    trunk (any part(s)) 911
    tunica vaginalis (and other part(s) of trunk) 911
    tympanum, tympanic membrane (and other part(s) of face, neck, or scalp, except eye) 910
    upper extremity NEC 913

◀ New   ◀|||| Revised   ~~deleted~~ Deleted   ● Use Additional Digit(s)   ▨ Omit code

Insufficiency, insufficient *(Continued)*
  cerebral (vascular) 437.9
  cerebrovascular 437.9
    with transient focal neurological
      signs and symptoms 435.9
    acute 437.1
      with transient focal neurological
        signs and symptoms 435.9
  circulatory NEC 459.9
    fetus or newborn 779.89
  convergence 378.83
  coronary (acute or subacute) 411.89
    chronic or with a stated duration of
      over 8 weeks 414.8
  corticoadrenal 255.41
  dietary 269.9
  divergence 378.85
  food 994.2
  gastroesophageal 530.89
  gonadal
    ovary 256.39
    testis 257.2
  gonadotropic hormone secretion 253.4
  heart - *see also* Insufficiency, myocardial
    fetus or newborn 779.89
    valve (*see also* Endocarditis) 424.90
      congenital NEC 746.89
  hepatic 573.8
  idiopathic autonomic 333.0
  interocclusal distance of teeth (ridge)
    524.36
  kidney
    acute 593.9
    chronic 585.9
  labyrinth, labyrinthine (function)
    386.53
    bilateral 386.54
    unilateral 386.53
  lacrimal 375.15
  liver 573.8
  lung (acute) (*see also* Insufficiency,
    pulmonary) 518.82
    following trauma, surgery, or shock
      518.5
    newborn 770.89
  mental (congenital) (*see also*
    Retardation, mental) 319
  mesenteric 557.1
  mitral (valve) 424.0
    with
      aortic (valve) disease 396.3
        insufficiency, incompetence, or
          regurgitation 396.3
        stenosis or obstruction 396.2
      obstruction or stenosis 394.2
        with aortic valve disease 396.8
    congenital 746.6
    rheumatic 394.1
      with
        aortic (valve) disease 396.3
          insufficiency, incompetence,
            or regurgitation 396.3
          stenosis or obstruction 396.2
        obstruction or stenosis 394.2
          with aortic valve disease
            396.8
      active or acute 391.1
        with chorea, rheumatic
          (Sydenham's) 392.0
    specified cause, except rheumatic
      424.0
  muscle
    heart - *see* Insufficiency, myocardial
  ocular (*see also* Strabismus) 378.9

Insufficiency, insufficient *(Continued)*
  myocardial, myocardium (with
    arteriosclerosis) 428.0
    with rheumatic fever (conditions
      classifiable to 390)
      active, acute, or subacute 391.2
        with chorea 392.0
      inactive or quiescent (with
        chorea) 398.0
    congenital 746.89
    due to presence of (cardiac)
      prosthesis 429.4
    fetus or newborn 779.89
    following cardiac surgery 429.4
    hypertensive (*see also* Hypertension,
      heart) 402.91
      benign 402.11
      malignant 402.01
    postoperative 997.1
      long-term effect of cardiac
        surgery 429.4
    rheumatic 398.0
      active, acute, or subacute 391.2
        with chorea (Sydenham's)
          392.0
    syphilitic 093.82
  nourishment 994.2
  organic 799.89
  ovary 256.39
    postablative 256.2
  pancreatic 577.8
  parathyroid (gland) 252.1
  peripheral vascular (arterial) 443.9
  pituitary (anterior) 253.2
    posterior 253.5
  placental - *see* Placenta, insufficiency
  platelets 287.5
  prenatal care in current pregnancy
    V23.7
  progressive pluriglandular 258.9
  pseudocholinesterase 289.89
  pulmonary (acute) 518.82
    following
      shock 518.5
      surgery 518.5
      trauma 518.5
    newborn 770.89
    valve (*see also* Endocarditis,
      pulmonary) 424.3
      congenital 746.09
  pyloric 537.0
  renal 593.9
    acute 593.9
    chronic 585.9
    due to a procedure 997.5
  respiratory 786.09
    acute 518.82
      following shock, surgery, or
        trauma 518.5
    newborn 770.89
  rotation - *see* Malrotation
  suprarenal 255.41
    medulla 255.5
  tarso-orbital fascia, congenital 743.66
  tear film 375.15
  testis 257.2
  thyroid (gland) (acquired) - *see also*
    Hypothyroidism
    congenital 243
  tricuspid (*see also* Endocarditis,
    tricuspid) 397.0
    congenital 746.89
    syphilitic 093.23
  urethral sphincter 599.84

Insufficiency, insufficient *(Continued)*
  valve, valvular (heart) (*see also*
    Endocarditis) 424.90
  vascular 459.9
    intestine NEC 557.9
    mesenteric 557.1
    peripheral 443.9
    renal (*see also* Hypertension, kidney)
      403.90
  velopharyngeal
    acquired 528.9
    congenital 750.29
  venous (peripheral) 459.81
  ventricular - *see* Insufficiency,
    myocardial
  vertebral artery 435.1
  vertebrobasilar artery 435.3
  weight gain during pregnancy
    646.8●
  zinc 269.3
Insufflation
  fallopian
    fertility testing V26.21
    following sterilization reversal
      V26.22
  meconium 770.11
    with respiratory symptoms 770.12
Insular - *see* condition
Insulinoma (M8151/0)
  malignant (M8151/3)
    pancreas 157.4
    specified site - *see* Neoplasm, by site,
      malignant
    unspecified site 157.4
  pancreas 211.7
  specified site - *see* Neoplasm, by site,
    benign
  unspecified site 211.7
Insuloma - *see* Insulinoma
Insult
  brain 437.9
    acute 436
  cerebral 437.9
    acute 436
  cerebrovascular 437.9
    acute 436
  vascular NEC 437.9
    acute 436
Insurance examination (certification)
  V70.3
Intemperance (*see also* Alcoholism)
  303.9●
Interception of pregnancy (menstrual
  extraction) V25.3
Interference
  balancing side 524.56
  non-working side 524.56
Intermenstrual
  bleeding 626.6
    irregular 626.6
    regular 626.5
  hemorrhage 626.6
    irregular 626.6
    regular 626.5
  pain(s) 625.2
Intermittent - *see* condition
Internal - *see* condition
Interproximal wear 521.10
Interruption
  aortic arch 747.11
  bundle of His 426.50
  fallopian tube (for sterilization) V25.2
  phase-shift, sleep cycle 307.45
  repeated REM-sleep 307.48

Interruption (Continued)
  sleep
    due to perceived environmental
        disturbances 307.48
    phase-shift, of 24-hour sleep-wake
        cycle 307.45
    repeated REM-sleep type 307.48
  vas deferens (for sterilization) V25.2
Intersexuality 752.7
Interstitial - *see* condition
Intertrigo 695.89
  labialis 528.5
Intervertebral disc - *see* condition
Intestine, intestinal - *see also* condition
  flu 487.8
Intolerance
  carbohydrate NEC 579.8
  cardiovascular exercise, with pain (at
      rest) (with less than ordinary
      activity) (with ordinary activity)
      V47.2
  cold 780.99
  dissacharide (hereditary) 271.3
  drug
    correct substance properly
        administered 995.27
    wrong substance given or taken in
        error 977.9
      specified drug - *see* Table of
          Drugs and Chemicals
  effort 306.2
  fat NEC 579.8
  foods NEC 579.8
  fructose (hereditary) 271.2
  glucose (-galactose) (congenital) 271.3
  gluten 579.0
  lactose (hereditary) (infantile) 271.3
  lysine (congenital) 270.7
  milk NEC 579.8
  protein (familial) 270.7
  starch NEC 579.8
  sucrose (-isomaltose) (congenital) 271.3
Intoxicated NEC (*see also* Alcoholism)
    305.0●
Intoxication
  acid 276.2
  acute
    alcoholic 305.0●
      with alcoholism 303.0●
      hangover effects 305.0●
    caffeine 305.9●
    hallucinogenic (*see also* Abuse,
        drugs, nondependent) 305.3●
  alcohol (acute) 305.0●
    with alcoholism 303.0●
    hangover effects 305.0●
    idiosyncratic 291.4
    pathological 291.4
  alimentary canal 558.2
  ammonia (hepatic) 572.2
  caffeine 305.9●
  chemical - *see also* Table of Drugs and
      Chemicals
    via placenta or breast milk 760.70
      alcohol 760.71
      anticonvulsants 760.77
      antifungals 760.74
      anti-infective agents 760.74
      antimetabolics 760.78
      cocaine 760.75
      "crack" 760.75
      hallucinogenic agents NEC 760.73
      medicinal agents NEC 760.79
      narcotics 760.72

Intoxication (Continued)
  chemical (Continued)
    via placenta or breast milk
        (Continued)
      obstetric anesthetic or analgesic
          drug 763.5
      specified agent NEC 760.79
      suspected, affecting
          management of
          pregnancy 655.5●
  cocaine, through placenta or breast
      milk 760.75
  delirium
    alcohol 291.0
    drug 292.81
  drug 292.89
    with delirium 292.81
    correct substance properly
        administered (*see also* Allergy,
        drug) 995.27
    newborn 779.4
    obstetric anesthetic or sedation
        668.9●
      affecting fetus or newborn 763.5
    overdose or wrong substance given
        or taken - *see* Table of Drugs
        and Chemicals
    pathologic 292.2
    specific to newborn 779.4
    via placenta or breast milk 760.70
      alcohol 760.71
      anticonvulsants 760.77
      antifungals 760.74
      anti-infective agents 760.74
      antimetabolics 760.78
      cocaine 760.75
      "crack" 760.75
      hallucinogenic agents 760.73
      medicinal agents NEC 760.79
      narcotics 760.72
      obstetric anesthetic or analgesic
          drug 763.5
      specified agent NEC 760.79
      suspected, affecting
          management of
          pregnancy 655.5●
  enteric - *see* Intoxication, intestinal
  fetus or newborn, via placenta or breast
      milk 760.70
    alcohol 760.71
    anticonvulsants 760.77
    antifungals 760.74
    anti-infective agents 760.74
    antimetabolics 760.78
    cocaine 760.75
    "crack" 760.75
    hallucinogenic agents 760.73
    medicinal agents NEC 760.79
    narcotics 760.72
    obstetric anesthetic or analgesic
        drug 763.5
    specified agent NEC 760.79
    suspected, affecting management of
        pregnancy 655.5●
  food - *see* Poisoning, food
  gastrointestinal 558.2
  hallucinogenic (acute) 305.3●
  hepatocerebral 572.2
  idiosyncratic alcohol 291.4
  intestinal 569.89
    due to putrefaction of food 005.9
  methyl alcohol (*see also* Alcoholism)
      305.0●
    with alcoholism 303.0●

Intoxication (Continued)
  non-foodborne due to toxins of
      Clostridium botulinum
      [C. botulinum] - *see* Botulism
  pathologic 291.4
    drug 292.2
  potassium (K) 276.7
  septic
    with
      abortion - *see* Abortion, by type,
          with sepsis
      ectopic pregnancy (*see also*
          categories 633.0–633.9) 639.0
      molar pregnancy (*see also*
          categories 630–632) 639.0
    during labor 659.3●
    following
      abortion 639.0
      ectopic or molar pregnancy 639.0
    generalized - *see* Septicemia
    puerperal, postpartum,
        childbirth 670.2●
  serum (prophylactic) (therapeutic) 999.5
  uremic - *see* Uremia
  water 276.69 ◄▦
Intracranial - *see* condition
Intrahepatic gallbladder 751.69
Intraligamentous - *see also* condition
  pregnancy - *see* Pregnancy, cornual
Intraocular - *see also* condition
  sepsis 360.00
Intrathoracic - *see also* condition
  kidney 753.3
  stomach - *see* Hernia, diaphragm
Intrauterine contraceptive device
  checking V25.42
  insertion V25.11 ◄▦
  in situ V45.51
  management V25.42
  prescription V25.02
    repeat V25.42
  reinsertion V25.13 ◄▦
    and reinsertion V25.13 ◄
  removal V25.12 ◄▦
  replacement V25.13 ◄
Intraventricular - *see* condition
Intrinsic deformity - *see* Deformity
Intruded tooth 524.34
Intrusion, repetitive, of sleep (due to
    environmental disturbances) (with
    atypical polysomnographic features)
    307.48
Intumescent, lens (eye) NEC 366.9
  senile 366.12
Intussusception (colon) (enteric)
    (intestine) (rectum) 560.0
  appendix 543.9
  congenital 751.5
  fallopian tube 620.8
  ileocecal 560.0
  ileocolic 560.0
  ureter (obstruction) 593.4
Invagination
  basilar 756.0
  colon or intestine 560.0
Invalid (since birth) 799.89
Invalidism (chronic) 799.89
Inversion
  albumin-globulin (A-G) ratio 273.8
  bladder 596.8
  cecum (*see also* Intussusception) 560.0
  cervix 622.8
  nipple 611.79
    congenital 757.6
    puerperal, postpartum 676.3●

Inversion *(Continued)*
  optic papilla 743.57
  organ or site, congenital NEC - *see*
      Anomaly, specified type NEC
  sleep rhythm 327.39
    nonorganic origin 307.45
  testis (congenital) 752.51
  uterus (postinfectional) (postpartal,
      old) 621.7
    chronic 621.7
      complicating delivery 665.2●
        affecting fetus or newborn 763.89
  vagina - *see* Prolapse, vagina
Investigation
  allergens V72.7
  clinical research (control) (normal
      comparison) (participant) V70.7
Inviability - *see* Immaturity
Involuntary movement, abnormal 781.0
Involution, involutional - *see also*
      condition
  breast, cystic or fibrocystic 610.1
  depression *(see also* Psychosis, affective)
      296.2●
    recurrent episode 296.3●
    single episode 296.2●
  melancholia *(see also* Psychosis,
      affective) 296.2●
    recurrent episode 296.3●
    single episode 296.2●
  ovary, senile 620.3
  paranoid state (reaction) 297.2
  paraphrenia (climacteric) (menopause)
      297.2
  psychosis 298.8
  thymus failure 254.8
IQ
  under 20 318.2
  20–34 318.1
  35–49 318.0
  50–70 317
IRDS 769
Irideremia 743.45
Iridis rubeosis 364.42
  diabetic 250.5● *[364.42]*
    due to secondary diabetes 249.5●
        [364.42]
Iridochoroiditis (panuveitis) 360.12
Iridocyclitis NEC 364.3
  acute 364.00
    primary 364.01
    recurrent 364.02
  chronic 364.10
    in
        lepromatous leprosy 030.0
            [364.11]
        sarcoidosis 135 *[364.11]*
        tuberculosis *(see also* Tuberculosis)
            017.3● *[364.11]*
  due to allergy 364.04
  endogenous 364.01
  gonococcal 098.41
  granulomatous 364.10
  herpetic (simplex) 054.44
    zoster 053.22
  hypopyon 364.05
  lens induced 364.23
  nongranulomatous 364.00
  primary 364.01
  recurrent 364.02
  rheumatic 364.10
  secondary 364.04
    infectious 364.03
    noninfectious 364.04

Iridocyclitis NEC *(Continued)*
  subacute 364.00
    primary 364.01
    recurrent 364.02
  sympathetic 360.11
  syphilitic (secondary) 091.52
  tuberculous (chronic) *(see also*
      Tuberculosis) 017.3● *[364.11]*
Iridocyclochoroiditis (panuveitis)
      360.12
Iridodialysis 364.76
Iridodonesis 364.89
Iridoplegia (complete) (partial) (reflex)
      379.49
Iridoschisis 364.52
Iris - *see* condition
Iritis 364.3
  acute 364.00
    primary 364.01
    recurrent 364.02
  chronic 364.10
    in
        sarcoidosis 135 *[364.11]*
        tuberculosis *(see also*
            Tuberculosis) 017.3●
            [364.11]
  diabetic 250.5● *[364.42]*
    due to secondary diabetes 249.5●
        [364.42]
  due to
    allergy 364.04
    herpes simplex 054.44
    leprosy 030.0 *[364.11]*
  endogenous 364.01
  gonococcal 098.41
  gouty 274.89 *[364.11]*
  granulomatous 364.10
  hypopyon 364.05
  lens induced 364.23
  nongranulomatous 364.00
  papulosa 095.8 *[364.11]*
  primary 364.01
  recurrent 364.02
  rheumatic 364.10
  secondary 364.04
    infectious 364.03
    noninfectious 364.04
  subacute 364.00
    primary 364.01
    recurrent 364.02
  sympathetic 360.11
  syphilitic (secondary) 091.52
    congenital 090.0 *[364.11]*
    late 095.8 *[364.11]*
  tuberculous *(see also* Tuberculosis)
      017.3● *[364.11]*
  uratic 274.89 *[364.11]*
Iron
  deficiency anemia 280.9
  metabolism disease 275.09 ◀▥
  storage disease 275.09 ◀▥
Iron-miners' lung 503
Irradiated enamel (tooth, teeth) 521.89
Irradiation
  burn - *see* Burn, by site
  effects, adverse 990
Irreducible, irreducibility - *see*
      condition
Irregular, irregularity
  action, heart 427.9
  alveolar process 525.8
  bleeding NEC 626.4
  breathing 786.09
  colon 569.89

Irregular, irregularity *(Continued)*
  contour
    of cornea 743.41
      acquired 371.70
    reconstructed breast 612.0
  dentin in pulp 522.3
  eye movements NEC 379.59
  menstruation (cause unknown) 626.4
  periods 626.4
  prostate 602.9
  pupil 364.75
  respiratory 786.09
  septum (nasal) 470
  shape, organ or site, congenital NEC -
      see Distortion
  sleep-wake rhythm (non-24-hour)
      327.39
    nonorganic origin 307.45
  vertebra 733.99
Irritability 799.22
  bladder 596.8
    neurogenic 596.54
      with cauda equina syndrome
          344.61
  bowel (syndrome) 564.1
  bronchial *(see also* Bronchitis) 490
  cerebral, newborn 779.1
  colon 564.1
    psychogenic 306.4
  duodenum 564.89
  heart (psychogenic) 306.2
  ileum 564.89
  jejunum 564.89
  myocardium 306.2
  nervousness 799.21
  rectum 564.89
  stomach 536.9
    psychogenic 306.4
  sympathetic (nervous system) *(see also*
      Neuropathy, peripheral,
      autonomic) 337.9
  urethra 599.84
  ventricular (heart) (psychogenic) 306.2
Irritable *(see also* Irritability) 799.22
Irritation
  anus 569.49
  axillary nerve 353.0
  bladder 596.8
  brachial plexus 353.0
  brain (traumatic) *(see also* Injury,
      intracranial) 854.0●
    nontraumatic - *see* Encephalitis
  bronchial *(see also* Bronchitis) 490
  cerebral (traumatic) *(see also* Injury,
      intracranial) 854.0●
    nontraumatic - *see* Encephalitis
  cervical plexus 353.2
  cervix *(see also* Cervicitis) 616.0
  choroid, sympathetic 360.11
  cranial nerve - *see* Disorder, nerve,
      cranial
  digestive tract 536.9
    psychogenic 306.4
  gastric 536.9
    psychogenic 306.4
  gastrointestinal (tract) 536.9
    functional 536.9
    psychogenic 306.4
  globe, sympathetic 360.11
  intestinal (bowel) 564.9
  labyrinth 386.50
  lumbosacral plexus 353.1
  meninges (traumatic) *(see also* Injury,
      intracranial) 854.0●
    nontraumatic - *see* Meningitis

Irritation *(Continued)*
 myocardium 306.2
 nerve - *see* Disorder, nerve
 nervous 799.21
 nose 478.19
 penis 607.89
 perineum 709.9
 peripheral
  autonomic nervous system *(see also*
   Neuropathy, peripheral,
   autonomic)* 337.9
  nerve - *see* Disorder, nerve
 peritoneum *(see also* Peritonitis) 567.9
 pharynx 478.29
 plantar nerve 355.6
 spinal (cord) (traumatic) - *see also*
  Injury, spinal, by site
  nerve - *see also* Disorder, nerve
   root NEC 724.9
   traumatic - *see* Injury, nerve,
    spinal
  nontraumatic - *see* Myelitis
 stomach 536.9
  psychogenic 306.4
 sympathetic nerve NEC *(see also*
  Neuropathy, peripheral,
  autonomic)* 337.9
 ulnar nerve 354.2
 vagina 623.9
Isambert's disease 012.3●
Ischemia, ischemic 459.9
 basilar artery (with transient
  neurologic deficit) 435.0
 bone NEC 733.40
 bowel (transient) 557.9
  acute 557.0
  chronic 557.1
  due to mesenteric artery
   insufficiency 557.1
 brain - *see also* Ischemia, cerebral
  recurrent focal 435.9
 cardiac *(see also* Ischemia, heart) 414.9
 cardiomyopathy 414.8
 carotid artery (with transient
  neurologic deficit) 435.8
 cerebral (chronic) (generalized) 437.1
  arteriosclerotic 437.0
  intermittent (with transient
   neurologic deficit) 435.9
  newborn 779.2
  puerperal, postpartum, childbirth
   674.0●
  recurrent focal (with transient
   neurologic deficit) 435.9
  transient (with transient neurologic
   deficit) 435.9
 colon 557.9
  acute 557.0
  chronic 557.1
  due to mesenteric artery
   insufficiency 557.1
 coronary (chronic) *(see also* Ischemia,
  heart) 414.9
 demand 411.89 ◀

Ischemia, ischemic *(Continued)*
 heart (chronic or with a stated duration
  of over 8 weeks) 414.9
  acute or with a stated duration
   of 8 weeks or less *(see also*
   Infarct, myocardium)
   410.9●
   without myocardial infarction
    411.89
    with coronary (artery)
     occlusion 411.81
  subacute 411.89
 intestine (transient) 557.9
  acute 557.0
  chronic 557.1
  due to mesenteric artery
   insufficiency 557.1
 kidney 593.81
 labyrinth 386.50
 muscles, leg 728.89
 myocardium, myocardial (chronic or
  with a stated duration of over 8
  weeks) 414.8
  acute *(see also* Infarct, myocardium)
   410.9●
   without myocardial infarction
    411.89
    with coronary (artery)
     occlusion 411.81
 renal 593.81
 retina, retinal 362.84
 small bowel 557.9
  acute 557.0
  chronic 557.1
  due to mesenteric artery
   insufficiency 557.1
 spinal cord 336.1
 subendocardial *(see also* Insufficiency,
  coronary) 411.89
 supply *(see also* Angina) 414.9 ◀
 vertebral artery (with transient
  neurologic deficit) 435.1
Ischialgia *(see also* Sciatica) 724.3
Ischiopagus 759.4
Ischium, ischial - *see* condition
Ischomenia 626.8
Ischuria 788.5
Iselin's disease or osteochondrosis
 732.5
Islands of
 parotid tissue in
  lymph nodes 750.26
  neck structures 750.26
 submaxillary glands in
  fascia 750.26
  lymph nodes 750.26
  neck muscles 750.26
Islet cell tumor, pancreas (M8150/0) 211.7
Isoimmunization NEC *(see also*
 Incompatibility) 656.2●
 anti-E 656.2●
 fetus or newborn 773.2
  ABO blood groups 773.1
  Rhesus (Rh) factor 773.0

Isolation V07.0
 social V62.4
Isosporosis 007.2
Issue
 medical certificate NEC V68.09
  cause of death V68.09
  disability examination V68.01
  fitness V68.09
  incapacity V68.09
 repeat prescription NEC V68.1
  appliance V68.1
  contraceptive V25.40
   device NEC V25.49
    intrauterine V25.42
    specified type NEC V25.49
   pill V25.41
  glasses V68.1
  medicinal substance V68.1
Itch *(see also* Pruritus) 698.9
 bakers' 692.89
 barbers' 110.0
 bricklayers' 692.89
 cheese 133.8
 clam diggers' 120.3
 coolie 126.9
 copra 133.8
 Cuban 050.1
 dew 126.9
 dhobie 110.3
 eye 379.99
 filarial *(see also* Infestation, filarial)
  125.9
 grain 133.8
 grocers' 133.8
 ground 126.9
 harvest 133.8
 jock 110.3
 Malabar 110.9
  beard 110.0
  foot 110.4
  scalp 110.0
 meaning scabies 133.0
 Norwegian 133.0
 perianal 698.0
 poultrymen's 133.8
 sarcoptic 133.0
 scrub 134.1
 seven year V61.10
  meaning scabies 133.0
 straw 133.8
 swimmers' 120.3
 washerwoman's 692.4
 water 120.3
 winter 698.8
Itsenko-Cushing syndrome (pituitary
 basophilism) 255.0
Ivemark's syndrome (asplenia with
 congenital heart disease) 759.0
Ivory bones 756.52
Ixodes 134.8
Ixodiasis 134.8

J

Jaccoud's nodular fibrositis, chronic (Jaccoud's syndrome) 714.4
Jackson's
　membrane 751.4
　paralysis or syndrome 344.89
　veil 751.4
Jacksonian
　epilepsy (*see also* Epilepsy) 345.5●
　seizures (focal) (*see also* Epilepsy) 345.5●
Jacob's ulcer (M8090/3) - *see* Neoplasm, skin, malignant, by site
Jacquet's dermatitis (diaper dermatitis) 691.0
Jadassohn's
　blue nevus (M8780/0) - *see* Neoplasm, skin, benign
　disease (maculopapular erythroderma) 696.2
　intraepidermal epithelioma (M8096/0) - *see* Neoplasm, skin, benign
Jadassohn-Lewandowski syndrome (pachyonychia congenita) 757.5
Jadassohn-Pellizari's disease (anetoderma) 701.3
Jadassohn-Tièche nevus (M8780/0) - *see* Neoplasm, skin, benign
Jaffe-Lichtenstein (-Uehlinger) syndrome 252.01
Jahnke's syndrome (encephalocutaneous angiomatosis) 759.6
Jakob-Creutzfeldt disease (CJD) (syndrome) 046.19
　with dementia
　　with behavioral disturba nce 046.19 [294.11]
　　without behavioral disturbance 046.19 [294.10]
　familial 046.19
　iatrogenic 046.19
　specified NEC 046.19
　sporadic 046.19
　variant (vCJD) 046.11
　　with dementia
　　　with behavioral disturbance 046.11 [294.11]
　　　without behavioral disturbance 046.11 [294.10]
Jaksch (-Luzet) disease or syndrome (pseudoleukemia infantum) 285.8
Jamaican
　neuropathy 349.82
　paraplegic tropical ataxic-spastic syndrome 349.82
Janet's disease (psychasthenia) 300.89
Janiceps 759.4
Jansky-Bielschowsky amaurotic familial idiocy 330.1
Japanese
　B-type encephalitis 062.0
　river fever 081.2
　seven-day fever 100.89
Jaundice (yellow) 782.4
　acholuric (familial) (splenomegalic) (*see also* Spherocytosis) 282.0
　　acquired 283.9
　breast milk 774.39
　catarrhal (acute) 070.1
　　with hepatic coma 070.0
　　chronic 571.9
　　epidemic - *see* Jaundice, epidemic
　cholestatic (benign) 782.4
　chronic idiopathic 277.4

Jaundice (*Continued*)
　epidemic (catarrhal) 070.1
　　with hepatic coma 070.0
　　leptospiral 100.0
　　spirochetal 100.0
　febrile (acute) 070.1
　　with hepatic coma 070.0
　　leptospiral 100.0
　　spirochetal 100.0
　fetus or newborn 774.6
　　due to or associated with
　　　ABO
　　　　antibodies 773.1
　　　　incompatibility, maternal/fetal 773.1
　　　　isoimmunization 773.1
　　　absence or deficiency of enzyme system for bilirubin conjugation (congenital) 774.39
　　　blood group incompatibility NEC 773.2
　　　breast milk inhibitors to conjugation 774.39
　　　　associated with preterm delivery 774.2
　　　bruising 774.1
　　　Crigler-Najjar syndrome 277.4 [774.31]
　　　delayed conjugation 774.30
　　　　associated with preterm delivery 774.2
　　　　development 774.39
　　　drugs or toxins transmitted from mother 774.1
　　　G-6-PD deficiency 282.2 [774.0]
　　　galactosemia 271.1 [774.5]
　　　Gilbert's syndrome 277.4 [774.31]
　　　hepatocellular damage 774.4
　　　hereditary hemolytic anemia (*see also* Anemia, hemolytic) 282.9 [774.0]
　　　hypothyroidism, congenital 243 [774.31]
　　　incompatibility, maternal/fetal NEC 773.2
　　　infection 774.1
　　　inspissated bile syndrome 774.4
　　　isoimmunization NEC 773.2
　　　mucoviscidosis 277.01 [774.5]
　　　obliteration of bile duct, congenital 751.61 [774.5]
　　　polycythemia 774.1
　　　preterm delivery 774.2
　　　red cell defect 282.9 [774.0]
　　　Rh
　　　　antibodies 773.0
　　　　incompatibility, maternal/fetal 773.0
　　　　isoimmunization 773.0
　　　spherocytosis (congenital) 282.0 [774.0]
　　　swallowed maternal blood 774.1
　　physiological NEC 774.6
　from injection, inoculation, infusion, or transfusion (blood) (plasma) (serum) (other substance) (onset within 8 months after administration) - *see* Hepatitis, viral
　Gilbert's (familial nonhemolytic) 277.4
　hematogenous 283.9
　hemolytic (acquired) 283.9
　　congenital (*see also* Spherocytosis) 282.0

Jaundice (*Continued*)
　hemorrhagic (acute) 100.0
　　leptospiral 100.0
　　newborn 776.0
　　spirochetal 100.0
　hepatocellular 573.8
　homologous (serum) - *see* Hepatitis, viral
　idiopathic, chronic 277.4
　infectious (acute) (subacute) 070.1
　　with hepatic coma 070.0
　　leptospiral 100.0
　　spirochetal 100.0
　leptospiral 100.0
　malignant (*see also* Necrosis, liver) 570
　newborn (physiological) (*see also* Jaundice, fetus or newborn) 774.6
　nonhemolytic, congenital familial (Gilbert's) 277.4
　nuclear, newborn (*see also* Kernicterus of newborn) 774.7
　obstructive NEC (*see also* Obstruction, biliary) 576.8
　postimmunization - *see* Hepatitis, viral
　posttransfusion - *see* Hepatitis, viral
　regurgitation (*see also* Obstruction, biliary) 576.8
　serum (homologous) (prophylactic) (therapeutic) - *see* Hepatitis, viral
　spirochetal (hemorrhagic) 100.0
　symptomatic 782.4
　　newborn 774.6
Jaw - *see* condition
Jaw-blinking 374.43
　congenital 742.8
Jaw-winking phenomenon or syndrome 742.8
Jealousy
　alcoholic 291.5
　childhood 313.3
　sibling 313.3
Jejunitis (*see also* Enteritis) 558.9
Jejunostomy status V44.4
Jejunum, jejunal - *see* condition
Jensen's disease 363.05
Jericho boil 085.1
Jerks, myoclonic 333.2
Jervell-Lange-Nielsen syndrome 426.82
Jeune's disease or syndrome (asphyxiating thoracic dystrophy) 756.4
Jigger disease 134.1
Job's syndrome (chronic granulomatous disease) 288.1
Jod-Basedow phenomenon 242.8●
Johnson-Stevens disease (erythema multiforme exudativum) 695.13
Joint - *see also* condition
　Charcôt's 094.0 [713.5]
　false 733.82
　flail - *see* Flail, joint
　mice - *see* Loose, body, joint, by site
　sinus to bone 730.9●
　von Gies' 095.8
Jordan's anomaly or syndrome 288.2
Josephs-Diamond-Blackfan anemia (congenital hypoplastic) 284.01
Joubert syndrome 759.89
Jumpers' knee 727.2
Jungle yellow fever 060.0
Jungling's disease (sarcoidosis) 135
Junin virus hemorrhagic fever 078.7
Juvenile - *see also* condition
　delinquent 312.9
　　group (*see also* Disturbance, conduct) 312.2●
　neurotic 312.4

K

Kabuki syndrome 759.89
Kahler (-Bozzolo) disease (multiple
    myeloma) (M9730/3) 203.0●
Kakergasia 300.9
Kakke 265.0
Kala-azar (Indian) (infantile)
    (Mediterranean) (Sudanese) 085.0
Kalischer's syndrome
    (encephalocutaneous angiomatosis)
    759.6
Kallmann's syndrome (hypogonadotropic
    hypogonadism with anosmia)
    253.4
Kanner's syndrome (autism) (see also
    Psychosis, childhood) 299.0●
Kaolinosis 502
Kaposi's
    disease 757.33
        lichen ruber 696.4
            acuminatus 696.4
            moniliformis 697.8
        xeroderma pigmentosum 757.33
    sarcoma (M9140/3) 176.9
        adipose tissue 176.1
        aponeurosis 176.1
        artery 176.1
        associated herpesvirus infection
            058.89
        blood vessel 176.1
        bursa 176.1
        connective tissue 176.1
        external genitalia 176.8
        fascia 176.1
        fatty tissue 176.1
        fibrous tissue 176.1
        gastrointestinal tract NEC 176.3
        ligament 176.1
        lung 176.4
        lymph
            gland(s) 176.5
            node(s) 176.5
        lymphatic(s) NEC 176.1
        muscle (skeletal) 176.1
        oral cavity NEC 176.8
        palate 176.2
        scrotum 176.8
        skin 176.0
        soft tissue 176.1
        specified site NEC 176.8
        subcutaneous tissue 176.1
        synovia 176.1
        tendon (sheath) 176.1
        vein 176.1
        vessel 176.1
        viscera NEC 176.9
        vulva 176.8
    varicelliform eruption 054.0
    vaccinia 999.0
Kartagener's syndrome or triad (sinusitis,
    bronchiectasis, situs inversus) 759.3
Kasabach-Merritt syndrome (capillary
    hemangioma associated with
    thrombocytopenic purpura) 287.39
Kaschin-Beck disease (endemic
    polyarthritis) - see Disease, Kaschin-
    Beck
Kast's syndrome (dyschondroplasia with
    hemangiomas) 756.4
Katatonia- see Catatonia
Katayama disease or fever 120.2
Kathisophobia 781.0
Kawasaki disease 446.1

Kayser-Fleischer ring (cornea)
    (pseudosclerosis) 275.1 [371.14]
Kaznelson's syndrome (congenital
    hypoplastic anemia) 284.01
Kearns-Sayre syndrome 277.87
Kedani fever 081.2
Kelis 701.4
Kelly (-Patterson) syndrome (sideropenic
    dysphagia) 280.8
Keloid, cheloid 701.4
    Addison's (morphea) 701.0
    cornea 371.00
    Hawkins' 701.4
    scar 701.4
Keloma 701.4
Kenya fever 082.1
Keratectasia 371.71
    congenital 743.41
Keratinization NEC
    alveolar ridge mucosa
        excessive 528.72
        minimal 528.71
Keratitis (nodular) (nonulcerative)
    (simple) (zonular) NEC 370.9
    with ulceration (see also Ulcer, cornea)
        370.00
    actinic 370.24
    arborescens 054.42
    areolar 370.22
    bullosa 370.8
    deep - see Keratitis, interstitial
    dendritic(a) 054.42
    desiccation 370.34
    diffuse interstitial 370.52
    disciform(is) 054.43
        varicella 052.7 [370.44]
    epithelialis vernalis 372.13 [370.32]
    exposure 370.34
    filamentary 370.23
    gonococcal (congenital) (prenatal)
        098.43
    herpes, herpetic (simplex) NEC 054.43
        zoster 053.21
    hypopyon 370.04
    in
        chickenpox 052.7 [370.44]
        exanthema (see also Exanthem) 057.9
            [370.44]
        paravaccinia (see also Paravaccinia)
            051.9 [370.44]
        smallpox (see also Smallpox) 050.9
            [370.44]
        vernal conjunctivitis 372.13 [370.32]
    interstitial (nonsyphilitic) 370.50
        with ulcer (see also Ulcer, cornea)
            370.00
        diffuse 370.52
        herpes, herpetic (simplex) 054.43
            zoster 053.21
        syphilitic (congenital) (hereditary)
            090.3
        tuberculous (see also Tuberculosis)
            017.3● [370.59]
    lagophthalmic 370.34
    macular 370.22
    neuroparalytic 370.35
    neurotrophic 370.35
    nummular 370.22
    oyster-shuckers' 370.8
    parenchymatous - see Keratitis,
        interstitial
    petrificans 370.8
    phlyctenular 370.31
    postmeasles 055.71

Keratitis (Continued)
    punctata, punctate 370.21
        leprosa 030.0 [370.21]
        profunda 090.3
        superficial (Thygeson's) 370.21
    purulent 370.8
    pustuliformis profunda 090.3
    rosacea 695.3 [370.49]
    sclerosing 370.54
    specified type NEC 370.8
    stellate 370.22
    striate 370.22
    superficial 370.20
        with conjunctivitis (see also
            Keratoconjunctivitis) 370.40
        punctate (Thygeson's) 370.21
    suppurative 370.8
    syphilitic (congenital) (prenatal)
        090.3
    trachomatous 076.1
        late effect 139.1
    tuberculous (phlyctenular) (see also
        Tuberculosis) 017.3● [370.31]
    ulcerated (see also Ulcer, cornea)
        370.00
    vesicular 370.8
    welders' 370.24
    xerotic (see also Keratomalacia)
        371.45
        vitamin A deficiency 264.4
Keratoacanthoma 238.2
Keratocele 371.72
Keratoconjunctivitis (see also Keratitis)
    370.40
    adenovirus type 8 077.1
    epidemic 077.1
    exposure 370.34
    gonococcal 098.43
    herpetic (simplex) 054.43
        zoster 053.21
    in
        chickenpox 052.7 [370.44]
        exanthema (see also Exanthem)
            057.9 [370.44]
        paravaccinia (see also Paravaccinia)
            051.9 [370.44]
        smallpox (see also Smallpox) 050.9
            [370.44]
    infectious 077.1
    neurotrophic 370.35
    phlyctenular 370.31
    postmeasles 055.71
    shipyard 077.1
    sicca (Sjögren's syndrome) 710.2
        not in Sjögren's syndrome 370.33
    specified type NEC 370.49
    tuberculous (phlyctenular) (see also
        Tuberculosis) 017.3● [370.31]
Keratoconus 371.60
    acute hydrops 371.62
    congenital 743.41
    stable 371.61
Keratocyst (dental) 526.0
Keratoderma, keratodermia (congenital)
    (palmaris et plantaris) (symmetrical)
    757.39
    acquired 701.1
    blennorrhagica 701.1
        gonococcal 098.81
    climacterium 701.1
    eccentrica 757.39
    gonorrheal 098.81
    punctata 701.1
    tylodes, progressive 701.1

◀ New   ◀▌ Revised   ~~deleted~~ Deleted   ● Use Additional Digit(s)   ▒ Omit code

Keratodermatocele 371.72
Keratoglobus 371.70
  congenital 743.41
    associated with buphthalmos 743.22
Keratohemia 371.12
Keratoiritis (*see also* Iridocyclitis) 364.3
  syphilitic 090.3
  tuberculous (*see also* Tuberculosis) 017.3● [364.11]
Keratolysis exfoliativa (congenital) 757.39
  acquired 695.89
  neonatorum 757.39
Keratoma 701.1
  congenital 757.39
  malignum congenitale 757.1
  palmaris et plantaris hereditarium 757.39
  senile 702.0
Keratomalacia 371.45
  vitamin A deficiency 264.4
Keratomegaly 743.41
Keratomycosis 111.1
  nigricans (palmaris) 111.1
Keratopathy 371.40
  band (*see also* Keratitis) 371.43
  bullous (*see also* Keratitis) 371.23
  degenerative (*see also* Degeneration, cornea) 371.40
    hereditary (*see also* Dystrophy, cornea) 371.50
  discrete colliquative 371.49
Keratoscleritis, tuberculous (*see also* Tuberculosis) 017.3● [370.31]
Keratosis 701.1
  actinic 702.0
  arsenical 692.4
  blennorrhagica 701.1
    gonococcal 098.81
  congenital (any type) 757.39
  ear (middle) (*see also* Cholesteatoma) 385.30
  female genital (external) 629.89
  follicular, vitamin A deficiency 264.8
  follicularis 757.39
    acquired 701.1
    congenital (acneiformis) (Siemens') 757.39
    spinulosa (decalvans) 757.39
    vitamin A deficiency 264.8
  gonococcal 098.81
  larynx, laryngeal 478.79
  male genital (external) 608.89
  middle ear (*see also* Cholesteatoma) 385.30
  nigricans 701.2
    congenital 757.39
  obturans 380.21
  oral epithelium
    residual ridge mucosa
      excessive 528.72
      minimal 528.71
  palmaris et plantaris (symmetrical) 757.39
  penile 607.89
  pharyngeus 478.29
  pilaris 757.39
    acquired 701.1
  punctata (palmaris et plantaris) 701.1
  scrotal 608.89
  seborrheic 702.19
    inflamed 702.11
  senilis 702.0
  solar 702.0

Keratosis (*Continued*)
  suprafollicularis 757.39
  tonsillaris 478.29
  vagina 623.1
  vegetans 757.39
  vitamin A deficiency 264.8
Kerato-uveitis (*see also* Iridocyclitis) 364.3
Keraunoparalysis 994.0
Kerion (celsi) 110.0
Kernicterus of newborn (not due to isoimmunization) 774.7
  due to isoimmunization (conditions classifiable to 773.0–773.2) 773.4
Ketoacidosis 276.2
  diabetic 250.1●
    due to secondary diabetes 249.1●
Ketonuria 791.6
  branched-chain, intermittent 270.3
Ketosis 276.2
  diabetic 250.1●
    due to secondary diabetes 249.1●
Kidney - *see* condition
Kienböck's
  disease 732.3
    adult 732.8
  osteochondrosis 732.3
Kimmelstiel (-Wilson) disease or syndrome (intercapillary glomerulosclerosis) 250.4● [581.81]
  due to secondary diabetes 249.4● [581.81]
Kink, kinking
  appendix 543.9
  artery 447.1
  cystic duct, congenital 751.61
  hair (acquired) 704.2
  ileum or intestine (*see also* Obstruction, intestine) 560.9
  Lane's (*see also* Obstruction, intestine) 560.9
  organ or site, congenital NEC - *see* Anomaly, specified type NEC, by site
  ureter (pelvic junction) 593.3
    congenital 753.20
  vein(s) 459.2
    caval 459.2
    peripheral 459.2
Kinnier Wilson's disease (hepatolenticular degeneration) 275.1
Kissing
  osteophytes 721.5
  spine 721.5
  vertebra 721.5
Klauder's syndrome (erythema multiforme exudativum) 695.19
Klebs' disease (*see also* Nephritis) 583.9
Klein-Waardenburg syndrome (ptosis-epicanthus) 270.2
Kleine-Levin syndrome 327.13
Kleptomania 312.32
Klinefelter's syndrome 758.7
Klinger's disease 446.4
Klippel's disease 723.8
Klippel-Feil disease or syndrome (brevicollis) 756.16
Klippel-Trenaunay syndrome 759.89
Klumpke (-Déjérine) palsy, paralysis (birth) (newborn) 767.6
Klüver-Bucy (-Terzian) syndrome 310.0
Knee - *see* condition

Knifegrinders' rot (*see also* Tuberculosis) 011.4●
Knock-knee (acquired) 736.41
  congenital 755.64
Knot
  intestinal, syndrome (volvulus) 560.2
  umbilical cord (true) 663.2●
    affecting fetus or newborn 762.5
Knots, surfer 919.8
  infected 919.9
Knotting (of)
  hair 704.2
  intestine 560.2
Knuckle pads (Garrod's) 728.79
Köbner's disease (epidermolysis bullosa) 757.39
Koch's
  infection (*see also* Tuberculosis, pulmonary) 011.9●
  relapsing fever 087.9
Koch-Weeks conjunctivitis 372.03
Koenig-Wichman disease (pemphigus) 694.4
Köhler's disease (osteochondrosis) 732.5
  first (osteochondrosis juvenilis) 732.5
  second (Freiburg's infarction, metatarsal head) 732.5
  patellar 732.4
  tarsal navicular (bone) (osteoarthrosis juvenilis) 732.5
Köhler-Mouchet disease (osteoarthrosis juvenilis) 732.5
Köhler-Pellegrini-Stieda disease or syndrome (calcification, knee joint) 726.62
Koilonychia 703.8
  congenital 757.5
Kojevnikov's, Kojewnikoff's epilepsy (*see also* Epilepsy) 345.7●
König's
  disease (osteochondritis dissecans) 732.7
  syndrome 564.89
Koniophthisis (*see also* Tuberculosis) 011.4●
Koplik's spots 055.9
Kopp's asthma 254.8
Korean hemorrhagic fever 078.6
Korsakoff (-Wernicke) disease, psychosis, or syndrome (nonalcoholic) 294.0
  alcoholic 291.1
Korsakov's disease - *see* Korsakoff's disease
Korsakow's disease - *see* Korsakoff's disease
Kostmann's disease or syndrome (infantile genetic agranulocytosis) 288.01
Krabbe's
  disease (leukodystrophy) 330.0
  syndrome
    congenital muscle hypoplasia 756.89
    cutaneocerebral angioma 759.6
Kraepelin-Morel disease (*see also* Schizophrenia) 295.9●
Kraft-Weber-Dimitri disease 759.6
Kraurosis
  ani 569.49
  penis 607.0
  vagina 623.8
  vulva 624.09
Kreotoxism 005.9

Krukenberg's
spindle 371.13
tumor (M8490/6) 198.6
Kufs' disease 330.1
Kugelberg-Welander disease 335.11
Kuhnt-Junius degeneration or disease
362.52
Kulchitsky's cell carcinoma (carcinoid
tumor of intestine) 259.2
Kümmell's disease or spondylitis 721.7
Kundrat's disease (lymphosarcoma)
200.1●
Kunekune - *see* Dermatophytosis
Kunkel syndrome (lupoid hepatitis)
571.49
Kupffer cell sarcoma (M9124/3) 155.0
Kuru 046.0
Kussmaul's
coma (diabetic) 250.3●
due to secondary diabetes
249.3●
disease (polyarteritis nodosa) 446.0
respiration (air hunger) 786.09
Kwashiorkor (marasmus type) 260
Kyasanur Forest disease 065.2

Kyphoscoliosis, kyphoscoliotic
(acquired) (*see also* Scoliosis)
737.30
congenital 756.19
due to radiation 737.33
heart (disease) 416.1
idiopathic 737.30
infantile
progressive 737.32
resolving 737.31
late effect of rickets 268.1 [737.43]
specified NEC 737.39
thoracogenic 737.34
tuberculous (*see also* Tuberculosis)
015.0● [737.43]
Kyphosis, kyphotic (acquired) (postural)
737.10
adolescent postural 737.0
congenital 756.19
dorsalis juvenilis 732.0
due to or associated with
Charcôt-Marie-Tooth disease 356.1
[737.41]
mucopolysaccharidosis 277.5
[737.41]

Kyphosis, kyphotic (*Continued***)**
due to or associated with (*Continued*)
neurofibromatosis 237.71 [737.41]
osteitis
deformans 731.0 [737.41]
fibrosa cystica 252.01 [737.41]
osteoporosis (*see also* Osteoporosis)
733.0 [737.41]
poliomyelitis (*see also* Poliomyelitis)
138 [737.41]
radiation 737.11
tuberculosis (*see also* Tuberculosis)
015.0● [737.41]
Kümmell's 721.7
late effect of rickets 268.1 [737.41]
Morquio-Brailsford type (spinal) 277.5
[737.41]
pelvis 738.6
postlaminectomy 737.12
specified cause NEC 737.19
syphilitic, congenital 090.5 [737.41]
tuberculous (*see also* Tuberculosis)
015.0● [737.41]
Kyrle's disease (hyperkeratosis
follicularis in cutem penetrans) 701.1

K

◀ New   ◀▥ Revised   ~~deleted~~ Deleted   ● Use Additional Digit(s)   ▨ Omit code

L

Labia, labium - *see* condition
Labiated hymen 752.49
Labile
  blood pressure 796.2
  emotions, emotionality 301.3
  vasomotor system 443.9
Lability, emotional 799.24
Labioglossal paralysis 335.22
Labium leporinum (*see also* Cleft, lip)
  749.10
Labor (*see also* Delivery)
  with complications - *see* Delivery,
    complicated
  abnormal NEC 661.9●
    affecting fetus or newborn 763.7
  arrested active phase 661.1●
    affecting fetus or newborn 763.7
  desultory 661.2●
    affecting fetus or newborn 763.7
  dyscoordinate 661.4●
    affecting fetus or newborn 763.7
  early onset (22–36 weeks gestation)
    644.2●
  failed
    induction 659.1●
      mechanical 659.0●
      medical 659.1●
      surgical 659.0●
    trial (vaginal delivery) 660.6●
  false 644.1●
  forced or induced, affecting fetus or
    newborn 763.89
  hypertonic 661.4●
    affecting fetus or newborn 763.7
  hypotonic 661.2●
    affecting fetus or newborn 763.7
    primary 661.0●
      affecting fetus or newborn 763.7
    secondary 661.1●
      affecting fetus or newborn 763.7
  incoordinate 661.4●
    affecting fetus or newborn 763.7
  irregular 661.2●
    affecting fetus or newborn 763.7
  long - *see* Labor, prolonged
  missed (at or near term) 656.4●
  obstructed NEC 660.9●
    affecting fetus or newborn 763.1
    due to female genital mutilation
      660.8●
    specified cause NEC 660.8●
      affecting fetus or newborn 763.1
  pains, spurious 644.1●
  precipitate 661.3●
    affecting fetus or newborn 763.6
  premature 644.2●
    threatened 644.0●
  prolonged or protracted 662.1●
    affecting fetus or newborn 763.89
    first stage 662.0●
      affecting fetus or newborn 763.89
    second stage 662.2●
      affecting fetus or newborn 763.89
  threatened NEC 644.1●
  undelivered 644.1●
Labored breathing (*see also*
  Hyperventilation) 786.09
Labyrinthitis (inner ear) (destructive)
  (latent) 386.30
  circumscribed 386.32
  diffuse 386.31
  focal 386.32
  purulent 386.33

Labyrinthitis (*Continued*)
  serous 386.31
  suppurative 386.33
  syphilitic 095.8
  toxic 386.34
  viral 386.35
Laceration - *see also* Wound, open, by site
  accidental, complicating surgery
    998.2
  Achilles tendon 845.09
    with open wound 892.2
  anus (sphincter) 879.6
    with
      abortion - *see* Abortion, by type,
        with damage to pelvic
        organs
      ectopic pregnancy (*see also*
        categories 633.0–633.9) 639.2
      molar pregnancy (*see also*
        categories 630–632) 639.2
    complicated 879.7
    complicating delivery (healed) (old)
      654.8●
      with laceration of anal or rectal
        mucosa 664.3●
      not associated with third-degree
        perineal laceration 664.6●
    following
      abortion 639.2
      ectopic or molar pregnancy 639.2
    nontraumatic, nonpuerperal
      (healed) (old) 569.43
  bladder (urinary)
    with
      abortion - *see* Abortion, by type,
        with damage to pelvic
        organs
      ectopic pregnancy (*see also*
        categories 633.0–633.9) 639.2
      molar pregnancy (*see also*
        categories 630–632) 639.2
    following
      abortion 639.2
      ectopic or molar pregnancy 639.2
    obstetrical trauma 665.5●
  blood vessel - *see* Injury, blood vessel,
    by site
  bowel
    with
      abortion - *see* Abortion, by type,
        with damage to pelvic
        organs
      ectopic pregnancy (*see also*
        categories 633.0–633.9) 639.2
      molar pregnancy (*see also*
        categories 630–632) 639.2
    following
      abortion 639.2
      ectopic or molar pregnancy 639.2
    obstetrical trauma 665.5●
  brain (cerebral) (membrane) (with
    hemorrhage) 851.8●

> Note: Use the following fifth-digit
> subclassification with categories
> 851–854:
>
> 0   unspecified state of
>   consciousness
> 1   with no loss of consciousness
> 2   with brief [less than one hour]
>   loss of consciousness
> 3   with moderate [1–24 hours] loss
>   of consciousness

Laceration (*Continued*)
  brain (*Continued*)

> 4   with prolonged [more than 24
>   hours] loss of consciousness
>   and return to pre-existing
>   conscious level
> 5   with prolonged [more than 24
>   hours] loss of
>   consciousness, without
>   return to pre-existing
>   conscious level
>
> Use fifth-digit 5 to designate when a
> patient is unconscious and dies before
> regaining consciousness, regardless of
> the duration of the loss of
> consciousness
>
> 6   with loss of consciousness of
>   unspecified duration
> 9   with concussion, unspecified

    with
      open intracranial wound 851.9●
      skull fracture - *see* Fracture, skull,
        by site
    cerebellum 851.6●
      with open intracranial wound
        851.7●
    cortex 851.2●
      with open intracranial wound
        851.3●
    during birth 767.0
    stem 851.6●
      with open intracranial wound
        851.7●
  broad ligament
    with
      abortion - *see* Abortion, by type,
        with damage to pelvic
        organs
      ectopic pregnancy (*see also*
        categories 633.0–633.9)
        639.2
      molar pregnancy (*see also*
        categories 630–632) 639.2
    following
      abortion 639.2
      ectopic or molar pregnancy
        639.2
    nontraumatic 620.6
    obstetrical trauma 665.6●
    syndrome (nontraumatic) 620.6
  capsule, joint - *see* Sprain, by site
  cardiac - *see* Laceration, heart
  causing eversion of cervix uteri (old)
    622.0
  central, complicating delivery 664.4●
  cerebellum - *see* Laceration, brain,
    cerebellum
  cerebral - *see also* Laceration, brain
    during birth 767.0
  cervix (uteri)
    with
      abortion - *see* Abortion, by type,
        with damage to pelvic
        organs
      ectopic pregnancy (*see also*
        categories 633.0–633.9)
        639.2
      molar pregnancy (*see also*
        categories 630–632) 639.2
    following
      abortion 639.2
      ectopic or molar pregnancy 639.2

Laceration *(Continued)*
  cervix *(Continued)*
    nonpuerperal, nontraumatic 622.3
    obstetrical trauma (current) 665.3●
    old (postpartal) 622.3
    traumatic - *see* Injury, internal, cervix
  chordae heart 429.5
  complicated 879.9
  cornea - *see* Laceration, eyeball
    superficial 918.1
  cortex (cerebral) - *see* Laceration, brain,
    cortex
  esophagus 530.89
  eye(s) - *see* Laceration, ocular
  eyeball NEC 871.4
    with prolapse or exposure of
      intraocular tissue 871.1
    penetrating - *see* Penetrating wound,
      eyeball
    specified as without prolapse of
      intraocular tissue 871.0
  eyelid NEC 870.8
    full thickness 870.1
      involving lacrimal passages 870.2
    skin (and periocular area) 870.0
      penetrating - *see* Penetrating
        wound, orbit
  fourchette
    with
      abortion - *see* Abortion, by type,
        with damage to pelvic
        organs
      ectopic pregnancy (*see also*
        categories 633.0–633.9) 639.2
      molar pregnancy (*see also*
        categories 630–632) 639.2
    complicating delivery 664.0●
    following
      abortion 639.2
      ectopic or molar pregnancy 639.2
  heart (without penetration of heart
    chambers) 861.02
    with
      open wound into thorax 861.12
      penetration of heart chambers
        861.03
        with open wound into thorax
          861.13
  hernial sac - *see* Hernia, by site
  internal organ (abdomen) (chest)
    (pelvis) NEC - *see* Injury, internal,
    by site
  kidney (parenchyma) 866.02
    with
      complete disruption of
        parenchyma (rupture)
        866.03
        with open wound into cavity
          866.13
      open wound into cavity 866.12
  labia
    complicating delivery 664.0●
  ligament - *see also* Sprain, by site
    with open wound - *see* Wound,
      open, by site
  liver 864.05
    with open wound into cavity 864.15
    major (disruption of hepatic
      parenchyma) 864.04
      with open wound into cavity
        864.14
    minor (capsule only) 864.02
      with open wound into cavity
        864.12

Laceration *(Continued)*
  liver *(Continued)*
    moderate (involving parenchyma
      without major disruption)
      864.03
      with open wound into cavity
        864.13
    multiple 864.04
      with open wound into cavity
        864.14
    stellate 864.04
      with open wound into cavity
        864.14
  lung 861.22
    with open wound into thorax
      861.32
  meninges - *see* Laceration, brain
  meniscus (knee) (*see also* Tear,
    meniscus) 836.2
    old 717.5
    site other than knee - *see also* Sprain,
      by site
    old NEC (*see also* Disorder,
      cartilage, articular) 718.0●
  muscle - *see also* Sprain, by site
    with open wound - *see* Wound,
      open, by site
  myocardium - *see* Laceration, heart
  nerve - *see* Injury, nerve, by site
  ocular NEC (*see also* Laceration,
    eyeball) 871.4
    adnexa NEC 870.8
      penetrating 870.3
        with foreign body 870.4
  orbit (eye) 870.8
    penetrating 870.3
      with foreign body 870.4
  pelvic
    floor (muscles)
      with
        abortion - *see* Abortion, by type,
          with damage to pelvic
          organs
        ectopic pregnancy (*see also*
          categories 633.0–633.9)
          639.2
        molar pregnancy (*see also*
          categories 630–632)
          639.2
      complicating delivery 664.1●
      following
        abortion 639.2
        ectopic or molar pregnancy
          639.2
      nonpuerperal 618.7
      old (postpartal) 618.7
    organ NEC
      with
        abortion - *see* Abortion, by type,
          with damage to pelvic
          organs
        ectopic pregnancy (*see also*
          categories 633.0–633.9)
          639.2
        molar pregnancy (*see also*
          categories 630–632) 639.2
      complicating delivery 665.5●
        affecting fetus or newborn
          763.89
      following
        abortion 639.2
        ectopic or molar pregnancy
          639.2
      obstetrical trauma 665.5●

Laceration *(Continued)*
  perineum, perineal (old) (postpartal)
    618.7
    with
      abortion - *see* Abortion, by type,
        with damage to pelvic floor
      ectopic pregnancy (*see also*
        categories 633.0–633.9) 639.2
      molar pregnancy (*see also*
        categories 630–632) 639.2
    complicating delivery 664.4●
      first degree 664.0●
      second degree 664.1●
      third degree 664.2●
      fourth degree 664.3●
      central 664.4●
      involving
        anal sphincter (healed) (old)
          654.8●
          fourchette 664.0●
          hymen 664.0●
          labia 664.0●
          not associated with third-
            degree perineal
            laceration 664.6●
        pelvic floor 664.1●
        perineal muscles 664.1●
        rectovaginal with septum
          664.2●
          with anal mucosa 664.3●
        skin 664.0●
        sphincter (anal) (healed) (old)
          654.8●
          with anal mucosa 664.3●
          not associated with third-
            degree perineal
            laceration 664.6●
        vagina 664.0●
        vaginal muscles 664.1●
        vulva 664.0●
      secondary 674.2●
    following
      abortion 639.2
      ectopic or molar pregnancy 639.2
    male 879.6
      complicated 879.7
    muscles, complicating delivery
      664.1●
    nonpuerperal, current injury 879.6
      complicated 879.7
    secondary (postpartal) 674.2●
  peritoneum
    with
      abortion - *see* Abortion, by type,
        with damage to pelvic
        organs
      ectopic pregnancy (*see also*
        categories 633.0–633.9)
        639.2
      molar pregnancy (*see also*
        categories 630–632) 639.2
    following
      abortion 639.2
      ectopic or molar pregnancy 639.2
    obstetrical trauma 665.5●
  periurethral tissue
    with
      abortion - *see* Abortion, by type,
        with damage to pelvic
        organs
      ectopic pregnancy (*see also*
        categories 633.0–633.9) 639.2
      molar pregnancy (*see also*
        categories 630–632) 639.2

◀ New   ◀▥ Revised   ~~deleted~~ Deleted   ● Use Additional Digit(s)   ▨ Omit code

Laceration *(Continued)*
  periurethral tissue *(Continued)*
    following
      abortion 639.2
      ectopic or molar pregnancy 639.2
    obstetrical trauma 664.8● ◀▥
  rectovaginal (septum)
    with
      abortion - *see* Abortion, by type,
        with damage to pelvic
        organs
      ectopic pregnancy *(see also*
        categories 633.0–633.9) 639.2
      molar pregnancy *(see also*
        categories 630–632) 639.2
    complicating delivery 665.4●
      with perineum 664.2●
        involving anal or rectal
          mucosa 664.3●
    following
      abortion 639.2
      ectopic or molar pregnancy
        639.2
    nonpuerperal 623.4
    old (postpartal) 623.4
  spinal cord (meninges) - *see also* Injury,
    spinal, by site
    due to injury at birth 767.4
    fetus or newborn 767.4
  spleen 865.09
    with
      disruption of parenchyma
        (massive) 865.04
        with open wound into cavity
          865.14
      open wound into cavity 865.19
    capsule (without disruption of
      parenchyma) 865.02
      with open wound into cavity
        865.12
    parenchyma 865.03
      with open wound into cavity
        865.13
      massive disruption (rupture)
        865.04
        with open wound into cavity
          865.14
  tendon 848.9
    with open wound - *see* Wound,
      open, by site
    Achilles 845.09
      with open wound 892.2
    lower limb NEC 844.9
      with open wound NEC 894.2
    upper limb NEC 840.9
      with open wound NEC 884.2
  tentorium cerebelli - *see* Laceration,
    brain, cerebellum
  tongue 873.64
    complicated 873.74
  urethra
    with
      abortion - *see* Abortion, by type,
        with damage to pelvic
        organs
      ectopic pregnancy *(see also*
        categories 633.0–633.9) 639.2
      molar pregnancy *(see also*
        categories 630–632) 639.2
    following
      abortion 639.2
      ectopic or molar pregnancy 639.2
    nonpuerperal, nontraumatic 599.84
    obstetrical trauma 665.5●

Laceration *(Continued)*
  uterus
    with
      abortion - *see* Abortion, by type,
        with damage to pelvic
        organs
      ectopic pregnancy *(see also*
        categories 633.0–633.9) 639.2
      molar pregnancy *(see also*
        categories 630–632) 639.2
    following
      abortion 639.2
      ectopic or molar pregnancy 639.2
    nonpuerperal, nontraumatic 621.8
    obstetrical trauma NEC 665.5●
    old (postpartal) 621.8
  vagina
    with
      abortion - *see* Abortion, by type,
        with damage to pelvic
        organs
      ectopic pregnancy *(see also*
        categories 633.0–633.9) 639.2
      molar pregnancy *(see also*
        categories 630–632) 639.2
      perineal involvement,
        complicating delivery
        664.0●
    complicating delivery 665.4●
      first degree 664.0●
      second degree 664.1●
      third degree 664.2●
      fourth degree 664.3●
      high 665.4●
      muscles 664.1●
      sulcus 665.4●
      wall 665.4●
    following
      abortion 639.2
      ectopic or molar pregnancy 639.2
    nonpuerperal, nontraumatic 623.4
    old (postpartal) 623.4
  valve, heart - *see* Endocarditis
  vulva
    with
      abortion - *see* Abortion, by type,
        with damage to pelvic
        organs
      ectopic pregnancy *(see also*
        categories 633.0–633.9) 639.2
      molar pregnancy *(see also*
        categories 630–632) 639.2
    complicating delivery 664.0●
    following
      abortion 639.2
      ectopic or molar pregnancy 639.2
    nonpuerperal, nontraumatic 624.4
    old (postpartal) 624.4
Lachrymal - *see* condition
Lachrymonasal duct - *see* condition
Lack of
  adequate intermaxillary vertical
    dimension 524.36
  appetite *(see also* Anorexia) 783.0
  care
    in home V60.4
    of adult 995.84
    of infant (at or after birth) 995.52
  coordination 781.3
  development - *see also* Hypoplasia
    physiological in childhood 783.40
  education V62.3
  energy 780.79
  financial resources V60.2

Lack of *(Continued)*
  food 994.2
    in environment V60.89
  growth in childhood 783.43
  heating V60.1
  housing (permanent) (temporary)
    V60.0
    adequate V60.1
  material resources V60.2
  medical attention 799.89
  memory *(see also* Amnesia) 780.93
    mild, following organic brain
      damage 310.8
  ovulation 628.0
  person able to render necessary care
    V60.4
  physical exercise V69.0
  physiologic development in childhood
    783.40
  posterior occlusal support 524.57
  prenatal care in current pregnancy
    V23.7
  shelter V60.0
  sleep V69.4
  water 994.3
Lacrimal - *see* condition
Lacrimation, abnormal *(see also* Epiphora)
  375.20
Lacrimonasal duct - *see* condition
Lactation, lactating (breast) (puerperal)
  (postpartum)
  defective 676.4●
  disorder 676.9●
    specified type NEC 676.8●
  excessive 676.6●
  failed 676.4●
  mastitis NEC 675.2●
  mother (care and/or examination)
    V24.1
  nonpuerperal 611.6
  suppressed 676.5●
Lacticemia 271.3
  excessive 276.2
Lactosuria 271.3
Lacunar skull 756.0
Laennec's cirrhosis (alcoholic) 571.2
  nonalcoholic 571.5
Lafora's disease 333.2
Lag, lid (nervous) 374.41
Lagleyze-von Hippel disease
  (retinocerebral angiomatosis) 759.6
Lagophthalmos (eyelid) (nervous)
  374.20
  cicatricial 374.23
  keratitis *(see also* Keratitis) 370.34
  mechanical 374.22
  paralytic 374.21
La grippe - *see* Influenza
Lahore sore 085.1
Lakes, venous (cerebral) 437.8
Laki-Lorand factor deficiency *(see also*
  Defect, coagulation) 286.3
Lalling 307.9
Lambliasis 007.1
Lame back 724.5
Lancereaux's diabetes (diabetes mellitus
  with marked emaciation) 250.8●
  [261]
  due to secondary diabetes 249.8●
  [261]
Landau-Kleffner syndrome 345.8●
Landouzy-Déjérine dystrophy
  (fascioscapulohumeral atrophy)
  359.1

Landry's disease or paralysis 357.0
Landry-Guillain-Barré syndrome 357.0
Lane's
  band 751.4
  disease 569.89
  kink (see also Obstruction, intestine)
    560.9
Langdon Down's syndrome (mongolism)
  758.0
Language abolition 784.69
Lanugo (persistent) 757.4
Laparoscopic surgical procedure
  converted to open procedure V64.41
Lardaceous
  degeneration (any site) 277.39
  disease 277.39
  kidney 277.39 [583.81]
  liver 277.39
Large
  baby (regardless of gestational age) 766.1
    exceptionally (weight of 4500 grams
      or more) 766.0
    of diabetic mother 775.0
  ear 744.22
  fetus - see also Oversize, fetus
    causing disproportion 653.5●
      with obstructed labor 660.1●
    for dates
      fetus or newborn (regardless of
        gestational age) 766.1
        affecting management of
          pregnancy 656.6●
        exceptionally (weight of 4500
          grams or more) 766.0
  physiological cup 743.57
  stature 783.9
  waxy liver 277.39
  white kidney - see Nephrosis
Larsen's syndrome (flattened facies and
  multiple congenital dislocations)
  755.8
Larsen-Johansson disease (juvenile
  osteopathia patellae) 732.4
Larva migrans
  cutaneous NEC 126.9
    ancylostoma 126.9
  of Diptera in vitreous 128.0
  visceral NEC 128.0
Laryngeal - see also condition
  syncope 786.2
Laryngismus (acute) (infectious)
  (stridulous) 478.75
  congenital 748.3
  diphtheritic 032.3
Laryngitis (acute) (edematous) (fibrinous)
  (gangrenous) (infective) (infiltrative)
  (malignant) (membranous)
  (phlegmonous) (pneumococcal)
  (pseudomembranous) (septic)
  (subglottic) (suppurative) (ulcerative)
  (viral) 464.00
  with
    influenza, flu, or grippe (see also
      Influenza) 487.1 ◀
    obstruction 464.01
    tracheitis (see also Laryngotracheitis)
      464.00
      with obstruction 464.21
      acute 464.20
        with obstruction 464.21
      chronic 476.1
  atrophic 476.0
  Borrelia vincentii 101
  catarrhal 476.0

Laryngitis (Continued)
  chronic 476.0
    with tracheitis (chronic) 476.1
    due to external agent - see
      Condition, respiratory, chronic,
      due to
  diphtheritic (membranous) 032.3
  due to external agent - see
    Inflammation, respiratory, upper,
    due to
  H. influenzae 464.00
    with obstruction 464.01
  Hemophilus influenzae 464.00
    with obstruction 464.01
  hypertrophic 476.0
  influenzal (see also Influenza) 487.1 ◀
  pachydermic 478.79
  sicca 476.0
  spasmodic 478.75
    acute 464.00
      with obstruction 464.01
  streptococcal 034.0
  stridulous 478.75
  syphilitic 095.8
    congenital 090.5
  tuberculous (see also Tuberculosis,
    larynx) 012.3●
  Vincent's 101
Laryngocele (congenital) (ventricular)
  748.3
Laryngofissure 478.79
  congenital 748.3
Laryngomalacia (congenital) 748.3
Laryngopharyngitis (acute) 465.0
  chronic 478.9
    due to external agent - see
      Condition, respiratory, chronic,
      due to
  due to external agent - see
    Inflammation, respiratory, upper,
    due to
  septic 034.0
Laryngoplegia (see also Paralysis, vocal
  cord) 478.30
Laryngoptosis 478.79
Laryngospasm 478.75
  due to external agent - see Condition,
    respiratory, acute, due to
Laryngostenosis 478.74
  congenital 748.3
Laryngotracheitis (acute) (infectional)
  (viral) (see also Laryngitis) 464.20
  with obstruction 464.21
  atrophic 476.1
  Borrelia vincentii 101
  catarrhal 476.1
  chronic 476.1
    due to external agent - see
      Condition, respiratory, chronic,
      due to
  diphtheritic (membranous) 032.3
  due to external agent - see
    Inflammation, respiratory, upper,
    due to
  H. influenzae 464.20
    with obstruction 464.21
  hypertrophic 476.1
  influenzal (see also Influenza) 487.1 ◀
  pachydermic 478.75
  sicca 476.1
  spasmodic 478.75
    acute 464.20
      with obstruction 464.21
  streptococcal 034.0

Laryngotracheitis (Continued)
  stridulous 478.75
  syphilitic 095.8
    congenital 090.5
  tuberculous (see also Tuberculosis,
    larynx) 012.3●
  Vincent's 101
Laryngotracheobronchitis (see also
  Bronchitis) 490
  acute 466.0
  chronic 491.8
  viral 466.0
Laryngotracheobronchopneumonitis - see
  Pneumonia, broncho-
Larynx, laryngeal - see condition
Lasègue's disease (persecution mania)
  297.9
Lassa fever 078.89
Lassitude (see also Weakness) 780.79
Late - see also condition
  effect(s) (of) - see also condition
    abscess
      intracranial or intraspinal
        (conditions classifiable to
        324) - see category 326
    adverse effect of drug, medicinal or
      biological substance 909.5
    allergic reaction 909.9
    amputation
      postoperative (late) 997.60
      traumatic (injury classifiable to
        885–887 and 895–897)
        905.9
    burn (injury classifiable to 948–949)
      906.9
      extremities NEC (injury
        classifiable to 943 or 945)
        906.7
      hand or wrist (injury
        classifiable to 944) 906.6
      eye (injury classifiable to 940)
        906.5
      face, head, and neck (injury
        classifiable to 941) 906.5
      specified site NEC (injury
        classifiable to 942 and
        946–947) 906.8
    cerebrovascular disease (conditions
      classifiable to 430–437) 438.9
      with
        alterations of sensations
          438.6
        aphasia 438.11
        apraxia 438.81
        ataxia 438.84
        cognitive deficits 438.0
        disturbances of vision 438.7
        dysarthria 438.13
        dysphagia 438.82
        dysphasia 438.12
        facial droop 438.83
        facial weakness 438.83
        fluency disorder 438.14
        hemiplegia/hemiparesis
          affecting
            dominant side 438.21
            nondominant side 438.22
            unspecified side 438.20
        monoplegia of lower limb
          affecting
            dominant side 438.41
            nondominant side
              438.42
            unspecified side 438.40

◀ New   ◀ Revised   deleted Deleted   ● Use Additional Digit(s)   Omit code

Late *(Continued)*
  effect(s) (of) *(Continued)*
    cerebrovascular disease *(Continued)*
      with *(Continued)*
        monoplegia of upper limb
          affecting
            dominant side 438.31
            nondominant side 438.32
            unspecified side 438.30
        paralytic syndrome NEC
          affecting
            bilateral 438.53
            dominant side 438.51
            nondominant side
              438.52
            unspecified side 438.50
        speech and language deficit
          438.10
        specified type NEC
          438.19
        stuttering 438.14
        vertigo 438.85
      specified type NEC 438.89
    childbirth complication(s) 677
    complication(s) of
      childbirth 677
      delivery 677
      pregnancy 677
      puerperium 677
      surgical and medical care
        (conditions classifiable to
        996–999) 909.3
      trauma (conditions classifiable to
        958) 908.6
    contusion (injury classifiable to
      920–924) 906.3
    crushing (injury classifiable to
      925–929) 906.4
    delivery complication(s) 677
    dislocation (injury classifiable to
      830–839) 905.6
    encephalitis or encephalomyelitis
      (conditions classifiable to
      323) - *see* category 326
      in infectious diseases 139.8
      viral (conditions classifiable to
        049.8, 049.9, 062–064)
        139.0
    external cause NEC (conditions
      classifiable to 995) 909.9
      certain conditions classifiable to
        categories 991–994 909.4
    foreign body in orifice (injury
      classifiable to 930–939) 908.5
    fracture (multiple) (injury
      classifiable to 828–829) 905.5
      extremity
        lower (injury classifiable to
          821–827) 905.4
        neck of femur (injury
          classifiable to 820)
          905.3
        upper (injury classifiable to
          810–819) 905.2
      face and skull (injury classifiable
        to 800–804) 905.0
      skull and face (injury classifiable
        to 800–804) 905.0
      spine and trunk (injury
        classifiable to 805 and
        807–809) 905.1
        with spinal cord lesion (injury
          classifiable to 806)
          907.2

Late *(Continued)*
  effect(s) (of) *(Continued)*
    infection
      pyogenic, intracranial - *see*
        category 326
    infectious diseases (conditions
      classifiable to 001–136) NEC
      139.8
    injury (injury classifiable to 959)
      908.9
      blood vessel 908.3
        abdomen and pelvis (injury
          classifiable to 902) 908.4
        extremity (injury classifiable to
          903–904) 908.3
        head and neck (injury
          classifiable to 900) 908.3
        intracranial (injury
          classifiable to 850–854)
          907.0
          with skull fracture 905.0
        thorax (injury classifiable to
          901) 908.4
      internal organ NEC (injury
        classifiable to 867 and 869)
        908.2
        abdomen (injury classifiable to
          863–866 and 868) 908.1
        thorax (injury classifiable to
          860–862) 908.0
      intracranial (injury classifiable to
        850–854) 907.0
        with skull fracture (injury
          classifiable to 800–801
          and 803–804) 905.0
      nerve NEC (injury classifiable to
        957) 907.9
        cranial (injury classifiable to
          950–951) 907.1
        peripheral NEC (injury
          classifiable to 957)
          907.9
          lower limb and pelvic
            girdle (injury
            classifiable to 956)
            907.5
          upper limb and shoulder
            girdle (injury
            classifiable to 955)
            907.4
      roots and plexus(es), spinal
        (injury classifiable to 953)
        907.3
      trunk (injury classifiable to
        954) 907.3
      spinal
        cord (injury classifiable to 806
          and 952) 907.2
        nerve root(s) and plexus(es)
          (injury classifiable to 953)
          907.3
      superficial (injury classifiable to
        910–919) 906.2
      tendon (tendon injury classifiable
        to 840–848, 880–884 with .2,
        and 890–894 with .2) 905.8
    meningitis
      bacterial (conditions classifiable
        to 320) - *see* category 326
      unspecified cause (conditions
        classifiable to 322) - *see*
        category 326
    myelitis (*see also* Late, effect(s) (of),
      encephalitis) - *see* category 326

Late *(Continued)*
  effect(s) (of) *(Continued)*
    parasitic diseases (conditions
      classifiable to 001–136 NEC)
      139.8
    phlebitis or thrombophlebitis of
      intracranial venous sinuses
      (conditions classifiable to
      325) - *see* category 326
    poisoning due to drug, medicinal or
      biological substance
      (conditions classifiable to
      960–979) 909.0
    poliomyelitis, acute (conditions
      classifiable to 045) 138
    pregnancy complication(s) 677
    puerperal complication(s) 677
    radiation (conditions classifiable to
      990) 909.2
    rickets 268.1
    sprain and strain without mention
      of tendon injury (injury
      classifiable to 840–848, except
      tendon injury) 905.7
      tendon involvement 905.8
    toxic effect of
      drug, medicinal or biological
        substance (conditions
        classifiable to 960–979)
        909.0
      nonmedical substance
        (conditions classifiable
        to 980–989) 909.1
    trachoma (conditions classifiable
      to 076) 139.1
    tuberculosis 137.0
      bones and joints (conditions
        classifiable to 015) 137.3
      central nervous system
        (conditions classifiable to
        013) 137.1
      genitourinary (conditions
        classifiable to 016) 137.2
      pulmonary (conditions
        classifiable to 010–012)
        137.0
      specified organs NEC (conditions
        classifiable to 014, 017–018)
        137.4
    viral encephalitis (conditions
      classifiable to 049.8, 049.9,
      062–064) 139.0
    wound, open
      extremity (injury classifiable to
        880–884 and 890–894,
        except .2) 906.1
        tendon (injury classifiable to
          880–884 with .2 and
          890–894 with .2) 905.8
      head, neck, and trunk (injury
        classifiable to 870–879)
        906.0
  infant
    post-term (gestation period
      over 40 completed weeks
      to 42 completed weeks)
      766.21
    prolonged gestation (period
      over 42 completed weeks)
      766.22
Latent - *see* condition
Lateral - *see* condition
Laterocession - *see* Lateroversion
Lateroflexion - *see* Lateroversion

Lateroversion
  cervix - *see* Lateroversion, uterus
  uterus, uterine (cervix) (postinfectional) (postpartal, old) 621.6
    congenital 752.39 ◀▥
    in pregnancy or childbirth 654.4●
      affecting fetus or newborn 763.89
Lathyrism 988.2
Launois' syndrome (pituitary gigantism) 253.0
Launois-Bensaude's lipomatosis 272.8
Launois-Cleret syndrome (adiposogenital dystrophy) 253.8
Laurence-Moon-Biedl syndrome (obesity, polydactyly, and mental retardation) 759.89
LAV (disease) (illness) (infection) - *see* Human immunodeficiency virus (disease) (illness) (infection)
LAV/HTLV-III (disease) (illness) (infection) - *see* Human immunodeficiency virus (disease) (illness) (infection)
Lawford's syndrome (encephalocutaneous angiomatosis) 759.6
Lax, laxity - *see also* Relaxation
  ligament 728.4
  skin (acquired) 701.8
    congenital 756.83
Laxative habit (*see also* Abuse, drugs, nondependent) 305.9●
Lazy leukocyte syndrome 288.09
LCAD (long chain/very long chain acyl CoA dehydrogenase deficiency, VLCAD) 277.85
LCHAD (long chain 3-hydroxyacyl CoA dehydrogenase deficiency) 277.85
Lead - *see also* condition
  exposure (suspected) to V15.86
  incrustation of cornea 371.15
  poisoning 984.9
    specified type of lead - *see* Table of Drugs and Chemicals
Lead miners' lung 503
Leakage
  amniotic fluid 658.1●
    with delayed delivery 658.2●
    affecting fetus or newborn 761.1
  bile from drainage tube (T tube) 997.4
  blood (microscopic), fetal, into maternal circulation 656.0●
    affecting management of pregnancy or puerperium 656.0●
  device, implant, or graft - *see* Complications, mechanical
  spinal fluid at lumbar puncture site 997.09
  urine, continuous 788.37
Leaky heart - *see* Endocarditis
Learning defect, specific NEC (strephosymbolia) 315.2
Leather bottle stomach (M8142/3) 151.9
Leber's
  congenital amaurosis 362.76
  optic atrophy (hereditary) 377.16
Lederer's anemia or disease (acquired infectious hemolytic anemia) 283.19
Lederer-Brill syndrome (acquired infectious hemolytic anemia) 283.19
Leeches (aquatic) (land) 134.2
Left-sided neglect 781.8
Leg - *see* condition
Legal investigation V62.5

Legg (-Calvé)-Perthes disease or syndrome (osteochondrosis, femoral capital) 732.1
Legionnaires' disease 482.84
Leigh's disease 330.8
Leiner's disease (exfoliative dermatitis) 695.89
Leiofibromyoma (M8890/0) - *see also* Leiomyoma
  uterus (cervix) (corpus) (*see also* Leiomyoma, uterus) 218.9
Leiomyoblastoma (M8891/1) - *see* Neoplasm, connective tissue, uncertain behavior
Leiomyofibroma (M8890/0) - *see also* Neoplasm, connective tissue, benign
  uterus (cervix) (corpus) (*see also* Leiomyoma, uterus) 218.9
Leiomyoma (M8890/0) - *see also* Neoplasm, connective tissue, benign
  bizarre (M8893/0) - *see* Neoplasm, connective tissue, benign
  cellular (M8892/1) - *see* Neoplasm, connective tissue, uncertain behavior
  epithelioid (M8891/1) - *see* Neoplasm, connective tissue, uncertain behavior
  prostate (polypoid) 600.20
    with
      other lower urinary tract symptoms (LUTS) 600.21
      urinary
        obstruction 600.21
        retention 600.21
  uterus (cervix) (corpus) 218.9
    interstitial 218.1
    intramural 218.1
    submucous 218.0
    subperitoneal 218.2
    subserous 218.2
  vascular (M8894/0) - *see* Neoplasm, connective tissue, benign
Leiomyomatosis (intravascular) (M8890/1) - *see* Neoplasm, connective tissue, uncertain behavior
Leiomyosarcoma (M8890/3) - *see also* Neoplasm, connective tissue, malignant
  epithelioid (M8891/3) - *see* Neoplasm, connective tissue, malignant
Leishmaniasis 085.9
  American 085.5
    cutaneous 085.4
    mucocutaneous 085.5
  Asian desert 085.2
  Brazilian 085.5
  cutaneous 085.9
    acute necrotizing 085.2
    American 085.4
    Asian desert 085.2
    diffuse 085.3
    dry form 085.1
    Ethiopian 085.3
    eyelid 085.5 [373.6]
    late 085.1
    lepromatous 085.3
    recurrent 085.1
    rural 085.2
    ulcerating 085.1
    urban 085.1
    wet form 085.2
    zoonotic form 085.2

Leishmaniasis (*Continued*)
  dermal - *see also* Leishmaniasis, cutaneous
    post kala-azar 085.0
  eyelid 085.5 [373.6]
  infantile 085.0
  Mediterranean 085.0
  mucocutaneous (American) 085.5
  naso-oral 085.5
  nasopharyngeal 085.5
  Old World 085.1
  tegumentaria diffusa 085.4
  vaccination, prophylactic (against) V05.2
  visceral (Indian) 085.0
Leishmanoid, dermal - *see also* Leishmaniasis, cutaneous
  post kala-azar 085.0
Leloir's disease 695.4
Lemiere syndrome 451.89
Lenegre's disease 426.0
Lengthening, leg 736.81
Lennox-Gastaut syndrome 345.0●
  with tonic seizures 345.1●
Lennox's syndrome (*see also* Epilepsy) 345.0●
Lens - *see* condition
Lenticonus (anterior) (posterior) (congenital) 743.36
Lenticular degeneration, progressive 275.1
Lentiglobus (posterior) (congenital) 743.36
Lentigo (congenital) 709.09
  juvenile 709.09
  Maligna (M8742/2) - *see also* Neoplasm, skin, in situ
    melanoma (M8742/3) - *see* Melanoma
  senile 709.09
Leonine leprosy 030.0
Leontiasis
  ossium 733.3
  syphilitic 095.8
    congenital 090.5
Léopold-Lévi's syndrome (paroxysmal thyroid instability) 242.9●
Lepore hemoglobin syndrome 282.49
Lepothrix 039.0
Lepra 030.9
  Willan's 696.1
Leprechaunism 259.8
Lepromatous leprosy 030.0
Leprosy 030.9
  anesthetic 030.1
  beriberi 030.1
  borderline (group B) (infiltrated) (neuritic) 030.3
  cornea (*see also* Leprosy, by type) 030.9 [371.89]
  dimorphous (group B) (infiltrated) (lepromatous) (neuritic) (tuberculoid) 030.3
  eyelid 030.0 [373.4]
  indeterminate (group I) (macular) (neuritic) (uncharacteristic) 030.2
  leonine 030.0
  lepromatous (diffuse) (infiltrated) (macular) (neuritic) (nodular) (type L) 030.0
  macular (early) (neuritic) (simple) 030.2
  maculoanesthetic 030.1
  mixed 030.0
  neuro 030.1
  nodular 030.0

◀ New   ◀▥ Revised   ~~deleted~~ Deleted   ● Use Additional Digit(s)   ▩ Omit code

Leprosy (Continued)
    primary neuritic 030.3
    specified type or group NEC 030.8
    tubercular 030.1
    tuberculoid (macular)
        (maculoanesthetic) (major)
        (minor) (neuritic) (type T)
        030.1
Leptocytosis, hereditary 282.49
Leptomeningitis (chronic)
        (circumscribed) (hemorrhagic)
        (nonsuppurative) (see also
        Meningitis) 322.9
    aseptic 047.9
        adenovirus 049.1
        Coxsackie virus 047.0
        ECHO virus 047.1
        enterovirus 047.9
        lymphocytic choriomeningitis
            049.0
    epidemic 036.0
    late effect - see category 326
    meningococcal 036.0
    pneumococcal 320.1
    syphilitic 094.2
    tuberculous (see also Tuberculosis,
        meninges) 013.0●
Leptomeningopathy (see also Meningitis)
        322.9
Leptospiral - see condition
Leptospirochetal - see condition
Leptospirosis 100.9
    autumnalis 100.89
    canicula 100.89
    grippotyphosa 100.89
    hebdomadis 100.89
    icterohemorrhagica 100.0
    nanukayami 100.89
    pomona 100.89
    Weil's disease 100.0
Leptothricosis - see Actinomycosis
Leptothrix infestation - see
        Actinomycosis
Leptotricosis - see Actinomycosis
Leptus dermatitis 133.8
Léris pleonosteosis 756.89
Léri-Weill syndrome 756.59
Leriche's syndrome (aortic bifurcation
        occlusion) 444.0
Lermoyez's syndrome (see also Disease,
        Ménière's) 386.00
Lesbianism - omit code
    ego-dystonic 302.0
    problems with 302.0
Lesch-Nyhan syndrome (hypoxanthine-
        guanine-phosphoribosyltransferase
        deficiency) 277.2
Lesion(s)
    abducens nerve 378.54
    alveolar process 525.8
    anorectal 569.49
    aortic (valve) - see Endocarditis, aortic
    auditory nerve 388.5
    basal ganglion 333.90
    bile duct (see also Disease, biliary)
        576.8
    bladder 596.9
    bone 733.90
    brachial plexus 353.0
    brain 348.89
        congenital 742.9
        vascular (see also Lesion,
            cerebrovascular) 437.9
            degenerative 437.1

Lesion(s) (Continued)
    brain (Continued)
        vascular (Continued)
            healed or old without residuals
                V12.54
            hypertensive 437.2
            late effect - see Late effect(s) (of)
                cerebrovascular disease
    buccal 528.9
    calcified - see Calcification
    canthus 373.9
    carate - see Pinta, lesions
    cardia 537.89
    cardiac - see also Disease, heart
        congenital 746.9
        valvular - see Endocarditis
    cauda equina 344.60
        with neurogenic bladder 344.61
    cecum 569.89
    cerebral - see Lesion, brain
    cerebrovascular (see also Disease,
        cerebrovascular NEC) 437.9
        degenerative 437.1
        healed or old without residuals
            V12.54
        hypertensive 437.2
        specified type NEC 437.8
    cervical root (nerve) NEC 353.2
    chiasmal 377.54
        associated with
            inflammatory disorders
                377.54
            neoplasm NEC 377.52
                pituitary 377.51
            pituitary disorders 377.51
            vascular disorders 377.53
    chorda tympani 351.8
    coin, lung 793.1
    colon 569.89
    congenital - see Anomaly
    conjunctiva 372.9
    coronary artery (see also Ischemia,
        heart) 414.9
    cranial nerve 352.9
        first 352.0
        second 377.49
        third
            partial 378.51
            total 378.52
        fourth 378.53
        fifth 350.9
        sixth 378.54
        seventh 351.9
        eighth 388.5
        ninth 352.2
        tenth 352.3
        eleventh 352.4
        twelfth 352.5
    cystic - see Cyst
    degenerative - see Degeneration
    dermal (skin) 709.9
    Dieulafoy (hemorrhagic)
        of
            duodenum 537.84
            intestine 569.86
            stomach 537.84
    duodenum 537.89
        with obstruction 537.3
    eyelid 373.9
    gasserian ganglion 350.8
    gastric 537.89
    gastroduodenal 537.89
    gastrointestinal 569.89
    glossopharyngeal nerve 352.2

Lesion(s) (Continued)
    heart (organic) - see also Disease, heart
        vascular - see Disease,
            cardiovascular
    helix (ear) 709.9
    high grade myelodysplastic syndrome
        238.73
    hyperchromic, due to pinta (carate)
        103.1
    hyperkeratotic (see also Hyperkeratosis)
        701.1
    hypoglossal nerve 352.5
    hypopharynx 478.29
    hypothalamic 253.9
    ileocecal coil 569.89
    ileum 569.89
    iliohypogastric nerve 355.79
    ilioinguinal nerve 355.79
    in continuity - see Injury, nerve, by site
    inflammatory - see Inflammation
    intestine 569.89
    intracerebral - see Lesion, brain
    intrachiasmal (optic) (see also Lesion,
        chiasmal) 377.54
    intracranial, space-occupying NEC 784.2
    joint 719.90
        ankle 719.97
        elbow 719.92
        foot 719.97
        hand 719.94
        hip 719.95
        knee 719.96
        multiple sites 719.99
        pelvic region 719.95
        sacroiliac (old) 724.6
        shoulder (region) 719.91
        specified site NEC 719.98
        wrist 719.93
    keratotic (see also Keratosis) 701.1
    kidney (see also Disease, renal) 593.9
    laryngeal nerve (recurrent) 352.3
    leonine 030.0
    lip 528.5
    liver 573.8
    low grade myelodysplastic syndrome
        238.72
    lumbosacral
        plexus 353.1
        root (nerve) NEC 353.4
    lung 518.89
        coin 793.1
    maxillary sinus 473.0
    mitral - see Endocarditis, mitral
    Morel Lavallée - see Hematoma,
        by site
    motor cortex 348.89
    nerve (see also Disorder, nerve) 355.9
    nervous system 349.9
        congenital 742.9
    nonallopathic NEC 739.9
        in region (of)
            abdomen 739.9
            acromioclavicular 739.7
            cervical, cervicothoracic 739.1
            costochondral 739.8
            costovertebral 739.8
            extremity
                lower 739.6
                upper 739.7
            head 739.0
            hip 739.5
            lower extremity 739.6
            lumbar, lumbosacral 739.3
            occipitocervical 739.0

Lesion(s) *(Continued)*
  nonallopathic NEC *(Continued)*
    in region (of) *(Continued)*
      pelvic 739.5
      pubic 739.5
      rib cage 739.8
      sacral, sacrococcygeal, sacroiliac
        739.4
      sternochondral 739.8
      sternoclavicular 739.7
      thoracic, thoracolumbar 739.2
      upper extremity 739.7
  nose (internal) 478.19
  obstructive - *see* Obstruction
  obturator nerve 355.79
  occlusive
    artery - *see* Embolism, artery
  organ or site NEC - *see* Disease, by
    site
  osteolytic 733.90
  paramacular, of retina 363.32
  peptic 537.89
  periodontal, due to traumatic occlusion
    523.8
  perirectal 569.49
  peritoneum (granulomatous)
    568.89
  pigmented (skin) 709.00
  pinta - *see* Pinta, lesions
  polypoid - *see* Polyp
  prechiasmal (optic) *(see also* Lesion,
    chiasmal) 377.54
  primary - *see also* Syphilis, primary
    carate 103.0
    pinta 103.0
    yaws 102.0
  pulmonary 518.89
    valve *(see also* Endocarditis,
      pulmonary) 424.3
  pylorus 537.89
  radiation NEC 990
  radium NEC 990
  rectosigmoid 569.89
  retina, retinal - *see also* Retinopathy
    vascular 362.17
  retroperitoneal 568.89
  romanus 720.1
  sacroiliac (joint) 724.6
  salivary gland 527.8
    benign lymphoepithelial 527.8
  saphenous nerve 355.79
  secondary - *see* Syphilis, secondary
  sigmoid 569.89
  sinus (accessory) (nasal) *(see also*
    Sinusitis) 473.9
  skin 709.9
    suppurative 686.00
  SLAP (superior glenoid labrum)
    840.7
  space-occupying, intracranial NEC
    784.2
  spinal cord 336.9
    congenital 742.9
    traumatic (complete) (incomplete)
      (transverse) - *see also* Injury,
      spinal, by site
      with
        broken
          back - *see* Fracture, vertebra,
            by site, with spinal
            cord injury
          neck - *see* Fracture, vertebra,
            cervical, with spinal
            cord injury

Lesion(s) *(Continued)*
  spinal cord *(Continued)*
    traumatic *(Continued)*
      with *(Continued)*
        fracture, vertebra - *see*
          Fracture, vertebra, by
          site, with spinal cord
          injury
  spleen 289.50
  stomach 537.89
  superior glenoid labrum (SLAP)
    840.7
  syphilitic - *see* Syphilis
  tertiary - *see* Syphilis, tertiary
  thoracic root (nerve) 353.3
  tonsillar fossa 474.9
  tooth, teeth 525.8
    white spot 521.01
  traumatic NEC *(see also* nature and site
    of injury) 959.9
  tricuspid (valve) - *see* Endocarditis,
    tricuspid
  trigeminal nerve 350.9
  ulcerated or ulcerative - *see* Ulcer
  uterus NEC 621.9
  vagina 623.8
  vagus nerve 352.3
  valvular - *see* Endocarditis
  vascular 459.9
    affecting central nervous system *(see
      also* Lesion, cerebrovascular)
      437.9
    following trauma *(see also* Injury,
      blood vessel, by site) 904.9
    retina 362.17
    traumatic - *see* Injury, blood vessel,
      by site
    umbilical cord 663.6●
      affecting fetus or newborn
        762.6
  visual
    cortex NEC *(see also* Disorder, visual,
      cortex) 377.73
    pathway NEC *(see also* Disorder,
      visual, pathway) 377.63
  warty - *see* Verruca
  white spot, on teeth 521.01
  x-ray NEC 990
Lethargic - *see* condition
Lethargy 780.79
Letterer-Siwe disease (acute histiocytosis
  X) (M9722/3) 202.5●
Leucinosis 270.3
Leucocoria 360.44
Leucosarcoma (M9850/3) 207.8●
Leukasmus 270.2
Leukemia, leukemic (congenital)
  (M9800/3) 208.9●

> Note: Use the following fifth-digit
> subclassification for categories 203–208:
>
> 0   without mention of having
>   achieved remission
>   failed remission
> 1   with remission
> 2   in relapse

  acute NEC (M9801/3) 208.0●
  aleukemic NEC (M9804/3) 208.8●
    granulocytic (M9864/3) 205.8●
  basophilic (M9870/3) 205.1●
  blast (cell) (M9801/3) 208.0●
  blastic (M9801/3) 208.0●
    granulocytic (M9861/3)
      205.0●

Leukemia, leukemic *(Continued)*
  chronic NEC (M9803/3) 208.1●
  compound (M9810/3) 207.8●
  eosinophilic (M9880/3) 205.1●
  giant cell (M9910/3) 207.2●
  granulocytic (M9860/3) 205.9●
    acute (M9861/3) 205.0●
    aleukemic (M9864/3) 205.8●
    blastic (M9861/3) 205.0●
    chronic (M9863/3) 205.1●
    subacute (M9862/3) 205.2●
    subleukemic (M9864/3) 205.8●
  hairy cell (M9940/3) 202.4●
  hemoblastic (M9801/3) 208.0●
  histiocytic (M9890/3) 206.9●
  lymphatic (M9820/3) 204.9●
    acute (M9821/3) 204.0●
    aleukemic (M9824/3) 204.8●
    chronic (M9823/3) 204.1●
    subacute (M9822/3) 204.2●
    subleukemic (M9824/3) 204.8●
  lymphoblastic (M9821/3) 204.0●
  lymphocytic (M9820/3) 204.9●
    acute (M9821/3) 204.0●
    aleukemic (M9824/3) 204.8●
    chronic (M9823/3) 204.1●
    granular
      large T-cell 204.8 ●
    subacute (M9822/3) 204.2●
    subleukemic (M9824/3) 204.8●
  lymphogenous (M9820/3) - *see*
    Leukemia, lymphoid
  lymphoid (M9820/3) 204.9●
    acute (M9821/3) 204.0●
    aleukemic (M9824/3) 204.8●
    blastic (M9821/3) 204.0●
    chronic (M9823/3) 204.1●
    subacute (M9822/3) 204.2●
    subleukemic (M9824/3) 204.8●
  lymphosarcoma cell (M9850/3)
    207.8●
  mast cell (M9900/3) 207.8●
  megakaryocytic (M9910/3) 207.2●
  megakaryocytoid (M9910/3) 207.2●
  mixed (cell) (M9810/3) 207.8●
  monoblastic (M9891/3) 206.0●
  monocytic (Schilling-type) (M9890/3)
    206.9●
    acute (M9891/3) 206.0●
    aleukemic (M9894/3) 206.8●
    chronic (M9893/3) 206.1●
    Naegeli-type (M9863/3) 205.1●
    subacute (M9892/3) 206.2●
    subleukemic (M9894/3) 206.8●
  monocytoid (M9890/3) 206.9●
    acute (M9891/3) 206.0●
    aleukemic (M9894/3) 206.8●
    chronic (M9893/3) 206.1●
    myelogenous (M9863/3) 205.1●
    subacute (M9892/3) 206.2●
    subleukemic (M9894/3) 206.8●
  monomyelocytic (M9860/3) - *see*
    Leukemia, myelomonocytic
  myeloblastic (M9861/3) 205.0●
  myelocytic (M9863/3) 205.1●
    acute (M9861/3) 205.0●
  myelogenous (M9860/3) 205.9●
    acute (M9861/3) 205.0●
    aleukemic (M9864/3) 205.8●
    chronic (M9863/3) 205.1●
    monocytoid (M9863/3) 205.1●
    subacute (M9862/3) 205.2●
    subleukemic (M9864) 205.8●
  myeloid (M9860/3) 205.9●
    acute (M9861/3) 205.0●

◄ New   ◄▦ Revised   ~~deleted~~ Deleted   ● Use Additional Digit(s)   ▦ Omit code

Leukemia, leukemic *(Continued)*
  myeloid *(Continued)*
    aleukemic (M9864/3) 205.8●
    chronic (M9863/3) 205.1●
    subacute (M9862/3) 205.2●
    subleukemic (M9864/3) 205.8●
  myelomonocytic (M9860/3) 205.9●
    acute (M9861/3) 205.0●
    chronic (M9863/3) 205.1●
  Naegeli-type monocytic (M9863/3)
    205.1●
  neutrophilic (M9865/3) 205.1●
  plasma cell (M9830/3) 203.1●
  plasmacytic (M9830/3) 203.1●
  prolymphocytic (M9825/3) - *see*
    Leukemia, lymphoid
  promyelocytic, acute (M9866/3)
    205.0●
  Schilling-type monocytic (M9890/3) -
    see Leukemia, monocytic
  stem cell (M9801/3) 208.0●
  subacute NEC (M9802/3) 208.2●
  subleukemic NEC (M9804/3) 208.8●
  thrombocytic (M9910/3) 207.2●
  undifferentiated (M9801/3) 208.0●
Leukemoid reaction (basophilic)
  (lymphocytic) (monocytic)
  (myelocytic) (neutrophilic) 288.62
Leukoaraiosis (hypertensive) 437.1
Leukoariosis - *see* Leukoaraiosis
Leukoclastic vasculitis 446.29
Leukocoria 360.44
Leukocythemia - *see* Leukemia
Leukocytopenia 288.50
Leukocytosis 288.60
  basophilic 288.8
  eosinophilic 288.3
  lymphocytic 288.8
  monocytic 288.8
  neutrophilic 288.8
Leukoderma 709.09
  syphilitic 091.3
    late 095.8
Leukodermia (*see also* Leukoderma)
  709.09
Leukodystrophy (cerebral) (globoid cell)
  (metachromatic) (progressive)
  (sudanophilic) 330.0
Leukoedema, mouth or tongue 528.79
Leukoencephalitis
  acute hemorrhagic (postinfectious)
    NEC 136.9 *[323.61]*
    postimmunization or postvaccinal
      323.51
  subacute sclerosing 046.2
  van Bogaert's 046.2
  van Bogaert's (sclerosing) 046.2
Leukoencephalopathy (*see also*
  Encephalitis) 323.9
  acute necrotizing hemorrhagic
    (postinfectious) 136.9 *[323.61]*
    postimmunization or postvaccinal
      323.51
  Binswanger's 290.12
  metachromatic 330.0
  multifocal (progressive) 046.3
  progressive multifocal 046.3
  reversible, posterior 348.5
Leukoerythroblastosis 289.9
Leukoerythrosis 289.0
Leukokeratosis (*see also* Leukoplakia)
  702.8
  mouth 528.6
  nicotina palati 528.79
  tongue 528.6

Leukokoria 360.44
Leukokraurosis vulva, vulvae 624.09
Leukolymphosarcoma (M9850/3)
  207.8●
Leukoma (cornea) (interfering with
  central vision) 371.03
  adherent 371.04
Leukomalacia, periventricular 779.7
Leukomelanopathy, hereditary 288.2
Leukonychia (punctata) (striata) 703.8
  congenital 757.5
Leukopathia
  unguium 703.8
    congenital 757.5
Leukopenia 288.50
  basophilic 288.59
  cyclic 288.02
  eosinophilic 288.59
  familial 288.59
  malignant (*see also* Agranulocytosis)
    288.09
  periodic 288.02
  transitory neonatal 776.7
Leukopenic - *see* condition
Leukoplakia 702.8
  anus 569.49
  bladder (postinfectional) 596.8
  buccal 528.6
  cervix (uteri) 622.2
  esophagus 530.83
  gingiva 528.6
  kidney (pelvis) 593.89
  larynx 478.79
  lip 528.6
  mouth 528.6
  oral soft tissue (including tongue)
    (mucosa) 528.6
  palate 528.6
  pelvis (kidney) 593.89
  penis (infectional) 607.0
  rectum 569.49
  syphilitic 095.8
  tongue 528.6
  tonsil 478.29
  ureter (postinfectional) 593.89
  urethra (postinfectional) 599.84
  uterus 621.8
  vagina 623.1
  vesical 596.8
  vocal cords 478.5
  vulva 624.09
Leukopolioencephalopathy 330.0
Leukorrhea (vagina) 623.5
  due to Trichomonas (vaginalis)
    131.00
  trichomonal (Trichomonas vaginalis)
    131.00
Leukosarcoma (M9850/3) 207.8●
Leukosis (M9800/3) - *see* Leukemia
Lev's disease or syndrome (acquired
  complete heart block) 426.0
Levi's syndrome (pituitary dwarfism)
  253.3
Levocardia (isolated) 746.87
  with situs inversus 759.3
Levulosuria 271.2
Lewandowski's disease (primary) (*see
  also* Tuberculosis) 017.0●
Lewandowski-Lutz disease
  (epidermodysplasia verruciformis)
  078.19
Lewy body dementia 331.82
Lewy body disease 331.82
Leyden's disease (periodic vomiting)
  536.2

Leyden-Möbius dystrophy 359.1
Leydig cell
  carcinoma (M8650/3)
    specified site - *see* Neoplasm, by site,
      malignant
    unspecified site
      female 183.0
      male 186.9
  tumor (M8650/1)
    benign (M8650/0)
      specified site - *see* Neoplasm, by
        site, benign
      unspecified site
        female 220
        male 222.0
    malignant (M8650/3)
      specified site - *see* Neoplasm, by
        site, malignant
      unspecified site
        female 183.0
        male 186.9
    specified site - *see* Neoplasm, by site,
      uncertain behavior
    unspecified site
      female 236.2
      male 236.4
Leydig-Sertoli cell tumor (M8631/0)
  specified site - *see* Neoplasm, by site,
    benign
  unspecified site
    female 220
    male 222.0
LGSIL (low grade squamous
  intraepithelial lesion)
  anus 796.73
  cervix 795.03
  vagina 795.13
Liar, pathologic 301.7
Libman-Sacks disease or syndrome
  710.0 *[424.91]*
Lice (infestation) 132.9
  body (pediculus corporis) 132.1
  crab 132.2
  head (pediculus capitis) 132.0
  mixed (classifiable to more than one
    of the categories 132.0–132.2)
    132.3
  pubic (pediculus pubis) 132.2
Lichen 697.9
  albus 701.0
  annularis 695.89
  atrophicus 701.0
  corneus obtusus 698.3
  myxedematous 701.8
  nitidus 697.1
  pilaris 757.39
    acquired 701.1
  planopilaris 697.0
  planus (acute) (chronicus)
    (hypertrophic) (verrucous)
    697.0
    morphoeicus 701.0
    sclerosus (et atrophicus) 701.0
  ruber 696.4
    acuminatus 696.4
    moniliformis 697.8
    obtusus corneus 698.3
    of Wilson 697.0
    planus 697.0
  sclerosus (et atrophicus) 701.0
  scrofulosus (primary) (*see also*
    Tuberculosis) 017.0●
  simplex (Vidal's) 698.3
    chronicus 698.3
    circumscriptus 698.3

Lichen (*Continued*)
  spinulosus 757.39
    mycotic 117.9
  striata 697.8
  urticatus 698.2
Lichenification 698.3
  nodular 698.3
Lichenoides tuberculosis (primary) (*see also* Tuberculosis) 017.0
Lichtheim's disease or syndrome (subacute combined sclerosis with pernicious anemia) 281.0 [*336.2*]
Lien migrans 289.59
Lientery (*see also* Diarrhea) 787.91
  infectious 009.2
Life circumstance problem NEC V62.89
Li-Fraumeni cancer syndrome V84.01
Ligament - *see* condition
Light-for-dates (infant) 764.0●
  with signs of fetal malnutrition 764.1●
  affecting management of pregnancy 656.5●
Light-headedness 780.4
Lightning (effects) (shock) (stroke) (struck by) 994.0
  burn - *see* Burn, by site
  foot 266.2
Lightwood's disease or syndrome (renal tubular acidosis) 588.89
Lignac's disease (cystinosis) 270.0
Lignac (-de Toni) (-Fanconi) (-Debré) syndrome (cystinosis) 270.0
Lignac (-Fanconi) syndrome (cystinosis) 270.0
Ligneous thyroiditis 245.3
Likoff's syndrome (angina in menopausal women) 413.9
Limb - *see* condition
Limitation of joint motion (*see also* Stiffness, joint) 719.5●
  sacroiliac 724.6
Limit dextrinosis 271.0
Limited
  cardiac reserve - *see* Disease, heart
  duction, eye NEC 378.63
  mandibular range of motion 524.52
Lindau's disease (retinocerebral angiomatosis) 759.6
Lindau (-von Hippel) disease (angiomatosis retinocerebellosa) 759.6
Linea corneae senilis 371.41
Lines
  Beau's (transverse furrows on fingernails) 703.8
  Harris' 733.91
  Hudson-Stähli 371.11
  Stähli's 371.11
Lingua
  geographical 529.1
  nigra (villosa) 529.3
  plicata 529.5
    congenital 750.13
  tylosis 528.6
Lingual (tongue) - *see also* condition
  thyroid 759.2
Linitis (gastric) 535.4●
  plastica (M8142/3) 151.9
Lioderma essentialis (cum melanosis et telangiectasia) 757.33
Lip - *see also* condition
  biting 528.9
Lipalgia 272.8
Lipedema - *see* Edema

Lipemia (*see also* Hyperlipidemia) 272.4
  retina, retinalis 272.3
Lipidosis 272.7
  cephalin 272.7
  cerebral (infantile) (juvenile) (late) 330.1
  cerebroretinal 330.1 [*362.71*]
  cerebroside 272.7
  cerebrospinal 272.7
  chemically-induced 272.7
  cholesterol 272.7
  diabetic 250.8● [*272.7*]
    due to secondary diabetes 249.8● [*272.7*]
  dystopic (hereditary) 272.7
  glycolipid 272.7
  hepatosplenomegalic 272.3
  hereditary, dystopic 272.7
  sulfatide 330.0
Lipoadenoma (M8324/0 - *see* Neoplasm, by site, benign
Lipoblastoma (M8881/0) - *see* Lipoma, by site
Lipoblastomatosis (M8881/0) - *see* Lipoma, by site
Lipochondrodystrophy 277.5
Lipochrome histiocytosis (familial) 288.1
Lipodystrophia progressiva 272.6
Lipodystrophy (progressive) 272.6
  insulin 272.6
  intestinal 040.2
  mesenteric 567.82
Lipofibroma (M8851/0) - *see* Lipoma, by site
Lipoglycoproteinosis 272.8
Lipogranuloma, sclerosing 709.8
Lipogranulomatosis (disseminated) 272.8
  kidney 272.8
Lipoid - *see also* condition
  histiocytosis 272.7
    essential 272.7
  nephrosis (*see also* Nephrosis) 581.3
  proteinosis of Urbach 272.8
Lipoidemia (*see also* Hyperlipidemia) 272.4
Lipoidosis (*see also* Lipidosis) 272.7
Lipoma (M8850/0) 214.9
  breast (skin) 214.1
  face 214.0
  fetal (M8881/0) - *see also* Lipoma, by site
    fat cell (M8880/0) - *see* Lipoma, by site
  infiltrating (M8856/0) - *see* Lipoma, by site
  intra-abdominal 214.3
  intramuscular (M8856/0) - *see* Lipoma, by site
  intrathoracic 214.2
  kidney 214.3
  mediastinum 214.2
  muscle 214.8
  peritoneum 214.3
  retroperitoneum 214.3
  skin 214.1
    face 214.0
  spermatic cord 214.4
  spindle cell (M8857/0) - *see* Lipoma, by site
  stomach 214.3
  subcutaneous tissue 214.1
    face 214.0
  thymus 214.2
  thyroid gland 214.2

Lipomatosis (dolorosa) 272.8
  epidural 214.8
  fetal (M8881/0) - *see* Lipoma, by site
  Launois-Bensaude's 272.8
Lipomyohemangioma (M8860/0)
  specified site - *see* Neoplasm, connective tissue, benign
  unspecified site 223.0
Lipomyoma (M8860/0)
  specified site - *see* Neoplasm, connective tissue, benign
  unspecified site 223.0
Lipomyxoma (M8852/0) - *see* Lipoma, by site
Lipomyxosarcoma (M8852/3) - *see* Neoplasm, connective tissue, malignant
Lipophagocytosis 289.89
Lipoproteinemia (alpha) 272.4
  broad-beta 272.2
  floating-beta 272.2
  hyper-pre-beta 272.1
Lipoproteinosis (Rossle-Urbach-Wiethe) 272.8
Liposarcoma (M8850/3) - *see also* Neoplasm, connective tissue, malignant
  differentiated type (M8851/3) - *see* Neoplasm, connective tissue, malignant
  embryonal (M8852/3) - *see* Neoplasm, connective tissue, malignant
  mixed type (M8855/3) - *see* Neoplasm, connective tissue, malignant
  myxoid (M8852/3) - *see* Neoplasm, connective tissue, malignant
  pleomorphic (M8854/3) - *see* Neoplasm, connective tissue, malignant
  round cell (M8853/3) - *see* Neoplasm, connective tissue, malignant
  well differentiated type (M8851/3) - *see* Neoplasm, connective tissue, malignant
Liposynovitis prepatellaris 272.8
Lipping
  cervix 622.0
  spine (*see also* Spondylosis) 721.90
  vertebra (*see also* Spondylosis) 721.90
Lip pits (mucus), congenital 750.25
Lipschütz disease or ulcer 616.50
Lipuria 791.1
  bilharziasis 120.0
Liquefaction, vitreous humor 379.21
Lisping 307.9
Lissauer's paralysis 094.1
Lissencephalia, lissencephaly 742.2
Listerellose 027.0
Listeriose 027.0
Listeriosis 027.0
  congenital 771.2
  fetal 771.2
  suspected fetal damage affecting management of pregnancy 655.4●
Listlessness 780.79
Lithemia 790.6
Lithiasis - *see also* Calculus
  hepatic (duct) - *see* Choledocholithiasis
  urinary 592.9
Lithopedion 779.9
  affecting management of pregnancy 656.8●

◀ New   ◀ Revised   ~~deleted~~ Deleted   ● Use Additional Digit(s)   Omit code

Lithosis (occupational) 502
  with tuberculosis - *see* Tuberculosis,
    pulmonary
Lithuria 791.9
Litigation V62.5
Little
  league elbow 718.82
  stroke syndrome 435.9
Little's disease - *see* Palsy, cerebral
Littre's
  gland - *see* condition
  hernia - *see* Hernia, Littre's
Littritis (*see also* Urethritis) 597.89
Livedo 782.61
  annularis 782.61
  racemose 782.61
  reticularis 782.61
Live flesh 781.0
Liver - *see also* condition
  donor V59.6
Livida, asphyxia
  newborn 768.6
Living
  alone V60.3
    with handicapped person V60.4
Lloyd's syndrome 258.1
Loa loa 125.2
Loasis 125.2
Lobe, lobar - *see* condition
Lobo's disease or blastomycosis
    116.2
Lobomycosis 116.2
Lobotomy syndrome 310.0
Lobstein's disease (brittle bones and
    blue sclera) 756.51
Lobster-claw hand 755.58
Lobulation (congenital) - *see also*
    Anomaly, specified type NEC, by
    site
  kidney, fetal 753.3
  liver, abnormal 751.69
  spleen 759.0
Lobule, lobular - *see* condition
Local, localized - *see* condition
Locked bowel or intestine (*see also*
    Obstruction, intestine) 560.9
Locked-in state 344.81
Locked twins 660.5●
  affecting fetus or newborn 763.1
Locking
  joint (*see also* Derangement, joint)
    718.90
  knee 717.9
Lockjaw (*see also* Tetanus) 037
Locomotor ataxia (progressive) 094.0
Löffler's
  endocarditis 421.0
  eosinophilia or syndrome 518.3
  pneumonia 518.3
  syndrome (eosinophilic
    pneumonitis) 518.3
Löfgren's syndrome (sarcoidosis)
    135
Loiasis 125.2
  eyelid 125.2 *[373.6]*
Loneliness V62.89
Lone Star fever 082.8
Long labor 662.1●
  affecting fetus or newborn 763.89
  first stage 662.0●
  second stage 662.2●
Longitudinal stripes or grooves, nails
    703.8
  congenital 757.5

Long-term (current) (prophylactic) drug
    use V58.69 ◀▥
  antibiotics V58.62
  anticoagulants V58.61
  anti-inflammatories, non-steroidal
    (NSAID) V58.64
  antiplatelets/antithrombotics V58.63
  aspirin V58.66
  high-risk medications NEC V58.69
  insulin V58.67
  methadone V58.69
  opiate analgesic V58.69
  pain killers V58.69
    anti-inflammatories, non-steroidal
      (NSAID) V58.64
    aspirin V58.66
  steroids V58.65
  tamoxifen V07.51
Loop
  intestine (*see also* Volvulus) 560.2
  intrascleral nerve 379.29
  vascular on papilla (optic) 743.57
Loose - *see also* condition
  body
    in tendon sheath 727.82
    joint 718.10
      ankle 718.17
      elbow 718.12
      foot 718.17
      hand 718.14
      hip 718.15
      knee 717.6
      multiple sites 718.19
      pelvic region 718.15
      prosthetic implant - *see*
        Complications, mechanical
      shoulder (region) 718.11
      specified site NEC 718.18
      wrist 718.13
    cartilage (joint) (*see also* Loose, body,
      joint) 718.1●
      knee 717.6
    facet (vertebral) 724.9
    prosthetic implant - *see* Complications,
      mechanical
    sesamoid, joint (*see also* Loose, body,
      joint) 718.1●
    tooth, teeth 525.8
Loosening epiphysis 732.9
Looser (-Debray)-Milkman syndrome
    (osteomalacia with
    pseudofractures) 268.2
Lop ear (deformity) 744.29
Lorain's disease or syndrome (pituitary
    dwarfism) 253.3
Lorain-Levi syndrome (pituitary
    dwarfism) 253.3
Lordosis (acquired) (postural) 737.20
  congenital 754.2
  due to or associated with
    Charcôt-Marie-Tooth disease 356.1
      [737.42]
    mucopolysaccharidosis 277.5
      [737.42]
    neurofibromatosis 237.71 *[737.42]*
    osteitis
      deformans 731.0 *[737.42]*
      fibrosa cystica 252.01 *[737.42]*
    osteoporosis (*see also* Osteoporosis)
      733.00 *[737.42]*
    poliomyelitis (*see also* Poliomyelitis)
      138 *[737.42]*
    tuberculosis (*see also* Tuberculosis)
      015.0● *[737.42]*

Lordosis (*Continued*)
  late effect of rickets 268.1 *[737.42]*
  postlaminectomy 737.21
  postsurgical NEC 737.22
  rachitic 268.1 *[737.42]*
  specified NEC 737.29
  tuberculous (*see also* Tuberculosis)
    015.0● *[737.42]*
Loss
  appetite 783.0
    hysterical 300.11
    nonorganic origin 307.59
    psychogenic 307.59
  blood - *see* Hemorrhage
  central vision 368.41
  consciousness 780.09
    transient 780.2
  control, sphincter, rectum 787.60 ◀▥
    nonorganic origin 307.7
  ear ossicle, partial 385.24
  elasticity, skin 782.8
  extremity or member, traumatic,
    current - *see* Amputation,
    traumatic
  fluid (acute) 276.50
    with
      hypernatremia 276.0
      hyponatremia 276.1
    fetus or newborn 775.5
  hair 704.00
  hearing - *see also* Deafness
    central 389.14
    conductive (air) 389.00
      with sensorineural hearing loss
        389.20
        bilateral 389.22
        unilateral 389.21
      bilateral 389.06
      combined types 389.08
      external ear 389.01
      inner ear 389.04
      middle ear 389.03
      multiple types 389.08
      tympanic membrane 389.02
      unilateral 389.05
    mixed conductive and sensorineural
      389.20
      bilateral 389.22
      unilateral 389.21
    mixed type 389.20
      bilateral 389.22
      unilateral 389.21
    nerve
      bilateral 389.12
      unilateral 389.13
    neural
      bilateral 389.12
      unilateral 389.13
    noise-induced 388.12
    perceptive NEC (*see also* Loss,
      hearing, sensorineural)
      389.10
    sensorineural 389.10
      with conductive hearing loss
        389.20
        bilateral 389.22
        unilateral 389.21
      asymmetrical 389.16
      bilateral 389.18
      central 389.14
      neural
        bilateral 389.12
        unilateral 389.13

Loss (Continued)
  hearing (Continued)
    sensorineural (Continued)
      sensory
        bilateral 389.11
          unilateral 389.17
        unilateral 389.15
      sensory
        bilateral 389.11
        unilateral 389.17
    specified type NEC 389.8
    sudden NEC 388.2
  height 781.91
  labyrinthine reactivity (unilateral) 386.55
    bilateral 386.56
  memory (see also Amnesia) 780.93
    mild, following organic brain
      damage 310.8
  mind (see also Psychosis) 298.9
  occlusal vertical dimension 524.37
  organ or part - see Absence, by site,
    acquired
  recurrent pregnancy - see Pregnancy,
    management affected by,
    abortion, habitual ◄
  sensation 782.0
  sense of
    smell (see also Disturbance,
      sensation) 781.1
    taste (see also Disturbance, sensation)
      781.1
    touch (see also Disturbance,
      sensation) 781.1
  sight (acquired) (complete)
    (congenital) - see Blindness
  spinal fluid
    headache 349.0
  substance of
    bone (see also Osteoporosis) 733.00
    cartilage 733.99
      ear 380.32
    vitreous (humor) 379.26
  tooth, teeth
    acquired 525.10
      due to
        caries 525.13
        extraction 525.10
        periodontal disease 525.12
        specified NEC 525.19
        trauma 525.11
  vision, visual (see also Blindness) 369.9
    both eyes (see also Blindness, both
      eyes) 369.3
    complete (see also Blindness, both
      eyes) 369.00
    one eye 369.8
      sudden 368.11
      transient 368.12
  vitreous 379.26
  voice (see also Aphonia) 784.41
  weight (cause unknown) 783.21
Lou Gehrig's disease 335.20
Louis-Bar syndrome (ataxia-
  telangiectasia) 334.8
Louping ill 063.1
Lousiness - see Lice
Low
  back syndrome 724.2
  basal metabolic rate (BMR) 794.7
  birthweight 765.1●
    extreme (less than 1000 grams) 765.0●
    for gestational age 764.0●
    status (see also Status, low birth
      weight) V21.30

Low (Continued)
  bladder compliance 596.52
  blood pressure (see also Hypotension)
    458.9
    reading (incidental) (isolated)
      (nonspecific) 796.3
  cardiac reserve - see Disease, heart
  compliance bladder 596.52
  frequency deafness - see Disorder,
    hearing
  function - see also Hypofunction
    kidney (see also Disease, renal) 593.9
    liver 573.9
  hemoglobin 285.9
  implantation, placenta - see Placenta,
    previa
  insertion, placenta - see Placenta, previa
  lying
    kidney 593.0
    organ or site, congenital - see
      Malposition, congenital
    placenta - see Placenta, previa
  output syndrome (cardiac) (see also
    Failure, heart) 428.9
  platelets (blood) (see also
    Thrombocytopenia) 287.5
  reserve, kidney (see also Disease, renal)
    593.9
  risk
    human papillomavirus (HPV) DNA
      test positive
        anal 796.79
        cervical 795.09
        vaginal 795.19
  salt syndrome 593.9
  tension glaucoma 365.12
  vision 369.9
    both eyes 369.20
    one eye 369.70
Lowe (-Terrey-MacLachlan) syndrome
  (oculocerebrorenal dystrophy)
  270.8
Lower extremity - see condition
Lown (-Ganong)-Levine syndrome (short
  P-R interval, normal QRS complex,
  and paroxysmal supraventricular
  tachycardia) 426.81
LSD reaction (see also Abuse, drugs,
  nondependent) 305.3●
L-shaped kidney 753.3
Lucas-Championnière disease (fibrinous
  bronchitis) 466.0
Lucey-Driscoll syndrome (jaundice due
  to delayed conjugation) 774.30
Ludwig's
  angina 528.3
  disease (submaxillary cellulitis) 528.3
Lues (venerea), luetic - see Syphilis
Luetscher's syndrome (dehydration)
  276.51
Lumbago 724.2
  due to displacement, intervertebral
    disc 722.10
Lumbalgia 724.2
  due to displacement, intervertebral
    disc 722.10
Lumbar - see condition
Lumbarization, vertebra 756.15
Lumbermen's itch 133.8
Lump - see also Mass
  abdominal 789.3●
  breast 611.72
  chest 786.6
  epigastric 789.3●

Lump (Continued)
  head 784.2
  kidney 753.3
  liver 789.1
  lung 786.6
  mediastinal 786.6
  neck 784.2
  nose or sinus 784.2
  pelvic 789.3●
  skin 782.2
  substernal 786.6
  throat 784.2
  umbilicus 789.3●
Lunacy (see also Psychosis) 298.9
Lunatomalacia 732.3
Lung - see also condition
  donor V59.8
  drug addict's 417.8
  mainliners' 417.8
  vanishing 492.0
Lupoid (miliary) of Boeck 135
Lupus 710.0
  anticoagulant 289.81
  Cazenave's (erythematosus) 695.4
  discoid (local) 695.4
  disseminated 710.0
  erythematodes (discoid) (local) 695.4
  erythematosus (discoid) (local) 695.4
    disseminated 710.0
    eyelid 373.34
    systemic 710.0
      with
        encephalitis 710.0 [323.81]
        lung involvement 710.0
          [517.8]
      inhibitor (presence of) 286.5
  exedens 017.0●
  eyelid (see also Tuberculosis) 017.0●
    [373.4]
  Hilliard's 017.0●
  hydralazine
    correct substance properly
      administered 695.4
    overdose or wrong substance given
      or taken 972.6
  miliaris disseminatus faciei 017.0●
  nephritis 710.0 [583.81]
    acute 710.0 [580.81]
    chronic 710.0 [582.81]
  nontuberculous, not disseminated
    695.4
  pernio (Besnier) 135
  tuberculous (see also Tuberculosis)
    017.0●
    eyelid (see also Tuberculosis) 017.0●
      [373.4]
  vulgaris 017.0●
Luschka's joint disease 721.90
Luteinoma (M8610/0) 220
Lutembacher's disease or syndrome
  (atrial septal defect with mitral
  stenosis) 745.5
Luteoma (M8610/0) 220
Lutz-Miescher disease (elastosis
  perforans serpiginosa) 701.1
Lutz-Splendore-de Almeida disease
  (Brazilian blastomycosis) 116.1
Luxatio
  bulbi due to birth injury 767.8
  coxae congenita (see also Dislocation,
    hip, congenital) 754.30
  erecta - see Dislocation, shoulder
  imperfecta - see Sprain, by site
  perinealis - see Dislocation, hip

◄ New ◄||| Revised ~~deleted~~ Deleted ● Use Additional Digit(s) ▓ Omit code

Luxation - *see also* Dislocation, by site
  eyeball 360.81
    due to birth injury 767.8
    lateral 376.36
  genital organs (external) NEC - *see*
    Wound, open, genital organs
  globe (eye) 360.81
    lateral 376.36
  lacrimal gland (postinfectional) 375.16
  lens (old) (partial) 379.32
    congenital 743.37
      syphilitic 090.49 [379.32]
    Marfan's disease 090.49
    spontaneous 379.32
  penis - *see* Wound, open, penis
  scrotum - *see* Wound, open, scrotum
  testis - *see* Wound, open, testis
L-xyloketosuria 271.8
Lycanthropy (*see also* Psychosis) 298.9
Lyell's disease or syndrome (toxic
    epidermal necrolysis) 695.15
  due to drug
    correct substance properly
      administered 695.15
    overdose or wrong substance given
      or taken 977.9
      specified drug - *see* Table of
        Drugs and Chemicals
Lyme disease 088.81
Lymph
  gland or node - *see* condition
  scrotum (*see also* Infestation, filarial)
    125.9
Lymphadenitis 289.3
  with
    abortion - *see* Abortion, by type,
      with sepsis
    ectopic pregnancy (*see also*
      categories 633.0–633.9)
      639.0
    molar pregnancy (*see also* categories
      630–632) 639.0
  acute 683
    mesenteric 289.2
  any site, except mesenteric 289.3
    acute 683
    chronic 289.1
    mesenteric (acute) (chronic)
      (nonspecific) (subacute)
      289.2
    subacute 289.1
      mesenteric 289.2
  breast, puerperal, postpartum
    675.2●
  chancroidal (congenital) 099.0
  chronic 289.1
    mesenteric 289.2
  dermatopathic 695.89
  due to
    anthracosis (occupational) 500
    Brugia (Wuchereria) malayi
      125.1
    diphtheria (toxin) 032.89
    lymphogranuloma venereum
      099.1
    Wuchereria bancrofti 125.0
  following
    abortion 639.0
    ectopic or molar pregnancy
      639.0
  generalized 289.3
  gonorrheal 098.89
  granulomatous 289.1
  infectional 683

Lymphadenitis (*Continued*)
  mesenteric (acute) (chronic)
    (nonspecific) (subacute) 289.2
    due to Bacillus typhi 002.0
    tuberculous (*see also* Tuberculosis)
      014.8●
  mycobacterial 031.8
  purulent 683
  pyogenic 683
  regional 078.3
  septic 683
  streptococcal 683
  subacute, unspecified site 289.1
  suppurative 683
  syphilitic (early) (secondary) 091.4
    late 095.8
  tuberculous - *see* Tuberculosis, lymph
    gland
  venereal 099.1
Lymphadenoid goiter 245.2
Lymphadenopathy (general) 785.6
  due to toxoplasmosis (acquired)
    130.7
    congenital (active) 771.2
Lymphadenopathy-associated virus
    (disease) (illness) (infection) - *see*
    Human immunodeficiency virus
    (disease) (illness) (infection)
Lymphadenosis 785.6
  acute 075
Lymphangiectasis 457.1
  conjunctiva 372.89
  postinfectional 457.1
  scrotum 457.1
Lymphangiectatic elephantiasis,
    nonfilarial 457.1
Lymphangioendothelioma (M9170/0)
    228.1
  malignant (M9170/3) - *see* Neoplasm,
    connective tissue, malignant
Lymphangioma (M9170/0) 228.1
  capillary (M9171/0) 228.1
  cavernous (M9172/0) 228.1
  cystic (M9173/0) 228.1
  malignant (M9170/3) - *see* Neoplasm,
    connective tissue, malignant
Lymphangiomyoma (M9174/0) 228.1
Lymphangiomyomatosis (M9174/1) - *see*
    Neoplasm, connective tissue,
    uncertain behavior
Lymphangiosarcoma (M9170/3) - *see*
    Neoplasm, connective tissue,
    malignant
Lymphangitis 457.2
  with
    abortion - *see* Abortion, by type,
      with sepsis
    abscess - *see* Abscess, by site
    cellulitis - *see* Abscess, by site
    ectopic pregnancy (*see also*
      categories 633.0–633.9)
      639.0
    molar pregnancy (*see also* categories
      630–632) 639.0
  acute (with abscess or cellulitis)
    682.9
    specified site - *see* Abscess, by site
  breast, puerperal, postpartum
    675.2●
  chancroidal 099.0
  chronic (any site) 457.2
  due to
    Brugia (Wuchereria) malayi 125.1
    Wuchereria bancrofti 125.0

Lymphangitis (*Continued*)
  following
    abortion 639.0
    ectopic or molar pregnancy
      639.0
  gangrenous 457.2
  penis
    acute 607.2
    gonococcal (acute) 098.0
      chronic or duration of 2 months
        or more 098.2
  puerperal, postpartum,
    childbirth 670.8●
  strumous, tuberculous (*see also*
    Tuberculosis) 017.2●
  subacute (any site) 457.2
  tuberculous - *see* Tuberculosis, lymph
    gland
Lymphatic (vessel) - *see* condition
Lymphatism 254.8
  scrofulous (*see also* Tuberculosis)
    017.2●
Lymphectasia 457.1
Lymphedema (*see also* Elephantiasis)
    457.1
  acquired (chronic) 457.1
  chronic hereditary 757.0
  congenital 757.0
  idiopathic hereditary 757.0
  praecox 457.1
  secondary 457.1
  surgical NEC 997.99
    postmastectomy (syndrome) 457.0
Lymph-hemangioma (M9120/0) - *see*
    Hemangioma, by site
Lymphoblastic - *see* condition
Lymphoblastoma (diffuse) (M9630/3)
    200.1●
  giant follicular (M9690/3) 202.0●
  macrofollicular (M9690/3) 202.0●
Lymphoblastosis, acute benign 075
Lymphocele 457.8
Lymphocythemia 288.51
Lymphocytic - *see also* condition
  chorioencephalitis (acute) (serous)
    049.0
  choriomeningitis (acute) (serous)
    049.0
Lymphocytoma (diffuse) (malignant)
    (M9620/3) 200.1●
Lymphocytomatosis (M9620/3) 200.1●
Lymphocytopenia 288.51
Lymphocytosis (symptomatic) 288.61
  infectious (acute) 078.89
Lymphoepithelioma (M8082/3) - *see*
    Neoplasm, by site, malignant
Lymphogranuloma (malignant)
    (M9650/3) 201.9●
  inguinale 099.1
  venereal (any site) 099.1
    with stricture of rectum 099.1
  venereum 099.1
Lymphogranulomatosis (malignant)
    (M9650/3) 201.9●
  benign (Boeck's sarcoid) (Schaumann's)
    135
  Hodgkin's (M9650/3) 201.9●
Lymphohistiocytosis, familial
    hemophagocytic 288.4
Lymphoid - *see* condition
Lympholeukoblastoma (M9850/3)
    207.8●
Lympholeukosarcoma (M9850/3)
    207.8●

Lymphoma (malignant) (M9590/3) 202.8●

> Note: Use the following fifth-digit subclassification with categories 200–202:
>
> 0 unspecified site, extranodal and solid organ sites
> 1 lymph nodes of head, face, and neck
> 2 intrathoracic lymph nodes
> 3 intra-abdominal lymph nodes
> 4 lymph nodes of axilla and upper limb
> 5 lymph nodes of inguinal region and lower limb
> 6 intrapelvic lymph nodes
> 7 spleen
> 8 lymph nodes of multiple sites

benign (M9590/0) - *see* Neoplasm, by site, benign
Burkitt's type (lymphoblastic) (undifferentiated) (M9750/3) 200.2●
Castleman's (mediastinal lymph node hyperplasia) 785.6
centroblastic-centrocytic
  diffuse (M9614/3) 202.8●
  follicular (M9692/3) 202.0●
centroblastic type (diffuse) (M9632/3) 202.8●
  follicular (M9697/3) 202.0●
centrocytic (M9622/3) 202.8●
compound (M9613/3) 200.8●
convoluted cell type (lymphoblastic) (M9602/3) 202.8●
diffuse NEC (M9590/3) 202.8●
  large B cell 202.8●
follicular (giant) (M9690/3) 202.0●
  center cell (diffuse) (M9615/3) 202.8●
  cleaved (diffuse) (M9623/3) 202.8●
    follicular (M9695/3) 202.0●
  non-cleaved (diffuse) (M9633/3) 202.8●
    follicular (M9698/3) 202.0●
  centroblastic-centrocytic (M9692/3) 202.0●
  centroblastic type (M9697/3) 202.0●
  large cell 202.0●
  lymphocytic
    intermediate differentiation (M9694/3) 202.0●
    poorly differentiated (M9696/3) 202.0●
  mixed (cell type) (lymphocytic-histiocytic) (small cell and large cell) (M9691/3) 202.0●
germinocytic (M9622/3) 202.8●
giant, follicular or follicle (M9690/3) 202.0●

Lymphoma (*Continued*)
histiocytic (diffuse) (M9640/3) 200.0●
  nodular (M9642/3) 200.0●
  pleomorphic cell type (M9641/3) 200.0●
Hodgkin's (M9650/3) (*see also* Disease, Hodgkin's) 201.9●
immunoblastic (type) (M9612/3) 200.8●
large cell (M9640/3) 200.7●
  anaplastic 200.6●
  nodular (M9642/3) 202.0●
  pleomorphic cell type (M9641/3) 200.0●
lymphoblastic (diffuse) (M9630/3) 200.1●
  Burkitt's type (M9750/3) 200.2●
  convoluted cell type (M9602/3) 202.8●
lymphocytic (cell type) (diffuse) (M9620/3) 200.1●
  with plasmacytoid differentiation, diffuse (M9611/3) 200.8●
  intermediate differentiation (diffuse) (M9621/3) 200.1●
    follicular (M9694/3) 202.0●
    nodular (M9694/3) 202.0●
  nodular (M9690/3) 202.0●
  poorly differentiated (diffuse) (M9630/3) 200.1●
    follicular (M9696/3) 202.0●
    nodular (M9696/3) 202.0●
  well differentiated (diffuse) (M9620/3) 200.1●
    follicular (M9693/3) 202.0●
    nodular (M9693/3) 202.0●
lymphocytic-histiocytic, mixed (diffuse) (M9613/3) 200.8●
  follicular (M9691/3) 202.0●
  nodular (M9691/3) 202.0●
lymphoplasmacytoid type (M9611/3) 200.8●
lymphosarcoma type (M9610/3) 200.1●
macrofollicular (M9690/3) 202.0●
mantle cell 200.4●
marginal zone 200.3●
  extranodal B-cell 200.3●
  nodal B-cell 200.3●
  splenic B-cell 200.3●
mixed cell type (diffuse) (M9613/3) 200.8●
  follicular (M9691/3) 202.0●
  nodular (M9691/3) 202.0●
nodular (M9690/3) 202.0●
  histiocytic (M9642/3) 200.0●
  lymphocytic (M9690/3) 202.0●
    intermediate differentiation (M9694/3) 202.0●
    poorly differentiated (M9696/3) 202.0●
  mixed (cell type) (lymphocytic-histiocytic) (small cell and large cell) (M9691/3) 202.0●
non-Hodgkin's type NEC (M9591/3) 202.8●

Lymphoma (*Continued*)
peripheral T-cell 202.7●
primary central nervous system 200.5●
reticulum cell (type) (M9640/3) 200.0●
small cell and large cell, mixed (diffuse) (M9613/3) 200.8●
  follicular (M9691/3) 202.0●
  nodular (9691/3) 202.0●
stem cell (type) (M9601/3) 202.8●
T-cell 202.1●
  peripheral 202.7●
undifferentiated (cell type) (non-Burkitt's) (M9600/3) 202.8●
  Burkitt's type (M9750/3) 200.2●
Lymphomatosis (M9590/3) - *see also* Lymphoma
  granulomatous 099.1
Lymphopathia
  venereum 099.1
  veneris 099.1
Lymphopenia 288.51
  familial 279.2
Lymphoreticulosis, benign (of inoculation) 078.3
Lymphorrhea 457.8
Lymphosarcoma (M9610/3) 200.1●
  diffuse (M9610/3) 200.1●
    with plasmacytoid differentiation (M9611/3) 200.8●
    lymphoplasmacytic (M9611/3) 200.8●
  follicular (giant) (M9690/3) 202.0●
    lymphoblastic (M9696/3) 202.0●
    lymphocytic, intermediate differentiation (M9694/3) 202.0●
    mixed cell type (M9691/3) 202.0●
  giant follicular (M9690/3) 202.0●
  Hodgkin's (M9650/3) 201.9●
  immunoblastic (M9612/3) 200.8●
  lymphoblastic (diffuse) (M9630/3) 200.1●
    follicular (M9696/3) 202.0●
    nodular (M9696/3) 202.0●
  lymphocytic (diffuse) (M9620/3) 200.1●
    intermediate differentiation (diffuse) (M9621/3) 200.1●
      follicular (M9694/3) 202.0●
      nodular (M9694/3) 202.0●
  mixed cell type (diffuse) (M9613/3) 200.8●
    follicular (M9691/3) 202.0●
    nodular (M9691/3) 202.0●
  nodular (M9690/3) 202.0●
    lymphoblastic (M9696/3) 202.0●
    lymphocytic, intermediate differentiation (M9694/3) 202.0●
    mixed cell type (M9691/3) 202.0●
  prolymphocytic (M9631/3) 200.1●
  reticulum cell (M9640/3) 200.0●
Lymphostasis 457.8
Lypemania (*see also* Melancholia) 296.2●
Lyssa 071

M

Macacus ear 744.29
Maceration
  fetus (cause not stated) 779.9
  wet feet, tropical (syndrome) 991.4
Machado-Joseph disease 334.8
Machupo virus hemorrhagic fever 078.7
Macleod's syndrome (abnormal
  transradiancy, one lung) 492.8
Macrocephalia, macrocephaly 756.0
Macrocheilia (congenital) 744.81
Macrochilia (congenital) 744.81
Macrocolon (congenital) 751.3
Macrocornea 743.41
  associated with buphthalmos 743.22
Macrocytic - see condition
Macrocytosis 289.89
Macrodactylia, macrodactylism (fingers)
  (thumbs) 755.57
  toes 755.65
Macrodontia 520.2
Macroencephaly 742.4
Macrogenia 524.05
Macrogenitosomia (female) (male)
  (praecox) 255.2
Macrogingivae 523.8
Macroglobulinemia (essential)
  (idiopathic) (monoclonal) (primary)
  (syndrome) (Waldenström's) 273.3
Macroglossia (congenital) 750.15
  acquired 529.8
Macrognathia, macrognathism
  (congenital) 524.00
  mandibular 524.02
    alveolar 524.72
  maxillary 524.01
    alveolar 524.71
Macrogyria (congenital) 742.4
Macrohydrocephalus (see also
  Hydrocephalus) 331.4
Macromastia (see also Hypertrophy,
  breast) 611.1
Macrophage activation syndrome 288.4
Macropsia 368.14
Macrosigmoid 564.7
  congenital 751.3
Macrospondylitis, acromegalic 253.0
Macrostomia (congenital) 744.83
Macrotia (external ear) (congenital)
  744.22
Macula
  cornea, corneal
    congenital 743.43
      interfering with vision 743.42
      interfering with central vision 371.03
      not interfering with central vision
        371.02
  degeneration (see also Degeneration,
    macula) 362.50
  hereditary (see also Dystrophy,
    retina) 362.70
  edema, cystoid 362.53
Maculae ceruleae 132.1
Macules and papules 709.8
Maculopathy, toxic 362.55
Madarosis 374.55
Madelung's
  deformity (radius) 755.54
  disease (lipomatosis) 272.8
  lipomatosis 272.8
Madness (see also Psychosis) 298.9
  myxedema (acute) 293.0
    subacute 293.1

Madura
  disease (actinomycotic) 039.9
    mycotic 117.4
  foot (actinomycotic) 039.4
    mycotic 117.4
Maduromycosis (actinomycotic) 039.9
  mycotic 117.4
Maffucci's syndrome (dyschondroplasia
  with hemangiomas) 756.4
Magenblase syndrome 306.4
Main en griffe (acquired) 736.06
  congenital 755.59
Maintenance
  chemotherapy regimen or treatment
    V58.11
  dialysis regimen or treatment
    extracorporeal (renal) V56.0
    peritoneal V56.8
    renal V56.0
  drug therapy or regimen
    chemotherapy, antineoplastic
      V58.11
    immunotherapy, antineoplastic
      V58.12
  external fixation NEC V54.89
  radiotherapy V58.0
  traction NEC V54.89
Majocchi's
  disease (purpura annularis
    telangiectodes) 709.1
  granuloma 110.6
Major - see condition
Mal
  cerebral (idiopathic) (see also Epilepsy)
    345.9●
  comital (see also Epilepsy) 345.9●
  de los pintos (see also Pinta) 103.9
  de Meleda 757.39
  de mer 994.6
  lie - see Presentation, fetal
  perforant (see also Ulcer, lower
    extremity) 707.15
Malabar itch 110.9
  beard 110.0
  foot 110.4
  scalp 110.0
Malabsorption 579.9
  calcium 579.8
  carbohydrate 579.8
  disaccharide 271.3
  drug-induced 579.8
  due to bacterial overgrowth 579.8
  fat 579.8
  folate, congenital 281.2
  galactose 271.1
  glucose-galactose (congenital) 271.3
  intestinal 579.9
  isomaltose 271.3
  lactose (hereditary) 271.3
  methionine 270.4
  monosaccharide 271.8
  postgastrectomy 579.3
  postsurgical 579.3
  protein 579.8
  sucrose (-isomaltose) (congenital)
    271.3
  syndrome 579.9
    postgastrectomy 579.3
    postsurgical 579.3
Malacia, bone 268.2
  juvenile (see also Rickets) 268.0
  Kienböck's (juvenile) (lunate) (wrist)
    732.3
    adult 732.8

Malacoplakia
  bladder 596.8
  colon 569.89
  pelvis (kidney) 593.89
  ureter 593.89
  urethra 599.84
Malacosteon 268.2
  juvenile (see also Rickets) 268.0
Maladaptation - see Maladjustment
Maladie de Roger 745.4
Maladjustment
  conjugal V61.10
    involving
      divorce V61.03
      estrangement V61.09
  educational V62.3
  family V61.9
    specified circumstance NEC
      V61.8
  marital V61.10
    involving
      divorce V61.03
      estrangement V61.09
  occupational V62.29
    current military deployment status
      V62.21
  simple, adult (see also Reaction,
    adjustment) 309.9
  situational acute (see also Reaction,
    adjustment) 309.9
  social V62.4
Malaise 780.79
Malakoplakia - see Malacoplakia
Malaria, malarial (fever) 084.6
  algid 084.9
  any type, with
    algid malaria 084.9
    blackwater fever 084.8
    fever
      blackwater 084.8
      hemoglobinuric (bilious)
        084.8
    hemoglobinuria, malarial 084.8
    hepatitis 084.9 [573.2]
    nephrosis 084.9 [581.81]
    pernicious complication NEC
      084.9
      cardiac 084.9
      cerebral 084.9
  cardiac 084.9
  carrier (suspected) of V02.9
  cerebral 084.9
  complicating pregnancy, childbirth,
    or puerperium 647.4●
  congenital 771.2
  congestion, congestive 084.6
    brain 084.9
  continued 084.0
  estivo-autumnal 084.0
  falciparum (malignant tertian)
    084.0
  hematinuria 084.8
  hematuria 084.8
  hemoglobinuria 084.8
  hemorrhagic 084.6
  induced (therapeutically) 084.7
    accidental - see Malaria, by type
  liver 084.9 [573.2]
  malariae (quartan) 084.2
  malignant (tertian) 084.0
  mixed infections 084.5
  monkey 084.4
  ovale 084.3
  pernicious, acute 084.0

Malaria, malarial *(Continued)*
  Plasmodium, P.
    falciparum 084.0
    malariae 084.2
    ovale 084.3
    vivax 084.1
  quartan 084.2
  quotidian 084.0
  recurrent 084.6
    induced (therapeutically) 084.7
      accidental - *see* Malaria, by type
  remittent 084.6
  specified types NEC 084.4
  spleen 084.6
  subtertian 084.0
  tertian (benign) 084.1
    malignant 084.0
  tropical 084.0
  typhoid 084.6
  vivax (benign tertian) 084.1
Malassez's disease (testicular cyst)
  608.89
Malassimilation 579.9
Maldescent, testis 752.51
Maldevelopment - *see also* Anomaly, by
  site
  brain 742.9
  colon 751.5
  hip (joint) 755.63
    congenital dislocation (*see also*
      Dislocation, hip, congenital)
      754.30
  mastoid process 756.0
  middle ear, except ossicles 744.03
    ossicles 744.04
  newborn (not malformation) 764.9●
  ossicles, ear 744.04
  spine 756.10
  toe 755.66
Male type pelvis 755.69
  with disproportion (fetopelvic) 653.2●
    affecting fetus or newborn 763.1
    causing obstructed labor 660.1●
      affecting fetus or newborn
      763.1
Malformation (congenital) - *see also*
  Anomaly
  bone 756.9
  bursa 756.9
  Chiari
    type I 348.4
    type II (*see also* Spina bifida)
      741.0●
    type III 742.0
    type IV 742.2
  circulatory system NEC 747.9
    specified type NEC 747.89
  cochlea 744.05
  digestive system NEC 751.9
    lower 751.5
    specified type NEC 751.8
    upper 750.9
  eye 743.9
  gum 750.9
  heart NEC 746.9
    specified type NEC 746.89
    valve 746.9
  internal ear 744.05
  joint NEC 755.9
    specified type NEC 755.8
  Mondini's (congenital) (malformation,
    cochlea) 744.05
  muscle 756.9
  nervous system (central) 742.9

Malformation *(Continued)*
  pelvic organs or tissues
    in pregnancy or childbirth 654.9●
      affecting fetus or newborn
      763.89
      causing obstructed labor 660.2●
        affecting fetus or newborn
        763.1
  placenta (*see also* Placenta, abnormal)
    656.7●
  respiratory organs 748.9
    specified type NEC 748.8
  Rieger's 743.44
  sense organs NEC 742.9
    specified type NEC 742.8
  skin 757.9
    specified type NEC 757.8
  spinal cord 742.9
  teeth, tooth NEC 520.9
  tendon 756.9
  throat 750.9
  umbilical cord (complicating delivery)
    663.9●
    affecting fetus or newborn 762.6
  umbilicus 759.9
  urinary system NEC 753.9
    specified type NEC 753.8
  venous - *see* Anomaly, vein
Malfunction - *see also* Dysfunction
  arterial graft 996.1
  cardiac pacemaker 996.01
  catheter device - *see* Complications,
    mechanical, catheter
  colostomy 569.62
    valve 569.62
  cystostomy 997.5
  device, implant, or graft NEC - *see*
    Complications, mechanical
  enteric stoma 569.62
  enterostomy 569.62
  esophagostomy 530.87
  gastroenteric 536.8
  gastrostomy 536.42
  ileostomy
    valve 569.62
  nephrostomy 997.5
  pacemaker - *see* Complications,
    mechanical, pacemaker
  prosthetic device, internal - *see*
    Complications, mechanical
  tracheostomy 519.02
  valve
    colostomy 569.62
    ileostomy 569.62
  vascular graft or shunt 996.1
Malgaigne's fracture (closed) 808.43
  open 808.53
Malherbe's
  calcifying epithelioma (M8110/0) - *see*
    Neoplasm, skin, benign
  tumor (M8110/0) - *see* Neoplasm, skin,
    benign
Malibu disease 919.8
  infected 919.9
Malignancy (M8000/3) - *see* Neoplasm,
  by site, malignant
Malignant - *see* condition
Malingerer, malingering V65.2
Mallet, finger (acquired) 736.1
  congenital 755.59
  late effect of rickets 268.1
Malleus 024
Mallory's bodies 034.1
Mallory-Weiss syndrome 530.7

Malnutrition (calorie) 263.9
  complicating pregnancy 648.9●
  degree
    first 263.1
    second 263.0
    third 262
    mild (protein) 263.1 ◀▥
    moderate (protein) 263.0 ◀▥
    severe 261
      protein-calorie 262
  fetus 764.2●
    "light-for-dates" 764.1●
  following gastrointestinal surgery 579.3
  intrauterine or fetal 764.2●
    fetus or infant "light-for-dates"
      764.1●
  lack of care, or neglect (child) (infant)
    995.52
    adult 995.84
  malignant 260
  mild (protein) 263.1 ◀▥
  moderate (protein) 263.0 ◀▥
  protein 260
  protein-calorie 263.9
    mild 263.1 ◀
    moderate 263.0 ◀
    severe 262
    specified type NEC 263.8
  severe 261
    protein-calorie NEC 262
Malocclusion (teeth) 524.4
  angle's class I 524.21
  angle's class II 524.22
  angle's class III 524.23
  due to
    abnormal swallowing 524.59
    accessory teeth (causing crowding)
      524.31
    dentofacial abnormality NEC 524.89
    impacted teeth (causing crowding)
      520.6
    missing teeth 524.30
    mouth breathing 524.59
    sleep postures 524.59
    supernumerary teeth (causing
      crowding) 524.31
    thumb sucking 524.59
    tongue, lip, or finger habits 524.59
  temporomandibular (joint) 524.69
Malposition
  cardiac apex (congenital) 746.87
  cervix - *see* Malposition, uterus
  congenital
    adrenal (gland) 759.1
    alimentary tract 751.8
      lower 751.5
      upper 750.8
    aorta 747.21
    appendix 751.5
    arterial trunk 747.29
    artery (peripheral) NEC (*see also*
      Malposition, congenital,
      peripheral vascular system)
      747.60
      coronary 746.85
      pulmonary 747.3
    auditory canal 744.29
      causing impairment of hearing
      744.02
    auricle (ear) 744.29
      causing impairment of hearing
      744.02
      cervical 744.43
    biliary duct or passage 751.69
    bladder (mucosa) 753.8
      exteriorized or extroverted 753.5

◀ New   ◀▥ Revised   ~~deleted~~ Deleted   ● Use Additional Digit(s)   ▬ Omit code

Malposition (Continued)
  congenital (Continued)
    brachial plexus 742.8
    brain tissue 742.4
    breast 757.6
    bronchus 748.3
    cardiac apex 746.87
    cecum 751.5
    clavicle 755.51
    colon 751.5
    digestive organ or tract NEC 751.8
      lower 751.5
      upper 750.8
    ear (auricle) (external) 744.29
      ossicles 744.04
    endocrine (gland) NEC 759.2
    epiglottis 748.3
    Eustachian tube 744.24
    eye 743.8
    facial features 744.89
    fallopian tube 752.19
    finger(s) 755.59
      supernumerary 755.01
    foot 755.67
    gallbladder 751.69
    gastrointestinal tract 751.8
    genitalia, genital organ(s) or tract
      female 752.89
        external 752.49
        internal NEC 752.89
      male 752.89
        penis 752.69
        scrotal transposition 752.81
    glottis 748.3
    hand 755.59
    heart 746.87
      dextrocardia 746.87
        with complete transposition of
          viscera 759.3
    hepatic duct 751.69
    hip (joint) (see also Dislocation, hip,
      congenital) 754.30
    intestine (large) (small) 751.5
      with anomalous adhesions,
        fixation, or malrotation
        751.4
    joint NEC 755.8
    kidney 753.3
    larynx 748.3
    limb 755.8
      lower 755.69
      upper 755.59
    liver 751.69
    lung (lobe) 748.69
    nail(s) 757.5
    nerve 742.8
    nervous system NEC 742.8
    nose, nasal (septum) 748.1
    organ or site NEC - see Anomaly,
      specified type NEC, by site
    ovary 752.0
    pancreas 751.7
    parathyroid (gland) 759.2
    patella 755.64
    peripheral vascular system 747.60
      gastrointestinal 747.61
      lower limb 747.64
      renal 747.62
      specified NEC 747.69
      spinal 747.82
      upper limb 747.63
    pituitary (gland) 759.2
    respiratory organ or system NEC
      748.9

Malposition (Continued)
  congenital (Continued)
    rib (cage) 756.3
      supernumerary in cervical region
        756.2
    scapula 755.59
    shoulder 755.59
    spinal cord 742.59
    spine 756.19
    spleen 759.0
    sternum 756.3
    stomach 750.7
    symphysis pubis 755.69
    testis (undescended) 752.51
    thymus (gland) 759.2
    thyroid (gland) (tissue) 759.2
      cartilage 748.3
    toe(s) 755.66
      supernumerary 755.02
    tongue 750.19
    trachea 748.3
    uterus 752.39 ◄▥
    vein(s) (peripheral) NEC (see also
      Malposition, congenital,
      peripheral vascular system)
      747.60
      great 747.49
      portal 747.49
      pulmonary 747.49
    vena cava (inferior) (superior)
      747.49
  device, implant, or graft - see
    Complications, mechanical
  fetus NEC (see also Presentation, fetal)
    652.9●
    with successful version 652.1●
    affecting fetus or newborn 763.1
    before labor, affecting fetus or
      newborn 761.7
    causing obstructed labor 660.0●
    in multiple gestation (one fetus or
      more) 652.6●
      with locking 660.5●
      causing obstructed labor 660.0●
  gallbladder (see also Disease,
    gallbladder) 575.8
  gastrointestinal tract 569.89
    congenital 751.8
  heart (see also Malposition, congenital,
    heart) 746.87
  intestine 569.89
    congenital 751.5
  pelvic organs or tissues
    in pregnancy or childbirth 654.4●
      affecting fetus or newborn
        763.89
      causing obstructed labor 660.2●
        affecting fetus or newborn
          763.1
  placenta - see Placenta, previa
  stomach 537.89
    congenital 750.7
  tooth, teeth 524.30
    with impaction 520.6
  uterus (acquired) (acute) (adherent)
    (any degree) (asymptomatic)
    (postinfectional) (postpartal, old)
    621.6
    anteflexion or anteversion (see also
      Anteversion, uterus) 621.6
    congenital 752.39 ◄▥
    flexion 621.6
      lateral (see also Lateroversion,
        uterus) 621.6

Malposition (Continued)
  uterus (Continued)
    in pregnancy or childbirth 654.4●
      affecting fetus or newborn
        763.89
      causing obstructed labor 660.2●
        affecting fetus or newborn
          763.1
    inversion 621.6
    lateral (flexion) (version) (see also
      Lateroversion, uterus) 621.6
    lateroflexion (see also Lateroversion,
      uterus) 621.6
    lateroversion (see also Lateroversion,
      uterus) 621.6
    retroflexion or retroversion (see also
      Retroversion, uterus) 621.6
Malposture 729.90
Malpresentation, fetus (see also
  Presentation, fetal) 652.9●
Malrotation
  cecum 751.4
  colon 751.4
  intestine 751.4
  kidney 753.3
MALT (mucosa associated lymphoid
  tissue) 200.3●
Malt workers' lung 495.4
Malta fever (see also Brucellosis) 023.9
Maltosuria 271.3
Maltreatment (of)
  adult 995.80
    emotional 995.82
    multiple forms 995.85
    neglect (nutritional) 995.84
    physical 995.81
    psychological 995.82
    sexual 995.83
  child 995.50
    emotional 995.51
    multiple forms 995.59
    neglect (nutritional) 995.52
    physical 995.54
    shaken infant syndrome 995.55
    psychological 995.51
    sexual 995.53
  spouse (see also Maltreatment, adult)
    995.80
Malum coxae senilis 715.25
Malunion, fracture 733.81
Mammillitis (see also Mastitis) 611.0
  puerperal, postpartum 675.2●
Mammitis (see also Mastitis) 611.0
  puerperal, postpartum 675.2●
Mammographic
  calcification 793.89
  calculus 793.89
  microcalcification 793.81
Mammoplasia 611.1
Management
  contraceptive V25.9
    specified type NEC V25.8
  procreative V26.9
    specified type NEC V26.89
Mangled NEC (see also nature and site of
  injury) 959.9
Mania (monopolar) (see also Psychosis,
  affective) 296.0●
  alcoholic (acute) (chronic) 291.9
  Bell's - see Mania, chronic
  chronic 296.0●
    recurrent episode 296.1●
    single episode 296.0●
  compulsive 300.3

M

Mania *(Continued)*
  delirious (acute) 296.0●
    recurrent episode 296.1●
    single episode 296.0●
  epileptic *(see also* Epilepsy) 345.4●
  hysterical 300.10
  inhibited 296.89
  puerperal (after delivery) 296.0●
    recurrent episode 296.1●
    single episode 296.0●
  recurrent episode 296.1●
  senile 290.8
  single episode 296.0●
  stupor 296.89
  stuporous 296.89
  unproductive 296.89
Manic-depressive insanity, psychosis,
    reaction, or syndrome *(see also*
    Psychosis, affective) 296.80
  circular (alternating) 296.7
    currently
      depressed 296.5●
      episode unspecified 296.7
      hypomanic, previously depressed
        296.4●
      manic 296.4●
      mixed 296.6●
  depressed (type), depressive 296.2●
    atypical 296.82
    recurrent episode 296.3●
    single episode 296.2●
  hypomanic 296.0●
    recurrent episode 296.1●
    single episode 296.0●
  manic 296.0●
    atypical 296.81
    recurrent episode 296.1●
    single episode 296.0●
  mixed NEC 296.89
  perplexed 296.89
  stuporous 296.89
Manifestations, rheumatoid
  lungs 714.81
  pannus - *see* Arthritis, rheumatoid
  subcutaneous nodules - *see* Arthritis,
    rheumatoid
Mankowsky's syndrome (familial
    dysplastic osteopathy) 731.2
Mannoheptulosuria 271.8
Mannosidosis 271.8
Manson's
  disease (schistosomiasis) 120.1
  pyosis (pemphigus contagiosus) 684
  schistosomiasis 120.1
Mansonellosis 125.5
Manual - *see* condition
Maple bark disease 495.6
Maple bark-strippers' lung 495.6
Maple syrup (urine) disease or syndrome
  270.3
Marable's syndrome (celiac artery
    compression) 447.4
Marasmus 261
  brain 331.9
  due to malnutrition 261
  intestinal 569.89
  nutritional 261
  senile 797
  tuberculous NEC *(see also* Tuberculosis)
    011.9●
Marble
  bones 756.52
  skin 782.61
Marburg disease (virus) 078.89

March
  foot 733.94
  hemoglobinuria 283.2
Marchand multiple nodular hyperplasia
    (liver) 571.5
Marchesani (-Weill) syndrome
    (brachymorphism and ectopia
    lentis) 759.89
Marchiafava (-Bignami) disease or
    syndrome 341.8
Marchiafava-Micheli syndrome
    (paroxysmal nocturnal
    hemoglobinuria) 283.2
Marcus Gunn's syndrome (jaw-winking
    syndrome) 742.8
Marfan's
  congenital syphilis 090.49
  disease 090.49
  syndrome (arachnodactyly) 759.82
    meaning congenital syphilis
      090.49
    with luxation of lens 090.49
      [379.32]
Marginal
  implantation, placenta - *see* Placenta,
    previa
  placenta - *see* Placenta, previa
  sinus (hemorrhage) (rupture) 641.2●
    affecting fetus or newborn 762.1
Marie's
  cerebellar ataxia 334.2
  syndrome (acromegaly) 253.0
Marie-Bamberger disease or syndrome
    (hypertrophic) (pulmonary)
    (secondary) 731.2
  idiopathic (acropachyderma) 757.39
  primary (acropachyderma) 757.39
Marie-Charcôt-Tooth neuropathic
    atrophy, muscle 356.1
Marie-Strümpell arthritis or disease
    (ankylosing spondylitis) 720.0
Marihuana, marijuana
  abuse *(see also* Abuse, drugs,
    nondependent) 305.2●
  dependence *(see also* Dependence)
    304.3●
Marion's disease (bladder neck
    obstruction) 596.0
Marital conflict V61.10
Mark
  port wine 757.32
  raspberry 757.32
  strawberry 757.32
  stretch 701.3
  tattoo 709.09
Maroteaux-Lamy syndrome
    (mucopolysaccharidosis VI) 277.5
Marriage license examination V70.3
Marrow (bone)
  arrest 284.9
  megakaryocytic 287.30
  poor function 289.9
Marseilles fever 082.1
Marsh's disease (exophthalmic goiter)
    242.0●
Marshall's (hidrotic) ectodermal
    dysplasia 757.31
Marsh fever *(see also* Malaria) 084.6
Martin's disease 715.27
Martin-Albright syndrome
    (pseudohypoparathyroidism)
    275.49
Martorell-Fabre syndrome (pulseless
    disease) 446.7

Masculinization, female, with adrenal
    hyperplasia 255.2
Masculinovoblastoma (M8670/0)
    220
Masochism 302.83
Masons' lung 502
Mass
  abdominal 789.3●
  anus 787.99
  bone 733.90
  breast 611.72
  cheek 784.2
  chest 786.6
  cystic - *see* Cyst
  ear 388.8
  epigastric 789.3●
  eye 379.92
  female genital organ 625.8
  gum 784.2
  head 784.2
  intracranial 784.2
  joint 719.60
    ankle 719.67
    elbow 719.62
    foot 719.67
    hand 719.64
    hip 719.65
    knee 719.66
    multiple sites 719.69
    pelvic region 719.65
    shoulder (region) 719.61
    specified site NEC 719.68
    wrist 719.63
  kidney *(see also* Disease, kidney)
    593.9
  lung 786.6
  lymph node 785.6
  malignant (M8000/3) - *see* Neoplasm,
    by site, malignant
  mediastinal 786.6
  mouth 784.2
  muscle (limb) 729.89
  neck 784.2
  nose or sinus 784.2
  palate 784.2
  pelvis, pelvic 789.3●
  penis 607.89
  perineum 625.8
  rectum 787.99
  scrotum 608.89
  skin 782.2
  specified organ NEC - *see* Disease of
    specified organ or site
  splenic 789.2
  substernal 786.6
    thyroid *(see also* Goiter) 240.9
  superficial (localized) 782.2
  testes 608.89
  throat 784.2
  tongue 784.2
  umbilicus 789.3●
  uterus 625.8
  vagina 625.8
  vulva 625.8
Massive - *see* condition
Mastalgia 611.71
  psychogenic 307.89
Mast cell
  disease 757.33
    systemic (M9741/3) 202.6●
  leukemia (M9900/3) 207.8●
  sarcoma (M9742/3) 202.6●
  tumor (M9740/1) 238.5
    malignant (M9740/3) 202.6●

◀ New   ◀⁞⁞ Revised   ~~deleted~~ Deleted   ● Use Additional Digit(s)   ▧ Omit code

Masters-Allen syndrome 620.6
Mastitis (acute) (adolescent)
  (diffuse) (interstitial) (lobular)
  (nonpuerperal) (nonsuppurative)
  (parenchymatous) (phlegmonous)
  (simple) (subacute) (suppurative)
  611.0
  chronic (cystic) (fibrocystic) 610.1
  cystic 610.1
    Schimmelbusch's type 610.1
  fibrocystic 610.1
  infective 611.0
  lactational 675.2●
  lymphangitis 611.0
  neonatal (noninfective) 778.7
    infective 771.5
  periductal 610.4
  plasma cell 610.4
  puerperal, postpartum, (interstitial)
    (nonpurulent) (parenchymatous)
    675.2●
    purulent 675.1●
    stagnation 676.2●
  puerperalis 675.2●
  retromammary 611.0
    puerperal, postpartum 675.1●
  submammary 611.0
    puerperal, postpartum 675.1●
Mastocytoma (M9740/1) 238.5
  malignant (M9740/3) 202.6●
Mastocytosis 757.33
  malignant (M9741/3) 202.6●
  systemic (M9741/3) 202.6●
Mastodynia 611.71
  psychogenic 307.89
Mastoid - see condition
Mastoidalgia (see also Otalgia) 388.70
Mastoiditis (coalescent) (hemorrhagic)
  (pneumococcal) (streptococcal)
  (suppurative) 383.9
  acute or subacute 383.00
    with
      Gradenigo's syndrome 383.02
      petrositis 383.02
      specified complication NEC
        383.02
      subperiosteal abscess 383.01
  chronic (necrotic) (recurrent) 383.1
  tuberculous (see also Tuberculosis)
    015.6●
Mastopathy, mastopathia 611.9
  chronica cystica 610.1
  diffuse cystic 610.1
  estrogenic 611.89
  ovarian origin 611.89
Mastoplasia 611.1
Masturbation 307.9
Maternal condition, affecting fetus or
  newborn
  acute yellow atrophy of liver 760.8
  albuminuria 760.1
  anesthesia or analgesia 763.5
  blood loss 762.1
  chorioamnionitis 762.7
  circulatory disease, chronic
    (conditions classifiable
    to 390–459, 745–747) 760.3
  congenital heart disease (conditions
    classifiable to 745–746) 760.3
  cortical necrosis of kidney 760.1
  death 761.6
  diabetes mellitus 775.0
    manifest diabetes in the infant
      775.1

Maternal condition, affecting fetus or
  newborn (Continued)
  disease NEC 760.9
    circulatory system, chronic
      (conditions classifiable to
      390–459, 745–747) 760.3
    genitourinary system (conditions
      classifiable to 580–599)
      760.1
    respiratory (conditions classifiable
      to 490–519, 748) 760.3
  eclampsia 760.0
  hemorrhage NEC 762.1
  hepatitis acute, malignant, or subacute
    760.8
  hyperemesis (gravidarum) 761.8
  hypertension (arising during
    pregnancy) (conditions
    classifiable to 642) 760.0
  infection
    disease classifiable to 001–136
      760.2
    genital tract NEC 760.8
    urinary tract 760.1
  influenza 760.2
    manifest influenza in the infant
      771.2
  injury (conditions classifiable to
    800–996) 760.5
  malaria 760.2
    manifest malaria in infant or fetus
      771.2
  malnutrition 760.4
  necrosis of liver 760.8
  nephritis (conditions classifiable to
    580–583) 760.1
  nephrosis (conditions classifiable to
    581) 760.1
  noxious substance transmitted via
    breast milk or placenta 760.70
    alcohol 760.71
    anticonvulsants 760.77
    antifungals 760.74
    anti-infective agents 760.74
    antimetabolics 760.78
    cocaine 760.75
    "crack" 760.75
    diethylstilbestrol [DES] 760.76
    hallucinogenic agents 760.73
    medicinal agents NEC 760.79
    narcotics 760.72
    obstetric anesthetic or analgesic
      drug 760.72
    specified agent NEC 760.79
  nutritional disorder (conditions
    classifiable to 260–269) 760.4
  operation unrelated to current delivery
    (see also Newborn, affected by)
    760.64
  pre-eclampsia 760.0
  pyelitis or pyelonephritis, arising
    during pregnancy (conditions
    classifiable to 590) 760.1
  renal disease or failure 760.1
  respiratory disease, chronic
    (conditions classifiable to
    490–519, 748) 760.3
  rheumatic heart disease (chronic)
    (conditions classifiable to 393–
    398) 760.3
  rubella (conditions classifiable to 056)
    760.2
    manifest rubella in the infant or
      fetus 771.0

Maternal condition, affecting fetus or
  newborn (Continued)
  surgery unrelated to current delivery
    (see also Newborn, affected by)
    760.64
    to uterus or pelvic organs 760.64
  syphilis (conditions classifiable to 090–
    097) 760.2
    manifest syphilis in the infant or
      fetus 090.0
  thrombophlebitis 760.3
  toxemia (of pregnancy) 760.0
    pre-eclamptic 760.0
  toxoplasmosis (conditions classifiable
    to 130) 760.2
    manifest toxoplasmosis in the infant
      or fetus 771.2
  transmission of chemical substance
    through the placenta 760.70
    alcohol 760.71
    anticonvulsants 760.77
    antifungals 760.74
    anti-infective 760.74
    antimetabolics 760.78
    cocaine 760.75
    "crack" 760.75
    diethylstilbestrol [DES] 760.76
    hallucinogenic agents 760.73
    narcotics 760.72
    specified substance NEC 760.79
  uremia 760.1
  urinary tract conditions (conditions
    classifiable to 580–599) 760.1
  vomiting (pernicious) (persistent)
    (vicious) 761.8
Maternity - see Delivery
Matheiu's disease (leptospiral jaundice)
  100.0
Mauclaire's disease or osteochondrosis
  732.3
Maxcy's disease 081.0
Maxilla, maxillary - see condition
May (-Hegglin) anomaly or syndrome 288.2
Mayaro fever 066.3
Mazoplasia 610.8
MBD (minimal brain dysfunction), child
  (see also Hyperkinesia) 314.9
MCAD (medium chain acyl CoA
  dehydrogenase deficiency) 277.85
McArdle (-Schmid-Pearson) disease or
  syndrome (glycogenosis V) 271.0
McCune-Albright syndrome (osteitis
  fibrosa disseminata) 756.59
MCLS (mucocutaneous lymph node
  syndrome) 446.1
McQuarrie's syndrome (idiopathic
  familial hypoglycemia) 251.2
Measles (black) (hemorrhagic)
  (suppressed) 055.9
  with
    encephalitis 055.0
    keratitis 055.71
    keratoconjunctivitis 055.71
    otitis media 055.2
    pneumonia 055.1
  complication 055.8
    specified type NEC 055.79
  encephalitis 055.0
  French 056.9
  German 056.9
  keratitis 055.71
  keratoconjunctivitis 055.71
  liberty 056.9
  otitis media 055.2

Measles (*Continued*)
pneumonia 055.1
specified complications NEC 055.79
vaccination, prophylactic (against)
V04.2
Meatitis, urethral (*see also* Urethritis)
597.89
Meat poisoning - *see* Poisoning, food
Meatus, meatal - *see* condition
Meat-wrappers' asthma 506.9
Meckel's
diverticulitis 751.0
diverticulum (displaced)
(hypertrophic) 751.0
Meconium
aspiration 770.11
with
pneumonia 770.12
pneumonitis 770.12
respiratory symptoms 770.12
below vocal cords 770.11
with respiratory symptoms
770.12
syndrome 770.12
delayed passage in newborn 777.1
ileus 777.1
due to cystic fibrosis 277.01
in liquor 792.3
noted during delivery - 656.8●
insufflation 770.11
with respiratory symptoms 770.12
obstruction
fetus or newborn 777.1
in mucoviscidosis 277.01
passage of 792.3
noted during delivery 763.84
peritonitis 777.6
plug syndrome (newborn) NEC
777.1
staining 779.84
Median - *see also* condition
arcuate ligament syndrome 447.4
bar (prostate) 600.90
with
other lower urinary tract
symptoms (LUTS)
600.91
urinary
obstruction 600.91
retention 600.91
rhomboid glossitis 529.2
vesical orifice 600.90
with
other lower urinary tract
symptoms (LUTS)
600.91
urinary
obstruction 600.91
retention 600.91
Mediastinal shift 793.2
Mediastinitis (acute) (chronic) 519.2
actinomycotic 039.8
syphilitic 095.8
tuberculous (*see also* Tuberculosis)
012.8●
Mediastinopericarditis (*see also*
Pericarditis) 423.9
acute 420.90
chronic 423.8
rheumatic 393
rheumatic, chronic 393
Mediastinum, mediastinal - *see* condition
Medical services provided for - *see* Health,
services provided because (of)

Medicine poisoning (by overdose)
(wrong substance given or taken in
error) 977.9
specified drug or substance - *see* Table
of Drugs and Chemicals
Medin's disease (poliomyelitis) 045.9●
Mediterranean
anemia (with other hemoglobinopathy)
282.49
disease or syndrome (hemipathic)
282.49
fever (*see also* Brucellosis) 023.9
familial 277.31
kala-azar 085.0
leishmaniasis 085.0
tick fever 082.1
Medulla - *see* condition
Medullary
cystic kidney 753.16
sponge kidney 753.17
Medullated fibers
optic (nerve) 743.57
retina 362.85
Medulloblastoma (M9470/3)
desmoplastic (M9471/3) 191.6
specified site - *see* Neoplasm, by site,
malignant
unspecified site 191.6
Medulloepithelioma (M9501/3) - *see also*
Neoplasm, by site, malignant
teratoid (M9502/3) - *see* Neoplasm, by
site, malignant
Medullomyoblastoma (M9472/3)
specified site - *see* Neoplasm, by site,
malignant
unspecified site 191.6
Meekeren-Ehlers-Danlos syndrome
756.83
Megacaryocytic - *see* condition
Megacolon (acquired) (functional) (not
Hirschsprung's disease) 564.7
aganglionic 751.3
congenital, congenitum 751.3
Hirschsprung's (disease) 751.3
psychogenic 306.4
toxic (*see also* Colitis, ulcerative) 556.9
Megaduodenum 537.3
Megaesophagus (functional) 530.0
congenital 750.4
Megakaryocytic - *see* condition
Megalencephaly 742.4
Megalerythema (epidermicum)
(infectiosum) 057.0
Megalia, cutis et ossium 757.39
Megaloappendix 751.5
Megalocephalus, megalocephaly NEC
756.0
Megalocornea 743.41
associated with buphthalmos 743.22
Megalocytic anemia 281.9
Megalodactylia (fingers) (thumbs) 755.57
toes 755.65
Megaloduodenum 751.5
Megaloesophagus (functional) 530.0
congenital 750.4
Megalogastria (congenital) 750.7
Megalomania 307.9
Megalophthalmos 743.8
Megalopsia 368.14
Megalosplenia (*see also* Splenomegaly)
789.2
Megaloureter 593.89
congenital 753.22
Megarectum 569.49

Megasigmoid 564.7
congenital 751.3
Megaureter 593.89
congenital 753.22
Megrim 346.9●
Meibomian
cyst 373.2
infected 373.12
gland - *see* condition
infarct (eyelid) 374.85
stye 373.11
Meibomitis 373.12
Meige
-Milroy disease (chronic hereditary
edema) 757.0
syndrome (blepharospasm-
oromandibular dystonia) 333.82
Melalgia, nutritional 266.2
Melancholia (*see also* Psychosis, affective)
296.90
climacteric 296.2●
recurrent episode 296.3●
single episode 296.2●
hypochondriac 300.7
intermittent 296.2●
recurrent episode 296.3●
single episode 296.2●
involutional 296.2●
recurrent episode 296.3●
single episode 296.2●
menopausal 296.2●
recurrent episode 296.3●
single episode 296.2●
puerperal 296.2●
reactive (from emotional stress,
psychological trauma) 298.0
recurrent 296.3●
senile 290.21
stuporous 296.2●
recurrent episode 296.3●
single episode 296.2●
Melanemia 275.09 ◀▥
Melanoameloblastoma (M9363/0) - *see*
Neoplasm, bone, benign
Melanoblastoma (M8720/3) - *see*
Melanoma
Melanoblastosis
Block-Sulzberger 757.33
cutis linearis sive systematisata 757.33
Melanocarcinoma (M8720/3) - *see*
Melanoma
Melanocytoma, eyeball (M8726/0) 224.0
Melanoderma, melanodermia 709.09
Addison's (primary adrenal
insufficiency) 255.41
Melanodontia, infantile 521.05
Melanodontoclasia 521.05
Melanoepithelioma (M8720/3) - *see*
Melanoma
Melanoma (malignant) (M8720/3) 172.9

Note: Except where otherwise
indicated, the morphological varieties
of melanoma in the list below should
be coded by site as for "Melanoma
(malignant)." Internal sites should be
coded to malignant neoplasm of those
sites.

abdominal wall 172.5
ala nasi 172.3
amelanotic (M8730/3) - *see* Melanoma,
by site

◀ New   ▥ Revised   ~~deleted~~ Deleted   ● Use Additional Digit(s)   ▥ Omit code

Melanoma *(Continued)*
ankle 172.7
anus, anal 154.3
  canal 154.2
arm 172.6
auditory canal (external) 172.2
auricle (ear) 172.2
auricular canal (external) 172.2
axilla 172.5
axillary fold 172.5
back 172.5
balloon cell (M8722/3) - *see* Melanoma,
  by site
benign (M8720/0) - *see* Neoplasm, skin,
  benign
breast (female) (male) 172.5
brow 172.3
buttock 172.5
canthus (eye) 172.1
cheek (external) 172.3
chest wall 172.5
chin 172.3
choroid 190.6
conjunctiva 190.3
ear (external) 172.2
epithelioid cell (M8771/3) - *see also*
  Melanoma, by site
  and spindle cell, mixed (M8775/3) -
    see Melanoma, by site
external meatus (ear) 172.2
eye 190.9
eyebrow 172.3
eyelid (lower) (upper) 172.1
face NEC 172.3
female genital organ (external) NEC
  184.4
finger 172.6
flank 172.5
foot 172.7
forearm 172.6
forehead 172.3
foreskin 187.1
gluteal region 172.5
groin 172.5
hand 172.6
heel 172.7
helix 172.2
hip 172.7
in
  giant pigmented nevus (M8761/3) -
    see Melanoma, by site
  Hutchinson's melanotic freckle
    (M8742/3) - *see* Melanoma, by
    site
  junctional nevus (M8740/3) - *see*
    Melanoma, by site
  precancerous melanosis (M8741/3) -
    see Melanoma, by site
in situ - *see* Melanoma, by site
  skin 172.9
interscapular region 172.5
iris 190.0
jaw 172.3
juvenile (M8770/0) - *see* Neoplasm,
  skin, benign
knee 172.7
labium
  majus 184.1
  minus 184.2
lacrimal gland 190.2
leg 172.7
lip (lower) (upper) 172.0
liver 197.7
lower limb NEC 172.7

Melanoma *(Continued)*
male genital organ (external) NEC
  187.9
meatus, acoustic (external) 172.2
meibomian gland 172.1
metastatic
  of or from specified site - *see*
    Melanoma, by site
  site not of skin - *see* Neoplasm, by
    site, malignant, secondary
  to specified site - *see* Neoplasm, by
    site, malignant, secondary
  unspecified site 172.9
nail 172.9
  finger 172.6
  toe 172.7
neck 172.4
nodular (M8721/3) - *see* Melanoma, by
  site
nose, external 172.3
orbit 190.1
penis 187.4
perianal skin 172.5
perineum 172.5
pinna 172.2
popliteal (fossa) (space) 172.7
prepuce 187.1
pubes 172.5
pudendum 184.4
retina 190.5
scalp 172.4
scrotum 187.7
septum nasal (skin) 172.3
shoulder 172.6
skin NEC 172.8
  in situ 172.9
spindle cell (M8772/3) - *see also*
  Melanoma, by site
  type A (M8773/3) 190.0
  type B (M8774/3) 190.0
submammary fold 172.5
superficial spreading (M8743/3) - *see*
  Melanoma, by site
temple 172.3
thigh 172.7
toe 172.7
trunk NEC 172.5
umbilicus 172.5
upper limb NEC 172.6
vagina vault 184.0
vulva 184.4
Melanoplakia 528.9
Melanosarcoma (M8720/3) - *see also*
  Melanoma
  epithelioid cell (M8771/3) - *see*
    Melanoma
Melanosis 709.09
addisonian (primary adrenal
  insufficiency) 255.41
  tuberculous (*see also* Tuberculosis)
    017.6●
adrenal 255.41
colon 569.89
conjunctiva 372.55
  congenital 743.49
corii degenerativa 757.33
cornea (presenile) (senile) 371.12
  congenital 743.43
    interfering with vision 743.42
  prenatal 743.43
    interfering with vision 743.42
eye 372.55
  congenital 743.49
jute spinners' 709.09

Melanosis *(Continued)*
lenticularis progressiva 757.33
liver 573.8
precancerous (M8741/2) - *see also*
  Neoplasm, skin, in situ
  malignant melanoma in (M8741/3) -
    see Melanoma
Riehl's 709.09
sclera 379.19
  congenital 743.47
suprarenal 255.41
tar 709.09
toxic 709.09
Melanuria 791.9
MELAS syndrome (mitochondrial
  encephalopathy, lactic acidosis and
  stroke-like episodes) 277.87
Melasma 709.09
adrenal (gland) 255.41
suprarenal (gland) 255.41
Melena 578.1
due to
  swallowed maternal blood 777.3
  ulcer - *see* Ulcer, by site, with
    hemorrhage
newborn 772.4
  due to swallowed maternal blood
    777.3
Meleney's
gangrene (cutaneous) 686.09
ulcer (chronic undermining) 686.09
Melioidosis 025
Melitensis, febris 023.0
Melitococcosis 023.0
Melkersson (-Rosenthal) syndrome
  351.8
Mellitus, diabetes - *see* Diabetes
Melorheostosis (bone) (leri) 733.99
Meloschisis 744.83
Melotia 744.29
Membrana
capsularis lentis posterior 743.39
epipapillaris 743.57
Membranacea placenta - *see* Placenta,
  abnormal
Membranaceous uterus 621.8
Membrane, membranous - *see also*
  condition
folds, congenital - *see* Web
Jackson's 751.4
over face (causing asphyxia), fetus or
  newborn 768.9
premature rupture - *see* Rupture,
  membranes, premature
pupillary 364.74
  persistent 743.46
retained (complicating delivery)
  (with hemorrhage) 666.2●
  without hemorrhage 667.1●
secondary (eye) 366.50
unruptured (causing asphyxia)
  768.9
vitreous humor 379.25
Membranitis, fetal 658.4●
affecting fetus or newborn 762.7
Memory disturbance, loss or lack (*see also*
  Amnesia) 780.93
mild, following organic brain damage
  310.8
MEN (multiple endocrine neoplasia)
  syndromes
type I 258.01
type IIA 258.02
type IIB 258.03

Menadione (vitamin K) deficiency 269.0
Menarche, precocious 259.1
Mendacity, pathologic 301.7
Mende's syndrome (ptosis-epicanthus) 270.2
Mendelson's syndrome (resulting from a procedure) 997.39
  obstetric 668.0●
Ménétrier's disease or syndrome (hypertrophic gastritis) 535.2●
Ménière's disease, syndrome, or vertigo 386.00
  cochlear 386.02
  cochleovestibular 386.01
  inactive 386.04
  in remission 386.04
  vestibular 386.03
Meninges, meningeal - see condition
Meningioma (M9530/0) - see also
  Neoplasm, meninges, benign
  angioblastic (M9535/0) - see Neoplasm, meninges, benign
  angiomatous (M9534/0) - see Neoplasm, meninges, benign
  endotheliomatous (M9531/0) - see Neoplasm, meninges, benign
  fibroblastic (M9532/0) - see Neoplasm, meninges, benign
  fibrous (M9532/0) - see Neoplasm, meninges, benign
  hemangioblastic (M9535/0) - see Neoplasm, meninges, benign
  hemangiopericytic (M9536/0) - see Neoplasm, meninges, benign
  malignant (M9530/3) - see Neoplasm, meninges, malignant
  meningiothelial (M9531/0) - see Neoplasm, meninges, benign
  meningotheliomatous (M9531/0) - see Neoplasm, meninges, benign
  mixed (M9537/0) - see Neoplasm, meninges, benign
  multiple (M9530/1) 237.6
  papillary (M9538/1) 237.6
  psammomatous (M9533/0) - see Neoplasm, meninges, benign
  syncytial (M9531/0) - see Neoplasm, meninges, benign
  transitional (M9537/0) - see Neoplasm, meninges, benign
Meningiomatosis (diffuse) (M9530/1) 237.6
Meningism (see also Meningismus) 781.6
Meningismus (infectional) (pneumococcal) 781.6
  due to serum or vaccine 997.09 [321.8]
  influenzal NEC (see also Influenza) 487.8 ◀▥
Meningitis (basal) (basic) (basilar) (brain) (cerebral) (cervical) (congestive) (diffuse) (hemorrhagic) (infantile) (membranous) (metastatic) (nonspecific) (pontine) (progressive) (simple) (spinal) (subacute) (sympathetica) (toxic) 322.9
  abacterial NEC (see also Meningitis, aseptic) 047.9
  actinomycotic 039.8 [320.7]
  adenoviral 049.1
  aerobacter aerogenes 320.82
  anaerobes (cocci) (gram-negative) (gram-positive) (mixed) (NEC) 320.81
  arbovirus NEC 066.9 [321.2]
    specified type NEC 066.8 [321.2]

Meningitis (Continued)
  aseptic (acute) NEC 047.9
    adenovirus 049.1
    Coxsackie virus 047.0
    due to
      adenovirus 049.1
      Coxsackie virus 047.0
      ECHO virus 047.1
      enterovirus 047.9
      mumps 072.1
      poliovirus (see also Poliomyelitis) 045.2● [321.2]
    ECHO virus 047.1
    herpes (simplex) virus 054.72
    zoster 053.0
    leptospiral 100.81
    lymphocytic choriomeningitis 049.0
    noninfective 322.0
  Bacillus pyocyaneus 320.89
  bacterial NEC 320.9
    anaerobic 320.81
    gram-negative 320.82
      anaerobic 320.81
  Bacteroides (fragilis) (oralis) (melaninogenicus) 320.81
  cancerous (M8000/6) 198.4
  candidal 112.83
  carcinomatous (M8010/6) 198.4
  caseous (see also Tuberculosis, meninges) 013.0●
  cerebrospinal (acute) (chronic) (diplococcal) (endemic) (epidemic) (fulminant) (infectious) (malignant) (meningococcal) (sporadic) 036.0
    carrier (suspected) of V02.59
  chronic NEC 322.2
  clear cerebrospinal fluid NEC 322.0
  Clostridium (haemolyticum) (novyi) NEC 320.81
  coccidioidomycosis 114.2
  Coxsackie virus 047.0
  cryptococcal 117.5 [321.0]
  diplococcal 036.0
    gram-negative 036.0
    gram-positive 320.1
  Diplococcus pneumoniae 320.1
  due to
    actinomycosis 039.8 [320.7]
    adenovirus 049.1
    coccidiomycosis 114.2
    enterovirus 047.9
      specified NEC 047.8
    histoplasmosis (see also Histoplasmosis) 115.91
    Listerosis 027.0 [320.7]
    Lyme disease 088.81 [320.7]
    moniliasis 112.83
    mumps 072.1
    neurosyphilis 094.2
    nonbacterial organisms NEC 321.8
    oidiomycosis 112.83
    poliovirus (see also Poliomyelitis) 045.2● [321.2]
    preventive immunization, inoculation, or vaccination 997.09 [321.8]
    sarcoidosis 135 [321.4]
    sporotrichosis 117.1 [321.1]
    syphilis 094.2
      acute 091.81
      congenital 090.42
      secondary 091.81

Meningitis (Continued)
  due to (Continued)
    trypanosomiasis (see also Trypanosomiasis) 086.9 [321.3]
    whooping cough 033.9 [320.7]
  E. coli 320.82
  ECHO virus 047.1
  endothelial-leukocytic, benign, recurrent 047.9
  Enterobacter aerogenes 320.82
  enteroviral 047.9
    specified type NEC 047.8
  enterovirus 047.9
    specified NEC 047.8
  eosinophilic 322.1
  epidemic NEC 036.0
  Escherichia coli (E. coli) 320.82
  Eubacterium 320.81
  fibrinopurulent NEC 320.9
    specified type NEC 320.89
  Friedländer (bacillus) 320.82
  fungal NEC 117.9 [321.1]
  Fusobacterium 320.81
  gonococcal 098.82
  gram-negative bacteria NEC 320.82
    anaerobic 320.81
    cocci 036.0
      specified NEC 320.82
  gram-negative cocci NEC 036.0
    specified NEC 320.82
  gram-positive cocci NEC 320.9
  H. influenzae 320.0
  herpes (simplex) virus 054.72
    zoster 053.0
  infectious NEC 320.9
  influenzal 320.0
  Klebsiella pneumoniae 320.82
  late effect - see Late, effect, meningitis
  leptospiral (aseptic) 100.81
  Listerella (monocytogenes) 027.0 [320.7]
  Listeria monocytogenes 027.0 [320.7]
  lymphocytic (acute) (benign) (serous) 049.0
    choriomeningitis virus 049.0
  meningococcal (chronic) 036.0
  Mima polymorpha 320.82
  Mollaret's 047.9
  monilial 112.83
  mumps (virus) 072.1
  mycotic NEC 117.9 [321.1]
  Neisseria 036.0
  neurosyphilis 094.2
  nonbacterial NEC (see also Meningitis, aseptic) 047.9
  nonpyogenic NEC 322.0
  oidiomycosis 112.83
  ossificans 349.2
  Peptococcus 320.81
  PeptoStreptococcus 320.81
  pneumococcal 320.1
  poliovirus (see also Poliomyelitis) 045.2● [321.2]
  Proprionibacterium 320.81
  Proteus morganii 320.82
  Pseudomonas (aeruginosa) (pyocyaneus) 320.82
  purulent NEC 320.9
    specified organism NEC 320.89
  pyogenic NEC 320.9
    specified organism NEC 320.89
  Salmonella 003.21
  septic NEC 320.9
    specified organism NEC 320.89

◀ New   ◀▥ Revised   ~~deleted~~ Deleted   ● Use Additional Digit(s)   Omit code

Meningitis (Continued)
serosa circumscripta NEC 322.0
serous NEC (see also Meningitis, aseptic) 047.9
lymphocytic 049.0
syndrome 348.2
Serratia (marcescens) 320.82
specified organism NEC 320.89
sporadic cerebrospinal 036.0
sporotrichosis 117.1 [321.1]
staphylococcal 320.3
sterile 997.09
streptococcal (acute) 320.2
suppurative 320.9
specified organism NEC 320.89
syphilitic 094.2
acute 091.81
congenital 090.42
secondary 091.81
torula 117.5 [321.0]
traumatic (complication of injury) 958.8
Treponema (denticola) (macrodenticum) 320.81
trypanosomiasis 086.1 [321.3]
tuberculous (see also Tuberculosis, meninges) 013.0●
typhoid 002.0 [320.7]
Veillonella 320.81
Vibrio vulnificus 320.82
viral, virus NEC (see also Meningitis, aseptic) 047.9
Wallgren's (see also Meningitis, aseptic) 047.9
Meningocele (congenital) (spinal) (see also Spina bifida) 741.9●
acquired (traumatic) 349.2
cerebral 742.0
cranial 742.0
Meningocerebritis - see Meningoencephalitis
Meningococcemia (acute) (chronic) 036.2
Meningococcus, meningococcal (see also condition) 036.9
adrenalitis, hemorrhagic 036.3
carditis 036.40
carrier (suspected) of V02.59
cerebrospinal fever 036.0
encephalitis 036.1
endocarditis 036.42
exposure to V01.84
infection NEC 036.9
meningitis (cerebrospinal) 036.0
myocarditis 036.43
optic neuritis 036.81
pericarditis 036.41
septicemia (chronic) 036.2
Meningoencephalitis (see also Encephalitis) 323.9
acute NEC 048
bacterial, purulent, pyogenic, or septic - see Meningitis
chronic NEC 094.1
diffuse NEC 094.1
diphasic 063.2
due to
actinomycosis 039.8 [320.7]
blastomycosis NEC (see also Blastomycosis) 116.0 [323.41]
free-living amebae 136.29
Listeria monocytogenes 027.0 [320.7]
Lyme disease 088.81 [320.7]
mumps 072.2

Meningoencephalitis (Continued)
due to (Continued)
Naegleria (amebae) (gruberi) (organisms) 136.29
rubella 056.01
sporotrichosis 117.1 [321.1]
toxoplasmosis (acquired) 130.0
congenital (active) 771.2 [323.41]
Trypanosoma 086.1 [323.2]
epidemic 036.0
herpes 054.3
herpetic 054.3
H. influenzae 320.0
infectious (acute) 048
influenzal 320.0
late effect - see category 326
Listeria monocytogenes 027.0 [320.7]
lymphocytic (serous) 049.0
mumps 072.2
parasitic NEC 123.9 [323.41]
pneumococcal 320.1
primary amebic 136.29
rubella 056.01
serous 048
lymphocytic 049.0
specific 094.2
staphylococcal 320.3
streptococcal 320.2
syphilitic 094.2
toxic NEC 989.9 [323.71]
due to
carbon tetrachloride (vapor) 987.8 [323.71]
hydroxyquinoline derivatives poisoning 961.3 [323.71]
lead 984.9 [323.71]
mercury 985.0 [323.71]
thallium 985.8 [323.71]
toxoplasmosis (acquired) 130.0
trypanosomic 086.1 [323.2]
tuberculous (see also Tuberculosis, meninges) 013.0●
virus NEC 048
Meningoencephalocele 742.0
syphilitic 094.89
congenital 090.49
Meningoencephalomyelitis (see also Meningoencephalitis) 323.9
acute NEC 048
disseminated (postinfectious) 136.9 [323.61]
postimmunization or postvaccination 323.51
due to
actinomycosis 039.8 [320.7]
torula 117.5 [323.41]
toxoplasma or toxoplasmosis (acquired) 130.0
congenital (active) 771.2 [323.41]
late effect - see category 326
Meningoencephalomyelopathy (see also Meningoencephalomyelitis) 349.9
Meningoencephalopathy (see also Meningoencephalitis) 348.39
Meningoencephalopoliomyelitis (see also Poliomyelitis, bulbar) 045.0●
late effect 138
Meningomyelitis (see also Meningoencephalitis) 323.9
blastomycotic NEC (see also Blastomycosis) 116.0 [323.41]

Meningomyelitis (Continued)
due to
actinomycosis 039.8 [320.7]
blastomycosis (see also Blastomycosis) 116.0 [323.41]
Meningococcus 036.0
sporotrichosis 117.1 [323.41]
torula 117.5 [323.41]
late effect - see category 326
lethargic 049.8
meningococcal 036.0
syphilitic 094.2
tuberculous (see also Tuberculosis, meninges) 013.0●
Meningomyelocele (see also Spina bifida) 741.9●
syphilitic 094.89
Meningomyeloneuritis - see Meningoencephalitis
Meningoradiculitis - see Meningitis
Meningovascular - see condition
Meniscocytosis 282.60
Menkes' syndrome - see Syndrome, Menkes'
Menolipsis 626.0
Menometrorrhagia 626.2
Menopause, menopausal (symptoms) (syndrome) 627.2
arthritis (any site) NEC 716.3●
artificial 627.4
bleeding 627.0
crisis 627.2
depression (see also Psychosis, affective) 296.2●
agitated 296.2●
recurrent episode 296.3●
single episode 296.2●
psychotic 296.2●
recurrent episode 296.3●
single episode 296.2●
recurrent episode 296.3●
single episode 296.2●
melancholia (see also Psychosis, affective) 296.2●
recurrent episode 296.3●
single episode 296.2●
paranoid state 297.2
paraphrenia 297.2
postsurgical 627.4
premature 256.31
postirradiation 256.2
postsurgical 256.2
psychoneurosis 627.2
psychosis NEC 298.8
surgical 627.4
toxic polyarthritis NEC 716.39
Menorrhagia (primary) 626.2
climacteric 627.0
menopausal 627.0
postclimacteric 627.1
postmenopausal 627.1
preclimacteric 627.0
premenopausal 627.0
puberty (menses retained) 626.3
Menorrhalgia 625.3
Menoschesis 626.8
Menostaxis 626.2
Menses, retention 626.8
Menstrual - see also Menstruation
cycle, irregular 626.4
disorders NEC 626.9
extraction V25.3
fluid, retained 626.8
molimen 625.4

Menstrual (*Continued*)
  period, normal V65.5
  regulation V25.3
Menstruation
  absent 626.0
  anovulatory 628.0
  delayed 626.8
  difficult 625.3
  disorder 626.9
    psychogenic 306.52
    specified NEC 626.8
  during pregnancy 640.8●
  excessive 626.2
  frequent 626.2
  infrequent 626.1
  irregular 626.4
  latent 626.8
  membranous 626.8
  painful (primary) (secondary) 625.3
    psychogenic 306.52
  passage of clots 626.2
  precocious 259.1◀▥
  protracted 626.8
  retained 626.8
  retrograde 626.8
  scanty 626.1
  suppression 626.8
  vicarious (nasal) 625.8
Mentagra (*see also* Sycosis) 704.8
Mental - *see also* condition
  deficiency (*see also* Retardation, mental)
    319
  deterioration (*see also* Psychosis) 298.9
  disorder (*see also* Disorder, mental)
    300.9
  exhaustion 300.5
  insufficiency (congenital) (*see also*
    Retardation, mental) 319
  observation without need for further
    medical care NEC V71.09
  retardation (*see also* Retardation,
    mental) 319
  subnormality (*see also* Retardation,
    mental) 319
    mild 317
    moderate 318.0
    profound 318.2
    severe 318.1
  upset (*see also* Disorder, mental)
    300.9
Meralgia paresthetica 355.1
Mercurial - *see* condition
Mercurialism NEC 985.0
Merergasia 300.9
Merkel cell tumor - *see* Carcinoma,
    Merkel cell
Merocele (*see also* Hernia, femoral) 553.00
Meromelia 755.4
  lower limb 755.30
    intercalary 755.32
      femur 755.34
        tibiofibular (complete)
          (incomplete) 755.33
      fibula 755.37
      metatarsal(s) 755.38
      tarsal(s) 755.38
      tibia 755.36
      tibiofibular 755.35
    terminal (complete) (partial)
      (transverse) 755.31
    longitudinal 755.32
      metatarsal(s) 755.38
      phalange(s) 755.39
      tarsal(s) 755.38
    transverse 755.31

Meromelia (*Continued*)
  upper limb 755.20
    intercalary 755.22
      carpal(s) 755.28
      humeral 755.24
        radioulnar (complete)
          (incomplete) 755.23
      metacarpal(s) 755.28
      phalange(s) 755.29
      radial 755.26
      radioulnar 755.25
      ulnar 755.27
    terminal (complete) (partial)
      (transverse) 755.21
    longitudinal 755.22
      carpal(s) 755.28
      metacarpal(s) 755.28
      phalange(s) 755.29
    transverse 755.21
Merosmia 781.1
MERRF syndrome (myoclonus with
    epilepsy and with ragged red fibers)
    277.87
Merycism - *see also* Vomiting
  psychogenic 307.53
Merzbacher-Pelizaeus disease 330.0
Mesaortitis - *see* Aortitis
Mesarteritis - *see* Arteritis
Mesencephalitis (*see also* Encephalitis)
    323.9
  late effect - *see* category 326
Mesenchymoma (M8990/1) - *see also*
    Neoplasm, connective tissue,
    uncertain behavior
  benign (M8990/0) - *see* Neoplasm,
    connective tissue, benign
  malignant (M8990/3) - *see* Neoplasm,
    connective tissue, malignant
Mesenteritis
  retractile 567.82
  sclerosing 567.82
Mesentery, mesenteric - *see* condition
Mesiodens, mesiodentes 520.1
  causing crowding 524.31
Mesio-occlusion 524.23
Mesocardia (with asplenia) 746.87
Mesocolon - *see* condition
Mesonephroma (malignant) (M9110/3) -
    see also Neoplasm, by site,
    malignant
  benign (M9110/0) - *see* Neoplasm, by
    site, benign
Mesophlebitis - *see* Phlebitis
Mesostromal dysgenesis 743.51
Mesothelioma (malignant) (M9050/3) -
    see also Neoplasm, by site,
    malignant
  benign (M9050/0) - *see* Neoplasm, by
    site, benign
  biphasic type (M9053/3) - *see also*
    Neoplasm, by site, malignant
    benign (M9053/0) - *see* Neoplasm,
      by site, benign
  epithelioid (M9052/3) - *see also*
    Neoplasm, by site, malignant
    benign (M9052/0) - *see* Neoplasm,
      by site, benign
  fibrous (M9051/3) - *see also* Neoplasm,
    by site, malignant
    benign (M9051/0) - *see* Neoplasm,
      by site, benign
Metabolic syndrome 277.7
Metabolism disorder 277.9
  specified type NEC 277.89
Metagonimiasis 121.5

Metagonimus infestation (small
    intestine) 121.5
Metal
  pigmentation (skin) 709.00
    polishers' disease 502
Metalliferous miners' lung 503
Metamorphopsia 368.14
Metaplasia
  bone, in skin 709.3
  breast 611.89
  cervix - *omit code*
  endometrium (squamous) 621.8
  esophagus 530.85
  intestinal, of gastric mucosa 537.89
  kidney (pelvis) (squamous) (*see also*
    Disease, renal) 593.89
  myelogenous 289.89
  myeloid 289.89
    agnogenic 238.76
    megakaryocytic 238.76
  spleen 289.59
  squamous cell
    amnion 658.8●
    bladder 596.8
    cervix - *see* condition
    trachea 519.19
    tracheobronchial tree 519.19
    uterus 621.8
      cervix - *see* condition
Metastasis, metastatic
  abscess - *see* Abscess
  calcification 275.40
  cancer, neoplasm, or disease
    from specified site (M8000/3) - *see*
      Neoplasm, by site, malignant
    to specified site (M8000/6) - *see*
      Neoplasm, by site, secondary
  deposits (in) (M8000/6) - *see* Neoplasm,
    by site, secondary
  mesentery, of neuroendocrine tumor
    209.71
  pneumonia 038.8 [484.8]
  spread (to) (M8000/6) - *see* Neoplasm,
    by site, secondary
Metatarsalgia 726.70
  anterior 355.6
  due to Freiberg's disease 732.5
  Morton's 355.6
Metatarsus, metatarsal - *see also*
    condition
  abductus valgus (congenital) 754.60
  adductus varus (congenital) 754.53
    primus varus 754.52
  valgus (adductus) (congenital) 754.60
  varus (abductus) (congenital) 754.53
    primus 754.52
Methadone use 304.00
Methemoglobinemia 289.7
  acquired (with sulfhemoglobinemia)
    289.7
  congenital 289.7
  enzymatic 289.7
  Hb-M disease 289.7
  hereditary 289.7
  toxic 289.7
Methemoglobinuria (*see also*
    Hemoglobinuria) 791.2
Methicillin
  resistant staphylococcus aureus
    (MRSA) 041.12
    colonization V02.54
    personal history of V12.04
  susceptible staphylococcus aureus
    (MSSA) 041.11
    colonization V02.53

Methioninemia 270.4
Metritis (catarrhal) (septic) (suppurative)
    (see also Endometritis) 615.9
  blennorrhagic 098.16
    chronic or duration of 2 months or
      over 098.36
  cervical (see also Cervicitis) 616.0
  gonococcal 098.16
    chronic or duration of 2 months or
      over 098.36
  hemorrhagic 626.8
  puerperal, postpartum, childbirth
    670.1●
  septic 670.2●
  tuberculous (see also Tuberculosis)
    016.7●
Metropathia hemorrhagica 626.8
Metroperitonitis (see also Peritonitis,
    pelvic, female) 614.5
Metrorrhagia 626.6
  arising during pregnancy - see
    Hemorrhage, pregnancy
  postpartum NEC 666.2●
  primary 626.6
  psychogenic 306.59
  puerperal 666.2●
Metrorrhexis - see Rupture, uterus
Metrosalpingitis (see also Salpingo-
    oophoritis) 614.2
Metrostaxis 626.6
Metrovaginitis (see also Endometritis) 615.9
  gonococcal (acute) 098.16
    chronic or duration of 2 months or
      over 098.36
Mexican fever - see Typhus, Mexican
Meyenburg-Altherr-Uehlinger syndrome
    733.99
Meyer-Schwickerath and Weyers
    syndrome (dysplasia
    oculodentodigitalis) 759.89
Meynert's amentia (nonalcoholic) 294.0
  alcoholic 291.1
Mibelli's disease 757.39
Mice, joint (see also Loose, body, joint)
    718.1●
  knee 717.6
Micheli-Rietti syndrome (thalassemia
    minor) 282.49
Michotte's syndrome 721.5
Micrencephalon, micrencephaly 742.1
Microalbuminuria 791.0
Microaneurysm, retina 362.14
  diabetic 250.5● [362.01]
    due to secondary diabetes 249.5●
      [362.01]
Microangiopathy 443.9
  diabetic (peripheral) 250.7●
      [443.81]
    due to secondary diabetes 249.7●
      [443.81]
    retinal 250.5● [362.01]
      due to secondary diabetes 249.5●
        [362.01]
  peripheral 443.9
    diabetic 250.7● [443.81]
      due to secondary diabetes 249.7●
        [443.81]
  retinal 362.18
    diabetic 250.5● [362.01]
      due to secondary diabetes 249.5●
        [362.01]
  thrombotic 446.6
    Moschcowitz's (thrombotic
      thrombocytopenic purpura)
      446.6

Microcalcification, mammographic
    793.81
Microcephalus, microcephalic,
    microcephaly 742.1
  due to toxoplasmosis (congenital)
    771.2
Microcheilia 744.82
Microcolon (congenital) 751.5
Microcornea (congenital) 743.41
Microcytic - see condition
Microdeletions NEC 758.33
Microdontia 520.2
Microdrepanocytosis (thalassemia-Hb-S
    disease) 282.49
Microembolism
  atherothrombotic - see
    Atheroembolism
  retina 362.33
Microencephalon 742.1
Microfilaria streptocerca infestation 125.3
Microgastria (congenital) 750.7
Microgenia 524.06
Microgenitalia (congenital) 752.89
  penis 752.64
Microglioma (M9710/3)
  specified site - see Neoplasm, by site,
    malignant
  unspecified site 191.9
Microglossia (congenital) 750.16
Micrognathia, micrognathism
    (congenital) 524.00
  mandibular 524.04
    alveolar 524.74
  maxillary 524.03
    alveolar 524.73
Microgyria (congenital) 742.2
Microinfarct, heart (see also Insufficiency,
    coronary) 411.89
Microlithiasis, alveolar, pulmonary
    516.2
Micromastia 611.82
Micromyelia (congenital) 742.59
Micropenis 752.64
Microphakia (congenital) 743.36
Microphthalmia (congenital) (see also
    Microphthalmos) 743.10
Microphthalmos (congenital) 743.10
  associated with eye and adnexal
    anomalies NEC 743.12
  due to toxoplasmosis (congenital)
    771.2
  isolated 743.11
  simple 743.11
  syndrome 759.89
Micropsia 368.14
Microsporidiosis 136.8
Microsporosis (see also Dermatophytosis)
    110.9
  nigra 111.1
Microsporum furfur infestation 111.0
Microstomia (congenital) 744.84
Microthelia 757.6
Microthromboembolism - see Embolism
Microtia (congenital) (external ear) 744.23
Microtropia 378.34
Microvillus inclusion disease (MVD)
    751.5 ◄
Micturition
  disorder NEC 788.69
    psychogenic 306.53
  frequency 788.41
    psychogenic 306.53
  nocturnal 788.43
  painful 788.1
    psychogenic 306.53

Middle
  ear - see condition
  lobe (right) syndrome 518.0
Midplane - see condition
Miescher's disease 709.3
  cheilitis 351.8
  granulomatosis disciformis 709.3
Miescher-Leder syndrome or
    granulomatosis 709.3
Mieten's syndrome 759.89
Migraine (idiopathic) 346.9●

Note: The following fifth digit
subclassification is for use with
category 346:

  0   without mention of intractable
        migraine without mention
        of status migrainosus
  1   with intractable migraine, so
        stated, without mention of
        status migrainosus
  2   without mention of intractable
        migraine with status
        migrainosus
  3   with intractable migraine, so
        stated, with status
        migrainosus

  with aura (acute-onset) (without
      headache) (prolonged) (typical)
      346.0●
  without aura 346.1●
    chronic 346.7●
    transformed 346.7●
  abdominal (syndrome) 346.2●
  allergic (histamine) 346.2●
  atypical 346.8●
  basilar 346.0●
  chronic without aura 346.7●
  classic(al) 346.0●
  common 346.1●
  hemiplegic 346.3●
    familial 346.3●
    sporadic 346.3●
  lower-half 339.00
  menstrual 346.4●
  menstrually related 346.4●
  ophthalmic 346.8●
  ophthalmoplegic 346.2●
  premenstrual 346.4●
  pure menstrual 346.4●
  retinal 346.0●
  specified form NEC 346.8●
  transformed without aura 346.7●
  variant 346.2●
Migrant, social V60.0
Migratory, migrating - see also condition
  person V60.0
  testis, congenital 752.52
Mikulicz's disease or syndrome (dryness
    of mouth, absent or decreased
    lacrimation) 527.1
Milian atrophia blanche 701.3
Miliaria (crystallina) (rubra) (tropicalis)
    705.1
  apocrine 705.82
Miliary - see condition
Milium (see also Cyst, sebaceous)
    706.2
  colloid 709.3
  eyelid 374.84
Milk
  crust 690.11
  excess secretion 676.6●

Milk *(Continued)*
   fever, female 672●
   poisoning 988.8
   retention 676.2●
   sickness 988.8
   spots 423.1
Milkers' nodes 051.1
Milk-leg (deep vessels) 671.4●
   complicating pregnancy 671.3●
   nonpuerperal 451.19
   puerperal, postpartum, childbirth 671.4●
Milkman (-Looser) disease or syndrome (osteomalacia with pseudofractures) 268.2
Milky urine *(see also* Chyluria) 791.1
Millar's asthma (laryngismus stridulus) 478.75
Millard-Gubler paralysis or syndrome 344.89
Millard-Gubler-Foville paralysis 344.89
Miller-Dieker syndrome 758.33
Miller's disease (osteomalacia) 268.2
Miller Fisher's syndrome 357.0
Milles' syndrome (encephalocutaneous angiomatosis) 759.6
Mills' disease 335.29
Millstone makers' asthma or lung 502
Milroy's disease (chronic hereditary edema) 757.0
Miners' - *see also* condition
   asthma 500
   elbow 727.2
   knee 727.2
   lung 500
   nystagmus 300.89
   phthisis *(see also* Tuberculosis) 011.4●
   tuberculosis *(see also* Tuberculosis) 011.4●
Minkowski-Chauffard syndrome *(see also* Spherocytosis) 282.0
Minor - *see* condition
Minor's disease 336.1
Minot's disease (hemorrhagic disease, newborn) 776.0
Minot-von Willebrand (-Jürgens) disease or syndrome (angiohemophilia) 286.4
Minus (and plus) hand (intrinsic) 736.09
Miosis (persistent) (pupil) 379.42
Mirizzi's syndrome (hepatic duct stenosis) *(see also* Obstruction, biliary) 576.2
   with calculus, cholelithiasis, or stones - *see* Choledocholithiasis
Mirror writing 315.09
   secondary to organic lesion 784.69
Misadventure (prophylactic) (therapeutic) *(see also* Complications) 999.9
   administration of insulin 962.3
   infusion - *see* Complications, infusion
   local applications (of fomentations, plasters, etc.) 999.9
      burn or scald - *see* Burn, by site
   medical care (early) (late) NEC 999.9
      adverse effect of drugs or chemicals - *see* Table of Drugs and Chemicals
      burn or scald - *see* Burn, by site
   radiation NEC 990
   radiotherapy NEC 990
   surgical procedure (early) (late) - *see* Complications, surgical procedure

Misadventure *(Continued)*
   transfusion - *see* Complications, transfusion
   vaccination or other immunological procedure - *see* Complications, vaccination
Misanthropy 301.7
Miscarriage - *see* Abortion, spontaneous
Mischief, malicious, child *(see also* Disturbance, conduct) 312.0●
Misdirection
   aqueous 365.83
Mismanagement, feeding 783.3
Misplaced, misplacement
   kidney *(see also* Disease, renal) 593.0
      congenital 753.3
   organ or site, congenital NEC - *see* Malposition, congenital
Missed
   abortion 632
   delivery (at or near term) 656.4●
   labor (at or near term) 656.4●
Misshapen reconstructed breast 612.0
Missing - *see also* Absence
   teeth (acquired) 525.10
      congenital *(see also* Anodontia) 520.0
      due to
         caries 525.13
         extraction 525.10
         periodontal disease 525.12
         specified NEC 525.19
         trauma 525.11
   vertebrae (congenital) 756.13
Misuse of drugs NEC *(see also* Abuse, drug, nondependent) 305.9●
Mitchell's disease (erythromelalgia) 443.82
Mite(s)
   diarrhea 133.8
   grain (itch) 133.8
   hair follicle (itch) 133.8
   in sputum 133.8
Mitochondrial encephalopathy, lactic acidosis and stroke-like episodes (MELAS syndrome) 277.87
Mitochondrial neurogastrointestinal encephalopathy syndrome (MNGIE) 277.87
Mitral - *see* condition
Mittelschmerz 625.2
Mixed - *see* condition
Mljet disease (mal de Meleda) 757.39
Mobile, mobility
   cecum 751.4
   coccyx 733.99
   excessive - *see* Hypermobility
   gallbladder 751.69
   kidney 593.0
      congenital 753.3
   organ or site, congenital NEC - *see* Malposition, congenital
   spleen 289.59
Mobitz heart block (atrioventricular) 426.10
   type I (Wenckebach's) 426.13
   type II 426.12
Möbius'
   disease 346.2●
   syndrome
      congenital oculofacial paralysis 352.6
      ophthalmoplegic migraine 346.2●

Moeller (-Barlow) disease (infantile scurvy) 267
   glossitis 529.4
Mohr's syndrome (types I and II) 759.89
Mola destruens (M9100/1) 236.1
Molarization, premolars 520.2
Molar pregnancy 631
   hydatidiform (delivered) (undelivered) 630
Mold(s) in vitreous 117.9
Molding, head (during birth) - omit code
Mole (pigmented) (M8720/0) - *see also* Neoplasm, skin, benign
   blood 631
   Breus' 631
   cancerous (M8720/3) - *see* Melanoma
   carneous 631
   destructive (M9100/1) 236.1
   ectopic - *see* Pregnancy, ectopic
   fleshy 631
   hemorrhagic 631
   hydatid, hydatidiform (benign) (complicating pregnancy) (delivered) (undelivered) *(see also* Hydatidiform mole) 630
      invasive (M9100/1) 236.1
      malignant (M9100/1) 236.1
      previous, affecting management of pregnancy V23.1
   invasive (hydatidiform) (M9100/1) 236.1
   malignant
      meaning
         malignant hydatidiform mole (9100/1) 236.1
         melanoma (M8720/3) - *see* Melanoma
   nonpigmented (M8730/0) - *see* Neoplasm, skin, benign
   pregnancy NEC 631
   skin (M8720/0) - *see* Neoplasm, skin, benign
   tubal - *see* Pregnancy, tubal
   vesicular *(see also* Hydatidiform mole) 630
Molimen, molimina (menstrual) 625.4
Mollaret's meningitis 047.9
Mollities (cerebellar) (cerebral) 437.8
   ossium 268.2
Molluscum
   contagiosum 078.0
   epitheliale 078.0
   fibrosum (M8851/0) - *see* Lipoma, by site
   pendulum (M8851/0) - *see* Lipoma, by site
Mönckeberg's arteriosclerosis, degeneration, disease, or sclerosis *(see also* Arteriosclerosis, extremities) 440.20
Monday fever 504
Monday morning dyspnea or asthma 504
Mondini's malformation (cochlea) 744.05
Mondor's disease (thrombophlebitis of breast) 451.89
Mongolian, mongolianism, mongolism, mongoloid 758.0
   spot 757.33
Monilethrix (congenital) 757.4
Monilia infestation - *see* Candidiasis
Moniliasis - *see also* Candidiasis
   neonatal 771.7
   vulvovaginitis 112.1

Monkeypox 059.01
Monoarthritis 716.60
  ankle 716.67
  arm 716.62
    lower (and wrist) 716.63
    upper (and elbow) 716.62
  foot (and ankle) 716.67
  forearm (and wrist) 716.63
  hand 716.64
  leg 716.66
    lower 716.66
    upper 716.65
  pelvic region (hip) (thigh) 716.65
  shoulder (region) 716.61
  specified site NEC 716.68
Monoblastic - see condition
Monochromatism (cone) (rod)
  368.54
Monocytic - see condition
Monocytopenia 288.59
Monocytosis (symptomatic) 288.63
Monofixation syndrome 378.34
Monomania (see also Psychosis) 298.9
Mononeuritis 355.9
  cranial nerve - see Disorder, nerve,
    cranial
  femoral nerve 355.2
  lateral
    cutaneous nerve of thigh 355.1
    popliteal nerve 355.3
  lower limb 355.8
    specified nerve NEC 355.79
  medial popliteal nerve 355.4
  median nerve 354.1
  multiplex 354.5
  plantar nerve 355.6
  posterior tibial nerve 355.5
  radial nerve 354.3
  sciatic nerve 355.0
  ulnar nerve 354.2
  upper limb 354.9
    specified nerve NEC 354.8
  vestibular 388.5
Mononeuropathy (see also Mononeuritis)
  355.9
  diabetic NEC 250.6● [355.9]
    due to secondary diabetes 249.6●
      [355.9]
    lower limb 250.6● [355.8]
      due to secondary diabetes 249.6●
        [355.8]
    upper limb 250.6● [354.9]
      due to secondary diabetes 249.6●
        [354.9]
  iliohypogastric nerve 355.79
  ilioinguinal nerve 355.79
  obturator nerve 355.79
  saphenous nerve 355.79
Mononucleosis, infectious 075
  with hepatitis 075 [573.1]
Monoplegia 344.5
  brain (current episode) (see also
    Paralysis, brain) 437.8
    fetus or newborn 767.8
  cerebral (current episode) (see also
    Paralysis, brain) 437.8
  congenital or infantile (cerebral)
    (spastic) (spinal) 343.3
  embolic (current) (see also Embolism,
    brain) 434.1●
    late effect - see Late effect(s) (of)
      cerebrovascular disease
  infantile (cerebral) (spastic) (spinal)
    343.3

Monoplegia (Continued)
  lower limb 344.30
    affecting
      dominant side 344.31
      nondominant side 344.32
    due to late effect of cerebrovascular
      accident - see Late effect(s) (of)
      cerebrovascular accident
  newborn 767.8
  psychogenic 306.0
    specified as conversion reaction
      300.11
  thrombotic (current) (see also
    Thrombosis, brain) 434.0●
    late effect - see Late effect(s) (of)
      cerebrovascular disease
  transient 781.4
  upper limb 344.40
    affecting
      dominant side 344.41
      nondominant side 344.42
    due to late effect of cerebrovascular
      accident - see Late effect(s) (of)
      cerebrovascular accident
Monorchism, monorchidism 752.89
Monteggia's fracture (closed) 813.03
  open 813.13
Mood swings
  brief compensatory 296.99
  rebound 296.99
Moore's syndrome (see also Epilepsy)
  345.5●
Mooren's ulcer (cornea) 370.07
Mooser-Neill reaction 081.0
Mooser bodies 081.0
Moral
  deficiency 301.7
  imbecility 301.7
Morax-Axenfeld conjunctivitis 372.03
Morbilli (see also Measles) 055.9
Morbus
  anglicus, anglorum 268.0
  Beigel 111.2
  caducus (see also Epilepsy) 345.9●
  caeruleus 746.89
  celiacus 579.0
  comitialis (see also Epilepsy) 345.9●
  cordis - see also Disease, heart
    valvulorum - see Endocarditis
  coxae 719.95
    tuberculous (see also Tuberculosis)
      015.1●
  hemorrhagicus neonatorum 776.0
  maculosus neonatorum 772.6
  renum 593.0
  senilis (see also Osteoarthrosis) 715.9●
Morel-Kraepelin disease (see also
  Schizophrenia) 295.9●
Morel-Moore syndrome (hyperostosis
  frontalis interna) 733.3
Morel-Morgagni syndrome (hyperostosis
  frontalis interna) 733.3
Morgagni
  cyst, organ, hydatid, or appendage
    752.89
    fallopian tube 752.11
  disease or syndrome (hyperostosis
    frontalis interna) 733.3
Morgagni-Adams-Stokes syndrome
  (syncope with heart block) 426.9
Morgagni-Stewart-Morel syndrome
  (hyperostosis frontalis interna) 733.3
Moria (see also Psychosis) 298.9
Morning sickness 643.0●

Moron 317
Morphea (guttate) (linear) 701.0
Morphine dependence (see also
  Dependence) 304.0●
Morphinism (see also Dependence)
  304.0●
Morphinomania (see also Dependence)
  304.0●
Morphoea 701.0
Morquio (-Brailsford) (-Ullrich) disease or
  syndrome (mucopolysaccharidosis
  IV) 277.5
  kyphosis 277.5
Morris syndrome (testicular feminization)
  259.51
Morsus humanus (open wound) - see also
  Wound, open, by site
  skin surface intact - see Contusion
Mortification (dry) (moist) (see also
  Gangrene) 785.4
Morton's
  disease 355.6
  foot 355.6
  metatarsalgia (syndrome) 355.6
  neuralgia 355.6
  neuroma 355.6
  syndrome (metatarsalgia) (neuralgia)
    355.6
  toe 355.6
Morvan's disease 336.0
Mosaicism, mosaic (chromosomal) 758.9
  autosomal 758.5
  sex 758.81
Moschcowitz's syndrome (thrombotic
  thrombocytopenic purpura) 446.6
Mother yaw 102.0
Motion sickness (from travel, any
  vehicle) (from roundabouts or
  swings) 994.6
Mottled teeth (enamel) (endemic)
  (nonendemic) 520.3
Mottling enamel (endemic) (nonendemic)
  (teeth) 520.3
Mouchet's disease 732.5
Mould(s) (in vitreous) 117.9
Moulders'
  bronchitis 502
  tuberculosis (see also Tuberculosis)
    011.4●
Mounier-Kuhn syndrome 748.3
  with
    acute exacerbation 494.1
    bronchiectasis 494.0
      with (acute) exacerbation 494.1
  acquired 519.19
    with bronchiectasis 494.0
      with (acute) exacerbation 494.1
Mountain
  fever - see Fever, mountain
  sickness 993.2
    with polycythemia, acquired 289.0
    acute 289.0
  tick fever 066.1
Mouse, joint (see also Loose, body, joint)
  718.1●
  knee 717.6
Mouth - see condition
Movable
  coccyx 724.71
  kidney (see also Disease, renal) 593.0
    congenital 753.3
  organ or site, congenital NEC - see
    Malposition, congenital
  spleen 289.59

M

Movement
  abnormal (dystonic) (involuntary)
    781.0
    decreased fetal 655.7●
    paradoxical facial 374.43
Moya Moya disease 437.5
Mozart's ear 744.29
MRSA (methicillin resistant
    staphylococcus aureus) 041.12
  colonization V02.54
  personal history of V12.04
MSSA (methicillin susceptible
    staphylococcus aureus) 041.11
  colonization V02.53
Mucha's disease (acute parapsoriasis
    varioliformis) 696.2
Mucha-Haberman syndrome (acute
    parapsoriasis varioliformis) 696.2
Mu-chain disease 273.2
Mucinosis (cutaneous) (papular) 701.8
Mucocele
  appendix 543.9
  buccal cavity 528.9
  gallbladder (see also Disease,
    gallbladder) 575.3
  lacrimal sac 375.43
  orbit (eye) 376.81
  salivary gland (any) 527.6
  sinus (accessory) (nasal) 478.19
  turbinate (bone) (middle) (nasal)
    478.19
  uterus 621.8
Mucocutaneous lymph node syndrome
    (acute) (febrile) (infantile) 446.1
Mucoenteritis 564.9
Mucolipidosis I, II, III 272.7
Mucopolysaccharidosis (types 1–6) 277.5
  cardiopathy 277.5 [425.7]
Mucormycosis (lung) 117.7
Mucosa associated lymphoid tissue
    (MALT) 200.3●
Mucositis - see also Inflammation, by site
    528.00
  cervix (ulcerative) 616.81
  due to
    antineoplastic therapy (ulcerative)
      528.01
    other drugs (ulcerative) 528.02
    specified NEC 528.09
  gastrointestinal (ulcerative) 538
  nasal (ulcerative) 478.11
  necroticans agranulocytica (see also
    Agranulocytosis) 288.09
  ulcerative 528.00
  vagina (ulcerative) 616.81
  vulva (ulcerative) 616.81
Mucous - see also condition
  patches (syphilitic) 091.3
    congenital 090.0
Mucoviscidosis 277.00
  with meconium obstruction 277.01
Mucus
  asphyxia or suffocation (see also
    Asphyxia, mucus) 933.1
    newborn 770.18
  in stool 792.1
  plug (see also Asphyxia, mucus) 933.1
    aspiration, of newborn 770.17
    tracheobronchial 519.19
      newborn 770.18
Muguet 112.0
Mulberry molars 090.5
Müllerian mixed tumor (M8950/3) - see
    Neoplasm, by site, malignant

Multicystic kidney 753.19
Multilobed placenta - see Placenta,
    abnormal
Multinodular prostate 600.10
  with
    urinary
      obstruction 600.11
      retention 600.11
Multiparity V61.5
  affecting
    fetus or newborn 763.89
    management of
      labor and delivery 659.4●
      pregnancy V23.3
  requiring contraceptive management
    (see also Contraception) V25.9
Multipartita placenta - see Placenta,
    abnormal
Multiple, multiplex - see also condition
  birth
    affecting fetus or newborn 761.5
    healthy liveborn - see Newborn,
      multiple
  digits (congenital) 755.00
    fingers 755.01
    toes 755.02
  organ or site NEC - see Accessory
  personality 300.14
  renal arteries 747.62
Mumps 072.9
  with complication 072.8
    specified type NEC 072.79
  encephalitis 072.2
  hepatitis 072.71
  meningitis (aseptic) 072.1
  meningoencephalitis 072.2
  oophoritis 072.79
  orchitis 072.0
  pancreatitis 072.3
  polyneuropathy 072.72
  vaccination, prophylactic (against)
    V04.6
Mumu (see also Infestation, filarial)
    125.9
Münchausen syndrome 301.51
Münchmeyer's disease or syndrome
    (exostosis luxurians) 728.11
Mural - see condition
Murmur (cardiac) (heart) (nonorganic)
    (organic) 785.2
  abdominal 787.5
  aortic (valve) (see also Endocarditis,
    aortic) 424.1
  benign - omit code
  cardiorespiratory 785.2
  diastolic - see condition
  Flint (see also Endocarditis, aortic) 424.1
  functional - omit code
  Graham Steell (pulmonic regurgitation)
    (see also Endocarditis, pulmonary)
    424.3
  innocent - omit code
  insignificant - omit code
  midsystolic 785.2
  mitral (valve) - see Stenosis
  physiologic - see condition
  presystolic, mitral - see Insufficiency,
    mitral
  pulmonic (valve) (see also Endocarditis,
    pulmonary) 424.3
  Still's (vibratory) - omit code
  systolic (valvular) - see condition
  tricuspid (valve) - see Endocarditis,
    tricuspid

Murmur (Continued)
  undiagnosed 785.2
  valvular - see condition
  vibratory - omit code
Murri's disease (intermittent
    hemoglobinuria) 283.2
Muscae volitantes 379.24
Muscle, muscular - see condition
Musculoneuralgia 729.1
Mushrooming hip 718.95
Mushroom workers' (pickers') lung 495.5
Mutation
  factor V leiden 289.81
  prothrombin gene 289.81
Mutism (see also Aphasia) 784.3
  akinetic 784.3
  deaf (acquired) (congenital) 389.7
  hysterical 300.11
  selective (elective) 313.23
    adjustment reaction 309.83
MVD (microvillus inclusion disease)
    751.5 ◀
Myà's disease (congenital dilation, colon)
    751.3
Myalgia (intercostal) 729.1
  eosinophilia syndrome 710.5
  epidemic 074.1
    cervical 078.89
  psychogenic 307.89
  traumatic NEC 959.9
Myasthenia 358.00
  cordis - see Failure, heart
  gravis 358.00
    with exacerbation (acute) 358.01
      in crisis 358.01
    neonatal 775.2
    pseudoparalytica 358.00
  stomach 536.8
    psychogenic 306.4
  syndrome
    in
      botulism 005.1 [358.1]
      diabetes mellitus 250.6● [358.1]
        due to secondary diabetes
          249.6● [358.1]
      hypothyroidism (see also
        Hypothyroidism) 244.9
        [358.1]
      malignant neoplasm NEC 199.1
        [358.1]
      pernicious anemia 281.0 [358.1]
      thyrotoxicosis (see also
        Thyrotoxicosis) 242.9●
        [358.1]
Myasthenic 728.87
Mycelium infection NEC 117.9
Mycetismus 988.1
Mycetoma (actinomycotic) 039.9
  bone 039.8
    mycotic 117.4
  foot 039.4
    mycotic 117.4
  madurae 039.9
    mycotic 117.4
  maduromycotic 039.9
    mycotic 117.4
  mycotic 117.4
  nocardial 039.9
Mycobacteriosis - see Mycobacterium
Mycobacterium, mycobacterial
    (infection) 031.9
  acid-fast (bacilli) 031.9
  anonymous (see also Mycobacterium,
    atypical) 031.9

◀ New   ◀▥ Revised   ~~deleted~~ Deleted   ● Use Additional Digit(s)   ▨ Omit code

Mycobacterium, mycobacterial
(*Continued*)
atypical (acid-fast bacilli) 031.9
cutaneous 031.1
pulmonary 031.0
tuberculous (*see also* Tuberculosis,
pulmonary) 011.9●
specified site NEC 031.8
avium 031.0
intracellulare complex bacteremia
(MAC) 031.2
balnei 031.1
Battey 031.0
cutaneous 031.1
disseminated 031.2
avium-intracellulare complex
(DMAC) 031.2
fortuitum 031.0
intracellulare (battey bacillus) 031.0
kakerifu 031.8
kansasii 031.0
kasongo 031.8
leprae - *see* Leprosy
luciflavum 031.0
marinum 031.1
pulmonary 031.0
tuberculous (*see also* Tuberculosis,
pulmonary) 011.9●
scrofulaceum 031.1
tuberculosis (human, bovine) - *see also*
Tuberculosis
avian type 031.0
ulcerans 031.1
xenopi 031.0
Mycosis, mycotic 117.9
cutaneous NEC 111.9
ear 111.8 [380.15]
fungoides (M9700/3) 202.1●
mouth 112.0
pharynx 117.9
skin NEC 111.9
stomatitis 112.0
systemic NEC 117.9
tonsil 117.9
vagina, vaginitis 112.1
Mydriasis (persistent) (pupil)
379.43
Myelatelia 742.59
Myelinoclasis, perivascular, acute
(postinfectious) NEC 136.9
[323.61]
postimmunization or postvaccinal
323.51
Myelinosis, central pontine 341.8
Myelitis (ascending) (cerebellar)
(childhood) (chronic) (descending)
(diffuse) (disseminated) (pressure)
(progressive) (spinal cord)
(subacute) (*see also* Encephalitis)
323.9
acute (transverse) 341.20
idiopathic 341.22
in conditions classified elsewhere
341.21
due to
infection classified elsewhere 136.9
[323.42]
specified cause NEC 323.82
vaccination (any) 323.52
viral diseases classified elsewhere
323.02
herpes simplex 054.74
herpes zoster 053.14
late effect - *see* category 326

Myelitis (*Continued*)
optic neuritis in 341.0
postchickenpox 052.2
postimmunization 323.52
postinfectious 136.9 [323.63]
postvaccinal 323.52
postvaricella 052.2
syphilitic (transverse) 094.89
toxic 989.9 [323.72]
transverse 323.82
acute 341.20
idiopathic 341.22
in conditions classified elsewhere
341.21
idiopathic 341.22
tuberculous (*see also* Tuberculosis)
013.6●
virus 049.9
Myeloblastic - *see* condition
Myelocele (*see also* Spina bifida) 741.9●
with hydrocephalus 741.0●
Myelocystocele (*see also* Spina bifida)
741.9●
Myelocytic - *see* condition
Myelocytoma 205.1●
Myelodysplasia (spinal cord) 742.59
meaning myelodysplastic syndrome -
see Syndrome, myelodysplastic
Myeloencephalitis - *see* Encephalitis
Myelofibrosis 289.83
with myeloid metaplasia 238.76
idiopathic (chronic) 238.76
megakaryocytic 238.79
primary 238.76
secondary 289.83
Myelogenous - *see* condition
Myeloid - *see* condition
Myelokathexis 288.09
Myeloleukodystrophy 330.0
Myelolipoma (M8870/0) - *see* Neoplasm,
by site, benign
Myeloma (multiple) (plasma cell)
(plasmacytic) (M9730/3) 203.0●
monostotic (M9731/1) 238.6
solitary (M9731/1) 238.6
Myelomalacia 336.8
Myelomata, multiple (M9730/3) 203.0●
Myelomatosis (M9730/3) 203.0●
Myelomeningitis - *see*
Meningoencephalitis
Myelomeningocele (spinal cord) (*see also*
Spina bifida) 741.9●
fetal, causing fetopelvic disproportion
653.7●
Myelo-osteo-musculodysplasia
hereditaria 756.89
Myelopathic - *see* condition
Myelopathy (spinal cord) 336.9
cervical 721.1
diabetic 250.6● [336.3]
due to secondary diabetes 249.6●
[336.3]
drug-induced 336.8
due to or with
carbon tetrachloride 987.8
[323.72]
degeneration or displacement,
intervertebral disc 722.70
cervical, cervicothoracic 722.71
lumbar, lumbosacral 722.73
thoracic, thoracolumbar 722.72
hydroxyquinoline derivatives 961.3
[323.72]
infection - *see* Encephalitis

Myelopathy (*Continued*)
due to or with (*Continued*)
intervertebral disc disorder
722.70
cervical, cervicothoracic
722.71
lumbar, lumbosacral 722.73
thoracic, thoracolumbar
722.72
lead 984.9 [323.72]
mercury 985.0 [323.72]
neoplastic disease (*see also*
Neoplasm, by site) 239.9
[336.3]
pernicious anemia 281.0 [336.3]
spondylosis 721.91
cervical 721.1
lumbar, lumbosacral 721.42
thoracic 721.41
thallium 985.8 [323.72]
lumbar, lumbosacral 721.42
necrotic (subacute) 336.1
radiation-induced 336.8
spondylogenic NEC 721.91
cervical 721.1
lumbar, lumbosacral 721.42
thoracic 721.41
thoracic 721.41
toxic NEC 989.9 [323.72]
transverse (*see also* Myelitis) 323.82
vascular 336.1
Myelophthisis 284.2
Myeloproliferative disease (M9960/1)
238.79
Myeloradiculitis (*see also*
Polyneuropathy) 357.0
Myeloradiculodysplasia (spinal)
742.59
Myelosarcoma (M9930/3) 205.3●
Myelosclerosis 289.89
with myeloid metaplasia (M9961/1)
238.76
disseminated, of nervous system
340
megakaryocytic (M9961/1) 238.79
Myelosis (M9860/3) (*see also* Leukemia,
myeloid) 205.9●
acute (M9861/3) 205.0●
aleukemic (M9864/3) 205.8●
chronic (M9863/3) 205.1●
erythremic (M9840/3) 207.0●
acute (M9841/3) 207.0●
megakaryocytic (M9920/3) 207.2●
nonleukemic (chronic) 288.8
subacute (M9862/3) 205.2●
Myesthenia - *see* Myasthenia
Myiasis (cavernous) 134.0
orbit 134.0 [376.13]
Myoadenoma, prostate 600.20
with
other lower urinary tract symptoms
(LUTS) 600.21
urinary
obstruction 600.21
retention 600.21
Myoblastoma
granular cell (M9580/0) - *see also*
Neoplasm, connective tissue,
benign
malignant (M9580/3) - *see*
Neoplasm, connective tissue,
malignant
tongue (M9580/0) 210.1
Myocardial - *see* condition

Myocardiopathy (congestive)
        (constrictive) (familial)
        (hypertrophic nonobstructive)
        (idiopathic) (infiltrative)
        (obstructive) (primary) (restrictive)
        (sporadic) 425.4
    alcoholic 425.5
    amyloid 277.39 [425.7]
    beriberi 265.0 [425.7]
    cobalt-beer 425.5
    due to
        amyloidosis 277.39 [425.7]
        beriberi 265.0 [425.7]
        cardiac glycogenosis 271.0 [425.7]
        Chagas' disease 086.0
        Friedreich's ataxia 334.0 [425.8]
        influenza (see also Influenza) 487.8
            [425.8] ◀▥
        mucopolysaccharidosis 277.5 [425.7]
        myotonia atrophica 359.21 [425.8]
        progressive muscular dystrophy
            359.1 [425.8]
        sarcoidosis 135 [425.8]
    glycogen storage 271.0 [425.7]
    hypertrophic obstructive 425.1
    metabolic NEC 277.9 [425.7]
    nutritional 269.9 [425.7]
    obscure (African) 425.2
    peripartum 674.5●
    postpartum 674.5●
    secondary 425.9
    thyrotoxic (see also Thyrotoxicosis)
        242.9 ● [425.7]
    toxic NEC 425.9
Myocarditis (fibroid) (interstitial) (old)
        (progressive) (senile) (with
        arteriosclerosis) 429.0
    with
        rheumatic fever (conditions
            classifiable to 390) 398.0
            active (see also Myocarditis, acute,
                rheumatic) 391.2
            inactive or quiescent (with
                chorea) 398.0
    active (nonrheumatic) 422.90
        rheumatic 391.2
            with chorea (acute) (rheumatic)
                (Sydenham's) 392.0
    acute or subacute (interstitial) 422.90
        due to Streptococcus (beta-
            hemolytic) 391.2
        idiopathic 422.91
        rheumatic 391.2
            with chorea (acute) (rheumatic)
                (Sydenham's) 392.0
        specified type NEC 422.99
    aseptic of newborn 074.23
    bacterial (acute) 422.92
    chagasic 086.0
    chronic (interstitial) 429.0
    congenital 746.89
    constrictive 425.4
    Coxsackie (virus) 074.23
    diphtheritic 032.82
    due to or in
        Coxsackie (virus) 074.23
        diphtheria 032.82
        epidemic louse-borne typhus 080
            [422.0]
        influenza (see also Influenza) 487.8
            [422.0] ◀▥
        Lyme disease 088.81 [422.0]
        scarlet fever 034.1 [422.0]
        toxoplasmosis (acquired) 130.3

Myocarditis (Continued)
    due to or in (Continued)
        tuberculosis (see also Tuberculosis)
            017.9● [422.0]
        typhoid 002.0 [422.0]
        typhus NEC 081.9 [422.0]
    eosinophilic 422.91
    epidemic of newborn 074.23
    Fiedler's (acute) (isolated) (subacute)
        422.91
    giant cell (acute) (subacute) 422.91
    gonococcal 098.85
    granulomatous (idiopathic) (isolated)
        (nonspecific) 422.91
    hypertensive (see also Hypertension,
        heart) 402.90
    idiopathic 422.91
        granulomatous 422.91
    infective 422.92
    influenzal (see also Influenza) 487.8
        [422.0] ◀▥
    isolated (diffuse) (granulomatous)
        422.91
    malignant 422.99
    meningococcal 036.43
    nonrheumatic, active 422.90
    parenchymatous 422.90
    pneumococcal (acute) (subacute) 422.92
    rheumatic (chronic) (inactive) (with
        chorea) 398.0
        active or acute 391.2
            with chorea (acute) (rheumatic)
                (Sydenham's) 392.0
    septic 422.92
    specific (giant cell) (productive)
        422.91
    staphylococcal (acute) (subacute)
        422.92
    suppurative 422.92
    syphilitic (chronic) 093.82
    toxic 422.93
        rheumatic (see also Myocarditis,
            acute rheumatic) 391.2
    tuberculous (see also Tuberculosis)
        017.9● [422.0]
    typhoid 002.0 [422.0]
    valvular - see Endocarditis
    viral, except Coxsackie 422.91
        Coxsackie 074.23
        of newborn (Coxsackie) 074.23
Myocardium, myocardial - see condition
Myocardosis (see also Cardiomyopathy)
    425.4
Myoclonia (essential) 333.2
    epileptica 345.1●
    Friedrich's 333.2
    massive 333.2
Myoclonic
    epilepsy, familial (progressive)
        345.1●
    jerks 333.2
Myoclonus (familial essential)
        (multifocal) (simplex) 333.2
    with epilepsy and with ragged red
        fibers (MERRF syndrome)
        277.87
    facial 351.8
    massive (infantile) 333.2
    palatal 333.2
    pharyngeal 333.2
Myocytolysis 429.1
Myodiastasis 728.84
Myoendocarditis - see also Endocarditis
    acute or subacute 421.9

Myoepithelioma (M8982/0) - see
    Neoplasm, by site, benign
Myofascitis (acute) 729.1
    low back 724.2
Myofibroma (M8890/0) - see also
    Neoplasm, connective tissue, benign
    uterus (cervix) (corpus) (see also
        Leiomyoma) 218.9
Myofibromatosis
    infantile 759.89
Myofibrosis 728.2
    heart (see also Myocarditis) 429.0
    humeroscapular region 726.2
    scapulohumeral 726.2
Myofibrositis (see also Myositis) 729.1
    scapulohumeral 726.2
Myogelosis (occupational) 728.89
Myoglobinuria 791.3
Myoglobulinuria, primary 791.3
Myokymia - see also Myoclonus
    facial 351.8
Myolipoma (M8860/0)
    specified site - see Neoplasm,
        connective tissue, benign
    unspecified site 223.0
Myoma (M8895/0) - see also Neoplasm,
        connective tissue, benign
    cervix (stump) (uterus) (see also
        Leiomyoma) 218.9
    malignant (M8895/3) - see Neoplasm,
        connective tissue, malignant
    prostate 600.20
        with
            other lower urinary tract
                symptoms (LUTS) 600.21
            urinary
                obstruction 600.21
                retention 600.21
    uterus (cervix) (corpus) (see also
        Leiomyoma) 218.9
    in pregnancy or childbirth 654.1●
        affecting fetus or newborn 763.89
        causing obstructed labor 660.2●
            affecting fetus or newborn
                763.1
Myomalacia 728.9
    cordis, heart (see also Degeneration,
        myocardial) 429.1
Myometritis (see also Endometritis)
    615.9
Myometrium - see condition
Myonecrosis, clostridial 040.0
Myopathy 359.9
    alcoholic 359.4
    amyloid 277.39 [359.6]
    benign, congenital 359.0
    central core 359.0
    centronuclear 359.0
    congenital (benign) 359.0
    critical illness 359.81
    distal 359.1
    due to drugs 359.4
    endocrine 259.9 [359.5]
        specified type NEC 259.8 [359.5]
    extraocular muscles 376.82
    facioscapulohumeral 359.1
    in
        Addison's disease 255.41 [359.5]
        amyloidosis 277.39 [359.6]
        cretinism 243 [359.5]
        Cushing's syndrome 255.0 [359.5]
        disseminated lupus erythematosus
            710.0 [359.6]
        giant cell arteritis 446.5 [359.6]

◀ New   ◀▥ Revised   deleted Deleted   ● Use Additional Digit(s)   ▥ Omit code

Myopathy (Continued)
  in (Continued)
    hyperadrenocorticism NEC 255.3
      [359.5]
    hyperparathyroidism 252.01 *[359.5]*
    hypopituitarism 253.2 *[359.5]*
    hypothyroidism (*see also*
      Hypothyroidism) 244.9 *[359.5]*
    malignant neoplasm NEC
      (M8000/3) 199.1 *[359.6]*
    myxedema (*see also* Myxedema)
      244.9 *[359.5]*
    polyarteritis nodosa 446.0 *[359.6]*
    rheumatoid arthritis 714.0 *[359.6]*
    sarcoidosis 135 *[359.6]*
    scleroderma 710.1 *[359.6]*
    Sjögren's disease 710.2 *[359.6]*
    thyrotoxicosis (*see also*
      Thyrotoxicosis) 242.9● *[359.5]*
  inflammatory 359.79
    immune NEC 359.79
    specified NEC 359.79
  intensive care (ICU) 359.81
  limb-girdle 359.1
  myotubular 359.0
  necrotizing, acute 359.81
  nemaline 359.0
  ocular 359.1
  oculopharyngeal 359.1
  of critical illness 359.81
  primary 359.89
  progressive NEC 359.89
  proximal myotonic (PROMM) 359.21
  quadriplegic, acute 359.81
  rod body 359.0
  scapulohumeral 359.1
  specified type NEC 359.89
  toxic 359.4
Myopericarditis (*see also* Pericarditis)
  423.9
Myopia (axial) (congenital) (increased
  curvature or refraction, nucleus of
  lens) 367.1
  degenerative, malignant 360.21
  malignant 360.21
  progressive high (degenerative) 360.21

Myosarcoma (M8895/3) - *see* Neoplasm,
  connective tissue, malignant
Myosis (persistent) 379.42
  stromal (endolymphatic) (M8931/1)
    236.0
Myositis 729.1
  clostridial 040.0
  due to posture 729.1
  epidemic 074.1
  fibrosa or fibrous (chronic) 728.2
    Volkmann's (complicating trauma)
      958.6
  inclusion body (IBM) 359.71
  infective 728.0
  interstitial 728.81
  multiple - *see* Polymyositis
  occupational 729.1
  orbital, chronic 376.12
  ossificans 728.12
    circumscribed 728.12
    progressive 728.11
    traumatic 728.12
  progressive fibrosing 728.11
  purulent 728.0
  rheumatic 729.1
  rheumatoid 729.1
  suppurative 728.0
  syphilitic 095.6
  traumatic (old) 729.1
Myospasia impulsiva 307.23
Myotonia (acquisita) (intermittens) 728.85
  atrophica 359.21
  congenita 359.22
    acetazolamide responsive 359.22
    dominant form 359.22
    recessive form 359.22
  drug-induced 359.24
  dystrophica 359.21
  fluctuans 359.29
  levior 359.22
  permanens 359.29
Myotonic pupil 379.46
Myriapodiasis 134.1

Myringitis
  with otitis media - *see* Otitis media
  acute 384.00
    specified type NEC 384.09
  bullosa hemorrhagica 384.01
  bullous 384.01
  chronic 384.1
Mysophobia 300.29
Mytilotoxism 988.0
Myxadenitis labialis 528.5
Myxedema (adult) (idiocy) (infantile)
  (juvenile) (thyroid gland) (*see also*
  Hypothyroidism) 244.9
  circumscribed 242.9●
  congenital 243
  cutis 701.8
  localized (pretibial) 242.9●
  madness (acute) 293.0
    subacute 293.1
  papular 701.8
  pituitary 244.8
  postpartum 674.8●
  pretibial 242.9●
  primary 244.9
Myxochondrosarcoma (M9220/3) -
  see Neoplasm, cartilage,
  malignant
Myxofibroma (M8811/0) - *see also*
  Neoplasm, connective tissue,
  benign
  odontogenic (M9320/0) 213.1
    upper jaw (bone) 213.0
Myxofibrosarcoma (M8811/3) - *see*
  Neoplasm, connective tissue,
  malignant
Myxolipoma (M8852/0) (*see also* Lipoma,
  by site) 214.9
Myxoliposarcoma (M8852/3) - *see*
  Neoplasm, connective tissue,
  malignant
Myxoma (M8840/0) - *see also* Neoplasm,
  connective tissue, benign
  odontogenic (M9320/0) 213.1
    upper jaw (bone) 213.0
Myxosarcoma (M8840/3) - *see* Neoplasm,
  connective tissue, malignant

M

N

Naegeli's
  disease (hereditary hemorrhagic
      thrombasthenia) 287.1
  leukemia, monocytic (M9863/3)
      205.1●
  syndrome (incontinentia pigmenti)
      757.33
Naffziger's syndrome 353.0
Naga sore (*see* also Ulcer, skin) 707.9
Nägele's pelvis 738.6
  with disproportion (fetopelvic)
      653.0●
      affecting fetus or newborn 763.1
      causing obstructed labor 660.1●
          affecting fetus or newborn 763.1
Nager-de Reynier syndrome (dysostosis
      mandibularis) 756.0
Nail - *see* also condition
  biting 307.9
  patella syndrome (hereditary
      osteoonychodysplasia) 756.89
Nanism, nanosomia (*see* also Dwarfism)
      259.4
  hypophyseal 253.3
  pituitary 253.3
  renis, renalis 588.0
Nanukayami 100.89
Napkin rash 691.0
Narcissism 301.81
Narcolepsy 347.00
  with cataplexy 347.01
  in conditions classified elsewhere
      347.10
      with cataplexy 347.11
Narcosis
  carbon dioxide (respiratory) 786.09
  due to drug
      correct substance properly
          administered 780.09
      overdose or wrong substance given
          or taken 977.9
      specified drug - *see* Table of
          Drugs and Chemicals
Narcotism (chronic) (*see* also Dependence)
      304.9●
  acute
      correct substance properly
          administered 349.82
      overdose or wrong substance given
          or taken 967.8
      specified drug - *see* Table of
          Drugs and Chemicals
NARP (ataxia and retinitis pigmentosa
      syndrome) 277.87
Narrow
  anterior chamber angle 365.02
  pelvis (inlet) (outlet) - *see* Contraction,
      pelvis
Narrowing
  artery NEC 447.1
      auditory, internal 433.8●
      basilar 433.0●
          with other precerebral artery
              433.3●
          bilateral 433.3●
      carotid 433.1●
          with other precerebral artery
              433.3●
          bilateral 433.3●
      cerebellar 433.8●
      choroidal 433.8●
      communicating posterior 433.8●

Narrowing (*Continued*)
  artery NEC (*Continued*)
      coronary - *see* also Arteriosclerosis,
          coronary
          congenital 746.85
              due to syphilis 090.5
      hypophyseal 433.8●
      pontine 433.8●
      precerebral NEC 433.9●
          multiple or bilateral 433.3●
          specified NEC 433.8●
      vertebral 433.2●
          with other precerebral artery
              433.3●
          bilateral 433.3●
  auditory canal (external) (*see* also
      Stricture, ear canal, acquired)
      380.50
  cerebral arteries 437.0
  cicatricial - *see* Cicatrix
  congenital - *see* Anomaly, congenital
  coronary artery - *see* Narrowing, artery,
      coronary
  ear, middle 385.22
  Eustachian tube (*see* also Obstruction,
      Eustachian tube) 381.60
  eyelid 374.46
      congenital 743.62
  intervertebral disc or space NEC - *see*
      Degeneration, intervertebral disc
  joint space, hip 719.85
  larynx 478.74
  lids 374.46
      congenital 743.62
  mesenteric artery (with gangrene) 557.0
  palate 524.89
  palpebral fissure 374.46
  retinal artery 362.13
  ureter 593.3
  urethra (*see* also Stricture, urethra) 598.9
Narrowness, abnormal, eyelid 743.62
Nasal - *see* condition
Nasolacrimal - *see* condition
Nasopharyngeal - *see* also condition
  bursa 478.29
  pituitary gland 759.2
  torticollis 723.5
Nasopharyngitis (acute) (infective)
      (subacute) 460
  chronic 472.2
      due to external agent - *see*
          Condition, respiratory, chronic,
          due to
  due to external agent - *see* Condition,
      respiratory, due to
  septic 034.0
  streptococcal 034.0
  suppurative (chronic) 472.2
  ulcerative (chronic) 472.2
Nasopharynx, nasopharyngeal - *see*
      condition
Natal tooth, teeth 520.6
Nausea (*see* also Vomiting) 787.02
  with vomiting 787.01
  epidemic 078.82
  gravidarum - *see* Hyperemesis,
      gravidarum
  marina 994.6
Naval - *see* condition
Neapolitan fever (*see* also Brucellosis)
      023.9
Near drowning 994.1
Nearsightedness 367.1
Near-syncope 780.2

Nebécourt's syndrome 253.3
Nebula, cornea (eye) 371.01
  congenital 743.43
      interfering with vision 743.42
Necator americanus infestation 126.1
Necatoriasis 126.1
Neck - *see* condition
Necrencephalus (*see* also Softening, brain)
      437.8
Necrobacillosis 040.3
Necrobiosis 799.89
  brain or cerebral (*see* also Softening,
      brain) 437.8
  lipoidica 709.3
      diabeticorum 250.8● [709.3]
          due to secondary diabetes 249.8●
              [709.3]
Necrodermolysis 695.15
Necrolysis, toxic epidermal 695.15
  due to drug
      correct substance properly
          administered 695.15
      overdose or wrong substance given
          or taken 977.9
      specified drug - *see* Table of
          Drugs and Chemicals
  Stevens-Johnson syndrome overlap
      (SJS-TEN overlap syndrome)
      695.14
Necrophilia 302.89
Necrosis, necrotic
  adrenal (capsule) (gland) 255.8
  antrum, nasal sinus 478.19
  aorta (hyaline) (*see* also Aneurysm,
      aorta) 441.9
      cystic medial 441.00
          abdominal 441.02
          thoracic 441.01
          thoracoabdominal 441.03
      ruptured 441.5
  arteritis 446.0
  artery 447.5
  aseptic, bone 733.40
      femur (head) (neck) 733.42
          medial condyle 733.43
      humoral head 733.41
      jaw 733.45
      medial femoral condyle 733.43
      specific site NEC 733.49
      talus 733.44
  avascular, bone NEC (*see* also Necrosis,
      aseptic, bone) 733.40
  bladder (aseptic) (sphincter) 596.8
  bone (*see* also Osteomyelitis) 730.1●
      acute 730.0●
      aseptic or avascular 733.40
          femur (head) (neck) 733.42
              medial condyle 733.43
          humoral head 733.41
          jaw 733.45
          medial femoral condyle 733.43
          specified site NEC 733.49
          talus 733.44
      ethmoid 478.19
      ischemic 733.40
      jaw 526.4
          aseptic 733.45
      marrow 289.89
      Paget's (osteitis deformans) 731.0
      tuberculous - *see* Tuberculosis, bone
  brain (softening) (*see* also Softening,
      brain) 437.8
  breast (aseptic) (fat) (segmental)
      611.3

◀ New   ◀▥ Revised   ~~deleted~~ Deleted   ● Use Additional Digit(s)   ▨ Omit code

Necrosis, necrotic *(Continued)*
   bronchus, bronchi 519.19
   central nervous system NEC *(see also*
         Softening, brain) 437.8
   cerebellar *(see also* Softening, brain) 437.8
   cerebral (softening) *(see also* Softening,
         brain) 437.8
   cerebrospinal (softening) *(see also*
         Softening, brain) 437.8
   colon 557.0
   cornea *(see also* Keratitis) 371.40
   cortical, kidney 583.6
   cystic medial (aorta) 441.00
      abdominal 441.02
         thoracic 441.01
         thoracoabdominal 441.03
   dental 521.09
      pulp 522.1
   due to swallowing corrosive
         substance - *see* Burn, by site
   ear (ossicle) 385.24
   esophagus 530.89
   ethmoid (bone) 478.19
   eyelid 374.50
   fat, fatty (generalized) *(see also*
         Degeneration, fatty) 272.8
      abdominal wall 567.82
      breast (aseptic) (segmental) 611.3
      intestine 569.89
      localized - *see* Degeneration, by site,
         fatty
      mesentery 567.82
      omentum 567.82
      pancreas 577.8
      peritoneum 567.82
      skin (subcutaneous) 709.3
         newborn 778.1
   femur (aseptic) (avascular) 733.42
      head 733.42
      medial condyle 733.43
      neck 733.42
   gallbladder *(see also* Cholecystitis,
         acute) 575.0
   gangrenous 785.4
   gastric 537.89
   glottis 478.79
   heart (myocardium) - *see* Infarct,
         myocardium
   hepatic *(see also* Necrosis, liver) 570
   hip (aseptic) (avascular) 733.42
   intestine (acute) (hemorrhagic)
         (massive) 557.0
   ischemic 785.4
   jaw 526.4
      aseptic 733.45
   kidney (bilateral) 583.9
      acute 584.9
      cortical 583.6
         acute 584.6
            with
               abortion - *see* Abortion, by
                  type, with renal
                  failure
               ectopic pregnancy *(see also*
                  categories 633.0–633.9)
                  639.3
               molar pregnancy *(see also*
                  categories 630–632)
                  639.3
            complicating pregnancy 646.2●
               affecting fetus or newborn
                  760.1
            following labor and delivery
               669.3●

Necrosis, necrotic *(Continued)*
   kidney *(Continued)*
      medullary (papillary) *(see also*
            Pyelitis) 590.80
         in
            acute renal failure 584.7
            nephritis, nephropathy 583.7
      papillary *(see also* Pyelitis) 590.80
         in
            acute renal failure 584.7
            nephritis, nephropathy 583.7
      tubular 584.5
         with
            abortion - *see* Abortion, by
               type, with renal failure
            ectopic pregnancy *(see also*
               categories 633.0–633.9)
               639.3
            molar pregnancy *(see also*
               categories 630–632)
               639.3
         complicating
            abortion 639.3
            ectopic or molar pregnancy
               639.3
            pregnancy 646.2●
               affecting fetus or newborn
                  760.1
         following labor and delivery
            669.3●
         traumatic 958.5
   larynx 478.79
   liver (acute) (congenital) (diffuse)
         (massive) (subacute) 570
      with
         abortion - *see* Abortion, by type,
            with specified complication
            NEC
         ectopic pregnancy *(see also*
            categories 633.0–633.9)
            639.8
         molar pregnancy *(see also*
            categories 630–632) 639.8
      complicating pregnancy 646.7●
         affecting fetus or newborn
            760.8
      following
         abortion 639.8
         ectopic or molar pregnancy
            639.8
      obstetrical 646.7●
      postabortal 639.8
      puerperal, postpartum 674.8●
      toxic 573.3
   lung 513.0
   lymphatic gland 683
   mammary gland 611.3
   mastoid (chronic) 383.1
   mesentery 557.0
      fat 567.82
   mitral valve - *see* Insufficiency, mitral
   myocardium, myocardial - *see* Infarct,
         myocardium
   nose (septum) 478.19
   omentum 557.0
      with mesenteric infarction 557.0
      fat 567.82
   orbit, orbital 376.10
   ossicles, ear (aseptic) 385.24
   ovary *(see also* Salpingo-oophoritis)
         614.2
   pancreas (aseptic) (duct) (fat) 577.8
      acute 577.0
      infective 577.0

Necrosis, necrotic *(Continued)*
   papillary, kidney *(see also* Pyelitis)
         590.80
   perineum 624.8
   peritoneum 557.0
      with mesenteric infarction 557.0
      fat 567.82
   pharynx 462
      in granulocytopenia 288.09
   phosphorus 983.9
   pituitary (gland) (postpartum)
         (Sheehan) 253.2
   placenta *(see also* Placenta, abnormal)
         656.7●
   pneumonia 513.0
   pulmonary 513.0
   pulp (dental) 522.1
   pylorus 537.89
   radiation - *see* Necrosis, by site
   radium - *see* Necrosis, by site
   renal - *see* Necrosis, kidney
   sclera 379.19
   scrotum 608.89
   skin or subcutaneous tissue 709.8
      due to burn - *see* Burn, by site
      gangrenous 785.4
   spine, spinal (column) 730.18
      acute 730.18
      cord 336.1
   spleen 289.59
   stomach 537.89
   stomatitis 528.1
   subcutaneous fat 709.3
      fetus or newborn 778.1
   subendocardial - *see* Infarct, myocardium
   suprarenal (capsule) (gland) 255.8
   teeth, tooth 521.09
   testis 608.89
   thymus (gland) 254.8
   tonsil 474.8
   trachea 519.19
   tuberculous NEC - *see* Tuberculosis
   tubular (acute) (anoxic) (toxic) 584.5
      due to a procedure 997.5
   umbilical cord, affecting fetus or
         newborn 762.6
   vagina 623.8
   vertebra (lumbar) 730.18
      acute 730.18
      tuberculous *(see also* Tuberculosis)
         015.0● [730.8]
   vesical (aseptic) (bladder) 596.8
   vulva 624.8
   x-ray - *see* Necrosis, by site
Necrospermia 606.0
Necrotizing angiitis 446.0
Negativism 301.7
Neglect (child) (newborn) NEC 995.52
   adult 995.84
   after or at birth 995.52
   hemispatial 781.8
   left-sided 781.8
   sensory 781.8
   visuospatial 781.8
Negri bodies 071
   Neill-Dingwall syndrome
         (microcephaly and dwarfism)
         759.89
Neisserian infection NEC - *see*
         Gonococcus
Nematodiasis NEC *(see also* Infestation,
         Nematode) 127.9
   ancylostoma *(see also* Ancylostomiasis)
         126.9

Neoformans cryptococcus infection 117.5
Neonatal - *see also* condition
   abstinence syndrome 779.5
   adrenoleukodystrophy 277.86
   teeth, tooth 520.6
Neonatorum - *see* condition
Neoplasia
   anal intraepithelial I (AIN I)
      (histologically confirmed)
      569.44 ◀▥
   anal intraepithelial II (AIN II)
      (histologically confirmed)
      569.44 ◀▥

Neoplasia *(Continued)*
   anal intraepithelial III (AIN III)
      230.6 ◀▥
     anal canal 230.5
   endometrial intraepithelial
      [EIN] 621.35
   multiple endocrine (MEN) ◀▥
      type I 258.01
      type IIA 258.02
      type IIB 258.03
   vaginal intraepithelial I (VAIN I)
      623.0 ◀▥

Neoplasia *(Continued)*
   vaginal intraepithelial II (VAIN II)
      623.0 ◀▥
   vaginal intraepithelial III (VAIN III)
      233.31 ◀▥
   vulvar intraepithelial I (VIN I)
      624.01 ◀▥
   vulvar intraepithelial II (VIN II)
      624.02 ◀▥
   vulvar intraepithelial III (VIN III)
      233.32 ◀▥
Neoplasm, neoplastic - *see* pages 365–409

◀ New   ◀▥ Revised   ~~deleted~~ Deleted   ● Use Additional Digit(s)   ▨ Omit code

	Malignant					
	Primary	Secondary	Ca in situ	Benign	Uncertain Behavior	Unspecified
Neoplasm, neoplastic	199.1	199.1	234.9	229.9	238.9	239.9

Notes — 1. The list below gives the code numbers for neoplasms by anatomical site. For each site there are six possible code numbers according to whether the neoplasm in question is malignant, benign, in situ, of uncertain behavior, or of unspecified nature. The description of the neoplasm will often indicate which of the six columns is appropriate; e.g., malignant melanoma of skin, benign fibroadenoma of breast, carcinoma in situ of cervix uteri.

Where such descriptors are not present, the remainder of the Index should be consulted where guidance is given to the appropriate column for each morphological (histological) variety listed; e.g., Mesonephroma — see Neoplasm, malignant; Embryoma — see also Neoplasm, uncertain behavior; Disease, Bowen's — see Neoplasm, skin, in situ. However, the guidance in the Index can be overridden if one of the descriptors mentioned above is present; e.g., malignant adenoma of colon is coded to 153.9 and not to 211.3 as the adjective "malignant" overrides the Index entry "Adenoma - see also Neoplasm, benign."

2. Sites marked with the sign * (e.g., face NEC*) should be classified to malignant neoplasm of skin of these sites if the variety of neoplasm is a squamous cell carcinoma or an epidermoid carcinoma and to benign neoplasm of skin of these sites if the variety of neoplasm is a papilloma (any type).

	Primary	Secondary	Ca in situ	Benign	Uncertain Behavior	Unspecified
abdomen, abdominal	195.2	198.89	234.8	229.8	238.8	239.89
cavity	195.2	198.89	234.8	229.8	238.8	239.89
organ	195.2	198.89	234.8	229.8	238.8	239.89
viscera	195.2	198.89	234.8	229.8	238.8	239.89
wall	173.5	198.2	232.5	216.5	238.2	239.2
connective tissue	171.5	198.89	—	215.5	238.1	239.2
abdominopelvic	195.8	198.89	234.8	229.8	238.8	239.89
accessory sinus - see Neoplasm, sinus						
acoustic nerve	192.0	198.4	—	225.1	237.9	239.7
acromion (process)	170.4	198.5	—	213.4	238.0	239.2
adenoid (pharynx) (tissue)	147.1	198.89	230.0	210.7	235.1	239.0
adipose tissue (see also Neoplasm, connective tissue)	171.9	198.89	—	215.9	238.1	239.2
adnexa (uterine)	183.9	198.82	233.39	221.8	236.3	239.5
adrenal (cortex) (gland) (medulla)	194.0	198.7	234.8	227.0	237.2	239.7
ala nasi (external)	173.3	198.2	232.3	216.3	238.2	239.2
alimentary canal or tract NEC	159.9	197.8	230.9	211.9	235.5	239.0
alveolar	143.9	198.89	230.0	210.4	235.1	239.0
mucosa	143.9	198.89	230.0	210.4	235.1	239.0
lower	143.1	198.89	230.0	210.4	235.1	239.0
upper	143.0	198.89	230.0	210.4	235.1	239.0
ridge or process	170.1	198.5	—	213.1	238.0	239.2
carcinoma	143.9	—	—	—	—	—
lower	143.1	—	—	—	—	—
upper	143.0	—	—	—	—	—
lower	170.1	198.5	—	213.1	238.0	239.2
mucosa	143.9	198.89	230.0	210.4	235.1	239.0
lower	143.1	198.89	230.0	210.4	235.1	239.0
upper	143.0	198.89	230.0	210.4	235.1	239.0
upper	170.0	198.5	—	213.0	238.0	239.2
sulcus	145.1	198.89	230.0	210.4	235.1	239.0

	Malignant			Benign	Uncertain Behavior	Unspecified
	Primary	Secondary	Ca in situ			
Neoplasm *(Continued)*						
alveolus	143.9	198.89	230.0	210.4	235.1	239.0
lower	143.1	198.89	230.0	210.4	235.1	239.0
upper	143.0	198.89	230.0	210.4	235.1	239.0
ampulla of Vater	156.2	197.8	230.8	211.5	235.3	239.0
ankle NEC*	195.5	198.89	232.7	229.8	238.8	239.89
anorectum, anorectal (junction)	154.8	197.5	230.7	211.4	235.2	239.0
antecubital fossa or space*	195.4	198.89	232.6	229.8	238.8	239.89
antrum (Highmore) (maxillary)	160.2	197.3	231.8	212.0	235.9	239.1
pyloric	151.2	197.8	230.2	211.1	235.2	239.0
tympanicum	160.1	197.3	231.8	212.0	235.9	239.1
anus, anal	154.3	197.5	230.6	211.4	235.5	239.0
canal	154.2	197.5	230.5	211.4	235.5	239.0
contiguous sites with rectosigmoid junction or rectum	154.8	—	—	—	—	—
margin	173.5	198.2	232.5	216.5	238.2	239.2
skin	173.5	198.2	232.5	216.5	238.2	239.2
sphincter	154.2	197.5	230.5	211.4	235.5	239.0
aorta (thoracic)	171.4	198.89	—	215.4	238.1	239.2
abdominal	171.5	198.89	—	215.5	238.1	239.2
aortic body	194.6	198.89	—	227.6	237.3	239.7
aponeurosis	171.9	198.89	—	215.9	238.1	239.2
palmar	171.2	198.89	—	215.2	238.1	239.2
plantar	171.3	198.89	—	215.3	238.1	239.2
appendix	153.5	197.5	230.3	211.3	235.2	239.0
arachnoid (cerebral)	192.1	198.4	—	225.2	237.6	239.7
spinal	192.3	198.4	—	225.4	237.6	239.7
areola (female)	174.0	198.81	233.0	217	238.3	239.3
male	175.0	198.81	233.0	217	238.3	239.3
arm NEC*	195.4	198.89	232.6	229.8	238.8	239.89
artery - *see* Neoplasm, connective tissue						
aryepiglottic fold	148.2	198.89	230.0	210.8	235.1	239.0
hypopharyngeal aspect	148.2	198.89	230.0	210.8	235.1	239.0
laryngeal aspect	161.1	197.3	231.0	212.1	235.6	239.1
marginal zone	148.2	198.89	230.0	210.8	235.1	239.0
arytenoid (cartilage)	161.3	197.3	231.0	212.1	235.6	239.1
fold - *see* Neoplasm, aryepiglottic						
associated with transplanted organ	199.2	—	—	—	—	—
atlas	170.2	198.5	—	213.2	238.0	239.2
atrium, cardiac	164.1	198.89	—	212.7	238.8	239.89
auditory						
canal (external) (skin)	173.2	198.2	232.2	216.2	238.2	239.2
internal	160.1	197.3	231.8	212.0	235.9	239.1

◀ New   ◀ Revised   ~~deleted~~ Deleted   ● Use Additional Digit(s)   ▨ Omit code

	Malignant					
	Primary	Secondary	Ca in situ	Benign	Uncertain Behavior	Unspecified
Neoplasm *(Continued)*						
auditory *(Continued)*						
nerve	192.0	198.4	—	225.1	237.9	239.7
tube	160.1	197.3	231.8	212.0	235.9	239.1
opening	147.2	198.89	230.0	210.7	235.1	239.0
auricle, ear	173.2	198.2	232.2	216.2	238.2	239.2
cartilage	171.0	198.89	—	215.0	238.1	239.2
auricular canal (external)	173.2	198.2	232.2	216.2	238.2	239.2
internal	160.1	197.3	231.8	212.0	235.9	239.1
autonomic nerve or nervous system NEC	171.9	198.89	—	215.9	238.1	239.2
axilla, axillary	195.1	198.89	234.8	229.8	238.8	239.89
fold	173.5	198.2	232.5	216.5	238.2	239.2
back NEC*	195.8	198.89	232.5	229.8	238.8	239.89
Bartholin's gland	184.1	198.82	233.39	221.2	236.3	239.5
basal ganglia	191.0	198.3	—	225.0	237.5	239.6
basis pedunculi	191.7	198.3	—	225.0	237.5	239.6
bile or biliary (tract)	156.9	197.8	230.8	211.5	235.3	239.0
canaliculi (biliferi) (intrahepatic)	155.1	197.8	230.8	211.5	235.3	239.0
canals, interlobular	155.1	197.8	230.8	211.5	235.3	239.0
contiguous sites	156.8	—	—	—	—	—
duct or passage (common) (cystic) (extrahepatic)	156.1	197.8	230.8	211.5	235.3	239.0
contiguous sites						
with gallbladder	156.8	—	—	—	—	—
interlobular	155.1	197.8	230.8	211.5	235.3	239.0
intrahepatic	155.1	197.8	230.8	211.5	235.3	239.0
and extrahepatic	156.9	197.8	230.8	211.5	235.3	239.0
bladder (urinary)	188.9	198.1	233.7	223.3	236.7	239.4
contiguous sites	188.8	—	—	—	—	—
dome	188.1	198.1	233.7	223.3	236.7	239.4
neck	188.5	198.1	233.7	223.3	236.7	239.4
orifice	188.9	198.1	233.7	223.3	236.7	239.4
ureteric	188.6	198.1	233.7	223.3	236.7	239.4
urethral	188.5	198.1	233.7	223.3	236.7	239.4
sphincter	188.8	198.1	233.7	223.3	236.7	239.4
trigone	188.0	198.1	233.7	223.3	236.7	239.4
urachus	188.7	—	233.7	223.3	236.7	239.4
wall	188.9	198.1	233.7	223.3	236.7	239.4
anterior	188.3	198.1	233.7	223.3	236.7	239.4
lateral	188.2	198.1	233.7	223.3	236.7	239.4
posterior	188.4	198.1	233.7	223.3	236.7	239.4
blood vessel - *see* Neoplasm, connective tissue						

	Malignant			Benign	Uncertain Behavior	Unspecified
	Primary	Secondary	Ca in situ			
Neoplasm *(Continued)*						
bone (periosteum)	170.9	198.5	—	213.9	238.0	239.2
Note — Carcinomas and adenocarcinomas, of any type other than intraosseous or odontogenic, of the sites listed under "Neoplasm, bone" should be considered as constituting metastatic spread from an unspecified primary site and coded to 198.5 for morbidity coding.						
acetabulum	170.6	198.5	—	213.6	238.0	239.2
acromion (process)	170.4	198.5	—	213.4	238.0	239.2
ankle	170.8	198.5	—	213.8	238.0	239.2
arm NEC	170.4	198.5	—	213.4	238.0	239.2
astragalus	170.8	198.5	—	213.8	238.0	239.2
atlas	170.2	198.5	—	213.2	238.0	239.2
axis	170.2	198.5	—	213.2	238.0	239.2
back NEC	170.2	198.5	—	213.2	238.0	239.2
calcaneus	170.8	198.5	—	213.8	238.0	239.2
calvarium	170.0	198.5	—	213.0	238.0	239.2
carpus (any)	170.5	198.5	—	213.5	238.0	239.2
cartilage NEC	170.9	198.5	—	213.9	238.0	239.2
clavicle	170.3	198.5	—	213.3	238.0	239.2
clivus	170.0	198.5	—	213.0	238.0	239.2
coccygeal vertebra	170.6	198.5	—	213.6	238.0	239.2
coccyx	170.6	198.5	—	213.6	238.0	239.2
costal cartilage	170.3	198.5	—	213.3	238.0	239.2
costovertebral joint	170.3	198.5	—	213.3	238.0	239.2
cranial	170.0	198.5	—	213.0	238.0	239.2
cuboid	170.8	198.5	—	213.8	238.0	239.2
cuneiform	170.9	198.5	—	213.9	238.0	239.2
ankle	170.8	198.5	—	213.8	238.0	239.2
wrist	170.5	198.5	—	213.5	238.0	239.2
digital	170.9	198.5	—	213.9	238.0	239.2
finger	170.5	198.5	—	213.5	238.0	239.2
toe	170.8	198.5	—	213.8	238.0	239.2
elbow	170.4	198.5	—	213.4	238.0	239.2
ethmoid (labyrinth)	170.0	198.5	—	213.0	238.0	239.2
face	170.0	198.5	—	213.0	238.0	239.2
lower jaw	170.1	198.5	—	213.1	238.0	239.2
femur (any part)	170.7	198.5	—	213.7	238.0	239.2
fibula (any part)	170.7	198.5	—	213.7	238.0	239.2
finger (any)	170.5	198.5	—	213.5	238.0	239.2
foot	170.8	198.5	—	213.8	238.0	239.2
forearm	170.4	198.5	—	213.4	238.0	239.2
frontal	170.0	198.5	—	213.0	238.0	239.2
hand	170.5	198.5	—	213.5	238.0	239.2

◀ New ◀▦ Revised ~~deleted~~ Deleted ● Use Additional Digit(s) ▨ Omit code

	Malignant			Benign	Uncertain Behavior	Unspecified
	Primary	Secondary	Ca in situ			
Neoplasm *(Continued)*						
bone *(Continued)*						
heel	170.8	198.5	—	213.8	238.0	239.2
hip	170.6	198.5	—	213.6	238.0	239.2
humerus (any part)	170.4	198.5	—	213.4	238.0	239.2
hyoid	170.0	198.5	—	213.0	238.0	239.2
ilium	170.6	198.5	—	213.6	238.0	239.2
innominate	170.6	198.5	—	213.6	238.0	239.2
intervertebral cartilage or disc	170.2	198.5	—	213.2	238.0	239.2
ischium	170.6	198.5	—	213.6	238.0	239.2
jaw (lower)	170.1	198.5	—	213.1	238.0	239.2
upper	170.0	198.5	—	213.0	238.0	239.2
knee	170.7	198.5	—	213.7	238.0	239.2
leg NEC	170.7	198.5	—	213.7	238.0	239.2
limb NEC	170.9	198.5	—	213.9	238.0	239.2
lower (long bones)	170.7	198.5	—	213.7	238.0	239.2
short bones	170.8	198.5	—	213.8	238.0	239.2
upper (long bones)	170.4	198.5	—	213.4	238.0	239.2
short bones	170.5	198.5	—	213.5	238.0	239.2
long	170.9	198.5	—	213.9	238.0	239.2
lower limbs NEC	170.7	198.5	—	213.7	238.0	239.2
upper limbs NEC	170.4	198.5	—	213.4	238.0	239.2
malar	170.0	198.5	—	213.0	238.0	239.2
mandible	170.1	198.5	—	213.1	238.0	239.2
marrow NEC	202.9 ●	198.5	—	—	—	238.79
mastoid	170.0	198.5	—	213.0	238.0	239.2
maxilla, maxillary (superior)	170.0	198.5	—	213.0	238.0	239.2
inferior	170.1	198.5	—	213.1	238.0	239.2
metacarpus (any)	170.5	198.5	—	213.5	238.0	239.2
metatarsus (any)	170.8	198.5	—	213.8	238.0	239.2
navicular (ankle)	170.8	198.5	—	213.8	238.0	239.2
hand	170.5	198.5	—	213.5	238.0	239.2
nose, nasal	170.0	198.5	—	213.0	238.0	239.2
occipital	170.0	198.5	—	213.0	238.0	239.2
orbit	170.0	198.5	—	213.0	238.0	239.2
parietal	170.0	198.5	—	213.0	238.0	239.2
patella	170.8	198.5	—	213.8	238.0	239.2
pelvic	170.6	198.5	—	213.6	238.0	239.2
phalanges	170.9	198.5	—	213.9	238.0	239.2
foot	170.8	198.5	—	213.8	238.0	239.2
hand	170.5	198.5	—	213.5	238.0	239.2

◀ New　◀▥ Revised　deleted Deleted　● Use Additional Digit(s)　▨ Omit code

	Malignant			Benign	Uncertain Behavior	Unspecified
	Primary	Secondary	Ca in situ			
Neoplasm *(Continued)*						
bone *(Continued)*						
pubic	170.6	198.5	—	213.6	238.0	239.2
radius (any part)	170.4	198.5	—	213.4	238.0	239.2
rib	170.3	198.5	—	213.3	238.0	239.2
sacral vertebra	170.6	198.5	—	213.6	238.0	239.2
sacrum	170.6	198.5	—	213.6	238.0	239.2
scaphoid (of hand)	170.5	198.5	—	213.5	238.0	239.2
of ankle	170.8	198.5	—	213.8	238.0	239.2
scapula (any part)	170.4	198.5	—	213.4	238.0	239.2
sella turcica	170.0	198.5	—	213.0	238.0	239.2
short	170.9	198.5	—	213.9	238.0	239.2
lower limb	170.8	198.5	—	213.8	238.0	239.2
upper limb	170.5	198.5	—	213.5	238.0	239.2
shoulder	170.4	198.5	—	213.4	238.0	239.2
skeleton, skeletal NEC	170.9	198.5	—	213.9	238.0	239.2
skull	170.0	198.5	—	213.0	238.0	239.2
sphenoid	170.0	198.5	—	213.0	238.0	239.2
spine, spinal (column)	170.2	198.5	—	213.2	238.0	239.2
coccyx	170.6	198.5	—	213.6	238.0	239.2
sacrum	170.6	198.5	—	213.6	238.0	239.2
sternum	170.3	198.5	—	213.3	238.0	239.2
tarsus (any)	170.8	198.5	—	213.8	238.0	239.2
temporal	170.0	198.5	—	213.0	238.0	239.2
thumb	170.5	198.5	—	213.5	238.0	239.2
tibia (any part)	170.7	198.5	—	213.7	238.0	239.2
toe (any)	170.8	198.5	—	213.8	238.0	239.2
trapezium	170.5	198.5	—	213.5	238.0	239.2
trapezoid	170.5	198.5	—	213.5	238.0	239.2
turbinate	170.0	198.5	—	213.0	238.0	239.2
ulna (any part)	170.4	198.5	—	213.4	238.0	239.2
unciform	170.5	198.5	—	213.5	238.0	239.2
vertebra (column)	170.2	198.5	—	213.2	238.0	239.2
coccyx	170.6	198.5	—	213.6	238.0	239.2
sacrum	170.6	198.5	—	213.6	238.0	239.2
vomer	170.0	198.5	—	213.0	238.0	239.2
wrist	170.5	198.5	—	213.5	238.0	239.2
xiphoid process	170.3	198.5	—	213.3	238.0	239.2
zygomatic	170.0	198.5	—	213.0	238.0	239.2
book-leaf (mouth)	145.8	198.89	230.0	210.4	235.1	239.0
bowel - *see* Neoplasm, intestine						

◄ New　◄ Revised　deleted Deleted　● Use Additional Digit(s)　Omit code

	Malignant					
	Primary	Secondary	Ca in situ	Benign	Uncertain Behavior	Unspecified
Neoplasm *(Continued)*						
brachial plexus	171.2	198.89	—	215.2	238.1	239.2
brain NEC	191.9	198.3	—	225.0	237.5	239.6
basal ganglia	191.0	198.3	—	225.0	237.5	239.6
cerebellopontine angle	191.6	198.3	—	225.0	237.5	239.6
cerebellum NOS	191.6	198.3	—	225.0	237.5	239.6
cerebrum	191.0	198.3	—	225.0	237.5	239.6
choroid plexus	191.5	198.3	—	225.0	237.5	239.6
contiguous sites	191.8	—	—	—	—	—
corpus callosum	191.8	198.3	—	225.0	237.5	239.6
corpus striatum	191.0	198.3	—	225.0	237.5	239.6
cortex (cerebral)	191.0	198.3	—	225.0	237.5	239.6
frontal lobe	191.1	198.3	—	225.0	237.5	239.6
globus pallidus	191.0	198.3	—	225.0	237.5	239.6
hippocampus	191.2	198.3	—	225.0	237.5	239.6
hypothalamus	191.0	198.3	—	225.0	237.5	239.6
internal capsule	191.0	198.3	—	225.0	237.5	239.6
medulla oblongata	191.7	198.3	—	225.0	237.5	239.6
meninges	192.1	198.4	—	225.2	237.6	239.7
midbrain	191.7	198.3	—	225.0	237.5	239.6
occipital lobe	191.4	198.3	—	225.0	237.5	239.6
parietal lobe	191.3	198.3	—	225.0	237.5	239.6
peduncle	191.7	198.3	—	225.0	237.5	239.6
pons	191.7	198.3	—	225.0	237.5	239.6
stem	191.7	198.3	—	225.0	237.5	239.6
tapetum	191.8	198.3	—	225.0	237.5	239.6
temporal lobe	191.2	198.3	—	225.0	237.5	239.6
thalamus	191.0	198.3	—	225.0	237.5	239.6
uncus	191.2	198.3	—	225.0	237.5	239.6
ventricle (floor)	191.5	198.3	—	225.0	237.5	239.6
branchial (cleft) (vestiges)	146.8	198.89	230.0	210.6	235.1	239.0
breast (connective tissue) (female) (glandular tissue) (soft parts)	174.9	198.81	233.0	217	238.3	239.3
areola	174.0	198.81	233.0	217	238.3	239.3
male	175.0	198.81	233.0	217	238.3	239.3
axillary tail	174.6	198.81	233.0	217	238.3	239.3
central portion	174.1	198.81	233.0	217	238.3	239.3
contiguous sites	174.8	—	—	—	—	—
ectopic sites	174.8	198.81	233.0	217	238.3	239.3
inner	174.8	198.81	233.0	217	238.3	239.3
lower	174.8	198.81	233.0	217	238.3	239.3
lower-inner quadrant	174.3	198.81	233.0	217	238.3	239.3

	Malignant					
	Primary	Secondary	Ca in situ	Benign	Uncertain Behavior	Unspecified
Neoplasm *(Continued)*						
breast *(Continued)*						
lower-outer quadrant	174.5	198.81	233.0	217	238.3	239.3
male	175.9	198.81	233.0	217	238.3	239.3
areola	175.0	198.81	233.0	217	238.3	239.3
ectopic tissue	175.9	198.81	233.0	217	238.3	239.3
nipple	175.0	198.81	233.0	217	238.3	239.3
mastectomy site (skin)	173.5	198.2	—	—	—	—
specified as breast tissue	174.8	198.81	—	—	—	—
midline	174.8	198.81	233.0	217	238.3	239.3
nipple	174.0	198.81	233.0	217	238.3	239.3
male	175.0	198.81	233.0	217	238.3	239.3
outer	174.8	198.81	233.0	217	238.3	239.3
skin	173.5	198.2	232.5	216.5	238.2	239.2
tail (axillary)	174.6	198.81	233.0	217	238.3	239.3
upper	174.8	198.81	233.0	217	238.3	239.3
upper-inner quadrant	174.2	198.81	233.0	217	238.3	239.3
upper-outer quadrant	174.4	198.81	233.0	217	238.3	239.3
broad ligament	183.3	198.82	233.39	221.0	236.3	239.5
bronchiogenic, bronchogenic (lung)	162.9	197.0	231.2	212.3	235.7	239.1
bronchiole	162.9	197.0	231.2	212.3	235.7	239.1
bronchus	162.9	197.0	231.2	212.3	235.7	239.1
carina	162.2	197.0	231.2	212.3	235.7	239.1
contiguous sites with lung or trachea	162.8	—	—	—	—	—
lower lobe of lung	162.5	197.0	231.2	212.3	235.7	239.1
main	162.2	197.0	231.2	212.3	235.7	239.1
middle lobe of lung	162.4	197.0	231.2	212.3	235.7	239.1
upper lobe of lung	162.3	197.0	231.2	212.3	235.7	239.1
brow	173.3	198.2	232.3	216.3	238.2	239.2
buccal (cavity)	145.9	198.89	230.0	210.4	235.1	239.0
commissure	145.0	198.89	230.0	210.4	235.1	239.0
groove (lower) (upper)	145.1	198.89	230.0	210.4	235.1	239.0
mucosa	145.0	198.89	230.0	210.4	235.1	239.0
sulcus (lower) (upper)	145.1	198.89	230.0	210.4	235.1	239.0
bulbourethral gland	189.3	198.1	233.9	223.81	236.99	239.5
bursa - *see* Neoplasm, connective tissue						
buttock NEC*	195.3	198.89	232.5	229.8	238.8	239.89
calf*	195.5	198.89	232.7	229.8	238.8	239.89
calvarium	170.0	198.5	—	213.0	238.0	239.2
calyx, renal	189.1	198.0	233.9	223.1	236.91	239.5

◀ New   ◀║ Revised   ~~deleted~~ Deleted   ● Use Additional Digit(s)   ▨ Omit code

| | Malignant | | | | | |
	Primary	Secondary	Ca in situ	Benign	Uncertain Behavior	Unspecified
Neoplasm *(Continued)*						
canal						
anal	154.2	197.5	230.5	211.4	235.5	239.0
auditory (external)	173.2	198.2	232.2	216.2	238.2	239.2
auricular (external)	173.2	198.2	232.2	216.2	238.2	239.2
canaliculi, biliary (biliferi) (intrahepatic)	155.1	197.8	230.8	211.5	235.3	239.0
canthus (eye) (inner) (outer)	173.1	198.2	232.1	216.1	238.2	239.2
capillary - *see* Neoplasm, connective tissue						
caput coli	153.4	197.5	230.3	211.3	235.2	239.0
cardia (gastric)	151.0	197.8	230.2	211.1	235.2	239.0
cardiac orifice (stomach)	151.0	197.8	230.2	211.1	235.2	239.0
cardio-esophageal junction	151.0	197.8	230.2	211.1	235.2	239.0
cardio-esophagus	151.0	197.8	230.2	211.1	235.2	239.0
carina (bronchus) (trachea)	162.2	197.0	231.2	212.3	235.7	239.1
carotid (artery)	171.0	198.89	—	215.0	238.1	239.2
body	194.5	198.89	—	227.5	237.3	239.7
carpus (any bone)	170.5	198.5	—	213.5	238.0	239.2
cartilage (articular) (joint) NEC - *see also* Neoplasm, bone	170.9	198.5	—	213.9	238.0	239.2
arytenoid	161.3	197.3	231.0	212.1	235.6	239.1
auricular	171.0	198.89	—	215.0	238.1	239.2
bronchi	162.2	197.3	—	212.3	235.7	239.1
connective tissue - *see* Neoplasm, connective tissue						
costal	170.3	198.5	—	213.3	238.0	239.2
cricoid	161.3	197.3	231.0	212.1	235.6	239.1
cuneiform	161.3	197.3	231.0	212.1	235.6	239.1
ear (external)	171.0	198.89	—	215.0	238.1	239.2
ensiform	170.3	198.5	—	213.3	238.0	239.2
epiglottis	161.1	197.3	231.0	212.1	235.6	239.1
anterior surface	146.4	198.89	230.0	210.6	235.1	239.0
eyelid	171.0	198.89	—	215.0	238.1	239.2
intervertebral	170.2	198.5	—	213.2	238.0	239.2
larynx, laryngeal	161.3	197.3	231.0	212.1	235.6	239.1
nose, nasal	160.0	197.3	231.8	212.0	235.9	239.1
pinna	171.0	198.89	—	215.0	238.1	239.2
rib	170.3	198.5	—	213.3	238.0	239.2
semilunar (knee)	170.7	198.5	—	213.7	238.0	239.2
thyroid	161.3	197.3	231.0	212.1	235.6	239.1
trachea	162.0	197.3	231.1	212.2	235.7	239.1
cauda equina	192.2	198.3	—	225.3	237.5	239.7

◀ New   ◀▥ Revised   ~~deleted~~ Deleted   ● Use Additional Digit(s)   ▦ Omit code

	Malignant					
	Primary	Secondary	Ca in situ	Benign	Uncertain Behavior	Unspecified
Neoplasm *(Continued)*						
cavity						
buccal	145.9	198.89	230.0	210.4	235.1	239.0
nasal	160.0	197.3	231.8	212.0	235.9	239.1
oral	145.9	198.89	230.0	210.4	235.1	239.0
peritoneal	158.9	197.6	—	211.8	235.4	239.0
tympanic	160.1	197.3	231.8	212.0	235.9	239.1
cecum	153.4	197.5	230.3	211.3	235.2	239.0
central						
nervous system - *see* Neoplasm, nervous system						
white matter	191.0	198.3	—	225.0	237.5	239.6
cerebellopontine (angle)	191.6	198.3	—	225.0	237.5	239.6
cerebellum, cerebellar	191.6	198.3	—	225.0	237.5	239.6
cerebrum, cerebral (cortex) (hemisphere) (white matter)	191.0	198.3	—	225.0	237.5	239.6
meninges	192.1	198.4	—	225.2	237.6	239.7
peduncle	191.7	198.3	—	225.0	237.5	239.6
ventricle (any)	191.5	198.3	—	225.0	237.5	239.6
cervical region	195.0	198.89	234.8	229.8	238.8	239.89
cervix (cervical) (uteri) (uterus)	180.9	198.82	233.1	219.0	236.0	239.5
canal	180.0	198.82	233.1	219.0	236.0	239.5
contiguous sites	180.8	—	—	—	—	—
endocervix (canal) (gland)	180.0	198.82	233.1	219.0	236.0	239.5
exocervix	180.1	198.82	233.1	219.0	236.0	239.5
external os	180.1	198.82	233.1	219.0	236.0	239.5
nabothian gland	180.0	198.82	233.1	219.0	236.0	239.5
squamocolumnar junction	180.8	198.82	233.1	219.0	236.0	239.5
stump	180.8	198.82	233.1	219.0	236.0	239.5
cheek	195.0	198.89	234.8	229.8	238.8	239.89
external	173.3	198.2	232.3	216.3	238.2	239.2
inner aspect	145.0	198.89	230.0	210.4	235.1	239.0
internal	145.0	198.89	230.0	210.4	235.1	239.0
mucosa	145.0	198.89	230.0	210.4	235.1	239.0
chest (wall) NEC	195.1	198.89	234.8	229.8	238.8	239.89
chiasma opticum	192.0	198.4	—	225.1	237.9	239.7
chin	173.3	198.2	232.3	216.3	238.2	239.2
choana	147.3	198.89	230.0	210.7	235.1	239.0
cholangiole	155.1	197.8	230.8	211.5	235.3	239.0
choledochal duct	156.1	197.8	230.8	211.5	235.3	239.0
choroid	190.6	198.4	234.0	224.6	238.8	239.81
plexus	191.5	198.3	—	225.0	237.5	239.6
ciliary body	190.0	198.4	234.0	224.0	238.8	239.89

◀ New ◀▥ Revised ~~deleted~~ Deleted ● Use Additional Digit(s) ▨ Omit code

	Malignant			Benign	Uncertain Behavior	Unspecified
	Primary	Secondary	Ca in situ			
Neoplasm *(Continued)*						
clavicle	170.3	198.5	—	213.3	238.0	239.2
clitoris	184.3	198.82	233.32	221.2	236.3	239.5
clivus	170.0	198.5	—	213.0	238.0	239.2
cloacogenic zone	154.8	197.5	230.7	211.4	235.5	239.0
coccygeal						
body or glomus	194.6	198.89	—	227.6	237.3	239.7
vertebra	170.6	198.5	—	213.6	238.0	239.2
coccyx	170.6	198.5	—	213.6	238.0	239.2
~~colon - *see also* Neoplasm, intestine, large and rectum~~	~~154.0~~	~~197.5~~	~~230.4~~	~~211.4~~	~~235.2~~	~~239.0~~
colon - *see also* Neoplasm, intestine, large	153.9	197.5	230.3	211.3	235.2	239.0 ◄
with rectum	154.0	197.5	230.4	211.4	235.2	239.0 ◄
column, spinal - *see* Neoplasm, spine						
columnella	173.3	198.2	232.3	216.3	238.2	239.2
commissure						
labial, lip	140.6	198.89	230.0	210.4	235.1	239.0
laryngeal	161.0	197.3	231.0	212.1	235.6	239.1
common (bile) duct	156.1	197.8	230.8	211.5	235.3	239.0
concha	173.2	198.2	232.2	216.2	238.2	239.2
nose	160.0	197.3	231.8	212.0	235.9	239.1
conjunctiva	190.3	198.4	234.0	224.3	238.8	239.89
connective tissue NEC	171.9	198.89	—	215.9	238.1	239.2

Note — For neoplasms of connective tissue (blood vessel, bursa, fascia, ligament, muscle, peripheral nerves, sympathetic and parasympathetic nerves and ganglia, synovia, tendon, etc.) or of morphological types that indicate connective tissue, code according to the list under "Neoplasm, connective tissue;" for sites that do not appear in this list, code to neoplasm of that site; e.g.,

      liposarcoma, shoulder 171.2

      leiomyosarcoma, stomach 151.9

      neurofibroma, chest wall 215.4

Morphological types that indicate connective tissue appear in their proper place in the alphabetic index with the instruction "see Neoplasm, connective tissue ...."

abdomen	171.5	198.89	—	215.5	238.1	239.2
abdominal wall	171.5	198.89	—	215.5	238.1	239.2
ankle	171.3	198.89	—	215.3	238.1	239.2
antecubital fossa or space	171.2	198.89	—	215.2	238.1	239.2
arm	171.2	198.89	—	215.2	238.1	239.2
auricle (ear)	171.0	198.89	—	215.0	238.1	239.2
axilla	171.4	198.89	—	215.4	238.1	239.2
back	171.7	198.89	—	215.7	238.1	239.2
breast (female) (*see also* Neoplasm, breast)	174.9	198.81	233.0	217	238.3	239.3
male	175.9	198.81	233.0	217	238.3	239.3
buttock	171.6	198.89	—	215.6	238.1	239.2
calf	171.3	198.89	—	215.3	238.1	239.2
cervical region	171.0	198.89	—	215.0	238.1	239.2

| | Malignant | | | | | |
	Primary	Secondary	Ca in situ	Benign	Uncertain Behavior	Unspecified
Neoplasm *(Continued)*						
connective tissue NEC *(Continued)*						
cheek	171.0	198.89	—	215.0	238.1	239.2
chest (wall)	171.4	198.89	—	215.4	238.1	239.2
chin	171.0	198.89	—	215.0	238.1	239.2
contiguous sites	171.8	—		—	—	—
diaphragm	171.4	198.89	—	215.4	238.1	239.2
ear (external)	171.0	198.89	—	215.0	238.1	239.2
elbow	171.2	198.89	—	215.2	238.1	239.2
extrarectal	171.6	198.89	—	215.6	238.1	239.2
extremity	171.8	198.89	—	215.8	238.1	239.2
lower	171.3	198.89	—	215.3	238.1	239.2
upper	171.2	198.89	—	215.2	238.1	239.2
eyelid	171.0	198.89	—	215.0	238.1	239.2
face	171.0	198.89	—	215.0	238.1	239.2
finger	171.2	198.89	—	215.2	238.1	239.2
flank	171.7	198.89	—	215.7	238.1	239.2
foot	171.3	198.89	—	215.3	238.1	239.2
forearm	171.2	198.89	—	215.2	238.1	239.2
forehead	171.0	198.89	—	215.0	238.1	239.2
gastric	171.5	198.89	—	215.5	238.1	—
gastrointestinal	171.5	198.89	—	215.5	238.1	—
gluteal region	171.6	198.89	—	215.6	238.1	239.2
great vessels NEC	171.4	198.89	—	215.4	238.1	239.2
groin	171.6	198.89	—	215.6	238.1	239.2
hand	171.2	198.89	—	215.2	238.1	239.2
head	171.0	198.89	—	215.0	238.1	239.2
heel	171.3	198.89	—	215.3	238.1	239.2
hip	171.3	198.89	—	215.3	238.1	239.2
hypochondrium	171.5	198.89	—	215.5	238.1	239.2
iliopsoas muscle	171.6	198.89	—	215.5	238.1	239.2
infraclavicular region	171.4	198.89	—	215.4	238.1	239.2
inguinal (canal) (region)	171.6	198.89	—	215.6	238.1	239.2
intestine	171.5	198.89	—	215.5	238.1	—
intrathoracic	171.4	198.89	—	215.4	238.1	239.2
ischorectal fossa	171.6	198.89	—	215.6	238.1	239.2
jaw	143.9	198.89	230.0	210.4	235.1	239.0
knee	171.3	198.89	—	215.3	238.1	239.2
leg	171.3	198.89	—	215.3	238.1	239.2
limb NEC	171.9	198.89	—	215.8	238.1	239.2
lower	171.3	198.89	—	215.3	238.1	239.2
upper	171.2	198.89	—	215.2	238.1	239.2

◀ New   ◀▥ Revised   ~~deleted~~ Deleted   ● Use Additional Digit(s)   ▨ Omit code

	Malignant					
	Primary	Secondary	Ca in situ	Benign	Uncertain Behavior	Unspecified
Neoplasm *(Continued)*						
connective tissue NEC *(Continued)*						
nates	171.6	198.89	—	215.6	238.1	239.2
neck	171.0	198.89	—	215.0	238.1	239.2
orbit	190.1	198.4	234.0	224.1	238.8	239.89
pararectal	171.6	198.89	—	215.6	238.1	239.2
para-urethral	171.6	198.89	—	215.6	238.1	239.2
paravaginal	171.6	198.89	—	215.6	238.1	239.2
pelvis (floor)	171.6	198.89	—	215.6	238.1	239.2
pelvo-abdominal	171.8	198.89	—	215.8	238.1	239.2
perineum	171.6	198.89	—	215.6	238.1	239.2
perirectal (tissue)	171.6	198.89	—	215.6	238.1	239.2
periurethral (tissue)	171.6	198.89	—	215.6	238.1	239.2
popliteal fossa or space	171.3	198.89	—	215.3	238.1	239.2
presacral	171.6	198.89	—	215.6	238.1	239.2
psoas muscle	171.5	198.89	—	215.5	238.1	239.2
pterygoid fossa	171.0	198.89	—	215.0	238.1	239.2
rectovaginal septum or wall	171.6	198.89	—	215.6	238.1	239.2
rectovesical	171.6	198.89	—	215.6	238.1	239.2
retroperitoneum	158.0	197.6	—	211.8	235.4	239.0
sacrococcygeal region	171.6	198.89	—	215.6	238.1	239.2
scalp	171.0	198.89	—	215.0	238.1	239.2
scapular region	171.4	198.89	—	215.4	238.1	239.2
shoulder	171.2	198.89	—	215.2	238.1	239.2
skin (dermis) NEC	173.9	198.2	232.9	216.9	238.2	239.2
stomach	171.5	198.89	—	215.5	238.1	—
submental	171.0	198.89	—	215.0	238.1	239.2
supraclavicular region	171.0	198.89	—	215.0	238.1	239.2
temple	171.0	198.89	—	215.0	238.1	239.2
temporal region	171.0	198.89	—	215.0	238.1	239.2
thigh	171.3	198.89	—	215.3	238.1	239.2
thoracic (duct) (wall)	171.4	198.89	—	215.4	238.1	239.2
thorax	171.4	198.89	—	215.4	238.1	239.2
thumb	171.2	198.89	—	215.2	238.1	239.2
toe	171.3	198.89	—	215.3	238.1	239.2
trunk	171.7	198.89	—	215.7	238.1	239.2
umbilicus	171.5	198.89	—	215.5	238.1	239.2
vesicorectal	171.6	198.89	—	215.6	238.1	239.2
wrist	171.2	198.89	—	215.2	238.1	239.2
conus medullaris	192.2	198.3	—	225.3	237.5	239.7

	Malignant					
	Primary	Secondary	Ca in situ	Benign	Uncertain Behavior	Unspecified
Neoplasm *(Continued)*						
cord (true) (vocal)	161.0	197.3	231.0	212.1	235.6	239.1
false	161.1	197.3	231.0	212.1	235.6	239.1
spermatic	187.6	198.82	233.6	222.8	236.6	239.5
spinal (cervical) (lumbar) (thoracic)	192.2	198.3	—	225.3	237.5	239.7
cornea (limbus)	190.4	198.4	234.0	224.4	238.8	239.89
corpus						
albicans	183.0	198.6	233.39	220	236.2	239.5
callosum, brain	191.8	198.3	—	225.0	237.5	239.6
cavernosum	187.3	198.82	233.5	222.1	236.6	239.5
gastric	151.4	197.8	230.2	211.1	235.2	239.0
penis	187.3	198.82	233.5	222.1	236.6	239.5
striatum, cerebrum	191.0	198.3	—	225.0	237.5	239.6
uteri	182.0	198.82	233.2	219.1	236.0	239.5
isthmus	182.1	198.82	233.2	219.1	236.0	239.5
cortex						
adrenal	194.0	198.7	234.8	227.0	237.2	239.7
cerebral	191.0	198.3	—	225.0	237.5	239.6
costal cartilage	170.3	198.5	—	213.3	238.0	239.2
costovertebral joint	170.3	198.5	—	213.3	238.0	239.2
Cowper's gland	189.3	198.1	233.9	223.81	236.99	239.5
cranial (fossa, any)	191.9	198.3	—	225.0	237.5	239.6
meninges	192.1	198.4	—	225.2	237.6	239.7
nerve (any)	192.0	198.4	—	225.1	237.9	239.7
craniobuccal pouch	194.3	198.89	234.8	227.3	237.0	239.7
craniopharyngeal (duct) (pouch)	194.3	198.89	234.8	227.3	237.0	239.7
cricoid	148.0	198.89	230.0	210.8	235.1	239.0
cartilage	161.3	197.3	231.0	212.1	235.6	239.1
cricopharynx	148.0	198.89	230.0	210.8	235.1	239.0
crypt of Morgagni	154.8	197.5	230.7	211.4	235.2	239.0
crystalline lens	190.0	198.4	234.0	224.0	238.8	239.89
cul-de-sac (Douglas')	158.8	197.6	—	211.8	235.4	239.0
cuneiform cartilage	161.3	197.3	231.0	212.1	235.6	239.1
cutaneous - *see* Neoplasm, skin						
cutis - *see* Neoplasm, skin						
cystic (bile) duct (common)	156.1	197.8	230.8	211.5	235.3	239.0
dermis - *see* Neoplasm, skin						
diaphragm	171.4	198.89	—	215.4	238.1	239.2
digestive organs, system, tube, or tract NEC	159.9	197.8	230.9	211.9	235.5	239.0
contiguous sites with peritoneum	159.8	—	—	—	—	—
disc, intervertebral	170.2	198.5	—	213.2	238.0	239.2

◀ New   ◀▥ Revised   ~~deleted~~ Deleted   ● Use Additional Digit(s)   ▨ Omit code

	Malignant					
	Primary	Secondary	Ca in situ	Benign	Uncertain Behavior	Unspecified
Neoplasm *(Continued)*						
disease, generalized	199.0	199.0	234.9	229.9	238.9	199.0
disseminated	199.0	199.0	234.9	229.9	238.9	199.0
Douglas' cul-de-sac or pouch	158.8	197.6	—	211.8	235.4	239.0
duodenojejunal junction	152.8	197.4	230.7	211.2	235.2	239.0
duodenum	152.0	197.4	230.7	211.2	235.2	239.0
dura (cranial) (mater)	192.1	198.4	—	225.2	237.6	239.7
cerebral	192.1	198.4	—	225.2	237.6	239.7
spinal	192.3	198.4	—	225.4	237.6	239.7
ear (external)	173.2	198.2	232.2	216.2	238.2	239.2
auricle or auris	173.2	198.2	232.2	216.2	238.2	239.2
canal, external	173.2	198.2	232.2	216.2	238.2	239.2
cartilage	171.0	198.89	—	215.0	238.1	239.2
external meatus	173.2	198.2	232.2	216.2	238.2	239.2
inner	160.1	197.3	231.8	212.0	235.9	239.89
lobule	173.2	198.2	232.2	216.2	238.2	239.2
middle	160.1	197.3	231.8	212.0	235.9	239.89
contiguous sites with accessory sinuses or nasal cavities	160.8	—	—	—	—	—
skin	173.2	198.2	232.2	216.2	238.2	239.2
earlobe	173.2	198.2	232.2	216.2	238.2	239.2
ejaculatory duct	187.8	198.82	233.6	222.8	236.6	239.5
elbow NEC*	195.4	198.89	232.6	229.8	238.8	239.89
endocardium	164.1	198.89	—	212.7	238.8	239.89
endocervix (canal) (gland)	180.0	198.82	233.1	219.0	236.0	239.5
endocrine gland NEC	194.9	198.89	—	227.9	237.4	239.7
pluriglandular NEC	194.8	198.89	234.8	227.8	237.4	239.7
endometrium (gland) (stroma)	182.0	198.82	233.2	219.1	236.0	239.5
ensiform cartilage	170.3	198.5	—	213.3	238.0	239.2
enteric - *see* Neoplasm, intestine						
ependyma (brain)	191.5	198.3	—	225.0	237.5	239.6
epicardium	164.1	198.89	—	212.7	238.8	239.89
epididymis	187.5	198.82	233.6	222.3	236.6	239.5
epidural	192.9	198.4	—	225.9	237.9	239.7
epiglottis	161.1	197.3	231.0	212.1	235.6	239.1
anterior aspect or surface	146.4	198.89	230.0	210.6	235.1	239.0
cartilage	161.3	197.3	231.0	212.1	235.6	239.1
free border (margin)	146.4	198.89	230.0	210.6	235.1	239.0
junctional region	146.5	198.89	230.0	210.6	235.1	239.0
posterior (laryngeal) surface	161.1	197.3	231.0	212.1	235.6	239.1
suprahyoid portion	161.1	197.3	231.0	212.1	235.6	239.1
esophagogastric junction	151.0	197.8	230.2	211.1	235.2	239.0

	Malignant					
	Primary	Secondary	Ca in situ	Benign	Uncertain Behavior	Unspecified
Neoplasm *(Continued)*						
esophagus	150.9	197.8	230.1	211.0	235.5	239.0
abdominal	150.2	197.8	230.1	211.0	235.5	239.0
cervical	150.0	197.8	230.1	211.0	235.5	239.0
contiguous sites	150.8	—	—	—	—	—
distal (third)	150.5	197.8	230.1	211.0	235.5	239.0
lower (third)	150.5	197.8	230.1	211.0	235.5	239.0
middle (third)	150.4	197.8	230.1	211.0	235.5	239.0
proximal (third)	150.3	197.8	230.1	211.0	235.5	239.0
specified part NEC	150.8	197.8	230.1	211.0	235.5	239.0
thoracic	150.1	197.8	230.1	211.0	235.5	239.0
upper (third)	150.3	197.8	230.1	211.0	235.5	239.0
ethmoid (sinus)	160.3	197.3	231.8	212.0	235.9	239.1
bone or labyrinth	170.0	198.5	—	213.0	238.0	239.2
Eustachian tube	160.1	197.3	231.8	212.0	235.9	239.1
exocervix	180.1	198.82	233.1	219.0	236.0	239.5
external						
meatus (ear)	173.2	198.2	232.2	216.2	238.2	239.2
os, cervix uteri	180.1	198.82	233.1	219.0	236.0	239.5
extradural	192.9	198.4	—	225.9	237.9	239.7
extrahepatic (bile) duct	156.1	197.8	230.8	211.5	235.3	239.0
contiguous sites with gallbladder	156.8	—	—	—	—	—
extraocular muscle	190.1	198.4	234.0	224.1	238.8	239.89
extrarectal	195.3	198.89	234.8	229.8	238.8	239.89
extremity*	195.8	198.89	232.8	229.8	238.8	239.89
lower*	195.5	198.89	232.7	229.8	238.8	239.89
upper*	195.4	198.89	232.6	229.8	238.8	239.89
eye NEC	190.9	198.4	234.0	224.9	238.8	239.89
contiguous sites	190.8	—	—	—	—	—
specified sites NEC	190.8	198.4	234.0	224.8	238.8	239.89
eyeball	190.0	198.4	234.0	224.0	238.8	239.89
eyebrow	173.3	198.2	232.3	216.3	238.2	239.2
eyelid (lower) (skin) (upper)	173.1	198.2	232.1	216.1	238.2	239.2
cartilage	171.0	198.89	—	215.0	238.1	239.2
face NEC*	195.0	198.89	232.3	229.8	238.8	239.89
Fallopian tube (accessory)	183.2	198.82	233.39	221.0	236.3	239.5
falx (cerebella) (cerebri)	192.1	198.4	—	225.2	237.6	239.7
fascia - *see also* Neoplasm, connective tissue						
palmar	171.2	198.89	—	215.2	238.1	239.2
plantar	171.3	198.89	—	215.3	238.1	239.2
fatty tissue - *see* Neoplasm, connective tissue						

◀ New ◀║ Revised ~~deleted~~ Deleted ● Use Additional Digit(s) ▨ Omit code

	Malignant					
	Primary	Secondary	Ca in situ	Benign	Uncertain Behavior	Unspecified
Neoplasm *(Continued)*						
fauces, faucial NEC	146.9	198.89	230.0	210.6	235.1	239.0
pillars	146.2	198.89	230.0	210.6	235.1	239.0
tonsil	146.0	198.89	230.0	210.5	235.1	239.0
femur (any part)	170.7	198.5	—	213.7	238.0	239.2
fetal membrane	181	198.82	233.2	219.8	236.1	239.5
fibrous tissue - *see* Neoplasm, connective tissue						
fibula (any part)	170.7	198.5	—	213.7	238.0	239.2
filum terminale	192.2	198.3	—	225.3	237.5	239.7
finger NEC*	195.4	198.89	232.6	229.8	238.8	239.89
flank NEC*	195.8	198.89	232.5	229.8	238.8	239.89
follicle, nabothian	180.0	198.82	233.1	219.0	236.0	239.5
foot NEC*	195.5	198.89	232.7	229.8	238.8	239.89
forearm NEC*	195.4	198.89	232.6	229.8	238.8	239.89
forehead (skin)	173.3	198.2	232.3	216.3	238.2	239.2
foreskin	187.1	198.82	233.5	222.1	236.6	239.5
fornix						
pharyngeal	147.3	198.89	230.0	210.7	235.1	239.0
vagina	184.0	198.82	233.31	221.1	236.3	239.5
fossa (of)						
anterior (cranial)	191.9	198.3	—	225.0	237.5	239.6
cranial	191.9	198.3	—	225.0	237.5	239.6
ischiorectal	195.3	198.89	234.8	229.8	238.8	239.89
middle (cranial)	191.9	198.3	—	225.0	237.5	239.6
pituitary	194.3	198.89	234.8	227.3	237.0	239.7
posterior (cranial)	191.9	198.3	—	225.0	237.5	239.6
pterygoid	171.0	198.89	—	215.0	238.1	239.2
pyriform	148.1	198.89	230.0	210.8	235.1	239.0
Rosenmüller	147.2	198.89	230.0	210.7	235.1	239.0
tonsillar	146.1	198.89	230.0	210.6	235.1	239.0
fourchette	184.4	198.82	233.32	221.2	236.3	239.5
frenulum						
labii - *see* Neoplasm, lip, internal						
linguae	141.3	198.89	230.0	210.1	235.1	239.0
frontal						
bone	170.0	198.5	—	213.0	238.0	239.2
lobe, brain	191.1	198.3	—	225.0	237.5	239.6
meninges	192.1	198.4	—	225.2	237.6	239.7
pole	191.1	198.3	—	225.0	237.5	239.6
sinus	160.4	197.3	231.8	212.0	235.9	239.1

	Malignant					
	Primary	Secondary	Ca in situ	Benign	Uncertain Behavior	Unspecified
Neoplasm *(Continued)*						
fundus						
stomach	151.3	197.8	230.2	211.1	235.2	239.0
uterus	182.0	198.82	233.2	219.1	236.0	239.5
gall duct (extrahepatic)	156.1	197.8	230.8	211.5	235.3	239.0
intrahepatic	155.1	197.8	230.8	211.5	235.3	239.0
gallbladder	156.0	197.8	230.8	211.5	235.3	239.0
contiguous sites with extrahepatic bile ducts	156.8	—	—	—	—	—
ganglia (*see also* Neoplasm, connective tissue)	171.9	198.89	—	215.9	238.1	239.2
basal	191.0	198.3	—	225.0	237.5	239.6
ganglion (*see also* Neoplasm, connective tissue)	171.9	198.89	—	215.9	238.1	239.2
cranial nerve	192.0	198.4	—	225.1	237.9	239.7
Gartner's duct	184.0	198.82	233.31	221.1	236.3	239.5
gastric - *see* Neoplasm, stomach						
gastrocolic	159.8	197.8	230.9	211.9	235.5	239.0
gastroesophageal junction	151.0	197.8	230.2	211.1	235.2	239.0
gastrointestinal (tract) NEC	159.9	197.8	230.9	211.9	235.5	239.0
generalized	199.0	199.0	234.9	229.9	238.9	199.0
genital organ or tract						
female NEC	184.9	198.82	233.39	221.9	236.3	239.5
contiguous sites	184.8					
specified site NEC	184.8	198.82	233.39	221.8	236.3	239.5
male NEC	187.9	198.82	233.6	222.9	236.6	239.5
contiguous sites	187.8	—	—	—	—	—
specified site NEC	187.8	198.82	233.6	222.8	236.6	239.5
genitourinary tract						
female	184.9	198.82	233.39	221.9	236.3	239.5
male	187.9	198.82	233.6	222.9	236.6	239.5
gingiva (alveolar) (marginal)	143.9	198.89	230.0	210.4	235.1	239.0
lower	143.1	198.89	230.0	210.4	235.1	239.0
mandibular	143.1	198.89	230.0	210.4	235.1	239.0
maxillary	143.0	198.89	230.0	210.4	235.1	239.0
upper	143.0	198.89	230.0	210.4	235.1	239.0
gland, glandular (lymphatic) (system) - *see also* Neoplasm, lymph gland						
endocrine NEC	194.9	198.89	—	227.9	237.4	239.7
salivary - *see* Neoplasm, salivary, gland						
glans penis	187.2	198.82	233.5	222.1	236.6	239.5
globus pallidus	191.0	198.3	—	225.0	237.5	239.6
glomus						
coccygeal	194.6	198.89	—	227.6	237.3	239.7
jugularis	194.6	198.89	—	227.6	237.3	239.7

◀ New   ◀▥ Revised   ~~deleted~~ Deleted   ● Use Additional Digit(s)   ▨ Omit code

	Malignant					
	Primary	Secondary	Ca in situ	Benign	Uncertain Behavior	Unspecified
Neoplasm *(Continued)*						
glosso-epiglottic fold(s)	146.4	198.89	230.0	210.6	235.1	239.0
glossopalatine fold	146.2	198.89	230.0	210.6	235.1	239.0
glossopharyngeal sulcus	146.1	198.89	230.0	210.6	235.1	239.0
glottis	161.0	197.3	231.0	212.1	235.6	239.1
gluteal region*	195.3	198.89	232.5	229.8	238.8	239.89
great vessels NEC	171.4	198.89	—	215.4	238.1	239.2
groin NEC	195.3	198.89	232.5	229.8	238.8	239.89
gum	143.9	198.89	230.0	210.4	235.1	239.0
contiguous sites	143.8	—	—	—	—	—
lower	143.1	198.89	230.0	210.4	235.1	239.0
upper	143.0	198.89	230.0	210.4	235.1	239.0
hand NEC*	195.4	198.89	232.6	229.8	238.8	239.89
head NEC*	195.0	198.89	232.4	229.8	238.8	239.89
heart	164.1	198.89	—	212.7	238.8	239.89
contiguous sites with mediastinum or thymus	164.8	—	—	—	—	—
heel NEC*	195.5	198.89	232.7	229.8	238.8	239.89
helix	173.2	198.2	232.2	216.2	238.2	239.2
hematopoietic, hemopoietic tissue NEC	202.8●	198.89	—	—	—	238.79
hemisphere, cerebral	191.0	198.3	—	225.0	237.5	239.6
hemorrhoidal zone	154.2	197.5	230.5	211.4	235.5	239.0
hepatic	155.2	197.7	230.8	211.5	235.3	239.0
duct (bile)	156.1	197.8	230.8	211.5	235.3	239.0
flexure (colon)	153.0	197.5	230.3	211.3	235.2	239.0
primary	155.0	—	—	—	—	—
hilus of lung	162.2	197.0	231.2	212.3	235.7	239.1
hip NEC*	195.5	198.89	232.7	229.8	238.8	239.89
hippocampus, brain	191.2	198.3	—	225.0	237.5	239.6
humerus (any part)	170.4	198.5	—	213.4	238.0	239.2
hymen	184.0	198.82	233.31	221.1	236.3	239.5
hypopharynx, hypopharyngeal NEC	148.9	198.89	230.0	210.8	235.1	239.0
contiguous sites	148.8	—	—	—	—	—
postcricoid region	148.0	198.89	230.0	210.8	235.1	239.0
posterior wall	148.3	198.89	230.0	210.8	235.1	239.0
pyriform fossa (sinus)	148.1	198.89	230.0	210.8	235.1	239.0
specified site NEC	148.8	198.89	230.0	210.8	235.1	239.0
wall	148.9	198.89	230.0	210.8	235.1	239.0
posterior	148.3	198.89	230.0	210.8	235.1	239.0
hypophysis	194.3	198.89	234.8	227.3	237.0	239.7
hypothalamus	191.0	198.3	—	225.0	237.5	239.6
ileocecum, ileocecal (coil) (junction) (valve)	153.4	197.5	230.3	211.3	235.2	239.0

	Malignant					
	Primary	Secondary	Ca in situ	Benign	Uncertain Behavior	Unspecified
Neoplasm *(Continued)*						
ileum	152.2	197.4	230.7	211.2	235.2	239.0
ilium	170.6	198.5	—	213.6	238.0	239.2
immunoproliferative NEC	203.8●	—	—	—	—	—
infraclavicular (region)*	195.1	198.89	232.5	229.8	238.8	239.89
inguinal (region)*	195.3	198.89	232.5	229.8	238.8	239.89
insula	191.0	198.3	—	225.0	237.5	239.6
insular tissue (pancreas)	157.4	197.8	230.9	211.7	235.5	239.0
brain	191.0	198.3	—	225.0	237.5	239.6
interarytenoid fold	148.2	198.89	230.0	210.8	235.1	239.0
hypopharyngeal aspect	148.2	198.89	230.0	210.8	235.1	239.0
laryngeal aspect	161.1	197.3	231.0	212.1	235.6	239.1
marginal zone	148.2	198.89	230.0	210.8	235.1	239.0
interdental papillae	143.9	198.89	230.0	210.4	235.1	239.0
lower	143.1	198.89	230.0	210.4	235.1	239.0
upper	143.0	198.89	230.0	210.4	235.1	239.0
internal						
capsule	191.0	198.3	—	225.0	237.5	239.6
os (cervix)	180.0	198.82	233.1	219.0	236.0	239.5
intervertebral cartilage or disc	170.2	198.5	—	213.2	238.0	239.2
intestine, intestinal	159.0	197.8	230.7	211.9	235.2	239.0
large	153.9	197.5	230.3	211.3	235.2	239.0
appendix	153.5	197.5	230.3	211.3	235.2	239.0
caput coli	153.4	197.5	230.3	211.3	235.2	239.0
cecum	153.4	197.5	230.3	211.3	235.2	239.0
colon	153.9	197.5	230.3	211.3	235.2	239.0
and rectum	154.0	197.5	230.4	211.4	235.2	239.0
ascending	153.6	197.5	230.3	211.3	235.2	239.0
caput	153.4	197.5	230.3	211.3	235.2	239.0
contiguous sites	153.8	—	—	—	—	—
descending	153.2	197.5	230.3	211.3	235.2	239.0
distal	153.2	197.5	230.3	211.3	235.2	239.0
left	153.2	197.5	230.3	211.3	235.2	239.0
pelvic	153.3	197.5	230.3	211.3	235.2	239.0
right	153.6	197.5	230.3	211.3	235.2	239.0
sigmoid (flexure)	153.3	197.5	230.3	211.3	235.2	239.0
transverse	153.1	197.5	230.3	211.3	235.2	239.0
contiguous sites	153.8	—	—	—	—	—
hepatic flexure	153.0	197.5	230.3	211.3	235.2	239.0
ileocecum, ileocecal (coil) (valve)	153.4	197.5	230.3	211.3	235.2	239.0
sigmoid flexure (lower) (upper)	153.3	197.5	230.3	211.3	235.2	239.0
splenic flexure	153.7	197.5	230.3	211.3	235.2	239.0

◀ New   ◀▦ Revised   deleted Deleted   ● Use Additional Digit(s)   ▦ Omit code

	Malignant			Benign	Uncertain Behavior	Unspecified
	Primary	Secondary	Ca in situ			
Neoplasm *(Continued)*						
intestine, intestinal *(Continued)*						
small	152.9	197.4	230.7	211.2	235.2	239.0
contiguous sites	152.8	—	—	—	—	—
duodenum	152.0	197.4	230.7	211.2	235.2	239.0
ileum	152.2	197.4	230.7	211.2	235.2	239.0
jejunum	152.1	197.4	230.7	211.2	235.2	239.0
tract NEC	159.0	197.8	230.7	211.9	235.2	239.0
intra-abdominal	195.2	198.89	234.8	229.8	238.8	239.89
intracranial NEC	191.9	198.3	—	225.0	237.5	239.6
intrahepatic (bile) duct	155.1	197.8	230.8	211.5	235.3	239.0
intraocular	190.0	198.4	234.0	224.0	238.8	239.89
intraorbital	190.1	198.4	234.0	224.1	238.8	239.89
intrasellar	194.3	198.89	234.8	227.3	237.0	239.7
intrathoracic (cavity) (organs NEC)	195.1	198.89	234.8	229.8	238.8	239.89
contiguous sites with respiratory organs	165.8	—	—	—	—	—
iris	190.0	198.4	234.0	224.0	238.8	239.89
ischiorectal (fossa)	195.3	198.89	234.8	229.8	238.8	239.89
ischium	170.6	198.5	—	213.6	238.0	239.2
island of Reil	191.0	198.3	—	225.0	237.5	239.6
islands or islets of Langerhans	157.4	197.8	230.9	211.7	235.5	239.0
isthmus uteri	182.1	198.82	233.2	219.1	236.0	239.5
jaw	195.0	198.89	234.8	229.8	238.8	239.89
bone	170.1	198.5	—	213.1	238.0	239.2
carcinoma	143.9	—	—	—	—	—
lower	143.1	—	—	—	—	—
upper	143.0	—	—	—	—	—
lower	170.1	198.5	—	213.1	238.0	239.2
upper	170.0	198.5	—	213.0	238.0	239.2
carcinoma (any type) (lower) (upper)	195.0	—	—	—	—	—
skin	173.3	198.2	232.3	216.3	238.2	239.2
soft tissues	143.9	198.89	230.0	210.4	235.1	239.0
lower	143.1	198.89	230.0	210.4	235.1	239.0
upper	143.0	198.89	230.0	210.4	235.1	239.0
jejunum	152.1	197.4	230.7	211.2	235.2	239.0
joint NEC *(see also* Neoplasm, bone)	170.9	198.5	—	213.9	238.0	239.2
acromioclavicular	170.4	198.5	—	213.4	238.0	239.2
bursa or synovial membrane - *see* Neoplasm, connective tissue						
costovertebral	170.3	198.5	—	213.3	238.0	239.2
sternocostal	170.3	198.5	—	213.3	238.0	239.2
temporomandibular	170.1	198.5	—	213.1	238.0	239.2

	Malignant					
	Primary	Secondary	Ca in situ	Benign	Uncertain Behavior	Unspecified
Neoplasm *(Continued)*						
junction						
anorectal	154.8	197.5	230.7	211.4	235.5	239.0
cardioesophageal	151.0	197.8	230.2	211.1	235.2	239.0
esophagogastric	151.0	197.8	230.2	211.1	235.2	239.0
gastroesophageal	151.0	197.8	230.2	211.1	235.2	239.0
hard and soft palate	145.5	198.89	230.0	210.4	235.1	239.0
ileocecal	153.4	197.5	230.3	211.3	235.2	239.0
pelvirectal	154.0	197.5	230.4	211.4	235.2	239.0
pelviureteric	189.1	198.0	233.9	223.1	236.91	239.5
rectosigmoid	154.0	197.5	230.4	211.4	235.2	239.0
squamocolumnar, of cervix	180.8	198.82	233.1	219.0	236.0	239.5
kidney (parenchymal)	189.0	198.0	233.9	223.0	236.91	239.5
calyx	189.1	198.0	233.9	223.1	236.91	239.5
hilus	189.1	198.0	233.9	223.1	236.91	239.5
pelvis	189.1	198.0	233.9	223.1	236.91	239.5
knee NEC*	195.5	198.89	232.7	229.8	238.8	239.89
labia (skin)	184.4	198.82	233.32	221.2	236.3	239.5
majora	184.1	198.82	233.32	221.2	236.3	239.5
minora	184.2	198.82	233.32	221.2	236.3	239.5
labial - *see also* Neoplasm, lip sulcus (lower) (upper)	145.1	198.89	230.0	210.4	235.1	239.0
labium (skin)	184.4	198.82	233.32	221.2	236.3	239.5
majus	184.1	198.82	233.32	221.2	236.3	239.5
minus	184.2	198.82	233.32	221.2	236.3	239.5
lacrimal						
canaliculi	190.7	198.4	234.0	224.7	238.8	239.89
duct (nasal)	190.7	198.4	234.0	224.7	238.8	239.89
gland	190.2	198.4	234.0	224.2	238.8	239.89
punctum	190.7	198.4	234.0	224.7	238.8	239.89
sac	190.7	198.4	234.0	224.7	238.8	239.89
Langerhans, islands or islets	157.4	197.8	230.9	211.7	235.5	239.0
laryngopharynx	148.9	198.89	230.0	210.8	235.1	239.0
larynx, laryngeal NEC	161.9	197.3	231.0	212.1	235.6	239.1
aryepiglottic fold	161.1	197.3	231.0	212.1	235.6	239.1
cartilage (arytenoid) (cricoid) (cuneiform) (thyroid)	161.3	197.3	231.0	212.1	235.6	239.1
commissure (anterior) (posterior)	161.0	197.3	231.0	212.1	235.6	239.1
contiguous sites	161.8	—	—	—	—	—
extrinsic NEC	161.1	197.3	231.0	212.1	235.6	239.1
meaning hypopharynx	148.9	198.89	230.0	210.8	235.1	239.0
interarytenoid fold	161.1	197.3	231.0	212.1	235.6	239.1
intrinsic	161.0	197.3	231.0	212.1	235.6	239.1

	Malignant					
	Primary	Secondary	Ca in situ	Benign	Uncertain Behavior	Unspecified
Neoplasm *(Continued)*						
larynx, laryngeal NEC *(Continued)*						
ventricular band	161.1	197.3	231.0	212.1	235.6	239.1
leg NEC*	195.5	198.89	232.7	229.8	238.8	239.89
lens, crystalline	190.0	198.4	234.0	224.0	238.8	239.89
lid (lower) (upper)	173.1	198.2	232.1	216.1	238.2	239.2
ligament - *see also* Neoplasm, connective tissue						
broad	183.3	198.82	233.39	221.0	236.3	239.5
Mackenrodt's	183.8	198.82	233.39	221.8	236.3	239.5
non-uterine - *see* Neoplasm, connective tissue						
round	183.5	198.82	—	221.0	236.3	239.5
sacro-uterine	183.4	198.82	—	221.0	236.3	239.5
uterine	183.4	198.82	—	221.0	236.3	239.5
utero-ovarian	183.8	198.82	233.39	221.8	236.3	239.5
uterosacral	183.4	198.82	—	221.0	236.3	239.5
limb*	195.8	198.89	232.8	229.8	238.8	239.89
lower*	195.5	198.89	232.7	229.8	238.8	239.89
upper*	195.4	198.89	232.6	229.8	238.8	239.89
limbus of cornea	190.4	198.4	234.0	224.4	238.8	239.89
lingual NEC (*see also* Neoplasm, tongue)	141.9	198.89	230.0	210.1	235.1	239.0
lingula, lung	162.3	197.0	231.2	212.3	235.7	239.1
lip (external) (lipstick area) (vermillion border)	140.9	198.89	230.0	210.0	235.1	239.0
buccal aspect - *see* Neoplasm, lip, internal						
commissure	140.6	198.89	230.0	210.4	235.1	239.0
contiguous sites	140.8	—	—	—	—	—
with oral cavity or pharynx	149.8	—	—	—	—	—
frenulum - *see* Neoplasm, lip, internal						
inner aspect - *see* Neoplasm, lip, internal						
internal (buccal) (frenulum) (mucosa) (oral)	140.5	198.89	230.0	210.0	235.1	239.0
lower	140.4	198.89	230.0	210.0	235.1	239.0
upper	140.3	198.89	230.0	210.0	235.1	239.0
lower	140.1	198.89	230.0	210.0	235.1	239.0
internal (buccal) (frenulum) (mucosa) (oral)	140.4	198.89	230.0	210.0	235.1	239.0
mucosa - *see* Neoplasm, lip, internal						
oral aspect - *see* Neoplasm, lip, internal						
skin (commissure) (lower) (upper)	173.0	198.2	232.0	216.0	238.2	239.2
upper	140.0	198.89	230.0	210.0	235.1	239.0
internal (buccal) (frenulum) (mucosa) (oral)	140.3	198.89	230.0	210.0	235.1	239.0
liver	155.2	197.7	230.8	211.5	235.3	239.0
primary	155.0	—	—	—	—	—

	Malignant			Benign	Uncertain Behavior	Unspecified
	Primary	Secondary	Ca in situ			
Neoplasm *(Continued)*						
lobe						
azygos	162.3	197.0	231.2	212.3	235.7	239.1
frontal	191.1	198.3	—	225.0	237.5	239.6
lower	162.5	197.0	231.2	212.3	235.7	239.1
middle	162.4	197.0	231.2	212.3	235.7	239.1
occipital	191.4	198.3	—	225.0	237.5	239.6
parietal	191.3	198.3	—	225.0	237.5	239.6
temporal	191.2	198.3	—	225.0	237.5	239.6
upper	162.3	197.0	231.2	212.3	235.7	239.1
lumbosacral plexus	171.6	198.4	—	215.6	238.1	239.2
lung	162.9	197.0	231.2	212.3	235.7	239.1
azygos lobe	162.3	197.0	231.2	212.3	235.7	239.1
carina	162.2	197.0	231.2	212.3	235.7	239.1
contiguous sites with bronchus or trachea	162.8	—	—	—	—	—
hilus	162.2	197.0	231.2	212.3	235.7	239.1
lingula	162.3	197.0	231.2	212.3	235.7	239.1
lobe NEC	162.9	197.0	231.2	212.3	235.7	239.1
lower lobe	162.5	197.0	231.2	212.3	235.7	239.1
main bronchus	162.2	197.0	231.2	212.3	235.7	239.1
middle lobe	162.4	197.0	231.2	212.3	235.7	239.1
upper lobe	162.3	197.0	231.2	212.3	235.7	239.1
lymph, lymphatic						
channel NEC (*see also* Neoplasm, connective tissue)	171.9	198.89	—	215.9	238.1	239.2
gland (secondary)	—	196.9	—	229.0	238.8	239.89
abdominal	—	196.2	—	229.0	238.8	239.89
aortic	—	196.2	—	229.0	238.8	239.89
arm	—	196.3	—	229.0	238.8	239.89
auricular (anterior) (posterior)	—	196.0	—	229.0	238.8	239.89
axilla, axillary	—	196.3	—	229.0	238.8	239.89
brachial	—	196.3	—	229.0	238.8	239.89
bronchial	—	196.1	—	229.0	238.8	239.89
bronchopulmonary	—	196.1	—	229.0	238.8	239.89
celiac	—	196.2	—	229.0	238.8	239.89
cervical	—	196.0	—	229.0	238.8	239.89
cervicofacial	—	196.0	—	229.0	238.8	239.89
Cloquet	—	196.5	—	229.0	238.8	239.89
colic	—	196.2	—	229.0	238.8	239.89
common duct	—	196.2	—	229.0	238.8	239.89
cubital	—	196.3	—	229.0	238.8	239.89
diaphragmatic	—	196.1	—	229.0	238.8	239.89

◀ New ◀▥ Revised ~~deleted~~ Deleted ● Use Additional Digit(s) ▨ Omit code

| | Malignant | | | | | |
	Primary	Secondary	Ca in situ	Benign	Uncertain Behavior	Unspecified
Neoplasm *(Continued)*						
lymph, lymphatic *(Continued)*						
gland *(Continued)*						
epigastric, inferior	—	196.6	—	229.0	238.8	239.89
epitrochlear	—	196.3	—	229.0	238.8	239.89
esophageal	—	196.1	—	229.0	238.8	239.89
face	—	196.0	—	229.0	238.8	239.89
femoral	—	196.5	—	229.0	238.8	239.89
gastric	—	196.2	—	229.0	238.8	239.89
groin	—	196.5	—	229.0	238.8	239.89
head	—	196.0	—	229.0	238.8	239.89
hepatic	—	196.2	—	229.0	238.8	239.89
hilar (pulmonary)	—	196.1	—	229.0	238.8	239.89
splenic	—	196.2	—	229.0	238.8	239.89
hypogastric	—	196.6	—	229.0	238.8	239.89
ileocolic	—	196.2	—	229.0	238.8	239.89
iliac	—	196.6	—	229.0	238.8	239.89
infraclavicular	—	196.3	—	229.0	238.8	239.89
inguina, inguinal	—	196.5	—	229.0	238.8	239.89
innominate	—	196.1	—	229.0	238.8	239.89
intercostal	—	196.1	—	229.0	238.8	239.89
intestinal	—	196.2	—	229.0	238.8	239.89
intrabdominal	—	196.2	—	229.0	238.8	239.89
intrapelvic	—	196.6	—	229.0	238.8	239.89
intrathoracic	—	196.1	—	229.0	238.8	239.9
jugular	—	196.0	—	229.0	238.8	239.89
leg	—	196.5	—	229.0	238.8	239.89
limb						
lower	—	196.5	—	229.0	238.8	239.89
upper	—	196.3	—	229.0	238.8	239.89
lower limb	—	196.5	—	229.0	238.8	239.9 ◀
lumbar	—	196.2	—	229.0	238.8	239.89
mandibular	—	196.0	—	229.0	238.8	239.89
mediastinal	—	196.1	—	229.0	238.8	239.89
mesenteric (inferior) (superior)	—	196.2	—	229.0	238.8	239.89
midcolic	—	196.2	—	229.0	238.8	239.89
multiple sites in categories 196.0–196.6	—	196.8	—	229.0	238.8	239.89
neck	—	196.0	—	229.0	238.8	239.89
obturator	—	196.6	—	229.0	238.8	239.89
occipital	—	196.0	—	229.0	238.8	239.89
pancreatic	—	196.2	—	229.0	238.8	239.89

◀ New   ◀▥ Revised   ~~deleted~~ Deleted   ● Use Additional Digit(s)   ▨ Omit code

	Malignant					
	Primary	Secondary	Ca in situ	Benign	Uncertain Behavior	Unspecified
Neoplasm *(Continued)*						
lymph, lymphatic *(Continued)*						
gland *(Continued)*						
para-aortic	—	196.2	—	229.0	238.8	239.89
paracervical	—	196.6	—	229.0	238.8	239.89
parametrial	—	196.6	—	229.0	238.8	239.89
parasternal	—	196.1	—	229.0	238.8	239.89
parotid	—	196.0	—	229.0	238.8	239.89
pectoral	—	196.3	—	229.0	238.8	239.89
pelvic	—	196.6	—	229.0	238.8	239.89
peri-aortic	—	196.2	—	229.0	238.8	239.89
peripancreatic	—	196.2	—	229.0	238.8	239.89
popliteal	—	196.5	—	229.0	238.8	239.89
porta hepatis	—	196.2	—	229.0	238.8	239.89
portal	—	196.2	—	229.0	238.8	239.89
preauricular	—	196.0	—	229.0	238.8	239.89
prelaryngeal	—	196.0	—	229.0	238.8	239.89
presymphysial	—	196.6	—	229.0	238.8	239.89
pretracheal	—	196.0	—	229.0	238.8	239.89
primary (any site) NEC	202.9●	—	—	—	—	—
pulmonary (hiler)	—	196.1	—	229.0	238.8	239.89
pyloric	—	196.2	—	229.0	238.8	239.89
retroperitoneal	—	196.2	—	229.0	238.8	239.89
retropharyngeal	—	196.0	—	229.0	238.8	239.89
Rosenmüller's	—	196.5	—	229.0	238.8	239.89
sacral	—	196.6	—	229.0	238.8	239.89
scalene	—	196.0	—	229.0	238.8	239.89
site NEC	—	196.9	—	229.0	238.8	239.89
splenic (hilar)	—	196.2	—	229.0	238.8	239.89
subclavicular	—	196.3	—	229.0	238.8	239.89
subinguinal	—	196.5	—	229.0	238.8	239.89
sublingual	—	196.0	—	229.0	238.8	239.89
submandibular	—	196.0	—	229.0	238.8	239.89
submaxillary	—	196.0	—	229.0	238.8	239.89
submental	—	196.0	—	229.0	238.8	239.89
subscapular	—	196.3	—	229.0	238.8	239.89
supraclavicular	—	196.0	—	229.0	238.8	239.89
thoracic	—	196.1	—	229.0	238.8	239.89
tibial	—	196.5	—	229.0	238.8	239.89
tracheal		196.1	—	229.0	238.8	239.89
tracheobronchial	—	196.1	—	229.0	238.8	239.89

◄ New   ◄||| Revised   ~~deleted~~ Deleted   ● Use Additional Digit(s)   ▨ Omit code

| | Malignant | | | | | |
	Primary	Secondary	Ca in situ	Benign	Uncertain Behavior	Unspecified
Neoplasm *(Continued)*						
lymph, lymphatic *(Continued)*						
gland *(Continued)*						
upper limb	—	196.3	—	229.0	238.8	239.89
Virchow's	—	196.0	—	229.0	238.8	239.89
node - *see also* Neoplasm, lymph gland	202.9●	—	—	—	—	—
primary NEC						
vessel (*see also* Neoplasm, connective tissue)	171.9	198.89	—	215.9	238.1	239.2
Mackenrodt's ligament	183.8	198.82	233.39	221.8	236.3	239.5
malar region - *see* Neoplasm, cheek	170.0	198.5	—	213.0	238.0	239.2
mammary gland - *see* Neoplasm, breast						
mandible	170.1	198.5	—	213.1	238.0	239.2
alveolar						
mucosa	143.1	198.89	230.0	210.4	235.1	239.0
ridge or process	170.1	198.5	—	213.1	238.0	239.2
carcinoma	143.1	—	—	—	—	—
carcinoma	143.1	—	—	—	—	—
marrow (bone) NEC	202.9●	198.5	—	—	—	238.79
mastectomy site (skin)	173.5	198.2	—	—	—	—
specified as breast tissue	174.8	198.81	—	—	—	—
mastoid (air cells) (antrum) (cavity)	160.1	197.3	231.8	212.0	235.9	239.1
bone or process	170.0	198.5	—	213.0	238.0	239.2
maxilla, maxillary (superior)	170.0	198.5	—	213.0	238.0	239.2
alveolar						
mucosa	143.0	198.89	230.0	210.4	235.1	239.0
ridge or process	170.0	198.5	—	213.0	238.0	239.2
carcinoma	143.0	—	—	—	—	—
antrum	160.2	197.3	231.8	212.0	235.9	239.1
carcinoma	143.0	—	—	—	—	—
inferior - *see* Neoplasm, mandible						
sinus	160.2	197.3	231.8	212.0	235.9	239.1
meatus						
external (ear)	173.2	198.2	232.2	216.2	238.2	239.2
Meckel's diverticulum	152.3	197.4	230.7	211.2	235.2	239.0
mediastinum, mediastinal	164.9	197.1	—	212.5	235.8	239.89
anterior	164.2	197.1	—	212.5	235.8	239.89
contiguous sites with heart and thymus	164.8	—	—	—	—	—
posterior	164.3	197.1	—	212.5	235.8	239.89
medulla						
adrenal	194.0	198.7	234.8	227.0	237.2	239.7
oblongata	191.7	198.3	—	225.0	237.5	239.6

	Malignant			Benign	Uncertain Behavior	Unspecified
	Primary	Secondary	Ca in situ	Benign	Uncertain Behavior	Unspecified
Neoplasm *(Continued)*						
meibomian gland	173.1	198.2	232.1	216.1	238.2	239.2
melanoma - *see* Melanoma						
meninges (brain) (cerebral) (cranial) (intracranial)	192.1	198.4	—	225.2	237.6	239.7
spinal (cord)	192.3	198.4	—	225.4	237.6	239.7
meniscus, knee joint (lateral) (medial)	170.7	198.5	—	213.7	238.0	239.2
mesentery, mesenteric	158.8	197.6	—	211.8	235.4	239.0
mesoappendix	158.8	197.6	—	211.8	235.4	239.0
mesocolon	158.8	197.6	—	211.8	235.4	239.0
mesopharynx - *see* Neoplasm, oropharynx						
mesosalpinx	183.3	198.82	233.39	221.0	236.3	239.5
mesovarium	183.3	198.82	233.39	221.0	236.3	239.5
metacarpus (any bone)	170.5	198.5	—	213.5	238.0	239.2
metastatic NEC - *see also* Neoplasm, by site, secondary	—	199.1	—	—	—	—
metatarsus (any bone)	170.8	198.5	—	213.8	238.0	239.2
midbrain	191.7	198.3	—	225.0	237.5	239.6
milk duct - *see* Neoplasm, breast						
mons						
pubis	184.4	198.82	233.32	221.2	236.3	239.5
veneris	184.4	198.82	233.32	221.2	236.3	239.5
motor tract	192.9	198.4	—	225.9	237.9	239.7
brain	191.9	198.3	—	225.0	237.5	239.6
spinal	192.2	198.3	—	225.3	237.5	239.7
mouth	145.9	198.89	230.0	210.4	235.1	239.0
contiguous sites	145.8	—	—	—	—	—
floor	144.9	198.89	230.0	210.3	235.1	239.0
anterior portion	144.0	198.89	230.0	210.3	235.1	239.0
contiguous sites	144.8	—	—	—	—	—
lateral portion	144.1	198.89	230.0	210.3	235.1	239.0
roof	145.5	198.89	230.0	210.4	235.1	239.0
specified part NEC	145.8	198.89	230.0	210.4	235.1	239.0
vestibule	145.1	198.89	230.0	210.4	235.1	239.0
mucosa						
alveolar (ridge or process)	143.9	198.89	230.0	210.4	235.1	239.0
lower	143.1	198.89	230.0	210.4	235.1	239.0
upper	143.0	198.89	230.0	210.4	235.1	239.0
buccal	145.0	198.89	230.0	210.4	235.1	239.0
cheek	145.0	198.89	230.0	210.4	235.1	239.0
lip - *see* Neoplasm, lip, internal						
nasal	160.0	197.3	231.8	212.0	235.9	239.1
oral	145.0	198.89	230.0	210.4	235.1	239.0

◀ New   ◀▥ Revised   ~~deleted~~ Deleted   ● Use Additional Digit(s)   Omit code

	Malignant					
	Primary	Secondary	Ca in situ	Benign	Uncertain Behavior	Unspecified
Neoplasm *(Continued)*						
Müllerian duct						
female	184.8	198.82	233.39	221.8	236.3	239.5
male	187.8	198.82	233.6	222.8	236.6	239.5
multiple sites NEC	199.0	199.0	234.9	229.9	238.9	199.0
muscle - *see also* Neoplasm, connective tissue extraocular	190.1	198.4	234.0	224.1	238.8	239.89
myocardium	164.1	198.89	—	212.7	238.8	239.89
myometrium	182.0	198.82	233.2	219.1	236.0	239.5
myopericardium	164.1	198.89	—	212.7	238.8	239.89
nabothian gland (follicle)	180.0	198.82	233.1	219.0	236.0	239.5
nail	173.9	198.2	232.9	216.9	238.2	239.2
finger	173.6	198.2	232.6	216.6	238.2	239.2
toe	173.7	198.2	232.7	216.7	238.2	239.2
nares, naris (anterior) (posterior)	160.0	197.3	231.8	212.0	235.9	239.1
nasal - *see* Neoplasm, nose						
nasolabial groove	173.3	198.2	232.3	216.3	238.2	239.2
nasolacrimal duct	190.7	198.4	234.0	224.7	238.8	239.89
nasopharynx, nasopharyngeal	147.9	198.89	230.0	210.7	235.1	239.0
contiguous sites	147.8	—	—	—	—	—
floor	147.3	198.89	230.0	210.7	235.1	239.0
roof	147.0	198.89	230.0	210.7	235.1	239.0
specified site NEC	147.8	198.89	230.0	210.7	235.1	239.0
wall	147.9	198.89	230.0	210.7	235.1	239.0
anterior	147.3	198.89	230.0	210.7	235.1	239.0
lateral	147.2	198.89	230.0	210.7	235.1	239.0
posterior	147.1	198.89	230.0	210.7	235.1	239.0
superior	147.0	198.89	230.0	210.7	235.1	239.0
nates	173.5	198.2	232.5	216.5	238.2	239.2
neck NEC*	195.0	198.89	234.8	229.8	238.8	239.89
nerve (autonomic) (ganglion) (parasympathetic) (peripheral) (sympathetic) - *see also* Neoplasm, connective tissue						
abducens	192.0	198.4	—	225.1	237.9	239.7
accessory (spinal)	192.0	198.4	—	225.1	237.9	239.7
acoustic	192.0	198.4	—	225.1	237.9	239.7
auditory	192.0	198.4	—	225.1	237.9	239.7
brachial	171.2	198.89	—	215.2	238.1	239.2
cranial (any)	192.0	198.4	—	225.1	237.9	239.7
facial	192.0	198.4	—	225.1	237.9	239.7
femoral	171.3	198.89	—	215.3	238.1	239.2
glossopharyngeal	192.0	198.4	—	225.1	237.9	239.7
hypoglossal	192.0	198.4	—	225.1	237.9	239.7

	Malignant			Benign	Uncertain Behavior	Unspecified
	Primary	Secondary	Ca in situ	Benign	Uncertain Behavior	Unspecified
Neoplasm *(Continued)*						
nerve *(Continued)*						
intercostal	171.4	198.89	—	215.4	238.1	239.2
lumbar	171.7	198.89	—	215.7	238.1	239.2
median	171.2	198.89	—	215.2	238.1	239.2
obturator	171.3	198.89	—	215.3	238.1	239.2
oculomotor	192.0	198.4	—	225.1	237.9	239.7
olfactory	192.0	198.4	—	225.1	237.9	239.7
optic	192.0	198.4	—	225.1	237.9	239.7
peripheral NEC	171.9	198.89	—	215.9	238.1	239.2
radial	171.2	198.89	—	215.2	238.1	239.2
sacral	171.6	198.89	—	215.6	238.1	239.2
sciatic	171.3	198.89	—	215.3	238.1	239.2
spinal NEC	171.9	198.89	—	215.9	238.1	239.2
trigeminal	192.0	198.4	—	225.1	237.9	239.7
trochlear	192.0	198.4	—	225.1	237.9	239.7
ulnar	171.2	198.89	—	215.2	238.1	239.2
vagus	192.0	198.4	—	225.1	237.9	239.7
nervous system (central) NEC	192.9	198.4	—	225.9	237.9	239.7
autonomic NEC	171.9	198.89	—	215.9	238.1	239.2
brain - *see also* Neoplasm, brain membrane or meninges	192.1	198.4	—	225.2	237.6	239.7
contiguous sites	192.8	—	—	—	—	—
parasympathetic NEC	171.9	198.89	—	215.9	238.1	239.2
sympathetic NEC	171.9	198.89	—	215.9	238.1	239.2
nipple (female)	174.0	198.81	233.0	217	238.3	239.3
male	175.0	198.81	233.0	217	238.3	239.3
nose, nasal	195.0	198.89	234.8	229.8	238.8	239.89
ala (external)	173.3	198.2	232.3	216.3	238.2	239.2
bone	170.0	198.5	—	213.0	238.0	239.2
cartilage	160.0	197.3	231.8	212.0	235.9	239.1
cavity	160.0	197.3	231.8	212.0	235.9	239.1
contiguous sites with accessory sinuses or middle ear	160.8	—	—	—	—	—
choana	147.3	198.89	230.0	210.7	235.1	239.0
external (skin)	173.3	198.2	232.3	216.3	238.2	239.2
fossa	160.0	197.3	231.8	212.0	235.9	239.1
internal	160.0	197.3	231.8	212.0	235.9	239.1
mucosa	160.0	197.3	231.8	212.0	235.9	239.1
septum	160.0	197.3	231.8	212.0	235.9	239.1
posterior margin	147.3	198.89	230.0	210.7	235.1	239.0
sinus - *see* Neoplasm, sinus						
skin	173.3	198.2	232.3	216.3	238.2	239.2

◀ New ◀◀ Revised ~~deleted~~ Deleted ● Use Additional Digit(s) ▨ Omit code

	Malignant					
	Primary	Secondary	Ca in situ	Benign	Uncertain Behavior	Unspecified
Neoplasm *(Continued)*						
nose, nasal *(Continued)*						
turbinate (mucosa)	160.0	197.3	231.8	212.0	235.9	239.1
bone	170.0	198.5	—	213.0	238.0	239.2
vestibule	160.0	197.3	231.8	212.0	235.9	239.1
nostril	160.0	197.3	231.8	212.0	235.9	239.1
nucleus pulposus	170.2	198.5	—	213.2	238.0	230.2
occipital						
bone	170.0	198.5	—	213.0	238.0	239.2
lobe or pole, brain	191.4	198.3	—	225.0	237.5	239.6
odontogenic - *see* Neoplasm, jaw bone						
oesophagus - *see* Neoplasm, esophagus						
olfactory nerve or bulb	192.0	198.4	—	225.1	237.9	239.7
olive (brain)	191.7	198.3	—	225.0	237.5	239.6
omentum	158.8	197.6	—	211.8	235.4	239.0
operculum (brain)	191.0	198.3	—	225.0	237.5	239.6
optic nerve, chiasm, or tract	192.0	198.4	—	225.1	237.9	239.7
oral (cavity)	145.9	198.89	230.0	210.4	235.1	239.0
contiguous sites with lip or pharynx	149.8	—	—	—	—	—
ill-defined	149.9	198.89	230.0	210.4	235.1	239.0
mucosa	145.9	198.89	230.0	210.4	235.1	239.0
orbit	190.1	198.4	234.0	224.1	238.8	239.89
bone	170.0	198.5	—	213.0	238.0	239.2
eye	190.1	198.4	234.0	224.1	238.8	239.89
soft parts	190.1	198.4	234.0	224.1	238.8	239.89
organ of Zuckerkandl	194.6	198.89	—	227.6	237.3	239.7
oropharynx	146.9	198.89	230.0	210.6	235.1	239.0
branchial cleft (vestige)	146.8	198.89	230.0	210.6	235.1	239.0
contiguous sites	146.8	—	—	—	—	—
junctional region	146.5	198.89	230.0	210.6	235.1	239.0
lateral wall	146.6	198.89	230.0	210.6	235.1	239.0
pillars of fauces	146.2	198.89	230.0	210.6	235.1	239.0
posterior wall	146.7	198.89	230.0	210.6	235.1	239.0
specified part NEC	146.8	198.89	230.0	210.6	235.1	239.0
vallecula	146.3	198.89	230.0	210.6	235.1	239.0
os						
external	180.1	198.82	233.1	219.0	236.0	239.5
internal	180.0	198.82	233.1	219.0	236.0	239.5
ovary	183.0	198.6	233.39	220	236.2	239.5
oviduct	183.2	198.82	233.39	221.0	236.3	239.5

◀ New   ◀||| Revised   ~~deleted~~ Deleted   ● Use Additional Digit(s)   ▭ Omit code

	Malignant					
	Primary	Secondary	Ca in situ	Benign	Uncertain Behavior	Unspecified
Neoplasm *(Continued)*						
palate	145.5	198.89	230.0	210.4	235.1	239.0
hard	145.2	198.89	230.0	210.4	235.1	239.0
junction of hard and soft palate	145.5	198.89	230.0	210.4	235.1	239.0
soft	145.3	198.89	230.0	210.4	235.1	239.0
nasopharyngeal surface	147.3	198.89	230.0	210.7	235.1	239.0
posterior surface	147.3	198.89	230.0	210.7	235.1	239.0
superior surface	147.3	198.89	230.0	210.7	235.1	239.0
palatoglossal arch	146.2	198.89	230.0	210.6	235.1	239.0
palatopharyngeal arch	146.2	198.89	230.0	210.6	235.1	239.0
pallium	191.0	198.3	—	225.0	237.5	239.6
palpebra	173.1	198.2	232.1	216.1	238.2	239.2
pancreas	157.9	197.8	230.9	211.6	235.5	239.0
body	157.1	197.8	230.9	211.6	235.5	239.0
contiguous sites	157.8	—	—	—	—	—
duct (of Santorini) (of Wirsung)	157.3	197.8	230.9	211.6	235.5	239.0
ectopic tissue	157.8	197.8				
head	157.0	197.8	230.9	211.6	235.5	239.0
islet cells	157.4	197.8	230.9	211.7	235.5	239.0
neck	157.8	197.8	230.9	211.6	235.5	239.0
tail	157.2	197.8	230.9	211.6	235.5	239.0
para-aortic body	194.6	198.89	—	227.6	237.3	239.7
paraganglion NEC	194.6	198.89	—	227.6	237.3	239.7
parametrium	183.4	198.82	—	221.0	236.3	239.5
paranephric	158.0	197.6	—	211.8	235.4	239.0
pararectal	195.3	198.89	—	229.8	238.8	239.89
parasagittal (region)	195.0	198.89	234.8	229.8	238.8	239.89
parasellar	192.9	198.4	—	225.9	237.9	239.7
parathyroid (gland)	194.1	198.89	234.8	227.1	237.4	239.7
paraurethral	195.3	198.89	—	229.8	238.8	239.89
gland	189.4	198.1	233.9	223.89	236.99	239.5
paravaginal	195.3	198.89	—	229.8	238.8	239.89
parenchyma, kidney	189.0	198.0	233.9	223.0	236.91	239.5
parietal						
bone	170.0	198.5	—	213.0	238.0	239.2
lobe, brain	191.3	198.3	—	225.0	237.5	239.6
paroophoron	183.3	198.82	233.39	221.0	236.3	239.5
parotid (duct) (gland)	142.0	198.89	230.0	210.2	235.0	239.0
parovarium	183.3	198.82	233.39	221.0	236.3	239.5
patella	170.8	198.5	—	213.8	238.0	239.2
peduncle, cerebral	191.7	198.3	—	225.0	237.5	239.6

◀ New   ◀ Revised   ~~deleted~~ Deleted   ● Use Additional Digit(s)   ▨ Omit code

Neoplasm (Continued)	Malignant			Benign	Uncertain Behavior	Unspecified
	Primary	Secondary	Ca in situ			
pelvirectal junction	154.0	197.5	230.4	211.4	235.2	239.0
pelvis, pelvic	195.3	198.89	234.8	229.8	238.8	239.89
bone	170.6	198.5	—	213.6	238.0	239.2
floor	195.3	198.89	234.8	229.8	238.8	239.89
renal	189.1	198.0	233.9	223.1	236.91	239.5
viscera	195.3	198.89	234.8	229.8	238.8	239.89
wall	195.3	198.89	234.8	229.8	238.8	239.89
pelvo-abdominal	195.8	198.89	234.8	229.8	238.8	239.89
penis	187.4	198.82	233.5	222.1	236.6	239.5
body	187.3	198.82	233.5	222.1	236.6	239.5
corpus (cavernosum)	187.3	198.82	233.5	222.1	236.6	239.5
glans	187.2	198.82	233.5	222.1	236.6	239.5
skin NEC	187.4	198.82	233.5	222.1	236.6	239.5
periadrenal (tissue)	158.0	197.6	—	211.8	235.4	239.0
perianal (skin)	173.5	198.2	232.5	216.5	238.2	239.2
pericardium	164.1	198.89	—	212.7	238.8	239.89
perinephric	158.0	197.6	—	211.8	235.4	239.0
perineum	195.3	198.89	234.8	229.8	238.8	239.89
periodontal tissue NEC	143.9	198.89	230.0	210.4	235.1	239.0
periosteum - see Neoplasm, bone						
peripancreatic	158.0	197.6	—	211.8	235.4	239.0
peripheral nerve NEC	171.9	198.89	—	215.9	238.1	239.2
perirectal (tissue)	195.3	198.89	—	229.8	238.8	239.89
perirenal (tissue)	158.0	197.6	—	211.8	235.4	239.0
peritoneum, peritoneal (cavity)	158.9	197.6	—	211.8	235.4	239.0
contiguous sites	158.8	—	—	—	—	—
with digestive organs	159.8	—	—	—	—	—
parietal	158.8	197.6	—	211.8	235.4	239.0
pelvic	158.8	197.6	—	211.8	235.4	239.0
specified part NEC	158.8	197.6	—	211.8	235.4	239.0
peritonsillar (tissue)	195.0	198.89	234.8	229.8	238.8	239.89
periurethral tissue	195.3	198.89	—	229.8	238.8	239.89
phalanges	170.9	198.5	—	213.9	238.0	239.2
foot	170.8	198.5	—	213.8	238.0	239.2
hand	170.5	198.5	—	213.5	238.0	239.2
pharynx, pharyngeal	149.0	198.89	230.0	210.9	235.1	239.0
bursa	147.1	198.89	230.0	210.7	235.1	239.0
fornix	147.3	198.89	230.0	210.7	235.1	239.0
recess	147.2	198.89	230.0	210.7	235.1	239.0
region	149.0	198.89	230.0	210.9	235.1	239.0

◀ New   ◀ᴵᴵᴵ Revised   deleted Deleted   ● Use Additional Digit(s)   ▨ Omit code

	Malignant			Benign	Uncertain Behavior	Unspecified
	Primary	Secondary	Ca in situ			
Neoplasm *(Continued)*						
pharynx, pharyngeal *(Continued)*						
tonsil	147.1	198.89	230.0	210.7	235.1	239.0
wall (lateral) (posterior)	149.0	198.89	230.0	210.9	235.1	239.0
pia mater (cerebral) (cranial)	192.1	198.4	—	225.2	237.6	239.7
spinal	192.3	198.4	—	225.4	237.6	239.7
pillars of fauces	146.2	198.89	230.0	210.6	235.1	239.0
pineal (body) (gland)	194.4	198.89	234.8	227.4	237.1	239.7
pinna (ear) NEC	173.2	198.2	232.2	216.2	238.2	239.2
cartilage	171.0	198.89	—	215.0	238.1	239.2
piriform fossa or sinus	148.1	198.89	230.0	210.8	235.1	239.0
pituitary (body) (fossa) (gland) (lobe)	194.3	198.89	234.8	227.3	237.0	239.7
placenta	181	198.82	233.2	219.8	236.1	239.5
pleura, pleural (cavity)	163.9	197.2	—	212.4	235.8	239.1
contiguous sites	163.8	—	—	—	—	—
parietal	163.0	197.2	—	212.4	235.8	239.1
visceral	163.1	197.2	—	212.4	235.8	239.1
plexus						
brachial	171.2	198.89	—	215.2	238.1	239.2
cervical	171.0	198.89	—	215.0	238.1	239.2
choroid	191.5	198.3	—	225.0	237.5	239.6
lumbosacral	171.6	198.89	—	215.6	238.1	239.2
sacral	171.6	198.89	—	215.6	238.1	239.2
pluri-endocrine	194.8	198.89	234.8	227.8	237.4	239.7
pole						
frontal	191.1	198.3	—	225.0	237.5	239.6
occipital	191.4	198.3	—	225.0	237.5	239.6
pons (varolii)	191.7	198.3	—	225.0	237.5	239.6
popliteal fossa or space*	195.5	198.89	234.8	229.8	238.8	239.89
postcricoid (region)	148.0	198.89	230.0	210.8	235.1	239.0
posterior fossa (cranial)	191.9	198.3	—	225.0	237.5	239.6
postnasal space	147.9	198.89	230.0	210.7	235.1	239.0
prepuce	187.1	198.82	233.5	222.1	236.6	239.5
prepylorus	151.1	197.8	230.2	211.1	235.2	239.0
presacral (region)	195.3	198.89	—	229.8	238.8	239.89
prostate (gland)	185	198.82	233.4	222.2	236.5	239.5
utricle	189.3	198.1	233.9	223.81	236.99	239.5
pterygoid fossa	171.0	198.89	—	215.0	238.1	239.2
pubic bone	170.6	198.5	—	213.6	238.0	239.2
pudenda, pudendum (female)	184.4	198.82	233.32	221.2	236.3	239.5
pulmonary	162.9	197.0	231.2	212.3	235.7	239.1

◄ New   ◄▥ Revised   ~~deleted~~ Deleted   ● Use Additional Digit(s)   ▤ Omit code

	Malignant					
	Primary	Secondary	Ca in situ	Benign	Uncertain Behavior	Unspecified
Neoplasm *(Continued)*						
putamen	191.0	198.3	—	225.0	237.5	239.6
pyloric						
antrum	151.2	197.8	230.2	211.1	235.2	239.0
canal	151.1	197.8	230.2	211.1	235.2	239.0
pylorus	151.1	197.8	230.2	211.1	235.2	239.0
pyramid (brain)	191.7	198.3	—	225.0	237.5	239.6
pyriform fossa or sinus	148.1	198.89	230.0	210.8	235.1	239.0
radius (any part)	170.4	198.5	—	213.4	238.0	239.2
Rathke's pouch	194.3	198.89	234.8	227.3	237.0	239.7
rectosigmoid (colon) (junction)	154.0	197.5	230.4	211.4	235.2	239.0
contiguous sites with anus or rectum	154.8	—	—	—	—	—
rectouterine pouch	158.8	197.6	—	211.8	235.4	239.0
rectovaginal septum or wall	195.3	198.89	234.8	229.8	238.8	239.89
rectovesical septum	195.3	198.89	234.8	229.8	238.8	239.89
rectum (ampulla)	154.1	197.5	230.4	211.4	235.2	239.0
and colon	154.0	197.5	230.4	211.4	235.2	239.0
contiguous sites with anus or rectosigmoid junction	154.8	—	—	—	—	—
renal	189.0	198.0	233.9	223.0	236.91	239.5
calyx	189.1	198.0	233.9	223.1	236.91	239.5
hilus	189.1	198.0	233.9	223.1	236.91	239.5
parenchyma	189.0	198.0	233.9	223.0	236.91	239.5
pelvis	189.1	198.0	233.9	223.1	236.91	239.5
respiratory						
organs or system NEC	165.9	197.3	231.9	212.9	235.9	239.1
contiguous sites with intrathoracic organs	165.8	—	—	—	—	—
specified sites NEC	165.8	197.3	231.8	212.8	235.9	239.1
tract NEC	165.9	197.3	231.9	212.9	235.9	239.1
upper	165.0	197.3	231.9	212.9	235.9	239.1
retina	190.5	198.4	234.0	224.5	238.8	239.81
retrobulbar	190.1	198.4	—	224.1	238.8	239.89
retrocecal	158.0	197.6	—	211.8	235.4	239.0
retromolar (area) (triangle) (trigone)	145.6	198.89	230.0	210.4	235.1	239.0
retro-orbital	195.0	198.89	234.8	229.8	238.8	239.89
retroperitoneal (space) (tissue)	158.0	197.6	—	211.8	235.4	239.0
contiguous sites	158.8	—	—	—	—	—
retroperitoneum	158.0	197.6	—	211.8	235.4	239.0
contiguous sites	158.8	—	—	—	—	—
retropharyngeal	149.0	198.89	230.0	210.9	235.1	239.0
retrovesical (septum)	195.3	198.89	234.8	229.8	238.8	239.89
rhinencephalon	191.0	198.3	—	225.0	237.5	239.6

◀ New   ◀‖‖ Revised   ~~deleted~~ Deleted   ● Use Additional Digit(s)   ▨ Omit code

	Malignant			Benign	Uncertain Behavior	Unspecified
	Primary	Secondary	Ca in situ			
Neoplasm *(Continued)*						
rib	170.3	198.5	—	213.3	238.0	239.2
Rosenmüller's fossa	147.2	198.89	230.0	210.7	235.1	239.0
round ligament	183.5	198.82	—	221.0	236.3	239.5
sacrococcyx, sacrococcygeal	170.6	198.5	—	213.6	238.0	239.2
region	195.3	198.89	234.8	229.8	238.8	239.89
sacrouterine ligament	183.4	198.82	—	221.0	236.3	239.5
sacrum, sacral (vertebra)	170.6	198.5	—	213.6	238.0	239.2
salivary gland or duct (major)	142.9	198.89	230.0	210.2	235.0	239.0
contiguous sites	142.8	—	—	—	—	—
minor NEC	145.9	198.89	230.0	210.4	235.1	239.0
parotid	142.0	198.89	230.0	210.2	235.0	239.0
pluriglandular	142.8	198.89	230.0	210.2	235.0	239.0
sublingual	142.2	198.89	230.0	210.2	235.0	239.0
submandibular	142.1	198.89	230.0	210.2	235.0	239.0
submaxillary	142.1	198.89	230.0	210.2	235.0	239.0
salpinx (uterine)	183.2	198.82	233.39	221.0	236.3	239.5
Santorini's duct	157.3	197.8	230.9	211.6	235.5	239.0
scalp	173.4	198.2	232.4	216.4	238.2	239.2
scapula (any part)	170.4	198.5	—	213.4	238.0	239.2
scapular region	195.1	198.89	234.8	229.8	238.8	239.89
scar NEC (*see also* Neoplasm, skin)	173.9	198.2	232.9	216.9	238.2	239.2
sciatic nerve	171.3	198.89	—	215.3	238.1	239.2
sclera	190.0	198.4	234.0	224.0	238.8	239.89
scrotum (skin)	187.7	198.82	233.6	222.4	236.6	239.5
sebaceous gland - *see* Neoplasm, skin						
sella turcica	194.3	198.89	234.8	227.3	237.0	239.7
bone	170.0	198.5	—	213.0	238.0	239.2
semilunar cartilage (knee)	170.7	198.5	—	213.7	238.0	239.2
seminal vesicle	187.8	198.82	233.6	222.8	236.6	239.5
septum						
nasal	160.0	197.3	231.8	212.0	235.9	239.1
posterior margin	147.3	198.89	230.0	210.7	235.1	239.0
rectovaginal	195.3	198.89	234.8	229.8	238.8	239.89
rectovesical	195.3	198.89	234.8	229.8	238.8	239.89
urethrovaginal	184.9	198.82	233.39	221.9	236.3	239.5
vesicovaginal	184.9	198.82	233.39	221.9	236.3	239.5
shoulder NEC*	195.4	198.89	232.6	229.8	238.8	239.89
sigmoid flexure (lower) (upper)	153.3	197.5	230.3	211.3	235.2	239.0
sinus (accessory)	160.9	197.3	231.8	212.0	235.9	239.1
bone (any)	170.0	198.5	—	213.0	238.0	239.2

◀ New   ◀▥ Revised   ~~deleted~~ Deleted   ● Use Additional Digit(s)   ▨ Omit code

	Malignant					
	Primary	Secondary	Ca in situ	Benign	Uncertain Behavior	Unspecified
Neoplasm *(Continued)*						
sinus *(Continued)*						
contiguous sites with middle ear or nasal cavities	160.8	—	—	—	—	—
ethmoidal	160.3	197.3	231.8	212.0	235.9	239.1
frontal	160.4	197.3	231.8	212.0	235.9	239.1
maxillary	160.2	197.3	231.8	212.0	235.9	239.1
nasal, paranasal NEC	160.9	197.3	231.8	212.0	235.9	239.1
pyriform	148.1	198.89	230.0	210.8	235.1	239.0
sphenoidal	160.5	197.3	231.8	212.0	235.9	239.1
skeleton, skeletal NEC	170.9	198.5	—	213.9	238.0	239.2
Skene's gland	189.4	198.1	233.9	223.89	236.99	239.5
skin NEC	173.9	198.2	232.9	216.9	238.2	239.2
abdominal wall	173.5	198.2	232.5	216.5	238.2	239.2
ala nasi	173.3	198.2	232.3	216.3	238.2	239.2
ankle	173.7	198.2	232.7	216.7	238.2	239.2
antecubital space	173.6	198.2	232.6	216.6	238.2	239.2
anus	173.5	198.2	232.5	216.5	238.2	239.2
arm	173.6	198.2	232.6	216.6	238.2	239.2
auditory canal (external)	173.2	198.2	232.2	216.2	238.2	239.2
auricle (ear)	173.2	198.2	232.2	216.2	238.2	239.2
auricular canal (external)	173.2	198.2	232.2	216.2	238.2	239.2
axilla, axillary fold	173.5	198.2	232.5	216.5	238.2	239.2
back	173.5	198.2	232.5	216.5	238.2	239.2
breast	173.5	198.2	232.5	216.5	238.2	239.2
brow	173.3	198.2	232.3	216.3	238.2	239.2
buttock	173.5	198.2	232.5	216.5	238.2	239.2
calf	173.7	198.2	232.7	216.7	238.2	239.2
canthus (eye) (inner) (outer)	173.1	198.2	232.1	216.1	238.2	239.2
cervical region	173.4	198.2	232.4	216.4	238.2	239.2
cheek (external)	173.3	198.2	232.3	216.3	238.2	239.2
chest (wall)	173.5	198.2	232.5	216.5	238.2	239.2
chin	173.3	198.2	232.3	216.3	238.2	239.2
clavicular area	173.5	198.2	232.5	216.5	238.2	239.2
clitoris	184.3	198.82	233.32	221.2	236.3	239.5
columnella	173.3	198.2	232.3	216.3	238.2	239.2
concha	173.2	198.2	232.2	216.2	238.2	239.2
contiguous sites	173.8	—	—	—	—	—
ear (external)	173.2	198.2	232.2	216.2	238.2	239.2
elbow	173.6	198.2	232.6	216.6	238.2	239.2
eyebrow	173.3	198.2	232.3	216.3	238.2	239.2
eyelid	173.1	198.2	232.1	216.1	238.2	239.2

| | Malignant | | | | | |
	Primary	Secondary	Ca in situ	Benign	Uncertain Behavior	Unspecified
Neoplasm *(Continued)*						
skin NEC *(Continued)*						
face NEC	173.3	198.2	232.3	216.3	238.2	239.2
female genital organs (external)	184.4	198.82	233.30	221.2	236.3	239.5
clitoris	184.3	198.82	233.32	221.2	236.3	239.5
labium NEC	184.4	198.82	233.32	221.2	236.3	239.5
majus	184.1	198.82	233.32	221.2	236.3	239.5
minus	184.2	198.82	233.32	221.2	236.3	239.5
pudendum	184.4	198.82	233.32	221.2	236.3	239.5
vulva	184.4	198.82	233.32	221.2	236.3	239.5
finger	173.6	198.2	232.6	216.6	238.2	239.2
flank	173.5	198.2	232.5	216.5	238.2	239.2
foot	173.7	198.2	232.7	216.7	238.2	239.2
forearm	173.6	198.2	232.6	216.6	238.2	239.2
forehead	173.3	198.2	232.3	216.3	238.2	239.2
glabella	173.3	198.2	232.3	216.3	238.2	239.2
gluteal region	173.5	198.2	232.5	216.5	238.2	239.2
groin	173.5	198.2	232.5	216.5	238.2	239.2
hand	173.6	198.2	232.6	216.6	238.2	239.2
head NEC	173.4	198.2	232.4	216.4	238.2	239.2
heel	173.7	198.2	232.7	216.7	238.2	239.2
helix	173.2	198.2	232.2	216.2	238.2	239.2
hip	173.7	198.2	232.7	216.7	238.2	239.2
infraclavicular region	173.5	198.2	232.5	216.5	238.2	239.2
inguinal region	173.5	198.2	232.5	216.5	238.2	239.2
jaw	173.3	198.2	232.3	216.3	238.2	239.2
knee	173.7	198.2	232.7	216.7	238.2	239.2
labia						
majora	184.1	198.82	233.32	221.2	236.3	239.5
minora	184.2	198.82	233.32	221.2	236.3	239.5
leg	173.7	198.2	232.7	216.7	238.2	239.2
lid (lower) (upper)	173.1	198.2	232.1	216.1	238.2	239.2
limb NEC	173.9	198.2	232.9	216.9	238.2	239.5
lower	173.7	198.2	232.7	216.7	238.2	239.2
upper	173.6	198.2	232.6	216.6	238.2	239.2
lip (lower) (upper)	173.0	198.2	232.0	216.0	238.2	239.2
male genital organs	187.9	198.82	233.6	222.9	236.6	239.5
penis	187.4	198.82	233.5	222.1	236.6	239.5
prepuce	187.1	198.82	233.5	222.1	236.6	239.5
scrotum	187.7	198.82	233.6	222.4	236.6	239.5

◀ New   ◀━ Revised   ~~deleted~~ Deleted   ● Use Additional Digit(s)   ▬ Omit code

	Malignant			Benign	Uncertain Behavior	Unspecified
	Primary	Secondary	Ca in situ			
Neoplasm *(Continued)*						
skin NEC *(Continued)*						
mastectomy site	173.5	198.2	—	—	—	—
specified as breast tissue	174.8	198.81	—	—	—	—
meatus, acoustic (external)	173.2	198.2	232.2	216.2	238.2	239.2
nates	173.5	198.2	232.5	216.5	238.2	239.2
neck	173.4	198.2	232.4	216.4	238.2	239.2
nose (external)	173.3	198.2	232.3	216.3	238.2	239.2
palm	173.6	198.2	232.6	216.6	238.2	239.2
palpebra	173.1	198.2	232.1	216.1	238.2	239.2
penis NEC	187.4	198.82	233.5	222.1	236.6	239.5
perianal	173.5	198.2	232.5	216.5	238.2	239.2
perineum	173.5	198.2	232.5	216.5	238.2	239.2
pinna	173.2	198.2	232.2	216.2	238.2	239.2
plantar	173.7	198.2	232.7	216.7	238.2	239.2
popliteal fossa or space	173.7	198.2	232.7	216.7	238.2	239.2
prepuce	187.1	198.82	233.5	222.1	236.6	239.5
pubes	173.5	198.2	232.5	216.5	238.2	239.2
sacrococcygeal region	173.5	198.2	232.5	216.5	238.2	239.2
scalp	173.4	198.2	232.4	216.4	238.2	239.2
scapular region	173.5	198.2	232.5	216.5	238.2	239.2
scrotum	187.7	198.82	233.6	222.4	236.6	239.5
shoulder	173.6	198.2	232.6	216.6	238.2	239.2
sole (foot)	173.7	198.2	232.7	216.7	238.2	239.2
specified sites NEC	173.8	198.2	232.8	216.8	232.8	239.2
submammary fold	173.5	198.2	232.5	216.5	238.2	239.2
supraclavicular region	173.4	198.2	232.4	216.4	238.2	239.2
temple	173.3	198.2	232.3	216.3	238.2	239.2
thigh	173.7	198.2	232.7	216.7	238.2	239.2
thoracic wall	173.5	198.2	232.5	216.5	238.2	239.2
thumb	173.6	198.2	232.6	216.6	238.2	239.2
toe	173.7	198.2	232.7	216.7	238.2	239.2
tragus	173.2	198.2	232.2	216.2	238.2	239.2
trunk	173.5	198.2	232.5	216.5	238.2	239.2
umbilicus	173.5	198.2	232.5	216.5	238.2	239.2
vulva	184.4	198.82	233.32	221.2	236.3	239.5
wrist	173.6	198.2	232.6	216.6	238.2	239.2
skull	170.0	198.5	—	213.0	238.0	239.2
soft parts or tissues - *see* Neoplasm, connective tissue						
specified site NEC	195.8	198.89	234.8	229.8	238.8	239.89

	Malignant					
	Primary	Secondary	Ca in situ	Benign	Uncertain Behavior	Unspecified
Neoplasm *(Continued)*						
spermatic cord	187.6	198.82	233.6	222.8	236.6	239.5
sphenoid	160.5	197.3	231.8	212.0	235.9	239.1
bone	170.0	198.5	—	213.0	238.0	239.2
sinus	160.5	197.3	231.8	212.0	235.9	239.1
sphincter						
anal	154.2	197.5	230.5	211.4	235.5	239.0
of Oddi	156.1	197.8	230.8	211.5	235.3	239.0
spine, spinal (column)	170.2	198.5	—	213.2	238.0	239.2
bulb	191.7	198.3	—	225.0	237.5	239.6
coccyx	170.6	198.5	—	213.6	238.0	239.2
cord (cervical) (lumbar) (sacral) (thoracic)	192.2	198.3	—	225.3	237.5	239.7
dura mater	192.3	198.4	—	225.4	237.6	239.7
lumbosacral	170.2	198.5	—	213.2	238.0	239.2
membrane	192.3	198.4	—	225.4	237.6	239.7
meninges	192.3	198.4	—	225.4	237.6	239.7
nerve (root)	171.9	198.89	—	215.9	238.1	239.2
pia mater	192.3	198.4	—	225.4	237.6	239.7
root	171.9	198.89	—	215.9	238.1	239.2
sacrum	170.6	198.5	—	213.6	238.0	239.2
spleen, splenic NEC	159.1	197.8	230.9	211.9	235.5	239.0
flexure (colon)	153.7	197.5	230.3	211.3	235.2	239.0
stem, brain	191.7	198.3	—	225.0	237.5	239.6
Stensen's duct	142.0	198.89	230.0	210.2	235.0	239.0
sternum	170.3	198.5	—	213.3	238.0	239.2
stomach	151.9	197.8	230.2	211.1	235.2	239.0
antrum (pyloric)	151.2	197.8	230.2	211.1	235.2	239.0
body	151.4	197.8	230.2	211.1	235.2	239.0
cardia	151.0	197.8	230.2	211.1	235.2	239.0
cardiac orifice	151.0	197.8	230.2	211.1	235.2	239.0
contiguous sites	151.8	—	—	—	—	—
corpus	151.4	197.8	230.2	211.1	235.2	239.0
fundus	151.3	197.8	230.2	211.1	235.2	239.0
greater curvature NEC	151.6	197.8	230.2	211.1	235.2	239.0
lesser curvature NEC	151.5	197.8	230.2	211.1	235.2	239.0
prepylorus	151.1	197.8	230.2	211.1	235.2	239.0
pylorus	151.1	197.8	230.2	211.1	235.2	239.0
wall NEC	151.9	197.8	230.2	211.1	235.2	239.0
anterior NEC	151.8	197.8	230.2	211.1	235.2	239.0
posterior NEC	151.8	197.8	230.2	211.1	235.2	239.0
stroma, endometrial	182.0	198.82	233.2	219.1	236.0	239.5

◀ New ◀▓ Revised ~~deleted~~ Deleted ● Use Additional Digit(s) ▓ Omit code

	Malignant					
	Primary	Secondary	Ca in situ	Benign	Uncertain Behavior	Unspecified
Neoplasm *(Continued)*						
stump, cervical	180.8	198.82	233.1	219.0	236.0	239.5
subcutaneous (nodule) (tissue) NEC - *see* Neoplasm, connective tissue						
subdural	192.1	198.4	—	225.2	237.6	239.7
subglottis, subglottic	161.2	197.3	231.0	212.1	235.6	239.1
sublingual	144.9	198.89	230.0	210.3	235.1	239.0
gland or duct	142.2	198.89	230.0	210.2	235.0	239.0
submandibular gland	142.1	198.89	230.0	210.2	235.0	239.0
submaxillary gland or duct	142.1	198.89	230.0	210.2	235.0	239.0
submental	195.0	198.89	234.8	229.8	238.8	239.89
subpleural	162.9	197.0	—	212.3	235.7	239.1
substernal	164.2	197.1	—	212.5	235.8	239.89
sudoriferous, sudoriparous gland, site unspecified	173.9	198.2	232.9	216.9	238.2	239.2
specified site - *see* Neoplasm, skin						
supraclavicular region	195.0	198.89	234.8	229.8	238.8	239.89
supraglottis	161.1	197.3	231.0	212.1	235.6	239.1
suprarenal (capsule) (cortex) (gland) (medulla)	194.0	198.7	234.8	227.0	237.2	239.7
suprasellar (region)	191.9	198.3	—	225.0	237.5	239.6
sweat gland (apocrine) (eccrine), site unspecified	173.9	198.2	232.9	216.9	238.2	239.2
specified site - *see* Neoplasm, skin						
sympathetic nerve or nervous system NEC	171.9	198.89	—	215.9	238.1	239.2
symphysis pubis	170.6	198.5	—	213.6	238.0	239.2
synovial membrane - *see* Neoplasm, connective tissue						
tapetum, brain	191.8	198.3	—	225.0	237.5	239.6
tarsus (any bone)	170.8	198.5	—	213.8	238.0	239.2
temple (skin)	173.3	198.2	232.3	216.3	238.2	239.2
temporal						
bone	170.0	198.5	—	213.0	238.0	239.2
lobe or pole	191.2	198.3	—	225.0	237.5	239.6
region	195.0	198.89	234.8	229.8	238.8	239.89
skin	173.3	198.2	232.3	216.3	238.2	239.2
tendon (sheath) - *see* Neoplasm, connective tissue						
tentorium (cerebelli)	192.1	198.4	—	225.2	237.6	239.7
testis, testes (descended) (scrotal)	186.9	198.82	233.6	222.0	236.4	239.5
ectopic	186.0	198.82	233.6	222.0	236.4	239.5
retained	186.0	198.82	233.6	222.0	236.4	239.5
undescended	186.0	198.82	233.6	222.0	236.4	239.5
thalamus	191.0	198.3	—	225.0	237.5	239.6
thigh NEC*	195.5	198.89	234.8	229.8	238.8	239.89
thorax, thoracic (cavity) (organs NEC)	195.1	198.89	234.8	229.8	238.8	239.89
duct	171.4	198.89	—	215.4	238.1	239.2
wall NEC	195.1	198.89	234.8	229.8	238.8	239.89

◄ New   ◄▮▮ Revised   ~~deleted~~ Deleted   ● Use Additional Digit(s)   ▮▮▮ Omit code

Neoplasm (Continued)	Malignant			Benign	Uncertain Behavior	Unspecified
	Primary	Secondary	Ca in situ	Benign	Uncertain Behavior	Unspecified
throat	149.0	198.89	230.0	210.9	235.1	239.0
thumb NEC*	195.4	198.89	232.6	229.8	238.8	239.89
thymus (gland)	164.0	198.89	—	212.6	235.8	239.89
contiguous sites with heart and mediastinum	164.8	—	—	—	—	—
thyroglossal duct	193	198.89	234.8	226	237.4	239.7
thyroid (gland)	193	198.89	234.8	226	237.4	239.7
cartilage	161.3	197.3	231.0	212.1	235.6	239.1
tibia (any part)	170.7	198.5	—	213.7	238.0	239.2
toe NEC*	195.5	198.89	232.7	229.8	238.8	239.89
tongue	141.9	198.89	230.0	210.1	235.1	239.0
anterior (two-thirds) NEC	141.4	198.89	230.0	210.1	235.1	239.0
dorsal surface	141.1	198.89	230.0	210.1	235.1	239.0
ventral surface	141.3	198.89	230.0	210.1	235.1	239.0
base (dorsal surface)	141.0	198.89	230.0	210.1	235.1	239.0
border (lateral)	141.2	198.89	230.0	210.1	235.1	239.0
contiguous sites	141.8	—	—	—	—	—
dorsal surface NEC	141.1	198.89	230.0	210.1	235.1	239.0
fixed part NEC	141.0	198.89	230.0	210.1	235.1	239.0
foramen cecum	141.1	198.89	230.0	210.1	235.1	239.0
frenulum linguae	141.3	198.89	230.0	210.1	235.1	239.0
junctional zone	141.5	198.89	230.0	210.1	235.1	239.0
margin (lateral)	141.2	198.89	230.0	210.1	235.1	239.0
midline NEC	141.1	198.89	230.0	210.1	235.1	239.0
mobile part NEC	141.4	198.89	230.0	210.1	235.1	239.0
posterior (third)	141.0	198.89	230.0	210.1	235.1	239.0
root	141.0	198.89	230.0	210.1	235.1	239.0
surface (dorsal)	141.1	198.89	230.0	210.1	235.1	239.0
base	141.0	198.89	230.0	210.1	235.1	239.0
ventral	141.3	198.89	230.0	210.1	235.1	239.0
tip	141.2	198.89	230.0	210.1	235.1	239.0
tonsil	141.6	198.89	230.0	210.1	235.1	239.0
tonsil	146.0	198.89	230.0	210.5	235.1	239.0
fauces, faucial	146.0	198.89	230.0	210.5	235.1	239.0
lingual	141.6	198.89	230.0	210.1	235.1	239.0
palatine	146.0	198.89	230.0	210.5	235.1	239.0
pharyngeal	147.1	198.89	230.0	210.7	235.1	239.0
pillar (anterior) (posterior)	146.2	198.89	230.0	210.6	235.1	239.0
tonsillar fossa	146.1	198.89	230.0	210.6	235.1	239.0
tooth socket NEC	143.9	198.89	230.0	210.4	235.1	239.0

◄ New   ◄ Revised   deleted Deleted   ● Use Additional Digit(s)   Omit code

	Malignant					
	Primary	Secondary	Ca in situ	Benign	Uncertain Behavior	Unspecified
Neoplasm *(Continued)*						
trachea (cartilage) (mucosa)	162.0	197.3	231.1	212.2	235.7	239.1
contiguous sites with bronchus or lung	162.8	—	—	—	—	—
tracheobronchial	162.8	197.3	231.1	212.2	235.7	239.1
contiguous sites with lung	162.8	—	—	—	—	—
tragus	173.2	198.2	232.2	216.2	238.2	239.2
trunk NEC*	195.8	198.89	232.5	229.8	238.8	239.89
tubo-ovarian	183.8	198.82	233.39	221.8	236.3	239.5
tunica vaginalis	187.8	198.82	233.6	222.8	236.6	239.5
turbinate (bone)	170.0	198.5	—	213.0	238.0	239.2
nasal	160.0	197.3	231.8	212.0	235.9	239.1
tympanic cavity	160.1	197.3	231.8	212.0	235.9	239.1
ulna (any part)	170.4	198.5	—	213.4	238.0	239.2
umbilicus, umbilical	173.5	198.2	232.5	216.5	238.2	239.2
uncus, brain	191.2	198.3	—	225.0	237.5	239.6
unknown site or unspecified	199.1	199.1	234.9	229.9	238.9	239.9
urachus	188.7	198.1	233.7	223.3	236.7	239.4
ureter, ureteral	189.2	198.1	233.9	223.2	236.91	239.5
orifice (bladder)	188.6	198.1	233.7	223.3	236.7	239.4
ureter-bladder (junction)	188.6	198.1	233.7	223.3	236.7	239.4
urethra, urethral (gland)	189.3	198.1	233.9	223.81	236.99	239.5
orifice, internal	188.5	198.1	233.7	223.3	236.7	239.4
urethrovaginal (septum)	184.9	198.82	233.39	221.9	236.3	239.5
urinary organ or system NEC	189.9	198.1	233.9	223.9	236.99	239.5
bladder - *see* Neoplasm, bladder						
contiguous sites	189.8	—	—	—	—	—
specified sites NEC	189.8	198.1	233.9	223.89	236.99	239.5
utero-ovarian	183.8	198.82	233.39	221.8	236.3	239.5
ligament	183.3	198.82	—	221.0	236.3	239.5
uterosacral ligament	183.4	198.82	—	221.0	236.3	239.5
uterus, uteri, uterine	179	198.82	233.2	219.9	236.0	239.5
adnexa NEC	183.9	198.82	233.39	221.8	236.3	239.5
contiguous sites	183.8	—	—	—	—	—
body	182.0	198.82	233.2	219.1	236.0	239.5
contiguous sites	182.8	—	—	—	—	—
cervix	180.9	198.82	233.1	219.0	236.0	239.5
cornu	182.0	198.82	233.2	219.1	236.0	239.5
corpus	182.0	198.82	233.2	219.1	236.0	239.5
endocervix (canal) (gland)	180.0	198.82	233.1	219.0	236.0	239.5
endometrium	182.0	198.82	233.2	219.1	236.0	239.5

| | Malignant | | | | | |
	Primary	Secondary	Ca in situ	Benign	Uncertain Behavior	Unspecified
Neoplasm *(Continued)*						
uterus, uteri, uterine *(Continued)*						
exocervix	180.1	198.82	233.1	219.0	236.0	239.5
external os	180.1	198.82	233.1	219.0	236.0	239.5
fundus	182.0	198.82	233.2	219.1	236.0	239.5
internal os	180.0	198.82	233.1	219.0	236.0	239.5
isthmus	182.1	198.82	233.2	219.1	236.0	239.5
ligament	183.4	198.82	—	221.0	236.3	239.5
broad	183.3	198.82	233.39	221.0	236.3	239.5
round	183.5	198.82	—	221.0	236.3	239.5
lower segment	182.1	198.82	233.2	219.1	236.0	239.5
myometrium	182.0	198.82	233.2	219.1	236.0	239.5
squamocolumnar junction	180.8	198.82	233.1	219.0	236.0	239.5
tube	183.2	198.82	233.39	221.0	236.3	239.5
utricle, prostatic	189.3	198.1	233.9	223.81	236.99	239.5
uveal tract	190.0	198.4	234.0	224.0	238.8	239.89
uvula	145.4	198.89	230.0	210.4	235.1	239.0
vagina, vaginal (fornix) (vault) (wall)	184.0	198.82	233.31	221.1	236.3	239.5
vaginovesical	184.9	198.82	233.39	221.9	236.3	239.5
septum	184.9	198.82	233.39	221.9	236.3	239.5
vallecula (epiglottis)	146.3	198.89	230.0	210.6	235.1	239.0
vascular - *see* Neoplasm, connective tissue						
vas deferens	187.6	198.82	233.6	222.8	236.6	239.5
Vater's ampulla	156.2	197.8	230.8	211.5	235.3	239.0
vein, venous - *see* Neoplasm, connective tissue						
vena cava (abdominal) (inferior)	171.5	198.89	—	215.5	238.1	239.2
superior	171.4	198.89	—	215.4	238.1	239.2
ventricle (cerebral) (floor) (fourth) (lateral) (third)	191.5	198.3	—	225.0	237.5	239.6
cardiac (left) (right)	164.1	198.89	—	212.7	238.8	239.89
ventricular band of larynx	161.1	197.3	231.0	212.1	235.6	239.1
ventriculus - *see* Neoplasm, stomach						
vermillion border - *see* Neoplasm, lip						
vermis, cerebellum	191.6	198.3	—	225.0	237.5	239.6
vertebra (column)	170.2	198.5	—	213.2	238.0	239.2
coccyx	170.6	198.5	—	213.6	238.0	239.2
sacrum	170.6	198.5	—	213.6	238.0	239.2
vesical - *see* Neoplasm, bladder						
vesicle, seminal	187.8	198.82	233.6	222.8	236.6	239.5
vesicocervical tissue	184.9	198.82	233.39	221.9	236.3	239.5
vesicorectal	195.3	198.89	234.8	229.8	238.8	239.89
vesicovaginal	184.9	198.82	233.39	221.9	236.3	239.5
septum	184.9	198.82	233.39	221.9	236.3	239.5

◀ New ◀▥ Revised ~~deleted~~ Deleted ● Use Additional Digit(s) ▭ Omit code

	Malignant					
	Primary	Secondary	Ca in situ	Benign	Uncertain Behavior	Unspecified
Neoplasm *(Continued)*						
vessel (blood) - *see* Neoplasm, connective tissue						
vestibular gland, greater	184.1	198.82	233.32	221.2	236.3	239.5
vestibule						
mouth	145.1	198.89	230.0	210.4	235.1	239.0
nose	160.0	197.3	231.8	212.0	235.9	239.1
Virchow's gland	—	196.0	—	229.0	238.8	239.89
viscera NEC	195.8	198.89	234.8	229.8	238.8	239.89
vocal cords (true)	161.0	197.3	231.0	212.1	235.6	239.1
false	161.1	197.3	231.0	212.1	235.6	239.1
vomer	170.0	198.5	—	213.0	238.0	239.2
vulva	184.4	198.82	233.32	221.2	236.3	239.5
vulvovaginal gland	184.4	198.82	233.32	221.2	236.3	239.5
Waldeyer's ring	149.1	198.89	230.0	210.9	235.1	239.0
Wharton's duct	142.1	198.89	230.0	210.2	235.0	239.0
white matter (central) (cerebral)	191.0	198.3	—	225.0	237.5	239.6
windpipe	162.0	197.3	231.1	212.2	235.7	239.1
Wirsung's duct	157.3	197.8	230.9	211.6	235.5	239.0
wolffian (body) (duct)						
female	184.8	198.82	233.39	221.8	236.3	239.5
male	187.8	198.82	233.6	222.8	236.6	239.5
womb - *see* Neoplasm, uterus						
wrist NEC*	195.4	198.89	232.6	229.8	238.8	239.89
xiphoid process	170.3	198.5	—	213.3	238.0	239.2
Zuckerkandl's organ	194.6	198.89	—	227.6	237.3	239.7

N

Neovascularization
  choroid 362.16
  ciliary body 364.42
  cornea 370.60
    deep 370.63
    localized 370.61
  iris 364.42
  retina 362.16
  subretinal 362.16
Nephralgia 788.0
Nephritis, nephritic (albuminuric)
  (azotemic) (congenital)
  (degenerative) (diffuse)
  (disseminated) (epithelial) (familial)
  (focal) (granulomatous)
  (hemorrhagic) (infantile)
  (nonsuppurative, excretory)
  (uremic) 583.9
  with
    edema - see Nephrosis
    lesion of
      glomerulonephritis
        hypocomplementemic
          persistent 583.2
          with nephrotic syndrome
            581.2
          chronic 582.2
        lobular 583.2
          with nephrotic syndrome
            581.2
          chronic 582.2
        membranoproliferative
          583.2
          with nephrotic syndrome
            581.2
          chronic 582.2
        membranous 583.1
          with nephrotic syndrome
            581.1
          chronic 582.1
        mesangiocapillary 583.2
          with nephrotic syndrome
            581.2
          chronic 582.2
        mixed membranous and
          proliferative 583.2
          with nephrotic syndrome
            581.2
          chronic 582.2
        proliferative (diffuse) 583.0
          with nephrotic syndrome
            581.0
          acute 580.0
          chronic 582.0
        rapidly progressive 583.4
          acute 580.4
          chronic 582.4
      interstitial nephritis (diffuse)
        (focal) 583.89
        with nephrotic syndrome
          581.89
        acute 580.89
        chronic 582.89
      necrotizing glomerulitis 583.4
        acute 580.4
        chronic 582.4
      renal necrosis 583.9
        cortical 583.6
        medullary 583.7
      specified pathology NEC 583.89
        with nephrotic syndrome
          581.89
        acute 580.89
        chronic 582.89

Nephritis, nephritic (Continued)
  with (Continued)
    necrosis, renal 583.9
      cortical 583.6
      medullary (papillary) 583.7
    nephrotic syndrome (see also
      Nephrosis) 581.9
    papillary necrosis 583.7
    specified pathology NEC 583.89
  acute 580.9
    extracapillary with epithelial
      crescents 580.4
    hypertensive (see also Hypertension,
      kidney) 403.90
    necrotizing 580.4
    poststreptococcal 580.0
    proliferative (diffuse) 580.0
    rapidly progressive 580.4
    specified pathology NEC 580.89
  amyloid 277.39 [583.81]
    chronic 277.39 [582.81]
  arteriolar (see also Hypertension,
    kidney) 403.90
  arteriosclerotic (see also Hypertension,
    kidney) 403.90
  ascending (see also Pyelitis) 590.80
  atrophic 582.9
  basement membrane NEC 583.89
    with pulmonary hemorrhage
      (Goodpasture's syndrome)
      446.21 [583.81]
  calculous, calculus 592.0
  cardiac (see also Hypertension, kidney)
    403.90
  cardiovascular (see also Hypertension,
    kidney) 403.90
  chronic 582.9
    arteriosclerotic (see also
      Hypertension, kidney) 403.90
    hypertensive (see also Hypertension,
      kidney) 403.90
  cirrhotic (see also Sclerosis, renal) 587
  complicating pregnancy, childbirth, or
    puerperium 646.2●
    with hypertension 642.1●
      affecting fetus or newborn 760.0
    affecting fetus or newborn 760.1
  croupous 580.9
  desquamative - see Nephrosis
  due to
    amyloidosis 277.39 [583.81]
      chronic 277.39 [582.81]
    arteriosclerosis (see also
      Hypertension, kidney) 403.90
    diabetes mellitus 250.4● [583.81]
      due to secondary diabetes 249.4●
        [583.81]
      with nephrotic syndrome 250.4●
        [581.81]
        due to secondary diabetes
          249.4● [581.81]
    diphtheria 032.89 [580.81]
    gonococcal infection (acute) 098.19
      [583.81]
      chronic or duration of 2 months
        or over 098.39 [583.81]
    gout 274.10
    infectious hepatitis 070.9 [580.81]
    mumps 072.79 [580.81]
    specified kidney pathology NEC
      583.89
      acute 580.89
      chronic 582.89
    streptotrichosis 039.8 [583.81]

Nephritis, nephritic (Continued)
  due to (Continued)
    subacute bacterial endocarditis 421.0
      [580.81]
    systemic lupus erythematosus 710.0
      [583.81]
      chronic 710.0 [582.81]
    typhoid fever 002.0 [580.81]
  endothelial 582.2
  end state (chronic) (terminal) NEC
    585.6
  epimembranous 581.1
  exudative 583.89
    with nephrotic syndrome 581.89
    acute 580.89
    chronic 582.89
  gonococcal (acute) 098.19 [583.81]
    chronic or duration of 2 months or
      over 098.39 [583.81]
  gouty 274.10
  hereditary (Alport's syndrome)
    759.89
  hydremic - see Nephrosis
  hypertensive (see also Hypertension,
    kidney) 403.90
  hypocomplementemic persistent
    583.2
    with nephrotic syndrome 581.2
    chronic 582.2
  immune complex NEC 583.89
  infective (see also Pyelitis) 590.80
  interstitial (diffuse) (focal) 583.89
    with nephrotic syndrome 581.89
    acute 580.89
    chronic 582.89
  latent or quiescent - see Nephritis,
    chronic
  lead 984.9
    specified type of lead - see Table of
      Drugs and Chemicals
  lobular 583.2
    with nephrotic syndrome
      581.2
    chronic 582.2
  lupus 710.0 [583.81]
    acute 710.0 [580.81]
    chronic 710.0 [582.81]
  membranoproliferative 583.2
    with nephrotic syndrome 581.2
    chronic 582.2
  membranous 583.1
    with nephrotic syndrome 581.1
    chronic 582.1
  mesangiocapillary 583.2
    with nephrotic syndrome 581.2
    chronic 582.2
  minimal change 581.3
  mixed membranous and proliferative
    583.2
    with nephrotic syndrome 581.2
    chronic 582.2
  necrotic, necrotizing 583.4
    acute 580.4
    chronic 582.4
  nephrotic - see Nephrosis
  old - see Nephritis, chronic
  parenchymatous 581.89
  polycystic 753.12
    adult type (APKD) 753.13
    autosomal dominant 753.13
    autosomal recessive 753.14
    childhood type (CPKD) 753.14
    infantile type 753.14
  poststreptococcal 580.0

Nephritis, nephritic (Continued)
  pregnancy - see Nephritis, complicating
    pregnancy
  proliferative 583.0
    with nephrotic syndrome 581.0
    acute 580.0
    chronic 582.0
  purulent (see also Pyelitis) 590.80
  rapidly progressive 583.4
    acute 580.4
    chronic 582.4
  salt-losing or salt-wasting (see also
    Disease, renal) 593.9
  saturnine 584.9
    specified type of lead - see Table of
      Drugs and Chemicals
  septic (see also Pyelitis) 590.80
  specified pathology NEC 583.89
    acute 580.89
    chronic 582.89
  staphylococcal (see also Pyelitis) 590.80
  streptotrichosis 039.8 [583.81]
  subacute (see also Nephrosis) 581.9
  suppurative (see also Pyelitis) 590.80
  syphilitic (late) 095.4
    congenital 090.5 [583.81]
    early 091.69 [583.81]
  terminal (chronic) (end-stage) NEC
    585.6
  toxic - see Nephritis, acute
  tubal, tubular - see Nephrosis, tubular
  tuberculous (see also Tuberculosis)
    016.0● [583.81]
  type II (Ellis) - see Nephrosis
  vascular - see also Hypertension, kidney
  war 580.9
Nephroblastoma (M8960/3) 189.0
  epithelial (M8961/3) 189.0
  mesenchymal (M8962/3) 189.0
Nephrocalcinosis 275.49
Nephrocystitis, pustular (see also Pyelitis)
  590.80
Nephrolithiasis (congenital) (pelvis)
  (recurrent) 592.0
  uric acid 274.11
Nephroma (M8960/3) 189.0
  mesoblastic (M8960/1) 236.9
Nephronephritis (see also Nephrosis)
  581.9
Nephronopthisis 753.16
Nephropathy (see also Nephritis) 583.9
  with
    exudative nephritis 583.89
    interstitial nephritis (diffuse) (focal)
      583.89
    medullary necrosis 583.7
    necrosis 583.9
      cortical 583.6
      medullary or papillary 583.7
    papillary necrosis 583.7
    specified lesion or cause NEC 583.89
  analgesic 583.89
    with medullary necrosis, acute 584.7
  arteriolar (see also Hypertension,
    kidney) 403.90
  arteriosclerotic (see also Hypertension,
    kidney) 403.90
  complicating pregnancy 646.2●
  diabetic 250.4● [583.81]
    due to secondary diabetes 249.4●
      [583.81]
  gouty 274.10
    specified type NEC 274.19
  hereditary amyloid 277.31

Nephropathy (Continued)
  hypercalcemic 588.89
  hypertensive (see also Hypertension,
    kidney) 403.90
  hypokalemic (vacuolar) 588.89
  IgA 583.9
  obstructive 593.89
    congenital 753.20
  phenacetin 584.7
  phosphate-losing 588.0
  potassium depletion 588.89
  proliferative (see also Nephritis,
    proliferative) 583.0
  protein-losing 588.89
  salt-losing or salt-wasting (see also
    Disease, renal) 593.9
  sickle-cell (see also Disease, sickle-cell)
    282.60 [583.81]
  toxic 584.5
  vasomotor 584.5
  water-losing 588.89
Nephroptosis (see also Disease, renal)
  593.0
  congenital (displaced) 753.3
Nephropyosis (see also Abscess, kidney)
  590.2
Nephrorrhagia 593.81
Nephrosclerosis (arteriolar)
  (arteriosclerotic) (chronic) (hyaline)
  (see also Hypertension, kidney)
  403.90
  gouty 274.10
  hyperplastic (arteriolar) (see also
    Hypertension, kidney) 403.90
  senile (see also Sclerosis, renal) 587
Nephrosis, nephrotic (Epstein's)
  (syndrome) 581.9
  with
    lesion of
      focal glomerulosclerosis 581.1
      glomerulonephritis
        endothelial 581.2
        hypocomplementemic
          persistent 581.2
        lobular 581.2
        membranoproliferative 581.2
        membranous 581.1
        mesangiocapillary 581.2
        minimal change 581.3
        mixed membranous and
          proliferative 581.2
        proliferative 581.0
      segmental hyalinosis 581.1
      specified pathology NEC 581.89
  acute - see Nephrosis, tubular
  anoxic - see Nephrosis, tubular
  arteriosclerotic (see also Hypertension,
    kidney) 403.90
  chemical - see Nephrosis, tubular
  cholemic 572.4
  complicating pregnancy, childbirth, or
    puerperium - see Nephritis,
    complicating pregnancy
  diabetic 250.4● [581.81]
    due to secondary diabetes 249.4●
      [581.81]
  Finnish type (congenital) 759.89
  hemoglobinuric - see Nephrosis,
    tubular
  in
    amyloidosis 277.39 [581.81]
    diabetes mellitus 250.4● [581.81]
      due to secondary diabetes 249.4●
        [581.81]

Nephrosis, nephrotic (Continued)
  in (Continued)
    epidemic hemorrhagic fever
      078.6
    malaria 084.9 [581.81]
    polyarteritis 446.0 [581.81]
    systemic lupus erythematosus
      710.0 [581.81]
  ischemic - see Nephrosis, tubular
  lipoid 581.3
  lower nephron - see Nephrosis,
    tubular
  lupoid 710.0 [581.81]
  lupus 710.0 [581.81]
  malarial 084.9 [581.81]
  minimal change 581.3
  necrotizing - see Nephrosis, tubular
  osmotic (sucrose) 588.89
  polyarteritic 446.0 [581.81]
  radiation 581.9
  specified lesion or cause NEC
    581.89
  syphilitic 095.4
  toxic - see Nephrosis, tubular
  tubular (acute) 584.5
    due to a procedure 997.5
    radiation 581.9
Nephrosonephritis hemorrhagic
  (endemic) 078.6
Nephrostomy status V44.6
  with complication 997.5
Nerve - see condition
Nerves 799.21
Nervous (see also condition) 799.21
  breakdown 300.9
  heart 306.2
  stomach 306.4
  tension 799.21
Nervousness 799.21
Nesidioblastoma (M8150/0)
  pancreas 211.7
  specified site NEC - see Neoplasm, by
    site, benign
  unspecified site 211.7
Netherton's syndrome (ichthyosiform
  erythroderma) 757.1
Nettle rash 708.8
Nettleship's disease (urticaria
  pigmentosa) 757.33
Neumann's disease (pemphigus
  vegetans) 694.4
Neuralgia, neuralgic (acute) (see also
  Neuritis) 729.2
  accessory (nerve) 352.4
  acoustic (nerve) 388.5
  ankle 355.8
  anterior crural 355.8
  anus 787.99
  arm 723.4
  auditory (nerve) 388.5
  axilla 353.0
  bladder 788.1
  brachial 723.4
  brain - see Disorder, nerve, cranial
  broad ligament 625.9
  cerebral - see Disorder, nerve, cranial
  ciliary 339.00
  cranial nerve - see also Disorder, nerve,
    cranial
    fifth or trigeminal (see also
      Neuralgia, trigeminal)
      350.1
  ear 388.71
    middle 352.1

Neuralgia, neuralgic *(Continued)*
  facial 351.8
  finger 354.9
  flank 355.8
  foot 355.8
  forearm 354.9
  Fothergill's *(see also* Neuralgia,
    trigeminal) 350.1
    postherpetic 053.12
  glossopharyngeal (nerve) 352.1
  groin 355.8
  hand 354.9
  heel 355.8
  Horton's 339.00
  Hunt's 053.11
  hypoglossal (nerve) 352.5
  iliac region 355.8
  infraorbital *(see also* Neuralgia,
    trigeminal) 350.1
  inguinal 355.8
  intercostal (nerve) 353.8
    postherpetic 053.19
  jaw 352.1
  kidney 788.0
  knee 355.8
  loin 355.8
  malarial *(see also* Malaria) 084.6
  mastoid 385.89
  maxilla 352.1
  median thenar 354.1
  metatarsal 355.6
  middle ear 352.1
  migrainous 339.00
  Morton's 355.6
  nerve, cranial - *see* Disorder, nerve,
    cranial
  nose 352.0
  occipital 723.8
  olfactory (nerve) 352.0
  ophthalmic 377.30
    postherpetic 053.19
  optic (nerve) 377.30
  penis 607.9
  perineum 355.8
  pleura 511.0
  postherpetic NEC 053.19
    geniculate ganglion 053.11
    ophthalmic 053.19
    trifacial 053.12
    trigeminal 053.12
  pubic region 355.8
  radial (nerve) 723.4
  rectum 787.99
  sacroiliac joint 724.3
  sciatic (nerve) 724.3
  scrotum 608.9
  seminal vesicle 608.9
  shoulder 354.9
  sluder's 337.09
  specified nerve NEC - *see* Disorder,
    nerve
  spermatic cord 608.9
  sphenopalatine (ganglion)
    337.09
  subscapular (nerve) 723.4
  suprascapular (nerve) 723.4
  testis 608.89
  thenar (median) 354.1
  thigh 355.8
  tongue 352.5
  trifacial (nerve) *(see also* Neuralgia,
    trigeminal) 350.1
  trigeminal (nerve) 350.1
    postherpetic 053.12
  tympanic plexus 388.71

Neuralgia, neuralgic *(Continued)*
  ulnar (nerve) 723.4
  vagus (nerve) 352.3
  wrist 354.9
  writers' 300.89
    organic 333.84
Neurapraxia - *see* Injury, nerve, by site
Neurasthenia 300.5
  cardiac 306.2
  gastric 306.4
  heart 306.2
  postfebrile 780.79
  postviral 780.79
Neurilemmoma (M9560/0) - *see also*
    Neoplasm, connective tissue,
    benign
  acoustic (nerve) 225.1
  malignant (M9560/3) - *see also*
    Neoplasm, connective tissue,
    malignant
    acoustic (nerve) 192.0
Neurilemmosarcoma (M9560/3) - *see*
    Neoplasm, connective tissue,
    malignant
Neurilemoma - *see* Neurilemmoma
Neurinoma (M9560/0) - *see*
    Neurilemmoma
Neurinomatosis (M9560/1) - *see also*
    Neoplasm, connective tissue,
    uncertain behavior
  centralis 759.5
Neuritis *(see also* Neuralgia) 729.2
  abducens (nerve) 378.54
  accessory (nerve) 352.4
  acoustic (nerve) 388.5
    syphilitic 094.86
  alcoholic 357.5
    with psychosis 291.1
  amyloid, any site 277.39 *[357.4]*
  anterior crural 355.8
  arising during pregnancy 646.4●
  arm 723.4
  ascending 355.2
  auditory (nerve) 388.5
  brachial (nerve) NEC 723.4
    due to displacement, intervertebral
      disc 722.0
  cervical 723.4
  chest (wall) 353.8
  costal region 353.8
  cranial nerve - *see also* Disorder, nerve,
    cranial
    first or olfactory 352.0
    second or optic 377.30
    third or oculomotor 378.52
    fourth or trochlear 378.53
    fifth or trigeminal *(see also*
      Neuralgia, trigeminal)
      350.1
    sixth or abducens 378.54
    seventh or facial 351.8
      newborn 767.5
    eighth or acoustic 388.5
    ninth or glossopharyngeal
      352.1
    tenth or vagus 352.3
    eleventh or accessory 352.4
    twelfth or hypoglossal 352.5
  Déjérine-Sottas 356.0
  diabetic 250.6● *[357.2]*
    due to secondary diabetes
      249.6● *[357.2]*
  diphtheritic 032.89 *[357.4]*

Neuritis *(Continued)*
  due to
    beriberi 265.0 *[357.4]*
    displacement, prolapse, protrusion,
      or rupture of intervertebral
      disc 722.2
      cervical 722.0
      lumbar, lumbosacral 722.10
      thoracic, thoracolumbar 722.11
    herniation, nucleus pulposus 722.2
      cervical 722.0
      lumbar, lumbosacral 722.10
      thoracic, thoracolumbar 722.11
  endemic 265.0 *[357.4]*
  facial (nerve) 351.8
    newborn 767.5
  general - *see* Polyneuropathy
  geniculate ganglion 351.1
    due to herpes 053.11
  glossopharyngeal (nerve) 352.1
  gouty 274.89 *[357.4]*
  hypoglossal (nerve) 352.5
  ilioinguinal (nerve) 355.8
  in diseases classified elsewhere - *see*
    Polyneuropathy, in
  infectious (multiple) 357.0
  intercostal (nerve) 353.8
  interstitial hypertrophic progressive
    NEC 356.9
  leg 355.8
  lumbosacral NEC 724.4
  median (nerve) 354.1
    thenar 354.1
  multiple (acute) (infective) 356.9
    endemic 265.0 *[357.4]*
  multiplex endemica 265.0 *[357.4]*
  nerve root *(see also* Radiculitis) 729.2
  oculomotor (nerve) 378.52
  olfactory (nerve) 352.0
  optic (nerve) 377.30
    in myelitis 341.0
    meningococcal 036.81
  pelvic 355.8
  peripheral (nerve) - *see also*
    Neuropathy, peripheral
    complicating pregnancy or
      puerperium 646.4●
    specified nerve NEC - *see*
      Mononeuritis
  pneumogastric (nerve) 352.3
  postchickenpox 052.7
  postherpetic 053.19
  progressive hypertrophic interstitial
    NEC 356.9
  puerperal, postpartum 646.4●
  radial (nerve) 723.4
  retrobulbar 377.32
    syphilitic 094.85
  rheumatic (chronic) 729.2
  sacral region 355.8
  sciatic (nerve) 724.3
    due to displacement of
      intervertebral disc 722.10
  serum 999.5
  specified nerve NEC - *see* Disorder,
    nerve
  spinal (nerve) 355.9
    root *(see also* Radiculitis) 729.2
  subscapular (nerve) 723.4
  suprascapular (nerve) 723.4
  syphilitic 095.8
  thenar (median) 354.1
  thoracic NEC 724.4
  toxic NEC 357.7
  trochlear (nerve) 378.53

◀ New   ◀▥ Revised   ~~deleted~~ Deleted   ● Use Additional Digit(s)   ▨ Omit code

Neuritis (*Continued*)
  ulnar (nerve) 723.4
  vagus (nerve) 352.3
Neuroangiomatosis, encephalofacial 759.6
Neuroastrocytoma (M9505/1) - *see*
    Neoplasm, by site, uncertain
    behavior
Neuro-avitaminosis 269.2
Neuroblastoma (M9500/3)
  olfactory (M9522/3) 160.0
  specified site - *see* Neoplasm, by site,
    malignant
  unspecified site 194.0
Neurochorioretinitis (*see also*
    Chorioretinitis) 363.20
Neurocirculatory asthenia 306.2
Neurocytoma (M9506/0) - *see* Neoplasm,
    by site, benign
Neurodermatitis (circumscribed)
    (circumscripta) (local) 698.3
  atopic 691.8
  diffuse (Brocq) 691.8
  disseminated 691.8
  nodulosa 698.3
Neuroencephalomyelopathy, optic 341.0
Neuroendocrine tumor - *see* Tumor,
    neuroendocrine
Neuroepithelioma (M9503/3) - *see also*
    Neoplasm, by site, malignant
  olfactory (M9521/3) 160.0
Neurofibroma (M9540/0) - *see also*
    Neoplasm, connective tissue, benign
  melanotic (M9541/0) - *see* Neoplasm,
    connective tissue, benign
  multiple (M9540/1) 237.70
    type 1 237.71
    type 2 237.72
  plexiform (M9550/0) - *see* Neoplasm,
    connective tissue, benign
Neurofibromatosis (multiple) (M9540/1)
    237.70
  acoustic 237.72
  malignant (M9540/3) - *see* Neoplasm,
    connective tissue, malignant
  Schwannomatosis 237.73 ◄
  specified type NEC 237.79 ◄
  type 1 237.71
  type 2 237.72
  von Recklinghausen's 237.71
Neurofibrosarcoma (M9540/3) - *see*
    Neoplasm, connective tissue,
    malignant
Neurogenic - *see also* condition
  bladder (atonic) (automatic)
    (autonomic) (flaccid) (hypertonic)
    (hypotonic) (inertia) (infranuclear)
    (irritable) (motor) (nonreflex)
    (nuclear) (paralysis) (reflex)
    (sensory) (spastic) (supranuclear)
    (uninhibited) 596.54
    with cauda equina syndrome 344.61
  bowel 564.81
  heart 306.2
Neuroglioma (M9505/1) - *see* Neoplasm,
    by site, uncertain behavior
Neurolabyrinthitis (of Dix and Hallpike)
    386.12
Neurolathyrism 988.2
Neuroleprosy 030.1
Neuroleptic malignant syndrome 333.92
Neurolipomatosis 272.8
Neuroma (M9570/0) - *see also* Neoplasm,
    connective tissue, benign
  acoustic (nerve) (M9560/0) 225.1
  amputation (traumatic) - *see also* Injury,
    nerve, by site
    surgical complication (late) 997.61

Neuroma (*Continued*)
  appendix 211.3
  auditory nerve 225.1
  digital 355.6
    toe 355.6
  interdigital (toe) 355.6
  intermetatarsal 355.6
  Morton's 355.6
  multiple 237.70
    type 1 237.71
    type 2 237.72
  nonneoplastic 355.9
    arm NEC 354.9
    leg NEC 355.8
    lower extremity NEC 355.8
    specified site NEC - *see*
      Mononeuritis, by site
    upper extremity NEC 354.9
  optic (nerve) 225.1
  plantar 355.6
  plexiform (M9550/0) - *see* Neoplasm,
    connective tissue, benign
  surgical (nonneoplastic) 355.9
    arm NEC 354.9
    leg NEC 355.8
    lower extremity NEC 355.8
    upper extremity NEC 354.9
  traumatic - *see also* Injury, nerve,
    by site old - *see* Neuroma,
    nonneoplastic
Neuromyalgia 729.1
Neuromyasthenia (epidemic) 049.8
Neuromyelitis 341.8
  ascending 357.0
  optica 341.0
Neuromyopathy NEC 358.9
Neuromyositis 729.1
Neuronevus (M8725/0) - *see* Neoplasm,
    skin, benign
Neuronitis 357.0
  ascending (acute) 355.2
  vestibular 386.12
Neuroparalytic - *see* condition
Neuropathy, neuropathic (*see also*
    Disorder, nerve) 355.9
  acute motor 357.82
  alcoholic 357.5
    with psychosis 291.1
  arm NEC 354.9
  ataxia and retinitis pigmentosa (NARP
    syndrome) 277.87
  autonomic (peripheral) - *see*
    Neuropathy, peripheral,
    autonomic
  axillary nerve 353.0
  brachial plexus 353.0
  cervical plexus 353.2
  chronic
    progressive segmentally
      demyelinating 357.89
    relapsing demyelinating 357.89
  congenital sensory 356.2
  Déjérine-Sottas 356.0
  diabetic 250.6● [357.2]
    autonomic (peripheral) 250.6
      [337.1]
    due to secondary diabetes 249.6●
      [357.2]
      autonomic (peripheral) 249.6
        [337.1]
  entrapment 355.9
    iliohypogastric nerve
      355.79
    ilioinguinal nerve 355.79

Neuropathy, neuropathic (*Continued*)
  entrapment (*Continued*)
    lateral cutaneous nerve of thigh
      355.1
    median nerve 354.0
    obturator nerve 355.79
    peroneal nerve 355.3
    posterior tibial nerve 355.5
    saphenous nerve 355.79
    ulnar nerve 354.2
  facial nerve 351.9
  hereditary 356.9
    peripheral 356.0
    sensory (radicular) 356.2
  hypertrophic
    Charcôt-Marie-Tooth 356.1
    Déjérine-Sottas 356.0
    interstitial 356.9
    Refsum 356.3
  intercostal nerve 354.8
  ischemic - *see* Disorder, nerve
  Jamaican (ginger) 357.7
  leg NEC 355.8
  lower extremity NEC 355.8
  lumbar plexus 353.1
  median nerve 354.1
  motor
    acute 357.82
  multiple (acute) (chronic) (*see also*
    Polyneuropathy) 356.9
  optic 377.39
    ischemic 377.41
    nutritional 377.33
    toxic 377.34
  peripheral (nerve) (*see also*
    Polyneuropathy) 356.9
    arm NEC 354.9
    autonomic 337.9
      amyloid 277.39 [337.1]
      idiopathic 337.00
      in
        amyloidosis 277.39 [337.1]
        diabetes (mellitus) 250.6●
          [337.1]
        due to secondary diabetes
          249.6● [337.1]
        diseases classified elsewhere
          337.1
        gout 274.89 [337.1]
        hyperthyroidism 242.9●
          [337.1]
    due to
      antitetanus serum 357.6
      arsenic 357.7
      drugs 357.6
      lead 357.7
      organophosphate compounds
        357.7
      toxic agent NEC 357.7
    hereditary 356.0
    idiopathic 356.9
      progressive 356.4
      specified type NEC 356.8
    in diseases classified elsewhere - *see*
      Polyneuropathy, in
    leg NEC 355.8
    lower extremity NEC 355.8
    upper extremity NEC 354.9
  plantar nerves 355.6
  progressive
    hypertrophic interstitial 356.9
    inflammatory 357.89
  radicular NEC 729.2
    brachial 723.4
    cervical NEC 723.4

Neuropathy, neuropathic *(Continued)*
  radicular NEC *(Continued)*
    hereditary sensory 356.2
      lumbar 724.4
      lumbosacral 724.4
      thoracic NEC 724.4
    sacral plexus 353.1
    sciatic 355.0
    spinal nerve NEC 355.9
      root *(see also* Radiculitis) 729.2
    toxic 357.7
    trigeminal sensory 350.8
    ulnar nerve 354.2
    upper extremity NEC 354.9
    uremic 585.9 *[357.4]*
    vitamin B$_{12}$ 266.2 *[357.4]*
      with anemia (pernicious) 281.0
        [357.4]
        due to dietary deficiency 281.1
          [357.4]
Neurophthisis - *see also* Disorder, nerve
  peripheral 356.9
    diabetic 250.6● *[357.2]*
      due to secondary diabetes 249.6●
        [357.2]
Neuropraxia - *see* Injury, nerve
Neuroretinitis 363.05
  syphilitic 094.85
Neurosarcoma (M9540/3) - *see* Neoplasm,
    connective tissue, malignant
Neurosclerosis - *see* Disorder, nerve
Neurosis, neurotic 300.9
  accident 300.16
  anancastic, anankastic 300.3
  anxiety (state) 300.00
    generalized 300.02
    panic type 300.01
  asthenic 300.5
  bladder 306.53
  cardiac (reflex) 306.2
  cardiovascular 306.2
  climacteric, unspecified type 627.2
  colon 306.4
  compensation 300.16
  compulsive, compulsion 300.3
  conversion 300.11
  craft 300.89
  cutaneous 306.3
  depersonalization 300.6
  depressive (reaction) (type) 300.4
  endocrine 306.6
  environmental 300.89
  fatigue 300.5
  functional *(see also* Disorder,
      psychosomatic) 306.9
  gastric 306.4
  gastrointestinal 306.4
  genitourinary 306.50
  heart 306.2
  hypochondriacal 300.7
  hysterical 300.10
    conversion type 300.11
    dissociative type 300.15
  impulsive 300.3
  incoordination 306.0
    larynx 306.1
    vocal cord 306.1
  intestine 306.4
  larynx 306.1
    hysterical 300.11
    sensory 306.1
  menopause, unspecified type
      627.2
  mixed NEC 300.89

Neurosis, neurotic *(Continued)*
  musculoskeletal 306.0
  obsessional 300.3
    phobia 300.3
  obsessive-compulsive 300.3
  occupational 300.89
  ocular 306.7
  oral *(see also* Disorder, fluency)
      315.35 ◀▥
  organ *(see also* Disorder,
      psychosomatic) 306.9
  pharynx 306.1
  phobic 300.20
  posttraumatic (acute) (situational)
      309.81
    chronic 309.81
  psychasthenic (type) 300.89
  railroad 300.16
  rectum 306.4
  respiratory 306.1
  rumination 306.4
  senile 300.89
  sexual 302.70
  situational 300.89
  specified type NEC 300.89
  state 300.9
    with depersonalization episode
        300.6
  stomach 306.4
  vasomotor 306.2
  visceral 306.4
  war 300.16
Neurospongioblastosis diffusa 759.5
Neurosyphilis (arrested) (early)
    (inactive) (late) (latent) (recurrent)
    094.9
  with ataxia (cerebellar) (locomotor)
      (spastic) (spinal) 094.0
  acute meningitis 094.2
  aneurysm 094.89
  arachnoid (adhesive) 094.2
  arteritis (any artery) 094.89
  asymptomatic 094.3
  congenital 090.40
  dura (mater) 094.89
  general paresis 094.1
  gumma 094.9
  hemorrhagic 094.9
  juvenile (asymptomatic) (meningeal)
      090.40
  leptomeninges (aseptic) 094.2
  meningeal 094.2
  meninges (adhesive) 094.2
  meningovascular (diffuse) 094.2
  optic atrophy 094.84
  parenchymatous (degenerative) 094.1
  paresis *(see also* Paresis, general) 094.1
  paretic *(see also* Paresis, general) 094.1
  relapse 094.9
  remission in (sustained) 094.9
  serological 094.3
  specified nature or site NEC 094.89
  tabes (dorsalis) 094.0
    juvenile 090.40
  tabetic 094.0
    juvenile 090.40
  taboparesis 094.1
    juvenile 090.40
  thrombosis 094.89
  vascular 094.89
Neurotic *(see also* Neurosis) 300.9
  excoriation 698.4
    psychogenic 306.3
Neurotmesis - *see* Injury, nerve, by site

Neurotoxemia - *see* Toxemia
Neutro-occlusion 524.21
Neutropenia, neutropenic (idiopathic)
    (pernicious) (primary) 288.00
  chronic 288.09
    hypoplastic 288.09
  congenital (nontransient) 288.01
  cyclic 288.02
  drug induced 288.03
  due to infection 288.04
  fever 288.00
  genetic 288.01
  immune 288.09
  infantile 288.01
  malignant 288.09
  neonatal, transitory (isoimmune)
      (maternal transfer) 776.7
  periodic 288.02
  splenic 289.53
  splenomegaly 289.53
  toxic 288.09
Neutrophilia, hereditary giant
    288.2
Nevocarcinoma (M8720/3) - *see*
    Melanoma
Nevus (M8720/0) - *see also* Neoplasm,
    skin, benign

> Note: Except where otherwise
> indicated, varieties of nevus in the list
> below that are followed by a
> morphology code number (M----/0)
> should be coded by site as for
> "Neoplasm, skin, benign."

  acanthotic 702.8
  achromic (M8730/0)
  amelanotic (M8730/0)
  anemic, anemicus 709.09
  angiomatous (M9120/0) *(see also*
      Hemangioma) 228.00
  araneus 448.1
  avasculosus 709.09
  balloon cell (M8722/0)
  bathing trunk (M8761/1) 238.2
  blue (M8780/0)
    cellular (M8790/0)
    giant (M8790/0)
    Jadassohn's (M8780/0)
    malignant (M8780/3) - *see*
        Melanoma
  capillary (M9131/0) *(see also*
      Hemangioma) 228.00
  cavernous (M9121/0) *(see also*
      Hemangioma) 228.00
  cellular (M8720/0)
    blue (M8790/0)
  comedonicus 757.33
  compound (M8760/0)
  conjunctiva (M8720/0) 224.3
  dermal (8750/0)
    and epidermal (M8760/0)
  epithelioid cell (and spindle cell)
      (M8770/0)
  flammeus 757.32
    osteohypertrophic 759.89
  hairy (M8720/0)
  halo (M8723/0)
  hemangiomatous (M9120/0) *(see also*
      Hemangioma) 228.00
  intradermal (M8750/0)
  intraepidermal (M8740/0)
  involuting (M8724/0)
  Jadassohn's (blue) (M8780/0)

◀ New   ◀▥ Revised   ~~deleted~~ Deleted   ● Use Additional Digit(s)   �▨ Omit code

Nevus *(Continued)*
 junction, junctional (M8740/0)
  malignant melanoma in (M8740/3) -
   see Melanoma
 juvenile (M8770/0)
 lymphatic (M9170/0) 228.1
 magnocellular (M8726/0)
  specified site - *see* Neoplasm, by site,
   benign
  unspecified site 224.0
 malignant (M8720/3) - *see* Melanoma
 meaning hemangioma (M9120/0) *(see
  also* Hemangioma) 228.00
 melanotic (pigmented) (M8720/0)
 multiplex 759.5
 nonneoplastic 448.1
 nonpigmented (M8730/0)
 nonvascular (M8720/0)
 oral mucosa, white sponge 750.26
 osteohypertrophic, flammeus
  759.89
 papillaris (M8720/0)
 papillomatosus (M8720/0)
 pigmented (M8720/0)
  giant (M8761/1) - *see also* Neoplasm,
   skin, uncertain behavior
   malignant melanoma in
    (M8761/3) - *see* Melanoma
  systematicus 757.33
 pilosus (M8720/0)
 port wine 757.32
 sanguineous 757.32
 sebaceous (senile) 702.8
 senile 448.1
 spider 448.1
 spindle cell (and epithelioid cell)
  (M8770/0)
 stellar 448.1
 strawberry 757.32
 syringocystadenomatous papilliferous
  (M8406/0)
 unius lateris 757.33
 Unna's 757.32
 vascular 757.32
 verrucous 757.33
 white sponge (oral mucosa) 750.26
Newborn (infant) (liveborn)
 abstinence syndrome 779.5
 affected by
  amniocentesis 760.61
  maternal abuse of drugs
   (gestational) (via placenta) (via
   breast milk) *(see also* Noxious,
   substances transmitted
   through placenta
   or breast milk (affecting fetus
   or newborn)) 760.70
   methamphetamine(s) 760.72
  procedure
   amniocentesis 760.61
   in utero NEC 760.62
   surgical on mother
    during pregnancy NEC
     760.63
    previous not associated with
     pregnancy 760.64
 apnea 770.81
  obstructive 770.82
  specified NEC 770.82
 breast buds 779.89
 cardiomyopathy 425.4
  congenital 425.3
 convulsion 779.0
 electrolyte imbalance NEC (transitory)
  775.5

Newborn *(Continued)*
 fever (environmentally-induced)
  778.4
 gestation
  24 completed weeks 765.22
  25–26 completed weeks 765.23
  27–28 completed weeks 765.24
  29–30 completed weeks 765.25
  31–32 completed weeks 765.26
  33–34 completed weeks 765.27
  35–36 completed weeks 765.28
  37 or more completed weeks 765.29
  less than 24 completed weeks
   765.21
  unspecified completed weeks
   765.20
 infection 771.89
  candida 771.7
  mastitis 771.5
  specified NEC 771.89
  urinary tract 771.82
 mastitis 771.5
 multiple NEC
  born in hospital (without mention of
   cesarean delivery or section)
   V37.00
   with cesarean delivery or section
    V37.01
  born outside hospital
   hospitalized V37.1●
   not hospitalized V37.2●
  mates all liveborn
   born in hospital (without
    mention of cesarean
    delivery or section)
    V34.00
    with cesarean delivery or
     section V34.01
   born outside hospital
    hospitalized V34.1●
    not hospitalized V34.2●
  mates all stillborn
   born in hospital (without
    mention of cesarean
    delivery or section)
    V35.00
    with cesarean delivery or
     section V35.01
   born outside hospital
    hospitalized V35.1●
    not hospitalized V35.2●
  mates liveborn and stillborn
   born in hospital (without
    mention of cesarean
    delivery or section)
    V36.00
    with cesarean delivery or
     section V36.01
   born outside hospital
    hospitalized V36.1●
    not hospitalized V36.2●
 omphalitis 771.4
 seizure 779.0
 sepsis 771.81
 single
  born in hospital (without mention of
   cesarean delivery or section)
   V30.00
   with cesarean delivery or section
    V30.01
  born outside hospital
   hospitalized V30.1●
   not hospitalized V30.2●
 specified condition NEC 779.89

Newborn *(Continued)*
 twin NEC
  born in hospital (without mention of
   cesarean delivery or section)
   V33.00
   with cesarean delivery or section
    V33.01
  born outside hospital
   hospitalized V33.1●
   not hospitalized V33.2●
  mate liveborn
   born in hospital V31.0●
   born outside hospital
    hospitalized V31.1●
    not hospitalized V31.2●
  mate stillborn
   born in hospital V32.0●
   born outside hospital
    hospitalized V32.1●
    not hospitalized V32.2●
 unspecified as to single or multiple
  birth
  born in hospital (without mention of
   cesarean delivery or section)
   V39.00
   with cesarean delivery or section
    V39.01
  born outside hospital
   hospitalized V39.1●
   not hospitalized V39.2●
 weight check V20.32
Newcastle's conjunctivitis or disease
 077.8
Nezelof's syndrome (pure
 alymphocytosis) 279.13
Niacin (amide) deficiency 265.2
Nicolas-Durand-Favre disease (climatic
 bubo) 099.1
Nicolas-Favre disease (climatic bubo)
 099.1
Nicotinic acid (amide) deficiency
 265.2
Niemann-Pick disease (lipid
 histiocytosis) (splenomegaly)
 272.7
Night
 blindness *(see also* Blindness, night)
  368.60
  congenital 368.61
  vitamin A deficiency 264.5
 cramps 729.82
 sweats 780.8
 terrors, child 307.46
Nightmare 307.47
 REM-sleep type 307.47
Nipple - *see* condition
Nisbet's chancre 099.0
Nishimoto (-Takeuchi) disease 437.5
Nitritoid crisis or reaction - *see* Crisis,
 nitritoid
Nitrogen retention, extrarenal 788.99
Nitrosohemoglobinemia 289.89
Njovera 104.0
No
 diagnosis 799.9
 disease (found) V71.9
 room at the inn V65.0
Nocardiasis - *see* Nocardiosis
Nocardiosis 039.9
 with pneumonia 039.1
 lung 039.1
 specified type NEC 039.8
Nocturia 788.43
 psychogenic 306.53

Nocturnal - *see also* condition
    dyspnea (paroxysmal) 786.09
    emissions 608.89
    enuresis 788.36
        psychogenic 307.6
    frequency (micturition) 788.43
        psychogenic 306.53
Nodal rhythm disorder 427.89
Nodding of head 781.0
Node(s) - *see also* Nodules
    Heberden's 715.04
    larynx 478.79
    lymph - *see* condition
    milkers' 051.1
    Osler's 421.0
    rheumatic 729.89
    Schmorl's 722.30
        lumbar, lumbosacral 722.32
        specified region NEC 722.39
        thoracic, thoracolumbar 722.31
    singers' 478.5
    skin NEC 782.2
    tuberculous - *see* Tuberculosis, lymph
        gland
    vocal cords 478.5
Nodosities, Haygarth's 715.04
Nodule(s), nodular
    actinomycotic (*see also* Actinomycosis)
        039.9
    arthritic - *see* Arthritis, nodosa
    breast 793.89
    cutaneous 782.2
    Haygarth's 715.04
    inflammatory - *see* Inflammation
    juxta-articular 102.7
        syphilitic 095.7
        yaws 102.7
    larynx 478.79
    lung, solitary 518.89
        emphysematous 492.8
    milkers' 051.1
    prostate 600.10
        with
            urinary
                obstruction 600.11
                retention 600.11
    retrocardiac 785.9
    rheumatic 729.89
    rheumatoid - *see* Arthritis rheumatoid
    scrotum (inflammatory) 608.4
    singers' 478.5
    skin NEC 782.2
    solitary, lung 518.89
        emphysematous 492.8
    subcutaneous 782.2
    thyroid (gland) (nontoxic) (uninodular)
        241.0
        with
            hyperthyroidism 242.1●
            thyrotoxicosis 242.1●
        toxic or with hyperthyroidism
            242.1●
    vocal cords 478.5
Noma (gangrenous) (hospital) (infective)
    528.1
    auricle (*see also* Gangrene) 785.4
    mouth 528.1
    pudendi (*see also* Vulvitis) 616.10
    vulvae (*see also* Vulvitis) 616.10
Nomadism V60.0
Non-adherence
    artificial skin graft 996.55
    decellularized allodermis graft
        996.55

Non-autoimmune hemolytic anemia
    NEC 283.10
Nonclosure - *see also* Imperfect, closure
    ductus
        arteriosus 747.0
        Botalli 747.0
    Eustachian valve 746.89
    foramen
        Botalli 745.5
        ovale 745.5
Noncompliance with medical treatment
    V15.81
    renal dialysis V45.12
Nondescent (congenital) - *see also*
    Malposition, congenital
    cecum 751.4
    colon 751.4
    testis 752.51
Nondevelopment
    brain 742.1
        specified part 742.2
    heart 746.89
    organ or site, congenital NEC - *see*
        Hypoplasia
Nonengagement
    head NEC 652.5●
        in labor 660.1●
            affecting fetus or newborn 763.1
Nonexanthematous tick fever 066.1
Nonexpansion, lung (newborn) NEC 770.4
Nonfunctioning
    cystic duct (*see also* Disease,
        gallbladder) 575.8
    gallbladder (*see also* Disease,
        gallbladder) 575.8
    kidney (*see also* Disease, renal) 593.9
    labyrinth 386.58
Nonhealing
    stump (surgical) 997.69
    wound, surgical 998.83
Nonimplantation of ovum, causing
    infertility 628.3
Noninsufflation, fallopian tube 628.2
Nonne-Milroy-Meige syndrome (chronic
    hereditary edema) 757.0
Nonovulation 628.0
Nonpatent fallopian tube 628.2
Nonpneumatization, lung NEC 770.4
Nonreflex bladder 596.54
    with cauda equina 344.61
Nonretention of food - *see* Vomiting
Nonrotation - *see* Malrotation
Nonsecretion, urine (*see also* Anuria)
    788.5
    newborn 753.3
Nonunion
    fracture 733.82
    organ or site, congenital NEC - *see*
        Imperfect, closure
    symphysis pubis, congenital 755.69
    top sacrum, congenital 756.19
Nonviability 765.0●
Nonvisualization, gallbladder 793.3
Nonvitalized tooth 522.9
Non-working side interference 524.56
Normal
    delivery - *see* category 650
    menses V65.5
    state (feared complaint unfounded)
        V65.5
Normoblastosis 289.89
Normocytic anemia (infectional) 285.9
    due to blood loss (chronic) 280.0
        acute 285.1

Norrie's disease (congenital) (progressive
    oculoacousticocerebral
    degeneration) 743.8
North American blastomycosis
    116.0
Norwegian itch 133.0
Nose, nasal - *see* condition
Nosebleed 784.7
Nosomania 298.9
Nosophobia 300.29
Nostalgia 309.89
Notch of iris 743.46
Notched lip, congenital (*see also* Cleft,
    lip) 749.10
Notching nose, congenital (tip) 748.1
Nothnagel's
    syndrome 378.52
    vasomotor acroparesthesia 443.89
Novy's relapsing fever (American)
    087.1
Noxious
    foodstuffs, poisoning by
        fish 988.0
        fungi 988.1
        mushrooms 988.1
        plants (food) 988.2
        shellfish 988.0
        specified type NEC 988.8
        toadstool 988.1
    substances transmitted through
        placenta or breast milk
        (affecting fetus or newborn)
        760.70
        acetretin 760.78
        alcohol 760.71
        aminopterin 760.78
        antiandrogens 760.79
        anticonvulsant 760.77
        antifungal 760.74
        anti-infective agents 760.74
        antimetabolic 760.78
        atorvastatin 760.78
        carbamazepine 760.77
        cocaine 760.75
        "crack" 760.75
        diethylstilbestrol (DES) 760.76
        divalproex sodium 760.77
        endocrine disrupting chemicals
        760.79
        estrogens 760.79
        etretinate 760.78
        fluconazole 760.74
        fluvastatin 760.78
        hallucinogenic agents NEC 760.73
        hormones 760.79
        lithium 760.79
        lovastatin 760.78
        medicinal agents NEC 760.79
        methotrexate 760.78
        misoprostil 760.79
        narcotics 760.72
        obstetric anesthetic or analgesic
        763.5
        phenobarbital 760.77
        phenytoin 760.77
        pravastatin 760.78
        progestins 760.79
        retinoic acid 760.78
        simvastatin 760.78
        solvents 760.79
        specified agent NEC 760.79
        statins 760.78
        suspected, affecting management of
            pregnancy 655.5●

◀ New   ◀▦ Revised   ~~deleted~~ Deleted   ● Use Additional Digit(s)   ▨ Omit code

Noxious *(Continued)*
  substances transmitted through placenta
    or breast milk *(Continued)*
    tetracycline 760.74
    thalidomide 760.79
    trimethadione 760.77
    valproate 760.77
    valproic acid 760.77
    vitamin A 760.78
NPDH (new persistent daily headache)
  339.42
Nuchal hitch (arm) 652.8●
Nucleus pulposus - *see* condition
Numbness 782.0
Nuns' knee 727.2
Nursemaid's
  elbow 832.2●
  shoulder 831.0●

Nutmeg liver 573.8
Nutrition, deficient or insufficient
  (particular kind of food)
  269.9
  due to
    insufficient food 994.2
    lack of
      care (child) (infant) 995.52
        adult 995.84
      food 994.2
Nyctalopia (*see also* Blindness, night)
  368.60
  vitamin A deficiency 264.5
Nycturia 788.43
  psychogenic 306.53
Nymphomania 302.89

Nystagmus 379.50
  associated with vestibular system
    disorders 379.54
  benign paroxysmal positional 386.11
  central positional 386.2
  congenital 379.51
  deprivation 379.53
  dissociated 379.55
  latent 379.52
  miners' 300.89
  positional
    benign paroxysmal 386.11
    central 386.2
  specified NEC 379.56
  vestibular 379.54
  visual deprivation 379.53

O

Oasthouse urine disease 270.2
Obermeyer's relapsing fever (European) 087.0
Obesity (constitutional) (exogenous) (familial) (nutritional) (simple) 278.00
   adrenal 255.8
   complicating pregnancy, childbirth, or puerperium 649.1●
   due to hyperalimentation 278.00
   endocrine NEC 259.9
   endogenous 259.9
   Fröhlich's (adiposogenital dystrophy) 253.8
   glandular NEC 259.9
   hypothyroid (see also Hypothyroidism) 244.9
   hypoventilation syndrome 278.03 ◀
   morbid 278.01
   of pregnancy 649.1●
   pituitary 253.8
   severe 278.01
   thyroid (see also Hypothyroidism) 244.9
Oblique - see also condition
   lie before labor, affecting fetus or newborn 761.7
Obliquity, pelvis 738.6
Obliteration
   abdominal aorta 446.7
   appendix (lumen) 543.9
   artery 447.1
   ascending aorta 446.7
   bile ducts 576.8
      with calculus, choledocholithiasis, or stones - see Choledocholithiasis
      congenital 751.61
         jaundice from 751.61 [774.5]
   common duct 576.8
      with calculus, choledocholithiasis, or stones - see Choledocholithiasis
      congenital 751.61
   cystic duct 575.8
      with calculus, choledocholithiasis, or stones - see Choledocholithiasis
   disease, arteriolar 447.1
   endometrium 621.8
   eye, anterior chamber 360.34
   fallopian tube 628.2
   lymphatic vessel 457.1
      postmastectomy 457.0
   organ or site, congenital NEC - see Atresia
   placental blood vessels - see Placenta, abnormal
   supra-aortic branches 446.7
   ureter 593.89
   urethra 599.84
   vein 459.9
   vestibule (oral) 525.8
Observation (for) V71.9
   without need for further medical care V71.9
   accident NEC V71.4
      at work V71.3
   criminal assault V71.6
   deleterious agent ingestion V71.89
   disease V71.9
      cardiovascular V71.7
      heart V71.7

Observation (Continued)
   disease (Continued)
      mental V71.09
         specified condition NEC V71.89
   foreign body ingestion V71.89
   growth and development variations V21.8
   injuries (accidental) V71.4
      inflicted NEC V71.6
         during alleged rape or seduction V71.5
   malignant neoplasm, suspected V71.1
   postpartum
      immediately after delivery V24.0
      routine follow-up V24.2
   pregnancy
      high-risk V23.9
         specified problem NEC V23.89
      normal (without complication) V22.1
         with nonobstetric complication V22.2
      first V22.0
   rape or seduction, alleged V71.5
      injury during V71.5
   suicide attempt, alleged V71.89
   suspected (undiagnosed) (unproven)
      abuse V71.81
      cardiovascular disease V71.7
      child or wife battering victim V71.6
      concussion (cerebral) V71.6
      condition NEC V71.89
         infant - see Observation, suspected, condition, newborn
        maternal and fetal
            amniotic cavity and membrane problem V89.01
            cervical shortening V89.05
            fetal anomaly V89.03
            fetal growth problem V89.04
            oligohydramnios V89.01
            other specified problem NEC V89.09
            placental problem V89.02
            polyhydramnios V89.01
        newborn V29.9
           cardiovascular disease V29.8
           congenital anomaly V29.8
           genetic V29.3
           infectious V29.0
           ingestion foreign object V29.8
           injury V29.8
           metabolic V29.3
           neoplasm V29.8
           neurological V29.1
           poison, poisoning V29.8
           respiratory V29.2
           specified NEC V29.8
      exposure
         anthrax V71.82
         biologic agent NEC V71.83
         SARS V71.83
      infectious disease not requiring isolation V71.89
      malignant neoplasm V71.1
      mental disorder V71.09
      neglect V71.81
      neoplasm
         benign V71.89
         malignant V71.1
      specified condition NEC V71.89
      tuberculosis V71.2
   tuberculosis, suspected V71.2

Obsession, obsessional 300.3
   ideas and mental images 300.3
   impulses 300.3
   neurosis 300.3
   phobia 300.3
   psychasthenia 300.3
   ruminations 300.3
   state 300.3
   syndrome 300.3
Obsessive-compulsive 300.3
   neurosis 300.3
   personality 301.4
   reaction 300.3
Obstetrical trauma NEC (complicating delivery) 665.9●
   with
      abortion - see Abortion, by type, with damage to pelvic organs
      ectopic pregnancy (see also categories 633.0-633.9) 639.2
      molar pregnancy (see also categories 630-632) 639.2
   affecting fetus or newborn 763.89
   following
      abortion 639.2
      ectopic or molar pregnancy 639.2
Obstipation (see also Constipation) 564.00
   psychogenic 306.4
Obstruction, obstructed, obstructive
   airway NEC 519.8
      with
         allergic alveolitis NEC 495.9
         asthma NEC (see also Asthma) 493.9●
         bronchiectasis 494.0
           with acute exacerbation 494.1
         bronchitis (see also Bronchitis, with, obstruction) 491.20
         emphysema NEC 492.8
   chronic 496
      with
         allergic alveolitis NEC 495.5
         asthma NEC (see also Asthma) 493.2●
         bronchiectasis 494.0
           with acute exacerbation 494.1
         bronchitis (chronic) (see also Bronchitis, chronic, obstructive) 491.20
         emphysema NEC 492.8
      due to
         bronchospasm 519.11
         foreign body 934.9
         inhalation of fumes or vapors 506.9
         laryngospasm 478.75
   alimentary canal (see also Obstruction, intestine) 560.9
   ampulla of Vater 576.2
      with calculus, cholelithiasis, or stones - see Choledocholithiasis
   aortic (heart) (valve) (see also Stenosis, aortic) 424.1
      rheumatic (see also Stenosis, aortic, rheumatic) 395.0
   aortoiliac 444.0
   aqueduct of Sylvius 331.4
      congenital 742.3
         with spina bifida (see also Spina bifida) 741.0●
   Arnold-Chiari (see also Spina bifida) 741.0●

◀ New   ◀‖‖ Revised   ~~deleted~~ Deleted   ● Use Additional Digit(s)   Omit code

Obstruction, obstructed, obstructive (*Continued*)
  lung (*Continued*)
    chronic NEC 496
      with
        asthma (chronic) (obstructive) 493.2●
    disease, chronic 496
      with
        asthma (chronic) (obstructive) 493.2●
    emphysematous 492.8
  lymphatic 457.1
  meconium
    fetus or newborn 777.1
      in mucoviscidosis 277.01
    newborn due to fecaliths 777.1
  mediastinum 519.3
  mitral (rheumatic) - *see* Stenosis, mitral
  nasal 478.19
    duct 375.56
      neonatal 375.55
    sinus - *see* Sinusitis
  nasolacrimal duct 375.56
    congenital 743.65
    neonatal 375.55
  nasopharynx 478.29
  nose 478.19
  organ or site, congenital NEC - *see* Atresia
  pancreatic duct 577.8
  parotid gland 527.8
  pelviureteral junction (*see also* Obstruction, ureter) 593.4
  pharynx 478.29
  portal (circulation) (vein) 452
  prostate 600.90
    with
      other lower urinary tract symptoms (LUTS) 600.91
      urinary
        obstruction 600.91
        retention 600.91
    valve (urinary) 596.0
  pulmonary
    valve (heart) (*see also* Endocarditis, pulmonary) 424.3
    vein, isolated 747.49
  pyemic - *see* Septicemia
  pylorus (acquired) 537.0
    congenital 750.5
    infantile 750.5
  rectosigmoid (*see also* Obstruction, intestine) 560.9
  rectum 569.49
  renal 593.89
  respiratory 519.8
    chronic 496
  retinal (artery) (vein) (central) (*see also* Occlusion, retina) 362.30
  salivary duct (any) 527.8
    with calculus 527.5
  sigmoid (*see also* Obstruction, intestine) 560.9
  sinus (accessory) (nasal) (*see also* Sinusitis) 473.9
  Stensen's duct 527.8
  stomach 537.89
    acute 536.1
    congenital 750.7
  submaxillary gland 527.8
    with calculus 527.5
  thoracic duct 457.1
  thrombotic - *see* Thrombosis
  tooth eruption 520.6

Obstruction, obstructed, obstructive (*Continued*)
  trachea 519.19
  tracheostomy airway 519.09
  tricuspid - *see* Endocarditis, tricuspid
  upper respiratory, congenital 748.8
  ureter (functional) 593.4
    congenital 753.20
    due to calculus 592.1
  ureteropelvic junction, congenital 753.21
  ureterovesical junction, congenital 753.22
  urethra 599.60
    congenital 753.6
  urinary (moderate) 599.60
    organ or tract (lower) 599.60
      due to
        benign prostatic hypertrophy (BPH) - *see* category 600
      specified NEC 599.69
        due to
          benign prostatic hypertrophy (BPH) - *see* category 600
    prostatic valve 596.0
    specified NEC 599.69
      due to
        benign prostatic hypertrophy (BPH) - *see* category 600
  uropathy 599.60
  uterus 621.8
  vagina 623.2
  valvular - *see* Endocarditis
  vascular graft or shunt 996.1
    atherosclerosis - *see* Arteriosclerosis, coronary
    embolism 996.74
    occlusion NEC 996.74
    thrombus 996.74
  vein, venous 459.2
    caval (inferior) (superior) 459.2
    thrombotic - *see* Thrombosis
  vena cava (inferior) (superior) 459.2
  ventricular shunt 996.2
  vesical 596.0
  vesicourethral orifice 596.0
  vessel NEC 459.9
Obturator - *see* condition
Occlusal
  plane deviation 524.76
  wear, teeth 521.10
Occlusion
  anus 569.49
    congenital 751.2
    infantile 751.2
  aortoiliac (chronic) 444.0
  aqueduct of Sylvius 331.4
    congenital 742.3
      with spina bifida (*see also* Spina bifida) 741.0●
  arteries of extremities, lower 444.22
    without thrombus or embolus (*see also* Arteriosclerosis, extremities) 440.20
    due to stricture or stenosis 447.1
    upper 444.21
      without thrombus or embolus (*see also* Arteriosclerosis, extremities) 440.20
      due to stricture or stenosis 447.1

Occlusion (*Continued*)
  artery NEC (*see also* Embolism, artery) 444.9
    auditory, internal 433.8●
    basilar 433.0●
      with other precerebral artery 433.3●
      bilateral 433.3●
    brain or cerebral (*see also* Infarct, brain) 434.9●
    carotid 433.1●
      with other precerebral artery 433.3●
      bilateral 433.3●
    cerebellar (anterior inferior) (posterior inferior) (superior) 433.8●
    cerebral (*see also* Infarct, brain) 434.9●
    choroidal (anterior) 433.8●
    chronic total
      coronary 414.2
      extremity(ies) 440.4
    communicating posterior 433.8●
    complete
      coronary 414.2
      extremity(ies) 440.4
    coronary (thrombotic) (*see also* Infarct, myocardium) 410.9●
      acute 410.9●
        without myocardial infarction 411.81
      chronic total 414.2
      complete 414.2
      healed or old 412
      total 414.2
    extremity(ies)
      chronic total 440.4
      complete 440.4
      total 440.4
    hypophyseal 433.8●
    iliac 444.81
    mesenteric (embolic) (thrombotic) (with gangrene) 557.0
    pontine 433.8●
    precerebral NEC 433.9●
      late effect - *see* Late effect(s) (of) cerebrovascular disease
      multiple or bilateral 433.3●
      puerperal, postpartum, childbirth 674.0●
      specified NEC 433.8●
    renal 593.81
    retinal - *see* Occlusion, retina, artery
    spinal 433.8●
    vertebral 433.2●
      with other precerebral artery 433.3●
      bilateral 433.3●
  basilar (artery) - *see* Occlusion, artery, basilar
  bile duct (any) (*see also* Obstruction, biliary) 576.2
  bowel (*see also* Obstruction, intestine) 560.9
  brain (artery) (vascular) (*see also* Infarct, brain) 434.9●
  breast (duct) 611.89
  carotid (artery) (common) (internal) - *see* Occlusion, artery, carotid
  cerebellar (anterior inferior) (artery) (posterior inferior) (superior) 433.8●
  cerebral (artery) (*see also* Infarct, brain) 434.9●

◀ New   ◀▌ Revised   ~~deleted~~ Deleted   ● Use Additional Digit(s)   ▧ Omit code

Occlusion *(Continued)*
  cerebrovascular *(see also* Infarct, brain)
      434.9 ●
    diffuse 437.0
  cervical canal *(see also* Stricture, cervix)
      622.4
    by falciparum malaria 084.0
  cervix (uteri) *(see also* Stricture, cervix)
      622.4
  choanal 748.0
  choroidal (artery) 433.8 ●
  colon *(see also* Obstruction, intestine)
      560.9
  communicating posterior artery 433.8 ●
  coronary (artery) (thrombotic) *(see also*
      Infarct, myocardium) 410.9 ●
    acute 410.9 ●
      without myocardial infarction
          411.81
    healed or old 412
  cystic duct *(see also* Obstruction,
      gallbladder) 575.2
    congenital 751.69
  disto
    division I 524.22
    division II 524.22
  embolic - *see* Embolism
  fallopian tube 628.2
    congenital 752.19
  gallbladder *(see also* Obstruction,
      gallbladder) 575.2
    congenital 751.69
      jaundice from 751.69 [744.5]
  gingiva, traumatic 523.8
  hymen 623.3
    congenital 752.42
  hypophyseal (artery) 433.8 ●
  iliac (artery) 444.81
  intestine *(see also* Obstruction, intestine)
      560.9
  kidney 593.89
  lacrimal apparatus - *see* Stenosis,
      lacrimal
  lung 518.89
  lymph or lymphatic channel 457.1
  mammary duct 611.89
  mesenteric artery (embolic)
      (thrombotic) (with gangrene)
      557.0
  nose 478.19
    congenital 748.0
  organ or site, congenital NEC - *see*
      Atresia
  oviduct 628.2
    congenital 752.19
  periodontal, traumatic 523.8
  peripheral arteries (lower extremity)
      444.22
    without thrombus or embolus *(see*
        also Arteriosclerosis,
        extremities) 440.20
    due to stricture or stenosis 447.1
    upper extremity 444.21
      without thrombus or embolus
          (see also Arteriosclerosis,
          extremities) 440.20
      due to stricture or stenosis 447.1
  pontine (artery) 433.8 ●
  posterior lingual, of mandibular teeth
      524.29
  precerebral artery - *see* Occlusion,
      artery, precerebral NEC
  puncta lacrimalia 375.52
  pupil 364.74
  pylorus *(see also* Stricture, pylorus)
      537.0

Occlusion *(Continued)*
  renal artery 593.81
  retina, retinal (vascular) 362.30
    artery, arterial 362.30
      branch 362.32
      central (total) 362.31
      partial 362.33
      transient 362.34
      tributary 362.32
    vein 362.30
      branch 362.36
      central (total) 362.35
      incipient 362.37
      partial 362.37
      tributary 362.36
  spinal artery 433.8 ●
  stent
    coronary 996.72
  teeth (mandibular) (posterior lingual)
      524.29
  thoracic duct 457.1
  tubal 628.2
  ureter (complete) (partial) 593.4
    congenital 753.29
  urethra *(see also* Stricture, urethra)
      598.9
    congenital 753.6
  uterus 621.8
  vagina 623.2
  vascular NEC 459.9
  vein - *see* Thrombosis
  vena cava
    inferior 453.2
    superior (acute) 453.87 ◀▥▥
      ~~acute 453.87~~
      chronic 453.77
  ventricle (brain) NEC 331.4
  vertebral (artery) - *see* Occlusion, artery,
      vertebral
  vessel (blood) NEC 459.9
  vulva 624.8
Occlusio pupillae 364.74
Occupational
  problems NEC V62.29
  therapy V57.21
Ochlophobia 300.29
Ochronosis (alkaptonuric) (congenital)
    (endogenous) 270.2
  with chloasma of eyelid 270.2
Ocular muscle - *see also* condition
  myopathy 359.1
  torticollis 781.93
Oculoauriculovertebral dysplasia 756.0
Oculogyric
  crisis or disturbance 378.87
    psychogenic 306.7
Oculomotor syndrome 378.81
Oddi's sphincter spasm 576.5
Odelberg's disease (juvenile
    osteochondrosis) 732.1
Odontalgia 525.9
Odontoameloblastoma (M9311/0) 213.1
  upper jaw (bone) 213.0
Odontoclasia 521.05
Odontoclasis 873.63
  complicated 873.73
Odontodysplasia, regional 520.4
Odontogenesis imperfecta 520.5
Odontoma (M9280/0) 213.1
  ameloblastic (M9311/0) 213.1
    upper jaw (bone) 213.0
  calcified (M9280/0) 213.1
    upper jaw (bone) 213.0
  complex (M9282/0) 213.1
    upper jaw (bone) 213.0

Odontoma *(Continued)*
  compound (M9281/0) 213.1
    upper jaw (bone) 213.0
  fibroameloblastic (M9290/0) 213.1
    upper jaw (bone) 213.0
  follicular 526.0
    upper jaw (bone) 213.0
Odontomyelitis (closed) (open) 522.0
Odontonecrosis 521.09
Odontorrhagia 525.8
Odontosarcoma, ameloblastic (M9290/3)
    170.1
  upper jaw (bone) 170.0
Odynophagia 787.20
Oesophagostomiasis 127.7
Oesophagostomum infestation 127.7
Oestriasis 134.0
Ogilvie's syndrome (sympathicotonic
    colon obstruction) 560.89
Oguchi's disease (retina) 368.61
Ohara's disease *(see also* Tularemia)
    021.9
Oidiomycosis *(see also* Candidiasis)
    112.9
Oidiomycotic meningitis 112.83
Oidium albicans infection *(see also*
    Candidiasis) 112.9
Old age 797
  dementia (of) 290.0
Olfactory - *see* condition
Oligemia 285.9
Oligergasia *(see also* Retardation, mental)
    319
Oligoamnios 658.0 ●
  affecting fetus or newborn 761.2
Oligoastrocytoma, mixed (M9382/3)
  specified site - *see* Neoplasm, by site,
      malignant
  unspecified site 191.9
Oligocythemia 285.9
Oligodendroblastoma (M9460/3)
  specified site - *see* Neoplasm, by site,
      malignant
  unspecified site 191.9
Oligodendroglioma (M9450/3)
  anaplastic type (M9451/3)
    specified site - *see* Neoplasm, by site,
        malignant
    unspecified site 191.9
  specified site - *see* Neoplasm, by site,
      malignant
  unspecified site 191.9
Oligodendroma - *see* Oligodendroglioma
Oligodontia *(see also* Anodontia) 520.0
Oligoencephalon 742.1
Oligohydramnios 658.0 ●
  affecting fetus or newborn 761.2
  due to premature rupture of
      membranes 658.1 ●
    affecting fetus or newborn 761.2
Oligohydrosis 705.0
Oligomenorrhea 626.1
Oligophrenia *(see also* Retardation,
    mental) 319
  phenylpyruvic 270.1
Oligospermia 606.1
Oligotrichia 704.09
  congenita 757.4
Oliguria 788.5
  with
    abortion - *see* Abortion, by type,
        with renal failure
    ectopic pregnancy *(see also*
        categories 633.0–633.9) 639.3
    molar pregnancy *(see also* categories
        630–632) 639.3

Oliguria (Continued)
  complicating
    abortion 639.3
    ectopic or molar pregnancy 639.3
    pregnancy 646.2●
      with hypertension - see Toxemia,
        of pregnancy
  due to a procedure 997.5
  following labor and delivery 669.3●
  heart or cardiac - see Failure, heart
  puerperal, postpartum 669.3●
  specified due to a procedure 997.5
Ollier's disease (chondrodysplasia)
  756.4
Omentitis (see also Peritonitis) 567.9
Omentocele (see also Hernia, omental)
  553.8
Omentum, omental - see condition
Omphalitis (congenital) (newborn)
  771.4
  not of newborn 686.9
  tetanus 771.3
Omphalocele 756.72
Omphalomesenteric duct, persistent
  751.0
Omphalorrhagia, newborn 772.3
Omsk hemorrhagic fever 065.1
Onanism 307.9
Onchocerciasis 125.3
  eye 125.3 [360.13]
Onchocercosis 125.3
Oncocytoma (M8290/0) - see Neoplasm,
  by site, benign
Ondine's curse 348.89
Oneirophrenia (see also Schizophrenia)
  295.4●
Onychauxis 703.8
  congenital 757.5
Onychia (with lymphangitis) 681.9
  dermatophytic 110.1
  finger 681.02
  toe 681.11
Onychitis (with lymphangitis) 681.9
  finger 681.02
  toe 681.11
Onychocryptosis 703.0
Onychodystrophy 703.8
  congenital 757.5
Onychogryphosis 703.8
Onychogryposis 703.8
Onycholysis 703.8
Onychomadesis 703.8
Onychomalacia 703.8
Onychomycosis 110.1
  finger 110.1
  toe 110.1
Onycho-osteodysplasia 756.89
Onychophagy 307.9
Onychoptosis 703.8
Onychorrhexis 703.8
  congenital 757.5
Onychoschizia 703.8
Onychotrophia (see also Atrophy, nail)
  703.8
O'Nyong Nyong fever 066.3
Onyxis (finger) (toe) 703.0
Onyxitis (with lymphangitis) 681.9
  finger 681.02
  toe 681.11
Oocyte (egg) (ovum)
  donor V59.70
    over age 35 V59.73
      anonymous recipient V59.73
      designated recipient V59.74

Oocyte (Continued)
  donor (Continued)
    under age 35 V59.71
      anonymous recipient V59.71
      designated recipient V59.72
Oophoritis (cystic) (infectional)
  (interstitial) (see also Salpingo-
  oophoritis) 614.2
  complicating pregnancy 646.6●
  fetal (acute) 752.0
  gonococcal (acute) 098.19
    chronic or duration of 2 months or
      over 098.39
  tuberculous (see also Tuberculosis)
    016.6●
Opacity, opacities
  cornea 371.00
    central 371.03
    congenital 743.43
      interfering with vision 743.42
    degenerative (see also Degeneration,
      cornea) 371.40
    hereditary (see also Dystrophy,
      cornea) 371.50
    inflammatory (see also Keratitis)
      370.9
    late effect of trachoma (healed) 139.1
    minor 371.01
    peripheral 371.02
  enamel (fluoride) (nonfluoride) (teeth)
    520.3
  lens (see also Cataract) 366.9
  snowball 379.22
  vitreous (humor) 379.24
    congenital 743.51
Opalescent dentin (hereditary) 520.5
Open, opening
  abnormal, organ or site, congenital - see
    Imperfect, closure
  angle with
    borderline intraocular pressure
      365.01
    cupping of discs 365.01
  bite
    anterior 524.24
    posterior 524.25
  false - see Imperfect, closure
  margin on tooth restoration 525.61
  restoration margins 525.61
  wound - see Wound, open, by site
Operation
  causing mutilation of fetus 763.89
  destructive, on live fetus, to facilitate
    birth 763.89
  for delivery, fetus or newborn 763.89
  maternal, unrelated to current
    delivery, affecting fetus or
    newborn (see also Newborn,
    affected by) 760.64
Operational fatigue 300.89
Operative - see condition
Operculitis (chronic) 523.40
  acute 523.30
Operculum, retina 361.32
  with detachment 361.01
Ophiasis 704.01
Ophthalmia (see also Conjunctivitis)
  372.30
  actinic rays 370.24
  allergic (acute) 372.05
    chronic 372.14
  blennorrhagic (neonatorum) 098.40
  catarrhal 372.03
  diphtheritic 032.81

Ophthalmia (Continued)
  Egyptian 076.1
  electric, electrica 370.24
  gonococcal (neonatorum) 098.40
  metastatic 360.11
  migraine 346.8●
  neonatorum, newborn 771.6
    gonococcal 098.40
  nodosa 360.14
  phlyctenular 370.31
    with ulcer (see also Ulcer, cornea)
      370.00
  sympathetic 360.11
Ophthalmitis - see Ophthalmia
Ophthalmocele (congenital) 743.66
Ophthalmoneuromyelitis 341.0
Ophthalmopathy, infiltrative with
  thyrotoxicosis 242.0●
Ophthalmoplegia (see also Strabismus)
  378.9
  anterior internuclear 378.86
  ataxia-areflexia syndrome 357.0
  bilateral 378.9
  diabetic 250.5● [378.86]
    due to secondary diabetes 249.5●
      [378.86]
  exophthalmic 242.0● [376.22]
  external 378.55
    progressive 378.72
    total 378.56
  internal (complete) (total) 367.52
  internuclear 378.86
  migraine 346.2●
  painful 378.55
  Parinaud's 378.81
  progressive external 378.72
  supranuclear, progressive 333.0
  total (external) 378.56
    internal 367.52
  unilateral 378.9
Opisthognathism 524.00
Opisthorchiasis (felineus) (tenuicollis)
  (viverrini) 121.0
Opisthotonos, opisthotonus 781.0
Opitz's disease (congestive
  splenomegaly) 289.51
Opiumism (see also Dependence) 304.0●
Oppenheim's disease 358.8
Oppenheim-Urbach disease or syndrome
  (necrobiosis lipoidica diabeticorum)
  250.8● [709.3]
  due to secondary diabetes 249.8● [709.3]
Opsoclonia 379.59
Optic nerve - see condition
Orbit - see condition
Orchioblastoma (M9071/3) 186.9
Orchitis (nonspecific) (septic) 604.90
  with abscess 604.0
  blennorrhagic (acute) 098.13
    chronic or duration of 2 months or
      over 098.33
  diphtheritic 032.89 [604.91]
  filarial 125.9 [604.91]
  gangrenous 604.99
  gonococcal (acute) 098.13
    chronic or duration of 2 months or
      over 098.33
  mumps 072.0
  parotidea 072.0
  suppurative 604.99
  syphilitic 095.8 [604.91]
  tuberculous (see also Tuberculosis)
    016.5● [608.81]
Orf 051.2

◄ New   ⏪ Revised   ~~deleted~~ Deleted   ● Use Additional Digit(s)   ▒ Omit code

Organic - *see also* condition
  heart - *see* Disease, heart
  insufficiency 799.89
Oriental
  bilharziasis 120.2
  schistosomiasis 120.2
  sore 085.1
Orientation
  ego-dystonic sexual 302.0
Orifice - *see* condition
Origin, both great vessels from right
    ventricle 745.11
Ormond's disease or syndrome 593.4
Ornithosis 073.9
  with
    complication 073.8
      specified NEC 073.7
    pneumonia 073.0
    pneumonitis (lobular) 073.0
Orodigitofacial dysostosis 759.89
Oropouche fever 066.3
Orotaciduria, oroticaciduria (congenital)
    (hereditary) (pyrimidine deficiency)
    281.4
Oroya fever 088.0
Orthodontics V58.5
  adjustment V53.4
  aftercare V58.5
  fitting V53.4
Orthopnea 786.02
Os, uterus - *see* condition
Osgood-Schlatter
  disease 732.4
  osteochondrosis 732.4
Osler's
  disease (M9950/1) (polycythemia vera)
    238.4
  nodes 421.0
Osler-Rendu disease (familial
    hemorrhagic telangiectasia) 448.0
Osler-Vaquez disease (M9950/1)
    (polycythemia vera) 238.4
Osler-Weber-Rendu syndrome (familial
    hemorrhagic telangiectasia) 448.0
Osmidrosis 705.89
Osseous - *see* condition
Ossification
  artery - *see* Arteriosclerosis
  auricle (ear) 380.39
  bronchus 519.19
  cardiac (*see also* Degeneration,
    myocardial) 429.1
  cartilage (senile) 733.99
  coronary - *see* Arteriosclerosis, coronary
  diaphragm 728.10
  ear 380.39
    middle (*see also* Otosclerosis) 387.9
  falx cerebri 349.2
  fascia 728.10
  fontanel
    defective or delayed 756.0
    premature 756.0
  heart (*see also* Degeneration,
    myocardial) 429.1
    valve - *see* Endocarditis
  larynx 478.79
  ligament
    posterior longitudinal 724.8
      cervical 723.7
  meninges (cerebral) 349.2
    spinal 336.8
  multiple, eccentric centers 733.99
  muscle 728.10
    heterotopic, postoperative 728.13

Ossification *(Continued)*
  myocardium, myocardial (*see also*
    Degeneration, myocardial) 429.1
  penis 607.81
  periarticular 728.89
  sclera 379.16
  tendon 727.82
  trachea 519.19
  tympanic membrane (*see also*
    Tympanosclerosis) 385.00
  vitreous (humor) 360.44
Osteitis (*see also* Osteomyelitis) 730.2●
  acute 730.0●
  alveolar 526.5
  chronic 730.1●
  condensans (ilii) 733.5
  deformans (Paget's) 731.0
    due to or associated with malignant
      neoplasm (*see also* Neoplasm,
      bone, malignant) 170.9 *[731.1]*
  due to yaws 102.6
  fibrosa NEC 733.29
    cystica (generalisata) 252.01
    disseminata 756.59
    osteoplastica 252.01
  fragilitans 756.51
  Garré's (sclerosing) 730.1●
  infectious (acute) (subacute) 730.0●
    chronic or old 730.1●
  jaw (acute) (chronic) (lower) (neonatal)
    (suppurative) (upper) 526.4
  parathyroid 252.01
  petrous bone (*see also* Petrositis) 383.20
  pubis 733.5
  sclerotic, nonsuppurative 730.1●
  syphilitic 095.5
  tuberculosa
    cystica (of Jüngling) 135
    multiplex cystoides 135
Osteoarthritica spondylitis (spine) (*see
    also* Spondylosis) 721.90
Osteoarthritis (*see also* Osteoarthrosis)
    715.9●
  distal interphalangeal 715.9●
  hyperplastic 731.2
  interspinalis (*see also* Spondylosis)
    721.90
  spine, spinal NEC (*see also* Spondylosis)
    721.90
Osteoarthropathy (*see also* Osteoarthrosis)
    715.9●
  chronic idiopathic hypertrophic 757.39
  familial idiopathic 757.39
  hypertrophic pulmonary 731.2
    secondary 731.2
  idiopathic hypertrophic 757.39
  primary hypertrophic 731.2
  pulmonary hypertrophic 731.2
  secondary hypertrophic 731.2
Osteoarthrosis (degenerative)
    (hypertrophic) (rheumatoid) 715.9●

> Note: Use the following fifth-digit
> subclassification with category 715:
>
> 0   site unspecified
> 1   shoulder region
> 2   upper arm
> 3   forearm
> 4   hand
> 5   pelvic region and thigh
> 6   lower leg
> 7   ankle and foot
> 8   other specified sites except spine
> 9   multiple sites

Osteoarthrosis *(Continued)*
  Deformans alkaptonurica 270.2
  generalized 715.09
  juvenilis (Köhler's) 732.5
  localized 715.3●
    idiopathic 715.1●
    primary 715.1●
    secondary 715.2●
  multiple sites, not specified as
    generalized 715.89
  polyarticular 715.09
  spine (*see also* Spondylosis) 721.90
  temporomandibular joint 524.69
Osteoblastoma (M9200/0) - *see*
    Neoplasm, bone, benign
Osteochondritis (*see also*
    Osteochondrosis) 732.9
  dissecans 732.7
    hip 732.7
  ischiopubica 732.1
  multiple 756.59
  syphilitic (congenital) 090.0
Osteochondrodermodysplasia 756.59
Osteochondrodystrophy 277.5
  deformans 277.5
  familial 277.5
  fetalis 756.4
Osteochondrolysis 732.7
Osteochondroma (M9210/0) - *see also*
    Neoplasm, bone, benign
  multiple, congenital 756.4
Osteochondromatosis (M9210/1) 238.0
  synovial 727.82
Osteochondromyxosarcoma (M9180/3) -
    see Neoplasm, bone, malignant
Osteochondropathy NEC 732.9
Osteochondrosarcoma (M9180/3) - *see*
    Neoplasm, bone, malignant
Osteochondrosis 732.9
  acetabulum 732.1
  adult spine 732.8
  astragalus 732.5
  Blount's 732.4
  Buchanan's (juvenile osteochondrosis
    of iliac crest) 732.1
  Buchman's (juvenile osteochondrosis)
    732.1
  Burns' 732.3
  calcaneus 732.5
  capitular epiphysis (femur) 732.1
  carpal
    lunate (wrist) 732.3
    scaphoid 732.3
  coxae juvenilis 732.1
  deformans juvenilis (coxae) (hip)
    732.1
    Scheuermann's 732.0
    spine 732.0
    tibia 732.4
    vertebra 732.0
  Diaz's (astragalus) 732.5
  dissecans (knee) (shoulder) 732.7
  femoral capital epiphysis 732.1
  femur (head) (juvenile) 732.1
  foot (juvenile) 732.5
  Freiberg's (disease) (second metatarsal)
    732.5
  Haas' 732.3
  Haglund's (os tibiale externum)
    732.5
  hand (juvenile) 732.3
  head of
    femur 732.1
    humerus (juvenile) 732.3

Osteochondrosis (Continued)
  hip (juvenile) 732.1
  humerus (juvenile) 732.3
  iliac crest (juvenile) 732.1
  ilium (juvenile) 732.1
  ischiopubic synchondrosis 732.1
  Iselin's (osteochondrosis fifth
      metatarsal) 732.5
  juvenile, juvenilis 732.6
    arm 732.3
    capital femoral epiphysis 732.1
    capitellum humeri 732.3
    capitular epiphysis 732.1
    carpal scaphoid 732.3
    clavicle, sternal epiphysis 732.6
    coxae 732.1
    deformans 732.1
    foot 732.5
    hand 732.3
    hip and pelvis 732.1
    lower extremity, except foot 732.4
    lunate, wrist 732.3
    medial cuneiform bone 732.5
    metatarsal (head) 732.5
    metatarsophalangeal 732.5
    navicular, ankle 732.5
    patella 732.4
    primary patellar center (of Köhler)
        732.4
    specified site NEC 732.6
    spine 732.0
    tarsal scaphoid 732.5
    tibia (epiphysis) (tuberosity) 732.4
    upper extremity 732.3
    vertebra (body) (Calvé) 732.0
      epiphyseal plates (of
          Scheuermann) 732.0
  Kienböck's (disease) 732.3
  Köhler's (disease) (navicular, ankle)
      732.5
    patellar 732.4
    tarsal navicular 732.5
  Legg-Calvé-Perthes (disease) 732.1
  lower extremity (juvenile) 732.4
  lunate bone 732.3
  Mauclaire's 732.3
  metacarpal heads (of Mauclaire) 732.3
  metatarsal (fifth) (head) (second) 732.5
  navicular, ankle 732.5
  os calcis 732.5
  Osgood-Schlatter 732.4
  os tibiale externum 732.5
  Panner's 732.3
  patella (juvenile) 732.4
  patellar center
    primary (of Köhler) 732.4
    secondary (of Sinding-Larsen) 732.4
  pelvis (juvenile) 732.1
  Pierson's 732.1
  radial head (juvenile) 732.3
  Scheuermann's 732.0
  Sever's (calcaneum) 732.5
  Sinding-Larsen (secondary patellar
      center) 732.4
  spine (juvenile) 732.0
    adult 732.8
  symphysis pubis (of Pierson) (juvenile)
      732.1
  syphilitic (congenital) 090.0
  tarsal (navicular) (scaphoid) 732.5
  tibia (proximal) (tubercle) 732.4
  tuberculous - see Tuberculosis, bone
  ulna 732.3
  upper extremity (juvenile) 732.3

Osteochondrosis (Continued)
  van Neck's (juvenile osteochondrosis)
      732.1
  vertebral (juvenile) 732.0
    adult 732.8
Osteoclastoma (M9250/1) 238.0
  malignant (M9250/3) - see Neoplasm,
      bone, malignant
Osteocopic pain 733.90
Osteodynia 733.90
Osteodystrophy
  azotemic 588.0
  chronica deformans hypertrophica
      731.0
  congenital 756.50
    specified type NEC 756.59
  deformans 731.0
  fibrosa localisata 731.0
  parathyroid 252.01
  renal 588.0
Osteofibroma (M9262/0) - see Neoplasm,
      bone, benign
Osteofibrosarcoma (M9182/3) - see
      Neoplasm, bone, malignant
Osteogenesis imperfecta 756.51
Osteogenic - see condition
Osteoma (M9180/0) - see also Neoplasm,
      bone, benign
  osteoid (M9191/0) - see also Neoplasm,
      bone, benign
    giant (M9200/0) - see Neoplasm,
        bone, benign
Osteomalacia 268.2
  chronica deformans hypertrophica
      731.0
  due to vitamin D deficiency 268.2
  infantile (see also Rickets) 268.0
  juvenile (see also Rickets) 268.0
  pelvis 268.2
  vitamin D-resistant 275.3
Osteomalacic bone 268.2
Osteomalacosis 268.2
Osteomyelitis (general) (infective)
    (localized) (neonatal) (purulent)
    (pyogenic) (septic) (staphylococcal)
    (streptococcal) (suppurative) (with
    periostitis) 730.2●

> Note: Use the following fifth-digit
> subclassification with category 730:
>
>   0   site unspecified
>   1   shoulder region
>   2   upper arm
>   3   forearm
>   4   hand
>   5   pelvic region and thigh
>   6   lower leg
>   7   ankle and foot
>   8   other specified sites
>   9   multiple sites

  acute or subacute 730.0●
  chronic or old 730.1●
  due to or associated with
    diabetes mellitus 250.8● [731.8]
      due to secondary diabetes 249.8●
          [731.8]
    tuberculosis (see also Tuberculosis,
        bone) 015.9● [730.8]●
      limb bones 015.5● [730.8]●
      specified bones NEC 015.7●
          [730.8]●
      spine 015.0● [730.8]●
    typhoid 002.0 [730.8]●

Osteomyelitis (Continued)
  Garré's 730.1●
  jaw (acute) (chronic) (lower) (neonatal)
      (suppurative) (upper) 526.4
  nonsuppurating 730.1●
  orbital 376.03
  petrous bone (see also Petrositis)
      383.20
  Salmonella 003.24
  sclerosing, nonsuppurative 730.1●
  sicca 730.1●
  syphilitic 095.5
    congenital 090.0 [730.8]●
  tuberculous - see Tuberculosis, bone
  typhoid 002.0 [730.8]●
Osteomyelofibrosis 289.89
Osteomyelosclerosis 289.89
Osteonecrosis 733.40
  meaning osteomyelitis 730.1●
Osteo-onycho-arthro dysplasia 756.89
Osteo-onychodysplasia, hereditary
      756.89
Osteopathia
  condensans disseminata 756.53
  hyperostotica multiplex infantilis
      756.59
  hypertrophica toxica 731.2
  striata 756.4
Osteopathy resulting from poliomyelitis
      (see also Poliomyelitis) 045.9●
      [730.7]
  familial dysplastic 731.2
Osteopecilia 756.53
Osteopenia 733.90
  borderline 733.90
Osteoperiostitis (see also Osteomyelitis)
      730.2●
  ossificans toxica 731.2
  toxica ossificans 731.2
Osteopetrosis (familial) 756.52
Osteophyte - see Exostosis
Osteophytosis - see Exostosis
Osteopoikilosis 756.53
Osteoporosis (generalized) 733.00
  circumscripta 731.0
  disuse 733.03
  drug-induced 733.09
  idiopathic 733.02
  postmenopausal 733.01
  posttraumatic 733.7
  screening V82.81
  senile 733.01
  specified type NEC 733.09
Osteoporosis-osteomalacia syndrome
      268.2
Osteopsathyrosis 756.51
Osteoradionecrosis, jaw 526.89
Osteosarcoma (M9180/3) - see also
      Neoplasm, bone, malignant
  chondroblastic (M9181/3) - see
      Neoplasm, bone, malignant
  fibroblastic (M9182/3) - see Neoplasm,
      bone, malignant
  in Paget's disease of bone (M9184/3) -
      see Neoplasm, bone, malignant
  juxtacortical (M9190/3) - see Neoplasm,
      bone malignant
  parosteal (M9190/3) - see Neoplasm,
      bone, malignant
  telangiectatic (M9183/3) - see
      Neoplasm, bone, malignant
Osteosclerosis 756.52
  fragilis (generalisata) 756.52
Osteosclerotic anemia 289.89

Osteosis
  acromegaloid 757.39
  cutis 709.3
  parathyroid 252.01
  renal fibrocystic 588.0
Österreicher-Turner syndrome 756.89
Ostium
  atrioventriculare commune 745.69
  primum (arteriosum) (defect)
      (persistent) 745.61
  secundum (arteriosum) (defect)
      (patent) (persistent) 745.5
Ostrum-Furst syndrome 756.59
Otalgia 388.70
  otogenic 388.71
  referred 388.72
Othematoma 380.31
Otitic hydrocephalus 348.2
Otitis 382.9
  with effusion 381.4
      purulent 382.4
      secretory 381.4
      serous 381.4
      suppurative 382.4
  acute 382.9
  adhesive (see also Adhesions, middle
      ear) 385.10
  chronic 382.9
      with effusion 381.3
      mucoid, mucous (simple) 381.20
      purulent 382.3
      secretory 381.3
      serous 381.10
      suppurative 382.3
  diffuse parasitic 136.8
  externa (acute) (diffuse) (hemorrhagica)
      380.10
      actinic 380.22
      candidal 112.82
      chemical 380.22
      chronic 380.23
          mycotic - see Otitis, externa,
              mycotic
          specified type NEC 380.23
      circumscribed 380.10
      contact 380.22
      due to
          erysipelas 035 [380.13]
          impetigo 684 [380.13]
          seborrheic dermatitis 690.10
              [380.13]
      eczematoid 380.22
      furuncular 680.0 [380.13]
      infective 380.10
          chronic 380.16
      malignant 380.14
      mycotic (chronic) 380.15
          due to
              aspergillosis 117.3 [380.15]
              moniliasis 112.82
              otomycosis 111.8 [380.15]
      reactive 380.22
      specified type NEC 380.22
      tropical 111.8 [380.15]
  insidiosa (see also Otosclerosis) 387.9
  interna (see also Labyrinthitis) 386.30
  media (hemorrhagic) (staphylococcal)
      (streptococcal) 382.9
      acute 382.9
          with effusion 381.00
          allergic 381.04
              mucoid 381.05
              sanguineous 381.06
              serous 381.04

Otitis (Continued)
  media (Continued)
      acute (Continued)
          catarrhal 381.00
          exudative 381.00
          mucoid 381.02
              allergic 381.05
          necrotizing 382.00
              with spontaneous rupture of
                  ear drum 382.01
              in
                  influenza (see also Influenza)
                      487.8 [382.02] ◀▥
                  measles 055.2
                  scarlet fever 034.1 [382.02]
          nonsuppurative 381.00
          purulent 382.00
              with spontaneous rupture of
                  ear drum 382.01
          sanguineous 381.03
              allergic 381.06
          secretory 381.01
          seromucinous 381.02
          serous 381.01
              allergic 381.04
          suppurative 382.00
              with spontaneous rupture of
                  ear drum 382.01
              due to
                  influenza (see also Influenza)
                      487.8 [382.02] ◀▥
                  scarlet fever 034.1 [382.02]
          transudative 381.00
      adhesive (see also Adhesions, middle
          ear) 385.10
      allergic 381.4
          acute 381.04
              mucoid 381.05
              sanguineous 381.06
              serous 381.04
          chronic 381.3
      catarrhal 381.4
          acute 381.00
          chronic (simple) 381.10
      chronic 382.9
          with effusion 381.3
          adhesive (see also Adhesions,
              middle ear) 385.10
          allergic 381.3
          atticoantral, suppurative (with
              posterior or superior
              marginal perforation of ear
              drum) 382.2
          benign suppurative (with
              anterior perforation of ear
              drum) 382.1
          catarrhal 381.10
          exudative 381.3
          mucinous 381.20
          mucoid, mucous (simple) 381.20
          mucosanguineous 381.29
          nonsuppurative 381.3
          purulent 382.3
          secretory 381.3
          seromucinous 381.3
          serosanguineous 381.19
          serous (simple) 381.10
          suppurative 382.3
              atticoantral (with posterior or
                  superior marginal
                  perforation of ear drum)
                  382.2
              benign (with anterior
                  perforation of ear drum)
                  382.1

Otitis (Continued)
  media (Continued)
      chronic (Continued)
          suppurative (Continued)
              tuberculous (see also
                  Tuberculosis) 017.4●
              tubotympanic 382.1
          transudative 381.3
      exudative 381.4
          acute 381.00
          chronic 381.3
      fibrotic (see also Adhesions, middle
          ear) 385.10
      mucoid, mucous 381.4
          acute 381.02
          chronic (simple) 381.20
      mucosanguineous, chronic 381.29
      nonsuppurative 381.4
          acute 381.00
          chronic 381.3
      postmeasles 055.2
      purulent 382.4
          acute 382.00
              with spontaneous rupture of
                  ear drum 382.01
          chronic 382.3
      sanguineous, acute 381.03
          allergic 381.06
      secretory 381.4
          acute or subacute 381.01
          chronic 381.3
      seromucinous 381.4
          acute or subacute 381.02
          chronic 381.3
      serosanguineous, chronic 381.19
      serous 381.4
          acute or subacute 381.01
          chronic (simple) 381.10
      subacute - see Otitis, media, acute
      suppurative 382.4
          acute 382.00
              with spontaneous rupture of
                  ear drum 382.01
          chronic 382.3
              atticoantral 382.2
              benign 382.1
              tuberculous (see also
                  Tuberculosis)
                  017.4●
              tubotympanic 382.1
      transudative 381.4
          acute 381.00
          chronic 381.3
      tuberculous (see also Tuberculosis)
          017.4●
      postmeasles 055.2
Otoconia 386.8
Otolith syndrome 386.19
Otomycosis 111.8 [380.15]
  in
      aspergillosis 117.3 [380.15]
      moniliasis 112.82
Otopathy 388.9
Otoporosis (see also Otosclerosis)
  387.9
Otorrhagia 388.69
  traumatic - see nature of injury
Otorrhea 388.60
  blood 388.69
  cerebrospinal (fluid) 388.61
Otosclerosis (general) 387.9
  cochlear (endosteal) 387.2
  involving
      otic capsule 387.2

Otosclerosis *(Continued)*
  involving *(Continued)*
    oval window
      nonobliterative 387.0
      obliterative 387.1
    round window 387.2
    nonobliterative 387.0
    obliterative 387.1
    specified type NEC 387.8
Otospongiosis *(see also* Otosclerosis) 387.9
Otto's disease or pelvis 715.35
Outburst, aggressive *(see also*
  Disturbance, conduct) 312.0●
  in children or adolescents 313.9
Outcome of delivery
  multiple birth NEC V27.9
    all liveborn V27.5
    all stillborn V27.7
    some liveborn V27.6
    unspecified V27.9
  single V27.9
    liveborn V27.0
    stillborn V27.1
  twins V27.9
    both liveborn V27.2
    both stillborn V27.4
    one liveborn, one stillborn V27.3
Outlet - *see also* condition
  syndrome (thoracic) 353.0
Outstanding ears (bilateral) 744.29
Ovalocytosis (congenital) (hereditary) *(see
  also* Elliptocytosis) 282.1
Ovarian - *see also* condition
  pregnancy - *see* Pregnancy, ovarian
  remnant syndrome 620.8
  vein syndrome 593.4
Ovaritis (cystic) *(see also* Salpingo-
  oophoritis) 614.2
Ovary, ovarian - *see* condition
Overactive - *see also* Hyperfunction
  bladder 596.51
  eye muscle *(see also* Strabismus) 378.9
  hypothalamus 253.8
  thyroid *(see also* Thyrotoxicosis) 242.9●
Overactivity, child 314.01
Overbite (deep) (excessive) (horizontal)
  (vertical) 524.29
Overbreathing *(see also* Hyperventilation)
  786.01
Overconscientious personality 301.4

Overdevelopment - *see also* Hypertrophy
  breast (female) (male) 611.1
  nasal bones 738.0
  prostate, congenital 752.89
Overdistention - *see* Distention
Overdose, overdosage (drug) 977.9
  specified drug or substance - *see* Table
    of Drugs and Chemicals
Overeating 783.6
  nonorganic origin 307.51
Overexertion (effects) (exhaustion)
  994.5
Overexposure (effects) 994.9
  exhaustion 994.4
Overfeeding *(see also* Overeating)
  783.6
Overfill, endodontic 526.62
Overgrowth, bone NEC 733.99
Overhanging
  tooth restoration 525.62
  unrepairable, dental restorative
    materials 525.62
Overheated (effects) (places) - *see* Heat
Overinhibited child 313.0
Overjet 524.29
  excessive horizontal 524.26
Overlaid, overlying (suffocation)
  994.7
Overlap
  excessive horizontal 524.26
Overlapping toe (acquired) 735.8
  congenital (fifth toe) 755.66
Overload
  fluid 276.69 ◀▥
    due to transfusion (blood) (blood
      components) 276.61 ◀
  iron, due to repeated red blood cell
    transfusions 275.02 ◀
  potassium (K) 276.7
  sodium (Na) 276.0
  transfusion associated circulatory
    (TACO) 276.61 ◀
Overnutrition *(see also*
  Hyperalimentation) 783.6
Overproduction - *see also* Hypersecretion
  ACTH 255.3
  cortisol 255.0
  growth hormone 253.0
  thyroid-stimulating hormone (TSH)
    242.8●

Overriding
  aorta 747.21
  finger (acquired) 736.29
    congenital 755.59
  toe (acquired) 735.8
    congenital 755.66
Oversize
  fetus (weight of 4500 grams or more)
    766.0
    affecting management of pregnancy
      656.6●
    causing disproportion 653.5●
      with obstructed labor 660.1●
      affecting fetus or newborn 763.1
Overstimulation, ovarian 256.1
Overstrained 780.79
  heart - *see* Hypertrophy, cardiac
Overweight *(see also* Obesity) 278.02
Overwork 780.79
Oviduct - *see* condition
Ovotestis 752.7
Ovulation (cycle)
  failure or lack of 628.0
  pain 625.2
Ovum
  blighted 631
  donor V59.70
    over age 35 V59.73
      anonymous recipient V59.73
      designated recipient V59.74
    under age 35 V59.71
      anonymous recipient V59.71
      designated recipient V59.72
  dropsical 631
  pathologic 631
Owren's disease or syndrome
  (parahemophilia) *(see also* Defect,
  coagulation) 286.3
Oxalosis 271.8
Oxaluria 271.8
Ox heart - *see* Hypertrophy, cardiac
OX syndrome 758.6
Oxycephaly, oxycephalic 756.0
  syphilitic, congenital 090.0
Oxyuriasis 127.4
Oxyuris vermicularis (infestation) 127.4
Ozena 472.0

◀ New   ◀▥ Revised   ~~deleted~~ Deleted   ● Use Additional Digit(s)   ▦ Omit code

P

Pacemaker syndrome 429.4
Pachyderma, pachydermia 701.8
  laryngis 478.5
  laryngitis 478.79
  larynx (verrucosa) 478.79
Pachydermatitis 701.8
Pachydermatocele (congenital) 757.39
  acquired 701.8
Pachydermatosis 701.8
Pachydermoperiostitis
  secondary 731.2
Pachydermoperiostosis
  primary idiopathic 757.39
  secondary 731.2
Pachymeningitis (adhesive) (basal)
    (brain) (cerebral) (cervical) (chronic)
    (circumscribed) (external) (fibrous)
    (hemorrhagic) (hypertrophic)
    (internal) (purulent) (spinal)
    (suppurative) (see also Meningitis)
    322.9
  gonococcal 098.82
Pachyonychia (congenital) 757.5
  acquired 703.8
Pachyperiosteodermia
  primary or idiopathic 757.39
  secondary 731.2
Pachyperiostosis
  primary or idiopathic 757.39
  secondary 731.2
Pacinian tumor (M9507/0) - see
    Neoplasm, skin, benign
Pads, knuckle or Garrod's 728.79
Paget's disease (osteitis deformans)
    731.0
  with infiltrating duct carcinoma of the
    breast (M8541/3) - see Neoplasm,
    breast, malignant
  bone 731.0
    osteosarcoma in (M9184/3) - see
      Neoplasm, bone, malignant
  breast (M8540/3) 174.0
  extramammary (M8542/3) - see also
    Neoplasm, skin, malignant
    anus 154.3
      skin 173.5
  malignant (M8540/3)
    breast 174.0
    specified site NEC (M8542/3) - see
      Neoplasm, skin, malignant
    unspecified site 174.0
  mammary (M8540/3) 174.0
  necrosis of bone 731.0
  nipple (M8540/3) 174.0
  osteitis deformans 731.0
Paget-Schroetter syndrome (intermittent
    venous claudication) 453.89
Pain(s) (see also Painful) 780.96
  abdominal 789.0●
  acute 338.19
    due to trauma 338.11
    postoperative 338.18
      post-thoracotomy 338.12
  adnexa (uteri) 625.9
  alimentary, due to vascular
    insufficiency 557.9
  anginoid (see also Pain, precordial)
    786.51
  anus 569.42
  arch 729.5
  arm 729.5
  axillary 729.5

Pain(s) (Continued)
  back (postural) 724.5
    low 724.2
    psychogenic 307.89
  bile duct 576.9
  bladder 788.99
  bone 733.90
  breast 611.71
    psychogenic 307.89
  broad ligament 625.9
  cancer associated 338.3
  cartilage NEC 733.90
  cecum 789.0●
  cervicobrachial 723.3
  chest (central) 786.50
    atypical 786.59
    midsternal 786.51
    musculoskeletal 786.59
    noncardiac 786.59
    substernal 786.51
    wall (anterior) 786.52
  chronic 338.29
    associated with significant
        psychosocial dysfunction
        338.4
    due to trauma 338.21
    postoperative 338.28
      post-thoracotomy 338.22
    syndrome 338.4
  coccyx 724.79
  colon 789.0●
  common duct 576.9
  coronary - see Angina
  costochondral 786.52
  diaphragm 786.52
  due to (presence of) any device,
      implant, or graft classifiable to
      996.0–996.5 - see Complications,
      due to (presence of) any device,
      implant, or graft classified to
      996.0–996.5 NEC
    malignancy (primary) (secondary)
      338.3
  ear (see also Otalgia) 388.70
  epigastric, epigastrium 789.06
  extremity (lower) (upper) 729.5
  eye 379.91
  face, facial 784.0
    atypical 350.2
    nerve 351.8
  false (labor) 644.1●
  female genital organ NEC 625.9
    psychogenic 307.89
  finger 729.5
  flank 789.0●
  foot 729.5
  gallbladder 575.9
  gas (intestinal) 787.3
  gastric 536.8
  generalized 780.96
  genital organ
    female 625.9
    male 608.9
    psychogenic 307.89
  groin 789.0●
  growing 781.99
  hand 729.5
  head (see also Headache) 784.0
  heart (see also Pain, precordial)
    786.51
  infraorbital (see also Neuralgia,
    trigeminal) 350.1
  intermenstrual 625.2
  jaw 784.92 ◀▥

Pain(s) (Continued)
  joint 719.40
    ankle 719.47
    elbow 719.42
    foot 719.47
    hand 719.44
    hip 719.45
    knee 719.46
    multiple sites 719.49
    pelvic region 719.45
    psychogenic 307.89
    shoulder (region) 719.41
    specified site NEC 719.48
    wrist 719.43
  kidney 788.0
  labor, false or spurious 644.1●
  laryngeal 784.1
  leg 729.5
  limb 729.5
  low back 724.2
  lumbar region 724.2
  mandible, mandibular 784.92 ◀
  mastoid (see also Otalgia) 388.70
  maxilla 784.92 ◀▥
  menstrual 625.3
  metacarpophalangeal (joint)
    719.44
  metatarsophalangeal (joint) 719.47
  mouth 528.9
  muscle 729.1
    intercostal 786.59
  musculoskeletal (see also Pain, by site)
    729.1
  nasal 478.19
  nasopharynx 478.29
  neck NEC 723.1
    psychogenic 307.89
  neoplasm related (acute) (chronic)
    338.3
  nerve NEC 729.2
  neuromuscular 729.1
  nose 478.19
  ocular 379.91
  ophthalmic 379.91
  orbital region 379.91
  osteocopic 733.90
  ovary 625.9
    psychogenic 307.89
  over heart (see also Pain, precordial)
    786.51
  ovulation 625.2
  pelvic (female) 625.9
    male NEC 789.0●
      psychogenic 307.89
    psychogenic 307.89
  penis 607.9
    psychogenic 307.89
  pericardial (see also Pain, precordial)
    786.51
  perineum
    female 625.9
    male 608.9
  pharynx 478.29
  pleura, pleural, pleuritic 786.52
  postoperative 338.18
    acute 338.18
    chronic 338.28
  post-thoracotomy 338.12
    acute 338.12
    chronic 338.22
  preauricular 388.70
  precordial (region) 786.51
    psychogenic 307.89
  premenstrual 625.4

Pain(s) *(Continued)*
   psychogenic 307.80
      cardiovascular system 307.89
      gastrointestinal system 307.89
      genitourinary system 307.89
      heart 307.89
      musculoskeletal system 307.89
      respiratory system 307.89
      skin 306.3
   radicular (spinal) *(see also* Radiculitis)
      729.2
   rectum 569.42
   respiration 786.52
   retrosternal 786.51
   rheumatic NEC 729.0
      muscular 729.1
   rib 786.50
   root (spinal) *(see also* Radiculitis)
      729.2
   round ligament (stretch) 625.9
   sacroiliac 724.6
   sciatic 724.3
   scrotum 608.9
      psychogenic 307.89
   seminal vesicle 608.9
   sinus 478.19
   skin 782.0
   spermatic cord 608.9
   spinal root *(see also* Radiculitis)
      729.2
   stomach 536.8
      psychogenic 307.89
   substernal 786.51
   temporomandibular (joint) 524.62
   temporomaxillary joint 524.62
   testis 608.9
      psychogenic 307.89
   thoracic spine 724.1
      with radicular and visceral pain
         724.4
   throat 784.1
   tibia 733.90
   toe 729.5
   tongue 529.6
   tooth 525.9
   trigeminal *(see also* Neuralgia,
      trigeminal) 350.1
   tumor associated 338.3
   umbilicus 789.05
   ureter 788.0
   urinary (organ) (system) 788.0
   uterus 625.9
      psychogenic 307.89
   vagina 625.9
   vertebrogenic (syndrome) 724.5
   vesical 788.99
   vulva 625.9
   xiphoid 733.90
Painful - *see also* Pain
   arc syndrome 726.19
   coitus
      female 625.0
      male 608.89
      psychogenic 302.76
   ejaculation (semen) 608.89
      psychogenic 302.79
   erection 607.3
   feet syndrome 266.2
   menstruation 625.3
      psychogenic 306.52
   micturition 788.1
   ophthalmoplegia 378.55
   respiration 786.52
   scar NEC 709.2

Painful *(Continued)*
   total hip replacement 996.77
   total knee replacement 996.77
   urination 788.1
   wire sutures 998.89
Painters' colic 984.9
   specified type of lead - *see* Table of
      Drugs and Chemicals
Palate - *see* condition
Palatoplegia 528.9
Palatoschisis *(see also* Cleft, palate) 749.00
Palilalia 784.69
Palindromic arthritis *(see also*
      Rheumatism, palindromic) 719.3●
Palliative care V66.7
Pallor 782.61
   temporal, optic disc 377.15
Palmar - *see also* condition
   fascia - *see* condition
Palpable
   cecum 569.89
   kidney 593.89
   liver 573.9
   lymph nodes 785.6
   ovary 620.8
   prostate 602.9
   spleen *(see also* Splenomegaly) 789.2
   uterus 625.8
Palpitation (heart) 785.1
   psychogenic 306.2
Palsy *(see also* Paralysis) 344.9
   atrophic diffuse 335.20
   Bell's 351.0
      newborn 767.5
   birth 767.7
   brachial plexus 353.0
      fetus or newborn 767.6
   brain - *see also* Palsy, cerebral
      noncongenital or noninfantile 344.89
         late effect - *see* Late effect(s) (of)
            cerebrovascular disease
      syphilitic 094.89
         congenital 090.49
   bulbar (chronic) (progressive) 335.22
      pseudo NEC 335.23
      supranuclear NEC 344.89
   cerebral (congenital) (infantile)
         (spastic) 343.9
      athetoid 333.71
      diplegic 343.0
         late effect - *see* Late effect(s) (of)
            cerebrovascular disease
      hemiplegic 343.1
      monoplegic 343.3
      noncongenital or noninfantile 437.8
         late effect - *see* Late effect(s) (of)
            cerebrovascular disease
      paraplegic 343.0
      quadriplegic 343.2
      spastic, not congenital or infantile
         344.89
      syphilitic 094.89
         congenital 090.49
      tetraplegic 343.2
   cranial nerve - *see also* Disorder, nerve,
      cranial
      multiple 352.6
   creeping 335.21
   divers' 993.3
   Erb's (birth injury) 767.6
   facial 351.0
      newborn 767.5
   glossopharyngeal 352.2
   Klumpke (-Déjérine) 767.6

Palsy *(Continued)*
   lead 984.9
      specified type of lead - *see* Table of
         Drugs and Chemicals
   median nerve (tardy) 354.0
   peroneal nerve (acute) (tardy) 355.3
   progressive supranuclear 333.0
   pseudobulbar NEC 335.23
   radial nerve (acute) 354.3
   seventh nerve 351.0
      newborn 767.5
   shaking *(see also* Parkinsonism)
      332.0
   spastic (cerebral) (spinal) 343.9
      hemiplegic 343.1
   specified nerve NEC - *see* Disorder,
      nerve
   supranuclear NEC 356.8
      progressive 333.0
   ulnar nerve (tardy) 354.2
   wasting 335.21
Paltauf-Sternberg disease 201.9●
Paludism - *see* Malaria
Panama fever 084.0
Panaris (with lymphangitis) 681.9
   finger 681.02
   toe 681.11
Panaritium (with lymphangitis) 681.9
   finger 681.02
   toe 681.11
Panarteritis (nodosa) 446.0
   brain or cerebral 437.4
Pancake heart 793.2
   with cor pulmonale (chronic) 416.9
Pancarditis (acute) (chronic) 429.89
   with
      rheumatic
         fever (active) (acute) (chronic)
            (subacute) 391.8
            inactive or quiescent 398.99
   rheumatic, acute 391.8
      chronic or inactive 398.99
Pancoast's syndrome or tumor
      (carcinoma, pulmonary apex)
      (M8010/3) 162.3
Pancoast-Tobias syndrome (M8010/3)
      (carcinoma, pulmonary apex)
      162.3
Pancolitis 556.6
Pancreas, pancreatic - *see* condition
Pancreatitis 577.0
   acute (edematous) (hemorrhagic)
      (recurrent) 577.0
   annular 577.0
   apoplectic 577.0
   calcereous 577.0
   chronic (infectious) 577.1
      recurrent 577.1
   cystic 577.2
   fibrous 577.8
   gangrenous 577.0
   hemorrhagic (acute) 577.0
   interstitial (chronic) 577.1
      acute 577.0
   malignant 577.0
   mumps 072.3
   painless 577.1
   recurrent 577.1
   relapsing 577.1
   subacute 577.0
   suppurative 577.0
   syphilitic 095.8
Pancreatolithiasis 577.8
Pancytolysis 289.9

◀ New   ◀▥ Revised   ~~deleted~~ Deleted   ● Use Additional Digit(s)   ▨ Omit code

Pancytopenia (acquired) 284.1
  with malformations 284.09
  congenital 284.09
Panencephalitis - *see also* Encephalitis
  subacute, sclerosing 046.2
Panhematopenia 284.81
  congenital 284.09
  constitutional 284.09
  splenic, primary 289.4
Panhemocytopenia 284.81
  congenital 284.09
  constitutional 284.09
Panhypogonadism 257.2
Panhypopituitarism 253.2
  prepubertal 253.3
Panic (attack) (state) 300.01
  reaction to exceptional stress (transient)
    308.0
Panmyelopathy, familial constitutional
  284.09
Panmyelophthisis 284.2
  acquired (secondary) 284.81
  congenital 284.2
  idiopathic 284.9
Panmyelosis (acute) (M9951/1) 238.79
Panner's disease 732.3
  capitellum humeri 732.3
  head of humerus 732.3
  tarsal navicular (bone)
    (osteochondrosis) 732.5
Panneuritis endemica 265.0 *[357.4]*
Panniculitis 729.30
  back 724.8
  knee 729.31
  mesenteric 567.82
  neck 723.6
  nodular, nonsuppurative 729.30
  sacral 724.8
  specified site NEC 729.39
Panniculus adiposus (abdominal)
  278.1
Pannus (corneal) 370.62
  abdominal (symptomatic) 278.1
  allergic eczematous 370.62
  degenerativus 370.62
  keratic 370.62
  rheumatoid - *see* Arthritis, rheumatoid
  trachomatosus, trachomatous (active)
    076.1 *[370.62]*
  late effect 139.1
Panophthalmitis 360.02
Panotitis - *see* Otitis media
Pansinusitis (chronic) (hyperplastic)
  (nonpurulent) (purulent) 473.8
  acute 461.8
  due to fungus NEC 117.9
  tuberculous (*see also* Tuberculosis)
    012.8●
Panuveitis 360.12
  sympathetic 360.11
Panvalvular disease - *see* Endocarditis,
  mitral
Papageienkrankheit 073.9
Papanicolaou smear
  anus 796.70
    with
      atypical squamous cells
        cannot exclude high grade
          squamous intraepithelial
          lesion (ASC-H) 796.72
        of undetermined significance
          (ASC-US) 796.71
      cytologic evidence of malignancy
        796.76

Papanicolaou smear *(Continued)*
  anus *(Continued)*
    with *(Continued)*
      high grade squamous
        intraepithelial lesion
        (HGSIL) 796.74
      low grade squamous
        intraepithelial lesion
        (LGSIL) 796.73
    glandular 796.70
    specified finding NEC 796.79
    unsatisfactory cytology 796.78
  cervix (screening test) V76.2
    as part of gynecological examination
      V72.31
    for suspected malignant neoplasm
      V76.2
    no disease found V71.1
    inadequate cytology sample
      795.08
    nonspecific abnormal finding
      795.00
      with
        atypical squamous cells
          cannot exclude high grade
            squamous
            intraepithelial lesion
            (ASC-H) 795.02
          of undetermined
            significance (ASC-US)
            795.01
        cytologic evidence of
          malignancy 795.06
        high grade squamous
          intraepithelial lesion
          (HGSIL) 795.04
        low grade squamous
          intraepithelial lesion
          (LGSIL) 795.03
        nonspecific finding NEC 795.09
        to confirm findings of recent
          normal smear following
          initial abnormal smear
          V72.32
    satisfactory smear but lacking
      transformation zone 795.07
    unsatisfactory cervical cytology
      795.08
  other specified site - *see also* Screening,
    malignant neoplasm
    for suspected malignant neoplasm -
      see also Screening, malignant
      neoplasm
    no disease found V71.1
    nonspecific abnormal finding
      796.9
    vagina V76.47
      with
        atypical squamous cells
          cannot exclude high grade
            squamous
            intraepithelial lesion
            (ASC-H) 795.12
          of undetermined
            significance (ASC-US)
            795.11
        cytologic evidence of
          malignancy 795.16
        high grade squamous
          intraepithelial lesion
          (HGSIL) 795.14
        low grade squamous
          intraepithelial lesion
          (LGSIL) 795.13

Papanicolaou smear *(Continued)*
  other specified site *(Continued)*
    vagina *(Continued)*
      abnormal NEC 795.19
      following hysterectomy for
        malignant condition V67.01
      inadequate cytology sample
        795.18
      unsatisfactory cytology 795.18
Papilledema 377.00
  associated with
    decreased ocular pressure 377.02
    increased intracranial pressure
      377.01
    retinal disorder 377.03
  choked disc 377.00
  infectional 377.00
Papillitis 377.31
  anus 569.49
  chronic lingual 529.4
  necrotizing, kidney 584.7
  optic 377.31
  rectum 569.49
  renal, necrotizing 584.7
  tongue 529.0
Papilloma (M8050/0) - *see also* Neoplasm,
  by site, benign

> Note: Except where otherwise
> indicated, the morphological varieties
> of papilloma in the list below should
> be coded by site as for "Neoplasm,
> benign".

  acuminatum (female) (male) 078.11
  bladder (urinary) (transitional cell)
    (M8120/1) 236.7
    benign (M8120/0) 223.3
  choroid plexus (M9390/0) 225.0
    anaplastic type (M9390/3) 191.5
    malignant (M9390/3) 191.5
  ductal (M8503/0)
  dyskeratotic (M8052/0)
  epidermoid (M8052/0)
  hyperkeratotic (M8052/0)
  intracystic (M8504/0)
  intraductal (M8503/0)
  inverted (M8053/0)
  keratotic (M8052/0)
  parakeratotic (M8052/0)
  pinta (primary) 103.0
  renal pelvis (transitional cell)
    (M8120/1) 236.99
    benign (M8120/0) 223.1
  Schneiderian (M8121/0)
    specified site - *see* Neoplasm, by site,
      benign
    unspecified site 212.0
  serous surface (M8461/0)
    borderline malignancy (M8461/1)
      specified site - *see* Neoplasm, by
        site, uncertain behavior
      unspecified site 236.2
    specified site - *see* Neoplasm, by site,
      benign
    unspecified site 220
  squamous (cell) (M8052/0)
  transitional (cell) (M8120/0)
    bladder (urinary) (M8120/1) 236.7
    inverted type (M8121/1) - *see*
      Neoplasm, by site, uncertain
      behavior
    renal pelvis (M8120/1) 236.91
    ureter (M8120/1) 236.91

Papilloma (*Continued*)
  ureter (transitional cell) (M8120/1) 236.91
    benign (M8120/0) 223.2
  urothelial (M8120/1) - *see* Neoplasm,
    by site, uncertain behavior
  verrucous (M8051/0)
  villous (M8261/1) - *see* Neoplasm, by
    site, uncertain behavior
  yaws, plantar or palmar 102.1
Papillomata, multiple, of yaws 102.1
Papillomatosis (M8060/0) - *see also*
    Neoplasm, by site, benign
  confluent and reticulate 701.8
  cutaneous 701.8
  ductal, breast 610.1
  Gougerot-Carteaud (confluent
    reticulate) 701.8
  intraductal (diffuse) (M8505/0) - *see*
    Neoplasm, by site, benign
  subareolar duct (M8506/0) 217
Papillon-Léage and Psaume syndrome
    (orodigitofacial dysostosis) 759.89
Papule 709.8
  carate (primary) 103.0
  fibrous, of nose (M8724/0) 216.3
  pinta (primary) 103.0
Papulosis, malignant 447.8 ◄▥
  lymphomatoid 709.8 ◄
  malignant 447.8 ◄
Papyraceous fetus 779.89
  complicating pregnancy 646.0●
Paracephalus 759.7
Parachute mitral valve 746.5
Paracoccidioidomycosis 116.1
  mucocutaneous-lymphangitic 116.1
  pulmonary 116.1
  visceral 116.1
Paracoccidiomycosis - *see*
    Paracoccidioidomycosis
Paracusis 388.40
Paradentosis 523.5
Paradoxical facial movements 374.43
Paraffinoma 999.9
Paraganglioma (M8680/1)
  adrenal (M8700/0) 227.0
    malignant (M8700/3) 194.0
  aortic body (M8691/1) 237.3
    malignant (M8691/3) 194.6
  carotid body (M8692/1) 237.3
    malignant (M8692/3) 194.5
  chromaffin (M8700/0) - *see also*
    Neoplasm, by site, benign
    malignant (M8700/3) - *see*
      Neoplasm, by site, malignant
  extra-adrenal (M8693/1)
    malignant (M8693/3)
      specified site - *see* Neoplasm, by
        site, malignant
      unspecified site 194.6
    specified site - *see* Neoplasm, by site,
      uncertain behavior
    unspecified site 237.3
  glomus jugulare (M8690/1) 237.3
    malignant (M8690/3) 194.6
  jugular (M8690/1) 237.3
  malignant (M8680/3)
    specified site - *see* Neoplasm, by site,
      malignant
    unspecified site 194.6
  nonchromaffin (M8693/1)
    malignant (M8693/3)
      specified site - *see* Neoplasm, by
        site, malignant
      unspecified site 194.6

Paraganglioma (*Continued*)
  nonchromaffin (*Continued*)
    specified site - *see* Neoplasm, by site,
      uncertain behavior
    unspecified site 237.3
  parasympathetic (M8682/1)
    specified site - *see* Neoplasm, by site,
      uncertain behavior
    unspecified site 237.3
  specified site - *see* Neoplasm, by site,
    uncertain behavior
  sympathetic (M8681/1)
    specified site - *see* Neoplasm, by site,
      uncertain behavior
    unspecified site 237.3
  unspecified site 237.3
Parageusia 781.1
  psychogenic 306.7
Paragonimiasis 121.2
Paragranuloma, Hodgkin's (M9660/3)
    201.0●
Parahemophilia (*see also* Defect,
    coagulation) 286.3
Parakeratosis 690.8
  psoriasiformis 696.2
  variegata 696.2
Paralysis, paralytic (complete)
    (incomplete) 344.9
  with
    broken
      back - *see* Fracture, vertebra, by
        site, with spinal cord injury
      neck - *see* Fracture, vertebra,
        cervical, with spinal cord
        injury
    fracture, vertebra - *see* Fracture,
      vertebra, by site, with spinal
      cord injury
    syphilis 094.89
  abdomen and back muscles 355.9
  abdominal muscles 355.9
  abducens (nerve) 378.54
  abductor 355.9
    lower extremity 355.8
    upper extremity 354.9
  accessory nerve 352.4
  accommodation 367.51
    hysterical 300.11
  acoustic nerve 388.5
  agitans 332.0
    arteriosclerotic 332.0
  alternating 344.89
    oculomotor 344.89
  amyotrophic 335.20
  ankle 355.8
  anterior serratus 355.9
  anus (sphincter) 569.49
  apoplectic (current episode) (*see also*
    Disease, cerebrovascular, acute)
    436
    late effect - *see* Late effect(s) (of)
      cerebrovascular disease
  arm 344.40
    affecting
      dominant side 344.41
      nondominant side 344.42
    both 344.2
    hysterical 300.11
    late effect - *see* Late effect(s) (of)
      cerebrovascular disease
    psychogenic 306.0
    transient 781.4
      traumatic NEC (*see also* Injury,
        nerve, upper limb) 955.9

Paralysis, paralytic (*Continued*)
  arteriosclerotic (current episode) 437.0
    late effect - *see* Late effect(s) (of)
      cerebrovascular disease
  ascending (spinal), acute 357.0
  associated, nuclear 344.89
  asthenic bulbar 358.00
  ataxic NEC 334.9
    general 094.1
  athetoid 333.71
  atrophic 356.9
    infantile, acute (*see also*
      Poliomyelitis, with paralysis)
      045.1●
    muscle NEC 355.9
    progressive 335.21
    spinal (acute) (*see also* Poliomyelitis,
      with paralysis) 045.1●
  attack (*see also* Disease, cerebrovascular,
    acute) 436
  axillary 353.0
  Babinski-Nageotte's 344.89
  Bell's 351.0
    newborn 767.5
  Benedikt's 344.89
  birth (injury) 767.7
    brain 767.0
      intracranial 767.0
    spinal cord 767.4
  bladder (sphincter) 596.53
    neurogenic 596.54
      with cauda equina syndrome
        344.61
    puerperal, postpartum, childbirth
      665.5●
    sensory 596.54
      with cauda equina 344.61
    spastic 596.54
      with cauda equina 344.61
  bowel, colon, or intestine (*see also* Ileus)
    560.1
  brachial plexus 353.0
    due to birth injury 767.6
    newborn 767.6
  brain
    congenital - *see* Palsy, cerebral
    current episode 437.8
    diplegia 344.2
      late effect - *see* Late effect(s) (of)
        cerebrovascular disease
    hemiplegia 342.9●
      late effect - *see* Late effect(s) (of)
        cerebrovascular disease
    infantile - *see* Palsy, cerebral
    monoplegia - *see also* Monoplegia
      late effect - *see* Late effect(s) (of)
        cerebrovascular disease
    paraplegia 344.1
    quadriplegia - *see* Quadriplegia
    syphilitic, congenital 090.49
    triplegia 344.89
  bronchi 519.19
  Brown-Séquard's 344.89
  bulbar (chronic) (progressive)
    335.22
    infantile (*see also* Poliomyelitis,
      bulbar) 045.0●
    poliomyelitic (*see also* Poliomyelitis,
      bulbar) 045.0●
    pseudo 335.23
    supranuclear 344.89
  bulbospinal 358.00
  cardiac (*see also* Failure, heart)
    428.9

◄ New   ◄▥ Revised   ~~deleted~~ Deleted   ● Use Additional Digit(s)   ▥ Omit code

Paralysis, paralytic (Continued)
  cerebral
    current episode 437.8
    spastic, infantile - see Palsy, cerebral
  cerebrocerebellar 437.8
    diplegic infantile 343.0
  cervical
    plexus 353.2
    sympathetic NEC 337.09
  Céstan-Chenais 344.89
  Charcôt-Marie-Tooth type 356.1
  childhood - see Palsy, cerebral
  Clark's 343.9
  colon (see also Ileus) 560.1
  compressed air 993.3
  compression
    arm NEC 354.9
    cerebral - see Paralysis, brain
    leg NEC 355.8
    lower extremity NEC 355.8
    upper extremity NEC 354.9
  congenital (cerebral) (spastic) (spinal) -
      see Palsy, cerebral
  conjugate movement (of eye) 378.81
    cortical (nuclear) (supranuclear)
        378.81
  convergence 378.83
  cordis (see also Failure, heart) 428.9
  cortical (see also Paralysis, brain)
      437.8
  cranial or cerebral nerve (see also
      Disorder, nerve, cranial) 352.9
  creeping 335.21
  crossed leg 344.89
  crutch 953.4
  deglutition 784.99
    hysterical 300.11
  dementia 094.1
  descending (spinal) NEC 335.9
  diaphragm (flaccid) 519.4
    due to accidental section of phrenic
        nerve during procedure 998.2
  digestive organs NEC 564.89
  diplegic - see Diplegia
  divergence (nuclear) 378.85
  divers' 993.3
  Duchenne's 335.22
  due to intracranial or spinal birth
      injury - see Palsy, cerebral
  embolic (current episode) (see also
      Embolism, brain) 434.1●
    late effect - see Late effect(s) (of)
        cerebrovascular disease
  enteric (see also Ileus) 560.1
    with hernia - see Hernia, by site,
        with obstruction
  Erb's syphilitic spastic spinal 094.89
  Erb (-Duchenne) (birth) (newborn)
      767.6
  esophagus 530.89
  essential, infancy (see also Poliomyelitis)
      045.9●
  extremity
    lower - see Paralysis, leg
    spastic (hereditary) 343.3
      noncongenital or noninfantile
          344.1
      transient (cause unknown) 781.4
    upper - see Paralysis, arm
  eye muscle (extrinsic) 378.55
    intrinsic 367.51
  facial (nerve) 351.0
    birth injury 767.5
    congenital 767.5

Paralysis, paralytic (Continued)
  facial (Continued)
    following operation NEC 998.2
    newborn 767.5
  familial 359.3
    periodic 359.3
    spastic 334.1
  fauces 478.29
  finger NEC 354.9
  foot NEC 355.8
  gait 781.2
  gastric nerve 352.3
  gaze 378.81
  general 094.1
    ataxic 094.1
    insane 094.1
    juvenile 090.40
    progressive 094.1
    tabetic 094.1
  glossopharyngeal (nerve) 352.2
  glottis (see also Paralysis, vocal cord)
      478.30
  gluteal 353.4
  Gubler (-Millard) 344.89
  hand 354.9
    hysterical 300.11
    psychogenic 306.0
  heart (see also Failure, heart) 428.9
  hemifacial, progressive 349.89
  hemiplegic - see Hemiplegia
  hyperkalemic periodic (familial) 359.3
  hypertensive (current episode) 437.8
  hypoglossal (nerve) 352.5
  hypokalemic periodic 359.3
  Hyrtl's sphincter (rectum) 569.49
  hysterical 300.11
  ileus (see also Ileus) 560.1
  infantile (see also Poliomyelitis) 045.9●
    atrophic acute 045.1●
    bulbar 045.0●
    cerebral - see Palsy, cerebral
    paralytic 045.1●
    progressive acute 045.9●
    spastic - see Palsy, cerebral
    spinal 045.9●
  infective (see also Poliomyelitis) 045.9●
  inferior nuclear 344.9
  insane, general or progressive 094.1
  internuclear 378.86
  interosseous 355.9
  intestine (see also Ileus) 560.1
  intracranial (current episode) (see also
      Paralysis, brain) 437.8
    due to birth injury 767.0
  iris 379.49
    due to diphtheria (toxin) 032.81
        [379.49]
  ischemic, Volkmann's (complicating
      trauma) 958.6
  isolated sleep, recurrent 327.43
  Jackson's 344.89
  jake 357.7
  Jamaica ginger (jake) 357.7
  juvenile general 090.40
  Klumpke (-Déjérine) (birth) (newborn)
      767.6
  labioglossal (laryngeal) (pharyngeal)
      335.22
  Landry's 357.0
  laryngeal nerve (recurrent) (superior)
      (see also Paralysis, vocal cord)
      478.30
  larynx (see also Paralysis, vocal cord)
      478.30
    due to diphtheria (toxin) 032.3

Paralysis, paralytic (Continued)
  late effect
    due to
      birth injury, brain or spinal
          (cord) - see Palsy, cerebral
      edema, brain or cerebral - see
          Paralysis, brain
      lesion
        late effect - see Late effect(s)
            (of) cerebrovascular
            disease
        spinal (cord) - see Paralysis,
            spinal
  lateral 335.24
  lead 984.9
    specified type of lead - see Table of
        Drugs and Chemicals
  left side - see Hemiplegia
  leg 344.30
    affecting
      dominant side 344.31
      nondominant side 344.32
    both (see also Paraplegia) 344.1
    crossed 344.89
    hysterical 300.11
    psychogenic 306.0
    transient or transitory 781.4
      traumatic NEC (see also
          Injury, nerve, lower limb)
          956.9
  levator palpebrae superioris 374.31
  limb NEC 344.5
    all four - see Quadriplegia
    quadriplegia - see Quadriplegia
  lip 528.5
  Lissauer's 094.1
  local 355.9
  lower limb - see also Paralysis,
      leg
    both (see also Paraplegia) 344.1
  lung 518.89
    newborn 770.89
  median nerve 354.1
  medullary (tegmental) 344.89
  mesencephalic NEC 344.89
    tegmental 344.89
  middle alternating 344.89
  Millard-Gubler-Foville 344.89
  monoplegic - see Monoplegia
  motor NEC 344.9
    cerebral - see Paralysis, brain
    spinal - see Paralysis, spinal
  multiple
    cerebral - see Paralysis, brain
    spinal - see Paralysis, spinal
  muscle (flaccid) 359.9
    due to nerve lesion NEC 355.9
    eye (extrinsic) 378.55
      intrinsic 367.51
      oblique 378.51
    iris sphincter 364.89
    ischemic (complicating trauma)
        (Volkmann's) 958.6
    pseudohypertrophic 359.1
  muscular (atrophic) 359.9
    progressive 335.21
  musculocutaneous nerve 354.9
  musculospiral 354.9
  nerve - see also Disorder, nerve
    third or oculomotor (partial)
        378.51
      total 378.52
    fourth or trochlear 378.53
    sixth or abducens 378.54

Paralysis, paralytic *(Continued)*
  nerve *(Continued)*
    seventh or facial 351.0
      birth injury 767.5
      due to
        injection NEC 999.9
        operation NEC 997.09
      newborn 767.5
    accessory 352.4
    auditory 388.5
    birth injury 767.7
    cranial or cerebral *(see also* Disorder,
        nerve, cranial) 352.9
    facial 351.0
      birth injury 767.5
      newborn 767.5
    laryngeal *(see also* Paralysis, vocal
        cord) 478.30
    newborn 767.7
    phrenic 354.8
      newborn 767.7
    radial 354.3
      birth injury 767.6
      newborn 767.6
    syphilitic 094.89
    traumatic NEC *(see also* Injury,
        nerve, by site) 957.9
    trigeminal 350.9
    ulnar 354.2
  newborn NEC 767.0
  normokalemic periodic 359.3
  obstetrical, newborn 767.7
  ocular 378.9
  oculofacial, congenital 352.6
  oculomotor (nerve) (partial) 378.51
    alternating 344.89
    external bilateral 378.55
    total 378.52
  olfactory nerve 352.0
  palate 528.9
  palatopharyngolaryngeal 352.6
  paratrigeminal 350.9
  periodic (familial) (hyperkalemic)
      (hypokalemic) (normokalemic)
      (potassium sensitive) (secondary)
      359.3
  peripheral
    autonomic nervous system - *see*
        Neuropathy, peripheral,
        autonomic
    nerve NEC 355.9
  peroneal (nerve) 355.3
  pharynx 478.29
  phrenic nerve 354.8
  plantar nerves 355.6
  pneumogastric nerve 352.3
  poliomyelitis (current) *(see also*
      Poliomyelitis, with paralysis)
      045.1●
    bulbar 045.0●
  popliteal nerve 355.3
  pressure *(see also* Neuropathy,
      entrapment) 355.9
  progressive 335.21
    atrophic 335.21
    bulbar 335.22
    general 094.1
    hemifacial 349.89
    infantile, acute *(see also*
        Poliomyelitis) 045.9●
    multiple 335.20
  pseudobulbar 335.23
  pseudohypertrophic 359.1
    muscle 359.1

Paralysis, paralytic *(Continued)*
  psychogenic 306.0
  pupil, pupillary 379.49
  quadriceps 355.8
  quadriplegic *(see also* Quadriplegia)
      344.0
  radial nerve 354.3
    birth injury 767.6
  rectum (sphincter) 569.49
  rectus muscle (eye) 378.55
  recurrent
    isolated sleep 327.43
    laryngeal nerve *(see also* Paralysis,
        vocal cord) 478.30
  respiratory (muscle) (system) (tract)
      786.09
    center NEC 344.89
      fetus or newborn 770.87
    congenital 768.9
    newborn 768.9
  right side - *see* Hemiplegia
  Saturday night 354.3
  saturnine 984.9
    specified type of lead - *see* Table of
        Drugs and Chemicals
  sciatic nerve 355.0
  secondary - *see* Paralysis, late effect
  seizure (cerebral) (current episode) *(see
      also* Disease, cerebrovascular,
      acute) 436
    late effect - *see* Late effect(s) (of)
        cerebrovascular disease
  senile NEC 344.9
  serratus magnus 355.9
  shaking *(see also* Parkinsonism) 332.0
  shock *(see also* Disease, cerebrovascular,
      acute) 436
    late effect - *see* Late effect(s) (of)
        cerebrovascular disease
  shoulder 354.9
  soft palate 528.9
  spasmodic - *see* Paralysis, spastic
  spastic 344.9
    cerebral infantile - *see* Palsy, cerebral
    congenital (cerebral) - *see* Palsy,
        cerebral
    familial 334.1
    hereditary 334.1
    infantile 343.9
    noncongenital or noninfantile,
        cerebral 344.9
    syphilitic 094.0
      spinal 094.89
  sphincter, bladder *(see also* Paralysis,
      bladder) 596.53
  spinal (cord) NEC 344.1
    accessory nerve 352.4
    acute *(see also* Poliomyelitis)
        045.9●
    ascending acute 357.0
    atrophic (acute) *(see also*
        Poliomyelitis, with paralysis)
        045.1●
      spastic, syphilitic 094.89
    congenital NEC 343.9
    hemiplegic - *see* Hemiplegia
    hereditary 336.8
    infantile *(see also* Poliomyelitis)
        045.9●
    late effect NEC 344.89
    monoplegic - *see* Monoplegia
    nerve 355.9
    progressive 335.10
    quadriplegic - *see* Quadriplegia

Paralysis, paralytic *(Continued)*
  spinal (cord) NEC *(Continued)*
    spastic NEC 343.9
      traumatic - *see* Injury, spinal, by site
  sternomastoid 352.4
  stomach 536.3
    diabetic 250.6● [536.3]
      due to secondary diabetes 249.6●
          [536.3]
    nerve (nondiabetic) 352.3
  stroke (current episode) - *see* Infarct,
      brain
    late effect - *see* Late effect(s) (of)
        cerebrovascular disease
  subscapularis 354.8
  superior nuclear NEC 334.9
  supranuclear 356.8
  sympathetic
    cervical NEC 337.09
    nerve NEC *(see also* Neuropathy,
        peripheral, autonomic) 337.9
    nervous system - *see* Neuropathy,
        peripheral, autonomic
  syndrome 344.9
    specified NEC 344.89
  syphilitic spastic spinal (Erb's) 094.89
  tabetic general 094.1
  thigh 355.8
  throat 478.29
    diphtheritic 032.0
    muscle 478.29
  thrombotic (current episode) *(see also*
      Thrombosis, brain) 434.0●
    late effect - *see* Late effect(s) (of)
        cerebrovascular disease
  thumb NEC 354.9
  tick (-bite) 989.5
  Todd's (postepileptic transitory
      paralysis) 344.89
  toe 355.6
  tongue 529.8
  transient
    arm or leg NEC 781.4
    traumatic NEC *(see also* Injury,
        nerve, by site) 957.9
  trapezius 352.4
  traumatic, transient NEC *(see also*
      Injury, nerve, by site) 957.9
  trembling *(see also* Parkinsonism)
      332.0
  triceps brachii 354.9
  trigeminal nerve 350.9
  trochlear nerve 378.53
  ulnar nerve 354.2
  upper limb - *see also* Paralysis, arm
    both *(see also* Diplegia) 344.2
  uremic - *see* Uremia
  uveoparotitic 135
  uvula 528.9
    hysterical 300.11
    postdiphtheritic 032.0
  vagus nerve 352.3
  vasomotor NEC 337.9
  velum palati 528.9
  vesical *(see also* Paralysis, bladder)
      596.53
  vestibular nerve 388.5
  visual field, psychic 368.16
  vocal cord 478.30
    bilateral (partial) 478.33
      complete 478.34
    complete (bilateral) 478.34
    unilateral (partial) 478.31
      complete 478.32

Paralysis, paralytic *(Continued)*
  Volkmann's (complicating trauma)
      958.6
  wasting 335.21
  Weber's 344.89
  wrist NEC 354.9
Paramedial orifice, urethrovesical 753.8
Paramenia 626.9
Parametritis (chronic) (*see also* Disease,
      pelvis, inflammatory) 614.4
  acute 614.3
  puerperal, postpartum,
      childbirth 670.8●
Parametrium, parametric - *see* condition
Paramnesia (*see also* Amnesia) 780.93
Paramolar 520.1
  causing crowding 524.31
Paramyloidosis 277.30
Paramyoclonus multiplex 333.2
Paramyotonia 359.29
  congenita (of von Eulenburg) 359.29
Paraneoplastic syndrome - *see* condition
Parangi (*see also* Yaws) 102.9
Paranoia 297.1
  alcoholic 291.5
  querulans 297.8
  senile 290.20
Paranoid
  dementia (*see also* Schizophrenia)
      295.3●
      praecox (acute) 295.3●
      senile 290.20
  personality 301.0
  psychosis 297.9
      alcoholic 291.5
      climacteric 297.2
      drug-induced 292.11
      involutional 297.2
      menopausal 297.2
      protracted reactive 298.4
      psychogenic 298.4
          acute 298.3
      senile 290.20
  reaction (chronic) 297.9
      acute 298.3
  schizophrenia (acute) (*see also*
      Schizophrenia) 295.3●
  state 297.9
      alcohol-induced 291.5
      climacteric 297.2
      drug-induced 292.11
      due to or associated with
          arteriosclerosis (cerebrovascular)
              290.42
          presenile brain disease 290.12
          senile brain disease 290.20
      involutional 297.2
      menopausal 297.2
      senile 290.20
      simple 297.0
      specified type NEC 297.8
  tendencies 301.0
  traits 301.0
  trends 301.0
  type, psychopathic personality 301.0
Paraparesis (*see also* Paraplegia) 344.1
Paraphasia 784.3
Paraphilia (*see also* Deviation, sexual) 302.9
Paraphimosis (congenital) 605
  chancroidal 099.0
Paraphrenia, paraphrenic (late) 297.2
  climacteric 297.2
  dementia (*see also* Schizophrenia)
      295.3●

Paraphrenia, paraphrenic *(Continued)*
  involutional 297.2
  menopausal 297.2
  schizophrenia (acute) (*see also*
      Schizophrenia) 295.3●
Paraplegia 344.1
  with
      broken back - *see* Fracture,
          vertebra, by site, with
          spinal cord injury
      fracture, vertebra - *see* Fracture,
          vertebra, by site, with spinal
          cord injury
  ataxic - *see* Degeneration, combined,
      spinal cord
  brain (current episode) (*see also*
      Paralysis, brain) 437.8
  cerebral (current episode) (*see also*
      Paralysis, brain) 437.8
  congenital or infantile (cerebral)
      (spastic) (spinal) 343.0
  cortical - *see* Paralysis, brain
  familial spastic 334.1
  functional (hysterical) 300.11
  hysterical 300.11
  infantile 343.0
  late effect 344.1
  Pott's (*see also* Tuberculosis) 015.0●
      [730.88]
  psychogenic 306.0
  spastic
      Erb's spinal 094.89
      hereditary 334.1
      not infantile or congenital
          344.1
  spinal (cord)
      traumatic NEC - *see* Injury, spinal,
          by site
  syphilitic (spastic) 094.89
  traumatic NEC - *see* Injury, spinal, by
      site
Paraproteinemia 273.2
  benign (familial) 273.1
  monoclonal 273.1
  secondary to malignant or
      inflammatory disease 273.1
Parapsoriasis 696.2
  en plaques 696.2
  guttata 696.2
  lichenoides chronica 696.2
  retiformis 696.2
  varioliformis (acuta) 696.2
Parascarlatina 057.8
Parasitic - *see also* condition
  disease NEC (*see also* Infestation,
      parasitic) 136.9
      contact V01.89
      exposure to V01.89
      intestinal NEC 129
      skin NEC 134.9
  stomatitis 112.0
  sycosis 110.0
      beard 110.0
      scalp 110.0
  twin 759.4
Parasitism NEC 136.9
  intestinal NEC 129
  skin NEC 134.9
  specified - *see* Infestation
Parasitophobia 300.29
Parasomnia 307.47
  alcohol induced 291.82
  drug induced 292.85
  nonorganic origin 307.47

Parasomnia *(Continued)*
  organic 327.40
      in conditions classified elsewhere
          327.44
      other 327.49
Paraspadias 752.69
Paraspasm facialis 351.8
Parathyroid gland - *see* condition
Parathyroiditis (autoimmune) 252.1
Parathyroprival tetany 252.1
Paratrachoma 077.0
Paratyphilitis (*see also* Appendicitis) 541
Paratyphoid (fever) - *see* Fever,
      paratyphoid
Paratyphus - *see* Fever, paratyphoid
Paraurethral duct 753.8
Para-urethritis 597.89
  gonococcal (acute) 098.0
      chronic or duration of 2 months or
          over 098.2
Paravaccinia NEC 051.9
  milkers' node 051.1
Paravaginitis (*see also* Vaginitis) 616.10
Parencephalitis (*see also* Encephalitis) 323.9
  late effect - *see* category 326
Parergasia 298.9
Paresis (*see also* Paralysis) 344.9
  accommodation 367.51
  bladder (spastic) (sphincter) (*see also*
      Paralysis, bladder) 596.53
      tabetic 094.0
  bowel, colon, or intestine (*see also* Ileus)
      560.1
  brain or cerebral - *see* Paralysis, brain
  extrinsic muscle, eye 378.55
  general 094.1
      arrested 094.1
      brain 094.1
      cerebral 094.1
      insane 094.1
      juvenile 090.40
          remission 090.49
      progressive 094.1
      remission (sustained) 094.1
      tabetic 094.1
  heart (*see also* Failure, heart) 428.9
  infantile (*see also* Poliomyelitis)
      045.9●
  insane 094.1
  juvenile 090.40
  late effect - *see* Paralysis, late effect
  luetic (general) 094.1
  peripheral progressive 356.9
  pseudohypertrophic 359.1
  senile NEC 344.9
  stomach 536.3
      diabetic 250.6● [536.3]
          due to secondary diabetes
              249.6● [536.3]
  syphilitic (general) 094.1
      congenital 090.40
  transient, limb 781.4
  vesical (sphincter) NEC 596.53
Paresthesia (*see also* Disturbance,
      sensation) 782.0
  Berger's (paresthesia of lower limb)
      782.0
  Bernhardt 355.1
  Magnan's 782.0
Paretic - *see* condition
Parinaud's
  conjunctivitis 372.02
  oculoglandular syndrome 372.02
  ophthalmoplegia 378.81

Parinaud's (Continued)
  syndrome (paralysis of conjugate
    upward gaze) 378.81
Parkes Weber and Dimitri syndrome
  (encephalocutaneous angiomatosis)
  759.6
Parkinson's disease, syndrome, or
  tremor - see Parkinsonism
Parkinsonism (arteriosclerotic)
  (idiopathic) (primary) 332.0
  associated with orthostatic hypotension
    (idiopathic) (symptomatic) 333.0
  due to drugs 332.1
  neuroleptic-induced 332.1
  secondary 332.1
  syphilitic 094.82
Parodontitis 523.40
Parodontosis 523.5
Paronychia (with lymphangitis) 681.9
  candidal (chronic) 112.3
  chronic 681.9
    candidal 112.3
    finger 681.02
    toe 681.11
  finger 681.02
  toe 681.11
  tuberculous (primary) (see also
    Tuberculosis) 017.0●
Parorexia NEC 307.52
  hysterical 300.11
Parosmia 781.1
  psychogenic 306.7
Parotid gland - see condition
Parotiditis (see also Parotitis) 527.2
  epidemic 072.9
  infectious 072.9
Parotitis 527.2
  allergic 527.2
  chronic 527.2
  epidemic (see also Mumps) 072.9
  infectious (see also Mumps) 072.9
  noninfectious 527.2
  nonspecific toxic 527.2
  not mumps 527.2
  postoperative 527.2
  purulent 527.2
  septic 527.2
  suppurative (acute) 527.2
  surgical 527.2
  toxic 527.2
Paroxysmal - see also condition
  dyspnea (nocturnal) 786.09
Parrot's disease (syphilitic
  osteochondritis) 090.0
Parrot fever 073.9
Parry's disease or syndrome
  (exophthalmic goiter) 242.0●
Parry-Romberg syndrome 349.89
Parson's disease (exophthalmic goiter)
  242.0●
Parsonage-Aldren-Turner syndrome 353.5
Parsonage-Turner syndrome 353.5
Pars planitis 363.21
Particolored infant 757.39
Parturition - see Delivery
Parvovirus 079.83
  B19 079.83
  human 079.83
Passage
  false, urethra 599.4
  meconium noted during delivery
    763.84
  of sounds or bougies (see also Attention
    to artificial opening) V55.9

Passive - see condition
Pasteurella septica 027.2
Pasteurellosis (see also Infection,
  Pasteurella) 027.2
PAT (paroxysmal atrial tachycardia)
  427.0
Patau's syndrome (trisomy D1) 758.1
Patch
  herald 696.3
Patches
  mucous (syphilitic) 091.3
    congenital 090.0
  smokers' (mouth) 528.6
Patellar - see condition
Patellofemoral syndrome 719.46
Patent - see also Imperfect closure
  atrioventricular ostium 745.69
  canal of Nuck 752.41
  cervix 622.5
    complicating pregnancy 654.5●
      affecting fetus or newborn 761.0
  ductus arteriosus or Botalli 747.0
  Eustachian
    tube 381.7
    valve 746.89
  foramen
    Botalli 745.5
    ovale 745.5
  interauricular septum 745.5
  interventricular septum 745.4
  omphalomesenteric duct 751.0
  os (uteri) - see Patent, cervix
  ostium secundum 745.5
  urachus 753.7
  vitelline duct 751.0
Paternity testing V70.4
Paterson's syndrome (sideropenic
  dysphagia) 280.8
Paterson (-Brown) (-Kelly) syndrome
  (sideropenic dysphagia) 280.8
Paterson-Kelly syndrome or web
  (sideropenic dysphagia) 280.8
Pathologic, pathological - see also
  condition
  asphyxia 799.01
  drunkenness 291.4
  emotionality 301.3
  fracture - see Fracture, pathologic
  liar 301.7
  personality 301.9
  resorption, tooth 521.40
    external 521.42
    internal 521.41
    specified NEC 521.49
  sexuality (see also Deviation, sexual)
    302.9
Pathology (of) - see also Disease
  periradicular, associated with previous
    endodontic treatment 526.69
Patterned motor discharge, idiopathic
  (see also Epilepsy) 345.5●
Patulous - see also Patent
  anus 569.49
  Eustachian tube 381.7
Pause, sinoatrial 427.81
Pavor nocturnus 307.46
Pavy's disease 593.6
Paxton's disease (white piedra) 111.2
Payr's disease or syndrome (splenic
  flexure syndrome) 569.89
PBA (pseudobulbar affect) 310.8
Pearls
  Elschnig 366.51
  enamel 520.2

Pearl-workers' disease (chronic
  osteomyelitis) (see also
  Osteomyelitis) 730.1●
Pectenitis 569.49
Pectenosis 569.49
Pectoral - see condition
Pectus
  carinatum (congenital) 754.82
    acquired 738.3
    rachitic (see also Rickets) 268.0
  excavatum (congenital) 754.81
    acquired 738.3
    rachitic (see also Rickets) 268.0
  recurvatum (congenital) 754.81
    acquired 738.3
Pedatrophia 261
Pederosis 302.2
Pediculosis (infestation) 132.9
  capitis (head louse) (any site) 132.0
  corporis (body louse) (any site) 132.1
  eyelid 132.0 [373.6]
  mixed (classifiable to more than one
    category in 132.0–132.2) 132.3
  pubis (pubic louse) (any site) 132.2
  vestimenti 132.1
  vulvae 132.2
Pediculus (infestation) - see Pediculosis
Pedophilia 302.2
Peg-shaped teeth 520.2
Pel's crisis 094.0
Pel-Ebstein disease - see Disease,
  Hodgkin's
Pelade 704.01
Pelger-Huët anomaly or syndrome
  (hereditary hyposegmentation) 288.2
Peliosis (rheumatica) 287.0
Pelizaeus-Merzbacher
  disease 330.0
  sclerosis, diffuse cerebral 330.0
Pellagra (alcoholic or with alcoholism)
  265.2
  with polyneuropathy 265.2 [357.4]
Pellagra-cerebellar-ataxia-renal
  aminoaciduria syndrome 270.0
Pellegrini's disease (calcification, knee
  joint) 726.62
Pellegrini (-Stieda) disease or syndrome
  (calcification, knee joint) 726.62
Pellizzi's syndrome (pineal) 259.8
Pelvic - see also condition
  congestion-fibrosis syndrome 625.5
  kidney 753.3
Pelvioectasis 591
Pelviolithiasis 592.0
Pelviperitonitis
  female (see also Peritonitis, pelvic,
    female) 614.5
  male (see also Peritonitis) 567.21
Pelvis, pelvic - see also condition or type
  infantile 738.6
  Nägele's 738.6
  obliquity 738.6
  Robert's 755.69
Pemphigoid 694.5
  benign, mucous membrane 694.60
    with ocular involvement 694.61
  bullous 694.5
  cicatricial 694.60
    with ocular involvement 694.61
  juvenile 694.2
Pemphigus 694.4
  benign 694.5
    chronic familial 757.39
  Brazilian 694.4

◀ New   ◀‖‖‖ Revised   ~~deleted~~ Deleted   ● Use Additional Digit(s)   ▨ Omit code

Pemphigus *(Continued)*
circinatus 694.0
congenital, traumatic 757.39
conjunctiva 694.61
contagiosus 684
erythematodes 694.4
erythematosus 694.4
foliaceus 694.4
frambesiodes 694.4
gangrenous *(see also* Gangrene) 785.4
malignant 694.4
neonatorum, newborn 684
ocular 694.61
papillaris 694.4
seborrheic 694.4
South American 694.4
syphilitic (congenital) 090.0
vegetans 694.4
vulgaris 694.4
wildfire 694.4
Pendred's syndrome (familial goiter with deaf-mutism) 243
Pendulous
abdomen 701.9
in pregnancy or childbirth 654.4●
affecting fetus or newborn 763.89
breast 611.89
Penetrating wound - *see also* Wound, open, by site
with internal injury - *see* Injury, internal, by site, with open wound
eyeball 871.7
with foreign body (nonmagnetic) 871.6
magnetic 871.5
ocular *(see also* Penetrating wound, eyeball) 871.7
adnexa 870.3
with foreign body 870.4
orbit 870.3
with foreign body 870.4
Penetration, pregnant uterus by instrument
with
abortion - *see* Abortion, by type, with damage to pelvic organs
ectopic pregnancy *(see also* categories 633.0–633.9) 639.2
molar pregnancy *(see also* categories 630–632) 639.2
complication of delivery 665.1●
affecting fetus or newborn 763.89
following
abortion 639.2
ectopic or molar pregnancy 639.2
Penfield's syndrome *(see also* Epilepsy) 345.5●
Penicilliosis of lung 117.3
Penis - *see* condition
Penitis 607.2
Penta X syndrome 758.81
Pentalogy (of Fallot) 745.2
Pentosuria (benign) (essential) 271.8
Peptic acid disease 536.8
Peregrinating patient V65.2
Perforated - *see* Perforation
Perforation, perforative (nontraumatic)
antrum *(see also* Sinusitis, maxillary) 473.0
appendix 540.0
with peritoneal abscess 540.1
atrial septum, multiple 745.5

Perforation, perforative *(Continued)*
attic, ear 384.22
healed 384.81
bile duct, except cystic *(see also* Disease, biliary) 576.3
cystic 575.4
bladder (urinary) 596.6
with
abortion - *see* Abortion, by type, with damage to pelvic organs
ectopic pregnancy *(see also* categories 633.0–633.9) 639.2
molar pregnancy *(see also* categories 630–632) 639.2
following
abortion 639.2
ectopic or molar pregnancy 639.2
obstetrical trauma 665.5●
bowel 569.83
with
abortion - *see* Abortion, by type, with damage to pelvic organs
ectopic pregnancy *(see also* categories 633.0–633.9) 639.2
molar pregnancy *(see also* categories 630–632) 639.2
fetus or newborn 777.6
following
abortion 639.2
ectopic or molar pregnancy 639.2
obstetrical trauma 665.5●
broad ligament
with
abortion - *see* Abortion, by type, with damage to pelvic organs
ectopic pregnancy *(see also* categories 633.0–633.9) 639.2
molar pregnancy *(see also* categories 630–632) 639.2
following
abortion 639.2
ectopic or molar pregnancy 639.2
obstetrical trauma 665.6●
by
device, implant, or graft - *see* Complications, mechanical
foreign body left accidentally in operation wound 998.4
instrument (any) during a procedure, accidental 998.2
cecum 540.0
with peritoneal abscess 540.1
cervix (uteri) - *see also* Injury, internal, cervix
with
abortion - *see* Abortion, by type, with damage to pelvic organs
ectopic pregnancy *(see also* categories 633.0–633.9) 639.2
molar pregnancy *(see also* categories 630–632) 639.2
following
abortion 639.2
ectopic or molar pregnancy 639.2
obstetrical trauma 665.3●
colon 569.83
common duct (bile) 576.3
cornea *(see also* Ulcer, cornea) 370.00
due to ulceration 370.06
cystic duct 575.4

Perforation, perforative *(Continued)*
diverticulum *(see also* Diverticula) 562.10
small intestine 562.00
duodenum, duodenal (ulcer) - *see* Ulcer, duodenum, with perforation
ear drum - *see* Perforation, tympanum
enteritis - *see* Enteritis
esophagus 530.4
ethmoidal sinus *(see also* Sinusitis, ethmoidal) 473.2
foreign body (external site) - *see also* Wound, open, by site, complicated
internal site, by ingested object - *see* Foreign body
frontal sinus *(see also* Sinusitis, frontal) 473.1
gallbladder or duct *(see also* Disease, gallbladder) 575.4
gastric (ulcer) - *see* Ulcer, stomach, with perforation
heart valve - *see* Endocarditis
ileum *(see also* Perforation, intestine) 569.83
instrumental
external - *see* Wound, open, by site
pregnant uterus, complicating delivery 665.9●
surgical (accidental) (blood vessel) (nerve) (organ) 998.2
intestine 569.83
with
abortion - *see* Abortion, by type, with damage to pelvic organs
ectopic pregnancy *(see also* categories 633.0–633.9) 639.2
molar pregnancy *(see also* categories 630–632) 639.2
fetus or newborn 777.6
obstetrical trauma 665.5●
ulcerative NEC 569.83
jejunum, jejunal 569.83
ulcer - *see* Ulcer, gastrojejunal, with perforation
mastoid (antrum) (cell) 383.89
maxillary sinus *(see also* Sinusitis, maxillary) 473.0
membrana tympani - *see* Perforation, tympanum
nasal
septum 478.19
congenital 748.1
syphilitic 095.8
sinus *(see also* Sinusitis) 473.9
congenital 748.1
palate (hard) 526.89
soft 528.9
syphilitic 095.8
syphilitic 095.8
palatine vault 526.89
syphilitic 095.8
congenital 090.5
pelvic
floor
with
abortion - *see* Abortion, by type, with damage to pelvic organs
ectopic pregnancy *(see also* categories 633.0–633.9) 639.2

Perforation, perforative (*Continued*)
  pelvic (*Continued*)
    floor (*Continued*)
      with (*Continued*)
        molar pregnancy (*see also*
          categories 630–632)
          639.2
        obstetrical trauma 664.1●
    organ
      with
        abortion - *see* Abortion, by
          type, with damage to
          pelvic organs
        ectopic pregnancy (*see also*
          categories 633.0–633.9)
          639.2
        molar pregnancy (*see also*
          categories 630–632)
          639.2
      following
        abortion 639.2
        ectopic or molar pregnancy
          639.2
      obstetrical trauma 665.5●
  perineum - *see* Laceration, perineum
  periurethral tissue
    with
      abortion - *see* Abortion, by type,
        with damage to pelvic
        organs
      ectopic pregnancy (*see also*
        categories 630–632) 639.2
      molar pregnancy (*see also*
        categories 630–632) 639.2
  pharynx 478.29
  pylorus, pyloric (ulcer) - *see* Ulcer,
    stomach, with perforation
  rectum 569.49
  root canal space 526.61
  sigmoid 569.83
  sinus (accessory) (chronic) (nasal) (*see
    also* Sinusitis) 473.9
  sphenoidal sinus (*see also* Sinusitis,
    sphenoidal) 473.3
  stomach (due to ulcer) - *see* Ulcer,
    stomach, with perforation
  surgical (accidental) (by instrument)
    (blood vessel) (nerve) (organ)
    998.2
  traumatic
    external - *see* Wound, open, by
      site
    eye (*see also* Penetrating wound,
      ocular) 871.7
    internal organ - *see* Injury, internal,
      by site
  tympanum (membrane) (persistent
    posttraumatic)
    (postinflammatory) 384.20
    with
      otitis media - *see* Otitis media
    attic 384.22
    central 384.21
    healed 384.81
    marginal NEC 384.23
    multiple 384.24
    pars flaccida 384.22
    total 384.25
    traumatic - *see* Wound, open, ear,
      drum
  typhoid, gastrointestinal 002.0
  ulcer - *see* Ulcer, by site, with
    perforation
  ureter 593.89

Perforation, perforative (*Continued*)
  urethra
    with
      abortion - *see* Abortion, by type,
        with damage to pelvic
        organs
      ectopic pregnancy (*see also*
        categories 633.0–633.9) 639.2
      molar pregnancy (*see also*
        categories 630–632) 639.2
    following
      abortion 639.2
      ectopic or molar pregnancy 639.2
    obstetrical trauma 665.5●
  uterus - *see also* Injury, internal, uterus
    with
      abortion - *see* Abortion, by type,
        with damage to pelvic
        organs
      ectopic pregnancy (*see also*
        categories 633.0–633.9) 639.2
      molar pregnancy (*see also*
        categories 630–632) 639.2
    by intrauterine contraceptive device
      996.32
    following
      abortion 639.2
      ectopic or molar pregnancy 639.2
    obstetrical trauma - *see* Injury,
      internal, uterus, obstetrical
      trauma
  uvula 528.9
    syphilitic 095.8
  vagina - *see* Laceration, vagina
  viscus NEC 799.89
    traumatic 868.00
      with open wound into cavity
        868.10
Periadenitis mucosa necrotica recurrens
  528.2
Periangiitis 446.0
Periantritis 535.4●
Periappendicitis (acute) (*see also*
  Appendicitis) 541
Periarteritis (disseminated) (infectious)
  (necrotizing) (nodosa) 446.0
Periarthritis (joint) 726.90
  Duplay's 726.2
  gonococcal 098.50
  humeroscapularis 726.2
  scapulohumeral 726.2
  shoulder 726.2
  wrist 726.4
Periarthrosis (angioneural) - *see*
  Periarthritis
Peribronchitis 491.9
  tuberculous (*see also* Tuberculosis)
    011.3●
Pericapsulitis, adhesive (shoulder) 726.0
Pericarditis (granular) (with
  decompensation) (with effusion)
  423.9
  with
    rheumatic fever (conditions
      classifiable to 390)
      active (*see also* Pericarditis,
        rheumatic) 391.0
      inactive or quiescent 393
  actinomycotic 039.8 *[420.0]*
  acute (nonrheumatic) 420.90
    with chorea (acute) (rheumatic)
      (Sydenham's) 392.0
    bacterial 420.99
    benign 420.91

Pericarditis (*Continued*)
  acute (*Continued*)
    hemorrhagic 420.90
    idiopathic 420.91
    infective 420.90
    nonspecific 420.91
    rheumatic 391.0
      with chorea (acute) (rheumatic)
        (Sydenham's) 392.0
    sicca 420.90
    viral 420.91
  adhesive or adherent (external)
    (internal) 423.1
    acute - *see* Pericarditis, acute
    rheumatic (external) (internal) 393
  amebic 006.8 *[420.0]*
  bacterial (acute) (subacute) (with
    serous or seropurulent effusion)
    420.99
  calcareous 423.2
  cholesterol (chronic) 423.8
    acute 420.90
  chronic (nonrheumatic) 423.8
    rheumatic 393
  constrictive 423.2
  Coxsackie 074.21
  due to
    actinomycosis 039.8 *[420.0]*
    amebiasis 006.8 *[420.0]*
    Coxsackie (virus) 074.21
    histoplasmosis (*see also*
      Histoplasmosis) 115.93
    nocardiosis 039.8 *[420.0]*
    tuberculosis (*see also* Tuberculosis)
      017.9● *[420.0]*
  fibrinocaseous (*see also* Tuberculosis)
    017.9● *[420.0]*
  fibrinopurulent 420.99
  fibrinous - *see* Pericarditis, rheumatic
  fibropurulent 420.99
  fibrous 423.1
  gonococcal 098.83
  hemorrhagic 423.0
  idiopathic (acute) 420.91
  infective (acute) 420.90
  meningococcal 036.41
  neoplastic (chronic) 423.8
    acute 420.90
  nonspecific 420.91
  obliterans, obliterating 423.1
  plastic 423.1
  pneumococcal (acute) 420.99
  postinfarction 411.0
  purulent (acute) 420.99
  rheumatic (active) (acute) (with
    effusion) (with pneumonia)
    391.0
    with chorea (acute) (rheumatic)
      (Sydenham's) 392.0
    chronic or inactive (with chorea)
      393
  septic (acute) 420.99
  serofibrinous - *see* Pericarditis,
    rheumatic
  staphylococcal (acute) 420.99
  streptococcal (acute) 420.99
  suppurative (acute) 420.99
  syphilitic 093.81
  tuberculous (acute) (chronic) (*see also*
    Tuberculosis) 017.9● *[420.0]*
  uremic 585.9 *[420.0]*
  viral (acute) 420.91
Pericardium, pericardial - *see* condition
Pericellulitis (*see also* Cellulitis) 682.9

Pericementitis 523.40
  acute 523.30
  chronic (suppurative) 523.40
Pericholecystitis (see also Cholecystitis) 575.10
Perichondritis
  auricle 380.00
    acute 380.01
    chronic 380.02
  bronchus 491.9
  ear (external) 380.00
    acute 380.01
    chronic 380.02
  larynx 478.71
    syphilitic 095.8
    typhoid 002.0 [478.71]
  nose 478.19
  pinna 380.00
    acute 380.01
    chronic 380.02
  trachea 478.9
Periclasia 523.5
Pericolitis 569.89
Pericoronitis (chronic) 523.40
  acute 523.33
Pericystitis (see also Cystitis) 595.9
Pericytoma (M9150/1) - see also
    Neoplasm, connective tissue, uncertain behavior
  benign (M9150/0) - see Neoplasm, connective tissue, benign
  malignant (M9150/3) - see Neoplasm, connective tissue, malignant
Peridacryocystitis, acute 375.32
Peridiverticulitis (see also Diverticulitis) 562.11
Periduodenitis 535.6●
Periendocarditis (see also Endocarditis) 424.90
  acute or subacute 421.9
Periepididymitis (see also Epididymitis) 604.90
Perifolliculitis (abscedens) 704.8
  capitis, abscedens et suffodiens 704.8
  dissecting, scalp 704.8
  scalp 704.8
  superficial pustular 704.8
Perigastritis (acute) 535.0●
Perigastrojejunitis (acute) 535.0●
Perihepatitis (acute) 573.3
  chlamydial 099.56
  gonococcal 098.86
Peri-ileitis (subacute) 569.89
Perilabyrinthitis (acute) - see Labyrinthitis
Perimeningitis - see Meningitis
Perimetritis (see also Endometritis) 615.9
Perimetrosalpingitis (see also Salpingo-oophoritis) 614.2
Perineocele 618.05
Perinephric - see condition
Perinephritic - see condition
Perinephritis (see also Infection, kidney) 590.9
  purulent (see also Abscess, kidney) 590.2
Perineum, perineal - see condition
Perineuritis NEC 729.2
Periodic - see also condition
  disease (familial) 277.31
  edema 995.1
    hereditary 277.6
  fever 277.31
  headache syndromes in child or adolescent 346.2●

Periodic (Continued)
  limb movement disorder 327.51
  paralysis (familial) 359.3
  peritonitis 277.31
  polyserositis 277.31
  somnolence (see also Narcolepsy) 347.00
Periodontal
  cyst 522.8
  pocket 523.8
Periodontitis (chronic) (complex) (compound) (simplex) 523.40
  acute 523.33
  aggressive 523.30
    generalized 523.32
    localized 523.31
  apical 522.6
    acute (pulpal origin) 522.4
  generalized 523.42
  localized 523.41
Periodontoclasia 523.5
Periodontosis 523.5
Periods - see also Menstruation
  heavy 626.2
  irregular 626.4
Perionychia (with lymphangitis) 681.9
  finger 681.02
  toe 681.11
Perioophoritis (see also Salpingo-oophoritis) 614.2
Periorchitis (see also Orchitis) 604.90
Periosteum, periosteal - see condition
Periostitis (circumscribed) (diffuse) (infective) 730.3●

> Note: Use the following fifth-digit subclassification with category 730:
> 0 site unspecified
> 1 shoulder region
> 2 upper arm
> 3 forearm
> 4 hand
> 5 pelvic region and thigh
> 6 lower leg
> 7 ankle and foot
> 8 other specified sites
> 9 multiple sites

  with osteomyelitis (see also Osteomyelitis) 730.2●
    acute or subacute 730.0●
    chronic or old 730.1●
  albuminosa, albuminosus 730.3●
  alveolar 526.5
  alveolodental 526.5
  dental 526.5
  gonorrheal 098.89
  hyperplastica, generalized 731.2
  jaw (lower) (upper) 526.4
  monomelic 733.99
  orbital 376.02
  syphilitic 095.5
    congenital 090.0 [730.8]●
    secondary 091.61
  tuberculous (see also Tuberculosis, bone) 015.9● [730.8]●
  yaws (early) (hypertrophic) (late) 102.6
Periostosis (see also Periostitis) 730.3●
  with osteomyelitis (see also Osteomyelitis) 730.2●
    acute or subacute 730.0●
    chronic or old 730.1●
  hyperplastic 756.59
Peripartum cardiomyopathy 674.5●

Periphlebitis (see also Phlebitis) 451.9
  lower extremity 451.2
    deep (vessels) 451.19
    superficial (vessels) 451.0
  portal 572.1
  retina 362.18
  superficial (vessels) 451.0
  tuberculous (see also Tuberculosis) 017.9●
    retina 017.3● [362.18]
Peripneumonia - see Pneumonia
Periproctitis 569.49
Periprostatitis (see also Prostatitis) 601.9
Perirectal - see condition
Perirenal - see condition
Perisalpingitis (see also Salpingo-oophoritis) 614.2
Perisigmoiditis 569.89
Perisplenitis (infectional) 289.59
Perispondylitis - see Spondylitis
Peristalsis reversed or visible 787.4
Peritendinitis (see also Tenosynovitis) 726.90
  adhesive (shoulder) 726.0
Perithelioma (M9150/1) - see Pericytoma
Peritoneum, peritoneal - see also condition
  equilibration test V56.32
Peritonitis (acute) (adhesive) (fibrinous) (hemorrhagic) (idiopathic) (localized) (perforative) (primary) (with adhesions) (with effusion) 567.9
  with or following
    abortion - see Abortion, by type, with sepsis
    abscess 567.21
    appendicitis 540.0
      with peritoneal abscess 540.1
    ectopic pregnancy (see also categories 633.0-633.9) 639.0
    molar pregnancy (see also categories 630-632) 639.0
  aseptic 998.7
  bacterial 567.29
    spontaneous 567.23
  bile, biliary 567.81
  chemical 998.7
  chlamydial 099.56
  chronic proliferative 567.89
  congenital NEC 777.6
  diaphragmatic 567.22
  diffuse NEC 567.29
  diphtheritic 032.83
  disseminated NEC 567.29
  due to
    bile 567.81
    foreign
      body or object accidentally left during a procedure (instrument) (sponge) (swab) 998.4
      substance accidentally left during a procedure (chemical) (powder) (talc) 998.7
    talc 998.7
    urine 567.89
  fibrinopurulent 567.29
  fibrinous 567.29
  fibrocaseous (see also Tuberculosis) 014.0●
  fibropurulent 567.29
  general, generalized (acute) 567.21
  gonococcal 098.86
  in infective disease NEC 136.9 [567.0]

Peritonitis (Continued)
  meconium (newborn) 777.6
  pancreatic 577.8
  paroxysmal, benign 277.31
  pelvic
    female (acute) 614.5
      chronic NEC 614.7
        with adhesions 614.6
      puerperal, postpartum, childbirth 670.8●
    male (acute) 567.21
  periodic (familial) 277.31
  phlegmonous 567.29
  pneumococcal 567.1
  postabortal 639.0
  proliferative, chronic 567.89
  puerperal, postpartum, childbirth 670.8●
  purulent 567.29
  septic 567.29
  spontaneous bacterial 567.23
  staphylococcal 567.29
  streptococcal 567.29
  subdiaphragmatic 567.29
  subphrenic 567.29
  suppurative 567.29
  syphilitic 095.2
    congenital 090.0 [567.0]
  talc 998.7
  tuberculous (see also Tuberculosis) 014.0●
  urine 567.89
Peritonsillar - see condition
Peritonsillitis 475
Perityphlitis (see also Appendicitis) 541
Periureteritis 593.89
Periurethral - see condition
Periurethritis (gangrenous) 597.89
Periuterine - see condition
Perivaginitis (see also Vaginitis) 616.10
Perivasculitis, retinal 362.18
Perivasitis (chronic) 608.4
Periventricular leukomalacia 779.7
Perivesiculitis (seminal) (see also Vesiculitis) 608.0
Perlèche 686.8
  due to
    moniliasis 112.0
    riboflavin deficiency 266.0
Pernicious - see condition
Pernio, perniosis 991.5
Persecution
  delusion 297.9
  social V62.4
Perseveration (tonic) 784.69
Persistence, persistent (congenital) 759.89
  anal membrane 751.2
  arteria stapedia 744.04
  atrioventricular canal 745.69
  bloody ejaculate 792.2
  branchial cleft 744.41
  bulbus cordis in left ventricle 745.8
  canal of Cloquet 743.51
  capsule (opaque) 743.51
  cilioretinal artery or vein 743.51
  cloaca 751.5
  communication - see Fistula, congenital
  convolutions
    aortic arch 747.21
    fallopian tube 752.19
    oviduct 752.19
    uterine tube 752.19
  double aortic arch 747.21

Persistence, persistent (Continued)
  ductus
    arteriosus 747.0
    Botalli 747.0
  fetal
    circulation 747.83
    form of cervix (uteri) 752.49
    hemoglobin (hereditary) ("Swiss variety") 282.7
    pulmonary hypertension 747.83
  foramen
    Botalli 745.5
    ovale 745.5
  Gartner's duct 752.41
  hemoglobin, fetal (hereditary) (HPFH) 282.7
  hyaloid
    artery (generally incomplete) 743.51
    system 743.51
  hymen (tag)
    in pregnancy or childbirth 654.8●
      causing obstructed labor 660.2●
  lanugo 757.4
  left
    posterior cardinal vein 747.49
    root with right arch of aorta 747.21
    superior vena cava 747.49
  Meckel's diverticulum 751.0
  mesonephric duct 752.89
    fallopian tube 752.11
  mucosal disease (middle ear) (with posterior or superior marginal perforation of ear drum) 382.2
  nail(s), anomalous 757.5
  occiput, anterior or posterior 660.3●
    fetus or newborn 763.1
  omphalomesenteric duct 751.0
  organ or site NEC - see Anomaly, specified type NEC
  ostium
    atrioventriculare commune 745.69
    primum 745.61
    secundum 745.5
  ovarian rests in fallopian tube 752.19
  pancreatic tissue in intestinal tract 751.5
  primary (deciduous)
    teeth 520.6
    vitreous hyperplasia 743.51
  pulmonary hypertension 747.83
  pupillary membrane 743.46
    iris 743.46
  Rhesus (Rh) titer (see also Complications, transfusion) 999.70 ◀▥
  right aortic arch 747.21
  sinus
    urogenitalis 752.89
    venosus with imperfect incorporation in right auricle 747.49
  thymus (gland) 254.8
    hyperplasia 254.0
  thyroglossal duct 759.2
  thyrolingual duct 759.2
  truncus arteriosus or communis 745.0
  tunica vasculosa lentis 743.39
  umbilical sinus 753.7
  urachus 753.7
  vegetative state 780.03
  vitelline duct 751.0
  wolffian duct 752.89

Person (with)
  admitted for clinical research, as participant or control subject V70.7
  affected by
    family member
      currently on deployment (military) V61.01
      returned from deployment (military) (current or past conflict) V61.02
  awaiting admission to adequate facility elsewhere V63.2
    undergoing social agency investigation V63.8
  concern (normal) about sick person in family V61.49
  consulting on behalf of another V65.19
    pediatric
      pre-adoption visit for adoptive parents V65.11
      pre-birth visit for expectant parents V65.11
  currently deployed in theater or in support of military war, peacekeeping and humanitarian operations V62.21
  feared
    complaint in whom no diagnosis was made V65.5
    condition not demonstrated V65.5
  feigning illness V65.2
  healthy, accompanying sick person V65.0
  history of military war, peacekeeping and humanitarian deployment (current or past conflict) V62.22
  living (in)
    alone V60.3
    boarding school V60.6
    residence remote from hospital or medical care facility V63.0
    residential institution V60.6
    without
      adequate
        financial resources V60.2
        housing (heating) (space) V60.1
      housing (permanent) (temporary) V60.0
      material resources V60.2
      person able to render necessary care V60.4
      shelter V60.0
  medical services in home not available V63.1
  on waiting list V63.2
    undergoing social agency investigation V63.8
  sick or handicapped in family V61.49
  "worried well" V65.5
Personality
  affective 301.10
  aggressive 301.3
  amoral 301.7
  anancastic, anankastic 301.4
  antisocial 301.7
  asocial 301.7
  asthenic 301.6
  avoidant 301.82
  borderline 301.83
  change 310.1
  compulsive 301.4

◀ New ◀▥ Revised ~~deleted~~ Deleted ● Use Additional Digit(s) ▥ Omit code

Personality *(Continued)*
  cycloid 301.13
  cyclothymic 301.13
  dependent 301.6
  depressive (chronic) 301.12
  disorder, disturbance NEC 301.9
    with
      antisocial disturbance 301.7
      pattern disturbance NEC 301.9
      sociopathic disturbance 301.7
      trait disturbance 301.9
  dual 300.14
  dyssocial 301.7
  eccentric 301.89
    "haltlose" type 301.89
  emotionally unstable 301.59
  epileptoid 301.3
  explosive 301.3
  fanatic 301.0
  histrionic 301.50
  hyperthymic 301.11
  hypomanic 301.11
  hypothymic 301.12
  hysterical 301.50
  immature 301.89
  inadequate 301.6
  labile 301.59
  masochistic 301.89
  morally defective 301.7
  multiple 300.14
  narcissistic 301.81
  obsessional 301.4
  obsessive-compulsive 301.4
  overconscientious 301.4
  paranoid 301.0
  passive (-dependent) 301.6
  passive-aggressive 301.84
  pathologic NEC 301.9
  pattern defect or disturbance 301.9
  pseudosocial 301.7
  psychoinfantile 301.59
  psychoneurotic NEC 301.89
  psychopathic 301.9
    with
      amoral trend 301.7
      antisocial trend 301.7
      asocial trend 301.7
      pathologic sexuality *(see also* Deviation, sexual) 302.9
    mixed types 301.9
  schizoid 301.20
    introverted 301.21
    schizotypal 301.22
  type A 301.4
  unstable (emotional) 301.59
Perthes' disease (capital femoral osteochondrosis) 732.1
Pertussis *(see also* Whooping cough) 033.9
  vaccination, prophylactic (against) V03.6
Peruvian wart 088.0
Perversion, perverted
  appetite 307.52
    hysterical 300.11
  function
    pineal gland 259.8
    pituitary gland 253.9
      anterior lobe
        deficient 253.2
        excessive 253.1
      posterior lobe 253.6
    placenta - *see* Placenta, abnormal
  sense of smell or taste 781.1
    psychogenic 306.7
  sexual *(see also* Deviation, sexual) 302.9

Pervious, congenital - *see also* Imperfect, closure
  ductus arteriosus 747.0
Pes (congenital) *(see also* Talipes) 754.70
  abductus (congenital) 754.60
    acquired 736.79
  acquired NEC 736.79
    planus 734
  adductus (congenital) 754.79
    acquired 736.79
  cavus 754.71
    acquired 736.73
  planovalgus (congenital) 754.69
    acquired 736.79
  planus (acquired) (any degree) 734
    congenital 754.61
    rachitic 268.1
  valgus (congenital) 754.61
    acquired 736.79
  varus (congenital) 754.50
    acquired 736.79
Pest *(see also* Plague) 020.9
Pestis *(see also* Plague) 020.9
  bubonica 020.0
  fulminans 020.0
  minor 020.8
  pneumonica - *see* Plague, pneumonic
Petechia, petechiae 782.7
  fetus or newborn 772.6
Petechial
  fever 036.0
  typhus 081.9
Petges-Cléjat or Petges-Clégat syndrome (poikilodermatomyositis) 710.3
Petit's
  disease *(see also* Hernia, lumbar) 553.8
Petit mal (idiopathic) *(see also* Epilepsy) 345.0●
  status 345.2
Petrellidosis 117.6
Petrositis 383.20
  acute 383.21
  chronic 383.22
Peutz-Jeghers disease or syndrome 759.6
Peyronie's disease 607.85
Pfeiffer's disease 075
Phacentocele 379.32
  traumatic 921.3
Phacoanaphylaxis 360.19
Phacocele (old) 379.32
  traumatic 921.3
Phaehyphomycosis 117.8
Phagedena (dry) (moist) *(see also* Gangrene) 785.4
  arteriosclerotic 440.24
  geometric 686.09
  penis 607.89
  senile 440.24
  sloughing 785.4
  tropical *(see also* Ulcer, skin) 707.9
  vulva 616.50
Phagedenic - *see also* condition
  abscess - *see also* Abscess
    chancroid 099.0
  bubo NEC 099.8
  chancre 099.0
  ulcer (tropical) *(see also* Ulcer, skin) 707.9
Phagomania 307.52
Phakoma 362.89
Phantom limb (syndrome) 353.6
Pharyngeal - *see also* condition
  arch remnant 744.41
  pouch syndrome 279.11

Pharyngitis (acute) (catarrhal) (gangrenous) (infective) (malignant) (membranous) (phlegmonous) (pneumococcal) (pseudomembranous) (simple) (staphylococcal) (subacute) (suppurative) (ulcerative) (viral) 462
  with influenza, flu, or grippe *(see also* Influenza) 487.1 ◀▬
  aphthous 074.0
  atrophic 472.1
  chlamydial 099.51
  chronic 472.1
  Coxsackie virus 074.0
  diphtheritic (membranous) 032.0
  follicular 472.1
  fusospirochetal 101
  gonococcal 098.6
  granular (chronic) 472.1
  herpetic 054.79
  hypertrophic 472.1
  infectional, chronic 472.1
  influenzal *(see also* Influenza) 487.1 ◀▬
  lymphonodular, acute 074.8
  septic 034.0
  streptococcal 034.0
  tuberculous *(see also* Tuberculosis) 012.8●
  vesicular 074.0
Pharyngoconjunctival fever 077.2
Pharyngoconjunctivitis, viral 077.2
Pharyngolaryngitis (acute) 465.0
  chronic 478.9
  septic 034.0
Pharyngoplegia 478.29
Pharyngotonsillitis 465.8
  tuberculous 012.8●
Pharyngotracheitis (acute) 465.8
  chronic 478.9
Pharynx, pharyngeal - *see* condition
Phase of life problem NEC V62.89
Phenomenon
  Arthus 995.21
  flashback (drug) 292.89
  jaw-winking 742.8
  Jod-Basedow 242.8●
  L. E. cell 710.0
  lupus erythematosus cell 710.0
  Pelger-Huët (hereditary hyposegmentation) 288.2
  Raynaud's (paroxysmal digital cyanosis) (secondary) 443.0
  Reilly's *(see also* Neuropathy, peripheral, autonomic) 337.9
  vasomotor 780.2
  vasospastic 443.9
  vasovagal 780.2
  Wenckebach's, heart block (second degree) 426.13
Phenylketonuria (PKU) 270.1
Phenylpyruvicaciduria 270.1
Pheochromoblastoma (M8700/3)
  specified site - *see* Neoplasm, by site, malignant
  unspecified site 194.0
Pheochromocytoma (M8700/0)
  malignant (M8700/3)
    specified site - *see* Neoplasm, by site, malignant
    unspecified site 194.0
  specified site - *see* Neoplasm, by site, benign
  unspecified site 227.0

Phimosis (congenital) 605
  chancroidal 099.0
  due to infection 605
Phlebectasia (*see also* Varicose, vein)
    454.9
  congenital NEC 747.60
  esophagus (*see also* Varix, esophagus)
    456.1
    with hemorrhage (*see also* Varix,
      esophagus, bleeding) 456.0
Phlebitis (infective) (pyemic) (septic)
    (suppurative) 451.9
  antecubital vein 451.82
  arm NEC 451.84
    axillary vein 451.89
    basilic vein 451.82
    deep 451.83
    superficial 451.82
  axillary vein 451.89
  basilic vein 451.82
  blue 451.9
  brachial vein 451.83
  breast, superficial 451.89
  cavernous (venous) sinus - *see*
      Phlebitis, intracranial sinus
  cephalic vein 451.82
  cerebral (venous) sinus - *see* Phlebitis,
      intracranial sinus
  chest wall, superficial 451.89
  complicating pregnancy or puerperium
      671.2●
    affecting fetus or newborn 760.3
  cranial (venous) sinus - *see* Phlebitis,
      intracranial sinus
  deep (vessels) 451.19
    femoral vein 451.11
    specified vessel NEC 451.19
  due to implanted device - *see*
      Complications, due to (presence
      of) any device, implant, or graft
      classified to 996.0–996.5 NEC
  during or resulting from a procedure
      997.2
  femoral vein (deep) (superficial)
      451.11
  femoropopliteal 451.19
  following infusion, perfusion, or
      transfusion 999.2
  gouty 274.89 [451.9]
  hepatic veins 451.89
  iliac vein 451.81
  iliofemoral 451.11
  intracranial sinus (any) (venous) 325
    late effect - *see* category 326
    nonpyogenic 437.6
      in pregnancy or puerperium
        671.5●
  jugular vein 451.89
  lateral (venous) sinus - *see* Phlebitis,
      intracranial sinus
  leg 451.2
    deep (vessels) 451.19
      specified vessel NEC 451.19
    superficial (vessels) 451.0
      femoral vein 451.11
  longitudinal sinus - *see* Phlebitis,
      intracranial sinus
  lower extremity 451.2
    deep (vessels) 451.19
      specified vessel NEC 451.19
    superficial (vessels) 451.0
      femoral vein 451.11
  migrans, migrating (superficial)
      453.1

Phlebitis (*Continued*)
  pelvic
    with
      abortion - *see* Abortion, by type,
        with sepsis
      ectopic pregnancy (*see also*
        categories 633.0–633.9)
        639.0
      molar pregnancy (*see also*
        categories 630–632)
        639.0
    following
      abortion 639.0
      ectopic or molar pregnancy
        639.0
    puerperal, postpartum 671.4●
  popliteal vein 451.19
  portal (vein) 572.1
  postoperative 997.2
  pregnancy 671.2●
    deep 671.3●
    specified type NEC 671.5●
    superficial 671.2●
  puerperal, postpartum, childbirth
      671.2●
    deep 671.4●
    lower extremities 671.2●
    pelvis 671.4●
    specified site NEC 671.5●
    superficial 671.2●
  radial vein 451.83
  retina 362.18
  saphenous (great) (long) 451.0
    accessory or small 451.0
  sinus (meninges) - *see* Phlebitis,
      intracranial sinus
  specified site NEC 451.89
  subclavian vein 451.89
  syphilitic 093.89
  tibial vein 451.19
  ulcer, ulcerative 451.9
    leg 451.2
      deep (vessels) 451.19
        specified vessel NEC 451.19
      superficial (vessels) 451.0
        femoral vein 451.11
    lower extremity 451.2
      deep (vessels) 451.19
        femoral vein 451.11
        specified vessel NEC
          451.19
      superficial (vessels) 451.0
  ulnar vein 451.83
  umbilicus 451.89
  upper extremity - *see* Phlebitis, arm
    deep (veins) 451.83
      brachial vein 451.83
      radial vein 451.83
      ulnar vein 451.83
    superficial (veins) 451.82
      antecubital vein 451.82
      basilic vein 451.82
      cephalic vein 451.82
  uterus (septic) (*see also* Endometritis)
      615.9
  varicose (leg) (lower extremity)
      (*see also* Varicose, vein)
      454.1
Phlebofibrosis 459.89
Phleboliths 459.89
Phlebosclerosis 459.89
Phlebothrombosis - *see* Thrombosis
Phlebotomus fever 066.0
Phlegm, choked on 933.1

Phlegmasia
  alba dolens (deep vessels) 451.19
    complicating pregnancy 671.3●
    nonpuerperal 451.19
    puerperal, postpartum, childbirth
      671.4●
  cerulea dolens 451.19
Phlegmon (*see also* Abscess) 682.9
  erysipelatous (*see also* Erysipelas) 035
  iliac 682.2
  fossa 540.1
  throat 478.29
Phlegmonous - *see* condition
Phlyctenulosis (allergic)
    (keratoconjunctivitis)
    (nontuberculous) 370.31
  cornea 370.31
    with ulcer (*see also* Ulcer, cornea)
      370.00
  tuberculous (*see also* Tuberculosis)
      017.3● [370.31]
Phobia, phobic (reaction) 300.20
  animal 300.29
  isolated NEC 300.29
  obsessional 300.3
  simple NEC 300.29
  social 300.23
  specified NEC 300.29
  state 300.20
Phocas' disease 610.1
Phocomelia 755.4
  lower limb 755.32
    complete 755.33
    distal 755.35
    proximal 755.34
  upper limb 755.22
    complete 755.23
    distal 755.25
    proximal 755.24
Phoria (*see also* Heterophoria) 378.40
Phosphate-losing tubular disorder 588.0
Phosphatemia 275.3
Phosphaturia 275.3
Photoallergic response 692.72
Photocoproporphyria 277.1
Photodermatitis (sun) 692.72
  light other than sun 692.82
Photokeratitis 370.24
Photo-ophthalmia 370.24
Photophobia 368.13
Photopsia 368.15
Photoretinitis 363.31
Photoretinopathy 363.31
Photosensitiveness (sun) 692.72
  light other than sun 692.82
Photosensitization skin (sun) 692.72
  light other than sun 692.82
Phototoxic response 692.72
Phrenitis 323.9
Phrynoderma 264.8
Phthiriasis (pubis) (any site) 132.2
  with any infestation classifiable to 132.0
    and 132.1 132.3
Phthirus infestation - *see* Phthiriasis
Phthisis (*see also* Tuberculosis) 011.9●
  bulbi (infectional) 360.41
  colliers' 011.4●
  cornea 371.05
  eyeball (due to infection) 360.41
  millstone makers' 011.4●
  miners' 011.4●
  potters' 011.4●
  sandblasters' 011.4●
  stonemasons' 011.4●

◀ New   ◀||||| Revised   ~~deleted~~ Deleted   ● Use Additional Digit(s)   ▨ Omit code

Phycomycosis 117.7
Physalopteriasis 127.7
Physical therapy NEC V57.1
  breathing exercises V57.0
Physiological cup, optic papilla
  borderline, glaucoma suspect 365.00
  enlarged 377.14
  glaucomatous 377.14
Phytobezoar 938
  intestine 936
  stomach 935.2
Pian (see also Yaws) 102.9
Pianoma 102.1
Piarhemia, piarrhemia (see also
    Hyperlipemia) 272.4
  bilharziasis 120.9
Pica 307.52
  hysterical 300.11
Pick's
  cerebral atrophy 331.11
    with dementia
      with behavioral disturbance
        331.11 [294.11]
      without behavioral disturbance
        331.11 [294.10]
  disease
    brain 331.11
      dementia in
        with behavioral disturbance
          331.11 [294.11]
        without behavioral
          disturbance 331.11
          [294.10]
    lipid histiocytosis 272.7
    liver (pericardial pseudocirrhosis of
      liver) 423.2
    pericardium (pericardial
      pseudocirrhosis of liver)
      423.2
  polyserositis (pericardial
    pseudocirrhosis of liver) 423.2
  syndrome
    heart (pericardial pseudocirrhosis of
      liver) 423.2
    liver (pericardial pseudocirrhosis of
      liver) 423.2
  tubular adenoma (M8640/0)
    specified site - see Neoplasm, by site,
      benign
    unspecified site
      female 220
      male 222.0
Pick-Herxheimer syndrome (diffuse
    idiopathic cutaneous atrophy) 701.8
Pick-Niemann disease (lipid
    histiocytosis) 272.7
Pickwickian syndrome (cardiopulmonary
    obesity) 278.03 ◀▥
Piebaldism, classic 709.09
Piedra 111.2
  beard 111.2
    black 111.3
    white 111.2
  black 111.3
  scalp 111.3
    black 111.3
    white 111.2
  white 111.2
Pierre Marie's syndrome (pulmonary
    hypertrophic osteoarthropathy)
    731.2
Pierre Marie-Bamberger syndrome
    (hypertrophic pulmonary
    osteoarthropathy) 731.2

Pierre Mauriac's syndrome (diabetes-
    dwarfism-obesity) 258.1
Pierre Robin deformity or syndrome
    (congenital) 756.0
Pierson's disease or osteochondrosis 732.1
Pigeon
  breast or chest (acquired) 738.3
    congenital 754.82
    rachitic (see also Rickets) 268.0
  breeders' disease or lung 495.2
  fanciers' disease or lung 495.2
  toe 735.8
Pigmentation (abnormal) 709.00
  anomalies NEC 709.00
    congenital 757.33
    specified NEC 709.09
  conjunctiva 372.55
  cornea 371.10
    anterior 371.11
    posterior 371.13
    stromal 371.12
  lids (congenital) 757.33
    acquired 374.52
  limbus corneae 371.10
  metals 709.00
  optic papilla, congenital 743.57
  retina (congenital) (grouped) (nevoid)
    743.53
    acquired 362.74
  scrotum, congenital 757.33
Piles - see Hemorrhoids
Pili
  annulati or torti (congenital) 757.4
  incarnati 704.8
Pill roller hand (intrinsic) 736.09
Pilomatrixoma (M8110/0) - see Neoplasm,
    skin, benign
Pilonidal - see condition
Pimple 709.8
PIN I (prostatic intraepithelial
    neoplasia I) 602.3
PIN II (prostatic intraepithelial
    neoplasia II) 602.3
PIN III (prostatic intraepithelial
    neoplasia III) 233.4
Pinched nerve - see Neuropathy,
    entrapment
Pineal body or gland - see condition
Pinealoblastoma (M9362/3) 194.4
Pinealoma (M9360/1) 237.1
  malignant (M9360/3) 194.4
Pineoblastoma (M9362/3) 194.4
Pineocytoma (M9361/1) 237.1
Pinguecula 372.51
Pingueculitis 372.34
Pinhole meatus (see also Stricture, urethra)
    598.9
Pink
  disease 985.0
  eye 372.03
  puffer 492.8
Pinkus' disease (lichen nitidus) 697.1
Pinpoint
  meatus (see also Stricture, urethra)
    598.9
  os (uteri) (see also Stricture, cervix)
    622.4
Pinselhaare (congenital) 757.4
Pinta 103.9
  cardiovascular lesions 103.2
  chancre (primary) 103.0
  erythematous plaques 103.1
  hyperchromic lesions 103.1
  hyperkeratosis 103.1

Pinta (Continued)
  lesions 103.9
    cardiovascular 103.2
    hyperchromic 103.1
    intermediate 103.1
    late 103.2
    mixed 103.3
    primary 103.0
    skin (achromic) (cicatricial)
      (dyschromic) 103.2
      hyperchromic 103.1
      mixed (achromic and
        hyperchromic) 103.3
  papule (primary) 103.0
  skin lesions (achromic) (cicatricial)
    (dyschromic) 103.2
    hyperchromic 103.1
    mixed (achromic and hyperchromic)
      103.3
  vitiligo 103.2
Pintid 103.0
Pinworms (disease) (infection)
    (infestation) 127.4
Piry fever 066.8
Pistol wound - see Gunshot wound
Pit, lip (mucus), congenital 750.25
Pitchers' elbow 718.82
Pithecoid pelvis 755.69
  with disproportion (fetopelvic)
    653.2●
    affecting fetus or newborn 763.1
    causing obstructed labor 660.1●
Pithiatism 300.11
Pitted - see also Pitting
  teeth 520.4
Pitting (edema) (see also Edema) 782.3
  lip 782.3
  nail 703.8
    congenital 757.5
Pituitary gland - see condition
Pituitary snuff-takers' disease 495.8
Pityriasis 696.5
  alba 696.5
  capitis 690.11
  circinata (et maculata) 696.3
  Hebra's (exfoliative dermatitis) 695.89
  lichenoides et varioliformis 696.2
  maculata (et circinata) 696.3
  nigra 111.1
  pilaris 757.39
    acquired 701.1
    Hebra's 696.4
  rosea 696.3
  rotunda 696.3
  rubra (Hebra) 695.89
    pilaris 696.4
  sicca 690.18
  simplex 690.18
  specified type NEC 696.5
  streptogenes 696.5
  versicolor 111.0
    scrotal 111.0
Placenta, placental
  ablatio 641.2●
    affecting fetus or newborn 762.1
  abnormal, abnormality 656.7●
    with hemorrhage 641.8●
      affecting fetus or newborn 762.1
    affecting fetus or newborn 762.2
  abruptio 641.2●
    affecting fetus or newborn 762.1
  accessory lobe - see Placenta, abnormal
  accreta (without hemorrhage) 667.0●
    with hemorrhage 666.0●

Placenta, placental (Continued)
 adherent (without hemorrhage) 667.0●
  with hemorrhage 666.0●
 apoplexy - see Placenta, separation
 battledore - see Placenta, abnormal
 bilobate - see Placenta, abnormal
 bipartita - see Placenta, abnormal
 carneous mole 631
 centralis - see Placenta, previa
 circumvallata - see Placenta, abnormal
 cyst (amniotic) - see Placenta, abnormal
 deficiency - see Placenta, insufficiency
 degeneration - see Placenta,
   insufficiency
 detachment (partial) (premature) (with
   hemorrhage) 641.2●
  affecting fetus or newborn 762.1
 dimidiata - see Placenta, abnormal
 disease 656.7●
  affecting fetus or newborn 762.2
 duplex - see Placenta, abnormal
 dysfunction - see Placenta,
   insufficiency
 fenestrata - see Placenta, abnormal
 fibrosis - see Placenta, abnormal
 fleshy mole 631
 hematoma - see Placenta, abnormal
 hemorrhage NEC - see Placenta,
   separation
 hormone disturbance or malfunction -
   see Placenta, abnormal
 hyperplasia - see Placenta, abnormal
 increta (without hemorrhage) 667.0●
  with hemorrhage 666.0●
 infarction 656.7●
  affecting fetus or newborn 762.2
 insertion, vicious - see Placenta, previa
 insufficiency
  affecting
    fetus or newborn 762.2
    management of pregnancy
     656.5●
 lateral - see Placenta, previa
 low implantation or insertion - see
   Placenta, previa
 low-lying - see Placenta, previa
 malformation - see Placenta, abnormal
 malposition - see Placenta, previa
 marginalis, marginata - see Placenta,
   previa
 marginal sinus (hemorrhage) (rupture)
   641.2●
  affecting fetus or newborn 762.1
 membranacea - see Placenta, abnormal
 multilobed - see Placenta, abnormal
 multipartita - see Placenta, abnormal
 necrosis - see Placenta, abnormal
 percreta (without hemorrhage) 667.0●
  with hemorrhage 666.0●
 polyp 674.4●
 previa (central) (centralis) (complete)
   (lateral) (marginal) (marginalis)
   (partial) (partialis) (total) (with
   hemorrhage) 641.1●
  affecting fetus or newborn 762.0
  noted
    before labor, without hemorrhage
     (with cesarean delivery)
     641.0●
    during pregnancy (without
     hemorrhage) 641.0●
   without hemorrhage (before labor
    and delivery) (during
    pregnancy) 641.0●

Placenta, placental (Continued)
 retention (with hemorrhage) 666.0●
  fragments, complicating
    puerperium (delayed
     hemorrhage) 666.2●
   without hemorrhage 667.1●
  postpartum, puerperal 666.2●
   without hemorrhage 667.0●
 separation (normally implanted)
   (partial) (premature) (with
   hemorrhage) 641.2●
  affecting fetus or newborn 762.1
 septuplex - see Placenta, abnormal
 small - see Placenta, insufficiency
 softening (premature) - see Placenta,
   abnormal
 spuria - see Placenta, abnormal
 succenturiata - see Placenta, abnormal
 syphilitic 095.8
 transfusion syndromes 762.3
 transmission of chemical substance -
   see Absorption, chemical, through
   placenta
 trapped (with hemorrhage) 666.0●
  without hemorrhage 667.0●
 trilobate - see Placenta, abnormal
 tripartita - see Placenta, abnormal
 triplex - see Placenta, abnormal
 varicose vessel - see Placenta, abnormal
 vicious insertion - see Placenta, previa
Placentitis
 affecting fetus or newborn 762.7
 complicating pregnancy 658.4●
Plagiocephaly (skull) 754.0
Plague 020.9
 abortive 020.8
 ambulatory 020.8
 bubonic 020.0
 cellulocutaneous 020.1
 lymphatic gland 020.0
 pneumonic 020.5
  primary 020.3
  secondary 020.4
 pulmonary - see Plague, pneumonic
 pulmonic - see Plague, pneumonic
 septicemic 020.2
 tonsillar 020.9
  septicemic 020.2
 vaccination, prophylactic (against)
   V03.3
Planning, family V25.09
 contraception V25.9
 natural
  procreative V26.41
  to avoid pregnancy V25.04
 procreation V26.49
  natural V26.41
Plaque
 artery, arterial - see Arteriosclerosis
 calcareous - see Calcification
 Hollenhorst's (retinal) 362.33
 tongue 528.6
Plasma cell myeloma 203.0●
Plasmacytoma, plasmocytoma (solitary)
   (M9731/1) 238.6
 benign (M9731/0) - see Neoplasm, by
   site, benign
 malignant (M9731/3) 203.8●
Plasmacytopenia 288.59
Plasmacytosis 288.64
Plaster ulcer (see also Ulcer, pressure)
   707.00
Plateau iris syndrome 364.82
Platybasia 756.0

Platyonychia (congenital) 757.5
 acquired 703.8
Platypelloid pelvis 738.6
 with disproportion (fetopelvic) 653.2●
  affecting fetus or newborn 763.1
  causing obstructed labor 660.1●
   affecting fetus or newborn 763.1
 congenital 755.69
Platyspondylia 756.19
Plethora 782.62
 newborn 776.4
Pleura, pleural - see condition
Pleuralgia 786.52
Pleurisy (acute) (adhesive) (chronic)
   (costal) (diaphragmatic) (double)
   (dry) (fetid) (fibrinous) (fibrous)
   (interlobar) (latent) (lung) (old)
   (plastic) (primary) (residual) (sicca)
   (sterile) (subacute) (unresolved)
   (with adherent pleura) 511.0
 with
  effusion (without mention of cause)
    511.9
   bacterial, nontuberculous 511.1
   nontuberculous NEC 511.9
    bacterial 511.1
   pneumococcal 511.1
   specified type NEC 511.89
   staphylococcal 511.1
   streptococcal 511.1
   tuberculous (see also Tuberculosis,
     pleura) 012.0●
    primary, progressive 010.1●
  influenza, flu, or grippe (see also
    Influenza) 487.1 ◀▥
  tuberculosis - see Pleurisy, tuberculous
 encysted 511.89
 exudative (see also Pleurisy, with
   effusion) 511.9
  bacterial, nontuberculous 511.1
 fibrinopurulent 510.9
  with fistula 510.0
 fibropurulent 510.9
  with fistula 510.0
 hemorrhagic 511.89
 influenzal (see also Influenza) 487.1 ◀▥
 pneumococcal 511.0
  with effusion 511.1
 purulent 510.9
  with fistula 510.0
 septic 510.9
  with fistula 510.0
 serofibrinous (see also Pleurisy, with
   effusion) 511.9
  bacterial, nontuberculous 511.1
 seropurulent 510.9
  with fistula 510.0
 serous (see also Pleurisy, with effusion)
   511.9
  bacterial, nontuberculous 511.1
 staphylococcal 511.0
  with effusion 511.1
 streptococcal 511.0
  with effusion 511.1
 suppurative 510.9
  with fistula 510.0
 traumatic (post) (current) 862.29
  with open wound into cavity 862.39
 tuberculous (with effusion) (see also
   Tuberculosis, pleura) 012.0●
  primary, progressive 010.1●
Pleuritis sicca - see Pleurisy
Pleurobronchopneumonia (see also
   Pneumonia, broncho-) 485

Pleurodynia 786.52
  epidemic 074.1
  viral 074.1
Pleurohepatitis 573.8
Pleuropericarditis (*see also* Pericarditis)
  423.9
  acute 420.90
Pleuropneumonia (acute) (bilateral)
  (double) (septic) (*see also*
  Pneumonia) 486
  chronic (*see also* Fibrosis, lung) 515
Pleurorrhea (*see also* Hydrothorax)
  511.89
Plexitis, brachial 353.0
Plica
  knee 727.83
  polonica 132.0
  tonsil 474.8
Plicae dysphonia ventricularis 784.49
Plicated tongue 529.5
  congenital 750.13
Plug
  bronchus NEC 519.19
  meconium (newborn) NEC 777.1
  mucus - *see* Mucus, plug
Plumbism 984.9
  specified type of lead - *see* Table of
    Drugs and Chemicals
Plummer's disease (toxic nodular goiter)
  242.3●
Plummer-Vinson syndrome (sideropenic
  dysphagia) 280.8
Pluricarential syndrome of infancy 260
Plurideficiency syndrome of infancy 260
Plus (and minus) hand (intrinsic) 736.09
PMDD (premenstrual dysphoric
  disorder) 625.4
PMS 625.4
Pneumathemia - *see* Air, embolism, by type
Pneumatic drill or hammer disease 994.9
Pneumatocele (lung) 518.89
  intracranial 348.89
  tension 492.0
Pneumatosis
  cystoides intestinalis 569.89
  peritonei 568.89
  pulmonum 492.8
Pneumaturia 599.84
Pneumoblastoma (M8981/3) - *see*
  Neoplasm, lung, malignant
Pneumocephalus 348.89
Pneumococcemia 038.2
Pneumococcus, pneumococcal - *see*
  condition
Pneumoconiosis (due to) (inhalation of)
  505
  aluminum 503
  asbestos 501
  bagasse 495.1
  bauxite 503
  beryllium 503
  carbon electrode makers' 503
  coal
    miners' (simple) 500
    workers' (simple) 500
  cotton dust 504
  diatomite fibrosis 502
  dust NEC 504
    inorganic 503
    lime 502
    marble 502
    organic NEC 504
  fumes or vapors (from silo) 506.9
  graphite 503

Pneumoconiosis (*Continued*)
  hard metal 503
  mica 502
  moldy hay 495.0
  rheumatoid 714.81
  silica NEC 502
    and carbon 500
  silicate NEC 502
  talc 502
Pneumocystis carinii pneumonia 136.3
Pneumocystis jiroveci pneumonia 136.3
Pneumocystosis 136.3
  with pneumonia 136.3
Pneumoenteritis 025
Pneumohemopericardium (*see also*
  Pericarditis) 423.9
Pneumohemothorax (*see also*
  Hemothorax) 511.89
  traumatic 860.4
    with open wound into thorax
      860.5
Pneumohydropericardium (*see also*
  Pericarditis) 423.9
Pneumohydrothorax (*see also*
  Hydrothorax) 511.89
Pneumomediastinum 518.1
  congenital 770.2
  fetus or newborn 770.2
Pneumomycosis 117.9
Pneumonia (acute) (Alpenstich) (benign)
  (bilateral) (brain) (cerebral)
  (circumscribed) (congestive)
  (creeping) (delayed resolution)
  (double) (epidemic) (fever) (flash)
  (fulminant) (fungoid)
  (granulomatous) (hemorrhagic)
  (incipient) (infantile) (infectious)
  (infiltration) (insular) (intermittent)
  (latent) (lobe) (migratory) (newborn)
  (organized) (overwhelming)
  (primary) (progressive)
  (pseudolobar) (purulent) (resolved)
  (secondary) (senile) (septic)
  (suppurative) (terminal) (true)
  (unresolved) (vesicular) 486
  with influenza, flu, or grippe 487.0
    due to ◄
      identified (virus) ◄
        avian 488.01 ◄
        novel H1N1 488.11 ◄
  adenoviral 480.0
  adynamic 514
  alba 090.0
  allergic 518.3
  alveolar - *see* Pneumonia, lobar
  anaerobes 482.81
  anthrax 022.1 [484.5]
  apex, apical - *see* Pneumonia, lobar
  ascaris 127.0 [484.8]
  aspiration 507.0
    due to
      aspiration of microorganisms
        bacterial 482.9
          specified type NEC 482.89
        specified organism NEC 483.8
          bacterial NEC 482.89
        viral 480.9
          specified type NEC 480.8
      food (regurgitated) 507.0
      gastric secretions 507.0
      milk 507.0
      oils, essences 507.1
      solids, liquids NEC 507.8
      vomitus 507.0

Pneumonia (*Continued*)
  aspiration (*Continued*)
    fetal 770.18
      due to
        blood 770.16
        clear amniotic fluid 770.14
        meconium 770.12
        postnatal stomach contents
          770.86
    newborn 770.18
      due to
        blood 770.16
        clear amniotic fluid 770.14
        meconium 770.12
        postnatal stomach contents
          770.86
  asthenic 514
  atypical (disseminated) (focal)
    (primary) 486
    with influenza (*see also* Influenza)
      487.0 ◄▥
  bacillus 482.9
    specified type NEC 482.89
  bacterial 482.9
    specified type NEC 482.89
  Bacteroides (fragilis) (oralis)
    (melaninogenicus) 482.81
  basal, basic, basilar - *see* Pneumonia, by
    type ◄▥
  bronchiolitis obliterans organized
    (BOOP) 516.8
  broncho-, bronchial (confluent)
    (croupous) (diffuse) (disseminated)
    (hemorrhagic) (involving lobes)
    (lobar) (terminal) 485
    with influenza 487.0
      due to ◄
        identified (virus) ◄
          avian 488.01 ◄
          novel H1N1 488.11 ◄
  allergic 518.3
  aspiration (*see also* Pneumonia,
    aspiration) 507.0
  bacterial 482.9
    specified type NEC 482.89
  capillary 466.19
    with bronchospasm or
      obstruction 466.19
  chronic (*see also* Fibrosis, lung) 515
  congenital (infective) 770.0
  diplococcal 481
  Eaton's agent 483.0
  Escherichia coli (E. coli) 482.82
  Friedländer's bacillus 482.0
  Hemophilus influenzae 482.2
  hiberno-vernal 083.0 [484.8]
  hypostatic 514
  influenzal (*see also* Influenza) 487.0 ◄▥
  inhalation (*see also* Pneumonia,
    aspiration) 507.0
    due to fumes or vapors
      (chemical) 506.0
  Klebsiella 482.0
  lipid 507.1
    endogenous 516.8
  Mycoplasma (pneumoniae) 483.0
  ornithosis 073.0
  pleuropneumonia-like organisms
    (PPLO) 483.0
  pneumococcal 481
  Proteus 482.83
  Pseudomonas 482.1
  specified organism NEC 483.8
    bacterial NEC 482.89

Pneumonia *(Continued)*
  broncho-, bronchial *(Continued)*
    staphylococcal 482.40
      aureus 482.41
        methicillin
          resistant (MRSA) 482.42
          susceptible (MSSA) 482.41
      specified type NEC 482.49
    streptococcal - *see* Pneumonia,
      streptococcal
    typhoid 002.0 *[484.8]*
    viral, virus *(see also* Pneumonia,
      viral) 480.9
  Butyrivibrio (fibriosolvens) 482.81
  Candida 112.4
  capillary 466.19
    with bronchospasm or obstruction
      466.19
  caseous *(see also* Tuberculosis) 011.6●
  catarrhal - *see* Pneumonia, broncho-
  central - *see* Pneumonia, lobar
  Chlamydia, chlamydial 483.1
    pneumoniae 483.1
    psittaci 073.0
    specified type NEC 483.1
    trachomatis 483.1
  cholesterol 516.8
  chronic *(see also* Fibrosis, lung) 515
  cirrhotic (chronic) *(see also* Fibrosis,
    lung) 515
  Clostridium (haemolyticum) (novyi)
    NEC 482.81
  confluent - *see* Pneumonia, broncho-
  congenital (infective) 770.0
    aspiration 770.18
  croupous - *see* Pneumonia, lobar
  cryptogenic organizing 516.8 ◀
  cytomegalic inclusion 078.5 *[484.1]*
  deglutition *(see also* Pneumonia,
    aspiration) 507.0
  desquamative interstitial 516.8
  diffuse - *see* Pneumonia, broncho-
  diplococcal, diplococcus (broncho-)
    (lobar) 481
  disseminated (focal) - *see* Pneumonia,
    broncho-
  due to
    adenovirus 480.0
    anaerobes 482.81
    Bacterium anitratum 482.83
    Chlamydia, chlamydial 483.1
      pneumoniae 483.1
      psittaci 073.0
      specified type NEC 483.1
      trachomatis 483.1
    coccidioidomycosis 114.0
    Diplococcus (pneumoniae) 481
    Eaton's agent 483.0
    Escherichia coli (E. coli) 482.82
    Friedländer's bacillus 482.0
    fumes or vapors (chemical)
      (inhalation) 506.0
    fungus NEC 117.9 *[484.7]*
      coccidioidomycosis 114.0
    Hemophilus influenzae (H.
      influenzae) 482.2
    Herellea 482.83
    influenza *(see also* Influenza) 487.0 ◀ⅲ
    Klebsiella pneumoniae 482.0
    Mycoplasma (pneumoniae) 483.0
    parainfluenza virus 480.2
    pleuropneumonia-like organism
      (PPLO) 483.0
    Pneumococcus 481
    Pneumocystis carinii 136.3

Pneumonia *(Continued)*
  due to *(Continued)*
    Pneumocystis jiroveci 136.3
    Proteus 482.83
    Pseudomonas 482.1
    respiratory syncytial virus 480.1
    rickettsia 083.9 *[484.8]*
    SARS-associated coronavirus 480.3
    specified
      bacteria NEC 482.89
      organism NEC 483.8
      virus NEC 480.8
    Staphylococcus 482.40
      aureus 482.41
        methicillin
          resistant (MRSA) 482.42
          susceptible (MSSA) 482.41
      specified type NEC 482.49
    Streptococcus - *see also* Pneumonia,
      streptococcal
      pneumoniae 481
    virus *(see also* Pneumonia, viral) 480.9
      SARS-associated coronavirus 480.3
  Eaton's agent 483.0
  embolic, embolism *(see* Embolism,
    pulmonary)
  eosinophilic 518.3
  Escherichia coli (E. coli) 482.82
  Eubacterium 482.81
  fibrinous - *see* Pneumonia, lobar
  fibroid (chronic) *(see also* Fibrosis, lung)
    515
  fibrous *(see also* Fibrosis, lung) 515
  Friedländer's bacillus 482.0
  fusobacterium (nucleatum) 482.81
  gangrenous 513.0
  giant cell *(see also* Pneumonia, viral) 480.9
  gram-negative bacteria NEC 482.83
    anaerobic 482.81
  grippal *(see also* Influenza) 487.0 ◀ⅲ
  Hemophilus influenzae (bronchial)
    (lobar) 482.2
  hypostatic (broncho-) (lobar) 514
  in
    actinomycosis 039.1
    anthrax 022.1 *[484.5]*
    aspergillosis 117.3 *[484.6]*
    candidiasis 112.4
    coccidioidomycosis 114.0
    cytomegalic inclusion disease 078.5
      [484.1]
    histoplasmosis *(see also*
      Histoplasmosis) 115.95
    infectious disease NEC 136.9 *[484.8]*
    measles 055.1
    mycosis, systemic NEC 117.9 *[484.7]*
    nocardiasis, nocardiosis 039.1
    ornithosis 073.0
    pneumocystosis 136.3
    psittacosis 073.0
    Q fever 083.0 *[484.8]*
    salmonellosis 003.22
    toxoplasmosis 130.4
    tularemia 021.2
    typhoid (fever) 002.0 *[484.8]*
    varicella 052.1
    whooping cough *(see also* Whooping
      cough) 033.9 *[484.3]*
  infective, acquired prenatally 770.0
  influenzal (broncho) (lobar) (virus) *(see*
    also Influenza) 487.0 ◀ⅲ
  inhalation *(see also* Pneumonia,
    aspiration) 507.0
    fumes or vapors (chemical) 506.0

Pneumonia *(Continued)*
  interstitial 516.8
    with influenzal *(see also* Influenza)
      487.0 ◀ⅲ
    acute 136.3
    chronic *(see also* Fibrosis, lung) 515
    desquamative 516.8
    hypostatic 514
    lipoid 507.1
    lymphoid 516.8
    plasma cell 136.3
    Pseudomonas 482.1
  intrauterine (infective) 770.0
    aspiration 770.18
    blood 770.16
    clear amniotic fluid 770.14
    meconium 770.12
    postnatal stomach contents 770.86
  Klebsiella pneumoniae 482.0
  Legionnaires' 482.84
  lipid, lipoid (exogenous) (interstitial)
    507.1
    endogenous 516.8
  lobar (diplococcal) (disseminated)
    (double) (interstitial)
    (pneumococcal, any type) 481
    with influenza *(see also* Influenza)
      487.0 ◀ⅲ
    bacterial 482.9
      specified type NEC 482.89
    chronic *(see also* Fibrosis, lung) 515
    Escherichia coli (E. coli) 482.82
    Friedländer's bacillus 482.0
    Hemophilus influenzae
      (H. influenzae) 482.2
    hypostatic 514
    influenzal *(see also* Influenza) 487.0 ◀ⅲ
    Klebsiella 482.0
    ornithosis 073.0
    Proteus 482.83
    Pseudomonas 482.1
    psittacosis 073.0
    specified organism NEC 483.8
      bacterial NEC 482.89
    staphylococcal 482.40
      aureus 482.41
        methicillin
          resistant (MRSA) 482.42
          susceptible (MSSA) 482.41
      specified type NEC 482.49
    streptococcal - *see* Pneumonia,
      streptococcal
    viral, virus *(see also* Pneumonia,
      viral) 480.9
  lobular (confluent) - *see* Pneumonia,
    broncho-
  Löffler's 518.3
  massive - *see* Pneumonia, lobar
  meconium aspiration 770.12
  metastatic NEC 038.8 *[484.8]*
  methicillin resistant Staphylococcus
    aureus (MRSA) 482.42
  methicillin susceptible Staphylococcus
    aureus (MSSA) 482.41
  MRSA (methicillin resistant
    Staphylococcus aureus) 482.42
  MSSA (methicillin susceptible
    Staphylococcus aureus) 482.41
  multilobar - *see* Pneumonia, by
    type ◀
  Mycoplasma (pneumoniae) 483.0
  necrotic 513.0
  nitrogen dioxide 506.9
  orthostatic 514
  parainfluenza virus 480.2

◀ New   ◀ⅲ Revised   ~~deleted~~ Deleted   ● Use Additional Digit(s)   Omit code

Poisoning *(Continued)*
  Bacillus, B. *(Continued)*
    paratyphosus *(see also* Infection,
      Salmonella) 003.9
    suipestifer *(see also* Infection,
      Salmonella) 003.9
  bacterial toxins NEC 005.9
  berries, noxious 988.2
  blood (general) - *see* Septicemia
  botulism 005.1
  bread, moldy, mouldy - *see* Poisoning,
    food
  Ciguatera 988.0
  damaged meat - *see* Poisoning, food
  death-cap (Amanita phalloides)
    (Amanita verna) 988.1
  decomposed food - *see* Poisoning, food
  diseased food - *see* Poisoning, food
  drug - *see* Table of Drugs and
    Chemicals
  epidemic, fish, meat, or other food - *see*
    Poisoning, food
  fava bean 282.2
  fish (bacterial) - *see also* Poisoning, food
    noxious 988.0
  food (acute) (bacterial) (diseased)
    (infected) NEC 005.9
    due to
      bacillus
        aertrycke *(see also* Poisoning,
          food, due to Salmonella)
          003.9
        botulinus 005.1
        cereus 005.89
        choleraesuis *(see also*
          Poisoning, food, due to
          Salmonella) 003.9
        paratyphosus *(see also*
          Poisoning, food, due to
          Salmonella) 003.9
        suipestifer *(see also* Poisoning,
          food, due to Salmonella)
          003.9
      Clostridium 005.3
        botulinum 005.1
        perfringens 005.2
        welchii 005.2
      Salmonella (aertrycke)
        (callinarum) (choleraesuis)
        (enteritidis) (paratyphi)
        (suipestifer) 003.9
        with
          gastroenteritis 003.0
          localized infection(s) *(see*
            also Infection,
            Salmonella) 003.20
          septicemia 003.1
          specified manifestation
            NEC 003.8
      specified bacterium NEC 005.89
      Staphylococcus 005.0
      Streptococcus 005.89
      Vibrio parahaemolyticus 005.4
      Vibrio vulnificus 005.81
    noxious or naturally toxic 988.0
      berries 988.2
      fish 988.0
      mushroom 988.1
      plants NEC 988.2
  ice cream - *see* Poisoning, food
  ichthyotoxism (bacterial) 005.9
  kreotoxism, food 005.9
  malarial - *see* Malaria
  meat - *see* Poisoning, food

Poisoning *(Continued)*
  mushroom (noxious) 988.1
  mussel - *see also* Poisoning, food
    noxious 988.0
  noxious foodstuffs *(see also* Poisoning,
    food, noxious) 988.9
    specified type NEC 988.8
  plants, noxious 988.2
  pork - *see also* Poisoning, food
    specified NEC 988.8
    Trichinosis 124
  ptomaine - *see* Poisoning, food
  putrefaction, food - *see* Poisoning, food
  radiation 508.0
  Salmonella *(see also* Infection,
    Salmonella) 003.9
  sausage - *see also* Poisoning, food
    Trichinosis 124
  saxitoxin 988.0
  shellfish - *see also* Poisoning, food
    noxious (amnesic) (azaspiracid)
      (diarrheic) (neurotoxic)
      (paralytic) 988.0
  Staphylococcus, food 005.0
  toxic, from disease NEC 799.89
  truffles - *see* Poisoning, food
  uremic - *see* Uremia
  uric acid 274.9
  water 276.69 ◀▥

Poison ivy, oak, sumac or other plant
  dermatitis 692.6
Poker spine 720.0
Policeman's disease 729.2
Polioencephalitis (acute) (bulbar) *(see also*
  Poliomyelitis, bulbar) 045.0 ●
  inferior 335.22
  influenzal *(see also* Influenza) 487.8 ◀▥
  superior hemorrhagic (acute)
    (Wernicke's) 265.1
  Wernicke's (superior hemorrhagic)
    265.1
Polioencephalomyelitis (acute) (anterior)
  (bulbar) *(see also* Polioencephalitis)
  045.0 ●
Polioencephalopathy, superior
  hemorrhagic 265.1
  with
    beriberi 265.0
    pellagra 265.2
Poliomeningoencephalitis - *see*
  Meningoencephalitis
Poliomyelitis (acute) (anterior)
  (epidemic) 045.9 ●

> Note: Use the following fifth-digit
> subclassification with category 045:
>
> 0   poliovirus, unspecified type
> 1   poliovirus, type I
> 2   poliovirus, type II
> 3   poliovirus, type III

  with
    paralysis 045.1 ●
      bulbar 045.0 ●
  abortive 045.2 ●
  ascending 045.9 ●
    progressive 045.9 ●
  bulbar 045.0 ●
  cerebral 045.0 ●
  chronic 335.21
  congenital 771.2
  contact V01.2
  deformities 138
  exposure to V01.2

Poliomyelitis *(Continued)*
  late effect 138
  nonepidemic 045.9 ●
  nonparalytic 045.2 ●
  old with deformity 138
  posterior, acute 053.19
  residual 138
  sequelae 138
  spinal, acute 045.9 ●
  syphilitic (chronic) 094.89
  vaccination, prophylactic (against)
    V04.0
Poliosis (eyebrow) (eyelashes)
  704.3
  circumscripta (congenital)
    757.4
    acquired 704.3
  congenital 757.4
Pollakiuria 788.41
  psychogenic 306.53
Pollinosis 477.0
Pollitzer's disease (hidradenitis
  suppurativa) 705.83
Polyadenitis *(see also* Adenitis) 289.3
  malignant 020.0
Polyalgia 729.99
Polyangiitis (essential) 446.0
Polyarteritis (nodosa) (renal) 446.0
Polyarthralgia 719.49
  psychogenic 306.0
Polyarthritis, polyarthropathy NEC
  716.59
  due to or associated with other
    specified conditions - *see*
    Arthritis, due to or associated
    with
  endemic *(see also* Disease, Kaschin-
    Beck) 716.0 ●
  inflammatory 714.9
    specified type NEC 714.89
  juvenile (chronic) 714.30
    acute 714.31
  migratory - *see* Fever, rheumatic
  rheumatic 714.0
    fever (acute) - *see* Fever, rheumatic
Polycarential syndrome of infancy 260
Polychondritis (atrophic) (chronic)
  (relapsing) 733.99
Polycoria 743.46
Polycystic (congenital) (disease) 759.89
  degeneration, kidney - *see* Polycystic,
    kidney
  kidney (congenital) 753.12
    adult type (APKD) 753.13
    autosomal dominant 753.13
    autosomal recessive 753.14
    childhood type (CPKD) 753.14
    infantile type 753.14
  liver 751.62
  lung 518.89
    congenital 748.4
  ovary, ovaries 256.4
  spleen 759.0
Polycythemia (primary) (rubra) (vera)
  (M9950/1) 238.4
  acquired 289.0
  benign 289.0
    familial 289.6
  due to
    donor twin 776.4
    fall in plasma volume 289.0
    high altitude 289.0
    maternal-fetal transfusion 776.4
    stress 289.0

◀ New   ◀▥ Revised   ~~deleted~~ Deleted   ● Use Additional Digit(s)   ▦ Omit code

Polycythemia (Continued)
emotional 289.0
erythropoietin 289.0
familial (benign) 289.6
Gaisböck's (hypertonica) 289.0
high altitude 289.0
hypertonica 289.0
hypoxemic 289.0
neonatorum 776.4
nephrogenous 289.0
relative 289.0
secondary 289.0
spurious 289.0
stress 289.0
Polycytosis cryptogenica 289.0
Polydactylism, polydactyly 755.00
fingers 755.01
toes 755.02
Polydipsia 783.5
Polydystrophic oligophrenia 277.5
Polyembryoma (M9072/3) - see
Neoplasm, by site, malignant
Polygalactia 676.6 ●
Polyglandular
deficiency 258.9
dyscrasia 258.9
dysfunction 258.9
syndrome 258.8
Polyhydramnios (see also Hydramnios)
657 ●
Polymastia 757.6
Polymenorrhea 626.2
Polymicrogyria 742.2
Polymyalgia 725
arteritica 446.5
rheumatica 725
Polymyositis (acute) (chronic)
(hemorrhagic) 710.4
with involvement of
lung 710.4 [517.8]
skin 710.3
ossificans (generalisata) (progressiva)
728.19
Wagner's (dermatomyositis) 710.3
Polyneuritis, polyneuritic (see also
Polyneuropathy) 356.9
alcoholic 357.5
with psychosis 291.1
cranialis 352.6
demyelinating, chronic inflammatory
(CIDP) 357.81
diabetic 250.6 ● [357.2]
due to secondary diabetes 249.6 ●
[357.2]
due to lack of vitamin NEC 269.2
[357.4]
endemic 265.0 [357.4]
erythredema 985.0
febrile 357.0
hereditary ataxic 356.3
idiopathic, acute 357.0
infective (acute) 357.0
nutritional 269.9 [357.4]
postinfectious 357.0
Polyneuropathy (peripheral) 356.9
alcoholic 357.5
amyloid 277.39 [357.4]
arsenical 357.7
critical illness 357.82
demyelinating, chronic inflammatory
(CIDP) 357.81
diabetic 250.6 ● [357.2]
due to secondary diabetes 249.6 ●
[357.2]

Polyneuropathy (Continued)
due to
antitetanus serum 357.6
arsenic 357.7
drug or medicinal substance 357.6
correct substance properly
administered 357.6
overdose or wrong substance
given or taken 977.9
specified drug - see Table of
Drugs and Chemicals
lack of vitamin NEC 269.2 [357.4]
lead 357.7
organophosphate compounds 357.7
pellagra 265.2 [357.4]
porphyria 277.1 [357.4]
serum 357.6
toxic agent NEC 357.7
hereditary 356.0
idiopathic 356.9
progressive 356.4
in
amyloidosis 277.39 [357.4]
avitaminosis 269.2 [357.4]
specified NEC 269.1 [357.4]
beriberi 265.0 [357.4]
collagen vascular disease NEC 710.9
[357.1]
deficiency
B-complex NEC 266.2 [357.4]
vitamin B 266.9 [357.4]
vitamin B₆ 266.1 [357.4]
diabetes 250.6 ● [357.2]
due to secondary diabetes 249.6 ●
[357.2]
diphtheria (see also Diphtheria)
032.89 [357.4]
disseminated lupus erythematosus
710.0 [357.1]
herpes zoster 053.13
hypoglycemia 251.2 [357.4]
malignant neoplasm (M8000/3)
NEC 199.1 [357.3]
mumps 072.72
pellagra 265.2 [357.4]
polyarteritis nodosa 446.0 [357.1]
porphyria 277.1 [357.4]
rheumatoid arthritis 714.0 [357.1]
sarcoidosis 135 [357.4]
uremia 585.9 [357.4]
lead 357.7
nutritional 269.9 [357.4]
specified NEC 269.8 [357.4]
postherpetic 053.13
progressive 356.4
sensory (hereditary) 356.2
specified NEC 356.8
Polyonychia 757.5
Polyopia 368.2
refractive 368.15
Polyorchism, polyorchidism (three testes)
752.89
Polyorrhymenitis (peritoneal) (see also
Polyserositis) 568.82
pericardial 423.2
Polyostotic fibrous dysplasia 756.54
Polyotia 744.1
Polyp, polypus

Note: Polyps of organs or sites that
do not appear in the list below should
be coded to the residual category for
diseases of the organ or site concerned.

Polyp, polypus (Continued)
accessory sinus 471.8
adenoid tissue 471.0
adenomatous (M8210/0) - see also
Neoplasm, by site, benign
adenocarcinoma in (M8210/3) - see
Neoplasm, by site, malignant
carcinoma in (M8210/3) - see
Neoplasm, by site, malignant
multiple (M8221/0) - see Neoplasm,
by site, benign
antrum 471.8
anus, anal (canal) (nonadenomatous)
569.0
adenomatous 211.4
Bartholin's gland 624.6
bladder (M8120/1) 236.7
broad ligament 620.8
cervix (uteri) 622.7
adenomatous 219.0
in pregnancy or childbirth 654.6 ●
affecting fetus or newborn
763.89
causing obstructed labor 660.2 ●
mucous 622.7
nonneoplastic 622.7
choanal 471.0
cholesterol 575.6
clitoris 624.6
colon (M8210/0) (see also Polyp,
adenomatous) 211.3
corpus uteri 621.0
dental 522.0
ear (middle) 385.30
endometrium 621.0
ethmoidal (sinus) 471.8
fallopian tube 620.8
female genital organs NEC 624.8
frontal (sinus) 471.8
gallbladder 575.6
gingiva 523.8
gum 523.8
labia 624.6
larynx (mucous) 478.4
malignant (M8000/3) - see Neoplasm,
by site, malignant
maxillary (sinus) 471.8
middle ear 385.30
myometrium 621.0
nares
anterior 471.9
posterior 471.0
nasal (mucous) 471.9
cavity 471.0
septum 471.9
nasopharyngeal 471.0
neoplastic (M8210/0) - see Neoplasm,
by site, benign
nose (mucous) 471.9
oviduct 620.8
paratubal 620.8
pharynx 478.29
congenital 750.29
placenta, placental 674.4 ●
prostate 600.20
with
other lower urinary tract
symptoms (LUTS) 600.21
urinary
obstruction 600.21
retention 600.21
pudenda 624.6
pulp (dental) 522.0
rectosigmoid 211.4

Polyp, polypus (Continued)
   rectum (nonadenomatous) 569.0
      adenomatous 211.4
   septum (nasal) 471.9
   sinus (accessory) (ethmoidal) (frontal)
      (maxillary) (sphenoidal) 471.8
   sphenoidal (sinus) 471.8
   stomach (M8210/0) 211.1
   tube, fallopian 620.8
   turbinate, mucous membrane 471.8
   ureter 593.89
   urethra 599.3
   uterine
      ligament 620.8
      tube 620.8
   uterus (body) (corpus) (mucous) 621.0
      in pregnancy or childbirth 654.1●
         affecting fetus or newborn 763.89
         causing obstructed labor 660.2●
   vagina 623.7
   vocal cord (mucous) 478.4
   vulva 624.6
Polyphagia 783.6
Polypoid - see condition
Polyposis - see also Polyp
   coli (adenomatous) (M8220/0) 211.3
      adenocarcinoma in (M8220/3) 153.9
      carcinoma in (M8220/3) 153.9
   familial (M8220/0) 211.3
   intestinal (adenomatous) (M8220/0)
      211.3
   multiple (M8221/0) - see Neoplasm, by
      site, benign
Polyradiculitis (acute) 357.0
Polyradiculoneuropathy (acute)
   (segmentally demyelinating) 357.0
Polysarcia 278.00
Polyserositis (peritoneal) 568.82
   due to pericarditis 423.2
   paroxysmal (familial) 277.31
   pericardial 423.2
   periodic (familial) 277.31
   pleural - see Pleurisy
   recurrent 277.31
   tuberculous (see also Tuberculosis,
      polyserositis) 018.9●
Polysialia 527.7
Polysplenia syndrome 759.0
Polythelia 757.6
Polytrichia (see also Hypertrichosis)
   704.1
Polyunguia (congenital) 757.5
   acquired 703.8
Polyuria 788.42
Pompe's disease (glycogenosis II) 271.0
Pompholyx 705.81
Poncet's disease (tuberculous
   rheumatism) (see also Tuberculosis)
   015.9●
Pond fracture - see Fracture, skull, vault
Ponos 085.0
Pons, pontine - see condition
Poor
   aesthetics of existing restoration of
      tooth 525.67
   contractions, labor 661.2●
      affecting fetus or newborn 763.7
   fetal growth NEC 764.9●
      affecting management of pregnancy
        656.5●
   incorporation
      artificial skin graft 996.55
      decellularized allodermis graft
        996.55

Poor (Continued)
   obstetrical history V13.29
      affecting management of current
        pregnancy V23.49
        pre-term labor V23.41
      pre-term labor V13.21
   sucking reflex (newborn) 796.1
   vision NEC 369.9
Poradenitis, nostras 099.1
Porencephaly (congenital)
   (developmental) (true) 742.4
   acquired 348.0
   nondevelopmental 348.0
   traumatic (post) 310.2
Porocephaliasis 134.1
Porokeratosis 757.39
   disseminated superficial actinic (DSAP)
      692.75
Poroma, eccrine (M8402/0) - see
   Neoplasm, skin, benign
Porphyria (acute) (congenital)
   (constitutional) (erythropoietic)
   (familial) (hepatica) (idiopathic)
   (idiosyncratic) (intermittent) (latent)
   (mixed hepatic) (photosensitive)
   (South African genetic) (Swedish)
   277.1
   acquired 277.1
   cutaneatarda
      hereditaria 277.1
      symptomatica 277.1
   due to drugs
      correct substance properly
        administered 277.1
      overdose or wrong substance given
        or taken 977.9
      specified drug - see Table of
        Drugs and Chemicals
   secondary 277.1
   toxic NEC 277.1
   variegata 277.1
Porphyrinuria (acquired) (congenital)
   (secondary) 277.1
Porphyruria (acquired) (congenital) 277.1
Portal - see condition
Port wine nevus or mark 757.32
Posadas-Wernicke disease 114.9
Position
   fetus, abnormal (see also Presentation,
      fetal) 652.9●
   teeth, faulty (see also Anomaly, position
      tooth) 524.30
Positive
   culture (nonspecific) 795.39
      AIDS virus V08
      blood 790.7
      HIV V08
      human immunodeficiency virus V08
      nose 795.39
        Staphylococcus - see Carrier
         (suspected) of,
         Staphylococcus
      skin lesion NEC 795.39
      spinal fluid 792.0
      sputum 795.39
      stool 792.1
      throat 795.39
      urine 791.9
      wound 795.39
   findings, anthrax 795.31
   HIV V08
   human immunodeficiency virus (HIV)
      V08
   PPD 795.5

Positive (Continued)
   serology
      AIDS virus V08
        inconclusive 795.71
      HIV V08
        inconclusive 795.71
      human immunodeficiency virus V08
        inconclusive 795.71
      syphilis 097.1
        with signs or symptoms - see
         Syphilis, by site and stage
        false 795.6
   skin test 795.7
      tuberculin (without active
        tuberculosis) 795.5
      VDRL 097.1
        with signs or symptoms - see
         Syphilis, by site and stage
        false 795.6
      Wassermann reaction 097.1
        false 795.6
Postcardiotomy syndrome 429.4
Postcaval ureter 753.4
Postcholecystectomy syndrome
   576.0
Postclimacteric bleeding 627.1
Postcommissurotomy syndrome
   429.4
Postconcussional syndrome 310.2
Postcontusional syndrome 310.2
Postcricoid region - see condition
Post-dates (pregnancy) - see Pregnancy
Postencephalitic - see also condition
   syndrome 310.8
Posterior - see condition
Posterolateral sclerosis (spinal cord) - see
   Degeneration, combined
Postexanthematous - see condition
Postfebrile - see condition
Postgastrectomy dumping syndrome
   564.2
Posthemiplegic chorea 344.89
Posthemorrhagic anemia (chronic) 280.0
   acute 285.1
   newborn 776.5
Posthepatitis syndrome 780.79
Postherpetic neuralgia (intercostal)
   (syndrome) (zoster) 053.19
   geniculate ganglion 053.11
   ophthalmica 053.19
   trigeminal 053.12
Posthitis 607.1
Postimmunization complication or
   reaction - see Complications,
   vaccination
Postinfectious - see condition
Postinfluenzal syndrome 780.79
Postlaminectomy syndrome 722.80
   cervical, cervicothoracic 722.81
   kyphosis 737.12
   lumbar, lumbosacral 722.83
   thoracic, thoracolumbar 722.82
Postleukotomy syndrome 310.0
Postlobectomy syndrome 310.0
Postmastectomy lymphedema
   (syndrome) 457.0
Postmaturity, postmature (fetus or
   newborn) (gestation period
   over 42 completed weeks)
   766.22
   affecting management of pregnancy
      post-term pregnancy 645.1●
      prolonged pregnancy 645.2●
   syndrome 766.22

◀ New   ◀▦ Revised   ~~deleted~~ Deleted   ● Use Additional Digit(s)   ▨ Omit code

Postmeasles - *see also* condition
 complication 055.8
  specified NEC 055.79
Postmenopausal
 endometrium (atrophic) 627.8
  suppurative (*see also* Endometritis)
   615.9
 hormone replacement therapy
  V07.4
 status (age related) (natural)
  V49.81
Postnasal drip 784.91
Postnatal - *see* condition
Postoperative - *see also* condition
 confusion state 293.9
 psychosis 293.9
 status NEC (*see also* Status (post))
  V45.89
Postpancreatectomy hyperglycemia
 251.3
Postpartum - *see also* condition
 anemia 648.2●
  cardiomyopathy 674.5●
 observation
  immediately after delivery
   V24.0
  routine follow-up V24.2
Postperfusion syndrome NEC
 999.89
 bone marrow 996.85
Postpoliomyelitic - *see* condition
Postsurgery status NEC (*see also* Status
 (post)) V45.89
Post-term (pregnancy) 645.1●
 infant (gestation period over 40
  completed weeks to 42
  completed weeks) 766.21
Post-transplant lymphoproliferative
 disorder (PTLD) 238.77
Posttraumatic - *see* condition
Posttraumatic brain syndrome,
 nonpsychotic 310.2
Post-Traumatic Stress Disorder (PTSD)
 309.81
Post-typhoid abscess 002.0
Postures, hysterical 300.11
Postvaccinal reaction or complication -
 see Complications, vaccination
Postvagotomy syndrome 564.2
Postvalvulotomy syndrome 429.4
Postvasectomy sperm count V25.8
Potain's disease (pulmonary edema)
 514
Potain's syndrome (gastrectasis with
 dyspepsia) 536.1
Pott's
 curvature (spinal) (*see also*
  Tuberculosis) 015.0● [737.43]
 disease or paraplegia (*see also*
  Tuberculosis) 015.0● [730.88]
 fracture (closed) 824.4
  open 824.5
 gangrene 440.24
 osteomyelitis (*see also* Tuberculosis)
  015.0● [730.88]
 spinal curvature (*see also* Tuberculosis)
  015.0● [737.43]
 tumor, puffy (*see also* Osteomyelitis)
  730.2●
Potter's
 asthma 502
 disease 753.0
 facies 754.0
 lung 502

Potter's *(Continued)*
 syndrome (with renal agenesis)
  753.0
Pouch
 bronchus 748.3
 Douglas' - *see* condition
 esophagus, esophageal (congenital)
  750.4
  acquired 530.6
 gastric 537.1
 Hartmann's (abnormal sacculation of
  gallbladder neck) 575.8
  of intestine V44.3
   attention to V55.3
 pharynx, pharyngeal (congenital)
  750.27
Pouchitis 569.71
Poulet's disease 714.2
Poultrymen's itch 133.8
Poverty V60.2
PPE (palmar plantar erythrodysesthesia)
 693.0
Prader-Labhart-Willi-Fanconi syndrome
 (hypogenital dystrophy with
 diabetic tendency) 759.81
Prader-Willi syndrome (hypogenital
 dystrophy with diabetic tendency)
 759.81
Preachers' voice 784.49
Pre-AIDS - *see* Human
 immunodeficiency virus
 (disease) (illness) (infection)
Preauricular appendage 744.1
Prebetalipoproteinemia (acquired)
 (essential) (familial) (hereditary)
 (primary) (secondary) 272.1
 with chylomicronemia 272.3
Precipitate labor 661.3●
 affecting fetus or newborn 763.6
Preclimacteric bleeding 627.0
 menorrhagia 627.0
Precocious
 adrenarche 259.1
 menarche 259.1
 menstruation 259.1 ◄▦
 pubarche 259.1
 puberty NEC 259.1
 sexual development NEC 259.1
 thelarche 259.1
Precocity, sexual (constitutional)
 (cryptogenic) (female) (idiopathic)
 (male) NEC 259.1
 with adrenal hyperplasia 255.2
Precordial pain 786.51
 psychogenic 307.89
Predeciduous teeth 520.2
Prediabetes, prediabetic 790.29
 complicating pregnancy, childbirth, or
  puerperium 648.8●
 fetus or newborn 775.89
Predislocation status of hip, at birth (*see
 also* Subluxation, congenital, hip)
 754.32
Pre-eclampsia (mild) 642.4●
 with pre-existing hypertension 642.7●
 affecting fetus or newborn 760.0
 severe 642.5●
 superimposed on pre-existing
  hypertensive disease 642.7●
Preeruptive color change, teeth, tooth
 520.8
Preexcitation 426.7
 atrioventricular conduction 426.7
 ventricular 426.7

Preglaucoma 365.00
Pregnancy (single) (uterine) (without
 sickness) V22.2

> Note: Use the following fifth-digit
> subclassification with categories
> 640–649, 651–679:
>
> 0 unspecified as to episode of care
> 1 delivered, with or without
>   mention of antepartum
>   condition
> 2 delivered, with mention of
>   postpartum complication
> 3 antepartum condition or
>   complication
> 4 postpartum condition or
>   complication

 abdominal (ectopic) 633.00
  with intrauterine pregnancy 633.01
  affecting fetus or newborn 761.4
 abnormal NEC 646.9●
 ampullar - *see* Pregnancy, tubal
 broad ligament - *see* Pregnancy, cornual
 cervical - *see* Pregnancy, cornual
 chemical 631
 combined (extrauterine and
  intrauterine) - *see* Pregnancy,
  cornual
 complicated (by) 646.9●
  abnormal, abnormality NEC 646.9●
   cervix 654.6●
   cord (umbilical) 663.9●
   glucose tolerance (conditions
    classifiable to 790.21–790.29)
    648.8●
   pelvic organs or tissues NEC
    654.9●
   pelvis (bony) 653.0●
   perineum or vulva 654.8●
   placenta, placental (vessel)
    656.7●
   position
    cervix 654.4●
    placenta 641.1●
     without hemorrhage 641.0●
    uterus 654.4●
   size, fetus 653.5●
   uterus (congenital) 654.0●
  abscess or cellulitis
   bladder 646.6●
   genitourinary tract (conditions
    classifiable to 590, 595,
    597, 599.0, 614.0–614.5,
    614.7–614.9, 615) 646.6●
   kidney 646.6●
   urinary tract NEC 646.6●
  adhesion, pelvic peritoneal 648.9●
  air embolism 673.0●
  albuminuria 646.2●
   with hypertension - *see* Toxemia,
    of pregnancy
  amnionitis 658.4●
  amniotic fluid embolism 673.1●
  anemia (conditions classifiable to
   280–285) 648.2●
  appendicitis 648.9●
  atrophy, yellow (acute) (liver)
   (subacute) 646.7●
  bacilluria, asymptomatic 646.5●
  bacteriuria, asymptomatic 646.5●
  bariatric surgery status 649.2●
  bicornis or bicornuate uterus
   654.0●
  biliary problems 646.8●

Pregnancy (Continued)
  complicated (Continued)
    bone and joint disorders
      (conditions classifiable to
      720–724 or conditions
      affecting lower limbs
      classifiable to 711–719,
      725–738) 648.7●
    breech presentation (buttocks)
      (complete) (frank) 652.2●
      with successful version 652.1●
    cardiovascular disease (conditions
      classifiable to 390–398, 410–
      429) 648.6●
      congenital (conditions classifiable
        to 745–747) 648.5●
    cerebrovascular disorders
      (conditions classifiable to
      430–434, 436–437) 674.0●
    cervicitis (conditions classifiable to
      616.0) 646.6●
    chloasma (gravidarum) 646.8●
    cholelithiasis 646.8●
    chorea (gravidarum) - see Eclampsia,
      pregnancy
    coagulation defect 649.3●
    conjoined twins 678.1●
    contraction, pelvis (general)
      653.1●
      inlet 653.2●
      outlet 653.3●
    convulsions (eclamptic) (uremic)
      642.6●
      with pre-existing hypertension
        642.7●
    current disease or condition
      (nonobstetric)
      abnormal glucose tolerance
        648.8●
      anemia 648.2●
      bone and joint (lower limb)
        648.7●
      cardiovascular 648.6●
        congenital 648.5●
      cerebrovascular 674.0●
      diabetes (conditions
        classifiable to 249 and
        250) 648.0●
      drug dependence 648.3●
      female genital mutilation
        648.9●
      genital organ or tract 646.6●
      gonorrheal 647.1●
      hypertensive 642.2●
        chronic kidney 642.2●
        renal 642.1●
      infectious 647.9●
        specified type NEC 647.8●
      liver 646.7●
      malarial 647.4●
      nutritional deficiency 648.9●
      parasitic NEC 647.8●
      periodontal disease 648.9●
      renal 646.2●
        hypertensive 642.1●
      rubella 647.5●
      specified condition NEC
        648.9●
      syphilitic 647.0●
      thyroid 648.1●
      tuberculous 647.3●
      urinary 646.6●
      venereal 647.2●
      viral NEC 647.6●
    cystitis 646.6●
    cystocele 654.4●

Pregnancy (Continued)
  complicated (Continued)
    death of fetus (near term) 656.4●
      early pregnancy (before 22
        completed weeks'
        gestation) 632
    deciduitis 646.6●
    decreased fetal movements 655.7●
    diabetes (mellitus) (conditions
      classifiable to 249 and 250)
      648.0●
    disorders of liver 646.7●
    displacement, uterus NEC 654.4●
    disproportion - see Disproportion
    double uterus 654.0●
    drug dependence (conditions
      classifiable to 304) 648.3●
    dysplasia, cervix 654.6●
    early onset of delivery
      (spontaneous) 644.2●
    eclampsia, eclamptic (coma)
      (convulsions) (delirium)
      (nephritis) (uremia) 642.6●
      with pre-existing hypertension
        642.7●
    edema 646.1●
      with hypertension - see Toxemia,
        of pregnancy
    effusion, amniotic fluid 658.1●
      delayed delivery following
        658.2●
    embolism
      air 673.0●
      amniotic fluid 673.1●
      blood-clot 673.2●
      cerebral 674.0●
      pulmonary NEC 673.2●
      pyemic 673.3●
      septic 673.3●
    emesis (gravidarum) - see Pregnancy,
      complicated, vomiting
    endometritis (conditions classifiable
      to 615.0–615.9) 670.1●
    decidual 646.6●
    epilepsy 649.4●
    excessive weight gain NEC 646.1●
    face presentation 652.4●
    failure, fetal head to enter pelvic
      brim 652.5●
    false labor (pains) 644.1●
    fatigue 646.8●
    fatty metamorphosis of liver
      646.7●
    female genital mutilation 648.9●
    fetal
      anemia 678.0●
      complications from in utero
        procedure 679.1●
      conjoined twins 678.1●
      death (near term) 656.4●
        early (before 22 completed
        weeks' gestation) 632
      deformity 653.7●
      distress 656.8●
      hematologic conditions
        678.0●
      reduction of multiple fetuses
        reduced to single fetus
        651.7●
      thrombocytopenia 678.0●
      twin to twin transfusion
        678.0●
    fibroid (tumor) (uterus) 654.1●
    footling presentation 652.8●
      with successful version 652.1●
    gallbladder disease 646.8●

Pregnancy (Continued)
  complicated (Continued)
    gastric banding status 649.2●
    gastric bypass status for obesity
      649.2●
    genital herpes (asymptomatic)
      (history of) (inactive) 647.6 ◄
    goiter 648.1●
    gonococcal infection (conditions
      classifiable to 098) 647.1●
    gonorrhea (conditions classifiable to
      098) 647.1●
    hemorrhage 641.9●
      accidental 641.2●
      before 22 completed weeks'
        gestation NEC 640.9●
      cerebrovascular 674.0●
      due to
        afibrinogenemia or other
          coagulation defect
          (conditions classifiable
          to 286.0–286.9) 641.3●
        leiomyoma, uterine 641.8●
        marginal sinus (rupture) 641.2●
        premature separation, placenta
          641.2●
        trauma 641.8●
      early (before 22 completed weeks'
        gestation) 640.9●
      threatened abortion 640.0●
      unavoidable 641.1●
    hepatitis (acute) (malignant)
      (subacute) 646.7●
      viral 647.6●
    herniation of uterus 654.4●
    high head at term 652.5●
    hydatidiform mole (delivered)
      (undelivered) 630
    hydramnios 657●
    hydrocephalic fetus 653.6●
    hydrops amnii 657●
    hydrorrhea 658.1●
    hyperemesis (gravidarum) - see
      Hyperemesis, gravidarum
    hypertension - see Hypertension,
      complicating pregnancy
    hypertensive
      chronic kidney disease 642.2●
      heart and chronic kidney
        disease 642.2●
      heart and renal disease 642.2●
      heart disease 642.2●
      renal disease 642.2●
    hypertensive heart and chronic
      kidney disease 642.2●
    hyperthyroidism 648.1●
    hypothyroidism 648.1●
    hysteralgia 646.8●
    icterus gravis 646.7●
    incarceration, uterus 654.3●
    incompetent cervix (os)
      654.5●
    infection 647.9●
      amniotic fluid 658.4●
      bladder 646.6●
      genital organ (conditions
        classifiable to 614.0–
        614.5, 614.7–614.9, 615)
        646.6●
      kidney (conditions classifiable to
        590.0–590.9) 646.6●
      urinary (tract) 646.6●
        asymptomatic 646.5●
    infective and parasitic diseases NEC
      647.8●

Pregnancy *(Continued)*
  complicated *(Continued)*
    inflammation●
      bladder 646.6●
      genital organ (conditions
          classifiable to 614.0–614.5,
          614.7–614.9, 615) 646.6●
      urinary tract NEC 646.6●
    injury 648.9●
      obstetrical NEC 665.9●
    insufficient weight gain 646.8●
    intrauterine fetal death (near term)
        NEC 656.4●
      early (before 22 completed weeks'
          gestation) 632
    malaria (conditions classifiable to
        084) 647.4●
    malformation, uterus (congenital)
        654.0●
    malnutrition (conditions classifiable
        to 260–269) 648.9●
    malposition
      fetus - *see* Pregnancy,
          complicated,
          malpresentation
      uterus or cervix 654.4●
    malpresentation 652.9●
      with successful version 652.1●
      in multiple gestation 652.6●
      specified type NEC 652.8●
    marginal sinus hemorrhage or
        rupture 641.2●
    maternal complications from in
        utero procedure 679.0●
    maternal drug abuse 648.4●
    maternal obesity syndrome 646.1●
    menstruation 640.8●
    mental disorders (conditions
        classifiable to 290–303, 305.0,
        305.2–305.9, 306–316, 317–319)
        648.4●
    mentum presentation 652.4●
    missed
      abortion 632
      delivery (at or near term) 656.4●
      labor (at or near term) 656.4●
    necrosis
      genital organ or tract (conditions
          classifiable to 614.0–614.5,
          614.7–614.9, 615) 646.6●
      liver (conditions classifiable to
          570) 646.7●
      renal, cortical 646.2●
    nephritis or nephrosis (conditions
        classifiable to 580–589)
        646.2●
      with hypertension 642.1●
    nephropathy NEC 646.2●
    neuritis (peripheral) 646.4●
    nutritional deficiency (conditions
        classifiable to 260–269) 648.9●
    obesity 649.1●
      surgery status 649.2●
    oblique lie or presentation 652.3●
      with successful version 652.1●
    obstetrical trauma NEC 665.9●
    oligohydramnios NEC 658.0●
    onset of contractions before 37
        weeks 644.0●
    oversize fetus 653.5●
    papyraceous fetus 646.0●
    patent cervix 654.5●
    pelvic inflammatory disease
        (conditions classifiable to
        614.0–614.5, 614.7–614.9, 615)
        646.6●

Pregnancy *(Continued)*
  complicated *(Continued)*
    pelvic peritoneal adhesion 648.9●
    placenta, placental
      abnormality 656.7●
      abruptio or ablatio 641.2●
      detachment 641.2●
      disease 656.7●
      infarct 656.7●
      low implantation 641.1●
        without hemorrhage 641.0●
      malformation 656.7●
      malposition 641.1●
        without hemorrhage 641.0●
      marginal sinus hemorrhage
          641.2●
      previa 641.1●
        without hemorrhage 641.0●
      separation (premature)
          (undelivered) 641.2●
    placentitis 658.4●
    pneumonia 648.9 ◀
    polyhydramnios 657●
    postmaturity
      post-term 645.1●
      prolonged 645.2●
    prediabetes 648.8●
    pre-eclampsia (mild) 642.4●
      severe 642.5●
      superimposed on pre-existing
          hypertensive disease 642.7●
    premature rupture of membranes
        658.1●
      with delayed delivery 658.2●
    previous
      infertility V23.0
      in utero procedure during
          previous pregnancy
          V23.86
      nonobstetric condition V23.89
      poor obstetrical history V23.49
      premature delivery V23.41
      trophoblastic disease (conditions
          classifiable to 630) V23.1
    prolapse, uterus 654.4●
    proteinuria (gestational) 646.2●
      with hypertension - *see* Toxemia,
          of pregnancy
    pruritus (neurogenic) 646.8●
    psychosis or psychoneurosis 648.4●
    ptyalism 646.8●
    pyelitis (conditions classifiable to
        590.0–590.9) 646.6●
    renal disease or failure NEC 646.2●
      with secondary hypertension
          642.1●
      hypertensive 642.2●
    retention, retained dead ovum 631●
    retroversion, uterus 654.3●
    Rh immunization, incompatibility,
        or sensitization 656.1●
    rubella (conditions classifiable to
        056) 647.5●
    rupture
      amnion (premature) 658.1●
        with delayed delivery 658.2●
      marginal sinus (hemorrhage)
          641.2●
      membranes (premature) 658.1●
        with delayed delivery 658.2●
      uterus (before onset of labor)
          665.0●
    salivation (excessive) 646.8●
    salpingo-oophoritis (conditions
        classifiable to 614.0–614.2)
        646.6●

Pregnancy *(Continued)*
  complicated *(Continued)*
    septicemia (conditions classifiable to
        038.0–038.9) 647.8●
      postpartum 670.2●
      puerperal 670.2●
      smoking 649.0●
    spasms, uterus (abnormal) 646.8●
    specified condition NEC 646.8●
    spotting 649.5●
    spurious labor pains 644.1●
    status post
      bariatric surgery 649.2●
      gastric banding 649.2●
      gastric bypass for obesity
          649.2●
      obesity surgery 649.2●
    superfecundation 651.9●
    superfetation 651.9●
    syphilis (conditions classifiable to
        090–097) 647.0●
    threatened
      abortion 640.0●
      premature delivery 644.2●
      premature labor 644.0●
    thrombophlebitis (superficial)
        671.2●
      deep 671.3●
      septic 670.3●
    thrombosis 671.2●
      venous (superficial) 671.2●
      deep 671.3●
    thyroid dysfunction (conditions
        classifiable to 240–246) 648.1●
    thyroiditis 648.1●
    thyrotoxicosis 648.1●
    tobacco use disorder 649.0●
    torsion of uterus 654.4●
    toxemia - *see* Toxemia, of pregnancy
    transverse lie or presentation 652.3●
      with successful version 652.1●
    trauma 648.9●
      obstetrical 665.9●
    tuberculosis (conditions classifiable
        to 010–018) 647.3●
    tumor
      cervix 654.6●
      ovary 654.4●
      pelvic organs or tissue NEC
          654.4●
      uterus (body) 654.1●
        cervix 654.6●
      vagina 654.7●
      vulva 654.8●
    unstable lie 652.0●
    uremia - *see* Pregnancy, complicated,
        renal disease
    urethritis 646.6●
    vaginitis or vulvitis (conditions
        classifiable to 616.1) 646.6●
    varicose
      placental vessels 656.7●
      veins (legs) 671.0●
        perineum 671.1●
        vulva 671.1●
    varicosity, labia or vulva 671.1●
    venereal disease NEC (conditions
        classifiable to 099) 647.2●
    venous complication 671.9●
    viral disease NEC (conditions
        classifiable to 042, 050–055,
        057–079, 795.05, 795.15, 796.75)
        647.6●
    vomiting (incoercible) (pernicious)
        (persistent) (uncontrollable)
        (vicious) 643.9●

Pregnancy (Continued)
  complicated (Continued)
    vomiting (Continued)
      due to organic disease or other
        cause 643.8 ●
      early - see Hyperemesis,
        gravidarum
      late (after 22 completed weeks
        gestation) 643.2 ●
    young maternal age 659.8 ●
  complications NEC 646.9 ●
  cornual 633.80
    with intrauterine pregnancy 633.81
    affecting fetus or newborn 761.4
  death, maternal NEC 646.9 ●
  delivered - see Delivery
  ectopic (ruptured) NEC 633.90
    with intrauterine pregnancy 633.91
    abdominal - see Pregnancy,
      abdominal
    affecting fetus or newborn 761.4
    combined (extrauterine and
      intrauterine) - see Pregnancy,
      cornual
    ovarian - see Pregnancy, ovarian
    specified type NEC 633.80
      with intrauterine pregnancy
        633.81
      affecting fetus or newborn 761.4
    tubal - see Pregnancy, tubal
  examination, pregnancy
    negative result V72.41
    not confirmed V72.40
    positive result V72.42
  extrauterine - see Pregnancy, ectopic
  fallopian - see Pregnancy, tubal
  false 300.11
    labor (pains) 644.1 ●
  fatigue 646.8 ●
  illegitimate V61.6
  incidental finding V22.2
  in double uterus 654.0 ●
  interstitial - see Pregnancy, cornual
  intraligamentous - see Pregnancy,
    cornual
  intramural - see Pregnancy, cornual
  intraperitoneal - see Pregnancy,
    abdominal
  isthmian - see Pregnancy, tubal
  management affected by
    abnormal, abnormality
      fetus (suspected) 655.9 ●
        specified NEC 655.8 ●
      placenta 656.7 ●
    advanced maternal age NEC 659.6 ●
      multigravida 659.6 ●
      primigravida 659.5 ●
    antibodies (maternal)
      anti-c 656.1 ●
      anti-d 656.1 ●
      anti-e 656.1 ●
      blood group (ABO) 656.2 ●
        Rh(esus) 656.1 ●
    appendicitis 648.9 ●
    bariatric surgery status 649.2 ●
    coagulation defect 649.3 ●
    elderly multigravida 659.6 ●
    elderly primigravida 659.5 ●
    epilepsy 649.4 ●
    fetal (suspected) ●
      abnormality 655.9 ●
        abdominal 655.8 ●
        acid-base balance 656.8 ●
        cardiovascular 655.8 ●
        facial 655.8 ●
        gastrointestinal 655.8 ●

Pregnancy (Continued)
  management affected by (Continued)
    fetal (Continued)
      abnormality (Continued)
        genitourinary 655.8 ●
        heart rate or rhythm 659.7 ●
        limb 655.8 ●
        specified NEC 655.8 ●
      acidemia 656.3 ●
      anencephaly 655.0 ●
      aneuploidy 655.1 ●
      bradycardia 659.7 ●
      central nervous system
        malformation 655.0 ●
      chromosomal abnormalities
        (conditions classifiable to
        758.0–758.9) 655.1 ●
      damage from
        drugs 655.5 ●
          obstetric, anesthetic, or
            sedative 655.5 ●
        environmental toxins 655.8 ●
        intrauterine contraceptive
          device 655.8 ●
        maternal
          alcohol addiction 655.4 ●
          disease NEC 655.4 ●
          drug use 655.5 ●
          listeriosis 655.4 ●
          rubella 655.3 ●
          toxoplasmosis 655.4 ●
          viral infection 655.3 ●
        radiation 655.6 ●
      death (near term) 656.4 ●
        early (before 22 completed
          weeks' gestation) 632
      distress 656.8 ●
      excessive growth 656.6 ●
      growth retardation 656.5 ●
      hereditary disease 655.2 ●
      hydrocephalus 655.0 ●
      intrauterine death 656.4 ●
      poor growth 656.5 ●
      spina bifida (with
        myelomeningocele)
        655.0 ●
    fetal-maternal hemorrhage 656.0 ●
    gastric banding status 649.2 ●
    gastric bypass status for obesity
      649.2 ●
    hereditary disease in family
      (possibly) affecting fetus
      655.2 ●
    incompatibility, blood groups (ABO)
      656.2 ●
      Rh(esus) 656.1 ●
    insufficient prenatal care V23.7
    intrauterine death 656.4 ●
    isoimmunization (ABO) 656.2 ●
      Rh(esus) 656.1 ●
    large-for-dates fetus 656.6 ●
    light-for-dates fetus 656.5 ●
    meconium in liquor 656.8 ●
    mental disorder (conditions
      classifiable to 290–303, 305.0,
      305.2–305.9, 306–316, 317–319)
      648.4 ●
    multiparity (grand) 659.4 ●
    obesity 649.1 ●
      surgery status 649.2 ●
    poor obstetric history V23.49
      pre-term labor V23.41
    postmaturity
      post-term 645.1 ●
      prolonged 645.2 ●
    post-term pregnancy 645.1 ●

Pregnancy (Continued)
  management affected by (Continued)
    previous
      abortion V23.2
        habitual 646.3 ●
      cesarean delivery 654.2 ●
      difficult delivery V23.49
      forceps delivery V23.49
      habitual abortions 646.3 ●
      hemorrhage, antepartum or
        postpartum V23.49
      hydatidiform mole V23.1
      infertility V23.0
      in utero procedure during
        previous pregnancy V23.86
      malignancy NEC V23.89
      nonobstetrical conditions V23.89
      premature delivery V23.41
      recurrent pregnancy loss 646.3 ◄
      trophoblastic disease (conditions
        in 630) V23.1
      vesicular mole V23.1
    prolonged pregnancy 645.2 ●
    recurrent pregnancy loss 646.3 ◄
    small-for-dates fetus 656.5 ●
    smoking 649.0 ●
    spotting 649.5 ●
    suspected conditions not found
      amniotic cavity and membrane
        problem V89.01
      cervical shortening V89.05
      fetal anomaly V89.03
      fetal growth problem V89.04
      oligohydramnios V89.01
      other specified problem NEC
        V89.09
      placental problem V89.02
      polyhydramnios V89.01
    tobacco use disorder 649.0 ●
    venous complication 671.9 ●
    young maternal age 659.8 ●
  maternal death NEC 646.9 ●
  mesometric (mural) - see Pregnancy,
    cornual
  molar 631
    hydatidiform (see also Hydatidiform
      mole) 630
      previous, affecting management
        of pregnancy V23.1
    previous, affecting management of
      pregnancy V23.49
  multiple NEC 651.9 ●
    with fetal loss and retention of one
      or more fetus(es) 651.6 ●
    affecting fetus or newborn 761.5
    following (elective) fetal reduction
      651.7 ●
    specified type NEC 651.8 ●
      with fetal loss and retention of one
        or more fetus(es) 651.6 ●
      following (elective) fetal
        reduction 651.7 ●
  mural - see Pregnancy, cornual
  observation NEC V22.1
    first pregnancy V22.0
    high-risk V23.9
      specified problem NEC V23.89
  ovarian 633.20
    with intrauterine pregnancy 633.21
    affecting fetus or newborn 761.4
  possible, not (yet) confirmed V72.40
  postmature
    post-term 645.1 ●
    prolonged 645.2 ●
  post-term 645.1 ●

◄ New   ◄▦ Revised   ~~deleted~~ Deleted   ● Use Additional Digit(s)   ▨ Omit code

Pressure (*Continued*)
  birth, fetus or newborn NEC 767.9
  brachial plexus 353.0
  brain 348.4
    injury at birth 767.0
  cerebral - *see* Pressure, brain
  chest 786.59
  cone, tentorial 348.4
    injury at birth 767.0
  funis - *see* Compression, umbilical cord
  hyposystolic (*see also* Hypotension)
    458.9
  increased
    intracranial 781.99
      due to
        benign intracranial
          hypertension 348.2
        hydrocephalus - *see*
          hydrocephalus
        injury at birth 767.8
    intraocular 365.00
  lumbosacral plexus 353.1
  mediastinum 519.3
  necrosis (chronic) (skin) (*see also*
    Decubitus) 707.00
  nerve - *see* Compression, nerve
  paralysis (*see also* Neuropathy,
    entrapment) 355.9
  pre-ulcer skin changes limited to
    persistent focal erythema (*see also*
    Ulcer, pressure) 707.21
  sore (chronic) (*see also* Ulcer, pressure)
    707.00
  spinal cord 336.9
  ulcer (chronic) (*see also* Ulcer, pressure)
    707.00
  umbilical cord - *see* Compression,
    umbilical cord
  venous, increased 459.89
Pre-syncope 780.2
Preterm infant NEC 765.1●
  extreme 765.0●
Priapism (penis) 607.3
Prickling sensation (*see also* Disturbance,
  sensation) 782.0
Prickly heat 705.1
Primary - *see* condition
Primigravida, elderly
  affecting
    fetus or newborn 763.89
    management of pregnancy, labor,
      and delivery 659.5●
Primipara, old
  affecting
    fetus or newborn 763.89
    management of pregnancy, labor,
      and delivery 659.5●
Primula dermatitis 692.6
Primus varus (bilateral) (metatarsus) 754.52
PRIND (prolonged reversible ischemic
  neurologic deficit) 434.91
  history of (personal) V12.54
Pringle's disease (tuberous sclerosis) 759.5
Prinzmetal's angina 413.1
Prinzmetal-Massumi syndrome (anterior
  chest wall) 786.52
Prizefighter ear 738.7
Problem (with) V49.9
  academic V62.3
  acculturation V62.4
  adopted child V61.24
  aged
    in-law V61.3
    parent V61.3
    person NEC V61.8

Problem (*Continued*)
  alcoholism in family V61.41
  anger reaction (*see also* Disturbance,
    conduct) 312.0●
  behavior, child 312.9
  behavioral V40.9
    specified NEC V40.3
  betting V69.3
  biological child V61.23
  cardiorespiratory NEC V47.2
  care of sick or handicapped person in
    family or household V61.49
  career choice V62.29
  communication V40.1
  conscience regarding medical care
    V62.6
  delinquency (juvenile) 312.9
  diet, inappropriate V69.1
  digestive NEC V47.3
  ear NEC V41.3
  eating habits, inappropriate V69.1
  economic V60.2
    affecting care V60.9
    specified type NEC V60.89
  educational V62.3
  enuresis, child 307.6
  exercise, lack of V69.0
  eye NEC V41.1
  family V61.9
    specified circumstance NEC
      V61.8
  fear reaction, child 313.0
  feeding (elderly) (infant) 783.3
    newborn 779.31
    nonorganic 307.59
  fetal, affecting management of
    pregnancy 656.9●
    specified type NEC 656.8●
  financial V60.2
  foster child V61.25
  functional V41.9
    specified type NEC V41.8
  gambling V69.3
  genital NEC V47.5
  head V48.9
    deficiency V48.0
    disfigurement V48.6
    mechanical V48.2
    motor V48.2
    movement of V48.2
    sensory V48.4
    specified condition NEC V48.8
  hearing V41.2
  high-risk sexual behavior V69.2
  identity 313.82
  influencing health status
    NEC V49.89
  internal organ NEC V47.9
    deficiency V47.0
    mechanical or motor V47.1
  interpersonal NEC V62.81
  jealousy, child 313.3
  learning V40.0
  legal V62.5
  life circumstance NEC V62.89
  lifestyle V69.9
    specified NEC V69.8
  limb V49.9
    deficiency V49.0
    disfigurement V49.4
    mechanical V49.1
    motor V49.2
    movement, involving
      musculoskeletal system V49.1
      nervous system V49.2

Problem (*Continued*)
  limb (*Continued*)
    sensory V49.3
    specified condition NEC V49.5
  litigation V62.5
  living alone V60.3
  loneliness NEC V62.89
  marital V61.10
    involving
      divorce V61.03
      estrangement V61.09
      psychosexual disorder 302.9
      sexual function V41.7
    relationship V61.10
  mastication V41.6
  medical care, within family V61.49
  mental V40.9
    specified NEC V40.2
  mental hygiene, adult V40.9
  multiparity V61.5
  nail biting, child 307.9
  neck V48.9
    deficiency V48.1
    disfigurement V48.7
    mechanical V48.3
    motor V48.3
    movement V48.3
    sensory V48.5
    specified condition NEC V48.8
  neurological NEC 781.99
  none (feared complaint unfounded)
    V65.5
  occupational V62.29
  parent-child V61.20
    adopted child V61.24
    biological child V61.23
    foster child V61.25
    relationship V61.20
  partner V61.10
    relationship V61.10
  personal NEC V62.89
    interpersonal conflict NEC
      V62.81
  personality (*see also* Disorder,
    personality) 301.9
  phase of life V62.89
  placenta, affecting management of
    pregnancy 656.9●
    specified type NEC 656.8●
  poverty V60.2
  presence of sick or handicapped
    person in family or household
    V61.49
  psychiatric 300.9
  psychosocial V62.9
    specified type NEC V62.89
  relational NEC V62.81
  relationship, childhood 313.3
  religious or spiritual belief
    other than medical care V62.89
    regarding medical care V62.6
  self-damaging behavior V69.8
  sexual
    behavior, high-risk V69.2
    function NEC V41.7
  sibling
    relational V61.8
    relationship V61.8
  sight V41.0
  sleep, lack of V69.4
  sleep disorder, child 307.40
  smell V41.5
  speech V40.1
  spite reaction, child (*see also*
    Disturbance, conduct) 312.0●

◀ New ◀▥ Revised ~~deleted~~ Deleted ● Use Additional Digit(s) ▦ Omit code

Problem *(Continued)*
  spoiled child reaction *(see also*
      Disturbance, conduct) 312.1●
  substance abuse in family V61.42
  swallowing V41.6
  tantrum, child *(see also* Disturbance,
      conduct) 312.1●
  taste V41.5
  thumb sucking, child 307.9
  tic (child) 307.21
  trunk V48.9
    deficiency V48.1
    disfigurement V48.7
    mechanical V48.3
    motor V48.3
    movement V48.3
    sensory V48.5
    specified condition NEC V48.8
  unemployment V62.0
  urinary NEC V47.4
  voice production V41.4
Procedure (surgical) not done NEC
    V64.3
  because of
    contraindication V64.1
    patient's decision V64.2
      for reasons of conscience or
          religion V62.6
    specified reason NEC V64.3
Procidentia
  anus (sphincter) 569.1
  rectum (sphincter) 569.1
  stomach 537.89
  uteri 618.1
Proctalgia 569.42
  fugax 564.6
  spasmodic 564.6
    psychogenic 307.89
Proctitis 569.49
  amebic 006.8
  chlamydial 099.52
  gonococcal 098.7
  granulomatous 555.1
  idiopathic 556.2
    with ulcerative sigmoiditis
        556.3
  tuberculous *(see also* Tuberculosis)
      014.8●
  ulcerative (chronic) (nonspecific)
      556.2
    with ulcerative sigmoiditis 556.3
Proctocele
  female (without uterine prolapse)
      618.04
    with uterine prolapse 618.4
      complete 618.3
      incomplete 618.2
  male 569.49
Proctocolitis, idiopathic 556.2
  with ulcerative sigmoiditis 556.3
Proctoptosis 569.1
Proctosigmoiditis 569.89
  ulcerative (chronic) 556.3
Proctospasm 564.6
  psychogenic 306.4
Prodromal-AIDS - *see* Human
    immunodeficiency virus (disease)
    (illness) (infection)
Profichet's disease or syndrome
    729.90
Progeria (adultorum) (syndrome) 259.8
Prognathism (mandibular) (maxillary)
    524.00
Progonoma (melanotic) (M9363/0) - *see*
    Neoplasm, by site, benign

Progressive - *see* condition
Prolapse, prolapsed
  anus, anal (canal) (sphincter) 569.1
  arm or hand, complicating delivery
      652.7●
    causing obstructed labor 660.0●
      affecting fetus or newborn
          763.1
    fetus or newborn 763.1
  bladder (acquired) (mucosa)
      (sphincter)
    congenital (female) (male) 756.71
    female *(see also* Cystocele, female)
        618.01
    male 596.8
  breast implant (prosthetic) 996.54
  cecostomy 569.69
  cecum 569.89
  cervix, cervical (hypertrophied) 618.1
    anterior lip, obstructing labor
        660.2●
      affecting fetus or newborn 763.1
    congenital 752.49
    postpartal (old) 618.1
    stump 618.84
  ciliary body 871.1
  colon (pedunculated) 569.89
  colostomy 569.69
  conjunctiva 372.73
  cord - *see* Prolapse, umbilical cord
  disc (intervertebral) - *see* Displacement,
      intervertebral disc
  duodenum 537.89
  eye implant (orbital) 996.59
    lens (ocular) 996.53
  fallopian tube 620.4
  fetal extremity, complicating delivery
      652.8●
    causing obstructed labor 660.0●
    fetus or newborn 763.1
  funis - *see* Prolapse, umbilical cord
  gastric (mucosa) 537.89
  genital, female 618.9
    specified NEC 618.89
  globe 360.81
  ileostomy bud 569.69
  intervertebral disc - *see* Displacement,
      intervertebral disc
  intestine (small) 569.89
  iris 364.89
    traumatic 871.1
  kidney *(see also* Disease, renal) 593.0
    congenital 753.3
  laryngeal muscles or ventricle
      478.79
  leg, complicating delivery 652.8●
    causing obstructed labor 660.0●
    fetus or newborn 763.1
  liver 573.8
  meatus urinarius 599.5
  mitral valve 424.0
  ocular lens implant 996.53
  organ or site, congenital NEC - *see*
      Malposition, congenital
  ovary 620.4
  pelvic (floor), female 618.89
  perineum, female 618.89
  pregnant uterus 654.4●
  rectum (mucosa) (sphincter) 569.1
    due to Trichuris trichiuria 127.3
  spleen 289.59
  stomach 537.89
  umbilical cord
    affecting fetus or newborn 762.4
    complicating delivery 663.0●

Prolapse, prolapsed *(Continued)*
  ureter 593.89
    with obstruction 593.4
  ureterovesical orifice 593.89
  urethra (acquired) (infected) (mucosa)
      599.5
    congenital 753.8
  uterovaginal 618.4
    complete 618.3
    incomplete 618.2
    specified NEC 618.89
  uterus (first degree) (second degree)
      (third degree) (complete)
      (without vaginal wall prolapse)
      618.1
    with mention of vaginal wall
        prolapse - *see* Prolapse,
        uterovaginal
    congenital 752.39 ◀▥
    in pregnancy or childbirth
        654.4●
      affecting fetus or newborn
          763.1
      causing obstructed labor
          660.2●
        affecting fetus or newborn
            763.1
    postpartal (old) 618.1
  uveal 871.1
  vagina (anterior) (posterior) (vault)
      (wall) (without uterine prolapse)
      618.00
    with uterine prolapse 618.4
      complete 618.3
      incomplete 618.2
    paravaginal 618.02
    posthysterectomy 618.5
    specified NEC 618.09
  vitreous (humor) 379.26
    traumatic 871.1
  womb - *see* Prolapse, uterus
Prolapsus, female 618.9
Proliferative - *see* condition
Prolinemia 270.8
Prolinuria 270.8
Prolonged, prolongation
  bleeding time *(see also* Defect,
      coagulation) 790.92
  "idiopathic" (in von Willebrand's
      disease) 286.4
  coagulation time *(see also* Defect,
      coagulation) 790.92
  gestation syndrome 766.22
  labor 662.1●
    affecting fetus or newborn
        763.89
    first stage 662.0●
    second stage 662.2●
  PR interval 426.11
  pregnancy 645.2●
  prothrombin time *(see also* Defect,
      coagulation) 790.92
  QT interval 794.31
    syndrome 426.82
  rupture of membranes (24 hours or
      more prior to onset of labor)
      658.2●
  uterine contractions in labor
      661.4●
    affecting fetus or newborn
        763.7
Prominauris 744.29
Prominence
  auricle (ear) (congenital) 744.29
    acquired 380.32

Prominence *(Continued)*
  ischial spine or sacral promontory
      with disproportion (fetopelvic)
          653.3●
      affecting fetus or newborn
          763.1
      causing obstructed labor 660.1●
          affecting fetus or newborn
              763.1
  nose (congenital) 748.1
      acquired 738.0
PROMM (proximal myotonic myotonia)
    359.21
Pronation
  ankle 736.79
  foot 736.79
      congenital 755.67
Prophylactic
  administration of
      ~~agents affecting estrogen receptors~~
          ~~and estrogen levels NEC~~
          ~~V07.59~~
      ~~anastrozole (Arimidex) V07.52~~
      antibiotics, long-term V58.62 ◀▥
          short-term - *omit code* ◀
      antitoxin, any V07.2
      antivenin V07.2
      ~~aromatase inhibitors V07.52~~
      chemotherapeutic agent NEC V07.39
          fluoride V07.31
      diphtheria antitoxin V07.2
      drug V07.39
      ~~estrogen receptor downregulators~~
          ~~V07.59~~
      ~~exemestane (Aromasin) V07.52~~
      ~~fulvestrant (Faslodex) V07.59~~
      gamma globulin V07.2
      ~~gonadotropin-releasing hormone~~
          ~~(GnRH) agonist V07.59~~
      ~~goserelin acetate (Zoladex) V07.59~~
      immune sera (gamma globulin)
          V07.2
      ~~letrozole (Femara) V07.52~~
      ~~leuprolide acetate (leuprorelin)~~
          ~~(Lupron) V07.59~~
      ~~megestrol acetate (Megace)~~
          ~~V07.59~~
      ~~raloxifene (Evista) V07.51~~
      RhoGAM V07.2
      ~~selective estrogen receptor~~
          ~~modulators (SERMs)~~
          ~~V07.51~~
      ~~tamoxifen (Nolvadex) V07.51~~
      tetanus antitoxin V07.2
      ~~toremifene (Fareston) V07.51~~
  chemotherapy NEC V07.39
      fluoride V07.31
  hormone replacement
      (postmenopausal) V07.4
  immunotherapy V07.2
  measure V07.9
      specified type NEC V07.8
  medication V07.39
  postmenopausal hormone replacement
      V07.4
  sterilization V25.2
Proptosis (ocular) *(see also* Exophthalmos)
    376.30
  thyroid 242.0●
Propulsion
  eyeball 360.81
Prosecution, anxiety concerning V62.5
Prosopagnosia 368.16
Prostate, prostatic - *see* condition

Prostatism 600.90
  with
      other lower urinary tract symptoms
          (LUTS) 600.91
      urinary
          obstruction 600.91
          retention 600.91
Prostatitis (congestive) (suppurative)
    601.9
  acute 601.0
  cavitary 601.8
  chlamydial 099.54
  chronic 601.1
  diverticular 601.8
  due to Trichomonas (vaginalis) 131.03
  fibrous 600.90
      with
          other lower urinary tract
              symptoms (LUTS) 600.91
          urinary
              obstruction 600.91
              retention 600.91
  gonococcal (acute) 098.12
      chronic or duration of 2 months or
          over 098.32
  granulomatous 601.8
  hypertrophic 600.00
      with
          other lower urinary tract
              symptoms (LUTS) 600.01
          urinary
              obstruction 600.01
              retention 600.01
  specified type NEC 601.8
  subacute 601.1
  trichomonal 131.03
  tuberculous *(see also* Tuberculosis)
    016.5● *[601.4]*
Prostatocystitis 601.3
Prostatorrhea 602.8
Prostatoseminovesiculitis, trichomonal
    131.03
Prostration 780.79
  heat 992.5
      anhydrotic 992.3
      due to
          salt (and water) depletion
              992.4
          water depletion 992.3
  nervous 300.5
  newborn 779.89
  senile 797
Protanomaly 368.51
Protanopia (anomalous trichromat)
    (complete) (incomplete) 368.51
Protection (against) (from) - *see*
    Prophylactic
Protein
  deficiency 260
  malnutrition 260
  sickness (prophylactic) (therapeutic)
    999.5
Proteinemia 790.99
Proteinosis
  alveolar, lung or pulmonary 516.0
  lipid 272.8
  lipoid (of Urbach) 272.8
Proteinuria *(see also* Albuminuria) 791.0
  Bence-Jones NEC 791.0
  gestational 646.2●
      with hypertension - *see* Toxemia, of
          pregnancy
  orthostatic 593.6
  postural 593.6

Proteolysis, pathologic 286.6
Protocoproporphyria 277.1
Protoporphyria (erythrohepatic)
    (erythropoietic) 277.1
Protrusio acetabuli 718.65
Protrusion
  acetabulum (into pelvis) 718.65
  device, implant, or graft - *see*
      Complications, mechanical
  ear, congenital 744.29
  intervertebral disc - *see* Displacement,
      intervertebral disc
  nucleus pulposus - *see* Displacement,
      intervertebral disc
Proud flesh 701.5
Prune belly (syndrome) 756.71
Prurigo (ferox) (gravis) (Hebra's) (hebrae)
    (mitis) (simplex) 698.2
  agria 698.3
  asthma syndrome 691.8
  Besnier's (atopic dermatitis) (infantile
      eczema) 691.8
  eczematodes allergicum 691.8
  estivalis (Hutchinson's) 692.72
  Hutchinson's 692.72
  nodularis 698.3
  psychogenic 306.3
Pruritus, pruritic 698.9
  ani 698.0
      psychogenic 306.3
  conditions NEC 698.9
      psychogenic 306.3
  due to Onchocerca volvulus 125.3
  ear 698.9
  essential 698.9
  genital organ(s) 698.1
      psychogenic 306.3
  gravidarum 646.8●
  hiemalis 698.8
  neurogenic (any site) 306.3
  perianal 698.0
  psychogenic (any site) 306.3
  scrotum 698.1
      psychogenic 306.3
  senile, senilis 698.8
  Trichomonas 131.9
  vulva, vulvae 698.1
      psychogenic 306.3
Psammocarcinoma (M8140/3) - *see*
    Neoplasm, by site, malignant
Pseudarthrosis, pseudoarthrosis (bone)
    733.82
  joint following fusion V45.4
Pseudoacanthosis
  nigricans 701.8
Pseudoaneurysm - *see* Aneurysm
Pseudoangina (pectoris) - *see* Angina
Pseudoangioma 452
Pseudo-Argyll-Robertson pupil
    379.45
Pseudoarteriosus 747.89
Pseudoarthrosis - *see* Pseudarthrosis
Pseudoataxia 799.89
Pseudobulbar affect (PBA) 310.8
Pseudobursa 727.89
Pseudocholera 025
Pseudochromidrosis 705.89
Pseudocirrhosis, liver, pericardial
    423.2
Pseudocoarctation 747.21
Pseudocowpox 051.1
Pseudocoxalgia 732.1
Pseudocroup 478.75
Pseudocyesis 300.11

◀ New   ◀▥ Revised   ~~deleted~~ Deleted   ● Use Additional Digit(s)   � Omit code

Pseudocyst
  lung 518.89
  pancreas 577.2
  retina 361.19
Pseudodementia 300.16
Pseudoelephantiasis neuroarthritica 757.0
Pseudoemphysema 518.89
Pseudoencephalitis
  superior (acute) hemorrhagic 265.1
Pseudoerosion cervix, congenital 752.49
Pseudoexfoliation, lens capsule 366.11
Pseudofracture (idiopathic) (multiple)
    (spontaneous) (symmetrical) 268.2
Pseudoglanders 025
Pseudoglioma 360.44
Pseudogout - see Chondrocalcinosis
Pseudohallucination 780.1
Pseudohemianesthesia 782.0
Pseudohemophilia (Bernuth's)
    (hereditary) (type B) 286.4
  type A 287.8
  vascular 287.8
Pseudohermaphroditism 752.7
  with chromosomal anomaly - see
    Anomaly, chromosomal
  adrenal 255.2
  female (without adrenocortical
    disorder) 752.7
    with adrenocortical disorder
      255.2
    adrenal 255.2
  male (without gonadal disorder)
    752.7
    with
      adrenocortical disorder 255.2
      cleft scrotum 752.7
      feminizing testis 259.51
      gonadal disorder 257.9
    adrenal 255.2
Pseudohole, macula 362.54
Pseudo-Hurler's disease (mucolipidosis
    III) 272.7
Pseudohydrocephalus 348.2
Pseudohypertrophic muscular dystrophy
    (Erb's) 359.1
Pseudohypertrophy, muscle 359.1
Pseudohypoparathyroidism 275.49
Pseudoinfluenza (see also Influenza)
    487.1 ◀▥
Pseudoinsomnia 307.49
Pseudoleukemia 288.8
  infantile 285.8
Pseudomembranous - see condition
Pseudomeningocele (cerebral) (infective)
    349.2
  postprocedural 997.01
  spinal 349.2
Pseudomenstruation 626.8
Pseudomucinous
  cyst (ovary) (M8470/0) 220
  peritoneum 568.89
Pseudomyeloma 273.1
Pseudomyxoma peritonei (M8480/6)
    197.6
Pseudoneuritis optic (nerve) 377.24
  papilla 377.24
    congenital 743.57
Pseudoneuroma - see Injury, nerve, by site
Pseudo-obstruction
  intestine (chronic) (idiopathic)
      (intermittent secondary)
      (primary) 564.89
    acute 560.89
Pseudopapilledema 377.24

Pseudoparalysis
  arm or leg 781.4
  atonic, congenital 358.8
Pseudopelade 704.09
Pseudophakia V43.1
Pseudopolycythemia 289.0
Pseudopolyposis, colon 556.4
Pseudoporencephaly 348.0
Pseudopseudohypoparathyroidism 275.49
Pseudopsychosis 300.16
Pseudopterygium 372.52
Pseudoptosis (eyelid) 374.34
Pseudorabies 078.89
Pseudoretinitis, pigmentosa 362.65
Pseudorickets 588.0
  senile (Pozzi's) 731.0
Pseudorubella 057.8
Pseudoscarlatina 057.8
Pseudosclerema 778.1
Pseudosclerosis (brain)
  Jakob's 046.19
  of Westphal (-Strümpell)
      (hepatolenticular degeneration)
      275.1
  spastic 046.19
    with dementia
      with behavioral disturbance
        046.19 [294.11]
      without behavioral disturbance
        046.19 [294.10]
Pseudoseizure 780.39
  non-psychiatric 780.39
  psychiatric 300.11
Pseudotabes 799.89
  diabetic 250.6 ● [337.1]
    due to secondary diabetes 249.6 ●
      [337.1]
Pseudotetanus (see also Convulsions)
    780.39
Pseudotetany 781.7
  hysterical 300.11
Pseudothalassemia 285.0
Pseudotrichinosis 710.3
Pseudotruncus arteriosus 747.29
Pseudotuberculosis, pasteurella
    (infection) 027.2
Pseudotumor
  cerebri 348.2
  orbit (inflammatory) 376.11
Pseudo-Turner's syndrome 759.89
Pseudoxanthoma elasticum 757.39
Psilosis (sprue) (tropical) 579.1
  Monilia 112.89
  nontropical 579.0
  not sprue 704.00
Psittacosis 073.9
Psoitis 728.89
Psora NEC 696.1
Psoriasis 696.1
  any type, except arthropathic 696.1
  arthritic, arthropathic 696.0
  buccal 528.6
  flexural 696.1
  follicularis 696.1
  guttate 696.1
  inverse 696.1
  mouth 528.6
  nummularis 696.1
  psychogenic 316 [696.1]
  punctata 696.1
  pustular 696.1
  rupioides 696.1
  vulgaris 696.1
Psorospermiasis 136.4

Psorospermosis 136.4
  follicularis (vegetans) 757.39
Psychalgia 307.80
Psychasthenia 300.89
  compulsive 300.3
  mixed compulsive states 300.3
  obsession 300.3
Psychiatric disorder or problem NEC
    300.9
Psychogenic - see also condition
  factors associated with physical
      conditions 316
Psychoneurosis, psychoneurotic (see also
    Neurosis) 300.9
  anxiety (state) 300.00
  climacteric 627.2
  compensation 300.16
  compulsion 300.3
  conversion hysteria 300.11
  depersonalization 300.6
  depressive type 300.4
  dissociative hysteria 300.15
  hypochondriacal 300.7
  hysteria 300.10
    conversion type 300.11
    dissociative type 300.15
  mixed NEC 300.89
  neurasthenic 300.5
  obsessional 300.3
  obsessive-compulsive 300.3
  occupational 300.89
  personality NEC 301.89
  phobia 300.20
  senile NEC 300.89
Psychopathic - see also condition
  constitution, posttraumatic 310.2
    with psychosis 293.9
  personality 301.9
    amoral trends 301.7
    antisocial trends 301.7
    asocial trends 301.7
    mixed types 301.7
  state 301.9
Psychopathy, sexual (see also Deviation,
    sexual) 302.9
Psychophysiologic, psychophysiological
    condition - see Reaction,
    psychophysiologic
Psychose passionelle 297.8
Psychosexual identity disorder 302.6
  adult-life 302.85
  childhood 302.6
Psychosis 298.9
  acute hysterical 298.1
  affecting management of pregnancy,
      childbirth, or puerperium 648.4 ●
  affective (see also Disorder, mood) 296.90

Note: Use the following fifth-digit
subclassification with categories
296.0–296.6:

  0   unspecified
  1   mild
  2   moderate
  3   severe, without mention of
        psychotic behavior
  4   severe, specified as with
        psychotic behavior
  5   in partial or unspecified remission
  6   in full remission

  drug-induced 292.84
  due to or associated with physical
      condition 293.9

Psychosis *(Continued)*
  affective *(Continued)*
    involutional 293.83
      recurrent episode 296.3●
      single episode 296.2●
    manic-depressive 296.80
      circular (alternating) 296.7
        currently depressed 296.5●
        currently manic 296.4●
      depressed type 296.2●
        atypical 296.82
        recurrent episode 296.3●
        single episode 296.2●
      manic 296.0●
        atypical 296.81
        recurrent episode 296.1●
        single episode 296.0●
      mixed type NEC 296.89
      specified type NEC 296.89
    senile 290.21
    specified type NEC 296.99
  alcoholic 291.9
    with
      anxiety 291.89
      delirium tremens 291.0
      delusions 291.5
      dementia 291.2
      hallucinosis 291.3
      jealousy 291.5
      mood disturbance 291.89
      paranoia 291.5
      persisting amnesia 291.1
      sexual dysfunction 291.89
      sleep disturbance 291.89
    amnestic confabulatory 291.1
    delirium tremens 291.0
    hallucinosis 291.3
    Korsakoff's, Korsakov's, Korsakow's
      291.1
    paranoid type 291.5
    pathological intoxication 291.4
    polyneuritic 291.1
    specified type NEC 291.89
  alternating *(see also* Psychosis, manic-
    depressive, circular) 296.7
  anergastic *(see also* Psychosis, organic)
    294.9
  arteriosclerotic 290.40
    with
      acute confusional state 290.41
      delirium 290.41
      delusions 290.42
      depressed mood 290.43
    depressed type 290.43
    paranoid type 290.42
    simple type 290.40
    uncomplicated 290.40
  atypical 298.9
    depressive 296.82
    manic 296.81
  borderline (schizophrenia) *(see also*
    Schizophrenia) 295.5●
    of childhood *(see also* Psychosis,
      childhood) 299.8●
      prepubertal 299.8●
  brief reactive 298.8
  childhood, with origin specific to
    299.9●

> Note: Use the following fifth-digit subclassification with category 299:
>
> 0   current or active state
> 1   residual state

Psychosis *(Continued)*
  childhood, with origin specific to
    (Continued)
    atypical 299.8●
    specified type NEC 299.8●
  circular *(see also* Psychosis, manic-
    depressive, circular) 296.7
  climacteric *(see also* Psychosis,
    involutional) 298.8
  confusional 298.9
    acute 293.0
    reactive 298.2
    subacute 293.1
  depressive *(see also* Psychosis, affective)
    296.2●
    atypical 296.82
    involutional 296.2●
      with hypomania (bipolar II)
        296.89
      recurrent episode 296.3●
      single episode 296.2●
    psychogenic 298.0
    reactive (emotional stress)
      (psychological trauma) 298.0
    recurrent episode 296.3●
      with hypomania (bipolar II)
        296.89
    single episode 296.2●
  disintegrative, childhood *(see also*
    Psychosis, childhood) 299.1●
  drug 292.9
    with
      affective syndrome 292.84
      amnestic syndrome 292.83
      anxiety 292.89
      delirium 292.81
        withdrawal 292.0
      delusions 292.11
      dementia 292.82
      depressive state 292.84
      hallucinations 292.12
      hallucinosis 292.12
      mood disorder 292.84
      mood disturbance 292.84
      organic personality syndrome
        NEC 292.89
      sexual dysfunction 292.89
      sleep disturbance 292.89
      withdrawal syndrome (and
        delirium) 292.0
    affective syndrome 292.84
    delusions 292.11
    hallucinatory state 292.12
    hallucinosis 292.12
    paranoid state 292.11
    specified type NEC 292.89
    withdrawal syndrome (and
      delirium) 292.0
  due to or associated with physical
    condition *(see also* Psychosis,
    organic) 294.9
  epileptic NEC 293.9
  excitation (psychogenic) (reactive) 298.1
  exhaustive *(see also* Reaction, stress,
    acute) 308.9
  hypomanic *(see also* Psychosis,
    affective) 296.0●
    recurrent episode 296.1●
    single episode 296.0●
  hysterical 298.8
    acute 298.1
  incipient 298.8
    schizophrenic *(see also*
      Schizophrenia) 295.5●

Psychosis *(Continued)*
  induced 297.3
  infantile *(see also* Psychosis, childhood)
    299.0●
  infective 293.9
    acute 293.0
    subacute 293.1
  in
    conditions classified elsewhere
      with
        delusions 293.81
        hallucinations 293.82
    pregnancy, childbirth, or
      puerperium 648.4●
  interactional (childhood) *(see also*
    Psychosis, childhood)
    299.1●
  involutional 298.8
    depressive *(see also* Psychosis,
      affective) 296.2●
      recurrent episode 296.3●
      single episode 296.2●
    melancholic 296.2●
      recurrent episode 296.3●
      single episode 296.2●
    paranoid state 297.2
    paraphrenia 297.2
  Korsakoff's, Korakov's, Korsakow's
    (nonalcoholic) 294.0
    alcoholic 291.1
  mania (phase) *(see also* Psychosis,
    affective) 296.0●
    recurrent episode 296.1●
    single episode 296.0●
  manic *(see also* Psychosis, affective)
    296.0●
    atypical 296.81
    recurrent episode 296.1●
    single episode 296.0●
  manic-depressive 296.80
    circular 296.7
      currently
        depressed 296.5●
        manic 296.4●
      mixed 296.6●
    depressive 296.2●
      recurrent episode 296.3●
        with hypomania (bipolar II)
          296.89
      single episode 296.2●
    hypomanic 296.0●
      recurrent episode 296.1●
      single episode 296.0●
    manic 296.0●
      atypical 296.81
      recurrent episode 296.1●
      single episode 296.0●
    mixed NEC 296.89
    perplexed 296.89
    stuporous 296.89
  menopausal *(see also* Psychosis,
    involutional) 298.8
  mixed schizophrenic and affective *(see*
    also Schizophrenia) 295.7●
  multi-infarct (cerebrovascular) *(see also*
    Psychosis, arteriosclerotic)
    290.40
  organic NEC 294.9
    due to or associated with
      addiction
        alcohol *(see also* Psychosis,
          alcoholic) 291.9
        drug *(see also* Psychosis, drug)
          292.9

◀ New   ◀░ Revised   ~~deleted~~ Deleted   ● Use Additional Digit(s)   ▒ Omit code

Psychosis *(Continued)*
  organic NEC *(Continued)*
    due to or associated with *(Continued)*
      alcohol intoxication, acute *(see also Psychosis, alcoholic)* 291.9
      alcoholism *(see also Psychosis, alcoholic)* 291.9
      arteriosclerosis (cerebral) *(see also Psychosis, arteriosclerotic)* 290.40
      cerebrovascular disease
        acute (psychosis) 293.0
        arteriosclerotic *(see also Psychosis, arteriosclerotic)* 290.40
      childbirth - *see* Psychosis, puerperal
      dependence
        alcohol *(see also Psychosis, alcoholic)* 291.9
        drug 292.9
      disease
        alcoholic liver *(see also Psychosis, alcoholic)* 291.9
        brain
          arteriosclerotic *(see also Psychosis, arteriosclerotic)* 290.40
          cerebrovascular
            acute (psychosis) 293.0
            arteriosclerotic *(see also Psychosis, arteriosclerotic)* 290.40
          endocrine or metabolic 293.9
            acute (psychosis) 293.0
            subacute (psychosis) 293.1
          Jakob-Creutzfeldt 046.19
            with behavioral disturbance 046.19 *[294.11]*
            without behavioral disturbance 046.19 *[294.10]*
            familial 046.19
            iatrogenic 046.19
            specified NEC 046.19
            sporadic 046.19
            variant 046.11
              with dementia
                with behavioral disturbance 046.11 *[294.11]*
                without behavioral disturbance 046.11 *[294.10]*
          liver, alcoholic *(see also Psychosis, alcoholic)* 291.9
      disorder
        cerebrovascular
          acute (psychosis) 293.0
          endocrine or metabolic 293.9
            acute (psychosis) 293.0
            subacute (psychosis) 293.1
      epilepsy
        with behavioral disturbance 345.9 *[294.11]*●
        without behavioral disturbance 345.9 *[294.10]*●
        transient (acute) 293.0

Psychosis *(Continued)*
  organic NEC *(Continued)*
    due to or associated with *(Continued)*
      Huntington's chorea
        with behavioral disturbance 333.4 *[294.11]*
        without behavioral disturbance 333.4 *[294.10]*
      infection
        brain 293.9
          acute (psychosis) 293.0
          chronic 294.8
          subacute (psychosis) 293.1
        intracranial NEC 293.9
          acute (psychosis) 293.0
          chronic 294.8
          subacute (psychosis) 293.1
      intoxication
        alcoholic (acute) *(see also Psychosis, alcoholic)* 291.9
        pathological 291.4
      drug *(see also Psychosis, drug)* 292.9
      ischemia
        cerebrovascular (generalized) *(see also Psychosis, arteriosclerotic)* 290.40
      Jakob-Creutzfeldt disease (syndrome) 046.19
        with behavioral disturbance 046.19 *[294.11]*
        without behavioral disturbance 046.19 *[294.10]*
        variant 046.11
          with dementia
            with behavioral disturbance 046.11 *[294.11]*
            without behavioral disturbance 046.11 *[294.10]*
      multiple sclerosis
        with behavioral disturbance 340 *[294.11]*
        without behavioral disturbance 340 *[294.10]*
      physical condition NEC 293.9
        with
          delusions 293.81
          hallucinations 293.82
      presenility 290.10
      puerperium - *see* Psychosis, puerperal
      sclerosis, multiple
        with behavioral disturbance 340 *[294.11]*
        without behavioral disturbance 340 *[294.10]*
      senility 290.20
      status epilepticus
        with behavioral disturbance 345.3 *[294.11]*
        without behavioral disturbance 345.3 *[294.10]*
      trauma
        brain (birth) (from electrical current) (surgical) 293.9
          acute (psychosis) 293.0
          chronic 294.8
          subacute (psychosis) 293.1

Psychosis *(Continued)*
  organic NEC *(Continued)*
    due to or associated with *(Continued)*
      unspecified physical condition 293.9
        with
          delusions 293.81
          hallucinations 293.82
      infective 293.9
        acute (psychosis) 293.0
        subacute 293.1
      posttraumatic 293.9
        acute 293.0
        subacute 293.1
      specified type NEC 294.8
      transient 293.9
        with
          anxiety 293.84
          delusions 293.81
          depression 293.83
          hallucinations 293.82
          depressive type 293.83
          hallucinatory type 293.82
          paranoid type 293.81
          specified type NEC 293.89
  paranoic 297.1
  paranoid (chronic) 297.9
    alcoholic 291.5
    chronic 297.1
    climacteric 297.2
    involutional 297.2
    menopausal 297.2
    protracted reactive 298.4
    psychogenic 298.4
      acute 298.3
    schizophrenic *(see also Schizophrenia)* 295.3●
    senile 290.20
  paroxysmal 298.9
    senile 290.20
  polyneuritic, alcoholic 291.1
  postoperative 293.9
  postpartum - *see* Psychosis, puerperal
  prepsychotic *(see also Schizophrenia)* 295.5●
  presbyophrenic (type) 290.8
  presenile *(see also Dementia, presenile)* 290.10
  prison 300.16
  psychogenic 298.8
    depressive 298.0
    paranoid 298.4
      acute 298.3
  puerperal
    specified type - *see* categories 295–298
    unspecified type 293.89
      acute 293.0
      chronic 293.89
      subacute 293.1
  reactive (emotional stress) (psychological trauma) 298.8
    brief 298.8
    confusion 298.2
    depressive 298.0
    excitation 298.1
  schizo-affective (depressed) (excited) *(see also Schizophrenia)* 295.7●
  schizophrenia, schizophrenic *(see also Schizophrenia)* 295.9●
    borderline type 295.5●
      of childhood *(see also Psychosis, childhood)* 299.8●

Psychosis (Continued)
schizophrenia, schizophrenic
(Continued)
catatonic (excited) (withdrawn)
295.2 ●
childhood type (see also Psychosis,
childhood) 299.9 ●
hebephrenic 295.1 ●
incipient 295.5 ●
latent 295.5 ●
paranoid 295.3 ●
prepsychotic 295.5 ●
prodromal 295.5 ●
pseudoneurotic 295.5 ●
pseudopsychopathic 295.5 ●
schizophreniform 295.4 ●
simple 295.0 ●
undifferentiated type 295.9 ●
schizophreniform 295.4 ●
senile NEC 290.20
with
delusional features 290.20
depressive features 290.21
depressed type 290.21
paranoid type 290.20
simple deterioration 290.20
specified type - see categories 295–298
shared 297.3
situational (reactive) 298.8
symbiotic (childhood) (see also
Psychosis, childhood) 299.1 ●
toxic (acute) 293.9
Psychotic (see also condition) 298.9
episode 298.9
due to or associated with physical
conditions (see also Psychosis,
organic) 293.9
Pterygium (eye) 372.40
central 372.43
colli 744.5
double 372.44
peripheral (stationary) 372.41
progressive 372.42
recurrent 372.45
Ptilosis 374.55
PTLD (post-transplant
lymphoproliferative disorder)
238.77
Ptomaine (poisoning) (see also Poisoning,
food) 005.9
Ptosis (adiposa) 374.30
breast 611.81
cecum 569.89
colon 569.89
congenital (eyelid) 743.61
specified site NEC - see Anomaly,
specified type NEC
epicanthus syndrome 270.2
eyelid 374.30
congenital 743.61
mechanical 374.33
myogenic 374.32
paralytic 374.31
gastric 537.5
intestine 569.89
kidney (see also Disease, renal) 593.0
congenital 753.3
liver 573.8
renal (see also Disease, renal) 593.0
congenital 753.3
splanchnic 569.89
spleen 289.59
stomach 537.5
viscera 569.89

PTP (posttransfusion purpura) 287.41 ◀
PTSD (Post-Traumatic Stress Disorder)
309.81
Ptyalism 527.7
hysterical 300.11
periodic 527.2
pregnancy 646.8 ●
psychogenic 306.4
Ptyalolithiasis 527.5
Pubalgia 848.8
Pubarche, precocious 259.1
Pubertas praecox 259.1
Puberty V21.1
abnormal 259.9
bleeding 626.3
delayed 259.0
precocious (constitutional) (cryptogenic)
(idiopathic) NEC 259.1
due to
adrenal
cortical hyperfunction 255.2
hyperplasia 255.2
cortical hyperfunction 255.2
ovarian hyperfunction 256.1
estrogen 256.0
pineal tumor 259.8
testicular hyperfunction 257.0
premature 259.1
due to
adrenal cortical hyperfunction
255.2
pineal tumor 259.8
pituitary (anterior) hyperfunction
253.1
Puckering, macula 362.56
Pudenda, pudendum - see condition
Puente's disease (simple glandular
cheilitis) 528.5
Puerperal
abscess
areola 675.1 ●
Bartholin's gland 646.6 ●
breast 675.1 ●
cervix (uteri) 670.8 ●
fallopian tube 670.8 ●
genital organ 670.8 ●
kidney 646.6 ●
mammary 675.1 ●
mesosalpinx 670.8 ●
nabothian 646.6 ●
nipple 675.0 ●
ovary, ovarian 670.8 ●
oviduct 670.8 ●
parametric 670.8 ●
para-uterine 670.8 ●
pelvic 670.8 ●
perimetric 670.8 ●
periuterine 670.8 ●
retro-uterine 670.8 ●
subareolar 675.1 ●
suprapelvic 670.8 ●
tubal (ruptured) 670.8 ●
tubo-ovarian 670.8 ●
urinary tract NEC 646.6 ●
uterine, uterus 670.8 ●
vagina (wall) 646.6 ●
vaginorectal 646.6 ●
vulvovaginal gland 646.6 ●
accident 674.9 ●
adnexitis 670.8 ●
afibrinogenemia, or other coagulation
defect 666.3 ●
albuminuria (acute) (subacute) 646.2 ●
pre-eclamptic 642.4 ●

Puerperal (Continued)
anemia (conditions classifiable to
280–285) 648.2 ●
anuria 669.3 ●
apoplexy 674.0 ●
asymptomatic bacteriuria 646.5 ●
atrophy, breast 676.3 ●
blood dyscrasia 666.3 ●
caked breast 676.2 ●
cardiomyopathy 674.5 ●
cellulitis - see Puerperal, abscess
cerebrovascular disorder (conditions
classifiable to 430–434, 436–437)
674.0 ●
cervicitis (conditions classifiable to
616.0) 646.6 ●
coagulopathy (any) 666.3 ●
complications 674.9 ●
specified type NEC 674.8 ●
convulsions (eclamptic) (uremic)
642.6 ●
with pre-existing hypertension
642.7 ●
cracked nipple 676.1 ●
cystitis 646.6 ●
cystopyelitis 646.6 ●
deciduitis (acute) 670.8 ●
delirium NEC 293.9
diabetes (mellitus) (conditions
classifiable to 249 and 250)
648.0 ●
disease 674.9 ●
breast NEC 676.3 ●
cerebrovascular (acute) 674.0 ●
nonobstetric NEC (see also
Pregnancy, complicated,
current disease or condition)
648.9 ●
pelvis inflammatory 670.8 ●
renal NEC 646.2 ●
tubo-ovarian 670.8 ●
Valsuani's (progressive pernicious
anemia) 648.2 ●
disorder
lactation 676.9 ●
specified type NEC 676.8 ●
nonobstetric NEC (see also
Pregnancy, complicated,
current disease or condition)
648.9 ●
disruption
cesarean wound 674.1 ●
episiotomy wound 674.2 ●
perineal laceration wound 674.2 ●
drug dependence (conditions
classifiable to 304) 648.3 ●
eclampsia 642.6 ●
with pre-existing hypertension
642.7 ●
embolism (pulmonary) 673.2 ●
air 673.0 ●
amniotic fluid 673.1 ●
blood clot 673.2 ●
brain or cerebral 674.0 ●
cardiac 674.8 ●
fat 673.8 ●
intracranial sinus (venous) 671.5 ●
pyemic 673.3 ●
septic 673.3 ●
spinal cord 671.5 ●
endometritis (conditions classifiable to
615.0–615.9) 670.1 ●
endophlebitis - see Puerperal, phlebitis
endotrachelitis 646.6 ●

◀ New   ◀▥ Revised   deleted Deleted   ● Use Additional Digit(s)   ▦ Omit code

Puerperal (Continued)
  engorgement, breasts 676.2●
  erysipelas 670.8●
  failure
    lactation 676.4●
    renal, acute 669.3●
  fever 672● ◀▥
    meaning pyrexia (of unknown
        origin) 672●
    meaning sepsis 670.2●
    fissure, nipple 676.1●
  fistula
    breast 675.1●
    mammary gland 675.1●
    nipple 675.0●
  galactophoritis 675.2●
  galactorrhea 676.6●
  gangrene
    gas 670.8●
      with sepsis 670.2●
    uterus 670.8●
  gonorrhea (conditions classifiable to
      098) 647.1●
  hematoma, subdural 674.0●
  hematosalpinx, infectional 670.8●
  hemiplegia, cerebral 674.0●
  hemorrhage 666.1●
    brain 674.0●
    bulbar 674.0●
    cerebellar 674.0●
    cerebral 674.0●
    cortical 674.0●
    delayed (after 24 hours) (uterine)
        666.2●
    extradural 674.0●
    internal capsule 674.0●
    intracranial 674.0●
    intrapontine 674.0●
    meningeal 674.0●
    pontine 674.0●
    subarachnoid 674.0●
    subcortical 674.0●
    subdural 674.0●
    uterine, delayed 666.2●
    ventricular 674.0●
  hemorrhoids 671.8●
  hepatorenal syndrome 674.8●
  hypertrophy
    breast 676.3●
    mammary gland 676.3●
  induration breast (fibrous) 676.3●
  infarction
    lung - see Puerperal, embolism
    pulmonary - see Puerperal,
        embolism
  infection
    Bartholin's gland 646.6●
    breast 675.2●
      with nipple 675.9●
        specified type NEC 675.8●
    cervix 646.6●
    endocervix 646.6●
    fallopian tube 670.8●
    generalized 670.0●
    genital tract (major) 670.0●
      minor or localized 646.6●
    kidney (bacillus coli) 646.6●
    mammary gland 675.2●
      with nipple 675.9●
        specified type NEC 675.8●
    nipple 675.0●
      with breast 675.9●
        specified type NEC 675.8●
    ovary 670.8●

Puerperal (Continued)
  infection (Continued)
    pelvic 670.8●
    peritoneum 670.8●
    renal 646.6●
    tubo-ovarian 670.8●
    urinary (tract) NEC 646.6●
      asymptomatic 646.5●
    uterus, uterine 670.8●
    vagina 646.6●
  inflammation - see also Puerperal,
      infection
    areola 675.1●
    Bartholin's gland 646.6●
    breast 675.2●
    broad ligament 670.8●
    cervix (uteri) 646.6●
    fallopian tube 670.8●
    genital organs 670.8●
      localized 646.6●
    mammary gland 675.2●
    nipple 675.0●
    ovary 670.8●
    oviduct 670.8●
    pelvis 670.8●
    periuterine 670.8●
    tubal 670.8●
    vagina 646.6●
    vein - see Puerperal, phlebitis●
  inversion, nipple 676.3●
  ischemia, cerebral 674.0●
  lymphangitis 670.8●
    breast 675.2●
  malaria (conditions classifiable to 084)
      647.4●
  malnutrition 648.9●
  mammillitis 675.0●
  mammitis 675.2●
  mania 296.0●
    recurrent episode 296.1●
    single episode 296.0●
  mastitis 675.2●
    purulent 675.1●
    retromammary 675.1●
    submammary 675.1●
  melancholia 296.2●
    recurrent episode 296.3●
    single episode 296.2●
  mental disorder (conditions
      classifiable to 290–303, 305.0,
      305.2–305.9, 306–316, 317–319)
      648.4●
  metritis (suppurative) 670.1●
    septic 670.2●
  metroperitonitis 670.8●
  metrorrhagia 666.2●
  metrosalpingitis 670.8●
  metrovaginitis 670.8●
  milk leg 671.4●
  monoplegia, cerebral 674.0●
  necrosis
    kidney, tubular 669.3●
    liver (acute) (subacute) (conditions
        classifiable to 570) 674.8●
    ovary 670.8●
    renal cortex 669.3●
  nephritis or nephrosis (conditions
      classifiable to 580–589) 646.2●
    with hypertension 642.1●
  nutritional deficiency (conditions
      classifiable to 260–269) 648.9●
  occlusion, precerebral artery 674.0●
  oliguria 669.3●
  oophoritis 670.8●
  ovaritis 670.8●

Puerperal (Continued)
  paralysis●
    bladder (sphincter) 665.5●
    cerebral 674.0●
  paralytic stroke 674.0●
  parametritis 670.8●
  paravaginitis 646.6●
  pelviperitonitis 670.8●
  perimetritis 670.8●
  perimetrosalpingitis 670.8●
  perinephritis 646.6●
  perioophoritis 670.8●
  periphlebitis - see Puerperal, phlebitis
  perisalpingitis 670.8●
  peritoneal infection 670.8●
  peritonitis (pelvic) 670.8●
  perivaginitis 646.6●
  phlebitis 671.2●
    deep 671.4●
    intracranial sinus (venous) 671.5●
    pelvic 671.4●
    specified site NEC 671.5●
    superficial 671.2●
  phlegmasia alba dolens 671.4●
  placental polyp 674.4●
  pneumonia, embolic - see Puerperal,
      embolism
  prediabetes 648.8●
  pre-eclampsia (mild) 642.4●
    with pre-existing hypertension
        642.7●
    severe 642.5●
  psychosis, unspecified (see also
      Psychosis, puerperal) 293.89●
  pyelitis 646.6●
  pyelocystitis 646.6●
  pyelohydronephrosis 646.6●
  pyelonephritis 646.6●
  pyelonephrosis 646.6●
  pyemia 670.2●
  pyocystitis 646.6●
  pyohemia 670.2●
  pyometra 670.8●
  pyonephritis 646.6●
  pyonephrosis 646.6●
  pyo-oophoritis 670.8●
  pyosalpingitis 670.8●
  pyosalpinx 670.8●
  pyrexia (of unknown origin) 672●
  renal
    disease NEC 646.2●
    failure, acute 669.3●
  retention
    decidua (fragments) (with delayed
        hemorrhage) 666.2●
      without hemorrhage 667.1●
    placenta (fragments) (with delayed
        hemorrhage) 666.2●
      without hemorrhage 667.1●
    secundines (fragments) (with
        delayed hemorrhage) 666.2●
      without hemorrhage 667.1●
  retracted nipple 676.0●
  rubella (conditions classifiable to 056)
      647.5●
  salpingitis 670.8●
  salpingo-oophoritis 670.8●
  salpingo-ovaritis 670.8●
  salpingoperitonitis 670.8●
  sapremia 670.2●
  secondary perineal tear 674.2●
  sepsis (pelvic) 670.2●
  septicemia 670.2●
  subinvolution (uterus) 674.8●

Puerperal *(Continued)*
  sudden death (cause unknown) 674.9●
  suppuration - *see* Puerperal, abscess
  syphilis (conditions classifiable to 090–097) 647.0●
  tetanus 670.8●
  thelitis 675.0●
  thrombocytopenia 666.3●
  thrombophlebitis (superficial) 671.2●
    deep 671.4●
    pelvic 671.4●
    septic 670.3●
    specified site NEC 671.5●
  thrombosis (venous) - *see* Thrombosis, puerperal
  thyroid dysfunction (conditions classifiable to 240–246) 648.1●
  toxemia (*see also* Toxemia, of pregnancy) 642.4●
    eclamptic 642.6●
      with pre-existing hypertension 642.7●
    pre-eclamptic (mild) 642.4●
      with
        convulsions 642.6●
        pre-existing hypertension 642.7●
      severe 642.5●
  tuberculosis (conditions classifiable to 010–018) 647.3●
  uremia 669.3●
  vaginitis (conditions classifiable to 616.1) 646.6●
  varicose veins (legs) 671.0●
    vulva or perineum 671.1●
  venous complication 671.9●
  vulvitis (conditions classifiable to 616.1) 646.6●
  vulvovaginitis (conditions classifiable to 616.1) 646.6●
  white leg 671.4●
Pulled muscle - *see* Sprain, by site
Pulmolithiasis 518.89
Pulmonary - *see* condition
Pulmonitis (unknown etiology) 486
Pulpitis (acute) (anachoretic) (chronic) (hyperplastic) (putrescent) (suppurative) (ulcerative) 522.0
Pulpless tooth 522.9
Pulse
  alternating 427.89
    psychogenic 306.2
  bigeminal 427.89
  fast 785.0
  feeble, rapid, due to shock following injury 958.4
  rapid 785.0
  slow 427.89
  strong 785.9
  trigeminal 427.89
  water-hammer (*see also* Insufficiency, aortic) 424.1
  weak 785.9
Pulseless disease 446.7
Pulsus
  alternans or trigeminy 427.89
    psychogenic 306.2
Punch drunk 310.2
Puncta lacrimalia occlusion 375.52
Punctiform hymen 752.49
Puncture (traumatic) - *see also* Wound, open, by site
  accidental, complicating surgery 998.2
  bladder, nontraumatic 596.6

Puncture *(Continued)*
  by
    device, implant, or graft - *see* Complications, mechanical
    foreign body
      internal organs - *see also* Injury, internal, by site
      by ingested object - *see* Foreign body
      left accidentally in operation wound 998.4
    instrument (any) during a procedure, accidental 998.2
  internal organs, abdomen, chest, or pelvis - *see* Injury, internal, by site
  kidney, nontraumatic 593.89
Pupil - *see* condition
Pupillary membrane 364.74
  persistent 743.46
Pupillotonia 379.46
  pseudotabetic 379.46
Purpura 287.2
  abdominal 287.0
  allergic 287.0
  anaphylactoid 287.0
  annularis telangiectodes 709.1
  arthritic 287.0
  autoerythrocyte sensitization 287.2
  autoimmune 287.0
  bacterial 287.0
  Bateman's (senile) 287.2
  capillary fragility (hereditary) (idiopathic) 287.8
  cryoglobulinemic 273.2
  devil's pinches 287.2
  fibrinolytic (*see also* Fibrinolysis) 286.6
  fulminans, fulminous 286.6
  gangrenous 287.0
  hemorrhagic (*see also* Purpura, thrombocytopenic) 287.39
    nodular 272.7
    nonthrombocytopenic 287.0
    thrombocytopenic 287.39
  Henoch's (purpura nervosa) 287.0
  Henoch-Schönlein (allergic) 287.0
  hypergammaglobulinemic (benign primary) (Waldenström's) 273.0
  idiopathic 287.31
    nonthrombocytopenic 287.0
    thrombocytopenic 287.31
  immune thrombocytopenic 287.31
  infectious 287.0
  malignant 287.0
  neonatorum 772.6
  nervosa 287.0
  newborn NEC 772.6
  nonthrombocytopenic 287.2
    hemorrhagic 287.0
    idiopathic 287.0
  nonthrombopenic 287.2
  peliosis rheumatica 287.0
  pigmentaria, progressiva 709.09
  posttransfusion (PTP) 287.41 ◄▥
    from whole blood (fresh) or blood products 287.41 ◄
  primary 287.0
  primitive 287.0
  red cell membrane sensitivity 287.2
  rheumatica 287.0
  Schönlein (-Henoch) (allergic) 287.0
  scorbutic 267
  senile 287.2
  simplex 287.2
  symptomatica 287.0
  telangiectasia annularis 709.1

Purpura *(Continued)*
  thrombocytopenic (*see also* Thrombocytopenia) 287.30
    congenital 287.33
    essential 287.30
    hereditary 287.31
    idiopathic 287.31
    immune 287.31
    neonatal, transitory (*see also* Thrombocytopenia, neonatal transitory) 776.1
    primary 287.30
    puerperal, postpartum 666.3●
    thrombotic 446.6
  thrombohemolytic (*see also* Fibrinolysis) 286.6
  thrombopenic (*see also* Thrombocytopenia) 287.30
    congenital 287.33
    essential 287.30
  thrombotic 446.6
    thrombocytic 446.6
    thrombocytopenic 446.6
  toxic 287.0
  variolosa 050.0
  vascular 287.0
  visceral symptoms 287.0
  Werlhof's (*see also* Purpura, thrombocytopenic) 287.39
Purpuric spots 782.7
Purulent - *see* condition
Pus
  absorption, general - *see* Septicemia
  in
    stool 792.1
    urine 791.9
  tube (rupture) (*see also* Salpingo-oophoritis) 614.2
Pustular rash 782.1
Pustule 686.9
  malignant 022.0
  nonmalignant 686.9
Putnam's disease (subacute combined sclerosis with pernicious anemia) 281.0 *[336.2]*
Putnam-Dana syndrome (subacute combined sclerosis with pernicious anemia) 281.0 *[336.2]*
Putrefaction, intestinal 569.89
Putrescent pulp (dental) 522.1
Pyarthritis - *see* Pyarthrosis
Pyarthrosis (*see also* Arthritis, pyogenic) 711.0●
  tuberculous - *see* Tuberculosis, joint
Pycnoepilepsy, pycnolepsy (idiopathic) (*see also* Epilepsy) 345.0●
Pyelectasia 593.89
Pyelectasis 593.89
Pyelitis (congenital) (uremic) 590.80
  with
    abortion - *see* Abortion, by type, with specified complication NEC
    contracted kidney 590.00
    ectopic pregnancy (*see also* categories 633.0–633.9) 639.8
    molar pregnancy (*see also* categories 630–632) 639.8
  acute 590.10
    with renal medullary necrosis 590.11
  chronic 590.00
    with
      renal medullary necrosis 590.01

◄ New   ◄▥ Revised   ~~deleted~~ Deleted   ● Use Additional Digit(s)   ▨ Omit code

Pyelitis (Continued)
  complicating pregnancy, childbirth, or
      puerperium 646.6●
    affecting fetus or newborn 760.1
  cystica 590.3
  following
    abortion 639.8
    ectopic or molar pregnancy 639.8
  gonococcal 098.19
    chronic or duration of 2 months or
        over 098.39
  tuberculous (see also Tuberculosis)
      016.0● [590.81]
Pyelocaliectasis 593.89
Pyelocystitis (see also Pyelitis) 590.80
Pyelohydronephrosis 591
Pyelonephritis (see also Pyelitis) 590.80
  acute 590.10
    with renal medullary necrosis 590.11
  chronic 590.00
  syphilitic (late) 095.4
  tuberculous (see also Tuberculosis)
      016.0● [590.81]
Pyelonephrosis (see also Pyelitis) 590.80
  chronic 590.00
Pyelophlebitis 451.89
Pyelo-ureteritis cystica 590.3
Pyemia, pyemic (purulent) (see also
    Septicemia) 038.9
  abscess - see Abscess
  arthritis (see also Arthritis, pyogenic)
      711.0●
  Bacillus coli 038.42
  embolism (see also Septicemia) 415.12
  fever 038.9
  infection 038.9
  joint (see also Arthritis, pyogenic)
      711.0●
  liver 572.1
  meningococcal 036.2
  newborn 771.81
  phlebitis - see Phlebitis
  pneumococcal 038.2
  portal 572.1
  postvaccinal 999.39
  puerperal 670.2●
  specified organism NEC 038.8
  staphylococcal 038.10
    aureus 038.11
      methicillin
        resistant 038.12
        susceptible 038.11
    specified organism NEC 038.19

Pyemia, pyemic (Continued)
  streptococcal 038.0
  tuberculous - see Tuberculosis,
      miliary
Pygopagus 759.4
Pykno-epilepsy, pyknolepsy
    (idiopathic) (see also Epilepsy)
    345.0●
Pyle (-Cohn) disease (craniometaphyseal
    dysplasia) 756.89
Pylephlebitis (suppurative) 572.1
Pylethrombophlebitis 572.1
Pylethrombosis 572.1
Pyloritis (see also Gastritis) 535.5●
Pylorospasm (reflex) 537.81
  congenital or infantile 750.5
  neurotic 306.4
  newborn 750.5
  psychogenic 306.4
Pylorus, pyloric - see condition
Pyoarthrosis - see Pyarthrosis
Pyocele
  mastoid 383.00
  sinus (accessory) (nasal) (see also
      Sinusitis) 473.9
  turbinate (bone) 473.9
  urethra (see also Urethritis) 597.0
Pyococcal dermatitis 686.00
Pyococcide, skin 686.00
Pyocolpos (see also Vaginitis)
    616.10
Pyocyaneus dermatitis 686.09
Pyocystitis (see also Cystitis) 595.9
Pyoderma, pyodermia 686.00
  gangrenosum 686.01
  specified type NEC 686.09
  vegetans 686.8
Pyodermatitis 686.00
  vegetans 686.8
Pyogenic - see condition
Pyohemia - see Septicemia
Pyohydronephrosis (see also Pyelitis)
    590.80
Pyometra 615.9
Pyometritis (see also Endometritis)
    615.9
Pyometrium (see also Endometritis)
    615.9
Pyomyositis 728.0
  ossificans 728.19
  tropical (bungpagga) 040.81
Pyonephritis (see also Pyelitis) 590.80
  chronic 590.00

Pyonephrosis (congenital) (see also
    Pyelitis) 590.80
  acute 590.10
Pyo-oophoritis (see also Salpingo-
    oophoritis) 614.2
Pyo-ovarium (see also Salpingo-
    oophoritis) 614.2
Pyopericarditis 420.99
Pyopericardium 420.99
Pyophlebitis - see Phlebitis
Pyopneumopericardium 420.99
Pyopneumothorax (infectional) 510.9
  with fistula 510.0
  subdiaphragmatic (see also Peritonitis)
      567.29
  subphrenic (see also Peritonitis)
      567.29
  tuberculous (see also Tuberculosis,
      pleura) 012.0●
Pyorrhea (alveolar) (alveolaris) 523.40
  degenerative 523.5
Pyosalpingitis (see also Salpingo-
    oophoritis) 614.2
Pyosalpinx (see also Salpingo-oophoritis)
    614.2
Pyosepticemia - see Septicemia
Pyosis
  Corlett's (impetigo) 684
  Manson's (pemphigus contagiosus)
      684
Pyothorax 510.9
  with fistula 510.0
  tuberculous (see also Tuberculosis,
      pleura) 012.0●
Pyoureter 593.89
  tuberculous (see also Tuberculosis)
      016.2●
Pyramidopallidonigral syndrome 332.0
Pyrexia (of unknown origin) (P.U.O.)
    780.60
  atmospheric 992.0
  during labor 659.2●
  environmentally-induced newborn
      778.4
  heat 992.0
  newborn, environmentally-induced
      778.4
  puerperal 672●
Pyroglobulinemia 273.8
Pyromania 312.33
Pyrosis 787.1
Pyrroloporphyria 277.1
Pyuria (bacterial) 791.9

Q

Q fever 083.0
   with pneumonia 083.0 [484.8]
Quadricuspid aortic valve 746.89
Quadrilateral fever 083.0
Quadriparesis - see Quadriplegia
   meaning muscle weakness 728.87
Quadriplegia 344.00
   with fracture, vertebra (process) - see
       Fracture, vertebra, cervical, with
       spinal cord injury
   brain (current episode) 437.8
   C_1–C_4
      complete 344.01
      incomplete 344.02
   C_5–C_7
      complete 344.03
      incomplete 344.04
   cerebral (current episode) 437.8
   congenital or infantile (cerebral)
      (spastic) (spinal) 343.2
   cortical 437.8
   embolic (current episode) (see also
      Embolism, brain) 434.1 ●
   functional 780.72

Quadriplegia (Continued)
   infantile (cerebral) (spastic) (spinal)
      343.2
   newborn NEC 767.0
   specified NEC 344.09
   thrombotic (current episode) (see also
      Thrombosis, brain) 434.0 ●
   traumatic - see Injury, spinal, cervical
Quadruplet
   affected by maternal complications of
      pregnancy 761.5
   healthy liveborn - see Newborn,
      multiple
   pregnancy (complicating delivery)
      NEC 651.8 ●
      with fetal loss and retention
         of one or more fetus(es)
         651.5 ●
      following (elective) fetal reduction
         651.7 ●
Quarrelsomeness 301.3
Quartan
   fever 084.2
   malaria (fever) 084.2
Queensland fever 083.0
   coastal 083.0
   seven-day 100.89

Quervain's disease 727.04
   thyroid (subacute granulomatous
      thyroiditis) 245.1
Queyrat's erythroplasia (M8080/2)
   specified site - see Neoplasm, skin, in
      situ
   unspecified site 233.5
Quincke's disease or edema - see Edema,
   angioneurotic
Quinquaud's disease (acne decalvans)
   704.09
Quinsy (gangrenous) 475
Quintan fever 083.1
Quintuplet
   affected by maternal complications of
      pregnancy 761.5
   healthy liveborn - see Newborn,
      multiple
   pregnancy (complicating delivery)
      NEC 651.2 ●
      with fetal loss and retention of one
         or more fetus(es) 651.6 ●
      following (elective) fetal reduction
         651.7 ●
Quotidian
   fever 084.0
   malaria (fever) 084.0

◀ New   ◀▥ Revised   ~~deleted~~ Deleted   ● Use Additional Digit(s)   ▭ Omit code

R

Rabbia 071
Rabbit fever (*see also* Tularemia) 021.9
Rabies 071
  contact V01.5
  exposure to V01.5
  inoculation V04.5
    reaction - *see* Complications,
      vaccination
  vaccination, prophylactic (against)
    V04.5
Rachischisis (*see also* Spina bifida) 741.9●
Rachitic - *see also* condition
  deformities of spine 268.1
  pelvis 268.1
    with disproportion (fetopelvic)
      653.2●
      affecting fetus or newborn 763.1
      causing obstructed labor 660.1●
        affecting fetus or newborn
          763.1
Rachitis, rachitism - *see also* Rickets
  acute 268.0
  fetalis 756.4
  renalis 588.0
  tarda 268.0
Racket nail 757.5
Radial nerve - *see* condition
Radiation effects or sickness - *see also*
    Effect, adverse, radiation
  cataract 366.46
  dermatitis 692.82
    sunburn (*see also* Sunburn) 692.71
Radiculitis (pressure) (vertebrogenic)
    729.2
  accessory nerve 723.4
  anterior crural 724.4
  arm 723.4
  brachial 723.4
  cervical NEC 723.4
  due to displacement of intervertebral
    disc - *see* Neuritis, due to,
    displacement intervertebral disc
  leg 724.4
  lumbar NEC 724.4
  lumbosacral 724.4
  rheumatic 729.2
  syphilitic 094.89
  thoracic (with visceral pain) 724.4
Radiculomyelitis 357.0
  toxic, due to
    Clostridium tetani 037
    corynebacterium diphtheriae 032.89
Radiculopathy (*see also* Radiculitis) 729.2
Radioactive substances, adverse effect -
    see Effect, adverse, radioactive
    substance
Radiodermal burns (acute) (chronic)
    (occupational) - *see* Burn, by site
Radiodermatitis 692.82
Radionecrosis - *see* Effect, adverse,
    radiation
Radiotherapy session V58.0
Radium, adverse effect - *see* Effect,
    adverse, radioactive substance
Raeder-Harbitz syndrome (pulseless
    disease) 446.7
Rage (*see also* Disturbance, conduct)
    312.0●
  meaning rabies 071
Rag sorters' disease 022.1
Raillietiniasis 123.8
Railroad neurosis 300.16

Railway spine 300.16
Raised - *see* Elevation
Raiva 071
Rake teeth, tooth 524.39
Rales 786.7
Ramifying renal pelvis 753.3
Ramsay Hunt syndrome (herpetic
    geniculate ganglionitis) 053.11
  meaning dyssynergia cerebellaris
    myoclonica 334.2
Ranke's primary infiltration (*see also*
    Tuberculosis) 010.0●
Ranula 527.6
  congenital 750.26
Rape
  adult 995.83
  alleged, observation or examination
    V71.5
  child 995.53
Rapid
  feeble pulse, due to shock, following
    injury 958.4
  heart (beat) 785.0
    psychogenic 306.2
  respiration 786.06
    psychogenic 306.1
  second stage (delivery) 661.3●
    affecting fetus or newborn 763.6
  time-zone change syndrome 327.35
Rarefaction, bone 733.99
Rash 782.1
  canker 034.1
  diaper 691.0
  drug (internal use) 693.0
    contact 692.3
  ECHO 9 virus 078.89
  enema 692.89
  food (*see also* Allergy, food) 693.1
  heat 705.1
  napkin 691.0
  nettle 708.8
  pustular 782.1
  rose 782.1
    epidemic 056.9
    of infants 057.8
  scarlet 034.1
  serum (prophylactic) (therapeutic)
    999.5
  toxic 782.1
  wandering tongue 529.1
Rasmussen's aneurysm (*see also*
    Tuberculosis) 011.2●
Rat-bite fever 026.9
  due to Streptobacillus moniliformis
    026.1
  spirochetal (morsus muris) 026.0
Rathke's pouch tumor (M9350/1) 237.0
Raymond (-Céstan) syndrome 433.8●
Raynaud's
  disease or syndrome (paroxysmal
    digital cyanosis) 443.0
  gangrene (symmetric) 443.0 [785.4]
  phenomenon (paroxysmal digital
    cyanosis) (secondary) 443.0
RDS 769
Reaction
  acute situational maladjustment (*see
    also* Reaction, adjustment) 309.9
  adaptation (*see also* Reaction,
    adjustment) 309.9
  adjustment 309.9
    with
      anxious mood 309.24
        with depressed mood 309.28

Reaction (*Continued*)
  adjustment (*Continued*)
    with (*Continued*)
      conduct disturbance 309.3
        combined with disturbance of
          emotions 309.4
      depressed mood 309.0
        brief 309.0
          with anxious mood 309.28
        prolonged 309.1
      elective mutism 309.83
      mixed emotions and conduct
        309.4
      mutism, elective 309.83
      physical symptoms 309.82
      predominant disturbance (of)
        conduct 309.3
        emotions NEC 309.29
          mixed 309.28
        mixed, emotions and conduct
          309.4
        specified type NEC 309.89
      specific academic or work
        inhibition 309.23
      withdrawal 309.83
    depressive 309.0
      with conduct disturbance 309.4
      brief 309.0
      prolonged 309.1
    specified type NEC 309.89
  adverse food NEC 995.7
  affective (*see also* Psychosis, affective)
    296.90
    specified type NEC 296.99
  aggressive 301.3
    unsocialized (*see also* Disturbance,
      conduct) 312.0●
  allergic (*see also* Allergy) 995.3
    drug, medicinal substance, and
      biological - *see* Allergy, drug
    due to correct medical substance
      properly administered
      995.27 ◄
    food - *see* Allergy, food
    serum 999.5
  anaphylactic - *see* Shock, anaphylactic
  anesthesia - *see* Anesthesia,
    complication
  anger 312.0●
  antisocial 301.7
  antitoxin (prophylactic) (therapeutic) -
    see Complications, vaccination
  anxiety 300.00
  Arthus 995.21
  asthenic 300.5
  compulsive 300.3
  conversion (anesthetic) (autonomic)
    (hyperkinetic) (mixed paralytic)
    (paresthetic) 300.11
  deoxyribonuclease (DNA) (DNase)
    hypersensitivity NEC 287.2
  depressive 300.4
    acute 309.0
    affective (*see also* Psychosis,
      affective) 296.2●
      recurrent episode 296.3●
      single episode 296.2●
    brief 309.0
    manic (*see also* Psychosis, affective)
      296.80
    neurotic 300.4
    psychoneurotic 300.4
    psychotic 298.0
  dissociative 300.15

Reaction (*Continued*)
  drug NEC (*see also* Table of Drugs and
      Chemicals) 995.20
    allergic - *see also* Allergy, drug 995.27
    correct substance properly
        administered 995.20
    obstetric anesthetic or analgesic
        NEC 668.9●
      affecting fetus or newborn 763.5
      specified drug - *see* Table of
          Drugs and Chemicals
    overdose or poisoning 977.9
      specified drug - *see* Table of
          Drugs and Chemicals
    specific to newborn 779.4
    transmitted via placenta or breast
        milk - *see* Absorption, drug,
        through placenta
    withdrawal NEC 292.0
      infant of dependent mother 779.5
    wrong substance given or taken in
        error 977.9
      specified drug - *see* Table of
          Drugs and Chemicals
  dyssocial 301.7
  dystonic, acute, due to drugs 333.72
  erysipeloid 027.1
  fear 300.20
    child 313.0
  fluid loss, cerebrospinal 349.0
  food - *see also* Allergy, food
    adverse NEC 995.7
    anaphylactic shock - *see*
        Anaphylactic shock, due to,
        food
  foreign
    body NEC 728.82
      in operative wound
          (inadvertently left) 998.4
        due to surgical material
            intentionally left - *see*
            Complications, due to
            (presence of) any device,
            implant, or graft classified
            to 996.0–996.5 NEC
      substance accidentally left during a
          procedure (chemical) (powder)
          (talc) 998.7
        body or object (instrument)
            (sponge) (swab) 998.4
  graft-versus-host (GVH) 279.50
  grief (acute) (brief) 309.0
    prolonged 309.1
  gross stress (*see also* Reaction, stress,
      acute) 308.9
  group delinquent (*see also* Disturbance,
      conduct) 312.2●
  Herxheimer's 995.0
  hyperkinetic (*see also* Hyperkinesia) 314.9
  hypochondriacal 300.7
  hypoglycemic, due to insulin 251.0
    therapeutic misadventure 962.3
  hypomanic (*see also* Psychosis,
      affective) 296.0●
    recurrent episode 296.1●
    single episode 296.0●
  hysterical 300.10
    conversion type 300.11
    dissociative 300.15
  id (bacterial cause) 692.89
  immaturity NEC 301.89
    aggressive 301.3
    emotional instability 301.59
  immunization - *see* Complications,
      vaccination

Reaction (*Continued*)
  incompatibility
    blood group (*see also* Complications,
        transfusion) 999.80 ◀▥
      ABO (due to transfusion of blood
          or blood products) (*see also*
          Complications, transfusion)
          999.60 ◀
        minor blood group 999.89 ◀
        non-ABO (*see also* Complications,
            transfusion) 999.75 ◀
      ABO 999.6
      minor blood group 999.89
      Rh antigen (C) (c) (D) (E) (e) (factor)
          (infusion) (transfusion) (*see*
          also Complications,
          transfusion) 999.70 ◀▥
    inflammatory - *see* Infection
    infusion - *see* Complications, infusion
    inoculation (immune serum) - *see*
        Complications, vaccination
  insulin 995.23
  involutional
    paranoid 297.2
    psychotic (*see also* Psychosis,
        affective, depressive) 296.2●
  leukemoid (basophilic) (lymphocytic)
      (monocytic) (myelocytic)
      (neutrophilic) 288.62
  LSD (*see also* Abuse, drugs,
      nondependent) 305.3●
  lumbar puncture 349.0
  manic-depressive (*see also* Psychosis,
      affective) 296.80
    depressed 296.2●
      recurrent episode 296.3●
      single episode 296.2●
    hypomanic 296.0●
  neurasthenic 300.5
  neurogenic (*see also* Neurosis) 300.9
  neurotic NEC 300.9
  neurotic-depressive 300.4
  nitritoid - *see* Crisis, nitritoid
  obsessive-compulsive 300.3
  organic 293.9
    acute 293.0
    subacute 293.1
  overanxious, child or adolescent 313.0
  paranoid (chronic) 297.9
    acute 298.3
    climacteric 297.2
    involutional 297.2
    menopausal 297.2
    senile 290.20
    simple 297.0
  passive
    aggressive 301.84
    dependency 301.6
  personality (*see also* Disorder,
      personality) 301.9
  phobic 300.20
  postradiation - *see* Effect, adverse,
      radiation
  psychogenic NEC 300.9
  psychoneurotic (*see also* Neurosis) 300.9
    anxiety 300.00
    compulsive 300.3
    conversion 300.11
    depersonalization 300.6
    depressive 300.4
    dissociative 300.15
    hypochondriacal 300.7
    hysterical 300.10
      conversion type 300.11
      dissociative type 300.15
    neurasthenic 300.5
    obsessive 300.3

Reaction (*Continued*)
  psychoneurotic (*Continued*)
    obsessive-compulsive 300.3
    phobic 300.20
    tension state 300.9
  psychophysiologic NEC (*see also*
      Disorder, psychosomatic) 306.9
    cardiovascular 306.2
    digestive 306.4
    endocrine 306.6
    gastrointestinal 306.4
    genitourinary 306.50
    heart 306.2
    hemic 306.8
    intestinal (large) (small) 306.4
    laryngeal 306.1
    lymphatic 306.8
    musculoskeletal 306.0
    pharyngeal 306.1
    respiratory 306.1
    skin 306.3
    special sense organs 306.7
  psychosomatic (*see also* Disorder,
      psychosomatic) 306.9
  psychotic (*see also* Psychosis) 298.9
    depressive 298.0
    due to or associated with physical
        condition (*see also* Psychosis,
        organic) 293.9
    involutional (*see also* Psychosis,
        affective) 296.2●
      recurrent episode 296.3●
      single episode 296.2●
  pupillary (myotonic) (tonic) 379.46
  radiation - *see* Effect, adverse, radiation
  runaway - *see also* Disturbance, conduct
    socialized 312.2●
    undersocialized, unsocialized 312.1●
  scarlet fever toxin - *see* Complications,
      vaccination
  schizophrenic (*see also* Schizophrenia)
      295.9●
    latent 295.5●
  serological for syphilis - *see* Serology
      for syphilis
  serum (prophylactic) (therapeutic)
      999.5
    immediate 999.4
  situational (*see also* Reaction,
      adjustment) 309.9
    acute, to stress 308.3
    adjustment (*see also* Reaction,
        adjustment) 309.9
  somatization (*see also* Disorder,
      psychosomatic) 306.9
  spinal puncture 349.0
  spite, child (*see also* Disturbance,
      conduct) 312.0●
  stress, acute 308.9
    with predominant disturbance (of)
      consciousness 308.1
      emotions 308.0
      mixed 308.4
      psychomotor 308.2
      specified type NEC 308.3
    bone or cartilage - *see* Fracture, stress
  surgical procedure - *see* Complications,
      surgical procedure
  tetanus antitoxin - *see* Complications,
      vaccination
  toxin-antitoxin - *see* Complications,
      vaccination
  transfusion (blood) (bone marrow)
      (lymphocytes) (allergic) (*see also*
      Complications, transfusion)
      999.80 ◀▥

◀ New   ◀▥ Revised   ~~deleted~~ Deleted   ● Use Additional Digit(s)   ▥ Omit code

Reaction *(Continued)*
  tuberculin skin test, nonspecific
      (without active tuberculosis)
      795.5
    positive (without active
        tuberculosis) 795.5
  ultraviolet - *see* Effect, adverse,
      ultraviolet
  undersocialized, unsocialized - *see also*
      Disturbance, conduct
    aggressive (type) 312.0●
    unaggressive (type) 312.1●
  vaccination (any) - *see* Complications,
      vaccination
  white graft (skin) 996.52
  withdrawing, child or adolescent 313.22
  x-ray - *see* Effect, adverse, x-rays
Reactive depression *(see also* Reaction,
    depressive) 300.4
  neurotic 300.4
  psychoneurotic 300.4
  psychotic 298.0
Rebound tenderness 789.6●
Recalcitrant patient V15.81
Recanalization, thrombus - *see*
    Thrombosis
Recession, receding
  chamber angle (eye) 364.77
  chin 524.06
  gingival (postinfective) (postoperative)
      523.20
    generalized 523.25
    localized 523.24
    minimal 523.21
    moderate 523.22
    severe 523.23
Recklinghausen's disease (M9540/1)
    237.71
  bones (osteitis fibrosa cystica) 252.01
Recklinghausen-Applebaum disease
    (hemochromatosis) 275.03 ◀▥
Reclus' disease (cystic) 610.1
Recrudescent typhus (fever) 081.1
Recruitment, auditory 388.44
Rectalgia 569.42
Rectitis 569.49
Rectocele
  female (without uterine prolapse)
      618.04
    with uterine prolapse 618.4
      complete 618.3
      incomplete 618.2
  in pregnancy or childbirth 654.4●
    causing obstructed labor 660.2●
      affecting fetus or newborn 763.1
  male 569.49
  vagina, vaginal (outlet) 618.04
Rectosigmoiditis 569.89
  ulcerative (chronic) 556.3
Rectosigmoid junction - *see* condition
Rectourethral - *see* condition
Rectovaginal - *see* condition
Rectovesical - *see* condition
Rectum, rectal - *see* condition
Recurrent - *see* condition
  pregnancy loss - *see* Pregnancy,
      management affected by,
      abortion, habitual ◀
Red bugs 133.8
Red cedar asthma 495.8
Redness
  conjunctiva 379.93
  eye 379.93
  nose 478.19

Reduced ventilatory or vital capacity
    794.2
Reduction
  function
    kidney *(see also* Disease, renal) 593.9
    liver 573.8
  ventilatory capacity 794.2
  vital capacity 794.2
Redundant, redundancy
  abdomen 701.9
  anus 751.5
  cardia 537.89
  clitoris 624.2
  colon (congenital) 751.5
  foreskin (congenital) 605
  intestine 751.5
  labia 624.3
  organ or site, congenital NEC - *see*
      Accessory
  panniculus (abdominal) 278.1
  prepuce (congenital) 605
  pylorus 537.89
  rectum 751.5
  scrotum 608.89
  sigmoid 751.5
  skin (of face) 701.9
    eyelids 374.30
  stomach 537.89
  uvula 528.9
  vagina 623.8
Reduplication - *see* Duplication
Referral
  adoption (agency) V68.89
  nursing care V63.8
  patient without examination or
      treatment V68.81
  social services V63.8
Reflex - *see also* condition
  blink, deficient 374.45
  hyperactive gag 478.29
  neurogenic bladder NEC 596.54
    atonic 596.54
      with cauda equina syndrome
          344.61
  vasoconstriction 443.9
  vasovagal 780.2
Reflux 530.81
  acid 530.81
  esophageal 530.81
    with esophagitis 530.11
  esophagitis 530.11
  gastroesophageal 530.81
  mitral - *see* Insufficiency, mitral
  ureteral - *see* Reflux, vesicoureteral
  vesicoureteral 593.70
    with
      reflux nephropathy 593.73
        bilateral 593.72
        unilateral 593.71
Reformed gallbladder 576.0
Reforming, artificial openings *(see also*
    Attention to, artificial, opening) V55.9
Refractive error *(see also* Error, refractive)
    367.9
Refsum's disease or syndrome
    (heredopathia atactica
    polyneuritiformis) 356.3
Refusal of
  food 307.59
    hysterical 300.11
  treatment because of, due to
    patient's decision NEC V64.2
    reason of conscience or religion
        V62.6

Regaud
  tumor (M8082/3) - *see* Neoplasm,
      nasopharynx, malignant
  type carcinoma (M8082/3) - *see*
      Neoplasm, nasopharynx,
      malignant
Regional - *see* condition
Regulation feeding (elderly) (infant) 783.3
  newborn 779.31
Regurgitated
  food, choked on 933.1
  stomach contents, choked on 933.1
Regurgitation 787.03
  aortic (valve) *(see also* Insufficiency,
      aortic) 424.1
    congenital 746.4
    syphilitic 093.22
  food - *see also* Vomiting
    with reswallowing - *see* Rumination
    newborn 779.33
  gastric contents - *see* Vomiting
  heart - *see* Endocarditis
  mitral (valve) - *see also* Insufficiency,
      mitral
    congenital 746.6
  myocardial - *see* Endocarditis
  pulmonary (heart) (valve) *(see also*
      Endocarditis, pulmonary) 424.3
  stomach - *see* Vomiting
  tricuspid - *see* Endocarditis, tricuspid
  valve, valvular - *see* Endocarditis
  vesicoureteral - *see* Reflux,
      vesicoureteral
Rehabilitation V57.9
  multiple types V57.89
  occupational V57.21
  specified type NEC V57.89
  speech (-language) V57.3
  vocational V57.22
Reichmann's disease or syndrome
    (gastrosuccorrhea) 536.8
Reifenstein's syndrome (hereditary
    familial hypogonadism, male)
    259.52
Reilly's syndrome or phenomenon *(see
    also* Neuropathy, peripheral,
    autonomic) 337.9
Reimann's periodic disease 277.31
Reinsertion, contraceptive device V25.42
  intrauterine V25.13 ◀
Reiter's disease, syndrome, or urethritis
    099.3 *[711.1]*●
Rejection
  food, hysterical 300.11
  transplant 996.80
    bone marrow 996.85
    corneal 996.51
    organ (immune or nonimmune
        cause) 996.80
      bone marrow 996.85
      heart 996.83
      intestines 996.87
      kidney 996.81
      liver 996.82
      lung 996.84
      pancreas 996.86
      specified NEC 996.89
    skin 996.52
      artificial 996.55
      decellularized allodermis 996.55
Relapsing fever 087.9
  Carter's (Asiatic) 087.0
  Dutton's (West African) 087.1
  Koch's 087.9

R

Relapsing fever *(Continued)*
 louse-borne (epidemic) 087.0
 Novy's (American) 087.1
 Obermeyer's (European) 087.0
 Spirillum 087.9
 tick-borne (endemic) 087.1
Relaxation
 anus (sphincter) 569.49
  due to hysteria 300.11
 arch (foot) 734
  congenital 754.61
 back ligaments 728.4
 bladder (sphincter) 596.59
 cardio-esophageal 530.89
 cervix (*see also* Incompetency, cervix)
  622.5
 diaphragm 519.4
 inguinal rings - *see* Hernia, inguinal
 joint (capsule) (ligament) (paralytic) (*see
  also* Derangement, joint) 718.90
  congenital 755.8
 lumbosacral joint 724.6
 pelvic floor 618.89
 pelvis 618.89
 perineum 618.89
 posture 729.90
 rectum (sphincter) 569.49
 sacroiliac (joint) 724.6
 scrotum 608.89
 urethra (sphincter) 599.84
 uterus (outlet) 618.89
 vagina (outlet) 618.89
 vesical 596.59
Remains
 canal of Cloquet 743.51
 capsule (opaque) 743.51
Remittent fever (malarial) 084.6
Remnant
 canal of Cloquet 743.51
 capsule (opaque) 743.51
 cervix, cervical stump (acquired)
  (postoperative) 622.8
 cystic duct, postcholecystectomy 576.0
 fingernail 703.8
  congenital 757.5
 meniscus, knee 717.5
 thyroglossal duct 759.2
 tonsil 474.8
  infected 474.00
 urachus 753.7
Remote effect of cancer - *see* condition
Removal (of)
 catheter (urinary) (indwelling) V53.6
  from artificial opening - *see*
   Attention to, artificial, opening
  non-vascular V58.82
  vascular V58.81
 cerebral ventricle (communicating)
  shunt V53.01
 device - *see also* Fitting (of)
  contraceptive V25.12 ◀▥
   with reinsertion V25.13 ◀
  fixation
   external V54.89
   internal V54.01
  traction V54.89
 drains V58.49
 dressing
  wound V58.30
   nonsurgical V58.30
   surgical V58.31
 ileostomy V55.2
 Kirschner wire V54.89
 non-vascular catheter V58.82

Removal (of) *(Continued)*
 pin V54.01
 plaster cast V54.89
 plate (fracture) V54.01
 rod V54.01
 screw V54.01
 splint, external V54.89
 staples V58.32
 subdermal implantable contraceptive
  V25.43
 sutures V58.32
 traction device, external V54.89
 vascular catheter V58.81
 wound packing V58.30
  nonsurgical V58.30
  surgical V58.31
Ren
 arcuatus 753.3
 mobile, mobilis (*see also* Disease, renal)
  593.0
  congenital 753.3
 unguliformis 753.3
Renal - *see also* condition
 glomerulohyalinosis-diabetic
  syndrome 250.4● *[581.81]*
  due to secondary diabetes 249.4●
   [581.81]
Rendu-Osler-Weber disease or syndrome
  (familial hemorrhagic telangiectasia)
  448.0
Reninoma (M8361/1) 236.91
Rénon-Delille syndrome 253.8
Repair
 pelvic floor, previous, in pregnancy or
  childbirth 654.4●
  affecting fetus or newborn 763.89
 scarred tissue V51.8
Replacement by artificial or mechanical
  device or prosthesis of (*see also*
  Fitting (of))
 artificial skin V43.83
 bladder V43.5
 blood vessel V43.4
 breast V43.82
 eye globe V43.0
 heart
  with
   assist device V43.21
   fully implantable artificial heart
    V43.22
  valve V43.3
 intestine V43.89
 joint V43.60
  ankle V43.66
  elbow V43.62
  finger V43.69
  hip (partial) (total) V43.64
  knee V43.65
  shoulder V43.61
  specified NEC V43.69
  wrist V43.63
 kidney V43.89
 larynx V43.81
 lens V43.1
 limb(s) V43.7
 liver V43.89
 lung V43.89
 organ NEC V43.89
 pancreas V43.89
 skin (artificial) V43.83
 tissue NEC V43.89
Reprogramming
 cardiac pacemaker V53.31
Request for expert evidence V68.2

Reserve, decreased or low
 cardiac - *see* Disease, heart
  kidney (*see also* Disease, renal) 593.9
Residual - *see also* condition
 bladder 596.8
 foreign body - *see* Retention, foreign
  body
 state, schizophrenic (*see also*
  Schizophrenia) 295.6●
 urine 788.69
Resistance, resistant (to)
 activated protein C 289.81

Note: Use the following subclassification for categories V09.5, V09.7, V09.8, V09.9
0 without mention of resistance to multiple drugs
1 with resistance to multiple drugs
V09.5 quinolones and fluoro-quinolones
V09.7 antimycobacterial agents
V09.8 specified drugs NEC
V09.9 unspecified drugs

 drugs by microorganisms V09.90
  amikacin V09.4
  aminoglycosides V09.4
  amodiaquine V09.5●
  amoxicillin V09.0
  ampicillin V09.0
  antimycobacterial agents V09.7●
  azithromycin V09.2
  azlocillin V09.0
  aztreonam V09.1
  B-lactam antibiotics V09.1
  bacampicillin V09.0
  bacitracin V09.8●
  benznidazole V09.8●
  capreomycin V09.7●
  carbenicillin V09.0
  cefaclor V09.1
  cefadroxil V09.1
  cefamandole V09.1
  cefatetan V09.1
  cefazolin V09.1
  cefixime V09.1
  cefonicid V09.1
  cefoperazone V09.1
  ceforanide V09.1
  cefotaxime V09.1
  cefoxitin V09.1
  ceftazidine V09.1
  ceftizoxime V09.1
  ceftriaxone V09.1
  cefuroxime V09.1
  cephalexin V09.1
  cephaloglycin V09.1
  cephaloridine V09.1
  cephalosporins V09.1
  cephalothin V09.1
  cephapirin V09.1
  cephradine V09.1
  chloramphenicol V09.8●
  chloraquine V09.5●
  chlorguanide V09.8●
  chlorproguanil V09.8●
  chlortetracycline V09.3
  cinoxacin V09.5●
  ciprofloxacin V09.5●
  clarithromycin V09.2
  clindamycin V09.8●
  clioquinol V09.5●
  clofazimine V09.7●

◀ New   ◀▥ Revised   ~~deleted~~ Deleted   ● Use Additional Digit(s)   ▨ Omit code

Resistance, resistant *(Continued)*
  drugs by microorganisms *(Continued)*
    cloxacillin V09.0
    cyclacillin V09.0
    cycloserine V09.7●
    dapsone [Dz] V09.7●
    demeclocycline V09.3
    dicloxacillin V09.0
    doxycycline V09.3
    enoxacin V09.5●
    erythromycin V09.2
    ethambutol [EMB] V09.7●
    ethionamide [ETA] V09.7●
    fluoroquinolones NEC V09.5●
    gentamicin V09.4
    halofantrine V09.8●
    imipenem V09.1
    iodoquinol V09.5●
    isoniazid [INH] V09.7●
    kanamycin V09.4
    macrolides V09.2
    mafenide V09.6
    MDRO (multiple drug resistant
        organisms) NOS V09.91
    mefloquine V09.8●
    melarsoprol V09.8●
    methicillin - see Infection,
        Methicillin
    methacycline V09.3
    methenamine V09.8●
    metronidazole V09.8●
    mezlocillin V09.0
    minocycline V09.3
    multiple drug resistant organisms
        NOS V09.91
    nafcillin V09.0
    nalidixic acid V09.5●
    natamycin V09.2
    neomycin V09.4
    netilmicin V09.4
    nimorazole V09.8●
    nitrofurantoin V09.8●
    norfloxacin V09.5●
    nystatin V09.2
    ofloxacin V09.5●
    oleandomycin V09.2
    oxacillin V09.0
    oxytetracycline V09.3
    para-amino salicyclic acid [PAS]
        V09.7●
    paromomycin V09.4
    penicillin (G) (V) (Vk) V09.0
    penicillins V09.0
    pentamidine V09.8●
    piperacillin V09.0
    primaquine V09.5●
    proguanil V09.8●
    pyrazinamide [PZA] V09.7●
    pyrimethamine/sulfalene V09.8●
    pyrimethamine/sulfodoxine V09.8●
    quinacrine V09.5●
    quinidine V09.8●
    quinine V09.8●
    quinolones V09.5●
    rifabutin V09.7●
    rifampin [Rif] V09.7●
    rifamycin V09.7●
    rolitetracycline V09.3
    specified drugs NEC V09.8●
    spectinomycin V09.8●
    spiramycin V09.2
    streptomycin [Sm] V09.4
    sulfacetamide V09.6
    sulfacytine V09.6

Resistance, resistant *(Continued)*
  drugs by microorganisms *(Continued)*
    sulfadiazine V09.6
    sulfadoxine V09.6
    sulfamethoxazole V09.6
    sulfapyridine V09.6
    sulfasalizine V09.6
    sulfasoxazone V09.6
    sulfonamides V09.6
    sulfoxone V09.7●
    tetracycline V09.3
    tetracyclines V09.3
    thiamphenicol V09.8●
    ticarcillin V09.0
    tinidazole V09.8●
    tobramycin V09.4
    triamphenicol V09.8●
    trimethoprim V09.8●
    vancomycin V09.8●
  insulin 277.7
  thyroid hormone 246.8
Resorption
  biliary 576.8
    purulent or putrid *(see also*
        Cholecystitis) 576.8
  dental (roots) 521.40
    alveoli 525.8
    pathological
        external 521.42
        internal 521.41
        specified NEC 521.49
  septic - *see* Septicemia
  teeth (roots) 521.40
    pathological
        external 521.42
        internal 521.41
        specified NEC 521.49
Respiration
  asymmetrical 786.09
  bronchial 786.09
  Cheyne-Stokes (periodic respiration)
      786.04
  decreased, due to shock following
      injury 958.4
  disorder of 786.00
    psychogenic 306.1
    specified NEC 786.09
  failure 518.81
    acute 518.81
    acute and chronic 518.84
    chronic 518.83
    newborn 770.84
  insufficiency 786.09
    acute 518.82
    newborn NEC 770.89
  Kussmaul (air hunger) 786.09
  painful 786.52
  periodic 786.09
  high altitude 327.22
  poor 786.09
    newborn NEC 770.89
  sighing 786.7
    psychogenic 306.1
  wheezing 786.07
Respiratory - *see also* condition
  distress 786.09
    acute 518.82
    fetus or newborn NEC 770.89
    syndrome (newborn) 769
      adult (following shock,
          surgery, or trauma)
          518.5
        specified NEC 518.82

Respiratory *(Continued)*
  failure 518.81
    acute 518.81
    acute and chronic 518.84
    chronic 518.83
Respiratory syncytial virus (RSV) 079.6
  bronchiolitis 466.11
  pneumonia 480.1
  vaccination, prophylactic (against)
      V04.82
Response
  photoallergic 692.72
  phototoxic 692.72
Rest, rests
  mesonephric duct 752.89
    fallopian tube 752.11
  ovarian, in fallopian tubes 752.19
  wolffian duct 752.89
Restless legs syndrome (RLS) 333.94
Restlessness 799.29
Restoration of organ continuity from
    previous sterilization (tuboplasty)
    (vasoplasty) V26.0
Restriction of housing space V60.1
Restzustand, schizophrenic *(see also*
    Schizophrenia) 295.6●
Retained - *see* Retention
Retardation
  development, developmental, specific
      (see also Disorder, development,
      specific) 315.9
    learning, specific 315.2
      arithmetical 315.1
      language (skills) 315.31
        expressive 315.31
        mixed receptive-expressive
            315.32
      mathematics 315.1
      reading 315.00
        phonological 315.39
      written expression 315.2
    motor 315.4
  endochondral bone growth 733.91
  growth (physical) in childhood 783.43
    due to malnutrition 263.2
    fetal (intrauterine) 764.9●
      affecting management of
          pregnancy 656.5●
  intrauterine growth 764.9●
    affecting management of pregnancy
        656.5●
  mental 319
    borderline V62.89
    mild, IQ 50–70 317
    moderate, IQ 35–49 318.0
    profound, IQ under 20 318.2
    severe, IQ 20–34 318.1
  motor, specific 315.4
  physical 783.43
    child 783.43
    due to malnutrition 263.2
    fetus (intrauterine) 764.9●
      affecting management of
          pregnancy 656.5●
  psychomotor NEC 307.9
  reading 315.00
Retching - *see* Vomiting
Retention, retained
  bladder *(see also* Retention, urine)
      788.20
    psychogenic 306.53
  carbon dioxide 276.2
  cholelithisis 997.4
  cyst - *see* Cyst

Retention, retained *(Continued)*
  dead
    fetus (after 22 completed weeks'
      gestation) 656.4●
      early fetal death (before 22
        completed weeks'
        gestation) 632
    ovum 631
  decidua (following delivery)
    (fragments) (with hemorrhage)
    666.2●
    without hemorrhage 667.1●
  deciduous tooth 520.6
  dental root 525.3
  fecal (*see also* Constipation) 564.00
  fluid 276.69 ◀▥●
  foreign body - *see also* Foreign body,
    retained
    bone 733.99
    current trauma - *see* Foreign body,
      by site or type
    middle ear 385.83
    muscle 729.6
    soft tissue NEC 729.6
  gallstones 997.4
  gastric 536.8
  membranes (following delivery) (with
    hemorrhage) 666.2●
    with abortion - *see* Abortion, by type
    without hemorrhage 667.1●
  menses 626.8
  milk (puerperal) 676.2●
  nitrogen, extrarenal 788.99
  placenta (total) (with hemorrhage)
    666.0●
    with abortion - *see* Abortion, by type
    portions or fragments 666.2●
      without hemorrhage 667.1●
    without hemorrhage 667.0●
  products of conception
    early pregnancy (fetal death before
      22 completed weeks'
      gestation) 632
    following
      abortion - *see* Abortion, by type
      delivery 666.2●
        with hemorrhage 666.2●
        without hemorrhage 667.1●
  secundines (following delivery) (with
    hemorrhage) 666.2●
    with abortion - *see* Abortion, by type
    complicating puerperium (delayed
      hemorrhage) 666.2●
    without hemorrhage 667.1●
  smegma, clitoris 624.8
  urine NEC 788.20
    bladder, incomplete emptying
      788.21
      due to
        benign prostatic hypertrophy
          (BPH) - *see* category 600
    due to
      benign prostatic hypertrophy
        (BPH) - *see* category 600
    psychogenic 306.53
    specified NEC 788.29
  water (in tissue) (*see also* Edema) 782.3
Reticulation, dust (occupational) 504
Reticulocytosis NEC 790.99
Reticuloendotheliosis
  acute infantile (M9722/3) 202.5●
  leukemic (M9940/3) 202.4●
  malignant (M9720/3) 202.3●
  nonlipid (M9722/3) 202.5●

Reticulohistiocytoma (giant cell) 277.89
Reticulohistiocytosis, multicentric
  272.8
Reticulolymphosarcoma (diffuse)
  (M9613/3) 200.8●
  follicular (M9691/3) 202.0●
  nodular (M9691/3) 202.0●
Reticulosarcoma (M9640/3) 200.0●
  nodular (M9642/3) 200.0●
  pleomorphic cell type (M9641/3)
    200.0●
Reticulosis (skin)
  acute of infancy (M9722/3) 202.5●
  familial hemophagocytic 288.4
  histiocytic medullary (M9721/3)
    202.3●
  lipomelanotic 695.89
  malignant (M9720/3) 202.3●
  Sézary's (M9701/3) 202.2● ◀▥
Retina, retinal - *see* condition
Retinitis (*see also* Chorioretinitis) 363.20
  albuminurica 585.9 *[363.10]*
  arteriosclerotic 440.8 *[362.13]*
  central angiospastic 362.41
  Coat's 362.12
  diabetic 250.5● *[362.01]*
    due to secondary diabetes 249.5●
      [362.01]
  disciformis 362.52
  disseminated 363.10
    metastatic 363.14
    neurosyphilitic 094.83
    pigment epitheliopathy 363.15
  exudative 362.12
  focal 363.00
    in histoplasmosis 115.92
      capsulatum 115.02
      duboisii 115.12
    juxtapapillary 363.05
    macular 363.06
    paramacular 363.06
    peripheral 363.08
    posterior pole NEC 363.07
  gravidarum 646.8●
  hemorrhagica externa 362.12
  juxtapapillary (Jensen's) 363.05
  luetic - *see* Retinitis, syphilitic
  metastatic 363.14
  pigmentosa 362.74
  proliferans 362.29
  proliferating 362.29
  punctata albescens 362.76
  renal 585.9 *[363.13]*
  syphilitic (secondary) 091.51
    congenital 090.0 *[363.13]*
    early 091.51
    late 095.8 *[363.13]*
  syphilitica, central, recurrent 095.8
    [363.13]
  tuberculous (*see also* Tuberculous)
    017.3● *[363.13]*
Retinoblastoma (M9510/3) 190.5
  differentiated type (M9511/3) 190.5
  undifferentiated type (M9512/3) 190.5
Retinochoroiditis (*see also* Chorioretinitis)
  363.20
  central angiospastic 362.41
  disseminated 363.10
    metastatic 363.14
    neurosyphilitic 094.83
    pigment epitheliopathy 363.15
    syphilitic 094.83
  due to toxoplasmosis (acquired) (focal)
    130.2

Retinochoroiditis *(Continued)*
  focal 363.00
    in histoplasmosis 115.92
      capsulatum 115.02
      duboisii 115.12
    juxtapapillary (Jensen's) 363.05
    macular 363.06
    paramacular 363.06
    peripheral 363.08
    posterior pole NEC 363.07
  juxtapapillaris 363.05
  syphilitic (disseminated) 094.83
Retinopathy (background) 362.10
  arteriosclerotic 440.8 *[362.13]*
  atherosclerotic 440.8 *[362.13]*
  central serous 362.41
  circinate 362.10
  Coat's 362.12
  diabetic 250.5● *[362.01]*
    due to secondary diabetes 249.5●
      [362.01]
    nonproliferative 250.5● *[362.03]*
      due to secondary diabetes
        249.5● *[362.03]*
      mild 250.5● *[362.04]*
        due to secondary diabetes
          249.5● *[362.04]*
      moderate 250.5● *[362.05]*
        due to secondary diabetes
          249.5● *[362.05]*
      severe 250.5● *[362.06]*
        due to secondary diabetes
          249.5● *[362.06]*
    proliferative 250.5● *[362.02]*
      due to secondary diabetes 249.5●
        [362.02]
  exudative 362.12
  hypertensive 362.11
  nonproliferative
    diabetic 250.5● *[362.03]*
      due to secondary diabetes 249.5●
        [362.03]
      mild 250.5● *[362.04]*
        due to secondary diabetes
          249.5● *[362.04]*
      moderate 250.5● *[362.05]*
        due to secondary diabetes
          249.5● *[362.05]*
      severe 250.5● *[362.06]*
        due to secondary diabetes
          249.5● *[362.06]*
  of prematurity 362.20
    cicatricial 362.21
    stage
      0 362.22
      1 362.23
      2 362.24
      3 362.25
      4 362.26
      5 362.27
  pigmentary, congenital 362.74
  proliferative 362.29
    diabetic 250.5● *[362.02]*
      due to secondary diabetes
        249.5● *[362.02]*
    sickle-cell 282.60 *[362.29]*
  solar 363.31
Retinoschisis 361.10
  bullous 361.12
  congenital 743.56
  flat 361.11
  juvenile 362.73
Retractile testis 752.52

◀ New   ◀▥ Revised   ~~deleted~~ Deleted   ● Use Additional Digit(s)   ▨ Omit code

Retraction
cervix *see* Retraction, uterus
drum (membrane) 384.82
eyelid 374.41
finger 736.29
head 781.0
lid 374.41
lung 518.89
mediastinum 519.3
nipple 611.79
   congenital 757.6
   puerperal, postpartum 676.0●
palmar fascia 728.6
pleura (*see also* Pleurisy) 511.0
ring, uterus (Bandl's) (pathological)
   661.4●
   affecting fetus or newborn 763.7
sternum (congenital) 756.3
   acquired 738.3
   during respiration 786.9
substernal 738.3
supraclavicular 738.8
syndrome (Duane's) 378.71
uterus 621.6
valve (heart) - *see* Endocarditis
Retrobulbar - *see* condition
Retrocaval ureter 753.4
Retrocecal - *see also* condition
appendix (congenital) 751.5
Retrocession - *see* Retroversion
Retrodisplacement - *see* Retroversion
Retroflection, retroflexion - *see*
   Retroversion
Retrognathia, retrognathism
   (mandibular) (maxillary) 524.10
Retrograde
ejaculation 608.87
menstruation 626.8
Retroiliac ureter 753.4
Retroperineal - *see* condition
Retroperitoneal - *see* condition
Retroperitonitis 567.39
Retropharyngeal - *see* condition
Retroplacental - *see* condition
Retroposition - *see* Retroversion
Retroprosthetic membrane 996.51 ◀
Retrosternal thyroid (congenital) 759.2
Retroversion, retroverted
cervix - *see* Retroversion, uterus
female NEC (*see also* Retroversion,
   uterus) 621.6
iris 364.70
testis (congenital) 752.51
uterus, uterine (acquired) (acute)
   (adherent) (any degree)
   (asymptomatic) (cervix)
   (postinfectional) (postpartal, old)
   621.6
   congenital 752.39 ◀▥
   in pregnancy or childbirth 654.3●
      affecting fetus or newborn
       763.89
      causing obstructed labor
       660.2●
       affecting fetus or newborn
        763.1
Retrusion, premaxilla (developmental)
   524.04
Rett's syndrome 330.8
Reverse, reversed
peristalsis 787.4
Reye's syndrome 331.81
Reye-Sheehan syndrome (postpartum
   pituitary necrosis) 253.2

Rh antigen (C) (c) (D) (E) (e) (factor) ◀▥
hemolytic disease 773.0
incompatibility, immunization, or
   sensitization
      affecting management of pregnancy
       656.1●
      fetus or newborn 773.0
      transfusion reaction (*see also*
       Complications, transfusion)
       999.70 ◀▥
negative mother, affecting fetus or
   newborn 773.0
titer elevated (*see also* Complications,
   transfusion) 999.70 ◀▥
transfusion reaction (*see also*
   Complications, transfusion)
   999.70 ◀▥
Rhabdomyolysis (idiopathic) 728.88
Rhabdomyoma (M8900/0) - *see also*
   Neoplasm, connective tissue, benign
adult (M8904/0) - *see* Neoplasm,
   connective tissue, benign
fetal (M8903/0) - *see* Neoplasm,
   connective tissue, benign
glycogenic (M8904/0) - *see* Neoplasm,
   connective tissue, benign
Rhabdomyosarcoma (M8900/3) - *see also*
   Neoplasm, connective tissue,
   malignant
alveolar (M8920/3) - *see* Neoplasm,
   connective tissue, malignant
embryonal (M8910/3) - *see* Neoplasm,
   connective tissue, malignant
mixed type (M8902/3) - *see* Neoplasm,
   connective tissue, malignant
pleomorphic (M8901/3) - *see* Neoplasm,
   connective tissue, malignant
Rhabdosarcoma (M8900/3) - *see*
   Rhabdomyosarcoma
Rhesus (factor) (Rh) incompatibility - *see*
   Rh, incompatibility
Rheumaticosis - *see* Rheumatism
Rheumatism, rheumatic (acute NEC) 729.0
adherent pericardium 393
arthritis
   acute or subacute - *see* Fever,
      rheumatic
   chronic 714.0
      spine 720.0
articular (chronic) NEC (*see also*
   Arthritis) 716.9●
   acute or subacute - *see* Fever,
      rheumatic
back 724.9
blennorrhagic 098.59
carditis - *see* Disease, heart, rheumatic
cerebral - *see* Fever, rheumatic
chorea (acute) - *see* Chorea, rheumatic
chronic NEC 729.0
coronary arteritis 391.9
   chronic 398.99
degeneration, myocardium (*see also*
   Degeneration, myocardium, with
   rheumatic fever) 398.0
desert 114.0
febrile - *see* Fever, rheumatic
fever - *see* Fever, rheumatic
gonococcal 098.59
gout 714.0 ◀▥
heart
   disease (*see also* Disease, heart,
      rheumatic) 398.90
   failure (chronic) (congestive)
      (inactive) 398.91

Rheumatism, rheumatic (*Continued*)
hemopericardium - *see* Rheumatic,
   pericarditis
hydropericardium - *see* Rheumatic,
   pericarditis
inflammatory (acute) (chronic)
   (subacute) - *see* Fever, rheumatic
intercostal 729.0
   meaning Tietze's disease 733.6
joint (chronic) NEC (*see also* Arthritis)
   716.9●
   acute - *see* Fever, rheumatic
mediastinopericarditis - *see* Rheumatic,
   pericarditis
muscular 729.0
myocardial degeneration (*see also*
   Degeneration, myocardium, with
   rheumatic fever) 398.0
myocarditis (chronic) (inactive) (with
   chorea) 398.0
   active or acute 391.2
      with chorea (acute) (rheumatic)
       (Sydenham's) 392.0
myositis 729.1
neck 724.9
neuralgic 729.0
neuritis (acute) (chronic) 729.2
neuromuscular 729.0
nodose - *see* Arthritis, nodosa
nonarticular 729.0
palindromic 719.30
   ankle 719.37
   elbow 719.32
   foot 719.37
   hand 719.34
   hip 719.35
   knee 719.36
   multiple sites 719.39
   pelvic region 719.35
   shoulder (region) 719.31
   specified site NEC 719.38
   wrist 719.33
pancarditis, acute 391.8
   with chorea (acute) (rheumatic)
      (Sydenham's) 392.0
   chronic or inactive 398.99
pericarditis (active) (acute) (with
   effusion) (with pneumonia) 391.0
   with chorea (acute) (rheumatic)
      (Sydenham's) 392.0
   chronic or inactive 393
pericardium - *see* Rheumatic, pericarditis
pleuropericarditis - *see* Rheumatic,
   pericarditis
pneumonia 390 [517.1]
pneumonitis 390 [517.1]
pneumopericarditis - *see* Rheumatic,
   pericarditis
polyarthritis
   acute or subacute - *see* Fever,
      rheumatic
   chronic 714.0
polyarticular NEC (*see also* Arthritis)
   716.9●
psychogenic 306.0
radiculitis 729.2
sciatic 724.3
septic - *see* Fever, rheumatic
spine 724.9
subacute NEC 729.0
torticollis 723.5
tuberculous NEC (*see also* Tuberculosis)
   015.9●
typhoid fever 002.0

Rheumatoid - *see also* condition
  lungs 714.81
Rhinitis (atrophic) (catarrhal) (chronic)
    (croupous) (fibrinous) (hyperplastic)
    (hypertrophic) (membranous)
    (purulent) (suppurative) (ulcerative)
    472.0
  with
    hay fever (*see also* Fever, hay) 477.9
      with asthma (bronchial) 493.0●
    sore throat - *see* Nasopharyngitis
  acute 460
  allergic (nonseasonal) (seasonal) (*see
    also* Fever, hay) 477.9
    with asthma (*see also* Asthma)
      493.0●
    due to food 477.1
  granulomatous 472.0
  infective 460
  obstructive 472.0
  pneumococcal 460
  syphilitic 095.8
    congenital 090.0
  tuberculous (*see also* Tuberculosis)
    012.8●
  vasomotor (*see also* Fever, hay) 477.9
Rhinoantritis (chronic) 473.0
  acute 461.0
Rhinodacryolith 375.57
Rhinolalia (aperta) (clausa) (open)
  784.43
Rhinolith 478.19
  nasal sinus (*see also* Sinusitis) 473.9
Rhinomegaly 478.19
Rhinopharyngitis (acute) (subacute) (*see
  also* Nasopharyngitis) 460
  chronic 472.2
  destructive ulcerating 102.5
  mutilans 102.5
Rhinophyma 695.3
Rhinorrhea 478.19
  cerebrospinal (fluid) 349.81
  paroxysmal (*see also* Fever, hay) 477.9
  spasmodic (*see also* Fever, hay) 477.9
Rhinosalpingitis 381.50
  acute 381.51
  chronic 381.52
Rhinoscleroma 040.1
Rhinosporidiosis 117.0
Rhinovirus infection 079.3
Rhizomelic chrondrodysplasia punctata
  277.86
Rhizomelique, pseudopolyarthritic 446.5
Rhoads and Bomford anemia (refractory)
  238.72
Rhus
  diversiloba dermatitis 692.6
  radicans dermatitis 692.6
  toxicodendron dermatitis 692.6
  venenata dermatitis 692.6
  verniciflua dermatitis 692.6
Rhythm
  atrioventricular nodal 427.89
  disorder 427.9
    coronary sinus 427.89
    ectopic 427.89
    nodal 427.89
  escape 427.89
  heart, abnormal 427.9
    fetus or newborn - *see* Abnormal,
      heart rate
  idioventricular 426.89
    accelerated 427.89
  nodal 427.89

Rhythm (*Continued*)
  sleep, inversion 327.39
    nonorganic origin 307.45
Rhytidosis facialis 701.8
Rib - *see also* condition
  cervical 756.2
Riboflavin deficiency 266.0
Rice bodies (*see also* Loose, body, joint)
  718.1●
  knee 717.6
Richter's hernia - *see* Hernia, Richter's
Ricinism 988.2
Rickets (active) (acute) (adolescent)
  (adult) (chest wall) (congenital)
  (current) (infantile) (intestinal) 268.0
  celiac 579.0
  fetal 756.4
  hemorrhagic 267
  hypophosphatemic with nephrotic-
    glycosuric dwarfism 270.0
  kidney 588.0
  late effect 268.1
  renal 588.0
  scurvy 267
  vitamin D-resistant 275.3
Rickettsial disease 083.9
  specified type NEC 083.8
Rickettsialpox 083.2
Rickettsiosis NEC 083.9
  specified type NEC 083.8
  tick-borne 082.9
    specified type NEC 082.8
  vesicular 083.2
Ricord's chancre 091.0
Riddoch's syndrome (visual
  disorientation) 368.16
Rider's
  bone 733.99
  chancre 091.0
Ridge, alveolus - *see also* condition
  edentulous
    atrophy 525.20
      mandible 525.20
        minimal 525.21
        moderate 525.22
        severe 525.23
      maxilla 525.20
        minimal 525.24
        moderate 525.25
        severe 525.26
    flabby 525.20
Ridged ear 744.29
Riedel's
  disease (ligneous thyroiditis) 245.3
  lobe, liver 751.69
  struma (ligneous thyroiditis) 245.3
  thyroiditis (ligneous) 245.3
Rieger's anomaly or syndrome
  (mesodermal dysgenesis, anterior
  ocular segment) 743.44
Riehl's melanosis 709.09
Rietti-Greppi-Micheli anemia or
  syndrome 282.49
Rieux's hernia - *see* Hernia, Rieux's
Rift Valley fever 066.3
Riga's disease (cachectic aphthae) 529.0
Riga-Fede disease (cachectic aphthae)
  529.0
Riggs' disease (compound periodontitis)
  523.40
Right middle lobe syndrome 518.0
Rigid, rigidity - *see also* condition
  abdominal 789.4●
  articular, multiple congenital 754.89

Rigid, rigidity (*Continued*)
  back 724.8
  cervix uteri
    in pregnancy or childbirth 654.6●
      affecting fetus or newborn 763.89
      causing obstructed labor 660.2●
        affecting fetus or newborn
          763.1
  hymen (acquired) (congenital) 623.3
  nuchal 781.6
  pelvic floor
    in pregnancy or childbirth 654.4●
      affecting fetus or newborn 763.89
      causing obstructed labor 660.2●
        affecting fetus or newborn
          763.1
  perineum or vulva
    in pregnancy or childbirth 654.8●
      affecting fetus or newborn 763.89
      causing obstructed labor 660.2●
        affecting fetus or newborn
          763.1
  spine 724.8
  vagina
    in pregnancy or childbirth 654.7●
      affecting fetus or newborn 763.89
      causing obstructed labor 660.2●
        affecting fetus or newborn 763.1
Rigors 780.99
Riley-Day syndrome (familial
  dysautonomia) 742.8
RIND (reversible ischemic neurological
  deficit) 434.91
  history of (personal) V12.54
Ring(s)
  aorta 747.21
  Bandl's, complicating delivery 661.4●
    affecting fetus or newborn 763.7
  contraction, complicating delivery
    661.4●
    affecting fetus or newborn 763.7
  esophageal (congenital) 750.3
  Fleischer (-Kayser) (cornea) 275.1
    [371.14]
  hymenal, tight (acquired) (congenital)
    623.3
  Kayser-Fleischer (cornea) 275.1 [371.14]
  retraction, uterus, pathological 661.4●
    affecting fetus or newborn 763.7
  Schatzki's (esophagus) (congenital)
    (lower) 750.3
    acquired 530.3
  Soemmering's 366.51
  trachea, abnormal 748.3
  vascular (congenital) 747.21
  Vossius' 921.3
    late effect 366.21
Ringed hair (congenital) 757.4
Ringing in the ear (*see also* Tinnitus)
  388.30
Ringworm 110.9
  beard 110.0
  body 110.5
  Burmese 110.9
  corporeal 110.5
  foot 110.4
  groin 110.3
  hand 110.2
  honeycomb 110.0
  nails 110.1
  perianal (area) 110.3
  scalp 110.0
  specified site NEC 110.8
  Tokelau 110.5

◄ New   ◄▥ Revised   ~~deleted~~ Deleted   ● Use Additional Digit(s)   ▨ Omit code

Rise, venous pressure 459.89
Risk
   factor - *see* Problem
   falling V15.88
   suicidal 300.9
Ritter's disease (dermatitis exfoliativa
   neonatorum) 695.81
Rivalry, sibling 313.3
Rivalta's disease (cervicofacial
   actinomycosis) 039.3
River blindness 125.3 *[360.13]*
Robert's pelvis 755.69
   with disproportion (fetopelvic)
      653.0●
      affecting fetus or newborn 763.1
      causing obstructed labor 660.1●
         affecting fetus or newborn
            763.1
Robin's syndrome 756.0
Robinson's (hidrotic) ectodermal
   dysplasia 757.31
Robles' disease (onchocerciasis) 125.3
   [360.13]
Rochalimea - *see* Rickettsial disease
Rocky Mountain fever (spotted) 082.0
Rodent ulcer (M8090/3) - *see also*
   Neoplasm, skin, malignant
   cornea 370.07
Roentgen ray, adverse effect - *see* Effect,
   adverse, x-ray
Roetheln 056.9
Roger's disease (congenital
   interventricular septal defect) 745.4
Rokitansky's
   disease (*see also* Necrosis, liver) 570
   tumor 620.2
Rokitansky-Aschoff sinuses (mucosal
   outpouching of gallbladder) (*see also*
   Disease, gallbladder) 575.8
Rokitansky-Kuster-Hauser syndrome
   (congenital absence vagina)
   752.45 ◀▥
Rollet's chancre (syphilitic) 091.0
Rolling of head 781.0
Romano-Ward syndrome (prolonged QT
   interval syndrome) 426.82
Romanus lesion 720.1
Romberg's disease or syndrome
   349.89
Roof, mouth - *see* condition
Rosacea 695.3
   acne 695.3
   keratitis 695.3 *[370.49]*
Rosary, rachitic 268.0
Rose
   cold 477.0
   fever 477.0
   rash 782.1
      epidemic 056.9
      of infants 057.8
Rosen-Castleman-Liebow syndrome
   (pulmonary proteinosis) 516.0
Rosenbach's erysipelatoid or erysipeloid
   027.1
Rosenthal's disease (factor XI deficiency)
   286.2
Roseola 057.8
   infantum, infantilis (*see also* Exanthem
      subitum) 058.10
Rossbach's disease (hyperchlorhydria)
   536.8
   psychogenic 306.4
Rossle-Urbach-Wiethe lipoproteinosis
   272.8

Ross river fever 066.3
Rostan's asthma (cardiac) (*see also* Failure,
   ventricular, left) 428.1
Rot
   Barcoo (*see also* Ulcer, skin) 707.9
   knife-grinders' (*see also* Tuberculosis)
      011.4●
Rot-Bernhardt disease 355.1
Rotation
   anomalous, incomplete or insufficient -
      see Malrotation
   cecum (congenital) 751.4
   colon (congenital) 751.4
   manual, affecting fetus or newborn
      763.89
   spine, incomplete or insufficient
      737.8
   tooth, teeth 524.35
   vertebra, incomplete or insufficient
      737.8
Röteln 056.9
Roth's disease or meralgia 355.1
Roth-Bernhardt disease or syndrome
   355.1
Rothmund (-Thomson) syndrome 757.33
Rotor's disease or syndrome (idiopathic
   hyperbilirubinemia) 277.4
Rotundum ulcus - *see* Ulcer, stomach
Round
   back (with wedging of vertebrae)
      737.10
      late effect of rickets 268.1
   hole, retina 361.31
      with detachment 361.01
   ulcer (stomach) - *see* Ulcer, stomach
   worms (infestation) (large) NEC
      127.0
Roussy-Lévy syndrome 334.3
Routine postpartum follow-up V24.2
Roy (-Jutras) syndrome (acropachyderma)
   757.39
Rubella (German measles) 056.9
   complicating pregnancy, childbirth, or
      puerperium 647.5●
   complication 056.8
      neurological 056.00
         encephalomyelitis 056.01
         specified type NEC 056.09
      specified type NEC 056.79
   congenital 771.0
   contact V01.4
   exposure to V01.4
   maternal
      with suspected fetal damage
         affecting management of
            pregnancy 655.3●
      affecting fetus or newborn 760.2
         manifest rubella in infant 771.0
   specified complications NEC 056.79
   vaccination, prophylactic (against)
      V04.3
Rubeola (measles) (*see also* Measles) 055.9
   complicated 055.8
   meaning rubella (*see also* Rubella) 056.9
   scarlatinosis 057.8
Rubeosis iridis 364.42
   diabetica 250.5● *[364.42]*
      due to secondary diabetes 249.5●
         [364.42]
Rubinstein-Taybi's syndrome
   (brachydactylia, short stature and
   mental retardation) 759.89
Rud's syndrome (mental deficiency,
   epilepsy, and infantilism) 759.89

Rudimentary (congenital) - *see also*
   Agenesis
   arm 755.22
   bone 756.9
   cervix uteri 752.43 ◀▥
   eye (*see also* Microphthalmos) 743.10
   fallopian tube 752.19
   leg 755.32
   lobule of ear 744.21
   patella 755.64
   respiratory organs in thoracopagus
      759.4
   tracheal bronchus 748.3
   uterine horn 752.39 ◀▥
   uterus 752.39 ◀▥
      in male 752.7
      solid or with cavity 752.39 ◀▥
   vagina 752.45 ◀▥
Ruiter-Pompen (-Wyers) syndrome
   (angiokeratoma corporis diffusum)
   272.7
Ruled out condition (*see also* Observation,
   suspected) V71.9
Rumination - *see also* Vomiting
   disorder 307.53
   neurotic 300.3
   obsessional 300.3
   psychogenic 307.53
Runaway reaction - *see also* Disturbance,
   conduct
   socialized 312.2●
   undersocialized, unsocialized 312.1●
Runeberg's disease (progressive
   pernicious anemia) 281.0
Runge's syndrome (postmaturity)
   766.22
Runny nose 784.99
Rupia 091.3
   congenital 090.0
   tertiary 095.9
Rupture, ruptured 553.9
   abdominal viscera NEC 799.89
      obstetrical trauma 665.5●
   abscess (spontaneous) - *see* Abscess, by
      site
   amnion - *see* Rupture, membranes
   aneurysm - *see* Aneurysm
   anus (sphincter) - *see* Laceration, anus
   aorta, aortic 441.5
      abdominal 441.3
      arch 441.1
      ascending 441.1
      descending 441.5
         abdominal 441.3
         thoracic 441.1
      syphilitic 093.0
      thoracoabdominal 441.6
      thorax, thoracic 441.1
      transverse 441.1
      traumatic (thoracic) 901.0
         abdominal 902.0
      valve or cusp (*see also* Endocarditis,
         aortic) 424.1
   appendix (with peritonitis) 540.0
      with peritoneal abscess 540.1
      traumatic - *see* Injury, internal,
         gastrointestinal tract
   arteriovenous fistula, brain (congenital)
      430
   artery 447.2
      brain (*see also* Hemorrhage, brain)
         431
      coronary (*see also* Infarct,
         myocardium) 410.9●

Rupture, ruptured *(Continued)*
  artery *(Continued)*
    heart *(see also* Infarct, myocardium)
      410.9●
    pulmonary 417.8
    traumatic (complication) *(see also*
      Injury, blood vessel, by site)
      904.9
  bile duct, except cystic *(see also* Disease,
    biliary) 576.3
    cystic 575.4
    traumatic - *see* Injury, internal, intra-
      abdominal
  bladder (sphincter) 596.6
    with
      abortion - *see* Abortion, by type,
        with damage to pelvic
        organs
      ectopic pregnancy *(see also*
        categories 633.0–633.9)
        639.2
      molar pregnancy *(see also*
        categories 630–632) 639.2
    following
      abortion 639.2
      ectopic or molar pregnancy
        639.2
    nontraumatic 596.6
    obstetrical trauma 665.5●
    spontaneous 596.6
    traumatic - *see* Injury, internal,
      bladder
  blood vessel *(see also* Hemorrhage)
    459.0
  brain *(see also* Hemorrhage, brain)
    431
    heart *(see also* Infarct, myocardium)
      410.9●
    traumatic (complication) *(see also*
      Injury, blood vessel, by site)
      904.9
  bone - *see* Fracture, by site
  bowel 569.89
    traumatic - *see* Injury, internal,
      intestine
  Bowman's membrane 371.31
  brain
    aneurysm (congenital) *(see also*
      Hemorrhage, subarachnoid)
      430
      late effect - *see* Late effect(s) (of)
        cerebrovascular disease
      syphilitic 094.87
    hemorrhagic *(see also* Hemorrhage,
      brain) 431
    injury at birth 767.0
    syphilitic 094.89
  capillaries 448.9
  cardiac *(see also* Infarct, myocardium)
    410.9●
  cartilage (articular) (current) - *see also*
    Sprain, by site
    knee - *see* Tear, meniscus
    semilunar - *see* Tear, meniscus
  cecum (with peritonitis) 540.0
    with peritoneal abscess 540.1
    traumatic 863.89
      with open wound into cavity
        863.99
  cerebral aneurysm (congenital) *(see
    also* Hemorrhage, subarachnoid)
    430
    late effect - *see* Late effect(s) (of)
      cerebrovascular disease

Rupture, ruptured *(Continued)*
  cervix (uteri)
    with
      abortion - *see* Abortion, by type,
        with damage to pelvic
        organs
      ectopic pregnancy *(see also*
        categories 633.0–633.9) 639.2
      molar pregnancy *(see also*
        categories 630–632) 639.2
    following
      abortion 639.2
      ectopic or molar pregnancy 639.2
    obstetrical trauma 665.3●
    traumatic - *see* Injury, internal, cervix
  chordae tendineae 429.5
  choroid (direct) (indirect) (traumatic)
    363.63
  circle of Willis *(see also* Hemorrhage,
    subarachnoid) 430
    late effect - *see* Late effect(s) (of)
      cerebrovascular disease
  colon 569.89
    traumatic - *see* Injury, internal, colon
  cornea (traumatic) - *see also* Rupture,
    eye
    due to ulcer 370.00
  coronary (artery) (thrombotic) *(see also*
    Infarct, myocardium) 410.9●
  corpus luteum (infected) (ovary) 620.1
  cyst - *see* Cyst
  cystic duct *(see also* Disease,
    gallbladder) 575.4
  Descemet's membrane 371.33
    traumatic - *see* Rupture, eye
  diaphragm - *see also* Hernia, diaphragm
    traumatic - *see* Injury, internal,
      diaphragm
  diverticulum
    bladder 596.3
    intestine (large) *(see also* Diverticula)
      562.10
      small 562.00
  duodenal stump 537.89
  duodenum (ulcer) - *see* Ulcer,
    duodenum, with perforation
  ear drum *(see also* Perforation,
    tympanum) 384.20
    with otitis media - *see* Otitis media
    traumatic - *see* Wound, open, ear
  esophagus 530.4
    traumatic 862.22
      with open wound into cavity
        862.32
      cervical region - *see* Wound, open,
        esophagus
  eye (without prolapse of intraocular
    tissue) 871.0
    with
      exposure of intraocular tissue
        871.1
      partial loss of intraocular tissue
        871.2
      prolapse of intraocular tissue
        871.1
    due to burn 940.5
  fallopian tube 620.8
    due to pregnancy - *see* Pregnancy,
      tubal
    traumatic - *see* Injury, internal,
      fallopian tube
  fontanel 767.3
  free wall (ventricle) *(see also* Infarct,
    myocardium) 410.9●

Rupture, ruptured *(Continued)*
  gallbladder or duct *(see also* Disease,
    gallbladder) 575.4
    traumatic - *see* Injury, internal,
      gallbladder
  gastric *(see also* Rupture, stomach)
    537.89
    vessel 459.0
  globe (eye) (traumatic) - *see* Rupture,
    eye
  graafian follicle (hematoma) 620.0
  heart (auricle) (ventricle) *(see also*
    Infarct, myocardium) 410.9●
    infectional 422.90
    traumatic - *see* Rupture,
      myocardium, traumatic
  hymen 623.8
  internal
    organ, traumatic - *see also* Injury,
      internal, by site
      heart - *see* Rupture, myocardium,
        traumatic
      kidney - *see* Rupture, kidney
      liver - *see* Rupture, liver
      spleen - *see* Rupture, spleen,
        traumatic
    semilunar cartilage - *see* Tear,
      meniscus
  intervertebral disc - *see* Displacement,
    intervertebral disc
    traumatic (current) - *see* Dislocation,
      vertebra
  intestine 569.89
    traumatic - *see* Injury, internal,
      intestine
  intracranial, birth injury 767.0
  iris 364.76
    traumatic - *see* Rupture, eye
  joint capsule - *see* Sprain, by site
  kidney (traumatic) 866.03
    with open wound into cavity
      866.13
    due to birth injury 767.8
    nontraumatic 593.89
  lacrimal apparatus (traumatic) 870.2
  lens (traumatic) 366.20
  ligament - *see also* Sprain, by site
    with open wound - *see* Wound,
      open, by site
    old *(see also* Disorder, cartilage,
      articular) 718.0●
  liver (traumatic) 864.04
    with open wound into cavity
      864.14
    due to birth injury 767.8
    nontraumatic 573.8
  lymphatic (node) (vessel) 457.8
  marginal sinus (placental) (with
    hemorrhage) 641.2●
    affecting fetus or newborn 762.1
  meaning hernia - *see* Hernia
  membrana tympani *(see also*
    Perforation, tympanum) 384.20
    with otitis media - *see* Otitis media
    traumatic - *see* Wound, open, ear
  membranes (spontaneous)
    artificial
      delayed delivery following
        658.3●
        affecting fetus or newborn
          761.1
      fetus or newborn 761.1
    delayed delivery following 658.2●
      affecting fetus or newborn 761.1

◄ New   ◄▮▮ Revised   ~~deleted~~ Deleted   ● Use Additional Digit(s)   ▨ Omit code

Rupture, ruptured (Continued)
  membranes (Continued)
    premature (less than 24 hours prior
        to onset of labor) 658.1●
    affecting fetus or newborn 761.1
    delayed delivery following
        658.2●
      affecting fetus or newborn
          761.1
  meningeal artery (see also Hemorrhage,
      subarachnoid) 430
    late effect - see Late effect(s) (of)
        cerebrovascular disease
  meniscus (knee) - see also Tear,
      meniscus
    old (see also Derangement, meniscus)
        717.5
      site other than knee - see Disorder,
          cartilage, articular
      site other than knee - see Sprain, by
          site
  mesentery 568.89
    traumatic - see Injury, internal,
        mesentery
  mitral - see Insufficiency, mitral
  muscle (traumatic) NEC - see also
      Sprain, by site
    with open wound - see Wound,
        open, by site
    nontraumatic 728.83
  musculotendinous cuff (nontraumatic)
      (shoulder) 840.4
  mycotic aneurysm, causing cerebral
      hemorrhage (see also
      Hemorrhage, subarachnoid) 430
    late effect - see Late effect(s) (of)
        cerebrovascular disease
  myocardium, myocardial (see also
      Infarct, myocardium) 410.9●
    traumatic 861.03
      with open wound into thorax
          861.13
  nontraumatic (meaning hernia) (see also
      Hernia, by site) 553.9
  obstructed (see also Hernia, by site, with
      obstruction) 552.9
    gangrenous (see also Hernia, by site,
        with gangrene) 551.9
  operation wound (see also Dehiscence)
      998.32
    internal 998.31
  ovary, ovarian 620.8
    corpus luteum 620.1
    follicle (graafian) 620.0
  oviduct 620.8
    due to pregnancy - see Pregnancy,
        tubal
  pancreas 577.8
    traumatic - see Injury, internal,
        pancreas
  papillary muscle (ventricular) 429.6
  pelvic
    floor, complicating delivery
        664.1●
    organ NEC - see Injury, pelvic,
        organs
  penis (traumatic) - see Wound, open,
      penis
  perineum 624.8
    during delivery (see also Laceration,
        perineum, complicating
        delivery) 664.4●
  pharynx (nontraumatic) (spontaneous)
      478.29

Rupture, ruptured (Continued)
  pregnant uterus (before onset of labor)
      665.0●
  prostate (traumatic) - see Injury,
      internal, prostate
  pulmonary
    artery 417.8
    valve (heart) (see also Endocarditis,
        pulmonary) 424.3
    vein 417.8
    vessel 417.8
  pupil, sphincter 364.75
  pus tube (see also Salpingo-oophoritis)
      614.2
  pyosalpinx (see also Salpingo-
      oophoritis) 614.2
  rectum 569.49
    traumatic - see Injury, internal,
        rectum
  retina, retinal (traumatic) (without
      detachment) 361.30
    with detachment (see also
        Detachment, retina, with
        retinal defect) 361.00
  rotator cuff (capsule) (traumatic) 840.4
    nontraumatic, complete 727.61
  sclera 871.0
  semilunar cartilage, knee (see also Tear,
      meniscus) 836.2
    old (see also Derangement, meniscus)
        717.5
  septum (cardiac) 410.8●
  sigmoid 569.89
    traumatic - see Injury, internal, colon,
        sigmoid
  sinus of Valsalva 747.29
  spinal cord - see also Injury, spinal, by
      site
    due to injury at birth 767.4
    fetus or newborn 767.4
    syphilitic 094.89
    traumatic - see also Injury, spinal, by
        site
      with fracture - see Fracture,
          vertebra, by site, with
          spinal cord injury
  spleen 289.59
    congenital 767.8
    due to injury at birth 767.8
    malarial 084.9
    nontraumatic 289.59
    spontaneous 289.59
    traumatic 865.04
      with open wound into cavity
          865.14
  splenic vein 459.0
  stomach 537.89
    due to injury at birth 767.8
    traumatic - see Injury, internal,
        stomach
    ulcer - see Ulcer, stomach, with
        perforation
  synovium 727.50
    specified site NEC 727.59
  tendon (traumatic) - see also Sprain, by
      site
    with open wound - see Wound,
        open, by site
    Achilles 845.09
      nontraumatic 727.67
    ankle 845.09
      nontraumatic 727.68
    biceps (long bead) 840.8
      nontraumatic 727.62

Rupture, ruptured (Continued)
  tendon (Continued)
    foot 845.10
      interphalangeal (joint) 845.13
      metatarsophalangeal (joint)
          845.12
      nontraumatic 727.68
      specified site NEC 845.19
      tarsometatarsal (joint) 845.11
    hand 842.10
      carpometacarpal (joint) 842.11
      interphalangeal (joint) 842.13
      metacarpophalangeal (joint)
          842.12
      nontraumatic 727.63
        extensors 727.63
        flexors 727.64
      specified site NEC 842.19
    nontraumatic 727.60
      specified site NEC 727.69
    patellar 844.8
      nontraumatic 727.66
    quadriceps 844.8
      nontraumatic 727.65
    rotator cuff (capsule) 840.4
      nontraumatic, complete
          727.61
    wrist 842.00
      carpal (joint) 842.01
      nontraumatic 727.63
        extensors 727.63
        flexors 727.64
      radiocarpal (joint) (ligament)
          842.02
      radioulnar (joint), distal
          842.09
      specified site NEC 842.09
  testis (traumatic) 878.2
    complicated 878.3
    due to syphilis 095.8
  thoracic duct 457.8
  tonsil 474.8
  traumatic
    with open wound - see Wound,
        open, by site
    aorta - see Rupture, aorta, traumatic
    ear drum - see Wound, open, ear,
        drum
    external site - see Wound, open, by
        site
    eye 871.2
    globe (eye) - see Wound, open,
        eyeball
    internal organ (abdomen, chest, or
        pelvis) - see also Injury,
        internal, by site
      heart - see Rupture, myocardium,
          traumatic
      kidney - see Rupture, kidney
      liver - see Rupture, liver
      spleen - see Rupture, spleen,
          traumatic
    ligament, muscle, or tendon - see also
        Sprain, by site
      with open wound - see Wound,
          open, by site
    meaning hernia - see Hernia
  tricuspid (heart) (valve) - see
      Endocarditis, tricuspid
  tube, tubal 620.8
    abscess (see also Salpingo-oophoritis)
        614.2
    due to pregnancy - see Pregnancy,
        tubal

Rupture, ruptured (Continued)
    tympanum, tympanic (membrane) (see
        also Perforation, tympanum)
        384.20
        with otitis media - see Otitis media
        traumatic - see Wound, open, ear,
            drum
    umbilical cord 663.8●
        fetus or newborn 772.0
    ureter (traumatic) (see also Injury,
        internal, ureter) 867.2
        nontraumatic 593.89
    urethra 599.84
        with
            abortion - see Abortion, by type,
                with damage to pelvic
                organs
            ectopic pregnancy (see also
                categories 633.0–633.9)
                639.2
            molar pregnancy (see also
                categories 630–632)
                639.2
        following
            abortion 639.2
            ectopic or molar pregnancy
                639.2

Rupture, ruptured (Continued)
    urethra (Continued)
        obstetrical trauma 665.5●
        traumatic - see Injury, internal
            urethra
    uterosacral ligament 620.8
    uterus (traumatic) - see also Injury,
        internal uterus
        affecting fetus or newborn 763.89
        during labor 665.1●
        nonpuerperal, nontraumatic 621.8
        nontraumatic 621.8
        pregnant (during labor) 665.1●
            before labor 665.0●
    vagina 878.6
        complicated 878.7
        complicating delivery - see
            Laceration, vagina,
            complicating delivery
    valve, valvular (heart) - see
        Endocarditis
    varicose vein - see Varicose, vein
    varix - see Varix
    vena cava 459.0
    ventricle (free wall) (left) (see also
        Infarct, myocardium)
        410.9●

Rupture, ruptured (Continued)
    vesical (urinary) 596.6
        traumatic - see Injury, internal,
            bladder
    vessel (blood) 459.0
        pulmonary 417.8
    viscus 799.89
    vulva 878.4
        complicated 878.5
        complicating delivery 664.0●
Russell's dwarf (uterine dwarfism and
    craniofacial dysostosis) 759.89
Russell's dysentery 004.8
Russell (-Silver) syndrome (congenital
    hemihypertrophy and short stature)
    759.89
Russian spring-summer type
    encephalitis 063.0
Rust's disease (tuberculous spondylitis)
    015.0● [720.81]
Rustitskii's disease (multiple myeloma)
    (M9730/3) 203.0●
Ruysch's disease (Hirschsprung's
    disease) 751.3
Rytand-Lipsitch syndrome (complete
    atrioventricular block) 426.0

◀ New   ◀▥ Revised   ~~deleted~~ Deleted   ● Use Additional Digit(s)   ▨ Omit code

S

Saber
shin 090.5
tibia 090.5
Sac, lacrimal - *see* condition
Saccharomyces infection (*see also*
Candidiasis) 112.9
Saccharopinuria 270.7
Saccular - *see* condition
Sacculation
aorta (nonsyphilitic) (*see also*
Aneurysm, aorta) 441.9
ruptured 441.5
syphilitic 093.0
bladder 596.3
colon 569.89
intralaryngeal (congenital)
(ventricular) 748.3
larynx (congenital) (ventricular)
748.3
organ or site, congenital - *see*
Distortion
pregnant uterus, complicating delivery
654.4●
affecting fetus or newborn 763.1
causing obstructed labor
660.2●
affecting fetus or newborn
763.1
rectosigmoid 569.89
sigmoid 569.89
ureter 593.89
urethra 599.2
vesical 596.3
Sachs (-Tay) disease (amaurotic familial
idiocy) 330.1
Sacks-Libman disease 710.0 *[424.91]*
Sacralgia 724.6
Sacralization
fifth lumbar vertebra 756.15
incomplete (vertebra) 756.15
Sacrodynia 724.6
Sacroiliac joint - *see* condition
Sacroiliitis NEC 720.2
Sacrum - *see* condition
Saddle
back 737.8
embolus, aorta 444.0
nose 738.0
congenital 754.0
due to syphilis 090.5
Sadism (sexual) 302.84
Saemisch's ulcer 370.04
Saenger's syndrome 379.46
Sago spleen 277.39
Sailors' skin 692.74
Saint
Anthony's fire (*see also* Erysipelas)
035
Guy's dance - *see* Chorea
Louis-type encephalitis 062.3
triad (*see also* Hernia, diaphragm)
553.3
Vitus' dance - *see* Chorea
Salicylism
correct substance properly
administered 535.4●
overdose or wrong substance given or
taken 965.1
Salivary duct or gland - *see also* condition
virus disease 078.5
Salivation (excessive) (*see also* Ptyalism)
527.7

Salmonella (aertrycke) (choleraesuis)
(enteritidis) (gallinarum)
(suipestifer) (typhimurium) (*see also*
Infection, Salmonella) 003.9
arthritis 003.23
carrier (suspected) of V02.3
meningitis 003.21
osteomyelitis 003.24
pneumonia 003.22
septicemia 003.1
typhosa 002.0
carrier (suspected) of V02.1
Salmonellosis 003.0
with pneumonia 003.22
Salpingitis (catarrhal) (fallopian tube)
(nodular) (pseudofollicular)
(purulent) (septic) (*see also* Salpingo-
oophoritis) 614.2
ear 381.50
acute 381.51
chronic 381.52
Eustachian (tube) 381.50
acute 381.51
chronic 381.52
follicularis 614.1
gonococcal (chronic) 098.37
acute 098.17
interstitial, chronic 614.1
isthmica nodosa 614.1
old - *see* Salpingo-oophoritis, chronic
puerperal, postpartum, childbirth
670.8●
specific (chronic) 098.37
acute 098.17
tuberculous (acute) (chronic) (*see also*
Tuberculosis) 016.6●
venereal (chronic) 098.37
acute 098.17
Salpingocele 620.4
Salpingo-oophoritis (catarrhal) (purulent)
(ruptured) (septic) (suppurative)
614.2
acute 614.0
with
abortion - *see* Abortion, by type,
with sepsis
ectopic pregnancy (*see also*
categories 633.0–633.9)
639.0
molar pregnancy (*see also*
categories 630–632) 639.0
following
abortion 639.0
ectopic or molar pregnancy
639.0
gonococcal 098.17
puerperal, postpartum, childbirth
670.8●
tuberculous (*see also* Tuberculosis)
016.6●
chronic 614.1
gonococcal 098.37
tuberculous (*see also* Tuberculosis)
016.6●
complicating pregnancy 646.6●
affecting fetus or newborn 760.8
gonococcal (chronic) 098.37
acute 098.17
old - *see* Salpingo-oophoritis, chronic
puerperal 670.8●
specific - *see* Salpingo-oophoritis,
gonococcal
subacute (*see also* Salpingo-oophoritis,
acute) 614.0

Salpingo-oophoritis (*Continued*)
tuberculous (acute) (chronic) (*see also*
Tuberculosis) 016.6●
venereal - *see* Salpingo-oophoritis,
gonococcal
Salpingo-ovaritis (*see also* Salpingo-
oophoritis) 614.2
Salpingoperitonitis (*see also* Salpingo-
oophoritis) 614.2
Salt-losing
nephritis (*see also* Disease, renal)
593.9
syndrome (*see also* Disease, renal)
593.9
Salt-rheum (*see also* Eczema) 692.9
Salzmann's nodular dystrophy 371.46
Sampling
chorionic villus V28.89
Sampson's cyst or tumor 617.1
Sandblasters'
asthma 502
lung 502
Sander's disease (paranoia) 297.1
Sandfly fever 066.0
Sandhoff's disease 330.1
Sanfilippo's syndrome
(mucopolysaccharidosis III) 277.5
Sanger-Brown's ataxia 334.2
San Joaquin Valley fever 114.0
Sao Paulo fever or typhus 082.0
Saponification, mesenteric 567.89
Sapremia - *see* Septicemia
Sarcocele (benign)
syphilitic 095.8
congenital 090.5
Sarcoepiplocele (*see also* Hernia) 553.9
Sarcoepiplomphalocele (*see also* Hernia,
umbilicus) 553.1
Sarcoid (any site) 135
with lung involvement 135 *[517.8]*
Boeck's 135
Darier-Roussy 135
Spiegler-Fendt 686.8
Sarcoidosis 135
cardiac 135 *[425.8]*
lung 135 *[517.8]*
Sarcoma (M8800/3) - *see also* Neoplasm,
connective tissue, malignant
alveolar soft part (M9581/3) - *see*
Neoplasm, connective tissue,
malignant
ameloblastic (M9330/3) 170.1
upper jaw (bone) 170.0
botryoid (M8910/3) - *see* Neoplasm,
connective tissue, malignant
botryoides (M8910/3) - *see* Neoplasm,
connective tissue, malignant
cerebellar (M9480/3) 191.6
circumscribed (arachnoidal)
(M9471/3) 191.6
circumscribed (arachnoidal) cerebellar
(M9471/3) 191.6
clear cell, of tendons and aponeuroses
(M9044/3) - *see* Neoplasm,
connective tissue, malignant
embryonal (M8991/3) - *see* Neoplasm,
connective tissue, malignant
endometrial (stromal) (M8930/3) 182.0
isthmus 182.1
endothelial (M9130/3) - *see also*
Neoplasm, connective tissue,
malignant
bone (M9260/3) - *see* Neoplasm,
bone, malignant

Sarcoma (Continued)
   epithelioid cell (M8804/3) - see
      Neoplasm, connective tissue,
      malignant
   Ewing's (M9260/3) - see Neoplasm,
      bone, malignant
   follicular dendritic cell 202.9 ●
   germinoblastic (diffuse) (M9632/3)
      202.8 ●
      follicular (M9697/3) 202.0 ●
   giant cell (M8802/3) - see also
      Neoplasm, connective tissue,
      malignant
      bone (M9250/3) - see Neoplasm,
         bone, malignant
   glomoid (M8710/3) - see Neoplasm,
      connective tissue, malignant
   granulocytic (M9930/3) 205.3 ●
   hemangioendothelial (M9130/3) - see
      Neoplasm, connective tissue,
      malignant
   hemorrhagic, multiple (M9140/3) - see
      Kaposi's, sarcoma
   Hodgkin's (M9662/3) 201.2 ●
   immunoblastic (M9612/3) 200.8 ●
   interdigitating dendritic cell 202.9 ●
   Kaposi's (M9140/3) - see Kaposi's,
      sarcoma
   Kupffer cell (M9124/3) 155.0
   Langerhans cell 202.9 ●
   leptomeningeal (M9530/3) - see
      Neoplasm, meninges,
      malignant
   lymphangioendothelial (M9170/3) - see
      Neoplasm, connective tissue,
      malignant
   lymphoblastic (M9630/3) 200.1 ●
   lymphocytic (M9620/3) 200.1 ●
   mast cell (M9740/3) 202.6 ●
   melanotic (M8720/3) - see Melanoma
   meningeal (M9530/3) - see Neoplasm,
      meninges, malignant
   meningothelial (M9530/3) - see
      Neoplasm, meninges,
      malignant
   mesenchymal (M8800/3) - see also
      Neoplasm, connective tissue,
      malignant
      mixed (M8990/3) - see Neoplasm,
         connective tissue, malignant
   mesothelial (M9050/3) - see Neoplasm,
      by site, malignant
   monstrocellular (M9481/3)
      specified site - see Neoplasm, by site,
         malignant
      unspecified site 191.9
   myeloid (M9930/3) 205.3 ●
   neurogenic (M9540/3) - see Neoplasm,
      connective tissue, malignant
   odontogenic (M9270/3) 170.1
      upper jaw (bone) 170.0
   osteoblastic (M9180/3) - see Neoplasm,
      bone, malignant
   osteogenic (M9180/3) - see also
      Neoplasm, bone, malignant
      juxtacortical (M9190/3) - see
         Neoplasm, bone, malignant
      periosteal (M9190/3) - see
         Neoplasm, bone, malignant
   periosteal (M8812/3) - see also
      Neoplasm, bone, malignant
      osteogenic (M9190/3) - see
         Neoplasm, bone, malignant
   plasma cell (M9731/3) 203.8 ●

Sarcoma (Continued)
   pleomorphic cell (M8802/3) - see
      Neoplasm, connective tissue,
      malignant
   reticuloendothelial (M9720/3)
      202.3 ●
   reticulum cell (M9640/3) 200.0 ●
      nodular (M9642/3) 200.0 ●
      pleomorphic cell type (M9641/3)
         200.0 ●
   round cell (M8803/3) - see
      Neoplasm, connective
      tissue, malignant
   small cell (M8803/3) - see
      Neoplasm, connective
      tissue, malignant
   spindle cell (M8801/3) - see
      Neoplasm, connective
      tissue, malignant
   stromal (endometrial) (M8930/3)
      182.0
      isthmus 182.1
   synovial (M9040/3) - see also
      Neoplasm, connective tissue,
      malignant
      biphasic type (M9043/3) - see
         Neoplasm, connective tissue,
         malignant
      epithelioid cell type (M9042/3) - see
         Neoplasm, connective tissue,
         malignant
      spindle cell type (M9041/3) - see
         Neoplasm, connective tissue,
         malignant
Sarcomatosis
   meningeal (M9539/3) - see Neoplasm,
      meninges, malignant
   specified site NEC (M8800/3) - see
      Neoplasm, connective tissue,
      malignant
   unspecified site (M8800/6) 171.9
Sarcosinemia 270.8
Sarcosporidiosis 136.5
Satiety, early 780.94
Satisfactory smear but lacking
     transformation zone
   anal 796.77
   cervical 795.07
Saturnine - see condition
Saturnism 984.9
   specified type of lead - see Table of
      Drugs and Chemicals
Satyriasis 302.89
Sauriasis - see Ichthyosis
Sauriderma 757.39
Sauriosis - see Ichthyosis
Savill's disease (epidemic exfoliative
      dermatitis) 695.89
SBE (subacute bacterial endocarditis)
      421.0
Scabies (any site) 133.0
Scabs 782.8
Scaglietti-Dagnini syndrome
      (acromegalic macrospondylitis)
      253.0
Scald, scalded - see also Burn, by site
   skin syndrome 695.81
Scalenus anticus (anterior) syndrome
      353.0
Scales 782.8
Scalp - see condition
Scaphocephaly 756.0
Scaphoiditis, tarsal 732.5
Scapulalgia 733.90

Scapulohumeral myopathy 359.1
Scar, scarring (see also Cicatrix) 709.2
   adherent 709.2
   atrophic 709.2
   cervix
      in pregnancy or childbirth 654.6 ●
         affecting fetus or newborn
            763.89
         causing obstructed labor 660.2 ●
           affecting fetus or newborn
             763.1
   cheloid 701.4
   chorioretinal 363.30
      disseminated 363.35
      macular 363.32
      peripheral 363.34
      posterior pole NEC 363.33
   choroid (see also Scar, chorioretinal)
      363.30
   compression, pericardial 423.9
   congenital 757.39
   conjunctiva 372.64
   cornea 371.00
      xerophthalmic 264.6
   due to previous cesarean delivery,
      complicating pregnancy or
      childbirth 654.2 ●
      affecting fetus or newborn 763.89
   duodenal (bulb) (cap) 537.3
   hypertrophic 701.4
   keloid 701.4
   labia 624.4
   lung (base) 518.89
   macula 363.32
      disseminated 363.35
      peripheral 363.34
   muscle 728.89
   myocardium, myocardial 412
   painful 709.2
   papillary muscle 429.81
   posterior pole NEC 363.33
      macular - see Scar, macula
   postnecrotic (hepatic) (liver) 571.9
   psychic V15.49
   retina (see also Scar, chorioretinal)
      363.30
   trachea 478.9
   uterus 621.8
      in pregnancy or childbirth NEC
         654.9 ●
         affecting fetus or newborn
           763.89
         from previous cesarean delivery
           654.2 ●
   vulva 624.4
Scarabiasis 134.1
Scarlatina 034.1
   anginosa 034.1
   maligna 034.1
   myocarditis, acute 034.1 [422.0]
      old (see also Myocarditis) 429.0
   otitis media 034.1 [382.02]
   ulcerosa 034.1
Scarlatinella 057.8
Scarlet fever (albuminuria) (angina)
      (convulsions) (lesions of lid) (rash)
      034.1
Schamberg's disease, dermatitis, or
     dermatosis (progressive pigmentary
      dermatosis) 709.09
Schatzki's ring (esophagus) (lower)
      (congenital) 750.3
   acquired 530.3
Schaufenster krankheit 413.9

◀ New   ◀ Revised   ~~deleted~~ Deleted   ● Use Additional Digit(s)   Omit code

Schaumann's
  benign lymphogranulomatosis 135
  disease (sarcoidosis) 135
  syndrome (sarcoidosis) 135
Scheie's syndrome
  (mucopolysaccharidosis IS) 277.5
Schenck's disease (sporotrichosis) 117.1
Scheuermann's disease or
  osteochondrosis 732.0
Scheuthauer-Marie-Sainton syndrome
  (cleidocranialis dysostosis) 755.59
Schilder (-Flatau) disease 341.1
Schilling-type monocytic leukemia
  (M9890/3) 206.9●
Schimmelbusch's disease, cystic mastitis,
  or hyperplasia 610.1
Schirmer's syndrome
  (encephalocutaneous angiomatosis)
  759.6
Schistocelia 756.79
Schistoglossia 750.13
Schistosoma infestation - see Infestation,
  Schistosoma
Schistosomiasis 120.9
  Asiatic 120.2
  bladder 120.0
  chestermani 120.8
  colon 120.1
  cutaneous 120.3
  due to
    S. hematobium 120.0
    S. japonicum 120.2
    S. mansoni 120.1
    S. mattheii 120.8
  eastern 120.2
  genitourinary tract 120.0
  intestinal 120.1
  lung 120.2
  Manson's (intestinal) 120.1
  Oriental 120.2
  pulmonary 120.2
  specified type NEC 120.8
  vesical 120.0
Schizencephaly 742.4
Schizo-affective psychosis (see also
  Schizophrenia) 295.7●
Schizodontia 520.2
Schizoid personality 301.20
  introverted 301.21
  schizotypal 301.22
Schizophrenia, schizophrenic (reaction)
  295.9●

Note: Use the following fifth-digit
subclassification with category 295:

0   unspecified
1   subchronic
2   chronic
3   subchronic with acute
     exacerbation
4   chronic with acute exacerbation
5   in remission

  acute (attack) NEC 295.8●
    episode 295.4●
  atypical form 295.8●
  borderline 295.5●
  catalepsy 295.2●
  catatonic (type) (acute) (excited)
    (withdrawn) 295.2●
  childhood (type) (see also Psychosis,
    childhood) 299.9●
  chronic NEC 295.6●
  coenesthesiopathic 295.8●

Schizophrenia, schizophrenic (Continued)
  cyclic (type) 295.7●
  disorganized (type) 295.1●
  flexibilitas cerea 295.2●
  hebephrenic (type) (acute) 295.1●
  incipient 295.5●
  latent 295.5●
  paranoid (type) (acute) 295.3●
  paraphrenic (acute) 295.3●
  prepsychotic 295.5●
  primary (acute) 295.0●
  prodromal 295.5●
  pseudoneurotic 295.5●
  pseudopsychopathic 295.5●
  reaction 295.9●
  residual type (state) 295.6●
  restzustand 295.6●
  schizo-affective (type) (depressed)
    (excited) 295.7●
  schizophreniform type 295.4●
  simple (type) (acute) 295.0●
  simplex (acute) 295.0●
  specified type NEC 295.8●
  syndrome of childhood NEC (see also
    Psychosis, childhood) 299.9●
  undifferentiated type 295.9●
    acute 295.8●
    chronic 295.6●
Schizothymia 301.20
  introverted 301.21
  schizotypal 301.22
Schlafkrankheit 086.5
Schlatter's tibia (osteochondrosis) 732.4
Schlatter-Osgood disease
  (osteochondrosis, tibial tubercle)
  732.4
Schloffer's tumor (see also Peritonitis) 567.29
Schmidt's syndrome
  sphallo-pharyngo-laryngeal
    hemiplegia 352.6
  thyroid-adrenocortical insufficiency
    258.1
  vagoaccessory 352.6
Schmincke
  carcinoma (M8082/3) - see Neoplasm,
    nasopharynx, malignant
  tumor (M8082/3) - see Neoplasm,
    nasopharynx, malignant
Schmitz (-Stutzer) dysentery 004.0
Schmorl's disease or nodes 722.30
  lumbar, lumbosacral 722.32
  specified region NEC 722.39
  thoracic, thoracolumbar 722.31
Schneider's syndrome 047.9
Schneiderian
  carcinoma (M8121/3)
    specified site - see Neoplasm, by site,
      malignant
    unspecified site 160.0
  papilloma (M8121/0)
    specified site - see Neoplasm, by site,
      benign
    unspecified site 212.0
Schnitzler syndrome 273.1
Schoffer's tumor (see also Peritonitis) 567.29
Scholte's syndrome (malignant carcinoid)
  259.2
Scholz's disease 330.0
Scholz (-Bielschowsky-Henneberg)
  syndrome 330.0
Schönlein (-Henoch) disease (primary)
  (purpura) (rheumatic) 287.0
School examination V70.3
  following surgery V67.09

Schottmüller's disease (see also Fever,
  paratyphoid) 002.9
Schroeder's syndrome (endocrine-
  hypertensive) 255.3
Schüller-Christian disease or syndrome
  (chronic histiocytosis X) 277.89
Schultz's disease or syndrome
  (agranulocytosis) 288.09
Schultze's acroparesthesia, simple 443.89
Schwalbe-Ziehen-Oppenheimer disease
  333.6
Schwannoma (M9560/0) - see also
  Neoplasm, connective tissues,
  benign
  malignant (M9560/3) - see Neoplasm,
    connective tissue, malignant
Schwannomatosis 237.73 ◄
Schwartz (-Jampel) syndrome 359.23
Schwartz-Bartter syndrome
  (inappropriate secretion of
  antidiuretic hormone) 253.6
Schweninger-Buzzi disease (macular
  atrophy) 701.3
Sciatic - see condition
Sciatica (infectional) 724.3
  due to
    displacement of intervertebral disc
      722.10
    herniation, nucleus pulposus 722.10
  wallet 724.3
Scimitar syndrome (anomalous venous
  drainage, right lung to inferior vena
  cava) 747.49
Sclera - see condition
Sclerectasia 379.11
Scleredema
  adultorum 710.1
  Buschke's 710.1
  newborn 778.1
Sclerema
  adiposum (newborn) 778.1
  adultorum 710.1
  edematosum (newborn) 778.1
  neonatorum 778.1
  newborn 778.1
Scleriasis - see Scleroderma
Scleritis 379.00
  with corneal involvement 379.05
  anterior (annular) (localized) 379.03
  brawny 379.06
  granulomatous 379.09
  posterior 379.07
  specified NEC 379.09
  suppurative 379.09
  syphilitic 095.0
  tuberculous (nodular) (see also
    Tuberculosis) 017.3● [379.09]
Sclerochoroiditis (see also Scleritis) 379.00
Scleroconjunctivitis (see also Scleritis)
  379.00
Sclerocystic ovary (syndrome) 256.4
Sclerodactylia 701.0
Scleroderma, sclerodermia (acrosclerotic)
  (diffuse) (generalized) (progressive)
  (pulmonary) 710.1
  circumscribed 701.0
  linear 701.0
  localized (linear) 701.0
  newborn 778.1
Sclerokeratitis 379.05
  meaning sclerosing keratitis 370.54
  tuberculous (see also Tuberculosis)
    017.3● [379.09]
Scleroma, trachea 040.1

S

Scleromalacia
  multiple 731.0
  perforans 379.04
Scleromyxedema 701.8
Scleroperikeratitis 379.05
Sclerose en plaques 340
Sclerosis, sclerotic
  adrenal (gland) 255.8
  Alzheimer's 331.0
    with dementia - *see* Alzheimer's,
      dementia
  amyotrophic (lateral) 335.20
  annularis fibrosi
    aortic 424.1
    mitral 424.0
  aorta, aortic 440.0
    valve (*see also* Endocarditis, aortic)
      424.1
  artery, arterial, arteriolar,
    arteriovascular - *see*
    Arteriosclerosis
  ascending multiple 340
  Balo's (concentric) 341.1
  basilar - *see* Sclerosis, brain
  bone (localized) NEC 733.99
  brain (general) (lobular) 348.89
    Alzheimer's - *see* Alzheimer's,
      dementia
    artery, arterial 437.0
    atrophic lobar 331.0
      with dementia
        with behavioral disturbance
          331.0 [294.11]
        without behavioral
          disturbance 331.0
          [294.10]
    diffuse 341.1
      familial (chronic) (infantile) 330.0
      infantile (chronic) (familial) 330.0
      Pelizaeus-Merzbacher type 330.0
    disseminated 340
    hereditary 334.2
    hippocampal 348.81
    infantile (degenerative) (diffuse) 330.0
    insular 340
    Krabbe's 330.0
    mesial temporal 348.81
    miliary 340
    multiple 340
    Pelizaeus-Merzbacher 330.0
    progressive familial 330.0
    senile 437.0
    temporal 348.81
      mesial 348.81
    tuberous 759.5
  bulbar, progressive 340
  bundle of His 426.50
    left 426.3
    right 426.4
  cardiac - *see* Arteriosclerosis, coronary
  cardiorenal (*see also* Hypertension,
    cardiorenal) 404.90
  cardiovascular (*see also* Disease,
    cardiovascular) 429.2
    renal (*see also* Hypertension,
      cardiorenal) 404.90
  centrolobar, familial 330.0
  cerebellar - *see* Sclerosis, brain
  cerebral - *see* Sclerosis, brain
  cerebrospinal 340
    disseminated 340
    multiple 340
  cerebrovascular 437.0
  choroid 363.40
    diffuse 363.56

Sclerosis, sclerotic (*Continued*)
  combined (spinal cord) - *see also*
    Degeneration, combined
    multiple 340
  concentric, Balo's 341.1
  cornea 370.54
  coronary (artery) - *see* Arteriosclerosis,
    coronary
  corpus cavernosum
    female 624.8
    male 607.89
  Dewitzky's
    aortic 424.1
    mitral 424.0
  diffuse NEC 341.1
  disease, heart - *see* Arteriosclerosis,
    coronary
  disseminated 340
  dorsal 340
  dorsolateral (spinal cord) - *see*
    Degeneration, combined
  endometrium 621.8
  extrapyramidal 333.90
  eye, nuclear (senile) 366.16
  Friedreich's (spinal cord) 334.0
  funicular (spermatic cord) 608.89
  gastritis 535.4●
  general (vascular) - *see* Arteriosclerosis
  gland (lymphatic) 457.8
  hepatic 571.9
  hereditary
    cerebellar 334.2
    spinal 334.0
  hippocampal 348.81
  idiopathic cortical (Garre's) (*see also*
    Osteomyelitis) 730.1●
  ilium, piriform 733.5
  insular 340
    pancreas 251.8
  Islands of Langerhans 251.8
  kidney - *see* Sclerosis, renal
  larynx 478.79
  lateral 335.24
    amyotrophic 335.20
    descending 335.24
    primary 335.24
    spinal 335.24
  liver 571.9
  lobar, atrophic (of brain) 331.0
    with dementia
      with behavioral disturbance 331.0
        [294.11]
      without behavioral disturbance
        331.0 [294.10]
  lung (*see also* Fibrosis, lung) 515
  mastoid 383.1
  mesial temporal 348.81
  mitral - *see* Endocarditis, mitral
  Mönckeberg's (medial) (*see also*
    Arteriosclerosis, extremities)
    440.20
  multiple (brain stem) (cerebral)
    (generalized) (spinal cord) 340
  myocardium, myocardial - *see*
    Arteriosclerosis, coronary
  nuclear (senile), eye 366.16
  ovary 620.8
  pancreas 577.8
  penis 607.89
  peripheral arteries (*see also*
    Arteriosclerosis, extremities)
    440.20
  plaques 340
  pluriglandular 258.8
  polyglandular 258.8

Sclerosis, sclerotic (*Continued*)
  posterior (spinal cord) (syphilitic) 094.0
  posterolateral (spinal cord) - *see*
    Degeneration, combined
  prepuce 607.89
  primary lateral 335.24
  progressive systemic 710.1
  pulmonary (*see also* Fibrosis, lung) 515
    artery 416.0
    valve (heart) (*see also* Endocarditis,
      pulmonary) 424.3
  renal 587
    with
      cystine storage disease 270.0
      hypertension (*see also*
        Hypertension, kidney)
        403.90
      hypertensive heart disease
        (conditions classifiable to
        402) (*see also* Hypertension,
        cardiorenal) 404.90
      arteriolar (hyaline) (*see also*
        Hypertension, kidney) 403.90
      hyperplastic (*see also*
        Hypertension, kidney)
        403.90
  retina (senile) (vascular) 362.17
  rheumatic
    aortic valve 395.9
    mitral valve 394.9
  Schilder's 341.1
  senile - *see* Arteriosclerosis
  spinal (cord) (general) (progressive)
    (transverse) 336.8
    ascending 357.0
    combined - *see also* Degeneration,
      combined
      multiple 340
      syphilitic 094.89
    disseminated 340
    dorsolateral - *see* Degeneration,
      combined
    hereditary (Friedreich's) (mixed
      form) 334.0
    lateral (amyotrophic) 335.24
    multiple 340
    posterior (syphilitic) 094.0
  stomach 537.89
  subendocardial, congenital 425.3
  systemic (progressive) 710.1
    with lung involvement 710.1 [517.2]
  temporal 348.81
    mesial 348.81
  tricuspid (heart) (valve) - *see*
    Endocarditis, tricuspid
  tuberous (brain) 759.5
  tympanic membrane (*see also*
    Tympanosclerosis) 385.00
  valve, valvular (heart) - *see*
    Endocarditis
  vascular - *see* Arteriosclerosis
  vein 459.89
Sclerotenonitis 379.07
Sclerotitis (*see also* Scleritis) 379.00
  syphilitic 095.0
  tuberculous (*see also* Tuberculosis) 017.3
    ● [379.09]
Scoliosis (acquired) (postural) 737.30
  congenital 754.2
  due to or associated with
    Charcôt-Marie-Tooth disease 356.1
      [737.43]
    mucopolysaccharidosis 277.5
      [737.43]
    neurofibromatosis 237.71 [737.43]

◄ New ◄▥ Revised ~~deleted~~ Deleted ● Use Additional Digit(s) ▨ Omit code

Scoliosis *(Continued)*
  due to or associated with *(Continued)*
    osteitis
      deformans 731.0 *[737.43]*
      fibrosa cystica 252.01 *[737.43]*
    osteoporosis *(see also* Osteoporosis) 733.00 *[737.43]*
    poliomyelitis 138 *[737.43]*
    radiation 737.33
    tuberculosis *(see also* Tuberculosis) 015.0● *[737.43]*
  idiopathic 737.30
    infantile
      progressive 737.32
      resolving 737.31
  paralytic 737.39
  rachitic 268.1
  sciatic 724.3
  specified NEC 737.39
  thoracogenic 737.34
  tuberculous *(see also* Tuberculosis) 015.0● *[737.43]*
Scoliotic pelvis 738.6
  with disproportion (fetopelvic) 653.0●
    affecting fetus or newborn 763.1
    causing obstructed labor 660.1●
      affecting fetus or newborn 763.1
Scorbutus, scorbutic 267
  anemia 281.8
Scotoma (ring) 368.44
  arcuate 368.43
  Bjerrum 368.43
  blind spot area 368.42
  central 368.41
  centrocecal 368.41
  paracecal 368.42
  paracentral 368.41
  scintillating 368.12
  Seidel 368.43
Scratch - *see* Injury, superficial, by site
Scratchy throat 784.99
Screening (for) V82.9
  alcoholism V79.1
  anemia, deficiency NEC V78.1
    iron V78.0
  anomaly, congenital V82.89
  antenatal, of mother V28.9
    alphafetoprotein levels, raised V28.1
    based on amniocentesis V28.2
      chromosomal anomalies V28.0
      raised alphafetoprotein levels V28.1
    fetal growth retardation using ultrasonics V28.4
    genomic V28.89
    isoimmunization V28.5
    malformations using ultrasonics V28.3
    proteomic V28.89
    raised alphafetoprotein levels V28.1
    risk
      pre-term labor V28.82
    specified condition NEC V28.89
    Streptococcus B V28.6
  arterial hypertension V81.1
  arthropod-borne viral disease NEC V73.5
  asymptomatic bacteriuria V81.5
  bacterial
    and spirochetal sexually transmitted diseases V74.5
    conjunctivitis V74.4
    disease V74.9
      sexually transmitted V74.5
      specified condition NEC V74.8

Screening *(Continued)*
  bacteriuria, asymptomatic V81.5
  blood disorder NEC V78.9
    specified type NEC V78.8
  bronchitis, chronic V81.3
  brucellosis V74.8
  cancer - *see* Screening, malignant neoplasm
  cardiovascular disease NEC V81.2
  cataract V80.2
  Chagas' disease V75.3
  chemical poisoning V82.5
  cholera V74.0
  cholesterol level V77.91
  chromosomal
    anomalies
      by amniocentesis, antenatal V28.0
      maternal postnatal V82.4
    athletes V70.3
  colonoscopy V76.51 ◀
  condition
    cardiovascular NEC V81.2
    eye NEC V80.2
    genitourinary NEC V81.6
    neurological NEC V80.09
    respiratory NEC V81.4
    skin V82.0
    specified NEC V82.89
  congenital
    anomaly V82.89
      eye V80.2
    dislocation of hip V82.3
    eye condition or disease V80.2
  conjunctivitis, bacterial V74.4
  contamination NEC *(see also* Poisoning) V82.5
  coronary artery disease V81.0
  cystic fibrosis V77.6
  deficiency anemia NEC V78.1
    iron V78.0
  dengue fever V73.5
  depression V79.0
  developmental handicap V79.9
    in early childhood V79.3
    specified type NEC V79.8
  diabetes mellitus V77.1
  diphtheria V74.3
  disease or disorder V82.9
    bacterial V74.9
      specified NEC V74.8
    blood V78.9
      specified type NEC V78.8
    blood-forming organ V78.9
      specified type NEC V78.8
    cardiovascular NEC V81.2
      hypertensive V81.1
      ischemic V81.0
    Chagas' V75.3
    chlamydial V73.98
      specified NEC V73.88
    ear NEC V80.3
    endocrine NEC V77.99
    eye NEC V80.2
    genitourinary NEC V81.6
    heart NEC V81.2
      hypertensive V81.1
      ischemic V81.0
    HPV (human papillomavirus) V73.81
    human papillomavirus (HPV) V73.81
    immunity NEC V77.99
    infectious NEC V75.9
    lipoid NEC V77.91
    mental V79.9
      specified type NEC V79.8

Screening *(Continued)*
  disease or disorder *(Continued)*
    metabolic NEC V77.99
      inborn NEC V77.7
    neurological NEC V80.09
    nutritional NEC V77.99
    rheumatic NEC V82.2
    rickettsial V75.0
    sexually transmitted V74.5
      bacterial V74.5
      spirochetal V74.5
    sickle-cell V78.2
      trait V78.2
    specified type NEC V82.89
    thyroid V77.0
    vascular NEC V81.2
      ischemic V81.0
    venereal V74.5
    viral V73.99
      arthropod-borne NEC V73.5
      specified type NEC V73.89
  dislocation of hip, congenital V82.3
  drugs in athletes V70.3
  elevated titer V82.9
  emphysema (chronic) V81.3
  encephalitis, viral (mosquito or tick borne) V73.5
  endocrine disorder NEC V77.99
  eye disorder NEC V80.2
    congenital V80.2
  fever
    dengue V73.5
    hemorrhagic V73.5
    yellow V73.4
  filariasis V75.6
  galactosemia V77.4
  genetic V82.79
    disease carrier status V82.71
  genitourinary condition NEC V81.6
  glaucoma V80.1
  gonorrhea V74.5
  gout V77.5
  Hansen's disease V74.2
  heart disease NEC V81.2
    hypertensive V81.1
    ischemic V81.0
  heavy metal poisoning V82.5
  helminthiasis, intestinal V75.7
  hematopoietic malignancy V76.89
  hemoglobinopathies NEC V78.3
  hemorrhagic fever V73.5
  Hodgkin's disease V76.89
  hormones in athletes V70.3
  HPV (human papillomavirus) V73.81
  human papillomavirus (HPV) V73.81
  hypercholesterolemia V77.91
  hyperlipidemia V77.91
  hypertension V81.1
  immunity disorder NEC V77.99
  inborn errors of metabolism NEC V77.7
  infection
    bacterial V74.9
      specified type NEC V74.8
    mycotic V75.4
    parasitic NEC V75.8
  infectious disease V75.9
    specified type NEC V75.8
  ingestion of radioactive substance V82.5
  intestinal helminthiasis V75.7
  iron deficiency anemia V78.0
  ischemic heart disease V81.0
  lead poisoning V82.5
  leishmaniasis V75.2

Screening *(Continued)*
leprosy V74.2
leptospirosis V74.8
leukemia V76.89
lipoid disorder NEC V77.91
lymphoma V76.89
malaria V75.1
malignant neoplasm (of) V76.9
  bladder V76.3
  blood V76.89
  breast V76.10
    mammogram NEC V76.12
      for high-risk patient V76.11
    specified type NEC V76.19
  cervix V76.2
  colon V76.51
  colorectal V76.51
  hematopoietic system V76.89
  intestine V76.50
    colon V76.51
    small V76.52
  lung V76.0
  lymph (glands) V76.89
  nervous system V76.81
  oral cavity V76.42
  other specified neoplasm NEC
      V76.89
  ovary V76.46
  prostate V76.44
  rectum V76.41
  respiratory organs V76.0
  skin V76.43
  specified sites NEC V76.49
  testis V76.45
  vagina V76.47
    following hysterectomy for
        malignant condition
        V67.01
malnutrition V77.2
mammogram NEC V76.12
  for high-risk patient V76.11
maternal postnatal chromosomal
    anomalies V82.4
measles V73.2
mental
  disorder V79.9
    specified type NEC V79.8
  retardation V79.2
metabolic disorder NEC V77.99
metabolic errors, inborn V77.7
mucoviscidosis V77.6
multiphasic V82.6
mycosis V75.4
mycotic infection V75.4
nephropathy V81.5
neurological condition NEC V80.09
nutritional disorder NEC V77.99
obesity V77.8
osteoporosis V82.81
parasitic infection NEC V75.8
phenylketonuria V77.3
plague V74.8
poisoning
  chemical NEC V82.5
    contaminated water supply V82.5
  heavy metal V82.5
poliomyelitis V73.0
postnatal chromosomal anomalies,
    maternal V82.4
prenatal - *see* Screening, antenatal
pulmonary tuberculosis V74.1
radiation exposure V82.5
renal disease V81.5
respiratory condition NEC V81.4

Screening *(Continued)*
rheumatic disorder NEC V82.2
rheumatoid arthritis V82.1
rickettsial disease V75.0
rubella V73.3
schistosomiasis V75.5
senile macular lesions of eye V80.2
sexually transmitted diseases V74.5
  bacterial V74.5
  spirochetal V74.5
sickle-cell anemia, disease, or trait
    V78.2
skin condition V82.0
sleeping sickness V75.3
smallpox V73.1
special V82.9
  specified condition NEC V82.89
specified type NEC V82.89
spirochetal disease V74.9
  sexually transmitted V74.5
  specified type NEC V74.8
stimulants in athletes V70.3
syphilis V74.5
tetanus V74.8
thyroid disorder V77.0
trachoma V73.6
traumatic brain injury V80.01
trypanosomiasis V75.3
tuberculosis, pulmonary V74.1
venereal disease V74.5
viral encephalitis
  mosquito-borne V73.5
  tick-borne V73.5
whooping cough V74.8
worms, intestinal V75.7
yaws V74.6
yellow fever V73.4
Scrofula *(see also* Tuberculosis) 017.2●
Scrofulide (primary) *(see also*
    Tuberculosis) 017.0●
Scrofuloderma, scrofulodermia
    (any site) (primary) *(see also*
    Tuberculosis) 017.0●
Scrofulosis (universal) *(see also*
    Tuberculosis) 017.2●
Scrofulosis lichen (primary) *(see also*
    Tuberculosis) 017.0●
Scrofulous - *see* condition
Scrotal tongue 529.5
  congenital 750.13
Scrotum - *see* condition
Scurvy (gum) (infantile) (rickets)
    (scorbutic) 267
Sea-blue histiocyte syndrome 272.7
Seabright-Bantam syndrome
    (pseudohypoparathyroidism) 275.49
Sealpox 059.12
Seasickness 994.6
Seatworm 127.4
Sebaceous
  cyst *(see also* Cyst, sebaceous)
    706.2
  gland disease NEC 706.9
Sebocystomatosis 706.2
Seborrhea, seborrheic 706.3
  adiposa 706.3
  capitis 690.11
  congestiva 695.4
  corporis 706.3
  dermatitis 690.10
    infantile 690.12
  diathesis in infants 695.89
  eczema 690.18
    infantile 690.12

Seborrhea, seborrheic *(Continued)*
  keratosis 702.19
    inflamed 702.11
  nigricans 759.89
  sicca 690.18
  wart 702.19
    inflamed 702.11
Seckel's syndrome 759.89
Seclusion pupil 364.74
Seclusiveness, child 313.22
Secondary - *see also* condition
  neoplasm - *see* Neoplasm, by site,
      malignant, secondary
Secretan's disease or syndrome
    (posttraumatic edema) 782.3
Secretion
  antidiuretic hormone, inappropriate
      (syndrome) 253.6
  catecholamine, by pheochromocytoma
      255.6
  hormone
    antidiuretic, inappropriate
        (syndrome) 253.6
    by
      carcinoid tumor 259.2
      pheochromocytoma 255.6
    ectopic NEC 259.3
  urinary
    excessive 788.42
    suppression 788.5
Section
  cesarean
    affecting fetus or newborn 763.4
    post mortem, affecting fetus or
        newborn 761.6
    previous, in pregnancy or childbirth
        654.2●
      affecting fetus or newborn 763.89
  nerve, traumatic - *see* Injury, nerve, by
      site
Seeligmann's syndrome (ichthyosis
    congenita) 757.1
Segmentation, incomplete (congenital) -
    see also Fusion
  bone NEC 756.9
  lumbosacral (joint) 756.15
  vertebra 756.15
    lumbosacral 756.15
Seizure(s) 780.39
  akinetic (idiopathic) *(see also* Epilepsy)
      345.0●
    psychomotor 345.4●
  apoplexy, apoplectic *(see also* Disease,
      cerebrovascular, acute) 436
  atonic *(see also* Epilepsy) 345.0●
  autonomic 300.11
  brain or cerebral *(see also* Disease,
      cerebrovascular, acute) 436
  convulsive *(see also* Convulsions)
      780.39
  cortical (focal) (motor) *(see also*
      Epilepsy) 345.5●
  disorder *(see also* Epilepsy) 345.9
  due to stroke 438.89
  epilepsy, epileptic (cryptogenic) *(see
      also* Epilepsy) 345.9●
  epileptiform, epileptoid 780.39
    focal *(see also* Epilepsy) 345.5●
  febrile (simple) 780.31
    with status epilepticus 345.3
    atypical 780.32
    complex 780.32
    complicated 780.32
  heart - *see* Disease, heart
  hysterical 300.11

◄ New　◄▦ Revised　~~deleted~~ Deleted　● Use Additional Digit(s)　▨ Omit code

Seizure(s) *(Continued)*
Jacksonian (focal) *(see also* Epilepsy)
345.5●
motor type 345.5●
sensory type 345.5●
migraine triggered 346.0●
newborn 779.0
paralysis *(see also* Disease,
cerebrovascular, acute) 436
post traumatic 780.33 ◀
recurrent 345.9●
epileptic - *see* Epilepsy
repetitive 780.39
epileptic - *see* Epilepsy
salaam *(see also* Epilepsy) 345.6●
uncinate *(see also* Epilepsy) 345.4●
Self-mutilation 300.9
Semicoma 780.09
Semiconsciousness 780.09
Seminal
vesicle - *see* condition
vesiculitis *(see also* Vesiculitis) 608.0
Seminoma (M9061/3)
anaplastic type (M9062/3)
specified site - *see* Neoplasm, by site,
malignant
unspecified site 186.9
specified site - *see* Neoplasm, by site,
malignant
spermatocytic (M9063/3)
specified site - *see* Neoplasm, by site,
malignant
unspecified site 186.9
unspecified site 186.9
Semliki Forest encephalitis 062.8
Senear-Usher disease or syndrome
(pemphigus erythematosus) 694.4
Senecio jacobae dermatitis 692.6
Senectus 797
Senescence 797
Senile *(see also* condition) 797
cervix (atrophic) 622.8
degenerative atrophy, skin 701.3
endometrium (atrophic) 621.8
fallopian tube (atrophic) 620.3
heart (failure) 797
lung 492.8
ovary (atrophic) 620.3
syndrome 259.8
vagina, vaginitis (atrophic) 627.3
wart 702.0
Senility 797
with
acute confusional state 290.3
delirium 290.3
mental changes 290.9
psychosis NEC *(see also* Psychosis,
senile) 290.20
premature (syndrome) 259.8
Sensation
burning *(see also* Disturbance,
sensation) 782.0
tongue 529.6
choking 784.99
loss of *(see also* Disturbance, sensation)
782.0
prickling *(see also* Disturbance,
sensation) 782.0
tingling *(see also* Disturbance,
sensation) 782.0
Sense loss (touch) *(see also* Disturbance,
sensation) 782.0
smell 781.1
taste 781.1

Sensibility disturbance NEC (cortical)
(deep) (vibratory) *(see also*
Disturbance, sensation) 782.0
Sensitive dentine 521.89
Sensitiver Beziehungswahn 297.8
Sensitivity, sensitization - *see also*
Allergy
autoerythrocyte 287.2
carotid sinus 337.01
child (excessive) 313.21
cold, autoimmune 283.0
methemoglobin 289.7
suxamethonium 289.89
tuberculin, without clinical or
radiological symptoms 795.5
Sensory
extinction 781.8
neglect 781.8
Separation
acromioclavicular - *see* Dislocation,
acromioclavicular
anxiety, abnormal 309.21
apophysis, traumatic - *see* Fracture, by
site
choroid 363.70
hemorrhagic 363.72
serous 363.71
costochondral (simple) (traumatic) - *see*
Dislocation, costochondral
delayed
umbilical cord 779.83
epiphysis, epiphyseal
nontraumatic 732.9
upper femoral 732.2
traumatic - *see* Fracture, by site
fracture - *see* Fracture, by site
infundibulum cardiac from right
ventricle by a partition 746.83
joint (current) (traumatic) - *see*
Dislocation, by site
placenta (normally implanted) - *see*
Placenta, separation
pubic bone, obstetrical trauma
665.6●
retina, retinal *(see also* Detachment,
retina) 361.9
layers 362.40
sensory *(see also* Retinoschisis)
361.10
pigment epithelium (exudative)
362.42
hemorrhagic 362.43
sternoclavicular (traumatic) - *see*
Dislocation, sternoclavicular
symphysis pubis, obstetrical trauma
665.6●
tracheal ring, incomplete (congenital)
748.3
Sepsis (generalized) 995.91
with
abortion - *see* Abortion, by type,
with sepsis
acute organ dysfunction 995.92
ectopic pregnancy *(see also*
categories 633.0–633.9) 639.0
molar pregnancy *(see also* categories
630–632) 639.0
multiple organ dysfunction (MOD)
995.92
buccal 528.3
complicating labor 659.3●
dental (pulpal origin) 522.4
female genital organ NEC 614.9
fetus (intrauterine) 771.81

Sepsis *(Continued)*
following
abortion 639.0
ectopic or molar pregnancy 639.0
infusion, perfusion, or transfusion
999.39
Friedländer's 038.49
intraocular 360.00
localized
in operation wound 998.59
skin *(see also* Abscess) 682.9
malleus 024
nadir 038.9
newborn (organism unspecified) NEC
771.81
oral 528.3
puerperal, postpartum, childbirth
(pelvic) 670.2●
resulting from infusion, injection,
transfusion, or vaccination
999.39
severe 995.92
skin, localized *(see also* Abscess) 682.9
umbilical (newborn) (organism
unspecified) 771.89
tetanus 771.3
urinary 599.0
meaning sepsis 995.91
meaning urinary tract infection
599.0
Septate - *see also* Septum
Septic - *see also* condition
adenoids 474.01
and tonsils 474.02
arm (with lymphangitis) 682.3
embolus - *see* Embolism
finger (with lymphangitis) 681.00
foot (with lymphangitis) 682.7
gallbladder *(see also* Cholecystitis)
575.8
hand (with lymphangitis) 682.4
joint *(see also* Arthritis, septic) 711.0●
kidney *(see also* Infection, kidney)
590.9
leg (with lymphangitis) 682.6
mouth 528.3
nail 681.9
finger 681.02
toe 681.11
shock (endotoxic) 785.52
sore *(see also* Abscess) 682.9
throat 034.0
milk-borne 034.0
streptococcal 034.0
spleen (acute) 289.59
teeth (pulpal origin) 522.4
throat 034.0
thrombus - *see* Thrombosis
toe (with lymphangitis) 681.10
tonsils 474.00
and adenoids 474.02
umbilical cord (newborn) (organism
unspecified) 771.89
uterus *(see also* Endometritis) 615.9
Septicemia, septicemic (generalized)
(suppurative) 038.9
with
abortion - *see* Abortion, by type,
with sepsis
ectopic pregnancy *(see also*
categories 633.0–633.9) 639.0
molar pregnancy *(see also* categories
630–632) 639.0
Aerobacter aerogenes 038.49

Septicemia, septicemic (*Continued*)
anaerobic 038.3
anthrax 022.3
Bacillus coli 038.42
Bacteroides 038.3
Clostridium 038.3
complicating labor 659.3●
cryptogenic 038.9
enteric gram-negative bacilli
038.40
Enterobacter aerogenes 038.49
Erysipelothrix (insidiosa)
(rhusiopathiae) 027.1
Escherichia coli 038.42
following
abortion 639.0
ectopic or molar pregnancy
639.0
infusion, injection, transfusion, or
vaccination 999.39
Friedländer's (bacillus) 038.49
gangrenous 038.9
gonococcal 098.89
gram-negative (organism)
038.40
anaerobic 038.3
Hemophilus influenzae 038.41
herpes (simplex) 054.5
herpetic 054.5
Listeria monocytogenes 027.0
meningeal - *see* Meningitis
meningococcal (chronic) (fulminating)
036.2
methicillin
resistant Staphylococcus aureus
(MRSA) 038.12
susceptible Staphylococcus aureus
(MSSA) 038.11
MRSA (methicillin resistant
Staphylococcus aureus)
038.12
MSSA (methicillin susceptible
Staphylococcus aureus) 038.11
navel, newborn (organism unspecified)
771.89
newborn (organism unspecified)
771.81
plague 020.2
pneumococcal 038.2
postabortal 639.0
postoperative 998.59
Proteus vulgaris 038.49
Pseudomonas (aeruginosa) 038.43
puerperal, postpartum 670.2●
Salmonella (aertrycke) (callinarum)
(choleraesuis) (enteritidis)
(suipestifer) 003.1
Serratia 038.44
Shigella (*see also* Dysentery, bacillary)
004.9
specified organism NEC 038.8
staphylococcal 038.10
aureus 038.11
methicillin
resistant (MRSA) 038.12
susceptible (MSSA) 038.11
specified organism NEC 038.19
streptococcal (anaerobic) 038.0
Streptococcus pneumoniae 038.2
suipestifer 003.1
umbilicus, newborn (organism
unspecified) 771.89
viral 079.99
Yersinia enterocolitica 038.49

Septum, septate (congenital) - *see also*
Anomaly, specified type NEC
anal 751.2
aqueduct of Sylvius 742.3
with spina bifida (*see also* Spina
bifida) 741.0●
hymen 752.49
uterus (*see also* Double, uterus)
(complete) (partial) 752.35 ◄▦
vagina 752.49 ◄▦
in pregnancy or childbirth 654.7●
affecting fetus or newborn 763.89
causing obstructed labor
660.2●
affecting fetus or newborn
763.1
longitudinal (with or without
obstruction) 752.47 ◄
transverse 752.46 ◄
Sequestration
lung (congenital) (extralobar)
(intralobar) 748.5
orbit 376.10
pulmonary artery (congenital) 747.3
splenic 289.52
Sequestrum
bone (*see also* Osteomyelitis) 730.1●
jaw 526.4
dental 525.8
jaw bone 526.4
sinus (accessory) (nasal) (*see also*
Sinusitis) 473.9
maxillary 473.0
Sequoiosis asthma 495.8
Serology for syphilis
doubtful
with signs or symptoms - *see*
Syphilis, by site and stage
follow-up of latent syphilis - *see*
Syphilis, latent
false positive 795.6
negative, with signs or symptoms - *see*
Syphilis, by site and stage
positive 097.1
with signs or symptoms - *see*
Syphilis, by site and stage
false 795.6
follow-up of latent syphilis - *see*
Syphilis, latent
only finding - *see* Syphilis, latent
reactivated 097.1
Seroma - (postoperative) (non-infected)
998.13
infected 998.51
post-traumatic 729.91
Seropurulent - *see* condition
Serositis, multiple 569.89
pericardial 423.2
peritoneal 568.82
pleural - *see* Pleurisy
Serotonin syndrome 333.99
Serous - *see* condition
Sertoli cell
adenoma (M8640/0)
specified site - *see* Neoplasm, by site,
benign
unspecified site
female 220
male 222.0
carcinoma (M8640/3)
specified site - *see* Neoplasm, by site,
malignant
unspecified site 186.9
syndrome (germinal aplasia) 606.0

Sertoli cell (*Continued*)
tumor (M8640/0)
with lipid storage (M8641/0)
specified site - *see* Neoplasm, by
site, benign
unspecified site
female 220
male 222.0
specified site - *see* Neoplasm, by site,
benign
unspecified site
female 220
male 222.0
Sertoli-Leydig cell tumor (M8631/0)
specified site - *see* Neoplasm, by site,
benign
unspecified site
female 220
male 222.0
Serum
allergy, allergic reaction 999.5
shock 999.4
arthritis 999.5 [713.6]
complication or reaction NEC 999.5
disease NEC 999.5
hepatitis 070.3●
intoxication 999.5
jaundice (homologous) - *see* Hepatitis,
viral, type B
neuritis 999.5
poisoning NEC 999.5
rash NEC 999.5
reaction NEC 999.5
sickness NEC 999.5
Sesamoiditis 733.99
Seven-day fever 061
of
Japan 100.89
Queensland 100.89
Sever's disease or osteochondrosis
(calcaneum) 732.5
Sex chromosome mosaics 758.81
Sex reassignment surgery status (*see also*
Trans-sexualism) 302.50
Sextuplet
affected by maternal complication of
pregnancy 761.5
healthy liveborn - *see* Newborn,
multiple
pregnancy (complicating delivery)
NEC 651.8●
with fetal loss and retention of one
or more fetus(es) 651.6●
following (elective) fetal reduction
651.7●
Sexual
anesthesia 302.72
deviation (*see also* Deviation, sexual)
302.9
disorder (*see also* Deviation, sexual)
302.9
frigidity (female) 302.72
function, disorder of (psychogenic)
302.70
specified type NEC 302.79
immaturity (female) (male) 259.0
impotence 607.84
organic origin NEC 607.84
psychogenic 302.72
precocity (constitutional) (cryptogenic)
(female) (idiopathic) (male) NEC
259.1
with adrenal hyperplasia 255.2
sadism 302.84

◄ New   ◄▦ Revised   ~~deleted~~ Deleted   ● Use Additional Digit(s)   ▦ Omit code

Sexuality, pathological (*see also* Deviation, sexual) 302.9

Sézary's disease, reticulosis, or syndrome (M9701/3) 202.2●

Shadow, lung 793.1

Shaken infant syndrome 995.55

Shaking
  head (tremor) 781.0
  palsy or paralysis (*see also* Parkinsonism) 332.0

Shallowness, acetabulum 736.39

Shaver's disease or syndrome (bauxite pneumoconiosis) 503

Shearing
  artificial skin graft 996.55
  decellularized allodermis graft 996.55

Sheath (tendon) - *see* condition

Shedding
  nail 703.8
  teeth, premature, primary (deciduous) 520.6

Sheehan's disease or syndrome (postpartum pituitary necrosis) 253.2

Shelf, rectal 569.49

Shell
  shock (current) (*see also* Reaction, stress, acute) 308.9
    lasting state 300.16
  teeth 520.5

Shield kidney 753.3

Shift, mediastinal 793.2

Shifting
  pacemaker 427.89
  sleep-work schedule (affecting sleep) 327.36

Shiga's
  bacillus 004.0
  dysentery 004.0

Shigella (dysentery) (*see also* Dysentery, bacillary) 004.9
  carrier (suspected) of V02.3

Shigellosis (*see also* Dysentery, bacillary) 004.9

Shingles (*see also* Herpes, zoster) 053.9
  eye NEC 053.29

Shin splints 844.9

Shipyard eye or disease 077.1

Shirodkar suture, in pregnancy 654.5●

Shock 785.50
  with
    abortion - *see* Abortion, by type, with shock
    ectopic pregnancy (*see also* categories 633.0–633.9) 639.5
    molar pregnancy (*see also* categories 630–632) 639.5
  allergic - *see* Shock, anaphylactic
  anaclitic 309.21
  anaphylactic 995.0
    chemical - *see* Table of Drugs and Chemicals
    correct medicinal substance properly administered 995.0
    drug or medicinal substance
      correct substance properly administered 995.0
      overdose or wrong substance given or taken 977.9
      specified drug - *see* Table of Drugs and Chemicals
    following sting(s) 989.5

Shock (*Continued*)
  anaphylactic (*Continued*)
    food - *see* Anaphylactic shock, due to, food
    immunization 999.4
    serum 999.4
  anaphylactoid - *see* Shock, anaphylactic
  anesthetic
    correct substance properly administered 995.4
    overdose or wrong substance given 968.4
      specified anesthetic - *see* Table of Drugs and Chemicals
  birth, fetus or newborn NEC 779.89
  cardiogenic 785.51
  chemical substance - *see* Table of Drugs and Chemicals
  circulatory 785.59
  complicating
    abortion - *see* Abortion, by type, with shock
    ectopic pregnancy - (*see also* categories 633.0–633.9) 639.5
    labor and delivery 669.1●
    molar pregnancy (*see also* categories 630–632) 639.5
  culture 309.29
  due to
    drug 995.0
      correct substance properly administered 995.0
      overdose or wrong substance given or taken 977.9
      specified drug - *see* Table of Drugs and Chemicals
    food - *see* Anaphylactic shock, due to, food
  during labor and delivery 669.1●
  electric 994.8
    from electroshock gun (taser) 994.8
  endotoxic 785.52
    due to surgical procedure 998.0
  following
    abortion 639.5
    ectopic or molar pregnancy 639.5
    injury (immediate) (delayed) 958.4
    labor and delivery 669.1●
  gram-negative 785.52
  hematogenic 785.59
  hemorrhagic
    due to
      disease 785.59
      surgery (intraoperative) (postoperative) 998.0
      trauma 958.4
  hypovolemic NEC 785.59
    surgical 998.0
    traumatic 958.4
  insulin 251.0
    therapeutic misadventure 962.3
  kidney 584.5
    traumatic (following crushing) 958.5
  lightning 994.0
  lung 518.5
  nervous (*see also* Reaction, stress, acute) 308.9

Shock (*Continued*)
  obstetric 669.1●
    with
      abortion - *see* Abortion, by type, with shock
      ectopic pregnancy (*see also* categories 633.0–633.9) 639.5
      molar pregnancy (*see also* categories 630–632) 639.5
    following
      abortion 639.5
      ectopic or molar pregnancy 639.5
  paralysis, paralytic (*see also* Disease, cerebrovascular, acute) 436
    late effect - *see* Late effect(s) (of) cerebrovascular disease
  pleural (surgical) 998.0
    due to trauma 958.4
  postoperative 998.0
    with
      abortion - *see* Abortion, by type, with shock
      ectopic pregnancy (*see also* categories 633.0–633.9) 639.5
      molar pregnancy (*see also* categories 630–632) 639.5
    following
      abortion 639.5
      ectopic or molar pregnancy 639.5
  psychic (*see also* Reaction, stress, acute) 308.9
    past history (of) V15.49
  psychogenic (*see also* Reaction, stress, acute) 308.9
  septic 785.52
    with
      abortion - *see* Abortion, by type, with shock
      ectopic pregnancy (*see also* categories 633.0–633.9) 639.5
      molar pregnancy (*see also* categories 630–632) 639.5
    due to
      surgical procedure 998.0
      transfusion NEC 999.89
        bone marrow 996.85
    following
      abortion 639.5
      ectopic or molar pregnancy 639.5
      surgical procedure 998.0
      transfusion NEC 999.89
        bone marrow 996.85
  spinal - *see also* Injury, spinal, by site
    with spinal bone injury - *see* Fracture, vertebra, by site, with spinal cord injury
  surgical 998.0
  therapeutic misadventure NEC (*see also* Complications) 998.89
  thyroxin 962.7
  toxic 040.82
  transfusion - *see* Complications, transfusion
  traumatic (immediate) (delayed) 958.4

Shoemakers' chest 738.3

Short, shortening, shortness
  Achilles tendon (acquired) 727.81
  arm 736.89
    congenital 755.20
  back 737.9
  bowel syndrome 579.3
  breath 786.05

Short, shortening, shortness *(Continued)*
  cervical, cervix 649.7●
    gravid uterus 649.7●
    non-gravid uterus 622.5
      acquired 622.5
      congenital 752.49
  chain acyl CoA dehydrogenase
    deficiency (SCAD) 277.85
  common bile duct, congenital 751.69
  cord (umbilical) 663.4●
    affecting fetus or newborn 762.6
  cystic duct, congenital 751.69
  esophagus (congenital) 750.4
  femur (acquired) 736.81
    congenital 755.34
  frenulum linguae 750.0
  frenum, lingual 750.0
  hamstrings 727.81
  hip (acquired) 736.39
    congenital 755.63
  leg (acquired) 736.81
    congenital 755.30
  metatarsus (congenital) 754.79
    acquired 736.79
  organ or site, congenital NEC - *see*
    Distortion
  palate (congenital) 750.26
  P-R interval syndrome 426.81
  radius (acquired) 736.09
    congenital 755.26
  round ligament 629.89
  sleeper 307.49
  stature, constitutional (hereditary)
    (idiopathic) 783.43
  tendon 727.81
    Achilles (acquired) 727.81
      congenital 754.79
    congenital 756.89
  thigh (acquired) 736.81
    congenital 755.34
  tibialis anticus 727.81
  umbilical cord 663.4●
    affecting fetus or newborn 762.6
  urethra 599.84
  uvula (congenital) 750.26
  vagina 623.8
Shortsightedness 367.1
Shoshin (acute fulminating beriberi) 265.0
Shoulder - *see* condition
Shovel-shaped incisors 520.2
Shower, thromboembolic - *see* Embolism
Shunt (status)
  aortocoronary bypass V45.81
  arterial-venous (dialysis) V45.11
  arteriovenous, pulmonary (acquired)
    417.0
    congenital 747.3
    traumatic (complication) 901.40
  cerebral ventricle (communicating) in
    situ V45.2
  coronary artery bypass V45.81
  surgical, prosthetic, with
    complications - *see*
    Complications, shunt
  vascular NEC V45.89
Shutdown
  renal 586
    with
      abortion - *see* Abortion, by type,
        with renal failure
      ectopic pregnancy (*see also*
        categories 633.0–633.9) 639.3
      molar pregnancy (*see also*
        categories 630–632) 639.3

Shutdown *(Continued)*
  complicating
    abortion 639.3
    ectopic or molar pregnancy 639.3
  following labor and delivery 669.3●
Shwachman's syndrome 288.02
Shy-Drager syndrome (orthostatic
  hypotension with multisystem
  degeneration) 333.0
Sialadenitis (any gland) (chronic)
  (supportive) 527.2
  epidemic - *see* Mumps
Sialadenosis, periodic 527.2
Sialaporia 527.7
Sialectasia 527.8
Sialitis 527.2
Sialoadenitis (*see also* Sialadenitis) 527.2
Sialoangitis 527.2
Sialodochitis (fibrinosa) 527.2
Sialodocholithiasis 527.5
Sialolithiasis 527.5
Sialorrhea (*see also* Ptyalism) 527.7
  periodic 527.2
Sialosis 527.8
  rheumatic 710.2
Siamese twin 759.4
  complicating pregnancy 678.1●
Sicard's syndrome 352.6
Sicca syndrome (keratoconjunctivitis)
  710.2
Sick 799.9
  cilia syndrome 759.89
  or handicapped person in family
    V61.49
Sickle-cell
  anemia (*see also* Disease, sickle-cell)
    282.60
  disease (*see also* Disease, sickle-cell)
    282.60
  hemoglobin
    C disease (without crisis) 282.63
      with
        crisis 282.64
          vaso-occlusive pain 282.64
    D disease (without crisis) 282.68
      with crisis 282.69
    E disease (without crisis) 282.68
      with crisis 282.69
    thalassemia (without crisis) 282.41
      with
        crisis 282.42
          vaso-occlusive pain 282.42
  trait 282.5
Sicklemia (*see also* Disease, sickle-cell)
  282.60
  trait 282.5
Sickness
  air (travel) 994.6
  airplane 994.6
  alpine 993.2
  altitude 993.2
  Andes 993.2
  aviators' 993.2
  balloon 993.2
  car 994.6
  compressed air 993.3
  decompression 993.3
  green 280.9
  harvest 100.89
  milk 988.8
  morning 643.0●
  motion 994.6
  mountain 993.2
    acute 289.0

Sickness *(Continued)*
  protein (*see also* Complications,
    vaccination) 999.5
  radiation NEC 990
  roundabout (motion) 994.6
  sea 994.6
  serum NEC 999.5
  sleeping (African) 086.5
    by Trypanosoma 086.5
      gambiense 086.3
      rhodesiense 086.4
    Gambian 086.3
    late effect 139.8
    Rhodesian 086.4
  sweating 078.2
  swing (motion) 994.6
  train (railway) (travel) 994.6
  travel (any vehicle) 994.6
Sick sinus syndrome 427.81
Sideropenia (*see also* Anemia, iron
  deficiency) 280.9
Siderosis (lung) (occupational) 503
  cornea 371.15
  eye (bulbi) (vitreous) 360.23
  lens 360.23
Siegal-Cattan-Mamou disease (periodic)
  277.31
Siemens' syndrome
  ectodermal dysplasia 757.31
  keratosis follicularis spinulosa
    (decalvans) 757.39
Sighing respiration 786.7
Sigmoid
  flexure - *see* condition
  kidney 753.3
Sigmoiditis - *see* Enteritis
Silfverskiöld's syndrome 756.50
Silicosis, silicotic (complicated)
  (occupational) (simple) 502
  fibrosis, lung (confluent) (massive)
    (occupational) 502
  non-nodular 503
  pulmonum 502
Silicotuberculosis (*see also* Tuberculosis)
  011.4●
Silo fillers' disease 506.9
Silver's syndrome (congenital
  hemihypertrophy and short
  stature) 759.89
Silver wire arteries, retina 362.13
Silvestroni-Bianco syndrome
  (thalassemia minima) 282.49
Simian crease 757.2
Simmonds' cachexia or disease
  (pituitary cachexia) 253.2
Simons' disease or syndrome
  (progressive lipodystrophy)
  272.6
Simple, simplex - *see* condition
Sinding-Larsen disease (juvenile
  osteopathia patellae) 732.4
Singapore hemorrhagic fever 065.4
Singers' node or nodule 478.5
Single
  atrium 745.69
  coronary artery 746.85
  umbilical artery 747.5
  ventricle 745.3
Singultus 786.8
  epidemicus 078.89
Sinus - *see also* Fistula
  abdominal 569.81
  arrest 426.6
  arrhythmia 427.89

◀ New   ◀▮▮▮ Revised   ~~deleted~~ Deleted   ● Use Additional Digit(s)   ▨ Omit code

Sinus *(Continued)*
bradycardia 427.89
   chronic 427.81
branchial cleft (external) (internal)
   744.41
coccygeal (infected) 685.1
   with abscess 685.0
dental 522.7
dermal (congenital) 685.1
   with abscess 685.0
draining - *see* Fistula
infected, skin NEC 686.9
marginal, rupture or bleeding
   641.2●
   affecting fetus or newborn
      762.1
pause 426.6
pericranii 742.0
pilonidal (infected) (rectum) 685.1
   with abscess 685.0
preauricular 744.46
rectovaginal 619.1
sacrococcygeal (dermoid) (infected)
   685.1
   with abscess 685.0
skin
   infected NEC 686.9
   noninfected- *see* Ulcer, skin
tachycardia 427.89
tarsi syndrome 726.79
testis 608.89
tract (postinfectional) - *see* Fistula
urachus 753.7
Sinuses, Rokitansky-Aschoff *(see also*
   Disease, gallbladder) 575.8
Sinusitis (accessory) (chronic)
   (hyperplastic) (nasal)
   (nonpurulent) (purulent) 473.9
with influenza, flu, or grippe *(see also*
   Influenza) 487.1 ◀▥
acute 461.9
   ethmoidal 461.2
   frontal 461.1
   maxillary 461.0
   specified type NEC 461.8
   sphenoidal 461.3
allergic *(see also* Fever, hay) 477.9
antrum - *see* Sinusitis, maxillary
due to
   fungus, any sinus 117.9
   high altitude 993.1
ethmoidal 473.2
   acute 461.2
frontal 473.1
   acute 461.1
influenzal *(see also* Influenza)
   487.1 ◀▥
maxillary 473.0
   acute 461.0
specified site NEC 473.8
sphenoidal 473.3
   acute 461.3
syphilitic, any sinus 095.8
tuberculous, any sinus *(see also*
   Tuberculosis) 012.8●
Sinusitis-bronchiectasis-situs inversus
   (syndrome) (triad) 759.3
Sipple's syndrome (medullary thyroid
   carcinoma-pheochromocytoma)
   258.02
Sirenomelia 759.89
Siriasis 992.0
Sirkari's disease 085.0

SIRS (systemic inflammatory response
   syndrome) 995.90
due to
   infectious process 995.91
      with acute organ dysfunction
         995.92
   non-infectious process 995.93
      with acute organ dysfunction
         995.94
Siti 104.0
Sitophobia 300.29
Situation, psychiatric 300.9
Situational
disturbance (transient) *(see also*
   Reaction, adjustment) 309.9
   acute 308.3
maladjustment, acute *(see also* Reaction,
   adjustment) 309.9
reaction *(see also* Reaction, adjustment)
   309.9
   acute 308.3
Situs inversus or transversus 759.3
abdominalis 759.3
thoracis 759.3
Sixth disease
due to
   human herpesvirus 6 058.11
   human herpesvirus 7 058.12
Sjögren (-Gougerot) syndrome or disease
   (keratoconjunctivitis sicca) 710.2
   with lung involvement 710.2 *[517.8]*
Sjögren-Larsson syndrome (ichthyosis
   congenita) 757.1
SJS-TEN (Stevens-Johnson syndrome-
   toxic epidermal necrolysis overlap
   syndrome) 695.14
Skeletal - *see* condition
Skene's gland - *see* condition
Skenitis *(see also* Urethritis) 597.89
gonorrheal (acute) 098.0
   chronic or duration of 2 months or
      over 098.2
Skerljevo 104.0
Skevas-Zerfus disease 989.5
Skin - *see also* condition
donor V59.1
hidebound 710.9
SLAP lesion (superior glenoid labrum)
   840.7
Slate-dressers' lung 502
Slate-miners' lung 502
Sleep
deprivation V69.4
disorder 780.50
   with apnea - *see* Apnea, sleep
   child 307.40
   movement, unspecified 780.58
   nonorganic origin 307.40
      specified type NEC 307.49
disturbance 780.50
   with apnea - *see* Apnea, sleep
   nonorganic origin 307.40
      specified type NEC 307.49
drunkenness 307.47
movement disorder, unspecified
   780.58
paroxysmal *(see also* Narcolepsy)
   347.00
related movement disorder,
   unspecified 780.58
rhythm inversion 327.39
   nonorganic origin 307.45
walking 307.46
   hysterical 300.13

Sleeping sickness 086.5
late effect 139.8
Sleeplessness *(see also* Insomnia) 780.52
menopausal 627.2
nonorganic origin 307.41
Slipped, slipping
epiphysis (postinfectional) 732.9
   traumatic (old) 732.9
      current - *see* Fracture, by site
   upper femoral (nontraumatic)
      732.2
intervertebral disc - *see* Displacement,
   intervertebral disc
ligature, umbilical 772.3
patella 717.89
rib 733.99
sacroiliac joint 724.6
tendon 727.9
ulnar nerve, nontraumatic 354.2
vertebra NEC *(see also*
   Spondylolisthesis) 756.12
Slocumb's syndrome 255.3
Sloughing (multiple) (skin) 686.9
abscess - *see* Abscess, by site
appendix 543.9
bladder 596.8
fascia 728.9
graft - *see* Complications, graft
phagedena *(see also* Gangrene) 785.4
reattached extremity *(see also*
   Complications, reattached
   extremity) 996.90
rectum 569.49
scrotum 608.89
tendon 727.9
transplanted organ *(see also* Rejection,
   transplant, organ, by site)
   996.80
ulcer *(see also* Ulcer, skin) 707.9
Slow
feeding newborn 779.31
fetal, growth NEC 764.9●
   affecting management of pregnancy
      656.5●
Slowing
heart 427.89
urinary stream 788.62
Sluder's neuralgia or syndrome 337.09
Slurred, slurring, speech 784.59
Small, smallness
cardia reserve - *see* Disease, heart
for dates
   fetus or newborn 764.0●
      with malnutrition 764.1●
      affecting management of
         pregnancy 656.5●
infant, term 764.0●
   with malnutrition 764.1●
   affecting management of pregnancy
      656.5●
introitus, vagina 623.3
kidney, unknown cause 589.9
   bilateral 589.1
   unilateral 589.0
ovary 620.8
pelvis
   with disproportion (fetopelvic)
      653.1●
      affecting fetus or newborn 763.1
      causing obstructed labor 660.1●
         affecting fetus or newborn 763.1
placenta - *see* Placenta, insufficiency
uterus 621.8
white kidney 582.9

Small-for-dates (see also Light-for-dates)
764.0●
  affecting management of pregnancy
    656.5●
Smallpox 050.9
  contact V01.3
  exposure to V01.3
  hemorrhagic (pustular) 050.0
  malignant 050.0
  modified 050.2
  vaccination
    complications - see Complications,
      vaccination
    prophylactic (against) V04.1
Smearing, fecal 787.62 ◀
Smith's fracture (separation) (closed) 813.41
  open 813.51
Smith-Lemli-Opitz syndrome
  (cerebrohepatorenal syndrome) 759.89
Smith-Magenis syndrome 758.33
Smith-Strang disease (oasthouse urine)
  270.2
Smokers'
  bronchitis 491.0
  cough 491.0
  syndrome (see also Abuse, drugs,
    nondependent) 305.1
  throat 472.1
  tongue 528.6
Smoking complicating pregnancy,
  childbirth, or the puerperium 649.0●
Smothering spells 786.09
Snaggle teeth, tooth 524.39
Snapping
  finger 727.05
  hip 719.65
  jaw 524.69
    temporomandibular joint sounds on
      opening or closing 524.64
  knee 717.9
  thumb 727.05
Sneddon-Wilkinson disease or
  syndrome (subcorneal pustular
    dermatosis) 694.1
Sneezing 784.99
  intractable 478.19
Sniffing
  cocaine (see also Dependence) 304.2●
  either (see also Dependence) 304.6●
  glue (airplane) (see also Dependence)
    304.6●
Snoring 786.09
Snow blindness 370.24
Snuffles (nonsyphilitic) 460
  syphilitic (infant) 090.0
Social migrant V60.0
Sodoku 026.0
Soemmering's ring 366.51
Soft - see also condition
  enlarged prostate 600.00
    with
      other lower urinary tract
        symptoms (LUTS) 600.01
      urinary
        obstruction 600.01
        retention 600.01
  nails 703.8
Softening
  bone 268.2
  brain (necrotic) (progressive) 348.89 ◀▥
    arteriosclerotic 437.0
    congenital 742.4
    due to cerebrovascular accident
      438.89 ◀

Softening (Continued)
  brain (Continued)
    embolic (see also Embolism, brain)
      434.1●
    hemorrhagic (see also Hemorrhage,
      brain) 431
    occlusive 434.9●
    thrombotic (see also Thrombosis,
      brain) 434.0●
  cartilage 733.92
  cerebellar - see Softening, brain
  cerebral - see Softening, brain
  cerebrospinal - see Softening, brain
  myocardial, heart (see also
    Degeneration, myocardial) 429.1
  nails 703.8
  spinal cord 336.8
  stomach 537.89
Soiling, fecal 787.62 ◀
Solar fever 061
Soldier's
  heart 306.2
  patches 423.1
Solitary
  cyst
    bone 733.21
    kidney 593.2
  kidney (congenital) 753.0
  tubercle, brain (see also Tuberculosis,
    brain) 013.2●
  ulcer, bladder 596.8
Somatization reaction, somatic reaction (see
  also Disorder, psychosomatic) 306.9
  disorder 300.81
Somatoform disorder 300.82
  atypical 300.82
  severe 300.81
  undifferentiated 300.82
Somnambulism 307.46
  hysterical 300.13
Somnolence 780.09
  nonorganic origin 307.43
  periodic 349.89
Sonne dysentery 004.3
Soor 112.0
Sore
  Delhi 085.1
  desert (see also Ulcer, skin) 707.9
  eye 379.99
  Lahore 085.1
  mouth 528.9
    canker 528.2
    due to dentures 528.9
  muscle 729.1
  naga (see also Ulcer, skin) 707.9
  oriental 085.1
  pressure (see also Ulcer, pressure) 707.00
    with gangrene (see also Ulcer,
      pressure) 707.00 [785.4]
  skin NEC 709.9
  soft 099.0
  throat 462
    with influenza, flu, or grippe (see
      also Influenza) 487.1 ◀▥
    acute 462
    chronic 472.1
    clergyman's 784.49
    Coxsackie (virus) 074.0
    diphtheritic 032.0
    epidemic 034.0
    gangrenous 462
    herpetic 054.79
    influenzal (see also Influenza) 487.1 ◀▥
    malignant 462

Sore (Continued)
  throat (Continued)
    purulent 462
    putrid 462
    septic 034.0
    streptococcal (ulcerative) 034.0
    ulcerated 462
    viral NEC 462
      Coxsackie 074.0
    tropical (see also Ulcer, skin) 707.9
    veldt (see also Ulcer, skin) 707.9
Sotos' syndrome (cerebral gigantism)
  253.0
Sounds
  friction, pleural 786.7
  succussion, chest 786.7
  temporomandibular joint
    on opening or closing 524.64
South African cardiomyopathy
  syndrome 425.2
South American
  blastomycosis 116.1
  trypanosomiasis - see Trypanosomiasis
Southeast Asian hemorrhagic fever 065.4
Spacing, teeth, abnormal 524.30
  excessive 524.32
Spade-like hand (congenital) 754.89
Spading nail 703.8
  congenital 757.5
Spanemia 285.9
Spanish collar 605
Sparganosis 123.5
Spasm, spastic, spasticity (see also
  condition) 781.0
  accommodation 367.53
  ampulla of Vater (see also Disease,
    gallbladder) 576.8
  anus, ani (sphincter) (reflex) 564.6
    psychogenic 306.4
  artery NEC 443.9
    basilar 435.0
    carotid 435.8
    cerebral 435.9
      specified artery NEC 435.8
    retinal (see also Occlusion, retinal,
      artery) 362.30
    vertebral 435.1
    vertebrobasilar 435.3
  Bell's 351.0
  bladder (sphincter, external or internal)
    596.8
  bowel 564.9
    psychogenic 306.4
  bronchus, bronchiole 519.11
  cardia 530.0
  cardiac - see Angina
  carpopedal (see also Tetany) 781.7
  cecum 564.9
    psychogenic 306.4
  cerebral (arteries) (vascular) 435.9
    specified artery NEC 435.8
  cerebrovascular 435.9
  cervix, complicating delivery 661.4●
    affecting fetus or newborn 763.7
  ciliary body (of accommodation)
    367.53
  colon 564.1
    psychogenic 306.4
  common duct (see also Disease, biliary)
    576.8
  compulsive 307.22
  conjugate 378.82
  convergence 378.84
  coronary (artery) - see Angina

◀ New   ◀▥ Revised   d̶e̶l̶e̶t̶e̶d̶ Deleted   ● Use Additional Digit(s)   ▥ Omit code

Spasm, spastic, spasticity *(Continued)*
diaphragm (reflex) 786.8
  psychogenic 306.1
duodenum, duodenal (bulb) 564.89
esophagus (diffuse) 530.5
  psychogenic 306.4
facial 351.8
fallopian tube 620.8
gait 781.2
gastrointestinal (tract) 536.8
  psychogenic 306.4
glottis 478.75
  hysterical 300.11
  psychogenic 306.1
    specified as conversion reaction 300.11
  reflex through recurrent laryngeal nerve 478.75
habit 307.20
  chronic 307.22
  transient (of childhood) 307.21
heart - *see* Angina
hourglass - *see* Contraction, hourglass
hysterical 300.11
infantile (*see also* Epilepsy) 345.6●
internal oblique, eye 378.51
intestinal 564.9
  psychogenic 306.4
larynx, laryngeal 478.75
  hysterical 300.11
  psychogenic 306.1
    specified as conversion reaction 300.11
levator palpebrae superioris 333.81
lightning (*see also* Epilepsy) 345.6●
mobile 781.0
muscle 728.85
  back 724.8
  psychogenic 306.0
nerve, trigeminal 350.1
nervous 306.0
nodding 307.3
  infantile (*see also* Epilepsy) 345.6●
occupational 300.89
oculogyric 378.87
ophthalmic artery 362.30
orbicularis 781.0
perineal 625.8
peroneo-extensor (*see also* Flat, foot) 734
pharynx (reflex) 478.29
  hysterical 300.11
  psychogenic 306.1
    specified as conversion reaction 300.11
pregnant uterus, complicating delivery 661.4●
psychogenic 306.0
pylorus 537.81
  adult hypertrophic 537.0
  congenital or infantile 750.5
  psychogenic 306.4
rectum (sphincter) 564.6
  psychogenic 306.4
retinal artery NEC (*see also* Occlusion, retina, artery) 362.30
sacroiliac 724.6
salaam (infantile) (*see also* Epilepsy) 345.6●
saltatory 781.0
sigmoid 564.9
  psychogenic 306.4
sphincter of Oddi (*see also* Disease, gallbladder) 576.5

Spasm, spastic, spasticity *(Continued)*
stomach 536.8
  neurotic 306.4
throat 478.29
  hysterical 300.11
  psychogenic 306.1
    specified as conversion reaction 300.11
tic 307.20
  chronic 307.22
  transient (of childhood) 307.21
tongue 529.8
torsion 333.6
trigeminal nerve 350.1
  postherpetic 053.12
ureter 593.89
urethra (sphincter) 599.84
uterus 625.8
  complicating labor 661.4●
    affecting fetus or newborn 763.7
vagina 625.1
  psychogenic 306.51
vascular NEC 443.9
vasomotor NEC 443.9
vein NEC 459.89
vesical (sphincter, external or internal) 596.8
viscera 789.0●
Spasmodic - *see* condition
Spasmophilia (*see also* Tetany) 781.7
Spasmus nutans 307.3
Spastic - *see also* Spasm
  child 343.9
Spasticity - *see also* Spasm
  cerebral, child 343.9
Speakers' throat 784.49
Specific, specified - *see* condition
Speech
  defect, disorder, disturbance, impediment NEC 784.59
    psychogenic 307.9
  (language) therapy V57.3
Spells 780.39
  breath-holding 786.9
Spencer's disease (epidemic vomiting) 078.82
Spens' syndrome (syncope with heart block) 426.9
Spermatic cord - *see* condition
Spermatocele 608.1
  congenital 752.89
Spermatocystitis 608.4
Spermatocytoma (M9063/3)
  specified site - *see* Neoplasm, by site, malignant
  unspecified site 186.9
Spermatorrhea 608.89
Sperm counts
  fertility testing V26.21
  following sterilization reversal V26.22
  postvasectomy V25.8
Sphacelus (*see also* Gangrene) 785.4
Sphenoidal - *see* condition
Sphenoiditis (chronic) (*see also* Sinusitis, sphenoidal) 473.3
Sphenopalatine ganglion neuralgia 337.09
Sphericity, increased, lens 743.36
Spherocytosis (congenital) (familial) (hereditary) 282.0
  hemoglobin disease 282.7
  sickle-cell (disease) 282.60
Spherophakia 743.36

Sphincter - *see* condition
Sphincteritis, sphincter of Oddi (*see also* Cholecystitis) 576.8
Sphingolipidosis 272.7
Sphingolipodystrophy 272.7
Sphingomyelinosis 272.7
Spicule tooth 520.2
Spider
  finger 755.59
  nevus 448.1
  vascular 448.1
Spiegler-Fendt sarcoid 686.8
Spielmeyer-Stock disease 330.1
Spielmeyer-Vogt disease 330.1
Spina bifida (aperta) 741.9●

Note: Use the following fifth-digit subclassification with category 741:
  0 unspecified region
  1 cervical region
  2 dorsal [thoracic] region
  3 lumbar region

with hydrocephalus 741.0●
  fetal (suspected), affecting management of pregnancy 655.0●
occulta 756.17
Spindle, Krukenberg's 371.13
Spine, spinal - *see* condition
Spiradenoma (eccrine) (M8403/0) - *see* Neoplasm, skin, benign
Spirillosis NEC (*see also* Fever, relapsing) 087.9
Spirillum minus 026.0
Spirillum obermeieri infection 087.0
Spirochetal - *see* condition
Spirochetosis 104.9
  arthritic, arthritica 104.9 *[711.8]*●
  bronchopulmonary 104.8
  icterohemorrhagica 100.0
  lung 104.8
Spitting blood (*see also* Hemoptysis) 786.30 ◀
Splanchnomegaly 569.89
Splanchnoptosis 569.89
Spleen, splenic - *see also* condition
  agenesis 759.0
  flexure syndrome 569.89
  neutropenia syndrome 289.53
  sequestration syndrome 289.52
Splenectasis (*see also* Splenomegaly) 789.2
Splenitis (interstitial) (malignant) (nonspecific) 289.59
  malarial (*see also* Malaria) 084.6
  tuberculous (*see also* Tuberculosis) 017.7●
Splenocele 289.59
Splenomegalia - *see* Splenomegaly
Splenomegalic - *see* condition
Splenomegaly 789.2
  Bengal 789.2
  cirrhotic 289.51
  congenital 759.0
  congestive, chronic 289.51
  cryptogenic 789.2
  Egyptian 120.1
  Gaucher's (cerebroside lipidosis) 272.7
  idiopathic 789.2
  malarial (*see also* Malaria) 084.6
  neutropenic 289.53
  Niemann-Pick (lipid histiocytosis) 272.7
  siderotic 289.51

Splenomegaly *(Continued)*
  syphilitic 095.8
    congenital 090.0
  tropical (Bengal) (idiopathic) 789.2
Splenopathy 289.50
Splenopneumonia - *see* Pneumonia
Splenoptosis 289.59
Splinter - *see* Injury, superficial, by site
Split, splitting
  heart sounds 427.89
  lip, congenital (*see also* Cleft, lip)
    749.10
  nails 703.8
  urinary stream 788.61
Spoiled child reaction (*see also*
    Disturbance, conduct) 312.1●
Spondylarthritis (*see also* Spondylosis)
    721.90
Spondylarthrosis (*see also* Spondylosis)
    721.90
Spondylitis 720.9
  ankylopoietica 720.0
  ankylosing (chronic) 720.0
  atrophic 720.9
    ligamentous 720.9
  chronic (traumatic) (*see also*
    Spondylosis) 721.90
  deformans (chronic) (*see also*
    Spondylosis) 721.90
  gonococcal 098.53
  gouty 274.00
  hypertrophic (*see also* Spondylosis)
    721.90
  infectious NEC 720.9
  juvenile (adolescent) 720.0
  Kummell's 721.7
  Marie-Strümpell (ankylosing) 720.0
  muscularis 720.9
  ossificans ligamentosa 721.6
  osteoarthritica (*see also* Spondylosis)
    721.90
  posttraumatic 721.7
  proliferative 720.0
  rheumatoid 720.0
  rhizomelica 720.0
  sacroiliac NEC 720.2
  senescent (*see also* Spondylosis)
    721.90
  senile (*see also* Spondylosis) 721.90
  static (*see also* Spondylosis) 721.90
  traumatic (chronic) (*see also*
    Spondylosis) 721.90
  tuberculous (*see also* Tuberculosis)
    015.0● [720.81]
  typhosa 002.0 [720.81]
Spondyloarthrosis (*see also* Spondylosis)
    721.90
Spondylolisthesis (congenital)
    (lumbosacral) 756.12
  with disproportion (fetopelvic)
    653.3●
    affecting fetus or newborn
      763.1
    causing obstructed labor
      660.1●
      affecting fetus or newborn
        763.1
  acquired 738.4
  degenerative 738.4
  traumatic 738.4
    acute (lumbar) - *see* Fracture,
      vertebra, lumbar
    site other than lumbosacral - *see*
      Fracture, vertebra, by site

Spondylolysis (congenital) 756.11
  acquired 738.4
  cervical 756.19
  lumbosacral region 756.11
    with disproportion (fetopelvic)
      653.3●
      affecting fetus or newborn
        763.1
      causing obstructed labor 660.1●
        affecting fetus or newborn
          763.1
Spondylopathy
  inflammatory 720.9
    specified type NEC 720.89
  traumatic 721.7
Spondylose rhizomelique 720.0
Spondylosis 721.90
  with
    disproportion 653.3●
      affecting fetus or newborn
        763.1
      causing obstructed labor 660.1●
        affecting fetus or newborn
          763.1
    myelopathy NEC 721.91
  cervical, cervicodorsal 721.0
    with myelopathy 721.1
  inflammatory 720.9
  lumbar, lumbosacral 721.3
    with myelopathy 721.42
  sacral 721.3
    with myelopathy 721.42
  thoracic 721.2
    with myelopathy 721.41
  traumatic 721.7
Sponge
  divers' disease 989.5
  inadvertently left in operation wound
    998.4
  kidney (medullary) 753.17
Spongioblastoma (M9422/3)
  multiforme (M9440/3)
    specified site - *see* Neoplasm, by site,
      malignant
    unspecified site 191.9
  polare (M9423/3)
    specified site - *see* Neoplasm, by site,
      malignant
    unspecified site 191.9
  primitive polar (M9443/3)
    specified site - *see* Neoplasm, by site,
      malignant
    unspecified site 191.9
  specified site - *see* Neoplasm, by site,
    malignant
  unspecified site 191.9
Spongiocytoma (M9400/3)
  specified site - *see* Neoplasm, by site,
    malignant
  unspecified site 191.9
Spongioneuroblastoma (M9504/3) - *see*
    Neoplasm, by site, malignant
Spontaneous - *see also* condition
  fracture - *see* Fracture, pathologic
Spoon nail 703.8
  congenital 757.5
Sporadic - *see* condition
Sporotrichosis (bones) (cutaneous)
    (disseminated) (epidermal)
    (lymphatic) (lymphocutaneous)
    (mucous membranes) (pulmonary)
    (skeletal) (visceral) 117.1
Sporotrichum schenckii infection
    117.1

Spots, spotting
  atrophic (skin) 701.3
  Bitôt's (in the young child) 264.1
  café au lait 709.09
  cayenne pepper 448.1
  complicating pregnancy 649.5●
  cotton wool (retina) 362.83
  de Morgan's (senile angiomas) 448.1
  Fúchs' black (myopic) 360.21
  intermenstrual
    irregular 626.6
    regular 626.5
  interpalpebral 372.53
  Koplik's 055.9
  liver 709.09
  Mongolian (pigmented) 757.33
  of pregnancy 649.5●
  purpuric 782.7
  ruby 448.1
Spotted fever - *see* Fever, spotted
Sprain, strain (joint) (ligament) (muscle)
    (tendon) 848.9
  abdominal wall (muscle) 848.8
  Achilles tendon 845.09
  acromioclavicular 840.0
  ankle 845.00
    and foot 845.00
  anterior longitudinal, cervical 847.0
  arm 840.9
    upper 840.9
      and shoulder 840.9
  astragalus 845.00
  atlanto-axial 847.0
  atlanto-occipital 847.0
  atlas 847.0
  axis 847.0
  back (*see also* Sprain, spine) 847.9
  breast bone 848.40
  broad ligaments - *see* Injury, internal,
    broad ligament
  calcaneofibular 845.02
  carpal 842.01
  carpometacarpal 842.11
  cartilage
    costal, without mention of injury to
      sternum 848.3
      involving sternum 848.42
    ear 848.8
    knee 844.9
      with current tear (*see also* Tear,
        meniscus) 836.2
    semilunar (knee) 844.8
      with current tear (*see also* Tear,
        meniscus) 836.2
    septal, nose 848.0
    thyroid region 848.2
    xiphoid 848.49
  cervical, cervicodorsal, cervicothoracic
    847.0
  chondrocostal, without mention of
    injury to sternum 848.3
    involving sternum 848.42
  chondrosternal 848.42
  chronic (joint) - *see* Derangement,
    joint
  clavicle 840.9
  coccyx 847.4
  collar bone 840.9
  collateral, knee (medial) (tibial)
    844.1
    lateral (fibular) 844.0
    recurrent or old 717.89
      lateral 717.81
      medial 717.82

◀ New   ◀▥ Revised   ~~deleted~~ Deleted   ● Use Additional Digit(s)   ▨ Omit code

Sprain, strain *(Continued)*
  coracoacromial 840.8
  coracoclavicular 840.1
  coracohumeral 840.2
  coracoid (process) 840.9
  coronary, knee 844.8
  costal cartilage, without mention of
      injury to sternum 848.3
    involving sternum 848.42
  cricoarytenoid articulation 848.2
  cricothyroid articulation 848.2
  cruciate
    knee 844.2
    old 717.89
      anterior 717.83
      posterior 717.84
  deltoid
    ankle 845.01
    shoulder 840.8
  dorsal (spine) 847.1
  ear cartilage 848.8
  elbow 841.9
    and forearm 841.9
    specified site NEC 841.8
  femur (proximal end) 843.9
    distal end 844.9
  fibula (proximal end) 844.9
    distal end 845.00
  fibulocalcaneal 845.02
  finger(s) 842.10
  foot 845.10
    and ankle 845.00
  forearm 841.9
    and elbow 841.9
    specified site NEC 841.8
  glenoid (shoulder) - *(see also* SLAP
      lesion) 840.8
  hand 842.10
  hip 843.9
    and thigh 843.9
  humerus (proximal end) 840.9
    distal end 841.9
  iliofemoral 843.0
  infraspinatus 840.3
  innominate
    acetabulum 843.9
    pubic junction 848.5
    sacral junction 846.1
  internal
    collateral, ankle 845.01
    semilunar cartilage 844.8
      with current tear *(see also* Tear,
        meniscus) 836.2
      old 717.5
  interphalangeal
    finger 842.13
    toe 845.13
  ischiocapsular 843.1
  jaw (cartilage) (meniscus) 848.1
    old 524.69
  knee 844.9
    and leg 844.9
    old 717.5
      collateral
        lateral 717.81
        medial 717.82
      cruciate
        anterior 717.83
        posterior 717.84
  late effect - *see* Late, effects (of), sprain
  lateral collateral, knee 844.0
    old 717.81
  leg 844.9
    and knee 844.9

Sprain, strain *(Continued)*
  ligamentum teres femoris 843.8
  low back 846.9
  lumbar (spine) 847.2
  lumbosacral 846.0
    chronic or old 724.6
  mandible 848.1
    old 524.69
  maxilla 848.1
  medial collateral, knee 844.1
    old 717.82
  meniscus
    jaw 848.1
      old 524.69
    knee 844.8
      with current tear *(see also* Tear,
        meniscus) 836.2
      old 717.5
    mandible 848.1
      old 524.69
    specified site NEC 848.8
  metacarpal 842.10
    distal 842.12
    proximal 842.11
  metacarpophalangeal 842.12
  metatarsal 845.10
  metatarsophalangeal 845.12
  midcarpal 842.19
  midtarsal 845.19
  multiple sites, except fingers alone or
      toes alone 848.8
  neck 847.0
  nose (septal cartilage) 848.0
  occiput from atlas 847.0
  old - *see* Derangement, joint
  orbicular, hip 843.8
  patella(r) 844.8
    old 717.89
  pelvis 848.5
  phalanx
    finger 842.10
    toe 845.10
  radiocarpal 842.02
  radiohumeral 841.2
  radioulnar 841.9
    distal 842.09
  radius, radial (proximal end) 841.9
    and ulna 841.9
      distal 842.09
    collateral 841.0
    distal end 842.00
  recurrent - *see* Sprain, by site
  rib (cage), without mention of injury to
      sternum 848.3
    involving sternum 848.42
  rotator cuff (capsule) 840.4
  round ligament - *see also* Injury,
      internal, round ligament
    femur 843.8
  sacral (spine) 847.3
  sacrococcygeal 847.3
  sacroiliac (region) 846.9
    chronic or old 724.6
    ligament 846.1
    specified site NEC 846.8
  sacrospinatus 846.2
  sacrospinous 846.2
  sacrotuberous 846.3
  scaphoid bone, ankle 845.00
  scapula(r) 840.9
  semilunar cartilage (knee) 844.8
    with current tear *(see also* Tear,
      meniscus) 836.2
    old 717.5

Sprain, strain *(Continued)*
  septal cartilage (nose) 848.0
  shoulder 840.9
    and arm, upper 840.9
    blade 840.9
  specified site NEC 848.8
  spine 847.9
    cervical 847.0
    coccyx 847.4
    dorsal 847.1
    lumbar 847.2
    lumbosacral 846.0
      chronic or old 724.6
    sacral 847.3
    sacroiliac *(see also* Sprain, sacroiliac)
      846.9
      chronic or old 724.6
    thoracic 847.1
  sternoclavicular 848.41
  sternum 848.40
  subglenoid - *(see also* SLAP lesion)
      840.8
  subscapularis 840.5
  supraspinatus 840.6
  symphysis
    jaw 848.1
      old 524.69
    mandibular 848.1
      old 524.69
    pubis 848.5
  talofibular 845.09
  tarsal 845.10
  tarsometatarsal 845.11
  temporomandibular 848.1
    old 524.69
  teres
    ligamentum femoris 843.8
    major or minor 840.8
  thigh (proximal end) 843.9
    and hip 843.9
    distal end 844.9
  thoracic (spine) 847.1
  thorax 848.8
  thumb 842.10
  thyroid cartilage or region 848.2
  tibia (proximal end) 844.9
    distal end 845.00
  tibiofibular
    distal 845.03
    superior 844.3
  toe(s) 845.10
  trachea 848.8
  trapezoid 840.8
  ulna, ulnar (proximal end) 841.9
    collateral 841.1
    distal end 842.00
  ulnohumeral 841.3
  vertebrae *(see also* Sprain, spine)
      847.9
    cervical, cervicodorsal,
        cervicothoracic 847.0
  wrist (cuneiform) (scaphoid)
      (semilunar) 842.00
  xiphoid cartilage 848.49
Sprengel's deformity (congenital)
    755.52
Spring fever 309.23
Sprue 579.1
  celiac 579.0
  idiopathic 579.0
  meaning thrush 112.0
  nontropical 579.0
  tropical 579.1

Spur - *see also* Exostosis
　bone 726.91
　　calcaneal 726.73
　calcaneal 726.73
　iliac crest 726.5
　nose (septum) 478.19
　　bone 726.91
　septal 478.19
Spuria placenta - *see* Placenta, abnormal
Spurway's syndrome (brittle bones and
　　blue sclera) 756.51
Sputum, abnormal (amount) (color)
　　(excessive) (odor) (purulent) 786.4
　bloody 786.30 ◀▦
Squamous - *see also* condition
　cell metaplasia
　　bladder 596.8
　　cervix - *see* condition
　epithelium in
　　cervical canal (congenital) 752.49
　　uterine mucosa (congenital)
　　　752.39 ◀▦
　metaplasia
　　bladder 596.8
　　cervix - *see* condition
Squashed nose 738.0
　congenital 754.0
Squeeze, divers' 993.3
Squint (*see also* Strabismus) 378.9
　accommodative (*see also* Esotropia)
　　378.00
　concomitant (*see also* Heterotropia)
　　378.30
Stab - *see also* Wound, open, by site
　internal organs - *see* Injury, internal, by
　　site, with open wound
Staggering gait 781.2
　hysterical 300.11
Staghorn calculus 592.0
Stähl's
　ear 744.29
　pigment line (cornea) 371.11
Stähli's pigment lines (cornea) 371.11
Stain, staining
　meconium 779.84
　port wine 757.32
　tooth, teeth (hard tissues) 521.7
　　due to
　　　accretions 523.6
　　　deposits (betel) (black) (green)
　　　　(materia alba) (orange)
　　　　(tobacco) 523.6
　　　metals (copper) (silver) 521.7
　　　nicotine 523.6
　　　pulpal bleeding 521.7
　　　tobacco 523.6
Stammering (*see also* Disorder, fluency)
　　315.35 ◀▦
Standstill
　atrial 426.6
　auricular 426.6
　cardiac (*see also* Arrest, cardiac) 427.5
　sinoatrial 426.6
　sinus 426.6
　ventricular (*see also* Arrest, cardiac)
　　427.5
Stannosis 503
Stanton's disease (melioidosis) 025
Staphylitis (acute) (catarrhal) (chronic)
　　(gangrenous) (membranous)
　　(suppurative) (ulcerative) 528.3
Staphylococcemia 038.10
　aureus 038.11
　specified organism NEC 038.19

Staphylococcus, staphylococcal - *see*
　condition
Staphyloderma (skin) 686.00
Staphyloma 379.11
　anterior, localized 379.14
　ciliary 379.11
　cornea 371.73
　equatorial 379.13
　posterior 379.12
　posticum 379.12
　ring 379.15
　sclera NEC 379.11
Starch eating 307.52
Stargardt's disease 362.75
Starvation (inanition) (due to lack of
　　food) 994.2
　edema 262
　voluntary NEC 307.1
Stasis
　bile (duct) (*see also* Disease, biliary)
　　576.8
　bronchus (*see also* Bronchitis) 490
　cardiac (*see also* Failure, heart)
　　428.0
　cecum 564.89
　colon 564.89
　dermatitis (*see also* Varix, with stasis
　　dermatitis) 454.1
　duodenal 536.8
　eczema (*see also* Varix, with stasis
　　dermatitis) 454.1
　edema (*see also* Hypertension, venous)
　　459.30
　foot 991.4
　gastric 536.3
　ileocecal coil 564.89
　ileum 564.89
　intestinal 564.89
　jejunum 564.89
　kidney 586
　liver 571.9
　　cirrhotic - *see* Cirrhosis, liver
　lymphatic 457.8
　pneumonia 514
　portal 571.9
　pulmonary 514
　rectal 564.89
　renal 586
　　tubular 584.5
　stomach 536.3
　ulcer
　　with varicose veins 454.0
　　without varicose veins 459.81
　urine NEC (*see also* Retention, urine)
　　788.20
　venous 459.81
State
　affective and paranoid, mixed, organic
　　psychotic 294.8
　agitated 307.9
　　acute reaction to stress 308.2
　anxiety (neurotic) (*see also* Anxiety)
　　300.00
　　specified type NEC 300.09
　apprehension (*see also* Anxiety) 300.00
　　specified type NEC 300.09
　climacteric, female 627.2
　　following induced menopause 627.4
　clouded
　　epileptic (*see also* Epilepsy) 345.9●
　　paroxysmal (idiopathic) (*see also*
　　　Epilepsy) 345.9●
　compulsive (mixed) (with obsession)
　　300.3

State (*Continued*)
　confusional 298.9
　　acute 293.0
　　　with
　　　　arteriosclerotic dementia
　　　　　290.41
　　　　presenile brain disease 290.11
　　　　senility 290.3
　　alcoholic 291.0
　　drug-induced 292.81
　　epileptic 293.0
　　postoperative 293.9
　　reactive (emotional stress)
　　　(psychological trauma) 298.2
　　subacute 293.1
　constitutional psychopathic 301.9
　convulsive (*see also* Convulsions) 780.39
　depressive NEC 311
　　induced by drug 292.84
　　neurotic 300.4
　dissociative 300.15
　hallucinatory 780.1
　　induced by drug 292.12
　hypercoagulable (primary) 289.81
　　secondary 289.82
　hyperdynamic beta-adrenergic
　　circulatory 429.82
　locked-in 344.81
　menopausal 627.2
　　artificial 627.4
　　following induced menopause 627.4
　neurotic NEC 300.9
　　with depersonalization episode 300.6
　obsessional 300.3
　oneiroid (*see also* Schizophrenia) 295.4●
　panic 300.01
　paranoid 297.9
　　alcohol-induced 291.5
　　arteriosclerotic 290.42
　　climacteric 297.2
　　drug-induced 292.11
　　in
　　　presenile brain disease 290.12
　　　senile brain disease 290.20
　　involutional 297.2
　　menopausal 297.2
　　senile 290.20
　　simple 297.0
　postleukotomy 310.0
　pregnant (*see also* Pregnancy) V22.2
　psychogenic, twilight 298.2
　psychotic, organic (*see also* Psychosis,
　　organic) 294.9
　　mixed paranoid and affective 294.8
　　senile or presenile NEC 290.9
　　transient NEC 293.9
　　　with
　　　　anxiety 293.84
　　　　delusions 293.81
　　　　depression 293.83
　　　　hallucinations 293.82
　residual schizophrenic (*see also*
　　Schizophrenia) 295.6●
　tension (*see also* Anxiety) 300.9
　transient organic psychotic 293.9
　　anxiety type 293.84
　　depressive type 293.83
　　hallucinatory type 293.83
　　paranoid type 293.81
　　specified type NEC 293.89
　twilight
　　epileptic 293.0
　　psychogenic 298.2
　vegetative (persistent) 780.03

◀ New　　◀▦ Revised　　deleted Deleted　　● Use Additional Digit(s)　　▦ Omit code

Status (post)
  absence
    epileptic (*see also* Epilepsy) 345.2
    of organ, acquired (postsurgical) - *see* Absence, by site, acquired
  administration of tPA (rtPA) in a different institution within the last 24 hours prior to admission to facility V45.88
  anastomosis of intestine (for bypass) V45.3
  anginosus 413.9
  angioplasty, percutaneous transluminal coronary V45.82
  ankle prosthesis V43.66
  aortocoronary bypass or shunt V45.81
  arthrodesis V45.4
  artificially induced condition NEC V45.89
  artificial opening (of) V44.9
    gastrointestinal tract NEC V44.4
    specified site NEC V44.8
    urinary tract NEC V44.6
    vagina V44.7
  aspirator V46.0
  asthmaticus (*see also* Asthma) 493.9●
  awaiting organ transplant V49.83
  bariatric surgery V45.86
    complicating pregnancy, childbirth, or the puerperium 649.2●
  bed confinement V49.84
  breast
    correction V43.82
    implant removal V45.83
    reconstruction V43.82
  cardiac
    device (in situ) V45.00
      carotid sinus V45.09
        fitting or adjustment V53.39
      defibrillator, automatic implantable (with synchronous cardiac pacemaker) V45.02 ◀▥
      pacemaker V45.01
        fitting or adjustment V53.31
  carotid sinus stimulator V45.09
  cataract extraction V45.61
  chemotherapy V66.2
    current V58.69
  circumcision, female 629.20
  clitorectomy (female genital mutilation type I) 629.21
    with excision of labia minora (female genital mutilation type II) 629.22
  colonization - *see* Carrier (suspected) of
  colostomy V44.3
  contraceptive device V45.59
    intrauterine V45.51
    subdermal V45.52
  convulsivus idiopathicus (*see also* Epilepsy) 345.3
  coronary artery bypass or shunt V45.81
  cutting
    female genital 629.20
      specified NEC 629.29
      type I 629.21
      type II 629.22
      type III 629.23
      type IV 629.29

State (*Continued*)
  cystostomy V44.50
    appendico-vesicostomy V44.52
    cutaneous-vesicostomy V44.51
    specifed type NEC V44.59
  defibrillator, automatic implantable cardiac (with synchronous cardiac pacemaker) V45.02 ◀▥
  delinquent immunization V15.83
  dental crowns V45.84
  dental fillings V45.84
  dental restoration V45.84
  dental sealant V49.82
  dialysis (hemo) (peritoneal) V45.11
  donor V59.9
  do not resuscitate V49.86 ◀
  drug therapy or regimen V67.59
    high-risk medication NEC V67.51
  elbow prosthesis V43.62
  embedded ◀
    fragment - *see* Foreign body, retained ◀
    splinter - *see* Foreign body, retained ◀
  enterostomy V44.4
  epileptic, epilepticus (absence) (grand mal) (*see also* Epilepsy) 345.3
    focal motor 345.7●
    partial 345.7●
    petit mal 345.2
    psychomotor 345.7●
    temporal lobe 345.7●
  estrogen receptor
    negative [ER-] V86.1
    positive [ER+] V86.0
  eye (adnexa) surgery V45.69
  female genital
    cutting 629.20
      specified NEC 629.29
      type I 629.21
      type II 629.22
      type III 629.23
      type IV 629.29
    mutilation 629.20
      type I 629.21
      type II 629.22
      type III 629.23
      type IV 629.29
  filtering bleb (eye) (postglaucoma) V45.69
    with rupture or complication 997.99
    postcataract extraction (complication) 997.99
  finger joint prosthesis V43.69
  foster care V60.81
  gastric
    banding V45.86
      complicating pregnancy, childbirth, or the puerperium 649.2●
    bypass for obesity V45.86
      complicating pregnancy, childbirth, or the puerperium 649.2●
  gastrostomy V44.1
  grand mal 345.3
  heart valve prosthesis V43.3
  hemodialysis V45.11
  hip prosthesis (joint) (partial) (total) V43.64
  hysterectomy V88.01
    partial with remaining cervical stump V88.02
    total V88.01
  ileostomy V44.2

Status (*Continued*)
  infibulation (female genital mutilation type III) 629.23
  insulin pump V45.85
  intestinal bypass V45.3
  intrauterine contraceptive device V45.51
  jejunostomy V44.4
  knee joint prosthesis V43.65
  lacunaris 437.8
  lacunosis 437.8
  lapsed immunization schedule V15.83
  low birth weight V21.30
    less than 500 grams V21.31
    500–999 grams V21.32
    1000–1499 grams V21.33
    1500–1999 grams V21.34
    2000–2500 grams V21.35
  lymphaticus 254.8
  malignant neoplasm, ablated or excised - *see* History, malignant neoplasm
  marmoratus 333.79
  military deployment V62.22
  mutilation, female 629.20
    type I 629.21
    type II 629.22
    type III 629.23
    type IV 629.29
  nephrostomy V44.6
  neuropacemaker NEC V45.89
    brain V45.89
    carotid sinus V45.09
    neurologic NEC V45.89
  obesity surgery V45.86
    complicating pregnancy, childbirth, or the puerperium 649.2●
  organ replacement
    by artificial or mechanical device or prosthesis of
      artery V43.4
      artificial skin V43.83
      bladder V43.5
      blood vessel V43.4
      breast V43.82
      eye globe V43.0
      heart
        assist device V43.21
        fully implantable artificial heart V43.22
        valve V43.3
      intestine V43.89
      joint V43.60
        ankle V43.66
        elbow V43.62
        finger V43.69
        hip (partial) (total) V43.64
        knee V43.65
        shoulder V43.61
        specified NEC V43.69
        wrist V43.63
      kidney V43.89
      larynx V43.81
      lens V43.1
      limb(s) V43.7
      liver V43.89
      lung V43.89
      organ NEC V43.89
      pancreas V43.89
      skin (artificial) V43.83
      tissue NEC V43.89
      vein V43.4
    by organ transplant (heterologous) (homologous) - *see* Status, transplant

Status *(Continued)*
  pacemaker
    brain V45.89
    cardiac V45.01
    carotid sinus V45.09
    neurologic NEC V45.89
    specified site NEC V45.89
  percutaneous transluminal coronary
    angioplasty V45.82
  peritoneal dialysis V45.11
  petit mal 345.2
  physical restraints V49.87 ◄
  postcommotio cerebri 310.2
  postmenopausal (age related) (natural)
    V49.81
  postoperative NEC V45.89
  postpartum NEC V24.2
    care immediately following delivery
      V24.0
    routine follow-up V24.2
  postsurgical NEC V45.89
  renal dialysis V45.11
    noncompliance V45.12
  respirator [ventilator] V46.11
    encounter
      during
        mechanical failure V46.14
        power failure V46.12
      for weaning V46.13
  retained foreign body - *see* Foreign
    body, retained ◄
  reversed jejunal transposition (for
    bypass) V45.3
  sex reassignment surgery *(see also*
    Trans-sexualism) 302.50
  shoulder prosthesis V43.61
  shunt
    aortocoronary bypass V45.81
    arteriovenous (for dialysis) V45.11
    cerebrospinal fluid V45.2
    vascular NEC V45.89
      aortocoronary (bypass) V45.81
    ventricular (communicating) (for
      drainage) V45.2
  sterilization
    tubal ligation V26.51
    vasectomy V26.52
  subdermal contraceptive device V45.52
  thymicolymphaticus 254.8
  thymicus 254.8
  thymolymphaticus 254.8
  tooth extraction 525.10
  tracheostomy V44.0
  transplant
    blood vessel V42.89
    bone V42.4
      marrow V42.81
    cornea V42.5
    heart V42.1
      valve V42.2
    intestine V42.84
    kidney V42.0
    liver V42.7
    lung V42.6
    organ V42.9
      removal (due to complication,
        failure, rejection or
        infection) V45.87
      specified site NEC V42.89
    pancreas V42.83
    peripheral stem cells V42.82
    skin V42.3
    stem cells, peripheral V42.82
    tissue V42.9
      specified type NEC V42.89
    vessel, blood V42.89

Status *(Continued)*
  tubal ligation V26.51
  underimmunization V15.83
  ureterostomy V44.6
  urethrostomy V44.6
  vagina, artificial V44.7
  vascular shunt NEC V45.89
    aortocoronary (bypass) V45.81
  vasectomy V26.52
  ventilator [respirator] V46.11
    encounter
      during
        mechanical failure V46.14
        power failure V46.12
      for weaning V46.13
  wheelchair confinement V46.3
  wrist prosthesis V43.63
Stave fracture - *see* Fracture, metacarpus,
  metacarpal bone(s)
Steal
  subclavian artery 435.2
  vertebral artery 435.1
Stealing, solitary, child problem *(see also*
  Disturbance, conduct) 312.1●
Steam burn - *see* Burn, by site
Steatocystoma multiplex 706.2
Steatoma (infected) 706.2
  eyelid (cystic) 374.84
    infected 373.13
Steatorrhea (chronic) 579.8
  with lacteal obstruction 579.2
  idiopathic 579.0
    adult 579.0
    infantile 579.0
  pancreatic 579.4
  primary 579.0
  secondary 579.8
  specified cause NEC 579.8
  tropical 579.1
Steatosis 272.8
  heart *(see also* Degeneration,
    myocardial) 429.1
  kidney 593.89
  liver 571.8
Steele-Richardson (-Olszewski)
  syndrome 333.0
Stein's syndrome (polycystic ovary) 256.4
Stein-Leventhal syndrome (polycystic
  ovary) 256.4
Steinbrocker's syndrome *(see also*
  Neuropathy, peripheral, autonomic)
  337.9
Steinert's disease 359.21
STEMI (ST elevation myocardial
  infarction) *(see also* - Infarct,
  myocardium, ST elevation) 410.9●
Stenocardia *(see also* Angina) 413.9
Stenocephaly 756.0
Stenosis (cicatricial) - *see also* Stricture
  ampulla of Vater 576.2
    with calculus, cholelithiasis, or
      stones - *see* Choledocholithiasis
  anus, anal (canal) (sphincter) 569.2
    congenital 751.2
  aorta (ascending) 747.22
    arch 747.10
    arteriosclerotic 440.0
    calcified 440.0
  aortic (valve) 424.1
    with
      mitral (valve)
        insufficiency or incompetence
          396.2
        stenosis or obstruction 396.0

Stenosis *(Continued)*
  aortic *(Continued)*
    atypical 396.0
    congenital 746.3
    rheumatic 395.0
      with
        insufficiency, incompetency or
          regurgitation 395.2
          with mitral (valve) disease
            396.8
        mitral (valve)
          disease (stenosis) 396.0
          insufficiency or
            incompetence 396.2
          stenosis or obstruction 396.0
    specified cause, except rheumatic
      424.1
    syphilitic 093.22
  aqueduct of Sylvius (congenital) 742.3
    with spina bifida *(see also* Spina
      bifida) 741.0●
    acquired 331.4
  artery NEC *(see also* Arteriosclerosis)
    447.1
    basilar - *see* Narrowing, artery,
      basilar
    carotid (common) (internal) - *see*
      Narrowing, artery, carotid
    celiac 447.4
    cerebral 437.0
      due to
        embolism *(see also* Embolism,
          brain) 434.1●
        thrombus *(see also* Thrombosis,
          brain) 434.0●
    extremities 440.20
    precerebral - *see* Narrowing, artery,
      precerebral
    pulmonary (congenital) 747.3
      acquired 417.8
    renal 440.1
    vertebral - *see* Narrowing, artery,
      vertebral
  bile duct or biliary passage *(see also*
    Obstruction, biliary) 576.2
    congenital 751.61
  bladder neck (acquired) 596.0
    congenital 753.6
  brain 348.89
  bronchus 519.19
    syphilitic 095.8
  cardia (stomach) 537.89
    congenital 750.7
  cardiovascular *(see also* Disease,
    cardiovascular) 429.2
  carotid artery - *see* Narrowing, artery,
    carotid
  cervix, cervical (canal) 622.4
    congenital 752.49
    in pregnancy or childbirth 654.6●
      affecting fetus or newborn
        763.89
      causing obstructed labor 660.2●
        affecting fetus or newborn
        763.1
  colon *(see also* Obstruction, intestine)
    560.9
    congenital 751.2
  colostomy 569.62
  common bile duct *(see also* Obstruction,
    biliary) 576.2
    congenital 751.61
  coronary (artery) - *see* Arteriosclerosis,
    coronary

Stenosis *(Continued)*
  cystic duct (*see also* Obstruction,
    gallbladder) 575.2
    congenital 751.61
  due to (presence of) any device, implant,
    or graft classifiable to 996.0–996.5 -
    see Complications, due to
    (presence of) any device, implant,
    or graft classified to 996.0–996.5
    NEC
  duodenum 537.3
    congenital 751.1
  ejaculatory duct NEC 608.89
  endocervical os - *see* Stenosis, cervix
  enterostomy 569.62
  esophagostomy 530.87
  esophagus 530.3
    congenital 750.3
    syphilitic 095.8
      congenital 090.5
  external ear canal 380.50
    secondary to
      inflammation 380.53
      surgery 380.52
      trauma 380.51
  gallbladder (*see also* Obstruction,
    gallbladder) 575.2
  glottis 478.74
  heart valve (acquired) - *see also*
    Endocarditis
    congenital NEC 746.89
      aortic 746.3
      mitral 746.5
      pulmonary 746.02
      tricuspid 746.1
  hepatic duct (*see also* Obstruction,
    biliary) 576.2
  hymen 623.3
  hypertrophic subaortic (idiopathic)
    425.1
  infundibulum cardiac 746.83
  intestine (*see also* Obstruction, intestine)
    560.9
    congenital (small) 751.1
      large 751.2
  lacrimal
    canaliculi 375.53
    duct 375.56
      congenital 743.65
    punctum 375.52
      congenital 743.65
    sac 375.54
      congenital 743.65
  lacrimonasal duct 375.56
    congenital 743.65
    neonatal 375.55
  larynx 478.74
    congenital 748.3
    syphilitic 095.8
      congenital 090.5
  mitral (valve) (chronic) (inactive) 394.0
    with
      aortic (valve)
        disease (insufficiency) 396.1
        insufficiency or incompetence
          396.1
        stenosis or obstruction 396.0
      incompetency, insufficiency or
        regurgitation 394.2
        with aortic valve disease
          396.8
    active or acute 391.1
      with chorea (acute) (rheumatic)
        (Sydenham's) 392.0

Stenosis *(Continued)*
  mitral *(Continued)*
    congenital 746.5
    specified cause, except rheumatic
      424.0
    syphilitic 093.21
  myocardium, myocardial (*see also*
    Degeneration, myocardial) 429.1
    hypertrophic subaortic (idiopathic)
      425.1
  nares (anterior) (posterior) 478.19
    congenital 748.0
  nasal duct 375.56
    congenital 743.65
  nasolacrimal duct 375.56
    congenital 743.65
    neonatal 375.55
  organ or site, congenital NEC - *see*
    Atresia
  papilla of Vater 576.2
    with calculus, cholelithiasis, or
      stones - *see* Choledocholithiasis
  pulmonary (artery) (congenital) 747.3
    with ventricular septal defect,
      dextraposition of aorta and
      hypertrophy of right ventricle
      745.2
    acquired 417.8
    infundibular 746.83
    in tetralogy of Fallot 745.2
    subvalvular 746.83
    valve (*see also* Endocarditis,
      pulmonary) 424.3
      congenital 746.02
    vein 747.49
      acquired 417.8
    vessel NEC 417.8
  pulmonic (congenital) 746.02
    infundibular 746.83
    subvalvular 746.83
  pylorus (hypertrophic) 537.0
    adult 537.0
    congenital 750.5
    infantile 750.5
  rectum (sphincter) (*see also* Stricture,
    rectum) 569.2
  renal artery 440.1
  salivary duct (any) 527.8
  sphincter of Oddi (*see also* Obstruction,
    biliary) 576.2
  spinal 724.00
    cervical 723.0
    lumbar, lumbosacral (without
      neurogenic claudication)
      724.02 ◄▥
    with neurogenic claudication
      724.03 ◄
    nerve (root) NEC 724.9
    specified region NEC 724.09
    thoracic, thoracolumbar 724.01
  stomach, hourglass 537.6
  subaortic 746.81
    hypertrophic (idiopathic) 425.1
  supra (valvular)-aortic 747.22
  trachea 519.19
    congenital 748.3
    syphilitic 095.8
    tuberculous (*see also* Tuberculosis)
      012.8 ●
  tracheostomy 519.02
  tricuspid (valve) (*see also* Endocarditis,
    tricuspid) 397.0
    congenital 746.1
    nonrheumatic 424.2

Stenosis *(Continued)*
  tubal 628.2
  ureter (*see also* Stricture, ureter) 593.3
    congenital 753.29
  urethra (*see also* Stricture, urethra) 598.9
  vagina 623.2
    congenital 752.49
    in pregnancy or childbirth 654.7●
      affecting fetus or newborn
        763.89
      causing obstructed labor 660.2●
        affecting fetus or newborn 763.1
  valve (cardiac) (heart) (*see also*
    Endocarditis) 424.90
    congenital NEC 746.89
      aortic 746.3
      mitral 746.5
      pulmonary 746.02
      tricuspid 746.1
      urethra 753.6
  valvular (*see also* Endocarditis) 424.90
    congenital NEC 746.89
      urethra 753.6
  vascular graft or shunt 996.1
    atherosclerosis - *see* Arteriosclerosis,
      extremities
    embolism 996.74
    occlusion NEC 996.74
    thrombus 996.74
  vena cava (inferior) (superior) 459.2
    congenital 747.49
  ventricular shunt 996.2
  vulva 624.8
Stercolith (*see also* Fecalith) 560.32 ◄▥
  appendix 543.9
Stercoraceous, stercoral ulcer 569.82
  anus or rectum 569.41
Stereopsis, defective
  with fusion 368.33
  without fusion 368.32
Stereotypies NEC 307.3
Sterility
  female - *see* Infertility, female
  male (*see also* Infertility, male) 606.9
Sterilization, admission for V25.2
  status
    tubal ligation V26.51
    vasectomy V26.52
Sternalgia (*see also* Angina) 413.9
Sternopagus 759.4
Sternum bifidum 756.3
Sternutation 784.99
Steroid
  effects (adverse) (iatrogenic)
    cushingoid
      correct substance properly
        administered 255.0
      overdose or wrong substance
        given or taken 962.0
    diabetes - *see* Diabetes, secondary
      correct substance properly
        administered 251.8
      overdose or wrong substance
        given or taken 962.0
    due to
      correct substance properly
        administered 255.8
      overdose or wrong substance
        given or taken 962.0
    fever
      correct substance properly
        administered 780.60
      overdose or wrong substance
        given or taken 962.0

Steroid (*Continued*)
  effects (*Continued*)
    withdrawal
      correct substance properly
        administered 255.41
      overdose or wrong substance
        given or taken 962.0
  responder 365.03
Stevens-Johnson disease or syndrome
    (erythema multiforme exudativum)
    695.13
  toxic epidermal necrolysis overlap
    (SJS-TEN overlap syndrome)
    695.14
Stewart-Morel syndrome (hyperostosis
    frontalis interna) 733.3
Sticker's disease (erythema infectiosum)
    057.0
Stickler syndrome 759.89
Sticky eye 372.03
Stieda's disease (calcification, knee joint)
    726.62
Stiff
  back 724.8
  neck (*see also* Torticollis) 723.5
Stiff-baby 759.89
Stiff-man syndrome 333.91
Stiffness, joint NEC 719.50
  ankle 719.57
  back 724.8
  elbow 719.52
  finger 719.54
  hip 719.55
  knee 719.56
  multiple sites 719.59
  sacroiliac 724.6
  shoulder 719.51
  specified site NEC 719.58
  spine 724.9
  surgical fusion V45.4
  wrist 719.53
Stigmata, congenital syphilis 090.5
Still's disease or syndrome 714.30
  adult onset 714.2
Still-Felty syndrome (rheumatoid
    arthritis with splenomegaly and
    leukopenia) 714.1
Stillbirth, stillborn NEC 779.9
Stiller's disease (asthenia) 780.79
Stilling-Türk-Duane syndrome (ocular
    retraction syndrome) 378.71
Stimulation, ovary 256.1
Sting (animal) (bee) (fish) (insect)
    (jellyfish) (Portuguese man-o-war)
    (wasp) (venomous) 989.5
  anaphylactic shock or reaction
    989.5
  plant 692.6
Stippled epiphyses 756.59
Stitch
  abscess 998.59
  burst (in external operation
    wound) (*see also* Dehiscence)
    998.32
    internal 998.31
  in back 724.5
Stojano's (subcostal) syndrome 098.86
Stokes' disease (exophthalmic goiter)
    242.0●
Stokes-Adams syndrome (syncope with
    heart block) 426.9
Stokvis' (-Talma) disease (enterogenous
    cyanosis) 289.7
Stomach - *see* condition

Stoma malfunction
  colostomy 569.62
  cystostomy 997.5
  enterostomy 569.62
  esophagostomy 530.87
  gastrostomy 536.42
  ileostomy 569.62
  nephrostomy 997.5
  tracheostomy 519.02
  ureterostomy 997.5
Stomatitis 528.00
  angular 528.5
    due to dietary or vitamin deficiency
      266.0
  aphthous 528.2
  bovine 059.11
  candidal 112.0
  catarrhal 528.00
  denture 528.9
  diphtheritic (membranous) 032.0
  due to
    dietary deficiency 266.0
    thrush 112.0
    vitamin deficiency 266.0
  epidemic 078.4
  epizootic 078.4
  follicular 528.00
  gangrenous 528.1
  herpetic 054.2
  herpetiformis 528.2
  malignant 528.00
  membranous acute 528.00
  monilial 112.0
  mycotic 112.0
  necrotic 528.1
    ulcerative 101
  necrotizing ulcerative 101
  parasitic 112.0
  septic 528.00
  specified NEC 528.09
  spirochetal 101
  suppurative (acute) 528.00
  ulcerative 528.00
    necrotizing 101
  ulceromembranous 101
  vesicular 528.00
    with exanthem 074.3
  Vincent's 101
Stomatocytosis 282.8
Stomatomycosis 112.0
Stomatorrhagia 528.9
Stone(s) - *see also* Calculus
  bladder 594.1
    diverticulum 594.0
  cystine 270.0
  heart syndrome (*see also* Failure,
    ventricular, left) 428.1
  kidney 592.0
  prostate 602.0
  pulp (dental) 522.2
  renal 592.0
  salivary duct or gland (any) 527.5
  ureter 592.1
  urethra (impacted) 594.2
  urinary (duct) (impacted) (passage)
    592.9
    bladder 594.1
      diverticulum 594.0
    lower tract NEC 594.9
    specified site 594.8
  xanthine 277.2
Stonecutters' lung 502
  tuberculous (*see also* Tuberculosis)
    011.4●

Stonemasons'
  asthma, disease, or lung 502
    tuberculous (*see also* Tuberculosis)
      011.4●
  phthisis (*see also* Tuberculosis) 011.4●
Stoppage
  bowel (*see also* Obstruction, intestine)
    560.9
  heart (*see also* Arrest, cardiac) 427.5
  intestine (*see also* Obstruction, intestine)
    560.9
  urine NEC (*see also* Retention, urine)
    788.20
Storm, thyroid (apathetic) (*see also*
    Thyrotoxicosis) 242.9●
Strabismus (alternating) (congenital)
    (nonparalytic) 378.9
  concomitant (*see also* Heterotropia)
    378.30
    convergent (*see also* Esotropia)
      378.00
    divergent (*see also* Exotropia)
      378.10
  convergent (*see also* Esotropia) 378.00
  divergent (*see also* Exotropia) 378.10
  due to adhesions, scars - *see*
    Strabismus, mechanical
  in neuromuscular disorder NEC
    378.73
    intermittent 378.20
      vertical 378.31
  latent 378.40
    convergent (esophoria) 378.41
    divergent (exophoria) 378.42
    vertical 378.43
  mechanical 378.60
    due to
      Brown's tendon sheath syndrome
        378.61
      specified musculofascial disorder
        NEC 378.62
  paralytic 378.50
    third or oculomotor nerve (partial)
      378.51
      total 378.52
    fourth or trochlear nerve 378.53
    sixth or abducens nerve 378.54
  specified type NEC 378.73
  vertical (hypertropia) 378.31
Strain - *see also* Sprain, by site
  eye NEC 368.13
  heart - *see* Disease, heart
  meaning gonorrhea - *see* Gonorrhea
  on urination 788.65
  physical NEC V62.89
  postural 729.90
  psychological NEC V62.89
Strands
  conjunctiva 372.62
  vitreous humor 379.25
Strangulation, strangulated 994.7
  appendix 543.9
  asphyxiation or suffocation by 994.7
  bladder neck 596.0
  bowel - *see* Strangulation, intestine
  colon - *see* Strangulation, intestine
  cord (umbilical) - *see* Compression,
    umbilical cord
  due to birth injury 767.8
  food or foreign body (*see also* Asphyxia,
    food) 933.1
  hemorrhoids 455.8
    external 455.5
    internal 455.2

Strangulation, strangulated *(Continued)*
  hernia - *see also* Hernia, by site, with
      obstruction
    gangrenous - *see* Hernia, by site,
        with gangrene
    intestine (large) (small) 560.2
      with hernia - *see also* Hernia, by site,
          with obstruction
        gangrenous - *see* Hernia, by site,
            with gangrene
      congenital (small) 751.1
        large 751.2
    mesentery 560.2
    mucus (*see also* Asphyxia, mucus)
        933.1
      newborn 770.18
    omentum 560.2
    organ or site, congenital NEC - *see*
        Atresia
    ovary 620.8
      due to hernia 620.4
    penis 607.89
      foreign body 939.3
    rupture (*see also* Hernia, by site, with
        obstruction) 552.9
      gangrenous (*see also* Hernia, by site,
          with gangrene) 551.9
    stomach, due to hernia (*see also*
        Hernia, by site, with obstruction)
        552.9
      with gangrene (*see also* Hernia, by
          site, with gangrene) 551.9
    umbilical cord - *see* Compression,
        umbilical cord
    vesicourethral orifice 596.0
Strangury 788.1
Strawberry
  gallbladder (*see also* Disease,
      gallbladder) 575.6
  mark 757.32
  tongue (red) (white) 529.3
Straw itch 133.8
Streak, ovarian 752.0
Strephosymbolia 315.01
  secondary to organic lesion 784.69
Streptobacillary fever 026.1
Streptobacillus moniliformis 026.1
Streptococcemia 038.0
Streptococcicosis - *see* Infection,
    streptococcal
Streptococcus, streptococcal - *see*
    condition
Streptoderma 686.00
Streptomycosis - *see* Actinomycosis
Streptothricosis - *see* Actinomycosis
Streptothrix - *see* Actinomycosis
Streptotrichosis - *see* Actinomycosis
Stress 308.9
  fracture - *see* Fracture, stress
  polycythemia 289.0
  reaction (gross) (*see also* Reaction,
      stress, acute) 308.9
Stretching, nerve - *see* Injury, nerve, by
    site
Striae (albicantes) (atrophicae) (cutis
    distensae) (distensae) 701.3
Striations of nails 703.8
Stricture (*see also* Stenosis) 799.89
  ampulla of Vater 576.2
    with calculus, cholelithiasis, or
        stones - *see* Choledocholithiasis
  anus (sphincter) 569.2
    congenital 751.2
    infantile 751.2

Stricture *(Continued)*
  aorta (ascending) 747.22
    arch 747.10
    arteriosclerotic 440.0
    calcified 440.0
  aortic (valve) (*see also* Stenosis, aortic)
      424.1
    congenital 746.3
  aqueduct of Sylvius (congenital)
      742.3
    with spina bifida (*see also* Spina
        bifida) 741.0●
    acquired 331.4
  artery 447.1
    basilar - *see* Narrowing, artery,
        basilar
    carotid (common) (internal) - *see*
        Narrowing, artery, carotid
    celiac 447.4
    cerebral 437.0
      congenital 747.81
      due to
        embolism (*see also* Embolism,
            brain) 434.1●
        thrombus (*see also* Thrombosis,
            brain) 434.0●
    congenital (peripheral) 747.60
      cerebral 747.81
      coronary 746.85
      gastrointestinal 747.61
      lower limb 747.64
      renal 747.62
      retinal 743.58
      specified NEC 747.69
      spinal 747.82
      umbilical 747.5
      upper limb 747.63
    coronary - *see* Arteriosclerosis,
        coronary
      congenital 746.85
    precerebral - *see* Narrowing, artery,
        precerebral NEC
    pulmonary (congenital) 747.3
      acquired 417.8
    renal 440.1
    vertebral - *see* Narrowing, artery,
        vertebral
  auditory canal (congenital) (external)
      744.02
    acquired (*see also* Stricture, ear canal,
        acquired) 380.50
  bile duct or passage (any)
      (postoperative) (*see also*
      Obstruction, biliary) 576.2
    congenital 751.61
  bladder 596.8
    congenital 753.6
    neck 596.0
      congenital 753.6
  bowel (*see also* Obstruction, intestine)
      560.9
  brain 348.89
  bronchus 519.19
    syphilitic 095.8
  cardia (stomach) 537.89
    congenital 750.7
  cardiac - *see also* Disease, heart orifice
      (stomach) 537.89
  cardiovascular (*see also* Disease,
      cardiovascular) 429.2
  carotid artery - *see* Narrowing, artery,
      carotid
  cecum (*see also* Obstruction, intestine)
      560.9

Stricture *(Continued)*
  cervix, cervical (canal) 622.4
    congenital 752.49
    in pregnancy or childbirth
        654.6●
      affecting fetus or newborn
          763.89
      causing obstructed labor
          660.2●
        affecting fetus or newborn
            763.1
  colon (*see also* Obstruction, intestine)
      560.9
    congenital 751.2
  colostomy 569.62
  common bile duct (*see also* Obstruction,
      biliary) 576.2
    congenital 751.61
  coronary (artery) - *see* Arteriosclerosis,
      coronary
    congenital 746.85
  cystic duct (*see also* Obstruction,
      gallbladder) 575.2
    congenital 751.61
  cystostomy 997.5
  digestive organs NEC, congenital
      751.8
  duodenum 537.3
    congenital 751.1
  ear canal (external) (congenital)
      744.02
    acquired 380.50
      secondary to
        inflammation 380.53
        surgery 380.52
        trauma 380.51
  ejaculatory duct 608.85
  enterostomy 569.62
  esophagostomy 530.87
  esophagus (corrosive) (peptic)
      530.3
    congenital 750.3
    syphilitic 095.8
      congenital 090.5
  Eustachian tube (*see also* Obstruction,
      Eustachian tube) 381.60
    congenital 744.24
  fallopian tube 628.2
    gonococcal (chronic) 098.37
      acute 098.17
    tuberculous (*see also* Tuberculosis)
        016.6●
  gallbladder (*see also* Obstruction,
      gallbladder) 575.2
    congenital 751.69
  glottis 478.74
  heart - *see also* Disease, heart
    congenital NEC 746.89
    valve - *see also* Endocarditis
      congenital NEC 746.89
        aortic 746.3
        mitral 746.5
        pulmonary 746.02
        tricuspid 746.1
  hepatic duct (*see also* Obstruction,
      biliary) 576.2
  hourglass, of stomach 537.6
  hymen 623.3
  hypopharynx 478.29
  intestine (*see also* Obstruction, intestine)
      560.9
    congenital (small) 751.1
      large 751.2
    ischemic 557.1

Stricture *(Continued)*
  lacrimal
    canaliculi 375.53
      congenital 743.65
    punctum 375.52
      congenital 743.65
    sac 375.54
      congenital 743.65
  lacrimonasal duct 375.56
    congenital 743.65
    neonatal 375.55
  larynx 478.79
    congenital 748.3
    syphilitic 095.8
      congenital 090.5
  lung 518.89
  meatus
    ear (congenital) 744.02
      acquired *(see also* Stricture, ear
        canal, acquired) 380.50
      osseous (congenital) (ear) 744.03
        acquired *(see also* Stricture, ear
          canal, acquired) 380.50
    urinarius *(see also* Stricture, urethra)
      598.9
      congenital 753.6
  mitral (valve) *(see also* Stenosis, mitral)
    394.0
    congenital 746.5
    specified cause, except rheumatic
      424.0
  myocardium, myocardial *(see also*
    Degeneration, myocardial)
    429.1
    hypertrophic subaortic (idiopathic)
      425.1
  nares (anterior) (posterior) 478.19
    congenital 748.0
  nasal duct 375.56
    congenital 743.65
    neonatal 375.55
  nasolacrimal duct 375.56
    congenital 743.65
    neonatal 375.55
  nasopharynx 478.29
    syphilitic 095.8
  nephrostomy 997.5
  nose 478.19
    congenital 748.0
  nostril (anterior) (posterior) 478.19
    congenital 748.0
  organ or site, congenital NEC - *see*
    Atresia
  osseous meatus (congenital) (ear)
    744.03
    acquired *(see also* Stricture, ear canal,
      acquired) 380.50
  os uteri *(see also* Stricture, cervix)
    622.4
  oviduct - *see* Stricture, fallopian tube
  pelviureteric junction 593.3
  pharynx (dilation) 478.29
  prostate 602.8
  pulmonary, pulmonic
    artery (congenital) 747.3
      acquired 417.8
      noncongenital 417.8
    infundibulum (congenital) 746.83
    valve *(see also* Endocarditis,
      pulmonary) 424.3
      congenital 746.02
    vein (congenital) 747.49
      acquired 417.8
    vessel NEC 417.8

Stricture *(Continued)*
  punctum lacrimale 375.52
    congenital 743.65
  pylorus (hypertrophic) 537.0
    adult 537.0
    congenital 750.5
    infantile 750.5
  rectosigmoid 569.89
  rectum (sphincter) 569.2
    congenital 751.2
    due to
      chemical burn 947.3
      irradiation 569.2
      lymphogranuloma venereum
        099.1
    gonococcal 098.7
    inflammatory 099.1
    syphilitic 095.8
    tuberculous *(see also* Tuberculosis)
      014.8●
  renal artery 440.1
  salivary duct or gland (any) 527.8
  sigmoid (flexure) *(see also* Obstruction,
    intestine) 560.9
  spermatic cord 608.85
  stoma (following) (of)
    colostomy 569.62
    cystostomy 997.5
    enterostomy 569.62
    esophagostomy 530.87
    gastrostomy 536.42
    ileostomy 569.62
    nephrostomy 997.5
    tracheostomy 519.02
    ureterostomy 997.5
  stomach 537.89
    congenital 750.7
    hourglass 537.6
  subaortic 746.81
    hypertrophic (acquired) (idiopathic)
      425.1
  subglottic 478.74
  syphilitic NEC 095.8
  tendon (sheath) 727.81
  trachea 519.19
    congenital 748.3
    syphilitic 095.8
    tuberculous *(see also* Tuberculosis)
      012.8●
  tracheostomy 519.02
  tricuspid (valve) *(see also* Endocarditis,
    tricuspid) 397.0
    congenital 746.1
    nonrheumatic 424.2
  tunica vaginalis 608.85
  ureter (postoperative) 593.3
    congenital 753.29
    tuberculous *(see also* Tuberculosis)
      016.2●
  ureteropelvic junction 593.3
    congenital 753.21
  ureterovesical orifice 593.3
    congenital 753.22
  urethra (anterior) (meatal) (organic)
    (posterior) (spasmodic) 598.9
    associated with schistosomiasis *(see
      also* Schistosomiasis) 120.9
      [598.01]
    congenital (valvular) 753.6
    due to
      infection 598.00
        syphilis 095.8 *[598.01]*
      trauma 598.1
    gonococcal 098.2 *[598.01]*

Stricture *(Continued)*
  urethra *(Continued)*
    gonorrheal 098.2 *[598.01]*
    infective 598.00
    late effect of injury 598.1
    postcatheterization 598.2
    postobstetric 598.1
    postoperative 598.2
    specified cause NEC 598.8
    syphilitic 095.8 *[598.01]*
    traumatic 598.1
    valvular, congenital 753.6
  urinary meatus *(see also* Stricture,
    urethra) 598.9
    congenital 753.6
  uterus, uterine 621.5
    os (external) (internal) - *see* Stricture,
      cervix
  vagina (outlet) 623.2
    congenital 752.49
  valve (cardiac) (heart) *(see also*
    Endocarditis) 424.90
    congenital (cardiac) (heart) NEC
      746.89
      aortic 746.3
      mitral 746.5
      pulmonary 746.02
      tricuspid 746.1
      urethra 753.6
  valvular *(see also* Endocarditis)
    424.90
  vascular graft or shunt 996.1
    atherosclerosis - *see* Arteriosclerosis,
      extremities
    embolism 996.74
    occlusion NEC 996.74
    thrombus 996.74
  vas deferens 608.85
    congenital 752.89
  vein 459.2
  vena cava (inferior) (superior) NEC
    459.2
    congenital 747.49
  ventricular shunt 996.2
  vesicourethral orifice 596.0
    congenital 753.6
  vulva (acquired) 624.8
Stridor 786.1
  congenital (larynx) 748.3
Stridulous - *see* condition
Strippling of nails 703.8
Stroke 434.91
  apoplectic *(see also* Disease,
    cerebrovascular, acute) 436
  brain - *see* Infarct, brain
  embolic 434.11
  epileptic - *see* Epilepsy
  healed or old V12.54
  heart - *see* Disease, heart
  heat 992.0
  hemorrhagic - *see* Hemorrhage, brain
  iatrogenic 997.02
  in evolution 434.91
  ischemic 434.91
  late effect - *see* Late effect(s) (of)
    cerebrovascular disease
  lightning 994.0
  paralytic - *see* Infarct, brain
  postoperative 997.02
  progressive 435.9
  thrombotic 434.01
Stromatosis, endometrial (M8931/1)
  236.0
Strong pulse 785.9

◀ New   ◀||| Revised   ~~deleted~~ Deleted   ● Use Additional Digit(s)   ▨ Omit code

Strongyloides stercoralis infestation 127.2
Strongyloidiasis 127.2
Strongyloidosis 127.2
Strongylus (gibsoni) infestation 127.7
Strophulus (newborn) 779.89
    pruriginosus 698.2
Struck by lighting 994.0
Struma (see also Goiter) 240.9
    fibrosa 245.3
    Hashimoto (struma lymphomatosa)
        245.2
    lymphomatosa 245.2
    nodosa (simplex) 241.9
        endemic 241.9
        multinodular 241.1
        sporadic 241.9
        toxic or with hyperthyroidism
            242.3●
            multinodular 242.2●
            uninodular 242.1●
        toxicosa 242.3●
            multinodular 242.2●
            uninodular 242.1●
        uninodular 241.0
    ovarii (M9090/0) 220
        and carcinoid (M9091/1) 236.2
        malignant (M9090/3) 183.0
    Riedel's (ligneous thyroiditis) 245.3
    scrofulous (see also Tuberculosis) 017.2●
    tuberculous (see also Tuberculosis)
        017.2●
        abscess 017.2●
        adenitis 017.2●
        lymphangitis 017.2●
        ulcer 017.2●
Strumipriva cachexia (see also
    Hypothyroidism) 244.9
Strümpell-Marie disease or spine
    (ankylosing spondylitis) 720.0
Strümpell-Westphal pseudosclerosis
    (hepatolenticular degeneration) 275.1
Stuart's disease (congenital factor X
    deficiency) (see also Defect,
    coagulation) 286.3
Stuart-Prower factor deficiency
    (congenital factor X deficiency) (see
    also Defect, coagulation) 286.3
Students' elbow 727.2
Stuffy nose 478.19
Stump - see also Amputation
    cervix, cervical (healed) 622.8
Stupor 780.09
    catatonic (see also Schizophrenia)
        295.2●
    circular (see also Psychosis, manic-
        depressive, circular) 296.7
    manic 296.89
    manic-depressive (see also Psychosis,
        affective) 296.89
    mental (anergic) (delusional) 298.9
    psychogenic 298.8
    reaction to exceptional stress (transient)
        308.2
    traumatic NEC - see also Injury,
        intracranial
        with spinal (cord)
            lesion - see Injury, spinal, by site
            shock - see Injury, spinal, by site
Sturge (-Weber) (-Dimitri) disease or
    syndrome (encephalocutaneous
    angiomatosis) 759.6
Sturge-Kalischer-Weber syndrome
    (encephalocutaneous angiomatosis)
    759.6

Stuttering 315.35 ◀▥
    adult onset 307.0 ◀
    childhood onset 315.35 ◀
    due to late effect of cerebrovascular
        disease (see also Late effect(s) (of)
        cerebrovascular disease) 438.14
    in conditions classified elsewhere
        784.52 ◀
Sty, stye 373.11
    external 373.11
    internal 373.12
    meibomian 373.12
Subacidity, gastric 536.8
    psychogenic 306.4
Subacute - see condition
Subarachnoid - see condition
Subclavian steal syndrome 435.2
Subcortical - see condition
Subcostal syndrome 098.86
    nerve compression 354.8
Subcutaneous, subcuticular - see condition
Subdelirium 293.1
Subdural - see condition
Subendocardium - see condition
Subependymoma (M9383/1) 237.5
Suberosis 495.3
Subglossitis - see Glossitis
Subhemophilia 286.0
Subinvolution (uterus) 621.1
    breast (postlactational) (postpartum)
        611.89
    chronic 621.1
    puerperal, postpartum 674.8●
Sublingual - see condition
Sublinguitis 527.2
Subluxation - see also Dislocation, by site
    congenital NEC - see also Malposition,
        congenital
        hip (unilateral) 754.32
            with dislocation of other hip
                754.35
            bilateral 754.33
        joint
            lower limb 755.69
            shoulder 755.59
            upper limb 755.59
        lower limb (joint) 755.69
        shoulder (joint) 755.59
        upper limb (joint) 755.59
    lens 379.32
        anterior 379.33
        posterior 379.34
    radial head 832.2
    rotary, cervical region of spine - see
        Fracture, vertebra, cervical
Submaxillary - see condition
Submersion (fatal) (nonfatal) 994.1
Submissiveness (undue), in child 313.0
Submucous - see condition
Subnormal, subnormality
    accommodation (see also Disorder,
        accommodation) 367.9
    mental (see also Retardation, mental) 319
        mild 317
        moderate 318.0
        profound 318.2
        severe 318.1
    temperature (accidental) 991.6
        not associated with low
            environmental temperature
            780.99
Subphrenic - see condition
Subscapular nerve - see condition
Subseptus uterus 752.35 ◀▥

Subsiding appendicitis 542
Substance abuse in family V61.42
Substernal thyroid (see also Goiter) 240.9
    congenital 759.2
Substitution disorder 300.11
Subtentorial - see condition
Subtertian
    fever 084.0
    malaria (fever) 084.0
Subthyroidism (acquired) (see also
    Hypothyroidism) 244.9
    congenital 243
Succenturiata placenta - see Placenta,
    abnormal
Succussion sounds, chest 786.7
Sucking thumb, child 307.9
Sudamen 705.1
Sudamina 705.1
Sudanese kala-azar 085.0
Sudden
    death, cause unknown (less than 24
        hours) 798.1
        cardiac (SCD)
            family history of V17.41
            personal history of, successfully
                resuscitated V12.53
        during childbirth 669.9●
        infant 798.0
        puerperal, postpartum 674.9●
    hearing loss NEC 388.2
    heart failure (see also Failure, heart)
        428.9
    infant death syndrome 798.0
Sudeck's atrophy, disease, or syndrome
    733.7
SUDS (Sudden unexplained death) 798.2
Suffocation (see also Asphyxia) 799.01
    by
        bed clothes 994.7
        bunny bag 994.7
        cave-in 994.7
        constriction 994.7
        drowning 994.1
        inhalation
            food or foreign body (see also
                Asphyxia, food or foreign
                body) 933.1
            oil or gasoline (see also Asphyxia,
                food or foreign body) 933.1
        overlying 994.7
        plastic bag 994.7
        pressure 994.7
        strangulation 994.7
    during birth 768.1
    mechanical 994.7
Sugar
    blood
        high 790.29
        low 251.2
    in urine 791.5
Suicide, suicidal (attempted)
    by poisoning - see Table of Drugs and
        Chemicals
    ideation V62.84
    risk 300.9
    tendencies 300.9
    trauma NEC (see also nature and site of
        injury) 959.9
Suipestifer infection (see also Infection,
    Salmonella) 003.9
Sulfatidosis 330.0
Sulfhemoglobinemia,
    sulphemoglobinemia (acquired)
    (congenital) 289.7

S

Sumatran mite fever 081.2
Summer - *see* condition
Sunburn 692.71
   dermatitis 692.71
   due to
      other ultraviolet radiation
         692.82
      tanning bed 692.82
   first degree 692.71
   second degree 692.76
   third degree 692.77
SUNCT (short lasting unilateral
   neuralgiform headache with
   conjunctival injection and tearing)
   339.05
Sunken
   acetabulum 718.85
   fontanels 756.0
Sunstroke 992.0
Superfecundation 651.9●
   with fetal loss and retention of one or
      more fetus(es) 651.6●
   following (elective) fetal reduction
      651.7●
Superfetation 651.9●
   with fetal loss and retention of one or
      more fetus(es) 651.6●
   following (elective) fetal reduction
      651.7●
Superinvolution uterus 621.8
Supernumerary (congenital)
   aortic cusps 746.89
   auditory ossicles 744.04
   bone 756.9
   breast 757.6
   carpal bones 755.56
   cusps, heart valve NEC 746.89
      mitral 746.5
      pulmonary 746.09
   digit(s) 755.00
      finger 755.01
      toe 755.02
   ear (lobule) 744.1
   fallopian tube 752.19
   finger 755.01
   hymen 752.49
   kidney 753.3
   lacrimal glands 743.64
   lacrimonasal duct 743.65
   lobule (ear) 744.1
   mitral cusps 746.5
   muscle 756.82
   nipples 757.6
   organ or site NEC - *see* Accessory
   ossicles, auditory 744.04
   ovary 752.0
   oviduct 752.19
   pulmonic cusps 746.09
   rib 756.3
      cervical or first 756.2
         syndrome 756.2
   roots (of teeth) 520.2
   spinal vertebra 756.19
   spleen 759.0
   tarsal bones 755.67
   teeth 520.1
      causing crowding 524.31
   testis 752.89
   thumb 755.01
   toe 755.02
   uterus 752.2
   vagina 752.49
   vertebra 756.19

Supervision (of)
   contraceptive method previously
      prescribed V25.40
      intrauterine device V25.42
      oral contraceptive (pill) V25.41
      specified type NEC V25.49
      subdermal implantable
         contraceptive V25.43
   dietary (for) V65.3
      allergy (food) V65.3
      colitis V65.3
      diabetes mellitus V65.3
      food allergy intolerance V65.3
      gastritis V65.3
      hypercholesterolemia V65.3
      hypoglycemia V65.3
      intolerance (food) V65.3
      obesity V65.3
      specified NEC V65.3
   lactation V24.1
   newborn health
      8 to 28 days old V20.32
      under 8 days old V20.31
   pregnancy - *see* Pregnancy,
      supervision of
Supplemental teeth 520.1
   causing crowding 524.31
Suppression
   binocular vision 368.31
   lactation 676.5●
   menstruation 626.8
   ovarian secretion 256.39
   renal 586
   urinary secretion 788.5
   urine 788.5
Suppuration, suppurative - *see also*
      condition
   accessory sinus (chronic) (*see also*
      Sinusitis) 473.9
   adrenal gland 255.8
   antrum (chronic) (*see also* Sinusitis,
      maxillary) 473.0
   bladder (*see also* Cystitis) 595.89
   bowel 569.89
   brain 324.0
      late effect 326
   breast 611.0
      puerperal, postpartum 675.1●
   dental periosteum 526.5
   diffuse (skin) 686.00
   ear (middle) (*see also* Otitis media)
      382.4
      external (*see also* Otitis, externa)
         380.10
      internal 386.33
   ethmoidal (sinus) (chronic) (*see also*
      Sinusitis, ethmoidal) 473.2
   fallopian tube (*see also* Salpingo-
      oophoritis) 614.2
   frontal (sinus) (chronic) (*see also*
      Sinusitis, frontal) 473.1
   gallbladder (*see also* Cholecystitis,
      acute) 575.0
   gum 523.30
   hernial sac - *see* Hernia, by site
   intestine 569.89
   joint (*see also* Arthritis, suppurative)
      711.0●
   labyrinthine 386.33
   lung 513.0
   mammary gland 611.0
      puerperal, postpartum 675.1●
   maxilla, maxillary 526.4
      sinus (chronic) (*see also* Sinusitis,
         maxillary) 473.0
   muscle 728.0

Suppuration, suppurative (*Continued*)
   nasal sinus (chronic) (*see also* Sinusitis)
      473.9
   pancreas 577.0
   parotid gland 527.2
   pelvis, pelvic
      female (*see also* Disease, pelvis,
         inflammatory) 614.4
         acute 614.3
      male (*see also* Peritonitis) 567.21
   pericranial (*see also* Osteomyelitis)
      730.2●
   salivary duct or gland (any) 527.2
   sinus (nasal) (*see also* Sinusitis) 473.9
   sphenoidal (sinus) (chronic) (*see also*
      Sinusitis, sphenoidal) 473.3
   thymus (gland) 254.1
   thyroid (gland) 245.0
   tonsil 474.8
   uterus (*see also* Endometritis) 615.9
   vagina 616.10
   wound - *see also* Wound, open, by site,
      complicated
      dislocation - *see* Dislocation, by site,
         compound
      fracture - *see* Fracture, by site, open
      scratch or other superficial injury -
         see Injury, superficial, by site
Supraeruption, teeth 524.34
Supraglottitis 464.50
   with obstruction 464.51
Suprapubic drainage 596.8
Suprarenal (gland) - *see* condition
Suprascapular nerve - *see* condition
Suprasellar - *see* condition
Supraspinatus syndrome 726.10
Surfer knots 919.8
   infected 919.9
Surgery
   cosmetic NEC V50.1
      breast reconstruction following
         mastectomy V51.0
      following healed injury or operation
         V51.8
      hair transplant V50.0
   elective V50.9
      breast
         augmentation or reduction
            V50.1
         reconstruction following
            mastectomy V51.0
      circumcision, ritual or routine (in
         absence of medical indication)
         V50.2
      cosmetic NEC V50.1
      ear piercing V50.3
      face-lift V50.1
      following healed injury or operation
         V51.8
      hair transplant V50.0
   not done because of
      contraindication V64.1
      patient's decision V64.2
      specified reason NEC V64.3
   plastic
      breast
         augmentation or reduction
            V50.1
         reconstruction following
            mastectomy V51.0
      cosmetic V50.1
      face-lift V50.1
      following healed injury or operation
         V51.8

◀ New   ◀ Revised   ~~deleted~~ Deleted   ● Use Additional Digit(s)   ▧ Omit code

Surgery *(Continued)*
    plastic *(Continued)*
        repair of scarred tissue (following healed injury or operation) V51.8
            specified type NEC V50.8
        previous, in pregnancy or childbirth
            cervix 654.6●
                affecting fetus or newborn *(see also* Newborn, affected by) 760.63
                causing obstructed labor 660.2●
                    affecting fetus or newborn 763.1
            pelvic soft tissues NEC 654.9●
                affecting fetus or newborn *(see also* Newborn, affected by) 760.63
                causing obstructed labor 660.2●
                    affecting fetus or newborn 763.1
            perineum or vulva 654.8●
            uterus NEC 654.9●
                affecting fetus or newborn *(see also* Newborn, affected by) 760.63
                causing obstructed labor 660.2●
                    affecting fetus or newborn 763.1
                from previous cesarean delivery 654.2●
            vagina 654.7●
Surgical
    abortion - *see* Abortion, legal
    emphysema 998.81
    kidney *(see also* Pyelitis) 590.80
    operation NEC 799.9
    procedures, complication or misadventure - *see* Complications, surgical procedure
    shock 998.0
Survey
    fetal anatomic V28.81
Susceptibility
    genetic
        to
            MEN (multiple endocrine neoplasia) V84.81
            neoplasia
                multiple endocrine (MEN) V84.81 ◀▥
            neoplasm
                malignant, of
                    breast V84.01
                    endometrium V84.04
                    other V84.09
                    ovary V84.02
                    prostate V84.03
                    specified disease NEC V84.89
Suspected condition, ruled out *(see also* Observation, suspected) V71.9
    specified condition NEC V71.89
Suspended uterus, in pregnancy or childbirth 654.4●
    affecting fetus or newborn 763.89
    causing obstructed labor 660.2●
        affecting fetus or newborn 763.1
Sutton's disease 709.09
Sutton and Gull's disease (arteriolar nephrosclerosis) *(see also* Hypertension, kidney) 403.90

Suture
    burst (in external operation wound) *(see also* Dehiscence) 998.32
        internal 998.31
    inadvertently left in operation wound 998.4
    removal V58.32
    Shirodkar, in pregnancy (with or without cervical incompetence) 654.5●
Swab inadvertently left in operation wound 998.4
Swallowed, swallowing
    difficulty *(see also* Dysphagia) 787.20
    foreign body NEC *(see also* Foreign body) 938
Swamp fever 100.89
Swan neck hand (intrinsic) 736.09
Sweat(s), sweating
    disease or sickness 078.2
    excessive *(see also* Hyperhidrosis) 780.8
    fetid 705.89
    fever 078.2
    gland disease 705.9
        specified type NEC 705.89
    miliary 078.2
    night 780.8
Sweeley-Klionsky disease (angiokeratoma corporis diffusum) 272.7
Sweet's syndrome (acute febrile neutrophilic dermatosis) 695.89
Swelling 782.3
    abdominal (not referable to specific organ) 789.3●
    adrenal gland, cloudy 255.8
    ankle 719.07
    anus 787.99
    arm 729.81
    breast 611.72
    Calabar 125.2
    cervical gland 785.6
    cheek 784.2
    chest 786.6
    ear 388.8
    epigastric 789.3●
    extremity (lower) (upper) 729.81
    eye 379.92
    female genital organ 625.8
    finger 729.81
    foot 729.81
    glands 785.6
    gum 784.2
    hand 729.81
    head 784.2
    inflammatory - *see* Inflammation
    joint *(see also* Effusion, joint) 719.0●
        tuberculous - *see* Tuberculosis, joint
    kidney, cloudy 593.89
    leg 729.81
    limb 729.81
    liver 573.8
    lung 786.6
    lymph nodes 785.6
    mediastinal 786.6
    mouth 784.2
    muscle (limb) 729.81
    neck 784.2
    nose or sinus 784.2
    palate 784.2
    pelvis 789.3●
    penis 607.83
    perineum 625.8

Swelling *(Continued)*
    rectum 787.99
    scrotum 608.86
    skin 782.2
    splenic *(see also* Splenomegaly) 789.2
    substernal 786.6
    superficial, localized (skin) 782.2
    testicle 608.86
    throat 784.2
    toe 729.81
    tongue 784.2
    tubular *(see also* Disease, renal) 593.9
    umbilicus 789.3●
    uterus 625.8
    vagina 625.8
    vulva 625.8
    wandering, due to Gnathostoma (spinigerum) 128.1
    white - *see* Tuberculosis, arthritis
Swift's disease 985.0
Swimmers'
    ear (acute) 380.12
    itch 120.3
Swimming in the head 780.4
Swollen - *see also* Swelling
    glands 785.6
Swyer-James syndrome (unilateral hyperlucent lung) 492.8
Swyer's syndrome (XY pure gonadal dysgenesis) 752.7
Sycosis 704.8
    barbae (not parasitic) 704.8
    contagiosa 110.0
    lupoid 704.8
    mycotic 110.0
    parasitic 110.0
    vulgaris 704.8
Sydenham's chorea - *see* Chorea, Sydenham's
Sylvatic yellow fever 060.0
Sylvest's disease (epidemic pleurodynia) 074.1
Symblepharon 372.63
    congenital 743.62
Symonds' syndrome 348.2
Sympathetic - *see* condition
Sympatheticotonia *(see also* Neuropathy, peripheral, autonomic) 337.9
Sympathicoblastoma (M9500/3)
    specified site - *see* Neoplasm, by site, malignant
    unspecified site 194.0
Sympathicogonioma (M9500/3) - *see* Sympathicoblastoma
Sympathoblastoma (M9500/3) - *see* Sympathicoblastoma
Sympathogonioma (M9500/3) - *see* Sympathicoblastoma
Symphalangy *(see also* Syndactylism) 755.10
Symptoms, specified (general) NEC 780.99
    abdomen NEC 789.9
    bone NEC 733.90
    breast NEC 611.79
    cardiac NEC 785.9
    cardiovascular NEC 785.9
    chest NEC 786.9
    cognition 799.59 ◀
    development NEC 783.9
    digestive system NEC 787.99
    emotional state NEC 799.29
    eye NEC 379.99
    gastrointestinal tract NEC 787.99
    genital organs NEC
        female 625.9
        male 608.9

Symptoms, specified (Continued)
head and neck NEC 784.99
heart NEC 785.9
jaw 784.92 ◀
joint NEC 719.60
  ankle 719.67
  elbow 719.62
  foot 719.67
  hand 719.64
  hip 719.65
  knee 719.66
  multiple sites 719.69
  pelvic region 719.65
  shoulder (region) 719.61
  specified site NEC 719.68
  temporomandibular 524.69 ◀
  wrist 719.63
larynx NEC 784.99
limbs NEC 729.89
lymphatic system NEC 785.9
maxilla 784.92 ◀
menopausal 627.2
metabolism NEC 783.9
mouth NEC 528.9
muscle NEC 728.9
musculoskeletal NEC 781.99
  limbs NEC 729.89
nervous system NEC 781.99
neurotic NEC 300.9
nutrition, metabolism, and
    development NEC 783.9
pelvis NEC 789.9
  female 625.9
peritoneum NEC 789.9
respiratory system NEC 786.9
skin and integument NEC 782.9
subcutaneous tissue NEC 782.9
throat NEC 784.99
tonsil NEC 784.99
urinary system NEC 788.99
vascular NEC 785.9
Sympus 759.89
Synarthrosis 719.80
ankle 719.87
elbow 719.82
foot 719.87
hand 719.84
hip 719.85
knee 719.86
multiple sites 719.89
pelvic region 719.85
shoulder (region) 719.81
specified site NEC 719.88
wrist 719.83
Syncephalus 759.4
Synchondrosis 756.9
abnormal (congenital) 756.9
ischiopubic (van Neck's) 732.1
Synchysis (senile) (vitreous humor) 379.21
scintillans 379.22
Syncope (near) (pre-) 780.2
anginosa 413.9
bradycardia 427.89
cardiac 780.2
carotid sinus 337.01
complicating delivery 669.2●
due to lumbar puncture 349.0
fatal 798.1
heart 780.2
heat 992.1
laryngeal 786.2
tussive 786.2
vasoconstriction 780.2
vasodepressor 780.2
vasomotor 780.2
vasovagal 780.2

Syncytial infarct - see Placenta, abnormal
Syndactylism, syndactyly (multiple sites)
755.10
  fingers (without fusion of bone) 755.11
    with fusion of bone 755.12
  toes (without fusion of bone) 755.13
    with fusion of bone 755.14
Syndrome - see also Disease
5q minus 238.74
abdominal
  acute 789.0●
  migraine 346.2●
  muscle deficiency 756.79
Abercrombie's (amyloid degeneration)
    277.39
abnormal innervation 374.43
abstinence
  alcohol 291.81
  drug 292.0
  neonatal 779.5
Abt-Letterer-Siwe (acute histiocytosis
    X) (M9722/3) 202.5●
Achard-Thiers (adrenogenital) 255.2
acid pulmonary aspiration 997.39
  obstetric (Mendelson's) 668.0●
acquired immune deficiency 042
acquired immunodeficiency 042
acrocephalosyndactylism 755.55
acute abdominal 789.0●
acute chest 517.3
acute coronary 411.1
Adair-Dighton (brittle bones and blue
    sclera, deafness) 756.51
Adams-Stokes (-Morgagni) (syncope
    with heart block) 426.9
Addisonian 255.41
Adie (-Holmes) (pupil) 379.46
adiposogenital 253.8
adrenal
  hemorrhage 036.3
  meningococcic 036.3
adrenocortical 255.3
adrenogenital (acquired) (congenital)
    255.2
  feminizing 255.2
  iatrogenic 760.79
  virilism (acquired) (congenital) 255.2
affective organic NEC 293.89
  drug-induced 292.84
afferent loop NEC 537.89
African macroglobulinemia 273.3
Ahumada-Del Castillo (nonpuerperal
    galactorrhea and amenorrhea)
    253.1
air blast concussion - see Injury,
    internal, by site
Alagille 759.89
Albright (-Martin)
    (pseudohypoparathyroidism)
    275.49
Albright-McCune-Sternberg (osteitis
    fibrosa disseminata) 756.59
alcohol withdrawal 291.81
Alder's (leukocyte granulation
    anomaly) 288.2
Aldrich (-Wiskott) (eczema-
    thrombocytopenia) 279.12
Alibert-Bazin (mycosis fungoides)
    (M9700/3) 202.1●
Alice in Wonderland 293.89
alien hand 781.8
Allen-Masters 620.6
Alligator baby (ichthyosis congenita)
    757.1

Syndrome (Continued)
Alport's (hereditary hematuria-
    nephropathy-deafness) 759.89
Alvarez (transient cerebral ischemia)
    435.9
alveolar capillary block 516.3
Alzheimer's 331.0
  with dementia - see Alzheimer's,
    dementia
amnestic (confabulatory) 294.0
  alcohol-induced persisting 291.1
  drug-induced 292.83
  posttraumatic 294.0
amotivational 292.89
amyostatic 275.1
amyotrophic lateral sclerosis 335.20
androgen insensitivity 259.51
  partial 259.52
Angelman 759.89
angina (see also Angina) 413.9
ankyloglossia superior 750.0
anterior
  chest wall 786.52
  compartment (tibial) 958.8
  spinal artery 433.8●
    compression 721.1
  tibial (compartment) 958.8
antibody deficiency 279.00
  agammaglobulinemic 279.00
  congenital 279.04
  hypogammaglobulinemic 279.00
anticardiolipin antibody 289.81
antimongolism 758.39
antiphospholipid antibody 289.81
Anton (-Babinski)
    (hemiasomatognosia) 307.9
anxiety (see also Anxiety) 300.00
  organic 293.84
aortic
  arch 446.7
  bifurcation (occlusion) 444.0
  ring 747.21
Apert's (acrocephalosyndactyly)
    755.55
Apert-Gallais (adrenogenital) 255.2
aphasia-apraxia-alexia 784.69
apical ballooning 429.83
"approximate answers" 300.16
arcuate ligament (-celiac axis) 447.4
arcus aortae 446.7
arc welders' 370.24
argentaffin, argentaffinoma 259.2
Argonz-Del Castillo (nonpuerperal
    galactorrhea and amenorrhea)
    253.1
Argyll Robertson's (syphilitic) 094.89
  nonsyphilitic 379.45
Armenian 277.31
arm-shoulder (see also Neuropathy,
    peripheral, autonomic) 337.9
Arnold-Chiari (see also Spina bifida)
    741.0●
  type I 348.4
  type II 741.0●
  type III 742.0
  type IV 742.2
Arrillaga-Ayerza (pulmonary artery
    sclerosis with pulmonary
    hypertension) 416.0
arteriomesenteric duodenum occlusion
    537.89
arteriovenous steal 996.73
arteritis, young female (obliterative
    brachiocephalic) 446.7

◀ New   ◀▥ Revised   ~~deleted~~ Deleted   ● Use Additional Digit(s)   ▨ Omit code

Syndrome (*Continued*)
  aseptic meningitis - *see* Meningitis, aseptic
  Asherman's 621.5
  Asperger's 299.8●
  asphyctic (*see also* Anxiety) 300.00
  aspiration, of newborn (massive 770.18)
    meconium 770.12
  ataxia-telangiectasia 334.8
  Audry's (acropachyderma) 757.39
  auriculotemporal 350.8
  autoimmune lymphoproliferative (ALPS) 279.41
  autosomal - *see also* Abnormal, autosomes NEC
    deletion 758.39
      5p 758.31
      22q11.2 758.32
  Avellis' 344.89
  Axenfeld's 743.44
  Ayerza (-Arrillaga) (pulmonary artery sclerosis with pulmonary hypertension) 416.0
  Baader's (erythema multiforme exudativum) 695.19
  Baastrup's 721.5
  Babinski (-Vaquez) (cardiovascular syphilis) 093.89
  Babinski-Fröhlich (adiposogenital dystrophy) 253.8
  Babinski-Nageotte 344.89
  Bagratuni's (temporal arteritis) 446.5
  Bakwin-Krida (craniometaphyseal dysplasia) 756.89
  Balint's (psychic paralysis of visual disorientation) 368.16
  Ballantyne (-Runge) (postmaturity) 766.22
  ballooning posterior leaflet 424.0
  Banti's - *see* Cirrhosis, liver
  Bard-Pic's (carcinoma, head of pancreas) 157.0
  Bardet-Biedl (obesity, polydactyly, and mental retardation) 759.89
  Barlow's (mitral valve prolapse) 424.0
  Barlow (-Möller) (infantile scurvy) 267
  Baron Munchausen's 301.51
  Barré-Guillain 357.0
  Barré-Liéou (posterior cervical sympathetic) 723.2
  Barrett's (chronic peptic ulcer of esophagus) 530.85
  Bársony-Pólgar (corkscrew esophagus) 530.5
  Bársony-Teschendorf (corkscrew esophagus) 530.5
  Barth 759.89
  Bartter's (secondary hyperaldosteronism with juxtaglomerular hyperplasia) 255.13
  basal cell nevus 759.89
  Basedow's (exophthalmic goiter) 242.0●
  basilar artery 435.0
  basofrontal 377.04
  Bassen-Kornzweig (abetalipoproteinemia) 272.5
  Batten-Steinert 359.21
  battered
    adult 995.81
    baby or child 995.54
    spouse 995.81
  Baumgarten-Cruveilhier (cirrhosis of liver) 571.5

Syndrome (*Continued*)
  Beals 759.82
  Bearn-Kunkel (-Slater) (lupoid hepatitis) 571.49
  Beau's (*see also* Degeneration, myocardial) 429.1
  Bechterew-Strümpell-Marie (ankylosing spondylitis) 720.0
  Beck's (anterior spinal artery occlusion) 433.8●
  Beckwith (-Wiedemann) 759.89
  Behçet's 136.1
  Bekhterev-Strümpell-Marie (ankylosing spondylitis) 720.0
  Benedikt's 344.89
  Béquez César (-Steinbrinck-Chédiak-Higashi) (congenital gigantism of peroxidase granules) 288.2
  Bernard-Horner (*see also* Neuropathy, peripheral, autonomic) 337.9
  Bernard-Sergent (acute adrenocortical insufficiency) 255.41
  Bernhardt-Roth 355.1
  Bernheim's (*see also* Failure, heart) 428.0
  Bertolotti's (sacralization of fifth lumbar vertebra) 756.15
  Besnier-Boeck-Schaumann (sarcoidosis) 135
  Bianchi's (aphasia-apraxia-alexia syndrome) 784.69
  Biedl-Bardet (obesity, polydactyly, and mental retardation) 759.89
  Biemond's (obesity, polydactyly, and mental retardation) 759.89
  big spleen 289.4
  bilateral polycystic ovarian 256.4
  Bing-Horton's 339.00
  Biörck (-Thorson) (malignant carcinoid) 259.2
  Birt-Hogg-Dube 759.89
  Blackfan-Diamond (congenital hypoplastic anemia) 284.01
  black lung 500
  black widow spider bite 989.5
  bladder neck (*see also* Incontinence, urine) 788.30
  blast (concussion) - *see* Blast, injury
  blind loop (postoperative) 579.2
  Block-Siemens (incontinentia pigmenti) 757.33
  Bloch-Sulzberger (incontinentia pigmenti) 757.33
  Bloom (-Machacek) (-Torre) 757.39
  Blount-Barber (tibia vara) 732.4
  blue
    bloater 491.20
      with
        acute bronchitis 491.22
        exacerbation (acute) 491.21
    diaper 270.0
    drum 381.02
    sclera 756.51
    toe 445.02
  Boder-Sedgwick (ataxia-telangiectasia) 334.8
  Boerhaave's (spontaneous esophageal rupture) 530.4
  Bonnevie-Ullrich 758.6
  Bonnier's 386.19
  Borjeson-Forssman-Lehmann 759.89
  Bouillaud's (rheumatic heart disease) 391.9
  Bourneville (-Pringle) (tuberous sclerosis) 759.5

Syndrome (*Continued*)
  Bouveret (-Hoffmann) (paroxysmal tachycardia) 427.2
  brachial plexus 353.0
  Brachman-de Lange (Amsterdam dwarf, mental retardation, and brachycephaly) 759.89
  bradycardia-tachycardia 427.81
  Brailsford-Morquio (dystrophy) (mucopolysaccharidosis IV) 277.5
  brain (acute) (chronic) (nonpsychotic) (organic) (with behavioral reaction) (with neurotic reaction) 310.9
    with
      presenile brain disease (*see also* Dementia, presenile) 290.10
      psychosis, psychotic reaction (*see also* Psychosis, organic) 294.9
    chronic alcoholic 291.2
    congenital (*see also* Retardation, mental) 319
    postcontusional 310.2
    posttraumatic
      nonpsychotic 310.2
      psychotic 293.9
        acute 293.0
        chronic (*see also* Psychosis, organic) 294.8
        subacute 293.1
    psycho-organic (*see also* Syndrome, psycho-organic) 310.9
    psychotic (*see also* Psychosis, organic) 294.9
    senile (*see also* Dementia, senile) 290.0
  branchial arch 744.41
  Brandt's (acrodermatitis enteropathica) 686.8
  Brennemann's 289.2
  Briquet's 300.81
  Brissaud-Meige (infantile myxedema) 244.9
  broad ligament laceration 620.6
  Brock's (atelectasis due to enlarged lymph nodes) 518.0
  broken heart 429.83
  Brown's tendon sheath 378.61
  Brown-Séquard 344.89
  brown spot 756.59
  Brugada 746.89
  Brugsch's (acropachyderma) 757.39
  bubbly lung 770.7
  Buchem's (hyperostosis corticalis) 733.3
  Budd-Chiari (hepatic vein thrombosis) 453.0
  Büdinger-Ludloff-Läwen 717.89
  bulbar 335.22
    lateral (*see also* Disease, cerebrovascular, acute) 436
  Bullis fever 082.8
  bundle of Kent (anomalous atrioventricular excitation) 426.7
  Bürger-Grutz (essential familial hyperlipemia) 272.3
  Burke's (pancreatic insufficiency and chronic neutropenia) 577.8
  Burnett's (milk-alkali) 275.42
  Burnier's (hypophyseal dwarfism) 253.3
  burning feet 266.2
  Bywaters' 958.5

S

Syndrome *(Continued)*
  Caffey's (infantile cortical hyperostosis) 756.59
  Calvé-Legg-Perthes (osteochrondrosis, femoral capital) 732.1
  Caplan (-Colinet) syndrome 714.81
  capsular thrombosis *(see also* Thrombosis, brain) 434.0●
  carbohydrate-deficient glycoprotein (CDGS) 271.8
  carcinogenic thrombophlebitis 453.1
  carcinoid 259.2
  cardiac asthma *(see also* Failure, ventricular, left) 428.1
  cardiacos negros 416.0
  cardiofaciocutaneous 759.89
  cardiopulmonary obesity 278.03 ◄▥
  cardiorenal *(see also* Hypertension, cardiorenal) 404.90
  cardiorespiratory distress (idiopathic), newborn 769
  cardiovascular renal *(see also* Hypertension, cardiorenal) 404.90
  cardiovasorenal 272.7
  Carini's (ichthyosis congenita) 757.1
  carotid
    artery (internal) 435.8
    body or sinus 337.01
  carpal tunnel 354.0
  Carpenter's 759.89
  Cassidy (-Scholte) (malignant carcinoid) 259.2
  cat-cry 758.31
  cauda equina 344.60
  causalgia 355.9
    lower limb 355.71
    upper limb 354.4
  cavernous sinus 437.6
  celiac 579.0
    artery compression 447.4
    axis 447.4
  central pain 338.0
  cerebellomedullary malformation *(see also* Spina bifida) 741.0●
  cerebral gigantism 253.0
  cerebrohepatorenal 759.89
  cervical (root) (spine) NEC 723.8
    disc 722.71
    posterior, sympathetic 723.2
    rib 353.0
    sympathetic paralysis 337.09
    traumatic (acute) NEC 847.0
  cervicobrachial (diffuse) 723.3
  cervicocranial 723.2
  cervicodorsal outlet 353.2
  Céstan's 344.89
  Céstan (-Raymond) 433.8●
  Céstan-Chenais 344.89
  chancriform 114.1
  Charcôt's (intermittent claudication) 443.9
    angina cruris 443.9
    due to atherosclerosis 440.21
  Charcôt-Marie-Tooth 356.1
  Charcôt-Weiss-Baker 337.01
  CHARGE association 759.89
  Cheadle (-Möller) (-Barlow) (infantile scurvy) 267
  Chédiak-Higashi (-Steinbrinck) (congenital gigantism of peroxidase granules) 288.2
  chest wall 786.52
  Chiari's (hepatic vein thrombosis) 453.0
  Chiari-Frommel 676.6●

Syndrome *(Continued)*
  chiasmatic 368.41
  Chilaiditi's (subphrenic displacement, colon) 751.4
  chondroectodermal dysplasia 756.55
  chorea-athetosis-agitans 275.1
  Christian's (chronic histiocytosis X) 277.89
  chromosome 4 short arm deletion 758.39
  chronic pain 338.4
  Churg-Strauss 446.4
  Clarke-Hadfield (pancreatic infantilism) 577.8
  Claude's 352.6
  Claude Bernard-Horner *(see also* Neuropathy, peripheral, autonomic) 337.9
  Clérambault's
    automatism 348.89
    erotomania 297.8
  Clifford's (postmaturity) 766.22
  climacteric 627.2
  Clouston's (hidrotic ectodermal dysplasia) 757.31
  clumsiness 315.4
  Cockayne's (microencephaly and dwarfism) 759.89
  Cockayne-Weber (epidermolysis bullosa) 757.39
  Coffin-Lowry 759.89
  Cogan's (nonsyphilitic interstitial keratitis) 370.52
  cold injury (newborn) 778.2
  Collet (-Sicard) 352.6
  combined immunity deficiency 279.2
  compartment(al) (anterior) (deep) (posterior) 958.8
    nontraumatic
      abdomen 729.73
      arm 729.71
      buttock 729.72
      fingers 729.71
      foot 729.72
      forearm 729.71
      hand 729.71
      hip 729.72
      leg 729.72
      lower extremity 729.72
      shoulder 729.71
      specified site NEC 729.79
      thigh 729.72
      toes 729.72
      upper extremity 729.71
      wrist 729.71
    post-surgical *(see also* Syndrome, compartment, non-traumatic) 998.89
    traumatic 958.90
      abdomen 958.93
      arm 958.91
      buttock 958.92
      fingers 958.91
      foot 958.92
      forearm 958.91
      hand 958.91
      hip 958.92
      leg 958.92
      lower extremity 958.92
      shoulder 958.91
      specified site NEC 958.99
      thigh 958.92
      tibial 958.92

Syndrome *(Continued)*
  compartment(al) *(Continued)*
    traumatic *(Continued)*
      toes 958.92
      upper extremity 958.91
      wrist 958.91
  complex regional pain - *see also* Dystrophy, sympathetic
    type I - *see* Dystrophy, sympathetic (posttraumatic) (reflex)
    type II - *see* Causalgia
  compression 958.5
    cauda equina 344.60
      with neurogenic bladder 344.61
  concussion 310.2
  congenital
    affecting more than one system 759.7
      specified type NEC 759.89
    congenital central alveolar hypoventilation 327.25
    facial diplegia 352.6
    muscular hypertrophy-cerebral 759.89
  congestion-fibrosis (pelvic) 625.5
  conjunctivourethrosynovial 099.3
  Conn (-Louis) (primary aldosteronism) 255.12
  Conradi (-Hünermann) (chondrodysplasia calcificans congenita) 756.59
  conus medullaris 336.8
  Cooke-Apert-Gallais (adrenogenital) 255.2
  Cornelia de Lange's (Amsterdam dwarf, mental retardation, and brachycephaly) 759.8
  coronary insufficiency or intermediate 411.1
  cor pulmonale 416.9
  corticosexual 255.2
  Costen's (complex) 524.60
  costochondral junction 733.6
  costoclavicular 353.0
  costovertebral 253.0
  Cotard's (paranoia) 297.1
  Cowden 759.6
  craniovertebral 723.2
  Creutzfeldt-Jakob 046.19
    with dementia
      with behavioral disturbance 046.19 *[294.11]*
      without behavioral disturbance 046.19 *[294.10]*
    variant 046.11
      with dementia
        with behavioral disturbance 046.11 *[294.11]*
        without behavioral disturbance 046.11 *[294.10]*
  crib death 798.0
  cricopharyngeal 787.20
  cri-du-chat 758.31
  Crigler-Najjar (congenital hyperbilirubinemia) 277.4
  crocodile tears 351.8
  Cronkhite-Canada 211.3
  croup 464.4
  CRST (cutaneous systemic sclerosis) 710.1
  crush 958.5
  crushed lung *(see also* Injury, internal, lung) 861.20

◄ New   ◄▥ Revised   ~~deleted~~ Deleted   ● Use Additional Digit(s)   ▥ Omit code

Syndrome (*Continued*)
Cruveilhier-Baumgarten (cirrhosis of liver) 571.5
cubital tunnel 354.2
Cuiffini-Pancoast (M8010/3) (carcinoma, pulmonary apex) 162.3
Curschmann (-Batten) (-Steinert) 359.21
Cushing's (iatrogenic) (idiopathic) (pituitary basophilism) (pituitary-dependent) 255.0
  overdose or wrong substance given or taken 962.0
Cyriax's (slipping rib) 733.99
cystic duct stump 576.0
Da Costa's (neurocirculatory asthenia) 306.2
Dameshek's (erythroblastic anemia) 282.49
Dana-Putnam (subacute combined sclerosis with pernicious anemia) 281.0 [336.2]
Danbolt (-Closs) (acrodermatitis enteropathica) 686.8
Dandy-Walker (atresia, foramen of Magendie) 742.3
  with spina bifida (*see also* Spina bifida) 741.0●
Danlos' 756.83
Davies-Colley (slipping rib) 733.99
dead fetus 641.3●
defeminization 255.2
defibrination (*see also* Fibrinolysis) 286.6
Degos' 447.8
Deiters' nucleus 386.19
Déjérine-Roussy 338.0
Déjérine-Thomas 333.0
de Lange's (Amsterdam dwarf, mental retardation, and brachycephaly) (Cornelia) 759.89
Del Castillo's (germinal aplasia) 606.0
deletion chromosomes 758.39
delusional
  induced by drug 292.11
dementia-aphonia, of childhood (*see also* Psychosis, childhood) 299.1●
demyelinating NEC 341.9
denial visual hallucination 307.9
depersonalization 300.6
de Quervain's 259.51
Dercum's (adiposis dolorosa) 272.8
de Toni-Fanconi (-Debre) (cystinosis) 270.0
diabetes-dwarfism-obesity (juvenile) 258.1
diabetes mellitus-hypertension-nephrosis 250.4● [581.81]
  due to secondary diabetes 249.4● [581.81]
diabetes mellitus in newborn infant 775.1
diabetes-nephrosis 250.4● [581.81]
  due to secondary diabetes 249.4● [581.81]
diabetic amyotrophy 250.6● [353.5]
  due to secondary diabetes 249.6● [353.5]
Diamond-Blackfan (congenital hypoplastic anemia) 284.01
Diamond-Gardner (autoerythrocyte sensitization) 287.2

Syndrome (*Continued*)
DIC (diffuse or disseminated intravascular coagulopathy) (*see also* Fibrinolysis) 286.6
diencephalohypophyseal NEC 253.8
diffuse cervicobrachial 723.3
diffuse obstructive pulmonary 496
DiGeorge's (thymic hypoplasia) 279.11
Dighton's 756.51
Di Guglielmo's (erythremic myelosis) (M9841/3) 207.0●
disequilibrium 276.9
disseminated platelet thrombosis 446.6
Ditthomska 307.81
Doan-Wiseman (primary splenic neutropenia) 289.53
Döhle body-panmyelopathic 288.2
Donohue's (leprechaunism) 259.8
dorsolateral medullary (*see also* Disease, cerebrovascular, acute) 436
double athetosis 333.71
double whammy 360.81
Down's (mongolism) 758.0
Dresbach's (elliptocytosis) 282.1
Dressler's (postmyocardial infarction) 411.0
  hemoglobinuria 283.2
  postcardiotomy 429.4
drug withdrawal, infant, of dependent mother 779.5
dry skin 701.1
  eye 375.15
DSAP (disseminated superficial actinic porokeratosis) 692.75
Duane's (retraction) 378.71
Duane-Stilling-Türk (ocular retraction syndrome) 378.71
Dubin-Johnson (constitutional hyperbilirubinemia) 277.4
Dubin-Sprinz (constitutional hyperbilirubinemia) 277.4
Duchenne's 335.22
due to abnormality
  autosomal NEC (*see also* Abnormal, autosomes NEC) 758.5
    13 758.1
    18 758.2
    21 or 22 758.0
    D_1 758.1
    E_3 758.2
    G 758.0
  chromosomal 758.89
    sex 758.81
dumping 564.2
  nonsurgical 536.8
Duplay's 726.2
Dupré's (meningism) 781.6
Dyke-Young (acquired macrocytic hemolytic anemia) 283.9
dyspraxia 315.4
dystocia, dystrophia 654.9●
Eagle-Barret 756.71
Eales' 362.18
Eaton-Lambert (*see also* Neoplasm, by site, malignant) 199.1 [358.1]
Ebstein's (downward displacement, tricuspid valve into right ventricle) 746.2
ectopic ACTH secretion 255.0
eczema-thrombocytopenia 279.12
Eddowes' (brittle bones and blue sclera) 756.51

Syndrome (*Continued*)
Edwards' 758.2
efferent loop 537.89
effort (aviators') (psychogenic) 306.2
Ehlers-Danlos 756.83
Eisenmenger's (ventricular septal defect) 745.4
Ekbom's (restless legs) 333.94
Ekman's (brittle bones and blue sclera) 756.51
electric feet 266.2
Elephant man 237.71
Ellison-Zollinger (gastric hypersecretion with pancreatic islet cell tumor) 251.5
Ellis-van Creveld (chondroectodermal dysplasia) 756.55
embryonic fixation 270.2
empty sella (turcica) 253.8
endocrine-hypertensive 255.3
Engel-von Recklinghausen (osteitis fibrosa cystica) 252.01
enteroarticular 099.3
entrapment - *see* Neuropathy, entrapment
eosinophilia myalgia 710.5
epidemic vomiting 078.82
Epstein's - *see* Nephrosis
Erb (-Oppenheim)-Goldflam 358.00
Erdheim-Chester 277.89
Erdheim's (acromegalic macrospondylitis) 253.0
Erlacher-Blount (tibia vara) 732.4
erythrocyte fragmentation 283.19
euthyroid sick 790.94
Evans' (thrombocytopenic purpura) 287.32
excess cortisol, iatrogenic 255.0
exhaustion 300.5
extrapyramidal 333.90
eyelid-malar-mandible 756.0
eye retraction 378.71
Faber's (achlorhydric anemia) 280.9
Fabry (-Anderson) (angiokeratoma corporis diffusum) 272.7
facet 724.8
Fallot's 745.2
falx (*see also* Hemorrhage, brain) 431
familial eczema-thrombocytopenia 279.12
Fanconi's (anemia) (congenital pancytopenia) 284.09
Fanconi (-de Toni) (-Debré) (cystinosis) 270.0
Farber (-Uzman) (disseminated lipogranulomatosis) 272.8
fatigue NEC 300.5
  chronic 780.71
faulty bowel habit (idiopathic megacolon) 564.7
FDH (focal dermal hypoplasia) 757.39
fecal reservoir 560.39
Feil-Klippel (brevicollis) 756.16
Felty's (rheumatoid arthritis with splenomegaly and leukopenia) 714.1
fertile eunuch 257.2
fetal alcohol 760.71
  late effect 760.71
fibrillation-flutter 427.32
fibrositis (periarticular) 729.0
Fiedler's (acute isolated myocarditis) 422.91
Fiessinger-Leroy (-Reiter) 099.3

Syndrome (Continued)

Fiessinger-Rendu (erythema multiforme exudativum) 695.19
first arch 756.0
Fisher's 357.0
fish odor 270.8
Fitz's (acute hemorrhagic pancreatitis) 577.0
Fitz-Hugh and Curtis 098.86
  due to
    Chlamydia trachomatis 099.56
    Neisseria gonorrhoeae (gonococcal peritonitis) 098.86
Flajani (-Basedow) (exophthalmic goiter) 242.0●
flat back
  acquired 737.29
  postprocedural 738.5
floppy
  infant 781.99
  iris 364.81
  valve (mitral) 424.0
flush 259.2
Foix-Alajouanine 336.1
Fong's (hereditary osteo-onychodysplasia) 756.89
foramen magnum 348.4
Forbes-Albright (nonpuerperal amenorrhea and lactation associated with pituitary tumor) 253.1
Foster-Kennedy 377.04
Foville's (peduncular) 344.89
fragile X 759.83
Franceschetti's (mandibulofacial dysostosis) 756.0
Fraser's 759.89
Freeman-Sheldon 759.89
Frey's (auriculotemporal) 705.22
Friderichsen-Waterhouse 036.3
Friedrich-Erb-Arnold (acropachyderma) 757.39
Fröhlich's (adiposogenital dystrophy) 253.8
Froin's 336.8
Frommel-Chiari 676.6●
frontal lobe 310.0
Fukuhara 277.87
Fuller Albright's (osteitis fibrosa disseminata) 756.59
functional
  bowel 564.9
  prepubertal castrate 752.89
Gaisböck's (polycythemia hypertonica) 289.0
ganglion (basal, brain) 333.90
  geniculi 351.1
Ganser's, hysterical 300.16
Gardner-Diamond (autoerythrocyte sensitization) 287.2
gastroesophageal junction 530.0
gastroesophageal laceration-hemorrhage 530.7
gastrojejunal loop obstruction 537.89
Gayet-Wernicke's (superior hemorrhagic polioencephalitis) 265.1
Gee-Herter-Heubner (nontropical sprue) 579.0
Gélineau's (see also Narcolepsy) 347.00
genito-anorectal 099.1

Syndrome (Continued)

Gerhardt's (vocal cord paralysis) 478.30
Gerstmann's (finger agnosia) 784.69
Gerstmann-Sträussler-Scheinker (GSS) 046.71
Gianotti Crosti 057.8
  due to known virus - see Infection, virus
  due to unknown virus 057.8
Gilbert's 277.4
Gilford (-Hutchinson) (progeria) 259.8
Gilles de la Tourette's 307.23
Gillespie's (dysplasia oculodentodigitalis) 759.89
Glénard's (enteroptosis) 569.89
Glinski-Simmonds (pituitary cachexia) 253.2
glucuronyl transferase 277.4
glue ear 381.20
Goldberg (-Maxwell) (-Morris) (testicular feminization) 259.51
Goldenhar's (oculoauriculovertebral dysplasia) 756.0
Goldflam-Erb 358.00
Goltz-Gorlin (dermal hypoplasia) 757.39
Goodpasture's (pneumorenal) 446.21
Good's 279.06
Gopalan's (burning feet) 266.2
Gorlin-Chaudhry-Moss 759.89
Gorlin's 759.89
Gougerot (-Houwer)-Sjögren (keratoconjunctivitis sicca) 710.2
Gougerot-Blum (pigmented purpuric lichenoid dermatitis) 709.1
Gougerot-Carteaud (confluent reticulate papillomatosis) 701.8
Gouley's (constrictive pericarditis) 423.2
Gowers' (vasovagal attack) 780.2
Gowers-Paton-Kennedy 377.04
Gradenigo's 383.02
Gray or grey (chloramphenicol) (newborn) 779.4
Greig's (hypertelorism) 756.0
GSS (Gerstmann-Sträussler-Scheinker) 046.71
Gubler-Millard 344.89
Guérin-Stern (arthrogryposis multiplex congenita) 754.89
Guillain-Barré (-Strohl) 357.0
Gunn's (jaw-winking syndrome) 742.8
Günther's (congenital erythropoietic porphyria) 277.1
gustatory sweating 350.8
H₂O 759.81
Hadfield-Clarke (pancreatic infantilism) 577.8
Haglund-Läwen-Fründ 717.89
hair tourniquet - see also Injury, superficial, by site
  finger 915.8
    infected 915.9
  penis 911.8
    infected 911.9
  toe 917.8
    infected 917.9
hairless women 257.8
Hallermann-Strieff 756.0
Hallervorden-Spatz 333.0
Hamman's (spontaneous mediastinal emphysema) 518.1

Syndrome (Continued)

Hamman-Rich (diffuse interstitial pulmonary fibrosis) 516.3
Hand-Schüller-Christian (chronic histiocytosis X) 277.89
hand-foot 693.0
Hanot-Chauffard (-Troisier) (bronze diabetes) 275.01 ◀▥
Harada's 363.22
Hare's (M8010/3) (carcinoma, pulmonary apex) 162.3
Harkavy's 446.0
harlequin color change 779.89
Harris' (organic hyperinsulinism) 251.1
Hart's (pellagra-cerebellar ataxia-renal aminoaciduria) 270.0
Hayem-Faber (achlorhydric anemia) 280.9
Hayem-Widal (acquired hemolytic jaundice) 283.9
headache - see Headache, syndrome
Heberden's (angina pectoris) 413.9
Hedinger's (malignant carcinoid) 259.2
Hegglin's 288.2
Heller's (infantile psychosis) (see also Psychosis, childhood) 299.1●
H.E.L.L.P. 642.5●
hemolytic-uremic (adult) (child) 283.11
hemophagocytic 288.4
  infection-associated 288.4
Hench-Rosenberg (palindromic arthritis) (see also Rheumatism, palindromic) 719.3●
Henoch-Schönlein (allergic purpura) 287.0
hepatic flexure 569.89
hepatorenal 572.4
  due to a procedure 997.4
  following delivery 674.8●
hepatourologic 572.4
Herrick's (hemoglobin S disease) 282.61
Herter (-Gee) (nontropical sprue) 579.0
Heubner-Herter (nontropical sprue) 579.0
Heyd's (hepatorenal) 572.4
HHHO 759.81
high grade myelodysplastic 238.73
  with 5q deletion 238.73
Hilger's 337.09
histiocytic 288.4
Hoffa (-Kastert) (liposynovitis prepatellaris) 272.8
Hoffmann's 244.9 [359.5]
Hoffmann-Bouveret (paroxysmal tachycardia) 427.2
Hoffmann-Werdnig 335.0
Holländer-Simons (progressive lipodystrophy) 272.6
Holmes' (visual disorientation) 368.16
Holmes-Adie 379.46
Hoppe-Goldflam 358.00
Horner's (see also Neuropathy, peripheral, autonomic) 337.9
  traumatic - see Injury, nerve, cervical sympathetic
hospital addiction 301.51
hungry bone 275.5
Hunt's (herpetic geniculate ganglionitis) 053.11
  dyssynergia cerebellaris myoclonica 334.2

◀ New   ◀▥ Revised   ~~deleted~~ Deleted   ● Use Additional Digit(s)   ▬ Omit code

Syndrome *(Continued)*
Hunter (-Hurler)
(mucopolysaccharidosis II) 277.5
hunterian glossitis 529.4
Hurler (-Hunter)
(mucopolysaccharidosis II)
277.5
Hutchinson's incisors or teeth 090.5
Hutchinson-Boeck (sarcoidosis) 135
Hutchinson-Gilford (progeria) 259.8
hydralazine
correct substance properly
administered 695.4
overdose or wrong substance given
or taken 972.6
hydraulic concussion (abdomen) *(see
also* Injury, internal, abdomen)
868.00
hyperabduction 447.8
hyperactive bowel 564.9
hyperaldosteronism with hypokalemic
alkalosis (Bartter's) 255.13
hypercalcemic 275.42
hypercoagulation NEC 289.89
hypereosinophilic (idiopathic) 288.3
hyperkalemic 276.7
hyperkinetic - *see also* Hyperkinesia,
heart 429.82
hyperlipemia-hemolytic anemia-icterus
571.1
hypermobility 728.5
hypernatremia 276.0
hyperosmolarity 276.0
hyperperfusion 997.01
hypersomnia-bulimia 349.89
hypersplenic 289.4
hypersympathetic *(see also* Neuropathy,
peripheral, autonomic) 337.9
hypertransfusion, newborn 776.4
hyperventilation, psychogenic 306.1
hyperviscosity (of serum) NEC 273.3
polycythemic 289.0
sclerothymic 282.8
hypoglycemic (familial) (neonatal)
251.2
functional 251.1
hypokalemic 276.8
hypophyseal 253.8
hypophyseothalamic 253.8
hypopituitarism 253.2
hypoplastic left heart 746.7
hypopotassemia 276.8
hyposmolality 276.1
hypotension, maternal 669.2 ●
hypothenar hammer 443.89
hypotonia-hypomentia-hypogonadism-
obesity 759.81
ICF (intravascular coagulation-
fibrinolysis) *(see also* Fibrinolysis)
286.6
idiopathic cardiorespiratory distress,
newborn 769
idiopathic nephrotic (infantile) 581.9
iliotibial band 728.89
Imerslund (-Gräsbeck) (anemia due to
familial selective vitamin B_{12}
malabsorption) 281.1
immobility (paraplegic) 728.3
immunity deficiency, combined
279.2
impending coronary 411.1
impingement
shoulder 726.2
vertebral bodies 724.4

Syndrome *(Continued)*
inappropriate secretion of antidiuretic
hormone (ADH) 253.6
incomplete
mandibulofacial 756.0
infant
death, sudden (SIDS) 798.0
Hercules 255.2
of diabetic mother 775.0
shaken 995.55
infantilism 253.3
inferior vena cava 459.2
influenza-like *(see also* Influenza)
487.1 ◀▥
inspissated bile, newborn 774.4
insufficient sleep 307.44
intermediate coronary (artery) 411.1
internal carotid artery *(see also*
Occlusion, artery, carotid)
433.1 ●
interspinous ligament 724.8
intestinal
carcinoid 259.2
gas 787.3
knot 560.2
intraoperative floppy iris (IFIS) 364.81
intravascular
coagulation-fibrinolysis (ICF) *(see
also* Fibrinolysis) 286.6
coagulopathy *(see also* Fibrinolysis)
286.6
inverted Marfan's 759.89
IRDS (idiopathic respiratory distress,
newborn) 769
irritable
bowel 564.1
heart 306.2
weakness 300.5
ischemic bowel (transient) 557.9
chronic 557.1
due to mesenteric artery
insufficiency 557.1
Itsenko-Cushing (pituitary
basophilism) 255.0
IVC (intravascular coagulopathy) *(see
also* Fibrinolysis) 286.6
Ivemark's (asplenia with congenital
heart disease) 759.0
Jaccoud's 714.4
Jackson's 344.89
Jadassohn-Lewandowski (pachyonchia
congenita) 757.5
Jaffe-Lichtenstein (-Uehlinger) 252.01
Jahnke's (encephalocutaneous
angiomatosis) 759.6
Jakob-Creutzfeldt 046.19
with dementia
with behavioral disturbance
046.19 *[294.11]*
without behavioral disturbance
046.19 *[294.10]*
variant 046.11
with dementia
with behavioral disturbance
046.11 *[294.11]*
without behavioral
disturbance 046.11
[294.10]
Jaksch's (pseudoleukemia infantum)
285.8
Jaksch-Hayem (-Luzet)
(pseudoleukemia infantum) 285.8
jaw-winking 742.8
jejunal 564.2

Syndrome *(Continued)*
Jervell-Lange-Nielsen 426.82
jet lag 327.35
Jeune's (asphyxiating thoracic
dystrophy of newborn) 756.4
Job's (chronic granulomatous disease)
288.1
Jordan's 288.2
Joseph-Diamond-Blackfan (congenital
hypoplastic anemia) 284.01
Joubert 759.89
jugular foramen 352.6
Kabuki 759.89
Kahler's (multiple myeloma)
(M9730/3) 203.0 ●
Kalischer's (encephalocutaneous
angiomatosis) 759.6
Kallmann's (hypogonadotropic
hypogonadism with anosmia)
253.4
Kanner's (autism) *(see also* Psychosis,
childhood) 299.0 ●
Kartagener's (sinusitis, bronchiectasis,
situs inversus) 759.3
Kasabach-Merritt (capillary
hemangioma associated with
thrombocytopenic purpura)
287.39
Kast's (dyschondroplasia with
hemangiomas) 756.4
Kaznelson's (congenital hypoplastic
anemia) 284.01
Kearns-Sayre 277.87
Kelly's (sideropenic dysphagia) 280.8
Kimmelstiel-Wilson (intercapillary
glomerulosclerosis) 250.4 ●
[581.81]
due to secondary diabetes 249.4 ●
[581.81]
Klauder's (erythema multiforme
exudativum) 695.19
Klein-Waardenburg (ptosis-epicanthus)
270.2
Kleine-Levin 327.13
Klinefelter's 758.7
Klippel-Feil (brevicollis) 756.16
Klippel-Trenaunay 759.89
Klumpke (-Déjérine) (injury to brachial
plexus at birth) 767.6
Klüver-Bucy (-Terzian) 310.0
Köhler-Pellgrini-Stieda (calcification,
knee joint) 726.62
König's 564.89
Korsakoff's (nonalcoholic) 294.0
alcoholic 291.1
Korsakoff (-Wernicke) (nonalcoholic)
294.0
alcoholic 291.1
Kostmann's (infantile genetic
agranulocytosis) 288.01
Krabbe's
congenital muscle hypoplasia 756.89
cutaneocerebral angioma 759.6
Kunkel (lupoid hepatitis) 571.49
labyrinthine 386.50
laceration, broad ligament 620.6
Landau-Kleffner 345.8 ●
Langdon Down (mongolism) 758.0
Larsen's (flattened facies and multiple
congenital dislocations) 755.8
lateral
cutaneous nerve of thigh 355.1
medullary *(see also* Disease,
cerebrovascular, acute) 436

Syndrome (Continued)
   Launois' (pituitary gigantism) 253.0
   Launois-Cléret (adiposogenital
         dystrophy) 253.8
   Laurence-Moon (-Bardet)-Biedl
         (obesity, polydactyly, and mental
         retardation) 759.89
   Lawford's (encephalocutaneous
         angiomatosis) 759.6
   lazy
      leukocyte 288.09
      posture 728.3
   Lederer-Brill (acquired infectious
         hemolytic anemia) 283.19
   Legg-Calvé-Perthes (osteochondrosis
         capital femoral) 732.1
   Lemiere 451.89
   Lennox-Gastaut syndrome 345.0●
      with tonic seizures 345.1●
   Lennox's (see also Epilepsy) 345.0●
   lenticular 275.1
   Léopold-Lévi's (paroxysmal thyroid
         instability) 242.9●
   Lepore hemoglobin 282.49
   Léri-Weill 756.59
   Leriche's (aortic bifurcation occlusion)
         444.0
   Lermoyez's (see also Disease, Ménière's)
         386.00
   Lesch-Nyhan (hypoxanthine-guanine-
         phosphoribosyltransferase
         deficiency) 277.2
   leukoencephalopathy, reversible,
         posterior 348.5
   Lev's (acquired complete heart block)
         426.0
   Levi's (pituitary dwarfism) 253.3
   Lévy-Roussy 334.3
   Lichtheim's (subacute combined
         sclerosis with pernicious anemia)
         281.0 [336.2]
   Li-Fraumeni V84.01
   Lightwood's (renal tubular acidosis)
         588.89
   Lignac (-de Toni) (-Fanconi) (-Debré)
         (cystinosis) 270.0
   Likoff's (angina in menopausal
         women) 413.9
   liver-kidney 572.4
   Lloyd's 258.1
   lobotomy 310.0
   Löffler's (eosinophilic pneumonitis)
         518.3
   Löfgren's (sarcoidosis) 135
   long arm 18 or 21 deletion 758.39
   Looser (-Debray)-Milkman
         (osteomalacia with
         pseudofractures) 268.2
   Lorain-Levi (pituitary dwarfism)
         253.3
   Louis-Bar (ataxia-telangiectasia)
         334.8
   low
      atmospheric pressure 993.2
      back 724.2
         psychogenic 306.0
      output (cardiac) (see also Failure,
            heart) 428.9
   Lowe's (oculocerebrorenal dystrophy)
         270.8
   Lowe-Terrey-MacLachlan
         (oculocerebrorenal
         dystrophy) 270.8
   lower radicular, newborn 767.4

Syndrome (Continued)
   Lown (-Ganong)-Levine (short P-R
         internal, normal QRS complex,
         and supraventricular tachycardia)
         426.81
   Lucey-Driscoll (jaundice due to
         delayed conjugation) 774.30
   Luetscher's (dehydration) 276.51
   lumbar vertebral 724.4
   Lutembacher's (atrial septal defect
         with mitral stenosis) 745.5
   Lyell's (toxic epidermal necrolysis)
         695.15
      due to drug
         correct substance properly
               administered 695.15
         overdose or wrong substance
               given or taken 977.9
         specified drug - see Table of
               Drugs and Chemicals
   MacLeod's 492.8
   macrogenitosomia praecox 259.8
   macroglobulinemia 273.3
   macrophage activation 288.4
   Maffucci's (dyschondroplasia with
         hemangiomas) 756.4
   Magenblase 306.4
   magnesium-deficiency 781.7
   malabsorption 579.9
      postsurgical 579.3
      spinal fluid 331.3
   Mal de Debarquement 780.4
   malignant carcinoid 259.2
   Mallory-Weiss 530.7
   mandibulofacial dysostosis 756.0
   manic-depressive (see also Psychosis,
         affective) 296.80
   Mankowsky's (familial dysplastic
         osteopathy) 731.2
   maple syrup (urine) 270.3
   Marable's (celiac artery compression)
         447.4
   Marchesani (-Weill) (brachymorphism
         and ectopia lentis) 759.89
   Marchiafava-Bignami 341.8
   Marchiafava-Micheli (paroxysmal
         nocturnal hemoglobinuria)
         283.2
   Marcus Gunn's (jaw-winking
         syndrome) 742.8
   Marfan's (arachnodactyly) 759.82
      meaning congenital syphilis 090.49
         with luxation of lens 090.49
               [379.32]
   Marie's (acromegaly) 253.0
      primary or idiopathic
            (acropachyderma) 757.39
      secondary (hypertrophic pulmonary
            osteoarthropathy) 731.2
   Markus-Adie 379.46
   Maroteaux-Lamy
         (mucopolysaccharidosis VI)
         277.5
   Martin's 715.27
   Martin-Albright
         (pseudohypoparathyroidism)
         275.49
   Martorell-Fabré (pulseless disease)
         446.7
   massive aspiration of newborn 770.18
   Masters-Allen 620.6
   mastocytosis 757.33
   maternal hypotension 669.2●
   maternal obesity 646.1●

Syndrome (Continued)
   May (-Hegglin) 288.2
   McArdle (-Schmid) (-Pearson)
         (glycogenosis V) 271.0
   McCune-Albright (osteitis fibrosa
         disseminata) 756.59
   McQuarrie's (idiopathic familial
         hypoglycemia) 251.2
   meconium
      aspiration 770.12
      plug (newborn) NEC 777.1
   median arcuate ligament 447.4
   mediastinal fibrosis 519.3
   Meekeren-Ehlers-Danlos 756.83
   Meige (blepharospasm-oromandibular
         dystonia) 333.82
      -Milroy (chronic hereditary edema)
            757.0
   MELAS (mitochondrial
         encephalopathy, lactic acidosis
         and stroke-like episodes)
         277.87
   Melkersson (-Rosenthal) 351.8
   MEN (multiple endocrine neoplasia)
      type I 258.01
      type IIA 258.02
      type IIB 258.03
   Mende's (ptosis-epicanthus) 270.2
   Mendelson's (resulting from a
         procedure) 997.39
      during labor 668.0●
      obstetric 668.0●
   Ménétrier's (hypertrophic gastritis)
         535.2●
   Ménière's (see also Disease, Ménière's)
         386.00
   meningo-eruptive 047.1
   Menkes' 759.89
      glutamic acid 759.89
      maple syrup (urine) disease 270.3
   menopause 627.2
      postartificial 627.4
   menstruation 625.4
   MERRF (myoclonus with epilepsy and
         with ragged red fibers) 277.87
   mesenteric
      artery, superior 557.1
      vascular insufficiency (with
            gangrene) 557.1
   metabolic 277.7
   metastatic carcinoid 259.2
   Meyenburg-Altherr-Uehlinger 733.99
   Meyer-Schwickerath and Weyers
         (dysplasia oculodentodigitalis)
         759.89
   Micheli-Rietti (thalassemia minor)
         282.49
   Michotte's 721.5
   micrognathia-glossoptosis 756.0
   microphthalmos (congenital) 759.89
   midbrain 348.89
   middle
      lobe (lung) (right) 518.0
      radicular 353.0
   Miescher's
      familial acanthosis nigricans 701.2
      granulomatosis disciformis 709.3
   Mieten's 759.89
   migraine 346.0●
   Mikity-Wilson (pulmonary
         dysmaturity) 770.7
   Mikulicz's (dryness of mouth, absent
         or decreased lacrimation) 527.1
   milk alkali (milk drinkers') 275.42

◀ New   ◀▥ Revised   deleted Deleted   ● Use Additional Digit(s)   ▨ Omit code

Syndrome *(Continued)*
Milkman (-Looser) (osteomalacia with pseudofractures) 268.2
Millard-Gubler 344.89
Miller-Dieker 758.33
Miller Fisher's 357.0
Milles' (encephalocutaneous angiomatosis) 759.6
Minkowski-Chauffard *(see also* Spherocytosis) 282.0
Mirizzi's (hepatic duct stenosis) 576.2
    with calculus, cholelithiasis, or stones - *see* Choledocholithiasis
mitochondrial neurogastrointestinal encephalopathy (MNGIE) 277.87
mitral
    click (-murmur) 785.2
    valve prolapse 424.0
MNGIE (mitochondrial neurogastrointestinal encephalopathy) 277.87
Möbius'
    congenital oculofacial paralysis 352.6
    ophthalmoplegic migraine 346.2 ●
Mohr's (types I and II) 759.89
monofixation 378.34
Moore's *(see also* Epilepsy) 345.5 ●
Morel-Moore (hyperostosis frontalis interna) 733.3
Morel-Morgagni (hyperostosis frontalis interna) 733.3
Morgagni (-Stewart-Morel) (hyperostosis frontalis interna) 733.3
Morgagni-Adams-Stokes (syncope with heart block) 426.9
Morquio (-Brailsford) (-Ullrich) (mucopolysaccharidosis IV) 277.5
Morris (testicular feminization) 259.51
Morton's (foot) (metatarsalgia) (metatarsal neuralgia) (neuralgia) (neuroma) (toe) 355.6
Moschcowitz (-Singer-Symmers) (thrombotic thrombocytopenic purpura) 446.6
Mounier-Kuhn 748.3
    with
        acute exacerbation 494.1
        bronchiectasis 494.0
            with (acute) exacerbation 494.1
    acquired 519.19
        with bronchiectasis 494.0
            with (acute) exacerbation 494.1
Mucha-Haberman (acute parapsoriasis varioliformis) 696.2
mucocutaneous lymph node (acute) (febrile) (infantile) (MCLS) 446.1
multiple
    deficiency 260
    endocrine neoplasia (MEN)
        type I 258.01
        type IIA 258.02
        type IIB 258.03
        operations 301.51
Munchausen's 301.51
Munchmeyer's (exostosis luxurians) 728.11
Murchison-Sanderson - *see* Disease, Hodgkin's
myasthenic - *see* Myasthenia, syndrome

Syndrome *(Continued)*
myelodysplastic 238.75
    with 5q deletion 238.74
    high grade with 5q deletion 238.73
    therapy-related 289.83
myeloproliferative (chronic) (M9960/1) 238.79
myofascial pain NEC 729.1
Naffziger's 353.0
Nager-de Reynier (dysostosis mandibularis) 756.0
nail-patella (hereditary osteo-onychodysplasia) 756.89
NARP (neuropathy, ataxia and retinitis pigmentosa) 277.87
Nebécourt's 253.3
Neill Dingwall (microencephaly and dwarfism) 759.89
nephrotic *(see also* Nephrosis) 581.9
    diabetic 250.4 ● *[581.81]*
        due to secondary diabetes 249.4 ● *[581.81]*
Netherton's (ichthyosiform erythroderma) 757.1
neurocutaneous 759.6
neuroleptic malignant 333.92
Nezelof's (pure alymphocytosis) 279.13
Niemann-Pick (lipid histiocytosis) 272.7
Nonne-Milroy-Meige (chronic hereditary edema) 757.0
nonsense 300.16
Noonan's 759.89
Nothnagel's
    ophthalmoplegia-cerebellar ataxia 378.52
    vasomotor acroparesthesia 443.89
nucleus ambiguous-hypoglossal 352.6
OAV (oculoauriculovertebral dysplasia) 756.0
obesity hypoventilation 278.03 ◄
obsessional 300.3
oculocutaneous 364.24
oculomotor 378.81
oculourethroarticular 099.3
Ogilvie's (sympathicotonic colon obstruction) 560.89
ophthalmoplegia-cerebellar ataxia 378.52
Oppenheim-Urbach (necrobiosis lipoidica diabeticorum) 250.8 ● *[709.3]*
    due to secondary diabetes 249.8 ● *[709.3]*
oral-facial-digital 759.89
organic
    affective NEC 293.83
        drug-induced 292.84
    anxiety 293.84
    delusional 293.81
        alcohol-induced 291.5
        drug-induced 292.11
        due to or associated with arteriosclerosis 290.42
            presenile brain disease 290.12
            senility 290.20
    depressive 293.83
        drug-induced 292.84
        due to or associated with arteriosclerosis 290.43
            presenile brain disease 290.13
            senile brain disease 290.21
    hallucinosis 293.82
        drug-induced 292.84

Syndrome *(Continued)*
organic affective 293.83
    induced by drug 292.84
organic personality 310.1
    induced by drug 292.89
Ormond's 593.4
orodigitofacial 759.89
orthostatic hypotensive-dysautonomic-dyskinetic 333.0
Osler-Weber-Rendu (familial hemmorrhagic telangiectasia) 448.0
osteodermopathic hyperostosis 757.39
osteoporosis-osteomalacia 268.2
Österreicher-Turner (hereditary osteo-onychodysplasia) 756.89
os trigonum 755.69
Ostrum-Furst 756.59
otolith 386.19
otopalatodigital 759.89
outlet (thoracic) 353.0
ovarian remnant 620.8
Owren's *(see also* Defect, coagulation) 286.3
OX 758.6
pacemaker 429.4
Paget-Schroetter (intermittent venous claudication) 453.89
pain - *see also* Pain
    central 338.0
    chronic 338.4
    complex regional 355.9
        type I 337.20
            lower limb 337.22
            specified site NEC 337.29
            upper limb 337.21
        type II
            lower limb 355.71
            upper limb 354.4
    myelopathic 338.0
    thalamic (hyperesthetic) 338.0
painful
    apicocostal vertebral (M8010/3) 162.3
    arc 726.19
    bruising 287.2
    feet 266.2
Pancoast's (carcinoma, pulmonary apex) (M8010/3) 162.3
panhypopituitary (postpartum) 253.2
papillary muscle 429.81
    with myocardial infarction 410.8 ●
Papillon-Léage and Psaume (orodigitofacial dysostosis) 759.89
parabiotic (transfusion)
    donor (twin) 772.0
    recipient (twin) 776.4
paralysis agitans 332.0
paralytic 344.9
    specified type NEC 344.89
paraneoplastic - *see* Condition
Parinaud's (paralysis of conjugate upward gaze) 378.81
    oculoglandular 372.02
Parkes Weber and Dimitri (encephalocutaneous angiomatosis) 759.6
Parkinson's *(see also* Parkinsonism) 332.0
parkinsonian *(see also* Parkinsonism) 332.0
Parry's (exophthalmic goiter) 242.0 ●
Parry-Romberg 349.89

Syndrome *(Continued)*
  Parsonage-Aldren-Turner 353.5
  Parsonage-Turner 353.5
  Patau's (trisomy D_1) 758.1
  patella clunk 719.66
  patellofemoral 719.46
  Paterson (-Brown) (-Kelly) (sideropenic dysphagia) 280.8
  Payr's (splenic flexure syndrome) 569.89
  pectoral girdle 447.8
  pectoralis minor 447.8
  Pelger-Huët (hereditary hyposegmentation) 288.2
  pellagra-cerebellar ataxia-renal aminoaciduria 270.0
  Pellegrini-Stieda 726.62
  pellagroid 265.2
  Pellizzi's (pineal) 259.8
  pelvic congestion (-fibrosis) 625.5
  Pendred's (familial goiter with deaf-mutism) 243
  Penfield's *(see also* Epilepsy) 345.5 ●
  Penta X 758.81
  peptic ulcer - *see* Ulcer, peptic 533.9
  perabduction 447.8
  periodic 277.31
  periurethral fibrosis 593.4
  persistent fetal circulation 747.83
  Petges-Cléjat (poikilodermatomyositis) 710.3
  Peutz-Jeghers 759.6
  Pfeiffer (acrocephalosyndactyly) 755.55
  phantom limb 353.6
  pharyngeal pouch 279.11
  Pick's (pericardial pseudocirrhosis of liver) 423.2
    heart 423.2
    liver 423.2
  Pick-Herxheimer (diffuse idiopathic cutaneous atrophy) 701.8
  Pickwickian (cardiopulmonary obesity) 278.03 ◄||||
  PIE (pulmonary infiltration with eosinophilia) 518.3
  Pierre Marie-Bamberger (hypertrophic pulmonary osteoarthropathy) 731.2
  Pierre Mauriac's (diabetes-dwarfism-obesity) 258.1
  Pierre Robin 756.0
  pigment dispersion, iris 364.53
  pineal 259.8
  pink puffer 492.8
  pituitary 253.0
  placental
    dysfunction 762.2
    insufficiency 762.2
    transfusion 762.3
  plantar fascia 728.71
  plateau iris 364.82
  plica knee 727.83
  Plummer-Vinson (sideropenic dysphagia) 280.8
  pluricarential of infancy 260
  plurideficiency of infancy 260
  pluriglandular (compensatory) 258.8
  Poland 756.81 ◄
  polycarential of infancy 260
  polyglandular 258.8
  polysplenia 759.0
  pontine 433.8 ●
  popliteal
    artery entrapment 447.8
    web 756.89

Syndrome *(Continued)*
  postartificial menopause 627.4
  postcardiac injury
    postcardiotomy 429.4
    postmyocardial infarction 411.0
  postcardiotomy 429.4
  postcholecystectomy 576.0
  postcommissurotomy 429.4
  postconcussional 310.2
  postcontusional 310.2
  postencephalitic 310.8
  posterior
    cervical sympathetic 723.2
    fossa compression 348.4
    inferior cerebellar artery *(see also* Disease, cerebrovascular, acute) 436
    reversible encephalopathy (PRES) 348.39
  postgastrectomy (dumping) 564.2
  post-gastric surgery 564.2
  posthepatitis 780.79
  postherpetic (neuralgia) (zoster) 053.19
    geniculate ganglion 053.11
    ophthalmica 053.19
  postimmunization - *see* Complications, vaccination
  postinfarction 411.0
  postinfluenza (asthenia) 780.79
  postirradiation 990
  postlaminectomy 722.80
    cervical, cervicothoracic 722.81
    lumbar, lumbosacral 722.83
    thoracic, thoracolumbar 722.82
  postleukotomy 310.0
  postlobotomy 310.0
  postmastectomy lymphedema 457.0
  postmature (of newborn) 766.22
  postmyocardial infarction 411.0
  postoperative NEC 998.9
    blind loop 579.2
  postpartum panhypopituitary 253.2
  postperfusion NEC 999.89
    bone marrow 996.85
  postpericardiotomy 429.4
  postphlebitic (asymptomatic) 459.10
    with
      complications NEC 459.19
      inflammation 459.12
        and ulcer 459.13
      stasis dermatitis 459.12
        with ulcer 459.13
      ulcer 459.11
        with inflammation 459.13
  postpolio (myelitis) 138
  postvagotomy 564.2
  postvalvulotomy 429.4
  postviral (asthenia) NEC 780.79
  Potain's (gastrectasis with dyspepsia) 536.1
  potassium intoxication 276.7
  Potter's 753.0
  Prader (-Labhart)-Willi (-Fanconi) 759.81
  preinfarction 411.1
  preleukemic 238.75
  premature senility 259.8
  premenstrual 625.4
  premenstrual tension 625.4
  pre ulcer 536.9

Syndrome *(Continued)*
  Prinzmetal-Massumi (anterior chest wall syndrome) 786.52
  Profichet's 729.90
  progeria 259.8
  progressive pallidal degeneration 333.0
  prolonged gestation 766.22
  Proteus (dermal hypoplasia) 757.39
  prune belly 756.71
  prurigo-asthma 691.8
  pseudocarpal tunnel (sublimis) 354.0
  pseudohermaphroditism-virilism hirsutism 255.2
  pseudoparalytica 358.00
  pseudo-Turner's 759.89
  psycho-organic 293.9
    acute 293.0
    anxiety type 293.84
    depressive type 293.83
    hallucinatory type 293.82
    nonpsychotic severity 310.1
      specified focal (partial) NEC 310.8
    paranoid type 293.81
    specified type NEC 293.89
    subacute 293.1
  pterygolymphangiectasia 758.6
  ptosis-epicanthus 270.2
  pulmonary
    arteriosclerosis 416.0
    hypoperfusion (idiopathic) 769
    renal (hemorrhagic) 446.21
  pulseless 446.7
  Putnam-Dana (subacute combined sclerosis with pernicious anemia) 281.0 *[336.2]*
  pyloroduodenal 537.89
  pyramidopallidonigral 332.0
  pyriformis 355.0
  QT interval prolongation 426.82
  radicular NEC 729.2
    lower limbs 724.4
    upper limbs 723.4
    newborn 767.4
  Raeder-Harbitz (pulseless disease) 446.7
  Ramsay Hunt's
    dyssynergia cerebellaris myoclonica 334.2
    herpetic geniculate ganglionitis 053.11
  rapid time-zone change 327.35
  Raymond (-Céstan) 433.8 ●
  Raynaud's (paroxysmal digital cyanosis) 443.0
  RDS (respiratory distress syndrome, newborn) 769
  Refsum's (heredopathia atactica polyneuritiformis) 356.3
  Reichmann's (gastrosuccorrhea) 536.8
  Reifenstein's (hereditary familial hypogonadism, male) 259.52
  Reilly's *(see also* Neuropathy, peripheral, autonomic 337.9
  Reiter's 099.3
  renal glomerulohyalinosis-diabetic 250.4 ● *[581.81]*
    due to secondary diabetes 249.4 ● *[581.81]*
  Rendu-Osler-Weber (familial hemorrhagic telangiectasia) 448.0
  renofacial (congenital biliary fibroangiomatosis) 753.0
  Rénon-Delille 253.8

◄ New   ◄|||| Revised   ~~deleted~~ Deleted   ● Use Additional Digit(s)   Omit code

Syndrome *(Continued)*
  respiratory distress (idiopathic)
      (newborn) 769
    adult (following shock, surgery, or
        trauma) 518.5
      specified NEC 518.82
      type II 770.6
  restless legs (RLS) 333.94
  retinoblastoma (familial) 190.5
  retraction (Duane's) 378.71
  retroperitoneal fibrosis 593.4
  retroviral seroconversion (acute) V08
  Rett's 330.8
  Reye's 331.81
  Reye-Sheehan (postpartum pituitary
      necrosis) 253.2
  Riddoch's (visual disorientation) 368.16
  Ridley's (*see also* Failure, ventricular,
      left) 428.1
  Rieger's (mesodermal dysgenesis,
      anterior ocular segment) 743.44
  Rietti-Greppi-Micheli (thalassemia
      minor) 282.49
  right ventricular obstruction - *see*
      Failure, heart
  Riley-Day (familial dysautonomia)
      742.8
  Robin's 756.0
  Rokitansky-Kuster-Hauser (congenital
      absence, vagina) 752.45 ◀▥
  Romano-Ward (prolonged QT interval
      syndrome) 426.82
  Romberg's 349.89
  Rosen-Castleman-Liebow (pulmonary
      proteinosis) 516.0
  rotator cuff, shoulder 726.10
  Roth's 355.1
  Rothmund's (congenital poikiloderma)
      757.33
  Rotor's (idiopathic hyperbilirubinemia)
      277.4
  Roussy-Lévy 334.3
  Roy (-Jutras) (acropachyderma)
      757.39
  rubella (congenital) 771.0
  Rubinstein-Taybi's (brachydactylia,
      short stature, and mental
      retardation) 759.89
  Rud's (mental deficiency, epilepsy, and
      infantilism) 759.89
  Ruiter-Pompen (-Wyers)
      (angiokeratoma corporis
      diffusum) 272.7
  Runge's (postmaturity) 766.22
  Russell (-Silver) (congenital
      hemihypertrophy and short
      stature) 759.89
  Rytand-Lipsitch (complete
      atrioventricular block) 426.0
  sacralization-scoliosis-sciatica 756.15
  sacroiliac 724.6
  Saenger's 379.46
  salt
    depletion (*see also* Disease, renal)
        593.9
      due to heat NEC 992.8
        causing heat exhaustion or
            prostration 992.4
    low (*see also* Disease, renal) 593.9
  salt-losing (*see also* Disease, renal) 593.9
  Sanfilippo's (mucopolysaccharidosis
      III) 277.5
  Scaglietti-Dagnini (acromegalic
      macrospondylitis) 253.0

Syndrome *(Continued)*
  scalded skin 695.81
  scalenus anticus (anterior) 353.0
  scapulocostal 354.8
  scapuloperoneal 359.1
  scapulovertebral 723.4
  Schaumann's (sarcoidosis) 135
  Scheie's (mucopolysaccharidosis IS)
      277.5
  Scheuthauer-Marie-Sainton
      (cleidocranialis dysostosis) 755.59
  Schirmer's (encephalocutaneous
      angiomatosis) 759.6
  schizophrenic, of childhood NEC (*see
      also* Psychosis, childhood) 299.9●
  Schmidt's
    sphallo-pharyngo-laryngeal
        hemiplegia 352.6
    thyroid-adrenocortical insufficiency
        258.1
    vagoaccessory 352.6
  Schneider's 047.9
  Schnitzler 273.1
  Scholte's (malignant carcinoid) 259.2
  Scholz (-Bielschowsky-Henneberg)
      330.0
  Schroeder's (endocrine-hypertensive)
      255.3
  Schüller-Christian (chronic
      histiocytosis X) 277.89
  Schultz's (agranulocytosis) 288.09
  Schwachman's - *see* Syndrome,
      Shwachman's
  Schwartz (-Jampel) 359.23
  Schwartz-Bartter (inappropriate
      secretion of antidiuretic hormone)
      253.6
  Scimitar (anomalous venous drainage,
      right lung to inferior vena cava)
      747.49
  sclerocystic ovary 256.4
  sea-blue histiocyte 272.7
  Seabright-Bantam
      (pseudohypoparathyroidism)
      275.49
  Seckel's 759.89
  Secretan's (posttraumatic edema) 782.3
  secretoinhibitor (keratoconjunctivitis
      sicca) 710.2
  Seeligmann's (ichthyosis congenita)
      757.1
  Senear-Usher (pemphigus
      erythematosus) 694.4
  senilism 259.8
  seroconversion, retroviral (acute) V08
  serotonin 333.99
  serous meningitis 348.2
  Sertoli cell (germinal aplasia) 606.0
  sex chromosome mosaic 758.81
  Sézary's (reticulosis) (M9701/3) 202.2●
  shaken infant 995.55
  Shaver's (bauxite pneumoconiosis) 503
  Sheehan's (postpartum pituitary
      necrosis) 253.2
  shock (traumatic) 958.4
    kidney 584.5
      following crush injury 958.5
    lung 518.5
    neurogenic 308.9
    psychic 308.9
  Shone's 746.84
  short
    bowel 579.3
    P-R interval 426.81

Syndrome *(Continued)*
  shoulder-arm (*see also* Neuropathy,
      peripheral, autonomic) 337.9
  shoulder-girdle 723.4
  shoulder-hand (*see also* Neuropathy,
      peripheral, autonomic) 337.9
  Shwachman's 288.02
  Shy-Drager (orthostatic hypotension
      with multisystem degeneration)
      333.0
  Sicard's 352.6
  sicca (keratoconjunctivitis) 710.2
  sick
    cell 276.1
    cilia 759.89
    sinus 427.81
  sideropenic 280.8
  Siemens'
    ectodermal dysplasia 757.31
    keratosis follicularis spinulosa
        (decalvans) 757.39
  Silfverskiöld's (osteochondrodystrophy,
      extremities) 756.50
  Silver's (congenital hemihypertrophy
      and short stature) 759.89
  Silvestroni-Bianco (thalassemia
      minima) 282.49
  Simons' (progressive lipodystrophy)
      272.6
  sinus tarsi 726.79
  sinusitis-bronchiectasis-situs inversus
      759.3
  Sipple's (medullary thyroid carcinoma-
      pheochromocytoma) 258.02
  Sjögren (-Gougerot)
      (keratoconjunctivitis sicca) 710.2
    with lung involvement 710.2 *[517.8]*
  Sjögren-Larsson (ichthyosis congenita)
      757.1
  SJS-TEN (Stevens-Johnson syndrome-
      toxic epidermal necrolysis
      overlap) 695.14
  Slocumb's 255.3
  Sluder's 337.09
  Smith-Lemli-Opitz (cerebrohepatorenal
      syndrome) 759.89
  Smith-Magenis 758.33
  smokers' 305.1
  Sneddon-Wilkinson (subcorneal
      pustular dermatosis) 694.1
  Sotos' (cerebral gigantism) 253.0
  South African cardiomyopathy 425.2
  spasmodic
    upward movement, eye(s) 378.82
    winking 307.20
  Spens' (syncope with heart block) 426.9
  spherophakia-brachymorphia 759.89
  spinal cord injury - *see also* Injury,
      spinal, by site
    with fracture, vertebra - *see* Fracture,
        vertebra, by site, with spinal
        cord injury
    cervical - *see* Injury, spinal, cervical
    fluid malabsorption (acquired)
        331.3
  splenic
    agenesis 759.0
    flexure 569.89
    neutropenia 289.53
    sequestration 289.52
  Spurway's (brittle bones and blue
      sclera) 756.51
  staphylococcal scalded skin 695.81
  Stein's (polycystic ovary) 256.4

Syndrome *(Continued)*
  Stein-Leventhal (polycystic ovary) 256.4
  Steinbrocker's (*see also* Neuropathy, peripheral, autonomic) 337.9
  Stevens-Johnson (erythema multiforme exudativum) 695.13
    toxic epidermal necrolysis overlap (SJS-TEN overlap syndrome) 695.14
  Stewart-Morel (hyperostosis frontalis interna) 733.3
  Stickler 759.89
  stiff-baby 759.89
  stiff-man 333.91
  Still's (juvenile rheumatoid arthritis) 714.30
  Still-Felty (rheumatoid arthritis with splenomegaly and leukopenia) 714.1
  Stilling-Türk-Duane (ocular retraction syndrome) 378.71
  Stojano's (subcostal) 098.86
  Stokes (-Adams) (syncope with heart block) 426.9
  Stokvis-Talma (enterogenous cyanosis) 289.7
  stone heart (*see also* Failure, ventricular, left) 428.1
  straight-back 756.19
  stroke (*see also* Disease, cerebrovascular, acute) 436
    little 435.9
  Sturge-Kalischer-Weber (encephalotrigeminal angiomatosis) 759.6
  Sturge-Weber (-Dimitri) (encephalocutaneous angiomatosis) 759.6
  subclavian-carotid obstruction (chronic) 446.7
  subclavian steal 435.2
  subcoracoid-pectoralis minor 447.8
  subcostal 098.86
    nerve compression 354.8
  subperiosteal hematoma 267
  subphrenic interposition 751.4
  sudden infant death (SIDS) 798.0
  Sudeck's 733.7
  Sudeck-Leriche 733.7
  superior
    cerebellar artery (*see also* Disease, cerebrovascular, acute) 436
    mesenteric artery 557.1
    pulmonary sulcus (tumor) (M8010/3) 162.3
    vena cava 459.2
  suprarenal cortical 255.3
  supraspinatus 726.10
  Susac 348.39
  swallowed blood 777.3
  sweat retention 705.1
  Sweet's (acute febrile neutrophilic dermatosis) 695.89
  Swyer-James (unilateral hyperlucent lung) 492.8
  Swyer's (XY pure gonadal dysgenesis) 752.7
  Symonds' 348.2
  sympathetic
    cervical paralysis 337.09
    pelvic 625.5
  syndactylic oxycephaly 755.55
  syphilitic-cardiovascular 093.89

Syndrome *(Continued)*
  systemic
    fibrosclerosing 710.8
    inflammatory response (SIRS) 995.90
      due to
        infectious process 995.91
          with acute organ dysfunction 995.92
        non-infectious process 995.93
          with acute organ dysfunction 995.94
  systolic click (-murmur) 785.2
  Tabagism 305.1
  tachycardia-bradycardia 427.81
  Takayasu (-Onishi) (pulseless disease) 446.7
  Takotsubo 429.83
  Tapia's 352.6
  tarsal tunnel 355.5
  Taussig-Bing (transposition, aorta and overriding pulmonary artery) 745.11
  Taybi's (otopalatodigital) 759.89
  Taylor's 625.5
  teething 520.7
  tegmental 344.89
  telangiectasis-pigmentation-cataract 757.33
  temporal 383.02
    lobectomy behavior 310.0
  temporomandibular joint-pain-dysfunction [TMJ] NEC 524.60
    specified NEC 524.69
  Terry's (*see also* Retinopathy of prematurity) 362.21
  testicular feminization 259.51
  testis, nonvirilizing 257.8
  tethered (spinal) cord 742.59
  thalamic 338.0
  Thibierge-Weissenbach (cutaneous systemic sclerosis) 710.1
  Thiele 724.6
  thoracic outlet (compression) 353.0
  thoracogenous rheumatic (hypertrophic pulmonary osteoarthropathy) 731.2
  Thorn's (*see also* Disease, renal) 593.9
  Thorson-Biörck (malignant carcinoid) 259.2
  thrombopenia-hemangioma 287.39
  thyroid-adrenocortical insufficiency 258.1
  Tietze's 733.6
  time-zone (rapid) 327.35
  Tobias' (carcinoma, pulmonary apex) (M8010/3) 162.3
  toilet seat 926.0
  Tolosa-Hunt 378.55
  Toni-Fanconi (cystinosis) 270.0
  Touraine's (hereditary osteo-onychodysplasia) 756.89
  Touraine-Solente-Golé (acropachyderma) 757.39
  toxic
    oil 710.5
    shock 040.82
  transfusion
    fetal-maternal 772.0
    twin
      donor (infant) 772.0
      recipient (infant) 776.4
  transient left ventricular apical ballooning 429.83

Syndrome *(Continued)*
  Treacher Collins' (incomplete mandibulofacial dysostosis) 756.0
  trigeminal plate 259.8
  triplex X female 758.81
  trisomy NEC 758.5
    13 or D₁ 758.1
    16–18 or E 758.2
    18 or E₃ 758.2
    20 758.5
    21 or G (mongolism) 758.0
    22 or G (mongolism) 758.0
    G 758.0
  Troisier-Hanot-Chauffard (bronze diabetes) 275.01 ◀▥
  tropical wet feet 991.4
  Trousseau's (thrombophlebitis migrans visceral cancer) 453.1
  tumor lysis (following antineoplastic drug therapy) (spontaneous) 277.88
  Türk's (ocular retraction syndrome) 378.71
  Turner's 758.6
  Turner-Varny 758.6
  Twiddler's (due to)
    automatic implantable defibrillator 996.04
    pacemaker 996.01
  twin-to-twin transfusion 762.3
    recipient twin 776.4
  Uehlinger's (acropachyderma) 757.39
  Ullrich (-Bonnevie) (-Turner) 758.6
  Ullrich-Feichtiger 759.89
  underwater blast injury (abdominal) (*see also* Injury, internal, abdomen) 868.00
  universal joint, cervix 620.6
  Unverricht (-Lundborg) 345.1●
  Unverricht-Wagner (dermatomyositis) 710.3
  upward gaze 378.81
  Urbach-Oppenheim (necrobiosis lipoidica diabeticorum) 250.8● [709.3]
    due to secondary diabetes 249.8● [709.3]
  Urbach-Wiethe (lipoid proteinosis) 272.8
  uremia, chronic 585.9
  urethral 597.81
  urethro-oculoarticular 099.3
  urethro-oculosynovial 099.3
  urohepatic 572.4
  uveocutaneous 364.24
  uveomeningeal, uveomeningitis 363.22
  vagohypoglossal 352.6
  vagovagal 780.2
  van Buchem's (hyperostosis corticalis) 733.3
  van der Hoeve's (brittle bones and blue sclera, deafness) 756.51
  van der Hoeve-Halbertsma-Waardenburg (ptosis-epicanthus) 270.2
  van der Hoeve-Waarderburg-Gualdi (ptosis-epicanthus) 270.2
  vanishing twin 651.33
  van Neck-Odelberg (juvenile osteochondrosis) 732.1
  vascular splanchnic 557.0
  vasomotor 443.9
  vasovagal 780.2

◀ New   ◀▥ Revised   ~~deleted~~ Deleted   ● Use Additional Digit(s)   ▥ Omit code

Syndrome (*Continued*)
VATER 759.89
Velo-cardio-facial 758.32
vena cava (inferior) (superior) (obstruction) 459.2
Verbiest's (claudicatio intermittens spinalis) 435.1
Vernet's 352.6
vertebral
  artery 435.1
    compression 721.1
    lumbar 724.4
    steal 435.1
vertebrogenic (pain) 724.5
vertiginous NEC 386.9
video display tube 723.8
Villaret's 352.6
Vinson-Plummer (sideropenic dysphagia) 280.8
virilizing adrenocortical hyperplasia, congenital 255.2
virus, viral 079.99
visceral larval migrans 128.0
visual disorientation 368.16
vitamin B$_6$ deficiency 266.1
vitreous touch 997.99
Vogt's (corpus striatum) 333.71
Vogt-Koyanagi 364.24
Volkmann's 958.6
von Bechterew-Stumpell (ankylosing spondylitis) 720.0
von Graefe's 378.72
von Hippel-Lindau (angiomatosis retinocerebellosa) 759.6
von Schroetter's (intermittent venous claudication) 453.89
von Willebrand (-Jürgens) (angiohemophilia) 286.4
Waardenburg-Klein (ptosis epicanthus) 270.2
Wagner (-Unverricht) (dermatomyositis) 710.3
Waldenström's (macroglobulinemia) 273.3
Waldenström-Kjellberg (sideropenic dysphagia) 280.8
Wallenberg's (posterior inferior cerebellar artery) (*see also* Disease, cerebrovascular, acute) 436
Waterhouse (-Friderichsen) 036.3
water retention 276.69
Weber's 344.89
Weber-Christian (nodular nonsuppurative panniculitis) 729.30
Weber-Cockayne (epidermolysis bullosa) 757.39
Weber-Dimitri (encephalocutaneous angiomatosis) 759.6
Weber-Gubler 344.89
Weber-Leyden 344.89
Weber-Osler (familial hemorrhagic telangiectasia) 448.0
Wegener's (necrotizing respiratory granulomatosis) 446.4
Weill-Marchesani (brachymorphism and ectopia lentis) 759.89
Weingarten's (tropical eosinophilia) 518.3
Weiss-Baker (carotid sinus syncope) 337.01
Weissenbach-Thibierge (cutaneous systemic sclerosis) 710.1
Werdnig-Hoffmann 335.0

Syndrome (*Continued*)
Werlhof-Wichmann (*see also* Purpura, thrombocytopenic) 287.39
Wermer's (polyendocrine adenomatosis) 258.01
Werner's (progeria adultorum) 259.8
Wernicke's (nonalcoholic) (superior hemorrhagic polioencephalitis) 265.1
Wernicke-Korsakoff (nonalcoholic) 294.0
  alcoholic 291.1
Westphal-Strümpell (hepatolenticular degeneration) 275.1
wet
  brain (alcoholic) 303.9●
  feet (maceration) (tropical) 991.4
  lung
    adult 518.5
    newborn 770.6
whiplash 847.0
Whipple's (intestinal lipodystrophy) 040.2
"whistling face" (craniocarpotarsal dystrophy) 759.89
Widal (-Abrami) (acquired hemolytic jaundice) 283.9
Wilkie's 557.1
Wilkinson-Sneddon (subcorneal pustular dermatosis) 694.1
Willan-Plumbe (psoriasis) 696.1
Willebrand (-Jürgens) (angiohemophilia) 286.4
Willi-Prader (hypogenital dystrophy with diabetic tendency) 759.81
Wilson's (hepatolenticular degeneration) 275.1
Wilson-Mikity 770.7
Wiskott-Aldrich (eczema-thrombocytopenia) 279.12
withdrawal
  alcohol 291.81
  drug 292.0
    infant of dependent mother 779.5
Woakes' (ethmoiditis) 471.1
Wolff-Parkinson-White (anomalous atrioventricular excitation) 426.7
Wright's (hyperabduction) 447.8
X
  cardiac 413.9
  dysmetabolic 277.7
xiphoidalgia 733.99
XO 758.6
XXX 758.81
XXXXY 758.81
XXY 758.7
yellow vernix (placental dysfunction) 762.2
Zahorsky's 074.0
Zellweger 277.86
Zieve's (jaundice, hyperlipemia and hemolytic anemia) 571.1
Zollinger-Ellison (gastric hypersecretion with pancreatic islet cell tumor) 251.5
Zuelzer-Ogden (nutritional megaloblastic anemia) 281.2
Synechia (iris) (pupil) 364.70
anterior 364.72
  peripheral 364.73
intrauterine (traumatic) 621.5
posterior 364.71
vulvae, congenital 752.49

Synesthesia (*see also* Disturbance, sensation) 782.0
Synodontia 520.2
Synophthalmus 759.89
Synorchidism 752.89
Synorchism 752.89
Synostosis (congenital) 756.59
astragaloscaphoid 755.67
radioulnar 755.53
talonavicular (bar) 755.67
tarsal 755.67
Synovial - *see* condition
Synovioma (M9040/3) - *see also* Neoplasm, connective tissue, malignant
benign (M9040/0) - *see* Neoplasm, connective tissue, benign
Synoviosarcoma (M9040/3) - *see* Neoplasm, connective tissue, malignant
Synovitis (*see also* Tenosynovitis) 727.00
chronic crepitant, wrist 727.2
due to crystals - *see* Arthritis, due to crystals
gonococcal 098.51
gouty 274.00
specified NEC 727.09
syphilitic 095.7
  congenital 090.0
traumatic, current - *see* Sprain, by site
tuberculous - *see* Tuberculosis, synovitis
villonodular 719.20
  ankle 719.27
  elbow 719.22
  foot 719.27
  hand 719.24
  hip 719.25
  knee 719.26
  multiple sites 719.29
  pelvic region 719.25
  shoulder (region) 719.21
  specified site NEC 719.28
  wrist 719.23
Syphilide 091.3
congenital 090.0
newborn 090.0
tubercular 095.8
  congenital 090.0
Syphilis, syphilitic (acquired) 097.9
with lung involvement 095.1
abdomen (late) 095.2
acoustic nerve 094.86
adenopathy (secondary) 091.4
adrenal (gland) 095.8
  with cortical hypofunction 095.8
age under 2 years NEC (*see also* Syphilis, congenital) 090.9
  acquired 097.9
alopecia (secondary) 091.82
anemia 095.8
aneurysm (artery) (ruptured) 093.89
  aorta 093.0
  central nervous system 094.89
  congenital 090.5
anus 095.8
  primary 091.1
  secondary 091.3
aorta, aortic (arch) (abdominal) (insufficiency) (pulmonary) (regurgitation) (stenosis) (thoracic) 093.89
  aneurysm 093.0

Syphilis, syphilitic (Continued)
arachnoid (adhesive) 094.2
artery 093.89
    cerebral 094.89
    spinal 094.89
arthropathy (neurogenic) (tabetic) 094.0
    [713.5]
asymptomatic - see Syphilis, latent
ataxia, locomotor (progressive) 094.0
atrophoderma maculatum 091.3
auricular fibrillation 093.89
Bell's palsy 094.89
bladder 095.8
bone 095.5
    secondary 091.61
brain 094.89
breast 095.8
bronchus 095.8
bubo 091.0
bulbar palsy 094.89
bursa (late) 095.7
cardiac decompensation 093.89
cardiovascular (early) (late) (primary)
        (secondary) (tertiary) 093.9
    specified type and site NEC 093.89
causing death under 2 years of age (see
        also Syphilis, congenital) 090.9
    stated to be acquired NEC 097.9
central nervous system (any site) (early)
        (late) (latent) (primary) (recurrent)
        (relapse) (secondary) (tertiary)
        094.9
    with
        ataxia 094.0
        paralysis, general 094.1
            juvenile 090.40
        paresis (general) 094.1
            juvenile 090.40
        tabes (dorsalis) 094.0
            juvenile 090.40
        taboparesis 094.1
            juvenile 090.40
    aneurysm (ruptured) 094.87
    congenital 090.40
    juvenile 090.40
    remission in (sustained) 094.9
    serology doubtful, negative, or
        positive 094.9
    specified nature or site NEC 094.89
    vascular 094.89
cerebral 094.89
    meningovascular 094.2
    nerves 094.89
    sclerosis 094.89
    thrombosis 094.89
cerebrospinal 094.89
    tabetic 094.0
cerebrovascular 094.89
cervix 095.8
chancre (multiple) 091.0
    extragenital 091.2
    Rollet's 091.2
Charcôt's joint 094.0 [713.5]
choked disc 094.89 [377.00]
chorioretinitis 091.51
    congenital 090.0 [363.13]
    late 094.83
choroiditis 091.51
    congenital 090.0 [363.13]
    late 094.83
    prenatal 090.0 [363.13]
choroidoretinitis (secondary) 091.51
    congenital 090.0 [363.13]
    late 094.83

Syphilis, syphilitic (Continued)
ciliary body (secondary) 091.52
    late 095.8 [364.11]
colon (late) 095.8
combined sclerosis 094.89
complicating pregnancy, childbirth, or
        puerperium 647.0●
    affecting fetus or newborn 760.2
condyloma (latum) 091.3
congenital 090.9
    with
        encephalitis 090.41
        paresis (general) 090.40
        tabes (dorsalis) 090.40
        taborparesis 090.40
    chorioretinitis, choroiditis 090.0
        [363.13]
    early or less than 2 years after birth
        NEC 090.2
        with manifestations 090.0
        latent (without manifestations)
            090.1
            negative spinal fluid test
                090.1
            serology, positive 090.1
        symptomatic 090.0
    interstitial keratitis 090.3
    juvenile neurosyphilis 090.40
    late or 2 years or more after birth
        NEC 090.7
        chorioretinitis, choroiditis 090.5
            [363.13]
        interstitial keratitis 090.3
        juvenile neurosyphilis NEC
            090.40
        latent (without manifestations)
            090.6
            negative spinal fluid test
                090.6
            serology, positive 090.6
        symptomatic or with
                manifestations NEC 090.5
            interstitial keratitis 090.3
conjugal 097.9
    tabes 094.0
conjunctiva 095.8 [372.10]
contact V01.6
cord, bladder 094.0
cornea, late 095.8 [370.59]
coronary (artery) 093.89
    sclerosis 093.89
coryza 095.8
    congenital 090.0
cranial nerve 094.89
cutaneous - see Syphilis, skin
dacryocystitis 095.8
degeneration, spinal cord 094.89
d'emblée 095.8
dementia 094.1
    paralytica 094.1
        juvenilis 090.40
destruction of bone 095.5
dilatation, aorta 093.0
due to blood transfusion 097.9
dura mater 094.89
ear 095.8
    inner 095.8
        nerve (eighth) 094.86
        neurorecurrence 094.86
early NEC 091.0
    cardiovascular 093.9
    central nervous system 094.9
        paresis 094.1
        tabes 094.0

Syphilis, syphilitic (Continued)
early NEC (Continued)
    latent (without manifestations) (less
            than 2 years after infection)
            092.9
        negative spinal fluid test 092.9
        serological relapse following
            treatment 092.0
        serology positive 092.9
    paresis 094.1
    relapse (treated, untreated) 091.7
    skin 091.3
    symptomatic NEC 091.89
        extragenital chancre 091.2
        primary, except extragenital
            chancre 091.0
        secondary (see also Syphilis,
            secondary) 091.3
            relapse (treated, untreated)
                091.7
    tabes 094.0
    ulcer 091.3
eighth nerve 094.86
endemic, nonveneral 104.0
endocarditis 093.20
    aortic 093.22
    mitral 093.21
    pulmonary 093.24
    tricuspid 093.23
epididymis (late) 095.8
epiglottis 095.8
epiphysitis (congenital) 090.0
esophagus 095.8
Eustachian tube 095.8
exposure to V01.6
eye 095.8 [363.13]
    neuromuscular mechanism
        094.85
eyelid 095.8 [373.5]
    with gumma 095.8 [373.5]
    ptosis 094.89
fallopian tube 095.8
fracture 095.5
gallbladder (late) 095.8
gastric 095.8
    crisis 094.0
    polyposis 095.8
general 097.9
    paralysis 094.1
        juvenile 090.40
genital (primary) 091.0
glaucoma 095.8
gumma (late) NEC 095.9
    cardiovascular system 093.9
    central nervous system 094.9
    congenital 090.5
    heart or artery 093.89
heart 093.89
    block 093.89
    decompensation 093.89
    disease 093.89
    failure 093.89
    valve (see also Syphilis, endocarditis)
        093.20
hemianesthesia 094.89
hemianopsia 095.8
hemiparesis 094.89
hemiplegia 094.89
hepatic artery 093.89
hepatitis 095.3
hepatomegaly 095.3
    congenital 090.0
hereditaria tarda (see also Syphilis,
        congenital, late) 090.7

◀ New   ◀▥ Revised   ~~deleted~~ Deleted   ● Use Additional Digit(s)   ▭ Omit code

Syphilis, syphilitic *(Continued)*
  hereditary *(see also* Syphilis, congenital)
      090.9
    interstitial keratitis 090.3
  Hutchinson's teeth 090.5
  hyalitis 095.8
  inactive - *see* Syphilis, latent
  infantum NEC *(see also* Syphilis,
      congenital) 090.9
  inherited - *see* Syphilis, congenital
  internal ear 095.8
  intestine (late) 095.8
  iris, iritis (secondary) 091.52
    late 095.8 *[364.11]*
  joint (late) 095.8
  keratitis (congenital) (early)
      (interstitial) (late)
      (parenchymatous) (punctata
      profunda) 090.3
  kidney 095.4
  lacrimal apparatus 095.8
  laryngeal paralysis 095.8
  larynx 095.8
  late 097.0
    cardiovascular 093.9
    central nervous system 094.9
    latent or 2 years or more after
        infection (without
        manifestation) 096
      negative spinal fluid test 096
      serology positive 096
    paresis 094.1
    specified site NEC 095.8
    symptomatic or with symptoms
        095.9
    tabes 094.0
  latent 097.1
    central nervous system 094.9
    date of infection unspecified
        097.1
    early or less than 2 years after
        infection 092.9
    late or 2 years or more after infection
        096
    serology
      doubtful
        follow-up of latent syphilis
            097.1
          central nervous system
              094.9
          date of infection unspecified
              097.1
          early or less than 2 years
              after infection 092.9
          late or 2 years or more after
              infection 096
      positive, only finding 097.1
        date of infection unspecified
            097.1
        early or less than 2 years after
            infection 097.1
        late or 2 years or more after
            infection 097.1
  lens 095.8
  leukoderma 091.3
    late 095.8
  lienis 095.8
  lip 091.3
    chancre 091.2
    late 095.8
    primary 091.2
  Lissauer's paralysis 094.1
  liver 095.3
    secondary 091.62

Syphilis, syphilitic *(Continued)*
  locomotor ataxia 094.0
  lung 095.1
  lymphadenitis (secondary) 091.4
  lymph gland (early) (secondary) 091.4
    late 095.8
  macular atrophy of skin 091.3
    striated 095.8
  maternal, affecting fetus or newborn
      760.2
    manifest syphilis in newborn - *see*
        Syphilis, congenital
  mediastinum (late) 095.8
  meninges (adhesive) (basilar) (brain)
      (spinal cord) 094.2
  meningitis 094.2
    acute 091.81
    congenital 090.42
  meningoencephalitis 094.2
  meningovascular 094.2
    congenital 090.49
  mesarteritis 093.89
    brain 094.89
    spine 094.89
  middle ear 095.8
  mitral stenosis 093.21
  monoplegia 094.89
  mouth (secondary) 091.3
    late 095.8
  mucocutaneous 091.3
    late 095.8
  mucous
    membrane 091.3
      late 095.8
    patches 091.3
      congenital 090.0
  mulberry molars 090.5
  muscle 095.6
  myocardium 093.82
  myositis 095.6
  nasal sinus 095.8
  neonatorum NEC *(see also* Syphilis,
      congenital) 090.9
  nerve palsy (any cranial nerve)
      094.89
  nervous system, central 094.9
  neuritis 095.8
    acoustic nerve 094.86
  neurorecidive of retina 094.83
  neuroretinitis 094.85
  newborn *(see also* Syphilis, congenital)
      090.9
  nodular superficial 095.8
  nonvenereal, endemic 104.0
  nose 095.8
    saddle back deformity 090.5
    septum 095.8
      perforated 095.8
  occlusive arterial disease 093.89
  ophthalmic 095.8 *[363.13]*
  ophthalmoplegia 094.89
  optic nerve (atrophy) (neuritis)
      (papilla) 094.84
  orbit (late) 095.8
  orchitis 095.8
  organic 097.9
  osseous (late) 095.5
  osteochondritis (congenital) 090.0
  osteoporosis 095.5
  ovary 095.8
  oviduct 095.8
  palate 095.8
    gumma 095.8
    perforated 090.5

Syphilis, syphilitic *(Continued)*
  pancreas (late) 095.8
  pancreatitis 095.8
  paralysis 094.89
    general 094.1
    juvenile 090.40
  paraplegia 094.89
  paresis (general) 094.1
    juvenile 090.40
  paresthesia 094.89
  Parkinson's disease or syndrome
      094.82
  paroxysmal tachycardia 093.89
  pemphigus (congenital) 090.0
  penis 091.0
    chancre 091.0
    late 095.8
  pericardium 093.81
  perichondritis, larynx 095.8
  periosteum 095.5
    congenital 090.0
    early 091.61
    secondary 091.61
  peripheral nerve 095.8
  petrous bone (late) 095.5
  pharynx 095.8
    secondary 091.3
  pituitary (gland) 095.8
  placenta 095.8
  pleura (late) 095.8
  pneumonia, white 090.0
  pontine (lesion) 094.89
  portal vein 093.89
  primary NEC 091.2
    anal 091.1
    and secondary *(see also* Syphilis,
        secondary) 091.9
    cardiovascular 093.9
    central nervous system 094.9
    extragenital chancre NEC 091.2
    fingers 091.2
    genital 091.0
    lip 091.2
    specified site NEC 091.2
    tonsils 091.2
  prostate 095.8
  psychosis (intracranial gumma) 094.89
  ptosis (eyelid) 094.89
  pulmonary (late) 095.1
    artery 093.89
  pulmonum 095.1
  pyelonephritis 095.4
  recently acquired, symptomatic NEC
      091.89
  rectum 095.8
  respiratory tract 095.8
  retina
    late 094.83
    neurorecidive 094.83
  retrobulbar neuritis 094.85
  salpingitis 095.8
  sclera (late) 095.0
  sclerosis
    cerebral 094.89
    coronary 093.89
    multiple 094.89
    subacute 094.89
  scotoma (central) 095.8
  scrotum 095.8
  secondary (and primary) 091.9
    adenopathy 091.4
    anus 091.3
    bone 091.61
    cardiovascular 093.9

S

Syphilis, syphilitic (Continued)
  secondary (Continued)
    central nervous system 094.9
    chorioretinitis, choroiditis 091.51
    hepatitis 091.62
    liver 091.62
    lymphadenitis 091.4
    meningitis, acute 091.81
    mouth 091.3
    mucous membranes 091.3
    periosteum 091.61
    periostitis 091.61
    pharynx 091.3
    relapse (treated) (untreated) 091.7
    skin 091.3
    specified form NEC 091.89
    tonsil 091.3
    ulcer 091.3
    viscera 091.69
    vulva 091.3
  seminal vesicle (late) 095.8
  seronegative
    with signs or symptoms - see
        Syphilis, by site and stage
  seropositive
    with signs or symptoms - see
        Syphilis, by site or stage
    follow-up of latent syphilis - see
        Syphilis, latent
    only finding - see Syphilis, latent
  seventh nerve (paralysis) 094.89
  sinus 095.8
  sinusitis 095.8
  skeletal system 095.5
  skin (early) (secondary) (with
      ulceration) 091.3
    late or tertiary 095.8
  small intestine 095.8
  spastic spinal paralysis 094.0
  spermatic cord (late) 095.8
  spinal (cord) 094.89
    with
        paresis 094.1
        tabes 094.0
  spleen 095.8
  splenomegaly 095.8
  spondylitis 095.5
  staphyloma 095.8
  stigmata (congenital) 090.5
  stomach 095.8
  synovium (late) 095.7

Syphilis, syphilitic (Continued)
  tabes dorsalis (early) (late) 094.0
    juvenile 090.40
  tabetic type 094.0
    juvenile 090.40
  taboparesis 094.1
    juvenile 090.40
  tachycardia 093.89
  tendon (late) 095.7
  tertiary 097.0
    with symptoms 095.8
    cardiovascular 093.9
    central nervous system 094.9
    multiple NEC 095.8
    specified site NEC 095.8
  testis 095.8
  thorax 095.8
  throat 095.8
  thymus (gland) 095.8
  thyroid (late) 095.8
  tongue 095.8
  tonsil (lingual) 095.8
    primary 091.2
    secondary 091.3
  trachea 095.8
  tricuspid valve 093.23
  tumor, brain 094.89
  tunica vaginalis (late) 095.8
  ulcer (any site) (early) (secondary)
      091.3
    late 095.9
    perforating 095.9
        foot 094.0
  urethra (stricture) 095.8
  urogenital 095.8
  uterus 095.8
  uveal tract (secondary) 091.50
    late 095.8 [363.13]
  uveitis (secondary) 091.50
    late 095.8 [363.13]
  uvula (late) 095.8
    perforated 095.8
  vagina 091.0
    late 095.8
  valvulitis NEC 093.20
  vascular 093.89
    brain or cerebral 094.89
  vein 093.89
    cerebral 094.89
  ventriculi 095.8
  vesicae urinariae 095.8

Syphilis, syphilitic (Continued)
  viscera (abdominal) 095.2
    secondary 091.69
  vitreous (hemorrhage) (opacities) 095.8
  vulva 091.0
    late 095.8
    secondary 091.3
Syphiloma 095.9
  cardiovascular system 093.9
  central nervous system 094.9
  circulatory system 093.9
  congenital 090.5
Syphilophobia 300.29
Syringadenoma (M8400/0) - see also
    Neoplasm, skin, benign
  papillary (M8406/0) - see Neoplasm,
      skin, benign
Syringobulbia 336.0
Syringocarcinoma (M8400/3) - see
    Neoplasm, skin, malignant
Syringocystadenoma (M8400/0) - see also
    Neoplasm, skin, benign
  papillary (M8406/0) - see Neoplasm,
      skin, benign
Syringocystoma (M8407/0) - see
    Neoplasm, skin, benign
Syringoma (M8407/0) - see also
    Neoplasm, skin, benign
  chondroid (M8940/0) - see Neoplasm,
      by site, benign
Syringomyelia 336.0
Syringomyelitis 323.9
  late effect - see category 326
Syringomyelocele (see also Spina bifida)
    741.9●
Syringopontia 336.0
System, systemic - see also condition
  disease, combined - see Degeneration,
      combined
  fibrosclerosing syndrome 710.8
  inflammatory response syndrome
      (SIRS) 995.90
    due to
        infectious process 995.91
            with acute organ dysfunction
                995.92
        non-infectious process 995.93
            with acute organ dysfunction
                995.94
  lupus erythematosus 710.0
    inhibitor 286.5

◀ New   ◀||||| Revised   ~~deleted~~ Deleted   ● Use Additional Digit(s)   ▓ Omit code

T

Tab - *see* Tag
Tabacism 989.84
Tabacosis 989.84
Tabardillo 080
   flea-borne 081.0
   louse-borne 080
Tabes, tabetic
   with
      central nervous system syphilis
        094.0
      Charcôt's joint 094.0 [713.5]
      cord bladder 094.0
      crisis, viscera (any) 094.0
      paralysis, general 094.1
      paresis (general) 094.1
      perforating ulcer 094.0
   arthropathy 094.0 [713.5]
   bladder 094.0
   bone 094.0
   cerebrospinal 094.0
   congenital 090.40
   conjugal 094.0
   dorsalis 094.0
      neurosyphilis 094.0
   early 094.0
   juvenile 090.40
   latent 094.0
   mesenterica (*see also* Tuberculosis)
      014.8●
   paralysis insane, general 094.1
   peripheral (nonsyphilitic) 799.89
   spasmodic 094.0
      not dorsal or dorsalis 343.9
   syphilis (cerebrospinal) 094.0
Taboparalysis 094.1
Taboparesis (remission) 094.1
   with
      Charcôt's joint 094.1 [713.5]
      cord bladder 094.1
      perforating ulcer 094.1
   juvenile 090.40
Tache noir 923.20
Tachyalimentation 579.3
Tachyarrhythmia, tachyrhythmia - *see also*
   Tachycardia
   paroxysmal with sinus bradycardia
      427.81
Tachycardia 785.0
   atrial 427.89
   auricular 427.89
   AV nodal re-entry (re-entrant)
      427.89
   junctional ectopic 427.0
   newborn 779.82
   nodal 427.89
      nonparoxysmal atrioventricular
        426.89
      nonparoxysmal atrioventricular (nodal)
        426.89
   nonsustained 427.2
   paroxysmal 427.2
      with sinus bradycardia 427.81
      atrial (PAT) 427.0
        psychogenic 316 [427.0]
      atrioventricular (AV) 427.0
        psychogenic 316 [427.0]
      essential 427.2
      junctional 427.0
      nodal 427.0
      psychogenic 316 [427.2]
        atrial 316 [427.0]
        supraventricular 316 [427.0]
        ventricular 316 [427.1]

Tachycardia (*Continued*)
   paroxysmal (*Continued*)
      supraventricular 427.0
        psychogenic 316 [427.0]
      ventricular 427.1
        psychogenic 316 [427.1]
   postoperative 997.1
   psychogenic 306.2
   sick sinus 427.81
   sinoauricular 427.89
   sinus 427.89
   supraventricular 427.89
   sustained 427.2
      supraventricular 427.0
      ventricular 427.1
   ventricular (paroxysmal) 427.1
      psychogenic 316 [427.1]
Tachygastria 536.8
Tachypnea 786.06
   hysterical 300.11
   newborn (idiopathic) (transitory) 770.6
   psychogenic 306.1
   transitory, of newborn 770.6
TACO (transfusion associated circulatory
   overload) 276.61 ◀
Taenia (infection) (infestation) (*see also*
   Infestation, taenia) 123.3
   diminuta 123.6
   echinococcal infestation (*see also*
      Echinococcus) 122.9
   nana 123.6
   saginata infestation 123.2
   solium (intestinal form) 123.0
      larval form 123.1
Taeniasis (intestine) (*see also* Infestation,
   taenia) 123.3
   saginata 123.2
   solium 123.0
Taenzer's disease 757.4
Tag (hypertrophied skin) (infected) 701.9
   adenoid 474.8
   anus 455.9
   endocardial (*see also* Endocarditis) 424.90
   hemorrhoidal 455.9
   hymen 623.8
   perineal 624.8
   preauricular 744.1
   rectum 455.9
   sentinel 455.9
   skin 701.9
      accessory 757.39
      anus 455.9
      congenital 757.39
      preauricular 744.1
      rectum 455.9
   tonsil 474.8
   urethra, urethral 599.84
   vulva 624.8
Tahyna fever 062.5
Takayasu (-Onishi) disease or syndrome
   (pulseless disease) 446.7
Takotsubo syndrome 429.83
Talc granuloma 728.82
   in operation wound 998.7
Talcosis 502
Talipes (congenital) 754.70
   acquired NEC 736.79
      planus 734
   asymmetric 754.79
      acquired 736.79
   calcaneovalgus 754.62
      acquired 736.76
   calcaneovarus 754.59
      acquired 736.76
   calcaneus 754.79
      acquired 736.76

Talipes (*Continued*)
   cavovarus 754.59
      acquired 736.75
   cavus 754.71
      acquired 736.73
   equinovalgus 754.69
      acquired 736.72
   equinovarus 754.51
      acquired 736.71
   equinus 754.79
      acquired, NEC 736.72
   percavus 754.71
      acquired 736.73
   planovalgus 754.69
      acquired 736.79
   planus (acquired) (any degree) 734
      congenital 754.61
      due to rickets 268.1
   valgus 754.60
      acquired 736.79
   varus 754.50
      acquired 736.79
Talma's disease 728.85
Talon noir 924.20
   hand 923.20
   heel 924.20
   toe 924.3
Tamponade heart (Rose's) (*see also*
   Pericarditis) 423.3
Tanapox 059.21
Tangier disease (familial high-density
   lipoprotein deficiency) 272.5
Tank ear 380.12
Tantrum (childhood) (*see also* Disturbance,
   conduct) 312.1●
Tapeworm (infection) (infestation) (*see
   also* Infestation, tapeworm) 123.9
Tapia's syndrome 352.6
Tarantism 297.8
Target-oval cell anemia 282.49
Tarlov's cyst 355.9
Tarral-Besnier disease (pityriasis rubra
   pilaris) 696.4
Tarsalgia 729.2
Tarsal tunnel syndrome 355.5
Tarsitis (eyelid) 373.00
   syphilitic 095.8 [373.00]
   tuberculous (*see also* Tuberculosis)
      017.0● [373.4]
Tartar (teeth) 523.6
Tattoo (mark) 709.09
Taurodontism 520.2
Taussig-Bing defect, heart, or syndrome
   (transposition, aorta and overriding
   pulmonary artery) 745.11
Tay's choroiditis 363.41
Tay-Sachs
   amaurotic familial idiocy 330.1
   disease 330.1
Taybi's syndrome (otopalatodigital)
   759.89
Taylor's
   disease (diffuse idiopathic cutaneous
      atrophy) 701.8
   syndrome 625.5
TBI (traumatic brain injury) (*see also*
   Injury, intracranial) 854.0●
   with skull fracture - *see* Fracture,
      skull, by site
Tear, torn (traumatic) - *see also* Wound,
   open, by site
   anus, anal (sphincter) 863.89
      with open wound in cavity 863.99
      complicating delivery (healed) (old)
        654.8●
        with mucosa 664.3●

Tear, torn *(Continued)*
  anus, anal *(Continued)*
    complicating delivery *(Continued)*
      not associated with third-degree
        perineal laceration 664.6●
    nontraumatic, nonpuerperal
      (healed) (old) 569.43
  articular cartilage, old *(see also*
    Disorder, cartilage, articular)
    718.0●
  bladder
    with
      abortion - *see* Abortion, by type,
        with damage to pelvic
        organs
      ectopic pregnancy *(see also*
        categories 633.0–633.9)
        639.2
      molar pregnancy *(see also*
        categories 630–632) 639.2
    following
      abortion 639.2
      ectopic or molar pregnancy 639.2
    obstetrical trauma 665.5●
  bowel
    with
      abortion - *see* Abortion, by type,
        with damage to pelvic
        organs
      ectopic pregnancy *(see also*
        categories 633.0–633.9) 639.2
      molar pregnancy *(see also*
        categories 630–632) 639.2
    following
      abortion 639.2
      ectopic or molar pregnancy
        639.2
    obstetrical trauma 665.5●
  broad ligament
    with
      abortion - *see* Abortion, by type,
        with damage to pelvic
        organs
      ectopic pregnancy *(see also*
        categories 633.0–633.9)
        639.2
      molar pregnancy *(see also*
        categories 630–632) 639.2
    following
      abortion 639.2
      ectopic or molar pregnancy
        639.2
    obstetrical trauma 665.6●
  bucket handle (knee) (meniscus) - *see*
    Tear, meniscus
  capsule
    joint - *see* Sprain, by site
    spleen - *see* Laceration, spleen,
      capsule
  cartilage - *see also* Sprain, by site
    articular, old *(see also* Disorder,
      cartilage, articular) 718.0●
    knee - *see* Tear, meniscus
    semilunar (knee) (current injury) -
      see Tear, meniscus
  cervix
    with
      abortion - *see* Abortion, by type,
        with damage to pelvic
        organs
      ectopic pregnancy *(see also*
        categories 633.0–633.9)
        639.2
      molar pregnancy *(see also*
        categories 630–632) 639.2

Tear, torn *(Continued)*
  cervix *(Continued)*
    following
      abortion 639.2
      ectopic or molar pregnancy 639.2
    obstetrical trauma (current) 665.3●
    old 622.3
  dural 349.31
    accidental puncture or laceration
      during a procedure 349.31
    incidental (inadvertent) 349.31
    nontraumatic NEC 349.39
  internal organ (abdomen, chest, or
    pelvis) - *see* Injury, internal, by
    site
  ligament - *see also* Sprain, by site
    with open wound - *see* Wound,
      open, by site
  meniscus (knee) (current injury) 836.2
    bucket handle 836.0
      old 717.0
    lateral 836.1
      anterior horn 836.1
        old 717.42
      bucket handle 836.1
        old 717.41
      old 717.40
      posterior horn 836.1
        old 717.43
      specified site NEC 836.1
        old 717.49
    medial 836.0
      anterior horn 836.0
        old 717.1
      bucket handle 836.0
        old 717.0
      old 717.3
      posterior horn 836.0
        old 717.2
    old NEC 717.5
    site other than knee - *see* Sprain, by
      site
  muscle - *see also* Sprain, by site
    with open wound - *see* Wound,
      open, by site
  pelvic
    floor, complicating delivery 664.1●
    organ NEC
      with
        abortion - *see* Abortion, by
          type, with damage to
          pelvic organs
        ectopic pregnancy *(see also*
          categories 633.0–633.9)
          639.2
        molar pregnancy *(see also*
          categories 630–632) 639.2
      following
        abortion 639.2
        ectopic or molar pregnancy
          639.2
      obstetrical trauma 665.5●
  perineum - *see also* Laceration,
    perineum
    obstetrical trauma 665.5●
  periurethral tissue
    with
      abortion - *see* Abortion, by type,
        with damage to pelvic
        organs
      ectopic pregnancy *(see also*
        categories 633.0–633.9) 639.2
      molar pregnancy *(see also*
        categories 630–632) 639.2
    following
      abortion 639.2
      ectopic or molar pregnancy 639.2

Tear, torn *(Continued)*
  periurethral tissue *(Continued)*
    obstetrical trauma 664.8● ◀▥
  rectovaginal septum - *see* Laceration,
    rectovaginal septum
  retina, retinal (recent) (with
    detachment) 361.00
    without detachment 361.30
    dialysis (juvenile) (with detachment)
      361.04
    giant (with detachment) 361.03
    horseshoe (without detachment)
      361.32
    multiple (with detachment) 361.02
      without detachment 361.33
    old
      delimited (partial) 361.06
      partial 361.06
      total or subtotal 361.07
    partial (without detachment)
      giant 361.03
      multiple defects 361.02
      old (delimited) 361.06
      single defect 361.01
    round hole (without detachment)
      361.31
    single defect (with detachment)
      361.01
    total or subtotal (recent) 361.05
      old 361.07
  rotator cuff (traumatic) 840.4
    current injury 840.4
    degenerative 726.10
    nontraumatic 727.61
  semilunar cartilage, knee *(see also* Tear,
    meniscus) 836.2
    old 717.5
  tendon - *see also* Sprain, by site
    with open wound - *see* Wound,
      open, by site
  tentorial, at birth 767.0
  umbilical cord
    affecting fetus or newborn 772.0
    complicating delivery 663.8●
  urethra
    with
      abortion - *see* Abortion, by type,
        with damage to pelvic
        organs
      ectopic pregnancy *(see also*
        categories 633.0–633.9) 639.2
      molar pregnancy *(see also*
        categories 630–632) 639.2
    following
      abortion 639.2
      ectopic or molar pregnancy
        639.2
    obstetrical trauma 665.5●
  uterus - *see* Injury, internal, uterus
  vagina - *see* Laceration, vagina
  vessel, from catheter 998.2
  vulva, complicating delivery
    664.0●
Tear stone 375.57
Teeth, tooth - *see also* condition
  grinding 306.8
  prenatal 520.6
Teething 520.7
  syndrome 520.7
Tegmental syndrome 344.89
Telangiectasia, telangiectasis (verrucous)
  448.9
  ataxic (cerebellar) 334.8
  familial 448.0
  hemorrhagic, hereditary (congenital)
    (senile) 448.0

Telangiectasia, telangiectasis (Continued)
   hereditary hemorrhagic 448.0
   retina 362.15
   spider 448.1
Telecanthus (congenital) 743.63
Telescoped bowel or intestine (see also
   Intussusception) 560.0
Teletherapy, adverse effect NEC 990
Telogen effluvium 704.02
Temperature
   body, high (of unknown origin) (see also
     Pyrexia) 780.60
   cold, trauma from 991.9
     newborn 778.2
     specified effect NEC 991.8
   high
     body (of unknown origin) (see also
      Pyrexia) 780.60
     trauma from - see Heat
Temper tantrum (childhood) (see also
   Disturbance, conduct) 312.1●
Temple - see condition
Temporal - see also condition
   lobe syndrome 310.0
Temporomandibular joint-pain-
   dysfunction syndrome 524.60
Temporosphenoidal - see condition
Tendency
   bleeding (see also Defect, coagulation)
     286.9
   homosexual, ego-dystonic
     302.0
   paranoid 301.0
   suicide 300.9
Tenderness
   abdominal (generalized) (localized)
     789.6●
   rebound 789.6●
   skin 782.0
Tendinitis, tendonitis (see also
   Tenosynovitis) 726.90
   Achilles 726.71
   adhesive 726.90
     shoulder 726.0
   calcific 727.82
     shoulder 726.11
   gluteal 726.5
   patellar 726.64
   peroneal 726.79
   pes anserinus 726.61
   psoas 726.5
   tibialis (anterior) (posterior) 726.72
   trochanteric 726.5
Tendon - see condition
Tendosynovitis - see Tenosynovitis
Tendovaginitis - see Tenosynovitis
Tenesmus 787.99
   rectal 787.99
   vesical 788.99
Tenia - see Taenia
Teniasis - see Taeniasis
Tennis elbow 726.32
Tenonitis - see also Tenosynovitis
   eye (capsule) 376.04
Tenontosynovitis - see Tenosynovitis
Tenontothecitis - see Tenosynovitis
Tenophyte 727.9
Tenosynovitis (see also Synovitis) 727.00
   adhesive 726.90
     shoulder 726.0
   ankle 727.06
   bicipital (calcifying) 726.12
   buttock 727.09
   due to crystals - see Arthritis, due to
     crystals
   elbow 727.09

Tenosynovitis (Continued)
   finger 727.05
   foot 727.06
   gonococcal 098.51
   hand 727.05
   hip 727.09
   knee 727.09
   radial styloid 727.04
   shoulder 726.10
     adhesive 726.0
   specified NEC 727.09
   spine 720.1
   supraspinatus 726.10
   toe 727.06
   tuberculous - see Tuberculosis,
     tenosynovitis
   wrist 727.05
Tenovaginitis - see Tenosynovitis
Tension
   arterial, high (see also Hypertension)
     401.9
     without diagnosis of hypertension
      796.2
   headache 307.81
   intraocular (elevated) 365.00
   nervous 799.21
   ocular (elevated) 365.00
   pneumothorax 512.0
     iatrogenic 512.1
     postoperative 512.1
     spontaneous 512.0
   premenstrual 625.4
   state 300.9
Tentorium - see condition
Teratencephalus 759.89
Teratism 759.7
Teratoblastoma (malignant)
   (M9080/3) - see Neoplasm,
   by site, malignant
Teratocarcinoma (M9081/3) - see also
   Neoplasm, by site, malignant
   liver 155.0
Teratoma (solid) (M9080/1) - see also
   Neoplasm, by site, uncertain
   behavior
   adult (cystic) (M9080/0) - see
     Neoplasm, by site, benign
   and embryonal carcinoma, mixed
     (M9081/3) - see Neoplasm, by
     site, malignant
   benign (M9080/0) - see Neoplasm, by
     site, benign
   combined with choriocarcinoma
     (M9101/3) - see Neoplasm, by
     site, malignant
   cystic (adult) (M9080/0) - see
     Neoplasm, by site, benign
   differentiated type (M9080/0) - see
     Neoplasm, by site, benign
   embryonal (M9080/3) - see also
     Neoplasm, by site, malignant
     liver 155.0
   fetal
     sacral, causing fetopelvic
      disproportion 653.7●
   immature (M9080/3) - see Neoplasm,
     by site, malignant
   liver (M9080/3) 155.0
     adult, benign, cystic, differentiated
      type, or mature (M9080/0)
      211.5
   malignant (M9080/3) - see also
     Neoplasm, by site, malignant
     anaplastic type (M9082/3) - see
      Neoplasm, by site, malignant

Teratoma (Continued)
   malignant (Continued)
     intermediate type (M9083/3) -
      see Neoplasm, by site,
      malignant
     liver (M9080/3) 155.0
     trophoblastic (M9102/3)
      specified site - see Neoplasm, by
       site, malignant
      unspecified site 186.9
     undifferentiated type (M9082/3) -
      see Neoplasm, by site,
      malignant
   mature (M9080/0) - see Neoplasm, by
     site, benign
   malignant (M9080/3) - see
     Neoplasm, by site,
     malignant
   ovary (M9080/0) 220
     embryonal, immature, or
      malignant (M9080/3)
      183.0
   suprasellar (M9080/3) - see
     Neoplasm, by site,
     malignant
   testis (M9080/3) 186.9
     adult, benign, cystic, differentiated
      type or mature (M9080/0)
      222.0
   undescended 186.0
Terminal care V66.7
Termination
   anomalous - see also Malposition,
     congenital
     portal vein 747.49
     right pulmonary vein 747.42
   pregnancy (legal) (therapeutic) (see
     Abortion, legal) 635.9●
     fetus NEC 779.6
     illegal (see also Abortion, illegal)
      636.9●
Ternidens diminutus infestation
   127.7
Terrors, night (child) 307.46
Terry's syndrome (see also
   Retinopathy of prematurity)
   362.21
Tertiary - see condition
Tessellated fundus, retina (tigroid)
   362.89
Test(s)
   adequacy
     hemodialysis V56.31
     peritoneal dialysis V56.32
   AIDS virus V72.69
   allergen V72.7
   bacterial disease NEC (see also
     Screening, by name of disease)
     V74.9
   basal metabolic rate V72.69
   blood
     alcohol V70.4
     drug V70.4
      for therapeutic drug monitoring
       V58.83
      for routine general physical
       examination V72.62
      prior to treatment or procedure
       V72.63
      typing V72.86
       Rh typing V72.86
   developmental, infant or child
     V20.2
   Dick V74.8
   fertility V26.21

Test(s) *(Continued)*
  genetic
    female V26.32
    for genetic disease carrier status
      female V26.31
      male V26.34
    male V26.39
  hearing V72.19
    following failed hearing screening
      V72.11
    routine, for infant and child V20.2
  HIV V72.69
  human immunodeficiency virus V72.69
  immunity status V72.61
  Kveim V82.89
  laboratory V72.60
    for medicolegal reason V70.4
    ordered as part of a routine
      general medical
      examination V72.62
    pre-operative V72.63
    pre-procedural V72.63
    specified NEC V72.69
  male partner of female with recurrent
    pregnancy loss V26.35 ◀
  Mantoux (for tuberculosis) V74.1
  mycotic organism V75.4
  nuchal translucency V28.89
  parasitic agent NEC V75.8
  paternity V70.4
  peritoneal equilibration V56.32
  pregnancy
    negative result V72.41
    positive result V72.42
      first pregnancy V72.42
    unconfirmed V72.40
  preoperative V72.84
    cardiovascular V72.81
    respiratory V72.82
    specified NEC V72.83
  procreative management NEC V26.29
    genetic disease carrier status
      female V26.31
      male V26.34
  Rh typing V72.86
  sarcoidosis V82.89
  Schick V74.3
  Schultz-Charlton V74.8
  skin, diagnostic
    allergy V72.7
    bacterial agent NEC *(see also*
      Screening, by name of
      disease) V74.9
    Dick V74.8
    hypersensitivity V72.7
    Kveim V82.89
    Mantoux V74.1
    mycotic organism V75.4
    parasitic agent NEC V75.8
    sarcoidosis V82.89
    Schick V74.3
    Schultz-Charlton V74.8
    tuberculin V74.1
  specified type NEC V72.85
  tuberculin V74.1
  vision V72.0
    routine, for infant and child
      V20.2
  Wassermann
    positive *(see also* Serology for
      syphilis, positive) 097.1
    false 795.6
Testicle, testicular, testis - *see also*
  condition
  feminization (syndrome) 259.51
Tetanus, tetanic (cephalic) (convulsions)
  037

Tetanus, tetanic *(Continued)*
  with
    abortion - *see* Abortion, by type,
      with sepsis
    ectopic pregnancy *(see also*
      categories 633.0–633.9) 639.0
    molar pregnancy *(see* categories
      630–632) 639.0
  following
    abortion 639.0
    ectopic or molar pregnancy 639.0
  inoculation V03.7
    reaction (due to serum) - *see*
      Complications, vaccination
  neonatorum 771.3
  puerperal, postpartum, childbirth
    670.8●
Tetany, tetanic 781.7
  alkalosis 276.3
  associated with rickets 268.0
  convulsions 781.7
    hysterical 300.11
  functional (hysterical) 300.11
  hyperkinetic 781.7
    hysterical 300.11
  hyperpnea 786.01
    hysterical 300.11
    psychogenic 306.1
  hyperventilation 786.01
    hysterical 300.11
    psychogenic 306.1
  hypocalcemic, neonatal 775.4
  hysterical 300.11
  neonatal 775.4
  parathyroid (gland) 252.1
  parathyroprival 252.1
  postoperative 252.1
  postthyroidectomy 252.1
  pseudotetany 781.7
    hysterical 300.11
  psychogenic 306.1
    specified as conversion reaction
      300.11
Tetralogy of Fallot 745.2
Tetraplegia - *see* Quadriplegia
Thailand hemorrhagic fever 065.4
Thalassanemia 282.49
Thalassemia (alpha) (beta) (disease)
  (Hb-C) (Hb-D) (Hb-E) (Hb-H)
  (Hb-I) (high fetal gene) (high fetal
  hemoglobin) (intermedia) (major)
  (minima) (minor) (mixed) (trait)
  (with other hemoglobinopathy)
  282.49
  Hb-S (without crisis) 282.41
    with
      crisis 282.42
      vaso-occlusive pain 282.42
  sickle-cell (without crisis) 282.41
    with
      crisis 282.42
      vaso-occlusive pain 282.42
Thalassemic variants 282.49
Thaysen-Gee disease (nontropical
  sprue) 579.0
Thecoma (M8600/0) 220
  malignant (M8600/3) 183.0
Thelarche, precocious 259.1
Thelitis 611.0
  puerperal, postpartum 675.0●
Therapeutic - *see* condition
Therapy V57.9
  blood transfusion, without reported
    diagnosis V58.2
  breathing V57.0
  chemotherapy, antineoplastic
    V58.11

Therapy *(Continued)*
  chemotherapy, antineoplastic
    (Continued)
    fluoride V07.31
    prophylactic NEC V07.39
  dialysis (intermittent) (treatment)
    extracorporeal V56.0
    peritoneal V56.8
    renal V56.0
    specified type NEC V56.8
  exercise NEC V57.1
    breathing V57.0
  extracorporeal dialysis (renal) V56.0
  fluoride prophylaxis V07.31
  hemodialysis V56.0
  hormone replacement
    (postmenopausal) V07.4
  immunotherapy antineoplastic V58.12
  long term oxygen therapy V46.2
  occupational V57.21
  orthoptic V57.4
  orthotic V57.81
  peritoneal dialysis V56.8
  physical NEC V57.1
  postmenopausal hormone replacement
    V07.4
  radiation V58.0
  speech (-language) V57.3
  vocational V57.22
Thermalgesia 782.0
Thermalgia 782.0
Thermanalgesia 782.0
Thermanesthesia 782.0
Thermic - *see* condition
Thermography (abnormal) 793.99
  breast 793.89
Thermoplegia 992.0
Thesaurismosis
  amyloid 277.39
  bilirubin 277.4
  calcium 275.40
  cystine 270.0
  glycogen *(see also* Disease, glycogen
    storage) 271.0
  kerasin 272.7
  lipoid 272.7
  melanin 255.41
  phosphatide 272.7
  urate 274.9
Thiaminic deficiency 265.1
  with beriberi 265.0
Thibierge-Weissenbach syndrome
  (cutaneous systemic sclerosis) 710.1
Thickened endometrium 793.5
Thickening
  bone 733.99
    extremity 733.99
  breast 611.79
  hymen 623.3
  larynx 478.79
  nail 703.8
    congenital 757.5
  periosteal 733.99
  pleura *(see also* Pleurisy) 511.0
  skin 782.8
  subepiglottic 478.79
  tongue 529.8
  valve, heart - *see* Endocarditis
Thiele syndrome 724.6
Thigh - *see* condition
Thinning vertebra *(see also* Osteoporosis)
  733.00
Thirst, excessive 783.5
  due to deprivation of water 994.3
Thomsen's disease 359.22
Thomson's disease (congenital
  poikiloderma) 757.33

◀ New   ◀ Revised   ~~deleted~~ Deleted   ● Use Additional Digit(s)   Omit code

Thoracic - *see also* condition
  kidney 753.3
  outlet syndrome 353.0
  stomach - *see* Hernia, diaphragm
Thoracogastroschisis (congenital) 759.89
Thoracopagus 759.4
Thoracoschisis 756.3
Thoracoscopic surgical procedure
    converted to open procedure V64.42
Thorax - *see* condition
Thorn's syndrome (*see also* Disease, renal)
  593.9
Thornwaldt's, Tornwaldt's
  bursitis (pharyngeal) 478.29
  cyst 478.26
  disease (pharyngeal bursitis) 478.29
Thorson-Biörck syndrome (malignant
    carcinoid) 259.2
Threadworm (infection) (infestation) 127.4
Threatened
  abortion or miscarriage 640.0●
    with subsequent abortion (*see also*
      Abortion, spontaneous) 634.9●
      affecting fetus 762.1
    labor 644.1●
      affecting fetus or newborn 761.8
      premature 644.0●
    miscarriage 640.0●
      affecting fetus 762.1
    premature
      delivery 644.2●
        affecting fetus or newborn 761.8
      labor 644.0●
        before 22 completed weeks
          gestation 640.0●
Three-day fever 066.0
Threshers' lung 495.0
Thrix annulata (congenital) 757.4
Throat - *see* condition
Thrombasthenia (Glanzmann's)
  (hemorrhagic) (hereditary) 287.1
Thromboangiitis 443.1
  obliterans (general) 443.1
    cerebral 437.1
    vessels
      brain 437.1
      spinal cord 437.1
Thromboarteritis - *see* Arteritis
Thromboasthenia (Glanzmann's)
  (hemorrhagic) (hereditary) 287.1
Thrombocytasthenia (Glanzmann's) 287.1
Thrombocythemia (primary) (M9962/1)
  238.71
  essential 238.71
  hemorrhagic 238.71
  idiopathic (hemorrhagic) (M9962/1)
    238.71
Thrombocytopathy (dystrophic)
  (granulopenic) 287.1
Thrombocytopenia, thrombocytopenic
  287.5
  with
    absent radii (TAR) syndrome 287.33
    giant hemangioma 287.39
  amegakaryocytic, congenital 287.33
  congenital 287.33
  cyclic 287.39
  dilutional 287.49 ◀▥
  due to
    drugs 287.49 ◀▥
    extracorporeal circulation of blood
      287.49 ◀▥
    massive blood transfusion 287.49 ◀▥
    platelet alloimmunization 287.49 ◀▥
  essential 287.30
  fetal 678.0●
  heparin-induced (HIT) 289.84

Thrombocytopenia,
  thrombocytopenic (*Continued*)
  hereditary 287.33
  Kasabach-Merritt 287.39
  neonatal, transitory 776.1
    due to
      exchange transfusion 776.1
      idiopathic maternal
        thrombocytopenia 776.1
      isoimmunization 776.1
  primary 287.30
  puerperal, postpartum 666.3●
  purpura (*see also* Purpura,
    thrombocytopenic) 287.30
    thrombotic 446.6
  secondary NEC 287.49 ◀▥
  sex-linked 287.39
Thrombocytosis 238.71
  essential 238.71
  primary 238.71
Thromboembolism - *see* Embolism
Thrombopathy (Bernard-Soulier)
  287.1
  constitutional 286.4
  Willebrand-Jürgens (angiohemophilia)
    286.4
Thrombopenia (*see also*
  Thrombocytopenia) 287.5
Thrombophlebitis 451.9
  antecubital vein 451.82
  antepartum (superficial) 671.2●
    affecting fetus or newborn 760.3
    deep 671.3●
  arm 451.89
    deep 451.83
    superficial 451.82
  breast, superficial 451.89
  cavernous (venous) sinus - *see*
    Thrombophlebitis, intracranial
    venous sinus
  cephalic vein 451.82
  cerebral (sinus) (vein) 325
    late effect - *see* category 326
    nonpyogenic 437.6
      in pregnancy or puerperium
        671.5●
      late effect - *see* Late effect(s) (of)
        cerebrovascular disease
  due to implanted device - *see*
    Complications, due to (presence
    of) any device, implant, or graft
    classified to 996.0–996.5 NEC
  during or resulting from a procedure
    NEC 997.2
  femoral 451.11
  femoropopliteal 451.19
  following infusion, perfusion, or
    transfusion 999.2
  hepatic (vein) 451.89
  idiopathic, recurrent 453.1
  iliac vein 451.81
  iliofemoral 451.11
  intracranial venous sinus (any) 325
    late effect - *see* category 326
    nonpyogenic 437.6
      in pregnancy or puerperium
        671.5●
      late effect - *see* Late effect(s) (of)
        cerebrovascular disease
  jugular vein 451.89
  lateral (venous) sinus - *see*
    Thrombophlebitis, intracranial
    venous sinus
  leg 451.2
    deep (vessels) 451.19
      femoral vein 451.11
      specified vessel NEC 451.19

Thrombophlebitis (*Continued*)
  leg (*Continued*)
    superficial (vessels) 451.0
      femoral vein 451.11
  longitudinal (venous) sinus - *see*
    Thrombophlebitis, intracranial
    venous sinus
  lower extremity 451.2
    deep (vessels) 451.19
      femoral vein 451.11
      specified vessel NEC 451.19
    superficial (vessels) 451.0
  migrans, migrating 453.1
  pelvic
    with
      abortion - *see* Abortion, by type,
        with sepsis
      ectopic pregnancy (*see also*
        categories 633.0–633.9) 639.0
      molar pregnancy (*see also*
        categories 630–632) 639.0
    following
      abortion 639.0
      ectopic or molar pregnancy 639.0
    puerperal 671.4●
  popliteal vein 451.19
  portal (vein) 572.1
  postoperative 997.2
  pregnancy (superficial) 671.2●
    affecting fetus or newborn 760.3
    deep 671.3●
  puerperal, postpartum, childbirth
    (extremities) (superficial)
    671.2●
    deep 671.4●
    pelvic 671.4●
    septic 670.3●
    specified site NEC 671.5●
  radial vein 451.82
  saphenous (greater) (lesser) 451.0
  sinus (intracranial) - *see*
    Thrombophlebitis, intracranial
    venous sinus
  specified site NEC 451.89
  tibial vein 451.19
Thrombosis, thrombotic (marantic)
  (multiple) (progressive) (vein)
  (vessel) 453.9
  with childbirth or during the
    puerperium - see Thrombosis,
    puerperal, postpartum
  antepartum - *see* Thrombosis,
    pregnancy
  aorta, aortic 444.1
    abdominal 444.0
    bifurcation 444.0
    saddle 444.0
    terminal 444.0
    thoracic 444.1
    valve - *see* Endocarditis, aortic
  apoplexy (*see also* Thrombosis, brain)
    434.0●
    late effect - *see* Late effect(s) (of)
      cerebrovascular disease
  appendix, septic - *see* Appendicitis,
    acute
  arteriolar-capillary platelet,
    disseminated 446.6
  artery, arteries (postinfectional) 444.9
    auditory, internal 433.8●
    basilar (*see also* Occlusion, artery,
      basilar) 433.0●
    carotid (common) (internal) (*see also*
      Occlusion, artery, carotid)
      433.1●
      with other precerebral artery
        433.3●

Thrombosis, thrombotic (Continued)
  artery, arteries (Continued)
    cerebellar (anterior inferior)
        (posterior inferior) (superior)
        433.8●
    cerebral (see also Thrombosis, brain)
        434.0●
    choroidal (anterior) 433.8●
    communicating posterior 433.8●
    coronary (see also Infarct,
        myocardium) 410.9●
      without myocardial infarction
          411.81
      due to syphilis 093.89
      healed or specified as old 412
    extremities 444.22
      lower 444.22
      upper 444.21
    femoral 444.22
    hepatic 444.89
    hypophyseal 433.8●
    meningeal, anterior or posterior
        433.8●
    mesenteric (with gangrene) 557.0
    ophthalmic (see also Occlusion,
        retina) 362.30
    pontine 433.8●
    popliteal 444.22
    precerebral - see Occlusion, artery,
        precerebral NEC
    pulmonary 415.19
      iatrogenic 415.11
      personal history of V12.51
      postoperative 415.11
      septic 415.12
    renal 593.81
    retinal (see also Occlusion, retina)
        362.30
    specified site NEC 444.89
    spinal, anterior or posterior 433.8●
    traumatic (complication) (early) (see
        also Injury, blood vessel, by
        site) 904.9
    vertebral (see also Occlusion, artery,
        vertebral) 433.2●
      with other precerebral artery
          433.3●
  atrial (endocardial) 424.90
    without endocarditis 429.89
    due to syphilis 093.89
  auricular (see also Infarct, myocardium)
      410.9●
  axillary (acute) (vein) 453.84
    chronic 453.74
    personal history of V12.51
  basilar (artery) (see also Occlusion,
      artery, basilar) 433.0●
  bland NEC 453.9
  brain (artery) (stem) 434.0●
    due to syphilis 094.89
    iatrogenic 997.02
    late effect - see Late effect(s) (of)
        cerebrovascular disease
    postoperative 997.02
    puerperal, postpartum, childbirth
        674.0●
    sinus (see also Thrombosis,
        intracranial venous sinus)
        325
  capillary 448.9
    arteriolar, generalized 446.6
  cardiac (see also Infarct, myocardium)
      410.9●
    due to syphilis 093.89
    healed or specified as old 412
    valve - see Endocarditis

Thrombosis, thrombotic (Continued)
  carotid (artery) (common) (internal)
      (see also Occlusion, artery, carotid)
      433.1●
    with other precerebral artery
        433.3●
  cavernous sinus (venous) - see
      Thrombosis, intracranial venous
      sinus
  cerebellar artery (anterior inferior)
      (posterior inferior) (superior)
      433.8●
    late effect - see Late effect(s) (of)
        cerebrovascular disease
  cerebral (arteries) (see also Thrombosis,
      brain) 434.0●
    late effect - see Late effect(s) (of)
        cerebrovascular disease
  coronary (artery) (see also Infarct,
      myocardium) 410.9●
    without myocardial infarction
        411.81
    due to syphilis 093.89
    healed or specified as old 412
  corpus cavernosum 607.82
  cortical (see also Thrombosis, brain)
      434.0●
  due to (presence of) any device,
      implant, or graft classifiable to
      996.0–996.5 - see Complications,
      due to (presence of) any device,
      implant, or graft classified to
      996.0–996.5 NEC
  effort 453.89
  endocardial - see Infarct, myocardium
  eye (see also Occlusion, retina)
      362.30
  femoral (vein) 453.6
    with inflammation or phlebitis
        451.11
    artery 444.22
    deep 453.41
    personal history of V12.51
  genital organ, male 608.83
  heart (chamber) (see also Infarct,
      myocardium) 410.9●
  hepatic (vein) 453.0
    artery 444.89
    infectional or septic 572.1
  iliac (acute) (vein) 453.89◀▥
    with inflammation or phlebitis
        451.81
    artery (common) (external)
        (internal) 444.81
    chronic 453.79 ◀
    personal history of V12.51
  inflammation, vein - see
      Thrombophlebitis
  internal carotid artery (see also
      Occlusion, artery, carotid) 433.1●
    with other precerebral artery
        433.3●
  intestine (with gangrene) 557.0
  intracranial (see also Thrombosis, brain)
      434.0●
    venous sinus (any) 325
      nonpyogenic origin 437.6
        in pregnancy or puerperium
            671.5●
  intramural (see also Infarct,
      myocardium) 410.9●
    without
      cardiac condition 429.89
      coronary artery disease 429.89
      myocardial infarction 429.89
    healed or specified as old 412

Thrombosis, thrombotic (Continued)
  jugular (bulb)
    external (acute) 453.89 ◀▥
      acute 453.89
      chronic 453.79
    internal (acute) 453.86 ◀▥
      acute 453.86
      chronic 453.76
  kidney 593.81
    artery 593.81
  lateral sinus (venous) - see
      Thrombosis, intracranial
      venous sinus
  leg (see also Thrombosis, lower
      extremity) 453.6
    with inflammation or phlebitis - see
        Thrombophlebitis
    deep (vessels) 453.40
      acute 453.40
        lower (distal) 453.42
        upper (proximal) 453.41
      chronic 453.50
        lower (distal) 453.52
        upper (proximal) 453.51
      lower (distal) 453.42
      upper (proximal) 453.41
    personal history of V12.51
    superficial (vessels) 453.6
  liver (venous) 453.0
    artery 444.89
    infectional or septic 572.1
    portal vein 452
  longitudinal sinus (venous) - see
      Thrombosis, intracranial venous
      sinus
  lower extremity (superficial)
      453.6
    deep vessels 453.40
      acute 453.40
        calf 453.42
        distal (lower leg)
            453.42
        femoral 453.41
        iliac 453.41
        lower leg 453.42
        peroneal 453.42
        popliteal 453.41
        proximal (upper leg)
            453.41
        thigh 453.41
        tibial 453.42
      chronic 453.50
        calf 453.52
        distal (lower leg)
            453.52
        femoral 453.51
        iliac 453.51
        lower leg 453.52
        peroneal 453.52
        popliteal 453.51
        proximal (upper leg)
            453.51
        thigh 453.51
        tibial 453.52
    personal history of V12.51
    saphenous (greater) (lesser)
        453.6
    superficial 453.6
  lung 415.19
    iatrogenic 415.11
    personal history of V12.51
    postoperative 415.11
    septic 415.12
  marantic, dural sinus 437.6

◀ New   ◀▥ Revised   ~~deleted~~ Deleted   ● Use Additional Digit(s)   ▥ Omit code

Thrombosis, thrombotic (*Continued*)
 meninges (brain) (*see also* Thrombosis, brain) 434.0●
 mesenteric (artery) (with gangrene) 557.0
  vein (inferior) (superior) 557.0
 mitral - *see* Insufficiency, mitral
 mural (heart chamber) (*see also* Infarct, myocardium) 410.9●
  without
   cardiac condition 429.89
   coronary artery disease 429.89
   myocardial infarction 429.89
  due to syphilis 093.89
  following myocardial infarction 429.79
  healed or specified as old 412
 omentum (with gangrene) 557.0
 ophthalmic (artery) (*see also* Occlusion, retina) 362.30
 pampiniform plexus (male) 608.83
  female 620.8
 parietal (*see also* Infarct, myocardium) 410.9●
 penis, penile 607.82
 peripheral arteries 444.22
  lower 444.22
  upper 444.21
 platelet 446.6
 portal 452
  due to syphilis 093.89
  infectional or septic 572.1
 precerebral artery - *see also* Occlusion, artery, precerebral NEC
 pregnancy 671.2●
  deep (vein) 671.3●
  superficial (vein) 671.2●
 puerperal, postpartum, childbirth 671.2●
  brain (artery) 674.0●
   venous 671.5●
  cardiac 674.8●
  cerebral (artery) 674.0●
   venous 671.5●
  deep (vein) 671.4●
  intracranial sinus (nonpyogenic) (venous) 671.5●
  pelvic 671.4●
  pulmonary (artery) 673.2●
  specified site NEC 671.5●
  superficial 671.2●
 pulmonary (artery) (vein) 415.19
  iatrogenic 415.11
  personal history of V12.51
  postoperative 415.11
  septic 415.12
 renal (artery) 593.81
  vein 453.3
 resulting from presence of shunt or other internal prosthetic device - *see* Complications, due to (presence of) any device, implant, or graft classifiable to 996.0–996.5 NEC
 retina, retinal (artery) 362.30
  arterial branch 362.32
  central 362.31
  partial 362.33
  vein
   central 362.35
   tributary (branch) 362.36
 saphenous vein (greater) (lesser) 453.6
 scrotum 608.83
 seminal vesicle 608.83

Thrombosis, thrombotic (*Continued*)
 sigmoid (venous) sinus (*see* Thrombosis, intracranial venous sinus) 325
 silent NEC 453.9
 sinus, intracranial (venous) (any) (*see also* Thrombosis, intracranial venous sinus) 325
 softening, brain (*see also* Thrombosis, brain) 434.0●
 specified site NEC (acute) 453.89
  chronic 453.79
 spermatic cord 608.83
 spinal cord 336.1
  due to syphilis 094.89
  in pregnancy or puerperium 671.5●
  pyogenic origin 324.1
   late effect - *see* category 326
 spleen, splenic 289.59
  artery 444.89
 testis 608.83
 traumatic (complication) (early) (*see also* Injury, blood vessel, by site) 904.9
 tricuspid - *see* Endocarditis, tricuspid
 tumor - *see* Neoplasm, by site
 tunica vaginalis 608.83
 umbilical cord (vessels) 663.6●
  affecting fetus or newborn 762.6
 upper extremity 453.83
  acute 453.83
   deep 453.82
   superficial 453.81
  chronic 453.73
   deep 453.72
   superficial 453.71
 vas deferens 608.83
 vein
  antecubital (acute) 453.81 ◄▥
   acute 453.81
   chronic 453.71
  axillary (acute) 453.84 ◄▥
   acute 453.84
   chronic 453.74
  basilic (acute) 453.81 ◄▥
   acute 453.81
   chronic 453.71
  brachial (acute) 453.82 ◄▥
   acute 453.82
   chronic 453.72
  brachiocephalic (innominate) (acute) 453.87 ◄▥
   acute 453.87
   chronic 453.77
  cephalic (acute) 453.81 ◄▥
   acute 453.81
   chronic 453.71
  deep 453.40
   personal history of V12.51
  internal jugular (acute) 453.86 ◄▥
   acute 453.86
   chronic 453.76
  lower extremity - *see* Thrombosis, lower extremity
  personal history of V12.51
  radial (acute) 453.82 ◄▥
   acute 453.82
   chronic 453.72
  saphenous (greater) (lesser) 453.6
  specified site NEC (acute) 453.89 ◄▥
   acute 453.89
   chronic 453.79
  subclavian (acute) 453.85 ◄▥
   acute 453.85
   chronic 453.75

Thrombosis, thrombotic (*Continued*)
 vein (*Continued*)
  superior vena cava (acute) 453.87 ◄▥
   acute 453.87
   chronic 453.77
  thoracic (acute) 453.87 ◄▥
   acute 453.87
   chronic 453.77
  ulnar (acute) 453.82 ◄▥
   acute 453.82
   chronic 453.72
  upper extremity - *see* Thrombosis, upper extremity
 vena cava
  inferior 453.2
  personal history of V12.51
  superior (acute) 453.87 ◄▥
   acute 453.87
   chronic 453.77
Thrombus - *see* Thrombosis
Thrush 112.0
 newborn 771.7
Thumb - *see also* condition
 gamekeeper's 842.12
 sucking (child problem) 307.9
Thygeson's superficial punctate keratitis 370.21
Thymergasia (*see also* Psychosis, affective) 296.80
Thymitis 254.8
Thymoma (benign) (M8580/0) 212.6
 malignant (M8580/3) 164.0
Thymus, thymic (gland) - *see* condition
Thyrocele (*see also* Goiter) 240.9
Thyroglossal - *see also* condition
 cyst 759.2
 duct, persistent 759.2
Thyroid (body) (gland) - *see also* condition
 hormone resistance 246.8
 lingual 759.2
Thyroiditis 245.9
 acute (pyogenic) (suppurative) 245.0
  nonsuppurative 245.0
 autoimmune 245.2
 chronic (nonspecific) (sclerosing) 245.8
  fibrous 245.3
  lymphadenoid 245.2
  lymphocytic 245.2
  lymphoid 245.2
 complicating pregnancy, childbirth, or puerperium 648.1●
 de Quervain's (subacute granulomatous) 245.1
 fibrous (chronic) 245.3
 giant (cell) (follicular) 245.1
 granulomatous (de Quervain's) (subacute) 245.1
 Hashimoto's (struma lymphomatosa) 245.2
 iatrogenic 245.4
 invasive (fibrous) 245.3
 ligneous 245.3
 lymphocytic (chronic) 245.2
 lymphoid 245.2
 lymphomatous 245.2
 pseudotuberculous 245.1
 pyogenic 245.0
 radiation 245.4
 Riedel's (ligneous) 245.3
 subacute 245.1
 suppurative 245.0

Thyroiditis *(Continued)*
  tuberculous *(see also* Tuberculosis)
      017.5●
  viral 245.1
  woody 245.3
Thyrolingual duct, persistent
      759.2
Thyromegaly 240.9
Thyrotoxic
  crisis or storm *(see also* Thyrotoxicosis)
      242.9●
  heart failure *(see also* Thyrotoxicosis)
      242.9● *[425.7]*
Thyrotoxicosis 242.9●

> Note: Use the following fifth-digit
> subclassification with category 242:
>
> 0   without mention of thyrotoxic
>   crisis or storm
> 1   with mention of thyrotoxic crisis
>   or storm

  with
      goiter (diffuse) 242.0●
          adenomatous 242.3●
              multinodular 242.2●
              uninodular 242.1●
          nodular 242.3●
              multinodular 242.2●
              uninodular 242.1●
      infiltrative●
          dermopathy 242.0●
          ophthalmopathy 242.0●
          thyroid acropachy 242.0●
  complicating pregnancy, childbirth, or
          puerperium 648.1●
  due to
      ectopic thyroid nodule 242.4●
      ingestion of (excessive) thyroid
          material 242.8●
      specified cause NEC 242.8●
  factitia 242.8●
  heart 242.9● *[425.7]*
  neonatal (transient) 775.3
TIA (transient ischemic attack) 435.9
  with transient neurologic deficit
      435.9
  late effect - *see* Late effect(s) (of)
      cerebrovascular disease
Tibia vara 732.4
Tic 307.20
  breathing 307.20
  child problem 307.21
  compulsive 307.22
  convulsive 307.20
  degenerative (generalized) (localized)
      333.3
      facial 351.8
  douloureux *(see also* Neuralgia,
      trigeminal) 350.1
      atypical 350.2
  habit 307.20
      chronic (motor or vocal) 307.22
      transient (of childhood) 307.21
  lid 307.20
      transient (of childhood) 307.21
  motor-verbal 307.23
  occupational 300.89
  orbicularis 307.20
      transient (of childhood) 307.21
  organic origin 333.3
  postchoreic - *see* Chorea
  psychogenic 307.20
      compulsive 307.22
  salaam 781.0

Tic *(Continued)*
  spasm 307.20
      chronic (motor or vocal) 307.22
      transient (of childhood) 307.21
Tick (-borne) fever NEC 066.1
  American mountain 066.1
  Colorado 066.1
  hemorrhagic NEC 065.3
      Crimean 065.0
      Kyasanur Forest 065.2
      Omsk 065.1
  mountain 066.1
  nonexanthematous 066.1
Tick-bite fever NEC 066.1
  African 087.1
  Colorado (virus) 066.1
  Rocky Mountain 082.0
Tick paralysis 989.5
Tics and spasms, compulsive 307.22
Tietze's disease or syndrome 733.6
Tight, tightness
  anus 564.89
  chest 786.59
  fascia (lata) 728.9
  foreskin (congenital) 605
  hymen 623.3
  introitus (acquired) (congenital) 623.3
  rectal sphincter 564.89
  tendon 727.81
      Achilles (heel) 727.81
  urethral sphincter 598.9
Tilting vertebra 737.9
Timidity, child 313.21
Tinea (intersecta) (tarsi) 110.9
  amiantacea 110.0
  asbestina 110.0
  barbae 110.0
  beard 110.0
  black dot 110.0
  blanca 111.2
  capitis 110.0
  corporis 110.5
  cruris 110.3
  decalvans 704.09
  flava 111.0
  foot 110.4
  furfuracea 111.0
  imbricata (Tokelau) 110.5
  lepothrix 039.0
  manuum 110.2
  microsporic *(see also*
      Dermatophytosis) 110.9
  nigra 111.1
  nodosa 111.2
  pedis 110.4
  scalp 110.0
  specified site NEC 110.8
  sycosis 110.0
  tonsurans 110.0
  trichophytic *(see also*
      Dermatophytosis) 110.9
  unguium 110.1
  versicolor 111.0
Tingling sensation *(see also*
      Disturbance, sensation)
      782.0
Tin-miners' lung 503
Tinnitus (aurium) 388.30
  audible 388.32
  objective 388.32
  subjective 388.31
Tipped, teeth 524.33
Tipping
  pelvis 738.6
      with disproportion (fetopelvic)
          653.0●

Tipping *(Continued)*
  pelvis *(Continued)*
      with disproportion *(Continued)*
          affecting fetus or newborn 763.1
          causing obstructed labor
              660.1●
              affecting fetus or newborn
                  763.1
  teeth 524.33
Tiredness 780.79
Tissue - *see* condition
Tobacco
  abuse (affecting health) NEC *(see also*
      Abuse, drugs, nondependent)
      305.1
  heart 989.84
  use disorder complicating pregnancy,
      childbirth, or the puerperium
      649.0●
Tobias' syndrome (carcinoma,
      pulmonary apex) (M8010/3) 162.3
Tocopherol deficiency 269.1
Todd's
  cirrhosis - *see* Cirrhosis, biliary
  paralysis (postepileptic transitory
      paralysis) 344.89
Toe - *see* condition
Toilet, artificial opening *(see also*
      Attention to, artificial, opening)
      V55.9
Tokelau ringworm 110.5
Tollwut 071
Tolosa-Hunt syndrome 378.55
Tommaselli's disease
  correct substance properly
      administered 599.70
  overdose or wrong substance given or
      taken 961.4
Tongue - *see also* condition
  worms 134.1
Tongue tie 750.0
Toni-Fanconi syndrome (cystinosis)
      270.0
Tonic pupil 379.46
Tonsil - *see* condition
Tonsillitis (acute) (catarrhal) (croupous)
      (follicular) (gangrenous) (infective)
      (lacunar) (lingual) (malignant)
      (membranous) (phlegmonous)
      (pneumococcal)
      (pseudomembranous) (purulent)
      (septic) (staphylococcal) (subacute)
      (suppurative) (toxic) (ulcerative)
      (vesicular) (viral) 463
  with influenza, flu, or grippe *(see also*
      Influenza) 487.1 ◀▥
  chronic 474.00
  diphtheritic (membranous) 032.0
  hypertrophic 474.00
  influenzal *(see also* Influenza) 487.1 ◀▥
  parenchymatous 475
  streptococcal 034.0
  tuberculous *(see also* Tuberculosis)
      012.8●
  Vincent's 101
Tonsillopharyngitis 465.8
Tooth, teeth - *see* condition
Toothache 525.9
Topagnosis 782.0
Tophi (gouty) 274.03
  ear 274.81
  heart 274.82
  specified site NEC 274.82
TORCH infection - *(see also* Infection,
      congenital) 760.2
Torn - *see* Tear, torn

Tornwaldt's bursitis (disease)
  (pharyngeal bursitis) 478.29
  cyst 478.26
Torpid liver 573.9
Torsion
  accessory tube 620.5
  adnexa (female) 620.5
  aorta (congenital) 747.29
    acquired 447.1
  appendix
    epididymis 608.24
    testis 608.23
  bile duct 576.8
    with calculus, choledocholithiasis
      or stones - see
      Choledocholithiasis
    congenital 751.69
  bowel, colon, or intestine 560.2
  cervix - see Malposition, uterus
  duodenum 537.3
  dystonia - see Dystonia, torsion
  epididymis 608.24
    appendix 608.24
  fallopian tube 620.5
  gallbladder (see also Disease,
    gallbladder) 575.8
    congenital 751.69
  gastric 537.89
  hydatid of Morgagni (female)
    620.5
  kidney (pedicle) 593.89
  Meckel's diverticulum (congenital)
    751.0
  mesentery 560.2
  omentum 560.2
  organ or site, congenital NEC - see
    Anomaly, specified type NEC
  ovary (pedicle) 620.5
    congenital 752.0
  oviduct 620.5
  penis 607.89
    congenital 752.69
  renal 593.89
  spasm - see Dystonia, torsion
  spermatic cord 608.22
    extravaginal 608.21
    intravaginal 608.22
  spleen 289.59
  testicle, testis 608.20
    appendix 608.23
  tibia 736.89
  umbilical cord - see Compression,
    umbilical cord
  uterus (see also Malposition, uterus)
    621.6
Torticollis (intermittent) (spastic) 723.5
  congenital 754.1
    sternomastoid 754.1
  due to birth injury 767.8
  hysterical 300.11
  ocular 781.93
  psychogenic 306.0
    specified as conversion reaction
      300.11
  rheumatic 723.5
  rheumatoid 714.0
  spasmodic 333.83
  traumatic, current NEC 847.0
Tortuous
  artery 447.1
  fallopian tube 752.19
  organ or site, congenital NEC - see
    Distortion
  renal vessel (congenital) 747.62
  retina vessel (congenital) 743.58
    acquired 362.17

Tortuous (Continued)
  ureter 593.4
  urethra 599.84
  vein - see Varicose, vein
Torula, torular (infection) 117.5
  histolytica 117.5
  lung 117.5
Torulosis 117.5
Torus
  fracture
    fibula 823.41
      with tibia 823.42
    humerus 812.49
    radius (alone) 813.45
      with ulna 813.47
    tibia 823.40
      with fibula 823.42
    ulna (alone) 813.46
      with radius 813.47
  mandibularis 526.81
  palatinus 526.81
Touch, vitreous 997.99
Touraine's syndrome (hereditary osteo-
  onychodysplasia) 756.89
Touraine-Solente-Golé syndrome
  (acropachyderma) 757.39
Tourette's disease (motor-verbal tic)
  307.23
Tower skull 756.0
  with exophthalmos 756.0
Toxemia 799.89
  with
    abortion - see Abortion, by type,
      with toxemia
    bacterial - see Septicemia
    biliary (see also Disease, biliary)
      576.8
    burn - see Burn, by site
    congenital NEC 779.89
    eclamptic 642.6●
      with pre-existing hypertension
        642.7●
    erysipelatous (see also Erysipelas) 035
    fatigue 799.89
    fetus or newborn NEC 779.89
    food (see also Poisoning, food) 005.9
    gastric 537.89
    gastrointestinal 558.2
    intestinal 558.2
    kidney (see also Disease, renal) 593.9
    lung 518.89
    malarial NEC (see also Malaria) 084.6
    maternal (of pregnancy), affecting fetus
      or newborn 760.0
    myocardial - see Myocarditis, toxic
    of pregnancy (mild) (pre-eclamptic)
      642.4●
      with
        convulsions 642.6●
        pre-existing hypertension
          642.7●
      affecting fetus or newborn 760.0
      severe 642.5●
    pre-eclamptic - see Toxemia, of
      pregnancy
    puerperal, postpartum - see Toxemia, of
      pregnancy
    pulmonary 518.89
    renal (see also Disease, renal) 593.9
    septic (see also Septicemia) 038.9
    small intestine 558.2
    staphylococcal 038.10
      aureus 038.11
      due to food 005.0
      specified organism NEC 038.19
    stasis 799.89

Toxemia (Continued)
  stomach 537.89
  uremic (see also Uremia) 586
  urinary 586
Toxemica cerebropathia psychica
  (nonalcoholic) 294.0
  alcoholic 291.1
Toxic (poisoning) - see also condition
  from drug or poison - see Table of
    Drugs and Chemicals
  oil syndrome 710.5
  shock syndrome 040.82
  thyroid (gland) (see also Thyrotoxicosis)
    242.9●
Toxicemia - see Toxemia
Toxicity
  dilantin
    asymptomatic 796.0
    symptomatic -see Table of Drugs and
      Chemicals
  drug
    asymptomatic 796.0
    symptomatic - see Table of Drugs
      and Chemicals
  fava bean 282.2
  from drug or poison
    asymptomatic 796.0
    symptomatic - see Table of Drugs
      and Chemicals
Toxicosis (see also Toxemia) 799.89
  capillary, hemorrhagic 287.0
Toxinfection 799.89
  gastrointestinal 558.2
Toxocariasis 128.0
Toxoplasma infection, generalized
  130.9
Toxoplasmosis (acquired) 130.9
  with pneumonia 130.4
  congenital, active 771.2
  disseminated (multisystemic) 130.8
  maternal
    with suspected damage to fetus
      affecting management of
        pregnancy 655.4●
    affecting fetus or newborn
      760.2
    manifest toxoplasmosis in fetus
      or newborn 771.2
  multiple sites 130.8
  multisystemic disseminated 130.8
  specified site NEC 130.7
Trabeculation, bladder 596.8
Trachea - see condition
Tracheitis (acute) (catarrhal) (infantile)
  (membranous) (plastic)
  (pneumococcal) (septic)
  (suppurative) (viral) 464.10
  with
    bronchitis 490
      acute or subacute 466.0
      chronic 491.8
      tuberculosis - see Tuberculosis,
        pulmonary
    laryngitis (acute) 464.20
      with obstruction 464.21
      chronic 476.1
      tuberculous (see also Tuberculosis,
        larynx) 012.3●
    obstruction 464.11
  chronic 491.8
    with
      bronchitis (chronic) 491.8
      laryngitis (chronic) 476.1
      due to external agent - see
        Condition, respiratory, chronic,
        due to

◀ New   ◀▥ Revised   ~~deleted~~ Deleted   ● Use Additional Digit(s)   ▨ Omit code

Transposition (*Continued*)
heart 746.87
with complete transposition of viscera 759.3
intestine (large) (small) 751.5
pulmonary veins 747.49
reversed jejunal (for bypass) (status) V45.3
scrotal 752.81
stomach 750.7
with general transposition of viscera 759.3
teeth, tooth 524.30
vessels (complete) 745.10
partial 745.11
viscera (abdominal) (thoracic) 759.3
Trans-sexualism 302.50
with
asexual history 302.51
heterosexual history 302.53
homosexual history 302.52
Transverse - *see also* condition
arrest (deep), in labor 660.3 ●
affecting fetus or newborn 763.1
lie 652.3 ●
before labor, affecting fetus or newborn 761.7
causing obstructed labor 660.0 ●
affecting fetus or newborn 763.1
during labor, affecting fetus or newborn 763.1
Transvestism, transvestitism (transvestic fetishism) 302.3
Trapped placenta (with hemorrhage) 666.0 ●
without hemorrhage 667.0 ●
Trauma, traumatism (*see also* Injury, by site) 959.9
birth - *see* Birth, injury NEC
causing hemorrhage of pregnancy or delivery 641.8 ●
complicating
abortion - *see* Abortion, by type, with damage to pelvic organs
ectopic pregnancy (*see also* categories 633.0–633.9) 639.2
molar pregnancy (*see also* categories 630–632) 639.2
during delivery NEC 665.9 ●
following
abortion 639.2
ectopic or molar pregnancy 639.2
maternal, during pregnancy, affecting fetus or newborn 760.5
neuroma - *see* Injury, nerve, by site
previous major, affecting management of pregnancy, childbirth, or puerperium V23.89
psychic (current) - *see also* Reaction, adjustment
previous (history) V15.49
psychologic, previous (affecting health) V15.49
transient paralysis - *see* Injury, nerve, by site
Traumatic - *see also* condition
brain injury (TBI) (*see also* Injury, intracranial) 854.0 ●
with skull fracture - *see* Fracture, skull, by site
Treacher Collins' syndrome (incomplete facial dysostosis) 756.0
Treitz's hernia - *see* Hernia, Treitz's
Trematode infestation NEC 121.9
Trematodiasis NEC 121.9
Trembles 988.8

Trembling paralysis (*see also* Parkinsonism) 332.0
Tremor 781.0
essential (benign) 333.1
familial 333.1
flapping (liver) 572.8
hereditary 333.1
hysterical 300.11
intention 333.1
medication-induced postural 333.1
mercurial 985.0
muscle 728.85
Parkinson's (*see also* Parkinsonism) 332.0
psychogenic 306.0
specified as conversion reaction 300.11
senilis 797
specified type NEC 333.1
Trench
fever 083.1
foot 991.4
mouth 101
nephritis - *see* Nephritis, acute
Treponema pallidum infection (*see also* Syphilis) 097.9
Treponematosis 102.9
due to
T. pallidum - *see* Syphilis
T. pertenue (yaws) (*see also* Yaws) 102.9
Triad
Kartagener's 759.3
Reiter's (complete) (incomplete) 099.3
Saint's (*see also* Hernia, diaphragm) 553.3
Trichiasis 704.2
cicatricial 704.2
eyelid 374.05
with entropion (*see also* Entropion) 374.00
Trichinella spiralis (infection) (infestation) 124
Trichinelliasis 124
Trichinellosis 124
Trichiniasis 124
Trichinosis 124
Trichobezoar 938
intestine 936
stomach 935.2
Trichocephaliasis 127.3
Trichocephalosis 127.3
Trichocephalus infestation 127.3
Trichoclasis 704.2
Trichoepithelioma (M8100/0) - *see also* Neoplasm, skin, benign
breast 217
genital organ NEC - *see* Neoplasm, by site, benign
malignant (M8100/3) - *see* Neoplasm, skin, malignant
Trichofolliculoma (M8101/0) - *see* Neoplasm, skin, benign
Tricholemmoma (M8102/0) - *see* Neoplasm, skin, benign
Trichomatosis 704.2
Trichomoniasis 131.9
bladder 131.09
cervix 131.09
intestinal 007.3
prostate 131.03
seminal vesicle 131.09
specified site NEC 131.8
urethra 131.02
urogenitalis 131.00

Trichomoniasis (*Continued*)
vagina 131.01
vulva 131.01
vulvovaginal 131.01
Trichomycosis 039.0
axillaris 039.0
nodosa 111.2
nodularis 111.2
rubra 039.0
Trichonocardiosis (axillaris) (palmellina) 039.0
Trichonodosis 704.2
Trichophytid, trichophyton infection (*see also* Dermatophytosis) 110.9
Trichophytide - *see* Dermatophytosis
Trichophytobezoar 938
intestine 936
stomach 935.2
Trichophytosis - *see* Dermatophytosis
Trichoptilosis 704.2
Trichorrhexis (nodosa) 704.2
Trichosporosis nodosa 111.2
Trichostasis spinulosa (congenital) 757.4
Trichostrongyliasis (small intestine) 127.6
Trichostrongylosis 127.6
Trichostrongylus (instabilis) infection 127.6
Trichotillomania 312.39
Trichromat, anomalous (congenital) 368.59
Trichromatopsia, anomalous (congenital) 368.59
Trichuriasis 127.3
Trichuris trichiuria (any site) (infection) (infestation) 127.3
Tricuspid (valve) - *see* condition
Trifid - *see also* Accessory
kidney (pelvis) 753.3
tongue 750.13
Trigeminal neuralgia (*see also* Neuralgia, trigeminal) 350.1
Trigeminoencephaloangiomatosis 759.6
Trigeminy 427.89
postoperative 997.1
Trigger finger (acquired) 727.03
congenital 756.89
Trigonitis (bladder) (chronic) (pseudomembranous) 595.3
tuberculous (*see also* Tuberculosis) 016.1 ●
Trigonocephaly 756.0
Trihexosidosis 272.7
Trilobate placenta - *see* Placenta, abnormal
Trilocular heart 745.8
Trimethylaminuria 270.8
Tripartita placenta - *see* Placenta, abnormal
Triple - *see also* Accessory
kidneys 753.3
uteri 752.2
X female 758.81
Triplegia 344.89
congenital or infantile 343.8
Triplet
affected by maternal complications of pregnancy 761.5
healthy liveborn - *see* Newborn, multiple
pregnancy (complicating delivery) NEC 651.1 ●
with fetal loss and retention of one or more fetus(es) 651.4 ●
following (elective) fetal reduction 651.7 ●
Triplex placenta - *see* Placenta, abnormal

Triplication - *see* Accessory
Trismus 781.0
  neonatorum 771.3
  newborn 771.3
Trisomy (syndrome) NEC 758.5
  13 (partial) 758.1
  16–18 758.2
  18 (partial) 758.2
  21 (partial) 758.0
  22 758.0
  autosomes NEC 758.5
  D_1 758.1
  E_3 758.2
  G (group) 758.0
  group D_1 758.1
  group E 758.2
  group G 758.0
Tritanomaly 368.53
Tritanopia 368.53
Troisier-Hanot-Chauffard syndrome
    (bronze diabetes) 275.01 ◀▥
Trombidiosis 133.8
Trophedema (hereditary) 757.0
  congenital 757.0
Trophoblastic disease (*see also*
    Hydatidiform mole) 630
  previous, affecting management of
    pregnancy V23.1
Tropholymphedema 757.0
Trophoneurosis NEC 356.9
  arm NEC 354.9
  disseminated 710.1
  facial 349.89
  leg NEC 355.8
  lower extremity NEC 355.8
  upper extremity NEC 354.9
Tropical - *see also* condition
  maceration feet (syndrome) 991.4
  wet foot (syndrome) 991.4
Trouble - *see also* Disease
  bowel 569.9
  heart - *see* Disease, heart
  intestine 569.9
  kidney (*see also* Disease, renal)
    593.9
  nervous 799.21
  sinus (*see also* Sinusitis) 473.9
Trousseau's syndrome (thrombophlebitis
    migrans) 453.1
Truancy, childhood - *see also* Disturbance,
    conduct
  socialized 312.2 ●
  undersocialized, unsocialized 312.1 ●
Truncus
  arteriosus (persistent) 745.0
  common 745.0
  communis 745.0
Trunk - *see* condition
Trychophytide - *see* Dermatophytosis
Trypanosoma infestation - *see*
    Trypanosomiasis
Trypanosomiasis 086.9
  with meningoencephalitis 086.9
    [323.2]
  African 086.5
    due to Trypanosoma 086.5
      gambiense 086.3
      rhodesiense 086.4
  American 086.2
    with
      heart involvement 086.0
      other organ involvement 086.1
    without mention of organ
      involvement 086.2
  Brazilian - *see* Trypanosomiasis,
    American

Trypanosomiasis (*Continued*)
  Chagas' - *see* Trypanosomiasis,
    American
  due to Trypanosoma
    cruzi - *see* Trypanosomiasis,
      American
    gambiense 086.3
    rhodesiense 086.4
  gambiensis, Gambian 086.3
  North American - *see* Trypanosomiasis,
    American
  rhodesiensis, Rhodesian 086.4
  South American - *see* Trypanosomiasis,
    American
T-shaped incisors 520.2
Tsutsugamushi fever 081.2
Tube, tubal, tubular - *see also* condition
  ligation, admission for V25.2
Tubercle - *see also* Tuberculosis
  brain, solitary 013.2 ●
  Darwin's 744.29
  epithelioid noncaseating 135
  Ghon, primary infection 010.0 ●
Tuberculid, tuberculide (indurating)
    (lichenoid) (miliary)
    (papulonecrotic) (primary) (skin)
    (subcutaneous) (*see also*
    Tuberculosis) 017.0 ●
Tuberculoma - *see also* Tuberculosis
  brain (any part) 013.2 ●
  meninges (cerebral) (spinal) 013.1 ●
  spinal cord 013.4 ●
Tuberculosis, tubercular, tuberculous
    (calcification) (calcified) (caseous)
    (chromogenic acid-fast bacilli)
    (congenital) (degeneration) (disease)
    (fibrocaseous) (fistula) (gangrene)
    (interstitial) (isolated circumscribed
    lesions) (necrosis) (parenchymatous)
    (ulcerative) 011.9 ●

> Note: Use the following fifth-digit
> subclassification with categories
> 010–018:
>
> 0   unspecified
> 1   bacteriological or histological
>   examination not done
> 2   bacteriological or histological
>   examination unknown (at
>   present)
> 3   tubercle bacilli found (in sputum)
>   by microscopy
> 4   tubercle bacilli not found (in
>   sputum) by microscopy, but
>   found by bacterial culture
> 5   tubercle bacilli not found by
>   bacteriological examination,
>   but tuberculosis confirmed
>   histologically
> 6   tubercle bacilli not found by
>   bacteriological or
>   histological examination,
>   but tuberculosis confirmed
>   by other methods
>   [inoculation of animals]
>
> For tuberculous conditions specified as
> late effects or sequelae, *see* category
> 137.

  abdomen 014.8 ●
    lymph gland 014.8 ●
  abscess 011.9 ●
    arm 017.9
    bone (*see also* Osteomyelitis, due to,
      tuberculosis) 015.9 ● [730.8] ●
      hip 015.1 ● [730.85]

Tuberculosis, tubercular, tuberculous
    (*Continued*)
  abscess (*Continued*)
    bone (*Continued*)
      knee 015.2 ● [730.86]
      sacrum 015.0 ● [730.88]
      specified site NEC 015.7 ●
        [730.88]
      spinal 015.0 ● [730.88]
      vertebra 015.0 ● [730.88]
    brain 013.3 ●
    breast 017.9 ●
    Cowper's gland 016.5 ●
    dura (mater) 013.8 ●
      brain 013.3 ●
      spinal cord 013.5 ●
    epidural 013.8 ●
      brain 013.3 ●
      spinal cord 013.5 ●
    frontal sinus - *see* Tuberculosis, sinus
    genital organs NEC 016.9 ●
      female 016.7 ●
      male 016.5 ●
    genitourinary NEC 016.9 ●
    gland (lymphatic) - *see* Tuberculosis,
      lymph gland
    hip 015.1 ●
    iliopsoas 015.0 ● [730.88]
    intestine 014.8 ●
    ischiorectal 014.8 ●
    joint 015.9 ●
      hip 015.1 ●
      knee 015.2 ●
      specified joint NEC 015.8 ●
      vertebral 015.0 ● [730.88]
    kidney 016.0 ● [590.81]
    knee 015.2 ●
    lumbar 015.0 ● [730.88]
    lung 011.2 ●
      primary, progressive 010.8 ●
    meninges (cerebral) (spinal) 013.0 ●
    pelvic 016.9 ●
      female 016.7 ●
      male 016.5 ●
    perianal 014.8 ●
      fistula 014.8 ●
    perinephritic 016.0 ● [590.81]
    perineum 017.9 ●
    perirectal 014.8 ●
    psoas 015.0 ● [730.88]
    rectum 014.8 ●
    retropharyngeal 012.8 ●
    sacrum 015.0 ● [730.88]
    scrofulous 017.2 ●
    scrotum 016.5 ●
    skin 017.0 ●
      primary 017.0 ●
    spinal cord 013.5 ●
    spine or vertebra (column) 015.0 ●
      [730.88]
    strumous 017.2 ●
    subdiaphragmatic 014.8 ●
    testis 016.5 ●
    thigh 017.9 ●
    urinary 016.3 ●
      kidney 016.0 ● [590.81]
    uterus 016.7 ●
  accessory sinus - *see* Tuberculosis, sinus
  Addison's disease 017.6 ●
  adenitis (*see also* Tuberculosis, lymph
    gland) 017.2 ●
  adenoids 012.8 ●
  adenopathy (*see also* Tuberculosis,
    lymph gland) 017.2 ●
    tracheobronchial 012.1 ●
      primary progressive 010.8 ●

◀ New   ◀▥ Revised   ~~deleted~~ Deleted   ● Use Additional Digit(s)   ▥ Omit code

Tuberculosis, tubercular, tuberculous
(Continued)
   adherent pericardium 017.9● [420.0]
   adnexa (uteri) 016.7●
   adrenal (capsule) (gland) 017.6●
   air passage NEC 012.8●
   alimentary canal 014.8●
   anemia 017.9●
   ankle (joint) 015.8●
      bone 015.5● [730.87]
   anus 014.8●
   apex (see also Tuberculosis, pulmonary)
      011.9●
   apical (see also Tuberculosis,
      pulmonary) 011.9●
   appendicitis 014.8●
   appendix 014.8●
   arachnoid 013.0●
   artery 017.9●
   arthritis (chronic) (synovial) 015.9●
      [711.40]
      ankle 015.8● [730.87]
      hip 015.1● [711.45]
      knee 015.2 [711.46]
      specified site NEC 015.8● [711.48]
      spine or vertebra (column) 015.0●
         [720.81]
      wrist 015.8● [730.83]
   articular - see Tuberculosis, joint
   ascites 014.0●
   asthma (see also Tuberculosis,
      pulmonary) 011.9●
   axilla, axillary 017.2●
      gland 017.2●
   bilateral (see also Tuberculosis,
      pulmonary) 011.9●
   bladder 016.1●
   bone (see also Osteomyelitis, due to,
      tuberculosis) 015.9● [730.8]
      hip 015.1● [730.85]
      knee 015.2● [730.86]
      limb NEC 015.5● [730.88]
      sacrum 015.0● [730.88]
      specified site NEC 015.7● [730.88]
      spinal or vertebral column 015.0●
         [730.88]
   bowel 014.8●
      miliary 018.9●
   brain 013.2●
   breast 017.9●
   broad ligament 016.7●
   bronchi, bronchial, bronchus 011.3●
      ectasia, ectasis 011.5●
      fistula 011.3●
         primary, progressive 010.8●
      gland 012.1●
         primary, progressive 010.8●
      isolated 012.2●
      lymph gland or node 012.1●
         primary, progressive 010.8●
   bronchiectasis 011.5●
   bronchitis 011.3●
   bronchopleural 012.0●
   bronchopneumonia,
      bronchopneumonic 011.6●
   bronchorrhagia 011.3●
   bronchotracheal 011.3●
      isolated 012.2●
   bronchus - see Tuberculosis, bronchi
   bronze disease (Addison's) 017.6●
   buccal cavity 017.9●
   bulbourethral gland 016.5●
   bursa (see also Tuberculosis, joint)
      015.9●
   cachexia NEC (see also Tuberculosis,
      pulmonary) 011.9●

Tuberculosis, tubercular, tuberculous
(Continued)
   cardiomyopathy 017.9● [425.8]
   caries (see also Tuberculosis, bone)
      015.9● [730.8]●
   cartilage (see also Tuberculosis, bone)
      015.9● [730.8]●
      intervertebral 015.0● [730.88]
   catarrhal (see also Tuberculosis,
      pulmonary) 011.9●
   cecum 014.8●
   cellular tissue (primary) 017.0●
   cellulitis (primary) 017.0●
   central nervous system 013.9●
      specified site NEC 013.8●
   cerebellum (current) 013.2●
   cerebral (current) 013.2●
      meninges 013.0●
   cerebrospinal 013.6●
      meninges 013.0●
   cerebrum (current) 013.2●
   cervical 017.2●
      gland 017.2●
      lymph nodes 017.2●
   cervicitis (uteri) 016.7●
   cervix 016.7●
   chest (see also Tuberculosis, pulmonary)
      011.9●
   childhood type or first infection
      010.0●
   choroid 017.3● [363.13]
   choroiditis 017.3● [363.13]
   ciliary body 017.3● [364.11]
   colitis 014.8●
   colliers' 011.4●
   colliquativa (primary) 017.0●
   colon 014.8●
      ulceration 014.8●
   complex, primary 010.0●
   complicating pregnancy, childbirth, or
      puerperium 647.3●
      affecting fetus or newborn 760.2
   congenital 771.2
   conjunctiva 017.3● [370.31]
   connective tissue 017.9●
      bone - see Tuberculosis, bone
   contact V01.1
   converter (tuberculin skin test)
      (without disease) 795.5
   cornea (ulcer) 017.3● [370.31]
   Cowper's gland 016.5●
   coxae 015.1● [730.85]
   coxalgia 015.1● [730.85]
   cul-de-sac of Douglas 014.8●
   curvature, spine 015.0● [737.40]
   cutis (colliquativa) (primary) 017.0●
   cyst, ovary 016.6●
   cystitis 016.1●
   dacryocystitis 017.3● [375.32]
   dactylitis 015.5●
   diarrhea 014.8●
   diffuse (see also Tuberculosis, miliary)
      018.9●
      lung - see Tuberculosis, pulmonary
      meninges 013.0●
   digestive tract 014.8●
   disseminated (see also Tuberculosis,
      miliary) 018.9●
      meninges 013.0●
   duodenum 014.8●
   dura (mater) 013.9●
      abscess 013.8●
         cerebral 013.3●
         spinal 013.5●
   dysentery 014.8●

Tuberculosis, tubercular, tuberculous
(Continued)
   ear (inner) (middle) 017.4●
      bone 015.6●
      external (primary) 017.0●
      skin (primary) 017.0●
   elbow 015.8●
   emphysema - see Tuberculosis,
      pulmonary
   empyema 012.0●
   encephalitis 013.6●
   endarteritis 017.9●
   endocarditis (any valve) 017.9●
      [424.91]
   endocardium (any valve) 017.9●
      [424.91]
   endocrine glands NEC 017.9●
   endometrium 016.7●
   enteric, enterica 014.8●
   enteritis 014.8●
   enterocolitis 014.8●
   epididymis 016.4●
   epididymitis 016.4●
   epidural abscess 013.8●
      brain 013.3●
      spinal cord 013.5●
   epiglottis 012.3●
   episcleritis 017.3● [379.00]
   erythema (induratum) (nodosum)
      (primary) 017.1●
   esophagus 017.8●
   Eustachian tube 017.4●
   exposure to V01.1
   exudative 012.0●
      primary, progressive 010.1●
   eye 017.3●
   eyelid (primary) 017.0●
      lupus 017.0● [373.4]
   fallopian tube 016.6●
   fascia 017.9●
   fauces 012.8●
   finger 017.9●
   first infection 010.0●
   fistula, perirectal 014.8●
   Florida 011.6●
   foot V01.9●
   funnel pelvis 137.3
   gallbladder 017.9●
   galloping (see also Tuberculosis,
      pulmonary) 011.9●
   ganglionic 015.9●
   gastritis 017.9●
   gastrocolic fistula 014.8●
   gastroenteritis 014.8●
   gastrointestinal tract 014.8●
   general, generalized 018.9●
      acute 018.0●
      chronic 018.8●
   genital organs NEC 016.9●
      female 016.7●
      male 016.5●
   genitourinary NEC 016.9●
   genu 015.2●
   glandulae suprarenalis 017.6●
   glandular, general 017.2●
   glottis 012.3●
   grinders' 011.4●
   groin 017.2●
   gum 017.9●
   hand 017.9●
   heart 017.9 [425.8]●
   hematogenous - see Tuberculosis,
      miliary

Tuberculosis, tubercular, tuberculous
(*Continued*)
hemoptysis (*see also* Tuberculosis,
   pulmonary) 011.9 ●
hemorrhage NEC (*see also* Tuberculosis,
   pulmonary) 011.9 ●
hemothorax 012.0 ●
hepatitis 017.9 ●
hilar lymph nodes 012.1 ●
   primary, progressive 010.8 ●
hip (disease) (joint) 015.1 ●
   bone 015.1 ● [730.85]
hydrocephalus 013.8 ●
hydropneumothorax 012.0 ●
hydrothorax 012.0 ●
hypoadrenalism 017.6 ●
hypopharynx 012.8 ●
ileocecal (hyperplastic) 014.8 ●
ileocolitis 014.8 ●
ileum 014.8 ●
iliac spine (superior) 015.0 ● [730.88]
incipient NEC (*see also* Tuberculosis,
   pulmonary) 011.9 ●
indurativa (primary) 017.1 ●
infantile 010.0 ●
infection NEC 011.9 ●
   without clinical manifestation
      010.0 ●
infraclavicular gland 017.2 ●
inguinal gland 017.2 ●
inguinalis 017.2 ●
intestine (any part) 014.8 ●
iris 017.3 ● [364.11]
iritis 017.3 ● [364.11]
ischiorectal 014.8 ●
jaw 015.7 ● [730.88]
jejunum 014.8 ●
joint 015.9 ●
   hip 015.1 ●
   knee 015.2 ●
   specified site NEC 015.8 ●
   vertebral 015.0 ● [730.88]
keratitis 017.3 ● [370.31]
   interstitial 017.3 ● [370.59]
keratoconjunctivitis 017.3 ● [370.31]
kidney 016.0 ●
knee (joint) 015.2 ●
kyphoscoliosis 015.0 ● [737.43]
kyphosis 015.0 ● [737.41]
lacrimal apparatus, gland 017.3 ●
laryngitis 012.3 ●
larynx 012.3 ●
leptomeninges, leptomeningitis
   (cerebral) (spinal) 013.0 ●
lichenoides (primary) 017.0 ●
linguae 017.9 ●
lip 017.9 ●
liver 017.9 ●
lordosis 015.0 ● [737.42]
lung - *see* Tuberculosis, pulmonary ●
luposa 017.0 ●
   eyelid 017.0 ● [373.4]
lymphadenitis - *see* Tuberculosis,
   lymph gland
lymphangitis - *see* Tuberculosis, lymph
   gland
lymphatic (gland) (vessel) - *see*
   Tuberculosis, lymph gland
lymph gland or node (peripheral)
   017.2 ●
   abdomen 014.8 ●
   bronchial 012.1 ●
      primary, progressive 010.8 ●
   cervical 017.2 ●

Tuberculosis, tubercular, tuberculous
(*Continued*)
lymph gland or node (*Continued*)
   hilar 012.1 ●
      primary, progressive 010.8 ●
   intrathoracic 012.1 ●
      primary, progressive 010.8 ●
   mediastinal 012.1 ●
      primary, progressive 010.8 ●
   mesenteric 014.8 ●
   peripheral 017.2 ●
   retroperitoneal 014.8 ●
   tracheobronchial 012.1 ●
      primary, progressive 010.8 ●
malignant NEC (*see also* Tuberculosis,
   pulmonary) 011.9 ●
mammary gland 017.9 ●
marasmus NEC (*see also* Tuberculosis,
   pulmonary) 011.9 ●
mastoiditis 015.6 ●
maternal, affecting fetus or newborn
   760.2
mediastinal (lymph) gland or node
   012.1 ●
   primary, progressive 010.8 ●
mediastinitis 012.8 ●
   primary, progressive 010.8 ●
mediastinopericarditis 017.9 ●
   [420.0]
mediastinum 012.8 ●
   primary, progressive 010.8 ●
medulla 013.9 ●
   brain 013.2 ●
   spinal cord 013.4 ●
melanosis, Addisonian 017.6 ●
membrane, brain 013.0 ●
meninges (cerebral) (spinal) 013.0 ●
meningitis (basilar) (brain) (cerebral)
   (cerebrospinal) (spinal) 013.0 ●
meningoencephalitis 013.0 ●
mesentery, mesenteric 014.8 ●
   lymph gland or node 014.8 ●
miliary (any site) 018.9 ●
   acute 018.0 ●
   chronic 018.8 ●
   specified type NEC 018.8 ●
millstone makers' 011.4 ●
miners' 011.4 ●
moulders' 011.4 ●
mouth 017.9 ●
multiple 018.9 ●
   acute 018.0 ●
   chronic 018.8 ●
muscle 017.9 ●
myelitis 013.6 ●
myocarditis 017.9 ● [422.0]
myocardium 017.9 ● [422.0]
nasal (passage) (sinus) 012.8 ●
nasopharynx 012.8 ●
neck gland 017.2 ●
nephritis 016.0 ● [583.81]
nerve 017.9 ●
nose (septum) 012.8 ●
ocular 017.3 ●
old NEC 137.0
   without residuals V12.01
omentum 014.8 ●
oophoritis (acute) (chronic) 016.6 ●
optic 017.3 ● [377.39]
   nerve trunk 017.3 ● [377.39]
   papilla, papillae 017.3 ● [377.39]
orbit 017.3 ●
orchitis 016.5 ● [608.81]
organ, specified NEC 017.9 ●

Tuberculosis, tubercular, tuberculous
(*Continued*)
orificialis (primary) 017.0 ●
osseous (*see also* Tuberculosis, bone)
   015.9 ● [730.8]
osteitis (*see also* Tuberculosis, bone)
   015.9 ● [730.8]
osteomyelitis (*see also* Tuberculosis,
   bone) 015.9 ● [730.8]
otitis (media) 017.4 ●
ovaritis (acute) (chronic) 016.6 ●
ovary (acute) (chronic) 016.6 ●
oviducts (acute) (chronic) 016.6 ●
pachymeningitis 013.0 ●
palate (soft) 017.9 ●
pancreas 017.9 ●
papulonecrotic (primary) 017.0 ●
parathyroid glands 017.9 ●
paronychia (primary) 017.0 ●
parotid gland or region 017.9 ●
pelvic organ NEC 016.9 ●
   female 016.7 ●
   male 016.5 ●
pelvis (bony) 015.7 ● [730.85]
penis 016.5 ●
peribronchitis 011.3 ●
pericarditis 017.9 ● [420.0]
pericardium 017.9 ● [420.0]
perichondritis, larynx 012.3 ●
perineum 017.9 ●
periostitis (*see also* Tuberculosis, bone)
   015.9 ● [730.8]
periphlebitis 017.9 ●
   eye vessel 017.3 ● [362.18]
   retina 017.3 ● [362.18]
perirectal fistula 014.8 ●
peritoneal gland 014.8 ●
peritoneum 014.0 ●
peritonitis 014.0 ●
pernicious NEC (*see also* Tuberculosis,
   pulmonary) 011.9 ●
pharyngitis 012.8 ●
pharynx 012.8 ●
phlyctenulosis (conjunctiva) 017.3 ●
   [370.31]
phthisis NEC (*see also* Tuberculosis,
   pulmonary) 011.9 ●
pituitary gland 017.9 ●
placenta 016.7 ●
pleura, pleural, pleurisy, pleuritis
   (fibrinous) (obliterative)
   (purulent) (simple plastic) (with
   effusion) 012.0 ●
   primary, progressive 010.1 ●
pneumonia, pneumonic 011.6 ●
pneumothorax 011.7 ●
polyserositis 018.9 ●
   acute 018.0 ●
   chronic 018.8 ●
potters' 011.4 ●
prepuce 016.5 ●
primary 010.9 ●
   complex 010.0 ●
   complicated 010.8 ●
      with pleurisy or effusion 010.1 ●
   progressive 010.8 ●
      with pleurisy or effusion
         010.1 ●
   skin 017.0 ●
proctitis 014.8 ●
prostate 016.5 ● [601.4]
prostatitis 016.5 ● [601.4]
pulmonaris (*see also* Tuberculosis,
   pulmonary) 011.9 ●

◀ New   ◀⃒ Revised   ~~deleted~~ Deleted   ● Use Additional Digit(s)   ▨ Omit code

Tuberculosis, tubercular, tuberculous
  (Continued)
  pulmonary (artery) (incipient)
      (malignant) (multiple round foci)
      (pernicious) (reinfection stage)
      011.9●
    cavitated or with cavitation 011.2●
      primary, progressive 010.8●
    childhood type or first infection
      010.0●
    chromogenic acid-fast bacilli 795.39
    fibrosis or fibrotic 011.4●
    infiltrative 011.0●
      primary, progressive 010.9●
    nodular 011.1●
    specified NEC 011.8●
    sputum positive only 795.39●
    status following surgical collapse of
      lung NEC 011.9●
  pyelitis 016.0● [590.81]
  pyelonephritis 016.0● [590.81]
  pyemia - see Tuberculosis, miliary
  pyonephrosis 016.0●
  pyopneumothorax 012.0●
  pyothorax 012.0●
  rectum (with abscess) 014.8●
    fistula 014.8●
  reinfection stage (see also Tuberculosis,
      pulmonary) 011.9●
  renal 016.0●
  renis 016.0●
  reproductive organ 016.7●
  respiratory NEC (see also Tuberculosis,
      pulmonary) 011.9●
    specified site NEC 012.8●
  retina 017.3● [363.13]
  retroperitoneal (lymph gland or node)
      014.8●
    gland 014.8●
  retropharyngeal abscess 012.8●
  rheumatism 015.9●
  rhinitis 012.8●
  sacroiliac (joint) 015.8●
  sacrum 015.0● [730.88]
  salivary gland 017.9●
  salpingitis (acute) (chronic) 016.6●
  sandblasters' 011.4●
  sclera 017.3● [379.09]
  scoliosis 015.0● [737.43]
  scrofulous 017.2●
  scrotum 016.5●
  seminal tract or vesicle 016.5●
      [608.81]
  senile NEC (see also Tuberculosis,
      pulmonary) 011.9●
  septic NEC (see also Tuberculosis,
      miliary) 018.9●
  shoulder 015.8●
    blade 015.7● [730.8] ●
  sigmoid 014.8●
  sinus (accessory) (nasal) 012.8●
    bone 015.7● [730.88]
    epididymis 016.4●
  skeletal NEC (see also Osteomyelitis,
      due to tuberculosis) 015.9●
      [730.8] ●
  skin (any site) (primary) 017.0●
  small intestine 014.8●
  soft palate 017.9●
  spermatic cord 016.5●
  spinal
    column 015.0● [730.88]
    cord 013.4●
    disease 015.0● [730.88]

Tuberculosis, tubercular, tuberculous
  (Continued)
  spinal (Continued)
    medulla 013.4●
    membrane 013.0●●
    meninges 013.0●
  spine 015.0● [730.88]
  spleen 017.7●
  splenitis 017.7●
  spondylitis 015.0● [720.81]
  spontaneous pneumothorax - see
      Tuberculosis, pulmonary
  sternoclavicular joint 015.8●
  stomach 017.9●
  stonemasons' 011.4●
  struma 017.2●
  subcutaneous tissue (cellular)
      (primary) 017.0●
  subcutis (primary) 017.0●
  subdeltoid bursa 017.9●
  submaxillary 017.9●
    region 017.9●
  supraclavicular gland 017.2●
  suprarenal (capsule) (gland) 017.6●
  swelling, joint (see also Tuberculosis,
      joint) 015.9●
  symphysis pubis 015.7● [730.88]
  synovitis 015.9● [727.01]
    hip 015.1● [727.01]
    knee 015.2● [727.01]
    specified site NEC 015.8●
      [727.01]
    spine or vertebra 015.0● [727.01]
  systemic - see Tuberculosis, miliary
  tarsitis (eyelid) 017.0● [373.4]
    ankle (bone) 015.5● [730.87]
  tendon (sheath) - see Tuberculosis,
      tenosynovitis
  tenosynovitis 015.9● [727.01]
    hip 015.1● [727.01]
    knee 015.2● [727.01]
    specified site NEC 015.8● [727.01]
    spine or vertebra 015.0● [727.01]
  testis 016.5● [608.81]
  throat 012.8●
  thymus gland 017.9●
  thyroid gland 017.5●
  toe 017.9●
  tongue 017.9●
  tonsil (lingual) 012.8●
  tonsillitis 012.8●
  trachea, tracheal 012.8●
    gland 012.1●
      primary, progressive 010.8●
    isolated 012.2●
  tracheobronchial 011.3●
    glandular 012.1●
      primary, progressive 010.8●
    isolated 012.2●
    lymph gland or node 012.1●
      primary, progressive 010.8●
  tubal 016.6●
  tunica vaginalis 016.5●
  typhlitis 014.8●
  ulcer (primary) (skin) 017.0●
    bowel or intestine 014.8●
    specified site NEC - see Tuberculosis,
      by site
  unspecified site - see Tuberculosis,
      pulmonary
  ureter 016.2●
  urethra, urethral 016.3●
  urinary organ or tract 016.3●
    kidney 016.0●

Tuberculosis, tubercular, tuberculous
  (Continued)
  uterus 016.7●
  uveal tract 017.3● [363.13]
  uvula 017.9●
  vaccination, prophylactic (against)
      V03.2
  vagina 016.7●
  vas deferens 016.5●
  vein 017.9●
  verruca (primary) 017.0●
  verrucosa (cutis) (primary) 017.0●
  vertebra (column) 015.0● [730.88]
  vesiculitis 016.5● [608.81]
  viscera NEC 014.8●
  vulva 016.7● [616.51]
  wrist (joint) 015.8●
    bone 015.5● [730.83]
Tuberculum
  auriculae 744.29
  occlusal 520.2
  paramolare 520.2
Tuberosity
  jaw, excessive 524.07
  maxillary, entire 524.07
Tuberous sclerosis (brain) 759.5
Tubo-ovarian - see condition
Tuboplasty, after previous sterilization
      V26.0
Tubotympanitis 381.10
Tularemia 021.9
  with
    conjunctivitis 021.3
    pneumonia 021.2
  bronchopneumonic 021.2
  conjunctivitis 021.3
  cryptogenic 021.1
  disseminated 021.8
  enteric 021.1
  generalized 021.8
  glandular 021.8
  intestinal 021.1
  oculoglandular 021.3
  ophthalmic 021.3
  pneumonia 021.2
  pulmonary 021.2
  specified NEC 021.8
  typhoidal 021.1
  ulceroglandular 021.0
  vaccination, prophylactic (against)
      V03.4
Tularensis conjunctivitis 021.3
Tumefaction - see also Swelling
  liver (see also Hypertrophy, liver) 789.1
Tumor (M8000/1) - see also Neoplasm,
      by site, unspecified nature
  Abrikossov's (M9580/0) - see also
      Neoplasm, connective tissue,
      benign
    malignant (M9580/3) - see
      Neoplasm, connective tissue,
      malignant
  acinar cell (M8550/1) - see
      Neoplasm, by site,
      uncertain behavior
  acinic cell (M8550/1) - see
      Neoplasm, by site,
      uncertain behavior
  adenomatoid (M9054/0) - see also
      Neoplasm, by site, benign
    odontogenic (M9300/0) 213.1
      upper jaw (bone) 213.0
  adnexal (skin) (M8390/0) - see
      Neoplasm, skin, benign

Tumor *(Continued)*
  adrenal
    cortical (benign) (M8370/0) 227.0
      malignant (M8370/3) 194.0
    rest (M8671/0) - *see* Neoplasm, by
        site, benign
  alpha cell (M8152/0)
    malignant (M8152/3)
      pancreas 157.4
      specified site NEC - *see*
          Neoplasm, by site,
          malignant
      unspecified site 157.4
    pancreas 211.7
    specified site NEC - *see* Neoplasm,
        by site, benign
    unspecified site 211.7
  aneurysmal (*see also* Aneurysm)
      442.9
  aortic body (M8691/1) 237.3
    malignant (M8691/3) 194.6
  argentaffin (M8241/1) - *see* Neoplasm,
      by site, uncertain behavior
  basal cell (M8090/1) - *see also*
      Neoplasm, skin, uncertain
      behavior
  benign (M8000/0) - *see* Neoplasm, by
      site, benign
  beta cell (M8151/0)
    malignant (M8151/3)
      pancreas 157.4
      specified site - *see* Neoplasm, by
          site, malignant
      unspecified site 157.4
    pancreas 211.7
    specified site NEC - *see* Neoplasm,
        by site, benign
    unspecified site 211.7
  blood - *see* Hematoma
  brenner (M9000/0) 220
    borderline malignancy (M9000/1)
        236.2
    malignant (M9000/3) 183.0
    proliferating (M9000/1) 236.2
  Brooke's (M8100/0) - *see* Neoplasm,
      skin, benign
  brown fat (M8880/0) - *see* Lipoma, by
      site
  Burkitt's (M9750/3) 200.2●
  calcifying epithelial odontogenic
      (M9340/0) 213.1
    upper jaw (bone) 213.0
  carcinoid (M8240/1) 209.60
    benign 209.60
      appendix 209.51
      ascending colon 209.53
      bronchus 209.61
      cecum 209.52
      colon 209.50
      descending colon 209.55
      duodenum 209.41
      foregut 209.65
      hindgut 209.67
      ileum 209.43
      jejunum 209.42
      kidney 209.64
      large intestine 209.50
      lung 209.61
      midgut 209.66
      rectum 209.57
      sigmoid colon 209.56
      small intestine 209.40
      specified NEC 209.69
      stomach 209.63

Tumor *(Continued)*
  carcinoid *(Continued)*
    benign *(Continued)*
      thymus 209.62
      transverse colon 209.54
    malignant (of) 209.20
      appendix 209.11
      ascending colon 209.13
      bronchus 209.21
      cecum 209.12
      colon 209.10
      descending colon 209.15
      duodenum 209.01
      foregut 209.25
      hindgut 209.27
      ileum 209.03
      jejunum 209.02
      kidney 209.24
      large intestine 209.10
      lung 209.21
      midgut 209.26
      rectum 209.17
      sigmoid colon 209.16
      small intestine 209.00
      specified NEC 209.29
      stomach 209.23
      thymus 209.22
      transverse colon 209.14
    secondary - *see* Tumor,
        neuroendocrine, secondary
  carotid body (M8692/1) 237.3
    malignant (M8692/3) 194.5
  Castleman's (mediastinal lymph node
      hyperplasia) 785.6
  cells (M8001/1) - *see also* Neoplasm, by
      site, unspecified nature
    benign (M8001/0) - *see* Neoplasm,
        by site, benign
    malignant (M8001/3) - *see*
        Neoplasm, by site, malignant
    uncertain whether benign or
        malignant (M8001/1) - *see*
        Neoplasm, by site, uncertain
        nature
  cervix
    in pregnancy or childbirth 654.6●
      affecting fetus or newborn 763.89
      causing obstructed labor 660.2●
        affecting fetus or newborn
            763.1
  chondromatous giant cell (M9230/0) -
      see Neoplasm, bone, benign
  chromaffin (M8700/0) - *see also*
      Neoplasm, by site, benign
    malignant (M8700/3) - *see*
        Neoplasm, by site, malignant
  Cock's peculiar 706.2
  Codman's (benign chondroblastoma)
      (M9230/0) - *see* Neoplasm, bone,
      benign
  dentigerous, mixed (M9282/0)
      213.1
    upper jaw (bone) 213.0
  dermoid (M9084/0) - *see* Neoplasm, by
      site, benign
    with malignant transformation
        (M9084/3) 183.0
  desmoid (extra-abdominal)
      (M8821/1) - *see also* Neoplasm,
      connective tissue, uncertain
      behavior
    abdominal (M8822/1) - *see*
        Neoplasm, connective tissue,
        uncertain behavior

Tumor *(Continued)*
  embryonal (mixed) (M9080/1) - *see also*
      Neoplasm, by site, uncertain
      behavior
    liver (M9080/3) 155.0
  endodermal sinus (M9071/3)
    specified site - *see* Neoplasm, by site,
        malignant
    unspecified site
      female 183.0
      male 186.9
  epithelial
    benign (M8010/0) - *see* Neoplasm,
        by site, benign
    malignant (M8010/3) - *see*
        Neoplasm, by site, malignant
  Ewing's (M9260/3) - *see* Neoplasm,
      bone, malignant
  fatty - *see* Lipoma
  fetal, causing disproportion 653.7●
    causing obstructed labor 660.1●
  fibroid (M8890/0) - *see* Leiomyoma
  G cell (M8153/1)
    malignant (M8153/3)
      pancreas 157.4
      specified site NEC - *see* Neoplasm,
          by site, malignant
      unspecified site 157.4
    specified site - *see* Neoplasm, by site,
        uncertain behavior
    unspecified site 235.5
  giant cell (type) (M8003/1) - *see also*
      Neoplasm, by site, unspecified
      nature
    bone (M9250/1) 238.0
      malignant (M9250/3) - *see*
          Neoplasm, bone, malignant
    chondromatous (M9230/0) - *see*
        Neoplasm, bone, benign
    malignant (M8003/3) - *see*
        Neoplasm, by site, malignant
    peripheral (gingiva) 523.8
    soft parts (M9251/1) - *see also*
        Neoplasm, connective tissue,
        uncertain behavior
      malignant (M9251/3) - *see*
          Neoplasm, connective
          tissue, malignant
    tendon sheath 727.02
  glomus (M8711/0) - *see also*
      Hemangioma, by site
    jugulare (M8690/1) 237.3
      malignant (M8690/3) 194.6
  gonadal stromal (M8590/1) - *see*
      Neoplasm, by site, uncertain
      behavior
  granular cell (M9580/0) - *see also*
      Neoplasm, connective tissue,
      benign
    malignant (M9580/3) - *see*
        Neoplasm, connective tissue,
        malignant
  granulosa cell (M8620/1) 236.2
    malignant (M8620/3) 183.0
  granulosa cell-theca cell (M8621/1) 236.2
    malignant (M8621/3) 183.0
  Grawitz's (hypernephroma) (M8312/3)
      189.0
  hazard-crile (M8350/3) 193
  hemorrhoidal - *see* Hemorrhoids
  hilar cell (M8660/0) 220
  Hürthle cell (benign) (M8290/0) 226
    malignant (M8290/3) 193
  hydatid (*see also* Echinococcus) 122.9

Tumor (Continued)
  hypernephroid (M8311/1) - see also
      Neoplasm, by site, uncertain
      behavior
  interstitial cell (M8650/1) - see also
      Neoplasm, by site, uncertain
      behavior
    benign (M8650/0) - see Neoplasm,
        by site, benign
    malignant (M8650/3) - see
        Neoplasm, by site, malignant
  islet cell (M8150/0)
    malignant (M8150/3)
      pancreas 157.4
      specified site - see Neoplasm, by
          site, malignant
      unspecified site 157.4
    pancreas 211.7
    specified site NEC - see Neoplasm,
        by site, benign
    unspecified site 211.7
  juxtaglomerular (M8361/1) 236.91
  Krukenberg's (M8490/6) 198.6
  Leydig cell (M8650/1)
    benign (M8650/0)
      specified site - see Neoplasm, by
          site, benign
      unspecified site
        female 220
        male 222.0
    malignant (M8650/3)
      specified site - see Neoplasm, by
          site, malignant
      unspecified site
        female 183.0
        male 186.9
    specified site - see Neoplasm, by site,
        uncertain behavior
    unspecified site
      female 236.2
      male 236.4
  lipid cell, ovary (M8670/0) 220
  lipoid cell, ovary (M8670/0) 220
  lymphomatous, benign (M9590/0) - see
      also Neoplasm, by site, benign
  lysis syndrome (following
      antineoplastic drug therapy)
      (spontaneous) 277.88
  Malherbe's (M8110/0) - see Neoplasm,
      skin, benign
  malignant (M8000/3) - see also
      Neoplasm, by site, malignant
    fusiform cell (type) (M8004/3) - see
        Neoplasm, by site, malignant
    giant cell (type) (M8003/3) - see
        Neoplasm, by site, malignant
    mixed NEC (M8940/3) - see
        Neoplasm, by site, malignant
    small cell (type) (M8002/3) - see
        Neoplasm, by site, malignant
    spindle cell (type) (M8004/3) - see
        Neoplasm, by site, malignant
  mast cell (M9740/1) 238.5
    malignant (M9740/3) 202.6●
  melanotic, neuroectodermal
      (M9363/0) - see Neoplasm, by site,
      benign
  Merkel cell - see Carcinoma, Merkel
      cell
  mesenchymal
    malignant (M8800/3) - see
        Neoplasm, connective tissue,
        malignant
    mixed (M8990/1) - see Neoplasm,
        connective tissue, uncertain
        behavior

Tumor (Continued)
  mesodermal, mixed (M8951/3) - see
      also Neoplasm, by site, malignant
    liver 155.0
  mesonephric (M9110/1) - see also
      Neoplasm, by site, uncertain
      behavior
    malignant (M9110/3) - see
        Neoplasm, by site, malignant
  metastatic
    from specified site (M8000/3) - see
        Neoplasm, by site, malignant
    to specified site (M8000/6) - see
        Neoplasm, by site, malignant,
        secondary
  mixed NEC (M8940/0) - see also
      Neoplasm, by site, benign
    malignant (M8940/3) - see
        Neoplasm, by site, malignant
  mucocarcinoid, malignant (M8243/3) -
      see Neoplasm, by site, malignant
  mucoepidermoid (M8430/1) - see
      Neoplasm, by site, uncertain
      behavior
  Müllerian, mixed (M8950/3) - see
      Neoplasm, by site, malignant
  myoepithelial (M8982/0) - see
      Neoplasm, by site, benign
  neuroendocrine 209.60
    malignant poorly differentiated
        209.30
    secondary 209.70
      bone 209.73
      distant lymph nodes 209.71
      liver 209.72
      peritoneum 209.74
      site specified NEC 209.79
  neurogenic olfactory (M9520/3) 160.0
  nonencapsulated sclerosing (M8350/3)
      193
  odontogenic (M9270/1) 238.0
    adenomatoid (M9300/0) 213.1
      upper jaw (bone) 213.0
    benign (M9270/0) 213.1
      upper jaw (bone) 213.0
    calcifying epithelial (M9340/0)
        213.1
      upper jaw (bone) 213.0
    malignant (M9270/3) 170.1
      upper jaw (bone) 170.0
    squamous (M9312/0) 213.1
      upper jaw (bone) 213.0
  ovarian stromal (M8590/1) 236.2
  ovary
    in pregnancy or childbirth 654.4●
      affecting fetus or newborn
          763.89
      causing obstructed labor 660.2●
        affecting fetus or newborn
            763.1
  pacinian (M9507/0) - see Neoplasm,
      skin, benign
  Pancoast's (M8010/3) 162.3
  papillary - see Papilloma
  pelvic, in pregnancy or childbirth
      654.9●
    affecting fetus or newborn 763.89
    causing obstructed labor 660.2●
      affecting fetus or newborn 763.1
  phantom 300.11
  plasma cell (M9731/1) 238.6
    benign (M9731/0) - see Neoplasm,
        by site, benign
    malignant (M9731/3) 203.8●

Tumor (Continued)
  polyvesicular vitelline (M9071/3)
    specified site - see Neoplasm, by site,
        malignant
    unspecified site
      female 183.0
      male 186.9
  Pott's puffy (see also Osteomyelitis)
      730.2●
  Rathke's pouch (M9350/1) 237.0
  regaud's (M8082/3) - see Neoplasm,
      nasopharynx, malignant
  rete cell (M8140/0) 222.0
  retinal anlage (M9363/0) - see
      Neoplasm, by site, benign
  Rokitansky's 620.2
  salivary gland type, mixed (M8940/0) -
      see also Neoplasm, by site,
      benign
    malignant (M8940/3) - see
        Neoplasm, by site, malignant
  Sampson's 617.1
  Schloffer's (see also Peritonitis) 567.29
  Schmincke (M8082/3) - see Neoplasm,
      nasopharynx, malignant
  sebaceous (see also Cyst, sebaceous)
      706.2
  secondary (M8000/6) - see Neoplasm,
      by site, secondary
    carcinoid - see Tumor,
        neuroendocrine, secondary
    neuroendocrine - see Tumor,
        neuroendocrine, secondary
  Sertoli cell (M8640/0)
    with lipid storage (M8641/0)
      specified site, - see Neoplasm, by
          site, benign
      unspecified site
        female 220
        male 222.0
    specified site - see Neoplasm, by site,
        benign
    unspecified site
      female 220
      male 222.0
  Sertoli-Leydig cell (M8631/0)
    specified site - see Neoplasm, by site,
        benign
    unspecified site
      female 220
      male 222.0
  sex cord (-stromal) (M8590/1) - see
      Neoplasm, by site, uncertain
      behavior
  skin appendage (M8390/0) - see
      Neoplasm, skin, benign
  soft tissue
    benign (M8800/0) - see Neoplasm,
        connective tissue, benign
    malignant (M8800/3) - see
        Neoplasm, connective tissue,
        malignant
  sternomastoid 754.1
  stromal
    abdomen
      benign 215.5
      malignant NEC 171.5
      uncertain behavior 238.1
    digestive system 238.1
      benign 215.5
      malignant NEC 171.5
      uncertain behavior 238.1
    endometrium (endometrial)
        236.0 ◄

Tumor (Continued)
  stromal (Continued)
    gastric 238.1
      benign 215.5
      malignant 151.9
      uncertain behavior 238.1
    gastrointestinal 238.1
      benign 215.5
      malignant NEC 171.5
      uncertain behavior 238.1
    intestine (small) 238.1
      benign 215.5
      malignant 152.9
      uncertain behavior 238.1
    stomach 238.1
      benign 215.5
      malignant 151.9
      uncertain behavior 238.1
  superior sulcus (lung) (pulmonary)
      (syndrome) (M8010/3) 162.3
  suprasulcus (M8010/3) 162.3
  sweat gland (M8400/1) - see also
      Neoplasm, skin, uncertain
      behavior
    benign (M8400/0) - see Neoplasm,
        skin, benign
    malignant (M8400/3) - see
        Neoplasm, skin, malignant
  syphilitic brain 094.89
    congenital 090.49
  testicular stromal (M8590/1) 236.4
  theca cell (M8600/0) 220
  theca cell-granulosa cell (M8621/1)
      236.2
  theca-lutein (M8610/0) 220
  turban (M8200/0) 216.4
  uterus
    in pregnancy or childbirth 654.1●
      affecting fetus or newborn
          763.89
      causing obstructed labor
          660.2●
        affecting fetus or newborn
            763.1
  vagina
    in pregnancy or childbirth 654.7●
      affecting fetus or newborn
          763.89
      causing obstructed labor 660.2●
        affecting fetus or newborn
            763.1
  varicose (see also Varicose, vein) 454.9
  von Recklinghausen's (M9540/1)
      237.71
  vulva
    in pregnancy or childbirth 654.8●
      affecting fetus or newborn
          763.89
      causing obstructed labor
          660.2●
        affecting fetus or newborn
            763.1
  Warthin's (salivary gland) (M8561/0)
      210.2
  white - see also Tuberculosis, arthritis
  White-Darier 757.39
  Wilms' (nephroblastoma) (M8960/3)
      189.0
  yolk sac (M9071/3)
    specified site - see Neoplasm, by site,
        malignant
    unspecified site
      female 183.0
      male 186.9

Tumorlet (M8040/1) - see Neoplasm, by
    site, uncertain behavior
Tungiasis 134.1
Tunica vasculosa lentis 743.39
Tunnel vision 368.45
Turban tumor (M8200/0) 216.4
Türck's trachoma (chronic catarrhal
    laryngitis) 476.0
Türk's syndrome (ocular retraction
    syndrome) 378.71
Turner's
  hypoplasia (tooth) 520.4
  syndrome 758.6
  tooth 520.4
Turner-Kieser syndrome (hereditary
    osteo-onychodysplasia) 756.89
Turner-Varny syndrome 758.6
Turricephaly 756.0
Tussis convulsiva (see also Whooping
    cough) 033.9
Twiddler's syndrome (due to)
  automatic implantable defibrillator
      996.04
  pacemaker 996.01
Twin
  affected by maternal complications of
      pregnancy 761.5
  conjoined 759.4
    fetal 678.1●
  healthy liveborn - see Newborn, twin
  pregnancy (complicating delivery)
      NEC 651.0●
    with fetal loss and retention of one
        fetus 651.3●
    conjoined 678.1●
    following (elective) fetal reduction
        651.7●
Twinning, teeth 520.2
Twist, twisted
  bowel, colon, or intestine 560.2
  hair (congenital) 757.4
  mesentery 560.2
  omentum 560.2
  organ or site, congenital NEC - see
      Anomaly, specified type NEC
  ovarian pedicle 620.5
    congenital 752.0
  umbilical cord - see Compression,
      umbilical cord
Twitch 781.0
Tylosis 700
  buccalis 528.6
  gingiva 523.8
  linguae 528.6
  palmaris et plantaris 757.39
Tympanism 787.3
Tympanites (abdominal) (intestine)
    787.3
Tympanitis - see Myringitis
Tympanosclerosis 385.00
  involving
    combined sites NEC 385.09
      with tympanic membrane 385.03
    tympanic membrane 385.01
      with ossicles 385.02
        and middle ear 385.03
Tympanum - see condition
Tympany
  abdomen 787.3
  chest 786.7
Typhlitis (see also Appendicitis) 541
Typhoenteritis 002.0
Typhogastric fever 002.0

Typhoid (abortive) (ambulant) (any site)
    (fever) (hemorrhagic) (infection)
    (intermittent) (malignant)
    (rheumatic) 002.0
  with pneumonia 002.0 [484.8]
  abdominal 002.0
  carrier (suspected) of V02.1
  cholecystitis (current) 002.0
  clinical (Widal and blood test negative)
      002.0
  endocarditis 002.0 [421.1]
  inoculation reaction - see
      Complications, vaccination
  meningitis 002.0 [320.7]
  mesenteric lymph nodes 002.0
  myocarditis 002.0 [422.0]
  osteomyelitis (see also Osteomyelitis,
      due to, typhoid) 002.0 [730.8]●
  perichondritis, larynx 002.0 [478.71]
  pneumonia 002.0 [484.8]
  spine 002.0 [720.81]
  ulcer (perforating) 002.0
  vaccination, prophylactic (against)
      V03.1
  Widal negative 002.0
Typhomalaria (fever) (see also Malaria)
    084.6
Typhomania 002.0
Typhoperitonitis 002.0
Typhus (fever) 081.9
  abdominal, abdominalis 002.0
  African tick 082.1
  amarillic (see also Fever, Yellow)
      060.9
  brain 081.9
  cerebral 081.9
  classical 080
  endemic (flea-borne) 081.0
  epidemic (louse-borne) 080
  exanthematic NEC 080
  exanthematicus SAI 080
    brillii SAI 081.1
    Mexicanus SAI 081.0
    pediculo vestimenti causa 080
    typhus murinus 081.0
  flea-borne 081.0
  Indian tick 082.1
  Kenya tick 082.1
  louse-borne 080
  Mexican 081.0
    flea-borne 081.0
    louse-borne 080
    tabardillo 080
  mite-borne 081.2
  murine 081.0
  North Asian tick-borne 082.2
  petechial 081.9
  Queensland tick 082.3
  rat 081.0
  recrudescent 081.1
  recurrent (see also Fever, relapsing)
      087.9
  São Paulo 082.0
  scrub (China) (India) (Malaya) (New
      Guinea) 081.2
  shop (of Malaya) 081.0
  Siberian tick 082.2
  tick-borne NEC 082.9
  tropical 081.2
  vaccination, prophylactic (against)
      V05.8
Tyrosinemia 270.2
  neonatal 775.89
Tyrosinosis (Medes) (Sakai) 270.2
Tyrosinuria 270.2
Tyrosyluria 270.2

◀ New   ◀▥ Revised   ~~deleted~~ Deleted   ● Use Additional Digit(s)   Omit code

U

Uehlinger's syndrome (acropachyderma) 757.39

Uhl's anomaly or disease (hypoplasia of myocardium, right ventricle) 746.84

Ulcer, ulcerated, ulcerating, ulceration, ulcerative 707.9
 with gangrene 707.9 [785.4]
 abdomen (wall) (see also Ulcer, skin) 707.8
 ala, nose 478.19
 alveolar process 526.5
 amebic (intestine) 006.9
  skin 006.6
 anastomotic - see Ulcer, gastrojejunal
 anorectal 569.41
 antral - see Ulcer, stomach
 anus (sphincter) (solitary) 569.41
  varicose - see Varicose, ulcer, anus
 aorta - see Aneurysm
 aphthous (oral) (recurrent) 528.2
   genital organ(s)
    female 616.50
    male 608.89
   mouth 528.2
 arm (see also Ulcer, skin) 707.8
 arteriosclerotic plaque - see Arteriosclerosis, by site
 artery NEC 447.2
  without rupture 447.8
 atrophic NEC - see Ulcer, skin
 Barrett's (chronic peptic ulcer of esophagus) 530.85
 bile duct 576.8
 bladder (solitary) (sphincter) 596.8
   bilharzial (see also Schistosomiasis) 120.9 [595.4]
   submucosal (see also Cystitis) 595.1
   tuberculous (see also Tuberculosis) 016.1 ●
 bleeding NEC - see Ulcer, peptic, with hemorrhage
 bone 730.9 ●
 bowel (see also Ulcer, intestine) 569.82
 breast 611.0
 bronchitis 491.8
 bronchus 519.19
 buccal (cavity) (traumatic) 528.9
 burn (acute) - see Ulcer, duodenum
 Buruli 031.1
 buttock (see also Ulcer, skin) 707.8
   decubitus (see also Ulcer, pressure) 707.00
 cancerous (M8000/3) - see Neoplasm, by site, malignant
 cardia - see Ulcer, stomach
 cardio-esophageal (peptic) 530.20
  with bleeding 530.21
 cecum (see also Ulcer, intestine) 569.82
 cervix (uteri) (trophic) 622.0
  with mention of cervicitis 616.0
 chancroidal 099.0
 chest (wall) (see also Ulcer, skin) 707.8
 Chiclero 085.4
 chin (pyogenic) (see also Ulcer, skin) 707.8
 chronic (cause unknown) - see also Ulcer, skin
  penis 607.89
 Cochin-China 085.1
 colitis - see Colitis, ulcerative
 colon (see also Ulcer, intestine) 569.82

Ulcer, ulcerated, ulcerating, ulceration, ulcerative (Continued)
 conjunctiva (acute) (postinfectional) 372.00
 cornea (infectional) 370.00
   with perforation 370.06
   annular 370.02
   catarrhal 370.01
   central 370.03
   dendritic 054.42
   marginal 370.01
   mycotic 370.05
   phlyctenular, tuberculous (see also Tuberculosis) 017.3 ● [370.31]
   ring 370.02
   rodent 370.07
   serpent, serpiginous 370.04
   superficial marginal 370.01
   tuberculous (see also Tuberculosis) 017.3 ● [370.31]
 corpus cavernosum (chronic) 607.89
 crural - see Ulcer, lower extremity
 Curling's - see Ulcer, duodenum
 Cushing's - see Ulcer, peptic
 cystitis (interstitial) 595.1
 decubitus (unspecified site) (see also Ulcer, pressure) 707.00
   with gangrene 707.00 [785.4]
   ankle 707.06
   back
    lower 707.03
    upper 707.02
   buttock 707.05
   coccyx 707.03
   elbow 707.01
   head 707.09
   heel 707.07
   hip 707.04
   other site 707.09
   sacrum 707.03
   shoulder blades 707.02
 dendritic 054.42
 diabetes, diabetic (mellitus) 250.8 ● [707.9]
   due to secondary diabetes 249.8 ● [707.9]
   lower limb 250.8 ● [707.10]
    due to secondary diabetes 249.8 ● [707.10]
    ankle 250.8 ● [707.13]
     due to secondary diabetes 249.8 ● [707.13]
    calf 250.8 ● [707.12]
     due to secondary diabetes 249.8 ● [707.12]
    foot 250.8 ● [707.15]
     due to secondary diabetes 249.8 ● [707.15]
    heel 250.8 ● [707.14]
     due to secondary diabetes 249.8 ● [707.14]
    knee 250.8 ● [707.19]
     due to secondary diabetes 249.8 ● [707.19]
    specified site NEC 250.8 ● [707.19]
     due to secondary diabetes 249.8 ● [707.19]
    thigh 250.8 ● [707.11]
     due to secondary diabetes 249.8 ● [707.11]
    toes 250.8 ● [707.15]
     due to secondary diabetes 249.8 ● [707.15]

Ulcer, ulcerated, ulcerating, ulceration, ulcerative (Continued)
 diabetes, diabetic (Continued)
  lower limb (Continued)
   specified site NEC 250.8 ● [707.8]
    due to secondary diabetes 249.8 ● [707.8]
 Dieulafoy - see Lesion, Dieulafoy
  due to
   infection NEC - see Ulcer, skin
   radiation, radium - see Ulcer, by site
   trophic disturbance (any region) - see Ulcer, skin
   x-ray - see Ulcer, by site
 duodenum, duodenal (eroded) (peptic) 532.9 ●

> Note: Use the following fifth-digit subclassification with categories 531–534:
>
> 0 without mention of obstruction
> 1 with obstruction

   with
    hemorrhage (chronic) 532.4 ●
     and perforation 532.6 ●
    perforation (chronic) 532.5 ●
     and hemorrhage 532.6 ●
   acute 532.3 ●
    with
     hemorrhage 532.0 ●
      and perforation 532.2 ●
     perforation 532.1 ●
      and hemorrhage 532.2 ●
   bleeding (recurrent) - see Ulcer, duodenum, with hemorrhage
   chronic 532.7 ●
    with
     hemorrhage 532.4 ●
      and perforation 532.6 ●
     perforation 532.5 ●
      and hemorrhage 532.6 ●
   penetrating - see Ulcer, duodenum, with perforation
   perforating - see Ulcer, duodenum, with perforation
 dysenteric NEC 009.0
 elusive 595.1
 endocarditis (any valve) (acute) (chronic) (subacute) 421.0
 enteritis - see Colitis, ulcerative
 enterocolitis 556.0
 epiglottis 478.79
 esophagus (peptic) 530.20
   with bleeding 530.21
   due to ingestion
    aspirin 530.20
    chemicals 530.20
    medicinal agents 530.20
   fungal 530.20
   infectional 530.20
   varicose (see also Varix, esophagus) 456.1
    bleeding (see also Varix, esophagus, bleeding) 456.0
 eye NEC 360.00
  dendritic 054.42
 eyelid (region) 373.01
 face (see also Ulcer, skin) 707.8
 fauces 478.29
 Fenwick (-Hunner) (solitary) (see also Cystitis) 595.1

Ulcer, ulcerated, ulcerating, ulceration, ulcerative *(Continued)*
fistulous NEC - *see* Ulcer, skin
foot (indolent) *(see also* Ulcer, lower extremity) 707.15
   perforating 707.15
     leprous 030.1
     syphilitic 094.0
   trophic 707.15
   varicose 454.0
     inflamed or infected 454.2
frambesial, initial or primary 102.0
gallbladder or duct 575.8
gall duct 576.8
gangrenous *(see also* Gangrene) 785.4
gastric - *see* Ulcer, stomach
gastrocolic - *see* Ulcer, gastrojejunal
gastroduodenal - *see* Ulcer, peptic
gastroesophageal - *see* Ulcer, stomach
gastrohepatic - *see* Ulcer, stomach
gastrointestinal - *see* Ulcer, gastrojejunal
gastrojejunal (eroded) (peptic) 534.9

> Note: Use the following fifth-digit subclassification with categories 531–534:
>
> 0   without mention of obstruction
> 1   with obstruction

   with
     hemorrhage (chronic) 534.4 ●
       and perforation 534.6 ●
     perforation 534.5 ●
       and hemorrhage 534.6 ●
   acute 534.3 ●
     with
       hemorrhage 534.0 ●
         and perforation 534.2 ●
       perforation 534.1 ●
        and hemorrhage 534.2 ●
   bleeding (recurrent) - *see* Ulcer, gastrojejunal, with hemorrhage
   chronic 534.7 ●
     with
       hemorrhage 534.4 ●
         and perforation 534.6 ●
       perforation 534.5 ●
        and hemorrhage 534.6 ●
   penetrating - *see* Ulcer, gastrojejunal, with perforation
   perforating - *see* Ulcer, gastrojejunal, with perforation
gastrojejunocolic - *see* Ulcer, gastrojejunal
genital organ
   female 629.89
   male 608.89
gingiva 523.8
gingivitis 523.10
glottis 478.79
granuloma of pudenda 099.2
groin *(see also* Ulcer, skin) 707.8
gum 523.8
gumma, due to yaws 102.4
hand *(see also* Ulcer, skin) 707.8
hard palate 528.9
heel *(see also* Ulcer, lower extremity) 707.14
   decubitus *(see also* Ulcer, pressure) 707.07
hemorrhoids 455.8
   external 455.5
   internal 455.2

Ulcer, ulcerated, ulcerating, ulceration, ulcerative *(Continued)*
hip *(see also* Ulcer, skin) 707.8
   decubitus *(see also* Ulcer, pressure) 707.04
Hunner's 595.1
hypopharynx 478.29
hypopyon (chronic) (subacute) 370.04
hypostaticum - *see* Ulcer, varicose
ileocolitis 556.1
ileum *(see also* Ulcer, intestine) 569.82
intestine, intestinal 569.82
   with perforation 569.83
   amebic 006.9
   duodenal - *see* Ulcer, duodenum
   granulocytopenic (with hemorrhage) 288.09
   marginal 569.82
   perforating 569.83
   small, primary 569.82
   stercoraceous 569.82
   stercoral 569.82
   tuberculous *(see also* Tuberculosis) 014.8 ●
   typhoid (fever) 002.0
   varicose 456.8
ischemic 707.9
   lower extremity *(see also* Ulcer, lower extremity) 707.10
     ankle 707.13
     calf 707.12
     foot 707.15
     heel 707.14
     knee 707.19
     specified site NEC 707.19
     thigh 707.11
     toes 707.15
jejunum, jejunal - *see* Ulcer, gastrojejunal
keratitis *(see also* Ulcer, cornea) 370.00
knee - *see* Ulcer, lower extremity
labium (majus) (minus) 616.50
laryngitis *(see also* Laryngitis) 464.00
   with obstruction 464.01
larynx (aphthous) (contact) 478.79
   diphtheritic 032.3
leg - *see* Ulcer, lower extremity
lip 528.5
Lipschütz's 616.50
lower extremity (atrophic) (chronic) (neurogenic) (perforating) (pyogenic) (trophic) (tropical) 707.10
   with gangrene *(see also* Ulcer, lower extremity) 707.10 *[785.4]*
     arteriosclerotic 440.24
   ankle 707.13
   arteriosclerotic 440.23
     with gangrene 440.24
   calf 707.12
   decubitus *(see also* Ulcer, pressure) 707.00
     with gangrene 707.00 *[785.4]*
     ankle 707.06
     buttock 707.05
     heel 707.07
     hip 707.04
   foot 707.15
   heel 707.14
   knee 707.19
   specified site NEC 707.19
   thigh 707.11

Ulcer, ulcerated, ulcerating, ulceration, ulcerative *(Continued)*
lower extremity *(Continued)*
   toes 707.15
   varicose 454.0
     inflamed or infected 454.2
luetic - *see* Ulcer, syphilitic
lung 518.89
   tuberculous *(see also* Tuberculosis) 011.2 ●
malignant (M8000/3) - *see* Neoplasm, by site, malignant
marginal NEC - *see* Ulcer, gastrojejunal
meatus (urinarius) 597.89
Meckel's diverticulum 751.0
Meleney's (chronic undermining) 686.09
Mooren's (cornea) 370.07
mouth (traumatic) 528.9
mycobacterial (skin) 031.1
nasopharynx 478.29
navel cord (newborn) 771.4
neck *(see also* Ulcer, skin) 707.8
   uterus 622.0
neurogenic NEC - *see* Ulcer, skin
nose, nasal (infectional) (passage) 478.19
   septum 478.19
     varicose 456.8
   skin - *see* Ulcer, skin
   spirochetal NEC 104.8
oral mucosa (traumatic) 528.9
palate (soft) 528.9
penetrating NEC - *see* Ulcer, peptic, with perforation
penis (chronic) 607.89
peptic (site unspecified) 533.9

> Note: Use the following fifth-digit subclassification with categories 531–534:
>
> 0   without mention of obstruction
> 1   with obstruction

   with
     hemorrhage 533.4 ●
       and perforation 533.6 ●
     perforation (chronic) 533.5 ●
       and hemorrhage 533.6 ●
   acute 533.3 ●
     with
       hemorrhage 533.0 ●
         and perforation 533.2 ●
       perforation 533.1 ●
        and hemorrhage 533.2 ●
   bleeding (recurrent) - *see* Ulcer, peptic, with hemorrhage
   chronic 533.7 ●
     with
       hemorrhage 533.4 ●
         and perforation 533.6 ●
       perforation 533.5 ●
        and hemorrhage 533.6 ●
   penetrating - *see* Ulcer, peptic, with perforation
   perforating NEC *(see also* Ulcer, peptic, with perforation) 533.5 ●
   skin 707.9
perineum *(see also* Ulcer, skin) 707.8
peritonsillar 474.8
phagedenic (tropical) NEC - *see* Ulcer, skin
pharynx 478.29
phlebitis - *see* Phlebitis

◀ New   ◀ Revised   ~~deleted~~ Deleted   ● Use Additional Digit(s)   ▢ Omit code

Ulcer, ulcerated, ulcerating, ulceration, ulcerative (Continued)
plaster (see also Ulcer, pressure) 707.00
popliteal space - see Ulcer, lower extremity
postpyloric - see Ulcer, duodenum
prepuce 607.89
prepyloric - see Ulcer, stomach
pressure 707.00
  with
    abrasion, blister, partial thickness skin loss involving epidermis and/or dermis 707.22
    full thickness skin loss involving damage or necrosis of subcutaneous tissue 707.23
    gangrene 707.00 [785.4]
    necrosis of soft tissues through to underlying muscle, tendon, or bone 707.24
  ankle 707.06
  back
    lower 707.03
    upper 707.02
  buttock 707.05
  coccyx 707.03
  elbow 707.01
  head 707.09
  healed - omit code
  healing - code to Ulcer, pressure, by stage
  heel 707.07
  hip 707.04
  other site 707.09
  sacrum 707.03
  shoulder blades 707.02
  stage
    I (healing) 707.21
    II (healing) 707.22
    III (healing) 707.23
    IV (healing) 707.24
    unspecified (healing) 707.20
  unstageable 707.25
primary of intestine 569.82
  with perforation 569.83
proctitis 556.2
  with ulcerative sigmoiditis 556.3
prostate 601.8
pseudopeptic - see Ulcer, peptic
pyloric - see Ulcer, stomach
rectosigmoid 569.82
  with perforation 569.83
rectum (sphincter) (solitary) 569.41
  stercoraceous, stercoral 569.41
  varicose - see Varicose, ulcer, anus
retina (see also Chorioretinitis) 363.20
rodent (M8090/3) - see also Neoplasm, skin, malignant
  cornea 370.07
round - see Ulcer, stomach
sacrum (region) (see also Ulcer, skin) 707.8
Saemisch's 370.04
scalp (see also Ulcer, skin) 707.8
sclera 379.09
scrofulous (see also Tuberculosis) 017.2●
scrotum 608.89
  tuberculous (see also Tuberculosis) 016.5●
  varicose 456.4
seminal vesicle 608.89

Ulcer, ulcerated, ulcerating, ulceration, ulcerative (Continued)
sigmoid 569.82
  with perforation 569.83
skin (atrophic) (chronic) (neurogenic) (non-healing) (perforating) (pyogenic) (trophic) 707.9
  with gangrene 707.9 [785.4]
  amebic 006.6
  decubitus (see also Ulcer, pressure) 707.00
    with gangrene 707.00 [785.4]
  in granulocytopenia 288.09
  lower extremity (see also Ulcer, lower extremity) 707.10
    with gangrene 707.10 [785.4]
    arteriosclerotic 440.24
    ankle 707.13
    arteriosclerotic 440.23
      with gangrene 440.24
    calf 707.12
    foot 707.15
    heel 707.14
    knee 707.19
    specified site NEC 707.19
    thigh 707.11
    toes 707.15
  mycobacterial 031.1
  syphilitic (early) (secondary) 091.3
  tuberculous (primary) (see also Tuberculosis) 017.0●
  varicose - see Ulcer, varicose
sloughing NEC - see Ulcer, skin
soft palate 528.9
solitary, anus or rectum (sphincter) 569.41
sore throat 462
  streptococcal 034.0
spermatic cord 608.89
spine (tuberculous) 015.0● [730.88]
stasis (leg) (venous) 454.0
  with varicose veins 454.0
  without varicose veins 459.81
  inflamed or infected 454.2
stercoral, stercoraceous 569.82
  with perforation 569.83
  anus or rectum 569.41
stoma, stomal - see Ulcer, gastrojejunal
stomach (eroded) (peptic) (round) 531.9●

Note: Use the following fifth-digit subclassification with categories 531–534:
  0 without mention of obstruction
  1 with obstruction

  with
    hemorrhage 531.4●
      and perforation 531.6●
    perforation (chronic) 531.5●
      and hemorrhage 531.6●
  acute 531.3●
    with
      hemorrhage 531.0●
        and perforation 531.2●
      perforation 531.1●
        and hemorrhage 531.2●
  bleeding (recurrent) - see Ulcer, stomach, with hemorrhage

Ulcer, ulcerated, ulcerating, ulceration, ulcerative (Continued)
stomach (Continued)
  chronic 531.7●
    with
      hemorrhage 531.4●
        and perforation 531.6●
      perforation 531.5●
        and hemorrhage 531.6●
  penetrating - see Ulcer, stomach, with perforation
  perforating - see Ulcer, stomach, with perforation
stomatitis 528.00
stress - see Ulcer, peptic
strumous (tuberculous) (see also Tuberculosis) 017.2●
submental (see also Ulcer, skin) 707.8
submucosal, bladder 595.1
syphilitic (any site) (early) (secondary) 091.3
  late 095.9
  perforating 095.9
    foot 094.0
testis 608.89
thigh - see Ulcer, lower extremity
throat 478.29
  diphtheritic 032.0
toe - see Ulcer, lower extremity
tongue (traumatic) 529.0
tonsil 474.8
  diphtheritic 032.0
trachea 519.19
trophic - see Ulcer, skin
tropical NEC (see also Ulcer, skin) 707.9
tuberculous - see Tuberculosis, ulcer
tunica vaginalis 608.89
turbinate 730.9●
typhoid (fever) 002.0
  perforating 002.0
umbilicus (newborn) 771.4
unspecified site NEC - see Ulcer, skin
urethra (meatus) (see also Urethritis) 597.89
uterus 621.8
  cervix 622.0
    with mention of cervicitis 616.0
  neck 622.0
    with mention of cervicitis 616.0
vagina 616.89
valve, heart 421.0
varicose (lower extremity, any part) 454.0
  anus - see Varicose, ulcer, anus
  broad ligament 456.5
  esophagus (see also Varix, esophagus) 456.1
    bleeding (see also Varix, esophagus, bleeding) 456.0
  inflamed or infected 454.2
  nasal septum 456.8
  perineum 456.6
  rectum - see Varicose, ulcer, anus
  scrotum 456.4
  specified site NEC 456.8
  sublingual 456.3
  vulva 456.6
vas deferens 608.89
vesical (see also Ulcer, bladder) 596.8
vulva (acute) (infectional) 616.50
  Behçet's syndrome 136.1 [616.51]
  herpetic 054.12
  tuberculous 016.7● [616.51]
vulvobuccal, recurring 616.50
x-ray - see Ulcer, by site
yaws 102.4

Ulcerosa scarlatina 034.1
Ulcus - *see also* Ulcer
  cutis tuberculosum (*see also*
      Tuberculosis) 017.0 ●
  duodeni - *see* Ulcer, duodenum
  durum 091.0
      extragenital 091.2
  gastrojejunale - *see* Ulcer, gastrojejunal
  hypostaticum - *see* Ulcer, varicose
  molle (cutis) (skin) 099.0
  serpens corneae (pneumococcal) 370.04
  ventriculi - *see* Ulcer, stomach
Ulegyria 742.4
Ulerythema
  acneiforma 701.8
  centrifugum 695.4
  ophryogenes 757.4
Ullrich (-Bonnevie) (-Turner) syndrome
    758.6
Ullrich-Feichtiger syndrome 759.89
Ulnar - *see* condition
Ulorrhagia 523.8
Ulorrhea 523.8
Umbilicus, umbilical - *see also* condition
  cord necrosis, affecting fetus or
      newborn 762.6
Unacceptable
  existing dental restoration
      contours 525.65
      morphology 525.65
Unavailability of medical facilities (at)
    V63.9
  due to
      investigation by social service
          agency V63.8
      lack of services at home V63.1
      remoteness from facility V63.0
      waiting list V63.2
  home V63.1
  outpatient clinic V63.0
  specified reason NEC V63.8
Uncinaria americana infestation 126.1
Uncinariasis (*see also* Ancylostomiasis)
    126.9
Unconscious, unconsciousness 780.09
Underdevelopment - *see also*
      Undeveloped sexual 259.0
Underfill, endodontic 526.63
Undernourishment 269.9
Undernutrition 269.9
Under observation - *see* Observation
Underweight 783.22
  for gestational age - *see* Light-for-dates
Underwood's disease (sclerema
    neonatorum) 778.1
Undescended - *see also* Malposition,
      congenital
  cecum 751.4
  colon 751.4
  testis 752.51
Undetermined diagnosis or cause 799.9
Undeveloped, undevelopment - *see also*
      Hypoplasia
  brain (congenital) 742.1
  cerebral (congenital) 742.1
  fetus or newborn 764.9 ●
  heart 746.89
  lung 748.5
  testis 257.2
  uterus 259.0
Undiagnosed (disease) 799.9
Undulant fever (*see also* Brucellosis) 023.9
Unemployment, anxiety concerning V62.0
Unequal leg (acquired) (length) 736.81
  congenital 755.30
Unerupted teeth, tooth 520.6
Unextracted dental root 525.3

Unguis incarnatus 703.0
Unicornis uterus 752.33 ◀━
Unicornuate uterus (with or without a
    separate uterine horn) 752.33 ◀
Unicorporeus uterus 752.39 ◀━
Uniformis uterus 752.39 ◀━
Unilateral - *see also* condition
  development, breast 611.89
  organ or site, congenital NEC - *see*
      Agenesis
  vagina 752.49
Unilateralis uterus 752.39 ◀━
Unilocular heart 745.8
Uninhibited bladder 596.54
  with cauda equina syndrome 344.61
  neurogenic (*see also* Neurogenic,
      bladder) 596.54
Union, abnormal - *see also* Fusion
  divided tendon 727.89
  larynx and trachea 748.3
Universal
  joint, cervix 620.6
  mesentery 751.4
Unknown
  cause of death 799.9
  diagnosis 799.9
Unna's disease (seborrheic dermatitis)
    690.10
Unresponsiveness, adrenocorticotropin
    (ACTH) 255.41
Unsatisfactory
  cytology smear
      anal 796.78
      cervical 795.08
      vaginal 795.18
  restoration, tooth (existing) 525.60
      specified NEC 525.69
Unsoundness of mind (*see also* Psychosis)
    298.9
Unspecified cause of death 799.9
Unstable
  back NEC 724.9
  colon 569.89
  joint - *see* Instability, joint
  lie 652.0 ●
      affecting fetus or newborn (before
          labor) 761.7
      causing obstructed labor 660.0 ●
          affecting fetus or newborn 763.1
  lumbosacral joint (congenital) 756.19
      acquired 724.6
  sacroiliac 724.6
  spine NEC 724.9
Untruthfulness, child problem (*see also*
    Disturbance, conduct) 312.0 ●
Unverricht (-Lundborg) disease,
    syndrome, or epilepsy 345.1 ●
Unverricht-Wagner syndrome
    (dermatomyositis) 710.3
Upper respiratory - *see* condition
Upset
  gastric 536.8
      psychogenic 306.4
  gastrointestinal 536.8
      psychogenic 306.4
      virus (*see also* Enteritis, viral) 008.8
  intestinal (large) (small) 564.9
      psychogenic 306.4
  menstruation 626.9
  mental 300.9
  stomach 536.8
      psychogenic 306.4
Urachus - *see also* condition
  patent 753.7
  persistent 753.7

Uratic arthritis 274.00
Urbach's lipoid proteinosis 272.8
Urbach-Oppenheim disease or syndrome
    (necrobiosis lipoidica diabeticorum)
    250.8 ● [709.3]
  due to secondary diabetes 249.8 ●
    [709.3]
Urbach-Wiethe disease or syndrome
    (lipoid proteinosis) 272.8
Urban yellow fever 060.1
Urea, blood, high - *see* Uremia
Uremia, uremic (absorption) (amaurosis)
    (amblyopia) (aphasia) (apoplexy)
    (coma) (delirium) (dementia)
    (dropsy) (dyspnea) (fever)
    (intoxication) (mania) (paralysis)
    (poisoning) (toxemia) (vomiting)
    586
  with
    abortion - *see* Abortion, by type,
        with renal failure
    ectopic pregnancy (*see also*
        categories 633.0–633.9) 639.3
    hypertension (*see also* Hypertension,
        kidney) 403.91
    molar pregnancy (*see also* categories
        630–632) 639.3
  chronic 585.9
  complicating
    abortion 639.3
    ectopic or molar pregnancy 639.3
    hypertension (*see also* Hypertension,
        kidney) 403.91
    labor and delivery 669.3 ●
  congenital 779.89
  extrarenal 788.99
  hypertensive (chronic) (*see also*
        Hypertension, kidney)
        403.91
  maternal NEC, affecting fetus or
        newborn 760.1
  neuropathy 585.9 [357.4]
  pericarditis 585.9 [420.0]
  prerenal 788.99
  pyelitic (*see also* Pyelitis) 590.80
Ureter, ureteral - *see* condition
Ureteralgia 788.0
Ureterectasis 593.89
Ureteritis 593.89
  cystica 590.3
  due to calculus 592.1
  gonococcal (acute) 098.19
    chronic or duration of 2 months or
        over 098.39
  nonspecific 593.89
Ureterocele (acquired) 593.89
  congenital 753.23
Ureterolith 592.1
Ureterolithiasis 592.1
Ureterostomy status V44.6
  with complication 997.5
Urethra, urethral - *see* condition
Urethralgia 788.99
Urethritis (abacterial) (acute) (allergic)
    (anterior) (chronic) (nonvenereal)
    (posterior) (recurrent) (simple)
    (subacute) (ulcerative)
    (undifferentiated) 597.80
  diplococcal (acute) 098.0
    chronic or duration of 2 months or
        over 098.2
  due to Trichomonas (vaginalis) 131.02
  gonococcal (acute) 098.0
    chronic or duration of 2 months or
        over 098.2

◀ New   ◀━ Revised   ~~deleted~~ Deleted   ● Use Additional Digit(s)   ▨ Omit code

Urethritis (*Continued*)
nongonococcal (sexually transmitted) 099.40
Chlamydia trachomatis 099.41
Reiter's 099.3
specified organism NEC 099.49
nonspecific (sexually transmitted) (*see also* Urethritis, nongonococcal) 099.40
not sexually transmitted 597.80
Reiter's 099.3
trichomonal or due to Trichomonas (vaginalis) 131.02
tuberculous (*see also* Tuberculosis) 016.3●
venereal NEC (*see also* Urethritis, nongonococcal) 099.40
Urethrocele
female 618.03
with uterine prolapse 618.4
complete 618.3
incomplete 618.2
male 599.5
Urethrolithiasis 594.2
Urethro-oculoarticular syndrome 099.3
Urethro-oculosynovial syndrome 099.3
Urethrorectal - *see* condition
Urethrorrhagia 599.84
Urethrorrhea 788.7
Urethrostomy status V44.6
with complication 997.5
Urethrotrigonitis 595.3
Urethrovaginal - *see* condition
Urgency ◀
fecal 787.63 ◀
hypertensive - *see* Hypertension ◀
Urhidrosis, uridrosis 705.89
Uric acid
diathesis 274.9
in blood 790.6
Uricacidemia 790.6
Uricemia 790.6
Uricosuria 791.9
Urination
frequent 788.41
painful 788.1
urgency 788.63
Urine, urinary - *see also* condition
abnormality NEC 788.69
blood in (*see also* Hematuria) 599.70
discharge, excessive 788.42
enuresis 788.30
nonorganic origin 307.6
extravasation 788.8
frequency 788.41
hesitancy 788.64
incontinence 788.30
active 788.30
female 788.30
stress 625.6
and urge 788.33
male 788.30
stress 788.32
and urge 788.33
mixed (stress and urge) 788.33
neurogenic 788.39
nonorganic origin 307.6
overflow 788.38
stress (female) 625.6
male NEC 788.32
intermittent stream 788.61
pus in 791.9

Urine, urinary (*Continued*)
retention or stasis NEC 788.20
bladder, incomplete emptying 788.21
psychogenic 306.53
specified NEC 788.29
secretion
deficient 788.5
excessive 788.42
frequency 788.41
strain 788.65
stream
intermittent 788.61
slowing 788.62
splitting 788.61
weak 788.62
urgency 788.63
Urinemia - *see* Uremia
Urinoma NEC 599.9
bladder 596.8
kidney 593.89
renal 593.89
ureter 593.89
urethra 599.84
Uroarthritis, infectious 099.3
Urodialysis 788.5
Urolithiasis 592.9
Uronephrosis 593.89
Uropathy 599.9
obstructive 599.60
Urosepsis 599.0
meaning sepsis 995.91
meaning urinary tract infection 599.0
Urticaria 708.9
with angioneurotic edema 995.1
hereditary 277.6
allergic 708.0
cholinergic 708.5
chronic 708.8
cold, familial 708.2
dermatographic 708.3
due to
cold or heat 708.2
drugs 708.0
food 708.0
inhalants 708.0
plants 708.8
serum 999.5
factitial 708.3
giant 995.1
hereditary 277.6
gigantea 995.1
hereditary 277.6
idiopathic 708.1
larynx 995.1
hereditary 277.6
neonatorum 778.8
nonallergic 708.1
papulosa (Hebra) 698.2
perstans hemorrhagica 757.39
pigmentosa 757.33
recurrent periodic 708.8
serum 999.5
solare 692.72
specified type NEC 708.8
thermal (cold) (heat) 708.2
vibratory 708.4
Urticarioides acarodermatitis 133.9
Use of
agents affecting estrogen receptors and estrogen levels NEC V07.59 ◀
anastrozole (Arimidex) V07.52 ◀
aromatase inhibitors V07.52 ◀
estrogen receptor downregulators V07.59 ◀

Urticaria (*Continued*)
exemestane (Aromasin) V07.52 ◀
fulvestrant (Faslodex) V07.59 ◀
gonadotropin-releasing hormone (GnRH) agonist V07.59 ◀
goserelin acetate (Zoladex) V07.59 ◀
letrozole (Femara) V07.52 ◀
leuprolide acetate (leuprorelin) (Lupron) V07.59 ◀
megestrol acetate (Megace) V07.59 ◀
methadone 304.00
nonprescribed drugs (*see also* Abuse, drugs, nondependent) 305.9●
patent medicines (*see also* Abuse, drugs, nondependent) 305.9●
raloxifene (Evista) V07.51 ◀
selective estrogen receptor modulators (SERMs) V07.51 ◀
tamoxifen (Nolvadex) V07.51 ◀
toremifene (Fareston) V07.51 ◀
Usher-Senear disease (pemphigus erythematosus) 694.4
Uta 085.5
Uterine size-date discrepancy 649.6●
Uteromegaly 621.2
Uterovaginal - *see* condition
Uterovesical - *see* condition
Uterus - *see also* condition ◀▥
with only one functioning horn 752.33 ◀
Utriculitis (utriculus prostaticus) 597.89
Uveal - *see* condition
Uveitis (anterior) (*see also* Iridocyclitis) 364.3
acute or subacute 364.00
due to or associated with
gonococcal infection 098.41
herpes (simplex) 054.44
zoster 053.22
primary 364.01
recurrent 364.02
secondary (noninfectious) 364.04
infectious 364.03
allergic 360.11
chronic 364.10
due to or associated with
sarcoidosis 135 [364.11]
tuberculosis (*see also* Tuberculosis) 017.3● [364.11]
due to
operation 360.11
toxoplasmosis (acquired) 130.2
congenital (active) 771.2
granulomatous 364.10
heterochromic 364.21
lens-induced 364.23
nongranulomatous 364.00
posterior 363.20
disseminated - *see* Chorioretinitis, disseminated
focal - *see* Chorioretinitis, focal
recurrent 364.02
sympathetic 360.11
syphilitic (secondary) 091.50
congenital 090.0 [363.13]
late 095.8 [363.13]
tuberculous (*see also* Tuberculosis) 017.3● [364.11]
Uveoencephalitis 363.22
Uveokeratitis (*see also* Iridocyclitis) 364.3
Uveoparotid fever 135
Uveoparotitis 135
Uvula - *see* condition
Uvulitis (acute) (catarrhal) (chronic) (gangrenous) (membranous) (suppurative) (ulcerative) 528.3

V

Vaccination
complication or reaction - *see*
    Complications, vaccination
delayed V64.00
not carried out V64.00
    because of
        acute illness V64.01
        allergy to vaccine or component
            V64.04
        caregiver refusal V64.05
        chronic illness V64.02
        guardian refusal V64.05
        immune compromised state
            V64.03
        parent refusal V64.05
        patient had disease being
            vaccinated against
            V64.08
        patient refusal V64.06
        reason NEC V64.09
        religious reasons V64.07
prophylactic (against) V05.9
    arthropod-borne viral
        disease NEC V05.1
        encephalitis V05.0
    chicken pox V05.4
    cholera (alone) V03.0
        with typhoid-paratyphoid
            (cholera + TAB) V06.0
    common cold V04.7
    diphtheria (alone) V03.5
        with
            poliomyelitis (DTP + polio)
                V06.3
            tetanus V06.5
                pertussis combined [DTP]
                    (DTaP) V06.1
                typhoid-paratyphoid (DTP +
                    TAB) V06.2
    disease (single) NEC V05.9
        bacterial NEC V03.9
            specified type NEC V03.89
        combination NEC V06.9
            specified type NEC V06.8
        specified type NEC V05.8
    encephalitis, viral, arthropod-borne
        V05.0
    Hemophilus influenzae, type B
        [Hib] V03.81
    hepatitis, viral V05.3
    influenza V04.81
        with
            Streptococcus pneumoniae
                [pneumococcus] V06.6
    leishmaniasis V05.2
    measles (alone) V04.2
        with mumps-rubella (MMR)
            V06.4
    mumps (alone) V04.6
        with measles and rubella (MMR)
            V06.4
    pertussis alone V03.6
    plague V03.3
    poliomyelitis V04.0
        with diphtheria-tetanus-pertussis
            (DTP polio) V06.3
    rabies V04.5
    respiratory syncytial virus (RSV)
        V04.82
    rubella (alone) V04.3
        with measles and mumps (MMR)
            V06.4

Vaccination *(Continued)*
    prophylactic *(Continued)*
        smallpox V04.1
        Streptococcus pneumoniae
            [pneumococcus] V03.82
            with
                influenza V06.6
        tetanus toxoid (alone) V03.7
            with diphtheria [Td] [DT] V06.5
                with
                    pertussis (DTP) (DTaP)
                        V06.1
                        with poliomyelitis (DTP
                            + polio) V06.3
        tuberculosis (BCG) V03.2
        tularemia V03.4
        typhoid-paratyphoid (TAB) (alone)
            V03.1
            with diphtheria-tetanus-pertussis
                (TAB + DTP) V06.2
        varicella V05.4
        viral
            disease NEC V04.89
            encephalitis, arthropod-borne
                V05.0
            hepatitis V05.3
        yellow fever V04.4
Vaccinia (generalized) 999.0
    congenital 771.2
    conjunctiva 999.39
    eyelids 999.3 [373.5]
    localized 999.39
    nose 999.39
    not from vaccination 051.02
        eyelid 051.02 [373.5]
    sine vaccinatione 051.02
    without vaccination 051.02
Vacuum
    extraction of fetus or newborn 763.3
    in sinus (accessory) (nasal) *(see also*
        Sinusitis) 473.9
Vagabond V60.0
Vagabondage V60.0
Vagabonds' disease 132.1
Vagina, vaginal - *see also* condition
    high risk human papillomavirus (HPV)
        DNA test positive 795.15
    low risk human papillomavirus (HPV)
        DNA test positive 795.19
Vaginalitis (tunica) 608.4
Vaginismus (reflex) 625.1
    functional 306.51
    hysterical 300.11
    psychogenic 306.51
Vaginitis (acute) (chronic)
        (circumscribed) (diffuse)
        (emphysematous) (Hemophilus
        vaginalis) (nonspecific)
        (nonvenereal) (ulcerative) 616.10
    with
        abortion - *see* Abortion, by type,
            with sepsis
        ectopic pregnancy *(see also*
            categories 633.0–633.9)
            639.0
        molar pregnancy *(see also* categories
            630–632) 639.0
    adhesive, congenital 752.49
    atrophic, postmenopausal 627.3
    bacterial 616.10
    blennorrhagic (acute) 098.0
        chronic or duration of 2 months or
            over 098.2
    candidal 112.1

Vaginitis *(Continued)*
    chlamydial 099.53
    complicating pregnancy or puerperium
        646.6●
        affecting fetus or newborn 760.8
    congenital (adhesive) 752.49
    due to
        C. albicans 112.1
        Trichomonas (vaginalis) 131.01
    following
        abortion 639.0
        ectopic or molar pregnancy 639.0
    gonococcal (acute) 098.0
        chronic or duration of 2 months or
            over 098.2
    granuloma 099.2
    Monilia 112.1
    mycotic 112.1
    pinworm 127.4 [616.11]
    postirradiation 616.10
    postmenopausal atrophic 627.3
    senile (atrophic) 627.3
    syphilitic (early) 091.0
        late 095.8
    trichomonal 131.01
    tuberculous *(see also* Tuberculosis)
        016.7●
    venereal NEC 099.8
Vaginosis - *see* Vaginitis
Vagotonia 352.3
Vagrancy V60.0
VAIN I (vaginal intraepithelial neoplasia
    I) 623.0
VAIN II (vaginal intraepithelial neoplasia
    II) 623.0
VAIN III (vaginal intraepithelial
    neoplasia III) 233.31
Vallecula - *see* condition
Valley fever 114.0
Valsuani's disease (progressive
    pernicious anemia, puerperal)
    648.2●
Valve, valvular (formation) - *see also*
    condition
    cerebral ventricle (communicating) in
        situ V45.2
    cervix, internal os 752.49
    colon 751.5
    congenital NEC - *see* Atresia
    formation congenital NEC - *see* Atresia
    heart defect - *see* Anomaly, heart, valve
    ureter 753.29
        pelvic junction 753.21
        vesical orifice 753.22
    urethra 753.6
Valvulitis (chronic) *(see also* Endocarditis)
    424.90
    rheumatic (chronic) (inactive) (with
        chorea) 397.9
        active or acute (aortic) (mitral)
            (pulmonary) (tricuspid)
            391.1
    syphilitic NEC 093.20
        aortic 093.22
        mitral 093.21
        pulmonary 093.24
        tricuspid 093.23
Valvulopathy - *see* Endocarditis
van Bogaert's leukoencephalitis
    (sclerosing) (subacute) 046.2
van Bogaert-Nijssen (-Peiffer) **disease**
    330.0
van Buchem's syndrome (hyperostosis
    corticalis) 733.3

Vancomycin (glycopeptide)
  intermediate staphylococcus aureus
    (VISA/GISA) V09.8
  resistant
    enterococcus (VRE) V09.8
    staphylococcus aureus (VRSA/
      GRSA) V09.8
van Creveld-von Gierke disease
  (glycogenosis I) 271.0
van den Bergh's disease (enterogenous
  cyanosis) 289.7
van der Hoeve's syndrome (brittle bones
  and blue sclera, deafness) 756.51
van der Hoeve-Halbertsma-
  Waardenburg syndrome (ptosis-
  epicanthus) 270.2
van der Hoeve-Waardenburg-Gualdi
  syndrome (ptosis-epicanthus) 270.2
Vanillism 692.89
Vanishing lung 492.0
Vanishing twin 651.33
van Neck (-Odelberg) disease or
  syndrome (juvenile osteochondrosis)
  732.1
Vapor asphyxia or suffocation NEC 987.9
  specified agent - see Table of Drugs and
    Chemicals
Vaquez's disease (M9950/1) 238.4
Vaquez-Osler disease (polycythemia
  vera) (M9950/1) 238.4
Variance, lethal ball, prosthetic heart
  valve 996.02
Variants, thalassemic 282.49
Variations in hair color 704.3
Varicella 052.9
  with
    complication 052.8
      specified NEC 052.7
    pneumonia 052.1
  exposure to V01.71
  vaccination and inoculation (against)
    (prophylactic) V05.4
Varices - see Varix
Varicocele (scrotum) (thrombosed) 456.4
  ovary 456.5
  perineum 456.6
  spermatic cord (ulcerated) 456.4
Varicose
  aneurysm (ruptured) (see also
    Aneurysm) 442.9
  dermatitis (lower extremity) - see
    Varicose, vein, inflamed or
    infected
  eczema - see Varicose, vein
  phlebitis - see Varicose, vein, inflamed
    or infected
  placental vessel - see Placenta,
    abnormal
  tumor - see Varicose, vein
  ulcer (lower extremity, any part) 454.0
    anus 455.8
      external 455.5
      internal 455.2
    esophagus (see also Varix,
      esophagus) 456.1
      bleeding (see also Varix,
        esophagus, bleeding)
        456.0
    inflamed or infected 454.2
    nasal septum 456.8
    perineum 456.6
    rectum - see Varicose, ulcer, anus
    scrotum 456.4
    specified site NEC 456.8

Varicose (Continued)
  vein (lower extremity) (ruptured) (see
    also Varix) 454.9
    with
      complications NEC 454.8
      edema 454.8
      inflammation or infection 454.1
        ulcerated 454.2
      pain 454.8
      stasis dermatitis 454.1
        with ulcer 454.2
      swelling 454.8
      ulcer 454.0
        inflamed or infected 454.2
    anus - see Hemorrhoids
    broad ligament 456.5
    congenital (peripheral) 747.60
      gastrointestinal 747.61
      lower limb 747.64
      renal 747.62
      specified NEC 747.69
      upper limb 747.63
    esophagus (ulcerated (see also Varix,
      esophagus) 456.1
      bleeding (see also Varix,
        esophagus, bleeding)
        456.0
    inflamed or infected 454.1
      with ulcer 454.2
    in pregnancy or puerperium
      671.0●
      vulva or perineum 671.1●
    nasal septum (with ulcer) 456.8
    pelvis 456.5
    perineum 456.6
      in pregnancy, childbirth, or
        puerperium 671.1●
    rectum - see Hemorrhoids
    scrotum (ulcerated) 456.4
    specified site NEC 456.8
    sublingual 456.3
    ulcerated 454.0
      inflamed or infected 454.2
    umbilical cord, affecting fetus or
      newborn 762.6
    urethra 456.8
    vulva 456.6
      in pregnancy, childbirth, or
        puerperium 671.1●
  vessel - see also Varix
    placenta - see Placenta, abnormal
Varicosis, varicosities, varicosity (see also
  Varix) 454.9
Variola 050.9
  hemorrhagic (pustular) 050.0
  major 050.0
  minor 050.1
  modified 050.2
Varioloid 050.2
Variolosa, purpura 050.0
Varix (lower extremity) (ruptured)
  454.9
  with
    complications NEC 454.8
    edema 454.8
    inflammation or infection 454.1
      with ulcer 454.2
    pain 454.8
    stasis dermatitis 454.1
      with ulcer 454.2
    swelling 454.8
    ulcer 454.0
      with inflammation or infection
        454.2

Varix (Continued)
  aneurysmal (see also Aneurysm)
    442.9
  anus - see Hemorrhoids
  arteriovenous (congenital) (peripheral)
    NEC 747.60
    gastrointestinal 747.61
    lower limb 747.64
    renal 747.62
    specified NEC 747.69
    spinal 747.82
    upper limb 747.63
  bladder 456.5
  broad ligament 456.5
  congenital (peripheral) 747.60
  esophagus (ulcerated) 456.1
    bleeding 456.0
      in
        cirrhosis of liver 571.5
          [456.20]
        portal hypertension 572.3
          [456.20]
    congenital 747.69
    in
      cirrhosis of liver 571.5 [456.21]
        with bleeding 571.5 [456.20]
      portal hypertension 572.3 [456.21]
        with bleeding 572.3 [456.20]
  gastric 456.8
  inflamed or infected 454.1
    ulcerated 454.2
  in pregnancy or puerperium 671.0●
    perineum 671.1●
    vulva 671.1●
  labia (majora) 456.6
  orbit 456.8
    congenital 747.69
  ovary 456.5
  papillary 448.1
  pelvis 456.5
  perineum 456.6
    in pregnancy or puerperium
      671.1●
  pharynx 456.8
  placenta - see Placenta, abnormal
  prostate 456.8
  rectum - see Hemorrhoids
  renal papilla 456.8
  retina 362.17
  scrotum (ulcerated) 456.4
  sigmoid colon 456.8
  specified site NEC 456.8
  spinal (cord) (vessels) 456.8
  spleen, splenic (vein) (with phlebolith)
    456.8
  sublingual 456.3
  ulcerated 454.0
    inflamed or infected 454.2
  umbilical cord, affecting fetus or
    newborn 762.6
  uterine ligament 456.5
  vocal cord 456.8
  vulva 456.6
    in pregnancy, childbirth, or
      puerperium 671.1●
Vasa previa 663.5●
  affecting fetus or newborn 762.6
  hemorrhage from, affecting fetus or
    newborn 772.0
Vascular - see also condition
  loop on papilla (optic) 743.57
  sheathing, retina 362.13
  spasm 443.9
  spider 448.1

Vascularity, pulmonary, congenital 747.3
Vascularization
    choroid 362.16
    cornea 370.60
        deep 370.63
        localized 370.61
    retina 362.16
    subretinal 362.16
Vasculitis 447.6
    allergic 287.0
    cryoglobulinemic 273.2
    disseminated 447.6
    kidney 447.8
    leukocytoclastic 446.29
    nodular 695.2
    retinal 362.18
    rheumatic - see Fever, rheumatic
Vasculopathy
    cardiac allograft 996.83
Vas deferens - see condition
Vas deferentitis 608.4
Vasectomy, admission for V25.2
Vasitis 608.4
    nodosa 608.4
    scrotum 608.4
    spermatic cord 608.4
    testis 608.4
    tuberculous (see also Tuberculosis)
        016.5●
    tunica vaginalis 608.4
    vas deferens 608.4
Vasodilation 443.9
Vasomotor - see condition
Vasoplasty, after previous sterilization
    V26.0
Vasoplegia, splanchnic (see also
    Neuropathy, peripheral, autonomic)
    337.9
Vasospasm 443.9
    cerebral (artery) 435.9
        with transient neurologic deficit
            435.9
    coronary 413.1
    nerve
        arm NEC 354.9
        autonomic 337.9
        brachial plexus 353.0
        cervical plexus 353.2
        leg NEC 355.8
        lower extremity NEC 355.8
        peripheral NEC 335.9
        spinal NEC 355.9
        sympathetic 337.9
        upper extremity NEC 354.9
    peripheral NEC 443.9
    retina (artery) (see also Occlusion,
        retinal, artery) 362.30
Vasospastic - see condition
Vasovagal attack (paroxysmal) 780.2
    psychogenic 306.2
Vater's ampulla - see condition
VATER syndrome 759.89
vCJD (variant Creutzfeldt-Jakob disease)
    046.11
Vegetation, vegetative
    adenoid (nasal fossa) 474.2
    consciousness (persistent) 780.03
    endocarditis (acute) (any valve)
        (chronic) (subacute) 421.0
    heart (mycotic) (valve) 421.0
    state (persistent) 780.03
Veil
    Jackson's 751.4
    over face (causing asphyxia) 768.9

Vein, venous - see condition
Veldt sore (see also Ulcer, skin) 707.9
Velo-cardio-facial syndrome 758.32
Velpeau's hernia - see Hernia, femoral
Venereal
    balanitis NEC 099.8
    bubo 099.1
    disease 099.9
        specified nature or type NEC 099.8
    granuloma inguinale 099.2
    lymphogranuloma (Durand-Nicolas-
        Favre), any site 099.1
    salpingitis 098.37
    urethritis (see also Urethritis,
        nongonococcal) 099.40
    vaginitis NEC 099.8
    warts 078.11
Vengefulness, in child (see also
    Disturbance, conduct) 312.0●
Venofibrosis 459.89
Venom, venomous
    bite or sting (animal or insect) 989.5
    poisoning 989.5
Venous - see condition
Ventouse delivery NEC 669.5●
    affecting fetus or newborn 763.3
Ventral - see condition
Ventricle, ventricular - see also condition
    escape 427.69
    standstill (see also Arrest, cardiac)
        427.5
Ventriculitis, cerebral (see also Meningitis)
    322.9
Ventriculostomy status V45.2
Verbiest's syndrome (claudicatio
    intermittens spinalis) 435.1
Vernet's syndrome 352.6
Verneuil's disease (syphilitic bursitis)
    095.7
Verruca (filiformis) 078.10
    acuminata (any site) 078.11
    necrogenica (primary) (see also
        Tuberculosis) 017.0●
    peruana 088.0
    peruviana 088.0
    plana (juvenilis) 078.19
    plantaris 078.12
    seborrheica 702.19
        inflamed 702.11
    senilis 702.0
    tuberculosa (primary) (see also
        Tuberculosis) 017.0●
    venereal 078.11
    viral 078.10
        specified NEC 078.19
    vulgaris 078.10
Verrucosities (see also Verruca) 078.10
Verrucous endocarditis (acute) (any
    valve) (chronic) (subacute) 710.0
    [424.91]
    nonbacterial 710.0 [424.91]
Verruga
    peruana 088.0
    peruviana 088.0
Verse's disease (calcinosis
    intervertebralis) 275.49 [722.90]
Version
    before labor, affecting fetus or newborn
        761.7
    cephalic (correcting previous
        malposition) 652.1●
        affecting fetus or newborn
            763.1
    cervix - see Version, uterus

Version (Continued)
    uterus (postinfectional) (postpartal,
        old) (see also Malposition, uterus)
        621.6
        forward - see Anteversion, uterus
        lateral - see Lateroversion, uterus
Vertebra, vertebral - see condition
Vertigo 780.4
    auditory 386.19
    aural 386.19
    benign paroxysmal positional 386.11
    central origin 386.2
    cerebral 386.2
    Dix and Hallpike (epidemic) 386.12
    endemic paralytic 078.81
    epidemic 078.81
        Dix and Hallpike 386.12
        Gerlier's 078.81
        Pedersen's 386.12
        vestibular neuronitis 386.12
    epileptic - see Epilepsy
    Gerlier's (epidemic) 078.81
    hysterical 300.11
    labyrinthine 386.10
    laryngeal 786.2
    malignant positional 386.2
    Ménière's (see also Disease, Ménière's)
        386.00
    menopausal 627.2
    otogenic 386.19
    paralytic 078.81
    paroxysmal positional, benign
        386.11
    Pedersen's (epidemic) 386.12
    peripheral 386.10
        specified type NEC 386.19
    positional
        benign paroxysmal 386.11
        malignant 386.2
Verumontanitis (chronic) (see also
    Urethritis) 597.89
Vesania (see also Psychosis) 298.9
Vesical - see condition
Vesicle
    cutaneous 709.8
    seminal - see condition
    skin 709.8
Vesicocolic - see condition
Vesicoperineal - see condition
Vesicorectal - see condition
Vesicourethrorectal - see condition
Vesicovaginal - see condition
Vesicular - see condition
Vesiculitis (seminal) 608.0
    amebic 006.8
    gonorrheal (acute) 098.14
        chronic or duration of 2 months or
            over 098.34
    trichomonal 131.09
    tuberculous (see also Tuberculosis)
        016.5● [608.81]
Vestibulitis (ear) (see also Labyrinthitis)
    386.30
    nose (external) 478.19
    vulvar 625.71
Vestibulopathy, acute peripheral
    (recurrent) 386.12
Vestige, vestigial - see also Persistence
    branchial 744.41
    structures in vitreous 743.51
Vibriosis NEC 027.9
Vidal's disease (lichen simplex chronicus)
    698.3
Video display tube syndrome 723.8

◄ New   ◄▥ Revised   ~~deleted~~ Deleted   ● Use Additional Digit(s)   ▨ Omit code

Vienna-type encephalitis 049.8
Villaret's syndrome 352.6
Villous - *see* condition
VIN I (vulvar intraepithelial neoplasia I) 624.01
VIN II (vulvar intraepithelial neoplasia II) 624.02
VIN III (vulvar intraepithelial neoplasia III) 233.32
Vincent's
  angina 101
  bronchitis 101
  disease 101
  gingivitis 101
  infection (any site) 101
  laryngitis 101
  stomatitis 101
  tonsillitis 101
Vinson-Plummer syndrome (sideropenic dysphagia) 280.8
Viosterol deficiency (*see also* Deficiency, calciferol) 268.9
Virchow's disease 733.99
Viremia 790.8
Virilism (adrenal) (female) NEC 255.2
  with
    3-beta-hydroxysteroid dehydrogenase defect 255.2
    11-hydroxylase defect 255.2
    21-hydroxylase defect 255.2
    adrenal
      hyperplasia 255.2
      insufficiency (congenital) 255.2
    cortical hyperfunction 255.2
Virilization (female) (suprarenal) (*see also* Virilism) 255.2
  isosexual 256.4
Virulent bubo 099.0
Virus, viral - *see also* condition
  infection NEC (*see also* Infection, viral) 079.99
  septicemia 079.99
  yaba monkey tumor 059.22
VISA (vancomycin intermediate staphylococcus aureus) V09.8
Viscera, visceral - *see* condition
Visceroptosis 569.89
Visible peristalsis 787.4
Vision, visual
  binocular, suppression 368.31
  blurred, blurring 368.8
    hysterical 300.11
  defect, defective (*see also* Impaired, vision) 369.9
  disorientation (syndrome) 368.16
  disturbance NEC (*see also* Disturbance, vision) 368.9
    hysterical 300.11
  examination V72.0
  field, limitation 368.40
  fusion, with defective steropsis 368.33
  hallucinations 368.16
  halos 368.16
  loss 369.9
    both eyes (*see also* Blindness, both eyes) 369.3
    complete (*see also* Blindness, both eyes) 369.00
    one eye 369.8
    sudden 368.16
  low (both eyes) 369.20
    one eye (other eye normal) (*see also* Impaired, vision) 369.70
      blindness, other eye 369.10

Vision, visual (*Continued*)
  perception, simultaneous without fusion 368.32
  tunnel 368.45
Vitality, lack or want of 780.79
  newborn 779.89
Vitamin deficiency NEC (*see also* Deficiency, vitamin) 269.2
Vitelline duct, persistent 751.0
Vitiligo 709.01
  due to pinta (carate) 103.2
  eyelid 374.53
  vulva 624.8
Vitium cordis - *see* Disease, heart
Vitreous - *see also* condition
  touch syndrome 997.99
VLCAD (long chain/very long chain acyl CoA dehydrogenase deficiency, LCAD) 277.85
Vocal cord - *see* condition
Vocational rehabilitation V57.22
Vogt's (Cecile) disease or syndrome 333.7
Vogt-Koyanagi syndrome 364.24
Vogt-Spielmeyer disease (amaurotic familial idiocy) 330.1
Voice
  change (*see also* Dysphonia) 784.49
  loss (*see also* Aphonia) 784.41
Volhard-Fahr disease (malignant nephrosclerosis) 403.00
Volhynian fever 083.1
Volkmann's ischemic contracture or paralysis (complicating trauma) 958.6
Voluntary starvation 307.1
Volvulus (bowel) (colon) (intestine) 560.2
  with
    hernia - *see also* Hernia, by site, with obstruction
      gangrenous - *see* Hernia, by site, with gangrene
    perforation 560.2
  congenital 751.5
  duodenum 537.3
  fallopian tube 620.5
  oviduct 620.5
  stomach (due to absence of gastrocolic ligament) 537.89
Vomiting 787.03
  with nausea 787.01
  allergic 535.4●
  asphyxia 933.1
  bilious (cause unknown) 787.04
    following gastrointestinal surgery 564.3
    newborn 779.32
  blood (*see also* Hematemesis) 578.0
  causing asphyxia, choking, or suffocation (*see also* Asphyxia, food) 933.1
  cyclical 536.2
    associated with migraine 346.2●
    psychogenic 306.4
  epidemic 078.82
  fecal matter 569.87
  following gastrointestinal surgery 564.3
  functional 536.8
    psychogenic 306.4
  habit 536.2
  hysterical 300.11
  nervous 306.4
  neurotic 306.4
  newborn 779.33
    bilious 779.32 ⬅

Vomiting (*Continued*)
  of or complicating pregnancy 643.9●
    due to
      organic disease 643.8●
      specific cause NEC 643.8●
    early - *see* Hyperemesis, gravidarum
    late (after 22 completed weeks of gestation) 643.2●
  pernicious or persistent 536.2
    complicating pregnancy - *see* Hyperemesis, gravidarum
  psychogenic 306.4
  physiological 787.03
    bilious 787.04
  psychic 306.4
  psychogenic 307.54
  stercoral 569.89
  uncontrollable 536.2
    psychogenic 306.4
  uremic - *see* Uremia
  winter 078.82
von Bechterew (-Strümpell) disease or syndrome (ankylosing spondylitis) 720.0
von Bezold's abscess 383.01
von Economo's disease (encephalitis lethargica) 049.8
von Eulenburg's disease (congenital paramyotonia) 359.29
von Gierke's disease (glycogenosis I) 271.0
von Gies' joint 095.8
von Graefe's disease or syndrome 378.72
von Hippel (-Lindau) disease or syndrome (retinocerebral angiomatosis) 759.6
von Jaksch's anemia or disease (pseudoleukemia infantum) 285.8
von Recklinghausen's
  disease or syndrome (nerves) (skin) (M9540/1) 237.71
    bones (osteitis fibrosa cystica) 252.01
  tumor (M9540/1) 237.71
von Recklinghausen-Applebaum disease (hemochromatosis) (*see also* Hemochromatosis) 275.03 ⬅
von Schroetter's syndrome (intermittent venous claudication) 453.89
von Willebrand (-Jürgens) (-Minot) disease or syndrome (angiohemophilia) 286.4
von Zambusch's disease (lichen sclerosus et atrophicus) 701.0
Voorhoeve's disease or dyschondroplasia 756.4
Vossius' ring 921.3
  late effect 366.21
Voyeurism 302.82
VRE (vancomycin resistant enterococcus) V09.8
Vrolik's disease (osteogenesis imperfecta) 756.51
VRSA (vancomycin resistant staphylococcus aureus) V09.8
Vulva - *see* condition
Vulvismus 625.1
Vulvitis (acute) (allergic) (chronic) (gangrenous) (hypertrophic) (intertriginous) 616.10
  with
    abortion - *see* Abortion, by type, with sepsis
    ectopic pregnancy (*see also* categories 633.0–633.9) 639.0
    molar pregnancy (*see also* categories 630–632) 639.0

Vulvitis *(Continued)*
    adhesive, congenital 752.49
    blennorrhagic (acute) 098.0
        chronic or duration of 2 months or
            over 098.2
    chlamydial 099.53
    complicating pregnancy or puerperium
        646.6●
    due to Ducrey's bacillus 099.0
    following
        abortion 639.0
        ectopic or molar pregnancy
            639.0

Vulvitis *(Continued)*
    gonococcal (acute) 098.0
        chronic or duration of
            2 months or over
            098.2
    herpetic 054.11
    leukoplakic 624.09
    monilial 112.1
    puerperal, postpartum, childbirth
        646.6●
    syphilitic (early) 091.0
        late 095.8
    trichomonal 131.01

Vulvodynia 625.70
    specified NEC 625.79
Vulvorectal - *see* condition
Vulvovaginitis *(see also* Vulvitis) 616.10
    amebic 006.8
    chlamydial 099.53
    gonococcal (acute) 098.0
        chronic or duration of 2 months or
            over 098.2
    herpetic 054.11
    monilial 112.1
    trichomonal (Trichomonas vaginalis)
        131.01

◀ New   ◀⃛ Revised   ~~deleted~~ Deleted   ● Use Additional Digit(s)   Omit code

W

Waardenburg's syndrome 756.89
  meaning ptosis-epicanthus 270.2
Waardenburg-Klein syndrome (ptosis-epicanthus) 270.2
Wagner's disease (colloid milium) 709.3
Wagner (-Unverricht) syndrome (dermatomyositis) 710.3
Waiting list, person on V63.2
  undergoing social agency investigation V63.8
Wakefulness disorder (*see also* Hypersomnia) 780.54
  nonorganic origin 307.43
Waldenström's
  disease (osteochondrosis, capital femoral) 732.1
  hepatitis (lupoid hepatitis) 571.49
  hypergammaglobulinemia 273.0
  macroglobulinemia 273.3
  purpura, hypergammaglobulinemic 273.0
  syndrome (macroglobulinemia) 273.3
Waldenström-Kjellberg syndrome (sideropenic dysphagia) 280.8
Walking
  difficulty 719.7
    psychogenic 307.9
  sleep 307.46
    hysterical 300.13
Wall, abdominal - *see* condition
Wallenberg's syndrome (posterior inferior cerebellar artery) (*see also* Disease, cerebrovascular, acute) 436
Wallgren's
  disease (obstruction of splenic vein with collateral circulation) 459.89
  meningitis (*see also* Meningitis, aseptic) 047.9
Wandering
  acetabulum 736.39
  gallbladder 751.69
  kidney, congenital 753.3
  organ or site, congenital NEC - *see* Malposition, congenital
  pacemaker (atrial) (heart) 427.89
  spleen 289.59
Wardrop's disease (with lymphangitis) 681.9
  finger 681.02
  toe 681.11
War neurosis 300.16
Wart (digitate) (filiform) (infectious) (viral) 078.10
  common 078.19
  external genital organs (venereal) 078.11
  fig 078.19
  flat 078.19
  genital 078.11
  Hassall-Henle's (of cornea) 371.41
  Henle's (of cornea) 371.41
  juvenile 078.19
  moist 078.10
  Peruvian 088.0
  plantar 078.12
  prosector (*see also* Tuberculosis) 017.0●
  seborrheic 702.19
    inflamed 702.11
  senile 702.0

Wart (*Continued*)
  specified NEC 078.19
  syphilitic 091.3
  tuberculous (*see also* Tuberculosis) 017.0●
  venereal (female) (male) 078.11
Warthin's tumor (salivary gland) (M8561/0) 210.2
Washerwoman's itch 692.4
Wassilieff's disease (leptospiral jaundice) 100.0
Wasting
  disease 799.4
    due to malnutrition 261
  extreme (due to malnutrition) 261
  muscular NEC 728.2
  palsy, paralysis 335.21
  pelvic muscle 618.83
Water
  clefts 366.12
  deprivation of 994.3
  in joint (*see also* Effusion, joint) 719.0●
  intoxication 276.69 ◀▬
  itch 120.3
  lack of 994.3
  loading 276.69 ◀▬
  on
    brain - *see* Hydrocephalus
    chest 511.89
  poisoning 276.69 ◀▬
Waterbrash 787.1
Water-hammer pulse (*see also* Insufficiency, aortic) 424.1
Waterhouse (-Friderichsen) disease or syndrome 036.3
Water-losing nephritis 588.89
Watermelon stomach 537.82
  with hemorrhage 537.83
  without hemorrhage 537.82
Wax in ear 380.4
Waxy
  degeneration, any site 277.39
  disease 277.39
  kidney 277.39 [583.81]
  liver (large) 277.39
  spleen 277.39
Weak, weakness (generalized) 780.79
  arches (acquired) 734
    congenital 754.61
  bladder sphincter 596.59
  congenital 779.89
  eye muscle - *see* Strabismus
  facial 781.94
  foot (double) - *see* Weak, arches
  heart, cardiac (*see also* Failure, heart) 428.9
    congenital 746.9
  mind 317
  muscle (generalized) 728.87
  myocardium (*see also* Failure, heart) 428.9
  newborn 779.89
  pelvic fundus
    pubocervical tissue 618.81
    rectovaginal tissue 618.82
  pulse 785.9
  senile 797
  urinary stream 788.62
  valvular - *see* Endocarditis
Wear, worn, tooth, teeth (approximal) (hard tissues) (interproximal) (occlusal) - *see also* Attrition, teeth 521.10

Weather, weathered
  effects of
    cold NEC 991.9
      specified effect NEC 991.8
    hot (*see also* Heat) 992.9
  skin 692.74
Web, webbed (congenital) - *see also* Anomaly, specified type NEC
  canthus 743.63
  digits (*see also* Syndactylism) 755.10
  duodenal 751.5
  esophagus 750.3
  fingers (*see also* Syndactylism, fingers) 755.11
  larynx (glottic) (subglottic) 748.2
  neck (pterygium colli) 744.5
  Paterson-Kelly (sideropenic dysphagia) 280.8
  popliteal syndrome 756.89
  toes (*see also* Syndactylism, toes) 755.13
Weber's paralysis or syndrome 344.89
Weber-Christian disease or syndrome (nodular nonsuppurative panniculitis) 729.30
Weber-Cockayne syndrome (epidermolysis bullosa) 757.39
Weber-Dimitri syndrome 759.6
Weber-Gubler syndrome 344.89
Weber-Leyden syndrome 344.89
Weber-Osler syndrome (familial hemorrhagic telangiectasia) 448.0
Wedge-shaped or wedging vertebra (*see also* Osteoporosis) 733.00
Wegener's granulomatosis or syndrome 446.4
Wegner's disease (syphilitic osteochondritis) 090.0
Weight
  gain (abnormal) (excessive) 783.1
    during pregnancy 646.1●
      insufficient 646.8●
  less than 1000 grams at birth 765.0●
  loss (cause unknown) 783.21
Weightlessness 994.9
Weil's disease (leptospiral jaundice) 100.0
Weill-Marchesani syndrome (brachymorphism and ectopia lentis) 759.89
Weingarten's syndrome (tropical eosinophilia) 518.3
Weir Mitchell's disease (erythromelalgia) 443.82
Weiss-Baker syndrome (carotid sinus syncope) 337.01
Weissenbach-Thibierge syndrome (cutaneous systemic sclerosis) 710.1
Wen (*see also* Cyst, sebaceous) 706.2
Wenckebach's phenomenon, heart block (second degree) 426.13
Werdnig-Hoffmann syndrome (muscular atrophy) 335.0
Werlhof's disease (*see also* Purpura, thrombocytopenic) 287.39
Werlhof-Wichmann syndrome (*see also* Purpura, thrombocytopenic) 287.39
Wermer's syndrome or disease (polyendocrine adenomatosis) 258.01
Werner's disease or syndrome (progeria adultorum) 259.8
Werner-His disease (trench fever) 083.1

Werner-Schultz disease (agranulocytosis) 288.09

Wernicke's encephalopathy, disease, or syndrome (superior hemorrhagic polioencephalitis) 265.1

Wernicke-Korsakoff syndrome or psychosis (nonalcoholic) 294.0
  alcoholic 291.1

Wernicke-Posadas disease (*see also* Coccidioidomycosis) 114.9

Wesselsbron fever 066.3

West African fever 084.8

West Nile
  encephalitis 066.41
  encephalomyelitis 066.41
  fever 066.40
    with
      cranial nerve disorders 066.42
      encephalitis 066.41
      optic neuritis 066.42
      other complications 066.49
      other neurologic manifestations 066.42
      polyradiculitis 066.42
    virus 066.40

Westphal-Strümpell syndrome (hepatolenticular degeneration) 275.1

Wet
  brain (alcoholic) (*see also* Alcoholism) 303.9●
  feet, tropical (syndrome) (maceration) 991.4
  lung (syndrome)
    adult 518.5
    newborn 770.6

Wharton's duct - *see* condition

Wheal 709.8

Wheelchair confinement status V46.3

Wheezing 786.07

Whiplash injury or syndrome 847.0

Whipple's disease or syndrome (intestinal lipodystrophy) 040.2

Whipworm 127.3

"Whistling face" syndrome (craniocarpotarsal dystrophy) 759.89

White - *see also* condition
  kidney
    large - *see* Nephrosis
    small 582.9
  leg, puerperal, postpartum, childbirth 671.4●
    nonpuerperal 451.19
  mouth 112.0
  patches of mouth 528.6
  sponge nevus of oral mucosa 750.26
  spot lesions, teeth 521.01

White's disease (congenital) (keratosis follicularis) 757.39

Whitehead 706.2

Whitlow (with lymphangitis) 681.01
  herpetic 054.6

Whitmore's disease or fever (melioidosis) 025

Whooping cough 033.9
  with pneumonia 033.9 [484.3]
  due to
    Bordetella
      bronchoseptica 033.8
        with pneumonia 033.8 [484.3]
      parapertussis 033.1
        with pneumonia 033.1 [484.3]

Whooping cough (*Continued*)
  due to (*Continued*)
    Bordetella (*Continued*)
      pertussis 033.0
        with pneumonia 033.0 [484.3]
      specified organism NEC 033.8
        with pneumonia 033.8 [484.3]
    vaccination, prophylactic (against) V03.6

Wichmann's asthma (laryngismus stridulus) 478.75

Widal (-Abrami) syndrome (acquired hemolytic jaundice) 283.9

Widening aorta (see also Aneurysm, aorta) 441.9 (*see also* Ectasia, aortic) 447.70 ◄⃫
  with aneurysm 441.9 ◄
  ruptured 441.5

Wilkie's disease or syndrome 557.1

Wilkinson-Sneddon disease or syndrome (subcorneal pustular dermatosis) 694.1

Willan's lepra 696.1

Willan-Plumbe syndrome (psoriasis) 696.1

Willebrand (-Jürgens) syndrome or thrombopathy (angiohemophilia) 286.4

Willi-Prader syndrome (hypogenital dystrophy with diabetic tendency) 759.81

Willis' disease (diabetes mellitus) (*see also* Diabetes) 250.0●
  due to secondary diabetes 249.0●

Wilms' tumor or neoplasm (nephroblastoma) (M8960/3) 189.0

Wilson's
  disease or syndrome (hepatolenticular degeneration) 275.1
  hepatolenticular degeneration 275.1
  lichen ruber 697.0

Wilson-Brocq disease (dermatitis exfoliativa) 695.89

Wilson-Mikity syndrome 770.7

Window - *see also* Imperfect, closure
  aorticopulmonary 745.0

Winged scapula 736.89

Winter - *see also* condition
  vomiting disease 078.82

Wise's disease 696.2

Wiskott-Aldrich syndrome (eczema-thrombocytopenia) 279.12

Withdrawal symptoms, syndrome
  alcohol 291.81
    delirium (acute) 291.0
      chronic 291.1
      newborn 760.71
  drug or narcotic 292.0
  newborn, infant of dependent mother 779.5
  steroid NEC
    correct substance properly administered 255.41
    overdose or wrong substance given or taken 962.0

Withdrawing reaction, child or adolescent 313.22

Witts' anemia (achlorhydric anemia) 280.9

Witzelsucht 301.9

Woakes' syndrome (ethmoiditis) 471.1

Wohlfart-Kugelberg-Welander disease 335.11

Woillez's disease (acute idiopathic pulmonary congestion) 518.5

Wolff-Parkinson-White syndrome (anomalous atrioventricular excitation) 426.7

Wolhynian fever 083.1

Wolman's disease (primary familial xanthomatosis) 272.7

Wood asthma 495.8

Woolly, wooly hair (congenital) (nevus) 757.4

Wool-sorters' disease 022.1

Word
  blindness (congenital) (developmental) 315.01
    secondary to organic lesion 784.61
  deafness (secondary to organic lesion) 784.69
    developmental 315.31

Worm(s) (colic) (fever) (infection) (infestation) (*see also* Infestation) 128.9
  guinea 125.7
  in intestine NEC 127.9

Worm-eaten soles 102.3

Worn out (*see also* Exhaustion) 780.79
  artificial heart valve 996.02
  cardiac defibrillator (with synchronous cardiac pacemaker) V53.32 ◄⃫
  cardiac pacemaker lead or battery V53.31
  joint prosthesis (*see also* Complications, mechanical, device NEC, prosthetic NEC, joint) 996.46

"Worried well" V65.5

Wound, open (by cutting or piercing instrument) (by firearms) (cut) (dissection) (incised) (laceration) (penetration) (perforating) (puncture) (with initial hemorrhage, not internal) 879.8

> Note: For fracture with open wound, see Fracture.
>
> For laceration, traumatic rupture, tear, or penetrating wound of internal organs, such as heart, lung, liver, kidney, pelvic organs, etc., whether or not accompanied by open wound or fracture in the same region, see Injury, internal. For contused wound, see Contusion. For crush injury, see Crush. For abrasion, insect bite (nonvenomous), blister, or scratch, see Injury, superficial.
>
> Complicated includes wounds with:
>
>   delayed healing
>   delayed treatment
>   foreign body
>   primary infection
>
> For late effect of open wound, see Late, effect, wound, open, by site.

  abdomen, abdominal (external) (muscle) 879.2
    complicated 879.3
    wall (anterior) 879.2
      complicated 879.3
      lateral 879.4
        complicated 879.5
  alveolar (process) 873.62
    complicated 873.72
  ankle 891.0
    with tendon involvement 891.2
    complicated 891.1
  anterior chamber, eye (*see also* Wound, open, intraocular) 871.9

◄ New   ◄⃫ Revised   ~~deleted~~ Deleted   ● Use Additional Digit(s)   ▒ Omit code

Wound, open *(Continued)*
anus 879.6
  complicated 879.7
arm 884.0
  with tendon involvement 884.2
  complicated 884.1
  forearm 881.00
    with tendon involvement 881.20
    complicated 881.10
  multiple sites - *see* Wound, open,
    multiple, upper limb
  upper 880.03
    with tendon involvement
      880.23
    complicated 880.13
    multiple sites (with axillary or
      shoulder regions) 880.09
      with tendon involvement
        880.29
      complicated 880.19
artery - *see* Injury, blood vessel, by site
auditory
  canal (external) (meatus) 872.02
    complicated 872.12
  ossicles (incus) (malleus) (stapes)
    872.62
    complicated 872.72
auricle, ear 872.01
  complicated 872.11
axilla 880.02
  with tendon involvement 880.22
  complicated 880.12
    with tendon involvement
      880.29
  involving other sites of upper arm
    880.09
    complicated 880.19
back 876.0
  complicated 876.1
bladder - *see* Injury, internal, bladder
blood vessel - *see* Injury, blood vessel,
  by site
brain - *see* Injury, intracranial, with
  open intracranial wound
breast 879.0
  complicated 879.1
brow 873.42
  complicated 873.52
buccal mucosa 873.61
  complicated 873.71
buttock 877.0
  complicated 877.1
calf 891.0
  with tendon involvement 891.2
  complicated 891.1
canaliculus lacrimalis 870.8
  with laceration of eyelid 870.2
canthus, eye 870.8
  laceration - *see* Laceration, eyelid
cavernous sinus - *see* Injury,
  intracranial
cerebellum - *see* Injury, intracranial
cervical esophagus 874.4
  complicated 874.5
cervix - *see* Injury, internal, cervix
cheek(s) (external) 873.41
  complicated 873.51
  internal 873.61
    complicated 873.71
chest (wall) (external) 875.0
  complicated 875.1
chin 873.44
  complicated 873.54
choroid 363.63
ciliary body (eye) (*see also* Wound,
  open, intraocular) 871.9

Wound, open *(Continued)*
clitoris 878.8
  complicated 878.9
cochlea 872.64
  complicated 872.74
complicated 879.9
conjunctiva - *see* Wound, open,
  intraocular
cornea (nonpenetrating) (*see also*
  Wound, open, intraocular)
  871.9
costal region 875.0
  complicated 875.1
Descemet's membrane (*see also* Wound,
  open, intraocular) 871.9
digit(s)
  foot 893.0
    with tendon involvement
      893.2
    complicated 893.1
  hand 883.0
    with tendon involvement
      883.2
    complicated 883.1
drumhead, ear 872.61
  complicated 872.71
ear 872.8
  canal 872.02
    complicated 872.12
  complicated 872.9
  drum 872.61
    complicated 872.71
  external 872.00
    complicated 872.10
  multiple sites 872.69
    complicated 872.79
  ossicles (incus) (malleus) (stapes)
    872.62
    complicated 872.72
  specified part NEC 872.69
    complicated 872.79
elbow 881.01
  with tendon involvement 881.21
  complicated 881.11
epididymis 878.2
  complicated 878.3
epigastric region 879.2
  complicated 879.3
epiglottis 874.01
  complicated 874.11
esophagus (cervical) 874.4
  complicated 874.5
  thoracic - *see* Injury, internal,
    esophagus
Eustachian tube 872.63
  complicated 872.73
extremity
  lower (multiple) NEC 894.0
    with tendon involvement 894.2
    complicated 894.1
  upper (multiple) NEC 884.0
    with tendon involvement 884.2
    complicated 884.1
eye(s) (globe) - *see* Wound, open,
  intraocular
eyeball NEC 871.9
  laceration (*see also* Laceration,
    eyeball) 871.4
  penetrating (*see also* Penetrating
    wound, eyeball) 871.7
eyebrow 873.42
  complicated 873.52
eyelid NEC 870.8
  laceration - *see* Laceration, eyelid

Wound, open *(Continued)*
face 873.40
  complicated 873.50
  multiple sites 873.49
    complicated 873.59
  specified part NEC 873.49
    complicated 873.59
fallopian tube - *see* Injury, internal,
  fallopian tube
finger(s) (nail) (subungual) 883.0
  with tendon involvement 883.2
  complicated 883.1
flank 879.4
  complicated 879.5
foot (any part, except toe(s) alone)
  892.0
  with tendon involvement 892.2
  complicated 892.1
forearm 881.00
  with tendon involvement 881.20
  complicated 881.10
forehead 873.42
  complicated 873.52
genital organs (external) NEC 878.8
  complicated 878.9
  internal - *see* Injury, internal, by site
globe (eye) (*see also* Wound, open,
  eyeball) 871.9
groin 879.4
  complicated 879.5
gum(s) 873.62
  complicated 873.72
hand (except finger(s) alone) 882.0
  with tendon involvement 882.2
  complicated 882.1
head NEC 873.8
  with intracranial injury - *see* Injury,
    intracranial
    due to or associated with skull
      fracture - *see* Fracture,
      skull
  complicated 873.9
  scalp - *see* Wound, open, scalp
heel 892.0
  with tendon involvement 892.2
  complicated 892.1
high-velocity (grease gun) - *see*
  Wound, open, complicated,
  by site
hip 890.0
  with tendon involvement 890.2
  complicated 890.1
hymen 878.6
  complicated 878.7
hypochondrium 879.4
  complicated 879.5
hypogastric region 879.2
  complicated 879.3
iliac (region) 879.4
  complicated 879.5
incidental to
  dislocation - *see* Dislocation, open,
    by site
  fracture - *see* Fracture, open, by site
  intracranial injury - *see* Injury,
    intracranial, with open
    intracranial wound
  nerve injury - *see* Injury, nerve, by
    site
inguinal region 879.4
  complicated 879.5
instep 892.0
  with tendon involvement 892.2
  complicated 892.1

Wound, open (*Continued*)
  interscapular region 876.0
    complicated 876.1
  intracranial - *see* Injury, intracranial,
      with open intracranial wound
  intraocular 871.9
    with
        partial loss (of intraocular tissue)
            871.2
        prolapse or exposure (of
            intraocular tissue) 871.1
      laceration (*see also* Laceration,
          eyeball) 871.4
      penetrating 871.7
        with foreign body (nonmagnetic)
            871.6
          magnetic 871.5
      without prolapse (of intraocular
          tissue) 871.0
  iris (*see also* Wound, open, eyeball)
      871.9
  jaw (fracture not involved) 873.44
    with fracture - *see* Fracture, jaw
    complicated 873.54
  knee 891.0
    with tendon involvement 891.2
    complicated 891.1
  labium (majus) (minus) 878.4
    complicated 878.5
  lacrimal apparatus, gland, or sac
      870.8
    with laceration of eyelid 870.2
  larynx 874.01
    with trachea 874.00
      complicated 874.10
    complicated 874.11
  leg (multiple) 891.0
    with tendon involvement 891.2
    complicated 891.1
    lower 891.0
      with tendon involvement 891.2
      complicated 891.1
    thigh 890.0
      with tendon involvement 890.2
      complicated 890.1
    upper 890.0
      with tendon involvement 890.2
      complicated 890.1
  lens (eye) (alone) (*see also* Cataract,
      traumatic) 366.20
    with involvement of other eye
        structures - *see* Wound, open,
        eyeball
  limb
    lower (multiple) NEC 894.0
      with tendon involvement 894.2
      complicated 894.1
    upper (multiple) NEC 884.0
      with tendon involvement 884.2
      complicated 884.1
  lip 873.43
    complicated 873.53
  loin 876.0
    complicated 876.1
  lumbar region 876.0
    complicated 876.1
  malar region 873.41
    complicated 873.51
  mastoid region 873.49
    complicated 873.59
  mediastinum - *see* Injury, internal,
      mediastinum
  midthoracic region 875.0
    complicated 875.1

Wound, open (*Continued*)
  mouth 873.60
    complicated 873.70
    floor 873.64
      complicated 873.74
    multiple sites 873.69
      complicated 873.79
    specified site NEC 873.69
      complicated 873.79
  multiple, unspecified site(s) 879.8

> Note: Multiple open wounds of sites
> classifiable to the same four-digit
> category should be classified to that
> category unless they are in different
> limbs.
>
> Multiple open wounds of sites
> classifiable to different four-digit
> categories, or to different limbs, should
> be coded separately.

    complicated 879.9
    lower limb(s) (one or both) (sites
        classifiable to more than one
        three-digit category in 890–
        893) 894.0
      with tendon involvement 894.2
      complicated 894.1
    upper limb(s) (one or both) (sites
        classifiable to more than one
        three-digit category in 880–
        883) 884.0
      with tendon involvement
          884.2
      complicated 884.1
  muscle - *see* Sprain, by site
  nail
    finger(s) 883.0
      complicated 883.1
    thumb 883.0
      complicated 883.1
    toe(s) 893.0
      complicated 893.1
  nape (neck) 874.8
    complicated 874.9
    specified part NEC 874.8
      complicated 874.9
  nasal - *see also* Wound, open, nose
    cavity 873.22
      complicated 873.32
    septum 873.21
      complicated 873.31
    sinuses 873.23
      complicated 873.33
  nasopharynx 873.22
    complicated 873.32
  neck 874.8
    complicated 874.9
    nape 874.8
      complicated 874.9
    specified part NEC 874.8
      complicated 874.9
  nerve - *see* Injury, nerve, by site
  non-healing surgical 998.83
  nose 873.20
    complicated 873.30
    multiple sites 873.29
      complicated 873.39
    septum 873.21
      complicated 873.31
    sinuses 873.23
      complicated 873.33
  occipital region - *see* Wound, open,
      scalp

Wound, open (*Continued*)
  ocular NEC 871.9
    adnexa 870.9
        specified region NEC 870.8
    laceration (*see also* Laceration,
        ocular) 871.4
    muscle (extraocular) 870.3
      with foreign body 870.4
        eyelid 870.1
        intraocular - *see* Wound, open,
            eyeball
    penetrating (*see also* Penetrating
        wound, ocular) 871.7
  orbit 870.8
    penetrating 870.3
      with foreign body 870.4
  orbital region 870.9
  ovary - *see* Injury, internal, pelvic
      organs
  palate 873.65
    complicated 873.75
  palm 882.0
    with tendon involvement 882.2
    complicated 882.1
  parathyroid (gland) 874.2
    complicated 874.3
  parietal region - *see* Wound, open,
      scalp
  pelvic floor or region 879.6
    complicated 879.7
  penis 878.0
    complicated 878.1
  perineum 879.6
    complicated 879.7
  periocular area 870.8
    laceration of skin 870.0
  pharynx 874.4
    complicated 874.5
  pinna 872.01
    complicated 872.11
  popliteal space 891.0
    with tendon involvement 891.2
    complicated 891.1
  prepuce 878.0
    complicated 878.1
  pubic region 879.2
    complicated 879.3
  pudenda 878.8
    complicated 878.9
  rectovaginal septum 878.8
    complicated 878.9
  sacral region 877.0
    complicated 877.1
  sacroiliac region 877.0
    complicated 877.1
  salivary (ducts) (glands) 873.69
    complicated 873.79
  scalp 873.0
    complicated 873.1
  scalpel, fetus or newborn 767.8
  scapular region 880.01
    with tendon involvement 880.21
    complicated 880.11
    involving other sites of upper arm
        880.09
      with tendon involvement
          880.29
      complicated 880.19
  sclera (*see also* Wound, open,
      intraocular) 871.9
  scrotum 878.2
    complicated 878.3
  seminal vesicle - *see* Injury, internal,
      pelvic organs

◀ New   ◀▥ Revised   ~~deleted~~ Deleted   ● Use Additional Digit(s)   ▭ Omit code

Wound, open (Continued)
shin 891.0
with tendon involvement 891.2
complicated 891.1
shoulder 880.00
with tendon involvement 880.20
complicated 880.10
involving other sites of upper arm
880.09
with tendon involvement 880.29
complicated 880.19
skin NEC 879.8
complicated 879.9
skull - see also Injury, intracranial, with
open intracranial wound
with skull fracture - see Fracture,
skull
spermatic cord (scrotal) 878.2
complicated 878.3
pelvic region - see Injury, internal,
spermatic cord
spinal cord - see Injury, spinal
sternal region 875.0
complicated 875.1
subconjunctival - see Wound, open,
intraocular
subcutaneous NEC 879.8
complicated 879.9
submaxillary region 873.44
complicated 873.54
submental region 873.44
complicated 873.54
subungual
finger(s) (thumb) - see Wound, open,
finger
toe(s) - see Wound, open, toe
supraclavicular region 874.8
complicated 874.9
supraorbital 873.42
complicated 873.52

Wound, open (Continued)
surgical, non-healing 998.83
temple 873.49
complicated 873.59
temporal region 873.49
complicated 873.59
testis 878.2
complicated 878.3
thigh 890.0
with tendon involvement 890.2
complicated 890.1
thorax, thoracic (external) 875.0
complicated 875.1
throat 874.8
complicated 874.9
thumb (nail) (subungual) 883.0
with tendon involvement 883.2
complicated 883.1
thyroid (gland) 874.2
complicated 874.3
toe(s) (nail) (subungual) 893.0
with tendon involvement 893.2
complicated 893.1
tongue 873.64
complicated 873.74
tonsil - see Wound, open, neck
trachea (cervical region) 874.02
with larynx 874.00
complicated 874.10
complicated 874.12
intrathoracic - see Injury, internal,
trachea
trunk (multiple) NEC 879.6
complicated 879.7
specified site NEC 879.6
complicated 879.7
tunica vaginalis 878.2
complicated 878.3
tympanic membrane 872.61
complicated 872.71

Wound, open (Continued)
tympanum 872.61
complicated 872.71
umbilical region 879.2
complicated 879.3
ureter - see Injury, internal, ureter
urethra - see Injury, internal, urethra
uterus - see Injury, internal, uterus
uvula 873.69
complicated 873.79
vagina 878.6
complicated 878.7
vas deferens - see Injury, internal, vas
deferens
vitreous (humor) 871.2
vulva 878.4
complicated 878.5
wrist 881.02
with tendon involvement 881.22
complicated 881.12
Wright's syndrome (hyperabduction)
447.8
pneumonia 390 [517.1]
Wringer injury - see Crush injury, by site
Wrinkling of skin 701.8
Wrist - see also condition
drop (acquired) 736.05
Wrong drug (given in error) NEC 977.9
specified drug or substance - see Table
of Drugs and Chemicals
Wry neck - see also Torticollis
congenital 754.1
Wuchereria infestation 125.0
bancrofti 125.0
Brugia malayi 125.1
malayi 125.1
Wuchereriasis 125.0
Wuchereriosis 125.0
Wuchernde struma langhans (M8332/3)
193

X

Xanthelasma 272.2
    eyelid 272.2 [374.51]
    palpebrarum 272.2 [374.51]
Xanthelasmatosis (essential) 272.2
Xanthelasmoidea 757.33
Xanthine stones 277.2
Xanthinuria 277.2
Xanthofibroma (M8831/0) - see
    Neoplasm, connective tissue, benign
Xanthoma(s), xanthomatosis 272.2
    with
        hyperlipoproteinemia
            type I 272.3
            type III 272.2
            type IV 272.1
            type V 272.3
    bone 272.7
    craniohypophyseal 277.89
    cutaneotendinous 272.7
    diabeticorum 250.8● [272.2]
        due to secondary diabetes
            249.8● [272.2]
    disseminatum 272.7
    eruptive 272.2
    eyelid 272.2 [374.51]
    familial 272.7
    hereditary 272.7
    hypercholesterinemic 272.0

Xanthoma(s) (Continued)
    hypercholesterolemic 272.0
    hyperlipemic 272.4
    hyperlipidemic 272.4
    infantile 272.7
    joint 272.7
    juvenile 272.7
    multiple 272.7
    multiplex 272.7
    primary familial 272.7
    tendon (sheath) 272.7
    tuberosum 272.2
    tuberous 272.2
    tubo-eruptive 272.2
Xanthosis 709.09
    surgical 998.81
Xenophobia 300.29
Xeroderma (congenital) 757.39
    acquired 701.1
        eyelid 373.33
    eyelid 373.33
    pigmentosum 757.33
    vitamin A deficiency 264.8
Xerophthalmia 372.53
    vitamin A deficiency 264.7
Xerosis
    conjunctiva 372.53
        with Bitôt's spot 372.53
            vitamin A deficiency 264.1
        vitamin A deficiency 264.0

Xerosis (Continued)
    cornea 371.40
        with corneal ulceration
            370.00
            vitamin A deficiency
                264.3
        vitamin A deficiency
            264.2
    cutis 706.8
    skin 706.8
Xerostomia 527.7
Xiphodynia 733.90
Xiphoidalgia 733.90
Xiphoiditis 733.99
Xiphopagus 759.4
XO syndrome 758.6
X-ray
    effects, adverse, NEC 990
    of chest
        for suspected tuberculosis
            V71.2
        routine V72.5
XXX syndrome 758.81
XXXXY syndrome 758.81
XXY syndrome 758.7
Xyloketosuria 271.8
Xylosuria 271.8
Xylulosuria 271.8
XYY syndrome 758.81

◀ New   ◀⁞⁞⁞ Revised   deleted Deleted   ● Use Additional Digit(s)   ▨ Omit code

Y

Yaba monkey tumor virus 059.22
Yawning 786.09
    psychogenic 306.1
Yaws 102.9
    bone or joint lesions 102.6
    butter 102.1
    chancre 102.0
    cutaneous, less than five years after
        infection 102.2
    early (cutaneous) (macular)
        (maculopapular) (micropapular)
        (papular) 102.2
      frambeside 102.2
      skin lesions NEC 102.2
    eyelid 102.9 [373.4]
    ganglion 102.6
    gangosis, gangosa 102.5
    gumma, gummata 102.4
      bone 102.6

Yaws (Continued)
    gummatous
      frambeside 102.4
      osteitis 102.6
      periostitis 102.6
    hydrarthrosis 102.6
    hyperkeratosis (early) (late) (palmar)
        (plantar) 102.3
    initial lesions 102.0
    joint lesions 102.6
    juxta-articular nodules 102.7
    late nodular (ulcerated) 102.4
    latent (without clinical
        manifestations) (with
        positive serology) 102.8
    mother 102.0
    mucosal 102.7
    multiple papillomata 102.1
    nodular, late (ulcerated) 102.4
    osteitis 102.6

Yaws (Continued)
    papilloma, papillomata (palmar)
        (plantar) 102.1
    periostitis (hypertrophic) 102.6
    ulcers 102.4
    wet crab 102.1
Yeast infection (see also Candidiasis)
    112.9
Yellow
    atrophy (liver) 570
      chronic 571.8
      resulting from administration of
        blood, plasma, serum, or other
        biological substance (within 8
        months of administration) - see
        Hepatitis, viral
    fever - see Fever, yellow
    jack (see also Fever, yellow) 060.9
    jaundice (see also Jaundice) 782.4
Yersinia septica 027.8

Z

Zagari's disease (xerostomia) 527.7
Zahorsky's disease (exanthema subitum)
(*see also* Exanthem subitum)
058.10
   syndrome (herpangina) 074.0
Zellweger syndrome 277.86
Zenker's diverticulum (esophagus) 530.6
Ziehen-Oppenheim disease 333.6

Zieve's syndrome (jaundice, hyperlipemia, and hemolytic anemia) 571.1
Zika fever 066.3
Zollinger-Ellison syndrome (gastric hypersecretion with pancreatic islet cell tumor) 251.5
Zona (*see also* Herpes, zoster) 053.9
Zoophilia (erotica) 302.1
Zoophobia 300.29

Zoster (herpes) (*see also* Herpes, zoster) 053.9
Zuelzer (-Ogden) anemia or syndrome (nutritional megaloblastic anemia) 281.2
Zygodactyly (*see also* Syndactylism) 755.10
Zygomycosis 117.7
Zymotic - *see* condition

◄ New   ◄▥ Revised   ~~deleted~~ Deleted   ● Use Additional Digit(s)   ▨ Omit code

ALPHABETIC INDEX TO POISONING AND EXTERNAL CAUSES OF ADVERSE EFFECTS OF DRUGS AND OTHER CHEMICAL SUBSTANCES

This table contains a classification of drugs and other chemical substances to identify poisoning states and external causes of adverse effects.

Each of the listed substances in the table is assigned a code according to the poisoning classification (960–989). These codes are used when there is a statement of poisoning, overdose, wrong substance given or taken, or intoxication.

The table also contains a listing of external causes of adverse effects. An adverse effect is a pathologic manifestation due to ingestion or exposure to drugs or other chemical substances (e.g., dermatitis, hypersensitivity reaction, aspirin gastritis). The adverse effect is to be identified by the appropriate code found in Section I, Index to Diseases and Injuries. An external cause code can then be used to identify the circumstances involved. The table headings pertaining to external causes are defined below:

Accidental poisoning (E850–E869)-accidental overdose of drug, wrong substance given or taken, drug taken inadvertently, accidents in the usage of drugs and biologicals in medical and surgical procedures, and to show external causes of poisonings classifiable to 980–989.

Therapeutic use (E930–E949)-a correct substance properly administered in therapeutic or prophylactic dosage as the external cause of adverse effects.

Suicide attempt (E950–E952)-instances in which self-inflicted injuries or poisonings are involved.

Assault (E961–E962)-injury or poisoning inflicted by another person with the intent to injure or kill.

Undetermined (E980–E982)-to be used when the intent of the poisoning or injury cannot be determined whether it was intentional or accidental.

The American Hospital Formulary Service (AHFS) list numbers are included in the table to help classify new drugs not identified in the table by name. The AHFS list numbers are keyed to the continually revised AHFS (American Hospital Formulary Service, 2 vol. Washington, D.C.: American Society of Hospital Pharmacists, 1959-). These listings are found in the table under the main term **Drug.**

Excluded from the table are radium and other radioactive substances. The classification of adverse effects and complications pertaining to these substances will be found in Index to Diseases and Injuries, and Index to External Causes of Injuries.

Although certain substances are indexed with one or more subentries, the majority are listed according to one use or state. It is recognized that many substances may be used in various ways, in medicine and in industry, and may cause adverse effects whatever the state of the agent (solid, liquid, or fumes arising from a liquid). In cases in which the reported data indicate a use or state not in the table, or which is clearly different from the one listed, an attempt should be made to classify the substance in the form which most nearly expresses the reported facts.

TABLE OF DRUGS AND CHEMICALS

Substance	Poisoning	External Cause (E Code)				
		Accident	Therapeutic Use	Suicide Attempt	Assault	Undetermined
1-propanol	980.3	E860.4	—	E950.9	E962.1	E980.9
2-propanol	980.2	E860.3	—	E950.9	E962.1	E980.9
2,4-D (dichlorophenoxyacetic acid)	989.4	E863.5	—	E950.6	E962.1	E980.7
2,4-toluene diisocyanate	983.0	E864.0	—	E950.7	E962.1	E980.6
2,4,5-T (trichlorophenoxyacetic acid)	989.2	E863.5	—	E950.6	E962.1	E980.7
14-hydroxydihydromorphinone	965.09	E850.2	E935.2	E950.0	E962.0	E980.0
ABOB	961.7	E857	E931.7	E950.4	E962.0	E980.4
Abrus (seed)	988.2	E865.3	—	E950.9	E962.1	E980.9
Absinthe	980.0	E860.1	—	E950.9	E962.1	E980.9
beverage	980.0	E860.0	—	E950.9	E962.1	E980.9
Acenocoumarin, acenocoumarol	964.2	E858.2	E934.2	E950.4	E962.0	E980.4
Acepromazine	969.1	E853.0	E939.1	E950.3	E962.0	E980.3
Acetal	982.8	E862.4	—	E950.9	E962.1	E980.9
Acetaldehyde (vapor)	987.8	E869.8	—	E952.8	E962.2	E982.8
liquid	989.89	E866.8	—	E950.9	E962.1	E980.9
Acetaminophen	965.4	E850.4	E935.4	E950.0	E962.0	E980.0
Acetaminosalol	965.1	E850.3	E935.3	E950.0	E962.0	E980.0
Acetanilid(e)	965.4	E850.4	E935.4	E950.0	E962.0	E980.0
Acetarsol, acetarsone	961.1	E857	E931.1	E950.4	E962.0	E980.4
Acetazolamide	974.2	E858.5	E944.2	E950.4	E962.0	E980.4
Acetic	—	—	—	—	—	—
acid	983.1	E864.1	—	E950.7	E962.1	E980.6
with sodium acetate (ointment)	976.3	E858.7	E946.3	E950.4	E962.0	E980.4
irrigating solution	974.5	E858.5	E944.5	E950.4	E962.0	E980.4
lotion	976.2	E858.7	E946.2	E950.4	E962.0	E980.4
anhydride	983.1	E864.1	—	E950.7	E962.1	E980.6
ether (vapor)	982.8	E862.4	—	E950.9	E962.1	E980.9
Acetohexamide	962.3	E858.0	E932.3	E950.4	E962.0	E980.4
Acetomenaphthone	964.3	E858.2	E934.3	E950.4	E962.0	E980.4
Acetomorphine	965.01	E850.0	E935.0	E950.0	E962.0	E980.0
Acetone (oils) (vapor)	982.8	E862.4	—	E950.9	E962.1	E980.9
Acetophenazine (maleate)	969.1	E853.0	E939.1	E950.3	E962.0	E980.3
Acetophenetidin	965.4	E850.4	E935.4	E950.0	E962.0	E980.0
Acetophenone	982.0	E862.4	—	E950.9	E962.1	E980.9
Acetorphine	965.09	E850.2	E935.2	E950.0	E962.0	E980.0
Acetosulfone (sodium)	961.8	E857	E931.8	E950.4	E962.0	E980.4
Acetrizoate (sodium)	977.8	E858.8	E947.8	E950.4	E962.0	E980.4
Acetylcarbromal	967.3	E852.2	E937.3	E950.2	E962.0	E980.2

◀ New   ◀▥ Revised   deleted Deleted   ● Use Additional Digit(s)

Substance	Poisoning	External Cause (E Code)				
		Accident	Therapeutic Use	Suicide Attempt	Assault	Undetermined
Acetylcholine (chloride)	971.0	E855.3	E941.0	E950.4	E962.0	E980.4
Acetylcysteine	975.5	E858.6	E945.5	E950.4	E962.0	E980.4
Acetyldigitoxin	972.1	E858.3	E942.1	E950.4	E962.0	E980.4
Acetyldihydrocodeine	965.09	E850.2	E935.2	E950.0	E962.0	E980.0
Acetyldihydrocodeinone	965.09	E850.2	E935.2	E950.0	E962.0	E980.0
Acetylene (gas) (industrial)	987.1	E868.1	—	E951.8	E962.2	E981.8
incomplete combustion of - *see* Carbon monoxide, fuel, utility	—	—	—	—	—	—
tetrachloride (vapor)	982.3	E862.4	—	E950.9	E962.1	E980.9
Acetyliodosalicylic acid	965.1	E850.3	E935.3	E950.0	E962.0	E980.0
Acetylphenylhydrazine	965.8	E850.8	E935.8	E950.0	E962.0	E980.0
Acetylsalicylic acid	965.1	E850.3	E935.3	E950.0	E962.0	E980.0
Achromycin	960.4	E856	E930.4	E950.4	E962.0	E980.4
ophthalmic preparation	976.5	E858.7	E946.5	E950.4	E962.0	E980.4
topical NEC	976.0	E858.7	E946.0	E950.4	E962.0	E980.4
Acidifying agents	963.2	E858.1	E933.2	E950.4	E962.0	E980.4
Acids (corrosive) NEC	983.1	E864.1	—	E950.7	E962.1	E980.6
Aconite (wild)	988.2	E865.4	—	E950.9	E962.1	E980.9
Aconitine (liniment)	976.8	E858.7	E946.8	E950.4	E962.0	E980.4
Aconitum ferox	988.2	E865.4	—	E950.9	E962.1	E980.9
Acridine	983.0	E864.0	—	E950.7	E962.1	E980.6
vapor	987.8	E869.8	—	E952.8	E962.2	E982.8
Acriflavine	961.9	E857	E931.9	E950.4	E962.0	E980.4
Acrisorcin	976.0	E858.7	E946.0	E950.4	E962.0	E980.4
Acrolein (gas)	987.8	E869.8	—	E952.8	E962.2	E982.8
liquid	989.89	E866.8	—	E950.9	E962.1	E980.9
Actaea spicata	988.2	E865.4	—	E950.9	E962.1	E980.9
Acterol	961.5	E857	E931.5	E950.4	E962.0	E980.4
ACTH	962.4	E858.0	E932.4	E950.4	E962.0	E980.4
Acthar	962.4	E858.0	E932.4	E950.4	E962.0	E980.4
Actinomycin (C) (D)	960.7	E856	E930.7	E950.4	E962.0	E980.4
Adalin (acetyl)	967.3	E852.2	E937.3	E950.2	E962.0	E980.2
Adenosine (phosphate)	977.8	E858.8	E947.8	E950.4	E962.0	E980.4
Adhesives	989.89	E866.6	—	E950.9	E962.1	E980.9
ADH	962.5	E858.0	E932.5	E950.4	E962.0	E980.4
Adicillin	960.0	E856	E930.0	E950.4	E962.0	E980.4
Adiphenine	975.1	E855.6	E945.1	E950.4	E962.0	E980.4
Adjunct, pharmaceutical	977.4	E858.8	E947.4	E950.4	E962.0	E980.4

TABLE OF DRUGS AND CHEMICALS

Substance	Poisoning	External Cause (E Code)				
		Accident	Therapeutic Use	Suicide Attempt	Assault	Undetermined
Adrenal (extract, cortex or medulla) (glucocorticoids) (hormones) (mineralocorticoids)	962.0	E858.0	E932.0	E950.4	E962.0	E980.4
ENT agent	976.6	E858.7	E946.6	E950.4	E962.0	E980.4
ophthalmic preparation	976.5	E858.7	E946.5	E950.4	E962.0	E980.4
topical NEC	976.0	E858.7	E946.0	E950.4	E962.0	E980.4
Adrenalin	971.2	E855.5	E941.2	E950.4	E962.0	E980.4
Adrenergic blocking agents	971.3	E855.6	E941.3	E950.4	E962.0	E980.4
Adrenergics	971.2	E855.5	E941.2	E950.4	E962.0	E980.4
Adrenochrome (derivatives)	972.8	E858.3	E942.8	E950.4	E962.0	E980.4
Adrenocorticotropic hormone	962.4	E858.0	E932.4	E950.4	E962.0	E980.4
Adrenocorticotropin	962.4	E858.0	E932.4	E950.4	E962.0	E980.4
Adriamycin	960.7	E856	E930.7	E950.4	E962.0	E980.4
Aerosol spray - *see* Sprays	—	—	—	—	—	—
Aerosporin	960.8	E856	E930.8	E950.4	E962.0	E980.4
ENT agent	976.6	E858.7	E946.6	E950.4	E962.0	E980.4
ophthalmic preparation	976.5	E858.7	E946.5	E950.4	E962.0	E980.4
topical NEC	976.0	E858.7	E946.0	E950.4	E962.0	E980.4
Aethusa cynapium	988.2	E865.4	—	E950.9	E962.1	E980.9
Afghanistan black	969.6	E854.1	E939.6	E950.3	E962.0	E980.3
Aflatoxin	989.7	E865.9	—	E950.9	E962.1	E980.9
African boxwood	988.2	E865.4	—	E950.9	E962.1	E980.9
Agar (-agar)	973.3	E858.4	E943.3	E950.4	E962.0	E980.4
Agricultural agent NEC	989.89	E863.9	—	E950.6	E962.1	E980.7
Agrypnal	967.0	E851	E937.0	E950.1	E962.0	E980.1
Air contaminant(s), source or type not specified	—	—	—	—	—	—
specified type - *see* specific substance	987.9	E869.9	—	E952.9	E962.2	E982.9
Akee	988.2	E865.4	—	E950.9	E962.1	E980.9
Akrinol	976.0	E858.7	E946.0	E950.4	E962.0	E980.4
Alantolactone	961.6	E857	E931.6	E950.4	E962.0	E980.4
Albamycin	960.8	E856	E930.8	E950.4	E962.0	E980.4
Albumin (normal human serum)	964.7	E858.2	E934.7	E950.4	E962.0	E980.4
Albuterol	975.7	E858.6	E945.7	E950.4	E962.0	E980.4
Alcohol	980.9	E860.9	—	E950.9	E962.1	E980.9
absolute	980.0	E860.1	—	E950.9	E962.1	E980.9
beverage	980.0	E860.0	E947.8	E950.9	E962.1	E980.9
amyl	980.3	E860.4	—	E950.9	E962.1	E980.9
antifreeze	980.1	E860.2	—	E950.9	E962.1	E980.9
butyl	980.3	E860.4	—	E950.9	E962.1	E980.9

◀ New   ◀ Revised   ~~deleted~~ Deleted   ● Use Additional Digit(s)

Substance	Poisoning	External Cause (E Code)				
		Accident	Therapeutic Use	Suicide Attempt	Assault	Undetermined
Alcohol *(Continued)*						
dehydrated	980.0	E860.1	—	E950.9	E862.1	E980.9
beverage	980.0	E860.0	E947.8	E950.9	E962.1	E980.9
denatured	980.0	E860.1	—	E950.9	E962.1	E980.9
deterrents	977.3	E858.8	E947.3	E950.4	E962.0	E980.4
diagnostic (gastric function)	977.8	E858.8	E947.8	E950.4	E962.0	E980.4
ethyl	980.0	E860.1	—	E950.9	E962.1	E980.9
beverage	980.0	E860.0	E947.8	E950.9	E962.1	E980.9
grain	980.0	E860.1	—	E950.9	E962.1	E980.9
beverage	980.0	E860.0	E947.8	E950.9	E962.1	E980.9
industrial	980.9	E860.9	—	E950.9	E962.1	E980.9
isopropyl	980.2	E860.3	—	E950.9	E962.1	E980.9
methyl	980.1	E860.2	—	E950.9	E962.1	E980.9
preparation for consumption	980.0	E860.0	E947.8	E950.9	E962.1	E980.9
propyl	980.3	E860.4	—	E950.9	E962.1	E980.9
secondary	980.2	E860.3	—	E950.9	E962.1	E980.9
radiator	980.1	E860.2	—	E950.9	E962.1	E980.9
rubbing	980.2	E860.3	—	E950.9	E962.1	E980.9
specified type NEC	980.8	E860.8	—	E950.9	E962.1	E980.9
surgical	980.9	E860.9	—	E950.9	E962.1	E980.9
vapor (from any type of alcohol)	987.8	E869.8	—	E952.8	E962.2	E982.8
wood	980.1	E860.2	—	E950.9	E962.1	E980.9
Alcuronium chloride	975.2	E858.6	E945.2	E950.4	E962.0	E980.4
Aldactone	974.4	E858.5	E944.4	E950.4	E962.0	E980.4
Aldicarb	989.3	E863.2	—	E950.6	E962.1	E980.7
Aldomet	972.6	E858.3	E942.6	E950.4	E962.0	E980.4
Aldosterone	962.0	E858.0	E932.0	E950.4	E962.0	E980.4
Aldrin (dust)	989.2	E863.0	—	E950.6	E962.1	E980.7
Aleve - *see* Naproxen	—	—	—	—	—	—
Algeldrate	973.0	E858.4	E943.0	E950.4	E962.0	E980.4
Alidase	963.4	E858.1	E933.4	E950.4	E962.0	E980.4
Aliphatic thiocyanates	989.0	E866.8	—	E950.9	E962.1	E980.9
Alkaline antiseptic solution (aromatic)	976.6	E858.7	E946.6	E950.4	E962.0	E980.4
Alkalinizing agents (medicinal)	963.3	E858.1	E933.3	E950.4	E962.0	E980.4
Alkalis, caustic	983.2	E864.2	—	E950.7	E962.1	E980.6
Alkalizing agents (medicinal)	963.3	E858.1	E933.3	E950.4	E962.0	E980.4
Alka-seltzer	965.1	E850.3	E935.3	E950.0	E962.0	E980.0
Alkavervir	972.6	E858.3	E942.6	E950.4	E962.0	E980.4

◀ New   ◀▦ Revised   ~~deleted~~ Deleted   ● Use Additional Digit(s)

TABLE OF DRUGS AND CHEMICALS

Substance	Poisoning	External Cause (E Code)				
		Accident	Therapeutic Use	Suicide Attempt	Assault	Undetermined
Allegron	969.05	E854.0	E939.0	E950.3	E962.0	E980.3
Allobarbital, allobarbitone	967.0	E851	E937.0	E950.1	E962.0	E980.1
Allopurinol	974.7	E858.5	E944.7	E950.4	E962.0	E980.4
Allylestrenol	962.2	E858.0	E932.2	E950.4	E962.0	E980.4
Allylisopropylacetylurea	967.8	E852.8	E937.8	E950.2	E962.0	E980.2
Allylisopropylmalonylurea	967.0	E851	E937.0	E950.1	E962.0	E980.1
Allyltribromide	967.3	E852.2	E937.3	E950.2	E962.0	E980.2
Aloe, aloes, aloin	973.1	E858.4	E943.1	E950.4	E962.0	E980.4
Alosetron	973.8	E858.4	E943.8	E950.4	E962.0	E980.4
Aloxidone	966.0	E855.0	E936.0	E950.4	E962.0	E980.4
Aloxiprin	965.1	E850.3	E935.3	E950.0	E962.0	E980.0
Alpha amylase	963.4	E858.1	E933.4	E950.4	E962.0	E980.4
Alpha-1 blockers	971.3	E855.6	E941.3	E950.4	E962.0	E980.4
Alphaprodine (hydrochloride)	965.09	E850.2	E935.2	E950.0	E962.0	E980.0
Alpha tocopherol	963.5	E858.1	E933.5	E950.4	E962.0	E980.4
Alseroxylon	972.6	E858.3	E942.6	E950.4	E962.0	E980.4
Alum (ammonium) (potassium)	983.2	E864.2	—	E950.7	E962.1	E980.6
medicinal (astringent) NEC	976.2	E858.7	E946.2	E950.4	E962.0	E980.4
Aluminium, aluminum (gel) (hydroxide)	973.0	E858.4	E943.0	E950.4	E962.0	E980.4
acetate solution	976.2	E858.7	E946.2	E950.4	E962.0	E980.4
aspirin	965.1	E850.3	E935.3	E950.0	E962.0	E980.0
carbonate	973.0	E858.4	E943.0	E950.4	E962.0	E980.4
glycinate	973.0	E858.4	E943.0	E950.4	E962.0	E980.4
nicotinate	972.2	E858.3	E942.2	E950.4	E962.0	E980.4
ointment (surgical) (topical)	976.3	E858.7	E946.3	E950.4	E962.0	E980.4
phosphate	973.0	E858.4	E943.0	E950.4	E962.0	E980.4
subacetate	976.2	E858.7	E946.2	E950.4	E962.0	E980.4
topical NEC	976.3	E858.7	E946.3	E950.4	E962.0	E980.4
Alurate	967.0	E851	E937.0	E950.1	E962.0	E980.1
Alverine (citrate)	975.1	E858.6	E945.1	E950.4	E962.0	E980.4
Alvodine	965.09	E850.2	E935.2	E950.0	E962.0	E980.0
Amanita phalloides	988.1	E865.5	—	E950.9	E962.1	E980.9
Amantadine (hydrochloride)	966.4	E855.0	E936.4	E950.4	E962.0	E980.4
Ambazone	961.9	E857	E931.9	E950.4	E962.0	E980.4
Ambenonium	971.0	E855.3	E941.0	E950.4	E962.0	E980.4
Ambutonium bromide	971.1	E855.4	E941.1	E950.4	E962.0	E980.4
Ametazole	977.8	E858.8	E947.8	E950.4	E962.0	E980.4
Amethocaine (infiltration) (topical)	968.5	E855.2	E938.5	E950.4	E962.0	E980.4
nerve block (peripheral) (plexus)	968.6	E855.2	E938.6	E950.4	E962.0	E980.4
spinal	968.7	E855.2	E938.7	E950.4	E962.0	E980.4

◀ New   ◀ Revised   deleted Deleted   ● Use Additional Digit(s)

Substance	Poisoning	External Cause (E Code)				
		Accident	Therapeutic Use	Suicide Attempt	Assault	Undetermined
Amethopterin	963.1	E858.1	E933.1	E950.4	E962.0	E980.4
Amfepramone	977.0	E858.8	E947.0	E950.4	E962.0	E980.4
Amidone	965.02	E850.1	E935.1	E950.0	E962.0	E980.0
Amidopyrine	965.5	E850.5	E935.5	E950.0	E962.0	E980.0
Aminacrine	976.0	E858.7	E946.0	E950.4	E962.0	E980.4
Aminitrozole	961.5	E857	E931.5	E950.4	E962.0	E980.4
Aminoacetic acid	974.5	E858.5	E944.5	E950.4	E962.0	E980.4
Amino acids	974.5	E858.5	E944.5	E950.4	E962.0	E980.4
Aminocaproic acid	964.4	E858.2	E934.4	E950.4	E962.0	E980.4
Aminoethylisothiourium	963.8	E858.1	E933.8	E950.4	E962.0	E980.4
Aminoglutethimide	966.3	E855.0	E936.3	E950.4	E962.0	E980.4
Aminometradine	974.3	E858.5	E944.3	E950.4	E962.0	E980.4
Aminopentamide	971.1	E855.4	E941.1	E950.4	E962.0	E980.4
Aminophenazone	965.5	E850.5	E935.5	E950.0	E962.0	E980.0
Aminophenol	983.0	E864.0	—	E950.7	E962.1	E980.6
Aminophenylpyridone	969.5	E853.8	E939.5	E950.3	E962.0	E980.3
Aminophylline	975.7	E858.6	E945.7	E950.4	E962.0	E980.4
Aminopterin	963.1	E858.1	E933.1	E950.4	E962.0	E980.4
Aminopyrine	965.5	E850.5	E935.5	E950.0	E962.0	E980.0
Aminosalicylic acid	961.8	E857	E931.8	E950.4	E962.0	E980.4
Amiphenazole	970.1	E854.3	E940.1	E950.4	E962.0	E980.4
Amiquinsin	972.6	E858.3	E942.6	E950.4	E962.0	E980.4
Amisometradine	974.3	E858.5	E944.3	E950.4	E962.0	E980.4
Amitriptyline	969.05	E854.0	E939.0	E950.3	E962.0	E980.3
Ammonia (fumes) (gas) (vapor)	987.8	E869.8	—	E952.8	E962.2	E982.8
liquid (household) NEC	983.2	E861.4	—	E950.7	E962.1	E980.6
spirit, aromatic	970.89 ◄ⅢⅢ	E854.3	E940.8	E950.4	E962.0	E980.4
Ammoniated mercury	976.0	E858.7	E946.0	E950.4	E962.0	E980.4
Ammonium	—	—	—	—	—	—
carbonate	983.2	E864.2	—	E950.7	E962.1	E980.6
chloride (acidifying agent)	963.2	E858.1	E933.2	E950.4	E962.0	E980.4
expectorant	975.5	E858.6	E945.5	E950.4	E962.0	E980.4
compounds (household) NEC	983.2	E861.4	—	E950.7	E962.1	E980.6
fumes (any usage)	987.8	E869.8	—	E952.8	E962.2	E982.8
industrial	983.2	E864.2	—	E950.7	E962.1	E980.6
ichthosulfonate	976.4	E858.7	E946.4	E950.4	E962.0	E980.4
mandelate	961.9	E857	E931.9	E950.4	E962.0	E980.4
Amobarbital	967.0	E851	E937.0	E950.1	E962.0	E980.1
Amodiaquin(e)	961.4	E857	E931.4	E950.4	E962.0	E980.4
Amopyroquin(e)	961.4	E857	E931.4	E950.4	E962.0	E980.4

◄ New   ◄ⅢⅢ Revised   ~~deleted~~ Deleted   ● Use Additional Digit(s)

Substance	Poisoning	External Cause (E Code)				
		Accident	Therapeutic Use	Suicide Attempt	Assault	Undetermined
Amphenidone	969.5	E853.8	E939.5	E950.3	E962.0	E980.3
Amphetamine	969.72	E854.2	E939.7	E950.3	E962.0	E980.3
Amphomycin	960.8	E856	E930.8	E950.4	E962.0	E980.4
Amphotericin B	960.1	E856	E930.1	E950.4	E962.0	E980.4
topical	976.0	E858.7	E946.0	E950.4	E962.0	E980.4
Ampicillin	960.0	E856	E930.0	E950.4	E962.0	E980.4
Amprotropine	971.1	E855.4	E941.1	E950.4	E962.0	E980.4
Amygdalin	977.8	E858.8	E947.8	E950.4	E962.0	E980.4
Amyl	—	—	—	—	—	—
acetate (vapor)	982.8	E862.4	—	E950.9	E962.1	E980.9
alcohol	980.3	E860.4	—	E950.9	E962.1	E980.9
nitrite (medicinal)	972.4	E858.3	E942.4	E950.4	E962.0	E980.4
Amylase (alpha)	963.4	E858.1	E933.4	E950.4	E962.0	E980.4
Amylene hydrate	980.8	E860.8	—	E950.9	E962.1	E980.9
Amylobarbitone	967.0	E851	E937.0	E950.1	E962.0	E980.1
Amylocaine	968.9	E855.2	E938.9	E950.4	E962.0	E980.4
infiltration (subcutaneous)	968.5	E855.2	E938.5	E950.4	E962.0	E980.4
nerve block (peripheral) (plexus)	968.6	E855.2	E938.6	E950.4	E962.0	E980.4
spinal	968.7	E855.2	E938.7	E950.4	E962.0	E980.4
topical (surface)	968.5	E855.2	E938.5	E950.4	E962.0	E980.4
Amytal (sodium)	967.0	E851	E937.0	E950.1	E962.0	E980.1
Analeptics	970.0	E854.3	E940.0	E950.4	E962.0	E980.4
Analgesics	965.9	E850.9	E935.9	E950.0	E962.0	E980.0
aromatic NEC	965.4	E850.4	E935.4	E950.0	E962.0	E980.0
non-narcotic NEC	965.7	E850.7	E935.7	E950.0	E962.0	E980.0
specified NEC	965.8	E850.8	E935.8	E950.0	E962.0	E980.0
Anamirta cocculus	988.2	E865.3	—	E950.9	E962.1	E980.9
Ancillin	960.0	E856	E930.0	E950.4	E962.0	E980.4
Androgens (anabolic congeners)	962.1	E858.0	E932.1	E950.4	E962.0	E980.4
Androstalone	962.1	E858.0	E932.1	E950.4	E962.0	E980.4
Androsterone	962.1	E858.0	E932.1	E950.4	E962.0	E980.4
Anemone pulsatilia	988.2	E865.4	—	E950.9	E962.1	E980.9
Anesthesia, anesthetic (general) NEC	968.4	E855.1	E938.4	E950.4	E962.0	E980.4
block (nerve) (plexus)	968.6	E855.2	E938.6	E950.4	E962.0	E980.4
gaseous NEC	968.2	E855.1	E938.2	E950.4	E962.0	E980.4
halogenated hydrocarbon derivatives NEC	968.2	E855.1	E938.2	E950.4	E962.0	E980.4
infiltration (intradermal) (subcutaneous) (submucosal)	968.5	E855.2	E938.5	E950.4	E962.0	E980.4
intravenous	968.3	E855.1	E938.3	E950.4	E962.0	E980.4
local NEC	968.9	E855.2	E938.9	E950.4	E962.0	E980.4

◀ New ◀▦ Revised ~~deleted~~ Deleted ● Use Additional Digit(s)

Substance	Poisoning	External Cause (E Code)				
		Accident	Therapeutic Use	Suicide Attempt	Assault	Undetermined
Anesthesia *(Continued)*						
nerve blocking (peripheral) (plexus)	968.6	E855.2	E938.6	E950.4	E962.0	E980.4
rectal NEC	968.3	E855.1	E938.3	E950.4	E962.0	E980.4
spinal	968.7	E855.2	E938.7	E950.4	E962.0	E980.4
surface	968.5	E855.2	E938.5	E950.4	E962.0	E980.4
topical	968.5	E855.2	E938.5	E950.4	E962.0	E980.4
Aneurine	963.5	E858.1	E933.5	E950.4	E962.0	E980.4
Anginine - *see* Glyceryl trinitrate	971.2	E855.5	E941.2	E950.4	E962.0	E980.4
Angio-Conray	977.8	E858.8	E947.8	E950.4	E962.0	E980.4
Angiotensin	971.2	E855.5	E941.2	E950.4	E962.0	E980.4
Anhydrohydroxyprogesterone	962.2	E858.0	E932.2	E950.4	E962.0	E980.4
Anhydron	974.3	E858.5	E944.3	E950.4	E962.0	E980.4
Anileridine	965.09	E850.2	E935.2	E950.0	E962.0	E980.0
Aniline (dye) (liquid)	983.0	E864.0	—	E950.7	E962.1	E980.6
analgesic	965.4	E850.4	E935.4	E950.0	E962.0	E980.0
derivatives, therapeutic NEC	965.4	E850.4	E935.4	E950.0	E962.0	E980.0
vapor	987.8	E869.8	—	E952.8	E962.2	E982.8
Aniscoropine	971.1	E855.4	E941.1	E950.4	E962.0	E980.4
Anisindione	964.2	E858.2	E934.2	E950.4	E962.0	E980.4
Anorexic agents	977.0	E858.8	E947.0	E950.4	E962.0	E980.4
Ant (bite) (sting)	989.5	E905.5	—	E950.9	E962.1	E980.9
Antabuse	977.3	E858.8	E947.3	E950.4	E962.0	E980.4
Antacids	973.0	E858.4	E943.0	E950.4	E962.0	E980.4
Antazoline	963.0	E858.1	E933.0	E950.4	E962.0	E980.4
Anthelmintics	961.6	E857	E931.6	E950.4	E962.0	E980.4
Anthralin	976.4	E858.7	E946.4	E950.4	E962.0	E980.4
Anthramycin	960.7	E856	E930.7	E950.4	E962.0	E980.4
Antiadrenergics	971.3	E855.6	E941.3	E950.4	E962.0	E980.4
Antiallergic agents	963.0	E858.1	E933.0	E950.4	E962.0	E980.4
Antianemic agents NEC	964.1	E858.2	E934.1	E950.4	E962.0	E980.4
Antiaris toxicaria	988.2	E865.4	—	E950.9	E962.1	E980.9
Antiarteriosclerotic agents	972.2	E858.3	E942.2	E950.4	E962.0	E980.4
Antiasthmatics	975.7	E858.6	E945.7	E950.4	E962.0	E980.4
Antibiotics	960.9	E856	E930.9	E950.4	E962.0	E980.4
antifungal	960.1	E856	E930.1	E950.4	E962.0	E980.4
antimycobacterial	960.6	E856	E930.6	E950.4	E962.0	E980.4
antineoplastic	960.7	E856	E930.7	E950.4	E962.0	E980.4
cephalosporin (group)	960.5	E856	E930.5	E950.4	E962.0	E980.4
chloramphenicol (group)	960.2	E856	E930.2	E950.4	E962.0	E980.4
macrolides	960.3	E856	E930.3	E950.4	E962.0	E980.4

◀ New ◀━ Revised ~~deleted~~ Deleted ● Use Additional Digit(s)

TABLE OF DRUGS AND CHEMICALS

Substance	Poisoning	External Cause (E Code)				
		Accident	Therapeutic Use	Suicide Attempt	Assault	Undetermined
Antibiotics *(Continued)*						
specified NEC	960.8	E856	E930.8	E950.4	E962.0	E980.4
tetracycline (group)	960.4	E856	E930.4	E950.4	E962.0	E980.4
Anticancer agents NEC	963.1	E858.1	E933.1	E950.4	E962.0	E980.4
antibiotics	960.7	E856	E930.7	E950.4	E962.0	E980.4
Anticholinergics	971.1	E855.4	E941.1	E950.4	E962.0	E980.4
Anticholinesterase (organophosphorus) (reversible)	971.0	E855.3	E941.0	E950.4	E962.0	E980.4
Anticoagulants	964.2	E858.2	E934.2	E950.4	E962.0	E980.4
antagonists	964.5	E858.2	E934.5	E950.4	E962.0	E980.4
Anti-common cold agents NEC	975.6	E858.6	E945.6	E950.4	E962.0	E980.4
Anticonvulsants NEC	966.3	E855.0	E936.3	E950.4	E962.0	E980.4
Antidepressants	969.00	E854.0	E939.0	E950.3	E962.0	E980.3
monoamine oxidase inhibitors (MAOI)	969.01	E854.0	E939.0	E950.3	E962.0	E980.3
specified type NEC	969.09	E854.0	E939.0	E950.3	E962.0	E980.3
SSNRI (selective serotonin and norepinephrine reuptake inhibitors)	969.02	E854.0	E939.0	E950.3	E962.0	E980.3
SSRI (selective serotonin reuptake inhibitors)	969.03	E854.0	E939.0	E950.3	E962.0	E980.3
tetracyclic	969.04	E854.0	E939.0	E950.3	E962.0	E980.3
tricyclic	969.05	E854.0	E939.0	E950.3	E962.0	E980.3
Antidiabetic agents	962.3	E858.0	E932.3	E950.4	E962.0	E980.4
Antidiarrheal agents	973.5	E858.4	E943.5	E950.4	E962.0	E980.4
Antidiuretic hormone	962.5	E858.0	E932.5	E950.4	E962.0	E980.4
Antidotes NEC	977.2	E858.8	E947.2	E950.4	E962.0	E980.4
Antiemetic agents	963.0	E858.1	E933.0	E950.4	E962.0	E980.4
Antiepilepsy agent NEC	966.3	E855.0	E936.3	E950.4	E962.0	E980.4
Antifertility pills	962.2	E858.0	E932.2	E950.4	E962.0	E980.4
Antiflatulents	973.8	E858.4	E943.8	E950.4	E962.0	E980.4
Antifreeze	989.89	E866.8	—	E950.9	E962.1	E980.9
alcohol	980.1	E860.2	—	E950.9	E962.1	E980.9
ethylene glycol	982.8	E862.4	—	E950.9	E962.1	E980.9
Antifungals (nonmedicinal) (sprays)	989.4	E863.6	—	E950.6	E962.1	E980.7
medicinal NEC	961.9	E857	E931.9	E950.4	E962.0	E980.4
antibiotic	960.1	E856	E930.1	E950.4	E962.0	E980.4
topical	976.0	E858.7	E946.0	E950.4	E962.0	E980.4
Antigastric secretion agents	973.0	E858.4	E943.0	E950.4	E962.0	E980.4
Antihelmintics	961.6	E857	E931.6	E950.4	E962.0	E980.4
Antihemophilic factor (human)	964.7	E858.2	E934.7	E950.4	E962.0	E980.4
Antihistamine	963.0	E858.1	E933.0	E950.4	E962.0	E980.4
Antihypertensive agents NEC	972.6	E858.3	E942.6	E950.4	E962.0	E980.4

◀ New　◀▥ Revised　~~deleted~~ Deleted　● Use Additional Digit(s)

Substance	Poisoning	External Cause (E Code) Accident	Therapeutic Use	Suicide Attempt	Assault	Undetermined
Anti-infectives NEC	961.9	E857	E931.9	E950.4	E962.0	E980.4
antibiotics	960.9	E856	E930.9	E950.4	E962.0	E980.4
specified NEC	960.8	E856	E930.8	E950.4	E962.0	E980.4
anthelmintic	961.6	E857	E931.6	E950.4	E962.0	E980.4
antimalarial	961.4	E857	E931.4	E950.4	E962.0	E980.4
antimycobacterial NEC	961.8	E857	E931.8	E950.4	E962.0	E980.4
antibiotics	960.6	E856	E930.6	E950.4	E962.0	E980.4
antiprotozoal NEC	961.5	E857	E931.5	E950.4	E962.0	E980.4
blood	961.4	E857	E931.4	E950.4	E962.0	E980.4
antiviral	961.7	E857	E931.7	E950.4	E962.0	E980.4
arsenical	961.1	E857	E931.1	E950.4	E962.0	E980.4
ENT agents	976.6	E858.7	E946.6	E950.4	E962.0	E980.4
heavy metals NEC	961.2	E857	E931.2	E950.4	E962.0	E980.4
local	976.0	E858.7	E946.0	E950.4	E962.0	E980.4
ophthalmic preparation	976.5	E858.7	E946.5	E950.4	E962.0	E980.4
topical NEC	976.0	E858.7	E946.0	E950.4	E962.0	E980.4
Anti-inflammatory agents (topical)	976.0	E858.7	E946.0	E950.4	E962.0	E980.4
Antiknock (tetraethyl lead)	984.1	E862.1	—	E950.9	E962.1	E980.9
Antilipemics	972.2	E858.3	E942.2	E950.4	E962.0	E980.4
Antimalarials	961.4	E857	E931.4	E950.4	E962.0	E980.4
Antimony (compounds) (vapor) NEC	985.4	E866.2	—	E950.9	E962.1	E980.9
anti-infectives	961.2	E857	E931.2	E950.4	E962.0	E980.4
pesticides (vapor)	985.4	E863.4	—	E950.6	E962.2	E980.7
potassium tartrate	961.2	E857	E931.2	E950.4	E962.0	E980.4
tartrated	961.2	E857	E931.2	E950.4	E962.0	E980.4
Antimuscarinic agents	971.1	E855.4	E941.1	E950.4	E962.0	E980.4
Antimycobacterials NEC	961.8	E857	E931.8	E950.4	E962.0	E980.4
antibiotics	960.6	E856	E930.6	E950.4	E962.0	E980.4
Antineoplastic agents	963.1	E858.1	E933.1	E950.4	E962.0	E980.4
antibiotics	960.7	E856	E930.7	E950.4	E962.0	E980.4
Anti-Parkinsonism agents	966.4	E855.0	E936.4	E950.4	E962.0	E980.4
Antiphlogistics	965.69	E850.6	E935.6	E950.0	E962.0	E980.0
Antiprotozoals NEC	961.5	E857	E931.5	E950.4	E962.0	E980.4
blood	961.4	E857	E931.4	E950.4	E962.0	E980.4
Antipruritics (local)	976.1	E858.7	E946.1	E950.4	E962.0	E980.4
Antipsychotic agents NEC	969.3	E853.8	E939.3	E950.3	E962.0	E980.3
Antipyretics	965.9	E850.9	E935.9	E950.0	E962.0	E980.0
specified NEC	965.8	E850.8	E935.8	E950.0	E962.0	E980.0
Antipyrine	965.5	E850.5	E935.5	E950.0	E962.0	E980.0
Antirabies serum (equine)	979.9	E858.8	E949.9	E950.4	E962.0	E980.4

Substance	Poisoning	External Cause (E Code)				
		Accident	Therapeutic Use	Suicide Attempt	Assault	Undetermined
Antirheumatics	965.69	E850.6	E935.6	E950.0	E962.0	E980.0
Antiseborrheics	976.4	E858.7	E946.4	E950.4	E962.0	E980.4
Antiseptics (external) (medicinal)	976.0	E858.7	E946.0	E950.4	E962.0	E980.4
Antistine	963.0	E858.1	E933.0	E950.4	E962.0	E980.4
Antithyroid agents	962.8	E858.0	E932.8	E950.4	E962.0	E980.4
Antitoxin, any	979.9	E858.8	E949.9	E950.4	E962.0	E980.4
Antituberculars	961.8	E857	E931.8	E950.4	E962.0	E980.4
antibiotics	960.6	E856	E930.6	E950.4	E962.0	E980.4
Antitussives	975.4	E858.6	E945.4	E950.4	E962.0	E980.4
Antivaricose agents (sclerosing)	972.7	E858.3	E942.7	E950.4	E962.0	E980.4
Antivenin (crotaline) (spider-bite)	979.9	E858.8	E949.9	E950.4	E962.0	E980.4
Antivert	963.0	E858.1	E933.0	E950.4	E962.0	E980.4
Antivirals NEC	961.7	E857	E931.7	E950.4	E962.0	E980.4
Ant poisons - *see* Pesticides	—	—	—	—	—	—
Antrol	989.4	E863.4	—	E950.6	E962.1	E980.7
fungicide	989.4	E863.6	—	E950.6	E962.1	E980.7
Apomorphine hydrochloride (emetic)	973.6	E858.4	E943.6	E950.4	E962.0	E980.4
Appetite depressants, central	977.0	E858.8	E947.0	E950.4	E962.0	E980.4
Apresoline	972.6	E858.3	E942.6	E950.4	E962.0	E980.4
Aprobarbital, aprobarbitone	967.0	E851	E937.0	E950.1	E962.0	E980.1
Apronalide	967.8	E852.8	E937.8	E950.2	E962.0	E980.2
Aqua fortis	983.1	E864.1	—	E950.7	E962.1	E980.6
Arachis oil (topical)	976.3	E858.7	E946.3	E950.4	E962.0	E980.4
cathartic	973.2	E858.4	E943.2	E950.4	E962.0	E980.4
Aralen	961.4	E857	E931.4	E950.4	E962.0	E980.4
Arginine salts	974.5	E858.5	E944.5	E950.4	E962.0	E980.4
Argyrol	976.0	E858.7	E946.0	E950.4	E962.0	E980.4
ENT agent	976.6	E858.7	E946.6	E950.4	E962.0	E980.4
ophthalmic preparation	976.5	E858.7	E946.5	E950.4	E962.0	E980.4
Aristocort	962.0	E858.0	E932.0	E950.4	E962.0	E980.4
ENT agent	976.6	E858.7	E946.6	E950.4	E962.0	E980.4
ophthalmic preparation	976.5	E858.7	E946.5	E950.4	E962.0	E980.4
topical NEC	976.0	E858.7	E946.0	E950.4	E962.0	E980.4
Aromatics, corrosive	983.0	E864.0	—	E950.7	E962.1	E980.6
disinfectants	983.0	E861.4	—	E950.7	E962.1	E980.6
Arsenate of lead (insecticide)	985.1	E863.4	—	E950.8	E962.1	E980.8
herbicide	985.1	E863.5	—	E950.8	E962.1	E980.8
Arsenic, arsenicals (compounds) (dust) (fumes) (vapor) NEC	985.1	E866.3	—	E950.8	E962.1	E980.8
anti-infectives	961.1	E857	E931.1	E950.4	E962.0	E980.4
pesticide (dust) (fumes)	985.1	E863.4	—	E950.8	E962.1	E980.8

◀ New   ◀▬ Revised   ~~deleted~~ Deleted   ● Use Additional Digit(s)

Substance	Poisoning	External Cause (E Code)				
		Accident	Therapeutic Use	Suicide Attempt	Assault	Undetermined
Arsine (gas)	985.1	E866.3	—	E950.8	E962.1	E980.8
Arsphenamine (silver)	961.1	E857	E931.1	E950.4	E962.0	E980.4
Arsthinol	961.1	E857	E931.1	E950.4	E962.0	E980.4
Artane	971.1	E855.4	E941.1	E950.4	E962.0	E980.4
Arthropod (venomous) NEC	989.5	E905.5	—	E950.9	E962.1	E980.9
Asbestos	989.81	E866.8	—	E950.9	E962.1	E980.9
Ascaridole	961.6	E857	E931.6	E950.4	E962.0	E980.4
Ascorbic acid	963.5	E858.1	E933.5	E950.4	E962.0	E980.4
Asiaticoside	976.0	E858.7	E946.0	E950.4	E962.0	E980.4
Aspidium (oleoresin)	961.6	E857	E931.6	E950.4	E962.0	E980.4
Aspirin	965.1	E850.3	E935.3	E950.0	E962.0	E980.0
Astringents (local)	976.2	E858.7	E946.2	E950.4	E962.0	E980.4
Atabrine	961.3	E857	E931.3	E950.4	E962.0	E980.4
Ataractics	969.5	E853.8	E939.5	E950.3	E962.0	E980.3
Atonia drug, intestinal	973.3	E858.4	E943.3	E950.4	E962.0	E980.4
Atophan	974.7	E858.5	E944.7	E950.4	E962.0	E980.4
Atropine	971.1	E855.4	E941.1	E950.4	E962.0	E980.4
Attapulgite	973.5	E858.4	E943.5	E950.4	E962.0	E980.4
Attenuvax	979.4	E858.8	E949.4	E950.4	E962.0	E980.4
Aureomycin	960.4	E856	E930.4	E950.4	E962.0	E980.4
ophthalmic preparation	976.5	E858.7	E946.5	E950.4	E962.0	E980.4
topical NEC	976.0	E858.7	E946.0	E950.4	E962.0	E980.4
Aurothioglucose	965.69	E850.6	E935.6	E950.0	E962.0	E980.0
Aurothioglycanide	965.69	E850.6	E935.6	E950.0	E962.0	E980.0
Aurothiomalate	965.69	E850.6	E935.6	E950.0	E962.0	E980.0
Automobile fuel	981	E862.1	—	E950.9	E962.1	E980.9
Autonomic nervous system agents NEC	971.9	E855.9	E941.9	E950.4	E962.0	E980.4
Avlosulfon	961.8	E857	E931.8	E950.4	E962.0	E980.4
Avomine	967.8	E852.8	E937.8	E950.2	E962.0	E980.2
Azacyclonol	969.5	E853.8	E939.5	E950.3	E962.0	E980.3
Azapetine	971.3	E855.6	E941.3	E950.4	E962.0	E980.4
Azaribine	963.1	E858.1	E933.1	E950.4	E962.0	E980.4
Azaserine	960.7	E856	E930.7	E950.4	E962.0	E980.4
Azathioprine	963.1	E858.1	E933.1	E950.4	E962.0	E980.4
Azosulfamide	961.0	E857	E931.0	E950.4	E962.0	E980.4
Azulfidine	961.0	E857	E931.0	E950.4	E962.0	E980.4
Azuresin	977.8	E858.8	E947.8	E950.4	E962.0	E980.4
Bacimycin	976.0	E858.7	E946.0	E950.4	E962.0	E980.4
ophthalmic preparation	976.5	E858.7	E946.5	E950.4	E962.0	E980.4

◀ New   ◀▥ Revised   ~~deleted~~ Deleted   ● Use Additional Digit(s)

TABLE OF DRUGS AND CHEMICALS

Substance	Poisoning	External Cause (E Code)				
		Accident	Therapeutic Use	Suicide Attempt	Assault	Undetermined
Bacitracin	960.8	E856	E930.8	E950.4	E962.0	E980.4
ENT agent	976.6	E858.7	E946.6	E950.4	E962.0	E980.4
ophthalmic preparation	976.5	E858.7	E946.5	E950.4	E962.0	E980.4
topical NEC	976.0	E858.7	E946.0	E950.4	E962.0	E980.4
Baking soda	963.3	E858.1	E933.3	E950.4	E962.0	E980.4
BAL	963.8	E858.1	E933.8	E950.4	E962.0	E980.4
Bamethan (sulfate)	972.5	E858.3	E942.5	E950.4	E962.0	E980.4
Bamipine	963.0	E858.1	E933.0	E950.4	E962.0	E980.4
Baneberry	988.2	E865.4	—	E950.9	E962.1	E980.9
Banewort	988.2	E865.4	—	E950.9	E962.1	E980.9
Barbenyl	967.0	E851	E937.0	E950.1	E962.0	E980.1
Barbital, barbitone	967.0	E851	E937.0	E950.1	E962.0	E980.1
Barbiturates, barbituric acid	967.0	E851	E937.0	E950.1	E962.0	E980.1
anesthetic (intravenous)	968.3	E855.1	E938.3	E950.4	E962.0	E980.4
Barium (carbonate) (chloride) (sulfate)	985.8	E866.4	—	E950.9	E962.1	E980.9
diagnostic agent	977.8	E858.8	E947.8	E950.4	E962.0	E980.4
pesticide	985.8	E863.4	—	E950.6	E962.1	E980.7
rodenticide	985.8	E863.7	—	E950.6	E962.1	E980.7
Barrier cream	976.3	E858.7	E946.3	E950.4	E962.0	E980.4
Battery acid or fluid	983.1	E864.1	—	E950.7	E962.1	E980.6
Bay rum	980.8	E860.8	—	E950.9	E962.1	E980.9
BCG vaccine	978.0	E858.8	E948.0	E950.4	E962.0	E980.4
Bearsfoot	988.2	E865.4	—	E950.9	E962.1	E980.9
Beclamide	966.3	E855.0	E936.3	E950.4	E962.0	E980.4
Bee (sting) (venom)	989.5	E905.3	—	E950.9	E962.1	E980.9
Belladonna (alkaloids)	971.1	E855.4	E941.1	E950.4	E962.0	E980.4
Bemegride	970.0	E854.3	E940.0	E950.4	E962.0	E980.4
Benactyzine	969.8	E855.8	E939.8	E950.3	E962.0	E980.3
Benadryl	963.0	E858.1	E933.0	E950.4	E962.0	E980.4
Bendrofluazide	974.3	E858.5	E944.3	E950.4	E962.0	E980.4
Bendroflumethiazide	974.3	E858.5	E944.3	E950.4	E962.0	E980.4
Benemid	974.7	E858.5	E944.7	E950.4	E962.0	E980.4
Benethamine penicillin G	960.0	E856	E930.0	E950.4	E962.0	E980.4
Benisone	976.0	E858.7	E946.0	E950.4	E962.0	E980.4
Benoquin	976.8	E858.7	E946.8	E950.4	E962.0	E980.4
Benoxinate	968.5	E855.2	E938.5	E950.4	E962.0	E980.4
Bentonite	976.3	E858.7	E946.3	E950.4	E962.0	E980.4
Benzalkonium (chloride)	976.0	E858.7	E946.0	E950.4	E962.0	E980.4
ophthalmic preparation	976.5	E858.7	E946.5	E950.4	E962.0	E980.4
Benzamidosalicylate (calcium)	961.8	E857	E931.8	E950.4	E962.0	E980.4

◀ New ◀ Revised ~~deleted~~ Deleted ● Use Additional Digit(s)

Substance	Poisoning	External Cause (E Code)				
		Accident	Therapeutic Use	Suicide Attempt	Assault	Undetermined
Benzathine penicillin	960.0	E856	E930.0	E950.4	E962.0	E980.4
Benzcarbimine	963.1	E858.1	E933.1	E950.4	E962.0	E980.4
Benzedrex	971.2	E855.5	E941.2	E950.4	E962.0	E980.4
Benzedrine (amphetamine)	969.72	E854.2	E939.7	E950.3	E962.0	E980.3
Benzene (acetyl) (dimethyl) (methyl) (solvent) (vapor)	982.0	E862.4	—	E950.9	E962.1	E980.9
hexachloride (gamma) (insecticide) (vapor)	989.2	E863.0	—	E950.6	E962.1	E980.7
Benzethonium	976.0	E858.7	E946.0	E950.4	E962.0	E980.4
Benzhexol (chloride)	966.4	E855.0	E936.4	E950.4	E962.0	E980.4
Benzilonium	971.1	E855.4	E941.1	E950.4	E962.0	E980.4
Benzin(e) - see Ligroin	—	—	—	—	—	—
Benziodarone	972.4	E858.3	E942.4	E950.4	E962.0	E980.4
Benzocaine	968.5	E855.2	E938.5	E950.4	E962.0	E980.4
Benzodiapin	969.4	E853.2	E939.4	E950.3	E962.0	E980.3
Benzodiazepines (tranquilizers) NEC	969.4	E853.2	E939.4	E950.3	E962.0	E980.3
Benzoic acid (with salicylic acid) (anti-infective)	976.0	E858.7	E946.0	E950.4	E962.0	E980.4
Benzoin	976.3	E858.7	E946.3	E950.4	E962.0	E980.4
Benzol (vapor)	982.0	E862.4	—	E950.9	E962.1	E980.9
Benzomorphan	965.09	E850.2	E935.2	E950.0	E962.0	E980.0
Benzonatate	975.4	E858.6	E945.4	E950.4	E962.0	E980.4
Benzothiadiazides	974.3	E858.5	E944.3	E950.4	E962.0	E980.4
Benzoylpas	961.8	E857	E931.8	E950.4	E962.0	E980.4
Benzperidol	969.5	E853.8	E939.5	E950.3	E962.0	E980.3
Benzphetamine	977.0	E858.8	E947.0	E950.4	E962.0	E980.4
Benzpyrinium	971.0	E855.3	E941.0	E950.4	E962.0	E980.4
Benzquinamide	963.0	E858.1	E933.0	E950.4	E962.0	E980.4
Benzthiazide	974.3	E858.5	E944.3	E950.4	E962.0	E980.4
Benztropine	971.1	E855.4	E941.1	E950.4	E962.0	E980.4
Benzyl	—	—	—	—	—	—
acetate	982.8	E862.4	—	E950.9	E962.1	E980.9
benzoate (anti-infective)	976.0	E858.7	E946.0	E950.4	E962.0	E980.4
morphine	965.09	E850.2	E935.2	E950.0	E962.0	E980.0
penicillin	960.0	E856	E930.0	E950.4	E962.0	E980.4
Bephenium	—	—	—	—	—	—
hydroxynapthoate	961.6	E857	E931.6	E950.4	E962.0	E980.4
Bergamot oil	989.89	E866.8	—	E950.9	E962.1	E980.9
Berries, poisonous	988.2	E865.3	—	E950.9	E962.1	E980.9
Beryllium (compounds) (fumes)	985.3	E866.4	—	E950.9	E962.1	E980.9
Beta-carotene	976.3	E858.7	E946.3	E950.4	E962.0	E980.4
Beta-Chlor	967.1	E852.0	E937.1	E950.2	E962.0	E980.2

◀ New　◀▥ Revised　~~deleted~~ Deleted　● Use Additional Digit(s)

TABLE OF DRUGS AND CHEMICALS

Substance	Poisoning	External Cause (E Code) Accident	Therapeutic Use	Suicide Attempt	Assault	Undetermined
Betamethasone	962.0	E858.0	E932.0	E950.4	E962.0	E980.4
topical	976.0	E858.7	E946.0	E950.4	E962.0	E980.4
Betazole	977.8	E858.8	E947.8	E950.4	E962.0	E980.4
Bethanechol	971.0	E855.3	E941.0	E950.4	E962.0	E980.4
Bethanidine	972.6	E858.3	E942.6	E950.4	E962.0	E980.4
Betula oil	976.3	E858.7	E946.3	E950.4	E962.0	E980.4
Bhang	969.6	E854.1	E939.6	E950.3	E962.0	E980.3
Bialamicol	961.5	E857	E931.5	E950.4	E962.0	E980.4
Bichloride of mercury - see Mercury, chloride	—	—	—	—	—	—
Bichromates (calcium) (crystals) (potassium) (sodium)	983.9	E864.3	—	E950.7	E962.1	E980.6
fumes	987.8	E869.8	—	E952.8	E962.2	E982.8
Biguanide derivatives, oral	962.3	E858.0	E932.3	E950.4	E962.0	E980.4
Biligrafin	977.8	E858.8	E947.8	E950.4	E962.0	E980.4
Bilopaque	977.8	E858.8	E947.8	E950.4	E962.0	E980.4
Bioflavonoids	972.8	E858.3	E942.8	E950.4	E962.0	E980.4
Biological substance NEC	979.9	E858.8	E949.9	E950.4	E962.0	E980.4
Biperiden	966.4	E855.0	E936.4	E950.4	E962.0	E980.4
Bisacodyl	973.1	E858.4	E943.1	E950.4	E962.0	E980.4
Bishydroxycoumarin	964.2	E858.2	E934.2	E950.4	E962.0	E980.4
Bismarsen	961.1	E857	E931.1	E950.4	E962.0	E980.4
Bismuth (compounds) NEC	985.8	E866.4	—	E950.9	E962.1	E980.9
anti-infectives	961.2	E857	E931.2	E950.4	E962.0	E980.4
subcarbonate	973.5	E858.4	E943.5	E950.4	E962.0	E980.4
sulfarsphenamine	961.1	E857	E931.1	E950.4	E962.0	E980.4
Bisphosphonates	—	—	—	—	—	—
intravenous	963.1	E858.1	E933.7	E950.4	E962.0	E980.4
oral	963.1	E858.1	E933.6	E950.4	E962.0	E980.4
Bithionol	961.6	E857	E931.6	E950.4	E962.0	E980.4
Bitter almond oil	989.0	E866.8	—	E950.9	E962.1	E980.9
Bittersweet	988.2	E865.4	—	E950.9	E962.1	E930.9
Black	—	—	—	—	—	—
flag	989.4	E863.4	—	E950.6	E962.1	E980.7
henbane	988.2	E865.4	—	E950.9	E962.1	E980.9
leaf (40)	989.4	E863.4	—	E950.6	E962.1	E980.7
widow spider (bite)	989.5	E905.1	—	E950.9	E962.1	E980.9
antivenin	979.9	E858.8	E949.9	E950.4	E962.0	E980.4
Blast furnace gas (carbon monoxide from)	986	E868.8	—	E952.1	E962.2	E982.1
Bleach NEC	983.9	E864.3	—	E950.7	E962.1	E980.6
Bleaching solutions	983.9	E864.3	—	E950.7	E962.1	E980.6
Bleomycin (sulfate)	960.7	E856	E930.7	E950.4	E962.0	E980.4

◀ New   ◀ Revised   ~~deleted~~ Deleted   ● Use Additional Digit(s)

Substance	Poisoning	External Cause (E Code)				
		Accident	Therapeutic Use	Suicide Attempt	Assault	Undetermined
Blockain	968.9	E855.2	E938.9	E950.4	E962.0	E980.4
infiltration (subcutaneous)	968.5	E855.2	E938.5	E950.4	E962.0	E980.4
nerve block (peripheral) (plexus)	968.6	E855.2	E938.6	E950.4	E962.0	E980.4
topical (surface)	968.5	E855.2	E938.5	E950.4	E962.0	E980.4
Blood (derivatives) (natural) (plasma) (whole)	964.7	E858.2	E934.7	E950.4	E962.0	E980.4
affecting agent	964.9	E858.2	E934.9	E950.4	E962.0	E980.4
specified NEC	964.8	E858.2	E934.8	E950.4	E962.0	E980.4
substitute (macromolecular)	964.8	E858.2	E934.8	E950.4	E962.0	E980.4
Blue velvet	965.09	E850.2	E935.2	E950.0	E962.0	E980.0
Bone meal	989.89	E866.5	—	E950.9	E962.1	E980.9
Bonine	963.0	E858.1	E933.0	E950.4	E962.0	E980.4
Boracic acid	976.0	E858.7	E946.0	E950.4	E962.0	E980.4
ENT agent	976.6	E858.7	E946.6	E950.4	E962.0	E980.4
ophthalmic preparation	976.5	E858.7	E946.5	E950.4	E962.0	E980.4
Borate (cleanser) (sodium)	989.6	E861.3	—	E950.9	E962.1	E980.9
Borax (cleanser)	989.6	E861.3	—	E950.9	E962.1	E980.9
Boric acid	976.0	E858.7	E946.0	E950.4	E962.0	E980.4
ENT agent	976.6	E858.7	E946.6	E950.4	E962.0	E980.4
ophthalmic preparation	976.5	E858.7	E946.5	E950.4	E962.0	E980.4
Boron hydride NEC	989.89	E866.8	—	E950.9	E962.1	E980.9
fumes or gas	987.8	E869.8	—	E952.8	E962.2	E982.8
Botox	975.3	E858.6	E945.3	E950.4	E962.0	E980.4
Brake fluid vapor	987.8	E869.8	—	E952.8	E962.2	E982.8
Brass (compounds) (fumes)	985.8	E866.4	—	E950.9	E962.1	E980.9
Brasso	981	E861.3	—	E950.9	E962.1	E980.9
Bretylium (tosylate)	972.6	E858.3	E942.6	E950.4	E962.0	E980.4
Brevital (sodium)	968.3	E855.1	E938.3	E950.4	E962.0	E980.4
British antilewisite	963.8	E858.1	E933.8	E950.4	E962.0	E980.4
Bromal (hydrate)	967.3	E852.2	E937.3	E950.2	E962.0	E980.2
Bromelains	963.4	E858.1	E933.4	E950.4	E962.0	E980.4
Bromides NEC	967.3	E852.2	E937.3	E950.2	E962.0	E980.2
Bromine (vapor)	987.8	E869.8	—	E952.8	E962.2	E982.8
compounds (medicinal)	967.3	E852.2	E937.3	E950.2	E962.0	E980.2
Bromisovalum	967.3	E852.2	E937.3	E950.2	E962.0	E980.2
Bromobenzyl cyanide	987.5	E869.3	—	E952.8	E962.2	E982.8
Bromodiphenhydramine	963.0	E858.1	E933.0	E950.4	E962.0	E980.4
Bromoform	967.3	E852.2	E937.3	E950.2	E962.0	E980.2
Bromophenol blue reagent	977.8	E858.8	E947.8	E950.4	E962.0	E980.4
Bromosalicylhydroxamic acid	961.8	E857	E931.8	E950.4	E962.0	E980.4
Bromo-seltzer	965.4	E850.4	E935.4	E950.0	E962.0	E980.0

◀ New   ⬅ Revised   ~~deleted~~ Deleted   ● Use Additional Digit(s)

TABLE OF DRUGS AND CHEMICALS

Substance	Poisoning	External Cause (E Code)				
		Accident	Therapeutic Use	Suicide Attempt	Assault	Undetermined
Brompheniramine	963.0	E858.1	E933.0	E950.4	E962.0	E980.4
Bromural	967.3	E852.2	E937.3	E950.2	E962.0	E980.2
Brown spider (bite) (venom)	989.5	E905.1	—	E950.9	E962.1	E980.9
Brucia	988.2	E865.3	—	E950.9	E962.1	E980.9
Brucine	989.1	E863.7	—	E950.6	E962.1	E980.7
Brunswick green - see Copper	—	—	—	—	—	—
Bruten - see Ibuprofen	—	—	—	—	—	—
Bryonia (alba) (dioica)	988.2	E865.4	—	E950.9	E962.1	E980.9
Buclizine	969.5	E853.8	E939.5	E950.3	E962.0	E980.3
Bufferin	965.1	E850.3	E935.3	E950.0	E962.0	E980.0
Bufotenine	969.6	E854.1	E939.6	E950.3	E962.0	E980.3
Buphenine	971.2	E855.5	E941.2	E950.4	E962.0	E980.4
Bupivacaine	968.9	E855.2	E938.9	E950.4	E962.0	E980.4
infiltration (subcutaneous)	968.5	E855.2	E938.5	E950.4	E962.0	E980.4
nerve block (peripheral) (plexus)	968.6	E855.2	E938.6	E950.4	E962.0	E980.4
Busulfan	963.1	E858.1	E933.1	E950.4	E962.0	E980.4
Butabarbital (sodium)	967.0	E851	E937.0	E950.1	E962.0	E980.1
Butabarbitone	967.0	E851	E937.0	E950.1	E962.0	E980.1
Butabarpal	967.0	E851	E937.0	E950.1	E962.0	E980.1
Butacaine	968.5	E855.2	E938.5	E950.4	E962.0	E980.4
Butallylonal	967.0	E851	E937.0	E950.1	E962.0	E980.1
Butane (distributed in mobile container)	987.0	E868.0	—	E951.1	E962.2	E981.1
distributed through pipes	987.0	E867	—	E951.0	E962.2	E981.0
incomplete combustion of - see Carbon monoxide, butane	—	—	—	—	—	—
Butanol	980.3	E860.4	—	E950.9	E962.1	E980.9
Butanone	982.8	E862.4	—	E950.9	E962.1	E980.9
Butaperazine	969.1	E853.0	E939.1	E950.3	E962.0	E980.3
Butazolidin	965.5	E850.5	E935.5	E950.0	E962.0	E980.0
Butethal	967.0	E851	E937.0	E950.1	E962.0	E980.1
Butethamate	971.1	E855.4	E941.1	E950.4	E962.0	E980.4
Buthalitone (sodium)	968.3	E855.1	E938.3	E950.4	E962.0	E980.4
Butisol (sodium)	967.0	E851	E937.0	E950.1	E962.0	E980.1
Butobarbital, butobarbitone	967.0	E851	E937.0	E950.1	E962.0	E980.1
Butriptyline	969.05	E854.0	E939.0	E950.3	E962.0	E980.3
Buttercups	988.2	E865.4	—	E950.9	E962.1	E980.9
Butter of antimony - see Antimony	—	—	—	—	—	—
Butyl	—	—	—	—	—	—
acetate (secondary)	982.8	E862.4	—	E950.9	E962.1	E980.9
alcohol	980.3	E860.4	—	E950.9	E962.1	E980.9

◀ New   ◀▥▥ Revised   ~~deleted~~ Deleted   ● Use Additional Digit(s)

Substance	Poisoning	External Cause (E Code) Accident	Therapeutic Use	Suicide Attempt	Assault	Undetermined
Butyl *(Continued)*						
carbinol	980.8	E860.8	—	E950.9	E962.1	E980.9
carbitol	982.8	E862.4	—	E950.9	E962.1	E980.9
cellosolve	982.8	E862.4	—	E950.9	E962.1	E980.9
chloral (hydrate)	967.1	E852.0	E937.1	E950.2	E962.0	E980.2
formate	982.8	E862.4	—	E950.9	E962.1	E980.9
scopolammonium bromide	971.1	E855.4	E941.1	E950.4	E962.0	E980.4
Butyn	968.5	E855.2	E938.5	E950.4	E962.0	E980.4
Butyrophenone (-based tranquilizers)	969.2	E853.1	E939.2	E950.3	E962.0	E980.3
Cacodyl, cacodylic acid - *see* Arsenic	—	—	—	—	—	—
Cactinomycin	960.7	E856	E930.7	E950.4	E962.0	E980.4
Cade oil	976.4	E858.7	E946.4	E950.4	E962.0	E980.4
Cadmium (chloride) (compounds) (dust) (fumes) (oxide)	985.5	E866.4	—	E950.9	E962.1	E980.9
sulfide (medicinal) NEC	976.4	E858.7	E946.4	E950.4	E962.0	E980.4
Caffeine	969.71	E854.2	E939.7	E950.3	E962.0	E980.3
Calabar bean	988.2	E865.4	—	E950.9	E962.1	E980.9
Caladium seguinium	988.2	E865.4	—	E950.9	E962.1	E980.9
Calamine (liniment) (lotion)	976.3	E858.7	E946.3	E950.4	E962.0	E980.4
Calciferol	963.5	E858.1	E933.5	E950.4	E962.0	E980.4
Calcium (salts) NEC	974.5	E858.5	E944.5	E950.4	E962.0	E980.4
acetylsalicylate	965.1	E850.3	E935.3	E950.0	E962.0	E980.0
benzamidosalicylate	961.8	E857	E931.8	E950.4	E962.0	E980.4
carbaspirin	965.1	E850.3	E935.3	E950.0	E962.0	E980.0
carbimide (citrated)	977.3	E858.8	E947.3	E950.4	E962.0	E980.4
carbonate (antacid)	973.0	E858.4	E943.0	E950.4	E962.0	E980.4
cyanide (citrated)	977.3	E858.8	E947.3	E950.4	E962.0	E980.4
dioctyl sulfosuccinate	973.2	E858.4	E943.2	E950.4	E962.0	E980.4
disodium edathamil	963.8	E858.1	E933.8	E950.4	E962.0	E980.4
disodium edetate	963.8	E858.1	E933.8	E950.4	E962.0	E980.4
EDTA	963.8	E858.1	E933.8	E950.4	E962.0	E980.4
hydrate, hydroxide	983.2	E864.2	—	E950.7	E962.1	E980.6
mandelate	961.9	E857	E931.9	E950.4	E962.0	E980.4
oxide	983.2	E864.2	—	E950.7	E962.1	E980.6
Calomel - *see* Mercury, chloride	—	—	—	—	—	—
Caloric agents NEC	974.5	E858.5	E944.5	E950.4	E962.0	E980.4
Calusterone	963.1	E858.1	E933.1	E950.4	E962.0	E980.4
Camoquin	961.4	E857	E931.4	E950.4	E962.0	E980.4
Camphor (oil)	976.1	E858.7	E946.1	E950.4	E962.0	E980.4
Candeptin	976.0	E858.7	E946.0	E950.4	E962.0	E980.4

TABLE OF DRUGS AND CHEMICALS

Substance	Poisoning	External Cause (E Code) Accident	Therapeutic Use	Suicide Attempt	Assault	Undetermined
Candicidin	976.0	E858.7	E946.0	E950.4	E962.0	E980.4
Cannabinols	969.6	E854.1	E939.6	E950.3	E962.0	E980.3
Cannabis (derivatives) (indica) (sativa)	969.6	E854.1	E939.6	E950.3	E962.0	E980.3
Canned heat	980.1	E860.2	—	E950.9	E962.1	E980.9
Cantharides, cantharidin, cantharis	976.8	E858.7	E946.8	E950.4	E962.0	E980.4
Capillary agents	972.8	E858.3	E942.8	E950.4	E962.0	E980.4
Capreomycin	960.6	E856	E930.6	E950.4	E962.0	E980.4
Captodiame, captodiamine	969.5	E853.8	E939.5	E950.3	E962.0	E980.3
Caramiphen (hydrochloride)	971.1	E855.4	E941.1	E950.4	E962.0	E980.4
Carbachol	971.0	E855.3	E941.0	E950.4	E962.0	E980.4
Carbacrylamine resins	974.5	E858.5	E944.5	E950.4	E962.0	E980.4
Carbamate (sedative)	967.8	E852.8	E937.8	E950.2	E962.0	E980.2
herbicide	989.3	E863.5	—	E950.6	E962.1	E980.7
insecticide	989.3	E863.2	—	E950.6	E962.1	E980.7
Carbamazepine	966.3	E855.0	E936.3	E950.4	E962.0	E980.4
Carbamic esters	967.8	E852.8	E937.8	E950.2	E962.0	E980.2
Carbamide	974.4	E858.5	E944.4	E950.4	E962.0	E980.4
topical	976.8	E858.7	E946.8	E950.4	E962.0	E980.4
Carbamylcholine chloride	971.0	E855.3	E941.0	E950.4	E962.0	E980.4
Carbarsone	961.1	E857	E931.1	E950.4	E962.0	E980.4
Carbaryl	989.3	E863.2	—	E950.6	E962.1	E980.7
Carbaspirin	965.1	E850.3	E935.3	E950.0	E962.0	E980.0
Carbazochrome	972.8	E858.3	E942.8	E950.4	E962.0	E980.4
Carbenicillin	960.0	E856	E930.0	E950.4	E962.0	E980.4
Carbenoxolone	973.8	E858.4	E943.8	E950.4	E962.0	E980.4
Carbetapentane	975.4	E858.6	E945.4	E950.4	E962.0	E980.4
Carbimazole	962.8	E858.0	E932.8	E950.4	E962.0	E980.4
Carbinol	980.1	E860.2	—	E950.9	E962.1	E980.9
Carbinoxamine	963.0	E858.1	E933.0	E950.4	E962.0	E980.4
Carbitol	982.8	E862.4	—	E950.9	E962.1	E980.9
Carbocaine	968.9	E855.2	E938.9	E950.4	E962.0	E980.4
infiltration (subcutaneous)	968.5	E855.2	E938.5	E950.4	E962.0	E980.4
nerve block (peripheral) (plexus)	968.6	E855.2	E938.6	E950.4	E962.0	E980.4
topical (surface)	968.5	E855.2	E938.5	E950.4	E962.0	E980.4
Carbol-fuchsin solution	976.0	E858.7	E946.0	E950.4	E962.0	E980.4
Carbolic acid (see also Phenol)	983.0	E864.0	—	E950.7	E962.1	E980.6
Carbomycin	960.8	E856	E930.8	E950.4	E962.0	E980.4
Carbon	—	—	—	—	—	—
bisulfide (liquid) (vapor)	982.2	E862.4	—	E950.9	E962.1	E980.9

◄ New   ◄‖ Revised   ~~deleted~~ Deleted   ● Use Additional Digit(s)

		External Cause (E Code)				
Substance	Poisoning	Accident	Therapeutic Use	Suicide Attempt	Assault	Undetermined
Carbon *(Continued)*						
dioxide (gas)	987.8	E869.8	—	E952.8	E962.2	E982.8
disulfide (liquid) (vapor)	982.2	E862.4	—	E950.9	E962.1	E980.9
monoxide (from incomplete combustion of) (in) NEC	986	E868.9	—	E952.1	E962.2	E982.1
blast furnace gas	986	E868.8	—	E952.1	E962.2	E982.1
butane (distributed in mobile container)	986	E868.0	—	E951.1	E962.2	E981.1
distributed through pipes	986	E867	—	E951.0	E962.2	E981.0
charcoal fumes	986	E868.3	—	E952.1	E962.2	E982.1
coal						
gas (piped)	986	E867	—	E951.0	E962.2	E981.0
solid (in domestic stoves, fireplaces)	986	E868.3	—	E952.1	E962.2	E982.1
coke (in domestic stoves, fireplaces)	986	E868.3	—	E952.1	E962.2	E982.1
exhaust gas (motor) not in transit	986	E868.2	—	E952.0	E962.2	E982.0
combustion engine, any not in watercraft	986	E868.2	—	E952.0	E962.2	E982.0
farm tractor, not in transit	986	E868.2	—	E952.0	E962.2	E982.0
gas engine	986	E868.2	—	E952.0	E962.2	E982.0
motor pump	986	E868.2	—	E952.0	E962.2	E982.0
motor vehicle, not in transit	986	E868.2	—	E952.0	E962.2	E982.0
fuel (in domestic use)	986	E868.3	—	E952.1	E962.2	E982.1
gas (piped)	986	E867	—	E951.0	E962.2	E981.0
in mobile container	986	E868.0	—	E951.1	E962.2	E981.1
utility	986	E868.1	—	E951.8	E962.2	E981.1
in mobile container	986	E868.0	—	E951.1	E962.2	E981.1
piped (natural)	986	E867	—	E951.0	E962.2	E981.0
illuminating gas	986	E868.1	—	E951.8	E962.2	E981.8
industrial fuels or gases, any	986	E868.8	—	E952.1	E962.2	E982.1
kerosene (in domestic stoves, fireplaces)	986	E868.3	—	E952.1	E962.2	E982.1
kiln gas or vapor	986	E868.8	—	E952.1	E962.2	E982.1
motor exhaust gas, not in transit	986	E868.2	—	E952.0	E962.2	E982.0
piped gas (manufactured) (natural)	986	E867	—	E951.0	E962.2	E981.0
producer gas	986	E868.8	—	E952.1	E962.2	E982.1
propane (distributed in mobile container)	986	E868.0	—	E951.1	E962.2	E981.1
distributed through pipes	986	E867	—	E951.0	E962.2	E981.0
specified source NEC	986	E868.8	—	E952.1	E962.2	E982.1
stove gas	986	E868.1	—	E951.8	E962.2	E981.8
piped	986	E867	—	E951.0	E962.2	E981.0
utility gas	986	E868.1	—	E951.8	E962.2	E981.8
piped	986	E867	—	E951.0	E962.2	E981.0

◀ New　◀▥ Revised　d̶e̶l̶e̶t̶e̶d̶ Deleted　● Use Additional Digit(s)

TABLE OF DRUGS AND CHEMICALS

Substance	Poisoning	External Cause (E Code)				
		Accident	Therapeutic Use	Suicide Attempt	Assault	Undetermined
Carbon (Continued)						
monoxide (from incomplete combustion of) (in) NEC (Continued)						
water gas	986	E868.1	—	E951.8	E962.2	E981.8
wood (in domestic stoves, fireplaces)	986	E868.3	—	E952.1	E962.2	E982.1
tetrachloride (vapor) NEC	987.8	E869.8	—	E952.8	E962.2	E982.8
liquid (cleansing agent) NEC	982.1	E861.3	—	E950.9	E962.1	E980.9
solvent	982.1	E862.4	—	E950.9	E962.1	E980.9
Carbonic acid (gas)	987.8	E869.8	—	E952.8	E962.2	E982.8
anhydrase inhibitors	974.2	E858.5	E944.2	E950.4	E962.0	E980.4
Carbowax	976.3	E858.7	E946.3	E950.4	E962.0	E980.4
Carbrital	967.0	E851	E937.0	E950.1	E962.0	E980.1
Carbromal (derivatives)	967.3	E852.2	E937.3	E950.2	E962.0	E980.2
Cardiac	—	—	—	—	—	—
depressants	972.0	E858.3	E942.0	E950.4	E962.0	E980.4
rhythm regulators	972.0	E858.3	E942.0	E950.4	E962.0	E980.4
Cardiografin	977.8	E858.8	E947.8	E950.4	E962.0	E980.4
Cardio-green	977.8	E858.8	E947.8	E950.4	E962.0	E980.4
Cardiotonic glycosides	972.1	E858.3	E942.1	E950.4	E962.0	E980.4
Cardiovascular agents NEC	972.9	E858.3	E942.9	E950.4	E962.0	E980.4
Cardrase	974.2	E858.5	E944.2	E950.4	E962.0	E980.4
Carfusin	976.0	E858.7	E946.0	E950.4	E962.0	E980.4
Carisoprodol	968.0	E855.1	E938.0	E950.4	E962.0	E980.4
Carmustine	963.1	E858.1	E933.1	E950.4	E962.0	E980.4
Carotene	963.5	E858.1	E933.5	E950.4	E962.0	E980.4
Carphenazine (maleate)	969.1	E853.0	E939.1	E950.3	E962.0	E980.3
Carter's Little Pills	973.1	E858.4	E943.1	E950.4	E962.0	E980.4
Cascara (sagrada)	973.1	E858.4	E943.1	E950.4	E962.0	E980.4
Cassava	988.2	E865.4	—	E950.9	E962.1	E980.9
Castellani's paint	976.0	E858.7	E946.0	E950.4	E962.0	E980.4
Castor	—	—	—	—	—	—
bean	988.2	E865.3	—	E950.9	E962.1	E980.9
oil	973.1	E858.4	E943.1	E950.4	E962.0	E980.4
Caterpillar (sting)	989.5	E905.5	—	E950.9	E962.1	E980.9
Catha (edulis)	970.89 ◀▥	E854.3	E940.8	E950.4	E962.0	E980.4
Cathartics NEC	973.3	E858.4	E943.3	E950.4	E962.0	E980.4
contact	973.1	E858.4	E943.1	E950.4	E962.0	E980.4
emollient	973.2	E858.4	E943.2	E950.4	E962.0	E980.4
intestinal irritants	973.1	E858.4	E943.1	E950.4	E962.0	E980.4
saline	973.3	E858.4	E943.3	E950.4	E962.0	E980.4
Cathomycin	960.8	E856	E930.8	E950.4	E962.0	E980.4

◀ New　◀▥ Revised　~~deleted~~ Deleted　● Use Additional Digit(s)

Substance	Poisoning	External Cause (E Code)				
		Accident	Therapeutic Use	Suicide Attempt	Assault	Undetermined
Caustic(s)	983.9	E864.4	—	E950.7	E962.1	E980.6
alkali	983.2	E864.2	—	E950.7	E962.1	E980.6
hydroxide	983.2	E864.2	—	E950.7	E962.1	E980.6
potash	983.2	E864.2	—	E950.7	E962.1	E980.6
soda	983.2	E864.2	—	E950.7	E962.1	E980.6
specified NEC	983.9	E864.3	—	E950.7	E962.1	E980.6
Ceepryn	976.0	E858.7	E946.0	E950.4	E962.0	E980.4
ENT agent	976.6	E858.7	E946.6	E950.4	E962.0	E980.4
lozenges	976.6	E858.7	E946.6	E950.4	E962.0	E980.4
Celestone	962.0	E858.0	E932.0	E950.4	E962.0	E980.4
topical	976.0	E858.7	E946.0	E950.4	E962.0	E980.4
Cellosolve	982.8	E862.4	—	E950.9	E962.1	E980.9
Cell stimulants and proliferants	976.8	E858.7	E946.8	E950.4	E962.0	E980.4
Cellulose derivatives, cathartic	973.3	E858.4	E943.3	E950.4	E962.0	E980.4
nitrates (topical)	976.3	E858.7	E946.3	E950.4	E962.0	E980.4
Centipede (bite)	989.5	E905.4	—	E950.9	E962.1	E980.9
Central nervous system	—	—	—	—	—	—
depressants	968.4	E855.1	E938.4	E950.4	E962.0	E980.4
anesthetic (general) NEC	968.4	E855.1	E938.4	E950.4	E962.0	E980.4
gases NEC	968.2	E855.1	E938.2	E950.4	E962.0	E980.4
intravenous	968.3	E855.1	E938.3	E950.4	E962.0	E980.4
barbiturates	967.0	E851	E937.0	E950.1	E962.0	E980.1
bromides	967.3	E852.2	E937.3	E950.2	E962.0	E980.2
cannabis sativa	969.6	E854.1	E939.6	E950.3	E962.0	E980.3
chloral hydrate	967.1	E852.0	E937.1	E950.2	E962.0	E980.2
hallucinogenics	969.6	E854.1	E939.6	E950.3	E962.0	E980.3
hypnotics	967.9	E852.9	E937.9	E950.2	E962.0	E980.2
specified NEC	967.8	E852.8	E937.8	E950.2	E962.0	E980.2
muscle relaxants	968.0	E855.1	E938.0	E950.4	E962.0	E980.4
paraldehyde	967.2	E852.1	E937.2	E950.2	E962.0	E980.2
sedatives	967.9	E852.9	E937.9	E950.2	E962.0	E980.2
mixed NEC	967.6	E852.5	E937.6	E950.2	E962.0	E980.2
specified NEC	967.8	E852.8	E937.8	E950.2	E962.0	E980.2
muscle-tone depressants	968.0	E855.1	E938.0	E950.4	E962.0	E980.4
stimulants	970.9	E854.3	E940.9	E950.4	E962.0	E980.4
amphetamines	969.72	E854.2	E939.7	E950.3	E962.0	E980.3
analeptics	970.0	E854.3	E940.0	E950.4	E962.0	E980.4
antidepressants	969.00	E854.0	E939.0	E950.3	E962.0	E980.3
opiate antagonists	970.1	E854.3	E940.0	E950.4	E962.0	E980.4
specified NEC	970.89 ◀	E854.3	E940.8	E950.4	E962.0	E980.4

◀ New　◀ Revised　deleted Deleted　● Use Additional Digit(s)

Substance	Poisoning	External Cause (E Code) Accident	Therapeutic Use	Suicide Attempt	Assault	Undetermined
Cephalexin	960.5	E856	E930.5	E950.4	E962.0	E980.4
Cephaloglycin	960.5	E856	E930.5	E950.4	E962.0	E980.4
Cephaloridine	960.5	E856	E930.5	E950.4	E962.0	E980.4
Cephalosporins NEC	960.5	E856	E930.5	E950.4	E962.0	E980.4
N (adicillin)	960.0	E856	E930.0	E950.4	E962.0	E980.4
Cephalothin (sodium)	960.5	E856	E930.5	E950.4	E962.0	E980.4
Cerbera (odallam)	988.2	E865.4	—	E950.9	E962.1	E980.9
Cerberin	972.1	E858.3	E942.1	E950.4	E962.0	E980.4
Cerebral stimulants	970.9	E854.3	E940.9	E950.4	E962.0	E980.4
psychotherapeutic	969.79	E854.2	E939.7	E950.3	E962.0	E980.3
specified NEC	970.89 ◄▥	E854.3	E940.8	E950.4	E962.0	E980.4
Cetalkonium (chloride)	976.0	E858.7	E946.0	E950.4	E962.0	E980.4
Cetoxime	963.0	E858.1	E933.0	E950.4	E962.0	E980.4
Cetrimide	976.2	E858.7	E946.2	E950.4	E962.0	E980.4
Cetylpyridinium	976.0	E858.7	E946.0	E950.4	E962.0	E980.4
ENT agent	976.6	E858.7	E946.6	E950.4	E962.0	E980.4
lozenges	976.6	E858.7	E946.6	E950.4	E962.0	E980.4
Cevadilla - see Sabadilla	—	—	—	—	—	—
Cevitamic acid	963.5	E858.1	E933.5	E950.4	E962.0	E980.4
Chalk, precipitated	973.0	E858.4	E943.0	E950.4	E962.0	E980.4
Charcoal	—	—	—	—	—	—
fumes (carbon monoxide)	986	E868.3	—	E952.1	E962.2	E982.1
industrial	986	E868.8	—	E952.1	E962.2	E982.1
medicinal (activated)	973.0	E858.4	E943.0	E950.4	E962.0	E980.4
Chelating agents NEC	977.2	E858.8	E947.2	E950.4	E962.0	E980.4
Chelidonium majus	988.2	E865.4	—	E950.9	E962.1	E980.9
Chemical substance	989.9	E866.9	—	E950.9	E962.1	E980.9
specified NEC	989.89	E866.8	—	E950.9	E962.1	E980.9
Chemotherapy, antineoplastic	963.1	E858.1	E933.1	E950.4	E962.0	E980.4
Chenopodium (oil)	961.6	E857	E931.6	E950.4	E962.0	E980.4
Cherry laurel	988.2	E865.4	—	E950.9	E962.1	E980.9
Chiniofon	961.3	E857	E931.3	E950.4	E962.0	E980.4
Chlophedianol	975.4	E858.6	E945.4	E950.4	E962.0	E980.4
Chloral (betaine) (formamide) (hydrate)	967.1	E852.0	E937.1	E950.2	E962.0	E980.2
Chloralamide	967.1	E852.0	E937.1	E950.2	E962.0	E980.2
Chlorambucil	963.1	E858.1	E933.1	E950.4	E962.0	E980.4
Chloramphenicol	960.2	E856	E930.2	E950.4	E962.0	E980.4
ENT agent	976.6	E858.7	E946.6	E950.4	E962.0	E980.4
ophthalmic preparation	976.5	E858.7	E946.5	E950.4	E962.0	E980.4
topical NEC	976.0	E858.7	E946.0	E950.4	E962.0	E980.4

◄ New ◄▥ Revised ~~deleted~~ Deleted ● Use Additional Digit(s)

| | External Cause (E Code) | | | | | |
Substance	Poisoning	Accident	Therapeutic Use	Suicide Attempt	Assault	Undetermined
Chlorate(s) (potassium) (sodium) NEC	983.9	E864.3	—	E950.7	E962.1	E980.6
herbicides	989.4	E863.5	—	E950.6	E962.1	E980.7
Chlorcyclizine	963.0	E858.1	E933.0	E950.4	E962.0	E980.4
Chlordan(e) (dust)	989.2	E863.0	—	E950.6	E962.1	E980.7
Chlordantoin	976.0	E858.7	E946.0	E950.4	E962.0	E980.4
Chlordiazepoxide	969.4	E853.2	E939.4	E950.3	E962.0	E980.3
Chloresium	976.8	E858.7	E946.8	E950.4	E962.0	E980.4
Chlorethiazol	967.1	E852.0	E937.1	E950.2	E962.0	E980.2
Chlorethyl - see Ethyl, chloride	—	—	—	—	—	—
Chloretone	967.1	E852.0	E937.1	E950.2	E962.0	E980.2
Chlorex	982.3	E862.4	—	E950.9	E962.1	E980.9
Chlorhexadol	967.1	E852.0	E937.1	E950.2	E962.0	E980.2
Chlorhexidine (hydrochloride)	976.0	E858.7	E946.0	E950.4	E962.0	E980.4
Chlorhydroxyquinolin	976.0	E858.7	E946.0	E950.4	E962.0	E980.4
Chloride of lime (bleach)	983.9	E864.3	—	E950.7	E962.1	E980.6
Chlorinated	—	—	—	—	—	—
camphene	989.2	E863.0	—	E950.6	E962.1	E980.7
diphenyl	989.89	E866.8	—	E950.9	E962.1	E980.9
hydrocarbons NEC	989.2	E863.0	—	E950.6	E962.1	E980.7
solvent	982.3	E862.4	—	E950.9	E962.1	E980.9
lime (bleach)	983.9	E864.3	—	E950.7	E962.1	E980.6
naphthalene - see Naphthalene	—	—	—	—	—	—
pesticides NEC	989.2	E863.0	—	E950.6	E962.1	E980.7
soda - see Sodium, hypochlorite	—	—	—	—	—	—
Chlorine (fumes) (gas)	987.6	E869.8	—	E952.8	E962.2	E982.8
bleach	983.9	E864.3	—	E950.7	E962.1	E980.6
compounds NEC	983.9	E864.3	—	E950.7	E962.1	E980.6
disinfectant	983.9	E861.4	—	E950.7	E962.1	E980.6
releasing agents NEC	983.9	E864.3	—	E950.7	E962.1	E980.6
Chlorisondamine	972.3	E858.3	E942.3	E950.4	E962.0	E980.4
Chlormadinone	962.2	E858.0	E932.2	E950.4	E962.0	E980.4
Chlormerodrin	974.0	E858.5	E944.0	E950.4	E962.0	E980.4
Chlormethiazole	967.1	E852.0	E937.1	E950.2	E962.0	E980.2
Chlormethylenecycline	960.4	E856	E930.4	E950.4	E962.0	E980.4
Chlormezanone	969.5	E853.8	E939.5	E950.3	E962.0	E980.3
Chloroacetophenone	987.5	E869.3	—	E952.8	E962.2	E982.8
Chloroaniline	983.0	E864.0	—	E950.7	E962.1	E980.6
Chlorobenzene, chlorobenzol	982.0	E862.4	—	E950.9	E962.1	E980.9
Chlorobutanol	967.1	E852.0	E937.1	E950.2	E962.0	E980.2

TABLE OF DRUGS AND CHEMICALS

Substance	Poisoning	External Cause (E Code)				
		Accident	Therapeutic Use	Suicide Attempt	Assault	Undetermined
Chlorodinitrobenzene	983.0	E864.0	—	E950.7	E962.1	E980.6
dust or vapor	987.8	E869.8	—	E952.8	E962.2	E982.8
Chloroethane - *see* Ethyl, chloride	—	—	—	—	—	—
Chloroform (fumes) (vapor)	987.8	E869.8	—	E952.8	E962.2	E982.8
anesthetic (gas)	968.2	E855.1	E938.2	E950.4	E962.0	E980.4
liquid NEC	968.4	E855.1	E938.4	E950.4	E962.0	E980.4
solvent	982.3	E862.4	—	E950.9	E962.1	E980.9
Chloroguanide	961.4	E857	E931.4	E950.4	E962.0	E980.4
Chloromycetin	960.2	E856	E930.2	E950.4	E962.0	E980.4
ENT agent	976.6	E858.7	E946.6	E950.4	E962.0	E980.4
ophthalmic preparation	976.5	E858.7	E946.5	E950.4	E962.0	E980.4
otic solution	976.6	E858.7	E946.6	E950.4	E962.0	E980.4
topical NEC	976.0	E858.7	E946.0	E950.4	E962.0	E980.4
Chloronitrobenzene	983.0	E864.0	—	E950.7	E962.1	E980.6
dust or vapor	987.8	E869.8	—	E952.8	E962.2	E982.8
Chlorophenol	983.0	E864.0	—	E950.7	E962.1	E980.6
Chlorophenothane	989.2	E863.0	—	E950.6	E962.1	E980.7
Chlorophyll (derivatives)	976.8	E858.7	E946.8	E950.4	E962.0	E980.4
Chloropicrin (fumes)	987.8	E869.8	—	E952.8	E962.2	E982.8
fumigant	989.4	E863.8	—	E950.6	E962.1	E980.7
fungicide	989.4	E863.6	—	E950.6	E962.1	E980.7
pesticide (fumes)	989.4	E863.4	—	E950.6	E962.1	E980.7
Chloroprocaine	968.9	E855.2	E938.9	E950.4	E962.0	E980.4
infiltration (subcutaneous)	968.5	E855.2	E938.5	E950.4	E962.0	E980.4
nerve block (peripheral) (plexus)	968.6	E855.2	E938.6	E950.4	E962.0	E980.4
Chloroptic	976.5	E858.7	E946.5	E950.4	E962.0	E980.4
Chloropurine	963.1	E858.1	E933.1	E950.4	E962.0	E980.4
Chloroquine (hydrochloride) (phosphate)	961.4	E857	E931.4	E950.4	E962.0	E980.4
Chlorothen	963.0	E858.1	E933.0	E950.4	E962.0	E980.4
Chlorothiazide	974.3	E858.5	E944.3	E950.4	E962.0	E980.4
Chlorotrianisene	962.2	E858.0	E932.2	E950.4	E962.0	E980.4
Chlorovinyldichloroarsine	985.1	E866.3	—	E950.8	E962.1	E980.8
Chloroxylenol	976.0	E858.7	E946.0	E950.4	E962.0	E980.4
Chlorphenesin (carbamate)	968.0	E855.1	E938.0	E950.4	E962.0	E980.4
topical (antifungal)	976.0	E858.7	E946.0	E950.4	E962.0	E980.4
Chlorpheniramine	963.0	E858.1	E933.0	E950.4	E962.0	E980.4
Chlorphenoxamine	966.4	E855.0	E936.4	E950.4	E962.0	E980.4
Chlorphentermine	977.0	E858.8	E947.0	E950.4	E962.0	E980.4
Chlorproguanil	961.4	E857	E931.4	E950.4	E962.0	E980.4

◄ New   ◄▬ Revised   ~~deleted~~ Deleted   ● Use Additional Digit(s)

	External Cause (E Code)					
Substance	Poisoning	Accident	Therapeutic Use	Suicide Attempt	Assault	Undetermined
Chlorpromazine	969.1	E853.0	E939.1	E950.3	E962.0	E980.3
Chlorpropamide	962.3	E858.0	E932.3	E950.4	E962.0	E980.4
Chlorprothixene	969.3	E853.8	E939.3	E950.3	E962.0	E980.3
Chlorquinaldol	976.0	E858.7	E946.0	E950.4	E962.0	E980.4
Chlortetracycline	960.4	E856	E930.4	E950.4	E962.0	E980.4
Chlorthalidone	974.4	E858.5	E944.4	E950.4	E962.0	E980.4
Chlortrianisene	962.2	E858.0	E932.2	E950.4	E962.0	E980.4
Chlor-Trimeton	963.0	E858.1	E933.0	E950.4	E962.0	E980.4
Chlorzoxazone	968.0	E855.1	E938.0	E950.4	E962.0	E980.4
Choke damp	987.8	E869.8	—	E952.8	E962.2	E982.8
Cholebrine	977.8	E858.8	E947.8	E950.4	E962.0	E980.4
Cholera vaccine	978.2	E858.8	E948.2	E950.4	E962.0	E980.4
Cholesterol-lowering agents	972.2	E858.3	E942.2	E950.4	E962.0	E980.4
Cholestyramine (resin)	972.2	E858.3	E942.2	E950.4	E962.0	E980.4
Cholic acid	973.4	E858.4	E943.4	E950.4	E962.0	E980.4
Choline	—	—	—	—	—	—
dihydrogen citrate	977.1	E858.8	E947.1	E950.4	E962.0	E980.4
salicylate	965.1	E850.3	E935.3	E950.0	E962.0	E980.0
theophyllinate	974.1	E858.5	E944.1	E950.4	E962.0	E980.4
Cholinergics	971.0	E855.3	E941.0	E950.4	E962.0	E980.4
Cholografin	977.8	E858.8	E947.8	E950.4	E962.0	E980.4
Chorionic gonadotropin	962.4	E858.0	E932.4	E950.4	E962.0	E980.4
Chromates	983.9	E864.3	—	E950.7	E962.1	E980.6
dust or mist	987.8	E869.8	—	E952.8	E962.2	E982.8
lead	984.0	E866.0	—	E950.9	E962.1	E980.9
paint	984.0	E861.5	—	E950.9	E962.1	E980.9
Chromic acid	983.9	E864.3	—	E950.7	E962.1	E980.6
dust or mist	987.8	E869.8	—	E952.8	E962.2	E982.8
Chromium	985.6	E866.4	—	E950.9	E962.1	E980.9
compounds - see Chromates	—	—	—	—	—	—
Chromonar	972.4	E858.3	E942.4	E950.4	E962.0	E980.4
Chromyl chloride	983.9	E864.3	—	E950.7	E962.1	E980.6
Chrysarobin (ointment)	976.4	E858.7	E946.4	E950.4	E962.0	E980.4
Chrysazin	973.1	E858.4	E943.1	E950.4	E962.0	E980.4
Chymar	963.4	E858.1	E933.4	E950.4	E962.0	E980.4
ophthalmic preparation	976.5	E858.7	E946.5	E950.4	E962.0	E980.4
Chymotrypsin	963.4	E858.1	E933.4	E950.4	E962.0	E980.4
ophthalmic preparation	976.5	E858.7	E946.5	E950.4	E962.0	E980.4
Cicuta maculata or virosa	988.2	E865.4	—	E950.9	E962.1	E980.9

◀ New   ◀▯ Revised   ~~deleted~~ Deleted   ● Use Additional Digit(s)

Substance	Poisoning	External Cause (E Code)				
		Accident	Therapeutic Use	Suicide Attempt	Assault	Undetermined
Cigarette lighter fluid	981	E862.1	—	E950.9	E962.1	E980.9
Cinchocaine (spinal)	968.7	E855.2	E938.7	E950.4	E962.0	E980.4
topical (surface)	968.5	E855.2	E938.5	E950.4	E962.0	E980.4
Cinchona	961.4	E857	E931.4	E950.4	E962.0	E980.4
Cinchonine alkaloids	961.4	E857	E931.4	E950.4	E962.0	E980.4
Cinchophen	974.7	E858.5	E944.7	E950.4	E962.0	E980.4
Cinnarizine	963.0	E858.1	E933.0	E950.4	E962.0	E980.4
Citanest	968.9	E855.2	E938.9	E950.4	E962.0	E980.4
infiltration (subcutaneous)	968.5	E855.2	E938.5	E950.4	E962.0	E980.4
nerve block (peripheral) (plexus)	968.6	E855.2	E938.6	E950.4	E962.0	E980.4
Citric acid	989.89	E866.8	—	E950.9	E962.1	E980.9
Citrovorum factor	964.1	E858.2	E934.1	E950.4	E962.0	E980.4
Claviceps purpurea	988.2	E865.4	—	E950.9	E962.1	E980.9
Cleaner, cleansing agent NEC	989.89	E861.3	—	E950.9	E962.1	E980.9
of paint or varnish	982.8	E862.9	—	E950.9	E962.1	E980.9
Clematis vitalba	988.2	E865.4	—	E950.9	E962.1	E980.9
Clemizole	963.0	E858.1	E933.0	E950.4	E962.0	E980.4
penicillin	960.0	E856	E930.0	E950.4	E962.0	E980.4
Clidinium	971.1	E855.4	E941.1	E950.4	E962.0	E980.4
Clindamycin	960.8	E856	E930.8	E950.4	E962.0	E980.4
Cliradon	965.09	E850.2	E935.2	E950.0	E962.0	E980.0
Clocortolone	962.0	E858.0	E932.0	E950.4	E962.0	E980.4
Clofedanol	975.4	E858.6	E945.4	E950.4	E962.0	E980.4
Clofibrate	972.2	E858.3	E942.2	E950.4	E962.0	E980.4
Clomethiazole	967.1	E852.0	E937.1	E950.2	E962.0	E980.2
Clomiphene	977.8	E858.8	E947.8	E950.4	E962.0	E980.4
Clonazepam	969.4	E853.2	E939.4	E950.3	E962.0	E980.3
Clonidine	972.6	E858.3	E942.6	E950.4	E962.0	E980.4
Clopamide	974.3	E858.5	E944.3	E950.4	E962.0	E980.4
Clorazepate	969.4	E853.2	E939.4	E950.3	E962.0	E980.3
Clorexolone	974.4	E858.5	E944.4	E950.4	E962.0	E980.4
Clorox (bleach)	983.9	E864.3	—	E950.7	E962.1	E980.6
Clortermine	977.0	E858.8	E947.0	E950.4	E962.0	E980.4
Clotrimazole	976.0	E858.7	E946.0	E950.4	E962.0	E980.4
Cloxacillin	960.0	E856	E930.0	E950.4	E962.0	E980.4
Coagulants NEC	964.5	E858.2	E934.5	E950.4	E962.0	E980.4
Coal (carbon monoxide from) - see also Carbon, monoxide, coal	—	—	—	—	—	—
oil - see Kerosene	—	—	—	—	—	—

◀ New   ◀▥ Revised   ~~deleted~~ Deleted   ● Use Additional Digit(s)

Substance	Poisoning	External Cause (E Code)				
		Accident	Therapeutic Use	Suicide Attempt	Assault	Undetermined
Coal (carbon monoxide from) *(Continued)*						
tar NEC	983.0	E864.0	—	E950.7	E962.1	E980.6
fumes	987.8	E869.8	—	E952.8	E962.2	E982.8
medicinal (ointment)	976.4	E858.7	E946.4	E950.4	E962.0	E980.4
analgesics NEC	965.5	E850.5	E935.5	E950.0	E962.0	E980.0
naphtha (solvent)	981	E862.0	—	E950.9	E962.1	E980.9
Cobalt (fumes) (industrial)	985.8	E866.4	—	E950.9	E962.1	E980.9
Cobra (venom)	989.5	E905.0	—	E950.9	E962.1	E980.9
Coca (leaf)	970.81 ◀▥	E854.3	E940.8	E950.4	E962.0	E980.4
Cocaine (hydrochloride) (salt)	970.81 ◀▥	E854.3	E940.8	E950.4	E962.0	E980.4
topical anesthetic	968.5	E855.2	E938.5	E950.4	E962.0	E980.4
Coccidioidin	977.8	E858.8	E947.8	E950.4	E962.0	E980.4
Cocculus indicus	988.2	E865.3	—	E950.9	E962.1	E980.9
Cochineal	989.89	E866.8	—	E950.9	E962.1	E980.9
medicinal products	977.4	E858.8	E947.4	E950.4	E962.0	E980.4
Codeine	965.09	E850.2	E935.2	E950.0	E962.0	E980.0
Coffee	989.89	E866.8	—	E950.9	E962.1	E980.9
Cogentin	971.1	E855.4	E941.1	E950.4	E962.0	E980.4
Coke fumes or gas (carbon monoxide)	986	E868.3	—	E952.1	E962.2	E982.1
industrial use	986	E868.8	—	E952.1	E962.2	E982.1
Colace	973.2	E858.4	E943.2	E950.4	E962.0	E980.4
Colchicine	974.7	E858.5	E944.7	E950.4	E962.0	E980.4
Colchicum	988.2	E865.3	—	E950.9	E962.1	E980.9
Cold cream	976.3	E858.7	E946.3	E950.4	E962.0	E980.4
Colestipol	972.2	E858.3	E942.2	E950.4	E962.0	E980.4
Colistimethate	960.8	E856	E930.8	E950.4	E962.0	E980.4
Colistin	960.8	E856	E930.8	E950.4	E962.0	E980.4
Collagen	977.8	E866.8	E947.8	E950.9	E962.1	E980.9
Collagenase	976.8	E858.7	E946.8	E950.4	E962.0	E980.4
Collodion (flexible)	976.3	E858.7	E946.3	E950.4	E962.0	E980.4
Colocynth	973.1	E858.4	E943.1	E950.4	E962.0	E980.4
Coloring matter - *see* Dye(s)	—	—	—	—	—	—
Combustion gas - *see* Carbon, monoxide	—	—	—	—	—	—
Compazine	969.1	E853.0	E939.1	E950.3	E962.0	E980.3
Compound	—	—	—	—	—	—
42 (warfarin)	989.4	E863.7	—	E950.6	E962.1	E980.7
269 (endrin)	989.2	E863.0	—	E950.6	E962.1	E980.7
497 (dieldrin)	989.2	E863.0	—	E950.6	E962.1	E980.7

◀ New　◀▥ Revised　~~deleted~~ Deleted　● Use Additional Digit(s)

Substance	Poisoning	External Cause (E Code)				
		Accident	Therapeutic Use	Suicide Attempt	Assault	Undetermined
Compound *(Continued)*						
1080 (sodium fluoroacetate)	989.4	E863.7	—	E950.6	E962.1	E980.7
3422 (parathion)	989.3	E863.1	—	E950.6	E962.1	E980.7
3911 (phorate)	989.3	E863.1	—	E950.6	E962.1	E980.7
3956 (toxaphene)	989.2	E863.0	—	E950.6	E962.1	E980.7
4049 (malathion)	989.3	E863.1	—	E950.6	E962.1	E980.7
4124 (dicapthon)	989.4	E863.4	—	E950.6	E962.1	E980.7
E (cortisone)	962.0	E858.0	E932.0	E950.4	E962.0	E980.4
F (hydrocortisone)	962.0	E858.0	E932.0	E950.4	E962.0	E980.4
Congo red	977.8	E858.8	E947.8	E950.4	E962.0	E980.4
Coniine, conine	965.7	E850.7	E935.7	E950.0	E962.0	E980.0
Conium (maculatum)	988.2	E865.4	—	E950.9	E962.1	E980.9
Conjugated estrogens (equine)	962.2	E858.0	E932.2	E950.4	E962.0	E980.4
Contac	975.6	E858.6	E945.6	E950.4	E962.0	E980.4
Contact lens solution	976.5	E858.7	E946.5	E950.4	E962.0	E980.4
Contraceptives (oral)	962.2	E858.0	E932.2	E950.4	E962.0	E980.4
vaginal	976.8	E858.7	E946.8	E950.4	E962.0	E980.4
Contrast media (roentgenographic)	977.8	E858.8	E947.8	E950.4	E962.0	E980.4
Convallaria majalis	988.2	E865.4	—	E950.9	E962.1	E980.9
Copper (dust) (fumes) (salts) NEC	985.8	E866.4	—	E950.9	E962.1	E980.9
arsenate, arsenite	985.1	E866.3	—	E950.8	E962.1	E980.8
insecticide	985.1	E863.4	—	E950.8	E962.1	E980.8
emetic	973.6	E858.4	E943.6	E950.4	E962.0	E980.4
fungicide	985.8	E863.6	—	E950.6	E962.1	E980.7
insecticide	985.8	E863.4	—	E950.6	E962.1	E980.7
oleate	976.0	E858.7	E946.0	E950.4	E962.0	E980.4
sulfate	983.9	E864.3	—	E950.7	E962.1	E980.6
fungicide	983.9	E863.6	—	E950.7	E962.1	E980.6
cupric	973.6	E858.4	E943.6	E950.4	E962.0	E980.4
cuprous	983.9	E864.3	—	E950.7	E962.1	E980.6
Copperhead snake (bite) (venom)	989.5	E905.0	—	E950.9	E962.1	E980.9
Coral (sting)	989.5	E905.6	—	E950.9	E962.1	E980.9
snake (bite) (venom)	989.5	E905.0	—	E950.9	E962.1	E980.9
Cordran	976.0	E858.7	E946.0	E950.4	E962.0	E980.4
Corn cures	976.4	E858.7	E946.4	E950.4	E962.0	E980.4
Cornhusker's lotion	976.3	E858.7	E946.3	E950.4	E962.0	E980.4
Corn starch	976.3	E858.7	E946.3	E950.4	E962.0	E980.4
Corrosive	983.9	E864.4	—	E950.7	E962.1	E980.6
acids NEC	983.1	E864.1	—	E950.7	E962.1	E980.6

◄ New   ◄▥▥ Revised   ~~deleted~~ Deleted   ● Use Additional Digit(s)

Substance	Poisoning	External Cause (E Code)				
		Accident	Therapeutic Use	Suicide Attempt	Assault	Undetermined
Corrosive *(Continued)*						
aromatics	983.0	E864.0	—	E950.7	E962.1	E980.6
disinfectant	983.0	E861.4	—	E950.7	E962.1	E980.6
fumes NEC	987.9	E869.9	—	E952.9	E962.2	E982.9
specified NEC	983.9	E864.3	—	E950.7	E962.1	E980.6
sublimate - *see* Mercury, chloride	—	—	—	—	—	—
Cortate	962.0	E858.0	E932.0	E950.4	E962.0	E980.4
Cort-Dome	962.0	E858.0	E932.0	E950.4	E962.0	E980.4
ENT agent	976.6	E858.7	E946.6	E950.4	E962.0	E980.4
ophthalmic preparation	976.5	E858.7	E946.5	E950.4	E962.0	E980.4
topical NEC	976.0	E858.7	E946.0	E950.4	E962.0	E980.4
Cortef	962.0	E858.0	E932.0	E950.4	E962.0	E980.4
ENT agent	976.6	E858.7	E946.6	E950.4	E962.0	E980.4
ophthalmic preparation	976.5	E858.7	E946.5	E950.4	E962.0	E980.4
topical NEC	976.0	E858.7	E946.0	E950.4	E962.0	E980.4
Corticosteroids (fluorinated)	962.0	E858.0	E932.0	E950.4	E962.0	E980.4
ENT agent	976.6	E858.7	E946.6	E950.4	E962.0	E980.4
ophthalmic preparation	976.5	E858.7	E946.5	E950.4	E962.0	E980.4
topical NEC	976.0	E858.7	E946.0	E950.4	E962.0	E980.4
Corticotropin	962.4	E858.0	E932.4	E950.4	E962.0	E980.4
Cortisol	962.0	E858.0	E932.0	E950.4	E962.0	E980.4
ENT agent	976.6	E858.7	E946.6	E950.4	E962.0	E980.4
ophthalmic preparation	976.5	E858.7	E946.5	E950.4	E962.0	E980.4
topical NEC	976.0	E858.7	E946.0	E950.4	E962.0	E980.4
Cortisone derivatives (acetate)	962.0	E858.0	E932.0	E950.4	E962.0	E980.4
ENT agent	976.6	E858.7	E946.6	E950.4	E962.0	E980.4
ophthalmic preparation	976.5	E858.7	E946.5	E950.4	E962.0	E980.4
topical NEC	976.0	E858.7	E946.0	E950.4	E962.0	E980.4
Cortogen	962.0	E858.0	E932.0	E950.4	E962.0	E980.4
ENT agent	976.6	E858.7	E946.6	E950.4	E962.0	E980.4
ophthalmic preparation	976.5	E858.7	E946.5	E950.4	E962.0	E980.4
Cortone	962.0	E858.0	E932.0	E950.4	E962.0	E980.4
ENT agent	976.6	E858.7	E946.6	E950.4	E962.0	E980.4
ophthalmic preparation	976.5	E858.7	E946.5	E950.4	E962.0	E980.4
Cortril	962.0	E858.0	E932.0	E950.4	E962.0	E980.4
ENT agent	976.6	E858.7	E946.6	E950.4	E962.0	E980.4
ophthalmic preparation	976.5	E858.7	E946.5	E950.4	E962.0	E980.4
topical NEC	976.0	E858.7	E946.0	E950.4	E962.0	E980.4
Cosmetics	989.89	E866.7	—	E950.9	E962.1	E980.9

TABLE OF DRUGS AND CHEMICALS

Substance	Poisoning	External Cause (E Code)				
		Accident	Therapeutic Use	Suicide Attempt	Assault	Undetermined
Cosyntropin	977.8	E858.8	E947.8	E950.4	E962.0	E980.4
Cotarnine	964.5	E858.2	E934.5	E950.4	E962.0	E980.4
Cottonseed oil	976.3	E858.7	E946.3	E950.4	E962.0	E980.4
Cough mixtures (antitussives)	975.4	E858.6	E945.4	E950.4	E962.0	E980.4
containing opiates	965.09	E850.2	E935.2	E950.0	E962.0	E980.0
expectorants	975.5	E858.6	E945.5	E950.4	E962.0	E980.4
Coumadin	964.2	E858.2	E934.2	E950.4	E962.0	E980.4
rodenticide	989.4	E863.7	—	E950.6	E962.1	E980.7
Coumarin	964.2	E858.2	E934.2	E950.4	E962.0	E980.4
Coumetarol	964.2	E858.2	E934.2	E950.4	E962.0	E980.4
Cowbane	988.2	E865.4	—	E950.9	E962.1	E980.9
Cozyme	963.5	E858.1	E933.5	E950.4	E962.0	E980.4
Crack	970.81	E854.3	E940.8	E950.4	E962.0	E980.4
Creolin	983.0	E864.0	—	E950.7	E962.1	E980.6
disinfectant	983.0	E861.4	—	E950.7	E962.1	E980.6
Creosol (compound)	983.0	E864.0	—	E950.7	E962.1	E980.6
Creosote (beechwood) (coal tar)	983.0	E864.0	—	E950.7	E962.1	E980.6
medicinal (expectorant)	975.5	E858.6	E945.5	E950.4	E962.0	E980.4
syrup	975.5	E858.6	E945.5	E950.4	E962.0	E980.4
Cresol	983.0	E864.0	—	E950.7	E962.1	E980.6
disinfectant	983.0	E861.4	—	E950.7	E962.1	E980.6
Cresylic acid	983.0	E864.0	—	E950.7	E962.1	E980.6
Cropropamide	965.7	E850.7	E935.7	E950.0	E962.0	E980.0
with crotethamide	970.0	E854.3	E940.0	E950.4	E962.0	E980.4
Crotamiton	976.0	E858.7	E946.0	E950.4	E962.0	E980.4
Crotethamide	965.7	E850.7	E935.7	E950.0	E962.0	E980.0
with cropropamide	970.0	E854.3	E940.0	E950.4	E962.0	E980.4
Croton (oil)	973.1	E858.4	E943.1	E950.4	E962.0	E980.4
chloral	967.1	E852.0	E937.1	E950.2	E962.0	E980.2
Crude oil	981	E862.1	—	E950.9	E962.1	E980.9
Cryogenine	965.8	E850.8	E935.8	E950.0	E962.0	E980.0
Cryolite (pesticide)	989.4	E863.4	—	E950.6	E962.1	E980.7
Cryptenamine	972.6	E858.3	E942.6	E950.4	E962.0	E980.4
Crystal violet	976.0	E858.7	E946.0	E950.4	E962.0	E980.4
Cuckoopint	988.2	E865.4	—	E950.9	E962.1	E980.9
Cumetharol	964.2	E858.2	E934.2	E950.4	E962.0	E980.4
Cupric sulfate	973.6	E858.4	E943.6	E950.4	E962.0	E980.4
Cuprous sulfate	983.9	E864.3	—	E950.7	E962.1	E980.6
Curare, curarine	975.2	E858.6	E945.2	E950.4	E962.0	E980.4

◀ New   ⬅ Revised   ~~deleted~~ Deleted   ● Use Additional Digit(s)

Substance	Poisoning	External Cause (E Code)				
		Accident	Therapeutic Use	Suicide Attempt	Assault	Undetermined
Cyanic acid - *see* Cyanide(s)	—	—	—	—	—	—
Cyanide(s) (compounds) (hydrogen) (potassium) (sodium) NEC	989.0	E866.8	—	E950.9	E962.1	E980.9
dust or gas (inhalation) NEC	987.7	E869.8	—	E952.8	E962.2	E982.8
fumigant	989.0	E863.8	—	E950.6	E962.1	E980.7
mercuric - *see* Mercury	—	—	—	—	—	—
pesticide (dust) (fumes)	989.0	E863.4	—	E950.6	E962.1	E980.7
Cyanocobalamin	964.1	E858.2	E934.1	E950.4	E962.0	E980.4
Cyanogen (chloride) (gas)	—	—	—	—	—	—
NEC	987.8	E869.8	—	E952.8	E962.2	E982.8
Cyclaine	968.5	E855.2	E938.5	E950.4	E962.0	E980.4
Cyclamen europaeum	988.2	E865.4	—	E950.9	E962.1	E980.9
Cyclandelate	972.5	E858.3	E942.5	E950.4	E962.0	E980.4
Cyclazocine	965.09	E850.2	E935.2	E950.0	E962.0	E980.0
Cyclizine	963.0	E858.1	E933.0	E950.4	E962.0	E980.4
Cyclobarbital, cyclobarbitone	967.0	E851	E937.0	E950.1	E962.0	E980.1
Cycloguanil	961.4	E857	E931.4	E950.4	E962.0	E980.4
Cyclohexane	982.0	E862.4	—	E950.9	E962.1	E980.9
Cyclohexanol	980.8	E860.8	—	E950.9	E962.1	E980.9
Cyclohexanone	982.8	E862.4	—	E950.9	E962.1	E980.9
Cyclomethycaine	968.5	E855.2	E938.5	E950.4	E962.0	E980.4
Cyclopentamine	971.2	E855.5	E941.2	E950.4	E962.0	E980.4
Cyclopenthiazide	974.3	E858.5	E944.3	E950.4	E962.0	E980.4
Cyclopentolate	971.1	E855.4	E941.1	E950.4	E962.0	E980.4
Cyclophosphamide	963.1	E858.1	E933.1	E950.4	E962.0	E980.4
Cyclopropane	968.2	E855.1	E938.2	E950.4	E962.0	E980.4
Cycloserine	960.6	E856	E930.6	E950.4	E962.0	E980.4
Cyclothiazide	974.3	E858.5	E944.3	E950.4	E962.0	E980.4
Cycrimine	966.4	E855.0	E936.4	E950.4	E962.0	E980.4
Cymarin	972.1	E858.3	E942.1	E950.4	E962.0	E980.4
Cyproheptadine	963.0	E858.1	E933.0	E950.4	E962.0	E980.4
Cyprolidol	969.09	E854.0	E939.0	E950.3	E962.0	E980.3
Cytarabine	963.1	E858.1	E933.1	E950.4	E962.0	E980.4
Cytisus	—	—	—	—	—	—
laburnum	988.2	E865.4	—	E950.9	E962.1	E980.9
scoparius	988.2	E865.4	—	E950.9	E962.1	E980.9
Cytomel	962.7	E858.0	E932.7	E950.4	E962.0	E980.4
Cytosine (antineoplastic)	963.1	E858.1	E933.1	E950.4	E962.0	E980.4
Cytoxan	963.1	E858.1	E933.1	E950.4	E962.0	E980.4
Dacarbazine	963.1	E858.1	E933.1	E950.4	E962.0	E980.4

◀ New ◀▥ Revised ~~deleted~~ Deleted ● Use Additional Digit(s)

Substance	Poisoning	External Cause (E Code)				
		Accident	Therapeutic Use	Suicide Attempt	Assault	Undetermined
Dactinomycin	960.7	E856	E930.7	E950.4	E962.0	E980.4
DADPS	961.8	E857	E931.8	E950.4	E962.0	E980.4
Dakin's solution (external)	976.0	E858.7	E946.0	E950.4	E962.0	E980.4
Dalmane	969.4	E853.2	E939.4	E950.3	E962.0	E980.3
DAM	977.2	E858.8	E947.2	E950.4	E962.0	E980.4
Danilone	964.2	E858.2	E934.2	E950.4	E962.0	E980.4
Danthron	973.1	E858.4	E943.1	E950.4	E962.0	E980.4
Dantrolene	975.2	E858.6	E945.2	E950.4	E962.0	E980.4
Daphne (gnidium) (mezereum)	988.2	E865.4	—	E950.9	E962.1	E980.9
berry	988.2	E865.3	—	E950.9	E962.1	E980.9
Dapsone	961.8	E857	E931.8	E950.4	E962.0	E980.4
Daraprim	961.4	E857	E931.4	E950.4	E962.0	E980.4
Darnel	988.2	E865.3	—	E950.9	E962.1	E980.9
Darvon	965.8	E850.8	E935.8	E950.0	E962.0	E980.0
Daunorubicin	960.7	E856	E930.7	E950.4	E962.0	E980.4
DBI	962.3	E858.0	E932.3	E950.4	E962.0	E980.4
D-Con (rodenticide)	989.4	E863.7	—	E950.6	E962.1	E980.7
DDS	961.8	E857	E931.8	E950.4	E962.0	E980.4
DDT	989.2	E863.0		E950.6	E962.1	E980.7
Deadly nightshade	988.2	E865.4	—	E950.9	E962.1	E980.9
berry	988.2	E865.3	—	E950.9	E962.1	E980.9
Deanol	969.79	E854.2	E939.7	E950.3	E962.0	E980.3
Debrisoquine	972.6	E858.3	E942.6	E950.4	E962.0	E980.4
Decaborane	989.89	E866.8	—	E950.9	E962.1	E980.9
fumes	987.8	E869.8	—	E952.8	E962.2	E982.8
Decadron	962.0	E858.0	E932.0	E950.4	E962.0	E980.4
ENT agent	976.6	E858.7	E946.6	E950.4	E962.0	E980.4
ophthalmic preparation	976.5	E858.7	E946.5	E950.4	E962.0	E980.4
topical NEC	976.0	E858.7	E946.0	E950.4	E962.0	E980.4
Decahydronaphthalene	982.0	E862.4	—	E950.9	E962.1	E980.9
Decalin	982.0	E862.4	—	E950.9	E962.1	E980.9
Decamethonium	975.2	E858.6	E945.2	E950.4	E962.0	E980.4
Decholin	973.4	E858.4	E943.4	E950.4	E962.0	E980.4
sodium (diagnostic)	977.8	E858.8	E947.8	E950.4	E962.0	E980.4
Declomycin	960.4	E856	E930.4	E950.4	E962.0	E980.4
Deferoxamine	963.8	E858.1	E933.8	E950.4	E962.0	E980.4
Dehydrocholic acid	973.4	E858.4	E943.4	E950.4	E962.0	E980.4
Dekalin ◄ⁱⁱⁱⁱ	982.0	E862.4	—	E950.9	E962.1	E980.9
Delalutin	962.2	E858.0	E932.2	E950.4	E962.0	E980.4

◄ New   ◄ⁱⁱⁱⁱ Revised   deleted Deleted   ● Use Additional Digit(s)

Substance	Poisoning	External Cause (E Code)				
		Accident	Therapeutic Use	Suicide Attempt	Assault	Undetermined
Delphinium	988.2	E865.3	—	E950.9	E962.1	E980.9
Deltasone	962.0	E858.0	E932.0	E950.4	E962.0	E980.4
Deltra	962.0	E858.0	E932.0	E950.4	E962.0	E980.4
Delvinal	967.0	E851	E937.0	E950.1	E962.0	E980.1
Demecarium (bromide)	971.0	E855.3	E941.0	E950.4	E962.0	E980.4
Demeclocycline	960.4	E856	E930.4	E950.4	E962.0	E980.4
Demecolcine	963.1	E858.1	E933.1	E950.4	E962.0	E980.4
Demelanizing agents	976.8	E858.7	E946.8	E950.4	E962.0	E980.4
Demerol	965.09	E850.2	E935.2	E950.0	E962.0	E980.0
Demethylchlortetracycline	960.4	E856	E930.4	E950.4	E962.0	E980.4
Demethyltetracycline	960.4	E856	E930.4	E950.4	E962.0	E980.4
Demeton	989.3	E863.1	—	E950.6	E962.1	E980.7
Demulcents	976.3	E858.7	E946.3	E950.4	E962.0	E980.4
Demulen	962.2	E858.0	E932.2	E950.4	E962.0	E980.4
Denatured alcohol	980.0	E860.1	—	E950.9	E962.1	E980.9
Dendrid	976.5	E858.7	E946.5	E950.4	E962.0	E980.4
Dental agents, topical	976.7	E858.7	E946.7	E950.4	E962.0	E980.4
Deodorant spray (feminine hygiene)	976.8	E858.7	E946.8	E950.4	E962.0	E980.4
Deoxyribonuclease	963.4	E858.1	E933.4	E950.4	E962.0	E980.4
Depressants	—	—	—	—	—	—
appetite, central	977.0	E858.8	E947.0	E950.4	E962.0	E980.4
cardiac	972.0	E858.3	E942.0	E950.4	E962.0	E980.4
central nervous system (anesthetic)	968.4	E855.1	E938.4	E950.4	E962.0	E980.4
psychotherapeutic	969.5	E853.9	E939.5	E950.3	E962.0	E980.3
Dequalinium	976.0	E858.7	E946.0	E950.4	E962.0	E980.4
Dermolate	976.2	E858.7	E946.2	E950.4	E962.0	E980.4
DES	962.2	E858.0	E932.2	E950.4	E962.0	E980.4
Desenex	976.0	E858.7	E946.0	E950.4	E962.0	E980.4
Deserpidine	972.6	E858.3	E942.6	E950.4	E962.0	E980.4
Desipramine	969.05	E854.0	E939.0	E950.3	E962.0	E980.3
Deslanoside	972.1	E858.3	E942.1	E950.4	E962.0	E980.4
Desocodeine	965.09	E850.2	E935.2	E950.0	E962.0	E980.0
Desomorphine	965.09	E850.2	E935.2	E950.0	E962.0	E980.0
Desonide	976.0	E858.7	E946.0	E950.4	E962.0	E980.4
Desoxycorticosterone derivatives	962.0	E858.0	E932.0	E950.4	E962.0	E980.4
Desoxyephedrine	969.72	E854.2	E939.7	E950.3	E962.0	E980.3
DET	969.6	E854.1	E939.6	E950.3	E962.0	E980.3
Detergents (ingested) (synthetic)	989.6	E861.0	—	E950.9	E962.1	E980.9
external medication	976.2	E858.7	E946.2	E950.4	E962.0	E980.4

◀ New   ◀▥ Revised   ~~deleted~~ Deleted   ● Use Additional Digit(s)

Substance	Poisoning	External Cause (E Code)				
		Accident	Therapeutic Use	Suicide Attempt	Assault	Undetermined
Deterrent, alcohol	977.3	E858.8	E947.3	E950.4	E962.0	E980.4
Detrothyronine	962.7	E858.0	E932.7	E950.4	E962.0	E980.4
Dettol (external medication)	976.0	E858.7	E946.0	E950.4	E962.0	E980.4
Dexamethasone	962.0	E858.0	E932.0	E950.4	E962.0	E980.4
ENT agent	976.6	E858.7	E946.6	E950.4	E962.0	E980.4
ophthalmic preparation	976.5	E858.7	E946.5	E950.4	E962.0	E980.4
topical NEC	976.0	E858.7	E946.0	E950.4	E962.0	E980.4
Dexamphetamine	969.72	E854.2	E939.7	E950.3	E962.0	E980.3
Dexedrine	969.72	E854.2	E939.7	E950.3	E962.0	E980.3
Dexpanthenol	963.5	E858.1	E933.5	E950.4	E962.0	E980.4
Dextran	964.8	E858.2	E934.8	E950.4	E962.0	E980.4
Dextriferron	964.0	E858.2	E934.0	E950.4	E962.0	E980.4
Dextroamphetamine	969.72	E854.2	E939.7	E950.3	E962.0	E980.3
Dextro calcium pantothenate	963.5	E858.1	E933.5	E950.4	E962.0	E980.4
Dextromethorphan	975.4	E858.6	E945.4	E950.4	E962.0	E980.4
Dextromoramide	965.09	E850.2	E935.2	E950.0	E962.0	E980.0
Dextro pantothenyl alcohol	963.5	E858.1	E933.5	E950.4	E962.0	E980.4
topical	976.8	E858.7	E946.8	E950.4	E962.0	E980.4
Dextropropoxyphene (hydrochloride)	965.8	E850.8	E935.8	E950.0	E962.0	E980.0
Dextrorphan	965.09	E850.2	E935.2	E950.0	E962.0	E980.0
Dextrose NEC	974.5	E858.5	E944.5	E950.4	E962.0	E980.4
Dextrothyroxine	962.7	E858.0	E932.7	E950.4	E962.0	E980.4
DFP	971.0	E855.3	E941.0	E950.4	E962.0	E980.4
DHE-45	972.9	E858.3	E942.9	E950.4	E962.0	E980.4
Diabinese	962.3	E858.0	E932.3	E950.4	E962.0	E980.4
Diacetyl monoxime	977.2	E858.8	E947.2	E950.4	E962.0	E980.4
Diacetylmorphine	965.01	E850.0	E935.0	E950.0	E962.0	E980.0
Diagnostic agents	977.8	E858.8	E947.8	E950.4	E962.0	E980.4
Dial (soap)	976.2	E858.7	E946.2	E950.4	E962.0	E980.4
sedative	967.0	E851	E937.0	E950.1	E962.0	E980.1
Diallylbarbituric acid	967.0	E851	E937.0	E950.1	E962.0	E980.1
Diaminodiphenyisulfone	961.8	E857	E931.8	E950.4	E962.0	E980.4
Diamorphine	965.01	E850.0	E935.0	E950.0	E962.0	E980.0
Diamox	974.2	E858.5	E944.2	E950.4	E962.0	E980.4
Diamthazole	976.0	E858.7	E946.0	E950.4	E962.0	E980.4
Diaphenyisulfone	961.8	E857	E931.8	E950.4	E962.0	E980.4
Diasone (sodium)	961.8	E857	E931.8	E950.4	E962.0	E980.4
Diazepam	969.4	E853.2	E939.4	E950.3	E962.0	E980.3
Diazinon	989.3	E863.1	—	E950.6	E962.1	E980.7

◀ New   ◀▥ Revised   ~~deleted~~ Deleted   ● Use Additional Digit(s)

Substance	Poisoning	External Cause (E Code)				
		Accident	Therapeutic Use	Suicide Attempt	Assault	Undetermined
Diazomethane (gas)	987.8	E869.8	—	E952.8	E962.2	E982.8
Diazoxide	972.5	E858.3	E942.5	E950.4	E962.0	E980.4
Dibenamine	971.3	E855.6	E941.3	E950.4	E962.0	E980.4
Dibenzheptropine	963.0	E858.1	E933.0	E950.4	E962.0	E980.4
Dibenzyline	971.3	E855.6	E941.3	E950.4	E962.0	E980.4
Diborane (gas)	987.8	E869.8	—	E952.8	E962.2	E982.8
Dibromomannitol	963.1	E858.1	E933.1	E950.4	E962.0	E980.4
Dibucaine (spinal)	968.7	E855.2	E938.7	E950.4	E962.0	E980.4
topical (surface)	968.5	E855.2	E938.5	E950.4	E962.0	E980.4
Dibunate sodium	975.4	E858.6	E945.4	E950.4	E962.0	E980.4
Dibutoline	971.1	E855.4	E941.1	E950.4	E962.0	E980.4
Dicapthon	989.4	E863.4	—	E950.6	E962.1	E980.7
Dichloralphenazone	967.1	E852.0	E937.1	E950.2	E962.0	E980.2
Dichlorodifluoromethane	987.4	E869.2	—	E952.8	E962.2	E982.8
Dichloroethane	982.3	E862.4	—	E950.9	E962.1	E980.9
Dichloroethylene	982.3	E862.4	—	E950.9	E962.1	E980.9
Dichloroethyl sulfide	987.8	E869.8	—	E952.8	E962.2	E982.8
Dichlorohydrin	982.3	E862.4	—	E950.9	E962.1	E980.9
Dichloromethane (solvent) (vapor)	982.3	E862.4	—	E950.9	E962.1	E980.9
Dichlorophen(e)	961.6	E857	E931.6	E950.4	E962.0	E980.4
Dichlorphenamide	974.2	E858.5	E944.2	E950.4	E962.0	E980.4
Dichlorvos	989.3	E863.1	—	E950.6	E962.1	E980.7
Diclofenac sodium	965.69	E850.6	E935.6	E950.0	E962.0	E980.0
Dicoumarin, dicumarol	964.2	E858.2	E934.2	E950.4	E962.0	E980.4
Dicyanogen (gas)	987.8	E869.8	—	E952.8	E962.2	E982.8
Dicyclomine	971.1	E855.4	E941.1	E950.4	E962.0	E980.4
Dieldrin (vapor)	989.2	E863.0	—	E950.6	E962.1	E980.7
Dienestrol	962.2	E858.0	E932.2	E950.4	E962.0	E980.4
Dietetics	977.0	E858.8	E947.0	E950.4	E962.0	E980.4
Diethazine	966.4	E855.0	E936.4	E950.4	E962.0	E980.4
Diethyl	—	—	—	—	—	—
barbituric acid	967.0	E851	E937.0	E950.1	E962.0	E980.1
carbamazine	961.6	E857	E931.6	E950.4	E962.0	E980.4
carbinol	980.8	E860.8	—	E950.9	E962.1	E980.9
carbonate	982.8	E862.4	—	E950.9	E962.1	E980.9
ether (vapor) - see Ether(s)	—	—	—	—	—	—
propion	977.0	E858.8	E947.0	E950.4	E962.0	E980.4
stilbestrol	962.2	E858.0	E932.2	E950.4	E962.0	E980.4

TABLE OF DRUGS AND CHEMICALS

Substance	Poisoning	External Cause (E Code) Accident	Therapeutic Use	Suicide Attempt	Assault	Undetermined
Diethylene	—	—	—	—	—	—
dioxide	982.8	E862.4	—	E950.9	E962.1	E980.9
glycol (monoacetate) (monoethyl ether)	982.8	E862.4	—	E950.9	E962.1	E980.9
Diethylsulfone-diethylmethane	967.8	E852.8	E937.8	E950.2	E962.0	E980.2
Difencloxazine	965.09	E850.2	E935.2	E950.0	E962.0	E980.0
Diffusin	963.4	E858.1	E933.4	E950.4	E962.0	E980.4
Diflos	971.0	E855.3	E941.0	E950.4	E962.0	E980.4
Digestants	973.4	E858.4	E943.4	E950.4	E962.0	E980.4
Digitalin(e)	972.1	E858.3	E942.1	E950.4	E962.0	E980.4
Digitalis glycosides	972.1	E858.3	E942.1	E950.4	E962.0	E980.4
Digitoxin	972.1	E858.3	E942.1	E950.4	E962.0	E980.4
Digoxin	972.1	E858.3	E942.1	E950.4	E962.0	E980.4
Dihydrocodeine	965.09	E850.2	E935.2	E950.0	E962.0	E980.0
Dihydrocodeinone	965.09	E850.2	E935.2	E950.0	E962.0	E980.0
Dihydroergocristine	972.9	E858.3	E942.9	E950.4	E962.0	E980.4
Dihydroergotamine	972.9	E858.3	E942.9	E950.4	E962.0	E980.4
Dihydroergotoxine	972.9	E858.3	E942.9	E950.4	E962.0	E980.4
Dihydrohydroxycodeinone	965.09	E850.2	E935.2	E950.0	E962.0	E980.0
Dihydrohydroxymorphinone	965.09	E850.2	E935.2	E950.0	E962.0	E980.0
Dihydroisocodeine	965.09	E850.2	E935.2	E950.0	E962.0	E980.0
Dihydromorphine	965.09	E850.2	E935.2	E950.0	E962.0	E980.0
Dihydromorphinone	965.09	E850.2	E935.2	E950.0	E962.0	E980.0
Dihydrostreptomycin	960.6	E856	E930.6	E950.4	E962.0	E980.4
Dihydrotachysterol	962.6	E858.0	E932.6	E950.4	E962.0	E980.4
Dihydroxyanthraquinone	973.1	E858.4	E943.1	E950.4	E962.0	E980.4
Dihydroxycodeinone	965.09	E850.2	E935.2	E950.0	E962.0	E980.0
Diiodohydroxyquin	961.3	E857	E931.3	E950.4	E962.0	E980.4
topical	976.0	E858.7	E946.0	E950.4	E962.0	E980.4
Diiodohydroxyquinoline	961.3	E857	E931.3	E950.4	E962.0	E980.4
Dilantin	966.1	E855.0	E936.1	E950.4	E962.0	E980.4
Dilaudid	965.09	E850.2	E935.2	E950.0	E962.0	E980.0
Diloxanide	961.5	E857	E931.5	E950.4	E962.0	E980.4
Dimefline	970.0	E854.3	E940.0	E950.4	E962.0	E980.4
Dimenhydrinate	963.0	E858.1	E933.0	E950.4	E962.0	E980.4
Dimercaprol	963.8	E858.1	E933.8	E950.4	E962.0	E980.4
Dimercaptopropanol	963.8	E858.1	E933.8	E950.4	E962.0	E980.4
Dimetane	963.0	E858.1	E933.0	E950.4	E962.0	E980.4
Dimethicone	976.3	E858.7	E946.3	E950.4	E962.0	E980.4
Dimethindene	963.0	E858.1	E933.0	E950.4	E962.0	E980.4

◀ New ◀ Revised ~~deleted~~ Deleted ● Use Additional Digit(s)

Substance	Poisoning	External Cause (E Code)				
		Accident	Therapeutic Use	Suicide Attempt	Assault	Undetermined
Dimethisoquin	968.5	E855.2	E938.5	E950.4	E962.0	E980.4
Dimethisterone	962.2	E858.0	E932.2	E950.4	E962.0	E980.4
Dimethoxanate	975.4	E858.6	E945.4	E950.4	E962.0	E980.4
Dimethyl	—	—	—	—	—	—
arsine, arsinic acid - see Arsenic	—	—	—	—	—	—
carbinol	980.2	E860.3	—	E950.9	E962.1	E980.9
diguanide	962.3	E858.0	E932.3	E950.4	E962.0	E980.4
ketone	982.8	E862.4	—	E950.9	E962.1	E980.9
vapor	987.8	E869.8	—	E952.8	E962.2	E982.8
meperidine	965.09	E850.2	E935.2	E950.0	E962.0	E980.0
parathion	989.3	E863.1	—	E950.6	E962.1	E980.7
polysiloxane	973.8	E858.4	E943.8	E950.4	E962.0	E980.4
sulfate (fumes)	987.8	E869.8	—	E952.8	E962.2	E982.8
liquid	983.9	E864.3	—	E950.7	E962.1	E980.6
sulfoxide NEC	982.8	E862.4	—	E950.9	E962.1	E980.9
medicinal	976.4	E858.7	E946.4	E950.4	E962.0	E980.4
triptamine	969.6	E854.1	E939.6	E950.3	E962.0	E980.3
tubocurarine	975.2	E858.6	E945.2	E950.4	E962.0	E980.4
Dindevan	964.2	E858.2	E934.2	E950.4	E962.0	E980.4
Dinitro (-ortho-) cresol (herbicide) (spray)	989.4	E863.5	—	E950.6	E962.1	E980.7
insecticide	989.4	E863.4	—	E950.6	E962.1	E980.7
Dinitrobenzene	983.0	E864.0	—	E950.7	E962.1	E980.6
vapor	987.8	E869.8	—	E952.8	E962.2	E982.8
Dinitro-orthocresol (herbicide)	989.4	E863.5	—	E950.6	E962.1	E980.7
insecticide	989.4	E863.4	—	E950.6	E962.1	E980.7
Dinitrophenol (herbicide) (spray)	989.4	E863.5	—	E950.6	E962.1	E980.7
insecticide	989.4	E863.4	—	E950.6	E962.1	E980.7
Dinoprost	975.0	E858.6	E945.0	E950.4	E962.0	E980.4
Dioctyl sulfosuccinate (calcium) (sodium)	973.2	E858.4	E943.2	E950.4	E962.0	E980.4
Diodoquin	961.3	E857	E931.3	E950.4	E962.0	E980.4
Dione derivatives NEC	966.3	E855.0	E936.3	E950.4	E962.0	E980.4
Dionin	965.09	E850.2	E935.2	E950.0	E962.0	E980.0
Dioxane	982.8	E862.4	—	E950.9	E962.1	E980.9
Dioxin - see herbicide	—	—	—	—	—	—
Dioxyline	972.5	E858.3	E942.5	E950.4	E962.0	E980.4
Dipentene	982.8	E862.4	—	E950.9	E962.1	E980.9
Diphemanil	971.1	E855.4	E941.1	E950.4	E962.0	E980.4
Diphenadione	964.2	E858.2	E934.2	E950.4	E962.0	E980.4
Diphenhydramine	963.0	E858.1	E933.0	E950.4	E962.0	E980.4

◀ New   ◀▥ Revised   ~~deleted~~ Deleted   ● Use Additional Digit(s)

TABLE OF DRUGS AND CHEMICALS

Substance	Poisoning	External Cause (E Code)				
		Accident	Therapeutic Use	Suicide Attempt	Assault	Undetermined
Diphenidol	963.0	E858.1	E933.0	E950.4	E962.0	E980.4
Diphenoxylate	973.5	E858.4	E943.5	E950.4	E962.0	E980.4
Diphenylchlorarsine	985.1	E866.3	—	E950.8	E962.1	E980.8
Diphenylhydantoin (sodium)	966.1	E855.0	E936.1	E950.4	E962.0	E980.4
Diphenylpyraline	963.0	E858.1	E933.0	E950.4	E962.0	E980.4
Diphtheria	—	—	—	—	—	—
antitoxin	979.9	E858.8	E949.9	E950.4	E962.0	E980.4
toxoid	978.5	E858.8	E948.5	E950.4	E962.0	E980.4
with tetanus toxoid	978.9	E858.8	E948.9	E950.4	E962.0	E980.4
with pertussis component	978.6	E858.8	E948.6	E950.4	E962.0	E980.4
vaccine	978.5	E858.8	E948.5	E950.4	E962.0	E980.4
Dipipanone	965.09	E850.2	E935.2	E950.0	E962.0	E980.0
Diplovax	979.5	E858.8	E949.5	E950.4	E962.0	E980.4
Diprophylline	975.1	E858.6	E945.1	E950.4	E962.0	E980.4
Dipyridamole	972.4	E858.3	E942.4	E950.4	E962.0	E980.4
Dipyrone	965.5	E850.5	E935.5	E950.0	E962.0	E980.0
Diquat	989.4	E863.5	—	E950.6	E962.1	E980.7
Disinfectant NEC	983.9	E861.4	—	E950.7	E962.1	E980.6
alkaline	983.2	E861.4	—	E950.7	E962.1	E980.6
aromatic	983.0	E861.4	—	E950.7	E962.1	E980.6
Disipal	966.4	E855.0	E936.4	E950.4	E962.0	E980.4
Disodium edetate	963.8	E858.1	E933.8	E950.4	E962.0	E980.4
Disulfamide	974.4	E858.5	E944.4	E950.4	E962.0	E980.4
Disulfanilamide	961.0	E857	E931.0	E950.4	E962.0	E980.4
Disulfiram	977.3	E858.8	E947.3	E950.4	E962.0	E980.4
Dithiazanine	961.6	E857	E931.6	E950.4	E962.0	E980.4
Dithioglycerol	963.8	E858.1	E933.8	E950.4	E962.0	E980.4
Dithranol	976.4	E858.7	E946.4	E950.4	E962.0	E980.4
Diucardin	974.3	E858.5	E944.3	E950.4	E962.0	E980.4
Diupres	974.3	E858.5	E944.3	E950.4	E962.0	E980.4
Diuretics NEC	974.4	E858.5	E944.4	E950.4	E962.0	E980.4
carbonic acid anhydrase inhibitors	974.2	E858.5	E944.2	E950.4	E962.0	E980.4
mercurial	974.0	E858.5	E944.0	E950.4	E962.0	E980.4
osmotic	974.4	E858.5	E944.4	E950.4	E962.0	E980.4
purine derivatives	974.1	E858.5	E944.1	E950.4	E962.0	E980.4
saluretic	974.3	E858.5	E944.3	E950.4	E962.0	E980.4
Diuril	974.3	E858.5	E944.3	E950.4	E962.0	E980.4
Divinyl ether	968.2	E855.1	E938.2	E950.4	E962.0	E980.4
D-lysergic acid diethylamide	969.6	E854.1	E939.6	E950.3	E962.0	E980.3

◀ New   ◀▥▥ Revised   ~~deleted~~ Deleted   ● Use Additional Digit(s)

TABLE OF DRUGS AND CHEMICALS

Substance	Poisoning	External Cause (E Code)				
		Accident	Therapeutic Use	Suicide Attempt	Assault	Undetermined
DMCT	960.4	E856	E930.4	E950.4	E962.0	E980.4
DMSO	982.8	E862.4	—	E950.9	E962.1	E980.9
DMT	969.6	E854.1	E939.6	E950.3	E962.0	E980.3
DNOC	989.4	E863.5	—	E950.6	E962.1	E980.7
DOCA	962.0	E858.0	E932.0	E950.4	E962.0	E980.4
Dolophine	965.02	E850.1	E935.1	E950.0	E962.0	E980.0
Doloxene	965.8	E850.8	E935.8	E950.0	E962.0	E980.0
DOM	969.6	E854.1	E939.6	E950.3	E962.0	E980.3
Domestic gas - *see* Gas, utility	—	—	—	—	—	—
Domiphen (bromide) (lozenges)	976.6	E858.7	E946.6	E950.4	E962.0	E980.4
Dopa (levo)	966.4	E855.0	E936.4	E950.4	E962.0	E980.4
Dopamine	971.2	E855.5	E941.2	E950.4	E962.0	E980.4
Doriden	967.5	E852.4	E937.5	E950.2	E962.0	E980.2
Dormiral	967.0	E851	E937.0	E950.1	E962.0	E980.1
Dormison	967.8	E852.8	E937.8	E950.2	E962.0	E980.2
Dornase	963.4	E858.1	E933.4	E950.4	E962.0	E980.4
Dorsacaine	968.5	E855.2	E938.5	E950.4	E962.0	E980.4
Dothiepin hydrochloride	969.05	E854.0	E939.0	E950.3	E962.0	E980.3
Doxapram	970.0	E854.3	E940.0	E950.4	E962.0	E980.4
Doxepin	969.05	E854.0	E939.0	E950.3	E962.0	E980.3
Doxorubicin	960.7	E856	E930.7	E950.4	E962.0	E980.4
Doxycycline	960.4	E856	E930.4	E950.4	E962.0	E980.4
Doxylamine	963.0	E858.1	E933.0	E950.4	E962.0	E980.4
Dramamine	963.0	E858.1	E933.0	E950.4	E962.0	E980.4
Drano (drain cleaner)	983.2	E864.2	—	E950.7	E962.1	E980.6
Dromoran	965.09	E850.2	E935.2	E950.0	E962.0	E980.0
Dromostanolone	962.1	E858.0	E932.1	E950.4	E962.0	E980.4
Droperidol	969.2	E853.1	E939.2	E950.3	E962.0	E980.3
Drotrecogin alfa	964.2	E858.2	E934.2	E950.4	E962.0	E980.4
Drug	977.9	E858.9	E947.9	E950.5	E962.0	E980.5
specified NEC	977.8	E858.8	E947.8	E950.4	E962.0	E980.4
AHFS List	—	—	—	—	—	—
4:00 antihistamine drugs	963.0	E858.1	E933.0	E950.4	E962.0	E980.4
8:04 amebacides	961.5	E857	E931.5	E950.4	E962.0	E980.4
arsenical anti-infectives	961.1	E857	E931.1	E950.4	E962.0	E980.4
quinoline derivatives	961.3	E857	E931.3	E950.4	E962.0	E980.4
8:08 anthelmintics	961.6	E857	E931.6	E950.4	E962.0	E980.4
quinoline derivatives	961.3	E857	E931.3	E950.4	E962.0	E980.4
8:12.04 antifungal antibiotics	960.1	E856	E930.1	E950.4	E962.0	E980.4

TABLE OF DRUGS AND CHEMICALS

Substance	Poisoning	External Cause (E Code)				
		Accident	Therapeutic Use	Suicide Attempt	Assault	Undetermined
Drug (Continued)						
8:12.06 cephalosporins	960.5	E856	E930.5	E950.4	E962.0	E980.4
8:12.08 chloramphenicol	960.2	E856	E930.2	E950.4	E962.0	E980.4
8:12.12 erythromycins	960.3	E856	E930.3	E950.4	E962.0	E980.4
8:12.16 penicillins	960.0	E856	E930.0	E950.4	E962.0	E980.4
8:12.20 streptomycins	960.6	E856	E930.6	E950.4	E962.0	E980.4
8:12.24 tetracyclines	960.4	E856	E930.4	E950.4	E962.0	E980.4
8:12.28 other antibiotics	960.8	E856	E930.8	E950.4	E962.0	E980.4
antimycobacterial	960.6	E856	E930.6	E950.4	E962.0	E980.4
macrolides	960.3	E856	E930.3	E950.4	E962.0	E980.4
8:16 antituberculars	961.8	E857	E931.8	E950.4	E962.0	E980.4
antibiotics	960.6	E856	E930.6	E950.4	E962.0	E980.4
8:18 antivirals	961.7	E857	E931.7	E950.4	E962.0	E980.4
8:20 plasmodicides (antimalarials)	961.4	E857	E931.4	E950.4	E962.0	E980.4
8:24 sulfonamides	961.0	E857	E931.0	E950.4	E962.0	E980.4
8:26 sulfones	961.8	E857	E931.8	E950.4	E962.0	E980.4
8:28 treponemicides	961.2	E857	E931.2	E950.4	E962.0	E980.4
8:32 trichomonacides	961.5	E857	E931.5	E950.4	E962.0	E980.4
quinoline derivatives	961.3	E857	E931.3	E950.4	E962.0	E980.4
nitrofuran derivatives	961.9	E857	E931.9	E950.4	E962.0	E980.4
8:36 urinary germicides	961.9	E857	E931.9	E950.4	E962.0	E980.4
quinoline derivatives	961.3	E857	E931.3	E950.4	E962.0	E980.4
8:40 other anti-infectives	961.9	E857	E931.9	E950.4	E962.0	E980.4
10:00 antineoplastic agents	963.1	E858.1	E933.1	E950.4	E962.0	E980.4
antibiotics	960.7	E856	E930.7	E950.4	E962.0	E980.4
progestogens	962.2	E858.0	E932.2	E950.4	E962.0	E980.4
12:04 parasympathomimetic (cholinergic) agents	971.0	E855.3	E941.0	E950.4	E962.0	E980.4
12:08 parasympatholytic (cholinergic-blocking) agents	971.1	E855.4	E941.1	E950.4	E962.0	E980.4
12:12 sympathomimetic (adrenergic) agents	971.2	E855.5	E941.2	E950.4	E962.0	E980.4
12:16 sympatholytic (adrenergic-blocking) agents	971.3	E855.6	E941.3	E950.4	E962.0	E980.4
12:20 skeletal muscle relaxants	—	—	—	—	—	—
central nervous system muscle-tone depressants	968.0	E855.1	E938.0	E950.4	E962.0	E980.4
myoneural blocking agents	975.2	E858.6	E945.2	E950.4	E962.0	E980.4
16:00 blood derivatives	964.7	E858.2	E934.7	E950.4	E962.0	E980.4
20:04 antianemia drugs	964.1	E858.2	E934.1	E950.4	E962.0	E980.4
20:04.04 iron preparations	964.0	E858.2	E934.0	E950.4	E962.0	E980.4
20:04.08 liver and stomach preparations	964.1	E858.2	E934.1	E950.4	E962.0	E980.4
20:12.04 anticoagulants	964.2	E858.2	E934.2	E950.4	E962.0	E980.4
20:12.08 antiheparin agents	964.5	E858.2	E934.5	E950.4	E962.0	E980.4

◀ New   ◀▥ Revised   ~~deleted~~ Deleted   ● Use Additional Digit(s)

Substance	Poisoning	External Cause (E Code)				
		Accident	Therapeutic Use	Suicide Attempt	Assault	Undetermined
Drug *(Continued)*						
20:12.12 coagulants	964.5	E858.2	E934.5	E950.4	E962.0	E980.4
20:12.16 hemostatics NEC	964.5	E858.2	E934.5	E950.4	E962.0	E980.4
capillary active drugs	972.8	E858.3	E942.8	E950.4	E962.0	E980.4
24:04 cardiac drugs	972.9	E858.3	E942.9	E950.4	E962.0	E980.4
cardiotonic agents	972.1	E858.3	E942.1	E950.4	E962.0	E980.4
rhythm regulators	972.0	E858.3	E942.0	E950.4	E962.0	E980.4
24:06 antilipemic agents	972.2	E858.3	E942.2	E950.4	E962.0	E980.4
thyroid derivatives	962.7	E858.0	E932.7	E950.4	E962.0	E980.4
24:08 hypotensive agents	972.6	E858.3	E942.6	E950.4	E962.0	E980.4
adrenergic blocking agents	971.3	E855.6	E941.3	E950.4	E962.0	E980.4
ganglion blocking agents	972.3	E858.3	E942.3	E950.4	E962.0	E980.4
vasodilators	972.5	E858.3	E942.5	E950.4	E962.0	E980.4
24:12 vasodilating agents NEC	972.5	E858.3	E942.5	E950.4	E962.0	E980.4
coronary	972.4	E858.3	E942.4	E950.4	E962.0	E980.4
nicotinic acid derivatives	972.2	E858.3	E942.2	E950.4	E962.0	E980.4
24:16 sclerosing agents	972.7	E858.3	E942.7	E950.4	E962.0	E980.4
28:04 general anesthetics	968.4	E855.1	E938.4	E950.4	E962.0	E980.4
gaseous anesthetics	968.2	E855.1	E938.2	E950.4	E962.0	E980.4
halothane	968.1	E855.1	E938.1	E950.4	E962.0	E980.4
intravenous anesthetics	968.3	E855.1	E938.3	E950.4	E962.0	E980.4
28:08 analgesics and antipyretics	965.9	E850.9	E935.9	E950.0	E962.0	E980.0
antirheumatics	965.69	E850.6	E935.6	E950.0	E962.0	E980.0
aromatic analgesics	965.4	E850.4	E935.4	E950.0	E962.0	E980.0
non-narcotic NEC	965.7	E850.7	E935.7	E950.0	E962.0	E980.0
opium alkaloids	965.00	E850.2	E935.2	E950.0	E962.0	E980.0
heroin	965.01	E850.0	E935.0	E950.0	E962.0	E980.0
methadone	965.02	E850.1	E935.1	E950.0	E962.0	E980.0
specified type NEC	965.09	E850.2	E935.2	E950.0	E962.0	E980.0
pyrazole derivatives	965.5	E850.5	E935.5	E950.0	E962.0	E980.0
salicylates	965.1	E850.3	E935.3	E950.0	E962.0	E980.0
specified NEC	965.8	E850.8	E935.8	E950.0	E962.0	E980.0
28:10 narcotic antagonists	970.1	E854.3	E940.1	E950.4	E962.0	E980.4
28:12 anticonvulsants	966.3	E855.0	E936.3	E950.4	E962.0	E980.4
barbiturates	967.0	E851	E937.0	E950.1	E962.0	E980.1
benzodiazepine-based tranquilizers	969.4	E853.2	E939.4	E950.3	E962.0	E980.3
bromides	967.3	E852.2	E937.3	E950.2	E962.0	E980.2
hydantoin derivatives	966.1	E855.0	E936.1	E950.4	E962.0	E980.4
oxazolidine (derivatives)	966.0	E855.0	E936.0	E950.4	E962.0	E980.4
succinimides	966.2	E855.0	E936.2	E950.4	E962.0	E980.4

◀ New　◀▥ Revised　deleted Deleted　● Use Additional Digit(s)

TABLE OF DRUGS AND CHEMICALS

Substance	Poisoning	External Cause (E Code)				
		Accident	Therapeutic Use	Suicide Attempt	Assault	Undetermined
Drug *(Continued)*						
28:16.04 antidepressants	969.00	E854.0	E939.0	E950.3	E962.0	E980.3
28:16.08 tranquilizers	969.5	E853.9	E939.5	E950.3	E962.0	E980.3
benzodiazepine-based	969.4	E853.2	E939.4	E950.3	E962.0	E980.3
butyrophenone-based	969.2	E853.1	E939.2	E950.3	E962.0	E980.3
major NEC	969.3	E853.8	E939.3	E950.3	E962.0	E980.3
phenothiazine-based	969.1	E853.0	E939.1	E950.3	E962.0	E980.3
28:16.12 other psychotherapeutic agents	969.8	E855.8	E939.8	E950.3	E962.0	E980.3
28:20 respiratory and cerebral stimulants	970.9	E854.3	E940.9	E950.4	E962.0	E980.4
analeptics	970.0	E854.3	E940.0	E950.4	E962.0	E980.4
anorexigenic agents	977.0	E858.8	E947.0	E950.4	E962.0	E980.4
psychostimulants	969.70	E854.2	E939.7	E950.3	E962.0	E980.3
specified NEC	970.89	E854.3	E940.8	E950.4	E962.0	E980.4
28:24 sedatives and hypnotics	967.9	E852.9	E937.9	E950.2	E962.0	E980.2
barbiturates	967.0	E851	E937.0	E950.1	E962.0	E980.1
benzodiazepine-based tranquilizers	969.4	E853.2	E939.4	E950.3	E962.0	E980.3
chloral hydrate (group)	967.1	E852.0	E937.1	E950.2	E962.0	E980.2
glutethimide group	967.5	E852.4	E937.5	E950.2	E962.0	E980.2
intravenous anesthetics	968.3	E855.1	E938.3	E950.4	E962.0	E980.4
methaqualone (compounds)	967.4	E852.3	E937.4	E950.2	E962.0	E980.2
paraldehyde	967.2	E852.1	E937.2	E950.2	E962.0	E980.2
phenothiazine-based tranquilizers	969.1	E853.0	E939.1	E950.3	E962.0	E980.3
specified NEC	967.8	E852.8	E937.8	E950.2	E962.0	E980.2
thiobarbiturates	968.3	E855.1	E938.3	E950.4	E962.0	E980.4
tranquilizer NEC	969.5	E853.9	E939.5	E950.3	E962.0	E980.3
36:04 to 36:88 diagnostic agents	977.8	E858.8	E947.8	E950.4	E962.0	E980.4
40:00 electrolyte, caloric, and water balance agents NEC	974.5	E858.5	E944.5	E950.4	E962.0	E980.4
40:04 acidifying agents	963.2	E858.1	E933.2	E950.4	E962.0	E980.4
40:08 alkalinizing agents	963.3	E858.1	E933.3	E950.4	E962.0	E980.4
40:10 ammonia detoxicants	974.5	E858.5	E944.5	E950.4	E962.0	E980.4
40:12 replacement solutions	974.5	E858.5	E944.5	E950.4	E962.0	E980.4
plasma expanders	964.8	E858.2	E934.8	E950.4	E962.0	E980.4
40:16 sodium-removing resins	974.5	E858.5	E944.5	E950.4	E962.0	E980.4
40:18 potassium-removing resins	974.5	E858.5	E944.5	E950.4	E962.0	E980.4
40:20 caloric agents	974.5	E858.5	E944.5	E950.4	E962.0	E980.4
40:24 salt and sugar substitutes	974.5	E858.5	E944.5	E950.4	E962.0	E980.4
40:28 diuretics NEC	974.4	E858.5	E944.4	E950.4	E962.0	E980.4
carbonic acid anhydrase inhibitors	974.2	E858.5	E944.2	E950.4	E962.0	E980.4

◀ New　◀▐ Revised　~~deleted~~ Deleted　● Use Additional Digit(s)

Substance	Poisoning	External Cause (E Code)				
		Accident	Therapeutic Use	Suicide Attempt	Assault	Undetermined
Drug *(Continued)*						
40:28 diuretics NEC *(Continued)*						
mercurials	974.0	E858.5	E944.0	E950.4	E962.0	E980.4
purine derivatives	974.1	E858.5	E944.1	E950.4	E962.0	E980.4
saluretics	974.3	E858.5	E944.3	E950.4	E962.0	E980.4
thiazides	974.3	E858.5	E944.3	E950.4	E962.0	E980.4
40:36 irrigating solutions	974.5	E858.5	E944.5	E950.4	E962.0	E980.4
40:40 uricosuric agents	974.7	E858.5	E944.7	E950.4	E962.0	E980.4
44:00 enzymes	963.4	E858.1	E933.4	E950.4	E962.0	E980.4
fibrinolysis-affecting agents	964.4	E858.2	E934.4	E950.4	E962.0	E980.4
gastric agents	973.4	E858.4	E943.4	E950.4	E962.0	E980.4
48:00 expectorants and cough preparations	—	—	—	—	—	—
antihistamine agents	963.0	E858.1	E933.0	E950.4	E962.0	E980.4
antitussives	975.4	E858.6	E945.4	E950.4	E962.0	E980.4
codeine derivatives	965.09	E850.2	E935.2	E950.0	E962.0	E980.0
expectorants	975.5	E858.6	E945.5	E950.4	E962.0	E980.4
narcotic agents NEC	965.09	E850.2	E935.2	E950.0	E962.0	E980.0
52:04 anti-infectives (EENT)	—	—	—	—	—	—
ENT agent	976.6	E858.7	E946.6	E950.4	E962.0	E980.4
ophthalmic preparation	976.5	E858.7	E946.5	E950.4	E962.0	E980.4
52:04.04 antibiotics (EENT)	—	—	—	—	—	—
ENT agent	976.6	E858.7	E946.6	E950.4	E962.0	E980.4
ophthalmic preparation	976.5	E858.7	E946.5	E950.4	E962.0	E980.4
52:04.06 antivirals (EENT)	—	—	—	—	—	—
ENT agent	976.6	E858.7	E946.6	E950.4	E962.0	E980.4
ophthalmic preparation	976.5	E858.7	E946.5	E950.4	E962.0	E980.4
52:04.08 sulfonamides (EENT)	—	—	—	—	—	—
ENT agent	976.6	E858.7	E946.6	E950.4	E962.0	E980.4
ophthalmic preparation	976.5	E858.7	E946.5	E950.4	E962.0	E980.4
52:04.12 miscellaneous anti-infectives (EENT)	—	—	—	—	—	—
ENT agent	976.6	E858.7	E946.6	E950.4	E962.0	E980.4
ophthalmic preparation	976.5	E858.7	E946.5	E950.4	E962.0	E980.4
52:08 anti-inflammatory agents (EENT)	—	—	—	—	—	—
ENT agent	976.6	E858.7	E946.6	E950.4	E962.0	E980.4
ophthalmic preparation	976.5	E858.7	E946.5	E950.4	E962.0	E980.4
52:10 carbonic anhydrase inhibitors	974.2	E858.5	E944.2	E950.4	E962.0	E980.4
52:12 contact lens solutions	976.5	E858.7	E946.5	E950.4	E962.0	E980.4
52:16 local anesthetics (EENT)	968.5	E855.2	E938.5	E950.4	E962.0	E980.4

◀ New   ◀▥ Revised   ~~deleted~~ Deleted   ● Use Additional Digit(s)

Substance	Poisoning	External Cause (E Code)				
		Accident	Therapeutic Use	Suicide Attempt	Assault	Undetermined
Drug *(Continued)*						
52:20 miotics	971.0	E855.3	E941.0	E950.4	E962.0	E980.4
52:24 mydriatics	—	—	—	—	—	—
adrenergics	971.2	E855.5	E941.2	E950.4	E962.0	E980.4
anticholinergics	971.1	E855.4	E941.1	E950.4	E962.0	E980.4
antimuscarinics	971.1	E855.4	E941.1	E950.4	E962.0	E980.4
parasympatholytics	971.1	E855.4	E941.1	E950.4	E962.0	E980.4
spasmolytics	971.1	E855.4	E941.1	E950.4	E962.0	E980.4
sympathomimetics	971.2	E855.5	E941.2	E950.4	E962.0	E980.4
52:28 mouth washes and gargles	976.6	E858.7	E946.6	E950.4	E962.0	E980.4
52:32 vasoconstrictors (EENT)	971.2	E855.5	E941.2	E950.4	E962.0	E980.4
52:36 unclassified agents (EENT)	—	—	—	—	—	—
ENT agent	976.6	E858.7	E946.6	E950.4	E962.0	E980.4
ophthalmic preparation	976.5	E858.7	E946.5	E950.4	E962.0	E980.4
56:04 antacids and adsorbents	973.0	E858.4	E943.0	E950.4	E962.0	E980.4
56:08 antidiarrhea agents	973.5	E858.4	E943.5	E950.4	E962.0	E980.4
56:10 antiflatulents	973.8	E858.4	E943.8	E950.4	E962.0	E980.4
56:12 cathartics NEC	973.3	E858.4	E943.3	E950.4	E962.0	E980.4
emollients	973.2	E858.4	E943.2	E950.4	E962.0	E980.4
irritants	973.1	E858.4	E943.1	E950.4	E962.0	E980.4
56:16 digestants	973.4	E858.4	E943.4	E950.4	E962.0	E980.4
56:20 emetics and antiemetics	—	—	—	—	—	—
antiemetics	963.0	E858.1	E933.0	E950.4	E962.0	E980.4
emetics	973.6	E858.4	E943.6	E950.4	E962.0	E980.4
56:24 lipotropic agents	977.1	E858.8	E947.1	E950.4	E962.0	E980.4
56:40 miscellaneous G.I. drugs	973.8	E858.4	E943.8	E950.4	E962.0	E980.4
60:00 gold compounds	965.69	E850.6	E935.6	E950.0	E962.0	E980.0
64:00 heavy metal antagonists	963.8	E858.1	E933.8	E950.4	E962.0	E980.4
68:04 adrenals	962.0	E858.0	E932.0	E950.4	E962.0	E980.4
68:08 androgens	962.1	E858.0	E932.1	E950.4	E962.0	E980.4
68:12 contraceptives, oral	962.2	E858.0	E932.2	E950.4	E962.0	E980.4
68:16 estrogens	962.2	E858.0	E932.2	E950.4	E962.0	E980.4
68:18 gonadotropins	962.4	E858.0	E932.4	E950.4	E962.0	E980.4
68:20 insulins and antidiabetic agents	962.3	E858.0	E932.3	E950.4	E962.0	E980.4
68:20.08 insulins	962.3	E858.0	E932.3	E950.4	E962.0	E980.4
68:24 parathyroid	962.6	E858.0	E932.6	E950.4	E962.0	E980.4
68:28 pituitary (posterior)	962.5	E858.0	E932.5	E950.4	E962.0	E980.4
anterior	962.4	E858.0	E932.4	E950.4	E962.0	E980.4
68:32 progestogens	962.2	E858.0	E932.2	E950.4	E962.0	E980.4

◀ New   ◀▥ Revised   ~~deleted~~ Deleted   ● Use Additional Digit(s)

Substance	Poisoning	External Cause (E Code)				
		Accident	Therapeutic Use	Suicide Attempt	Assault	Undetermined
Drug (Continued)						
68:34 other corpus luteum hormones NEC	962.2	E858.0	E932.2	E950.4	E962.0	E980.4
68:36 thyroid and antithyroid	—	—	—	—	—	—
antithyroid	962.8	E858.0	E932.8	E950.4	E962.0	E980.4
thyroid (derivatives)	962.7	E858.0	E932.7	E950.4	E962.0	E980.4
72:00 local anesthetics NEC	968.9	E855.2	E938.9	E950.4	E962.0	E980.4
topical (surface)	968.5	E855.2	E938.5	E950.4	E962.0	E980.4
infiltration (intradermal) (subcutaneous) (submucosal)	968.5	E855.2	E938.5	E950.4	E962.0	E980.4
nerve blocking (peripheral) (plexus) (regional)	968.6	E855.2	E938.6	E950.4	E962.0	E980.4
spinal	968.7	E855.2	E938.7	E950.4	E962.0	E980.4
76:00 oxytocics	975.0	E858.6	E945.0	E950.4	E962.0	E980.4
78:00 radioactive agents	990	—	—	—	—	—
80:04 serums NEC	979.9	E858.8	E949.9	E950.4	E962.0	E980.4
immune gamma globulin (human)	964.6	E858.2	E934.6	E950.4	E962.0	E980.4
80:08 toxoids NEC	978.8	E858.8	E948.8	E950.4	E962.0	E980.4
diphtheria	978.5	E858.8	E948.5	E950.4	E962.0	E980.4
and tetanus	978.9	E858.8	E948.9	E950.4	E962.0	E980.4
with pertussis component	978.6	E858.8	E948.6	E950.4	E962.0	E980.4
tetanus	978.4	E858.8	E948.4	E950.4	E962.0	E980.4
and diphtheria	978.9	E858.8	E948.9	E950.4	E962.0	E980.4
with pertussis component	978.6	E858.8	E948.6	E950.4	E962.0	E980.4
80:12 vaccines	979.9	E858.8	E949.9	E950.4	E962.0	E980.4
bacterial NEC	978.8	E858.8	E948.8	E950.4	E962.0	E980.4
with	—	—	—	—	—	—
other bacterial components	978.9	E858.8	E948.9	E950.4	E962.0	E980.4
pertussis component	978.6	E858.8	E948.6	E950.4	E962.0	E980.4
viral and rickettsial components	979.7	E858.8	E949.7	E950.4	E962.0	E980.4
rickettsial NEC	979.6	E858.8	E949.6	E950.4	E962.0	E980.4
with	—	—	—	—	—	—
bacterial component	979.7	E858.8	E949.7	E950.4	E962.0	E980.4
pertussis component	978.6	E858.8	E948.6	E950.4	E962.0	E980.4
viral component	979.7	E858.8	E949.7	E950.4	E962.0	E980.4
viral NEC	979.6	E858.8	E949.6	E950.4	E962.0	E980.4
with	—	—	—	—	—	—
bacterial component	979.7	E858.8	E949.7	E950.4	E962.0	E980.4
pertussis component	978.6	E858.8	E948.6	E950.4	E962.0	E980.4
rickettsial component	979.7	E858.8	E949.7	E950.4	E962.0	E980.4
84:04.04 antibiotics (skin and mucous membrane)	976.0	E858.7	E946.0	E950.4	E962.0	E980.4
84:04.08 fungicides (skin and mucous membrane)	976.0	E858.7	E946.0	E950.4	E962.0	E980.4

◄ New ◄⊪ Revised ~~deleted~~ Deleted ● Use Additional Digit(s)

Substance	Poisoning	External Cause (E Code) Accident	Therapeutic Use	Suicide Attempt	Assault	Undetermined
Drug *(Continued)*						
84:04.12 scabicides and pediculicides (skin and mucous membrane)	976.0	E858.7	E946.0	E950.4	E962.0	E980.4
84:04.16 miscellaneous local anti-infectives (skin and mucous membrane)	976.0	E858.7	E946.0	E950.4	E962.0	E980.4
84:06 anti-inflammatory agents (skin and mucous membrane)	976.0	E858.7	E946.0	E950.4	E962.0	E980.4
84:08 antipruritics and local anesthetics	—	—	—	—	—	—
antipruritics	976.1	E858.7	E946.1	E950.4	E962.0	E980.4
local anesthetics	968.5	E855.2	E938.5	E950.4	E962.0	E980.4
84:12 astringents	976.2	E858.7	E946.2	E950.4	E962.0	E980.4
84:16 cell stimulants and proliferants	976.8	E858.7	E946.8	E950.4	E962.0	E980.4
84:20 detergents	976.2	E858.7	E946.2	E950.4	E962.0	E980.4
84:24 emollients, demulcents, and protectants	976.3	E858.7	E946.3	E950.4	E962.0	E980.4
84:28 keratolytic agents	976.4	E858.7	E946.4	E950.4	E962.0	E980.4
84:32 keratoplastic agents	976.4	E858.7	E946.4	E950.4	E962.0	E980.4
84:36 miscellaneous agents (skin and mucous membrane)	976.8	E858.7	E946.8	E950.4	E962.0	E980.4
86:00 spasmolytic agents	975.1	E858.6	E945.1	E950.4	E962.0	E980.4
antiasthmatics	975.7	E858.6	E945.7	E950.4	E962.0	E980.4
papaverine	972.5	E858.3	E942.5	E950.4	E962.0	E980.4
theophylline	974.1	E858.5	E944.1	E950.4	E962.0	E980.4
88:04 vitamin A	963.5	E858.1	E933.5	E950.4	E962.0	E980.4
88:08 vitamin B complex	963.5	E858.1	E933.5	E950.4	E962.0	E980.4
hematopoietic vitamin	964.1	E858.2	E934.1	E950.4	E962.0	E980.4
nicotinic acid derivatives	972.2	E858.3	E942.2	E950.4	E962.0	E980.4
88:12 vitamin C	963.5	E858.1	E933.5	E950.4	E962.0	E980.4
88:16 vitamin D	963.5	E858.1	E933.5	E950.4	E962.0	E980.4
88:20 vitamin E	963.5	E858.1	E933.5	E950.4	E962.0	E980.4
88:24 vitamin K activity	964.3	E858.2	E934.3	E950.4	E962.0	E980.4
88:28 multivitamin preparations	963.5	E858.1	E933.5	E950.4	E962.0	E980.4
92:00 unclassified therapeutic agents	977.8	E858.8	E947.8	E950.4	E962.0	E980.4
Duboisine	971.1	E855.4	E941.1	E950.4	E962.0	E980.4
Dulcolax	973.1	E858.4	E943.1	E950.4	E962.0	E980.4
Duponol (C) (EP)	976.2	E858.7	E946.2	E950.4	E962.0	E980.4
Durabolin	962.1	E858.0	E932.1	E950.4	E962.0	E980.4
Dyclone	968.5	E855.2	E938.5	E950.4	E962.0	E980.4
Dyclonine	968.5	E855.2	E938.5	E950.4	E962.0	E980.4
Dydrogesterone	962.2	E858.0	E932.2	E950.4	E962.0	E980.4
Dyes NEC	989.89	E866.8	—	E950.9	E962.1	E980.9
diagnostic agents	977.8	E858.8	E947.8	E950.4	E962.0	E980.4
pharmaceutical NEC	977.4	E858.8	E947.4	E950.4	E962.0	E980.4
Dyflos	971.0	E855.3	E941.0	E950.4	E962.0	E980.4

◀ New ◀‖ Revised deleted Deleted ● Use Additional Digit(s)

		External Cause (E Code)				
Substance	Poisoning	Accident	Therapeutic Use	Suicide Attempt	Assault	Undetermined
Dymelor	962.3	E858.0	E932.3	E950.4	E962.0	E980.4
Dynamite	989.89	E866.8	—	E950.9	E962.1	E980.9
fumes	987.8	E869.8	—	E952.8	E962.2	E982.8
Dyphylline	975.1	E858.6	E945.1	E950.4	E962.0	E980.4
Ear preparations	976.6	E858.7	E946.6	E950.4	E962.0	E980.4
Echothiopate, ecothiopate	971.0	E855.3	E941.0	E950.4	E962.0	E980.4
Ecstasy	969.72	E854.2	E939.7	E950.3	E962.0	E980.3
Ectylurea	967.8	E852.8	E937.8	E950.2	E962.0	E980.2
Edathamil disodium	963.8	E858.1	E933.8	E950.4	E962.0	E980.4
Edecrin	974.4	E858.5	E944.4	E950.4	E962.0	E980.4
Edetate, disodium (calcium)	963.8	E858.1	E933.8	E950.4	E962.0	E980.4
Edrophonium	971.0	E855.3	E941.0	E950.4	E962.0	E980.4
Elase	976.8	E858.7	E946.8	E950.4	E962.0	E980.4
Elaterium	973.1	E858.4	E943.1	E950.4	E962.0	E980.4
Elder	988.2	E865.4	—	E950.9	E962.1	E980.9
berry (unripe)	988.2	E865.3	—	E950.9	E962.1	E980.9
Electrolytes NEC	974.5	E858.5	E944.5	E950.4	E962.0	E980.4
Electrolytic agent NEC	974.5	E858.5	E944.5	E950.4	E962.0	E980.4
Embramine	963.0	E858.1	E933.0	E950.4	E962.0	E980.4
Emetics	973.6	E858.4	E943.6	E950.4	E962.0	E980.4
Emetine (hydrochloride)	961.5	E857	E931.5	E950.4	E962.0	E980.4
Emollients	976.3	E858.7	E946.3	E950.4	E962.0	E980.4
Emylcamate	969.5	E853.8	E939.5	E950.3	E962.0	E980.3
Encyprate	969.09	E854.0	E939.0	E950.3	E962.0	E980.3
Endocaine	968.5	E855.2	E938.5	E950.4	E962.0	E980.4
Endrin	989.2	E863.0	—	E950.6	E962.1	E980.7
Enflurane	968.2	E855.1	E938.2	E950.4	E962.0	E980.4
Enovid	962.2	E858.0	E932.2	E950.4	E962.0	E980.4
ENT preparations (anti-infectives)	976.6	E858.7	E946.6	E950.4	E962.0	E980.4
Enzodase	963.4	E858.1	E933.4	E950.4	E962.0	E980.4
Enzymes NEC	963.4	E858.1	E933.4	E950.4	E962.0	E980.4
Epanutin	966.1	E855.0	E936.1	E950.4	E962.0	E980.4
Ephedra (tincture)	971.2	E855.5	E941.2	E950.4	E962.0	E980.4
Ephedrine	971.2	E855.5	E941.2	E950.4	E962.0	E980.4
Epiestriol	962.2	E858.0	E932.2	E950.4	E962.0	E980.4
Epilim - see Sodium valproate	—	—	—	—	—	—
Epinephrine	971.2	E855.5	E941.2	E950.4	E962.0	E980.4
Epsom salt	973.3	E858.4	E943.3	E950.4	E962.0	E980.4
Equanil	969.5	E853.8	E939.5	E950.3	E962.0	E980.3

◀ New   ◀Ⅲ Revised   deleted Deleted   ● Use Additional Digit(s)

TABLE OF DRUGS AND CHEMICALS

Substance	Poisoning	External Cause (E Code)				
		Accident	Therapeutic Use	Suicide Attempt	Assault	Undetermined
Equisetum (diuretic)	974.4	E858.5	E944.4	E950.4	E962.0	E980.4
Ergometrine	975.0	E858.6	E945.0	E950.4	E962.0	E980.4
Ergonovine	975.0	E858.6	E945.0	E950.4	E962.0	E980.4
Ergot NEC	988.2	E865.4	—	E950.9	E962.1	E980.9
medicinal (alkaloids)	975.0	E858.6	E945.0	E950.4	E962.0	E980.4
Ergotamine (tartrate) (for migraine) NEC	972.9	E858.3	E942.9	E950.4	E962.0	E980.4
Ergotrate	975.0	E858.6	E945.0	E950.4	E962.0	E980.4
Erythrityl tetranitrate	972.4	E858.3	E942.4	E950.4	E962.0	E980.4
Erythrol tetranitrate	972.4	E858.3	E942.4	E950.4	E962.0	E980.4
Erythromycin	960.3	E856	E930.3	E950.4	E962.0	E980.4
ophthalmic preparation	976.5	E858.7	E946.5	E950.4	E962.0	E980.4
topical NEC	976.0	E858.7	E946.0	E950.4	E962.0	E980.4
Eserine	971.0	E855.3	E941.0	E950.4	E962.0	E980.4
Eskabarb	967.0	E851	E937.0	E950.1	E962.0	E980.1
Eskalith	969.8	E855.8	E939.8	E950.3	E962.0	E980.3
Estradiol (cypionate) (dipropionate) (valerate)	962.2	E858.0	E932.2	E950.4	E962.0	E980.4
Estriol	962.2	E858.0	E932.2	E950.4	E962.0	E980.4
Estrogens (with progestogens)	962.2	E858.0	E932.2	E950.4	E962.0	E980.4
Estrone	962.2	E858.0	E932.2	E950.4	E962.0	E980.4
Etafedrine	971.2	E855.5	E941.2	E950.4	E962.0	E980.4
Ethacrynate sodium	974.4	E858.5	E944.4	E950.4	E962.0	E980.4
Ethacrynic acid	974.4	E858.5	E944.4	E950.4	E962.0	E980.4
Ethambutol	961.8	E857	E931.8	E950.4	E962.0	E980.4
Ethamide	974.2	E858.5	E944.2	E950.4	E962.0	E980.4
Ethamivan	970.0	E854.3	E940.0	E950.4	E962.0	E980.4
Ethamsylate	964.5	E858.2	E934.5	E950.4	E962.0	E980.4
Ethanol	980.0	E860.1	—	E950.9	E962.1	E980.9
beverage	980.0	E860.0	—	E950.9	E962.1	E980.9
Ethchlorvynol	967.8	E852.8	E937.8	E950.2	E962.0	E980.2
Ethebenecid	974.7	E858.5	E944.7	E950.4	E962.0	E980.4
Ether(s) (diethyl) (ethyl) (vapor)	987.8	E869.8	—	E952.8	E962.2	E982.8
anesthetic	968.2	E855.1	E938.2	E950.4	E962.0	E980.4
petroleum - see Ligroin solvent	982.8	E862.4	—	E950.9	E962.1	E980.9
Ethidine chloride (vapor)	987.8	E869.8	—	E952.8	E962.2	E982.8
liquid (solvent)	982.3	E862.4	—	E950.9	E962.1	E980.9
Ethinamate	967.8	E852.8	E937.8	E950.2	E962.0	E980.2
Ethinylestradiol	962.2	E858.0	E932.2	E950.4	E962.0	E980.4
Ethionamide	961.8	E857	E931.8	E950.4	E962.0	E980.4
Ethisterone	962.2	E858.0	E932.2	E950.4	E962.0	E980.4

◀ New ◀▪▪▪ Revised ~~deleted~~ Deleted ● Use Additional Digit(s)

Substance	Poisoning	External Cause (E Code)				
		Accident	Therapeutic Use	Suicide Attempt	Assault	Undetermined
Ethobral	967.0	E851	E937.0	E950.1	E962.0	E980.1
Ethocaine (infiltration) (topical)	968.5	E855.2	E938.5	E950.4	E962.0	E980.4
nerve block (peripheral) (plexus)	968.6	E855.2	E938.6	E950.4	E962.0	E980.4
spinal	968.7	E855.2	E938.7	E950.4	E962.0	E980.4
Ethoheptazine (citrate)	965.7	E850.7	E935.7	E950.0	E962.0	E980.0
Ethopropazine	966.4	E855.0	E936.4	E950.4	E962.0	E980.4
Ethosuximide	966.2	E855.0	E936.2	E950.4	E962.0	E980.4
Ethotoin	966.1	E855.0	E936.1	E950.4	E962.0	E980.4
Ethoxazene	961.9	E857	E931.9	E950.4	E962.0	E980.4
Ethoxzolamide	974.2	E858.5	E944.2	E950.4	E962.0	E980.4
Ethyl	—	—	—	—	—	—
acetate (vapor)	982.8	E862.4	—	E950.9	E962.1	E980.9
alcohol	980.0	E860.1	—	E950.9	E962.1	E980.9
beverage	980.0	E860.0	—	E950.9	E962.1	E980.9
aldehyde (vapor)	987.8	E869.8	—	E952.8	E962.2	E982.8
liquid	989.89	E866.8	—	E950.9	E962.1	E980.9
aminobenzoate	968.5	E855.2	E938.5	E950.4	E962.0	E980.4
biscoumacetate	964.2	E858.2	E934.2	E950.4	E962.0	E980.4
bromide (anesthetic)	968.2	E855.1	E938.2	E950.4	E962.0	E980.4
carbamate (antineoplastic)	963.1	E858.1	E933.1	E950.4	E962.0	E980.4
carbinol	980.3	E860.4	—	E950.9	E962.1	E980.9
chaulmoograte	961.8	E857	E931.8	E950.4	E962.0	E980.4
chloride (vapor)	987.8	E869.8	—	E952.8	E962.2	E982.8
anesthetic (local)	968.5	E855.2	E938.5	E950.4	E962.0	E980.4
inhaled	968.2	E855.1	E938.2	E950.4	E962.0	E980.4
solvent	982.3	E862.4	—	E950.9	E962.1	E980.9
estranol	962.1	E858.0	E932.1	E950.4	E962.0	E980.4
ether - see Ether(s)	—	—	—	—	—	—
formate (solvent) NEC	982.8	E862.4	—	E950.9	E962.1	E980.9
iodoacetate	987.5	E869.3	—	E952.8	E962.2	E982.8
lactate (solvent) NEC	982.8	E862.4	—	E950.9	E962.1	E980.9
methylcarbinol	980.8	E860.8	—	E950.9	E962.1	E980.9
morphine	965.09	E850.2	E935.2	E950.0	E962.0	E980.0
Ethylene (gas)	987.1	E869.8	—	E952.8	E962.2	E982.8
anesthetic (general)	968.2	E855.1	E938.2	E950.4	E962.0	E980.4
chlorohydrin (vapor)	982.3	E862.4	—	E950.9	E962.1	E980.9
dichloride (vapor)	982.3	E862.4	—	E950.9	E962.1	E980.9
glycol(s) (any) (vapor)	982.8	E862.4	—	E950.9	E962.1	E980.9

◀ New   ◀▥ Revised   ~~deleted~~ Deleted   ● Use Additional Digit(s)

Substance	Poisoning	External Cause (E Code)				
		Accident	Therapeutic Use	Suicide Attempt	Assault	Undetermined
Ethylidene	—	—	—	—	—	—
chloride NEC	982.3	E862.4	—	E950.9	E962.1	E980.9
diethyl ether	982.8	—	E862.4	E950.9	E962.1	E980.9
Ethynodiol	962.2	E858.0	E932.2	E950.4	E962.0	E980.4
Etidocaine	968.9	E855.2	E938.9	E950.4	E962.0	E980.4
infiltration (subcutaneous)	968.5	E855.2	E938.5	E950.4	E962.0	E980.4
nerve (peripheral) (plexus)	968.6	E855.2	E938.6	E950.4	E962.0	E980.4
Etilfen	967.0	E851	E937.0	E950.1	E962.0	E980.1
Etomide	965.7	E850.7	E935.7	E950.0	E962.0	E980.0
Etorphine	965.09	E850.2	E935.2	E950.0	E962.0	E980.0
Etoval	967.0	E851	E937.0	E950.1	E962.0	E980.1
Etryptamine	969.01	E854.0	E939.0	E950.3	E962.0	E980.3
Eucaine	968.5	E855.2	E938.5	E950.4	E962.0	E980.4
Eucalyptus (oil) NEC	975.5	E858.6	E945.5	E950.4	E962.0	E980.4
Eucatropine	971.1	E855.4	E941.1	E950.4	E962.0	E980.4
Eucodal	965.09	E850.2	E935.2	E950.0	E962.0	E980.0
Euneryl	967.0	E851	E937.0	E950.1	E962.0	E980.1
Euphthalmine	971.1	E855.4	E941.1	E950.4	E962.0	E980.4
Eurax	976.0	E858.7	E946.0	E950.4	E962.0	E980.4
Euresol	976.4	E858.7	E946.4	E950.4	E962.0	E980.4
Euthroid	962.7	E858.0	E932.7	E950.4	E962.0	E980.4
Evans blue	977.8	E858.8	E947.8	E950.4	E962.0	E980.4
Evipal	967.0	E851	E937.0	E950.1	E962.0	E980.1
sodium	968.3	E855.1	E938.3	E950.4	E962.0	E980.4
Evipan	967.0	E851	E937.0	E950.1	E962.0	E980.1
sodium	968.3	E855.1	E938.3	E950.4	E962.0	E980.4
Exalgin	965.4	E850.4	E935.4	E950.0	E962.0	E980.0
Excipients, pharmaceutical	977.4	E858.8	E947.4	E950.4	E962.0	E980.4
Exhaust gas - see Carbon, monoxide	—	—	—	—	—	—
Ex-Lax (phenolphthalein)	973.1	E858.4	E943.1	E950.4	E962.0	E980.4
Expectorants	975.5	E858.6	E945.5	E950.4	E962.0	E980.4
External medications (skin) (mucous membrane)	976.9	E858.7	E946.9	E950.4	E962.0	E980.4
dental agent	976.7	E858.7	E946.7	E950.4	E962.0	E980.4
ENT agent	976.6	E858.7	E946.6	E950.4	E962.0	E980.4
ophthalmic preparation	976.5	E858.7	E946.5	E950.4	E962.0	E980.4
specified NEC	976.8	E858.7	E946.8	E950.4	E962.0	E980.4
Eye agents (anti-infective)	976.5	E858.7	E946.5	E950.4	E962.0	E980.4
Factor IX complex (human)	964.5	E858.2	E934.5	E950.4	E962.0	E980.4
Fecal softeners	973.2	E858.4	E943.2	E950.4	E962.0	E980.4

◄ New ◄▥ Revised ~~deleted~~ Deleted ● Use Additional Digit(s)

Substance	Poisoning	External Cause (E Code)				
		Accident	Therapeutic Use	Suicide Attempt	Assault	Undetermined
Fenbutrazate	977.0	E858.8	E947.0	E950.4	E962.0	E980.4
Fencamfamin	970.89 ◄▥	E854.3	E940.8	E950.4	E962.0	E980.4
Fenfluramine	977.0	E858.8	E947.0	E950.4	E962.0	E980.4
Fenoprofen	965.61	E850.6	E935.6	E950.0	E962.0	E980.0
Fentanyl	965.09	E850.2	E935.2	E950.0	E962.0	E980.0
Fentazin	969.1	E853.0	E939.1	E930.3	E962.0	E980.3
Fenticlor, fentichlor	976.0	E858.7	E946.0	E950.4	E962.0	E980.4
Fer de lance (bite) (venom)	989.5	E905.0	—	E950.9	E962.1	E980.9
Ferric - *see* Iron	—	—	—	—	—	—
Ferrocholinate	964.0	E858.2	E934.0	E950.4	E962.0	E980.4
Ferrous fumerate, gluconate, lactate, salt NEC, sulfate (medicinal)	964.0	E858.2	E934.0	E950.4	E962.0	E980.4
Ferrum - *see* Iron	—	—	—	—	—	—
Fertilizers NEC	989.89	E866.5	—	E950.9	E962.1	E980.4
with herbicide mixture	989.4	E863.5	—	E950.6	E962.1	E980.7
Fibrinogen (human)	964.7	E858.2	E934.7	E950.4	E962.0	E980.4
Fibrinolysin	964.4	E858.2	E934.4	E950.4	E962.0	E980.4
Fibrinolysis-affecting agents	964.4	E858.2	E934.4	E950.4	E962.0	E980.4
Filix mas	961.6	E857	E931.6	E950.4	E962.0	E980.4
Fiorinal	965.1	E850.3	E935.3	E950.0	E962.0	E980.0
Fire damp	987.1	E869.8	—	E952.8	E962.2	E982.8
Fish, nonbacterial or noxious	988.0	E865.2	—	E950.9	E962.1	E980.9
shell	988.0	E865.1	—	E950.9	E962.1	E980.9
Flagyl	961.5	E857	E931.5	E950.4	E962.0	E980.4
Flavoxate	975.1	E858.6	E945.1	E950.4	E962.0	E980.4
Flaxedil	975.2	E858.6	E945.2	E950.4	E962.0	E980.4
Flaxseed (medicinal)	976.3	E858.7	E946.3	E950.4	E962.0	E980.4
Flomax	971.3	E855.6	E941.3	E950.4	E962.0	E980.4
Florantyrone	973.4	E858.4	E943.4	E950.4	E962.0	E980.4
Floraquin	961.3	E857	E931.3	E950.4	E962.0	E980.4
Florinef	962.0	E858.0	E932.0	E950.4	E962.0	E980.4
ENT agent	976.6	E858.7	E946.6	E950.4	E962.0	E980.4
ophthalmic preparation	976.5	E858.7	E946.5	E950.4	E962.0	E980.4
topical NEC	976.0	E858.7	E946.0	E950.4	E962.0	E980.4
Flowers of sulfur	976.4	E858.7	E946.4	E950.4	E962.0	E980.4
Floxuridine	963.1	E858.1	E933.1	E950.4	E962.0	E980.4
Flucytosine	961.9	E857	E931.9	E950.4	E962.0	E980.4
Fludrocortisone	962.0	E858.0	E932.0	E950.4	E962.0	E980.4
ENT agent	976.6	E858.7	E946.6	E950.4	E962.0	E980.4
ophthalmic preparation	976.5	E858.7	E946.5	E950.4	E962.0	E980.4

Substance	Poisoning	External Cause (E Code)				
		Accident	Therapeutic Use	Suicide Attempt	Assault	Undetermined
Fludrocortisone *(Continued)*						
topical NEC	976.0	E858.7	E946.0	E950.4	E962.0	E980.4
Flumethasone	976.0	E858.7	E946.0	E950.4	E962.0	E980.4
Flumethiazide	974.3	E858.5	E944.3	E950.4	E962.0	E980.4
Flumidin	961.7	E857	E931.7	E950.4	E962.0	E980.4
Flunitrazepam	969.4	E853.2	E939.4	E950.3	E962.0	E980.3
Fluocinolone	976.0	E858.7	E946.0	E950.4	E962.0	E980.4
Fluocortolone	962.0	E858.0	E932.0	E950.4	E962.0	E980.4
Fluohydrocortisone	962.0	E858.0	E932.0	E950.4	E962.0	E980.4
ENT agent	976.6	E858.7	E946.6	E950.4	E962.0	E980.4
ophthalmic preparation	976.5	E858.7	E946.5	E950.4	E962.0	E980.4
topical NEC	976.0	E858.7	E946.0	E950.4	E962.0	E980.4
Fluonid	976.0	E858.7	E946.0	E950.4	E962.0	E980.4
Fluopromazine	969.1	E853.0	E939.1	E950.3	E962.0	E980.3
Fluoracetate	989.4	E863.7	—	E950.6	E962.1	E980.7
Fluorescein (sodium)	977.8	E858.8	E947.8	E950.4	E962.0	E980.4
Fluoride(s) (pesticides) (sodium) NEC	989.4	E863.4	—	E950.6	E962.1	E980.7
hydrogen - *see* Hydrofluoric acid	—	—	—	—	—	—
medicinal	976.7	E858.7	E946.7	E950.4	E962.0	E980.4
not pesticide NEC	983.9	E864.4	—	E950.7	E962.1	E980.6
stannous	976.7	E858.7	E946.7	E950.4	E962.0	E980.4
Fluorinated corticosteroids	962.0	E858.0	E932.0	E950.4	E962.0	E980.4
Fluorine (compounds) (gas)	987.8	E869.8	—	E952.8	E962.2	E982.8
salt - *see* Fluoride(s)	—	—	—	—	—	—
Fluoristan	976.7	E858.7	E946.7	E950.4	E962.0	E980.4
Fluoroacetate	989.4	E863.7	—	E950.6	E962.1	E980.7
Fluorodeoxyuridine	963.1	E858.1	E933.1	E950.4	E962.0	E980.4
Fluorometholone (topical) NEC	976.0	E858.7	E946.0	E950.4	E962.0	E980.4
ophthalmic preparation	976.5	E858.7	E946.5	E950.4	E962.0	E980.4
Fluorouracil	963.1	E858.1	E933.1	E950.4	E962.0	E980.4
Fluothane	968.1	E855.1	E938.1	E950.4	E962.0	E980.4
Fluoxetine hydrochloride	969.03	E854.0	E939.0	E950.3	E962.0	E980.3
Fluoxymesterone	962.1	E858.0	E932.1	E950.4	E962.0	E980.4
Fluphenazine	969.1	E853.0	E939.1	E950.3	E962.0	E980.3
Fluprednisolone	962.0	E858.0	E932.0	E950.4	E962.0	E980.4
Flurandrenolide	976.0	E858.7	E946.0	E950.4	E962.0	E980.4
Flurazepam (hydrochloride)	969.4	E853.2	E939.4	E950.3	E962.0	E980.3
Flurbiprofen	965.61	E850.6	E935.6	E950.0	E962.0	E980.0

◀ New   ◀▦ Revised   ~~deleted~~ Deleted   ● Use Additional Digit(s)

TABLE OF DRUGS AND CHEMICALS

Substance	Poisoning	External Cause (E Code)				
		Accident	Therapeutic Use	Suicide Attempt	Assault	Undetermined
Flurobate	976.0	E858.7	E946.0	E950.4	E962.0	E980.4
Flurothyl	969.8	E855.8	E939.8	E950.3	E962.0	E980.3
Fluroxene	968.2	E855.1	E938.2	E950.4	E962.0	E980.4
Folacin	964.1	E858.2	E934.1	E950.4	E962.0	E980.4
Folic acid	964.1	E858.2	E934.1	E950.4	E962.0	E980.4
Follicle stimulating hormone	962.4	E858.0	E932.4	E950.4	E962.0	E980.4
Food, foodstuffs, nonbacterial or noxious	988.9	E865.9	—	E950.9	E962.1	E980.9
berries, seeds	988.2	E865.3	—	E950.9	E962.1	E980.9
fish	988.0	E865.2	—	E950.9	E962.1	E980.9
mushrooms	988.1	E865.5	—	E950.9	E962.1	E980.9
plants	988.2	E865.9	—	E950.9	E962.1	E980.9
specified type NEC	988.2	E865.4	—	E950.9	E962.1	E980.9
shellfish	988.0	E865.1	—	E950.9	E962.1	E980.9
specified NEC	988.8	E865.8	—	E950.9	E962.1	E980.9
Fool's parsley	988.2	E865.4	—	E950.9	E962.1	E980.9
Formaldehyde (solution)	989.89	E861.4	—	E950.9	E962.1	E980.9
fungicide	989.4	E863.6	—	E950.6	E962.1	E980.7
gas or vapor	987.8	E869.8	—	E952.8	E962.2	E982.8
Formalin	989.89	E861.4	—	E950.9	E962.1	E980.9
fungicide	989.4	E863.6	—	E950.6	E962.1	E980.7
vapor	987.8	E869.8	—	E952.8	E962.2	E982.8
Formic acid	983.1	E864.1	—	E950.7	E962.1	E980.6
vapor	987.8	E869.8	—	E952.8	E962.2	E982.8
Fowler's solution	985.1	E866.3	—	E950.8	E962.1	E980.8
Foxglove	988.2	E865.4	—	E950.9	E962.1	E980.9
Fox green	977.8	E858.8	E947.8	E950.4	E962.0	E980.4
Framycetin	960.8	E856	E930.8	E950.4	E962.0	E980.4
Frangula (extract)	973.1	E858.4	E943.1	E950.4	E962.0	E980.4
Frei antigen	977.8	E858.8	E947.8	E950.4	E962.0	E980.4
Freons	987.4	E869.2	—	E952.8	E962.2	E982.8
Fructose	974.5	E858.5	E944.5	E950.4	E962.0	E980.4
Frusemide	974.4	E858.5	E944.4	E950.4	E962.0	E980.4
FSH	962.4	E858.0	E932.4	E950.4	E962.0	E980.4
Fuel	—	—	—	—	—	—
automobile	981	E862.1	—	E950.9	E962.1	E980.9
exhaust gas, not in transit	986	E868.2	—	E952.0	E962.2	E982.0
vapor NEC	987.1	E869.8	—	E952.8	E962.2	E982.8

TABLE OF DRUGS AND CHEMICALS

Substance	External Cause (E Code)					
	Poisoning	Accident	Therapeutic Use	Suicide Attempt	Assault	Undetermined
Fuel *(Continued)*						
gas (domestic use) - *see also* Carbon, monoxide, fuel	—	—	—	—	—	—
utility	987.1	E868.1	—	E951.8	E962.2	E981.8
incomplete combustion of - *see* Carbon, monoxide, fuel, utility	—	—	—	—	—	—
in mobile container	987.0	E868.0	—	E951.1	E962.2	E981.1
piped (natural)	987.1	E867	—	E951.0	E962.2	E981.0
industrial, incomplete combustion	986	E868.3	—	E952.1	E962.2	E982.1
Fugillin	960.8	E856	E930.8	E950.4	E962.0	E980.4
Fulminate of mercury	985.0	E866.1	—	E950.9	E962.1	E980.9
Fulvicin	960.1	E856	E930.1	E950.4	E962.0	E980.4
Fumadil	960.8	E856	E930.8	E950.4	E962.0	E980.4
Fumagillin	960.8	E856	E930.8	E950.4	E962.0	E980.4
Fumes (from)	987.9	E869.9	—	E952.9	E962.2	E982.9
carbon monoxide - *see* Carbon, monoxide	—	—	—	—	—	—
charcoal (domestic use)	986	E868.3	—	E952.1	E962.2	E982.1
chloroform - *see* Chloroform						
coke (in domestic stoves, fireplaces)	986	E868.3	—	E952.1	E962.2	E982.1
corrosive NEC	987.8	E869.8	—	E952.8	E962.2	E982.8
ether - *see* Ether(s)						
freons	987.4	E869.2	—	E952.8	E962.2	E982.8
hydrocarbons	987.1	E869.8	—	E952.8	E962.2	E982.8
petroleum (liquefied)	987.0	E868.0	—	E951.1	E962.2	E981.1
distributed through pipes (pure or mixed with air)	987.0	E867	—	E951.0	E962.2	E981.0
lead - *see* Lead	—	—	—	—	—	—
metals - *see* specified metal	—	—	—	—	—	—
nitrogen dioxide	987.2	E869.0	—	E952.8	E962.2	E982.8
pesticides - *see* Pesticides	—	—	—	—	—	—
petroleum (liquefied)	987.0	E868.0	—	E951.1	E962.2	E981.1
distributed through pipes (pure or mixed with air)	987.0	E867	—	E951.0	E962.2	E981.0
polyester	987.8	E869.8	—	E952.8	E962.2	E982.8
specified source, other (*see also* substance specified)	987.8	E869.8	—	E952.8	E962.2	E982.8
sulfur dioxide	987.3	E869.1	—	E952.8	E962.2	E982.8
Fumigants	989.4	E863.8	—	E950.6	E962.1	E980.7
Fungi, noxious, used as food	988.1	E865.5	—	E950.9	E962.1	E980.9
Fungicides (*see also* Antifungals)	989.4	E863.6	—	E950.6	E962.1	E980.7
Fungizone	960.1	E856	E930.1	E950.4	E962.0	E980.4
topical	976.0	E858.7	E946.0	E950.4	E962.0	E980.4
Furacin	976.0	E858.7	E946.0	E950.4	E962.0	E980.4

◄ New   ◄▦ Revised   ~~deleted~~ Deleted   ● Use Additional Digit(s)

Substance	Poisoning	External Cause (E Code)				
		Accident	Therapeutic Use	Suicide Attempt	Assault	Undetermined
Furadantin	961.9	E857	E931.9	E950.4	E962.0	E980.4
Furazolidone	961.9	E857	E931.9	E950.4	E962.0	E980.4
Furnace (coal burning) (domestic), gas from	986	E868.3	—	E952.1	E962.2	E982.1
industrial	986	E868.8	—	E952.1	E962.2	E982.1
Furniture polish	989.89	E861.2	—	E950.9	E962.1	E980.9
Furosemide	974.4	E858.5	E944.4	E950.4	E962.0	E980.4
Furoxone	961.9	E857	E931.9	E950.4	E962.0	E980.4
Fusel oil (amyl) (butyl) (propyl)	980.3	E860.4	—	E950.9	E962.1	E980.9
Fusidic acid	960.8	E856	E930.8	E950.4	E962.0	E980.4
Gallamine	975.2	E858.6	E945.2	E950.4	E962.0	E980.4
Gallotannic acid	976.2	E858.7	E946.2	E950.4	E962.0	E980.4
Gamboge	973.1	E858.4	E943.1	E950.4	E962.0	E980.4
Gamimune	964.6	E858.2	E934.6	E950.4	E962.0	E980.4
Gamma-benzene hexachloride (vapor)	989.2	E863.0	—	E950.6	E962.1	E980.7
Gamma globulin	964.6	E858.2	E934.6	E950.4	E962.0	E980.4
Gamma hydroxy butyrate (GHB)	968.4	E855.1	E938.4	E950.4	E962.0	E980.4
Gamulin	964.6	E858.2	E934.6	E950.4	E962.0	E980.4
Ganglionic blocking agents	972.3	E858.3	E942.3	E950.4	E962.0	E980.4
Ganja	969.6	E854.1	E939.6	E950.3	E962.0	E980.3
Garamycin	960.8	E856	E930.8	E950.4	E962.0	E980.4
ophthalmic preparation	976.5	E858.7	E946.5	E950.4	E962.0	E980.4
topical NEC	976.0	E858.7	E946.0	E950.4	E962.0	E980.4
Gardenal	967.0	E851	E937.0	E950.1	E962.0	E980.1
Gardepanyl	967.0	E851	E937.0	E950.1	E962.0	E980.1
Gas	987.9	E869.9	—	E952.9	E962.2	E982.9
acetylene	987.1	E868.1	—	E951.8	E962.2	E981.8
incomplete combustion of - see Carbon, monoxide, fuel, utility	—	—	—	—	—	—
air contaminants, source or type not specified	987.9	E869.9	—	E952.9	E962.2	E982.9
anesthetic (general) NEC	968.2	E855.1	E938.2	E950.4	E962.0	E980.4
blast furnace	986	E868.8	—	E952.1	E962.2	E982.1
butane - see Butane	—	—	—	—	—	—
carbon monoxide - see Carbon, monoxide, chlorine	987.6	E869.8	—	E952.8	E962.2	E982.8
coal - see Carbon, monoxide, coal	—	—	—	—	—	—
cyanide	987.7	E869.8	—	E952.8	E962.2	E982.8
dicyanogen	987.8	E869.8	—	E952.8	E962.2	E982.8
domestic - see Gas, utility	—	—	—	—	—	—
exhaust - see Carbon, monoxide, exhaust gas	—	—	—	—	—	—
from wood- or coal-burning stove or fireplace	986	E868.3	—	E952.1	E962.2	E982.1

Substance	Poisoning	External Cause (E Code)				
		Accident	Therapeutic Use	Suicide Attempt	Assault	Undetermined
Gas *(Continued)*						
fuel (domestic use) - *see also* Carbon, monoxide, fuel	—	—	—	—	—	—
industrial use	986	E868.8	—	E952.1	E962.2	E982.1
utility	987.1	E868.1	—	E951.8	E962.2	E981.8
incomplete combustion of - *see* Carbon, monoxide, fuel, utility	—	—	—	—	—	—
in mobile container	987.0	E868.0	—	E951.1	E962.2	E981.1
piped (natural)	987.1	E867	—	E951.0	E962.2	E981.0
garage	986	E868.2	—	E952.0	E962.2	E982.0
hydrocarbon NEC	987.1	E869.8	—	E952.8	E962.2	E982.8
incomplete combustion of - *see* Carbon, monoxide, fuel, utility	—	—	—	—	—	—
liquefied (mobile container)	987.0	E868.0	—	E951.1	E962.2	E981.1
piped	987.0	E867	—	E951.0	E962.2	E981.0
hydrocyanic acid	987.7	E869.8	—	E952.8	E962.2	E982.8
illuminating - *see* Gas, utility	—	—	—	—	—	—
incomplete combustion, any - *see* Carbon, monoxide	—	—	—	—	—	—
kiln	986	E868.8	—	E952.1	E962.2	E982.1
lacrimogenic	987.5	E869.3	—	E952.8	E962.2	E982.8
marsh	987.1	E869.8	—	E952.8	E962.2	E982.8
motor exhaust, not in transit	986	E868.8	—	E952.1	E962.2	E982.1
mustard - *see* Mustard, gas	—	—	—	—	—	—
natural	987.1	E867	—	E951.0	E962.2	E981.0
nerve (war)	987.9	E869.9	—	E952.9	E962.2	E982.9
oils	981	E862.1	—	E950.9	E962.1	E980.9
petroleum (liquefied) (distributed in mobile containers)	987.0	E868.0	—	E951.1	E962.2	E981.1
piped (pure or mixed with air)	987.0	E867	—	E951.1	E962.2	E981.1
piped (manufactured) (natural) NEC	987.1	E867	—	E951.0	E962.2	E981.0
producer	986	E868.8	—	E952.1	E962.2	E982.1
propane - *see* Propane	—	—	—	—	—	—
refrigerant (freon)	987.4	E869.2	—	E952.8	E962.2	E982.8
not freon	987.9	E869.9	—	E952.9	E962.2	E982.9
sewer	987.8	E869.8	—	E952.8	E962.2	E982.8
specified source NEC (*see also* substance specified)	987.8	E869.8	—	E952.8	E962.2	E982.8
stove - *see* Gas, utility	—	—	—	—	—	—
tear	987.5	E869.3	—	E952.8	E962.2	E982.8
utility (for cooking, heating, or lighting) (piped) NEC	987.1	E868.1	—	E951.8	E962.2	E981.8
incomplete combustion of - *see* Carbon, monoxide, fuel, utility ◀▬	—	—	—	—	—	—
in mobile container	987.0	E868.0	—	E951.1	E962.2	E981.1
piped (natural)	987.1	E867	—	E951.0	E962.2	E981.0
water	987.1	E868.1	—	E951.8	E962.2	E981.8
incomplete combustion of - *see* Carbon, monoxide, fuel, utility	—	—	—	—	—	—

◀ New   ◀▬ Revised   ~~deleted~~ Deleted   ● Use Additional Digit(s)

TABLE OF DRUGS AND CHEMICALS

Substance	Poisoning	External Cause (E Code)				
		Accident	Therapeutic Use	Suicide Attempt	Assault	Undetermined
Gaseous substance - *see* Gas	—	—	—	—	—	—
Gasoline, gasolene	981	E862.1	—	E950.9	E962.1	E980.9
vapor	987.1	E869.8	—	E952.8	E962.2	E982.8
Gastric enzymes	973.4	E858.4	E943.4	E950.4	E962.0	E980.4
Gastrografin	977.8	E858.8	E947.8	E950.4	E962.0	E980.4
Gastrointestinal agents	973.9	E858.4	E943.9	E950.4	E962.0	E980.4
specified NEC	973.8	E858.4	E943.8	E950.4	E962.0	E980.4
Gaultheria procumbens	988.2	E865.4	—	E950.9	E962.1	E980.9
Gelatin (intravenous)	964.8	E858.2	E934.8	E950.4	E962.0	E980.4
absorbable (sponge)	964.5	E858.2	E934.5	E950.4	E962.0	E980.4
Gelfilm	976.8	E858.7	E946.8	E950.4	E962.0	E980.4
Gelfoam	964.5	E858.2	E934.5	E950.4	E962.0	E980.4
Gelsemine	970.89 ◀▥	E854.3	E940.8	E950.4	E962.0	E980.4
Gelsemium (sempervirens)	988.2	E865.4	—	E950.9	E962.1	E980.9
Gemonil	967.0	E851	E937.0	E950.1	E962.0	E980.1
Gentamicin	960.8	E856	E930.8	E950.4	E962.0	E980.4
ophthalmic preparation	976.5	E858.7	E946.5	E950.4	E962.0	E980.4
topical NEC	976.0	E858.7	E946.0	E950.4	E962.0	E980.4
Gentian violet	976.0	E858.7	E946.0	E950.4	E962.0	E980.4
Gexane	976.0	E858.7	E946.0	E950.4	E962.0	E980.4
Gila monster (venom)	989.5	E905.0	—	E950.9	E962.1	E980.9
Ginger, Jamaica	989.89	E866.8	—	E950.9	E962.1	E980.9
Gitalin	972.1	E858.3	E942.1	E950.4	E962.0	E980.4
Gitoxin	972.1	E858.3	E942.1	E950.4	E962.0	E980.4
Glandular extract (medicinal) NEC	977.9	E858.9	E947.9	E950.5	E962.0	E980.5
Glaucarubin	961.5	E857	E931.5	E950.4	E962.0	E980.4
Globin zinc insulin	962.3	E858.0	E932.3	E950.4	E962.0	E980.4
Glucagon	962.3	E858.0	E932.3	E950.4	E962.0	E980.4
Glucochloral	967.1	E852.0	E937.1	E950.2	E962.0	E980.2
Glucocorticoids	962.0	E858.0	E932.0	E950.4	E962.0	E980.4
Glucose	974.5	E858.5	E944.5	E950.4	E962.0	E980.4
oxidase reagent	977.8	E858.8	E947.8	E950.4	E962.0	E980.4
Glucosulfone sodium	961.8	E857	E931.8	E950.4	E962.0	E980.4
Glue(s)	989.89	E866.6	—	E950.9	E962.1	E980.9
Glutamic acid (hydrochloride)	973.4	E858.4	E943.4	E950.4	E962.0	E980.4
Glutaraldehyde	989.89	E861.4	—	E950.9	E962.1	E980.9
Glutathione	963.8	E858.1	E933.8	E950.4	E962.0	E980.4
Glutethimide (group)	967.5	E852.4	E937.5	E950.2	E962.0	E980.2
Glycerin (lotion)	976.3	E858.7	E946.3	E950.4	E962.0	E980.4
Glycerol (topical)	976.3	E858.7	E946.3	E950.4	E962.0	E980.4

◀ New   ◀▥ Revised   ~~deleted~~ Deleted   ● Use Additional Digit(s)

Substance	Poisoning	External Cause (E Code)				
		Accident	Therapeutic Use	Suicide Attempt	Assault	Undetermined
Glyceryl	—	—	—	—	—	—
guaiacolate	975.5	E858.6	E945.5	E950.4	E962.0	E980.4
triacetate (topical)	976.0	E858.7	E946.0	E950.4	E962.0	E980.4
trinitrate	972.4	E858.3	E942.4	E950.4	E962.0	E980.4
Glycine	974.5	E858.5	E944.5	E950.4	E962.0	E980.4
Glycobiarsol	961.1	E857	E931.1	E950.4	E962.0	E980.4
Glycols (ether)	982.8	E862.4	—	E950.9	E962.1	E980.9
Glycopyrrolate	971.1	E855.4	E941.1	E950.4	E962.0	E980.4
Glymidine	962.3	E858.0	E932.3	E950.4	E962.0	E980.4
Gold (compounds) (salts)	965.69	E850.6	E935.6	E950.0	E962.0	E980.0
Golden sulfide of antimony	985.4	E866.2	—	E950.9	E962.1	E980.9
Goldylocks	988.2	E865.4	—	E950.9	E962.1	E980.9
Gonadal tissue extract	962.9	E858.0	E932.9	E950.4	E962.0	E980.4
female	962.2	E858.0	E932.2	E950.4	E962.0	E980.4
male	962.1	E858.0	E932.1	E950.4	E962.0	E980.4
Gonadotropin	962.4	E858.0	E932.4	E950.4	E962.0	E980.4
Grain alcohol	980.0	E860.1	—	E950.9	E962.1	E980.9
beverage	980.0	E860.0	—	E950.9	E962.1	E980.9
Gramicidin	960.8	E856	E930.8	E950.4	E962.0	E980.4
Gratiola officinalis	988.2	E865.4	—	E950.9	E962.1	E980.9
Grease	989.89	E866.8	—	E950.9	E962.1	E980.9
Green hellebore	988.2	E865.4	—	E950.9	E962.1	E980.9
Green soap	976.2	E858.7	E946.2	E950.4	E962.0	E980.4
Grifulvin	960.1	E856	E930.1	E950.4	E962.0	E980.4
Griseofulvin	960.1	E856	E930.1	E950.4	E962.0	E980.4
Growth hormone	962.4	E858.0	E932.4	E950.4	E962.0	E980.4
Guaiacol	975.5	E858.6	E945.5	E950.4	E962.0	E980.4
Giuaiac reagent	977.8	E858.8	E947.8	E950.4	E962.0	E980.4
Guaifenesin	975.5	E858.6	E945.5	E950.4	E962.0	E980.4
Guaiphenesin	975.5	E858.6	E945.5	E950.4	E962.0	E980.4
Guanatol	961.4	E857	E931.4	E950.4	E962.0	E980.4
Guanethidine	972.6	E858.3	E942.6	E950.4	E962.0	E980.4
Guano	989.89	E866.5	—	E950.9	E962.1	E980.9
Guanochlor	972.6	E858.3	E942.6	E950.4	E962.0	E980.4
Guanoctine	972.6	E858.3	E942.6	E950.4	E962.0	E980.4
Guanoxan	972.6	E858.3	E942.6	E950.4	E962.0	E980.4
Hair treatment agent NEC	976.4	E858.7	E946.4	E950.4	E962.0	E980.4
Halcinonide	976.0	E858.7	E946.0	E950.4	E962.0	E980.4
Halethazole	976.0	E858.7	E946.0	E950.4	E962.0	E980.4

◀ New   ◀ Revised   ~~deleted~~ Deleted   ● Use Additional Digit(s)

	External Cause (E Code)					
Substance	Poisoning	Accident	Therapeutic Use	Suicide Attempt	Assault	Undetermined
Hallucinogens	969.6	E854.1	E939.6	E950.3	E962.0	E980.3
Haloperidol	969.2	E853.1	E939.2	E950.3	E962.0	E980.3
Haloprogin	976.0	E858.7	E946.0	E950.4	E962.0	E980.4
Halotex	976.0	E858.7	E946.0	E950.4	E962.0	E980.4
Halothane	968.1	E855.1	E938.1	E950.4	E962.0	E980.4
Halquinols	976.0	E858.7	E946.0	E950.4	E962.0	E980.4
Hand sanitizer	976.0	E858.7	E946.0	E950.4	E962.0	E980.4
Harmonyl	972.6	E858.3	E942.6	E950.4	E962.0	E980.4
Hartmann's solution	974.5	E858.5	E944.5	E950.4	E962.0	E980.4
Hashish	969.6	E854.1	E939.6	E950.3	E962.0	E980.3
Hawaiian wood rose seeds	969.6	E854.1	E939.6	E950.3	E962.0	E980.3
Headache cures, drugs, powders NEC	977.9	E858.9	E947.9	E950.5	E962.0	E980.9
Heavenly Blue (morning glory)	969.6	E854.1	E939.6	E950.3	E962.0	E980.3
Heavy metal antagonists	963.8	E858.1	E933.8	E950.4	E962.0	E980.4
anti-infectives	961.2	E857	E931.2	E950.4	E962.0	E980.4
Hedaquinium	976.0	E858.7	E946.0	E950.4	E962.0	E980.4
Hedge hyssop	988.2	E865.4	—	E950.9	E962.1	E980.9
Heet	976.8	E858.7	E946.8	E950.4	E962.0	E980.4
Helenin	961.6	E857	E931.6	E950.4	E962.0	E980.4
Hellebore (black) (green) (white)	988.2	E865.4	—	E950.9	E962.1	E980.9
Hemlock	988.2	E865.4	—	E950.9	E962.1	E980.9
Hemostatics	964.5	E858.2	E934.5	E950.4	E962.0	E980.4
capillary active drugs	972.8	E858.3	E942.8	E950.4	E962.0	E980.4
Henbane	988.2	E865.4	—	E950.9	E962.1	E980.9
Heparin (sodium)	964.2	E858.2	E934.2	E950.4	E962.0	E980.4
Heptabarbital, heptabarbitone	967.0	E851	E937.0	E950.1	E962.0	E980.1
Heptachlor	989.2	E863.0	—	E950.6	E962.1	E980.7
Heptalgin	965.09	E850.2	E935.2	E950.0	E962.0	E980.0
Herbicides	989.4	E863.5	—	E950.6	E962.1	E980.7
Heroin	965.01	E850.0	E935.0	E950.0	E962.0	E980.0
Herplex	976.5	E858.7	E946.5	E950.4	E962.0	E980.4
HES	964.8	E858.2	E934.8	E950.4	E962.0	E980.4
Hetastarch	964.8	E858.2	E934.8	E950.4	E962.0	E980.7
Hexachlorocyclohexane	989.2	E863.0	—	E950.6	E962.1	E980.7
Hexachlorophene	976.2	E858.7	E946.2	E950.4	E962.0	E980.4
Hexadimethrine (bromide)	964.5	E858.2	E934.5	E950.4	E962.0	E980.4
Hexafluorenium	975.2	E858.6	E945.2	E950.4	E962.0	E980.4
Hexa-germ	976.2	E858.7	E946.2	E950.4	E962.0	E980.4
Hexahydrophenol	980.8	E860.8	—	E950.9	E962.1	E980.9

◀ New   ◀▥ Revised   ~~deleted~~ Deleted   ● Use Additional Digit(s)

Substance	Poisoning	External Cause (E Code) Accident	Therapeutic Use	Suicide Attempt	Assault	Undetermined
Hexalen	980.8	E860.8	—	E950.9	E962.1	E980.9
Hexamethonium	972.3	E858.3	E942.3	E950.4	E962.0	E980.4
Hexamethylenamine	961.9	E857	E931.9	E950.4	E962.0	E980.4
Hexamine	961.9	E857	E931.9	E950.4	E962.0	E980.4
Hexanone	982.8	E862.4	—	E950.9	E962.1	E980.9
Hexapropymate	967.8	E852.8	E937.8	E950.2	E962.0	E980.2
Hexestrol	962.2	E858.0	E932.2	E950.4	E962.0	E980.4
Hexethal (sodium)	967.0	E851	E937.0	E950.1	E962.0	E980.1
Hexetidine	976.0	E858.7	E946.0	E950.4	E962.0	E980.4
Hexobarbital, hexobarbitone	967.0	E851	E937.0	E950.1	E962.0	E980.1
sodium (anesthetic)	968.3	E855.1	E938.3	E950.4	E962.0	E980.4
soluble	968.3	E855.1	E938.3	E950.4	E962.0	E980.4
Hexocyclium	971.1	E855.4	E941.1	E950.4	E962.0	E980.4
Hexoestrol	962.2	E858.0	E932.2	E950.4	E962.0	E980.4
Hexone	982.8	E862.4	—	E950.9	E962.1	E980.9
Hexylcaine	968.5	E855.2	E938.5	E950.4	E962.0	E980.4
Hexylresorcinol	961.6	E857	E931.6	E950.4	E962.0	E980.4
Hinkle's pills	973.1	E858.4	E943.1	E950.4	E962.0	E980.4
Histalog	977.8	E858.8	E947.8	E950.4	E962.0	E980.4
Histamine (phosphate)	972.5	E858.3	E942.5	E950.4	E962.0	E980.4
Histoplasmin	977.8	E858.8	E947.8	E950.4	E962.0	E980.4
Holly berries	988.2	E865.3	—	E950.9	E962.1	E980.9
Homatropine	971.1	E855.4	E941.1	E950.4	E962.0	E980.4
Homo-tet	964.6	E858.2	E934.6	E950.4	E962.0	E980.4
Hormones (synthetic substitute) NEC	962.9	E858.0	E932.9	E950.4	E962.0	E980.4
adrenal cortical steroids	962.0	E858.0	E932.0	E950.4	E962.0	E980.4
antidiabetic agents	962.3	E858.0	E932.3	E950.4	E962.0	E980.4
follicle stimulating	962.4	E858.0	E932.4	E950.4	E962.0	E980.4
gonadotropic	962.4	E858.0	E932.4	E950.4	E962.0	E980.4
growth	962.4	E858.0	E932.4	E950.4	E962.0	E980.4
ovarian (substitutes)	962.2	E858.0	E932.2	E950.4	E962.0	E980.4
parathyroid (derivatives)	962.6	E858.0	E932.6	E950.4	E962.0	E980.4
pituitary (posterior)	962.5	E858.0	E932.5	E950.4	E962.0	E980.4
anterior	962.4	E858.0	E932.4	E950.4	E962.0	E980.4
thyroid (derivative)	962.7	E858.0	E932.7	E950.4	E962.0	E980.4
Hornet (sting)	989.5	E905.3	—	E950.9	E962.1	E980.9
Horticulture agent NEC	989.4	E863.9	—	E950.6	E962.1	E980.7
Hyaluronidase	963.4	E858.1	E933.4	E950.4	E962.0	E980.4
Hyazyme	963.4	E858.1	E933.4	E950.4	E962.0	E980.4

New ◀ Revised ◀ deleted Deleted ● Use Additional Digit(s)

Substance	Poisoning	External Cause (E Code)				
		Accident	Therapeutic Use	Suicide Attempt	Assault	Undetermined
Hycodan	965.09	E850.2	E935.2	E950.0	E962.0	E980.0
Hydantoin derivatives	966.1	E855.0	E936.1	E950.4	E962.0	E980.4
Hydeltra	962.0	E858.0	E932.0	E950.4	E962.0	E980.4
Hydergine	971.3	E855.6	E941.3	E950.4	E962.0	E980.4
Hydrabamine penicillin	960.0	E856	E930.0	E950.4	E962.0	E980.4
Hydralazine, hydrallazine	972.6	E858.3	E942.6	E950.4	E962.0	E980.4
Hydrargaphen	976.0	E858.7	E946.0	E950.4	E962.0	E980.4
Hydrazine	983.9	E864.3	—	E950.7	E962.1	E980.6
Hydriodic acid	975.5	E858.6	E945.5	E950.4	E962.0	E980.4
Hydrocarbon gas	987.1	E869.8	—	E952.8	E962.2	E982.8
incomplete combustion of - *see* Carbon, monoxide, fuel, utility	—	—	—	—	—	—
liquefied (mobile container)	987.0	E868.0	—	E951.1	E962.2	E981.1
piped (natural)	987.0	E867	—	E951.0	E962.2	E981.0
Hydrochloric acid (liquid)	983.1	E864.1	—	E950.7	E962.1	E980.6
medicinal	973.4	E858.4	E943.4	E950.4	E962.0	E980.4
vapor	987.8	E869.8	—	E952.8	E962.2	E982.8
Hydrochlorothiazide	974.3	E858.5	E944.3	E950.4	E962.0	E980.4
Hydrocodone	965.09	E850.2	E935.2	E950.0	E962.0	E980.0
Hydrocortisone	962.0	E858.0	E932.0	E950.4	E962.0	E980.4
ENT agent	976.6	E858.7	E946.6	E950.4	E962.0	E980.4
ophthalmic preparation	976.5	E858.7	E946.5	E950.4	E962.0	E980.4
topical NEC	976.0	E858.7	E946.0	E950.4	E962.0	E980.4
Hydrocortone	962.0	E858.0	E932.0	E950.4	E962.0	E980.4
ENT agent	976.6	E858.7	E946.6	E950.4	E962.0	E980.4
ophthalmic preparation	976.5	E858.7	E946.5	E950.4	E962.0	E980.4
topical NEC	976.0	E858.7	E946.0	E950.4	E962.0	E980.4
Hydrocyanic acid - *see* Cyanide(s)	—	—	—	—	—	—
Hydroflumethiazide	974.3	E858.5	E944.3	E950.4	E962.0	E980.4
Hydrofluoric acid (liquid)	983.1	E864.1	—	E950.7	E962.1	E980.6
vapor	987.8	E869.8	—	E952.8	E962.2	E982.8
Hydrogen	987.8	E869.8	—	E952.8	E962.2	E982.8
arsenide	985.1	E866.3	—	E950.8	E962.1	E980.8
arseniurated	985.1	E866.3	—	E950.8	E962.1	E980.8
cyanide (salts)	989.0	E866.8	—	E950.9	E962.1	E980.9
gas	987.7	E869.8	—	E952.8	E962.2	E982.8
fluoride (liquid)	983.1	E864.1	—	E950.7	E962.1	E980.6
vapor	987.8	E869.8	—	E952.8	E962.2	E982.8
peroxide (solution)	976.6	E858.7	E946.6	E950.4	E962.0	E980.4
phosphorated	987.8	E869.8	—	E952.8	E962.2	E982.8

◀ New ◀▏▏ Revised ~~deleted~~ Deleted ● Use Additional Digit(s)

TABLE OF DRUGS AND CHEMICALS

Substance	Poisoning	External Cause (E Code)				
		Accident	Therapeutic Use	Suicide Attempt	Assault	Undetermined
Hydrogen *(Continued)*						
sulfide (gas)	987.8	E869.8	—	E952.8	E962.2	E982.8
arseniurated	985.1	E866.3	—	E950.8	E962.1	E980.8
sulfureted	987.8	E869.8	—	E952.8	E962.2	E982.8
Hydromorphinol	965.09	E850.2	E935.2	E950.0	E962.0	E980.0
Hydromorphinone	965.09	E850.2	E935.2	E950.0	E962.0	E980.0
Hydromorphone	965.09	E850.2	E935.2	E950.0	E962.0	E980.0
Hydromox	974.3	E858.5	E944.3	E950.4	E962.0	E980.4
Hydrophilic lotion	976.3	E858.7	E946.3	E950.4	E962.0	E980.4
Hydroquinone	983.0	E864.0	—	E950.7	E962.1	E980.6
vapor	987.8	E869.8	—	E952.8	E962.2	E982.8
Hydrosulfuric acid (gas)	987.8	E869.8	—	E952.8	E962.2	E982.8
Hydrous wool fat (lotion)	976.3	E858.7	E946.3	E950.4	E962.0	E980.4
Hydroxide, caustic	983.2	E864.2	—	E950.7	E962.1	E980.6
Hydroxocobalamin	964.1	E858.2	E934.1	E950.4	E962.0	E980.4
Hydroxyamphetamine	971.2	E858.5	E941.2	E950.4	E962.0	E980.4
Hydroxychloroquine	961.4	E857	E931.4	E950.4	E962.0	E980.4
Hydroxydihydrocodeinone	965.09	E850.2	E935.2	E950.0	E962.0	E980.0
Hydroxyethyl starch	964.8	E858.2	E934.8	E950.4	E962.0	E980.4
Hydroxyphenamate	969.5	E853.8	E939.5	E950.3	E962.0	E980.3
Hydroxyphenylbutazone	965.5	E850.5	E935.5	E950.0	E962.0	E980.0
Hydroxyprogesterone	962.2	E858.0	E932.2	E950.4	E962.0	E980.4
Hydroxyquinoline derivatives	961.3	E857	E931.3	E950.4	E962.0	E980.4
Hydroxystilbamidine	961.5	E857	E931.5	E950.4	E962.0	E980.4
Hydroxyurea	963.1	E858.1	E933.1	E950.4	E962.0	E980.4
Hydroxyzine	969.5	E853.8	E939.5	E950.3	E962.0	E980.3
Hyoscine (hydrobromide)	971.1	E855.4	E941.1	E950.4	E962.0	E980.4
Hyoscyamine	971.1	E855.4	E941.1	E950.4	E962.0	E980.4
Hyoscyamus (albus) (niger)	988.2	E865.4	—	E950.9	E962.1	E980.9
Hypaque	977.8	E858.8	E947.8	E950.4	E962.0	E980.4
Hypertussis	964.6	E858.2	E934.6	E950.4	E962.0	E980.4
Hypnotics NEC	967.9	E852.9	E937.9	E950.2	E962.0	E980.2
Hypochlorites - *see* Sodium, hypochlorite	—	—	—	—	—	—
Hypotensive agents NEC	972.6	E858.3	E942.6	E950.4	E962.0	E980.4
Ibufenac	965.69	E850.6	E935.6	E950.0	E962.0	E980.0
Ibuprofen	965.61	E850.6	E935.6	E950.0	E962.0	E980.0
ICG	977.8	E858.8	E947.8	E950.4	E962.0	E980.4
Ichthammol	976.4	E858.7	E946.4	E950.4	E962.0	E980.4

◀ New   ◀▥ Revised   ~~deleted~~ Deleted   ● Use Additional Digit(s)

Substance	Poisoning	External Cause (E Code)				
		Accident	Therapeutic Use	Suicide Attempt	Assault	Undetermined
Ichthyol	976.4	E858.7	E946.4	E950.4	E962.0	E980.4
Idoxuridine	976.5	E858.7	E946.5	E950.4	E962.0	E980.4
IDU	976.5	E858.7	E946.5	E950.4	E962.0	E980.4
Iletin	962.3	E858.0	E932.3	E950.4	E962.0	E980.4
Ilex	988.2	E865.4	—	E950.9	E962.1	E980.9
Illuminating gas - *see* Gas, utility	—	—	—	—	—	—
Ilopan	963.5	E858.1	E933.5	E950.4	E962.0	E980.4
Ilotycin	960.3	E856	E930.3	E950.4	E962.0	E980.4
ophthalmic preparation	976.5	E858.7	E946.5	E950.4	E962.0	E980.4
topical NEC	976.0	E858.7	E946.0	E950.4	E962.0	E980.4
Imipramine	969.05	E854.0	E939.0	E950.3	E962.0	E980.3
Immu-G	964.6	E858.2	E934.6	E950.4	E962.0	E980.4
Immuglobin	964.6	E858.2	E934.6	E950.4	E962.0	E980.4
Immune serum globulin	964.6	E858.2	E934.6	E950.4	E962.0	E980.4
Immunosuppressive agents	963.1	E858.1	E933.1	E950.4	E962.0	E980.4
Immu-tetanus	964.6	E858.2	E934.6	E950.4	E962.0	E980.4
Indandione (derivatives)	964.2	E858.2	E934.2	E950.4	E962.0	E980.4
Inderal	972.0	E858.3	E942.0	E950.4	E962.0	E980.4
Indian	—	—	—	—	—	—
hemp	969.6	E854.1	E939.6	E950.3	E962.0	E980.3
tobacco	988.2	E865.4	—	E950.9	E962.1	E980.9
Indigo carmine	977.8	E858.8	E947.8	E950.4	E962.0	E980.4
Indocin	965.69	E850.6	E935.6	E950.0	E962.0	E980.0
Indocyanine green	977.8	E858.8	E947.8	E950.4	E962.0	E980.4
Indomethacin	965.69	E850.6	E935.6	E950.0	E962.0	E980.0
Industrial	—	—	—	—	—	—
alcohol	980.9	E860.9	—	E950.9	E962.1	E980.9
fumes	987.8	E869.8	—	E952.8	E962.2	E982.8
solvents (fumes) (vapors)	982.8	E862.9	—	E950.9	E962.1	E980.9
Influenza vaccine	979.6	E858.8	E949.6	E950.4	E962.0	E982.8
Ingested substances NEC	989.9	E866.9	—	E950.9	E962.1	E980.9
INH (isoniazid)	961.8	E857	E931.8	E950.4	E962.0	E980.4
Inhalation, gas (noxious) - *see* Gas	—	—	—	—	—	—
Ink	989.89	E866.8	—	E950.9	E962.1	E980.9
Innovar	967.6	E852.5	E937.6	E950.2	E962.0	E980.2
Inositol niacinate	972.2	E858.3	E942.2	E950.4	E962.0	E980.4
Inproquone	963.1	E858.1	E933.1	E950.4	E962.0	E980.4
Insect (sting), venomous	989.5	E905.5	—	E950.9	E962.1	E980.9

TABLE OF DRUGS AND CHEMICALS

TABLE OF DRUGS AND CHEMICALS

Substance	Poisoning	External Cause (E Code)				
		Accident	Therapeutic Use	Suicide Attempt	Assault	Undetermined
Insecticides (*see also* Pesticides)	989.4	E863.4	—	E950.6	E962.1	E980.7
chlorinated	989.2	E863.0	—	E950.6	E962.1	E980.7
mixtures	989.4	E863.3	—	E950.6	E962.1	E980.7
organochlorine (compounds)	989.2	E863.0	—	E950.6	E962.1	E980.7
organophosphorus (compounds)	989.3	E863.1	—	E950.6	E962.1	E980.7
Insular tissue extract	962.3	E858.0	E932.3	E950.4	E962.0	E980.4
Insulin (amorphous) (globin) (isophane) (Lente) (NPH) (Protamine) (Semilente) (Ultralente) (zinc)	962.3	E858.0	E932.3	E950.4	E962.0	E980.4
Intranarcon	968.3	E855.1	E938.3	E950.4	E962.0	E980.4
Inulin	977.8	E858.8	E947.8	E950.4	E962.0	E980.4
Invert sugar	974.5	E858.5	E944.5	E950.4	E962.0	E980.4
Inza - see Naproxen	—	—	—	—	—	—
Iodide NEC (*see also* Iodine)	976.0	E858.7	E946.0	E950.4	E962.0	E980.4
mercury (ointment)	976.0	E858.7	E946.0	E950.4	E962.0	E980.4
methylate	976.0	E858.7	E946.0	E950.4	E962.0	E980.4
potassium (expectorant) NEC	975.5	E858.6	E945.5	E950.4	E962.0	E980.4
Iodinated glycerol	975.5	E858.6	E945.5	E950.4	E962.0	E980.4
Iodine (antiseptic, external) (tincture) NEC	976.0	E858.7	E946.0	E950.4	E962.0	E980.4
diagnostic	977.8	E858.8	E947.8	E950.4	E962.0	E980.4
for thyroid conditions (antithyroid)	962.8	E858.0	E932.8	E950.4	E962.0	E980.4
vapor	987.8	E869.8	—	E952.8	E962.2	E982.8
Iodized oil	977.8	E858.8	E947.8	E950.4	E962.0	E980.4
Iodobismitol	961.2	E857	E931.2	E950.4	E962.0	E980.4
Iodochlorhydroxyquin	961.3	E857	E931.3	E950.4	E962.0	E980.4
topical	976.0	E858.7	E946.0	E950.4	E962.0	E980.4
Iodoform	976.0	E858.7	E946.0	E950.4	E962.0	E980.4
Iodopanoic acid	977.8	E858.8	E947.8	E950.4	E962.0	E980.4
Iodophthalein	977.8	E858.8	E947.8	E950.4	E962.0	E980.4
Ion exchange resins	974.5	E858.5	E944.5	E950.4	E962.0	E980.4
Iopanoic acid	977.8	E858.8	E947.8	E950.4	E962.0	E980.4
Iophendylate	977.8	E858.8	E947.8	E950.4	E962.0	E980.4
Iothiouracil	962.8	E858.0	E932.8	E950.4	E962.0	E980.4
Ipecac	973.6	E858.4	E943.6	E950.4	E962.0	E980.4
Ipecacuanha	973.6	E858.4	E943.6	E950.4	E962.0	E980.4
Ipodate	977.8	E858.8	E947.8	E950.4	E962.0	E980.4
Ipral	967.0	E851	E937.0	E950.1	E962.0	E980.1
Ipratropium	975.1	E858.6	E945.1	E950.4	E962.0	E980.4
Iproniazid	969.01	E854.0	E939.0	E950.3	E962.0	E980.3

◄ New ◄◄◄ Revised ~~deleted~~ Deleted ● Use Additional Digit(s)

Substance	Poisoning	External Cause (E Code)				
		Accident	Therapeutic Use	Suicide Attempt	Assault	Undetermined
Iron (compounds) (medicinal) (preparations)	964.0	E858.2	E934.0	E950.4	E962.0	E980.4
dextran	964.0	E858.2	E934.0	E950.4	E962.0	E980.4
nonmedicinal (dust) (fumes) NEC	985.8	E866.4	—	E950.9	E962.1	E980.9
Irritant drug	977.9	E858.9	E947.9	E950.5	E962.0	E980.5
Ismelin	972.6	E858.3	E942.6	E950.4	E962.0	E980.4
Isoamyl nitrite	972.4	E858.3	E942.4	E950.4	E962.0	E980.4
Isobutyl acetate	982.8	E862.4	—	E950.9	E962.1	E980.9
Isocarboxazid	969.01	E854.0	E939.0	E950.3	E962.0	E980.3
Isoephedrine	971.2	E855.5	E941.2	E950.4	E962.0	E980.4
Isoetharine	971.2	E855.5	E941.2	E950.4	E962.0	E980.4
Isofluorophate	971.0	E855.3	E941.0	E950.4	E962.0	E980.4
Isoniazid (INH)	961.8	E857	E931.8	E950.4	E962.0	E980.4
Isopentaquine	961.4	E857	E931.4	E950.4	E962.0	E980.4
Isophane insulin	962.3	E858.0	E932.3	E950.4	E962.0	E980.4
Isopregnenone	962.2	E858.0	E932.2	E950.4	E962.0	E980.4
Isoprenaline	971.2	E855.5	E941.2	E950.4	E962.0	E980.4
Isopropamide	971.1	E855.4	E941.1	E950.4	E962.0	E980.4
Isopropanol	980.2	E860.3	—	E950.9	E962.1	E980.9
topical (germicide)	976.0	E858.7	E946.0	E950.4	E962.0	E980.4
Isopropyl	—	—	—	—	—	—
acetate	982.8	E862.4	—	E950.9	E962.1	E980.9
alcohol	980.2	E860.3	—	E950.9	E962.1	E980.9
topical (germicide)	976.0	E858.7	E946.0	E950.4	E962.0	E980.4
ether	982.8	E862.4	—	E950.9	E962.1	E980.9
Isoproterenol	971.2	E855.5	E941.2	E950.4	E962.0	E980.4
Isosorbide dinitrate	972.4	E858.3	E942.4	E950.4	E962.0	E980.4
Isothipendyl	963.0	E858.1	E933.0	E950.4	E962.0	E980.4
Isoxazolyl penicillin	960.0	E856	E930.0	E950.4	E962.0	E980.4
Isoxsuprine hydrochloride	972.5	E858.3	E942.5	E950.4	E962.0	E980.4
l-thyroxine sodium	962.7	E858.0	E932.7	E950.4	E962.0	E980.4
Jaborandi (pilocarpus) (extract)	971.0	E855.3	E941.0	E950.4	E962.0	E980.4
Jalap	973.1	E858.4	E943.1	E950.4	E962.0	E980.4
Jamaica	—	—	—	—	—	—
dogwood (bark)	965.7	E850.7	E935.7	E950.0	E962.0	E980.0
ginger	989.89	E866.8	—	E950.9	E962.1	E980.9
Jatropha	988.2	E865.4	—	E950.9	E962.1	E980.9
curcas	988.2	E865.3	—	E950.9	E962.1	E980.9
Jectofer	964.0	E858.2	E934.0	E950.4	E962.0	E980.4

◀ New ◀ Revised ~~deleted~~ Deleted ● Use Additional Digit(s)

Substance	Poisoning	External Cause (E Code)				
		Accident	Therapeutic Use	Suicide Attempt	Assault	Undetermined
Jellyfish (sting)	989.5	E905.6	—	E950.9	E962.1	E980.9
Jequirity (bean)	988.2	E865.3	—	E950.9	E962.1	E980.9
Jimson weed	988.2	E865.4	—	E950.9	E962.1	E980.9
seeds	988.2	E865.3	—	E950.9	E962.1	E980.9
Juniper tar (oil) (ointment)	976.4	E858.7	E946.4	E950.4	E962.0	E980.4
Kallikrein	972.5	E858.3	E942.5	E950.4	E962.0	E980.4
Kanamycin	960.6	E856	E930.6	E950.4	E962.0	E980.4
Kantrex	960.6	E856	E930.6	E950.4	E962.0	E980.4
Kaolin	973.5	E858.4	E943.5	E950.4	E962.0	E980.4
Karaya (gum)	973.3	E858.4	E943.3	E950.4	E962.0	E980.4
Kemithal	968.3	E855.1	E938.3	E950.4	E962.0	E980.4
Kenacort	962.0	E858.0	E932.0	E950.4	E962.0	E980.4
Keratolytics	976.4	E858.7	E946.4	E950.4	E962.0	E980.4
Keratoplastics	976.4	E858.7	E946.4	E950.4	E962.0	E980.4
Kerosene, kerosine (fuel) (solvent) NEC	981	E862.1	—	E950.9	E962.1	E980.9
insecticide	981	E863.4	—	E950.6	E962.1	E980.7
vapor	987.1	E869.8	—	E952.8	E962.2	E982.8
Ketamine	968.3	E855.1	E938.3	E950.4	E962.0	E980.4
Ketobemidone	965.09	E850.2	E935.2	E950.0	E962.0	E980.0
Ketols	982.8	E862.4	—	E950.9	E962.1	E980.9
Ketone oils	982.8	E862.4	—	E950.9	E962.1	E980.9
Ketoprofen	965.61	E850.6	E935.6	E950.0	E962.0	E980.0
Kiln gas or vapor (carbon monoxide)	986	E868.8	—	E952.1	E962.2	E982.1
Konsyl	973.3	E858.4	E943.3	E950.4	E962.0	E980.4
Kosam seed	988.2	E865.3	—	E950.9	E962.1	E980.9
Krait (venom)	989.5	E905.0	—	E950.9	E962.1	E980.9
Kwell (insecticide)	989.2	E863.0	—	E950.6	E962.1	E980.7
anti-infective (topical)	976.0	E858.7	E946.0	E950.4	E962.0	E980.4
Laburnum (flowers) (seeds)	988.2	E865.3	—	E950.9	E962.1	E980.9
leaves	988.2	E865.4	—	E950.9	E962.1	E980.9
Lacquers	989.89	E861.6	—	E950.9	E962.1	E980.9
Lacrimogenic gas	987.5	E869.3	—	E952.8	E962.2	E982.8
Lactic acid	983.1	E864.1	—	E950.7	E962.1	E980.6
Lactobacillus acidophilus	973.5	E858.4	E943.5	E950.4	E962.0	E980.4
Lactoflavin	963.5	E858.1	E933.5	E950.4	E962.0	E980.4
Lactuca (virosa) (extract)	967.8	E852.8	E937.8	E950.2	E962.0	E980.2
Lactucarium	967.8	E852.8	E937.8	E950.2	E962.0	E980.2
Laevulose	974.5	E858.5	E944.5	E950.4	E962.0	E980.4
Lanatoside (C)	972.1	E858.3	E942.1	E950.4	E962.0	E980.4
Lanolin (lotion)	976.3	E858.7	E946.3	E950.4	E962.0	E980.4

◄ New   ◄ Revised   ~~deleted~~ Deleted   ● Use Additional Digit(s)

Substance	Poisoning	External Cause (E Code)				
		Accident	Therapeutic Use	Suicide Attempt	Assault	Undetermined
Largactil	969.1	E853.0	E939.1	E950.3	E962.0	E980.3
Larkspur	988.2	E865.3	—	E950.9	E962.1	E980.9
Laroxyl	969.05	E854.0	E939.0	E950.3	E962.0	E980.3
Lasix	974.4	E858.5	E944.4	E950.4	E962.0	E980.4
Latex	989.82	E866.8	—	E950.9	E962.1	E980.9
Lathyrus (seed)	988.2	E865.3	—	E950.9	E962.1	E980.9
Laudanum	965.09	E850.2	E935.2	E950.0	E962.0	E980.0
Laudexium	975.2	E858.6	E945.2	E950.4	E962.0	E980.4
Laurel, black or cherry	988.2	E865.4	—	E950.9	E962.1	E980.9
Laurolinium	976.0	E858.7	E946.0	E950.4	E962.0	E980.4
Lauryl sulfoacetate	976.2	E858.7	E946.2	E950.4	E962.0	E980.4
Laxatives NEC	973.3	E858.4	E943.3	E950.4	E962.0	E980.4
emollient	973.2	E858.4	E943.2	E950.4	E962.0	E980.4
L-dopa	966.4	E855.0	E936.4	E950.4	E962.0	E980.4
L-Tryptophan - see amino acid	—	—	—	—	—	—
Lead (dust) (fumes) (vapor) NEC	984.9	E866.0	—	E950.9	E962.1	E980.9
acetate (dust)	984.1	E866.0	—	E950.9	E962.1	E980.9
anti-infectives	961.2	E857	E931.2	E950.4	E962.0	E980.4
antiknock compound (tetra-ethyl)	984.1	E862.1	—	E950.9	E962.1	E980.9
arsenate, arsenite (dust) (insecticide) (vapor)	985.1	E863.4	—	E950.8	E962.1	E980.8
herbicide	985.1	E863.5	—	E950.8	E962.1	E980.8
carbonate	984.0	E866.0	—	E950.9	E962.1	E980.9
paint	984.0	E861.5	—	E950.9	E962.1	E980.9
chromate	984.0	E866.0	—	E950.9	E962.1	E980.9
paint	984.0	E861.5	—	E950.9	E962.1	E980.9
dioxide	984.0	E866.0	—	E950.9	E962.1	E980.9
inorganic (compound)	984.0	E866.0	—	E950.9	E962.1	E980.9
paint	984.0	E861.5	—	E950.9	E962.1	E980.9
iodide	984.0	E866.0	—	E950.9	E962.1	E980.9
pigment (paint)	984.0	E861.5	—	E950.9	E962.1	E980.9
monoxide (dust)	984.0	E866.0	—	E950.9	E962.1	E980.9
paint	984.0	E861.5	—	E950.9	E962.1	E980.9
organic	984.1	E866.0	—	E950.9	E962.1	E980.9
oxide	984.0	E866.0	—	E950.9	E962.1	E980.9
paint	984.0	E861.5	—	E950.9	E962.1	E980.9
paint	984.0	E861.5	—	E950.9	E962.1	E980.9
salts	984.0	E866.0	—	E950.9	E962.1	E980.9
specified compound NEC	984.8	E866.0	—	E950.9	E962.1	E980.9
tetra-ethyl	984.1	E862.1	—	E950.9	E962.1	E980.9
Lebanese red	969.6	E854.1	E939.6	E950.3	E962.0	E980.3

◀ New ◀▏▏▏ Revised ~~deleted~~ Deleted ● Use Additional Digit(s)

Substance	Poisoning	External Cause (E Code)				
		Accident	Therapeutic Use	Suicide Attempt	Assault	Undetermined
Lente Iletin (insulin)	962.3	E858.0	E932.3	E950.4	E962.0	E980.4
Leptazol	970.0	E854.3	E940.0	E950.4	E962.0	E980.4
Leritine	965.09	E850.2	E935.2	E950.0	E962.0	E980.0
Letter	962.7	E858.0	E932.7	E950.4	E962.0	E980.4
Lettuce opium	967.8	E852.8	E937.8	E950.2	E962.0	E980.2
Leucovorin (factor)	964.1	E858.2	E934.1	E950.4	E962.0	E980.4
Leukeran	963.1	E858.1	E933.1	E950.4	E962.0	E980.4
Levalbuterol	975.7	E858.6	E945.7	E950.4	E962.0	E980.4
Levallorphan	970.1	E854.3	E940.1	E950.4	E962.0	E980.4
Levanil	967.8	E852.8	E937.8	E950.2	E962.0	E980.2
Levarterenol	971.2	E855.5	E941.2	E950.4	E962.0	E980.4
Levodopa	966.4	E855.0	E936.4	E950.4	E962.0	E980.4
Levo-dromoran	965.09	E850.2	E935.2	E950.0	E962.0	E980.0
Levoid	962.7	E858.0	E932.7	E950.4	E962.0	E980.4
Levo-iso-methadone	965.02	E850.1	E935.1	E950.0	E962.0	E980.0
Levomepromazine	967.8	E852.8	E937.8	E950.2	E962.0	E980.2
Levoprome	967.8	E852.8	E937.8	E950.2	E962.0	E980.2
Levopropoxyphene	975.4	E858.6	E945.4	E950.4	E962.0	E980.4
Levorphan, levophanol	965.09	E850.2	E935.2	E950.0	E962.0	E980.0
Levothyroxine (sodium)	962.7	E858.0	E932.7	E950.4	E962.0	E980.4
Levsin	971.1	E855.4	E941.1	E950.4	E962.0	E980.4
Levulose	974.5	E858.5	E944.5	E950.4	E962.0	E980.4
Lewisite (gas)	985.1	E866.3	—	E950.8	E962.1	E980.8
Librium	969.4	E853.2	E939.4	E950.3	E962.0	E980.3
Lidex	976.0	E858.7	E946.0	E950.4	E962.0	E980.4
Lidocaine (infiltration) (topical)	968.5	E855.2	E938.5	E950.4	E962.0	E980.4
nerve block (peripheral) (plexus)	968.6	E855.2	E938.6	E950.4	E962.0	E980.4
spinal	968.7	E855.2	E938.7	E950.4	E962.0	E980.4
Lighter fluid	981	E862.1	—	E950.9	E962.1	E980.9
Lignocaine (infiltration) (topical)	968.5	E855.2	E938.5	E950.4	E962.0	E980.4
nerve block (peripheral) (plexus)	968.6	E855.2	E938.6	E950.4	E962.0	E980.4
spinal	968.7	E855.2	E938.7	E950.4	E962.0	E980.4
Ligroin(e) (solvent)	981	E862.0	—	E950.9	E962.1	E980.9
vapor	987.1	E869.8	—	E952.8	E962.2	E982.8
Ligustrum vulgare	988.2	E865.3	—	E950.9	E962.1	E980.9
Lily of the valley	988.2	E865.4	—	E950.9	E962.1	E980.9
Lime (chloride)	983.2	E864.2	—	E950.7	E962.1	E980.6
solution, sulferated	976.4	E858.7	E946.4	E950.4	E962.0	E980.4
Limonene	982.8	E862.4	—	E950.9	E962.1	E980.9

◄ New   ◄▦ Revised   ~~deleted~~ Deleted   ● Use Additional Digit(s)

Substance	Poisoning	External Cause (E Code)				
		Accident	Therapeutic Use	Suicide Attempt	Assault	Undetermined
Lincomycin	960.8	E856	E930.8	E950.4	E962.0	E980.4
Lindane (insecticide) (vapor)	989.2	E863.0	—	E950.6	E962.1	E980.7
anti-infective (topical)	976.0	E858.7	E946.0	E950.4	E962.0	E980.4
Liniments NEC	976.9	E858.7	E946.9	E950.4	E962.0	E980.4
Linoleic acid	972.2	E858.3	E942.2	E950.4	E962.0	E980.4
Liothyronine	962.7	E858.0	E932.7	E950.4	E962.0	E980.4
Liotrix	962.7	E858.0	E932.7	E950.4	E962.0	E980.4
Lipancreatin	973.4	E858.4	E943.4	E950.4	E962.0	E980.4
Lipo-Lutin	962.2	E858.0	E932.2	E950.4	E962.0	E980.4
Lipotropic agents	977.1	E858.8	E947.1	E950.4	E962.0	E980.4
Liquefied petroleum gases	987.0	E868.0	—	E951.1	E962.2	E981.1
piped (pure or mixed with air)	987.0	E867	—	E951.0	E962.2	E981.0
Liquid petrolatum	973.2	E858.4	E943.2	E950.4	E962.0	E980.4
substance	989.9	E866.9	—	E950.9	E962.1	E980.9
specified NEC	989.89	E866.8	—	E950.9	E962.1	E980.9
Lirugen	979.4	E858.8	E949.4	E950.4	E962.0	E980.4
Lithane	969.8	E855.8	E939.8	E950.3	E962.0	E980.3
Lithium	985.8	E866.4	—	E950.9	E962.1	E980.9
carbonate	969.8	E855.8	E939.8	E950.3	E962.0	E980.3
Lithonate	969.8	E855.8	E939.8	E950.3	E962.0	E980.3
Liver (extract) (injection) (preparations)	964.1	E858.2	E934.1	E950.4	E962.0	E980.4
Lizard (bite) (venom)	989.5	E905.0	—	E950.9	E962.1	E980.9
LMD	964.8	E858.2	E934.8	E950.4	E962.0	E980.4
Lobelia	988.2	E865.4	—	E950.9	E962.1	E980.9
Lobeline	970.0	E854.3	E940.0	E950.4	E962.0	E980.4
Locorten	976.0	E858.7	E946.0	E950.4	E962.0	E980.4
Lolium temulentum	988.2	E865.3	—	E950.9	E962.1	E980.9
Lomotil	973.5	E858.4	E943.5	E950.4	E962.0	E980.4
Lomustine	963.1	E858.1	E933.1	E950.4	E962.0	E980.4
Lophophora williamsii	969.6	E854.1	E939.6	E950.3	E962.0	E980.3
Lorazepam	969.4	E853.2	E939.4	E950.3	E962.0	E980.3
Lotions NEC	976.9	E858.7	E946.9	E950.4	E962.0	E980.4
Lotronex	973.8	E858.4	E943.8	E950.4	E962.0	E980.4
Lotusate	967.0	E851	E937.0	E950.1	E962.0	E980.1
Lowila	976.2	E858.7	E946.2	E950.4	E962.0	E980.4
Loxapine	969.3	E853.8	E939.3	E950.3	E962.0	E980.3
Lozenges (throat)	976.6	E858.7	E946.6	E950.4	E962.0	E980.4
LSD (25)	969.6	E854.1	E939.6	E950.3	E962.0	E980.3
Lubricating oil NEC	981	E862.2	—	E950.9	E962.1	E980.9

◀ New   ◀▥ Revised   ~~deleted~~ Deleted   ● Use Additional Digit(s)

TABLE OF DRUGS AND CHEMICALS

Substance	Poisoning	External Cause (E Code)				
		Accident	Therapeutic Use	Suicide Attempt	Assault	Undetermined
Lucanthone	961.6	E857	E931.6	E950.4	E962.0	E980.4
Luminal	967.0	E851	E937.0	E950.1	E962.0	E980.1
Lung irritant (gas) NEC	987.9	E869.9	—	E952.9	E962.2	E982.9
Lutocylol	962.2	E858.0	E932.2	E950.4	E962.0	E980.4
Lutromone	962.2	E858.0	E932.2	E950.4	E962.0	E980.4
Lututrin	975.0	E858.6	E945.0	E950.4	E962.0	E980.4
Lye (concentrated)	983.2	E864.2	—	E950.7	E962.1	E980.6
Lygranum (skin test)	977.8	E858.8	E947.8	E950.4	E962.0	E980.4
Lymecycline	960.4	E856	E930.4	E950.4	E962.0	E980.4
Lymphogranuloma venereum antigen	977.8	E858.8	E947.8	E950.4	E962.0	E980.4
Lynestrenol	962.2	E858.0	E932.2	E950.4	E962.0	E980.4
Lyovac Sodium Edecrin	974.4	E858.5	E944.4	E950.4	E962.0	E980.4
Lypressin	962.5	E858.0	E932.5	E950.4	E962.0	E980.4
Lysergic acid (amide) (diethylamide)	969.6	E854.1	E939.6	E950.3	E962.0	E980.3
Lysergide	969.6	E854.1	E939.6	E950.3	E962.0	E980.3
Lysine vasopressin	962.5	E858.0	E932.5	E950.4	E962.0	E980.4
Lysol	983.0	E864.0	—	E950.7	E962.1	E980.6
Lytta (vitatta)	976.8	E858.7	E946.8	E950.4	E962.0	E980.4
Mace	987.5	E869.3	—	E952.8	E962.2	E982.8
Macrolides (antibiotics)	960.3	E856	E930.3	E950.4	E962.0	E980.4
Mafenide	976.0	E858.7	E946.0	E950.4	E962.0	E980.4
Magaldrate	973.0	E858.4	E943.0	E950.4	E962.0	E980.4
Magic mushroom	969.6	E854.1	E939.6	E950.3	E962.0	E980.3
Magnamycin	960.8	E856	E930.8	E950.4	E962.0	E980.4
Magnesia magma	973.0	E858.4	E943.0	E950.4	E962.0	E980.4
Magnesium (compounds) (fumes) NEC	985.8	E866.4	—	E950.9	E962.1	E980.9
antacid	973.0	E858.4	E943.0	E950.4	E962.0	E980.4
carbonate	973.0	E858.4	E943.0	E950.4	E962.0	E980.4
cathartic	973.3	E858.4	E943.3	E950.4	E962.0	E980.4
citrate	973.3	E858.4	E943.3	E950.4	E962.0	E980.4
hydroxide	973.0	E858.4	E943.0	E950.4	E962.0	E980.4
oxide	973.0	E858.4	E943.0	E950.4	E962.0	E980.4
sulfate (oral)	973.3	E858.4	E943.3	E950.4	E962.0	E980.4
intravenous	966.3	E855.0	E936.3	E950.4	E962.0	E980.4
trisilicate	973.0	E858.4	E943.0	E950.4	E962.0	E980.4
Malathion (insecticide)	989.3	E863.1	—	E950.6	E962.1	E980.7
Male fern (oleoresin)	961.6	E857	E931.6	E950.4	E962.0	E980.4
Mandelic acid	961.9	E857	E931.9	E950.4	E962.0	E980.4
Manganese compounds (fumes) NEC	985.2	E866.4	—	E950.9	E962.1	E980.9

◀ New   ⬅ Revised   ~~deleted~~ Deleted   ● Use Additional Digit(s)

Substance	Poisoning	External Cause (E Code)				
		Accident	Therapeutic Use	Suicide Attempt	Assault	Undetermined
Mannitol (diuretic) (medicinal) NEC	974.4	E858.5	E944.4	E950.4	E962.0	E980.4
hexanitrate	972.4	E858.3	E942.4	E950.4	E962.0	E980.4
mustard	963.1	E858.1	E933.1	E950.4	E962.0	E980.4
Mannomustine	963.1	E858.1	E933.1	E950.4	E962.0	E980.4
MAO inhibitors	969.01	E854.0	E939.0	E950.3	E962.0	E980.3
Mapharsen	961.1	E857	E931.1	E950.4	E962.0	E980.4
Marcaine	968.9	E855.2	E938.9	E950.4	E962.0	E980.4
infiltration (subcutaneous)	968.5	E855.2	E938.5	E950.4	E962.0	E980.4
nerve block (peripheral) (plexus)	968.6	E855.2	E938.6	E950.4	E962.0	E980.4
Marezine	963.0	E858.1	E933.0	E950.4	E962.0	E980.4
Marihuana, marijuana (derivatives)	969.6	E854.1	E939.6	E950.3	E962.0	E980.3
Marine animals or plants (sting)	989.5	E905.6	—	E950.9	E962.1	E980.9
Marplan	969.01	E854.0	E939.0	E950.3	E962.0	E980.3
Marsh gas	987.1	E869.8	—	E952.8	E962.2	E982.8
Marsilid	969.01	E854.0	E939.0	E950.3	E962.0	E980.3
Matulane	963.1	E858.1	E933.1	E950.4	E962.0	E980.4
Mazindol	977.0	E858.8	E947.0	E950.4	E962.0	E980.4
MDMA	969.72	E854.2	E939.7	E950.3	E962.0	E980.3
Meadow saffron	988.2	E865.3	—	E950.9	E962.1	E980.9
Measles vaccine	979.4	E858.8	E949.4	E950.4	E962.0	E980.4
Meat, noxious or nonbacterial	988.8	E865.0	—	E950.9	E962.1	E980.9
Mebanazine	969.01	E854.0	E939.0	E950.3	E962.0	E980.3
Mebaral	967.0	E851	E937.0	E950.1	E962.0	E980.1
Mebendazole	961.6	E857	E931.6	E950.4	E962.0	E980.4
Mebeverine	975.1	E858.6	E945.1	E950.4	E962.0	E980.4
Mebhydroline	963.0	E858.1	E933.0	E950.4	E962.0	E980.4
Mebrophenhydramine	963.0	E858.1	E933.0	E950.4	E962.0	E980.4
Mebutamate	969.5	E853.8	E939.5	E950.3	E962.0	E980.3
Mecamylamine (chloride)	972.3	E858.3	E942.3	E950.4	E962.0	E980.4
Mechlorethamine hydrochloride	963.1	E858.1	E933.1	E950.4	E962.0	E980.4
Meclizene (hydrochloride)	963.0	E858.1	E933.0	E950.4	E962.0	E980.4
Meclofenoxate	970.0	E854.3	E940.0	E950.4	E962.0	E980.4
Meclozine (hydrochloride)	963.0	E858.1	E933.0	E950.4	E962.0	E980.4
Medazepam	969.4	E853.2	E939.4	E950.3	E962.0	E980.3
Medicine, medicinal substance	977.9	E858.9	E947.9	E950.5	E962.0	E980.5
specified NEC	977.8	E858.8	E947.8	E950.4	E962.0	E980.4
Medinal	967.0	E851	E937.0	E950.1	E962.0	E980.1
Medomin	967.0	E851	E937.0	E950.1	E962.0	E980.1
Medroxyprogesterone	962.2	E858.0	E932.2	E950.4	E962.0	E980.4

TABLE OF DRUGS AND CHEMICALS

Substance	Poisoning	External Cause (E Code)				
		Accident	Therapeutic Use	Suicide Attempt	Assault	Undetermined
Medrysone	976.5	E858.7	E946.5	E950.4	E962.0	E980.4
Mefenamic acid	965.7	E850.7	E935.7	E950.0	E962.0	E980.0
Megahallucinogen	969.6	E854.1	E939.6	E950.3	E962.0	E980.3
Megestrol	962.2	E858.0	E932.2	E950.4	E962.0	E980.4
Meglumine	977.8	E858.8	E947.8	E950.4	E962.0	E980.4
Meladinin	976.3	E858.7	E946.3	E950.4	E962.0	E980.4
Melanizing agents	976.3	E858.7	E946.3	E950.4	E962.0	E980.4
Melarsoprol	961.1	E857	E931.1	E950.4	E962.0	E980.4
Melia azedarach	988.2	E865.3	—	E950.9	E962.1	E980.9
Mellaril	969.1	E853.0	E939.1	E950.3	E962.0	E980.3
Meloxine	976.3	E858.7	E946.3	E950.4	E962.0	E980.4
Melphalan	963.1	E858.1	E933.1	E950.4	E962.0	E980.4
Memantine hydrochloride	969.8	E854.8	E939.8	E950.3	E962.0	E980.3
Menadiol sodium diphosphate	964.3	E858.2	E934.3	E950.4	E962.0	E980.4
Menadione (sodium bisulfite)	964.3	E858.2	E934.3	E950.4	E962.0	E980.4
Menaphthone	964.3	E858.2	E934.3	E950.4	E962.0	E980.4
Meningococcal vaccine	978.8	E858.8	E948.8	E950.4	E962.0	E980.4
Menningovax-C	978.8	E858.8	E948.8	E950.4	E962.0	E980.4
Menotropins	962.4	E858.0	E932.4	E950.4	E962.0	E980.4
Menthol NEC	976.1	E858.7	E946.1	E950.4	E962.0	E980.4
Mepacrine	961.3	E857	E931.3	E950.4	E962.0	E980.4
Meparfynol	967.8	E852.8	E937.8	E950.2	E962.0	E980.2
Mepazine	969.1	E853.0	E939.1	E950.3	E962.0	E980.3
Mepenzolate	971.1	E855.4	E941.1	E950.4	E962.0	E980.4
Meperidine	965.09	E850.2	E935.2	E950.0	E962.0	E980.0
Mephenamin(e)	966.4	E855.0	E936.4	E950.4	E962.0	E980.4
Mephenesin (carbamate)	968.0	E855.1	E938.0	E950.4	E962.0	E980.4
Mephenoxalone	969.5	E853.8	E939.5	E950.3	E962.0	E980.3
Mephentermine	971.2	E855.5	E941.2	E950.4	E962.0	E980.4
Mephenytoin	966.1	E855.0	E936.1	E950.4	E962.0	E980.4
Mephobarbital	967.0	E851	E937.0	E950.1	E962.0	E980.1
Mepiperphenidol	971.1	E855.4	E941.1	E950.4	E962.0	E980.4
Mepivacaine	968.9	E855.2	E938.9	E950.4	E962.0	E980.4
infiltration (subcutaneous)	968.5	E855.2	E938.5	E950.4	E962.0	E980.4
nerve block (peripheral) (plexus)	968.6	E855.2	E938.6	E950.4	E962.0	E980.4
topical (surface)	968.5	E855.2	E938.5	E950.4	E962.0	E980.4
Meprednisone	962.0	E858.0	E932.0	E950.4	E962.0	E980.4
Meprobam	969.5	E853.8	E939.5	E950.3	E962.0	E980.3
Meprobamate	969.5	E853.8	E939.5	E950.3	E962.0	E980.3

◀ New   ◀▥ Revised   ~~deleted~~ Deleted   ● Use Additional Digit(s)

Substance	Poisoning	External Cause (E Code)				
		Accident	Therapeutic Use	Suicide Attempt	Assault	Undetermined
Mepyramine (maleate)	963.0	E858.1	E933.0	E950.4	E962.0	E980.4
Meralluride	974.0	E858.5	E944.0	E950.4	E962.0	E980.4
Merbaphen	974.0	E858.5	E944.0	E950.4	E962.0	E980.4
Merbromin	976.0	E858.7	E946.0	E950.4	E962.0	E980.4
Mercaptomerin	974.0	E858.5	E944.0	E950.4	E962.0	E980.4
Mercaptopurine	963.1	E858.1	E933.1	E950.4	E962.0	E980.4
Mercumatilin	974.0	E858.5	E944.0	E950.4	E962.0	E980.4
Mercuramide	974.0	E858.5	E944.0	E950.4	E962.0	E980.4
Mercuranin	976.0	E858.7	E946.0	E950.4	E962.0	E980.4
Mercurochrome	976.0	E858.7	E946.0	E950.4	E962.0	E980.4
Mercury, mercuric, mercurous (compounds) (cyanide) (fumes) (nonmedicinal) (vapor) NEC	985.0	E866.1	—	E950.9	E962.1	E980.9
ammoniated	976.0	E858.7	E946.0	E950.4	E962.0	E980.4
anti-infective	961.2	E857	E931.2	E950.4	E962.0	E980.4
topical	976.0	E858.7	E946.0	E950.4	E962.0	E980.4
chloride (antiseptic) NEC	976.0	E858.7	E946.0	E950.4	E962.0	E980.4
fungicide	985.0	E863.6	—	E950.6	E962.1	E980.7
diuretic compounds	974.0	E858.5	E944.0	E950.4	E962.0	E980.4
fungicide	985.0	E863.6	—	E950.6	E962.1	E980.7
organic (fungicide)	985.0	E863.6	—	E950.6	E962.1	E980.7
Merethoxylline	974.0	E858.5	E944.0	E950.4	E962.0	E980.4
Mersalyl	974.0	E858.5	E944.0	E950.4	E962.0	E980.4
Merthiolate (topical)	976.0	E858.7	E946.0	E950.4	E962.0	E980.4
ophthalmic preparation	976.5	E858.7	E946.5	E950.4	E962.0	E980.4
Meruvax	979.4	E858.8	E949.4	E950.4	E962.0	E980.4
Mescal buttons	969.6	E854.1	E939.6	E950.3	E962.0	E980.3
Mescaline (salts)	969.6	E854.1	E939.6	E950.3	E962.0	E980.3
Mesoridazine besylate	969.1	E853.0	E939.1	E950.3	E962.0	E980.3
Mestanolone	962.1	E858.0	E932.1	E950.4	E962.0	E980.4
Mestranol	962.2	E858.0	E932.2	E950.4	E962.0	E980.4
Metactesylacetate	976.0	E858.7	E946.0	E950.4	E962.0	E980.4
Metaldehyde (snail killer) NEC	989.4	E863.4	—	E950.6	E962.1	E980.7
Metals (heavy) (nonmedicinal) NEC	985.9	E866.4	—	E950.9	E962.1	E980.9
dust, fumes, or vapor NEC	985.9	E866.4	—	E950.9	E962.1	E980.9
light NEC	985.9	E866.4	—	E950.9	E962.1	E980.9
dust, fumes, or vapor NEC	985.9	E866.4	—	E950.9	E962.1	E980.9
pesticides (dust) (vapor)	985.9	E863.4	—	E950.6	E962.1	E980.7
Metamucil	973.3	E858.4	E943.3	E950.4	E962.0	E980.4
Metaphen	976.0	E858.7	E946.0	E950.4	E962.0	E980.4

TABLE OF DRUGS AND CHEMICALS

Substance	Poisoning	External Cause (E Code)				
		Accident	Therapeutic Use	Suicide Attempt	Assault	Undetermined
Metaproterenol	975.1	E858.6	E945.1	E950.4	E962.0	E980.4
Metaraminol	972.8	E858.3	E942.8	E950.4	E962.0	E980.4
Metaxalone	968.0	E855.1	E938.0	E950.4	E962.0	E980.4
Metformin	962.3	E858.0	E932.3	E950.4	E962.0	E980.4
Methacycline	960.4	E856	E930.4	E950.4	E962.0	E980.4
Methadone	965.02	E850.1	E935.1	E950.0	E962.0	E980.0
Methallenestril	962.2	E858.0	E932.2	E950.4	E962.0	E980.4
Methamphetamine	969.72	E854.2	E939.7	E950.3	E962.0	E980.3
Methandienone	962.1	E858.0	E932.1	E950.4	E962.0	E980.4
Methandriol	962.1	E858.0	E932.1	E950.4	E962.0	E980.4
Methandrostenolone	962.1	E858.0	E932.1	E950.4	E962.0	E980.4
Methane gas	987.1	E869.8	—	E952.8	E962.2	E982.8
Methanol	980.1	E860.2	—	E950.9	E962.1	E980.9
vapor	987.8	E869.8	—	E952.8	E962.2	E982.8
Methantheline	971.1	E855.4	E941.1	E950.4	E962.0	E980.4
Methaphenilene	963.0	E858.1	E933.0	E950.4	E962.0	E980.4
Methapyrilene	963.0	E858.1	E933.0	E950.4	E962.0	E980.4
Methaqualone (compounds)	967.4	E852.3	E937.4	E950.2	E962.0	E980.2
Metharbital, metharbitone	967.0	E851	E937.0	E950.1	E962.0	E980.1
Methazolamide	974.2	E858.5	E944.2	E950.4	E962.0	E980.4
Methdilazine	963.0	E858.1	E933.0	E950.4	E962.0	E980.4
Methedrine	969.72	E854.2	E939.7	E950.3	E962.0	E980.3
Methenamine (mandelate)	961.9	E857	E931.9	E950.4	E962.0	E980.4
Methenolone	962.1	E858.0	E932.1	E950.4	E962.0	E980.4
Methergine	975.0	E858.6	E945.0	E950.4	E962.0	E980.4
Methiacil	962.8	E858.0	E932.8	E950.4	E962.0	E980.4
Methicillin (sodium)	960.0	E856	E930.0	E950.4	E962.0	E980.4
Methimazole	962.8	E858.0	E932.8	E950.4	E962.0	E980.4
Methionine	977.1	E858.8	E947.1	E950.4	E962.0	E980.4
Methisazone	961.7	E857	E931.7	E950.4	E962.0	E980.4
Methitural	967.0	E851	E937.0	E950.1	E962.0	E980.1
Methixene	971.1	E855.4	E941.1	E950.4	E962.0	E980.4
Methobarbital, methobarbitone	967.0	E851	E937.0	E950.1	E962.0	E980.1
Methocarbamol	968.0	E855.1	E938.0	E950.4	E962.0	E980.4
Methohexital, methohexitone (sodium)	968.3	E855.1	E938.3	E950.4	E962.0	E980.4
Methoin	966.1	E855.0	E936.1	E950.4	E962.0	E980.4
Methopholine	965.7	E850.7	E935.7	E950.0	E962.0	E980.0
Methorate	975.4	E858.6	E945.4	E950.4	E962.0	E980.4
Methoserpidine	972.6	E858.3	E942.6	E950.4	E962.0	E980.4

◀ New   ◀▥ Revised   ~~deleted~~ Deleted   ● Use Additional Digit(s)

TABLE OF DRUGS AND CHEMICALS

Substance	Poisoning	External Cause (E Code)				
		Accident	Therapeutic Use	Suicide Attempt	Assault	Undetermined
Methotrexate	963.1	E858.1	E933.1	E950.4	E962.0	E980.4
Methotrimeprazine	967.8	E852.8	E937.8	E950.2	E962.0	E980.2
Methoxa-Dome	976.3	E858.7	E946.3	E950.4	E962.0	E980.4
Methoxamine	971.2	E855.5	E941.2	E950.4	E962.0	E980.4
Methoxsalen	976.3	E858.7	E946.3	E950.4	E962.0	E980.4
Methoxybenzyl penicillin	960.0	E856	E930.0	E950.4	E962.0	E980.4
Methoxychlor	989.2	E863.0	—	E950.6	E962.1	E980.7
Methoxyflurane	968.2	E855.1	E938.2	E950.4	E962.0	E980.4
Methoxyphenamine	971.2	E855.5	E941.2	E950.4	E962.0	E980.4
Methoxypromazine	969.1	E853.0	E939.1	E950.3	E962.0	E980.3
Methoxypsoralen	976.3	E858.7	E946.3	E950.4	E962.0	E980.4
Methscopolamine (bromide)	971.1	E855.4	E941.1	E950.4	E962.0	E980.4
Methsuximide	966.2	E855.0	E936.2	E950.4	E962.0	E980.4
Methyclothiazide	974.3	E858.5	E944.3	E950.4	E962.0	E980.4
Methyl	—	—	—	—	—	—
acetate	982.8	E862.4	—	E950.9	E962.1	E980.9
acetone II	982.8	E862.4	—	E950.9	E962.1	E980.9
alcohol	980.1	E860.2	—	E950.9	E962.1	E980.9
amphetamine	969.72	E854.2	E939.7	E950.3	E962.0	E980.3
androstanolone	962.1	E858.0	E932.1	E950.4	E962.0	E980.4
atropine	971.1	E855.4	E941.1	E950.4	E962.0	E980.4
benzene	982.0	E862.4	—	E950.9	E962.1	E980.9
bromide (gas)	987.8	E869.8	—	E952.8	E962.2	E982.8
fumigant	987.8	E863.8	—	E950.6	E962.2	E980.7
butanol	980.8	E860.8	—	E950.9	E962.1	E980.9
carbinol	980.1	E860.2	—	E950.9	E962.1	E980.9
cellosolve	982.8	E862.4	—	E950.9	E962.1	E980.9
cellulose	973.3	E858.4	E943.3	E950.4	E962.0	E980.4
chloride (gas)	987.8	E869.8	—	E952.8	E962.2	E982.8
cyclohexane	982.8	E862.4	—	E950.9	E962.1	E980.9
cyclohexanone	982.8	E862.4	—	E950.9	E962.1	E980.9
dihydromorphinone	965.09	E850.2	E935.2	E950.0	E962.0	E980.0
ergometrine	975.0	E858.6	E945.0	E950.4	E962.0	E980.4
ergonovine	975.0	E858.6	E945.0	E950.4	E962.0	E980.4
ethyl ketone	982.8	E862.4	—	E950.9	E962.1	E980.9
hydrazine	983.9	E864.3	—	E950.7	E962.1	E980.6
isobutyl ketone	982.8	E862.4	—	E950.9	E962.1	E980.9
morphine NEC	965.09	E850.2	E935.2	E950.0	E962.0	E980.0
parafynol	967.8	E852.8	E937.8	E950.2	E962.0	E980.2

Substance	Poisoning	External Cause (E Code)				
		Accident	Therapeutic Use	Suicide Attempt	Assault	Undetermined
Methyl *(Continued)*						
parathion	989.3	E863.1	—	E950.6	E962.1	E980.7
pentynol NEC	967.8	E852.8	E937.8	E950.2	E962.0	E980.2
peridol	969.2	E853.1	E939.2	E950.3	E962.0	E980.3
phenidate	969.73	E854.2	E939.7	E950.3	E962.0	E980.3
prednisolone	962.0	E858.0	E932.0	E950.4	E962.0	E980.4
ENT agent	976.6	E858.7	E946.6	E950.4	E962.0	E980.4
ophthalmic preparation	976.5	E858.7	E946.5	E950.4	E962.0	E980.4
topical NEC	976.0	E858.7	E946.0	E950.4	E962.0	E980.4
propylcarbinol	980.8	E860.8	—	E950.9	E962.1	E980.9
rosaniline NEC	976.0	E858.7	E946.0	E950.4	E962.0	E980.4
salicylate NEC	976.3	E858.7	E946.3	E950.4	E962.0	E980.4
sulfate (fumes)	987.8	E869.8	—	E952.8	E962.2	E982.8
liquid	983.9	E864.3	—	E950.7	E962.1	E980.6
sulfonal	967.8	E852.8	E937.8	E950.2	E962.0	E980.2
testosterone	962.1	E858.0	E932.1	E950.4	E962.0	E980.4
thiouracil	962.8	E858.0	E932.8	E950.4	E962.0	E980.4
Methylated spirit	980.0	E860.1	—	E950.9	E962.1	E980.9
Methyldopa	972.6	E858.3	E942.6	E950.4	E962.0	E980.4
Methylene blue	961.9	E857	E931.9	E950.4	E962.0	E980.4
chloride or dichloride (solvent) NEC	982.3	E862.4	—	E950.9	E962.1	E980.9
Methylhexabital	967.0	E851	E937.0	E950.1	E962.0	E980.1
Methylparaben (ophthalmic)	976.5	E858.7	E946.5	E950.4	E962.0	E980.4
Methyprylon	967.5	E852.4	E937.5	E950.2	E962.0	E980.2
Methysergide	971.3	E855.6	E941.3	E950.4	E962.0	E980.4
Metoclopramide	963.0	E858.1	E933.0	E950.4	E962.0	E980.4
Metofoline	965.7	E850.7	E935.7	E950.0	E962.0	E980.0
Metopon	965.09	E850.2	E935.2	E950.0	E962.0	E980.0
Metronidazole	961.5	E857	E931.5	E950.4	E962.0	E980.4
Metycaine	968.9	E855.2	E938.9	E950.4	E962.0	E980.4
infiltration (subcutaneous)	968.5	E855.2	E938.5	E950.4	E962.0	E980.4
nerve block (peripheral) (plexus)	968.6	E855.2	E938.6	E950.4	E962.0	E980.4
topical (surface)	968.5	E855.2	E938.5	E950.4	E962.0	E980.4
Metyrapone	977.8	E858.8	E947.8	E950.4	E962.0	E980.4
Mevinphos	989.3	E863.1	—	E950.6	E962.1	E980.7
Mezereon (berries)	988.2	E865.3	—	E950.9	E962.1	E980.9
Micatin	976.0	E858.7	E946.0	E950.4	E962.0	E980.4
Miconazole	976.0	E858.7	E946.0	E950.4	E962.0	E980.4
Midol	965.1	E850.3	E935.3	E950.0	E962.0	E980.0

◀ New ◀▥ Revised ~~deleted~~ Deleted ● Use Additional Digit(s)

Substance	Poisoning	External Cause (E Code)				
		Accident	Therapeutic Use	Suicide Attempt	Assault	Undetermined
Mifepristone	962.9	E858.0	E932.9	E950.4	E962.0	E980.4
Milk of magnesia	973.0	E858.4	E943.0	E950.4	E962.0	E980.4
Millipede (tropical) (venomous)	989.5	E905.4	—	E950.9	E962.1	E980.9
Miltown	969.5	E853.8	E939.5	E950.3	E962.0	E980.3
Mineral	—	—	—	—	—	—
oil (medicinal)	973.2	E858.4	E943.2	E950.4	E962.0	E980.4
nonmedicinal	981	E862.1	—	E950.9	E962.1	E980.9
topical	976.3	E858.7	E946.3	E950.4	E962.0	E980.4
salts NEC	974.6	E858.5	E944.6	E950.4	E962.0	E980.4
spirits	981	E862.0	—	E950.9	E962.1	E980.9
Minocycline	960.4	E856	E930.4	E950.4	E962.0	E980.4
Mithramycin (antineoplastic)	960.7	E856	E930.7	E950.4	E962.0	E980.4
Mitobronitol	963.1	E858.1	E933.1	E950.4	E962.0	E980.4
Mitomycin (antineoplastic)	960.7	E856	E930.7	E950.4	E962.0	E980.4
Mitotane	963.1	E858.1	E933.1	E950.4	E962.0	E980.4
Moderil	972.6	E858.3	E942.6	E950.4	E962.0	E980.4
Mogadon - *see* Nitrazepam	—	—	—	—	—	—
Molindone	969.3	E853.8	E939.3	E950.3	E962.0	E980.3
Monistat	976.0	E858.7	E946.0	E950.4	E962.0	E980.4
Monkshood	988.2	E865.4	—	E950.9	E962.1	E980.9
Monoamine oxidase inhibitors	969.01	E854.0	E939.0	E950.3	E962.0	E980.3
Monochlorobenzene	982.0	E862.4	—	E950.9	E962.1	E980.9
Monosodium glutamate	989.89	E866.8	—	E950.9	E962.1	E980.9
Monoxide, carbon - *see* Carbon, monoxide	—	—	—	—	—	—
Moperone	969.2	E853.1	E939.2	E950.3	E962.0	E980.3
Morning glory seeds	969.6	E854.1	E939.6	E950.3	E962.0	E980.3
Moroxydine (hydrochloride)	961.7	E857	E931.7	E950.4	E962.0	E980.4
Morphazinamide	961.8	E857	E931.8	E950.4	E962.0	E980.4
Morphinans	965.09	E850.2	E935.2	E950.0	E962.0	E980.0
Morphine NEC	965.09	E850.2	E935.2	E950.0	E962.0	E980.0
antagonists	970.1	E854.3	E940.1	E950.4	E962.0	E980.4
Morpholinylethyl morphine	965.09	E850.2	E935.2	E950.0	E962.0	E980.0
Morrhuate sodium	972.7	E858.3	E942.7	E950.4	E962.0	E980.4
Moth balls (*see also* Pesticides)	989.4	E863.4	—	E950.6	E962.1	E980.7
naphthalene	983.0	E863.4	—	E950.7	E962.1	E980.6
Motor exhaust gas - *see* Carbon, monoxide, exhaust gas	—	—	—	—	—	—
Mouth wash	976.6	E858.7	E946.6	E950.4	E962.0	E980.4
Mucolytic agent	975.5	E858.6	E945.5	E950.4	E962.0	E980.4
Mucomyst	975.5	E858.6	E945.5	E950.4	E962.0	E980.4

◀ New   ◀◊ Revised   ~~deleted~~ Deleted   ● Use Additional Digit(s)

Substance	Poisoning	External Cause (E Code)				
		Accident	Therapeutic Use	Suicide Attempt	Assault	Undetermined
Mucous membrane agents (external)	976.9	E858.7	E946.9	E950.4	E962.0	E980.4
specified NEC	976.8	E858.7	E946.8	E950.4	E962.0	E980.4
Mumps	—	—	—	—	—	—
immune globulin (human)	964.6	E858.2	E934.6	E950.4	E962.0	E980.4
skin test antigen	977.8	E858.8	E947.8	E950.4	E962.0	E980.4
vaccine	979.6	E858.8	E949.6	E950.4	E962.0	E980.4
Mumpsvax	979.6	E858.8	E949.6	E950.4	E962.0	E980.4
Muriatic acid - see Hydrochloric acid	—	—	—	—	—	—
Muscarine	971.0	E855.3	E941.0	E950.4	E962.0	E980.4
Muscle affecting agents NEC	975.3	E858.6	E945.3	E950.4	E962.0	E980.4
oxytocic	975.0	E858.6	E945.0	E950.4	E962.0	E980.4
relaxants	975.3	E858.6	E945.3	E950.4	E962.0	E980.4
central nervous system	968.0	E855.1	E938.0	E950.4	E962.0	E980.4
skeletal	975.2	E858.6	E945.2	E950.4	E962.0	E980.4
smooth	975.1	E858.6	E945.1	E950.4	E962.0	E980.4
Mushrooms, noxious	988.1	E865.5	—	E950.9	E962.1	E980.9
Mussel, noxious	988.0	E865.1	—	E950.9	E962.1	E980.9
Mustard (emetic)	973.6	E858.4	E943.6	E950.4	E962.0	E980.4
gas	987.8	E869.8	—	E952.8	E962.2	E982.8
nitrogen	963.1	E858.1	E933.1	E950.4	E962.0	E980.4
Mustine	963.1	E858.1	E933.1	E950.4	E962.0	E980.4
M-vac	979.4	E858.8	E949.4	E950.4	E962.0	E980.4
Mycifradin	960.8	E856	E930.8	E950.4	E962.0	E980.4
topical	976.0	E858.7	E946.0	E950.4	E962.0	E980.4
Mycitracin	960.8	E856	E930.8	E950.4	E962.0	E980.4
ophthalmic preparation	976.5	E858.7	E946.5	E950.4	E962.0	E980.4
Mycostatin	960.1	E856	E930.1	E950.4	E962.0	E980.4
topical	976.0	E858.7	E946.0	E950.4	E962.0	E980.4
Mydriacyl	971.1	E855.4	E941.1	E950.4	E962.0	E980.4
Myelobromal	963.1	E858.1	E933.1	E950.4	E962.0	E980.4
Myleran	963.1	E858.1	E933.1	E950.4	E962.0	E980.4
Myochrysin(e)	965.69	E850.6	E935.6	E950.0	E962.0	E980.0
Myoneural blocking agents	975.2	E858.6	E945.2	E950.4	E962.0	E980.4
Myristica fragrans	988.2	E865.3	—	E950.9	E962.1	E980.9
Myristicin	988.2	E865.3	—	E950.9	E962.1	E980.9
Mysoline	966.3	E855.0	E936.3	E950.4	E962.0	E980.4
Nafcillin (sodium)	960.0	E856	E930.0	E950.4	E962.0	E980.4
Nail polish remover	982.8	E862.4	—	E950.9	E962.1	E980.9
Nalidixic acid	961.9	E857	E931.9	E950.4	E962.0	E980.4

◀ New ◀▥▥ Revised ~~deleted~~ Deleted ● Use Additional Digit(s)

Substance	Poisoning	External Cause (E Code)				
		Accident	Therapeutic Use	Suicide Attempt	Assault	Undetermined
Nalorphine	970.1	E854.3	E940.1	E950.4	E962.0	E980.4
Naloxone	970.1	E854.3	E940.1	E950.4	E962.0	E980.4
Namenda	969.8	E854.8	E939.8	E950.3	E962.0	E980.3
Nandrolone (decanoate) (phenpropionate)	962.1	E858.0	E932.1	E950.4	E962.0	E980.4
Naphazoline	971.2	E855.5	E941.2	E950.4	E962.0	E980.4
Naphtha (painter's) (petroleum)	981	E862.0	—	E950.9	E962.1	E980.9
solvent	981	E862.0	—	E950.9	E962.1	E980.9
vapor	987.1	E869.8	—	E952.8	E962.2	E982.8
Naphthalene (chlorinated)	983.0	E864.0	—	E950.7	E962.1	E980.6
insecticide or moth repellent	983.0	E863.4	—	E950.7	E962.1	E980.6
vapor	987.8	E869.8	—	E952.8	E962.2	E982.8
Naphthol	983.0	E864.0	—	E950.7	E962.1	E980.6
Naphthylamine	983.0	E864.0	—	E950.7	E962.1	E980.6
Naprosyn - see Naproxen	—	—	—	—	—	—
Naproxen	965.61	E850.6	E935.6	E950.0	E962.0	E980.0
Narcotic (drug)	967.9	E852.9	E937.9	E950.2	E962.0	E980.2
analgesic NEC	965.8	E850.8	E935.8	E950.0	E962.0	E980.0
antagonist	970.1	E854.3	E940.1	E950.4	E962.0	E980.4
specified NEC	967.8	E852.8	E937.8	E950.2	E962.0	E980.2
Narcotine	975.4	E858.6	E945.4	E950.4	E962.0	E980.4
Nardil	969.01	E854.0	E939.0	E950.3	E962.0	E980.3
Natrium cyanide - see Cyanide(s)	—	—	—	—	—	—
Natural	—	—	—	—	—	—
blood (product)	964.7	E858.2	E934.7	E950.4	E962.0	E980.4
gas (piped)	987.1	E867	—	E951.0	E962.2	E981.0
incomplete combustion	986	E867	—	E951.0	E962.2	E981.0
Nealbarbital, nealbarbitone	967.0	E851	E937.0	E950.1	E962.0	E980.1
Nectadon	975.4	E858.6	E945.4	E950.4	E962.0	E980.4
Nematocyst (sting)	989.5	E905.6	—	E950.9	E962.1	E980.9
Nembutal	967.0	E851	E937.0	E950.1	E962.0	E980.1
Neoarsphenamine	961.1	E857	E931.1	E950.4	E962.0	E980.4
Neocinchophen	974.7	E858.5	E944.7	E950.4	E962.0	E980.4
Neomycin	960.8	E856	E930.8	E950.4	E962.0	E980.4
ENT agent	976.6	E858.7	E946.6	E950.4	E962.0	E980.4
ophthalmic preparation	976.5	E858.7	E946.5	E950.4	E962.0	E980.4
topical NEC	976.0	E858.7	E946.0	E950.4	E962.0	E980.4
Neonal	967.0	E851	E937.0	E950.1	E962.0	E980.1
Neoprontosil	961.0	E857	E931.0	E950.4	E962.0	E980.4
Neosalvarsan	961.1	E857	E931.1	E950.4	E962.0	E980.4

TABLE OF DRUGS AND CHEMICALS

TABLE OF DRUGS AND CHEMICALS

Substance	Poisoning	External Cause (E Code)				
		Accident	Therapeutic Use	Suicide Attempt	Assault	Undetermined
Neosilversalvarsan	961.1	E857	E931.1	E950.4	E962.0	E980.4
Neosporin	960.8	E856	E930.8	E950.4	E962.0	E980.4
ENT agent	976.6	E858.7	E946.6	E950.4	E962.0	E980.4
ophthalmic preparation	976.5	E858.7	E946.5	E950.4	E962.0	E980.4
topical NEC	976.0	E858.7	E946.0	E950.4	E962.0	E980.4
Neostigmine	971.0	E855.3	E941.0	E950.4	E962.0	E980.4
Neraval	967.0	E851	E937.0	E950.1	E962.0	E980.1
Neravan	967.0	E851	E937.0	E950.1	E962.0	E980.1
Nerium oleander	988.2	E865.4	—	E950.9	E962.1	E980.9
Nerve gases (war)	987.9	E869.9	—	E952.9	E962.2	E982.9
Nesacaine	968.9	E855.2	E938.9	E950.4	E962.0	E980.4
infiltration (subcutaneous)	968.5	E855.2	E938.5	E950.4	E962.0	E980.4
nerve block (peripheral) (plexus)	968.6	E855.2	E938.6	E950.4	E962.0	E980.4
Neurobarb	967.0	E851	E937.0	E950.1	E962.0	E980.1
Neuroleptics NEC	969.3	E853.8	E939.3	E950.3	E962.0	E980.3
Neuroprotective agent	977.8	E858.8	E947.8	E950.4	E962.0	E980.4
Neutral spirits	980.0	E860.1	—	E950.9	E962.1	E980.9
beverage	980.0	E860.0	—	E950.9	E962.1	E980.9
Niacin, niacinamide	972.2	E858.3	E942.2	E950.4	E962.0	E980.4
Nialamide	969.01	E854.0	E939.0	E950.3	E962.0	E980.3
Nickle (carbonyl) (compounds) (fumes) (tetracarbonyl) (vapor)	985.8	E866.4	—	E950.9	E962.1	E980.9
Niclosamide	961.6	E857	E931.6	E950.4	E962.0	E980.4
Nicomorphine	965.09	E850.2	E935.2	E950.0	E962.0	E980.0
Nicotinamide	972.2	E858.3	E942.2	E950.4	E962.0	E980.4
Nicotine (insecticide) (spray) (sulfate) NEC	989.4	E863.4	—	E950.6	E962.1	E980.7
not insecticide	989.89	E866.8	—	E950.9	E962.1	E980.9
Nicotinic acid (derivatives)	972.2	E858.3	E942.2	E950.4	E962.0	E980.4
Nicotinyl alcohol	972.2	E858.3	E942.2	E950.4	E962.0	E980.4
Nicoumalone	964.2	E858.2	E934.2	E950.4	E962.0	E980.4
Nifenazone	965.5	E850.5	E935.5	E950.0	E962.0	E980.0
Nifuraldezone	961.9	E857	E931.9	E950.4	E962.0	E980.4
Nightshade (deadly)	988.2	E865.4	—	E950.9	E962.1	E980.9
Nikethamide	970.0	E854.3	E940.0	E950.4	E962.0	E980.4
Nilstat	960.1	E856	E930.1	E950.4	E962.0	E980.4
topical	976.0	E858.7	E946.0	E950.4	E962.0	E980.4
Nimodipine	977.8	E858.8	E947.8	E950.4	E962.0	E980.4
Niridazole	961.6	E857	E931.6	E950.4	E962.0	E980.4
Nisentil	965.09	E850.2	E935.2	E950.0	E962.0	E980.0
Nitrates	972.4	E858.3	E942.4	E950.4	E962.0	E980.4

◀ New ◀░ Revised ~~deleted~~ Deleted ● Use Additional Digit(s)

Substance	Poisoning	External Cause (E Code)				
		Accident	Therapeutic Use	Suicide Attempt	Assault	Undetermined
Nitrazepam	969.4	E853.2	E939.4	E950.3	E962.0	E980.3
Nitric	—	—	—	—	—	—
acid (liquid)	983.1	E864.1	—	E950.7	E962.1	E980.6
vapor	987.8	E869.8	—	E952.8	E962.2	E982.8
oxide (gas)	987.2	E869.0	—	E952.8	E962.2	E982.8
Nitrite, amyl (medicinal) (vapor)	972.4	E858.3	E942.4	E950.4	E962.0	E980.4
Nitroaniline	983.0	E864.0	—	E950.7	E962.1	E980.6
vapor	987.8	E869.8	—	E952.8	E962.2	E982.8
Nitrobenzene, nitrobenzol	983.0	E864.0	—	E950.7	E962.1	E980.6
vapor	987.8	E869.8	—	E952.8	E962.2	E982.8
Nitrocellulose	976.3	E858.7	E946.3	E950.4	E962.0	E980.4
Nitrofuran derivatives	961.9	E857	E931.9	E950.4	E962.0	E980.4
Nitrofurantoin	961.9	E857	E931.9	E950.4	E962.0	E980.4
Nitrofurazone	976.0	E858.7	E946.0	E950.4	E962.0	E980.4
Nitrogen (dioxide) (gas) (oxide)	987.2	E869.0	—	E952.8	E962.2	E982.8
mustard (antineoplastic)	963.1	E858.1	E933.1	E950.4	E962.0	E980.4
Nitroglycerin, nitroglycerol (medicinal)	972.4	E858.3	E942.4	E950.4	E962.0	E980.4
nonmedicinal	989.89	E866.8	—	E950.9	E962.1	E980.9
fumes	987.8	E869.8	—	E952.8	E962.2	E982.8
Nitrohydrochloric acid	983.1	E864.1	—	E950.7	E962.1	E980.6
Nitromersol	976.0	E858.7	E946.0	E950.4	E962.0	E980.4
Nitronaphthalene	983.0	E864.0	—	E950.7	E962.2	E980.6
Nitrophenol	983.0	E864.0	—	E950.7	E962.2	E980.6
Nitrothiazol	961.6	E857	E931.6	E950.4	E962.0	E980.4
Nitrotoluene, nitrotoluol	983.0	E864.0	—	E950.7	E962.1	E980.6
vapor	987.8	E869.8	—	E952.8	E962.2	E982.8
Nitrous	968.2	E855.1	E938.2	E950.4	E962.0	E980.4
acid (liquid)	983.1	E864.1	—	E950.7	E962.1	E980.6
fumes	987.2	E869.0	—	E952.8	E962.2	E982.8
oxide (anesthetic) NEC	968.2	E855.1	E938.2	E950.4	E962.0	E980.4
Nitrozone	976.0	E858.7	E946.0	E950.4	E962.0	E980.4
Noctec	967.1	E852.0	E937.1	E950.2	E962.0	E980.2
Noludar	967.5	E852.4	E937.5	E950.2	E962.0	E980.2
Noptil	967.0	E851	E937.0	E950.1	E962.0	E980.1
Noradrenalin	971.2	E855.5	E941.2	E950.4	E962.0	E980.4
Noramidopyrine	965.5	E850.5	E935.5	E950.0	E962.0	E980.0
Norepinephrine	971.2	E855.5	E941.2	E950.4	E962.0	E980.4
Norethandrolone	962.1	E858.0	E932.1	E950.4	E962.0	E980.4
Norethindrone	962.2	E858.0	E932.2	E950.4	E962.0	E980.4

◀ New　◀▥ Revised　~~deleted~~ Deleted　● Use Additional Digit(s)

Substance	Poisoning	External Cause (E Code)				
		Accident	Therapeutic Use	Suicide Attempt	Assault	Undetermined
Norethisterone	962.2	E858.0	E932.2	E950.4	E962.0	E980.4
Norethynodrel	962.2	E858.0	E932.2	E950.4	E962.0	E980.4
Norlestrin	962.2	E858.0	E932.2	E950.4	E962.0	E980.4
Norlutin	962.2	E858.0	E932.2	E950.4	E962.0	E980.4
Normison - *see* Benzodiazepines	—	—	—	—	—	—
Normorphine	965.09	E850.2	E935.2	E950.0	E962.0	E980.0
Nortriptyline	969.05	E854.0	E939.0	E950.3	E962.0	E980.3
Noscapine	975.4	E858.6	E945.4	E950.4	E962.0	E980.4
Nose preparations	976.6	E858.7	E946.6	E950.4	E962.0	E980.4
Novobiocin	960.8	E856	E930.8	E950.4	E962.0	E980.4
Novocain (infiltration) (topical)	968.5	E855.2	E938.5	E950.4	E962.0	E980.4
nerve block (peripheral) (plexus)	968.6	E855.2	E938.6	E950.4	E962.0	E980.4
spinal	968.7	E855.2	E938.7	E950.4	E962.0	E980.4
Noxythiolin	961.9	E857	E931.9	E950.4	E962.0	E980.4
NPH Iletin (insulin)	962.3	E858.0	E932.3	E950.4	E962.0	E980.4
Numorphan	965.09	E850.2	E935.2	E950.0	E962.0	E980.0
Nunol	967.0	E851	E937.0	E950.1	E962.0	E980.1
Nupercaine (spinal anesthetic)	968.7	E855.2	E938.7	E950.4	E962.0	E980.4
topical (surface)	968.5	E855.2	E938.5	E950.4	E962.0	E980.4
Nutmeg oil (liniment)	976.3	E858.7	E946.3	E950.4	E962.0	E980.4
Nux vomica	989.1	E863.7	—	E950.6	E962.1	E980.7
Nydrazid	961.8	E857	E931.8	E950.4	E962.0	E980.4
Nylidrin	971.2	E855.5	E941.2	E950.4	E962.0	E980.4
Nystatin	960.1	E856	E930.1	E950.4	E962.0	E980.4
topical	976.0	E858.7	E946.0	E950.4	E962.0	E980.4
Nytol	963.0	E858.1	E933.0	E950.4	E962.0	E980.4
Oblivion	967.8	E852.8	E937.8	E950.2	E962.0	E980.2
Octyl nitrite	972.4	E858.3	E942.4	E950.4	E962.0	E980.4
Oestradiol (cypionate) (dipropionate) (valerate)	962.2	E858.0	E932.2	E950.4	E962.0	E980.4
Oestriol	962.2	E858.0	E932.2	E950.4	E962.0	E980.4
Oestrone	962.2	E858.0	E932.2	E950.4	E962.0	E980.4
Oil (of) NEC	989.89	E866.8	—	E950.9	E962.1	E980.9
bitter almond	989.0	E866.8	—	E950.9	E962.1	E980.9
camphor	976.1	E858.7	E946.1	E950.4	E962.0	E980.4
colors	989.89	E861.6	—	E950.9	E962.1	E980.9
fumes	987.8	E869.8	—	E952.8	E962.2	E982.8
lubricating	981	E862.2	—	E950.9	E962.1	E980.9
specified source, other - *see* substance specified	—	—	—	—	—	—

◀ New ◀▦ Revised ~~deleted~~ Deleted ● Use Additional Digit(s)

Substance	Poisoning	External Cause (E Code)				
		Accident	Therapeutic Use	Suicide Attempt	Assault	Undetermined
Oil (of) NEC *(Continued)*						
vitriol (liquid)	983.1	E864.1	—	E950.7	E962.1	E980.6
fumes	987.8	E869.8	—	E952.8	E962.2	E982.8
wintergreen (bitter) NEC	976.3	E858.7	E946.3	E950.4	E962.0	E980.4
Ointments NEC	976.9	E858.7	E946.9	E950.4	E962.0	E980.4
Oleander	988.2	E865.4	—	E950.9	E962.1	E980.9
Oleandomycin	960.3	E856	E930.3	E950.4	E962.0	E980.4
Oleovitamin A	963.5	E858.1	E933.5	E950.4	E962.0	E980.4
Oleum ricini	973.1	E858.4	E943.1	E950.4	E962.0	E980.4
Olive oil (medicinal) NEC	973.2	E858.4	E943.2	E950.4	E962.0	E980.4
OMPA	989.3	E863.1	—	E950.6	E962.1	E980.7
Oncovin	963.1	E858.1	E933.1	E950.4	E962.0	E980.4
Ophthaine	968.5	E855.2	E938.5	E950.4	E962.0	E980.4
Ophthetic	968.5	E855.2	E938.5	E950.4	E962.0	E980.4
Opiates, opioids, opium NEC	965.00	E850.2	E935.2	E950.0	E962.0	E980.0
antagonists	970.1	E854.3	E940.1	E950.4	E962.0	E980.4
Oracon	962.2	E858.0	E932.2	E950.4	E962.0	E980.4
Oragrafin	977.8	E858.8	E947.8	E950.4	E962.0	E980.4
Oral contraceptives	962.2	E858.0	E932.2	E950.4	E962.0	E980.4
Orciprenaline	975.1	E858.6	E945.1	E950.4	E962.0	E980.4
Organidin	975.5	E858.6	E945.5	E950.4	E962.0	E980.4
Organophosphates	989.3	E863.1	—	E950.6	E962.1	E980.7
Orimune	979.5	E858.8	E949.5	E950.4	E962.0	E980.4
Orinase	962.3	E858.0	E932.3	E950.4	E962.0	E980.4
Orphenadrine	966.4	E855.0	E936.4	E950.4	E962.0	E980.4
Ortal (sodium)	967.0	E851	E937.0	E950.1	E962.0	E980.1
Orthoboric acid	976.0	E858.7	E946.0	E950.4	E962.0	E980.4
ENT agent	976.6	E858.7	E946.6	E950.4	E962.0	E980.4
ophthalmic preparation	976.5	E858.7	E946.5	E950.4	E962.0	E980.4
Orthocaine	968.5	E855.2	E938.5	E950.4	E962.0	E980.4
Ortho-Novum	962.2	E858.0	E932.2	E950.4	E962.0	E980.4
Orthotolidine (reagent)	977.8	E858.8	E947.8	E950.4	E962.0	E980.4
Osmic acid (liquid)	983.1	E864.1	—	E950.7	E962.1	E980.6
fumes	987.8	E869.8	—	E952.8	E962.2	E982.8
Osmotic diuretics	974.4	E858.5	E944.4	E950.4	E962.0	E980.4
Ouabain	972.1	E858.3	E942.1	E950.4	E962.0	E980.4
Ovarian hormones (synthetic substitutes)	962.2	E858.0	E932.2	E950.4	E962.0	E980.4
Ovral	962.2	E858.0	E932.2	E950.4	E962.0	E980.4

TABLE OF DRUGS AND CHEMICALS

Substance	Poisoning	External Cause (E Code)				
		Accident	Therapeutic Use	Suicide Attempt	Assault	Undetermined
Ovulation suppressants	962.2	E858.0	E932.2	E950.4	E962.0	E980.4
Ovulen	962.2	E858.0	E932.2	E950.4	E962.0	E980.4
Oxacillin (sodium)	960.0	E856	E930.0	E950.4	E962.0	E980.4
Oxalic acid	983.1	E864.1	—	E950.7	E962.1	E980.6
Oxanamide	969.5	E853.8	E939.5	E950.3	E962.0	E980.3
Oxandrolone	962.1	E858.0	E932.1	E950.4	E962.0	E980.4
Oxaprozin	965.61	E850.6	E935.6	E950.0	E962.0	E980.0
Oxazepam	969.4	E853.2	E939.4	E950.3	E962.0	E980.3
Oxazolidine derivatives	966.0	E855.0	E936.0	E950.4	E962.0	E980.4
Ox bile extract	973.4	E858.4	E943.4	E950.4	E962.0	E980.4
Oxedrine	971.2	E855.5	E941.2	E950.4	E962.0	E980.4
Oxeladin	975.4	E858.6	E945.4	E950.4	E962.0	E980.4
Oxethazaine NEC	968.5	E855.2	E938.5	E950.4	E962.0	E980.4
Oxidizing agents NEC	983.9	E864.3	—	E950.7	E962.1	E980.6
Oxolinic acid	961.3	E857	E931.3	E950.4	E962.0	E980.4
Oxophenarsine	961.1	E857	E931.1	E950.4	E962.0	E980.4
Oxsoralen	976.3	E858.7	E946.3	E950.4	E962.0	E980.4
Oxtriphylline	976.7	E858.6	E945.7	E950.4	E962.0	E980.4
Oxybuprocaine	968.5	E855.2	E938.5	E950.4	E962.0	E980.4
Oxybutynin	975.1	E858.6	E945.1	E950.4	E962.0	E980.4
Oxycodone	965.09	E850.2	E935.2	E950.0	E962.0	E980.0
Oxygen	987.8	E869.8	—	E952.8	E962.2	E982.8
Oxylone	976.0	E858.7	E946.0	E950.4	E962.0	E980.4
ophthalmic preparation	976.5	E858.7	E946.5	E950.4	E962.0	E980.4
Oxymesterone	962.1	E858.0	E932.1	E950.4	E962.0	E980.4
Oxymetazoline	971.2	E855.5	E941.2	E950.4	E962.0	E980.4
Oxymetholone	962.1	E858.0	E932.1	E950.4	E962.0	E980.4
Oxymorphone	965.09	E850.2	E935.2	E950.0	E962.0	E980.0
Oxypertine	969.09	E854.0	E939.0	E950.3	E962.0	E980.3
Oxyphenbutazone	965.5	E850.5	E935.5	E950.0	E962.0	E980.0
Oxyphencyclimine	971.1	E855.4	E941.1	E950.4	E962.0	E980.4
Oxyphenisatin	973.1	E858.4	E943.1	E950.4	E962.0	E980.4
Oxyphenonium	971.1	E855.4	E941.1	E950.4	E962.0	E980.4
Oxyquinoline	961.3	E857	E931.3	E950.4	E962.0	E980.4
Oxytetracycline	960.4	E856	E930.4	E950.4	E962.0	E980.4
Oxytocics	975.0	E858.6	E945.0	E950.4	E962.0	E980.4
Oxytocin	975.0	E858.6	E945.0	E950.4	E962.0	E980.4
Ozone	987.8	E869.8	—	E952.8	E962.2	E982.8
PABA	976.3	E858.7	E946.3	E950.4	E962.0	E980.4

◄ New ◄▮▮ Revised ~~deleted~~ Deleted ● Use Additional Digit(s)

Substance	Poisoning	External Cause (E Code)				
		Accident	Therapeutic Use	Suicide Attempt	Assault	Undetermined
Packed red cells	964.7	E858.2	E934.7	E950.4	E962.0	E980.4
Paint NEC	989.89	E861.6	—	E950.9	E962.1	E980.9
cleaner	982.8	E862.9	—	E950.9	E962.1	E980.9
fumes NEC	987.8	E869.8	—	E952.8	E962.1	E982.8
lead (fumes)	984.0	E861.5	—	E950.9	E962.1	E980.9
solvent NEC	982.8	E862.9	—	E950.9	E962.1	E980.9
stripper	982.8	E862.9	—	E950.9	E962.1	E980.9
Palfium	965.09	E850.2	E935.2	E950.0	E962.0	E980.0
Palivizumab	979.9	E858.8	E949.6	E950.4	E962.0	E980.4
Paludrine	961.4	E857	E931.4	E950.4	E962.0	E980.4
PAM	977.2	E855.8	E947.2	E950.4	E962.0	E980.4
Pamaquine (napthoate)	961.4	E857	E931.4	E950.4	E962.0	E980.4
Pamprin	965.1	E850.3	E935.3	E950.0	E962.0	E980.0
Panadol	965.4	E850.4	E935.4	E950.0	E962.0	E980.0
Pancreatic dornase (mucolytic)	963.4	E858.1	E933.4	E950.4	E962.0	E980.4
Pancreatin	973.4	E858.4	E943.4	E950.4	E962.0	E980.4
Pancrelipase	973.4	E858.4	E943.4	E950.4	E962.0	E980.4
Pangamic acid	963.5	E858.1	E933.5	E950.4	E962.0	E980.4
Panthenol	963.5	E858.1	E933.5	E950.4	E962.0	E980.4
topical	976.8	E858.7	E946.8	E950.4	E962.0	E980.4
Pantopaque	977.8	E858.8	E947.8	E950.4	E962.0	E980.4
Pantopon	965.00	E850.2	E935.2	E950.0	E962.0	E980.0
Pantothenic acid	963.5	E858.1	E933.5	E950.4	E962.0	E980.4
Panwarfin	964.2	E858.2	E934.2	E950.4	E962.0	E980.4
Papain	973.4	E858.4	E943.4	E950.4	E962.0	E980.4
Papaverine	972.5	E858.3	E942.5	E950.4	E962.0	E980.4
Para-aminobenzoic acid	976.3	E858.7	E946.3	E950.4	E962.0	E980.4
Para-aminophenol derivatives	965.4	E850.4	E935.4	E950.0	E962.0	E980.0
Para-aminosalicylic acid (derivatives)	961.8	E857	E931.8	E950.4	E962.0	E980.4
Paracetaldehyde (medicinal)	967.2	E852.1	E937.2	E950.2	E962.0	E980.2
Paracetamol	965.4	E850.4	E935.4	E950.0	E962.0	E980.0
Paracodin	965.09	E850.2	E935.2	E950.0	E962.0	E980.0
Paradione	966.0	E855.0	E936.0	E950.4	E962.0	E980.4
Paraffin(s) (wax)	981	E862.3	—	E950.9	E962.1	E980.9
liquid (medicinal)	973.2	E858.4	E943.2	E950.4	E962.0	E980.4
nonmedicinal (oil)	981	E962.1	—	E950.9	E962.1	E980.9
Paraldehyde (medicinal)	967.2	E852.1	E937.2	E950.2	E962.0	E980.2
Paramethadione	966.0	E855.0	E936.0	E950.4	E962.0	E980.4
Paramethasone	962.0	E858.0	E932.0	E950.4	E962.0	E980.4

Substance	Poisoning	External Cause (E Code)				
		Accident	Therapeutic Use	Suicide Attempt	Assault	Undetermined
Paraquat	989.4	E863.5	—	E950.6	E962.1	E980.7
Parasympatholytics	971.1	E855.4	E941.1	E950.4	E962.0	E980.4
Parasympathomimetics	971.0	E855.3	E941.0	E950.4	E962.0	E980.4
Parathion	989.3	E863.1	—	E950.6	E962.1	E980.7
Parathormone	962.6	E858.0	E932.6	E950.4	E962.0	E980.4
Parathyroid (derivatives)	962.6	E858.0	E932.6	E950.4	E962.0	E980.4
Paratyphoid vaccine	978.1	E858.8	E948.1	E950.4	E962.0	E980.4
Paredrine	971.2	E855.5	E941.2	E950.4	E962.0	E980.4
Paregoric	965.00	E850.2	E935.2	E950.0	E962.0	E980.0
Pargyline	972.3	E858.3	E942.3	E950.4	E962.0	E980.4
Paris green	985.1	E866.3	—	E950.8	E962.1	E980.8
insecticide	985.1	E863.4	—	E950.8	E962.1	E980.8
Parnate	969.01	E854.0	E939.0	E950.3	E962.0	E980.3
Paromomycin	960.8	E856	E930.8	E950.4	E962.0	E980.4
Paroxypropione	963.1	E858.1	E933.1	E950.4	E962.0	E980.4
Parzone	965.09	E850.2	E935.2	E950.0	E962.0	E980.0
PAS	961.8	E857	E931.8	E950.4	E962.0	E980.4
PCBs	981	E862.3	—	E950.9	E962.1	E980.9
PCP (pentachlorophenol)	989.4	E863.6	—	E950.6	E962.1	E980.7
herbicide	989.4	E863.5	—	E950.6	E962.1	E980.7
insecticide	989.4	E863.4	—	E950.6	E962.1	E980.7
phencyclidine	968.3	E855.1	E938.3	E950.4	E962.0	E980.4
Peach kernel oil (emulsion)	973.2	E858.4	E943.2	E950.4	E962.0	E980.4
Peanut oil (emulsion) NEC	973.2	E858.4	E943.2	E950.4	E962.0	E980.4
topical	976.3	E858.7	E946.3	E950.4	E962.0	E980.4
Pearly Gates (morning glory seeds)	969.6	E854.1	E939.6	E950.3	E962.0	E980.3
Pecazine	969.1	E853.0	E939.1	E950.3	E962.0	E980.3
Pecilocin	960.1	E856	E930.1	E950.4	E962.0	E980.4
Pectin (with kaolin) NEC	973.5	E858.4	E943.5	E950.4	E962.0	E980.4
Pelletierine tannate	961.6	E857	E931.6	E950.4	E962.0	E980.4
Pemoline	969.79	E854.2	E939.7	E950.3	E962.0	E980.3
Pempidine	972.3	E858.3	E942.3	E950.4	E962.0	E980.4
Penamecillin	960.0	E856	E930.0	E950.4	E962.0	E980.4
Penethamate hydriodide	960.0	E856	E930.0	E950.4	E962.0	E980.4
Penicillamine	963.8	E858.1	E933.8	E950.4	E962.0	E980.4
Penicillin (any type)	960.0	E856	E930.0	E950.4	E962.0	E980.4
Penicillinase	963.4	E858.1	E933.4	E950.4	E962.0	E980.4
Pentachlorophenol (fungicide)	989.4	E863.6	—	E950.6	E962.1	E980.7
herbicide	989.4	E863.5	—	E950.6	E962.1	E980.7
insecticide	989.4	E863.4	—	E950.6	E962.1	E980.7

◀ New   ◀▥ Revised   ~~deleted~~ Deleted   ● Use Additional Digit(s)

Substance	Poisoning	External Cause (E Code)				
		Accident	Therapeutic Use	Suicide Attempt	Assault	Undetermined
Pentaerythritol	972.4	E858.3	E942.4	E950.4	E962.0	E980.4
chloral	967.1	E852.0	E937.1	E950.2	E962.0	E980.2
tetranitrate NEC	972.4	E858.3	E942.4	E950.4	E962.0	E980.4
Pentagastrin	977.8	E858.8	E947.8	E950.4	E962.0	E980.4
Pentalin	982.3	E862.4	—	E950.9	E962.1	E980.9
Pentamethonium (bromide)	972.3	E858.3	E942.3	E950.4	E962.0	E980.4
Pentamidine	961.5	E857	E931.5	E950.4	E962.0	E980.4
Pentanol	980.8	E860.8	—	E950.9	E962.1	E980.9
Pentaquine	961.4	E857	E931.4	E950.4	E962.0	E980.4
Pentazocine	965.8	E850.8	E935.8	E950.0	E962.0	E980.0
Penthienate	971.1	E855.4	E941.1	E950.4	E962.0	E980.4
Pentobarbital, pentobarbitone (sodium)	967.0	E851	E937.0	E950.1	E962.0	E980.1
Pentolinium (tartrate)	972.3	E858.3	E942.3	E950.4	E962.0	E980.4
Pentothal	968.3	E855.1	E938.3	E950.4	E962.0	E980.4
Pentylenetetrazol	970.0	E854.3	E940.0	E950.4	E962.0	E980.4
Pentylsalicylamide	961.8	E857	E931.8	E950.4	E962.0	E980.4
Pepsin	973.4	E858.4	E943.4	E950.4	E962.0	E980.4
Peptavlon	977.8	E858.8	E947.8	E950.4	E962.0	E980.4
Percaine (spinal)	968.7	E855.2	E938.7	E950.4	E962.0	E980.4
topical (surface)	968.5	E855.2	E938.5	E950.4	E962.0	E980.4
Perchloroethylene (vapor)	982.3	E862.4	—	E950.9	E962.1	E980.9
medicinal	961.6	E857	E931.6	E950.4	E962.0	E980.4
Percodan	965.09	E850.2	E935.2	E950.0	E962.0	E980.0
Percogesic	965.09	E850.2	E935.2	E950.0	E962.0	E980.0
Percorten	962.0	E858.0	E932.0	E950.4	E962.0	E980.4
Pergonal	962.4	E858.0	E932.4	E950.4	E962.0	E980.4
Perhexiline	972.4	E858.3	E942.4	E950.4	E962.0	E980.4
Periactin	963.0	E858.1	E933.0	E950.4	E962.0	E980.4
Periclor	967.1	E852.0	E937.1	E950.2	E962.0	E980.2
Pericyazine	969.1	E853.0	E939.1	E950.3	E962.0	E980.3
Peritrate	972.4	E858.3	E942.4	E950.4	E962.0	E980.4
Permanganates NEC	983.9	E864.3	—	E950.7	E962.1	E980.6
potassium (topical)	976.0	E858.7	E946.0	E950.4	E962.0	E980.4
Pernocton	967.0	E851	E937.0	E950.1	E962.0	E980.1
Pernoston	967.0	E851	E937.0	E950.1	E962.0	E980.1
Peronin(e)	965.09	E850.2	E935.2	E950.0	E962.0	E980.0
Perphenazine	969.1	E853.0	E939.1	E950.3	E962.0	E980.3
Pertofrane	969.05	E854	E939.0	E950.3	E962.0	E980.3

◄ New   ⬅ Revised   ~~deleted~~ Deleted   ● Use Additional Digit(s)

Substance	Poisoning	External Cause (E Code)				
		Accident	Therapeutic Use	Suicide Attempt	Assault	Undetermined
Pertussis	—	—	—	—	—	—
immune serum (human)	964.6	E858.2	E934.6	E950.4	E962.0	E980.4
vaccine (with diphtheria toxoid) (with tetanus toxoid)	978.6	E858.8	E948.6	E950.4	E962.0	E980.4
Peruvian balsam	976.8	E858.7	E946.8	E950.4	E962.0	E980.4
Pesticides (dust) (fumes) (vapor)	989.4	E863.4	—	E950.6	E962.1	E980.7
arsenic	985.1	E863.4	—	E950.8	E962.1	E980.8
chlorinated	989.2	E863.0	—	E950.6	E962.1	E980.7
cyanide	989.0	E863.4	—	E950.6	E962.1	E980.7
kerosene	981	E863.4	—	E950.6	E962.1	E980.7
mixture (of compounds)	989.4	E863.3	—	E950.6	E962.1	E980.7
naphthalene	983.0	E863.4	—	E950.7	E962.1	E980.6
organochlorine (compounds)	989.2	E863.0	—	E950.6	E962.1	E980.7
petroleum (distillate) (products) NEC	981	E863.4	—	E950.6	E962.1	E980.7
specified ingredient NEC	989.4	E863.4	—	E950.6	E962.1	E980.7
strychnine	989.1	E863.4	—	E950.6	E962.1	E980.7
thallium	985.8	E863.7	—	E950.6	E962.1	E980.7
Pethidine (hydrochloride)	965.09	E850.2	E935.2	E950.0	E962.0	E980.0
Petrichloral	967.1	E852.0	E937.1	E950.2	E962.0	E980.2
Petrol	981	E862.1	—	E950.9	E962.1	E980.9
vapor	987.1	E869.8	—	E952.8	E962.2	E982.8
Petrolatum (jelly) (ointment)	976.3	E858.7	E946.3	E950.4	E962.0	E980.4
hydrophilic	976.3	E858.7	E946.3	E950.4	E962.0	E980.4
liquid	973.2	E858.4	E943.2	E950.4	E962.0	E980.4
topical	976.3	E858.7	E946.3	E950.4	E962.0	E980.4
nonmedicinal	981	E862.1	—	E950.9	E962.1	E980.9
Petroleum (cleaners) (fuels) (products) NEC	981	E862.1	—	E950.9	E962.1	E980.9
benzin(e) - *see* Ligroin	—	—	—	—	—	—
ether - *see* Ligroin	—	—	—	—	—	—
jelly - *see* Petrolatum	—	—	—	—	—	—
aphtha - *see* Ligroin	—	—	—	—	—	—
pesticide	981	E863.4	—	E950.6	E962.1	E980.7
solids	981	E862.3	—	E950.9	E962.1	E980.9
solvents	981	E862.0	—	E950.9	E962.1	E980.9
vapor	987.1	E869.8	—	E952.8	E962.2	E982.8
Peyote	969.6	E854.1	E939.6	E950.3	E962.0	E980.3
Phanodorm, phanodorn	967.0	E851	E937.0	E950.1	E962.0	E980.1
Phanquinone, phanquone	961.5	E857	E931.5	E950.4	E962.0	E980.4
Pharmaceutical excipient or adjunct	977.4	E858.8	E947.4	E950.4	E962.0	E980.4
Phenacemide	966.3	E855.0	E936.3	E950.4	E962.0	E980.4

◀ New   ◀▥ Revised   ~~deleted~~ Deleted   ● Use Additional Digit(s)

Substance	Poisoning	External Cause (E Code)				
		Accident	Therapeutic Use	Suicide Attempt	Assault	Undetermined
Phenacetin	965.4	E850.4	E935.4	E950.0	E962.0	E980.0
Phenadoxone	965.09	E850.2	E935.2	E950.0	E962.0	E980.0
Phenaglycodol	969.5	E853.8	E939.5	E950.3	E962.0	E980.3
Phenantoin	966.1	E855.0	E936.1	E950.4	E962.0	E980.4
Phenaphthazine reagent	977.8	E858.8	E947.8	E950.4	E962.0	E980.4
Phenazocine	965.09	E850.2	E935.2	E950.0	E962.0	E980.0
Phenazone	965.5	E850.5	E935.5	E950.0	E962.0	E980.0
Phenazopyridine	976.1	E858.7	E946.1	E950.4	E962.0	E980.4
Phenbenicillin	960.0	E856	E930.0	E950.4	E962.0	E980.4
Phenbutrazate	977.0	E858.8	E947.0	E950.4	E962.0	E980.4
Phencyclidine	968.3	E855.1	E938.3	E950.4	E962.0	E980.4
Phendimetrazine	977.0	E858.8	E947.0	E950.4	E962.0	E980.4
Phenelzine	969.01	E854.0	E939.0	E950.3	E962.0	E980.3
Phenergan	967.8	E852.8	E937.8	E950.2	E962.0	E980.2
Phenethicillin (potassium)	960.0	E856	E930.0	E950.4	E962.0	E980.4
Phenetsal	965.1	E850.3	E935.3	E950.0	E962.0	E980.0
Pheneturide	966.3	E855.0	E936.3	E950.4	E962.0	E980.4
Phenformin	962.3	E858.0	E932.3	E950.4	E962.0	E980.4
Phenglutarimide	971.1	E855.4	E941.1	E950.4	E962.0	E980.4
Phenicarbazide	965.8	E850.8	E935.8	E950.0	E962.0	E980.0
Phenindamine (tartrate)	963.0	E858.1	E933.0	E950.4	E962.0	E980.4
Phenindione	964.2	E858.2	E934.2	E950.4	E962.0	E980.4
Pheniprazine	969.01	E854.0	E939.0	E950.3	E962.0	E980.3
Pheniramine (maleate)	963.0	E858.1	E933.0	E950.4	E962.0	E980.4
Phenmetrazine	977.0	E858.8	E947.0	E950.4	E962.0	E980.4
Phenobal	967.0	E851	E937.0	E950.1	E962.0	E980.1
Phenobarbital	967.0	E851	E937.0	E950.1	E962.0	E980.1
Phenobarbitone	967.0	E851	E937.0	E950.1	E962.0	E980.1
Phenoctide	976.0	E858.7	E946.0	E950.4	E962.0	E980.4
Phenol (derivatives) NEC	983.0	E864.0	—	E950.7	E962.1	E980.6
disinfectant	983.0	E864.0	—	E950.7	E962.1	E980.6
pesticide	989.4	E863.4	—	E950.6	E962.1	E980.7
red	977.8	E858.8	E947.8	E950.4	E962.0	E980.4
Phenolphthalein	973.1	E858.4	E943.1	E950.4	E962.0	E980.4
Phenolsulfonphthalein	977.8	E858.8	E947.8	E950.4	E962.0	E980.4
Phenomorphan	965.09	E850.2	E935.2	E950.0	E962.0	E980.0
Phenonyl	967.0	E851	E937.0	E950.1	E962.0	E980.1
Phenoperidine	965.09	E850.2	E935.2	E950.0	E962.0	E980.0
Phenoquin	974.7	E858.5	E944.7	E950.4	E962.0	E980.4

◀ New   ◀▥ Revised   ~~deleted~~ Deleted   ● Use Additional Digit(s)

Substance	Poisoning	External Cause (E Code)				
		Accident	Therapeutic Use	Suicide Attempt	Assault	Undetermined
Phenothiazines (tranquilizers) NEC	969.1	E853.0	E939.1	E950.3	E962.0	E980.3
insecticide	989.3	E863.4	—	E950.6	E962.1	E980.7
Phenoxybenzamine	971.3	E855.6	E941.3	E950.4	E962.0	E980.4
Phenoxymethyl penicillin	960.0	E856	E930.0	E950.4	E962.0	E980.4
Phenprocoumon	964.2	E858.2	E934.2	E950.4	E962.0	E980.4
Phensuximide	966.2	E855.0	E936.2	E950.4	E962.0	E980.4
Phentermine	977.0	E858.8	E947.0	E950.4	E962.0	E980.4
Phentolamine	971.3	E855.6	E941.3	E950.4	E962.0	E980.4
Phenyl	—	—	—	—	—	—
butazone	965.5	E850.5	E935.5	E950.0	E962.0	E980.0
enediamine	983.0	E864.0	—	E950.7	E962.1	E980.6
hydrazine	983.0	E864.0	—	E950.7	E962.1	E980.6
antineoplastic	963.1	E858.1	E933.1	E950.4	E962.0	E980.4
mercuric compounds - see Mercury	—	—	—	—	—	—
salicylate	976.3	E858.7	E946.3	E950.4	E962.0	E980.4
Phenylephrine	971.2	E855.5	E941.2	E950.4	E962.0	E980.4
Phenylethylbiguanide	962.3	E858.0	E932.3	E950.4	E962.0	E980.4
Phenylpropanolamine	971.2	E855.5	E941.2	E950.4	E962.0	E980.4
Phenylsulfthion	989.3	E863.1	—	E950.6	E962.1	E980.7
Phenyramidol, phenyramidon	965.7	E850.7	E935.7	E950.0	E962.0	E980.0
Phenytoin	966.1	E855.0	E936.1	E950.4	E962.0	E980.4
pHisoHex	976.2	E858.7	E946.2	E950.4	E962.0	E980.4
Pholcodine	965.09	E850.2	E935.2	E950.0	E962.0	E980.0
Phorate	989.3	E863.1	—	E950.6	E962.1	E980.7
Phosdrin	989.3	E863.1	—	E950.6	E962.1	E980.7
Phosgene (gas)	987.8	E869.8	—	E952.8	E962.2	E982.8
Phosphate (tricresyl)	989.89	E866.8	—	E950.9	E962.1	E980.9
organic	989.3	E863.1	—	E950.6	E962.1	E980.7
solvent	982.8	E862.4	—	E950.9	E962.1	E980.9
Phosphine	987.8	E869.8	—	E952.8	E962.2	E982.8
fumigant	987.8	E863.8	—	E950.6	E962.2	E980.7
Phospholine	971.0	E855.3	E941.0	E950.4	E962.0	E980.4
Phosphoric acid	983.1	E864.1	—	E950.7	E962.1	E980.6
Phosphorus (compounds) NEC	983.9	E864.3	—	E950.7	E962.1	E980.6
rodenticide	983.9	E863.7	—	E950.7	E962.1	E980.6
Phthalimidoglutarimide	967.8	E852.8	E937.8	E950.2	E962.0	E980.2
Phthalylsulfathiazole	961.0	E857	E931.0	E950.4	E962.0	E980.4
Phylloquinone	964.3	E858.2	E934.3	E950.4	E962.0	E980.4
Physeptone	965.02	E850.1	E935.1	E950.0	E962.0	E980.0

◀ New ◀▥ Revised ~~deleted~~ Deleted ● Use Additional Digit(s)

Substance	Poisoning	External Cause (E Code)				
		Accident	Therapeutic Use	Suicide Attempt	Assault	Undetermined
Physostigma venenosum	988.2	E865.4	—	E950.9	E962.1	E980.9
Physostigmine	971.0	E855.3	E941.0	E950.4	E962.0	E980.4
Phytolacca decandra	988.2	E865.4	—	E950.9	E962.1	E980.9
Phytomenadione	964.3	E858.2	E934.3	E950.4	E962.0	E980.4
Phytonadione	964.3	E858.2	E934.3	E950.4	E962.0	E980.4
Picric (acid)	983.0	E864.0	—	E950.7	E962.1	E980.6
Picrotoxin	970.0	E854.3	E940.0	E950.4	E962.0	E980.4
Pilocarpine	971.0	E855.3	E941.0	E950.4	E962.0	E980.4
Pilocarpus (jaborandi) extract	971.0	E855.3	E941.0	E950.4	E962.0	E980.4
Pimaricin	960.1	E856	E930.1	E950.4	E962.0	E980.4
Piminodine	965.09	E850.2	E935.2	E950.0	E962.0	E980.0
Pine oil, pinesol (disinfectant)	983.9	E861.4	—	E950.7	E962.1	E980.6
Pinkroot	961.6	E857	E931.6	E950.4	E962.0	E980.4
Pipadone	965.09	E850.2	E935.2	E950.0	E962.0	E980.0
Pipamazine	963.0	E858.1	E933.0	E950.4	E962.0	E980.4
Pipazethate	975.4	E858.6	E945.4	E950.4	E962.0	E980.4
Pipenzolate	971.1	E855.4	E941.1	E950.4	E962.0	E980.4
Piperacetazine	969.1	E853.0	E939.1	E950.3	E962.0	E980.3
Piperazine NEC	961.6	E857	E931.6	E950.4	E962.0	E980.4
estrone sulfate	962.2	E858.0	E932.2	E950.4	E962.0	E980.4
Piper cubeba	988.2	E865.4	—	E950.9	E962.1	E980.9
Piperidione	975.4	E858.6	E945.4	E950.4	E962.0	E980.4
Piperidolate	971.1	E855.4	E941.1	E950.4	E962.0	E980.4
Piperocaine	968.9	E855.2	E938.9	E950.4	E962.0	E980.4
infiltration (subcutaneous)	968.5	E855.2	E938.5	E950.4	E962.0	E980.4
nerve block (peripheral) (plexus)	968.6	E855.2	E938.6	E950.4	E962.0	E980.4
topical (surface)	968.5	E855.2	E938.5	E950.4	E962.0	E980.4
Pipobroman	963.1	E858.1	E933.1	E950.4	E962.0	E980.4
Pipradrol	970.89 ◀ⅢⅢ	E854.3	E940.8	E950.4	E962.0	E980.4
Piscidia (bark) (erythrina)	965.7	E850.7	E935.7	E950.0	E962.0	E980.0
Pitch	983.0	E864.0	—	E950.7	E962.1	E980.6
Pitkin's solution	968.7	E855.2	E938.7	E950.4	E962.0	E980.4
Pitocin	975.0	E858.6	E945.0	E950.4	E962.0	E980.4
Pitressin (tannate)	962.5	E858.0	E932.5	E950.4	E962.0	E980.4
Pituitary extracts (posterior)	962.5	E858.0	E932.5	E950.4	E962.0	E980.4
anterior	962.4	E858.0	E932.4	E950.4	E962.0	E980.4
Pituitrin	962.5	E858.0	E932.5	E950.4	E962.0	E980.4
Placental extract	962.9	E858.0	E932.9	E950.4	E962.0	E980.4
Placidyl	967.8	E852.8	E937.8	E950.2	E962.0	E980.2

◀ New   ◀ⅢⅢ Revised   ~~deleted~~ Deleted   ● Use Additional Digit(s)

TABLE OF DRUGS AND CHEMICALS

Substance	Poisoning	External Cause (E Code)				
		Accident	Therapeutic Use	Suicide Attempt	Assault	Undetermined
Plague vaccine	978.3	E858.8	E948.3	E950.4	E962.0	E980.4
Plant foods or fertilizers NEC	989.89	E866.5	—	E950.9	E962.1	E980.9
mixed with herbicides	989.4	E863.5	—	E950.6	E962.1	E930.7
Plants, noxious, used as food	988.2	E865.9	—	E950.9	E962.1	E980.9
berries and seeds	988.2	E865.3	—	E950.9	E962.1	E980.9
specified type NEC	988.2	E865.4	—	E950.9	E962.1	E980.9
Plasma (blood)	964.7	E858.2	E934.7	E950.4	E962.0	E980.4
expanders	964.8	E858.2	E934.8	E950.4	E962.0	E980.4
Plasmanate	964.7	E858.2	E934.7	E950.4	E962.0	E980.4
Plegicil	969.1	E853.0	E939.1	E950.3	E962.0	E980.3
Podophyllin	976.4	E858.7	E946.4	E950.4	E962.0	E980.4
Podophyllum resin	976.4	E858.7	E946.4	E950.4	E962.0	E980.4
Poison NEC	989.9	E866.9	—	E950.9	E962.1	E980.9
Poisonous berries	988.2	E865.3	—	E950.9	E962.1	E980.9
Pokeweed (any part)	988.2	E865.4	—	E950.9	E962.1	E980.9
Poldine	971.1	E855.4	E941.1	E950.4	E962.0	E980.4
Poliomyelitis vaccine	979.5	E858.8	E949.5	E950.4	E962.0	E980.4
Poliovirus vaccine	979.5	E858.8	E949.5	E950.4	E962.0	E980.4
Polish (car) (floor) (furniture) (metal) (silver)	989.89	E861.2	—	E950.9	E962.1	E980.9
abrasive	989.89	E861.3	—	E950.9	E962.1	E980.9
porcelain	989.89	E861.3	—	E950.9	E962.1	E980.9
Poloxalkol	973.2	E858.4	E943.2	E950.4	E962.0	E980.4
Polyaminostyrene resins	974.5	E858.5	E944.5	E950.4	E962.0	E980.4
Polychlorinated biphenyl - see PCBs	—	—	—	—	—	—
Polycycline	960.4	E856	E930.4	E950.4	E962.0	E980.4
Polyester resin hardener	982.8	E862.4	—	E950.9	E962.1	E980.9
fumes	987.8	E869.8	—	E952.8	E962.2	E982.8
Polyestradiol (phosphate)	962.2	E858.0	E932.2	E950.4	E962.0	E980.4
Polyethanolamine alkyl sulfate	976.2	E858.7	E946.2	E950.4	E962.0	E980.4
Polyethylene glycol	976.3	E858.7	E946.3	E950.4	E962.0	E980.4
Polyferose	964.0	E858.2	E934.0	E950.4	E962.0	E980.4
Polymyxin B	960.8	E856	E930.8	E950.4	E962.0	E980.4
ENT agent	976.6	E858.7	E946.6	E950.4	E962.0	E980.4
ophthalmic preparation	976.5	E858.7	E946.5	E950.4	E962.0	E980.4
topical NEC	976.0	E858.7	E946.0	E950.4	E962.0	E980.4
Polynoxylin(e)	976.0	E858.7	E946.0	E950.4	E962.0	E980.4
Polyoxymethyleneurea	976.0	E858.7	E946.0	E950.4	E962.0	E980.4
Polytetrafluoroethylene (inhaled)	987.8	E869.8	—	E952.8	E962.2	E982.8
Polythiazide	974.3	E858.5	E944.3	E950.4	E962.0	E980.4

◀ New　◀ Revised　deleted Deleted　● Use Additional Digit(s)

Substance	Poisoning	External Cause (E Code)				
		Accident	Therapeutic Use	Suicide Attempt	Assault	Undetermined
Polyvinylpyrrolidone	964.8	E858.2	E934.8	E950.4	E962.0	E980.4
Pontocaine (hydrochloride) (infiltration) (topical)	968.5	E855.2	E938.5	E950.4	E962.0	E980.4
nerve block (peripheral) (plexus)	968.6	E855.2	E938.6	E950.4	E962.0	E980.4
spinal	968.7	E855.2	E938.7	E950.4	E962.0	E980.4
Pot	969.6	E854.1	E939.6	E950.3	E962	E980.3
Potash (caustic)	983.2	E864.2	—	E950.7	E962.1	E980.6
Potassic saline injection (lactated)	974.5	E858.5	E944.5	E950.4	E962.0	E980.4
Potassium (salts) NEC	974.5	E858.5	E944.5	E950.4	E962.0	E980.4
aminosalicylate	961.8	E857	E931.8	E950.4	E962.0	E980.4
arsenite (solution)	985.1	E866.3	—	E950.8	E962.1	E980.8
bichromate	983.9	E864.3	—	E950.7	E962.1	E980.6
bisulfate	983.9	E864.3	—	E950.7	E962.1	E980.6
bromide (medicinal) NEC	967.3	E852.2	E937.3	E950.2	E962.0	E980.2
carbonate	983.2	E864.2	—	E950.7	E962.1	E980.6
chlorate NEC	983.9	E864.3	—	E950.7	E962.1	E980.6
cyanide - *see* Cyanide	—	—	—	—	—	—
hydroxide	983.2	E864.2	—	E950.7	E962.1	E980.6
iodide (expectorant) NEC	975.5	E858.6	E945.5	E950.4	E962.0	E980.4
nitrate	989.89	E866.8	—	E950.9	E962.1	E980.9
oxalate	983.9	E864.3	—	E950.7	E962.1	E980.6
perchlorate NEC	977.8	E858.8	E947.8	E950.4	E962.0	E980.4
antithyroid	962.8	E858.0	E932.8	E950.4	E962.0	E980.4
permanganate	976.0	E858.7	E946.0	E950.4	E962.0	E980.4
nonmedicinal	983.9	E864.3	—	E950.7	E962.1	E980.6
Povidone-iodine (anti-infective) NEC	976.0	E858.7	E946.0	E950.4	E962.0	E980.4
Practolol	972.0	E858.3	E942.0	E950.4	E962.0	E980.4
Pralidoxime (chloride)	977.2	E858.8	E947.2	E950.4	E962.0	E980.4
Pramoxine	968.5	E855.2	E938.5	E950.4	E962.0	E980.4
Prazosin	972.6	E858.3	E942.6	E950.4	E962.0	E980.4
Prednisolone	962.0	E858.0	E932.0	E950.4	E962.0	E980.4
ENT agent	976.6	E858.7	E946.6	E950.4	E962.0	E980.4
ophthalmic preparation	976.5	E858.7	E946.5	E950.4	E962.0	E980.4
topical NEC	976.0	E858.7	E946.0	E950.4	E962.0	E980.4
Prednisone	962.0	E858.0	E932.0	E950.4	E962.0	E980.4
Pregnanediol	962.2	E858.0	E932.2	E950.4	E962.0	E980.4
Pregneninolone	962.2	E858.0	E932.2	E950.4	E962.0	E980.4
Preludin	977.0	E858.8	E947.0	E950.4	E962.0	E980.4
Premarin	962.2	E858.0	E932.2	E950.4	E962.0	E980.4
Prenylamine	972.4	E858.3	E942.4	E950.4	E962.0	E980.4

◀ New　◀▥ Revised　~~deleted~~ Deleted　● Use Additional Digit(s)

Substance	Poisoning	External Cause (E Code)				
		Accident	Therapeutic Use	Suicide Attempt	Assault	Undetermined
Preparation H	976.8	E858.7	E946.8	E950.4	E962.0	E980.4
Preservatives	989.89	E866.8	—	E950.9	E962.1	E980.9
Pride of China	988.2	E865.3	—	E950.9	E962.1	E980.9
Prilocaine	968.9	E855.2	E938.9	E950.4	E962.0	E980.4
infiltration (subcutaneous)	968.5	E855.2	E938.5	E950.4	E962.0	E980.4
nerve block (peripheral) (plexus)	968.6	E855.2	E938.6	E950.4	E962.0	E980.4
Primaquine	961.4	E857	E931.4	E950.4	E962.0	E980.4
Primidone	966.3	E855.0	E936.3	E950.4	E962.0	E980.4
Primula (veris)	988.2	E865.4	—	E950.9	E962.1	E980.9
Prinodol	965.09	E850.2	E935.2	E950.0	E962.0	E980.0
Priscol, Priscoline	971.3	E855.6	E941.3	E950.4	E962.0	E980.4
Privet	988.2	E865.4	—	E950.9	E962.1	E980.9
Privine	971.2	E855.5	E941.2	E950.4	E962.0	E980.4
Pro-Banthine	971.1	E855.4	E941.1	E950.4	E962.0	E980.4
Probarbital	967.0	E851	E937.0	E950.1	E962.0	E980.1
Probenecid	974.7	E858.5	E944.7	E950.4	E962.0	E980.4
Procainamide (hydrochloride)	972.0	E858.3	E942.0	E950.4	E962.0	E980.4
Procaine (hydrochloride) (infiltration) (topical)	968.5	E855.2	E938.5	E950.4	E962.0	E980.4
nerve block (periphreal) (plexus)	968.6	E855.2	E938.6	E950.4	E962.0	E980.4
penicillin G	960.0	E856	E930.0	E950.4	E962.0	E980.4
spinal	968.7	E855.2	E938.7	E950.4	E962.0	E980.4
Procalmidol	969.5	E853.8	E939.5	E950.3	E962.0	E980.3
Procarbazine	963.1	E858.1	E933.1	E950.4	E962.0	E980.4
Prochlorperazine	969.1	E853.0	E939.1	E950.3	E962.0	E980.3
Procyclidine	966.4	E855.0	E936.4	E950.4	E962.0	E980.4
Producer gas	986	E868.8	—	E952.1	E962.2	E982.1
Profenamine	966.4	E855.0	E936.4	E950.4	E962.0	E980.4
Profenil	975.1	E858.6	E945.1	E950.4	E962.0	E980.4
Progesterones	962.2	E858.0	E932.2	E950.4	E962.0	E980.4
Progestin	962.2	E858.0	E932.2	E950.4	E962.0	E980.4
Progestogens (with estrogens)	962.2	E858.0	E932.2	E950.4	E962.0	E980.4
Progestone	962.2	E858.0	E932.2	E950.4	E962.0	E980.4
Proguanil	961.4	E857	E931.4	E950.4	E962.0	E980.4
Prolactin	962.4	E858.0	E932.4	E950.4	E962.0	E980.4
Proloid	962.7	E858.0	E932.7	E950.4	E962.0	E980.4
Proluton	962.2	E858.0	E932.2	E950.4	E962.0	E980.4
Promacetin	961.8	E857	E931.8	E950.4	E962.0	E980.4
Promazine	969.1	E853.0	E939.1	E950.3	E962.0	E980.3
Promedrol	965.09	E850.2	E935.2	E950.0	E962.0	E980.0

◀ New ◀ Revised ~~deleted~~ Deleted ● Use Additional Digit(s)

TABLE OF DRUGS AND CHEMICALS

Substance	External Cause (E Code)					
	Poisoning	Accident	Therapeutic Use	Suicide Attempt	Assault	Undetermined
Promethazine	967.8	E852.8	E937.8	E950.2	E962.0	E980.2
Promine	961.8	E857	E931.8	E950.4	E962.0	E980.4
Pronestyl (hydrochloride)	972.0	E858.3	E942.0	E950.4	E962.0	E980.4
Pronetalol, pronethalol	972.0	E858.3	E942.0	E950.4	E962.0	E980.4
Prontosil	961.0	E857	E931.0	E950.4	E962.0	E980.4
Propamidine isethionate	961.5	E857	E931.5	E950.4	E962.0	E980.4
Propanal (medicinal)	967.8	E852.8	E937.8	E950.2	E962.0	E980.2
Propane (gas) (distributed in mobile container)	987.0	E868.0	—	E951.1	E962.2	E981.1
distributed through pipes	987.0	E867	—	E951.0	E962.2	E981.0
incomplete combustion of - see Carbon monoxide, Propane	—	—	—	—	—	—
Propanidid	968.3	E855.1	E938.3	E950.4	E962.0	E980.4
Propanol	980.3	E860.4	—	E950.9	E962.1	E980.9
Propantheline	971.1	E855.4	E941.1	E950.4	E962.0	E980.4
Proparacaine	968.5	E855.2	E938.5	E950.4	E962.0	E980.4
Propatyl nitrate	972.4	E858.3	E942.4	E950.4	E962.0	E980.4
Propicillin	960.0	E856	E930.0	E950.4	E962.0	E980.4
Propiolactone (vapor)	987.8	E869.8	—	E952.8	E962.2	E982.8
Propiomazine	967.8	E852.8	E937.8	E950.2	E962.0	E980.2
Propionaldehyde (medicinal)	967.8	E852.8	E937.8	E950.2	E962.0	E980.2
Propionate compound	976.0	E858.7	E946.0	E950.4	E962.0	E980.4
Propion gel	976.0	E858.7	E946.0	E950.4	E962.0	E980.4
Propitocaine	968.9	E855.2	E938.9	E950.4	E962.0	E980.4
infiltration (subcutaneous)	968.5	E855.2	E938.5	E950.4	E962.0	E980.4
nerve block (peripheral) (plexus)	968.6	E855.2	E938.6	E950.4	E962.0	E980.4
Propoxur	989.3	E863.2	—	E950.6	E962.1	E980.7
Propoxycaine	968.9	E855.2	E938.9	E950.4	E962.0	E980.4
infiltration (subcutaneous)	968.5	E855.2	E938.5	E950.4	E962.0	E980.4
nerve block (peripheral) (plexus)	968.6	E855.2	E938.6	E950.4	E962.0	E980.4
topical (surface)	968.5	E855.2	E938.5	E950.4	E962.0	E980.4
Propoxyphene (hydrochloride)	965.8	E850.8	E935.8	E950.0	E962.0	E980.0
Propranolol	972.0	E858.3	E942.0	E950.4	E962.0	E980.4
Propyl	—	—	—	—	—	—
alcohol	980.3	E860.4	—	E950.9	E962.1	E980.9
carbinol	980.3	E860.4	—	E950.9	E962.1	E980.9
hexadrine	971.2	E855.5	E941.2	E950.4	E962.0	E980.4
iodone	977.8	E858.8	E947.8	E950.4	E962.0	E980.4
thiouracil	962.8	E858.0	E932.8	E950.4	E962.0	E980.4
Propylene	987.1	E869.8	—	E952.8	E962.2	E982.8
Propylparaben (ophthalmic)	976.5	E858.7	E946.5	E950.4	E962.0	E980.4

◀ New   ◀▥ Revised   ~~deleted~~ Deleted   ● Use Additional Digit(s)   649

TABLE OF DRUGS AND CHEMICALS

Substance	Poisoning	External Cause (E Code) Accident	Therapeutic Use	Suicide Attempt	Assault	Undetermined
Proscillaridin	972.1	E858.3	E942.1	E950.4	E962.0	E980.4
Prostaglandins	975.0	E858.6	E945.0	E950.4	E962.0	E980.4
Prostigmin	971.0	E855.3	E941.0	E950.4	E962.0	E980.4
Protamine (sulfate)	964.5	E858.2	E934.5	E950.4	E962.0	E980.4
zinc insulin	962.3	E858.0	E932.3	E950.4	E962.0	E980.4
Protectants (topical)	976.3	E858.7	E946.3	E950.4	E962.0	E980.4
Protein hydrolysate	974.5	E858.5	E944.5	E950.4	E962.0	E980.4
Prothiaden - *see* Dothiepin hydrochloride	—	—	—	—	—	—
Prothionamide	961.8	E857	E931.8	E950.4	E962.0	E980.4
Prothipendyl	969.5	E853.8	E939.5	E950.3	E962.0	E980.3
Protokylol	971.2	E855.5	E941.2	E950.4	E962.0	E980.4
Protopam	977.2	E858.8	E947.2	E950.4	E962.0	E980.4
Protoveratrine(s) (A) (B)	972.6	E858.3	E942.6	E950.4	E962.0	E980.4
Protriptyline	969.05	E854.0	E939.0	E950.3	E962.0	E980.3
Provera	962.2	E858.0	E932.2	E950.4	E962.0	E980.4
Provitamin A	963.5	E858.1	E933.5	E950.4	E962.0	E980.4
Proxymetacaine	968.5	E855.2	E938.5	E950.4	E962.0	E980.4
Proxyphylline	975.1	E858.6	E945.1	E950.4	E962.0	E980.4
Prozac - *see* Fluoxetine hydrochloride	—	—	—	—	—	—
Prunus	—	—	—	—	—	—
laurocerasus	988.2	E865.4	—	E950.9	E962.1	E980.9
virginiana	988.2	E865.4	—	E950.9	E962.1	E980.9
Prussic acid	989.0	E866.8	—	E950.9	E962.1	E980.9
vapor	987.7	E869.8	—	E952.8	E962.2	E982.8
Pseudoephedrine	971.2	E855.5	E941.2	E950.4	E962.0	E980.4
Psilocin	969.6	E854.1	E939.6	E950.3	E962.0	E980.3
Psilocybin	969.6	E854.1	E939.6	E950.3	E962.0	E980.3
PSP	977.8	E858.8	E947.8	E950.4	E962.0	E980.4
Psychedelic agents	969.6	E854.1	E939.6	E950.3	E962.0	E980.3
Psychodysleptics	969.6	E854.1	E939.6	E950.3	E962.0	E980.3
Psychostimulants	969.70	E854.2	E939.7	E950.3	E962.0	E980.3
Psychotherapeutic agents	969.9	E855.9	E939.9	E950.3	E962.0	E980.3
antidepressants	969.00	E854.0	E939.0	E950.3	E962.0	E980.3
specified NEC	969.8	E855.8	E939.8	E950.3	E962.0	E980.3
tranquilizers NEC	969.5	E853.9	E939.5	E950.3	E962.0	E980.3
Psychotomimetic agents	969.6	E854.1	E939.6	E950.3	E962.0	E980.3
Psychotropic agents	969.9	E854.8	E939.9	E950.3	E962.0	E980.3
specified NEC	969.8	E854.8	E939.8	E950.3	E962.0	E980.3
Psyllium	973.3	E858.4	E943.3	E950.4	E962.0	E980.4

◄ New ◄▥ Revised ~~deleted~~ Deleted ● Use Additional Digit(s)

Substance	Poisoning	External Cause (E Code)				
		Accident	Therapeutic Use	Suicide Attempt	Assault	Undetermined
Pteroylglutamic acid	964.1	E858.2	E934.1	E950.4	E962.0	E980.4
Pteroyltriglutamate	963.1	E858.1	E933.1	E950.4	E962.0	E980.4
PTFE	987.8	E869.8	—	E952.8	E962.2	E982.8
Pulsatilla	988.2	E865.4	—	E950.9	E962.1	E980.9
Purex (bleach)	983.9	E864.3	—	E950.7	E962.1	E980.6
Purine diuretics	974.1	E858.5	E944.1	E950.4	E962.0	E980.4
Purinethol	963.1	E858.1	E933.1	E950.4	E962.0	E980.4
PVP	964.8	E858.2	E934.8	E950.4	E962.0	E980.4
Pyrabital	965.7	E850.7	E935.7	E950.0	E962.0	E980.0
Pyramidon	965.5	E850.5	E935.5	E950.0	E962.0	E980.0
Pyrantel (pamoate)	961.6	E857	E931.6	E950.4	E962.0	E980.4
Pyrathiazine	963.0	E858.1	E933.0	E950.4	E962.0	E980.4
Pyrazinamide	961.8	E857	E931.8	E950.4	E962.0	E980.4
Pyrazinoic acid (amide)	961.8	E857	E931.8	E950.4	E962.0	E980.4
Pyrazole (derivatives)	965.5	E850.5	E935.5	E950.0	E962.0	E980.0
Pyrazolone (analgesics)	965.5	E850.5	E935.5	E950.0	E962.0	E980.0
Pyrethrins, pyrethrum	989.4	E863.4	—	E950.6	E962.1	E980.7
Pyribenzamine	963.0	E858.1	E933.0	E950.4	E962.0	E980.4
Pyridine (liquid) (vapor)	982.0	E862.4	—	E950.9	E962.1	E980.9
aldoxime chloride	977.2	E858.8	E947.2	E950.4	E962.0	E980.4
Pyridium	976.1	E858.7	E946.1	E950.4	E962.0	E980.4
Pyridostigmine	971.0	E855.3	E941.0	E950.4	E962.0	E980.4
Pyridoxine	963.5	E858.1	E933.5	E950.4	E962.0	E980.4
Pyrilamine	963.0	E858.1	E933.0	E950.4	E962.0	E980.4
Pyrimethamine	961.4	E857	E931.4	E950.4	E962.0	E980.4
Pyrogallic acid	983.0	E864.0	—	E950.7	E962.1	E980.6
Pyroxylin	976.3	E858.7	E946.3	E950.4	E962.0	E980.4
Pyrrobutamine	963.0	E858.1	E933.0	E950.4	E962.0	E980.4
Pyrrocitine	968.5	E855.2	E938.5	E950.4	E962.0	E980.4
Pyrvinium (pamoate)	961.6	E857	E931.6	E950.4	E962.0	E980.4
PZI	962.3	E858.0	E932.3	E950.4	E962.0	E980.4
Quaalude	967.4	E852.3	E937.4	E950.2	E962.0	E980.2
Quaternary ammonium derivatives	971.1	E855.4	E941.1	E950.4	E962.0	E980.4
Quicklime	983.2	E864.2	—	E950.7	E962.1	E980.6
Quinacrine	961.3	E857	E931.3	E950.4	E962.0	E980.4
Quinaglute	972.0	E858.3	E942.0	E950.4	E962.0	E980.4
Quinalbarbitone	967.0	E851	E937.0	E950.1	E962.0	E980.1
Quinestradiol	962.2	E858.0	E932.2	E950.4	E962.0	E980.4
Quinethazone	974.3	E858.5	E944.3	E950.4	E962.0	E980.4

◄ New   ◄▥ Revised   ~~deleted~~ Deleted   ● Use Additional Digit(s)

TABLE OF DRUGS AND CHEMICALS

Substance	Poisoning	External Cause (E Code)				
		Accident	Therapeutic Use	Suicide Attempt	Assault	Undetermined
Quinidine (gluconate) (polygalacturonate) (salts) (sulfate)	972.0	E858.3	E942.0	E950.4	E962.0	E980.4
Quinine	961.4	E857	E931.4	E950.4	E962.0	E980.4
Quiniobine	961.3	E857	E931.3	E950.4	E962.0	E980.4
Quinolines	961.3	E857	E931.3	E950.4	E962.0	E980.4
Quotane	968.5	E855.2	E938.5	E950.4	E962.0	E980.4
Rabies	—	—	—	—	—	—
immune globulin (human)	964.6	E858.2	E934.6	E950.4	E962.0	E980.4
vaccine	979.1	E858.8	E949.1	E950.4	E962.0	E980.4
Racemoramide	965.09	E850.2	E935.2	E950.0	E962.0	E980.0
Racemorphan	965.09	E850.2	E935.2	E950.0	E962.0	E980.0
Radiator alcohol	980.1	E860.2	—	E950.9	E962.1	E980.9
Radio-opaque (drugs) (materials)	977.8	E858.8	E947.8	E950.4	E962.0	E980.4
Ranunculus	988.2	E865.4	—	E950.9	E962.1	E980.9
Rat poison	989.4	E863.7	—	E950.6	E962.1	E980.7
Rattlesnake (venom)	989.5	E905.0	—	E950.9	E962.1	E980.9
Raudixin	972.6	E858.3	E942.6	E950.4	E962.0	E980.4
Rautensin	972.6	E858.3	E942.6	E950.4	E962.0	E980.4
Rautina	972.6	E858.3	E942.6	E950.4	E962.0	E980.4
Rautotal	972.6	E858.3	E942.6	E950.4	E962.0	E980.4
Rauwiloid	972.6	E858.3	E942.6	E950.4	E962.0	E980.4
Rauwoldin	972.6	E858.3	E942.6	E950.4	E962.0	E980.4
Rauwolfia (alkaloids)	972.6	E858.3	E942.6	E950.4	E962.0	E980.4
Realgar	985.1	E866.3	—	E950.8	E962.1	E980.8
Red cells, packed	964.7	E858.2	E934.7	E950.4	E962.0	E980.4
Reducing agents, industrial NEC	983.9	E864.3	—	E950.7	E962.1	E980.6
Refrigerant gas (freon)	987.4	E869.2	—	E952.8	E962.2	E982.8
not freon	987.9	E869.9	—	E952.9	E962.2	E982.9
Regroton	974.4	E858.5	E944.4	E950.4	E962.0	E980.4
Rela	968.0	E855.1	E938.0	E950.4	E962.0	E980.4
Relaxants, skeletal muscle (autonomic)	975.2	E858.6	E945.2	E950.4	E962.0	E980.4
central nervous system	968.0	E855.1	E938.0	E950.4	E962.0	E980.4
Renese	974.3	E858.5	E944.3	E950.4	E962.0	E980.4
Renografin	977.8	E858.8	E947.8	E950.4	E962.0	E980.4
Replacement solutions	974.5	E858.5	E944.5	E950.4	E962.0	E980.4
Rescinnamine	972.6	E858.3	E942.6	E950.4	E962.0	E980.4
Reserpine	972.6	E858.3	E942.6	E950.4	E962.0	E980.4
Resorcin, resorcinol	976.4	E858.7	E946.4	E950.4	E962.0	E980.4
Respaire	975.5	E858.6	E945.5	E950.4	E962.0	E980.4
Respiratory agents NEC	975.8	E858.6	E945.8	E950.4	E962.0	E980.4

◀ New   ◀▦ Revised   ~~deleted~~ Deleted   ● Use Additional Digit(s)

Substance	Poisoning	External Cause (E Code)				
		Accident	Therapeutic Use	Suicide Attempt	Assault	Undetermined
Retinoic acid	976.8	E858.7	E946.8	E950.4	E962.0	E980.4
Retinol	963.5	E858.1	E933.5	E950.4	E962.0	E980.4
Rh (D) immune globulin (human)	964.6	E858.2	E934.6	E950.4	E962.0	E980.4
Rhodine	965.1	E850.3	E935.3	E950.0	E962.0	E980.0
RhoGAM	964.6	E858.2	E934.6	E950.4	E962.0	E980.4
Riboflavin	963.5	E858.1	E933.5	E950.4	E962.0	E980.4
Ricin	989.89	E866.8	—	E950.9	E962.1	E980.9
Ricinus communis	988.2	E865.3	—	E950.9	E962.1	E980.9
Rickettsial vaccine NEC	979.6	E858.8	E949.6	E950.4	E962.0	E980.4
with viral and bacterial vaccine	979.7	E858.8	E949.7	E950.4	E962.0	E980.4
Rifampin	960.6	E856	E930.6	E950.4	E962.0	E980.4
Rimifon	961.8	E857	E931.8	E950.4	E962.0	E980.4
Ringer's injection (lactated)	974.5	E858.5	E944.5	E950.4	E962.0	E980.4
Ristocetin	960.8	E856	E930.8	E950.4	E962.0	E980.4
Ritalin	969.73	E854.2	E939.7	E950.3	E962.0	E980.3
Roach killers - see Pesticides	—	—	—	—	—	—
Rocky Mountain spotted fever vaccine	979.6	E858.8	E949.6	E950.4	E962.0	E980.4
Rodenticides	989.4	E863.7	—	E950.6	E962.1	E980.7
Rohypnol	969.4	E853.2	E939.4	E950.3	E962.0	E980.3
Rolaids	973.0	E858.4	E943.0	E950.4	E962.0	E980.4
Rolitetracycline	960.4	E856	E930.4	E950.4	E962.0	E980.4
Romilar	975.4	E858.6	E945.4	E950.4	E962.0	E980.4
Rose water ointment	976.3	E858.7	E946.3	E950.4	E962.0	E980.4
Rotenone	989.4	E863.7	—	E950.6	E962.1	E980.7
Rotoxamine	963.0	E858.1	E933.0	E950.4	E962.0	E980.4
Rough-on-rats	989.4	E863.7	—	E950.6	E962.1	E980.7
RU486	962.9	E858.0	E932.9	E950.4	E962.0	E980.4
Rubbing alcohol	980.2	E860.3	—	E950.9	E962.1	E980.9
Rubella virus vaccine	979.4	E858.8	E949.4	E950.4	E962.0	E980.4
Rubelogen	979.4	E858.8	E949.4	E950.4	E962.0	E980.4
Rubeovax	979.4	E858.8	E949.4	E950.4	E962.0	E980.4
Rubidomycin	960.7	E856	E930.7	E950.4	E962.0	E980.4
Rue	988.2	E865.4	—	E950.9	E962.1	E980.9
Ruta	988.2	E865.4	—	E950.9	E962.1	E980.9
Sabadilla (medicinal)	976.0	E858.7	E946.0	E950.4	E962.0	E980.4
pesticide	989.4	E863.4	—	E950.6	E962.1	E980.7
Sabin oral vaccine	979.5	E858.8	E949.5	E950.4	E962.0	E980.4
Saccharated iron oxide	964.0	E858.2	E934.0	E950.4	E962.0	E980.4
Saccharin	974.5	E858.5	E944.5	E950.4	E962.0	E980.4

Substance	Poisoning	External Cause (E Code) Accident	External Cause (E Code) Therapeutic Use	External Cause (E Code) Suicide Attempt	External Cause (E Code) Assault	External Cause (E Code) Undetermined
Safflower oil	972.2	E858.3	E942.2	E950.4	E962.0	E980.4
Salbutamol sulfate	975.7	E858.6	E945.7	E950.4	E962.0	E980.4
Salicylamide	965.1	E850.3	E935.3	E950.0	E962.0	E980.0
Salicylate(s)	965.1	E850.3	E935.3	E950.0	E962.0	E980.0
methyl	976.3	E858.7	E946.3	E950.4	E962.0	E980.4
theobromine calcium	974.1	E858.5	E944.1	E950.4	E962.0	E980.4
Salicylazosulfapyridine	961.0	E857	E931.0	E950.4	E962.0	E980.4
Salicylhydroxamic acid	976.0	E858.7	E946.0	E950.4	E962.0	E980.4
Salicylic acid (keratolytic) NEC	976.4	E858.7	E946.4	E950.4	E962.0	E980.4
congeners	965.1	E850.3	E935.3	E950.0	E962.0	E980.0
salts	965.1	E850.3	E935.3	E950.0	E962.0	E980.0
Saliniazid	961.8	E857	E931.8	E950.4	E962.0	E980.4
Salol	976.3	E858.7	E946.3	E950.4	E962.0	E980.4
Salt (substitute) NEC	974.5	E858.5	E944.5	E950.4	E962.0	E980.4
Saluretics	974.3	E858.5	E944.3	E950.4	E962.0	E980.4
Saluron	974.3	E858.5	E944.3	E950.4	E962.0	E980.4
Salvarsan 606 (neosilver) (silver)	961.1	E857	E931.1	E950.4	E962.0	E980.4
Sambucus canadensis	988.2	E865.4	—	E950.9	E962.1	E980.9
berry	988.2	E865.3	—	E950.9	E962.1	E980.9
Sandril	972.6	E858.3	E942.6	E950.4	E962.0	E980.4
Sanguinaria canadensis	988.2	E865.4	—	E950.9	E962.1	E980.9
Saniflush (cleaner)	983.9	E861.3	—	E950.7	E962.1	E980.6
Santonin	961.6	E857	E931.6	E950.4	E962.0	E980.4
Santyl	976.8	E858.7	E946.8	E950.4	E962.0	E980.4
Sarkomycin	960.7	E856	E930.7	E950.4	E962.0	E980.4
Saroten	969.05	E854.0	E939.0	E950.3	E962.0	E980.3
Saturnine - see Lead	—	—	—	—	—	—
Savin (oil)	976.4	E858.7	E946.4	E950.4	E962.0	E980.4
Scammony	973.1	E858.4	E943.1	E950.4	E962.0	E980.4
Scarlet red	976.8	E858.7	E946.8	E950.4	E962.0	E980.4
Scheele's green	985.1	E866.3	—	E950.8	E962.1	E980.8
insecticide	985.1	E863.4	—	E950.8	E962.1	E980.8
Schradan	989.3	E863.1	—	E950.6	E962.1	E980.7
Schweinfurt(h) green	985.1	E866.3	—	E950.8	E962.1	E980.8
insecticide	985.1	E863.4	—	E950.8	E962.1	E980.8
Scilla - see Squill	—	—	—	—	—	—
Sclerosing agents	972.7	E858.3	E942.7	E950.4	E962.0	E980.4
Scopolamine	971.1	E855.4	E941.1	E950.4	E962.0	E980.4
Scouring powder	989.89	E861.3	—	E950.9	E962.1	E980.9

◀ New　◀▥ Revised　~~deleted~~ Deleted　● Use Additional Digit(s)

Substance	Poisoning	External Cause (E Code)				
		Accident	Therapeutic Use	Suicide Attempt	Assault	Undetermined
Sea	—	—	—	—	—	—
anemone (sting)	989.5	E905.6	—	E950.9	E962.1	E980.9
cucumber (sting)	989.5	E905.6	—	E950.9	E962.1	E980.9
snake (bite) (venom)	989.5	E905.0	—	E950.9	E962.1	E980.9
urchin spine (puncture)	989.5	E905.6	—	E950.9	E962.1	E980.9
Secbutabarbital	967.0	E851	E937.0	E950.1	E962.0	E980.1
Secbutabarbitone	967.0	E851	E937.0	E950.1	E962.0	E980.1
Secobarbital	967.0	E851	E937.0	E950.1	E962.0	E980.1
Seconal	967.0	E851	E937.0	E950.1	E962.0	E980.1
Secretin	977.8	E858.8	E947.8	E950.4	E962.0	E980.4
Sedatives, nonbarbiturate	967.9	E852.9	E937.9	E950.2	E962.0	E980.2
specified NEC	967.8	E852.8	E937.8	E950.2	E962.0	E980.2
Sedormid	967.8	E852.8	E937.8	E950.2	E962.0	E980.2
Seed (plant)	988.2	E865.3	—	E950.9	E962.1	E980.9
disinfectant or dressing	989.89	E866.5	—	E950.9	E962.1	E980.9
Selective serotonin and norepinephrine reuptake inhibitors (SSNRI)	969.02	E854.0	E939.0	E950.3	E962.0	E980.3
Selective serotonin reuptake inhibitors (SSRI)	969.03	E854.0	E939.0	E950.3	E962.0	E980.3
Selenium (fumes) NEC	985.8	E866.4	—	E950.9	E962.1	E980.9
disulfide or sulfide	976.4	E858.7	E946.4	E950.4	E962.0	E980.4
Selsun	976.4	E858.7	E946.4	E950.4	E962.0	E980.4
Senna	973.1	E858.4	E943.1	E950.4	E962.0	E980.4
Septisol	976.2	E858.7	E946.2	E950.4	E962.0	E980.4
Serax	969.4	E853.2	E939.4	E950.3	E962.0	E980.3
Serenesil	967.8	E852.8	E937.8	E950.2	E962.0	E980.2
Serenium (hydrochloride)	961.9	E857	E931.9	E950.4	E962.0	E980.4
Serepax - *see* Oxazepam	—	—	—	—	—	—
Sernyl	968.3	E855.1	E938.3	E950.4	E962.0	E980.4
Serotonin	977.8	E858.8	E947.8	E950.4	E962.0	E980.4
Serpasil	972.6	E858.3	E942.6	E950.4	E962.0	E980.4
Sewer gas	987.8	E869.8	—	E952.8	E962.2	E982.8
Shampoo	989.6	E861.0	—	E950.9	E962.1	E980.9
Shellfish, nonbacterial or noxious	988.0	E865.1	—	E950.9	E962.1	E980.9
Silicones NEC	989.83	E866.8	E947.8	E950.9	E962.1	E980.9
Silvadene	976.0	E858.7	E946.0	E950.4	E962.0	E980.4
Silver (compound) (medicinal) NEC	976.0	E858.7	E946.0	E950.4	E962.0	E980.4
anti-infectives	976.0	E858.7	E946.0	E950.4	E962.0	E980.4
arsphenamine	961.1	E857	E931.1	E950.4	E962.0	E980.4
nitrate	976.0	E858.7	E946.0	E950.4	E962.0	E980.4
ophthalmic preparation	976.5	E858.7	E946.5	E950.4	E962.0	E980.4
toughened (keratolytic)	976.4	E858.7	E946.4	E950.4	E962.0	E980.4

TABLE OF DRUGS AND CHEMICALS

Substance	Poisoning	External Cause (E Code)				
		Accident	Therapeutic Use	Suicide Attempt	Assault	Undetermined
Silver (compound) (medicinal) NEC *(Continued)*						
nonmedicinal (dust)	985.8	E866.4	—	E950.9	E962.1	E980.9
protein (mild) (strong)	976.0	E858.7	E946.0	E950.4	E962.0	E980.4
salvarsan	961.1	E857	E931.1	E950.4	E962.0	E980.4
Simethicone	973.8	E858.4	E943.8	E950.4	E962.0	E980.4
Sinequan	969.05	E854.0	E939.0	E950.3	E962.0	E980.3
Singoserp	972.6	E858.3	E942.6	E950.4	E962.0	E980.4
Sintrom	964.2	E858.2	E934.2	E950.4	E962.0	E980.4
Sitosterols	972.2	E858.3	E942.2	E950.4	E962.0	E980.4
Skeletal muscle relaxants	975.2	E858.6	E945.2	E950.4	E962.0	E980.4
Skin	—	—	—	—	—	—
agents (external)	976.9	E858.7	E946.9	E950.4	E962.0	E980.4
specified NEC	976.8	E858.7	E946.8	E950.4	E962.0	E980.4
test antigen	977.8	E858.8	E947.8	E950.4	E962.0	E980.4
Sleep-eze	963.0	E858.1	E933.0	E950.4	E962.0	E980.4
Sleeping draught (drug) (pill) (tablet)	967.9	E852.9	E937.9	E950.2	E962.0	E980.2
Smallpox vaccine	979.0	E858.8	E949.0	E950.4	E962.0	E980.4
Smelter fumes NEC	985.9	E866.4	—	E950.9	E962.1	E980.9
Smog	987.3	E869.1	—	E952.8	E962.2	E982.8
Smoke NEC	987.9	E869.9	—	E952.9	E962.2	E982.9
Smooth muscle relaxant	975.1	E858.6	E945.1	E950.4	E962.0	E980.4
Snail killer	989.4	E863.4	—	E950.6	E962.1	E980.7
Snake (bite) (venom)	989.5	E905.0	—	E950.9	E962.1	E980.9
Snuff	989.89	E866.8	—	E950.9	E962.1	E980.9
Soap (powder) (product)	989.6	E861.1	—	E950.9	E962.1	E980.9
medicinal, soft	976.2	E858.7	E946.2	E950.4	E962.0	E980.4
Soda (caustic)	983.2	E864.2	—	E950.7	E962.1	E980.6
bicarb	963.3	E858.1	E933.3	E950.4	E962.0	E980.4
chlorinated - *see* Sodium, hypochlorite	—	—	—	—	—	—
Sodium	—	—	—	—	—	—
acetosulfone	961.8	E857	E931.8	E950.4	E962.0	E980.4
acetrizoate	977.8	E858.8	E947.8	E950.4	E962.0	E980.4
amytal	967.0	E851	E937.0	E950.1	E962.0	E980.1
arsenate - *see* Arsenic	—	—	—	—	—	—
bicarbonate	963.3	E858.1	E933.3	E950.4	E962.0	E980.4
bichromate	983.9	E864.3	—	E950.7	E962.1	E980.6
biphosphate	963.2	E858.1	E933.2	E950.4	E962.0	E980.4
bisulfate	983.9	E864.3	—	E950.7	E962.1	E980.6
borate (cleanser)	989.6	E861.3	—	E950.9	E962.1	E980.9
bromide NEC	967.3	E852.2	E937.3	E950.2	E962.0	E980.2

◄ New   ◀▥ Revised   ~~deleted~~ Deleted   ● Use Additional Digit(s)

	External Cause (E Code)					
Substance	Poisoning	Accident	Therapeutic Use	Suicide Attempt	Assault	Undetermined
Sodium *(Continued)*						
cacodylate (nonmedicinal) NEC	978.8	E858.8	E948.8	E950.4	E962.0	E980.4
anti-infective	961.1	E857	E931.1	E950.4	E962.0	E980.4
herbicide	989.4	E863.5	—	E950.6	E962.1	E980.7
calcium edetate	963.8	E858.1	E933.8	E950.4	E962.0	E980.4
carbonate NEC	983.2	E864.2	—	E950.7	E962.1	E980.6
chlorate NEC	983.9	E864.3	—	E950.7	E962.1	E980.6
herbicide	983.9	E863.5	—	E950.7	E962.1	E980.6
chloride NEC	974.5	E858.5	E944.5	E950.4	E962.0	E980.4
chromate	983.9	E864.3	—	E950.7	E962.1	E980.6
citrate	963.3	E858.1	E933.3	E950.4	E962.0	E980.4
cyanide - *see* Cyanide(s)	—	—	—	—	—	—
cyclamate	974.5	E858.5	E944.5	E950.4	E962.0	E980.4
diatrizoate	977.8	E858.8	E947.8	E950.4	E962.0	E980.4
dibunate	975.4	E858.6	E945.4	E950.4	E962.0	E980.4
dioctyl sulfosuccinate	973.2	E858.4	E943.2	E950.4	E962.0	E980.4
edetate	963.8	E858.1	E933.8	E950.4	E962.0	E980.4
ethacrynate	974.4	E858.5	E944.4	E950.4	E962.0	E980.4
fluoracetate (dust) (rodenticide)	989.4	E863.7	—	E950.6	E962.1	E980.7
fluoride - *see* Fluoride(s)	—	—	—	—	—	—
free salt	974.5	E858.5	E944.5	E950.4	E962.0	E980.4
glucosulfone	961.8	E857	E931.8	E950.4	E962.0	E980.4
hydroxide	983.2	E864.2	—	E950.7	E962.1	E980.6
hypochlorite (bleach) NEC	983.9	E864.3	—	E950.7	E962.1	E980.6
disinfectant	983.9	E861.4	—	E950.7	E962.1	E980.6
medicinal (anti-infective) (external)	976.0	E858.7	E946.0	E950.4	E962.0	E980.4
vapor	987.8	E869.8	—	E952.8	E962.2	E982.8
hyposulfite	976.0	E858.7	E946.0	E950.4	E962.0	E980.4
indigotindisulfonate	977.8	E858.8	E947.8	E950.4	E962.0	E980.4
iodide	977.8	E858.8	E947.8	E950.4	E962.0	E980.4
iothalamate	977.8	E858.8	E947.8	E950.4	E962.0	E980.4
iron edetate	964.0	E858.2	E934.0	E950.4	E962.0	E980.4
lactate	963.3	E858.1	E933.3	E950.4	E962.0	E980.4
lauryl sulfate	976.2	E858.7	E946.2	E950.4	E962.0	E980.4
L-triiodothyronine	962.7	E858.0	E932.7	E950.4	E962.0	E980.4
metrizoate	977.8	E858.8	E947.8	E950.4	E962.0	E980.4
monofluoracetate (dust) (rodenticide)	989.4	E863.7	—	E950.6	E962.1	E980.7
morrhuate	972.7	E858.3	E942.7	E950.4	E962.0	E980.4
nafcillin	960.0	E856	E930.0	E950.4	E962.0	E980.4

Substance	Poisoning	External Cause (E Code)				
		Accident	Therapeutic Use	Suicide Attempt	Assault	Undetermined
Sodium (Continued)						
nitrate (oxidizing agent)	983.9	E864.3	—	E950.7	E962.1	E980.6
nitrite (medicinal)	972.4	E858.3	E942.4	E950.4	E962.0	E980.4
nitroferricyanide	972.6	E858.3	E942.6	E950.4	E962.0	E980.4
nitroprusside	972.6	E858.3	E942.6	E950.4	E962.0	E980.4
para-aminohippurate	977.8	E858.8	E947.8	E950.4	E962.0	E980.4
perborate (nonmedicinal) NEC	989.89	E866.8	—	E950.9	E962.1	E980.9
medicinal	976.6	E858.7	E946.6	E950.4	E962.0	E980.4
soap	989.6	E861.1	—	E950.9	E962.1	E980.9
percarbonate - see Sodium, perborate	—	—	—	—	—	—
phosphate	973.3	E858.4	E943.3	E950.4	E962.0	E980.4
polystyrene sulfonate	974.5	E858.5	E944.5	E950.4	E962.0	E980.4
propionate	976.0	E858.7	E946.0	E950.4	E962.0	E980.4
psylliate	972.7	E858.3	E942.7	E950.4	E962.0	E980.4
removing resins	974.5	E858.5	E944.5	E950.4	E962.0	E980.4
salicylate	965.1	E850.3	E935.3	E950.0	E962.0	E980.0
sulfate	973.3	E858.4	E943.3	E950.4	E962.0	E980.4
sulfoxone	961.8	E857	E931.8	E950.4	E962.0	E980.4
tetradecyl sulfate	972.7	E858.3	E942.7	E950.4	E962.0	E980.4
thiopental	968.3	E855.1	E938.3	E950.4	E962.0	E980.4
thiosalicylate	965.1	E850.3	E935.3	E950.0	E962.0	E980.0
thiosulfate	976.0	E858.7	E946.0	E950.4	E962.0	E980.4
tolbutamide	977.8	E858.8	E947.8	E950.4	E962.0	E980.4
tyropanoate	977.8	E858.8	E947.8	E950.4	E962.0	E980.4
valproate	966.3	E855.0	E936.3	E950.4	E962.0	E980.4
Solanine	977.8	E858.8	E947.8	E950.4	E962.0	E980.4
Solanum dulcamara	988.2	E865.4	—	E950.9	E962.1	E980.9
Solapsone	961.8	E857	E931.8	E950.4	E962.0	E980.4
Solasulfone	961.8	E857	E931.8	E950.4	E962.0	E980.4
Soldering fluid	983.1	E864.1	—	E950.7	E962.1	E980.6
Solid substance	989.9	E866.9	—	E950.9	E962.1	E980.9
specified NEC	989.9	E866.8	—	E950.9	E962.1	E980.9
Solvents, industrial	982.8	E862.9	—	E950.9	E962.1	E980.9
naphtha	981	E862.0	—	E950.9	E962.1	E980.9
petroleum	981	E862.0	—	E950.9	E962.1	E980.9
specified NEC	982.8	E862.4	—	E950.9	E962.1	E980.9
Soma	968.0	E855.1	E938.0	E950.4	E962.0	E980.4
Somatotropin	962.4	E858.0	E932.4	E950.4	E962.0	E980.4
Sominex	963.0	E858.1	E933.0	E950.4	E962.0	E980.4

◀ New   ◀⁞⁞⁞ Revised   ~~deleted~~ Deleted   ● Use Additional Digit(s)

Substance	Poisoning	External Cause (E Code)				
		Accident	Therapeutic Use	Suicide Attempt	Assault	Undetermined
Somnos	967.1	E852.0	E937.1	E950.2	E962.0	E980.2
Somonal	967.0	E851	E937.0	E950.1	E962.0	E980.1
Soneryl	967.0	E851	E937.0	E950.1	E962.0	E980.1
Soothing syrup	977.9	E858.9	E947.9	E950.5	E962.0	E980.5
Sopor	967.4	E852.3	E937.4	E950.2	E962.0	E980.2
Soporific drug	967.9	E852.9	E937.9	E950.2	E962.0	E980.2
specified type NEC	967.8	E852.8	E937.8	E950.2	E962.0	E980.2
Sorbitol NEC	977.4	E858.8	E947.4	E950.4	E962.0	E980.4
Sotradecol	972.7	E858.3	E942.7	E950.4	E962.0	E980.4
Spacoline	975.1	E858.6	E945.1	E950.4	E962.0	E980.4
Spanish fly	976.8	E858.7	E946.8	E950.4	E962.0	E980.4
Sparine	969.1	E853.0	E939.1	E950.3	E962.0	E980.3
Sparteine	975.0	E858.6	E945.0	E950.4	E962.0	E980.4
Spasmolytics	975.1	E858.6	E945.1	E950.4	E962.0	E980.4
anticholinergics	971.1	E855.4	E941.1	E950.4	E962.0	E980.4
Spectinomycin	960.8	E856	E930.8	E950.4	E962.0	E980.4
Speed	969.72	E854.2	E939.7	E950.3	E962.0	E980.3
Spermicides	976.8	E858.7	E946.8	E950.4	E962.0	E980.4
Spider (bite) (venom)	989.5	E905.1	—	E950.9	E962.1	E980.9
antivenin	979.9	E858.8	E949.9	E950.4	E962.0	E980.4
Spigelia (root)	961.6	E857	E931.6	E950.4	E962.0	E980.4
Spiperone	969.2	E853.1	E939.2	E950.3	E962.0	E980.3
Spiramycin	960.3	E856	E930.3	E950.4	E962.0	E980.4
Spirilene	969.5	E853.8	E939.5	E950.3	E962.0	E980.3
Spirit(s) (neutral) NEC	980.0	E860.1	—	E950.9	E962.1	E980.9
beverage	980.0	E860.0	—	E950.9	E962.1	E980.9
industrial	980.9	E860.9	—	E950.9	E962.1	E980.9
mineral	981	E862.0	—	E950.9	E962.1	E980.9
of salt - *see* Hydrochloric acid	—	—	—	—	—	—
surgical	980.9	E860.9	—	E950.9	E962.1	E980.9
Spironolactone	974.4	E858.5	E944.4	E950.4	E962.0	E980.4
Sponge, absorbable (gelatin)	964.5	E858.2	E934.5	E950.4	E962.0	E980.4
Sporostacin	976.0	E858.7	E946.0	E950.4	E962.0	E980.4
Sprays (aerosol)	989.89	E866.8	—	E950.9	E962.1	E980.9
cosmetic	989.89	E866.7	—	E950.9	E962.1	E980.9
medicinal NEC	977.9	E858.9	E947.9	E950.5	E962.0	E980.5
pesticides - *see* Pesticides	—	—	—	—	—	—
specified content - *see* substance specified	—	—	—	—	—	—
Spurge flax	988.2	E865.4	—	E950.9	E962.1	E980.9

TABLE OF DRUGS AND CHEMICALS

TABLE OF DRUGS AND CHEMICALS

Substance	Poisoning	External Cause (E Code)				
		Accident	Therapeutic Use	Suicide Attempt	Assault	Undetermined
Spurges	988.2	E865.4	—	E950.9	E962.1	E980.9
Squill (expectorant) NEC	975.5	E858.6	E945.5	E950.4	E962.0	E980.4
rat poison	989.4	E863.7	—	E950.6	E962.1	E980.7
Squirting cucumber (cathartic)	973.1	E858.4	E943.1	E950.4	E962.0	E980.4
SSNRI (selective serotonin and norepinephrine reuptake inhibitors)	969.02	E854.0	E939.0	E950.3	E962.0	E980.3
SSRI (selective serotonin reuptake inhibitors)	969.03	E854.0	E939.0	E950.3	E962.0	E980.3
Stains	989.89	E866.8	—	E950.9	E962.1	E980.9
Stannous - see also Tin fluoride	976.7	E858.7	E946.7	E950.4	E962.0	E980.4
Stanolone	962.1	E858.0	E932.1	E950.4	E962.0	E980.4
Stanozolol	962.1	E858.0	E932.1	E950.4	E962.0	E980.4
Staphisagria or stavesacre (pediculicide)	976.0	E858.7	E946.0	E950.4	E962.0	E980.4
Stelazine	969.1	E853.0	E939.1	E950.3	E962.0	E980.3
Stemetil	969.1	E853.0	E939.1	E950.3	E962.0	E980.3
Sterculia (cathartic) (gum)	973.3	E858.4	E943.3	E950.4	E962.0	E980.4
Sternutator gas	987.8	E869.8	—	E952.8	E962.2	E982.8
Steroids NEC	962.0	E858.0	E932.0	E950.4	E962.0	E980.4
ENT agent	976.6	E858.7	E946.6	E950.4	E962.0	E980.4
ophthalmic preparation	976.5	E858.7	E946.5	E950.4	E962.0	E980.4
topical NEC	976.0	E858.7	E946.0	E950.4	E962.0	E980.4
Stibine	985.8	E866.4	—	E950.9	E962.1	E980.9
Stibophen	961.2	E857	E931.2	E950.4	E962.0	E980.4
Stilbamide, stilbamidine	961.5	E857	E931.5	E950.4	E962.0	E980.4
Stilbestrol	962.2	E858.0	E932.2	E950.4	E962.0	E980.4
Stimulants (central nervous system)	970.9	E854.3	E940.9	E950.4	E962.0	E980.4
analeptics	970.0	E854.3	E940.0	E950.4	E962.0	E980.4
opiate antagonist	970.1	E854.3	E940.1	E950.4	E962.0	E980.4
psychotherapeutic NEC	969.09	E854.0	E939.0	E950.3	E962.0	E980.3
specified NEC	970.89 ◀▥	E854.3	E940.8	E950.4	E962.0	E980.4
Storage batteries (acid) (cells)	983.1	E864.1	—	E950.7	E962.1	E980.6
Stovaine	968.9	E855.2	E938.9	E950.4	E962.0	E980.4
infiltration (subcutaneous)	968.5	E855.2	E938.5	E950.4	E962.0	E980.4
nerve block (peripheral) (plexus)	968.6	E855.2	E938.6	E950.4	E962.0	E980.4
spinal	968.7	E855.2	E938.7	E950.4	E962.0	E980.4
topical (surface)	968.5	E855.2	E938.5	E950.4	E962.0	E980.4
Stovarsal	961.1	E857	E931.1	E950.4	E962.0	E980.4
Stove gas - see Gas, utility	—	—	—	—	—	—
Stoxil	976.5	E858.7	E946.5	E950.4	E962.0	E980.4
STP	969.6	E854.1	E939.6	E950.3	E962.0	E980.3
Stramonium (medicinal) NEC	971.1	E855.4	E941.1	E950.4	E962.0	E980.4
natural state	988.2	E865.4	—	E950.9	E962.1	E980.9

◀ New ◀▥ Revised ~~deleted~~ Deleted ● Use Additional Digit(s)

Substance	Poisoning	External Cause (E Code)				
		Accident	Therapeutic Use	Suicide Attempt	Assault	Undetermined
Streptodornase	964.4	E858.2	E934.4	E950.4	E962.0	E980.4
Streptoduocin	960.6	E856	E930.6	E950.4	E962.0	E980.4
Streptokinase	964.4	E858.2	E934.4	E950.4	E962.0	E980.4
Streptomycin	960.6	E856	E930.6	E950.4	E962.0	E980.4
Streptozocin	960.7	E856	E930.7	E950.4	E962.0	E980.4
Stripper (paint) (solvent)	982.8	E862.9	—	E950.9	E962.1	E980.9
Strobane	989.2	E863.0	—	E950.6	E962.1	E980.7
Strophanthin	972.1	E858.3	E942.1	E950.4	E962.0	E980.4
Strophanthus hispidus or kombe	988.2	E865.4	—	E950.9	E962.1	E980.9
Strychnine (rodenticide) (salts)	989.1	E863.7	—	E950.6	E962.1	E980.7
medicinal NEC	970.89 ◀━	E854.3	E940.8	E950.4	E962.0	E980.4
Strychnos (ignatii) - *see* Strychnine	—	—	—	—	—	—
Styramate	968.0	E855.1	E938.0	E950.4	E962.0	E980.4
Styrene	983.0	E864.0	—	E950.7	E962.1	E980.6
Succinimide (anticonvulsant)	966.2	E855.0	E936.2	E950.4	E962.0	E980.4
mercuric - *see* Mercury	—	—	—	—	—	—
Succinylcholine	975.2	E858.6	E945.2	E950.4	E962.0	E980.4
Succinylsulfathiazole	961.0	E857	E931.0	E950.4	E962.0	E980.4
Sucrose	974.5	E858.5	E944.5	E950.4	E962.0	E980.4
Sulfacetamide	961.0	E857	E931.0	E950.4	E962.0	E980.4
ophthalmic preparation	976.5	E858.7	E946.5	E950.4	E962.0	E980.4
Sulfachlorpyridazine	961.0	E857	E931.0	E950.4	E962.0	E980.4
Sulfacytine	961.0	E857	E931.0	E950.4	E962.0	E980.4
Sulfadiazine	961.0	E857	E931.0	E950.4	E962.0	E980.4
silver (topical)	976.0	E858.7	E946.0	E950.4	E962.0	E980.4
Sulfadimethoxine	961.0	E857	E931.0	E950.4	E962.0	E980.4
Sulfadimidine	961.0	E857	E931.0	E950.4	E962.0	E980.4
Sulfaethidole	961.0	E857	E931.0	E950.4	E962.0	E980.4
Sulfafurazole	961.0	E857	E931.0	E950.4	E962.0	E980.4
Sulfaguanidine	961.0	E857	E931.0	E950.4	E962.0	E980.4
Sulfamerazine	961.0	E857	E931.0	E950.4	E962.0	E980.4
Sulfameter	961.0	E857	E931.0	E950.4	E962.0	E980.4
Sulfamethizole	961.0	E857	E931.0	E950.4	E962.0	E980.4
Sulfamethoxazole	961.0	E857	E931.0	E950.4	E962.0	E980.4
Sulfamethoxydiazine	961.0	E857	E931.0	E950.4	E962.0	E980.4
Sulfamethoxypyridazine	961.0	E857	E931.0	E950.4	E962.0	E980.4
Sulfamethylthiazole	961.0	E857	E931.0	E950.4	E962.0	E980.4
Sulfamylon	976.0	E858.7	E946.0	E950.4	E962.0	E980.4
Sulfan blue (diagnostic dye)	977.8	E858.8	E947.8	E950.4	E962.0	E980.4
Sulfanilamide	961.0	E857	E931.0	E950.4	E962.0	E980.4

TABLE OF DRUGS AND CHEMICALS

Substance	Poisoning	External Cause (E Code)				
		Accident	Therapeutic Use	Suicide Attempt	Assault	Undetermined
Sulfanilylguanidine	961.0	E857	E931.0	E950.4	E962.0	E980.4
Sulfaphenazole	961.0	E857	E931.0	E950.4	E962.0	E980.4
Sulfaphenylthiazole	961.0	E857	E931.0	E950.4	E962.0	E980.4
Sulfaproxyline	961.0	E857	E931.0	E950.4	E962.0	E980.4
Sulfapyridine	961.0	E857	E931.0	E950.4	E962.0	E980.4
Sulfapyrimidine	961.0	E857	E931.0	E950.4	E962.0	E980.4
Sulfarsphenamine	961.1	E857	E931.1	E950.4	E962.0	E980.4
Sulfasalazine	961.0	E857	E931.0	E950.4	E962.0	E980.4
Sulfasomizole	961.0	E857	E931.0	E950.4	E962.0	E980.4
Sulfasuxidine	961.0	E857	E931.0	E950.4	E962.0	E980.4
Sulfinpyrazone	974.7	E858.5	E944.7	E950.4	E962.0	E980.4
Sulfisoxazole	961.0	E857	E931.0	E950.4	E962.0	E980.4
ophthalmic preparation	976.5	E858.7	E946.5	E950.4	E962.0	E980.4
Sulfomyxin	960.8	E856	E930.8	E950.4	E962.0	E980.4
Sulfonal	967.8	E852.8	E937.8	E950.2	E962.0	E980.2
Sulfonamides (mixtures)	961.0	E857	E931.0	E950.4	E962.0	E980.4
Sulfones	961.8	E857	E931.8	E950.4	E962.0	E980.4
Sulfonethylmethane	967.8	E852.8	E937.8	E950.2	E962.0	E980.2
Sulfonmethane	967.8	E852.8	E937.8	E950.2	E962.0	E980.2
Sulfonphthal, sulfonphthol	977.8	E858.8	E947.8	E950.4	E962.0	E980.4
Sulfonylurea derivatives, oral	962.3	E858.0	E932.3	E950.4	E962.0	E980.4
Sulfoxone	961.8	E857	E931.8	E950.4	E962.0	E980.4
Sulfur, sulfureted, sulfuric, sulfurous, sulfuryl (compounds) NEC	989.89	E866.8	—	E950.9	E962.1	E980.9
acid	983.1	E864.1	—	E950.7	E962.1	E980.6
dioxide	987.3	E869.1	—	E952.8	E962.2	E982.8
ether - see Ether(s)	—	—	—	—	—	—
hydrogen	987.8	E869.8	—	E952.8	E962.2	E982.8
medicinal (keratolytic) (ointment) NEC	976.4	E858.7	E946.4	E950.4	E962.0	E980.4
pesticide (vapor)	989.4	E863.4	—	E950.6	E962.1	E980.7
vapor NEC	987.8	E869.8	—	E952.8	E962.2	E982.8
Sulkowitch's reagent	977.8	E858.8	E947.8	E950.4	E962.0	E980.4
Sulph - see also Sulf-	—	—	—	—	—	—
Sulphadione	961.8	E857	E931.8	E950.4	E962.0	E980.4
Sulthiame, sultiame	966.3	E855.0	E936.3	E950.4	E962.0	E980.4
Superinone	975.5	E858.6	E945.5	E950.4	E962.0	E980.4
Suramin	961.5	E857	E931.5	E950.4	E962.0	E980.4
Surfacaine	968.5	E855.2	E938.5	E950.4	E962.0	E980.4
Surital	968.3	E855.1	E938.3	E950.4	E962.0	E980.4
Sutilains	976.8	E858.7	E946.8	E950.4	E962.0	E980.4

◀ New   ◀||| Revised   ~~deleted~~ Deleted   ● Use Additional Digit(s)

TABLE OF DRUGS AND CHEMICALS

Substance	Poisoning	External Cause (E Code)				
		Accident	Therapeutic Use	Suicide Attempt	Assault	Undetermined
Suxamethonium (bromide) (chloride) (iodide)	975.2	E858.6	E945.2	E950.4	E962.0	E980.4
Suxethonium (bromide)	975.2	E858.6	E945.2	E950.4	E962.0	E980.4
Sweet oil (birch)	976.3	E858.7	E946.3	E950.4	E962.0	E980.4
Sym-dichloroethyl ether	982.3	E862.4	—	E950.9	E962.1	E980.9
Sympatholytics	971.3	E855.6	E941.3	E950.4	E962.0	E980.4
Sympathomimetics	971.2	E855.5	E941.2	E950.4	E962.0	E980.4
Synagis	979.6	E858.8	E949.6	E950.4	E962.0	E980.4
Synalar	976.0	E858.7	E946.0	E950.4	E962.0	E980.4
Synthroid	962.7	E858.0	E932.7	E950.4	E962.0	E980.4
Syntocinon	975.0	E858.6	E945.0	E950.4	E962.0	E950.4
Syrosingopine	972.6	E858.3	E942.6	E950.4	E962.0	E980.4
Systemic agents (primarily)	963.9	E858.1	E933.9	E950.4	E962.0	E980.4
specified NEC	963.8	E858.1	E933.8	E950.4	E962.0	E980.4
Tablets (*see also* specified substance)	977.9	E858.9	E947.9	E950.5	E962.0	E980.5
Tace	962.2	E858.0	E932.2	E950.4	E962.0	E980.4
Tacrine	971.0	E855.3	E941.0	E950.4	E962.0	E980.4
Talbutal	967.0	E851	E937.0	E950.1	E962.0	E980.1
Talc	976.3	E858.7	E946.3	E950.4	E962.0	E980.4
Talcum	976.3	E858.7	E946.3	E950.4	E962.0	E980.4
Tamsulosin	971.3	E855.6	E941.3	E950.4	E962.0	E980.4
Tandearil, tanderil	965.5	E850.5	E935.5	E950.0	E962.0	E980.0
Tannic acid	983.1	E864.1	—	E950.7	E962.1	E980.6
medicinal (astringent)	976.2	E858.7	E946.2	E950.4	E962.0	E980.4
Tannin - *see* Tannic acid	—	—	—	—	—	—
Tansy	988.2	E865.4	—	E950.9	E962.1	E980.9
TAO	960.3	E856	E930.3	E950.4	E962.0	E980.4
Tapazole	962.8	E858.0	E932.8	E950.4	E962.0	E980.4
Tar NEC	983.0	E864.0	—	E950.7	E962.1	E980.6
camphor - *see* Naphthalene	—	—	—	—	—	—
fumes	987.8	E869.8	—	E952.8	E962.2	E982.8
Taractan	969.3	E853.8	E939.3	E950.3	E962.0	E980.3
Tarantula (venomous)	989.5	E905.1	—	E950.9	E962.1	E980.9
Tartar emetic (anti-infective)	961.2	E857	E931.2	E950.4	E962.0	E980.4
Tartaric acid	983.1	E864.1	—	E950.7	E962.1	E980.6
Tartrated antimony (anti-infective)	961.2	E857	E931.2	E950.4	E962.0	E980.4
TCA - *see* Trichloroacetic acid	—	—	—	—	—	—
TDI	983.0	E864.0		E950.7	E962.1	E980.6
vapor	987.8	E869.8	—	E952.8	E962.2	E982.8
Tear gas	987.5	E869.3	—	E952.8	E962.2	E982.8

◀ New   ◀◀ Revised   ~~deleted~~ Deleted   ● Use Additional Digit(s)

TABLE OF DRUGS AND CHEMICALS

Substance	Poisoning	External Cause (E Code)				
		Accident	Therapeutic Use	Suicide Attempt	Assault	Undetermined
Teclothiazide	974.3	E858.5	E944.3	E950.4	E962.0	E980.4
Tegretol	966.3	E855.0	E936.3	E950.4	E962.0	E980.4
Telepaque	977.8	E858.8	E947.8	E950.4	E962.0	E980.4
Tellurium	985.8	E866.4	—	E950.9	E962.1	E980.9
fumes	985.8	E866.4	—	E950.9	E962.1	E980.9
TEM	963.1	E858.1	E933.1	E950.4	E962.0	E980.4
Temazepam - see Benzodiazepines	—	—	—	—	—	—
TEPA	963.1	E858.1	E933.1	E950.4	E962.0	E980.4
TEPP	989.3	E863.1	—	E950.6	E962.1	E980.7
Terbutaline	971.2	E855.5	E941.2	E950.4	E962.0	E980.4
Teroxalene	961.6	E857	E931.6	E950.4	E962.0	E980.4
Terpin hydrate	975.5	E858.6	E945.5	E950.4	E962.0	E980.4
Terramycin	960.4	E856	E930.4	E950.4	E962.0	E980.4
Tessalon	975.4	E858.6	E945.4	E950.4	E962.0	E980.4
Testosterone	962.1	E858.0	E932.1	E950.4	E962.0	E980.4
Tetanus (vaccine)	978.4	E858.8	E948.4	E950.4	E962.0	E980.4
antitoxin	979.9	E858.8	E949.9	E950.4	E962.0	E980.4
immune globulin (human)	964.6	E858.2	E934.6	E950.4	E962.0	E980.4
toxoid	978.4	E858.8	E948.4	E950.4	E962.0	E980.4
with diphtheria toxoid	978.9	E858.8	E948.9	E950.4	E962.0	E980.4
with pertussis	978.6	E858.8	E948.6	E950.4	E962.0	E980.4
Tetrabenazine	969.5	E853.8	E939.5	E950.3	E962.0	E980.3
Tetracaine (infiltration) (topical)	968.5	E855.2	E938.5	E950.4	E962.0	E980.4
nerve block (peripheral) (plexus)	968.6	E855.2	E938.6	E950.4	E962.0	E980.4
spinal	968.7	E855.2	E938.7	E950.4	E962.0	E980.4
Tetrachlorethylene - see Tetrachloroethylene	—	—	—	—	—	—
Tetrachlormethiazide	974.3	E858.5	E944.3	E950.4	E962.0	E980.4
Tetrachloroethane (liquid) (vapor)	982.3	E862.4	—	E950.9	E962.1	E980.9
paint or varnish	982.3	E861.6	—	E950.9	E962.1	E980.9
Tetrachloroethylene (liquid) (vapor)	982.3	E862.4	—	E950.9	E962.1	E980.9
medicinal	961.6	E857	E931.6	E950.4	E962.0	E980.4
Tetrachloromethane - see Carbon, tetrachloride	—	—	—	—	—	—
Tetracycline	960.4	E856	E930.4	E950.4	E962.0	E980.4
ophthalmic preparation	976.5	E858.7	E946.5	E950.4	E962.0	E980.4
topical NEC	976.0	E858.7	E946.0	E950.4	E962.0	E980.4
Tetraethylammonium chloride	972.3	E858.3	E942.3	E950.4	E962.0	E980.4
Tetraethyl lead (antiknock compound)	984.1	E862.1	—	E950.9	E962.1	E980.9
Tetraethyl pyrophosphate	989.3	E863.1	—	E950.6	E962.1	E980.7
Tetraethylthiuram disulfide	977.3	E858.8	E947.3	E950.4	E962.0	E980.4

◀ New   ◀▥ Revised   ~~deleted~~ Deleted   ● Use Additional Digit(s)

Substance	Poisoning	External Cause (E Code)				
		Accident	Therapeutic Use	Suicide Attempt	Assault	Undetermined
Tetrahydroaminoacridine	971.0	E855.3	E941.0	E950.4	E962.0	E980.4
Tetrahydrocannabinol	969.6	E854.1	E939.6	E950.3	E962.0	E980.3
Tetrahydronaphthalene	982.0	E862.4	—	E950.9	E962.1	E980.9
Tetrahydrozoline	971.2	E855.5	E941.2	E950.4	E962.0	E980.4
Tetralin	982.0	E862.4	—	E950.9	E962.1	E980.9
Tetramethylthiuram (disulfide) NEC	989.4	E863.6	—	E950.6	E962.1	E980.7
medicinal	976.2	E858.7	E946.2	E950.4	E962.0	E980.4
Tetronal	967.8	E852.8	E937.8	E950.2	E962.0	E980.2
Tetryl	983.0	E864.0	—	E950.7	E962.1	E980.6
Thalidomide	967.8	E852.8	E937.8	E950.2	E962.0	E980.2
Thallium (compounds) (dust) NEC	985.8	E866.4	—	E950.9	E962.1	E980.9
pesticide (rodenticide)	985.8	E863.7	—	E950.6	E962.1	E980.7
THC	969.6	E854.1	E939.6	E950.3	E962.0	E980.3
Thebacon	965.09	E850.2	E935.2	E950.0	E962.0	E980.0
Thebaine	965.09	E850.2	E935.2	E950.0	E962.0	E980.0
Theobromine (calcium salicylate)	974.1	E858.5	E944.1	E950.4	E962.0	E980.4
Theophylline (diuretic)	974.1	E858.5	E944.1	E950.4	E962.0	E980.4
ethylenediamine	975.7	E858.6	E945.7	E950.4	E962.0	E980.4
Thiabendazole	961.6	E857	E931.6	E950.4	E962.0	E980.4
Thialbarbital, thialbarbitone	968.3	E855.1	E938.3	E950.4	E962.0	E980.4
Thiamine	963.5	E858.1	E933.5	E950.4	E962.0	E980.4
Thiamylal (sodium)	968.3	E855.1	E938.3	E950.4	E962.0	E980.4
Thiazesim	969.09	E854.0	E939.0	E950.3	E962.0	E980.3
Thiazides (diuretics)	974.3	E858.5	E944.3	E950.4	E962.0	E980.4
Thiethylperazine	963.0	E858.1	E933.0	E950.4	E962.0	E980.4
Thimerosal (topical)	976.0	E858.7	E946.0	E950.4	E962.0	E980.4
ophthalmic preparation	976.5	E858.7	E946.5	E950.4	E962.0	E980.4
Thioacetazone	961.8	E857	E931.8	E950.4	E962.0	E980.4
Thiobarbiturates	968.3	E855.1	E938.3	E950.4	E962.0	E980.4
Thiobismol	961.2	E857	E931.2	E950.4	E962.0	E980.4
Thiocarbamide	962.8	E858.0	E932.8	E950.4	E962.0	E980.4
Thiocarbarsone	961.1	E857	E931.1	E950.4	E962.0	E980.4
Thiocarlide	961.8	E857	E931.8	E950.4	E962.0	E980.4
Thioguanine	963.1	E858.1	E933.1	E950.4	E962.0	E980.4
Thiomercaptomerin	974.0	E858.5	E944.0	E950.4	E962.0	E980.4
Thiomerin	974.0	E858.5	E944.0	E950.4	E962.0	E980.4
Thiopental, thiopentone (sodium)	968.3	E855.1	E938.3	E950.4	E962.0	E980.4
Thiopropazate	969.1	E853.0	E939.1	E950.3	E962.0	E980.3
Thioproperazine	969.1	E853.0	E939.1	E950.3	E962.0	E980.3

Substance	Poisoning	External Cause (E Code) Accident	Therapeutic Use	Suicide Attempt	Assault	Undetermined
Thioridazine	969.1	E853.0	E939.1	E950.3	E962.0	E980.3
Thio-TEPA, thiotepa	963.1	E858.1	E933.1	E950.4	E962.0	E980.4
Thiothixene	969.3	E853.8	E939.3	E950.3	E962.0	E980.3
Thiouracil	962.8	E858.0	E932.8	E950.4	E962.0	E980.4
Thiourea	962.8	E858.0	E932.8	E950.4	E962.0	E980.4
Thiphenamil	971.1	E855.4	E941.1	E950.4	E962.0	E980.4
Thiram NEC	989.4	E863.6	—	E950.6	E962.1	E980.7
medicinal	976.2	E858.7	E946.2	E950.4	E962.0	E980.4
Thonzylamine	963.0	E858.1	E933.0	E950.4	E962.0	E980.4
Thorazine	969.1	E853.0	E939.1	E950.3	E962.0	E980.3
Thornapple	988.2	E865.4	—	E950.9	E962.1	E980.9
Throat preparation (lozenges) NEC	976.6	E858.7	E946.6	E950.4	E962.0	E980.4
Thrombin	964.5	E858.2	E934.5	E950.4	E962.0	E980.4
Thrombolysin	964.4	E858.2	E934.4	E950.4	E962.0	E980.4
Thymol	983.0	E864.0	—	E950.7	E962.1	E980.6
Thymus extract	962.9	E858.0	E932.9	E950.4	E962.0	E980.4
Thyroglobulin	962.7	E858.0	E932.7	E950.4	E962.0	E980.4
Thyroid (derivatives) (extract)	962.7	E858.0	E932.7	E950.4	E962.0	E980.4
Thyrolar	962.7	E858.0	E932.7	E950.4	E962.0	E980.4
Thyrotrophin, thyrotropin	977.8	E858.8	E947.8	E950.4	E962.0	E980.4
Thyroxin(e)	962.7	E858.0	E932.7	E950.4	E962.0	E980.4
Tigan	963.0	E858.1	E933.0	E950.4	E962.0	E980.4
Tigloidine	968.0	E855.1	E938.0	E950.4	E962.0	E980.4
Tin (chloride) (dust) (oxide) NEC	985.8	E866.4	—	E950.9	E962.1	E980.9
anti-infectives	961.2	E857	E931.2	E950.4	E962.0	E980.4
Tinactin	976.0	E858.7	E946.0	E950.4	E962.0	E980.4
Tincture, iodine - see Iodine	—	—	—	—	—	—
Tindal	969.1	E853.0	E939.1	E950.3	E962.0	E980.3
Titanium (compounds) (vapor)	985.8	E866.4	—	E950.9	E962.1	E980.9
ointment	976.3	E858.7	E946.3	E950.4	E962.0	E980.4
Titroid	962.7	E858.0	E932.7	E950.4	E962.0	E980.4
TMTD - see Tetramethylthiuram disulfide	—	—	—	—	—	—
TNT	989.89	E866.8	—	E950.9	E962.1	E980.9
fumes	987.8	E869.8	—	E952.8	E962.2	E982.8
Toadstool	988.1	E865.5	—	E950.9	E962.1	E980.9
Tobacco NEC	989.84	E866.8	—	E950.9	E962.1	E980.9
Indian	988.2	E865.4	—	E950.9	E962.1	E980.9
smoke, second-hand	987.8	E869.4	—	—	—	—

◀ New   ◀▭ Revised   ~~deleted~~ Deleted   ● Use Additional Digit(s)

Substance	Poisoning	External Cause (E Code)				
		Accident	Therapeutic Use	Suicide Attempt	Assault	Undetermined
Tocopherol	963.5	E858.1	E933.5	E950.4	E962.0	E980.4
Tocosamine	975.0	E858.6	E945.0	E950.4	E962.0	E980.4
Tofranil	969.05	E854.0	E939.0	E950.3	E962.0	E980.3
Toilet deodorizer	989.89	E866.8	—	E950.9	E962.1	E980.9
Tolazamide	962.3	E858.0	E932.3	E950.4	E962.0	E980.4
Tolazoline	971.3	E855.6	E941.3	E950.4	E962.0	E980.4
Tolbutamide	962.3	E858.0	E932.3	E950.4	E962.0	E980.4
sodium	977.8	E858.8	E947.8	E950.4	E962.0	E980.4
Tolmetin	965.69	E850.6	E935.6	E950.0	E962.0	E980.0
Tolnaftate	976.0	E858.7	E946.0	E950.4	E962.0	E980.4
Tolpropamine	976.1	E858.7	E946.1	E950.4	E962.0	E980.4
Tolserol	968.0	E855.1	E938.0	E950.4	E962.0	E980.4
Toluene (liquid) (vapor)	982.0	E862.4	—	E950.9	E962.1	E980.9
diisocyanate	983.0	E864.0	—	E950.7	E962.1	E980.6
Toluidine	983.0	E864.0	—	E950.7	E962.1	E980.6
vapor	987.8	E869.8	—	E952.8	E962.2	E982.8
Toluol (liquid) (vapor)	982.0	E862.4	—	E950.9	E962.1	E980.9
Tolylene-2,4-diisocyanate	983.0	E864.0	—	E950.7	E962.1	E980.6
Tonics, cardiac	972.1	E858.3	E942.1	E950.4	E962.0	E980.4
Toxaphene (dust) (spray)	989.2	E863.0	—	E950.6	E962.1	E980.7
Toxoids NEC	978.8	E858.8	E948.8	E950.4	E962.0	E980.4
Tractor fuel NEC	981	E862.1	—	E950.9	E962.1	E980.9
Tragacanth	973.3	E858.4	E943.3	E950.4	E962.0	E980.4
Tramazoline	971.2	E855.5	E941.2	E950.4	E962.0	E980.4
Tranquilizers	969.5	E853.9	E939.5	E950.3	E962.0	E980.3
benzodiazepine-based	969.4	E853.2	E939.4	E950.3	E962.0	E980.3
butyrophenone-based	969.2	E853.1	E939.2	E950.3	E962.0	E980.3
major NEC	969.3	E853.8	E939.3	E950.3	E962.0	E980.3
phenothiazine-based	969.1	E853.0	E939.1	E950.3	E962.0	E980.3
specified NEC	969.5	E853.8	E939.5	E950.3	E962.0	E980.3
Trantoin	961.9	E857	E931.9	E950.4	E962.0	E980.4
Tranxene	969.4	E853.2	E939.4	E950.3	E962.0	E980.3
Tranylcypromine (sulfate)	969.01	E854.0	E939.0	E950.3	E962.0	E980.3
Trasentine	975.1	E858.6	E945.1	E950.4	E962.0	E980.4
Travert	974.5	E858.5	E944.5	E950.4	E962.0	E980.4
Trecator	961.8	E857	E931.8	E950.4	E962.0	E980.4
Tretinoin	976.8	E858.7	E946.8	E950.4	E962.0	E980.4
Triacetin	976.0	E858.7	E946.0	E950.4	E962.0	E980.4

◀ New   ◀▥ Revised   deleted Deleted   ● Use Additional Digit(s)

Substance	Poisoning	External Cause (E Code)				
		Accident	Therapeutic Use	Suicide Attempt	Assault	Undetermined
Triacetyloleandomycin	960.3	E856	E930.3	E950.4	E962.0	E980.4
Triamcinolone	962.0	E858.0	E932.0	E950.4	E962.0	E980.4
ENT agent	976.6	E858.7	E946.6	E950.4	E962.0	E980.4
ophthalmic preparation	976.5	E858.7	E946.5	E950.4	E962.0	E980.4
topical NEC	976.0	E858.7	E946.0	E950.4	E962.0	E980.4
Triamterene	974.4	E858.5	E944.4	E950.4	E962.0	E980.4
Triaziquone	963.1	E858.1	E933.1	E950.4	E962.0	E980.4
Tribromacetaldehyde	967.3	E852.2	E937.3	E950.2	E962.0	E980.2
Tribromoethanol	968.2	E855.1	E938.2	E950.4	E962.0	E980.4
Tribromomethane	967.3	E852.2	E937.3	E950.2	E962.0	E980.2
Trichlorethane	982.3	E862.4	—	E950.9	E962.1	E980.9
Trichlormethiazide	974.3	E858.5	E944.3	E950.4	E962.0	E980.4
Trichloroacetic acid	983.1	E864.1	—	E950.7	E962.1	E980.6
medicinal (keratolytic)	976.4	E858.7	E946.4	E950.4	E962.0	E980.4
Trichloroethanol	967.1	E852.0	E937.1	E950.2	E962.0	E980.2
Trichloroethylene (liquid) (vapor)	982.3	E862.4	—	E950.9	E962.1	E980.9
anesthetic (gas)	968.2	E855.1	E938.2	E950.4	E962.0	E980.4
Trichloroethyl phosphate	967.1	E852.0	E937.1	E950.2	E962.0	E980.2
Trichlorofluoromethane NEC	987.4	E869.2	—	E952.8	E962.2	E982.8
Trichlorotriethylamine	963.1	E858.1	E933.1	E950.4	E962.0	E980.4
Trichomonacides NEC	961.5	E857	E931.5	E950.4	E962.0	E980.4
Trichomycin	960.1	E856	E930.1	E950.4	E962.0	E980.4
Triclofos	967.1	E852.0	E937.1	E950.2	E962.0	E980.2
Tricresyl phosphate	989.89	E866.8	—	E950.9	E962.1	E980.9
solvent	982.8	E862.4	—	E950.9	E962.1	E980.9
Tricyclamol	966.4	E855.0	E936.4	E950.4	E962.0	E980.4
Tridesilon	976.0	E858.7	E946.0	E950.4	E962.0	E980.4
Tridihexethyl	971.1	E855.4	E941.1	E950.4	E962.0	E980.4
Tridione	966.0	E855.0	E936.0	E950.4	E962.0	E980.4
Triethanolamine NEC	983.2	E864.2	—	E950.7	E962.1	E980.6
detergent	983.2	E861.0	—	E950.7	E962.1	E980.6
trinitrate	972.4	E858.3	E942.4	E950.4	E962.0	E980.4
Triethanomelamine	963.1	E858.1	E933.1	E950.4	E962.0	E980.4
Triethylene melamine	963.1	E858.1	E933.1	E950.4	E962.0	E980.4
Triethylenephosphoramide	963.1	E858.1	E933.1	E950.4	E962.0	E980.4
Triethylenethiophosphoramide	963.1	E858.1	E933.1	E950.4	E962.0	E980.4
Trifluoperazine	969.1	E853.0	E939.1	E950.3	E962.0	E980.3
Trifluperidol	969.2	E853.1	E939.2	E950.3	E962.0	E980.3
Triflupromazine	969.1	E853.0	E939.1	E950.3	E962.0	E980.3

◄ New   ◄ Revised   ~~deleted~~ Deleted   ● Use Additional Digit(s)

Substance	Poisoning	External Cause (E Code)				
		Accident	Therapeutic Use	Suicide Attempt	Assault	Undetermined
Trihexyphenidyl	971.1	E855.4	E941.1	E950.4	E962.0	E980.4
Triiodothyronine	962.7	E858.0	E932.7	E950.4	E962.0	E980.4
Trilene	968.2	E855.1	E938.2	E950.4	E962.0	E980.4
Trimeprazine	963.0	E858.1	E933.0	E950.4	E962.0	E980.4
Trimetazidine	972.4	E858.3	E942.4	E950.4	E962.0	E980.4
Trimethadione	966.0	E855.0	E936.0	E950.4	E962.0	E980.4
Trimethaphan	972.3	E858.3	E942.3	E950.4	E962.0	E980.4
Trimethidinium	972.3	E858.3	E942.3	E950.4	E962.0	E980.4
Trimethobenzamide	963.0	E858.1	E933.0	E950.4	E962.0	E980.4
Trimethylcarbinol	980.8	E860.8	—	E950.9	E962.1	E980.9
Trimethylpsoralen	976.3	E858.7	E946.3	E950.4	E962.0	E980.4
Trimeton	963.0	E858.1	E933.0	E950.4	E962.0	E980.4
Trimipramine	969.05	E854.0	E939.0	E950.3	E962.0	E980.3
Trimustine	963.1	E858.1	E933.1	E950.4	E962.0	E980.4
Trinitrin	972.4	E858.3	E942.4	E950.4	E962.0	E980.4
Trinitrophenol	983.0	E864.0	—	E950.7	E962.1	E980.6
Trinitrotoluene	989.89	E866.8	—	E950.9	E962.1	E980.9
fumes	987.8	E869.8	—	E952.8	E962.2	E982.8
Trional	967.8	E852.8	E937.8	E950.2	E962.0	E980.2
Trioxide of arsenic - *see* Arsenic	—	—	—	—	—	—
Trioxsalen	976.3	E858.7	E946.3	E950.4	E962.0	E980.4
Tripelennamine	963.0	E858.1	E933.0	E950.4	E962.0	E980.4
Triperidol	969.2	E853.1	E939.2	E950.3	E962.0	E980.3
Triprolidine	963.0	E858.1	E933.0	E950.4	E962.0	E980.4
Trisoralen	976.3	E858.7	E946.3	E950.4	E962.0	E980.4
Troleandomycin	960.3	E856	E930.3	E950.4	E962.0	E980.4
Trolnitrate (phosphate)	972.4	E858.3	E942.4	E950.4	E962.0	E980.4
Trometamol	963.3	E858.1	E933.3	E950.4	E962.0	E980.4
Tromethamine	963.3	E858.1	E933.3	E950.4	E962.0	E980.4
Tronothane	968.5	E855.2	E938.5	E950.4	E962.0	E980.4
Tropicamide	971.1	E855.4	E941.1	E950.4	E962.0	E980.4
Troxidone	966.0	E855.0	E936.0	E950.4	E962.0	E980.4
Tryparsamide	961.1	E857	E931.1	E950.4	E962.0	E980.4
Trypsin	963.4	E858.1	E933.4	E950.4	E962.0	E980.4
Tryptizol	969.05	E854.0	E939.0	E950.3	E962.0	E980.3
Tuaminoheptane	971.2	E855.5	E941.2	E950.4	E962.0	E980.4
Tuberculin (old)	977.8	E858.8	E947.8	E950.4	E962.0	E980.4
Tubocurare	975.2	E858.6	E945.2	E950.4	E962.0	E980.4
Tubocurarine	975.2	E858.6	E945.2	E950.4	E962.0	E980.4

◀ New ◀▥ Revised ~~deleted~~ Deleted ● Use Additional Digit(s)

Substance	Poisoning	External Cause (E Code)				
		Accident	Therapeutic Use	Suicide Attempt	Assault	Undetermined
Turkish green	969.6	E854.1	E939.6	E950.3	E962.0	E980.3
Turpentine (spirits of) (liquid) (vapor)	982.8	E862.4	—	E950.9	E962.1	E980.9
Tybamate	969.5	E853.8	E939.5	E950.3	E962.0	E980.3
Tyloxapol	975.5	E858.6	E945.5	E950.4	E962.0	E980.4
Tymazoline	971.2	E855.5	E941.2	E950.4	E962.0	E980.4
Typhoid vaccine	978.1	E858.8	E948.1	E950.4	E962.0	E980.4
Typhus vaccine	979.2	E858.8	E949.2	E950.4	E962.0	E980.4
Tyrothricin	976.0	E858.7	E946.0	E950.4	E962.0	E980.4
ENT agent	976.6	E858.7	E946.6	E950.4	E962.0	E980.4
ophthalmic preparation	976.5	E858.7	E946.5	E950.4	E962.0	E980.4
Undecenoic acid	976.0	E858.7	E946.0	E950.4	E962.0	E980.4
Undecylenic acid	976.0	E858.7	E946.0	E950.4	E962.0	E980.4
Unna's boot	976.3	E858.7	E946.3	E950.4	E962.0	E980.4
Uracil mustard	963.1	E858.1	E933.1	E950.4	E962.0	E980.4
Uramustine	963.1	E858.1	E933.1	E950.4	E962.0	E980.4
Urari	975.2	E858.6	E945.2	E950.4	E962.0	E980.4
Urea	974.4	E858.5	E944.4	E950.4	E962.0	E980.4
topical	976.8	E858.7	E946.8	E950.4	E962.0	E980.4
Urethan(e) (antineoplastic)	963.1	E858.1	E933.1	E950.4	E962.0	E980.4
Urginea (maritima) (scilla) - see Squill	—	—	—	—	—	—
Uric acid metabolism agents NEC	974.7	E858.5	E944.7	E950.4	E962.0	E980.4
Urokinase	964.4	E858.2	E934.4	E950.4	E962.0	E980.4
Urokon	977.8	E858.8	E947.8	E950.4	E962.0	E980.4
Urotropin	961.9	E857	E931.9	E950.4	E962.0	E980.4
Urtica	988.2	E865.4	—	E950.9	E962.1	E980.9
Utility gas - see Gas, utility	—	—	—	—	—	—
Vaccine NEC	979.9	E858.8	E949.9	E950.4	E962.0	E980.4
bacterial NEC	978.8	E858.8	E948.8	E950.4	E962.0	E980.4
with	—	—	—	—	—	—
other bacterial component	978.9	E858.8	E948.9	E950.4	E962.0	E980.4
pertussis component	978.6	E858.8	E948.6	E950.4	E962.0	E980.4
viral-rickettsial component	979.7	E858.8	E949.7	E950.4	E962.0	E980.4
mixed NEC	978.9	E858.8	E948.9	E950.4	E962.0	E980.4
BCG	978.0	E858.8	E948.0	E950.4	E962.0	E980.4
cholera	978.2	E858.8	E948.2	E950.4	E962.0	E980.4
diphtheria	978.5	E858.8	E948.5	E950.4	E962.0	E980.4
influenza	979.6	E858.8	E949.6	E950.4	E962.0	E980.4

◄ New ◄▥ Revised ~~deleted~~ Deleted ● Use Additional Digit(s)

Substance	Poisoning	External Cause (E Code)				
		Accident	Therapeutic Use	Suicide Attempt	Assault	Undetermined
Vaccine NEC *(Continued)*						
measles	979.4	E858.8	E949.4	E950.4	E962.0	E980.4
meningococcal	978.8	E858.8	E948.8	E950.4	E962.0	E980.4
mumps	979.6	E858.8	E949.6	E950.4	E962.0	E980.4
paratyphoid	978.1	E858.8	E948.1	E950.4	E962.0	E980.4
pertussis (with diphtheria toxoid) (with tetanus toxoid)	978.6	E858.8	E948.6	E950.4	E962.0	E980.4
plague	978.3	E858.8	E948.3	E950.4	E962.0	E980.4
poliomyelitis	979.5	E858.8	E949.5	E950.4	E962.0	E980.4
poliovirus	979.5	E858.8	E949.5	E950.4	E962.0	E980.4
rabies	979.1	E858.8	E949.1	E950.4	E962.0	E980.4
respiratory syncytial virus	979.6	E858.8	E949.6	E950.4	E962.0	E980.4
rickettsial NEC	979.6	E858.8	E949.6	E950.4	E962.0	E980.4
with	—	—	—	—	—	—
bacterial component	979.7	E858.8	E949.7	E950.4	E962.0	E980.4
pertussis component	978.6	E858.8	E948.6	E950.4	E962.0	E980.4
viral component	979.7	E858.8	E949.7	E950.4	E962.0	E980.4
Rocky Mountain spotted fever	979.6	E858.8	E949.6	E950.4	E962.0	E980.4
rotavirus	979.6	E858.8	E949.6	E950.4	E962.0	E980.4
rubella virus	979.4	E858.8	E949.4	E950.4	E962.0	E980.4
sabin oral	979.5	E858.8	E949.5	E950.4	E962.0	E980.4
smallpox	979.0	E858.8	E949.0	E950.4	E962.0	E980.4
tetanus	978.4	E858.8	E948.4	E950.4	E962.0	E980.4
typhoid	978.1	E858.8	E948.1	E950.4	E962.0	E980.4
typhus	979.2	E858.8	E949.2	E950.4	E962.0	E980.4
viral NEC	979.6	E858.8	E949.6	E950.4	E962.0	E980.4
with	—	—	—	—	—	—
bacterial component	979.7	E858.8	E949.7	E950.4	E962.0	E980.4
pertussis component	978.6	E858.8	E948.6	E950.4	E962.0	E980.4
rickettsial component	979.7	E858.8	E949.7	E950.4	E962.0	E980.4
yellow fever	979.3	E858.8	E949.3	E950.4	E962.0	E980.4
Vaccinia immune globulin (human)	964.6	E858.2	E934.6	E950.4	E962.0	E980.4
Vaginal contraceptives	976.8	E858.7	E946.8	E950.4	E962.0	E980.4
Valethamate	971.1	E855.4	E941.1	E950.4	E962.0	E980.4
Valisone	976.0	E858.7	E946.0	E950.4	E962.0	E980.4
Valium	969.4	E853.2	E939.4	E950.3	E962.0	E980.3
Valmid	967.8	E852.8	E937.8	E950.2	E962.0	E980.2
Vanadium	985.8	E866.4	—	E950.9	E962.1	E980.9
Vancomycin	960.8	E856	E930.8	E950.4	E962.0	E980.4

TABLE OF DRUGS AND CHEMICALS

Substance	Poisoning	External Cause (E Code)				
		Accident	Therapeutic Use	Suicide Attempt	Assault	Undetermined
Vapor (see also Gas)	987.9	E869.9	—	E952.9	E962.2	E982.9
kiln (carbon monoxide)	986	E868.8	—	E952.1	E962.2	E982.1
lead - see Lead	—	—	—	—	—	—
specified source NEC - (see also specific substance)	987.8	E869.8	—	E952.8	E962.2	E982.8
Varidase	964.4	E858.2	E934.4	E950.4	E962.0	E980.4
Varnish	989.89	E861.6	—	E950.9	E962.1	E980.9
cleaner	982.8	E862.9	—	E950.9	E962.1	E980.9
Vaseline	976.3	E858.7	E946.3	E950.4	E962.0	E980.4
Vasodilan	972.5	E858.3	E942.5	E950.4	E962.0	E980.4
Vasodilators NEC	972.5	E858.3	E942.5	E950.4	E962.0	E980.4
coronary	972.4	E858.3	E942.4	E950.4	E962.0	E980.4
Vasopressin	962.5	E858.0	E932.5	E950.4	E962.0	E980.4
Vasopressor drugs	962.5	E858.0	E932.5	E950.4	E962.0	E980.4
Venom, venomous (bite) (sting)	989.5	E905.9	—	E950.9	E962.1	E980.9
arthropod NEC	989.5	E905.5	—	E950.9	E962.1	E980.9
bee	989.5	E905.3	—	E950.9	E962.1	E980.9
centipede	989.5	E905.4	—	E950.9	E962.1	E980.9
hornet	989.5	E905.3	—	E950.9	E962.1	E980.9
lizard	989.5	E905.0	—	E950.9	E962.1	E980.9
marine animals or plants	989.5	E905.6	—	E950.9	E962.1	E980.9
millipede (tropical)	989.5	E905.4	—	E950.9	E962.1	E980.9
plant NEC	989.5	E905.7	—	E950.9	E962.1	E980.9
marine	989.5	E905.6	—	E950.9	E962.1	E980.9
scorpion	989.5	E905.2	—	E950.9	E962.1	E980.9
snake	989.5	E905.0	—	E950.9	E962.1	E980.9
specified NEC	989.5	E905.8	—	E950.9	E962.1	E980.9
spider	989.5	E905.1	—	E950.9	E962.1	E980.9
wasp	989.5	E905.3	—	E950.9	E962.1	E980.9
Ventolin - see Salbutamol sulfate	—	—	—	—	—	—
Veramon	967.0	E851	E937.0	E950.1	E962.0	E980.1
Veratrum	—	—	—	—	—	—
album	988.2	E865.4	—	E950.9	E962.1	E980.9
alkaloids	972.6	E858.3	E942.6	E950.4	E962.0	E980.4
viride	988.2	E865.4	—	E950.9	E962.1	E980.9
Verdigris (see also Copper)	985.8	E866.4	—	E950.9	E962.1	E980.9
Veronal	967.0	E851	E937.0	E950.1	E962.0	E980.1
Veroxil	961.6	E857	E931.6	E950.4	E962.0	E980.4
Versidyne	965.7	E850.7	E935.7	E950.0	E962.0	E980.0
Viagra	972.5	E858.3	E942.5	E950.4	E962.0	E980.4

◀ New ◀▥ Revised ~~deleted~~ Deleted ● Use Additional Digit(s)

Substance	External Cause (E Code)					
	Poisoning	Accident	Therapeutic Use	Suicide Attempt	Assault	Undetermined
Vienna	—	—	—	—	—	—
green	985.1	E866.3	—	E950.8	E962.1	E980.8
insecticide	985.1	E863.4	—	E950.6	E962.1	E980.7
red	989.89	E866.8	—	E950.9	E962.1	E980.9
pharmaceutical dye	977.4	E858.8	E947.4	E950.4	E962.0	E980.4
Vinbarbital, vinbarbitone	967.0	E851	E937.0	E950.1	E962.0	E980.1
Vinblastine	963.1	E858.1	E933.1	E950.4	E962.0	E980.4
Vincristine	963.1	E858.1	E933.1	E950.4	E962.0	E980.4
Vinesthene, vinethene	968.2	E855.1	E938.2	E950.4	E962.0	E980.4
Vinyl	—	—	—	—	—	—
bital	967.0	E851	E937.0	E950.1	E962.0	E980.1
ether	968.2	E855.1	E938.2	E950.4	E962.0	E980.4
Vioform	961.3	E857	E931.3	E950.4	E962.0	E980.4
topical	976.0	E858.7	E946.0	E950.4	E962.0	E980.4
Viomycin	960.6	E856	E930.6	E950.4	E962.0	E980.4
Viosterol	963.5	E858.1	E933.5	E950.4	E962.0	E980.4
Viper (venom)	989.5	E905.0	—	E950.9	E962.1	E980.9
Viprynium (embonate)	961.6	E857	E931.6	E950.4	E962.0	E980.4
Virugon	961.7	E857	E931.7	E950.4	E962.0	E980.4
Visine	976.5	E858.7	E946.5	E950.4	E962.0	E980.4
Vitamins NEC	963.5	E858.1	E933.5	E950.4	E962.0	E980.4
B_{12}	964.1	E858.2	E934.1	E950.4	E962.0	E980.4
hematopoietic	964.1	E858.2	E934.1	E950.4	E962.0	E980.4
K	964.3	E858.2	E934.3	E950.4	E962.0	E980.4
Vleminckx's solution	976.4	E858.7	E946.4	E950.4	E962.0	E980.4
Voltaren - *see* Diclofenac sodium	—	—	—	—	—	—
Warfarin (potassium) (sodium)	964.2	E858.2	E934.2	E950.4	E962.0	E980.4
rodenticide	989.4	E863.7	—	E950.6	E962.1	E980.7
Wasp (sting)	989.5	E905.3	—	E950.9	E962.1	E980.9
Water	—	—	—	—	—	—
balance agents NEC	974.5	E858.5	E944.5	E950.4	E962.0	E980.4
gas	987.1	E868.1	—	E951.8	E962.2	E981.8
incomplete combustion of - *see* Carbon, monoxide, fuel, utility	—	—	—	—	—	—
hemlock	988.2	E865.4	—	E950.9	E962.1	E980.9
moccasin (venom)	989.5	E905.0	—	E950.9	E962.1	E980.9
Wax (paraffin) (petroleum)	981	E862.3	—	E950.9	E962.1	E980.9
automobile	989.89	E861.2	—	E950.9	E962.1	E980.9
floor	981	E862.0	—	E950.9	E962.1	E980.9
Weed killers NEC	989.4	E863.5	—	E950.6	E962.1	E980.7

TABLE OF DRUGS AND CHEMICALS

◀ New   ◀▥ Revised   deleted Deleted   ● Use Additional Digit(s)

TABLE OF DRUGS AND CHEMICALS

Substance	Poisoning	External Cause (E Code)				
		Accident	Therapeutic Use	Suicide Attempt	Assault	Undetermined
Welldorm	967.1	E852.0	E937.1	E950.2	E962.0	E980.2
White	—	—	—	—	—	—
arsenic - *see* Arsenic	—	—	—	—	—	—
hellebore	988.2	E865.4	—	E950.9	E962.1	E980.9
lotion (keratolytic)	976.4	E858.7	E946.4	E950.4	E962.0	E980.4
spirit	981	E862.0	—	E950.9	E962.1	E980.9
Whitewashes	989.89	E861.6	—	E950.9	E962.1	E980.9
Whole blood	964.7	E858.2	E934.7	E950.4	E962.0	E980.4
Wild	—	—	—	—	—	—
black cherry	988.2	E865.4	—	E950.9	E962.1	E980.9
poisonous plants NEC	988.2	E865.4	—	E950.9	E962.1	E980.9
Window cleaning fluid	989.89	E861.3	—	E950.9	E962.1	E980.9
Wintergreen (oil)	976.3	E858.7	E946.3	E950.4	E962.0	E980.4
Witch hazel	976.2	E858.7	E946.2	E950.4	E962.0	E980.4
Wood	—	—	—	—	—	—
alcohol	980.1	E860.2	—	E950.9	E962.1	E980.9
spirit	980.1	E860.2	—	E950.9	E962.1	E980.9
Woorali	975.2	E858.6	E945.2	E950.4	E962.0	E980.4
Wormseed, American	961.6	E857	E931.6	E950.4	E962.0	E980.4
Xanthine diuretics	974.1	E858.5	E944.1	E950.4	E962.0	E980.4
Xanthocillin	960.0	E856	E930.0	E950.4	E962.0	E980.4
Xanthotoxin	976.3	E858.7	E946.3	E950.4	E962.0	E980.4
Xigris	964.2	E858.2	E934.2	E950.4	E962.0	E980.4
Xylene (liquid) (vapor)	982.0	E862.4	—	E950.9	E962.1	E980.9
Xylocaine (infiltration) (topical)	968.5	E855.2	E938.5	E950.4	E962.0	E980.4
nerve block (peripheral) (plexus)	968.6	E855.2	E938.6	E950.4	E962.0	E980.4
spinal	968.7	E855.2	E938.7	E950.4	E962.0	E980.4
Xylol (liquid) (vapor)	982.0	E862.4	—	E950.9	E962.1	E980.9
Xylometazoline	971.2	E855.5	E941.2	E950.4	E962.0	E980.4
Yellow	—	—	—	—	—	—
fever vaccine	979.3	E858.8	E949.3	E950.4	E962.0	E980.4
jasmine	988.2	E865.4	—	E950.9	E962.1	E980.9
Yew	988.2	E865.4	—	E950.9	E962.1	E980.9
Zactane	965.7	E850.7	E935.7	E950.0	E962.0	E980.0
Zaroxolyn	974.3	E858.5	E944.3	E950.4	E962.0	E980.4
Zephiran (topical)	976.0	E858.7	E946.0	E950.4	E962.0	E980.4
ophthalmic preparation	976.5	E858.7	E946.5	E950.4	E962.0	E980.4
Zerone	980.1	E860.2	—	E950.9	E962.1	E980.9

◀ New   ◀▥ Revised   ~~deleted~~ Deleted   ● Use Additional Digit(s)

Substance	Poisoning	External Cause (E Code)				
		Accident	Therapeutic Use	Suicide Attempt	Assault	Undetermined
Zinc (compounds) (fumes) (salts) (vapor) NEC	985.8	E866.4	—	E950.9	E962.1	E980.9
anti-infectives	976.0	E858.7	E946.0	E950.4	E962.0	E980.4
antivaricose	972.7	E858.3	E942.7	E950.4	E962.0	E980.4
bacitracin	976.0	E858.7	E946.0	E950.4	E962.0	E980.4
chloride	976.2	E858.7	E946.2	E950.4	E962.0	E980.4
gelatin	976.3	E858.7	E946.3	E950.4	E962.0	E980.4
oxide	976.3	E858.7	E946.3	E950.4	E962.0	E980.4
peroxide	976.0	E858.7	E946.0	E950.4	E962.0	E980.4
pesticides	985.8	E863.4	—	E950.6	E962.1	E980.7
phosphide (rodenticide)	985.8	E863.7	—	E950.6	E962.1	E980.7
stearate	976.3	E858.7	E946.3	E950.4	E962.0	E980.4
sulfate (antivaricose)	972.7	E858.3	E942.7	E950.4	E962.0	E980.4
ENT agent	976.6	E858.7	E946.6	E950.4	E962.0	E980.4
ophthalmic solution	976.5	E858.7	E946.5	E950.4	E962.0	E980.4
topical NEC	976.0	E858.7	E946.0	E950.4	E962.0	E980.4
undecylenate	976.0	E858.7	E946.0	E950.4	E962.0	E980.4
Zovant	964.2	E858.2	E934.2	E950.4	E962.0	E980.4
Zoxazolamine	968.0	E855.1	E938.0	E950.4	E962.0	E980.4
Zygadenus (venenosus)	988.2	E865.4	—	E950.9	E962.1	E980.9
Zyprexa	969.3	E853.8	E939.3	E950.3	E962.0	E980.3

◄ New   ◄||| Revised   ~~deleted~~ Deleted   ● Use Additional Digit(s)

INDEX TO EXTERNAL CAUSES OF INJURY (E CODE)

This section contains the index to the codes which classify environmental events, circumstances, and other conditions as the cause of injury and other adverse effects. Where a code from the section Supplementary Classification of External Causes of Injury and Poisoning (E800–E998) is applicable, it is intended that the E code shall be used in addition to a code from the main body of the classification, Chapters 1 to 17.

The alphabetic index to the E codes is organized by main terms which describe the accident, circumstance, event, or specific agent which caused the injury or other adverse effect.

Note: Transport accidents (E800–E848) include accidents involving:

> aircraft and spacecraft (E840–E845)
> watercraft (E830–E838)
> motor vehicle (E810–E825)
> railway (E800–E807)
> other road vehicles (E826–E829)

For definitions and examples related to transport accidents - see Supplementary Classification of External Causes of Injury and Poisoning (E800–E999).

The fourth-digit subdivisions for use with categories E800–E848 to identify the injured person are found at the end of this section.

For identifying the place in which an accident or poisoning occurred (circumstances classifiable to categories E850–E869 and E880–E928) - see the listing in this section under "Accident, occurring."

See the Table of Drugs and Chemicals (Section 2 of this volume) for identifying the specific agent involved in drug overdose or a wrong substance given or taken in error, and for intoxication or poisoning by a drug or other chemical substance.

The specific adverse effect, reaction, or localized toxic effect to a correct drug or substance properly administered in therapeutic or prophylactic dosage should be classified according to the nature of the adverse effect (e.g., allergy, dermatitis, tachycardia) listed in Section I of this volume.

E CODES

E CODES

Accident *(Continued)*
  caused by, due to *(Continued)*
    saw E920.4
      band E919.4
      bench E919.4
      chain E920.1
      circular E919.4
      hand E920.4
        powered E920.1
      powered, except hand E919.4
      radial E919.4
    sawing machine, metal E919.3
    shaft
      hoist E919.1
      lift E919.1
      transmission E919.6
    shears E920.4
      hand E920.4
        powered E920.1
      mechanical E919.3
    shovel E920.4
      steam E919.7
    spinning machine E919.8
    steam - *see also* Burning, steam
      engine E919.5
      shovel E919.7
    thresher E919.0
    thunderbolt NEC E907
    tractor E919.0
      when in transport under its own power - *see* categories E810–E825
    transmission belt, cable, chain, gear, pinion, pulley, shaft E919.6
    turbine (gas) (water driven) E919.5
    under-cutter E919.1
    weaving machine E919.8
    winch E919.2
      agricultural operations E919.0
      mining operations E919.1
  diving E883.0
    with insufficient air supply E913.2
  glider (hang) (*see also* Collision, aircraft, unpowered) E842 ●
  hovercraft
    on
      land - *see* Accident, motor vehicle
      water - *see* Accident, watercraft
  ice yacht (*see also* Accident, vehicle NEC) E848
  in
    medical, surgical procedure
      as, or due to misadventure - *see* Misadventure
      causing an abnormal reaction or later complication without mention of misadventure - *see* Reaction, abnormal
  kite carrying a person (*see also* Collision, involving aircraft, unpowered) E842 ●
  land yacht (*see also* Accident, vehicle NEC) E848
  late effect of - *see* Late effect
  launching pad E845 ●
  machine, machinery (*see also* Accident, caused by, due to, by specific type of machine) E919.9
    agricultural including animal-powered premises E919.0
    earth-drilling E919.1
    earth moving or scraping E919.7
    excavating E919.7

Accident *(Continued)*
  machine, machinery *(Continued)*
    involving transport under own power on highway or transport vehicle - *see* categories E810-E825, E840-E845
    lifting (appliances) E919.2
    metalworking E919.3
    mining E919.1
    prime movers, except electric motors E919.5
      electric motors - *see* Accident, machine, by specific type of machine
    recreational E919.8
    specified type NEC E919.8
    transmission E919.6
    watercraft (deck) (engine room) (galley) (laundry) (loading) E836 ●
    woodworking or forming E919.4
  motor vehicle (on public highway) (traffic) E819 ●
    due to cataclysm - *see* categories E908, E909
    involving
      collision (*see also* Collision, motor vehicle) E812 ●
    nontraffic, not on public highway - *see* categories E820–E825
    not involving collision - *see* categories E816–E819
  nonmotor vehicle NEC E829 ●
    nonroad - *see* Accident, vehicle NEC
    road, except pedal cycle, animal-drawn vehicle, or animal being ridden E829 ●
  nonroad vehicle NEC - *see* Accident, vehicle NEC
  not elsewhere classifiable involving
    cable car (not on rails) E847
      on rails E829 ●
    coal car in mine E846
    hand truck - *see* Accident, vehicle NEC
    logging car E846
    sled(ge), meaning snow or ice vehicle E848
    tram, mine or quarry E846
    truck
      mine or quarry E846
      self-propelled, industrial E846
      station baggage E846
    tub, mine or quarry E846
    vehicle NEC E848
      snow and ice E848
      used only on industrial premises E846
    wheelbarrow E848
  occurring (at) (in)
    apartment E849.0
    baseball field, diamond E849.4
    construction site, any E849.3
    dock E849.8
      yard E849.3
    dormitory E849.7
    factory (building) (premises) E849.3
    farm E849.1
      buildings E849.1
      house E849.0
    football field E849.4
    forest E849.8
    garage (place of work) E849.3
      private (home) E849.0

Accident *(Continued)*
  occurring *(Continued)*
    gravel pit E849.2
    gymnasium E849.4
    highway E849.5
    home (private) (residential) E849.0
      institutional E849.7
    hospital E849.7
    hotel E849.6
    house (private) (residential) E849.0
      movie E849.6
      public E849.6
    institution, residential E849.7
    jail E849.7
    mine E849.2
    motel E849.6
    movie house E849.6
    office (building) E849.6
    orphanage E849.7
    park (public) E849.4
      mobile home E849.8
      trailer E849.8
    parking lot or place E849.8
    place
      industrial NEC E849.3
      parking E849.8
      public E849.8
        specified place NEC E849.5
      recreational NEC E849.4
      sport NEC E849.4
    playground (park) (school) E849.4
    prison E849.6
    public building NEC E849.6
    quarry E849.2
    railway
      line NEC E849.8
      yard E849.3
    residence
      home (private) E849.0
    resort (beach) (lake) (mountain) (seashore) (vacation) E849.4
    restaurant E849.6
    sand pit E849.2
    school (building) (private) (public) (state) E849.6
      reform E849.7
      riding E849.4
    seashore E849.8
      resort E849.4
    shop (place of work) E849.3
      commercial E849.6
    skating rink E849.4
    sports palace E849.4
    stadium E849.4
    store E849.6
    street E849.5
    swimming pool (public) E849.4
      private home or garden E849.0
    tennis court E849.4
    theatre, theater E849.6
    trailer court E849.8
    tunnel E849.8
      under construction E849.2
    warehouse E849.3
    yard
      dock E849.3
      industrial E849.3
      private (home) E849.0
      railway E849.3
  off-road type motor vehicle (not on public highway) NEC E821 ●
  on public highway - *see* categories E810–E819
  pedal cycle E826 ●

◀ New   ◀||| Revised   ~~deleted~~ Deleted   ● Use Additional Digit(s)   ▨ Omit code

Accident *(Continued)*
    railway E807 ●
        due to cataclysm - *see* categories
            E908, E909
        involving
            burning by engine, locomotive,
                train *(see also* Explosion,
                railway engine) E803 ●
            collision *(see also* Collision,
                railway) E800 ●
            derailment *(see also* Derailment,
                railway) E802 ●
            explosion *(see also* Explosion,
                railway engine) E803 ●
            fall *(see also* Fall, from, railway
                rolling stock) E804 ●
            fire *(see also* Explosion, railway
                engine) E803 ●
            hitting by, being struck by
                object falling in, on, from,
                    rolling stock, train,
                    vehicle E806 ●
                rolling stock, train, vehicle
                    E805 ●
            overturning, railway rolling
                stock, train, vehicle *(see also*
                Derailment, railway) E802 ●
            running off rails, railway *(see also*
                Derailment, railway) E802 ●
            specified circumstances NEC
                E806 ●
            train or vehicle hit by
                avalanche E909.2
                falling object (earth, rock, tree)
                    E806 ●
                    due to cataclysm - *see*
                        categories E908, E909
                landslide E909.2
    roller skate E885.1
    scooter (nonmotorized) E885.0
    skateboard E885.2
    ski(ing) E885.3
        jump E884.9
        lift or tow (with chair or gondola) E847
    snow vehicle, motor driven (not on
        public highway) E820 ●
        on public highway - *see* categories
            E810–E819
    snowboard E885.4
    spacecraft E845 ●
    specified cause NEC E928.8
    street car E829 ●
    traffic NEC E819 ●
    vehicle NEC (with pedestrian) E848
        battery powered
            airport passenger vehicle E846
            truck (baggage) (mail) E846
        powered commercial or industrial
            (with other vehicle or object
            within commercial or
            industrial premises) E846
    watercraft E838 ●
        with
            drowning or submersion
                resulting from
                accident other than to
                    watercraft E832 ●
                accident to watercraft E830 ●
            injury, except drowning or
                submersion, resulting from
                accident other than to
                    watercraft - *see* categories
                    E833–E838
                accident to watercraft E831 ●

Accident *(Continued)*
    watercraft *(Continued)*
        due to, caused by cataclysm - *see*
            categories E908, E909
        machinery E836 ●
Acid throwing E961
Acosta syndrome E902.0
Activity (involving) E030
    aerobic and step exercise (class)
        E009.2
    alpine skiing E003.2
    animal care NEC E019.9
    arts and handcrafts NEC E012.9
    athletics NEC E008.9
        played
            as a team or group NEC E007.9
            individually NEC E006.9
    baking E015.2
    ballet E005.0
    barbells E010.2
    BASE (Building, Antenna, Span,
        Earth) jumping E004.2
    baseball E007.3
    basketball E007.6
    bathing (personal) E013.0
    beach volleyball E007.7
    bike riding E006.4
    boogie boarding E002.7
    bowling E006.3
    boxing E008.0
    brass instrument playing E018.3
    building and construction E016.2
    bungee jumping E004.3
    calisthenics E009.1
    canoeing (in calm and turbulent
        water) E002.5
    capture the flag E007.8
    cardiorespiratory exercise
        NEC E009.9
    caregiving (providing) NEC E014.9
        bathing E014.0
        lifting E014.1
    cellular
        communication device E011.1
        telephone E011.1
    challenge course E009.4
    cheerleading E005.4
    circuit training E009.3
    cleaning
        floor E013.4
    climbing NEC E004.9
        mountain E004.0
        rock E004.0
        wall climbing E004.0
    combatives E008.4
    computer
        keyboarding E011.0
        technology NEC E011.9
    confidence course E009.4
    construction (building) E016.2
    cooking and baking E015.2
    cooking and grilling NEC E015.9
    cool down exercises E009.1
    cricket E007.9
    crocheting E012.0
    cross country skiing E003.3
    dancing (all types) E005.0
    digging
        dirt E016.0
    dirt digging E016.0
    dishwashing E015.0
    diving (platform) (springboard)
        E002.1
        underwater E002.4

Activity *(Continued)*
    dodge ball E007.8
    downhill skiing E003.2
    drum playing E018.1
    dumbbells E010.2
    electronic
        devices NEC E011.9
            hand held interactive E011.1
        game playing (using) (with)
            interactive device E011.1
            keyboard or other stationary
                device E011.0
    elliptical machine E009.0
    exercise(s)
        machines ((primarily) for)
            cardiorespiratory conditioning
                E009.0
            muscle strengthening E010.0
        muscle strengthening
            (non-machine) NEC
            E010.9
    external motion NEC E017.9
        roller coaster E017.0 ◀▥
    field hockey E007.4
    figure skating (pairs) (singles)
        E003.0
    flag football E007.1
    floor mopping and cleaning E013.4
    food preparation and clean up
        E015.0
    football (American) NOS E007.0
        flag E007.1
        tackle E007.0
        touch E007.1
    four square E007.8
    free weights E010.2
    frisbee (ultimate) E008.3
    furniture
        building E012.2
        finishing E012.2
        repair E012.2
    game playing (electronic)
        using
            interactive device E011.1
            keyboard or other stationary
                device E011.0
    gardening E016.1
    golf E006.2
    grass drills E009.5
    grilling and smoking food
        E015.1
    grooming and shearing an animal
        E019.2
    guerilla drills E009.5
    gymnastics (rhythmic) E005.2
    handball E008.2
    handcrafts NEC E012.9
    hand held interactive electronic
        device E011.1
    hang gliding E004.4
    hiking (on level or elevated
        terrain) E001.0
    hockey (ice) E003.1
        field E007.4
    horseback riding E006.1
    household maintenance
        NEC E013.9
    ice NEC E003.9
        dancing E003.0
        hockey E003.1
        skating E003.0
    inline roller skating E006.0
    ironing E013.3
    judo E008.4

Activity *(Continued)*
jumping (off) NEC E004.9
    BASE (Building, Antenna, Span,
        Earth) E004.2
    bungee E004.3
    jacks E009.1
    rope E006.5
jumping jacks E009.1
jumping rope E006.5
karate E008.4
kayaking (in calm and turbulent
    water) E002.5
keyboarding (computer) E011.0
kickball E007.8
knitting E012.0
lacrosse E007.4
land maintenance NEC E016.9
landscaping E016.1
laundry E013.1
machines (exercise) primarily for
    cardiorespiratory conditioning
    E009.0
maintenance
    building E016.9
    household NEC E013.9
    land E016.9
    property E016.9
marching (on level or elevated
    terrain) E001.0
martial arts E008.4
microwave oven E015.2
mopping (floor) E013.4
mountain climbing E004.0
milking an animal E019.1
muscle strengthening
    exercises (non-machine)
        NEC E010.9
    machines E010.0
musical keyboard (electronic)
    playing E018.0
nordic skiing E003.3
obstacle course E009.4
oven (microwave) E015.2
packing up and unpacking in moving
    to a new residence E013.5
parasailing E002.9
percussion instrument playing NEC
    E018.1
personal
    bathing and showering E013.0
    hygiene NEC E013.8
    showering E013.0
physical
    games generally associated with
        school recess, summer camp
        and children 007.8
    training NEC E009.9
piano playing E018.0
pilates E010.3
platform diving E002.1
playing musical instrument
    brass instrument E018.3
    drum E018.1
    musical keyboard (electronic)
        E018.0
    percussion instrument NEC
        E018.1
    piano E018.0
    string instrument E018.2
    wind instrument E018.3
property maintenance NEC E016.9
pruning (garden and lawn) E016.1
pull-ups E010.1
push-ups E010.1
racquetball E008.2

Activity *(Continued)*
rafting (in calm and turbulent
    water) E002.5
raking (leaves) E016.0
rappelling E004.1
refereeing a sports activity E029.0
residential relocation E013.5
rhythmic
    gymnastics E005.2
    movement NEC E005.9
riding
    horseback E006.1
    roller coaster E017.0 ◄▥
rock climbing E004.0
roller coaster riding E017.0 ◄▥
roller skating (inline) E006.0
rough housing and horseplay E029.2
rowing (in calm and turbulent
    water) E002.5
rugby E007.2
running E001.1
SCUBA diving E002.4
sewing E012.1
shoveling E016.0
    dirt E016.0
    snow E016.0
showering (personal) E013.0
sit-ups E010.1
skateboarding E006.0
skating (ice) E003.0
    roller E006.0
skiing (alpine) (downhill) E003.2
    cross country E003.3
    nordic E003.3
sledding (snow) E003.2
smoking and grilling food E015.1
snorkeling E002.4
snow NEC E003.9
    boarding E003.2
    shoveling E016.0
    sledding E003.2
    tubing E003.2
soccer E007.5
softball E007.3
specified NEC E029.9
spectator at an event E029.1
sports NEC E008.9
sports played as a team or group
    NEC E007.9
sports played individually NEC E006.9
springboard diving E002.1
squash E008.2
stationary bike E009.0
step (stepping) exercise (class) E009.2
stepper machine E009.0
stove E015.2
string instrument playing E018.2
surfing E002.7
swimming E002.0
tackle football E007.0
tap dancing E005.0
tennis E008.2
tobogganing E003.2
touch football E007.1
track and field events
    (non-running) E006.6
    running E001.1
trampoline E005.3
treadmill E009.0
trimming shrubs E016.1
tubing (in calm and turbulent water)
    E002.5
    snow E003.2
ultimate frisbee E008.3
underwater diving E002.4

Activity *(Continued)*
unpacking in moving to a new
    residence E013.5
use of stove, oven and microwave
    oven E015.2
vacuuming E013.2
volleyball (beach) (court) E007.7
wake boarding E002.6
walking an animal E019.0
walking (on level or elevated
    terrain) E001.0
    an animal E019.0
wall climbing E004.0
warm up and cool down
    exercises E009.1
water NEC E002.9
    aerobics E002.3
    craft NEC E002.9
    exercise E002.3
    polo E002.2
    skiing E002.6
    sliding E002.8
    survival training and testing E002.9
weeding (garden and lawn) E016.1
wind instrument playing E018.3
windsurfing E002.7
wrestling E008.1
yoga E005.1
Activity status E000.9
child assisting in compensated work of
    other family member E000.8 ◄
civilian
    done for
        financial or other compensation
        E000.0
        pay or income E000.0
family member assisting in
    compensated work of other
    family member E000.8 ◄
for income E000.0
hobby or leisure E000.8
off duty military E000.8
military E000.1
    off duty E000.8
recreation E000.8
specified NEC E000.8
sport not for income E000.8
student E000.8
volunteer E000.2 ◄▥
Aeroneurosis E902.1
Aero-otitis media - *see* Effects of, air
    pressure
Aerosinusitis - *see* Effects of, air pressure
After-effect, late - *see* Late effect
Air
blast
    in
        terrorism E979.2
        war operations E993.9
embolism (traumatic) NEC E928.9
    in
        infusion or transfusion E874.1
        perfusion E874.2
sickness E903
Alpine sickness E902.0
Altitude sickness - *see* Effects of, air
    pressure
Anaphylactic shock, anaphylaxis *(see also*
    Table of Drugs and Chemicals) E947.9
due to bite or sting (venomous) - *see*
    Bite, venomous
Andes disease E902.0
Apoplexy
heat - *see* Heat
Arachnidism E905.1

E CODES

◄ New   ◄▥ Revised   ~~deleted~~ Deleted   ● Use Additional Digit(s)   ▨ Omit code

Arson E968.0
Asphyxia, asphyxiation
  by
    chemical
      in
        terrorism E979.7
        war operations E997.2
    explosion - *see* Explosion E965.8
    food (bone) (regurgitated food)
      (seed) E911
    foreign object, except food E912
    fumes
      in
        terrorism (chemical weapons)
          E979.7
        war operations E997.2
    gas - *see also* Table of Drugs and
      Chemicals
      in
        terrorism E979.7
        war operations E997.2
      legal
        execution E978
        intervention (tear) E972
      tear E972
    mechanical means (*see also*
      Suffocation) E913.9
  from
    conflagration - *see* Conflagration
    fire - *see also* Fire E899
      in
        terrorism E979.3
        war operations E990.9
    ignition - *see* Ignition
Aspiration
  foreign body - *see* Foreign body,
    aspiration
  mucus, not of newborn (with asphyxia,
    obstruction respiratory passage,
    suffocation) E912
  phlegm (with asphyxia, obstruction
    respiratory passage, suffocation)
    E912
  vomitus (with asphyxia, obstruction
    respiratory passage, suffocation)
    (*see also* Foreign body, aspiration,
    food) E911
Assassination (attempt) (*see also* Assault)
  E968.9
Assault (homicidal) (by) (in) E968.9
  acid E961
    swallowed E962.1
  air gun E968.6
  BB gun E968.6
  bite NEC E968.8
    of human being E968.7
  bomb ((placed in) car or house) E965.8
    antipersonnel E965.5
    letter E965.7
    petrol E965.6
  brawl (hand) (fists) (foot) E960.0
  burning, burns (by fire) E968.0
    acid E961
      swallowed E962.1
    caustic, corrosive substance E961
      swallowed E962.1
    chemical from swallowing caustic,
      corrosive substance NEC E962.1
    hot liquid E968.3
    scalding E968.3
    vitriol E961
      swallowed E962.1
  caustic, corrosive substance E961
    swallowed E962.1
  cut, any part of body E966
  dagger E966
  drowning E964

Assault (*Continued*)
  explosives E965.9
    bomb (*see also* Assault, bomb) E965.8
    dynamite E965.8
  fight (hand) (fists) (foot) E960.0
    with weapon E968.9
      blunt or thrown E968.2
      cutting or piercing E966
      firearm - *see* Shooting, homicide
    fire E968.0
  firearm(s) - *see* Shooting, homicide
  garrotting E963
  gunshot (wound) - *see* Shooting,
    homicide
  hanging E963
  injury NEC E968.9
  knife E966
  late effect of E969
  ligature E963
  poisoning E962.9
    drugs or medicinals E962.0
    gas(es) or vapors, except drugs and
      medicinals E962.2
    solid or liquid substances, except
      drugs and medicinals E962.1
  puncture, any part of body E966
  pushing
    before moving object, train, vehicle
      E968.5
    from high place E968.1
  rape E960.1
  scalding E968.3
  shooting - *see* Shooting, homicide
  sodomy E960.1
  stab, any part of body E966
  strangulation E963
  submersion E964
  suffocation E963
  transport vehicle E968.5
  violence NEC E968.9
  vitriol E961
    swallowed E962.1
  weapon E968.9
    blunt or thrown E968.2
    cutting or piercing E966
    firearm - *see* Shooting, homicide
  wound E968.9
    cutting E966
    gunshot - *see* Shooting, homicide
    knife E966
    piercing E966
    puncture E966
    stab E966
Attack by animal NEC E906.9
Avalanche E909.2
  falling on or hitting
    motor vehicle (in motion) (on public
      highway) E909.2
    railway train E909.2
Aviators' disease E902.1

B

Barotitis, barodontalgia, berosinusitis,
  barotrauma (otitic) (sinus) - *see*
  Effects of, air pressure
Battered
  baby or child (syndrome) - *see* Abuse,
    child; category E967
  person other than baby or child - *see*
    Assault
Bayonet wound (*see also* Cut, by bayonet)
  E920.3
  in
    legal intervention E974
    terrorism E979.8
    war operations E995.2

Bean in nose E912
Bed set on fire NEC E898.0
Beheading (by guillotine)
  homicide E966
  legal execution E978
Bending, injury ~~in E927.8~~ ◀▥
  due to ◀
    repetitive movement E927.3 ◀
    sudden strenuous movement
      E927.0 ◀
Bends E902.0
Bite
  animal NEC E906.5
    other specified (except arthropod)
      E906.3
    venomous NEC E905.9
  arthropod (nonvenomous) NEC E906.4
    venomous - *see* Sting
  black widow spider E905.1
  cat E906.3
  centipede E905.4
  cobra E905.0
  copperhead snake E905.0
  coral snake E905.0
  dog E906.0
  fer de lance E905.0
  gila monster E905.0
  human being
    accidental E928.3
    assault E968.7
  insect (nonvenomous) E906.4
    venomous - *see* Sting
  krait E905.0
  late effect of - *see* Late effect
  lizard E906.2
    venomous E905.0
  mamba E905.0
  marine animal
    nonvenomous E906.3
      snake E906.2
    venomous E905.6
      snake E905.0
  millipede E906.4
    venomous E905.4
  moray eel E906.3
  rat E906.1
  rattlesnake E905.0
  rodent, except rat E906.3
  serpent - *see* Bite, snake
  shark E906.3
  snake (venomous) E905.0
    nonvenomous E906.2
    sea E905.0
  spider E905.1
    nonvenomous E906.4
  tarantula (venomous) E905.1
  venomous NEC E905.9
    by specific animal - *see* category
      E905
  viper E905.0
  water moccasin E905.0
Blast (air)
  in
    terrorism E979.2
      from nuclear explosion E979.5
      underwater E979.0
    war operations E993.9
      from nuclear explosion ~~(see~~
        ~~also War operations,~~
        ~~injury due to, nuclear~~
        ~~weapons) E996.0~~ - *see* War
        operation, injury due to,
        nuclear weapons ◀▥
      underwater E992.9
Blizzard E908.3

E CODES

E CODES

Blow E928.9
  by law-enforcing agent, police (on
      duty) E975
    with blunt object (baton)
        (nightstick) (stave)
        (truncheon) E973
Blowing up (see also Explosion) E923.9
Brawl (hand) (fists) (foot) E960.0
Breakage (accidental)
  cable of cable car not on rails E847
  ladder (causing fall) E881.0
  part (any) of
    animal-drawn vehicle E827●
    ladder (causing fall) E881.0
    motor vehicle
      in motion (on public highway)
          E818●
        not on public highway
            E825●
    nonmotor road vehicle, except
        animal-drawn vehicle or pedal
        cycle E829●
    off-road type motor vehicle (not
        on public highway)
        NEC E821●
      on public highway E818●
    pedal cycle E826●
    scaffolding (causing fall) E881.1
    snow vehicle, motor-driven (not on
        public highway) E820●
      on public highway E818●
    vehicle NEC - see Accident, vehicle
Broken
  glass
    fall on E888.0
    injury by E920.8
  power line (causing electric shock)
      E925.1
Bumping against, into (accidentally)
  object (moving) E917.9
    caused by crowd E917.1
      with subsequent fall E917.6
    furniture E917.3
      with subsequent fall E917.7
    in
      running water E917.2
      sports E917.0
        with subsequent fall E917.5
    stationary E917.4
      with subsequent fall E917.8
  person(s) E917.9
    with fall E886.9
      in sports E886.0
    as, or caused by, a crowd E917.1
      with subsequent fall E917.6
    in sports E917.0
      with fall E886.0
Burning, burns (accidental) (by) (from)
    (on) E899
  acid (any kind) E924.1
    swallowed - see Table of Drugs and
        Chemicals
  airgun E928.7
  bedclothes (see also Fire, specified NEC)
      E898.0
  blowlamp (see also Fire, specified NEC)
      E898.1
  blowtorch (see also Fire, specified NEC)
      E898.1
  boat, ship, watercraft - see categories
      E830, E831, E837
  bonfire (controlled) E897
    uncontrolled E892
  candle (see also Fire, specified NEC)
      E898.1

Burning, burns (Continued)
  caustic liquid, substance E924.1
    swallowed - see Table of Drugs and
        Chemicals
  chemical E924.1
    from swallowing caustic, corrosive
        substance - see Table of Drugs
        and Chemicals
    in
      terrorism E979.7
      war operations E997.2
  cigar(s) or cigarette(s) (see also Fire,
      specified NEC) E898.1
  clothes, clothing, nightdress - see
      Ignition, clothes
    with conflagration - see
        Conflagration
  conflagration - see Conflagration
  corrosive liquid, substance
      E924.1
    swallowed - see Table of Drugs
        and Chemicals
  electric current (see also Electric shock)
      E925.9
  fire, flames (see also Fire) E899
  firearm E928.7
  flare, Verey pistol E922.8
  heat
    from appliance (electrical) E924.8
    in local application, or packing
        during medical or surgical
        procedure E873.5
  homicide (attempt) (see also Assault,
      burning) E968.0
  hot
    liquid E924.0
      caustic or corrosive E924.1
    object (not producing fire or flames)
        E924.8
    substance E924.9
      caustic or corrosive E924.1
      liquid (metal) NEC E924.0
      specified type NEC E924.8
    tap water E924.2
  ignition - see also Ignition
    clothes, clothing, nightdress - see also
        Ignition, clothes
      with conflagration - see
          Conflagration
    highly inflammable material
        (benzine) (fat) (gasoline)
        (kerosine) (paraffin) (petrol)
        E894
  inflicted by other person
    stated as
      homicidal, intentional (see also
          Assault, burning) E968.0
      undetermined whether
          accidental or intentional
          (see also Burn, stated as
          undetermined whether
          accidental or intentional)
          E988.1
  internal, from swallowed caustic,
      corrosive liquid, substance - see
      Table of Drugs and Chemicals
  in
    terrorism E979.3
      from nuclear explosion E979.5
      petrol bomb E979.3
    war operations (from fire-producing
        device or conventional
        weapon) E990.9
      from nuclear explosion (see
          also War operations,
          injury due to, nuclear
          weapons) E996.2

Burning, burns (Continued)
  in (Continued)
    war operations (Continued)
      incendiary bomb E990.0
      petrol bomb E990.0
  lamp (see also Fire, specified NEC)
      E898.1
  late effect of NEC E929.4
  lighter (cigar) (cigarette) (see also Fire,
      specified NEC) E898.1
  lightning E907
  liquid (boiling) (hot) (molten)
      E924.0
    caustic, corrosive (external)
        E924.1
      swallowed - see Table of Drugs
          and Chemicals
  local application of externally applied
      substance in medical or surgical
      care E873.5
  machinery - see Accident, machine
  matches (see also Fire, specified NEC)
      E898.1
  medicament, externally applied
      E873.5
  metal, molten E924.0
  object (hot) E924.8
    producing fire or flames - see Fire
  oven (electric) (gas) E924.8
  pipe (smoking) (see also Fire, specified
      NEC) E898.1
  radiation - see Radiation
  railway engine, locomotive, train (see
      also Explosion, railway engine)
      E803●
  self-inflicted (unspecified whether
      accidental or intentional)
      E988.1
    caustic or corrosive substance NEC
        E988.7
    stated as intentional, purposeful
        E958.1
      caustic or corrosive substance
          NEC E958.7
    stated as undetermined whether
        accidental or intentional
        E988.1
      caustic or corrosive substance NEC
          E988.7
  steam E924.0
    pipe E924.8
  substance (hot) E924.9
    boiling or molten E924.0
    caustic, corrosive (external)
        E924.1
      swallowed - see Table of Drugs
          and Chemicals
  suicidal (attempt) NEC E958.1
    caustic substance E958.7
    late effect of E959
  tanning bed E926.2
  therapeutic misadventure
    overdose of radiation E873.2
  torch, welding (see also Fire, specified
      NEC) E898.1
  trash fire (see also Burning, bonfire)
      E897
  vapor E924.0
  vitriol E924.1
  x-rays E926.3
    in medical, surgical procedure - see
        Misadventure, failure, in
        dosage, radiation
        operations
Butted by animal E906.8

◀ New   ◀▦▦ Revised   ~~deleted~~ Deleted   ● Use Additional Digit(s)   ▦▦ Omit code

C

Cachexia, lead or saturnine E866.0
  from pesticide NEC (*see also* Table
    of Drugs and Chemicals)
    E863.4
Caisson disease E902.2
Capital punishment (any means) E978
Car sickness E903
Casualty (not due to war) NEC E928.9
  terrorism E979.8
  war (*see also* War operations) E995.9
Cat
  bite E906.3
  scratch E906.8
Cataclysmic (any injury)
  earth surface movement or eruption
    E909.9
    specified type NEC E909.8
  storm or flood resulting from storm
    E908.9
    specified type NEC E909.8
Catching fire - *see* Ignition
Caught
  between
    objects (moving) (stationary and
      moving) E918
      and machinery - *see* Accident,
        machine
  by cable car, not on rails E847
  in
    machinery (moving parts of) - *see*
      Accident, machine
    object E918
Cave-in (causing asphyxia, suffocation
  (by pressure)) (*see also* Suffocation,
  due to, cave-in) E913.3
  with injury other than asphyxia or
    suffocation E916
  with asphyxia or suffocation (*see
    also* Suffocation, due to,
    cave-in) E913.3
  struck or crushed by E916
    with asphyxia or suffocation (*see also*
      Suffocation, due to, cave-in)
      E913.3
Change(s) in air pressure - *see also* Effects
  of, air pressure
  sudden, in aircraft (ascent) (descent)
    (causing aeroneurosis or aviators'
    disease) E902.1
Chilblains E901.0
  due to manmade conditions E901.1
Choking (on) (any object except food or
  vomitus) E912
  apple E911
  bone E911
  food, any type (regurgitated) E911
  mucus or phlegm E912
  seed E911
Civil insurrection - *see* War operations
Cloudburst E908.8
Cold, exposure to (accidental) (excessive)
  (extreme) (place) E901.9
  causing chilblains or immersion foot
    E901.0
  due to
    manmade conditions E901.1
    specified cause NEC E901.8
    weather (conditions) E901.0
  late effect of NEC E929.5
  self-inflicted (undetermined whether
    accidental or intentional)
    E988.3
    suicidal E958.3
  suicide E958.3

Colic, lead, painters', or saturnine - *see*
  category E866
Collapse
  building E916
    burning (uncontrolled fire) E891.8
      in terrorism E979.3
      private E890.8
  dam E909.3
  due to heat - *see* Heat
  machinery - *see* Accident, machine or
    vehicle
  man-made structure E909.3
  postoperative NEC E878.9
  structure
    burning (uncontrolled fire) NEC
      E891.8
      in terrorism E979.3
Collision (accidental)

Note: In the case of collisions
between different types of vehicles,
persons and objects, priority in
classification is in the following order:

    Aircraft
    Watercraft
    Motor vehicle
    Railway vehicle
    Pedal cycle
    Animal-drawn vehicle
    Animal being ridden
    Streetcar or other
      nonmotor road vehicle
    Other vehicle
    Pedestrian or person using
      pedestrian conveyance
    Object (except where falling from
      or set in motion by vehicle, etc.
      listed above)

In the listing below, the combinations
are listed only under the vehicle, etc.,
having priority. For definitions, *see*
Supplementary Classification of
External Causes of Injury and
Poisoning (E800–E999).

---

  aircraft (with object or vehicle) (fixed)
    (movable) (moving) E841●
    with
      person (while landing, taking off)
        (without accident to
        aircraft) E844●
      powered (in transit) (with
        unpowered aircraft) E841●
      while landing, taking off E840●
      unpowered E842●
      while landing, taking off E840●
  animal being ridden (in sport or
    transport) E828●
    and
      animal (being ridden) (herded)
        (unattended) E828●
      nonmotor road vehicle, except
        pedal cycle or animal-
        drawn vehicle E828●
      object (fallen) (fixed) (movable)
        (moving) not falling from or
        set in motion by vehicle of
        higher priority E828●
      pedestrian (conveyance or
        vehicle) E828●
  animal-drawn vehicle E827●
    and
      animal (being ridden) (herded)
        (unattended) E827●

Collision (Continued)
  animal-drawn vehicle (Continued)
    and (Continued)
      nonmotor road vehicle, except
        pedal cycle E827●
      object (fallen) (fixed) (movable)
        (moving) not falling from or
        set in motion by vehicle of
        higher priority E827●
      pedestrian (conveyance or
        vehicle) E827●
      streetcar E827●
  motor vehicle (on public highway)
    (traffic accident) E812●
    after leaving, running off, public
      highway (without antecedent
      collision) (without re-entry)
      E816●
    with antecedent collision on
      public highway - *see*
      categories E810–E815
    with re-entrance collision with
      another motor vehicle
      E811●
    and
      abutment (bridge) (overpass)
        E815●
      animal (herded) (unattended)
        E815●
        carrying person, property
          E813●
      animal-drawn vehicle E813●
      another motor vehicle
        (abandoned) (disabled)
        (parked) (stalled) (stopped)
        E812●
        with, involving re-entrance (on
          same roadway) (across
          median strip) E811●
      any object, person, or vehicle off
        the public highway
        resulting from a
        noncollision motor vehicle
        nontraffic accident E816●
      avalanche, fallen or not moving
        E815●
        falling E909.2
      boundary fence E815●
      culvert E815●
      fallen
        stone E815●
        tree E815●
      guard post or guard rail E815●
      inter-highway divider E815●
      landslide, fallen or not moving
        E815●
        moving E909.2
      machinery (road) E815●
      nonmotor road vehicle NEC
        E813●
      object (any object, person, or
        vehicle off the public
        highway resulting from a
        noncollision motor vehicle
        nontraffic accident) E815●
      off, normally not on, public
        highway resulting from a
        noncollision motor
        vehicle traffic accident
        E816●
      pedal cycle E813●
      pedestrian (conveyance)
        E814●
      person (using pedestrian
        conveyance) E814●

E CODES

E CODES

E CODES

Cut, cutting *(Continued)*
  by *(Continued)*
    hand saw or tool (not powered)
      E920.4
      powered E920.1
    hedge clipper E920.4
      powered E920.1
    hoe E920.4
    ice pick E920.4
    knife E920.3
      electric E920.2
      in war operations E995.2
    lathe turnings E920.8
    lawn mower E920.4
      powered E920.0
      riding E919.8
    machine - *see* Accident, machine
    meat
      grinder E919.8
      slicer E919.8
    nails E920.8
    needle E920.4
      hypodermic E920.5
    object, edged, pointed, sharp - *see*
      category E920
      following fall E888.0
    paper cutter E920.4
    piercing instrument - *see also*
      category E920
      late effect of E929.8
    pitchfork E920.4
    powered
      can opener E920.2
      garden cultivator E920.1
        riding E919.8
      hand saw E920.1
      hand tool NEC E920.1
      hedge clipper E920.1
      household appliance or
        implement E920.2
      lawn mower (hand) E920.0
        riding E919.8
      rivet gun E920.1
      staple gun E920.1
    rake E920.4
    saw
      circular E919.4
      hand E920.4
    scissors E920.4
    screwdriver E920.4
    sewing machine (electric) (powered)
      E920.2
      not powered E920.4
    shears E920.4
    shovel E920.4
    slide trigger mechanism, scope or
      other part of gun E928.7
    spade E920.4
    splinters E920.8
    sword E920.3
      in war operations E995.2
    tin can lid E920.8
    wood slivers E920.8
  homicide (attempt) E966
  inflicted by other person
    stated as
      intentional, homicidal E966
      undetermined whether accidental
        or intentional E986
  late effect of NEC E929.8
  legal
    execution E978
    intervention E974

Cut, cutting *(Continued)*
  self-inflicted (unspecified whether
    accidental or intentional) E986
    stated as intentional, purposeful
      E956
    stated as undetermined whether
      accidental or intentional E986
  suicidal (attempt) E956
  terrorism E979.8
  war operations E995.2
Cyclone E908.1

D

Death due to injury occurring one year
  or more previous - *see* Late effect
Decapitation (accidental circumstances)
  NEC E928.9
  homicidal E966
  legal execution (by guillotine) E978
Deprivation - *see also* Privation action
  E913.3
  homicidal intent E968.4
Derailment (accidental)
  railway (rolling stock) (train) (vehicle)
    (with subsequent collision)
    E802 ●
    with
      collision (antecedent) (*see also*
        Collision, railway)
        E800 ●
      explosion (subsequent) (without
        antecedent collision)
        E802 ●
        antecedent collision E803 ●
      fall (without collision
        (antecedent)) E802 ●
      fire (without collision
        (antecedent)) E802 ●
  street car E829 ●
Descent
  parachute (voluntary) (without
    accident to aircraft) E844 ●
    due to accident to aircraft - *see*
      categories E840–E842
Desertion
  child, with intent to injure or kill E968.4
  helpless person, infant, newborn
    E904.0
    with intent to injure or kill E968.4
Destitution - *see* Privation
Dirty bomb (*see also* War operations,
  injury due to, nuclear weapons)
  E996.9
Disability, late effect or sequela of
  injury - *see* Late effect
Disease
  Andes E902.0
  aviators' E902.1
  caisson E902.2
  range E902.0
Divers' disease, palsy, paralysis, squeeze
  E902.0
Dog bite E906.0
Dragged by
  cable car (not on rails) E847
    on rails E829 ●
  motor vehicle (on highway) E814 ●
    not on highway, nontraffic accident
      E825 ●
  street car E829 ●
Drinking poison (accidental) - *see* Table of
  Drugs and Chemicals
Drowning - *see* Submersion
Dust in eye E914

E

Earth falling (on) (with asphyxia or
  suffocation (by pressure)) (*see also*
  Suffocation, due to, cave-in) E913.3
  as, or due to, a cataclysm (involving
    any transport vehicle) - *see*
    categories E908, E909
  not due to cataclysmic action E913.3
    motor vehicle (in motion) (on public
      highway) E813 ●
      not on public highway E825 ●
      nonmotor road vehicle NEC E829 ●
      pedal cycle E826 ●
      railway rolling stock, train, vehicle
        E806 ●
      street car E829 ●
    struck or crushed by E916
      with asphyxiation or suffocation
        E913.3
      with injury other than asphyxia,
        suffocation E916
Earthquake (any injury) E909.0
Effect(s) (adverse) of
  air pressure E902.9
    at high altitude E902.9
      in aircraft E902.1
      residence or prolonged visit
        (causing conditions
        classifiable to E902.0)
        E902.0
    due to
      diving E902.2
      specified cause NEC E902.8
    in aircraft E902.1
  cold, excessive (exposure to) (*see also*
    Cold, exposure to) E901.9
  heat (excessive) (*see also* Heat) E900.9
  hot
    place - *see* Heat
    weather E900.0
  insulation - *see* Heat
  late - *see* Late effect of
  motion E903
  nuclear explosion or weapon
    in
      terrorism E979.5
      war operations (*see also* War
        operations, injury due
        to, nuclear weapons)
        E996.9
  radiation - *see* Radiation
  terrorism, secondary E979.9
  travel E903
Electric shock, electrocution (accidental)
  (from exposed wire, faulty
  appliance, high voltage cable, live
  rail, open socket) (by) (in) E925.9
  appliance or wiring
    domestic E925.0
    factory E925.2
    farm (building) E925.8
      house E925.0
    home E925.0
    industrial (conductor) (control
      apparatus) (transformer)
      E925.2
    outdoors E925.8
    public building E925.8
    residential institution E925.8
    school E925.8
    specified place NEC E925.8
  caused by other person
    stated as
      intentional, homicidal E968.8
      undetermined whether accidental
        or intentional E988.4

◀ New   ◀▏▏ Revised   ~~deleted~~ Deleted   ● Use Additional Digit(s)   ▨ Omit code

Electric shock, electrocution (*Continued*)
electric power generating plant,
  distribution station E925.1
electroshock gun (taser) (stun gun)
  E925.8
  caused by other person E968.8
    legal intervention E975
    stated as accidental E925.8
    stated as intentional E968.8
  due to legal intervention E975
  stated as intentional self-harm
    (suicidal (attempt)) E958.4
  stated as undetermined whether
    accidental or intentional
    E988.4
  suicide (attempt) E958.4
  homicidal (attempt) E968.8
  legal execution E978
  lightning E907
  machinery E925.9
    domestic E925.0
    factory E925.2
    farm E925.8
    home E925.0
  misadventure in medical or surgical
    procedure
    in electroshock therapy E873.4
  self-inflicted (undetermined whether
    accidental or intentional)
    E988.4
  stated as intentional E958.4
  stated as undetermined whether
    accidental or intentional
    E988.4
  suicidal (attempt) E958.4
  transmission line E925.1
Electrocution - *see* Electric shock
Embolism E921.1
  air (traumatic) NEC - *see* Air, embolism
Encephalitis
  lead or saturnine E866.0
    from pesticide NEC E863.4
Entanglement
  in
    bedclothes, causing suffocation
      E913.0
    wheel of pedal cycle E826●
Entry of foreign body, material, any - *see*
  Foreign body
Execution, legal (any method) E978
Exertion, excessive physical, from
  prolonged activity E927.2
Exhaustion
  cold - *see* Cold, exposure to
  due to excessive exertion E927.2 ◀▥
  heat - *see* Heat
Explosion (accidental) (in) (of) (on) E923.9
  acetylene E923.2
  aerosol can E921.8
  aircraft (in transit) (powered) E841●
    at landing, take-off E840●
    in
      terrorism E979.1
      war operations
        from
          enemy fire or explosive(s)
            (device placed on
            aircraft) E994.0
          own onboard explosives
            E994.1
    unpowered E842●
  air tank (compressed) (in machinery)
    E921.1
  anesthetic gas in operating theatre
    E923.2

Explosion (*Continued*)
  automobile tire NEC E921.8
    causing transport accident - *see*
      categories E810-E825
  blasting (cap) (materials) E923.1
  boiler (machinery), not on transport
    vehicle E921.0
    steamship - *see* Explosion, watercraft
  bomb E923.8
    in
      terrorism E979.2
      war operations E993.8
        after cessation of hostilities
          E998.1
        atom, hydrogen or nuclear
          (*see also* War operations,
          injury due to, nuclear
          weapons) E996.9
        injury by fragments from
          E991.9
          antipersonnel bomb E991.3
  butane E923.2
  caused by
    other person
      stated as
        intentional, homicidal - *see*
          Assault, explosive
        undetermined whether
          accidental or homicidal
          E985.5
  coal gas E923.2
  detonator E923.1
  dynamite E923.1
  explosive (material) NEC E923.9
    gas(es) E923.2
    missile E923.8
      in
        terrorism E979.2
        war operations E993.1
          injury by fragments from
            E991.9
            antipersonnel bomb
              E991.3
    used in blasting operations E923.1
  fire-damp E923.2
  fireworks E923.0
  gas E923.2
    cylinder (in machinery) E921.1
    pressure tank (in machinery)
      E921.1
  gasoline (fumes) (tank) not in moving
    motor vehicle E923.2
  grain store (military) (munitions)
    E923.8
  grenade E923.8
    in
      terrorism E979.2
      war operations E993.8
        injury by fragments from
          E991.4
  homicide (attempt) - *see* Assault,
    explosive
  hot water heater, tank (in machinery)
    E921.0
  in mine (of explosive gases) NEC
    E923.2
  late effect of NEC E929.8
  machinery - *see also* Accident, machine
  pressure vessel - *see* Explosion,
    pressure vessel
  methane E923.2
  missile E923.8
    in
      terrorism E979.2
      war operations E993.1
        injury by fragments from
          E991.4

Explosion (*Continued*)
  motor vehicle (part of)
    in motion (on public highway)
      E818●
    not on public highway E825●
  munitions (dump) (factory) E923.8
    in
      terrorism E979.2
      war operations E993.9
  of mine E923.8
    in
      terrorism
        at sea or in harbor E979.0
        land E979.2
        marine E979.0
      war operations
        after cessation of hostilities
          E998.0
        at sea or in harbor E992.2
        land E993.8
          after cessation of hostilities
            E998.0
          injury by fragments from
            E991.4
        marine E992.2
  own weapons
    in
      terrorism (*see also* Suicide)
        E979.2
      war operations E993.7
        injury by fragments from
          E991.9
          antipersonnel bomb
            E991.3
  pressure
    cooker E921.8
    gas tank (in machinery) E921.1
    vessel (in machinery) E921.9
      on transport vehicle - *see*
        categories E800-E848
    specified type NEC E921.8
  propane E923.2
  railway engine, locomotive, train
    (boiler) (with subsequent
    collision, derailment, fall)
    E803●
    with
      collision (antecedent) (*see also*
        Collision, railway)
        E800●
      derailment (antecedent) E802●
      fire (without antecedent collision
        or derailment) E803●
  secondary fire resulting from - *see* Fire
  self-inflicted (unspecified whether
    accidental or intentional) E985.5
    stated as intentional, purposeful
      E955.5
  shell (artillery) E923.8
    in
      terrorism E979.2
      war operations E993.2
        injury by fragments from
          E991.4
  stated as undetermined whether
    caused accidentally or purposely
    inflicted E985.5
  steam or water lines (in machinery)
    E921.0
  suicide (attempted) E955.5
  terrorism - *see* Terrorism, explosion
  torpedo E923.8
    in
      terrorism E979.0
      war operations E992.0

E CODES

Explosion (Continued)
transport accident - *see* categories E800–E848
war operations - *see* War operations, explosion
watercraft (boiler) E837●
causing drowning, submersion (after jumping from watercraft) E830●
Exposure (weather) (conditions) (rain) (wind) E904.3
with homicidal intent E968.4
environmental
to
algae bloom E928.6
blue-green algae bloom E928.6
brown tide E928.6
cyanobacteria bloom E928.6
Florida red tide E928.6
harmful algae
and toxins E928.6
bloom E928.6
pfiesteria piscicida E928.6
red tide E928.6
excessive E904.3
cold (*see also* Cold, exposure to) E901.9
self-inflicted - *see* Cold, exposure to, self-inflicted
heat (*see also* Heat) E900.9
helpless person, infant, newborn due to abandonment or neglect E904.0
noise E928.1
prolonged in deep-freeze unit or refrigerator E901.1
radiation - *see* Radiation
resulting from transport accident - *see* categories E800–E848
smoke from, due to
fire - *see* Fire
tobacco, second-hand E869.4
vibration E928.2
External cause status E000.9
child assisting in compensated work of other family member E000.8 ◀
civilian
done for
financial or other compensation E000.0
pay or income E000.0
family member assisting in compensated work of other family member E000.8 ◀
for income E000.0
hobby or leisure E000.8
off duty military E000.8
military E000.1
off duty E000.8
recreation E000.8
specified NEC E000.8
sport not for income E000.8
student E000.8
volunteer E000.2 ◀▥

F

Fall, falling (accidental) E888.9
building E916
burning E891.8
private E890.8
down
escalator E880.0
ladder E881.0
in boat, ship, watercraft E833●
staircase E880.9
stairs, steps - *see* Fall, from, stairs

Fall, falling (Continued)
earth (with asphyxia or suffocation (by pressure)) (*see also* Earth, falling) E913.3
from, off
aircraft (at landing, take-off) (in-transit) (while alighting, boarding) E843●
resulting from accident to aircraft - *see* categories E840–E842
animal (in sport or transport) E828●
animal-drawn vehicle E827●
balcony E882
bed E884.4
bicycle E826●
boat, ship, watercraft (into water) E832●
after accident to, collision, fire on E830●
and subsequently struck by (part of) boat E831●
and subsequently struck by (part of) while alighting, boat E838●
burning, crushed, sinking E830●
and subsequently struck by (part of) boat E831●
bridge E882
building E882
burning (uncontrolled fire) E891.8
in terrorism E979.3
private E890.8
bunk in boat, ship, watercraft E834●
due to accident to watercraft E831●
cable car (not on rails) E847
on rails E829●
car - *see* Fall from motor vehicle E884.9
chair E884.2
cliff E884.1
commode E884.6
curb (sidewalk) E880.1
elevation aboard ship E834●
due to accident to ship E831●
embankment E884.9
escalator E880.0
fire escape E882
flagpole E882
furniture NEC E884.5
gangplank (into water) (*see also* Fall, from, boat) E832●
to deck, dock E834●
hammock on ship E834●
due to accident to watercraft E831●
haystack E884.9
heelies E885.1
high place NEC E884.9
stated as undetermined whether accidental or intentional - *see* Jumping, from, high place
horse (in sport or transport) E828●
in-line skates E885.1
ladder E881.0
in boat, ship, watercraft E833●
due to accident to watercraft E831●
machinery - *see also* Accident, machine
not in operation E884.9

Fall, falling (Continued)
from, off (Continued)
motor vehicle (in motion) (on public highway) E818●
not on public highway E825●
stationary, except while alighting, boarding, entering, leaving E884.9
while alighting, boarding, entering, leaving E824●
stationary, except while alighting, boarding, entering, leaving E884.9
while alighting, boarding, entering, leaving, except off-road type motor vehicle E817●
off-road type - *see* Fall, from, off-road type motor vehicle
motorized ◀
mobility scooter E884.3 ◀
wheelchair E884.3 ◀
nonmotor road vehicle (while alighting, boarding) NEC E829●
stationary, except while alighting, boarding, entering, leaving E884.9
off road type motor vehicle (not on public highway) NEC E821●
on public highway E818●
while alighting, boarding, entering, leaving E817●
snow vehicle - *see* Fall from snow vehicle, motor-driven
one
deck to another on ship E834●
due to accident to ship E831●
level to another NEC E884.9
boat, ship, or watercraft E834●
due to accident to watercraft E831●
pedal cycle E826●
playground equipment E884.0
railway rolling stock, train, vehicle (while alighting, boarding) E804●
with
collision (*see also* Collision, railway) E800●
derailment (*see also* Derailment, railway) E802●
explosion (*see also* Explosion, railway engine) E803●
rigging (aboard ship) E834●
due to accident to watercraft E831●
roller skates E885.1
scaffolding E881.1
scooter (nonmotorized) E885.0
motorized mobility E884.3 ◀
sidewalk (curb) E880.1
moving E885.9
skateboard E885.2
skis E885.3
snow vehicle, motor-driven (not on public highway) E820●
on public highway E818●
while alighting, boarding, entering, leaving E817●
snowboard E885.4

◀ New   ◀▥ Revised   ~~deleted~~ Deleted   ● Use Additional Digit(s)   ▥ Omit code

Fall, falling *(Continued)*
  from, off *(Continued)*
    stairs, steps E880.9
      boat, ship, watercraft E833●
        due to accident to watercraft
          E831●
      motor bus, motor vehicle - *see*
        Fall, from, motor vehicle,
        while alighting, boarding
      street car E829●
    stationary vehicle NEC E884.9
    stepladder E881.0
    street car (while boarding, alighting)
      E829●
      stationary, except while boarding
        or alighting E884.9
    structure NEC E882
      burning (uncontrolled fire) E891.8
        in terrorism E979.3
    table E884.9
    toilet E884.6
    tower E882
    tree E884.9
    turret E882
    vehicle NEC - *see also* Accident,
      vehicle NEC
      stationary E884.9
    viaduct E882
    wall E882
    wheelchair (electric) (motorized)
      E884.3 ◀║║║
    wheelies E885.1
    window E882
  in, on
    aircraft (at landing, take-off)
      (in-transit) E843●
      resulting from accident to
        aircraft - *see* categories
        E840–E842
    boat, ship, watercraft E835●
      due to accident to watercraft
        E831●
      one level to another NEC
        E834●
      on ladder, stairs E833●
    cutting or piercing instrument
      machine E888.0
    deck (of boat, ship, watercraft)
      E835●
      due to accident to watercraft
        E831●
    escalator E880.0
    gangplank E835●
    glass, broken E888.0
    knife E888.0
    ladder E881.0
      in boat, ship, watercraft E833●
        due to accident to watercraft
          E831●
    object
      edged, pointed or sharp E888.0
      other E888.1
    pitchfork E888.0
    railway rolling stock, train, vehicle
      (while alighting, boarding)
      E804●
      with
        collision (*see also* Collision,
          railway) E800●
        derailment (*see also*
          Derailment, railway)
          E802●
        explosion (*see also* Explosion,
          railway engine) E803●

Fall, falling *(Continued)*
  in, on *(Continued)*
    scaffolding E881.1
    scissors E888.0
    staircase, stairs, steps (*see also* Fall,
      from, stairs) E880.9
    street car E829●
    water transport (*see also* Fall, in,
      boat) E835●
  into
    cavity E883.9
    dock E883.9
      from boat, ship, watercraft (*see
        also* Fall, from, boat)
        E832●
    hold (of ship) E834●
      due to accident to watercraft
        E831●
    hole E883.9
    manhole E883.2
    moving part of machinery - *see*
      Accident, machine
    opening in surface NEC E883.9
    pit E883.9
    quarry E883.9
    shaft E883.9
    storm drain E883.2
    tank E883.9
    water (with drowning or
      submersion) E910.9
    well E883.1
  late effect of NEC E929.3
  object (*see also* Hit by, object, falling)
    E916
  other E888.8
  over
    animal E885.9
    cliff E884.1
    embankment E884.9
    small object E885.9
  overboard (*see also* Fall, from, boat)
    E832●
  resulting in striking against object
    E888.1
    sharp E888.0
  rock E916
  same level NEC E888.9
    aircraft (any kind) E843●
      resulting from accident to
        aircraft - *see* categories
        E840–E842
    boat, ship, watercraft E835●
      due to accident to, collision,
        watercraft E831●
    from
      collision, pushing, shoving, by
        or with other person(s)
        E886.9
        as, or caused by, a crowd
          E917.6
        in sports E886.0
      in-line skates E885.1
      roller skates E885.1
      scooter (nonmotorized)
        E885.0
      skateboard E885.2
      skis E885.3
      slipping, stumbling, tripping
        E885.9
      snowboard E885.4
  snowslide E916
    as avalanche E909.2
  stone E916

Fall, falling *(Continued)*
  through
    hatch (on ship) E834●
      due to accident to watercraft
        E831●
    roof E882
    window E882
  timber E916
  while alighting from, boarding,
    entering, leaving
    aircraft (any kind) E843●
    motor bus, motor vehicle - *see* Fall,
      from, motor vehicle, while
      alighting, boarding
    nonmotor road vehicle NEC E829●
    railway train E804●
    street car E829●
Fallen on by
  animal (horse) (not being ridden)
    E906.8
    being ridden (in sport or transport)
      E828●
**Fell or jumped from high place, so
  stated** - *see* Jumping, from, high
  place
Felo-de-se (*see also* Suicide) E958.9
Fever
  heat - *see* Heat
  thermic - *see* Heat
Fight (hand) (fist) (foot) (*see also* Assault,
  fight) E960.0
Fire (accidental) (caused by great heat
  from appliance (electrical), hot
  object, or hot substance) (secondary,
  resulting from explosion) E899
  conflagration - *see* Conflagration E892
  controlled, normal (in brazier,
    fireplace, furnace, or stove)
    (charcoal) (coal) (coke) (electric)
    (gas) (wood)
    bonfire E897
    brazier, not in building or structure
      E897
    in building or structure, except
      private dwelling (barn) (church)
      (convalescent or residential
      home) (factory) (farm
      outbuilding) (hospital) (hotel)
      (institution (educational)
      (dormitory) (residential)
      (private garage) (school) (shop)
      (store) (theatre) E896
    in private dwelling (apartment)
      (boarding house) (camping
      place) (caravan) (farmhouse)
      (home (private) (house)
      (lodging house) (rooming
      house) (tenement) E895
    not in building or structure E897
    trash E897
  forest (uncontrolled) E892
  grass (uncontrolled) E892
  hay (uncontrolled) E892
  homicide (attempt) E968.0
    late effect of E969
  in, of, on, starting in E892
    aircraft (in transit) (powered) E841●
      at landing, take-off E840●
      stationary E892
      unpowered (balloon) (glider)
        E842●
    balloon E842●
    boat, ship, watercraft - *see* categories
      E830, E831, E837

Fire *(Continued)*
in, of, on, starting in *(Continued)*
building or structure, except private dwelling (barn) (church) (convalescent or residential home) (factory) (farm outbuilding) (hospital) (hotel) (institution) (educational) (dormitory) (residential)) (school) (shop) (store) (theatre) *(see also* Conflagration, building or structure, except private dwelling) E891.9
forest (uncontrolled) E892
glider E842●
grass (uncontrolled) E892
hay (uncontrolled) E892
lumber (uncontrolled) E892
machinery - *see* Accident, machine
mine (uncontrolled) E892
motor vehicle (in motion) (on public highway) E818●
not on public highway E825●
stationary E892
prairie (uncontrolled) E892
private dwelling (apartment) (boarding house) (camping place) (caravan) (farmhouse) (home (private)) (house) (lodging house) (private garage) (rooming house) (tenement) *(see also* Conflagration, private dwelling) E890.9
railway rolling stock, train, vehicle *(see also* Explosion, railway engine) E803●
stationary E892
room NEC E898.1
street car (in motion) E829●
stationary E892
terrorism (by fire-producing device) E979.3
fittings or furniture (burning building) (uncontrolled fire) E979.3
from nuclear explosion E979.5
transport vehicle, stationary NEC E892
tunnel (uncontrolled) E892
war operations (by fire-producing device or conventional weapon) E990.9
from nuclear explosion *(see also* War operations, injury due to, nuclear weapons) E996.2
incendiary bomb E990.0
petrol bomb E990.0
late effect of NEC E929.4
lumber (uncontrolled) E892
mine (uncontrolled) E892
prairie (uncontrolled) E892
self-inflicted (unspecified whether accidental or intentional) E988.1
stated as intentional, purposeful E958.1
specified NEC E898.1
with
conflagration - *see* Conflagration
ignition (of)
clothing - *see* Ignition, clothes
highly inflammable material (benzine) (fat) (gasoline) (kerosene) (paraffin) (petrol) E894

Fire *(Continued)*
started by other person
stated as
with intent to injure or kill E968.0
undetermined whether or not with intent to injure or kill E988.1
suicide (attempted) E958.1
late effect of E959
tunnel (uncontrolled) E892
Fireball effects from nuclear explosion in
terrorism E979.5
war operations *(see also* War operations, injury due to, nuclear weapons) E996.2
Fireworks (explosion) E923.0
Flash burns from explosion *(see also* Explosion) E923.9
Flood (any injury) (resulting from storm) E908.2
caused by collapse of dam or manmade structure E909.3
Forced landing (aircraft) E840●
Foreign body, object or material (entrance into (accidental))
air passage (causing injury) E915
with asphyxia, obstruction, suffocation E912
food or vomitus E911
nose (with asphyxia, obstruction, suffocation) E912
causing injury without asphyxia, obstruction, suffocation E915
alimentary canal (causing injury) (with obstruction) E915
with asphyxia, obstruction respiratory passage, suffocation E912
food E911
mouth E915
with asphyxia, obstruction, suffocation E912
food E911
pharynx E915
with asphyxia, obstruction, suffocation E912
food E911
aspiration (with asphyxia, obstruction respiratory passage, suffocation) E912
causing injury without asphyxia, obstruction respiratory passage, suffocation E915
food (regurgitated) (vomited) E911
causing injury without asphyxia, obstruction respiratory passage, suffocation E915
mucus (not of newborn) E912
phlegm E912
bladder (causing injury or obstruction) E915
bronchus, bronchi - *see* Foreign body, air passages
conjunctival sac E914
digestive system - *see* Foreign body, alimentary canal
ear (causing injury or obstruction) E915
esophagus (causing injury or obstruction) *(see also* Foreign body, alimentary canal) E915
eye (any part) E914
eyelid E914

Foreign body, object or material *(Continued)*
hairball (stomach) (with obstruction) E915
ingestion - *see* Foreign body, alimentary canal
inhalation - *see* Foreign body, aspiration
intestine (causing injury or obstruction) E915
iris E914
lacrimal apparatus E914
larynx - *see* Foreign body, air passage
late effect of NEC E929.8
lung - *see* Foreign body, air passage
mouth - *see* Foreign body, alimentary canal, mouth
nasal passage - *see* Foreign body, air passage, nose
nose - *see* Foreign body, air passage, nose
ocular muscle E914
operation wound (left in) - *see* Misadventure, foreign object
orbit E914
pharynx - *see* Foreign body, alimentary canal, pharynx
rectum (causing injury or obstruction) E915
stomach (hairball) (causing injury or obstruction) E915
tear ducts or glands E914
trachea - *see* Foreign body, air passage
urethra (causing injury or obstruction) E915
vagina (causing injury or obstruction) E915
Found dead, injured
from exposure (to) - *see* Exposure
on
public highway E819●
railway right of way E807●
Fracture (circumstances unknown or unspecified) E887
due to specified external means - *see* manner of accident
late effect of NEC E929.3
occurring in water transport NEC E835●
Freezing - *see* Cold, exposure to
Frostbite E901.0
due to manmade conditions E901.1
Frozen - *see* Cold, exposure to

G

Garrotting, homicidal (attempted) E963
Gored E906.8
Gunshot wound *(see also* Shooting) E922.9

H

Hailstones, injury by E904.3
Hairball (stomach) (with obstruction) E915
Hanged himself *(see also* Hanging, self-inflicted) E983.0
Hang gliding E842●
Hanging (accidental) E913.8
caused by other person
in accidental circumstances E913.8

◄ New   ◄ Revised   ~~deleted~~ Deleted   ● Use Additional Digit(s)   ▚ Omit code

Hanging *(Continued)*
  caused by other person *(Continued)*
    stated as
      intentional, homicidal E963
      undetermined whether accidental
        or intentional E983.0
  homicide (attempt) E963
  in bed or cradle E913.0
  legal execution E978
  self-inflicted (unspecified whether
    accidental or intentional)
    E983.0
    in accidental circumstances E913.8
    stated as intentional, purposeful
      E953.0
    stated as undetermined whether
      accidental or intentional E983.0
  suicidal (attempt) E953.0
Heat (apoplexy) (collapse) (cramps)
  (effects of) (excessive) (exhaustion)
  (fever) (prostration) (stroke) E900.9
  due to
    manmade conditions (as listed in
      E900.1, except boat, ship,
      watercraft) E900.1
    weather (conditions) E900.0
  from
    electric heating apparatus causing
      burning E924.8
    nuclear explosion
      in
        terrorism E979.5
        war operations *(see also* War
          operations, injury due
          to, nuclear weapons)
          E996.2
  generated in, boiler, engine,
    evaporator, fire room of boat,
    ship, watercraft E838●
  inappropriate in local application or
    packing in medical or surgical
    procedure E873.5
  late effect of NEC E989
Hemorrhage
  delayed following medical or surgical
    treatment without mention of
    misadventure - *see* Reaction,
    abnormal
  during medical or surgical treatment as
    misadventure - *see* Misadventure,
    cut
High
  altitude, effects E902.9
  level of radioactivity, effects - *see*
    Radiation
  pressure effects - *see also* Effects of, air
    pressure
    from rapid descent in water
      (causing caisson or divers'
      disease, palsy, or paralysis)
      E902.2
  temperature, effects - *see* Heat
Hit, hitting (accidental) by
  aircraft (propeller) (without accident to
    aircraft) E844●
    unpowered E842●
  avalanche E909.2
  being thrown against object in or
    part of
    motor vehicle (in motion) (on public
      highway) E818●
      not on public highway E825●
    nonmotor road vehicle NEC
      E829●
    street car E829●

Hit, hitting *(Continued)*
  boat, ship, watercraft
    after fall from watercraft E838●
      damaged, involved in accident
        E831●
    while swimming, water skiing
      E838●
  bullet *(see also* Shooting) E922.9
    from air gun E922.4
    in
      terrorism E979.4
    war operations E991.2
      rubber E991.0
  flare, Verey pistol *(see also* Shooting)
    E922.8
  hailstones E904.3
  landslide E909.2
  law-enforcing agent (on duty) E975
    with blunt object (baton) (night
      stick) (stave) (truncheon)
      E973
  machine - *see* Accident, machine
  missile
    firearm *(see also* Shooting)
      E922.9
    in
      terrorism - *see* Terrorism,
        missile
      war operations - *see* War
        operations, missile
  motor vehicle (on public highway)
    (traffic accident) E814●
    not on public highway, nontraffic
      accident E822●
  nonmotor road vehicle NEC E829●
  object
    falling E916
      from, in, on
        aircraft E844●
          due to accident to aircraft -
            see categories
            E840–E842
          unpowered E842●
        boat, ship, watercraft E838●
          due to accident to
            watercraft E831●
        building E916
          burning E891.8
            in terrorism E979.3
            private E890.8
        cataclysmic
          earth surface movement or
            eruption E909.9
          storm E908.9
        cave-in E916
          with asphyxiation or
            suffocation *(see also*
            Suffocation, due to,
            cave-in) E913.3
        earthquake E909.0
        motor vehicle (in motion)
          (on public highway)
          E818●
          not on public highway
            E825●
          stationary E916
        nonmotor road vehicle NEC
          E829●
        pedal cycle E826●
        railway rolling stock, train,
          vehicle E806●
        street car E829●
        structure, burning NEC
          E891.8
        vehicle, stationary E916

Hit, hitting *(Continued)*
  object *(Continued)*
    moving NEC - *see* Striking against,
      object
    projected NEC - *see* Striking against,
      object
    set in motion by
      compressed air or gas, spring,
        striking, throwing - *see*
        Striking against, object
      explosion - *see* Explosion
    thrown into, on, or towards
      motor vehicle (in motion) (on
        public highway) E818●
        not on public highway E825●
      nonmotor road vehicle NEC
        E829●
      pedal cycle E826●
      street car E829●
    off-road type motor vehicle (not on
      public highway) E821●
      on public highway E814●
    other person(s) E917.9
      with blunt or thrown object
        E917.9
        in sports E917.0
          with subsequent fall E917.5
        intentionally, homicidal E968.2
      as, or caused by, a crowd E917.1
        with subsequent fall E917.6
      in sports E917.0
    pedal cycle E826●
    police (on duty) E975
      with blunt object (baton)
        (nightstick) (stave)
        (truncheon) E973
    railway, rolling stock, train, vehicle
      (part of) E805●
    shot - *see* Shooting
    snow vehicle, motor-driven (not on
      public highway) E820●
      on public highway E814●
    street car E829●
    vehicle NEC - *see* Accident, vehicle
      NEC
Homicide, homicidal (attempt)
  (justifiable) *(see also* Assault) E968.9
Hot
  liquid, object, substance, accident
    caused by - *see also* Accident,
    caused by, hot, by type of
    substance
    late effect of E929.8
  place, effects - *see* Heat
  weather, effects E900.0
Humidity, causing problem E904.3
Hunger E904.1
  resulting from
    abandonment or neglect E904.0
    transport accident - *see* categories
      E800–E848
Hurricane (any injury) E908.0
Hypobarism, hypobaropathy - *see* Effects
  of, air pressure
Hypothermia - *see* Cold, exposure to

I

Ictus
  caloris - *see* Heat
  solaris E900.0
Ignition (accidental)
  anesthetic gas in operating theatre
    E923.2

Ignition (Continued)
  bedclothes
    with
      conflagration - *see* Conflagration
      ignition (of)
        clothing - *see* Ignition, clothes
        highly inflammable material
          obstruction (benzine)
            (fat) (gasoline) (kerosene)
            (paraffin) (petrol) E894
  benzine E894
  clothes, clothing (from controlled fire)
    (in building) E893.9
    with conflagration - *see*
      Conflagration
    from
      bonfire E893.2
      highly inflammable material
        E894
      sources or material as listed in
        E893.8
      trash fire E893.2
      uncontrolled fire - *see*
        Conflagration
    in
      private dwelling E893.0
      specified building or structure,
        except of private dwelling
        E893.1
    not in building or structure E893.2
  explosive material - *see* Explosion
  fat E894
  gasoline E894
  kerosene E894
  material
    explosive - *see* Explosion
    highly inflammable E894
      with conflagration - *see*
        Conflagration
      with explosion E923.2
  nightdress - *see* Ignition, clothes
  paraffin E894
  petrol E894
Immersion - *see* Submersion
Implantation of quills of porcupine
  E906.8
Inanition (from) E904.9
  hunger - *see* Lack of, food
  resulting from homicidal intent
    E968.4
  thirst - *see* Lack of, water
Inattention after, at birth E904.0
  homicidal, infanticidal intent E968.4
Infanticide (*see also* Assault)
Ingestion
  foreign body (causing injury) (with
    obstruction) - *see* Foreign body,
    alimentary canal
  poisonous substance NEC - *see* Table of
    Drugs and Chemicals
Inhalation
  excessively cold substance, manmade
    E901.1
  foreign body - *see* Foreign body,
    aspiration
  liquid air, hydrogen, nitrogen E901.1
  mucus, not of newborn (with asphyxia,
    obstruction respiratory passage,
    suffocation) E912
  phlegm (with asphyxia, obstruction
    respiratory passage, suffocation)
    E912
  poisonous gas - *see* Table of Drugs and
    Chemicals

Inhalation (Continued)
  smoke from, due to
    fire - *see* Fire
    tobacco, second-hand E869.4
  vomitus (with asphyxia, obstruction
    respiratory passage, suffocation)
    E911
Injury, injured (accidental(ly)) NEC
  E928.9
  by, caused by, from
    air rifle (B-B gun) E922.4
    animal (not being ridden) NEC E906.9
      being ridden (in sport or
        transport) E828●
    assault (*see also* Assault) E968.9
    avalanche E909.2
    bayonet (*see also* Bayonet wound)
      E920.3
    being thrown against some part of,
      or object in
      motor vehicle (in motion) (on
        public highway) E818●
      not on public highway E825●
      nonmotor road vehicle NEC
        E829●
      off-road motor vehicle NEC E821●
      railway train E806●
      snow vehicle, motor-driven E820●
      street car E829●
    bending E927.8 ◀▥▥
      due to ◀
        repetitive movement E927.3 ◀
        sudden strenuous movement
          E927.0 ◀
    bite, human E928.3
    broken glass E920.8
    bullet - *see* Shooting
    cave-in (*see also* Suffocation, due to,
      cave-in) E913.3
      earth surface movement or
        eruption E909.9
      storm E908.9
      without asphyxiation or
        suffocation E916
    cloudburst E908.8
    component of firearm or air gun
      E928.7
    cutting or piercing instrument (*see
      also* Cut) E920.9
    cyclone E908.1
    earth surface movement or eruption
      E909.9
    earthquake E909.0
    electric current (*see also* Electric
      shock) E925.9
    explosion (*see also* Explosion) E923.9
      of gun part E928.7
    fire - *see* Fire
    flare, Verey pistol E922.8
    flood E908.2
    foreign body - *see* Foreign body
    gun recoil E928.7
    hailstones E904.3
    hurricane E908.0
    landslide E909.2
    law-enforcing agent, police, in
      course of legal intervention -
      see Legal intervention
    lightning E907
    live rail or live wire - *see* Electric shock
    machinery - *see also* Accident,
      machine aircraft, without
      accident to aircraft E844●
      boat, ship, watercraft (deck)
        (engine room) (galley)
        (laundry) (loading) E836●

Injury, injured (Continued)
  by, caused by, from (Continued)
    mechanism of firearm or air gun
      E928.7
    missile
      explosive E923.8
      firearm - *see* Shooting
      in
        terrorism - *see* Terrorism,
          missile
        war operations - *see* War
          operations, missile
    moving part of motor vehicle (in
      motion) (on public highway)
      E818●
      not on public highway, nontraffic
        accident E825●
      while alighting, boarding,
        entering, leaving - *see* Fall,
        from, motor vehicle, while
        alighting, boarding
    nail E920.8
    needle (sewing) E920.4
      hypodermic E920.5
    noise E928.1
    object
      fallen on
        motor vehicle (in motion) (on
          public highway) E818●
        not on public highway
          E825●
      falling - *see* Hit by, object, falling
    paintball gun E922.5
    radiation - *see* Radiation
    railway rolling stock, train, vehicle
      (part of) E805●
      door or window E806●
    recoil of firearm E928.7
    rotating propeller, aircraft E844●
    rough landing of off-road type motor
      vehicle (after leaving ground
      or rough terrain) E821●
    snow vehicle E820●
    saber (*see also* Wound, saber) E920.3
    shot - *see* Shooting
    sound waves E928.1
    splinter or sliver, wood E920.8
    straining E927.8 ◀▥▥
      due to ◀
        repetitive movement E927.3 ◀
        sudden strenuous movement
          E927.0 ◀
    street car (door) E829●
    suicide (attempt) E958.9
    sword E920.3
    terrorism - *see* Terrorism
    third rail - *see* Electric shock
    thunderbolt E907
    tidal wave E909.4
      caused by storm E908.0
    tornado E908.1
    torrential rain E908.2
    twisting E927.8 ◀▥▥
      due to ◀
        repetitive movement E927.3 ◀
        sudden strenuous movement
          E927.0 ◀
    vehicle NEC - *see* Accident, vehicle
      NEC
    vibration E928.2
    volcanic eruption E909.1
    weapon burst, in war operations
      E993.9
    weightlessness (in spacecraft, real or
      simulated) E928.0
    wood splinter or sliver E920.8

◀ New   ◀▥▥ Revised   ~~deleted~~ Deleted   ● Use Additional Digit(s)   ▥▥ Omit code

Injury, injured *(Continued)*
　due to
　　civil insurrection - *see* War operations
　　　occurring after cessation of
　　　　hostilities E993.9
　　terrorism - *see* Terrorism
　　war operations - *see* War operations
　　　occurring after cessation of
　　　　hostilities E993.9
　　weapon of mass destruction
　　　[WMD] E997.3
　homicidal *(see also* Assault) E968.9
　in, on
　　civil insurrection - *see* War
　　　operations
　　fight E960.0
　　parachute descent (voluntary)
　　　(without accident to aircraft)
　　　E844●
　　　with accident to aircraft - *see*
　　　　categories E840-E842
　　public highway E819●
　　railway right of way E807●
　　terrorism - *see* Terrorism
　　war operations - *see* War operations
　inflicted (by)
　　in course of arrest (attempted),
　　　suppression of disturbance,
　　　maintenance of order, by law
　　　enforcing agents - *see* Legal
　　　intervention
　　law-enforcing agent (on duty) - *see*
　　　Legal intervention
　　other person
　　　stated as
　　　　accidental E928.9
　　　　homicidal, intentional - *see*
　　　　　Assault
　　　　undetermined whether
　　　　　accidental or intentional -
　　　　　see Injury, stated as
　　　　　undetermined
　　police (on duty) - *see* Legal
　　　intervention
　late effect of E929.9
　purposely (inflicted) by other
　　person(s) - *see* Assault
　self-inflicted (unspecified whether
　　accidental or intentional) E988.9
　　stated as
　　　accidental E928.9
　　　intentionally, purposely E958.9
　specified cause NEC E928.8
　stated as
　　undetermined whether accidentally
　　　or purposely inflicted (by)
　　　E988.9
　　cut (any part of body) E986
　　cutting or piercing instrument
　　　(classifiable to E920) E986
　　drowning E984
　　explosive(s) (missile) E985.5
　　falling from high place E987.9
　　　manmade structure, except
　　　　residential E987.1
　　　natural site E987.2
　　　residential premises E987.0
　　hanging E983.0
　　knife E986
　　late effect of E989
　　puncture (any part of body) E986
　　shooting - *see* Shooting, stated as
　　　undetermined whether
　　　accidental or intentional
　　specified means NEC E988.8
　　stab (any part of body) E986

Injury, injured *(Continued)*
　stated as *(Continued)*
　　strangulation - *see* Suffocation,
　　　stated as undetermined
　　　whether accidental or
　　　intentional
　　submersion E984
　　suffocation - *see* Suffocation, stated
　　　as undetermined whether
　　　accidental or intentional
　to child due to criminal abortion
　　E968.8
Insufficient nourishment - *see also* Lack
　of, food
　homicidal intent E968.4
Insulation, effects - *see* Heat
Interruption of respiration by
　food lodged in esophagus E911
　foreign body, except food, in
　　esophagus E912
Intervention, legal - *see* Legal
　intervention
Intoxication, drug or poison - *see* Table
　of Drugs and Chemicals
Irradiation - *see* Radiation

J

Jammed (accidentally)
　between objects (moving) (stationary
　　and moving) E918
　in object E918
Jumped or fell from high place, so
　stated - *see* Jumping, from, high
　place, stated as
　in undetermined circumstances
Jumping
　before train, vehicle or other moving
　　object (unspecified whether
　　accidental or intentional) E988.0
　　stated as
　　　intentional, purposeful E958.0
　　　suicidal (attempt) E958.0
　from
　　aircraft
　　　by parachute (voluntarily)
　　　　(without accident to
　　　　aircraft) E844●
　　　due to accident to aircraft - *see*
　　　　categories E840–E842
　　boat, ship, watercraft (into water)
　　　after accident to, fire on,
　　　　watercraft E830●
　　　and subsequently struck by
　　　　(part of) boat E831●
　　　burning, crushed, sinking E830●
　　　and subsequently struck by
　　　　(part of) boat E831●
　　　voluntarily, without accident (to
　　　　boat) with injury other than
　　　　drowning or submersion
　　　　E883.0
　　building - *see also* Jumping, from,
　　　high place
　　　burning (uncontrolled fire) E891.8
　　　　in terrorism E979.3
　　　private E890.8
　　cable car (not on rails) E847
　　　on rails E829●
　　high place
　　　in accidental circumstances or
　　　　in sport - *see* categories
　　　　E880–E884

Jumping *(Continued)*
　from *(Continued)*
　　high place *(Continued)*
　　　stated as
　　　　with intent to injure self E957.9
　　　　　man-made structures NEC
　　　　　　E957.1
　　　　　natural sites E957.2
　　　　　residential premises E957.0
　　　　in undetermined
　　　　　circumstances E987.9
　　　　　man-made structures NEC
　　　　　　E987.1
　　　　　natural sites E987.2
　　　　　residential premises E987.0
　　　　suicidal (attempt) E957.9
　　　　　man-made structures NEC
　　　　　　E957.1
　　　　　natural sites E957.1
　　　　　residential premises E957.0
　　motor vehicle (in motion) (on public
　　　highway) - *see* Fall, from,
　　　motor vehicle
　　nonmotor road vehicle NEC E829●
　　street car E829●
　　structure - *see also* Jumping, from,
　　　high place
　　　burning NEC (uncontrolled fire)
　　　　E891.8
　　　in terrorism E979.3
　into water
　　with injury other than drowning or
　　　submersion E883.0
　　drowning or submersion - *see*
　　　Submersion
　　from, off, watercraft - *see* Jumping,
　　　from, boat
Justifiable homicide - *see* Assault

K

Kicked by
　animal E906.8
　person(s) (accidentally) E917.9
　　with intent to injure or kill E960.0
　　as, or caused by a crowd E917.1
　　　with subsequent fall E917.6
　　in fight E960.0
　　in sports E917.0
　　　with subsequent fall E917.5
Kicking against
　object (moving) E917.9
　　in sports E917.0
　　　with subsequent fall E917.5
　　stationary E917.4
　　　with subsequent fall E917.8
　person - *see* Striking against, person
Killed, killing (accidentally) NEC *(see also*
　Injury) E928.9
　in
　　action - *see* War operations
　　brawl, fight (hand) (fists) (foot)
　　　E960.0
　　　by weapon - *see also* Assault
　　　　cutting, piercing E966
　　　　firearm - *see* Shooting,
　　　　　homicide
　self
　　stated as
　　　accident E928.9
　　　suicide - *see* Suicide
　　　unspecified whether accidental or
　　　　suicidal E988.9

E CODES

Knocked down (accidentally) (by) NEC
E928.9
  animal (not being ridden) E906.8
    being ridden (in sport or transport)
     E828●
  blast from explosion (see also
    Explosion) E923.9
  crowd, human stampede E917.6
  late effect of - see Late effect
  person (accidentally) E917.9
    in brawl, fight E960.0
    in sports E917.5
  transport vehicle - see vehicle involved
    under Hit by
  while boxing E917.5

L

Laceration NEC E928.9
Lack of
  air (refrigerator or closed place),
    suffocation by E913.2
  care (helpless person) (infant)
    (newborn) E904.0
    homicidal intent E968.4
  food except as result of transport
    accident E904.1
    helpless person, infant, newborn
     due to abandonment or
     neglect E904.0
  water except as result of transport
    accident E904.2
    helpless person, infant, newborn
     due to abandonment or
     neglect E904.0
Landslide E909.2
  falling on, hitting
    motor vehicle (any) (in motion) (on
     or off public highway) E909.2
    railway rolling stock, train, vehicle
     E909.2
Late effect of
  accident NEC (accident classifiable to
    E928.9) E929.9
    specified NEC (accident classifiable
     to E910–E928.8) E929.8
  assault E969
  fall, accidental (accident classifiable to
    E880–E888) E929.3
  fire, accident caused by (accident
    classifiable to E890–E899) E929.4
  homicide, attempt (any means) E969
  injury due to terrorism E999.1
  injury undetermined whether
    accidentally or purposely
    inflicted (injury classifiable to
    E980–E988) E989
  legal intervention (injury classifiable to
    E970–E976) E977
  medical or surgical procedure, test or
    therapy
    as, or resulting in, or from
     abnormal or delayed reaction or
     complication - see Reaction,
     abnormal
     misadventure - see Misadventure
  motor vehicle accident (accident
    classifiable to E810–E825)
    E929.0
  natural or environmental factor,
    accident due to (accident
    classifiable to E900–E909)
    E929.5

Late effect of (Continued)
  poisoning, accidental (accident
    classifiable to E850–E858,
    E860–E869) E929.2
  suicide, attempt (any means) E959
  transport accident NEC (accident
    classifiable to E800–E807,
    E826–E838, E840–E848) E929.1
  war operations, injury due to (injury
    classifiable to E990–E998) E999.0
Launching pad accident E845●
Legal
  execution, any method E978
  intervention (by) (injury from) E976
    baton E973
    bayonet E974
    blow E975
    blunt object (baton) (nightstick)
     (stave) (truncheon) E973
    cutting or piercing instrument E974
    dynamite E971
    execution, any method E973
    explosive(s) (shell) E971
    firearm(s) E970
    gas (asphyxiation) (poisoning)
     (tear) E972
    grenade E971
    late effect of E977
    machine gun E970
    manhandling E975
    mortar bomb E971
    nightstick E973
    revolver E970
    rifle E970
    specified means NEC E975
    stabbing E974
    stave E973
    truncheon E973
Lifting, injury in E927.8 ◀▥
  due to ◀
    repetitive movement E927.3 ◀
    sudden strenuous movement
     E927.0 ◀
Lightning (shock) (stroke) (struck by)
  E907
Liquid (noncorrosive) in eye E914
  corrosive E924.1
Loss of control
  motor vehicle (on public highway)
    (without antecedent collision)
    E816●
    with
     antecedent collision on public
      highway - see Collision,
      motor vehicle
     involving any object, person or
      vehicle not on public
      highway E816●
     on public highway - see
      Collision, motor vehicle
     not on public highway,
      nontraffic accident E825●
      with antecedent collision -
       see Collision, motor
       vehicle, not on public
       highway
    off-road type motor vehicle (not on
     public highway) E821●
     on public highway - see Loss of
      control, motor vehicle
    snow vehicle, motor-driven (not on
     public highway) E820●
     on public highway - see Loss of
      control, motor vehicle

Lost at sea E832●
  with accident to watercraft E830●
  in war operations E995.8
Low
  pressure, effects - see Effects of, air
    pressure
  temperature, effects - see Cold
    exposure to
Lying before train, vehicle or other
  moving object (unspecified
  whether accidental or intentional)
  E988.0
  stated as intentional, purposeful,
    suicidal (attempt) E958.0
Lynching (see also Assault) E968.9

M

Malfunction, atomic power plant in
  water transport E838●
Mangled (accidentally) NEC E928.9
Manhandling (in brawl, fight) E960.0
  legal intervention E975
Manslaughter (nonaccidental) - see
  Assault
Marble in nose E912
Mauled by animal E906.8
Medical procedure, complication of
  delayed or as an abnormal reaction
    without mention of
    misadventure - see Reaction,
    abnormal
  due to or as a result of misadventure -
    see Misadventure
Melting of fittings and furniture in
  burning
  in terrorism E979.3
Minamata disease E865.2
Misadventure(s) to patient(s) during
  surgical or medical care E876.9
  contaminated blood, fluid, drug or
    biological substance (presence of
    agents and toxins as listed in
    E875) E875.9
    administered (by) NEC E875.9
     infusion E875.0
     injection E875.1
     specified means NEC E875.2
     transfusion E875.0
     vaccination E875.1
  cut, cutting, puncture, perforation or
    hemorrhage (accidental)
    (inadvertent) (inappropriate)
    (during) E870.9
    aspiration of fluid or tissue (by
     puncture or catheterization,
     except heart) E870.5
    biopsy E870.8
     needle (aspirating) E870.5
    blood sampling E870.5
    catheterization E870.5
     heart E870.6
    dialysis (kidney) E870.2
    endoscopic examination E870.4
    enema E870.7
    infusion E870.1
    injection E870.3
    lumbar puncture E870.5
    needle biopsy E870.5
    paracentesis, abdominal E870.5
    perfusion E870.2
    specified procedure NEC E870.8
    surgical operation E870.0

◀ New   ◀▥ Revised   ~~deleted~~ Deleted   ● Use Additional Digit(s)   ▥ Omit code

Misadventure(s) to patient(s) during surgical or medical care *(Continued)*
cut, cutting, puncture, perforation or hemorrhage *(Continued)*
  thoracentesis E870.5
  transfusion E870.1
  vaccination E870.3
excessive amount of blood or other fluid during transfusion or infusion E873.0
failure
  in dosage E873.9
  electroshock therapy E873.4
  inappropriate temperature (too hot or too cold) in local application and packing E873.5
  infusion
    excessive amount of fluid E873.0
    incorrect dilution of fluid E873.1
  insulin-shock therapy E873.4
  nonadministration of necessary drug or medicinal E873.6
  overdose - *see also* Overdose
  radiation, in therapy E873.2
  radiation
    inadvertent exposure of patient (receiving radiation for test or therapy) E873.3
    not receiving radiation for test or therapy - *see* Radiation
    overdose E873.2
  specified procedure NEC E873.8
  transfusion
    excessive amount of blood E873.0
mechanical, of instrument or apparatus (during procedure) E874.9
  aspiration of fluid or tissue (by puncture or catheterization, except of heart) E874.4
  biopsy E874.8
    needle (aspirating) E874.4
  blood sampling E874.4
  catheterization E874.4
    heart E874.5
  dialysis (kidney) E874.2
  endoscopic examination E874.3
  enema E874.8
  infusion E874.1
  injection E874.8
  lumbar puncture E874.4
  needle biopsy E874.4
  paracentesis, abdominal E874.4
  perfusion E874.2
  specified procedure NEC E874.8
  surgical operation E874.0
  thoracentesis E874.4
  transfusion E874.1
  vaccination E874.8
sterile precautions (during procedure) E872.9
  aspiration of fluid or tissue (by puncture or catheterization, except heart) E872.5
  biopsy E872.8
    needle (aspirating) E872.5

Misadventure(s) to patient(s) during surgical or medical care *(Continued)*
failure *(Continued)*
  sterile precautions *(Continued)*
    blood sampling E872.5
    catheterization E872.5
      heart E872.6
    dialysis (kidney) E872.2
    endoscopic examination E872.4
    enema E872.8
    infusion E872.1
    injection E872.3
    lumbar puncture E872.5
    needle biopsy E872.5
    paracentesis, abdominal E872.5
    perfusion E872.2
    removal of catheter or packing E872.8
    specified procedure NEC E872.8
    surgical operation E872.0
    thoracentesis E872.5
    transfusion E872.1
    vaccination E872.3
  suture or ligature during surgical procedure E876.2
  to introduce or to remove tube or instrument E876.4
  foreign object left in body - *see* Misadventure, foreign object
foreign object left in body (during procedure) E871.9
  aspiration of fluid or tissue (by puncture or catheterization, except heart) E871.5
  biopsy E871.8
    needle (aspirating) E871.5
  blood sampling E871.5
  catheterization E871.5
    heart E871.6
  dialysis (kidney) E871.2
  endoscopic examination E871.4
  enema E871.8
  infusion E871.1
  injection E871.3
  lumbar puncture E871.5
  needle biopsy E871.5
  paracentesis, abdominal E871.5
  perfusion E871.2
  removal of catheter or packing E871.7
  specified procedure NEC E871.8
  surgical operation E871.0
  thoracentesis E871.5
  transfusion E871.1
  vaccination E871.3
hemorrhage - *see* Misadventure, cut
inadvertent exposure of patient to radiation (being received for test or therapy) E873.3
inappropriate
  temperature (too hot or too cold) in local application or packing E873.5
infusion - *see also* Misadventure, by specific type, infusion
  excessive amount of fluid E873.0
  incorrect dilution of fluid E873.1
  wrong fluid E876.1
mismatched blood in transfusion E876.0

Misadventure(s) to patient(s) during surgical or medical care *(Continued)*
nonadministration of necessary drug or medicinal E873.6
overdose - *see also* Overdose
  radiation, in therapy E873.2
perforation - *see* Misadventure, cut
performance of correct operation (procedure) on wrong
  body part E876.7
  side E876.7
  site E876.7
performance of operation (procedure)
  intended for another patient E876.6
  on patient not scheduled for surgery E876.6
  on wrong patient E876.6
performance of wrong operation on correct patient E876.5
puncture - *see* Misadventure, cut
specified type NEC E876.8
  failure
    suture or ligature during surgical operation E876.2
    to introduce or to remove tube or instrument E876.4
    foreign object left in body E871.9
  infusion of wrong fluid E876.1
  transfusion of mismatched blood E876.0
  wrong
    fluid in infusion E876.1
    placement of endotracheal tube during anesthetic procedure E876.3
transfusion - *see also* Misadventure, by specific type, transfusion
  excessive amount of blood E873.0
  mismatched blood E876.0
wrong
  device implanted into correct surgical site E876.5
  drug given in error - *see* Table of Drugs and Chemicals
  fluid in infusion E876.1
  placement of endotracheal tube during anesthetic procedure E876.3
  procedure (operation) performed on the correct patient E876.5
Motion (effects) E903
  sickness E903
Mountain sickness E902.0
Mucus aspiration or inhalation, not of newborn (with asphyxia, obstruction respiratory passage, suffocation) E912
Mudslide of cataclysmic nature E909.2
Murder (attempt) (*see also* Assault) E968.9

N

Nail, injury by E920.8
Needlestick (sewing needle) E920.4
  hypodermic E920.5

E CODES

Neglect - *see also* Privation
  criminal E968.4
  homicidal intent E968.4
Noise (causing injury) (pollution) E928.1
Nuclear weapon (*see also* War
  operations, injury due to,
  nuclear weapons) E996.9

O

Object
  falling
    from, in, on, hitting
      aircraft E844●
        due to accident to aircraft - *see*
          categories E840–E842
      machinery - *see also* Accident,
        machine
        not in operation E916
      motor vehicle (in motion) (on
        public highway) E818●
        not on public highway E825●
        stationary E916
      nonmotor road vehicle NEC
        E829●
      pedal cycle E826●
      person E916
      railway rolling stock, train,
        vehicle E806●
      street car E829●
      watercraft E838●
        due to accident to
          watercraft E831●
  set in motion by
    accidental explosion of pressure
      vessel - *see* category E921
    firearm - *see* category E922
    machine(ry) - *see* Accident,
      machine
    transport vehicle - *see* categories
      E800–E848
  thrown from, in, on, towards
    aircraft E844●
    cable car (not on rails) E847
      on rails E829●
    motor vehicle (in motion) (on public
      highway) E818●
      not on public highway E825●
    nonmotor road vehicle NEC E829●
    pedal cycle E826●
    street car E829●
    vehicle NEC - *see* Accident, vehicle
      NEC
Obstruction
  air passages, larynx, respiratory
    passages
    by
      external means NEC - *see*
        Suffocation
      food, any type (regurgitated)
        (vomited) E911
      material or object, except food
        E912
      mucus E912
      phlegm E912
      vomitus E911
  digestive tract, except mouth or
    pharynx
    by
      food, any type E915
      foreign body (any) E915
  esophagus
    food E911
    foreign body, except food E912
    without asphyxia or obstruction of
      respiratory passage E915

Obstruction (*Continued*)
  mouth or pharynx
    by
      food, any type E911
      material or object, except food
        E912
  respiration - *see* Obstruction, air
    passages
Oil in eye E914
Overdose
  anesthetic (drug) - *see* Table of Drugs
    and Chemicals
  drug - *see* Table of Drugs and
    Chemicals
Overexertion E927.9
  from
    lifting E927.8 ◀▥
      repetitive movement E927.3 ◀
      sudden strenuous movement
        E927.0 ◀
    maintaining prolonged positions
      E927.1
      holding E927.1
      sitting E927.1
      standing E927.1
    prolonged static position E927.1
    pulling E927.8 ◀▥
      repetitive movement E927.3 ◀
      sudden strenuous movement
        E927.0 ◀
    pushing E927.8 ◀▥
      repetitive movement E927.3 ◀
      sudden strenuous movement
        E927.0 ◀
    specified NEC E927.8 ◀
    sudden strenuous movement E927.0
Overexposure (accidental) (to)
  cold (*see also* Cold, exposure to) E901.9
    due to manmade conditions E901.1
  heat (*see also* Heat) E900.9
  radiation - *see* Radiation
  radioactivity - *see* Radiation
  sun, except sunburn E900.0
  weather - *see* Exposure
  wind - *see* Exposure
Overheated (*see also* Heat) E900.9
Overlaid E913.0
Overturning (accidental)
  animal-drawn vehicle E827●
  boat, ship, watercraft
    causing
      drowning, submersion E830●
      injury except drowning,
        submersion E831●
  machinery - *see* Accident, machine
  motor vehicle (*see also* Loss of control,
    motor vehicle) E816●
    with antecedent collision on public
      highway - *see* Collision, motor
      vehicle
    not on public highway, nontraffic
      accident E825●
      with antecedent collision - *see*
        Collision, motor vehicle, not
        on public highway
  nonmotor road vehicle NEC E829●
  off-road type motor vehicle - *see* Loss of
    control, off-road type motor
    vehicle
  pedal cycle E826●
  railway rolling stock, train, vehicle
    (*see also* Derailment, railway)
    E802●
  street car E829●
  vehicle NEC - *see* Accident, vehicle NEC

P

Palsy, divers' E902.2
Parachuting (voluntary) (without
  accident to aircraft) E844●
  due to accident to aircraft - *see*
    categories E840–E842
Paralysis
  divers' E902.2
  lead or saturnine E866.0
    from pesticide NEC E863.4
Pecked by bird E906.8
Performance of correct operation
  (procedure) on wrong
  body part E876.7
  side E876.7
  site E876.7
Performance of operation (procedure)
  intended for another patient E876.6
  on patient not scheduled for surgery
    E876.6
  on wrong patient E876.6
Performance of wrong operation on
  correct patient E876.5
Phlegm aspiration or inhalation (with
  asphyxia, obstruction respiratory
  passage, suffocation) E912
Piercing (*see also* Cut) E920.9
  by slide trigger mechanism, scope
    or other part of gun E928.7
Pinched
  between objects (moving) (stationary
    and moving) E918
  by slide trigger mechanism, scope
    or other part of gun E928.7
  in object E918
Pinned under
  machine(ry) - *see* Accident, machine
Place of occurrence of accident - *see*
  Accident (to), occurring (at) (in)
Plumbism E866.0
  from insecticide NEC E863.4
Poisoning (accidental) (by) - *see also* Table
  of Drugs and Chemicals
  carbon monoxide
    generated by
      aircraft in transit E844●
      motor vehicle
        in motion (on public highway)
          E818●
        not on public highway
          E825●
      watercraft (in transit) (not in
        transit) E838●
  caused by injection of poisons or toxins
    into or through skin by plant
    thorns, spines, or other
    mechanism E905.7
    marine or sea plants E905.6
  fumes or smoke due to
    conflagration - *see* Conflagration
    explosion or fire - *see* Fire
    ignition - *see* Ignition
  gas
    in legal intervention E972
    legal execution, by E978
    on watercraft E838●
    used as anesthetic - *see* Table of
      Drugs and Chemicals
  in
    terrorism (chemical weapons) E979.7
    war operations E997.2
  late effect of - *see* Late effect
  legal
    execution E978
    intervention
      by gas E972

Pressure, external, causing asphyxia, suffocation (*see also* Suffocation) E913.9
Privation E904.9
   food (*see also* Lack of, food) E904.1
   helpless person, infant, newborn due to abandonment or neglect E904.0
   late effect of NEC E929.5
   resulting from transport accident - *see* categories E800–E848
   water (*see also* Lack of, water) E904.2
Projected objects, striking against or struck by - *see* Striking against, object
Prolonged stay in
   high altitude (causing conditions as listed in E902.0) E902.0
   weightless environment E928.0
Prostration
   heat - *see* Heat
Pulling, injury in E927.8 ◄▥
   due to ◄
      repetitive movement E927.3 ◄
      sudden strenuous movement E927.0 ◄
Puncture, puncturing (*see also* Cut) E920.9
   by
      plant thorns or spines E920.8
         toxic reaction E905.7
            marine or sea plants E905.6
      sea-urchin spine E905.6
Pushing (injury in) (overexertion) E927.8
   by other person(s) (accidental) E917.9
      as, or caused by, a crowd, human stampede E917.1
         with subsequent fall E917.6
      before moving vehicle or object
         stated as
            intentional, homicidal E968.5
            undetermined whether accidental or intentional E988.8
      from
         high place
            in accidental circumstances - *see* categories E880–E884
            stated as
               intentional, homicidal E968.1
               undetermined whether accidental or intentional E987.9
               man-made structure, except residential E987.1
               natural site E987.2
               residential E987.0
         motor vehicle (*see also* Fall, from, motor vehicle) E818●
            stated as
               intentional, homicidal E968.5
               undetermined whether accidental or intentional E988.8
      in sports E917.0
         with fall E886.0
      with fall E886.9
         in sports E886.0
   due to ◄
      repetitive movement E927.3 ◄
      sudden strenuous movement E927.0 ◄

R

Radiation (exposure to) E926.9
   abnormal reaction to medical test or therapy E879.2
   arc lamps E926.2
   atomic power plant (malfunction) NEC E926.9
      in water transport E838●
   electromagnetic, ionizing E926.3
   gamma rays E926.3
   in
      terrorism (from or following nuclear explosion) (direct) (secondary) E979.5
         laser E979.8
      war operations (*see also* War operations, injury due to, nuclear weapons) E996.3
         laser(s) E997.0
         water transport E838●
   inadvertent exposure of patient (receiving test or therapy) E873.3
   infrared (heaters and lamps) E926.1
      excessive heat E900.1
   ionized, ionizing (particles, artificially accelerated) E926.8
      electromagnetic E926.3
   isotopes, radioactive - *see* Radiation, radioactive isotopes
   laser(s) E926.4
      in
         terrorism E979.8
         war operations E997.0
      misadventure in medical care - *see* Misadventure, failure, in dosage, radiation
   late effect of NEC E929.8
      excessive heat from - *see* Heat
   light sources (visible) (ultraviolet) E926.2
   misadventure in medical or surgical procedure - *see* Misadventure, failure, in dosage, radiation
   overdose (in medical or surgical pacemaker procedure) E873.2
   radar E926.0
   radioactive isotopes E926.5
      atomic power plant malfunction E926.5
      in water transport E838●
      misadventure in medical or surgical treatment - *see* Misadventure, failure, in dosage, radiation
   radiobiologicals - *see* Radiation, radioactive isotopes
   radiofrequency E926.0
   radiopharmaceuticals - *see* Radiation, radioactive isotopes
   radium NEC E926.9
   sun E926.2
      excessive heat from E900.0
   tanning bed E926.2
   welding arc or torch E926.2
      excessive heat from E900.1
   x-rays (hard) (soft) E926.3
      misadventure in medical or surgical treatment - *see* Misadventure, failure, in dosage, radiation

Rape E960.1
Reaction, abnormal to or following
   (medical or surgical procedure) E879.9
   amputation (of limbs) E878.5
   anastomosis (arteriovenous) (blood vessel) (gastrojejunal) (skin) (tendon) (natural, artificial material, tissue) E878.2
      external stoma, creation of E878.3
   aspiration (of fluid) E879.4
      tissue E879.8
   biopsy E879.8
   blood
      sampling E879.7
      transfusion
         procedure E879.8
   bypass - *see* Reaction, abnormal, anastomosis
   catheterization
      cardiac E879.0
      urinary E879.6
   colostomy E878.3
   cystostomy E878.3
   dialysis (kidney) E879.1
   drugs or biologicals - *see* Table of Drugs and Chemicals
   duodenostomy E878.3
   electroshock therapy E879.3
   formation of external stoma E878.3
   gastrostomy E878.3
   graft - *see* Reaction, abnormal, anastomosis
   hypothermia E879.8
   implant, implantation (of)
      artificial
         internal device (cardiac pacemaker) (electrodes in brain) (heart valve prosthesis) (orthopedic) E878.1
         material or tissue (for anastomosis or bypass) E878.2
            with creation of external stoma E878.3
         natural tissues (for anastomosis or bypass) E878.2
            as transplantion - *see* Reaction, abnormal, transplant
            with creation of external stoma E878.3
   infusion
      procedure E879.8
   injection
      procedure E879.8
   insertion of gastric or duodenal sound E879.5
   insulin-shock therapy E879.3
   lumbar puncture E879.4
   perfusion E879.1
   procedures other than surgical operation (*see also* Reaction, abnormal, by specific type of procedure) E879.9
      specified procedure NEC E879.8
   radiological procedure or therapy E879.2
   removal of organ (partial) (total) NEC E878.6
      with
         anastomosis, bypass or graft E878.2
         formation of external stoma E878.3

E CODES

E CODES

Reaction, abnormal to or
  following *(Continued)*
  removal of organ NEC *(Continued)*
    with *(Continued)*
      implant of artificial internal
        device E878.1
      transplant(ation)
        partial organ E878.4
        whole organ E878.0
  sampling
    blood E879.7
    fluid NEC E879.4
    tissue E879.8
  shock therapy E879.3
  surgical operation *(see also* Reaction,
    abnormal, by specified type of
    operation) E878.9
  restorative NEC E878.4
    with
      anastomosis, bypass or graft
        E878.2
      formation of external stoma
        E878.3
      implant(ation) - *see* Reaction,
        abnormal, implant
      transplantation - *see*
        Reaction, abnormal,
        transplant
    specified operation NEC
      E878.8
  thoracentesis E879.4
  transfusion
    procedure E879.8
  transplant, transplantation (heart)
    (kidney) (liver) E878.0
    partial organ E878.4
  ureterostomy E878.3
  vaccination E879.8
Reduction in
  atmospheric pressure - *see also* Effects
    of, air pressure
    while surfacing from
      deep water diving causing
        caisson or divers' disease,
        palsy or paralysis E902.2
      underground E902.8
Repetitive movements NEC E927.8 ◀
Residual (effect) - *see* Late effect
Rock falling on or hitting (accidentally)
  motor vehicle (in motion) (on public
    highway) E818●
    not on public highway E825●
  nonmotor road vehicle NEC
    E829●
  pedal cycle E826●
  person E916
  railway rolling stock, train, vehicle
    E806●
Running off, away
  animal (being ridden) (in sport or
    transport) E828●
    not being ridden E906.8
  animal-drawn vehicle E827●
  rails, railway *(see also* Derailment)
    E802●
  roadway
    motor vehicle (without antecedent
      collision) E816●
      nontraffic accident E825●
        with antecedent collision - *see*
          categories Collision,
          motor vehicle, not on
          public highway

Running off, away *(Continued)*
  roadway *(Continued)*
    motor vehicle *(Continued)*
      with
        antecedent collision - *see*
          Collision motor vehicle
        subsequent collision
          involving any object, person
            or vehicle not on
            public highway E816●
          on public highway E811●
      nonmotor road vehicle NEC E829●
      pedal cycle E826●
Run over (accidentally) (by)
  animal (not being ridden) E906.8
    being ridden (in sport or transport)
      E828●
  animal-drawn vehicle E827●
  machinery - *see* Accident, machine
  motor vehicle (on public highway) - *see*
    Hit by, motor vehicle
  nonmotor road vehicle NEC E829●
  railway train E805●
  street car E829●
  vehicle NEC E848

S

Saturnism E866.0
  from insecticide NEC E863.4
Scald, scalding (accidental) (by) (from)
  (in) E924.0
  acid - *see* Scald, caustic
  boiling tap water E924.2
  caustic or corrosive liquid, substance
    E924.1
    swallowed - *see* Table of Drugs and
      Chemicals
  homicide (attempt) - *see* Assault,
    burning
  inflicted by other person
    stated as
      intentional or homicidal E968.3
      undetermined whether
        accidental or intentional
        E988.2
  late effect of NEC E929.8
  liquid (boiling) (hot) E924.0
  local application of externally applied
    substance in medical or surgical
    care E873.5
  molten metal E924.0
  self-inflicted (unspecified whether
    accidental or intentional)
    E988.2
    stated as intentional, purposeful
      E958.2
  stated as undetermined whether
    accidental or intentional
    E988.2
  steam E924.0
  tap water (boiling) E924.2
  transport accident - *see* categories
    E800–E848
  vapor E924.0
Scratch, cat E906.8
Sea
  sickness E903
Self-mutilation - *see* Suicide
Sequelae (of)
  in
    terrorism E999.1
    war operations E999.0

Shock
  anaphylactic *(see also* Table of Drugs
    and Chemicals) E947.9
    due to
      bite (venomous) - *see* Bite,
        venomous NEC
      sting - *see* Sting
  electric *(see also* Electric shock) E925.9
  from electric appliance or current *(see
    also* Electric shock) E925.9
Shooting, shot (accidental(ly)) E922.9
  air gun E922.4
  BB gun E922.4
  hand gun (pistol) (revolver) E922.0
  himself *(see also* Shooting, self-
    inflicted) E985.4
    hand gun (pistol) (revolver) E985.0
    military firearm, except hand gun
      E985.3
      hand gun (pistol) (revolver) E985.0
    rifle (hunting) E985.2
      military E985.3
    shotgun (automatic) E985.1
    specified firearm NEC E985.4
    Verey pistol E985.4
  homicide (attempt) E965.4
    air gun E968.6
    BB gun E968.6
    hand gun (pistol) (revolver) E965.0
    military firearm, except hand gun
      E965.3
      hand gun (pistol) (revolver)
        E965.0
    paintball gun E965.4
    rifle (hunting) E965.2
      military E965.3
    shotgun (automatic) E965.1
    specified firearm NEC E965.4
    Verey pistol E965.4
  inflicted by other person
    in accidental circumstances E922.9
      hand gun (pistol) (revolver)
        E922.0
      military firearm, except hand gun
        E922.3
        hand gun (pistol) (revolver)
          E922.0
      rifle (hunting) E922.2
        military E922.3
      shotgun (automatic) E922.1
      specified firearm NEC E922.8
      Verey pistol E922.8
    stated as
      intentional, homicidal E965.4
        hand gun (pistol) (revolver)
          E965.0
        military firearm, except hand
          gun E965.3
          hand gun (pistol) (revolver)
            E965.0
        paintball gun E965.4
        rifle (hunting) E965.2
          military E965.3
        shotgun (automatic) E965.1
        specified firearm E965.4
        Verey pistol E965.4
      undetermined whether accidental
        or intentional E985.4
        air gun E985.6
        BB gun E985.6
        hand gun (pistol) (revolver)
          E985.0
        military firearm, except hand
          gun E985.3

◀ New   ◀▥ Revised   ~~deleted~~ Deleted   ● Use Additional Digit(s)   ▥ Omit code

Shooting, shot *(Continued)*
  inflicted by other person *(Continued)*
    stated as *(Continued)*
      undetermined whether accidental
        or intentional *(Continued)*
        hand gun (pistol) (revolver)
          E985.0
        paintball gun E985.7
        rifle (hunting) E985.2
        shotgun (automatic) E985.1
        specified firearm NEC
          E985.4
        Verey pistol E985.4
  in
    terrorism - *see* Terrorism, shooting
    war operations - *see* War operations,
      shooting
  legal
    execution E978
    intervention E970
  military firearm, except hand gun
    E922.3
    hand gun (pistol) (revolver)
      E922.0
  paintball gun E922.5
  rifle (hunting) E922.2
    military E922.3
  self-inflicted (unspecified whether
    accidental or intentional)
    E985.4
    air gun E985.6
    BB gun E985.6
    hand gun (pistol) (revolver)
      E985.0
    military firearm, except hand gun
      E985.3
      hand gun (pistol) (revolver)
        E985.0
    paintball gun E985.7
    rifle (hunting) E985.2
      military E985.3
    shotgun (automatic) E985.1
    specified firearm NEC E985.4
    stated as
      accidental E922.9
        hand gun (pistol) (revolver)
          E922.0
        military firearm, except hand
          gun E922.3
          hand gun (pistol) (revolver)
            E922.0
        paintball gun E922.5
        rifle (hunting) E922.2
          military E922.3
        shotgun (automatic) E922.1
        specified firearm NEC
          E922.8
        Verey pistol E922.8
      intentional, purposeful E955.4
        hand gun (pistol) (revolver)
          E955.0
        military firearm, except hand
          gun E955.3
          hand gun (pistol) (revolver)
            E955.0
        paintball gun E955.7
        rifle (hunting) E955.2
          military E955.3
        shotgun (automatic) E955.1
        specified firearm NEC
          E955.4
        Verey pistol E955.4
  shotgun (automatic) E922.1
  specified firearm NEC E922.8

Shooting, shot *(Continued)*
  stated as undetermined whether
    accidental or intentional E985.4
    hand gun (pistol) (revolver) E985.0
    military firearm, except hand gun
      E985.3
      hand gun (pistol) (revolver)
        E985.0
    paintball gun E985.7
    rifle (hunting) E985.2
      military E985.3
    shotgun (automatic) E985.1
    specified firearm NEC E985.4
    Verey pistol E985.4
  suicidal (attempt) E955.4
    air gun E985.6
    BB gun E985.6
    hand gun (pistol) (revolver) E955.0
    military firearm, except hand gun
      E955.3
      hand gun (pistol) (revolver)
        E955.0
    paintball gun E955.7
    rifle (hunting) E955.2
      military E955.3
    shotgun (automatic) E955.1
    specified firearm NEC E955.4
    Verey pistol E955.4
  Verey pistol E922.8
Shoving (accidentally) by other person
  (see also Pushing by other person)
  E917.9
Sickness
  air E903
  alpine E902.0
  car E903
  motion E903
  mountain E902.0
  sea E903
  travel E903
Sinking (accidental)
  boat, ship, watercraft (causing
    drowning, submersion) E830 ●
    causing injury except drowning,
      submersion E831 ●
Siriasis E900.0
Skydiving E844 ●
Slashed wrists *(see also* Cut, self-inflicted)
  E986
Slipping (accidental)
  on
    deck (of boat, ship, watercraft) (icy)
      (oily) (wet) E835 ●
    ice E885.9
    ladder of ship E833 ●
      due to accident to watercraft
        E831 ●
    mud E885.9
    oil E885.9
    snow E885.9
    stairs of ship E833 ●
      due to accident to watercraft
        E831 ●
    surface
      slippery E885.9
      wet E885.9
Sliver, wood, injury by E920.8
Smothering, smothered *(see also*
  Suffocation) E913.9
Smouldering building or structure in
  terrorism E979.3
Sodomy (assault) E960.1
Solid substance in eye (any part) or
  adnexa E914

Sound waves (causing injury) E928.1
Splinter, injury by E920.8
Stab, stabbing E966
  accidental - *see* Cut
Starvation E904.1
  helpless person, infant, newborn - *see*
    Lack of food
  homicidal intent E968.4
  late effect of NEC E929.5
  resulting from accident connected
    with transport - *see* categories
    E800-E848
Stepped on
  by
    animal (not being ridden) E906.8
      being ridden (in sport or
        transport) E828 ●
    crowd E917.1
    person E917.9
      in sports E917.0
  in sports E917.0
Stepping on
  object (moving) E917.9
    in sports E917.0
      with subsequent fall E917.5
    stationary E917.4
      with subsequent fall E917.8
  person E917.9
    as, or caused by a crowd E917.1
      with subsequent fall E917.6
    in sports E917.0
Sting E905.9
  ant E905.5
  bee E905.3
  caterpillar E905.5
  coral E905.6
  hornet E905.3
  insect NEC E905.5
  jelly fish E905.6
  marine animal or plant E905.6
  nematocysts E905.6
  scorpion E905.2
  sea anemone E905.6
  sea cucumber E905.6
  wasp E905.3
  yellow jacket E905.3
Storm E908.9
  specified type NEC E908.8
Straining, injury ~~in E927.8~~ ◀▥
  due to ◀
    repetitive movement E927.3 ◀
    sudden strenuous movement
      E927.0 ◀
Strangling - *see* Suffocation
Strangulation - *see* Suffocation
Strenuous movements (in recreational or
  other activities) NEC E927.8 ◀▥
Striking against
  bottom (when jumping or diving into
    water) E883.0
  object (moving) E917.9
    caused by crowd E917.1
      with subsequent fall E917.6
    furniture E917.3
      with subsequent fall E917.7
    in
      running water E917.2
        with drowning or submersion -
          see Submersion
      sports E917.0
        with subsequent fall E917.5
    stationary E917.4
      with subsequent fall E917.8

E CODES

Striking against (Continued)
  person(s) E917.9
    with fall E886.9
      in sports E886.0
    as, or caused by, a crowd E917.1
      with subsequent fall E917.6
        in sports E917.0
          with fall E886.0
Stroke
  heat - *see* Heat
  lightning E907
Struck by - *see also* Hit by
  bullet
    in
      terrorism E979.4
      war operations E991.2
        rubber E991.0
  lightning E907
  missile
    in terrorism - *see* Terrorism, missile
  object
    falling
      from, in, on
        building
          burning (uncontrolled fire)
            in terrorism E979.3
  thunderbolt E907
Stumbling over animal, carpet, curb, rug or (small) object (with fall) E885.9
  without fall - *see* Striking against, object
Submersion (accidental) E910.8
  boat, ship, watercraft (causing drowning, submersion) E830 ●
    causing injury except drowning, submersion E831 ●
  by other person
    in accidental circumstances - *see* category E910
    intentional, homicidal E964
    stated as undetermined whether accidental or intentional E984
  due to
    accident
      machinery - *see* Accident, machine
      to boat, ship, watercraft E830 ●
      transport - *see* categories E800-E848
    avalanche E909.2
    cataclysmic
      earth surface movement or eruption E909.9
      storm E908.9
    cloudburst E908.8
    cyclone E908.1
    fall
      from
        boat, ship, watercraft (not involved in accident) E832 ●
          burning, crushed E830 ●
          involved in accident, collision E830 ●
        gangplank (into water) E832 ●
        overboard NEC E832 ●
    flood E908.2
    hurricane E908.0
    jumping into water E910.8
      from boat, ship, watercraft
        burning, crushed, sinking E830 ●
        involved in accident, collision E830 ●
        not involved in accident, for swim E910.2

Submersion (Continued)
  due to (Continued)
    jumping into water (Continued)
      in recreational activity (without diving equipment) E910.2
        with or using diving equipment E910.1
      to rescue another person E910.3
    homicide (attempt) E964
    in
      bathtub E910.4
      specified activity, not sport, transport or recreational E910.3
      sport or recreational activity (without diving equipment) E910.2
        with or using diving equipment E910.1
        water skiing E910.0
      swimming pool NEC E910.8
      terrorism E979.8
      war operations E995.4
        intentional E995.3
      water transport E832 ●
        due to accident to boat, ship, watercraft E830 ●
    landslide E909.2
      overturning boat, ship, watercraft E909.2
      sinking boat, ship, watercraft E909.2
      submersion boat, ship, watercraft E909.2
    tidal wave E909.4
      caused by storm E908.0
    torrential rain E908.2
  late effect of NEC E929.8
  quenching tank E910.8
  self-inflicted (unspecified whether accidental or intentional) E984
    in accidental circumstances - *see* category E910
    stated as intentional, purposeful E954
  stated as undetermined whether accidental or intentional E984
  suicidal (attempted) E954
  while
    attempting rescue of another person E910.3
    engaged in
      marine salvage E910.3
      underwater construction or repairs E910.3
    fishing, not from boat E910.2
    hunting, not from boat E910.2
    ice skating E910.2
    pearl diving E910.3
    placing fishing nets E910.3
    playing in water E910.2
    scuba diving E910.1
      nonrecreational E910.3
    skin diving E910.1
    snorkel diving E910.2
    spear fishing underwater E910.1
    surfboarding E910.2
    swimming (swimming pool) E910.2
    wading (in water) E910.2
    water skiing E910.0
Sucked
  into
    jet (aircraft) E844 ●

Suffocation (accidental) (by external means) (by pressure) (mechanical) E913.9
  caused by other person
    in accidental circumstances - *see* category E913
    stated as
      intentional, homicidal E963
      undetermined whether accidental or intentional E983.9
        by, in
          hanging E983.0
          plastic bag E983.1
          specified means NEC E983.8
  due to, by
    avalanche E909.2
    bedclothes E913.0
    bib E913.0
    blanket E913.0
    cave-in E913.3
      caused by cataclysmic earth surface movement or eruption E909.9
    conflagration - *see* Conflagration E983.8
    explosion - *see* Explosion
    falling earth, other substance E913.3
    fire - *see* Fire
    food, any type (ingestion) (inhalation) (regurgitated) (vomited) E911
    foreign body, except food (ingestion) (inhalation) E912
    ignition - *see* Ignition
    landslide E909.2
    machine(ry) - *see* Accident, machine
    material, object except food entering by nose or mouth, ingested, inhaled E912
    mucus (aspiration) (inhalation), not of newborn E912
    phlegm (aspiration) (inhalation) E912
    pillow E913.0
    plastic bag - *see* Suffocation, in, plastic bag
    sheet (plastic) E913.0
    specified means NEC E913.8
    vomitus (aspiration) (inhalation) E911
  homicidal (attempt) E963
    in war operations E995.3
  in
    airtight enclosed place E913.2
    baby carriage E913.0
    bed E913.0
    closed place E913.2
    cot, cradle E913.0
    perambulator E913.0
    plastic bag (in accidental circumstances) E913.1
      homicidal, purposely inflicted by other person E963
      self-inflicted (unspecified whether accidental or intentional) E983.1
      in accidental circumstances E913.1
      intentional, suicidal E953.1
      stated as undetermined whether accidentally or purposely inflicted E983.1

◀ New   ⬅ Revised   ~~deleted~~ Deleted   ● Use Additional Digit(s)   Omit code

E CODES

Suffocation *(Continued)*
  in *(Continued)*
    plastic bag *(Continued)*
      suicidal, purposely self-inflicted
        E953.1
    refrigerator E913.2
    war operations E995.3
    self-inflicted - *see also* Suffocation,
        stated as undetermined whether
        accidental or intentional E953.9
      in accidental circumstances - *see*
        category E913
      stated as intentional, purposeful - *see*
        Suicide, suffocation
    stated as undetermined whether
        accidental or intentional E983.9
      by, in
        hanging E983.0
        plastic bag E983.1
        specified means NEC E983.8
    suicidal - *see* Suicide, suffocation
Suicide, suicidal (attempted) (by)
    E958.9
  burning, burns E958.1
  caustic substance E958.7
    poisoning E950.7
    swallowed E950.7
  cold, extreme E958.3
  cut (any part of body) E956
  cutting or piercing instrument
    (classifiable to E920) E956
  drowning E954
  electrocution E958.4
  explosive(s) (classifiable to E923)
    E955.5
  fire E958.1
  firearm (classifiable to E922) - *see*
    Shooting, suicidal
  hanging E953.0
  jumping
    before moving object, train, vehicle
      E958.0
    from high place - *see* Jumping,
      from, high place, stated as,
      suicidal
  knife E956
  late effect of E959
  motor vehicle, crashing of E958.5
  poisoning - *see* Table of Drugs and
    Chemicals
  puncture (any part of body) E956
  scald E958.2
  shooting - *see* Shooting, suicidal
  specified means NEC E958.8
  stab (any part of body) E956
  strangulation - *see* Suicide,
    suffocation
  submersion E954
  suffocation E953.9
    by, in
      hanging E953.0
      plastic bag E953.1
      specified means NEC E953.8
  wound NEC E958.9
Sunburn E926.2
Sunstroke E900.0
Supersonic waves (causing injury)
    E928.1
Surgical procedure, complication of
  delayed or as an abnormal reaction
    without mention of
    misadventure, *see* Reaction,
    abnormal
  due to or as a result of misadventure -
    see Misadventure

Swallowed, swallowing
  foreign body - *see* Foreign body,
    alimentary canal
  poison - *see* Table of Drugs and
    Chemicals
  substance
    caustic - *see* Table of Drugs and
      Chemicals drugs
    corrosive - *see* Table of Drugs and
      Chemicals
    poisonous - *see* Table of Drugs and
      Chemicals
Swimmers' cramp (*see also* category
    E910) E910.2
  not in recreation or sport E910.3
Syndrome, battered
  baby or child - *see* Abuse, child
  wife - *see* Assault

T

Tackle in sport E886.0
Terrorism (by) (in) (injury) E979.8
  air blast E979.2
  aircraft burned, destroyed, exploded,
    shot down E979.1
    used as a weapon E979.1
  anthrax E979.6
  asphyxia from
    chemical (weapons) E979.7
    fire, conflagration (caused by fire-
      producing device) E979.3
      from nuclear explosion
        E979.5
    gas or fumes E979.7
  bayonet E979.8
  biological agents E979.6
  blast (air) (effects) E979.2
    from nuclear explosion E979.5
    underwater E979.0
  bomb (antipersonnel) (mortar)
    (explosion) (fragments)
    E979.2
  bullet(s) (from carbine, machine gun,
    pistol, rifle, shotgun)
    E979.4
  burn from
    chemical E979.7
    fire, conflagration (caused by fire-
      producing device) E979.3
      from nuclear explosion E979.5
    gas E979.7
  burning aircraft E979.1
  chemical E979.7
  cholera E979.6
  conflagration E979.3
  crushed by falling aircraft E979.1
  depth-charge E979.0
  destruction of aircraft E979.1
  disability, as sequelae one year or more
    after injury E999.1
  drowning E979.8
  effect
    of nuclear weapon (direct)
      (secondary) E979.5
    secondary NEC E979.9
    sequelae E999.1
  explosion (artillery shell) (breech-
    block) (cannon block) E979.2
    aircraft E979.1
    bomb (antipersonnel) (mortar)
      E979.2
    nuclear (atom) (hydrogen)
      E979.5

Terrorism *(Continued)*
  explosion *(Continued)*
    depth-charge E979.0
    grenade E979.2
    injury by fragments from E979.2
    land-mine E979.2
    marine weapon E979.0
    mine (land) E979.2
      at sea or in harbor E979.0
      marine E979.0
    missile (explosive) NEC E979.2
    munitions (dump) (factory)
      E979.2
    nuclear (weapon) E979.5
      other direct and secondary effects
        of E979.5
    sea-based artillery shell
      E979.0
    torpedo E979.0
  exposure to ionizing radiation from
    nuclear explosion E979.5
  falling aircraft E979.1
  fire or fire-producing device E979.3
  firearms E979.4
  fireball effects from nuclear explosion
    E979.5
  fragments from artillery shell, bomb
    NEC, grenade, guided missile,
    land-mine, rocket, shell, shrapnel
    E979.2
  gas or fumes E979.7
  grenade (explosion) (fragments)
    E979.2
  guided missile (explosion) (fragments)
    E979.2
    nuclear E979.5
  heat from nuclear explosion E979.5
  hot substances E979.3
  hydrogen cyanide E979.7
  land-mine (explosion) (fragments)
    E979.2
  laser(s) E979.8
  late effect of E999.1
  lewisite E979.7
  lung irritant (chemical) (fumes) (gas)
    E979.7
  marine mine E979.0
  mine E979.2
    at sea E979.0
    in harbor E979.0
    land (explosion) (fragments)
      E979.2
    marine E979.0
  missile (explosion) (fragments)
    (guided) E979.2
    marine E979.0
    nuclear weapons E979.5
  mortar bomb (explosion) (fragments)
    E979.2
  mustard gas E979.7
  nerve gas E979.7
  nuclear weapons E979.5
  pellets (shotgun) E979.4
  petrol bomb E979.3
  phosgene E979.7
  piercing object E979.8
  poisoning (chemical) (fumes) (gas)
    E979.7
  radiation, ionizing from nuclear
    explosion E979.5
  rocket (explosion) (fragments)
    E979.2
  saber, sabre E979.8
  sarin E979.7
  screening smoke E979.7

E CODES

◄ New   ◄▥ Revised   ~~deleted~~ Deleted   ● Use Additional Digit(s)   ▨ Omit code

E CODES

War operations *(Continued)*
    explosion *(Continued)*
        aircraft *(Continued)*
            due to
                enemy fire or explosives
                    E994.0
                own onboard explosives
                    E994.1
            artillery shell E993.2
            bomb (mortar) E993.2
                aerial E993.0
                atom (*see also* War operations,
                    injury due to, nuclear
                    weapons) E996.9
                hydrogen (*see also* War
                    operations, injury due to,
                    nuclear weapons) E996.9
                injury by fragments from E991.4
                    antipersonnel E991.3
                nuclear (*see also* War operations,
                    injury due to, nuclear
                    weapons) E996.9
            depth charge E992.1
            injury by fragments from E991.4
                antipersonnel E991.3
            marine weapon NEC E992.8
            mine
                at sea or in harbor E992.2
                land E993.8
                    injury by fragments from
                        E991.4
                marine E992.2
            missile, guided E993.1
            mortar E993.2
            munitions (accidental) (being used
                in war) (dump) (factory)
                E993.9
                own E993.7
                    ammunition (artillery)
                        (mortars) E993.6
                    launch device (autocannons)
                        (automatic grenade
                        launchers) (missile
                        launchers) (small arms)
                        E993.7
            nuclear (weapon) (*see also* War
                operations, injury due to,
                nuclear weapons) E996.9
            own weapons (accidental) E993.7
                injury by fragments from E991.9
                    antipersonnel E991.3
            sea-based artillery shell E992.3
            specified NEC E993.8
            torpedo E992.0
        exposure to ionizing radiation from
            nuclear explosion (*see also* War
            operations, injury due to, nuclear
            weapons) E996.3
        falling aircraft E994.8
        fire or fire-producing device E990.9
            flamethrower E990.1
            incendiary bomb E990.0
            incendiary bullet E990.2
            indirectly caused from conventional
                weapon E990.3
            petrol bomb E990.0
        fireball effects from nuclear explosion
            E996.2
        fragments from
            antipersonnel bomb E991.3
            artillery shell E991.4
            bomb NEC E991.4
            grenade E991.4
            guided missile E991.4

War operations *(Continued)*
    fragments from *(Continued)*
        land mine E991.4
        rocket E991.4
        shell E991.4
        shrapnel E991.9
    fumes E997.2
    gas E997.2
    grenade (explosion) E993.8
        fragments, injury by E991.4
    guided missile (explosion) E993.1
        fragments, injury by E991.4
        nuclear (*see also* War operations,
            injury due to, nuclear
            weapons) E996.9
    heat from nuclear explosion
        E996.2
    injury due to
        aerial bomb E993.0
        air blast E993.9
        aircraft shot down E994.0
        artillery shell E993.2
        blast E993.9
            wave E993.9
            wind E993.9
        bomb E993.8
        but occurring after cessation of
            hostilities E998.9
            explosion of bombs E998.1
            explosion of mines E998.0
            specified NEC E998.8
        conventional warfare E995.9
            specified form NEC E995.8
        depth charge E992.1
        destruction of aircraft E994.9
            due to
                air to air missile E994.0
                collision with other aircraft
                    E994.2
                enemy fire or explosives
                    E994.0
                on board explosion
                    (explosives) E994.1
                on board fire E994.3
                rocket propelled grenade
                    [RPG] E994.0
                small arms fire E994.0
                surface to air missile E994.0
            specified NEC E994.8
        dirty bomb (*see also* War
            operations, injury due to,
            nuclear weapons) E996.9
        drowning E995.4
        explosion (direct pressure)
            (indirect pressure)
            (due to) E993.9
            depth charge E992.1
            improvised explosive device
                [IED]
                person borne E993.3
                roadside E993.5
                specified NEC E993.5
                transport vehicle (air) (land)
                    (water) borne E993.4
                vehicle (air) (land) (water)
                    borne E993.4
            marine mines (in harbor)
                (at sea) E992.2
            marine weapons E992.9
                specified NEC E992.8
            sea based artillery shell
                E992.3
            specified NEC E993.8
            torpedo E992.0

War operations *(Continued)*
    injury due to *(Continued)*
        explosion *(Continued)*
            unintentional (of own)
                autocannons E993.7
                automatic grenade launchers
                    E993.7
                launch device discharge
                    E993.7
                munitions detonation
                    (ammunition) (artillery)
                    (mortars) E993.6
                missile launchers E993.7
                small arms E993.7
        fragments (from) E991.9
            artillery E991.8
            artillery shells E991.4
            autocannons E991.8
            automatic grenade launchers
                [AGL] E991.8
            bombs E991.4
                antipersonnel E991.3
            detonation of unexploded
                ordnance [UXO] E991.4
            grenade E991.4
            guided missile E991.4
            improvised explosive device
                [IED]
                person borne E991.5
                roadside E991.7
                specified NEC E991.7
                transport vehicle (air) (land)
                    (water) borne E991.6
                vehicle (air) (land) (water)
                    borne E991.6
            land mine E991.4
            missile launchers E991.8
            mortars E991.8
            munitions (artillery shells)
                (bombs) (grenades)
                (rockets) (shells) E991.4
            rockets E991.4
            shells E991.4
            small arms E991.8
            specified NEC E991.9
            weapons (artillery)
                (autocannons) (mortars)
                (small arms) E991.8
        grenade E993.8
        guided missile E993.1
        hand to hand combat,
            unarmed E995.0
        improvised explosive device
            [IED]
            person borne E993.3
            roadside E993.5
            specified NEC E993.5
            transport vehicle (air) (land)
                (water) borne E993.4
            vehicle (air) (land) (water) borne
                E993.4
        inability to surface or obtain air
            E995.4
        land mine E993.8
        marine mines (in harbor) (at sea)
            E992.2
        marine weapons E992.9
            specified NEC E992.8
        mortar E993.2
        nuclear weapons E996.9
            beta burns E996.3
            blast debris E996.1
            blast pressure E996.0
            burns due to thermal radiation
                E996.2

E CODES

E CODES

War operations *(Continued)*
  injury due to *(Continued)*
    nuclear weapons *(Continued)*
      direct blast effect E996.0
      fallout exposure E996.3
      fireball effect E996.2
      flash burns E996.2
      heat effect E996.2
      indirect blast effect E996.1
      nuclear radiation effects
        E996.3
      radiation exposure (acute)
        E996.3
      radiation sickness E996.3
      secondary effects E996.3
      specified effects NEC E996.8
      thermal radiation effect E996.2
    piercing object E995.2
    restriction of airway, intentional
      E995.3
    sea based artillery shell E992.3
    shrapnel E991.9
    stave E995.1
    strangulation E995.3
    strike by blunt object (baton)
      (nightstick) (stave) E995.1
    submersion (accidental)
      (unintentional) E995.4
      intentional E995.3
    suffocation E995.3
      accidental E995.4
    torpedo E992.0
    underwater blast E992.9
    weapon of mass destruction
      [WMD] E997.3
  knife E995.2
  lacrimator (gas) (chemical) E997.2
  land mine (explosion) E993.8
    after cessation of hostilities
      E998.0
    fragments, injury by E991.4
  laser(s) E997.0
  late effect of E999.0
  lewisite E997.2
  lung irritant (chemical) (fumes)
    (gas) E997.2
  marine mine E992.2
  mine
    after cessation of hostilities
      E998.0
    at sea E992.2

War operations *(Continued)*
  mine *(Continued)*
    in harbor E992.2
    land (explosion) E993.8
      fragments, injury by E991.4
    marine E992.2
  missile (guided) (explosion) E993.1
    fragments, injury by E991.4
    marine E992.8
    nuclear (*see also* War operations,
      injury due to, nuclear
      weapons) E996.9
  mortar bomb (explosion) E993.2
    fragments, injury by E991.4
  mustard gas E997.2
  nerve gas E997.2
  phosgene E997.2
  piercing object E995.2
  poisoning (chemical) (fumes) (gas)
    E997.2
  radiation, ionizing from nuclear
    explosion (*see also* War
    operations, injury due to,
    nuclear weapons) E996.3
  rocket (explosion) E993.8
    fragments, injury by E991.4
  saber, sabre E995.2
  screening smoke E997.8
  shell (aircraft) (artillery) (cannon)
    (land based) (explosion)
    E993.2
    fragments, injury by E991.4
    sea-based E992.3
  shooting E991.2
    after cessation of hostilities
      E998.8
    bullet(s) E991.2
      rubber E991.0
    pellet(s) (rifle) E991.1
    shrapnel E991.9
  stave E995.2
  strike by blunt object (baton)
    (nightstick) (stave)
    E995.1
  submersion E995.4
    intentional E995.3
  sword E995.2
  torpedo E992.0
  unconventional warfare, except by
    nuclear weapon E997.9
    biological (warfare) E997.1

War operations *(Continued)*
  unconventional warfare *(Continued)*
    gas, fumes, chemicals E997.2
    laser(s) E997.0
    specified type NEC E997.8
  underwater blast E992.9
  vesicant (chemical) (fumes) (gas)
    E997.2
  weapon burst E993.9
Washed
  away by flood - *see* Flood
  away by tidal wave - *see* Tidal wave
  off road by storm (transport vehicle)
    E908.9
  overboard E832●
Weapon of mass destruction [WMD]
  E997.3
Weather exposure - *see also* Exposure
  cold E901.0
  hot E900.0
Weightlessness (causing injury) (effects
  of) (in spacecraft, real or simulated)
  E928.0
Wound (accidental) NEC (*see also* Injury)
  E928.9
  battle (*see also* War operations)
    E995.9
  bayonet E920.3
    in
      legal intervention E974
      war operations E995.2
  gunshot - *see* Shooting
  incised - *see* Cut
  saber, sabre E920.3
    in war operations E995.2
Wrong
  body part, performance of correct
    operation (procedure) on
    E876.7
  device implanted into correct
    surgical site E876.5
  patient, performance of operation
    (procedure) on E876.6
  procedure (operation) performed
    on correct patient E876.5
  side, performance of correct
    operation (procedure) on
    E876.7
  site, performance of correct operation
    (procedure) on E876.7

◀ New   ⇐ Revised   ~~deleted~~ Deleted   ● Use Additional Digit(s)   ▨ Omit code

PART III

Diseases: Tabular List Volume 1

1. INFECTIOUS AND PARASITIC DISEASES (001–139)

> **Note:** Categories for "late effects" of infectious and parasitic diseases are to be found at 137–139.

> **Includes**   diseases generally recognized as communicable or transmissible as well as a few diseases of unknown but possibly infectious origin

>> **Excludes**   *acute respiratory infections (460–466)*
>> *carrier or suspected carrier of infectious organism (V02.0–V02.9)*
>> *certain localized infections*
>> *influenza (487.0–487.8, 488.01–488.19)* ◀━━

INTESTINAL INFECTIOUS DISEASES (001–009)

> **Excludes**   *helminthiases (120.0–129)*
>> *Diseases or infestations caused by parasitic worms*

● **001** **Cholera**
A serious, often deadly, infectious disease of the small intestine

   001.0 **Due to Vibrio cholerae**

   001.1 **Due to Vibrio cholerae el tor**

   001.9 **Cholera, unspecified**

● **002** **Typhoid and paratyphoid fevers**
Caused by Salmonella typhi and Salmonella paratyphi A, B, and C bacteria

   002.0 **Typhoid fever**
       Typhoid (fever) (infection) [any site]

   002.1 **Paratyphoid fever A**

   002.2 **Paratyphoid fever B**

   002.3 **Paratyphoid fever C**

   002.9 **Paratyphoid fever, unspecified**

Item 1–1 **Salmonella** is a bacterium that lives in the intestines of fowl and mammals and can spread to humans through improper food preparation and cooking. Salmonellosis is an infection with the bacterium. Symptoms include diarrhea, fever, and abdominal cramps 12 to 72 hours after infection. The illness usually lasts 4 to 7 days, and most persons recover without treatment. The diarrhea may be so severe that the patient needs to be hospitalized. Patients with immunocompromised systems in chronic, ill health are more likely to have the infection invade their bloodstream with life-threatening results. For example, patients with sickle cell disease are more prone to salmonella osteomyelitis than others.

● **003** **Other salmonella infections**

> **Includes**   infection or food poisoning by Salmonella [any serotype]

   003.0 **Salmonella gastroenteritis**
       Salmonellosis

   003.1 **Salmonella septicemia**

● **003.2** **Localized salmonella infections**

      003.20 **Localized salmonella infection, unspecified**
          Specified in the documentation as localized, but unspecified as to type

      003.21 **Salmonella meningitis**
          Specified as localized in the meninges

      003.22 **Salmonella pneumonia**
          Specified as localized in the lungs

      003.23 **Salmonella arthritis**
          Specified as localized in the joints

      003.24 **Salmonella osteomyelitis**
          Specified as localized in bone

      003.29 **Other**
          Specified as localized (because it is still under localized heading) but does not assign into any of the above codes

---

◀ New   ◀━ Revised   ~~deleted~~ Deleted | Excludes | | Includes | Use additional   Code first   Omit code   **705**
● Unacceptable Principal Diagnosis   ● Use Additional Digit(s)   **OGCR** Official Guidelines   **Coding Clinic**

003.8 **Other specified salmonella infections**
Any specified salmonella infection which does NOT assign into any of the above codes (not specified as localized)

003.9 **Salmonella infection, unspecified**
Unspecified in the documentation as to specific type of salmonella

● 004 **Shigellosis**
An infectious disease caused by a group of bacteria (Shigella)
| **Includes** | bacillary dysentery |

004.0 **Shigella dysenteriae**
Infection by group A Shigella (Schmitz) (Shiga)

004.1 **Shigella flexneri**
Infection by group B Shigella

004.2 **Shigella boydii**
Infection by group C Shigella

004.3 **Shigella sonnei**
Infection by group D Shigella

004.8 **Other specified shigella infections**

004.9 **Shigellosis, unspecified**

● 005 **Other food poisoning (bacterial)**
See Table A, Table of Bacterial Food Poisoning, pg. 1118
Excludes	*salmonella infections (003.0–003.9)*
	toxic effect of:
	food contaminants (989.7)
	noxious foodstuffs (988.0–988.9)

005.0 **Staphylococcal food poisoning**
Staphylococcal toxemia specified as due to food

005.1 **Botulism food poisoning**
Botulism NOS
Food poisoning due to Clostridium botulinum
| **Excludes** | *infant botulism (040.41)* |
| | *wound botulism (040.42)* |

005.2 **Food poisoning due to Clostridium perfringens [C. welchii]**
Enteritis necroticans

005.3 **Food poisoning due to other Clostridia**

005.4 **Food poisoning due to Vibrio parahaemolyticus**

● 005.8 **Other bacterial food poisoning**
| **Excludes** | *salmonella food poisoning (003.0–003.9)* |

005.81 **Food poisoning due to Vibrio vulnificus**

005.89 **Other bacterial food poisoning**
Food poisoning due to Bacillus cereus

005.9 **Food poisoning, unspecified**

● 006 **Amebiasis**
An intestinal illness caused by the microscopic parasite Entamoeba histolytica
| **Includes** | infection due to Entamoeba histolytica |
| **Excludes** | *amebiasis due to organisms other than Entamoeba histolytica (007.8)* |

006.0 **Acute amebic dysentery without mention of abscess**
Acute amebiasis

006.1 **Chronic intestinal amebiasis without mention of abscess**
Chronic:
amebiasis
amebic dysentery

006.2 **Amebic nondysenteric colitis**

006.3 **Amebic liver abscess**
Hepatic amebiasis

006.4 **Amebic lung abscess**
Amebic abscess of lung (and liver)

006.5 **Amebic brain abscess**
Amebic abscess of brain (and liver) (and lung)

006.6 **Amebic skin ulceration**
Cutaneous amebiasis

006.8 **Amebic infection of other sites**
Amebic:
appendicitis
balanitis
Ameboma
| **Excludes** | *specific infections by free-living amebae (136.21–136.29)* |

006.9 **Amebiasis, unspecified**
Amebiasis NOS

● 007 **Other protozoal intestinal diseases**
Includes	protozoal:
	colitis
	diarrhea
	dysentery

007.0 **Balantidiasis**
Infection by Balantidium coli

007.1 **Giardiasis**
Infection by Giardia lamblia
Lambliasis

007.2 **Coccidiosis**
Infection by Isospora belli and Isospora hominis
Isosporiasis

007.3 **Intestinal trichomoniasis**

007.4 **Cryptosporidiosis**
Coding Clinic: 1997, Q4, P30-31

007.5 **Cyclosporiasis**

007.8 **Other specified protozoal intestinal diseases**
Amebiasis due to organisms other than Entamoeba histolytica

007.9 **Unspecified protozoal intestinal disease**
Flagellate diarrhea
Protozoal dysentery NOS

● 008 **Intestinal infections due to other organisms**
| **Includes** | any condition classifiable to 009.0–009.3 with mention of the responsible organisms |
| **Excludes** | *food poisoning by these organisms (005.0–005.9)* |

● 008.0 **Escherichia coli [E. coli]**
Coding Clinic: 1988, Q2, P10

008.00 **E. coli, unspecified**
E. coli enteritis NOS

008.01 **Enteropathogenic E. coli**

008.02 **Enterotoxigenic E. coli**

008.03 **Enteroinvasive E. coli**

008.04 **Enterohemorrhagic E. coli**

008.09 **Other intestinal E. coli infections**

Figure 1–1 Electron micrograph of escherichia coli *(E. coli)* expressing P fimbriae. (From Mandell, Bennett, & Dolin: Principles and Practice of Infectious Diseases, 6th ed. 2005, Churchill Livingstone, An Imprint of Elsevier.)

Item 1–2 *Escherichia coli [E. coli]* is a gram-negative bacterium found in the intestinal tracts of humans and animals and is usually nonpathogenic. Pathogenic strains can cause diarrhea or pyogenic (pus-producing) infections. Can be a threat to food safety.

◀ New   ◀▦ Revised   ~~deleted~~ Deleted   Excludes   Includes   Use additional   Code first   Omit code
● Unacceptable Principal Diagnosis   ● Use Additional Digit(s)   OGCR Official Guidelines   Coding Clinic

008.1 Arizona group of paracolon bacilli

008.2 Aerobacter aerogenes
Enterobacter aerogenes

008.3 Proteus (mirabilis) (morganii)

● **008.4 Other specified bacteria**

008.41 Staphylococcus
Staphylococcal enterocolitis

008.42 Pseudomonas
Coding Clinic: 1989, Q2, P10

008.43 Campylobacter

008.44 Yersinia enterocolitica

008.45 Clostridium difficile
Pseudomembranous colitis

008.46 Other anaerobes
Anaerobic enteritis NOS
Bacteroides (fragilis)
Gram-negative anaerobes

008.47 Other gram-negative bacteria
Gram-negative enteritis NOS
| Excludes | *gram-negative anaerobes (008.46)* |

008.49 Other
Coding Clinic: 1989, Q2, P10

008.5 Bacterial enteritis, unspecified

● **008.6 Enteritis due to specified virus**

008.61 Rotavirus

008.62 Adenovirus

008.63 Norwalk virus
Norovirus
Norwalk-like agent

008.64 Other small round viruses [SRV's]
Small round virus NOS

008.65 Calicivirus

008.66 Astrovirus

008.67 Enterovirus NEC
Coxsackie virus
Echovirus
| Excludes | *poliovirus (045.0–045.9)* |

008.69 Other viral enteritis
Torovirus
Coding Clinic: 2003, Q1, P10-11

008.8 Other organism, not elsewhere classified
Viral:
enteritis NOS
gastroenteritis
| Excludes | *influenza with involvement of gastrointestinal tract (487.8, 488.09, 488.19)* ◀||| |

● **009 Ill-defined intestinal infections**
Excludes	*diarrheal disease or intestinal infection due to specified organism (001.0–008.8)*
	diarrhea following gastrointestinal surgery (564.4)
	intestinal malabsorption (579.0–579.9)
	ischemic enteritis (557.0–557.9)
	other noninfectious gastroenteritis and colitis (558.1–558.9)
	regional enteritis (555.0–555.9)
	ulcerative colitis (556)

009.0 Infectious colitis, enteritis, and gastroenteritis
Colitis (septic)   Enteritis (septic)
Dysentery: Gastroenteritis (septic)
  NOS
  catarrhal
  hemorrhagic
Coding Clinic: 1988, Q2, P10

009.1 Colitis, enteritis, and gastroenteritis of presumed infectious origin
Excludes	*colitis NOS (558.9)*
	enteritis NOS (558.9)
	gastroenteritis NOS (558.9)
Coding Clinic: 1999, Q3, P6-7

009.2 Infectious diarrhea
Diarrhea:
  dysenteric
  epidemic
Infectious diarrheal disease NOS

009.3 Diarrhea of presumed infectious origin
| Excludes | *diarrhea NOS (787.91)* |
Coding Clinic: 1987, Nov-Dec, P7

TUBERCULOSIS (010–018)

| Includes | infection by Mycobacterium tuberculosis (human) (bovine) |

| Excludes | *congenital tuberculosis (771.2)* |
| | *late effects of tuberculosis (137.0–137.4)* |

The following fifth-digit subclassification is for use with categories 010–018:

> 0 unspecified
> 1 bacteriological or histological examination not done
> 2 bacteriological or histological examination unknown (at present)
> 3 tubercle bacilli found (in sputum) by microscopy
> 4 tubercle bacilli not found (in sputum) by microscopy, but found by bacterial culture
> 5 tubercle bacilli not found by bacteriological examination, but tuberculosis confirmed histologically
> 6 tubercle bacilli not found by bacteriological or histological examination, but tuberculosis confirmed by other methods [inoculation of animals]

● **010 Primary tuberculous infection**
Requires fifth digit. See beginning of section 010–018 for codes and definitions.

● **010.0 Primary tuberculous infection**
[0-6]
Excludes	*nonspecific reaction to tuberculin skin test without active tuberculosis (795.5)*
	positive PPD (795.5)
	positive tuberculin skin test without active tuberculosis (795.5)

● **010.1 Tuberculous pleurisy in primary progressive**
[0-6] **tuberculosis**

Figure 1-2 Far advanced bilateral pulmonary tuberculosis before and after 8 months of treatment with streptomycin, PAS, and isoniazid. (From Hinshaw HC, Garland LH: Diseases of the Chest, 2nd ed. Philadelphia, WB Saunders, 1963, p. 538.)

Item 1–3 Tuberculosis is a common and deadly infectious disease caused by the *Mycobacterium tuberculosis* organism. The first tuberculosis infection is called the **primary infection** and most commonly attacks the lungs but can affect the central nervous system, lymphatic system, circulatory system, genitourinary system, bones, joints, and even the skin. A **Ghon** lesion is the **initial lesion.** A **secondary lesion** occurs when the tubercle bacilli are carried to other areas.

Item 1–4 Although it primarily affects the lungs, the bacteria ***Mycobacterium tuberculosis*** can travel from the pulmonary circulation to virtually any organ in the body, much as a cancer metastasizes to a secondary site. If the immune system becomes compromised by age or disease, what would otherwise be a self-limiting primary tuberculosis in the lungs will develop in other organs. These are known as extrapulmonary sites.

● **010.8 Other primary progressive tuberculosis**
[0-6]   Excludes   *tuberculous erythema nodosum (017.1)*

● **010.9 Primary tuberculous infection, unspecified**
[0-6]

● **011 Pulmonary tuberculosis**

Requires fifth digit. See beginning of section 010–018 for codes and definitions.

Use additional code to identify any associated silicosis (502)

● **011.0 Tuberculosis of lung, infiltrative**
[0-6]

● **011.1 Tuberculosis of lung, nodular**
[0-6]

● **011.2 Tuberculosis of lung with cavitation**
[0-6]   *Cavitation = pitting*
       Coding Clinic: 1994, Q4, P36

● **011.3 Tuberculosis of bronchus**
[0-6]   Excludes   *isolated bronchial tuberculosis (012.2)*

● **011.4 Tuberculous fibrosis of lung**
[0-6]

● **011.5 Tuberculous bronchiectasis**
[0-6]

● **011.6 Tuberculous pneumonia [any form]**
[0-6]

● **011.7 Tuberculous pneumothorax**
[0-6]

● **011.8 Other specified pulmonary tuberculosis**
[0-6]

● **011.9 Pulmonary tuberculosis, unspecified**
[0-6]   Respiratory tuberculosis NOS
       Tuberculosis of lung NOS

● **012 Other respiratory tuberculosis**

Requires fifth digit. See beginning of section 010–018 for codes and definitions.

Excludes   *respiratory tuberculosis, unspecified (011.9)*

● **012.0 Tuberculous pleurisy**
[0-6]   Tuberculosis of pleura
       Tuberculous empyema
       Tuberculous hydrothorax

       Excludes   *pleurisy with effusion without mention of cause (511.9)*
           tuberculous pleurisy in primary progressive tuberculosis (010.1)

● **012.1 Tuberculosis of intrathoracic lymph nodes**
[0-6]   Tuberculosis of lymph nodes:
       hilar
       mediastinal
       tracheobronchial
       Tuberculous tracheobronchial adenopathy
       Excludes   *that specified as primary (010.0–010.9)*

● **012.2 Isolated tracheal or bronchial tuberculosis**
[0-6]

● **012.3 Tuberculous laryngitis**
[0-6]   Tuberculosis of glottis

● **012.8 Other specified respiratory tuberculosis**
[0-6]   Tuberculosis of:
       mediastinum
       nasopharynx
       nose (septum)
       sinus [any nasal]

● **013 Tuberculosis of meninges and central nervous system**

Requires fifth digit. See beginning of section 010–018 for codes and definitions.

● **013.0 Tuberculous meningitis**
[0-6]   Tuberculosis of meninges (cerebral) (spinal)
       Tuberculous:
       leptomeningitis
       meningoencephalitis

       Excludes   *tuberculoma of meninges (013.1)*

● **013.1 Tuberculoma of meninges**
[0-6]

● **013.2 Tuberculoma of brain**
[0-6]   Tuberculosis of brain (current disease)

● **013.3 Tuberculous abscess of brain**
[0-6]

● **013.4 Tuberculoma of spinal cord**
[0-6]

● **013.5 Tuberculous abscess of spinal cord**
[0-6]

● **013.6 Tuberculous encephalitis or myelitis**
[0-6]

● **013.8 Other specified tuberculosis of central nervous**
[0-6] **system**

● **013.9 Unspecified tuberculosis of central nervous**
[0-6] **system**
       Tuberculosis of central nervous system NOS

● **014 Tuberculosis of intestines, peritoneum, and mesenteric glands**

Requires fifth digit. See beginning of section 010–018 for codes and definitions.

● **014.0 Tuberculous peritonitis**
[0-6]   Tuberculous ascites

● **014.8 Other**
[0-6]   Tuberculosis (of):
       anus
       intestine (large) (small)
       mesenteric glands
       rectum
       retroperitoneal (lymph nodes)
       Tuberculous enteritis

◀ New   ◀▐▐ Revised   ~~deleted~~ Deleted   Excludes   Includes   Use additional   Code first   Omit code
● Unacceptable Principal Diagnosis   ● Use Additional Digit(s)   OGCR Official Guidelines   Coding Clinic

● **015 Tuberculosis of bones and joints**

Requires fifth digit. See beginning of section 010–018 for codes and definitions.

Use additional code to identify manifestation, as:
tuberculous:
arthropathy (711.4)
necrosis of bone (730.8)
osteitis (730.8)
osteomyelitis (730.8)
synovitis (727.01)
tenosynovitis (727.01)

● **015.0 Vertebral column**
[0-6] Pott's disease

Use additional code to identify manifestation, as:
curvature of spine [Pott's] (737.4)
kyphosis (737.4)
spondylitis (720.81)

● **015.1 Hip**
[0-6]

● **015.2 Knee**
[0-6]

● **015.5 Limb bones**
[0-6] Tuberculous dactylitis

● **015.6 Mastoid**
[0-6] Tuberculous mastoiditis

● **015.7 Other specified bone**
[0-6]

● **015.8 Other specified joint**
[0-6]

● **015.9 Tuberculosis of unspecified bones and joints**
[0-6]

● **016 Tuberculosis of genitourinary system**

Requires fifth digit. See beginning of section 010–018 for codes and definitions.

● **016.0 Kidney**
[0-6] Renal tuberculosis

Use additional code to identify manifestation, as:
tuberculous:
nephropathy (583.81)
pyelitis (590.81)
pyelonephritis (590.81)

● **016.1 Bladder**
[0-6]

● **016.2 Ureter**
[0-6]

● **016.3 Other urinary organs**
[0-6]

● **016.4 Epididymis**
[0-6]

● **016.5 Other male genital organs**
[0-6] Use additional code to identify manifestation, as:
tuberculosis of:
prostate (601.4)
seminal vesicle (608.81)
testis (608.81)

● **016.6 Tuberculous oophoritis and salpingitis**
[0-6] *Oophoritis = inflammation of ovary*
Salpingitis = inflammation of fallopian tube

● **016.7 Other female genital organs**
[0-6] Tuberculous:
cervicitis
endometritis

● **016.9 Genitourinary tuberculosis, unspecified**
[0-6]

● **017 Tuberculosis of other organs**

Requires fifth digit. See beginning of section 010–018 for codes and definitions.

● **017.0 Skin and subcutaneous cellular tissue**
[0-6] Lupus: Tuberculosis:
exedens   colliquativa
vulgaris   cutis
Scrofuloderma   lichenoides
                 papulonecrotica
                 verrucosa cutis

Excludes *lupus erythematosus (695.4)*
disseminated (710.0)
lupus NOS (710.0)
nonspecific reaction to tuberculin skin test
without active tuberculosis (795.5)
positive PPD (795.5)
positive tuberculin skin test without active
tuberculosis (795.5)

● **017.1 Erythema nodosum with hypersensitivity reaction in**
[0-6] **tuberculosis**
Bazin's disease
Erythema:
induratum
nodosum, tuberculous
Tuberculosis indurativa

Excludes *erythema nodosum NOS (695.2)*

● **017.2 Peripheral lymph nodes**
[0-6] Scrofula
Scrofulous abscess
Tuberculous adenitis

Excludes *tuberculosis of lymph nodes:*
bronchial and mediastinal (012.1)
mesenteric and retroperitoneal (014.8)
tuberculous tracheobronchial adenopathy
(012.1)

● **017.3 Eye**
[0-6] Use additional code to identify manifestation, as:
tuberculous:
episcleritis (379.09)
interstitial keratitis (370.59)
iridocyclitis, chronic (364.11)
keratoconjunctivitis (phlyctenular) (370.31)

● **017.4 Ear**
[0-6] Tuberculosis of ear
Tuberculous otitis media

Excludes *tuberculous mastoiditis (015.6)*

● **017.5 Thyroid gland**
[0-6]

● **017.6 Adrenal glands**
[0-6] Addison's disease, tuberculous

● **017.7 Spleen**
[0-6]

● **017.8 Esophagus**
[0-6]

● **017.9 Other specified organs**
[0-6] Use additional code to identify manifestation, as:
tuberculosis of:
endocardium [any valve] (424.91)
myocardium (422.0)
pericardium (420.0)

Item 1–5 Miliary tuberculosis can be a life-threatening condition. If a tuberculous lesion enters a blood vessel, immense dissemination of tuberculous organisms can occur if the immune system is weak. High-risk populations—children under 4 years of age, the elderly, or the immunocompromised—are particularly prone to this type of infection. The lesions will have a millet seed-like appearance on chest x-ray. Bronchial washings and biopsy may aid in diagnosis.

INFECTIOUS AND PARASITIC DISEASES (001–139)

● **018   Miliary tuberculosis**

Requires fifth digit. See beginning of section 010–018 for codes and definitions.

> **Includes**   tuberculosis:
> disseminated
> generalized
> miliary, whether of a single specified site, multiple sites, or unspecified site
> polyserositis

● **018.0   Acute miliary tuberculosis**
[0-6]

● **018.8   Other specified miliary tuberculosis**
[0-6]

● **018.9   Miliary tuberculosis, unspecified**
[0-6]

ZOONOTIC BACTERIAL DISEASES (020–027)

● **020   Plague**

Infectious disease caused by Yersinia pestis bacterium, transmitted by rodent flea bite or handling infected animal

> **Includes**   infection by Yersinia [Pasteurella] pestis

020.0   Bubonic

020.1   Cellulocutaneous

020.2   Septicemic

020.3   Primary pneumonic

020.4   Secondary pneumonic

020.5   Pneumonic, unspecified

020.8   Other specified types of plague
Abortive plague
Ambulatory plague
Pestis minor

020.9   Plague, unspecified

● **021   Tularemia**

Caused by Francisella tularensis bacterium found in rodents, rabbits, and hares; transmitted by contact with infected animal tissues or ticks, biting flies, and mosquitoes

> **Includes**   deerfly fever
> infection by Francisella [Pasteurella] tularensis
> rabbit fever

021.0   Ulceroglandular tularemia

021.1   Enteric tularemia
Tularemia:
cryptogenic
intestinal
typhoidal

021.2   Pulmonary tularemia
Bronchopneumonic tularemia

021.3   Oculoglandular tularemia

021.8   Other specified tularemia
Tularemia:
generalized or disseminated
glandular

021.9   Unspecified tularemia

● **022   Anthrax**

An acute infectious disease caused by the spore-forming Bacillus anthracis; it may occur in humans exposed to infected animals or tissue from infected animals

022.0   Cutaneous anthrax
Malignant pustule

022.1   Pulmonary anthrax
Respiratory anthrax
Wool-sorters' disease

022.2   Gastrointestinal anthrax

022.3   Anthrax septicemia

022.8   Other specified manifestations of anthrax

022.9   Anthrax, unspecified

● **023   Brucellosis**

Infectious disease caused by bacterium Brucella. Humans are infected by contact with contaminated animals or animal products. Brucellosis symptoms are similar to flu.

> **Includes**   fever:
> Malta
> Mediterranean
> undulant
> *Rising and falling*

023.0   Brucella melitensis

023.1   Brucella abortus

023.2   Brucella suis

023.3   Brucella canis

023.8   Other brucellosis
Infection by more than one organism

023.9   Brucellosis, unspecified

024   Glanders
Infection by:
Actinobacillus mallei
Malleomyces mallei
Pseudomonas mallei
Farcy
Malleus

025   Melioidosis
Infection by:
Malleomyces pseudomallei
Pseudomonas pseudomallei
Whitmore's bacillus
Pseudoglanders

● **026   Rat-bite fever**

RBF is an infectious disease caused by Streptobacillus moniliformis or Spirillum minus.

026.0   Spirillary fever
Rat-bite fever due to Spirillum minor [S. minus]
Sodoku

026.1   Streptobacillary fever
Epidemic arthritic erythema
Haverhill fever
Rat-bite fever due to Streptobacillus moniliformis

026.9   Unspecified rat-bite fever

● **027   Other zoonotic bacterial diseases**

027.0   Listeriosis
Infection by Listeria monocytogenes
Septicemia by Listeria monocytogenes

> Use additional code to identify manifestations, as meningitis (320.7)

> **Excludes**   *congenital listeriosis (771.2)*

027.1   Erysipelothrix infection
Erysipeloid (of Rosenbach)
Infection by Erysipelothrix insidiosa [E. rhusiopathiae]
Septicemia by Erysipelothrix insidiosa [E. rhusiopathiae]

027.2 Pasteurellosis
Pasteurella pseudotuberculosis infection by
Pasteurella multocida [P. septica]
Mesenteric adenitis by Pasteurella multocida
[P. septica]
Septic infection (cat bite) (dog bite) by Pasteurella
multocida [P. septica]

> **Excludes** *infection by:*
> *Francisella [Pasteurella] tularensis*
> *(021.0–021.9)*
> *Yersinia [Pasteurella] pestis*
> *(020.0–020.9)*

027.8 Other specified zoonotic bacterial diseases

027.9 Unspecified zoonotic bacterial disease

OTHER BACTERIAL DISEASES (030–041)

> **Excludes** *bacterial venereal diseases (098.0–099.9)*
> *bartonellosis (088.0)*

● **030 Leprosy**
*Also known as Hansen's disease; chronic infectious disease
attacking skin, peripheral nerves, and mucous
membranes*

> **Includes** Hansen's disease
> infection by Mycobacterium leprae

030.0 Lepromatous [type L]
Lepromatous leprosy (macular) (diffuse)
(infiltrated) (nodular) (neuritic)

030.1 Tuberculoid [type T]
Tuberculoid leprosy (macular) (maculoanesthetic)
(major) (minor) (neuritic)

030.2 Indeterminate [group I]
Indeterminate [uncharacteristic] leprosy (macular)
(neuritic)

030.3 Borderline [group B]
Borderline or dimorphous leprosy (infiltrated)
(neuritic)

030.8 Other specified leprosy

030.9 Leprosy, unspecified

● **031 Diseases due to other mycobacteria**

031.0 Pulmonary
Battey disease
Infection by Mycobacterium:
avium
intracellulare [Battey bacillus]
kansasii

031.1 Cutaneous
Buruli ulcer
Infection by Mycobacterium:
marinum [M. balnei]
ulcerans

031.2 Disseminated
Disseminated mycobacterium avium-intracellulare
complex (DMAC)
Mycobacterium avium-intracellulare complex
(MAC) bacteremia
Coding Clinic: 1997, Q4, P31

031.8 Other specified mycobacterial diseases

031.9 Unspecified diseases due to mycobacteria
Atypical mycobacterium infection NOS

● **032 Diphtheria**
*Highly contagious bacterial disease that results in formation
of an adherent membrane in the throat that may lead to
suffocation. It may attack the heart and lungs. The exact
location is specified in the codes.*

> **Includes** infection by Corynebacterium diphtheriae

032.0 Faucial diphtheria
Membranous angina, diphtheritic

032.1 Nasopharyngeal diphtheria

032.2 Anterior nasal diphtheria

032.3 Laryngeal diphtheria
Laryngotracheitis, diphtheritic

● **032.8 Other specified diphtheria**
032.81 Conjunctival diphtheria
Pseudomembranous diphtheritic
conjunctivitis

032.82 Diphtheritic myocarditis

032.83 Diphtheritic peritonitis

032.84 Diphtheritic cystitis

032.85 Cutaneous diphtheria

032.89 Other

032.9 Diphtheria, unspecified

● **033 Whooping cough**
*Pertussis (whooping cough) is a highly contagious disease
caused by the bacterium Bordetella pertussis and results
in a whooping sound.*

> **Includes** pertussis

Use additional code to identify any associated
pneumonia (484.3)

033.0 Bordetella pertussis [B. pertussis]

033.1 Bordetella parapertussis [B. parapertussis]

033.8 Whooping cough due to other specified organism
Bordetella bronchiseptica [B. bronchiseptica]

033.9 Whooping cough, unspecified organism

● **034 Streptococcal sore throat and scarlet fever**

034.0 Streptococcal sore throat

Septic:	Streptococcal:
angina	angina
sore throat	laryngitis
	pharyngitis
	tonsillitis

Coding Clinic: 1985, Sept-Oct, P9

034.1 Scarlet fever
Scarlatina

> **Excludes** *parascarlatina (057.8)*

035 Erysipelas

> **Excludes** *postpartum or puerperal erysipelas (670.8)*

Item 1–6 034.0 is the common **"strep throat"** (sore throat with
strep infection). It is grouped in the same three-digit category with scarlet
fever. If a patient has both scarlet fever and the strep throat, use both
codes. "Streptococcal" must be indicated on the laboratory report to use
034.0; otherwise use 462 for "sore throat" (pharyngitis).

● **036 Meningococcal infection**

Most commonly caused by bacteria Streptococcus pneumoniae and Neisseria meningitidis

036.0 Meningococcal meningitis
Cerebrospinal fever (meningococcal)
Meningitis:
  cerebrospinal
  epidemic

036.1 Meningococcal encephalitis

036.2 Meningococcemia
Meningococcal septicemia

036.3 Waterhouse-Friderichsen syndrome, meningococcal
Meningococcal hemorrhagic adrenalitis
Meningococcic adrenal syndrome
Waterhouse-Friderichsen syndrome NOS

● **036.4 Meningococcal carditis**

036.40 Meningococcal carditis, unspecified

036.41 Meningococcal pericarditis

036.42 Meningococcal endocarditis

036.43 Meningococcal myocarditis

● **036.8 Other specified meningococcal infections**

036.81 Meningococcal optic neuritis

036.82 Meningococcal arthropathy

036.89 Other

036.9 Meningococcal infection, unspecified
Meningococcal infection NOS

037 Tetanus

Also indexed as "lockjaw." Do not confuse tetanus with tetany, which is severe muscle twitches, cramps, and spasms (781.7).

Excludes *tetanus:*
  complicating:
    abortion (634–638 with .0, 639.0)
    ectopic or molar pregnancy (639.0)
  neonatorum (771.3)
  puerperal (670.8)

● **038 Septicemia**

Blood poisoning/bacteremia, often associated with serious illness.

Use additional code for systemic inflammatory response syndrome (SIRS) (995.91–995.92).

Excludes *bacteremia (790.7)*
  septicemia (sepsis) of newborn (771.81)
Coding Clinic: 2004, Q2, P16; 1994, Q2, P13; 1993, Q3, P6; 1988, Q2, P12

038.0 Streptococcal septicemia
Coding Clinic: 1996, Q2, P5

● **038.1 Staphylococcal septicemia**

038.10 Staphylococcal septicemia, unspecified

038.11 Methicillin susceptible Staphylococcus aureus septicemia
MSSA septicemia
Staphylococcus aureus septicemia NOS
Coding Clinic: 2008, Q4, P69-73; 1998, Q4, P41-42

038.12 Methicillin resistant Staphylococcus aureus septicemia
Coding Clinic: 2008, Q4, P69-73

038.19 Other staphylococcal septicemia

038.2 Pneumococcal septicemia [Streptococcus pneumoniae septicemia]
Coding Clinic: 1996, Q2, P5; 1991, Q1, P13

038.3 Septicemia due to anaerobes
Septicemia due to bacteroides

Excludes *gas gangrene (040.0)*
  that due to anaerobic streptococci (038.0)

● **038.4 Septicemia due to other gram-negative organisms**

038.40 Gram-negative organism, unspecified
Gram-negative septicemia NOS
Coding Clinic: 2007, Q4, P84-86

038.41 Hemophilus influenzae [H. influenzae]

038.42 Escherichia coli [E. coli]
Coding Clinic: 2003, Q4, P73

038.43 Pseudomonas

038.44 Serratia

038.49 Other

038.8 Other specified septicemias

Excludes *septicemia (due to):*
  anthrax (022.3)
  gonococcal (098.89)
  herpetic (054.5)
  meningococcal (036.2)
  septicemic plague (020.2)

038.9 Unspecified septicemia
Septicemia NOS

Excludes *bacteremia NOS (790.7)*

Coding Clinic: 2007, Q4, P96-97; 2005, Q2, P18-20; 2004, Q2, P16; 1999, Q3, P9; Q3, P5-6; 1998, Q1, P5; 1996, Q3, P16; Q2, P6; 1995, Q2, P7

● **039 Actinomycotic infections**

Includes actinomycotic mycetoma
infection by Actinomycetales, such as
  species of Actinomyces, Actinomadura, Nocardia, Streptomyces
maduromycosis (actinomycotic)
schizomycetoma (actinomycotic)

039.0 Cutaneous
Erythrasma
Trichomycosis axillaris

039.1 Pulmonary
Thoracic actinomycosis

039.2 Abdominal

039.3 Cervicofacial

039.4 Madura foot

Excludes *madura foot due to mycotic infection (117.4)*

039.8 Of other specified sites

039.9 Of unspecified site
Actinomycosis NOS
Maduromycosis NOS
Nocardiosis NOS

● **040 Other bacterial diseases**

Excludes *bacteremia NOS (790.7)*
  bacterial infection NOS (041.9)

040.0 Gas gangrene
Gas bacillus infection or gangrene
Infection by Clostridium:
  histolyticum
  oedematiens
  perfringens [welchii]
  septicum
  sordellii
Malignant edema
Myonecrosis, clostridial
Myositis, clostridial
Coding Clinic: 1995, Q1, P11

◄ New   ◄◄ Revised   ~~deleted~~ Deleted   Excludes   Includes   Use additional   Code first   Omit code
● Unacceptable Principal Diagnosis   ● Use Additional Digit(s)   OGCR Official Guidelines   Coding Clinic

Item 1–7 Gas gangrene is a necrotizing subcutaneous infection that will cause tissue death. Patients with poor circulation (e.g., diabetes, peripheral nephropathy) will have low oxygen content in their tissues (hypoxia), which allows the Clostridium bacteria to flourish. Gas gangrene often occurs at the site of a surgical wound or trauma. Onset is sudden and dramatic. Treatment can include debridement, amputation, and/or hyperbaric oxygen treatments.

040.1 Rhinoscleroma

040.2 Whipple's disease
Intestinal lipodystrophy

040.3 Necrobacillosis
Coding Clinic: 2007, Q4, P84-86

● **040.4 Other specified botulism**
Non-foodborne intoxication due to toxins of Clostridium botulinum [C. botulinum]

> **Excludes** botulism NOS (005.1)
> food poisoning due to toxins of Clostridium botulinum (005.1)

040.41 Infant botulism
Coding Clinic: 2007, Q4, P60-61

040.42 Wound botulism
Non-foodborne botulism NOS

> **Use additional** code to identify complicated open wound
> Coding Clinic: 2007, Q4, P60-61; 2006, Q2, P7

● **040.8 Other specified bacterial diseases**

040.81 Tropical pyomyositis

040.82 Toxic shock syndrome

> **Use additional** code to identify the organism
> Coding Clinic: 2002, Q4, P44

040.89 Other
Coding Clinic: 1986, Nov-Dec, P7

● **041 Bacterial infection in conditions classified elsewhere and of unspecified site**

Note: This category is provided to be used as an additional code to identify the bacterial agent in diseases classified elsewhere. This category will also be used to classify bacterial infections of unspecified nature or site.
Report the disease first, then the bacterium.

> **Excludes** septicemia (038.0–038.9)

Coding Clinic: 2001, Q2, P12; 1984, July-Aug, P19

● **041.0 Streptococcus**
Gram-positive bacteria that is the primary cause of strep throat

041.00 Streptococcus, unspecified
Specified in documentation as streptococcus, but unspecified as to Group

041.01 Group A
Specified as Group A
Coding Clinic: 2002, Q1, P3-4

041.02 Group B
Specified as Group B

041.03 Group C
Specified as Group C

041.04 Group D [Enterococcus]
Specified as Group D

041.05 Group G
Specified as Group G

041.09 Other Streptococcus
Streptococcus that is documented but not specified as Group A, B, C, D, or G

● **041.1 Staphylococcus**
"Staph" infections caused by Staphylococcus aureus bacteria and range from common skin infections (pimples and boils) to serious infection of surgical wounds, bloodstream infections, and pneumonia.
Coding Clinic: 1987, Jan-Feb, P14-15

041.10 Staphylococcus, unspecified
Coding Clinic: 2006, Q2, P15

041.11 Methicillin susceptible Staphylococcus aureus
MSSA
Staphylococcus aureus NOS
Coding Clinic: 2008, Q4, P69-73; 2006, Q2, P16-17; 2003, Q4, P104-107; 2001, Q2, P11; 1998, Q4, P42-44, 54.55; 1994, Q3, P6

041.12 Methicillin resistant Staphylococcus aureus
Methicillin-resistant staphylococcus aureus (MRSA)
Coding Clinic: 2009, Q4, P74; 2008, Q4, P69-73

041.19 Other Staphylococcus
Coding Clinic: 2008, Q2, P3

041.2 Pneumococcus

041.3 Klebsiella pneumoniae
Coding Clinic: 2008, Q4, P148-149

041.4 Escherichia coli [E. coli]
Coding Clinic: 1984, July-Aug, P19

041.5 Hemophilus influenzae [H. influenzae]

041.6 Proteus (mirabilis) (morganii)

041.7 Pseudomonas
Coding Clinic: 1988, Q4, P10

● **041.8 Other specified bacterial infections**

041.81 Mycoplasma
Eaton's agent
Pleuropneumonia-like organisms [PPLO]

041.82 Bacteroides fragilis

041.83 Clostridium perfringens

041.84 Other anaerobes
Gram-negative anaerobes

> **Excludes** Helicobacter pylori (041.86)

041.85 Other gram-negative organisms
Aerobacter aerogenes
Gram-negative bacteria NOS
Mima polymorpha
Serratia

> **Excludes** gram-negative anaerobes (041.84)

Coding Clinic: 1994, Q1, P18

041.86 Helicobacter pylori [H. pylori]

041.89 Other specified bacteria
Coding Clinic: 2006, Q2, P7; 2003, Q2, P7-8

041.9 Bacterial infection, unspecified
Coding Clinic: 1991, Q2, P9

INFECTIOUS AND PARASITIC DISEASES (001–139)

Item 1–8 **AIDS** (acquired immune deficiency syndrome) is caused by **HIV** (human immunodeficiency virus). HIV affects certain white blood cells (T-4 lymphocytes) and destroys the ability of the cells to fight infections, making patients susceptible to a host of infectious diseases (e.g., *Pneumocystis carinii* pneumonia **(PCP)**, **Kaposi's sarcoma,** and **lymphoma). AIDS-related complex (ARC)** is an early stage of AIDS in which tests for HIV are positive but the symptoms are mild.

Figure 1–3 Kaposi's sarcoma. There are large confluent hyperpigmented patch-stage lesions with lymphedema. (From Cohen & Powderly: Infectious Diseases, 2nd ed. 2004, Mosby, An Imprint of Elsevier.)

OGCR Section I.C.1.a and b

If a patient is admitted for an HIV-related condition, the principal diagnosis should be 042, followed by additional diagnosis codes for all reported HIV-related conditions. If a patient with HIV disease is admitted for an unrelated condition (such as a traumatic injury), the code for the unrelated condition (e.g., the nature of injury code) should be the principal diagnosis. Other diagnoses would be 042 followed by additional diagnosis codes for all reported HIV-related conditions.

HUMAN IMMUNODEFICIENCY VIRUS (HIV) INFECTION (042)

042 Human immunodeficiency virus [HIV] disease
Acquired immune deficiency syndrome
Acquired immunodeficiency syndrome
AIDS
AIDS-like syndrome
AIDS-related complex
ARC
HIV infection, symptomatic

Use additional code(s) to identify all manifestations of HIV

Use additional code to identify HIV-2 infection (079.53)

Excludes   *asymptomatic HIV infection status (V08)*
exposure to HIV virus (V01.79)
nonspecific serologic evidence of HIV (795.71)

Coding Clinic: 2007, Q4, P61-64; 2006, Q3, P14-15; 2004, Q2, P11-12; Q1, P5; 2003, Q1, P10-11,15; 1999, Q1, P14; 1997, Q4, P30-31; 1994, Q4, P35-36x2; 1993, Q3, P9; Q1, P20-22; 1990, Q3, P17; 1989, Q1, P9

POLIOMYELITIS AND OTHER NON-ARTHROPOD-BORNE VIRAL DISEASES AND PRION DISEASES OF CENTRAL NERVOUS SYSTEM (045–049)

● **045 Acute poliomyelitis**
Also called infantile paralysis caused by poliovirus, which enters the body orally and infects the intestinal wall and then enters the bloodstream and central nervous system, causing muscle weakness and paralysis.

Excludes   *late effects of acute poliomyelitis (138)*

The following fifth-digit subclassification is for use with category 045:

> 0   poliovirus, unspecified type
> 1   poliovirus type I
> 2   poliovirus type II
> 3   poliovirus type III

● **045.0 Acute paralytic poliomyelitis specified as bulbar**
[0-3]   Infantile paralysis (acute) specified as bulbar
Poliomyelitis (acute) (anterior) specified as bulbar
Polioencephalitis (acute) (bulbar)
Polioencephalomyelitis (acute) (anterior) (bulbar)

● **045.1 Acute poliomyelitis with other paralysis**
[0-3]   Paralysis:
acute atrophic, spinal
infantile, paralytic
Poliomyelitis (acute) with paralysis except bulbar
anterior with paralysis except bulbar
epidemic with paralysis except bulbar

● **045.2 Acute nonparalytic poliomyelitis**
[0-3]   Poliomyelitis (acute) specified as nonparalytic
anterior specified as nonparalytic
epidemic specified as nonparalytic

● **045.9 Acute poliomyelitis, unspecified**
[0-3]   Infantile paralysis unspecified whether paralytic or nonparalytic
Poliomyelitis (acute) unspecified whether paralytic or nonparalytic
anterior unspecified whether paralytic or nonparalytic
epidemic unspecified whether paralytic or nonparalytic

● **046 Slow virus infections and prion diseases of central nervous system**

046.0 Kuru

● **046.1 Jakob-Creutzfeldt disease** *(JCD)*

Use additional code to identify dementia:
with behavioral disturbance (294.11)
without behavioral disturbance (294.10)

046.11 Variant Creutzfeldt-Jakob disease
vCJD

046.19 Other and unspecified Creutzfeldt-Jakob disease
CJD
Familial Creutzfeldt-Jakob disease
Iatrogenic Creutzfeldt-Jakob disease
Jakob-Creutzfeldt disease, unspecified
Sporadic Creutzfeldt-Jakob disease
Subacute spongiform encephalopathy

Excludes   *variant Creutzfeldt-Jakob disease (vCJD) (046.11)*

046.2 Subacute sclerosing panencephalitis
Dawson's inclusion body encephalitis
Van Bogaert's sclerosing leukoencephalitis

046.3 Progressive multifocal leukoencephalopathy
Multifocal leukoencephalopathy NOS

● **046.7 Other specified prion diseases of central nervous system**

Excludes   *Creutzfeldt-Jakob disease (046.11-046.19)*
Jakob-Creutzfeldt disease (046.11-046.19)
kuru (046.0)
variant Creutzfeldt-Jakob disease (vCJD) (046.11)

046.71 Gerstmann-Sträussler-Scheinker syndrome
GSS syndrome

046.72 Fatal familial insomnia
FFI

046.79 Other and unspecified prion disease of central nervous system

046.8 Other specified slow virus infection of central nervous system

046.9 Unspecified slow virus infection of central nervous system

◄ New   ◄▥ Revised   ~~deleted~~ Deleted   Excludes   Includes   Use additional   Code first   Omit code
● Unacceptable Principal Diagnosis   ● Use Additional Digit(s)   OGCR Official Guidelines   Coding Clinic

●047 **Meningitis due to enterovirus**

| Includes | meningitis:
abacterial
aseptic
viral |

| Excludes | meningitis due to:
adenovirus (049.1)
arthropod-borne virus (060.0–066.9)
leptospira (100.81)
virus of:
  herpes simplex (054.72)
  herpes zoster (053.0)
  lymphocytic choriomeningitis (049.0)
  mumps (072.1)
  poliomyelitis (045.0–045.9)
any other infection specifically classified
  elsewhere |

047.0 **Coxsackie virus**

047.1 **ECHO virus**
  Meningo-eruptive syndrome

047.8 **Other specified viral meningitis**

047.9 **Unspecified viral meningitis**
  Viral meningitis NOS

048 **Other enterovirus diseases of central nervous system**
  Boston exanthem

●049 **Other non-arthropod-borne viral diseases of central nervous system**

| Excludes | late effects of viral encephalitis (139.0) |

049.0 **Lymphocytic choriomeningitis**
  Lymphocytic:
    meningitis (serous) (benign)
    meningoencephalitis (serous) (benign)

049.1 **Meningitis due to adenovirus**

049.8 **Other specified non-arthropod-borne viral diseases of central nervous system**
  Encephalitis:
  acute:
    inclusion body
    necrotizing
    epidemic
    lethargica
    Rio Bravo
  von Economo's disease

| Excludes | human herpesvirus 6 encephalitis (058.21)
other human herpesvirus encephalitis
  (058.29) |

049.9 **Unspecified non-arthropod-borne viral diseases of central nervous system**
  Viral encephalitis NOS

VIRAL DISEASES GENERALLY ACCOMPANIED BY EXANTHEM (050–059)

| Excludes | arthropod-borne viral diseases (060.0–066.9)
Boston exanthem (048) |

●050 **Smallpox**
  Caused by variola virus and is a serious, contagious, and sometimes fatal infectious disease

050.0 **Variola major**
  Hemorrhagic (pustular) smallpox
  Malignant smallpox
  Purpura variolosa

050.1 **Alastrim**
  Variola minor

050.2 **Modified smallpox**
  Varioloid

050.9 **Smallpox, unspecified**

●051 **Cowpox and paravaccinia**

●051.0 **Cowpox and vaccinia not from vaccination**
  Coding Clinic: 2008, Q4, P76-78

051.01 **Cowpox**

051.02 **Vaccinia not from vaccination**

| Excludes | vaccinia (generalized) (from
vaccination) (999.0) |

051.1 **Pseudocowpox**
  Milkers' node

051.2 **Contagious pustular dermatitis**
  Ecthyma contagiosum
  Orf

051.9 **Paravaccinia, unspecified**

●052 **Chickenpox**
  Very contagious disease caused by varicella zoster virus; results in itchy outbreak of skin blisters (varicella). The same virus causes shingles (zoster). The Varicella zoster virus is a member of the herpes virus family.

052.0 **Postvaricella encephalitis**
  Postchickenpox encephalitis

052.1 **Varicella (hemorrhagic) pneumonitis**

052.2 **Postvaricella myelitis**
  Postchickenpox myelitis

052.7 **With other specified complications**
  Coding Clinic: 2002, Q1, P3-4

052.8 **With unspecified complication**

052.9 **Varicella without mention of complication**
  Chickenpox NOS
  Varicella NOS

●053 **Herpes zoster**
  *Also known as **shingles,** caused by same virus as chickenpox. After exposure, the virus lies dormant in nerve tissue and is activated by factors including aging, stress, suppression of the immune system, and certain medication. Begins as a unilateral rash that leads to blisters and sores on skin. Chickenpox NOS is reported with 052.9.*

| Includes | shingles
zona |

053.0 **With meningitis**

●053.1 **With other nervous system complications**

053.10 **With unspecified nervous system complication**

053.11 **Geniculate herpes zoster**
  Herpetic geniculate ganglionitis

053.12 **Postherpetic trigeminal neuralgia**

053.13 **Postherpetic polyneuropathy**

053.14 **Herpes zoster myelitis**

053.19 **Other**

Figure 1–4 Primary herpes simplex in and around the mouth. The infection is usually acquired from siblings or parents and is readily transmitted to other direct contacts. (From Forbes, Jackson: Colour Atlas and Text of Clinical Medicine, International Edition. 2002, Mosby.)

Item 1–9 **Herpes** is a viral disease for which there is no cure. There are two types of the herpes simplex virus: **Type I** causes **cold sores** or **fever blisters,** and **Type II** causes **genital herpes.** The virus can be spread from a sore on the lips to the genitals or from the genitals to the lips.

INFECTIOUS AND PARASITIC DISEASES (001–139)

● 053.2 **With ophthalmic complications**

    053.20 **Herpes zoster dermatitis of eyelid**
       Herpes zoster ophthalmicus

    053.21 **Herpes zoster keratoconjunctivitis**

    053.22 **Herpes zoster iridocyclitis**

    053.29 **Other**

● 053.7 **With other specified complications**

    053.71 **Otitis externa due to herpes zoster**

    053.79 **Other**

  053.8 **With unspecified complication**

  053.9 **Herpes zoster without mention of complication**
    Herpes zoster NOS

● 054 **Herpes simplex**
    Excludes *congenital herpes simplex (771.2)*

  054.0 **Eczema herpeticum**
    Kaposi's varicelliform eruption

● 054.1 **Genital herpes**

    054.10 **Genital herpes, unspecified**
       Herpes progenitalis
       Coding Clinic: 2007, Q4, P61-64; 1985, Jan-Feb, P15-16

    054.11 **Herpetic vulvovaginitis**

    054.12 **Herpetic ulceration of vulva**

    054.13 **Herpetic infection of penis**

    054.19 **Other**

  054.2 **Herpetic gingivostomatitis**

  054.3 **Herpetic meningoencephalitis**
    Herpes encephalitis   Simian B disease

    Excludes *human herpesvirus 6 encephalitis (058.21)*
       other human herpesvirus encephalitis
       (058.29)

● 054.4 **With ophthalmic complications**

    054.40 **With unspecified ophthalmic complication**

    054.41 **Herpes simplex dermatitis of eyelid**

    054.42 **Dendritic keratitis**

    054.43 **Herpes simplex disciform keratitis**

    054.44 **Herpes simplex iridocyclitis**

    054.49 **Other**

  054.5 **Herpetic septicemia**

  054.6 **Herpetic whitlow**
    Herpetic felon

● 054.7 **With other specified complications**

    054.71 **Visceral herpes simplex**

    054.72 **Herpes simplex meningitis**

    054.73 **Herpes simplex otitis externa**

    054.74 **Herpes simplex myelitis**

    054.79 **Other**

  054.8 **With unspecified complication**

  054.9 **Herpes simplex without mention of complication**

● 055 **Measles**
    Includes morbilli
           rubeola
    The first four combination codes specify condition(s)/
    complication(s) manifesting after measles.

  055.0 **Postmeasles encephalitis**

  055.1 **Postmeasles pneumonia**

  055.2 **Postmeasles otitis media**

Item 1–10 **Rubeola** (055) and **rubella** (056) are medical terms for two different strains of measles. The MMR (measles, mumps, and rubella) vaccination is an attempt to eradicate these childhood diseases.

● 055.7 **With other specified complications**

    055.71 **Measles keratoconjunctivitis**
       Measles keratitis

    055.79 **Other**

  055.8 **With unspecified complication**

  055.9 **Measles without mention of complication**

● 056 **Rubella**
    Includes German measles
    Excludes *congenital rubella (771.0)*

● 056.0 **With neurological complications**

    056.00 **With unspecified neurological complication**

    056.01 **Encephalomyelitis due to rubella**
       Encephalitis due to rubella
       Meningoencephalitis due to rubella

    056.09 **Other**

● 056.7 **With other specified complications**

    056.71 **Arthritis due to rubella**

    056.79 **Other**

  056.8 **With unspecified complications**

  056.9 **Rubella without mention of complication**

● 057 **Other viral exanthemata**

  057.0 **Erythema infectiosum [fifth disease]**

  057.8 **Other specified viral exanthemata**
    Dukes (-Filatow) disease   Parascarlatina
    Fourth disease   Pseudoscarlatina

    Excludes *exanthema subitum [sixth disease]*
       (058.10–058.12)
       roseola infantum (058.10–058.12)

  057.9 **Viral exanthem, unspecified**

● 058 **Other human herpesvirus**
    Excludes *congenital herpes (771.2)*
       cytomegalovirus (078.5)
       Epstein-Barr virus (075)
       herpes NOS (054.0–054.9)
       herpes simplex (054.0–054.9)
       herpes zoster (053.0–053.9)
       human herpesvirus NOS (054.0–054.9)
       human herpesvirus 1 (054.0–054.9)
       human herpesvirus 2 (054.0–054.9)
       human herpesvirus 3 (052.0–053.9)
       human herpesvirus 4 (075)
       human herpesvirus 5 (078.5)
       varicella (052.0–052.9)
       varicella-zoster virus (052.0–053.9)

● 058.1 **Roseola infantum**
    Exanthema subitum [sixth disease]

    058.10 **Roseola infantum, unspecified**
       Exanthema subitum [sixth disease],
       unspecified

    058.11 **Roseola infantum due to human herpesvirus 6**
       Exanthema subitum [sixth disease]
       due to human herpesvirus 6

    058.12 **Roseola infantum due to human herpesvirus 7**
       Exanthema subitum [sixth disease] due to
       human herpesvirus 7

● **058.2 Other human herpesvirus encephalitis**

> | Excludes | *herpes encephalitis NOS (054.3)* |
> |---|---|

herpes simplex encephalitis (054.3)
human herpesvirus encephalitis NOS (054.3)
simian B herpes virus encephalitis (054.3)
Coding Clinic: 2007, Q4, P61-64

058.21 Human herpesvirus 6 encephalitis

058.29 Other human herpesvirus encephalitis
Human herpesvirus 7 encephalitis

● **058.8 Other human herpesvirus infections**

058.81 Human herpesvirus 6 infection

058.82 Human herpesvirus 7 infection

058.89 Other human herpesvirus infection
Human herpesvirus 8 infection
Kaposi's sarcoma-associated herpesvirus infection
Coding Clinic: 2007, Q4, P61-64

● **059 Other poxvirus infections**

> | Excludes | *contagious pustular dermatitis (051.2)* |
> |---|---|

cowpox (051.01)
ecthyma contagiosum (051.2)
milker's nodule (051.1)
orf (051.2)
paravaccinia NOS (051.9)
pseudocowpox (051.1)
smallpox (050.0-050.9)
vaccinia (generalized) (from vaccination) (999.0)
vaccinia not from vaccination (051.02)
Coding Clinic: 2008, Q4, P76-78

● **059.0 Other orthopoxvirus infections**

059.00 Orthopoxvirus infection, unspecified

059.01 Monkeypox

059.09 Other orthopoxvirus infection

● **059.1 Other parapoxvirus infections**

059.10 Parapoxvirus infection, unspecified

059.11 Bovine stomatitis

059.12 Sealpox

059.19 Other parapoxvirus infections

● **059.2 Yatapoxvirus infections**

059.20 Yatapoxvirus infection, unspecified

059.21 Tanapox

059.22 Yaba monkey tumor virus

059.8 Other poxvirus infections

059.9 Poxvirus infections, unspecified

ARTHROPOD-BORNE VIRAL DISEASES (060–066)

Use additional code to identify any associated meningitis (321.2)

> | Excludes | *late effects of viral encephalitis (139.0)* |
> |---|---|

● **060 Yellow fever**

060.0 Sylvatic
Yellow fever:
jungle
sylvan

060.1 Urban

060.9 Yellow fever, unspecified

061 Dengue
Breakbone fever

> | Excludes | *hemorrhagic fever caused by dengue virus (065.4)* |
> |---|---|

● **062 Mosquito-borne viral encephalitis**
Inflammation of the brain caused most commonly by Herpes Simplex virus. It may be a complication of Lyme disease and is often transmitted by mosquitoes, ticks, or rabid animals.

062.0 Japanese encephalitis
Japanese B encephalitis

062.1 Western equine encephalitis

062.2 Eastern equine encephalitis

> | Excludes | *Venezuelan equine encephalitis (066.2)* |
> |---|---|

062.3 St. Louis encephalitis

062.4 Australian encephalitis
Australian arboencephalitis
Australian X disease
Murray Valley encephalitis

062.5 California virus encephalitis
Encephalitis: Encephalitis:
California   Tahyna fever
La Crosse

062.8 Other specified mosquito-borne viral encephalitis
Encephalitis by Ilheus virus

> | Excludes | *West Nile virus (066.40–066.49)* |
> |---|---|

062.9 Mosquito-borne viral encephalitis, unspecified

● **063 Tick-borne viral encephalitis**

> | Includes | diphasic meningoencephalitis |
> |---|---|

063.0 Russian spring-summer [taiga] encephalitis

063.1 Louping ill

063.2 Central European encephalitis

063.8 Other specified tick-borne viral encephalitis
Langat encephalitis
Powassan encephalitis

063.9 Tick-borne viral encephalitis, unspecified

064 Viral encephalitis transmitted by other and unspecified arthropods
Arthropod-borne viral encephalitis, vector unknown
Negishi virus encephalitis

> | Excludes | *viral encephalitis NOS (049.9)* |
> |---|---|

● **065 Arthropod-borne hemorrhagic fever**

065.0 Crimean hemorrhagic fever [CHF Congo virus]
Central Asian hemorrhagic fever

065.1 Omsk hemorrhagic fever

065.2 Kyasanur Forest disease

065.3 Other tick-borne hemorrhagic fever

065.4 Mosquito-borne hemorrhagic fever
Chikungunya hemorrhagic fever
Dengue hemorrhagic fever

> | Excludes | *Chikungunya fever (066.3)* |
> |---|---|

dengue (061)
yellow fever (060.0–060.9)

065.8 Other specified arthropod-borne hemorrhagic fever
Mite-borne hemorrhagic fever

065.9 Arthropod-borne hemorrhagic fever, unspecified
Arbovirus hemorrhagic fever NOS

INFECTIOUS AND PARASITIC DISEASES (001–139)

● **066 Other arthropod-borne viral diseases**

  066.0 Phlebotomus fever
    Changuinola fever
    Sandfly fever

  066.1 Tick-borne fever
    Nairobi sheep disease
    Tick fever:
        American mountain
        Colorado
        Kemerovo
        Quaranfil

  066.2 Venezuelan equine fever
    Venezuelan equine encephalitis

  066.3 Other mosquito-borne fever
    Fever (viral):   Fever (viral):
        Bunyamwera   Oropouche
        Bwamba   Pixuna
        Chikungunya   Rift valley
        Guama   Ross river
        Mayaro   Wesselsbron
        Mucambo   Zika
        O' Nyong-Nyong

    Excludes *dengue (061)*
              yellow fever (060.0–060.9)

● **066.4 West Nile fever**
    Also indexed as West Nile virus
    Coding Clinic: 2004, Q4, P50-52; 2002, Q4, P44

  066.40 West Nile fever, unspecified
    West Nile fever NOS
    West Nile fever without complications
    West Nile virus NOS

  066.41 West Nile fever with encephalitis
    West Nile encephalitis
    West Nile encephalomyelitis

  066.42 West Nile fever with other neurologic manifestation
      Use additional code to specify the neurologic manifestation

  066.49 West Nile fever with other complications
      Use additional code to specify the other conditions

  066.8 Other specified arthropod-borne viral diseases
    Chandipura fever
    Piry fever

  066.9 Arthropod-borne viral disease, unspecified
    Arbovirus infection NOS

OTHER DISEASES DUE TO VIRUSES AND CHLAMYDIAE (070–079)

● **070 Viral hepatitis**

    Includes viral hepatitis (acute) (chronic)

    Excludes *cytomegalic inclusion virus hepatitis (078.5)*

    The following fifth-digit subclassification is for use with categories 070.2 and 070.3:

    > **0 acute or unspecified, without mention of hepatitis delta**
    > **1 acute or unspecified, with hepatitis delta**
    > **2 chronic, without mention of hepatitis delta**
    > **3 chronic, with hepatitis delta**

    Coding Clinic: 2007, Q2, P6-7x3; 2004, Q4, P52-53

  070.0 Viral hepatitis A with hepatic coma

  070.1 Viral hepatitis A without mention of hepatic coma
    Infectious hepatitis

● **070.2 Viral hepatitis B with hepatic coma**
    [0-3]

Figure 1–5 Hepatitis B viral infection. **A.** Liver parenchyma showing hepatocytes with diffuse granular cytoplasm, so-called ground glass hepatocytes (H&E). **B.** Immunoperoxidase stains from the same case, showing cytoplasmic inclusions of viral particles. (From Kumar: Robbins and Cotran: Pathologic Basis of Disease, 7th ed. 2005, Saunders, An Imprint of Elsevier.)

Item 1–11 Hepatitis A (HAV) was formerly called epidemic, infectious, short-incubation, or acute catarrhal jaundice hepatitis. The primary transmission mode is the oral–fecal route. **Hepatitis B (HBV)** was formerly called long-incubation period, serum, or homologous serum hepatitis. Transmission modes are through blood from infected persons and from body fluids of infected mother to neonate. **Hepatitis C (HCV),** caused by the hepatitis C virus, is primarily transfusion associated. **Hepatitis D (HDV),** also called delta hepatitis, is caused by the hepatitis D virus in patients formerly or currently infected with hepatitis B. **Hepatitis E (HEV)** is also called enterically transmitted non-A, non-B hepatitis. The primary transmission mode is the oral–fecal route, usually through contaminated water.

● **070.3 Viral hepatitis B without mention of hepatic coma**
    [0-3]   Serum hepatitis
          Coding Clinic: 1993, Q1, P28

● **070.4 Other specified viral hepatitis with hepatic coma**

  070.41 Acute hepatitis C with hepatic coma

  070.42 Hepatitis delta without mention of active hepatitis B disease with hepatic coma
    Hepatitis delta with hepatitis B carrier state

  070.43 Hepatitis E with hepatic coma

  070.44 Chronic hepatitis C with hepatic coma

  070.49 Other specified viral hepatitis with hepatic coma

● **070.5 Other specified viral hepatitis without mention of hepatic coma**

  070.51 Acute hepatitis C without mention of hepatic coma

  070.52 Hepatitis delta without mention of active hepatitis B disease or hepatic coma

  070.53 Hepatitis E without mention of hepatic coma

  070.54 Chronic hepatitis C without mention of hepatic coma
          Coding Clinic: 2008, Q4, P120; 2007, Q3, P9; 2006, Q2, P13

  070.59 Other specified viral hepatitis without mention of hepatic coma

  070.6 Unspecified viral hepatitis with hepatic coma
      Excludes *unspecified viral hepatitis C with hepatic coma (070.71)*

● **070.7 Unspecified viral hepatitis C**

  070.70 Unspecified viral hepatitis C without hepatic coma
    Unspecified viral hepatitis C NOS

  070.71 Unspecified viral hepatitis C with hepatic coma

  070.9 Unspecified viral hepatitis without mention of hepatic coma
    Viral hepatitis NOS
      Excludes *unspecified viral hepatitis C without hepatic coma (070.70)*

071 Rabies
Viral disease affecting central nervous system and transmitted from infected mammals.
Hydrophobia
Lyssa

● 072 Mumps
An acute, contagious, viral disease that causes painful enlargement of the salivary or parotid glands and is spread by respiratory droplets or direct contact. The following combination codes are specific diseases as an existing complication of mumps.

072.0 **Mumps orchitis**

072.1 **Mumps meningitis**

072.2 **Mumps encephalitis**
Mumps meningoencephalitis

072.3 **Mumps pancreatitis**

● 072.7 **Mumps with other specified complications**
- 072.71 **Mumps hepatitis**
- 072.72 **Mumps polyneuropathy**
- 072.79 **Other**

072.8 **Mumps with unspecified complication**

072.9 **Mumps without mention of complication**
Epidemic parotitis
Infectious parotitis

● 073 Ornithosis
Includes parrot fever
psittacosis

073.0 **With pneumonia**
Lobular pneumonitis due to ornithosis

073.7 **With other specified complications**

073.8 **With unspecified complication**

073.9 **Ornithosis, unspecified**

● 074 Specific diseases due to Coxsackie virus
Excludes *Coxsackie virus:*
infection NOS (079.2)
meningitis (047.0)

074.0 **Herpangina**
Vesicular pharyngitis

074.1 **Epidemic pleurodynia**
Bornholm disease   Epidemic:
Devil's grip   myalgia
                          myositis

● 074.2 **Coxsackie carditis**
- 074.20 **Coxsackie carditis, unspecified**
- 074.21 **Coxsackie pericarditis**
- 074.22 **Coxsackie endocarditis**
- 074.23 **Coxsackie myocarditis**
Aseptic myocarditis of newborn

074.3 **Hand, foot, and mouth disease**
Vesicular stomatitis and exanthem
Check your documentation—this code is HAND, foot, and mouth disease. Code 078.4 is foot and mouth disease.

074.8 **Other specified diseases due to Coxsackie virus**
Acute lymphonodular pharyngitis

075 Infectious mononucleosis
Glandular fever
Monocytic angina
Pfeiffer's disease
Coding Clinic: 2001, Q3, P13-14x2

● 076 Trachoma
Excludes *late effect of trachoma (139.1)*

076.0 **Initial stage**
Trachoma dubium

076.1 **Active stage**
Granular conjunctivitis (trachomatous)
Trachomatous:
follicular conjunctivitis
pannus

076.9 **Trachoma, unspecified**
Trachoma NOS

● 077 Other diseases of conjunctiva due to viruses and Chlamydiae
Excludes *ophthalmic complications of viral diseases classified elsewhere*

077.0 **Inclusion conjunctivitis**
Paratrachoma
Swimming pool conjunctivitis
Excludes *inclusion blennorrhea (neonatal) (771.6)*

077.1 **Epidemic keratoconjunctivitis**
Shipyard eye

077.2 **Pharyngoconjunctival fever**
Viral pharyngoconjunctivitis

077.3 **Other adenoviral conjunctivitis**
Acute adenoviral follicular conjunctivitis

077.4 **Epidemic hemorrhagic conjunctivitis**
Apollo:
conjunctivitis
disease
Conjunctivitis due to enterovirus type 70
Hemorrhagic conjunctivitis (acute) (epidemic)

077.8 **Other viral conjunctivitis**
Newcastle conjunctivitis

● 077.9 **Unspecified diseases of conjunctiva due to viruses and Chlamydiae**
- 077.98 **Due to Chlamydiae**
- 077.99 **Due to viruses**
Viral conjunctivitis NOS

● 078 Other diseases due to viruses and Chlamydiae
Excludes *viral infection NOS (079.0–079.9)*
viremia NOS (790.8)

078.0 **Molluscum contagiosum**

● 078.1 **Viral warts**
Viral warts due to human papillomavirus
Coding Clinic: 1997, Q2, P9
- 078.10 **Viral warts, unspecified**
Verruca:
NOS
Vulgaris
Warts (infectious)
- 078.11 **Condyloma acuminatum**
Condyloma NOS
Genital warts NOS
- 078.12 **Plantar wart**
Verruca plantaris
Coding Clinic: 2008, Q4, P78-79
- 078.19 **Other specified viral warts**
Common wart
Flat wart
Verruca plana

078.2 **Sweating fever**
Miliary fever
Sweating disease

INFECTIOUS AND PARASITIC DISEASES (001–139)

078.3 Cat-scratch disease
Benign lymphoreticulosis (of inoculation)
Cat-scratch fever

078.4 Foot and mouth disease
Aphthous fever
Epizootic:
aphthae
stomatitis
Check your documentation. Code 074.3 is for HAND, foot, and mouth disease.

078.5 Cytomegaloviral disease
Cytomegalic inclusion disease
Salivary gland virus disease
Use additional code to identify manifestation, as:
cytomegalic inclusion virus:
hepatitis (573.1)
pneumonia (484.1)
Excludes *congenital cytomegalovirus infection (771.1)*
Coding Clinic: 2003, Q1, P11; 1993, Q3, P13; Q2, P11; Q1, P24; 1989, Q1, P9

078.6 Hemorrhagic nephrosonephritis
Hemorrhagic fever:
epidemic
Korean
Russian with renal syndrome

078.7 Arenaviral hemorrhagic fever
Hemorrhagic fever:
Argentine
Bolivian
Junin virus
Machupo virus

●**078.8 Other specified diseases due to viruses and Chlamydiae**
Excludes *epidemic diarrhea (009.2)*
lymphogranuloma venereum (099.1)

078.81 Epidemic vertigo

078.82 Epidemic vomiting syndrome
Winter vomiting disease

078.88 Other specified diseases due to Chlamydiae

078.89 Other specified diseases due to viruses
Epidemic cervical myalgia
Marburg disease

●**079 Viral and chlamydial infection in conditions classified elsewhere and of unspecified site**
Note: This category is provided to be used as an additional code to identify the viral agent in diseases classifiable elsewhere. This category will also be used to classify virus infection of unspecified nature or site.

079.0 Adenovirus

079.1 ECHO virus

079.2 Coxsackie virus

079.3 Rhinovirus

079.4 Human papillomavirus
Coding Clinic: 1997, Q2, P9

●**079.5 Retrovirus**
Excludes *human immunodeficiency virus, type 1 [HIV-1] (042)*
human T-cell lymphotrophic virus, type III [HTLV-III] (042)
lymphadenopathy-associated virus [LAV] (042)

079.50 Retrovirus, unspecified

079.51 Human T-cell lymphotrophic virus, type I [HTLV-I]

Item 1–12 Retrovirus develops by copying its RNA, genetic materials, into the DNA, which then produces new virus particles. It is from the Retroviridae virus family.
Human T-cell lymphotropic virus, Type I (HTLV-I) is also called human T-cell leukemia virus, Type I, and is a retrovirus thought to cause T-cell leukemia/lymphoma.
Human T-cell lymphotropic virus, Type II (HTLV-II), is also called human T-cell leukemia virus, Type II, and is a retrovirus associated with hematologic disorders.
HIV-2 is one of the serotypes of HIV and is usually confined to West Africa, whereas HIV-1 is found worldwide.

079.52 Human T-cell lymphotrophic virus, type II [HTLV-II]

079.53 Human immunodeficiency virus, type 2 [HIV-2]

079.59 Other specified retrovirus

079.6 Respiratory syncytial virus (RSV)
Coding Clinic: 1996, Q4, P27-28

●**079.8 Other specified viral and chlamydial infections**
Coding Clinic: 1988, Q1, P12; Q1, P12

079.81 Hantavirus

079.82 SARS-associated coronavirus
Coding Clinic: 2003, Q4, P46-48

079.83 Parvovirus B19
Human parvovirus
Parvovirus NOS
Excludes *erythema infectiosum [fifth disease] (057.0)*
Coding Clinic: 2007, Q4, P64

079.88 Other specified chlamydial infection

079.89 Other specified viral infection
Coding Clinic: 1995, Q1, P7

●**079.9 Unspecified viral and chlamydial infections**
Excludes *viremia NOS (790.8)*
Coding Clinic: 1988, Q4, P10; 1987, Jan-Feb, P16

079.98 Unspecified chlamydial infection
Chlamydial infection NOS

079.99 Unspecified viral infection
Viral infection NOS
Coding Clinic: 1991, Q2, P8

RICKETTSIOSES AND OTHER ARTHROPOD-BORNE DISEASES (080–088)
Excludes *arthropod-borne viral diseases (060.0–066.9)*

080 Louse-borne [epidemic] typhus
Typhus (fever):
classical
epidemic
Infecting a large number of individuals at the same time
exanthematic NOS
louse-borne

●**081 Other typhus**

081.0 Murine [endemic] typhus
Typhus (fever):
endemic
Restricted to a particular region
flea-borne

081.1 Brill's disease
Brill-Zinsser disease
Recrudescent typhus (fever)

081.2 Scrub typhus
Japanese river fever   Mite-borne typhus
Kedani fever   Tsutsugamushi

081.9 Typhus, unspecified
Typhus (fever) NOS

◄ New   ◄▥ Revised   ~~deleted~~ Deleted   Excludes   Includes   Use additional   Code first   Omit code
● Unacceptable Principal Diagnosis   ● Use Additional Digit(s)   OGCR Official Guidelines   Coding Clinic

Item 1–13 Rickettsioses are diseases spread from ticks, lice, fleas, or mites to humans.
Typhus is spread to humans chiefly by the fleas of rats.
Endemic identifies a disease as being present in low numbers of humans at all times, whereas **epidemic** identifies a disease as being present in high numbers of humans at a specific time. Morbidity (death) is higher in epidemic diseases.
Brill's disease, also known as **Brill-Zinsser disease,** is spread from human to human by body lice and also from the lice of flying squirrels. **Scrub typhus** is spread in the same ways as Brill's disease.
Malaria is spread to humans by mosquitoes.

● **082 Tick-borne rickettsioses**

    082.0 Spotted fevers
        Rocky mountain spotted fever
        Sao Paulo fever

    082.1 Boutonneuse fever
        African tick typhus   Marseilles fever
        India tick typhus   Mediterranean tick fever
        Kenya tick typhus

    082.2 North Asian tick fever
        Siberian tick typhus

    082.3 Queensland tick typhus

  ● **082.4 Ehrlichiosis**

      082.40 Ehrlichiosis, unspecified

      082.41 Ehrlichiosis chaffeensis [E. chaffeensis]

      082.49 Other ehrlichiosis

    082.8 Other specified tick-borne rickettsioses
        Lone star fever
        Coding Clinic: 1999, Q4, P19

    082.9 Tick-borne rickettsiosis, unspecified
        Tick-borne typhus NOS

● **083 Other rickettsioses**

    083.0 Q fever

    083.1 Trench fever
        Quintan fever
        Wolhynian fever

    083.2 Rickettsialpox
        Vesicular rickettsiosis

    083.8 Other specified rickettsioses

    083.9 Rickettsiosis, unspecified

● **084 Malaria**
    Mosquito-borne disease caused by parasite. Left untreated, severe complications and death may result.

    Note: Subcategories 084.0–084.6 exclude the listed conditions with mention of pernicious complications (084.8–084.9).

    Excludes *congenital malaria (771.2)*

    084.0 Falciparum malaria [malignant tertian]
        Malaria (fever):
          by Plasmodium falciparum
          subtertian

    084.1 Vivax malaria [benign tertian]
        Malaria (fever) by Plasmodium vivax

    084.2 Quartan malaria
        Malaria (fever) by Plasmodium malariae
        Malariae malaria

    084.3 Ovale malaria
        Malaria (fever) by Plasmodium ovale

    084.4 Other malaria
        Monkey malaria

    084.5 Mixed malaria
        Malaria (fever) by more than one parasite

    084.6 Malaria, unspecified
        Malaria (fever) NOS

    084.7 Induced malaria
        Therapeutically induced malaria

      Excludes *accidental infection from syringe, blood transfusion, etc. (084.0–084.6, above, according to parasite species)*
        transmission from mother to child during delivery (771.2)

    084.8 Blackwater fever
        Hemoglobinuric:
          fever (bilious)
          malaria
        Malarial hemoglobinuria

    084.9 Other pernicious complications of malaria
        Algid malaria
        Cerebral malaria

      Use additional code to identify complication, as:
        malarial:
          hepatitis (573.2)
          nephrosis (581.81)

● **085 Leishmaniasis**

    085.0 Visceral [kala-azar]
        Dumdum fever
        Infection by Leishmania:
          donovani
          infantum
        Leishmaniasis:
          dermal, post-kala-azar
          Mediterranean
          visceral (Indian)

    085.1 Cutaneous, urban
        Aleppo boil
        Baghdad boil
        Delhi boil
        Infection by Leishmania tropica (minor)
        Leishmaniasis, cutaneous:
          dry form
          late
          recurrent
          ulcerating
        Oriental sore

    085.2 Cutaneous, Asian desert
        Infection by Leishmania tropica major
        Leishmaniasis, cutaneous:
          acute necrotizing
          rural
          wet form
          zoonotic form

    085.3 Cutaneous, Ethiopian
        Infection by Leishmania ethiopica
        Leishmaniasis, cutaneous:
          diffuse
          lepromatous

    085.4 Cutaneous, American
        Chiclero ulcer
        Infection by Leishmania mexicana
        Leishmaniasis tegumentaria diffusa

    085.5 Mucocutaneous (American)
        Espundia
        Infection by Leishmania braziliensis
        Uta

    085.9 Leishmaniasis, unspecified

INFECTIOUS AND PARASITIC DISEASES (001–139)

◀ New   ◀▦▦ Revised   ~~deleted~~ Deleted   Excludes   Includes   Use additional   Code first   Omit code
● Unacceptable Principal Diagnosis   ● Use Additional Digit(s)   OGCR Official Guidelines   Coding Clinic

INFECTIOUS AND PARASITIC DISEASES (001–139)

● **086 Trypanosomiasis**

Human African trypanosomiasis (HAT) is transmitted by fly bites that transmit either Trypanosoma brucei gambiense (causes a chronic infection lasting years) or Trypanosoma brucei rhodesiense (causes acute illness lasting several weeks).

Use additional code to identify manifestations, as:
trypanosomiasis:
encephalitis (323.2)
meningitis (321.3)

086.0 Chagas' disease with heart involvement
American trypanosomiasis with heart involvement
Infection by Trypanosoma cruzi with heart involvement
Any condition classifiable to 086.2 with heart involvement

086.1 Chagas' disease with other organ involvement
American trypanosomiasis with involvement of organ other than heart
Infection by Trypanosoma cruzi with involvement of organ other than heart
Any condition classifiable to 086.2 with involvement of organ other than heart

086.2 Chagas' disease without mention of organ involvement
American trypanosomiasis
Infection by Trypanosoma cruzi

086.3 Gambian trypanosomiasis
Gambian sleeping sickness
Infection by Trypanosoma gambiense

086.4 Rhodesian trypanosomiasis
Infection by Trypanosoma rhodesiense
Rhodesian sleeping sickness

086.5 African trypanosomiasis, unspecified
Sleeping sickness NOS

086.9 Trypanosomiasis, unspecified

● **087 Relapsing fever**

Includes recurrent fever

087.0 Louse-borne

087.1 Tick-borne

087.9 Relapsing fever, unspecified

● **088 Other arthropod-borne diseases**

088.0 Bartonellosis
Carrión's disease
Oroya fever
Verruga peruana

● **088.8 Other specified arthropod-borne diseases**

088.81 Lyme disease
Erythema chronicum migrans
Coding Clinic: 1990, Q3, P14; 1989, Q2, P10

088.82 Babesiosis
Babesiasis

088.89 Other

088.9 Arthropod-borne disease, unspecified

Figure 1–6 Chancre of primary syphilis. (From Mandell, Bennett, & Dolin: Principles and Practice of Infectious Diseases, 6th ed. 2005, Churchill Livingstone, An Imprint of Elsevier.)

Item 1–14 Syphilis, also known as lues, is the most serious of the venereal diseases caused by *Treponema pallidum.* The **primary** stage is characterized by an ulceration known as **chancre,** which usually appears on the genitals but can also develop on the anus, lips, tonsils, breasts, or fingers. Syphilis is easy to cure in its early stages. A single intramuscular injection of penicillin will usually cure a person who has had syphilis for less than a year.

The **secondary** stage is characterized by a rash that can affect any area of the body. **Latent** syphilis is divided into **early,** which is diagnosed within two years of infection, and **late,** which is diagnosed two years or more after infection. Additional doses of penicillin or another antibiotic are needed to treat someone who has had syphilis for longer than a year. For those allergic to penicillin, there are other antibiotic treatments. **Congenital** syphilis is also labeled **early** or **late** based on the time of diagnosis.

SYPHILIS AND OTHER VENEREAL DISEASES (090–099)

Excludes *nonvenereal endemic syphilis (104.0)*
urogenital trichomoniasis (131.0)

● **090 Congenital syphilis**

090.0 Early congenital syphilis, symptomatic
Congenital syphilitic:
choroiditis
coryza (chronic)
hepatomegaly
mucous patches
periostitis
splenomegaly
Syphilitic (congenital):
epiphysitis
osteochondritis
pemphigus
Any congenital syphilitic condition specified as early or manifest less than two years after birth

090.1 Early congenital syphilis, latent
Congenital syphilis without clinical manifestations, with positive serological reaction and negative spinal fluid test, less than two years after birth

090.2 Early congenital syphilis, unspecified
Congenital syphilis NOS, less than two years after birth

090.3 Syphilitic interstitial keratitis
Syphilitic keratitis:
parenchymatous
punctata profunda
Excludes *interstitial keratitis NOS (370.50)*

● **090.4 Juvenile neurosyphilis**

Use additional code to identify any associated mental disorder

090.40 Juvenile neurosyphilis, unspecified
Congenital neurosyphilis
Dementia paralytica juvenilis
Juvenile:
general paresis
tabes
taboparesis

◄ New ◄⚡ Revised ~~deleted~~ Deleted Excludes Includes Use additional Code first Omit code
● Unacceptable Principal Diagnosis ● Use Additional Digit(s) OGCR Official Guidelines Coding Clinic

090.41 **Congenital syphilitic encephalitis**

090.42 **Congenital syphilitic meningitis**

090.49 **Other**

090.5 **Other late congenital syphilis, symptomatic**
Gumma due to congenital syphilis
Hutchinson's teeth
Syphilitic saddle nose
Any congenital syphilitic condition specified as late
or manifest two years or more after birth

090.6 **Late congenital syphilis, latent**
Congenital syphilis without clinical manifestations,
with positive serological reaction and
negative spinal fluid test, two years or more
after birth

090.7 **Late congenital syphilis, unspecified**
Congenital syphilis NOS, two years or more after
birth

090.9 **Congenital syphilis, unspecified**

● 091 **Early syphilis, symptomatic**

> **Excludes** *early cardiovascular syphilis (093.0–093.9)*
> *early neurosyphilis (094.0–094.9)*

091.0 **Genital syphilis (primary)**
Genital chancre

091.1 **Primary anal syphilis**

091.2 **Other primary syphilis**
Primary syphilis of:
breast
fingers
lip
tonsils

091.3 **Secondary syphilis of skin or mucous membranes**
Condyloma latum
Secondary syphilis of:
anus
mouth
pharynx
skin
tonsils
vulva

091.4 **Adenopathy due to secondary syphilis**
Syphilitic adenopathy (secondary)
Syphilitic lymphadenitis (secondary)

● 091.5 **Uveitis due to secondary syphilis**

091.50 **Syphilitic uveitis, unspecified**

091.51 **Syphilitic chorioretinitis (secondary)**

091.52 **Syphilitic iridocyclitis (secondary)**

● 091.6 **Secondary syphilis of viscera and bone**

091.61 **Secondary syphilitic periostitis**

091.62 **Secondary syphilitic hepatitis**
Secondary syphilis of liver

091.69 **Other viscera**

091.7 **Secondary syphilis, relapse**
Secondary syphilis, relapse (treated) (untreated)

● 091.8 **Other forms of secondary syphilis**

091.81 **Acute syphilitic meningitis (secondary)**

091.82 **Syphilitic alopecia**

091.89 **Other**

091.9 **Unspecified secondary syphilis**

● 092 **Early syphilis, latent**
Early syphilis is the disease, latent is the characteristic.

> **Includes** syphilis (acquired) without clinical
> manifestations, with positive serological
> reaction and negative spinal fluid test,
> less than two years after infection

092.0 **Early syphilis, latent, serological relapse after treatment**

092.9 **Early syphilis, latent, unspecified**

● 093 **Cardiovascular syphilis**

093.0 **Aneurysm of aorta, specified as syphilitic**
Dilatation of aorta, specified as syphilitic

093.1 **Syphilitic aortitis**

● 093.2 **Syphilitic endocarditis**
Check documentation for documentation of a specific valve.

093.20 **Valve, unspecified**
Syphilitic ostial coronary disease

093.21 **Mitral valve**

093.22 **Aortic valve**
Syphilitic aortic incompetence or stenosis

093.23 **Tricuspid valve**

093.24 **Pulmonary valve**

● 093.8 **Other specified cardiovascular syphilis**

093.81 **Syphilitic pericarditis**

093.82 **Syphilitic myocarditis**

093.89 **Other**

093.9 **Cardiovascular syphilis, unspecified**

● 094 **Neurosyphilis**

> Use additional code to identify any associated mental disorder

094.0 **Tabes dorsalis**
Locomotor ataxia (progressive)
Posterior spinal sclerosis (syphilitic)
Tabetic neurosyphilis

> Use additional code to identify manifestation, as:
> neurogenic arthropathy [Charcot's joint disease] (713.5)

094.1 **General paresis**
Dementia paralytica
General paralysis (of the insane) (progressive)
Paretic neurosyphilis
Taboparesis

094.2 **Syphilitic meningitis**
Meningovascular syphilis

> **Excludes** *acute syphilitic meningitis (secondary)*
> *(091.81)*

094.3 **Asymptomatic neurosyphilis**

● 094.8 **Other specified neurosyphilis**

094.81 **Syphilitic encephalitis**

094.82 **Syphilitic Parkinsonism**

094.83 **Syphilitic disseminated retinochoroiditis**

094.84 **Syphilitic optic atrophy**

094.85 **Syphilitic retrobulbar neuritis**

094.86 **Syphilitic acoustic neuritis**

094.87 **Syphilitic ruptured cerebral aneurysm**

094.89 **Other**

094.9 **Neurosyphilis, unspecified**
Gumma (syphilitic) of central nervous system NOS
Syphilis (early) (late) of central nervous system NOS
Syphiloma of central nervous system NOS

Item 1–15 Notice the placement of 091.4 combination code in with the Infectious and Parasitic Disease codes (syphilis). This uveitis does not appear in the eye code section because it is a manifestation of the underlying disease of syphilis.

INFECTIOUS AND PARASITIC DISEASES (001–139)

◄ New   ◄■■ Revised   ~~deleted~~ Deleted   Excludes   Includes   Use additional   Code first   Omit code

● Unacceptable Principal Diagnosis   ● Use Additional Digit(s)   OGCR Official Guidelines   **Coding Clinic**

● **095 Other forms of late syphilis, with symptoms**
In the late stages, syphilis can damage organs and body systems.

Includes gumma (syphilitic)
Destructive lesions of syphilis
tertiary, or unspecified stage

095.0 Syphilitic episcleritis

095.1 Syphilis of lung

095.2 Syphilitic peritonitis

095.3 Syphilis of liver

095.4 Syphilis of kidney

095.5 Syphilis of bone

095.6 Syphilis of muscle
Syphilitic myositis

095.7 Syphilis of synovium, tendon, and bursa
Syphilitic:
bursitis
synovitis

095.8 Other specified forms of late symptomatic syphilis
Excludes *cardiovascular syphilis (093.0–093.9)*
neurosyphilis (094.0–094.9)

095.9 Late symptomatic syphilis, unspecified

096 Late syphilis, latent
Syphilis (acquired) without clinical manifestations, with positive serological reaction and negative spinal fluid test, two years or more after infection

● **097 Other and unspecified syphilis**

097.0 Late syphilis, unspecified

097.1 Latent syphilis, unspecified
Positive serological reaction for syphilis

097.9 Syphilis, unspecified
Syphilis (acquired) NOS
Excludes *syphilis NOS causing death under two years of age (090.9)*

● **098 Gonococcal infections**
STD (sexually transmitted disease) caused by Neisseria gonorrhoeae that flourishes in the warm, moist areas of the reproductive tract. Untreated gonorrhea spreads to other parts of the body, causing inflammation of the testes or prostate or pelvic inflammatory disease (PID).

098.0 Acute, of lower genitourinary tract
Gonococcal:
Bartholinitis (acute)
Female only: Bartholin gland
urethritis (acute)
vulvovaginitis (acute)
Gonorrhea (acute):
NOS
genitourinary (tract) NOS

● **098.1 Acute, of upper genitourinary tract**

098.10 Gonococcal infection (acute) of upper genitourinary tract, site unspecified

098.11 Gonococcal cystitis (acute)
Gonorrhea (acute) of bladder

098.12 Gonococcal prostatitis (acute)

098.13 Gonococcal epididymo-orchitis (acute)
Gonococcal orchitis (acute)

098.14 Gonococcal seminal vesiculitis (acute)
Gonorrhea (acute) of seminal vesicle

098.15 Gonococcal cervicitis (acute)
Gonorrhea (acute) of cervix

098.16 Gonococcal endometritis (acute)
Gonorrhea (acute) of uterus

098.17 Gonococcal salpingitis, specified as acute

098.19 Other

098.2 Chronic, of lower genitourinary tract
Gonococcal specified as chronic or with duration of two months or more:
Bartholinitis specified as chronic or with duration of two months or more
urethritis specified as chronic or with duration of two months or more
vulvovaginitis specified as chronic or with duration of two months or more
Gonorrhea specified as chronic or with duration of two months or more:
NOS specified as chronic or with duration of two months or more
genitourinary (tract) specified as chronic or with duration of two months or more
Any condition classifiable to 098.0 specified as chronic or with duration of two months or more

● **098.3 Chronic, of upper genitourinary tract**
Any condition classifiable to 098.1 stated as chronic or with a duration of two months or more

098.30 Chronic gonococcal infection of upper genitourinary tract, site unspecified

098.31 Gonococcal cystitis, chronic
Any condition classifiable to 098.11, specified as chronic
Gonorrhea of bladder, chronic

098.32 Gonococcal prostatitis, chronic
Any condition classifiable to 098.12, specified as chronic

098.33 Gonococcal epididymo-orchitis, chronic
Any condition classifiable to 098.13, specified as chronic
Chronic gonococcal orchitis

098.34 Gonococcal seminal vesiculitis, chronic
Any condition classifiable to 098.14, specified as chronic
Gonorrhea of seminal vesicle, chronic

098.35 Gonococcal cervicitis, chronic
Any condition classifiable to 098.15, specified as chronic
Gonorrhea of cervix, chronic

098.36 Gonococcal endometritis, chronic
Any condition classifiable to 098.16, specified as chronic

098.37 Gonococcal salpingitis (chronic)

098.39 Other

● **098.4 Gonococcal infection of eye**

098.40 Gonococcal conjunctivitis (neonatorum)
Neonate = newborn
Gonococcal ophthalmia (neonatorum)

098.41 Gonococcal iridocyclitis

098.42 Gonococcal endophthalmia

098.43 Gonococcal keratitis

098.49 Other

● **098.5 Gonococcal infection of joint**

098.50 Gonococcal arthritis
Gonococcal infection of joint NOS

098.51 Gonococcal synovitis and tenosynovitis

098.52 Gonococcal bursitis

098.53 Gonococcal spondylitis

098.59 Other
Gonococcal rheumatism

098.6 Gonococcal infection of pharynx

098.7 Gonococcal infection of anus and rectum
Gonococcal proctitis

◀ New   ◀▥ Revised   ~~deleted~~ Deleted   Excludes   Includes   Use additional   Code first   Omit code
● Unacceptable Principal Diagnosis   ● Use Additional Digit(s)   OGCR Official Guidelines   Coding Clinic

● **098.8 Gonococcal infection of other specified sites**

098.81 Gonococcal keratosis (blennorrhagica)

098.82 Gonococcal meningitis

098.83 Gonococcal pericarditis

098.84 Gonococcal endocarditis

098.85 Other gonococcal heart disease

098.86 Gonococcal peritonitis

098.89 Other
Gonococcemia
Blood condition

● **099 Other venereal diseases**

099.0 Chancroid
*Sexually transmitted infection caused by bacteria
    (Haemophilus ducreyi).*
Bubo (inguinal):
    chancroidal
    due to Hemophilus ducreyi
Chancre:
    Ducrey's simple soft
    Ulcus molle (cutis) (skin)

099.1 Lymphogranuloma venereum
Climatic or tropical bubo
(Durand-) Nicolas-Favre disease
Esthiomene
Lymphogranuloma inguinale

099.2 Granuloma inguinale
Donovanosis
Granuloma pudendi (ulcerating)
Granuloma venereum
Pudendal ulcer

099.3 Reiter's disease
Reiter's syndrome

Use additional code for associated:
    arthropathy (711.1)
    conjunctivitis (372.33)

● **099.4 Other nongonococcal urethritis [NGU]**

099.40 Unspecified
Nonspecific urethritis

099.41 Chlamydia trachomatis

099.49 Other specified organism

● **099.5 Other venereal diseases due to Chlamydia trachomatis**

Excludes *Chlamydia trachomatis infection of
    conjunctiva (076.0–076.9, 077.0,
    077.9)
    Lymphogranuloma venereum (099.1)*

099.50 Unspecified site

099.51 Pharynx

099.52 Anus and rectum

099.53 Lower genitourinary sites

Excludes *urethra (099.41)*

Use additional code to specify site of
    infection, such as:
        bladder (595.4)
        cervix (616.0)
        vagina and vulva (616.11)

099.54 Other genitourinary sites

Use additional code to specify site of
    infection, such as:
        pelvic inflammatory disease NOS (614.9)
        testis and epididymis (604.91)

099.55 Unspecified genitourinary site

099.56 Peritoneum
Perihepatitis

099.59 Other specified site

099.8 Other specified venereal diseases

099.9 Venereal disease, unspecified

OTHER SPIROCHETAL DISEASES (100–104)

● **100 Leptospirosis**

100.0 Leptospirosis icterohemorrhagica
Leptospiral or spirochetal jaundice (hemorrhagic)
Weil's disease

● **100.8 Other specified leptospiral infections**

100.81 Leptospiral meningitis (aseptic)

100.89 Other
Fever:
    Fort Bragg
    pretibial
    swamp
Infection by Leptospira:
    australis
    bataviae
    pyrogenes

100.9 Leptospirosis, unspecified

101 Vincent's angina
Acute necrotizing ulcerative:
    gingivitis
    stomatitis
Fusospirochetal pharyngitis
Spirochetal stomatitis
Trench mouth
Vincent's:
    gingivitis
    infection [any site]

● **102 Yaws**

Includes frambesia
          pian

102.0 Initial lesions
Chancre of yaws
Frambesia, initial or primary
Initial frambesial ulcer
Mother yaw

102.1 Multiple papillomata and wet crab yaws
Butter yaws
Frambesioma
Pianoma
Plantar or palmar papilloma of yaws

102.2 Other early skin lesions
Cutaneous yaws, less than five years after infection
Early yaws (cutaneous) (macular) (papular)
    (maculopapular) (micropapular)
Frambeside of early yaws

102.3 Hyperkeratosis
Ghoul hand
Hyperkeratosis, palmar or plantar (early) (late) due
    to yaws
Worm-eaten soles

102.4 Gummata and ulcers
Nodular late yaws (ulcerated)
Gummatous frambeside

102.5 Gangosa
Rhinopharyngitis mutilans

102.6 Bone and joint lesions
Goundou of yaws (late)
Gumma, bone of yaws (late)
Gummatous osteitis or periostitis of yaws (late)
Hydrarthrosis of yaws (early) (late)
Osteitis of yaws (early) (late)
Periostitis (hypertrophic) of yaws (early) (late)

102.7 Other manifestations
Juxta-articular nodules of yaws
Mucosal yaws

102.8 Latent yaws
Yaws without clinical manifestations, with positive
serology

102.9 Yaws, unspecified

● **103 Pinta**

103.0 Primary lesions
Chancre (primary) of pinta [carate]
Papule (primary) of pinta [carate]
Pintid of pinta [carate]

103.1 Intermediate lesions
Erythematous plaques of pinta [carate]
Hyperchromic lesions of pinta [carate]
Hyperkeratosis of pinta [carate]

103.2 Late lesions
Cardiovascular lesions of pinta [carate]
Skin lesions of pinta [carate]:
achromic of pinta [carate]
cicatricial of pinta [carate]
dyschromic of pinta [carate]
Vitiligo of pinta [carate]

103.3 Mixed lesions
Achromic and hyperchromic skin lesions of pinta
[carate]

103.9 Pinta, unspecified

● **104 Other spirochetal infection**

104.0 Nonvenereal endemic syphilis
Bejel
Njovera

104.8 Other specified spirochetal infections

> **Excludes** *relapsing fever (087.0–087.9)*
> *syphilis (090.0–097.9)*

104.9 Spirochetal infection, unspecified

MYCOSES (110–118)

Use additional code to identify manifestation, as:
arthropathy (711.6)
meningitis (321.0–321.1)
otitis externa (380.15)

> **Excludes** *infection by Actinomycetales, such as species of*
> *Actinomyces, Actinomadura, Nocardia,*
> *Streptomyces (039.0–039.9)*

● **110 Dermatophytosis**
Also known as tinea or ringworm; condition of scalp, glabrous
skin, and/or nails. Caused by fungi (dermatophytes).

> **Includes** infection by species of Epidermophyton,
> Microsporum, and Trichophyton
> tinea, any type except those in 111

110.0 Of scalp and beard
Kerion
Sycosis, mycotic
Trichophytic tinea [black dot tinea], scalp

110.1 Of nail
Dermatophytic onychia
Onychomycosis
Tinea unguium

110.2 Of hand
Tinea manuum

110.3 Of groin and perianal area
Dhobie itch
Eczema marginatum
Tinea cruris

110.4 Of foot
Athlete's foot
Tinea pedis

110.5 Of the body
Herpes circinatus
Tinea imbricata [Tokelau]

110.6 Deep seated dermatophytosis
Granuloma trichophyticum
Majocchi's granuloma

110.8 Of other specified sites

110.9 Of unspecified site
Favus NOS
Microsporic tinea NOS
Ringworm NOS

● **111 Dermatomycosis, other and unspecified**

111.0 Pityriasis versicolor
Infection by Malassezia [Pityrosporum] furfur
Tinea flava
Tinea versicolor

111.1 Tinea nigra
Infection by Cladosporium species
Keratomycosis nigricans
Microsporosis nigra
Pityriasis nigra
Tinea palmaris nigra

111.2 Tinea blanca
Infection by Trichosporon (beigelii) cutaneum
White piedra

111.3 Black piedra
Infection by Piedraia hortai

111.8 Other specified dermatomycoses

111.9 Dermatomycosis, unspecified

● **112 Candidiasis**

> **Includes** infection by Candida species
> moniliasis

> **Excludes** *neonatal monilial infection (771.7)*

112.0 Of mouth
Thrush (oral)

112.1 Of vulva and vagina
Candidal vulvovaginitis
Monilial vulvovaginitis
Coding Clinic: 1994, Q1, P21

112.2 Of other urogenital sites
Candidal balanitis
Male condition only
Coding Clinic: 2003, Q4, P105-106; 1996, Q4, P33

Figure 1–7 Oral candidiasis (thrush).
(Courtesy of Stephen Raffanti, MD,
MPH.) (From Mandell, Bennett, & Dolin:
Principles and Practice of Infectious
Diseases, 6th ed. 2005, Churchill
Livingstone, An Imprint of Elsevier.)

Item 1–16 Candidiasis, also called oidiomycosis or moniliasis, is a
fungal infection. It most often appears on moist cutaneous areas of the
body but can also be responsible for a variety of systemic infections such
as endocarditis, meningitis, arthritis, and myositis. Antifungal medications
cure most yeast infections.

◀ New   ◀▥ Revised   ~~deleted~~ Deleted   Excludes   Includes   Use additional   Code first   Omit code
● Unacceptable Principal Diagnosis   ● Use Additional Digit(s)   OGCR Official Guidelines   Coding Clinic

112.3 Of skin and nails
Candidal intertrigo
Candidal onychia
Candidal perionyxis [paronychia]

112.4 Of lung
Candidal pneumonia
Coding Clinic: 1998, Q2, P7

112.5 Disseminated
Systemic candidiasis
Coding Clinic: 1989, Q2, P10

● **112.8 Of other specified sites**

112.81 Candidal endocarditis

112.82 Candidal otitis externa
Otomycosis in moniliasis

112.83 Candidal meningitis

112.84 Candidal esophagitis

112.85 Candidal enteritis

112.89 Other
Coding Clinic: 1992, Q1, P17; 1991, Q3, P20

112.9 Of unspecified site
Coding Clinic: 1996, Q4, P33

● **114 Coccidioidomycosis**
Includes infection by Coccidioides (immitis)
Posada-Wernicke disease

114.0 Primary coccidioidomycosis (pulmonary)
Acute pulmonary coccidioidomycosis
Coccidioidomycotic pneumonitis
Desert rheumatism
Pulmonary coccidioidomycosis
San Joaquin Valley fever

114.1 Primary extrapulmonary coccidioidomycosis
Chancriform syndrome
Primary cutaneous coccidioidomycosis

114.2 Coccidioidal meningitis

114.3 Other forms of progressive coccidioidomycosis
Coccidioidal granuloma
Disseminated coccidioidomycosis

114.4 Chronic pulmonary coccidioidomycosis

114.5 Pulmonary coccidioidomycosis, unspecified

114.9 Coccidioidomycosis, unspecified

● **115 Histoplasmosis**
The following fifth-digit subclassification is for use with
category 115:

0 without mention of manifestation
1 meningitis
2 retinitis
3 pericarditis
4 endocarditis
5 pneumonia
9 other

● **115.0 Infection by Histoplasma capsulatum**
[0-5,9] American histoplasmosis
Darling's disease
Reticuloendothelial cytomycosis
Small form histoplasmosis

● **115.1 Infection by Histoplasma duboisii**
[0-5,9] African histoplasmosis
Large form histoplasmosis

● **115.9 Histoplasmosis, unspecified**
[0-5,9] Histoplasmosis NOS

Item 1-17 Bird and bat droppings that fall into the soil give rise to a fungus that can spread airborne spores. When inhaled into the lungs, these spores divide and multiply into lesions. Histoplasmosis capsulatum takes three forms: primary (lodged in the lungs only), chronic (resembles TB), and disseminated (infection has moved to other organs). This is an opportunistic infection in immunosuppressed patients.

● **116 Blastomycotic infection**
Rare and potentially fatal infections caused by fungus B. dermatitidis inhaled and found in moist soil in temperate climates.

116.0 Blastomycosis
Blastomycotic dermatitis
Chicago disease
Cutaneous blastomycosis
Disseminated blastomycosis
Gilchrist's disease
Infection by Blastomyces [Ajellomyces] dermatitidis
North American blastomycosis
Primary pulmonary blastomycosis

116.1 Paracoccidioidomycosis
Brazilian blastomycosis
Infection by Paracoccidioides [Blastomyces] brasiliensis
Lutz-Splendore-Almeida disease
Mucocutaneous-lymphangitic paracoccidioidomycosis
Pulmonary paracoccidioidomycosis
South American blastomycosis
Visceral paracoccidioidomycosis

116.2 Lobomycosis
Infections by Loboa [Blastomyces] loboi
Keloidal blastomycosis
Lobo's disease

● **117 Other mycoses**
117.0 Rhinosporidiosis
Infection by Rhinosporidium seeberi

117.1 Sporotrichosis
Cutaneous sporotrichosis
Disseminated sporotrichosis
Infection by Sporothrix [Sporotrichum] schenckii
Lymphocutaneous sporotrichosis
Pulmonary sporotrichosis
Sporotrichosis of the bones

117.2 Chromoblastomycosis
Chromomycosis
Infection by Cladosporidium carrionii, Fonsecaea compactum, Fonsecaea pedrosoi, Phialophora verrucosa

117.3 Aspergillosis
Infection by Aspergillus species, mainly A. fumigatus, A. flavus group, A. terreus group
Coding Clinic: 1997, Q4, P40

117.4 Mycotic mycetomas
Infection by various genera and species of Ascomycetes and Deuteromycetes, such as Acremonium [Cephalosporium] falciforme, Neotestudina rosatii, Madurella grisea, Madurella mycetomii, Pyrenochaeta romeroi, Zopfia [Leptosphaeria] senegalensis
Madura foot, mycotic
Maduromycosis, mycotic
Excludes *actinomycotic mycetomas (039.0–039.9)*

117.5 Cryptococcosis
Busse-Buschke's disease
European cryptococcosis
Infection by Cryptococcus neoformans
Pulmonary cryptococcosis
Systemic cryptococcosis
Torula

117.6 Allescheriosis [Petriellidosis]
Infections by Allescheria [Petriellidium] boydii
[Monosporium apiospermum]

    Excludes   *mycotic mycetoma (117.4)*

117.7 Zygomycosis [Phycomycosis or Mucormycosis]
Infection by species of Absidia, Basidiobolus,
Conidiobolus, Cunninghamella,
Entomophthora, Mucor, Rhizopus, Saksenaea

**117.8 Infection by dematiacious fungi
[Phaehyphomycosis]**
Infection by dematiacious fungi, such as
Cladosporium trichoides [bantianum],
Dreschlera hawaiiensis, Phialophora
gougerotii, Phialophora jeanselmi

117.9 Other and unspecified mycoses
Coding Clinic: 1995, Q2, P7

118 Opportunistic mycoses
Infection of skin, subcutaneous tissues, and/or organs by
a wide variety of fungi generally considered to be
pathogenic to compromised hosts only (e.g., infection
by species of Alternaria, Dreschlera, Fusarium)

    Use additional code to identify manifestation, such as:
keratitis (370.8)

HELMINTHIASES (120–129)

● **120 Schistosomiasis [bilharziasis]**
Parasitic disease (worm induced) that leads to chronic illness

120.0 Schistosoma haematobium
Vesical schistosomiasis NOS

120.1 Schistosoma mansoni
Intestinal schistosomiasis NOS

120.2 Schistosoma japonicum
Asiatic schistosomiasis NOS
Katayama disease or fever

120.3 Cutaneous
Cercarial dermatitis
Infection by cercariae of Schistosoma
Schistosome dermatitis
Swimmers' itch

120.8 Other specified schistosomiasis
Infection by Schistosoma:
bovis
intercalatum
mattheii
Infection by Schistosoma spindale
Schistosomiasis chestermani

120.9 Schistosomiasis, unspecified
Blood flukes NOS   Hemic distomiasis

● **121 Other trematode infections**

121.0 Opisthorchiasis
Infection by:
cat liver fluke
Opisthorchis (felineus) (tenuicollis) (viverrini)

121.1 Clonorchiasis
Biliary cirrhosis due to clonorchiasis
Chinese liver fluke disease
Hepatic distomiasis due to Clonorchis sinensis
Oriental liver fluke disease

121.2 Paragonimiasis
Infection by Paragonimus
Lung fluke disease (oriental)
Pulmonary distomiasis

121.3 Fascioliasis
Infection by Fasciola:
gigantica
hepatica
Liver flukes NOS
Sheep liver fluke infection

121.4 Fasciolopsiasis
Infection by Fasciolopsis (buski)
Intestinal distomiasis

121.5 Metagonimiasis
Infection by Metagonimus yokogawai

121.6 Heterophyiasis
Infection by:
Heterophyes heterophyes
Stellantchasmus falcatus

121.8 Other specified trematode infections
Infection by:
Dicrocoelium dendriticum
Echinostoma ilocanum
Gastrodiscoides hominis

121.9 Trematode infection, unspecified
Distomiasis NOS
Fluke disease NOS

● **122 Echinococcosis**
*Also known as hydatid disease; caused by Echinococcus
granulosus, E. multilocularis, and E. vogeli tapeworms;
and is contracted from infected food.*

    Includes   echinococciasis
hydatid disease
hydatidosis

122.0 Echinococcus granulosus infection of liver

122.1 Echinococcus granulosus infection of lung

122.2 Echinococcus granulosus infection of thyroid

122.3 Echinococcus granulosus infection, other

122.4 Echinococcus granulosus infection, unspecified

122.5 Echinococcus multilocularis infection of liver

122.6 Echinococcus multilocularis infection, other

122.7 Echinococcus multilocularis infection, unspecified

122.8 Echinococcosis, unspecified, of liver

122.9 Echinococcosis, other and unspecified

● **123 Other cestode infection**

123.0 Taenia solium infection, intestinal form
Pork tapeworm (adult) (infection)

123.1 Cysticercosis
Cysticerciasis
Infection by Cysticercus cellulosae [larval form of
Taenia solium]
Coding Clinic: 1997, Q2, P8

123.2 Taenia saginata infection
Beef tapeworm (infection)
Infection by Taeniarhynchus saginatus

123.3 Taeniasis, unspecified

123.4 Diphyllobothriasis, intestinal
Diphyllobothrium (adult) (latum) (pacificum)
infection
Fish tapeworm (infection)

123.5 Sparganosis [larval diphyllobothriasis]
Infection by:
Diphyllobothrium larvae
Sparganum (mansoni) (proliferum)
Spirometra larvae

123.6 Hymenolepiasis
Dwarf tapeworm (infection)
Hymenolepis (diminuta) (nana) infection
Rat tapeworm (infection)

123.8 Other specified cestode infection
Diplogonoporus (grandis) infection
Dipylidium (caninum) infection
Dog tapeworm (infection)

123.9 Cestode infection, unspecified
Tapeworm (infection) NOS

124 Trichinosis
Trichinella spiralis infection
Trichinellosis
Trichiniasis

● **125 Filarial infection and dracontiasis**

125.0 Bancroftian filariasis
Chyluria due to Wuchereria bancrofti
Elephantiasis due to Wuchereria bancrofti
Infection due to Wuchereria bancrofti
Lymphadenitis due to Wuchereria bancrofti
Lymphangitis due to Wuchereria bancrofti
Wuchereriasis

125.1 Malayan filariasis
Brugia filariasis due to Brugia [Wuchereria] malayi
Chyluria due to Brugia [Wuchereria] malayi
Elephantiasis due to Brugia [Wuchereria] malayi
Infection due to Brugia [Wuchereria] malayi
Lymphadenitis due to Brugia [Wuchereria] malayi
Lymphangitis due to Brugia [Wuchereria] malayi

125.2 Loiasis
Eyeworm disease of Africa
Loa loa infection

125.3 Onchocerciasis
Onchocerca volvulus infection
Onchocercosis

125.4 Dipetalonemiasis
Infection by:
Acanthocheilonema perstans
Dipetalonema perstans

125.5 Mansonella ozzardi infection
Filariasis ozzardi

125.6 Other specified filariasis
Dirofilaria infection
Infection by:
Acanthocheilonema streptocerca
Dipetalonema streptocerca

125.7 Dracontiasis
Guinea-worm infection
Infection by Dracunculus medinensis

125.9 Unspecified filariasis

● **126 Ancylostomiasis and necatoriasis**

| Includes | cutaneous larva migrans due to Ancylostoma hookworm (disease) (infection) uncinariasis |

126.0 Ancylostoma duodenale

126.1 Necator americanus

126.2 Ancylostoma braziliense

126.3 Ancylostoma ceylanicum

126.8 Other specified Ancylostoma

126.9 Ancylostomiasis and necatoriasis, unspecified
Creeping eruption NOS
Cutaneous larva migrans NOS

● **127 Other intestinal helminthiases**

127.0 Ascariasis
Ascaridiasis
Infection by Ascaris lumbricoides
Roundworm infection

127.1 Anisakiasis
Infection by Anisakis larva

127.2 Strongyloidiasis
Infection by Strongyloides stercoralis
| Excludes | *trichostrongyliasis (127.6)* |

127.3 Trichuriasis
Infection by Trichuris trichiuria
Trichocephaliasis
Whipworm (disease) (infection)

127.4 Enterobiasis
Infection by Enterobius vermicularis
Oxyuriasis
Oxyuris vermicularis infection
Pinworm (disease) (infection)
Threadworm infection

127.5 Capillariasis
Infection by Capillaria philippinensis
| Excludes | *infection by Capillaria hepatica (128.8)* |

127.6 Trichostrongyliasis
Infection by Trichostrongylus species

127.7 Other specified intestinal helminthiasis
Infection by:
Oesophagostomum apiostomum and related species
Ternidens diminutus
other specified intestinal helminth
Physalopteriasis

127.8 Mixed intestinal helminthiasis
Infection by intestinal helminths classified to more than one of the categories 120.0–127.7
Mixed helminthiasis NOS

127.9 Intestinal helminthiasis, unspecified

● **128 Other and unspecified helminthiases**

128.0 Toxocariasis
Larva migrans visceralis
Toxocara (canis) (cati) infection
Visceral larva migrans syndrome

128.1 Gnathostomiasis
Infection by Gnathostoma spinigerum and related species

128.8 Other specified helminthiasis
Infection by:
Angiostrongylus cantonensis
Capillaria hepatica
other specified helminth

128.9 Helminth infection, unspecified
Helminthiasis NOS
Worms NOS

129 Intestinal parasitism, unspecified

OTHER INFECTIOUS AND PARASITIC DISEASES (130–136)

● **130 Toxoplasmosis**

| Includes | infection by toxoplasma gondii toxoplasmosis (acquired) |

| Excludes | *congenital toxoplasmosis (771.2)* |

130.0 Meningoencephalitis due to toxoplasmosis
Encephalitis due to acquired toxoplasmosis

130.1 Conjunctivitis due to toxoplasmosis

INFECTIOUS AND PARASITIC DISEASES (001–139)

◀ New ◀▥ Revised ~~deleted~~ Deleted [Excludes] [Includes] Use additional Code first Omit code
● Unacceptable Principal Diagnosis ● Use Additional Digit(s) OGCR Official Guidelines Coding Clinic

729

INFECTIOUS AND PARASITIC DISEASES (001–139)

Item 1–18 Toxoplasmosis is caused by the protozoa **Toxoplasma gondii,** of which the house cat can be a host. Human infection occurs when contact is made with materials containing the pathogen, such as feces, contaminated soil, or ingestion of infected lamb, goat, or pork. Of the infected, very few have symptoms because a healthy person's immune system keeps the parasite from causing illness. When the immune system is compromised, symptoms may occur. Clinical symptoms include flu-like symptoms, but the disease progresses to include the eyes and the brain in babies.

130.2 Chorioretinitis due to toxoplasmosis
　　Focal retinochoroiditis due to acquired toxoplasmosis

130.3 Myocarditis due to toxoplasmosis

130.4 Pneumonitis due to toxoplasmosis

130.5 Hepatitis due to toxoplasmosis

130.7 Toxoplasmosis of other specified sites

130.8 Multisystemic disseminated toxoplasmosis
　　Toxoplasmosis of multiple sites

130.9 Toxoplasmosis, unspecified

● **131 Trichomoniasis**
　　A common STD caused by a parasite, Trichomonas vaginalis, affecting both women and men.

　　Includes infection due to Trichomonas (vaginalis)

● **131.0 Urogenital trichomoniasis**

　　131.00 Urogenital trichomoniasis, unspecified
　　　Fluor (vaginalis) trichomonal or due to Trichomonas (vaginalis)
　　　Leukorrhea (vaginalis) trichomonal or due to Trichomonas (vaginalis)

　　131.01 Trichomonal vulvovaginitis
　　　Vaginitis, trichomonal or due to Trichomonas (vaginalis)

　　131.02 Trichomonal urethritis

　　131.03 Trichomonal prostatitis

　　131.09 Other

131.8 Other specified sites
　　Excludes intestinal (007.3)

131.9 Trichomoniasis, unspecified

● **132 Pediculosis and phthirus infestation**
　　Infestation of lice, Pediculus humanus, specifically capitis infest the head, corporis infest the body-trunk area, and pubis infest the pubic region.

132.0 Pediculus capitis [head louse]

132.1 Pediculus corporis [body louse]

132.2 Phthirus pubis [pubic louse]
　　Pediculus pubis

132.3 Mixed infestation
　　This is a combination code.
　　Infestation classifiable to more than one of the categories 132.0–132.2

132.9 Pediculosis, unspecified

● **133 Acariasis**

133.0 Scabies
　　Infestation by Sarcoptes scabiei
　　Norwegian scabies
　　Sarcoptic itch

133.8 Other acariasis
　　Chiggers
　　Infestation by:
　　　Demodex folliculorum
　　　Trombicula

133.9 Acariasis, unspecified
　　Infestation by mites NOS

● **134 Other infestation**

134.0 Myiasis
　　Infestation by:
　　　Dermatobia (hominis)
　　　fly larvae
　　　Gasterophilus (intestinalis)
　　　maggots
　　　Oestrus ovis

134.1 Other arthropod infestation
　　Infestation by:
　　　chigoe
　　　Jigger disease
　　　sand flea
　　　Scarabiasis
　　　Tunga penetrans
　　　Tungiasis

134.2 Hirudiniasis
　　Hirudiniasis (external) (internal)
　　Leeches (aquatic) (land)

134.8 Other specified infestations

134.9 Infestation, unspecified
　　Infestation (skin) NOS
　　Skin parasites NOS

135 Sarcoidosis
　　Symptom of an inflammation producing tiny lumps of cells (granulomas) in various organs, most commonly the lungs and lymph nodes, that affect organ function.
　　Besnier-Boeck-Schaumann disease
　　Lupoid (miliary) of Boeck
　　Lupus pernio (Besnier)
　　Lymphogranulomatosis, benign (Schaumann's)
　　Sarcoid (any site):
　　　NOS
　　　Boeck
　　　Darier-Roussy
　　Uveoparotid fever

● **136 Other and unspecified infectious and parasitic diseases**

136.0 Ainhum
　　Dactylolysis spontanea

136.1 Behçet's syndrome

● **136.2 Specific infections by free-living amebae**

　　136.21 Specific infection due to acanthamoeba
　　　Use additional code to identify manifestation, such as:
　　　keratitis (370.8)
　　　Coding Clinic: 2008, Q4, P79-81

　　136.29 Other specific infections by free-living amebae
　　　Meningoencephalitis due to Naegleria
　　　Coding Clinic: 2008, Q4, P79-81

136.3 Pneumocystosis
　　Pneumonia due to Pneumocystis carinii
　　Pneumonia due to Pneumocystis jiroveci
　　Coding Clinic: 2003, Q1, P15; 1987, Nov-Dec, P5-6

136.4 Psorospermiasis

136.5 Sarcosporidiosis
　　Infection by Sarcocystis lindemanni

136.8 Other specified infectious and parasitic diseases
　　Candiru infestation

136.9 Unspecified infectious and parasitic diseases
　　Infectious disease NOS
　　Parasitic disease NOS
　　Coding Clinic: 1991, Q2, P8

◀ New ⫸ Revised ~~deleted~~ Deleted [Excludes] [Includes] [Use additional] [Code first] [Omit code]
● Unacceptable Principal Diagnosis ● Use Additional Digit(s) OGCR Official Guidelines Coding Clinic

LATE EFFECTS OF INFECTIOUS AND PARASITIC DISEASES (137–139)

● **137** **Late effects of tuberculosis**

> **Note:** This category is to be used to indicate conditions classifiable to 010–018 as the cause of late effects, which are themselves classified elsewhere. The "late effects" include those specified as such, as sequelae, or as due to old or inactive tuberculosis, without evidence of active disease.

> **137.0** **Late effects of respiratory or unspecified tuberculosis**

> **137.1** **Late effects of central nervous system tuberculosis**

> **137.2** **Late effects of genitourinary tuberculosis**

> **137.3** **Late effects of tuberculosis of bones and joints**

> **137.4** **Late effects of tuberculosis of other specified organs**

138 **Late effects of acute poliomyelitis**

> **Note:** This category is to be used to indicate conditions classifiable to 045 as the cause of late effects, which are themselves classified elsewhere. The "late effects" include conditions specified as such, or as sequelae, or as due to old or inactive poliomyelitis, without evidence of active disease.

Item 1–19 Before you assign the late code 137.X, check your documentation. The original problem (tuberculosis, TB) that is causing the current late effect (necrosis) must have been attributable to categories 010–018. A patient who originally had TB of a joint (015.2X) now has a late effect (137.3), which is necrosis of bone (730.8). Because there is no active TB, 015.2X is not coded but serves as an authorization to use the late effect code. Remember to code the manifestation of the late effect, which is the current problem (necrosis).

● **139** **Late effects of other infectious and parasitic diseases**

> **Note:** This category is to be used to indicate conditions classifiable to categories 001–009, 020–041, 046–136 as the cause of late effects, which are themselves classified elsewhere. The "late effects" include conditions specified as such; they also include sequela of diseases classifiable to the above categories if there is evidence that the disease itself is no longer present.

> **139.0** **Late effects of viral encephalitis**
> Late effects of conditions classifiable to 049.8–049.9, 062–064

> **139.1** **Late effects of trachoma**
> Late effects of conditions classifiable to 076

> **139.8** **Late effects of other and unspecified infectious and parasitic diseases**
> Coding Clinic: 2006, Q2, P17-18; 1990, Q3, P14

INFECTIOUS AND PARASITIC DISEASES (001–139)

NEOPLASMS (140–239)

Item 2–1 Neoplasm: Neo = new, plasm = growth, development, formation. This new growth (mass, tumor) can be malignant or benign, which is confirmed by the pathology report. Do not assign a code to a neoplasm until you review the pathology report. Certain CPT codes will specify benign or malignant lesion, so be certain the diagnosis code supports the procedure code.

2.   NEOPLASMS (140–239)

1. Content:
   This chapter contains the following broad groups:
   - 140–195 Malignant neoplasms, stated or presumed to be primary, of specified sites, except of lymphatic and hematopoietic tissue
   - 196–198 Malignant neoplasms, stated or presumed to be secondary, of specified sites
   - 199 Malignant neoplasms, without specification of site
   - 200–208 Malignant neoplasms, stated or presumed to be primary, of lymphatic and hematopoietic tissue
   - 209 Neuroendocrine tumors
   - 210–229 Benign neoplasms
   - 230–234 Carcinoma in situ
   - 235–238 Neoplasms of uncertain behavior [see Note, at beginning of section 235–238]
   - 239 Neoplasms of unspecified nature

2. Functional activity
   All neoplasms are classified in this chapter, whether or not functionally active. An additional code from Chapter 3 may be used to identify such functional activity associated with any neoplasm, e.g.:
   catecholamine-producing malignant pheochromocytoma of adrenal:
      code 194.0, additional code 255.6
   basophil adenoma of pituitary with Cushing's syndrome:
      code 227.3, additional code 255.0

3. Morphology [Histology]
   For those wishing to identify the histological type of neoplasms, a comprehensive coded nomenclature, which comprises the morphology rubrics of the ICD-Oncology, is given after the E-code chapter.

4. Malignant neoplasms overlapping site boundaries
   Categories 140–195 are for the classification of primary malignant neoplasms according to their point of origin. A malignant neoplasm that overlaps two or more subcategories within a three-digit rubric and whose point of origin cannot be determined should be classified to the subcategory .8 "Other." For example, "carcinoma involving tip and ventral surface of tongue" should be assigned to 141.8. On the other hand, "carcinoma of tip of tongue, extending to involve the ventral surface" should be coded to 141.2, as the point of origin, the tip, is known. Three subcategories (149.8, 159.8, 165.8) have been provided for malignant neoplasms that overlap the boundaries of three-digit rubrics within certain systems. Overlapping malignant neoplasms that cannot be classified as indicated above should be assigned to the appropriate subdivision of category 195 (Malignant neoplasm of other and ill-defined sites).

MALIGNANT NEOPLASM OF LIP, ORAL CAVITY, AND PHARYNX (140–149)

> **Excludes**   carcinoma in situ (230.0)

● **140   Malignant neoplasm of lip**
Malignant neoplasm is a general term used to describe a cancerous growth or tumor.

> **Excludes**   skin of lip (173.0)

140.0   Upper lip, vermilion border
Upper lip:	Upper lip:
NOS	lipstick area
external	

140.1   Lower lip, vermilion border
Lower lip:	Lower lip:
NOS	lipstick area
external	

140.3   Upper lip, inner aspect
Upper lip:	Upper lip:
buccal aspect	mucosa
frenulum	oral aspect

140.4   Lower lip, inner aspect
Lower lip:	Lower lip:
buccal aspect	mucosa
frenulum	oral aspect

140.5   Lip, unspecified, inner aspect
Lip, not specified whether upper or lower:
buccal aspect
frenulum
mucosa
oral aspect

140.6   Commissure of lip
Labial commissure

140.8   Other sites of lip
Malignant neoplasm of contiguous or overlapping sites of lip whose point of origin cannot be determined

140.9   Lip, unspecified, vermilion border
Lip, not specified as upper or lower:
NOS
external
lipstick area

● **141   Malignant neoplasm of tongue**

141.0   Base of tongue
Dorsal surface of base of tongue
Fixed part of tongue NOS
Coding Clinic: 2006, Q4, P88-91

141.1   Dorsal surface of tongue
Anterior two-thirds of tongue, dorsal surface
Dorsal tongue NOS
Midline of tongue

> **Excludes**   dorsal surface of base of tongue (141.0)

141.2   Tip and lateral border of tongue

141.3   Ventral surface of tongue
Anterior two-thirds of tongue, ventral surface
Frenulum linguae

Figure 2–1 Anatomical structures of the mouth and lips. **A.** Transitional or vermilion borders. Lips are connected to the gums by frenulum. **B.** Dorsal surface. **C.** Ventral surface.

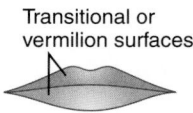
Transitional or vermilion surfaces

Lips are connected to
A   the gums by frenulum

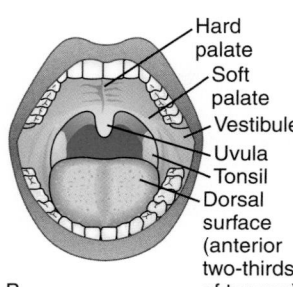
Hard palate
Soft palate
Vestibule
Uvula
Tonsil
Dorsal surface (anterior two-thirds of tongue)
B

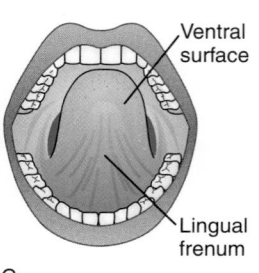
Ventral surface
Lingual frenum
C

◀ New   ◀▦ Revised   ~~deleted~~ Deleted   Excludes   Includes   Use additional   Code first   Omit code
● Unacceptable Principal Diagnosis   ● Use Additional Digit(s)   **OGCR** Official Guidelines   **Coding Clinic**

Figure 2–2 Major salivary glands.

Parotid gland
Sublingual gland
Submandibular gland

141.4 Anterior two-thirds of tongue, part unspecified
Mobile part of tongue NOS

141.5 Junctional zone
Border of tongue at junction of fixed and mobile parts at insertion of anterior tonsillar pillar

141.6 Lingual tonsil

141.8 Other sites of tongue
Malignant neoplasm of contiguous or overlapping sites of tongue whose point of origin cannot be determined

141.9 Tongue, unspecified
Tongue NOS

● **142 Malignant neoplasm of major salivary glands**

| Includes | salivary ducts |

| Excludes | malignant neoplasm of minor salivary glands: |
NOS (145.9)
buccal mucosa (145.0)
soft palate (145.3)
tongue (141.0–141.9)
tonsil, palatine (146.0)

142.0 Parotid gland

142.1 Submandibular gland
Submaxillary gland

142.2 Sublingual gland

142.8 Other major salivary glands
Malignant neoplasm of contiguous or overlapping sites of salivary glands and ducts whose point of origin cannot be determined

142.9 Salivary gland, unspecified
Salivary gland (major) NOS

● **143 Malignant neoplasm of gum**

| Includes | alveolar (ridge) mucosa |
gingiva (alveolar) (marginal)
interdental papillae

| Excludes | malignant odontogenic neoplasms (170.0–170.1) |

143.0 Upper gum

143.1 Lower gum

143.8 Other sites of gum
Malignant neoplasm of contiguous or overlapping sites of gum whose point of origin cannot be determined

143.9 Gum, unspecified

● **144 Malignant neoplasm of floor of mouth**

144.0 Anterior portion
Anterior to the premolar-canine junction

144.1 Lateral portion

144.8 Other sites of floor of mouth
Malignant neoplasm of contiguous or overlapping sites of floor of mouth whose point of origin cannot be determined

144.9 Floor of mouth, part unspecified

● **145 Malignant neoplasm of other and unspecified parts of mouth**

| Excludes | mucosa of lips (140.0–140.9) |

145.0 Cheek mucosa
Buccal mucosa
Cheek, inner aspect

145.1 Vestibule of mouth
Buccal sulcus (upper) (lower)
Labial sulcus (upper) (lower)

145.2 Hard palate

145.3 Soft palate

| Excludes | nasopharyngeal [posterior] [superior] surface of soft palate (147.3) |
Coding Clinic: 1993, 5th Issue, P16

145.4 Uvula

145.5 Palate, unspecified
Junction of hard and soft palate
Roof of mouth

145.6 Retromolar area

145.8 Other specified parts of mouth
Malignant neoplasm of contiguous or overlapping sites of mouth whose point of origin cannot be determined

145.9 Mouth, unspecified
Buccal cavity NOS
Minor salivary gland, unspecified site
Oral cavity NOS

● **146 Malignant neoplasm of oropharynx**

146.0 Tonsil
Tonsil: Tonsil:
NOS   palatine
faucial

| Excludes | lingual tonsil (141.6) |
pharyngeal tonsil (147.1)
Coding Clinic: 1987, Sept-Oct, P8

146.1 Tonsillar fossa

146.2 Tonsillar pillars (anterior) (posterior)
Faucial pillar
Glossopalatine fold
Palatoglossal arch
Palatopharyngeal arch

146.3 Vallecula
Anterior and medial surface of the pharyngoepiglottic fold

146.4 Anterior aspect of epiglottis
Epiglottis, free border [margin]
Glossoepiglottic fold(s)

| Excludes | epiglottis: |
NOS (161.1)
suprahyoid portion (161.1)

146.5 Junctional region
Junction of the free margin of the epiglottis, the aryepiglottic fold, and the pharyngoepiglottic fold

146.6 Lateral wall of oropharynx

146.7 Posterior wall of oropharynx

146.8 Other specified sites of oropharynx
Branchial cleft
Malignant neoplasm of contiguous or overlapping sites of oropharynx whose point of origin cannot be determined

146.9 Oropharynx, unspecified
Coding Clinic: 2002, Q2, P6

NEOPLASMS (140–239)

◀ New   ⇐ Revised   ~~deleted~~ Deleted   Excludes   Includes   Use additional   Code first   Omit code
● Unacceptable Principal Diagnosis   ● Use Additional Digit(s)   OGCR Official Guidelines   Coding Clinic

● **147 Malignant neoplasm of nasopharynx**

147.0 Superior wall
Roof of nasopharynx

147.1 Posterior wall
Adenoid   Pharyngeal tonsil

147.2 Lateral wall
Fossa of Rosenmüller   Pharyngeal recess
Opening of auditory tube

147.3 Anterior wall
Floor of nasopharynx
Nasopharyngeal [posterior] [superior] surface of
     soft palate
Posterior margin of nasal septum and choanae

147.8 Other specified sites of nasopharynx
Malignant neoplasm of contiguous or overlapping
     sites of nasopharynx whose point of origin
     cannot be determined

147.9 Nasopharynx, unspecified
Nasopharyngeal wall NOS

● **148 Malignant neoplasm of hypopharynx**

148.0 Postcricoid region
Behind the cricoid cartilage of neck

148.1 Pyriform sinus
Pyriform fossa

148.2 Aryepiglottic fold, hypopharyngeal aspect
Aryepiglottic fold or interarytenoid fold:
     NOS
     marginal zone

Excludes	*aryepiglottic fold or interarytenoid fold,*
	laryngeal aspect (161.1)

148.3 Posterior hypopharyngeal wall

148.8 Other specified sites of hypopharynx
Malignant neoplasm of contiguous or overlapping
     sites of hypopharynx whose point of origin
     cannot be determined

148.9 Hypopharynx, unspecified
Hypopharyngeal wall NOS
Hypopharynx NOS

● **149 Malignant neoplasm of other and ill-defined sites within the lip, oral cavity, and pharynx**

149.0 Pharynx, unspecified

149.1 Waldeyer's ring

149.8 Other
Malignant neoplasms of lip, oral cavity, and
     pharynx whose point of origin cannot be
     assigned to any one of the categories 140–148

Excludes	*"book leaf" neoplasm [ventral surface of*
	tongue and floor of mouth] (145.8)

149.9 Ill-defined

MALIGNANT NEOPLASM OF DIGESTIVE ORGANS AND PERITONEUM (150–159)

Excludes	*carcinoma in situ (230.1–230.9)*

● **150 Malignant neoplasm of esophagus**

150.0 Cervical esophagus

150.1 Thoracic esophagus

150.2 Abdominal esophagus

Excludes	*adenocarcinoma (151.0)*
	cardio-esophageal junction (151.0)

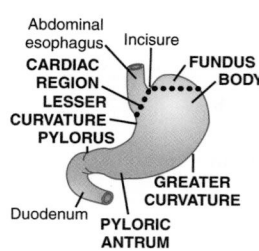

CERVICAL ESOPHAGUS
Left subclavian artery
First rib
Arch of aorta
Diaphragm
THORACIC ESOPHAGUS
ABDOMINAL ESOPHAGUS
Stomach

Figure 2–3 The esophagus is the muscular tube that connects the pharynx and the stomach. The 10 inch (25 cm) long esophagus is divided into three parts: **cervical, thoracic,** and **abdominal.**

150.3 Upper third of esophagus
Proximal third of esophagus

150.4 Middle third of esophagus

150.5 Lower third of esophagus
Distal third of esophagus

Excludes	*adenocarcinoma (151.0)*
	cardio-esophageal junction (151.0)

150.8 Other specified part
Malignant neoplasm of contiguous or overlapping
     sites of esophagus whose point of origin
     cannot be determined

150.9 Esophagus, unspecified

● **151 Malignant neoplasm of stomach**

Excludes	*benign carcinoid tumor of stomach (209.63)*
	malignant carcinoid tumor of stomach (209.23)

151.0 Cardia
Cardiac orifice
Cardio-esophageal junction

Excludes	*squamous cell carcinoma (150.2, 150.5)*

151.1 Pylorus
Prepylorus
Pyloric canal

151.2 Pyloric antrum
Antrum of stomach NOS

151.3 Fundus of stomach

151.4 Body of stomach

151.5 Lesser curvature, unspecified
Lesser curvature, not classifiable to 151.1–151.4

151.6 Greater curvature, unspecified
Greater curvature, not classifiable to 151.0–151.4

Abdominal esophagus   Incisure
CARDIAC REGION
LESSER CURVATURE
PYLORUS
FUNDUS
BODY
GREATER CURVATURE
Duodenum
PYLORIC ANTRUM

Figure 2–4 Parts of the stomach.

Item 2–2 The esophagus opens into the stomach through the **cardiac orifice,** also called the **cardioesophageal junction.** The **cardia** is adjacent to the cardiac orifice. The stomach widens into the **greater** and **lesser curvatures.** The **pyloric antrum** precedes the **pylorus,** which opens to the duodenum.

◀ New   ⬱ Revised   ~~deleted~~ Deleted   Excludes   Includes   Use additional   Code first   Omit code
● Unacceptable Principal Diagnosis   ● Use Additional Digit(s)   OGCR Official Guidelines   Coding Clinic

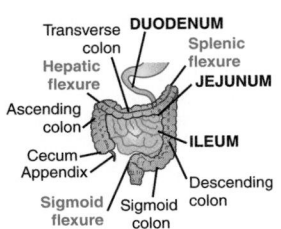

Transverse colon — **DUODENUM**
Hepatic flexure — Splenic flexure
Ascending colon — **JEJUNUM**
Cecum — **ILEUM**
Appendix — Descending colon
Sigmoid flexure — Sigmoid colon

Figure 2–5   Small intestine and colon.

151.8 Other specified sites of stomach
Anterior wall, not classifiable to 151.0–151.4
Posterior wall, not classifiable to 151.0–151.4
Malignant neoplasm of contiguous or overlapping sites of stomach whose point of origin cannot be determined

151.9 Stomach, unspecified
Carcinoma ventriculi
Gastric cancer
Coding Clinic: 2001, Q2, P17-18; 1988, Q2, P11

● **152 Malignant neoplasm of small intestine, including duodenum**
   Excludes *benign carcinoid tumor of small intestine and duodenum (209.40-209.43)*
malignant carcinoid tumor of small intestine and duodenum (209.00-209.03)

152.0 Duodenum

152.1 Jejunum

152.2 Ileum
   Excludes *ileocecal valve (153.4)*

152.3 Meckel's diverticulum

152.8 Other specified sites of small intestine
Duodenojejunal junction
Malignant neoplasm of contiguous or overlapping sites of small intestine whose point of origin cannot be determined

152.9 Small intestine, unspecified

● **153 Malignant neoplasm of colon**
   Excludes *benign carcinoid tumor of colon (209.50-209.56)*
malignant carcinoid tumor of colon (209.10-209.16)

153.0 Hepatic flexure
Flexure is a bending in a structure or organ. Note the three flexures illustrated in Figure 2–5. Hepatic = liver, sigmoid = colon, splenic = spleen.

153.1 Transverse colon

153.2 Descending colon
Left colon
Coding Clinic: 1995, Q1, P4

153.3 Sigmoid colon
Sigmoid (flexure)
   Excludes *rectosigmoid junction (154.0)*
Flexure is a bending in a structure or organ. Note the three flexures illustrated in Figure 2–5. Hepatic = liver, sigmoid = colon, splenic = spleen.

153.4 Cecum
Ileocecal valve

153.5 Appendix

153.6 Ascending colon
Right colon

153.7 Splenic flexure
Flexure is a bending in a structure or organ. Note the three flexures illustrated in Figure 2–5. Hepatic = liver, sigmoid = colon, splenic = spleen.

153.8 Other specified sites of large intestine
Malignant neoplasm of contiguous or overlapping sites of colon whose point of origin cannot be determined
   Excludes *ileocecal valve (153.4)*
rectosigmoid junction (154.0)

153.9 Colon, unspecified
Large intestine NOS

● **154 Malignant neoplasm of rectum, rectosigmoid junction, and anus**
   Excludes *benign carcinoid tumor of rectum (209.57)*
malignant carcinoid tumor of rectum (209.17)

154.0 Rectosigmoid junction
Colon with rectum
Rectosigmoid (colon)

154.1 Rectum
Rectal ampulla

154.2 Anal canal
Anal sphincter
   Excludes *skin of anus (172.5, 173.5)*
Coding Clinic: 2001, Q1, P8

154.3 Anus, unspecified
   Excludes *anus:*
margin (172.5, 173.5)
skin (172.5, 173.5)
perianal skin (172.5, 173.5)

154.8 Other
Anorectum
Cloacogenic zone
Malignant neoplasm of contiguous or overlapping sites of rectum, rectosigmoid junction, and anus whose point of origin cannot be determined

● **155 Malignant neoplasm of liver and intrahepatic bile ducts**

155.0 Liver, primary
Carcinoma:
liver, specified as primary
hepatocellular
liver cell
Hepatoblastoma
Coding Clinic: 2008, Q4, P82-83

155.1 Intrahepatic bile ducts
Canaliculi biliferi   Intrahepatic:
Interlobular: biliary passages
   bile ducts   canaliculi
   biliary canals   gall duct
   Excludes *hepatic duct (156.1)*

155.2 Liver, not specified as primary or secondary
Stated as a liver neoplasm, but not specific as to type

NEOPLASMS (140–239)

◀ New   ◀━ Revised   ~~deleted~~ Deleted   Excludes   Includes   Use additional   Code first   Omit code
● Unacceptable Principal Diagnosis   ● Use Additional Digit(s)   OGCR Official Guidelines   Coding Clinic
735

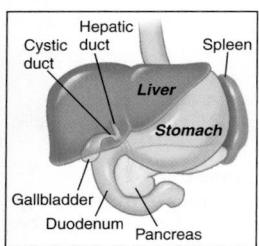

Figure 2–6 Diagram of liver, gallbladder, hepatic duct, pancreas, and spleen. (From Thibodeau and Patton: Anatomy and Physiology, 6th ed. 2007, Mosby.)

● 156 **Malignant neoplasm of gallbladder and extrahepatic bile ducts**
   Extrahepatic = outside the liver

   156.0 **Gallbladder**

   156.1 **Extrahepatic bile ducts**
   Biliary duct or passage   Cystic duct
   NOS   Hepatic duct
   Common bile duct   Sphincter of Oddi

   156.2 **Ampulla of Vater**

   156.8 **Other specified sites of gallbladder and extrahepatic bile ducts**
   Malignant neoplasm of contiguous or overlapping sites of gallbladder and extrahepatic bile ducts whose point of origin cannot be determined

   156.9 **Biliary tract, part unspecified**
   Malignant neoplasm involving both intrahepatic and extrahepatic bile ducts
   Intra = inside; extra = outside

● 157 **Malignant neoplasm of pancreas**
   Check documentation for specific site.

   157.0 **Head of pancreas**
   Coding Clinic: 2005, Q2, P9-10; 2000, Q4, P39-40

   157.1 **Body of pancreas**

   157.2 **Tail of pancreas**

   157.3 **Pancreatic duct**
   Duct of:
      Santorini
      Wirsung

   157.4 **Islets of Langerhans**
   Islets of Langerhans, any part of pancreas
   Use additional code to identify any functional activity
   Coding Clinic: 2007, Q4, P70-72

   157.8 **Other specified sites of pancreas**
   Ectopic pancreatic tissue
   Malignant neoplasm of contiguous or overlapping sites of pancreas whose point of origin cannot be determined

   157.9 **Pancreas, part unspecified**
   Coding Clinic: 1989, Q4, P11

● 158 **Malignant neoplasm of retroperitoneum and peritoneum**

   158.0 **Retroperitoneum**
   Periadrenal tissue   Perirenal tissue
   Perinephric tissue   Retrocecal tissue

   158.8 **Specified parts of peritoneum**
   Cul-de-sac (of Douglas)
   Mesentery
   Mesocolon
   Omentum
   Peritoneum:
     parietal
     pelvic
   Rectouterine pouch
   Malignant neoplasm of contiguous or overlapping sites of retroperitoneum and peritoneum whose point of origin cannot be determined

   158.9 **Peritoneum, unspecified**

● 159 **Malignant neoplasm of other and ill-defined sites within the digestive organs and peritoneum**

   159.0 **Intestinal tract, part unspecified**
   Intestine NOS

   159.1 **Spleen, not elsewhere classified**
   Angiosarcoma of spleen
   Fibrosarcoma of spleen

Excludes	*Hodgkin's disease (201.0–201.9)*
	lymphosarcoma (200.1)
	reticulosarcoma (200.0)

   159.8 **Other sites of digestive system and intra-abdominal organs**
   Malignant neoplasm of digestive organs and peritoneum whose point of origin cannot be assigned to any one of the categories 150–158

Excludes	*anus and rectum (154.8)*
	cardio-esophageal junction (151.0)
	colon and rectum (154.0)

   159.9 **Ill-defined**
   Alimentary canal or tract NOS
   Gastrointestinal tract NOS

Excludes	*abdominal NOS (195.2)*
	intra-abdominal NOS (195.2)

MALIGNANT NEOPLASM OF RESPIRATORY AND INTRATHORACIC ORGANS (160–165)

Excludes	*carcinoma in situ (231.0–231.9)*

● 160 **Malignant neoplasm of nasal cavities, middle ear, and accessory sinuses**

   160.0 **Nasal cavities**
   Cartilage of nose   Septum of nose
   Conchae, nasal   Vestibule of nose
   Internal nose

Excludes	*nasal bone (170.0)*
	nose NOS (195.0)
	olfactory bulb (192.0)
	posterior margin of septum and choanae (147.3)
	skin of nose (172.3, 173.3)
	turbinates (170.0)

   160.1 **Auditory tube, middle ear, and mastoid air cells**
   Antrum tympanicum
   Eustachian tube
   Tympanic cavity

Excludes	*auditory canal (external) (172.2, 173.2)*
	bone of ear (meatus) (170.0)
	cartilage of ear (171.0)
	ear (external) (skin) (172.2, 173.2)

Item 2–3 Islets of Langerhans (endocrine producing cells comprising 1% to 2% of the pancreatic mass) make and secrete hormones that regulate the body's production of insulin, glucagon, and stomach acid. Breakdown of the insulin-producing cells can cause diabetes mellitus. Islet cell tumors can be benign or malignant and include glucagonomas, insulinomas, gastrinomas, and neuroendocrine tumor. The neoplasm table must be consulted for the correct neoplasm code.

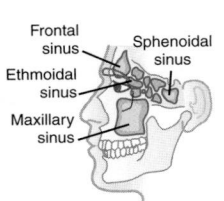

Figure 2-7　Paranasal sinuses. (From Buck CJ: Step-by-Step Medical Coding, 2006 ed. Philadelphia, WB Saunders, 2006.)

Frontal sinus
Sphenoidal sinus
Ethmoidal sinus
Maxillary sinus

160.2　Maxillary sinus
　　　　Antrum (Highmore) (maxillary)

160.3　Ethmoidal sinus

160.4　Frontal sinus

160.5　Sphenoidal sinus

160.8　Other
　　　　Malignant neoplasm of contiguous or overlapping sites of nasal cavities, middle ear, and accessory sinuses whose point of origin cannot be determined

160.9　Accessory sinus, unspecified

● **161　Malignant neoplasm of larynx**

161.0　Glottis
　　　　Intrinsic larynx
　　　　Laryngeal commissure (anterior) (posterior)
　　　　True vocal cord
　　　　　*True vocal cords (lower vocal folds) produce vocalization when air from lungs passes between them. Check your documentation. Code 161.1 is for malignant neoplasm of **false** vocal cords.*
　　　　Vocal cord NOS

161.1　Supraglottis
　　　　Aryepiglottic fold or interarytenoid fold, laryngeal aspect
　　　　Epiglottis (suprahyoid portion) NOS
　　　　Extrinsic larynx
　　　　False vocal cords
　　　　　False vocal cords (upper vocal folds) are not involved in vocalization. Check your documentation. Code 161.0 is for true vocal cords.
　　　　Posterior (laryngeal) surface of epiglottis
　　　　Ventricular bands
　　　　| Excludes | *anterior aspect of epiglottis (146.4)*
　　　　　　　　　aryepiglottic fold or interarytenoid fold:
　　　　　　　　　　NOS (148.2)
　　　　　　　　　　hypopharyngeal aspect (148.2)
　　　　　　　　　　marginal zone (148.2)

161.2　Subglottis

161.3　Laryngeal cartilages
　　　　Cartilage:　　　　　　Cartilage:
　　　　　arytenoid　　　　　　cuneiform
　　　　　cricoid　　　　　　　thyroid

161.8　Other specified sites of larynx
　　　　Malignant neoplasm of contiguous or overlapping sites of larynx whose point of origin cannot be determined
　　　　Coding Clinic: 2007, Q3, P8-9

161.9　Larynx, unspecified

● **162　Malignant neoplasm of trachea, bronchus, and lung**
　　　| Excludes | *benign carcinoid tumor of bronchus (209.61)*
　　　　　　　　malignant carcinoid tumor of bronchus (209.21)
　　　Coding Clinic: 2006, Q3, P7-8

162.0　Trachea
　　　　Cartilage of trachea
　　　　Mucosa of trachea

162.2　Main bronchus
　　　　Carina
　　　　Hilus of lung

162.3　Upper lobe, bronchus or lung
　　　Coding Clinic: 2004, Q1, P4-5

162.4　Middle lobe, bronchus or lung

162.5　Lower lobe, bronchus or lung

162.8　Other parts of bronchus or lung
　　　　Malignant neoplasm of contiguous or overlapping sites of bronchus or lung whose point of origin cannot be determined
　　　Coding Clinic: 2006, Q3, P7-8

162.9　Bronchus and lung, unspecified
　　　Coding Clinic: 2006, Q3, P14-15; 1997, Q2, P3; 1996, Q4, P47-48; 1993, Q4, P 36;1988, Q2, P10; 1984, May-June, P11, 14

● **163　Malignant neoplasm of pleura**
　　　Pleura are comprised of serous membrane that lines thoracic cavity (parietal) and covers lungs (visceral).

163.0　Parietal pleura

163.1　Visceral pleura

163.8　Other specified sites of pleura
　　　　Malignant neoplasm of contiguous or overlapping sites of pleura whose point of origin cannot be determined

163.9　Pleura, unspecified

● **164　Malignant neoplasm of thymus, heart, and mediastinum**
164.0　Thymus
　　　| Excludes | *benign carcinoid tumor of the thymus (209.62)*
　　　　　　　　malignant carcinoid tumor of the thymus (209.22)

164.1　Heart
　　　　Endocardium　　　　　Myocardium
　　　　Epicardium　　　　　　Pericardium
　　　| Excludes | *great vessels (171.4)*

164.2　Anterior mediastinum

164.3　Posterior mediastinum

164.8　Other
　　　　Malignant neoplasm of contiguous or overlapping sites of thymus, heart, and mediastinum whose point of origin cannot be determined

164.9　Mediastinum, part unspecified

● **165　Malignant neoplasm of other and ill-defined sites within the respiratory system and intrathoracic organs**

165.0　Upper respiratory tract, part unspecified

165.8　Other
　　　　Malignant neoplasm of respiratory and intrathoracic organs whose point of origin cannot be assigned to any one of the categories 160–164

165.9　Ill-defined sites within the respiratory system
　　　　Respiratory tract NOS
　　　| Excludes | *intrathoracic NOS (195.1)*
　　　　　　　　thoracic NOS (195.1)

NEOPLASMS (140–239)

◀ New　　◀▥▥ Revised　　~~deleted~~ Deleted　　| Excludes |　| Includes |　　Use additional　　Code first　　Omit code
● Unacceptable Principal Diagnosis　　● Use Additional Digit(s)　　OGCR Official Guidelines　　Coding Clinic

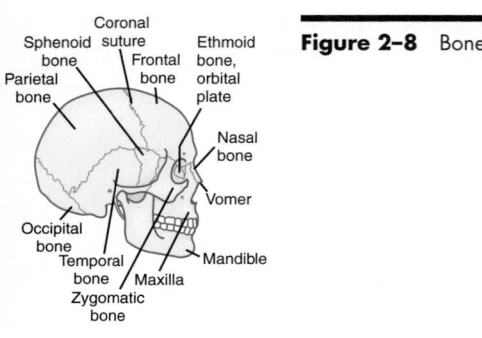

Figure 2-8 Bones of the skull.

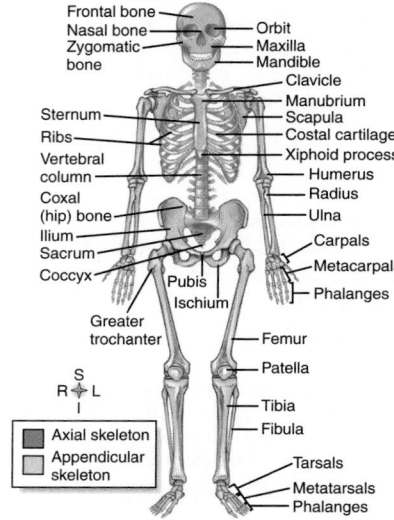

Figure 2-9 Diagram of skeleton of trunk and limbs with bones labeled. (From Thibodeau and Patton: Anatomy and Physiology, 6th ed. 2007, Mosby.)

MALIGNANT NEOPLASM OF BONE, CONNECTIVE TISSUE, SKIN, AND BREAST (170–176)

| Excludes | carcinoma in situ:
breast (233.0)
skin (232.0–232.9) |

● **170 Malignant neoplasm of bone and articular cartilage**

| Includes | cartilage (articular) (joint)
periosteum |

| Excludes | bone marrow NOS (202.9)
cartilage:
ear (171.0)
eyelid (171.0)
larynx (161.3)
nose (160.0)
synovia (171.0–171.9) |

170.0 Bones of skull and face, except mandible
Mandible = lower jaw

Bone:
ethmoid
frontal
malar
nasal
occipital
orbital
parietal

Bone:
sphenoid
temporal
zygomatic
Maxilla (superior)
Turbinate
Upper jaw bone
Vomer

| Excludes | carcinoma, any type except intraosseous or
odontogenic:
maxilla, maxillary (sinus) (160.2)
upper jaw bone (143.0)
jaw bone (lower) (170.1) |

170.1 Mandible
Inferior maxilla
Jaw bone NOS
Lower jaw bone

| Excludes | carcinoma, any type except intraosseous or
odontogenic:
jaw bone NOS (143.9)
lower (143.1)
upper jaw bone (170.0) |

170.2 Vertebral column, excluding sacrum and coccyx
Spinal column
Spine
Vertebra

| Excludes | sacrum and coccyx (170.6) |

170.3 Ribs, sternum, and clavicle
Costal cartilage
Costovertebral joint
Xiphoid process

170.4 Scapula and long bones of upper limb
Acromion
Bones NOS of upper limb
Humerus
Radius
Ulna
Coding Clinic: 1999, Q2, P9

170.5 Short bones of upper limb
Carpal
Cuneiform, wrist
Metacarpal
Navicular, of hand
Phalanges of hand
Pisiform
Scaphoid (of hand)
Semilunar or lunate
Trapezium
Trapezoid
Unciform

170.6 Pelvic bones, sacrum, and coccyx
Coccygeal vertebra
Ilium
Ischium
Pubic bone
Sacral vertebra

170.7 Long bones of lower limb
Bones NOS of lower limb
Femur
Fibula
Tibia

170.8 Short bones of lower limb
Astragalus [talus]
Calcaneus
Cuboid
Cuneiform, ankle
Metatarsal
Navicular (of ankle)
Patella
Phalanges of foot
Tarsal

170.9 Bone and articular cartilage, site unspecified

● **171 Malignant neoplasm of connective and other soft tissue**

|Includes| blood vessel
bursa
fascia
fat
ligament, except uterine
muscle
peripheral, sympathetic, and parasympathetic
  nerves and ganglia
synovia
tendon (sheath)

|Excludes| *cartilage (of):*
  articular (170.0–170.9)
  larynx (161.3)
  nose (160.0)
connective tissue:
  breast (174.0–175.9)
  internal organs—code to malignant neoplasm of
    the site [e.g., leiomyosarcoma of stomach,
    151.9]
    heart (164.1)
    uterine ligament (183.4)

171.0 Head, face, and neck
Cartilage of:
  ear
  eyelid
Coding Clinic: 1999, Q2, P6-7

171.2 Upper limb, including shoulder
Arm   Forearm
Finger   Hand

171.3 Lower limb, including hip
Foot
Leg
Popliteal space
  Popliteal space = popliteal cavity, popliteal fossa.
  Depression in posterior aspect of knee (behind
  knee).
Thigh
Toe

171.4 Thorax
Axilla
Diaphragm
Great vessels

|Excludes| *heart (164.1)*
mediastinum (164.2–164.9)
thymus (164.0)

171.5 Abdomen
Abdominal wall
Hypochondrium

|Excludes| *peritoneum (158.8)*
retroperitoneum (158.0)

171.6 Pelvis
Buttock   Inguinal region
Groin   Perineum

|Excludes| *pelvic peritoneum (158.8)*
retroperitoneum (158.0)
uterine ligament, any (183.3–183.5)

171.7 Trunk, unspecified
Back NOS
Flank NOS

171.8 Other specified sites of connective and other soft tissue
Malignant neoplasm of contiguous or overlapping
  sites of connective tissue whose point of
  origin cannot be determined

171.9 Connective and other soft tissue, site unspecified

● **172 Malignant melanoma of skin**

|Includes| melanocarcinoma
melanoma in situ of skin
melanoma (skin) NOS

|Excludes| *skin of genital organs (184.0–184.9, 187.1–187.9)*
sites other than skin - code to malignant neoplasm
  of the site

172.0 Lip

|Excludes| *vermilion border of lip (140.0–140.1, 140.9)*

172.1 Eyelid, including canthus

172.2 Ear and external auditory canal
Auricle (ear)
Auricular canal, external
External [acoustic] meatus
Pinna

172.3 Other and unspecified parts of face
Cheek (external)   Forehead
Chin   Nose, external
Eyebrow   Temple

172.4 Scalp and neck

172.5 Trunk, except scrotum
Axilla   Perianal skin
Breast   Perineum
Buttock   Umbilicus
Groin

|Excludes| *anal canal (154.2)*
anus NOS (154.3)
scrotum (187.7)

172.6 Upper limb, including shoulder
Arm   Forearm
Finger   Hand

172.7 Lower limb, including hip
Ankle   Leg
Foot   Popliteal area
Heel   Thigh
Knee   Toe

172.8 Other specified sites of skin
Malignant melanoma of contiguous or overlapping
  sites of skin whose point of origin cannot be
  determined

172.9 Melanoma of skin, site unspecified

● **173 Other malignant neoplasm of skin**

|Includes| malignant neoplasm of:
  sebaceous glands
  sudoriferous, sudoriparous glands
  sweat glands

|Excludes| *Kaposi's sarcoma (176.0–176.9)*
malignant melanoma of skin (172.0–172.9)
skin of genital organs (184.0–184.9, 187.1–187.9)
Coding Clinic: 2000, Q1, P8; 1996, Q2, P12

173.0 Skin of lip

|Excludes| *vermilion border of lip (140.0–140.1, 140.9)*

173.1 Eyelid, including canthus

|Excludes| *cartilage of eyelid (171.0)*

173.2 Skin of ear and external auditory canal
Auricle (ear)
Auricular canal, external
External meatus
Pinna

|Excludes| *cartilage of ear (171.0)*

NEOPLASMS (140–239)

Item 2–4 Malignant melanoma is a serious form of skin cancer that affects the melanocytes (pigment-forming cells) and is caused by ultraviolet (UV) rays from the sun that damage skin. It is most commonly seen in the 40- to 60-year-olds with fair skin, blue or green eyes, and red or blond hair who sunburn easily. Melanoma can spread very rapidly and is the most deadly form of skin cancer. It is less common than other types of skin cancer. The rate of melanoma is increasing and currently is the leading cause of death from skin disease.

Figure 2–10 Malignant melanoma of skin. (From Goldman: Cecil Textbook of Medicine, 22nd ed. 2004, Saunders.)

173.3 Skin of other and unspecified parts of face

Cheek, external	Forehead
Chin	Nose, external
Eyebrow	Temple

Coding Clinic: 2000, Q1, P3

173.4 Scalp and skin of neck

173.5 Skin of trunk, except scrotum
Axillary fold
Perianal skin
Skin of:
    abdominal wall
    anus
    back
    breast
    buttock
    chest wall
    groin
    perineum
Umbilicus

Excludes anal canal (154.2)
          anus NOS (154.3)
          skin of scrotum (187.7)
Coding Clinic: 2001, Q1, P8

173.6 Skin of upper limb, including shoulder

Arm	Forearm
Finger	Hand

173.7 Skin of lower limb, including hip

Ankle	Leg
Foot	Popliteal area
Heel	Thigh
Knee	Toe

173.8 Other specified sites of skin
Malignant neoplasm of contiguous or overlapping sites of skin whose point of origin cannot be determined

173.9 Skin, site unspecified

● **174 Malignant neoplasm of female breast**
This code is for female breast; see 175 for male breast.

Includes breast (female)
              connective tissue
              soft parts
          Paget's disease of:
              breast
              nipple

Use additional code to identify estrogen receptor status (V86.0, V86.1)

Excludes skin of breast (172.5, 173.5)

174.0 Nipple and areola

174.1 Central portion

174.2 Upper-inner quadrant
Coding Clinic: 1989, Q4, P11

Figure 2–11 Female breast quadrants and axillary tail.

174.3 Lower-inner quadrant
Coding Clinic: 1989, Q4, P11

174.4 Upper-outer quadrant
Coding Clinic: 2008, Q4, P152-155; 2004, Q1, P3-4; 1997, Q3, P8; 1984, May-June, P11

174.5 Lower-outer quadrant

174.6 Axillary tail

174.8 Other specified sites of female breast
Ectopic sites
Inner breast
Lower breast
Malignant neoplasm of contiguous or overlapping sites of breast whose point of origin cannot be determined
Midline of breast
Outer breast
Upper breast
Coding Clinic: 1985, July-Aug, P11

174.9 Breast (female), unspecified
Coding Clinic: 2009, Q3, P4; 2005, Q3, P11-12; 1994, Q2, P10x2

● **175 Malignant neoplasm of male breast**

Use additional code to identify estrogen receptor status (V86.0, V86.1)

Excludes skin of breast (172.5, 173.5)

175.0 Nipple and areola

175.9 Other and unspecified sites of male breast
Ectopic breast tissue, male

● **176 Kaposi's sarcoma**

176.0 Skin
Coding Clinic: 2007, Q4, P61-64

176.1 Soft tissue

Blood vessel	Ligament
Connective tissue	Lymphatic(s) NEC
Fascia	Muscle

Excludes lymph glands and nodes (176.5)

176.2 Palate

176.3 Gastrointestinal sites

176.4 Lung

176.5 Lymph nodes

176.8 Other specified sites
Oral cavity NEC

176.9 Unspecified
Viscera NOS

Item 2–5 Kaposi's sarcoma is a cancer that causes patches of abnormal tissue to grow under the skin; in the lining of the mouth, nose, and throat; or in other organs, often beginning and spreading to other organs. Patients who have had organ transplants or patients with AIDS are at high risk for this malignancy.

NEOPLASMS (140–239)

◀ New   ◀||| Revised   ~~deleted~~ Deleted   Excludes   Includes   Use additional   Code first   Omit code
● Unacceptable Principal Diagnosis   ● Use Additional Digit(s)   OGCR Official Guidelines   Coding Clinic

Figure 2-12   Cervix uteri.

MALIGNANT NEOPLASM OF GENITOURINARY ORGANS (179–189)

| Excludes | *carcinoma in situ (233.1–233.9)*

179   Malignant neoplasm of uterus, part unspecified

● **180   Malignant neoplasm of cervix uteri**

| Includes | invasive malignancy [carcinoma]

| Excludes | *carcinoma in situ (233.1)*

180.0   Endocervix
Inside the cervix
Cervical canal NOS
Endocervical canal
Endocervical gland

180.1   Exocervix
Outside the cervix

180.8   Other specified sites of cervix
Cervical stump
Squamocolumnar junction of cervix
Malignant neoplasm of contiguous or overlapping sites of cervix uteri whose point of origin cannot be determined

180.9   Cervix uteri, unspecified

181   Malignant neoplasm of placenta
Choriocarcinoma NOS
Chorioepithelioma NOS

| Excludes | *chorioadenoma (destruens) (236.1)*
hydatidiform mole (630)
  malignant (236.1)
invasive mole (236.1)
male choriocarcinoma NOS (186.0–186.9)

● **182   Malignant neoplasm of body of uterus**

| Excludes | *carcinoma in situ (233.2)*

182.0   Corpus uteri, except isthmus
Cornu   Fundus
Endometrium   Myometrium
Coding Clinic: 2009, Q3, P4

182.1   Isthmus
Lower uterine segment

182.8   Other specified sites of body of uterus
Malignant neoplasm of contiguous or overlapping sites of body of uterus whose point of origin cannot be determined

| Excludes | *uterus NOS (179)*

● **183   Malignant neoplasm of ovary and other uterine adnexa**

| Excludes | *Douglas' cul-de-sac (158.8)*

183.0   Ovary
Use additional code to identify any functional activity
Coding Clinic: 2007, Q4, P95-96

183.2   Fallopian tube
Oviduct
Uterine tube

183.3   Broad ligament
Mesovarium
Parovarian region

183.4   Parametrium
Uterine ligament NOS
Uterosacral ligament

183.5   Round ligament

183.8   Other specified sites of uterine adnexa
Tubo-ovarian
Utero-ovarian
Malignant neoplasm of contiguous or overlapping sites of ovary and other uterine adnexa whose point of origin cannot be determined

183.9   Uterine adnexa, unspecified

● **184   Malignant neoplasm of other and unspecified female genital organs**

| Excludes | *carcinoma in situ (233.30–233.39)*

184.0   Vagina
Gartner's duct   Vaginal vault

184.1   Labia majora
Greater vestibular [Bartholin's] gland

184.2   Labia minora

184.3   Clitoris

184.4   Vulva, unspecified
External female genitalia NOS
Pudendum

184.8   Other specified sites of female genital organs
Malignant neoplasm of contiguous or overlapping sites of female genital organs whose point of origin cannot be determined

184.9   Female genital organ, site unspecified
Female genitourinary tract NOS

185   Malignant neoplasm of prostate

| Excludes | *seminal vesicles (187.8)*
Coding Clinic: 2003, Q3, P13; 1999, Q3, P5; 1994, Q1, P20; 1992, Q3, P7

● **186   Malignant neoplasm of testis**
Use additional code to identify any functional activity

186.0   Undescended testis
Ectopic testis   Retained testis

186.9   Other and unspecified testis
Testis: Testis:
  NOS   scrotal
  descended

● **187   Malignant neoplasm of penis and other male genital organs**

187.1   Prepuce
Foreskin

187.2   Glans penis

187.3   Body of penis
Corpus cavernosum

187.4   Penis, part unspecified
Skin of penis NOS

187.5   Epididymis

Figure 2-13   Penis and other male genital organs.

NEOPLASMS (140–239)

NEOPLASMS (140–239)

187.6 Spermatic cord
Vas deferens

187.7 Scrotum
Skin of scrotum

187.8 Other specified sites of male genital organs
Seminal vesicle
Tunica vaginalis
Malignant neoplasm of contiguous or overlapping sites of penis and other male genital organs whose point of origin cannot be determined

187.9 Male genital organ, site unspecified
Male genital organ or tract NOS

●**188 Malignant neoplasm of bladder**
| Excludes | carcinoma in situ (233.7)

188.0 Trigone of urinary bladder

188.1 Dome of urinary bladder

188.2 Lateral wall of urinary bladder

188.3 Anterior wall of urinary bladder

188.4 Posterior wall of urinary bladder

188.5 Bladder neck
Internal urethral orifice

188.6 Ureteric orifice

188.7 Urachus

188.8 Other specified sites of bladder
Malignant neoplasm of contiguous or overlapping sites of bladder whose point of origin cannot be determined

188.9 Bladder, part unspecified
Bladder wall NOS
Coding Clinic: 2000, Q1, P5

●**189 Malignant neoplasm of kidney and other and unspecified urinary organs**
| Excludes | benign carcinoid tumor of kidney (209.64)
malignant carcinoid tumor of kidney (209.24)◄▥

189.0 Kidney, except pelvis
Kidney NOS   Kidney parenchyma
Coding Clinic: 2005, Q2, P4-5; 2004, Q2, P4

189.1 Renal pelvis
Renal calyces   Ureteropelvic junction

189.2 Ureter
| Excludes | ureteric orifice of bladder (188.6)

189.3 Urethra
| Excludes | urethral orifice of bladder (188.5)

189.4 Paraurethral glands

189.8 Other specified sites of urinary organs
Malignant neoplasm of contiguous or overlapping sites of kidney and other urinary organs whose point of origin cannot be determined

189.9 Urinary organ, site unspecified
Urinary system NOS
| Excludes | carcinoma in situ (234.0–234.9)

MALIGNANT NEOPLASM OF OTHER AND UNSPECIFIED SITES (190–199)
| Excludes | carcinoma in situ (234.0-234.9)

●**190 Malignant neoplasm of eye**
| Excludes | carcinoma in situ (234.0)
dark area on retina and choroid (239.81)
eyelid (skin) (172.1, 173.1)
cartilage (171.0)
optic nerve (192.0)
orbital bone (170.0)
retinal freckle (239.81)

190.0 Eyeball, except conjunctiva, cornea, retina, and choroid
Note the use of "except" in this code.
Ciliary body   Sclera
Crystalline lens   Uveal tract
Iris

190.1 Orbit
Connective tissue of orbit
Extraocular muscle
Retrobulbar
| Excludes | bone of orbit (170.0)

190.2 Lacrimal gland

190.3 Conjunctiva

190.4 Cornea

190.5 Retina

190.6 Choroid

190.7 Lacrimal duct
Lacrimal sac   Nasolacrimal duct

190.8 Other specified sites of eye
Malignant neoplasm of contiguous or overlapping sites of eye whose point of origin cannot be determined

190.9 Eye, part unspecified

●**191 Malignant neoplasm of brain**
| Excludes | cranial nerves (192.0)
retrobulbar area (190.1)

191.0 Cerebrum, except lobes and ventricles
Basal ganglia   Globus pallidus
Cerebral cortex   Hypothalamus
Corpus striatum   Thalamus

191.1 Frontal lobe
Coding Clinic: 2005, Q4, P117-119; 1993, Q4, P33

191.2 Temporal lobe
Hippocampus   Uncus
Coding Clinic: 2009, Q3, P4; 2006, Q4, P122-123

191.3 Parietal lobe

191.4 Occipital lobe

191.5 Ventricles
Choroid plexus
Floor of ventricle

191.6 Cerebellum NOS
Cerebellopontine angle

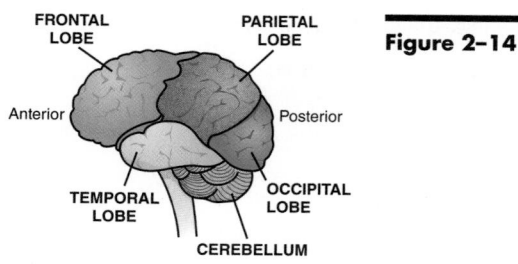

Figure 2-14 The brain.

◄ New   ◀▥ Revised   ~~deleted~~ Deleted | Excludes | Includes   Use additional   Code first   Omit code
● Unacceptable Principal Diagnosis   ● Use Additional Digit(s)   OGCR Official Guidelines   Coding Clinic

191.7 **Brain stem**
  Cerebral peduncle   Midbrain
  Medulla oblongata   Pons

191.8 **Other parts of brain**
  Corpus callosum
  Tapetum
  Malignant neoplasm of contiguous or overlapping sites of brain whose point of origin cannot be determined
  Coding Clinic: 2007, Q4, P103-104

191.9 **Brain, unspecified**
  Cranial fossa NOS
  Coding Clinic: 2009, Q4, P78; 1994, Q2, P8

● 192 **Malignant neoplasm of other and unspecified parts of nervous system**
  Excludes *peripheral, sympathetic, and parasympathetic nerves and ganglia (171.0–171.9)*

192.0 **Cranial nerves**
  Olfactory bulb

192.1 **Cerebral meninges**
  Dura (mater)
  Falx (cerebelli) (cerebri)
  Meninges NOS
  Tentorium

192.2 **Spinal cord**
  Cauda equina

192.3 **Spinal meninges**

192.8 **Other specified sites of nervous system**
  Malignant neoplasm of contiguous or overlapping sites of other parts of nervous system whose point of origin cannot be determined

192.9 **Nervous system, part unspecified**
  Nervous system (central) NOS
  Excludes *meninges NOS (192.1)*

193 **Malignant neoplasm of thyroid gland**
  Thyroglossal duct
  Use additional code to identify any functional activity

● 194 **Malignant neoplasm of other endocrine glands and related structures**
  Excludes *islets of Langerhans (157.4)*
  neuroendocrine tumors (209.00–209.69)
  ovary (183.0)
  testis (186.0–186.9)
  thymus (164.0)

194.0 **Adrenal gland**
  Adrenal cortex   Suprarenal gland
  Adrenal medulla

194.1 **Parathyroid gland**

194.3 **Pituitary gland and craniopharyngeal duct**
  Craniobuccal pouch   Rathke's pouch
  Hypophysis   Sella turcica
  Coding Clinic: 1985, July-Aug, P9

194.4 **Pineal gland**

194.5 **Carotid body**

194.6 **Aortic body and other paraganglia**
  Coccygeal body   Para-aortic body
  Glomus jugulare

194.8 **Other**
  Pluriglandular involvement NOS
  Note: If the sites of multiple involvements are known, they should be coded separately.

194.9 **Endocrine gland, site unspecified**

● 195 **Malignant neoplasm of other and ill-defined sites**
  Includes malignant neoplasms of contiguous sites, not elsewhere classified, whose point of origin cannot be determined
  Excludes *malignant neoplasm:*
  lymphatic and hematopoietic tissue (200.0–208.9)
  secondary sites (196.0–198.8)
  unspecified site (199.0–199.1)

195.0 **Head, face, and neck**
  Cheek NOS
  Jaw NOS
  Nose NOS
  Supraclavicular region NOS
  Coding Clinic: 2003, Q4, P107

195.1 **Thorax**
  Axilla   Intrathoracic NOS
  Chest (wall) NOS

195.2 **Abdomen**
  Intra-abdominal NOS
  Coding Clinic: 1997, Q2, P3

195.3 **Pelvis**
  Groin
  Inguinal region NOS
  Presacral region
  Sacrococcygeal region
  Sites overlapping systems within pelvis, as:
    rectovaginal (septum)
    rectovesical (septum)

195.4 **Upper limb**

195.5 **Lower limb**

195.8 **Other specified sites**
  Back NOS   Trunk NOS
  Flank NOS

(See Plate 315 on page NAP-1.)

● 196 **Secondary and unspecified malignant neoplasm of lymph nodes**
  Excludes *any malignant neoplasm of lymph nodes, specified as primary (200.0–202.9)*
  Hodgkin's disease (201.0–201.9)
  lymphosarcoma (200.1)
  other forms of lymphoma (202.0–202.9)
  reticulosarcoma (200.0)
  secondary neuroendocrine tumor of (distant) lymph nodes (209.71)
  Coding Clinic: 1992, Q2, P3-4

196.0 **Lymph nodes of head, face, and neck**
  Cervical   Scalene
  Cervicofacial   Supraclavicular
  Coding Clinic: 2007, Q3, P8-9

196.1 **Intrathoracic lymph nodes**
  Bronchopulmonary   Mediastinal
  Intercostal   Tracheobronchial
  Coding Clinic: 2006, Q3, P7-8

196.2 **Intra-abdominal lymph nodes**
  Intestinal   Retroperitoneal
  Mesenteric
  Coding Clinic: 2003, Q4, P111

196.3 **Lymph nodes of axilla and upper limb**
  Brachial   Infraclavicular
  Epitrochlear   Pectoral

196.5 **Lymph nodes of inguinal region and lower limb**
  Femoral   Popliteal
  Groin   Tibial

NEOPLASMS (140–239)

◀ New   ◀▥ Revised   ~~deleted~~ Deleted   Excludes   Includes   Use additional   Code first   Omit code
● Unacceptable Principal Diagnosis   ● Use Additional Digit(s)   OGCR Official Guidelines   Coding Clinic

743

NEOPLASMS (140–239)

196.6 **Intrapelvic lymph nodes**
    Hypogastric   Obturator
    Iliac   Parametrial

196.8 **Lymph nodes of multiple sites**

196.9 **Site unspecified**
    Lymph nodes NOS

● 197 **Secondary malignant neoplasm of respiratory and digestive systems**

   Excludes *lymph node metastasis (196.0–196.9)*
   secondary neuroendocrine tumor of liver (209.72)
   secondary neuroendocrine tumor of respiratory organs (209.79)

197.0 **Lung**
    Bronchus
    Coding Clinic: 2006, Q1, P4-5; 1999, Q2, P9

197.1 **Mediastinum**
    Coding Clinic: 2006, Q3, P7-8

197.2 **Pleura**
    Coding Clinic: 2008, Q1, P16-17; 2007, Q3, P3; 2003, Q4, P110; 1989, Q4, P11

197.3 **Other respiratory organs**
    Trachea

197.4 **Small intestine, including duodenum**

197.5 **Large intestine and rectum**

197.6 **Retroperitoneum and peritoneum**
    Coding Clinic: 2004, Q2, P4; 1989, Q4, P11

197.7 **Liver, specified as secondary**
    Coding Clinic: 2006, Q1, P4-5; 2005, Q2, P9-10; 1984, May-June, P11

197.8 **Other digestive organs and spleen**
    Coding Clinic: 1997, Q2, P3

● 198 **Secondary malignant neoplasm of other specified sites**

   Excludes *lymph node metastasis (196.0–196.9)*
   secondary neuroendocrine tumor of other specified sites (209.79)

198.0 **Kidney**

198.1 **Other urinary organs**

198.2 **Skin**
    Skin of breast

198.3 **Brain and spinal cord**
    Coding Clinic: 2007, Q3, P4; 1999, Q3, P7-8; 1984, May-June, P14

198.4 **Other parts of nervous system**
    Meninges (cerebral) (spinal)

198.5 **Bone and bone marrow**
    Coding Clinic: 2007, Q1, P3-8; 2003, Q4, P110; 1999, Q3, P5; 1989, Q4, P12; 1984, May-June, P14

198.6 **Ovary**

198.7 **Adrenal gland**
    Suprarenal gland
    Coding Clinic: 1988, Q2, P10

● 198.8 **Other specified sites**

   198.81 **Breast**
       Excludes *skin of breast (198.2)*

   198.82 **Genital organs**

   198.89 **Other**
       Excludes *retroperitoneal lymph nodes (196.2)*
       Coding Clinic: 2005, Q2, P4-5; 1997, Q2, P4

● 199 **Malignant neoplasm without specification of site**

   Excludes *malignant carcinoid tumor of unknown primary site (209.20)*
   malignant (poorly differentiated) neuroendocrine carcinoma, any site (209.30)
   malignant (poorly differentiated) neuroendocrine tumor, any site (209.30)
   neuroendocrine carcinoma (high grade), any site (209.30)

199.0 **Disseminated**
    Carcinomatosis unspecified site (primary) (secondary)
    Generalized:
        cancer unspecified site (primary) (secondary)
        malignancy unspecified site (primary) (secondary)
    Multiple cancer unspecified site (primary) (secondary)
    Coding Clinic: 1989, Q4, P10; 1988, Q2, P11

199.1 **Other**
    Cancer unspecified site (primary) (secondary)
    Carcinoma unspecified site (primary) (secondary)
    Malignancy unspecified site (primary) (secondary)
    Coding Clinic: 2006, Q3, P14-15; Q1, P4-5

● 199.2 **Malignant neoplasm associated with transplanted organ**

   Code first *complication of transplanted organ (996.80-996.89)*

   Use additional code for specific malignancy
   Coding Clinic: 2008, Q4, P82-83

MALIGNANT NEOPLASM OF LYMPHATIC AND HEMATOPOIETIC TISSUE (200–208)

   Excludes *autoimmune lymphoproliferative syndrome (279.41)*
   secondary neoplasm of:
       bone marrow (198.5)
       spleen (197.8)
   secondary and unspecified neoplasm of lymph nodes (196.0–196.9)

The following fifth-digit subclassification is for use with categories 200–202:

   0 unspecified site, extranodal and solid organ sites
   1 lymph nodes of head, face, and neck
   2 intrathoracic lymph nodes
   3 intra-abdominal lymph nodes
   4 lymph nodes of axilla and upper limb
   5 lymph nodes of inguinal region and lower limb
   6 intrapelvic lymph nodes
   7 spleen
   8 lymph nodes of multiple sites

● 200 **Lymphosarcoma and reticulosarcoma and other specified malignant tumors of lymphatic tissue**

   Requires fifth digit. See note before section 200 for codes and definitions.
   Coding Clinic: 2007, Q4, P65-67

● 200.0 **Reticulosarcoma**
[0-8]   Lymphoma (malignant):
            histiocytic (diffuse):
                nodular
                pleomorphic cell type
            reticulum cell type
        Reticulum cell sarcoma:
            NOS
            pleomorphic cell type
        Coding Clinic: 2006, Q4, P135-136; 2001, Q3, P12-13

Item 2-6 Lymphosarcoma, also known as malignant lymphoma, is a cancer of the lymph system exhibiting abnormal cells encompassing an entire lymph node creating a diffuse pattern without any definite organization. Diffuse pattern lymphoma has a more unfavorable survival outlook than those with a follicular or nodular pattern. Reticulosarcoma is the most common aggressive form of non-Hodgkin's lymphoma.

● **200.1 Lymphosarcoma**
  [0-8]   Lymphoblastoma (diffuse)
          Lymphoma (malignant):
              lymphoblastic (diffuse)
              lymphocytic (cell type) (diffuse)
              lymphosarcoma type
          Lymphosarcoma:
              NOS
              diffuse NOS
              lymphoblastic (diffuse)
              lymphocytic (diffuse)
              prolymphocytic

     Excludes   lymphosarcoma:
                   follicular or nodular (202.0)
                   mixed cell type (200.8)
                   lymphosarcoma cell leukemia (207.8)

● **200.2 Burkitt's tumor or lymphoma**
  [0-8]   Malignant lymphoma, Burkitt's type

● **200.3 Marginal zone lymphoma**
  [0-8]   Extranodal marginal zone B-cell lymphoma
          Mucosa associated lymphoid tissue [MALT]
          Nodal marginal zone B-cell lymphoma
          Splenic marginal zone B-cell lymphoma

● **200.4 Mantle cell lymphoma**
  [0-8]

● **200.5 Primary central nervous system lymphoma**
  [0-8]

● **200.6 Anaplastic large cell lymphoma**
  [0-8]

● **200.7 Large cell lymphoma**
  [0-8]

● **200.8 Other named variants**
  [0-8]   Lymphoma (malignant):
              lymphoplasmacytoid type
              mixed lymphocytic-histiocytic (diffuse)
          Lymphosarcoma, mixed cell type (diffuse)
          Reticulolymphosarcoma (diffuse)

● **201 Hodgkin's disease**
          Also known as malignant lymphoma/lymphosarcoma and is
          cancer of the lymphatic system including the lymph
          nodes and related structures

          Requires fifth digit. See note before section 200 for codes
             and definitions.

● **201.0 Hodgkin's paragranuloma**
  [0-8]

● **201.1 Hodgkin's granuloma**
  [0-8]

● **201.2 Hodgkin's sarcoma**
  [0-8]

● **201.4 Lymphocytic-histiocytic predominance**
  [0-8]

● **201.5 Nodular sclerosis**
  [0-8]   Hodgkin's disease, nodular sclerosis:
              NOS
              cellular phase

● **201.6 Mixed cellularity**
  [0-8]

● **201.7 Lymphocytic depletion**
  [0-8]   Hodgkin's disease, lymphocytic depletion:
              NOS
              diffuse fibrosis
              reticular type

● **201.9 Hodgkin's disease, unspecified**
  [0-8]   Hodgkin's:
              disease NOS
              lymphoma NOS
          Malignant:
              lymphogranuloma
              lymphogranulomatosis

● **202 Other malignant neoplasms of lymphoid and histiocytic tissue**
          Requires fifth digit. See note before section 200 for codes
             and definitions.

● **202.0 Nodular lymphoma**
  [0-8]   Brill-Symmers disease
          Lymphoma:
              follicular (giant) (large cell)
              lymphocytic, nodular
          Lymphosarcoma:
              follicular (giant)
              nodular
          Coding Clinic: 2009, Q3, P5x2

● **202.1 Mycosis fungoides**
  [0-8]   Excludes   *peripheral T-cell lymphoma (202.7)*
          Coding Clinic: 1999, Q2, P7-8; 1992, Q2, P4

● **202.2 Sézary's disease**
  [0-8]   **Coding Clinic: 1999, Q2, P7-8**

● **202.3 Malignant histiocytosis**
  [0-8]   Histiocytic medullary reticulosis
          Malignant:
              reticuloendotheliosis
              reticulosis

● **202.4 Leukemic reticuloendotheliosis**
  [0-8]   Hairy-cell leukemia

● **202.5 Letterer-Siwe disease**
  [0-8]   Acute:
              differentiated progressive histiocytosis
              histiocytosis X (progressive)
              infantile reticuloendotheliosis
              reticulosis of infancy

     Excludes   *Hand-Schüller-Christian disease (277.89)*
                histiocytosis (acute) (chronic) (277.89)
                histiocytosis X (chronic) (277.89)

● **202.6 Malignant mast cell tumors**
  [0-8]   Malignant:
              mastocytoma
              mastocytosis
          Mast cell sarcoma
          Systemic tissue mast cell disease

     Excludes   *mast cell leukemia (207.8)*

● **202.7 Peripheral T cell lymphoma**
  [0-8]

● **202.8 Other lymphomas**
  [0-8]   Lymphoma (malignant):
              NOS
              diffuse

     Excludes   *benign lymphoma (229.0)*

          Coding Clinic: 2008, Q4, P82-83; Q1, P16-17; 2007, Q3, P3; 2006,
            Q4, P135-136; Q2, P20-22; 1993, Q4, P33; 1992, Q2, P3-4

● **202.9 Other and unspecified malignant neoplasms of**
  [0-8] **lymphoid and histiocytic tissue**
              Follicular dendritic cell sarcoma
              Interdigitating dendritic cell sarcoma
              Langerhans cell sarcoma
              Malignant neoplasm of bone marrow NOS

NEOPLASMS (140-239)

● **203 Multiple myeloma and immunoproliferative neoplasms**
  *Multiple myeloma is cancer of plasma cell (type of white
  blood cell) and is incurable but treatable disease.
  Immunoproliferative neoplasm is term for diseases (mostly
  cancers) in which immune system cells proliferate.*

The following fifth-digit subclassification is for use with
category 203:

> **0 without mention of having achieved remission**
>   **failed remission**
> **1 in remission**
> **2 in relapse**

  Coding Clinic: 2008, Q4, P83-85

● **203.0 Multiple myeloma**
  [0-2]   Kahler's disease   Myelomatosis
          | **Excludes** | solitary myeloma (238.6)
          Coding Clinic: 2008, Q4, P90-91; 2007, Q2, P9-10; 1999, Q4, P10;
          1996, Q1, P16

● **203.1 Plasma cell leukemia**
  [0-2]   Plasmacytic leukemia

● **203.8 Other immunoproliferative neoplasms**
  [0-2]   Coding Clinic: 1990, Q4, P26

● **204 Lymphoid leukemia**
  | **Includes** | leukemia: leukemia:
               lymphatic   lymphocytic
               lymphoblastic   lymphogenous

The following fifth-digit subclassification is for use with
category 204:

> **0 without mention of having achieved remission**
>   **failed remission**
> **1 in remission**
> **2 in relapse**

  Coding Clinic: 2008, Q4, P83-85

● **204.0 Acute**
  [0-2] | **Excludes** | acute exacerbation of chronic lymphoid
                          leukemia (204.1)
          Coding Clinic: 1999, Q3, P4, 6-7; 1993, Q3, P4x2; 1985, May-June,
          P18-19

● **204.1 Chronic**
  [0-2]

● **204.2 Subacute**
  [0-2]

● **204.8 Other lymphoid leukemia**
  [0-2]   Aleukemic leukemia:
              lymphatic
              lymphocytic
              lymphoid
          Coding Clinic: 2009, Q3, P6

● **204.9 Unspecified lymphoid leukemia**
  [0-2]

● **205 Myeloid leukemia**
  | **Includes** | leukemia: leukemia:
               granulocytic   myelomonocytic
               myeloblastic   myelosclerotic
               myelocytic   myelosis
               myelogenous

The following fifth-digit subclassification is for use with
category 205:

> **0 without mention of having achieved remission**
>   **failed remission**
> **1 in remission**
> **2 in relapse**

  Coding Clinic: 2008, Q4, P83-85

● **205.0 Acute**
  [0-2]   Acute promyelocytic leukemia
          | **Excludes** | acute exacerbation of chronic myeloid
                          leukemia (205.1)
          Coding Clinic: 2009, Q4, P78; 2006, Q2, P20-22; 2002, Q1, P11-12;
          1993, Q3, P3-4x2

● **205.1 Chronic**
  [0-2]   Eosinophilic leukemia
          Neutrophilic leukemia
          Coding Clinic: 2008, Q4, P140-143; 2000, Q1, P6; 1995, Q2, P12;
          1985, July-Aug, P13

● **205.2 Subacute**
  [0-2]

● **205.3 Myeloid sarcoma**
  [0-2]   Chloroma
          Granulocytic sarcoma

● **205.8 Other myeloid leukemia**
  [0-2]   Aleukemic leukemia:
              granulocytic
              myelogenous
              myeloid
          Aleukemic myelosis

● **205.9 Unspecified myeloid leukemia**
  [0-2]   Coding Clinic: 1985, May-June, P18-19

● **206 Monocytic leukemia**
  | **Includes** | leukemia:
               histiocytic
               monoblastic
               monocytoid

The following fifth-digit subclassification is for use with
category 206:

> **0 without mention of having achieved remission**
>   **failed remission**
> **1 in remission**
> **2 in relapse**

  Coding Clinic: 2008, Q4, P83-85

● **206.0 Acute**
  [0-2] | **Excludes** | acute exacerbation of chronic monocytic
                          leukemia (206.1)

● **206.1 Chronic**
  [0-2]

● **206.2 Subacute**
  [0-2]

● **206.8 Other monocytic leukemia**
  [0-2]   Aleukemic:
              monocytic leukemia
              monocytoid leukemia

● **206.9 Unspecified monocytic leukemia**
  [0-2]

Item 2-7   Leukemia is a cancer (acute or chronic) of the blood-forming
tissues of the bone marrow. Blood cells all start out as stem cells. They
mature and become red cells, white cells, or platelets. There are three
main types of leukocytes (white cells that fight infection): monocytes,
lymphocytes, and granulocytes. **Acute monocytic leukemia**
(AML) affects monocytes. **Acute lymphoid leukemia** (ALL) affects
lymphocytes, and **acute myeloid leukemia** (AML) affects cells that
typically develop into white blood cells (not lymphocytes), though it may
develop in other blood cells.

◄ New   ◄ Revised   ~~deleted~~ Deleted | Excludes | | Includes | | Use additional | | Code first | | Omit code |
● Unacceptable Principal Diagnosis   ● Use Additional Digit(s)   OGCR Official Guidelines   Coding Clinic

NEOPLASMS (140-239)

● **207 Other specified leukemia**

> **Excludes** *leukemic reticuloendotheliosis (202.4)*
> *plasma cell leukemia (203.1)*

The following fifth-digit subclassification is for use with category 207:

> **0 without mention of having achieved remission**
>   **failed remission**
> **1 in remission**
> **2 in relapse**

Coding Clinic: 2008, Q4, P83-85

● **207.0 Acute erythremia and erythroleukemia**
[0-2]   Acute erythremic myelosis
       Di Guglielmo's disease
       Erythremic myelosis

● **207.1 Chronic erythremia**
[0-2]   Heilmeyer-Schöner disease

● **207.2 Megakaryocytic leukemia**
[0-2]   Megakaryocytic myelosis
       Thrombocytic leukemia

● **207.8 Other specified leukemia**
[0-2]   Lymphosarcoma cell leukemia

● **208 Leukemia of unspecified cell type**

The following fifth-digit subclassification is for use with category 208:

> **0 without mention of having achieved remission**
>   **failed remission**
> **1 in remission**
> **2 in relapse**

Coding Clinic: 2008, Q4, P83-85

● **208.0 Acute**
[0-2]   Acute leukemia NOS
       Blast cell leukemia
       Stem cell leukemia

> **Excludes** *acute exacerbation of chronic unspecified leukemia (208.1)*
> Coding Clinic: 1987, Mar-April, P12

● **208.1 Chronic**
[0-2]   Chronic leukemia NOS

● **208.2 Subacute**
[0-2]   *Somewhat acute, between acute and chronic*
       Subacute leukemia NOS

● **208.8 Other leukemia of unspecified cell type**
[0-2]   Coding Clinic: 1987, Mar-April, P12

● **208.9 Unspecified leukemia**
[0-2]   Leukemia NOS

NEUROENDOCRINE TUMORS (209)

● **209 Neuroendocrine tumors**

> *Code first any associated multiple endocrine neoplasia syndrome (258.01-258.03)*

> Use additional code to identify associated endocrine syndrome, such as:
>   carcinoid syndrome (259.2)

> **Excludes** *benign pancreatic islet cell tumors (211.7)*
> *malignant pancreatic islet cell tumors (157.4)*
> Coding Clinic: 2009, Q4, P78; 2008, Q4, P85-90

● **209.0 Malignant carcinoid tumors of the small intestine**

    209.00 Malignant carcinoid tumor of the small intestine, unspecified portion

    209.01 Malignant carcinoid tumor of the duodenum

    209.02 Malignant carcinoid tumor of the jejunum

    209.03 Malignant carcinoid tumor of the ileum

● **209.1 Malignant carcinoid tumors of the appendix, large intestine, and rectum**

    209.10 Malignant carcinoid tumor of the large intestine, unspecified portion
        Malignant carcinoid tumor of the colon NOS

    209.11 Malignant carcinoid tumor of the appendix

    209.12 Malignant carcinoid tumor of the cecum

    209.13 Malignant carcinoid tumor of the ascending colon

    209.14 Malignant carcinoid tumor of the transverse colon

    209.15 Malignant carcinoid tumor of the descending colon

    209.16 Malignant carcinoid tumor of the sigmoid colon

    209.17 Malignant carcinoid tumor of the rectum

● **209.2 Malignant carcinoid tumors of other and unspecified sites**

    209.20 Malignant carcinoid tumor of unknown primary site

    209.21 Malignant carcinoid tumor of the bronchus and lung

    209.22 Malignant carcinoid tumor of the thymus

    209.23 Malignant carcinoid tumor of the stomach
        Coding Clinic: 2008, Q4, P85-90

    209.24 Malignant carcinoid tumor of the kidney

    209.25 Malignant carcinoid tumor of the foregut NOS

    209.26 Malignant carcinoid tumor of the midgut NOS

    209.27 Malignant carcinoid tumor of the hindgut NOS

    209.29 Malignant carcinoid tumors of other sites

● **209.3 Malignant poorly differentiated neuroendocrine tumors**

    209.30 Malignant poorly differentiated neuroendocrine carcinoma, any site
        High grade neuroendocrine carcinoma, any site
        Malignant poorly differentiated neuroendocrine tumor NOS

> **Excludes** *Merkel cell carcinoma (209.31-209.36)*

    209.31 Merkel cell carcinoma of the face
        Merkel cell carcinoma of the ear
        Merkel cell carcinoma of the eyelid, including canthus
        Merkel cell carcinoma of the lip

    209.32 Merkel cell carcinoma of the scalp and neck

    209.33 Merkel cell carcinoma of the upper limb

    209.34 Merkel cell carcinoma of the lower limb

    209.35 Merkel cell carcinoma of the trunk

    209.36 Merkel cell carcinoma of other sites
        Merkel cell carcinoma of the buttock
        Merkel cell carcinoma of the genitals
        Merkel cell carcinoma NOS
        Coding Clinic: 2009, Q4, P79

NEOPLASMS (140–239)

● **209.4 Benign carcinoid tumors of the small intestine**

   209.40 Benign carcinoid tumor of the small intestine, unspecified portion

   209.41 Benign carcinoid tumor of the duodenum

   209.42 Benign carcinoid tumor of the jejunum

   209.43 Benign carcinoid tumor of the ileum

● **209.5 Benign carcinoid tumors of the appendix, large intestine, and rectum**

   209.50 Benign carcinoid tumor of the large intestine, unspecified portion
      Benign carcinoid tumor of the colon NOS

   209.51 Benign carcinoid tumor of the appendix

   209.52 Benign carcinoid tumor of the cecum

   209.53 Benign carcinoid tumor of the ascending colon

   209.54 Benign carcinoid tumor of the transverse colon

   209.55 Benign carcinoid tumor of the descending colon

   209.56 Benign carcinoid tumor of the sigmoid colon

   209.57 Benign carcinoid tumor of the rectum

● **209.6 Benign carcinoid tumors of other and unspecified sites**

   209.60 Benign carcinoid tumor of unknown primary site
      Carcinoid tumor NOS
      Neuroendocrine tumor NOS

   209.61 Benign carcinoid tumor of the bronchus and lung
      Coding Clinic: 2009, Q4, P79

   209.62 Benign carcinoid tumor of the thymus

   209.63 Benign carcinoid tumor of the stomach

   209.64 Benign carcinoid tumor of the kidney

   209.65 Benign carcinoid tumor of the foregut NOS

   209.66 Benign carcinoid tumor of the midgut NOS

   209.67 Benign carcinoid tumor of the hindgut NOS

   209.69 Benign carcinoid tumors of other sites

● **209.7 Secondary neuroendocrine tumors**
      Secondary carcinoid tumors

   209.70 Secondary neuroendocrine tumor, unspecified site

   209.71 Secondary neuroendocrine tumor of distant lymph nodes
      Mesentery metastasis of neuroendocrine tumor

   209.72 Secondary neuroendocrine tumor of liver

   209.73 Secondary neuroendocrine tumor of bone

   209.74 Secondary neuroendocrine tumor of peritoneum
      Coding Clinic: 2009, Q4, P79

   209.75 Secondary Merkel cell carcinoma
      Merkel cell carcinoma nodal presentation
      Merkel cell carcinoma visceral metastatic presentation
      Secondary Merkel cell carcinoma, any site

   209.79 Secondary neuroendocrine tumor of other sites

BENIGN NEOPLASMS (210–229)

Benign neoplasm: Tumor that does not metastasize to other parts of body and is caused by cell overgrowth, differentiating it from cyst or abscess

● **210 Benign neoplasm of lip, oral cavity, and pharynx**

   Excludes *cyst (of):*
      jaw (526.0–526.2, 526.89)
      oral soft tissue (528.4)
      radicular (522.8)

   210.0 Lip
      Frenulum labii
      Lip (inner aspect) (mucosa) (vermilion border)

      Excludes *labial commissure (210.4)*
         skin of lip (216.0)

   210.1 Tongue
      Lingual tonsil

   210.2 Major salivary glands
      Gland: Gland:
         parotid   submandibular
         sublingual

      Excludes *benign neoplasms of minor salivary glands:*
         NOS (210.4)
         buccal mucosa (210.4)
         lips (210.0)
         palate (hard) (soft) (210.4)
         tongue (210.1)
         tonsil, palatine (210.5)

   210.3 Floor of mouth

   210.4 Other and unspecified parts of mouth
      Gingiva   Oral mucosa
      Gum (upper) (lower)   Palate (hard) (soft)
      Labial commissure   Uvula
      Oral cavity NOS

      Excludes *benign odontogenic neoplasms of bone (213.0–213.1)*
         developmental odontogenic cysts (526.0)
         mucosa of lips (210.0)
         nasopharyngeal [posterior] [superior] surface of soft palate (210.7)

   210.5 Tonsil
      Tonsil (faucial) (palatine)

      Excludes *lingual tonsil (210.1)*
         pharyngeal tonsil (210.7)
         tonsillar:
            fossa (210.6)
            pillars (210.6)

   210.6 Other parts of oropharynx
      Branchial cleft or vestiges
      Epiglottis, anterior aspect
      Fauces NOS
      Mesopharynx NOS
      Tonsillar:
         fossa
         pillars
      Vallecula

      Excludes *epiglottis:*
         NOS (212.1)
         suprahyoid portion (212.1)

   210.7 Nasopharynx
      Adenoid tissue   Pharyngeal tonsil
      Lymphadenoid tissue   Posterior nasal septum

   210.8 Hypopharynx
      Arytenoid fold   Postcricoid region
      Laryngopharynx   Pyriform fossa

   210.9 Pharynx, unspecified
      Throat NOS

● 211 **Benign neoplasm of other parts of digestive system**

> **Excludes** benign stromal tumors of digestive system (215.5)

211.0 **Esophagus**

211.1 **Stomach**
> Body of stomach   Cardiac orifice
> Cardia of stomach   Pylorus
> Fundus of stomach
>
> > **Excludes** benign carcinoid tumors of the stomach
> > (209.63)

211.2 **Duodenum, jejunum, and ileum**
> Small intestine NOS
>
> > **Excludes** ampulla of Vater (211.5)
> > benign carcinoid tumors of the small
> > intestine (209.40-209.43)
> > ileocecal valve (211.3)

211.3 **Colon**
> Appendix   Ileocecal valve
> Cecum   Large intestine NOS
>
> > **Excludes** benign carcinoid tumors of the large
> > intestine (209.50-209.56)
> > rectosigmoid junction (211.4)
>
> Coding Clinic: 2005, Q3, P17-18; Q2, P16-17; 2001, Q4, P55-56x2; 1995, Q1, P4; 1992, Q3, P11

211.4 **Rectum and anal canal**
> Anal canal or sphincter
> Anus NOS
> Rectosigmoid junction
>
> > **Excludes** anus:
> > margin (216.5)
> > perianal skin (216.5)
> > skin (216.5)
> > benign carcinoid tumors of the rectum
> > (209.57)

211.5 **Liver and biliary passages**
> Ampulla of Vater   Gallbladder
> Common bile duct   Hepatic duct
> Cystic duct   Sphincter of Oddi

211.6 **Pancreas, except islets of Langerhans**

211.7 **Islets of Langerhans**
> Islet cell tumor
>
> > Use additional code to identify any functional
> > activity

211.8 **Retroperitoneum and peritoneum**
> Mesentery   Omentum
> Mesocolon   Retroperitoneal tissue

211.9 **Other and unspecified site**
> Alimentary tract NOS
> Digestive system NOS
> Gastrointestinal tract NOS
> Intestinal tract NOS
> Intestine NOS
> Spleen, not elsewhere classified

● 212 **Benign neoplasm of respiratory and intrathoracic organs**

212.0 **Nasal cavities, middle ear, and accessory sinuses**
> Cartilage of nose
> Eustachian tube
> Nares
> Septum of nose
> Sinus: Sinus:
>   ethmoidal   maxillary
>   frontal   sphenoidal
>
> > **Excludes** auditory canal (external) (216.2)
> > bone of:
> > ear (213.0)
> > nose [turbinates] (213.0)
> > cartilage of ear (215.0)
> > ear (external) (skin) (216.2)
> > nose NOS (229.8)
> > skin (216.3)
> > olfactory bulb (225.1)
> > polyp of:
> > accessory sinus (471.8)
> > ear (385.30–385.35)
> > nasal cavity (471.0)
> > posterior margin of septum and choanae
> > (210.7)
>
> Coding Clinic: 2000, Q3, P10-11

212.1 **Larynx**
> Cartilage:
>   arytenoid
>   cricoid
>   cuneiform
>   thyroid
> Epiglottis (suprahyoid portion) NOS
> Glottis
> Vocal cords (false) (true)
>
> > **Excludes** epiglottis, anterior aspect (210.6)
> > polyp of vocal cord or larynx (478.4)

212.2 **Trachea**

212.3 **Bronchus and lung**
> Carina
> Hilus of lung
>
> > **Excludes** benign carcinoid tumors of bronchus and
> > lung (209.61)

212.4 **Pleura**

212.5 **Mediastinum**

212.6 **Thymus**
> > **Excludes** benign carcinoid tumors of thymus (209.62)

212.7 **Heart**
> > **Excludes** great vessels (215.4)

212.8 **Other specified sites**

212.9 **Site unspecified**
> Respiratory organ NOS
> Upper respiratory tract NOS
>
> > **Excludes** intrathoracic NOS (229.8)
> > thoracic NOS (229.8)

NEOPLASMS (140–239)

◀ New   ◀▥ Revised   ~~deleted~~ Deleted   Excludes   Includes   Use additional   Code first   Omit code
● Unacceptable Principal Diagnosis   ● Use Additional Digit(s)   OGCR Official Guidelines   Coding Clinic

749

● **213 Benign neoplasm of bone and articular cartilage**

> **Includes** cartilage (articular) (joint)
> periosteum

> **Excludes** *cartilage of:*
> *ear (215.0)*
> *eyelid (215.0)*
> *larynx (212.1)*
> *nose (212.0)*
> *exostosis NOS (726.91)*
> *synovia (215.0–215.9)*

213.0 **Bones of skull and face**

> **Excludes** *lower jaw bone (213.1)*

213.1 **Lower jaw bone**

213.2 **Vertebral column, excluding sacrum and coccyx**

213.3 **Ribs, sternum, and clavicle**

213.4 **Scapula and long bones of upper limb**

213.5 **Short bones of upper limb**

213.6 **Pelvic bones, sacrum, and coccyx**

213.7 **Long bones of lower limb**

213.8 **Short bones of lower limb**

213.9 **Bone and articular cartilage, site unspecified**

● **214 Lipoma**

> *Slow growing benign tumors (discrete rubbery masses) of mature fat cells enclosed in a thin fibrous capsule found in subcutaneous tissues of trunk and proximal extremities and in internal organs*

> **Includes** angiolipoma
> fibrolipoma
> hibernoma
> lipoma (fetal) (infiltrating) (intramuscular)
> myelolipoma
> myxolipoma

214.0 **Skin and subcutaneous tissue of face**

214.1 **Other skin and subcutaneous tissue**

214.2 **Intrathoracic organs**

214.3 **Intra-abdominal organs**

214.4 **Spermatic cord**

214.8 **Other specified sites**
Coding Clinic: 1994, Q3, P7

214.9 **Lipoma, unspecified site**

● **215 Other benign neoplasm of connective and other soft tissue**

> **Includes** blood vessel
> bursa
> fascia
> ligament
> muscle
> peripheral, sympathetic, and parasympathetic nerves and ganglia
> synovia
> tendon (sheath)

> **Excludes** *cartilage:*
> *articular (213.0–213.9)*
> *larynx (212.1)*
> *nose (212.0)*
> *connective tissue of:*
> *breast (217)*
> *internal organ, except lipoma and hemangioma-code to benign neoplasm of the site*
> *lipoma (214.0–214.9)*

215.0 **Head, face, and neck**

215.2 **Upper limb, including shoulder**

215.3 **Lower limb, including hip**

215.4 **Thorax**

> **Excludes** *heart (212.7)*
> *mediastinum (212.5)*
> *thymus (212.6)*

215.5 **Abdomen**
Abdominal wall
Benign stromal tumors of abdomen
Hypochondrium

215.6 **Pelvis**
Buttock   Inguinal region
Groin   Perineum

> **Excludes** *uterine:*
> *leiomyoma (218.0–218.9)*
> *ligament, any (221.0)*

215.7 **Trunk, unspecified**
Back NOS
Flank NOS

215.8 **Other specified sites**

215.9 **Site unspecified**

● **216 Benign neoplasm of skin**

> **Includes** blue nevus
> dermatofibroma
> hydrocystoma
> pigmented nevus
> syringoadenoma
> syringoma

> **Excludes** *skin of genital organs (221.0–222.9)*
> Coding Clinic: 2000, Q1, P21-22

216.0 **Skin of lip**

> **Excludes** *vermilion border of lip (210.0)*

216.1 **Eyelid, including canthus**

> **Excludes** *cartilage of eyelid (215.0)*

216.2 **Ear and external auditory canal**
Auricle (ear)
Auricular canal, external
External meatus
Pinna

> **Excludes** *cartilage of ear (215.0)*

216.3 **Skin of other and unspecified parts of face**
Cheek, external   Nose, external
Eyebrow   Temple

216.4 **Scalp and skin of neck**

216.5 **Skin of trunk, except scrotum**
Axillary fold
Perianal skin
Skin of: Skin of:
  abdominal wall   chest wall
  anus   groin
  back   perineum
  breast
  buttock
Umbilicus

> **Excludes** *anal canal (211.4)*
> *anus NOS (211.4)*
> *skin of scrotum (222.4)*

216.6 **Skin of upper limb, including shoulder**

216.7 **Skin of lower limb, including hip**

216.8 **Other specified sites of skin**

216.9 **Skin, site unspecified**

217 Benign neoplasm of breast
Note no gender difference for this code.
Breast (male) (female)
   connective tissue
   glandular tissue
   soft parts

> | Excludes | *adenofibrosis (610.2)*
> | | *benign cyst of breast (610.0)*
> | | *fibrocystic disease (610.1)*
> | | *skin of breast (216.5)*

Coding Clinic: 2000, Q1, P4

● **218 Uterine leiomyoma**
Benign tumors or nodules of the uterine wall

> | Includes | fibroid (bleeding) (uterine)
> | | uterine:
> | | fibromyoma
> | | myoma

218.0 Submucous leiomyoma of uterus

218.1 Intramural leiomyoma of uterus
   Interstitial leiomyoma of uterus

218.2 Subserous leiomyoma of uterus
   Subperitoneal leiomyoma of uterus

218.9 Leiomyoma of uterus, unspecified
Coding Clinic: 2003, Q1, P4-5; 1995, Q4, P50

● **219 Other benign neoplasm of uterus**

219.0 Cervix uteri

219.1 Corpus uteri
   Endometrium   Myometrium
   Fundus

219.8 Other specified parts of uterus

219.9 Uterus, part unspecified

220 Benign neoplasm of ovary
Use additional code to identify any functional activity (256.0–256.1)

> | Excludes | *cyst:*
> | | *corpus albicans (620.2)*
> | | *corpus luteum (620.1)*
> | | *endometrial (617.1)*
> | | *follicular (atretic) (620.0)*
> | | *graafian follicle (620.0)*
> | | *ovarian NOS (620.2)*
> | | *retention (620.2)*

Coding Clinic: 2009, Q4, P79, 82

● **221 Benign neoplasm of other female genital organs**

> | Includes | adenomatous polyp
> | | benign teratoma

> | Excludes | *cyst:*
> | | *epoophoron (752.11)*
> | | *fimbrial (752.11)*
> | | *Gartner's duct (752.11)*
> | | *parovarian (752.11)*

221.0 Fallopian tube and uterine ligaments
   Oviduct
   Parametrium
   Uterine ligament (broad) (round) (uterosacral)
   Uterine tube

221.1 Vagina

221.2 Vulva
   Clitoris
   External female genitalia NOS
   Greater vestibular [Bartholin's] gland
   Labia (majora) (minora)
   Pudendum

> | Excludes | *Bartholin's (duct) (gland) cyst (616.2)*

221.8 Other specified sites of female genital organs

221.9 Female genital organ, site unspecified
   Female genitourinary tract NOS

● **222 Benign neoplasm of male genital organs**

222.0 Testis
Use additional code to identify any functional activity

222.1 Penis
   Corpus cavernosum
   Glans penis
   Prepuce

222.2 Prostate

> | Excludes | *adenomatous hyperplasia of prostate (600.20–600.21)*
> | | *prostatic:*
> | | *adenoma (600.20–600.21)*
> | | *enlargement (600.00–600.01)*
> | | *hypertrophy (600.00–600.01)*

222.3 Epididymis

222.4 Scrotum
   Skin of scrotum

222.8 Other specified sites of male genital organs
   Seminal vesicle
   Spermatic cord

222.9 Male genital organ, site unspecified
   Male genitourinary tract NOS

● **223 Benign neoplasm of kidney and other urinary organs**

223.0 Kidney, except pelvis
   Kidney NOS

> | Excludes | *benign carcinoid tumors of kidney (209.64)*
> | | *renal:*
> | | *calyces (223.1)*
> | | *pelvis (223.1)*

223.1 Renal pelvis

223.2 Ureter

> | Excludes | *ureteric orifice of bladder (223.3)*

223.3 Bladder

● **223.8 Other specified sites of urinary organs**

223.81 Urethra

> | Excludes | *urethral orifice of bladder (223.3)*

223.89 Other
   Paraurethral glands

223.9 Urinary organ, site unspecified
   Urinary system NOS

● **224 Benign neoplasm of eye**

> | Excludes | *cartilage of eyelid (215.0)*
> | | *eyelid (skin) (216.1)*
> | | *optic nerve (225.1)*
> | | *orbital bone (213.0)*

224.0 Eyeball, except conjunctiva, cornea, retina, and choroid
   Ciliary body   Sclera
   Iris   Uveal tract

Item 2–8 Teratoma: terat = monster, oma = mass, tumor. Alternate terms: dermoid cyst of the ovary, ovarian teratoma. Teratomas are neoplasms and arise from germ cells (ovaries in female and testes in male) and can be benign or malignant. Teratomas have been known to contain hair, nails, and teeth, giving them a bizarre ("monster") appearance.

NEOPLASMS (140–239)

NEOPLASMS (140–239)

224.1 Orbit

> **Excludes** *bone of orbit (213.0)*

224.2 Lacrimal gland

224.3 Conjunctiva

224.4 Cornea

224.5 Retina

> **Excludes** *hemangioma of retina (228.03)*

224.6 Choroid

224.7 Lacrimal duct
Lacrimal sac
Nasolacrimal duct

224.8 Other specified parts of eye

224.9 Eye, part unspecified

● **225 Benign neoplasm of brain and other parts of nervous system**

> **Excludes** *hemangioma (228.02)*
> *neurofibromatosis (237.70-237.79)* ◀▥
> *peripheral, sympathetic, and parasympathetic*
>   *nerves and ganglia (215.0–215.9)*
> *retrobulbar (224.1)*

225.0 Brain

225.1 Cranial nerves
Coding Clinic: 2004, Q4, P111-113

225.2 Cerebral meninges
Meninges NOS
Meningioma (cerebral)

225.3 Spinal cord
Cauda equina

225.4 Spinal meninges
Spinal meningioma

225.8 Other specified sites of nervous system

225.9 Nervous system, part unspecified
Nervous system (central) NOS

> **Excludes** *meninges NOS (225.2)*

226 Benign neoplasm of thyroid glands

> **Use additional** code to identify any functional activity

● **227 Benign neoplasm of other endocrine glands and related structures**

> **Use additional** code to identify any functional activity

> **Excludes** *ovary (220)*
> *pancreas (211.6)*
> *testis (222.0)*

227.0 Adrenal gland
Suprarenal gland

227.1 Parathyroid gland

227.3 Pituitary gland and craniopharyngeal duct (pouch)
Craniobuccal pouch   Rathke's pouch
Hypophysis   Sella turcica

227.4 Pineal gland
Pineal body

227.5 Carotid body

227.6 Aortic body and other paraganglia
Coccygeal body
Glomus jugulare
Para-aortic body
Coding Clinic: 1984, Nov-Dec, P17

227.8 Other

227.9 Endocrine gland, site unspecified

Item 2–9 Hemangiomas are abnormally dense collections of dilated capillaries that occur on the skin or in internal organs. Hemangiomas are both deep and superficial and undergo a rapid growth phase when the size increases rapidly, followed by a rest phase, in which the tumor changes very little, followed by an involutional phase in which the tumor begins to and can disappear altogether. **Lymphangiomas** or cystic hygroma are benign collections of overgrown lymph vessels and, although rare, may occur anywhere but most commonly on the head and neck of children and infants. Visceral organs, lungs, and gastrointestinal tract may also be involved.

Figure 2–15 Hemangioma of skin and subcutaneous tissue. (From Yanoff: Ophthalmology, 2nd ed. 2004, Mosby, Inc.)

● **228 Hemangioma and lymphangioma, any site**

> **Includes** *angioma (benign) (cavernous) (congenital)*
>   *NOS*
> *cavernous nevus*
> *glomus tumor*
> *hemangioma (benign) (congenital)*

> **Excludes** *benign neoplasm of spleen, except hemangioma and*
>   *lymphangioma (211.9)*
> *glomus jugulare (227.6)*
> *nevus:*
>   *NOS (216.0–216.9)*
>   *blue or pigmented (216.0–216.9)*
>   *vascular (757.32)*

● **228.0 Hemangioma, any site**
Coding Clinic: 2001, Q1, P18; 1999, Q2, P9

228.00 Of unspecified site

228.01 Of skin and subcutaneous tissue
Coding Clinic: 1988, Q4, P6

228.02 Of intracranial structures
Coding Clinic: 1988, Q4, P6; 1985, Jan-Feb, P15

228.03 Of retina

228.04 Of intra-abdominal structures
Peritoneum
Retroperitoneal tissue
Coding Clinic: 1988, Q4, P6

228.09 Of other sites
Systemic angiomatosis
Coding Clinic: 1991, Q3, P20

228.1 Lymphangioma, any site
Congenital lymphangioma
Lymphatic nevus

● **229 Benign neoplasm of other and unspecified sites**

229.0 Lymph nodes

> **Excludes** *lymphangioma (228.1)*

229.8 Other specified sites
Intrathoracic NOS
Thoracic NOS

229.9 Site unspecified

◀ New   ◀▥ Revised   ~~deleted~~ Deleted   Excludes   Includes   Use additional   Code first   Omit code
● Unacceptable Principal Diagnosis   ● Use Additional Digit(s)   OGCR Official Guidelines   Coding Clinic

CARCINOMA IN SITU (230–234)

Includes   Bowen's disease
erythroplasia
Queyrat's erythroplasia

Excludes   *leukoplakia - see Alphabetic Index*

● **230 Carcinoma in situ of digestive organs**
*Cancer involving cells in localized tissues that has not spread
to nearby tissues*

230.0 Lip, oral cavity, and pharynx

Gingiva	Oropharynx
Hypopharynx	Salivary gland or duct
Mouth [any part]	Tongue
Nasopharynx	

Excludes   *aryepiglottic fold or interarytenoid fold,
laryngeal aspect (231.0)
epiglottis:
NOS (231.0)
suprahyoid portion (231.0)
skin of lip (232.0)*

230.1 Esophagus

230.2 Stomach

Body of stomach	Cardiac orifice
Cardia of stomach	Pylorus
Fundus of stomach	

230.3 Colon

Appendix	Ileocecal valve
Cecum	Large intestine NOS

Excludes   *rectosigmoid junction (230.4)*

230.4 Rectum
Rectosigmoid junction

230.5 Anal canal
Anal sphincter

230.6 Anus, unspecified

Excludes   *anus:
margin (232.5)
skin (232.5)
perianal skin (232.5)*

230.7 Other and unspecified parts of intestine

Duodenum	Jejunum
Ileum	Small intestine NOS

Excludes   *ampulla of Vater (230.8)*

230.8 Liver and biliary system

Ampulla of Vater	Gallbladder
Common bile duct	Hepatic duct
Cystic duct	Sphincter of Oddi

230.9 Other and unspecified digestive organs
Digestive organ NOS
Gastrointestinal tract NOS
Pancreas
Spleen

● **231 Carcinoma in situ of respiratory system**

231.0 Larynx

Cartilage:	Epiglottis:
arytenoid	NOS
cricoid	posterior surface
cuneiform	suprahyoid portion
thyroid	Vocal cords (false) (true)

Excludes   *aryepiglottic fold or interarytenoid fold:
NOS (230.0)
hypopharyngeal aspect (230.0)
marginal zone (230.0)*

231.1 Trachea

231.2 Bronchus and lung
Carina
Hilus of lung

231.8 Other specified parts of respiratory system

Accessory sinuses	Nasal cavities
Middle ear	Pleura

Excludes   *ear (external) (skin) (232.2)
nose NOS (234.8)
skin (232.3)*

231.9 Respiratory system, part unspecified
Respiratory organ NOS

● **232 Carcinoma in situ of skin**

Includes   pigment cells

Excludes   *melanoma in situ of skin (172.0-172.9)*

232.0 Skin of lip

Excludes   *vermilion border of lip (230.0)*

232.1 Eyelid, including canthus

232.2 Ear and external auditory canal

232.3 Skin of other and unspecified parts of face

232.4 Scalp and skin of neck

232.5 Skin of trunk, except scrotum

Anus, margin	Skin of:
Axillary fold	breast
Perianal skin	buttock
Skin of:	chest wall
abdominal wall	groin
anus	perineum
back	Umbilicus

Excludes   *anal canal (230.5)
anus NOS (230.6)
skin of genital organs (233.30–233.39,
233.5–233.6)*

232.6 Skin of upper limb, including shoulder

232.7 Skin of lower limb, including hip

232.8 Other specified sites of skin

232.9 Skin, site unspecified

● **233 Carcinoma in situ of breast and genitourinary system**
*This category incorporates specific male and female
genitourinary designations (233.0–233.6), while codes
233.7 and 233.9 apply to either male or female organs.*

233.0 Breast

Excludes   *Paget's disease (174.0–174.9)
skin of breast (232.5)*

233.1 Cervix uteri
Adenocarcinoma in situ of cervix
Cervical intraepithelial glandular neoplasia,
grade III
Cervical intraepithelial neoplasia III [CIN III]
Severe dysplasia of cervix

Excludes   *cervical intraepithelial neoplasia II [CIN II]
(622.12)
cytologic evidence of malignancy without
histologic confirmation (795.06)
high grade squamous intraepithelial lesion
(HGSIL) (795.04)
moderate dysplasia of cervix (622.12)*
Coding Clinic: 1992, Q3, P7-8; 1991, Q1, P11

233.2 Other and unspecified parts of uterus

NEOPLASMS (140–239)

● 233.3 Other and unspecified female genital organs
Coding Clinic: 2007, Q4, P67-68

　233.30 **Unspecified female genital organ**

　233.31 **Vagina**
　　Severe dysplasia of vagina
　　Vaginal intraepithelial neoplasia [VAIN III]

　233.32 **Vulva**
　　Severe dysplasia of vulva
　　Vulvar intraepithelial neoplasia [VIN III]
　　Coding Clinic: 1995, Q1, P8

　233.39 **Other female genital organ**

233.4 **Prostate**

233.5 **Penis**

233.6 **Other and unspecified male genital organs**

233.7 **Bladder**

233.9 **Other and unspecified urinary organs**

● 234 Carcinoma in situ of other and unspecified sites

234.0 **Eye**

Excludes *cartilage of eyelid (234.8)*
eyelid (skin) (232.1)
optic nerve (234.8)
orbital bone (234.8)

234.8 **Other specified sites**
　Endocrine gland [any]

234.9 **Site unspecified**
　Carcinoma in situ NOS

NEOPLASMS OF UNCERTAIN BEHAVIOR (235–238)

Note: Categories 235–238 classify by site certain histo-morphologically well-defined neoplasms, the subsequent behavior of which cannot be predicted from the present appearance.

● 235 Neoplasm of uncertain behavior of digestive and respiratory systems

Excludes *stromal tumors of uncertain behavior of digestive system (238.1)*

235.0 **Major salivary glands**
　Gland:
　　parotid
　　sublingual
　　submandibular

Excludes *minor salivary glands (235.1)*

235.1 **Lip, oral cavity, and pharynx**
　Gingiva　　　　Nasopharynx
　Hypopharynx　　Oropharynx
　Minor salivary glands　Tongue
　Mouth

Excludes *aryepiglottic fold or interarytenoid fold, laryngeal aspect (235.6)*
epiglottis:
NOS (235.6)
suprahyoid portion (235.6)
skin of lip (238.2)

235.2 **Stomach, intestines, and rectum**

235.3 **Liver and biliary passages**
　Ampulla of Vater　　Gallbladder
　Bile ducts [any]　　Liver

235.4 **Retroperitoneum and peritoneum**

235.5 **Other and unspecified digestive organs**
　Anal:　　　　　Esophagus
　　canal　　　　Pancreas
　　sphincter　　Spleen
　Anus NOS

Excludes *anus:*
margin (238.2)
skin (238.2)
perianal skin (238.2)

235.6 **Larynx**

Excludes *aryepiglottic fold or interarytenoid fold:*
NOS (235.1)
hypopharyngeal aspect (235.1)
marginal zone (235.1)

235.7 **Trachea, bronchus, and lung**

235.8 **Pleura, thymus, and mediastinum**

235.9 **Other and unspecified respiratory organs**
　Accessory sinuses
　Middle ear
　Nasal cavities
　Respiratory organ NOS

Excludes *ear (external) (skin) (238.2)*
nose (238.8)
skin (238.2)

● 236 Neoplasm of uncertain behavior of genitourinary organs

236.0 **Uterus**

236.1 **Placenta**
　Chorioadenoma (destruens)
　Invasive mole
　Malignant hydatid(iform) mole

236.2 **Ovary**
　Use additional code to identify any functional activity

236.3 **Other and unspecified female genital organs**

236.4 **Testis**
　Use additional code to identify any functional activity

236.5 **Prostate**

236.6 **Other and unspecified male genital organs**

236.7 **Bladder**

● 236.9 Other and unspecified urinary organs

　236.90 **Urinary organ, unspecified**

　236.91 **Kidney and ureter**

　236.99 **Other**

● 237 Neoplasm of uncertain behavior of endocrine glands and nervous system

237.0 **Pituitary gland and craniopharyngeal duct**
　Use additional code to identify any functional activity

237.1 **Pineal gland**

237.2 **Adrenal gland**
　Suprarenal gland
　Use additional code to identify any functional activity
　Pair of glands situated on top of or above each kidney ("suprarenal") responsible for regulating stress response through corticosteroids.

237.3 **Paraganglia**
　Aortic body　　　Coccygeal body
　Carotid body　　　Glomus jugulare
　Coding Clinic: 1984, Nov-Dec, P17

◀ New　◀▦ Revised　~~deleted~~ Deleted　Excludes　Includes　Use additional　Code first　Omit code
● Unacceptable Principal Diagnosis　● Use Additional Digit(s)　OGCR Official Guidelines　Coding Clinic

237.4 Other and unspecified endocrine glands
Parathyroid gland
Thyroid gland

237.5 Brain and spinal cord

237.6 Meninges
Meninges:
NOS
cerebral
spinal

● **237.7 Neurofibromatosis**
Disorder of nervous system that causes tumors to grow around nerves.
~~von Recklinghausen's disease~~

  237.70 Neurofibromatosis, unspecified

  237.71 Neurofibromatosis, type 1 [von Recklinghausen's disease]

  237.72 Neurofibromatosis, type 2 [acoustic neurofibromatosis]

  237.73 Schwannomatosis ◀

  237.79 Other neurofibromatosis ◀

237.9 Other and unspecified parts of nervous system
Cranial nerves

| Excludes | *peripheral, sympathetic, and parasympathetic nerves and ganglia (238.1)* |

● **238 Neoplasm of uncertain behavior of other and unspecified sites and tissues**

  238.0 Bone and articular cartilage

Excludes	*cartilage:*
	ear (238.1)
	eyelid (238.1)
	larynx (235.6)
	nose (235.9)
	synovia (238.1)

Coding Clinic: 2004, Q4, P128-129

  238.1 Connective and other soft tissue
Peripheral, sympathetic, and parasympathetic nerves and ganglia
Stromal tumors of digestive system

Excludes	*cartilage (of):*
	articular (238.0)
	larynx (235.6)
	nose (235.9)
	connective tissue of breast (238.3)

  238.2 Skin

Excludes	*anus NOS (235.5)*
	skin of genital organs (236.3, 236.6)
	vermilion border of lip (235.1)

  238.3 Breast

| Excludes | *skin of breast (238.2)* |

  238.4 Polycythemia vera
Primary polycythemia. Secondary polycythemia is 289.0. Check your documentation. Polycythemia is caused by too many red blood cells, which increase thickness of blood (viscosity). This can cause engorgement of the spleen (splenomegaly) with extra RBCs and potential clot formation.

  238.5 Histiocytic and mast cells
Mast cell tumor NOS
Mastocytoma NOS

  238.6 Plasma cells
Plasmacytoma NOS
Solitary myeloma

● **238.7 Other lymphatic and hematopoietic tissues**

Excludes	*acute myelogenous leukemia (205.0)*
	chronic myelomonocytic leukemia (205.1)
	myelosclerosis NOS (289.89)
	myelosis:
	NOS (205.9)
	megakaryocytic (207.2)

Coding Clinic: 2006, Q4, P63-66; 2001, Q3, P13-14; 1997, Q1, P5-6

  238.71 Essential thrombocythemia
Essential hemorrhagic thrombocythemia
Essential thrombocytosis
Idiopathic (hemorrhagic) thrombocythemia
Primary thrombocytosis
Coding Clinic: 2006, Q4, P64

  238.72 Low grade myelodysplastic syndrome lesions
Refractory anemia with excess blasts-1 (RAEB-1)
Refractory anemia (RA)
Refractory anemia with ringed sideroblasts (RARS)
Refractory cytopenia with multilineage dysplasia (RCMD)
Refractory cytopenia with multilineage dysplasia and ringed sideroblasts (RCMD-RS)

  238.73 High grade myelodysplastic syndrome lesions
Refractory anemia with excess blasts-2 (RAEB-2)

  238.74 Myelodysplastic syndrome with 5q deletion
5q minus syndrome NOS

| Excludes | *constitutional 5q deletion (758.39)* |
| | *high grade myelodysplastic syndrome with 5q deletion (238.73)* |

  238.75 Myelodysplastic syndrome, unspecified

  238.76 Myelofibrosis with myeloid metaplasia
Agnogenic myeloid metaplasia
Idiopathic myelofibrosis (chronic)
Myelosclerosis with myeloid metaplasia
Primary myelofibrosis

Excludes	*myelofibrosis NOS (289.83)*
	myelophthisic anemia (284.2)
	myelophthisis (284.2)
	secondary myelofibrosis (289.83)

●   **238.77 Post-transplant lymphoproliferative disorder (PTLD)**

Code first complications of transplant (996.80-996.89)
Coding Clinic: 2008, Q4, P90-91

  238.79 Other lymphatic and hematopoietic tissues
Lymphoproliferative disease (chronic) NOS
Megakaryocytic myelosclerosis
Myeloproliferative disease (chronic) NOS
Panmyelosis (acute)

  238.8 Other specified sites
Eye
Heart

| Excludes | *eyelid (skin) (238.2)* |
| | *cartilage (238.1)* |

  238.9 Site unspecified

NEOPLASMS (140–239)

NEOPLASMS OF UNSPECIFIED NATURE (239)

● **239   Neoplasms of unspecified nature**

   Note: Category 239 classifies by site neoplasms of
   unspecified morphology and behavior. The term
   "mass," unless otherwise stated, is not to be
   regarded as a neoplastic growth.

   Includes   "growth" NOS
                  neoplasm NOS
                  new growth NOS
                  tumor NOS

   239.0 Digestive system

   Excludes   *anus:*
                      margin (239.2)
                      skin (239.2)
                  perianal skin (239.2)

   239.1 Respiratory system

   239.2 Bone, soft tissue, and skin

   Excludes   *anal canal (239.0)*
                  anus NOS (239.0)
                  bone marrow (202.9)
                  cartilage:
                      larynx (239.1)
                      nose (239.1)
                  connective tissue of breast (239.3)
                  skin of genital organs (239.5)
                  vermilion border of lip (239.0)

   239.3 Breast

   Excludes   *skin of breast (239.2)*

   239.4 Bladder

   239.5 Other genitourinary organs

   239.6 Brain

   Excludes   *cerebral meninges (239.7)*
                  cranial nerves (239.7)

   239.7 Endocrine glands and other parts of nervous system

   Excludes   *peripheral, sympathetic, and
                  parasympathetic nerves and ganglia
                  (239.2)*

● **239.8 Other specified sites**

   Excludes   *eyelid (skin) (239.2)*
                  cartilage (239.2)
                  great vessels (239.2)
                  optic nerve (239.7)

   239.81 Retina and choroid
            Dark area on retina
            Retinal freckle

   239.89 Other specified sites

   239.9 Site unspecified

NEOPLASMS (140–239)

◀ New   ◀▥ Revised   ~~deleted~~ Deleted   Excludes   Includes   Use additional   Code first   Omit code
● Unacceptable Principal Diagnosis   ● Use Additional Digit(s)   OGCR Official Guidelines   Coding Clinic

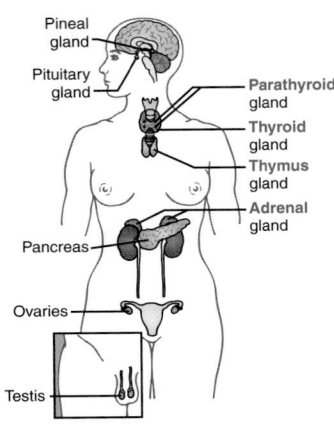

Figure 3–1 The endocrine system. (From Buck CJ: Step-by-Step Medical Coding, 2006 ed. Philadelphia, WB Saunders, 2006.)

Item 3–1 **Simple** goiter indicates no nodules are present. The most common type of goiter is a **diffuse colloidal,** also called a **nontoxic** or **endemic** goiter. Goiters classifiable to 240.0 or 240.9 are those goiters without mention of nodules.

Figure 3–2 **Goiter** is an enlargement of the thyroid gland.

3. ENDOCRINE, NUTRITIONAL AND METABOLIC DISEASES, AND IMMUNITY DISORDERS (240–279)

Excludes *endocrine and metabolic disturbances specific to the fetus and newborn (775.0–775.9)*

Note: All neoplasms, whether functionally active or not, are classified in Chapter 2. Codes in Chapter 3 (i.e., 242.8, 246.0, 251–253, 255–259) may be used to identify such functional activity associated with any neoplasm, or by ectopic endocrine tissue.

DISORDERS OF THYROID GLAND (240–246)

● **240 Simple and unspecified goiter**

240.0 Goiter, specified as simple
Any condition classifiable to 240.9, specified as simple

240.9 Goiter, unspecified
Enlargement of thyroid
Goiter or struma:
   NOS
   diffuse colloid
   endemic
Goiter or struma:
   hyperplastic
   nontoxic (diffuse)
   parenchymatous
   sporadic

Excludes *congenital (dyshormonogenic) goiter (246.1)*

● **241 Nontoxic nodular goiter**

Excludes *adenoma of thyroid (226)*
cystadenoma of thyroid (226)

241.0 Nontoxic uninodular goiter
Thyroid nodule
Uninodular goiter (nontoxic)

241.1 Nontoxic multinodular goiter
Multinodular goiter (nontoxic)

241.9 Unspecified nontoxic nodular goiter
Adenomatous goiter
Nodular goiter (nontoxic) NOS
Struma nodosa (simplex)

Figure 3–3 Graves' disease. In Graves' disease, exophthalmos often looks more pronounced than it actually is because of the extreme lid retraction that may occur. This patient, for instance, had minimal proptosis of the left eye but marked lid retraction. (Courtesy Dr. HG Scheie. From Yanoff M, Fine BS: Ocular Pathology, ed 5. St. Louis, Mosby, 2002.)

Item 3–2 **Thyrotoxicosis** is a condition caused by excessive amounts of the thyroid hormone thyroxine production or hyperthyroidism. **Graves' disease is associated with hyperthyroidism** (known as **Basedow's disease** in Europe).

● **242 Thyrotoxicosis with or without goiter**

Excludes *neonatal thyrotoxicosis (775.3)*

The following fifth-digit subclassification is for use with category 242:

> **0 without mention of thyrotoxic crisis or storm**
> **1 with mention of thyrotoxic crisis or storm**

● **242.0 Toxic diffuse goiter**
[0-1] Basedow's disease
Exophthalmic or toxic goiter NOS
Graves' disease
Primary thyroid hyperplasia

● **242.1 Toxic uninodular goiter**
[0-1] Thyroid nodule, toxic or with hyperthyroidism
Uninodular goiter, toxic or with hyperthyroidism

● **242.2 Toxic multinodular goiter**
[0-1] Secondary thyroid hyperplasia

● **242.3 Toxic nodular goiter, unspecified**
[0-1] Adenomatous goiter, toxic or with hyperthyroidism
Nodular goiter, toxic or with hyperthyroidism
Struma nodosa, toxic or with hyperthyroidism
Any condition classifiable to 241.9 specified as toxic or with hyperthyroidism

● **242.4 Thyrotoxicosis from ectopic thyroid nodule**
[0-1]

● **242.8 Thyrotoxicosis of other specified origin**
[0-1] Overproduction of thyroid-stimulating hormone [TSH]
Thyrotoxicosis:
   factitia from ingestion of excessive thyroid material

Use additional E code to identify cause, if drug-induced

● **242.9 Thyrotoxicosis without mention of goiter or other**
[0-1] **cause**
Hyperthyroidism NOS
Thyrotoxicosis NOS
Thyrotoxicosis is also known as thyroid storm.

243 Congenital hypothyroidism
Congenital thyroid insufficiency
Cretinism (athyrotic) (endemic)

Use additional code to identify associated mental retardation

Excludes *congenital (dyshormonogenic) goiter (246.1)*

Figure 3–4 Typical appearance of patients with moderately severe primary hypothyroidism or myxedema. (From Larsen: Williams Textbook of Endocrinology, 10th ed. 2003, Saunders, An Imprint of Elsevier.)

Item 3–3 Hypothyroidism is a condition in which there are insufficient levels of thyroxine.
Cretinism is congenital hypothyroidism, which can result in mental and physical retardation.

● **244 Acquired hypothyroidism**
> **Includes** athyroidism (acquired)
> hypothyroidism (acquired)
> myxedema (adult) (juvenile)
> thyroid (gland) insufficiency (acquired)

244.0 Postsurgical hypothyroidism

244.1 Other postablative hypothyroidism
> Hypothyroidism following therapy, such as irradiation

244.2 Iodine hypothyroidism
> Hypothyroidism resulting from administration or ingestion of iodide
>
> **Use additional** E code to identify drug
>
> **Excludes** *hypothyroidism resulting from administration of radioactive iodine (244.1)* ◄

244.3 Other iatrogenic hypothyroidism
> Hypothyroidism resulting from:
> P-aminosalicylic acid [PAS]
> Phenylbutazone
> Resorcinol
> Iatrogenic hypothyroidism NOS
>
> **Use additional** E code to identify drug

244.8 Other specified acquired hypothyroidism
> Secondary hypothyroidism NEC
> Coding Clinic: 1985, July-Aug, P9

244.9 Unspecified hypothyroidism
> Hypothyroidism, primary or NOS
> Myxedema, primary or NOS
> Coding Clinic: 1999, Q3, P19-20; 1996, Q4, P29

● **245 Thyroiditis**
> *Inflammation of thyroid gland, results in inability to convert iodine into thyroid hormone. Common types are autoimmune or chronic lymphatic thyroiditis.*

245.0 Acute thyroiditis
> Abscess of thyroid
> Thyroiditis: Thyroiditis:
> nonsuppurative, acute   suppurative
> pyogenic
>
> **Use additional** code to identify organism

245.1 Subacute thyroiditis
> Thyroiditis: Thyroiditis:
> de Quervain's   granulomatous
> giant cell   viral

245.2 Chronic lymphocytic thyroiditis
> Hashimoto's disease   Thyroiditis:
> Struma lymphomatosa   autoimmune
>   lymphocytic (chronic)

245.3 Chronic fibrous thyroiditis
> Struma fibrosa
> Thyroiditis: Thyroiditis:
> invasive (fibrous)   Riedel's
> ligneous

245.4 Iatrogenic thyroiditis
> **Use additional** E to identify cause

245.8 Other and unspecified chronic thyroiditis
> Chronic thyroiditis:
> NOS
> nonspecific

245.9 Thyroiditis, unspecified
> Thyroiditis NOS

● **246 Other disorders of thyroid**

246.0 Disorders of thyrocalcitonin secretion
> Hypersecretion of calcitonin or thyrocalcitonin

246.1 Dyshormonogenic goiter
> Congenital (dyshormonogenic) goiter
> Goiter due to enzyme defect in synthesis of thyroid hormone
> Goitrous cretinism (sporadic)

246.2 Cyst of thyroid
> **Excludes** *cystadenoma of thyroid (226)*

246.3 Hemorrhage and infarction of thyroid

246.8 Other specified disorders of thyroid
> Abnormality of thyroid-binding globulin
> Atrophy of thyroid
> Hyper-TBG-nemia
> Hypo-TBG-nemia
> Coding Clinic: 2006, Q2, P5

246.9 Unspecified disorder of thyroid

DISEASES OF OTHER ENDOCRINE GLANDS (249–259)

OGCR Section I.C.3.a.2
If the type of diabetes mellitus is not documented in the medical record the default is type II.

● **249 Secondary diabetes mellitus**
> **Includes** diabetes mellitus (due to) (in) (secondary) (with):
> drug-induced or chemical induced
> infection
>
> **Excludes** *gestational diabetes (648.8)*
> *hyperglycemia NOS (790.29)*
> *neonatal diabetes mellitus (775.1)*
> *nonclinical diabetes (790.29)*
> *Type I diabetes – see category 250*
> *Type II diabetes – see category 250*

The following fifth-digit subclassification is for use with category 249:

> **0 not stated as uncontrolled**
> **1 uncontrolled**

> **Use additional** code to identify any associated insulin use (V58.67)
> Coding Clinic: 2008, Q4, P91-95

● **249.0 Secondary diabetes mellitus without mention of**
[0-1] **complication**
> Secondary diabetes mellitus without mention of complication or manifestation classifiable to 249.1-249.9
> Secondary diabetes mellitus NOS

● **249.1** **Secondary diabetes mellitus with ketoacidosis**
[0-1]   Secondary diabetes mellitus with diabetic
     acidosis without mention of coma
   Secondary diabetes mellitus with diabetic
     ketosis without mention of coma

● **249.2** **Secondary diabetes mellitus with**
[0-1] **hyperosmolarity**
   Secondary diabetes mellitus with hyperosmolar
     (nonketotic) coma

● **249.3** **Secondary diabetes mellitus with other coma**
[0-1]   Secondary diabetes mellitus with diabetic coma
     (with ketoacidosis)
   Secondary diabetes mellitus with diabetic
     hypoglycemic coma
   Secondary diabetes mellitus with insulin coma
     NOS

> | Excludes | secondary diabetes mellitus with
>   hyperosmolar coma (249.2)

● **249.4** **Secondary diabetes mellitus with renal**
[0-1] **manifestations**
   Use additional code to identify manifestation, as:
     chronic kidney disease (585.1-585.9)
     diabetic nephropathy NOS (583.81)
     diabetic nephrosis (581.81)
     intercapillary glomerulosclerosis (581.81)
     Kimmelstiel-Wilson syndrome (581.81)

● **249.5** **Secondary diabetes mellitus with ophthalmic**
[0-1] **manifestations**
   Use additional code to identify manifestation, as:
     diabetic blindness (369.00-369.9)
     diabetic cataract (366.41)
     diabetic glaucoma (365.44)
     diabetic macular edema (362.07)
     diabetic retinal edema (362.07)
     diabetic retinopathy (362.01-362.07)

● **249.6** **Secondary diabetes mellitus with neurological**
[0-1] **manifestations**
   Use additional code to identify manifestation, as:
     diabetic amyotrophy (353.5)
     diabetic gastroparalysis (536.3)
     diabetic gastroparesis (536.3)
     diabetic mononeuropathy (354.0-355.9)
     diabetic neurogenic arthropathy (713.5)
     diabetic peripheral autonomic neuropathy
       (337.1)
     diabetic polyneuropathy (357.2)
   Coding Clinic: 2008, Q4, P91-95

● **249.7** **Secondary diabetes mellitus with peripheral**
[0-1] **circulatory disorders**
   Use additional code to identify manifestation, as:
     diabetic gangrene (785.4)
     diabetic peripheral angiopathy (443.81)

● **249.8** **Secondary diabetes mellitus with other specified**
[0-1] **manifestations**
   Secondary diabetic hypoglycemia in diabetes
     mellitus
   Secondary hypoglycemic shock in diabetes
     mellitus
   Use additional code to identify manifestation, as:
     any associated ulceration (707.10-707.9)
     diabetic bone changes (731.8)

● **249.9** **Secondary diabetes mellitus with unspecified**
[0-1] **complication**

● **250** **Diabetes mellitus**
   Metabolic disease that results in persistent hyperglycemia.
   The three primary forms of diabetes mellitus are
   differentiated by patterns of pancreatic failure—type 1,
   type 2 and 3.

> | Excludes | *gestational diabetes (648.8)*
>   *hyperglycemia NOS (790.29)*
>   *neonatal diabetes mellitus (775.1)*
>   *nonclinical diabetes (790.29)*
>   *secondary diabetes (249.0–249.9)*

The following fifth-digit subclassification is for use with
category 250:

> **0**   **type II or unspecified type, not stated as**
>   **uncontrolled**
>   Fifth-digit 0 is for use for type II patients, even if
>   the patient requires insulin
>
>   Use additional code, if applicable, for associated
>   long-term (current) insulin use V58.67
> **1**   **type I [juvenile type], not stated as uncontrolled**
> **2**   **type II or unspecified type, uncontrolled**
>   Fifth-digit 2 is for use for type II patients, even if
>   the patient requires insulin
>
>   Use additional code, if applicable, for associated
>   long-term (current) insulin use V58.67
> **3**   **type I [juvenile type], uncontrolled**

   Coding Clinic: 2006, Q1, P14; 1996, Q3, P5
OGCR   Section I.C.3.a.3
   If the documentation in a medical record does not indicate
   the type of diabetes but does indicate that the patient uses
   insulin, the appropriate fifth-digit for type II must be used.

● **250.0** **Diabetes mellitus without mention of complication**
[0-3]   Diabetes mellitus without mention of complication
     or manifestation classifiable to 250.1–250.9
   Diabetes (mellitus) NOS
   Coding Clinic: 2009, Q4, P81-82; 2005, Q2, P21-22; Q1, P15; 2004,
     Q2, P17; 2003, Q4, P105-106, 108-109, P110; Q2, P6-7, 16;
     Q1, P5; 2002, Q2, P13; Q1, P7-8; 2001, Q2, P16; 1997, Q4,
     P33; 1994, Q1, P16-17, 21; 1993, Q4, P42; 5th Issue, P15;
     1992, Q2, P15; 1990, Q2, P22; 1985, Nov-Dec, P11; Sept-Oct,
     P11; Mar-April, P12

● **250.1** **Diabetes with ketoacidosis**
[0-3]   Diabetic:
     acidosis without mention of coma
     ketosis without mention of coma
   Coding Clinic: 2006, Q2, P19-20; 2003, Q4, P81-82; 1987, Jan-Feb,
     P15

● **250.2** **Diabetes with hyperosmolarity**
[0-3]   Hyperosmolar (nonketotic) coma

● **250.3** **Diabetes with other coma**
[0-3]   Diabetic coma (with ketoacidosis)
   Diabetic hypoglycemic coma
   Insulin coma NOS

> | Excludes | *diabetes with hyperosmolar coma (250.2)*

● **250.4** **Diabetes with renal manifestations**
[0-3]   Use additional code to identify manifestation, as:
     chronic kidney disease (585.1–585.9) diabetic:
       nephropathy NOS (583.81)
       nephrosis (581.81)
       intercapillary glomerulosclerosis (581.81)
       Kimmelstiel-Wilson syndrome (581.81)
   Coding Clinic: 2003, Q1, P20-21; 1987, Sept-Oct, P9

ENDOCRINE, NUTRITIONAL AND METABOLIC DISEASES, AND IMMUNITY DISORDERS (240–279)

● **250.5 Diabetes with ophthalmic manifestations**
[0-3]   Use additional code to identify manifestation, as:
       diabetic:
          blindness (369.00–369.9)
          cataract (366.41)
          glaucoma (365.44)
          macular edema (362.07)
          retinal edema (362.07)
          retinopathy (362.01–362.07)
       Coding Clinic: 2005, Q4, P65-67; 1993, Q4, P38; 1985, Sept-Oct, P11

● **250.6 Diabetes with neurological manifestations**
[0-3]   Use additional code to identify manifestation, as:
       diabetic:
          amyotrophy (353.5)
          gastroparalysis (536.3)
          gastroparesis (536.3)
          mononeuropathy (354.0–355.9)
          neurogenic arthropathy (713.5)
          peripheral autonomic neuropathy (337.1)
          polyneuropathy (357.2)
       Coding Clinic: 2009, Q4, P81; Q2, P13, 15; 2008, Q3, P5-6; 2004, Q2, P7; 2003, Q4, P105; 1993, Q2, P6; 5th Issue, P15; 1984, Nov-Dec, P9

● **250.7 Diabetes with peripheral circulatory disorders**
[0-3]   Use additional code to identify manifestation, as:
       diabetic:
          gangrene (785.4)
          peripheral angiopathy (443.81)
       Coding Clinic: 2004, Q1, P14-15; 2002, Q1, P7-8; 1996, Q1, P10; 1994, Q3, P5; Q2, P17; 1990, Q3, P15; 1986, Mar-April, P12

● **250.8 Diabetes with other specified manifestations**
[0-3]   Diabetic hypoglycemia NOS
       Hypoglycemic shock NOS

     Use additional code to identify manifestation, as:
       any associated ulceration (707.10–707.9)
       diabetic bone changes (731.8)
       Coding Clinic: 1997, Q4, P43; 1994, Q2, P13

● **250.9 Diabetes with unspecified complication**
[0-3]   Coding Clinic: 2006, Q1, P14; 1993, Q4, P38; 5th Issue, P15; 5th Issue, P11; 1985, Nov-Dec, P11

● **251 Other disorders of pancreatic internal secretion**

   251.0 Hypoglycemic coma
       Iatrogenic hyperinsulinism
       Non-diabetic insulin coma

      Use additional E code to identify cause, if
       drug-induced

      Excludes   *hypoglycemic coma in diabetes mellitus*
           (249.3, 250.3)
       Coding Clinic: 1985, Mar-April, P8-9

   251.1 Other specified hypoglycemia
       Hyperinsulinism:
         NOS
         ectopic
         functional
       Hyperplasia of pancreatic islet beta cells NOS

      Excludes   *hypoglycemia in diabetes mellitus*
           (249.8, 250.8)
        hypoglycemia in infant of diabetic
           mother (775.0)
        hypoglycemic coma (251.0)
        neonatal hypoglycemia (775.6)

      Use additional E code to identify cause, if
       drug-induced
       Coding Clinic: 2003, Q1, P10

   251.2 Hypoglycemia, unspecified
       Hypoglycemia:
         NOS
         reactive
         spontaneous

      Excludes   *hypoglycemia:*
           with coma (251.0)
           in diabetes mellitus (249.8, 250.8)
           leucine-induced (270.3)
       Coding Clinic: 1985, Mar-April, P8-9

   251.3 Postsurgical hypoinsulinemia
       Hypoinsulinemia following complete or partial
         pancreatectomy
       Postpancreatectomy hyperglycemia

      Use additional code to identify (any associated):
       acquired absence of pancreas
         (V88.11-V88.12) ◀▥
       insulin use (V58.67)
       secondary diabetes mellitus (249.00-249.91)

      Excludes   *transient hyperglycemia post procedure*
           (790.29)
        transient hypoglycemia post procedure
           (251.2)

   251.4 Abnormality of secretion of glucagon
       Hyperplasia of pancreatic islet alpha cells with
         glucagon excess

   251.5 Abnormality of secretion of gastrin
       Hyperplasia of pancreatic alpha cells with gastrin
         excess
       Zollinger-Ellison syndrome

   **251.8 Other specified disorders of pancreatic internal
       secretion**
       Coding Clinic: 1998, Q2, P15

   251.9 Unspecified disorder of pancreatic internal secretion
       Islet cell hyperplasia NOS

● **252 Disorders of parathyroid gland**

      Excludes   *hungry bone syndrome (275.5)*

● **252.0 Hyperparathyroidism**

      Excludes   *ectopic hyperparathyroidism (259.3)*
       Coding Clinic: 2004, Q4, P57-59

     252.00 Hyperparathyroidism, unspecified

     252.01 Primary hyperparathyroidism
         Hyperplasia of parathyroid

     252.02 Secondary hyperparathyroidism, non-renal

      Excludes   *secondary hyperparathyroidism (of*
           renal origin) (588.81)

     252.08 Other hyperparathyroidism
         Tertiary hyperparathyroidism

Figure 3–5   Tetany caused by hypoparathyroidism.

Item 3–4   Hyperparathyroidism is an overactive parathyroid gland that secretes excessive parathormone, causing increased levels of circulating calcium. This results in a loss of calcium in the bone (osteoporosis).

Hypoparathyroidism is an underactive parathyroid gland that results in decreased levels of circulating calcium. The primary manifestation is **tetany,** a continuous muscle spasm.

◀ New   ◀▥ Revised   ~~deleted~~ Deleted   Excludes   Includes   Use additional   Code first   Omit code
● Unacceptable Principal Diagnosis   ● Use Additional Digit(s)   OGCR Official Guidelines   Coding Clinic

252.1 Hypoparathyroidism
Parathyroiditis (autoimmune)
Tetany:
  parathyroid
  parathyroprival

> | Excludes | *pseudohypoparathyroidism (275.49)*
> *pseudopseudohypoparathyroidism (275.49)*
> *tetany NOS (781.7)*
> *transitory neonatal hypoparathyroidism*
>   *(775.4)*

252.8 Other specified disorders of parathyroid gland
Cyst of parathyroid gland
Hemorrhage of parathyroid gland

252.9 Unspecified disorder of parathyroid gland

● **253 Disorders of the pituitary gland and its hypothalamic control**

> | Includes | the listed conditions whether the disorder is in the pituitary or the hypothalamus

> | Excludes | *Cushing's syndrome (255.0)*

253.0 Acromegaly and gigantism
Overproduction of growth hormone

253.1 Other and unspecified anterior pituitary hyperfunction
Forbes-Albright syndrome

> | Excludes | *overproduction of:*
>   *ACTH (255.3)*
>   *thyroid-stimulating hormone [TSH]*
>   *(242.8)*

Coding Clinic: 1985, July-Aug, P9

253.2 Panhypopituitarism
Cachexia, pituitary
Necrosis of pituitary (postpartum)
Pituitary insufficiency NOS
Sheehan's syndrome
Simmonds' disease

> | Excludes | *iatrogenic hypopituitarism (253.7)*

253.3 Pituitary dwarfism
Isolated deficiency of (human) growth hormone
  [HGH]
Lorain-Levi dwarfism

253.4 Other anterior pituitary disorders
Isolated or partial deficiency of an anterior
  pituitary hormone, other than growth
  hormone
Prolactin deficiency
Coding Clinic: 1985, July-Aug, P9

253.5 Diabetes insipidus
Vasopressin deficiency

> | Excludes | *nephrogenic diabetes insipidus (588.1)*

253.6 Other disorders of neurohypophysis
Syndrome of inappropriate secretion of antidiuretic
  hormone [ADH]

> | Excludes | *ectopic antidiuretic hormone secretion*
>   *(259.3)*

Coding Clinic: 1993, 5th Issue, P8

253.7 Iatrogenic pituitary disorders
Hypopituitarism:
  hormone-induced
  hypophysectomy-induced
  postablative
  radiotherapy-induced

> Use additional E code to identify cause

253.8 Other disorders of the pituitary and other syndromes of diencephalohypophyseal origin
Abscess of pituitary
Adiposogenital dystrophy
Cyst of Rathke's pouch
Fröhlich's syndrome

> | Excludes | *craniopharyngioma (237.0)*

253.9 Unspecified
Dyspituitarism

● **254 Diseases of thymus gland**

> | Excludes | *aplasia or dysplasia with immunodeficiency*
>   *(279.2)*
> *hypoplasia with immunodeficiency (279.2)*
> *myasthenia gravis (358.00–358.01)*

254.0 Persistent hyperplasia of thymus
Hypertrophy of thymus

254.1 Abscess of thymus

254.8 Other specified diseases of thymus gland
Atrophy of thymus
Cyst of thymus

> | Excludes | *thymoma (212.6)*

254.9 Unspecified disease of thymus gland

● **255 Disorders of adrenal glands**

> | Includes | the listed conditions whether the basic disorder is in the adrenals or is pituitary-induced

255.0 Cushing's syndrome
Adrenal hyperplasia due to excess ACTH
Cushing's syndrome:
  NOS
  iatrogenic
  idiopathic
  pituitary-dependent
Ectopic ACTH syndrome
Iatrogenic syndrome of excess cortisol
Overproduction of cortisol

> Use additional E code to identify cause, if
>   drug-induced

> | Excludes | *congenital adrenal hyperplasia (255.2)*

Figure 3–6 Centripetal and generalized obesity and dorsal kyphosis in a 30-year-old woman with Cushing's disease. (From Larsen: Williams Textbook of Endocrinology, 10th ed. 2003, Saunders, An Imprint of Elsevier.)

Item 3–5 Hyperadrenalism is overactivity of the adrenal cortex, which secretes corticosterioid hormones. Excessive glucocorticoid hormone results in hyperglycemia **(Cushing's syndrome),** and excessive aldosterone results in **Conn's syndrome. Adrenogenital syndrome** is the result of excessive secretion of androgens, male hormones, which stimulates premature sexual development. **Hypoadrenalism, Addison's disease,** is a condition in which the adrenal glands atrophy.

● **255.1 Hyperaldosteronism**
Coding Clinic: 2003, Q4, P48-50

    255.10 Hyperaldosteronism, unspecified
        Aldosteronism NOS
        Primary aldosteronism, unspecified
        | Excludes | *Conn's syndrome (255.12)*

    255.11 Glucocorticoid-remediable aldosteronism
        Familial aldosteronism type I
        | Excludes | *Conn's syndrome (255.12)*

    255.12 Conn's syndrome

    255.13 Bartter's syndrome

    255.14 Other secondary aldosteronism
        Coding Clinic: 2006, Q3, P24

255.2 Adrenogenital disorders
    Achard-Thiers syndrome
    Adrenogenital syndromes, virilizing or feminizing,
        whether acquired or associated with
        congenital adrenal hyperplasia consequent on
        inborn enzyme defects in hormone synthesis
    Congenital adrenal hyperplasia
    Female adrenal pseudohermaphroditism
    Male:
        macrogenitosomia praecox
        sexual precocity with adrenal hyperplasia
    Virilization (female) (suprarenal)
    | Excludes | *adrenal hyperplasia due to excess ACTH*
        (255.0)
        isosexual virilization (256.4)

255.3 Other corticoadrenal overactivity
    Acquired benign adrenal androgenic overactivity
    Overproduction of ACTH

● **255.4 Corticoadrenal insufficiency**
    | Excludes | *tuberculous Addison's disease (017.6)*
    Coding Clinic: 2006, Q3, P24; 1985, July-Aug, P8

    255.41 Glucocorticoid deficiency
        Addisonian crisis
        Addison's disease NOS
        Adrenal atrophy (autoimmune)
        Adrenal calcification
        Adrenal crisis
        Adrenal hemorrhage
        Adrenal infarction
        Adrenal insufficiency NOS
        Combined glucocorticoid and
            mineralocorticoid deficiency
        Corticoadrenal insufficiency NOS
        Coding Clinic: 2007, Q4, P68-70

    255.42 Mineralocorticoid deficiency
        Hypoaldosteronism
        | Excludes | *combined glucocorticoid and*
        mineralocorticoid deficiency
        (255.41)
        Coding Clinic: 2006, Q3, P24

255.5 Other adrenal hypofunction
    Adrenal medullary insufficiency
    | Excludes | *Waterhouse-Friderichsen syndrome*
        (meningococcal) (036.3)

255.6 Medulloadrenal hyperfunction
    Catecholamine secretion by pheochromocytoma

255.8 Other specified disorders of adrenal glands
    Abnormality of cortisol-binding globulin
    Coding Clinic: 1985, July-Aug, P8

255.9 Unspecified disorder of adrenal glands

● **256 Ovarian dysfunction**

    256.0 Hyperestrogenism

    256.1 Other ovarian hyperfunction
        Hypersecretion of ovarian androgens
        Coding Clinic: 1995, Q3, P15

    256.2 Postablative ovarian failure
        Ovarian failure:
            iatrogenic
            postirradiation
            postsurgical
        Use additional code for states associated with
            artificial menopause (627.4)
        | Excludes | *acquired absence of ovary (V45.77)*
        asymptomatic age-related (natural)
        postmenopausal status (V49.81)
        Coding Clinic: 2002, Q2, P12-13

●   **256.3 Other ovarian failure**
        Use additional code for states associated with
            natural menopause (627.2)
        | Excludes | *asymptomatic age-related (natural)*
        postmenopausal status (V49.81)

        256.31 Premature menopause

        256.39 Other ovarian failure
            Delayed menarche
            Ovarian hypofunction
            Primary ovarian failure NOS

    256.4 Polycystic ovaries
        Isosexual virilization Stein-Leventhal syndrome

    256.8 Other ovarian dysfunction

    256.9 Unspecified ovarian dysfunction

● **257 Testicular dysfunction**

    257.0 Testicular hyperfunction
        Hypersecretion of testicular hormones

    257.1 Postablative testicular hypofunction
        Testicular hypofunction:
            iatrogenic
            postirradiation
            postsurgical

    257.2 Other testicular hypofunction
        Defective biosynthesis of testicular androgen
        Eunuchoidism:
            NOS
            hypogonadotropic
        Failure:
            Leydig's cell, adult
            seminiferous tubule, adult
        Testicular hypogonadism
        | Excludes | *azoospermia (606.0)*

    257.8 Other testicular dysfunction
        | Excludes | *androgen insensitivity syndrome*
        (259.50–259.52)

    257.9 Unspecified testicular dysfunction

● **258 Polyglandular dysfunction and related disorders**

●   **258.0 Polyglandular activity in multiple endocrine adenomatosis**
        Multiple endocrine neoplasia [MEN] syndromes
        Use additional codes to identify any malignancies
            and other conditions associated with the
            syndromes
        Coding Clinic: 2009, Q4, P84x2

        258.01 Multiple endocrine neoplasia [MEN] type I
            Wermer's syndrome
            Coding Clinic: 2008, Q4, P85-90; 2007, Q4, P70-72

◀ New   ⬅ Revised   ~~deleted~~ Deleted | Excludes | | Includes | Use additional   Code first   Omit code
● Unacceptable Principal Diagnosis   ● Use Additional Digit(s)   OGCR Official Guidelines   Coding Clinic

258.02 Multiple endocrine neoplasia [MEN] type IIA
Sipple's syndrome

258.03 Multiple endocrine neoplasia [MEN] type IIB

258.1 Other combinations of endocrine dysfunction
Lloyd's syndrome
Schmidt's syndrome

258.8 Other specified polyglandular dysfunction

258.9 Polyglandular dysfunction, unspecified

● **259 Other endocrine disorders**

259.0 Delay in sexual development and puberty, not elsewhere classified
Delayed puberty

259.1 Precocious sexual development and puberty, not elsewhere classified
Sexual precocity:
NOS
constitutional
cryptogenic
idiopathic

259.2 Carcinoid syndrome
Hormone secretion by carcinoid tumors
Coding Clinic: 2008, Q4, P85-90

259.3 Ectopic hormone secretion, not elsewhere classified
Ectopic:
antidiuretic hormone secretion [ADH]
hyperparathyroidism

Excludes ectopic ACTH syndrome (255.0)

259.4 Dwarfism, not elsewhere classified
Dwarfism:
NOS
constitutional

Excludes dwarfism:
achondroplastic (756.4)
intrauterine (759.7)
nutritional (263.2)
pituitary (253.3)
renal (588.0)
progeria (259.8)

● **259.5 Androgen insensitivity syndrome**
Coding Clinic: 2008, Q4, P95-96; 2005, Q4, P53-54

259.50 Androgen insensitivity, unspecified

259.51 Androgen insensitivity syndrome
Complete androgen insensitivity
de Quervain's syndrome
Goldberg-Maxwell Syndrome

259.52 Partial androgen insensitivity
Partial androgen insensitivity syndrome
Reifenstein syndrome

259.8 Other specified endocrine disorders
Pineal gland dysfunction
Progeria
Werner's syndrome

259.9 Unspecified endocrine disorder
Disturbance:
endocrine NOS
hormone NOS
Infantilism NOS

NUTRITIONAL DEFICIENCIES (260–269)

Excludes deficiency anemias (280.0–281.9)

260 Kwashiorkor
Nutritional edema with dyspigmentation of skin and hair
Coding Clinic: 2009, Q3, P6

261 Nutritional marasmus
Nutritional atrophy
Severe calorie deficiency
Severe malnutrition NOS
Coding Clinic: 2007, Q4, P96-97; 2006, Q3, P14-15; Q2, P12

262 Other severe protein-calorie malnutrition
Nutritional edema without mention of dyspigmentation of skin and hair
Coding Clinic: 1985, July-Aug, P12-13

● **263 Other and unspecified protein-calorie malnutrition**

263.0 Malnutrition of moderate degree
Coding Clinic: 2009, Q3, P6; 1985, July-Aug, P12-13

263.1 Malnutrition of mild degree
Coding Clinic: 1985, July-Aug, P12-13

263.2 Arrested development following protein-calorie malnutrition
Nutritional dwarfism
Physical retardation due to malnutrition

263.8 Other protein-calorie malnutrition

263.9 Unspecified protein-calorie malnutrition
Dystrophy due to malnutrition
Malnutrition (calorie) NOS

Excludes nutritional deficiency NOS (269.9)

Coding Clinic: 2006, Q2, P12; 2003, Q4, P109-110; 1984, Nov-Dec, P19

● **264 Vitamin A deficiency**

264.0 With conjunctival xerosis

264.1 With conjunctival xerosis and Bitot's spot
Bitot's spot in the young child

264.2 With corneal xerosis

264.3 With corneal ulceration and xerosis

264.4 With keratomalacia

264.5 With night blindness

264.6 With xerophthalmic scars of cornea

264.7 Other ocular manifestations of vitamin A deficiency
Xerophthalmia due to vitamin A deficiency

264.8 Other manifestations of vitamin A deficiency
Follicular keratosis due to vitamin A deficiency
Xeroderma due to vitamin A deficiency

264.9 Unspecified vitamin A deficiency
Hypovitaminosis A NOS

Figure 3–7   Bitot's spot on the conjunctiva.

Item 3–6   **Bitot's spots** are the result of a buildup of keratin debris found on the superficial surface the conjunctiva; oval, triangular, or irregular in shape; and a sign of vitamin A deficiency and associated with night blindness. The disease may progress to **keratomalacia,** which can result in eventual prolapse of the iris and loss of the lens.

ENDOCRINE, NUTRITIONAL AND METABOLIC DISEASES, AND IMMUNITY DISORDERS (240–279)

Figure 3–8 The sharply demarcated, characteristic scaling dermatitis of pellagra. (From Kumar: Robbins and Cotran: Pathologic Basis of Disease, 7th ed. 2005, Saunders, An Imprint of Elsevier.)

Item 3–7 Pellagra is associated with a deficiency of niacin and its precursor, **tryptophan.** Characteristics of the condition include diarrhea, dermatitis on exposed skin surfaces, dementia, and death. It is prevalent in developing countries where nutrition is inadequate. **Beriberi** is associated with thiamine deficiency.

● **265 Thiamine and niacin deficiency states**

265.0 Beriberi

265.1 Other and unspecified manifestations of thiamine deficiency
Other vitamin B$_1$ deficiency states

265.2 Pellagra
Deficiency:
niacin (-tryptophan)
nicotinamide
nicotinic acid
vitamin PP
Pellagra (alcoholic)

● **266 Deficiency of B-complex components**

266.0 Ariboflavinosis
Riboflavin [vitamin B$_2$] deficiency
Coding Clinic: 1986, Sept-Oct, P10

266.1 Vitamin B$_6$ deficiency
Deficiency:
pyridoxal
pyridoxamine
pyridoxine
Vitamin B$_6$ deficiency syndrome
Excludes *vitamin B$_6$-responsive sideroblastic anemia (285.0)*

266.2 Other B-complex deficiencies
Deficiency:
cyanocobalamin
folic acid
vitamin B$_{12}$
Excludes *combined system disease with anemia (281.0–281.1)*
deficiency anemias (281.0–281.9)
subacute degeneration of spinal cord with anemia (281.0–281.1)

266.9 Unspecified vitamin B deficiency

267 Ascorbic acid deficiency
Deficiency of vitamin C
Scurvy
Excludes *scorbutic anemia (281.8)*

● **268 Vitamin D deficiency**
Excludes *vitamin D-resistant:*
osteomalacia (275.3)
rickets (275.3)

268.0 Rickets, active
Excludes *celiac rickets (579.0)*
renal rickets (588.0)

268.1 Rickets, late effect
Any condition specified as due to rickets and stated to be a late effect or sequela of rickets
Code first the nature of late effect

268.2 Osteomalacia, unspecified
Softening of bone

268.9 Unspecified vitamin D deficiency
Avitaminosis D

● **269 Other nutritional deficiencies**

269.0 Deficiency of vitamin K
Excludes *deficiency of coagulation factor due to vitamin K deficiency (286.7)*
vitamin K deficiency of newborn (776.0)

269.1 Deficiency of other vitamins
Deficiency:
vitamin E
vitamin P

269.2 Unspecified vitamin deficiency
Multiple vitamin deficiency NOS

269.3 Mineral deficiency, not elsewhere classified
Deficiency:
calcium, dietary
iodine
Excludes *deficiency:*
calcium NOS (275.40)
potassium (276.8)
sodium (276.1)

269.8 Other nutritional deficiency
Excludes *adult failure to thrive (783.7)*
failure to thrive in childhood (783.41)
feeding problems (783.3)
newborn (779.31–779.34)

269.9 Unspecified nutritional deficiency

OTHER METABOLIC AND IMMUNITY DISORDERS (270–279)

Use additional code to identify any associated mental retardation

● **270 Disorders of amino-acid transport and metabolism**
Excludes *abnormal findings without manifest disease (790.0–796.9)*
disorders of purine and pyrimidine metabolism (277.1–277.2)
gout (274.00–274.9)

270.0 Disturbances of amino-acid transport
Cystinosis
Cystinuria
Fanconi (-de Toni) (-Debré) syndrome
Glycinuria (renal)
Hartnup disease

270.1 Phenylketonuria [PKU]
Hyperphenylalaninemia

270.2 Other disturbances of aromatic amino-acid metabolism
Albinism
Alkaptonuria
Alkaptonuric ochronosis
Disturbances of metabolism of tyrosine and tryptophan
Homogentisic acid defects
Hydroxykynureninuria
Hypertyrosinemia
Indicanuria
Kynureninase defects
Oasthouse urine disease
Ochronosis
Tyrosinosis
Tyrosinuria
Waardenburg syndrome
Excludes *vitamin B$_6$-deficiency syndrome (266.1)*
Coding Clinic: 1999, Q3, P20-21

◄ New   ◄▬ Revised   ~~deleted~~ Deleted   Excludes   Includes   Use additional   Code first   Omit code
● Unacceptable Principal Diagnosis   ● Use Additional Digit(s)   OGCR Official Guidelines   Coding Clinic

Item 3–8 Any term ending with "emia" will be a blood condition. Any term ending with "uria" will have to do with urine. A term ending with "opathy" is a disease condition. Check for laboratory work.

270.3 Disturbances of branched-chain amino-acid metabolism
    Disturbances of metabolism of leucine, isoleucine, and valine
    Hypervalinemia
    Intermittent branched-chain ketonuria
    Leucine-induced hypoglycemia
    Leucinosis
    Maple syrup urine disease
    Coding Clinic: 2000, Q3, P8

270.4 Disturbances of sulphur-bearing amino-acid metabolism
    Cystathioninemia
    Cystathioninuria
    Disturbances of metabolism of methionine, homocystine, and cystathionine
    Homocystinuria
    Hypermethioninemia
    Methioninemia
    Coding Clinic: 2007, Q2, P9; 2004, Q1, P6

270.5 Disturbances of histidine metabolism
    Carnosinemia   Hyperhistidinemia
    Histidinemia   Imidazole aminoaciduria

270.6 Disorders of urea cycle metabolism
    Argininosuccinic aciduria
    Citrullinemia
    Disorders of metabolism of ornithine, citrulline, argininosuccinic acid, arginine, and ammonia
    Hyperammonemia
    Hyperornithinemia

270.7 Other disturbances of straight-chain amino-acid metabolism
    Glucoglycinuria
    Glycinemia (with methylmalonic acidemia)
    Hyperglycinemia
    Hyperlysinemia
    Pipecolic acidemia
    Saccharopinuria
    Other disturbances of metabolism of glycine, threonine, serine, glutamine, and lysine
    Coding Clinic: 2000, Q3, P8

270.8 Other specified disorders of amino-acid metabolism
    Alaninemia   Iminoacidopathy
    Ethanolaminuria   Prolinemia
    Glycoprolinuria   Prolinuria
    Hydroxyprolinemia   Sarcosinemia
    Hyperprolinemia

270.9 Unspecified disorder of amino-acid metabolism

● **271 Disorders of carbohydrate transport and metabolism**
    Excludes *abnormality of secretion of glucagon (251.4)*
    diabetes mellitus (249.0–249.9, 250.0–250.9)
    hypoglycemia NOS (251.2)
    mucopolysaccharidosis (277.5)

271.0 Glycogenosis
    Amylopectinosis
    Glucose-6-phosphatase deficiency
    Glycogen storage disease
    McArdle's disease
    Pompe's disease
    von Gierke's disease
    Coding Clinic: 1998, Q1, P5-6

271.1 Galactosemia
    Galactose-1-phosphate uridyl transferase deficiency
    Galactosuria

271.2 Hereditary fructose intolerance
    Essential benign fructosuria
    Fructosemia

271.3 Intestinal disaccharidase deficiencies and disaccharide malabsorption
    Intolerance or malabsorption (congenital) (of):
        glucose-galactose
        lactose
        sucrose-isomaltose

271.4 Renal glycosuria
    Renal diabetes

271.8 Other specified disorders of carbohydrate transport and metabolism
    Essential benign pentosuria   Mannosidosis
    Fucosidosis   Oxalosis
    Glycolic aciduria   Xylosuria
    Hyperoxaluria (primary)   Xylulosuria

271.9 Unspecified disorder of carbohydrate transport and metabolism

● **272 Disorders of lipoid metabolism**
    Excludes *localized cerebral lipidoses (330.1)*

272.0 Pure hypercholesterolemia
    Familial hypercholesterolemia
    Fredrickson Type IIa hyperlipoproteinemia
    Hyperbetalipoproteinemia
    Hyperlipidemia, Group A
    Low-density-lipoid-type [LDL] hyperlipoproteinemia
    Coding Clinic: 2005, Q4, P68-69

272.1 Pure hyperglyceridemia
    Endogenous hyperglyceridemia
    Fredrickson Type IV hyperlipoproteinemia
    Hyperlipidemia, Group B
    Hyperprebetalipoproteinemia
    Hypertriglyceridemia, essential
    Very-low-density-lipoid-type [VLDL] hyperlipoproteinemia
    Coding Clinic: 1985, Jan-Feb, P15

272.2 Mixed hyperlipidemia
    Broad- or floating-betalipoproteinemia
    Combined hyperlipidemia
    Elevated cholesterol with elevated triglycerides NEC
    Fredrickson Type IIb or III hyperlipoproteinemia
    Hypercholesterolemia with endogenous hyperglyceridemia
    Hyperbetalipoproteinemia with prebetalipoproteinemia
    Tubo-eruptive xanthoma
    Xanthoma tuberosum

272.3 Hyperchylomicronemia
    Bürger-Grütz syndrome
    Fredrickson type I or V hyperlipoproteinemia
    Hyperlipidemia, Group D
    Mixed hyperglyceridemia

272.4 Other and unspecified hyperlipidemia
    Alpha-lipoproteinemia
    Hyperlipidemia NOS
    Hyperlipoproteinemia NOS
    Coding Clinic: 2005, Q1, P17

272.5 Lipoprotein deficiencies
    Abetalipoproteinemia
    Bassen-Kornzweig syndrome
    High-density lipoid deficiency
    Hypoalphalipoproteinemia
    Hypobetalipoproteinemia (familial)

ENDOCRINE, NUTRITIONAL AND METABOLIC DISEASES, AND IMMUNITY DISORDERS (240–279)

272.6 Lipodystrophy
Barraquer-Simons disease
Progressive lipodystrophy
Use additional E code to identify cause, if iatrogenic
Excludes intestinal lipodystrophy (040.2)

272.7 Lipidoses
Chemically induced lipidosis
Disease:
  Anderson's
  Fabry's
  Gaucher's
  I cell [mucolipidosis I]
  lipoid storage NOS
  Niemann-Pick
  pseudo-Hurler's or mucolipidosis III
  triglyceride storage, Type I or II
  Wolman's or triglyceride storage, Type III
Mucolipidosis II
Primary familial xanthomatosis
Excludes cerebral lipidoses (330.1)
    Tay-Sachs disease (330.1)

272.8 Other disorders of lipoid metabolism
Hoffa's disease or liposynovitis prepatellaris
Launois-Bensaude's lipomatosis
Lipoid dermatoarthritis

272.9 Unspecified disorder of lipoid metabolism

273 Disorders of plasma protein metabolism
Excludes agammaglobulinemia and hypogammaglobulinemia (279.0–279.2)
    coagulation defects (286.0–286.9)
    hereditary hemolytic anemias (282.0–282.9)

273.0 Polyclonal hypergammaglobulinemia
Hypergammaglobulinemic purpura:
  benign primary
  Waldenström's

273.1 Monoclonal paraproteinemia
Benign monoclonal hypergammaglobulinemia [BMH]
Monoclonal gammopathy:
  NOS
  associated with lymphoplasmacytic dyscrasias
  benign
Paraproteinemia:
  benign (familial)
  secondary to malignant or inflammatory disease

273.2 Other paraproteinemias
Cryoglobulinemic:
  purpura
  vasculitis
Mixed cryoglobulinemia
Coding Clinic: 2008, Q2, P17

273.3 Macroglobulinemia
Macroglobulinemia (idiopathic) (primary)
Waldenström's macroglobulinemia

273.4 Alpha-1-antitrypsin deficiency
AAT deficiency
Coding Clinic: 2004, Q4, P59-60

273.8 Other disorders of plasma protein metabolism
Abnormality of transport protein
Bisalbuminemia
Coding Clinic: 1998, Q2, P11

273.9 Unspecified disorder of plasma protein metabolism
Coding Clinic: 1998, Q2, P11

274 Gout
Result of accumulation of uric acid caused by either too much production, or insufficient natural removal of uric acid from body. Results in swollen, red, hot, painful, stiff joints. Also called gouty arthritis.
Excludes lead gout (984.0–984.9)

274.0 Gouty arthropathy
274.00 Gouty arthropathy, unspecified
274.01 Acute gouty arthropathy
  Acute gout   Gout flare
  Gout attack   Podagra
274.02 Chronic gouty arthropathy without mention of tophus (tophi)
  Chronic gout
274.03 Chronic gouty arthropathy with tophus (tophi)
  Chronic tophaceous gout
  Gout with tophi NOS
  Coding Clinic: 2009, Q4, P84

274.1 Gouty nephropathy
274.10 Gouty nephropathy, unspecified
  Coding Clinic: 1985, Nov-Dec, P15
274.11 Uric acid nephrolithiasis
274.19 Other

274.8 Gout with other specified manifestations
Tophi = chalky deposit of sodium urate occurring in gout
274.81 Gouty tophi of ear
274.82 Gouty tophi of other sites
  Gouty tophi of heart
  Excludes gout with tophi NOS (274.03)
    gouty arthropathy with tophi (274.03)
274.89 Other
  Use additional code to identify manifestations, as:
  gouty:
    iritis (364.11)
    neuritis (357.4)

274.9 Gout, unspecified

275 Disorders of mineral metabolism
Excludes abnormal findings without manifest disease (790.0–796.9)

275.0 Disorders of iron metabolism
Bronzed diabetes
Hemochromatosis
Pigmentary cirrhosis (of liver)
Excludes anemia:
  iron deficiency (280.0–280.9)
  sideroblastic (285.0)
Coding Clinic: 1997, Q2, P11
275.01 Hereditary hemochromatosis ◄
  Bronzed diabetes ◄
  Pigmentary cirrhosis (of liver) ◄
  Primary (hereditary) hemochromatosis ◄
275.02 Hemochromatosis due to repeated red blood cell transfusions ◄
  Iron overload due to repeated red blood cell transfusions ◄
  Transfusion (red blood cell) associated hemochromatosis ◄
275.03 Other hemochromatosis ◄
  Hemochromatosis NOS ◄
275.09 Other disorders of iron metabolism ◄

275.1 Disorders of copper metabolism
Hepatolenticular degeneration
Wilson's disease

275.2 Disorders of magnesium metabolism
Hypermagnesemia   Hypomagnesemia
Coding Clinic: 2010, Q1, P3-4; 2009, Q3, P6

275.3 Disorders of phosphorus metabolism
Familial hypophosphatemia
Hypophosphatasia
Vitamin D-resistant:
   osteomalacia
   rickets

● **275.4 Disorders of calcium metabolism**

Excludes	*hungry bone syndrome (275.5)*
	parathyroid disorders (252.00–252.9)
	vitamin D deficiency (268.0–268.9)

275.40 Unspecified disorder of calcium metabolism

275.41 Hypocalcemia
Coding Clinic: 2007, Q3, P5-6

275.42 Hypercalcemia
Coding Clinic: 2003, Q4, P110

275.49 Other disorders of calcium metabolism
Nephrocalcinosis
Pseudohypoparathyroidism
Pseudopseudohypoparathyroidism

275.5 Hungry bone syndrome
Coding Clinic: 2008, Q4, P96-97

275.8 Other specified disorders of mineral metabolism

275.9 Unspecified disorder of mineral metabolism

● **276 Disorders of fluid, electrolyte, and acid-base balance**

Excludes	*diabetes insipidus (253.5)*
	familial periodic paralysis (359.3)

276.0 Hyperosmolality and/or hypernatremia
Sodium [Na] excess   Sodium [Na] overload

276.1 Hyposmolality and/or hyponatremia
Sodium [Na] deficiency

276.2 Acidosis
Acidosis:
   NOS   metabolic
   lactic   respiratory

Excludes	*diabetic acidosis (249.1, 250.1)*

Coding Clinic: 1987, Jan-Feb, P15

276.3 Alkalosis
Alkalosis:
   NOS   respiratory
   metabolic

276.4 Mixed acid-base balance disorder
Hypercapnia with mixed acid-base disorder

● **276.5 Volume depletion**

Excludes	*hypovolemic shock:*
	postoperative (998.0)
	traumatic (958.4)

Coding Clinic: 2005, Q4, P54-55; Q2, P9-10; 2003, Q1, P5, 20-22;
    2002, Q3, P21x2; 1997, Q4, P30-31; 1993, 5th Issue, P1;
    1988, Q2, P9-11; 1984, July-Aug, P19-20

276.50 Volume depletion, unspecified

276.51 Dehydration
Coding Clinic: 2008, Q1, P10-11

276.52 Hypovolemia
Depletion of volume of plasma

Item 3–9 Circulating fluid volume is regulated by the amount of water and sodium ingested, excreted by the kidneys into the urine, and lost through the gastrointestinal tract, lungs, and skin. To maintain blood volume within a normal range, the kidneys regulate the amount of water and sodium lost into the urine. Too much (**fluid overload**) or too little fluid volume (**volume depletion**) will affect blood pressure. Severe cases of vomiting, diarrhea, bleeding, and burns (fluid loss through exposed burn surface area) can contribute to fluid loss. Internal body environment must maintain a precise balance (homeostasis) between too much fluid and too little fluid. This complex balancing mechanism is critical to good health.

● **276.6 Fluid overload** ◀▦
~~Fluid retention~~

Excludes	*ascites (789.51–789.59)*
	localized edema (782.3)

Coding Clinic: 2007, Q3, P11; 2006, Q4, P136; 1987, Sept-Oct, P9

276.61 Transfusion associated circulatory overload ◀
Fluid overload due to transfusion (blood)
   (blood components) ◀
TACO ◀

276.69 Other fluid overload ◀
Fluid retention ◀

276.7 Hyperpotassemia
Hyperkalemia
Potassium [K]:   Potassium [K]:
   excess   overload
   intoxication
Coding Clinic: 2005, Q1, P9-10; 2001, Q2, P12-13

276.8 Hypopotassemia
Hypokalemia
Potassium [K] deficiency

276.9 Electrolyte and fluid disorders not elsewhere classified
Electrolyte imbalance
Hyperchloremia
Hypochloremia

Excludes	*electrolyte imbalance:*
	associated with hyperemesis gravidarum (643.1)
	complicating labor and delivery (669.0)
	following abortion and ectopic or molar pregnancy (634–638 with .4, 639.4)

Coding Clinic: 1987, Jan-Feb, P15

● **277 Other and unspecified disorders of metabolism**

● **277.0 Cystic fibrosis**
Fibrocystic disease of the pancreas
Mucoviscidosis
Coding Clinic: 2002, Q4, P45-46; 1994, Q3, P7; 1990, Q3, P18

277.00 Without mention of meconium ileus
Cystic fibrosis NOS
Coding Clinic: 2003, Q2, P12

277.01 With meconium ileus
Meconium:
   ileus (of newborn)
   obstruction of intestine in mucoviscidosis

277.02 With pulmonary manifestations
Cystic fibrosis with pulmonary exacerbation
Use additional code to identify any
      infectious organism present, such as:
   pseudomonas (041.7)
Coding Clinic: 2002, Q4, P46

277.03 With gastrointestinal manifestations

Excludes	*with meconium ileus (277.01)*

277.09 With other manifestations

ENDOCRINE, NUTRITIONAL AND METABOLIC DISEASES, AND IMMUNITY DISORDERS (240–279)

277.1 Disorders of porphyrin metabolism
Hematoporphyria   Porphyrinuria
Hematoporphyrinuria   Protocoproporphyria
Hereditary coproporphyria   Protoporphyria
Porphyria   Pyrroloporphyria

277.2 Other disorders of purine and pyrimidine metabolism
Hypoxanthine-guanine-phosphoribosyltransferase deficiency [HG-PRT deficiency]
Lesch-Nyhan syndrome
Xanthinuria

> **Excludes** *gout (274.00–274.9)*
> *orotic aciduric anemia (281.4)*

● **277.3 Amyloidosis**
Disorder resulting from abnormal deposition of particular protein (amyloid) into tissues.
Coding Clinic: 2006, Q4, P66-67; 1997, Q2, P12-13; 1996, Q1, P16; 1985, July-Aug, P9

277.30 Amyloidosis, unspecified
Amyloidosis NOS

277.31 Familial Mediterranean fever
Benign paroxysmal peritonitis
Hereditary amyloid nephropathy
Periodic familial polyserositis
Recurrent polyserositis

277.39 Other amyloidosis
Hereditary cardiac amyloidosis
Inherited systemic amyloidosis
Neuropathic (Portuguese) (Swiss) amyloidosis
Secondary amyloidosis
Coding Clinic: 2009, Q1, P17; 2008, Q2, P8-9

277.4 Disorders of bilirubin excretion
Hyperbilirubinemia: Syndrome:
  congenital   Crigler-Najjar
  constitutional   Dubin-Johnson
                  Gilbert's
                  Rotor's

> **Excludes** *hyperbilirubinemias specific to the perinatal period (774.0–774.7)*

277.5 Mucopolysaccharidosis
Gargoylism
Hunter's syndrome
Hurler's syndrome
Lipochondrodystrophy
Maroteaux-Lamy syndrome
Morquio-Brailsford disease
Osteochondrodystrophy
Sanfilippo's syndrome
Scheie's syndrome

277.6 Other deficiencies of circulating enzymes
Hereditary angioedema
Coding Clinic: 2004, Q4, P59-60

277.7 Dysmetabolic syndrome X
Use additional code for associated manifestation, such as:
cardiovascular disease (414.00–414.07)
obesity (278.00–278.03) ◀▥
Coding Clinic: 2001, Q4, P42

● **277.8 Other specified disorders of metabolism**
Coding Clinic: 2003, Q4, P50-51; 2001, Q2, P18-20

277.81 Primary carnitine deficiency

277.82 Carnitine deficiency due to inborn errors of metabolism

277.83 Iatrogenic carnitine deficiency
Carnitine deficiency due to:
Hemodialysis
Valproic acid therapy

277.84 Other secondary carnitine deficiency

277.85 Disorders of fatty acid oxidation
Carnitine palmitoyltransferase deficiencies (CPT1, CPT2)
Glutaric aciduria type II (type IIA, IIB, IIC)
Long chain 3-hydroxyacyl CoA dehydrogenase deficiency (LCHAD)
Long chain/very long chain acyl CoA dehydrogenase deficiency (LCAD, VLCAD)
Medium chain acyl CoA dehydrogenase deficiency (MCAD)
Short chain acyl CoA dehydrogenase deficiency (SCAD)

> **Excludes** *primary carnitine deficiency (277.81)*

Coding Clinic: 2004, Q4, P60-61

277.86 Peroxisomal disorders
Adrenomyeloneuropathy
Neonatal adrenoleukodystrophy
Rhizomelic chondrodysplasia punctata
X-linked adrenoleukodystrophy
Zellweger syndrome

> **Excludes** *infantile Refsum disease (356.3)*

Coding Clinic: 2004, Q4, P61-62

277.87 Disorders of mitochondrial metabolism
Kearns-Sayre syndrome
Mitochondrial Encephalopathy, Lactic Acidosis and Stroke-like episodes (MELAS syndrome)
Mitochondrial Neurogastrointestinal Encephalopathy syndrome (MNGIE)
Myoclonus with Epilepsy and with Ragged Red Fibers (MERRF syndrome)
Neuropathy, Ataxia and Retinitis Pigmentosa (NARP syndrome)

Use additional code for associated conditions

> **Excludes** *disorders of pyruvate metabolism (271.8)*
> *Leber's optic atrophy (377.16)*
> *Leigh's subacute necrotizing encephalopathy (330.8)*
> *Reye's syndrome (331.81)*

Coding Clinic: 2004, Q4, P62-63

277.88 Tumor lysis syndrome
Spontaneous tumor lysis syndrome
Tumor lysis syndrome following antineoplastic drug therapy

Use additional E code to identify cause, if drug-induced
Coding Clinic: 2009, Q4, P84

277.89 Other specified disorders of metabolism
Hand-Schüller-Christian disease
Histiocytosis (acute) (chronic)
Histiocytosis X (chronic)

> **Excludes** *histiocytosis:*
> *acute differentiated progressive (202.5)*
> *X, acute (progressive) (202.5)*

277.9 Unspecified disorder of metabolism
Enzymopathy NOS
Coding Clinic: 1987, Sept-Oct, P9

● **278 Overweight, obesity and other hyperalimentation**

     Excludes   *hyperalimentation NOS (783.6)*
                       poisoning by vitamins NOS (963.5)
                       polyphagia (783.6)

● **278.0 Overweight and obesity**

     Excludes   *adiposogenital dystrophy (253.8)*
                       obesity of endocrine origin NOS (259.9)

     Use additional code to identify Body Mass Index
         (BMI), if known (V85.0–V85.54)
         Coding Clinic: 2005, Q4, P55

     278.00 Obesity, unspecified
          Obesity NOS
          Coding Clinic: 2001, Q4, P42; 1999, Q1, P5-6

     278.01 Morbid obesity
          Severe obesity
          Coding Clinic: 2009, Q2, P11; 2006, Q2, P5-6; 2003, Q3,
          P3-8

     278.02 Overweight

     278.03 Obesity hypoventilation syndrome ◄
          Pickwickian syndrome ◄

   278.1 Localized adiposity
        Fat pad
        Coding Clinic: 2006, Q2, P10-11

   278.2 Hypervitaminosis A

   278.3 Hypercarotinemia

   278.4 Hypervitaminosis D

   278.8 Other hyperalimentation
        Coding Clinic: 2009, Q2, P11

● **279 Disorders involving the immune mechanism**

     Use additional code for associated manifestations ◄

● **279.0 Deficiency of humoral immunity**

     279.00 Hypogammaglobulinemia, unspecified
          Agammaglobulinemia NOS

     279.01 Selective IgA immunodeficiency

     279.02 Selective IgM immunodeficiency

     **279.03 Other selective immunoglobulin
           deficiencies**
          Selective deficiency of IgG

     279.04 Congenital hypogammaglobulinemia
          Agammaglobulinemia:
             Bruton's type
             X-linked

     279.05 Immunodeficiency with increased IgM
          Immunodeficiency with hyper-IgM:
             autosomal recessive
             X-linked

     279.06 Common variable immunodeficiency
          Dysgammaglobulinemia (acquired)
             (congenital) (primary)
          Hypogammaglobulinemia:
             acquired primary
             congenital non-sex-linked
             sporadic

     279.09 Other
          Transient hypogammaglobulinemia of
             infancy

● **279.1 Deficiency of cell-mediated immunity**

     **279.10 Immunodeficiency with predominant T-cell
           defect, unspecified**
          Coding Clinic: 1987, Sept-Oct, P10; 1985, Mar-April, P7

     279.11 DiGeorge's syndrome
          Pharyngeal pouch syndrome
          Thymic hypoplasia

     279.12 Wiskott-Aldrich syndrome

     279.13 Nezelof's syndrome
          Cellular immunodeficiency with abnormal
             immunoglobulin deficiency

     279.19 Other

          Excludes   *ataxia-telangiectasia (334.8)*

          Coding Clinic: 1985, Mar-April, P7

   279.2 Combined immunity deficiency
        Agammaglobulinemia:
           autosomal recessive
           Swiss-type
           X-linked recessive
        Severe combined immunodeficiency [SCID]
        Thymic:
           alymphoplasia
           aplasia or dysplasia with immunodeficiency

        Excludes   *thymic hypoplasia (279.11)*

   279.3 Unspecified immunity deficiency

● **279.4 Autoimmune disease, not elsewhere classified**

        Excludes   *transplant failure or rejection*
                          (996.80–996.89)

        Coding Clinic: 2008, Q3, P5

     **279.41 Autoimmune lymphoproliferative
           syndrome**
          ALPS

     **279.49 Autoimmune disease, not elsewhere
           classified**
          Autoimmune disease NOS

● **279.5 Graft-versus-host disease**

     Code first *underlying cause, such as:*
          complication of blood transfusion (999.89)
          complication of transplanted organ
             (996.80-996.89)

     Use additional code to identify associated
          manifestations, such as:
          desquamative dermatitis (695.89)
          diarrhea (787.91)
          elevated bilirubin (782.4)
          hair loss (704.09)
     Coding Clinic: 2008, Q4, P97-100

    ● **279.50 Graft-versus-host disease, unspecified**

    ● **279.51 Acute graft-versus-host disease**

    ● **279.52 Chronic graft-versus-host disease**

    ● **279.53 Acute on chronic graft-versus-host
           disease**

   **279.8 Other specified disorders involving the immune
        mechanism**
        Single complement $[C_1-C_9]$ deficiency or dysfunction

   279.9 Unspecified disorder of immune mechanism
        Coding Clinic: 1996, Q2, P12; 1992, Q3, P13-14

ENDOCRINE, NUTRITIONAL AND METABOLIC DISEASES, AND IMMUNITY DISORDERS (240–279)

DISEASES OF THE BLOOD AND BLOOD-FORMING ORGANS (280–289)

4. DISEASES OF THE BLOOD AND BLOOD-FORMING ORGANS (280–289)

● **280 Iron deficiency anemias**

Disease characterized by decrease in number of red cells (hemoglobin) in blood, diminishing body's ability to carry adequate amounts of oxygen to cells.

Includes   anemia:
    asiderotic
    hypochromic-microcytic
    sideropenic

Excludes *familial microcytic anemia (282.49)*

280.0 Secondary to blood loss (chronic)
    Normocytic anemia due to blood loss

    Excludes *acute posthemorrhagic anemia (285.1)*
    Coding Clinic: 1993, Q4, P34; 1985, July-Aug, P13

280.1 Secondary to inadequate dietary iron intake

280.8 Other specified iron deficiency anemias
    Paterson-Kelly syndrome
    Plummer-Vinson syndrome
    Sideropenic dysphagia

280.9 Iron deficiency anemia, unspecified
    Anemia:
        achlorhydric
        chlorotic
        idiopathic hypochromic
        iron [Fe] deficiency NOS

● **281 Other deficiency anemias**

281.0 Pernicious anemia
    Anemia:
        Addison's
        Biermer's
        congenital pernicious
    Congenital intrinsic factor [Castle's] deficiency

    Excludes *combined system disease without mention of anemia (266.2)*
          subacute degeneration of spinal cord without mention of anemia (266.2)

281.1 Other vitamin B$_{12}$ deficiency anemia
    Anemia:
        vegan's
        vitamin B$_{12}$ deficiency (dietary)
        due to selective vitamin B$_{12}$ malabsorption with proteinuria
    Syndrome:
        Imerslund's
        Imerslund-Gräsbeck

    Excludes *combined system disease without mention of anemia (266.2)*
          subacute degeneration of spinal cord without mention of anemia (266.2)

281.2 Folate-deficiency anemia
    Congenital folate malabsorption
    Folate or folic acid deficiency anemia:
        NOS
        dietary
        drug-induced
    Goat's milk anemia
    Nutritional megaloblastic anemia (of infancy)

    Use additional E code to identify drug

281.3 Other specified megaloblastic anemias, not elsewhere classified
    Combined B$_{12}$ and folate-deficiency anemia

281.4 Protein-deficiency anemia
    Amino-acid-deficiency anemia

281.8 Anemia associated with other specified nutritional deficiency
    Scorbutic anemia

281.9 Unspecified deficiency anemia
    Anemia:
        dimorphic
        macrocytic
        megaloblastic NOS
        nutritional NOS
        simple chronic
    Coding Clinic: 1984, Sept-Oct, P16

● **282 Hereditary hemolytic anemias**

Genetic condition in which bone marrow is unable to compensate for premature destruction of red blood cells

282.0 Hereditary spherocytosis
    Acholuric (familial) jaundice
    Congenital hemolytic anemia (spherocytic)
    Congenital spherocytosis
    Minkowski-Chauffard syndrome
    Spherocytosis (familial)

    Excludes *hemolytic anemia of newborn (773.0–773.5)*

282.1 Hereditary elliptocytosis
    Elliptocytosis (congenital)
    Ovalocytosis (congenital) (hereditary)

282.2 Anemias due to disorders of glutathione metabolism
    Anemia:
        6-phosphogluconic dehydrogenase deficiency
        enzyme deficiency, drug-induced
        erythrocytic glutathione deficiency
        glucose-6-phosphate dehydrogenase [G-6-PD] deficiency
        glutathione-reductase deficiency
        hemolytic nonspherocytic (hereditary), type I
    Disorder of pentose phosphate pathway
    Favism

282.3 Other hemolytic anemias due to enzyme deficiency
    Anemia:
        hemolytic nonspherocytic (hereditary), type II
        hexokinase deficiency
        pyruvate kinase [PK] deficiency
        triosephosphate isomerase deficiency

● **282.4 Thalassemias**

Hereditary disorders characterized by low production of hemoglobin or excessive destruction of red blood cells

    Excludes *sickle-cell:*
        disease (282.60–282.69)
        trait (282.5)
    Coding Clinic: 2003, Q4, P51-56

282.41 Sickle-cell thalassemia without crisis
    Sickle-cell thalassemia NOS
    Thalassemia Hb-S disease without crisis

282.42 Sickle-cell thalassemia with crisis
    Sickle-cell thalassemia with vaso-occlusive pain
    Thalassemia Hb-S disease with crisis

    Use additional code for type of crisis, such as:
        Acute chest syndrome (517.3)
        Splenic sequestration (289.52)
        Occurs when sickled red blood cells become entrapped in spleen, causing splenomegaly (enlargement) and decreased circulating blood volume.

◄ New   ◄▪▪ Revised   ~~deleted~~ Deleted   Excludes   Includes   Use additional   Code first   Omit code
● Unacceptable Principal Diagnosis   ● Use Additional Digit(s)   OGCR Official Guidelines   Coding Clinic

282.49 Other thalassemia
Cooley's anemia
Hb-Bart's disease
Hereditary leptocytosis
Mediterranean anemia (with other
 hemoglobinopathy)
Microdrepanocytosis
Thalassemia (alpha) (beta) (intermedia)
 (major) (minima) (minor) (mixed)
 (trait) (with other hemoglobinopathy)
Thalassemia NOS

282.5 Sickle-cell trait
Hb-AS genotype
Hemoglobin S [Hb-S] trait
Heterozygous:
 hemoglobin S
 Hb-S

> **Excludes** *that with other hemoglobinopathy*
> *(282.60–282.69)*
> *that with thalassemia (282.49)*
> Coding Clinic: 2003, Q4, P51-56

● **282.6 Sickle-cell disease**
*Inherited disease in which red blood cells, normally
disc-shaped, become crescent shaped. Small blood
clots form, resulting in painful episodes called
sickle cell crises.*
Sickle-cell anemia

> **Excludes** *sickle-cell thalassemia (282.41–282.42)*
> *sickle-cell trait (282.5)*

282.60 Sickle-cell disease, unspecified
Sickle-cell anemia NOS
Coding Clinic: 1997, Q2, P11

282.61 Hb-SS disease without crisis
Coding Clinic: 2007, Q2, P9-10

282.62 Hb-SS disease with crisis
Hb-SS disease with vaso-occlusive pain
Sickle-cell crisis NOS
> Use additional code for type of crisis, such
> as:
> Acute chest syndrome (517.3)
> Splenic sequestration (289.52)
> Coding Clinic: 2003, Q4, P51-56; 1998, Q2, P8; 1991, Q2,
> P15

282.63 Sickle-cell/Hb-C disease without crisis
Hb-S/Hb-C disease without crisis

282.64 Sickle-cell/Hb-C disease with crisis
Hb-S/Hb-C disease with crisis
Sickle-cell/Hb-C disease with
 vaso-occlusive pain
> Use additional code for types of crisis,
> such as:
> Acute chest syndrome (517.3)
> Splenic sequestration (289.52)

282.68 Other sickle-cell disease without crisis
Hb-S/Hb-D disease without crisis
Hb-S/Hb-E disease without crisis
Sickle-cell/Hb-D disease without crisis
Sickle-cell/Hb-E disease without crisis

282.69 Other sickle-cell disease with crisis
Hb-S/Hb-D disease with crisis
Hb-S/Hb-E disease with crisis
Other sickle-cell disease with vaso-occlusive
 pain
Sickle-cell/Hb-D disease with crisis
Sickle-cell/Hb-E disease with crisis
> Use additional code for type of crisis, such
> as:
> Acute chest syndrome (517.3)
> Splenic sequestration (289.52)

282.7 Other hemoglobinopathies
Abnormal hemoglobin NOS
Congenital Heinz-body anemia
Disease:
 hemoglobin C [Hb-C]
 hemoglobin D [Hb-D]
 hemoglobin E [Hb-E]
 hemoglobin Zurich [Hb-Zurich]
Hemoglobinopathy NOS
Hereditary persistence of fetal hemoglobin
 [HPFH]
Unstable hemoglobin hemolytic disease
> **Excludes** *familial polycythemia (289.6)*
> *hemoglobin M [Hb-M] disease (289.7)*
> *high-oxygen-affinity hemoglobin (289.0)*

282.8 Other specified hereditary hemolytic anemias
Stomatocytosis

282.9 Hereditary hemolytic anemia, unspecified
Hereditary hemolytic anemia NOS

● **283 Acquired hemolytic anemias**
*Also known as autoimmune hemolytic or Coombs positive
hemolytic anemia. The red blood cells produced are
healthy but are destroyed when trapped in the spleen by
infection or certain drugs.*

283.0 Autoimmune hemolytic anemias
Autoimmune hemolytic disease (cold type) (warm
 type)
Chronic cold hemagglutinin disease
Cold agglutinin disease or hemoglobinuria
Hemolytic anemia:
 cold type (secondary) (symptomatic)
 drug-induced
 warm type (secondary) (symptomatic)
> Use additional E code to identify cause, if
> drug-induced
> **Excludes** *Evans' syndrome (287.32)*
> *hemolytic disease of newborn (773.0–773.5)*
> Coding Clinic: 2008, Q3, P5

● **283.1 Non-autoimmune hemolytic anemias**

**283.10 Non-autoimmune hemolytic anemia,
unspecified**

283.11 Hemolytic-uremic syndrome

283.19 Other non-autoimmune hemolytic anemias
Hemolytic anemia:
 mechanical
 microangiopathic
 toxic
> Use additional E code to identify cause

**283.2 Hemoglobinuria due to hemolysis from external
causes**
Acute intravascular hemolysis
Hemoglobinuria:
 from exertion
 march
 paroxysmal (cold) (nocturnal)
 due to other hemolysis
Marchiafava-Micheli syndrome
> Use additional E code to identify cause

283.9 Acquired hemolytic anemia, unspecified
Acquired hemolytic anemia NOS
Chronic idiopathic hemolytic anemia

DISEASES OF THE BLOOD AND BLOOD-FORMING ORGANS (280–289)

DISEASES OF THE BLOOD AND BLOOD-FORMING ORGANS (280–289)

● **284 Aplastic anemia and other bone marrow failure syndromes**
Coding Clinic: 2006, Q4, P67-69

● **284.0 Constitutional aplastic anemia**
Coding Clinic: 1991, Q1, P14

284.01 Constitutional red blood cell aplasia
Aplasia, (pure) red cell:
congenital
of infants
primary
Blackfan-Diamond syndrome
Familial hypoplastic anemia

284.09 Other constitutional aplastic anemia
Fanconi's anemia
Pancytopenia with malformations

284.1 Pancytopenia
Marked deficiency of all the blood elements: Red blood cells (erythrocytes), white blood cells (leukocytes), and platelets (thrombocytes). Check laboratory results.

Excludes *pancytopenia (due to) (with):*
aplastic anemia NOS (284.9)
bone marrow infiltration (284.2)
constitutional red blood cell aplasia (284.01)
drug induced (284.89)
hairy cell leukemia (202.4)
human immunodeficiency virus disease (042)
leukoerythroblastic anemia (284.2)
malformations (284.09)
myelodysplastic syndromes (238.72–238.75)
myeloproliferative disease (238.79)
other constitutional aplastic anemia (284.09)
Coding Clinic: 2005, Q3, P11-12

284.2 Myelophthisis
Leukoerythroblastic anemia
Myelophthisic anemia

Code first the underlying disorder, such as:
malignant neoplasm of breast (174.0–174.9, 175.0–175.9)
tuberculosis (015.0–015.9)

Excludes *idiopathic myelofibrosis (238.76)*
myelofibrosis NOS (289.83)
myelofibrosis with myeloid metaplasia (238.76)
primary myelofibrosis (238.76)
secondary myelofibrosis (289.83)

● **284.8 Other specified aplastic anemias**
Coding Clinic: 2007, Q4, P72-73; 2005, Q3, P11-12; 1997, Q1, P5-6; 1991, Q1, P14; 1984, Sept-Oct, P16

284.81 Red cell aplasia (acquired) (adult) (with thymoma)
Red cell aplasia NOS

284.89 Other specified aplastic anemias
Aplastic anemia (due to):
chronic systemic disease
drugs
infection
radiation
toxic (paralytic)
Use additional E code to identify cause
Coding Clinic: 2009, Q1, P17; 2008, Q2, P6

284.9 Aplastic anemia, unspecified
Anemia:
aplastic (idiopathic) NOS
aregenerative
hypoplastic NOS
nonregenerative
Medullary hypoplasia

Excludes *refractory anemia (238.72)*

● **285 Other and unspecified anemias**
Coding Clinic: 1990, Q3, P17

285.0 Sideroblastic anemia
Anemia:
hypochromic with iron loading
sideroachrestic
sideroblastic:
acquired
congenital
hereditary
primary
secondary (drug-induced) (due to disease)
sex-linked hypochromic
vitamin B_6-responsive
Pyridoxine-responsive (hypochromic) anemia

Excludes *refractory sideroblastic anemia (238.72)*

Use additional E code to identify cause, if drug-induced

285.1 Acute posthemorrhagic anemia
Anemia due to acute blood loss

Excludes *anemia due to chronic blood loss (280.0)*
blood loss anemia NOS (280.0)
Coding Clinic: 2007, Q1, P19; 2004, Q3, P4; 1993, Q4, P34; 1992, Q2, P15-16

● **285.2 Anemia of chronic disease**
Anemia in (due to) (with) chronic illness

285.21 Anemia in chronic kidney disease
Anemia in end stage renal disease
Erythropoietin-resistant anemia (EPO resistant anemia)
Coding Clinic: 2000, Q4, P39-40

285.22 Anemia in neoplastic disease

Excludes *anemia due to antineoplastic chemotherapy (285.3)*
aplastic anemia due to antineoplastic chemotherapy (284.89) ◄
Coding Clinic: 2009, Q4, P94x2; 2008, Q2, P6; 2000, Q4, P39-40

OGCR Section I.C.4.a.2

When assigning code 285.22, Anemia in neoplastic disease, it is also necessary to assign the neoplasm code that is responsible for the anemia. Code 285.22 is for use for anemia that is due to the malignancy, not for anemia due to antineoplastic chemotherapy drugs, assign code 285.3 for anemia due to antineoplastic chemotherapy.

285.29 Anemia of other chronic disease
Anemia in other chronic illness

285.3 Antineoplastic chemotherapy induced anemia
Anemia due to antineoplastic chemotherapy

Excludes *anemia due to drug NEC – code to type of anemia*
anemia in neoplastic disease (285.22)
aplastic anemia due to antineoplastic chemotherapy (284.89)
Coding Clinic: 2009, Q4, P94x2

◄ New   ◄▥ Revised   ~~deleted~~ Deleted   Excludes   Includes   Use additional   Code first   Omit code
● Unacceptable Principal Diagnosis   ● Use Additional Digit(s)   OGCR Official Guidelines   Coding Clinic

285.8 Other specified anemias
Anemia:
dyserythropoietic (congenital)
dyshematopoietic (congenital)
von Jaksch's
Infantile pseudoleukemia

285.9 Anemia, unspecified
Anemia:
NOS
essential
normocytic, not due to blood loss
profound
progressive
secondary
Oligocythemia

| **Excludes** | anemia (due to): |
blood loss:
acute (285.1)
chronic or unspecified (280.0)
iron deficiency (280.0–280.9)
Coding Clinic: 2009, Q1, P17x2; 2007, Q1, P19; 2002, Q1, P14; 1992, Q2, P15-16; 1985, Mar-April, P13

● **286 Coagulation defects**
Can be acquired or genetic and results in inability to control blood clotting. Most common genetic coagulation disorder is hemophilia.
Coding Clinic: 2006, Q2, P17; 1992, Q3, P15

286.0 Congenital factor VIII disorder
Antihemophilic globulin [AHG] deficiency
Factor VIII (functional) deficiency
Hemophilia:
NOS
A
classical
familial
hereditary
Subhemophilia

| **Excludes** | factor VIII deficiency with vascular defect (286.4)

286.1 Congenital factor IX disorder
Christmas disease
Deficiency:
factor IX (functional)
plasma thromboplastin component [PTC]
Hemophilia B

286.2 Congenital factor XI deficiency
Hemophilia C
Plasma thromboplastin antecedent [PTA] deficiency
Rosenthal's disease

286.3 Congenital deficiency of other clotting factors
Congenital afibrinogenemia
Deficiency:
AC globulin factor:
I [fibrinogen]
II [prothrombin]
V [labile]
VII [stable]
X [Stuart-Prower]
XII [Hageman]
XIII [fibrin stabilizing]
Laki-Lorand factor
proaccelerin
Disease:
Owren's
Stuart-Prower
Dysfibrinogenemia (congenital)
Dysprothrombinemia (constitutional)
Hypoproconvertinemia
Hypoprothrombinemia (hereditary)
Parahemophilia

286.4 von Willebrand's disease
Angiohemophilia (A) (B)
Constitutional thrombopathy
Factor VIII deficiency with vascular defect
Pseudohemophilia type B
Vascular hemophilia
von Willebrand's (-Jürgens') disease

| **Excludes** | factor VIII deficiency:
NOS (286.0)
with functional defect (286.0)
hereditary capillary fragility (287.8)

286.5 Hemorrhagic disorder due to intrinsic circulating anticoagulants
Antithrombinemia
Antithromboplastinemia
Antithromboplastino-genemia
Hyperheparinemia
Increase in:
anti-VIIIa
anti-IXa
anti-Xa
anti-XIa
antithrombin
Secondary hemophilia
Systemic lupus erythematosus [SLE] inhibitor
Coding Clinic: 2004, Q3, P7; 1994, Q1, P22; 1993, 5th Issue, P16; 1992, Q3, P15-16; 1990, Q3, P14

286.6 Defibrination syndrome
Afibrinogenemia, acquired
Consumption coagulopathy
Diffuse or disseminated intravascular coagulation [DIC syndrome]
Fibrinolytic hemorrhage, acquired
Hemorrhagic fibrinogenolysis
Pathologic fibrinolysis
Purpura:
fibrinolytic
fulminans

| **Excludes** | that complicating:
abortion (634–638 with .1, 639.1)
pregnancy or the puerperium (641.3, 666.3)
disseminated intravascular coagulation in newborn (776.2)

286.7 Acquired coagulation factor deficiency
Deficiency of coagulation factor due to:
liver disease
vitamin K deficiency
Hypoprothrombinemia, acquired

| **Excludes** | vitamin K deficiency of newborn (776.0)

Use additional E-code to identify cause, if drug-induced

286.9 Other and unspecified coagulation defects
Defective coagulation NOS
Deficiency, coagulation factor NOS
Delay, coagulation
Disorder:
coagulation
hemostasis

| **Excludes** | abnormal coagulation profile (790.92)
hemorrhagic disease of newborn (776.0)
that complicating:
abortion (634–638 with .1, 639.1)
pregnancy or the puerperium (641.3, 666.3)
Coding Clinic: 1999, Q4, P22-23

DISEASES OF THE BLOOD AND BLOOD-FORMING ORGANS (280–289)

DISEASES OF THE BLOOD AND BLOOD-FORMING ORGANS (280–289)

● 287 **Purpura and other hemorrhagic conditions**

| **Excludes** | *hemorrhagic thrombocythemia (238.79)* |
| | *purpura fulminans (286.6)* |

287.0 **Allergic purpura**
Peliosis rheumatica
Purpura:
anaphylactoid
autoimmune
Henoch's
nonthrombocytopenic:
hemorrhagic
idiopathic
rheumatica
Schönlein-Henoch
vascular
Vasculitis, allergic

| **Excludes** | *hemorrhagic purpura (287.39)* |
| | *purpura annularis telangiectodes (709.1)* |

287.1 **Qualitative platelet defects**
Thrombasthenia (hemorrhagic) (hereditary)
Thrombocytasthenia
Thrombocytopathy (dystrophic)
Thrombopathy (Bernard-Soulier)

| **Excludes** | *von Willebrand's disease (286.4)* |

287.2 **Other nonthrombocytopenic purpuras**
Purpura:
NOS
senile
simplex

● 287.3 **Primary thrombocytopenia**
Also known as idiopathic thrombocytopenia, may be acquired or congenital and is a common cause of coagulation disorders.

| **Excludes** | *thrombotic thrombocytopenic purpura (446.6)* |
| | *transient thrombocytopenia of newborn (776.1)* |

Thrombo = clot forming, cyto = cell, penia = deficiency of: deficiency of platelets.

287.30 **Primary thrombocytopenia unspecified**
Megakaryocytic hypoplasia

287.31 **Immune thrombocytopenic purpura**
Idiopathic thrombocytopenic purpura
Tidal platelet dysgenesis
Coding Clinic: 2005, Q4, P56-57

287.32 **Evans' syndrome**

287.33 **Congenital and hereditary thrombocytopenic purpura**
Congenital and hereditary thrombocytopenia
Thrombocytopenia with absent radii (TAR) syndrome

| **Excludes** | *Wiskott-Aldrich syndrome (279.12)* |

287.39 **Other primary thrombocytopenia**

● 287.4 **Secondary thrombocytopenia** ◀▥
~~Posttransfusion purpura~~
~~Thrombocytopenia (due to):~~
~~dilutional~~
~~drugs~~
~~extracorporeal circulation of blood~~
~~massive blood transfusion~~
~~platelet alloimmunization~~

Use additional E code to identify cause

| **Excludes** | *heparin-induced thrombocytopenia (HIT) (289.84)* |
| | *transient thrombocytopenia of newborn (776.1)* |

Coding Clinic: 1985, July-Aug, P13; Mar-April, P14

287.41 **Posttransfusion purpura** ◀
Posttransfusion purpura from whole blood (fresh) or blood products ◀
PTP ◀

287.49 **Other secondary thrombocytopenia** ◀
Thrombocytopenia (due to): ◀
dilutional ◀
drugs ◀
extracorporeal circulation of blood ◀
massive blood transfusion ◀
platelet alloimmunization ◀
secondary NOS ◀

287.5 **Thrombocytopenia, unspecified**

287.8 **Other specified hemorrhagic conditions**
Capillary fragility (hereditary)
Vascular pseudohemophilia
Coding Clinic: 1985, Mar-April, P14

287.9 **Unspecified hemorrhagic conditions**
Hemorrhagic diathesis (familial)

● 288 **Diseases of white blood cells**

| **Excludes** | *leukemia (204.0–208.9)* |

● 288.0 **Neutropenia**
Decreased Absolute Neutrophil Count (ANC)

Use additional code for any associated:
fever (780.61)
mucositis (478.11, 528.00–528.09, 538, 616.81)

| **Excludes** | *neutropenic splenomegaly (289.53)* |
| | *transitory neonatal neutropenia (776.7)* |

Coding Clinic: 2005, Q3, P11-12; 1999, Q3, P6-7; 1996, Q3, P16; Q2, P6; 1985, Mar-April, P14

288.00 **Neutropenia, unspecified**

288.01 **Congenital neutropenia**
Congenital agranulocytosis
Infantile genetic agranulocytosis
Kostmann's syndrome

288.02 **Cyclic neutropenia**
Cyclic hematopoiesis
Periodic neutropenia

288.03 **Drug induced neutropenia**
Use additional E code to identify drug
Coding Clinic: 2006, Q4, P69-73

288.04 **Neutropenia due to infection**

288.09 **Other neutropenia**
Agranulocytosis
Neutropenia:
immune
toxic

◀ New   ◀▥ Revised   ~~deleted~~ Deleted   Excludes   Includes   Use additional   Code first   Omit code
● Unacceptable Principal Diagnosis   ● Use Additional Digit(s)   OGCR Official Guidelines   Coding Clinic

288.1 Functional disorders of polymorphonuclear neutrophils
    Chronic (childhood) granulomatous disease
    Congenital dysphagocytosis
    Job's syndrome
    Lipochrome histiocytosis (familial)
    Progressive septic granulomatosis

288.2 Genetic anomalies of leukocytes
    Anomaly (granulation) (granulocyte) or syndrome:
      Alder's (-Reilly)
      Chédiak-Steinbrinck (-Higashi)
      Jordan's
      May-Hegglin
      Pelger-Huet
    Hereditary:
      hypersegmentation
      hyposegmentation
      leukomelanopathy

288.3 Eosinophilia
    Eosinophilia
      allergic
      hereditary
      idiopathic
      secondary
    Eosinophilic leukocytosis

    Excludes | *Löffler's syndrome (518.3)*
                    pulmonary eosinophilia (518.3)
    Coding Clinic: 2000, Q3, P11

288.4 Hemophagocytic syndromes
    Familial hemophagocytic lymphohistiocytosis
    Familial hemophagocytic reticulosis
    Hemophagocytic syndrome, infection-associated
    Histiocytic syndromes
    Macrophage activation syndrome

● **288.5 Decreased white blood cell count**
    Excludes | *neutropenia (288.01–288.09)*

    288.50 Leukocytopenia, unspecified
        Decreased leukocytes, unspecified
        Decreased white blood cell count, unspecified
        Leukopenia NOS

    288.51 Lymphocytopenia
        Decreased lymphocytes

    288.59 Other decreased white blood cell count
        Basophilic leukopenia
        Eosinophilic leukopenia
        Monocytopenia
        Plasmacytopenia

● **288.6 Elevated white blood cell count**
    Excludes | *eosinophilia (288.3)*

    288.60 Leukocytosis, unspecified
        Elevated leukocytes, unspecified
        Elevated white blood cell count, unspecified

    288.61 Lymphocytosis (symptomatic)
        Elevated lymphocytes

    288.62 Leukemoid reaction
        Basophilic leukemoid reaction
        Lymphocytic leukemoid reaction
        Monocytic leukemoid reaction
        Myelocytic leukemoid reaction
        Neutrophilic leukemoid reaction

    288.63 Monocytosis (symptomatic)
        Excludes | *infectious mononucleosis (075)*

    288.64 Plasmacytosis

    288.65 Basophilia

    288.66 Bandemia
        Bandemia without diagnosis of specific infection

        Excludes | *confirmed infection – code to infection*
                       leukemia (204.00–208.9)
        Coding Clinic: 2007, Q4, P73-74

    288.69 Other elevated white blood cell count

288.8 Other specified disease of white blood cells
    Excludes | *decreased white blood cell counts (288.50–288.59)*
             elevated white blood cell counts (288.60–288.69)
             immunity disorders (279.0–279.9)
    Coding Clinic: 1987, Mar-April, P12

288.9 Unspecified disease of white blood cells

● **289 Other diseases of blood and blood-forming organs**

  289.0 Polycythemia, secondary
    See 238.4 for primary polycythemia (polycythemia vera)
    High-oxygen-affinity hemoglobin
    Polycythemia:
      acquired
      benign
      due to:
        fall in plasma volume
        high altitude
      emotional
      erythropoietin
      hypoxemic
      nephrogenous
      relative
      spurious
      stress

    Excludes | *polycythemia:*
                neonatal (776.4)
                primary (238.4)
                vera (238.4)

  289.1 Chronic lymphadenitis
    Chronic:
      adenitis any lymph node, except mesenteric
      lymphadenitis any lymph node, except mesenteric

    Excludes | *acute lymphadenitis (683)*
                mesenteric (289.2)
                enlarged glands NOS (785.6)

  289.2 Nonspecific mesenteric lymphadenitis
    Mesenteric lymphadenitis (acute) (chronic)

  289.3 Lymphadenitis, unspecified, except mesenteric
    Coding Clinic: 1992, Q2, P8

  289.4 Hypersplenism
    "Big spleen" syndrome
    Dyssplenism
    Hypersplenia

    Excludes | *primary splenic neutropenia (289.53)*

● **289.5 Other diseases of spleen**

    289.50 Disease of spleen, unspecified

    289.51 Chronic congestive splenomegaly

    289.52 Splenic sequestration
        Code first sickle-cell disease in crisis (282.42, 282.62, 282.64, 282.69)
        Coding Clinic: 2003, Q4, P51-56

    289.53 Neutropenic splenomegaly

DISEASES OF THE BLOOD AND BLOOD-FORMING ORGANS (280–289)

289.59 Other
Lien migrans
Perisplenitis
Splenic:
  abscess
  atrophy
  cyst
Splenic:
  fibrosis
  infarction
  rupture, nontraumatic
Splenitis
Wandering spleen

Excludes *bilharzial splenic fibrosis*
(120.0–120.9)
hepatolienal fibrosis (571.5)
splenomegaly NOS (789.2)

289.6 Familial polycythemia
Familial:
  benign polycythemia
  erythrocytosis

289.7 Methemoglobinemia
Congenital NADH
  [DPNH]-methemoglobin-reductase deficiency
Hemoglobin M [Hb-M] disease
Methemoglobinemia:
  NOS
  acquired (with sulfhemoglobinemia)
  hereditary
  toxic
Stokvis' disease
Sulfhemoglobinemia

Use additional E code to identify cause

● **289.8 Other specified diseases of blood and blood-forming organs**
Coding Clinic: 2003, Q4, P56-57; 2002, Q1, P16-17; 1987, Mar-April, P12

289.81 Primary hypercoagulable state
Activated protein C resistance
Antithrombin III deficiency
Factor V Leiden mutation
Lupus anticoagulant
Protein C deficiency
Protein S deficiency
Prothrombin gene mutation
Coding Clinic: 2008, Q3, P16-17

289.82 Secondary hypercoagulable state
Excludes *heparin-induced thrombocytopenia (HIT) (289.84)*
Coding Clinic: 2008, Q3, P16-17

289.83 Myelofibrosis
Myelofibrosis NOS
Secondary myelofibrosis

Code first the underlying disorder, such as:
malignant neoplasm of breast
  (174.0–174.9, 175.0–175.9)

Excludes *idiopathic myelofibrosis (238.76)*
leukoerythroblastic anemia (284.2)
myelofibrosis with myeloid metaplasia (238.76)
myelophthisic anemia (284.2)
myelophthisis (284.2)
primary myelofibrosis (238.76)

Use additional code for associated therapy-related myelodysplastic syndrome, if applicable (238.72, 238.73)

Use additional external cause code if due to anti-neoplastic chemotherapy (E933.1)

289.84 Heparin-induced thrombocytopenia (HIT)
Coding Clinic: 2008, Q4, P100-101

289.89 Other specified diseases of blood and blood-forming organs
Hypergammaglobulinemia
Pseudocholinesterase deficiency

289.9 Unspecified diseases of blood and blood-forming organs
Blood dyscrasia NOS
Erythroid hyperplasia
Coding Clinic: 1985, Mar-April, P14

◀ New ◀▥ Revised ~~deleted~~ Deleted | Excludes | Includes | Use additional | Code first | Omit code
● Unacceptable Principal Diagnosis ● Use Additional Digit(s) OGCR Official Guidelines Coding Clinic

5.   MENTAL DISORDERS (290–319)

Item 5-1 Psychosis was a term formerly applied to any mental disorder but is now restricted to disturbances of a great magnitude in which there is a personality disintegration and loss of contact with reality.

PSYCHOSES (290–299)

Excludes	*mental retardation (317–319)*

ORGANIC PSYCHOTIC CONDITIONS (290–294)

Includes	psychotic organic brain syndrome
Excludes	*nonpsychotic syndromes of organic etiology (310.0–310.9)*

psychoses classifiable to 295–298 and without impairment of orientation, comprehension, calculation, learning capacity, and judgment, but associated with physical disease, injury, or condition affecting the brain [e.g., following childbirth] (295.0–298.8)

● 290   Dementias

Progressive decline in cognition along with a short- and long-term memory loss due to brain damage/disease.

Code first the associated neurological condition

Excludes	*dementia due to alcohol (291.0–291.2)*

dementia due to drugs (292.82)
dementia not classified as senile, presenile, or arteriosclerotic (294.10–294.11)
psychoses classifiable to 295–298 occurring in the senium without dementia or delirium (295.0–298.8)
senility with mental changes of nonpsychotic severity (310.1)
transient organic psychotic conditions (293.0–293.9)

290.0   Senile dementia, uncomplicated
Senile dementia:
  NOS
  simple type

Excludes	*mild memory disturbances, not amounting to dementia, associated with senile brain disease (310.8)*

senile dementia with:
delirium or confusion (290.3)
delusional [paranoid] features (290.20)
depressive features (290.21)
Coding Clinic: 1999, Q4, P4-5; 1994, Q1, P21

● 290.1   Presenile dementia

Brain syndrome with presenile brain disease

Excludes	*arteriosclerotic dementia (290.40–290.43)*

dementia associated with other cerebral conditions (294.10–294.11)

290.10   Presenile dementia, uncomplicated
Presenile dementia:
  NOS
  simple type
Coding Clinic: 1984, Nov-Dec, P20

290.11   Presenile dementia with delirium
Presenile dementia with acute confusional state
Coding Clinic: 1984, Nov-Dec, P20

290.12   Presenile dementia with delusional features
Presenile dementia, paranoid type
Coding Clinic: 1984, Nov-Dec, P20

290.13   Presenile dementia with depressive features
Presenile dementia, depressed type
Coding Clinic: 1984, Nov-Dec, P20

● 290.2   Senile dementia with delusional or depressive features

Excludes	*senile dementia:*

NOS (290.0)
with delirium and/or confusion (290.3)

290.20   Senile dementia with delusional features
Senile dementia, paranoid type
Senile psychosis NOS

290.21   Senile dementia with depressive features

290.3   Senile dementia with delirium
Senile dementia with acute confusional state

Excludes	*senile:*

dementia NOS (290.0)
psychosis NOS (290.20)
Coding Clinic: 2009, Q3, P6

● 290.4   Vascular dementia

Multi-infarct dementia or psychosis

Use additional code to identify cerebral atherosclerosis (437.0)

Excludes	*suspected cases with no clear evidence of arteriosclerosis (290.9)*

290.40   Vascular dementia, uncomplicated
Arteriosclerotic dementia:
  NOS
  simple type

290.41   Vascular dementia with delirium
Arteriosclerotic dementia with acute confusional state

290.42   Vascular dementia with delusions
Arteriosclerotic dementia, paranoid type

290.43   Vascular dementia with depressed mood
Arteriosclerotic dementia, depressed type

290.8   Other specified senile psychotic conditions
Presbyophrenic psychosis

290.9   Unspecified senile psychotic condition

● 291   Alcohol-induced mental disorders

Excludes	*alcoholism without psychosis (303.0–303.9)*

291.0   Alcohol withdrawal delirium
Alcoholic delirium
Delirium tremens

Excludes	*alcohol withdrawal (291.81)*

291.1   Alcohol-induced persisting amnestic disorder
Alcoholic polyneuritic psychosis
Korsakoff's psychosis, alcoholic
Wernicke-Korsakoff syndrome (alcoholic)

291.2   Alcohol-induced persisting dementia
Alcoholic dementia NOS
Alcoholism associated with dementia NOS
Chronic alcoholic brain syndrome

291.3   Alcohol-induced psychotic disorder with hallucinations
Alcoholic:
  hallucinosis (acute)
  psychosis with hallucinosis

Excludes	*alcohol withdrawal with delirium (291.0)*

schizophrenia (295.0–295.9) and paranoid states (297.0–297.9) taking the form of chronic hallucinosis with clear consciousness in an alcoholic

291.4   Idiosyncratic alcohol intoxication
Pathologic:
  alcohol intoxication
  drunkenness

Excludes	*acute alcohol intoxication (305.0)*

in alcoholism (303.0)
simple drunkenness (305.0)

MENTAL DISORDERS (290–319)

291.5 Alcohol-induced psychotic disorder with delusions
Alcoholic:
  paranoia
  psychosis, paranoid type

> **Excludes**   *nonalcoholic paranoid states (297.0–297.9)*
> *schizophrenia, paranoid type (295.3)*

● **291.8 Other specified alcohol-induced mental disorders**
Coding Clinic: 1989, Q2, P9

291.81 Alcohol withdrawal
Alcohol:
  abstinence syndrome or symptoms
  withdrawal syndrome or symptoms

> **Excludes**   *alcohol withdrawal:*
> *delirium (291.0)*
> *hallucinosis (291.3)*
> *delirium tremens (291.0)*

Coding Clinic: 1985, July-Aug, P10

291.82 Alcohol induced sleep disorders
Alcohol induced circadian rhythm sleep
  disorders
Alcohol induced hypersomnia
Alcohol induced insomnia
Alcohol induced parasomnia

291.89 Other
Alcohol-induced anxiety disorder
Alcohol-induced mood disorder
Alcohol-induced sexual dysfunction

291.9 Unspecified alcohol-induced mental disorders
Alcoholic:
  mania NOS
  psychosis NOS
Alcoholism (chronic) with psychosis
Alcohol-related disorder NOS

● **292 Drug-induced mental disorders**

> **Includes**   organic brain syndrome associated with
> consumption of drugs

> **Use additional** code for any associated drug dependence
> (304.0–304.9)

> **Use additional** E code to identify drug

Coding Clinic: 2004, Q3, P8

292.0 Drug withdrawal
Drug:
  abstinence syndrome or symptoms
  withdrawal syndrome or symptoms
Coding Clinic: 1997, Q1, P12-13

● **292.1 Drug-induced psychotic disorders**

292.11 Drug-induced psychotic disorder with delusions
Paranoid state induced by drugs

292.12 Drug-induced psychotic disorder with hallucinations
Hallucinatory state induced by drugs

> **Excludes**   *states following LSD or other*
> *hallucinogens, lasting only a*
> *few days or less ["bad trips"]*
> *(305.3)*

Coding Clinic: 2004, Q3, P8

292.2 Pathological drug intoxication
Drug reaction resulting in brief psychotic states
  NOS
  idiosyncratic
  pathologic

> **Excludes**   *expected brief psychotic reactions to*
> *hallucinogens ["bad trips"] (305.3)*
> *physiological side-effects of drugs (e.g.,*
> *dystonias)*

● **292.8 Other specified drug-induced mental disorders**

292.81 Drug-induced delirium

292.82 Drug-induced persisting dementia
Coding Clinic: 2004, Q3, P8

292.83 Drug-induced persisting amnestic disorder

292.84 Drug-induced mood disorder
Depressive state induced by drugs

292.85 Drug induced sleep disorders
Drug induced circadian rhythm sleep
  disorder
Drug induced hypersomnia
Drug induced insomnia
Drug induced parasomnia

292.89 Other
Drug-induced anxiety disorder
Drug-induced organic personality
  syndrome
Drug-induced sexual dysfunction
Drug intoxication

292.9 Unspecified drug-induced mental disorder
Drug-related disorder NOS
Organic psychosis NOS due to or associated with
  drugs

● **293 Transient mental disorders due to conditions classified elsewhere**

> **Includes**   transient organic mental disorders not
> associated with alcohol or drugs

> *Code first the associated physical or neurological condition*

> **Excludes**   *confusional state or delirium superimposed on*
> *senile dementia (290.3)*
> *dementia due to:*
> *alcohol (291.0–291.9)*
> *arteriosclerosis (290.40–290.43)*
> *drugs (292.82)*
> *senility (290.0)*

293.0 Delirium due to conditions classified elsewhere
Acute:
  confusional state
  infective psychosis
  organic reaction
  posttraumatic organic psychosis
  psycho-organic syndrome
Acute psychosis associated with endocrine,
  metabolic, or cerebrovascular disorder
Epileptic:
  confusional state
  twilight state
Coding Clinic: 1993, Q3, P11

293.1 Subacute delirium
Subacute:
  confusional state
  infective psychosis
  organic reaction
  posttraumatic organic psychosis
  psycho-organic syndrome
  psychosis associated with endocrine or
    metabolic disorder

● **293.8 Other specified transient mental disorders due to conditions classified elsewhere**

293.81 Psychotic disorder with delusions in conditions classified elsewhere
Transient organic psychotic condition,
  paranoid type

293.82 Psychotic disorder with hallucinations in conditions classified elsewhere
Transient organic psychotic condition,
  hallucinatory type

293.83 Mood disorder in conditions classified elsewhere
Transient organic psychotic condition, depressive type

293.84 Anxiety disorder in conditions classified elsewhere
Coding Clinic: 1996, Q4, P29

293.89 Other
Catatonic disorder in conditions classified elsewhere

293.9 Unspecified transient mental disorder in conditions classified elsewhere
Organic psychosis:
infective NOS
posttraumatic NOS
transient NOS
Psycho-organic syndrome

● **294 Persistent mental disorders due to conditions classified elsewhere**
| Includes | organic psychotic brain syndromes (chronic), not elsewhere classified |

294.0 Amnestic disorder in conditions classified elsewhere
Korsakoff's psychosis or syndrome (nonalcoholic)
Code first underlying condition
| Excludes | *alcoholic:* |
amnestic syndrome (291.1)
Korsakoff's psychosis (291.1)

● **294.1 Dementia in conditions classified elsewhere**
Dementia of the Alzheimer's type
Code first any underlying physical condition as:
dementia in:
Alzheimer's disease (331.0)
cerebral lipidoses (330.1)
dementia with Lewy bodies (331.82)
dementia with Parkinsonism (331.82)
epilepsy (345.0–345.9)
frontal dementia (331.19)
frontotemporal dementia (331.19)
general paresis [syphilis] (094.1)
hepatolenticular degeneration (275.1)
Huntington's chorea (333.4)
Jakob-Creutzfeldt disease (046.11--046.19)
multiple sclerosis (340)
Pick's disease of the brain (331.11)
polyarteritis nodosa (446.0)
syphilis (094.1)
| Excludes | *dementia:* |
arteriosclerotic (290.40–290.43)
presenile (290.10–290.13)
senile (290.0)
epileptic psychosis NOS (294.8)
Coding Clinic: 1999, Q1, P14; 1985, Sept-Oct, P12

294.10 Dementia in conditions classified elsewhere without behavioral disturbance
Dementia in conditions classified elsewhere NOS

294.11 Dementia in conditions classified elsewhere with behavioral disturbance
Aggressive behavior
Combative behavior
Violent behavior
Wandering off
Coding Clinic: 2000, Q4, P40-41

294.8 Other persistent mental disorders due to conditions classified elsewhere
Amnestic disorder NOS
Dementia NOS
Epileptic psychosis NOS
Mixed paranoid and affective organic psychotic states
| Use additional | code for associated epilepsy (345.0–345.9)
| Excludes | *mild memory disturbances, not amounting to dementia (310.8)*
Coding Clinic: 2009, Q3, P6x2; 2003, Q3, P14

294.9 Unspecified persistent mental disorders due to conditions classified elsewhere
Cognitive disorder NOS
Organic psychosis (chronic)
Coding Clinic: 2007, Q2, P5

OTHER PSYCHOSES (295–299)

| Use additional | code to identify any associated physical disease, injury, or condition affecting the brain with psychoses classifiable to 295–298

● **295 Schizophrenic disorders**
Personality disorders characterized by multiple mental and behavioral irregularities.
| Includes | schizophrenia of the types described in 295.0–295.9 occurring in children
| Excludes | *childhood type schizophrenia (299.9)*
infantile autism (299.0)

The following fifth-digit subclassification is for use with category 295:

> **0 unspecified**
> **1 subchronic**
> **2 chronic**
> **3 subchronic with acute exacerbation**
> **4 chronic with acute exacerbation**
> **5 in remission**

● **295.0 Simple type**
[0-5] Schizophrenia simplex
| Excludes | *latent schizophrenia (295.5)*

● **295.1 Disorganized type**
[0-5] Hebephrenia
Hebephrenic type schizophrenia

● **295.2 Catatonic type**
[0-5] Catatonic (schizophrenia):   Schizophrenic:
agitation   catalepsy
excitation   catatonia
excited type   flexibilitas cerea
stupor
withdrawn type

● **295.3 Paranoid type**
[0-5] Paraphrenic schizophrenia
| Excludes | *involutional paranoid state (297.2)*
paranoia (297.1)
paraphrenia (297.2)

● **295.4 Schizophreniform disorder**
[0-5] Oneirophrenia
Schizophreniform:
attack
psychosis, confusional type
| Excludes | *acute forms of schizophrenia of:*
catatonic type (295.2)
hebephrenic type (295.1)
paranoid type (295.3)
simple type (295.0)
undifferentiated type (295.8)

MENTAL DISORDERS (290–319)

● **295.5 Latent schizophrenia**
[0-5]   Latent schizophrenic reaction
Schizophrenia: Schizophrenia:
  borderline   prodromal
  incipient   pseudoneurotic
  prepsychotic   pseudopsychopathic
Excludes *schizoid personality (301.20–301.22)*

● **295.6 Residual type**
[0-5]   Chronic undifferentiated schizophrenia
Restzustand (schizophrenic)
Schizophrenic residual state
Coding Clinic: 2006, Q4, P76-78

● **295.7 Schizoaffective disorder**
[0-5]   Cyclic schizophrenia
Mixed schizophrenic and affective psychosis
Schizo-affective psychosis
Schizophreniform psychosis, affective type

● **295.8 Other specified types of schizophrenia**
[0-5]   Acute (undifferentiated) schizophrenia
Atypical schizophrenia
Cenesthopathic schizophrenia
Excludes *infantile autism (299.0)*

● **295.9 Unspecified schizophrenia**
[0-5]   Schizophrenia: Schizophrenia:
  NOS   undifferentiated NOS
  mixed NOS   undifferentiated type
Schizophrenic reaction NOS
Schizophreniform psychosis NOS
Coding Clinic: 1995, Q3, P6

● **296 Episodic mood disorders**

Includes episodic affective disorders

Excludes *neurotic depression (300.4)*
reactive depressive psychosis (298.0)
reactive excitation (298.1)

Coding Clinic: 1985, Mar-April, P14

The following fifth-digit subclassification is for use with
categories 296.0–296.6:

0 unspecified
1 mild
2 moderate
3 severe, without mention of psychotic behavior
4 severe, specified as with psychotic behavior
5 in partial or unspecified remission
6 in full remission

● **296.0 Bipolar I disorder, single manic episode**
[0-6]   *Manic depressive disorder, characterized by moods that
swing between periods of exaggerated euphoria,
irritability, or both (manic) and episodes of
depression.*
Hypomania (mild) NOS single episode or unspecified
Hypomanic psychosis single episode or unspecified
Mania (monopolar) NOS single episode or
  unspecified
Manic-depressive psychosis or reaction, single
  episode or unspecified:
  hypomanic, single episode or unspecified
  manic, single episode or unspecified
Excludes *circular type, if there was a previous attack
of depression (296.4)*

● **296.1 Manic disorder, recurrent episode**
[0-6]   Any condition classifiable to 296.0, stated to be
recurrent
Excludes *circular type, if there was a previous attack
of depression (296.4)*

● **296.2 Major depressive disorder, single episode**
[0-6]   Depressive psychosis, single episode or unspecified
Endogenous depression, single episode or
  unspecified
Involutional melancholia, single episode or
  unspecified
Manic-depressive psychosis or reaction, depressed
  type, single episode or unspecified
Monopolar depression, single episode or unspecified
Psychotic depression, single episode or unspecified
Excludes *circular type, if previous attack was of
manic type (296.5)*
depression NOS (311)
reactive depression (neurotic) (300.4)
psychotic (298.0)
Coding Clinic: 2009, Q3, P6x2, 7

● **296.3 Major depressive disorder, recurrent episode**
[0-6]   Any condition classifiable to 296.2, stated to be
recurrent
Excludes *circular type, if previous attack was of
manic type (296.5)*
depression NOS (311)
reactive depression (neurotic) (300.4)
psychotic (298.0)

● **296.4 Bipolar I disorder, most recent episode (or current)**
[0-6] **manic**
Bipolar disorder, now manic
Manic-depressive psychosis, circular type but
  currently manic
Excludes *brief compensatory or rebound mood swings
(296.99)*

● **296.5 Bipolar I disorder, most recent episode (or current)**
[0-6] **depressed**
Bipolar disorder, now depressed
Manic-depressive psychosis, circular type but
  currently depressed
Excludes *brief compensatory or rebound mood swings
(296.99)*
Coding Clinic: 2006, Q1, P10

● **296.6 Bipolar I disorder, most recent episode (or current)**
[0-6] **mixed**
Manic-depressive psychosis, circular type, mixed

**296.7 Bipolar I disorder, most recent episode (or current)
unspecified**
Atypical bipolar affective disorder NOS
Manic-depressive psychosis, circular type, current
  condition not specified as either manic or
  depressive

● **296.8 Other and unspecified bipolar disorders**

296.80 Bipolar disorder, unspecified
Bipolar disorder NOS
Manic-depressive:
  reaction NOS
  syndrome NOS

296.81 Atypical manic disorder

296.82 Atypical depressive disorder

296.89 Other
Bipolar II disorder
Manic-depressive psychosis, mixed type

● **296.9 Other and unspecified episodic mood disorder**

> **Excludes** *psychogenic affective psychoses (298.0–298.8)*

296.90 Unspecified episodic mood disorder
Affective psychosis NOS
Melancholia NOS
Mood disorder NOS
Coding Clinic: 1985, Mar-April, P14

296.99 Other specified episodic mood disorder
Mood swings:
brief compensatory
rebound

● **297 Delusional disorders**

> **Includes** paranoid disorders

> **Excludes** *acute paranoid reaction (298.3)*
> *alcoholic jealousy or paranoid state (291.5)*
> *paranoid schizophrenia (295.3)*

297.0 Paranoid state, simple

297.1 Delusional disorder
Chronic paranoid psychosis
Sander's disease
Systematized delusions

> **Excludes** *paranoid personality disorder (301.0)*

297.2 Paraphrenia
Involutional paranoid state
Late paraphrenia
Paraphrenia (involutional)

297.3 Shared psychotic disorder
Folie à deux
Induced psychosis or paranoid disorder

297.8 Other specified paranoid states
Paranoia querulans
Sensitiver Beziehungswahn

> **Excludes** *acute paranoid reaction or state (298.3)*
> *senile paranoid state (290.20)*

297.9 Unspecified paranoid state
Paranoid:
disorder NOS
psychosis NOS
reaction NOS
state NOS

● **298 Other nonorganic psychoses**

> **Includes** psychotic conditions due to or provoked by:
> emotional stress
> environmental factors as major part of
> etiology

298.0 Depressive type psychosis
Psychogenic depressive psychosis
Psychotic reactive depression
Reactive depressive psychosis

> **Excludes** *manic-depressive psychosis, depressed type (296.2–296.3)*
> *neurotic depression (300.4)*
> *reactive depression NOS (300.4)*

298.1 Excitative type psychosis
Acute hysterical psychosis
Psychogenic excitation
Reactive excitation

> **Excludes** *manic-depressive psychosis, manic type (296.0–296.1)*

298.2 Reactive confusion
Psychogenic confusion
Psychogenic twilight state

> **Excludes** *acute confusional state (293.0)*

Item 5-2 Anxiety is also known as **generalized disorder** and is evidenced by persistent, excessive, and unrealistic worry about everyday things. **Dissociative disorders** are characterized by a persistent disruption in the integration of memory, consciousness, or identity and a lack of mental connectedness to events. **Somatoform disorders** are characterized by unusual physical symptoms in the absence of any known physical pathology and may lead to unnecessary medical treatments.

298.3 Acute paranoid reaction
Acute psychogenic paranoid psychosis
Bouffée délirante

> **Excludes** *paranoid states (297.0–297.9)*

298.4 Psychogenic paranoid psychosis
Protracted reactive paranoid psychosis

298.8 Other and unspecified reactive psychosis
Brief psychotic disorder
Brief reactive psychosis NOS
Hysterical psychosis
Psychogenic psychosis NOS
Psychogenic stupor

> **Excludes** *acute hysterical psychosis (298.1)*

298.9 Unspecified psychosis
Atypical psychosis
Psychosis NOS
Psychotic disorder NOS
Coding Clinic: 2006, Q3, P22; 1993, Q3, P11

● **299 Pervasive developmental disorders**

> **Excludes** *adult type psychoses occurring in childhood, as:*
> *affective disorders (296.0–296.9)*
> *manic-depressive disorders (296.0–296.9)*
> *schizophrenia (295.0–295.9)*

The following fifth-digit subclassification is for use with category 299:

> **0 current or active state**
> **1 residual state**

● **299.0 Autistic disorder**
[0-1] Childhood autism
Infantile psychosis
Kanner's syndrome

> **Excludes** *disintegrative psychosis (299.1)*
> *Heller's syndrome (299.1)*
> *schizophrenic syndrome of childhood (299.9)*

● **299.1 Childhood disintegrative disorder**
[0-1] Heller's syndrome

> **Use additional** code to identify any associated neurological disorder

> **Excludes** *infantile autism (299.0)*
> *schizophrenic syndrome of childhood (299.9)*

● **299.8 Other specified pervasive developmental**
[0-1] **disorders**
Asperger's disorder
Atypical childhood psychosis
Borderline psychosis of childhood

> **Excludes** *simple stereotypes without psychotic disturbance (307.3)*

● **299.9 Unspecified pervasive developmental disorder**
[0-1] Child psychosis NOS
Pervasive developmental disorder NOS
Schizophrenia, childhood type NOS
Schizophrenic syndrome of childhood NOS

> **Excludes** *schizophrenia of adult type occurring in childhood (295.0–295.9)*

MENTAL DISORDERS (290–319)

◀ New ◀▥ Revised ~~deleted~~ Deleted | **Excludes** | **Includes** | **Use additional** | **Code first** | **Omit code**
● Unacceptable Principal Diagnosis ● Use Additional Digit(s) **OGCR** Official Guidelines **Coding Clinic**

781

NEUROTIC DISORDERS, PERSONALITY DISORDERS, AND OTHER NONPSYCHOTIC MENTAL DISORDERS (300–316)

● **300 Anxiety, dissociative and somatoform disorders**

  ● **300.0 Anxiety states**

    Excludes   *anxiety in:*
      acute stress reaction (308.0)
      transient adjustment reaction (309.24)
      neurasthenia (300.5)
      psychophysiological disorders (306.0–306.9)
      separation anxiety (309.21)

    300.00 Anxiety state, unspecified
      Anxiety:
        neurosis
        reaction
        state (neurotic)
      Atypical anxiety disorder

    300.01 Panic disorder without agoraphobia
      Panic:
        attack
        state

      Excludes   *panic disorder with agoraphobia (300.21)*

    300.02 Generalized anxiety disorder

    300.09 Other

  ● **300.1 Dissociative, conversion and factitious disorders**

    Excludes   *adjustment reaction (309.0–309.9)*
      anorexia nervosa (307.1)
      gross stress reaction (308.0–308.9)
      hysterical personality (301.50–301.59)
      psychophysiologic disorders (306.0–306.9)

    300.10 Hysteria, unspecified

    300.11 Conversion disorder
      Astasia-abasia, hysterical
      Conversion hysteria or reaction
      Hysterical:
        blindness
        deafness
        paralysis
      Coding Clinic: 1985, Nov-Dec, P15

    300.12 Dissociative amnesia
      Hysterical amnesia

    300.13 Dissociative fugue
      Hysterical fugue

    300.14 Dissociative identity disorder

    300.15 Dissociative disorder or reaction, unspecified

    300.16 Factitious disorder with predominantly psychological signs and symptoms
      Compensation neurosis
      Ganser's syndrome, hysterical

    300.19 Other and unspecified factitious illness
      Factitious disorder (with combined psychological and physical signs and symptoms) (with predominantly physical signs and symptoms) NOS

      Excludes   *multiple operations or hospital addiction syndrome (301.51)*

● **300.2 Phobic disorders**
  Irrational fear with avoidance of the feared subject, activity, or situation. Divided into 3 types: specific phobias, social phobias, and agoraphobia.

    Excludes   *anxiety state not associated with a specific situation or object (300.00–300.09)*
      obsessional phobias (300.3)

    300.20 Phobia, unspecified
      Anxiety-hysteria NOS
      Phobia NOS

    300.21 Agoraphobia with panic disorder
      Fear of:
        open spaces with panic attacks
        streets with panic attacks
        travel with panic attacks
      Panic disorder with agoraphobia

      Excludes   *agoraphobia without panic disorder (300.22)*
        panic disorder without agoraphobia (300.01)

    300.22 Agoraphobia without mention of panic attacks
      Any condition classifiable to 300.21 without mention of panic attacks

    300.23 Social phobia
      Fear of:
        eating in public
        public speaking
        washing in public

    300.29 Other isolated or specific phobias
      Acrophobia
        Fear of heights
      Animal phobias
      Claustrophobia
        Fear of closed spaces
      Fear of crowds

300.3 Obsessive-compulsive disorders *(OCD)*
  Anancastic neurosis
  Compulsive neurosis
  Obsessional phobia [any]

  Excludes   *obsessive-compulsive symptoms occurring in:*
    endogenous depression (296.2–296.3)
    organic states (e.g., encephalitis)
    schizophrenia (295.0–295.9)

300.4 Dysthymic disorder
  Anxiety depression
  Depression with anxiety
  Depressive reaction
  Neurotic depressive state
  Reactive depression

  Excludes   *adjustment reaction with depressive symptoms (309.0–309.1)*
    depression NOS (311)
    manic-depressive psychosis, depressed type (296.2–296.3)
    reactive depressive psychosis (298.0)

300.5 Neurasthenia
  Fatigue neurosis   Psychogenic:
  Nervous debility   asthenia
                     general fatigue

  Use additional code to identify any associated physical disorder

  Excludes   *anxiety state (300.00–300.09)*
    neurotic depression (300.4)
    psychophysiological disorders (306.0–306.9)
    specific nonpsychotic mental disorders following organic brain damage (310.0–310.9)

300.6 Depersonalization disorder
Derealization (neurotic)
Neurotic state with depersonalization episode

> **Excludes** *depersonalization associated with:*
> *anxiety (300.00–300.09)*
> *depression (300.4)*
> *manic-depressive disorder or psychosis*
> *(296.0–296.9)*
> *schizophrenia (295.0–295.9)*

300.7 Hypochondriasis
Hypochondriac
Body dysmorphic disorder

> **Excludes** *hypochondriasis in:*
> *hysteria (300.10–300.19)*
> *manic-depressive psychosis, depressed*
> *type (296.2–296.3)*
> *neurasthenia (300.5)*
> *obsessional disorder (300.3)*
> *schizophrenia (295.0–295.9)*

● **300.8 Somatoform disorders**

300.81 Somatization disorder
Briquet's disorder
Severe somatoform disorder

300.82 Undifferentiated somatoform disorder
Atypical somatoform disorder
Somatoform disorder NOS

300.89 Other somatoform disorders
Occupational neurosis, including writers' cramp
Psychasthenia
Psychasthenic neurosis

300.9 Unspecified nonpsychotic mental disorder
Psychoneurosis NOS

● **301 Personality disorders**
Long-term patterns of thoughts and behaviors causing serious problems with relationships and work.

> **Includes** character neurosis

> Use additional code to identify any associated neurosis or psychosis, or physical condition

> **Excludes** *nonpsychotic personality disorder associated with organic brain syndromes (310.0–310.9)*

301.0 Paranoid personality disorder
Fanatic personality
Paranoid personality (disorder)
Paranoid traits

> **Excludes** *acute paranoid reaction (298.3)*
> *alcoholic paranoia (291.5)*
> *paranoid schizophrenia (295.3)*
> *paranoid states (297.0–297.9)*

● **301.1 Affective personality disorder**

> **Excludes** *affective psychotic disorders (296.0–296.9)*
> *neurasthenia (300.5)*
> *neurotic depression (300.4)*

301.10 Affective personality disorder, unspecified

301.11 Chronic hypomanic personality disorder
Chronic hypomanic disorder
Hypomanic personality

301.12 Chronic depressive personality disorder
Chronic depressive disorder
Depressive character or personality

301.13 Cyclothymic disorder
Cycloid personality
Cyclothymia
Cyclothymic personality

● **301.2 Schizoid personality disorder**

> **Excludes** *schizophrenia (295.0–295.9)*

301.20 Schizoid personality disorder, unspecified

301.21 Introverted personality

301.22 Schizotypal personality disorder

301.3 Explosive personality disorder
Aggressive:
    personality
    reaction
Aggressiveness
Emotional instability (excessive)
Pathological emotionality
Quarrelsomeness

> **Excludes** *dyssocial personality (301.7)*
> *hysterical neurosis (300.10–300.19)*

301.4 Obsessive-compulsive personality disorder
Anancastic personality
Obsessional personality

> **Excludes** *obsessive-compulsive disorder (300.3)*
> *phobic state (300.20–300.29)*

● **301.5 Histrionic personality disorder**

> **Excludes** *hysterical neurosis (300.10–300.19)*

301.50 Histrionic personality disorder, unspecified
Hysterical personality NOS

301.51 Chronic factitious illness with physical symptoms
Hospital addiction syndrome
Multiple operations syndrome
Munchausen syndrome

301.59 Other histrionic personality disorder
Personality: Personality:
    emotionally unstable   psychoinfantile
    labile

301.6 Dependent personality disorder
Asthenic personality
Inadequate personality
Passive personality

> **Excludes** *neurasthenia (300.5)*
> *passive-aggressive personality (301.84)*

301.7 Antisocial personality disorder
Amoral personality
Asocial personality
Dyssocial personality
Personality disorder with predominantly sociopathic or asocial manifestation

> **Excludes** *disturbance of conduct without specifiable personality disorder (312.0–312.9)*
> *explosive personality (301.3)*

Coding Clinic: 1984, Sept-Oct, P16

● **301.8 Other personality disorders**

301.81 Narcissistic personality disorder

301.82 Avoidant personality disorder

301.83 Borderline personality disorder

301.84 Passive-aggressive personality

301.89 Other
Personality: Personality:
    eccentric   masochistic
    "haltlose" type   psychoneurotic
    immature

> **Excludes** *psychoinfantile personality (301.59)*

MENTAL DISORDERS (290–319)

MENTAL DISORDERS (290–319)

301.9 Unspecified personality disorder
Pathological personality NOS
Personality disorder NOS
Psychopathic:
  constitutional state
  personality (disorder)

● **302 Sexual and gender identity disorders**
Excludes *sexual disorder manifest in:*
  organic brain syndrome (290.0–294.9,
    310.0–310.9)
  psychosis (295.0–298.9)

302.0 Ego-dystonic sexual orientation
Ego-dystonic lesbianism
Sexual orientation conflict disorder
Excludes *homosexual pedophilia (302.2)*

302.1 Zoophilia
Bestiality

302.2 Pedophilia

302.3 Transvestic fetishism
Excludes *trans-sexualism (302.5)*

302.4 Exhibitionism

● **302.5 Trans-sexualism**
Sex reassignment surgery status
Excludes *transvestism (302.3)*

302.50 With unspecified sexual history

302.51 With asexual history

302.52 With homosexual history

302.53 With heterosexual history

302.6 Gender identity disorder in children
Check age: adolescents and adults separately classified
  under 302.85.
Feminism in boys
Gender identity disorder NOS
Excludes *gender identity disorder in adult (302.85)*
  trans-sexualism (302.50–302.53)
  transvestism (302.3)

● **302.7 Psychosexual dysfunction**
Excludes *decreased sexual desire NOS (799.81)*
  impotence of organic origin (607.84)
  normal transient symptoms from ruptured
    hymen
  transient or occasional failures of erection
    due to fatigue, anxiety, alcohol, or
    drugs

302.70 Psychosexual dysfunction, unspecified
Sexual dysfunction NOS

302.71 Hypoactive sexual desire disorder
Excludes *decreased sexual desire NOS*
  (799.81)

302.72 With inhibited sexual excitement
Female sexual arousal disorder
Frigidity
Impotence
Male erectile disorder

302.73 Female orgasmic disorder

302.74 Male orgasmic disorder

302.75 Premature ejaculation

302.76 Dyspareunia, psychogenic

302.79 With other specified psychosexual dysfunctions
Sexual aversion disorder

● **302.8 Other specified psychosexual disorders**
302.81 Fetishism

302.82 Voyeurism

302.83 Sexual masochism

302.84 Sexual sadism

302.85 Gender identity disorder in adolescents or adults
Use additional code to identify sex
  reassignment surgery status (302.5)
Excludes *gender identity disorder NOS*
  (302.6)
  gender identity disorder in children
    (302.6)

302.89 Other
Frotteurism
Nymphomania
Satyriasis

302.9 Unspecified psychosexual disorder
Paraphilia NOS
Pathologic sexuality NOS
Sexual deviation NOS
Sexual disorder NOS

● **303 Alcohol dependence syndrome**
Use additional code to identify any associated
  condition, as:
alcoholic psychoses (291.0–291.9)
drug dependence (304.0–304.9)
physical complications of alcohol, such as:
  cerebral degeneration (331.7)
  cirrhosis of liver (571.2)
  epilepsy (345.0–345.9)
  gastritis (535.3)
  hepatitis (571.1)
  liver damage NOS (571.3)
Excludes *drunkenness NOS (305.0)*
Coding Clinic: 2010, Q1, P3-4; 1995, Q3, P6

The following fifth-digit subclassification is for use with
category 303:

0	unspecified
1	continuous
2	episodic
3	in remission

● **303.0 Acute alcoholic intoxication**
[0-3] Acute drunkenness in alcoholism
Coding Clinic: 1985, July-Aug, P15

● **303.9 Other and unspecified alcohol dependence**
[0-3] Chronic alcoholism
Dipsomania
Coding Clinic: 2002, Q2, P4; Q1, P3-4; 1989, Q2, P9; 1985, Nov-Dec, P14

● **304 Drug dependence**

For some "dependence" codes there is a corresponding "abuse" code. There is a point at which drug use crosses from "dependence" to "abuse." Check documentation or query provider for patient status.

Excludes *nondependent abuse of drugs (305.1–305.9)*

Coding Clinic: 2010, Q1, P3

The following fifth-digit subclassification is for use with category 304:

> 0 unspecified
> 1 continuous
> 2 episodic
> 3 in remission

● **304.0 Opioid type dependence**
[0-3]   Heroin
            Meperidine
            Methadone
            Morphine
            Opium
            Opium alkaloids and their derivatives
            Synthetics with morphine-like effects
            Coding Clinic: 2006, Q2, P7; 1988, Q4, P8

● **304.1 Sedative, hypnotic or anxiolytic dependence**
[0-3]   Barbiturates
            Nonbarbiturate sedatives and tranquilizers with a
                similar effect:
                chlordiazepoxide
                diazepam
                glutethimide
                meprobamate
                methaqualone

● **304.2 Cocaine dependence**
[0-3]   Coca leaves and derivatives

● **304.3 Cannabis dependence**
[0-3]   *Code 305.2 is for abuse of cannabis.*
            Hashish
            Hemp
            Marihuana

● **304.4 Amphetamine and other psychostimulant**
[0-3] **dependence**
            Methylphenidate
            Phenmetrazine

● **304.5 Hallucinogen dependence**
[0-3]   Dimethyltryptamine [DMT]
            Lysergic acid diethylamide [LSD] and derivatives
            Mescaline
            Psilocybin

● **304.6 Other specified drug dependence**
[0-3]   Absinthe addiction
            Glue sniffing
            Inhalant dependence
            Phencyclidine dependence
            Excludes *tobacco dependence (305.1)*

● **304.7 Combinations of opioid type drug with any other**
[0-3]   Coding Clinic: 1986, Mar-April, P12

● **304.8 Combinations of drug dependence excluding opioid**
[0-3] **type drug**
            Coding Clinic: 1986, Mar-April, P12

● **304.9 Unspecified drug dependence**
[0-3]   Drug addiction NOS
            Drug dependence NOS
            Coding Clinic: 2003, Q4, P103-104

● **305 Nondependent abuse of drugs**

Note: Includes cases where a person, for whom no
        other diagnosis is possible, has come under
        medical care because of the maladaptive effect of
        a drug on which he is not dependent and that he
        has taken on his own initiative *(self-medicating)* to
        the detriment of his health or social functioning.

Excludes *alcohol dependence syndrome (303.0–303.9)*
            drug dependence (304.0–304.9)
            drug withdrawal syndrome (292.0)
            *poisoning by drugs or medicinal substances
                (960.0–979.9)*

Coding Clinic: 2010, Q1, P5

The following fifth-digit subclassification is for use with codes 305.0, 305.2–305.9:

> 0 unspecified
> 1 continuous
> 2 episodic
> 3 in remission

● **305.0 Alcohol abuse**
[0-3]   Drunkenness NOS
            Excessive drinking of alcohol NOS
            "Hangover" (alcohol)
            Inebriety NOS
            Excludes *acute alcohol intoxication in alcoholism
                (303.0)*
                alcoholic psychoses (291.0–291.9)
            Coding Clinic: 2009, Q4, P98; Q1, P8; 1996, Q3, P16; 1985, July-Aug, P15

● **305.1 Tobacco use disorder**
            Tobacco dependence
            Excludes *history of tobacco use (V15.82)*
                smoking complicating pregnancy (649.0)
                *tobacco use disorder complicating
                    pregnancy (649.0)*
            Coding Clinic: 2009, Q4, P98; Q1, P8; 1996, Q2, P10; 1984,
            Nov-Dec, P12

● **305.2 Cannabis abuse**
[0-3]   *Code 304.3 is for cannabis dependence.*

● **305.3 Hallucinogen abuse**
[0-3]   Acute intoxication from hallucinogens ["bad
                trips"]
            LSD reaction

● **305.4 Sedative, hypnotic or anxiolytic abuse**
[0-3]

● **305.5 Opioid abuse**
[0-3]

● **305.6 Cocaine abuse**
[0-3]   Coding Clinic: 1993, Q1, P25; Q1, P25; 1988, Q4, P8

● **305.7 Amphetamine or related acting sympathomimetic**
[0-3] **abuse**
            Coding Clinic: 2003, Q2, P10,11x2

● **305.8 Antidepressant type abuse**
[0-3]

● **305.9 Other, mixed, or unspecified drug abuse**
[0-3]   Caffeine intoxication
            Inhalant abuse
            "Laxative habit"
            Misuse of drugs NOS
            Nonprescribed use of drugs or patent medicinals
            Phencyclidine abuse
            Coding Clinic: 1999, Q3, P20; 1994, Q4, P36

MENTAL DISORDERS (290–319)

● **306 Physiological malfunction arising from mental factors**

     Includes   psychogenic:
        physical symptoms not involving tissue
          damage
        physiological manifestations not involving
          tissue damage

     Excludes   *hysteria (300.11–300.19)*
        physical symptoms secondary to a psychiatric
          disorder classified elsewhere
        psychic factors associated with physical conditions
          involving tissue damage classified elsewhere
          (316)
        specific nonpsychotic mental disorders following
          organic brain damage (310.0–310.9)

    306.0 Musculoskeletal
       Psychogenic paralysis
       Psychogenic torticollis

     Excludes   *Gilles de la Tourette's syndrome (307.23)*
        paralysis as hysterical or conversion
          reaction (300.11)
        tics (307.20–307.22)

    306.1 Respiratory
       Psychogenic: Psychogenic:
         air hunger   hyperventilation
         cough   yawning
         hiccough

     Excludes   *psychogenic asthma (316 and 493.9)*

    306.2 Cardiovascular
       Cardiac neurosis
       Cardiovascular neurosis
       Neurocirculatory asthenia
       Psychogenic cardiovascular disorder

     Excludes   *psychogenic paroxysmal tachycardia*
        (316 and 427.2)

     Coding Clinic: 1985, July-Aug, P14

    306.3 Skin
       Psychogenic pruritus

     Excludes   *psychogenic:*
        alopecia (316 and 704.00)
        dermatitis (316 and 692.9)
        eczema (316 and 691.8 or 692.9)
        urticaria (316 and 708.0–708.9)

    306.4 Gastrointestinal
       Aerophagy
       Cyclical vomiting, psychogenic
       Diarrhea, psychogenic
       Nervous gastritis
       Psychogenic dyspepsia

     Excludes   *cyclical vomiting NOS (536.2)*
        associated with migraine (346.2)
        globus hystericus (300.11)
        mucous colitis (316 and 564.9)
        psychogenic:
          cardiospasm (316 and 530.0)
          duodenal ulcer (316 and 532.0–532.9)
          gastric ulcer (316 and 531.0–531.9)
          peptic ulcer NOS (316 and 533.0–533.9)
        vomiting NOS (307.54)

     Coding Clinic: 1989, Q2, P11

● **306.5 Genitourinary**

     Excludes   *enuresis, psychogenic (307.6)*
        frigidity (302.72)
        impotence (302.72)
        psychogenic dyspareunia (302.76)

    **306.50 Psychogenic genitourinary malfunction,
        unspecified**

    306.51 Psychogenic vaginismus
       Functional vaginismus

    306.52 Psychogenic dysmenorrhea

    306.53 Psychogenic dysuria

    306.59 Other

    306.6 Endocrine

    306.7 Organs of special sense

     Excludes   *hysterical blindness or deafness (300.11)*
        psychophysical visual disturbances (368.16)

    306.8 Other specified psychophysiological malfunction
       Bruxism
       Sleep-related bruxism, 327.53
       Teeth grinding

    306.9 Unspecified psychophysiological malfunction
       Psychophysiologic disorder NOS
       Psychosomatic disorder NOS

● **307 Special symptoms or syndromes, not elsewhere classified**

    Note: This category is intended for use if the
       psychopathology is manifested by a single
       specific symptom or group of symptoms which
       is not part of an organic illness or other mental
       disorder classifiable elsewhere.

     Excludes   *those due to mental disorders classified elsewhere*
        those of organic origin

    307.0 ~~Stuttering~~ **Adult onset fluency disorder** ◀▥

     Excludes   *childhood onset fluency disorder (315.35)* ◀
        dysphasia (784.59)
        ~~stuttering~~ (fluency disorder) due to late effect
          of cerebrovascular accident (438.14) ◀▥
        fluency disorder in conditions classified
          elsewhere (784.52) ◀
        lisping or lalling (307.9)
        retarded development of speech
          (315.31–315.39)

    307.1 Anorexia nervosa

     Excludes   *eating disturbance NOS (307.50)*
        feeding problem (783.3)
        of nonorganic origin (307.59)
        loss of appetite (783.0)
        of nonorganic origin (307.59)

     Coding Clinic: 2006, Q2, P12; 1989, Q4, P11

● **307.2 Tics**

     Excludes   *nail-biting or thumb-sucking (307.9)*
        stereotypes occurring in isolation (307.3)
        tics of organic origin (333.3)

    307.20 Tic disorder, unspecified
       Tic disorder NOS

    307.21 Transient tic disorder

    307.22 Chronic motor or vocal tic disorder

    307.23 Tourette's disorder
       Motor-verbal tic disorder

    307.3 Stereotypic movement disorder
       Body-rocking   Spasmus nutans
       Head banging   Stereotypes NOS

     Excludes   *tics (307.20–307.23)*
        of organic origin (333.3)

● **307.4 Specific disorders of sleep of nonorganic origin**

> **Excludes**   *narcolepsy (347.00–347.11)*
> *organic hypersomnia (327.10–327.19)*
> *organic insomnia (327.00–327.09)*
> *those of unspecified cause (780.50–780.59)*

307.40 Nonorganic sleep disorder, unspecified

307.41 Transient disorder of initiating or maintaining sleep
> Adjustment insomnia
> Hyposomnia associated with acute or intermittent emotional reactions or conflicts
> Insomnia associated with acute or intermittent emotional reactions or conflicts
> Sleeplessness associated with acute or intermittent emotional reactions or conflicts

307.42 Persistent disorder of initiating or maintaining sleep
> Hyposomnia, insomnia, or sleeplessness associated with:
> > anxiety
> > conditioned arousal
> > depression (major) (minor)
> > psychosis
> Idiopathic insomnia
> Paradoxical insomnia
> Primary insomnia
> Psychophysiological insomnia

307.43 Transient disorder of initiating or maintaining wakefulness
> Hypersomnia associated with acute or intermittent emotional reactions or conflicts

307.44 Persistent disorder of initiating or maintaining wakefulness
> Hypersomnia associated with depression (major) (minor)
> Insufficient sleep syndrome
> Primary hypersomnia
> > **Excludes**   *sleep deprivation (V69.4)*

307.45 Circadian rhythm sleep disorder of nonorganic origin

307.46 Sleep arousal disorder
> Night terror disorder
> Night terrors
> Sleep terror disorder
> Sleepwalking
> Somnambulism

307.47 Other dysfunctions of sleep stages or arousal from sleep
> Nightmare disorder
> Nightmares:
> > NOS
> > REM-sleep type
> Sleep drunkenness

307.48 Repetitive intrusions of sleep
> Repetitive intrusion of sleep with:
> > atypical polysomnographic features
> > environmental disturbances
> > repeated REM-sleep interruptions

307.49 Other
> "Short-sleeper"
> Subjective insomnia complaint

● **307.5 Other and unspecified disorders of eating**

> **Excludes**   *anorexia:*
> > *nervosa (307.1)*
> > *of unspecified cause (783.0)*
> *overeating, of unspecified cause (783.6)*
> *vomiting:*
> > *NOS (787.03)*
> > *cyclical (536.2)*
> > > *associated with migraine (346.2)*
> > *psychogenic (306.4)*

307.50 Eating disorder, unspecified
> Eating disorder NOS

307.51 Bulimia nervosa
> Overeating of nonorganic origin

307.52 Pica
> Perverted appetite of nonorganic origin
> *Craving and eating substances such as paint, clay, or dirt to replace a nutritional deficit in the body.*

307.53 Rumination disorder
> Regurgitation, of nonorganic origin, of food with reswallowing
> > **Excludes**   *obsessional rumination (300.3)*

307.54 Psychogenic vomiting

307.59 Other
> Feeding disorder of infancy or early childhood of nonorganic origin
> Infantile feeding disturbances of nonorganic origin
> Loss of appetite of nonorganic origin

307.6 Enuresis
> Enuresis (primary) (secondary) of nonorganic origin
> > **Excludes**   *enuresis of unspecified cause (788.3)*

307.7 Encopresis
> Encopresis (continuous) (discontinuous) of nonorganic origin
> > **Excludes**   *encopresis of unspecified cause (787.60-787.63)* ◀

● **307.8 Pain disorders related to psychological factors**

307.80 Psychogenic pain, site unspecified

307.81 Tension headache
> > **Excludes**   *headache:*
> > > *migraine (346.0–346.9)*
> > > *NOS (784.0)*
> > > *syndromes (339.00–339.89)*
> > > *tension type (339.10–339.12)*
> > Coding Clinic: 1985, Nov-Dec, P16

307.89 Other
> *Code first* to type or site of pain
> > **Excludes**   *pain disorder exclusively attributed to psychological factors (307.80)*
> > *psychogenic pain (307.80)*

307.9 Other and unspecified special symptoms or syndromes, not elsewhere classified
> Communication disorder NOS
> Hair plucking
> Lalling
> Lisping
> Masturbation
> Nail-biting
> Thumb-sucking

Item 5–3 **Enuresis**: Bed wetting by children at night. Causes can be either psychological or medical (diabetes, urinary tract infections, or abnormalities). **Encopresis**: Overflow incontinence of bowels sometimes resulting from chronic constipation or fecal impaction. Check the documentation for additional diagnoses.

MENTAL DISORDERS (290–319)

MENTAL DISORDERS (290–319)

● **308 Acute reaction to stress**

     Includes   catastrophic stress
                   combat and operational stress reaction ◄
                   combat fatigue
                   gross stress reaction (acute)
                   transient disorders in response to exceptional physical or mental stress which usually subside within hours or days

     Excludes   *adjustment reaction or disorder (309.0–309.9)*
                      chronic stress reaction (309.1–309.9)

     308.0 Predominant disturbance of emotions
         Anxiety as acute reaction to exceptional [gross] stress
         Emotional crisis as acute reaction to exceptional [gross] stress
         Panic state as acute reaction to exceptional [gross] stress

     308.1 Predominant disturbance of consciousness
         Fugues as acute reaction to exceptional [gross] stress

     308.2 Predominant psychomotor disturbance
         Agitation states as acute reaction to exceptional [gross] stress
         Stupor as acute reaction to exceptional [gross] stress

     308.3 Other acute reactions to stress
         Acute situational disturbance
         Acute stress disorder

         Excludes   *prolonged posttraumatic emotional disturbance (309.81)*

     308.4 Mixed disorders as reaction to stress

     308.9 Unspecified acute reaction to stress

● **309 Adjustment reaction**

     Includes   adjustment disorders
                   reaction (adjustment) to chronic stress

     Excludes   *acute reaction to major stress (308.0–308.9)*
                      neurotic disorders (300.0–300.9)

     309.0 Adjustment disorder with depressed mood
         Grief reaction

         Excludes   *affective psychoses (296.0–296.9)*
                      neurotic depression (300.4)
                      prolonged depressive reaction (309.1)
                      psychogenic depressive psychosis (298.0)

     309.1 Prolonged depressive reaction

         Excludes   *affective psychoses (296.0–296.9)*
                      brief depressive reaction (309.0)
                      neurotic depression (300.4)
                      psychogenic depressive psychosis (298.0)

● **309.2 With predominant disturbance of other emotions**

     309.21 Separation anxiety disorder

     309.22 Emancipation disorder of adolescence and early adult life

     309.23 Specific academic or work inhibition

     309.24 Adjustment disorder with anxiety

     309.28 Adjustment disorder with mixed anxiety and depressed mood
         Adjustment reaction with anxiety and depression

     309.29 Other
         Culture shock

     309.3 Adjustment disorder with disturbance of conduct
         Conduct disturbance as adjustment reaction
         Destructiveness as adjustment reaction

         Excludes   *destructiveness in child (312.9)*
                      disturbance of conduct NOS (312.9)
                      dyssocial behavior without manifest psychiatric disorder (V71.01–V71.02)
                      personality disorder with predominantly sociopathic or asocial manifestations (301.7)

     309.4 Adjustment disorder with mixed disturbance of emotions and conduct

● **309.8 Other specified adjustment reactions**

     309.81 Posttraumatic stress disorder
         Chronic posttraumatic stress disorder
         Concentration camp syndrome
         Posttraumatic stress disorder NOS
         Post-Traumatic Stress Disorder (PTSD)

         Excludes   *acute stress disorder (308.3)*
                      posttraumatic brain syndrome:
                      nonpsychotic (310.2)
                      psychotic (293.0–293.9)

     309.82 Adjustment reaction with physical symptoms

     309.83 Adjustment reaction with withdrawal
         Elective mutism as adjustment reaction
         Hospitalism (in children) NOS

     309.89 Other

     309.9 Unspecified adjustment reaction
         Adaptation reaction NOS
         Adjustment reaction NOS

● **310 Specific nonpsychotic mental disorders due to brain damage**

     Excludes   *neuroses, personality disorders, or other nonpsychotic conditions occurring in a form similar to that seen with functional disorders but in association with a physical condition (300.0–300.9, 301.0–301.9)*

     310.0 Frontal lobe syndrome
         Lobotomy syndrome
         Postleucotomy syndrome [state]

         Excludes   *postcontusion syndrome (310.2)*

     310.1 Personality change due to conditions classified elsewhere
         Cognitive or personality change of other type, of nonpsychotic severity
         Organic psychosyndrome of nonpsychotic severity
         Presbyophrenia NOS
         Senility with mental changes of nonpsychotic severity

         Excludes   *mild cognitive impairment (331.83)*
                      postconcussion syndrome (310.2)
                      signs and symptoms involving emotional state (799.21-799.29)

     Coding Clinic: 2005, Q2, P6-7

     310.2 Postconcussion syndrome
         Postcontusion syndrome or encephalopathy
         Posttraumatic brain syndrome, nonpsychotic
         Status postcommotio cerebri

         Excludes   *any organic psychotic conditions following head injury (293.0–294.0)*
                      frontal lobe syndrome (310.0)
                      postencephalitic syndrome (310.8)

         Use additional code to identify associated post-traumatic headache, if applicable (339.20-339.22)

310.8 Other specified nonpsychotic mental disorders following organic brain damage
Mild memory disturbance
Postencephalitic syndrome
Other focal (partial) organic psychosyndromes

Excludes　*memory loss of unknown cause (780.93)*

310.9 Unspecified nonpsychotic mental disorder following organic brain damage
Coding Clinic: 2003, Q4, P103-104

311 Depressive disorder, not elsewhere classified
Depressive disorder NOS
Depressive state NOS
Depression NOS

Excludes　*acute reaction to major stress with depressive symptoms (308.0)*
affective personality disorder (301.10–301.13)
affective psychoses (296.0–296.9)
brief depressive reaction (309.0)
depressive states associated with stressful events (309.0–309.1)
disturbance of emotions specific to childhood and adolescence, with misery and unhappiness (313.1)
mixed adjustment reaction with depressive symptoms (309.4)
neurotic depression (300.4)
prolonged depressive adjustment reaction (309.1)
psychogenic depressive psychosis (298.0)

Coding Clinic: 2003, Q4, P75-76

●**312 Disturbance of conduct, not elsewhere classified**

Excludes　*adjustment reaction with disturbance of conduct (309.3)*
drug dependence (304.0–304.9)
dyssocial behavior without manifest psychiatric disorder (V71.01–V71.02)
personality disorder with predominantly sociopathic or asocial manifestations (301.7)
sexual deviations (302.0–302.9)

The following fifth-digit subclassification is for use with categories 312.0–312.2:

> 0　unspecified
> 1　mild
> 2　moderate
> 3　severe

●**312.0 Undersocialized conduct disorder, aggressive type**
[0-3]　Aggressive outburst
Anger reaction
Unsocialized aggressive disorder

●**312.1 Undersocialized conduct disorder, unaggressive type**
[0-3]　Childhood truancy, unsocialized
Solitary stealing
Tantrums

●**312.2 Socialized conduct disorder**
[0-3]　Childhood truancy, socialized
Group delinquency

Excludes　*gang activity without manifest psychiatric disorder (V71.01)*

●**312.3 Disorders of impulse control, not elsewhere classified**
　　312.30 Impulse control disorder, unspecified
　　312.31 Pathological gambling
　　312.32 Kleptomania *(stealing)*
　　312.33 Pyromania *(setting fires)*
　　312.34 Intermittent explosive disorder
　　312.35 Isolated explosive disorder

　　312.39 Other
　　　　Trichotillomania
　　　　Pulling or twisting hair until it falls out

312.4 Mixed disturbance of conduct and emotions
Neurotic delinquency

Excludes　*compulsive conduct disorder (312.3)*

●**312.8 Other specified disturbances of conduct, not elsewhere classified**
　　312.81 Conduct disorder, childhood onset type
　　312.82 Conduct disorder, adolescent onset type
　　312.89 Other conduct disorder
　　　　Conduct disorder of unspecified onset

312.9 Unspecified disturbance of conduct
Delinquency (juvenile)
Disruptive behavior disorder NOS

●**313 Disturbance of emotions specific to childhood and adolescence**

Excludes　*adjustment reaction (309.0–309.9)*
emotional disorder of neurotic type (300.0–300.9)
masturbation, nail-biting, thumb-sucking, and other isolated symptoms (307.0–307.9)

313.0 Overanxious disorder
Anxiety and fearfulness of childhood and adolescence
Overanxious disorder of childhood and adolescence

Excludes　*abnormal separation anxiety (309.21)*
anxiety states (300.00–300.09)
hospitalism in children (309.83)
phobic state (300.20–300.29)

313.1 Misery and unhappiness disorder

Excludes　*depressive neurosis (300.4)*

●**313.2 Sensitivity, shyness, and social withdrawal disorder**

Excludes　*infantile autism (299.0)*
schizoid personality (301.20–301.22)
schizophrenia (295.0–295.9)

　　313.21 Shyness disorder of childhood
　　　　Sensitivity reaction of childhood or adolescence
　　313.22 Introverted disorder of childhood
　　　　Social withdrawal of childhood or adolescence
　　　　Withdrawal reaction of childhood or adolescence
　　313.23 Selective mutism

Excludes　*elective mutism as adjustment reaction (309.83)*

313.3 Relationship problems
Sibling jealousy

Excludes　*relationship problems associated with aggression, destruction, or other forms of conduct disturbance (312.0–312.9)*

●**313.8 Other or mixed emotional disturbances of childhood or adolescence**
　　313.81 Oppositional defiant disorder
　　313.82 Identity disorder
　　　　Identity problem
　　313.83 Academic underachievement disorder
　　313.89 Other
　　　　Reactive attachment disorder of infancy or early childhood

313.9 Unspecified emotional disturbance of childhood or adolescence
Mental disorder of infancy, childhood or adolescence NOS

MENTAL DISORDERS (290–319)

MENTAL DISORDERS (290–319)

● 314 **Hyperkinetic syndrome of childhood**
- **Excludes** *hyperkinesis as symptom of underlying disorder-code the underlying disorder*

● 314.0 **Attention deficit disorder** *(ADD)*
Adult
Child

  314.00 **Without mention of hyperactivity**
  Predominantly inattentive type
  Coding Clinic: 1997, Q1, P8-9

  314.01 **With hyperactivity**
  Attention deficit disorder with hyperactivity = ADHD
  Combined type
  Overactivity NOS
  Predominantly hyperactive/impulsive type
  Simple disturbance of attention with overactivity
  Coding Clinic: 1997, Q1, P8-9

314.1 **Hyperkinesis with developmental delay**
Developmental disorder of hyperkinesis
  Use additional code to identify any associated neurological disorder

314.2 **Hyperkinetic conduct disorder**
Hyperkinetic conduct disorder without developmental delay
  Excludes *hyperkinesis with significant delays in specific skills (314.1)*

314.8 **Other specified manifestations of hyperkinetic syndrome**

314.9 **Unspecified hyperkinetic syndrome**
Hyperkinetic reaction of childhood or adolescence NOS
Hyperkinetic syndrome NOS

● 315 **Specific delays in development**
- **Excludes** *that due to a neurological disorder (320.0–389.9)*

● 315.0 **Specific reading disorder**
  315.00 **Reading disorder, unspecified**
  315.01 **Alexia**
  315.02 **Developmental dyslexia**
  315.09 **Other**
  Specific spelling difficulty

315.1 **Mathematics disorder**
Dyscalculia

315.2 **Other specific learning difficulties**
Disorder of written expression
  Excludes *specific arithmetical disorder (315.1)*
  specific reading disorder (315.00–315.09)

● 315.3 **Developmental speech or language disorder**
  315.31 **Expressive language disorder**
  Developmental aphasia
  Word deafness
  Excludes *acquired aphasia (784.3)*
  elective mutism (309.83, 313.0, 313.23)

  315.32 **Mixed receptive-expressive language disorder**
  Central auditory processing disorder
  Excludes *acquired auditory processing disorder (388.45)*
  Coding Clinic: 2005, Q2, P5-6

  315.34 **Speech and language developmental delay due to hearing loss**
  Coding Clinic: 2007, Q4, P80-81

315.35 **Childhood onset fluency disorder ◄**
Cluttering NOS ◄
Stuttering NOS ◄
  Excludes *adult onset fluency disorder (307.0) ◄*
  fluency disorder due to late effect of cerebrovascular accident (438.14) ◄
  fluency disorder in conditions classified elsewhere (784.52) ◄

315.39 **Other**
Developmental articulation disorder
Dyslalia
Phonological disorder
  Excludes *lisping and lalling (307.9)*
  stammering and stuttering (307.0)
  Coding Clinic: 2007, Q3, P9-10

315.4 **Developmental coordination disorder**
Clumsiness syndrome
Dyspraxia syndrome
Specific motor development disorder

315.5 **Mixed development disorder**
Coding Clinic: 2002, Q2, P11

315.8 **Other specified delays in development**

315.9 **Unspecified delay in development**
Developmental disorder NOS
Learning disorder NOS

316 **Psychic factors associated with diseases classified elsewhere**
Psychologic factors in physical conditions classified elsewhere
  Use additional code to identify the associated physical condition, as:
  psychogenic:
    asthma (493.9)
    dermatitis (692.9)
    duodenal ulcer (532.0–532.9)
    eczema (691.8, 692.9)
    gastric ulcer (531.0–531.9)
    mucous colitis (564.9)
    paroxysmal tachycardia (427.2)
    ulcerative colitis (556)
    urticaria (708.0–708.9)
  psychosocial dwarfism (259.4)
  Excludes *physical symptoms and physiological malfunctions, not involving tissue damage, of mental origin (306.0–306.9)*

MENTAL RETARDATION (317–319)

  Use additional code(s) to identify any associated psychiatric or physical condition(s)

317 **Mild mental retardation**
High-grade defect
IQ 50–70
Mild mental subnormality

● 318 **Other specified mental retardation**
  318.0 **Moderate mental retardation**
  IQ 35–49
  Moderate mental subnormality

  318.1 **Severe mental retardation**
  IQ 20–34
  Severe mental subnormality

  318.2 **Profound mental retardation**
  IQ under 20
  Profound mental subnormality

319 **Unspecified mental retardation**
Mental deficiency NOS
Mental subnormality NOS

◄ New   ◄▥ Revised   ~~deleted~~ Deleted   Excludes   Includes   Use additional   Code first   Omit code
● Unacceptable Principal Diagnosis   ● Use Additional Digit(s)   OGCR Official Guidelines   Coding Clinic

(See Plate 164 on page NAP-2.)

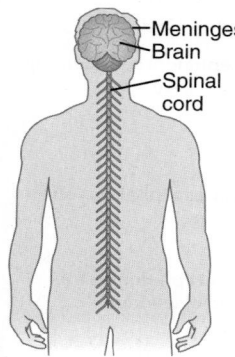
- Meninges
- Brain
- Spinal cord

Figure 6–1 The brain and spinal cord make up the central nervous system.

Item 6–1 The two major classifications of the nervous system are the peripheral nervous system and the central nervous system (CNS). The central nervous system is comprised of the brain and the spinal cord. The peripheral nervous system is comprised of the parasympathetic and sympathetic systems. **Encephalitis** is the swelling of the brain. **Meningitis** is swelling of the covering of the brain, the meninges. Types and causes of brain infections are:

Type	Cause
purulent	bacterial
aseptic/abacterial	viral
chronic meningitis	mycobacterial and fungal

6. DISEASES OF THE NERVOUS SYSTEM AND SENSE ORGANS (320–389)

INFLAMMATORY DISEASES OF THE CENTRAL NERVOUS SYSTEM (320–326)

● **320 Bacterial meningitis**
Infection of cerebrospinal fluid surrounding spinal cord and brain

Includes arachnoiditis bacterial
leptomeningitis bacterial
meningitis bacterial
meningoencephalitis bacterial
meningomyelitis bacterial
pachymeningitis bacterial

320.0 Hemophilus meningitis
Meningitis due to Hemophilus influenzae [H. influenzae]

320.1 Pneumococcal meningitis

320.2 Streptococcal meningitis

320.3 Staphylococcal meningitis

320.7 Meningitis in other bacterial diseases classified elsewhere
Code first underlying disease as:
actinomycosis (039.8)
listeriosis (027.0)
typhoid fever (002.0)
whooping cough (033.0–033.9)

Excludes *meningitis (in):*
epidemic (036.0)
gonococcal (098.82)
meningococcal (036.0)
salmonellosis (003.21)
syphilis:
NOS (094.2)
congenital (090.42)
meningovascular (094.2)
secondary (091.81)
tuberculosis (013.0)

● **320.8 Meningitis due to other specified bacteria**

320.81 Anaerobic meningitis
Bacteroides (fragilis)
Gram-negative anaerobes

320.82 Meningitis due to gram-negative bacteria, not elsewhere classified
Aerobacter aerogenes
Escherichia coli [E. coli]
Friedlander bacillus
Klebsiella pneumoniae
Proteus morganii
Pseudomonas
Excludes *gram-negative anaerobes (320.81)*

320.89 Meningitis due to other specified bacteria
Bacillus pyocyaneus

320.9 Meningitis due to unspecified bacterium
Meningitis: Meningitis:
bacterial NOS   pyogenic NOS
purulent NOS   suppurative NOS

● **321 Meningitis due to other organisms**
Includes arachnoiditis due to organisms other than bacteria
leptomeningitis due to organisms other than bacteria
meningitis due to organisms other than bacteria
pachymeningitis due to organisms other than bacteria

321.0 Cryptococcal meningitis
Code first underlying disease (117.5)

321.1 Meningitis in other fungal diseases
Code first underlying disease (110.0–118)
Excludes *meningitis in:*
candidiasis (112.83)
coccidioidomycosis (114.2)
histoplasmosis (115.01, 115.11, 115.91)

321.2 Meningitis due to viruses not elsewhere classified
Code first underlying disease, as:
meningitis due to arbovirus (060.0–066.9)
Excludes *meningitis (due to):*
abacterial (047.0–047.9)
adenovirus (049.1)
aseptic NOS (047.9)
Coxsackie (virus) (047.0)
ECHO virus (047.1)
enterovirus (047.0–047.9)
herpes simplex virus (054.72)
herpes zoster virus (053.0)
lymphocytic choriomeningitis virus (049.0)
mumps (072.1)
viral NOS (047.9)
meningo-eruptive syndrome (047.1)
Coding Clinic: 2004, Q4, P50-52

321.3 Meningitis due to trypanosomiasis
Code first underlying disease (086.0–086.9)

321.4 Meningitis in sarcoidosis
Code first underlying disease (135)

321.8 Meningitis due to other nonbacterial organisms classified elsewhere
Code first underlying disease
Excludes *leptospiral meningitis (100.81)*

● **322 Meningitis of unspecified cause**

> **Includes**   arachnoiditis with no organism specified as cause
>
> leptomeningitis with no organism specified as cause
>
> meningitis with no organism specified as cause
>
> pachymeningitis with no organism specified as cause

322.0 Nonpyogenic meningitis
    Meningitis with clear cerebrospinal fluid

322.1 Eosinophilic meningitis

322.2 Chronic meningitis

322.9 Meningitis, unspecified

● **323 Encephalitis, myelitis, and encephalomyelitis**

> **Includes**   acute disseminated encephalomyelitis
>
> meningoencephalitis, except bacterial
>
> meningomyelitis, except bacterial
>
> myelitis:
>   ascending
>   transverse

> **Excludes**   *acute transverse myelitis NOS (341.20)*
>
> *acute transverse myelitis in conditions classified elsewhere (341.21)*
>
> *bacterial:*
>   *meningoencephalitis (320.0–320.9)*
>   *meningomyelitis (320.0–320.9)*
>
> *idiopathic transverse myelitis (341.22)*

Coding Clinic: 2006, Q4, P58-63

● **323.0 Encephalitis, myelitis, and encephalomyelitis in viral diseases classified elsewhere**

> Code first *underlying disease, as:*
>   cat-scratch disease (078.3)
>   infectious mononucleosis (075)
>   ornithosis (073.7)

323.01 Encephalitis and encephalomyelitis in viral diseases classified elsewhere

> **Excludes**   *encephalitis (in):*
>   *arthropod-borne viral (062.0–064)*
>   *herpes simplex (054.3)*
>   *mumps (072.2)*
>   *other viral diseases of central nervous system (049.8–049.9)*
>   *poliomyelitis (045.0–045.9)*
>   *rubella (056.01)*
>   *slow virus infections of central nervous system (046.0–046.9)*
>   *viral NOS (049.9)*
>   *West Nile (066.41)*

323.02 Myelitis in viral diseases classified elsewhere

> **Excludes**   *myelitis (in):*
>   *herpes simplex (054.74)*
>   *herpes zoster (053.14)*
>   *other viral diseases of central nervous system (049.8–049.9)*
>   *poliomyelitis (045.0–045.9)*
>   *rubella (056.01)*

Item 6-2   Encephalitis is an inflammation of the brain most often caused by a virus but may also be caused by a bacteria and most commonly transmitted by a mosquito. **Myelitis** is an inflammation of the spinal cord that may disrupt CNS function. Untreated myelitis may rapidly lead to permanent damage to the spinal cord. **Encephalomyelitis** is a general term for an inflammation of the brain and spinal cord.

323.1 Encephalitis, myelitis, and encephalomyelitis in rickettsial diseases classified elsewhere

> Code first *underlying disease (080–083.9)*

323.2 Encephalitis, myelitis, and encephalomyelitis in protozoal diseases classified elsewhere

> Code first *underlying disease, as:*
>   malaria (084.0–084.9)
>   trypanosomiasis (086.0–086.9)

● **323.4 Other encephalitis, myelitis, and encephalomyelitis due to infection classified elsewhere**

> Code first *underlying disease*

323.41 Other encephalitis and encephalomyelitis due to infection classified elsewhere

> **Excludes**   *encephalitis (in):*
>   *meningococcal (036.1)*
>   *syphilis:*
>   *NOS (094.81)*
>   *congenital (090.41)*
>   *toxoplasmosis (130.0)*
>   *tuberculosis (013.6)*
>   *meningoencephalitis due to free-living ameba [Naegleria] (136.29)*

323.42 Other myelitis due to infection classified elsewhere

> **Excludes**   *myelitis (in):*
>   *syphilis (094.89)*
>   *tuberculosis (013.6)*

● **323.5 Encephalitis, myelitis, and encephalomyelitis following immunization procedures**

> Use additional E code to identify vaccine

323.51 Encephalitis and encephalomyelitis following immunization procedures
    Encephalitis postimmunization or postvaccinal
    Encephalomyelitis postimmunization or postvaccinal

323.52 Myelitis following immunization procedures
    Myelitis postimmunization or postvaccinal

● **323.6 Postinfectious encephalitis, myelitis, and encephalomyelitis**

> Code first *underlying disease*

323.61 Infectious acute disseminated encephalomyelitis (ADEM)
    Acute necrotizing hemorrhagic encephalopathy

> **Excludes**   *noninfectious acute disseminated encephalomyelitis (323.81)*

323.62 Other postinfectious encephalitis and encephalomyelitis

> **Excludes**   *encephalitis:*
>   *postchickenpox (052.0)*
>   *postmeasles (055.0)*

323.63 Postinfectious myelitis

● **323.7 Toxic encephalitis, myelitis, and encephalomyelitis**

> Code first *underlying cause, as:*
>   carbon tetrachloride (982.1)
>   hydroxyquinoline derivatives (961.3)
>   lead (984.0–984.9)
>   mercury (985.0)
>   thallium (985.8)

323.71 Toxic encephalitis and encephalomyelitis

323.72 Toxic myelitis

◀ New   ◀▦ Revised   ~~deleted~~ Deleted   Excludes   Includes   Use additional   Code first   Omit code
● Unacceptable Principal Diagnosis   ● Use Additional Digit(s)   **OGCR** Official Guidelines   **Coding Clinic**

● **323.8 Other causes of encephalitis, myelitis, and encephalomyelitis**
Coding Clinic: 1997, Q2, P8-9

  323.81 Other causes of encephalitis and encephalomyelitis
Noninfectious acute disseminated encephalomyelitis (ADEM)

  323.82 Other causes of myelitis
Transverse myelitis NOS

323.9 Unspecified cause of encephalitis, myelitis, and encephalomyelitis
Coding Clinic: 2006, Q1, P8

● **324 Intracranial and intraspinal abscess**
Accumulation of pus in either brain or spinal cord

  324.0 Intracranial abscess
Abscess (embolic):
cerebellar
cerebral
Abscess (embolic) of brain [any part]:
epidural
extradural
otogenic
subdural
> **Excludes** *tuberculous (013.3)*

  324.1 Intraspinal abscess
Abscess (embolic) of spinal cord [any part]:
epidural
extradural
subdural
> **Excludes** *tuberculous (013.5)*

  324.9 Of unspecified site
Extradural or subdural abscess NOS

325 Phlebitis and thrombophlebitis of intracranial venous sinuses
Embolism of cavernous, lateral, or other intracranial or unspecified intracranial venous sinus
Endophlebitis of cavernous, lateral, or other intracranial or unspecified intracranial venous sinus
Phlebitis, septic or suppurative of cavernous, lateral, or other intracranial or unspecified intracranial venous sinus
Thrombophlebitis of cavernous, lateral, or other intracranial or unspecified intracranial venous sinus
Thrombosis of cavernous, lateral, or other intracranial or unspecified intracranial venous sinus
> **Excludes** *that specified as:*
> *complicating pregnancy, childbirth, or the puerperium (671.5)*
> *of nonpyogenic origin (437.6)*

326 Late effects of intracranial abscess or pyogenic infection
Note: This category is to be used to indicate conditions whose primary classification is to 320–325 [excluding 320.7, 321.0–321.8, 323.01–323.42, 323.61–323.72] as the cause of late effects, themselves classifiable elsewhere. The "late effects" include conditions specified as such, or as sequelae, which may occur at any time after the resolution of the causal condition.
Use additional code to identify condition, as:
hydrocephalus (331.4)
paralysis (342.0–342.9, 344.0–344.9)

● **327 Organic sleep disorders**
Involve difficulties of sleep at all levels, including difficulty falling or staying asleep, falling asleep at inappropriate times, excessive total sleep time, or abnormal behaviors associated with sleep

● **327.0 Organic disorders of initiating and maintaining sleep [Organic insomnia]**
> **Excludes** *insomnia NOS (780.52)*
> *insomnia not due to a substance or known physiological condition (307.41–307.42)*
> *insomnia with sleep apnea NOS (780.51)*

  327.00 Organic insomnia, unspecified
  327.01 Insomnia due to medical condition classified elsewhere
  Code first underlying condition
  > **Excludes** *insomnia due to mental disorder (327.02)*

  327.02 Insomnia due to mental disorder
  Code first mental disorder
  > **Excludes** *alcohol induced insomnia (291.82)*
  > *drug induced insomnia (292.85)*

  327.09 Other organic insomnia

● **327.1 Organic disorder of excessive somnolence [Organic hypersomnia]**
> **Excludes** *hypersomnia NOS (780.54)*
> *hypersomnia not due to a substance or known physiological condition (307.43–307.44)*
> *hypersomnia with sleep apnea NOS (780.53)*

  327.10 Organic hypersomnia, unspecified
  327.11 Idiopathic hypersomnia with long sleep time
  327.12 Idiopathic hypersomnia without long sleep time
  327.13 Recurrent hypersomnia
  Kleine-Levin syndrome
  Menstrual related hypersomnia
  327.14 Hypersomnia due to medical condition classified elsewhere
  Code first underlying condition
  > **Excludes** *hypersomnia due to mental disorder (327.15)*

  327.15 Hypersomnia due to mental disorder
  Code first mental disorder
  > **Excludes** *alcohol induced insomnia (291.82)*
  > *drug induced insomnia (292.85)*

  327.19 Other organic hypersomnia

● **327.2 Organic sleep apnea**
Characterized by episodes in which breathing stops during sleep, resulting in a lack of prolonged deep sleep and excessive daytime sleepiness
> **Excludes** *Cheyne-Stokes breathing (786.04)*
> *hypersomnia with sleep apnea NOS (780.53)*
> *insomnia with sleep apnea NOS (780.51)*
> *sleep apnea in newborn (770.81–770.82)*
> *sleep apnea NOS (780.57)*

  327.20 Organic sleep apnea, unspecified
  327.21 Primary central sleep apnea
  327.22 High altitude periodic breathing
  327.23 Obstructive sleep apnea (adult) (pediatric)

327.24 Idiopathic sleep related nonobstructive alveolar hypoventilation
Sleep related hypoxia

327.25 Congenital central alveolar hypoventilation syndrome

327.26 Sleep related hypoventilation/hypoxemia in conditions classifiable elsewhere
Code first underlying condition

327.27 Central sleep apnea in conditions classified elsewhere
Code first underlying condition

327.29 Other organic sleep apnea

● **327.3 Circadian rhythm sleep disorder**
Involves one of the sleep/wake regulating hormones. The inability to sleep results from a mismatch between the body's internal clock and the external 24-hour schedule.
Organic disorder of sleep wake cycle
Organic disorder of sleep wake schedule

Excludes   *alcohol induced circadian rhythm sleep disorder (291.82)*
circadian rhythm sleep disorder of nonorganic origin (307.45)
disruption of 24 hour sleep wake cycle NOS (780.55)
drug induced circadian rhythm sleep disorder (292.85)

327.30 Circadian rhythm sleep disorder, unspecified

327.31 Circadian rhythm sleep disorder, delayed sleep phase type

327.32 Circadian rhythm sleep disorder, advanced sleep phase type

327.33 Circadian rhythm sleep disorder, irregular sleep-wake type

327.34 Circadian rhythm sleep disorder, free-running type

327.35 Circadian rhythm sleep disorder, jet lag type

327.36 Circadian rhythm sleep disorder, shift work type

327.37 Circadian rhythm sleep disorder in conditions classified elsewhere
Code first underlying condition

327.39 Other circadian rhythm sleep disorder

● **327.4 Organic parasomnia**

Excludes   *alcohol induced parasomnia (291.82)*
drug induced parasomnia (292.85)
parasomnia not due to a known physiological condition (307.47)

327.40 Organic parasomnia, unspecified

327.41 Confusional arousals

327.42 REM sleep behavior disorder

327.43 Recurrent isolated sleep paralysis

327.44 Parasomnia in conditions classified elsewhere
Code first underlying condition

327.49 Other organic parasomnia

● **327.5 Organic sleep related movement disorders**

Excludes   *restless legs syndrome (333.94)*
sleep related movement disorder NOS (780.58)

327.51 Periodic limb movement disorder
Periodic limb movement sleep disorder

327.52 Sleep related leg cramps

327.53 Sleep related bruxism

327.59 Other organic sleep related movement disorders

327.8 Other organic sleep disorders
Coding Clinic: 2007, Q2, P7-8

HEREDITARY AND DEGENERATIVE DISEASES OF THE CENTRAL NERVOUS SYSTEM (330–337)

Excludes   *hepatolenticular degeneration (275.1)*
multiple sclerosis (340)
other demyelinating diseases of central nervous system (341.0–341.9)

● **330 Cerebral degenerations usually manifest in childhood**
Use additional code to identify associated mental retardation

330.0 Leukodystrophy
Krabbe's disease
Leukodystrophy:
   NOS
   globoid cell
   metachromatic
   sudanophilic
Pelizaeus-Merzbacher disease
Sulfatide lipidosis

330.1 Cerebral lipidoses
Amaurotic (familial) idiocy
Disease:
   Batten
   Jansky-Bielschowsky
   Kufs'
   Spielmeyer-Vogt
   Tay-Sachs
Gangliosidosis

330.2 Cerebral degeneration in generalized lipidoses
Code first underlying disease, as:
   Fabry's disease (272.7)
   Gaucher's disease (272.7)
   Niemann-Pick disease (272.7)
   sphingolipidosis (272.7)

330.3 Cerebral degeneration of childhood in other diseases classified elsewhere
Code first underlying disease, as:
   Hunter's disease (277.5)
   mucopolysaccharidosis (277.5)

330.8 Other specified cerebral degenerations in childhood
Alpers' disease or gray-matter degeneration
Infantile necrotizing encephalomyelopathy
Leigh's disease
Subacute necrotizing encephalopathy or encephalomyelopathy
Coding Clinic: 1995, Q1, P9

330.9 Unspecified cerebral degeneration in childhood

Item 6-3 Leukodystrophy is characterized by degeneration and/or failure of the myelin formation of the central nervous system and sometimes of the peripheral nervous system. The disease is inherited and progressive.

◀ New   ◀║║║ Revised   ~~deleted~~ Deleted   Excludes   Includes   Use additional   Code first   Omit code
● Unacceptable Principal Diagnosis   ● Use Additional Digit(s)   OGCR   Official Guidelines   Coding Clinic

Item 6–4 Pick's disease is the atrophy of the frontal and temporal lobes, causing dementia; **Alzheimer's** is characterized by a more diffuse cerebral atrophy.

● **331 Other cerebral degenerations**

> Use additional code, where applicable, to identify dementia:
> with behavioral disturbance (294.11)
> without behavioral disturbance (294.10)

331.0 Alzheimer's disease
> Coding Clinic: 2000, Q4, P40-41; 1999, Q4, P7; 1994, Q2, P10-11; Q1, P21; 1984, Nov-Dec, P20

● **331.1 Frontotemporal dementia**

331.11 Pick's disease
> Coding Clinic: 2003, Q4, P57-58

331.19 Other frontotemporal dementia
> Frontal dementia
> Coding Clinic: 2003, Q4, P57-58

331.2 Senile degeneration of brain
> Excludes *senility NOS (797)*

331.3 Communicating hydrocephalus
> Secondary normal pressure hydrocephalus
> Excludes *congenital hydrocephalus (742.3)*
> *idiopathic normal pressure hydrocephalus (331.5)*
> *normal pressure hydrocephalus (331.5)*
> *spina bifida with hydrocephalus (741.0)*
> Coding Clinic: 2007, Q4, P74-75; 1985, Sept-Oct, P12

331.4 Obstructive hydrocephalus
> Acquired hydrocephalus NOS
> Excludes *congenital hydrocephalus (742.3)*
> *idiopathic normal pressure hydrocephalus (331.5)*
> *normal pressure hydrocephalus (331.5)*
> *spina bifida with hydrocephalus (741.0)*
> Coding Clinic: 2007, Q4, P74-75; 2003, Q4, P106-107; 1999, Q1, P9-10

331.5 Idiopathic normal pressure hydrocephalus (INPH)
> Normal pressure hydrocephalus NOS
> Excludes *congenital hydrocephalus (742.3)*
> *secondary normal pressure hydrocephalus (331.3)*
> *spina bifida with hydrocephalus (741.0)*
> Coding Clinic: 2007, Q4, P74-75

331.7 Cerebral degeneration in diseases classified elsewhere
> *Code first underlying disease, as:*
> alcoholism (303.0–303.9)
> beriberi (265.0)
> cerebrovascular disease (430–438)
> congenital hydrocephalus (741.0, 742.3)
> neoplastic disease (140.0–239.9)
> myxedema (244.0–244.9)
> vitamin B12 deficiency (266.2)
> Excludes *cerebral degeneration in:*
> *Jakob-Creutzfeldt disease (046.11–046.19)*
> *progressive multifocal leukoencephalopathy (046.3)*
> *subacute spongiform encephalopathy (046.1)*

● **331.8 Other cerebral degeneration**

331.81 Reye's syndrome

331.82 Dementia with Lewy bodies
> Dementia with Parkinsonism
> Lewy body dementia
> Lewy body disease
> Coding Clinic: 2003, Q4, P57-58

331.83 Mild cognitive impairment, so stated
> Excludes *altered mental status (780.97)*
> *cerebral degeneration (331.0–331.9)*
> *change in mental status (780.97)*
> *cognitive deficits following (late effects of) cerebral hemorrhage or infarction (438.0)*
> *cognitive impairment due to intracranial or head injury (850–854, 959.01)*
> *cognitive impairment due to late effect of intracranial injury (907.0)*
> *cognitive impairment due to skull fracture (800-801, 803-804)*
> *dementia (290.0–290.43, 294.8)*
> *mild memory disturbance (310.8)*
> *neurologic neglect syndrome (781.8)*
> *personality change, nonpsychotic (310.1)*
> Coding Clinic: 2006, Q4, P75-76

331.89 Other
> Cerebral ataxia

331.9 Cerebral degeneration, unspecified

● **332 Parkinson's disease**
> *Movement disorder (chronic or progressive); cause unknown, and no cure.*
> Excludes *dementia with Parkinsonism (331.82)*

332.0 Paralysis agitans
> Parkinsonism or Parkinson's disease:
> NOS
> idiopathic
> primary

332.1 Secondary Parkinsonism
> Neuroleptic-induced Parkinsonism
> Parkinsonism due to drugs
> Use additional E code to identify drug, if drug-induced
> Excludes *Parkinsonism (in):*
> *Huntington's disease (333.4)*
> *progressive supranuclear palsy (333.0)*
> *Shy-Drager syndrome (333.0)*
> *syphilitic (094.82)*

● **333 Other extrapyramidal disease and abnormal movement disorders**
> Includes other forms of extrapyramidal, basal ganglia, or striatopallidal disease
> Excludes *abnormal movements of head NOS (781.0)*
> *sleep related movement disorders (327.51–327.59)*

333.0 Other degenerative diseases of the basal ganglia
> Atrophy or degeneration:
> olivopontocerebellar [Déjérine-Thomas syndrome]
> pigmentary pallidal [Hallervorden-Spatz disease] striatonigral
> Parkinsonian syndrome associated with:
> idiopathic orthostatic hypotension
> symptomatic orthostatic hypotension
> Progressive supranuclear ophthalmoplegia
> Shy-Drager syndrome
> Coding Clinic: 1996, Q2, P8-9

Item 6–5 Huntington's chorea is an inherited degenerative disorder of the central nervous system and is characterized by ceaseless, jerky movements and progressive cognitive and behavioral deterioration.

333.1 Essential and other specified forms of tremor
Benign essential tremor
Familial tremor
Medication-induced postural tremor

Use additional E code to identify drug, if drug-induced

Excludes tremor NOS (781.0)

333.2 Myoclonus
Familial essential myoclonus
Palatal myoclonus

Excludes progressive myoclonic epilepsy (345.1)
Unverricht-Lundborg disease (345.1)

Use additional E code to identify drug, if drug-induced
Coding Clinic: 1997, Q3, P5; 1987, Mar-April, P12

333.3 Tics of organic origin

Excludes Gilles de la Tourette's syndrome (307.23)
habit spasm (307.22)
tic NOS (307.20)

Use additional E code to identify drug, if drug-induced

333.4 Huntington's chorea

333.5 Other choreas
Hemiballism(us)
Paroxysmal choreo-athetosis

Excludes Sydenham's or rheumatic chorea (392.0–392.9)

Use additional E code to identify drug, if drug-induced

333.6 Genetic torsion dystonia
Dystonia:
deformans progressiva
musculorum deformans
(Schwalbe-) Ziehen-Oppenheim disease
Coding Clinic: 2006, Q4, P76-78

● 333.7 Acquired torsion dystonia
Coding Clinic: 2006, Q4, P76-78

333.71 Athetoid cerebral palsy
Double athetosis (syndrome)
Vogt's disease

Excludes infantile cerebral palsy (343.0–343.9)

333.72 Acute dystonia due to drugs
Acute dystonic reaction due to drugs
Neuroleptic-induced acute dystonia

Use additional E code to identify drug

Excludes blepharospasm due to drugs (333.85)
orofacial dyskinesia due to drugs (333.85)
secondary Parkinsonism (332.1)
subacute dyskinesia due to drugs (333.85)
tardive dyskinesia (333.85)

333.79 Other acquired torsion dystonia

● 333.8 Fragments of torsion dystonia

Use additional E code to identify drug, if drug-induced

333.81 Blepharospasm

Excludes blepharospasm due to drugs (333.85)

333.82 Orofacial dyskinesia

Excludes orofacial dyskinesia due to drugs (333.85)

333.83 Spasmodic torticollis

Excludes torticollis:
NOS (723.5)
hysterical (300.11)
psychogenic (306.0)

333.84 Organic writers' cramp

Excludes psychogenic (300.89)

333.85 Subacute dyskinesia due to drugs
Blepharospasm due to drugs
Orofacial dyskinesia due to drugs
Tardive dyskinesia

Use additional E code to identify drug

Excludes acute dystonia due to drugs (333.72)
acute dystonic reaction due to drugs (333.72)
secondary Parkinsonism (332.1)
Coding Clinic: 2006, Q4, P76-78

333.89 Other

● 333.9 Other and unspecified extrapyramidal diseases and abnormal movement disorders

333.90 Unspecified extrapyramidal disease and abnormal movement disorder
Medication-induced movement disorders NOS

Use additional E code to identify drug, if drug-induced

333.91 Stiff-man syndrome

333.92 Neuroleptic malignant syndrome

Use additional E code to identify drug

Excludes neuroleptic induced Parkinsonism (332.1)

333.93 Benign shuddering attacks

333.94 Restless legs syndrome (RLS)
Coding Clinic: 2006, Q4, P79

333.99 Other
Neuroleptic-induced acute akathisia

Use additional E code to identify drug, if drug-induced
Coding Clinic: 2004, Q2, P12

● 334 Spinocerebellar disease
Group of degenerative disorders in which primary symptom is progressive ataxia (jerky, uncoordinated movements)

Excludes olivopontocerebellar degeneration (333.0)
peroneal muscular atrophy (356.1)

334.0 Friedreich's ataxia

334.1 Hereditary spastic paraplegia

334.2 Primary cerebellar degeneration
Cerebellar ataxia:
Marie's
Sanger-Brown
Dyssynergia cerebellaris myoclonica
Primary cerebellar degeneration:
NOS
hereditary
sporadic
Coding Clinic: 1987, Mar-April, P9

334.3 Other cerebellar ataxia
Cerebellar ataxia NOS

Use additional E code to identify drug, if drug-induced

334.4 Cerebellar ataxia in diseases classified elsewhere

Code first underlying disease, as:
alcoholism (303.0–303.9)
myxedema (244.0–244.9)
neoplastic disease (140.0–239.9)

334.8 Other spinocerebellar diseases
Ataxia-telangiectasia [Louis-Bar syndrome]
Corticostriatal-spinal degeneration

334.9 Spinocerebellar disease, unspecified

● **335 Anterior horn cell disease**

335.0 Werdnig-Hoffmann disease
Infantile spinal muscular atrophy
Progressive muscular atrophy of infancy

● **335.1 Spinal muscular atrophy**

335.10 Spinal muscular atrophy, unspecified

335.11 Kugelberg-Welander disease
Spinal muscular atrophy:
familial
juvenile

335.19 Other
Adult spinal muscular atrophy

● **335.2 Motor neuron disease**

335.20 Amyotrophic lateral sclerosis
Also listed in the Index as "Lou Gehrig's disease" (ALS)
Motor neuron disease (bulbar) (mixed type)
Coding Clinic: 1995, Q4, P81

335.21 Progressive muscular atrophy
Duchenne-Aran muscular atrophy
Progressive muscular atrophy (pure)

335.22 Progressive bulbar palsy

335.23 Pseudobulbar palsy

335.24 Primary lateral sclerosis

335.29 Other

335.8 Other anterior horn cell diseases
Coding Clinic: 2006, Q4, P76-78

335.9 Anterior horn cell disease, unspecified

● **336 Other diseases of spinal cord**

336.0 Syringomyelia and syringobulbia
Coding Clinic: 1989, Q1, P10

336.1 Vascular myelopathies
Acute infarction of spinal cord (embolic)
(nonembolic)
Arterial thrombosis of spinal cord
Edema of spinal cord
Hematomyelia
Subacute necrotic myelopathy

336.2 Subacute combined degeneration of spinal cord in diseases classified elsewhere

Code first underlying disease, as:
pernicious anemia (281.0)
other vitamin B12 deficiency anemia (281.1)
vitamin B12 deficiency (266.2)

336.3 Myelopathy in other diseases classified elsewhere

Code first underlying disease, as:
myelopathy in neoplastic disease (140.0–239.9)

| Excludes | *myelopathy in:*
intervertebral disc disorder (722.70–722.73)
spondylosis (721.1, 721.41–721.42, 721.91)

Coding Clinic: 1999, Q3, P5

336.8 Other myelopathy
Myelopathy:
drug-induced
radiation-induced

Use additional E code to identify cause

336.9 Unspecified disease of spinal cord
Cord compression NOS
Myelopathy NOS

| Excludes | *myelitis (323.02, 323.1, 323.2, 323.42, 323.52, 323.63, 323.72, 323.82, 323.9)*
spinal (canal) stenosis (723.0, 724.00–724.09)

● **337 Disorders of the autonomic nervous system**

| Includes | disorders of peripheral autonomic, sympathetic, parasympathetic, or vegetative system

| Excludes | *familial dysautonomia [Riley-Day syndrome] (742.8)*

● **337.0 Idiopathic peripheral autonomic neuropathy**

337.00 Idiopathic peripheral autonomic neuropathy, unspecified

337.01 Carotid sinus syndrome
Carotid sinus syncope
Coding Clinic: 2008, Q4, P101-102

337.09 Other idiopathic peripheral autonomic neuropathy
Cervical sympathetic dystrophy or paralysis

337.1 Peripheral autonomic neuropathy in disorders classified elsewhere

Code first underlying disease, as:
amyloidosis (277.30–277.39)
diabetes (249.6, 250.6)
Coding Clinic: 2009, Q2, P13; 1993, Q2, P6; 1984, Nov-Dec, P9

● **337.2 Reflex sympathetic dystrophy**

337.20 Reflex sympathetic dystrophy, unspecified
Complex regional pain syndrome type I, unspecified

337.21 Reflex sympathetic dystrophy of the upper limb
Complex regional pain syndrome type I of the upper limb

337.22 Reflex sympathetic dystrophy of the lower limb
Complex regional pain syndrome type I of the lower limb

337.29 Reflex sympathetic dystrophy of other specified site
Complex regional pain syndrome type I of other specified site

337.3 Autonomic dysreflexia

Use additional code to identify the cause, such as:
fecal impaction (560.32) ◀▥
pressure ulcer (707.00–707.09)
urinary tract infection (599.0)
Coding Clinic: 1998, Q4, P37-38

337.9 Unspecified disorder of autonomic nervous system

DISEASES OF THE NERVOUS SYSTEM AND SENSE ORGANS (320–389)

DISEASES OF THE NERVOUS SYSTEM AND SENSE ORGANS (320–389)

PAIN (338)

● **338 Pain, not elsewhere classified**

Use additional code to identify:
pain associated with psychological factors (307.89)

Excludes *generalized pain (780.96)*
headache syndromes (339.00-339.89)
localized pain, unspecified type - code to pain by site
migraines (346.0-346.9)
pain disorder exclusively attributed to psychological factors (307.80)
vulvar vestibulitis (625.71)
vulvodynia (625.70-625.79)

338.0 Central pain syndrome
Déjérine-Roussy syndrome
Myelopathic pain syndrome
Thalamic pain syndrome (hyperesthetic)

● **338.1 Acute pain**

338.11 Acute pain due to trauma
Coding Clinic: 2007, Q1, P3-8

338.12 Acute post-thoracotomy pain
Post-thoracotomy pain NOS

338.18 Other acute postoperative pain
Postoperative pain NOS
Coding Clinic: 2007, Q2, P13-15; 2003, Q1, P4-5, 8

338.19 Other acute pain

Excludes *neoplasm related acute pain (338.3)*

Coding Clinic: 2007, Q2, P13-15

● **338.2 Chronic pain**

Excludes *causalgia (355.9)*
lower limb (355.71)
upper limb (354.4)
chronic pain syndrome (338.4)
myofascial pain syndrome (729.1)
neoplasm related chronic pain (338.3)
reflex sympathetic dystrophy (337.20–337.29)

Coding Clinic: 2008, Q3, P4

338.21 Chronic pain due to trauma

338.22 Chronic post-thoracotomy pain

338.28 Other chronic postoperative pain
Coding Clinic: 2007, Q2, P13-15

338.29 Other chronic pain
Coding Clinic: 2007, Q2, P13-15

338.3 Neoplasm related pain (acute) (chronic)
Cancer associated pain
Pain due to malignancy (primary) (secondary)
Tumor associated pain
Coding Clinic: 2007, Q2, P13-15

338.4 Chronic pain syndrome
Chronic pain associated with significant psychosocial dysfunction
Coding Clinic: 2007, Q2, P13-15

OTHER HEADACHE SYNDROMES (339)

● **339 Other headache syndromes**

Excludes *headache:*
NOS (784.0)
due to lumbar puncture (349.0)
migraine (346.0-346.9)
Coding Clinic: 2008, Q4, P102-109

● **339.0 Cluster headaches and other trigeminal autonomic cephalgias**
TACS

339.00 Cluster headache syndrome, unspecified
Ciliary neuralgia
Cluster headache NOS
Histamine cephalgia
Lower half migraine
Migrainous neuralgia

339.01 Episodic cluster headache

339.02 Chronic cluster headache

339.03 Episodic paroxysmal hemicrania
Paroxysmal hemicrania NOS

339.04 Chronic paroxysmal hemicrania

339.05 Short lasting unilateral neuralgiform headache with conjunctival injection and tearing
SUNCT

339.09 Other trigeminal autonomic cephalgias

● **339.1 Tension type headache**

Excludes *tension headache NOS (307.81)*
tension headache related to psychological factors (307.81)

339.10 Tension type headache, unspecified

339.11 Episodic tension type headache

339.12 Chronic tension type headache

● **339.2 Post-traumatic headache**

339.20 Post-traumatic headache, unspecified
Coding Clinic: 2008, Q4, P102-109

339.21 Acute post-traumatic headache
Coding Clinic: 2008, Q4, P102-109

339.22 Chronic post-traumatic headache

339.3 Drug induced headache, not elsewhere classified
Medication overuse headache
Rebound headache

● **339.4 Complicated headache syndromes**

339.41 Hemicrania continua

339.42 New daily persistent headache
NDPH

339.43 Primary thunderclap headache

339.44 Other complicated headache syndrome

● **339.8 Other specified headache syndromes**

339.81 Hypnic headache

339.82 Headache associated with sexual activity
Orgasmic headache
Preorgasmic headache

339.83 Primary cough headache

339.84 Primary exertional headache

339.85 Primary stabbing headache

339.89 Other specified headache syndromes

◀ New   ◀▦ Revised   ~~deleted~~ Deleted   Excludes   Includes   Use additional   Code first   Omit code
● Unacceptable Principal Diagnosis   ● Use Additional Digit(s)   OGCR Official Guidelines   Coding Clinic

Item 6-6 Multiple sclerosis (MS) is a nervous system disease affecting the brain and spinal cord by damaging the myelin sheath surrounding and protecting nerve cells. The damage slows down/blocks messages between the brain and body. Symptoms are: visual disturbances, muscle weakness, coordination and balance issues, numbness, prickling, and thinking and memory problems. The cause is unknown, though it is thought that it may be an autoimmune disease. It affects women more than men, between 20 and 40 years of age. MS can be mild, but it may cause the loss of ability to write, walk, and speak. There is no cure, but medication may slow or control symptoms.

OTHER DISORDERS OF THE CENTRAL NERVOUS SYSTEM (340–349)

340 Multiple sclerosis *(MS)*

> Disseminated or multiple sclerosis:
>
> NOS   cord
> brain stem   generalized

● **341 Other demyelinating diseases of central nervous system**

341.0 Neuromyelitis optica

341.1 Schilder's disease
> Balo's concentric sclerosis
> Encephalitis periaxialis:
> concentrica [Balo's]
> diffusa [Schilder's]

● **341.2 Acute (transverse) myelitis**

> **Excludes** *acute (transverse) myelitis (in) (due to):*
> *following immunization procedures (323.52)*
> *infection classified elsewhere (323.42)*
> *postinfectious (323.63)*
> *protozoal diseases classified elsewhere (323.2)*
> *rickettsial diseases classified elsewhere (323.1)*
> *toxic (323.72)*
> *viral diseases classified elsewhere (323.02)*
> *transverse myelitis NOS (323.82)*

341.20 Acute (transverse) myelitis NOS

341.21 Acute (transverse) myelitis in conditions classified elsewhere

> *Code first* underlying condition

341.22 Idiopathic transverse myelitis

341.8 Other demyelinating diseases of central nervous system
> Central demyelination of corpus callosum
> Central pontine myelinosis
> Marchiafava (-Bignami) disease
> Coding Clinic: 1987, Nov-Dec, P6

341.9 Demyelinating disease of central nervous system, unspecified

● **342 Hemiplegia and hemiparesis**

> **Note:** This category is to be used when hemiplegia (complete) (incomplete) is reported without further specification, or is stated to be old or long-standing but of unspecified cause. The category is also for use in multiple coding to identify these types of hemiplegia resulting from any cause.

> **Excludes** *congenital (343.1)*
> *hemiplegia due to late effect of cerebrovascular accident (438.20–438.22)*
> *infantile NOS (343.4)*

The following fifth-digits are for use with codes 342.0–342.9

> 0 affecting unspecified side
> 1 affecting dominant side
> 2 affecting nondominant side

● **342.0 Flaccid hemiplegia**
> [0-2]

● **342.1 Spastic hemiplegia**
> [0-2]

● **342.8 Other specified hemiplegia**
> [0-2]

● **342.9 Hemiplegia, unspecified**
> [0-2]   Coding Clinic: 2006, Q3, P5; 1998, Q4, P87

● **343 Infantile cerebral palsy**

> **Includes** cerebral:
> palsy NOS
> spastic infantile paralysis
> congenital spastic paralysis (cerebral)
> Little's disease
> paralysis (spastic) due to birth injury:
> intracranial
> spinal

> **Excludes** *athetoid cerebral palsy (333.71)*
> *hereditary cerebral paralysis, such as:*
> *hereditary spastic paraplegia (334.1)*
> *Vogt's disease (333.71)*
> *spastic paralysis specified as noncongenital or noninfantile (344.0–344.9)*

343.0 Diplegic
> Congenital diplegia
> Congenital paraplegia

343.1 Hemiplegic
> Congenital hemiplegia
> **Excludes** *infantile hemiplegia NOS (343.4)*

343.2 Quadriplegic
> Tetraplegic

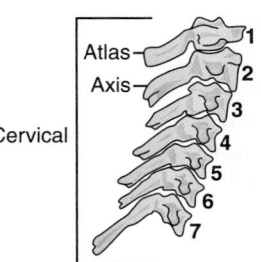

Figure 6–2 Cervical vertebrae.

Item 6–7 Hemiplegia is complete paralysis of one side of the body—arm, leg, and trunk. **Hemiparesis** is a generalized weakness or incomplete paralysis of one side of the body. If most activities (eating, writing) are performed with the right hand, the right is the dominant side, and the left is the nondominant side. **Quadriplegia,** also called tetraplegia, is the complete paralysis of all four limbs. **Quadriparesis** is the incomplete paralysis of all four limbs. Nerve damage in C1–C4 is associated with lower limb paralysis, and C5–C7 damage is associated with upper limb paralysis. **Diplegia** is the paralysis of the upper limbs. **Monoplegia** is the complete paralysis of one limb. There are separate codes for upper (344.4x) and lower (344.3x) limb. Dominant, nondominant, or unspecified side becomes the fifth digit. Dominant side (right/left) is the side that a person leads with for movement, such as in writing and sports.

Cauda equina syndrome is due to pressure on the roots of the spinal nerves and causes paresthesia (abnormal sensations).

DISEASES OF THE NERVOUS SYSTEM AND SENSE ORGANS (320–389)

343.3 **Monoplegic**

343.4 **Infantile hemiplegia**
Infantile hemiplegia (postnatal) NOS

343.8 **Other specified infantile cerebral palsy**

343.9 **Infantile cerebral palsy, unspecified**
Cerebral palsy NOS
Coding Clinic: 2005, Q4, P89-90

● 344 **Other paralytic syndromes**

Note: This category is to be used when the listed conditions are reported without further specification or are stated to be old or long-standing but of unspecified cause. The category is also for use in multiple coding to identify these conditions resulting from any cause.

Includes paralysis (complete) (incomplete), except as classifiable to 342 and 343

Excludes *congenital or infantile cerebral palsy (343.0–343.9)*
hemiplegia (342.0–342.9)
congenital or infantile (343.1, 343.4)

● 344.0 **Quadriplegia and quadriparesis**

344.00 **Quadriplegia, unspecified**
Coding Clinic: 2003, Q4, P103-104; 1998, Q4, P37-38

344.01 **C₁-C₄, complete**
344.02 **C₁-C₄, incomplete**
344.03 **C₅-C₇, complete**
344.04 **C₅-C₇, incomplete**
344.09 **Other**
Coding Clinic: 2001, Q1, P12; 1998, Q4, P39-40

344.1 **Paraplegia**
Paralysis of both lower limbs
Paraplegia (lower)
Coding Clinic: 2003, Q4, P110; 1987, Mar-April, P10-11

344.2 **Diplegia of upper limbs**
Diplegia (upper)
Paralysis of both upper limbs

● 344.3 **Monoplegia of lower limb**
Paralysis of lower limb

Excludes *monoplegia of lower limb due to late effect of cerebrovascular accident (438.40–438.42)*

344.30 **Affecting unspecified side**
344.31 **Affecting dominant side**
344.32 **Affecting nondominant side**

● 344.4 **Monoplegia of upper limb**
Paralysis of upper limb

Excludes *monoplegia of upper limb due to late effect of cerebrovascular accident (438.30–438.32)*

344.40 **Affecting unspecified side**
344.41 **Affecting dominant side**
344.42 **Affecting nondominant side**
344.5 **Unspecified monoplegia**

● 344.6 **Cauda equina syndrome**

344.60 **Without mention of neurogenic bladder**
344.61 **With neurogenic bladder**
Acontractile bladder
Autonomic hyperreflexia of bladder
Cord bladder
Detrusor hyperreflexia
Coding Clinic: 1987, Mar-April, P10-11

● 344.8 **Other specified paralytic syndromes**
344.81 **Locked-in state**
344.89 **Other specified paralytic syndrome**
Coding Clinic: 1999, Q2, P4

344.9 **Paralysis, unspecified**
Coding Clinic: 1994, Q3, P4

● 345 **Epilepsy and recurrent seizures**
The following fifth-digit subclassification is for use with categories 345.0, .1, .4–.9:

0 **without mention of intractable epilepsy**
1 **with intractable epilepsy**
pharmacoresistant (pharmacologically resistant)
poorly controlled
refractory (medically)
treatment resistant

Excludes *hippocampal sclerosis (348.81)*
mesial temporal sclerosis (348.81)
~~*progressive myoclonic epilepsy (333.2)*~~
temporal sclerosis (348.81)

● 345.0 **Generalized nonconvulsive epilepsy**
[0-1] Absences: Pykno-epilepsy
atonic   Seizures:
typical   akinetic
Minor epilepsy   atonic
Petit mal
Coding Clinic: 2004, Q1, P18; 1992, Q2, P8

● 345.1 **Generalized convulsive epilepsy**
[0-1] Epileptic seizures:
clonic
myoclonic
tonic
tonic-clonic
Grand mal
Major epilepsy
Progressive myoclonic epilepsy
Unverricht-Lundborg disease

Excludes *convulsions:*
NOS (780.39)
infantile (780.39)
newborn (779.0)
infantile spasms (345.6)
Coding Clinic: 1997, Q3, P5; 1994, Q3, P9

345.2 **Petit mal status**
Epileptic absence status
Temporary disturbance of brain function caused by abnormal electrical activity.

345.3 **Grand mal status**
Status epilepticus NOS
Grand mal seizure is a generalized tonic-clonic seizure involving the entire body, which involves muscle rigidity, violent muscle contractions, and loss of consciousness.

Excludes *epilepsia partialis continua (345.7) status:*
psychomotor (345.7)
temporal lobe (345.7)
Coding Clinic: 2005, Q3, P12-13

◀ New   ◀▬ Revised   ~~deleted~~ Deleted   Excludes   Includes   Use additional   Code first   Omit code
● Unacceptable Principal Diagnosis   ● Use Additional Digit(s)   OGCR Official Guidelines   Coding Clinic

● **345.4** **Localization-related (focal) (partial) epilepsy and**
[0-1] **epileptic syndromes with complex partial seizures**
Epilepsy:
limbic system
partial:
secondarily generalized
with impairment of consciousness
with memory and ideational disturbances
psychomotor
psychosensory
temporal lobe
Epileptic automatism
Coding Clinic: 2009, Q4, P98

● **345.5** **Localization-related (focal) (partial) epilepsy and**
[0-1] **epileptic syndromes with simple partial seizures**
Epilepsy:
Bravais-Jacksonian NOS
focal (motor) NOS
Jacksonian NOS
motor partial
partial NOS
without mention of impairment of
consciousness
sensory-induced
somatomotor
somatosensory
visceral
visual

● **345.6** **Infantile spasms**
[0-1] Hypsarrhythmia
Lightning spasms
Salaam attacks
Excludes salaam tic (781.0)
Coding Clinic: 1984, Nov-Dec, P11

● **345.7** **Epilepsia partialis continua**
[0-1] Kojevnikov's epilepsy

● **345.8** **Other forms of epilepsy and recurrent seizures**
[0-1] Epilepsy:
cursive [running]
gelastic
Recurrent seizures NOS
Seizure disorder NOS
Excludes convulsion (convulsive) disorder (780.39)
convulsive seizure or fit NOS (780.39)
recurrent convulsions (780.39)
Coding Clinic: 2009, Q2, P10; 2008, Q1, P17; 1993, Q1, P24; 1987, Nov-Dec, P12

● **345.9** **Epilepsy, unspecified**
[0-1] Epileptic convulsions, fits, or seizures NOS
Recurrent seizures NOS
Seizure disorder NOS

● **346** **Migraine**
Excludes headache:
NOS (784.0)
syndromes (339.00-339.89)
Coding Clinic: 2008, Q4, P102-109

The following fifth-digit subclassification is for use with category 346:

0 without mention of intractable migraine without
mention of status migrainosus
1 with intractable migraine, so stated, without
mention of status migrainosus
2 without mention of intractable migraine with
status migrainosus
3 with intractable migraine, so stated, with status
migrainosus

Intractable migraine: Not easily cured or managed; relentless pain from a migraine

Item 6-8 Migraine headache is described as an intense pulsing or throbbing pain in one area of the head. It can be accompanied by extreme sensitivity to light (photophoic) and sound and is three times more common in women than in men. Symptoms include nausea and vomiting. Research indicates migraine headaches are caused by inherited abnormalities in genes that control the activities of certain cell populations in the brain.

● **346.0** **Migraine with aura**
[0-3] Basilar migraine
Classic migraine
Migraine preceded or accompanied by transient
focal neurological phenomena
Migraine triggered seizures
Migraine with acute-onset aura
Migraine with aura without headache (migraine
equivalents)
Migraine with prolonged aura
Migraine with typical aura
Retinal migraine
Excludes persistent migraine aura (346.5, 346.6)

● **346.1** **Migraine without aura**
[0-3] Common migraine

● **346.2** **Variants of migraine, not elsewhere classified**
[0-3] Abdominal migraine
Cyclical vomiting associated with migraine
Ophthalmoplegic migraine
Periodic headache syndromes in child or
adolescent
Excludes cyclical vomiting NOS (536.2)
psychogenic cyclical vomiting (306.4)

● **346.3** **Hemiplegic migraine**
[0-3] Familial migraine
Sporadic migraine

● **346.4** **Menstrual migraine**
[0-3] Menstrual headache
Menstrually related migraine
Premenstrual headache
Premenstrual migraine
Pure menstrual migraine

● **346.5** **Persistent migraine aura without cerebral**
[0-3] **infarction**
Persistent migraine aura NOS

● **346.6** **Persistent migraine aura with cerebral**
[0-3] **infarction**

● **346.7** **Chronic migraine without aura**
[0-3] Transformed migraine without aura

● **346.8** **Other forms of migraine**
[0-3]

● **346.9** **Migraine, unspecified**
[0-3] Coding Clinic: 1985, Nov-Dec, P16

● **347** **Cataplexy and narcolepsy**
Cataplexy is a disorder evidenced by seizures. Narcolepsy is difficulty remaining awake during daytime.
Coding Clinic: 2004, Q4, P74-75

● **347.0** **Narcolepsy**
347.00 **Without cataplexy**
Narcolepsy NOS
347.01 **With cataplexy**

● **347.1** **Narcolepsy in conditions classified elsewhere**
Code first underlying condition
347.10 **Without cataplexy**
347.11 **With cataplexy**

◀ New ◀▥ Revised ~~deleted~~ Deleted Excludes Includes Use additional Code first Omit code
● Unacceptable Principal Diagnosis ● Use Additional Digit(s) OGCR Official Guidelines Coding Clinic

801

DISEASES OF THE NERVOUS SYSTEM AND SENSE ORGANS (320–389)

● **348　Other conditions of brain**

348.0　Cerebral cysts
Arachnoid cyst　　　　Porencephaly, acquired
Porencephalic cyst　　Pseudoporencephaly

348.1　Anoxic brain damage
Brain permanently damaged by lack of oxygen perfusion through brain tissues. This is the result of another problem, so use an additional E code to identify the cause.

| Excludes | *that occurring in:*
abortion (634–638 with .7, 639.8)
ectopic or molar pregnancy (639.8)
labor or delivery (668.2, 669.4)
*that of newborn (767.0, 768.0–768.9,
772.1–772.2)*

Use additional E code to identify cause

348.2　Benign intracranial hypertension
Pseudotumor cerebri

| Excludes | *hypertensive encephalopathy (437.2)*

● **348.3　Encephalopathy, not elsewhere classified**
A general term for any degenerative brain disease
Coding Clinic: 2003, Q4, P58-59; 1997, Q3, P5

348.30　Encephalopathy, unspecified

348.31　Metabolic encephalopathy
Septic encephalopathy

| Excludes | *toxic metabolic encephalopathy
(349.82)*

348.39　Other encephalopathy

| Excludes | *encephalopathy:
alcoholic (291.2)
hepatic (572.2)
hypertensive (437.2)
toxic (349.82)*

348.4　Compression of brain
Compression brain (stem)
Herniation brain (stem)
Posterior fossa compression syndrome

348.5　Cerebral edema
Coding Clinic: 2010, Q1, P6; 2009, Q3, P7

● **348.8　Other conditions of brain**
Coding Clinic: 1992, Q3, P8; 1987, Sept-Oct, P9

348.81　Temporal sclerosis
Hippocampal sclerosis
Mesial temporal sclerosis
Coding Clinic: 2009, Q4, P98

348.89　Other conditions of brain
Cerebral:
calcification
fungus

348.9　Unspecified condition of brain

● **349　Other and unspecified disorders of the nervous system**

349.0　Reaction to spinal or lumbar puncture
Headache following lumbar puncture
Cerebral spinal fluid (CSF) maintains a specific level of pressure inside brain and spinal cord. If this pressure does not return to normal after a puncture, headache will result.
Coding Clinic: 1999, Q2, P9-10; 1990, Q3, P18

349.1　Nervous system complications from surgically implanted device

| Excludes | *immediate postoperative complications
(997.00–997.09)
mechanical complications of nervous system
device (996.2)*

349.2　Disorders of meninges, not elsewhere classified
Adhesions, meningeal (cerebral) (spinal)
Cyst, spinal meninges
Meningocele, acquired
Pseudomeningocele, acquired
Coding Clinic: 2006, Q1, P15-16; 1998, Q2, P18; 1994, Q3, P4; Q1, P22-23

● **349.3　Dural tear**
Coding Clinic: 2008, Q4, P109-110

349.31　Accidental puncture or laceration of dura during a procedure
Incidental (inadvertent) durotomy

349.39　Other dural tear

● **349.8　Other specified disorders of nervous system**

349.81　Cerebrospinal fluid rhinorrhea

| Excludes | *cerebrospinal fluid otorrhea (388.61)*

349.82　Toxic encephalopathy
Toxic metabolic encephalopathy

Use additional E code to identify cause

349.89　Other

349.9　Unspecified disorders of nervous system
Disorder of nervous system (central) NOS

DISORDERS OF THE PERIPHERAL NERVOUS SYSTEM (350–359)

| Excludes | *diseases of:
acoustic [8th] nerve (388.5)
oculomotor [3rd, 4th, 6th] nerves (378.0–378.9)
optic [2nd] nerve (377.0–377.9)
peripheral autonomic nerves (337.0–337.9)
neuralgia NOS or "rheumatic" (729.2)
neuritis NOS or "rheumatic" (729.2)
radiculitis NOS or "rheumatic" (729.2)
peripheral neuritis in pregnancy (646.4)*

● **350　Trigeminal nerve disorders**

| Includes | disorders of 5th cranial nerve

350.1　Trigeminal neuralgia
Tic douloureux
Trifacial neuralgia
Trigeminal neuralgia NOS

| Excludes | *postherpetic (053.12)*

350.2　Atypical face pain

350.8　Other specified trigeminal nerve disorders

350.9　Trigeminal nerve disorder, unspecified

Item 6–9 The **peripheral nervous system** consists of 31 pairs of spinal nerves, 12 pairs of cranial nerves, and the autonomic nerves, which are divided into the parasympathetic and sympathetic nerves. The cranial nerves are: olfactory (I), optic (II), oculomotor (III), trochlear (IV), trigeminal (V), abducens (VI), facial (VII), vestibulocochlear (VIII), glossopharyngeal (IX), vagus (X), accessory (XI), and hypoglossal (XII).

Item 6-10　Trigeminal neuralgia, tic douloureux, is a pain syndrome diagnosed from the patient's history alone. The condition is characterized by pain and a brief facial spasm or tic. Pain is unilateral and follows the sensory distribution of cranial nerve V, typically radiating to the maxillary (V2) or mandibular (V3) area.

Item 6-11 The most common facial nerve disorder is **Bell's Palsy,** which occurs suddenly and results in facial drooping unilaterally. This disorder is the result of a reaction to a virus that causes the facial nerve in the ear to swell resulting in pressure in the bony canal.

◀ New　◀◀ Revised　~~deleted~~ Deleted　Excludes　Includes　Use additional　Code first　Omit code
● Unacceptable Principal Diagnosis　● Use Additional Digit(s)　OGCR Official Guidelines　Coding Clinic

● **351 Facial nerve disorders**

    Includes   disorders of 7th cranial nerve

    Excludes   *that in newborn (767.5)*

   351.0 Bell's palsy
     Facial palsy

   351.1 Geniculate ganglionitis
     Geniculate ganglionitis NOS

     Excludes   *herpetic (053.11)*

     Coding Clinic: 2002, Q2, P8

   351.8 Other facial nerve disorders
     Facial myokymia
     Melkersson's syndrome
     Coding Clinic: 2002, Q3, P12-13

   351.9 Facial nerve disorder, unspecified

● **352 Disorders of other cranial nerves**

   352.0 Disorders of olfactory [1st] nerve

   352.1 Glossopharyngeal neuralgia
     Coding Clinic: 1987, Jan-Feb, P14

   352.2 Other disorders of glossopharyngeal [9th] nerve

   352.3 Disorders of pneumogastric [10th] nerve
     Disorders of vagal nerve

     Excludes   *paralysis of vocal cords or larynx (478.30–478.34)*

   352.4 Disorders of accessory [11th] nerve

   352.5 Disorders of hypoglossal [12th] nerve

   352.6 Multiple cranial nerve palsies
     Collet-Sicard syndrome
     Polyneuritis cranialis

   352.9 Unspecified disorder of cranial nerves

● **353 Nerve root and plexus disorders**

    Excludes   *conditions due to:*
       intervertebral disc disorders (722.0–722.9)
       spondylosis (720.0–721.9)
       vertebrogenic disorders (723.0–724.9)

   353.0 Brachial plexus lesions
     Cervical rib syndrome
     Costoclavicular syndrome
     Scalenus anticus syndrome
     Thoracic outlet syndrome

     Excludes   *brachial neuritis or radiculitis NOS (723.4)*
       that in newborn (767.6)
     Coding Clinic: 2006, Q3, P12

   353.1 Lumbosacral plexus lesions

   353.2 Cervical root lesions, not elsewhere classified

   ● **353.3 Thoracic root lesions, not elsewhere classified**

   353.4 Lumbosacral root lesions, not elsewhere classified

   353.5 Neuralgic amyotrophy
     Parsonage-Aldren-Turner syndrome
     Phantom limb syndrome: Patients with amputated limbs feel sensations in a limb that no longer exists. There is no separate code for phantom limb pain, and the pain can be part of the syndrome.

     Code first *any associated underlying disease, such as:*
       diabetes mellitus (249.6, 250.6)

   353.6 Phantom limb (syndrome)

   353.8 Other nerve root and plexus disorders

   353.9 Unspecified nerve root and plexus disorder

● **354 Mononeuritis of upper limb and mononeuritis multiplex**

   354.0 Carpal tunnel syndrome *(CTS)*
     Of the wrist
     Median nerve entrapment
     Partial thenar atrophy

   354.1 Other lesion of median nerve
     Median nerve neuritis

   354.2 Lesion of ulnar nerve
     Cubital tunnel syndrome
     Tardy ulnar nerve palsy

   354.3 Lesion of radial nerve
     Acute radial nerve palsy
     Coding Clinic: 1987, Nov-Dec, P6

   354.4 Causalgia of upper limb
     Complex regional pain syndrome type II of the upper limb

     Excludes   *causalgia:*
       NOS (355.9)
       lower limb (355.71)
       complex regional pain syndrome type II of the lower limb (355.71)

   354.5 Mononeuritis multiplex
     Combinations of single conditions classifiable to 354 or 355

   354.8 Other mononeuritis of upper limb

   354.9 Mononeuritis of upper limb, unspecified

● **355 Mononeuritis of lower limb**
    Coding Clinic: 1989, Q2, P12

   355.0 Lesion of sciatic nerve

     Excludes   *sciatica NOS (724.3)*

     Coding Clinic: 1989, Q2, P12

   355.1 Meralgia paresthetica
     Lateral cutaneous femoral nerve of thigh compression or syndrome

   355.2 Other lesion of femoral nerve

   355.3 Lesion of lateral popliteal nerve
     Lesion of common peroneal nerve

   355.4 Lesion of medial popliteal nerve

   355.5 Tarsal tunnel syndrome
     Of the ankle

   355.6 Lesion of plantar nerve
     Morton's metatarsalgia, neuralgia, or neuroma

   ● **355.7 Other mononeuritis of lower limb**

     355.71 Causalgia of lower limb

       Excludes   *causalgia:*
         NOS (355.9)
         upper limb (354.4)
         complex regional pain syndrome type II of the upper limb (354.4)

     355.79 Other mononeuritis of lower limb

   355.8 Mononeuritis of lower limb, unspecified

   355.9 Mononeuritis of unspecified site
     Causalgia NOS
     Complex regional pain syndrome NOS

     Excludes   *causalgia:*
       lower limb (355.71)
       upper limb (354.4)
       complex regional pain syndrome:
       lower limb (355.71)
       upper limb (354.4)

DISEASES OF THE NERVOUS SYSTEM AND SENSE ORGANS (320–389)

● **356 Hereditary and idiopathic peripheral neuropathy**
Any disease that affects nervous system and of an unknown cause.

356.0 Hereditary peripheral neuropathy
Déjérine-Sottas disease

356.1 Peroneal muscular atrophy
Charcot-Marie-Tooth disease
Neuropathic muscular atrophy

356.2 Hereditary sensory neuropathy

356.3 Refsum's disease
Heredopathia atactica polyneuritiformis

356.4 Idiopathic progressive polyneuropathy

356.8 Other specified idiopathic peripheral neuropathy
Supranuclear paralysis

356.9 Unspecified

● **357 Inflammatory and toxic neuropathy**

357.0 Acute infective polyneuritis
Guillain-Barre syndrome
Postinfectious polyneuritis
Coding Clinic: 1998, Q2, P12

357.1 Polyneuropathy in collagen vascular disease
Code first underlying disease, as:
disseminated lupus erythematosus (710.0)
polyarteritis nodosa (446.0)
rheumatoid arthritis (714.0)

357.2 Polyneuropathy in diabetes
Code first underlying disease (249.6, 250.6)
Coding Clinic: 2009, Q4, P98; Q2, P13; 2008, Q3, P5-6; 2003, Q4, P105; 1992, Q2, P15

357.3 Polyneuropathy in malignant disease
Code first underlying disease (140.0–208.9)

357.4 Polyneuropathy in other diseases classified elsewhere
Code first underlying disease, as:
amyloidosis (277.30–277.39)
beriberi (265.0)
chronic uremia (585.9)
deficiency of B vitamins (266.0–266.9)
diphtheria (032.0–032.9)
hypoglycemia (251.2)
pellagra (265.2)
porphyria (277.1)
sarcoidosis (135)
uremia NOS (586)

Excludes *polyneuropathy in:*
herpes zoster (053.13)
mumps (072.72)
Coding Clinic: 2008, Q2, P8-9; 1998, Q2, P15

357.5 Alcoholic polyneuropathy

357.6 Polyneuropathy due to drugs
Use additional E code to identify drug

357.7 Polyneuropathy due to other toxic agents
Use additional E code to identify toxic agent

● **357.8 Other**
Coding Clinic: 2002, Q4, P47-48; 1998, Q2, P12

357.81 Chronic inflammatory demyelinating polyneuritis

357.82 Critical illness polyneuropathy
Acute motor neuropathy
Coding Clinic: 2003, Q4, P111

357.89 Other inflammatory and toxic neuropathy

357.9 Unspecified

● **358 Myoneural disorders**

● **358.0 Myasthenia gravis**
Acquired and results in fatigable muscle weakness exacerbated by activity and improved with rest. Caused by autoimmune assault against nerve-muscle junction.
Coding Clinic: 2003, Q4, P59-60

358.00 Myasthenia gravis without (acute) exacerbation

358.01 Myasthenia gravis with acute exacerbation
Myasthenia gravis in crisis
Coding Clinic: 2007, Q4, P108-109; 2004, Q4, P139

358.1 Myasthenic syndromes in diseases classified elsewhere
Eaton-Lambert syndrome from stated cause classified elsewhere

Code first underlying disease, as:
botulism (005.1, 040.41–040.42)
hypothyroidism (244.0–244.9)
malignant neoplasm (140.0–208.9)
pernicious anemia (281.0)
thyrotoxicosis (242.0–242.9)

358.2 Toxic myoneural disorders
Use additional E code to identify toxic agent

358.8 Other specified myoneural disorders

358.9 Myoneural disorders, unspecified
Coding Clinic: 2002, Q2, P16

● **359 Muscular dystrophies and other myopathies**
Excludes *idiopathic polymyositis (710.4)*

359.0 Congenital hereditary muscular dystrophy
Benign congenital myopathy
Central core disease
Centronuclear myopathy
Myotubular myopathy
Nemaline body disease
Excludes *arthrogryposis multiplex congenita (754.89)*

359.1 Hereditary progressive muscular dystrophy
Muscular dystrophy:
NOS
distal
Duchenne
Erb's
fascioscapulohumeral
Gower's
Landouzy-Déjérine
limb-girdle
ocular
oculopharyngeal

● **359.2 Myotonic disorders**
Excludes *periodic paralysis (359.3)*
Coding Clinic: 2007, Q4, P75-77

359.21 Myotonic muscular dystrophy
Dystrophia myotonica
Myotonia atrophica
Myotonic dystrophy
Proximal myotonic myopathy (PROMM)
Steinert's disease

359.22 Myotonia congenita
Acetazolamide responsive myotonia congenita
Dominant form (Thomsen's disease)
Myotonia levior
Recessive form (Becker's disease)

359.23 Myotonic chondrodystrophy
Congenital myotonic chondrodystrophy
Schwartz-Jampel disease

Item 6-12 Muscular dystrophies (MD) are a group of rare inherited muscle diseases. Voluntary muscles become progressively weaker. In the late stages of MD, fat and connective tissue replace muscle fibers. In some types of muscular dystrophy, heart muscles, other involuntary muscles, and other organs are affected. **Myopathies** is a general term for neuromuscular diseases in which the muscle fibers dysfunction for any one of many reasons, resulting in muscular weakness.

359.24 Drug-induced myotonia

Use additional E code to identify drug

359.29 Other specified myotonic disorder
Myotonia fluctuans
Myotonia permanens
Paramyotonia congenita
(of von Eulenburg)

359.3 Periodic paralysis
Familial periodic paralysis
Hyperkalemic periodic paralysis
Hypokalemic familial periodic paralysis
Hypokalemic periodic paralysis
Potassium sensitive periodic paralysis

Excludes paramyotonia congenita (of von Eulenburg) (359.29)

359.4 Toxic myopathy

Use additional E code to identify toxic agent

359.5 Myopathy in endocrine diseases classified elsewhere

Code first underlying disease, as:
Addison's disease (255.41)
Cushing's syndrome (255.0)
hypopituitarism (253.2)
myxedema (244.0–244.9)
thyrotoxicosis (242.0–242.9)

359.6 Symptomatic inflammatory myopathy in diseases classified elsewhere

Code first underlying disease, as:
amyloidosis (277.30–277.39)
disseminated lupus erythematosus (710.0)
malignant neoplasm (140.0–208.9)
polyarteritis nodosa (446.0)
rheumatoid arthritis (714.0)
sarcoidosis (135)
scleroderma (710.1)
Sjögren's disease (710.2)

●**359.7 Inflammatory and immune myopathies, NEC**

359.71 Inclusion body myositis
IBM

359.79 Other inflammatory and immune myopathies, NEC
Inflammatory myopathy NOS

●**359.8 Other myopathies**
Coding Clinic: 2002, Q4, P47-48; 1990, Q3, P17

359.81 Critical illness myopathy
Acute necrotizing myopathy
Acute quadriplegic myopathy
Intensive care (ICU) myopathy
Myopathy of critical illness

359.89 Other myopathies

359.9 Myopathy, unspecified

DISORDERS OF THE EYE AND ADNEXA (360–379)

Use additional external cause code, if applicable, to identify the cause of the eye condition

●360 **Disorders of the globe**
Includes disorders affecting multiple structures of eye

●**360.0 Purulent endophthalmitis**
Excludes bleb associated endophthalmitis (379.63)
360.00 Purulent endophthalmitis, unspecified
360.01 Acute endophthalmitis
360.02 Panophthalmitis
360.03 Chronic endophthalmitis
360.04 Vitreous abscess

●**360.1 Other endophthalmitis**
Excludes bleb associated endophthalmitis (379.63)
360.11 Sympathetic uveitis
360.12 Panuveitis
360.13 Parasitic endophthalmitis NOS
360.14 Ophthalmia nodosa
360.19 Other
Phacoanaphylactic endophthalmitis

●**360.2 Degenerative disorders of globe**
360.20 Degenerative disorder of globe, unspecified
360.21 Progressive high (degenerative) myopia
Malignant myopia
360.23 Siderosis
360.24 Other metallosis
Chalcosis
360.29 Other
Excludes xerophthalmia (264.7)

●**360.3 Hypotony of eye**
360.30 Hypotony, unspecified
360.31 Primary hypotony
360.32 Ocular fistula causing hypotony
360.33 Hypotony associated with other ocular disorders
360.34 Flat anterior chamber

●**360.4 Degenerated conditions of globe**
360.40 Degenerated globe or eye, unspecified
360.41 Blind hypotensive eye
Atrophy of globe
Phthisis bulbi
360.42 Blind hypertensive eye
Absolute glaucoma
360.43 Hemophthalmos, except current injury
Excludes traumatic (871.0–871.9, 921.0–921.9)
360.44 Leucocoria

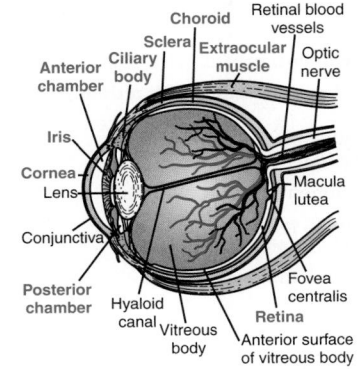

Figure 6–3 Eye and ocular adnexa. (From Buck CJ: Step-by-Step Medical Coding, 2005 ed. Philadelphia, WB Saunders, 2005.)

DISEASES OF THE NERVOUS SYSTEM AND SENSE ORGANS (320–389)

● **360.5 Retained (old) intraocular foreign body, magnetic**

Use additional code to identify foreign body (V90.11) ◄

> Excludes *current penetrating injury with magnetic foreign body (871.5)*
> *retained (old) foreign body of orbit (376.6)*

360.50 Foreign body, magnetic, intraocular, unspecified

360.51 Foreign body, magnetic, in anterior chamber

360.52 Foreign body, magnetic, in iris or ciliary body

360.53 Foreign body, magnetic, in lens

360.54 Foreign body, magnetic, in vitreous

360.55 Foreign body, magnetic, in posterior wall

360.59 Foreign body, magnetic, in other or multiple sites

● **360.6 Retained (old) intraocular foreign body, nonmagnetic**

Retained (old) foreign body:
   NOS
   nonmagnetic

Use additional code to identify foreign body (V90.01-V90.10, V90.12, V90.2-V90.9) ◄

> Excludes *current penetrating injury with (nonmagnetic) foreign body (871.6)*
> *retained (old) foreign body in orbit (376.6)*

360.60 Foreign body, intraocular, unspecified

360.61 Foreign body in anterior chamber

360.62 Foreign body in iris or ciliary body

360.63 Foreign body in lens

360.64 Foreign body in vitreous

360.65 Foreign body in posterior wall

360.69 Foreign body in other or multiple sites

● **360.8 Other disorders of globe**

360.81 Luxation of globe

360.89 Other

360.9 Unspecified disorder of globe

● **361 Retinal detachments and defects**

● **361.0 Retinal detachment with retinal defect**

Rhegmatogenous retinal detachment

> Excludes *detachment of retinal pigment epithelium (362.42–362.43)*
> *retinal detachment (serous) (without defect) (361.2)*

Coding Clinic: 1994, Q1, P17

361.00 Retinal detachment with retinal defect, unspecified

361.01 Recent detachment, partial, with single defect

361.02 Recent detachment, partial, with multiple defects

361.03 Recent detachment, partial, with giant tear

361.04 Recent detachment, partial, with retinal dialysis

Dialysis (juvenile) of retina (with detachment)

361.05 Recent detachment, total or subtotal

361.06 Old detachment, partial

Delimited old retinal detachment

361.07 Old detachment, total or subtotal

Item 6-13 Retinal detachments and defects are conditions of the eye in which the retina separates from the underlying tissue. Initial detachment may be localized, requiring rapid treatment (medical emergency) to avoid the entire retina from detaching, which leads to vision loss and blindness.

● **361.1 Retinoschisis and retinal cysts**

> Excludes *juvenile retinoschisis (362.73)*
> *microcystoid degeneration of retina (362.62)*
> *parasitic cyst of retina (360.13)*

361.10 Retinoschisis, unspecified

361.11 Flat retinoschisis

361.12 Bullous retinoschisis

361.13 Primary retinal cysts

361.14 Secondary retinal cysts

361.19 Other

Pseudocyst of retina

361.2 Serous retinal detachment

Retinal detachment without retinal defect

> Excludes *central serous retinopathy (362.41)*
> *retinal pigment epithelium detachment (362.42–362.43)*

● **361.3 Retinal defects without detachment**

> Excludes *chorioretinal scars after surgery for detachment (363.30–363.35)*
> *peripheral retinal degeneration without defect (362.60–362.66)*

361.30 Retinal defect, unspecified

Retinal break(s) NOS

361.31 Round hole of retina without detachment

361.32 Horseshoe tear of retina without detachment

Operculum of retina without mention of detachment

361.33 Multiple defects of retina without detachment

● **361.8 Other forms of retinal detachment**

361.81 Traction detachment of retina

Traction detachment with vitreoretinal organization

361.89 Other

Coding Clinic: 1999, Q3, P12

361.9 Unspecified retinal detachment

Coding Clinic: 1987, Nov-Dec, P10

● **362 Other retinal disorders**

> Excludes *chorioretinal scars (363.30–363.35)*
> *chorioretinitis (363.0–363.2)*

● **362.0 Diabetic retinopathy**

Code first diabetes (249.5, 250.5)

Most common diabetic eye disease and leading cause of blindness in adults. Caused by changes in the blood vessels of retina in which the blood vessels swell and leak fluid into retinal surface.

362.01 Background diabetic retinopathy

Diabetic retinal microaneurysms
Diabetic retinopathy NOS

362.02 Proliferative diabetic retinopathy

Coding Clinic: 1996, Q3, P5

362.03 Nonproliferative diabetic retinopathy NOS

362.04 Mild nonproliferative diabetic retinopathy

362.05 Moderate nonproliferative diabetic retinopathy

362.06 Severe nonproliferative diabetic retinopathy

Coding Clinic: 2005, Q4, P65-67

362.07 Diabetic macular edema
Diabetic retinal edema

Note: Code 362.07 must be used with a code for diabetic retinopathy (362.01–362.06)

● **362.1 Other background retinopathy and retinal vascular changes**

362.10 Background retinopathy, unspecified
Coding Clinic: 2006, Q1, P12

362.11 Hypertensive retinopathy
OGCR Section I.C.7.a.6

Two codes are necessary to identify the condition. First assign the code from subcategory 362.11, Hypertensive retinopathy, then the appropriate code from categories 401–405 to indicate the type of hypertension.

362.12 Exudative retinopathy
Coats' syndrome
Coding Clinic: 1999, Q3, P12

362.13 Changes in vascular appearance
Vascular sheathing of retina

Use additional code for any associated atherosclerosis (440.8)

362.14 Retinal microaneurysms NOS

362.15 Retinal telangiectasia

362.16 Retinal neovascularization NOS
Neovascularization:
choroidal
subretinal

362.17 Other intraretinal microvascular abnormalities
Retinal varices

362.18 Retinal vasculitis
Eales' disease
Retinal:
arteritis
endarteritis
perivasculitis
phlebitis

● **362.2 Other proliferative retinopathy**

362.20 Retinopathy of prematurity, unspecified
Retinopathy of prematurity NOS
Coding Clinic: 2008, Q4, P110-111

362.21 Retrolental fibroplasia
Cicatricial retinopathy of prematurity

362.22 Retinopathy of prematurity, stage 0

362.23 Retinopathy of prematurity, stage 1

362.24 Retinopathy of prematurity, stage 2

362.25 Retinopathy of prematurity, stage 3

362.26 Retinopathy of prematurity, stage 4

362.27 Retinopathy of prematurity, stage 5

362.29 Other nondiabetic proliferative retinopathy
Coding Clinic: 1996, Q3, P5

● **362.3 Retinal vascular occlusion**
Blockage in vessel of the retina

362.30 Retinal vascular occlusion, unspecified

362.31 Central retinal artery occlusion

362.32 Arterial branch occlusion

362.33 Partial arterial occlusion
Hollenhorst plaque
Retinal microembolism

362.34 Transient arterial occlusion
Amaurosis fugax
Coding Clinic: 2000, Q1, P16

362.35 Central retinal vein occlusion
Coding Clinic: 1993, Q2, P6

362.36 Venous tributary (branch) occlusion

362.37 Venous engorgement
Occlusion:
of retinal vein
incipient of retinal vein
partial of retinal vein

● **362.4 Separation of retinal layers**

Excludes *retinal detachment (serous) (361.2) rhegmatogenous (361.00–361.07)*

362.40 Retinal layer separation, unspecified

362.41 Central serous retinopathy

362.42 Serous detachment of retinal pigment epithelium
Exudative detachment of retinal pigment epithelium

362.43 Hemorrhagic detachment of retinal pigment epithelium

● **362.5 Degeneration of macula and posterior pole**

Excludes *degeneration of optic disc (377.21–377.24) hereditary retinal degeneration [dystrophy] (362.70–362.77)*

362.50 Macular degeneration (senile), unspecified

362.51 Nonexudative senile macular degeneration
Senile macular degeneration:
atrophic
dry

362.52 Exudative senile macular degeneration
Kuhnt-Junius degeneration
Senile macular degeneration:
disciform
wet

362.53 Cystoid macular degeneration
Cystoid macular edema

362.54 Macular cyst, hole, or pseudohole

362.55 Toxic maculopathy

Use additional E code to identify drug, if drug induced

362.56 Macular puckering
Preretinal fibrosis

362.57 Drusen (degenerative)

● **362.6 Peripheral retinal degenerations**

Excludes *hereditary retinal degeneration [dystrophy] (362.70–362.77) retinal degeneration with retinal defect (361.00–361.07)*

362.60 Peripheral retinal degeneration, unspecified

362.61 Paving stone degeneration

362.62 Microcystoid degeneration
Blessig's cysts
Iwanoff's cysts

362.63 Lattice degeneration
Palisade degeneration of retina

362.64 Senile reticular degeneration

362.65 Secondary pigmentary degeneration
Pseudoretinitis pigmentosa

362.66 Secondary vitreoretinal degenerations

Item 6-14 Macular degeneration is typically age-related, chronic, and is evidenced by deterioration of the macula (the part of the retina that provides for central field vision), resulting in blurred vision or a blind spot in the center of visual field while not affecting peripheral vision.

DISEASES OF THE NERVOUS SYSTEM AND SENSE ORGANS (320–389)

● **362.7 Hereditary retinal dystrophies**

   362.70 Hereditary retinal dystrophy, unspecified

   362.71 Retinal dystrophy in systemic or cerebroretinal lipidoses

     Code first underlying disease, as:
      cerebroretinal lipidoses (330.1)
      systemic lipidoses (272.7)

   362.72 Retinal dystrophy in other systemic disorders and syndromes

     Code first underlying disease, as:
      Bassen-Kornzweig syndrome (272.5)
      Refsum's disease (356.3)

   362.73 Vitreoretinal dystrophies
     Juvenile retinoschisis

   362.74 Pigmentary retinal dystrophy
     Retinal dystrophy, albipunctate
     Retinitis pigmentosa

   362.75 Other dystrophies primarily involving the sensory retina
     Progressive cone (-rod) dystrophy
     Stargardt's disease

   362.76 Dystrophies primarily involving the retinal pigment epithelium
     Fundus flavimaculatus
     Vitelliform dystrophy

   362.77 Dystrophies primarily involving Bruch's membrane
     Dystrophy:
      hyaline
      pseudoinflammatory foveal
     Hereditary drusen

● **362.8 Other retinal disorders**

   Excludes *chorioretinal inflammations (363.0–363.2)*
     chorioretinal scars (363.30–363.35)

   362.81 Retinal hemorrhage
     Hemorrhage:
      preretinal
      retinal (deep) (superficial)
      subretinal
     Coding Clinic: 1996, Q4, P43-44

   362.82 Retinal exudates and deposits

   362.83 Retinal edema
     Retinal:
      cotton wool spots
      edema (localized) (macular) (peripheral)

   362.84 Retinal ischemia

   362.85 Retinal nerve fiber bundle defects

   362.89 Other retinal disorders

  362.9 Unspecified retinal disorder

● **363 Chorioretinal inflammations, scars, and other disorders of choroid**

● **363.0 Focal chorioretinitis and focal retinochoroiditis**

   Excludes *focal chorioretinitis or retinochoroiditis in:*
     histoplasmosis (115.02, 115.12, 115.92)
     toxoplasmosis (130.2)
      congenital infection (771.2)

   363.00 Focal chorioretinitis, unspecified
     Focal:
      choroiditis or chorioretinitis NOS
      retinitis or retinochoroiditis NOS

   363.01 Focal choroiditis and chorioretinitis, juxtapapillary

   363.03 Focal choroiditis and chorioretinitis of other posterior pole

   363.04 Focal choroiditis and chorioretinitis, peripheral

   363.05 Focal retinitis and retinochoroiditis, juxtapapillary
     Neuroretinitis

   363.06 Focal retinitis and retinochoroiditis, macular or paramacular

   363.07 Focal retinitis and retinochoroiditis of other posterior pole

   363.08 Focal retinitis and retinochoroiditis, peripheral

● **363.1 Disseminated chorioretinitis and disseminated retinochoroiditis**

   Excludes *disseminated choroiditis or chorioretinitis in secondary syphilis (091.51)*
     neurosyphilitic disseminated retinitis or retinochoroiditis (094.83)
     retinal (peri) vasculitis (362.18)

   363.10 Disseminated chorioretinitis, unspecified
     Disseminated:
      choroiditis or chorioretinitis NOS
      retinitis or retinochoroiditis NOS

   363.11 Disseminated choroiditis and chorioretinitis, posterior pole

   363.12 Disseminated choroiditis and chorioretinitis, peripheral

   363.13 Disseminated choroiditis and chorioretinitis, generalized

     Code first any underlying disease, as:
      tuberculosis (017.3)

   363.14 Disseminated retinitis and retinochoroiditis, metastatic

   363.15 Disseminated retinitis and retinochoroiditis, pigment epitheliopathy
     Acute posterior multifocal placoid pigment epitheliopathy

● **363.2 Other and unspecified forms of chorioretinitis and retinochoroiditis**

   Excludes *panophthalmitis (360.02)*
     sympathetic uveitis (360.11)
     uveitis NOS (364.3)

   363.20 Chorioretinitis, unspecified
     Choroiditis NOS
     Retinitis NOS
     Uveitis, posterior NOS

   363.21 Pars planitis
     Posterior cyclitis

   363.22 Harada's disease

● **363.3 Chorioretinal scars**
     Scar (postinflammatory) (postsurgical) (posttraumatic):
     choroid
     retina

   363.30 Chorioretinal scar, unspecified

   363.31 Solar retinopathy

   363.32 Other macular scars

   363.33 Other scars of posterior pole

   363.34 Peripheral scars

   363.35 Disseminated scars

● **363.4 Choroidal degenerations**

   363.40 Choroidal degeneration, unspecified
     Choroidal sclerosis NOS

   363.41 Senile atrophy of choroid

   363.42 Diffuse secondary atrophy of choroid

   363.43 Angioid streaks of choroid

◀ New　◀◁▯ Revised　~~deleted~~ Deleted　Excludes　Includes　Use additional　Code first　Omit code
● Unacceptable Principal Diagnosis　● Use Additional Digit(s)　OGCR Official Guidelines　Coding Clinic

● **363.5 Hereditary choroidal dystrophies**
Hereditary choroidal atrophy:
partial [choriocapillaris]
total [all vessels]

363.50 Hereditary choroidal dystrophy or atrophy, unspecified

363.51 Circumpapillary dystrophy of choroid, partial

363.52 Circumpapillary dystrophy of choroid, total
Helicoid dystrophy of choroid

363.53 Central dystrophy of choroid, partial
Dystrophy, choroidal:
central areolar
circinate

363.54 Central choroidal atrophy, total
Dystrophy, choroidal:
central gyrate
serpiginous

363.55 Choroideremia

363.56 Other diffuse or generalized dystrophy, partial
Diffuse choroidal sclerosis

363.57 Other diffuse or generalized dystrophy, total
Generalized gyrate atrophy, choroid

● **363.6 Choroidal hemorrhage and rupture**

363.61 Choroidal hemorrhage, unspecified

363.62 Expulsive choroidal hemorrhage

363.63 Choroidal rupture

● **363.7 Choroidal detachment**

363.70 Choroidal detachment, unspecified

363.71 Serous choroidal detachment

363.72 Hemorrhagic choroidal detachment

363.8 Other disorders of choroid
Coding Clinic: 2006, Q1, P12

363.9 Unspecified disorder of choroid

● **364 Disorders of iris and ciliary body**

● **364.0 Acute and subacute iridocyclitis**
Anterior uveitis, acute, subacute
Cyclitis, acute, subacute
Iridocyclitis, acute, subacute
Iritis, acute, subacute

| Excludes | gonococcal (098.41)
herpes simplex (054.44)
herpes zoster (053.22) |

364.00 Acute and subacute iridocyclitis, unspecified

364.01 Primary iridocyclitis

364.02 Recurrent iridocyclitis

364.03 Secondary iridocyclitis, infectious

364.04 Secondary iridocyclitis, noninfectious
Aqueous:
cells
fibrin
flare

364.05 Hypopyon

● **364.1 Chronic iridocyclitis**

| Excludes | posterior cyclitis (363.21) |

364.10 Chronic iridocyclitis, unspecified

364.11 Chronic iridocyclitis in diseases classified elsewhere

Code first underlying disease, as:
sarcoidosis (135)
tuberculosis (017.3)

| Excludes | syphilitic iridocyclitis (091.52) |

● **364.2 Certain types of iridocyclitis**

| Excludes | posterior cyclitis (363.21)
sympathetic uveitis (360.11) |

364.21 Fuchs' heterochromic cyclitis

364.22 Glaucomatocyclitic crises

364.23 Lens-induced iridocyclitis

364.24 Vogt-Koyanagi syndrome

364.3 Unspecified iridocyclitis
Uveitis NOS

● **364.4 Vascular disorders of iris and ciliary body**

364.41 Hyphema
Hemorrhage of iris or ciliary body

364.42 Rubeosis iridis
Neovascularization of iris or ciliary body

● **364.5 Degenerations of iris and ciliary body**

364.51 Essential or progressive iris atrophy

364.52 Iridoschisis

364.53 Pigmentary iris degeneration
Acquired heterochromia of iris
Pigment dispersion syndrome of iris
Translucency of iris

364.54 Degeneration of pupillary margin
Atrophy of sphincter of iris
Ectropion of pigment epithelium of iris

364.55 Miotic cysts of pupillary margin

364.56 Degenerative changes of chamber angle

364.57 Degenerative changes of ciliary body

364.59 Other iris atrophy
Iris atrophy (generalized) (sector shaped)

● **364.6 Cysts of iris, ciliary body, and anterior chamber**

| Excludes | miotic pupillary cyst (364.55)
parasitic cyst (360.13) |

364.60 Idiopathic cysts

364.61 Implantation cysts
Epithelial down-growth, anterior chamber
Implantation cysts (surgical) (traumatic)

364.62 Exudative cysts of iris or anterior chamber

364.63 Primary cyst of pars plana

364.64 Exudative cyst of pars plana

● **364.7 Adhesions and disruptions of iris and ciliary body**

| Excludes | flat anterior chamber (360.34) |

364.70 Adhesions of iris, unspecified
Synechiae (iris) NOS

364.71 Posterior synechiae

364.72 Anterior synechiae

364.73 Goniosynechiae
Peripheral anterior synechiae

364.74 Pupillary membranes
Iris bombé
Pupillary:
occlusion
seclusion

364.75 Pupillary abnormalities
Deformed pupil
Ectopic pupil
Rupture of sphincter, pupil

364.76 Iridodialysis
Coding Clinic: 1985, July-Aug, P16

364.77 Recession of chamber angle

● **364.8 Other disorders of iris and ciliary body**
Coding Clinic: 2007, Q2, P11

    364.81 Floppy iris syndrome
Intraoperative floppy iris syndrome (IFIS)

Use additional E code to identify cause, such as:
sympatholytics [antiadrenergics] causing adverse effect in therapeutic use (E941.3)
Coding Clinic: 2007, Q4, P77-79

    364.82 Plateau iris syndrome
Coding Clinic: 2008, Q4, P112

    364.89 Other disorders of iris and ciliary body
Prolapse of iris NOS

Excludes   *prolapse of iris in recent wound (871.1)*

   364.9 Unspecified disorder of iris and ciliary body

● **365 Glaucoma**
Intraocular pressure (IOP) is too high. IOP is the result of too much aqueous humor because of excess production or inadequate drainage. Leads to optic nerve damage and vision loss.

Excludes   *blind hypertensive eye [absolute glaucoma] (360.42)*
congenital glaucoma (743.20–743.22)

● **365.0 Borderline glaucoma [glaucoma suspect]**

    365.00 Preglaucoma, unspecified
Coding Clinic: 1990, Q1, P8

    365.01 Open angle with borderline findings
Open angle with:
borderline intraocular pressure
cupping of optic discs

    365.02 Anatomical narrow angle

    365.03 Steroid responders

    365.04 Ocular hypertension

● **365.1 Open-angle glaucoma**

    365.10 Open-angle glaucoma, unspecified
Wide-angle glaucoma NOS

    365.11 Primary open angle glaucoma
Chronic simple glaucoma

    365.12 Low tension glaucoma

    365.13 Pigmentary glaucoma

    365.14 Glaucoma of childhood
Infantile or juvenile glaucoma

    365.15 Residual stage of open angle glaucoma

● **365.2 Primary angle-closure glaucoma**

    365.20 Primary angle-closure glaucoma, unspecified

    365.21 Intermittent angle-closure glaucoma
Angle-closure glaucoma:
interval   subacute

    365.22 Acute angle-closure glaucoma

    365.23 Chronic angle-closure glaucoma
Coding Clinic: 1998, Q2, P16

    365.24 Residual stage of angle-closure glaucoma

● **365.3 Corticosteroid-induced glaucoma**

    365.31 Glaucomatous stage

    365.32 Residual stage

● **365.4 Glaucoma associated with congenital anomalies, dystrophies, and systemic syndromes**

    365.41 Glaucoma associated with chamber angle anomalies

    365.42 Glaucoma associated with anomalies of iris

    365.43 Glaucoma associated with other anterior segment anomalies

    365.44 Glaucoma associated with systemic syndromes

Code first *associated disease, as:*
neurofibromatosis (237.70-237.79) ◀▥
Sturge-Weber (-Dimitri) syndrome (759.6)

● **365.5 Glaucoma associated with disorders of the lens**

    365.51 Phacolytic glaucoma

    365.52 Pseudoexfoliation glaucoma

    365.59 Glaucoma associated with other lens disorders

● **365.6 Glaucoma associated with other ocular disorders**

    365.60 Glaucoma associated with unspecified ocular disorder

    365.61 Glaucoma associated with pupillary block

    365.62 Glaucoma associated with ocular inflammations

    365.63 Glaucoma associated with vascular disorders

    365.64 Glaucoma associated with tumors or cysts

    365.65 Glaucoma associated with ocular trauma

● **365.8 Other specified forms of glaucoma**

    365.81 Hypersecretion glaucoma

    365.82 Glaucoma with increased episcleral venous pressure

    365.83 Aqueous misdirection
Malignant glaucoma
Coding Clinic: 2002, Q4, P48

    365.89 Other specified glaucoma
Coding Clinic: 1998, Q2, P16

   365.9 Unspecified glaucoma
Coding Clinic: 2003, Q3, P14; 2001, Q2, P16-17

● **366 Cataract**

Excludes   *congenital cataract (743.30–743.34)*

● **366.0 Infantile, juvenile, and presenile cataract**

    366.00 Nonsenile cataract, unspecified
Coding Clinic: 1987, Mar-April, P9

    366.01 Anterior subcapsular polar cataract

    366.02 Posterior subcapsular polar cataract

    366.03 Cortical, lamellar, or zonular cataract

    366.04 Nuclear cataract

    366.09 Other and combined forms of nonsenile cataract

Figure 6–4   Age-related cataract.
Nuclear sclerosis and cortical lens opacities are present. (From Yanoff: Ophthalmology, 2nd ed. 2004, Mosby, Inc.)

Item 6–15   **Senile** cataracts are linked to the aging process. The most common area for the formation of a cataract is the cortical area of the lens. **Polar cataracts** can be either anterior or posterior. **Anterior polar cataracts** are more common and are small, white, capsular cataracts located on the anterior portion of the lens. **Total cataracts,** also called **complete** or **mature,** cause an opacity of all fibers of the lens. **Hypermature** describes a mature cataract with a swollen, milky cortex that covers the entire lens. **Immature,** also called **incipient,** cataracts have a clear cortex and are only slightly opaque. Treatment for all cataracts is the removal of the lens.

◀ New   ◀▥ Revised   ~~deleted~~ Deleted   Excludes   Includes   Use additional   Code first   Omit code
● Unacceptable Principal Diagnosis   ● Use Additional Digit(s)   OGCR   Official Guidelines   Coding Clinic

366.1 Senile cataract

  366.10 Senile cataract, unspecified
    Coding Clinic: 2003, Q1, P5

  366.11 Pseudoexfoliation of lens capsule

  366.12 Incipient cataract
    Cataract:
     coronary
     immature NOS
     punctate
     Water clefts

  366.13 Anterior subcapsular polar senile cataract

  366.14 Posterior subcapsular polar senile cataract

  366.15 Cortical senile cataract

  366.16 Nuclear sclerosis
    Cataracta brunescens
    Nuclear cataract
    Coding Clinic: 2007, Q4, P77-79; 1985, Sept-Oct, P11

  366.17 Total or mature cataract

  366.18 Hypermature cataract
    Morgagni cataract

  366.19 Other and combined forms of senile cataract

366.2 Traumatic cataract

  366.20 Traumatic cataract, unspecified

  366.21 Localized traumatic opacities
    Vossius' ring

  366.22 Total traumatic cataract

  366.23 Partially resolved traumatic cataract

366.3 Cataract secondary to ocular disorders

  366.30 Cataracta complicata, unspecified

  366.31 Glaucomatous flecks (subcapsular)
    Code first underlying glaucoma (365.0–365.9)

  366.32 Cataract in inflammatory disorders
    Code first underlying condition, as:
    chronic choroiditis (363.0–363.2)

  366.33 Cataract with neovascularization
    Code first underlying condition, as:
    chronic iridocyclitis (364.10)

  366.34 Cataract in degenerative disorders
    Sunflower cataract
    Code first underlying condition, as:
    chalcosis (360.24)
    degenerative myopia (360.21)
    pigmentary retinal dystrophy (362.74)

366.4 Cataract associated with other disorders

  366.41 Diabetic cataract
    Code first diabetes (249.5, 250.5)
    Coding Clinic: 1985, Sept-Oct, P11

  366.42 Tetanic cataract
    Code first underlying disease as:
    calcinosis (275.40)
    hypoparathyroidism (252.1)

  366.43 Myotonic cataract
    Code first underlying disorder (359.21, 359.23)

  366.44 Cataract associated with other syndromes
    Code first underlying condition, as:
    craniofacial dysostosis (756.0)
    galactosemia (271.1)

  366.45 Toxic cataract
    Drug-induced cataract
    Use additional E code to identify drug or other toxic substance
    Coding Clinic: 1995, Q4, P51

  366.46 Cataract associated with radiation and other physical influences
    Use additional E code to identify cause

366.5 After-cataract

  366.50 After-cataract, unspecified
    Secondary cataract NOS

  366.51 Soemmering's ring

  366.52 Other after-cataract, not obscuring vision

  366.53 After-cataract, obscuring vision

366.8 Other cataract
  Calcification of lens
  Coding Clinic: 1994, Q1, P16

366.9 Unspecified cataract
  Coding Clinic: 2009, Q4, P101; 1985, Sept-Oct, P10

367 Disorders of refraction and accommodation

  367.0 Hypermetropia
    Far-sightedness
    Hyperopia

  367.1 Myopia
    Near-sightedness

  367.2 Astigmatism

    367.20 Astigmatism, unspecified

    367.21 Regular astigmatism

    367.22 Irregular astigmatism

  367.3 Anisometropia and aniseikonia

    367.31 Anisometropia

    367.32 Aniseikonia

  367.4 Presbyopia

  367.5 Disorders of accommodation

    367.51 Paresis of accommodation
     Cycloplegia

    367.52 Total or complete internal ophthalmoplegia

    367.53 Spasm of accommodation

  367.8 Other disorders of refraction and accommodation

    367.81 Transient refractive change

    367.89 Other
     Drug-induced disorders of refraction and accommodation
     Toxic disorders of refraction and accommodation

  367.9 Unspecified disorder of refraction and accommodation

Figure 6–5 Corneal perforation.
Preoperative appearance of a patient who has a small, 1.5 mm corneal perforation at the 10 o'clock limbus. *(Courtesy of Dr RK Forster.)* (From Yanoff: Ophthalmology, 2nd ed. 2004, Mosby, Inc.)

Item 6-16 Vossius' ring is the result of contusion-type traumatic injury and results in a ring of iris pigment pressed onto the anterior lens capsule.

Item 6-17 Disorders of refraction: **Hypermetropia**, or far-sightedness, means focus at a distance is adequate but not on close objects. **Myopia** is near-sightedness or short-sightedness and means the focus on nearby objects is clear but distant objects appear blurred. **Astigmatism** is warping of the curvature of the cornea so light rays entering do not meet a single focal point, resulting in a distorted image. **Anisometropia** is unequal refractive power in which one eye may be myopic (near-sighted) and the other hyperopic (far-sighted). **Presbyopia** is the loss of focus on near objects, which occurs with age because the lens loses elasticity.

DISEASES OF THE NERVOUS SYSTEM AND SENSE ORGANS (320–389)

● **368 Visual disturbances**

> **Excludes** *electrophysiological disturbances (794.11–794.14)*

● **368.0 Amblyopia ex anopsia**

368.00 Amblyopia, unspecified

368.01 Strabismic amblyopia
Suppression amblyopia

368.02 Deprivation amblyopia

368.03 Refractive amblyopia

● **368.1 Subjective visual disturbances**

368.10 Subjective visual disturbance, unspecified

368.11 Sudden visual loss

368.12 Transient visual loss
Concentric fading
Scintillating scotoma

368.13 Visual discomfort
Asthenopia
Eye strain
Photophobia

368.14 Visual distortions of shape and size
Macropsia
Metamorphopsia
Micropsia

368.15 Other visual distortions and entoptic phenomena
Photopsia
Refractive:
diplopia
polyopia
Visual halos

368.16 Psychophysical visual disturbances
Prosopagnosia
Visual:
agnosia
disorientation syndrome
hallucinations
object agnosia

368.2 Diplopia
Double vision

● **368.3 Other disorders of binocular vision**

368.30 Binocular vision disorder, unspecified

368.31 Suppression of binocular vision

368.32 Simultaneous visual perception without fusion

368.33 Fusion with defective stereopsis

368.34 Abnormal retinal correspondence

● **368.4 Visual field defects**

368.40 Visual field defect, unspecified

368.41 Scotoma involving central area
Scotoma:
central
centrocecal
paracentral

368.42 Scotoma of blind spot area
Enlarged:
angioscotoma
blind spot
Paracecal scotoma

368.43 Sector or arcuate defects
Scotoma:
arcuate
Bjerrum
Seidel

368.44 Other localized visual field defect

Scotoma:	Visual field defect:
NOS	nasal step
ring	peripheral

368.45 Generalized contraction or constriction

368.46 Homonymous bilateral field defects
Hemianopsia (altitudinal) (homonymous)
Quadrant anopia

368.47 Heteronymous bilateral field defects
Hemianopsia:
binasal
bitemporal

● **368.5 Color vision deficiencies**
Color blindness

368.51 Protan defect
Protanomaly
Protanopia

368.52 Deutan defect
Deuteranomaly
Deuteranopia

368.53 Tritan defect
Tritanomaly
Tritanopia

368.54 Achromatopsia
Monochromatism (cone) (rod)

368.55 Acquired color vision deficiencies

368.59 Other color vision deficiencies

● **368.6 Night blindness**

368.60 Night blindness, unspecified

368.61 Congenital night blindness
Hereditary night blindness
Oguchi's disease

368.62 Acquired night blindness

> **Excludes** *that due to vitamin A deficiency (264.5)*

368.63 Abnormal dark adaptation curve
Abnormal threshold of cones or rods
Delayed adaptation of cones or rods

368.69 Other night blindness

368.8 Other specified visual disturbances
Blurred vision NOS
Coding Clinic: 2002, Q4, P56

368.9 Unspecified visual disturbance
Coding Clinic: 2006, Q3, P22

● **369 Blindness and low vision**

> | Excludes | *correctable impaired vision due to refractive errors (367.0–367.9)*

> **Note:** Visual impairment refers to a functional limitation of the eye (e.g., limited visual acuity or visual field). It should be distinguished from visual disability, indicating a limitation of the abilities of the individual (e.g., limited reading skills, vocational skills), and from visual handicap, indicating a limitation of personal and socioeconomic independence (e.g., limited mobility, limited employability).

The levels of impairment defined in the table after 369.9 are based on the recommendations of the WHO Study Group on Prevention of Blindness (Geneva, November 6–10, 1972; WHO Technical Report Series 518), and of the International Council of Ophthalmology (1976).

Note that definitions of blindness vary in different settings.

For international reporting, WHO defines blindness as profound impairment. This definition can be applied to blindness of one eye (369.1, 369.6) and to blindness of the individual (369.0).

For determination of benefits in the U.S.A., the definition of legal blindness as severe impairment is often used. This definition applies to blindness of the individual only.

● **369.0 Profound impairment, both eyes**

     369.00 Impairment level not further specified
         Blindness:
           NOS according to WHO definition
           both eyes

     369.01 Better eye: total impairment; lesser eye: total impairment

     369.02 Better eye: near-total impairment; lesser eye: not further specified

     369.03 Better eye: near-total impairment; lesser eye: total impairment

     369.04 Better eye: near-total impairment; lesser eye: near-total impairment

     369.05 Better eye: profound impairment; lesser eye: not further specified

     369.06 Better eye: profound impairment; lesser eye: total impairment

     369.07 Better eye: profound impairment; lesser eye: near-total impairment

     369.08 Better eye: profound impairment; lesser eye: profound impairment

● **369.1 Moderate or severe impairment, better eye, profound impairment lesser eye**

     369.10 Impairment level not further specified
         Blindness, one eye, low vision other eye

     369.11 Better eye: severe impairment; lesser eye: blind, not further specified

     369.12 Better eye: severe impairment; lesser eye: total impairment

     369.13 Better eye: severe impairment; lesser eye: near-total impairment

     369.14 Better eye: severe impairment; lesser eye: profound impairment

     369.15 Better eye: moderate impairment; lesser eye: blind, not further specified

     369.16 Better eye: moderate impairment; lesser eye: total impairment

     369.17 Better eye: moderate impairment; lesser eye: near-total impairment

     369.18 Better eye: moderate impairment; lesser eye: profound impairment

● **369.2 Moderate or severe impairment, both eyes**

     369.20 Impairment level not further specified
         Low vision, both eyes NOS

     369.21 Better eye: severe impairment; lesser eye: not further specified

     369.22 Better eye: severe impairment; lesser eye: severe impairment

     369.23 Better eye: moderate impairment; lesser eye: not further specified

     369.24 Better eye: moderate impairment; lesser eye: severe impairment

     369.25 Better eye: moderate impairment; lesser eye: moderate impairment

   369.3 Unqualified visual loss, both eyes

> | Excludes | *blindness NOS:*
>   *legal [U.S.A. definition] (369.4)*
>   *WHO definition (369.00)*

   369.4 Legal blindness, as defined in U.S.A.
     Blindness NOS according to U.S.A. definition

> | Excludes | *legal blindness with specification of impairment level (369.01–369.08, 369.11–369.14, 369.21–369.22)*

● **369.6 Profound impairment, one eye**
     Coding Clinic: 2002, Q3, P20-21

     369.60 Impairment level not further specified
         Blindness, one eye

     369.61 One eye: total impairment; other eye: not specified

     369.62 One eye: total impairment; other eye: near-normal vision

     369.63 One eye: total impairment; other eye: normal vision

     369.64 One eye: near-total impairment; other eye: not specified

     369.65 One eye: near-total impairment; other eye: near-normal vision

     369.66 One eye: near-total impairment; other eye: normal vision

     369.67 One eye: profound impairment; other eye: not specified

     369.68 One eye: profound impairment; other eye: near-normal vision

     369.69 One eye: profound impairment; other eye: normal vision

● **369.7 Moderate or severe impairment, one eye**

     369.70 Impairment level not further specified
         Low vision, one eye

     369.71 One eye: severe impairment; other eye: not specified

     369.72 One eye: severe impairment; other eye: near-normal vision

     369.73 One eye: severe impairment; other eye: normal vision

     369.74 One eye: moderate impairment; other eye: not specified

     369.75 One eye: moderate impairment; other eye: near-normal vision

     369.76 One eye: moderate impairment; other eye: normal vision

   369.8 Unqualified visual loss, one eye

   369.9 Unspecified visual loss

DISEASES OF THE NERVOUS SYSTEM AND SENSE ORGANS (320–389)

Classification		Levels of Visual Impairment	Additional Descriptors Which May Be Encountered
"Legal"	WHO	Visual Acuity and/or Visual Field Limitation (Whichever Is Worse)	
	(Near-) normal vision	Range of Normal Vision 20/10 20/13 20/16 20/20 20/25 2.0 1.6 1.25 1.0 0.8	
		Near-Normal Vision 20/30 20/40 20/50 20/60 0.7 0.6 0.5 0.4 0.3	
	Low vision	Moderate Visual Impairment 20/70 20/80 20/100 20/125 20/160 0.25 0.20 0.16 0.12	Moderate low vision
Legal Blindness (U.S.A.) both eyes	Blindness (WHO) one or both eyes	Severe Visual Impairment 20/200 20/250 20/320 20/400 0.10 0.08 0.06 0.05 Visual field: 20 degrees or less	Severe low vision, "Legal" blindness
		Profound Visual Impairment 20/500 20/630 20/800 20/1000 0.04 0.03 0.025 0.02 Count fingers at: less than 3 m (10 ft) Visual field: 10 degrees or less	Profound low vision, Moderate blindness
		Near-Total Visual Impairment Visual acuity: less than 0.02 (20/1000) Count fingers: 1 m (3 ft) or less Hand movements: 5 m (15 ft) or less Light projection, light perception Visual field: 5 degrees or less	Severe blindness, Near-total blindness
		Total Visual Impairment No light perception (NLP)	Total blindness

Visual acuity refers to best achievable acuity with correction.
Non-listed Snellen fractions may be classified by converting to the nearest decimal equivalent, e.g., 10/200 = 0.05, 6/30 = 0.20.
CF (count fingers) without designation of distance, may be classified to profound impairment.
HM (hand motion) without designation of distance, may be classified to near-total impairment.
Visual field measurements refer to the largest field diameter for a 1/100 white test object.

| Marginal (catarrhal) ulcer | Ring ulcer | Central corneal ulcer | Rosacea ulcer | Mooren's (rodent) ulcer |

Figure 6–6 Corneal ulcers: marginal, ring, central corneal, rosacea, and Mooren's.

Item 6–18 An infected ulcer is usually called a **serpiginous** or **hypopyon** ulcer which is a pus sac in the anterior chamber of the eye.
Marginal ulcers are usually asymptomatic, not primary, and are often superficial and simple. More severe marginal ulcers spread to form a ring ulcer. **Ring** ulcers can extend around the entire corneal periphery.
Central corneal ulcers develop when there is an abrasion to the epithelium and an infection develops in the eroded area.
The **pyocyaneal** ulcer is the most serious corneal infection, which, if left untreated, can lead to loss of the eye.

370 Keratitis
- ● **370.0 Corneal ulcer**
  - Excludes | *that due to vitamin A deficiency (264.3)*
  - **370.00 Corneal ulcer, unspecified**
  - **370.01 Marginal corneal ulcer**
  - **370.02 Ring corneal ulcer**
  - **370.03 Central corneal ulcer**
  - **370.04 Hypopyon ulcer**
    - Serpiginous ulcer
  - **370.05 Mycotic corneal ulcer**
  - **370.06 Perforated corneal ulcer**
  - **370.07 Mooren's ulcer**
- ● **370.2 Superficial keratitis without conjunctivitis**
  - Excludes | *dendritic [herpes simplex] keratitis (054.42)*
  - **370.20 Superficial keratitis, unspecified**
  - **370.21 Punctate keratitis**
    - Thygeson's superficial punctate keratitis
  - **370.22 Macular keratitis**
    - Keratitis: Keratitis:
    - areolar   stellate
    - nummular   striate
  - **370.23 Filamentary keratitis**
  - **370.24 Photokeratitis**
    - Snow blindness
    - Welders' keratitis
    - Coding Clinic: 1996, Q3, P6
- ● **370.3 Certain types of keratoconjunctivitis**
  - **370.31 Phlyctenular keratoconjunctivitis**
    - Phlyctenulosis
    - Use additional code for any associated tuberculosis (017.3)
  - **370.32 Limbal and corneal involvement in vernal conjunctivitis**
    - Use additional code for vernal conjunctivitis (372.13)
  - **370.33 Keratoconjunctivitis sicca, not specified as Sjögren's**
    - Excludes | *Sjögren's syndrome (710.2)*
  - **370.34 Exposure keratoconjunctivitis**
    - Coding Clinic: 1996, Q3, P6
  - **370.35 Neurotrophic keratoconjunctivitis**
- ● **370.4 Other and unspecified keratoconjunctivitis**
  - **370.40 Keratoconjunctivitis, unspecified**
    - Superficial keratitis with conjunctivitis NOS
  - **370.44 Keratitis or keratoconjunctivitis in exanthema**
    - Code first underlying condition (050.0–052.9)
    - Excludes | *herpes simplex (054.43)*
    - *herpes zoster (053.21)*
    - *measles (055.71)*
  - **370.49 Other**
    - Excludes | *epidemic keratoconjunctivitis (077.1)*
- ● **370.5 Interstitial and deep keratitis**
  - **370.50 Interstitial keratitis, unspecified**
  - **370.52 Diffuse interstitial keratitis**
    - Cogan's syndrome
  - **370.54 Sclerosing keratitis**
  - **370.55 Corneal abscess**
  - **370.59 Other**
    - Excludes | *disciform herpes simplex keratitis (054.43)*
    - *syphilitic keratitis (090.3)*

◀ New   ◀▥ Revised   ~~deleted~~ Deleted   Excludes   Includes   Use additional   Code first   Omit code
● Unacceptable Principal Diagnosis   ● Use Additional Digit(s)   OGCR Official Guidelines   Coding Clinic

● **370.6 Corneal neovascularization**

  370.60 Corneal neovascularization, unspecified

  370.61 Localized vascularization of cornea

  370.62 Pannus (corneal)
    Coding Clinic: 2002, Q3, P20-21

  370.63 Deep vascularization of cornea

  370.64 Ghost vessels (corneal)

● **370.8 Other forms of keratitis**
  Code first underlying condition, such as:
    Acanthamoeba (136.21)
    Fusarium (118)
  Coding Clinic: 2008, Q4, P79-81; 1994, Q3, P5

  370.9 Unspecified keratitis

● **371 Corneal opacity and other disorders of cornea**

 ● **371.0 Corneal scars and opacities**
  Excludes *that due to vitamin A deficiency (264.6)*

  371.00 Corneal opacity, unspecified
    Corneal scar NOS

  371.01 Minor opacity of cornea
    Corneal nebula

  371.02 Peripheral opacity of cornea
    Corneal macula not interfering with central vision

  371.03 Central opacity of cornea
    Corneal:
     leucoma interfering with central vision
     macula interfering with central vision

  371.04 Adherent leucoma

  371.05 Phthisical cornea
  Code first underlying tuberculosis (017.3)

 ● **371.1 Corneal pigmentations and deposits**

  371.10 Corneal deposit, unspecified

  371.11 Anterior pigmentations
    Stähli's lines

  371.12 Stromal pigmentations
    Hematocornea

  371.13 Posterior pigmentations
    Krukenberg spindle

  371.14 Kayser-Fleischer ring

  371.15 Other deposits associated with metabolic disorders

  371.16 Argentous deposits

 ● **371.2 Corneal edema**

  371.20 Corneal edema, unspecified

  371.21 Idiopathic corneal edema

  371.22 Secondary corneal edema

  371.23 Bullous keratopathy

  371.24 Corneal edema due to wearing of contact lenses

 ● **371.3 Changes of corneal membranes**

  371.30 Corneal membrane change, unspecified

  371.31 Folds and rupture of Bowman's membrane

  371.32 Folds in Descemet's membrane

  371.33 Rupture in Descemet's membrane

● **371.4 Corneal degenerations**

  371.40 Corneal degeneration, unspecified

  371.41 Senile corneal changes
    Arcus senilis   Hassall-Henle bodies

  371.42 Recurrent erosion of cornea
    Excludes *Mooren's ulcer (370.07)*

  371.43 Band-shaped keratopathy

  371.44 Other calcerous degenerations of cornea

  371.45 Keratomalacia NOS
    Excludes *that due to vitamin A deficiency (264.4)*

  371.46 Nodular degeneration of cornea
    Salzmann's nodular dystrophy

  371.48 Peripheral degenerations of cornea
    Marginal degeneration of cornea [Terrien's]

  371.49 Other
    Discrete colliquative keratopathy

● **371.5 Hereditary corneal dystrophies**

  371.50 Corneal dystrophy, unspecified

  371.51 Juvenile epithelial corneal dystrophy

  371.52 Other anterior corneal dystrophies
    Corneal dystrophy:
     microscopic cystic
     ring-like

  371.53 Granular corneal dystrophy

  371.54 Lattice corneal dystrophy

  371.55 Macular corneal dystrophy

  371.56 Other stromal corneal dystrophies
    Crystalline corneal dystrophy

  371.57 Endothelial corneal dystrophy
    Combined corneal dystrophy
    Cornea guttata
    Fuchs' endothelial dystrophy

  371.58 Other posterior corneal dystrophies
    Polymorphous corneal dystrophy

● **371.6 Keratoconus**

  371.60 Keratoconus, unspecified

  371.61 Keratoconus, stable condition

  371.62 Keratoconus, acute hydrops

● **371.7 Other corneal deformities**

  371.70 Corneal deformity, unspecified

  371.71 Corneal ectasia

  371.72 Descemetocele

  371.73 Corneal staphyloma

Figure 6–7 Lateral view of the displacement of the cone apex in keratoconus. (From Yanoff: Ophthalmology, 2nd ed. 2004, Mosby, Inc.)

Item 6–19 Keratoconus results in corneal degeneration that begins in childhood, gradually changes the cornea from a round to cone shape, decreasing visual acuity. Treatment includes contact lenses. In severe cases the need for corneal transplant may be the treatment of choice; however, newer technologies may use high frequency radio energy to shrink the edges of the cornea, pulling the central area back to a more normal shape. It can help delay or avoid the need for a corneal transplantation.

DISEASES OF THE NERVOUS SYSTEM AND SENSE ORGANS (320–389)

● **371.8 Other corneal disorders**

371.81 Corneal anesthesia and hypoesthesia

371.82 Corneal disorder due to contact lens
Excludes | *corneal edema due to contact lens (371.24)*

371.89 Other
Coding Clinic: 1999, Q3, P12

371.9 Unspecified corneal disorder

● **372 Disorders of conjunctiva**
Excludes | *keratoconjunctivitis (370.3–370.4)*

● **372.0 Acute conjunctivitis**

372.00 Acute conjunctivitis, unspecified

372.01 Serous conjunctivitis, except viral
Excludes | *viral conjunctivitis NOS (077.9)*
Coding Clinic: 2008, Q3, P6-7

372.02 Acute follicular conjunctivitis
Conjunctival folliculosis NOS
Excludes | *conjunctivitis:*
adenoviral (acute follicular) (077.3)
epidemic hemorrhagic (077.4)
inclusion (077.0)
Newcastle (077.8)
epidemic keratoconjunctivitis (077.1)
pharyngoconjunctival fever (077.2)

372.03 Other mucopurulent conjunctivitis
Catarrhal conjunctivitis
Excludes | *blennorrhea neonatorum (gonococcal) (098.40)*
neonatal conjunctivitis (771.6)
ophthalmia neonatorum NOS (771.6)

372.04 Pseudomembranous conjunctivitis
Membranous conjunctivitis
Excludes | *diphtheritic conjunctivitis (032.81)*

372.05 Acute atopic conjunctivitis

372.06 Acute chemical conjunctivitis
Acute toxic conjunctivitis
Use additional E code to identify the chemical or toxic agent
Excludes | *burn of eye and adnexa (940.0–940.9)*
chemical corrosion injury of eye (940.2-940.3)

● **372.1 Chronic conjunctivitis**

372.10 Chronic conjunctivitis, unspecified

372.11 Simple chronic conjunctivitis

372.12 Chronic follicular conjunctivitis

372.13 Vernal conjunctivitis
Coding Clinic: 1996, Q3, P8

372.14 Other chronic allergic conjunctivitis
Coding Clinic: 1996, Q3, P8

372.15 Parasitic conjunctivitis
Code first *underlying disease as:*
filariasis (125.0–125.9)
mucocutaneous leishmaniasis (085.5)

● **372.2 Blepharoconjunctivitis**

372.20 Blepharoconjunctivitis, unspecified

372.21 Angular blepharoconjunctivitis

372.22 Contact blepharoconjunctivitis

● **372.3 Other and unspecified conjunctivitis**

372.30 Conjunctivitis, unspecified

372.31 Rosacea conjunctivitis
Code first *underlying rosacea dermatitis (695.3)*

372.33 Conjunctivitis in mucocutaneous disease
Code first *underlying disease as:*
erythema multiforme (695.10–695.19)
Reiter's disease (099.3)
Excludes | *ocular pemphigoid (694.61)*

372.34 Pingueculitis
Excludes | *pinguecula (372.51)*
Coding Clinic: 2008, Q4, P112-113

372.39 Other
Coding Clinic: 2007, Q2, P11

● **372.4 Pterygium**
Excludes | *pseudopterygium (372.52)*

372.40 Pterygium, unspecified

372.41 Peripheral pterygium, stationary

372.42 Peripheral pterygium, progressive

372.43 Central pterygium

372.44 Double pterygium

372.45 Recurrent pterygium

● **372.5 Conjunctival degenerations and deposits**

372.50 Conjunctival degeneration, unspecified

372.51 Pinguecula
Excludes | *pingueculitis (372.34)*

372.52 Pseudopterygium

372.53 Conjunctival xerosis
Excludes | *conjunctival xerosis due to vitamin A deficiency (264.0, 264.1, 264.7)*

372.54 Conjunctival concretions

372.55 Conjunctival pigmentations
Conjunctival argyrosis

372.56 Conjunctival deposits

● **372.6 Conjunctival scars**

372.61 Granuloma of conjunctiva

372.62 Localized adhesions and strands of conjunctiva

372.63 Symblepharon
Extensive adhesions of conjunctiva

372.64 Scarring of conjunctiva
Contraction of eye socket (after enucleation)

● **372.7 Conjunctival vascular disorders and cysts**

372.71 Hyperemia of conjunctiva

372.72 Conjunctival hemorrhage
Hyposphagma
Subconjunctival hemorrhage

Figure 6–8 Double pterygium. Note both nasal and temporal pterygia in a 57-year-old farmer. (From Yanoff: Ophthalmology, 2nd ed. 2004, Mosby, Inc.)

Item 6–20 Pterygium is Greek for batlike. The condition is characterized by a membrane that extends from the limbus to the center of the cornea and resembles a wing.

◀ New ◀ Revised ~~deleted~~ Deleted Excludes Includes Use additional Code first Omit code
● Unacceptable Principal Diagnosis ● Use Additional Digit(s) OGCR Official Guidelines Coding Clinic

372.73 Conjunctival edema
Chemosis of conjunctiva
Subconjunctival edema

372.74 Vascular abnormalities of conjunctiva
Aneurysm(ata) of conjunctiva

372.75 Conjunctival cysts

● **372.8 Other disorders of conjunctiva**

372.81 Conjunctivochalasis
Coding Clinic: 2000, Q4, P41

372.89 Other disorders of conjunctiva

372.9 Unspecified disorder of conjunctiva

● **373 Inflammation of eyelids**

● **373.0 Blepharitis**

Excludes blepharoconjunctivitis (372.20–372.22)

373.00 Blepharitis, unspecified

373.01 Ulcerative blepharitis

373.02 Squamous blepharitis

● **373.1 Hordeolum and other deep inflammation of eyelid**
Bacterial infection (staphylococcus) of sebaceous gland of eyelid (stye)

373.11 Hordeolum externum
Hordeolum NOS
Stye

373.12 Hordeolum internum
Infection of meibomian gland

373.13 Abscess of eyelid
Furuncle of eyelid

373.2 Chalazion
Most often caused by accumulation of meibomian gland secretions resulting from blockage of duct.
Meibomian (gland) cyst

Excludes *infected meibomian gland (373.12)*

● **373.3 Noninfectious dermatoses of eyelid**

373.31 Eczematous dermatitis of eyelid

373.32 Contact and allergic dermatitis of eyelid

373.33 Xeroderma of eyelid

373.34 Discoid lupus erythematosus of eyelid

373.4 Infective dermatitis of eyelid of types resulting in deformity

Code first *underlying disease, as:*
leprosy (030.0–030.9)
lupus vulgaris (tuberculous) (017.0)
yaws (102.0–102.9)

373.5 Other infective dermatitis of eyelid

Code first *underlying disease, as:*
actinomycosis (039.3)
impetigo (684)
mycotic dermatitis (110.0–111.9)
vaccinia (051.0)
postvaccination (999.0)

Excludes *herpes:*
simplex (054.41)
zoster (053.20)

Figure 6–9 Photograph of eyelids with marginal blepharitis. (From Mandell, Bennett, & Dolin: Principles and Practice of Infectious Diseases, 6th ed. 2005, Churchill Livingstone, An Imprint of Elsevier.)

Item 6–21 Blepharitis is a common condition in which the eyelid is swollen and yellow scaling and conjunctivitis develop. Usually the hair on the scalp and brow is involved.

Figure 6–10 Right lower eyelid entropion. Note the inward rotation of the tarsal plate about the horizontal axis and the resultant contact between the mucocutaneous junction and ocular surface. (From Yanoff: Ophthalmology, 2nd ed. 2004, Mosby, Inc.)

373.6 Parasitic infestation of eyelid

Code first *underlying disease, as:*
leishmaniasis (085.0–085.9)
loiasis (125.2)
onchocerciasis (125.3)
pediculosis (132.0)

373.8 Other inflammations of eyelids

373.9 Unspecified inflammation of eyelid

● **374 Other disorders of eyelids**

● **374.0 Entropion and trichiasis of eyelid**

374.00 Entropion, unspecified

374.01 Senile entropion

374.02 Mechanical entropion

374.03 Spastic entropion

374.04 Cicatricial entropion

374.05 Trichiasis without entropion

● **374.1 Ectropion**

374.10 Ectropion, unspecified

374.11 Senile ectropion

374.12 Mechanical ectropion

374.13 Spastic ectropion

374.14 Cicatricial ectropion

● **374.2 Lagophthalmos**

374.20 Lagophthalmos, unspecified

374.21 Paralytic lagophthalmos

374.22 Mechanical lagophthalmos

374.23 Cicatricial lagophthalmos

● **374.3 Ptosis of eyelid**
Falling forward, drooping, sagging of eyelid

374.30 Ptosis of eyelid, unspecified
Coding Clinic: 1996, Q2, P11

374.31 Paralytic ptosis

374.32 Myogenic ptosis

374.33 Mechanical ptosis

374.34 Blepharochalasis
Pseudoptosis

Item 6–22 Ptosis of eyelid is drooping of the upper eyelid over the pupil when the eyes are fully opened resulting from nerve or muscle damage, which may require surgical correction.

Figure 6–11 Ptosis of eyelid. (From Yanoff: Ophthalmology, 2nd ed. 2004, Mosby, Inc.)

DISEASES OF THE NERVOUS SYSTEM AND SENSE ORGANS (320–389)

● **374.4 Other disorders affecting eyelid function**

> | Excludes | blepharoclonus (333.81)
> blepharospasm (333.81)
> facial nerve palsy (351.0)
> third nerve palsy or paralysis
> (378.51–378.52)
> tic (psychogenic) (307.20–307.23)
> organic (333.3)

374.41 Lid retraction or lag

374.43 Abnormal innervation syndrome
Jaw-blinking
Paradoxical facial movements

374.44 Sensory disorders

374.45 Other sensorimotor disorders
Deficient blink reflex

374.46 Blepharophimosis
Ankyloblepharon

● **374.5 Degenerative disorders of eyelid and periocular area**

374.50 Degenerative disorder of eyelid, unspecified

374.51 Xanthelasma
Xanthoma (planum) (tuberosum) of eyelid
Code first underlying condition (272.0–272.9)

374.52 Hyperpigmentation of eyelid
Chloasma
Dyspigmentation

374.53 Hypopigmentation of eyelid
Vitiligo of eyelid

374.54 Hypertrichosis of eyelid

374.55 Hypotrichosis of eyelid
Madarosis of eyelid

374.56 Other degenerative disorders of skin affecting eyelid

● **374.8 Other disorders of eyelid**

374.81 Hemorrhage of eyelid
> | Excludes | black eye (921.0)

374.82 Edema of eyelid
Hyperemia of eyelid
Coding Clinic: 2008, Q4, P128-131

374.83 Elephantiasis of eyelid

374.84 Cysts of eyelids
Sebaceous cyst of eyelid

374.85 Vascular anomalies of eyelid

374.86 Retained foreign body of eyelid
Use additional code to identify foreign body (V90.01-V90.9) ◄

374.87 Dermatochalasis

374.89 Other disorders of eyelid

374.9 Unspecified disorder of eyelid

● **375 Disorders of lacrimal system**

● **375.0 Dacryoadenitis**

375.00 Dacryoadenitis, unspecified

375.01 Acute dacryoadenitis

375.02 Chronic dacryoadenitis

375.03 Chronic enlargement of lacrimal gland

● **375.1 Other disorders of lacrimal gland**

375.11 Dacryops

375.12 Other lacrimal cysts and cystic degeneration

375.13 Primary lacrimal atrophy

375.14 Secondary lacrimal atrophy

375.15 Tear film insufficiency, unspecified
Dry eye syndrome
Coding Clinic: 1996, Q3, P6

375.16 Dislocation of lacrimal gland

Figure 6–12 Lacrimal apparatus. (From Buck CJ: Step-by-Step Medical Coding. Philadelphia, WB Saunders, 2006, p 302.)

● **375.2 Epiphora**

375.20 Epiphora, unspecified as to cause

375.21 Epiphora due to excess lacrimation

375.22 Epiphora due to insufficient drainage

● **375.3 Acute and unspecified inflammation of lacrimal passages**
> | Excludes | neonatal dacryocystitis (771.6)

375.30 Dacryocystitis, unspecified

375.31 Acute canaliculitis, lacrimal

375.32 Acute dacryocystitis
Acute peridacryocystitis

375.33 Phlegmonous dacryocystitis

● **375.4 Chronic inflammation of lacrimal passages**

375.41 Chronic canaliculitis

375.42 Chronic dacryocystitis

375.43 Lacrimal mucocele

● **375.5 Stenosis and insufficiency of lacrimal passages**

375.51 Eversion of lacrimal punctum

375.52 Stenosis of lacrimal punctum

375.53 Stenosis of lacrimal canaliculi

375.54 Stenosis of lacrimal sac

375.55 Obstruction of nasolacrimal duct, neonatal
> | Excludes | congenital anomaly of nasolacrimal duct (743.65)

375.56 Stenosis of nasolacrimal duct, acquired

375.57 Dacryolith

● **375.6 Other changes of lacrimal passages**

375.61 Lacrimal fistula

375.69 Other

● **375.8 Other disorders of lacrimal system**

375.81 Granuloma of lacrimal passages

375.89 Other

375.9 Unspecified disorder of lacrimal system

● **376 Disorders of the orbit**

● **376.0 Acute inflammation of orbit**

376.00 Acute inflammation of orbit, unspecified

376.01 Orbital cellulitis
Abscess of orbit

376.02 Orbital periostitis

376.03 Orbital osteomyelitis

376.04 Tenonitis

● **376.1 Chronic inflammatory disorders of orbit**

376.10 Chronic inflammation of orbit, unspecified

376.11 Orbital granuloma
Pseudotumor (inflammatory) of orbit

376.12 Orbital myositis

376.13 Parasitic infestation of orbit
Code first underlying disease, as:
hydatid infestation of orbit (122.3, 122.6, 122.9)
myiasis of orbit (134.0)

◄ New   ◀▦ Revised   ~~deleted~~ Deleted | Excludes | Includes   Use additional   Code first   Omit code
● Unacceptable Principal Diagnosis   ● Use Additional Digit(s)   OGCR Official Guidelines   Coding Clinic

● 376.2 **Endocrine exophthalmos**
    Code first underlying thyroid disorder (242.0–242.9)
   376.21 **Thyrotoxic exophthalmos**
   376.22 **Exophthalmic ophthalmoplegia**

● 376.3 **Other exophthalmic conditions**
   376.30 **Exophthalmos, unspecified**
   376.31 **Constant exophthalmos**
   376.32 **Orbital hemorrhage**
   376.33 **Orbital edema or congestion**
   376.34 **Intermittent exophthalmos**
   376.35 **Pulsating exophthalmos**
   376.36 **Lateral displacement of globe**

● 376.4 **Deformity of orbit**
   376.40 **Deformity of orbit, unspecified**
   376.41 **Hypertelorism of orbit**
   376.42 **Exostosis of orbit**
   376.43 **Local deformities due to bone disease**
   376.44 **Orbital deformities associated with craniofacial deformities**
   376.45 **Atrophy of orbit**
   376.46 **Enlargement of orbit**
   376.47 **Deformity due to trauma or surgery**

● 376.5 **Enophthalmos**
   376.50 **Enophthalmos, unspecified as to cause**
   376.51 **Enophthalmos due to atrophy of orbital tissue**
   376.52 **Enophthalmos due to trauma or surgery**

  376.6 **Retained (old) foreign body following penetrating wound of orbit**
    Retrobulbar foreign body
    Use additional code to identify foreign body (V90.01-V90.9) ◄

● 376.8 **Other orbital disorders**
   376.81 **Orbital cysts**
     Encephalocele of orbit
     Coding Clinic: 1999, Q3, P13
   376.82 **Myopathy of extraocular muscles**
   376.89 **Other**

  376.9 **Unspecified disorder of orbit**

● 377 **Disorders of optic nerve and visual pathways**
● 377.0 **Papilledema**
   377.00 **Papilledema, unspecified**
   377.01 **Papilledema associated with increased intracranial pressure**
   377.02 **Papilledema associated with decreased ocular pressure**
   377.03 **Papilledema associated with retinal disorder**
   377.04 **Foster-Kennedy syndrome**

● 377.1 **Optic atrophy**
   377.10 **Optic atrophy, unspecified**
   377.11 **Primary optic atrophy**
     Excludes *neurosyphilitic optic atrophy (094.84)*
   377.12 **Postinflammatory optic atrophy**
   377.13 **Optic atrophy associated with retinal dystrophies**
   377.14 **Glaucomatous atrophy [cupping] of optic disc**
   377.15 **Partial optic atrophy**
     Temporal pallor of optic disc
   377.16 **Hereditary optic atrophy**
     Optic atrophy:
      dominant hereditary
      Leber's

● 377.2 **Other disorders of optic disc**
   377.21 **Drusen of optic disc**
   377.22 **Crater-like holes of optic disc**
   377.23 **Coloboma of optic disc**
   377.24 **Pseudopapilledema**

● 377.3 **Optic neuritis**
     Excludes *meningococcal optic neuritis (036.81)*
   377.30 **Optic neuritis, unspecified**
   377.31 **Optic papillitis**
   377.32 **Retrobulbar neuritis (acute)**
     Excludes *syphilitic retrobulbar neuritis (094.85)*
   377.33 **Nutritional optic neuropathy**
   377.34 **Toxic optic neuropathy**
     Toxic amblyopia
   377.39 **Other**
     Excludes *ischemic optic neuropathy (377.41)*

● 377.4 **Other disorders of optic nerve**
   377.41 **Ischemic optic neuropathy**
   377.42 **Hemorrhage in optic nerve sheaths**
   377.43 **Optic nerve hypoplasia**
     Coding Clinic: 2006, Q4, P81-82
   377.49 **Other**
     Compression of optic nerve

● 377.5 **Disorders of optic chiasm**
   377.51 **Associated with pituitary neoplasms and disorders**
   377.52 **Associated with other neoplasms**
   377.53 **Associated with vascular disorders**
   377.54 **Associated with inflammatory disorders**

● 377.6 **Disorders of other visual pathways**
   377.61 **Associated with neoplasms**
   377.62 **Associated with vascular disorders**
   377.63 **Associated with inflammatory disorders**

● 377.7 **Disorders of visual cortex**
     Excludes *visual:*
      agnosia (368.16)
      hallucinations (368.16)
      halos (368.15)
   377.71 **Associated with neoplasms**
   377.72 **Associated with vascular disorders**
   377.73 **Associated with inflammatory disorders**
   377.75 **Cortical blindness**

  377.9 **Unspecified disorder of optic nerve and visual pathways**

Item 6-23 Papilledema is swelling of the optic disc caused by increased intracranial pressure. It is most often bilateral and occurs quickly (hours) or over weeks of time. It is a common symptom of a brain tumor. The term should not be used to describe optic disc swelling with underlying infectious, infiltrative, or inflammatory etiologies.

● **378 Strabismus and other disorders of binocular eye movements**

  Excludes *nystagmus and other irregular eye movements (379.50–379.59)*

● **378.0 Esotropia**
  Convergent concomitant strabismus
  Excludes *intermittent esotropia (378.20–378.22)*

  378.00 Esotropia, unspecified
  378.01 Monocular esotropia
  378.02 Monocular esotropia with A pattern
  378.03 Monocular esotropia with V pattern
  378.04 Monocular esotropia with other noncomitancies
      Monocular esotropia with X or Y pattern
  378.05 Alternating esotropia
  378.06 Alternating esotropia with A pattern
  378.07 Alternating esotropia with V pattern
  378.08 Alternating esotropia with other noncomitancies
      Alternating esotropia with X or Y pattern

● **378.1 Exotropia**
  Misalignment in which one eye deviates outward (away from nose) while other fixates normally
  Divergent concomitant strabismus
  Excludes *intermittent exotropia (378.20, 378.23–378.24)*

  378.10 Exotropia, unspecified
  378.11 Monocular exotropia
  378.12 Monocular exotropia with A pattern
  378.13 Monocular exotropia with V pattern
  378.14 Monocular exotropia with other noncomitancies
      Monocular exotropia with X or Y pattern
  378.15 Alternating exotropia
  378.16 Alternating exotropia with A pattern
  378.17 Alternating exotropia with V pattern
  378.18 Alternating exotropia with other noncomitancies
      Alternating exotropia with X or Y pattern

● **378.2 Intermittent heterotropia**
  Displacement of an organ or part of an organ from normal position
  Excludes *vertical heterotropia (intermittent) (378.31)*

  378.20 Intermittent heterotropia, unspecified
      Intermittent:
        esotropia NOS
        exotropia NOS
  378.21 Intermittent esotropia, monocular
  378.22 Intermittent esotropia, alternating
  378.23 Intermittent exotropia, monocular
  378.24 Intermittent exotropia, alternating

● **378.3 Other and unspecified heterotropia**
  378.30 Heterotropia, unspecified
  378.31 Hypertropia
      Vertical heterotropia (constant) (intermittent)
  378.32 Hypotropia
  378.33 Cyclotropia
  378.34 Monofixation syndrome
      Microtropia
  378.35 Accommodative component in esotropia

Item 6-24 Strabismus or esotropia (crossed eyes) is a condition of the extraocular eye muscles, resulting in an inability of the eyes to focus and also affects depth perception.

Figure 6–13 A. Image of strabismus. **B.** Exotropia. (**A** from Yanoff: Ophthalmology, 2nd ed. 2004, Mosby, Inc. **B** from Rakel: Textbook of Family Practice, 7th ed. 2007, Saunders.)

● **378.4 Heterophoria**
  Condition in which one or both eyes wander away from position where both eyes are looking

  378.40 Heterophoria, unspecified
  378.41 Esophoria
      Eye deviates inward (toward nose)
  378.42 Exophoria
      Eye deviates outward (toward ear)
  378.43 Vertical heterophoria
  378.44 Cyclophoria
  378.45 Alternating hyperphoria

● **378.5 Paralytic strabismus**
  378.50 Paralytic strabismus, unspecified
  378.51 Third or oculomotor nerve palsy, partial
  378.52 Third or oculomotor nerve palsy, total
  378.53 Fourth or trochlear nerve palsy
      Coding Clinic: 2001, Q2, P21
  378.54 Sixth or abducens nerve palsy
  378.55 External ophthalmoplegia
      Coding Clinic: 1989, Q2, P12
  378.56 Total ophthalmoplegia

● **378.6 Mechanical strabismus**
  378.60 Mechanical strabismus, unspecified
  378.61 Brown's (tendon) sheath syndrome
  378.62 Mechanical strabismus from other musculofascial disorders
  378.63 Limited duction associated with other conditions

● **378.7 Other specified strabismus**
  378.71 Duane's syndrome
  378.72 Progressive external ophthalmoplegia
  378.73 Strabismus in other neuromuscular disorders

● **378.8 Other disorders of binocular eye movements**
  Excludes *nystagmus (379.50–379.56)*

  378.81 Palsy of conjugate gaze
  378.82 Spasm of conjugate gaze
  378.83 Convergence insufficiency or palsy
  378.84 Convergence excess or spasm
  378.85 Anomalies of divergence
  378.86 Internuclear ophthalmoplegia
  378.87 Other dissociated deviation of eye movements
      Skew deviation

378.9 Unspecified disorder of eye movements
  Ophthalmoplegia NOS
  Strabismus NOS
  Coding Clinic: 2001, Q2, P21

● 379 **Other disorders of eye**
  ● 379.0 **Scleritis and episcleritis**
    Inflammation of white (sclera and episclera) of eye.
    Autoimmune disorders are most common cause.

    | Excludes | *syphilitic episcleritis (095.0)*

    379.00 **Scleritis, unspecified**
      Episcleritis NOS
    379.01 **Episcleritis periodica fugax**
    379.02 **Nodular episcleritis**
    379.03 **Anterior scleritis**
    379.04 **Scleromalacia perforans**
    379.05 **Scleritis with corneal involvement**
      Scleroperikeratitis
    379.06 **Brawny scleritis**
    379.07 **Posterior scleritis**
      Sclerotenonitis
    379.09 **Other**
      Scleral abscess

  ● 379.1 **Other disorders of sclera**

    | Excludes | *blue sclera (743.47)*

    379.11 **Scleral ectasia**
      Scleral staphyloma NOS
    379.12 **Staphyloma posticum**
    379.13 **Equatorial staphyloma**
    379.14 **Anterior staphyloma, localized**
    379.15 **Ring staphyloma**
    379.16 **Other degenerative disorders of sclera**
    379.19 **Other**

  ● 379.2 **Disorders of vitreous body**
    379.21 **Vitreous degeneration**
      Vitreous:
        cavitation
        detachment
        liquefaction
    379.22 **Crystalline deposits in vitreous**
      Asteroid hyalitis
      Synchysis scintillans
    379.23 **Vitreous hemorrhage**
      Coding Clinic: 1991, Q3, P15-16
    379.24 **Other vitreous opacities**
      Vitreous floaters
      Small clumps of cells that float in vitreous of the
      eye, appearing as black specks or dots in
      field of vision.
      Coding Clinic: 1994, Q1, P16
    379.25 **Vitreous membranes and strands**
    379.26 **Vitreous prolapse**
    379.29 **Other disorders of vitreous**

      | Excludes | *vitreous abscess (360.04)*
      Coding Clinic: 1999, Q1, P11

  ● 379.3 **Aphakia and other disorders of lens**

    | Excludes | *after-cataract (366.50–366.53)*

    379.31 **Aphakia**

      | Excludes | *cataract extraction status (V45.61)*

    379.32 **Subluxation of lens**
      Coding Clinic: 1994, Q1, P16-17
    379.33 **Anterior dislocation of lens**
    379.34 **Posterior dislocation of lens**
    379.39 **Other disorders of lens**

  ● 379.4 **Anomalies of pupillary function**
    379.40 **Abnormal pupillary function, unspecified**
    379.41 **Anisocoria**
    379.42 **Miosis (persistent), not due to miotics**
    379.43 **Mydriasis (persistent), not due to mydriatics**
    379.45 **Argyll Robertson pupil, atypical**
      Argyll Robertson phenomenon or pupil,
      nonsyphilitic

      | Excludes | *Argyll Robertson pupil (syphilitic)*
      (094.89)

    379.46 **Tonic pupillary reaction**
      Adie's pupil or syndrome
    379.49 **Other**
      Hippus
      Pupillary paralysis

  ● 379.5 **Nystagmus and other irregular eye movements**
    Nystagmus is rapid, involuntary movements of eyes in
    horizontal or vertical direction.

    379.50 **Nystagmus, unspecified**
      Coding Clinic: 2002, Q4, P68; 2001, Q2, P21
    379.51 **Congenital nystagmus**
    379.52 **Latent nystagmus**
    379.53 **Visual deprivation nystagmus**
    379.54 **Nystagmus associated with disorders of the**
      vestibular system
    379.55 **Dissociated nystagmus**
    379.56 **Other forms of nystagmus**
    379.57 **Deficiencies of saccadic eye movements**
      Abnormal optokinetic response
    379.58 **Deficiencies of smooth pursuit movements**
    379.59 **Other irregularities of eye movements**
      Opsoclonus

  ● 379.6 **Inflammation (infection) of postprocedural bleb**
    Postprocedural blebitis
    379.60 **Inflammation (infection) of postprocedural**
      bleb, unspecified
    379.61 **Inflammation (infection) of postprocedural**
      bleb, stage 1
    379.62 **Inflammation (infection) of postprocedural**
      bleb, stage 2
      Coding Clinic: 2006, Q4, P82-83
    379.63 **Inflammation (infection) of postprocedural**
      bleb, stage 3
      Bleb associated endophthalmitis

  379.8 **Other specified disorders of eye and adnexa**

  ● 379.9 **Unspecified disorder of eye and adnexa**
    379.90 **Disorder of eye, unspecified**
    379.91 **Pain in or around eye**
    379.92 **Swelling or mass of eye**
    379.93 **Redness or discharge of eye**
    379.99 **Other ill-defined disorders of eye**

      | Excludes | *blurred vision NOS (368.8)*

DISEASES OF THE NERVOUS SYSTEM AND SENSE ORGANS (320–389)

◀ New   ⬱ Revised   ~~deleted~~ Deleted | Excludes | Includes   Use additional   Code first   Omit code
● Unacceptable Principal Diagnosis   ● Use Additional Digit(s)   OGCR Official Guidelines   Coding Clinic

821

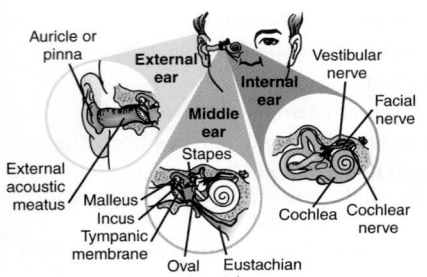

Figure 6–14
Auditory system.
(From Buck CJ:
Step-by-Step Medical
Coding, 2010 ed.
Philadelphia, WB
Saunders, 2010.)

DISEASES OF THE EAR AND MASTOID PROCESS (380–389)

Use additional external cause code, if applicable, to identify the cause of the ear condition

● **380 Disorders of external ear**

● **380.0 Perichondritis and chondritis of pinna**
Chondritis of auricle
Perichondritis of auricle

380.00 Perichondritis of pinna, unspecified

380.01 Acute perichondritis of pinna

380.02 Chronic perichondritis of pinna

380.03 Chondritis of pinna
Coding Clinic: 2004, Q4, P75-76

● **380.1 Infective otitis externa**

380.10 Infective otitis externa, unspecified
Otitis externa (acute):
NOS
circumscribed
diffuse
hemorrhagica
infective NOS

380.11 Acute infection of pinna
Excludes *furuncular otitis externa (680.0)*

380.12 Acute swimmers' ear
Beach ear
Tank ear

380.13 Other acute infections of external ear
Code first underlying disease, as:
erysipelas (035)
impetigo (684)
seborrheic dermatitis (690.10–690.18)
Excludes *herpes simplex (054.73)*
herpes zoster (053.71)

380.14 Malignant otitis externa

380.15 Chronic mycotic otitis externa
Code first underlying disease, as:
aspergillosis (117.3)
otomycosis NOS (111.9)
Excludes *candidal otitis externa (112.82)*

380.16 Other chronic infective otitis externa
Chronic infective otitis externa NOS

● **380.2 Other otitis externa**

380.21 Cholesteatoma of external ear
Keratosis obturans of external ear (canal)
Excludes *cholesteatoma NOS*
(385.30–385.35)
postmastoidectomy (383.32)

380.22 Other acute otitis externa
Acute otitis externa:
actinic
chemical
contact
eczematoid
reactive

380.23 Other chronic otitis externa
Chronic otitis externa NOS

● **380.3 Noninfectious disorders of pinna**

380.30 Disorder of pinna, unspecified

380.31 Hematoma of auricle or pinna

380.32 Acquired deformities of auricle or pinna
Excludes *cauliflower ear (738.7)*
Coding Clinic: 2003, Q3, P12-13

380.39 Other
Excludes *gouty tophi of ear (274.81)*

380.4 Impacted cerumen
Wax in ear

● **380.5 Acquired stenosis of external ear canal**
Collapse of external ear canal

380.50 Acquired stenosis of external ear canal, unspecified as to cause

380.51 Secondary to trauma

380.52 Secondary to surgery

380.53 Secondary to inflammation

● **380.8 Other disorders of external ear**

380.81 Exostosis of external ear canal

380.89 Other

380.9 Unspecified disorder of external ear

● **381 Nonsuppurative otitis media and Eustachian tube disorders**
Nonsuppurative: not producing pus.

● **381.0 Acute nonsuppurative otitis media**
Acute tubotympanic catarrh
Otitis media, acute or subacute:
catarrhal
exudative
transudative
with effusion
Excludes *otitic barotrauma (993.0)*

381.00 Acute nonsuppurative otitis media, unspecified

381.01 Acute serous otitis media
Acute or subacute secretory otitis media

381.02 Acute mucoid otitis media
Acute or subacute seromucinous otitis media
Blue drum syndrome

381.03 Acute sanguinous otitis media

381.04 Acute allergic serous otitis media

381.05 Acute allergic mucoid otitis media

381.06 Acute allergic sanguinous otitis media

● **381.1 Chronic serous otitis media**
Chronic tubotympanic catarrh

381.10 Chronic serous otitis media, simple or unspecified

381.19 Other
Serosanguinous chronic otitis media

● **381.2 Chronic mucoid otitis media**
    Glue ear
      Excludes *adhesive middle ear disease (385.10–385.19)*

    381.20 Chronic mucoid otitis media, simple or unspecified

    381.29 Other
        Mucosanguinous chronic otitis media

381.3 Other and unspecified chronic nonsuppurative otitis media

Otitis media, chronic:	Otitis media, chronic:
allergic	seromucinous
exudative	transudative
secretory	with effusion

381.4 Nonsuppurative otitis media, not specified as acute or chronic

Otitis media:	Otitis media:
allergic	seromucinous
catarrhal	serous
exudative	transudative
mucoid	with effusion
secretory	

● **381.5 Eustachian salpingitis**

    381.50 Eustachian salpingitis, unspecified

    381.51 Acute Eustachian salpingitis

    381.52 Chronic Eustachian salpingitis

● **381.6 Obstruction of Eustachian tube**
    Stenosis of Eustachian tube
    Stricture of Eustachian tube

    381.60 Obstruction of Eustachian tube, unspecified

    381.61 Osseous obstruction of Eustachian tube
        Obstruction of Eustachian tube from cholesteatoma, polyp, or other osseous lesion

    381.62 Intrinsic cartilaginous obstruction of Eustachian tube

    381.63 Extrinsic cartilaginous obstruction of Eustachian tube
        Compression of Eustachian tube

    381.7 Patulous Eustachian tube

● **381.8 Other disorders of Eustachian tube**

    381.81 Dysfunction of Eustachian tube

    381.89 Other

    381.9 Unspecified Eustachian tube disorder

● **382 Suppurative and unspecified otitis media**

● **382.0 Acute suppurative otitis media**
    Suppurative: Discharging pus
    Otitis media, acute:
      necrotizing NOS
      purulent
        pus-filled

    382.00 Acute suppurative otitis media without spontaneous rupture of ear drum

    382.01 Acute suppurative otitis media with spontaneous rupture of ear drum

    382.02 Acute suppurative otitis media in diseases classified elsewhere
        Code first underlying disease, as:
          influenza (487.8, 488.09, 488.19) ◀▥
          scarlet fever (034.1)
        Excludes *postmeasles otitis (055.2)*

382.1 Chronic tubotympanic suppurative otitis media
    Benign chronic suppurative otitis media (with anterior perforation of ear drum)
    Chronic tubotympanic disease (with anterior perforation of ear drum)

382.2 Chronic atticoantral suppurative otitis media
    Chronic atticoantral disease (with posterior or superior marginal perforation of ear drum)
    Persistent mucosal disease (with posterior or superior marginal perforation of ear drum)

382.3 Unspecified chronic suppurative otitis media
    Chronic purulent otitis media
      Excludes *tuberculous otitis media (017.4)*

382.4 Unspecified suppurative otitis media
    Purulent otitis media NOS

382.9 Unspecified otitis media
    Otitis media:
      NOS
      acute NOS
      chronic NOS

● **383 Mastoiditis and related conditions**

● **383.0 Acute mastoiditis**
    Abscess of mastoid
    Empyema of mastoid

    383.00 Acute mastoiditis without complications

    383.01 Subperiosteal abscess of mastoid

    383.02 Acute mastoiditis with other complications
        Gradenigo's syndrome

    383.1 Chronic mastoiditis
    Caries of mastoid
    Fistula of mastoid
      Excludes *tuberculous mastoiditis (015.6)*

● **383.2 Petrositis**
    Coalescing osteitis of petrous bone
    Inflammation of petrous bone
    Osteomyelitis of petrous bone

    383.20 Petrositis, unspecified

    383.21 Acute petrositis

    383.22 Chronic petrositis

● **383.3 Complications following mastoidectomy**

    383.30 Postmastoidectomy complication, unspecified

    383.31 Mucosal cyst of postmastoidectomy cavity

    383.32 Recurrent cholesteatoma of postmastoidectomy cavity

    383.33 Granulations of postmastoidectomy cavity
        Chronic inflammation of postmastoidectomy cavity

● **383.8 Other disorders of mastoid**

    383.81 Postauricular fistula

    383.89 Other

    383.9 Unspecified mastoiditis

● **384 Other disorders of tympanic membrane**

● **384.0 Acute myringitis without mention of otitis media**

    384.00 Acute myringitis, unspecified
        Acute tympanitis NOS

    384.01 Bullous myringitis
        Myringitis bullosa hemorrhagica

    384.09 Other

Item 6-25 Mastoiditis is an infection of the portion of the temporal bone of the skull that is behind the ear (mastoid process) caused by an untreated otitis media, leading to an infection of the surrounding structures which may include the brain.

DISEASES OF THE NERVOUS SYSTEM AND SENSE ORGANS (320–389)

384.1 Chronic myringitis without mention of otitis media
Chronic tympanitis

● **384.2 Perforation of tympanic membrane**
Perforation of ear drum:
NOS
persistent posttraumatic
postinflammatory

> Excludes   *otitis media with perforation of tympanic*
> *membrane (382.00–382.9)*
> *traumatic perforation [current injury]*
> *(872.61)*

384.20 Perforation of tympanic membrane, unspecified

384.21 Central perforation of tympanic membrane

384.22 Attic perforation of tympanic membrane
Pars flaccida

384.23 Other marginal perforation of tympanic membrane

384.24 Multiple perforations of tympanic membrane

384.25 Total perforation of tympanic membrane

● **384.8 Other specified disorders of tympanic membrane**

384.81 Atrophic flaccid tympanic membrane
Healed perforation of ear drum

384.82 Atrophic nonflaccid tympanic membrane

384.9 Unspecified disorder of tympanic membrane

● **385 Other disorders of middle ear and mastoid**

> Excludes   *mastoiditis (383.0–383.9)*

● **385.0 Tympanosclerosis**

385.00 Tympanosclerosis, unspecified as to involvement

385.01 Tympanosclerosis involving tympanic membrane only

385.02 Tympanosclerosis involving tympanic membrane and ear ossicles

385.03 Tympanosclerosis involving tympanic membrane, ear ossicles, and middle ear

385.09 Tympanosclerosis involving other combination of structures

● **385.1 Adhesive middle ear disease**
Adhesive otitis
Otitis media: Otitis media:
chronic adhesive   fibrotic

> Excludes   *glue ear (381.20–381.29)*

385.10 Adhesive middle ear disease, unspecified as to involvement

385.11 Adhesions of drum head to incus

385.12 Adhesions of drum head to stapes

385.13 Adhesions of drum head to promontorium

385.19 Other adhesions and combinations

● **385.2 Other acquired abnormality of ear ossicles**

385.21 Impaired mobility of malleus
Ankylosis of malleus

385.22 Impaired mobility of other ear ossicles
Ankylosis of ear ossicles, except malleus

385.23 Discontinuity or dislocation of ear ossicles

385.24 Partial loss or necrosis of ear ossicles

● **385.3 Cholesteatoma of middle ear and mastoid**
Cholesterosis of (middle) ear
Epidermosis of (middle) ear
Keratosis of (middle) ear
Polyp of (middle) ear

> Excludes   *cholesteatoma:*
> *external ear canal (380.21)*
> *recurrent of postmastoidectomy cavity*
> *(383.32)*

385.30 Cholesteatoma, unspecified

385.31 Cholesteatoma of attic

385.32 Cholesteatoma of middle ear

385.33 Cholesteatoma of middle ear and mastoid
Coding Clinic: 2000, Q3, P10-11

385.35 Diffuse cholesteatosis

● **385.8 Other disorders of middle ear and mastoid**

385.82 Cholesterin granuloma

385.83 Retained foreign body of middle ear

> Use additional code to identify foreign
> body (V90.01-V90.9) ◄
> Coding Clinic: 1987, Nov-Dec, P9

385.89 Other

385.9 Unspecified disorder of middle ear and mastoid

● **386 Vertiginous syndromes and other disorders of vestibular system**

> Excludes   *vertigo NOS (780.4)*

Coding Clinic: 1985, Mar-April, P12

● **386.0 Méniére's disease**
Vestibular disorder that produces recurring symptoms
including severe and intermittent hearing loss
including feeling of ear pressure or pain.
Endolymphatic hydrops
Lermoyez's syndrome
Méniére's syndrome or vertigo

386.00 Méniére's disease, unspecified
Méniére's disease (active)
Coding Clinic: 1985, Mar-April, P12

386.01 Active Méniére's disease, cochleovestibular

386.02 Active Méniére's disease, cochlear

386.03 Active Méniére's disease, vestibular

386.04 Inactive Méniére's disease
Méniére's disease in remission

● **386.1 Other and unspecified peripheral vertigo**

> Excludes   *epidemic vertigo (078.81)*

386.10 Peripheral vertigo, unspecified

386.11 Benign paroxysmal positional vertigo
Benign paroxysmal positional nystagmus

386.12 Vestibular neuronitis
Acute (and recurrent) peripheral
vestibulopathy

386.19 Other
Aural vertigo   Otogenic vertigo

386.2 Vertigo of central origin
Central positional nystagmus
Malignant positional vertigo

◄ New   ◄▥ Revised   ~~deleted~~ Deleted   Excludes   Includes   Use additional   Code first   Omit code
● Unacceptable Principal Diagnosis   ● Use Additional Digit(s)   OGCR Official Guidelines   Coding Clinic

● **386.3 Labyrinthitis**
Balance disorder that follows a URI or head injury. The inflammatory process affects the labyrinth that houses vestibular system (senses changes in head position) of inner ear.

386.30 Labyrinthitis, unspecified

386.31 Serous labyrinthitis
Diffuse labyrinthitis

386.32 Circumscribed labyrinthitis
Focal labyrinthitis

386.33 Suppurative labyrinthitis
Purulent labyrinthitis

386.34 Toxic labyrinthitis

386.35 Viral labyrinthitis

● **386.4 Labyrinthine fistula**

386.40 Labyrinthine fistula, unspecified

386.41 Round window fistula

386.42 Oval window fistula

386.43 Semicircular canal fistula

386.48 Labyrinthine fistula of combined sites

● **386.5 Labyrinthine dysfunction**

386.50 Labyrinthine dysfunction, unspecified

386.51 Hyperactive labyrinth, unilateral

386.52 Hyperactive labyrinth, bilateral

386.53 Hypoactive labyrinth, unilateral

386.54 Hypoactive labyrinth, bilateral

386.55 Loss of labyrinthine reactivity, unilateral

386.56 Loss of labyrinthine reactivity, bilateral

386.58 Other forms and combinations

386.8 Other disorders of labyrinth

386.9 Unspecified vertiginous syndromes and labyrinthine disorders

● **387 Otosclerosis**
Inherited middle ear spongelike bone growth causing hearing loss because growth prevents vibration from sound waves required for hearing.

| **Includes** | otospongiosis |

387.0 Otosclerosis involving oval window, nonobliterative

387.1 Otosclerosis involving oval window, obliterative

387.2 Cochlear otosclerosis
Otosclerosis involving:
otic capsule
round window

387.8 Other otosclerosis

387.9 Otosclerosis, unspecified

● **388 Other disorders of ear**

● **388.0 Degenerative and vascular disorders of ear**

388.00 Degenerative and vascular disorders, unspecified

388.01 Presbyacusis

388.02 Transient ischemic deafness

● **388.1 Noise effects on inner ear**

388.10 Noise effects on inner ear, unspecified

388.11 Acoustic trauma (explosive) to ear
Otitic blast injury

388.12 Noise-induced hearing loss

388.2 Sudden hearing loss, unspecified

● **388.3 Tinnitus**
Perception of sound in absence of external noise and may affect one or both ears and/or head

388.30 Tinnitus, unspecified

388.31 Subjective tinnitus

388.32 Objective tinnitus

● **388.4 Other abnormal auditory perception**

388.40 Abnormal auditory perception, unspecified

388.41 Diplacusis

388.42 Hyperacusis

388.43 Impairment of auditory discrimination

388.44 Recruitment

388.45 Acquired auditory processing disorder
Auditory processing disorder NOS

| **Excludes** | *central auditory processing disorder (315.32)* |

Coding Clinic: 2007, Q4, P79

388.5 Disorders of acoustic nerve
Acoustic neuritis
Degeneration of acoustic or eighth nerve
Disorder of acoustic or eighth nerve

| **Excludes** | *acoustic neuroma (225.1)* |
| | *syphilitic acoustic neuritis (094.86)* |

Coding Clinic: 1987, Mar-April, P8

● **388.6 Otorrhea**

388.60 Otorrhea, unspecified
Discharging ear NOS

388.61 Cerebrospinal fluid otorrhea

| **Excludes** | *cerebrospinal fluid rhinorrhea (349.81)* |

388.69 Other
Otorrhagia

● **388.7 Otalgia**

388.70 Otalgia, unspecified
Earache NOS

388.71 Otogenic pain

388.72 Referred pain
Pain from a diseased area of the body that is not felt directly in that area, but in another part of the body.

388.8 Other disorders of ear

388.9 Unspecified disorder of ear

● **389 Hearing loss**

● **389.0 Conductive hearing loss**
Conductive deafness

| **Excludes** | *mixed conductive and sensorineural hearing loss (389.20–389.22)* |

389.00 Conductive hearing loss, unspecified

389.01 Conductive hearing loss, external ear

389.02 Conductive hearing loss, tympanic membrane

389.03 Conductive hearing loss, middle ear

389.04 Conductive hearing loss, inner ear

389.05 Conductive hearing loss, unilateral

389.06 Conductive hearing loss, bilateral
Coding Clinic: 2007, Q4, P80-81

389.08 Conductive hearing loss of combined types

● 389.1 **Sensorineural hearing loss**
Perceptive hearing loss or deafness

> **Excludes** *abnormal auditory perception*
> *(388.40–388.44)*
> *mixed conductive and sensorineural hearing*
> *loss (389.20–389.22)*
> *psychogenic deafness (306.7)*
> Coding Clinic: 2007, Q4, P80-81; 2006, Q4, P84

389.10 **Sensorineural hearing loss, unspecified**
Coding Clinic: 1993, Q1, P29

389.11 **Sensory hearing loss, bilateral**

389.12 **Neural hearing loss, bilateral**

389.13 **Neural hearing loss, unilateral**

389.14 **Central hearing loss**

389.15 **Sensorineural hearing loss, unilateral**

389.16 **Sensorineural hearing loss, asymmetrical**

389.17 **Sensory hearing loss, unilateral**

389.18 **Sensorineural hearing loss, bilateral**

● 389.2 **Mixed conductive and sensorineural hearing loss**
Deafness or hearing loss of type classifiable
to 389.00–389.08 with type classifiable to
389.10–389.18
Coding Clinic: 2007, Q4, P80-81

389.20 **Mixed hearing loss, unspecified**

389.21 **Mixed hearing loss, unilateral**

389.22 **Mixed hearing loss, bilateral**

389.7 **Deaf nonspeaking, not elsewhere classifiable**

389.8 **Other specified forms of hearing loss**

389.9 **Unspecified hearing loss**
Deafness NOS
Coding Clinic: 2004, Q1, P15-16

Figure 7-1 Cardiovascular valves.

Item 7-1   Rheumatic fever is the inflammation of the valve(s) of the heart, usually the mitral or aortic, which leads to valve damage. Rheumatic heart inflammations are usually **pericarditis** (sac surrounding heart), **endocarditis** (heart cavity), or **myocarditis** (heart muscle).

7.   DISEASES OF THE CIRCULATORY SYSTEM (390–459)

ACUTE RHEUMATIC FEVER (390–392)

390   Rheumatic fever without mention of heart involvement
Arthritis, rheumatic, acute or subacute
Rheumatic fever (active) (acute)
Rheumatism, articular, acute or subacute
> **Excludes** *that with heart involvement (391.0–391.9)*

● **391   Rheumatic fever with heart involvement**
> **Excludes** *chronic heart diseases of rheumatic origin (393–398.99) unless rheumatic fever is also present or there is evidence of recrudescence or activity of the rheumatic process*

391.0   Acute rheumatic pericarditis
Rheumatic:
    fever (active) (acute) with pericarditis
    pericarditis (acute)
Any condition classifiable to 390 with pericarditis
> **Excludes** *that not specified as rheumatic (420.0–420.9)*

391.1   Acute rheumatic endocarditis
Rheumatic:
    endocarditis, acute
    fever (active) (acute) with endocarditis or valvulitis
    valvulitis acute
Any condition classifiable to 390 with endocarditis or valvulitis

391.2   Acute rheumatic myocarditis
Rheumatic fever (active) (acute) with myocarditis
Any condition classifiable to 390 with myocarditis

391.8   Other acute rheumatic heart disease
Rheumatic:
    fever (active) (acute) with other or multiple types of heart involvement
    pancarditis, acute
Any condition classifiable to 390 with other or multiple types of heart involvement

391.9   Acute rheumatic heart disease, unspecified
Rheumatic:
    carditis, acute
    fever (active) (acute) with unspecified type of heart involvement
    heart disease, active or acute
Any condition classifiable to 390 with unspecified type of heart involvement

Item 7-2   Rheumatic chorea, also called Sydenham's, juvenile, minor, simple, or St. Vitus' dance, is a major symptom of rheumatic fever and is characterized by ceaseless, involuntary, jerky, purposeless movements.

● **392   Rheumatic chorea**
> **Includes** Sydenham's chorea
> **Excludes** *chorea:*
>   *NOS (333.5)*
>   *Huntington's (333.4)*

392.0   With heart involvement
Rheumatic chorea with heart involvement of any type classifiable to 391

392.9   Without mention of heart involvement

CHRONIC RHEUMATIC HEART DISEASE (393–398)

393   Chronic rheumatic pericarditis
Adherent pericardium, rheumatic
Chronic rheumatic:
    mediastinopericarditis
    myopericarditis
> **Excludes** *pericarditis NOS or not specified as rheumatic (423.0–423.9)*

● **394   Diseases of mitral valve**
> **Excludes** *that with aortic valve involvement (396.0–396.9)*

394.0   Mitral stenosis
Mitral (valve):
    obstruction (rheumatic)
    stenosis NOS

394.1   Rheumatic mitral insufficiency
Rheumatic mitral:
    incompetence
    regurgitation
> **Excludes** *that not specified as rheumatic (424.0)*
> Coding Clinic: 2005, Q2, P14-15

394.2   Mitral stenosis with insufficiency
Mitral stenosis with incompetence or regurgitation
Coding Clinic: 2007, Q2, P11-12

394.9   Other and unspecified mitral valve diseases
Mitral (valve):
    disease (chronic)
    failure

● **395   Diseases of aortic valve**
> **Excludes** *that not specified as rheumatic (424.1)*
>   *that with mitral valve involvement (396.0–396.9)*

395.0   Rheumatic aortic stenosis
Rheumatic aortic (valve) obstruction
Coding Clinic: 1988, Q4, P8

395.1   Rheumatic aortic insufficiency
Rheumatic aortic:
    incompetence
    regurgitation

395.2   Rheumatic aortic stenosis with insufficiency
Rheumatic aortic stenosis with incompetence or regurgitation

395.9   Other and unspecified rheumatic aortic diseases
Rheumatic aortic (valve) disease

Item 7-3   Mitral stenosis is the narrowing of the mitral valve separating the left atrium from the left ventricle. **Mitral insufficiency** is the improper closure of the mitral valve which may lead to enlargement (hypertrophy) of the left atrium.

Item 7-4   Aortic stenosis is the narrowing of the aortic valve located between the left ventricle and the aorta. **Aortic insufficiency** is the improper closure of the aortic valve which may lead to enlargement (hypertrophy) of the left ventricle.

Item 7–5 Mitral and aortic valve stenosis is the narrowing of these valves, which leads to enlargement (hypertrophy) of the left atrium and left ventricle respectively, while **mitral and aortic insufficiency** is the improper closure of the mitral and aortic valves resulting in the same outcome as stenosis.

● **396 Diseases of mitral and aortic valves**
>   **Includes** involvement of both mitral and aortic valves, whether specified as rheumatic or not

  396.0 Mitral valve stenosis and aortic valve stenosis
>   Atypical aortic (valve) stenosis
>   Mitral and aortic (valve) obstruction (rheumatic)

  396.1 Mitral valve stenosis and aortic valve insufficiency

  396.2 Mitral valve insufficiency and aortic valve stenosis
>   Coding Clinic: 2009, Q2, P11; 2000, Q2, P16-17; 1987, Nov-Dec, P8

  396.3 Mitral valve insufficiency and aortic valve insufficiency
>   Mitral and aortic (valve):
>   incompetence
>   regurgitation
>   Coding Clinic: 2009, Q2, P11; Q1, P8; 1995, Q1, P6

  396.8 Multiple involvement of mitral and aortic valves
>   Stenosis and insufficiency of mitral or aortic valve with stenosis or insufficiency, or both, of the other valve

  396.9 Mitral and aortic valve diseases, unspecified

● **397 Diseases of other endocardial structures**
>   *Affects thin serous endothelial tissue that lines inside of heart*

  397.0 Diseases of tricuspid valve
>   Tricuspid (valve) (rheumatic):
>   disease
>   insufficiency
>   obstruction
>   regurgitation
>   stenosis
>   Coding Clinic: 2006, Q3, P7; 2000, Q2, P16-17

  397.1 Rheumatic diseases of pulmonary valve
>   **Excludes** that not specified as rheumatic (424.3)

  397.9 Rheumatic diseases of endocardium, valve unspecified
>   Rheumatic:
>   endocarditis (chronic)
>   valvulitis (chronic)
>   **Excludes** that not specified as rheumatic (424.90–424.99)

● **398 Other rheumatic heart disease**

  398.0 Rheumatic myocarditis
>   Rheumatic degeneration of myocardium
>   **Excludes** myocarditis not specified as rheumatic (429.0)

  ● **398.9 Other and unspecified rheumatic heart diseases**

    398.90 Rheumatic heart disease, unspecified
>   Rheumatic:
>   carditis
>   heart disease NOS
>   **Excludes** carditis not specified as rheumatic (429.89)
>   heart disease NOS not specified as rheumatic (429.9)

    398.91 Rheumatic heart failure (congestive)
>   Rheumatic left ventricular failure
>   Coding Clinic: 2005, Q2, P14-15; 1995, Q1, P6

    398.99 Other

Item 7–6 Hypertension is caused by high arterial blood pressure in the arteries. **Essential, primary,** or **idiopathic** hypertension occurs without identifiable organic cause.
Secondary hypertension is that which has an organic cause.
Malignant hypertension is severely elevated blood pressure. **Benign** hypertension is mildly elevated blood pressure.

HYPERTENSIVE DISEASE (401–405)
>   **Excludes** *that complicating pregnancy, childbirth, or the puerperium (642.0–642.9)*
>   *that involving coronary vessels (410.00–414.9)*

● **401 Essential hypertension**
>   **Includes** high blood pressure
>   hyperpiesia
>   hyperpiesis
>   hypertension (arterial) (essential) (primary) (systemic)
>   hypertensive vascular:
>   degeneration
>   disease
>   **Excludes** *elevated blood pressure without diagnosis of hypertension (796.2)*
>   *pulmonary hypertension (416.0–416.9)*
>   *that involving vessels of:*
>   *brain (430–438)*
>   *eye (362.11)*
>   Coding Clinic: 1992, Q2, P5

  401.0 Malignant
>   Coding Clinic: 1993, Q4, P37; 5th Issue, P9-10

  401.1 Benign

  401.9 Unspecified
>   Coding Clinic: 2009, Q4, P101-102; Q1, P6; 2008, Q2, P16; 2005, Q4, P68-69; Q3, P3-9; 2004, Q4, P77-78; 2003, Q4, P105-106,108, 111; Q3, P14-15; Q2, P16; 1997, Q4, P35-37; 1989, Q2, P12; 1987, Sept-Oct, P11

>   OGCR Section I.C.7.a.2
>   Heart conditions (425.8, 429.0-429.3, 429.8, 429.9) are assigned to a code from category 402 when a causal relationship is stated (due to hypertension) or implied (hypertensive). Use an additional code from category 428 to identify the type of heart failure in those patients with heart failure. More than one code from category 428 may be assigned if the patient has systolic or diastolic failure and congestive heart failure. The same heart conditions (425.8, 429.0-429.3, 429.8, 429.9) with hypertension, but without a stated causal relationship, are coded separately. Sequence according to the circumstances of the admission/encounter.

● **402 Hypertensive heart disease**
>   **Includes** hypertensive:
>   cardiomegaly
>   cardiopathy
>   cardiovascular disease
>   heart (disease) (failure)
>   any condition classifiable to 429.0–429.3, 429.8, 429.9 due to hypertension
>   Use additional code to specify type of heart failure (428.0–428.43), if known
>   Coding Clinic: 1993, Q2, P9; 1987, Nov-Dec, P9

  ● **402.0 Malignant**
    402.00 Without heart failure
>   Coding Clinic: 2008, Q4, P177-180
    402.01 With heart failure

  ● **402.1 Benign**
    402.10 Without heart failure
    402.11 With heart failure

● **402.9 Unspecified**
    Coding Clinic: 1993, Q2, P9

  402.90 Without heart failure

  402.91 With heart failure
      Coding Clinic: 2002, Q4, P52; 1993, Q1, P19-20; 1989, Q2,
      P12; 1984, Nov-Dec, P18

OGCR Section I.C.7.a.3
Assign codes from category 403, Hypertensive chronic kidney disease, when conditions classified to category 585 are present. Unlike hypertension with heart disease, ICD-9-CM presumes a cause-and-effect relationship and classifies chronic kidney disease (CKD) with hypertension as hypertensive chronic kidney disease.

● **403 Hypertensive chronic kidney disease**
    Includes arteriolar nephritis
            arteriosclerosis of:
                kidney
                renal arterioles
            arteriosclerotic nephritis (chronic) (interstitial)
            hypertensive:
                nephropathy
                renal failure
                uremia (chronic)
            nephrosclerosis
            renal sclerosis with hypertension
            any condition classifiable to 585 and 587 with
                any condition classifiable to 401 ◄▥

    Excludes *acute kidney failure (584.5–584.9)*
            renal disease stated as not due to hypertension
            renovascular hypertension (405.0–405.9 with
                fifth-digit 1)
    Coding Clinic: 2003, Q1, P20-21; 1992, Q2, P5

The following fifth-digit subclassification is for use with category 403:

    0 with chronic kidney disease stage I through stage IV, or unspecified
        Use additional code to identify the stage of chronic kidney disease (585.1–585.4, 585.9)

    1 with chronic kidney disease stage V or end stage renal disease
        Use additional code to identify the stage of chronic kidney disease (585.5, 585.6)

● **403.0 Malignant**
    [0-1]

● **403.1 Benign**
    [0-1]

● **403.9 Unspecified**
    [0-1]   Coding Clinic: 2008, Q1, P7-8, 10-11; 2007, Q2, P3; 2006, Q4,
            P84-86; 2005, Q4, P68-69; 2004, Q1, P14-15; 2001, Q2,
            P11; 1987, Sept-Oct, P9, 11; 1985, Nov-Dec, P15

OGCR Section I.C.7.a.4
Assign codes from combination category 404, Hypertensive heart and chronic kidney disease, when both hypertensive kidney disease and hypertensive heart disease are stated in the diagnosis. Assume a relationship between the hypertension and the chronic kidney disease, whether or not the condition is so designated. Assign an additional code from category 428, to identify the type of heart failure. More than one code from category 428 may be assigned if the patient has systolic or diastolic failure and congestive heart failure.

● **404 Hypertensive heart and chronic kidney disease**
    Includes disease:
            cardiorenal
            cardiovascular renal
        any condition classifiable to 402 with any
            condition classifiable to 403

    Use additional code to specify type of heart failure
        (428.0–428.43), if known
    Coding Clinic: 2006, Q4, P84-86; 2005, Q4, P68-69

The following fifth-digit subclassification is for use with category 404:

    0 without heart failure and with chronic kidney disease stage I through stage IV, or unspecified
        Use additional code to identify the stage of chronic kidney disease (585.1–585.4, 585.9)

    1 with heart failure and with chronic kidney disease stage I through stage IV, or unspecified
        Use additional code to identify the stage of chronic kidney disease (585.1–585.4, 585.9)

    2 without heart failure and with chronic kidney disease stage V or end stage renal disease
        Use additional code to identify the stage of chronic kidney disease (585.5, 585.6)

    3 with heart failure and chronic kidney disease stage V or end stage renal disease
        Use additional code to identify the stage of chronic kidney disease (585.5, 585.6)

● **404.0 Malignant**
    [0-3]

● **404.1 Benign**
    [0-3]

● **404.9 Unspecified**
    [0-3]

● **405 Secondary hypertension**
  ● **405.0 Malignant**
        405.01 Renovascular
        405.09 Other
  ● **405.1 Benign**
        405.11 Renovascular
        405.19 Other
  ● **405.9 Unspecified**
        405.91 Renovascular
        405.99 Other
            Coding Clinic: 2000, Q3, P4-5; 1987, Sept-Oct, P9, 11

DISEASES OF THE CIRCULATORY SYSTEM (390–459)

Zone of injury
Zone of infarction
Zone of ischemia

Figure 7–2 Myocardial infarction.

Item 7–7 Myocardial infarction is a sudden decrease in the coronary artery blood flow that results in death of the heart muscle. Classifications are based on the affected heart tissue.

ISCHEMIC HEART DISEASE (410–414)

Includes   that with mention of hypertension

Use additional code to identify presence of hypertension (401.0–405.9)

● **410 Acute myocardial infarction**

Includes   cardiac infarction
coronary (artery):
     embolism
     occlusion
     rupture
     thrombosis
infarction of heart, myocardium, or ventricle
rupture of heart, myocardium, or ventricle
ST elevation (STEMI) and non-ST elevation (NSTEMI) myocardial infarction
any condition classifiable to 414.1–414.9 specified as acute or with a stated duration of 8 weeks or less

Coding Clinic: 2006, Q2, P9; 1997, Q4, P37; 1994, Q4, P55; 1993, Q4, P39-41; 1992, Q1, P10; 1991, Q3, P18; 1986, Nov-Dec, P12

The following fifth-digit subclassification is for use with category 410:

> **0   episode of care unspecified**
>   Use when the source document does not contain sufficient information for the assignment of fifth-digit 1 or 2.
>
> **1   initial episode of care**
>   Use fifth-digit 1 to designate the first episode of care (regardless of facility site) for a newly diagnosed myocardial infarction. The fifth-digit 1 is assigned regardless of the number of times a patient may be transferred during the initial episode of care.
>
> **2   subsequent episode of care**
>   Use fifth-digit 2 to designate an episode of care following the initial episode when the patient is admitted for further observation, evaluation or treatment for a myocardial infarction that has received initial treatment, but is still less than 8 weeks old.

● **410.0 Of anterolateral wall**
     [0-2]   ST elevation myocardial infarction (STEMI) of anterolateral wall
            Coding Clinic: 2009, Q4, P102; 2008, Q4, P69-73; 2001, Q3, P21; 1998, Q3, P15; 1993, 5th Issue, P14, 17-24

● **410.1 Of other anterior wall**
     [0-2]   Infarction:
            anterior (wall) NOS (with contiguous portion of intraventricular septum)
            anteroapical (with contiguous portion of intraventricular septum)
            anteroseptal (with contiguous portion of intraventricular septum)
        ST elevation myocardial infarction (STEMI) of other anterior wall
            Coding Clinic: 2003, Q3, P10-11

● **410.2 Of inferolateral wall**
     [0-2]   ST elevation myocardial infarction (STEMI) of inferolateral wall
            Coding Clinic: 1993, 5th Issue, P17-24

● **410.3 Of inferoposterior wall**
     [0-2]   ST elevation myocardial infarction (STEMI) of inferoposterior wall

● **410.4 Of other inferior wall**
     [0-2]   Infarction:
            diaphragmatic wall NOS (with contiguous portion of intraventricular septum)
            inferior (wall) NOS (with contiguous portion of intraventricular septum)
        ST elevation myocardial infarction (STEMI) of other inferior wall
            Coding Clinic: 2009, Q3, P10; 2006, Q3, P8-9; 2001, Q2, P8-9; 2000, Q1, P7; 1997, Q3, P10; 1993, 5th Issue, P13-14x2

● **410.5 Of other lateral wall**
     [0-2]   Infarction:
            apical-lateral
            basal-lateral
            high lateral
            posterolateral
        ST elevation myocardial infarction (STEMI) of other lateral wall
            Coding Clinic: 2009, Q3, P7

● **410.6 True posterior wall infarction**
     [0-2]   Infarction:
            posterobasal
            strictly posterior
        ST elevation myocardial infarction (STEMI) of true posterior wall

● **410.7 Subendocardial infarction**
     [0-2]   Non-ST elevation myocardial infarction (NSTEMI)
        Nontransmural infarction
            Coding Clinic: 2005, Q4, P69-72; Q2, P19-20; 2000, Q1, P7

OGCR   Section I.C.7.e.1
The ICD-9-CM codes for acute myocardial infarction (AMI) identify the site, such as anterolateral wall or true posterior wall. Subcategories 410.0–410.6 and 410.8 are used for ST elevtion myocardial infarction (STEMI). Subcategory 410.7, Subendocardial infarction, is used for non ST elevation myocardial infarction (NSTEMI) and nontransmural MIs.

● **410.8 Of other specified sites**
     [0-2]   Infarction of:
            atrium
            papillary muscle
            septum alone
        ST elevation myocardial infarction (STEMI) of other specified sites

● **410.9 Unspecified site**
     [0-2]   Acute myocardial infarction NOS
        Coronary occlusion NOS
        Myocardial infarction NOS
            Coding Clinic: 2005, Q2, P18-19; 2002, Q3, P5; 1999, Q4, P9; 1993, 5th Issue, P13

OGCR   Section I.C.7.e.2
Subcategory 410.9 is the default for the unspecified term acute myocardial infarction. If only STEMI or transmural MI without the site is documented, query the provider as to the site, or assign a code from subcategory 410.9.

◄ New   ◄▥ Revised   ~~deleted~~ Deleted   Excludes   Includes   Use additional   Code first   Omit code
● Unacceptable Principal Diagnosis   ● Use Additional Digit(s)   OGCR Official Guidelines   Coding Clinic

● **411 Other acute and subacute forms of ischemic heart disease**
Coding Clinic: 1994, Q4, P55

411.0 Postmyocardial infarction syndrome
Dressler's syndrome

411.1 Intermediate coronary syndrome
Impending infarction
Preinfarction angina
Preinfarction syndrome
Unstable angina

> **Excludes** *angina (pectoris) (413.9)*
> *decubitus (413.0)*

Coding Clinic: 2005, Q4, P103-106; 2004, Q2, P3-4; 2003, Q1,
P12-13; 2001, Q3, P15; Q2, P7-9; 1998, Q4, P85-86; 1996,
Q2, P10; 1995, Q2, P18-19; 1993, Q4, P39-40; 5th Issue,
P17-24; 1991, Q1, P14; 1989, Q4, P10

● **411.8 Other**

411.81 Acute coronary occlusion without myocardial infarction
Acute coronary (artery):
embolism without or not resulting in
myocardial infarction
obstruction without or not resulting in
myocardial infarction
occlusion without or not resulting in
myocardial infarction
thrombosis without or not resulting in
myocardial infarction

> **Excludes** *obstruction without infarction*
> *due to atherosclerosis*
> *(414.00–414.07)*
> *occlusion without infarction*
> *due to atherosclerosis*
> *(414.00–414.07)*

Coding Clinic: 2001, Q2, P7-8; 1991, Q3, P18; Q1, P14

411.89 Other
Coronary insufficiency (acute)
Subendocardial ischemia
Coding Clinic: 2001, Q3, P14; 1992, Q1, P9-10;
1991, Q3, P18

412 Old myocardial infarction
Healed myocardial infarction
Past myocardial infarction diagnosed on ECG [EKG] or
other special investigation, but currently presenting
no symptoms
Coding Clinic: 2003, Q2, P10; 2001, Q3, P21; Q2, P9; 1998, Q3, P15; 1993,
5th Issue, P17-24

● **413 Angina pectoris**
Chest pain/discomfort due to lack of oxygen to heart muscle.
Principal symptom of myocardial infarction.

413.0 Angina decubitus
Nocturnal angina

413.1 Prinzmetal angina
Variant angina pectoris
Coding Clinic: 2006, Q3, P23

413.9 Other and unspecified angina pectoris

Angina:	Anginal syndrome
NOS	Status anginosus
cardiac	Stenocardia
equivalent	Syncope anginosa
of effort	

> **Excludes** *preinfarction angina (411.1)*

Use additional code(s) for symptoms associated
with angina equivalent
Coding Clinic: 2008, Q2, P16, 2003, Q1, P12-13; 2002, Q3, P4-5;
1995, Q2, P18; 1993, 5th Issue, P17-24; 1991, Q3, P16;
1985, Sept-Oct, P9

● **414 Other forms of chronic ischemic heart disease**

> **Excludes** *arteriosclerotic cardiovascular disease [ASCVD]*
> *(429.2)*
> *cardiovascular:*
> *arteriosclerosis or sclerosis (429.2)*
> *degeneration or disease (429.2)*

● **414.0 Coronary atherosclerosis**
Arteriosclerotic heart disease [ASHD]
Atherosclerotic heart disease
Coronary (artery):
arteriosclerosis
arteritis or endarteritis
atheroma
sclerosis
stricture

Use additional code, if applicable, to identify
chronic total occlusion of coronary artery
(414.2)

> **Excludes** *embolism of graft (996.72)*
> *occlusion NOS of graft (996.72)*
> *thrombus of graft (996.72)*

Coding Clinic: 2002, Q3, P3-9; 1994, Q2, P13, 15; Q1, P6-7; 1993,
Q1, P20; 5th Issue, P17-24; 5th Issue, P14; 1984, Nov-Dec, P18

414.00 Of unspecified type of vessel, native or graft
Coding Clinic: 2003, Q2, P16; 2001, Q3, P15; 1997, Q3,
P15; 1996, Q4, P31

414.01 Of native coronary artery
Coding Clinic: 2009, Q3, P8; 2008, Q3, P10-11; Q2, P16;
2006, Q3, P25; 2005, Q4, P68-69; 2004, Q2, P3-4;
2003, Q4, P105-106, 108-109; Q3, P9.10, 14;
2001, Q3, P15-16; Q2, P8-9; 1997, Q3, P15; 1996,
Q2, P10; 1995, Q2, P17-19

414.02 Of autologous biological bypass graft
Coding Clinic: 1995, Q2, P18-19

414.03 Of nonautologous biological bypass graft

414.04 Of artery bypass graft
Internal mammary artery

Figure 7–3 Atherosclerosis. (From Buck
CJ: Step-by-Step Medical Coding, 2008 ed.
Philadelphia, WB Saunders, 2008.)

Item 7–8 "Old" (healed) myocardial infarction: Code 412 cannot
be used if the patient is experiencing current ischemic heart disease
symptoms. Recent infarctions still under care cannot be coded to 412.
This code is only assigned if infarction has some impact on the current
episode of care—essentially, it is a history of (H/O) a past, healed MI.
(There is no V code for this status/post MI.)

Item 7–9 Classification is based on the location of the atherosclerosis.
"Of native coronary artery" indicates the atherosclerosis is within
an original heart artery. **"Of autologous vein bypass graft"**
indicates that the atherosclerosis is within a vein graft that was taken from
within the patient. **"Of nonautologous biological bypass graft"**
indicates the atherosclerosis is within a vessel grafted from other than the
patient. **"Of artery bypass graft"** indicates the atherosclerosis is
within an artery that was grafted from within the patient.

414.05 Of unspecified type of bypass graft
Bypass graft NOS
Coding Clinic: 1997, Q3, P15; 1996, Q4, P31

414.06 Of native coronary artery of transplanted heart
Coding Clinic: 2003, Q4, P60; 2002, Q4, P53-54; Q4, P53-54

414.07 Of bypass graft (artery) (vein) of transplanted heart
Coding Clinic: 2003, Q4, P60

● **414.1 Aneurysm and dissection of heart**

414.10 Aneurysm of heart (wall)
Aneurysm (arteriovenous):
mural
ventricular

414.11 Aneurysm of coronary vessels
Aneurysm (arteriovenous) of coronary vessels
Coding Clinic: 1999, Q1, P17-18

414.12 Dissection of coronary artery
Coding Clinic: 2002, Q4, P54-55

414.19 Other aneurysm of heart
Arteriovenous fistula, acquired, of heart

● **414.2 Chronic total occlusion of coronary artery**
Complete occlusion of coronary artery
Total occlusion of coronary artery

Code first coronary atherosclerosis (414.00–414.07)

Excludes *acute coronary occlusion with myocardial infarction (410.00–410.92)*
acute coronary occlusion without myocardial infarction (411.81)
Coding Clinic: 2007, Q4, P82

● **414.3 Coronary atherosclerosis due to lipid rich plaque**
Code first coronary atherosclerosis (414.00-414.07)
Coding Clinic: 2008, Q4, P113

414.8 Other specified forms of chronic ischemic heart disease
Chronic coronary insufficiency
Ischemia, myocardial (chronic)
Any condition classifiable to 410 specified as chronic, or presenting with symptoms after 8 weeks from date of infarction

Excludes *coronary insufficiency (acute) (411.89)*
Coding Clinic: 2003, Q2, P10; 2001, Q3, P15-16; 1992, Q1, P10; 1990, Q3, P15; Q2, P19; 1986, Nov-Dec, P12

414.9 Chronic ischemic heart disease, unspecified
Ischemic heart disease NOS
Coding Clinic: 2001, Q3, P15-16

DISEASES OF PULMONARY CIRCULATION (415–417)

● **415 Acute pulmonary heart disease**

415.0 Acute cor pulmonale
Excludes *cor pulmonale NOS (416.9)*

● **415.1 Pulmonary embolism and infarction**
Pulmonary (artery) (vein):
apoplexy   infarction (hemorrhagic)
embolism   thrombosis

Excludes *chronic pulmonary embolism (416.2)*
personal history of pulmonary embolism (V12.51)
that complicating:
abortion (634–638 with .6, 639.6)
ectopic or molar pregnancy (639.6)
pregnancy, childbirth, or the puerperium (673.0–673.8)

Item 7-10 Pulmonary heart disease or cor pulmonale is right ventricle hypertrophy or RVH as a result of a respiratory disorder increasing back flow pressure to the right ventricle. Left untreated, cor pulmonale leads to right-heart failure and death.

415.11 Iatrogenic pulmonary embolism and infarction
Use additional code for associated septic pulmonary embolism, if applicable, 415.12
Coding Clinic: 1990, Q4, P25

● **415.12 Septic pulmonary embolism**
Septic embolism NOS

Code first underlying infection, such as:
septicemia (038.0–038.9)

Excludes *septic arterial embolism (449)*
Coding Clinic: 2007, Q4, P84-86

415.19 Other
Coding Clinic: 1998, Q2, P8

● **416 Chronic pulmonary heart disease**

416.0 Primary pulmonary hypertension
Idiopathic pulmonary arteriosclerosis
Pulmonary hypertension (essential) (idiopathic) (primary)

Excludes *pulmonary hypertension NOS (416.8)* ◄
secondary pulmonary hypertension (416.8) ◄

416.1 Kyphoscoliotic heart disease

416.2 Chronic pulmonary embolism
Use additional code, if applicable, for associated long-term (current) use of anticoagulants (V58.61)

Excludes *personal history of pulmonary embolism (V12.51)*

416.8 Other chronic pulmonary heart diseases
Pulmonary hypertension NOS ◄
Pulmonary hypertension, secondary

416.9 Chronic pulmonary heart disease, unspecified
Chronic cardiopulmonary disease
Cor pulmonale (chronic) NOS

● **417 Other diseases of pulmonary circulation**

417.0 Arteriovenous fistula of pulmonary vessels
Excludes *congenital arteriovenous fistula (747.3)*

417.1 Aneurysm of pulmonary artery
Excludes *congenital aneurysm (747.3)*

417.8 Other specified diseases of pulmonary circulation
Pulmonary:
arteritis
endarteritis
Rupture of pulmonary vessel
Stricture of pulmonary vessel

417.9 Unspecified disease of pulmonary circulation

OTHER FORMS OF HEART DISEASE (420–429)

● **420 Acute pericarditis**

Inflammation of the sac surrounding the heart caused by infection. The chest pain is significant on inspiration, and onset is sudden and worst when lying down.

Includes acute:

    mediastinopericarditis
    myopericarditis
    pericardial effusion
    pleuropericarditis
    pneumopericarditis

Excludes *acute rheumatic pericarditis (391.0)*
    postmyocardial infarction syndrome [Dressler's] (411.0)

420.0 Acute pericarditis in diseases classified elsewhere

Code first underlying disease, as:
    actinomycosis (039.8)
    amebiasis (006.8)
    chronic uremia (585.9)
    nocardiosis (039.8)
    tuberculosis (017.9)
    uremia NOS (586)

Excludes *pericarditis (acute) (in):*
    Coxsackie (virus) (074.21)
    gonococcal (098.83)
    histoplasmosis (115.0–115.9 with fifth-digit 3)
    meningococcal infection (036.41)
    syphilitic (093.81)

● **420.9 Other and unspecified acute pericarditis**

420.90 Acute pericarditis, unspecified

Pericarditis (acute):
    NOS
    infective NOS
    sicca
Coding Clinic: 1989, Q2, P12

420.91 Acute idiopathic pericarditis

Pericarditis, acute:
    benign
    nonspecific
    viral

420.99 Other

Pericarditis (acute):
    pneumococcal
    purulent
    staphylococcal
    streptococcal
    suppurative
Pneumopyopericardium
Pyopericardium

Excludes *pericarditis in diseases classified elsewhere (420.0)*

● **421 Acute and subacute endocarditis**

Inflammation/infection of lining of heart, affecting heart valves, usually caused by bacterial infection

421.0 Acute and subacute bacterial endocarditis

Endocarditis (acute) (chronic) (subacute):
    bacterial
    infective NOS
    lenta
    malignant
    purulent
    septic
    ulcerative
    vegetative
Infective aneurysm
Subacute bacterial endocarditis [SBE]

Use additional code, if desired, to identify infectious organism [e.g., Streptococcus 041.0, Staphylococcus 041.1]
Coding Clinic: 2008, Q4, P69-73; 2006, Q2, P16-17; 1999, Q1, P12; 1991, Q1, P15

421.1 Acute and subacute infective endocarditis in diseases classified elsewhere

Code first underlying disease, as:
    blastomycosis (116.0)
    Q fever (083.0)
    typhoid (fever) (002.0)

Excludes *endocarditis (in):*
    Coxsackie (virus) (074.22)
    gonococcal (098.84)
    histoplasmosis (115.0–115.9 with fifth-digit 4)
    meningococcal infection (036.42)
    monilial (112.81)

421.9 Acute endocarditis, unspecified

Endocarditis, acute or subacute
Myoendocarditis, acute or subacute
Periendocarditis, acute or subacute

Excludes *acute rheumatic endocarditis (391.1)*

● **422 Acute myocarditis**

An inflammation of the heart muscle due to an infection (viral/bacterial).

Excludes *acute rheumatic myocarditis (391.2)*

422.0 Acute myocarditis in diseases classified elsewhere

Code first underlying disease, as:
    myocarditis (acute):
        influenzal (487.8, 488.09, 488.19) ◄▥
        tuberculous (017.9)

Excludes *myocarditis (acute) (due to):*
    aseptic, of newborn (074.23)
    Coxsackie (virus) (074.23)
    diphtheritic (032.82)
    meningococcal infection (036.43)
    syphilitic (093.82)
    toxoplasmosis (130.3)

● **422.9 Other and unspecified acute myocarditis**

422.90 Acute myocarditis, unspecified

Acute or subacute (interstitial) myocarditis

422.91 Idiopathic myocarditis

Myocarditis (acute or subacute):
    Fiedler's
    giant cell
    isolated (diffuse) (granulomatous)
    nonspecific granulomatous

DISEASES OF THE CIRCULATORY SYSTEM (390–459)

422.92 Septic myocarditis

Myocarditis, acute or subacute:
  pneumococcal
  staphylococcal

Use additional code to identify infectious organism [e.g., Staphylococcus 041.1]

Excludes *myocarditis, acute or subacute:*
  in bacterial diseases classified elsewhere (422.0)
  streptococcal (391.2)

422.93 Toxic myocarditis

422.99 Other

● **423 Other diseases of pericardium**

Excludes *that specified as rheumatic (393)*

423.0 Hemopericardium

423.1 Adhesive pericarditis

Adherent pericardium
Fibrosis of pericardium
Milk spots
Pericarditis:
  adhesive
  obliterative
Soldiers' patches

423.2 Constrictive pericarditis

Concato's disease
Pick's disease of heart (and liver)

● **423.3 Cardiac tamponade**

Code first the underlying cause
Coding Clinic: 2007, Q4, P86-87; 2007, Q2, P11-12

423.8 Other specified diseases of pericardium

Calcification of pericardium
Fistula of pericardium
Coding Clinic: 1989, Q2, P12

423.9 Unspecified disease of pericardium
Coding Clinic: 2007, Q2, P11-12

● **424 Other diseases of endocardium**

Excludes *bacterial endocarditis (421.0–421.9)*
  rheumatic endocarditis (391.1, 394.0–397.9)
  syphilitic endocarditis (093.20–093.24)

424.0 Mitral valve disorders

Mitral (valve):
  incompetence NOS of specified cause, except rheumatic
  insufficiency NOS of specified cause, except rheumatic
  regurgitation NOS of specified cause, except rheumatic

Excludes *mitral (valve):*
  disease (394.9)
  failure (394.9)
  stenosis (394.0)
  the listed conditions:
    specified as rheumatic (394.1)
    unspecified as to cause but with mention of:
      diseases of aortic valve (396.0–396.9)
      mitral stenosis or obstruction (394.2)
Coding Clinic: 2006, Q3, P7; 2000, Q2, P16-17; 1998, Q3, P11; 1987, Nov-Dec, P8

424.1 Aortic valve disorders

Aortic (valve):
  incompetence NOS of specified cause, except rheumatic
  insufficiency NOS of specified cause, except rheumatic
  regurgitation NOS of specified cause, except rheumatic
  stenosis NOS of specified cause, except rheumatic

Excludes *hypertrophic subaortic stenosis (425.1)*
  that specified as rheumatic (395.0–395.9)
  that of unspecified cause but with mention of diseases of mitral valve (396.0–396.9)
Coding Clinic: 2008, Q4, P177-180; 1988, Q4, P8; 1987, Nov-Dec, P8

424.2 Tricuspid valve disorders, specified as nonrheumatic

Tricuspid valve:
  incompetence of specified cause, except rheumatic
  insufficiency of specified cause, except rheumatic
  regurgitation of specified cause, except rheumatic
  stenosis of specified cause, except rheumatic

Excludes *rheumatic or of unspecified cause (397.0)*

424.3 Pulmonary valve disorders

Pulmonic:
  incompetence NOS
  insufficiency NOS
  regurgitation NOS
  stenosis NOS

Excludes *that specified as rheumatic (397.1)*

● **424.9 Endocarditis, valve unspecified**

424.90 Endocarditis, valve unspecified, unspecified cause

Endocarditis (chronic):
  NOS
  nonbacterial thrombotic
Valvular:
  incompetence of unspecified valve, unspecified cause
  insufficiency of unspecified valve, unspecified cause
  regurgitation of unspecified valve, unspecified cause
  stenosis of unspecified valve, unspecified cause
Valvulitis (chronic)

424.91 Endocarditis in diseases classified elsewhere

Code first underlying disease, as:
  atypical verrucous endocarditis [Libman-Sacks] (710.0)
  disseminated lupus erythematosus (710.0)
  tuberculosis (017.9)

Excludes *syphilitic (093.20–093.24)*

424.99 Other

Any condition classifiable to 424.90 with specified cause, except rheumatic

Excludes *endocardial fibroelastosis (425.3)*
  that specified as rheumatic (397.9)

● **425 Cardiomyopathy**
  Disease of the heart muscle resulting in abnormally enlarged,
  weakened, thickened, and/or stiffened muscle causing an
  inability to pump blood normally and leads to CHF.

  Includes myocardiopathy

425.0 Endomyocardial fibrosis

425.1 Hypertrophic obstructive cardiomyopathy
    Hypertrophic subaortic stenosis (idiopathic)

425.2 Obscure cardiomyopathy of Africa
    Becker's disease
    Idiopathic mural endomyocardial disease

425.3 Endocardial fibroelastosis
    Elastomyofibrosis

425.4 Other primary cardiomyopathies
    Cardiomyopathy:
      NOS
      congestive
      constrictive
      familial
      hypertrophic
      idiopathic
      nonobstructive
      obstructive
      restrictive
    Cardiovascular collagenosis
    Coding Clinic: 2009, Q4, P102; 2007, Q1, P20; 2005, Q2, P14-15;
        2000, Q1, P22; 1997, Q4, P54-55; 1990, Q2, P19; 1985,
        Sept-Oct, P15

425.5 Alcoholic cardiomyopathy
    Coding Clinic: 1985, Sept-Oct, P15; July-Aug, P15

425.7 Nutritional and metabolic cardiomyopathy
    Code first underlying disease, as:
      amyloidosis (277.30–277.39)
      beriberi (265.0)
      cardiac glycogenosis (271.0)
      mucopolysaccharidosis (277.5)
      thyrotoxicosis (242.0–242.9)
      Excludes *gouty tophi of heart (274.82)*

425.8 Cardiomyopathy in other diseases classified
elsewhere
    Code first underlying disease, as:
      Friedreich's ataxia (334.0)
      myotonia atrophica (359.21)
      progressive muscular dystrophy (359.1)
      sarcoidosis (135)
      Excludes *cardiomyopathy in Chagas' disease (086.0)*
    Coding Clinic: 1993, Q2, P9

425.9 Secondary cardiomyopathy, unspecified

● **426 Conduction disorders**
  Heart block or atrioventricular block (AV block) caused
  by conduction problem resulting in arrhythmias/
  dysrhythmias due to lack of electrical impulses being
  transmitted normally through heart.

426.0 Atrioventricular block, complete
    Third degree atrioventricular block
    Coding Clinic: 2006, Q2, P14

● **426.1 Atrioventricular block, other and unspecified**

  426.10 Atrioventricular block, unspecified
      Atrioventricular [AV] block (incomplete)
        (partial)

  426.11 First degree atrioventricular block
      Incomplete atrioventricular block, first
        degree
      Prolonged P-R interval NOS
      Coding Clinic: 2006, Q2, P14

  426.12 Mobitz (type) II atrioventricular block
      Incomplete atrioventricular block:
        Mobitz (type) II
        second degree, Mobitz (type) II
      Coding Clinic: 2006, Q2, P14

  426.13 Other second degree atrioventricular block
      Incomplete atrioventricular block:
        Mobitz (type) I [Wenckebach's]
        second degree:
          NOS
          Mobitz (type) I
          with 2:1 atrioventricular response [block]
      Wenckebach's phenomenon

426.2 Left bundle branch hemiblock
    Block:
      left anterior fascicular
      left posterior fascicular

426.3 Other left bundle branch block
    Left bundle branch block:
      NOS
      anterior fascicular with posterior fascicular
      complete
      main stem

426.4 Right bundle branch block
    Coding Clinic: 2000, Q3, P3

● **426.5 Bundle branch block, other and unspecified**

  426.50 Bundle branch block, unspecified

  426.51 Right bundle branch block and left posterior
  fascicular block

  426.52 Right bundle branch block and left anterior
  fascicular block

  426.53 Other bilateral bundle branch block
      Bifascicular block NOS
      Bilateral bundle branch block NOS
      Right bundle branch with left bundle
        branch block (incomplete) (main stem)

  426.54 Trifascicular block

426.6 Other heart block
    Intraventricular block: Sinoatrial block
      NOS   Sinoauricular block
      diffuse
      myofibrillar

426.7 Anomalous atrioventricular excitation
    Atrioventricular conduction:
      accelerated
      accessory
      pre-excitation
    Ventricular pre-excitation
    Wolff-Parkinson-White syndrome

● **426.8 Other specified conduction disorders**

  426.81 Lown-Ganong-Levine syndrome
      Syndrome of short P-R interval, normal
        QRS complexes, and supraventricular
        tachycardias

  426.82 Long QT syndrome
      Coding Clinic: 2005, Q4, P72-73

  426.89 Other
      Dissociation:
        atrioventricular [AV]
        interference
        isorhythmic
      Nonparoxysmal AV nodal tachycardia

426.9 Conduction disorder, unspecified
    Heart block NOS
    Stokes-Adams syndrome

DISEASES OF THE CIRCULATORY SYSTEM (390–459)

DISEASES OF THE CIRCULATORY SYSTEM (390–459)

● **427 Cardiac dysrhythmias**
Abnormality in rate, regularity, or sequence of cardiac activation.

Excludes *that complicating:*
abortion (634–638 with .7, 639.8)
ectopic or molar pregnancy (639.8)
labor or delivery (668.1, 669.4)

427.0 Paroxysmal supraventricular tachycardia
Paroxysmal tachycardia:
atrial [PAT]   junctional
atrioventricular [AV] nodal

427.1 Paroxysmal ventricular tachycardia
Ventricular tachycardia (paroxysmal)
Coding Clinic: 2008, Q1, P14-15; 2006, Q2, P15-16; 1995, Q3, P9;
Q1, P8; 1986, Mar-April, P11-12; 1985, July-Aug, P15

427.2 Paroxysmal tachycardia, unspecified
Bouveret-Hoffmann syndrome
Paroxysmal tachycardia:
NOS
essential

● **427.3 Atrial fibrillation and flutter**
427.31 Atrial fibrillation
Most common abnormal heart rhythm (arrhythmia) presenting as irregular, rapid beating (tachycardia) of the heart's upper chamber.
Coding Clinic: 2008, Q4, P134-136; 2005, Q3, P3-9; 2004,
Q4, P77-78, 121-122; Q3, P7; 2003, Q4, P93-95,
105-106; Q1, P8; 1999, Q2, P17; 1996, Q2, P7x2;
1995, Q3, P8; 1994, Q1, P22; 1985, July-Aug, P15

427.32 Atrial flutter
Rapid contractions of the upper heart chamber, but regular, rather than irregular, beats.
Coding Clinic: 2003, Q4, P93-95

● **427.4 Ventricular fibrillation and flutter**
427.41 Ventricular fibrillation
Coding Clinic: 2002, Q3, P5

427.42 Ventricular flutter

427.5 Cardiac arrest
Cardiorespiratory arrest
Coding Clinic: 2002, Q3, P5; 2000, Q2, P12; 1995, Q3, P9

● **427.6 Premature beats**
427.60 Premature beats, unspecified
Ectopic beats
Extrasystoles
Extrasystolic arrhythmia
Premature contractions or systoles NOS

427.61 Supraventricular premature beats
Atrial premature beats, contractions, or systoles
Coding Clinic: 1994, Q1, P20

427.69 Other
Ventricular premature beats, contractions, or systoles
Coding Clinic: 1993, Q4, P42-43

● **427.8 Other specified cardiac dysrhythmias**
427.81 Sinoatrial node dysfunction
Sinus bradycardia:
persistent
severe
Syndrome:
sick sinus
tachycardia-bradycardia

Excludes *sinus bradycardia NOS (427.89)*

427.89 Other
Rhythm disorder:
coronary sinus
ectopic
nodal
Wandering (atrial) pacemaker

Excludes *carotid sinus syncope (337.0)*
neonatal bradycardia (779.81)
neonatal tachycardia (779.82)
reflex bradycardia (337.0)
tachycardia NOS (785.0)
Coding Clinic: 2000, Q3, P8-9; 1985, July-Aug, P15

427.9 Cardiac dysrhythmia, unspecified
Arrhythmia (cardiac) NOS
Coding Clinic: 1989, Q2, P10

● **428 Heart failure**
Code, if applicable, heart failure due to hypertension first (402.0–402.9, with fifth-digit 1 or 404.0–404.9 with fifth-digit 1 or 3)

Excludes *rheumatic (398.91)*
that complicating:
abortion (634–638 with .7, 639.8)
ectopic or molar pregnancy (639.8)
labor or delivery (668.1, 669.4)
Coding Clinic: 2005, Q2, P14-15; 2002, Q4, P49-53

428.0 Congestive heart failure, unspecified
Congestive heart disease
Right heart failure (secondary to left heart failure)

Excludes *fluid overload NOS (276.69)* ◄▦

Coding Clinic: 2009, Q4, P106x2; Q1, P6x2; 2008, Q4, P69-73,
177-182; Q3, P12-13x2; 2007, Q3, P11; Q1, P20; 2006, Q3,
P7; 2005, Q4, P119-120; Q3, P3-9; Q1, P9; 2004, Q4, P140;
Q3, P7; 2003, Q4, P109-110; Q1, P9; 2002, Q4, P52-53; 2001,
Q2, P13; 2000, Q4, P47-48; Q2, P16-17; Q1, P22; 1999, Q4,
P13-14; Q1, P11, 1998, Q3, P5; 1997, Q4, P54-55; Q3, P10;
1996, Q3, P9; 1991, Q3, P18-20; 1990, Q2, P19; 1989, Q2,
P12; 1987, Sept-Oct, P11; 1985, Sept-Oct, P15; Nov-Dec, P14

428.1 Left heart failure
Acute edema of lung with heart disease NOS or heart failure
Acute pulmonary edema with heart disease NOS or heart failure
Cardiac asthma
Left ventricular failure
Coding Clinic: 1990, Q2, P19

● **428.2 Systolic heart failure**

Excludes *combined systolic and diastolic heart failure (428.40–428.43)*

428.20 Unspecified

428.21 Acute
Presenting a short and relatively severe episode

428.22 Chronic
Long-lasting, presenting over time
Coding Clinic: 2005, Q4, P119-120

428.23 Acute on chronic
Combination code. What was a chronic condition now has an acute exacerbation (to make more severe). Because two conditions are now present, the combination code reports both.
Coding Clinic: 2009, Q1, P10; 2003, Q1, P9

Item 7–11 Congestive heart failure (CHF) is a condition in which the left ventricle of the heart cannot pump enough blood to the body. The blood flow from the heart slows or returns to the heart from the venous system back flow resulting in congestion (fluid accumulation) particularly in the abdomen. Most commonly, fluid collects in the lungs and results in shortness of breath, especially when in a reclining position.

◄ New   ◄▦ Revised   ~~deleted~~ Deleted   Excludes   Includes   Use additional   Code first   Omit code
● Unacceptable Principal Diagnosis   ● Use Additional Digit(s)   OGCR Official Guidelines   Coding Clinic

● **428.3 Diastolic heart failure**

> | Excludes | *combined systolic and diastolic heart failure (428.40–428.43)*

428.30 Unspecified
> Coding Clinic: 2002, Q4, P52

428.31 Acute

428.32 Chronic
> Coding Clinic: 2008, Q3, P12-13

428.33 Acute on chronic
> Coding Clinic: 2009, Q4, P106; 2008, Q3, P12; 2007, Q1, P20

● **428.4 Combined systolic and diastolic heart failure**

428.40 Unspecified

428.41 Acute
> Coding Clinic: 2004, Q4, P140

428.42 Chronic

428.43 Acute on chronic
> Coding Clinic: 2006, Q3, P7; 2002, Q4, P52-53

428.9 Heart failure, unspecified
Cardiac failure NOS
Heart failure NOS
Myocardial failure NOS
Weak heart
> Coding Clinic: 1989, Q2, P10; 1985, Nov-Dec, P14

● **429 Ill-defined descriptions and complications of heart disease**

429.0 Myocarditis, unspecified
Myocarditis (with mention of arteriosclerosis):
  NOS (with mention of arteriosclerosis)
  chronic (interstitial) (with mention of
    arteriosclerosis)
  fibroid (with mention of arteriosclerosis)
  senile (with mention of arteriosclerosis)

> Use additional code to identify presence of arteriosclerosis

> | Excludes | *acute or subacute (422.0–422.9)*
>   *rheumatic (398.0)*
>   *acute (391.2)*
>   *that due to hypertension (402.0–402.9)*

429.1 Myocardial degeneration
Degeneration of heart or myocardium (with
  mention of arteriosclerosis):
  fatty (with mention of arteriosclerosis)
  mural (with mention of arteriosclerosis)
  muscular (with mention of arteriosclerosis)
Myocardial (with mention of arteriosclerosis):
  degeneration (with mention of arteriosclerosis)
  disease (with mention of arteriosclerosis)

> Use additional code to identify presence of arteriosclerosis

> | Excludes | *that due to hypertension (402.0–402.9)*

429.2 Cardiovascular disease, unspecified
Arteriosclerotic cardiovascular disease [ASCVD]
Cardiovascular arteriosclerosis
Cardiovascular:
  degeneration (with mention of arteriosclerosis)
  disease (with mention of arteriosclerosis)
  sclerosis (with mention of arteriosclerosis)

> Use additional code to identify presence of arteriosclerosis

> | Excludes | *that due to hypertension (402.0–402.9)*

429.3 Cardiomegaly
Cardiac:
  dilatation
  hypertrophy
Ventricular dilatation

> | Excludes | *that due to hypertension (402.0–402.9)*

429.4 Functional disturbances following cardiac surgery
Cardiac insufficiency following cardiac surgery or
  due to prosthesis
Heart failure following cardiac surgery or due to
  prosthesis
Postcardiotomy syndrome
Postvalvulotomy syndrome

> | Excludes | *cardiac failure in the immediate
>   postoperative period (997.1)*
> Coding Clinic: 2002, Q2, P12-13

429.5 Rupture of chordae tendineae

429.6 Rupture of papillary muscle

● **429.7 Certain sequelae of myocardial infarction, not
elsewhere classified**

> Use additional code to identify the associated
>   myocardial infarction:
>   with onset of 8 weeks or less (410.00–410.92)
>   with onset of more than 8 weeks (414.8)

> | Excludes | *congenital defects of heart (745, 746)*
>   *coronary aneurysm (414.11)*
>   *disorders of papillary muscle (429.6,
>   429.81)*
>   *postmyocardial infarction syndrome (411.0)*
>   *rupture of chordae tendineae (429.5)*

429.71 Acquired cardiac septal defect

> | Excludes | *acute septal infarction
>   (410.00–410.92)*

429.79 Other
Mural thrombus (atrial) (ventricular)
  acquired, following myocardial
  infarction
> Coding Clinic: 1992, Q1, P10

● **429.8 Other ill-defined heart diseases**

429.81 Other disorders of papillary muscle
Papillary muscle:
  atrophy
  degeneration
  dysfunction
  incompetence
  incoordination
  scarring

429.82 Hyperkinetic heart disease

429.83 Takotsubo syndrome
Broken heart syndrome
Reversible left ventricular dysfunction
  following sudden emotional stress
Stress induced cardiomyopathy
Transient left ventricular apical ballooning
  syndrome
> Coding Clinic: 2006, Q4, P87

429.89 Other
Carditis

> | Excludes | *that due to hypertension
>   (402.0–402.9)*
> Coding Clinic: 2006, Q2, P18-19; 2005, Q3, P14; 1992,
> Q1, P10

429.9 Heart disease, unspecified
Heart disease (organic) NOS
Morbus cordis NOS

> | Excludes | *that due to hypertension (402.0–402.9)*
> Coding Clinic: 2009, Q1, P10x2; 1993, Q1, P19-20

DISEASES OF THE CIRCULATORY SYSTEM (390–459)

CEREBROVASCULAR DISEASE (430–438)

| **Includes** | with mention of hypertension (conditions classifiable to 401–405) |

Use additional code to identify presence of hypertension

| **Excludes** | any condition classifiable to 430–434, 436, 437 occurring during pregnancy, childbirth, or the puerperium, or specified as puerperal (674.0) |
| | iatrogenic cerebrovascular infarction or hemorrhage (997.02) |

OGCR Section I.C.7.a.5

First assign codes from 430-438, Cerebrovascular disease, then the appropriate hypertension code from categories 401-405.

430 Subarachnoid hemorrhage
 Meningeal hemorrhage
 Ruptured:
  berry aneurysm
  (congenital) cerebral aneurysm NOS

| **Excludes** | syphilitic ruptured cerebral aneurysm (094.87) |

Coding Clinic: 2000, Q3, P16; 1991, Q3, P15-16

431 Intracerebral hemorrhage
 Hemorrhage (of):
  basilar
  bulbar
  cerebellar
  cerebral
  cerebromeningeal
  cortical
  internal capsule
  intrapontine
  pontine
  subcortical
  ventricular
 Rupture of blood vessel in brain
 Coding Clinic: 2010, Q1, P7; 2007, Q3, P4; 1997, Q3, P11

● **432 Other and unspecified intracranial hemorrhage**

 432.0 Nontraumatic extradural hemorrhage
  Nontraumatic epidural hemorrhage

 432.1 Subdural hemorrhage
  Subdural hematoma, nontraumatic

 432.9 Unspecified intracranial hemorrhage
  Intracranial hemorrhage NOS

● **433 Occlusion and stenosis of precerebral arteries**

 The following fifth-digit subclassification is for use with category 433:

| **0 without mention of cerebral infarction** |
| **1 with cerebral infarction** |

Includes	embolism of basilar, carotid, and vertebral arteries
	narrowing of basilar, carotid, and vertebral arteries
	obstruction of basilar, carotid, and vertebral arteries
	thrombosis of basilar, carotid, and vertebral arteries

| **Excludes** | insufficiency NOS of precerebral arteries (435.0–435.9) |

Use additional code, if applicable, to identify status post administration of tPA (rtPA) in a different facility within the last 24 hours prior to admission to current facility (V45.88)
Coding Clinic: 1995, Q2, P16; 1993, Q4, P38-39

● **433.0 Basilar artery**
 [0-1]

● **433.1 Carotid artery**
 [0-1]   Coding Clinic: 2006, Q1, P17; 2002, Q1, P7-8, 10-11; 2000, Q1, P16; 1995, Q2, P16

● **433.2 Vertebral artery**
 [0-1]

● **433.3 Multiple and bilateral**
 [0-1]   Coding Clinic: 2006, Q1, P17; 2002, Q1, P10-11

● **433.8 Other specified precerebral artery**
 [0-1]

● **433.9 Unspecified precerebral artery**
 [0-1]   Precerebral artery NOS

● **434 Occlusion of cerebral arteries**

 The following fifth-digit subclassification is for use with category 434:

| **0 without mention of cerebral infarction** |
| **1 with cerebral infarction** |

Use additional code, if applicable, to identify status post administration of tPA (rtPA) in a different facility within the last 24 hours prior to admission to current facility (V45.88)
Coding Clinic: 2007, Q3, P12; 1995, Q2, P16; 1993, Q4, P38-39

● **434.0 Cerebral thrombosis**
 [0-1]   Thrombosis of cerebral arteries

● **434.1 Cerebral embolism**
 [0-1]   Coding Clinic: 1997, Q3, P11

● **434.9 Cerebral artery occlusion, unspecified**
 [0-1]   Coding Clinic: 2008, Q4, P102-109; 2007, Q1, P23-24; 2004, Q4, P77-78; 1998, Q4, P87; 1996, Q2, P5

● **435 Transient cerebral ischemia**

Includes	cerebrovascular insufficiency (acute) with transient focal neurological signs and symptoms
	insufficiency of basilar, carotid, and vertebral arteries
	spasm of cerebral arteries

| **Excludes** | acute cerebrovascular insufficiency NOS (437.1) that due to any condition classifiable to 433 (433.0–433.9) |

 435.0 Basilar artery syndrome

 435.1 Vertebral artery syndrome

 435.2 Subclavian steal syndrome

 435.3 Vertebrobasilar artery syndrome

 435.8 Other specified transient cerebral ischemias

 435.9 Unspecified transient cerebral ischemia
  Impending cerebrovascular accident
  Intermittent cerebral ischemia
  Transient ischemic attack [TIA]
  Coding Clinic: 1985, Nov-Dec, P12

◀ New   ◀◀ Revised   ~~deleted~~ Deleted   Excludes   Includes   Use additional   Code first   Omit code
● Unacceptable Principal Diagnosis   ● Use Additional Digit(s)   OGCR Official Guidelines   Coding Clinic

436   Acute, but ill-defined, cerebrovascular disease
     Apoplexy, apoplectic:
         NOS
         attack
         cerebral
         seizure
     Cerebral seizure

> **Excludes**   *any condition classifiable to categories 430–435*
> *cerebrovascular accident (434.91)*
> *CVA (ischemic) (434.91)*
>   *embolic (434.11)*
>   *hemorrhagic (430, 431, 432.0–432.9)*
>   *thrombotic (434.01)*
> *postoperative cerebrovascular accident (997.02)*
> *stroke (ischemic) (434.91)*
>   *embolic (434.11)*
>   *hemorrhagic (430, 431, 432.0–432.9)*
>   *thrombotic (434.01)*

     Coding Clinic: 2004, Q4, P77-78; 1999, Q4, P3-4; 1993, Q4, P38-39; Q1, P27

OGCR   Section I.C.7.b

The terms stroke and CVA are often used interchangeably to refer to a cerebral vascular infarction. The terms stroke, CVA, and cerebral infarction NOS are all indexed to the default code 434.91, Cerebral artery occlusion, unspecified, with infarction. Code 436, Acute, but ill-defined, cerebrovascular disease, should not be used when the documentation states stroke or CVA.

● 437   Other and ill-defined cerebrovascular disease

     437.0   Cerebral atherosclerosis
         Atheroma of cerebral arteries
         Cerebral arteriosclerosis

     437.1   Other generalized ischemic cerebrovascular disease
         Acute cerebrovascular insufficiency NOS
         Cerebral ischemia (chronic)
         Coding Clinic: 2009, Q1, P10

     437.2   Hypertensive encephalopathy

     437.3   Cerebral aneurysm, nonruptured
         Internal carotid artery, intracranial portion
         Internal carotid artery NOS

> **Excludes**   *congenital cerebral aneurysm, nonruptured*
>   *(747.81)*
> *internal carotid artery, extracranial portion*
>   *(442.81)*

         Coding Clinic: 2009, Q2, P12

     437.4   Cerebral arteritis
         Coding Clinic: 1999, Q4, P21-22

     437.5   Moyamoya disease

     437.6   Nonpyogenic thrombosis of intracranial venous sinus

> **Excludes**   *pyogenic (325)*

     437.7   Transient global amnesia

     437.8   Other

     437.9   Unspecified
         Cerebrovascular disease or lesion NOS
         Coding Clinic: 2009, Q1, P16; 1986, Nov-Dec, P12

OGCR   Section I.C.7.d.3

Assign code V12.54, Transient ischemic attack (TIA), and cerebral infarction without residual deficits (and not a code from category 438) as an additional code for history of cerebrovascular disease when no neurologic deficits are present.

● 438   Late effects of cerebrovascular disease

     Note: This category is to be used to indicate conditions in 430–437 as the cause of late effects. The "late effects" include conditions specified as such, or as sequelae, which may occur at any time after the onset of the causal condition.

> **Excludes**   *personal history of:*
> *cerebral infarction without residual deficits*
>   *(V12.54)*
> *PRIND (Prolonged reversible ischemic*
>   *neurologic deficit) (V12.54)*
> *RIND (Reversible ischemic neurological deficit)*
>   *(V12.54)*
> *transient ischemic attack (TIA) (V12.54)*

     Coding Clinic: 2006, Q3, P3-4, 6; 1999, Q4, P6-8x2; Q4, P4-5; 1994, Q1,
     P22-23; 1993, Q1, P27

     438.0   Cognitive deficits
         Coding Clinic: 2007, Q2, P5

     ● 438.1   Speech and language deficits

         438.10   Speech and language deficit, unspecified

         438.11   Aphasia
            Coding Clinic: 2003, Q4, P105-106; 1997, Q4, P35-37

         438.12   Dysphasia
            Coding Clinic: 1999, Q4, P9; Q4, P3-4

         438.13   Dysarthria

         438.14   Fluency disorder
            Stuttering due to late effect of
                cerebrovascular accident ◀▥

         438.19   Other speech and language deficits

     ● 438.2   Hemiplegia/hemiparesis
         Coding Clinic: 2005, Q1, P13

         438.20   Hemiplegia affecting unspecified side
            Coding Clinic: 2007, Q4, P92-95; 2003, Q4, P105-106;
                1999, Q4, P9; Q4, P3-4

         438.21   Hemiplegia affecting dominant side

         438.22   Hemiplegia affecting nondominant side
            Coding Clinic: 2003, Q4, P105; 2002, Q1, P16

     ● 438.3   Monoplegia of upper limb

         438.30   Monoplegia of upper limb affecting unspecified side

         438.31   Monoplegia of upper limb affecting dominant side

         438.32   Monoplegia of upper limb affecting nondominant side

     ● 438.4   Monoplegia of lower limb

         438.40   Monoplegia of lower limb affecting unspecified side

         438.41   Monoplegia of lower limb affecting dominant side

         438.42   Monoplegia of lower limb affecting nondominant side

DISEASES OF THE CIRCULATORY SYSTEM (390–459)

● **438.5 Other paralytic syndrome**

Use additional code to identify type of paralytic
syndrome, such as:
locked-in state (344.81)
quadriplegia (344.00–344.09)

Excludes   *late effects of cerebrovascular accident with:*
hemiplegia/hemiparesis (438.20–438.22)
monoplegia of lower limb
(438.40–438.42)
monoplegia of upper limb
(438.40–438.42)

438.50 **Other paralytic syndrome affecting**
unspecified side

438.51 **Other paralytic syndrome affecting dominant**
side

438.52 **Other paralytic syndrome affecting**
nondominant side

438.53 **Other paralytic syndrome, bilateral**
Coding Clinic: 1998, Q4, P39-40

438.6 **Alterations of sensations**

Use additional code to identify the altered
sensation
Coding Clinic: 2002, Q4, P56

438.7 **Disturbances of vision**

Use additional code to identify the visual
disturbance
Coding Clinic: 2002, Q4, P56

● **438.8 Other late effects of cerebrovascular disease**
Coding Clinic: 2005, Q1, P13; 2002, Q4, P56

438.81 **Apraxia**

438.82 **Dysphagia**

Use additional code to identify the type of
dysphagia, if known (787.20–787.29)
Coding Clinic: 2007, Q4, P92-95

438.83 **Facial weakness**
Facial droop

438.84 **Ataxia**

438.85 **Vertigo**
Coding Clinic: 2002, Q4, P56

438.89 **Other late effects of cerebrovascular**
disease

Use additional code to identify the late
effect
Coding Clinic: 2009, Q2, P10; 2005, Q1, P13; 1998, Q4,
P39-40

438.9 **Unspecified late effects of cerebrovascular disease**

DISEASES OF ARTERIES, ARTERIOLES, AND CAPILLARIES (440–449)

● **440 Atherosclerosis**
Disease in which fatty deposits form on walls of arteries

Includes   arteriolosclerosis
arteriosclerosis (obliterans) (senile)
arteriosclerotic vascular disease
atheroma
degeneration:
arterial
arteriovascular
vascular
endarteritis deformans or obliterans
senile:
arteritis
endarteritis

Excludes   *atheroembolism (445.01–445.89)*
atherosclerosis of bypass graft of the extremities
(440.30–440.32)

440.0 Of aorta
Coding Clinic: 1993, Q2, P7-8; 1988, Q4, P8

440.1 Of renal artery

Excludes   *atherosclerosis of renal arterioles*
(403.00–403.91)

● **440.2 Of native arteries of the extremities**

Use additional code, if applicable, to identify
chronic total occlusion of artery of the
extremities (440.4)

Excludes   *atherosclerosis of bypass graft of the*
extremities (440.30–440.32)
Coding Clinic: 1994, Q3, P5; 1990, Q3, P15

440.20 **Atherosclerosis of the extremities,**
unspecified

440.21 **Atherosclerosis of the extremities with**
intermittent claudication

440.22 **Atherosclerosis of the extremities with rest**
pain
Any condition classifiable to 440.21

440.23 **Atherosclerosis of the extremities with**
ulceration
Any condition classifiable to 440.21–440.22

Use additional code for any associated
ulceration (707.10–707.9)

440.24 **Atherosclerosis of the extremities with**
gangrene
Any condition classifiable to 440.21, 440.22,
and 440.23 with ischemic gangrene
785.4

Use additional code for any associated
ulceration (707.10–707.9)

Excludes   *gas gangrene 040.0*

Coding Clinic: 2003, Q4, P109-110; Q3, P14x2; 1995, Q1,
P11; 1994, Q3, P5

440.29 **Other**
Coding Clinic: 1995, Q1, P11

● **440.3 Of bypass graft of the extremities**

Excludes   *atherosclerosis of native artery of the*
extremity (440.21–440.24)
embolism [occlusion NOS] [thrombus] of
graft (996.74)

440.30 **Of unspecified graft**

440.31 **Of autologous vein bypass graft**

440.32 **Of nonautologous vein bypass graft**

● **440.4 Chronic total occlusion of artery of the extremities**
Complete occlusion of artery of the extremities
Total occlusion of artery of the extremities

Code first atherosclerosis of arteries of the extremities
(440.20–440.29, 440.30–440.32)

Excludes   *acute occlusion of artery of extremity*
(444.21–444.22)
Coding Clinic: 2007, Q4, P82-83

Figure 7–4 Atherosclerotic plaque.

Atherosclerotic
plaque
(atheromas)

◀ New   ◀‖ Revised   ~~deleted~~ Deleted   Excludes   Includes   Use additional   Code first   Omit code
● Unacceptable Principal Diagnosis   ● Use Additional Digit(s)   OGCR Official Guidelines   Coding Clinic

440.8 Of other specified arteries

> **Excludes** | *basilar (433.0)*
> *carotid (433.1)*
> *cerebral (437.0)*
> *coronary (414.00–414.07)*
> *mesenteric (557.1)*
> *precerebral (433.0–433.9)*
> *pulmonary (416.0)*
> *vertebral (433.2)*

Coding Clinic: 2009, Q3, P9

440.9 Generalized and unspecified atherosclerosis
Arteriosclerotic vascular disease NOS

> **Excludes** | *arteriosclerotic cardiovascular disease*
> *[ASCVD] (429.2)*

● **441 Aortic aneurysm and dissection**

> **Excludes** | *aortic ectasia (447.70-447.73)* ◄
> *syphilitic aortic aneurysm (093.0)*
> *traumatic aortic aneurysm (901.0, 902.0)*

● **441.0 Dissection of aorta**
Coding Clinic: 1989, Q4, P10

441.00 Unspecified site

441.01 Thoracic
Coding Clinic: 2009, Q1, P16; 2007, Q4, P86-87

441.02 Abdominal

441.03 Thoracoabdominal

441.1 Thoracic aneurysm, ruptured
Coding Clinic: 1994, Q2, P15

441.2 Thoracic aneurysm without mention of rupture
Coding Clinic: 1992, Q3, P10-11

441.3 Abdominal aneurysm, ruptured

441.4 Abdominal aneurysm without mention of rupture
Coding Clinic: 2000, Q4, P63-64; 1999, Q1, P15-17x2; 1992, Q3, P10-11

441.5 Aortic aneurysm of unspecified site, ruptured
Rupture of aorta NOS

441.6 Thoracoabdominal aneurysm, ruptured

441.7 Thoracoabdominal aneurysm, without mention of rupture
Coding Clinic: 2006, Q2, P16-17

441.9 Aortic aneurysm of unspecified site without mention of rupture
Aneurysm
Dilatation of aorta
Hyaline necrosis of aorta
Coding Clinic: 1992, Q3, P10-11

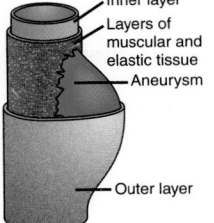
Inner layer
Layers of muscular and elastic tissue
Aneurysm
Outer layer

Figure 7–5 An aneurysm is an enclosed swelling on the wall of the vessel.

Item 7–12 Rupture is the tearing of the aneurysm.

● **442 Other aneurysm**

> **Includes** | aneurysm (ruptured) (cirsoid) (false) (varicose)
> aneurysmal varix

> **Excludes** | *arteriovenous aneurysm or fistula:*
> *acquired (447.0)*
> *congenital (747.60–747.69)*
> *traumatic (900.0–904.9)*

442.0 Of artery of upper extremity

442.1 Of renal artery

442.2 Of iliac artery
Coding Clinic: 1999, Q1, P16-17

442.3 Of artery of lower extremity
Aneurysm:
femoral artery
popliteal artery
Coding Clinic: 2008, Q2, P13; 2002, Q3, P24-27; 1999, Q1, P16

● **442.8 Of other specified artery**

442.81 Artery of neck
Aneurysm of carotid artery (common) (external) (internal, extracranial portion)

> **Excludes** | *internal carotid artery, intracranial portion (437.3)*

442.82 Subclavian artery

442.83 Splenic artery

442.84 Other visceral artery
Aneurysm:
celiac artery
gastroduodenal artery
gastroepiploic artery
hepatic artery
pancreaticoduodenal artery
superior mesenteric artery

442.89 Other
Aneurysm: Aneurysm:
mediastinal artery   spinal artery

> **Excludes** | *cerebral (nonruptured) (437.3)*
> *congenital (747.81)*
> *ruptured (430)*
> *coronary (414.11)*
> *heart (414.10)*
> *pulmonary (417.1)*

442.9 Of unspecified site

● **443 Other peripheral vascular disease**

443.0 Raynaud's syndrome
Resulting from a diminishing oxygen supply to fingers, toes, nose, and ears when exposed to temperature changes or stress with symptoms of pallor, numbness, and feeling cold
Raynaud's:
disease
phenomenon (secondary)
Use additional code to identify gangrene (785.4)

443.1 Thromboangiitis obliterans [Buerger's disease]
Inflammatory occlusive disease resulting in poor circulation to legs, feet, and sometimes hands due to progressive inflammatory narrowing of the small arteries
Presenile gangrene

DISEASES OF THE CIRCULATORY SYSTEM (390–459)

DISEASES OF THE CIRCULATORY SYSTEM (390–459)

● **443.2 Other arterial dissection**

> **Excludes** *dissection of aorta (441.00–441.03)*
> *dissection of coronary arteries (414.12)*
> Coding Clinic: 2002, Q4, P54-55

   443.21 Dissection of carotid artery

   443.22 Dissection of iliac artery

   443.23 Dissection of renal artery

   443.24 Dissection of vertebral artery

   443.29 Dissection of other artery

● **443.8 Other specified peripheral vascular diseases**

   443.81 Peripheral angiopathy in diseases classified elsewhere

   > Code first *underlying disease, as:*
   > diabetes mellitus (249.7, 250.7)
   > Coding Clinic: 2004, Q1, P14-15; 1996, Q1, P10

   443.82 Erythromelalgia
   > Coding Clinic: 2005, Q4, P73-74

   443.89 Other
   Acrocyanosis
   Acroparesthesia:
      simple [Schultze's type]
      vasomotor [Nothnagel's type]
   Erythrocyanosis

   > **Excludes** *chilblains (991.5)*
   > *frostbite (991.0–991.3)*
   > *immersion foot (991.4)*
   > Coding Clinic: 2007, Q4, P124

   443.9 Peripheral vascular disease, unspecified
   Intermittent claudication NOS
   Peripheral:
      angiopathy NOS
      vascular disease NOS
   Spasm of artery

   > **Excludes** *atherosclerosis of the arteries of the extremities (440.20–440.22)*
   > *spasm of cerebral artery (435.0–435.9)*

● **444 Arterial embolism and thrombosis**

   > **Includes** infarction:
   > embolic
   > thrombotic
   > occlusion

   > **Excludes** *atheroembolism (445.01–445.89)*
   > *septic arterial embolism (449)*
   > *that complicating:*
   > *abortion (634–638 with .6, 639.6)*
   > *ectopic or molar pregnancy (639.6)*
   > *pregnancy, childbirth, or the puerperium (673.0–673.8)*
   > Coding Clinic: 2003, Q1, P16-18x2; 1992, Q2, P10-11

   444.0 Of abdominal aorta
   Aortic bifurcation syndrome
   Aortoiliac obstruction
   Leriche's syndrome
   Saddle embolus
   Coding Clinic: 1990, Q4, P27

   444.1 Of thoracic aorta
   Embolism or thrombosis of aorta (thoracic)

● **444.2 Of arteries of the extremities**

   444.21 Upper extremity
   > Coding Clinic: 1990, Q3, P16

   444.22 Lower extremity
   Arterial embolism or thrombosis:
      femoral   popliteal
      peripheral NOS

   > **Excludes** *iliofemoral (444.81)*
   > Coding Clinic: 2007, Q4, P84-86; 2003, Q3, P10

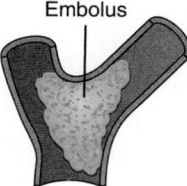

Embolus

Figure 7–6 An arterial embolus.

Item 7–13 An **embolus** is a mass of undissolved matter present in the blood that is transported by the blood current. A **thrombus** is a blood clot that occludes or shuts off a vessel. When a thrombus is dislodged, it becomes an embolus.

● **444.8 Of other specified artery**

   444.81 Iliac artery
   > Coding Clinic: 2003, Q1, P16-17

   444.89 Other

   > **Excludes** *basilar (433.0)*
   > *carotid (433.1)*
   > *cerebral (434.0–434.9)*
   > *coronary (410.00–410.92)*
   > *mesenteric (557.0)*
   > *ophthalmic (362.30–362.34)*
   > *precerebral (433.0–433.9)*
   > *pulmonary (415.19)*
   > *renal (593.81)*
   > *retinal (362.30–362.34)*
   > *vertebral (433.2)*

   444.9 Of unspecified artery

● **445 Atheroembolism**

   > **Includes** Atherothrombotic microembolism
   > Cholesterol embolism
   > Coding Clinic: 2002, Q4, P57-58

● **445.0 Of extremities**

   445.01 Upper extremity

   445.02 Lower extremity

● **445.8 Of other sites**

   445.81 Kidney

   > Use additional code for any associated acute
   > kidney failure or chronic kidney disease
   > (584, 585)

   445.89 Other site

● **446 Polyarteritis nodosa and allied conditions**

   446.0 Polyarteritis nodosa
   Disseminated necrotizing periarteritis
   Necrotizing angiitis
   Panarteritis (nodosa)
   Periarteritis (nodosa)

   446.1 Acute febrile mucocutaneous lymph node syndrome [MCLS]
   Kawasaki disease

● **446.2 Hypersensitivity angiitis**

   > **Excludes** *antiglomerular basement membrane disease*
   > *without pulmonary hemorrhage*
   > *(583.89)*

   446.20 Hypersensitivity angiitis, unspecified

   446.21 Goodpasture's syndrome
   Antiglomerular basement membrane
      antibody-mediated nephritis with
      pulmonary hemorrhage

   > Use additional code to identify renal
   > disease (583.81)

   446.29 Other specified hypersensitivity angiitis
   > Coding Clinic: 1995, Q1, P3

◀ New   ◀▥ Revised   ~~deleted~~ Deleted   Excludes   Includes   Use additional   Code first   Omit code
● Unacceptable Principal Diagnosis   ● Use Additional Digit(s)   OGCR Official Guidelines   Coding Clinic

446.3 Lethal midline granuloma
Malignant granuloma of face

446.4 Wegener's granulomatosis
Necrotizing respiratory granulomatosis
Wegener's syndrome
Coding Clinic: 2000, Q3, P11

446.5 Giant cell arteritis
Cranial arteritis
Horton's disease
Temporal arteritis

446.6 Thrombotic microangiopathy
Moschcowitz's syndrome
Thrombotic thrombocytopenic purpura

446.7 Takayasu's disease
Aortic arch arteritis
Pulseless disease

● **447 Other disorders of arteries and arterioles**

447.0 Arteriovenous fistula, acquired
Arteriovenous aneurysm, acquired
| Excludes | *cerebrovascular (437.3)*
coronary (414.19)
pulmonary (417.0)
surgically created arteriovenous shunt or
fistula:
complication (996.1, 996.61–996.62)
status or presence (V45.11)
traumatic (900.0–904.9)

447.1 Stricture of artery
Coding Clinic: 1993, Q2, P8; 1987, Jan-Feb, P14

447.2 Rupture of artery
Erosion of artery
Fistula, except arteriovenous of artery
Ulcer of artery
| Excludes | *traumatic rupture of artery (900.0–904.9)*

447.3 Hyperplasia of renal artery
Fibromuscular hyperplasia of renal artery

447.4 Celiac artery compression syndrome
Celiac axis syndrome
Marable's syndrome

447.5 Necrosis of artery

447.6 Arteritis, unspecified
Aortitis NOS
Endarteritis NOS
| Excludes | *arteritis, endarteritis:*
aortic arch (446.7)
cerebral (437.4)
coronary (414.00–414.07)
deformans (440.0–440.9)
obliterans (440.0–440.9)
pulmonary (417.8)
senile (440.0–440.9)
polyarteritis NOS (446.0)
syphilitic aortitis (093.1)
Coding Clinic: 1999, Q4, P21-22

● **447.7 Aortic ectasia ◄**
Ectasis aorta ◄
| Excludes | *aortic aneurysm and dissection*
(441.00-441.9) ◄

447.70 Aortic ectasia, unspecified site ◄

447.71 Thoracic aortic ectasia ◄

447.72 Abdominal aortic ectasia ◄

447.73 Thoracoabdominal aortic ectasia ◄

447.8 Other specified disorders of arteries and arterioles
Fibromuscular hyperplasia of arteries, except
renal

447.9 Unspecified disorders of arteries and arterioles

● **448 Disease of capillaries**

448.0 Hereditary hemorrhagic telangiectasia
Rendu-Osler-Weber disease

448.1 Nevus, non-neoplastic
Nevus:
araneus
senile
spider
stellar
| Excludes | *neoplastic (216.0–216.9)*
port wine (757.32)
strawberry (757.32)

448.9 Other and unspecified capillary diseases
Capillary:
hemorrhage
hyperpermeability
thrombosis
| Excludes | *capillary fragility (hereditary) (287.8)*

● **449 Septic arterial embolism**
Code first underlying infection, such as:
infective endocarditis (421.0)
lung abscess (513.0)
Use additional code to identify the site of the embolism
(433.0–433.9, 444.0–444.9)
| Excludes | *septic pulmonary embolism (415.12)*
Coding Clinic: 2007, Q4, P84-86

**DISEASES OF VEINS AND LYMPHATICS, AND OTHER DISEASES
OF CIRCULATORY SYSTEM (451–459)**

● **451 Phlebitis and thrombophlebitis**
*Inflammation of vein with infiltration of walls (phlebitis)
and, usually, formation of clot (thrombus) in vein
(thrombophlebitis)*

| Includes | endophlebitis
inflammation, vein
periphlebitis
suppurative phlebitis

Use additional E code to identify drug if drug-induced
| Excludes | *that complicating:*
abortion (634–638 with .7, 639.8)
ectopic or molar pregnancy (639.8)
pregnancy, childbirth, or the puerperium
(671.0–671.9)
that due to or following:
implant or catheter device (996.61–996.62)
infusion, perfusion, or transfusion (999.2)
Coding Clinic: 2004, Q4, P78-80; 1993, Q1, P26; 1992, Q1, P15-16

451.0 Of superficial vessels of lower extremities
Saphenous vein (greater) (lesser)

● **451.1 Of deep vessels of lower extremities**
Coding Clinic: 1991, Q3, P16

451.11 Femoral vein (deep) (superficial)

451.19 Other
Femoropopliteal vein
Popliteal vein
Tibial vein

451.2 Of lower extremities, unspecified
Coding Clinic: 2004, Q4, P78-80

DISEASES OF THE CIRCULATORY SYSTEM (390–459)

● **451.8 Of other sites**

> **Excludes** *intracranial venous sinus (325)*
> *nonpyogenic (437.6)*
> *portal (vein) (572.1)*

451.81 Iliac vein

451.82 Of superficial veins of upper extremities
Antecubital vein
Basilic vein
Cephalic vein

451.83 Of deep veins of upper extremities
Brachial vein
Radial vein
Ulnar vein

451.84 Of upper extremities, unspecified

451.89 Other
Axillary vein
Jugular vein
Subclavian vein
Thrombophlebitis of breast (Mondor's disease)

451.9 Of unspecified site

452 Portal vein thrombosis
Portal (vein) obstruction

> **Excludes** *hepatic vein thrombosis (453.0)*
> *phlebitis of portal vein (572.1)*

● **453 Other venous embolism and thrombosis**

> **Excludes** *that complicating:*
> *abortion (634–638 with .7, 639.8)*
> *ectopic or molar pregnancy (639.8)*
> *pregnancy, childbirth, or the puerperium (671.0–671.9)*

Coding Clinic: 2004, Q4, P78-80; 1992, Q1, P15-16

453.0 Budd-Chiari syndrome
Hepatic vein thrombosis

453.1 Thrombophlebitis migrans
"White leg" is the other term used to describe a migrating thrombus.

453.2 Of inferior vena cava

453.3 Of renal vein

● **453.4 Acute venous embolism and thrombosis of deep vessels of lower extremity**

453.40 Acute venous embolism and thrombosis of unspecified deep vessels of lower extremity
Deep vein thrombosis NOS
DVT NOS

453.41 Acute venous embolism and thrombosis of deep vessels of proximal lower extremity
Femoral   Thigh
Iliac   Upper leg NOS
Popliteal
Coding Clinic: 2004, Q4, P78-80

453.42 Acute venous embolism and thrombosis of deep vessels of distal lower extremity
Calf   Peroneal
Lower leg NOS Tibial

● **453.5 Chronic venous embolism and thrombosis of deep vessels of lower extremity**

> **Use additional** code, if applicable, for associated long-term (current) use of anticoagulants (V58.61)

> **Excludes** *personal history of venous thrombosis and embolism (V12.51)*

453.50 Chronic venous embolism and thrombosis of unspecified deep vessels of lower extremity

453.51 Chronic venous embolism and thrombosis of deep vessels of proximal lower extremity
Femoral ◄   Thigh ◄
Iliac ◄   Upper leg NOS ◄
Popliteal ◄

453.52 Chronic venous embolism and thrombosis of deep vessels of distal lower extremity
Calf ◄
Lower leg NOS ◄
Peroneal ◄
Tibial ◄

453.6 Venous embolism and thrombosis of superficial vessels of lower extremity
Saphenous vein (greater) (lesser)

> **Use additional** code, if applicable, for associated long-term (current) use of anticoagulants (V58.61) ◄

● **453.7 Chronic venous embolism and thrombosis of other specified vessels**

> **Use additional** code, if applicable, for associated long-term (current) use of anticoagulants (V58.61)

> **Excludes** *personal history of venous thrombosis and embolism (V12.51)*

453.71 Chronic venous embolism and thrombosis of superficial veins of upper extremity
Antecubital vein   Cephalic vein
Basilic vein

453.72 Chronic venous embolism and thrombosis of deep veins of upper extremity
Brachial vein   Ulnar vein
Radial vein

453.73 Chronic venous embolism and thrombosis of upper extremity, unspecified

453.74 Chronic venous embolism and thrombosis of axillary veins

453.75 Chronic venous embolism and thrombosis of subclavian veins

453.76 Chronic venous embolism and thrombosis of internal jugular veins

453.77 Chronic venous embolism and thrombosis of other thoracic veins
Brachiocephalic (innominate)
Superior vena cava

453.79 Chronic venous embolism and thrombosis of other specified veins

● **453.8 Acute venous embolism and thrombosis of other specified veins**

> **Excludes** *cerebral (434.0–434.9)*
> *coronary (410.00–410.92)*
> *intracranial venous sinus (325)*
> *nonpyogenic (437.6)*
> *mesenteric (557.0)*
> *portal (452)*
> *precerebral (433.0–433.9)*
> *pulmonary (415.19)*

Coding Clinic: 2004, Q4, P78-80; 1992, Q1, P15-16

453.81 Acute venous embolism and thrombosis of superficial veins of upper extremity
Antecubital vein   Cephalic vein
Basilic vein

453.82 Acute venous embolism and thrombosis of deep veins of upper extremity
Brachial vein   Ulnar vein
Radial vein

453.83 Acute venous embolism and thrombosis of upper extremity, unspecified

453.84 Acute venous embolism and thrombosis of axillary veins

DISEASES OF THE CIRCULATORY SYSTEM (390–459)

◄ New   ◄▮ Revised   ~~deleted~~ Deleted   Excludes   Includes   Use additional   Code first   Omit code
● Unacceptable Principal Diagnosis   ● Use Additional Digit(s)   OGCR Official Guidelines   Coding Clinic

453.85 Acute venous embolism and thrombosis of subclavian veins

453.86 Acute venous embolism and thrombosis of internal jugular veins

453.87 Acute venous embolism and thrombosis of other thoracic veins
   Brachiocephalic (innominate)
   Superior vena cava

453.89 Acute venous embolism and thrombosis of other specified veins

453.9 Of unspecified site
   Embolism of vein   Thrombosis (vein)

● **454 Varicose veins of lower extremities**
   | Excludes | *that complicating pregnancy, childbirth, or the puerperium (671.0)*

454.0 With ulcer
   Varicose ulcer (lower extremity, any part)
   Varicose veins with ulcer of lower extremity [any part] or of unspecified site
   Any condition classifiable to 454.9 with ulcer or specified as ulcerated
   Coding Clinic: 1999, Q4, P18

454.1 With inflammation
   Stasis dermatitis
   Varicose veins with inflammation of lower extremity [any part] or of unspecified site
   Any condition classifiable to 454.9 with inflammation or specified as inflamed
   Coding Clinic: 1991, Q2, P20

454.2 With ulcer and inflammation
   Varicose veins with ulcer and inflammation of lower extremity [any part] or of unspecified site
   Any condition classifiable to 454.9 with ulcer and inflammation
   Coding Clinic: 2004, Q3, P5-6; 1991, Q2, P20

454.8 With other complications
   Edema
   Pain
   Swelling
   Coding Clinic: 2002, Q4, P58-60

454.9 Asymptomatic varicose veins
   Phlebectasia of lower extremity [any part] or of unspecified site
   Varicose veins NOS
   Varicose veins of lower extremity [any part] or of unspecified site
   Varix of lower extremity [any part] or of unspecified site

Item 7–14 Varicose/Varicosities (varix = singular, varices = plural): Enlarged, engorged, tortuous, twisted vascular vessels (veins, arteries, lymphatics). As such, the condition can present in various parts of the body, although the most familiar locations are the lower extremities. A common complication of varices is thrombophlebitis. Varicosities of the anus and rectum are called hemorrhoids. There are additional codes for esophageal, sublingual (under the tongue), scrotal, pelvic, vulval, and nasal varices as well.

Figure 7–7 Varicose veins of the legs. (From Goldman: Cecil Medicine, 23rd ed. 2008, Saunders.)

● **455 Hemorrhoids**
   | Includes | hemorrhoids (anus) (rectum)
               piles
               varicose veins, anus or rectum
   | Excludes | *that complicating pregnancy, childbirth, or the puerperium (671.8)*

455.0 Internal hemorrhoids without mention of complication
   Coding Clinic: 2005, Q3, P17

455.1 Internal thrombosed hemorrhoids

455.2 Internal hemorrhoids with other complication
   Internal hemorrhoids:
      bleeding
      prolapsed
      strangulated
      ulcerated
   Coding Clinic: 2005, Q3, P17; 2003, Q1, P8

455.3 External hemorrhoids without mention of complication
   Coding Clinic: 2007, Q1, P13

455.4 External thrombosed hemorrhoids

455.5 External hemorrhoids with other complication
   External hemorrhoids:
      bleeding
      prolapsed
      strangulated
      ulcerated
   Coding Clinic: 2005, Q3, P17; 2003, Q1, P8

455.6 Unspecified hemorrhoids without mention of complication
   Hemorrhoids NOS

455.7 Unspecified thrombosed hemorrhoids
   Thrombosed hemorrhoids, unspecified whether internal or external

455.8 Unspecified hemorrhoids with other complication
   Hemorrhoids, unspecified whether internal or external:
      bleeding
      prolapsed
      strangulated
      ulcerated

455.9 Residual hemorrhoidal skin tags
   Skin tags, anus or rectum

● **456 Varicose veins of other sites**

456.0 Esophageal varices with bleeding

456.1 Esophageal varices without mention of bleeding

● **456.2 Esophageal varices in diseases classified elsewhere**
   Code first underlying disease, as:
      cirrhosis of liver (571.0–571.9)
      portal hypertension (572.3)

   456.20 With bleeding
      Coding Clinic: 1985, Nov-Dec, P14

   456.21 Without mention of bleeding
      Coding Clinic: 2005, Q3, P15-16; 2002, Q2, P4

456.3 Sublingual varices

456.4 Scrotal varices
   Varicocele

456.5 Pelvic varices
   Varices of broad ligament

456.6 Vulval varices
   Varices of perineum
   | Excludes | *that complicating pregnancy, childbirth, or the puerperium (671.1)*

456.8 Varices of other sites
Varicose veins of nasal septum (with ulcer)

> **Excludes** *placental varices (656.7)*
> *retinal varices (362.17)*
> *varicose ulcer of unspecified site (454.0)*
> *varicose veins of unspecified site (454.9)*

Coding Clinic: 2002, Q2, P4

● **457 Noninfectious disorders of lymphatic channels**

457.0 Postmastectomy lymphedema syndrome
Elephantiasis due to mastectomy
Obliteration of lymphatic vessel due to mastectomy
Coding Clinic: 2002, Q2, P12-13

457.1 Other lymphedema
Elephantiasis (nonfilarial) NOS
Lymphangiectasis
Lymphedema:
  acquired (chronic)
  praecox
  secondary
Obliteration, lymphatic vessel

> **Excludes** *elephantiasis (nonfilarial):*
> *congenital (757.0)*
> *eyelid (374.83)*
> *vulva (624.8)*

Coding Clinic: 2004, Q3, P5-6

457.2 Lymphangitis
Lymphangitis:
  NOS
  chronic
  subacute

> **Excludes** *acute lymphangitis (682.0–682.9)*

457.8 Other noninfectious disorders of lymphatic channels
Chylocele (nonfilarial)   Lymph node or vessel:
Chylous: fistula
  ascites   infarction
  cyst   rupture

> **Excludes** *chylocele:*
> *filarial (125.0–125.9)*
> *tunica vaginalis (nonfilarial) (608.84)*

Coding Clinic: 2004, Q1, P5; 2003, Q3, P16-17

457.9 Unspecified noninfectious disorder of lymphatic channels

● **458 Hypotension**
Subnormal arterial blood pressure

> **Includes** hypopiesis

> **Excludes** *cardiovascular collapse (785.50)*
> *maternal hypotension syndrome (669.2)*
> *shock (785.50–785.59)*
> *Shy-Drager syndrome (333.0)*

Coding Clinic: 1994, Q3, P9; 1993, 5th Issue, P6-7

458.0 Orthostatic hypotension
Hypotension:
  orthostatic (chronic)
  postural
    Moving from sitting or reclining position to
    standing position precipitates sudden drop
    in blood pressure.
Coding Clinic: 2000, Q3, P8-9

458.1 Chronic hypotension
Permanent idiopathic hypotension

● **458.2 Iatrogenic hypotension**
Coding Clinic: 2002, Q3, P12; 1993, Q4, P41-42

458.21 Hypotension of hemodialysis
Intra-dialytic hypotension
Coding Clinic: 2003, Q4, P60-61

458.29 Other iatrogenic hypotension
Postoperative hypotension
Coding Clinic: 1993, Q4, P41-42

458.8 Other specified hypotension
Coding Clinic: 1997. Q4, P37

458.9 Hypotension, unspecified
Hypotension (arterial) NOS

● **459 Other disorders of circulatory system**

459.0 Hemorrhage, unspecified
Rupture of blood vessel NOS
Spontaneous hemorrhage NEC

> **Excludes** *hemorrhage:*
> *gastrointestinal NOS (578.9)*
> *in newborn NOS (772.9)*
> *nontraumatic hematoma of soft tissue*
> *(729.92)*
> *secondary or recurrent following trauma*
> *(958.2)*
> *traumatic rupture of blood vessel*
> *(900.0–904.9)*

Coding Clinic: 1999, Q4, P18

● **459.1 Postphlebitic syndrome**
Chronic venous hypertension due to deep vein
  thrombosis

> **Excludes** *chronic venous hypertension without deep*
> *vein thrombosis (459.30–459.39)*

Coding Clinic: 2002, Q4, P58-60; 1991, Q2, P20

459.10 Postphlebitic syndrome without complications
Asymptomatic postphlebitic syndrome
Postphlebitic syndrome NOS

459.11 Postphlebitic syndrome with ulcer

459.12 Postphlebitic syndrome with inflammation

459.13 Postphlebitic syndrome with ulcer and inflammation

459.19 Postphlebitic syndrome with other complication

459.2 Compression of vein
Stricture of vein
Vena cava syndrome (inferior) (superior)

● **459.3 Chronic venous hypertension (idiopathic)**
Stasis edema

> **Excludes** *chronic venous hypertension due to deep*
> *vein thrombosis (459.10–459.19)*
> *varicose veins (454.0–454.9)*

Coding Clinic: 2002, Q4, P58-60

459.30 Chronic venous hypertension without complications
Asymptomatic chronic venous hypertension
Chronic venous hypertension NOS

459.31 Chronic venous hypertension with ulcer

459.32 Chronic venous hypertension with inflammation

459.33 Chronic venous hypertension with ulcer and inflammation

459.39 Chronic venous hypertension with other complication

● **459.8 Other specified disorders of circulatory system**

459.81 Venous (peripheral) insufficiency, unspecified
Chronic venous insufficiency NOS

Use additional code for any associated
  ulceration (707.10–707.9)
Coding Clinic: 2004, Q3, P5-6; 1991, Q2, P20

459.89 Other
Collateral circulation (venous), any site
Phlebosclerosis
Venofibrosis

459.9 Unspecified circulatory system disorder

◄ New   ◄▬ Revised   ~~deleted~~ Deleted   Excludes   Includes   Use additional   Code first   Omit code
● Unacceptable Principal Diagnosis   ● Use Additional Digit(s)   OGCR Official Guidelines   Coding Clinic

8. DISEASES OF THE RESPIRATORY SYSTEM (460–519)

Use additional code to identify infectious organism

ACUTE RESPIRATORY INFECTIONS (460–466)

| Excludes | *pneumonia and influenza (480.0-488.19)* ◀ⁿⁿⁿ |

460 Acute nasopharyngitis [common cold]
Coryza (acute)
Nasal catarrh, acute

Nasopharyngitis:	Rhinitis:
NOS	acute
acute	infective
infective NOS	

Excludes	*nasopharyngitis, chronic (472.2)*
	pharyngitis:
	acute or unspecified (462)
	chronic (472.1)
	rhinitis:
	allergic (477.0–477.9)
	chronic or unspecified (472.0)
	sore throat:
	acute or unspecified (462)
	chronic (472.1)

Coding Clinic: 1988, Q1, P12

● **461 Acute sinusitis**
Code to specific sinus if indicated in documentation.

Includes	abscess, acute, of sinus (accessory) (nasal)
	empyema, acute, of sinus (accessory) (nasal)
	infection, acute, of sinus (accessory) (nasal)
	inflammation, acute, of sinus (accessory) (nasal)
	suppuration, acute, of sinus (accessory) (nasal)

| Excludes | *chronic or unspecified sinusitis (473.0–473.9)* |

461.0 Maxillary
Acute antritis

461.1 Frontal

461.2 Ethmoidal

461.3 Sphenoidal

461.8 Other acute sinusitis
Acute pansinusitis

461.9 Acute sinusitis, unspecified
Acute sinusitis NOS

462 Acute pharyngitis
Acute sore throat NOS
Pharyngitis (acute):
  NOS
  gangrenous
  infective
  phlegmonous
  pneumococcal
  staphylococcal
  suppurative
  ulcerative
Sore throat (viral) NOS
Viral pharyngitis

Excludes	*abscess:*
	peritonsillar [quinsy] (475)
	pharyngeal NOS (478.29)
	retropharyngeal (478.24)
	chronic pharyngitis (472.1)
	infectious mononucleosis (075)
	that specified as (due to):
	Coxsackie (virus) (074.0)
	gonococcus (098.6)
	herpes simplex (054.79)
	influenza (487.1, 488.02, 488.12) ◀ⁿⁿⁿ
	septic (034.0)
	streptococcal (034.0)

Coding Clinic: 1985, Sept-Oct, P9

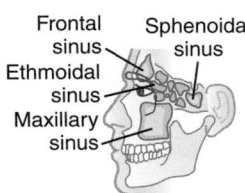

Figure 8-1 Respiratory system. (From Buck CJ: Step-by-Step Medical Coding, 2006 ed. Philadelphia, WB Saunders, 2006.)

Figure 8-2 Paranasal sinuses. (From Buck CJ: Step-by-Step Medical Coding, 2006 ed. Philadelphia, WB Saunders, 2006.)

Item 8-1 Pharyngitis is painful inflammation of the pharynx (sore throat). Ninety percent of the infections are caused by a virus with the remaining being bacterial and rarely a fungus (candidiasis). Other irritants such as pollutants, chemicals, or smoke may cause similar symptoms.

463 Acute tonsillitis
Inflammation of pharyngeal tonsils caused by virus/bacteria

Tonsillitis (acute):	Tonsillitis (acute):
NOS	septic
follicular	staphylococcal
gangrenous	suppurative
infective	ulcerative
pneumococcal	viral

Excludes	*chronic tonsillitis (474.0)*
	hypertrophy of tonsils (474.1)
	peritonsillar abscess [quinsy] (475)
	sore throat:
	acute or NOS (462)
	septic (034.0)
	streptococcal tonsillitis (034.0)

Coding Clinic: 1984, Nov-Dec, P16

● **464 Acute laryngitis and tracheitis**

Excludes	*that associated with influenza*
	(487.1, 488.02, 488.12) ◀ⁿⁿⁿ
	that due to Streptococcus (034.0)

● **464.0 Acute laryngitis**
Laryngitis (acute):
  NOS
  edematous
  Hemophilus influenzae [H. influenzae]
  pneumococcal
  septic
  suppurative
  ulcerative

Excludes	*chronic laryngitis (476.0–476.1)*
	influenzal laryngitis
	(487.1, 488.02, 488.12) ◀ⁿⁿⁿ

464.00 Without mention of obstruction

464.01 With obstruction

Item 8-2 Laryngitis is an inflammation of the larynx (voice box) resulting in hoarse voice or the complete loss of the voice. **Tracheitis** is an inflammation of the trachea (often following a URI) commonly caused by *staphylococcus aureus* resulting in inspiratory stridor (crowing sound on inspiration) and a croup-like cough.

● **464.1 Acute tracheitis**
Tracheitis (acute):   Tracheitis (acute):
  NOS   viral
  catarrhal

> Excludes   *chronic tracheitis (491.8)*

464.10 Without mention of obstruction

464.11 With obstruction

● **464.2 Acute laryngotracheitis**
Laryngotracheitis (acute)
Tracheitis (acute) with laryngitis (acute)

> Excludes   *chronic laryngotracheitis (476.1)*

464.20 Without mention of obstruction

464.21 With obstruction

● **464.3 Acute epiglottitis**
Viral epiglottitis

> Excludes   *epiglottitis, chronic (476.1)*

464.30 Without mention of obstruction

464.31 With obstruction

464.4 Croup
Croup syndrome

● **464.5 Supraglottitis, unspecified**

464.50 Without mention of obstruction
Coding Clinic: 2001, Q4, P42-43

464.51 With obstruction

● **465 Acute upper respiratory infections of multiple or
unspecified sites**

> Excludes   *upper respiratory infection due to:*
>   *influenza (487.1, 488.02, 488.12)* ◄▥
>   *Streptococcus (034.0)*

465.0 Acute laryngopharyngitis

465.8 Other multiple sites
Multiple URI
Coding Clinic: 2007, Q4, P84-86

465.9 Unspecified site
Acute URI NOS
Upper respiratory infection (acute)
Coding Clinic: 1990, Q1, P19

● **466 Acute bronchitis and bronchiolitis**

> Includes   that with:
>   bronchospasm
>   obstruction

466.0 Acute bronchitis
*Inflammation/irritation of bronchial tubes lasting 2-3
weeks, which is most commonly caused by a virus*
Bronchitis, acute or   Bronchitis, acute or
  subacute: subacute:
    fibrinous   septic
    membranous   viral
    pneumococcal   with tracheitis
    purulent
Croupous bronchitis
Tracheobronchitis, acute

> Excludes   *acute bronchitis with chronic obstructive
>   pulmonary disease (491.22)*
> Coding Clinic: 2004, Q4, P81-82,137; Q1, P3; 2002, Q4, P46; 1996,
>   Q4, P27-28; 1993, 5th Issue, P4x2; 1991, Q3, P17-18; 1988,
>   Q1, P12

OGCR   Section I.C.8.b.1
Acute bronchitis, 466.0, is due to an infectious organism. When
acute bronchitis is documented with COPD, code 491.22,
Obstructive chronic bronchitis with acute bronchitis, should
be assigned. It is not necessary to also assign code 466.0. If a
medical record documents acute bronchitis with COPD with
acute exacerbation, only code 491.22 should be assigned. The
acute bronchitis included in code 491.22 supersedes the acute
exacerbation. If a medical record documents COPD with acute
exacerbation without mention of acute bronchitis, only code
491.21 should be assigned.

● **466.1 Acute bronchiolitis**
Bronchiolitis (acute)
Capillary pneumonia
Coding Clinic: 1988, Q1, P12

**466.11 Acute bronchiolitis due to respiratory
syncytial virus (RSV)**
Coding Clinic: 2005, Q1, P10; 1996, Q4, P27-28

**466.19 Acute bronchiolitis due to other infectious
organisms**
> Use additional code to identify organism

OTHER DISEASES OF THE UPPER RESPIRATORY TRACT (470–478)

470 Deviated nasal septum
Deflected septum (nasal) (acquired)

> Excludes   *congenital (754.0)*

● **471 Nasal polyps**

> Excludes   *adenomatous polyps (212.0)*

471.0 Polyp of nasal cavity
Polyp:
  choanal
  nasopharyngeal

471.1 Polypoid sinus degeneration
Woakes' syndrome or ethmoiditis

471.8 Other polyp of sinus
Polyp of sinus:
  accessory
  ethmoidal
  maxillary
  sphenoidal

471.9 Unspecified nasal polyp
Nasal polyp NOS

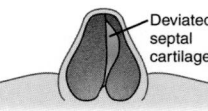
Deviated
septal
cartilage

Figure 8–3   Deviated nasal septum.

Item 8–3   A deviated nasal septum is the displacement of the septal
cartilage that separates the nares. This displacement causes obstructed
air flow through the nasal passages. A child can be born with this
displacement (congenital), or the condition may be acquired through
trauma, such as a sports injury. Symptoms include nasal block, sinusitis,
and related secondary infections. Septoplasty is surgical repair of this
condition.

Item 8-4   Nasal polyps are an abnormal growth of tissue (tumor)
projecting from a mucous membrane and attached to the surface by a
narrow elongated stalk (pedunculated). Nasal polyps usually originate
in the ethmoid sinus but also may occur in the maxillary sinus. Symptoms
are nasal block, sinusitis, anosmia, and secondary infections.

◄ New   ◄▥ Revised   ~~deleted~~ Deleted   Excludes   Includes   Use additional   Code first   Omit code
● Unacceptable Principal Diagnosis   ● Use Additional Digit(s)   OGCR Official Guidelines   Coding Clinic

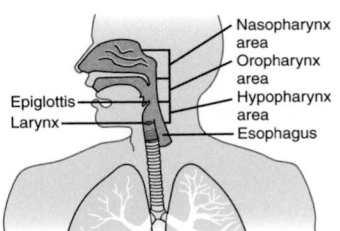

Nasopharynx area
Oropharynx area
Hypopharynx area
Esophagus
Epiglottis
Larynx

Figure 8-4   The pharynx.

Item 8-5   The **pharynx** is the passage for both food and air between the mouth and the esophagus and is divided into three areas: nasopharynx, oropharynx, and hypopharynx. The hypopharynx branches into the esophagus and the voice box.

● **472   Chronic pharyngitis and nasopharyngitis**

472.0   Chronic rhinitis
Ozena
Rhinitis: Rhinitis:
  NOS   obstructive
  atrophic   purulent
  granulomatous   ulcerative
  hypertrophic

Excludes   *allergic rhinitis (477.0–477.9)*

472.1   Chronic pharyngitis
Chronic sore throat
Pharyngitis: Pharyngitis:
  atrophic   hypertrophic
  granular (chronic)

472.2   Chronic nasopharyngitis
Excludes   *acute or unspecified nasopharyngitis (460)*

● **473   Chronic sinusitis**

Includes   abscess (chronic) of sinus (accessory) (nasal)
empyema (chronic) of sinus (accessory) (nasal)
infection (chronic) of sinus (accessory) (nasal)
suppuration (chronic) of sinus (accessory)
  (nasal)

Excludes   *acute sinusitis (461.0–461.9)*

473.0   Maxillary
Antritis (chronic)

473.1   Frontal

473.2   Ethmoidal
Excludes   *Woakes' ethmoiditis (471.1)*

473.3   Sphenoidal

473.8   Other chronic sinusitis
Pansinusitis (chronic)

473.9   Unspecified sinusitis (chronic)
Sinusitis (chronic) NOS

● **474   Chronic disease of tonsils and adenoids**

● **474.0   Chronic tonsillitis and adenoiditis**
Excludes   *acute or unspecified tonsillitis (463)*

474.00   Chronic tonsillitis
Coding Clinic: 1984, Nov-Dec, P16

474.01   Chronic adenoiditis

474.02   Chronic tonsillitis and adenoiditis

● **474.1   Hypertrophy of tonsils and adenoids**
Enlargement of tonsils or adenoids
Hyperplasia of tonsils or adenoids
Hypertrophy of tonsils or adenoids

Excludes   *that with:*
  adenoiditis (474.01)
  adenoiditis and tonsillitis (474.02)
  tonsillitis (474.00)

474.10   Tonsils with adenoids
Coding Clinic: 2005, Q2, P16

474.11   Tonsils alone
Coding Clinic: 1984, Nov-Dec, P16

474.12   Adenoids alone

474.2   Adenoid vegetations

474.8   Other chronic disease of tonsils and adenoids
Amygdalolith
Calculus, tonsil
Cicatrix of tonsil (and adenoid)
Tonsillar tag
Ulcer, tonsil

474.9   Unspecified chronic disease of tonsils and adenoids
Disease (chronic) of tonsils (and adenoids)

475   Peritonsillar abscess
Abscess of tonsil
Peritonsillar cellulitis
Quinsy

Excludes   *tonsillitis:*
  acute or NOS (463)
  chronic (474.0)

● **476   Chronic laryngitis and laryngotracheitis**

476.0   Chronic laryngitis
Laryngitis: Laryngitis:
  catarrhal   sicca
  hypertrophic

476.1   Chronic laryngotracheitis
Laryngitis, chronic, with tracheitis (chronic)
Tracheitis, chronic, with laryngitis

Excludes   *chronic tracheitis (491.8)*
  laryngitis and tracheitis, acute or
    unspecified (464.00–464.51)

● **477   Allergic rhinitis**

Includes   allergic rhinitis (nonseasonal) (seasonal)
hay fever
spasmodic rhinorrhea

Excludes   *allergic rhinitis with asthma (bronchial) (493.0)*

477.0   Due to pollen
Pollinosis

477.1   Due to food

477.2   Due to animal (cat) (dog) hair and dander

477.8   Due to other allergen

477.9   Cause unspecified
Coding Clinic: 1997, Q2, P9-10

● **478   Other diseases of upper respiratory tract**

478.0   Hypertrophy of nasal turbinates

● **478.1   Other diseases of nasal cavity and sinuses**
Excludes   *varicose ulcer of nasal septum (456.8)*
Coding Clinic: 1995, Q4, P50; 1990, Q1, P8

478.11   Nasal mucositis (ulcerative)
Use additional E code to identify adverse
  effects of therapy, such as:
  antineoplastic and immunosuppressive
    drugs (E930.7, E933.1)
  radiation therapy (E879.2)
Coding Clinic: 2006, Q4, P88-91

478.19   Other disease of nasal cavity and sinuses
Abscess of nose (septum)
Cyst or mucocele of sinus (nasal)
Necrosis of nose (septum)
Rhinolith
Ulcer of nose (septum)

DISEASES OF THE RESPIRATORY SYSTEM (460–519)

● **478.2 Other diseases of pharynx, not elsewhere classified**

     478.20 Unspecified disease of pharynx

     478.21 Cellulitis of pharynx or nasopharynx

     478.22 Parapharyngeal abscess

     478.24 Retropharyngeal abscess

     478.25 Edema of pharynx or nasopharynx

     478.26 Cyst of pharynx or nasopharynx

     478.29 Other
         Abscess of pharynx or nasopharynx

         Excludes *ulcerative pharyngitis (462)*

● **478.3 Paralysis of vocal cords or larynx**

     478.30 Paralysis, unspecified
         Laryngoplegia
         Paralysis of glottis

     478.31 Unilateral, partial

     478.32 Unilateral, complete

     478.33 Bilateral, partial

     478.34 Bilateral, complete

   478.4 Polyp of vocal cord or larynx

     Excludes *adenomatous polyps (212.1)*

   478.5 Other diseases of vocal cords
     Abscess of vocal cords
     Cellulitis of vocal cords
     Granuloma of vocal cords
     Leukoplakia of vocal cords
     Chorditis (fibrinous) (nodosa) (tuberosa)
     Singers' nodes

   478.6 Edema of larynx
     Edema (of):
       glottis
       subglottic
       supraglottic

● **478.7 Other diseases of larynx, not elsewhere classified**

     478.70 Unspecified disease of larynx

     478.71 Cellulitis and perichondritis of larynx

     478.74 Stenosis of larynx

     478.75 Laryngeal spasm
         Laryngismus (stridulus)

   478.79 Other
     Abscess of larynx
     Necrosis of larynx
     Obstruction of larynx
     Pachyderma of larynx
     Ulcer of larynx

     Excludes *ulcerative laryngitis (464.00–464.01)*
     Coding Clinic: 1991, Q3, P20

   478.8 Upper respiratory tract hypersensitivity reaction, site unspecified

     Excludes *hypersensitivity reaction of lower respiratory tract, as:*
         extrinsic allergic alveolitis (495.0–495.9)
         pneumoconiosis (500–505)

   478.9 Other and unspecified diseases of upper respiratory tract
     Abscess of trachea
     Cicatrix of trachea

PNEUMONIA AND INFLUENZA (480–488)

Excludes *pneumonia:*
     allergic or eosinophilic (518.3)
     aspiration:
         NOS (507.0)
         newborn (770.18)
         solids and liquids (507.0–507.8)
     congenital (770.0)
     lipoid (507.1)
     passive (514)
     rheumatic (390)
     ventilator-associated (997.31)

● **480 Viral pneumonia**

   480.0 Pneumonia due to adenovirus

   480.1 Pneumonia due to respiratory syncytial virus
     Coding Clinic: 1996, Q4, P27-28; 1988, Q1, P12

   480.2 Pneumonia due to parainfluenza virus

   480.3 Pneumonia due to SARS-associated coronavirus
     Coding Clinic: 2003, Q4, P46-48

   480.8 Pneumonia due to other virus not elsewhere classified

     Excludes *congenital rubella pneumonitis (771.0)*
         ~~*influenza with pneumonia, any form (487.0)*~~
         pneumonia complicating viral diseases classified elsewhere (484.1–484.8)

   480.9 Viral pneumonia, unspecified
     Coding Clinic: 1998, Q3, P5

481 Pneumococcal pneumonia [Streptococcus pneumoniae pneumonia]
     Lobar pneumonia, organism unspecified
     Coding Clinic: 2009, Q3, P9; 1998, Q2, P7; 1991, Q1, P13; 1988, Q1, P13; 1985, Mar-April, P6

● **482 Other bacterial pneumonia**

   482.0 Pneumonia due to Klebsiella pneumoniae

   482.1 Pneumonia due to Pseudomonas

   482.2 Pneumonia due to Hemophilus influenzae [H. influenzae]
     Coding Clinic: 2005, Q2, P19-20; 1993, Q4, P39

● **482.3 Pneumonia due to Streptococcus**

     Excludes *Streptococcus pneumoniae pneumonia (481)*
     Coding Clinic: 1988, Q1, P13

     482.30 Streptococcus, unspecified

     482.31 Group A

     482.32 Group B

     482.39 Other Streptococcus

Hyoid bone, greater cornu
Adipose tissue
Hyothyroid ligament
Vestibular fold
Thyroid cartilage
Vocal fold
Cartilages of trachea
Isthmus of thyroid gland

Tongue
Epiglottis
Aryepiglottic fold
Laryngeal sinus
Cuneiform cartilage
Corniculate cartilage
Arytenoid muscle
Vocal process of arytenoid cartilage
Cricoid cartilage
Muscularis of esophagus
Lumen of trachea

Figure 8–5 Coronal section of the larynx.

Item 8–6 The **larynx** extends from the tongue to the trachea and is divided into an upper and lower portion separated by folds. The framework of the larynx is cartilage composed of the single cricoid, thyroid, and epiglottic cartilages, and the paired arytenoid, cuneiform, and corniculate cartilages.

◄ New   ◄ Revised   ~~deleted~~ Deleted   Excludes   Includes   Use additional   Code first   Omit code
● Unacceptable Principal Diagnosis   ● Use Additional Digit(s)   OGCR Official Guidelines   Coding Clinic

Item 8-7 Pneumonia is an infection of the lungs, caused by a variety of microorganisms, including viruses, most commonly the *Streptococcus pneumoniae* (pneumococcus) bacteria, fungi, and parasites. Pneumonia occurs when the immune system is weakened, often by a URI or influenza.

● **482.4 Pneumonia due to Staphylococcus**
Coding Clinic: 1991, Q3, P16-17

482.40 Pneumonia due to Staphylococcus, unspecified

482.41 Methicillin susceptible pneumonia due to Staphylococcus aureus
MSSA pneumonia
Pneumonia due to Staphylococcus aureus NOS
Coding Clinic: 2008, Q4, P69-73

482.42 Methicillin resistant pneumonia due to Staphylococcus aureus
Coding Clinic: 2008, Q4, P69-73

482.49 Other Staphylococcus pneumonia

● **482.8 Pneumonia due to other specified bacteria**

Excludes   *pneumonia complicating infectious disease classified elsewhere (484.1–484.8)*
Coding Clinic: 1988, Q3, P11

482.81 Anaerobes
Bacteroides (melaninogenicus)
Gram-negative anaerobes

482.82 Escherichia coli [E. coli]

482.83 Other gram-negative bacteria
Gram-negative pneumonia NOS
Proteus
Serratia marcescens

Excludes   *gram-negative anaerobes (482.81)*
Legionnaires' disease (482.84)
Coding Clinic: 1998, Q2, P5; 1994, Q3, P9; 1993, Q4, P39

482.84 Legionnaires' disease

482.89 Other specified bacteria
Coding Clinic: 1998, Q2, P6; 1997, Q2, P6; 1994, Q1, P17-18

482.9 Bacterial pneumonia unspecified
Coding Clinic: 1998, Q2, P4, 6X2; 1997, Q2, P6; 1994, Q1, P17-18

● **483 Pneumonia due to other specified organism**

483.0 Mycoplasma pneumoniae
Eaton's agent
Pleuropneumonia-like organisms [PPLO]
Coding Clinic: 1987, Nov-Dec, P5-6

483.1 Chlamydia

483.8 Other specified organism

● **484 Pneumonia in infectious diseases classified elsewhere**

Excludes   *influenza with pneumonia, any form (487.0)*

484.1 Pneumonia in cytomegalic inclusion disease
Code first underlying disease, as: (078.5)

484.3 Pneumonia in whooping cough
Code first underlying disease, as: (033.0–033.9)

484.5 Pneumonia in anthrax
Code first underlying disease (022.1)

484.6 Pneumonia in aspergillosis
Code first underlying disease (117.3)
Coding Clinic: 1997, Q4, P40

484.7 Pneumonia in other systemic mycoses
Code first underlying disease
Excludes   *pneumonia in:*
candidiasis (112.4)
coccidioidomycosis (114.0)
histoplasmosis (115.0–115.9 with fifth-digit 5)

484.8 Pneumonia in other infectious diseases classified elsewhere

Code first underlying disease, as:
Q fever (083.0)
typhoid fever (002.0)

Excludes   *pneumonia in:*
actinomycosis (039.1)
measles (055.1)
nocardiosis (039.1)
ornithosis (073.0)
Pneumocystis carinii (136.3)
salmonellosis (003.22)
toxoplasmosis (130.4)
tuberculosis (011.6)
tularemia (021.2)
varicella (052.1)

485 Bronchopneumonia, organism unspecified
Bronchopneumonia: Pneumonia:
hemorrhagic   lobular
terminal   segmental
Pleurobronchopneumonia

Excludes   *bronchiolitis (acute) (466.11–466.19)*
chronic (491.8)
lipoid pneumonia (507.1)

486 Pneumonia, organism unspecified

Excludes   *hypostatic or passive pneumonia (514)*
influenza with pneumonia, any form (487.0)
inhalation or aspiration pneumonia due to foreign materials (507.0–507.8)
pneumonitis due to fumes and vapors (506.0)
Coding Clinic: 2010, Q1, P8; 2008, Q4, P140-143; 2006, Q2, P20; 1999, Q4, P6; Q3, P9; 1998, Q3, P7; Q2, P4-5; Q1, P8; 1997, Q3, P9; 1995, Q4, P52; 1994, Q1, P17-18; 1993, Q3, P9; Q1, P21; 1985, Mar-April, P6

● **487 Influenza**
Influenza caused by unspecified influenza virus

Excludes   *Hemophilus influenzae [H. influenzae]:*
infection NOS (041.5)
laryngitis (464.00–464.01)
meningitis (320.0)
influenza due to novel 2009 H1N1 [swine] influenza virus (488.11-488.19) ◀▥
influenza due to identified avian influenza virus (488.01-488.09) ◀▥
influenza due to identified novel H1N1 influenza virus (488.11-488.19) ◀▥

487.0 With pneumonia
Influenza with pneumonia, any form
Influenzal:
bronchopneumonia
pneumonia
Use additional code to identify the type of pneumonia (480.0–480.9, 481, 482.0–482.9, 483.0–483.8, 485)
Coding Clinic: 2010, Q1, P8; 2005, Q2, P18-19

487.1 With other respiratory manifestations
Influenza NEC ◀
Influenza NOS
Influenzal:
laryngitis
pharyngitis
respiratory infection (upper) (acute)
Coding Clinic: 2005, Q2, P18-19; 1999, Q4, P26; 1987, Jan-Feb, P16

487.8 With other manifestations
Encephalopathy due to influenza
Influenza with involvement of gastrointestinal tract

Excludes   *"intestinal flu" [viral gastroenteritis] (008.8)*

DISEASES OF THE RESPIRATORY SYSTEM (460–519)

DISEASES OF THE RESPIRATORY SYSTEM (460–519)

● 488 **Influenza due to certain identified influenza viruses**

> **Excludes** *influenza caused by unspecified influenza viruses (487.0–487.8)*

Coding Clinic: 2007, Q4, P87-88

● 488.0 **Influenza due to identified avian influenza virus** ◀▥
  Avian influenza
  Bird flu
  Influenza A/H5N1

  488.01 **Influenza due to identified avian influenza virus with pneumonia** ◀
    Avian influenzal: ◀
      bronchopneumonia ◀
      pneumonia ◀
    Influenza due to identified avian influenza virus with pneumonia, any form ◀

    > Use additional code to identify the type of pneumonia (480.0- 480.9, 481, 482.0-482.9, 483.0-483.8, 485) ◀

  488.02 **Influenza due to identified avian influenza virus with other respiratory manifestations** ◀
    Avian influenzal: ◀
      laryngitis ◀
      pharyngitis ◀
      respiratory infection (acute) (upper) ◀
    Identified avian influenza NOS ◀

  488.09 **Influenza due to identified avian influenza virus with other manifestations** ◀
    Avian influenza with involvement of gastrointestinal tract ◀
    Encephalopathy due to identified avian influenza ◀

    > **Excludes** *"intestinal flu" [viral gastroenteritis] (008.8)* ◀

● 488.1 **Influenza due to identified novel H1N1 influenza virus** ◀▥
  2009 H1N1 [swine] influenza virus
  Novel 2009 influenza H1N1
  Novel H1N1 influenza
  Novel influenza A/H1N1
  Swine flu

Coding Clinic: 2010, Q1, P8

  488.11 **Influenza due to identified novel H1N1 influenza virus with pneumonia** ◀
    Influenza due to identified novel H1N1 with pneumonia, any form ◀
    Novel H1N1 influenzal: ◀
      bronchopneumonia ◀
      pneumonia ◀

    > Use additional code to identify the type of pneumonia (480.0-480.9, 481, 482.0-482.9, 483.0-483.8, 485) ◀

  488.12 **Influenza due to identified novel H1N1 influenza virus with other respiratory manifestations** ◀
    Novel H1N1 influenza NOS ◀
    Novel H1N1 influenzal: ◀
      laryngitis ◀
      pharyngitis ◀
      respiratory infection (acute) (upper) ◀

  488.19 **Influenza due to identified novel H1N1 influenza virus with other manifestations** ◀
    Encephalopathy due to identified novel H1N1 influenza ◀
    Novel H1N1 influenza with involvement of gastrointestinal tract ◀

    > **Excludes** *"intestinal flu" [viral gastroenteritis] (008.8)* ◀

Item 8–8 Chronic bronchitis is usually defined as being present in any patient who has persistent cough with sputum production for at least three months in at least two consecutive years. **Simple chronic bronchitis** is marked by a productive cough but no pathological airflow obstruction. **Chronic obstructive pulmonary disease (COPD)** is a group of conditions—bronchitis, emphysema, asthma, bronchiectasis, allergic alveolitis—marked by dyspnea. **Catarrhal** bronchitis is an acute form of bronchitis marked by profuse mucus and pus production (**mucopurulent** discharge). **Croupous** bronchitis, also known as pseudomembranous, fibrinous, plastic, exudative, or membranous, is marked by a violent cough and dyspnea.

CHRONIC OBSTRUCTIVE PULMONARY DISEASE AND ALLIED CONDITIONS (490–496)

490 **Bronchitis, not specified as acute or chronic**

Bronchitis NOS:	Bronchitis NOS:
catarrhal	with tracheitis NOS
Tracheobronchitis NOS	

  > **Excludes** *bronchitis:*
  > *allergic NOS (493.9)*
  > *asthmatic NOS (493.9)*
  > *due to fumes and vapors (506.0)*

● 491 **Chronic bronchitis**

  > **Excludes** *chronic obstructive asthma (493.2)*

  491.0 **Simple chronic bronchitis**
    Catarrhal bronchitis, chronic
    Smokers' cough

  491.1 **Mucopurulent chronic bronchitis**
    Bronchitis (chronic) (recurrent):
      fetid   purulent
      mucopurulent
Coding Clinic: 1988, Q2, P11

● 491.2 **Obstructive chronic bronchitis**
    Bronchitis:
      emphysematous
      obstructive (chronic) (diffuse)
    Bronchitis with:
      chronic airway obstruction
      emphysema

    > **Excludes** *asthmatic bronchitis (acute) (NOS) 493.9*
    > *chronic obstructive asthma 493.2*

Coding Clinic: 2004, Q4, P81-82; 2002, Q3, P18, 19x2; 1991, Q2, P21; 1984, Nov-Dec, P17

  491.20 **Without exacerbation**
    Emphysema with chronic bronchitis
Coding Clinic: 1997, Q3, P9

  491.21 **With (acute) exacerbation**
    Acute exacerbation of chronic obstructive pulmonary disease [COPD]
    Decompensated chronic obstructive pulmonary disease [COPD]
    Decompensated chronic obstructive pulmonary disease [COPD] with exacerbation

    > **Excludes** *chronic obstructive asthma with acute exacerbation 493.22*

Coding Clinic: 2010, Q1, P9; 2004, Q1, P3; 1996, Q2, P10; 1993, 5th Issue, P5x2

491.22 With acute bronchitis
> Coding Clinic: 2006, Q3, P20; 2004, Q4, P80-81; Q1, P3

OGCR Section I.C.8.b.1
> When acute bronchitis, 466.0, is
> documented with COPD, code 491.22
> should be assigned. It is not necessary to
> also assign code 466.0. If a medical record
> documents acute bronchitis with COPD
> with acute exacerbation, only code 491.22
> should be assigned. The acute bronchitis
> included in code 491.22 supersedes the
> acute exacerbation. If a medical record
> documents COPD with acute exacerbation
> without mention of acute bronchitis, only
> code 491.21 should be assigned.

491.8 Other chronic bronchitis
Chronic: Chronic:
  tracheitis   tracheobronchitis

491.9 Unspecified chronic bronchitis
> Coding Clinic: 1991, Q3, P17-18

● **492 Emphysema**
> Coding Clinic: 1991, Q2, P21; 1984, Nov-Dec, P19

492.0 Emphysematous bleb
Giant bullous emphysema
Ruptured emphysematous bleb
Tension pneumatocele
Vanishing lung

492.8 Other emphysema
Emphysema (lung or pulmonary):
  NOS   panacinar
  centriacinar   panlobular
  centrilobular   unilateral
  obstructive   vesicular
MacLeod's syndrome
Swyer-James syndrome
Unilateral hyperlucent lung

| **Excludes** | emphysema: |
> *with chronic bronchitis 491.20–491.22)*
> *compensatory (518.2)*
> *due to fumes and vapors (506.4)*
> *interstitial (518.1)*
>   *newborn (770.2)*
> *mediastinal (518.1)*
> *surgical (subcutaneous) (998.81)*
> *traumatic (958.7)*
> Coding Clinic: 2008, Q4, P174-175; 1993, Q4, P41; 5th Issue, P4

● **493 Asthma**

| **Excludes** | *wheezing NOS (786.07)* |
> Coding Clinic: 2003, Q4, P62, 137; 1991, Q1, P13; 1985, July-Aug, P8

The following fifth-digit subclassification is for use with
category 493.0–493.2, 493.9:

> 0 **unspecified**
> 1 **with status asthmaticus**
> 2 **with (acute) exacerbation**

● **493.0 Extrinsic asthma**
[0-2] Asthma:
    allergic with stated cause
    atopic
    childhood
    hay
    platinum
  Hay fever with asthma

| **Excludes** | *asthma:* |
> *allergic NOS (493.9)*
> *detergent (507.8)*
> *miners' (500)*
> *wood (495.8)*
> Coding Clinic: 1990, Q2, P20

Item 8–9 **Asthma** is a bronchial condition marked by airway
obstruction, hyper-responsiveness, and inflammation. **Extrinsic**
asthma, also known as allergic asthma, is characterized by the
same symptoms that occur with exposure to allergens and is divided
into the following types: **atopic, occupational, and allergic
bronchopulmonary aspergillosis. Intrinsic** asthma occurs in
patients who have no history of allergy or sensitivities to allergens and is
divided into the following types: **nonreaginic and pharmacologic.
Status asthmaticus** is the most severe form of asthma attack and can
last for days or weeks.

● **493.1 Intrinsic asthma**
[0-2] Late-onset asthma
> Coding Clinic: 1990, Q2, P20

● **493.2 Chronic obstructive asthma**
[0-2] Asthma with chronic obstructive pulmonary
    disease [COPD]
Chronic asthmatic bronchitis

| **Excludes** | *acute bronchitis (466.0)* |
> *chronic obstructive bronchitis*
> *(491.20–491.22)*
> Coding Clinic: 2009, Q1, P16; 2006, Q3, P20; 2003, Q4, P108; 1993,
> 5th Issue, P4; 1991, Q2, P21; 1990, Q2, P20

● **493.8 Other forms of asthma**

493.81 Exercise induced bronchospasm
> Coding Clinic: 2003, Q4, P62

493.82 Cough variant asthma
> Coding Clinic: 2003, Q4, P62

● **493.9 Asthma, unspecified**
[0-2] Asthma (bronchial) (allergic NOS)
Bronchitis:
  allergic
  asthmatic
> Coding Clinic: 2004, Q4, P137; 2003, Q4, P108-109; Q1, P9; 1999,
> Q4, P25; 1997, Q4, P39-40; Q1, P7; 1996, Q3, P20; 1993,
> Q4, P32; 1992, Q1, P15; 1990, Q2, P20; 1984, Nov-Dec, P17

● **494 Bronchiectasis**
Bronchiectasis (fusiform) (postinfectious) (recurrent)
Bronchiolectasis

| **Excludes** | *congenital (748.61)* |
> *tuberculous bronchiectasis (current disease) (011.5)*

494.0 Bronchiectasis without acute exacerbation

494.1 Bronchiectasis with acute exacerbation

● **495 Extrinsic allergic alveolitis**

| **Includes** | allergic alveolitis and pneumonitis due to |
> inhaled organic dust particles of fungal,
> thermophilic actinomycete, or other origin

495.0 Farmers' lung

495.1 Bagassosis

495.2 Bird-fanciers' lung
Budgerigar-fanciers' disease or lung
Pigeon-fanciers' disease or lung

495.3 Suberosis
Cork-handlers' disease or lung

495.4 Malt workers' lung
Alveolitis due to Aspergillus clavatus

495.5 Mushroom workers' lung

495.6 Maple bark-strippers' lung
Alveolitis due to Cryptostroma corticale

495.7 "Ventilation" pneumonitis
Allergic alveolitis due to fungal, thermophilic
  actinomycete, and other organisms growing
  in ventilation [air conditioning] systems

◀ New ◀IIII Revised ~~deleted~~ Deleted | Excludes | Includes Use additional Code first Omit code   **853**
● Unacceptable Principal Diagnosis ● Use Additional Digit(s) OGCR Official Guidelines Coding Clinic

495.8 Other specified allergic alveolitis and pneumonitis
Cheese-washers' lung
Coffee workers' lung
Fish-meal workers' lung
Furriers' lung
Grain-handlers' disease or lung
Pituitary snuff-takers' disease
Sequoiosis or red-cedar asthma
Wood asthma

495.9 Unspecified allergic alveolitis and pneumonitis
Alveolitis, allergic (extrinsic)
Hypersensitivity pneumonitis

496 Chronic airway obstruction, not elsewhere classified
Chronic:
nonspecific lung disease
obstructive lung disease
obstructive pulmonary disease [COPD] NOS

Note: This code is not to be used with any code from categories 491–493.

Excludes *chronic obstructive lung disease [COPD] specified (as) (with):*
allergic alveolitis (495.0–495.9)
asthma (493.2)
bronchiectasis (494.0–494.1)
bronchitis (491.20–491.22)
with emphysema (491.20–491.22)
decompensated (491.21)
emphysema (492.0–492.8)
Coding Clinic: 2010, Q1, P9; 2009, Q1, P16; 2006, Q3, P20; 2003, Q4, P109-110; 2000, Q2, P15; 1994, Q1, P19; 1993, Q4, P43; 1992, Q2, P16-17; 1991, Q2, P21; 1988, Q2, P12

OGCR Section I.C.8.a.1

Code 496, Chronic airway obstruction, is a nonspecific code that should only be used when the documentation in a medical record does not specify the type of COPD being treated.

PNEUMOCONIOSES AND OTHER LUNG DISEASES DUE TO EXTERNAL AGENTS (500–508)

500 Coal workers' pneumoconiosis
Anthracosilicosis   Coal workers' lung
Anthracosis   Miners' asthma
Black lung disease

501 Asbestosis

502 Pneumoconiosis due to other silica or silicates
Pneumoconiosis due to talc
Silicotic fibrosis (massive) of lung
Silicosis (simple) (complicated)

503 Pneumoconiosis due to other inorganic dust
Aluminosis (of lung)   Graphite fibrosis (of lung)
Bauxite fibrosis (of lung)   Siderosis
Berylliosis   Stannosis

504 Pneumonopathy due to inhalation of other dust
Byssinosis
Cannabinosis
Flax-dressers' disease

Excludes *allergic alveolitis (495.0–495.9)*
asbestosis (501)
bagassosis (495.1)
farmers' lung (495.0)

505 Pneumoconiosis, unspecified

Figure 8–6 Progressive massive fibrosis superimposed on coal workers' pneumoconiosis. The large, blackened scars are located principally in the upper lobe. (From Cotran R, Kumar V, Collins T: Robbins Pathologic Basis of Disease, 6th ed. Philadelphia, WB Saunders, 1999, p 730. Courtesy of Dr. Warner Laquer, Dr. Jerome Kleinerman, and the National Institute of Occupational Safety and Health, Morgantown, WV.)

Item 8–10 Pneumoconiosis refers to a lung condition resulting from exposure to inorganic or organic airborne particles, such as coal dust or moldy hay, as well as chemical fumes and vapors, such as insecticides. In this condition, the lungs retain the airborne particles.

● **506 Respiratory conditions due to chemical fumes and vapors**

Use additional E code to identify cause

506.0 Bronchitis and pneumonitis due to fumes and vapors
Chemical bronchitis (acute)
Coding Clinic: 2008, Q3, P6-7

506.1 Acute pulmonary edema due to fumes and vapors
Chemical pulmonary edema (acute)

Excludes *acute pulmonary edema NOS (518.4)*
chronic or unspecified pulmonary edema (514)

506.2 Upper respiratory inflammation due to fumes and vapors
Coding Clinic: 2005, Q3, P10

506.3 Other acute and subacute respiratory conditions due to fumes and vapors

506.4 Chronic respiratory conditions due to fumes and vapors
Emphysema (diffuse) (chronic) due to inhalation of chemical fumes and vapors
Obliterative bronchiolitis (chronic) (subacute) due to inhalation of chemical fumes and vapors
Pulmonary fibrosis (chronic) due to inhalation of chemical fumes and vapors

506.9 Unspecified respiratory conditions due to fumes and vapors
Silo-fillers' disease

● **507 Pneumonitis due to solids and liquids**

Excludes *fetal aspiration pneumonitis (770.18)*
Coding Clinic: 1993, Q2, P9-10

507.0 Due to inhalation of food or vomitus
Aspiration pneumonia (due to):
NOS   milk
food (regurgitated) saliva
gastric secretions   vomitus
Coding Clinic: 2008, Q1, P18-19; Q1, P18-19; 1991, Q3, P16-17; 1989, Q1, P10

507.1 Due to inhalation of oils and essences
Lipoid pneumonia (exogenous)

Excludes *endogenous lipoid pneumonia (516.8)*
Coding Clinic: 1991, Q3, P16-17

507.8 Due to other solids and liquids
Detergent asthma
Coding Clinic: 1991, Q3, P16-17

◀ New   ◀ⁱⁱⁱⁱ Revised   ~~deleted~~ Deleted   Excludes   Includes   Use additional   Code first   Omit code
● Unacceptable Principal Diagnosis   ● Use Additional Digit(s)   OGCR Official Guidelines   Coding Clinic

● **508 Respiratory conditions due to other and unspecified external agents**

     Use additional E code to identify cause

   508.0 Acute pulmonary manifestations due to radiation
       Radiation pneumonitis

   508.1 Chronic and other pulmonary manifestations due to radiation
       Fibrosis of lung following radiation

   508.8 Respiratory conditions due to other specified external agents

   508.9 Respiratory conditions due to unspecified external agent

OTHER DISEASES OF RESPIRATORY SYSTEM (510–519)

● **510 Empyema**

     Use additional code to identify infectious organism (041.0–041.9)

     Excludes *abscess of lung (513.0)*

   510.0 With fistula
       Fistula:
         bronchocutaneous
         bronchopleural
         hepatopleural
         mediastinal
         pleural
         thoracic
       Any condition classifiable to 510.9 with fistula

   510.9 Without mention of fistula
       Abscess:
         pleura
         thorax
       Empyema (chest) (lung) (pleura)
       Fibrinopurulent pleurisy
       Pleurisy:
         purulent
         septic
         seropurulent
         suppurative
       Pyopneumothorax
       Pyothorax
       Coding Clinic: 2007, Q4, P109-113; 1994, Q3, P6

● **511 Pleurisy**

     Occurs when double membrane (pleura) lining chest cavity and lung surface becomes inflamed causing sharp pain on inspiration and expiration.

     Excludes *pleurisy with mention of tuberculosis, current disease (012.0)*

   511.0 Without mention of effusion or current tuberculosis
       Adhesion, lung or pleura
       Calcification of pleura
       Pleurisy (acute) (sterile):
         diaphragmatic
         fibrinous
         interlobar
       Pleurisy:
         NOS
         pneumococcal
         staphylococcal
         streptococcal
       Thickening of pleura
       Coding Clinic: 1994, Q3, P5

   511.1 With effusion, with mention of a bacterial cause other than tuberculosis
       Pleurisy with effusion (exudative) (serous):
         pneumococcal
         staphylococcal
         streptococcal
         other specified nontuberculous bacterial cause

Figure 8–7 Bullous emphysema with large subpleural bullae *(upper left)*. (From Kumar: Robbins and Cotran: Pathologic Basis of Disease, 7th ed. 2005, Saunders, An Imprint of Elsevier.)

Item 8–11 **Empyema** is a condition in which pus accumulates in a body cavity. Empyema **with fistula** occurs when the pus passes from one cavity to another organ or structure.

   ● **511.8 Other specified forms of effusion, except tuberculous**
       Excludes *traumatic (860.2–860.5, 862.29, 862.39)*
       Coding Clinic: 2008, Q1, P16-17; 1997, Q1, P10

     511.81 Malignant pleural effusion
         Code first malignant neoplasm, if known
         Coding Clinic: 2008, Q4, P113-114

     511.89 Other specified forms of effusion, except tuberculous
         Encysted pleurisy
         Hemopneumothorax
         Hemothorax
         Hydropneumothorax
         Hydrothorax

   511.9 Unspecified pleural effusion
       Pleural effusion NOS
       Pleurisy:
         exudative
         serofibrinous
         serous
         with effusion NOS
       Coding Clinic: 2003, Q2, P7-8; 1991, Q3, P19-20; 1989, Q4, P11; 1988, Q1, P9

● **512 Pneumothorax**
     Collapsed lung

   512.0 Spontaneous tension pneumothorax
       Tension pneumothorax (most serious type) occurs when air (positive pressure) collects in the pleural space

   512.1 Iatrogenic pneumothorax
       Postoperative pneumothorax
       Coding Clinic: 2003, Q3, P19

   512.8 Other spontaneous pneumothorax
       Pneumothorax: Pneumothorax:
         NOS   chronic
         acute
       Excludes *pneumothorax:*
         congenital (770.2)
         traumatic (860.0–860.1, 860.4–860.5)
         tuberculous, current disease (011.7)
       Coding Clinic: 1993, Q2, P3

● **513 Abscess of lung and mediastinum**

   513.0 Abscess of lung
       Abscess (multiple) of lung
       Gangrenous or necrotic pneumonia
       Pulmonary gangrene or necrosis
       Coding Clinic: 2007, Q4, P84-86; 2005, Q2, P14-15; 1998, Q2, P7

   513.1 Abscess of mediastinum

DISEASES OF THE RESPIRATORY SYSTEM (460–519)

514   Pulmonary congestion and hypostasis
Hypostatic:
  bronchopneumonia
  pneumonia
Passive pneumonia
Pulmonary congestion (chronic) (passive)
Pulmonary edema:
  NOS
  chronic

> **Excludes** *acute pulmonary edema:*
>   *NOS (518.4)*
>   *with mention of heart disease or failure (428.1)*
>   *hypostatic pneumonia due to or specified as a*
>   *specific type of pneumonia - code to the*
>   *type of pneumonia (480.0–480.9, 481,*
>   *482.0–482.9, 483.0–483.8, 485, 486, 487.0,*
>   *488.01, 488.11)* ◀▥

Coding Clinic: 1998, Q2, P6-7

515   Postinflammatory pulmonary fibrosis
Cirrhosis of lung chronic or unspecified
Fibrosis of lung (atrophic) (confluent) (massive)
  (perialveolar) (peribronchial) chronic or unspecified
Induration of lung chronic or unspecified

● **516   Other alveolar and parietoalveolar pneumonopathy**

516.0   Pulmonary alveolar proteinosis

516.1   Idiopathic pulmonary hemosiderosis
Essential brown induration of lung

Code first underlying disease (275.01-275.09) ◀▥

> **Excludes** *acute idiopathic pulmonary hemorrhage in*
>   *infants [AIPHI] (786.31)* ◀

516.2   Pulmonary alveolar microlithiasis

516.3   Idiopathic fibrosing alveolitis
Alveolar capillary block
Diffuse (idiopathic) (interstitial) pulmonary
  fibrosis
Hamman-Rich syndrome

516.8   Other specified alveolar and parietoalveolar pneumonopathies
Endogenous lipoid pneumonia
Interstitial pneumonia (desquamative) (lymphoid)

> **Excludes** *lipoid pneumonia, exogenous or unspecified*
>   *(507.1)*

Coding Clinic: 2010, Q1, P9; 2006, Q2, P20; 1992, Q1, P12

516.9   Unspecified alveolar and parietoalveolar pneumonopathy

● **517   Lung involvement in conditions classified elsewhere**

> **Excludes** *rheumatoid lung (714.81)*

517.1   Rheumatic pneumonia

Code first underlying disease (390)

517.2   Lung involvement in systemic sclerosis

Code first underlying disease (710.1)

517.3   Acute chest syndrome

Code first sickle-cell disease in crisis (282.42, 282.62,
282.64, 282.69)

Coding Clinic: 2003, Q4, P51-56; 1998, Q2, P8

517.8   Lung involvement in other diseases classified elsewhere

Code first underlying disease, as:
  amyloidosis (277.30–277.39)
  polymyositis (710.4)
  sarcoidosis (135)
  Sjögren's disease (710.2)
  systemic lupus erythematosus (710.0)

> **Excludes** *syphilis (095.1)*

Coding Clinic: 2003, Q2, P7-8

● **518   Other diseases of lung**

518.0   Pulmonary collapse
Atelectasis
Collapse of lung
Middle lobe syndrome

> **Excludes** *atelectasis:*
>   *congenital (partial) (770.5)*
>   *primary (770.4)*
>   *tuberculous, current disease (011.8)*

Coding Clinic: 1990, Q4, P25

518.1   Interstitial emphysema
Mediastinal emphysema

> **Excludes** *surgical (subcutaneous) emphysema*
>   *(998.81)*
>   *that in fetus or newborn (770.2)*
>   *traumatic emphysema (958.7)*

518.2   Compensatory emphysema

518.3   Pulmonary eosinophilia
Eosinophilic asthma
Löffler's syndrome
Pneumonia:
  allergic
  eosinophilic
Tropical eosinophilia

518.4   Acute edema of lung, unspecified
Acute pulmonary edema NOS
Pulmonary edema, postoperative

> **Excludes** *pulmonary edema:*
>   *acute, with mention of heart disease or*
>   *failure (428.1)*
>   *chronic or unspecified (514)*
>   *due to external agents (506.0–508.9)*

518.5   Pulmonary insufficiency following trauma and surgery
Adult respiratory distress syndrome
Pulmonary insufficiency following:
  shock
  surgery
  trauma
Shock lung

> **Excludes** *adult respiratory distress syndrome*
>   *associated with other conditions*
>   *(518.82)*
>   *pneumonia:*
>   *aspiration (507.0)*
>   *hypostatic (514)*
>   *respiratory failure in other conditions*
>   *(518.81, 518.83–518.84)*

Coding Clinic: 2004, Q4, P139

518.6   Allergic bronchopulmonary aspergillosis
Coding Clinic: 1997, Q4, P39-40

518.7   Transfusion related acute lung injury (TRALI)
Coding Clinic: 2006, Q4, P91-92

● **518.8   Other diseases of lung**

518.81   Acute respiratory failure
Respiratory failure NOS

> **Excludes** *acute and chronic respiratory failure*
>   *(518.84)*
>   *acute respiratory distress (518.82)*
>   *chronic respiratory failure (518.83)*
>   *respiratory arrest (799.1)*
>   *respiratory failure, newborn*
>   *(770.84)*

Coding Clinic: 2009, Q2, P11; 2008, Q1, P18-19; 2007, Q3,
P7-8; 2005, Q2, P19-20; Q1, P3-8; 2004, Q4, P139;
2003, Q2, P21-22; Q1, P15; 1993, Q1, P25; 1991,
Q3, P14; 1990, Q4, P25; 1987, Nov-Dec, P5-6

◀ New   ◀▥ Revised   ~~deleted~~ Deleted   **Excludes**   **Includes**   **Use additional**   **Code first**   **Omit code**
● Unacceptable Principal Diagnosis   ● Use Additional Digit(s)   **OGCR** Official Guidelines   **Coding Clinic**

518.82 Other pulmonary insufficiency, not elsewhere classified
Acute respiratory distress
Acute respiratory insufficiency
Adult respiratory distress syndrome NEC

> **Excludes** *adult respiratory distress syndrome associated with trauma or surgery (518.5)*
> *pulmonary insufficiency following trauma or surgery (518.5)*
> *respiratory distress:*
> *NOS (786.09)*
> *newborn (770.89)*
> *syndrome, newborn (769)*
> *shock lung (518.5)*

Coding Clinic: 2003, Q4, P105-106; 1995, Q1, P7; 1991, Q2, P21

518.83 Chronic respiratory failure
Coding Clinic: 2003, Q4, P103-104, 111

518.84 Acute and chronic respiratory failure
Acute on chronic respiratory failure

518.89 Other diseases of lung, not elsewhere classified
Broncholithiasis   Lung disease NOS
Calcification of lung   Pulmolithiasis
Coding Clinic: 1988, Q4, P6; 1987, Nov-Dec, P8; 1986, Sept-Oct, P10

● **519 Other diseases of respiratory system**

● **519.0 Tracheostomy complications**
These complications do not appear in the usual complication range of 996–999.

519.00 Tracheostomy complication, unspecified

519.01 Infection of tracheostomy

> **Use additional** code to identify type of infection, such as:
> abscess or cellulitis of neck (682.1)
> septicemia (038.0–038.9)

> **Use additional** code to identify organism (041.00–041.9)

Coding Clinic: 1998, Q4, P41-42

519.02 Mechanical complication of tracheostomy
Tracheal stenosis due to tracheostomy

519.09 Other tracheostomy complications
Hemorrhage due to tracheostomy
Tracheoesophageal fistula due to tracheostomy

● **519.1 Other diseases of trachea and bronchus, not elsewhere classified**
Coding Clinic: 2002, Q3, P18

519.11 Acute bronchospasm
Bronchospasm NOS

> **Excludes** *acute bronchitis with bronchospasm (466.0)*
> *asthma (493.00–493.92)*
> *exercise induced bronchospasm (493.81)*

Coding Clinic: 2006, Q4, P92-93

519.19 Other diseases of trachea and bronchus
Calcification of bronchus or trachea
Stenosis of bronchus or trachea
Ulcer of bronchus or trachea

519.2 Mediastinitis

519.3 Other diseases of mediastinum, not elsewhere classified
Fibrosis of mediastinum
Hernia of mediastinum
Retraction of mediastinum

519.4 Disorders of diaphragm
Diaphragmitis
Paralysis of diaphragm
Relaxation of diaphragm

> **Excludes** *congenital defect of diaphragm (756.6)*
> *diaphragmatic hernia (551–553 with .3)*
> *congenital (756.6)*

519.8 Other diseases of respiratory system, not elsewhere classified
Coding Clinic: 1989, Q4, P12

519.9 Unspecified disease of respiratory system
Respiratory disease (chronic) NOS

DISEASES OF THE RESPIRATORY SYSTEM (460–519)

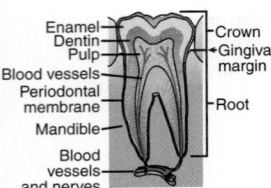

Enamel
Dentin
Pulp
Blood vessels
Periodontal
membrane
Mandible
Blood
vessels
and nerves
Crown
Gingival
margin
Root

Figure 9–1   Anatomy of a tooth.

Item 9–1   **Anodontia** is the congenital absence of teeth. **Hypodontia** is partial anodontia. **Oligodontia** is the congenital absence of some teeth, whereas **supernumerary** is having more teeth than the normal number. **Mesiodens** are small extra teeth that often appear in pairs, although single small teeth are not uncommon.

9.   DISEASES OF THE DIGESTIVE SYSTEM (520–579)

DISEASES OF ORAL CAVITY, SALIVARY GLANDS, AND JAWS (520–529)

● **520**   **Disorders of tooth development and eruption**

    520.0   **Anodontia**
       Absence of teeth (complete) (congenital) (partial)
       Hypodontia
       Oligodontia
       Excludes   *acquired absence of teeth (525.10–525.19)*

    520.1   **Supernumerary teeth**
       Distomolar   Paramolar
       Fourth molar   Supplemental teeth
       Mesiodens
       Excludes   *supernumerary roots (520.2)*

    520.2   **Abnormalities of size and form**
       Concrescence of teeth   Macrodontia
       Fusion of teeth   Microdontia
       Gemination of teeth   Peg-shaped [conical] teeth
       Dens evaginatus   Supernumerary roots
       Dens in dente   Taurodontism
       Dens invaginatus   Tuberculum paramolare
       Enamel pearls
       Excludes   *that due to congenital syphilis (090.5)*
                     tuberculum Carabelli, which is regarded as
                     a normal variation

    520.3   **Mottled teeth**
       Dental fluorosis
       Mottling of enamel
       Nonfluoride enamel opacities

    520.4   **Disturbances of tooth formation**
       Aplasia and hypoplasia of cementum
       Dilaceration of tooth
       Enamel hypoplasia (neonatal) (postnatal) (prenatal)
       Horner's teeth
       Hypocalcification of teeth
       Regional odontodysplasia
       Turner's tooth
       Excludes   *Hutchinson's teeth and mulberry molars in*
                     congenital syphilis (090.5)
                     mottled teeth (520.3)

    520.5   **Hereditary disturbances in tooth structure, not elsewhere classified**
       Amelogenesis imperfecta
       Dentinogenesis imperfecta
       Odontogenesis imperfecta
       Dentinal dysplasia
       Shell teeth

    520.6   **Disturbances in tooth eruption**
       Teeth:
         embedded
         impacted
         natal
         neonatal
         prenatal
         primary [deciduous]:
           persistent
           shedding, premature
       Tooth eruption:
         late
         obstructed
         premature
       Excludes   *exfoliation of teeth (attributable to disease of*
                     surrounding tissues) (525.0–525.19)
       Coding Clinic: 2006, Q1, P18; 2005, Q2, P15-16; 2004, Q1, P17

    520.7   **Teething syndrome**

    520.8   **Other specified disorders of tooth development and eruption**
       Color changes during tooth formation
       Pre-eruptive color changes
       Excludes   *posteruptive color changes (521.7)*

    520.9   **Unspecified disorder of tooth development and eruption**

● **521**   **Diseases of hard tissues of teeth**

   ● **521.0**   **Dental caries**

      521.00   **Dental caries, unspecified**

      521.01   **Dental caries limited to enamel**
         Initial caries
         White spot lesion

      521.02   **Dental caries extending into dentin**

      521.03   **Dental caries extending into pulp**

      521.04   **Arrested dental caries**

      521.05   **Odontoclasia**
         Infantile melanodontia
         Melanodontoclasia
         Excludes   *internal and external resorption of*
                     teeth (521.40–521.49)

      521.06   **Dental caries pit and fissure**
         Primary dental caries, pit and fissure
           origin

      521.07   **Dental caries of smooth surface**
         Primary dental caries, smooth surface
           origin

      521.08   **Dental caries of root surface**
         Primary dental caries, root surface

      521.09   **Other dental caries**
         Coding Clinic: 2002, Q3, P14

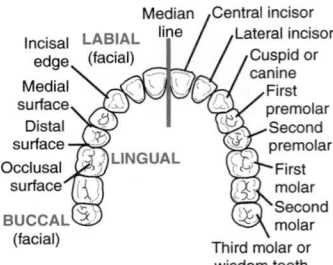

Median line
Central incisor
Incisal edge
LABIAL (facial)
Lateral incisor
Cuspid or canine
Medial surface
First premolar
Distal surface
Second premolar
Occlusal surface
LINGUAL
First molar
BUCCAL (facial)
Second molar
Third molar or wisdom tooth

Figure 9–2   The permanent teeth within the dental arch.

Item 9–2   Each dental arch (jaw) normally contains 16 teeth. Tooth decay or **dental caries** is a disease of the enamel, dentin, and cementum of the tooth and can result in a cavity.

◀ New   ◀▥ Revised   ~~deleted~~ Deleted   Excludes   Includes   Use additional   Code first   Omit code
● Unacceptable Principal Diagnosis   ● Use Additional Digit(s)   OGCR Official Guidelines   Coding Clinic

● **521.1 Excessive attrition (approximal wear) (occlusal wear)**

    521.10 Excessive attrition, unspecified

    521.11 Excessive attrition, limited to enamel

    521.12 Excessive attrition, extending into dentine

    521.13 Excessive attrition, extending into pulp

    521.14 Excessive attrition, localized

    521.15 Excessive attrition, generalized

● **521.2 Abrasion**
    Abrasion of teeth:
      dentifrice
      habitual
      occupational
      ritual
      traditional
    Wedge defect NOS of teeth

    521.20 Abrasion, unspecified

    521.21 Abrasion, limited to enamel

    521.22 Abrasion, extending into dentine

    521.23 Abrasion, extending into pulp

    521.24 Abrasion, localized

    521.25 Abrasion, generalized

● **521.3 Erosion**
    Erosion of teeth:
      NOS
      due to:
        medicine
        persistent vomiting
      idiopathic
      occupational

    521.30 Erosion, unspecified

    521.31 Erosion, limited to enamel

    521.32 Erosion, extending into dentine

    521.33 Erosion, extending into pulp

    521.34 Erosion, localized

    521.35 Erosion, generalized

● **521.4 Pathological resorption**

    521.40 Pathological resorption, unspecified

    521.41 Pathological resorption, internal

    521.42 Pathological resorption, external

    521.49 Other pathological resorption
        Internal granuloma of pulp

    521.5 Hypercementosis
        Cementation hyperplasia

    521.6 Ankylosis of teeth

    521.7 Intrinsic posteruptive color changes
        Staining [discoloration] of teeth:
          NOS
          due to:
            drugs
            metals
          pulpal bleeding

      Excludes *accretions [deposits] on teeth (523.6)*
              extrinsic color changes (523.6)
              pre-eruptive color changes (520.8)

● **521.8 Other specified diseases of hard tissues of teeth**

    521.81 Cracked tooth

      Excludes *asymptomatic craze lines in*
            enamel - omit code
            broken tooth due to trauma
               (873.63, 873.73)
            fractured tooth due to trauma
               (873.63, 873.73)

    521.89 Other specified diseases of hard tissues of teeth
        Irradiated enamel
        Sensitive dentin

    521.9 Unspecified disease of hard tissues of teeth

● **522 Diseases of pulp and periapical tissues**

    522.0 Pulpitis
        Pulpal:
          abscess
          polyp
        Pulpitis:
          acute
          chronic (hyperplastic) (ulcerative)
          suppurative

    522.1 Necrosis of the pulp
        Pulp gangrene

    522.2 Pulp degeneration
        Denticles   Pulp calcifications
        Pulp stones

    522.3 Abnormal hard tissue formation in pulp
        Secondary or irregular dentin

    522.4 Acute apical periodontitis of pulpal origin

    522.5 Periapical abscess without sinus
        Abscess:
          dental
          dentoalveolar

      Excludes *periapical abscess with sinus (522.7)*

    522.6 Chronic apical periodontitis
        Apical or periapical granuloma
        Apical periodontitis NOS

    522.7 Periapical abscess with sinus
        Fistula:
          alveolar process
          dental

    522.8 Radicular cyst
        Cyst:
          apical (periodontal)
          periapical
          radiculodental
          residual radicular

      Excludes *lateral developmental or lateral periodontal*
               cyst (526.0)

    522.9 Other and unspecified diseases of pulp and periapical tissues

● **523 Gingival and periodontal diseases**

  ● **523.0 Acute gingivitis**

      Excludes *acute necrotizing ulcerative gingivitis (101)*
               herpetic gingivostomatitis (054.2)

    523.00 Acute gingivitis, plaque induced
        Acute gingivitis NOS

    523.01 Acute gingivitis, non-plaque induced

Item 9–3 Acute gingivitis, also known as orilitis or ulitis, is the short-term, severe inflammation of the gums (gingiva) caused by bacteria. **Chronic gingivitis** is persistent inflammation of the gums. When the gingivitis moves into the periodontium it is called periodontitis, also known as paradentitis.

DISEASES OF THE DIGESTIVE SYSTEM (520–579)

DISEASES OF THE DIGESTIVE SYSTEM (520–579)

● **523.1 Chronic gingivitis**
Gingivitis (chronic):
   desquamative   simple marginal
   hyperplastic   ulcerative
   Excludes *herpetic gingivostomatitis (054.2)*

   523.10 Chronic gingivitis, plaque induced
      Chronic gingivitis NOS
      Gingivitis NOS

   523.11 Chronic gingivitis, non-plaque induced

● **523.2 Gingival recession**
Gingival recession (postinfective) (postoperative)

   523.20 Gingival recession, unspecified

   523.21 Gingival recession, minimal

   523.22 Gingival recession, moderate

   523.23 Gingival recession, severe

   523.24 Gingival recession, localized

   523.25 Gingival recession, generalized

● **523.3 Aggressive and acute periodontitis**
Acute:
   pericementitis
   pericoronitis
   Excludes *acute apical periodontitis (522.4)*
               periapical abscess (522.5, 522.7)

   523.30 Aggressive periodontitis, unspecified

   523.31 Aggressive periodontitis, localized
      Periodontal abscess

   523.32 Aggressive periodontitis, generalized

   523.33 Acute periodontitis

● **523.4 Chronic periodontitis**
Chronic pericoronitis
Pericementitis (chronic)
Periodontitis:
   NOS
   complex
   simplex
   Excludes *chronic apical periodontitis (522.6)*

   523.40 Chronic periodontitis, unspecified

   523.41 Chronic periodontitis, localized

   523.42 Chronic periodontitis, generalized

523.5 Periodontosis

523.6 Accretions on teeth
Dental calculus:
   subgingival
   supragingival
Deposits on teeth:
   betel
   materia alba
   soft
   tartar
   tobacco
Extrinsic discoloration of teeth
   Excludes *intrinsic discoloration of teeth (521.7)*

523.8 Other specified periodontal diseases
Giant cell:
   epulis
   peripheral granuloma
Gingival:
   cysts
   enlargement NOS
   fibromatosis
Gingival polyp
Periodontal lesions due to traumatic occlusion
Peripheral giant cell granuloma
   Excludes *leukoplakia of gingiva (528.6)*

523.9 Unspecified gingival and periodontal disease
Coding Clinic: 2002, Q3, P14

● **524 Dentofacial anomalies, including malocclusion**
 ● **524.0 Major anomalies of jaw size**
   Excludes *hemifacial atrophy or hypertrophy (754.0)*
               unilateral condylar hyperplasia or
               hypoplasia of mandible

   524.00 Unspecified anomaly

   524.01 Maxillary hyperplasia

   524.02 Mandibular hyperplasia

   524.03 Maxillary hypoplasia

   524.04 Mandibular hypoplasia

   524.05 Macrogenia

   524.06 Microgenia

   524.07 Excessive tuberosity of jaw
      Entire maxillary tuberosity

   524.09 Other specified anomaly

 ● **524.1 Anomalies of relationship of jaw to cranial base**
   524.10 Unspecified anomaly
      Prognathism   Retrognathism

   524.11 Maxillary asymmetry

   524.12 Other jaw asymmetry

   524.19 Other specified anomaly

 ● **524.2 Anomalies of dental arch relationship**
Anomaly of dental arch
   Excludes *hemifacial atrophy or hypertrophy (754.0)*
               soft tissue impingement (524.81–524.82)
               unilateral condylar hyperplasia or
               hypoplasia of mandible (526.89)

   524.20 Unspecified anomaly of dental arch relationship

   524.21 Malocclusion, Angle's class I
      Neutro-occlusion

   524.22 Malocclusion, Angle's class II
      Disto-occlusion Division I
      Disto-occlusion Division II

   524.23 Malocclusion, Angle's class III
      Mesio-occlusion

   524.24 Open anterior occlusal relationship
      Anterior open bite

   524.25 Open posterior occlusal relationship
      Posterior open bite

   524.26 Excessive horizontal overlap
      Excessive horizontal overjet

   524.27 Reverse articulation
      Anterior articulation
      Crossbite
      Posterior articulation

   524.28 Anomalies of interarch distance
      Excessive interarch distance
      Inadequate interarch distance

   524.29 Other anomalies of dental arch relationship
      Other anomalies of dental arch

Figure 9–3 Dentofacial malocclusion.

Item 9–4 **Hyperplasia** is a condition of overdevelopment, whereas **hypoplasia** is a condition of underdevelopment. **Macrogenia** is overdevelopment of the chin, whereas microgenia is underdevelopment of the chin.

◀ New   ◀◀◀ Revised   ~~deleted~~ Deleted   Excludes   Includes   Use additional   Code first   Omit code
● Unacceptable Principal Diagnosis   ● Use Additional Digit(s)   OGCR Official Guidelines   Coding Clinic

●**524.3 Anomalies of tooth position of fully erupted teeth**

> Excludes *impacted or embedded teeth with abnormal position of such teeth or adjacent teeth (520.6)*

Coding Clinic: 2004, Q1, P17

524.30 Unspecified anomaly of tooth position
Diastema of teeth NOS
Displacement of teeth NOS
Transposition of teeth NOS

524.31 Crowding of teeth

524.32 Excessive spacing of teeth

524.33 Horizontal displacement of teeth
Tipped teeth
Tipping of teeth

524.34 Vertical displacement of teeth
Extruded tooth
Infraeruption of teeth
Intruded tooth
Supraeruption of teeth

524.35 Rotation of tooth/teeth

524.36 Insufficient interocclusal distance of teeth (ridge)
Lack of adequate intermaxillary vertical dimension

524.37 Excessive interocclusal distance of teeth
Excessive intermaxillary vertical dimension
Loss of occlusal vertical dimension

524.39 Other anomalies of tooth position

524.4 Malocclusion, unspecified

●**524.5 Dentofacial functional abnormalities**

524.50 Dentofacial functional abnormality, unspecified

524.51 Abnormal jaw closure

524.52 Limited mandibular range of motion

524.53 Deviation in opening and closing of the mandible

524.54 Insufficient anterior guidance
Insufficient anterior occlusal guidance

524.55 Centric occlusion maximum intercuspation discrepancy
Centric occlusion of teeth discrepancy

524.56 Non-working side interference
Balancing side interference

524.57 Lack of posterior occlusal support

524.59 Other dentofacial functional abnormalities
Abnormal swallowing
Mouth breathing
Sleep postures
Tongue, lip, or finger habits

●**524.6 Temporomandibular joint disorders**

> Excludes *current temporomandibular joint: dislocation (830.0–830.1) strain (848.1)*

524.60 Temporomandibular joint disorders, unspecified
Temporomandibular joint-pain-dysfunction syndrome [TMJ]

524.61 Adhesions and ankylosis (bony or fibrous)

524.62 Arthralgia of temporomandibular joint

524.63 Articular disc disorder (reducing or nonreducing)

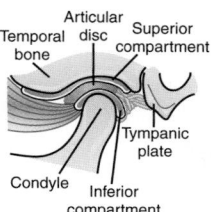

Figure 9–4 Temporomandibular joint.

Item 9–5 Dysfunction of the temporomandibular joint is termed **temporomandibular joint (TMJ) syndrome** and is characterized by pain and tenderness/spasm of the muscles of mastication, joint noise, and in the later stages, limited mandibular movement.

524.64 Temporomandibular joint sounds on opening and/or closing the jaw

524.69 Other specified temporomandibular joint disorders

●**524.7 Dental alveolar anomalies**

524.70 Unspecified alveolar anomaly

524.71 Alveolar maxillary hyperplasia

524.72 Alveolar mandibular hyperplasia

524.73 Alveolar maxillary hypoplasia

524.74 Alveolar mandibular hypoplasia

524.75 Vertical displacement of alveolus and teeth
Extrusion of alveolus and teeth

524.76 Occlusal plane deviation

524.79 Other specified alveolar anomaly

●**524.8 Other specified dentofacial anomalies**

524.81 Anterior soft tissue impingement

524.82 Posterior soft tissue impingement

524.89 Other specified dentofacial anomalies

524.9 Unspecified dentofacial anomalies

●**525 Other diseases and conditions of the teeth and supporting structures**

525.0 Exfoliation of teeth due to systemic causes

●**525.1 Loss of teeth due to trauma, extraction, or periodontal disease**

> *Code first class of edentulism (525.40–525.44, 525.50–525.54)*

525.10 Acquired absence of teeth, unspecified
Tooth extraction status, NOS

525.11 Loss of teeth due to trauma
Check for E code assignment.

525.12 Loss of teeth due to periodontal disease

525.13 Loss of teeth due to caries

525.19 Other loss of teeth

●**525.2 Atrophy of edentulous alveolar ridge**

525.20 Unspecified atrophy of edentulous alveolar ridge
Atrophy of the mandible NOS
Atrophy of the maxilla NOS

525.21 Minimal atrophy of the mandible

525.22 Moderate atrophy of the mandible

525.23 Severe atrophy of the mandible

525.24 Minimal atrophy of the maxilla

525.25 Moderate atrophy of the maxilla

525.26 Severe atrophy of the maxilla

DISEASES OF THE DIGESTIVE SYSTEM (520–579)

DISEASES OF THE DIGESTIVE SYSTEM (520–579)

525.3   **Retained dental root**

● 525.4   **Complete edentulism**

> Use additional code to identify cause of edentulism (525.10–525.19)

    525.40   **Complete edentulism, unspecified**
        Edentulism NOS

    525.41   **Complete edentulism, class I**

    525.42   **Complete edentulism, class II**

    525.43   **Complete edentulism, class III**

    525.44   **Complete edentulism, class IV**

● 525.5   **Partial edentulism**

> Use additional code to identify cause of edentulism (525.10–525.19)

    525.50   **Partial edentulism, unspecified**

    525.51   **Partial edentulism, class I**

    525.52   **Partial edentulism, class II**

    525.53   **Partial edentulism, class III**

    525.54   **Partial edentulism, class IV**

● 525.6   **Unsatisfactory restoration of tooth**
     Defective bridge, crown, fillings
     Defective dental restoration

> **Excludes**   *dental restoration status (V45.84)*
> *unsatisfactory endodontic treatment (526.61–526.69)*

    525.60   **Unspecified unsatisfactory restoration of tooth**
        Unspecified defective dental restoration

    525.61   **Open restoration margins**
        Dental restoration failure of marginal integrity
        Open margin on tooth restoration

    525.62   **Unrepairable overhanging of dental restorative materials**
        Overhanging of tooth restoration

    525.63   **Fractured dental restorative material without loss of material**

> **Excludes**   *cracked tooth (521.81)*
> *fractured tooth (873.63, 873.73)*

    525.64   **Fractured dental restorative material with loss of material**

> **Excludes**   *cracked tooth (521.81)*
> *fractured tooth (873.63, 873.73)*

    525.65   **Contour of existing restoration of tooth biologically incompatible with oral health**
        Dental restoration failure of periodontal anatomical integrity
        Unacceptable contours of existing restoration
        Unacceptable morphology of existing restoration

    525.66   **Allergy to existing dental restorative material**

> Use additional code to identify the specific type of allergy

    525.67   **Poor aesthetics of existing restoration**
        Dental restoration aesthetically inadequate or displeasing

    525.69   **Other unsatisfactory restoration of existing tooth**

● 525.7   **Endosseous dental implant failure**

    525.71   **Osseointegration failure of dental implant**
        Failure of dental implant due to infection
        Failure of dental implant due to unintentional loading
        Failure of dental implant osseointegration due to premature loading
        Failure of dental implant to osseointegrate prior to intentional prosthetic loading
        Hemorrhagic complications of dental implant placement
        Iatrogenic osseointegration failure of dental implant
        Osseointegration failure of dental implant due to complications of systemic disease
        Osseointegration failure of dental implant due to poor bone quality
        Pre-integration failure of dental implant NOS
        Pre-osseointegration failure of dental implant

    525.72   **Post-osseointegration biological failure of dental implant**
        Failure of dental implant due to lack of attached gingiva
        Failure of dental implant due to occlusal trauma (caused by poor prosthetic design)
        Failure of dental implant due to parafunctional habits
        Failure of dental implant due to periodontal infection (peri-implantitis)
        Failure of dental implant due to poor oral hygiene
        Failure of dental implant to osseointegrate following intentional prosthetic loading
        Iatrogenic post-osseointegration failure of dental implant
        Post-osseointegration failure of dental implant due to complications of systemic disease

    525.73   **Post-osseointegration mechanical failure of dental implant**
        Failure of dental prosthesis causing loss of dental implant
        Fracture of dental implant
        Mechanical failure of dental implant NOS

> **Excludes**   *cracked tooth (521.81)*
> *fractured dental restorative material with loss of material (525.64)*
> *fractured dental restorative material without loss of material (525.63)*
> *fractured tooth (873.63, 873.73)*

    525.79   Other endosseous dental implant failure
        Dental implant failure NOS

525.8   **Other specified disorders of the teeth and supporting structures**
     Enlargement of alveolar ridge NOS
     Irregular alveolar process

525.9   **Unspecified disorder of the teeth and supporting structures**

◀ New   ◀▦ Revised   ~~deleted~~ Deleted   Excludes   Includes   Use additional   Code first   Omit code
● Unacceptable Principal Diagnosis   ● Use Additional Digit(s)   OGCR Official Guidelines   Coding Clinic

● **526 Diseases of the jaws**

526.0 Developmental odontogenic cysts
Cyst:
  dentigerous
  eruption
  follicular
  lateral developmental
  lateral periodontal
  primordial
Keratocyst
| **Excludes** | radicular cyst (522.8) |

526.1 Fissural cysts of jaw
Cyst:
  globulomaxillary
  incisor canal
  median anterior maxillary
  median palatal
  nasopalatine
  palatine of papilla
| **Excludes** | cysts of oral soft tissues (528.4) |

526.2 Other cysts of jaws
Cyst of jaw: Cyst of jaw:
  NOS   hemorrhagic
  aneurysmal   traumatic

526.3 Central giant cell (reparative) granuloma
| **Excludes** | peripheral giant cell granuloma (523.8) |

526.4 Inflammatory conditions
Abscess of jaw (acute) (chronic) (suppurative)
Osteitis of jaw (acute) (chronic) (suppurative)
Osteomyelitis (neonatal) of jaw (acute) (chronic)
  (suppurative)
Periostitis of jaw (acute) (chronic) (suppurative)
Sequestrum of jaw bone
| **Excludes** | alveolar osteitis (526.5) |
| | osteonecrosis of jaw (733.45) |

526.5 Alveolitis of jaw
Alveolar osteitis
Dry socket

● **526.6 Periradicular pathology associated with previous endodontic treatment**

　526.61 Perforation of root canal space

　526.62 Endodontic overfill

　526.63 Endodontic underfill

　526.69 Other periradicular pathology associated with previous endodontic treatment

● **526.8 Other specified diseases of the jaws**

　526.81 Exostosis of jaw
　　Torus mandibularis
　　Torus palatinus

　526.89 Other
　　Cherubism
　　Fibrous dysplasia of jaw(s)
　　Latent bone cyst of jaw(s)
　　Osteoradionecrosis of jaw(s)
　　Unilateral condylar hyperplasia or
　　　hypoplasia of mandible

526.9 Unspecified disease of the jaws

● **527 Diseases of the salivary glands**

527.0 Atrophy

527.1 Hypertrophy

Figure 9–5   Major salivary glands.

Parotid gland
Sublingual gland
Submandibular gland

Item 9–6   **Atrophy** is wasting away of a tissue or organ, whereas **hypertrophy** is overdevelopment or enlargement of a tissue or organ. **Sialoadenitis** is salivary gland inflammation. **Parotitis** is the inflammation of the parotid gland. In the epidemic form, parotitis is also known as mumps. **Sialolithiasis** is the formation of calculus within a salivary gland. **Mucocele** is a polyp composed of mucus.

527.2 Sialoadenitis
Parotitis: Sialoangitis
  NOS   Sialodochitis
  allergic
  toxic
Excludes	epidemic or infectious parotitis
	(072.0–072.9)
	uveoparotid fever (135)

527.3 Abscess

527.4 Fistula
| **Excludes** | congenital fistula of salivary gland (750.24) |

527.5 Sialolithiasis
Calculus of salivary gland or duct
Stone of salivary gland or duct
Sialodocholithiasis

527.6 Mucocele
Mucous:
  extravasation cyst of salivary gland
  retention cyst of salivary gland
Ranula

527.7 Disturbance of salivary secretion
Hyposecretion   Sialorrhea
Ptyalism   Xerostomia

527.8 Other specified diseases of the salivary glands
Benign lymphoepithelial lesion of salivary gland
Sialectasia
Sialosis
Stenosis of salivary duct
Stricture of salivary duct

527.9 Unspecified disease of the salivary glands

● **528 Diseases of the oral soft tissues, excluding lesions specific for gingiva and tongue**

● **528.0 Stomatitis and mucositis (ulcerative)**
Excludes	Stevens-Johnson syndrome (695.13)
	stomatitis:
	acute necrotizing ulcerative (101)
	aphthous (528.2)
	cellulitis and abscess of mouth (528.3)
	diphtheritic stomatitis (032.0)
	epizootic stomatitis (078.4)
	gangrenous (528.1)
	gingivitis (523.0–523.1)
	herpetic (054.2)
	oral thrush (112.0)
	Vincent's (101)

Coding Clinic: 1999, Q2, P9

　528.00 Stomatitis and mucositis, unspecified
　　Mucositis NOS
　　Ulcerative mucositis NOS
　　Ulcerative stomatitis NOS
　　Vesicular stomatitis NOS

DISEASES OF THE DIGESTIVE SYSTEM (520–579)

Item 9–7 **Stomatitis** is the inflammation of the oral mucosa. **Cancrum oris,** also known as **noma** or **gangrenous stomatitis,** begins as an ulcer of the gingiva and results in a progressive gangrenous process. Mucositis is the inflammation of the mucous membranes lining the digestive tract from the mouth to the anus. It is a common side effect of chemotherapy and of radiotherapy that involves any part of the digestive tract.

528.01 Mucositis (ulcerative) due to antineoplastic therapy
> Use additional E code to identify adverse effects of therapy, such as:
> antineoplastic and immunosuppressive drugs (E930.7, E933.1)
> radiation therapy (E879.2)
> Coding Clinic: 2006, Q4, P88-91

528.02 Mucositis (ulcerative) due to other drugs
> Use additional E code to identify drug

528.09 Other stomatitis and mucositis (ulcerative)

528.1 Cancrum oris
> Gangrenous stomatitis
> Noma

528.2 Oral aphthae
> Aphthous stomatitis
> Canker sore
> Periadenitis mucosa necrotica recurrens
> Recurrent aphthous ulcer
> Stomatitis herpetiformis
> **Excludes** *herpetic stomatitis (054.2)*

528.3 Cellulitis and abscess
> Cellulitis of mouth (floor)
> Ludwig's angina
> Oral fistula
> **Excludes** *abscess of tongue (529.0)*
> *cellulitis or abscess of lip (528.5)*
> *fistula (of):*
> *dental (522.7)*
> *lip (528.5)*
> *gingivitis (523.00–523.11)*

528.4 Cysts
> Dermoid cyst of mouth
> Epidermoid cyst of mouth
> Epstein's pearl of mouth
> Lymphoepithelial cyst of mouth
> Nasoalveolar cyst of mouth
> Nasolabial cyst of mouth
> **Excludes** *cyst:*
> *gingiva (523.8)*
> *tongue (529.8)*

528.5 Diseases of lips

Abscess of lip(s)	Cheilitis:
Cellulitis of lip(s)	NOS
Fistula of lip(s)	angular
Hypertrophy of lip(s)	Cheilodynia
	Cheilosis

> **Excludes** *actinic cheilitis (692.79)*
> *congenital fistula of lip (750.25)*
> *leukoplakia of lips (528.6)*
> Coding Clinic: 1986, Sept-Oct, P10

528.6 Leukoplakia of oral mucosa, including tongue
> *Considered precancerous and evidenced by thickened white patches of epithelium on mucous membranes*
> Leukokeratosis of oral mucosa
> Leukoplakia of:
> gingiva
> lips
> tongue
> **Excludes** *carcinoma in situ (230.0, 232.0)*
> *leukokeratosis nicotina palati (528.79)*

Figure 9–6 Oral leukoplakia and associated squamous carcinoma. (From Feldman: Sleisenger & Fordtran's Gastrointestinal and Liver Disease, 8th ed. 2006, Saunders, An Imprint of Elsevier.)

● **528.7 Other disturbances of oral epithelium, including tongue**
> **Excludes** *carcinoma in situ (230.0, 232.0)*
> *leukokeratosis NOS (702.8)*

528.71 Minimal keratinized residual ridge mucosa
> Minimal keratinization of alveolar ridge mucosa

528.72 Excessive keratinized residual ridge mucosa
> Excessive keratinization of alveolar ridge mucosa

528.79 Other disturbances of oral epithelium, including tongue
> Erythroplakia of mouth or tongue
> Focal epithelial hyperplasia of mouth or tongue
> Leukoedema of mouth or tongue
> Leukokeratosis nicotina palati
> Other oral epithelium disturbances

528.8 Oral submucosal fibrosis, including of tongue

528.9 Other and unspecified diseases of the oral soft tissues
> Cheek and lip biting
> Denture sore mouth
> Denture stomatitis
> Melanoplakia
> Papillary hyperplasia of palate
> Eosinophilic granuloma of oral mucosa
> Irritative hyperplasia of oral mucosa
> Pyogenic granuloma of oral mucosa
> Ulcer (traumatic) of oral mucosa

● **529 Diseases and other conditions of the tongue**

529.0 Glossitis
> Abscess of tongue
> Ulceration (traumatic) of tongue
> **Excludes** *glossitis:*
> *benign migratory (529.1)*
> *Hunter's (529.4)*
> *median rhomboid (529.2)*
> *Moeller's (529.4)*

529.1 Geographic tongue
> Benign migratory glossitis
> Glossitis areata exfoliativa

529.2 Median rhomboid glossitis

529.3 Hypertrophy of tongue papillae
> Black hairy tongue
> Coated tongue
> Hypertrophy of foliate papillae
> Lingua villosa nigra

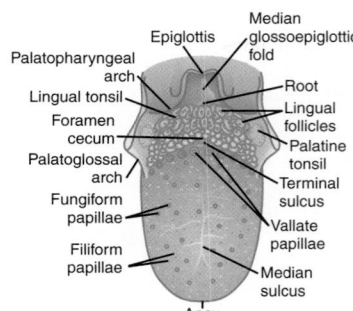

Palatopharyngeal arch
Lingual tonsil
Foramen cecum
Palatoglossal arch
Fungiform papillae
Filiform papillae
Apex
Epiglottis
Median glossoepiglottic fold
Root
Lingual follicles
Palatine tonsil
Terminal sulcus
Vallate papillae
Median sulcus

Figure 9–7 Structure of the tongue.

DISEASES OF THE DIGESTIVE SYSTEM (520–579)

529.4 Atrophy of tongue papillae
Bald tongue   Glossodynia exfoliativa
Glazed tongue   Smooth atrophic tongue
Glossitis:
Hunter's
Moeller's

529.5 Plicated tongue
Fissured tongue   Scrotal tongue
Furrowed tongue

> **Excludes** *fissure of tongue, congenital (750.13)*

529.6 Glossodynia
Glossopyrosis   Painful tongue

> **Excludes** *glossodynia exfoliativa (529.4)*

529.8 Other specified conditions of the tongue
Atrophy (of) tongue
Crenated (of) tongue
Enlargement (of) tongue
Hypertrophy (of) tongue
Glossocele
Glossoptosis

> **Excludes** *erythroplasia of tongue (528.79)*
> *leukoplakia of tongue (528.6)*
> *macroglossia (congenital) (750.15)*
> *microglossia (congenital) (750.16)*
> *oral submucosal fibrosis (528.8)*

529.9 Unspecified condition of the tongue

DISEASES OF ESOPHAGUS, STOMACH, AND DUODENUM (530–538)

● **530 Diseases of esophagus**

> **Excludes** *esophageal varices (456.0–456.2)*

530.0 Achalasia and cardiospasm
Achalasia (of cardia)
Aperistalsis of esophagus
Megaesophagus

> **Excludes** *congenital cardiospasm (750.7)*

● **530.1 Esophagitis**
Esophagitis: Esophagitis:
chemical   postoperative
peptic   regurgitant
Use additional E code to identify cause, if induced
by chemical

> **Excludes** *tuberculous esophagitis (017.8)*

Coding Clinic: 1985, Sept-Oct, P9

530.10 Esophagitis, unspecified
Esophagitis NOS
Coding Clinic: 2005, Q3, P17-18

530.11 Reflux esophagitis
Coding Clinic: 1995, Q4, P82

530.12 Acute esophagitis

530.13 Eosinophilic esophagitis
Coding Clinic: 2008, Q4, P115-116

530.19 Other esophagitis
Abscess of esophagus
Coding Clinic: 2001, Q3, P15

● **530.2 Ulcer of esophagus**
Ulcer of esophagus
fungal
peptic
Ulcer of esophagus due to ingestion of:
aspirin
chemicals
medicines
Use additional E code to identify cause, if induced
by chemical or drug

530.20 Ulcer of esophagus without bleeding
Ulcer of esophagus NOS

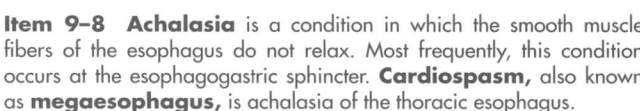

Figure 9–8 The esophagus is the muscular tube that connects the pharynx and the stomach. The 10 inch (25 cm) long esophagus is divided into three parts: **cervical, thoracic,** and **abdominal.**

Item 9–8 Achalasia is a condition in which the smooth muscle fibers of the esophagus do not relax. Most frequently, this condition occurs at the esophagogastric sphincter. **Cardiospasm,** also known as **megaesophagus,** is achalasia of the thoracic esophagus.

Item 9–9 Dyskinesia is difficulty in moving, and **diverticulum** is a sac or pouch.

530.21 Ulcer of esophagus with bleeding

> **Excludes** *bleeding esophageal varices (456.0, 456.20)*

530.3 Stricture and stenosis of esophagus
Compression of esophagus
Obstruction of esophagus

> **Excludes** *congenital stricture of esophagus (750.3)*

Coding Clinic: 2001, Q2, P4; 1997, Q2, P3; 1988, Q1, P13

530.4 Perforation of esophagus
Rupture of esophagus

> **Excludes** *traumatic perforation of esophagus (862.22, 862.32, 874.4–874.5)*

530.5 Dyskinesia of esophagus
Corkscrew esophagus
Curling esophagus
Esophagospasm
Spasm of esophagus

> **Excludes** *cardiospasm (530.0)*

Coding Clinic: 1988, Q1, P13; 1984, Nov-Dec, P19

Figure 9–9 A. Ulcer. **B.** Perforated ulcer. **C.** Laparoscopic view of a perforated duodenal ulcer *(arrow)* with fibrinous exudate on the adjacent peritoneum. (**C** from Feldman: Sleisenger & Fordtran's Gastrointestinal and Liver Disease, 8th ed. 2006, Saunders, An Imprint of Elsevier.)

Item 9–10 Gastric ulcers are lesions of the stomach that result in the death of the tissue and a defect of the surface. **Perforated ulcers** are those in which the lesion penetrates the gastric wall, leaving a hole. **Peptic ulcers** are lesions of the stomach or the duodenum. **Peptic** refers to the gastric juice, pepsin.

DISEASES OF THE DIGESTIVE SYSTEM (520–579)

530.6 Diverticulum of esophagus, acquired
Diverticulum, acquired:
   epiphrenic
   pharyngoesophageal
   pulsion
   subdiaphragmatic
   traction
   Zenker's (hypopharyngeal)
Esophageal pouch, acquired
Esophagocele, acquired

> **Excludes** *congenital diverticulum of esophagus*
> *(750.4)*

Coding Clinic: 1985, Mar-April, P15

530.7 Gastroesophageal laceration-hemorrhage syndrome
Mallory-Weiss syndrome

● **530.8 Other specified disorders of esophagus**

530.81 Esophageal reflux
Gastroesophageal reflux

> **Excludes** *reflux esophagitis (530.11)*

Coding Clinic: 2001, Q2, P4; 1995, Q1, P7

530.82 Esophageal hemorrhage

> **Excludes** *hemorrhage due to esophageal*
> *varices (456.0–456.2)*

Coding Clinic: 2005, Q1, P17-18

530.83 Esophageal leukoplakia

530.84 Tracheoesophageal fistula

> **Excludes** *congenital tracheoesophageal fistula*
> *(750.3)*

530.85 Barrett's esophagus
Coding Clinic: 2003, Q4, P63

530.86 Infection of esophagostomy

> Use additional code to specify infection
> Coding Clinic: 2004, Q4, P83

530.87 Mechanical complication of esophagostomy
Malfunction of esophagostomy
Coding Clinic: 2004, Q4, P83

530.89 Other

> **Excludes** *Paterson-Kelly syndrome (280.8)*

530.9 Unspecified disorder of esophagus

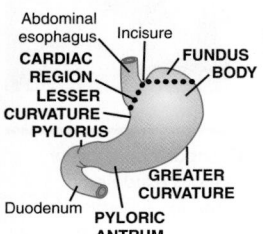

Abdominal esophagus
Incisure
CARDIAC REGION
FUNDUS
BODY
LESSER CURVATURE
PYLORUS
Duodenum
GREATER CURVATURE
PYLORIC ANTRUM

Figure 9–10   Parts of the stomach.

Item 9–11   **Esophageal reflux** is the return flow of the contents of the stomach to the esophagus and is referred to as GERD and/or "heartburn." **Gastroesophageal reflux** is the return flow of the contents of the stomach and duodenum to the esophagus. **Esophageal leukoplakia** are white areas on the mucous membrane of the esophagus for which no specific cause can be identified.

● **531 Gastric ulcer**

> **Includes**   ulcer (peptic):
>   prepyloric
>   pylorus
>   stomach

> Use additional E code to identify drug, if drug-induced

> **Excludes** *peptic ulcer NOS (533.0–533.9)*

Coding Clinic: 1990, Q4, P27

The following fifth-digit subclassification is for use with category 531:

0	without mention of obstruction
1	with obstruction

● **531.0 Acute with hemorrhage**
[0-1]   Coding Clinic: 1984, Nov-Dec, P15

● **531.1 Acute with perforation**
[0-1]

● **531.2 Acute with hemorrhage and perforation**
[0-1]

● **531.3 Acute without mention of hemorrhage or**
[0-1] **perforation**

● **531.4 Chronic or unspecified with hemorrhage**
[0-1]

● **531.5 Chronic or unspecified with perforation**
[0-1]

● **531.6 Chronic or unspecified with hemorrhage and**
[0-1] **perforation**

● **531.7 Chronic without mention of hemorrhage or**
[0-1] **perforation**

● **531.9 Unspecified as acute or chronic, without mention of**
[0-1] **hemorrhage or perforation**

● **532 Duodenal ulcer**

> **Includes**   erosion (acute) of duodenum
>   ulcer (peptic):
>   duodenum
>   postpyloric

> Use additional E code to identify drug, if drug-induced

> **Excludes** *peptic ulcer NOS (533.0–533.9)*

Coding Clinic: 1990, Q4, P27

The following fifth-digit subclassification is for use with category 532:

0	without mention of obstruction
1	with obstruction

● **532.0 Acute with hemorrhage**
[0-1]

● **532.1 Acute with perforation**
[0-1]

● **532.2 Acute with hemorrhage and perforation**
[0-1]

● **532.3 Acute without mention of hemorrhage or**
[0-1] **perforation**

● **532.4 Chronic or unspecified with hemorrhage**
[0-1]

● **532.5 Chronic or unspecified with perforation**
[0-1]

● **532.6 Chronic or unspecified with hemorrhage and**
[0-1] **perforation**

● **532.7 Chronic without mention of hemorrhage or**
[0-1] **perforation**

● **532.9 Unspecified as acute or chronic, without mention of**
[0-1] **hemorrhage or perforation**

◀ New   ◀▥ Revised   ~~deleted~~ Deleted   Excludes   Includes   Use additional   Code first   Omit code
● Unacceptable Principal Diagnosis   ● Use Additional Digit(s)   OGCR Official Guidelines   Coding Clinic

● **533 Peptic ulcer, site unspecified**

> **Includes** gastroduodenal ulcer NOS
> peptic ulcer NOS
> stress ulcer NOS

> Use additional E code to identify drug, if drug-induced

> **Excludes** *peptic ulcer:*
> *duodenal (532.0–532.9)*
> *gastric (531.0–531.9)*
> Coding Clinic: 1990, Q4, P27

The following fifth-digit subclassification is for use with category 533:

> 0 **without mention of obstruction**
> 1 **with obstruction**

● **533.0 Acute with hemorrhage**
[0-1]

● **533.1 Acute with perforation**
[0-1]

● **533.2 Acute with hemorrhage and perforation**
[0-1]

● **533.3 Acute without mention of hemorrhage and**
[0-1] **perforation**

● **533.4 Chronic or unspecified with hemorrhage**
[0-1]

● **533.5 Chronic or unspecified with perforation**
[0-1]

● **533.6 Chronic or unspecified with hemorrhage and**
[0-1] **perforation**

● **533.7 Chronic without mention of hemorrhage or**
[0-1] **perforation**
> Coding Clinic: 1989, Q2, P16

● **533.9 Unspecified as acute or chronic, without mention of**
[0-1] **hemorrhage or perforation**

● **534 Gastrojejunal ulcer**

> **Includes** ulcer (peptic) or erosion:
> anastomotic
> gastrocolic
> gastrointestinal
> gastrojejunal
> jejunal
> marginal
> stomal

> **Excludes** *primary ulcer of small intestine (569.82)*
> Coding Clinic: 1990, Q4, P27

The following fifth-digit subclassification is for use with category 534:

> 0 **without mention of obstruction**
> 1 **with obstruction**

● **534.0 Acute with hemorrhage**
[0-1]

● **534.1 Acute with perforation**
[0-1]

● **534.2 Acute with hemorrhage and perforation**
[0-1]

● **534.3 Acute without mention of hemorrhage or**
[0-1] **perforation**

● **534.4 Chronic or unspecified with hemorrhage**
[0-1]

● **534.5 Chronic or unspecified with perforation**
[0-1]

● **534.6 Chronic or unspecified with hemorrhage and**
[0-1] **perforation**

● **534.7 Chronic without mention of hemorrhage or**
[0-1] **perforation**

● **534.9 Unspecified as acute or chronic, without mention of**
[0-1] **hemorrhage or perforation**

Item 9–12 Gastritis is a severe inflammation of the stomach. **Atrophic gastritis** is a chronic inflammation of the stomach that results in destruction of the cells of the mucosa of the stomach. Duodenitis is an inflammation of the duodenum, the first section of the small intestine.

● **535 Gastritis and duodenitis**
> Coding Clinic: 2007, Q2, P13; 2005, Q3, P17-18

The following fifth-digit subclassification is for use with category 535:

> 0 **without mention of hemorrhage**
> 1 **with hemorrhage**

● **535.0 Acute gastritis**
[0-1] > Coding Clinic: 1992, Q2, P8-9; 1986, Nov-Dec, P9

● **535.1 Atrophic gastritis**
[0-1] Gastritis:
> atrophic-hyperplastic   chronic (atrophic)
> Coding Clinic: 1994, Q1, P18

● **535.2 Gastric mucosal hypertrophy**
[0-1] Hypertrophic gastritis

● **535.3 Alcoholic gastritis**
[0-1]

● **535.4 Other specified gastritis**
[0-1] Gastritis:
> allergic
> bile induced
> irritant
> superficial
> toxic

> **Excludes** *eosinophilic gastritis (535.7)*
> Coding Clinic: 1990, Q4, P27

● **535.5 Unspecified gastritis and gastroduodenitis**
[0-1] > Coding Clinic: 2005, Q3, P17-18; 1999, Q4, P25-26; 1992, Q3, P15

● **535.6 Duodenitis**
[0-1] > Coding Clinic: 2005, Q3, P17-18

● **535.7 Eosinophilic gastritis**
[0-1] > Coding Clinic: 2008, Q4, P115-116

● **536 Disorders of function of stomach**

> **Excludes** *functional disorders of stomach specified as*
> *psychogenic (306.4)*

536.0 Achlorhydria

536.1 Acute dilatation of stomach
> Acute distention of stomach

536.2 Persistent vomiting
> Cyclical vomiting
> Habit vomiting
> Persistent vomiting [not of pregnancy]
> Uncontrollable vomiting

> **Excludes** *bilious emesis (vomiting) (787.04)*
> *excessive vomiting in pregnancy*
> *(643.0–643.9)*
> *vomiting NOS (787.03)*
> *cyclical, associated with migraine*
> *(346.2)*
> *vomiting of fecal matter (569.87)*

536.3 Gastroparesis
> Gastroparalysis

> *Code first underlying disease, such as:*
> diabetes mellitus (249.6, 250.6)
> Coding Clinic: 2004, Q2, P7-8x2; 2001, Q2, P4

Item 9–13 Achlorhydria, also known as gastric anacidity, is the absence of gastric acid. **Gastroparesis** is paralysis of the stomach.

◀ New ◀▥▥ Revised ~~deleted~~ Deleted | Excludes | | Includes | | Use additional | | Code first | | Omit code |
● Unacceptable Principal Diagnosis ● Use Additional Digit(s) OGCR Official Guidelines Coding Clinic

867

● **536.4　Gastrostomy complications**

　　536.40　Gastrostomy complication, unspecified

　　536.41　Infection of gastrostomy

　　　　Use additional code to identify type of
　　　　　infection, such as:
　　　　abscess or cellulitis of abdomen (682.2)
　　　　septicemia (038.0–038.9)
　　　　Use additional code to identify organism
　　　　　(041.00–041.9)
　　　　Coding Clinic: 1998, Q4, P42-44

　　536.42　Mechanical complication of gastrostomy

　　536.49　Other gastrostomy complications
　　　　Coding Clinic: 1998, Q4, P42-44

536.8　Dyspepsia and other specified disorders of function of stomach

Achylia gastrica	Hyperchlorhydria
Hourglass contraction	Hypochlorhydria
of stomach	Indigestion
Hyperacidity	Tachygastria

　　Excludes *achlorhydria (536.0)*
　　　　　　heartburn (787.1)
　　Coding Clinic: 1993, Q2, P6; 1989, Q2, P16; 1984, Nov-Dec, P9

536.9　Unspecified functional disorder of stomach
　　Functional gastrointestinal:
　　　disorder
　　　disturbance
　　　irritation
　　Coding Clinic: 2007, Q1, P19

● **537　Other disorders of stomach and duodenum**

537.0　Acquired hypertrophic pyloric stenosis
　　Constriction of pylorus, acquired or adult
　　Obstruction of pylorus, acquired or adult
　　Stricture of pylorus, acquired or adult
　　Excludes *congenital or infantile pyloric stenosis (750.5)*
　　Coding Clinic: 2001, Q2, P17-18; 1985, Jan-Feb, P14-15

537.1　Gastric diverticulum
　　Excludes *congenital diverticulum of stomach (750.7)*

537.2　Chronic duodenal ileus

537.3　Other obstruction of duodenum
　　Cicatrix of duodenum
　　　Cicatrix = scar
　　Stenosis of duodenum
　　　Stenosis = narrowing
　　Stricture of duodenum
　　　Stricture = narrowing
　　Volvulus of duodenum
　　　Volvulus = twisting/knotting
　　Excludes *congenital obstruction of duodenum (751.1)*

537.4　Fistula of stomach or duodenum
　　Gastrocolic fistula
　　Gastrojejunocolic fistula

537.5　Gastroptosis

537.6　Hourglass stricture or stenosis of stomach
　　Cascade stomach
　　Excludes *congenital hourglass stomach (750.7)*
　　　　　　hourglass contraction of stomach (536.8)

● **537.8　Other specified disorders of stomach and duodenum**

　　537.81　Pylorospasm
　　　　Excludes *congenital pylorospasm (750.5)*

　　537.82　Angiodysplasia of stomach and duodenum without mention of hemorrhage
　　　　Coding Clinic: 2007, Q2, P9; 1996, Q3, P10

　　537.83　Angiodysplasia of stomach and duodenum with hemorrhage
　　　　Coding Clinic: 2007, Q2, P9

　　537.84　Dieulafoy lesion (hemorrhagic) of stomach and duodenum
　　　　Coding Clinic: 2002, Q4, P60-61

　　537.89　Other
　　　　Gastric or duodenal:
　　　　　prolapse
　　　　　rupture
　　　　Intestinal metaplasia of gastric mucosa
　　　　Passive congestion of stomach
　　　　Excludes *diverticula of duodenum (562.00–562.01)*
　　　　　　　gastrointestinal hemorrhage (578.0–578.9)
　　　　Coding Clinic: 2005, Q3, P15-16

537.9　Unspecified disorder of stomach and duodenum

● **538　Gastrointestinal mucositis (ulcerative)**
　　Use additional E code to identify adverse effects of therapy, such as:
　　antineoplastic and immunosuppressive drugs (E930.7, E933.1)
　　radiation therapy (E879.2)
　　Excludes *mucositis (ulcerative) of mouth and oral soft tissue (528.00–528.09)*

　　　　　　APPENDICITIS (540–543)

● **540　Acute appendicitis**

540.0　With generalized peritonitis
　　Appendicitis (acute) with: perforation, peritonitis (generalized), rupture:
　　　fulminating
　　　gangrenous
　　　obstructive
　　Cecitis (acute) with: perforation, peritonitis (generalized), rupture
　　Rupture of appendix
　　Excludes *acute appendicitis with peritoneal abscess (540.1)*
　　Coding Clinic: 1984, Nov-Dec, P19

540.1　With peritoneal abscess
　　Abscess of appendix
　　　With generalized peritonitis
　　Coding Clinic: 1984, Nov-Dec, P19

540.9　Without mention of peritonitis
　　Acute:
　　　appendicitis without mention of perforation, peritonitis, or rupture:
　　　　fulminating
　　　　gangrenous
　　　　inflamed
　　　　obstructive
　　　cecitis without mention of perforation, peritonitis, or rupture
　　Coding Clinic: 2001, Q1, P15-16; 1997, Q4, P52

● **541　Appendicitis, unqualified**
　　Coding Clinic: 1990, Q2, P26

● **542　Other appendicitis**
　　Appendicitis:
　　　chronic
　　　recurrent
　　　relapsing
　　　subacute
　　Excludes *hyperplasia (lymphoid) of appendix (543.0)*
　　Coding Clinic: 2001, Q1, P15-16

◀ New　⬅ Revised　~~deleted~~ Deleted　Excludes　Includes　Use additional　Code first　Omit code
● Unacceptable Principal Diagnosis　● Use Additional Digit(s)　OGCR Official Guidelines　Coding Clinic

DISEASES OF THE DIGESTIVE SYSTEM (520–579)

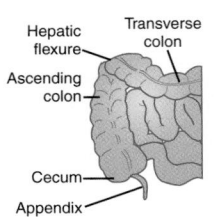

Hepatic flexure
Transverse colon
Ascending colon
Cecum
Appendix

Figure 9-11 Acute appendicitis is the inflammation of the appendix, usually associated with obstruction. Most often this is a disease of adolescents and young adults.

● **543 Other diseases of appendix**

543.0 Hyperplasia of appendix (lymphoid)

543.9 Other and unspecified diseases of appendix
Appendicular or appendiceal:
colic
concretion
fistula
Diverticulum of appendix
Fecalith of appendix
Intussusception of appendix
Mucocele of appendix
Stercolith of appendix

HERNIA OF ABDOMINAL CAVITY (550–553)

Includes   hernia:
acquired
congenital, except diaphragmatic or hiatal

● **550 Inguinal hernia**

Includes   bubonocele
inguinal hernia (direct) (double) (indirect) (oblique) (sliding)
scrotal hernia

The following fifth-digit subclassification is for use with category 550:

> 0 unilateral or unspecified (not specified as recurrent)
>   **Unilateral NOS**
> 1 unilateral or unspecified, recurrent
> 2 bilateral (not specified as recurrent)
>   **Bilateral NOS**
> 3 bilateral, recurrent

● **550.0 Inguinal hernia, with gangrene**
[0-3]   Inguinal hernia with gangrene (and obstruction)

Right Lumbar	Umbilical	Left Lumbar
RIGHT INGUINAL OR ILIAC	Hypogastric or pubic	LEFT INGUINAL OR ILIAC

Figure 9-12 Inguinal hernias are those that are located in the inguinal or iliac areas of the abdomen.

● **550.1 Inguinal hernia, with obstruction, without mention**
[0-3] **of gangrene**
Inguinal hernia with mention of incarceration, irreducibility, or strangulation

● **550.9 Inguinal hernia, without mention of obstruction or**
[0-3] **gangrene**
Inguinal hernia NOS
Coding Clinic: 2003, Q3, P10-11; 2003, Q1, P4; 1985, Nov-Dec, P12; 1984, May-June, P11

● **551 Other hernia of abdominal cavity, with gangrene**
Includes   that with gangrene (and obstruction)

● **551.0 Femoral hernia with gangrene**

551.00 Unilateral or unspecified (not specified as recurrent)
Femoral hernia NOS with gangrene

551.01 Unilateral or unspecified, recurrent

551.02 Bilateral (not specified as recurrent)

551.03 Bilateral, recurrent

551.1 Umbilical hernia with gangrene
Parumbilical hernia specified as gangrenous

● **551.2 Ventral hernia with gangrene**

551.20 Ventral, unspecified, with gangrene

551.21 Incisional, with gangrene
Hernia:
postoperative specified as gangrenous
recurrent, ventral specified as gangrenous

551.29 Other
Epigastric hernia specified as gangrenous

551.3 Diaphragmatic hernia with gangrene
Hernia:
hiatal (esophageal) (sliding) specified as gangrenous
paraesophageal specified as gangrenous
Thoracic stomach specified as gangrenous
Excludes   congenital diaphragmatic hernia (756.6)

551.8 Hernia of other specified sites, with gangrene
Any condition classifiable to 553.8 if specified as gangrenous

551.9 Hernia of unspecified site, with gangrene
Any condition classifiable to 553.9 if specified as gangrenous

● **552 Other hernia of abdominal cavity, with obstruction, but without mention of gangrene**
Excludes   that with mention of gangrene (551.0–551.9)

● **552.0 Femoral hernia with obstruction**
Femoral hernia specified as incarcerated, irreducible, strangulated, or causing obstruction

552.00 Unilateral or unspecified (not specified as recurrent)

552.01 Unilateral or unspecified, recurrent

552.02 Bilateral (not specified as recurrent)

552.03 Bilateral, recurrent

Item 9-14 Hernias of the groin are the most common type, accounting for 80 percent of all hernias. There are two major types of inguinal hernias: indirect (oblique) affecting men only and direct. **Indirect inguinal hernias** result when the intestines emerge through the abdominal wall in an indirect fashion through the inguinal canal. **Direct inguinal hernias** penetrate through the abdominal wall in a direct fashion. **Femoral hernias** occur at the femoral ring where the femoral vessels enter the thigh and is most common in women. An abdominal wall hernia is also called a ventral or epigastric hernia and occurs in both sexes. Classification is based on location of the hernia and whether there is obstruction or gangrene.

Item 9-15 Ventral, epigastric, or incisional hernia occurs on the abdominal surface caused by musculature weakness or a tear at a previous surgical site and is evidenced by a bulge that changes in size, becoming larger with exertion. An **incarcerated** hernia is one in which the intestines become trapped in the hernia. A **strangulated** hernia is one in which the blood supply to the intestines is lost. Hiatal hernia occurs when a loop of the stomach protrudes upward through the small opening in the diaphragm through which the esophagus passes, leaving the abdominal cavity and entering the chest. It occurs in both sexes.

DISEASES OF THE DIGESTIVE SYSTEM (520–579)

552.1 Umbilical hernia with obstruction
Parumbilical hernia specified as incarcerated, irreducible, strangulated, or causing obstruction

● **552.2 Ventral hernia with obstruction**
Ventral hernia specified as incarcerated, irreducible, strangulated, or causing obstruction

552.20 Ventral, unspecified, with obstruction

552.21 Incisional, with obstruction
Hernia:
postoperative specified as incarcerated, irreducible, strangulated, or causing obstruction
recurrent, ventral specified as incarcerated, irreducible, strangulated, or causing obstruction
Coding Clinic: 2003, Q3, P11

552.29 Other
Epigastric hernia specified as incarcerated, irreducible, strangulated, or causing obstruction

552.3 Diaphragmatic hernia with obstruction
Hernia:
hiatal (esophageal) (sliding) specified as incarcerated, irreducible, strangulated, or causing obstruction
paraesophageal specified as incarcerated, irreducible, strangulated, or causing obstruction
Thoracic stomach specified as incarcerated, irreducible, strangulated, or causing obstruction
Excludes *congenital diaphragmatic hernia (756.6)*

552.8 Hernia of other specified sites, with obstruction
Any condition classifiable to 553.8 if specified as incarcerated, irreducible, strangulated, or causing obstruction
Excludes ~~*hernia due to adhesion with obstruction (560.81)*~~
Coding Clinic: 2004, Q1, P10-11

552.9 Hernia of unspecified site, with obstruction
Any condition classifiable to 553.9 if specified as incarcerated, irreducible, strangulated, or causing obstruction

● **553 Other hernia of abdominal cavity without mention of obstruction or gangrene**
Excludes *the listed conditions with mention of:*
gangrene (and obstruction) (551.0–551.9)
obstruction (552.0–552.9)

● **553.0 Femoral hernia**

553.00 Unilateral or unspecified (not specified as recurrent)
Femoral hernia NOS

553.01 Unilateral or unspecified, recurrent

553.02 Bilateral (not specified as recurrent)

553.03 Bilateral, recurrent

553.1 Umbilical hernia
Parumbilical hernia

● **553.2 Ventral hernia**

553.20 Ventral, unspecified
Coding Clinic: 2006, Q2, P10-11; 2003, Q3, P6-7; 1996, Q3, P15

553.21 Incisional
Hernia:
postoperative
recurrent, ventral
Coding Clinic: 2003, Q3, P6

553.29 Other
Hernia:
epigastric
spigelian

553.3 Diaphragmatic hernia
Hernia:
hiatal (esophageal) (sliding)
paraesophageal
Thoracic stomach
Excludes *congenital:*
diaphragmatic hernia (756.6)
hiatal hernia (750.6)
esophagocele (530.6)
Coding Clinic: 2001, Q2, P6; 2000, Q1, P6

553.8 Hernia of other specified sites
Hernia:
ischiatic
ischiorectal
lumbar
obturator
pudendal
retroperitoneal
sciatic
Other abdominal hernia of specified site
Excludes *vaginal enterocele (618.6)*

553.9 Hernia of unspecified site
Enterocele   Rupture (nontraumatic)
Epiplocele   Sarcoepiplocele
Hernia:
NOS
interstitial
intestinal
intra-abdominal

NONINFECTIOUS ENTERITIS AND COLITIS (555–558)

● **555 Regional enteritis**
Includes Crohn's disease
Granulomatous enteritis
Excludes *ulcerative colitis (556)*

555.0 Small intestine
Ileitis:
regional
segmental
terminal
Regional enteritis or Crohn's disease of:
duodenum
ileum
jejunum

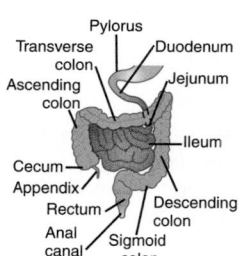

Figure 9–13 Small and large intestines.

Item 9–16 Crohn's disease, also known as **regional enteritis,** is a chronic inflammatory disease of the intestines. Classification is based on location in the small (duodenum, ileum, jejunum) or large (cecum, colon, rectum, anal canal) intestine.

◄ New   ◄▥ Revised   ~~deleted~~ Deleted   Excludes   Includes   Use additional   Code first   Omit code
● Unacceptable Principal Diagnosis   ● Use Additional Digit(s)   OGCR Official Guidelines   Coding Clinic

Item 9–17 Ulcerative colitis attacks the colonic mucosa and forms abscesses. The disease involves the intestines. Classification is based on the location:

Enterocolitis: large and small intestine
Ileocolitis: ileum and colon
Proctitis: rectum
Proctosigmoiditis: sigmoid colon and rectum

555.1 Large intestine
Colitis:
granulomatous
regional
transmural
Regional enteritis or Crohn's disease of:
colon
large bowel
rectum
Coding Clinic: 1999, Q3, P8

555.2 Small intestine with large intestine
Regional ileocolitis
Coding Clinic: 2003, Q1, P18

555.9 Unspecified site
Crohn's disease NOS
Regional enteritis NOS
Coding Clinic: 2009, Q1, P20; 2005, Q2, P11-12; 1999, Q3, P8-9; 1997, Q4, P37; Q2, P3; 1996, Q1, P13; 1988, Q2, P9-10

●**556 Ulcerative colitis**

556.0 Ulcerative (chronic) enterocolitis

556.1 Ulcerative (chronic) ileocolitis

556.2 Ulcerative (chronic) proctitis

556.3 Ulcerative (chronic) proctosigmoiditis

556.4 Pseudopolyposis of colon

556.5 Left-sided ulcerative (chronic) colitis

556.6 Universal ulcerative (chronic) colitis
Pancolitis

556.8 Other ulcerative colitis

556.9 Ulcerative colitis, unspecified
Ulcerative enteritis NOS
Coding Clinic: 2003, Q1, P10-11

●**557 Vascular insufficiency of intestine**
Excludes *necrotizing enterocolitis of the newborn (777.50–777.53)*

557.0 Acute vascular insufficiency of intestine
Acute:
hemorrhagic enterocolitis
ischemic colitis, enteritis, or enterocolitis
massive necrosis of intestine
Bowel infarction
Embolism of mesenteric artery
Fulminant enterocolitis
Hemorrhagic necrosis of intestine
Infarction of appendices epiploicae
Intestinal gangrene
Intestinal infarction (acute) (agnogenic) (hemorrhagic) (nonocclusive)
Mesenteric infarction (embolic) (thrombotic)
Necrosis of intestine
Terminal hemorrhagic enteropathy
Thrombosis of mesenteric artery
Coding Clinic: 2008, Q2, P15-16

557.1 Chronic vascular insufficiency of intestine
Angina, abdominal
Chronic ischemic colitis, enteritis, or enterocolitis
Ischemic stricture of intestine
Mesenteric:
angina
artery syndrome (superior)
vascular insufficiency
Coding Clinic: 1996, Q3, P9-10; 1986, Nov-Dec, P11; 1985, Sept-Oct, P9

557.9 Unspecified vascular insufficiency of intestine
Alimentary pain due to vascular insufficiency
Ischemic colitis, enteritis, or enterocolitis NOS

●**558 Other and unspecified noninfectious gastroenteritis and colitis**
Excludes *infectious:*
colitis, enteritis, or gastroenteritis (009.0–009.1)
diarrhea (009.2–009.3)

558.1 Gastroenteritis and colitis due to radiation
Radiation enterocolitis

558.2 Toxic gastroenteritis and colitis
Use additional E code to identify cause
Coding Clinic: 2008, Q2, P10-11

558.3 Allergic gastroenteritis and colitis
Use additional code to identify type of food allergy (V15.01–V15.05)
Coding Clinic: 2008, Q4, P115-116; 2003, Q1, P12

●**558.4 Eosinophilic gastroenteritis and colitis**

558.41 Eosinophilic gastroenteritis
Eosinophilic enteritis
Coding Clinic: 2008, Q4, P115-116

558.42 Eosinophilic colitis
Coding Clinic: 2008, Q4, P115-116

558.9 Other and unspecified noninfectious gastroenteritis and colitis
Colitis, NOS, dietetic, or noninfectious
Enteritis, NOS, dietetic, or noninfectious
Gastroenteritis, NOS, dietetic, or noninfectious
Ileitis, NOS, dietetic or noninfectious
Jejunitis, NOS, dietetic, or noninfectious
Sigmoiditis, NOS, dietetic, or noninfectious
Coding Clinic: 2008, Q2, P10-11; Q1, P10-12; 1999, Q3, P4-7; 1987, Nov-Dec, P7-8; 1984, July-Aug, P19-20

OTHER DISEASES OF INTESTINES AND PERITONEUM (560–569)

●**560 Intestinal obstruction without mention of hernia**
Excludes *duodenum (537.2–537.3)*
inguinal hernia with obstruction (550.1)
intestinal obstruction complicating hernia (552.0–552.9)
mesenteric:
embolism (557.0)
infarction (557.0)
thrombosis (557.0)
neonatal intestinal obstruction (277.01, 777.1–777.2, 777.4)

560.0 Intussusception
Intussusception (colon) (intestine) (rectum)
Invagination of intestine or colon
Excludes *intussusception of appendix (543.9)*
Coding Clinic: 1998, Q4, P82-83

Figure 9–14 Types of intussusception.

SIMPLE TYPES   DOUBLE TYPES

Cecum and appendix

Ileum
Ileocecal valve

Ileum Ileocecal
valve

ILEOCOLIC

ILEOCECAL

Item 9–18 Intussusception is the prolapse (telescoping) of a part of the intestine into another adjacent part of the intestine. Intussusception may be enteric (ileoileal, jejunoileal, jejunojejunal), colic (colocolic), or intracolic (ileocecal, ileocolic).

Item 9–19 Volvulus is the twisting of a segment of the intestine, resulting in obstruction. Paralytic ileus is paralysis of the intestine. It need not be a complete paralysis, but it must prohibit the passage of food through the intestine and lead to intestinal blockage. It is a common aftermath of some types of surgery.

560.1 **Paralytic ileus**
   Adynamic ileus
   Ileus (of intestine) (of bowel) (of colon)
   Paralysis of intestine or colon
   | Excludes | gallstone ileus (560.31)
   Coding Clinic: 1987, Jan-Feb, P13-14

560.2 **Volvulus**
   Knotting of intestine, bowel, or colon
   Strangulation of intestine, bowel, or colon
   Torsion of intestine, bowel, or colon
   Twist of intestine, bowel, or colon

● 560.3 **Impaction of intestine**

   560.30 **Impaction of intestine, unspecified**
      Impaction of colon

   560.31 **Gallstone ileus**
      Obstruction of intestine by gallstone

   560.32 **Fecal impaction** ◄
      | Excludes | constipation (564.00-564.09) ◄
                   incomplete defecation (787.61) ◄

   560.39 **Other**
      Concretion of intestine
      Enterolith
      ~~Fecal impaction~~
      Coding Clinic: 1998, Q4, P37-38

● 560.8 **Other specified intestinal obstruction**

   560.81 **Intestinal or peritoneal adhesions with obstruction (postoperative) (postinfection)**
      | Excludes | adhesions without obstruction
                   (568.0)
      Coding Clinic: 2010, Q1, P10-11; 1995, Q3, P6;
         1987, Nov-Dec, P9

   560.89 **Other**
      Acute pseudo-obstruction of intestine
      Mural thickening causing obstruction
      | Excludes | ischemic stricture of intestine
                   (557.1)
      Coding Clinic: 1997, Q2, P3

Item 9–20 Diverticula of the intestines are acquired herniations of the mucosa. Diverticulum (singular): Pocket or pouch that bulges outward through a weak spot (herniation) in the colon. Diverticula (plural). **Diverticulosis** is the condition of having diverticula. **Diverticulitis** is inflammation of these pouches or herniations. Classification is based on location (small intestine or colon) and whether it occurs with or without hemorrhage.

560.9 **Unspecified intestinal obstruction**
   Enterostenosis
   Obstruction of intestine or colon
   Occlusion of intestine or colon
   Stenosis of intestine or colon
   Stricture of intestine or colon
   | Excludes | congenital stricture or stenosis of intestine
                (751.1–751.2)

● 562 **Diverticula of intestine**
   Use additional code to identify any associated:
   peritonitis (567.0–567.9)
   | Excludes | congenital diverticulum of colon (751.5)
                diverticulum of appendix (543.9)
                Meckel's diverticulum (751.0)

● 562.0 **Small intestine**

   562.00 **Diverticulosis of small intestine (without mention of hemorrhage)**
      Diverticulosis:
         duodenum without mention of
            diverticulitis
         ileum without mention of diverticulitis
         jejunum without mention of diverticulitis

   562.01 **Diverticulitis of small intestine (without mention of hemorrhage)**
      Diverticulitis (with diverticulosis):
         duodenum
         ileum
         jejunum
         small intestine

   562.02 **Diverticulosis of small intestine with hemorrhage**

   562.03 **Diverticulitis of small intestine with hemorrhage**

● 562.1 **Colon**

   562.10 **Diverticulosis of colon (without mention of hemorrhage)**
      Diverticulosis without mention of
         diverticulitis:
         NOS
         intestine (large) without mention of
            diverticulitis
      Diverticular disease (colon) without
         mention of diverticulitis
      Coding Clinic: 2005, Q3, P17-18; 2002, Q3, P14-15

   562.11 **Diverticulitis of colon without mention of hemorrhage**
      Diverticulitis (with diverticulosis):
         NOS
         colon
         intestine (large)
      Coding Clinic: 1996, Q1, P13-14

   562.12 **Diverticulosis of colon with hemorrhage**

   562.13 **Diverticulitis of colon with hemorrhage**

● **564 Functional digestive disorders, not elsewhere classified**

     Excludes *functional disorders of stomach (536.0–536.9)*
         those specified as psychogenic (306.4)

   ● **564.0 Constipation**

     Excludes *fecal impaction (560.32)* ◄
         incomplete defecation (787.61) ◄
         psychogenic constipation (306.4)

     564.00 Constipation, unspecified

     564.01 Slow transit constipation

     564.02 Outlet dysfunction constipation

     564.09 Other constipation

   564.1 Irritable bowel syndrome
     Irritable colon
     Spastic colon

   564.2 Postgastric surgery syndromes
     Dumping syndrome
     Jejunal syndrome
     Postgastrectomy syndrome
     Postvagotomy syndrome

     Excludes *malnutrition following gastrointestinal*
         surgery (579.3)
         postgastrojejunostomy ulcer (534.0–534.9)
     Coding Clinic: 1995, Q1, P11

   564.3 Vomiting following gastrointestinal surgery
     Vomiting (bilious) following gastrointestinal
     surgery

   564.4 Other postoperative functional disorders
     Diarrhea following gastrointestinal surgery

     Excludes *colostomy and enterostomy complications*
         (569.60–569.69)

   564.5 Functional diarrhea

     Excludes *diarrhea:*
         NOS (787.91)
         psychogenic (306.4)
     Coding Clinic: 1988, Q2, P9-10

   564.6 Anal spasm
     Proctalgia fugax

   564.7 Megacolon, other than Hirschsprung's
     Dilatation of colon

     Excludes *megacolon:*
         congenital [Hirschsprung's] (751.3)
         toxic (556)

   ● **564.8 Other specified functional disorders of intestine**

     Excludes *malabsorption (579.0–579.9)*

     564.81 Neurogenic bowel
       Coding Clinic: 2001, Q1, P12

     564.89 Other functional disorders of intestine
       Atony of colon

   564.9 Unspecified functional disorder of intestine

● **565 Anal fissure and fistula**

   565.0 Anal fissure

     Excludes *anal sphincter tear (healed) (non-traumatic)*
         (old) (569.43)
         traumatic (863.89, 863.99)

   565.1 Anal fistula
     Fistula:
       anorectal
       rectal
       rectum to skin

     Excludes *fistula of rectum to internal organs - see*
         Alphabetic Index
         ischiorectal fistula (566)
         rectovaginal fistula (619.1)
     Coding Clinic: 2007, Q1, P13

Item 9–21   A **fissure** is a groove in the surface, whereas a **fistula** is an abnormal passage. An abscess is an accumulation of pus in a tissue cavity resulting from a bacterial or parasitic infection.

   566 Abscess of anal and rectal regions

Abscess:	Cellulitis:
ischiorectal	anal
perianal	perirectal
perirectal	rectal
	Ischiorectal fistula

     Coding Clinic: 1999, Q3, P8-9

● **567 Peritonitis and retroperitoneal infections**

     Excludes *peritonitis:*
         benign paroxysmal (277.31)
         pelvic, female (614.5, 614.7)
         periodic familial (277.31)
         puerperal (670.8)
         with or following:
         abortion (634–638 with .0, 639.0)
         appendicitis (540.0–540.1)
         ectopic or molar pregnancy (639.0)

   567.0 Peritonitis in infectious diseases classified elsewhere

     Code first underlying disease

     Excludes *peritonitis:*
         gonococcal (098.86)
         syphilitic (095.2)
         tuberculous (014.0)

   567.1 Pneumococcal peritonitis

   ● **567.2 Other suppurative peritonitis**
     Coding Clinic: 2005, Q4, P74-77; 1998, Q2, P19-20; 1996, Q1,
       P13-14; 1987, Jan-Feb, P14-15

     567.21 Peritonitis (acute) generalized
       Pelvic peritonitis, male

     567.22 Peritoneal abscess

Abscess (of):	Abscess (of):
abdominopelvic	retrocecal
mesenteric	subdiaphragmatic
omentum	subhepatic
peritoneum	subphrenic

     567.23 Spontaneous bacterial peritonitis

       Excludes *bacterial peritonitis NOS (567.29)*

     567.29 Other suppurative peritonitis
       Subphrenic peritonitis
       Coding Clinic: 2001, Q2, P11-12; 1999, Q3, P9; 1995,
       Q3, P5

   ● **567.3 Retroperitoneal infections**

     567.31 Psoas muscle abscess

     567.38 Other retroperitoneal abscess
       Coding Clinic: 2005, Q4, P74-77; 1998, Q2, P19-20

     567.39 Other retroperitoneal infections

Item 9-22   **Peritonitis** is an inflammation of the lining (peritoneum) of the abdominal cavity and surface of the intestines. **Retroperitoneal infections** occur between the posterior parietal peritoneum and posterior abdominal wall where the kidneys, adrenal glands, ureters, duodenum, ascending colon, descending colon, pancreas, and the large vessels and nerves are located. Both are caused by bacteria, parasites, injury, bleeding, or diseases such as systemic lupus erythematosus.

DISEASES OF THE DIGESTIVE SYSTEM (520–579)

● **567.8 Other specified peritonitis**

    567.81 Choleperitonitis
        Peritonitis due to bile

    567.82 Sclerosing mesenteritis
        Fat necrosis of peritoneum
        (Idiopathic) sclerosing mesenteric fibrosis
        Mesenteric lipodystrophy
        Mesenteric panniculitis
        Retractile mesenteritis
        Coding Clinic: 2005, Q4, P74-77

    567.89 Other specified peritonitis
        Chronic proliferative peritonitis
        Mesenteric saponification
        Peritonitis due to urine

567.9 Unspecified peritonitis
    Peritonitis: Peritonitis:
        NOS   of unspecified cause
    Coding Clinic: 2004, Q1, P10-11

● **568 Other disorders of peritoneum**

    568.0 Peritoneal adhesions (postoperative) (postinfection)
        Adhesions (of):   Adhesions (of):
           abdominal (wall)   mesenteric
           diaphragm   omentum
           intestine   stomach
           male pelvis
        Adhesive bands

        | Excludes | adhesions: |
                 pelvic, female (614.6)
                 with obstruction:
                      duodenum (537.3)
                      intestine (560.81)
        Coding Clinic: 2003, Q3, P7&11; 1995, Q3, P7; 1985, Sept-Oct, P11

● **568.8 Other specified disorders of peritoneum**

    568.81 Hemoperitoneum (nontraumatic)

    568.82 Peritoneal effusion (chronic)

        | Excludes | *ascites NOS (789.51–789.59)* |

    568.89 Other
        Peritoneal: Penitoneal:
           cyst   granuloma

    568.9 Unspecified disorder of peritoneum

● **569 Other disorders of intestine**

    569.0 Anal and rectal polyp
        Anal and rectal polyp NOS

        | Excludes | *adenomatous anal and rectal polyp (211.4)* |

    569.1 Rectal prolapse
        Procidentia: Prolapse:
           anus (sphincter)   anal canal
           rectum (sphincter)   rectal mucosa
        Proctoptosis

        | Excludes | *prolapsed hemorrhoids (455.2, 455.5)* |

    569.2 Stenosis of rectum and anus
        Stricture of anus (sphincter)

    569.3 Hemorrhage of rectum and anus

        | Excludes | *gastrointestinal bleeding NOS (578.9)* |
                   melena (578.1)
        Coding Clinic: 2005, Q3, P17

● **569.4 Other specified disorders of rectum and anus**

    569.41 Ulcer of anus and rectum
        Solitary ulcer of anus (sphincter) or rectum
           (sphincter)
        Stercoral ulcer of anus (sphincter) or rectum
           (sphincter)

    569.42 Anal or rectal pain
        Coding Clinic: 2003, Q1, P8; 1996, Q1, P13

    569.43 Anal sphincter tear (healed) (old)
        Tear of anus, nontraumatic

        Use additional code for any associated fecal
           incontinence (787.60-787.63) ◀▦

        | Excludes | *anal fissure (565.0)* |
                 anal sphincter tear (healed) (old)
                    complicating delivery (654.8)

    569.44 Dysplasia of anus
        Anal intraepithelial neoplasia I and II
           (AIN I and II) (histologically
           confirmed)
        Dysplasia of anus NOS
        Mild and moderate dysplasia of anus
           (histologically confirmed)

        | Excludes | *abnormal results from anal* |
                 cytologic examination
                 without histologic
                 confirmation (796.70-
                 796.79)
                 anal intraepithelial neoplasia III
                   (230.5, 230.6)
                 carcinoma in situ of anus
                   (230.5, 230.6)
                 HGSIL of anus (796.74)
                 severe dysplasia of anus
                   (230.5, 230.6)
        Coding Clinic: 2008, Q4, P117-119

    569.49 Other
        Granuloma of rectum (sphincter)
        Rupture of rectum (sphincter)
        Hypertrophy of anal papillae
        Proctitis NOS

        Use additional code for associated fecal
           incontinence (787.60-787.63) ◀

        | Excludes | *fistula of rectum to:* |
                 internal organs - see Alphabetic
                   Index
                 skin (565.1)
                 hemorrhoids (455.0–455.9)
                 ~~*incontinence of sphincter ani*~~
                   ~~*(787.6)*~~

    569.5 Abscess of intestine

        | Excludes | *appendiceal abscess (540.1)* |
        Coding Clinic: 1996, Q1, P13-14

● **569.6 Colostomy and enterostomy complications**

    **569.60 Colostomy and enterostomy complication,
        unspecified**

    569.61 Infection of colostomy and enterostomy

        Use additional code to specify type of
           infection, such as:
        abscess or cellulitis of abdomen (682.2)
        septicemia (038.0–038.9)

        Use additional code to identify organism
           (041.00–041.9)

    **569.62 Mechanical complication of colostomy and
        enterostomy**
        Malfunction of colostomy and enterostomy
        Coding Clinic: 2005, Q2, P11-12; 2003, Q1, P10

    569.69 Other complication
        Fistula   Prolapse
        Hernia

● **569.7 Complications of intestinal pouch**

    569.71 Pouchitis
        Inflammation of internal ileoanal pouch
        Coding Clinic: 2009, Q4, P106

    569.79 Other complications of intestinal pouch

● **569.8 Other specified disorders of intestine**

569.81 Fistula of intestine, excluding rectum and anus
Fistula:
abdominal wall
enterocolic
enteroenteric
ileorectal

> **Excludes** *fistula of intestine to internal organs - see Alphabetic Index*
> *persistent postoperative fistula (998.6)*

Coding Clinic: 1999, Q3, P8

569.82 Ulceration of intestine
Primary ulcer of intestine
Ulceration of colon

> **Excludes** *that with perforation (569.83)*

569.83 Perforation of intestine

569.84 Angiodysplasia of intestine (without mention of hemorrhage)
Coding Clinic: 1996, Q3, P9-10

569.85 Angiodysplasia of intestine with hemorrhage
Coding Clinic: 1996, Q3, P9-10

569.86 Dieulafoy lesion (hemorrhagic) of intestine
Coding Clinic: 2002, Q4, P60-61

569.87 Vomiting of fecal matter

569.89 Other
Enteroptosis   Pericolitis
Granuloma of intestine   Perisigmoiditis
Prolapse of intestine   Visceroptosis

> **Excludes** *gangrene of intestine, mesentery, or omentum (557.0)*
> *hemorrhage of intestine NOS (578.9)*
> *obstruction of intestine (560.0–560.9)*

569.9 Unspecified disorder of intestine

OTHER DISEASES OF DIGESTIVE SYSTEM (570–579)

570 Acute and subacute necrosis of liver
Acute hepatic failure
Acute or subacute hepatitis, not specified as infective
Necrosis of liver (acute) (diffuse) (massive) (subacute)
Parenchymatous degeneration of liver
Yellow atrophy (liver) (acute) (subacute)

> **Excludes** *icterus gravis of newborn (773.0–773.2)*
> *serum hepatitis (070.2–070.3)*
> *that with:*
>   *abortion (634–638 with .7, 639.8)*
>   *ectopic or molar pregnancy (639.8)*
>   *pregnancy, childbirth, or the puerperium (646.7)*
> *viral hepatitis (070.0–070.9)*

Coding Clinic: 2005, Q2, P9-10; 2000, Q1, P22

● **571 Chronic liver disease and cirrhosis**

571.0 Alcoholic fatty liver

571.1 Acute alcoholic hepatitis
Acute alcoholic liver disease
Coding Clinic: 2002, Q2, P4

571.2 Alcoholic cirrhosis of liver
Florid cirrhosis
Laennec's cirrhosis (alcoholic)
Coding Clinic: 2007, Q3, P9; Q2, P6-7x2; 2002, Q2, P4; Q1, P3; 1985, Nov-Dec, P14

571.3 Alcoholic liver damage, unspecified

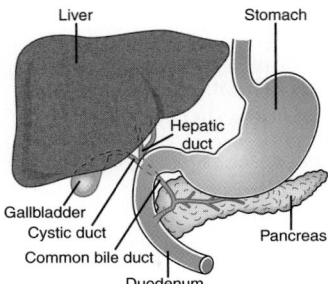

Figure 9–15 Liver and bile ducts.

Item 9–23   Cirrhosis is the progressive fibrosis of the liver resulting in loss of liver function. The main causes of cirrhosis of the liver are alcohol abuse, chronic hepatitis (inflammation of the liver), biliary disease, and excessive amounts of iron. **Alcoholic cirrhosis of the liver** is also called portal, Laënnec's, or fatty nutritional cirrhosis.

● **571.4 Chronic hepatitis**

> **Excludes** *viral hepatitis (acute) (chronic) (070.0–070.9)*

571.40 Chronic hepatitis, unspecified

571.41 Chronic persistent hepatitis

571.42 Autoimmune hepatitis
Coding Clinic: 2008, Q4, P120

571.49 Other
Chronic hepatitis:
active
aggressive
Recurrent hepatitis
Coding Clinic: 1999, Q3, P19

571.5 Cirrhosis of liver without mention of alcohol
Cirrhosis of liver: Cirrhosis of liver:
NOS   micronodular
cryptogenic   posthepatitic
macronodular   postnecrotic
Healed yellow atrophy (liver)
Portal cirrhosis

Code first, if applicable, viral hepatitis (acute) (chronic) (070.0–070.9)
Coding Clinic: 2007, Q3, P9

571.6 Biliary cirrhosis
Chronic nonsuppurative destructive cholangitis
Cirrhosis:
cholangitic
cholestatic

571.8 Other chronic nonalcoholic liver disease
Chronic yellow atrophy (liver)
Fatty liver, without mention of alcohol
Coding Clinic: 1996, Q2, P12

571.9 Unspecified chronic liver disease without mention of alcohol

● **572 Liver abscess and sequelae of chronic liver disease**

572.0 Abscess of liver

> **Excludes** *amebic liver abscess (006.3)*

572.1 Portal pyemia
Phlebitis of portal vein
Portal thrombophlebitis
Pylephlebitis
Pylethrombophlebitis

DISEASES OF THE DIGESTIVE SYSTEM (520–579)

572.2 Hepatic encephalopathy
Hepatic coma
Hepatocerebral intoxication
Portal-systemic encephalopathy

> **Excludes** *hepatic coma associated with viral hepatitis - see category 070*

Coding Clinic: 2007, Q2, P6; 2005, Q2, P9-10; 2002, Q1, P3; 1995, Q3, P14

572.3 Portal hypertension

Use additional code for any associated complications, such as: ◄
portal hypertensive gastropathy (537.89) ◄

Coding Clinic: 2005, Q3, P15-16

572.4 Hepatorenal syndrome

> **Excludes** *that following delivery (674.8)*

Coding Clinic: 1992, Q3, P15

572.8 Other sequelae of chronic liver disease

● **573 Other disorders of liver**

> **Excludes** *amyloid or lardaceous degeneration of liver (277.39)*
> *congenital cystic disease of liver (751.62)*
> *glycogen infiltration of liver (271.0)*
> *hepatomegaly NOS (789.1)*
> *portal vein obstruction (452)*

573.0 Chronic passive congestion of liver

573.1 Hepatitis in viral diseases classified elsewhere
Code first underlying disease, as:
Coxsackie virus disease (074.8)
cytomegalic inclusion virus disease (078.5)
infectious mononucleosis (075)

> **Excludes** *hepatitis (in):*
> *mumps (072.71)*
> *viral (070.0–070.9)*
> *yellow fever (060.0–060.9)*

573.2 Hepatitis in other infectious diseases classified elsewhere
Code first underlying disease, as:
malaria (084.9)

> **Excludes** *hepatitis in:*
> *late syphilis (095.3)*
> *secondary syphilis (091.62)*
> *toxoplasmosis (130.5)*

573.3 Hepatitis, unspecified
Toxic (noninfectious) hepatitis

Use additional E code to identify cause

Coding Clinic: 1998, Q3, P4; 1990, Q4, P26

573.4 Hepatic infarction

573.8 Other specified disorders of liver
Hepatoptosis

573.9 Unspecified disorder of liver

● **574 Cholelithiasis**
Presence or formation of gallstones
Coding Clinic: 1990, Q1, P19

The following fifth-digit subclassification is for use with category 574:

> 0   without mention of obstruction
> 1   with obstruction

Check documentation for acute/chronic gallbladder/common bile duct either with or without obstruction.

● **574.0 Calculus of gallbladder with acute cholecystitis**
[0-1]   Biliary calculus with acute cholecystitis
Calculus of cystic duct with acute cholecystitis
Cholelithiasis with acute cholecystitis
Any condition classifiable to 574.2 with acute cholecystitis
Coding Clinic: 1996, Q4, P32; 1984, Nov-Dec, P18

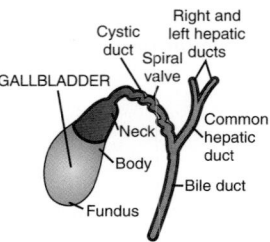

Figure 9–16 Gallbladder and bile ducts.

● **574.1 Calculus of gallbladder with other cholecystitis**
[0-1]   Biliary calculus with cholecystitis
Calculus of cystic duct with cholecystitis
Cholelithiasis with cholecystitis
Cholecystitis with cholelithiasis NOS
Any condition classifiable to 574.2 with cholecystitis (chronic)
Coding Clinic: 2003, Q1, P5; 1999, Q3, P9; 1996, Q4, P69; Q2, P13-15; Q1, P7

● **574.2 Calculus of gallbladder without mention of**
[0-1]   **cholecystitis**
Biliary:
calculus NOS
colic NOS
Calculus of cystic duct
Cholelithiasis NOS
Colic (recurrent) of gallbladder
Gallstone (impacted)
Coding Clinic: 1995, Q4, P51-52; 1988, Q1, P14

● **574.3 Calculus of bile duct with acute cholecystitis**
[0-1]   Calculus of bile duct [any] with acute cholecystitis
Choledocholithiasis with acute cholecystitis
Any condition classifiable to 574.5 with acute cholecystitis

● **574.4 Calculus of bile duct with other cholecystitis**
[0-1]   Calculus of bile duct [any] with cholecystitis (chronic)
Choledocholithiasis with cholecystitis (chronic)
Any condition classifiable to 574.5 with cholecystitis (chronic)
Coding Clinic: 1996, Q1, P7

● **574.5 Calculus of bile duct without mention of**
[0-1]   **cholecystitis**
Calculus of: Choledocholithiasis
bile duct [any]   Hepatic:
common duct   colic (recurrent)
hepatic duct   lithiasis
Coding Clinic: 1996, Q2, P13-15; 1994, Q3, P11

● **574.6 Calculus of gallbladder and bile duct with acute**
[0-1]   **cholecystitis**
Any condition classifiable to 574.0 and 574.3

● **574.7 Calculus of gallbladder and bile duct with other**
[0-1]   **cholecystitis**
Any condition classifiable to 574.1 and 574.4

● **574.8 Calculus of gallbladder and bile duct with acute and**
[0-1]   **chronic cholecystitis**
Any condition classifiable to 574.6 and 574.7
Coding Clinic: 1996, Q4, P32

● **574.9 Calculus of gallbladder and bile duct without**
[0-1]   **cholecystitis**
Any condition classifiable to 574.2 and 574.5

◄ New   ◄▯▯ Revised   ~~deleted~~ Deleted   Excludes   Includes   Use additional   Code first   Omit code
● Unacceptable Principal Diagnosis   ● Use Additional Digit(s)   OGCR Official Guidelines   Coding Clinic

● **575 Other disorders of gallbladder**
Cholecystitis is chronic or acute inflammation of gallbladder.

575.0 Acute cholecystitis
Abscess of gallbladder without mention of calculus
Angiocholecystitis without mention of calculus
Cholecystitis without mention of calculus:
emphysematous (acute)
gangrenous
suppurative
Empyema of gallbladder without mention of calculus
Gangrene of gallbladder without mention of calculus

Excludes	*that with:*

acute and chronic cholecystitis (575.12)
choledocholithiasis (574.3)
choledocholithiasis and cholelithiasis (574.6)
cholelithiasis (574.0)
Coding Clinic: 1991, Q3, P17-18

● **575.1 Other cholecystitis**
Cholecystitis without mention of calculus:
NOS without mention of calculus
chronic without mention of calculus

Excludes	*that with:*

choledocholithiasis (574.4)
choledocholithiasis and cholelithiasis (574.8)
cholelithiasis (574.1)
Coding Clinic: 1991, Q3, P17-18

575.10 Cholecystitis, unspecified
Cholecystitis NOS

575.11 Chronic cholecystitis

575.12 Acute and chronic cholecystitis
Coding Clinic: 1997, Q4, P52; 1996, Q4, P32

575.2 Obstruction of gallbladder
Occlusion of cystic duct or gallbladder without mention of calculus
Stenosis of cystic duct or gallbladder without mention of calculus
Stricture of cystic duct or gallbladder without mention of calculus

575.3 Hydrops of gallbladder
Mucocele of gallbladder

575.4 Perforation of gallbladder
Rupture of cystic duct or gallbladder

575.5 Fistula of gallbladder
Fistula: Fistula:
cholecystoduodenal cholecystoenteric

575.6 Cholesterolosis of gallbladder
Strawberry gallbladder

575.8 Other specified disorders of gallbladder
Adhesions (of) cystic duct gallbladder
Atrophy (of) cystic duct gallbladder
Cyst (of) cystic duct gallbladder
Hypertrophy (of) cystic duct gallbladder
Nonfunctioning (of) cystic duct gallbladder
Ulcer (of) cystic duct gallbladder
Biliary dyskinesia

Excludes	*Hartmann's pouch of intestine (V44.3)*

nonvisualization of gallbladder (793.3)
Coding Clinic: 1989, Q2, P13

575.9 Unspecified disorder of gallbladder

● **576 Other disorders of biliary tract**

Excludes	*that involving the:*

cystic duct (575.0–575.9)
gallbladder (575.0–575.9)

576.0 Postcholecystectomy syndrome
Coding Clinic: 1988, Q1, P10

576.1 Cholangitis
Cholangitis: Cholangitis:
NOS   recurrent
acute   sclerosing
ascending   secondary
chronic   stenosing
primary   suppurative
Coding Clinic: 1999, Q2, P13-14; 1995, Q2, P7

576.2 Obstruction of bile duct
Occlusion of bile duct, except cystic duct, without mention of calculus
Stenosis of bile duct, except cystic duct, without mention of calculus
Stricture of bile duct, except cystic duct, without mention of calculus

Excludes	*congenital (751.61)*

that with calculus (574.3–574.5 with fifth-digit 1)
Coding Clinic: 2003, Q3, P17-18; 2001, Q1, P8-9; 1999, Q2, P13-14

576.3 Perforation of bile duct
Rupture of bile duct, except cystic duct

576.4 Fistula of bile duct
Choledochoduodenal fistula

576.5 Spasm of sphincter of Oddi

576.8 Other specified disorders of biliary tract
Adhesions of bile duct [any]
Atrophy of bile duct [any]
Cyst of bile duct [any]
Hypertrophy of bile duct [any]
Stasis of bile duct [any]
Ulcer of bile duct [any]

Excludes	*congenital choledochal cyst (751.69)*

Coding Clinic: 2003, Q3, P17-18; 1999, Q2, P14

576.9 Unspecified disorder of biliary tract

● **577 Diseases of pancreas**
Pancreatitis is inflammatory process that may be acute or chronic.

577.0 Acute pancreatitis
Abscess of pancreas   Pancreatitis:
Necrosis of pancreas: NOS
acute   acute (recurrent)
infective   apoplectic
                         hemorrhagic
                         subacute
                         suppurative

Excludes	*mumps pancreatitis (072.3)*

Coding Clinic: 1999, Q3, P9; 1998, Q2, P19-20; 1996, Q2, P13-15; 1989, Q2, P9

577.1 Chronic pancreatitis
Chronic pancreatitis: Pancreatitis:
NOS   painless
infectious   recurrent
interstitial   relapsing
Coding Clinic: 2001, Q1, P8-9; 1996, Q2, P13-15; 1994, Q3, P11

Common bile duct
Accessory duct
Pancreatic duct
Ampulla of Vater

Figure 9-17 Pancreatic ductal system.

DISEASES OF THE DIGESTIVE SYSTEM (520–579)

ICD-9-CM

577.2 **Cyst and pseudocyst of pancreas**

577.8 **Other specified diseases of pancreas**
Atrophy of pancreas
Calculus of pancreas
Cirrhosis of pancreas
Fibrosis of pancreas
Pancreatic:
infantilism
necrosis:
NOS
aseptic
fat
Pancreatolithiasis

| Excludes | *fibrocystic disease of pancreas (277.00–277.09)*
islet cell tumor of pancreas (211.7)
pancreatic steatorrhea (579.4) |

Coding Clinic: 2001, Q1, P8-9

577.9 **Unspecified disease of pancreas**

● 578 **Gastrointestinal hemorrhage**

| Excludes | *that with mention of:*
angiodysplasia of stomach and duodenum (537.83)
angiodysplasia of intestine (569.85)
diverticulitis, intestine:
large (562.13)
small (562.03)
diverticulosis, intestine:
large (562.12)
small (562.02)
gastritis and duodenitis (535.0–535.6)
ulcer:
duodenal, gastric, gastrojejunal, or peptic (531.00–534.91) |

Coding Clinic: 2007, Q2, P13; 1992, Q2, P9-10; Q2, P8-9

578.0 **Hematemesis**
Vomiting of blood
Coding Clinic: 2002, Q2, P4

578.1 **Blood in stool**
Melena

| Excludes | *melena of the newborn (772.4, 777.3)*
occult blood (792.1) |

Coding Clinic: 2006, Q2, P17; 1992, Q2, P8-9

578.9 **Hemorrhage of gastrointestinal tract, unspecified**
Gastric hemorrhage   Intestinal hemorrhage
Coding Clinic: 2008, Q2, P15-16; 2006, Q4, P91-92; 2005, Q3,
P17-18; 1986, Nov-Dec, P9; 1985, Sept-Oct, P9

● 579 **Intestinal malabsorption**

579.0 **Celiac disease**
Celiac:
crisis
infantilism
rickets
Gee (-Herter) disease
Gluten enteropathy
Idiopathic steatorrhea
Nontropical sprue

579.1 **Tropical sprue**
Sprue:
NOS
tropical
Tropical steatorrhea

579.2 **Blind loop syndrome**
Postoperative blind loop syndrome

579.3 **Other and unspecified postsurgical nonabsorption**
Hypoglycemia following gastrointestinal surgery
Malnutrition following gastrointestinal surgery
Coding Clinic: 2003, Q4, P104-105

579.4 **Pancreatic steatorrhea**

579.8 **Other specified intestinal malabsorption**
Enteropathy:
exudative
protein-losing
Steatorrhea (chronic)
Coding Clinic: 2003, Q1, P12

579.9 **Unspecified intestinal malabsorption**
Malabsorption syndrome NOS
Coding Clinic: 2004, Q4, P57-59

◀ New   ◀▪▪▪ Revised   ~~deleted~~ Deleted   Excludes   Includes   Use additional   Code first   Omit code
● Unacceptable Principal Diagnosis   ● Use Additional Digit(s)   OGCR Official Guidelines   Coding Clinic

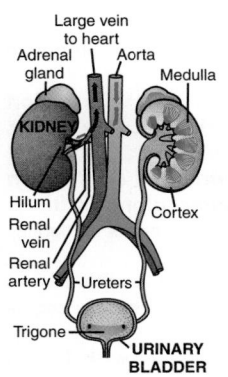

Figure 10-1 Kidneys within the urinary system.

Item 10-1 Glomerulonephritis is nephritis accompanied by inflammation of the glomeruli of the kidney, resulting in the degeneration of the glomeruli and the nephrons.
Acute glomerulonephritis primarily affects children and young adults and is usually a result of a streptococcal infection.
Proliferative glomerulonephritis is the acute form of the disease resulting from a streptococcal infection.
Rapidly progressive glomerulonephritis, also known as **crescentic** or **malignant glomerulonephritis,** is the acute form of the disease, which leads quickly to rapid and progressive decline in renal function.

10. DISEASES OF THE GENITOURINARY SYSTEM (580–629)

NEPHRITIS, NEPHROTIC SYNDROME, AND NEPHROSIS (580–589)

Excludes *hypertensive chronic kidney disease (403.00–403.91, 404.00–404.93)*

● **580 Acute glomerulonephritis**

   Includes acute nephritis

580.0 With lesion of proliferative glomerulonephritis
   Acute (diffuse) proliferative glomerulonephritis
   Acute poststreptococcal glomerulonephritis

580.4 With lesion of rapidly progressive glomerulonephritis
   Acute nephritis with lesion of necrotizing glomerulitis

● **580.8 With other specified pathological lesion in kidney**

   580.81 Acute glomerulonephritis in diseases classified elsewhere

     Code first underlying disease, as:
      infectious hepatitis (070.0–070.9)
      mumps (072.79)
      subacute bacterial endocarditis (421.0)
      typhoid fever (002.0)

   580.89 Other
     Glomerulonephritis, acute, with lesion of:
      exudative nephritis
      interstitial (diffuse) (focal) nephritis

580.9 Acute glomerulonephritis with unspecified pathological lesion in kidney
   Glomerulonephritis: specified as acute
     NOS specified as acute
     hemorrhagic specified as acute
   Nephritis specified as acute
   Nephropathy specified as acute

● **581 Nephrotic syndrome**

581.0 With lesion of proliferative glomerulonephritis

581.1 With lesion of membranous glomerulonephritis
   Epimembranous nephritis
   Idiopathic membranous glomerular disease
   Nephrotic syndrome with lesion of:
     focal glomerulosclerosis
     sclerosing membranous glomerulonephritis
     segmental hyalinosis

581.2 With lesion of membranoproliferative glomerulonephritis
   Nephrotic syndrome with lesion (of):
     endothelial glomerulonephritis
     hypocomplementemic glomerulonephritis
      persistent glomerulonephritis
     lobular glomerulonephritis
     mesangiocapillary glomerulonephritis
     mixed membranous and proliferative glomerulonephritis

581.3 With lesion of minimal change glomerulonephritis
   Foot process disease
   Lipoid nephrosis
   Minimal change:
     glomerular disease
     glomerulitis
     nephrotic syndrome
   Coding Clinic: 2007, Q1, P23

● **581.8 With other specified pathological lesion in kidney**

   581.81 Nephrotic syndrome in diseases classified elsewhere

     Code first underlying disease, as:
      amyloidosis (277.30–277.39)
      diabetes mellitus (249.4, 250.4)
      malaria (084.9)
      polyarteritis (446.0)
      systemic lupus erythematosus (710.0)

     Excludes *nephrosis in epidemic hemorrhagic fever (078.6)*

   581.89 Other
     Glomerulonephritis with edema and lesion of:
      exudative nephritis
      interstitial (diffuse) (focal) nephritis

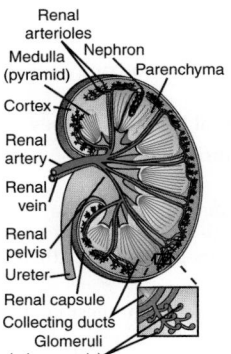

Figure 10-2 Kidney cross section.

Item 10-2 Nephrotic syndrome (NS) is marked by massive proteinuria (protein in the urine) and water retention. Patients with NS are particularly vulnerable to staphylococcal and pneumococcal infections. NS with lesion of proliferative glomerulonephritis results from a streptococcal infection. NS with lesion of membranous glomerulonephritis results in thickening of the capillary walls. NS with lesion of minimal change glomerulonephritis is usually a benign disorder that occurs mostly in children and requires electron microscopy (biopsy) to verify changes in the glomeruli.

Item 10–3 Chronic glomerulonephritis (GN) persists over a period of years, with remissions and exacerbation.

Chronic GN with lesion of proliferative glomerulonephritis results from a streptococcal infection.

Chronic GN with lesion of membranous glomerulonephritis, also known as membranous nephropathy, is characterized by deposits along the epithelial side of the basement membrane.

Chronic GN with lesion of membranoproliferative glomerulonephritis (MPGN) is a group of disorders characterized by alterations in the basement membranes of the kidney and the glomerular cells.

Chronic GN with lesion of rapidly progressive glomerulonephritis is characterized by necrosis, endothelial proliferation, and mesangial proliferation. The condition is marked by rapid and progressive decline in renal function.

> **581.9 Nephrotic syndrome with unspecified pathological lesion in kidney**
> Glomerulonephritis with edema NOS
> Nephritis:
>   nephrotic NOS
>   with edema NOS
> Nephrosis NOS
> Renal disease with edema NOS

● **582 Chronic glomerulonephritis**

> **Includes**   chronic nephritis

> **582.0 With lesion of proliferative glomerulonephritis**
> Chronic (diffuse) proliferative glomerulonephritis

> **582.1 With lesion of membranous glomerulonephritis**
> Chronic glomerulonephritis:
>   membranous
>   sclerosing
> Focal glomerulosclerosis
> Segmental hyalinosis
> **Coding Clinic: 1984, Sept-Oct, P16**

> **582.2 With lesion of membranoproliferative glomerulonephritis**
> Chronic glomerulonephritis:
>   endothelial
>   hypocomplementemic persistent
>   lobular
>   membranoproliferative
>   mesangiocapillary
>   mixed membranous and proliferative

> **582.4 With lesion of rapidly progressive glomerulonephritis**
> Chronic nephritis with lesion of necrotizing
>   glomerulitis

> ● **582.8 With other specified pathological lesion in kidney**

>> **582.81 Chronic glomerulonephritis in diseases classified elsewhere**
>> *Code first* underlying disease, as:
>>   amyloidosis (277.30–277.39)
>>   systemic lupus erythematosus (710.0)

>> **582.89 Other**
>> Chronic glomerulonephritis with lesion of:
>>   exudative nephritis
>>   interstitial (diffuse) (focal) nephritis

> **582.9 Chronic glomerulonephritis with unspecified pathological lesion in kidney**
> Glomerulonephritis: specified as chronic
>   NOS specified as chronic
>   hemorrhagic specified as chronic
> Nephritis specified as chronic
> Nephropathy specified as chronic
> **Coding Clinic: 2001, Q2, P12**

Item 10–4 Nephritis (inflammation) or **nephropathy** (disease) **with lesion of proliferative glomerulonephritis** results from a streptococcal infection.

Nephritis (inflammation) or **nephropathy** (disease) **with lesion of membranous glomerulonephritis** is characterized by deposits along the epithelial side of the basement membrane.

Nephritis (inflammation) or **nephropathy** (disease) **with lesion of membranoproliferative glomerulonephritis** is characterized by alterations in the basement membranes of the kidney and the glomerular cells.

Nephritis (inflammation) or **nephropathy** (disease) **with lesion of rapidly progressive glomerulonephritis** is characterized by rapid and progressive decline in renal function.

Nephritis (inflammation) or **nephropathy** (disease) **with lesion of renal cortical necrosis** is characterized by death of the cortical tissues.

Nephritis (inflammation) or **nephropathy** (disease) **with lesion of renal medullary necrosis** is characterized by death of the tissues that collect urine.

● **583 Nephritis and nephropathy, not specified as acute or chronic**

> **Includes**   "renal disease" so stated, not specified
>   as acute or chronic but with stated
>   pathology or cause

> **583.0 With lesion of proliferative glomerulonephritis**
> Proliferative:
>   glomerulonephritis (diffuse) NOS
>   nephritis NOS
>   nephropathy NOS

> **583.1 With lesion of membranous glomerulonephritis**
> Membranous:
>   glomerulonephritis NOS
>   nephritis NOS
> Membranous nephropathy NOS

> **583.2 With lesion of membranoproliferative glomerulonephritis**
> Membranoproliferative:
>   glomerulonephritis NOS
>   nephritis NOS
>   nephropathy NOS
> Nephritis NOS, with lesion of:
>   hypocomplementemic persistent
>   glomerulonephritis
>   lobular glomerulonephritis
>   mesangiocapillary glomerulonephritis
>   mixed membranous and proliferative
>   glomerulonephritis

> **583.4 With lesion of rapidly progressive glomerulonephritis**
> Necrotizing or rapidly progressive:
>   glomerulitis NOS
>   glomerulonephritis NOS
>   nephritis NOS
>   nephropathy NOS
> Nephritis, unspecified, with lesion of necrotizing
>   glomerulitis

> **583.6 With lesion of renal cortical necrosis**
> Nephritis NOS with (renal) cortical necrosis
> Nephropathy NOS with (renal) cortical necrosis ◄▥
> Renal cortical necrosis NOS

> **583.7 With lesion of renal medullary necrosis**
> Nephritis NOS with (renal) medullary [papillary]
>   necrosis
> Nephropathy NOS with (renal) medullary
>   [papillary] necrosis

◄ New   ◄▥ Revised   ~~deleted~~ Deleted   [Excludes]   Includes   Use additional   Code first   Omit code
● Unacceptable Principal Diagnosis   ● Use Additional Digit(s)   OGCR Official Guidelines   Coding Clinic

DISEASES OF THE GENITOURINARY SYSTEM (580–629)

● **583.8 With other specified pathological lesion in kidney**

    583.81 Nephritis and nephropathy, not specified as acute or chronic, in diseases classified elsewhere

        Code first underlying disease, as:
          amyloidosis (277.30–277.39)
          diabetes mellitus (249.4, 250.4)
          gonococcal infection (098.19)
          Goodpasture's syndrome (446.21)
          systemic lupus erythematosus (710.0)
          tuberculosis (016.0)

          | **Excludes** | *gouty nephropathy (274.10)* |
                   syphilitic nephritis (095.4)

        Coding Clinic: 2003, Q2, P7

    583.89 Other
        Glomerulitis with lesion of:
          exudative nephritis
          interstitial nephritis
        Glomerulonephritis with lesion of:
          exudative nephritis
          interstitial nephritis
        Nephritis with lesion of:
          exudative nephritis
          interstitial nephritis
        Nephropathy with lesion of:
          exudative nephritis
          interstitial nephritis
        Renal disease with lesion of:
          exudative nephritis
          interstitial nephritis

  583.9 With unspecified pathological lesion in kidney
    Glomerulitis NOS   Nephritis NOS
    Glomerulonephritis NOS   Nephropathy NOS

    | **Excludes** | *nephropathy complicating pregnancy, labor, or the puerperium (642.0–642.9, 646.2)* |
                renal disease NOS with no stated cause (593.9)

    Coding Clinic: 1994, Q4, P35

● **584 Acute kidney failure**

    | **Includes** | Acute renal failure |

    | **Excludes** | *following labor and delivery (669.3)* |
               posttraumatic (958.5)
               that complicating:
                 abortion (634–638 with .3, 639.3)
                 ectopic or molar pregnancy (639.3)

    Coding Clinic: 1992, Q2, P5x2

  584.5 Acute kidney failure with lesion of tubular necrosis
    Lower nephron nephrosis
    Renal failure with (acute) tubular necrosis
    Tubular necrosis:
      NOS
      acute

  584.6 Acute kidney failure with lesion of renal cortical necrosis

  584.7 Acute kidney failure with lesion of renal medullary [papillary] necrosis
    Necrotizing renal papillitis

  584.8 Acute kidney failure with other specified pathological lesion in kidney

  584.9 Acute kidney failure, unspecified
    Acute kidney injury (nontraumatic)

    | **Excludes** | *traumatic kidney injury (866.00-866.13)* |

    Coding Clinic: 2009, Q4, P106; 2008, Q4, P192-193; 2007, Q4, P96-97; 2005, Q2, P18-19; 2003, Q2, P7; 2003, Q1, P22; 2002, Q3, P21x2, 28x2; 2001, Q2, P14x2; 2000, Q3, P9; 2000, Q1, P22; 1996, Q3, P9; 1993, Q4, P34

Item 10–5 Decreased blood flow is the usual cause of **acute renal failure** that offers a good prognosis for recovery. **Chronic renal failure** is usually the result of long-standing kidney disease and is a very serious condition that generally results in death.

OGCR Section I.C.10.a.1

The ICD-9-CM classifies CKD based on severity. The severity of CKD is designated by stages I-V. Stage II, code 585.2, equates to mild CKD; stage III, code 585.3, equates to moderate CKD; and stage IV, code 585.4, equates to severe CKD. Code 585.6, End stage renal disease (ESRD), is assigned when the provider has documented end-stage-renal disease (ESRD). If both a stage of CKD and ESRD are documented, assign code 585.6 only.

● **585 Chronic kidney disease (CKD)**

    | **Includes** | Chronic uremia |

    Code first hypertensive chronic kidney disease, if applicable, (403.00–403.91, 404.00–404.93)

    Use additional code to identify:
      kidney transplant status, if applicable (V42.0)
      manifestation as:
        uremic:
          neuropathy (357.4)
          pericarditis (420.0)

  585.1 Chronic kidney disease, Stage I

  585.2 Chronic kidney disease, Stage II (mild)

  585.3 Chronic kidney disease, Stage III (moderate)
    Coding Clinic: 2005, Q4, P68-69

  585.4 Chronic kidney disease, Stage IV (severe)

  585.5 Chronic kidney disease, Stage V

    | **Excludes** | *chronic kidney disease, stage V requiring chronic dialysis (585.6)* |

  585.6 End stage renal disease
    Chronic kidney disease, stage V requiring chronic dialysis
    Coding Clinic: 2008, Q4, P193; Q1, P7-8; 2007, Q4, P84-86; Q3, P5-6; Q3, P11; 2006, Q4, P136; 2004, Q1, P5

  585.9 Chronic kidney disease, unspecified
    Chronic renal disease
    Chronic renal failure NOS
    Chronic renal insufficiency
    Coding Clinic: 2008, Q1, P7-8, 19; 2007, Q2, P3; 2006, Q4, P84-86; 2003, Q4, P60-61,111-112; 2001, Q2, P11-13x2; Q1, P3; 2000, Q4, P39-40; 1998, Q4, P54-55; Q3, P6-7; Q2, P20-21; 1996, Q3, P9; 1995, Q2, P10; 1987, Sept-Oct, P10; 1985, Nov-Dec, P15

586 Renal failure, unspecified

    | **Includes** | Uremia NOS |

    | **Excludes** | *following labor and delivery (669.3)* |
               posttraumatic renal failure (958.5)
               that complicating:
                 abortion (634–638 with .3, 639.3)
                 ectopic or molar pregnancy (639.3)
               uremia:
                 extrarenal (788.9)
                 prerenal (788.9)
    Coding Clinic: 1998, Q3, P6; 1984, Sept-Oct, P16

587 Renal sclerosis, unspecified

    | **Includes** | Atrophy of kidney |
                Contracted kidney
                Renal:
                  cirrhosis
                  fibrosis

DISEASES OF THE GENITOURINARY SYSTEM (580–629)

DISEASES OF THE GENITOURINARY SYSTEM (580–629)

● **588 Disorders resulting from impaired renal function**

588.0 Renal osteodystrophy
Azotemic osteodystrophy
Phosphate-losing tubular disorders
Renal:
dwarfism
infantilism
rickets

588.1 Nephrogenic diabetes insipidus
Excludes | *diabetes insipidus NOS (253.5)*

● **588.8 Other specified disorders resulting from impaired renal function**
Excludes | *secondary hypertension (405.0–405.9)*
Coding Clinic: 2004, Q4, P57-59

588.81 Secondary hyperparathyroidism (of renal origin)
Secondary hyperparathyroidism NOS

588.89 Other specified disorders resulting from impaired renal function
Hypokalemic nephropathy

588.9 Unspecified disorder resulting from impaired renal function

● **589 Small kidney of unknown cause**

589.0 Unilateral small kidney

589.1 Bilateral small kidneys

589.9 Small kidney, unspecified

OTHER DISEASES OF URINARY SYSTEM (590–599)

● **590 Infections of kidney**
Use additional code to identify organism, such as Escherichia coli [E. coli] (041.4)

● **590.0 Chronic pyelonephritis**
Chronic pyelitis   Chronic pyonephrosis
Code, if applicable, any causal condition first

590.00 Without lesion of renal medullary necrosis

590.01 With lesion of renal medullary necrosis

● **590.1 Acute pyelonephritis**
Acute pyelitis
Acute pyonephrosis

590.10 Without lesion of renal medullary necrosis

590.11 With lesion of renal medullary necrosis

590.2 Renal and perinephric abscess
Abscess:
kidney
nephritic
perirenal
Carbuncle of kidney

590.3 Pyeloureteritis cystica
Infection of renal pelvis and ureter
Ureteritis cystica
Cystica is an infection of the urinary bladder.

Figure 10–3 Acute pyelonephritis. Cortical surface exhibits grayish white areas of inflammation and abscess formation. (From Kumar: Robbins and Cotran: Pathologic Basis of Disease, 7th ed. 2005, Saunders, An Imprint of Elsevier.)

Item 10-6 Pyelonephritis is an infection of the kidneys and ureters and may be chronic or acute in one or both kidneys.

Figure 10–4 Hydronephrosis of the kidney, with marked dilatation of pelvis and calyces and thinning of renal parenchyma. (From Kumar: Robbins and Cotran: Pathologic Basis of Disease, 7th ed. 2005, Saunders, An Imprint of Elsevier.)

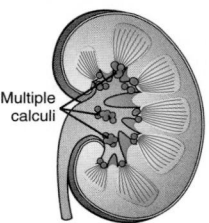
Figure 10–5 Multiple urinary calculi.
Multiple calculi

● **590.8 Other pyelonephritis or pyonephrosis, not specified as acute or chronic**

590.80 Pyelonephritis, unspecified
Pyelitis NOS
Pyelonephritis NOS
Coding Clinic: 1997, Q4, P40

590.81 Pyelitis or pyelonephritis in diseases classified elsewhere
Code first underlying disease, as:
tuberculosis (016.0)

590.9 Infection of kidney, unspecified
Excludes | *urinary tract infection NOS (599.0)*

591 Hydronephrosis
Hydrocalycosis   Hydroureteronephrosis
Hydronephrosis
Excludes | *congenital hydronephrosis (753.29)*
hydroureter (593.5)
Coding Clinic: 1998, Q2, P9

● **592 Calculus of kidney and ureter**
Excludes | *nephrocalcinosis (275.49)*

592.0 Calculus of kidney
Nephrolithiasis NOS   Staghorn calculus
Renal calculus or stone   Stone in kidney
Excludes | *uric acid nephrolithiasis (274.11)*
Coding Clinic: 2000, Q1, P4; 1993, Q2, P3

592.1 Calculus of ureter
Ureteric stone   Ureterolithiasis
Coding Clinic: 1998, Q2, P9; 1991, Q1, P11

592.9 Urinary calculus, unspecified
Coding Clinic: 1997, Q4, P40

● **593 Other disorders of kidney and ureter**

593.0 Nephroptosis
Floating kidney   Mobile kidney

593.1 Hypertrophy of kidney

593.2 Cyst of kidney, acquired
Cyst (multiple) (solitary) of kidney, not congenital
Peripelvic (lymphatic) cyst
Excludes | *calyceal or pyelogenic cyst of kidney (591)*
congenital cyst of kidney (753.1)
polycystic (disease of) kidney (753.1)

593.3 Stricture or kinking of ureter
Angulation of ureter (postoperative)
Constriction of ureter (postoperative)
Stricture of pelviureteric junction
Coding Clinic: 1994, Q3, P8

◄ New   ◄ Revised   ~~deleted~~ Deleted   Excludes   Includes   Use additional   Code first   Omit code
● Unacceptable Principal Diagnosis   ● Use Additional Digit(s)   OGCR Official Guidelines   Coding Clinic

593.4 Other ureteric obstruction
Idiopathic retroperitoneal fibrosis
Occlusion NOS of ureter
> **Excludes** *that due to calculus (592.1)*

Coding Clinic: 2010, Q1, P10; 1997, Q2, P4

593.5 Hydroureter
> **Excludes** *congenital hydroureter (753.22)*
> *hydroureteronephrosis (591)*

593.6 Postural proteinuria
Benign postural proteinuria
Orthostatic proteinuria
> **Excludes** *proteinuria NOS (791.0)*

● **593.7 Vesicoureteral reflux**
Occurs when urine flows from bladder back into ureters

593.70 Unspecified or without reflux nephropathy

593.71 With reflux nephropathy, unilateral

593.72 With reflux nephropathy, bilateral

593.73 With reflux nephropathy NOS

● **593.8 Other specified disorders of kidney and ureter**

593.81 Vascular disorders of kidney
Renal (artery):
embolism
hemorrhage
thrombosis
Renal infarction

593.82 Ureteral fistula
Intestinoureteral fistula
> **Excludes** *fistula between ureter and female*
> *genital tract (619.0)*

593.89 Other
Adhesions, kidney or ureter
Periureteritis
Polyp of ureter
Pyelectasia
Ureterocele
> **Excludes** *tuberculosis of ureter (016.2)*
> *ureteritis cystica (590.3)*

Coding Clinic: 1984, Nov-Dec, P17

593.9 Unspecified disorder of kidney and ureter
Acute renal disease
Acute renal insufficiency
Renal disease NOS
Salt-losing nephritis or syndrome
> **Excludes** *chronic renal insufficiency (585.9)*
> *cystic kidney disease (753.1)*
> *nephropathy, so stated (583.0–583.9)*
> *renal disease:*
> *arising in pregnancy or the puerperium*
> *(642.1–642.2, 642.4–642.7, 646.2)*
> *not specified as acute or chronic, but*
> *with stated pathology or cause*
> *(583.0–583.9)*

Coding Clinic: 2005, Q4, P79-80; 1998, Q2, P9

● **594 Calculus of lower urinary tract**

594.0 Calculus in diverticulum of bladder

594.1 Other calculus in bladder
Urinary bladder stone
> **Excludes** *staghorn calculus (592.0)*

594.2 Calculus in urethra

594.8 Other lower urinary tract calculus
Coding Clinic: 1985, Jan-Feb, P16

594.9 Calculus of lower urinary tract, unspecified
> **Excludes** *calculus of urinary tract NOS (592.9)*

● **595 Cystitis**
A general term used to describe an infection of the bladder and
irritations in the lower urinary tract
> **Excludes** *prostatocystitis (601.3)*

Use additional code to identify organism, such as
Escherichia coli [E. coli] (041.4)

595.0 Acute cystitis
> **Excludes** *trigonitis (595.3)*

Coding Clinic: 1999, Q2, P15-16; 1984, Nov-Dec, P15

595.1 Chronic interstitial cystitis
Describes an ongoing infection of the kidney glomeruli
and tubules
Hunner's ulcer
Panmural fibrosis of bladder
Submucous cystitis

595.2 Other chronic cystitis
Chronic cystitis NOS
Subacute cystitis
> **Excludes** *trigonitis (595.3)*

595.3 Trigonitis
Inflammation of triangular area of bladder (where
ureters and urethra come together)
Follicular cystitis
Trigonitis (acute) (chronic)
Urethrotrigonitis

595.4 Cystitis in diseases classified elsewhere
Code first *underlying disease, as:*
actinomycosis (039.8)
amebiasis (006.8)
bilharziasis (120.0–120.9)
Echinococcus infestation (122.3, 122.6)
> **Excludes** *cystitis:*
> *diphtheritic (032.84)*
> *gonococcal (098.11, 098.31)*
> *monilial (112.2)*
> *trichomonal (131.09)*
> *tuberculous (016.1)*

● **595.8 Other specified types of cystitis**

595.81 Cystitis cystica

595.82 Irradiation cystitis

Use additional E code to identify cause

595.89 Other
Abscess of bladder
Cystitis:
bullous
emphysematous
glandularis

595.9 Cystitis, unspecified

● **596 Other disorders of bladder**

Use additional code to identify urinary incontinence
(625.6, 788.30–788.39)

596.0 Bladder neck obstruction
Contracture (acquired) of bladder neck or
vesicourethral orifice
Obstruction (acquired) of bladder neck or
vesicourethral orifice
Stenosis (acquired) of bladder neck or
vesicourethral orifice
> **Excludes** *congenital (753.6)*

Coding Clinic: 2002, Q3, P28; 2001, Q2, P14; 1994, Q3, P12

DISEASES OF THE GENITOURINARY SYSTEM (580–629)

596.1 Intestinovesical fistula
Passage between bladder and the intestine
Fistula: Fistula:
   enterovesical   vesicoenteric
   vesicocolic   vesicorectal

596.2 Vesical fistula, not elsewhere classified
Fistula: Fistula:
   bladder NOS   vesicocutaneous
   urethrovesical   vesicoperineal
     Excludes *fistula between bladder and female genital tract (619.0)*

596.3 Diverticulum of bladder
Formation of a sac from a herniation of the wall of the bladder
Diverticulitis of bladder
Diverticulum (acquired) (false) of bladder
     Excludes *that with calculus in diverticulum of bladder (594.0)*

596.4 Atony of bladder
Diminished tone of bladder muscle
High compliance bladder
Hypotonicity of bladder
Inertia of bladder
     Excludes *neurogenic bladder (596.54)*

● **596.5 Other functional disorders of bladder**
     Excludes *cauda equina syndrome with neurogenic bladder (344.61)*

  596.51 Hypertonicity of bladder
    Hyperactivity   Overactive bladder

  596.52 Low bladder compliance

  596.53 Paralysis of bladder

  596.54 Neurogenic bladder NOS
    Coding Clinic: 2001, Q1, P12

  596.55 Detrusor sphincter dyssynergia

  596.59 Other functional disorder of bladder
    Detrusor instability
    Coding Clinic: 1995, Q4, P72-73

596.6 Rupture of bladder, nontraumatic

596.7 Hemorrhage into bladder wall
Hyperemia of bladder
     Excludes *acute hemorrhagic cystitis (595.0)*

596.8 Other specified disorders of bladder
Calcified   Hemorrhage
Contracted   Hypertrophy
     Excludes *cystocele, female (618.01–618.02, 618.09, 618.2–618.4)*
         hernia or prolapse of bladder, female (618.01–618.02, 618.09, 618.2–618.4)

596.9 Unspecified disorder of bladder

● **597 Urethritis, not sexually transmitted, and urethral syndrome**
Inflammation of urethra caused by bacteria or virus
     Excludes *nonspecific urethritis, so stated (099.4)*

597.0 Urethral abscess
Abscess of: Abscess:
   bulbourethral gland   periurethral
   Cowper's gland   urethral (gland)
   Littré's gland   Periurethral cellulitis
     Excludes *urethral caruncle (599.3)*

● **597.8 Other urethritis**

  597.80 Urethritis, unspecified

  597.81 Urethral syndrome NOS

  597.89 Other
    Adenitis, Skene's glands
    Cowperitis
    Meatitis, urethral
    Ulcer, urethra (meatus)
    Verumontanitis
     Excludes *trichomonal (131.02)*

● **598 Urethral stricture**
Narrowing of lumen of urethra caused by scarring from an infection or injury, which results in functional obstruction
    Includes pinhole meatus
         stricture of urinary meatus
    Use additional code to identify urinary incontinence (625.6, 788.30–788.39)
     Excludes *congenital stricture of urethra and urinary meatus (753.6)*

● **598.0 Urethral stricture due to infection**

  598.00 Due to unspecified infection

  598.01 Due to infective diseases classified elsewhere
    Code first underlying disease, as:
      gonococcal infection (098.2)
      schistosomiasis (120.0–120.9)
      syphilis (095.8)

598.1 Traumatic urethral stricture
Stricture of urethra:
   late effect of injury
   postobstetric
     Excludes *postoperative following surgery on genitourinary tract (598.2)*

598.2 Postoperative urethral stricture
Postcatheterization stricture of urethra
Coding Clinic: 1997, Q3, P6

598.8 Other specified causes of urethral stricture
Coding Clinic: 1984, Nov-Dec, P9

598.9 Urethral stricture, unspecified

● **599 Other disorders of urethra and urinary tract**

599.0 Urinary tract infection, site not specified
     Excludes *Candidiasis of urinary tract (112.2)*
         urinary tract infection of newborn (771.82)
    Use additional code to identify organism, such as Escherichia coli [E. coli] (041.4)
    Coding Clinic: 2010, Q1, P11; 2009, Q3, P10x2; 2005, Q3, P12-13; 2004, Q2, P13; 1999, Q4, P6; Q2, P15-16; 1998, Q1, P5; 1996, Q4, P33; 1995, Q2, P7; 1994, Q1, P21; 1992, Q1, P13; 1988, Q4, P10; 1984, Nov-Dec, P15; July-Aug, P19

599.1 Urethral fistula
Fistula:
   urethroperineal
   urethrorectal
Urinary fistula NOS
     Excludes *fistula:*
         urethroscrotal (608.89)
         urethrovaginal (619.0)
         urethrovesicovaginal (619.0)
    Coding Clinic: 1997, Q3, P6

◀ New   ◀▥ Revised   ~~deleted~~ Deleted   Excludes   Includes   Use additional   Code first   Omit code
● Unacceptable Principal Diagnosis   ● Use Additional Digit(s)   OGCR Official Guidelines   Coding Clinic

599.2 **Urethral diverticulum**

599.3 **Urethral caruncle**
Polyp of urethra

599.4 **Urethral false passage**

599.5 **Prolapsed urethral mucosa**
Prolapse of urethra   Urethrocele
> **Excludes** urethrocele, female (618.03, 618.09, 618.2–618.4)

● 599.6 **Urinary obstruction**
> Use additional code to identify urinary incontinence (625.6, 788.30–788.39)
> **Excludes** obstructive nephropathy NOS (593.89)

Coding Clinic: 2005, Q4, P80-81

599.60 **Urinary obstruction, unspecified**
Obstructive uropathy NOS
Urinary (tract) obstruction NOS

599.69 **Urinary obstruction, not elsewhere classified**
Code, if applicable, any causal condition first, such as:
hyperplasia of prostate (600.0–600.9 with fifth-digit 1)

● 599.7 **Hematuria**
Hematuria (benign) (essential)
> **Excludes** hemoglobinuria (791.2)

Coding Clinic: 2008, Q4, P121; 2000, Q1, P5; 1995, Q3, P8; 1993, Q1, P26; 5th Issue, P16; 1985, Nov-Dec, P15

599.70 **Hematuria, unspecified**

599.71 **Gross hematuria**

599.72 **Microscopic hematuria**

● 599.8 **Other specified disorders of urethra and urinary tract**
> Use additional code to identify urinary incontinence (625.6, 788.30–788.39)
> **Excludes** symptoms and other conditions classifiable to 788.0–788.2, 788.4–788.9, 791.0–791.9

599.81 **Urethral hypermobility**

599.82 **Intrinsic (urethral) sphincter deficiency [ISD]**

599.83 **Urethral instability**

599.84 **Other specified disorders of urethra**
Rupture of urethra (nontraumatic)
Urethral:
cyst
granuloma
Coding Clinic: 2009, Q1, P20

599.89 **Other specified disorders of urinary tract**

599.9 **Unspecified disorder of urethra and urinary tract**

(See Plates 366B and 387 on pages NAP-3 and NAP-5.)

DISEASES OF MALE GENITAL ORGANS (600–608)

● 600 **Hyperplasia of prostate**
Benign prostatic hyperplasia (BPH) and is an enlargement of prostate gland usually occurring with age and causing obstructed urine flow
> **Includes** Enlarged prostate

Coding Clinic: 2005, Q3, P20; 2003, Q4, P63-64; 2002, Q3, P28; 1994, Q3, P12-13; 1992, Q3, P7; 1986, Sept-Oct, P12; Nov-Dec, P10; 1984, Nov-Dec, P9

● 600.0 **Hypertrophy (benign) of prostate**
Benign prostatic hypertrophy
Enlargement of prostate
Smooth enlarged prostate
Soft enlarged prostate
Coding Clinic: 2003, Q1, P6; 2001, Q2, P14

600.00 **Hypertrophy (benign) of prostate without urinary obstruction and other lower urinary tract symptoms (LUTS)**
Hypertrophy (benign) of prostate NOS

600.01 **Hypertrophy (benign) of prostate with urinary obstruction and other lower urinary tract symptoms (LUTS)**
Hypertrophy (benign) of prostate with urinary retention

> Use additional code to identify symptoms:
> incomplete bladder emptying (788.21)
> nocturia (788.43)
> straining on urination (788.65)
> urinary frequency (788.41)
> urinary hesitancy (788.64)
> urinary incontinence (788.30–788.39)
> urinary obstruction (599.69)
> urinary retention (788.20)
> urinary urgency (788.63)
> weak urinary stream (788.62)

Coding Clinic: 2006, Q4, P93-95

● 600.1 **Nodular prostate**
Hard, firm prostate
Multinodular prostate
> **Excludes** malignant neoplasm of prostate (185)

600.10 **Nodular prostate without urinary obstruction**
Nodular prostate NOS

600.11 **Nodular prostate with urinary obstruction**
Nodular prostate with urinary retention

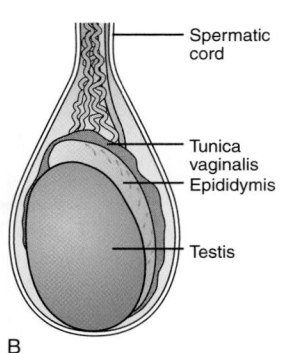

A. Sacrum, Rectum, SEMINAL VESICLE, Prostate gland, Anus, Bulbourethral gland, TUNICA VAGINALIS, Urinary bladder, Symphysis pubis, SPERMATIC CORD, VAS DEFERENS, PENIS, EPIDIDYMIS, GLANS PENIS, Urethra, Testis, SCROTUM

B. Spermatic cord, Tunica vaginalis, Epididymis, Testis

Figure 10–6 **A.** Male genital system. **B.** Testis.

● **600.2 Benign localized hyperplasia of prostate**
Adenofibromatous hypertrophy of prostate
Adenoma of prostate
Fibroadenoma of prostate
Fibroma of prostate
Myoma of prostate
Polyp of prostate

> **Excludes** *benign neoplasms of prostate (222.2)*
> *hypertrophy of prostate (600.00–600.01)*
> *malignant neoplasm of prostate (185)*

600.20 Benign localized hyperplasia of prostate without urinary obstruction and other lower urinary tract symptoms (LUTS)
Benign localized hyperplasia of prostate NOS

600.21 Benign localized hyperplasia of prostate with urinary obstruction and other lower urinary tract symptoms (LUTS)
Benign localized hyperplasia of prostate with urinary retention

> **Use additional** code to identify symptoms:
> incomplete bladder emptying (788.21)
> nocturia (788.43)
> straining on urination (788.65)
> urinary frequency (788.41)
> urinary hesitancy (788.64)
> urinary incontinence (788.30–788.39)
> urinary obstruction (599.69)
> urinary retention (788.20)
> urinary urgency (788.63)
> weak urinary stream (788.62)

600.3 Cyst of prostate

● **600.9 Hyperplasia of prostate, unspecified**
Median bar
Prostatic obstruction NOS

600.90 Hyperplasia of prostate, unspecified, without urinary obstruction and other lower urinary tract symptoms (LUTS)
Hyperplasia of prostate NOS

600.91 Hyperplasia of prostate, unspecified, with urinary obstruction and other lower urinary tract symptoms (LUTS)
Hyperplasia of prostate, unspecified, with urinary retention

> **Use additional** code to identify symptoms:
> incomplete bladder emptying (788.21)
> nocturia (788.43)
> straining on urination (788.65)
> urinary frequency (788.41)
> urinary hesitancy (788.64)
> urinary incontinence (788.30–788.39)
> urinary obstruction (599.69)
> urinary retention (788.20)
> urinary urgency (788.63)
> weak urinary stream (788.62)

● **601 Inflammatory diseases of prostate**

> **Use additional** code to identify organism, such as
> Staphylococcus (041.1), or Streptococcus (041.0)

601.0 Acute prostatitis

601.1 Chronic prostatitis

601.2 Abscess of prostate

601.3 Prostatocystitis

601.4 Prostatitis in diseases classified elsewhere

> *Code first underlying disease, as:*
> actinomycosis (039.8) syphilis (095.8)
> blastomycosis (116.0) tuberculosis (016.5)

> **Excludes** *prostatitis:*
> *gonococcal (098.12, 098.32)*
> *monilial (112.2)*
> *trichomonal (131.03)*

601.8 Other specified inflammatory diseases of prostate
Prostatitis:
cavitary
diverticular
granulomatous

601.9 Prostatitis, unspecified
Prostatitis NOS

● **602 Other disorders of prostate**

602.0 Calculus of prostate
Prostatic stone

602.1 Congestion or hemorrhage of prostate

602.2 Atrophy of prostate

602.3 Dysplasia of prostate
Prostatic intraepithelial neoplasia I (PIN I)
Prostatic intraepithelial neoplasia II (PIN II)

> **Excludes** *prostatic intraepithelial neoplasia III (PIN III) (233.4)*

602.8 Other specified disorders of prostate
Fistula of prostate   Stricture of prostate
Infarction of prostate   Periprostatic adhesions

602.9 Unspecified disorder of prostate

● **603 Hydrocele**

> **Includes** hydrocele of spermatic cord, testis, or tunica vaginalis

> **Excludes** *congenital (778.6)*

603.0 Encysted hydrocele

603.1 Infected hydrocele

> **Use additional** code to identify organism

603.8 Other specified types of hydrocele

603.9 Hydrocele, unspecified

● **604 Orchitis and epididymitis**

*An inflammation of one or both testes as a result of mumps or other infection, trauma, or metastasis. **Epididymitis** is an inflammation of the epididymis (the tubular structure that connects testicle with vas deferens).*

> **Use additional** code to identify organism such as
> Escherichia coli [E. coli] (041.4), Staphylococcus (041.1), or Streptococcus (041.0)

604.0 Orchitis, epididymitis, and epididymo-orchitis, with abscess
Abscess of epididymis or testis

Blood vessels
Vas deferens
Epididymis
Testis
Hydrocele
A   B

Figure 10–7 A. Hydrocele. **B.** Newborn with large right hydrocele. (**B** from Behrman: Nelson Textbook of Pediatrics, 17th ed. 2004, Saunders, An Imprint of Elsevier.)

Item 10–7 Hydrocele is a sac of fluid accumulating in the testes membrane.

◀ New   ◀▥ Revised   ~~deleted~~ Deleted   [Excludes]   Includes   Use additional   Code first   Omit code
● Unacceptable Principal Diagnosis   ● Use Additional Digit(s)   OGCR Official Guidelines   Coding Clinic

- **604.9 Other orchitis, epididymitis, and epididymo-orchitis, without mention of abscess**

   604.90 Orchitis and epididymitis, unspecified

   604.91 Orchitis and epididymitis in diseases classified elsewhere

   Code first underlying disease, as:
   diphtheria (032.89)
   filariasis (125.0–125.9)
   syphilis (095.8)

   | **Excludes** | *orchitis:* |

   gonococcal (098.13, 098.33)
   mumps (072.0)
   tuberculous (016.5)
   tuberculous epididymitis (016.4)

   604.99 Other

605 Redundant prepuce and phimosis
   Adherent prepuce   Phimosis (congenital)
   Paraphimosis   Tight foreskin
   Coding Clinic: 2008, Q3, P9

- **606 Infertility, male**
   Coding Clinic: 1996, Q2, P9

   606.0 Azoospermia
   Absolute infertility
   Infertility due to:
      germinal (cell) aplasia
      spermatogenic arrest (complete)

   606.1 Oligospermia
   Infertility due to:
      germinal cell desquamation
      hypospermatogenesis
      incomplete spermatogenic arrest

   606.8 Infertility due to extratesticular causes
   Infertility due to:
      drug therapy
      infection
      obstruction of efferent ducts
      radiation
      systemic disease

   606.9 Male infertility, unspecified

- **607 Disorders of penis**

   | **Excludes** | *phimosis (605)* |

   607.0 Leukoplakia of penis
   Kraurosis of penis

   | **Excludes** | *carcinoma in situ of penis (233.5)* |

   erythroplasia of Queyrat (233.5)

   607.1 Balanoposthitis
   Balanitis

   Use additional code to identify organism

   607.2 Other inflammatory disorders of penis
   Abscess of corpus cavernosum or penis
   Boil of corpus cavernosum or penis
   Carbuncle of corpus cavernosum or penis
   Cellulitis of corpus cavernosum or penis
   Cavernitis (penis)

   Use additional code to identify organism

   | **Excludes** | *herpetic infection (054.13)* |

   607.3 Priapism
   Painful erection

- **607.8 Other specified disorders of penis**

   607.81 Balanitis xerotica obliterans
   Induratio penis plastica

   607.82 Vascular disorders of penis
   Embolism of corpus cavernosum or penis
   Hematoma (nontraumatic) of corpus cavernosum or penis
   Hemorrhage of corpus cavernosum or penis
   Thrombosis of corpus cavernosum or penis

   607.83 Edema of penis

   607.84 Impotence of organic origin

   | **Excludes** | *nonorganic (302.72)* |

   Coding Clinic: 1985, July-Aug, P9

   607.85 Peyronie's disease
   Coding Clinic: 2003, Q4, P64-65

   607.89 Other
   Atrophy of corpus cavernosum or penis
   Fibrosis of corpus cavernosum or penis
   Hypertrophy of corpus cavernosum or penis
   Ulcer (chronic) of corpus cavernosum or penis

   607.9 Unspecified disorder of penis

- **608 Other disorders of male genital organs**

   608.0 Seminal vesiculitis
   Abscess of seminal vesicle
   Cellulitis of seminal vesicle
   Vesiculitis (seminal)

   Use additional code to identify organism

   | **Excludes** | *gonococcal infection (098.14, 098.34)* |

   608.1 Spermatocele

Rotation of spermatic cord

Epididymis

Testis

A   B

Figure 10–8 A. Torsion of testis. **B.** Torsion of the testis. (**B** from Kumar: Robbins and Cotran: Pathologic Basis of Disease, 7th ed. 2005, Saunders, An Imprint of Elsevier.)

Item 10-8 Male infertility is the inability of the female sex partner to conceive after one year of unprotected intercourse. **Azoospermia** is no sperm ejaculated and **oligospermia** is few sperm ejaculated—both resulting in infertility. Extratesticular causes such as injury, infections, radiation, and chemotherapy may also cause male infertility.

Item 10-9 Seminal vesiculitis is an inflammation of the seminal vesicle. Spermatocele is a benign cystic accumulation of sperm arising from the head of the epididymis. Torsion of the testis is a medical emergency occurring most commonly in boys 7 to 12 years of age and results from a congenital abnormality of the covering of the testis allowing the testis to twist within its sac and cutting off the blood supply to the testis.

DISEASES OF THE GENITOURINARY SYSTEM (580–629)

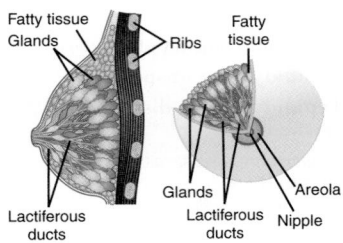

Figure 10–9 Breast.

DISEASES OF THE GENITOURINARY SYSTEM (580–629)

● **608.2 Torsion of testis**
  Coding Clinic: 2006, Q4, P95-96

  608.20 Torsion of testis, unspecified

  608.21 Extravaginal torsion of spermatic cord

  608.22 Intravaginal torsion of spermatic cord
    Torsion of spermatic cord NOS

  608.23 Torsion of appendix testis

  608.24 Torsion of appendix epididymis

  608.3 Atrophy of testis

  608.4 Other inflammatory disorders of male genital organs
    Abscess of scrotum, spermatic cord, testis [except abscess], tunica vaginalis, or vas deferens
    Boil of scrotum, spermatic cord, testis [except abscess], tunica vaginalis, or vas deferens
    Carbuncle of scrotum, spermatic cord, testis [except abscess], tunica vaginalis, or vas deferens
    Cellulitis of scrotum, spermatic cord, testis [except abscess], tunica vaginalis, or vas deferens
    Vasitis

    Use additional code to identify organism

    Excludes   *abscess of testis (604.0)*

● **608.8 Other specified disorders of male genital organs**

  608.81 Disorders of male genital organs in diseases classified elsewhere

    Code first *underlying disease, as:*
      filariasis (125.0–125.9)
      tuberculosis (016.5)

  608.82 Hematospermia

  608.83 Vascular disorders
    Hematoma (nontraumatic) of seminal vesicle, spermatic cord, testis, scrotum, tunica vaginalis, or vas deferens
    Hemorrhage of seminal vesicle, spermatic cord, testis, scrotum, tunica vaginalis, or vas deferens
    Thrombosis of seminal vesicle, spermatic cord, testis, scrotum, tunica vaginalis, or vas deferens
    Hematocele NOS, male
    Coding Clinic: 2003, Q4, P110

  608.84 Chylocele of tunica vaginalis

  608.85 Stricture
    Stricture of: Stricture of:
      spermatic cord   vas deferens
      tunica vaginalis

  608.86 Edema

  608.87 Retrograde ejaculation

  608.89 Other
    Atrophy of seminal vesicle, spermatic cord, testis, scrotum tunica vaginalis, or vas deferens
    Fibrosis of seminal vesicle, spermatic cord, testis, scrotum tunica vaginalis, or vas deferens
    Hypertrophy of seminal vesicle, spermatic cord, testis, scrotum tunica vaginalis, or vas deferens
    Ulcer of seminal vesicle, spermatic cord, testis, scrotum tunica vaginalis, or vas deferens

    Excludes   *atrophy of testis (608.3)*

  608.9 Unspecified disorder of male genital organs

DISORDERS OF BREAST (610–612)

● **610 Benign mammary dysplasias**
  Benign lumpiness of the breast.

  610.0 Solitary cyst of breast
    Cyst (solitary) of breast

  610.1 Diffuse cystic mastopathy
    Chronic cystic mastitis
    Cystic breast
    Fibrocystic disease of breast
    Coding Clinic: 2006, Q2, P10

  610.2 Fibroadenosis of breast
    Fibroadenosis of   Fibroadenosis of
      breast: breast:
      NOS   diffuse
      chronic   periodic
      cystic   segmental

  610.3 Fibrosclerosis of breast

  610.4 Mammary duct ectasia
    Comedomastitis
    Duct ectasia
    Mastitis:
      periductal
      plasma cell

  610.8 Other specified benign mammary dysplasias
    Mazoplasia
    Sebaceous cyst of breast
    Coding Clinic: 2009, Q2, P9

  610.9 Benign mammary dysplasia, unspecified

● **611 Other disorders of breast**

    Excludes   *that associated with lactation or the puerperium (675.0–676.9)*

  611.0 Inflammatory disease of breast
    Abscess (acute) (chronic) (nonpuerperal) of:
      areola
      breast
    Mammillary fistula
    Mastitis (acute) (subacute) (nonpuerperal):
      NOS
      infective
      retromammary
      submammary

    Excludes   *carbuncle of breast (680.2)*
      chronic cystic mastitis (610.1)
      neonatal infective mastitis (771.5)
      thrombophlebitis of breast [Mondor's disease] (451.89)

  611.1 Hypertrophy of breast
    Gynecomastia
    Hypertrophy of breast:
      NOS
      massive pubertal

    Excludes   *breast engorgement in newborn (778.7)*
      disproportion of reconstructed breast (612.1)

  611.2 Fissure of nipple

● **611.3 Fat necrosis of breast**
Fat necrosis (segmental) of breast
Code first breast necrosis due to breast graft (996.79)

611.4 Atrophy of breast

611.5 Galactocele

611.6 Galactorrhea not associated with childbirth
Excessive or spontaneous flow of milk
Coding Clinic: 1985, July-Aug, P9

● **611.7 Signs and symptoms in breast**

611.71 Mastodynia
Pain in breast

611.72 Lump or mass in breast
Coding Clinic: 2009, Q4, P108; 2003, Q2, P3-5

611.79 Other
Induration of breast
Inversion of nipple
Nipple discharge
Retraction of nipple

● **611.8 Other specified disorders of breast**
Coding Clinic: 2008, Q4, P121-122

611.81 Ptosis of breast
| Excludes | ptosis of native breast in relation to reconstructed breast (612.1) |

611.82 Hypoplasia of breast
Micromastia
| Excludes | congenital absence of breast (757.6) hypoplasia of native breast in relation to reconstructed breast (612.1) |

611.83 Capsular contracture of breast implant

611.89 Other specified disorders of breast
Hematoma (nontraumatic) of breast
Infarction of breast
Occlusion of breast duct
Subinvolution of breast (postlactational) (postpartum)

611.9 Unspecified breast disorder

● **612 Deformity and disproportion of reconstructed breast**
Coding Clinic: 2008, Q4, P123

612.0 Deformity of reconstructed breast
Contour irregularity in reconstructed breast
Excess tissue in reconstructed breast
Misshapen reconstructed breast

612.1 Disproportion of reconstructed breast
Breast asymmetry between native breast and reconstructed breast
Disproportion between native breast and reconstructed breast

(See Plate 366A on page NAP-3.)

INFLAMMATORY DISEASE OF FEMALE PELVIC ORGANS (614–616)

Use additional code to identify organism, such as Staphylococcus (041.1), or Streptococcus (041.0)
| Excludes | that associated with pregnancy, abortion, childbirth, or the puerperium (630–676.9) |

● **614 Inflammatory disease of ovary, fallopian tube, pelvic cellular tissue, and peritoneum**
| Excludes | endometritis (615.0–615.9) major infection following delivery (670.0-670.8) that complicating: abortion (634–638 with .0, 639.0) ectopic or molar pregnancy (639.0) pregnancy or labor (646.6) |

Fallopian tube (oviduct)
Corpus uteri
Cervix uteri
Rectum
Vagina
Ovary
Isthmus
Urinary bladder
Symphysis pubis
Clitoris
Urethra

*Mons veneris
*Labium majus
Urethra
*Labium minus
Introitus
Bartholin's glands
Perineum

A   Female Genital System   B   *The three parts of the vulva

Figure 10–10 A. Female genital system. **B.** External female genital system. (From Buck CJ: Step-by-Step Medical Coding, 2006 ed. Philadelphia, WB Saunders, 2006.)

Item 10-10 Salpingitis is an infection of one or both fallopian tubes. **Oophoritis** is an infection of one or both ovaries.

614.0 Acute salpingitis and oophoritis
Any condition classifiable to 614.2, specified as acute or subacute

614.1 Chronic salpingitis and oophoritis
Hydrosalpinx
Salpingitis:
follicularis
isthmica nodosa
Any condition classifiable to 614.2, specified as chronic

614.2 Salpingitis and oophoritis not specified as acute, subacute, or chronic
Abscess (of):
fallopian tube
ovary
tubo-ovarian
Oophoritis
Perioophoritis
Perisalpingitis
Pyosalpinx
Salpingitis
Salpingo-oophoritis
Tubo-ovarian inflammatory disease
| Excludes | gonococcal infection (chronic) (098.37) acute (098.17) tuberculous (016.6) |

614.3 Acute parametritis and pelvic cellulitis
Acute inflammatory pelvic disease
Any condition classifiable to 614.4, specified as acute

614.4 Chronic or unspecified parametritis and pelvic cellulitis
Abscess (of):
broad ligament chronic or NOS
parametrium chronic or NOS
pelvis, female chronic or NOS
pouch of Douglas chronic or NOS
Chronic inflammatory pelvic disease
Pelvic cellulitis, female
| Excludes | tuberculous (016.7) |

614.5 Acute or unspecified pelvic peritonitis, female

614.6 Pelvic peritoneal adhesions, female (postoperative) (postinfection)
Adhesions:
peritubal
tubo-ovarian
Use additional code to identify any associated infertility (628.2)
Coding Clinic: 2003, Q3, P6-7; Q1, P4-5; 1995, Q3, P7

614.7 Other chronic pelvic peritonitis, female
> Excludes *tuberculous (016.7)*

614.8 Other specified inflammatory disease of female pelvic organs and tissues

614.9 Unspecified inflammatory disease of female pelvic organs and tissues
Pelvic infection or inflammation, female NOS
Pelvic inflammatory disease [PID]

● **615 Inflammatory diseases of uterus, except cervix**
> Excludes *following delivery (670.0-670.8)*
> *hyperplastic endometritis (621.30–621.35)*
> *that complicating:*
> *abortion (634–638 with .0, 639.0)*
> *ectopic or molar pregnancy (639.0)*
> *pregnancy or labor (646.6)*

615.0 Acute
Any condition classifiable to 615.9, specified as acute or subacute

615.1 Chronic
Any condition classifiable to 615.9, specified as chronic

615.9 Unspecified inflammatory disease of uterus

Endometritis	Perimetritis
Endomyometritis	Pyometra
Metritis	Uterine abscess
Myometritis	

● **616 Inflammatory disease of cervix, vagina, and vulva**
> Excludes *that complicating:*
> *abortion (634–638 with .0, 639.0)*
> *ectopic or molar pregnancy (639.0)*
> *pregnancy, childbirth, or the puerperium (646.6)*

616.0 Cervicitis and endocervicitis
Cervicitis with or without mention of erosion or ectropion
Endocervicitis with or without mention of erosion or ectropion
Nabothian (gland) cyst or follicle
> Excludes *erosion or ectropion without mention of cervicitis (622.0)*

● **616.1 Vaginitis and vulvovaginitis**
> Excludes *vulvar vestibulitis (625.71)*

616.10 Vaginitis and vulvovaginitis, unspecified
Vaginitis:
  NOS
  postirradiation
Vulvitis NOS
Vulvovaginitis NOS
> Use additional code to identify organism, such as Escherichia coli [E. coli] (041.4), Staphylococcus (041.1), or Streptococcus (041.0)
> Excludes *noninfective leukorrhea (623.5)*
> *postmenopausal or senile vaginitis (627.3)*

616.11 Vaginitis and vulvovaginitis in diseases classified elsewhere
> Code first *underlying disease, as:*
> pinworm vaginitis (127.4)
> Excludes *herpetic vulvovaginitis (054.11)*
> *monilial vulvovaginitis (112.1)*
> *trichomonal vaginitis or vulvovaginitis (131.01)*

616.2 Cyst of Bartholin's gland
Cysts filled with liquid or semisolid material.
Bartholin's duct cyst

616.3 Abscess of Bartholin's gland
Localized collection of pus
Vulvovaginal gland abscess

616.4 Other abscess of vulva
Abscess of vulva
Carbuncle of vulva
Furuncle of vulva

● **616.5 Ulceration of vulva**

616.50 Ulceration of vulva, unspecified
Ulcer NOS of vulva

616.51 Ulceration of vulva in diseases classified elsewhere
> Code first *underlying disease, as:*
> Behçet's syndrome (136.1)
> tuberculosis (016.7)
> Excludes *vulvar ulcer (in):*
> *gonococcal (098.0)*
> *herpes simplex (054.12)*
> *syphilitic (091.0)*

● **616.8 Other specified inflammatory diseases of cervix, vagina, and vulva**
> Excludes *noninflammatory disorders of:*
> *cervix (622.0–622.9)*
> *vagina (623.0–623.9)*
> *vulva (624.0–624.9)*

616.81 Mucositis (ulcerative) of cervix, vagina, and vulva
> Use additional E code to identify adverse effects of therapy, such as:
> antineoplastic and immunosuppressive drugs (E930.7, E933.1)
> radiation therapy (E879.2)

616.89 Other inflammatory disease of cervix, vagina and vulva
Caruncle, vagina or labium
Ulcer, vagina

616.9 Unspecified inflammatory disease of cervix, vagina, and vulva

---

OTHER DISORDERS OF FEMALE GENITAL TRACT (617–629)

● **617 Endometriosis**
Coding Clinic: 1995, Q1, P7

617.0 Endometriosis of uterus
Adenomyosis
Endometriosis:
  cervix
  internal
  myometrium
> Excludes *stromal endometriosis (236.0)*
Coding Clinic: 1992, Q3, P7-8

617.1 Endometriosis of ovary
Chocolate cyst of ovary
Endometrial cystoma of ovary

617.2 Endometriosis of fallopian tube

617.3 Endometriosis of pelvic peritoneum
Endometriosis:
  broad ligament
  cul-de-sac (Douglas')
  parametrium
  round ligament

617.4 Endometriosis of rectovaginal septum and vagina

617.5 Endometriosis of intestine
Endometriosis:
  appendix
  colon
  rectum

◀ New   ◀▦ Revised   ~~deleted~~ Deleted | Excludes | | Includes | | Use additional | | Code first | | Omit code |
● Unacceptable Principal Diagnosis   ● Use Additional Digit(s)   OGCR Official Guidelines   Coding Clinic

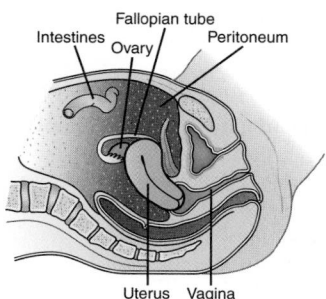

Figure 10–11 Intestines, Ovary, Fallopian tube, Peritoneum, Uterus, Vagina

Figure 10–11 Sites of potential endometrial implants.

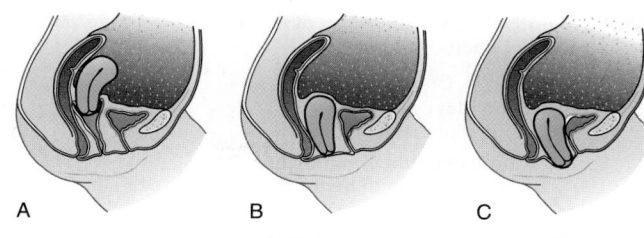

A   B   C

Figure 10–12 Three stages of uterine prolapse. **A.** Uterus is prolapsed. **B.** Vagina and uterus are prolapsed (incomplete uterovaginal prolapse). **C.** Vagina and uterus are completely prolapsed and are exposed through the external genitalia (complete uterovaginal prolapse).

Item 10–11 Endometriosis is a condition for which no clear cause has been identified. Endometrial tissue is expelled from the uterus into the abdominal cavity and can implant onto a variety of organs. Classification is based on the site of implant of the endometrial tissue.

617.6 Endometriosis in scar of skin

617.8 Endometriosis of other specified sites
> Endometriosis:
> bladder   umbilicus
> lung   vulva

617.9 Endometriosis, site unspecified

● **618 Genital prolapse**

> Use additional code to identify urinary incontinence (625.6, 788.31, 788.33–788.39)

> Excludes   *that complicating pregnancy, labor, or delivery (654.4)*

● **618.0 Prolapse of vaginal walls without mention of uterine prolapse**

> Excludes   *that with uterine prolapse (618.2–618.4)*
> *enterocele (618.6)*
> *vaginal vault prolapse following hysterectomy (618.5)*

> Coding Clinic: 2004, Q4, P83-85

> **618.00 Unspecified prolapse of vaginal walls**
> Vaginal prolapse NOS

> **618.01 Cystocele, midline**
> Cystocele NOS

> **618.02 Cystocele, lateral**
> Paravaginal

> **618.03 Urethrocele**

> **618.04 Rectocele**
> Proctocele
> > Use additional code for associated fecal incontinence (787.60-787.63) ◄

> **618.05 Perineocele**

> **618.09 Other prolapse of vaginal walls without mention of uterine prolapse**
> Cystourethrocele

618.1 Uterine prolapse without mention of vaginal wall prolapse
> Descensus uteri
> Uterine prolapse:
> NOS
> complete
> first degree
> second degree
> third degree

> Excludes   *that with mention of cystocele, urethrocele, or rectocele (618.2–618.4)*

618.2 Uterovaginal prolapse, incomplete

618.3 Uterovaginal prolapse, complete

618.4 Uterovaginal prolapse, unspecified

618.5 Prolapse of vaginal vault after hysterectomy

618.6 Vaginal enterocele, congenital or acquired
> Pelvic enterocele, congenital or acquired

618.7 Old laceration of muscles of pelvic floor

● **618.8 Other specified genital prolapse**

> **618.81 Incompetence or weakening of pubocervical tissue**

> **618.82 Incompetence or weakening of rectovaginal tissue**

> **618.83 Pelvic muscle wasting**
> Disuse atrophy of pelvic muscles and anal sphincter

> **618.84 Cervical stump prolapse**

> **618.89 Other specified genital prolapse**

618.9 Unspecified genital prolapse

● **619 Fistula involving female genital tract**

> Excludes   *vesicorectal and intestinovesical fistula (596.1)*

619.0 Urinary-genital tract fistula, female
> Fistula:
> cervicovesical
> ureterovaginal
> urethrovaginal
> urethrovesicovaginal
> uteroureteric
> uterovesical
> vesicocervicovaginal
> vesicovaginal

619.1 Digestive-genital tract fistula, female
> Fistula: Fistula:
> intestinouterine   rectovulval
> intestinovaginal   sigmoidovaginal
> rectovaginal   uterorectal

619.2 Genital tract-skin fistula, female
> Fistula:
> uterus to abdominal wall
> vaginoperineal

619.8 Other specified fistulas involving female genital tract
> Fistula:
> cervix
> cul-de-sac (Douglas')
> uterus
> vagina

619.9 Unspecified fistula involving female genital tract

● **620 Noninflammatory disorders of ovary, fallopian tube, and broad ligament**

> **Excludes** *hydrosalpinx (614.1)*

620.0 Follicular cyst of ovary
Cyst of graafian follicle

620.1 Corpus luteum cyst or hematoma
Corpus luteum hemorrhage or rupture
Lutein cyst

620.2 Other and unspecified ovarian cyst
Cyst of ovary:
　NOS
　corpus albicans
　retention NOS
　serous
　theca-lutein
Simple cystoma of ovary

> **Excludes** *cystadenoma (benign) (serous) (220)*
> *developmental cysts (752.0)*
> *neoplastic cysts (220)*
> *polycystic ovaries (256.4)*
> *Stein-Leventhal syndrome (256.4)*

620.3 Acquired atrophy of ovary and fallopian tube
Senile involution of ovary

620.4 Prolapse or hernia of ovary and fallopian tube
Displacement of ovary and fallopian tube
Salpingocele

620.5 Torsion of ovary, ovarian pedicle, or fallopian tube
Torsion:
　accessory tube
　hydatid of Morgagni

620.6 Broad ligament laceration syndrome
Masters-Allen syndrome

620.7 Hematoma of broad ligament
Hematocele, broad ligament

620.8 Other noninflammatory disorders of ovary, fallopian tube, and broad ligament
Cyst of broad ligament or fallopian tube
Polyp of broad ligament or fallopian tube
Infarction of ovary or fallopian tube
Rupture of ovary or fallopian tube
Hematosalpinx of ovary or fallopian tube

> **Excludes** *hematosalpinx in ectopic pregnancy (639.2)*
> *peritubal adhesions (614.6)*
> *torsion of ovary, ovarian pedicle, or fallopian tube (620.5)*

620.9 Unspecified noninflammatory disorder of ovary, fallopian tube, and broad ligament

● **621 Disorders of uterus, not elsewhere classified**

621.0 Polyp of corpus uteri
Polyp:
　endometrium
　uterus NOS

> **Excludes** *cervical polyp NOS (622.7)*

621.1 Chronic subinvolution of uterus

> **Excludes** *puerperal (674.8)*

621.2 Hypertrophy of uterus
Bulky or enlarged uterus

> **Excludes** *puerperal (674.8)*

● **621.3 Endometrial hyperplasia**
Coding Clinic: 2004, Q4, P85-86

621.30 Endometrial hyperplasia, unspecified
Endometrial hyperplasia NOS
Hyperplasia (adenomatous) (cystic) (glandular) of endometrium
Hyperplastic endometritis

621.31 Simple endometrial hyperplasia without atypia

> **Excludes** *benign endometrial hyperplasia (621.34)*

621.32 Complex endometrial hyperplasia without atypia

> **Excludes** *benign endometrial hyperplasia (621.34)*

621.33 Endometrial hyperplasia with atypia

> **Excludes** *endometrial intraepithelial neoplasia [EIN] (621.35)*

621.34 Benign endometrial hyperplasia

621.35 Endometrial intraepithelial neoplasia [EIN]

> **Excludes** *malignant neoplasm of endometrium with endometrium intraepithelial neoplasia [EIN] (182.0)*

621.4 Hematometra
Hemometra

> **Excludes** *that in congenital anomaly (752.2-752.39)* ◀▥

621.5 Intrauterine synechiae
Adhesions of uterus　　Band(s) of uterus

621.6 Malposition of uterus
Anteversion of uterus
Retroflexion of uterus
Retroversion of uterus

> **Excludes** *malposition complicating pregnancy, labor, or delivery (654.3–654.4)*
> *prolapse of uterus (618.1–618.4)*

621.7 Chronic inversion of uterus

> **Excludes** *current obstetrical trauma (665.2)*
> *prolapse of uterus (618.1–618.4)*

621.8 Other specified disorders of uterus, not elsewhere classified
Atrophy, acquired of uterus
Cyst of uterus
Fibrosis NOS of uterus
Old laceration (postpartum) of uterus
Ulcer of uterus

> **Excludes** *bilharzial fibrosis (120.0–120.9)*
> *endometriosis (617.0)*
> *fistulas (619.0–619.8)*
> *inflammatory diseases (615.0–615.9)*

621.9 Unspecified disorder of uterus

● **622 Noninflammatory disorders of cervix**

> **Excludes** *abnormality of cervix complicating pregnancy, labor, or delivery (654.5–654.6)*
> *fistula (619.0–619.8)*

622.0 Erosion and ectropion of cervix
Eversion of cervix
Ulcer of cervix

> **Excludes** *that in chronic cervicitis (616.0)*

● **622.1 Dysplasia of cervix (uteri)**

> **Excludes** *abnormal results from cervical cytologic examination without histologic confirmation (795.00–795.09)*
> *carcinoma in situ of cervix (233.1)*
> *cervical intraepithelial neoplasia III [CIN III] (233.1)*
> *HGSIL of cervix (795.04)*
> Coding Clinic: 2004, Q4, P86-88; 1991, Q1, P11

622.10 Dysplasia of cervix, unspecified
Anaplasia of cervix
Cervical atypism
Cervical dysplasia NOS

622.11 Mild dysplasia of cervix
Cervical intraepithelial neoplasia I [CIN I]

622.12 Moderate dysplasia of cervix
Cervical intraepithelial neoplasia II [CIN II]

> **Excludes** *carcinoma in situ of cervix (233.1)*
> *cervical intraepithelial neoplasia III*
> *[CIN III] (233.1)*
> *severe dysplasia (233.1)*

622.2 Leukoplakia of cervix (uteri)

> **Excludes** *carcinoma in situ of cervix (233.1)*

622.3 Old laceration of cervix
Adhesions of cervix
Band(s) of cervix
Cicatrix (postpartum) of cervix

> **Excludes** *current obstetrical trauma (665.3)*

622.4 Stricture and stenosis of cervix
Atresia (acquired) of cervix
Contracture of cervix
Occlusion of cervix
Pinpoint os uteri

> **Excludes** *congenital (752.49)*
> *that complicating labor (654.6)*

622.5 Incompetence of cervix

> **Excludes** *complicating pregnancy (654.5)*
> *that affecting fetus or newborn (761.0)*

622.6 Hypertrophic elongation of cervix

622.7 Mucous polyp of cervix
Polyp NOS of cervix

> **Excludes** *adenomatous polyp of cervix (219.0)*

622.8 Other specified noninflammatory disorders of cervix
Atrophy (senile) of cervix
Cyst of cervix
Fibrosis of cervix
Hemorrhage of cervix

> **Excludes** *endometriosis (617.0)*
> *fistula (619.0–619.8)*
> *inflammatory diseases (616.0)*

622.9 Unspecified noninflammatory disorder of cervix

● **623 Noninflammatory disorders of vagina**

> **Excludes** *abnormality of vagina complicating pregnancy,*
> *labor, or delivery (654.7)*
> *congenital absence of vagina (752.49)*
> *congenital diaphragm or bands (752.49)*
> *fistulas involving vagina (619.0–619.8)*

623.0 Dysplasia of vagina
Mild and moderate dysplasia of vagina
Vaginal intraepithelial neoplasia I and II [VAIN I
and II]

> **Excludes** *abnormal results from vaginal cytological*
> *examination without histologic*
> *confirmation (795.10-795.19)*
> *carcinoma in situ of vagina (233.31)*
> *HGSIL of vagina (795.14)*
> *severe dysplasia of vagina (233.31)*
> *vaginal intraepithelial neoplasia III [VAIN*
> *III] (233.31)*

623.1 Leukoplakia of vagina

623.2 Stricture or atresia of vagina
Adhesions (postoperative) (postradiation) of
vagina
Occlusion of vagina
Stenosis, vagina

Use additional E code to identify any external
cause

> **Excludes** *congenital atresia or stricture (752.49)*

623.3 Tight hymenal ring
Rigid hymen acquired or congenital
Tight hymenal ring acquired or congenital
Tight introitus acquired or congenital

> **Excludes** *imperforate hymen (752.42)*

623.4 Old vaginal laceration

> **Excludes** *old laceration involving muscles of pelvic*
> *floor (618.7)*

623.5 Leukorrhea, not specified as infective
Leukorrhea NOS of vagina
Vaginal discharge NOS

> **Excludes** *trichomonal (131.00)*

623.6 Vaginal hematoma

> **Excludes** *current obstetrical trauma (665.7)*

623.7 Polyp of vagina

**623.8 Other specified noninflammatory disorders of
vagina**
Cyst of vagina
Hemorrhage of vagina

623.9 Unspecified noninflammatory disorder of vagina

● **624 Noninflammatory disorders of vulva and perineum**

> **Excludes** *abnormality of vulva and perineum complicating*
> *pregnancy, labor, or delivery (654.8)*
> *condyloma acuminatum (078.11)*
> *fistulas involving:*
> *perineum - see Alphabetic Index*
> *vulva (619.0–619.8)*
> *vulval varices (456.6)*
> *vulvar involvement in skin conditions (690–709.9)*

● **624.0 Dystrophy of vulva**

> **Excludes** *carcinoma in situ of vulva (233.32)*
> *severe dysplasia of vulva (233.32)*
> *vulvar intraepithelial neoplasia III [VIN III]*
> *(233.32)*

624.01 Vulvar intraepithelial neoplasia I [VIN I]
Mild dysplasia of vulva

624.02 Vulvar intraepithelial neoplasia II [VIN II]
Moderate dysplasia of vulva
Coding Clinic: 2007, Q4, P90-91

624.09 Other dystrophy of vulva
Kraurosis of vulva
Leukoplakia of vulva

624.1 Atrophy of vulva

624.2 Hypertrophy of clitoris

> **Excludes** *that in endocrine disorders (255.2, 256.1)*

624.3 Hypertrophy of labia
Hypertrophy of vulva NOS

624.4 Old laceration or scarring of vulva

624.5 Hematoma of vulva

> **Excludes** *that complicating delivery (664.5)*

624.6 Polyp of labia and vulva

**624.8 Other specified noninflammatory disorders of vulva
and perineum**
Cyst of vulva
Edema of vulva
Stricture of vulva
Coding Clinic: 2003, Q1, P13-14; 1995, Q1, P8

**624.9 Unspecified noninflammatory disorder of vulva and
perineum**

● **625 Pain and other symptoms associated with female genital organs**

625.0 Dyspareunia
Painful intercourse/coitus

> **Excludes** *psychogenic dyspareunia (302.76)*

625.1 Vaginismus
Colpospasm
Vulvismus

> **Excludes** *psychogenic vaginismus (306.51)*

625.2 Mittelschmerz
Intermenstrual pain
Ovulation pain

625.3 Dysmenorrhea
Painful menstruation

> **Excludes** *psychogenic dysmenorrhea (306.52)*

Coding Clinic: 1994, Q2, P12

625.4 Premenstrual tension syndromes
Menstrual molimen
Premenstrual dysphoric disorder
Premenstrual syndrome
Premenstrual tension NOS

> **Excludes** *menstrual migraine (346.4)*

Coding Clinic: 2003, Q4, P116

625.5 Pelvic congestion syndrome
Congestion-fibrosis syndrome
Taylor's syndrome

625.6 Stress incontinence, female

> **Excludes** *mixed incontinence (788.33)*
> *stress incontinence, male (788.32)*

● **625.7 Vulvodynia**
Coding Clinic: 2008, Q4, P124

625.70 Vulvodynia, unspecified
Vulvodynia NOS

625.71 Vulvar vestibulitis

625.79 Other vulvodynia

625.8 Other specified symptoms associated with female genital organs
Coding Clinic: 1985, Nov-Dec, P16

625.9 Unspecified symptom associated with female genital organs
Coding Clinic: 2006, Q4, P109-110; 1994, Q2, P12; 1985, Nov-Dec, P16

● **626 Disorders of menstruation and other abnormal bleeding from female genital tract**

> **Excludes** *menopausal and premenopausal bleeding (627.0)*
> *pain and other symptoms associated with menstrual cycle (625.2–625.4)*
> *postmenopausal bleeding (627.1)*
> *precocious puberty (259.1)* ◄

626.0 Absence of menstruation
Amenorrhea (primary) (secondary)
Coding Clinic: 1985, July-Aug, P9

626.1 Scanty or infrequent menstruation
Hypomenorrhea
Oligomenorrhea

626.2 Excessive or frequent menstruation
Heavy periods   Menorrhagia
Menometrorrhagia   Polymenorrhea

> **Excludes** *premenopausal (627.0)*
> *that in puberty (626.3)*

Coding Clinic: 2006, Q4, P97-98; 2004, Q4, P88-90; 1994, Q2, P12

626.3 Puberty bleeding
Excessive bleeding associated with onset of menstrual periods
Pubertal menorrhagia

626.4 Irregular menstrual cycle
Irregular: Irregular:
  bleeding NOS   periods
  menstruation

626.5 Ovulation bleeding
Regular intermenstrual bleeding

626.6 Metrorrhagia
Bleeding unrelated to menstrual cycle
Irregular intermenstrual bleeding

626.7 Postcoital bleeding

626.8 Other
Dysfunctional or functional uterine hemorrhage NOS
Menstruation: Menstruation:
  retained   suppression of

626.9 Unspecified

● **627 Menopausal and postmenopausal disorders**

> **Excludes** *asymptomatic age-related (natural) postmenopausal status (V49.81)*

627.0 Premenopausal menorrhagia
Excessive bleeding associated with onset of menopause
Menorrhagia: Menorrhagia:
  climacteric   preclimacteric
  menopausal

627.1 Postmenopausal bleeding

627.2 Symptomatic menopausal or female climacteric states
Symptoms, such as flushing, sleeplessness, headache, lack of concentration, associated with the menopause

627.3 Postmenopausal atrophic vaginitis
Senile (atrophic) vaginitis

627.4 Symptomatic states associated with artificial menopause
Postartificial menopause syndromes
Any condition classifiable to 627.1, 627.2, or 627.3 which follows induced menopause

627.8 Other specified menopausal and postmenopausal disorders

> **Excludes** *premature menopause NOS (256.31)*

627.9 Unspecified menopausal and postmenopausal disorder

● **628 Infertility, female**

> **Includes** primary and secondary sterility

Coding Clinic: 1996, Q2, P9; 1995, Q1, P7

628.0 Associated with anovulation
Anovulatory cycle

> Use additional code for any associated Stein-Leventhal syndrome (256.4)

628.1 Of pituitary-hypothalamic origin

> *Code first underlying disease, as:*
> adiposogenital dystrophy (253.8)
> anterior pituitary disorder (253.0–253.4)

628.2 Of tubal origin
Infertility associated with congenital anomaly of tube
Tubal: Tubal:
  block   stenosis
  occlusion

> Use additional code for any associated peritubal adhesions (614.6)

628.3 Of uterine origin
Infertility associated with congenital anomaly of
    uterus
Nonimplantation

Use additional code for any associated tuberculous
    endometritis (016.7)

628.4 Of cervical or vaginal origin
Infertility associated with:
    anomaly or cervical mucus
    congenital structural anomaly
    dysmucorrhea

628.8 Of other specified origin

628.9 Of unspecified origin

● **629 Other disorders of female genital organs**

629.0 Hematocele, female, not elsewhere classified

Excludes *hematocele or hematoma:*
    broad ligament (620.7)
    fallopian tube (620.8)
    that associated with ectopic pregnancy
        (633.00–633.91)
    uterus (621.4)
    vagina (623.6)
    vulva (624.5)

629.1 Hydrocele, canal of Nuck
Cyst of canal of Nuck (acquired)

Excludes *congenital (752.41)*

● **629.2 Female genital multilation status**
Female circumcision status
Female genital cutting

629.20 Female genital mutilation status, unspecified
Female genital cutting status, unspecified
Female genital mutilation status NOS

629.21 Female genital mutilation Type I status
Clitorectomy status
Female genital cutting Type I status

629.22 Female genital mutilation Type II status
Clitorectomy with excision of labia minora
    status
Female genital cutting Type II status
Coding Clinic: 2004, Q4, P88-90

629.23 Female genital mutilation Type III status
Female genital cutting Type III status
Infibulation status

629.29 Other female genital mutilation status
Female genital cutting Type IV status
Female genital mutilation Type IV status
Other female genital cutting status

● **629.8 Other specified disorders of female genital organs**

**629.81 ~~Habitual aborter~~ Recurrent pregnancy loss
without current pregnancy** ◄

Excludes *~~habitual aborter~~ recurrent*
    pregnancy loss with current
    pregnancy (646.3) ◄
Coding Clinic: 2006, Q4, P98

**629.89 Other specified disorders of female genital
organs**

629.9 Unspecified disorder of female genital organs

DISEASES OF THE GENITOURINARY SYSTEM (580–629)

(See Plate 375 on page NAP-4.)

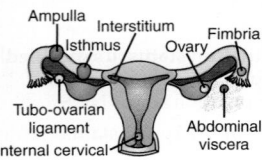

Figure 11–1 Implantation sites of ectopic pregnancy.

Item 11–1 Ectopic pregnancy most often occurs in the fallopian tube. Pregnancy outside the uterus may end in a life-threatening rupture.

Item 11–2 A hydatidiform mole is a benign tumor of the placenta. The tumor secretes a hormone, chorionic gonadotropic hormone (CGH), that indicates a positive pregnancy test.

OGCR Section I.C.11.a.1 and 2

> Obstetric cases require codes from chapter 11, codes in the range 630-679, Complications of Pregnancy, Childbirth, and the Puerperium. Chapter 11 codes have sequencing priority over codes from other chapters. Additional codes from other chapters may be used in conjunction with chapter 11 codes to further specify conditions. Should the provider document that the pregnancy is incidental to the encounter, then code V22.2 should be used in place of any chapter 11 codes. It is the provider's responsibility to state that the condition being treated is not affecting the pregnancy.

11. COMPLICATIONS OF PREGNANCY, CHILDBIRTH, AND THE PUERPERIUM (630–679)

ECTOPIC AND MOLAR PREGNANCY (630–633)

Use additional code from category 639 to identify any complications

630 Hydatidiform mole
Trophoblastic disease NOS
Vesicular mole

> Excludes   *chorioadenoma (destruens) (236.1)*
> *chorionepithelioma (181)*
> *malignant hydatidiform mole (236.1)*

631 Other abnormal product of conception
Blighted ovum
Mole:
  NOS
  carneous
  fleshy
  stone

632 Missed abortion
Early fetal death before completion of 22 weeks' gestation with retention of dead fetus
Retained products of conception, not following spontaneous or induced abortion or delivery

> Excludes   *failed induced abortion (638.0–638.9)*
> *fetal death (intrauterine) (late) (656.4)*
> *missed delivery (656.4)*
> *that with abnormal product of conception (630, 631)*

Coding Clinic: 2001, Q1, P5

633 Ectopic pregnancy

Includes   ruptured ectopic pregnancy

Coding Clinic: 2002, Q4, P61-62

● **633.0 Abdominal pregnancy**
Intraperitoneal pregnancy

  633.00 Abdominal pregnancy without intrauterine pregnancy

  633.01 Abdominal pregnancy with intrauterine pregnancy

● **633.1 Tubal pregnancy**
Fallopian pregnancy
Rupture of (fallopian) tube due to pregnancy
Tubal abortion

  633.10 Tubal pregnancy without intrauterine pregnancy

  633.11 Tubal pregnancy with intrauterine pregnancy

● **633.2 Ovarian pregnancy**

  633.20 Ovarian pregnancy without intrauterine pregnancy

  633.21 Ovarian pregnancy with intrauterine pregnancy

● **633.8 Other ectopic pregnancy**
Pregnancy:
  cervical
  combined
  cornual
  intraligamentous
  mesometric
  mural

  633.80 Other ectopic pregnancy without intrauterine pregnancy

  633.81 Other ectopic pregnancy with intrauterine pregnancy

● **633.9 Unspecified ectopic pregnancy**

  633.90 Unspecified ectopic pregnancy without intrauterine pregnancy

  633.91 Unspecified ectopic pregnancy with intrauterine pregnancy

OTHER PREGNANCY WITH ABORTIVE OUTCOME (634–639)

The following fourth digit subdivisions are for use with categories 634–638:

> **0 Complicated by genital tract and pelvic infection**
> Endometritis
> Salpingo-oophoritis
> Sepsis NOS
> Septicemia NOS
> Any condition classifiable to 639.0, with condition classifiable to 634–638
>
> > Excludes   *urinary tract infection (634–638 with .7)*
>
> **1 Complicated by delayed or excessive hemorrhage**
> Afibrinogenemia
> Defibrination syndrome
> Intravascular hemolysis
> Any condition classifiable to 639.1, with condition classifiable to 634–638
>
> **2 Complicated by damage to pelvic organs and tissues**
> Laceration, perforation, or tear of:
>   bladder
>   uterus
> Any condition classifiable to 639.2, with condition classifiable to 634–638

◄ New   ◄||||| Revised   ~~deleted~~ Deleted   Excludes   Includes   Use additional   Code first   Omit code
● Unacceptable Principal Diagnosis   ● Use Additional Digit(s)   **OGCR** Official Guidelines   **Coding Clinic**

3 Complicated by renal failure
   Oliguria
   Uremia
   Any condition classifiable to 639.3, with condition
      classifiable to 634–638
4 Complicated by metabolic disorder
   Electrolyte imbalance with conditions classifiable to
      634–638
5 Complicated by shock
   Circulatory collapse
   Shock (postoperative) (septic)
   Any condition classifiable to 639.5, with condition
      classifiable to 634–638
6 Complicated by embolism
   Embolism:
     NOS
     amniotic fluid
     pulmonary
   Any condition classifiable to 639.6, with condition
      classifiable to 634–638
7 With other specified complications
   Cardiac arrest or failure
   Urinary tract infection
   Any condition classifiable to 639.8, with condition
      classifiable to 634–638
8 With unspecified complications
9 Without mention of complication

OGCR Section I.C.11.k.1
Fifth-digits are required for abortion categories 634-637. Fifth digit assignment is based on the status of the patient at the beginning (or start) of the encounter. Fifth-digit 1, incomplete, indicates that all of the products of conception have not been expelled from the uterus. Fifth-digit 2, complete, indicates that all products of conception have been expelled from the uterus.

OGCR Section I.C.11.k.5
Subsequent admissions for retained products of conception following a spontaneous or legally induced abortion are assigned the appropriate code from category 634, Spontaneous abortion, or 635 Legally induced abortion, with a fifth digit of "1" (incomplete). This advice is appropriate even when the patient was discharged previously with a discharge diagnosis of complete abortion.

● **634 Spontaneous abortion**
   Requires fifth digit to identify stage:

> **0 unspecified**
> **1 incomplete**
> **2 complete**

   Includes miscarriage
             spontaneous abortion

● **634.0 Complicated by genital tract and pelvic**
  [0-2] **infection**
● **634.1 Complicated by delayed or excessive hemorrhage**
  [0-2]   Coding Clinic: 2003, Q1, P6
● **634.2 Complicated by damage to pelvic organs or**
  [0-2] **tissues**
● **634.3 Complicated by renal failure**
  [0-2]
● **634.4 Complicated by metabolic disorder**
  [0-2]
● **634.5 Complicated by shock**
  [0-2]
● **634.6 Complicated by embolism**
  [0-2]

● **634.7 With other specified complications**
  [0-2]
● **634.8 With unspecified complication**
  [0-2]
● **634.9 Without mention of complication**
  [0-2]

● **635 Legally induced abortion**
   Requires fifth digit to identify stage:

> **0 unspecified**
> **1 incomplete**
> **2 complete**

   Includes abortion or termination of pregnancy:
             elective
             legal
             therapeutic
   Excludes *menstrual extraction or regulation (V25.3)*

● **635.0 Complicated by genital tract and pelvic**
  [0-2] **infection**
● **635.1 Complicated by delayed or excessive hemorrhage**
  [0-2]
● **635.2 Complicated by damage to pelvic organs or**
  [0-2] **tissues**
● **635.3 Complicated by renal failure**
  [0-2]
● **635.4 Complicated by metabolic disorder**
  [0-2]
● **635.5 Complicated by shock**
  [0-2]
● **635.6 Complicated by embolism**
  [0-2]
● **635.7 With other specified complications**
  [0-2]
● **635.8 With unspecified complication**
  [0-2]
● **635.9 Without mention of complication**
  [0-2]   Coding Clinic: 1994, Q2, P14

● **636 Illegally induced abortion**
   Requires fifth digit to identify stage:

> **0 unspecified**
> **1 incomplete**
> **2 complete**

   Includes abortion:
             criminal
             illegal
             self-induced

● **636.0 Complicated by genital tract and pelvic**
  [0-2] **infection**
● **636.1 Complicated by delayed or excessive hemorrhage**
  [0-2]
● **636.2 Complicated by damage to pelvic organs or**
  [0-2] **tissues**
● **636.3 Complicated by renal failure**
  [0-2]
● **636.4 Complicated by metabolic disorder**
  [0-2]
● **636.5 Complicated by shock**
  [0-2]

COMPLICATIONS OF PREGNANCY, CHILDBIRTH, AND THE PUERPERIUM (630–679)

● **636.6 Complicated by embolism**
[0-2]

● **636.7 With other specified complications**
[0-2]

● **636.8 With unspecified complication**
[0-2]

● **636.9 Without mention of complication**
[0-2]

● **637 Unspecified abortion**
Requires following fifth digit to identify stage:
Coding Clinic: 1994, Q2, P14

> 0   **unspecified**
> 1   **incomplete**
> 2   **complete**

Includes   abortion NOS
retained products of conception following
abortion, not classifiable elsewhere

● **637.0 Complicated by genital tract and pelvic**
[0-2] **infection**

● **637.1 Complicated by delayed or excessive hemorrhage**
[0-2]

● **637.2 Complicated by damage to pelvic organs or**
[0-2] **tissues**

● **637.3 Complicated by renal failure**
[0-2]

● **637.4 Complicated by metabolic disorder**
[0-2]

● **637.5 Complicated by shock**
[0-2]

● **637.6 Complicated by embolism**
[0-2]

● **637.7 With other specified complications**
[0-2]

● **637.8 With unspecified complication**
[0-2]

● **637.9 Without mention of complication**
[0-2]

● **638 Failed attempted abortion**

Includes   failure of attempted induction of (legal)
abortion

Excludes   *incomplete abortion (634.0–637.9)*

638.0 Complicated by genital tract and pelvic infection

638.1 Complicated by delayed or excessive hemorrhage

638.2 Complicated by damage to pelvic organs or tissues

638.3 Complicated by renal failure

638.4 Complicated by metabolic disorder

638.5 Complicated by shock

638.6 Complicated by embolism

638.7 With other specified complications

638.8 With unspecified complication

638.9 Without mention of complication

● **639 Complications following abortion and ectopic and molar pregnancies**

Note: This category is provided for use when it is
required to classify separately the complications
classifiable to the fourth digit level in categories
634–638; for example:
a) when the complication itself was responsible
for an episode of medical care, the abortion,
ectopic or molar pregnancy itself having been
dealt with at a previous episode
b) when these conditions are immediate
complications of ectopic or molar pregnancies
classifiable to 630–633 where they cannot be
identified at fourth digit level.

OGCR   Section I.C.11.k.3
Code 639 is to be used for all complications following
abortion. Code 639 cannot be assigned with codes from
categories 634-638.

639.0 Genital tract and pelvic infection
Endometritis following conditions classifiable to
630–638
Parametritis following conditions classifiable to
630–638
Pelvic peritonitis following conditions classifiable
to 630–638
Salpingitis following conditions classifiable to
630–638
Salpingo-oophoritis following conditions
classifiable to 630–638
Sepsis NOS following conditions classifiable to
630–638
Septicemia NOS following conditions classifiable
to 630–638

Excludes   *urinary tract infection (639.8)*

639.1 Delayed or excessive hemorrhage
Afibrinogenemia following conditions classifiable
to 630–638
Defibrination syndrome following conditions
classifiable to 630–638
Intravascular hemolysis following conditions
classifiable to 630–638

639.2 Damage to pelvic organs and tissues
Laceration, perforation, or tear of:
bladder following conditions classifiable to
630–638
bowel following conditions classifiable to
630–638
broad ligament following conditions classifiable
to 630–638
cervix following conditions classifiable to
630–638
periurethral tissue following conditions
classifiable to 630–638
uterus following conditions classifiable to
630–638
vagina following conditions classifiable to
630–638

639.3 Kidney failure
Oliguria following conditions classifiable to 630–638
Renal (kidney):
failure (acute) following conditions classifiable
to 630–638
shutdown following conditions classifiable to
630–638
tubular necrosis following conditions classifiable
to 630–638
Uremia following conditions classifiable to 630–638

639.4 Metabolic disorders
Electrolyte imbalance following conditions
classifiable to 630–638

◀ New   ◀|||| Revised   ~~deleted~~ Deleted   Excludes   Includes   Use additional   Code first   Omit code
● Unacceptable Principal Diagnosis   ● Use Additional Digit(s)   OGCR Official Guidelines   Coding Clinic

639.5 Shock
    Circulatory collapse following conditions
        classifiable to 630–638
    Shock (postoperative) (septic) following conditions
        classifiable to 630–638

639.6 Embolism
    Embolism:
        NOS following conditions classifiable to 630–638
        air following conditions classifiable to 630–638
        amniotic fluid following conditions classifiable
            to 630–638
        blood-clot following conditions classifiable to
            630–638
        fat following conditions classifiable to 630–638
        pulmonary following conditions classifiable to
            630–638
        pyemic following conditions classifiable to
            630–638
        septic following conditions classifiable to 630–638
        soap following conditions classifiable to 630–638

**639.8 Other specified complications following abortion or
    ectopic and molar pregnancy**
    Acute yellow atrophy or necrosis of liver following
        conditions classifiable to 630–638
    Cardiac arrest or failure following conditions
        classifiable to 630–638
    Cerebral anoxia following conditions classifiable to
        630–638
    Urinary tract infection following conditions
        classifiable to 630–638

**639.9 Unspecified complication following abortion or
    ectopic and molar pregnancy**
    Complication(s) not further specified following
        conditions classifiable to 630–638

OGCR Section I.C.11.k.2

A code from categories 640-648 and 651-659 may be used
as additional codes with an abortion code to indicate the
complication leading to the abortion. Fifth digit 3 is assigned
with codes from these categories when used with an abortion
code because the other fifth digits will not apply. Codes from the
660-669 series are not to be used for complications of abortion.

COMPLICATIONS MAINLY RELATED TO PREGNANCY (640–649)

Includes   the listed conditions even if they arose or were
                present during labor, delivery, or the
                puerperium

The following fifth-digit subclassification is for use with
categories 640–649 to denote the current episode of care:

0 unspecified as to episode of care or not applicable
1 delivered, with or without mention of antepartum
condition
Antepartum condition with delivery
Delivery NOS (with mention of antepartum
complication during current episode of care)
Intrapartum
obstetric condition (with mention of antepartum
complication during current episode of care)
Pregnancy, delivered (with mention of antepartum
complication during current episode of care)
2 delivered, with mention of postpartum complication
Delivery with mention of puerperal complication
during current episode of care
3 antepartum condition or complication
Antepartum obstetric condition, not delivered
during the current episode of care
4 postpartum condition or complication
Postpartum or puerperal obstetric condition or
complication following delivery that occurred:
during previous episode of care
outside hospital, with subsequent admission for
observation or care

● **640 Hemorrhage in early pregnancy**
    Requires fifth digit; valid digits are in [brackets] under
        each code. See beginning of section 640–649 for
        definitions.

    Includes   hemorrhage before completion of 22 weeks'
                    gestation

● **640.0 Threatened abortion**
    [0,1,3]

● **640.8 Other specified hemorrhage in early pregnancy**
    [0,1,3]

● **640.9 Unspecified hemorrhage in early pregnancy**
    [0,1,3]

● **641 Antepartum hemorrhage, abruptio placentae, and placenta
    previa**
    Requires fifth digit; valid digits are in [brackets] under
        each code. See beginning of section 640–649 for
        definitions.

● **641.0 Placenta previa without hemorrhage**
    [0,1,3]   Low implantation of placenta without hemorrhage
            Placenta previa noted:
                during pregnancy without hemorrhage
                before labor (and delivered by cesarean delivery)
                    without hemorrhage

● **641.1 Hemorrhage from placenta previa**
    [0,1,3]   Low-lying placenta NOS or with hemorrhage
                (intrapartum)
            Placenta previa:
                incomplete NOS or with hemorrhage
                    (intrapartum)
                marginal NOS or with hemorrhage
                    (intrapartum)
                partial NOS or with hemorrhage (intrapartum)
                total NOS or with hemorrhage (intrapartum)

    Excludes   *hemorrhage from vasa previa (663.5)*

● **641.2 Premature separation of placenta**
    [0,1,3]   Ablatio placentae
            Abruptio placentae
            Accidental antepartum hemorrhage
            Couvelaire uterus
            Detachment of placenta (premature)
            Premature separation of normally implanted
                placenta

Item 11–3 Placenta previa is a condition in which the opening of the
cervix is obstructed by the displaced placenta. The three types, marginal,
partial, and total, are varying degrees of placenta displacement.
Placenta abruption is the premature breaking away of the placenta from
the site of the uterine implant before the delivery of the fetus.

Figure 11–2 Abruptio placentae is classified according to the
grade of separation of the placenta from the uterine wall. **A.** Mild
separation in which hemorrhage is internal. **B.** Moderate separation
in which there is external hemorrhage. **C.** Severe separation in
which there is external hemorrhage and extreme separation.

COMPLICATIONS OF PREGNANCY, CHILDBIRTH, AND THE PUERPERIUM (630–679)

● **641.3 Antepartum hemorrhage associated with coagulation**
[0,1,3] **defects**
> Antepartum or intrapartum hemorrhage associated
> with:
> > afibrinogenemia
> > hyperfibrinolysis
> > hypofibrinogenemia
>
> > **Excludes** *coagulation defects not associated with*
> > *antepartum hemorrhage (649.3)*

● **641.8 Other antepartum hemorrhage**
[0,1,3]   Antepartum or intrapartum hemorrhage associated
> with:
> > trauma
> > uterine leiomyoma

● **641.9 Unspecified antepartum hemorrhage**
[0,1,3]   Hemorrhage:
> > antepartum NOS
> > intrapartum NOS
> > of pregnancy NOS

● **642 Hypertension complicating pregnancy, childbirth, and the**
puerperium
> Requires fifth digit; valid digits are in [brackets] under
> each code. See beginning of section 640–649 for
> definitions.

● **642.0 Benign essential hypertension complicating**
[0-4] **pregnancy, childbirth, and the puerperium**
> Hypertension:
> > benign essential specified as complicating,
> > or as a reason for obstetric care during
> > pregnancy, childbirth, or the puerperium
> > chronic NOS specified as complicating, or as a
> > reason for obstetric care during pregnancy,
> > childbirth, or the puerperium
> > essential specified as complicating, or as a
> > reason for obstetric care during pregnancy,
> > childbirth, or the puerperium
> > pre-existing NOS specified as complicating,
> > or as a reason for obstetric care during
> > pregnancy, childbirth, or the puerperium

● **642.1 Hypertension secondary to renal disease,**
[0-4] **complicating pregnancy, childbirth, and the**
puerperium
> Hypertension secondary to renal disease, specified
> as complicating, or as a reason for obstetric
> care during pregnancy, childbirth, or the
> puerperium

● **642.2 Other pre-existing hypertension complicating**
[0-4] **pregnancy, childbirth, and the puerperium**
> Hypertensive:
> > chronic kidney disease specified as
> > complicating, or as a reason for obstetric
> > care during pregnancy, childbirth, or the
> > puerperium
> > heart and chronic kidney disease specified as
> > complicating, or as a reason for obstetric
> > care during pregnancy, childbirth, or the
> > puerperium
> > heart disease specified as complicating, or as a
> > reason for obstetric care during pregnancy,
> > childbirth, or the puerperium
> Malignant hypertension specified as complicating,
> > or as a reason for obstetric care during
> > pregnancy, childbirth, or the puerperium

● **642.3 Transient hypertension of pregnancy**
[0-4]   Gestational hypertension
> Transient hypertension, so described, in pregnancy,
> childbirth, or the puerperium

OGCR Section I.C.7.a.8
Assign code 796.2, Elevated blood pressure reading without
diagnosis of hypertension, unless patient has an established
diagnosis of hypertension. Assign code 642.3x for transient
hypertension of pregnancy.

● **642.4 Mild or unspecified pre-eclampsia**
[0-4]   Hypertension in pregnancy, childbirth, or the
> puerperium, not specified as pre-existing,
> with either albuminuria or edema, or both;
> mild or unspecified
> Pre-eclampsia:
> > NOS
> > mild
> Toxemia (pre-eclamptic):
> > NOS
> > mild
>
> > **Excludes** *albuminuria in pregnancy, without mention*
> > *of hypertension (646.2)*
> > *edema in pregnancy, without mention of*
> > *hypertension (646.1)*
> > Coding Clinic: 2009, Q4, P108

● **642.5 Severe pre-eclampsia**
[0-4]   Hypertension in pregnancy, childbirth, or the
> puerperium, not specified as pre-existing,
> with either albuminuria or edema, or both;
> specified as severe
> Pre-eclampsia, severe
> Toxemia (pre-eclamptic), severe

● **642.6 Eclampsia**
[0-4]   Toxemia:
> > eclamptic
> > with convulsions

● **642.7 Pre-eclampsia or eclampsia superimposed on pre-**
[0-4] **existing hypertension**
> Conditions classifiable to 642.4–642.6, with
> conditions classifiable to 642.0–642.2

● **642.9 Unspecified hypertension complicating pregnancy,**
[0-4] **childbirth, or the puerperium**
> Hypertension NOS, without mention of
> albuminuria or edema, complicating
> pregnancy, childbirth, or the puerperium
> Coding Clinic: 2009, Q1, P18

● **643 Excessive vomiting in pregnancy**
> Requires fifth digit; valid digits are in [brackets] under
> each code. See beginning of section 640–649 for
> definitions.
>
> > **Includes** hyperemesis arising during pregnancy
> > vomiting:
> > > persistent arising during pregnancy
> > > vicious arising during pregnancy
> > hyperemesis gravidarum

● **643.0 Mild hyperemesis gravidarum**
[0,1,3]   Hyperemesis gravidarum, mild or unspecified,
> starting before the end of the 22nd week of
> gestation

● **643.1 Hyperemesis gravidarum with metabolic**
[0,1,3] **disturbance**
> Hyperemesis gravidarum, starting before the end
> of the 22nd week of gestation, with metabolic
> disturbance, such as:
> > carbohydrate depletion
> > dehydration
> > electrolyte imbalance

● **643.2 Late vomiting of pregnancy**
[0,1,3]   Excessive vomiting starting after 22 completed
> weeks of gestation

● **643.8 Other vomiting complicating pregnancy**
[0,1,3]   Vomiting due to organic disease or other cause,
            specified as complicating pregnancy, or as a
            reason for obstetric care during pregnancy

      Use additional code to specify cause

● **643.9 Unspecified vomiting of pregnancy**
[0,1,3]   Vomiting as a reason for care during pregnancy,
            length of gestation unspecified

● **644 Early or threatened labor**

      Requires fifth digit; valid digits are in [brackets] under
            each code. See beginning of section 640–649 for
            definitions.

● **644.0 Threatened premature labor**
[0,3]   Premature labor after 22 weeks, but before 37
            completed weeks of gestation without
            delivery

      Excludes | *that occurring before 22 completed weeks of
                  gestation (640.0)*

● **644.1 Other threatened labor**
[0,3]   False labor:
              NOS without delivery
              after 37 completed weeks of gestation without
                delivery
            Threatened labor NOS without delivery

● **644.2 Early onset of delivery**
[0-1]   Onset (spontaneous) of delivery before 37
            completed weeks of gestation
            Premature labor with onset of delivery before 37
            completed weeks of gestation
            Coding Clinic: 1991, Q2, P16

      OGCR Section I.C.11.k.4

      When an attempted termination of pregnancy
      results in a liveborn fetus assign code 644.21, Early
      onset of delivery, with an appropriate code from
      category V27, Outcome of Delivery. The procedure
      code for the attempted termination of pregnancy
      should also be assigned.

● **645 Late pregnancy**

      Requires fifth digit; valid digits are in [brackets] under
            each code. See beginning of section 640–649 for
            definitions.
            Coding Clinic: 2000, Q1, P17-18

● **645.1 Post term pregnancy**
[0,1,3]   Pregnancy over 40 completed weeks to 42
            completed weeks gestation

● **645.2 Prolonged pregnancy**
[0,1,3]   Pregnancy which has advanced beyond 42
            completed weeks of gestation

● **646 Other complications of pregnancy, not elsewhere
        classified**

      Use additional code(s) to further specify complication

      Requires fifth digit; valid digits are in [brackets] under
            each code. See beginning of section 640–649 for
            definitions.

● **646.0 Papyraceous fetus**
[0,1,3]

● **646.1 Edema or excessive weight gain in pregnancy,**
[0-4]   **without mention of hypertension**
            Gestational edema
            Maternal obesity syndrome

      Excludes | *that with mention of hypertension
                  (642.0–642.9)*

● **646.2 Unspecified renal disease in pregnancy, without**
[0-4]   **mention of hypertension**
            Albuminuria in pregnancy or the puerperium,
              without mention of hypertension
            Nephropathy NOS in pregnancy or the
              puerperium, without mention of
              hypertension
            Renal disease NOS in pregnancy or the
              puerperium, without mention of
              hypertension
            Uremia in pregnancy or the puerperium, without
              mention of hypertension
            Gestational proteinuria in pregnancy or
              the puerperium, without mention of
              hypertension

      Excludes | *that with mention of hypertension
                  (642.0–642.9)*

● **646.3** ~~Habitual aborter~~ **Recurrent pregnancy loss** ◄▦
[0,1,3]   Excludes | *with current abortion (634.0–634.9)
                  without current pregnancy (629.81)*

● **646.4 Peripheral neuritis in pregnancy**
[0-4]

● **646.5 Asymptomatic bacteriuria in pregnancy**
[0-4]

● **646.6 Infections of genitourinary tract in**
[0-4]   **pregnancy**
            Conditions classifiable to 590, 595, 597, 599.0, 616
              complicating pregnancy, childbirth, or the
              puerperium
            Conditions classifiable to 614.0–614.5, 614.7–614.9,
              615 complicating pregnancy or labor

      Excludes | *major puerperal infection (670.0-670.8)*
            Coding Clinic: 2004, Q4, P88-90

      OGCR Section I.C.2.g.

      During pregnancy, childbirth or the puerperium,
      a patient admitted (or presenting for a health
      care encounter) because of an HIV-related illness
      should receive a principal diagnosis code of
      647.6X, Other specified infectious and parasitic
      diseases in the mother classifiable elsewhere, but
      complicating the pregnancy, childbirth or the
      puerperium, followed by 042 and the code(s) for
      the HIV-related illness(es). Codes from Chapter
      15 always take sequencing priority. Patients with
      asymptomatic HIV infection status admitted (or
      presenting for a health care encounter) during
      pregnancy, childbirth, or the puerperium should
      receive codes of 647.6X and V08.

● **646.7 Liver disorders in pregnancy**
[0,1,3]   Acute yellow atrophy of liver (obstetric) (true) of
              pregnancy
            Icterus gravis of pregnancy
            Necrosis of liver of pregnancy

      Excludes | *hepatorenal syndrome following delivery
                  (674.8)
                  viral hepatitis (647.6)*

● **646.8 Other specified complications of pregnancy**
[0-4]   Fatigue during pregnancy
            Herpes gestationis
            Insufficient weight gain of pregnancy
            Coding Clinic: 1998, Q3, P16; 1985, Jan-Feb, P15-16

● **646.9 Unspecified complication of pregnancy**
[0,1,3]

● **647 Infectious and parasitic conditions in the mother classifiable elsewhere, but complicating pregnancy, childbirth, or the puerperium**

Use additional code(s) to further specify complication

Requires fifth digit; valid digits are in [brackets] under each code. See beginning of section 640–649 for definitions.

Includes the listed conditions when complicating the pregnant state, aggravated by the pregnancy, or when a main reason for obstetric care

Excludes *those conditions in the mother known or suspected to have affected the fetus (655.0–655.9)*

● **647.0 Syphilis**
[0-4] Conditions classifiable to 090–097

● **647.1 Gonorrhea**
[0-4] Conditions classifiable to 098

● **647.2 Other venereal diseases**
[0-4] Conditions classifiable to 099

● **647.3 Tuberculosis**
[0-4] Conditions classifiable to 010–018

● **647.4 Malaria**
[0-4] Conditions classifiable to 084

● **647.5 Rubella**
[0-4] Conditions classifiable to 056

● **647.6 Other viral diseases**
[0-4] Conditions classifiable to 042, 050-055, 057-079, 795.05, 795.15, 796.75
Coding Clinic: 1985, Jan-Feb, P15-16

● **647.8 Other specified infectious and parasitic**
[0-4] **diseases**

● **647.9 Unspecified infection or infestation**
[0-4]

● **648 Other current conditions in the mother classifiable elsewhere, but complicating pregnancy, childbirth, or the puerperium**

Use additional code(s) to identify the condition

Requires fifth digit; valid digits are in [brackets] under each code. See beginning of section 640–649 for definitions.

Includes the listed conditions when complicating the pregnant state, aggravated by the pregnancy, or when a main reason for obstetric care

Excludes *those conditions in the mother known or suspected to have affected the fetus (655.0–655.9)*

● **648.0 Diabetes mellitus**
[0-4] Conditions classifiable to 249, 250
Excludes *gestational diabetes (648.8)*

● **648.1 Thyroid dysfunction**
[0-4] Conditions classifiable to 240–246

● **648.2 Anemia**
[0-4] Conditions classifiable to 280–285
Coding Clinic: 2002, Q1, P14

● **648.3 Drug dependence**
[0-4] Conditions classifiable to 304
Coding Clinic: 1998, Q2, P13-14; 1988, Q4, P8

● **648.4 Mental disorders**
[0-4] Conditions classifiable to 290–303, 305.0, 305.2–305.9, 306–316, 317–319
Coding Clinic: 1998, Q2, P13-14

● **648.5 Congenital cardiovascular disorders**
[0-4] Conditions classifiable to 745–747

● **648.6 Other cardiovascular diseases**
[0-4] Conditions classifiable to 390–398, 410–429
Excludes *cerebrovascular disorders in the puerperium (674.0)*
peripartum cardiomyopathy (674.5)
venous complications (671.0–671.9)
Coding Clinic: 1998, Q3, P11

● **648.7 Bone and joint disorders of back, pelvis, and lower**
[0-4] **limbs**
Conditions classifiable to 720–724, and those classifiable to 711–719 or 725–738, specified as affecting the lower limbs

● **648.8 Abnormal glucose tolerance**
[0-4] Conditions classifiable to 790.21–790.29
Gestational diabetes
Use additional code, if applicable, for associated long-term (current) insulin use V58.67
Coding Clinic: 2004, Q4, P53-56

● **648.9 Other current conditions classifiable elsewhere**
[0-4] Conditions classifiable to 440–459, 795.01–795.04, 795.06, 795.10–795.14, 795.16, 796.70–796.74, 796.76
Nutritional deficiencies [conditions classifiable to 260–269]
Coding Clinic: 2009, Q1, P17; 2006, Q3, P14; 2004, Q4, P88-90; 2002, Q1, P14-15; 1984, Nov-Dec, P18

● **649 Other conditions or status of the mother complicating pregnancy, childbirth, or the puerperium**

Requires fifth digit; valid digits are in [brackets] under each code. See beginning of section 640-649 for definitions.

● **649.0 Tobacco use disorder complicating pregnancy,**
[0-4] **childbirth, or the puerperium**
Smoking complicating pregnancy, childbirth, or the puerperium

● **649.1 Obesity complicating pregnancy, childbirth, or the**
[0-4] **puerperium**
Use additional code to identify the obesity (278.00-278.03) ◄▥

● **649.2 Bariatric surgery status complicating pregnancy,**
[0-4] **childbirth, or the puerperium**
Gastric banding status complicating pregnancy, childbirth, or the puerperium
Gastric bypass status for obesity complicating pregnancy, childbirth, or the puerperium
Obesity surgery status complicating pregnancy, childbirth, or the puerperium

● **649.3 Coagulation defects complicating pregnancy,**
[0-4] **childbirth, or the puerperium**
Conditions classifiable to 286, 287, 289
Use additional code to identify the specific coagulation defect (286.0–286.9, 287.0-287.9, 289.0-289.9)
Excludes *coagulation defects causing antepartum hemorrhage (641.3)*

● **649.4 Epilepsy complicating pregnancy, childbirth, or the**
[0-4] **puerperium**
Conditions classifiable to 345
Use additional code to identify the specific type of epilepsy (345.00–345.91)
Excludes *eclampsia (642.6)*

● **649.5 Spotting complicating pregnancy**
[0,1,3] **Excludes** *antepartum hemorrhage (641.0–641.9)*
hemorrhage in early pregnancy (640.0–640.9)

◄ New   ◄▥ Revised   ~~deleted~~ Deleted   Excludes   Includes   Use additional   Code first   Omit code
● Unacceptable Principal Diagnosis   ● Use Additional Digit(s)   OGCR Official Guidelines   Coding Clinic

● **649.6 Uterine size date discrepancy**
[0-4] **Excludes** *suspected problem with fetal growth not found (V89.04)*

● **649.7 Cervical shortening**
[0,1,3] **Excludes** *suspected cervical shortening not found (V89.05)*
Coding Clinic: 2008, Q4, P124-125

OGCR Section I.C.11.h.1
Code 650 is for use in cases when a woman is admitted for a full-term normal delivery and delivers a single, healthy infant without any complications antepartum, during the delivery, or postpartum during the delivery episode. Code 650 is always a principal diagnosis. It is not to be used if any other code from chapter 11 is needed to describe a current complication of the antenatal, delivery, or perinatal period. Additional codes from other chapters may be used with code 650 if they are not related to or are in any way complicating the pregnancy.

OGCR Section I.C.11.h.2
Code 650 may be used if the patient had a complication at some point during her pregnancy, but the complication is not present at the time of the admission for delivery.

OGCR Section I.C.11.h.3
V27.0, Single liveborn, is the only outcome of delivery code appropriate for use with 650.

OGCR Section I.C.11.i.1
The postpartum period begins immediately after delivery and continues for six weeks following delivery. The peripartum period is defined as the last month of pregnancy to five months postpartum.

NORMAL DELIVERY, AND OTHER INDICATIONS FOR CARE IN PREGNANCY, LABOR, AND DELIVERY (650–659)

The following fifth-digit subclassification is for use with categories 651–659 to denote the current episode of care:

0 unspecified as to episode of care or not applicable
1 delivered, with or without mention of antepartum condition
2 delivered, with mention of postpartum complication
3 antepartum condition or complication
4 postpartum condition or complication

650 Normal delivery
Delivery requiring minimal or no assistance, with or without episiotomy, without fetal manipulation [e.g., rotation version] or instrumentation [forceps] of a spontaneous, cephalic, vaginal, full-term, single, live-born infant. This code is for use as a single diagnosis code and is not to be used with any other code in the range 630–676.
Use additional code to indicate outcome of delivery (V27.0)
Excludes *breech delivery (assisted) (spontaneous) NOS (652.2)*
delivery by vacuum extractor, forceps, cesarean section, or breech extraction, without specified complication (669.5–669.7)
Coding Clinic: 2002, Q2, P10; 2001, Q3, P12; 2000, Q3, P5

● **651 Multiple gestation**
Requires fifth digit; valid digits are in [brackets] under each code. See beginning of section 650–659 for definitions.
Use additional code to specify placenta status (V91.00-V91.99) ◄
Excludes *fetal conjoined twins (678.1)*

● **651.0 Twin pregnancy**
[0,1,3] **Excludes** *fetal conjoined twins (678.1)*
Coding Clinic: 2006, Q3, P16-18; 1992, Q3, P10

● **651.1 Triplet pregnancy**
[0,1,3]

● **651.2 Quadruplet pregnancy**
[0,1,3]

● **651.3 Twin pregnancy with fetal loss and retention of one**
[0,1,3] **fetus**
OGCR Section I.C.11.k.2
A code from categories 640-648 and 651-659 may be used as additional codes with an abortion code to indicate the complication leading to the abortion. Fifth digit 3 is assigned with codes from these categories when used with an abortion code because the other fifth digits will not apply. Codes from the 660-669 series are not to be used for complications of abortion.

● **651.4 Triplet pregnancy with fetal loss and retention of**
[0,1,3] **one or more fetus(es)**

● **651.5 Quadruplet pregnancy with fetal loss and retention**
[0,1,3] **of one or more fetus(es)**

● **651.6 Other multiple pregnancy with fetal loss and**
[0,1,3] **retention of one or more fetus(es)**

● **651.7 Multiple gestation following (elective) fetal**
[0,1,3] **reduction**
Fetal reduction of multiple fetuses reduced to single fetus
Coding Clinic: 2006, Q3, P16-18; 2005, Q4, P81

● **651.8 Other specified multiple gestation**
[0,1,3]

● **651.9 Unspecified multiple gestation**
[0,1,3]

● **652 Malposition and malpresentation of fetus**
Requires fifth digit; valid digits are in [brackets] under each code. See beginning of section 650–659 for definitions.
Code first any associated obstructed labor (660.0)
Coding Clinic: 1995, Q3, P10

● **652.0 Unstable lie**
[0,1,3]

● **652.1 Breech or other malpresentation successfully**
[0,1,3] **converted to cephalic presentation**
Cephalic version NOS

● **652.2 Breech presentation without mention of version**
[0,1,3] Breech delivery (assisted) (spontaneous) NOS
Buttocks presentation
Complete breech
Frank breech
Excludes *footling presentation (652.8)*
incomplete breech (652.8)

● **652.3 Transverse or oblique presentation**
[0,1,3] Oblique lie
Transverse lie
Excludes *transverse arrest of fetal head (660.3)*

COMPLICATIONS OF PREGNANCY, CHILDBIRTH, AND THE PUERPERIUM (630–679)

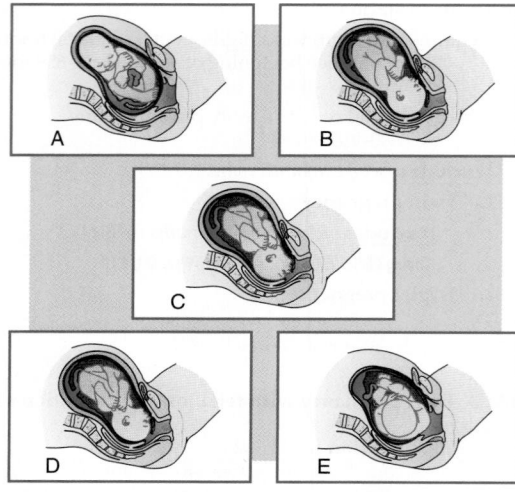

Figure 11–3 Five types of malposition and malpresentation of the fetus: **A.** Breech. **B.** Vertex. **C.** Face. **D.** Brow. **E.** Shoulder.

Figure 11–4 Hydrocephalic fetus causing disproportion.

● **652.4 Face or brow presentation**
[0,1,3]   Mentum presentation

● **652.5 High head at term**
[0,1,3]   Failure of head to enter pelvic brim

● **652.6 Multiple gestation with malpresentation of one**
[0,1,3] **fetus or more**

● **652.7 Prolapsed arm**
[0,1,3]

● **652.8 Other specified malposition or malpresentation**
[0,1,3]   Compound presentation

● **652.9 Unspecified malposition or malpresentation**
[0,1,3]

● **653   Disproportion**

Requires fifth digit; valid digits are in [brackets] under each code. See beginning of section 650–659 for definitions.

Code first any associated obstructed labor (660.1)

Coding Clinic: 1995, Q3, P10

● **653.0 Major abnormality of bony pelvis, not further**
[0,1,3] **specified**
          Pelvic deformity NOS

● **653.1 Generally contracted pelvis**
[0,1,3]   Contracted pelvis NOS

● **653.2 Inlet contraction of pelvis**
[0,1,3]   Inlet contraction (pelvis)

● **653.3 Outlet contraction of pelvis**
[0,1,3]   Outlet contraction (pelvis)

● **653.4 Fetopelvic disproportion**
[0,1,3]   Cephalopelvic disproportion NOS
          Disproportion of mixed maternal and fetal origin, with normally formed fetus

● **653.5 Unusually large fetus causing disproportion**
[0,1,3]   Disproportion of fetal origin with normally formed fetus
          Fetal disproportion NOS
          Excludes | *that when the reason for medical care was concern for the fetus (656.6)*

● **653.6 Hydrocephalic fetus causing disproportion**
[0,1,3]   **Excludes** | *that when the reason for medical care was concern for the fetus (655.0)*

● **653.7 Other fetal abnormality causing disproportion**
[0,1,3]   Fetal: Fetal:
          ascites   sacral teratoma
          hydrops   tumor
          myelomeningocele
          Excludes | *conjoined twins causing disporportion (678.1)*

● **653.8 Disproportion of other origin**
[0,1,3]   **Excludes** | *shoulder (girdle) dystocia (660.4)*

● **653.9 Unspecified disproportion**
[0,1,3]

● **654   Abnormality of organs and soft tissues of pelvis**

Requires fifth digit; valid digits are in [brackets] under each code. See beginning of section 650–659 for definitions.

Includes   the listed conditions during pregnancy, childbirth, or the puerperium

Code first any associated obstructed labor (660.2)

Excludes | *trauma to perineum and vulva complicating current delivery (664.0–664.9)*

Coding Clinic: 1995, Q3, P10

● **654.0 Congenital abnormalities of uterus**
[0-4]   Double uterus
          Uterus bicornis

● **654.1 Tumors of body of uterus**
[0-4]   Uterine fibroids
          Coding Clinic: 1994, Q2, P14

● **654.2 Previous cesarean delivery**
[0,1,3]   Uterine scar from previous cesarean delivery

● **654.3 Retroverted and incarcerated gravid uterus**
[0-4]

● **654.4 Other abnormalities in shape or position of**
[0-4] **gravid uterus and of neighboring structures**
          Cystocele
          Pelvic floor repair
          Pendulous abdomen
          Prolapse of gravid uterus
          Rectocele
          Rigid pelvic floor

● **654.5 Cervical incompetence**
[0-4]   Presence of Shirodkar suture with or without mention of cervical incompetence

● **654.6 Other congenital or acquired abnormality of**
[0-4] **cervix**
          Cicatricial cervix
          Polyp of cervix
          Previous surgery to cervix
          Rigid cervix (uteri)
          Stenosis or stricture of cervix
          Tumor of cervix

● **654.7 Congenital or acquired abnormality of vagina**
[0-4]   Previous surgery to vagina
          Septate vagina
          Stenosis of vagina (acquired) (congenital)
          Stricture of vagina
          Tumor of vagina

● **654.8 Congenital or acquired abnormality of vulva**
[0-4]   Anal sphincter tear (healed) (old) complicating
         delivery
         Fibrosis of perineum
         Persistent hymen
         Previous surgery to perineum or vulva
         Rigid perineum
         Tumor of vulva

    Excludes   *anal sphincter tear (healed) (old) not*
              associated with delivery (569.43)
              varicose veins of vulva (671.1)
    Coding Clinic: 2003, Q1, P14

● **654.9 Other and unspecified**
[0-4]   Uterine scar NEC
OGCR   Section I.C.11.c.2

In cases when in utero surgery is performed on the fetus, a diagnosis code from category 655, Known or suspected fetal abnormalities affecting management of the mother, should be assigned identifying the fetal condition. Procedure code 75.36, Correction of fetal defect, should be assigned on the hospital inpatient record. No code from Chapter 15, the perinatal codes, should be used on the mother's record to identify fetal conditions. Surgery performed in utero on a fetus is still to be coded as an obstetric encounter.

● **655 Known or suspected fetal abnormality affecting management of mother**
    Requires fifth digit; valid digits are in [brackets] under each code. See beginning of section 650–659 for definitions.

    Includes   the listed conditions in the fetus as a reason
              for observation or obstetrical care of the
              mother, or for termination of pregnancy

● **655.0 Central nervous system malformation in fetus**
[0,1,3]   Fetal or suspected fetal:
         anencephaly
         hydrocephalus
         spina bifida (with myelomeningocele)

● **655.1 Chromosomal abnormality in fetus**
[0,1,3]

● **655.2 Hereditary disease in family possibly affecting**
[0,1,3] **fetus**

● **655.3 Suspected damage to fetus from viral disease in the**
[0,1,3] **mother**
         Suspected damage to fetus from maternal rubella

● **655.4 Suspected damage to fetus from other disease in the**
[0,1,3] **mother**
         Suspected damage to fetus from maternal:
            alcohol addiction
            listeriosis
            toxoplasmosis

● **655.5 Suspected damage to fetus from drugs**
[0,1,3]

● **655.6 Suspected damage to fetus from radiation**
[0,1,3]

● **655.7 Decreased fetal movements**
[0,1,3]   Coding Clinic: 1997, Q4, P41

● **655.8 Other known or suspected fetal abnormality, not**
[0,1,3] **elsewhere classified**
         Suspected damage to fetus from:
            environmental toxins
            intrauterine contraceptive device
         Coding Clinic: 2006, Q3, P16-18x2

● **655.9 Unspecified**
[0,1,3]

● **656 Other known or suspected fetal and placental problems affecting management of mother**
    Requires fifth digit; valid digits are in [brackets] under each code. See beginning of section 650–659 for definitions.

    Excludes   *fetal hematologic conditions (678.0)*
            suspected placental problems not found
               (V89.02)

● **656.0 Fetal-maternal hemorrhage**
[0,1,3]   Leakage (microscopic) of fetal blood into maternal
         circulation

● **656.1 Rhesus isoimmunization**
[0,1,3]   Anti-D [Rh] antibodies
         Rh incompatibility

● **656.2 Isoimmunization from other and unspecified blood-**
[0,1,3] **group incompatibility**
         ABO isoimmunization
         Coding Clinic: 2006, Q4, P135

● **656.3 Fetal distress**
[0,1,3]   Fetal metabolic acidemia

    Excludes   *abnormal fetal acid-base balance (656.8)*
            abnormality in fetal heart rate or rhythm
               (659.7)
            fetal bradycardia (659.7)
            fetal tachycardia (659.7)
            meconium in liquor (656.8)

● **656.4 Intrauterine death**
[0,1,3]   Fetal death:
         NOS
         after completion of 22 weeks' gestation
         late
         Missed delivery

    Excludes   *missed abortion (632)*

● **656.5 Poor fetal growth**
[0,1,3]   "Light-for-dates"
         "Placental insufficiency"
         "Small-for-dates"

● **656.6 Excessive fetal growth**
[0,1,3]   "Large-for-dates"

● **656.7 Other placental conditions**
[0,1,3]   Abnormal placenta
         Placental infarct

    Excludes   *placental polyp (674.4)*
            placentitis (658.4)

● **656.8 Other specified fetal and placental problems**
[0,1,3]   Abnormal acid-base balance
         Intrauterine acidosis
         Lithopedian
         Meconium in liquor
         Subchorionic hematoma

● **656.9 Unspecified fetal and placental problem**
[0,1,3]

● **657 Polyhydramnios**
[0,1,3]   Hydramnios
    Requires fifth digit; valid digits are in [brackets] under each code. See beginning of section 650–659 for definitions.

    Use 0 as fourth digit for category 657

    Excludes   *suspected polyhydramnios not found (V89.01)*
    Coding Clinic: 2006, Q3, P16-18

COMPLICATIONS OF PREGNANCY, CHILDBIRTH, AND THE PUERPERIUM (630–679)

COMPLICATIONS OF PREGNANCY, CHILDBIRTH, AND THE PUERPERIUM (630–679)

● 658 **Other problems associated with amniotic cavity and membranes**

> Requires fifth digit; valid digits are in [brackets] under each code. See beginning of section 650–659 for definitions.

> **Excludes** *amniotic fluid embolism (673.1)*
> *suspected problems with amniotic cavity and membranes not found (V89.01)*

● 658.0 **Oligohydramnios**
[0,1,3] Oligohydramnios without mention of rupture of membranes
Coding Clinic: 2006, Q3, P16-18

● 658.1 **Premature rupture of membranes**
[0,1,3] Rupture of amniotic sac less than 24 hours prior to the onset of labor
Coding Clinic: 2001, Q1, P5; 1998, Q4, P76-77

● 658.2 **Delayed delivery after spontaneous or unspecified**
[0,1,3] **rupture of membranes**
Prolonged rupture of membranes NOS
Rupture of amniotic sac 24 hours or more prior to the onset of labor

● 658.3 **Delayed delivery after artificial rupture of**
[0,1,3] **membranes**

● 658.4 **Infection of amniotic cavity**
[0,1,3] Amnionitis   Membranitis
Chorioamnionitis   Placentitis

● 658.8 **Other**
[0,1,3] Amnion nodosum
Amniotic cyst

● 658.9 **Unspecified**
[0,1,3]

● 659 **Other indications for care or intervention related to labor and delivery, not elsewhere classified**

> Requires fifth digit; valid digits are in [brackets] under each code. See beginning of section 650–659 for definitions.

● 659.0 **Failed mechanical induction**
[0,1,3] Failure of induction of labor by surgical or other instrumental methods

● 659.1 **Failed medical or unspecified induction**
[0,1,3] Failed induction NOS
Failure of induction of labor by medical methods, such as oxytocic drugs

● 659.2 **Maternal pyrexia during labor, unspecified**
[0,1,3]

● 659.3 **Generalized infection during labor**
[0,1,3] Septicemia during labor

● 659.4 **Grand multiparity**
[0,1,3]
> **Excludes** *supervision only, in pregnancy (V23.3)*
> *without current pregnancy (V61.5)*

● 659.5 **Elderly primigravida**
[0,1,3] First pregnancy in a woman who will be 35 years of age or older at expected date of delivery
> **Excludes** *supervision only, in pregnancy (V23.81)*
Coding Clinic: 2001, Q3, P12

● 659.6 **Elderly multigravida**
[0,1,3] Second or more pregnancy in a woman who will be 35 years of age or older at expected date of delivery
> **Excludes** *elderly primigravida (659.5)*
> *supervision only, in pregnancy (V23.82)*
Coding Clinic: 2001, Q3, P12

● 659.7 **Abnormality in fetal heart rate or rhythm**
[0,1,3] Depressed fetal heart tones
Fetal:
bradycardia
tachycardia
Fetal heart rate decelerations
Non-reassuring fetal heart rate or rhythm
Coding Clinic: 1998, Q4, P47-48

● 659.8 **Other specified indications for care or intervention**
[0,1,3] **related to labor and delivery**
Pregnancy in a female less than 16 years of age at expected date of delivery
Very young maternal age
Coding Clinic: 2001, Q3, P12

● 659.9 **Unspecified indication for care or intervention**
[0,1,3] **related to labor and delivery**

OGCR Section I.C.11.k.2

Codes from the 660-669 series are not to be used for complications of abortion.

COMPLICATIONS OCCURRING MAINLY IN THE COURSE OF LABOR AND DELIVERY (660–669)

> The following fifth-digit subclassification is for use with categories 660–669 to denote the current episode of care:

> 0 unspecified as to episode of care or not applicable
> 1 delivered, with or without mention of antepartum condition
> 2 delivered, with mention of postpartum complication
> 3 antepartum condition or complication
> 4 postpartum condition or complication

● 660 **Obstructed labor**
> Requires fifth digit; valid digits are in [brackets] under each code. See beginning of section 660–669 for definitions.
Coding Clinic: 1995, Q3, P10

● 660.0 **Obstruction caused by malposition of fetus at onset**
[0,1,3] **of labor**
Any condition classifiable to 652, causing obstruction during labor
> Use additional code from 652.0–652.9 to identify condition
Coding Clinic: 1995, Q3, P10

● 660.1 **Obstruction by bony pelvis**
[0,1,3] Any condition classifiable to 653, causing obstruction during labor
> Use additional code from 653.0–653.9 to identify condition
Coding Clinic: 1995, Q3, P10

● 660.2 **Obstruction by abnormal pelvic soft tissues**
[0,1,3] Prolapse of anterior lip of cervix
Any condition classifiable to 654, causing obstruction during labor
> Use additional code from 654.0–654.9 to identify condition
Coding Clinic: 1995, Q3, P10

● 660.3 **Deep transverse arrest and persistent occipito-**
[0,1,3] **posterior position**

● 660.4 **Shoulder (girdle) dystocia**
[0,1,3] Impacted shoulders

● 660.5 **Locked twins**
[0,1,3]

● 660.6 **Failed trial of labor, unspecified**
[0,1,3] Failed trial of labor, without mention of condition or suspected condition

● **660.7 Failed forceps or vacuum extractor, unspecified**
[0,1,3]   Application of ventouse or forceps, without
            mention of condition

● **660.8 Other causes of obstructed labor**
[0,1,3]   Use additional code to identify condition

● **660.9 Unspecified obstructed labor**
[0,1,3]   Dystocia:
            NOS
            fetal NOS
            maternal NOS

● **661   Abnormality of forces of labor**

        Requires fifth digit; valid digits are in [brackets] under
            each code. See beginning of section 660–669 for
            definitions.

● **661.0 Primary uterine inertia**
[0,1,3]   Failure of cervical dilation
            Hypotonic uterine dysfunction, primary
            Prolonged latent phase of labor
            Coding Clinic: 1985, July-Aug, P11

● **661.1 Secondary uterine inertia**
[0,1,3]   Arrested active phase of labor
            Hypotonic uterine dysfunction, secondary
            Coding Clinic: 1985, July-Aug, P11

● **661.2 Other and unspecified uterine inertia**
[0,1,3]   Atony of uterus without hemorrhage
            Desultory labor
            Irregular labor
            Poor contractions
            Slow slope active phase of labor

        | **Excludes** | *atony of uterus with hemorrhage (666.1)* |

            postpartum atony of uterus without
            hemorrhage (669.8)
            Coding Clinic: 1985, July-Aug, P11

● **661.3 Precipitate labor**
[0,1,3]

● **661.4 Hypertonic, incoordinate, or prolonged uterine**
[0,1,3] **contractions**
            Cervical spasm
            Contraction ring (dystocia)
            Dyscoordinate labor
            Hourglass contraction of uterus
            Hypertonic uterine dysfunction
            Incoordinate uterine action
            Retraction ring (Bandl's) (pathological)
            Tetanic contractions
            Uterine dystocia NOS
            Uterine spasm

● **661.9 Unspecified abnormality of labor**
[0,1,3]

● **662   Long labor**

        Requires fifth digit; valid digits are in [brackets] under
            each code. See beginning of section 660–669 for
            definitions.

● **662.0 Prolonged first stage**
[0,1,3]

● **662.1 Prolonged labor, unspecified**
[0,1,3]

● **662.2 Prolonged second stage**
[0,1,3]

● **662.3 Delayed delivery of second twin, triplet, etc.**
[0,1,3]

● **663   Umbilical cord complications**

        Requires fifth digit; valid digits are in [brackets] under
            each code. See beginning of section 660–669 for
            definitions.

● **663.0 Prolapse of cord**
[0,1,3]   Presentation of cord

● **663.1 Cord around neck, with compression**
[0,1,3]   Cord tightly around neck

● **663.2 Other and unspecified cord entanglement, with**
[0,1,3] **compression**
            Entanglement of cords of twins in mono-amniotic
                sac
            Knot in cord (with compression)

● **663.3 Other and unspecified cord entanglement, without**
[0,1,3] **mention of compression**
            Coding Clinic: 2003, Q2, P9

● **663.4 Short cord**
[0,1,3]

● **663.5 Vasa previa**
[0,1,3]

● **663.6 Vascular lesions of cord**
[0,1,3]   Bruising of cord
            Hematoma of cord
            Thrombosis of vessels of cord

● **663.8 Other umbilical cord complications**
[0,1,3]   Velamentous insertion of umbilical cord

● **663.9 Unspecified umbilical cord complication**
[0,1,3]

● **664   Trauma to perineum and vulva during delivery**

        Requires fifth digit; valid digits are in [brackets] under
            each code. See beginning of section 660–669 for
            definitions.

        | **Includes** | damage from instruments |

                that from extension of episiotomy
        Coding Clinic: 2008, Q4, P192; 1992, Q1, P10-11

● **664.0 First-degree perineal laceration**
[0,1,4]   Perineal laceration, rupture, or tear involving:
            fourchette
            hymen
            labia vulva
            skin
            vagina
            Coding Clinic: 1984, Nov-Dec, P10

● **664.1 Second-degree perineal laceration**
[0,1,4]   Perineal laceration, rupture, or tear (following
                episiotomy) involving:
            pelvic floor
            perineal muscles
            vaginal muscles

        | **Excludes** | *that involving anal sphincter (664.2)* |

            Coding Clinic: 2008, Q4, P192; 1984, Nov-Dec, P10

● **664.2 Third-degree perineal laceration**
[0,1,4]   Perineal laceration, rupture, or tear (following
                episiotomy) involving:
            anal sphincter
            rectovaginal septum
            sphincter NOS

        | **Excludes** | *anal sphincter tear during delivery not* |

                associated with third-degree perineal
                laceration (664.6)
            that with anal or rectal mucosal laceration
                (664.3)
            Coding Clinic: 1984, Nov-Dec, P10

COMPLICATIONS OF PREGNANCY, CHILDBIRTH, AND THE PUERPERIUM (630–679)

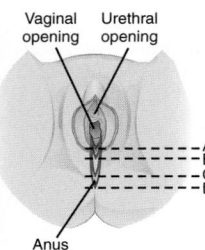

Vaginal opening   Urethral opening

A
B
C
D

Anus

Figure 11-5 Perineal lacerations: **A.** First-degree is laceration of superficial tissues. **B.** Second-degree is limited to the pelvic floor and may involve the perineal or vaginal muscles. **C.** Third-degree involves the anal sphincter. **D.** Fourth-degree involves anal or rectal mucosa.

COMPLICATIONS OF PREGNANCY, CHILDBIRTH, AND THE PUERPERIUM (630–679)

● **664.3 Fourth-degree perineal laceration**
[0,1,4]   Perineal laceration, rupture, or tear as classifiable to 664.2 and involving also:
         anal mucosa
         rectal mucosa
         Coding Clinic: 1984, Nov-Dec, P10

● **664.4 Unspecified perineal laceration**
[0,1,4]   Central laceration

● **664.5 Vulval and perineal hematoma**
[0,1,4]   Coding Clinic: 1984, Nov-Dec, P10

● **664.6 Anal sphincter tear complicating delivery, not**
[0,1,4] **associated with third-degree perineal laceration**
        Excludes   *third-degree perineal laceration (664.2)*
        Coding Clinic: 2007, Q4, P88-90

● **664.8 Other specified trauma to perineum and vulva**
[0,1,4]   Periurethral trauma ◀
        Coding Clinic: 2007, Q4, P125

● **664.9 Unspecified trauma to perineum and vulva**
[0,1,4]

● **665 Other obstetrical trauma**
       Requires fifth digit; valid digits are in [brackets] under each code. See beginning of section 660–669 for definitions.
       Includes   damage from instruments

● **665.0 Rupture of uterus before onset of labor**
[0,1,3]

● **665.1 Rupture of uterus during labor**
  [0,1]   Rupture of uterus NOS

● **665.2 Inversion of uterus**
[0,2,4]

● **665.3 Laceration of cervix**
[0,1,4]   Coding Clinic: 1984, Nov-Dec, P10

● **665.4 High vaginal laceration**
[0,1,4]   Laceration of vaginal wall or sulcus without mention of perineal laceration
        Coding Clinic: 1984, Nov-Dec, P10

● **665.5 Other injury to pelvic organs**
[0,1,4]   Injury to:
         bladder
         urethra
        Excludes   *periurethral trauma (664.8)* ◀
        Coding Clinic: 1984, Nov-Dec, P10, 12

● **665.6 Damage to pelvic joints and ligaments**
[0,1,4]   Avulsion of inner symphyseal cartilage
         Damage to coccyx
         Separation of symphysis (pubis)

● **665.7 Pelvic hematoma**
[0-2,4]   Hematoma of vagina
        Coding Clinic: 1984, Nov-Dec, P10

● **665.8 Other specified obstetrical trauma**
  [0-4]

● **665.9 Unspecified obstetrical trauma**
  [0-4]

● **666 Postpartum hemorrhage**
       Requires fifth digit; valid digits are in [brackets] under each code. See beginning of section 660–669 for definitions.

● **666.0 Third-stage hemorrhage**
[0,2,4]   Hemorrhage associated with retained, trapped, or adherent placenta
         Retained placenta NOS
        Coding Clinic: 1988, Q1, P14

● **666.1 Other immediate postpartum hemorrhage**
[0,2,4]   Atony of uterus with hemorrhage
         Hemorrhage within the first 24 hours following delivery of placenta
         Postpartum atony of uterus with hemorrhage
         Postpartum hemorrhage (atonic) NOS
         Excludes   *atony of uterus without hemorrhage (661.2)*
                   postpartum atony of uterus without hemorrhage (669.8)
        Coding Clinic: 1988, Q1, P14

● **666.2 Delayed and secondary postpartum**
[0,2,4] **hemorrhage**
         Hemorrhage:
           after the first 24 hours following delivery
           associated with retained portions of placenta or membranes
         Postpartum hemorrhage specified as delayed or secondary
         Retained products of conception NOS, following delivery
        Coding Clinic: 1988, Q1, P14

● **666.3 Postpartum coagulation defects**
[0,2,4]   Postpartum:
         afibrinogenemia
         fibrinolysis

● **667 Retained placenta without hemorrhage**
       Requires fifth digit; valid digits are in [brackets] under each code. See beginning of section 660–669 for definitions.

● **667.0 Retained placenta without hemorrhage**
[0,2,4]   Placenta accreta without hemorrhage
         Retained placenta:
           NOS without hemorrhage
           total without hemorrhage
        Coding Clinic: 1988, Q1, P14

● **667.1 Retained portions of placenta or membranes,**
[0,2,4] **without hemorrhage**
         Retained products of conception following delivery, without hemorrhage
        Coding Clinic: 1988, Q1, P14

● **668 Complications of the administration of anesthetic or other sedation in labor and delivery**
       Use additional code(s) to further specify complication
       Requires fifth digit; valid digits are in [brackets] under each code. See beginning of section 660–669 for definitions.
       Includes   complications arising from the administration of a general or local anesthetic, analgesic, or other sedation in labor and delivery
       Excludes   *reaction to spinal or lumbar puncture (349.0)*
                   spinal headache (349.0)

● **668.0 Pulmonary complications**
  [0-4]   Inhalation [aspiration] of stomach contents or secretions following anesthesia or other sedation in labor or delivery
         Mendelson's syndrome following anesthesia or other sedation in labor or delivery
         Pressure collapse of lung following anesthesia or other sedation in labor or delivery

◀ New   ◀▥ Revised   ~~deleted~~ Deleted   Excludes   Includes   Use additional   Code first   Omit code
● Unacceptable Principal Diagnosis   ● Use Additional Digit(s)   OGCR Official Guidelines   Coding Clinic

668.1 Cardiac complications
[0-4] Cardiac arrest or failure following anesthesia or other sedation in labor and delivery

668.2 Central nervous system complications
[0-4] Cerebral anoxia following anesthesia or other sedation in labor and delivery

668.8 Other complications of anesthesia or other sedation
[0-4] **in labor and delivery**
Coding Clinic: 1999, Q2, P9-10

668.9 Unspecified complication of anesthesia and other
[0-4] **sedation**

669 Other complications of labor and delivery, not elsewhere classified

Requires fifth digit; valid digits are in [brackets] under each code. See beginning of section 660–669 for definitions.

669.0 Maternal distress
[0-4] Metabolic disturbance in labor and delivery

669.1 Shock during or following labor and
[0-4] **delivery**
Obstetric shock

669.2 Maternal hypotension syndrome
[0-4]

669.3 Acute kidney failure following labor and
[0,2,4] **delivery**

669.4 Other complications of obstetrical surgery and
[0-4] **procedures**
Cardiac:
arrest following cesarean or other obstetrical surgery or procedure, including delivery NOS
failure following cesarean or other obstetrical surgery or procedure, including delivery NOS
Cerebral anoxia following cesarean or other obstetrical surgery or procedure, including delivery NOS

| Excludes | complications of obstetrical surgical wounds (674.1–674.3) |

669.5 Forceps or vacuum extractor delivery without
[0,1] **mention of indication**
Delivery by ventouse, without mention of indication

669.6 Breech extraction, without mention of indication
[0,1] | Excludes | breech delivery NOS (652.2) |

669.7 Cesarean delivery, without mention of indication
[0,1] Coding Clinic: 2001, Q1, P11-12

669.8 Other complications of labor and delivery
[0-4] Coding Clinic: 2006, Q4, P135

669.9 Unspecified complication of labor and delivery
[0-4]

COMPLICATIONS OF THE PUERPERIUM (670–677)

Note: Categories 671 and 673–676 include the listed conditions even if they occur during pregnancy or childbirth.

The following fifth-digit subclassification is for use with categories 670–676 to denote the current episode of care:

0 unspecified as to episode of care or not applicable
1 delivered, with or without mention of antepartum condition
2 delivered, with mention of postpartum complication
3 antepartum condition or complication
4 postpartum condition or complication

670 Major puerperal infection
Requires fifth digit; valid digits are in [brackets] under each code. See beginning of section 670–676 for definitions.

Excludes	infection following abortion (639.0)
	minor genital tract infection following delivery (646.6)
	puerperal fever NOS (672)
	puerperal pyrexia NOS (672)
	puerperal pyrexia of unknown origin (672)
	urinary tract infection following delivery (646.6)
Coding Clinic: 2007, Q3, P10

670.0 Major puerpal infection, unspecified
[0,2,4]

670.1 Puerpal endometritis
[0,2,4]

670.2 Puerpal sepsis
[0,2,4] Puerpal pyemia
Use additional code to identify severe sepsis (995.92) and any associated acute organ dysfunction, if applicable ◄
Coding Clinic: 2009, Q4, P108

670.3 Puerpal septic thrombophlebitis
[0,2,4]

670.8 Other major puerpal infection
[0,2,4] Puerpal:
pelvic cellulitis
peritonitis
salpingitis

671 Venous complications in pregnancy and the puerperium

Excludes	personal history of venous complications prior to pregnancy, such as:
	thrombophlebitis (V12.52)
	thrombosis and embolism (V12.51)

Requires fifth digit; valid digits are in [brackets] under each code. See beginning of section 670–676 for definitions.

671.0 Varicose veins of legs
[0-4] Varicose veins NOS

671.1 Varicose veins of vulva and perineum
[0-4]

671.2 Superficial thrombophlebitis
[0-4] Phlebitis NOS
Thrombophlebitis (superficial)
Thrombosis NOS
Use additional code to identify the superficial thrombophlebitis (453.6, 453.71, 453.81) ◄

671.3 Deep phlebothrombosis, antepartum
[0,1,3] Use additional code to identify the deep vein thrombosis (453.40-453.42, 453.50-453.52, 453.72-453.79, 453.82-453.89)
Use additional code for long-term (current) use of anticoagulants if applicable (V58.61)
Deep-vein thrombosis, antepartum

671.4 Deep phlebothrombosis, postpartum
[0,2,4] Deep-vein thrombosis, postpartum
Pelvic thrombophlebitis, postpartum
Phlegmasia alba dolens (puerperal)
Use additional code to identify the deep vein thrombosis (453.40-453.42, 453.50-453.52, 453.72-453.79, 453.82-453.89)
Use additional code for long-term (current) use of anticoagulants if applicable (V58.61)

671.5 Other phlebitis and thrombosis
[0-4] Cerebral venous thrombosis
Thrombosis of intracranial venous sinus

671.8 Other venous complications
[0-4] Hemorrhoids

671.9 Unspecified venous complication
[0-4]

●**672 Pyrexia of unknown origin during the**
[0,2,4] **puerperium**
   Postpartum fever NOS
   Puerperal fever NOS
   Puerperal pyrexia NOS

   Requires fifth digit; valid digits are in [brackets] under each code. See beginning of section 670–676 for definitions.

   Use 0 as fourth digit for category 672

●**673 Obstetrical pulmonary embolism**
   Requires fifth digit; valid digits are in [brackets] under each code. See beginning of section 670–676 for definitions.

   Includes pulmonary emboli in pregnancy, childbirth, or the puerperium, or specified as puerperal

   Excludes *embolism following abortion (639.6)*

●**673.0 Obstetrical air embolism**
[0-4]

●**673.1 Amniotic fluid embolism**
[0-4]

●**673.2 Obstetrical blood-clot embolism**
[0-4]   Puerperal pulmonary embolism NOS

●**673.3 Obstetrical pyemic and septic**
[0-4] **embolism**

●**673.8 Other pulmonary embolism**
[0-4]   Fat embolism

●**674 Other and unspecified complications of the puerperium, not elsewhere classified**
   Requires fifth digit; valid digits are in [brackets] under each code. See beginning of section 670–676 for definitions.

●**674.0 Cerebrovascular disorders in the**
[0-4] **puerperium**
   Any condition classifiable to 430–434, 436–437 occurring during pregnancy, childbirth, or the puerperium, or specified as puerperal

   Excludes *intracranial venous sinus thrombosis (671.5)*

●**674.1 Disruption of cesarean wound**
[0,2,4]   Dehiscence or disruption of uterine wound

   Excludes *uterine rupture before onset of labor (665.0)*
   uterine rupture during labor (665.1)

●**674.2 Disruption of perineal wound**
[0,2,4]   Breakdown of perineum
   Disruption of wound of:
      episiotomy
      perineal laceration
   Secondary perineal tear
   Coding Clinic: 1997, Q1, P9-10

●**674.3 Other complications of obstetrical surgical**
[0,2,4] **wounds**
   Hematoma of cesarean section or perineal wound
   Hemorrhage of cesarean section or perineal wound
   Infection of cesarean section or perineal wound

   Excludes *damage from instruments in delivery (664.0–665.9)*
   Coding Clinic: 2009, Q4, P108

●**674.4 Placental polyp**
[0,2,4]

●**674.5 Peripartum cardiomyopathy**
[0-4]   Postpartum cardiomyopathy
   Coding Clinic: 2003, Q4, P65

●**674.8 Other**
[0,2,4]   Hepatorenal syndrome, following delivery
   Postpartum:
      subinvolution of uterus
      uterine hypertrophy
   Coding Clinic: 1998, Q3, P16

●**674.9 Unspecified**
[0,2,4]   Sudden death of unknown cause during the puerperium

●**675 Infections of the breast and nipple associated with childbirth**
   Requires fifth digit; valid digits are in [brackets] under each code. See beginning of section 670–676 for definitions.

   Includes the listed conditions during pregnancy, childbirth, or the puerperium

●**675.0 Infections of nipple**
[0-4]   Abscess of nipple

●**675.1 Abscess of breast**
[0-4]   Abscess: Mastitis:
      mammary   purulent
      subareolar   retromammary
      submammary   submammary

●**675.2 Nonpurulent mastitis**
[0-4]   Lymphangitis of breast
   Mastitis:
      NOS
      interstitial
      parenchymatous

●**675.8 Other specified infections of the breast and**
[0-4] **nipple**

●**675.9 Unspecified infection of the breast and nipple**
[0-4]

●**676 Other disorders of the breast associated with childbirth and disorders of lactation**
   Requires fifth digit; valid digits are in [brackets] under each code. See beginning of section 670–676 for definitions.

   Includes the listed conditions during pregnancy, the puerperium, or lactation

●**676.0 Retracted nipple**
[0-4]

●**676.1 Cracked nipple**
[0-4]   Fissure of nipple

●**676.2 Engorgement of breasts**
[0-4]

●**676.3 Other and unspecified disorder of breast**
[0-4]

●**676.4 Failure of lactation**
[0-4]   Agalactia

●**676.5 Suppressed lactation**
[0-4]

●**676.6 Galactorrhea**
[0-4]   **Excludes** *galactorrhea not associated with childbirth (611.6)*
   Coding Clinic: 1985, July-Aug, P9

●**676.8 Other disorders of lactation**
[0-4]   Galactocele

●**676.9 Unspecified disorder of lactation**
[0-4]

OGCR Section I.C.11.j.1-3
1) **Code 677**
Code 677, Late effect of complication of pregnancy, childbirth, and the puerperium is for use in those cases when an initial complication of a pregnancy develops a sequelae requiring care or treatment at a future date.
2) **After the initial postpartum period**
This code may be used at any time after the initial postpartum period.
3) **Sequencing of Code 677**
This code, like all late effect codes, is to be sequenced following the code describing the sequelae of the complication.

677 Late effect of complication of pregnancy, childbirth, and the puerperium

Note: This category is to be used to indicate conditions in 632–648.9 and 651–676.9 as the cause of the late effect, themselves classifiable elsewhere. The "late effects" include conditions specified as such, or as sequelae, which may occur at any time after the puerperium.

Code first any sequelae

Coding Clinic: 1997, Q1, P9-10

OTHER MATERNAL AND FETAL COMPLICATIONS (678-679)

The following fifth-digit subclassification is for use with categories 678-679 to denote the current episode of care:

0 unspecified as to episode of care or not applicable
1 delivered, with or without mention of antepartum condition
2 delivered, with mention of postpartum complication
3 antepartum condition or complication
4 postpartum condition or complication

● **678 Other fetal conditions**
Requires fifth digit; valid digits are in [brackets] under each code. See beginning of section 678-679 for definitions.
Coding Clinic: 2008, Q4, P125-127

● **678.0 Fetal hematologic conditions**
[0,1,3] Fetal anemia
Fetal thrombocytopenia
Fetal twin to twin transfusion

Excludes | *fetal and neonatal hemorrhage (772.0-772.9)*
fetal hematologic disorders affecting newborn (776.0-776.9)
fetal-maternal hemorrhage (656.00-656.03)
isoimmunization incompatibility (656.10-656.13, 656.20-656.23)

● **678.1 Fetal conjoined twins**
[0,1,3]

● **679 Complications of in utero procedures**
Requires fifth digit; valid digits are in [brackets] under each code. See beginning of section 678-679 for definitions.
Coding Clinic: 2008, Q4, P127-128

● **679.0 Maternal complications from in utero procedure**
[0-4] Excludes | *maternal history of in utero procedure during previous pregnancy (V23.86)*

● **679.1 Fetal complications from in utero procedure**
[0-4] Fetal complications from amniocentesis

Excludes | *newborn affected by in utero procedure (760.61-760.64)*

COMPLICATIONS OF PREGNANCY, CHILDBIRTH, AND THE PUERPERIUM (630–679)

Carbuncle Furuncle Deep
                     folliculitis
                     Superficial
                     folliculitis

A   B

Figure 12–1 Furuncle, also known as a boil, is a staphylococcal infection. The organism enters the body through a hair follicle and so furuncles usually appear in hairy areas of the body. A cluster of furuncles is known as a carbuncle and involves infection into the deep subcutaneous fascia. These usually appear on the back and neck. (**B** from Habif: Clinical Dermatology, 4th ed. 2004, Mosby.)

12. DISEASES OF THE SKIN AND SUBCUTANEOUS TISSUE (680–709)

INFECTIONS OF SKIN AND SUBCUTANEOUS TISSUE (680–686)

Excludes *certain infections of skin classified under "Infectious and Parasitic Diseases," such as:*
erysipelas (035)
erysipeloid of Rosenbach (027.1)
herpes:
simplex (054.0–054.9)
zoster (053.0–053.9)
molluscum contagiosum (078.0)
viral warts (078.10-078.19)

● **680 Carbuncle and furuncle**

Includes boil
furunculosis

680.0 Face
Ear [any part]   Nose (septum)
Face [any part, except eye] Temple (region)

Excludes *eyelid (373.13)*
lacrimal apparatus (375.31)
orbit (376.01)

680.1 Neck

680.2 Trunk
Abdominal wall
Back [any part, except buttocks]
Breast
Chest wall
Flank
Groin
Pectoral region
Perineum
Umbilicus

Excludes *buttocks (680.5)*
external genital organs:
female (616.4)
male (607.2, 608.4)

680.3 Upper arm and forearm
Arm [any part, except hand]
Axilla
Shoulder

680.4 Hand
Finger [any]   Wrist
Thumb

680.5 Buttock
Anus   Gluteal region

680.6 Leg, except foot
Ankle   Knee
Hip   Thigh

680.7 Foot
Heel
Toe

680.8 Other specified sites
Head [any part, except face]
Scalp

Excludes *external genital organs:*
female (616.4)
male (607.2, 608.4)

680.9 Unspecified site
Boil NOS   Furuncle NOS
Carbuncle NOS

● **681 Cellulitis and abscess of finger and toe**

Includes that with lymphangitis

Use additional code to identify organism, such as:
Staphylococcus (041.1)

● **681.0 Finger**

681.00 Cellulitis and abscess, unspecified

681.01 Felon
Pulp abscess   Whitlow

Excludes *herpetic whitlow (054.6)*

681.02 Onychia and paronychia of finger
Panaritium of finger
Perionychia of finger

● **681.1 Toe**

681.10 Cellulitis and abscess, unspecified
Coding Clinic: 2005, Q1, P14

681.11 Onychia and paronychia of toe
Panaritium of toe
Perionychia of toe

681.9 Cellulitis and abscess of unspecified digit
Infection of nail NOS

● **682 Other cellulitis and abscess**

Includes abscess (acute) (with lymphangitis) except of finger or toe
cellulitis (diffuse) (with lymphangitis) except of finger or toe
lymphangitis, acute (with lymphangitis) except of finger or toe

Use additional code to identify organism, such as:
Staphylococcus (041.1)

Excludes *lymphangitis (chronic) (subacute) (457.2)*

682.0 Face
This code reports forehead but not head (682.8).
Cheek, external   Nose, external
Chin   Submandibular
Forehead   Temple (region)

Excludes *ear [any part] (380.10–380.16)*
eyelid (373.13)
lacrimal apparatus (375.31)
lip (528.5)
mouth (528.3)
nose (internal) (478.1)
orbit (376.01)

Item 12-1 **Cellulitis** is an acute spreading bacterial infection below the surface of the skin characterized by redness (erythema), warmth, swelling, pain, fever, chills, and enlarged lymph nodes ("swollen glands"). **Abscess** is a localized collection of pus in tissues or organs and is a sign of infection resulting in swelling and inflammation. **Onychia** is an inflammation of the tissue surrounding the nail with pus accumulation and loss of the nail, resulting from microscopic pathogens entering through small wounds. **Paronychia** is a nail disease also known as felon or whitlow and is a bacterial or fungal infection.

◄ New   ◄▥ Revised   ~~deleted~~ Deleted   Excludes   Includes   Use additional   Code first   Omit code
● Unacceptable Principal Diagnosis   ● Use Additional Digit(s)   OGCR Official Guidelines   Coding Clinic

682.1 Neck

682.2 Trunk
    Abdominal wall
    Back [any part, except buttock]
       Buttocks see 682.5
    Chest wall
    Flank
    Groin
    Pectoral region
    Perineum
    Umbilicus, except newborn

    | Excludes | *anal and rectal regions (566)* |
       breast:
         NOS (611.0)
         puerperal (675.1)
       external genital organs:
         female (616.3–616.4)
         male (604.0, 607.2, 608.4)
       umbilicus, newborn (771.4)

    Coding Clinic: 1993, Q1, P26

682.3 Upper arm and forearm
    Arm [any part, except hand]
    Axilla
    Shoulder

    | Excludes | *hand (682.4)* |

    Coding Clinic: 2003, Q2, P7-8; 1998, Q4, P42-44

682.4 Hand, except fingers and thumb
    Wrist

    | Excludes | *finger and thumb (681.00–681.02)* |

682.5 Buttock
    Gluteal region

    | Excludes | *anal and rectal regions (566)* |

682.6 Leg, except foot
    Ankle   Knee
    Hip   Thigh
    Coding Clinic: 2009, Q1, P18x2; 2004, Q3, P5-6; 2003, Q4, P108;
        1995, Q1, P3

682.7 Foot, except toes
    Heel

    | Excludes | *toe (681.10–681.11)* |

682.8 Other specified sites
    Head [except face]
    Scalp

    | Excludes | *face (682.0)* |

682.9 Unspecified site
    Abscess NOS
    Cellulitis NOS
    Lymphangitis, acute NOS

    | Excludes | *lymphangitis NOS (457.2)* |

683 Acute lymphadenitis
    Short term inflammation of lymph nodes which can be
       regionalized to involve a given area of lymph system or
       systemic involvement
    Abscess (acute) lymph gland or node, except mesenteric
    Adenitis, acute lymph gland or node, except mesenteric
    Lymphadenitis, acute lymph gland or node, except
       mesenteric

    Use additional code to identify organism such as
       Staphylococcus (041.1)

    | Excludes | *enlarged glands NOS (785.6)* |
       lymphadenitis:
         chronic or subacute, except mesenteric (289.1)
         mesenteric (acute) (chronic) (subacute) (289.2)
         unspecified (289.3)

684 Impetigo
    Contagious skin infection caused by streptococcus or
       staphylococcus aureus that produces blisters or sores on
       the face and hands
    Impetiginization of other dermatoses
    Impetigo (contagiosa) [any site] [any organism]:
       bullousneonatorum   simplex
       circinate
    Pemphigus neonatorum

    | Excludes | *impetigo herpetiformis (694.3)* |

● **685 Pilonidal cyst**
    | Includes | fistula, coccygeal or pilonidal |
               sinus, coccygeal or pilonidal

    685.0 With abscess

    685.1 Without mention of abscess

● **686 Other local infections of skin and subcutaneous tissue**
    Use additional code to identify any infectious organism
       (041.0–041.8)

   ● **686.0 Pyoderma**
       Dermatitis:
          purulent   suppurative
          septic

       686.00 Pyoderma, unspecified

       686.01 Pyoderma gangrenosum
          Coding Clinic: 1997, Q4, P42

       686.09 Other pyoderma

    686.1 Pyogenic granuloma
       Granuloma:
          septic   telangiectaticum
          suppurative

       | Excludes | *pyogenic granuloma of oral mucosa (528.9)* |

    686.8 Other specified local infections of skin and
       subcutaneous tissue
       Bacterid (pustular)   Ecthyma
       Dermatitis vegetans   Perlèche

       | Excludes | *dermatitis infectiosa eczematoides (690.8)* |
            panniculitis (729.30–729.39)

    686.9 Unspecified local infection of skin and subcutaneous
       tissue
       Fistula of skin NOS   Skin infection NOS

       | Excludes | *fistula to skin from internal organs—see* |
            Alphabetic Index

Figure 12–2   Impetigo. A thick, honey-yellow adherent crust covers the entire eroded surface. (From Habif: Clinical Dermatology, 4th ed. 2004, Mosby, Inc.)

Figure 12–3   Seborrheic dermatitis. (From Cohen BA: Atlas of Pediatric Dermatology. St. Louis, Mosby, 1993.)

Item 12–2   Pilonidal cyst, also called a coccygeal cyst, is the result of a disorder called pilonidal disease. The cyst usually contains hair and pus.

DISEASES OF THE SKIN AND SUBCUTANEOUS TISSUE (680–709)

◀ New   ◀|||| Revised   ~~deleted~~ Deleted | Excludes | | Includes | | Use additional | | Code first | | Omit code |
● Unacceptable Principal Diagnosis   ● Use Additional Digit(s)   OGCR Official Guidelines   Coding Clinic

DISEASES OF THE SKIN AND SUBCUTANEOUS TISSUE (680–709)

Item 12–3 Seborrheic dermatitis is characterized by greasy, scaly, red patches and is associated with oily skin and scalp.

OTHER INFLAMMATORY CONDITIONS OF SKIN AND SUBCUTANEOUS TISSUE (690–698)

> **Excludes** *panniculitis (729.30–729.39)*

● **690 Erythematosquamous dermatosis**

> **Excludes** *eczematous dermatitis of eyelid (373.31)*
> *parakeratosis variegata (696.2)*
> *psoriasis (696.0–696.1)*
> *seborrheic keratosis (702.11–702.19)*

● **690.1 Seborrheic dermatitis**

    690.10 Seborrheic dermatitis, unspecified
      Seborrheic dermatitis NOS

    690.11 Seborrhea capitis
      Cradle cap

    690.12 Seborrheic infantile dermatitis

    690.18 Other seborrheic dermatitis

    690.8 Other erythematosquamous dermatosis

● **691 Atopic dermatitis and related conditions**

    691.0 Diaper or napkin rash
      Ammonia dermatitis
      Diaper or napkin:
        dermatitis
        erythema
        rash
      Psoriasiform napkin eruption

    691.8 Other atopic dermatitis and related conditions
      Atopic dermatitis
      Besnier's prurigo
      Eczema:
        atopic
        flexural
        intrinsic (allergic)
      Neurodermatitis:
        atopic
        diffuse (of Brocq)

Figure 12–4 Atopic dermatitis. (From Moschella SL, Hurley HJ: Dermatology, 2nd ed. Philadelphia, WB Saunders, 1985, p 336.)

Item 12–4 Atopic dermatitis, also known as atopic eczema, infantile eczema, disseminated neurodermatitis, flexural eczema, and *prurigo diathesique* (Besnier), is characterized by intense itching and is often hereditary.

● **692 Contact dermatitis and other eczema**

> **Includes** dermatitis:
>   NOS
>   contact
>   occupational
>   venenata
> eczema (acute) (chronic):
>   NOS
>   allergic
>   erythematous
>   occupational

> **Excludes** *allergy NOS (995.3)*
> *contact dermatitis of eyelids (373.32)*
> *dermatitis due to substances taken internally (693.0–693.9)*
> *eczema of external ear (380.22)*
> *perioral dermatitis (695.3)*
> *urticarial reactions (708.0–708.9, 995.1)*

    692.0 Due to detergents

    692.1 Due to oils and greases

    692.2 Due to solvents
      Dermatitis due to solvents of:
        chlorocompound group
        cyclohexane group
        ester group
        glycol group
        hydrocarbon group
        ketone group

    692.3 Due to drugs and medicines in contact with skin
      Dermatitis (allergic) (contact) due to:
        arnica
        fungicides
        iodine
        keratolytics
        mercurials
        neomycin
        pediculocides
        phenols
        scabicides
        any drug applied to skin
      Dermatitis medicamentosa due to drug applied to skin

> Use additional E code to identify drug

> **Excludes** *allergy NOS due to drugs (995.27)*
> *dermatitis due to ingested drugs (693.0)*
> *dermatitis medicamentosa NOS (693.0)*

    692.4 Due to other chemical products

      Dermatitis due to: Dermatitis due to:
        acids   insecticide
        adhesive plaster   nylon
        alkalis   plastic
        caustics   rubber
        dichromate
      Coding Clinic: 2008, Q3, P6-7; 1989, Q2, P16

    692.5 Due to food in contact with skin
      Dermatitis, contact, due to:
        cereals
        fish
        flour
        fruit
        meat
        milk

> **Excludes** *dermatitis due to:*
> *dyes (692.89)*
> *ingested foods (693.1)*
> *preservatives (692.89)*

◀ New   ◀ Revised   ~~deleted~~ Deleted   Excludes   Includes   Use additional   Code first   Omit code
● Unacceptable Principal Diagnosis   ● Use Additional Digit(s)   OGCR Official Guidelines   Coding Clinic

692.6 Due to plants [except food]
Dermatitis due to:
   lacquer tree [Rhus verniciflua]
   poison:
      ivy [Rhus toxicodendron]
      oak [Rhus diversiloba]
      sumac [Rhus venenata]
      vine [Rhus radicans]
   primrose [Primula]
   ragweed [Senecio jacobae]
   other plants in contact with the skin

> **Excludes** *allergy NOS due to pollen (477.0)*
> *nettle rash (708.8)*

● **692.7 Due to solar radiation**

> **Excludes** *sunburn due to other ultraviolet radiation exposure (692.82)*

692.70 Unspecified dermatitis due to sun

692.71 Sunburn
First degree sunburn
See codes 692.76 and 692.77 for second and third degrees.
Sunburn NOS

692.72 Acute dermatitis due to solar radiation
Berloque dermatitis
Photoallergic response
Phototoxic response
Polymorphous light eruption
Acute solar skin damage NOS

> **Excludes** *sunburn (692.71, 692.76–692.77)*

Use additional E code to identify drug, if drug induced

692.73 Actinic reticuloid and actinic granuloma

692.74 Other chronic dermatitis due to solar radiation
Chronic solar skin damage NOS
Solar elastosis

> **Excludes** *actinic [solar] keratosis (702.0)*

692.75 Disseminated superficial actinic porokeratosis (DSAP)

692.76 Sunburn of second degree

692.77 Sunburn of third degree

692.79 Other dermatitis due to solar radiation
Hydroa aestivale
Photodermatitis (due to sun)
Photosensitiveness (due to sun)
Solar skin damage NOS

● **692.8 Due to other specified agents**

692.81 Dermatitis due to cosmetics

692.82 Dermatitis due to other radiation
Infrared rays
Light, except from sun
Radiation NOS
Tanning bed
Ultraviolet rays, except from sun
X-rays

> **Excludes** *that due to solar radiation (692.70–692.79)*

Coding Clinic: 2000, Q3, P5

692.83 Dermatitis due to metals
Jewelry

692.84 Due to animal (cat) (dog) dander
Due to animal (cat) (dog) hair
Coding Clinic: 2004, Q4, P90-91

692.89 Other
Dermatitis due to:
   cold weather
   dyes
   hot weather
   preservatives

> **Excludes** *allergy (NOS) (rhinitis) due to animal hair or dander (477.2)*
> *allergy to dust (477.8)*
> *sunburn (692.71, 692.76–692.77)*

692.9 Unspecified cause
Dermatitis:
   NOS
   contact NOS
   venenata NOS
Eczema NOS

● **693 Dermatitis due to substances taken internally**

> **Excludes** *adverse effect NOS of drugs and medicines (995.20)*
> *allergy NOS (995.3)*
> *contact dermatitis (692.0–692.9)*
> *urticarial reactions (708.0–708.9, 995.1)*

693.0 Due to drugs and medicines
Dermatitis medicamentosa NOS

Use additional E code to identify drug

> **Excludes** *that due to drugs in contact with skin (692.3)*

Coding Clinic: 2007, Q2, P9-10

693.1 Due to food

693.8 Due to other specified substances taken internally

693.9 Due to unspecified substance taken internally

> **Excludes** *dermatitis NOS (692.9)*

● **694 Bullous dermatoses**

694.0 Dermatitis herpetiformis
Dermatosis herpetiformis
Duhring's disease
Hydroa herpetiformis

> **Excludes** *herpes gestationis (646.8)*
> *dermatitis herpetiformis:*
>   *juvenile (694.2)*
>   *senile (694.5)*

694.1 Subcorneal pustular dermatosis
Sneddon-Wilkinson disease or syndrome

694.2 Juvenile dermatitis herpetiformis
Juvenile pemphigoid

694.3 Impetigo herpetiformis

694.4 Pemphigus
Pemphigus:
   NOS
   erythematosus
   foliaceus
   malignant
   vegetans
   vulgaris

> **Excludes** *pemphigus neonatorum (684)*

694.5 Pemphigoid
Benign pemphigus NOS
Bullous pemphigoid
Herpes circinatus bullosus
Senile dermatitis herpetiformis

DISEASES OF THE SKIN AND SUBCUTANEOUS TISSUE (680–709)

Figure 12–5 Dermatitis herpetiformis. (From Arnold HL, Odom RB, James WD: Andrews' Diseases of the Skin, Clinical Dermatology, 8th ed. Philadelphia, WB Saunders, 1990, p 553.)

Item 12–5 Dermatitis herpetiformis, also known as Duhring's disease, is a systemic disease characterized by small blisters (3 to 5 mm) and occasionally large bullae (+5 mm).

● **694.6 Benign mucous membrane pemphigoid**
    Cicatricial pemphigoid
    Mucosynechial atrophic bullous dermatitis

    694.60 Without mention of ocular involvement

    694.61 With ocular involvement
        Ocular pemphigus

    694.8 Other specified bullous dermatoses
        | **Excludes** | herpes gestationis (646.8) |

    694.9 Unspecified bullous dermatoses

● **695 Erythematous conditions**

    695.0 Toxic erythema
        Erythema venenatum

● **695.1 Erythema multiforme**

    Use additional code to identify associated
        manifestations, such as:
        arthropathy associated with dermatological
            disorders (713.3)
        conjunctival edema (372.73)
        conjunctivitis (372.04, 372.33)
        corneal scars and opacities (371.00-371.05)
        corneal ulcer (370.00-370.07)
        edema of eyelid (374.82)
        inflammation of eyelid (373.8)
        keratoconjunctivitis sicca (370.33)
        mechanical lagophthalmos (374.22)
        mucositis (478.11, 528.00, 538, 616.81)
        stomatitis (528.00)
        symblepharon (372.63)

    Use additional E-code to identify drug, if drug-
        induced

    Use additional code to identify percentage of skin
        exfoliation (695.50–695.59)

        | **Excludes** | (staphylococcal) scalded skin syndrome (695.81) |

    Coding Clinic: 2008, Q4, P128-131

    695.10 Erythema multiforme, unspecified
        Erythema iris
        Herpes iris

    695.11 Erythema multiforme minor

    695.12 Erythema multiforme major

    695.13 Stevens-Johnson syndrome

    695.14 Stevens-Johnson syndrome-toxic epidermal necrolysis overlap syndrome
        SJS-TEN overlap syndrome
        Coding Clinic: 2008, Q4, P128-131

    695.15 Toxic epidermal necrolysis
        Lyell's syndrome

    695.19 Other erythema multiforme

    695.2 Erythema nodosum
        | **Excludes** | tuberculous erythema nodosum (017.1) |

    695.3 Rosacea
        Acne: Perioral dermatitis
          erythematosa   Rhinophyma
          rosacea

    695.4 Lupus erythematosus
        *See 710.0 for designated as systemic lupus
            erythematosus (SLE).*
        Lupus:
          erythematodes (discoid)
          erythematosus (discoid), not disseminated

        | **Excludes** | lupus (vulgaris) NOS (017.0) |
                    systemic [disseminated] lupus erythematosus (710.0)

● **695.5 Exfoliation due to erythematous conditions according to extent of body surface involved**

    *Code first erythematous condition causing
        exfoliation, such as:*
    Ritter's disease (695.81)
    (Staphylococcal) scalded skin syndrome (695.81)
    Stevens-Johnson syndrome (695.13)
    Stevens-Johnson syndrome-toxic epidermal
        necrolysis overlap syndrome (695.14)
    toxic epidermal necrolysis (695.15)

  ● **695.50 Exfoliation due to erythematous condition involving less than 10 percent of body surface**
        Exfoliation due to erythematous condition NOS

  ● **695.51 Exfoliation due to erythematous condition involving 10-19 percent of body surface**

  ● **695.52 Exfoliation due to erythematous condition involving 20-29 percent of body surface**

  ● **695.53 Exfoliation due to erythematous condition involving 30-39 percent of body surface**
        Coding Clinic: 2008, Q4, P128-131

  ● **695.54 Exfoliation due to erythematous condition involving 40-49 percent of body surface**

  ● **695.55 Exfoliation due to erythematous condition involving 50-59 percent of body surface**

  ● **695.56 Exfoliation due to erythematous condition involving 60-69 percent of body surface**

  ● **695.57 Exfoliation due to erythematous condition involving 70-79 percent of body surface**

  ● **695.58 Exfoliation due to erythematous condition involving 80-89 percent of body surface**

  ● **695.59 Exfoliation due to erythematous condition involving 90 percent or more of body surface**

● **695.8 Other specified erythematous conditions**

    695.81 Ritter's disease
        Dermatitis exfoliativa neonatorum
        (Staphylococcal) Scalded skin syndrome

        Use additional code to identify percentage
          of skin exfoliation (695.50-695.59)

    695.89 Other
        Erythema intertrigo
        Intertrigo
        Pityriasis rubra (Hebra)

        | **Excludes** | mycotic intertrigo (111.0–111.9) |
        Coding Clinic: 1986, Sept-Oct, P10

    695.9 Unspecified erythematous condition
        Erythema NOS
        Erythroderma (secondary)

◄ New   ◄||||| Revised   ~~deleted~~ Deleted | Excludes | | Includes | | Use additional | | Code first | | Omit code |
● Unacceptable Principal Diagnosis   ● Use Additional Digit(s)   **OGCR** Official Guidelines   **Coding Clinic**

Figure 12–6 Erythematous plaques with silvery scales in a patient with psoriasis. (From Goldman: Cecil Textbook of Medicine, 22nd ed. 2004, Saunders.)

Item 12–6 Psoriasis is a chronic, recurrent inflammatory skin disease characterized by small patches covered with thick silvery scales. **Parapsoriasis** is a treatment-resistant erythroderma. **Pityriasis rosea** is characterized by a herald patch that is a single large lesion and that usually appears on the trunk and is followed by scattered, smaller lesions.

● **696 Psoriasis and similar disorders**

696.0 Psoriatic arthropathy

696.1 Other psoriasis
Acrodermatitis continua
Dermatitis repens
Psoriasis:
  NOS
  any type, except arthropathic
  | Excludes | *psoriatic arthropathy (696.0)*
  Coding Clinic: 1996, Q2, P12

696.2 Parapsoriasis
Parakeratosis variegata
Parapsoriasis lichenoides chronica
Pityriasis lichenoides et varioliformis

696.3 Pityriasis rosea
Pityriasis circinata (et maculata)

696.4 Pityriasis rubra pilaris
Devergie's disease
Lichen ruber acuminatus
  | Excludes | *pityriasis rubra (Hebra) (695.89)*

696.5 Other and unspecified pityriasis
Pityriasis:
  NOS
  alba
  streptogenes
  | Excludes | *pityriasis:*
    simplex (690.18)
    versicolor (111.0)

696.8 Other

● **697 Lichen**
  | Excludes | *lichen:*
    obtusus corneus (698.3)
    pilaris (congenital) (757.39)
    ruber acuminatus (696.4)
    sclerosus et atrophicus (701.0)
    scrofulosus (017.0)
    simplex chronicus (698.3)
    spinulosus (congenital) (757.39)
    urticatus (698.2)

697.0 Lichen planus
Lichen:
  planopilaris
  ruber planus

697.1 Lichen nitidus
Pinkus' disease

697.8 Other lichen, not elsewhere classified
Lichen:
  ruber moniliforme
  striata

697.9 Lichen, unspecified

● **698 Pruritus and related conditions**
  | Excludes | *pruritus specified as psychogenic (306.3)*

698.0 Pruritus ani
Perianal itch

698.1 Pruritus of genital organs

698.2 Prurigo
Lichen urticatus
Prurigo: Prurigo:
  NOS   mitis
  Hebra's   simplex
Urticaria papulosa (Hebra)
  | Excludes | *prurigo nodularis (698.3)*

698.3 Lichenification and lichen simplex chronicus
Hyde's disease
Neurodermatitis (circumscripta) (local)
Prurigo nodularis
  | Excludes | *neurodermatitis, diffuse (of Brocq) (691.8)*

698.4 Dermatitis factitia [artefacta]
Dermatitis ficta
Neurotic excoriation
  Use additional code to identify any associated
    mental disorder

698.8 Other specified pruritic conditions
Pruritus:
  hiemalis
  senilis
Winter itch

698.9 Unspecified pruritic disorder
Itch NOS
Pruritus NOS

OTHER DISEASES OF SKIN AND SUBCUTANEOUS TISSUE (700–709)
  | Excludes | *conditions confined to eyelids (373.0–374.9)*
    congenital conditions of skin, hair, and nails
      (757.0–757.9)

700 Corns and callosities
Callus
Clavus

● **701 Other hypertrophic and atrophic conditions of skin**
  | Excludes | *dermatomyositis (710.3)*
    hereditary edema of legs (757.0)
    scleroderma (generalized) (710.1)

701.0 Circumscribed scleroderma
Addison's keloid
Dermatosclerosis, localized
Lichen sclerosus et atrophicus
Morphea
Scleroderma, circumscribed or localized

701.1 Keratoderma, acquired
Acquired:
  ichthyosis
  keratoderma palmaris et plantaris
Elastosis perforans serpiginosa
Hyperkeratosis:
  NOS
  follicularis in cutem penetrans
  palmoplantaris climacterica
Keratoderma:
  climactericum
  tylodes, progressive
Keratosis (blennorrhagica)
  | Excludes | *Darier's disease [keratosis follicularis]*
    (congenital) (757.39)
    keratosis:
      arsenical (692.4)
      gonococcal (098.81)

DISEASES OF THE SKIN AND SUBCUTANEOUS TISSUE (680–709)

Item 12–7 Scleroderma means hard skin. It is a group of diseases that causes abnormal growth of connective tissues that support the skin and organs. There are two types: localized scleroderma affecting the skin and systemic scleroderma affecting blood vessels and internal organs and the skin. **Keratoderma** is characterized by firm horny papules that have a cobblestone appearance. **Keratoderma climactericum,** also known as endocrine keratoderma, is hyperkeratosis located on the palms and soles.

701.2 Acquired acanthosis nigricans
Keratosis nigricans

701.3 Striae atrophicae
Atrophic spots of skin
Atrophoderma maculatum
Atrophy blanche (of Milian)
Degenerative colloid atrophy
Senile degenerative atrophy
Striae distensae

701.4 Keloid scar
Cheloid
Hypertrophic scar
Keloid
Coding Clinic: 1995, Q3, P14

701.5 Other abnormal granulation tissue
Excessive granulation

701.8 Other specified hypertrophic and atrophic conditions of skin
Acrodermatitis atrophicans chronica
Atrophia cutis senilis
Atrophoderma neuriticum
Confluent and reticulate papillomatosis
Cutis laxa senilis
Elastosis senilis
Folliculitis ulerythematosa reticulata
Gougerot-Carteaud syndrome or disease
Coding Clinic: 2008, Q1, P7-8

701.9 Unspecified hypertrophic and atrophic conditions of skin
Atrophoderma

● **702 Other dermatoses**
        Excludes   carcinoma in situ (232.0–232.9)

702.0 Actinic keratosis

● **702.1 Seborrheic keratosis**

702.11 Inflamed seborrheic keratosis

702.19 Other seborrheic keratosis
Seborrheic keratosis NOS

702.8 Other specified dermatoses

● **703 Diseases of nail**
        Excludes   congenital anomalies (757.5)
                   onychia and paronychia (681.02, 681.11)

703.0 Ingrowing nail
Ingrowing nail with infection
Unguis incarnatus
        Excludes   infection, nail NOS (681.9)

703.8 Other specified diseases of nail
Dystrophia unguium
Hypertrophy of nail
Koilonychia
Leukonychia (punctata) (striata)
Onychauxis
Onychogryposis
Onycholysis

703.9 Unspecified disease of nail

● **704 Diseases of hair and hair follicles**
        Excludes   congenital anomalies (757.4)

● **704.0 Alopecia**
        Excludes   madarosis (374.55)
                   syphilitic alopecia (091.82)

704.00 Alopecia, unspecified
Baldness   Loss of hair

704.01 Alopecia areata
Ophiasis

704.02 Telogen effluvium

704.09 Other
Folliculitis decalvans
Hypotrichosis:
    NOS
    postinfectional NOS
Pseudopelade

704.1 Hirsutism
Excessive growth of hair
Hypertrichosis:
    NOS
    lanuginosa, acquired
Polytrichia
        Excludes   hypertrichosis of eyelid (374.54)

704.2 Abnormalities of the hair
Atrophic hair   Trichiasis:
Clastothrix   NOS
Fragilitas crinium   cicatrical
                       Trichorrhexis (nodosa)
        Excludes   trichiasis of eyelid (374.05)
        Coding Clinic: 2004, Q4, P91-92

704.3 Variations in hair color
Canities (premature)
Grayness, hair (premature)
Heterochromia of hair
Poliosis:
    NOS
    circumscripta, acquired

704.8 Other specified diseases of hair and hair follicles
Folliculitis:
    NOS
    abscedens et suffodiens
    pustular
Perifolliculitis:
    NOS
    capitis abscedens et suffodiens
    scalp
Sycosis:
    NOS
    barbae [not parasitic]
    lupoid
    vulgaris

704.9 Unspecified disease of hair and hair follicles

Item 12–8 Alopecia is lack of hair and takes many forms. The most common is male pattern alopecia, also known as **androgenetic alopecia. Telogen effluvium** is early and excessive loss of hair resulting from a trauma to the hair follicle (fever, drugs, surgery, etc.).

Figure 12–7 Male pattern alopecia.

◀ New   ◀▦ Revised   ~~deleted~~ Deleted | Excludes | | Includes | | Use additional | | Code first | | Omit code |
● Unacceptable Principal Diagnosis   ● Use Additional Digit(s)   OGCR Official Guidelines   Coding Clinic

● **705 Disorders of sweat glands**

705.0 Anhidrosis
    Hypohidrosis   Oligohidrosis

705.1 Prickly heat
    Heat rash   Sudamina
    Miliaria rubra (tropicalis)

● **705.2 Focal hyperhidrosis**
    Excludes *generalized (secondary) hyperhidrosis (780.8)*

    705.21 Primary focal hyperhidrosis
        Focal hyperhidrosis NOS
        Hyperhidrosis NOS
        Hyperhidrosis of:
            axilla   palms
            face   soles

    705.22 Secondary focal hyperhidrosis
        Frey's syndrome

● **705.8 Other specified disorders of sweat glands**

    705.81 Dyshidrosis
        Cheiropompholyx
        Pompholyx

    705.82 Fox-Fordyce disease

    705.83 Hidradenitis
        Hidradenitis suppurativa

    705.89 Other
        Bromhidrosis   Granulosis rubra nasi
        Chromhidrosis   Urhidrosis
        Excludes *hidrocystoma (216.0–216.9)*
                generalized hyperhidrosis (780.8)

705.9 Unspecified disorder of sweat glands
    Disorder of sweat glands NOS

● **706 Diseases of sebaceous glands**

706.0 Acne varioliformis
    Acne:
        frontalis
        necrotica

706.1 Other acne
    Acne:
        NOS
        conglobata
        cystic
        pustular
        vulgaris
    Blackhead
    Comedo
    Excludes *acne rosacea (695.3)*

706.2 Sebaceous cyst
    Atheroma, skin
    Keratin cyst
    Wen

706.3 Seborrhea
    Excludes *seborrhea:*
        capitis (690.11)
        sicca (690.18)
      seborrheic
        dermatitis (690.10)
        keratosis (702.11–702.19)

706.8 Other specified diseases of sebaceous glands
    Asteatosis (cutis)
    Xerosis cutis

706.9 Unspecified disease of sebaceous glands

● **707 Chronic ulcer of skin**
    Includes   non-infected sinus of skin
                non-healing ulcer
    Excludes *varicose ulcer (454.0, 454.2)*

● **707.0 Pressure ulcer**
    Bed sore
    Decubitus ulcer
    Plaster ulcer

    Use additional code to identify pressure ulcer stage (707.20–707.25)
    Coding Clinic: 2004, Q4, P92-93; Q1, P14-15; 2003, Q4, P110; 1999, Q4, P20; 1996, Q1, P15; 1990, Q3, P15; 1987, Nov-Dec, P9

    707.00 Unspecified site

    707.01 Elbow

    707.02 Upper back
        Shoulder blades

    707.03 Lower back
        Coccyx
        Sacrum
        Coding Clinic: 2008, Q3, P17; 2005, Q1, P16

    707.04 Hip

    707.05 Buttock

    707.06 Ankle

    707.07 Heel
        Coding Clinic: 2009, Q4, P108; 2005, Q1, P16

    707.09 Other site
        Head
        Coding Clinic: 2008, Q3, P17

● **707.1 Ulcer of lower limbs, except pressure ulcer**
    Ulcer, chronic, of lower limb:
        neurogenic of lower limb
        trophic of lower limb
    Code if applicable, any causal condition first:
        atherosclerosis of the extremities with ulceration (440.23)
        chronic venous hypertension with ulcer (459.31)
        chronic venous hypertension with ulcer and inflammation (459.33)
        diabetes mellitus (249.80–249.81, 250.80–250.83)
        postphlebitic syndrome with ulcer (459.11)
        postphlebitic syndrome with ulcer and inflammation (459.13)
    Coding Clinic: 2004, Q1, P14-15; 1999, Q4, P15; 1996, Q1, P10

    707.10 Ulcer of lower limb, unspecified
        Coding Clinic: 2004, Q3, P5-6

    707.11 Ulcer of thigh

    707.12 Ulcer of calf

    707.13 Ulcer of ankle

    707.14 Ulcer of heel and midfoot
        Plantar surface of midfoot

    707.15 Ulcer of other part of foot
        Toes

    707.19 Ulcer of other part of lower limb

● **707.2 Pressure ulcer stages**
    Code first site of pressure ulcer (707.00-707.09)
    Coding Clinic: 2008, Q4, P132-134

    707.20 Pressure ulcer, unspecified stage
        Healing pressure ulcer NOS
        Healing pressure ulcer, unspecified stage

    707.21 Pressure ulcer stage I
        Healing pressure ulcer, stage I
        Pressure pre-ulcer skin changes limited to persistent focal erythema

DISEASES OF THE SKIN AND SUBCUTANEOUS TISSUE (680–709)

707.22 Pressure ulcer stage II
Healing pressure ulcer, stage II
Pressure ulcer with abrasion, blister, partial
thickness skin loss involving
epidermis and/or dermis

707.23 Pressure ulcer stage III
Healing pressure ulcer, stage III
Pressure ulcer with full thickness skin loss
involving damage or necrosis of
subcutaneous tissue
Coding Clinic: 2009, Q4, P113

707.24 Pressure ulcer stage IV
Healing pressure ulcer, stage IV
Pressure ulcer with necrosis of soft tissues
through to underlying muscle, tendon,
or bone

707.25 Pressure ulcer, unstageable

707.8 Chronic ulcer of other specified sites
Ulcer, chronic, of other specified sites:
neurogenic of other specified sites
trophic of other specified sites

707.9 Chronic ulcer of unspecified site
Chronic ulcer NOS   Tropical ulcer NOS
Trophic ulcer NOS   Ulcer of skin NOS

● **708 Urticaria**
| Excludes | edema:
angioneurotic (995.1)
Quincke's (995.1)
hereditary angioedema (277.6)
urticaria:
giant (995.1)
papulosa (Hebra) (698.2)
pigmentosa (juvenile) (congenital) (757.33)

708.0 Allergic urticaria
Coding Clinic: 1984, May-June, P11

708.1 Idiopathic urticaria

708.2 Urticaria due to cold and heat
Thermal urticaria

708.3 Dermatographic urticaria
Dermatographia
Factitial urticaria

708.4 Vibratory urticaria

708.5 Cholinergic urticaria
Coding Clinic: 1995, Q4, P50

708.8 Other specified urticaria
Nettle rash
Urticaria:
chronic
recurrent periodic

708.9 Urticaria, unspecified
Hives NOS

Figure 12-8 Urticaria (hives). *(Courtesy of David Effron, MD.)* (From Marx: Rosen's Emergency Medicine: Concepts and Clinical Practice, 6th ed. 2006, Mosby, Inc.)

● **709 Other disorders of skin and subcutaneous tissue**
● **709.0 Dyschromia**
| Excludes | albinism (270.2)
pigmented nevus (216.0–216.9)
that of eyelid (374.52–374.53)

709.00 Dyschromia, unspecified

709.01 Vitiligo

709.09 Other

709.1 Vascular disorders of skin
Angioma serpiginosum
Purpura (primary) annularis telangiectodes

709.2 Scar conditions and fibrosis of skin
Adherent scar (skin)
Cicatrix
Disfigurement (due to scar)
Fibrosis, skin NOS
Scar NOS
| Excludes | keloid scar (701.4)
Coding Clinic: 1984, Nov-Dec, P19

709.3 Degenerative skin disorders
Calcinosis:
circumscripta
cutis
Colloid milium
Degeneration, skin
Deposits, skin
Senile dermatosis NOS
Subcutaneous calcification

709.4 Foreign body granuloma of skin and subcutaneous tissue
Use additional code to identify foreign body (V90.01-V90.9) ◄
| Excludes | residual foreign body without granuloma of
skin and subcutaneous tissue (729.6)
that of muscle (728.82)

709.8 Other specified disorders of skin
Epithelial hyperplasia
Menstrual dermatosis
Vesicular eruption
Coding Clinic: 1987, Nov-Dec, P6

709.9 Unspecified disorder of skin and subcutaneous tissue
Dermatosis NOS

Item 12–9 Urticaria is a vascular reaction in which wheals surrounded by a red halo appear and cause severe itching. The causes of urticaria or hives are extensive and varied (e.g., food, heat, cold, drugs, stress, infections). Dyschromia is any disorder of the pigmentation of the skin or hair.

13. **DISEASES OF THE MUSCULOSKELETAL SYSTEM AND CONNECTIVE TISSUE (710–739)**

Use additional external cause code, if applicable, to identify the cause of the musculoskeletal condition

The following fifth-digit subclassification is for use with categories 711–712, 715–716, 718–719, and 730:

0 site unspecified	6 lower leg
1 shoulder region	Fibula
Acromioclavicular	Knee joint
joint(s)	Patella
Clavicle	Tibia
Glenohumeral joint(s)	7 ankle and foot
Scapula	Ankle joint
Sternoclavicular joint(s)	Digits [toes]
2 upper arm	Metatarsus
Elbow joint	Phalanges, foot
Humerus	Tarsus
3 forearm	Other joints in foot
Radius	8 other specified sites
Ulna	Head
Wrist joint	Neck
4 hand	Ribs
Carpus	Skull
Metacarpus	Trunk
Phalanges [fingers]	Vertebral column
5 pelvic region and thigh	9 multiple sites
Buttock	
Femur	
Hip (joint)	

ARTHROPATHIES AND RELATED DISORDERS (710–719)

Excludes *disorders of spine (720.0–724.9)*

● **710 Diffuse diseases of connective tissue**

  Includes all collagen diseases whose effects are not mainly confined to a single system

  Excludes *those affecting mainly the cardiovascular system, i.e., polyarteritis nodosa and allied conditions (446.0–446.7)*

710.0 Systemic lupus erythematosus

  Autoimmune inflammatory connective tissue disease of unknown cause that occurs most often in women. See 695.4 for nonsystemic.

  Disseminated lupus erythematosus
  Libman-Sacks disease

  Use additional code to identify manifestation, as:
    endocarditis (424.91)
    nephritis (583.81)
      chronic (582.81)
    nephrotic syndrome (581.81)

  Excludes *lupus erythematosus (discoid) NOS (695.4)*

  Coding Clinic: 2003, Q2, P7x2; 1997, Q2, P8-9; 1987, Sept-Oct, P8

710.1 Systemic sclerosis
  Acrosclerosis
  CRST syndrome
  Progressive systemic sclerosis
  Scleroderma

  Use additional code to identify manifestation, as:
    lung involvement (517.2)
    myopathy (359.6)

  Excludes *circumscribed scleroderma (701.0)*

710.2 Sicca syndrome
  Keratoconjunctivitis sicca
  Sjögren's disease

710.3 Dermatomyositis
  Poikilodermatomyositis
  Polymyositis with skin involvement

710.4 Polymyositis

710.5 Eosinophilia myalgia syndrome
  Toxic oil syndrome

  Use additional E code to identify drug, if drug induced

710.8 Other specified diffuse diseases of connective tissue
  Multifocal fibrosclerosis (idiopathic) NEC
  Systemic fibrosclerosing syndrome
  Coding Clinic: 1987, Mar-April, P12

710.9 Unspecified diffuse connective tissue disease
  Collagen disease NOS

● **711 Arthropathy associated with infections**
  Abnormality of a joint

  Includes arthritis associated with conditions classifiable below
    arthropathy associated with conditions classifiable below
    polyarthritis associated with conditions classifiable below
    polyarthropathy associated with conditions classifiable below

  Excludes *rheumatic fever (390)*

  Coding Clinic: 1992, Q1, P16-17

The following fifth-digit subclassification is for use with category 711; valid digits are in [brackets] under each code. See list at beginning of chapter for definitions:

0 site unspecified	5 pelvic region and thigh
1 shoulder region	6 lower leg
2 upper arm	7 ankle and foot
3 forearm	8 other specified sites
4 hand	9 multiple sites

● **711.0 Pyogenic arthritis**
[0-9]   Arthritis or polyarthritis (due to):
    coliform [Escherichia coli]
    Hemophilus influenzae [H. influenzae]
    pneumococcal
    Pseudomonas
    staphylococcal
    streptococcal
  Pyarthrosis

  Use additional code to identify infectious organism (041.0–041.8)
  Coding Clinic: 1992, Q1, P16-17; 1991, Q1, P15

● **711.1 Arthropathy associated with Reiter's disease and**
[0-9] **nonspecific urethritis**

  Code first underlying disease, as:
    nonspecific urethritis (099.4)
    Reiter's disease (099.3)

● **711.2 Arthropathy in Behçet's syndrome**
[0-9]   *Code first* underlying disease (136.1)

● **711.3 Postdysenteric arthropathy**
[0-9]   *Code first* underlying disease, as:
    dysentery (009.0)
    enteritis, infectious (008.0–009.3)
    paratyphoid fever (002.1–002.9)
    typhoid fever (002.0)

  Excludes *salmonella arthritis (003.23)*

DISEASES OF THE MUSCULOSKELETAL SYSTEM AND CONNECTIVE TISSUE (710–739)

● **711.4 Arthropathy associated with other bacterial**
[0-9] **diseases**

> *Code first* underlying disease, as:
> diseases classifiable to 010–040, 090–099, except
> as in 711.1, 711.3, and 713.5
> leprosy (030.0–030.9)
> tuberculosis (015.0–015.9)
>
> **Excludes** *gonococcal arthritis (098.50)*
> *meningococcal arthritis (036.82)*

● **711.5 Arthropathy associated with other viral diseases**
[0-9]
> *Code first* underlying disease, as:
> diseases classifiable to 045–049, 050–079, 480, 487
> O'nyong-nyong (066.3)
>
> **Excludes** *that due to rubella (056.71)*

● **711.6 Arthropathy associated with mycoses**
[0-9]
> *Code first* underlying disease (110.0–118)

● **711.7 Arthropathy associated with helminthiasis**
[0-9]
> *Code first* underlying disease, as:
> filariasis (125.0–125.9)

● **711.8 Arthropathy associated with other infectious and**
[0-9] **parasitic diseases**

> *Code first* underlying disease, as:
> diseases classifiable to 080–088, 100–104,
> 130–136
>
> **Excludes** *arthropathy associated with sarcoidosis*
> *(713.7)*
>
> **Coding Clinic: 1990, Q3, P14**

● **711.9 Unspecified infective arthritis**
[0-9] Infective arthritis or polyarthritis (acute) (chronic)
(subacute) NOS

● **712 Crystal arthropathies**

> **Includes** crystal-induced arthritis and synovitis
>
> **Excludes** *gouty arthropathy (274.00-274.03)*

The following fifth-digit subclassification is for use with
category 712; valid digits are in [brackets] under each code.
See list at beginning of chapter for definitions:

0	site unspecified	5	pelvic region and thigh
1	shoulder region	6	lower leg
2	upper arm	7	ankle and foot
3	forearm	8	other specified sites
4	hand	9	multiple sites

● **712.1 Chondrocalcinosis due to dicalcium phosphate**
[0-9] **crystals**
Chondrocalcinosis due to dicalcium phosphate
crystals (with other crystals)

> *Code first* underlying disease (275.49)

● **712.2 Chondrocalcinosis due to pyrophosphate crystals**
[0-9]
> *Code first* underlying disease (275.49)

● **712.3 Chondrocalcinosis, unspecified**
[0-9]
> *Code first* underlying disease (275.49)

● **712.8 Other specified crystal arthropathies**
[0-9]

● **712.9 Unspecified crystal arthropathy**
[0-9]

● **713 Arthropathy associated with other disorders classified**
elsewhere

> **Includes** arthritis associated with conditions classifiable
> below
> arthropathy associated with conditions
> classifiable below
> polyarthritis associated with conditions
> classifiable below
> polyarthropathy associated with conditions
> classifiable below

713.0 Arthropathy associated with other endocrine and
metabolic disorders

> *Code first* underlying disease, as:
> acromegaly (253.0)
> hemochromatosis (275.01-275.09) ◄▥
> hyperparathyroidism (252.00–252.08)
> hypogammaglobulinemia (279.00–279.09)
> hypothyroidism (243–244.9)
> lipoid metabolism disorder (272.0–272.9)
> ochronosis (270.2)
>
> **Excludes** *arthropathy associated with:*
> *amyloidosis (713.7)*
> *crystal deposition disorders, except gout*
> *(712.1–712.9)*
> *diabetic neuropathy (713.5)*
> *gout (274.00-274.03)*

713.1 Arthropathy associated with gastrointestinal
conditions other than infections

> *Code first* underlying disease, as:
> regional enteritis (555.0–555.9)
> ulcerative colitis (556)

713.2 Arthropathy associated with hematological
disorders

> *Code first* underlying disease, as:
> hemoglobinopathy (282.4–282.7)
> hemophilia (286.0–286.2)
> leukemia (204.0–208.9)
> malignant reticulosis (202.3)
> multiple myelomatosis (203.0)
>
> **Excludes** *arthropathy associated with*
> *Henoch-Schönlein purpura (713.6)*

713.3 Arthropathy associated with dermatological
disorders

> *Code first* underlying disease, as:
> erythema multiforme (695.10–695.19)
> erythema nodosum (695.2)
>
> **Excludes** *psoriatic arthropathy (696.0)*

713.4 Arthropathy associated with respiratory disorders

> *Code first* underlying disease, as:
> diseases classifiable to 490–519
>
> **Excludes** *arthropathy associated with respiratory*
> *infections (711.0, 711.4–711.8)*

713.5 Arthropathy associated with neurological
disorders
Charcot's arthropathy associated with diseases
classifiable elsewhere
Neuropathic arthritis associated with diseases
classifiable elsewhere

> *Code first* underlying disease, as:
> neuropathic joint disease [Charcot's joints]:
> NOS (094.0)
> diabetic (249.6, 250.6)
> syringomyelic (336.0)
> tabetic [syphilitic] (094.0)

◄ New   ◄▥ Revised   ~~deleted~~ Deleted   Excludes   Includes   Use additional   Code first   Omit code
● Unacceptable Principal Diagnosis   ● Use Additional Digit(s)   OGCR Official Guidelines   Coding Clinic

713.6 Arthropathy associated with hypersensitivity reaction
> *Code first underlying disease, as:*
> Henoch-Schönlein purpura (287.0)
> serum sickness (999.5)
> Excludes *allergic arthritis NOS (716.2)*

713.7 Other general diseases with articular involvement
> *Code first underlying disease, as:*
> amyloidosis (277.30–277.39)
> familial Mediterranean fever (277.31)
> sarcoidosis (135)
> Coding Clinic: 1997, Q2, P12-13

713.8 Arthropathy associated with other conditions classifiable elsewhere
> *Code first underlying disease, as:*
> conditions classifiable elsewhere except as in 711.1–711.8, 712, and 713.0–713.7

● **714 Rheumatoid arthritis and other inflammatory polyarthropathies**
> Excludes *rheumatic fever (390)*
> *rheumatoid arthritis of spine NOS (720.0)*

714.0 Rheumatoid arthritis
> Arthritis or polyarthritis:
> atrophic
> rheumatic (chronic)
> Use additional code to identify manifestation, as:
> myopathy (359.6)
> polyneuropathy (357.1)
> Excludes *juvenile rheumatoid arthritis NOS (714.30)*
> Coding Clinic: 2006, Q2, P20; 1995, Q4, P51

714.1 Felty's syndrome
> Rheumatoid arthritis with splenoadenomegaly and leukopenia

714.2 Other rheumatoid arthritis with visceral or systemic involvement
> Rheumatoid carditis

● **714.3 Juvenile chronic polyarthritis**

> **714.30 Polyarticular juvenile rheumatoid arthritis, chronic or unspecified**
> Juvenile rheumatoid arthritis NOS
> Still's disease

> **714.31 Polyarticular juvenile rheumatoid arthritis, acute**

> **714.32 Pauciarticular juvenile rheumatoid arthritis**

> **714.33 Monoarticular juvenile rheumatoid arthritis**

714.4 Chronic postrheumatic arthropathy
> Chronic rheumatoid nodular fibrositis
> Jaccoud's syndrome

● **714.8 Other specified inflammatory polyarthropathies**

> **714.81 Rheumatoid lung**
> Caplan's syndrome
> Diffuse interstitial rheumatoid disease of lung
> Fibrosing alveolitis, rheumatoid

> **714.89 Other**

714.9 Unspecified inflammatory polyarthropathy
> Inflammatory polyarthropathy or polyarthritis NOS
> Excludes *polyarthropathy NOS (716.5)*

Item 13-1 Rheumatoid arthritis (RA) is a chronic systemic inflammatory disease of undetermined etiology involving primarily the synovial membranes and articular structures of multiple joints. The disease is often progressive and results in pain, stiffness, and swelling of joints. In late stages, deformity, ankylosis, and other **inflammatory polyarthropathies** develop.

● **715 Osteoarthrosis and allied disorders**
> *Degenerative joint disease with breaking down the cartilage causing pain, swelling, and reduced motion in the joints, affecting any joint.*

> **Note:** Localized, in the subcategories below, includes bilateral involvement of the same site.
> Includes arthritis or polyarthritis:
> degenerative
> hypertrophic
> degenerative joint disease
> osteoarthritis
> Excludes *Marie-Strümpell spondylitis (720.0)*
> *osteoarthrosis [osteoarthritis] of spine (721.0–721.9)*

The following fifth-digit subclassification is for use with category 715; valid digits are in [brackets] under each code. See list at beginning of chapter for definitions:

0	site unspecified	5	pelvic region and thigh
1	shoulder region	6	lower leg
2	upper arm	7	ankle and foot
3	forearm	8	other specified sites
4	hand	9	multiple sites

● **715.0 Osteoarthrosis, generalized**
[0,4,9] Degenerative joint disease, involving multiple joints
> Primary generalized hypertrophic osteoarthrosis
> Coding Clinic: 1995, Q2, P5

● **715.1 Osteoarthrosis, localized, primary**
[0-8] Localized osteoarthropathy, idiopathic

● **715.2 Osteoarthrosis, localized, secondary**
[0-8] Coxae malum senilis

● **715.3 Osteoarthrosis, localized, not specified whether**
[0-8] **primary or secondary**
> Otto's pelvis
> Coding Clinic: 2004, Q2, P15; 2003, Q2, P18; 1995, Q2, P5

● **715.8 Osteoarthrosis involving, or with mention of more**
[0,9] **than one site, but not specified as generalized**
> Coding Clinic: 1995, Q2, P5

● **715.9 Osteoarthrosis, unspecified whether generalized or**
[0-8] **localized**
> Coding Clinic: 2003, Q2, P18; 1997, Q2, P12-13; 1996, Q1, P16; 1995, Q2, P5

● **716 Other and unspecified arthropathies**
> Excludes *cricoarytenoid arthropathy (478.79)*

The following fifth-digit subclassification is for use with category 716; valid digits are in [brackets] under each code. See list at beginning of chapter for definitions:

0	site unspecified	5	pelvic region and thigh
1	shoulder region	6	lower leg
2	upper arm	7	ankle and foot
3	forearm	8	other specified sites
4	hand	9	multiple sites

● **716.0 Kaschin-Beck disease**
[0-9] Endemic polyarthritis

● **716.1 Traumatic arthropathy**
[0-9] Coding Clinic: 2009, Q2, P11; 2002, Q1, P9-10

● **716.2 Allergic arthritis**
[0-9] Excludes *arthritis associated with Henoch-Schönlein purpura or serum sickness (713.6)*

● **716.3 Climacteric arthritis**
[0-9]   Menopausal arthritis

● **716.4 Transient arthropathy**
[0-9]   **Excludes** *palindromic rheumatism (719.3)*

● **716.5 Unspecified polyarthropathy or polyarthritis**
[0-9]

● **716.6 Unspecified monoarthritis**
[0-8]   Coxitis

● **716.8 Other specified arthropathy**
[0-9]

● **716.9 Arthropathy, unspecified**
[0-9]   Arthritis (acute) (chronic) (subacute)
          Arthropathy (acute) (chronic) (subacute)
          Articular rheumatism (chronic)
          Inflammation of joint NOS

● **717 Internal derangement of knee**
Includes degeneration of articular cartilage or meniscus
              of knee
              rupture, old of articular cartilage or meniscus
              of knee
              tear, old of articular cartilage or meniscus of
              knee

Excludes *acute derangement of knee (836.0–836.6)*
              ankylosis (718.5)
              contracture (718.4)
              current injury (836.0–836.6)
              deformity (736.4–736.6)
              recurrent dislocation (718.3)

717.0 Old bucket handle tear of medial meniscus
        Old bucket handle tear of unspecified cartilage

717.1 Derangement of anterior horn of medial meniscus

717.2 Derangement of posterior horn of medial meniscus

717.3 Other and unspecified derangement of medial meniscus
        Degeneration of internal semilunar cartilage

● **717.4 Derangement of lateral meniscus**

    717.40 Derangement of lateral meniscus, unspecified

    717.41 Bucket handle tear of lateral meniscus

    717.42 Derangement of anterior horn of lateral meniscus

    717.43 Derangement of posterior horn of lateral meniscus

    717.49 Other

717.5 Derangement of meniscus, not elsewhere classified
        Congenital discoid meniscus
        Cyst of semilunar cartilage
        Derangement of semilunar cartilage NOS

717.6 Loose body in knee
        Joint mice, knee
        Rice bodies, knee (joint)

717.7 Chondromalacia of patella
        Chondromalacia patellae
        Degeneration [softening] of articular cartilage of
        patella
        Coding Clinic: 1985, July-Aug, P14; 1984, Nov-Dec, P9

● **717.8 Other internal derangement of knee**

    717.81 Old disruption of lateral collateral ligament

    717.82 Old disruption of medial collateral ligament

    717.83 Old disruption of anterior cruciate ligament

    717.84 Old disruption of posterior cruciate ligament

    717.85 Old disruption of other ligaments of knee
            Capsular ligament of knee

    717.89 Other
            Old disruption of ligaments of knee NOS

717.9 Unspecified internal derangement of knee
        Derangement NOS of knee

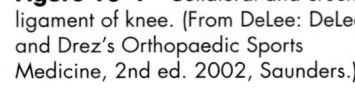

Figure 13–1 Collateral and cruciate ligament of knee. (From DeLee: DeLee and Drez's Orthopaedic Sports Medicine, 2nd ed. 2002, Saunders.)

● **718 Other derangement of joint**
Excludes *current injury (830.0–848.9)*
              jaw (524.60–524.69)

The following fifth-digit subclassification is for use with category 718; valid digits are in [brackets] under each code. See list at beginning of chapter for definitions:

0 site unspecified	5 pelvic region and thigh
1 shoulder region	6 lower leg
2 upper arm	7 ankle and foot
3 forearm	8 other specified sites
4 hand	9 multiple sites

● **718.0 Articular cartilage disorder**
[0-5,7-9] Meniscus:
              disorder
              rupture, old
              tear, old
           Old rupture of ligament(s) of joint NOS
           Excludes *articular cartilage disorder:*
                         in ochronosis (270.2)
                         knee (717.0–717.9)
                         chondrocalcinosis (275.49)
                         metastatic calcification (275.40)

● **718.1 Loose body in joint**
[0-5,7-9] Joint mice
           Excludes *knee (717.6)*
           Coding Clinic: 2001, Q2, P14-15

● **718.2 Pathological dislocation**
[0-9]   Dislocation or displacement of joint, not recurrent
          and not current

● **718.3 Recurrent dislocation of joint**
[0-9]   **Coding Clinic: 1987, Nov-Dec, P7**

● **718.4 Contracture of joint**
[0-9]   **Coding Clinic: 1998, Q4, P39-40**

● **718.5 Ankylosis of joint**
[0-9]   Ankylosis of joint (fibrous) (osseous)
          Excludes *spine (724.9)*
                        stiffness of joint without mention of
                        ankylosis (719.5)
          Coding Clinic: 1995, Q1, P10

● **718.6 Unspecified intrapelvic protrusion of acetabulum**
[0,5]   Protrusio acetabuli, unspecified

● **718.7 Developmental dislocation of joint**
[0-9]   **Excludes** *congenital dislocation of joint (754.0–755.8)*
                        traumatic dislocation of joint (830–839)

● **718.8 Other joint derangement, not elsewhere classified**
[0-9]   Flail joint (paralytic)
          Instability of joint
          Excludes *deformities classifiable to 736 (736.0–736.9)*
          Coding Clinic: 2000, Q2, P14-15

● **718.9 Unspecified derangement of joint**
[0-5,7-9] **Excludes** *knee (717.9)*

◀ New   ◀▦ Revised   ~~deleted~~ Deleted   Excludes   Includes   Use additional   Code first   Omit code
● Unacceptable Principal Diagnosis   ● Use Additional Digit(s)   **OGCR** Official Guidelines   **Coding Clinic**

● **719 Other and unspecified disorders of joint**

| **Excludes** | *jaw (524.60–524.69)* |

The following fifth-digit subclassification is for use with codes 719.0–719.6, 719.8–719.9; valid digits are in [brackets] under each code. See list at beginning of chapter for definitions:

0	site unspecified	5	pelvic region and thigh
1	shoulder region	6	lower leg
2	upper arm	7	ankle and foot
3	forearm	8	other specified sites
4	hand	9	multiple sites

● **719.0 Effusion of joint**
[0-9]   Hydrarthrosis
        Swelling of joint, with or without pain

| **Excludes** | *intermittent hydrarthrosis (719.3)* |

● **719.1 Hemarthrosis**
[0-9]

| **Excludes** | *current injury (840.0–848.9)* |

● **719.2 Villonodular synovitis**
[0-9]

● **719.3 Palindromic rheumatism**
[0-9]   Hench-Rosenberg syndrome
        Intermittent hydrarthrosis

● **719.4 Pain in joint**
[0-9]   Arthralgia
        Coding Clinic: 2001, Q1, P3-4

● **719.5 Stiffness of joint, not elsewhere classified**
[0-9]

● **719.6 Other symptoms referable to joint**
[0-9]   Joint crepitus
        Snapping hip
        Coding Clinic: 2007, Q2, P7; 1984, Sept-Oct, P15-16

719.7 Difficulty in walking

| **Excludes** | *abnormality of gait (781.2)* |

Coding Clinic: 2004, Q2, P15

● **719.8 Other specified disorders of joint**
[0-9]   Calcification of joint
        Fistula of joint

| **Excludes** | *temporomandibular joint-pain-dysfunction syndrome [Costen's syndrome] (524.60)* |

● **719.9 Unspecified disorder of joint**
[0-9]

DORSOPATHIES (720–724)

| **Excludes** | *curvature of spine (737.0–737.9)* *osteochondrosis of spine (juvenile) (732.0) adult (732.8)* |

● **720 Ankylosing spondylitis and other inflammatory spondylopathies**

720.0 Ankylosing spondylitis
        Rheumatoid arthritis of spine NOS
        Spondylitis:
            Marie-Strümpell
            rheumatoid

720.1 Spinal enthesopathy
        Disorder of peripheral ligamentous or muscular attachments of spine
        Romanus lesion

720.2 Sacroiliitis, not elsewhere classified
        Inflammation of sacroiliac joint NOS

Item 13-2 Ankylosis or arthrokleisis is a consolidation of a joint due to disease, injury, or surgical procedure. Spondylosis is the degeneration of the vertebral processes and formation of osteophytes and commonly occurs with age. **Spondylitis** or ankylosing spondylitis is a type of arthritis that affects the spine or backbone causing back pain and stiffness.

● **720.8 Other inflammatory spondylopathies**

720.81 Inflammatory spondylopathies in diseases classified elsewhere
        Code first underlying disease, as:
            tuberculosis (015.0)

720.89 Other

720.9 Unspecified inflammatory spondylopathy
        Spondylitis NOS

● **721 Spondylosis and allied disorders**
Coding Clinic: 1989, Q2, P14

721.0 Cervical spondylosis without myelopathy
        Cervical or cervicodorsal:
            arthritis
            osteoarthritis
            spondylarthritis

721.1 Cervical spondylosis with myelopathy
        Anterior spinal artery compression syndrome
        Spondylogenic compression of cervical spinal cord
        Vertebral artery compression syndrome

721.2 Thoracic spondylosis without myelopathy
        Thoracic:
            arthritis
            osteoarthritis
            spondylarthritis

721.3 Lumbosacral spondylosis without myelopathy
        Lumbar or lumbosacral:
            arthritis
            osteoarthritis
            spondylarthritis
        Coding Clinic: 2002, Q4, P107-108

● **721.4 Thoracic or lumbar spondylosis with myelopathy**

721.41 Thoracic region
        Spondylogenic compression of thoracic spinal cord

721.42 Lumbar region
        ~~Spondylogenic compression of lumbar spinal cord~~

721.5 Kissing spine
        Baastrup's syndrome

721.6 Ankylosing vertebral hyperostosis

721.7 Traumatic spondylopathy
        Kümmell's disease or spondylitis

721.8 Other allied disorders of spine

● **721.9 Spondylosis of unspecified site**

721.90 Without mention of myelopathy
        Spinal:
            arthritis (deformans) (degenerative) (hypertrophic)
            osteoarthritis NOS
        Spondylarthrosis NOS

721.91 With myelopathy
        Spondylogenic compression of spinal cord NOS

DISEASES OF THE MUSCULOSKELETAL SYSTEM AND CONNECTIVE TISSUE (710–739)

● 722 **Intervertebral disc disorders**
Coding Clinic: 1989, Q2, P14

722.0 **Displacement of cervical intervertebral disc without myelopathy**
Neuritis (brachial) or radiculitis due to displacement or rupture of cervical intervertebral disc
Any condition classifiable to 722.2 of the cervical or cervicothoracic intervertebral disc
Coding Clinic: 1988, Q1, P10

● 722.1 **Displacement of thoracic or lumbar intervertebral disc without myelopathy**

722.10 **Lumbar intervertebral disc without myelopathy**
Lumbago or sciatica due to displacement of intervertebral disc
Neuritis or radiculitis due to displacement or rupture of lumbar intervertebral disc
Any condition classifiable to 722.2 of the lumbar or lumbosacral intervertebral disc
Coding Clinic: 2008, Q4, P183-184; 2007, Q1, P9; 2003, Q3, P12; Q1, P7; 2002, Q4, P107-108; 1994, Q3, P14

722.11 **Thoracic intervertebral disc without myelopathy**
Any condition classifiable to 722.2 of thoracic intervertebral disc

722.2 **Displacement of intervertebral disc, site unspecified, without myelopathy**
Discogenic syndrome NOS
Herniation of nucleus pulposus NOS
Intervertebral disc NOS:
    extrusion
    prolapse
    protrusion
    rupture
Neuritis or radiculitis due to displacement or rupture of intervertebral disc
Coding Clinic: 1988, Q1, P10

● 722.3 **Schmorl's nodes**

722.30 **Unspecified region**

722.31 **Thoracic region**

722.32 **Lumbar region**

722.39 **Other**

722.4 **Degeneration of cervical intervertebral disc**
Degeneration of cervicothoracic intervertebral disc

● 722.5 **Degeneration of thoracic or lumbar intervertebral disc**

722.51 **Thoracic or thoracolumbar intervertebral disc**

722.52 **Lumbar or lumbosacral intervertebral disc**
Coding Clinic: 2006, Q2, P18; 2004, Q4, P129-133

722.6 **Degeneration of intervertebral disc, site unspecified**
Degenerative disc disease NOS
Narrowing of intervertebral disc or space NOS

● 722.7 **Intervertebral disc disorder with myelopathy**

722.70 **Unspecified region**

722.71 **Cervical region**

722.72 **Thoracic region**

722.73 **Lumbar region**

● 722.8 **Postlaminectomy syndrome**

722.80 **Unspecified region**

722.81 **Cervical region**

722.82 **Thoracic region**

722.83 **Lumbar region**
Coding Clinic: 1997, Q2, P15x2

● 722.9 **Other and unspecified disc disorder**
Calcification of intervertebral cartilage or disc
Discitis

722.90 **Unspecified region**
Coding Clinic: 1984, Nov-Dec, P19

722.91 **Cervical region**

722.92 **Thoracic region**

722.93 **Lumbar region**

● 723 **Other disorders of cervical region**
Excludes conditions due to:
    intervertebral disc disorders (722.0–722.9)
    spondylosis (721.0–721.9)
Coding Clinic: 1989, Q2, P14

723.0 **Spinal stenosis of cervical region**
Coding Clinic: 2003, Q4, P99-101

723.1 **Cervicalgia**
Pain in neck

723.2 **Cervicocranial syndrome**
Barré-Liéou syndrome
Posterior cervical sympathetic syndrome

723.3 **Cervicobrachial syndrome (diffuse)**
Coding Clinic: 1985, Nov-Dec, P12

723.4 **Brachia neuritis or radiculitis NOS**
Cervical radiculitis
Radicular syndrome of upper limbs

723.5 **Torticollis, unspecified**
Contracture of neck
Excludes congenital (754.1)
    due to birth injury (767.8)
    hysterical (300.11)
    ocular torticollis (781.93)
    psychogenic (306.0)
    spasmodic (333.83)
    traumatic, current (847.0)
Coding Clinic: 2001, Q2, P21; 1995, Q1, P7

723.6 **Panniculitis specified as affecting neck**

723.7 **Ossification of posterior longitudinal ligament in cervical region**

723.8 **Other syndromes affecting cervical region**
Cervical syndrome NEC
Klippel's disease
Occipital neuralgia
Coding Clinic: 2000, Q1, P7-8

723.9 **Unspecified musculoskeletal disorders and symptoms referable to neck**
Cervical (region) disorder NOS

● 724 **Other and unspecified disorders of back**
Excludes collapsed vertebra (code to cause, e.g., osteoporosis, 733.00–733.09)
    conditions due to:
        intervertebral disc disorders (722.0–722.9)
        spondylosis (721.0–721.9)
Coding Clinic: 1989, Q2, P14

● 724.0 **Spinal stenosis, other than cervical**

724.00 **Spinal stenosis, unspecified region**

724.01 **Thoracic region**

724.02 **Lumbar region, without neurogenic claudication ◀▥**
Lumbar region NOS ◀
Coding Clinic: 2008, Q4, P109-110; 2007, Q4, P116-120; Q1, P20-21; 1999, Q4, P13-14; 1994, Q3, P14

724.03 **Lumbar region, with neurogenic claudication ◀**

724.09 **Other**

◀ New   ◀▥ Revised   ~~deleted~~ Deleted   Excludes   Includes   Use additional   Code first   Omit code
● Unacceptable Principal Diagnosis   ● Use Additional Digit(s)   OGCR Official Guidelines   Coding Clinic

724.1 **Pain in thoracic spine**

724.2 **Lumbago**
Low back pain   Lumbalgia
Low back syndrome
Coding Clinic: 2007, Q2, P13-15; 1985, Nov-Dec, P12

724.3 **Sciatica**
Neuralgia or neuritis of sciatic nerve
Excludes *specified lesion of sciatic nerve (355.0)*
Coding Clinic: 1989, Q2, P12

724.4 **Thoracic or lumbosacral neuritis or radiculitis, unspecified**
Radicular syndrome of lower limbs
Coding Clinic: 1999, Q2, P3-4

724.5 **Backache, unspecified**
Vertebrogenic (pain) syndrome NOS

724.6 **Disorders of sacrum**
Ankylosis, lumbosacral or sacroiliac (joint)
Instability, lumbosacral or sacroiliac (joint)

● 724.7 **Disorders of coccyx**
724.70 **Unspecified disorder of coccyx**
724.71 **Hypermobility of coccyx**
724.79 **Other**
Coccygodynia

724.8 **Other symptoms referable to back**
Ossification of posterior longitudinal ligament NOS
Panniculitis specified as sacral or affecting back

724.9 **Other unspecified back disorders**
Ankylosis of spine NOS
Compression of spinal nerve root NEC
Spinal disorder NOS
Excludes *sacroiliitis (720.2)*

RHEUMATISM, EXCLUDING THE BACK (725–729)

Includes disorders of muscles and tendons and their attachments, and of other soft tissues

725 **Polymyalgia rheumatica**

● 726 **Peripheral enthesopathies and allied syndromes**
Note: Enthesopathies are disorders of peripheral ligamentous or muscular attachments.
Excludes *spinal enthesopathy (720.1)*

726.0 **Adhesive capsulitis of shoulder**

● 726.1 **Rotator cuff syndrome of shoulder and allied disorders**
726.10 **Disorders of bursae and tendons in shoulder region, unspecified**
Rotator cuff syndrome NOS
Supraspinatus syndrome NOS
Coding Clinic: 2001, Q2, P12

726.11 **Calcifying tendinitis of shoulder**
726.12 **Bicipital tenosynovitis**
726.19 **Other specified disorders**
Excludes *complete rupture of rotator cuff, nontraumatic (727.61)*
Coding Clinic: 2002, Q1, P9-10

726.2 **Other affections of shoulder region, not elsewhere classified**
Periarthritis of shoulder
Scapulohumeral fibrositis

● 726.3 **Enthesopathy of elbow region**
726.30 **Enthesopathy of elbow, unspecified**
726.31 **Medial epicondylitis**
726.32 **Lateral epicondylitis**
Epicondylitis NOS   Tennis elbow
Golfers' elbow
726.33 **Olecranon bursitis**
Bursitis of elbow
726.39 **Other**

726.4 **Enthesopathy of wrist and carpus**
Bursitis of hand or wrist
Periarthritis of wrist

726.5 **Enthesopathy of hip region**
Bursitis of hip   Psoas tendinitis
Gluteal tendinitis   Trochanteric tendinitis
Iliac crest spur

● 726.6 **Enthesopathy of knee**
726.60 **Enthesopathy of knee, unspecified**
Bursitis of knee NOS
726.61 **Pes anserinus tendinitis or bursitis**
726.62 **Tibial collateral ligament bursitis**
Pellegrini-Stieda syndrome
726.63 **Fibular collateral ligament bursitis**
726.64 **Patellar tendinitis**
726.65 **Prepatellar bursitis**
Coding Clinic: 2006, Q2, P15
726.69 **Other**
Bursitis:
infrapatellar
subpatellar

● 726.7 **Enthesopathy of ankle and tarsus**
726.70 **Enthesopathy of ankle and tarsus, unspecified**
Metatarsalgia NOS
Excludes *Morton's metatarsalgia (355.6)*
726.71 **Achilles bursitis or tendinitis**
726.72 **Tibialis tendinitis**
Tibialis (anterior) (posterior) tendinitis
726.73 **Calcaneal spur**
726.79 **Other**
Peroneal tendinitis

726.8 **Other peripheral enthesopathies**

● 726.9 **Unspecified enthesopathy**
726.90 **Enthesopathy of unspecified site**
Capsulitis NOS   Tendinitis NOS
Periarthritis NOS
726.91 **Exostosis of unspecified site**
Bone spur NOS
Coding Clinic: 2001, Q2, P13-15

● 727 **Other disorders of synovium, tendon, and bursa**
● 727.0 **Synovitis and tenosynovitis**
727.00 **Synovitis and tenosynovitis, unspecified**
Synovitis NOS
Tenosynovitis NOS
727.01 **Synovitis and tenosynovitis in diseases classified elsewhere**
Code first underlying disease, as:
tuberculosis (015.0–015.9)
Excludes *crystal-induced (275.49)*
gonococcal (098.51)
gout (274.00-274.03)
syphilitic (095.7)
727.02 **Giant cell tumor of tendon sheath**
727.03 **Trigger finger (acquired)**

Item 13-3 Polymyalgia rheumatica is a syndrome characterized by aching and morning stiffness and is related to aging and hereditary predisposition.

DISEASES OF THE MUSCULOSKELETAL SYSTEM AND CONNECTIVE TISSUE (710–739)

727.04 Radial styloid tenosynovitis
de Quervain's disease

727.05 Other tenosynovitis of hand and wrist

727.06 Tenosynovitis of foot and ankle

727.09 Other

727.1 Bunion

727.2 Specific bursitides often of occupational origin
Beat:
    elbow
    hand
    knee
Chronic crepitant synovitis of wrist
Miners':
    elbow
    knee

727.3 Other bursitis
Bursitis NOS

Excludes	bursitis:
	gonococcal (098.52)
	subacromial (726.19)
	subcoracoid (726.19)
	subdeltoid (726.19)
	syphilitic (095.7)
	"frozen shoulder" (726.0)

● **727.4 Ganglion and cyst of synovium, tendon, and bursa**

727.40 Synovial cyst, unspecified

Excludes	that of popliteal space (727.51)

Coding Clinic: 1997, Q2, P6

727.41 Ganglion of joint

727.42 Ganglion of tendon sheath

727.43 Ganglion, unspecified

727.49 Other
Cyst of bursa

● **727.5 Rupture of synovium**

727.50 Rupture of synovium, unspecified

727.51 Synovial cyst of popliteal space
Baker's cyst (knee)

727.59 Other

● **727.6 Rupture of tendon, nontraumatic**

727.60 Nontraumatic rupture of unspecified tendon

727.61 Complete rupture of rotator cuff

727.62 Tendons of biceps (long head)

727.63 Extensor tendons of hand and wrist

727.64 Flexor tendons of hand and wrist

727.65 Quadriceps tendon

727.66 Patellar tendon

727.67 Achilles tendon

727.68 Other tendons of foot and ankle

727.69 Other

Item 13-4 Synovitis is an inflammation of a synovial membrane resulting in pain on motion and is characterized by fluctuating swelling due to effusion in a synovial sac. **Tenosynovitis** is an inflammation of a tendon sheath and occurs most commonly in the wrists, hands, and feet. Bursitis is inflammation of a bursa (fluid filled sac) caused by repetitive use, trauma, infection, or systemic inflammatory disease. Bursae act as protectors and facilitate movement between bones and overlapping muscles (deep bursae) or between bones and tendons/skin (superficial bursae).

● **727.8 Other disorders of synovium, tendon, and bursa**

727.81 Contracture of tendon (sheath)
Short Achilles tendon (acquired)

727.82 Calcium deposits in tendon and bursa
Calcification of tendon NOS
Calcific tendinitis NOS

Excludes	peripheral ligamentous or muscular attachments (726.0–726.9)

727.83 Plica syndrome
Plica knee

727.89 Other
Abscess of bursa or tendon

Excludes	xanthomatosis localized to tendons (272.7)

Coding Clinic: 1989, Q2, P15; 1985, July-Aug, P14; 1984, Nov-Dec, P9

727.9 Unspecified disorder of synovium, tendon, and bursa

● **728 Disorders of muscle, ligament, and fascia**

Excludes	enthesopathies (726.0–726.9)
	muscular dystrophies (359.0–359.1)
	myoneural disorders (358.00–358.9)
	myopathies (359.2–359.9)
	nontraumatic hematoma of muscle (729.92)
	old disruption of ligaments of knee (717.81–717.89)

728.0 Infective myositis
Myositis:
    purulent   suppurative

Excludes	myositis:
	epidemic (074.1)
	interstitial (728.81)
	myoneural disorder (358.00–358.9)
	syphilitic (095.6)
	tropical (040.81)

● **728.1 Muscular calcification and ossification**

728.10 Calcification and ossification, unspecified
Massive calcification (paraplegic)

728.11 Progressive myositis ossificans

728.12 Traumatic myositis ossifications
Myositis ossificans (circumscripta)

728.13 Postoperative heterotopic calcification

728.19 Other
Polymyositis ossificans

728.2 Muscular wasting and disuse atrophy, not elsewhere classified
Amyotrophia NOS   Myofibrosis

Excludes	neuralgic amyotrophy (353.5)
	pelvic muscle wasting and disuse atrophy (618.83)
	progressive muscular atrophy (335.0–335.9)

728.3 Other specific muscle disorders
Arthrogryposis
Immobility syndrome (paraplegic)

Excludes	arthrogryposis multiplex congenita (754.89)
	stiff-man syndrome (333.91)

728.4 Laxity of ligament

728.5 Hypermobility syndrome

728.6 Contracture of palmar fascia
Dupuytren's contracture

● **728.7 Other fibromatoses**

728.71 Plantar fascial fibromatosis
Contracture of plantar fascia
Plantar fasciitis (traumatic)

728.79 Other
Garrod's or knuckle pads
Nodular fasciitis
Pseudosarcomatous Fibromatosis (proliferative) (subcutaneous)

◄ New   ◄▥▥ Revised   deleted Deleted | Excludes | | Includes | | Use additional | | Code first | | Omit code |
● Unacceptable Principal Diagnosis   ● Use Additional Digit(s)   OGCR Official Guidelines   Coding Clinic

● **728.8 Other disorders of muscle, ligament, and fascia**

    728.81 Interstitial myositis

    728.82 Foreign body granuloma of muscle
        Talc granuloma of muscle
        Use additional code to identify foreign
          body (V90.01-V90.9) ◀

    728.83 Rupture of muscle, nontraumatic

    728.84 Diastasis of muscle
        Diastasis recti (abdomen)
        Excludes   *diastasis recti complicating*
          pregnancy, labor, and delivery
          (665.8)

    728.85 Spasm of muscle

    728.86 Necrotizing fasciitis
        Use additional code to identify:
          infectious organism (041.00–041.89)
          gangrene (785.4), if applicable

    728.87 Muscle weakness (generalized)
        Excludes   *generalized weakness (780.79)*
        Coding Clinic: 2005, Q1, P13

    728.88 Rhabdomyolysis
        Coding Clinic: 2003, Q4, P66-67; 2001, Q2, P14

    728.89 Other
        Eosinophilic fasciitis
        Use additional E code to identify drug, if
          drug induced
        Coding Clinic: 2006, Q3, P13; 2002, Q3, P28; 2001, Q2, P15

    728.9 Unspecified disorder of muscle, ligament, and fascia

● **729 Other disorders of soft tissues**
    Excludes   *acroparesthesia (443.89)*
        carpal tunnel syndrome (354.0)
        disorders of the back (720.0–724.9)
        entrapment syndromes (354.0–355.9)
        palindromic rheumatism (719.3)
        periarthritis (726.0–726.9)
        psychogenic rheumatism (306.0)
    Coding Clinic: 1984, Nov-Dec, P17

    729.0 Rheumatism, unspecified and fibrositis

    729.1 Myalgia and myositis, unspecified
        Fibromyositis NOS
        Coding Clinic: 1984, Nov-Dec, P17

    729.2 Neuralgia, neuritis, and radiculitis, unspecified
        Excludes   *brachia radiculitis (723.4)*
          cervical radiculitis (723.4)
          lumbosacral radiculitis (724.4)
          mononeuritis (354.0–355.9)
          radiculitis due to intervertebral disc
            involvement (722.0–722.2, 722.7)
          sciatica (724.3)

● **729.3 Panniculitis, unspecified**
    Inflammation of adipose tissue of heel pad

    729.30 Panniculitis, unspecified site
        Weber-Christian disease

    729.31 Hypertrophy of fat pad, knee
        Hypertrophy of infrapatellar fat pad

    729.39 Other site
        Excludes   *panniculitis specified as (affecting):*
          back (724.8)
          neck (723.6)
          sacral (724.8)

    729.4 Fasciitis, unspecified
        Excludes   *necrotizing fasciitis (728.86)*
          nodular fasciitis (728.79)
        Coding Clinic: 1994, Q2, P13

    729.5 Pain in limb
        Coding Clinic: 2007, Q2, P13-15

    729.6 Residual foreign body in soft tissue
        Use additional code to identify foreign body
          (V90.01-V90.9) ◀
        Excludes   *foreign body granuloma:*
          muscle (728.82)
          skin and subcutaneous tissue (709.4)

● **729.7 Nontraumatic compartment syndrome**
    Excludes   *compartment syndrome NOS (958.90)*
        traumatic compartment syndrome
          (958.90–958.99)
    Code first, if applicable, postprocedural complication
      (998.89)

    729.71 Nontraumatic compartment syndrome of upper extremity
        Nontraumatic compartment syndrome of
          shoulder, arm, forearm, wrist, hand
          and fingers
        Coding Clinic: 2006, Q4, P100-102

    729.72 Nontraumatic compartment syndrome of lower extremity
        Nontraumatic compartment syndrome of
          hip, buttock, thigh, leg, foot and toes

    729.73 Nontraumatic compartment syndrome of abdomen

    729.79 Nontraumatic compartment syndrome of other sites

● **729.8 Other musculoskeletal symptoms referable to limbs**

    729.81 Swelling of limb
        Coding Clinic: 1988, Q4, P6

    729.82 Cramp

    729.89 Other
        Excludes   *abnormality of gait (781.2)*
          tetany (781.7)
          transient paralysis of limb (781.4)
        Coding Clinic: 1988, Q4, P12

● **729.9 Other and unspecified disorders of soft tissue**
    Coding Clinic: 2008, Q4, P134-136

    729.90 Disorders of soft tissue, unspecified

    729.91 Post-traumatic seroma
        Excludes   *seroma complicating a procedure*
          (998.13)

    729.92 Nontraumatic hematoma of soft tissue
        Nontraumatic hematoma of muscle

    729.99 Other disorders of soft tissue
        Polyalgia

DISEASES OF THE MUSCULOSKELETAL SYSTEM AND CONNECTIVE TISSUE (710–739)

OSTEOPATHIES, CHONDROPATHIES, AND ACQUIRED MUSCULOSKELETAL DEFORMITIES (730–739)

● **730 Osteomyelitis, periostitis, and other infections involving bone**

> **Excludes** *jaw (526.4–526.5)*
> *petrous bone (383.2)*

> **Use additional** code to identify organism, such as:
> Staphylococcus (041.1)
> Coding Clinic: 1997, Q4, P43; 1993, 5th Issue, P3

The following fifth-digit subclassification is for use with category 730; valid digits are in [brackets] under each code. See list at beginning of chapter for definitions:

> 0 site unspecified
> 1 shoulder region
> 2 upper arm
> 3 forearm
> 4 hand
> 5 pelvic region and thigh
> 6 lower leg
> 7 ankle and foot
> 8 other specified sites
> 9 multiple sites

● **730.0 Acute osteomyelitis**
  [0-9]   Abscess of any bone except accessory sinus, jaw, or mastoid
  Acute or subacute osteomyelitis, with or without mention of periostitis

> **Use additional** code to identify major osseous defect, if applicable (731.3)
> Coding Clinic: 2004, Q1, P14-15; 2002, Q1, P3-4

● **730.1 Chronic osteomyelitis**
  [0-9]   Brodie's abscess
  Chronic or old osteomyelitis, with or without mention of periostitis
  Sequestrum
  Sclerosing osteomyelitis of Garré

> **Use additional** code to identify major osseous defect, if applicable (731.3)

> **Excludes** *aseptic necrosis of bone (733.40–733.49)*
> Coding Clinic: 2000, Q3, P4

Figure 13–2 Osteomyelitis of the spine. A lateral view of the lower thoracic spine demonstrates destruction of the disk space *(arrow)* as well as destruction of the adjoining vertebral bodies. (From Mettler: Essentials of Radiology, 2nd ed. 2005, Saunders, An Imprint of Elsevier.)

Item 13–5 Osteomyelitis is an inflammation of the bone. **Acute osteomyelitis** is a rapidly destructive, pus-producing infection capable of causing severe bone destruction. **Chronic osteomyelitis** can remain long after the initial acute episode has passed and may lead to a recurrence of the acute phase. **Brodie's abscess** is an encapsulated focal abscess that must be surgically drained. Periostitis is an inflammation of the periosteum, a dense membrane composed of fibrous connective tissue that closely wraps all bone, except those with articulating surfaces in joints, which are covered by synovial membranes.

● **730.2 Unspecified osteomyelitis**
  [0-9]   Osteitis or osteomyelitis NOS, with or without mention of periostitis

> **Use additional** code to identify major osseous defect, if applicable (731.3)

● **730.3 Periostitis without mention of osteomyelitis**
  [0-9]   Abscess of periosteum, without mention of osteomyelitis
  Periostosis, without mention of osteomyelitis

> **Excludes** *that in secondary syphilis (091.61)*

● **730.7 Osteopathy resulting from poliomyelitis**
  [0-9]   *Code first* underlying disease (045.0–045.9)

● **730.8 Other infections involving bone in disease classified**
  [0-9] **elsewhere**

> *Code first* underlying disease, as:
> tuberculosis (015.0–015.9)
> typhoid fever (002.0)

> **Excludes** *syphilitis of bone NOS (095.5)*

● **730.9 Unspecified infection of bone**
  [0-9]

● **731 Osteitis deformans and osteopathies associated with other disorders classified elsewhere**
  Also known as Paget's Disease; chronic disorder that results in enlarged and deformed bones. The excessive breakdown and formation of bone tissue causes bones to weaken and results in bone pain, arthritis, deformities, and fractures.

731.0 Osteitis deformans without mention of bone tumor
  Paget's disease of bone
  Coding Clinic: 1994, Q2, P6-7

731.1 Osteitis deformans in diseases classified elsewhere
> *Code first* underlying disease, as:
> malignant neoplasm of bone (170.0–170.9)

731.2 Hypertrophic pulmonary osteoarthropathy
  Bamberger-Marie disease

731.3 Major osseous defects
> *Code first* underlying disease, if known, such as:
> aseptic necrosis (733.40–733.49)
> malignant neoplasm of bone (170.0–170.9)
> osteomyelitis (730.00–730.29)
> osteoporosis (733.00–733.09)
> peri-prosthetic osteolysis (996.45)
> Coding Clinic: 2006, Q4, P103-104

731.8 Other bone involvement in diseases classified elsewhere
> *Code first* underlying disease, as:
> diabetes mellitus (249.8, 250.8)

> **Use additional** code to specify bone condition, such as:
> acute osteomyelitis (730.00–730.09)
> Coding Clinic: 2004, Q1, P14-115; 1997, Q4, P43

● **732 Osteochondropathies**

732.0 Juvenile osteochondrosis of spine
  Juvenile osteochondrosis (of):
  marginal or vertebral ephiphysis (of Scheuermann) spine NOS
  Vertebral epiphysitis

> **Excludes** *adolescent postural kyphosis (737.0)*

732.1 Juvenile osteochondrosis of hip and pelvis
  Coxa plana
  Ischiopubic synchondrosis (of van Neck)
  Osteochondrosis (juvenile) of:
  acetabulum
  head of femur (of Legg-Calvé-Perthes)
  iliac crest (of Buchanan)
  symphysis pubis (of Pierson)
  Pseudocoxalgia

732.2 Nontraumatic slipped upper femoral epiphysis
Slipped upper femoral epiphysis NOS

732.3 Juvenile osteochondrosis of upper extremity
Osteochondrosis (juvenile) of:
    capitulum of humerus (of Panner)
    carpal lunate (of Kienbock)
    hand NOS
    head of humerus (of Haas)
    heads of metacarpals (of Mauclaire)
    lower ulna (of Burns)
    radial head (of Brailsford)
    upper extremity NOS

732.4 Juvenile osteochondrosis of lower extremity, excluding foot
Osteochondrosis (juvenile) of:
    lower extremity NOS
    primary patellar center (of Köhler)
    proximal tibia (of Blount)
    secondary patellar center (of Sinding-Larsen)
    tibial tubercle (of Osgood-Schlatter)
Tibia vara

732.5 Juvenile osteochondrosis of foot
Calcaneal apophysitis
Epiphysitis, os calcis
Osteochondrosis (juvenile) of:
    astragalus (of Diaz)
    calcaneum (of Sever)
    foot NOS
    metatarsal:
        second (of Freiberg)
        fifth (of Iselin)
    os tibiale externum (of Haglund)
    tarsal navicular (of Köhler)

732.6 Other juvenile osteochondrosis
Apophysis specified as juvenile, of other site, or site NOS
Epiphysitis specified as juvenile, of other site, or site NOS
Osteochondritis specified as juvenile, of other site, or site NOS
Osteochondrosis specified as juvenile, of other site, or site NOS

732.7 Osteochondritis dissecans

732.8 Other specified forms of osteochondropathy
Adult osteochondrosis of spine

732.9 Unspecified osteochondropathy
Apophysitis
    NOS
    not specified as adult or juvenile, of unspecified site
Epiphysitis
    NOS
    not specified as adult or juvenile, of unspecified site
Osteochondritis
    NOS
    not specified as adult or juvenile, of unspecified site
Osteochondrosis
    NOS
    not specified as adult or juvenile, of unspecified site

● **733 Other disorders of bone and cartilage**

> **Excludes** *bone spur (726.91)*
> *cartilage of, or loose body in, joint (717.0–717.9, 718.0–718.9)*
> *giant cell granuloma of jaw (526.3)*
> *osteitis fibrosa cystica generalisata (252.01)*
> *osteomalacia (268.2)*
> *polyostotic fibrous dysplasia of bone (756.54)*
> *prognathism, retrognathism (524.1)*
> *xanthomatosis localized to bone (272.7)*

● **733.0 Osteoporosis**
Condition of excessive skeletal fragility (porous bone) resulting in bone fractures

Use additional code to identify:
    major osseous defect, if applicable (731.3)
    personal history of pathologic (healed) fracture (V13.51)
Coding Clinic: 1993, Q4, P25-26

733.00 Osteoporosis, unspecified
Wedging of vertebra NOS
Coding Clinic: 2007, Q4, P91-92; Q1, P22; 2001, Q3, P19; 1998, Q2, P12

733.01 Senile osteoporosis
Postmenopausal osteoporosis
Coding Clinic: 2007, Q1, P3-8

733.02 Idiopathic osteoporosis

733.03 Disuse osteoporosis

733.09 Other
Drug-induced osteoporosis
Use additional E code to identify drug
Coding Clinic: 2003, Q4, P108-109

● **733.1 Pathologic fracture**
Chronic fracture
Spontaneous fracture

> **Excludes** *stress fracture (733.93–733.95)*
> *traumatic fractures (800–829)*
Coding Clinic: 1986, Nov-Dec, P10; 1985, Nov-Dec, P16

733.10 Pathologic fracture, unspecified site

733.11 Pathologic fracture of humerus

733.12 Pathologic fracture of distal radius and ulna
Wrist NOS

733.13 Pathologic fracture of vertebrae
Collapse of vertebra NOS
Coding Clinic: 2008, Q3, P4; 2007, Q1, P3-8,22; 1999, Q3, P5

733.14 Pathologic fracture of neck of femur
Femur NOS
Hip NOS
Coding Clinic: 2001, Q1, P10-11; 1996, Q1, P16; 1993, Q4, P25-26

733.15 Pathologic fracture of other specified part of femur
Coding Clinic: 1998, Q2, P12; 1994, Q2, P6-7

733.16 Pathologic fracture of tibia and fibula
Ankle NOS

733.19 Pathologic fracture of other specified site

DISEASES OF THE MUSCULOSKELETAL SYSTEM AND CONNECTIVE TISSUE (710–739)

● **733.2 Cyst of bone**

    733.20 Cyst of bone (localized), unspecified

    733.21 Solitary bone cyst
        Unicameral bone cyst

    733.22 Aneurysmal bone cyst

    733.29 Other
        Fibrous dysplasia (monostotic)
        Excludes *cyst of jaw (526.0–526.2, 526.89)*
                osteitis fibrosa cystica (252.01)
                polyostotic fibrous dysplasia of bone
                    (756.54)

733.3 Hyperostosis of skull
    Hyperostosis interna frontalis
    Leontiasis ossium

● **733.4 Aseptic necrosis of bone**

    Use additional code to identify major osseous
        defect, if applicable (731.3)
    Excludes *osteochondropathies (732.0–732.9)*
    Coding Clinic: 2007, Q4, P116-120

    733.40 Aseptic necrosis of bone, site unspecified

    733.41 Head of humerus

    733.42 Head and neck of femur
        Femur NOS
        Excludes *Legg-Calvé-Perthes disease (732.1)*

    733.43 Medial femoral condyle

    733.44 Talus

    733.45 Jaw
        Use additional E code to identify drug, if
           drug-induced
        Excludes *osteoradionecrosis of jaw (526.89)*
        Coding Clinic: 2007, Q4, P91-92

    733.49 Other

733.5 Osteitis condensans
    Piriform sclerosis of ilium

733.6 Tietze's disease
    Costochondral junction syndrome
    Costochondritis

733.7 Algoneurodystrophy
    Disuse atrophy of bone
    Sudeck's atrophy

● **733.8 Malunion and nonunion of fracture**

    733.81 Malunion of fracture
        Fracture ends do not heal together correctly.

    733.82 Nonunion of fracture
        Total failure of fracture healing
        Pseudoarthrosis (bone)
        Coding Clinic: 1994, Q2, P7; 1987, Jan-Feb, P13; 1984,
          Nov-Dec, P18

● **733.9 Other and unspecified disorders of bone and cartilage**
    Coding Clinic: 2008, Q4, P136-137

    733.90 Disorder of bone and cartilage, unspecified

    733.91 Arrest of bone development or growth
        Epiphyseal arrest

    733.92 Chondromalacia
        Chondromalacia:
          NOS
          localized, except patella
          systemic
          tibial plateau
        Excludes *chondromalacia of patella (717.7)*

    733.93 Stress fracture of tibia or fibula
        Stress reaction of tibia or fibula
        Use additional external cause code(s)
          to identify the cause of the stress
          fracture

    733.94 Stress fracture of the metatarsals
        Stress reaction of metatarsals
        Use additional external cause code(s)
          to identify the cause of the stress
          fracture
        Coding Clinic: 2001, Q4, P48-49

    733.95 Stress fracture of other bone
        Stress reaction of other bone
        Use additional external cause code(s)
          to identify the cause of the stress
          fracture
        Excludes *stress fracture of:*
              femoral neck (733.96)
              fibula (733.93)
               metatarsals (733.94)
              pelvis (733.98)
               shaft of femur (733.97)
               tibia (733.93)

    733.96 Stress fracture of femoral neck
        Stress reaction of femoral neck
        Use additional external cause code(s)
          to identify the cause of the stress
          fracture

    733.97 Stress fracture of shaft of femur
        Stress reaction of shaft of femur
        Use additional external cause code(s)
          to identify the cause of the stress
          fracture

    733.98 Stress fracture of pelvis
        Stress reaction of pelvis
        Use additional external cause code(s)
          to identify the cause of the stress
          fracture

    733.99 Other
        Diaphysitis
        Hypertrophy of bone
        Relapsing polychondritis
        Coding Clinic: 2000, Q3, P4; 1987, Jan-Feb, P14

734 Flat foot
    Pes planus (acquired)
    Talipes planus (acquired)
    Excludes *congenital (754.61)*
               rigid flat foot (754.61)
               spastic (everted) flat foot (754.61)

● **735 Acquired deformities of toe**
    Excludes *congenital (754.60–754.69, 755.65–755.66)*

    735.0 Hallux valgus (acquired)

    735.1 Hallux varus (acquired)

    735.2 Hallux rigidus

    735.3 Hallux malleus

    735.4 Other hammer toe (acquired)

    735.5 Claw toe (acquired)
        Coding Clinic: 2007, Q4, P123

    735.8 Other acquired deformities of toe

    735.9 Unspecified acquired deformity of toe

Figure 13-3 **A.** Claw toes, right foot, secondary to medial and lateral plantar nerve laceration. **B.** Metatarsophalangeal joints of second and third toes could not be flexed to neutral position and none could be flexed past neutral. **C.** Extension posture of claw toes increases plantar pressure on metatarsal heads. (From Canale: Campbell's Operative Orthopaedics, 10th ed. 2003, Mosby, Inc.)

Item 13-6   Claw toe is caused by a contraction of the flexor tendon producing a flexion deformity characterized by hyperextension of the big toe.

Figure 13-4   Hallux valgus or bunion.

Item 13-7   Hallux valgus, or bunion, is a bursa usually found along the medial aspect of the big toe. It is most often attributed to heredity or poorly fitted shoes.

Item 13-8   Hallux valgus or bunion is a sometimes painful structural deformity caused by an inflammation of the bursal sac at the base of the metatarsophalangeal joint (big toe). **Hallus varus** is a deviation of the great toe to the inner side of the foot or away from the next toe.

Item 13-9   Cubitus valgus is a deformity of the elbow resulting in an increased carrying angle in which the arm extends at the side and the palm faces forward, which results in the forearm and hand extended at greater than 15 degrees. **Cubitus varus** is a deformity of the elbow resulting in the arm extended at the side and the palm facing forward so that the forearm and hand are held at less than 5 degrees.

● **736   Other acquired deformities of limbs**
    Excludes   *congenital (754.3–755.9)*

● **736.0   Acquired deformities of forearm, excluding fingers**

736.00   Unspecified deformity
    Deformity of elbow, forearm, hand, or wrist (acquired) NOS

736.01   Cubitus valgus (acquired)

736.02   Cubitus varus (acquired)

736.03   Valgus deformity of wrist (acquired)

736.04   Varus deformity of wrist (acquired)

736.05   Wrist drop (acquired)

736.06   Claw hand (acquired)

736.07   Club hand (acquired)

736.09   Other

736.1   Mallet finger

● **736.2   Other acquired deformities of finger**

736.20   Unspecified deformity
    Deformity of finger (acquired) NOS

736.21   Boutonniere deformity

736.22   Swan-neck deformity

736.29   Other
    Excludes   *trigger finger (727.03)*
    Coding Clinic: 2005, Q2, P7; 1989, Q2, P13

● **736.3   Acquired deformities of hip**
    Coding Clinic: 2008, Q2, P3-4

736.30   Unspecified deformity
    Deformity of hip (acquired) NOS

736.31   Coxa valga (acquired)

736.32   Coxa vara (acquired)

736.39   Other

● **736.4   Genu valgum or varum (acquired)**

736.41   Genu valgum (acquired)

736.42   Genu varum (acquired)

736.5   Genu recurvatum (acquired)

736.6   Other acquired deformities of knee
    Deformity of knee (acquired) NOS

● **736.7   Other acquired deformities of ankle and foot**
    Excludes   *deformities of toe (acquired) (735.0–735.9)*
            pes planus (acquired) (734)

736.70   Unspecified deformity of ankle and foot, acquired

736.71   Acquired equinovarus deformity
    Clubfoot, acquired
    Excludes   *clubfoot not specified as acquired (754.5–754.7)*

736.72   Equinus deformity of foot, acquired

736.73   Cavus deformity of foot
    Excludes   *that with claw foot (736.74)*

736.74   Claw foot, acquired

736.75   Cavovarus deformity of foot, acquired

736.76   Other calcaneus deformity

736.79   Other
    Acquired:
        pes not elsewhere classified
        talipes not elsewhere classified

● **736.8   Acquired deformities of other parts of limbs**

736.81   Unequal leg length (acquired)
    Coding Clinic: 1995, Q1, P10

736.89   Other
    Deformity (acquired):
        arm or leg, not elsewhere classified
        shoulder
    Coding Clinic: 2008, Q2, P5-6

736.9   Acquired deformity of limb, site unspecified
    Coding Clinic: 2008, Q2, P3-4

Figure 13-5   Supination and cavus deformity of forefoot. *(Courtesy Jay Cummings, MD.)* (From Canale: Campbell's Operative Orthopaedics, 10th ed. 2003, Mosby, Inc.)

Item 13-10   Equinus foot is a term referring to the hoof of a horse. The deformity is usually congenital or spastic. Talipes equinovarus is referred to as clubfoot. The foot tends to be smaller than normal, with the heel pointing downward and the forefoot turning inward. The heel cord (Achilles tendon) is tight, causing the heel to be drawn up toward the leg.

◄ New   ◄▥ Revised   ~~deleted~~ Deleted   Excludes   Includes   Use additional   Code first   Omit code   **933**
● Unacceptable Principal Diagnosis   ● Use Additional Digit(s)   OGCR Official Guidelines   Coding Clinic

● **737 Curvature of spine**

> **Excludes** *congenital (754.2)*

    737.0 Adolescent postural kyphosis

> **Excludes** *osteochondrosis of spine (juvenile) (732.0)*
>   *adult (732.8)*

● **737.1 Kyphosis (acquired)**

    737.10 Kyphosis (acquired) (postural)

    737.11 Kyphosis due to radiation

    737.12 Kyphosis, postlaminectomy

    737.19 Other

> **Excludes** *that associated with conditions*
>   *classifiable elsewhere (737.41)*
>
> Coding Clinic: 2007, Q1, P20-21

● **737.2 Lordosis (acquired)**

    Abnormal increase in normal curvature of lumbar spine
    (sway back)

    737.20 Lordosis (acquired) (postural)

    737.21 Lordosis, postlaminectomy

    737.22 Other postsurgical lordosis

    737.29 Other

> **Excludes** *that associated with conditions*
>   *classifiable elsewhere (737.42)*

● **737.3 Kyphoscoliosis and scoliosis**

    737.30 Scoliosis [and kyphoscoliosis], idiopathic
        Coding Clinic: 2003, Q3, P19x2

    737.31 Resolving infantile idiopathic scoliosis

    737.32 Progressive infantile idiopathic scoliosis
        Coding Clinic: 2002, Q3, P12

    737.33 Scoliosis due to radiation

    737.34 Thoracogenic scoliosis

    737.39 Other

> **Excludes** *that associated with conditions*
>   *classifiable elsewhere (737.43)*
>   *that in kyphoscoliotic heart disease*
>   *(416.1)*
>
> Coding Clinic: 2002, Q2, P16

● **737.4 Curvature of spine associated with other conditions**

> *Code first associated condition, as:*
>   Charcot-Marie-Tooth disease (356.1)
>   mucopolysaccharidosis (277.5)
>   neurofibromatosis (237.70-237.79) ◀▥
>   osteitis deformans (731.0)
>   osteitis fibrosa cystica (252.01)
>   osteoporosis (733.00–733.09)
>   poliomyelitis (138)
>   tuberculosis [Pott's curvature] (015.0)

    737.40 Curvature of spine, unspecified

    737.41 Kyphosis

    737.42 Lordosis

    737.43 Scoliosis

    737.8 Other curvatures of spine

    737.9 Unspecified curvature of spine

        Curvature of spine (acquired) (idiopathic) NOS
        Hunchback, acquired

> **Excludes** *deformity of spine NOS (738.5)*

● **738 Other acquired deformity**

> **Excludes** *congenital (754.0–756.9, 758.0–759.9)*
>   *dentofacial anomalies (524.0–524.9)*

    738.0 Acquired deformity of nose

        Deformity of nose (acquired)
        Overdevelopment of nasal bones

> **Excludes** *deflected or deviated nasal septum (470)*

● **738.1 Other acquired deformity of head**

    738.10 Unspecified deformity

    738.11 Zygomatic hyperplasia

    738.12 Zygomatic hypoplasia

    738.19 Other specified deformity
        Coding Clinic: 2006, Q1, P6-7; 2003, Q2, P13

    738.2 Acquired deformity of neck

    738.3 Acquired deformity of chest and rib

        Deformity:
            chest (acquired)
            rib (acquired)
        Pectus:
            carinatum, acquired
            excavatum, acquired

    738.4 Acquired spondylolisthesis

        Degenerative spondylolisthesis
        Spondylolysis, acquired

> **Excludes** *congenital (756.12)*
>
> Coding Clinic: 2007, Q4, P116-120

    738.5 Other acquired deformity of back or spine

        Deformity of spine NOS

> **Excludes** *curvature of spine (737.0–737.9)*
>
> Coding Clinic: 2007, Q4, P116-120

    738.6 Acquired deformity of pelvis

        Pelvic obliquity

> **Excludes** *intrapelvic protrusion of acetabulum (718.6)*
>   *that in relation to labor and delivery*
>   *(653.0–653.4, 653.8–653.9)*

    738.7 Cauliflower ear

    738.8 Acquired deformity of other specified site

        Deformity of clavicle
        Coding Clinic: 2001, Q2, P14-15

    738.9 Acquired deformity of unspecified site

Item 13–11 Kyphosis is an abnormal curvature of the spine. **Senile kyphosis** is a result of disc degeneration causing ossification (turning to bone). **Adolescent** or **juvenile kyphosis** is also known as **Scheuermann's disease,** a condition in which the discs of the lower thoracic spine herniate, causing the disc space to narrow and the spine to tilt forward. This condition is attributed to poor posture. Lordosis or swayback is an abnormal curvature of the spine resulting in an inward curve of the lumbar spine just above the buttocks. Scoliosis causes a sideways curve to the spine. The curves are S- or C-shaped, and it is most commonly acquired in late childhood and early teen years, when growth is fast.

Item 13–12 Spondylolisthesis is a condition caused by the slipping forward of one disc over another.

Figure 13–6 Scoliosis is a lateral curvature of the spine.

◀ New   ◀▥ Revised   ~~deleted~~ Deleted   Excludes   Includes   Use additional   Code first   Omit code
● Unacceptable Principal Diagnosis   ● Use Additional Digit(s)   OGCR Official Guidelines   Coding Clinic

● **739 Nonallopathic lesions, not elsewhere classified**

　　Includes　segmental dysfunction
　　　　　　　somatic dysfunction
　　Coding Clinic: 1995, Q4, P51; 1990, Q1, P18

　739.0 Head region
　　　Occipitocervical region

　739.1 Cervical region
　　　Cervicothoracic region

　739.2 Thoracic region
　　　Thoracolumbar region

　739.3 Lumbar region
　　　Lumbosacral region

　739.4 Sacral region
　　　Sacrococcygeal region
　　　Sacroiliac region

　739.5 Pelvic region
　　　Hip region
　　　Pubic region

　739.6 Lower extremities

　739.7 Upper extremities
　　　Acromioclavicular region
　　　Sternoclavicular region

　739.8 Rib cage
　　　Costochondral region
　　　Costovertebral region
　　　Sternochondral region

　739.9 Abdomen and other

DISEASES OF THE MUSCULOSKELETAL SYSTEM AND CONNECTIVE TISSUE (710–739)

Figure 14–1   Generalized craniosynostosis in a 4-year-old girl without symptoms or signs of increased intracranial pressure. (From Bell WE, McCormick WF: Increased Intracranial Pressure in Children, 2nd ed. Philadelphia, WB Saunders, 1978, p 116.)

Item 14–1   Anencephalus is a congenital deformity of the cranial vault. **Craniosynostosis**, also known as craniostenosis and stenocephaly, signifies any form of congenital deformity of the skull that results from the premature closing of the sutures of the skull. **Iniencephaly** is a deformity in which the head and neck are flexed backward to a great extent and the head is very large in comparison to the shortened body.

14.   CONGENITAL ANOMALIES (740–759)

● **740   Anencephalus and similar anomalies**

 740.0   Anencephalus
  Acrania
  Amyelencephalus
  Hemianencephaly
  Hemicephaly

 740.1   Craniorachischisis

 740.2   Iniencephaly

● **741   Spina bifida**

 Excludes   *spina bifida occulta (756.17)*
  Coding Clinic: 1994, Q3, P7

The following fifth-digit subclassification is for use with category 741:

> 0   unspecified region
> 1   cervical region
> 2   dorsal (thoracic) region
> 3   lumbar region

● **741.0   With hydrocephalus**
 [0-3] Arnold-Chiari syndrome, type II
   Any condition classifiable to 741.9 with any
    condition classifiable to 742.3
   Chiari malformation, type II
   Coding Clinic: 1997, Q4, P51; 1987, Sept-Oct, P10

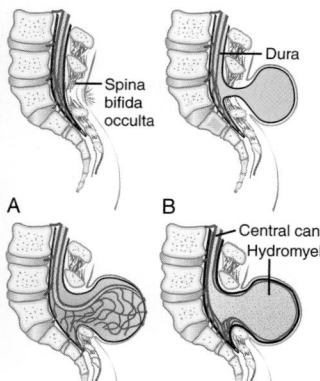

A
B
C
D

Figure 14–2
A. Spina bifida occulta.
B. Meningocele.
C. Myelomeningocele.
D. Myelocystocele (syringomyelocele) or hydromyelia.

Item 14–2   Spina bifida is a midline spinal defect in which one or more vertebrae fail to fuse, leaving an opening in the vertebral canal. When the defect is not visible, it is called spina bifida occulta, and when it is visible, it is called spina bifida cystica.

Figure 14–3   An infant with a large occipital encephalocele. The large skin-covered encephalocele is visible. (From Townsend: Sabiston Textbook of Surgery, 17th ed. 2004, Saunders, An Imprint of Elsevier.)

● **741.9   Without mention of hydrocephalus**
 [0-3] Hydromeningocele (spinal)
   Hydromyelocele
   Meningocele (spinal)
   Meningomyelocele
   Myelocele
   Myelocystocele
   Rachischisis
   Spina bifida (aperta)
   Syringomyelocele
   Coding Clinic: 1987, Sept-Oct, P10

● **742   Other congenital anomalies of nervous system**

 Excludes   *congenital central alveolar hypoventilation
    syndrome (327.25)*

 742.0   Encephalocele
  *Sac-like protrusions of brain and membranes visible
   through an opening in various locations in skull*
  Encephalocystocele
  Encephalomyelocele
  Hydroencephalocele
  Hydromeningocele, cranial
  Meningocele, cerebral
  Meningoencephalocele

 742.1   Microcephalus
  *Describes head size that measures significantly below
   normal based on standardized charts for age and
   sex*
  Hydromicrocephaly
  Micrencephaly

 742.2   Reduction deformities of brain
  Absence of part of brain
  Agenesis of part of brain
  Agyria
  Aplasia of part of brain
  Arhinencephaly
  Holoprosencephaly
  Hypoplasia of part of brain
  Microgyria
  Coding Clinic: 2003, Q3, P15-16

 742.3   Congenital hydrocephalus
  *An accumulation of cerebrospinal fluid in ventricles
   resulting in swelling and enlargement*
  Aqueduct of Sylvius:
   anomaly
   obstruction, congenital
   stenosis
  Atresia of foramina of Magendie and Luschka
  Hydrocephalus in newborn

  Excludes   *hydrocephalus:*
    acquired (331.3–331.4)
    due to congenital toxoplasmosis (771.2)
    *with any condition classifiable to 741.9
     (741.0)*
   Coding Clinic: 2005, Q4, P82-83

◀ New ⬅⫶ Revised ~~deleted~~ Deleted Excludes Includes Use additional Code first Omit code
● Unacceptable Principal Diagnosis ● Use Additional Digit(s) OGCR Official Guidelines Coding Clinic

742.4 Other specified anomalies of brain
Congenital cerebral cyst
Macroencephaly
Macrogyria
Megalencephaly
Multiple anomalies of brain NOS
Porencephaly
Ulegyria
Coding Clinic: 1999, Q1, P9-10; 1992, Q3, P12

● **742.5 Other specified anomalies of spinal cord**

    742.51 Diastematomyelia

    742.53 Hydromyelia
        Hydrorhachis

    742.59 Other
        Amyelia
        Atelomyelia
        Congenital anomaly of spinal meninges
        Defective development of cauda equina
        Hypoplasia of spinal cord
        Myelatelia
        Myelodysplasia
        Coding Clinic: 1991, Q2, P14; 1989, Q1, P10

742.8 Other specified anomalies of nervous system
Agenesis of nerve
Displacement of brachial plexus
Familial dysautonomia
Jaw-winking syndrome
Marcus-Gunn syndrome
Riley-Day syndrome
    | Excludes | *neurofibromatosis (237.70-237.79)* ◀▥

742.9 Unspecified anomaly of brain, spinal cord, and nervous system
Anomaly of brain, nervous system, and spinal cord
Congenital, of brain, nervous system, and spinal cord:
    disease of brain, nervous system, and spinal cord
    lesion of brain, nervous system, and spinal cord
Deformity of brain, nervous system, and spinal cord

● **743 Congenital anomalies of eye**

● **743.0 Anophthalmos**
    Absence of eye and optic pit

    743.00 Clinical anophthalmos, unspecified
        Agenesis
        Congenital absence of eye
        Anophthalmos NOS

    743.03 Cystic eyeball, congenital

    743.06 Cryptophthalmos

● **743.1 Microphthalmos**
    Partial absence of eye and optic pit
    Dysplasia of eye
    Hypoplasia of eye
    Rudimentary eye

    743.10 Microphthalmos, unspecified

    743.11 Simple microphthalmos

    743.12 Microphthalmos associated with other anomalies of eye and adnexa

Figure 14-4 Bilateral congenital **hydrophthalmia,** in which the eyes are very large in comparison to the other facial features due to glaucoma.

● **743.2 Buphthalmos**
    Also known as Sturge-Weber Syndrome and is congenital syndrome characterized by a port-wine nevus covering portions of face and cranium
    Glaucoma:
        congenital
        newborn
    Hydrophthalmos
    | Excludes | *glaucoma of childhood (365.14)*
                traumatic glaucoma due to birth injury (767.8)

    743.20 Buphthalmos, unspecified

    743.21 Simple buphthalmos

    743.22 Buphthalmos associated with other ocular anomalies
        Keratoglobus, congenital, associated with buphthalmos
        Megalocornea associated with buphthalmos

● **743.3 Congenital cataract and lens anomalies**
    | Excludes | *infantile cataract (366.00–366.09)*

    743.30 Congenital cataract, unspecified

    743.31 Capsular and subcapsular cataract

    743.32 Cortical and zonular cataract

    743.33 Nuclear cataract

    743.34 Total and subtotal cataract, congenital

    743.35 Congenital aphakia
        Congenital absence of lens

    743.36 Anomalies of lens shape
        Microphakia   Spherophakia

    743.37 Congenital ectopic lens

    743.39 Other

● **743.4 Coloboma and other anomalies of anterior segment**

    743.41 Anomalies of corneal size and shape
        Microcornea
        | Excludes | *that associated with buphthalmos (743.22)*

    743.42 Corneal opacities, interfering with vision, congenital

    743.43 Other corneal opacities, congenital

    743.44 Specified anomalies of anterior chamber, chamber angle, and related structures
        Anomaly:
            Axenfeld's
            Peters'
            Rieger's

    743.45 Aniridia
        Coding Clinic: 2002, Q3, P20-21

    743.46 Other specified anomalies of iris and ciliary body
        Anisocoria, congenital
        Atresia of pupil
        Coloboma of iris
        Corectopia

    743.47 Specified anomalies of sclera

    743.48 Multiple and combined anomalies of anterior segment

    743.49 Other

● **743.5 Congenital anomalies of posterior segment**

    743.51 Vitreous anomalies
        Congenital vitreous opacity

    743.52 Fundus coloboma

    743.53 Chorioretinal degeneration, congenital

    743.54 Congenital folds and cysts of posterior segment

CONGENITAL ANOMALIES (740–759)

743.55 **Congenital macular changes**

743.56 **Other retinal changes, congenital**
Coding Clinic: 1999, Q3, P12

743.57 **Specified anomalies of optic disc**
Coloboma of optic disc (congenital)

743.58 **Vascular anomalies**
Congenital retinal aneurysm

743.59 **Other**

● 743.6 **Congenital anomalies of eyelids, lacrimal system, and orbit**

743.61 **Congenital ptosis**

743.62 **Congenital deformities of eyelids**
Ablepharon
Absence of eyelid
Accessory eyelid
Congenital:
   ectropion
   entropion
Coding Clinic: 2000, Q1, P22-23

743.63 **Other specified congenital anomalies of eyelid**
Absence, agenesis, of cilia

743.64 **Specified congenital anomalies of lacrimal gland**

743.65 **Specified congenital anomalies of lacrimal passages**
Absence, agenesis of:
   lacrimal apparatus
   punctum lacrimale
Accessory lacrimal canal

743.66 **Specified congenital anomalies of orbit**

743.69 **Other**
Accessory eye muscles

743.8 **Other specified anomalies of eye**
Excludes	*congenital nystagmus (379.51)*
	ocular albinism (270.2)
	optic nerve hypoplasia (377.43)
	retinitis pigmentosa (362.74)

743.9 **Unspecified anomaly of eye**
Congenital:
   anomaly NOS of eye [any part]
   deformity NOS of eye [any part]

● 744 **Congenital anomalies of ear, face, and neck**
Excludes	*anomaly of:*
	cervical spine (754.2, 756.10–756.19)
	larynx (748.2–748.3)
	nose (748.0–748.1)
	parathyroid gland (759.2)
	thyroid gland (759.2)
	cleft lip (749.10–749.25)

● 744.0 **Anomalies of ear causing impairment of hearing**
Excludes	*congenital deafness without mention of cause (380.0–389.9)*

744.00 **Unspecified anomaly of ear with impairment of hearing**

744.01 **Absence of external ear**
Absence of:
   auditory canal (external)
   auricle (ear) (with stenosis or atresia of auditory canal)

744.02 **Other anomalies of external ear with impairment of hearing**
Atresia or stricture of auditory canal (external)

744.03 **Anomaly of middle ear, except ossicles**
Atresia or stricture of osseous meatus (ear)

744.04 **Anomalies of ear ossicles**
Fusion of ear ossicles

744.05 **Anomalies of inner ear**
Congenital anomaly of:
   membranous labyrinth
   organ of Corti

744.09 **Other**
Absence of ear, congenital

744.1 **Accessory auricle**
Accessory tragus	Supernumerary:
Polyotia	ear
Preauricular appendage	lobule

● 744.2 **Other specified anomalies of ear**
Excludes	*that with impairment of hearing (744.00–744.09)*

744.21 **Absence of ear lobe, congenital**

744.22 **Macrotia**
Enlarged ear

744.23 **Microtia**
Abnormally small ear

744.24 **Specified anomalies of Eustachian tube**
Absence of Eustachian tube

744.29 **Other**
Bat ear
Darwin's tubercle
Pointed ear
Prominence of auricle
Ridge ear
Excludes	*preauricular sinus (744.46)*

744.3 **Unspecified anomaly of ear**
Congenital:
   anomaly NOS of ear, NEC
   deformity NOS of ear, NEC

● 744.4 **Branchial cleft cyst or fistula; preauricular sinus**

744.41 **Branchial cleft sinus or fistula**
Branchial:
   sinus (external) (internal)
   vestige

744.42 **Branchial cleft cyst**

744.43 **Cervical auricle**

744.46 **Preauricular sinus or fistula**

744.47 **Preauricular cyst**

744.49 **Other**
Fistula (of):
   auricle, congenital
   cervicoaural

744.5 **Webbing of neck**
Pterygium colli

● 744.8 **Other specified anomalies of face and neck**

744.81 **Macrocheilia**
Hypertrophy of lip, congenital

744.82 **Microcheilia**

744.83 **Macrostomia**
Abnormally large mouth

744.84 **Microstomia**

744.89 **Other**
Excludes	*congenital fistula of lip (750.25)*
	musculoskeletal anomalies (754.0–754.1, 756.0)

744.9 **Unspecified anomalies of face and neck**
Congenital:
   anomaly NOS of face [any part] or neck [any part]
   deformity NOS of face [any part] or neck [any part]

◄ New   ◄ Revised   ~~deleted~~ Deleted   Excludes   Includes   Use additional   Code first   Omit code
● Unacceptable Principal Diagnosis   ● Use Additional Digit(s)   OGCR Official Guidelines   Coding Clinic

● **745 Bulbus cordis anomalies and anomalies of cardiac septal closure**

745.0 Common truncus
Absent septum between aorta and pulmonary artery
Communication (abnormal) between aorta and pulmonary artery
Aortic septal defect
Common aortopulmonary trunk
Persistent truncus arteriosus

● **745.1 Transposition of great vessels**

745.10 Complete transposition of great vessels
Transposition of great vessels:
NOS
classical

745.11 Double outlet right ventricle
Dextrotransposition of aorta
Incomplete transposition of great vessels
Origin of both great vessels from right ventricle
Taussig-Bing syndrome or defect

745.12 Corrected transposition of great vessels

745.19 Other

745.2 Tetralogy of Fallot
Fallot's pentalogy
Ventricular septal defect with pulmonary stenosis or atresia, dextroposition of aorta, and hypertrophy of right ventricle
| Excludes | *Fallot's triad (746.09)*

745.3 Common ventricle
Cor triloculare biatriatum
Single ventricle

745.4 Ventricular septal defect
Eisenmenger's defect or complex
Gerbode defect
Interventricular septal defect
Left ventricular-right atrial communication
Roger's disease
| Excludes | *common atrioventricular canal type (745.69)*
single ventricle (745.3)

745.5 Ostium secundum type atrial septal defect
Defect: Patent or persistent:
atrium secundum   foramen ovale
fossa ovalis   ostium secundum
Lutembacher's syndrome
Coding Clinic: 2009, Q3, P10

● **745.6 Endocardial cushion defects**

745.60 Endocardial cushion defect, unspecified type

745.61 Ostium primum defect
Persistent ostium primum

745.69 Other
Absence of atrial septum
Atrioventricular canal type ventricular septal defect
Common atrioventricular canal
Common atrium

745.7 Cor biloculare
Absence of atrial and ventricular septa

745.8 Other

745.9 Unspecified defect of septal closure
Septal defect NOS

● **746 Other congenital anomalies of heart**
| Excludes | *endocardial fibroelastosis (425.3)*
Coding Clinic: 2004, Q3, P4-5

● **746.0 Anomalies of pulmonary valve**
| Excludes | *infundibular or subvalvular pulmonic stenosis (746.83)*
tetralogy of Fallot (745.2)

746.00 Pulmonary valve anomaly, unspecified

746.01 Atresia, congenital
Congenital absence of pulmonary valve

746.02 Stenosis, congenital
Coding Clinic: 2004, Q1, P16-17

746.09 Other
Congenital insufficiency of pulmonary valve
Fallot's triad or trilogy

746.1 Tricuspid atresia and stenosis, congenital
Absence of tricuspid valve

746.2 Ebstein's anomaly

746.3 Congenital stenosis of aortic valve
Congenital aortic stenosis
| Excludes | *congenital:*
subaortic stenosis (746.81)
supravalvular aortic stenosis (747.22)
Coding Clinic: 1988, Q4, P8

746.4 Congenital insufficiency of aortic valve
Bicuspid aortic valve
Congenital aortic insufficiency

746.5 Congenital mitral stenosis
Fused commissure of mitral valve
Parachute deformity of mitral valve
Supernumerary cusps of mitral valve
Coding Clinic: 2007, Q3, P3

746.6 Congenital mitral insufficiency

746.7 Hypoplastic left heart syndrome
Atresia, or marked hypoplasia, of aortic orifice or valve, with hypoplasia of ascending aorta and defective development of left ventricle (with mitral valve atresia)

● **746.8 Other specified anomalies of heart**

746.81 Subaortic stenosis
Coding Clinic: 2007, Q3, P3

746.82 Cor triatriatum

746.83 Infundibular pulmonic stenosis
Subvalvular pulmonic stenosis

746.84 Obstructive anomalies of heart, NEC
Shone's syndrome
Uhl's disease
Use additional code for associated anomalies, such as:
coarctation of aorta (747.10)
congenital mitral stenosis (746.5)
subaortic stenosis (746.81)

746.85 Coronary artery anomaly
Anomalous origin or communication of coronary artery
Arteriovenous malformation of coronary artery
Coronary artery:
absence
arising from aorta or pulmonary trunk
single

746.86 Congenital heart block
Complete or incomplete atrioventricular [AV] block

CONGENITAL ANOMALIES (740–759)

746.87 Malposition of heart and cardiac apex
Abdominal heart
Dextrocardia
Ectopia cordis
Levocardia (isolated)
Mesocardia

> **Excludes** *dextrocardia with complete transposition of viscera (759.3)*

746.89 Other
Atresia of cardiac vein
Hypoplasia of cardiac vein
Congenital:
    cardiomegaly
    diverticulum, left ventricle
    pericardial defect
Coding Clinic: 2000, Q3, P3; 1999, Q1, P11; 1995, Q1, P8

746.9 Unspecified anomaly of heart
Congenital:
    anomaly of heart NOS
    heart disease NOS

● **747 Other congenital anomalies of circulatory system**

747.0 Patent ductus arteriosus *(PDA)*
Patent ductus Botalli
Persistent ductus arteriosus
Coding Clinic: 2009, Q3, P10-11x2

● **747.1 Coarctation of aorta**

747.10 Coarctation of aorta (preductal) (postductal)
Hypoplasia of aortic arch
Coding Clinic: 2007, Q3, P3; 1999, Q1, P11; 1988, Q4, P8

747.11 Interruption of aortic arch

● **747.2 Other anomalies of aorta**

747.20 Anomaly of aorta, unspecified

747.21 Anomalies of aortic arch
Anomalous origin, right subclavian artery
Dextroposition of aorta
Double aortic arch
Kommerell's diverticulum
Overriding aorta
Persistent:
    convolutions, aortic arch
    right aortic arch
Vascular ring

> **Excludes** *hypoplasia of aortic arch (747.10)*

Coding Clinic: 2003, Q1, P15-16

747.22 Atresia and stenosis of aorta
Absence of aorta
Aplasia of aorta
Hypoplasia of aorta
Stricture of aorta
Supra (valvular)-aortic stenosis

> **Excludes** *congenital aortic (valvular) stenosis or stricture, so stated (746.3)*
> *hypoplasia of aorta in hypoplastic left heart syndrome (746.7)*

Coding Clinic: 1988, Q4, P8

747.29 Other
Aneurysm of sinus of Valsalva
Congenital: Congenital:
    aneurysm of aorta   dilation of aorta

747.3 Anomalies of pulmonary artery
Agenesis of pulmonary artery
Anomaly of pulmonary artery
Atresia of pulmonary artery
Coarctation of pulmonary artery
Hypoplasia of pulmonary artery
Stenosis of pulmonary artery
Pulmonary arteriovenous aneurysm
Coding Clinic: 2009, Q3, P10x2; 2004, Q1, P16-17; 1994, Q1, P15

● **747.4 Anomalies of great veins**

747.40 Anomaly of great veins, unspecified
Anomaly NOS of: Anomaly NOS of:
    pulmonary veins   vena cava

747.41 Total anomalous pulmonary venous connection
Total anomalous pulmonary venous return [TAPVR]:
    subdiaphragmatic
    supradiaphragmatic

747.42 Partial anomalous pulmonary venous connection
Partial anomalous pulmonary venous return

747.49 Other anomalies of great veins
Absence of vena cava (inferior) (superior)
Congenital stenosis of vena cava (inferior) (superior)
Persistent:
    left posterior cardinal vein
    left superior vena cava
Scimitar syndrome
Transposition of pulmonary veins NOS

747.5 Absence or hypoplasia of umbilical artery
Single umbilical artery

● **747.6 Other anomalies of peripheral vascular system**
Absence of artery or vein, NEC
Anomaly of artery or vein, NEC
Atresia of artery or vein, NEC
Arteriovenous aneurysm (peripheral)
Arteriovenous malformation of the peripheral vascular system
Congenital: Congenital:
    aneurysm (peripheral)   stricture, artery
    phlebectasia   varix
Multiple renal arteries

> **Excludes** *anomalies of:*
> *cerebral vessels (747.81)*
> *pulmonary artery (747.3)*
> *congenital retinal aneurysm (743.58)*
> *hemangioma (228.00–228.09)*
> *lymphangioma (228.1)*

747.60 Anomaly of the peripheral vascular system, unspecified site

747.61 Gastrointestinal vessel anomaly
Coding Clinic: 1996, Q3, P10

747.62 Renal vessel anomaly

747.63 Upper limb vessel anomaly

747.64 Lower limb vessel anomaly

747.69 Anomalies of other specified sites of peripheral vascular system

● **747.8 Other specified anomalies of circulatory system**

747.81 Anomalies of cerebrovascular system
Arteriovenous malformation of brain
Cerebral arteriovenous aneurysm, congenital
Congenital anomalies of cerebral vessels

> **Excludes** *ruptured cerebral (arteriovenous) aneurysm (430)*

Coding Clinic: 1985, Jan-Feb, P15

◀ New   ◀▥ Revised   ~~deleted~~ Deleted   Excludes   Includes   Use additional   Code first   Omit code
● Unacceptable Principal Diagnosis   ● Use Additional Digit(s)   OGCR Official Guidelines   Coding Clinic

747.82 Spinal vessel anomaly
Arteriovenous malformation of spinal
vessel
Coding Clinic: 1995, Q3, P5-6

747.83 Persistent fetal circulation
Persistent pulmonary hypertension
Primary pulmonary hypertension of
newborn
Coding Clinic: 2002, Q4, P62-63

747.89 Other
Aneurysm, congenital, specified site not
elsewhere classified

> **Excludes** *congenital aneurysm:*
> *coronary (746.85)*
> *peripheral (747.6)*
> *pulmonary (747.3)*
> *retinal (743.58)*

747.9 Unspecified anomaly of circulatory system

● **748 Congenital anomalies of respiratory system**

> **Excludes** *congenital central alveolar hypoventilation*
> *syndrome (327.25)*
> *congenital defect of diaphragm (756.6)*

748.0 Choanal atresia
Atresia of nares (anterior) (posterior)
Congenital stenosis of nares (anterior) (posterior)

748.1 Other anomalies of nose
Absent nose
Accessory nose
Cleft nose
Deformity of wall of nasal sinus
Congenital:
deformity of nose
notching of tip of nose
perforation of wall of nasal sinus ◀▥

> **Excludes** *congenital deviation of nasal septum (754.0)*

748.2 Web of larynx
Web of larynx: Web of larynx:
  NOS   subglottic
  glottic

748.3 Other anomalies of larynx, trachea, and bronchus
Absence or agenesis of:
bronchus
larynx
trachea
Anomaly (of):   Anomaly (of):
  cricoid cartilage   thyroid cartilage
  epiglottis   tracheal cartilage
Atresia (of):   Atresia (of):
  epiglottis   larynx
  glottis   trachea
Cleft thyroid, cartilage, congenital
Congenital:
dilation, trachea
stenosis:
larynx
trachea
tracheocele
Diverticulum:
bronchus
trachea
Fissure of epiglottis
Laryngocele
Posterior cleft of cricoid cartilage (congenital)
Rudimentary tracheal bronchus
Stridor, laryngeal, congenital
Coding Clinic: 1999, Q1, P14

748.4 Congenital cystic lung
Disease, lung:
cystic, congenital
polycystic, congenital
Honeycomb lung, congenital

> **Excludes** *acquired or unspecified cystic lung (518.89)*

748.5 Agenesis, hypoplasia, and dysplasia of lung
Absence of lung (fissures) (lobe)
Aplasia of lung
Hypoplasia of lung (lobe)
Sequestration of lung

● **748.6 Other anomalies of lung**

  748.60 Anomaly of lung, unspecified

  748.61 Congenital bronchiectasis

  748.69 Other
Accessory lung (lobe)
Azygos lobe (fissure), lung

748.8 Other specified anomalies of respiratory system
Abnormal communication between pericardial and
pleural sacs
Anomaly, pleural folds
Atresia of nasopharynx
Congenital cyst of mediastinum

748.9 Unspecified anomaly of respiratory system
Anomaly of respiratory system NOS

● **749 Cleft palate and cleft lip**

● **749.0 Cleft palate**

  749.00 Cleft palate, unspecified

  749.01 Unilateral, complete

  749.02 Unilateral, incomplete
Cleft uvula

  749.03 Bilateral, complete

  749.04 Bilateral, incomplete

● **749.1 Cleft lip**
Cheiloschisis   Harelip
Congenital fissure of lip   Labium leporinum

  749.10 Cleft lip, unspecified

  749.11 Unilateral, complete

  749.12 Unilateral, incomplete

  749.13 Bilateral, complete

  749.14 Bilateral, incomplete

● **749.2 Cleft palate with cleft lip**
Cheilopalatoschisis

  749.20 Cleft palate with cleft lip, unspecified

  749.21 Unilateral, complete

  749.22 Unilateral, incomplete

  749.23 Bilateral, complete
Coding Clinic: 1996, Q1, P14

  749.24 Bilateral, incomplete

  749.25 Other combinations

Figure 14-5   Cleft palate.

CONGENITAL ANOMALIES (740–759)

● **750 Other congenital anomalies of upper alimentary tract**

> **Excludes** dentofacial anomalies (524.0–524.9)

750.0 Tongue tie
> Ankyloglossia

● **750.1 Other anomalies of tongue**

750.10 Anomaly of tongue, unspecified

750.11 Aglossia

750.12 Congenital adhesions of tongue

750.13 Fissure of tongue
> Bifid tongue
> Double tongue

750.15 Macroglossia
> Congenital hypertrophy of tongue

750.16 Microglossia
> Hypoplasia of tongue

750.19 Other

● **750.2 Other specified anomalies of mouth and pharynx**

750.21 Absence of salivary gland

750.22 Accessory salivary gland

750.23 Atresia, salivary gland
> Imperforate salivary duct

750.24 Congenital fistula of salivary gland

750.25 Congenital fistula of lip
> Congenital (mucus) lip pits

750.26 Other specified anomalies of mouth
> Absence of uvula

750.27 Diverticulum of pharynx
> Pharyngeal pouch

750.29 Other specified anomalies of pharynx
> Imperforate pharynx

750.3 Tracheoesophageal fistula, esophageal atresia and stenosis
> Absent esophagus
> Atresia of esophagus
> Congenital:
>> esophageal ring
>> stenosis of esophagus
>> stricture of esophagus
> Congenital fistula:
>> esophagobronchial
>> esophagotracheal
> Imperforate esophagus
> Webbed esophagus

750.4 Other specified anomalies of esophagus
> Dilatation, congenital, of esophagus
> Displacement, congenital, of esophagus
> Diverticulum of esophagus
> Duplication of esophagus
> Esophageal pouch
> Giant esophagus

> **Excludes** congenital hiatus hernia (750.6)

750.5 Congenital hypertrophic pyloric stenosis
> Congenital or infantile:
>> constriction of pylorus
>> hypertrophy of pylorus
>> spasm of pylorus
>> stenosis of pylorus
>> stricture of pylorus

750.6 Congenital hiatus hernia
> Displacement of cardia through esophageal hiatus

> **Excludes** congenital diaphragmatic hernia (756.6)

Item 14-3 A muscle thickening and pyloric stenosis overgrows the pyloric sphincter, resulting in a narrowing of the outlet between the stomach and small intestine. Infants with pyloric stenosis have projectile vomiting, leading to dehydration and electrolyte imbalance.

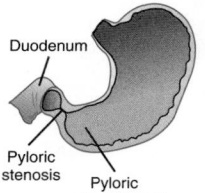

Duodenum

Pyloric stenosis

Pyloric part of stomach

Figure 14–6 Pyloric stenosis.

750.7 Other specified anomalies of stomach
> Congenital:
>> cardiospasm
>> hourglass stomach
> Displacement of stomach
> Diverticulum of stomach, congenital
> Duplication of stomach
> Megalogastria
> Microgastria
> Transposition of stomach

750.8 Other specified anomalies of upper alimentary tract

750.9 Unspecified anomaly of upper alimentary tract
> Congenital:
>> anomaly NOS of upper alimentary tract [any part, except tongue]
>> deformity NOS of upper alimentary tract [any part, except tongue]

● **751 Other congenital anomalies of digestive system**

751.0 Meckel's diverticulum
> Meckel's diverticulum (displaced) (hypertrophic)
> Persistent:
>> omphalomesenteric duct
>> vitelline duct
> **Coding Clinic: 2004, Q1, P10-11**

751.1 Atresia and stenosis of small intestine
> Atresia of:
>> duodenum
>> ileum
>> intestine NOS
> Congenital:
>> absence of small intestine or intestine NOS
>> obstruction of small intestine or intestine NOS
>> stenosis of small intestine or intestine NOS
>> stricture of small intestine or intestine NOS
> Imperforate jejunum

751.2 Atresia and stenosis of large intestine, rectum, and anal canal
> Absence:
>> anus (congenital)
>> appendix, congenital
>> large intestine, congenital ◄▬
>> rectum
> Atresia of:
>> anus
>> colon
>> rectum
> Congenital or infantile:
>> obstruction of large intestine
>> occlusion of anus
>> stricture of anus
> Imperforate:
>> anus
>> rectum
> Stricture of rectum, congenital
> **Coding Clinic: 1998, Q2, P16-17**

◄ New   ◄▬ Revised   ~~deleted~~ Deleted |Excludes| |Includes| Use additional   Code first   Omit code
● Unacceptable Principal Diagnosis   ● Use Additional Digit(s)   OGCR Official Guidelines   Coding Clinic

751.3 Hirschsprung's disease and other congenital functional disorders of colon

Absence of ganglion cells in distal colon resulting in functional obstruction.

Aganglionosis
Congenital dilation of colon
Congenital megacolon
Macrocolon ◀▥

751.4 Anomalies of intestinal fixation

Congenital adhesions:
    omental, anomalous
    peritoneal
Jackson's membrane
Malrotation of colon
Rotation of cecum or colon:
    failure of
    incomplete
    insufficient
Universal mesentery
Coding Clinic: 1985, Sept-Oct, P11

751.5 Other anomalies of intestine

Congenital diverticulum, colon	Megaloappendix
Dolichocolon	Megaloduodenum
Duplication of:	Microcolon
anus	Persistent cloaca
appendix	Transposition of:
cecum	appendix
intestine	colon
Ectopic anus	intestine

Coding Clinic: 2002, Q3, P11; 2001, Q3, P8-9

● **751.6 Anomalies of gallbladder, bile ducts, and liver**

  751.60 Unspecified anomaly of gallbladder, bile ducts, and liver

  751.61 Biliary atresia

Congenital:
    absence of bile duct (common) or passage
    hypoplasia of bile duct (common) or passage
    obstruction of bile duct (common) or passage
    stricture of bile duct (common) or passage
Coding Clinic: 1987, Sept-Oct, P8

  751.62 Congenital cystic disease of liver

Congenital polycystic disease of liver
Fibrocystic disease of liver

  751.69 Other anomalies of gallbladder, bile ducts, and liver

Absence of:
  gallbladder, congenital
  liver (lobe)
Accessory:
  hepatic ducts
  liver
Congenital:
  choledochal cyst
  hepatomegaly

Duplication of:	Duplication of:
biliary duct	gallbladder
cystic duct	liver
Floating:	Floating:
gallbladder	liver

Intrahepatic gallbladder
Coding Clinic: 1987, Sept-Oct, P8

751.7 Anomalies of pancreas

Absence of pancreas
Accessory pancreas
Agenesis of pancreas
Annular pancreas
Ectopic pancreatic tissue
Hypoplasia of pancreas
Pancreatic heterotopia

  Excludes *diabetes mellitus (249.0–249.9, (250.0–250.9)*
    fibrocystic disease of pancreas (277.00–277.09)
    neonatal diabetes mellitus (775.1)

751.8 Other specified anomalies of digestive system

Absence (complete) (partial) of alimentary tract NOS
Duplication of digestive organs NOS
Malposition, congenital of digestive organs NOS

  Excludes *congenital diaphragmatic hernia (756.6)*
    congenital hiatus hernia (750.6)

751.9 Unspecified anomaly of digestive system

Congenital:
  anomaly NOS of digestive system NOS
  deformity NOS of digestive system NOS

● **752 Congenital anomalies of genital organs**

  Excludes *syndromes associated with anomalies in the number and form of chromosomes (758.0–758.9)*

752.0 Anomalies of ovaries

Absence, congenital, of ovary
Accessory ovary
Ectopic ovary
Streak of ovary

● **752.1 Anomalies of fallopian tubes and broad ligaments**

  752.10 Unspecified anomaly of fallopian tubes and broad ligaments

  752.11 Embryonic cyst of fallopian tubes and broad ligaments

Cyst:
  epoophoron
  fimbrial
  parovarian
Coding Clinic: 1985, Sept-Oct, P13

  752.19 Other

Absence of fallopian tube or broad ligament
Accessory fallopian tube or broad ligament
Atresia of fallopian tube or broad ligament

752.2 Doubling of uterus

Didelphic uterus
Doubling of uterus [any degree] (associated with doubling of cervix and vagina)

● **752.3 Other anomalies of uterus** ◀▥

~~Absence, congenital, of uterus~~
~~Agenesis of uterus~~
~~Aplasia of uterus~~
~~Bicornuate uterus~~
~~Uterus unicornis~~
~~Uterus with only one functioning horn~~
Coding Clinic: 2006, Q3, P18-19

  752.31 Agenesis of uterus ◀

Congenital absence of uterus ◀

  752.32 Hypoplasia of uterus ◀

  752.33 Unicornuate uterus ◀

Unicornate uterus with or without a separate uterine horn ◀
Uterus with only one functioning horn ◀

752.34 Bicornuate uterus ◀
    Bicornuate uterus, complete or partial ◀

752.35 Septate uterus ◀
    Septate uterus, complete or partial ◀

752.36 Arcuate uterus ◀

752.39 Other anomalies of uterus ◀
    Aplasia of uterus NOS ◀
    Müllerian anomaly of the uterus, NEC ◀

> **Excludes** *anomaly of uterus due to exposure*
> *to diethylstilbestrol [DES] in*
> *utero (760.76)* ◀
> *didelphic uterus (752.2)* ◀
> *doubling of uterus (752.2)* ◀

● **752.4 Anomalies of cervix, vagina, and external female genitalia**

752.40 Unspecified anomaly of cervix, vagina, and external female genitalia

752.41 Embryonic cyst of cervix, vagina, and external female genitalia
    Cyst of:
        canal of Nuck, congenital
        Gartner's duct
        vagina, embryonal
        vulva, congenital

752.42 Imperforate hymen

752.43 Cervical agenesis ◀
    Cervical hypoplasia ◀

752.44 Cervical duplication ◀

752.45 Vaginal agenesis ◀
    Agenesis of vagina, total or partial ◀

752.46 Transverse vaginal septum ◀

752.47 Longitudinal vaginal septum ◀
    Longitudinal vaginal septum with or
        without obstruction ◀

752.49 Other anomalies of cervix, vagina, and external female genitalia
    Absence of ~~cervix,~~ clitoris, ~~vagina,~~ or vulva ◀▥
    Agenesis of ~~cervix,~~ clitoris, ~~vagina,~~ or vulva ◀▥
    Anomalies of cervix, NEC ◀
    Anomalies of hymen, NEC ◀
    Congenital stenosis or stricture of:
        cervical canal
        vagina
    Müllerian anomalies of the cervix and
        vagina, NEC ◀

> **Excludes** *double vagina associated with total*
> *duplication (752.2)*
> **Coding Clinic: 2006, Q3, P18-19**

● **752.5 Undescended and retractile testicle**

752.51 Undescended testis
    Cryptorchism
    Ectopic testis

752.52 Retractile testis

● **752.6 Hypospadias and epispadias and other penile anomalies**

752.61 Hypospadias
    **Coding Clinic: 2003, Q4, P67-68; 1997, Q3, P6; Q3, P6;
    1996, Q4, P34-35**

752.62 Epispadias
    Anaspadias

752.63 Congenital chordee
    Coding Clinic: 1996, Q4, P34-35

752.64 Micropenis

752.65 Hidden penis

752.69 Other penile anomalies

752.7 Indeterminate sex and pseudohermaphroditism
    Condition in which internal reproductive organs are
        opposite external physical characteristics.
    Gynandrism
    Hermaphroditism
    Ovotestis
    Pseudohermaphroditism (male) (female)
    Pure gonadal dysgenesis

> **Excludes** *androgen insensitivity (259.50–259.52)*
> *pseudohermaphroditism:*
>   *female, with adrenocortical disorder*
>   *(255.2)*
>   *male, with gonadal disorder (257.8)*
>   *with specified chromosomal anomaly*
>   *(758.0–758.9)*
> *testicular feminization syndrome*
>   *(259.50–259.52)*

● **752.8 Other specified anomalies of genital organs**

> **Excludes** *congenital hydrocele (778.6)*
> *penile anomalies (752.61–752.69)*
> *phimosis or paraphimosis (605)*

752.81 Scrotal transposition
    Coding Clinic: 2003, Q4, P67-68

752.89 Other specified anomalies of genital organs
    Absence of:
    Check Index for V codes for acquired or
        congenital.
        prostate
        spermatic cord
        vas deferens
    Anorchism
    Aplasia (congenital) of:
        prostate
        round ligament
        testicle
    Atresia of:
        ejaculatory duct
        vas deferens
    Fusion of testes
    Hypoplasia of testis
    Monorchism
    Polyorchism

752.9 Unspecified anomaly of genital organs
    Congenital:
        anomaly NOS of genital organ, NEC
        deformity NOS of genital organ, NEC

ECTOPIC TESTES	CRYPTORCHID TESTES
Penile	Abdominal
Superficial inguinal	Inguinal
(most common)	Prepubic
Femoral	(most common)

Figure 14–7 Undescended testes and the positions of the testes in various types of cryptorchidism or abnormal paths of descent.

Item 14–4 Testes form in the abdomen of the male and only descend into the scrotum during normal embryonic development. "Ectopic" testes are out of their normal place or "retained" (left behind) in the abdomen. Crypto (hidden) orchism (testicle) is a major risk factor for testicular cancer.

◀ New   ◀▥ Revised   ~~deleted~~ Deleted   Excludes   Includes   Use additional   Code first   Omit code
● Unacceptable Principal Diagnosis   ● Use Additional Digit(s)   **OGCR** Official Guidelines   **Coding Clinic**

● **753 Congenital anomalies of urinary system**

    753.0 Renal agenesis and dysgenesis
        Atrophy of kidney:
          congenital
          infantile
        Congenital absence of kidney(s)
        Hypoplasia of kidney(s)

● **753.1 Cystic kidney disease**
        | **Excludes** | *acquired cyst of kidney (593.2)* |

        753.10 Cystic kidney disease, unspecified

        753.11 Congenital single renal cyst

        753.12 Polycystic kidney, unspecified type
          PKD (polycystic kidney disease)

        753.13 Polycystic kidney, autosomal dominant

        753.14 Polycystic kidney, autosomal recessive

        753.15 Renal dysplasia

        753.16 Medullary cystic kidney
          Nephronophthisis

        753.17 Medullary sponge kidney

        753.19 Other specified cystic kidney disease
          Multicystic kidney

● **753.2 Obstructive defects of renal pelvis and ureter**

        753.20 Unspecified obstructive defect of renal pelvis and ureter

        753.21 Congenital obstruction of ureteropelvic junction

        753.22 Congenital obstruction of ureterovesical junction
          Adynamic ureter
          Congenital hydroureter

        753.23 Congenital ureterocele

        753.29 Other

    753.3 Other specified anomalies of kidney
        Accessory kidney
        Congenital:
          calculus of kidney
          displaced kidney
        Discoid kidney
        Double kidney with double pelvis
        Ectopic kidney
        Fusion of kidneys
        Giant kidney
        Horseshoe kidney
        Hyperplasia of kidney
        Lobulation of kidney
        Malrotation of kidney
        Trifid kidney (pelvis)
        Coding Clinic: 2007, Q1, P23

    753.4 Other specified anomalies of ureter
        Absent ureter
        Accessory ureter
        Deviation of ureter ◀▥
        Displaced ureteric orifice
        Double ureter
        Ectopic ureter
        Implantation, anomalous, of ureter

    753.5 Exstrophy of urinary bladder
        Ectopia vesicae   Extroversion of bladder

    753.6 Atresia and stenosis of urethra and bladder neck
        Congenital obstruction:
          bladder neck
          urethra
        Congenital stricture of:
          urethra (valvular)
          urinary meatus
          vesicourethral orifice
        Imperforate urinary meatus
        Impervious urethra
        Urethral valve formation

    753.7 Anomalies of urachus
        Cyst (of) urachus   Patent (of) urachus
        Fistula (of) urachus   Persistent umbilical sinus

    753.8 Other specified anomalies of bladder and urethra
        Absence, congenital of:
          bladder
          urethra
        Accessory:
          bladder
          urethra
        Congenital:
          diverticulum of bladder
          hernia of bladder
        Congenital urethrorectal fistula
        Congenital prolapse of:
          bladder (mucosa)
          urethra
        Double:
          urethra
          urinary meatus

    753.9 Unspecified anomaly of urinary system
        Congenital:
          anomaly NOS of urinary system [any part, except urachus]
          deformity NOS of urinary system [any part, except urachus]

● **754 Certain congenital musculoskeletal deformities**

    | **Includes** | nonteratogenic deformities which are considered to be due to intrauterine malposition and pressure |

    754.0 Of skull, face, and jaw
        Asymmetry of face
        Compression facies
        Depressions in skull
        Deviation of nasal septum, congenital
        Dolichocephaly
        Plagiocephaly
        Potter's facies
        Squashed or bent nose, congenital

        | **Excludes** | *dentofacial anomalies (524.0–524.9)* |
        | | *syphilitic saddle nose (090.5)* |

    754.1 Of sternocleidomastoid muscle
        Congenital sternomastoid torticollis
        Congenital wryneck
        Contracture of sternocleidomastoid (muscle)
        Sternomastoid tumor

    754.2 Of spine
        Congenital postural:
          lordosis
          scoliosis

CONGENITAL ANOMALIES (740–759)

Figure 14–8 Mild to moderate inbowing of the lower leg. (From Jones KL: Smith's Recognizable Patterns of Human Malformation, 4th ed. Philadelphia, Saunders, 1988, p 671.)

◀ New   ◀▥ Revised   ~~deleted~~ Deleted | Excludes | | Includes | | Use additional | | Code first | | Omit code |
● Unacceptable Principal Diagnosis   ● Use Additional Digit(s)   **OGCR** Official Guidelines   **Coding Clinic**

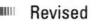

945

● 754.3 **Congenital dislocation of hip**

    754.30 **Congenital dislocation of hip, unilateral**
        Congenital dislocation of hip NOS

    754.31 **Congenital dislocation of hip, bilateral**

    754.32 **Congenital subluxation of hip, unilateral**
        Congenital flexion deformity, hip or thigh
        Predislocation status of hip at birth
        Preluxation of hip, congenital

    754.33 **Congenital subluxation of hip, bilateral**

    754.35 **Congenital dislocation of one hip with subluxation of other hip**

● 754.4 **Congenital genu recurvatum and bowing of long bones of leg**

    754.40 **Genu recurvatum**
        Hyperextension of knee resulting from hypermobility

    754.41 **Congenital dislocation of knee (with genu recurvatum)**

    754.42 **Congenital bowing of femur**

    754.43 **Congenital bowing of tibia and fibula**

    754.44 **Congenital bowing of unspecified long bones of leg**

● 754.5 **Varus deformities of feet**
    Foot deformity (pes equino varus) also known as club foot in which there is an inward angulation of distal segment of a bone or joint

     Excludes *acquired (736.71, 736.75, 736.79)*

    754.50 **Talipes varus**
        Congenital varus deformity of foot, unspecified
        Pes varus

    754.51 **Talipes equinovarus**
        Equinovarus (congenital)

    754.52 **Metatarsus primus varus**

    754.53 **Metatarsus varus**

    754.59 **Other**
        Talipes calcaneovarus

● 754.6 **Valgus deformities of feet**
    Inward angulation

     Excludes *valgus deformity of foot (acquired) (736.79)*

    754.60 **Talipes valgus**
        Congenital valgus deformity of foot, unspecified

    754.61 **Congenital pes planus**
        Congenital rocker bottom flat foot
        Flat foot, congenital

         Excludes *pes planus (acquired) (734)*

    754.62 **Talipes calcaneovalgus**

    754.69 **Other**
        Talipes:
          equinovalgus
          planovalgus

● 754.7 **Other deformities of feet**

     Excludes *acquired (736.70–736.79)*

    754.70 **Talipes, unspecified**
        Congenital deformity of foot NOS

    754.71 **Talipes cavus**
        Cavus foot (congenital)

    754.79 **Other**
        Asymmetric talipes
        Talipes:
          calcaneus
          equinus

● 754.8 **Other specified nonteratogenic anomalies**

    754.81 **Pectus excavatum**
        Congenital funnel chest

    754.82 **Pectus carinatum**
        Congenital pigeon chest [breast]

    754.89 **Other**
        Club hand (congenital)
        Congenital:
          deformity of chest wall
          dislocation of elbow
        Generalized flexion contractures of lower limb joints, congenital
        Spade-like hand (congenital)

● 755 **Other congenital anomalies of limbs**

     Excludes *those deformities classifiable to 754.0–754.8*

● 755.0 **Polydactyly**
    Also known as hyperdactyly, consists of duplicate fingers or toes

    755.00 **Polydactyly, unspecified digits**
        Supernumerary digits

    755.01 **Of fingers**
        Accessory fingers

    755.02 **Of toes**
        Accessory toes

● 755.1 **Syndactyly**
    Symphalangy
    Webbing of digits

    755.10 **Of multiple and unspecified sites**

    755.11 **Of fingers without fusion of bone**

    755.12 **Of fingers with fusion of bone**

    755.13 **Of toes without fusion of bone**

    755.14 **Of toes with fusion of bone**

● 755.2 **Reduction deformities of upper limb**

    755.20 **Unspecified reduction deformity of upper limb**
        Ectromelia NOS of upper limb
        Gross hypoplasia or aplasia of one or more long bones of one or more limbs
        Hemimelia NOS of upper limb
        Absence of one-half of long bone
        Shortening of arm, congenital

    755.21 **Transverse deficiency of upper limb**
        Amelia of upper limb
        Congenital absence of:
          fingers, all (complete or partial)
          forearm, including hand and fingers
          upper limb, complete
        Congenital amputation of upper limb
        Transverse hemimelia of upper limb

    755.22 **Longitudinal deficiency of upper limb, NEC**
        Phocomelia NOS of upper limb
        Absence/shortening of long bones primarily as a result of thalidomide
        Rudimentary arm

Figure 14–9 Polydactyly, congenital duplicated thumb. (From DeLee: DeLee and Drez's Orthopaedic Sports Medicine, 2nd ed. 2003, Saunders, An Imprint of Elsevier.)

755.23 Longitudinal deficiency, combined, involving humerus, radius, and ulna (complete or incomplete)
Congenital absence of arm and forearm (complete or incomplete) with or without metacarpal deficiency and/or phalangeal deficiency, incomplete
Phocomelia, complete, of upper limb

755.24 Longitudinal deficiency, humeral, complete or partial (with or without distal deficiencies, incomplete)
Congenital absence of humerus (with or without absence of some [but not all] distal elements)
Proximal phocomelia of upper limb

755.25 Longitudinal deficiency, radioulnar, complete or partial (with or without distal deficiencies, incomplete)
Congenital absence of radius and ulna (with or without absence of some [but not all] distal elements)
Distal phocomelia of upper limb

755.26 Longitudinal deficiency, radial, complete or partial (with or without distal deficiencies, incomplete)
Agenesis of radius
Congenital absence of radius (with or without absence of some [but not all] distal elements)

755.27 Longitudinal deficiency, ulnar, complete or partial (with or without distal deficiencies, incomplete)
Agenesis of ulna
Congenital absence of ulna (with or without absence of some [but not all] distal elements)

755.28 Longitudinal deficiency, carpals or metacarpals, complete or partial (with or without incomplete phalangeal deficiency)

755.29 Longitudinal deficiency, phalanges, complete or partial
Absence of finger, congenital
Aphalangia of upper limb, terminal, complete or partial
| Excludes | terminal deficiency of all five digits (755.21) |
transverse deficiency of phalanges (755.21)

● **755.3 Reduction deformities of lower limb**

755.30 Unspecified reduction deformity of lower limb
Ectromelia NOS of lower limb
Hemimelia NOS of lower limb
Shortening of leg, congenital

755.31 Transverse deficiency of lower limb
Amelia of lower limb
Congenital absence of:
foot
leg, including foot and toes
lower limb, complete
toes, all, complete
Transverse hemimelia of lower limb

755.32 Longitudinal deficiency of lower limb, NEC
Phocomelia NOS of lower limb

755.33 Longitudinal deficiency, combined, involving femur, tibia, and fibula (complete or incomplete)
Congenital absence of thigh and (lower) leg (complete or incomplete) with or without metacarpal deficiency and/or phalangeal deficiency, incomplete
Phocomelia, complete, of lower limb

755.34 Longitudinal deficiency, femoral, complete or partial (with or without distal deficiencies, incomplete)
Congenital absence of femur (with or without absence of some [but not all] distal elements)
Proximal phocomelia of lower limb

755.35 Longitudinal deficiency, tibiofibular, complete or partial (with or without distal deficiencies, incomplete)
Congenital absence of tibia and fibula (with or without absence of some [but not all] distal elements)
Distal phocomelia of lower limb

755.36 Longitudinal deficiency, tibia, complete or partial (with or without distal deficiencies, incomplete)
Agenesis of tibia
Congenital absence of tibia (with or without absence of some [but not all] distal elements)

755.37 Longitudinal deficiency, fibular, complete or partial (with or without distal deficiencies, incomplete)
Agenesis of fibula
Congenital absence of fibula (with or without absence of some [but not all] distal elements)

755.38 Longitudinal deficiency, tarsals or metatarsals, complete or partial (with or without incomplete phalangeal deficiency)

755.39 Longitudinal deficiency, phalanges, complete or partial
Absence of toe, congenital
Aphalangia of lower limb, terminal, complete or partial
| Excludes | terminal deficiency of all five digits (755.31) |
transverse deficiency of phalanges (755.31)

755.4 **Reduction deformities, unspecified limb**
Absence, congenital (complete or partial) of limb NOS
Amelia of unspecified limb
Ectromelia of unspecified limb
Hemimelia of unspecified limb
Phocomelia of unspecified limb

● **755.5 Other anomalies of upper limb, including shoulder girdle**

755.50 Unspecified anomaly of upper limb

755.51 Congenital deformity of clavicle

755.52 Congenital elevation of scapula
Sprengel's deformity

755.53 Radioulnar synostosis

755.54 Madelung's deformity

755.55 Acrocephalosyndactyly
Apert's syndrome

755.56 Accessory carpal bones

755.57 Macrodactylia (fingers)

755.58 Cleft hand, congenital
Lobster-claw hand

755.59 Other
Cleidocranial dysostosis
Cubitus:
valgus, congenital
varus, congenital
| Excludes | club hand (congenital) (754.89) |
congenital dislocation of elbow (754.89)

● **755.6 Other anomalies of lower limb, including pelvic girdle**

755.60 Unspecified anomaly of lower limb

755.61 Coxa valga, congenital

755.62 Coxa vara, congenital

755.63 Other congenital deformity of hip (joint)
Congenital anteversion of femur (neck)
> Excludes congenital dislocation of hip (754.30–754.35)

755.64 Congenital deformity of knee (joint)
Congenital:
absence of patella
genu valgum [knock-knee]
genu varum [bowleg]
Rudimentary patella
Coding Clinic: 1985, July-Aug, P14; 1984, Nov-Dec, P9

755.65 Macrodactylia of toes

755.66 Other anomalies of toes
Congenital:
hallux valgus
hallux varus
hammer toe

755.67 Anomalies of foot, NEC
Astragaloscaphoid synostosis
Calcaneonavicular bar
Coalition of calcaneus
Talonavicular synostosis
Tarsal coalitions

755.69 Other
Congenital:
angulation of tibia
deformity (of):
ankle (joint)
sacroiliac (joint)
fusion of sacroiliac joint

755.8 Other specified anomalies of unspecified limb

755.9 Unspecified anomaly of unspecified limb
Congenital:
anomaly NOS of unspecified limb
deformity NOS of unspecified limb
> Excludes reduction deformity of unspecified limb (755.4)

● **756 Other congenital musculoskeletal anomalies**
> Excludes congenital myotonic chondrodystrophy (359.23)
> those deformities classifiable to 754.0–754.8

756.0 Anomalies of skull and face bones
Absence of skull bones
Acrocephaly
Congenital deformity of forehead
Craniosynostosis
Crouzon's disease
Hypertelorism
Imperfect fusion of skull
Oxycephaly
Platybasia
Premature closure of cranial sutures
Tower skull
Trigonocephaly
> Excludes acrocephalosyndactyly [Apert's syndrome] (755.55)
> dentofacial anomalies (524.0–524.9)
> skull defects associated with brain anomalies, such as:
> anencephalus (740.0)
> encephalocele (742.0)
> hydrocephalus (742.3)
> microcephalus (742.1)
Coding Clinic: 1998, Q3, P9-10; 1996, Q3, P15

● **756.1 Anomalies of spine**

756.10 Anomaly of spine, unspecified

756.11 Spondylolysis, lumbosacral region
Prespondylolisthesis (lumbosacral)

756.12 Spondylolisthesis

756.13 Absence of vertebra, congenital

756.14 Hemivertebra

756.15 Fusion of spine [vertebra], congenital

756.16 Klippel-Feil syndrome

756.17 Spina bifida occulta
> Excludes spina bifida (aperta) (741.0–741.9)

756.19 Other
Platyspondylia
Supernumerary vertebra

756.2 Cervical rib
Supernumerary rib in the cervical region

756.3 Other anomalies of ribs and sternum
Congenital absence of:
rib
sternum
Congenital:
fissure of sternum
fusion of ribs
Sternum bifidum
> Excludes nonteratogenic deformity of chest wall (754.81–754.89)

756.4 Chondrodystrophy
Skeletal dysplasia (dwarfism) is caused by genetic mutations affecting hyaline cartilage capping long bones and vertebrae
Achondroplasia   Enchondromatosis
Chondrodystrophia (fetalis) Ollier's disease
Dyschondroplasia
> Excludes congenital myotonic chondrodystrophy (359.23)
> lipochondrodystrophy [Hurler's syndrome] (277.5)
> Morquio's disease (277.5)
Coding Clinic: 2002, Q2, P16-17; 1987, Sept-Oct, P10

● **756.5 Osteodystrophies**
Defective bone development; most commonly caused by renal disease or disturbances in calcium and phosphorus metabolism

756.50 Osteodystrophy, unspecified

756.51 Osteogenesis imperfecta
Fragilitas ossium
Osteopsathyrosis

756.52 Osteopetrosis

756.53 Osteopoikilosis

756.54 Polyostotic fibrous dysplasia of bone

756.55 Chondroectodermal dysplasia
Ellis-van Creveld syndrome

756.56 Multiple epiphyseal dysplasia

756.59 Other
Albright (-McCune)-Sternberg syndrome

756.6 Anomalies of diaphragm
Absence of diaphragm
Congenital hernia:
diaphragmatic
foramen of Morgagni
Eventration of diaphragm
> Excludes congenital hiatus hernia (750.6)

◀ New ◀▦ Revised ~~deleted~~ Deleted Excludes Includes Use additional Code first Omit code
● Unacceptable Principal Diagnosis ● Use Additional Digit(s) OGCR Official Guidelines Coding Clinic

● **756.7 Anomalies of abdominal wall**

  756.70 Anomaly of abdominal wall, unspecified

  756.71 Prune belly syndrome
    Eagle-Barrett syndrome
    Prolapse of bladder mucosa

  756.72 Omphalocele
    Exomphalos

  756.73 Gastroschisis

  756.79 Other congenital anomalies of abdominal wall

    Excludes   *umbilical hernia (551–553 with .1)*

● **756.8 Other specified anomalies of muscle, tendon, fascia, and connective tissue**

  756.81 Absence of muscle and tendon
    Absence of muscle (pectoral)
    Coding Clinic: 2010, Q1, P11

  756.82 Accessory muscle

  756.83 Ehlers-Danlos syndrome

  756.89 Other
    Amyotrophia congenita
    Congenital shortening of tendon
    Coding Clinic: 1999, Q3, P16-17

● **756.9 Other and unspecified anomalies of musculoskeletal system**
  Congenital:
    anomaly NOS of musculoskeletal system, NEC
    deformity NOS of musculoskeletal system, NEC

● **757 Congenital anomalies of the integument**

  Includes   anomalies of skin, subcutaneous tissue, hair, nails, and breast

  Excludes   *hemangioma (228.00–228.09)*
    pigmented nevus (216.0–216.9)

757.0 Hereditary edema of legs
  Congenital lymphedema
  Hereditary trophedema
  Milroy's disease

757.1 Ichthyosis congenita
  Congenital ichthyosis
  Harlequin fetus
  Ichthyosiform erythroderma

757.2 Dermatoglyphic anomalies
  Abnormal palmar creases

● **757.3 Other specified anomalies of skin**

  757.31 Congenital ectodermal dysplasia

  757.32 Vascular hamartomas
    Birthmarks
    Port-wine stain
    Strawberry nevus

  757.33 Congenital pigmentary anomalies of skin
    Congenital poikiloderma
    Urticaria pigmentosa
    Xeroderma pigmentosum

    Excludes   *albinism (270.2)*

  757.39 Other
    Accessory skin tags, congenital
    Congenital scar
    Epidermolysis bullosa
    Keratoderma (congenital)

    Excludes   *pilonidal cyst (685.0–685.1)*

757.4 Specified anomalies of hair
  Congenital:
    alopecia
    atrichosis
    beaded hair
    hypertrichosis
    monilethrix
  Persistent lanugo

757.5 Specified anomalies of nails
  Anonychia
  Congenital:
    clubnail
    koilonychia
    leukonychia
    onychauxis
    pachyonychia

757.6 Specified congenital anomalies of breast
  Congenital absent breast or nipple
  Accessory breast or nipple
  Supernumerary breast or nipple

  Excludes   *absence of pectoral muscle (756.81)*
    hypoplasia of breast (611.82)
    micromastia (611.82)

757.8 Other specified anomalies of the integument

757.9 Unspecified anomaly of the integument
  Congenital:
    anomaly NOS of integument
    deformity NOS of integument

● **758 Chromosomal anomalies**

  Includes   syndromes associated with anomalies in the number and form of chromosomes

  Use additional codes for conditions associated with the chromosomal anomalies

  758.0 Down's syndrome
    Mongolism
    Translocation Down's syndrome
    Trisomy:
      21 or 22
      G

  758.1 Patau's syndrome
    Trisomy:
      13
      D_1

  758.2 Edward's syndrome
    Trisomy:
      18
      E_3

● **758.3 Autosomal deletion syndromes**
    Coding Clinic: 2004, Q4, P93-95; 1995, Q2, P6-7, 11

  758.31 Cri-du-chat syndrome
    Deletion 5p

  758.32 Velo-cardio-facial syndrome
    Deletion 22q11.2

  758.33 Other microdeletions
    Miller-Dieker syndrome
    Smith-Magenis syndrome

  758.39 Other autosomal deletions

  758.4 Balanced autosomal translocation in normal individual

  758.5 Other conditions due to autosomal anomalies
    Accessory autosomes NEC

  758.6 Gonadal dysgenesis
    Ovarian dysgenesis
    Turner's syndrome
    XO syndrome

    Excludes   *pure gonadal dysgenesis (752.7)*

  758.7 Klinefelter's syndrome
    XXY syndrome

● **758.8 Other conditions due to chromosome anomalies**

  758.81 Other conditions due to sex chromosome anomalies

  758.89 Other

  758.9 Conditions due to anomaly of unspecified chromosome

CONGENITAL ANOMALIES (740–759)

CONGENITAL ANOMALIES (740–759)

● **759 Other and unspecified congenital anomalies**

759.0 Anomalies of spleen

Aberrant spleen	Congenital splenomegaly
Absent spleen	Ectopic spleen
Accessory spleen	Lobulation of spleen

759.1 Anomalies of adrenal gland

Aberrant adrenal gland
Absent adrenal gland
Accessory adrenal gland

Excludes *adrenogenital disorders (255.2)*
congenital disorders of steroid metabolism
(255.2)

759.2 Anomalies of other endocrine glands

Absent parathyroid gland
Accessory thyroid gland
Persistent thyroglossal or thyrolingual duct
Thyroglossal (duct) cyst

Excludes *congenital:*
goiter (246.1)
hypothyroidism (243)

759.3 Situs inversus

Situs inversus or transversus:
    abdominalis
    thoracis
Transposition of viscera:
    abdominal
    thoracic

Excludes *dextrocardia without mention of complete*
transposition (746.87)

759.4 Conjoined twins

Craniopagus	Thoracopagus
Dicephalus	Xiphopagus
Pygopagus	

759.5 Tuberous sclerosis

Bourneville's disease
Epiloia

759.6 Other hamartoses, NEC

Syndrome:
    Peutz-Jeghers
    Sturge-Weber (-Dimitri)
    von Hippel-Lindau

Excludes *neurofibromatosis (237.70-237.79)* ◀▥

Coding Clinic: 1992, Q3, P11

759.7 Multiple congenital anomalies, so described

Congenital:
    anomaly, multiple NOS
    deformity, multiple NOS

● **759.8 Other specified anomalies**

759.81 Prader-Willi syndrome

759.82 Marfan syndrome
Coding Clinic: 1993, Q3, P11

759.83 Fragile X syndrome

759.89 Other
Index directs coder to this code for Noonan's
syndrome.
Congenital malformation syndromes
    affecting multiple systems, NEC
Laurence-Moon-Biedl syndrome
Coding Clinic: 2008, Q3, P3-4; 2006, Q3, P21; 2005, Q2,
P17; 2004, Q2, P12; 2001, Q1, P3; 1999, Q3,
P17-19x2; 1998, Q3, P8; 1987, Sept-Oct, P9;
1985, Sept-Oct, P11

759.9 Congenital anomaly, unspecified

◀ New   ◀▥ Revised   ~~deleted~~ Deleted   Excludes   Includes   Use additional   Code first   Omit code
● Unacceptable Principal Diagnosis   ● Use Additional Digit(s)   OGCR Official Guidelines   Coding Clinic

OGCR Section I.C.15.a

For coding and reporting purposes the perinatal period is defined as before birth through the 28th day following birth. The following guidelines are provided for reporting purposes. Hospitals may record other diagnoses as needed for internal data use.

1) **Chapter 15 Codes**

They are <u>never</u> for use on the maternal record. Codes from Chapter 11, the obstetric chapter, are never permitted on the newborn record. Chapter 15 code may be used throughout the life of the patient if the condition is still present.

2) **Sequencing of perinatal codes**

Generally, codes from Chapter 15 should be sequenced as the principal/first-listed diagnosis on the newborn record, with the exception of the appropriate V30 code for the birth episode, followed by codes from any other chapter that provide additional detail. The "use additional code" note at the beginning of the chapter supports this guideline. If the index does not provide a specific code for a perinatal condition, assign code 779.89, Other specified conditions originating in the perinatal period, followed by the code from another chapter that specifies the condition. Codes for signs and symptoms may be assigned when a definitive diagnosis has not been established.

3) **Birth process or community acquired conditions**

If a newborn has a condition that may be either due to the birth process or community acquired and the documentation does not indicate which it is, the default is due to the birth process and the code from Chapter 15 should be used. If the condition is community-acquired, a code from Chapter 15 should not be assigned.

15. CERTAIN CONDITIONS ORIGINATING IN THE PERINATAL PERIOD (760–779)

> **Includes**   conditions which have their origin in the perinatal period, before birth through the first 28 days after birth, even though death or morbidity occurs later

> **Use additional** code(s) to further specify condition

MATERNAL CAUSES OF PERINATAL MORBIDITY AND MORTALITY (760–763)

● **760 Fetus or newborn affected by maternal conditions which may be unrelated to present pregnancy**

> **Includes**   the listed maternal conditions only when specified as a cause of mortality or morbidity of the fetus or newborn

> **Excludes**   *maternal endocrine and metabolic disorders affecting fetus or newborn (775.0–775.9)*

Coding Clinic: 1992, Q2, P12

760.0 Maternal hypertensive disorders
Fetus or newborn affected by maternal conditions classifiable to 642

760.1 Maternal renal and urinary tract diseases
Fetus or newborn affected by maternal conditions classifiable to 580–599

760.2 Maternal infections
Fetus or newborn affected by maternal infectious disease classifiable to 001–136 and 487, but fetus or newborn not manifesting that disease

> **Excludes**   *congenital infectious diseases (771.0–771.8) maternal genital tract and other localized infections (760.8)*

760.3 Other chronic maternal circulatory and respiratory diseases
Fetus or newborn affected by chronic maternal conditions classifiable to 390–459, 490–519, 745–748

760.4 Maternal nutritional disorders
Fetus or newborn affected by:
maternal disorders classifiable to 260–269
maternal malnutrition NOS

> **Excludes**   *fetal malnutrition (764.10–764.29)*

760.5 Maternal injury
Fetus or newborn affected by maternal conditions classifiable to 800–995

● **760.6 Surgical operation on mother and fetus**

> **Excludes**   *cesarean section for present delivery (763.4) damage to placenta from amniocentesis, cesarean section, or surgical induction (762.1)*

Coding Clinic: 2008, Q4, P137-138

760.61 Newborn affected by amniocentesis

> **Excludes**   *fetal complications from amniocentesis (679.1)*

760.62 Newborn affected by other in utero procedure

> **Excludes**   *fetal complications of in utero procedure (679.1)*

760.63 Newborn affected by other surgical operations on mother during pregnancy

> **Excludes**   *newborn affected by previous surgical procedure on mother not associated with pregnancy (760.64)*

760.64 Newborn affected by previous surgical procedure on mother not associated with pregnancy

● **760.7 Noxious influences affecting fetus or newborn via placenta or breast milk**
Fetus or newborn affected by noxious substance transmitted via placenta or breast milk

> **Excludes**   *anesthetic and analgesic drugs administered during labor and delivery (763.5) drug withdrawal syndrome in newborn (779.5)*

Coding Clinic: 1991, Q3, P21

760.70 Unspecified noxious substance
Fetus or newborn affected by:
drug NEC

760.71 Alcohol
Fetal alcohol syndrome

760.72 Narcotics

760.73 Hallucinogenic agents

760.74 Anti-infectives
Antibiotics
Antifungals

760.75 Cocaine
Coding Clinic: 1994, Q3, P6; 1992, Q2, P12

760.76 Diethylstilbestrol [DES]

760.77 Anticonvulsants
Carbamazepine   Phenytoin
Phenobarbital   Valproic acid
Coding Clinic: 2005, Q4, P82-83

760.78 Antimetabolic agents
Methotrexate
Retinoic acid
Statins
Coding Clinic: 2005, Q4, P82-83

CERTAIN CONDITIONS ORIGINATING IN THE PERINATAL PERIOD (760–779)

760.79 Other
> Fetus or newborn affected by:
>> immune sera transmitted via placenta or breast milk
>> medicinal agents NEC transmitted via placenta or breast milk
>> toxic substance NEC transmitted via placenta or breast milk
>
> Coding Clinic: 2010, Q1, P12; 2009, Q3, P12x3

760.8 Other specified maternal conditions affecting fetus or newborn
> Maternal genital tract and other localized infection affecting fetus or newborn, but fetus or newborn not manifesting that disease
>
> | Excludes | maternal urinary tract infection affecting fetus or newborn (760.1) |
> |---|---|

760.9 Unspecified maternal condition affecting fetus or newborn

● **761 Fetus or newborn affected by maternal complications of pregnancy**
> | Includes | the listed maternal conditions only when specified as a cause of mortality or morbidity of the fetus or newborn |
> |---|---|

761.0 Incompetent cervix

761.1 Premature rupture of membranes

761.2 Oligohydramnios
> *Scant volume of amniotic fluid*
>
> | Excludes | that due to premature rupture of membranes (761.1) |
> |---|---|

761.3 Polyhydramnios
> *Overabundance of amniotic fluid*
> Hydramnios (acute) (chronic)

761.4 Ectopic pregnancy
> Pregnancy:
>> abdominal
>> intraperitoneal
>> tubal

761.5 Multiple pregnancy
> Triplet (pregnancy)
> Twin (pregnancy)

761.6 Maternal death

761.7 Malpresentation before labor
> Breech presentation before labor
> External version before labor
> Oblique lie before labor
> Transverse lie before labor
> Unstable lie before labor

761.8 Other specified maternal complications of pregnancy affecting fetus or newborn
> Spontaneous abortion, fetus

761.9 Unspecified maternal complication of pregnancy affecting fetus or newborn

● **762 Fetus or newborn affected by complications of placenta, cord, and membranes**
> | Includes | the listed maternal conditions only when specified as a cause of mortality or morbidity in the fetus or newborn |
> |---|---|

762.0 Placenta previa

762.1 Other forms of placental separation and hemorrhage
> Abruptio placentae
> Antepartum hemorrhage
> Damage to placenta from amniocentesis, cesarean section, or surgical induction
> Maternal blood loss
> Premature separation of placenta
> Rupture of marginal sinus

762.2 Other and unspecified morphological and functional abnormalities of placenta
> Placental:
>> dysfunction
>> infarction
>> insufficiency

762.3 Placental transfusion syndromes
> Placental and cord abnormality resulting in twin-to-twin or other transplacental transfusion
>
> Use additional code to indicate resultant condition in newborn:
>> fetal blood loss (772.0)
>> polycythemia neonatorum (776.4)

762.4 Prolapsed cord
> Cord presentation

762.5 Other compression of umbilical cord
> Cord around neck   Knot in cord
> Entanglement of cord   Torsion of cord
> Coding Clinic: 2003, Q2, P9

762.6 Other and unspecified conditions of umbilical cord
> Short cord
> Thrombosis of umbilical cord
> Varices of umbilical cord
> Velamentous insertion of umbilical cord
> Vasa previa
>
> | Excludes | infection of umbilical cord (771.4) single umbilical artery (747.5) |
> |---|---|

762.7 Chorioamnionitis
> Amnionitis
> Membranitis
> Placentitis

762.8 Other specified abnormalities of chorion and amnion

762.9 Unspecified abnormality of chorion and amnion

● **763 Fetus or newborn affected by other complications of labor and delivery**
> | Includes | the listed conditions only when specified as a cause of mortality or morbidity in the fetus or newborn |
> |---|---|
>
> | Excludes | newborn affected by surgical procedures on mother (760.61-760.64) |
> |---|---|

763.0 Breech delivery and extraction

763.1 Other malpresentation, malposition, and disproportion during labor and delivery
> Fetus or newborn affected by:
>> abnormality of bony pelvis
>> contracted pelvis
>> persistent occipitoposterior position
>> shoulder presentation
>> transverse lie
>> conditions classifiable to 652, 653, and 660

763.2 Forceps delivery
> Fetus or newborn affected by forceps extraction

763.3 Delivery by vacuum extractor

763.4 Cesarean delivery
> | Excludes | placental separation or hemorrhage from cesarean section (762.1) |
> |---|---|

763.5 Maternal anesthesia and analgesia
> Reactions and intoxications from maternal opiates and tranquilizers during labor and delivery ◄
>
> | Excludes | drug withdrawal syndrome in newborn (779.5) |
> |---|---|

763.6 Precipitate delivery
> Rapid second stage

763.7 Abnormal uterine contractions
Fetus or newborn affected by:
contraction ring
hypertonic labor
hypotonic uterine dysfunction
uterine inertia or dysfunction
conditions classifiable to 661, except 661.3

● **763.8 Other specified complications of labor and delivery affecting fetus or newborn**

763.81 Abnormality in fetal heart rate or rhythm before the onset of labor

763.82 Abnormality in fetal heart rate or rhythm during labor
Coding Clinic: 1998, Q4, P46-47

763.83 Abnormality in fetal heart rate or rhythm, unspecified as to time of onset

763.84 Meconium passage during delivery

Excludes	meconium aspiration (770.11, 770.12)
	meconium staining (779.84)

Coding Clinic: 2005, Q4, P83-89

763.89 Other specified complications of labor and delivery affecting fetus or newborn
Fetus or newborn affected by:
abnormality of maternal soft tissues
destructive operation on live fetus to facilitate delivery
induction of labor (medical)
other conditions classifiable to 650–669
other procedures used in labor and delivery

763.9 Unspecified complication of labor and delivery affecting fetus or newborn

OTHER CONDITIONS ORIGINATING IN THE PERINATAL PERIOD (764–779)

The following fifth-digit subclassification is for use with category 764 and codes 765.0 and 765.1 to denote birthweight:

```
0  unspecified [weight]
1  less than 500 grams
2  500–749 grams
3  750–999 grams
4  1,000–1,249 grams
5  1,250–1,499 grams
6  1,500–1,749 grams
7  1,750–1,999 grams
8  2,000–2,499 grams
9  2,500 grams and over
```

● **764 Slow fetal growth and fetal malnutrition**
Requires fifth digit. See beginning of section 764–779 for codes and definitions.
Coding Clinic: 2009, Q1, P7; 2004, Q3, P4-5; 1994, Q1, P15; 1989, Q2, P15
OGCR Section I.C.15.i

Providers utilize different criteria in determining prematurity. A code for prematurity should not be assigned unless it is documented. The 5th digit assignment for codes from category 764 and subcategories 765.0 and 765.1 should be based on the recorded birth weight and estimated gestational age.

● **764.0 "Light-for-dates" without mention of fetal**
[0-9] **malnutrition**
Infants underweight for gestational age
"Small-for-dates"

● **764.1 "Light-for-dates" with signs of fetal malnutrition**
[0-9] Infants "light-for-dates" classifiable to 764.0, who in addition show signs of fetal malnutrition, such as dry peeling skin and loss of subcutaneous tissue

● **764.2 Fetal malnutrition without mention of**
[0-9] **"light-for-dates"**
Infants, not underweight for gestational age, showing signs of fetal malnutrition, such as dry peeling skin and loss of subcutaneous tissue
Intrauterine malnutrition

● **764.9 Fetal growth retardation, unspecified**
[0-9] Intrauterine growth retardation
Coding Clinic: 1997, Q1, P6

● **765 Disorders relating to short gestation and low birthweight**
Requires fifth digit. See beginning of section 764–779 for codes and definitions.

Includes	the listed conditions, without further specification, as causes of mortality, morbidity, or additional care, in fetus or newborn

Coding Clinic: 2002, Q4, P63-64; 1994, Q1, P15; 1991, Q2, P19, 1989, Q2, P15

● **765.0 Extreme immaturity**
[0-9] **Note:** Usually implies a birthweight of less than 1,000 grams

Use additional code for weeks of gestation (765.20–765.29)
Coding Clinic: 2009, Q1, P12; 2004, Q3, P4-5; 2001, Q4, P50-51
OGCR Section I.C.15.i

Providers utilize different criteria in determining prematurity. A code for prematurity should not be assigned unless it is documented. The 5th digit assignment for codes from subcategory 765.0 should be based on the recorded birth weight and estimated gestational age.

● **765.1 Other preterm infants**
[0-9] Prematurity NOS
Prematurity or small size, not classifiable to 765.0 or as "light-for-dates" in 764

Note: Usually implies birthweight of 1,000–2,499 grams

Use additional code for weeks of gestation (765.20–765.29)
Coding Clinic: 2009, Q1, P12; 2008, Q4, P138-140; 2004, Q3, P4-5; 2002, Q4, P64; 1997, Q1, P6; 1994, Q1, P14
OGCR Section I.C.15.i

Providers utilize different criteria in determining prematurity. A code for prematurity should not be assigned unless it is documented. The 5th digit assignment for codes from category 764 and subcategories 765.0 and 765.1 should be based on the recorded birth weight and estimated gestational age.

● **765.2 Weeks of gestation**
Coding Clinic: 2004, Q3, P4-5
OGCR Section I.C.15.i

A code from subcategory 765.2, Weeks of gestation, should be assigned as an additional code with category 764 and codes from 765.0 and 765.1 to specify weeks of gestation as documented by the provider in the record.

765.20 Unspecified weeks of gestation

765.21 Less than 24 completed weeks of gestation

765.22 24 weeks of gestation

765.23 25–26 weeks of gestation
Coding Clinic: 2009, Q1, P6

765.24 **27–28 weeks of gestation**

765.25 **29–30 weeks of gestation**

765.26 **31–32 weeks of gestation**
　　　Coding Clinic: 2009, Q1, P6; 2008, Q4, P138-140

765.27 **33–34 weeks of gestation**

765.28 **35–36 weeks of gestation**
　　　Coding Clinic: 2002, Q4, P64

765.29 **37 or more weeks of gestation**

● 766 **Disorders relating to long gestation and high birthweight**

　　　Includes the listed conditions, without further specification, as causes of mortality, morbidity, or additional care, in fetus or newborn

766.0 **Exceptionally large baby**

　　　Note: Usually implies a birthweight of 4,500 grams or more.

766.1 **Other "heavy-for-dates" infants**
　　　Other fetus or infant "heavy-" or "large-for-dates" regardless of period of gestation

● 766.2 **Late infant, not "heavy-for-dates"**
　　　Coding Clinic: 2006, Q2, P12-13; 2003, Q4, P69

　　766.21 **Post-term infant**
　　　　Infant with gestation period over 40 completed weeks to 42 completed weeks
　　　　Coding Clinic: 2009, Q1, P6; 2006, Q2, P12-13

　　766.22 **Prolonged gestation of infant**
　　　　Infant with gestation period over 42 completed weeks
　　　　Postmaturity NOS
　　　　Coding Clinic: 2009, Q1, P6; 2006, Q2, P12-13

● 767 **Birth trauma**

767.0 **Subdural and cerebral hemorrhage**
　　　Subdural and cerebral hemorrhage, whether described as due to birth trauma or to intrapartum anoxia or hypoxia
　　　Subdural hematoma (localized)
　　　Tentorial tear

　　　Use additional code to identify cause

　　　Excludes *intraventricular hemorrhage (772.10–772.14)*
　　　　subarachnoid hemorrhage (772.2)

● 767.1 **Injuries to scalp**
　　　Coding Clinic: 2003, Q4, P69-70

　　767.11 **Epicranial subaponeurotic hemorrhage (massive)**
　　　　Subgaleal hemorrhage

　　767.19 **Other injuries to scalp**
　　　　Caput succedaneum
　　　　Cephalhematoma
　　　　Chignon (from vacuum extraction)

767.2 **Fracture of clavicle**

767.3 **Other injuries to skeleton**
　　　Fracture of:
　　　　long bones
　　　　skull

　　　Excludes *congenital dislocation of hip (754.30–754.35)*
　　　　fracture of spine, congenital (767.4)

767.4 **Injury to spine and spinal cord**
　　　Dislocation of spine or spinal cord due to birth trauma
　　　Fracture of spine or spinal cord due to birth trauma
　　　Laceration of spine or spinal cord due to birth trauma
　　　Rupture of spine or spinal cord due to birth trauma

767.5 **Facial nerve injury**
　　　Facial palsy

767.6 **Injury to brachial plexus**
　　　Palsy or paralysis:
　　　　brachial
　　　　Erb (-Duchenne)
　　　　Klumpke (-Déjérine)

767.7 **Other cranial and peripheral nerve injuries**
　　　Phrenic nerve paralysis

767.8 **Other specified birth trauma**

Eye damage	Rupture of:
Hematoma of:	liver
liver (subcapsular)	spleen
testes	Scalpel wound
vulva	Traumatic glaucoma

　　　Excludes *hemorrhage classifiable to 772.0–772.9*

767.9 **Birth trauma, unspecified**
　　　Birth injury NOS

● 768 **Intrauterine hypoxia and birth asphyxia**
　　　Use only when associated with newborn morbidity classifiable elsewhere

　　　Excludes *acidemia NOS of newborn (775.81)*
　　　　acidosis NOS of newborn (775.81)
　　　　cerebral ischemia NOS (779.2)
　　　　hypoxia NOS of newborn (770.88)
　　　　mixed metabolic and respiratory acidosis of newborn (775.81)
　　　　respiratory arrest of newborn (770.87)

768.0 **Fetal death from asphyxia or anoxia before onset of labor or at unspecified time**

768.1 **Fetal death from asphyxia or anoxia during labor**

768.2 **Fetal distress before onset of labor, in liveborn infant**
　　　Fetal metabolic acidemia before onset of labor, in liveborn infant

768.3 **Fetal distress first noted during labor and delivery, in liveborn infant**
　　　Fetal metabolic acidemia first noted during labor and delivery, in liveborn infant

768.4 **Fetal distress, unspecified as to time of onset, in liveborn infant**
　　　Fetal metabolic acidemia unspecified as to time of onset, in liveborn infant
　　　Coding Clinic: 1986, Nov-Dec, P10

768.5 **Severe birth asphyxia**
　　　Birth asphyxia with neurologic involvement

　　　Excludes *hypoxic-ischemic encephalopathy (HIE) (768.70-768.73)*

768.6 **Mild or moderate birth asphyxia**
　　　Other specified birth asphyxia (without mention of neurologic involvement)

　　　Excludes *hypoxic-ischemic encephalopathy (HIE) (768.70-768.73)*

● **768.7 Hypoxic-ischemic encephalopathy (HIE)**
Coding Clinic: 2006, Q4, P104-106

768.70 Hypoxic-ischemic encephalopathy, unspecified

768.71 Mild hypoxic-ischemic encephalopathy

768.72 Moderate hypoxic-ischemic encephalopathy
Coding Clinic: 2009, Q4, P113

768.73 Severe hypoxic-ischemic encephalopathy

768.9 Unspecified birth asphyxia in liveborn infant
Anoxia NOS, in liveborn infant
Asphyxia NOS, in liveborn infant

769 Respiratory distress syndrome
Cardiorespiratory distress syndrome of newborn
Hyaline membrane disease (pulmonary)
Idiopathic respiratory distress syndrome [IRDS or RDS] of newborn
Pulmonary hypoperfusion syndrome

Excludes *transient tachypnea of newborn (770.6)*

Coding Clinic: 2009, Q3, P12; 1989, Q1, P10

● **770 Other respiratory conditions of fetus and newborn**

770.0 Congenital pneumonia
Infective pneumonia acquired prenatally

Excludes *pneumonia from infection acquired after birth (480.0–486)*

Coding Clinic: 2005, Q1, P10-11

● **770.1 Fetal and newborn aspiration**

Excludes *aspiration of postnatal stomach contents (770.85, 770.86)*
meconium passage during delivery (763.84)
meconium staining (779.84)

Coding Clinic: 2005, Q4, P83-89

770.10 Fetal and newborn aspiration, unspecified

770.11 Meconium aspiration without respiratory symptoms
Meconium aspiration NOS

770.12 Meconium aspiration with respiratory symptoms
Meconium aspiration pneumonia
Meconium aspiration pneumonitis
Meconium aspiration syndrome NOS

Use additional code to identify any secondary pulmonary hypertension (416.8), if applicable

770.13 Aspiration of clear amniotic fluid without respiratory symptoms
Aspiration of clear amniotic fluid NOS

770.14 Aspiration of clear amniotic fluid with respiratory symptoms
Aspiration of clear amniotic fluid with pneumonia
Aspiration of clear amniotic fluid with pneumonitis

Use additional code to identify any secondary pulmonary hypertension (416.8), if applicable

770.15 Aspiration of blood without respiratory symptoms
Aspiration of blood NOS

770.16 Aspiration of blood with respiratory symptoms
Aspiration of blood with pneumonia
Aspiration of blood with pneumonitis

Use additional code to identify any secondary pulmonary hypertension (416.8), if applicable

770.17 Other fetal and newborn aspiration without respiratory symptoms

770.18 Other fetal and newborn aspiration with respiratory symptoms
Other aspiration pneumonia
Other aspiration pneumonitis

Use additional code to identify any secondary pulmonary hypertension (416.8), if applicable

770.2 Interstitial emphysema and related conditions
Pneumomediastinum originating in the perinatal period
Pneumopericardium originating in the perinatal period
Pneumothorax originating in the perinatal period

770.3 Pulmonary hemorrhage
Hemorrhage:
alveolar (lung) originating in the perinatal period
intra-alveolar (lung) originating in the perinatal period
massive pulmonary originating in the perinatal period

770.4 Primary atelectasis
Failure of lungs to expand properly at birth
Pulmonary immaturity NOS

770.5 Other and unspecified atelectasis
Atelectasis:
NOS originating in the perinatal period
partial originating in the perinatal period
secondary originating in the perinatal period
Pulmonary collapse originating in the perinatal period

770.6 Transitory tachypnea of newborn
Idiopathic tachypnea of newborn
Wet lung syndrome

Excludes *respiratory distress syndrome (769)*

Coding Clinic: 2009, Q3, P17x2; 1993, Q3, P7x2; 1989, Q1, P10

770.7 Chronic respiratory disease arising in the perinatal period
Bronchopulmonary dysplasia
Interstitial pulmonary fibrosis of prematurity
Wilson-Mikity syndrome
Coding Clinic: 1991, Q2, P19; 1986, Nov-Dec, P11-12

● **770.8 Other respiratory problems after birth**

Excludes *mixed metabolic and respiratory acidosis of newborn (775.81)*
Coding Clinic: 2005, Q4, P83-89; 2002, Q4, P65-66; 1998, Q2, P10; 1996, Q2, P10-11

770.81 Primary apnea of newborn
Apneic spells of newborn NOS
Essential apnea of newborn
Sleep apnea of newborn

770.82 Other apnea of newborn
Obstructive apnea of newborn

770.83 Cyanotic attacks of newborn

770.84 Respiratory failure of newborn

Excludes *respiratory distress syndrome (769)*

CERTAIN CONDITIONS ORIGINATING IN THE PERINATAL PERIOD (760–779)

770.85 Aspiration of postnatal stomach contents without respiratory symptoms
Aspiration of postnatal stomach contents NOS

770.86 Aspiration of postnatal stomach contents with respiratory symptoms
Aspiration of postnatal stomach contents with pneumonia
Aspiration of postnatal stomach contents with pneumonitis
Use additional code to identify any secondary pulmonary hypertension (416.8), if applicable

770.87 Respiratory arrest of newborn

770.88 Hypoxemia of newborn
Hypoxia NOS, in liveborn infant

770.89 Other respiratory problems after birth
Coding Clinic: 2009, Q3, P17

770.9 Unspecified respiratory condition of fetus and newborn

● **771 Infections specific to the perinatal period**
Includes   infections acquired before or during birth or via the umbilicus or during the first 28 days after birth

Excludes   congenital pneumonia (770.0)
congenital syphilis (090.0–090.9)
infant botulism (040.41)
maternal infectious disease as a cause of mortality or morbidity in fetus or newborn, but fetus or newborn not manifesting the disease (760.2)
ophthalmia neonatorum due to gonococcus (098.40)
other infections not specifically classified to this category
Coding Clinic: 2005, Q1, P10

771.0 Congenital rubella
Congenital rubella pneumonitis

771.1 Congenital cytomegalovirus infection
Congenital cytomegalic inclusion disease

771.2 Other congenital infections
Congenital: Congenital:
herpes simplex   toxoplasmosis
listeriosis   tuberculosis
malaria

771.3 Tetanus neonatorum
Tetanus omphalitis
Excludes   hypocalcemic tetany (775.4)

771.4 Omphalitis of the newborn
Infection: Infection:
navel cord   umbilical stump
Excludes   tetanus omphalitis (771.3)
Coding Clinic: 2009, Q4, P113

771.5 Neonatal infective mastitis
Excludes   noninfective neonatal mastitis (778.7)

771.6 Neonatal conjunctivitis and dacryocystitis
Ophthalmia neonatorum NOS
Excludes   ophthalmia neonatorum due to gonococcus (098.40)

771.7 Neonatal Candida infection
Neonatal moniliasis
Thrush in newborn

● **771.8 Other infections specific to the perinatal period**
Use additional code to identify organism or specific infection (041.00–041.9) ◄

771.81 Septicemia [sepsis] of newborn
Use additional code to identify severe sepsis (995.92) and any associated acute organ dysfunction, if applicable
OGCR Section I.C.15.j
771.81 should be assigned with a secondary code from category 041, Bacterial infections in conditions classified elsewhere and of unspecified site, to identify the organism.

771.82 Urinary tract infection of newborn

771.83 Bacteremia of newborn

771.89 Other infections specific to the perinatal period
Intra-amniotic infection of fetus NOS
Infection of newborn NOS
Coding Clinic: 2005, Q1, P10

● **772 Fetal and neonatal hemorrhage**
Excludes   fetal hematologic conditions complicating pregnancy (678.0)
hematological disorders of fetus and newborn (776.0–776.9)

772.0 Fetal blood loss affecting newborn
Fetal blood loss from:
cut end of co-twin's cord
placenta
ruptured cord
vasa previa
Fetal exsanguination
Fetal hemorrhage into:
co-twin
mother's circulation

● **772.1 Intraventricular hemorrhage**
Intraventricular hemorrhage from any perinatal cause
Coding Clinic: 1992, Q3, P8; 1988, Q4, P8

772.10 Unspecified grade

772.11 Grade I
Bleeding into germinal matrix

772.12 Grade II
Bleeding into ventricle

772.13 Grade III
Bleeding with enlargement of ventricle
Coding Clinic: 2001, Q4, P50-51

772.14 Grade IV
Bleeding into cerebral cortex

772.2 Subarachnoid hemorrhage
Subarachnoid hemorrhage from any perinatal cause
Excludes   subdural and cerebral hemorrhage (767.0)

772.3 Umbilical hemorrhage after birth
Slipped umbilical ligature

772.4 Gastrointestinal hemorrhage
Excludes   swallowed maternal blood (777.3)

772.5 Adrenal hemorrhage

772.6 Cutaneous hemorrhage
Bruising in fetus or newborn
Ecchymoses in fetus or newborn
Petechiae in fetus or newborn
Superficial hematoma in fetus or newborn

772.8 Other specified hemorrhage of fetus or newborn

> Excludes | *hemorrhagic disease of newborn (776.0)*
> *pulmonary hemorrhage (770.3)*

772.9 Unspecified hemorrhage of newborn

● **773 Hemolytic disease of fetus or newborn, due to isoimmunization**

> *Also known as erythroblastosis fetalis as a result of Rh blood factor incompatibilities between mother (Rh negative) and fetus (Rh positive)*

773.0 Hemolytic disease due to Rh isoimmunization

Anemia due to RH:
   antibodies
   isoimmunization
   maternal/fetal incompatibility
Erythroblastosis (fetalis) due to RH:
   antibodies
   isoimmunization
   maternal/fetal incompatibility
Hemolytic disease (fetus) (newborn) due to RH:
   antibodies
   isoimmunization
   maternal/fetal incompatibility
Jaundice due to RH:
   antibodies
   isoimmunization
   maternal/fetal incompatibility
Rh hemolytic disease
Rh isoimmunization

773.1 Hemolytic disease due to ABO isoimmunization

ABO hemolytic disease
ABO isoimmunization
Anemia due to ABO:
   antibodies
   isoimmunization
   maternal/fetal incompatibility
Erythroblastosis (fetalis) due to ABO:
   antibodies
   isoimmunization
   maternal/fetal incompatibility
Hemolytic disease (fetus) (newborn) due to ABO:
   antibodies
   isoimmunization
   maternal/fetal incompatibility
Jaundice due to ABO:
   antibodies
   isoimmunization
   maternal/fetal incompatibility
Coding Clinic: 2003, Q2, P14-15; 1992, Q3, P8-9

773.2 Hemolytic disease due to other and unspecified isoimmunization

Erythroblastosis (fetalis) (neonatorum) NOS
Hemolytic disease (fetus) (newborn) NOS
Jaundice or anemia due to other and unspecified blood-group incompatibility
Coding Clinic: 1994, Q1, P13

773.3 Hydrops fetalis due to isoimmunization

> Use additional code, if desired, to identify type of isoimmunization (773.0–773.2)

773.4 Kernicterus due to isoimmunization

> Use additional code, if desired, to identify type of isoimmunization (773.0–773.2)

773.5 Late anemia due to isoimmunization

● **774 Other perinatal jaundice**

774.0 Perinatal jaundice from hereditary hemolytic anemias

> *Code first* underlying disease (282.0–282.9)

774.1 Perinatal jaundice from other excessive hemolysis

Fetal or neonatal jaundice from:
   bruising
   drugs or toxins transmitted from mother
   infection
   polycythemia
   swallowed maternal blood

> Use additional code to identify cause

> Excludes | *jaundice due to isoimmunization (773.0–773.2)*

774.2 Neonatal jaundice associated with preterm delivery

Hyperbilirubinemia of prematurity
Jaundice due to delayed conjugation associated with preterm delivery
Coding Clinic: 1994, Q1, P13; 1991, Q3, P21

● **774.3 Neonatal jaundice due to delayed conjugation from other causes**

   774.30 Neonatal jaundice due to delayed conjugation, cause unspecified

   774.31 Neonatal jaundice due to delayed conjugation in diseases classified elsewhere

> *Code first* underlying diseases, as:
>   congenital hypothyroidism (243)
>   Crigler-Najjar syndrome (277.4)
>   Gilbert's syndrome (277.4)

   774.39 Other

Jaundice due to delayed conjugation from causes, such as:
   breast milk inhibitors
   delayed development of conjugating system

774.4 Perinatal jaundice due to hepatocellular damage

Fetal or neonatal hepatitis
Giant cell hepatitis
Inspissated bile syndrome

774.5 Perinatal jaundice from other causes

> *Code first* underlying cause, as:
>   congenital obstruction of bile duct (751.61)
>   galactosemia (271.1)
>   mucoviscidosis (277.00–277.09)

774.6 Unspecified fetal and neonatal jaundice

Icterus neonatorum
Neonatal hyperbilirubinemia (transient)
Physiologic jaundice NOS in newborn

> Excludes | *that in preterm infants (774.2)*

Coding Clinic: 1994, Q1, P13

774.7 Kernicterus not due to isoimmunization

Bilirubin encephalopathy
Kernicterus of newborn NOS

> Excludes | *kernicterus due to isoimmunization (773.4)*

CERTAIN CONDITIONS ORIGINATING IN THE PERINATAL PERIOD (760–779)

● **775   Endocrine and metabolic disturbances specific to the fetus and newborn**

Includes   transitory endocrine and metabolic disturbances caused by the infant's response to maternal endocrine and metabolic factors, its removal from them, or its adjustment to extrauterine existence

775.0   Syndrome of "infant of a diabetic mother"
Maternal diabetes mellitus affecting fetus or newborn (with hypoglycemia)
Coding Clinic: 2004, Q1, P7-8x3

775.1   Neonatal diabetes mellitus
Diabetes mellitus syndrome in newborn infant

775.2   Neonatal myasthenia gravis

775.3   Neonatal thyrotoxicosis
Neonatal hyperthyroidism (transient)

775.4   Hypocalcemia and hypomagnesemia of newborn
Cow's milk hypocalcemia
Hypocalcemic tetany, neonatal
Neonatal hypoparathyroidism
Phosphate-loading hypocalcemia

775.5   Other transitory neonatal electrolyte disturbances
Dehydration, neonatal
Coding Clinic: 2010, Q1, P12; 2009, Q3, P18; 2008, Q4, P139-140; 2005, Q1, P9-10

775.6   Neonatal hypoglycemia
Excludes   *infant of mother with diabetes mellitus (775.0)*

775.7   Late metabolic acidosis of newborn

● **775.8   Other neonatal endocrine and metabolic disturbances**

775.81   Other acidosis of newborn
Acidemia NOS of newborn
Acidosis of newborn NOS
Mixed metabolic and respiratory acidosis of newborn

775.89   Other neonatal endocrine and metabolic disturbances
Amino-acid metabolic disorders described as transitory

775.9   Unspecified endocrine and metabolic disturbances specific to the fetus and newborn

● **776   Hematological disorders of newborn**
Includes   disorders specific to the newborn though possibly originating in utero
Excludes   *fetal hematologic conditions (678.0)*

776.0   Hemorrhagic disease of newborn
Hemorrhagic diathesis of newborn
Vitamin K deficiency of newborn
Excludes   *fetal or neonatal hemorrhage (772.0–772.9)*

776.1   Transient neonatal thrombocytopenia
Lack of sufficient numbers of circulating thrombocytes (platelets)
Neonatal thrombocytopenia due to:
exchange transfusion
idiopathic maternal thrombocytopenia
isoimmunization

776.2   Disseminated intravascular coagulation in newborn

776.3   Other transient neonatal disorders of coagulation
Transient coagulation defect, newborn

776.4   Polycythemia neonatorum
Excess number of thrombocytes (platelets)
Plethora of newborn
Polycythemia due to:
donor twin transfusion
maternal-fetal transfusion

776.5   Congenital anemia
Anemia following fetal blood loss
Excludes   *anemia due to isoimmunization (773.0–773.2, 773.5)*
hereditary hemolytic anemias (282.0–282.9)

776.6   Anemia of prematurity

776.7   Transient neonatal neutropenia
Isoimmune neutropenia
Low levels of white blood cells
Maternal transfer neutropenia
Excludes   *congenital neutropenia (nontransient) (288.01)*

776.8   Other specified transient hematological disorders

776.9   Unspecified hematological disorder specific to newborn

● **777   Perinatal disorders of digestive system**
Includes   disorders specific to the fetus and newborn
Excludes   *intestinal obstruction classifiable to 560.0–560.9*

777.1   Meconium obstruction
Congenital fecaliths
Stoney feces formations
Delayed passage of meconium
Meconium ileus NOS
Meconium plug syndrome
Excludes   *meconium ileus in cystic fibrosis (277.01)*

777.2   Intestinal obstruction due to inspissated milk
Being thickened, dried, or made less fluid

777.3   Hematemesis and melena due to swallowed maternal blood
Swallowed blood syndrome in newborn
Excludes   *that not due to swallowed maternal blood (772.4)*

777.4   Transitory ileus of newborn
Excludes   *Hirschsprung's disease (751.3)*

● **777.5   Necrotizing enterocolitis in newborn**

777.50   Necrotizing enterocolitis in newborn, unspecified
Necrotizing enterocolitis in newborn, NOS

777.51   Stage I necrotizing enterocolitis in newborn
Necrotizing enterocolitis without pneumatosis, without perforation

777.52   Stage II necrotizing enterocolitis in newborn
Necrotizing enterocolitis with pneumatosis, without perforation

777.53   Stage III necrotizing enterocolitis in newborn
Necrotizing enterocolitis with perforation
Necrotizing enterocolitis with pneumatosis and perforation
Coding Clinic: 2008, Q4, P138-140

777.6   Perinatal intestinal perforation
Meconium peritonitis

777.8   Other specified perinatal disorders of digestive system

777.9   Unspecified perinatal disorder of digestive system

◀ New   ◀▥ Revised   ~~deleted~~ Deleted | Excludes | | Includes | | Use additional | | Code first | | Omit code |
● Unacceptable Principal Diagnosis   ● Use Additional Digit(s)   **OGCR** Official Guidelines   **Coding Clinic**

● 778 **Conditions involving the integument and temperature regulation of fetus and newborn**

  778.0 **Hydrops fetalis not due to isoimmunization**
     Idiopathic hydrops
     Severe, life-threatening problem of edema (swelling) in fetus and newborn

     | Excludes | *hydrops fetalis due to isoimmunization (773.3)*

  778.1 **Sclerema neonatorum**

  778.2 **Cold injury syndrome of newborn**

  778.3 **Other hypothermia of newborn**

  778.4 **Other disturbances of temperature regulation of newborn**
     Dehydration fever in newborn
     Environmentally induced pyrexia
     Hyperthermia in newborn
     Transitory fever of newborn

  778.5 **Other and unspecified edema of newborn**
     Edema neonatorum

  778.6 **Congenital hydrocele**
     Congenital hydrocele of tunica vaginalis

  778.7 **Breast engorgement in newborn**
     Noninfective mastitis of newborn

     | Excludes | *infective mastitis of newborn (771.5)*

  778.8 **Other specified conditions involving the integument of fetus and newborn**
     Urticaria neonatorum
     Skin rash

     | Excludes | *impetigo neonatorum (684)*
                pemphigus neonatorum (684)

  778.9 **Unspecified condition involving the integument and temperature regulation of fetus and newborn**

● 779 **Other and ill-defined conditions originating in the perinatal period**

  779.0 **Convulsions in newborn**
     Fits in newborn
     Seizures in newborn
     Coding Clinic: 1984, Nov-Dec, P11

  779.1 **Other and unspecified cerebral irritability in newborn**

  779.2 **Cerebral depression, coma, and other abnormal cerebral signs**
     Cerebral ischemia NOS of newborn
     CNS dysfunction in newborn NOS

     | Excludes | *cerebral ischemia due to birth trauma (767.0)*
                intrauterine cerebral ischemia (768.2–768.9)
                intraventricular hemorrhage (772.10–772.14)

● 779.3 **Disorder of stomach function and feeding problems in newborn**
     Coding Clinic: 1989, Q2, P15

  779.31 **Feeding problems in newborn**
     Slow feeding in newborn

     | Excludes | *feeding problem in child over 28 days old (783.3)*
     Coding Clinic: 2009, Q4, P113

  779.32 **Bilious vomiting in newborn**

     | Excludes | *bilious vomiting in child over 28 days old (787.04)*

  779.33 **Other vomiting in newborn**
     Regurgitation of food in newborn

     | Excludes | *vomiting in child over 28 days old (536.2, 787.01-787.03, 787.04)*

  779.34 **Failure to thrive in newborn**

     | Excludes | *failure to thrive in child over 28 days old (783.41)*

  779.4 **Drug reactions and intoxications specific to newborn**
     Gray syndrome from chloramphenicol administration in newborn

     | Excludes | *fetal alcohol syndrome (760.71)*
                reactions and intoxications from maternal opiates and tranquilizers (763.5)

  779.5 **Drug withdrawal syndrome in newborn**
     Drug withdrawal syndrome in infant of dependent mother

     | Excludes | *fetal alcohol syndrome (760.71)*
     Coding Clinic: 1994, Q3, P6

  779.6 **Termination of pregnancy (fetus)**
     Fetal death due to:
        induced abortion
        termination of pregnancy

     | Excludes | *spontaneous abortion (fetus) (761.8)*

  779.7 **Periventricular leukomalacia**
     Coding Clinic: 2001, Q4, P50-51

● 779.8 **Other specified conditions originating in the perinatal period**
     Coding Clinic: 2006, Q1, P18; 2002, Q4, P67; 1994, Q1, P15

  779.81 **Neonatal bradycardia**

     | Excludes | *abnormality in fetal heart rate or rhythm complicating labor and delivery (763.81–763.83)*
                bradycardia due to birth asphyxia (768.5–768.9)

  779.82 **Neonatal tachycardia**

     | Excludes | *abnormality in fetal heart rate or rhythm complicating labor and delivery (763.81–763.83)*

  779.83 **Delayed separation of umbilical cord**
     Coding Clinic: 2003, Q4, P71

  779.84 **Meconium staining**

     | Excludes | *meconium aspiration (770.11, 770.12)*
                meconium passage during delivery (763.84)
     Coding Clinic: 2005, Q4, P83-89x2

  779.85 **Cardiac arrest of newborn**

  779.89 **Other specified conditions originating in the perinatal period**

     Use additional code to specify condition
     Coding Clinic: 2005, Q2, P15-16; Q1, P9
     OGCR Section I.C.15.a.2
        If the index does not provide a specific code for a perinatal condition, assign code 779.89 followed by the code from another chapter that specifies the condition.

  779.9 **Unspecified condition originating in the perinatal period**
     Congenital debility NOS
     Stillbirth NEC

◀ New   ◀┅ Revised   ~~deleted~~ Deleted | Excludes | Includes   Use additional   Code first   Omit code

● Unacceptable Principal Diagnosis   ● Use Additional Digit(s)   OGCR Official Guidelines   Coding Clinic

16. SYMPTOMS, SIGNS, AND ILL-DEFINED CONDITIONS (780–799)

This section includes symptoms, signs, abnormal results of laboratory or other investigative procedures, and ill-defined conditions regarding which no diagnosis classifiable elsewhere is recorded.

Signs and symptoms that point rather definitely to a given diagnosis are assigned to some category in the preceding part of the classification. In general, categories 780–796 include the more ill-defined conditions and symptoms that point with perhaps equal suspicion to two or more diseases or to two or more systems of the body, and without the necessary study of the case to make a final diagnosis. Practically all categories in this group could be designated as "not otherwise specified," or as "unknown etiology," or as "transient." The Alphabetic Index should be consulted to determine which symptoms and signs are to be allocated here and which to more specific sections of the classification; the residual subcategories numbered .9 are provided for other relevant symptoms which cannot be allocated elsewhere in the classification.

The conditions and signs or symptoms included in categories 780–796 consist of: (a) cases for which no more specific diagnosis can be made even after all facts bearing on the case have been investigated; (b) signs or symptoms existing at the time of initial encounter that proved to be transient and whose causes could not be determined; (c) provisional diagnoses in a patient who failed to return for further investigation or care; (d) cases referred elsewhere for investigation or treatment before the diagnosis was made; (e) cases in which a more precise diagnosis was not available for any other reason; (f) certain symptoms which represent important problems in medical care and which it might be desired to classify in addition to a known cause.

SYMPTOMS (780–789)

● **780　General symptoms**

● **780.0　Alteration of consciousness**

> **Excludes** alteration of consciousness due to:
> intracranial injuries (850.0-854.19)
> skull fractures (800.00-801.99, 803.00-804.99)
> coma:
> diabetic (249.2–249.3, 250.2–250.3)
> hepatic (572.2)
> originating in the perinatal period (779.2)

780.01　Coma
Coding Clinic: 1996, Q3, P16

780.02　Transient alteration of awareness

780.03　Persistent vegetative state

780.09　Other
Drowsiness　　　　Somnolence
Semicoma　　　　Stupor
　　　　　　　　　Unconsciousness

780.1　Hallucinations
Hallucinations:
NOS
auditory
gustatory
olfactory
tactile

> **Excludes** those associated with mental disorders, as functional psychoses (295.0–298.9)
> organic brain syndromes (290.0–294.9, 310.0–310.9)
> visual hallucinations (368.16)

780.2　Syncope and collapse
Blackout　　　　　(Near) (Pre)syncope
Fainting　　　　　Vasovagal attack

> **Excludes** carotid sinus syncope (337.0)
> heat syncope (992.1)
> neurocirculatory asthenia (306.2)
> orthostatic hypotension (458.0)
> shock NOS (785.50)

Coding Clinic: 2002, Q1, P6; 2000, Q3, P12; 1995, Q4, P50-51; Q3, P14; 1992, Q3, P16; 1990, Q1, P9; 1985, Nov-Dec, P12

● **780.3　Convulsions**

> **Excludes** convulsions:
> epileptic (345.10–345.91)
> in newborn (779.0)

Coding Clinic: 1984, Nov-Dec, P11

780.31　Febrile convulsions (simple), unspecified
Febrile seizures NOS
Coding Clinic: 2005, Q3, P12-13; 1987, Nov-Dec, P11

780.32　Complex febrile convulsions
Febrile seizure:
atypical
complex
complicated

> **Excludes** status epilepticus (345.3)

Coding Clinic: 2006, Q4, P106-107

780.33　Post traumatic seizures ◄

> **Excludes** post traumatic epilepsy (345.00-345.91) ◄

780.39　Other convulsions
Convulsive disorder NOS
Fits NOS
Recurrent convulsions NOS
Seizure NOS
Seizures NOS
Coding Clinic: 2008, Q1, P17; 2006, Q3, P22; 2004, Q4, P50-52; 2003, Q1, P7; 1998, Q4, P39-40; 1997, Q2, P8; Q1, P12-13; 1994, Q3, P9; 1993, Q1, P24; 1987, Nov-Dec, P12; 1985, July-Aug, P10; 1984, May-June, P14

780.4　Dizziness and giddiness
Light-headedness
Vertigo NOS

> **Excludes** Méniére's disease and other specified vertiginous syndromes (386.0–386.9)

Coding Clinic: 2003, Q2, P11; 2000, Q3, P12; 1997, Q2, P9-10; 1991, Q2, P17

● **780.5　Sleep disturbances**

> **Excludes** circadian rhythm sleep disorders (327.30–327.39)
> organic hypersomnia (327.10–327.19)
> organic insomnia (327.00–327.09)
> organic sleep apnea (327.20–327.29)
> organic sleep related movement disorders (327.51–327.59)
> parasomnias (327.40–327.49)
> that of nonorganic origin (307.40–307.49)

780.50　Sleep disturbance, unspecified

780.51　Insomnia with sleep apnea, unspecified
Coding Clinic: 1993, Q1, P28-29

780.52　Insomnia, unspecified

780.53　Hypersomnia with sleep apnea, unspecified
Coding Clinic: 1993, Q1, P28-29

780.54　Hypersomnia, unspecified

780.55　Disruptions of 24 hour sleep wake cycle, unspecified

◄ New　◄▥ Revised　~~deleted~~ Deleted　Excludes　Includes　Use additional　Code first　Omit code
● Unacceptable Principal Diagnosis　● Use Additional Digit(s)　OGCR Official Guidelines　Coding Clinic

780.56 Dysfunctions associated with sleep stages or arousal from sleep

780.57 Unspecified sleep apnea
Coding Clinic: 2001, Q1, P6-7; 1997, Q1, P5; 1993, Q1, P28-29

780.58 Sleep related movement disorder, unspecified
> Excludes | restless legs syndrome (333.94)

Coding Clinic: 2004, Q4, P95-96

780.59 Other

● **780.6 Fever and other physiologic disturbances of temperature regulation**
> Excludes | effects of reduced environmental
>   temperature (991.0-991.9)
> effects of heat and light (992.0-992.9)
> fever, chills or hypothermia associated with
>   confirmed infection – code to infection

Coding Clinic: 2008, Q4, P140-143; 2005, Q3, P16-17; 2000, Q3,
P13; 1991, Q2, P8x2; 1990, Q1, P8; 1985, July-Aug, P13

780.60 Fever, unspecified
Chills with fever
Fever NOS
Fever of unknown origin (FUO)
Hyperpyrexia NOS
Pyrexia NOS
Pyrexia of unknown origin
> Excludes | chills without fever (780.64)
> neonatal fever (778.4)
> pyrexia of unknown origin (during):
>   in newborn (778.4)
>   labor (659.2)
>   the puerperium (672)

780.61 Fever presenting with conditions classified elsewhere
> Code first underlying condition when associated
>   fever is present, such as with:
>   leukemia (conditions classifiable to
>   204-208)
>   neutropenia (288.00-288.09)
>   sickle-cell disease (282.60-282.69)

Coding Clinic: 2008, Q4, P140-143

780.62 Postprocedural fever
> Excludes | posttransfusion fever (780.66) ◄
> postvaccination fever (780.63)

780.63 Postvaccination fever
Postimmunization fever

780.64 Chills (without fever)
Chills NOS
> Excludes | chills with fever (780.60)

780.65 Hypothermia not associated with low environmental temperature
> Excludes | hypothermia:
>   associated with low environmental
>   temperature (991.6)
>   due to anesthesia (995.89)
>   of newborn (778.2, 778.3)

780.66 Febrile nonhemolytic transfusion reaction ◄
FNHTR ◄   Posttransfusion fever ◄

● **780.7 Malaise and fatigue**
> Excludes | debility, unspecified (799.3)
> fatigue (during):
>   combat (308.0–308.9)
>   heat (992.6)
>   pregnancy (646.8)
> neurasthenia (300.5)
> senile asthenia (797)

780.71 Chronic fatigue syndrome
Coding Clinic: 1998, Q4, P48-49

780.72 Functional quadriplegia
Complete immobility due to severe physical
disability or frailty
> Excludes | hysterical paralysis (300.11)
> immobility syndrome (728.3)
> neurologic quadriplegia
>   (344.00-344.09)
> quadriplegia NOS (344.00)

Coding Clinic: 2008, Q4, P143

780.79 Other malaise and fatigue
Asthenia NOS
Lethargy
Postviral (asthenic) syndrome
Tiredness
Coding Clinic: 2004, Q4, P77-78; 2000, Q1, P6

780.8 Generalized hyperhidrosis
Diaphoresis   Secondary hyperhidrosis
Excessive sweating
> Excludes | focal (localized) (primary) (secondary)
>   hyperhidrosis (705.21–705.22)
> Frey's syndrome (705.22)

● **780.9 Other general symptoms**
> Excludes | hypothermia:
>   NOS (accidental) (991.6)
>   due to anesthesia (995.89)
> memory disturbance as part of a pattern
>   of mental disorder
> of newborn (778.2–778.3)

Coding Clinic: 2002, Q4, P67-68

780.91 Fussy infant (baby)

780.92 Excessive crying of infant (baby)
> Excludes | excessive crying of child, adolescent
>   or adult (780.95)

Coding Clinic: 2005, Q4, P89-90

780.93 Memory loss
Amnesia (retrograde)
Memory loss NOS
> Excludes | memory loss due to:
>   intracranial injuries
>   (850.0-854.19)
>   skull fractures (800.00-801.99,
>   803.00-804.99)
> mild memory disturbance due to
>   organic brain damage (310.8)
> transient global amnesia (437.7)

Coding Clinic: 2003, Q4, P71

780.94 Early satiety
Coding Clinic: 2003, Q4, P72

780.95 Excessive crying of child, adolescent, or adult
> Excludes | excessive crying of infant (baby)
>   (780.92)

Coding Clinic: 2005, Q4, P89-90

780.96 Generalized pain
Pain NOS

780.97 Altered mental status
Change in mental status
> Excludes | altered level of consciousness
>   (780.01-780.09)
> altered mental status due to known
>   condition - code to condition
> delirium NOS (780.09)

Coding Clinic: 2006, Q4, P107-108; 1993, Q3, P11

780.99 Other general symptoms
Coding Clinic: 2003, Q4, P103-104; 1999, Q4, P10; 1985,
Nov-Dec, P12

SYMPTOMS, SIGNS, AND ILL-DEFINED CONDITIONS (780–799)

● **781 Symptoms involving nervous and musculoskeletal systems**

    Excludes *depression NOS (311)*
        disorders specifically relating to:
          back (724.0–724.9)
          hearing (388.0–389.9)
          joint (718.0–719.9)
          limb (729.0–729.9)
          neck (723.0–723.9)
          vision (368.0–369.9)
        pain in limb (729.5)

781.0 Abnormal involuntary movements
  Abnormal head movements
  Fasciculation
  Spasms NOS
  Tremor NOS

    Excludes *abnormal reflex (796.1)*
        chorea NOS (333.5)
        infantile spasms (345.60–345.61)
        spastic paralysis (342.1, 343.0–344.9)
        specified movement disorders classifiable to 333 (333.0–333.9)
        that of nonorganic origin (307.2–307.3)

781.1 Disturbances of sensation of smell and taste
  Anosmia   Parosmia
  Parageusia

781.2 Abnormality of gait
  Gait:
    ataxic
    paralytic
    spastic
    staggering

    Excludes *ataxia:*
        NOS (781.3)
        difficulty in walking (719.7)
        locomotor (progressive) (094.0)
  Coding Clinic: 2005, Q2, P6-7; 2004, Q2, P15

781.3 Lack of coordination
  Ataxia NOS
  Muscular incoordination

    Excludes *ataxic gait (781.2)*
        cerebellar ataxia (334.0–334.9)
        difficulty in walking (719.7)
        vertigo NOS (780.4)
  Coding Clinic: 2004, Q4, P50-52; 1997, Q3, P12-13

781.4 Transient paralysis of limb
  Monoplegia, transient NOS

    Excludes *paralysis (342.0–344.9)*

781.5 Clubbing of fingers

781.6 Meningismus
  Dupre's syndrome   Meningism
  Coding Clinic: 2000, Q3, P13

781.7 Tetany
  Carpopedal spasm

    Excludes *tetanus neonatorum (771.3)*
        tetany:
          hysterical (300.11)
          newborn (hypocalcemic) (775.4)
          parathyroid (252.1)
          psychogenic (306.0)

781.8 Neurologic neglect syndrome ◄▥
  Asomatognosia   Left-sided neglect
  Hemi-akinesia   Sensory extinction
  Hemi-inattention   Sensory neglect
  Hemispatial neglect   Visuospatial neglect

    Excludes *visuospatial deficit (799.53)* ◄

781.9 Other symptoms involving nervous and musculoskeletal systems

781.91 Loss of height

    Excludes *osteoporosis (733.00–733.09)*

781.92 Abnormal posture

781.93 Ocular torticollis
  Coding Clinic: 2002, Q4, P68; Q4, P68

781.94 Facial weakness
  Facial droop

    Excludes *facial weakness due to late effect of cerebrovascular accident (438.83)*
  Coding Clinic: 2003, Q4, P72

781.99 Other symptoms involving nervous and musculoskeletal systems

● **782 Symptoms involving skin and other integumentary tissue**

    Excludes *symptoms relating to breast (611.71–611.79)*

782.0 Disturbance of skin sensation
  Anesthesia of skin
  Burning or prickling sensation
  Hyperesthesia
  Hypoesthesia
  Numbness
  Paresthesia
  Tingling
  Coding Clinic: 2009, Q4, P113

782.1 Rash and other nonspecific skin eruption
  Exanthem

    Excludes *vesicular eruption (709.8)*

782.2 Localized superficial swelling, mass, or lump
  Subcutaneous nodules

    Excludes *localized adiposity (278.1)*

782.3 Edema
  Anasarca
  Dropsy
  Localized edema NOS

    Excludes *ascites (789.51–789.59)*
        edema of:
          newborn NOS (778.5)
          pregnancy (642.0–642.9, 646.1)
        fluid retention (276.69) ◄▥
        hydrops fetalis (773.3, 778.0)
        hydrothorax (511.81–511.89)
        nutritional edema (260, 262)
  Coding Clinic: 2000, Q2, P18

782.4 Jaundice, unspecified, not of newborn
  Cholemia NOS   Icterus NOS

    Excludes *due to isoimmunization (773.0–773.2, 773.4)*
        jaundice in newborn (774.0–774.7)

782.5 Cyanosis

    Excludes *newborn (770.83)*

● **782.6 Pallor and flushing**

782.61 Pallor

782.62 Flushing
  Excessive blushing

782.7 Spontaneous ecchymoses
  Petechiae

    Excludes *ecchymosis in fetus or newborn (772.6)*
        purpura (287.0–287.9)

782.8 Changes in skin texture
  Induration of skin   Thickening of skin

782.9 Other symptoms involving skin and integumentary tissues

◄ New   ◄▥ Revised   ~~deleted~~ Deleted   Excludes   Includes   Use additional   Code first   Omit code
● Unacceptable Principal Diagnosis   ● Use Additional Digit(s)   OGCR Official Guidelines   Coding Clinic

SYMPTOMS, SIGNS, AND ILL-DEFINED CONDITIONS (780–799)

● **783 Symptoms concerning nutrition, metabolism, and development**

  783.0 Anorexia
  Loss of appetite

  | Excludes | anorexia nervosa (307.1)
  loss of appetite of nonorganic origin (307.59) |

  783.1 Abnormal weight gain

  | Excludes | excessive weight gain in pregnancy (646.1)
  obesity (278.00)
  morbid (278.01) |

● **783.2 Abnormal loss of weight and underweight**
  Use additional code to identify Body Mass Index (BMI), if known (V85.0–V85.54)

    783.21 Loss of weight

    783.22 Underweight

  783.3 Feeding difficulties and mismanagement
  Feeding problem (elderly) (infant)

  | Excludes | feeding disturbance or problems:
  in newborn (779.31-779.34)
  of nonorganic origin (307.50–307.59) |

  Coding Clinic: 1997, Q3, P12-13; 1994, Q2, P10-11

● **783.4 Lack of expected normal physiological development in childhood**

  | Excludes | delay in sexual development and puberty (259.0)
  gonadal dysgenesis (758.6)
  pituitary dwarfism (253.3)
  slow fetal growth and fetal malnutrition (764.00–764.99)
  specific delays in mental development (315.0–315.9) |

  Coding Clinic: 1997, Q3, P5

    783.40 Lack of normal physiological development, unspecified
    Inadequate development
    Lack of development

    783.41 Failure to thrive
    Failure to gain weight

    | Excludes | failure to thrive in newborn (779.34) |

    Coding Clinic: 2003, Q1, P12

    783.42 Delayed milestones
    Late talker   Late walker

    783.43 Short stature
    Growth failure   Lack of growth
    Growth retardation   Physical retardation
    Coding Clinic: 2004, Q2, P3

  783.5 Polydipsia
  Excessive thirst

  783.6 Polyphagia
  Excessive eating
  Hyperalimentation NOS

  | Excludes | disorders of eating of nonorganic origin (307.50–307.59) |

  783.7 Adult failure to thrive

  783.9 Other symptoms concerning nutrition, metabolism, and development
  Hypometabolism

  | Excludes | abnormal basal metabolic rate (794.7)
  dehydration (276.51)
  other disorders of fluid, electrolyte, and acid-base balance (276.0–276.9) |

  Coding Clinic: 2004, Q2, P3

● **784 Symptoms involving head and neck**

  | Excludes | encephalopathy NOS (348.30)
  specific symptoms involving neck classifiable to 723 (723.0–723.9) |

  784.0 Headache
  Facial pain   Pain in head NOS

  | Excludes | atypical face pain (350.2)
  migraine (346.0–346.9)
  tension headache (307.81) |

  Coding Clinic: 2006, Q3, P22; Q2, P17-18; 2000, Q3, P13; 1992, Q3, P14; 1990, Q1, P9

  784.1 Throat pain

  | Excludes | dysphagia (787.20–787.29)
  neck pain (723.1)
  sore throat (462)
  chronic (472.1) |

  784.2 Swelling, mass, or lump in head and neck
  Space-occupying lesion, intracranial NOS
  Coding Clinic: 2003, Q1, P8

  784.3 Aphasia

  | Excludes | aphasia due to late effects of cerebrovascular disease (438.11)
  developmental aphasia (315.31) |

  Coding Clinic: 2004, Q4, P77-78; 1998, Q4, P87; 1997, Q3, P12-13

● **784.4 Voice and resonance disorders**

    784.40 Voice and resonance disorder, unspecified

    784.41 Aphonia
    Loss of voice

    784.42 Dysphonia
    Hoarseness

    784.43 Hypernasality

    784.44 Hyponasality

    784.49 Other voice and resonance disorders
    Change in voice

● **784.5 Other speech disturbance**

  | Excludes | speech disorder due to late effect of cerebrovascular accident (438.10-438.19)
  stammering and stuttering (315.35) ◄
  that of nonorganic origin (307.0, 307.9) |

    784.51 Dysarthria

    | Excludes | dysarthria due to late effect of cerebrovascular accident (438.13) |

    784.52 Fluency disorder in conditions classified elsewhere ◄
    Stuttering in conditions classified elsewhere ◄

    Code first underlying disease or condition, such as: ◄
    Parkinson's disease (332.0) ◄

    | Excludes | adult onset fluency disorder (307.0) ◄
    childhood onset fluency disorder (315.35) ◄
    fluency disorder due to late effect of cerebrovascular accident (438.14) ◄ |

    784.59 Other speech disturbance
    Dysphasia   Speech disturbance NOS
    Slurred speech

SYMPTOMS, SIGNS, AND ILL-DEFINED CONDITIONS (780–799)

● **784.6 Other symbolic dysfunction**

> **Excludes** *developmental learning delays (315.0–315.9)*

784.60 Symbolic dysfunction, unspecified

784.61 Alexia and dyslexia
Alexia (with agraphia)
Loss of ability to read

784.69 Other
Acalculia
Difficulty performing simple mathematical tasks
Agnosia
Loss of ability to recognize objects, persons, sounds, shapes, or smells
Agraphia NOS
Apraxia
Loss of the ability to execute or carry out movements

784.7 Epistaxis
Hemorrhage from nose
Nosebleed
Coding Clinic: 2004, Q3, P7; 1995, Q1, P5

784.8 Hemorrhage from throat

> **Excludes** *hemoptysis (786.30-786.39)* ◀▥
> *Spitting blood*

● **784.9 Other symptoms involving head and neck**

784.91 Postnasal drip

784.92 Jaw pain ◀
Mandibular pain ◀   Maxilla pain ◀

> **Excludes** *temporomandibular joint arthralgia (524.62)* ◀

784.99 Other symptoms involving head and neck
Choking sensation
Feeling of foreign body in throat
Halitosis
Bad breath
Mouth breathing
Sneezing

> **Excludes** *foreign body in throat (933.0)*

● **785 Symptoms involving cardiovascular system**

> **Excludes** *heart failure NOS (428.9)*

785.0 Tachycardia, unspecified
Rapid heart beat

> **Excludes** *neonatal tachycardia (779.82)*
> *paroxysmal tachycardia (427.0–427.2)*
> Coding Clinic: 2003, Q2, P11

785.1 Palpitations
Awareness of heart beat

> **Excludes** *specified dysrhythmias (427.0–427.9)*

785.2 Undiagnosed cardiac murmurs
Heart murmur NOS

785.3 Other abnormal heart sounds
Cardiac dullness, increased or decreased
Friction fremitus, cardiac
Precordial friction

785.4 Gangrene
Gangrene: Gangrene:
NOS   Gangrenous cellulitis
spreading cutaneous   Phagedena
Rapidly spreading destructive ulceration of soft tissue

> **Code first** *any associated underlying condition*

> **Excludes** *gangrene of certain sites-see Alphabetic Index*
> *gangrene with atherosclerosis of the extremities (440.24)*
> *gas gangrene (040.0)*
> Coding Clinic: 2004, Q1, P14-15; 1994, Q3, P5; 1990, Q3, P15; 1986, Mar-April, P12

● **785.5 Shock without mention of trauma**

785.50 Shock, unspecified
Failure of peripheral circulation
Resulting in significant blood pressure drop

785.51 Cardiogenic shock
Coding Clinic: 2008, Q4, P180-182; 2005, Q3, P14

785.52 Septic shock
Endotoxic   Gram-negative

> Code first:
> systemic inflammatory response syndrome due to infectious process with organ dysfunction (995.92)
> Coding Clinic: 2005, Q3, P23; Q2, P18-20x2; 2003, Q4, P73,79-81

785.59 Other
Shock:
hypovolemic
Decreased blood volume

> **Excludes** *shock (due to):*
> *anesthetic (995.4)*
> *anaphylactic (995.0)*
> *due to serum (999.4)*
> *electric (994.8)*
> *following abortion (639.5)*
> *lightning (994.0)*
> *obstetrical (669.1)*
> *postoperative (998.0)*
> *traumatic (958.4)*
> Coding Clinic: 2008, Q4, P97-100

785.6 Enlargement of lymph nodes
Lymphadenopathy   "Swollen glands"

> **Excludes** *lymphadenitis (chronic) (289.1–289.3)*
> *acute (683)*

785.9 Other symptoms involving cardiovascular system
Bruit (arterial)   Weak pulse

● **786 Symptoms involving respiratory system and other chest symptoms**

● **786.0 Dyspnea and respiratory abnormalities**

786.00 Respiratory abnormality, unspecified

786.01 Hyperventilation

> **Excludes** *hyperventilation, psychogenic (306.1)*

786.02 Orthopnea

786.03 Apnea

> **Excludes** *apnea of newborn (770.81, 770.82)*
> *sleep apnea (780.51, 780.53, 780.57)*
> Coding Clinic: 1998, Q2, P10

786.04 Cheyne-Stokes respiration
Abnormal pattern of breathing with gradually increasing and decreasing tidal volume with some periods of apnea

786.05 Shortness of breath
Coding Clinic: 1999, Q4, P25; Q1, P6

786.06 Tachypnea

> **Excludes** *transitory tachypnea of newborn (770.6)*

786.07 Wheezing

> **Excludes** *asthma (493.00–493.92)*

786.09 Other
Respiratory:
distress
insufficiency
> | Excludes | respiratory distress:
> following trauma and surgery
> (518.5)
> newborn (770.89)
> respiratory failure (518.81,
> 518.83–518.84)
> newborn (770.84)
> syndrome (newborn) (769)
> adult (518.5)
Coding Clinic: 1990, Q1, P9

786.1 Stridor
> | Excludes | congenital laryngeal stridor (748.3)

786.2 Cough
> | Excludes | cough:
> psychogenic (306.1)
> smokers' (491.0)
> with hemorrhage (786.39) ◀▥
Coding Clinic: 1995, Q4, P50; 1990, Q1, P8

● **786.3 Hemoptysis** ◀▥
~~Cough with hemorrhage~~
~~Pulmonary hemorrhage NOS~~
> | ~~Excludes~~ | ~~pulmonary hemorrhage of newborn (770.3)~~
Coding Clinic: 2006, Q2, P17

786.30 Hemoptysis, unspecified ◀
Pulmonary hemorrhage NOS ◀

786.31 Acute idiopathic pulmonary hemorrhage in infants [AIPHI] ◀
Acute idiopathic pulmonary hemorrhage in infant over 28 days old ◀
> | Excludes | pulmonary hemorrhage of newborn
> under 28 days old (770.3) ◀
> von Willebrand's disease (286.4) ◀

786.39 Other hemoptysis ◀
Cough with hemorrhage ◀

786.4 Abnormal sputum
Abnormal:
amount of sputum
color of sputum
odor of sputum
Excessive sputum

● **786.5 Chest pain**
786.50 Chest pain, unspecified
Coding Clinic: 2007, Q1, P19; 2006, Q2, P7-8; 2003, Q1, P6-7;
2002, Q1, P4-5; 1999, Q4, P25-26; 1993, Q1, P25

786.51 Precordial pain
Coding Clinic: 1984, May-June, P11

786.52 Painful respiration
Pain:
anterior chest wall
pleuritic
Pleurodynia
> | Excludes | epidemic pleurodynia (074.1)
Coding Clinic: 1984, Nov-Dec, P17

786.59 Other
Discomfort in chest
Pressure in chest
Tightness in chest
> | Excludes | pain in breast (611.71)
Coding Clinic: 2007, Q1, P19; 2002, Q1, P6

786.6 Swelling, mass, or lump in chest
> | Excludes | lump in breast (611.72)

786.7 Abnormal chest sounds
Abnormal percussion, chest
Friction sounds, chest
Rales
> *Wet rattling, clicking, crackling sounds on auscultation*
Tympany, chest
> | Excludes | wheezing (786.07)

786.8 Hiccough
> | Excludes | psychogenic hiccough (306.1)

786.9 Other symptoms involving respiratory system and chest
Breath-holding spell

● **787 Symptoms involving digestive system**
> | Excludes | constipation (564.0–564.9)
> pylorospasm (537.81)
> congenital (750.5)

● **787.0 Nausea and vomiting**
Emesis
> | Excludes | hematemesis NOS (578.0)
> vomiting:
> bilious, following gastrointestinal surgery
> (564.3)
> cyclical (536.2)
> associated with migraine (346.2)
> psychogenic (306.4)
> excessive, in pregnancy (643.0–643.9)
> fecal matter (569.87)
> habit (536.2)
> of newborn (779.32, 779.33)
> persistent (536.2)
> psychogenic NOS (307.54)

787.01 Nausea with vomiting
Concurrent conditions
Coding Clinic: 2003, Q1, P5

787.02 Nausea alone
Separate condition
Coding Clinic: 2000, Q3, P12; 1997, Q2, P9-10

787.03 Vomiting alone
Separate condition
Coding Clinic: 1985, Mar-April, P11

787.04 Bilious emesis
Bilious vomiting
> | Excludes | bilious emesis (vomiting) in
> newborn (779.32)

787.1 Heartburn
Pyrosis   Waterbrash
> | Excludes | dyspepsia or indigestion (536.8)
Coding Clinic: 2001, Q2, P6

● **787.2 Dysphagia**
> *Code first*, if applicable, dysphagia due to late effect of
> cerebrovascular accident (438.82)
Coding Clinic: 2007, Q3, P8-9; 2003, Q4, P103-104, 109-110; 2001,
Q2, P4-6; 1993, 5th Issue, P16; 1986, Nov-Dec, P10

787.20 Dysphagia, unspecified
Difficulty in swallowing NOS

787.21 Dysphagia, oral phase

787.22 Dysphagia, oropharyngeal phase
Coding Clinic: 2007, Q4, P92-95

787.23 Dysphagia, pharyngeal phase

787.24 Dysphagia, pharyngoesophageal phase

787.29 Other dysphagia
Cervical dysphagia
Neurogenic dysphagia

787.3 Flatulence, eructation, and gas pain
Abdominal distention (gaseous)
Bloating
Tympanites (abdominal) (intestinal)

> **Excludes** *aerophagy (306.4)*

787.4 Visible peristalsis
Hyperperistalsis

787.5 Abnormal bowel sounds
Absent bowel sounds
Hyperactive bowel sounds

● **787.6 Incontinence of feces** ◀▥
Encopresis NOS
Incontinence of sphincter ani

> **Excludes** *that of nonorganic origin (307.7)*

Coding Clinic: 1997, Q1, P9-10

787.60 Full incontinence of feces ◀
Fecal incontinence NOS ◀

787.61 Incomplete defecation ◀

> **Excludes** *constipation (564.00-564.09)* ◀
> *fecal impaction (560.32)* ◀

787.62 Fecal smearing ◀
Fecal soiling ◀

787.63 Fecal urgency ◀

787.7 Abnormal feces
Bulky stools

> **Excludes** *abnormal stool content (792.1)*
> *melena:*
> *NOS (578.1)*
> *newborn (772.4, 777.3)*

● **787.9 Other symptoms involving digestive system**

> **Excludes** *gastrointestinal hemorrhage (578.0–578.9)*
> *intestinal obstruction (560.0–560.9)*
> *specific functional digestive disorders:*
> *esophagus (530.0–530.9)*
> *stomach and duodenum (536.0–536.9)*
> *those not elsewhere classified*
> *(564.0–564.9)*

787.91 Diarrhea
Diarrhea NOS
Coding Clinic: 2008, Q4, P97-100

787.99 Other
Change in bowel habits
Tenesmus (rectal)

● **788 Symptoms involving urinary system**

> **Excludes** *hematuria (599.70–599.72)*
> *nonspecific findings on examination of the urine*
> *(791.0–791.9)*
> *small kidney of unknown cause (589.0–589.9)*
> *uremia NOS (586)*
> *urinary obstruction (599.60, 599.69)*

788.0 Renal colic
Colic (recurrent) of:
kidney
ureter
Coding Clinic: 2004, Q3, P8

788.1 Dysuria
Painful urination   Strangury

● **788.2 Retention of urine**

> *Code first, if applicable, hyperplasia of prostate*
> *(600.0–600.9 with fifth-digit 1)*
> Coding Clinic: 2003, Q3, P13; 1994, Q1, P20; 1986, Sept-Oct, P12

788.20 Retention of urine, unspecified
Coding Clinic: 2006, Q4, P93-95; 2004, Q2, P18; 2003, Q3, P12; Q1, P6; 1996, Q3, P10-11; 1994, Q3, P13

788.21 Incomplete bladder emptying

788.29 Other specified retention of urine

● **788.3 Urinary incontinence**

> **Excludes** *functional urinary incontinence (788.91)*
> *that of nonorganic origin (307.6)*
> *urinary incontinence associated with*
> *cognitive impairment (788.91)*
> *Code, if applicable, any causal condition first, such as:*
> congenital ureterocele (753.23)
> genital prolapse (618.00–618.9)
> hyperplasia of prostate (600.0–600.9 with
> fifth-digit 1)
> Coding Clinic: 2005, Q3, P20

788.30 Urinary incontinence, unspecified
Enuresis NOS
Coding Clinic: 2009, Q1, P18; 1995, Q4, P72-73

788.31 Urge incontinence
Coding Clinic: 2000, Q1, P19-20

788.32 Stress incontinence, male

> **Excludes** *stress incontinence, female (625.6)*
> Coding Clinic: 1995, Q4, P72-73

788.33 Mixed incontinence (female) (male)
Urge and stress

788.34 Incontinence without sensory awareness

788.35 Post-void dribbling

788.36 Nocturnal enuresis

788.37 Continuous leakage

788.38 Overflow incontinence
Coding Clinic: 2004, Q4, P96

788.39 Other urinary incontinence

● **788.4 Frequency of urination and polyuria**

> *Code first, if applicable, hyperplasia of prostate*
> *(600.0–600.9 with fifth-digit 1)*

788.41 Urinary frequency
Frequency of micturition

788.42 Polyuria

788.43 Nocturia

788.5 Oliguria and anuria
Deficient secretion of urine
Suppression of urinary secretion

> **Excludes** *that complicating:*
> *abortion (634–638 with .3, 639.3)*
> *ectopic or molar pregnancy (639.3)*
> *pregnancy, childbirth, or the puerperium*
> *(642.0–642.9, 646.2)*

● **788.6 Other abnormality of urination**

> *Code first, if applicable, hyperplasia of prostate*
> *(600.0–600.9 with fifth-digit 1)*

788.61 Splitting of urinary stream
Intermittent urinary stream

788.62 Slowing of urinary stream
Weak stream

788.63 Urgency of urination

> **Excludes** *urge incontinence (788.31, 788.33)*
> Coding Clinic: 2003, Q4, P74

788.64 Urinary hesitancy

788.65 Straining on urination

788.69 Other

788.7 Urethral discharge
Penile discharge   Urethrorrhea

788.8 Extravasation of urine
Leakage, discharge

● **788.9　Other symptoms involving urinary system**
　　Coding Clinic: 2005, Q1, P12-13

　　788.91　Functional urinary incontinence
　　　　Urinary incontinence due to cognitive
　　　　impairment, or severe physical
　　　　disability or immobility

　　　　| Excludes | urinary incontinence due to
　　　　　physiologic condition
　　　　　(788.30-788.39)
　　　　Coding Clinic: 2008, Q4, P144-145

　　788.99　Other symptoms involving urinary system
　　　　Extrarenal uremia
　　　　Vesical:
　　　　　pain
　　　　　tenesmus

● **789　Other symptoms involving abdomen and pelvis**
　　The following fifth-digit subclassification is to be used for
　　codes 789.0, 789.3, 789.4, 789.6

0	unspecified site	5	periumbilic
1	right upper quadrant	6	epigastric
2	left upper quadrant	7	generalized
3	right lower quadrant	9	other specified site
4	left lower quadrant		multiple sites

　　| Excludes | symptoms referable to genital organs:
　　　　female (625.0–625.9)
　　　　male (607.0–608.9)
　　　　psychogenic (302.70–302.79)

● **789.0　Abdominal pain**
　[0-7,9]　　Cramps, abdominal
　　　　Coding Clinic: 2002, Q1, P5; 1995, Q1, P3; 1990, Q2, P26

　789.1　Hepatomegaly
　　　Enlargement of liver

　789.2　Splenomegaly
　　　Enlargement of spleen

● **789.3　Abdominal or pelvic swelling, mass, or lump**
　[0-7,9]　　Diffuse or generalized swelling or mass:
　　　　abdominal NOS
　　　　umbilical

　　| Excludes | abdominal distention (gaseous) (787.3)
　　　　ascites (789.51–789.59)

● **789.4　Abdominal rigidity**
　[0-7,9]

● **789.5　Ascites**
　　　Fluid in peritoneal cavity
　　　Coding Clinic: 2008, Q1, P16-18; 2007, Q4, P95-96; 2005, Q2, P8;
　　　　1989, Q4, P11

　● **789.51　Malignant ascites**

　　　Code first malignancy, such as:
　　　　malignant neoplasm of ovary (183.0)
　　　　secondary malignant neoplasm of
　　　　　retroperitoneum and peritoneum
　　　　　(197.6)
　　　　Coding Clinic: 2008, Q1, P16-17

　　789.59　Other ascites

● **789.6　Abdominal tenderness**
　[0-7,9]　　Rebound tenderness

　789.7　Colic
　　　Colic NOS　　　　　　　Infantile colic

　　| Excludes | colic in adult and child over
　　　　12 months old (789.0)
　　　　renal colic (788.0)

　789.9　Other symptoms involving abdomen and pelvis
　　　Umbilical:　　　　　　Umbilical:
　　　　bleeding　　　　　　　discharge

NONSPECIFIC ABNORMAL FINDINGS (790–796)

● **790　Nonspecific findings on examination of blood**
　　| Excludes | abnormality of:
　　　　platelets (287.0–287.9)
　　　　thrombocytes (287.0–287.9)
　　　　white blood cells (288.00–288.9)

● **790.0　Abnormality of red blood cells**
　　| Excludes | anemia:
　　　　congenital (776.5)
　　　　newborn, due to isoimmunization
　　　　　(773.0–773.2, 773.5)
　　　　of premature infant (776.6)
　　　　other specified types (280.0–285.9)
　　　　hemoglobin disorders (282.5–282.7)
　　　　polycythemia:
　　　　　familial (289.6)
　　　　　neonatorum (776.4)
　　　　　secondary (289.0)
　　　　　vera (238.4)

　　790.01　Precipitous drop in hematocrit
　　　　Drop in hematocrit
　　　　Drop in hemoglobin
　　　　　Decrease in red blood cells

　　790.09　Other abnormality of red blood cells
　　　　Abnormal red cell morphology NOS
　　　　Abnormal red cell volume NOS
　　　　Anisocytosis
　　　　　Red blood cells of unequal size
　　　　Poikilocytosis
　　　　　Red blood cells of abnormal shape

　790.1　Elevated sedimentation rate

● **790.2　Abnormal glucose**
　　| Excludes | diabetes mellitus (249.00–249.91,
　　　　250.00–250.93)
　　　　dysmetabolic syndrome X (277.7)
　　　　gestational diabetes (648.8)
　　　　glycosuria (791.5)
　　　　hypoglycemia (251.2)
　　　　that complicating pregnancy, childbirth, or
　　　　　the puerperium (648.8)
　　　Coding Clinic: 2003, Q4, P74-75

　　790.21　Impaired fasting glucose
　　　　Elevated fasting glucose

　　790.22　Impaired glucose tolerance test (oral)
　　　　Elevated glucose tolerance test

　　790.29　Other abnormal glucose
　　　　Abnormal glucose NOS
　　　　Abnormal non-fasting glucose
　　　　Hyperglycemia NOS
　　　　Pre-diabetes NOS
　　　　Coding Clinic: 2009, Q3, P18; 2005, Q2, P21-22; 2004, Q4,
　　　　　P53-56

　790.3　Excessive blood level of alcohol
　　　Elevated blood-alcohol

　790.4　Nonspecific elevation of levels of transaminase or
　　　lactic acid dehydrogenase [LDH]

　790.5　Other nonspecific abnormal serum enzyme levels
　　　Abnormal serum level of:
　　　　acid phosphatase
　　　　alkaline phosphatase
　　　　amylase
　　　　lipase

　　| Excludes | deficiency of circulating enzymes (277.6)

SYMPTOMS, SIGNS, AND ILL-DEFINED CONDITIONS (780–799)

SYMPTOMS, SIGNS, AND ILL-DEFINED CONDITIONS (780–799)

790.6 Other abnormal blood chemistry
Abnormal blood levels of:
cobalt
copper
iron
lead
lithium
magnesium
mineral
zinc

> **Excludes** *abnormality of electrolyte or acid-base*
> *balance (276.0–276.9)*
> *hypoglycemia NOS (251.2)*
> *lead poisoning (984.0–984.9)*
> *specific finding indicating abnormality of:*
> *amino-acid transport and metabolism*
> *(270.0–270.9)*
> *carbohydrate transport and metabolism*
> *(271.0–271.9)*
> *lipid metabolism (272.0–272.9)*
> *uremia NOS (586)*

790.7 Bacteremia

> **Excludes** *bacteremia of newborn (771.83)*
> *septicemia (038)*

Use additional code to identify organism (041)
Coding Clinic: 2003, Q2, P7-8

790.8 Viremia, unspecified
Coding Clinic: 1988, Q4, P10

● **790.9 Other nonspecific findings on examination of blood**

    790.91 Abnormal arterial blood gases

    790.92 Abnormal coagulation profile
    Abnormal or prolonged:
    bleeding time
    coagulation time
    partial thromboplastin time [PTT]
    prothrombin time [PT]

> **Excludes** *coagulation (hemorrhagic) disorders*
> *(286.0–286.9)*

    Coding Clinic: 1994, Q1, P22

    790.93 Elevated prostate specific antigen [PSA]

    790.94 Euthyroid sick syndrome

    790.95 Elevated C-reactive protein (CRP)
    Coding Clinic: 2004, Q4, P96-97

    790.99 Other

● **791 Nonspecific findings on examination of urine**

> **Excludes** *hematuria NOS (599.70–599.72)*
> *specific findings indicating abnormality of:*
> *amino-acid transport and metabolism*
> *(270.0–270.9)*
> *carbohydrate transport and metabolism*
> *(271.0–271.9)*

791.0 Proteinuria
Albuminuria
Bence-Jones proteinuria

> **Excludes** *postural proteinuria (593.6)*
> *that arising during pregnancy or the*
> *puerperium (642.0–642.9, 646.2)*

791.1 Chyluria
White milky urine

> **Excludes** *filarial (125.0–125.9)*

791.2 Hemoglobinuria

791.3 Myoglobinuria

791.4 Biliuria

791.5 Glycosuria

> **Excludes** *renal glycosuria (271.4)*

791.6 Acetonuria
Ketonuria

791.7 Other cells and casts in urine

791.9 Other nonspecific findings on examination of urine
Crystalluria
Elevated urine levels of:
17-ketosteroids
catecholamines
indolacetic acid
vanillylmandelic acid [VMA]
Melanuria
Coding Clinic: 2005, Q1, P12

● **792 Nonspecific abnormal findings in other body substances**

> **Excludes** *that in chromosomal analysis (795.2)*

792.0 Cerebrospinal fluid

792.1 Stool contents
Abnormal stool color   Occult blood
Fat in stool   Pus in stool
Mucus in stool

> **Excludes** *blood in stool [melena] (578.1)*
> *newborn (772.4, 777.3)*

Coding Clinic: 1992, Q2, P9-10; Q2, P9

792.2 Semen
Abnormal spermatozoa

> **Excludes** *azoospermia (606.0)*
> *oligospermia (606.1)*

792.3 Amniotic fluid

792.4 Saliva

> **Excludes** *that in chromosomal analysis (795.2)*

792.5 Cloudy (hemodialysis) (peritoneal) dialysis effluent

792.9 Other nonspecific abnormal findings in body substances
Peritoneal fluid   Synovial fluid
Pleural fluid   Vaginal fluids

● **793 Nonspecific (abnormal) findings on radiological and other examination of body structure**

> **Includes** nonspecific abnormal findings of:
> thermography
> ultrasound examination [echogram]
> x-ray examination

> **Excludes** *abnormal results of function studies and*
> *radioisotope scans (794.0–794.9)*

793.0 Skull and head

> **Excludes** *nonspecific abnormal echoencephalogram*
> *(794.01)*

Coding Clinic: 2006, Q3, P22

793.1 Lung field
Coin lesion lung
Shadow, lung

793.2 Other intrathoracic organ
Abnormal:
echocardiogram
heart shadow
ultrasound cardiogram
Mediastinal shift

793.3 Biliary tract
Nonvisualization of gallbladder

793.4 Gastrointestinal tract

793.5 Genitourinary organs
Filling defect:
bladder
kidney
ureter

793.6 Abdominal area, including retroperitoneum

793.7 Musculoskeletal system

● 793.8 Breast

    793.80 Abnormal mammogram, unspecified

    793.81 Mammographic microcalcification

        Excludes *mammographic calcification (793.89)*
                mammographic calculus (793.89)

    793.82 Inconclusive mammogram
        Dense breasts NOS
        Inconclusive mammogram NEC
        Inconclusive mammography due to dense breasts
        Inconclusive mammography NEC
        Coding Clinic: 2009, Q4, P113

    793.89 Other (abnormal) findings on radiological examination of breast
        Mammographic calcification
        Mammographic calculus

● 793.9 Other

    Excludes *abnormal finding by radioisotope localization of placenta (794.9)*

    793.91 Image test inconclusive due to excess body fat
        Use additional code to identify Body Mass Index (BMI), if known (V85.0–V85.54)
        Coding Clinic: 2006, Q4, P109-110

    793.99 Other nonspecific (abnormal) findings on radiological and other examinations of body structure
        Abnormal:
           placental finding by x-ray or ultrasound method
           radiological findings in skin and subcutaneous tissue

● 794 Nonspecific abnormal results of function studies

    Includes radioisotope:
        scans
        uptake studies
        scintiphotography

● 794.0 Brain and central nervous system

    794.00 Abnormal function study, unspecified

    794.01 Abnormal echoencephalogram

    794.02 Abnormal electroencephalogram [EEG]

    794.09 Other
        Abnormal brain scan

● 794.1 Peripheral nervous system and special senses

    794.10 Abnormal response to nerve stimulation, unspecified

    794.11 Abnormal retinal function studies
        Abnormal electroretinogram [ERG]

    794.12 Abnormal electro-oculogram [EOG]

    794.13 Abnormal visually evoked potential

    794.14 Abnormal oculomotor studies

    794.15 Abnormal auditory function studies
        Coding Clinic: 2004, Q1, P15-16

    794.16 Abnormal vestibular function studies

    794.17 Abnormal electromyogram [EMG]
        Excludes *that of eye (794.14)*

    794.19 Other

794.2 Pulmonary
    Abnormal lung scan
    Reduced:
        ventilatory capacity
        vital capacity

● 794.3 Cardiovascular

    794.30 Abnormal function study, unspecified

    794.31 Abnormal electrocardiogram [ECG] [EKG]
        Excludes *long QT syndrome (426.82)*
        Coding Clinic: 1985, Mar-April, P13

    794.39 Other
        Abnormal:
           ballistocardiogram
           phonocardiogram
           vectorcardiogram

794.4 Kidney
    Abnormal renal function test

794.5 Thyroid
    Abnormal thyroid:
        scan
        uptake

794.6 Other endocrine function study

794.7 Basal metabolism
    Abnormal basal metabolic rate [BMR]

794.8 Liver
    Abnormal liver scan

794.9 Other
    Bladder   Placenta
    Pancreas   Spleen

● 795 Other and nonspecific abnormal cytological, histological, immunological, and DNA test findings

    Excludes *abnormal cytologic smear of anus and anal HPV (796.70-796.79)*
        nonspecific abnormalities of red blood cells (790.01–790.09)
    Coding Clinic: 2002, Q4, P69-70

● 795.0 Abnormal Papanicolaou smear of cervix and cervical HPV
    Abnormal thin preparation smear of cervix
    Abnormal cervical cytology

    Excludes *abnormal cytologic smear of vagina and vaginal HPV (795.10-795.19)*
        carcinoma in situ of cervix (233.1)
        cervical intraepithelial neoplasia I (CIN I) (622.11)
        cervical intraepithelial neoplasia II (CIN II) (622.12)
        cervical intraepithelial neoplasia III (CIN III) (233.1)
        dysplasia (histologically confirmed) of cervix (uteri) NOS (622.10)
        mild cervical dysplasia (histologically confirmed) (622.11)
        moderate cervical dysplasia (histologically confirmed) (622.12)
        severe cervical dysplasia (histologically confirmed) (233.1)
    Coding Clinic: 2008, Q4, P145-148; 2004, Q4, P97-99

    795.00 Abnormal glandular Papanicolaou smear of cervix
        Atypical endocervical cells NOS
        Atypical endometrial cells NOS
        Atypical cervical glandular cells NOS

    795.01 Papanicolaou smear of cervix with atypical squamous cells of undetermined significance (ASC-US)
        Coding Clinic: 2006, Q2, P3,4

    795.02 Papanicolaou smear of cervix with atypical squamous cells cannot exclude high grade squamous intraepithelial lesion (ASC-H)

    795.03 Papanicolaou smear of cervix with low grade squamous intraepithelial lesion (LGSIL)

SYMPTOMS, SIGNS, AND ILL-DEFINED CONDITIONS (780–799)

SYMPTOMS, SIGNS, AND ILL-DEFINED CONDITIONS (780–799)

795.04 Papanicolaou smear of cervix with high grade squamous intraepithelial lesion (HGSIL)

795.05 Cervical high risk human papillomavirus (HPV) DNA test positive

795.06 Papanicolaou smear of cervix with cytologic evidence of malignancy

795.07 Satisfactory cervical smear but lacking transformation zone

795.08 Unsatisfactory cervical cytology smear
Inadequate cervical cytology sample
Coding Clinic: 2006, Q2, P3,4

795.09 Other abnormal Papanicolaou smear of cervix and cervical HPV
Cervical low risk human papillomavirus (HPV) DNA test positive

Use additional code for associated human papillomavirus (079.4)

| Excludes | encounter for Papanicolaou cervical smear to confirm findings of recent normal smear following initial abnormal smear (V72.32) |

● **795.1 Abnormal Papanicolaou smear of vagina and vaginal HPV**
Abnormal thin preparation smear of vagina NOS
Abnormal vaginal cytology NOS

Use additional code to identify acquired absence of uterus and cervix, if applicable (V88.01-V88.03)

Excludes	abnormal cytologic smear of cervix and cervical HPV (795.00-795.09)
	carcinoma in situ of vagina (233.31)
	carcinoma in situ of vulva (233.32)
	dysplasia (histologically confirmed) of vagina NOS (623.0, 233.31)
	dysplasia (histologically confirmed) of vulva NOS (624.01, 624.02, 233.32)
	mild vaginal dysplasia (histologically confirmed) (623.0)
	mild vulvar dysplasia (histologically confirmed) (624.01)
	moderate vaginal dysplasia (histologically confirmed) (623.0)
	moderate vulvar dysplasia (histologically confirmed) (624.02)
	severe vaginal dysplasia (histologically confirmed) (233.31)
	severe vulvar dysplasia (histologically confirmed) (233.32)
	vaginal intraepithelial neoplasia I (VAIN I) (623.0)
	vaginal intraepithelial neoplasia II (VAIN II) (623.0)
	vaginal intraepithelial neoplasia III (VAIN III) (233.31)
	vulvar intraepithelial neoplasia I (VIN I) (624.01)
	vulvar intraepithelial neoplasia II (VIN II) (624.02)
	vulvar intraepithelial neoplasia III (VIN III) (233.32)

Coding Clinic: 2008, Q4, P145-148

795.10 Abnormal glandular Papanicolaou smear of vagina
Atypical vaginal glandular cells NOS

795.11 Papanicolaou smear of vagina with atypical squamous cells of undetermined significance (ASC-US)

795.12 Papanicolaou smear of vagina with atypical squamous cells cannot exclude high grade squamous intraepithelial lesion (ASC-H)

795.13 Papanicolaou smear of vagina with low grade squamous intraepithelial lesion (LGSIL)

795.14 Papanicolaou smear of vagina with high grade squamous intraepithelial lesion (HGSIL)

795.15 Vaginal high risk human papillomavirus (HPV) DNA test positive

| Excludes | condyloma acuminatum (078.11) |
| | genital warts (078.11) |

795.16 Papanicolaou smear of vagina with cytologic evidence of malignancy
Coding Clinic: 2004, Q2, P11

795.18 Unsatisfactory vaginal cytology smear
Inadequate vaginal cytology sample

795.19 Other abnormal Papanicolaou smear of vagina and vaginal HPV
Vaginal low risk human papillomavirus (HPV) DNA test positive

Use additional code for associated human papillomavirus (079.4)

795.2 Nonspecific abnormal findings on chromosomal analysis
Abnormal karyotype

● **795.3 Nonspecific positive culture findings**
Positive culture findings in:
   nose
   sputum
   throat
   wound

Excludes	that of:
	blood (790.7–790.8)
	urine (791.9)

795.31 Nonspecific positive findings for anthrax
Positive findings by nasal swab
Coding Clinic: 2002, Q4, P70

795.39 Other nonspecific positive culture findings

| Excludes | colonization status (V02.0-V02.9) |

795.4 Other nonspecific abnormal histological findings

795.5 Nonspecific reaction to tuberculin skin test without active tuberculosis
Abnormal result of Mantoux test
PPD positive
Tuberculin (skin test):
   positive
   reactor

795.6 False positive serological test for syphilis
False positive Wassermann reaction

◀ New   ◀▥ Revised   ~~deleted~~ Deleted   Excludes   Includes   Use additional   Code first   Omit code
● Unacceptable Principal Diagnosis   ● Use Additional Digit(s)   OGCR Official Guidelines   Coding Clinic

● **795.7 Other nonspecific immunological findings**

> **Excludes**   *abnormal tumor markers (795.81–795.89)*
> *elevated prostate specific antigen [PSA]*
> *(790.93)*
> *elevated tumor associated antigens*
> *(795.81–795.89)*
> *isoimmunization, in pregnancy*
> *(656.1–656.2)*
> *affecting fetus or newborn (773.0–773.2)*

795.71 Nonspecific serologic evidence of human immunodeficiency virus [HIV]
Inconclusive human immunodeficiency virus [HIV] test (adult) (infant)

Note: This code is ONLY to be used when a test finding is reported as nonspecific. Asymptomatic positive findings are coded to V08. If any HIV infection symptom or condition is present, see code 042. Negative findings are not coded.

> **Excludes**   *acquired immunodeficiency syndrome [AIDS] (042)*
> *asymptomatic human immunodeficiency virus [HIV] infection status (V08)*
> *HIV infection, symptomatic (042)*
> *human immunodeficiency virus [HIV] disease (042)*
> *positive (status) NOS (V08)*

OGCR Section I.C.1.a.2.e

Patients with inconclusive HIV serology, but no definitive diagnosis or manifestations of the illness, may be assigned code 795.71, Inconclusive serologic test for Human Immunodeficiency Virus [HIV].

795.79 Other and unspecified nonspecific immunological findings
Raised antibody titer
Raised level of immunoglobulins
Coding Clinic: 1993, Q2, P6

● **795.8 Abnormal tumor markers**
Elevated tumor associated antigens [TAA]
Elevated tumor specific antigens [TSA]

> **Excludes**   *elevated prostate specific antigen [PSA] (790.93)*

Coding Clinic: 2006, Q4, P111-112; 1993, Q1, P21-22; 1992, Q2, P11

795.81 Elevated carcinoembryonic antigen [CEA]

795.82 Elevated cancer antigen 125 [CA 125]

795.89 Other abnormal tumor markers

● **796 Other nonspecific abnormal findings**

796.0 Nonspecific abnormal toxicological findings
Abnormal levels of heavy metals or drugs in blood, urine, or other tissue

> Use additional code for retained foreign body, if applicable, (V90.01-V90.9) ◄

> **Excludes**   *excessive blood level of alcohol (790.3)*

Coding Clinic: 1997, Q1, P16

796.1 Abnormal reflex

796.2 Elevated blood pressure reading without diagnosis of hypertension

Note: This category is to be used to record an episode of elevated blood pressure in a patient in whom no formal diagnosis of hypertension has been made, or as an incidental finding.
Coding Clinic: 2003, Q2, P11; 1993, 5th Issue, P6-7

OGCR Section I.C.7.a.8

Assign code 796.2, Elevated blood pressure reading without diagnosis of hypertension, unless patient has an established diagnosis of hypertension. Assign code 642.3x for transient hypertension of pregnancy.

796.3 Nonspecific low blood pressure reading

796.4 Other abnormal clinical findings
Coding Clinic: 1995, Q3, P13

796.5 Abnormal finding on antenatal screening

796.6 Abnormal findings on neonatal screening

> **Excludes**   *nonspecific serologic evidence of human immunodeficiency virus [HIV] (795.71)*

Coding Clinic: 2004, Q4, P99-100

● **796.7 Abnormal cytologic smear of anus and anal HPV**

> **Excludes**   *abnormal cytologic smear of cervix and cervical HPV (795.00-795.09)*
> *abnormal cytologic smear of vagina and vaginal HPV (795.10-795.19)*
> *anal intraepithelial neoplasia I (AIN I) (569.44)*
> *anal intraepithelial neoplasia II (AIN II) (569.44)*
> *anal intraepithelial neoplasia III (AIN III) (230.5, 230.6)*
> *carcinoma in situ of anus (230.5, 230.6)*
> *dysplasia (histologically confirmed) of anus NOS (569.44)*
> *mild anal dysplasia (histologically confirmed) (569.44)*
> *moderate anal dysplasia (histologically confirmed) (569.44)*
> *severe anal dysplasia (histologically confirmed) (230.5, 230.6)*

Coding Clinic: 2008, Q4, P117-119

796.70 Abnormal glandular Papanicolaou smear of anus
Atypical anal glandular cells NOS

796.71 Papanicolaou smear of anus with atypical squamous cells of undetermined significance (ASC-US)

796.72 Papanicolaou smear of anus with atypical squamous cells cannot exclude high grade squamous intraepithelial lesion (ASC-H)

796.73 Papanicolaou smear of anus with low grade squamous intraepithelial lesion (LGSIL)

796.74 Papanicolaou smear of anus with high grade squamous intraepithelial lesion (HGSIL)

796.75 Anal high risk human papillomavirus (HPV) DNA test positive

796.76 Papanicolaou smear of anus with cytologic evidence of malignancy

796.77 Satisfactory anal smear but lacking transformation zone

796.78 Unsatisfactory anal cytology smear
Inadequate anal cytology sample

796.79 Other abnormal Papanicolaou smear of anus and anal HPV
Anal low risk human papillomavirus (HPV) DNA test positive

> Use additional code for associated human papillomavirus (079.4)

796.9 Other

SYMPTOMS, SIGNS, AND ILL-DEFINED CONDITIONS (780–799)

ILL-DEFINED AND UNKNOWN CAUSES OF MORBIDITY AND MORTALITY (797–799)

797 Senility without mention of psychosis
Frailty
Old age
Senescence
Senile asthenia

Senile:
  debility
  exhaustion

> **Excludes** *senile psychoses (290.0–290.9)*

● **798 Sudden death, cause unknown**

798.0 Sudden infant death syndrome *(SIDS)*
Cot death
Crib death
Sudden death of nonspecific cause in infancy

● **798.1 Instantaneous death**

● **798.2 Death occurring in less than 24 hours from onset of symptoms, not otherwise explained**
Death known not to be violent or instantaneous, for which no cause could be discovered
Died without sign of disease

● **798.9 Unattended death**
Death in circumstances where the body of the deceased was found and no cause could be discovered
Found dead

● **799 Other ill-defined and unknown causes of morbidity and mortality**

● **799.0 Asphyxia and hypoxemia**

> **Excludes** *asphyxia and hypoxemia (due to):*
> *carbon monoxide (986)*
> *hypercapnia (786.09)*
> *inhalation of food or foreign body (932–934.9)*
> *newborn (768.0–768.9)*
> *traumatic (994.7)*

Coding Clinic: 2005, Q4, P90; 1990, Q1, P20

799.01 Asphyxia

799.02 Hypoxemia
Coding Clinic: 2009, Q3, P18; 2006, Q2, P24,25

799.1 Respiratory arrest
Cardiorespiratory failure

> **Excludes** *cardiac arrest (427.5)*
> *failure of peripheral circulation (785.50)*
> *respiratory distress:*
> *NOS (786.09)*
> *acute (518.82)*
> *following trauma or surgery (518.5)*
> *newborn (770.89)*
> *syndrome (newborn) (769)*
> *adult (following trauma or surgery) (518.5)*
> *other (518.82)*
> *respiratory failure (518.81, 518.83–518.84)*
> *newborn (770.84)*
> *respiratory insufficiency (786.09)*
> *acute (518.82)*

● **799.2 Signs and symptoms involving emotional state**

> **Excludes** *anxiety (293.84, 300.00-300.09)*
> *depression (311)*

799.21 Nervousness
Nervous
Coding Clinic: 2009, Q4, P120

799.22 Irritability
Irritable
Coding Clinic: 2009, Q4, P120

799.23 Impulsiveness
Impulsive

> **Excludes** *impulsive neurosis (300.3)*

799.24 Emotional lability

799.25 Demoralization and apathy
Apathetic

799.29 Other signs and symptoms involving emotional state

799.3 Debility, unspecified

> **Excludes** *asthenia (780.79)*
> *nervous debility (300.5)*
> *neurasthenia (300.5)*
> *senile asthenia (797)*

Coding Clinic: 1997, Q3, P11-12

799.4 Cachexia
Wasting disease

Code first underlying condition, if known

Coding Clinic: 2006, Q3, P14-15x2; 1990, Q3, P17

● **799.5 Signs and symptoms involving cognition** ◄

> **Excludes** *amnesia (780.93)* ◄
> *amnestic syndrome (294.0)* ◄
> *attention deficit disorder (314.00-314.01)* ◄
> *late effects of cerebrovascular disease (438)* ◄
> *memory loss (780.93)* ◄
> *mild cognitive impairment, so stated (331.83)* ◄
> *specific problems in developmental delay (315.00-315.9)* ◄
> *transient global amnesia (437.7)* ◄
> *visuospatial neglect 781.8* ◄

799.51 Attention or concentration deficit ◄

799.52 Cognitive communication deficit ◄

799.53 Visuospatial deficit ◄

799.54 Psychomotor deficit ◄

799.55 Frontal lobe and executive function deficit ◄

799.59 Other signs and symptoms involving cognition ◄

● **799.8 Other ill-defined conditions**

799.81 Decreased libido
Decreased sexual desire

> **Excludes** *psychosexual dysfunction with inhibited sexual desire (302.71)*

Coding Clinic: 2003, Q4, P75-76; Q4, P75-76

799.82 Apparent life threatening event in infant
ALTE
Apparent life threatening event in newborn and infant

Code first confirmed diagnosis, if known ◄

Use additional code(s) for associated signs and symptoms if no confirmed diagnosis established, or if signs and symptoms are not associated routinely with confirmed diagnosis, or provide additional information for cause of ALTE ◄

> ~~**Excludes** signs and symptoms associated with a confirmed diagnosis--code to confirmed diagnosis~~

799.89 Other ill-defined conditions

799.9 Other unknown and unspecified cause
Undiagnosed disease, not specified as to site or system involved
Unknown cause of morbidity or mortality
Coding Clinic: 1998, Q1, P4; 1990, Q1, P22

◄ New   ⬅ Revised   ~~deleted~~ Deleted   Excludes   Includes   Use additional   Code first   Omit code
● Unacceptable Principal Diagnosis   ● Use Additional Digit(s)   OGCR Official Guidelines   Coding Clinic

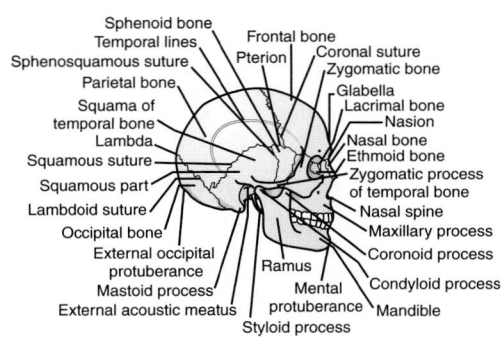

Figure 17-1 Lateral view of skull.

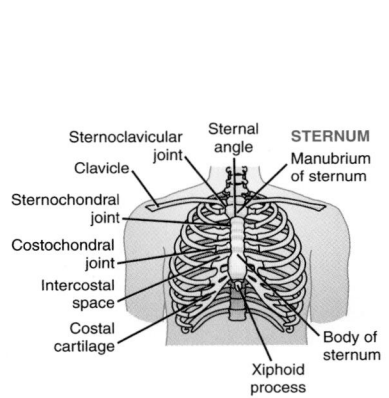

Figure 17-2 Frontal view of skull.

Figure 17-3 Anterior view of vertebral column.

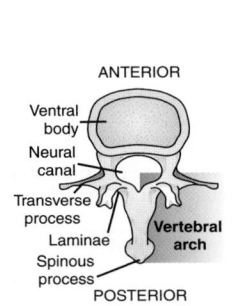

Figure 17-4 Vertebra viewed from above.

Figure 17-5 Anterior view of rib cage.

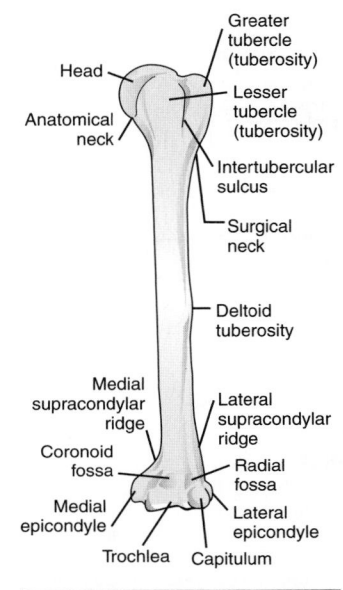

Figure 17-6 Anterior aspect of left humerus.

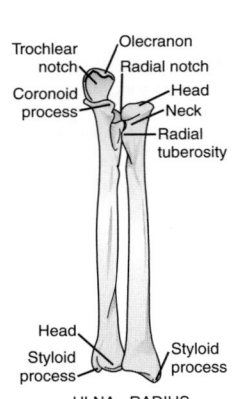

Figure 17-7 Anterior aspect of left radius and ulna.

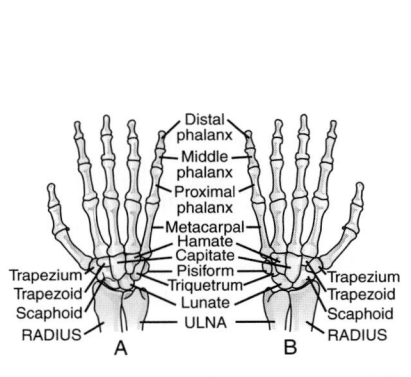

Figure 17-8 Right hand and wrist: **A.** Dorsal surface. **B.** Palmar surface.

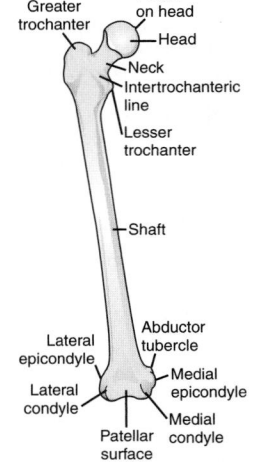

Figure 17-9 Anterior aspect of right femur.

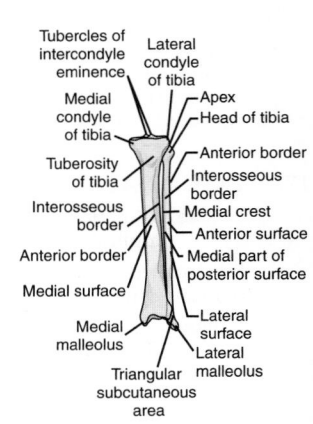

Figure 17-10 Anterior aspect of left tibia and fibula.

INJURY AND POISONING (800–999)

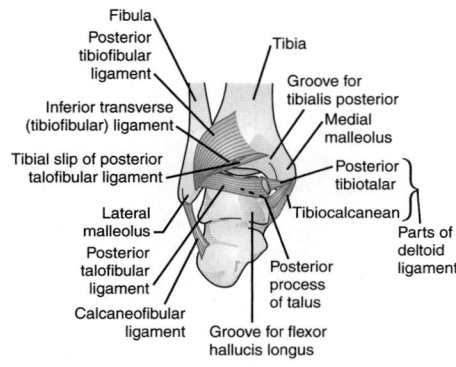

Figure 17–11 Posterior aspect of the left ankle joint.

Figure 17–12 Right foot viewed from above.

OGCR Section I.C.17.a

When coding injuries, assign separate codes for each injury unless a combination code is provided, in which case the combination code is assigned. Multiple injury codes are provided in ICD-9-CM, but should not be assigned unless information for a more specific code is not available. These traumatic injury codes are not to be used for normal, healing surgical wounds or to identify complications of surgical wounds.

The code for the most serious injury, as determined by the provider and the focus of treatment, is sequenced first.

1) **Superficial injuries:** Superficial injuries such as abrasions or contusions are not coded when associated with more severe injuries of the same site.

2) **Primary injury with damage to nerves/blood vessels:** When a primary injury results in minor damage to peripheral nerves or blood vessels, the primary injury is sequenced first with additional code(s) from categories 950-957, Injury to nerves and spinal cord, and/or 900-904, Injury to blood vessels. When the primary injury is to the blood vessels or nerves, that injury should be sequenced first.

17. INJURY AND POISONING (800–999)

Use additional code for retained foreign body, if applicable, V90.01-V90.9) ◄

Use E code(s) to identify the cause and intent of the injury or poisoning (E800–E999)

Note:

1. The principle of multiple coding of injuries should be followed wherever possible. Combination categories for multiple injuries are provided for use when there is insufficient detail as to the nature of the individual conditions, or for primary tabulation purposes when it is more convenient to record a single code; otherwise, the component injuries should be coded separately.

Where multiple sites of injury are specified in the titles, the word "with" indicates involvement of both sites, and the word "and" indicates involvement of either or both sites. The word "finger" includes thumb.

2. Categories for "late effect" of injuries are to be found at 905–909.

FRACTURES (800–829)

Excludes *malunion (733.81)*
nonunion (733.82)
pathologic or spontaneous fracture (733.10–733.19)
stress fracture (733.93–733.95)

The terms "condyle," "coronoid process," "ramus," and "symphysis" indicate the portion of the bone fractured, not the name of the bone involved.

The descriptions "closed" and "open" used in the fourth-digit subdivisions include the following terms:
closed (with or without delayed healing):
  comminuted
  depressed
  elevated
  fissured
  fracture NOS
  greenstick
  impacted
  linear
  simple
  slipped epiphysis
  spiral
open (with or without delayed healing):
  compound
  infected
  missile
  puncture
  with foreign body

Note: A fracture not indicated as closed or open should be classified as closed.

FRACTURE OF SKULL (800–804)

Includes *traumatic brain injury due to fracture of skull*

The following fifth-digit subclassification is for use with the appropriate codes in categories 800, 801, 803, and 804:

0 **unspecified state of consciousness**
1 **with no loss of consciousness**
2 **with brief [less than one hour] loss of consciousness**
3 **with moderate [1–24 hours] loss of consciousness**
4 **with prolonged [more than 24 hours] loss of consciousness and return to pre-existing conscious level**
5 **with prolonged [more than 24 hours] loss of consciousness, without return to pre-existing conscious level**
    Use fifth-digit 5 to designate when a patient is unconscious and dies before regaining consciousness, regardless of the duration of the loss of consciousness
6 **with loss of consciousness of unspecified duration**
9 **with concussion, unspecified**

◄ New   ◄ Revised   ~~deleted~~ Deleted   Excludes   Includes   Use additional   Code first   Omit code
● Unacceptable Principal Diagnosis   ● Use Additional Digit(s)   **OGCR** Official Guidelines   **Coding Clinic**

● 800 **Fracture of vault of skull**

Requires fifth digit. See beginning of section 800–804 for codes and definitions.

| **Includes** | frontal bone |
| | parietal bone |

● **800.0 Closed without mention of intracranial injury**
[0-6,9]

● **800.1 Closed with cerebral laceration and contusion**
[0-6,9]

● **800.2 Closed with subarachnoid, subdural, and extradural**
[0-6,9] **hemorrhage**

● **800.3 Closed with other and unspecified intracranial**
[0-6,9] **hemorrhage**

● **800.4 Closed with intracranial injury of other and**
[0-6,9] **unspecified nature**

● **800.5 Open without mention of intracranial injury**
[0-6,9]

● **800.6 Open with cerebral laceration and contusion**
[0-6,9]

● **800.7 Open with subarachnoid, subdural, and extradural**
[0-6,9] **hemorrhage**

● **800.8 Open with other and unspecified intracranial**
[0-6,9] **hemorrhage**

● **800.9 Open with intracranial injury of other and**
[0-6,9] **unspecified nature**

● 801 **Fracture of base of skull**

Requires fifth digit. See beginning of section 800–804 for codes and definitions.

Includes	fossa:
	anterior
	middle
	posterior
	occiput bone
	orbital roof
	sinus:
	ethmoid
	frontal
	sphenoid bone
	temporal bone

● **801.0 Closed without mention of intracranial**
[0-6,9] **injury**

● **801.1 Closed with cerebral laceration and contusion**
[0-6,9]   Coding Clinic: 1996, Q4, P36.37

● **801.2 Closed with subarachnoid, subdural, and extradural**
[0-6,9] **hemorrhage**

● **801.3 Closed with other and unspecified intracranial**
[0-6,9] **hemorrhage**

● **801.4 Closed with intracranial injury of other and**
[0-6,9] **unspecified nature**

● **801.5 Open without mention of intracranial injury**
[0-6,9]

● **801.6 Open with cerebral laceration and contusion**
[0-6,9]

● **801.7 Open with subarachnoid, subdural, and extradural**
[0-6,9] **hemorrhage**

● **801.8 Open with other and unspecified intracranial**
[0-6,9] **hemorrhage**

● **801.9 Open with intracranial injury of other and**
[0-6,9] **unspecified nature**

● 802 **Fracture of face bones**

802.0 Nasal bones, closed

802.1 Nasal bones, open

● **802.2 Mandible, closed**
Inferior maxilla
Lower jaw (bone)

    802.20 Unspecified site

    802.21 Condylar process

    802.22 Subcondylar

    802.23 Coronoid process

    802.24 Ramus, unspecified

    802.25 Angle of jaw

    802.26 Symphysis of body

    802.27 Alveolar border of body

    802.28 Body, other and unspecified

    802.29 Multiple sites

● **802.3 Mandible, open**

    802.30 Unspecified site

    802.31 Condylar process

    802.32 Subcondylar

    802.33 Coronoid process

    802.34 Ramus, unspecified

    802.35 Angle of jaw

    802.36 Symphysis of body

    802.37 Alveolar border of body

    802.38 Body, other and unspecified

    802.39 Multiple sites

    802.4 Malar and maxillary bones, closed
| Superior maxilla | Zygoma |
| Upper jaw (bone) | Zygomatic arch |

    802.5 Malar and maxillary bones, open

    802.6 Orbital floor (blow-out), closed

    802.7 Orbital floor (blow-out), open

    802.8 Other facial bones, closed
Alveolus
Orbit:
  NOS
  part other than roof or floor
Palate

Excludes	*orbital:*
	floor (802.6)
	roof (801.0–801.9)

    802.9 Other facial bones, open

● 803 **Other and unqualified skull fractures**

Requires fifth digit. See beginning of section 800–804 for codes and definitions.

| **Includes** | skull NOS |
| | skull multiple NOS |

● **803.0 Closed without mention of intracranial injury**
[0-6,9]

● **803.1 Closed with cerebral laceration and contusion**
[0-6,9]

● **803.2 Closed with subarachnoid, subdural, and extradural**
[0-6,9] **hemorrhage**

● **803.3 Closed with other and unspecified intracranial**
[0-6,9] **hemorrhage**

● **803.4 Closed with intracranial injury of other and**
[0-6,9] **unspecified nature**

● **803.5 Open without mention of intracranial injury**
[0-6,9]

● **803.6 Open with cerebral laceration and contusion**
[0-6,9]

● **803.7 Open with subarachnoid, subdural, and extradural**
[0-6,9] **hemorrhage**

INJURY AND POISONING (800–999)

● **803.8 Open with other and unspecified intracranial**
[0-6,9] **hemorrhage**

● **803.9 Open with intracranial injury of other and**
[0-6,9] **unspecified nature**

● **804 Multiple fractures involving skull or face with other bones**

Requires fifth digit. See beginning of section 800–804 for codes and definitions.

● **804.0 Closed without mention of intracranial injury**
[0-6,9]

● **804.1 Closed with cerebral laceration and contusion**
[0-6,9]   Coding Clinic: 2006, Q1, P6-7

● **804.2 Closed with subarachnoid, subdural, and extradural**
[0-6,9] **hemorrhage**

● **804.3 Closed with other and unspecified intracranial**
[0-6,9] **hemorrhage**

● **804.4 Closed with intracranial injury of other and**
[0-6,9] **unspecified nature**

● **804.5 Open without mention of intracranial injury**
[0-6,9]

● **804.6 Open with cerebral laceration and contusion**
[0-6,9]

● **804.7 Open with subarachnoid, subdural, and extradural**
[0-6,9] **hemorrhage**

● **804.8 Open with other and unspecified intracranial**
[0-6,9] **hemorrhage**

● **804.9 Open with intracranial injury of other and**
[0-6,9] **unspecified nature**

FRACTURE OF NECK AND TRUNK (805–809)

● **805 Fracture of vertebral column without mention of spinal cord injury**

> **Includes**   neural arch
>   spine
>   spinous process
>   transverse process
>   vertebra
> Coding Clinic: 1985, Nov-Dec, P16

The following fifth-digit subclassification is for use with codes 805.0–805.1:

> 0   **cervical vertebra, unspecified level**
> 1   **first cervical vertebra**
> 2   **second cervical vertebra**
> 3   **third cervical vertebra**
> 4   **fourth cervical vertebra**
> 5   **fifth cervical vertebra**
> 6   **sixth cervical vertebra**
> 7   **seventh cervical vertebra**
> 8   **multiple cervical vertebrae**

● **805.0 Cervical, closed**
[0-8]   Atlas
        Axis

● **805.1 Cervical, open**
[0-8]

805.2 Dorsal [thoracic], closed

805.3 Dorsal [thoracic], open

805.4 Lumbar, closed
      Coding Clinic: 2007, Q1, P3-8

805.5 Lumbar, open

805.6 Sacrum and coccyx, closed

805.7 Sacrum and coccyx, open

805.8 Unspecified, closed

805.9 Unspecified, open

● **806 Fracture of vertebral column with spinal cord injury**

> **Includes**   any condition classifiable to 805 with:
>   complete or incomplete transverse lesion (of cord)
>   hematomyelia
>   injury to:
>   cauda equina
>   nerve
>   paralysis
>   paraplegia
>   quadriplegia
>   spinal concussion

● **806.0 Cervical, closed**

806.00 C_1-C_4 level with unspecified spinal cord injury
> Cervical region NOS with spinal cord injury NOS

806.01 C_1-C_4 level with complete lesion of cord

806.02 C_1-C_4 level with anterior cord syndrome

806.03 C_1-C_4 level with central cord syndrome

806.04 C_1-C_4 level with other specified spinal cord injury
> C_1-C_4 level with:
>   incomplete spinal cord lesion NOS
>   posterior cord syndrome

806.05 C_5-C_7 level with unspecified spinal cord injury

806.06 C_5-C_7 level with complete lesion of cord

806.07 C_5-C_7 level with anterior cord syndrome

806.08 C_5-C_7 level with central cord syndrome

806.09 C_5-C_7 level with other specified spinal cord injury
> C_5-C_7 level with:
>   incomplete spinal cord lesion NOS
>   posterior cord syndrome

● **806.1 Cervical, open**

806.10 C_1-C_4 level with unspecified spinal cord injury

806.11 C_1-C_4 level with complete lesion of cord

806.12 C_1-C_4 level with anterior cord syndrome

806.13 C_1-C_4 level with central cord syndrome

806.14 C_1-C_4 level with other specified spinal cord injury
> C_1-C_4 level with:
>   incomplete spinal cord lesion NOS
>   posterior cord syndrome

806.15 C_5-C_7 level with unspecified spinal cord injury

806.16 C_5-C_7 level with complete lesion of cord

806.17 C_5-C_7 level with anterior cord syndrome

806.18 C_5-C_7 level with central cord syndrome

806.19 C_5-C_7 level with other specified spinal cord injury
> C_5-C_7 level with:
>   incomplete spinal cord lesion NOS
>   posterior cord syndrome

● **806.2 Dorsal [thoracic], closed**

806.20 T_1-T_6 level with unspecified spinal cord injury
> Thoracic region NOS with spinal cord injury NOS

806.21 T_1-T_6 level with complete lesion of cord

806.22 T_1-T_6 level with anterior cord syndrome

806.23 T_1-T_6 level with central cord syndrome

806.24 T_1-T_6 level with other specified spinal cord injury
> T_1-T_6 level with:
>> incomplete spinal cord lesion NOS
>> posterior cord syndrome

806.25 T_7-T_{12} level with unspecified spinal cord injury

806.26 T_7-T_{12} level with complete lesion of cord

806.27 T_7-T_{12} level with anterior cord syndrome

806.28 T_7-T_{12} level with central cord syndrome

806.29 T_7-T_{12} level with other specified spinal cord injury
> T_7-T_{12} level with:
>> incomplete spinal cord lesion NOS
>> posterior cord syndrome

● 806.3   **Dorsal [thoracic], open**

806.30 T_1-T_6 level with unspecified spinal cord injury

806.31 T_1-T_6 level with complete lesion of cord

806.32 T_1-T_6 level with anterior cord syndrome

806.33 T_1-T_6 level with central cord syndrome

806.34 T_1-T_6 level with other specified spinal cord injury
> T_1-T_6 level with:
>> incomplete spinal cord lesion NOS
>> posterior cord syndrome

806.35 T_7-T_{12} level with unspecified spinal cord injury

806.36 T_7-T_{12} level with complete lesion of cord

806.37 T_7-T_{12} level with anterior cord syndrome

806.38 T_7-T_{12} level with central cord syndrome

806.39 T_7-T_{12} level with other specified spinal cord injury
> T_7-T_{12} level with:
>> incomplete spinal cord lesion NOS
>> posterior cord syndrome

806.4   **Lumbar, closed**
> Coding Clinic: 1999, Q4, P11-13

806.5   **Lumbar, open**

● 806.6   **Sacrum and coccyx, closed**

806.60   With unspecified spinal cord injury

806.61   With complete cauda equina lesion

806.62   With other cauda equina injury

806.69   With other spinal cord injury

● 806.7   **Sacrum and coccyx, open**

806.70   With unspecified spinal cord injury

806.71   With complete cauda equina lesion

806.72   With other cauda equina injury

806.79   With other spinal cord injury

806.8   **Unspecified, closed**

806.9   **Unspecified, open**

● 807   **Fracture of rib(s), sternum, larynx, and trachea**

The following fifth-digit subclassification is for use with codes 807.0–807.1:

> 0   rib(s), unspecified
> 1   one rib
> 2   two ribs
> 3   three ribs
> 4   four ribs
> 5   five ribs
> 6   six ribs
> 7   seven ribs
> 8   eight or more ribs
> 9   multiple ribs, unspecified

● 807.0   **Rib(s), closed**
[0-9]

● 807.1   **Rib(s), open**
[0-9]

807.2   **Sternum, closed**

807.3   **Sternum, open**

807.4   **Flail chest**
> *Unstable chest due to sternum and/or rib fracture*

807.5   **Larynx and trachea, closed**
> Hyoid bone
> Thyroid cartilage
> Trachea

807.6   **Larynx and trachea, open**

● 808   **Fracture of pelvis**

808.0   **Acetabulum, closed**

808.1   **Acetabulum, open**

808.2   **Pubis, closed**
> Coding Clinic: 2008, Q1, P9-10

808.3   **Pubis, open**

● 808.4   **Other specified part, closed**

808.41   Ilium

808.42   Ischium

808.43   Multiple pelvic fractures with disruption of pelvic circle
> Coding Clinic: 2008, Q1, P9-10

808.49   Other
> Innominate bone
> Pelvic rim

● 808.5   **Other specified part, open**

808.51   Ilium

808.52   Ischium

808.53   Multiple pelvic fractures with disruption of pelvic circle

808.59   Other

808.8   **Unspecified, closed**

808.9   **Unspecified, open**

● 809   **Ill-defined fractures of bones of trunk**

> **Includes**   bones of trunk with other bones except those of skull and face
> multiple bones of trunk

> **Excludes**   *multiple fractures of:*
>> *pelvic bones alone (808.0–808.9)*
>> *ribs alone (807.0–807.1, 807.4)*
>> *ribs or sternum with limb bones (819.0–819.1, 828.0–828.1)*
>> *skull or face with other bones (804.0–804.9)*

809.0   **Fracture of bones of trunk, closed**

809.1   **Fracture of bones of trunk, open**

INJURY AND POISONING (800–999)

INJURY AND POISONING (800–999)

FRACTURE OF UPPER LIMB (810–819)

● **810 Fracture of clavicle**

     Includes   collar bone
                    interligamentous part of clavicle

The following fifth-digit subclassification is for use with category 810:

0 unspecified part	2 shaft of clavicle
Clavicle NOS	3 acromial end of clavicle
1 sternal end of clavicle	

● **810.0 Closed**
     [0-3]

● **810.1 Open**
     [0-3]

● **811 Fracture of scapula**

     Includes   shoulder blade

The following fifth-digit subclassification is for use with category 811:

0   unspecified part
1   acromial process
Acromion (process)
2   coracoid process
3   glenoid cavity and neck of scapula
9   other

● **811.0 Closed**
     [0-3,9]

● **811.1 Open**
     [0-3,9]

● **812 Fracture of humerus**

● **812.0 Upper end, closed**

     812.00 Upper end, unspecified part
            Proximal end   Shoulder

     812.01 Surgical neck
            Neck of humerus NOS

     812.02 Anatomical neck

     812.03 Greater tuberosity

     812.09 Other
            Head   Upper epiphysis

● **812.1 Upper end, open**

     812.10 Upper end, unspecified part

     812.11 Surgical neck

     812.12 Anatomical neck

     812.13 Greater tuberosity

     812.19 Other

● **812.2 Shaft or unspecified part, closed**

     812.20 Unspecified part of humerus
            Humerus NOS   Upper arm NOS

     812.21 Shaft of humerus
            Coding Clinic: 2005, Q4, P127-129; 1999, Q3, P14-15

● **812.3 Shaft or unspecified part, open**

     812.30 Unspecified part of humerus

     812.31 Shaft of humerus

● **812.4 Lower end, closed**
            Distal end of humerus   Elbow

     812.40 Lower end, unspecified part

     812.41 Supracondylar fracture of humerus

     812.42 Lateral condyle
            External condyle

     812.43 Medial condyle
            Internal epicondyle

     812.44 Condyle(s), unspecified
            Articular process NOS
            Lower epiphysis

     812.49 Other
            Multiple fractures of lower end
            Trochlea

● **812.5 Lower end, open**

     812.50 Lower end, unspecified part

     812.51 Supracondylar fracture of humerus

     812.52 Lateral condyle

     812.53 Medial condyle

     812.54 Condyle(s), unspecified

     812.59 Other

● **813 Fracture of radius and ulna**

● **813.0 Upper end, closed**
            Proximal end

     813.00 Upper end of forearm, unspecified

     813.01 Olecranon process of ulna

     813.02 Coronoid process of ulna

     813.03 Monteggia's fracture

     813.04 Other and unspecified fractures of proximal end of ulna (alone)
            Multiple fractures of ulna, upper end

     813.05 Head of radius

     813.06 Neck of radius

     813.07 Other and unspecified fractures of proximal end of radius (alone)
            Multiple fractures of radius, upper end

     813.08 Radius with ulna, upper end [any part]

● **813.1 Upper end, open**

     813.10 Upper end of forearm, unspecified

     813.11 Olecranon process of ulna

     813.12 Coronoid process of ulna

     813.13 Monteggia's fracture

     813.14 Other and unspecified fractures of proximal end of ulna (alone)

     813.15 Head of radius

     813.16 Neck of radius

     813.17 Other and unspecified fractures of proximal end of radius (alone)

     813.18 Radius with ulna, upper end [any part]

● **813.2 Shaft, closed**

     813.20 Shaft, unspecified

     813.21 Radius (alone)

     813.22 Ulna (alone)

     813.23 Radius with ulna
            Coding Clinic: 2009, Q4, P120

● **813.3 Shaft, open**

     813.30 Shaft, unspecified

     813.31 Radius (alone)

     813.32 Ulna (alone)

     813.33 Radius with ulna

● **813.4 Lower end, closed**
Distal end

   813.40 Lower end of forearm, unspecified

   813.41 Colles' fracture
      Smith's fracture

   813.42 Other fractures of distal end of radius (alone)
      Dupuytren's fracture, radius
      Radius, lower end

   813.43 Distal end of ulna (alone)

Ulna:	Ulna:
head	lower epiphysis
lower end	styloid process

   813.44 Radius with ulna, lower end
      Coding Clinic: 2007, Q1, P3-8

   813.45 Torus fracture of radius (alone)
      Excludes *torus fracture of radius and ulna (813.47)*
      Coding Clinic: 2002, Q4, P70-71

   813.46 Torus fracture of ulna (alone)
      Excludes *torus fracture of radius and ulna (813.47)*

   813.47 Torus fracture of radius and ulna

● **813.5 Lower end, open**

   813.50 Lower end of forearm, unspecified

   813.51 Colles' fracture

   813.52 Other fractures of distal end of radius (alone)

   813.53 Distal end of ulna (alone)

   813.54 Radius with ulna, lower end

● **813.8 Unspecified part, closed**

   813.80 Forearm, unspecified

   813.81 Radius (alone)
      Coding Clinic: 1998, Q2, P19

   813.82 Ulna (alone)

   813.83 Radius with ulna

● **813.9 Unspecified part, open**

   813.90 Forearm, unspecified

   813.91 Radius (alone)

   813.92 Ulna (alone)

   813.93 Radius with ulna

● **814 Fracture of carpal bone(s)**

The following fifth-digit subclassification is for use with category 814:

> 0 **carpal bone, unspecified**
>   Wrist NOS
> 1 **navicular [scaphoid] of wrist**
> 2 **lunate [semilunar] bone of wrist**
> 3 **triquetral [cuneiform] bone of wrist**
> 4 **pisiform**
> 5 **trapezium bone [larger multangular]**
> 6 **trapezoid bone [smaller multangular]**
> 7 **capitate bone [os magnum]**
> 8 **hamate [unciform] bone**
> 9 **other**

● **814.0 Closed**
[0-9]

● **814.1 Open**
[0-9]

● **815 Fracture of metacarpal bone(s)**

   Includes hand [except finger]
            metacarpus

The following fifth-digit subclassification is for use with category 815:

> 0 **metacarpal bone(s), site unspecified**
> 1 **base of thumb [first] metacarpal**
>   Bennett's fracture
> 2 **base of other metacarpal bone(s)**
> 3 **shaft of metacarpal bone(s)**
> 4 **neck of metacarpal bone(s)**
> 9 **multiple sites of metacarpus**

● **815.0 Closed**
[0-4,9]   Coding Clinic: 1994, Q2, P6

● **815.1 Open**
[0-4,9]

● **816 Fracture of one or more phalanges of hand**
   Includes finger(s)
            thumb

The following fifth-digit subclassification is for use with category 816:

> 0 **phalanx or phalanges, unspecified**
> 1 **middle or proximal phalanx or phalanges**
> 2 **distal phalanx or phalanges**
> 3 **multiple sites**

● **816.0 Closed**
[0-3]

● **816.1 Open**
[0-3]   Coding Clinic: 2003, Q4, P76-78

● **817 Multiple fractures of hand bones**
   Includes metacarpal bone(s) with phalanx or phalanges
            of same hand

   817.0 Closed

   817.1 Open

● **818 Ill-defined fractures of upper limb**
   Includes arm NOS
            multiple bones of same upper limb

   Excludes *multiple fractures of:*
      metacarpal bone(s) with phalanx or phalanges (817.0–817.1)
      phalanges of hand alone (816.0–816.1)
      radius with ulna (813.0–813.9)

   818.0 Closed

   818.1 Open
   OGCR Section I.C.17.b.4

> Multiple fracture categories 819 and 828 classify bilateral fractures of both upper limbs (819) and both lower limbs (828), but without any detail at the fourth-digit level other than open and closed type of fractures.

● **819 Multiple fractures involving both upper limbs, and upper limb with rib(s) and sternum**
   Includes arm(s) with rib(s) or sternum
            both arms [any bones]

   819.0 Closed

   819.1 Open

INJURY AND POISONING (800–999)

FRACTURE OF LOWER LIMB (820–829)

● **820　Fracture of neck of femur**

● **820.0　Transcervical fracture, closed**

820.00　Intracapsular section, unspecified

820.01　Epiphysis (separation) (upper)
　　　　Transepiphyseal
　　　　Fracture and separation across growth plate

820.02　Midcervical section
　　　　Transcervical NOS
　　　　Coding Clinic: 2003, Q3, P12-13

820.03　Base of neck
　　　　Cervicotrochanteric section

820.09　Other
　　　　Head of femur　　　Subcapital

● **820.1　Transcervical fracture, open**

820.10　Intracapsular section, unspecified

820.11　Epiphysis (separation) (upper)

820.12　Midcervical section

820.13　Base of neck

820.19　Other

● **820.2　Pertrochanteric fracture, closed**

820.20　Trochanteric section, unspecified
　　　　Trochanter:
　　　　　NOS
　　　　　greater
　　　　　lesser

820.21　Intertrochanteric section
　　　　Coding Clinic: 1994, Q2, P6; 1984, May-June, P11

820.22　Subtrochanteric section

● **820.3　Pertrochanteric fracture, open**

820.30　Trochanteric section, unspecified

820.31　Intertrochanteric section

820.32　Subtrochanteric section

820.8　Unspecified part of neck of femur, closed
　　　　Hip NOS　　　　　Neck of femur NOS
　　　　Coding Clinic: 1994, Q2, P9; 1985, Nov-Dec, P16

820.9　Unspecified part of neck of femur, open

● **821　Fracture of other and unspecified parts of femur**

● **821.0　Shaft or unspecified part, closed**

821.00　Unspecified part of femur
　　　　Thigh　　　　　　Upper leg
　　　　Excludes　*hip NOS (820.8)*

821.01　Shaft
　　　　Coding Clinic: 2007, Q1, P3-8; 1999, Q1, P5

● **821.1　Shaft or unspecified part, open**

821.10　Unspecified part of femur

821.11　Shaft

● **821.2　Lower end, closed**
　　　　Distal end

821.20　Lower end, unspecified part

821.21　Condyle, femoral

821.22　Epiphysis, lower (separation)

821.23　Supracondylar fracture of femur

821.29　Other
　　　　Multiple fractures of lower end

821.3　Lower end, open

821.30　Lower end, unspecified part

821.31　Condyle, femoral

821.32　Epiphysis, lower (separation)

821.33　Supracondylar fracture of femur

821.39　Other

● **822　Fracture of patella**

822.0　Closed

822.1　Open

● **823　Fracture of tibia and fibula**

　　Excludes　*Dupuytren's fracture (824.4–824.5)*
　　　　　　　　ankle (824.4–824.5)
　　　　　　　　radius (813.42, 813.52)
　　　　　　　Pott's fracture (824.4–824.5)
　　　　　　　that involving ankle (824.0–824.9)

The following fifth-digit subclassification is for use with category 823:

　　0　tibia alone
　　1　fibula alone
　　2　fibula with tibia

● **823.0　Upper end, closed**
[0-2]　　Head　　　　　　　Tibia:
　　　　Proximal end　　　　condyles
　　　　　　　　　　　　　tuberosity

● **823.1　Upper end, open**
[0-2]

● **823.2　Shaft, closed**
[0-2]

● **823.3　Shaft, open**
[0-2]

● **823.4　Torus fracture**
[0-2]　　Coding Clinic: 2002, Q4, P70-71

● **823.8　Unspecified part, closed**
[0-2]　　Lower leg NOS
　　　　Coding Clinic: 1997, Q1, P8

● **823.9　Unspecified part, open**
[0-2]

● **824　Fracture of ankle**

824.0　Medial malleolus, closed
　　　　Tibia involving:
　　　　　ankle　　　　　　malleolus
　　　　Coding Clinic: 2004, Q1, P9

824.1　Medial malleolus, open

824.2　Lateral malleolus, closed
　　　　Fibula involving:
　　　　　ankle　　　　　　malleolus
　　　　Coding Clinic: 2002, Q2, P3

824.3　Lateral malleolus, open

824.4　Bimalleolar, closed
　　　　Dupuytren's fracture, fibula
　　　　Pott's fracture

824.5　Bimalleolar, open

824.6　Trimalleolar, closed
　　　　Lateral and medial malleolus with anterior or
　　　　　posterior lip of tibia

824.7　Trimalleolar, open

824.8　Unspecified, closed
　　　　Ankle NOS
　　　　Coding Clinic: 2000, Q3, P12; 1994, Q2, P7

824.9　Unspecified, open

◄ New　　◄▥ Revised　　~~deleted~~ Deleted　　Excludes　　Includes　　Use additional　　Code first　　Omit code
● Unacceptable Principal Diagnosis　　● Use Additional Digit(s)　　OGCR Official Guidelines　　Coding Clinic

● 825 **Fracture of one or more tarsal and metatarsal bones**

   825.0 **Fracture of calcaneus, closed**
       Heel bone   Os calcis

   825.1 **Fracture of calcaneus, open**

● 825.2 **Fracture of other tarsal and metatarsal bones, closed**

   825.20 **Unspecified bone(s) of foot [except toes]**
       Instep

   825.21 **Astragalus**
       Talus

   825.22 **Navicular [scaphoid], foot**

   825.23 **Cuboid**

   825.24 **Cuneiform, foot**

   825.25 **Metatarsal bone(s)**

   825.29 **Other**
       Tarsal with metatarsal bone(s) only
       | Excludes | *calcaneus (825.0)*
       Coding Clinic: 1994, Q2, P5

● 825.3 **Fracture of other tarsal and metatarsal bones, open**

   825.30 **Unspecified bone(s) of foot [except toes]**

   825.31 **Astragalus**

   825.32 **Navicular [scaphoid], foot**

   825.33 **Cuboid**

   825.34 **Cuneiform, foot**

   825.35 **Metatarsal bone(s)**

   825.39 **Other**

● 826 **Fracture of one or more phalanges of foot**
   | Includes | toe(s)

   826.0 **Closed**

   826.1 **Open**

● 827 **Other, multiple, and ill-defined fractures of lower limb**
   | Includes | leg NOS
       multiple bones of same lower limb
   | Excludes | *multiple fractures of:*
       ankle bones alone (824.4–824.9)
       phalanges of foot alone (826.0–826.1)
       tarsal with metatarsal bones (825.29, 825.39)
       tibia with fibula (823.0–823.9 with fifth-digit 2)

   827.0 **Closed**

   827.1 **Open**

● 828 **Multiple fractures involving both lower limbs, lower with upper limb, and lower limb(s) with rib(s) and sternum**
   | Includes | arm(s) with leg(s) [any bones]
       both legs [any bones]
       leg(s) with rib(s) or sternum

   OGCR Section I.C.17.b.4
   Multiple fracture categories 819 and 828 classify bilateral fractures of both upper limbs (819) and both lower limbs (828), but without any detail at the fourth-digit level other than open and closed type of fractures.

   828.0 **Closed**

   828.1 **Open**

● 829 **Fracture of unspecified bones**
   829.0 **Unspecified bone, closed**
   829.1 **Unspecified bone, open**

DISLOCATION (830–839)

| Includes | displacement
    subluxation
    Out of position

| Excludes | *congenital dislocation (754.0–755.8)*
    pathological dislocation (718.2)
    recurrent dislocation (718.3)

The descriptions "closed" and "open," used in the fourth-digit subdivisions, include the following terms:

closed:	open:
complete	compound
dislocation NOS	infected
partial	with foreign body
simple	
uncomplicated	

Note: A dislocation not indicated as closed or open should be classified as closed.

● 830 **Dislocation of jaw**
   | Includes | jaw (cartilage) (meniscus)
       mandible
       maxilla (inferior)
       temporomandibular (joint)

   830.0 **Closed dislocation**

   830.1 **Open dislocation**

● 831 **Dislocation of shoulder**
   | Excludes | *sternoclavicular joint (839.61, 839.71)*
       sternum (839.61, 839.71)

   The following fifth-digit subclassification is for use with category 831:

   > 0 **shoulder, unspecified**
   >   Humerus NOS
   > 1 **anterior dislocation of humerus**
   > 2 **posterior dislocation of humerus**
   > 3 **inferior dislocation of humerus**
   > 4 **acromioclavicular (joint)**
   >   Clavicle
   > 9 **other**
   >   Scapula

● 831.0 **Closed dislocation**
   [0-4,9] Coding Clinic: 1987, Nov-Dec, P7

● 831.1 **Open dislocation**
   [0-4,9]

Figure 17–13 Dislocation including displacement and subluxation. (From Grainger & Allison's Diagnostic Radiology: A Textbook of Medical Imaging, 4th ed. 2001, Churchill Livingstone.)

A   B

◀ New   ◀╫ Revised   ~~deleted~~ Deleted | Excludes | Includes   Use additional   Code first   Omit code
● Unacceptable Principal Diagnosis   ● Use Additional Digit(s)   **OGCR** Official Guidelines   **Coding Clinic**
981

● **832 Dislocation of elbow**

The following fifth-digit subclassification is for use with subcategories 832.0 and 832.1:

> 0 elbow unspecified
> 1 anterior dislocation of elbow
> 2 posterior dislocation of elbow
> 3 medial dislocation of elbow
> 4 lateral dislocation of elbow
> 9 other

● **832.0 Closed dislocation**
[0-4,9]

● **832.1 Open dislocation**
[0-4,9]

832.2 Nursemaid's elbow
Subluxation of radial head

● **833 Dislocation of wrist**

The following fifth-digit subclassification is for use with category 833:

> 0 wrist, unspecified part
>   Carpal (bone)
>   Radius, distal end
> 1 radioulnar (joint), distal
> 2 radiocarpal (joint)
> 3 midcarpal (joint)
> 4 carpometacarpal (joint)
> 5 metacarpal (bone), proximal end
> 9 other
>   Ulna, distal end

● **833.0 Closed dislocation**
[0-5,9]

● **833.1 Open dislocation**
[0-5,9]

● **834 Dislocation of finger**

> **Includes** finger(s)
> phalanx of hand
> thumb

The following fifth-digit subclassification is for use with category 834:

> 0 finger, unspecified part
> 1 metacarpophalangeal (joint)
>   Metacarpal (bone), distal end
> 2 interphalangeal (joint), hand

● **834.0 Closed dislocation**
[0-2]

● **834.1 Open dislocation**
[0-2]

● **835 Dislocation of hip**

The following fifth-digit subclassification is for use with category 835:

> 0 dislocation of hip, unspecified
> 1 posterior dislocation
> 2 obturator dislocation
> 3 other anterior dislocation

● **835.0 Closed dislocation**
[0-3]

● **835.1 Open dislocation**
[0-3]

● **836 Dislocation of knee**

> **Excludes** dislocation of knee:
> old or pathological (718.2)
> recurrent (718.3)
> internal derangement of knee joint (717.0–717.5, 717.8–717.9)
> old tear of cartilage or meniscus of knee (717.0–717.5, 717.8–717.9)

836.0 Tear of medial cartilage or meniscus of knee, current
Bucket handle tear:
NOS current injury
medial meniscus current injury

836.1 Tear of lateral cartilage or meniscus of knee, current

836.2 Other tear of cartilage or meniscus of knee, current
Tear of:
cartilage (semilunar) current injury, not specified as medial or lateral
meniscus current injury, not specified as medial or lateral

836.3 Dislocation of patella, closed

836.4 Dislocation of patella, open

● **836.5 Other dislocation of knee, closed**

836.50 Dislocation of knee, unspecified

836.51 Anterior dislocation of tibia, proximal end
Posterior dislocation of femur, distal end, closed ◀▥

836.52 Posterior dislocation of tibia, proximal end
Anterior dislocation of femur, distal end, closed ◀▥

836.53 Medial dislocation of tibia, proximal end

836.54 Lateral dislocation of tibia, proximal end

836.59 Other

● **836.6 Other dislocation of knee, open**

836.60 Dislocation of knee, unspecified

836.61 Anterior dislocation of tibia, proximal end
Posterior dislocation of femur, distal end, open ◀

836.62 Posterior dislocation of tibia, proximal end
Anterior dislocation of femur, distal end, open ◀

836.63 Medial dislocation of tibia, proximal end

836.64 Lateral dislocation of tibia, proximal end

836.69 Other

● **837 Dislocation of ankle**

> **Includes** astragalus   scaphoid, foot
> fibula, distal end   tibia, distal end
> navicular, foot

837.0 Closed dislocation

837.1 Open dislocation

◀ New   ◀▥ Revised   ~~deleted~~ Deleted   Excludes   Includes   Use additional   Code first   Omit code
● Unacceptable Principal Diagnosis   ● Use Additional Digit(s)   OGCR Official Guidelines   Coding Clinic

● **838 Dislocation of foot**

The following fifth-digit subclassification is for use with category 838:

> 0 foot, unspecified
> 1 tarsal (bone), joint unspecified
> 2 midtarsal (joint)
> 3 tarsometatarsal (joint)
> 4 metatarsal (bone), joint unspecified
> 5 metatarsophalangeal (joint)
> 6 interphalangeal (joint), foot
> 9 other
> > Phalanx of foot
> > Toe(s)

● **838.0 Closed dislocation**
[0-6,9]

● **838.1 Open dislocation**
[0-6,9]

● **839 Other, multiple, and ill-defined dislocations**
Coding Clinic: 1995, Q4, P51

● **839.0 Cervical vertebra, closed**
Cervical spine
Neck

839.00 Cervical vertebra, unspecified
839.01 First cervical vertebra
839.02 Second cervical vertebra
839.03 Third cervical vertebra
839.04 Fourth cervical vertebra
839.05 Fifth cervical vertebra
839.06 Sixth cervical vertebra
839.07 Seventh cervical vertebra
839.08 Multiple cervical vertebrae

● **839.1 Cervical vertebra, open**
839.10 Cervical vertebra, unspecified
839.11 First cervical vertebra
839.12 Second cervical vertebra
839.13 Third cervical vertebra
839.14 Fourth cervical vertebra
839.15 Fifth cervical vertebra
839.16 Sixth cervical vertebra
839.17 Seventh cervical vertebra
839.18 Multiple cervical vertebrae

● **839.2 Thoracic and lumbar vertebra, closed**
839.20 Lumbar vertebra
839.21 Thoracic vertebra
Dorsal [thoracic] vertebra

● **839.3 Thoracic and lumbar vertebra, open**
839.30 Lumbar vertebra
839.31 Thoracic vertebra

● **839.4 Other vertebra, closed**
839.40 Vertebra, unspecified site
Spine NOS
839.41 Coccyx
839.42 Sacrum
Sacroiliac (joint)
839.49 Other

● **839.5 Other vertebra, open**
839.50 Vertebra, unspecified site
839.51 Coccyx
839.52 Sacrum
839.59 Other

● **839.6 Other location, closed**
839.61 Sternum
Sternoclavicular joint
839.69 Other
Pelvis

● **839.7 Other location, open**
839.71 Sternum
839.79 Other

839.8 Multiple and ill-defined, closed
Arm
Back
Hand
Multiple locations, except fingers or toes alone
Other ill-defined locations
Unspecified location

839.9 Multiple and ill-defined, open

SPRAINS AND STRAINS OF JOINTS AND ADJACENT MUSCLES (840–848)

Includes avulsion of joint capsule, ligament, muscle, tendon ◄
hemarthrosis of joint capsule, ligament, muscle, tendon ◄
Bleeding into joint space
laceration of joint capsule, ligament, muscle, tendon ◄
rupture of joint capsule, ligament, muscle, tendon ◄
sprain of joint capsule, ligament, muscle, tendon ◄
strain of joint capsule, ligament, muscle, tendon ◄
tear of joint capsule, ligament, muscle, tendon ◄

Excludes *laceration of tendon in open wounds (880–884 and 890–894 with .2)*

● **840 Sprains and strains of shoulder and upper arm**
Sprains are an injury to ligaments when one or more is stretched/torn and strains are caused by twisting or pulling a muscle(s) or tendon.

840.0 Acromioclavicular (joint) (ligament)
840.1 Coracoclavicular (ligament)
840.2 Coracohumeral (ligament)
840.3 Infraspinatus (muscle) (tendon)
840.4 Rotator cuff (capsule)
> **Excludes** *complete rupture of rotator cuff, nontraumatic (727.61)*
840.5 Subscapularis (muscle)
840.6 Supraspinatus (muscle) (tendon)
840.7 Superior glenoid labrum lesion
SLAP lesion
Coding Clinic: 2001, Q4, P52
840.8 Other specified sites of shoulder and upper arm
840.9 Unspecified site of shoulder and upper arm
Arm NOS   Shoulder NOS

INJURY AND POISONING (800–999)

INJURY AND POISONING (800–999)

- 841   **Sprains and strains of elbow and forearm**
  - 841.0   **Radial collateral ligament**
  - 841.1   **Ulnar collateral ligament**
  - 841.2   **Radiohumeral (joint)**
  - 841.3   **Ulnohumeral (joint)**
  - 841.8   **Other specified sites of elbow and forearm**
  - 841.9   **Unspecified site of elbow and forearm**
    Elbow NOS

- 842   **Sprains and strains of wrist and hand**
  - 842.0   **Wrist**
    - 842.00   **Unspecified site**
    - 842.01   **Carpal (joint)**
    - 842.02   **Radiocarpal (joint) (ligament)**
    - 842.09   **Other**
      Radioulnar joint, distal
  - 842.1   **Hand**
    - 842.10   **Unspecified site**
    - 842.11   **Carpometacarpal (joint)**
    - 842.12   **Metacarpophalangeal (joint)**
    - 842.13   **Interphalangeal (joint)**
    - 842.19   **Other**
      Midcarpal (joint)

- 843   **Sprains and strains of hip and thigh**
  - 843.0   **Iliofemoral (ligament)**
  - 843.1   **Ischiocapsular (ligament)**
  - 843.8   **Other specified sites of hip and thigh**
  - 843.9   **Unspecified site of hip and thigh**
    Hip NOS   Thigh NOS

- 844   **Sprains and strains of knee and leg**
  - 844.0   **Lateral collateral ligament of knee**
  - 844.1   **Medial collateral ligament of knee**
  - 844.2   **Cruciate ligament of knee**
  - 844.3   **Tibiofibular (joint) (ligament), superior**
  - 844.8   **Other specified sites of knee and leg**
  - 844.9   **Unspecified site of knee and leg**
    Knee NOS   Leg NOS

- 845   **Sprains and strains of ankle and foot**
  - 845.0   **Ankle**
    - 845.00   **Unspecified site**
      Coding Clinic: 2002, Q2, P3
    - 845.01   **Deltoid (ligament), ankle**
      Internal collateral (ligament), ankle
    - 845.02   **Calcaneofibular (ligament)**
    - 845.03   **Tibiofibular (ligament), distal**
      Coding Clinic: 2004, Q1, P9
    - 845.09   **Other**
      Achilles tendon
  - 845.1   **Foot**
    - 845.10   **Unspecified site**
    - 845.11   **Tarsometatarsal (joint) (ligament)**
    - 845.12   **Metatarsophalangeal (joint)**
    - 845.13   **Interphalangeal (joint), toe**
    - 845.19   **Other**

- 846   **Sprains and strains of sacroiliac region**
  - 846.0   **Lumbosacral (joint) (ligament)**
  - 846.1   **Sacroiliac ligament**
  - 846.2   **Sacrospinatus (ligament)**
  - 846.3   **Sacrotuberous (ligament)**
  - 846.8   **Other specified sites of sacroiliac region**
  - 846.9   **Unspecified site of sacroiliac region**

- 847   **Sprains and strains of other and unspecified parts of back**
  - **Excludes**   *lumbosacral (846.0)*
  - 847.0   **Neck**
    Anterior longitudinal (ligament), cervical
    Atlanto-axial (joints)
    Atlanto-occipital (joints)
    Whiplash injury
    - **Excludes**   *neck injury NOS (959.09)*
      thyroid region (848.2)
  - 847.1   **Thoracic**
  - 847.2   **Lumbar**
  - 847.3   **Sacrum**
    Sacrococcygeal (ligament)
  - 847.4   **Coccyx**
  - 847.9   **Unspecified site of back**
    Back NOS

- 848   **Other and ill-defined sprains and strains**
  - 848.0   **Septal cartilage of nose**
  - 848.1   **Jaw**
    Temporomandibular (joint) (ligament)
  - 848.2   **Thyroid region**
    Cricoarytenoid (joint) (ligament)
    Cricothyroid (joint) (ligament)
    Thyroid cartilage
  - 848.3   **Ribs**
    Chondrocostal (joint) without mention of injury to sternum
    Costal cartilage without mention of injury to sternum
  - 848.4   **Sternum**
    - 848.40   **Unspecified site**
    - 848.41   **Sternoclavicular (joint) (ligament)**
    - 848.42   **Chondrosternal (joint)**
    - 848.49   **Other**
      Xiphoid cartilage
  - 848.5   **Pelvis**
    Symphysis pubis
    - **Excludes**   *that in childbirth (665.6)*
  - 848.8   **Other specified sites of sprains and strains**
  - 848.9   **Unspecified site of sprain and strain**

◀ New   ◀▥ Revised   ~~deleted~~ Deleted   Excludes   Includes   Use additional   Code first   Omit code
● Unacceptable Principal Diagnosis   ● Use Additional Digit(s)   OGCR Official Guidelines   Coding Clinic

INTRACRANIAL INJURY, EXCLUDING THOSE WITH SKULL FRACTURE (850–854)

Includes traumatic brain injury without skull fracture

Excludes *intracranial injury with skull fracture (800–801 and 803–804, except .0 and .5)*
open wound of head without intracranial injury (870.0–873.9)
skull fracture alone (800–801 and 803–804 with .0, .5)

Note: The description "with open intracranial wound," used in the fourth-digit subdivisions, includes those specified as open or with mention of infection or foreign body.

The following fifth-digit subclassification is for use with categories 851–854:

> 0 unspecified state of consciousness
> 1 with no loss of consciousness
> 2 with brief [less than one hour] loss of consciousness
> 3 with moderate [1–24 hours] loss of consciousness
> 4 with prolonged [more than 24 hours] loss of consciousness and return to pre-existing conscious level
> 5 with prolonged [more than 24 hours] loss of consciousness without return to pre-existing conscious level
>
> > Use fifth-digit 5 to designate when a patient is unconscious and dies before regaining consciousness, regardless of the duration of the loss of consciousness
> 6 with loss of consciousness of unspecified duration
> 9 with concussion, unspecified

● **850 Concussion**

Includes commotio cerebri

Excludes *concussion with:*
cerebral laceration or contusion (851.0–851.9)
cerebral hemorrhage (852–853)
head injury NOS (959.01)
Coding Clinic: 1993, Q1, P22-23

● **850.0 With no loss of consciousness**
Concussion with mental confusion or disorientation, without loss of consciousness
Coding Clinic: 1992, Q2, P5-6

● **850.1 With brief loss of consciousness**
Loss of consciousness for less than one hour
Coding Clinic: 2003, Q4, P76; 1999, Q1, P10; 1992, Q2, P5-6

   850.11 With loss of consciousness of 30 minutes or less

   850.12 With loss of consciousness from 31 to 59 minutes

● **850.2 With moderate loss of consciousness**
Loss of consciousness for 1–24 hours

● **850.3 With prolonged loss of consciousness and return to pre-existing conscious level**
Loss of consciousness for more than 24 hours with complete recovery

● **850.4 With prolonged loss of consciousness, without return to pre-existing conscious level**

● **850.5 With loss of consciousness of unspecified duration**

● **850.9 Concussion, unspecified**

● **851 Cerebral laceration and contusion**
Cerebral lacerations are tears in brain tissue. Cerebral contusions are bruises on brain.

Requires fifth digit. See beginning of section 850–854 for codes and definitions.
Coding Clinic: 1993, Q1, P22-23

● **851.0** **Cortex (cerebral) contusion without mention of open intracranial wound**
[0-6,9]

● **851.1** **Cortex (cerebral) contusion with open intracranial wound**
[0-6,9]

● **851.2** **Cortex (cerebral) laceration without mention of open intracranial wound**
[0-6,9]

● **851.3** **Cortex (cerebral) laceration with open intracranial wound**
[0-6,9]

● **851.4** **Cerebellar or brain stem contusion without mention of open intracranial wound**
[0-6,9]

● **851.5** **Cerebellar or brain stem contusion with open intracranial wound**
[0-6,9]

● **851.6** **Cerebellar or brain stem laceration without mention of open intracranial wound**
[0-6,9]

● **851.7** **Cerebellar or brain stem laceration with open intracranial wound**
[0-6,9]

● **851.8** **Other and unspecified cerebral laceration and contusion, without mention of open intracranial wound**
[0-6,9]
Brain (membrane) NOS
Coding Clinic: 1996, Q4, P36.37

● **851.9** **Other and unspecified cerebral laceration and contusion, with open intracranial wound**
[0-6,9]

● **852 Subarachnoid, subdural, and extradural hemorrhage, following injury**

Requires fifth digit. See beginning of section 850–854 for codes and definitions.

Excludes *cerebral contusion or laceration (with hemorrhage) (851.0–851.9)*

● **852.0** **Subarachnoid hemorrhage following injury without mention of open intracranial wound**
[0-6,9]
Middle meningeal hemorrhage following injury
Coding Clinic: 1991, Q3, P15-16

● **852.1** **Subarachnoid hemorrhage following injury with open intracranial wound**
[0-6,9]
Coding Clinic: 1991, Q3, P15-16

● **852.2** **Subdural hemorrhage following injury without mention of open intracranial wound**
[0-6,9]
Coding Clinic: 2007, Q4, P105-107; 1996, Q4, P43-44

● **852.3** **Subdural hemorrhage following injury with open intracranial wound**
[0-6,9]

● **852.4** **Extradural hemorrhage following injury without mention of open intracranial wound**
[0-6,9]
Epidural hematoma following injury

● **852.5** **Extradural hemorrhage following injury with open intracranial wound**
[0-6,9]

● **853 Other and unspecified intracranial hemorrhage following injury**

Requires fifth digit. See beginning of section 850–854 for codes and definitions.

● **853.0** **Without mention of open intracranial wound**
[0-6,9]
Cerebral compression due to injury
Intracranial hematoma following injury
Traumatic cerebral hemorrhage
Coding Clinic: 1990, Q3, P14

● **853.1** **With open intracranial wound**
[0-6,9]

INJURY AND POISONING (800–999)

INJURY AND POISONING (800-999)

● **854　Intracranial injury of other and unspecified nature**

Requires fifth digit. See beginning of section 850-854 for codes and definitions.

Includes　injury:
　　　brain NOS
　　　cavernous sinus
　　　intracranial
　　　traumatic brain NOS

Excludes　any condition classifiable to 850–853
　　　head injury NOS (959.01)

Coding Clinic: 1999, Q1, P10; 1992, Q2, P5-6

● **854.0　Without mention of open intracranial wound**
[0-6,9]　Coding Clinic: 2009, Q4, P120; 2005, Q2, P6-7

● **854.1　With open intracranial wound**
[0-6,9]

INTERNAL INJURY OF THORAX, ABDOMEN, AND PELVIS (860–869)

Includes　blast injuries of internal organs
　　　blunt trauma of internal organs
　　　bruise of internal organs
　　　concussion injuries (except cerebral) of
　　　　internal organs
　　　crushing of internal organs
　　　hematoma of internal organs
　　　laceration of internal organs
　　　puncture of internal organs
　　　tear of internal organs
　　　traumatic rupture of internal organs

Excludes　concussion NOS (850.0–850.9)
　　　flail chest (807.4)
　　　foreign body entering through orifice
　　　　(930.0–939.9)
　　　injury to blood vessels (901.0–902.9)

Note:　The description "with open wound," used in the fourth-digit subdivisions, includes those with mention of infection or foreign body.

● **860　Traumatic pneumothorax and hemothorax**

860.0　Pneumothorax without mention of open wound into thorax
Coding Clinic: 1993, Q2, P4-5

860.1　Pneumothorax with open wound into thorax
Coding Clinic: 1995, Q3, P17; 1993, Q2, P4-5

860.2　Hemothorax without mention of open wound into thorax

860.3　Hemothorax with open wound into thorax
Coding Clinic: 1995, Q3, P17

860.4　Pneumohemothorax without mention of open wound into thorax

860.5　Pneumohemothorax with open wound into thorax
Coding Clinic: 1995, Q3, P17

● **861　Injury to heart and lung**

Excludes　injury to blood vessels of thorax (901.0–901.9)
Coding Clinic: 1992, Q1, P9-10

● **861.0　Heart, without mention of open wound into thorax**

861.00　Unspecified injury

861.01　Contusion
　　　Cardiac contusion
　　　Myocardial contusion

861.02　Laceration without penetration of heart chambers

861.03　Laceration with penetration of heart chambers

● **861.1　Heart, with open wound into thorax**

861.10　Unspecified injury

861.11　Contusion

861.12　Laceration without penetration of heart chambers

861.13　Laceration with penetration of heart chambers

● **861.2　Lung, without mention of open wound into thorax**

861.20　Unspecified injury

861.21　Contusion

861.22　Laceration

● **861.3　Lung, with open wound into thorax**

861.30　Unspecified injury

861.31　Contusion

861.32　Laceration

● **862　Injury to other and unspecified intrathoracic organs**

Excludes　injury to blood vessels of thorax (901.0–901.9)

862.0　Diaphragm, without mention of open wound into cavity

862.1　Diaphragm, with open wound into cavity

● **862.2　Other specified intrathoracic organs, without mention of open wound into cavity**

862.21　Bronchus

862.22　Esophagus

862.29　Other
　　　Pleura
　　　Thymus gland

● **862.3　Other specified intrathoracic organs, with open wound into cavity**

862.31　Bronchus

862.32　Esophagus

862.39　Other

862.8　Multiple and unspecified intrathoracic organs, without mention of open wound into cavity
　　　Crushed chest
　　　Multiple intrathoracic organs

862.9　Multiple and unspecified intrathoracic organs, with open wound into cavity

---

Item 17-1　Pneumothorax is a collection of gas (positive air pressure) in the pleural space resulting in the lung collapsing. A tension pneumothorax is life-threatening and is a result of air in the pleural space causing a displacement in the mediastinal structures and cardiopulmonary function compromise. A traumatic pneumothorax results from blunt or penetrating injury that disrupts the parietal/visceral pleura. **Hemothorax** is blood or bloody fluid in the pleural cavity as a result of traumatic blood vessel rupture or inflammation of the lungs from pneumonia.

◀ New　　◀▥ Revised　　~~deleted~~ Deleted　　Excludes　　Includes　　Use additional　　Code first　　Omit code
● Unacceptable Principal Diagnosis　　● Use Additional Digit(s)　　OGCR Official Guidelines　　Coding Clinic

● **863 Injury to gastrointestinal tract**
Trauma to any structure from the stomach to the anus

> Excludes   *anal sphincter laceration during delivery (664.2)*
> *bile duct (868.0–868.1 with fifth-digit 2)*
> *gallbladder (868.0–868.1 with fifth-digit 2)*

863.0 **Stomach, without mention of open wound into cavity**

863.1 **Stomach, with open wound into cavity**

● 863.2 **Small intestine, without mention of open wound into cavity**

    863.20 **Small intestine, unspecified site**

    863.21 **Duodenum**

    863.29 **Other**

● 863.3 **Small intestine, with open wound into cavity**

    863.30 **Small intestine, unspecified site**

    863.31 **Duodenum**

    863.39 **Other**

● 863.4 **Colon or rectum, without mention of open wound into cavity**

    863.40 **Colon, unspecified site**

    863.41 **Ascending [right] colon**

    863.42 **Transverse colon**

    863.43 **Descending [left] colon**

    863.44 **Sigmoid colon**

    863.45 **Rectum**

    863.46 **Multiple sites in colon and rectum**

    863.49 **Other**

● 863.5 **Colon or rectum, with open wound into cavity**

    863.50 **Colon, unspecified site**

    863.51 **Ascending [right] colon**

    863.52 **Transverse colon**

    863.53 **Descending [left] colon**

    863.54 **Sigmoid colon**

    863.55 **Rectum**

    863.56 **Multiple sites in colon and rectum**

    863.59 **Other**

● 863.8 **Other and unspecified gastrointestinal sites, without mention of open wound into cavity**

    863.80 **Gastrointestinal tract, unspecified site**

    863.81 **Pancreas, head**

    863.82 **Pancreas, body**

    863.83 **Pancreas, tail**

    863.84 **Pancreas, multiple and unspecified sites**

    863.85 **Appendix**

    863.89 **Other**
       Intestine NOS

● 863.9 **Other and unspecified gastrointestinal sites, with open wound into cavity**

    863.90 **Gastrointestinal tract, unspecified site**

    863.91 **Pancreas, head**

    863.92 **Pancreas, body**

    863.93 **Pancreas, tail**

    863.94 **Pancreas, multiple and unspecified sites**

    863.95 **Appendix**

    863.99 **Other**

● **864 Injury to liver**

The following fifth-digit subclassification is for use with category 864:

> 0 **unspecified injury**
> 1 **hematoma and contusion**
> 2 **laceration, minor**
>   Laceration involving capsule only, or without significant involvement of hepatic parenchyma [i.e., less than 1 cm deep]
> 3 **laceration, moderate**
>   Laceration involving parenchyma but without major disruption of parenchyma [i.e., less than 10 cm long and less than 3 cm deep]
> 4 **laceration, major**
>   Laceration with significant disruption of hepatic parenchyma [i.e., 10 cm long and 3 cm deep]
>   Multiple moderate lacerations, with or without hematoma
>   Stellate lacerations of liver
> 5 **laceration, unspecified**
> 9 **other**

● 864.0 **Without mention of open wound into**
[0-5,9] **cavity**

● 864.1 **With open wound into cavity**
[0-5,9]

● **865 Injury to spleen**

The following fifth-digit subclassification is for use with category 865:

> 0 **unspecified injury**
> 1 **hematoma without rupture of capsule**
> 2 **capsular tears, without major disruption of parenchyma**
> 3 **laceration extending into parenchyma**
> 4 **massive parenchymal disruption**
> 9 **other**

● 865.0 **Without mention of open wound into**
[0-4,9] **cavity**

● 865.1 **With open wound into cavity**
[0-4,9]

● **866 Injury to kidney**

The following fifth-digit subclassification is for use with category 866:

> 0 **unspecified injury**
> 1 **hematoma without rupture of capsule**
> 2 **laceration**
> 3 **complete disruption of kidney parenchyma**

> Excludes   *acute kidney injury (nontraumatic) (584.9)*

● 866.0 **Without mention of open wound into cavity**
[0-3]   Coding Clinic: 2008, Q4, P192-193

● 866.1 **With open wound into cavity**
[0-3]

● **867 Injury to pelvic organs**

> Excludes   *injury during delivery (664.0–665.9)*

867.0 **Bladder and urethra, without mention of open wound into cavity**
    Coding Clinic: 2009, Q1, P8; 1985, Nov-Dec, P15; 1984, Nov-Dec, P15

867.1 **Bladder and urethra, with open wound into cavity**
    Coding Clinic: 1984, Nov-Dec, P12

867.2 **Ureter, without mention of open wound into cavity**

867.3 **Ureter, with open wound into cavity**

INJURY AND POISONING (800–999)

867.4 Uterus, without mention of open wound into cavity

867.5 Uterus, with open wound into cavity

867.6 Other specified pelvic organs, without mention of open wound into cavity
Fallopian tube　　　Seminal vesicle
Ovary　　　　　　　Vas deferens
Prostate

867.7 Other specified pelvic organs, with open wound into cavity

867.8 Unspecified pelvic organ, without mention of open wound into cavity

867.9 Unspecified pelvic organ, with open wound into cavity

● **868 Injury to other intra-abdominal organs**
The following fifth-digit subclassification is for use with category 868:

> 0　unspecified intra-abdominal organ
> 1　adrenal gland
> 2　bile duct and gallbladder
> 3　peritoneum
> 4　retroperitoneum
> 9　other and multiple intra-abdominal organs

● **868.0 Without mention of open wound into cavity**
[0-4,9]

● **868.1 With open wound into cavity**
[0-4,9]

● **869 Internal injury to unspecified or ill-defined organs**
Includes internal injury NOS
multiple internal injury NOS

869.0 Without mention of open wound into cavity

869.1 With open wound into cavity

OPEN WOUNDS (870–897)

Includes animal bite
avulsion
cut
laceration
puncture wound
traumatic amputation

Excludes *burn (940.0–949.5)*
crushing (925–929.9)
puncture of internal organs (860.0–869.1)
superficial injury (910.0–919.9)
that incidental to:
dislocation (830.0–839.9)
fracture (800.0–829.1)
internal injury (860.0–869.1)
intracranial injury (851.0–854.1)

Note: The description "complicated" used in the fourth-digit subdivisions includes those with mention of delayed healing, delayed treatment, foreign body, or infection.

OPEN WOUND OF HEAD, NECK, AND TRUNK (870–879)

● **870 Open wound of ocular adnexa**

870.0 Laceration of skin of eyelid and periocular area

870.1 Laceration of eyelid, full-thickness, not involving lacrimal passages

870.2 Laceration of eyelid involving lacrimal passages

870.3 Penetrating wound of orbit, without mention of foreign body

870.4 Penetrating wound of orbit with foreign body
Excludes *retained (old) foreign body in orbit (376.6)*

870.8 Other specified open wounds of ocular adnexa

870.9 Unspecified open wound of ocular adnexa

● **871 Open wound of eyeball**
Excludes *2nd cranial nerve [optic] injury (950.0–950.9)*
3rd cranial nerve [oculomotor] injury (951.0)

871.0 Ocular laceration without prolapse of intraocular tissue
Coding Clinic: 1996, Q3, P7

871.1 Ocular laceration with prolapse or exposure of intraocular tissue

871.2 Rupture of eye with partial loss of intraocular tissue

871.3 Avulsion of eye
Traumatic enucleation

871.4 Unspecified laceration of eye

871.5 Penetration of eyeball with magnetic foreign body
Excludes *retained (old) magnetic foreign body in globe (360.50–360.59)*

871.6 Penetration of eyeball with (nonmagnetic) foreign body
Excludes *retained (old) (nonmagnetic) foreign body in globe (360.60–360.69)*

871.7 Unspecified ocular penetration

871.9 Unspecified open wound of eyeball

● **872 Open wound of ear**

● **872.0 External ear, without mention of complication**
872.00 External ear, unspecified site
872.01 Auricle, ear
Pinna
872.02 Auditory canal

● **872.1 External ear, complicated**
872.10 External ear, unspecified site
872.11 Auricle, ear
872.12 Auditory canal

● **872.6 Other specified parts of ear, without mention of complication**
872.61 Ear drum
Drumhead
Tympanic membrane
872.62 Ossicles
872.63 Eustachian tube
872.64 Cochlea
872.69 Other and multiple sites

● **872.7 Other specified parts of ear, complicated**
872.71 Ear drum
872.72 Ossicles
872.73 Eustachian tube
872.74 Cochlea
872.79 Other and multiple sites

872.8 Ear, part unspecified, without mention of complication
Ear NOS

872.9 Ear, part unspecified, complicated

● 873 Other open wound of head

  873.0 Scalp, without mention of complication

  873.1 Scalp, complicated

● 873.2 Nose, without mention of complication

    873.20 Nose, unspecified site

    873.21 Nasal septum

    873.22 Nasal cavity

    873.23 Nasal sinus

    873.29 Multiple sites

● 873.3 Nose, complicated

    873.30 Nose, unspecified site

    873.31 Nasal septum

    873.32 Nasal cavity

    873.33 Nasal sinus

    873.39 Multiple sites

● 873.4 Face, without mention of complication

    873.40 Face, unspecified site

    873.41 Cheek

    873.42 Forehead
            Eyebrow
            Coding Clinic: 1996, Q4, P43-44

    873.43 Lip

    873.44 Jaw

    873.49 Other and multiple sites

● 873.5 Face, complicated

    873.50 Face, unspecified site

    873.51 Cheek

    873.52 Forehead

    873.53 Lip

    873.54 Jaw

    873.59 Other and multiple sites

● 873.6 Internal structures of mouth, without mention of complication

    873.60 Mouth, unspecified site

    873.61 Buccal mucosa

    873.62 Gum (alveolar process)

    873.63 Tooth (broken) (fractured) (due to trauma)
            | Excludes | *cracked tooth (521.81)*
            Coding Clinic: 2004, Q1, P17

    873.64 Tongue and floor of mouth

    873.65 Palate

    873.69 Other and multiple sites

● 873.7 Internal structures of mouth, complicated

    873.70 Mouth, unspecified site

    873.71 Buccal mucosa

    873.72 Gum (alveolar process)

    873.73 Tooth (broken) (fractured) (due to trauma)
            | Excludes | *cracked tooth (521.81)*
            Coding Clinic: 2004, Q1, P17

    873.74 Tongue and floor of mouth

    873.75 Palate

    873.79 Other and multiple sites

  873.8 Other and unspecified open wound of head without mention of complication
         Head NOS

  873.9 Other and unspecified open wound of head, complicated

● 874 Open wound of neck

● 874.0 Larynx and trachea, without mention of complication

    874.00 Larynx with trachea

    874.01 Larynx

    874.02 Trachea

● 874.1 Larynx and trachea, complicated

    874.10 Larynx with trachea

    874.11 Larynx

    874.12 Trachea

  874.2 Thyroid gland, without mention of complication

  874.3 Thyroid gland, complicated

  874.4 Pharynx, without mention of complication
         Cervical esophagus

  874.5 Pharynx, complicated

  874.8 Other and unspecified parts, without mention of complication
         Nape of neck   Throat NOS
         Supraclavicular region

  874.9 Other and unspecified parts, complicated

● 875 Open wound of chest (wall)
       | Excludes | *open wound into thoracic cavity (860.0–862.9)*
                    traumatic pneumothorax and hemothorax (860.1, 860.3, 860.5)
       Coding Clinic: 1995, Q3, P17

  875.0 Without mention of complication

  875.1 Complicated

● 876 Open wound of back
       | Includes | loin
                    lumbar region
       | Excludes | *open wound into thoracic cavity (860.0–862.9)*
                    traumatic pneumothorax and hemothorax (860.1, 860.3, 860.5)
       Coding Clinic: 1995, Q3, P17

  876.0 Without mention of complication
         Coding Clinic: 1993, Q2, P4-5

  876.1 Complicated

● 877 Open wound of buttock
       | Includes | sacroiliac region

  877.0 Without mention of complication

  877.1 Complicated

● 878 Open wound of genital organs (external), including traumatic amputation
       | Excludes | *injury during delivery (664.0–665.9)*
                    internal genital organs (867.0–867.9)

  878.0 Penis, without mention of complication

  878.1 Penis, complicated

  878.2 Scrotum and testes, without mention of complication

  878.3 Scrotum and testes, complicated

  878.4 Vulva, without mention of complication
         Labium (majus) (minus)

  878.5 Vulva, complicated

  878.6 Vagina, without mention of complication

  878.7 Vagina, complicated

  878.8 Other and unspecified parts, without mention of complication

  878.9 Other and unspecified parts, complicated

INJURY AND POISONING (800–999)

INJURY AND POISONING (800–999)

● 879 **Open wound of other and unspecified sites, except limbs**

879.0 **Breast, without mention of complication**

879.1 **Breast, complicated**

879.2 **Abdominal wall, anterior, without mention of complication**
Abdominal wall NOS	Pubic region
Epigastric region	Umbilical region
Hypogastric region	

879.3 **Abdominal wall, anterior, complicated**

879.4 **Abdominal wall, lateral, without mention of complication**
Flank	Iliac (region)
Groin	Inguinal region
Hypochondrium	

879.5 **Abdominal wall, lateral, complicated**

879.6 **Other and unspecified parts of trunk, without mention of complication**
| Pelvic region | Trunk NOS |
| Perineum | |

879.7 **Other and unspecified parts of trunk, complicated**

879.8 **Open wound(s) (multiple) of unspecified site(s) without mention of complication**
Multiple open wounds NOS
Open wound NOS

879.9 **Open wound(s) (multiple) of unspecified site(s), complicated**

OPEN WOUND OF UPPER LIMB (880–887)

● 880 **Open wound of shoulder and upper arm**

The following fifth-digit subclassification is for use with category 880:

> 0 **shoulder region**
> 1 **scapular region**
> 2 **axillary region**
> 3 **upper arm**
> 9 **multiple sites**

● 880.0 **Without mention of complication**
[0-3,9]

● 880.1 **Complicated**
[0-3,9]   Coding Clinic: 2006, Q2, P7

● 880.2 **With tendon involvement**
[0-3,9]

● 881 **Open wound of elbow, forearm, and wrist**

The following fifth-digit subclassification is for use with category 881:

> 0 **forearm**
> 1 **elbow**
> 2 **wrist**

● 881.0 **Without mention of complication**
[0-2]

● 881.1 **Complicated**
[0-2]

● 881.2 **With tendon involvement**
[0-2]

● 882 **Open wound of hand except finger(s) alone**

882.0 **Without mention of complication**

882.1 **Complicated**
Coding Clinic: 2008, Q4, P149-152

882.2 **With tendon involvement**

● 883 **Open wound of finger(s)**

Includes fingernail
thumb (nail)

883.0 **Without mention of complication**
Avulsion of fingernail reported with this code

883.1 **Complicated**

883.2 **With tendon involvement**

● 884 **Multiple and unspecified open wound of upper limb**

Includes arm NOS
multiple sites of one upper limb
upper limb NOS

884.0 **Without mention of complication**

884.1 **Complicated**

884.2 **With tendon involvement**

● 885 **Traumatic amputation of thumb (complete) (partial)**

Includes thumb(s) (with finger(s) of either hand)

885.0 **Without mention of complication**
Coding Clinic: 2003, Q1, P7

885.1 **Complicated**

● 886 **Traumatic amputation of other finger(s) (complete) (partial)**

Includes finger(s) of one or both hands, without mention of thumb(s)

886.0 **Without mention of complication**

886.1 **Complicated**

● 887 **Traumatic amputation of arm and hand (complete) (partial)**

887.0 **Unilateral, below elbow, without mention of complication**

887.1 **Unilateral, below elbow, complicated**

887.2 **Unilateral, at or above elbow, without mention of complication**

887.3 **Unilateral, at or above elbow, complicated**

887.4 **Unilateral, level not specified, without mention of complication**

887.5 **Unilateral, level not specified, complicated**

887.6 **Bilateral [any level], without mention of complication**
One hand and other arm

887.7 **Bilateral [any level], complicated**

OPEN WOUND OF LOWER LIMB (890–897)

● 890 **Open wound of hip and thigh**

890.0 **Without mention of complication**

890.1 **Complicated**

890.2 **With tendon involvement**

● 891 **Open wound of knee, leg [except thigh], and ankle**

Includes leg NOS
multiple sites of leg, except thigh

Excludes *that of thigh (890.0–890.2)*
with multiple sites of lower limb (894.0–894.2)

891.0 **Without mention of complication**

891.1 **Complicated**

891.2 **With tendon involvement**

● 892 **Open wound of foot except toe(s) alone**

Includes heel

892.0 **Without mention of complication**

892.1 **Complicated**
Coding Clinic: 1985, Sept-Oct, P10

892.2 **With tendon involvement**

● **893 Open wound of toe(s)**
   Includes   toenail
   893.0 **Without mention of complication**
   893.1 **Complicated**
      Coding Clinic: 2008, Q4, P69-73
   893.2 **With tendon involvement**

● **894 Multiple and unspecified open wound of lower limb**
   Includes   lower limb NOS
             multiple sites of one lower limb, with thigh
   894.0 **Without mention of complication**
   894.1 **Complicated**
   894.2 **With tendon involvement**

● **895 Traumatic amputation of toe(s) (complete) (partial)**
   Includes   toe(s) of one or both feet
   895.0 **Without mention of complication**
   895.1 **Complicated**

● **896 Traumatic amputation of foot (complete) (partial)**
   896.0 **Unilateral, without mention of complication**
   896.1 **Unilateral, complicated**
   896.2 **Bilateral, without mention of complication**
      Excludes *one foot and other leg (897.6–897.7)*
   896.3 **Bilateral, complicated**

● **897 Traumatic amputation of leg(s) (complete) (partial)**
   897.0 **Unilateral, below knee, without mention of complication**
   897.1 **Unilateral, below knee, complicated**
   897.2 **Unilateral, at or above knee, without mention of complication**
   897.3 **Unilateral, at or above knee, complicated**
   897.4 **Unilateral, level not specified, without mention of complication**
   897.5 **Unilateral, level not specified, complicated**
   897.6 **Bilateral [any level], without mention of complication**
      One foot and other leg
   897.7 **Bilateral [any level], complicated**

INJURY TO BLOOD VESSELS (900–904)

   Includes   arterial hematoma of blood vessel, secondary to other injuries, e.g., fracture or open wound
      avulsion of blood vessel, secondary to other injuries, e.g., fracture or open wound
      cut of blood vessel, secondary to other injuries, e.g., fracture or open wound
      laceration of blood vessel, secondary to other injuries, e.g., fracture or open wound
      rupture of blood vessel, secondary to other injuries, e.g., fracture or open wound
      traumatic aneurysm or fistula (arteriovenous) of blood vessel, secondary to other injuries, e.g., fracture or open wound
   Excludes *accidental puncture or laceration during medical procedure (998.2)*
      intracranial hemorrhage following injury (851.0–854.1)

● **900 Injury to blood vessels of head and neck**
  ● **900.0 Carotid artery**
     900.00 **Carotid artery, unspecified**
     900.01 **Common carotid artery**
     900.02 **External carotid artery**
     900.03 **Internal carotid artery**

     900.1 **Internal jugular vein**
  ● **900.8 Other specified blood vessels of head and neck**
     900.81 **External jugular vein**
       Jugular vein NOS
     900.82 **Multiple blood vessels of head and neck**
     900.89 **Other**
     900.9 **Unspecified blood vessel of head and neck**

● **901 Injury to blood vessels of thorax**
   Excludes *traumatic hemothorax (860.2–860.5)*
   901.0 **Thoracic aorta**
   901.1 **Innominate and subclavian arteries**
   901.2 **Superior vena cava**
   901.3 **Innominate and subclavian veins**
  ● **901.4 Pulmonary blood vessels**
     901.40 **Pulmonary vessel(s), unspecified**
     901.41 **Pulmonary artery**
     901.42 **Pulmonary vein**
  ● **901.8 Other specified blood vessels of thorax**
     901.81 **Intercostal artery or vein**
     901.82 **Internal mammary artery or vein**
     901.83 **Multiple blood vessels of thorax**
     901.89 **Other**
       Azygos vein
       Hemiazygos vein
     901.9 **Unspecified blood vessel of thorax**

● **902 Injury to blood vessels of abdomen and pelvis**
   902.0 **Abdominal aorta**
  ● **902.1 Inferior vena cava**
     902.10 **Inferior vena cava, unspecified**
     902.11 **Hepatic veins**
     902.19 **Other**
  ● **902.2 Celiac and mesenteric arteries**
     902.20 **Celiac and mesenteric arteries, unspecified**
     902.21 **Gastric artery**
     902.22 **Hepatic artery**
     902.23 **Splenic artery**
     902.24 **Other specified branches of celiac axis**
     902.25 **Superior mesenteric artery (trunk)**
     902.26 **Primary branches of superior mesenteric artery**
       Ileo-colic artery
     902.27 **Inferior mesenteric artery**
     902.29 **Other**
  ● **902.3 Portal and splenic veins**
     902.31 **Superior mesenteric vein and primary subdivisions**
       Ileo-colic vein
     902.32 **Inferior mesenteric vein**
     902.33 **Portal vein**
     902.34 **Splenic vein**
     902.39 **Other**
       Cystic vein
       Gastric vein
  ● **902.4 Renal blood vessels**
     902.40 **Renal vessel(s), unspecified**
     902.41 **Renal artery**
     902.42 **Renal vein**
     902.49 **Other**
       Suprarenal arteries

INJURY AND POISONING (800–999)

● **902.5 Iliac blood vessels**

    902.50 Iliac vessel(s), unspecified

    902.51 Hypogastric artery

    902.52 Hypogastric vein

    902.53 Iliac artery

    902.54 Iliac vein

    902.55 Uterine artery

    902.56 Uterine vein

    902.59 Other

● **902.8 Other specified blood vessels of abdomen and pelvis**

    902.81 Ovarian artery

    902.82 Ovarian vein

    902.87 Multiple blood vessels of abdomen and pelvis

    902.89 Other

902.9 Unspecified blood vessel of abdomen and pelvis

● **903 Injury to blood vessels of upper extremity**

  ● **903.0 Axillary blood vessels**

    903.00 Axillary vessel(s), unspecified

    903.01 Axillary artery

    903.02 Axillary vein

  903.1 Brachial blood vessels

  903.2 Radial blood vessels

  903.3 Ulnar blood vessels

  903.4 Palmar artery

  903.5 Digital blood vessels

  903.8 Other specified blood vessels of upper extremity
    Multiple blood vessels of upper extremity

  903.9 Unspecified blood vessel of upper extremity

● **904 Injury to blood vessels of lower extremity and unspecified sites**

  904.0 Common femoral artery
    Femoral artery above profunda origin
    Profunda = deep and posterior

  904.1 Superficial femoral artery

  904.2 Femoral veins

  904.3 Saphenous veins
    Saphenous vein (greater) (lesser)

  ● **904.4 Popliteal blood vessels**

    904.40 Popliteal vessel(s), unspecified

    904.41 Popliteal artery

    904.42 Popliteal vein

  ● **904.5 Tibial blood vessels**

    904.50 Tibial vessel(s), unspecified

    904.51 Anterior tibial artery

    904.52 Anterior tibial vein

    904.53 Posterior tibial artery

    904.54 Posterior tibial vein

  904.6 Deep plantar blood vessels

  904.7 Other specified blood vessels of lower extremity
    Multiple blood vessels of lower extremity

  904.8 Unspecified blood vessel of lower extremity

  904.9 Unspecified site
    Injury to blood vessel NOS

LATE EFFECTS OF INJURIES, POISONINGS, TOXIC EFFECTS, AND OTHER EXTERNAL CAUSES (905–909)

Note: These categories are to be used to indicate conditions classifiable to 800–999 as the cause of late effects, which are themselves classified elsewhere. The "late effects" include those specified as such, or as sequelae, which may occur at any time after the acute injury.

● **905 Late effects of musculoskeletal and connective tissue injuries**

  905.0 Late effect of fracture of skull and face bones
    Late effect of injury classifiable to 800–804
    Coding Clinic: 1997, Q3, P12-13

  905.1 Late effect of fracture of spine and trunk without mention of spinal cord lesion
    Late effects of injury classifiable to 805, 807–809
    Coding Clinic: 2007, Q1, P20-21

  905.2 Late effect of fracture of upper extremities
    Late effect of injury classifiable to 810–819

  905.3 Late effect of fracture of neck of femur
    Late effect of injury classifiable to 820

  905.4 Late effect of fracture of lower extremities
    Late effect of injury classifiable to 821–827
    Coding Clinic: 1995, Q1, P10; 1994, Q2, P7

  905.5 Late effect of fracture of multiple and unspecified bones
    Late effect of injury classifiable to 828–829

  905.6 Late effect of dislocation
    Late effect of injury classifiable to 830–839

  905.7 Late effect of sprain and strain without mention of tendon injury
    Late effect of injury classifiable to 840–848, except tendon injury

  905.8 Late effect of tendon injury
    Late effect of tendon injury due to:
      open wound [injury classifiable to 880–884 with .2, 890–894 with .2]
      sprain and strain [injury classifiable to 840–848]
    Coding Clinic: 1989, Q2, P15; Q2, P13

  905.9 Late effect of traumatic amputation
    Late effect of injury classifiable to 885–887, 895–897

Excludes	*late amputation stump complication (997.60–997.69)*

● **906 Late effects of injuries to skin and subcutaneous tissues**

  906.0 Late effect of open wound of head, neck, and trunk
    Late effect of injury classifiable to 870–879

  906.1 Late effect of open wound of extremities without mention of tendon injury
    Late effect of injury classifiable to 880–884, 890–894 except .2
    Coding Clinic: 1993, 5th Issue, P3

  906.2 Late effect of superficial injury
    Late effect of injury classifiable to 910–919

  906.3 Late effect of contusion
    Late effect of injury classifiable to 920–924

  906.4 Late effect of crushing
    Late effect of injury classifiable to 925–929

  906.5 Late effect of burn of eye, face, head, and neck
    Late effect of injury classifiable to 940–941
    Coding Clinic: 2004, Q4, P75-76

  906.6 Late effect of burn of wrist and hand
    Late effect of injury classifiable to 944

906.7 Late effect of burn of other extremities
Late effect of injury classifiable to 943 or 945

906.8 Late effect of burns of other specified sites
Late effect of injury classifiable to 942, 946–947

906.9 Late effect of burn of unspecified site
Late effect of injury classifiable to 948–949
OGCR Section I.C.17.c.7
Encounters for the treatment of the late effects of burns (i.e., scars or joint contractures) should be coded to the residual condition (sequelae) followed by the appropriate late effect code (906.5–906.9). A late effect E code may also be used, if desired.

● **907 Late effects of injuries to the nervous system**

907.0 Late effect of intracranial injury without mention of skull fracture
Late effect of injury classifiable to 850–854
Coding Clinic: 2009, Q4, P120; 2008, Q4, P102-109; 2003, Q4, P103-104; 1987, Nov-Dec, P12

907.1 Late effect of injury to cranial nerve
Late effect of injury classifiable to 950–951

907.2 Late effect of spinal cord injury
Late effect of injury classifiable to 806, 952
Coding Clinic: 2003, Q4, P103-104; 1998, Q4, P37-38; 1994, Q3, P4

907.3 Late effect of injury to nerve root(s), spinal plexus(es), and other nerves of trunk
Late effect of injury classifiable to 953–954
Coding Clinic: 2007, Q2, P13-15

907.4 Late effect of injury to peripheral nerve of shoulder girdle and upper limb
Late effect of injury classifiable to 955

907.5 Late effect of injury to peripheral nerve of pelvic girdle and lower limb
Late effect of injury classifiable to 956

907.9 Late effect of injury to other and unspecified nerve
Late effect of injury classifiable to 957

● **908 Late effects of other and unspecified injuries**

908.0 Late effect of internal injury to chest
Late effect of injury classifiable to 860–862

908.1 Late effect of internal injury to intra-abdominal organs
Late effect of injury classifiable to 863–866, 868

908.2 Late effect of internal injury to other internal organs
Late effect of injury classifiable to 867 or 869

908.3 Late effect of injury to blood vessel of head, neck, and extremities
Late effect of injury classifiable to 900, 903–904

908.4 Late effect of injury to blood vessel of thorax, abdomen, and pelvis
Late effect of injury classifiable to 901–902

908.5 Late effect of foreign body in orifice
Late effect of injury classifiable to 930–939

908.6 Late effect of certain complications of trauma
Late effect of complications classifiable to 958

908.9 Late effect of unspecified injury
Late effect of injury classifiable to 959
Coding Clinic: 2000, Q3, P4

● **909 Late effects of other and unspecified external causes**

909.0 Late effect of poisoning due to drug, medicinal or biological substance
Late effect of conditions classifiable to 960–979
Excludes *Late effect of adverse effect of drug, medicinal or biological substance (909.5)*
Coding Clinic: 2003, Q4, P103-104; 1984, Sept-Oct, P16

909.1 Late effect of toxic effects of nonmedical substances
Late effect of conditions classifiable to 980–989

909.2 Late effect of radiation
Late effect of conditions classifiable to 990
Coding Clinic: 1984, Nov-Dec, P19

909.3 Late effect of complications of surgical and medical care
Late effect of conditions classifiable to 996–999
Coding Clinic: 1993, Q1, P29

909.4 Late effect of certain other external causes
Late effect of conditions classifiable to 991–994

909.5 Late effect of adverse effect of drug, medicinal or biological substance
Excludes *late effect of poisoning due to drug, medicinal or biological substances (909.0)*

909.9 Late effect of other and unspecified external causes

SUPERFICIAL INJURY (910–919)

Excludes *burn (blisters) (940.0–949.5)*
contusion (920–924.9)
foreign body:
   granuloma (728.82)
   inadvertently left in operative wound (998.4)
   residual, in soft tissue (729.6)
insect bite, venomous (989.5)
open wound with incidental foreign body (870.0–897.7)

● **910 Superficial injury of face, neck, and scalp except eye**

Includes	cheek	lip
	ear	nose
	gum	throat

Excludes *eye and adnexa (918.0–918.9)*

910.0 Abrasion or friction burn without mention of infection

910.1 Abrasion or friction burn, infected

910.2 Blister without mention of infection

910.3 Blister, infected

910.4 Insect bite, nonvenomous, without mention of infection

910.5 Insect bite, nonvenomous, infected

910.6 Superficial foreign body (splinter) without major open wound and without mention of infection

910.7 Superficial foreign body (splinter) without major open wound, infected

910.8 Other and unspecified superficial injury of face, neck, and scalp without mention of infection

910.9 Other and unspecified superficial injury of face, neck, and scalp, infected

INJURY AND POISONING (800–999)

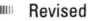

INJURY AND POISONING (800–999)

● 911   **Superficial injury of trunk**

     Includes   abdominal wall   interscapular region
                   anus   labium (majus) (minus)
                   back   penis
                   breast   perineum
                   buttock   scrotum
                   chest wall   testis
                   flank   vagina
                   groin   vulva

     Excludes   *hip (916.0–916.9)*
                   scapular region (912.0–912.9)

911.0   **Abrasion or friction burn without mention of infection**
        Coding Clinic: 2001, Q3, P10

911.1   **Abrasion or friction burn, infected**

911.2   **Blister without mention of infection**

911.3   **Blister, infected**

911.4   **Insect bite, nonvenomous, without mention of infection**

911.5   **Insect bite, nonvenomous, infected**

911.6   **Superficial foreign body (splinter) without major open wound and without mention of infection**

911.7   **Superficial foreign body (splinter) without major open wound, infected**

911.8   **Other and unspecified superficial injury of trunk without mention of infection**

911.9   **Other and unspecified superficial injury of trunk, infected**

● 912   **Superficial injury of shoulder and upper arm**

     Includes   axilla
                   scapular region

912.0   **Abrasion or friction burn without mention of infection**

912.1   **Abrasion or friction burn, infected**

912.2   **Blister without mention of infection**

912.3   **Blister, infected**

912.4   **Insect bite, nonvenomous, without mention of infection**

912.5   **Insect bite, nonvenomous, infected**

912.6   **Superficial foreign body (splinter) without major open wound and without mention of infection**

912.7   **Superficial foreign body (splinter) without major open wound, infected**

912.8   **Other and unspecified superficial injury of shoulder and upper arm without mention of infection**

912.9   **Other and unspecified superficial injury of shoulder and upper arm, infected**

● 913   **Superficial injury of elbow, forearm, and wrist**

913.0   **Abrasion or friction burn without mention of infection**

913.1   **Abrasion or friction burn, infected**

913.2   **Blister without mention of infection**

913.3   **Blister, infected**

913.4   **Insect bite, nonvenomous, without mention of infection**

913.5   **Insect bite, nonvenomous, infected**

913.6   **Superficial foreign body (splinter) without major open wound and without mention of infection**

913.7   **Superficial foreign body (splinter) without major open wound, infected**

913.8   **Other and unspecified superficial injury of elbow, forearm, and wrist without mention of infection**

913.9   **Other and unspecified superficial injury of elbow, forearm, and wrist, infected**

● 914   **Superficial injury of hand(s) except finger(s) alone**

914.0   **Abrasion or friction burn without mention of infection**

914.1   **Abrasion or friction burn, infected**

914.2   **Blister without mention of infection**

914.3   **Blister, infected**

914.4   **Insect bite, nonvenomous, without mention of infection**

914.5   **Insect bite, nonvenomous, infected**

914.6   **Superficial foreign body (splinter) without major open wound and without mention of infection**

914.7   **Superficial foreign body (splinter) without major open wound, infected**

914.8   **Other and unspecified superficial injury of hand without mention of infection**

914.9   **Other and unspecified superficial injury of hand, infected**

● 915   **Superficial injury of finger(s)**

     Includes   fingernail
                   thumb (nail)

915.0   **Abrasion or friction burn without mention of infection**

915.1   **Abrasion or friction burn, infected**

915.2   **Blister without mention of infection**

915.3   **Blister, infected**

915.4   **Insect bite, nonvenomous, without mention of infection**

915.5   **Insect bite, nonvenomous, infected**

915.6   **Superficial foreign body (splinter) without major open wound and without mention of infection**

915.7   **Superficial foreign body (splinter) without major open wound, infected**

915.8   **Other and unspecified superficial injury of fingers without mention of infection**
        Coding Clinic: 2001, Q3, P10

915.9   **Other and unspecified superficial injury of fingers, infected**

● 916   **Superficial injury of hip, thigh, leg, and ankle**

916.0   **Abrasion or friction burn without mention of infection**
        Coding Clinic: 2000, Q4, P61

916.1   **Abrasion or friction burn, infected**

916.2   **Blister without mention of infection**

916.3   **Blister, infected**

916.4   **Insect bite, nonvenomous, without mention of infection**

916.5   **Insect bite, nonvenomous, infected**

916.6   **Superficial foreign body (splinter) without major open wound and without mention of infection**

916.7   **Superficial foreign body (splinter) without major open wound, infected**

916.8   **Other and unspecified superficial injury of hip, thigh, leg, and ankle without mention of infection**

916.9   **Other and unspecified superficial injury of hip, thigh, leg, and ankle, infected**

◀ New   ◀⫴ Revised   ~~deleted~~ Deleted   Excludes   Includes   Use additional   Code first   Omit code
● Unacceptable Principal Diagnosis   ● Use Additional Digit(s)   **OGCR** Official Guidelines   **Coding Clinic**

● **917 Superficial injury of foot and toe(s)**

　　　Includes　heel
　　　　　　　　toenail

　　917.0 Abrasion or friction burn without mention of infection

　　917.1 Abrasion or friction burn, infected

　　917.2 Blister without mention of infection

　　917.3 Blister, infected

　　917.4 Insect bite, nonvenomous, without mention of infection

　　917.5 Insect bite, nonvenomous, infected

　　917.6 Superficial foreign body (splinter) without major open wound and without mention of infection

　　917.7 Superficial foreign body (splinter) without major open wound, infected

　　917.8 Other and unspecified superficial injury of foot and toes without mention of infection
　　　　　　　Coding Clinic: 2003, Q1, P13

　　917.9 Other and unspecified superficial injury of foot and toes, infected
　　　　　　　Coding Clinic: 2003, Q1, P13

● **918 Superficial injury of eye and adnexa**

　　　Excludes　burn (940.0–940.9)
　　　　　　　　foreign body on external eye (930.0–930.9)

　　918.0 Eyelids and periocular area
　　　　　　Abrasion
　　　　　　Insect bite
　　　　　　Superficial foreign body (splinter)

　　918.1 Cornea
　　　　　　Corneal abrasion
　　　　　　Superficial laceration

　　　　　　Excludes　corneal injury due to contact lens (371.82)

　　918.2 Conjunctiva

　　918.9 Other and unspecified superficial injuries of eye
　　　　　　Eye (ball) NOS

● **919 Superficial injury of other, multiple, and unspecified sites**

　　　Excludes　multiple sites classifiable to the same three-digit category (910.0–918.9)

　　919.0 Abrasion or friction burn without mention of infection

　　919.1 Abrasion or friction burn, infected

　　919.2 Blister without mention of infection

　　919.3 Blister, infected

　　919.4 Insect bite, nonvenomous, without mention of infection

　　919.5 Insect bite, nonvenomous, infected

　　919.6 Superficial foreign body (splinter) without major open wound and without mention of infection

　　919.7 Superficial foreign body (splinter) without major open wound, infected

　　919.8 Other and unspecified superficial injury without mention of infection

　　919.9 Other and unspecified superficial injury, infected

CONTUSION WITH INTACT SKIN SURFACE (920–924)

　　　Includes　bruise without fracture or open wound
　　　　　　　　hematoma without fracture or open wound

　　　Excludes　concussion (850.0–850.9)
　　　　　　　　hemarthrosis (840.0–848.9)
　　　　　　　　internal organs (860.0–869.1)
　　　　　　　　that incidental to:
　　　　　　　　　crushing injury (925–929.9)
　　　　　　　　　dislocation (830.0–839.9)
　　　　　　　　　fracture (800.0–829.1)
　　　　　　　　　internal injury (860.0–869.1)
　　　　　　　　　intracranial injury (850.0–854.1)
　　　　　　　　　nerve injury (950.0–957.9)
　　　　　　　　　open wound (870.0–897.7)

　　920 **Contusion of face, scalp, and neck except eye(s)**
　　　　　Cheek　　　　　　　　Mandibular joint area
　　　　　Ear (auricle)　　　　　Nose
　　　　　Gum　　　　　　　　　Throat
　　　　　Lip

● **921 Contusion of eye and adnexa**

　　921.0 Black eye, NOS

　　921.1 Contusion of eyelids and periocular area

　　921.2 Contusion of orbital tissues

　　921.3 Contusion of eyeball
　　　　　　　Coding Clinic: 1985, July-Aug, P16

　　921.9 Unspecified contusion of eye
　　　　　　Injury of eye NOS

● **922 Contusion of trunk**

　　922.0 Breast

　　922.1 Chest wall

　　922.2 Abdominal wall
　　　　　　Flank
　　　　　　Groin

● 　922.3 Back

　　　　922.31 Back

　　　　　　Excludes　interscapular region (922.33)
　　　　　　　Coding Clinic: 1999, Q3, P14-15

　　　　922.32 Buttock

　　　　922.33 Interscapular region

　　　　　　Excludes　scapular region (923.01)

　　922.4 Genital organs
　　　　　　Labium (majus) (minus)　　Testis
　　　　　　Penis　　　　　　　　　　Vagina
　　　　　　Perineum　　　　　　　　Vulva
　　　　　　Scrotum

　　922.8 Multiple sites of trunk

　　922.9 Unspecified part
　　　　　　Trunk NOS

● **923 Contusion of upper limb**

● 　923.0 Shoulder and upper arm

　　　　923.00 Shoulder region

　　　　923.01 Scapular region

　　　　923.02 Axillary region

　　　　923.03 Upper arm

　　　　923.09 Multiple sites

● 　923.1 Elbow and forearm

　　　　923.10 Forearm

　　　　923.11 Elbow

INJURY AND POISONING (800–999)

◀ New　　◀═ Revised　　~~deleted~~ Deleted　　Excludes　　Includes　　Use additional　　Code first　　Omit code
● Unacceptable Principal Diagnosis　　● Use Additional Digit(s)　　OGCR Official Guidelines　　Coding Clinic

995

INJURY AND POISONING (800–999)

● **923.2 Wrist and hand(s), except finger(s) alone**

　　923.20 Hand(s)

　　923.21 Wrist

　923.3 Finger
　　　Fingernail
　　　Thumb (nail)

　923.8 Multiple sites of upper limb

　923.9 Unspecified part of upper limb
　　　Arm NOS

● **924 Contusion of lower limb and of other and unspecified sites**

　● **924.0 Hip and thigh**

　　924.00 Thigh
　　　　Coding Clinic: 2009, Q1, P10x2

　　924.01 Hip

　● **924.1 Knee and lower leg**

　　924.10 Lower leg

　　924.11 Knee

　● **924.2 Ankle and foot, excluding toe(s)**

　　924.20 Foot
　　　　Heel

　　924.21 Ankle

　924.3 Toe
　　　Toenail

　924.4 Multiple sites of lower limb

　924.5 Unspecified part of lower limb
　　　Leg NOS

　924.8 Multiple sites, not elsewhere classified
　　　Coding Clinic: 2003, Q1, P7

　924.9 Unspecified site

CRUSHING INJURY (925–929)

Use additional code to identify any associated injuries, such as:
　　fractures (800–829)
　　internal injuries (860.0–869.1)
　　intracranial injury (850.0–854.1)

● **925 Crushing injury of face, scalp, and neck**
　　Cheek　　　　　Pharynx
　　Ear　　　　　　Throat
　　Larynx
　　Coding Clinic: 2003, Q4, P76-78

　925.1 Crushing injury of face and scalp
　　　Cheek
　　　Ear

　925.2 Crushing injury of neck
　　　Larynx
　　　Throat
　　　Pharynx

● **926 Crushing injury of trunk**
　　Coding Clinic: 2003, Q4, P76-78

　926.0 External genitalia
　　　Labium (majus) (minus)
　　　Penis
　　　Scrotum
　　　Testis
　　　Vulva

　● **926.1 Other specified sites**

　　926.11 Back

　　926.12 Buttock

　　926.19 Other
　　　　Breast

　926.8 Multiple sites of trunk

　926.9 Unspecified site
　　　Trunk NOS

● **927 Crushing injury of upper limb**

　● **927.0 Shoulder and upper arm**

　　927.00 Shoulder region

　　927.01 Scapular region

　　927.02 Axillary region

　　927.03 Upper arm

　　927.09 Multiple sites

　● **927.1 Elbow and forearm**

　　927.10 Forearm

　　927.11 Elbow

　● **927.2 Wrist and hand(s), except finger(s) alone**

　　927.20 Hand(s)

　　927.21 Wrist

　927.3 Finger(s)
　　　Coding Clinic: 2003, Q4, P76-78

　927.8 Multiple sites of upper limb

　927.9 Unspecified site
　　　Arm NOS

● **928 Crushing injury of lower limb**
　　Coding Clinic: 2003, Q4, P76-78

　● **928.0 Hip and thigh**

　　928.00 Thigh

　　928.01 Hip

　● **928.1 Knee and lower leg**

　　928.10 Lower leg

　　928.11 Knee

　● **928.2 Ankle and foot, excluding toe(s) alone**

　　928.20 Foot
　　　　Heel

　　928.21 Ankle

　928.3 Toe(s)

　928.8 Multiple sites of lower limb

　928.9 Unspecified site
　　　Leg NOS

● **929 Crushing injury of multiple and unspecified sites**
　　Coding Clinic: 2003, Q4, P76-78

　929.0 Multiple sites, not elsewhere classified

　929.9 Unspecified site

◄ New　　◀▥▥ Revised　　~~deleted~~ Deleted　　Excludes　　Includes　　Use additional　　Code first　　Omit code
　　● Unacceptable Principal Diagnosis　　● Use Additional Digit(s)　　OGCR Official Guidelines　　Coding Clinic

EFFECTS OF FOREIGN BODY ENTERING THROUGH ORIFICE (930–939)

Excludes *foreign body:*
    granuloma (728.82)
    inadvertently left in operative wound (998.4,
        998.7)
    in open wound (800–839, 851–897)
    residual, in soft tissues (729.6)
    superficial without major open wound
        (910–919 with .6 or .7)

● 930 **Foreign body on external eye**

Excludes *foreign body in penetrating wound of:*
    eyeball (871.5–871.6)
        retained (old) (360.5–360.6)
    ocular adnexa (870.4)
        retained (old) (376.6)

    930.0 **Corneal foreign body**

    930.1 **Foreign body in conjunctival sac**

    930.2 **Foreign body in lacrimal punctum**

    930.8 **Other and combined sites**

    930.9 **Unspecified site**
        External eye NOS

  931 **Foreign body in ear**
      Auditory canal
      Auricle

  932 **Foreign body in nose**
      Nasal sinus
      Nostril

● 933 **Foreign body in pharynx and larynx**

    933.0 **Pharynx**
        Nasopharynx
        Throat NOS

    933.1 **Larynx**
        Asphyxia due to foreign body
        Choking due to:
           food (regurgitated)
           phlegm

● 934 **Foreign body in trachea, bronchus, and lung**

    934.0 **Trachea**

    934.1 **Main bronchus**

    934.8 **Other specified parts**
        Bronchioles
        Lung

    934.9 **Respiratory tree, unspecified**
        Inhalation of liquid or vomitus, lower respiratory
          tract NOS

● 935 **Foreign body in mouth, esophagus, and stomach**

    935.0 **Mouth**

    935.1 **Esophagus**
        Coding Clinic: 1988, Q1, P13

    935.2 **Stomach**
        Coding Clinic: 1985, Jan-Feb, P14-15

  936 **Foreign body in intestine and colon**

  937 **Foreign body in anus and rectum**
      Rectosigmoid (junction)

  938 **Foreign body in digestive system, unspecified**
      Alimentary tract NOS
      Swallowed foreign body

● 939 **Foreign body in genitourinary tract**

    939.0 **Bladder and urethra**

    939.1 **Uterus, any part**

        Excludes *intrauterine contraceptive device:*
           complications from (996.32, 996.65)
           presence of (V45.51)

    939.2 **Vulva and vagina**

    939.3 **Penis**

    939.9 **Unspecified site**

OGCR Section I.C.17.c
Current burns (940-948) are classified by depth, extent and by
agent (E code). Burns are classified by depth as first degree
(erythema), second degree (blistering), and third degree
(full-thickness involvement).

OGCR Section I.C.17.c.1
Sequence first the code that reflects the highest degree of burn
when more than one burn is present.

OGCR Section I.C.17.c.2
Classify burns of the same local site (three-digit category level,
940-947) but of different degrees to the subcategory identifying
the highest degree recorded in the diagnosis.

BURNS (940–949)

Includes   burns from:
      electrical heating appliance
      electricity
      flame
      hot object
      lightning
      radiation
    chemical burns (external) (internal)
    scalds

Excludes *friction burns (910–919 with .0, .1)*
    sunburn (692.71, 692.76–692.77)

● 940 **Burn confined to eye and adnexa**

    940.0 **Chemical burn of eyelids and periocular area**

    940.1 **Other burns of eyelids and periocular area**

    940.2 **Alkaline chemical burn of cornea and conjunctival
        sac**

    940.3 **Acid chemical burn of cornea and conjunctival sac**

    940.4 **Other burn of cornea and conjunctival sac**

    940.5 **Burn with resulting rupture and destruction of
        eyeball**

    940.9 **Unspecified burn of eye and adnexa**

Figure 17–14 **A.** Second-degree burn.
B. Third-degree burn. (From Cummings:
Otolaryngology: Head & Neck Surgery,
4th ed. 2005, Mosby.)

INJURY AND POISONING (800–999)

● **941 Burn of face, head, and neck**

> **Excludes** *mouth (947.0)*

The following fifth-digit subclassification is for use with category 941:

> 0 face and head, unspecified site
> 1 ear [any part]
> 2 eye (with other parts of face, head, and neck)
> 3 lip(s)
> 4 chin
> 5 nose (septum)
> 6 scalp [any part]
>   Temple (region)
> 7 forehead and cheek
> 8 neck
> 9 multiple sites [except with eye] of face, head, and neck

● **941.0 Unspecified degree**
[0-9]

● **941.1 Erythema [first degree]**
[0-9]   Coding Clinic: 2005, Q3, P10-11

● **941.2 Blisters, epidermal loss [second degree]**
[0-9]

● **941.3 Full-thickness skin loss [third degree NOS]**
[0-9]

● **941.4 Deep necrosis of underlying tissues [deep third**
[0-9] **degree] without mention of loss of a body part**

● **941.5 Deep necrosis of underlying tissues [deep third**
[0-9] **degree] with loss of a body part**

● **942 Burn of trunk**

> **Excludes** *scapular region (943.0–943.5 with fifth-digit 6)*

The following fifth-digit subclassification is for use with category 942:

> 0 trunk, unspecified site
> 1 breast
> 2 chest wall, excluding breast and nipple
> 3 abdominal wall
>   Flank
>   Groin
> 4 back [any part]
>   Buttock
>   Interscapular region
> 5 genitalia
>   Labium (majus) (minus)   Scrotum
>   Penis   Testis
>   Perineum   Vulva
> 9 other and multiple sites of trunk

● **942.0 Unspecified degree**
[0-5,9]

● **942.1 Erythema [first degree]**
[0-5,9]

● **942.2 Blisters, epidermal loss [second degree]**
[0-5,9]   Coding Clinic: 1984, Nov-Dec, P13

● **942.3 Full-thickness skin loss [third degree NOS]**
[0-5,9]

● **942.4 Deep necrosis of underlying tissues [deep third**
[0-5,9] **degree] without mention of loss of a body part**

● **942.5 Deep necrosis of underlying tissues [deep third**
[0-5,9] **degree] with loss of a body part**

● **943 Burn of upper limb, except wrist and hand**

The following fifth-digit subclassification is for use with category 943:

> 0 upper limb, unspecified site
> 1 forearm
> 2 elbow
> 3 upper arm
> 4 axilla
> 5 shoulder
> 6 scapular region
> 9 multiple sites of upper limb, except wrist and hand

● **943.0 Unspecified degree**
[0-6,9]

● **943.1 Erythema [first degree]**
[0-6,9]

● **943.2 Blisters, epidermal loss [second degree]**
[0-6,9]

● **943.3 Full-thickness skin loss [third degree NOS]**
[0-6,9]

● **943.4 Deep necrosis of underlying tissues [deep third**
[0-6,9] **degree] without mention of loss of a body part**

● **943.5 Deep necrosis of underlying tissues [deep third**
[0-6,9] **degree] with loss of a body part**

● **944 Burn of wrist(s) and hand(s)**

The following fifth-digit subclassification is for use with category 944:

> 0 hand, unspecified site
> 1 single digit [finger (nail)] other than thumb
> 2 thumb (nail)
> 3 two or more digits, not including thumb
> 4 two or more digits including thumb
> 5 palm
> 6 back of hand
> 7 wrist
> 8 multiple sites of wrist(s) and hand(s)

● **944.0 Unspecified degree**
[0-8]

● **944.1 Erythema [first degree]**
[0-8]

● **944.2 Blisters, epidermal loss [second degree]**
[0-8]

● **944.3 Full-thickness skin loss [third degree NOS]**
[0-8]

● **944.4 Deep necrosis of underlying tissues [deep third**
[0-8] **degree] without mention of loss of a body part**

● **944.5 Deep necrosis of underlying tissues [deep third**
[0-8] **degree] with loss of a body part**

● **945 Burn of lower limb(s)**

The following fifth-digit subclassification is for use with category 945:

> 0 lower limb [leg], unspecified site
> 1 toe(s) (nail)
> 2 foot
> 3 ankle
> 4 lower leg
> 5 knee
> 6 thigh [any part]
> 9 multiple sites of lower limb(s)

● **945.0 Unspecified degree**
[0-6,9]

◀ New   ◀▥ Revised   ~~deleted~~ Deleted   Excludes   Includes   Use additional   Code first   Omit code
● Unacceptable Principal Diagnosis   ● Use Additional Digit(s)   OGCR Official Guidelines   Coding Clinic

● **945.1** Erythema [first degree]
[0–6,9]

● **945.2** Blisters, epidermal loss [second degree]
[0–6,9]

● **945.3** Full-thickness skin loss [third degree NOS]
[0–6,9]

● **945.4** Deep necrosis of underlying tissues [deep third
[0–6,9] degree] without mention of loss of a body
part

● **945.5** Deep necrosis of underlying tissues [deep third
[0–6,9] degree] with loss of a body part

OGCR Section I.C.17.c.5

When coding burns, assign separate codes for each burn
site. Category 946 should only be used if the location of
the burns are not documented.

● **946** **Burns of multiple specified sites**
Documented as multiple sites but not specified as to location

Includes burns of sites classifiable to more than one
three-digit category in 940–945

Excludes *multiple burns NOS (949.0–949.5)*

946.0 Unspecified degree

946.1 Erythema [first degree]

946.2 Blisters, epidermal loss [second degree]

946.3 Full-thickness skin loss [third degree NOS]

946.4 Deep necrosis of underlying tissues [deep third
degree] without mention of loss of a body part

946.5 Deep necrosis of underlying tissues [deep third
degree] with loss of a body part

● **947** **Burn of internal organs**

Includes burns from chemical agents (ingested)

947.0 Mouth and pharynx
Gum
Tongue

947.1 Larynx, trachea, and lung

947.2 Esophagus

947.3 Gastrointestinal tract
Colon
Rectum
Small intestine
Stomach

947.4 Vagina and uterus

947.8 Other specified sites

947.9 Unspecified site

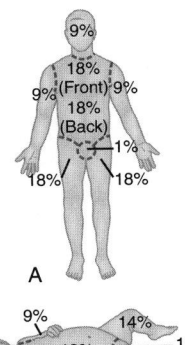

Figure 17–15 Rule of nines:
percentages of total body area. (From
Marx: Rosen's Emergency Medicine:
Concepts and Clinical Practice, 6th
ed. 2006, Mosby.)

OGCR Section I.C.17.c.6

Fourth-digit identifies percentage of **total body surface**
involved in a burn (all degrees). **Fifth-digit** identifies the
percentage of body surface involved in **third-degree burn.**
Fifth-digit zero (0) assigned when less than 10 percent or when
no body surface is involved in a third-degree burn.

Category 948 is based on the classic "rule of nines" in
estimating body surface involved: head and neck are assigned
nine percent, each arm nine percent, each leg 18 percent, the
anterior trunk 18 percent, posterior trunk 18 percent, and
genitalia one percent. Providers may change these percentage
assignments where necessary to accommodate infants and
children who have proportionately larger heads than adults
and patients who have large buttocks, thighs, or abdomen that
involve burns.

● **948** **Burns classified according to extent of body surface involved**

Excludes *sunburn (692.71, 692.76–692.77)*

Note: This category is to be used when the site of the
burn is unspecified, or with categories 940–947
when the site is specified.
Coding Clinic: 1984, Nov-Dec, P13

The following fifth-digit subclassification is for use with
category 948 to indicate the percent of body surface with third
degree burn; valid digits are in [brackets] under each code:

```
0  less than 10 percent or unspecified
1  10–19%
2  20–29%
3  30–39%
4  40–49%
5  50–59%
6  60–69%
7  70–79%
8  80–89%
9  90% or more of body surface
```

● **948.0** Burn [any degree] involving less than 10 percent of
[0] body surface

● **948.1** 10–19 percent of body surface
[0–1] Coding Clinic: 1984, Nov-Dec, P13

● **948.2** 20–29 percent of body surface
[0–2] Coding Clinic: 1984, Nov-Dec, P13

● **948.3** 30–39 percent of body surface
[0–3]

● **948.4** 40–49 percent of body surface
[0–4]

● **948.5** 50–59 percent of body surface
[0–5]

● **948.6** 60–69 percent of body surface
[0–6]

● **948.7** 70–79 percent of body surface
[0–7]

● **948.8** 80–89 percent of body surface
[0–8]

● **948.9** 90 percent or more of body surface
[0–9]

OGCR Section I.C.17.c.5

When coding burns, assign separate codes for each burn site.
Category 946 Burns of Multiple specified sites, should only be
used if the location of the burns are not documented. Category
949, Burn, unspecified, is extremely vague and should rarely be
used.

INJURY AND POISONING (800–999)

INJURY AND POISONING (800–999)

● **949 Burn, unspecified**

> **Includes** burn NOS
> multiple burns NOS

> **Excludes** *burn of unspecified site but with statement of the extent of body surface involved (948.0–948.9)*

949.0 Unspecified degree

949.1 Erythema [first degree]

949.2 Blisters, epidermal loss [second degree]

949.3 Full-thickness skin loss [third degree NOS]

949.4 Deep necrosis of underlying tissues [deep third degree] without mention of loss of a body part

949.5 Deep necrosis of underlying tissues [deep third degree] with loss of a body part

> **Includes** division of nerve
> lesion in continuity (with open wound)
> traumatic neuroma (with open wound)
> traumatic transient paralysis (with open wound)

> **Excludes** *accidental puncture or laceration during medical procedure (998.2)*

INJURY TO NERVES AND SPINAL CORD (950–957)

● **950 Injury to optic nerve and pathways**

950.0 Optic nerve injury
Second cranial nerve

950.1 Injury to optic chiasm

950.2 Injury to optic pathways

950.3 Injury to visual cortex

950.9 Unspecified
Traumatic blindness NOS

● **951 Injury to other cranial nerve(s)**

951.0 Injury to oculomotor nerve
Third cranial nerve

951.1 Injury to trochlear nerve
Fourth cranial nerve

951.2 Injury to trigeminal nerve
Fifth cranial nerve

951.3 Injury to abducens nerve
Sixth cranial nerve

951.4 Injury to facial nerve
Seventh cranial nerve

951.5 Injury to acoustic nerve
Auditory nerve
Eighth cranial nerve
Traumatic deafness NOS

951.6 Injury to accessory nerve
Eleventh cranial nerve

951.7 Injury to hypoglossal nerve
Twelfth cranial nerve

951.8 Injury to other specified cranial nerves
Glossopharyngeal [9th cranial] nerve
Olfactory [1st cranial] nerve
Pneumogastric [10th cranial] nerve
Traumatic anosmia NOS
Vagus [10th cranial] nerve

951.9 Injury to unspecified cranial nerve

● **952 Spinal cord injury without evidence of spinal bone injury**

● **952.0 Cervical**

952.00 C_1-C_4 level with unspecified spinal cord injury
Spinal cord injury, cervical region NOS

952.01 C_1-C_4 level with complete lesion of spinal cord

952.02 C_1-C_4 level with anterior cord syndrome

952.03 C_1-C_4 level with central cord syndrome

952.04 C_1-C_4 level with other specified spinal cord injury
Incomplete spinal cord lesion at C_1-C_4 level:
NOS
with posterior cord syndrome

952.05 C_5-C_7 level with unspecified spinal cord injury

952.06 C_5-C_7 level with complete lesion of spinal cord

952.07 C_5-C_7 level with anterior cord syndrome

952.08 C_5-C_7 level with central cord syndrome

952.09 C_5-C_7 level with other specified spinal cord injury
Incomplete spinal cord lesion at C_5-C_7 level:
NOS
with posterior cord syndrome

● **952.1 Dorsal [thoracic]**

952.10 T_1-T_6 level with unspecified spinal cord injury
Spinal cord injury, thoracic region NOS

952.11 T_1-T_6 level with complete lesion of spinal cord

952.12 T_1-T_6 level with anterior cord syndrome

952.13 T_1-T_6 level with central cord syndrome

952.14 T_1-T_6 level with other specified spinal cord injury
Incomplete spinal cord lesion at T_1-T_6 level:
NOS
with posterior cord syndrome

952.15 T_7-T_{12} level with unspecified spinal cord injury

952.16 T_7-T_{12} level with complete lesion of spinal cord

952.17 T_7-T_{12} level with anterior cord syndrome

952.18 T_7-T_{12} level with central cord syndrome

952.19 T_7-T_{12} level with other specified spinal cord injury
Incomplete spinal cord lesion at T_7-T_{12} level:
NOS
with posterior cord syndrome

952.2 Lumbar

952.3 Sacral

952.4 Cauda equina

952.8 Multiple sites of spinal cord

952.9 Unspecified site of spinal cord

● **953 Injury to nerve roots and spinal plexus**

953.0 Cervical root

953.1 Dorsal root

953.2 Lumbar root

953.3 Sacral root

953.4 Brachial plexus

◄ New   ◄▥ Revised   ~~deleted~~ Deleted   Excludes   Includes   Use additional   Code first   Omit code
● Unacceptable Principal Diagnosis   ● Use Additional Digit(s)   **OGCR** Official Guidelines   **Coding Clinic**

953.5 Lumbosacral plexus

953.8 Multiple sites

953.9 Unspecified site

● 954 Injury to other nerve(s) of trunk, excluding shoulder and pelvic girdles

954.0 Cervical sympathetic

954.1 Other sympathetic
Celiac ganglion or plexus   Splanchnic nerve(s)
Inferior mesenteric plexus   Stellate ganglion

954.8 Other specified nerve(s) of trunk

954.9 Unspecified nerve of trunk

● 955 Injury to peripheral nerve(s) of shoulder girdle and upper limb

955.0 Axillary nerve

955.1 Median nerve

955.2 Ulnar nerve

955.3 Radial nerve

955.4 Musculocutaneous nerve

955.5 Cutaneous sensory nerve, upper limb

955.6 Digital nerve

955.7 Other specified nerve(s) of shoulder girdle and upper limb

955.8 Multiple nerves of shoulder girdle and upper limb

955.9 Unspecified nerve of shoulder girdle and upper limb

● 956 Injury to peripheral nerve(s) of pelvic girdle and lower limb

956.0 Sciatic nerve

956.1 Femoral nerve

956.2 Posterior tibial nerve

956.3 Peroneal nerve

956.4 Cutaneous sensory nerve, lower limb

956.5 Other specified nerve(s) of pelvic girdle and lower limb

956.8 Multiple nerves of pelvic girdle and lower limb

956.9 Unspecified nerve of pelvic girdle and lower limb

● 957 Injury to other and unspecified nerves

957.0 Superficial nerves of head and neck

957.1 Other specified nerve(s)

957.8 Multiple nerves in several parts
Multiple nerve injury NOS

957.9 Unspecified site
Nerve injury NOS

CERTAIN TRAUMATIC COMPLICATIONS AND UNSPECIFIED INJURIES (958–959)

● 958 Certain early complications of trauma

Excludes *adult respiratory distress syndrome (518.5)*
flail chest (807.4)
post-traumatic seroma (729.91)
shock lung (518.5)
that occurring during or following medical procedures (996.0–999.9)

958.0 Air embolism
Pneumathemia

Excludes *that complicating:*
abortion (634–638 with .6, 639.6)
ectopic or molar pregnancy (639.6)
pregnancy, childbirth, or the puerperium (673.0)

958.1 Fat embolism

Excludes *that complicating:*
abortion (634–638 with .6, 639.6)
pregnancy, childbirth, or the puerperium (673.8)

958.2 Secondary and recurrent hemorrhage

958.3 Posttraumatic wound infection, not elsewhere classified

Excludes *infected open wounds - code to complicated open wound of site*
Coding Clinic: 1993, 5th Issue, P3; 1985, Sept-Oct, P10; 1984, Nov-Dec, P20

OGCR Section I.C.17.c.4
Assign code 958.3, Posttraumatic wound infection, not elsewhere classified, as an additional code for any documented infected burn site.

958.4 Traumatic shock
Shock (immediate) (delayed) following injury

Excludes *shock:*
anaphylactic (995.0)
due to serum (999.4)
anesthetic (995.4)
electric (994.8)
following abortion (639.5)
lightning (994.0)
nontraumatic NOS (785.50)
obstetric (669.1)
postoperative (998.0)

958.5 Traumatic anuria
Crush syndrome
Renal failure following crushing

Excludes *that due to a medical procedure (997.5)*

958.6 Volkmann's ischemic contracture
Posttraumatic muscle contracture

958.7 Traumatic subcutaneous emphysema

Excludes *subcutaneous emphysema resulting from a procedure (998.81)*

958.8 Other early complications of trauma
Coding Clinic: 1992, Q2, P13

● 958.9 Traumatic compartment syndrome

Excludes *nontraumatic compartment syndrome (729.71–729.79)*

958.90 Compartment syndrome, unspecified

958.91 Traumatic compartment syndrome of upper extremity
Traumatic compartment syndrome of shoulder, arm, forearm, wrist, hand, and fingers

958.92 Traumatic compartment syndrome of lower extremity
Traumatic compartment syndrome of hip, buttock, thigh, leg, foot, and toes

958.93 Traumatic compartment syndrome of abdomen
Coding Clinic: 2006, Q4, P100-102

958.99 Traumatic compartment syndrome of other sites

INJURY AND POISONING (800–999)

◀ New   ◀▥ Revised   ~~deleted~~ Deleted   Excludes   Includes   Use additional   Code first   Omit code
● Unacceptable Principal Diagnosis   ● Use Additional Digit(s)   OGCR Official Guidelines   Coding Clinic

1001

● **959 Injury, other and unspecified**

> **Includes**   injury NOS
>
> **Excludes**   *injury NOS of:*
> *blood vessels (900.0–904.9)*
> *eye (921.0–921.9)*
> *internal organs (860.0–869.1)*
> *intracranial sites (854.0–854.1)*
> *nerves (950.0–951.9, 953.0–957.9)*
> *spinal cord (952.0–952.9)*
>
> Coding Clinic: 1984, Nov-Dec, P9

● **959.0 Head, face, and neck**

> **959.01 Head injury, unspecified**
>
> > **Excludes**   *concussion (850.0–850.9)*
> > *with head injury NOS*
> > *(850.0–850.9)*
> > *head injury NOS with loss of*
> > *consciousness (850.1–850.5)*
> > *specified head injuries*
> > *(850.0–854.1)*
> >
> > Coding Clinic: 2008, Q4, P102-109; 1999, Q1, P10
>
> **959.09 Injury of face and neck**

● **959.1 Trunk**

> **Excludes**   *scapular region (959.2)*
>
> **959.11 Other injury of chest wall**
>
> **959.12 Other injury of abdomen**
>
> **959.13 Fracture of corpus cavernosum penis**
>
> **959.14 Other injury of external genitals**
>
> **959.19 Other injury of other sites of trunk**
> Injury of trunk NOS

959.2 Shoulder and upper arm
Axilla
Scapular region

959.3 Elbow, forearm, and wrist
Coding Clinic: 1997, Q1, P8

959.4 Hand, except finger

959.5 Finger
Fingernail
Thumb (nail)

959.6 Hip and thigh
Upper leg

959.7 Knee, leg, ankle, and foot

959.8 Other specified sites, including multiple

> **Excludes**   *multiple sites classifiable to the same*
> *four-digit category (959.0–959.7)*

959.9 Unspecified site
Coding Clinic: 1984, Nov-Dec, P9

POISONING BY DRUGS, MEDICINAL AND BIOLOGICAL SUBSTANCES (960–979)

> **Includes**   overdose of these substances
> wrong substance given or taken in error
>
> **Excludes**   *adverse effects ["hypersensitivity," "reaction,"*
> *etc.] of correct substance properly*
> *administered. Such cases are to be classified*
> *according to the nature of the adverse effect,*
> *such as:*
> *adverse effect NOS (995.20)*
> *allergic lymphadenitis (289.3)*
> *aspirin gastritis (535.4)*
> *blood disorders (280.0–289.9)*
> *dermatitis:*
> *contact (692.0–692.9)*
> *due to ingestion (693.0–693.9)*
> *nephropathy (583.9)*
> *[The drug giving rise to the adverse effect may be*
> *identified by use of categories E930–E949.]*
> *drug dependence (304.0–304.9)*
> *drug reaction and poisoning affecting the newborn*
> *(760.0–779.9)*
> *nondependent abuse of drugs (305.0–305.9)*
> *pathological drug intoxication (292.2)*
>
> Use additional code to specify the effects of the
> poisoning

● **960 Poisoning by antibiotics**

> **Excludes**   *antibiotics:*
> *ear, nose, and throat (976.6)*
> *eye (976.5)*
> *local (976.0)*

960.0 Penicillins

Ampicillin	Cloxacillin
Carbenicillin	Penicillin G

960.1 Antifungal antibiotics

Amphotericin B	Nystatin
Griseofulvin	Trichomycin

> **Excludes**   *preparations intended for topical use*
> *(976.0–976.9)*

960.2 Chloramphenicol group
Chloramphenicol
Thiamphenicol

960.3 Erythromycin and other macrolides
Oleandomycin
Spiramycin

OGCR Section I.C.17.e.2

Poisoning. Errors made in drug prescription or in the administration of the drug by provider, nurse, patient, or other person, use the appropriate poisoning code from the 960-979 series. If an overdose of a drug was **intentionally** taken or administered and resulted in drug toxicity, it would be coded as a poisoning (960-979 series). If a **nonprescribed** drug or medicinal agent was taken in combination with a correctly prescribed and properly administered drug, any drug toxicity or other reaction resulting from the interaction of the two drugs would be classified as a poisoning.

When a reaction results from the interaction of a drug(s) and alcohol, this would be classified as poisoning.

Sequencing of poisoning: When coding a poisoning or reaction to the improper use of a medication (e.g., wrong dose, wrong substance, wrong route of administration) the poisoning code is sequenced first, followed by a code for the manifestation. If there is also a diagnosis of drug abuse or dependence to the substance, the abuse or dependence is coded as an additional code.

See Section I.C.3.a.6.b. if poisoning is the result of insulin pump malfunctions and Section I.C.19 for general use of E-codes.

960.4 **Tetracycline group**
Doxycycline
Minocycline
Oxytetracycline

960.5 **Cephalosporin group**
Cephalexin   Cephaloridine
Cephaloglycin   Cephalothin

960.6 **Antimycobacterial antibiotics**
Cycloserine   Rifampin
Kanamycin   Streptomycin

960.7 **Antineoplastic antibiotics**
Actinomycin such as:
Bleomycin   Dactinomycin
Cactinomycin   Daunorubicin
Mitomycin

960.8 **Other specified antibiotics**

960.9 **Unspecified antibiotic**

● 961 **Poisoning by other anti-infectives**
| Excludes | *anti-infectives:*
ear, nose, and throat (976.6)
eye (976.5)
local (976.0)

961.0 **Sulfonamides**
Sulfadiazine
Sulfafurazole
Sulfamethoxazole

961.1 **Arsenical anti-infectives**

961.2 **Heavy metal anti-infectives**
Compounds of: Compounds of:
antimony   lead
bismuth   mercury
| Excludes | *mercurial diuretics (974.0)*

961.3 **Quinoline and hydroxyquinoline derivatives**
Chiniofon
Diiodohydroxyquin
| Excludes | *antimalarial drugs (961.4)*

961.4 **Antimalarials and drugs acting on other blood protozoa**
Chloroquine
Cycloguanil
Primaquine
Proguanil [chloroguanide]
Pyrimethamine
Quinine

961.5 **Other antiprotozoal drugs**
Emetine

961.6 **Anthelmintics**
Hexylresorcinol   Thiabendazole
Piperazine

961.7 **Antiviral drugs**
Methisazone
| Excludes | *amantadine (966.4)*
cytarabine (963.1)
idoxuridine (976.5)

961.8 **Other antimycobacterial drugs**
Ethambutol
Ethionamide
Isoniazid
Para-aminosalicylic acid derivatives
Sulfones

961.9 **Other and unspecified anti-infectives**
Flucytosine
Nitrofuran derivatives

● 962 **Poisoning by hormones and synthetic substitutes**
| Excludes | *oxytocic hormones (975.0)*

962.0 **Adrenal cortical steroids**
Cortisone derivatives
Desoxycorticosterone derivatives
Fluorinated corticosteroids

962.1 **Androgens and anabolic congeners**
Methandriol   Oxymetholone
Nandrolone   Testosterone

962.2 **Ovarian hormones and synthetic substitutes**
Contraceptives, oral
Estrogens
Estrogens and progestogens, combined
Progestogens

962.3 **Insulins and antidiabetic agents**
Acetohexamide
Biguanide derivatives, oral
Chlorpropamide
Glucagon
Insulin
Phenformin
Sulfonylurea derivatives, oral
Tolbutamide

962.4 **Anterior pituitary hormones**
Corticotropin
Gonadotropin
Somatotropin [growth hormone]

962.5 **Posterior pituitary hormones**
Vasopressin
| Excludes | *oxytocic hormones (975.0)*

962.6 **Parathyroid and parathyroid derivatives**

962.7 **Thyroid and thyroid derivatives**
Dextrothyroxin
Levothyroxine sodium
Liothyronine
Thyroglobulin

962.8 **Antithyroid agents**
Iodides
Thiouracil
Thiourea

962.9 **Other and unspecified hormones and synthetic substitutes**

● 963 **Poisoning by primarily systemic agents**
963.0 **Antiallergic and antiemetic drugs**
Antihistamines   Diphenylpyraline
Chlorpheniramine   Thonzylamine
Diphenhydramine   Tripelennamine
| Excludes | *phenothiazine-based tranquilizers (969.1)*

963.1 **Antineoplastic and immunosuppressive drugs**
Azathioprine   Cytarabine
Busulfan   Fluorouracil
Chlorambucil   Mercaptopurine
Cyclophosphamide   thio-TEPA
| Excludes | *antineoplastic antibiotics (960.7)*

963.2 **Acidifying agents**

963.3 **Alkalizing agents**

963.4 **Enzymes, not elsewhere classified**
Penicillinase

963.5 **Vitamins, not elsewhere classified**
Vitamin A
Vitamin D
| Excludes | *nicotinic acid (972.2)*
vitamin K (964.3)

963.8 **Other specified systemic agents**
Heavy metal antagonists

963.9 **Unspecified systemic agent**

INJURY AND POISONING (800–999)

- **964 Poisoning by agents primarily affecting blood constituents**
  - **964.0 Iron and its compounds**
    - Ferric salts
    - Ferrous sulfate and other ferrous salts
  - **964.1 Liver preparations and other antianemic agents**
    - Folic acid
  - **964.2 Anticoagulants**
    - Coumarin
    - Heparin
    - Phenindione
    - Warfarin sodium
    - Coding Clinic: 1994, Q1, P22
  - **964.3 Vitamin K [phytonadione]**
  - **964.4 Fibrinolysis-affecting drugs**
    - Aminocaproic acid
    - Streptodornase
    - Streptokinase
    - Urokinase
  - **964.5 Anticoagulant antagonists and other coagulants**
    - Hexadimethrine
    - Protamine sulfate
  - **964.6 Gamma globulin**
  - **964.7 Natural blood and blood products**
    - Blood plasma
    - Human fibrinogen
    - Packed red cells
    - Whole blood
    - **Excludes** transfusion reactions (999.4–999.8)
  - **964.8 Other specified agents affecting blood constituents**
    - Macromolecular blood substitutes
    - Plasma expanders
  - **964.9 Unspecified agents affecting blood constituents**

- **965 Poisoning by analgesics, antipyretics, and antirheumatics**
  - Use additional code to identify:
    - drug dependence (304.0–304.9)
    - nondependent abuse (305.0–305.9)
  - **965.0 Opiates and related narcotics**
    - **965.00 Opium (alkaloids), unspecified**
      - Coding Clinic: 2007, Q3, P7-8
    - **965.01 Heroin**
      - Diacetylmorphine
    - **965.02 Methadone**
    - **965.09 Other**
      - Codeine [methylmorphine]
      - Meperidine [pethidine]
      - Morphine
      - Coding Clinic: 2007, Q3, P7-8
  - **965.1 Salicylates**
    - Acetylsalicylic acid [aspirin]
    - Salicylic acid salts
    - Coding Clinic: 1984, Nov-Dec, P15
  - **965.4 Aromatic analgesics, not elsewhere classified**
    - Acetanilid
    - Paracetamol [acetaminophen]
    - Phenacetin [acetophenetidin]
  - **965.5 Pyrazole derivatives**
    - Aminophenazone [aminopyrine]
    - Phenylbutazone

  - **965.6 Antirheumatics [antiphlogistics]**
    - **Excludes** salicylates (965.1)
      - steroids (962.0–962.9)
    - **965.61 Propionic acid derivatives**
      - Fenoprofen
      - Flurbiprofen
      - Ibuprofen
      - Ketoprofen
      - Naproxen
      - Oxaprozin
      - Coding Clinic: 1998, Q4, P42-44
    - **965.69 Other antirheumatics**
      - Gold salts
      - Indomethacin
  - **965.7 Other non-narcotic analgesics**
    - Pyrabital
  - **965.8 Other specified analgesics and antipyretics**
    - Pentazocine
  - **965.9 Unspecified analgesic and antipyretic**

- **966 Poisoning by anticonvulsants and anti-Parkinsonism drugs**
  - **966.0 Oxazolidine derivatives**
    - Paramethadione
    - Trimethadione
  - **966.1 Hydantoin derivatives**
    - Phenytoin
  - **966.2 Succinimides**
    - Ethosuximide
    - Phensuximide
  - **966.3 Other and unspecified anticonvulsants**
    - Primidone
    - **Excludes** barbiturates (967.0)
      - sulfonamides (961.0)
  - **966.4 Anti-Parkinsonism drugs**
    - Amantadine
    - Ethopropazine [profenamine]
    - Levodopa [L-dopa]

- **967 Poisoning by sedatives and hypnotics**
  - Use additional code to identify:
    - drug dependence (304.0–304.9)
    - nondependent abuse (305.0–305.9)
  - **967.0 Barbiturates**
    - Amobarbital [amylobarbitone]
    - Barbital [barbitone]
    - Butabarbital [butabarbitone]
    - Pentobarbital [pentobarbitone]
    - Phenobarbital [phenobarbitone]
    - Secobarbital [quinalbarbitone]
    - **Excludes** thiobarbiturate anesthetics (968.3)
  - **967.1 Chloral hydrate group**
  - **967.2 Paraldehyde**
  - **967.3 Bromine compounds**
    - Bromide
    - Carbromal (derivatives)
  - **967.4 Methaqualone compounds**
  - **967.5 Glutethimide group**
  - **967.6 Mixed sedatives, not elsewhere classified**
  - **967.8 Other sedatives and hypnotics**
  - **967.9 Unspecified sedative or hypnotic**
    - Sleeping:
      - drug NOS
      - pill NOS
    - Sleeping:
      - tablet NOS

◄ New   ◄▥ Revised   ~~deleted~~ Deleted   Excludes   Includes   Use additional   Code first   Omit code
● Unacceptable Principal Diagnosis   ● Use Additional Digit(s)   OGCR Official Guidelines   Coding Clinic

● **968 Poisoning by other central nervous system depressants and anesthetics**

Use additional code to identify:
drug dependence (304.0–304.9)
nondependent abuse (305.0–305.9)

968.0 Central nervous system muscle-tone depressants
Chlorphenesin (carbamate)
Mephenesin
Methocarbamol

968.1 Halothane

968.2 Other gaseous anesthetics
Ether
Halogenated hydrocarbon derivatives, except halothane
Nitrous oxide

968.3 Intravenous anesthetics
Ketamine
Methohexital [methohexitone]
Thiobarbiturates, such as thiopental sodium

968.4 Other and unspecified general anesthetics

968.5 Surface [topical] and infiltration anesthetics
Cocaine   Procaine
Lidocaine [lignocaine]   Tetracaine
Coding Clinic: 1993, Q1, P25

968.6 Peripheral nerve- and plexus-blocking anesthetics

968.7 Spinal anesthetics

968.9 Other and unspecified local anesthetics

● **969 Poisoning by psychotropic agents**

Use additional code to identify:
drug dependence (304.0–304.9)
nondependent abuse (305.0–305.9)

● **969.0 Antidepressants**
Coding Clinic: 2007, Q3, P7-8; 1991, Q3, P14

969.00 Antidepressant, unspecified

969.01 Monoamine oxidase inhibitors
MAOI

969.02 Selective serotonin and norepinephrine reuptake inhibitors
SSNRI antidepressants

969.03 Selective serotonin reuptake inhibitors
SSRI antidepressants

969.04 Tetracyclic antidepressants

969.05 Tricyclic antidepressants
Coding Clinic: 2009, Q4, P129

969.09 Other antidepressants

969.1 Phenothiazine-based tranquilizers
Chlorpromazine   Prochlorperazine
Fluphenazine   Promazine

969.2 Butyrophenone-based tranquilizers
Haloperidol   Trifluperidol
Spiperone

969.3 Other antipsychotics, neuroleptics, and major tranquilizers

969.4 Benzodiazepine-based tranquilizers
Chlordiazepoxide   Lorazepam
Diazepam   Medazepam
Flurazepam   Nitrazepam
Coding Clinic: 2009, Q4, P129; 1991, Q3, P14

969.5 Other tranquilizers
Hydroxyzine
Meprobamate

969.6 Psychodysleptics [hallucinogens]
Cannabis (derivatives)
Lysergide [LSD]
Marihuana (derivatives)
Marijuana
Mescaline
Psilocin
Psilocybin

● **969.7 Psychostimulants**

Excludes *central appetite depressants (977.0)*
Coding Clinic: 2003, Q2, P11

969.70 Psychostimulant, unspecified

969.71 Caffeine

969.72 Amphetamines
Methamphetamines

969.73 Methylphenidate

969.79 Other psychostimulants

969.8 Other specified psychotropic agents

969.9 Unspecified psychotropic agent

● **970 Poisoning by central nervous system stimulants**

970.0 Analeptics
Lobeline
Nikethamide

970.1 Opiate antagonists
Levallorphan
Nalorphine
Naloxone

● **970.8 Other specified central nervous system stimulants** ◀▥

970.81 Cocaine ◀
Crack ◀

970.89 Other central nervous system stimulants ◀

970.9 Unspecified central nervous system stimulant

● **971 Poisoning by drugs primarily affecting the autonomic nervous system**

971.0 Parasympathomimetics [cholinergics]
Acetylcholine
Anticholinesterase:
organophosphorus
reversible
Pilocarpine

971.1 Parasympatholytics [anticholinergics and antimuscarinics] and spasmolytics
Atropine
Homatropine
Hyoscine [scopolamine]
Quaternary ammonium derivatives
Excludes *papaverine (972.5)*

971.2 Sympathomimetics [adrenergics]
Epinephrine [adrenalin]
Levarterenol [noradrenalin]

971.3 Sympatholytics [antiadrenergics]
Phenoxybenzamine
Tolazoline hydrochloride

971.9 Unspecified drug primarily affecting autonomic nervous system

INJURY AND POISONING (800–999)

● **972 Poisoning by agents primarily affecting the cardiovascular system**

  972.0 Cardiac rhythm regulators
    Practolol   Propranolol
    Procainamide   Quinidine
    | Excludes | *lidocaine (968.5)*

  972.1 Cardiotonic glycosides and drugs of similar action
    Digitalis glycosides   Strophanthins
    Digoxin

  972.2 Antilipemic and antiarteriosclerotic drugs
    Clofibrate
    Nicotinic acid derivatives

  972.3 Ganglion-blocking agents
    Pentamethonium bromide

  972.4 Coronary vasodilators
    Dipyridamole
    Nitrates [nitroglycerin]
    Nitrites

  972.5 Other vasodilators
    Cyclandelate
    Diazoxide
    Papaverine
    | Excludes | *nicotinic acid (972.2)*

  972.6 Other antihypertensive agents
    Clonidine   Rauwolfia alkaloids
    Guanethidine   Reserpine

  972.7 Antivaricose drugs, including sclerosing agents
    Sodium morrhuate
    Zinc salts

  972.8 Capillary-active drugs
    Adrenochrome derivatives
    Metaraminol

  972.9 Other and unspecified agents primarily affecting the cardiovascular system

● **973 Poisoning by agents primarily affecting the gastrointestinal system**

  973.0 Antacids and antigastric secretion drugs
    Aluminum hydroxide
    Magnesium trisilicate
    Coding Clinic: 2003, Q1, P19

  973.1 Irritant cathartics
    Bisacodyl
    Castor oil
    Phenolphthalein

  973.2 Emollient cathartics
    Dioctyl sulfosuccinates

  973.3 Other cathartics, including intestinal atonia drugs
    Magnesium sulfate

  973.4 Digestants
    Pancreatin   Pepsin
    Papain

  973.5 Antidiarrheal drugs
    Kaolin
    Pectin
    | Excludes | *anti-infectives (960.0–961.9)*

  973.6 Emetics

  973.8 Other specified agents primarily affecting the gastrointestinal system

  973.9 Unspecified agent primarily affecting the gastrointestinal system

● **974 Poisoning by water, mineral, and uric acid metabolism drugs**

  974.0 Mercurial diuretics
    Chlormerodrin
    Mercaptomerin
    Mersalyl

  974.1 Purine derivative diuretics
    Theobromine
    Theophylline
    | Excludes | *aminophylline [theophylline ethylenediamine] (975.7)*
                 caffeine (969.71)

  974.2 Carbonic acid anhydrase inhibitors
    Acetazolamide

  974.3 Saluretics
    Benzothiadiazides
    Chlorothiazide group

  974.4 Other diuretics
    Ethacrynic acid
    Furosemide

  974.5 Electrolytic, caloric, and water-balance agents

  974.6 Other mineral salts, not elsewhere classified

  974.7 Uric acid metabolism drugs
    Allopurinol
    Colchicine
    Probenecid

● **975 Poisoning by agents primarily acting on the smooth and skeletal muscles and respiratory system**

  975.0 Oxytocic agents
    Ergot alkaloids
    Oxytocin
    Prostaglandins

  975.1 Smooth muscle relaxants
    Adiphenine
    Metaproterenol [orciprenaline]
    | Excludes | *papaverine (972.5)*

  975.2 Skeletal muscle relaxants

  975.3 Other and unspecified drugs acting on muscles

  975.4 Antitussives
    Dextromethorphan
    Pipazethate

  975.5 Expectorants
    Acetylcysteine
    Guaifenesin
    Terpin hydrate

  975.6 Anti-common cold drugs

  975.7 Antiasthmatics
    Aminophylline [theophylline ethylenediamine]

  975.8 Other and unspecified respiratory drugs

● **976 Poisoning by agents primarily affecting skin and mucous membrane, ophthalmological, otorhinolaryngological, and dental drugs**

  976.0 Local anti-infectives and anti-inflammatory drugs

  976.1 Antipruritics

  976.2 Local astringents and local detergents

  976.3 Emollients, demulcents, and protectants

  976.4 Keratolytics, keratoplastics, other hair treatment drugs and preparations

  976.5 Eye anti-infectives and other eye drugs
    Idoxuridine

  976.6 Anti-infectives and other drugs and preparations for ear, nose, and throat

◀ New   ◀▥ Revised   ~~deleted~~ Deleted | Excludes | | Includes | Use additional   Code first   Omit code
● Unacceptable Principal Diagnosis   ● Use Additional Digit(s)   OGCR Official Guidelines   Coding Clinic

976.7 Dental drugs topically applied

> | Excludes | *anti-infectives (976.0)*
> *local anesthetics (968.5)*

976.8 Other agents primarily affecting skin and mucous membrane
Spermicides [vaginal contraceptives]

976.9 Unspecified agent primarily affecting skin and mucous membrane

● **977 Poisoning by other and unspecified drugs and medicinal substances**

977.0 Dietetics
Central appetite depressants

977.1 Lipotropic drugs

977.2 Antidotes and chelating agents, not elsewhere classified

977.3 Alcohol deterrents

977.4 Pharmaceutical excipients
Pharmaceutical adjuncts

977.8 Other specified drugs and medicinal substances
Contrast media used for diagnostic x-ray procedures
Diagnostic agents and kits

977.9 Unspecified drug or medicinal substance
Coding Clinic: 1986, Mar-April, P12

● **978 Poisoning by bacterial vaccines**

978.0 BCG

978.1 Typhoid and paratyphoid

978.2 Cholera

978.3 Plague

978.4 Tetanus

978.5 Diphtheria

978.6 Pertussis vaccine, including combinations with a pertussis component

978.8 Other and unspecified bacterial vaccines

978.9 Mixed bacterial vaccines, except combinations with a pertussis component

● **979 Poisoning by other vaccines and biological substances**

> | Excludes | *gamma globulin (964.6)*

979.0 Smallpox vaccine

979.1 Rabies vaccine

979.2 Typhus vaccine

979.3 Yellow fever vaccine

979.4 Measles vaccine

979.5 Poliomyelitis vaccine

979.6 Other and unspecified viral and rickettsial vaccines
Mumps vaccine

979.7 Mixed viral-rickettsial and bacterial vaccines, except combinations with a pertussis component

> | Excludes | *combinations with a pertussis component (978.6)*

979.9 Other and unspecified vaccines and biological substances

---

OGCR Section I.C.17.e.3

When a harmful substance is ingested or comes in contact with a person, this is classified as a toxic effect. The toxic effect codes are in categories 980-989. A toxic effect code should be sequenced first, followed by the code(s) that identify the result of the toxic effect. An external cause code from categories E860-E869 for accidental exposure, codes E950.6 or E950.7 for intentional self-harm, category E962 for assault, or categories E980-E982, for undetermined, should also be assigned to indicate intent.

TOXIC EFFECTS OF SUBSTANCES CHIEFLY NONMEDICINAL AS TO SOURCE (980–989)

> | Excludes | *burns from chemical agents (ingested)*
> *(947.0–947.9)*
> *localized toxic effects indexed elsewhere*
> *(001.0–799.9)*
> *respiratory conditions due to external agents*
> *(506.0–508.9)*

Use additional code to identify: ◄
personal history of retained foreign body fully removed (V15.53) ◄
retained foreign body status, if applicable (V90.01-V90.9) ◄

Use additional code to specify the nature of the toxic effect

● **980 Toxic effect of alcohol**

980.0 Ethyl alcohol
Denatured alcohol
Ethanol
Grain alcohol

Use additional code to identify any associated:
acute alcohol intoxication (305.0)
in alcoholism (303.0)
drunkenness (simple) (305.0)
pathological (291.4)
Coding Clinic: 2009, Q4, P129; 1996, Q3, P16; 1991, Q3, P14

980.1 Methyl alcohol
Methanol
Wood alcohol

980.2 Isopropyl alcohol
Dimethyl carbinol
Isopropanol
Rubbing alcohol

980.3 Fusel oil
Alcohol:
amyl
butyl
propyl

980.8 Other specified alcohols

980.9 Unspecified alcohol

981 Toxic effect of petroleum products
Benzine   Petroleum:
Gasoline   ether
Kerosene   naphtha
Paraffin wax   spirit

● **982 Toxic effect of solvents other than petroleum based**

982.0 Benzene and homologues

982.1 Carbon tetrachloride

982.2 Carbon disulfide
Carbon bisulfide

INJURY AND POISONING (800–999)

982.3 Other chlorinated hydrocarbon solvents
Tetrachloroethylene
Trichloroethylene

> **Excludes** *chlorinated hydrocarbon preparations other than solvents (989.2)*
>
> Coding Clinic: 2008, Q3, P6, 7×2

982.4 Nitroglycol

982.8 Other nonpetroleum-based solvents
Acetone

● **983 Toxic effect of corrosive aromatics, acids, and caustic alkalis**

983.0 Corrosive aromatics
Carbolic acid or phenol
Cresol

983.1 Acids
Acid:
  hydrochloric
  nitric
  sulfuric

983.2 Caustic alkalis
Lye
Potassium hydroxide
Sodium hydroxide

983.9 Caustic, unspecified

● **984 Toxic effect of lead and its compounds (including fumes)**

> **Includes**   that from all sources except medicinal substances

984.0 Inorganic lead compounds
Lead dioxide
Lead salts

984.1 Organic lead compounds
Lead acetate
Tetraethyl lead

984.8 Other lead compounds

984.9 Unspecified lead compound

● **985 Toxic effect of other metals**

> **Includes**   that from all sources except medicinal substances

985.0 Mercury and its compounds
Minamata disease

985.1 Arsenic and its compounds

985.2 Manganese and its compounds

985.3 Beryllium and its compounds

985.4 Antimony and its compounds

985.5 Cadmium and its compounds

985.6 Chromium

985.8 Other specified metals
Brass fumes   Iron compounds
Copper salts   Nickel compounds

985.9 Unspecified metal

986 Toxic effect of carbon monoxide

● **987 Toxic effect of other gases, fumes, or vapors**

987.0 Liquefied petroleum gases
Butane
Propane

987.1 Other hydrocarbon gas

987.2 Nitrogen oxides
Nitrogen dioxide
Nitrous fumes

987.3 Sulfur dioxide

987.4 Freon
Dichloromonofluoromethane

987.5 Lacrimogenic gas
Bromobenzyl cyanide
Chloroacetophenone
Ethyliodoacetate

987.6 Chlorine gas

987.7 Hydrocyanic acid gas

987.8 Other specified gases, fumes, or vapors
Phosgene
Polyester fumes

987.9 Unspecified gas, fume, or vapor
Coding Clinic: 2005, Q3, P10-11

● **988 Toxic effect of noxious substances eaten as food**

> **Excludes** *allergic reaction to food, such as:*
>   *gastroenteritis (558.3)*
>   *rash (692.5, 693.1)*
> *food poisoning (bacterial) (005.0–005.9)*
> *toxic effects of food contaminants, such as:*
>   *aflatoxin and other mycotoxin (989.7)*
>   *mercury (985.0)*

988.0 Fish and shellfish

988.1 Mushrooms

988.2 Berries and other plants

988.8 Other specified noxious substances eaten as food

988.9 Unspecified noxious substance eaten as food

● **989 Toxic effect of other substances, chiefly nonmedicinal as to source**

989.0 Hydrocyanic acid and cyanides
Potassium cyanide   Sodium cyanide

> **Excludes** *gas and fumes (987.7)*

989.1 Strychnine and salts

989.2 Chlorinated hydrocarbons
Aldrin   DDT
Chlordane   Dieldrin

> **Excludes** *chlorinated hydrocarbon solvents (982.0–982.3)*

989.3 Organophosphate and carbamate
Carbaryl   Parathion
Dichlorvos   Phorate
Malathion   Phosdrin

989.4 Other pesticides, not elsewhere classified
Mixtures of insecticides

989.5 Venom
Bites of venomous snakes, lizards, and spiders
Tick paralysis

989.6 Soaps and detergents

989.7 Aflatoxin and other mycotoxin [food contaminants]

● **989.8 Other substances, chiefly nonmedicinal as to source**

989.81 Asbestos

> **Excludes** *asbestosis (501)*
> *exposure to asbestos (V15.84)*

989.82 Latex

989.83 Silicone

> **Excludes** *silicone used in medical devices, implants and grafts (996.00–996.79)*

989.84 Tobacco

989.89 Other

989.9 Unspecified substance, chiefly nonmedicinal as to source

◀ New   ◀||| Revised   ~~deleted~~ Deleted   Excludes   Includes   Use additional   Code first   Omit code
● Unacceptable Principal Diagnosis   ● Use Additional Digit(s)   OGCR Official Guidelines   Coding Clinic

OTHER AND UNSPECIFIED EFFECTS OF EXTERNAL CAUSES (990–995)

990 Effects of radiation, unspecified
Complication of:
    phototherapy
    radiation therapy
Radiation sickness

> **Excludes** *specified adverse effects of radiation. Such*
> *conditions are to be classified according to*
> *the nature of the adverse effect, as:*
> *burns (940.0–949.5)*
> *dermatitis (692.7–692.8)*
> *leukemia (204.0–208.9)*
> *pneumonia (508.0)*
> *sunburn (692.71, 692.76–692.77)*
> *[The type of radiation giving rise to the adverse*
> *effect may be identified by use of the E codes.]*

● **991 Effects of reduced temperature**

991.0 Frostbite of face

991.1 Frostbite of hand

991.2 Frostbite of foot

991.3 Frostbite of other and unspecified sites

991.4 Immersion foot
Trench foot

991.5 Chilblains
Erythema pernio   Perniosis

991.6 Hypothermia
Hypothermia (accidental)

> **Excludes** *hypothermia following anesthesia (995.89)*
> *hypothermia not associated with low*
> *environmental temperature (780.65)*

991.8 Other specified effects of reduced temperature

991.9 Unspecified effect of reduced temperature
Effects of freezing or excessive cold NOS

● **992 Effects of heat and light**

> **Excludes** *burns (940.0–949.5)*
> *diseases of sweat glands due to heat (705.0–705.9)*
> *malignant hyperpyrexia following anesthesia*
> *(995.86)*
> *sunburn (692.71, 692.76–692.77)*

992.0 Heat stroke and sunstroke
Heat apoplexy   Siriasis
Heat pyrexia   Thermoplegia
Ictus solaris

Use additional code(s) to identify any associated
complication of heat stroke, such as: ◄
alterations of consciousness (780.01-780.09) ◄
systemic inflammatory response syndrome
    (995.93-995.94) ◄

992.1 Heat syncope
Heat collapse

992.2 Heat cramps

992.3 Heat exhaustion, anhydrotic
Heat prostration due to water depletion

> **Excludes** *that associated with salt depletion (992.4)*

992.4 Heat exhaustion due to salt depletion
Heat prostration due to salt (and water) depletion

992.5 Heat exhaustion, unspecified
Heat prostration NOS

992.6 Heat fatigue, transient

992.7 Heat edema

992.8 Other specified heat effects

992.9 Unspecified

● **993 Effects of air pressure**

993.0 Barotrauma, otitic
Aero-otitis media
Effects of high altitude on ears

993.1 Barotrauma, sinus
Aerosinusitis
Effects of high altitude on sinuses

993.2 Other and unspecified effects of high altitude
Alpine sickness
Andes disease
Anoxia due to high altitude
Hypobaropathy
Mountain sickness

993.3 Caisson disease
Bends
Compressed-air disease
Decompression sickness
Divers' palsy or paralysis

993.4 Effects of air pressure caused by explosion

993.8 Other specified effects of air pressure

993.9 Unspecified effect of air pressure

● **994 Effects of other external causes**

> **Excludes** *certain adverse effects not elsewhere classified*
> *(995.0–995.8)*

994.0 Effects of lightning
Shock from lightning
Struck by lightning NOS

> **Excludes** *burns (940.0–949.5)*

994.1 Drowning and nonfatal submersion
Bathing cramp
Immersion

994.2 Effects of hunger
Deprivation of food
Starvation

994.3 Effects of thirst
Deprivation of water

994.4 Exhaustion due to exposure

994.5 Exhaustion due to excessive exertion
Exhaustion due to overexertion

994.6 Motion sickness
Air sickness
Seasickness
Travel sickness

994.7 Asphyxiation and strangulation
Suffocation (by):
    bedclothes
    cave-in
    constriction
    mechanical
    plastic bag
    pressure
    strangulation

> **Excludes** *asphyxia from:*
> *carbon monoxide (986)*
> *inhalation of food or foreign body*
> *(932–934.9)*
> *other gases, fumes, and vapors*
> *(987.0–987.9)*

**994.8 Electrocution and nonfatal effects of electric
current**
Shock from electric current
Shock from electroshock gun (taser)

> **Excludes** *electric burns (940.0–949.5)*

994.9 Other effects of external causes
Effects of:
    abnormal gravitational [G] forces or states
    weightlessness

INJURY AND POISONING (800–999)

◄ New   ◄|||| Revised   ~~deleted~~ Deleted   Excludes   Includes   Use additional   Code first   Omit code
● Unacceptable Principal Diagnosis   ● Use Additional Digit(s)   OGCR Official Guidelines   Coding Clinic

● **995 Certain adverse effects not elsewhere classified**

> **Excludes** *complications of surgical and medical care (996.0–999.9)*

> Coding Clinic: 2008, Q1, P12-13

995.0 Other anaphylactic shock
　Allergic shock NOS or due to adverse effect of correct medicinal substance properly administered
　Anaphylactic reaction NOS or due to adverse effect of correct medicinal substance properly administered
　Anaphylaxis NOS or due to adverse effect of correct medicinal substance properly administered

> **Excludes** *anaphylactic reaction to serum (999.4)*
> *anaphylactic shock due to adverse food reaction (995.60–995.69)*

> Use additional E code to identify external cause, such as:
> adverse effects of correct medicinal substance properly administered [E930–E949]

995.1 Angioneurotic edema
　Giant urticaria

> **Excludes** *urticaria:*
> *due to serum (999.5)*
> *other specified (698.2, 708.0–708.9, 757.33)*

● **995.2 Other and unspecified adverse effect of drug, medicinal and biological substance** ~~(due) to correct medicinal substance properly administered~~ ◀▥

> ~~Adverse effect to correct medicinal substance properly administered~~
> ~~Allergic reaction to correct medicinal substance properly administered~~
> ~~Hypersensitivity to correct medicinal substance properly administered~~
> ~~Idiosyncrasy due to correct medicinal substance properly administered~~
> ~~Drug:~~
> 　~~hypersensitivity NOS~~
> 　~~reaction NOS~~

> **Excludes** *pathological drug intoxication (292.2)*

> Coding Clinic: 2006, Q4, P112-113; 1997, Q2, P12; 1995, Q3, P13; 1992, Q3, P16-17

995.20 Unspecified adverse effect of unspecified drug, medicinal and biological substance
　Unspecified adverse effect of unspecified medicinal substance properly administered ◀

995.21 Arthus phenomenon
　Arthus reaction
　Hypersensitivity reaction resulting from immune complex reactions

995.22 Unspecified adverse effect of anesthesia

995.23 Unspecified adverse effect of insulin

995.24 Failed moderate sedation during procedure
　Failed conscious sedation during procedure

995.27 Other drug allergy
　Allergic reaction NEC (due) to correct medical substance properly administered ◀
　Drug allergy NOS
　Drug hypersensitivity NOS
　Hypersensitivity (due) to correct medical substance properly administered ◀

995.29 Unspecified adverse effect of other drug, medicinal and biological substance
　Unspecified adverse effect of medicinal substance NEC properly administered ◀

995.3 Allergy, unspecified
　Allergic reaction NOS
　Hypersensitivity NOS
　Idiosyncrasy NOS

> **Excludes** *allergic reaction NOS to correct medicinal substance properly administered (995.27)*
> *allergy to existing dental restorative materials (525.66)*
> *specific types of allergic reaction, such as:*
> 　*allergic diarrhea (558.3)*
> 　*dermatitis (691.0–693.9)*
> 　*hayfever (477.0–477.9)*

995.4 Shock due to anesthesia
　Shock due to anesthesia in which the correct substance was properly administered

> **Excludes** *complications of anesthesia in labor or delivery (668.0–668.9)*
> *overdose or wrong substance given (968.0–969.9)*
> *postoperative shock NOS (998.0)*
> *specified adverse effects of anesthesia classified elsewhere, such as:*
> 　*anoxic brain damage (348.1)*
> 　*hepatitis (070.0–070.9), etc.*
> *unspecified adverse effect of anesthesia (995.22)*

● **995.5 Child maltreatment syndrome**

> Use additional code(s), if applicable, to identify any associated injuries

> Use additional E code to identify:
> nature of abuse (E960–E968)
> perpetrator (E967.0–E967.9)
> Coding Clinic: 1998, Q1, P11; 1984, Sept-Oct, P16; 1984, Nov-Dec, P9

995.50 Child abuse, unspecified

995.51 Child emotional/psychological abuse

995.52 Child neglect (nutritional)

> Use additional code to identify intent of neglect (E904.0,E968.4)

995.53 Child sexual abuse

995.54 Child physical abuse
　Battered baby or child syndrome

> **Excludes** *Shaken infant syndrome (995.55)*

> Coding Clinic: 1999, Q3, P14-15

995.55 Shaken infant syndrome

> Use additional code(s) to identify any associated injuries
> Coding Clinic: 1996, Q4, P43-44

995.59 Other child abuse and neglect
　Multiple forms of abuse

> Use additional code to identify intent of neglect (E904.0,E968.4)

● **995.6 Anaphylactic shock due to adverse food reaction**
　Anaphylactic reaction due to food
　Anaphylactic shock due to nonpoisonous foods

995.60 Due to unspecified food

995.61 Due to peanuts

995.62 Due to crustaceans

995.63 Due to fruits and vegetables

995.64 Due to tree nuts and seeds
> Coding Clinic: 2008, Q1, P12-13

995.65 **Due to fish**

995.66 **Due to food additives**

995.67 **Due to milk products**

995.68 **Due to eggs**

995.69 **Due to other specified food**

995.7 **Other adverse food reactions, not elsewhere classified**

> Use additional code to identify the type of reaction, such as:
> hives (708.0)
> wheezing (786.07)
>
> > **Excludes** *anaphylactic shock due to adverse food reaction (995.6)*
> > *asthma (493.0, 493.9)*
> > *dermatitis due to food (693.1)*
> > *in contact with the skin (692.5)*
> > *gastroenteritis and colitis due to food (558.3)*
> > *rhinitis due to food (477.1)*

● 995.8 **Other specified adverse effects, not elsewhere classified**

995.80 **Adult maltreatment, unspecified**
Abused person NOS

> Use additional code to identify:
> any associated injury
> nature of abuse (E960–E968)
> perpetrator (E967.0–E967.9)

995.81 **Adult physical abuse**
Battered:
person syndrome NEC
man
spouse
woman

> Use additional code to identify:
> any associated injury
> nature of abuse (E960–E968)
> perpetrator (E967.0–E967.9)
> Coding Clinic: 1996, Q4, P43-44; 1984, Sept-Oct, P16

995.82 **Adult emotional/psychological abuse**

> Use additional E code to identify
> perpetrator (E967.0–E967.9)

995.83 **Adult sexual abuse**

> Use additional code to identify:
> any associated injury
> perpetrator (E967.0–E967.9)

995.84 **Adult neglect (nutritional)**

> Use additional code to identify:
> intent of neglect (E904.0–E968.4)
> perpetrator (E967.0–E967.9)

995.85 **Other adult abuse and neglect**
Multiple forms of abuse and neglect

> Use additional code to identify:
> any associated injury
> intent of neglect (E904.0, E968.4)
> nature of abuse (E960–E968)
> perpetrator (E967.0–E967.9)

995.86 **Malignant hyperthermia**
Malignant hyperpyrexia due to anesthesia
Extremely high body temperature—greater than 106° F or 41.1° C

995.89 **Other**
Hypothermia due to anesthesia
Coding Clinic: 2004, Q2, P18; 2003, Q3, P12

● 995.9 **Systemic inflammatory response syndrome (SIRS)**
Coding Clinic: 2010, Q1, P12; 2006, Q4, P113-116; 2005, Q3, P23; 2004, Q2, P16; 2002, Q4, P71-73

995.90 **Systemic inflammatory response syndrome, unspecified SIRS NOS**

● 995.91 **Sepsis**
Systemic inflammatory response syndrome due to infectious process without acute organ dysfunction

> *Code first underlying infection*
>
> > **Excludes** *sepsis with acute organ dysfunction (995.92)*
> > *sepsis with multiple organ dysfunction (995.92)*
> > *severe sepsis (995.92)*
> > Coding Clinic: 2008, Q4, P69-73; 2007, Q4, P84-86; 2004, Q2, P16

OGCR Section I.C.1.b.2.12

Only one code from subcategory 995.9 should be assigned. Therefore, when a non-infectious condition leads to an infection resulting in sepsis or severe sepsis, assign either code 995.91 or 995.92. Do not additionally assign code 995.93, Systemic inflammatory response syndrome due to noninfectious process without acute organ dysfunctiion, or 995.94, Systemic inflammatory response syndrome with acute organ dysfunction.

995.92 **Severe sepsis**
Sepsis with acute organ dysfunction
Sepsis with multiple organ dysfunction (MOD)
Systemic inflammatory response syndrome due to infectious process with acute organ dysfunction

> *Code first underlying infection*
>
> Use additional code to specify acute organ dysfunction, such as:
> acute kidney failure (584.5–584.9)
> acute respiratory failure (518.81)
> critical illness myopathy (359.81)
> critical illness polyneuropathy (357.82)
> disseminated intravascular coagulopathy (DIC) syndrome (286.6)
> encephalopathy (348.31)
> hepatic failure (570)
> septic shock (785.52)
> Coding Clinic: 2009, Q4, P129; 2007, Q4, P96-97; 2005, Q2, P18-20x2; 2004, Q2, P16; 2003, Q4, P73, 79-81

995.93 **Systemic inflammatory response syndrome due to noninfectious process without acute organ dysfunction**

> *Code first underlying conditions, such as:*
> acute pancreatitis (577.0)
> trauma
>
> > **Excludes** *systemic inflammatory response syndrome due to noninfectious process with acute organ dysfunction (995.94)*
> > Coding Clinic: 2010, Q1, P12

INJURY AND POISONING (800–999)

995.94 Systemic inflammatory response syndrome due to non-infectious process with acute organ dysfunction

Code first underlying conditions, such as:
acute pancreatitis (577.0)
heat stroke (992.0) ◄
trauma

Use additional code to specify acute organ dysfunction, such as:
acute kidney failure (584.5–584.9)
acute respiratory failure (518.81)
critical illness myopathy (359.81)
critical illness polyneuropathy (357.82)
disseminated intravascular coagulopathy (DIC) syndrome (286.6)
encephalopathy (348.31)
hepatic failure (570)

Excludes   *severe sepsis (995.92)*

Coding Clinic: 2010, Q1, P12; 2005, Q2, P19-20

OGCR   Section I.C.19.a.7
An external cause code is not appropriate with a code from subcategory 995.9, unless the patient also has another condition for which an E code would be appropriate (such as an injury, poisoning, or adverse effect of drugs).

COMPLICATIONS OF SURGICAL AND MEDICAL CARE, NOT ELSEWHERE CLASSIFIED (996–999)

Excludes   *adverse effects of medicinal agents (001.0–799.9, 995.0–995.8)*
burns from local applications and irradiation (940.0–949.5)
complications of:
conditions for which the procedure was performed
surgical procedures during abortion, labor, and delivery (630–676.9)
poisoning and toxic effects of drugs and chemicals (960.0–989.9)
postoperative conditions in which no complications are present, such as:
artificial opening status (V44.0–V44.9)
closure of external stoma (V55.0–V55.9)
fitting of prosthetic device (V52.0–V52.9)
specified complications classified elsewhere:
anesthetic shock (995.4)
electrolyte imbalance (276.0–276.9)
postlaminectomy syndrome (722.80–722.83)
postmastectomy lymphedema syndrome (457.0)
postoperative psychosis (293.0–293.9)
any other condition classified elsewhere in the Alphabetic Index when described as due to a procedure

● **996 Complications peculiar to certain specified procedures**

Includes   complications, not elsewhere classified, in the use of artificial substitutes [e.g., Dacron, metal, Silastic, Teflon] or natural sources [e.g., bone] involving:
anastomosis (internal)
graft (bypass) (patch)
implant
internal device:
catheter
electronic
fixation
prosthetic
reimplant
transplant

Excludes   *accidental puncture or laceration during procedure (998.2)*
capsular contracture of breast implant (611.83)
complications of internal anastomosis of:
gastrointestinal tract (997.4)
urinary tract (997.5)
endosseous dental implant failures (525.71–525.79)
intraoperative floppy iris syndrome (IFIS) (364.81)
mechanical complication of respirator (V46.14)
other specified complications classified elsewhere, such as:
hemolytic anemia (283.1)
functional cardiac disturbances (429.4)
serum hepatitis (070.2–070.3)

● **996.0 Mechanical complication of cardiac device, implant, and graft**

Breakdown (mechanical)   Obstruction, mechanical
Displacement   Perforation
Leakage   Protrusion
Coding Clinic: 2007, Q3, P7-8

996.00 Unspecified device, implant, and graft

996.01 Due to cardiac pacemaker (electrode)
Coding Clinic: 2006, Q2, P15-16; 1999, Q2, P11-12

996.02 Due to heart valve prosthesis
Coding Clinic: 1999, Q2, P4

996.03 Due to coronary bypass graft

Excludes   *atherosclerosis of graft (414.02, 414.03)*
embolism [occlusion NOS] [thrombus] of graft (996.72)
Coding Clinic: 1993, Q4, P40-41

996.04 Due to automatic implantable cardiac defibrillator
Coding Clinic: 2005, Q2, P3

996.09 Other
Coding Clinic: 1993, Q2, P9

996.1 Mechanical complication of other vascular device, implant, and graft
    Mechanical complications involving:
        aortic (bifurcation) graft (replacement)
        arteriovenous:
            dialysis catheter
            fistula surgically created
            shunt surgically created
        balloon (counterpulsation) device, intra-aortic
        carotid artery bypass graft
        femoral-popliteal bypass graft
        umbrella device, vena cava

> **Excludes** *atherosclerosis of biological graft (440.30–440.32)*
> *embolism [occlusion NOS] [thrombus] of (biological) (synthetic) graft (996.74)*
> *peritoneal dialysis catheter (996.56)*

Coding Clinic: 2006, Q1, P10-11; 2005, Q2, P8; 2002, Q1, P13; 1995, Q1, P3

996.2 Mechanical complication of nervous system device, implant, and graft
    Mechanical complications involving:
        dorsal column stimulator
        electrodes implanted in brain [brain "pacemaker"]
        peripheral nerve graft
        ventricular (communicating) shunt
Coding Clinic: 1987, Sept-Oct, P10

● **996.3 Mechanical complication of genitourinary device, implant, and graft**

    996.30 Unspecified device, implant, and graft

    996.31 Due to urethral [indwelling] catheter

    996.32 Due to intrauterine contraceptive device

    996.39 Other
        Cystostomy catheter
        Prosthetic reconstruction of vas deferens
        Repair (graft) of ureter without mention of resection

> **Excludes** *complications due to:*
>   *external stoma of urinary tract (997.5)*
>   *internal anastomosis of urinary tract (997.5)*

● **996.4 Mechanical complication of internal orthopedic device, implant, and graft**
    Mechanical complications involving:
        external (fixation) device utilizing internal screw(s), pin(s) or other methods of fixation
        grafts of bone, cartilage, muscle, or tendon
        internal (fixation) device such as nail, plate, rod, etc.

Use additional code to identify prosthetic joint with mechanical complication (V43.60–V43.69)

> **Excludes** *complications of external orthopedic device, such as:*
>   *pressure ulcer due to cast (707.00–707.09)*

Coding Clinic: 2005, Q4, P91-93, 110-112; 1999, Q2, P10-11; 1998, Q2, P19; 1996, Q2, P11; 1985, Nov-Dec, P11; 1984, Nov-Dec, P18

    996.40 Unspecified mechanical complication of internal orthopedic device, implant, and graft

    996.41 Mechanical loosening of prosthetic joint
        Aseptic loosening
        Coding Clinic: 2005, Q4, P91-93

    996.42 Dislocation of prosthetic joint
        Instability of prosthetic joint
        Subluxation of prosthetic joint

    996.43 Broken prosthetic joint implant
        Breakage (fracture) of prosthetic joint

    996.44 Peri-prosthetic fracture around prosthetic joint
        Coding Clinic: 2005, Q4, P91-93

    996.45 Peri-prosthetic osteolysis
        Use additional code to identify major osseous defect, if applicable (731.3)
        Coding Clinic: 2006, Q4, P103-104

    996.46 Articular bearing surface wear of prosthetic joint

    996.47 Other mechanical complication of prosthetic joint implant
        Mechanical complication of prosthetic joint NOS
        Prosthetic joint implant failure NOS

    996.49 Other mechanical complication of other internal orthopedic device, implant, and graft
        Breakage of internal fixation device in bone
        Dislocation of internal fixation device in bone

> **Excludes** *mechanical complication of prosthetic joint implant (996.41–996.46)*

    Coding Clinic: 2010, Q1, P13

● **996.5 Mechanical complication of other specified prosthetic device, implant, and graft**
    Mechanical complications involving:
        prosthetic implant in:
            bile duct
            breast
            chin
            orbit of eye
        nonabsorbable surgical material NOS
        other graft, implant, and internal device, not elsewhere classified

    996.51 Due to corneal graft

    996.52 Due to graft of other tissue, not elsewhere classified
        Skin graft failure or rejection

> **Excludes** *failure of artificial skin graft (996.55)*
> *failure of decellularized allodermis (996.55)*
> *sloughing of temporary skin allografts or xenografts (pigskin)- omit code*

    Coding Clinic: 1996, Q1, P10; 1990, Q3, P15

    996.53 Due to ocular lens prosthesis

> **Excludes** *contact lenses—code to condition*

    Coding Clinic: 2000, Q1, P9-10

    996.54 Due to breast prosthesis
        Breast capsule (prosthesis)
        Mammary implant
        Coding Clinic: 1998, Q2, P14; 1992, Q3, P4-5

    996.55 Due to artificial skin graft and decellularized allodermis

Dislodgement	Non-adherence
Displacement	Poor incorporation
Failure	Shearing

        Coding Clinic: 1998, Q4, P52-53

    996.56 Due to peritoneal dialysis catheter

> **Excludes** *mechanical complication of arteriovenous dialysis catheter (996.1)*

    Coding Clinic: 1998, Q4, P54

INJURY AND POISONING (800–999)

996.57 Due to insulin pump
Coding Clinic: 2003, Q4, P81-82

OGCR Section I.C.3.a.6.a

An underdose of insulin due to an insulin pump failure should be assigned 996.57, Mechanical complication due to insulin pump, as the principal or first listed code, followed by the appropriate diabetes mellitus code based on documentation.

OGCR Section I.C.3.a.6.b

The principal or first listed code for an encounter due to an insulin pump malfunction resulting in an overdose of insulin, should also be 996.57, Mechanical complication due to insulin pump, followed by 962.3, Poisoning by insulins and antidiabetic agents, and the appropriate diabetes mellitus code based on documentation.

996.59 Due to other implant and internal device, not elsewhere classified
Nonabsorbable surgical material NOS
Prosthetic implant in:
    bile duct
    chin
    orbit of eye
Coding Clinic: 1999, Q2, P13-14; 1997, Q3, P7; 1994, Q3, P7x2

● **996.6 Infection and inflammatory reaction due to internal prosthetic device, implant, and graft**
Infection (causing obstruction) due to (presence of) any device, implant, and graft classifiable to 996.0–996.5
Inflammation due to (presence of) any device, implant, and graft classifiable to 996.0–996.5

Use additional code to identify specified infections
Coding Clinic: 2008, Q2, P9-10; 1987, Jan-Feb, P14-15

996.60 Due to unspecified device, implant and graft

996.61 Due to cardiac device, implant and graft
Cardiac pacemaker or defibrillator:
    electrode(s), lead(s)
    pulse generator
    subcutaneous pocket
Coronary artery bypass graft
Heart valve prosthesis

996.62 Due to vascular device, implant and graft
Arterial graft
Arteriovenous fistula or shunt
Infusion pump
Vascular catheter (arterial) (dialysis) (peripheral venous)

Excludes	*infection due to:*

central venous catheter (999.31)
Hickman catheter (999.31)
peripherally inserted central catheter (PICC) (999.31)
portacath (port-a-cath) (999.31)
triple lumen catheter (999.31)
umbilical venous catheter (999.31)
Coding Clinic: 2007, Q4, P84-86; 2004, Q2, P16; Q1, P5; 2003, Q4, P111-112; Q2, P7-8; 1994, Q2, P13

996.63 Due to nervous system device, implant and graft
Electrodes implanted in brain
Peripheral nerve graft
Spinal canal catheter
Ventricular (communicating) shunt (catheter)

996.64 Due to indwelling urinary catheter
Use additional code to identify specified infections, such as:
    cystitis (595.0–595.9)
    sepsis (038.0–038.9)
Coding Clinic: 2009, Q3, P18-19; 1993, Q3, P6

996.65 Due to other genitourinary device, implant and graft
Intrauterine contraceptive device
Coding Clinic: 2000, Q1, P15-16

996.66 Due to internal joint prosthesis
Use additional code to identify infected prosthetic joint (V43.60–V43.69)
Coding Clinic: 2008, Q2, P3-5x3; 2007, Q2, P8-9; 2005, Q4, P110-112; 1991, Q2, P18

996.67 Due to other internal orthopedic device, implant and graft
Bone growth stimulator (electrode)
Internal fixation device (pin) (rod) (screw)

996.68 Due to peritoneal dialysis catheter
Exit-site infection or inflammation
Coding Clinic: 2001, Q2, P11; 1998, Q4, P55

996.69 Due to other internal prosthetic device, implant, and graft
Breast prosthesis
Ocular lens prosthesis
Prosthetic orbital implant
Coding Clinic: 2008, Q2, P9-11; 2003, Q4, P108; 1998, Q4, P52-53

● **996.7 Other complications of internal (biological) (synthetic) prosthetic device, implant, and graft**
Complication NOS due to (presence of) any device, implant, and graft classifiable to 996.0–996.5
    occlusion NOS
Embolism due to (presence of) any device, implant, and graft classifiable to 996.0–996.5
Fibrosis due to (presence of) any device, implant, and graft classifiable to 996.0–996.5
Hemorrhage due to (presence of) any device, implant, and graft classifiable to 996.0–996.5
Pain due to (presence of) any device, implant, and graft classifiable to 996.0–996.5
Stenosis due to (presence of) any device, implant, and graft classifiable to 996.0–996.5
Thrombus due to (presence of) any device, implant, and graft classifiable to 996.0–996.5

Use additional code to identify complication, such as:
pain due to presence of device, implant or graft (338.18–338.19, 338.28–338.29)
venous embolism and thrombosis (453.2–453.9)

Excludes	*disruption (dehiscence) of internal suture material (998.31)*

transplant rejection (996.8)
Coding Clinic: 2007, Q2, P13-15; 2004, Q2, P7-8; 1989, Q1, P9&10; 1984, Nov-Dec, P18

996.70 Due to unspecified device, implant, and graft

996.71 Due to heart valve prosthesis
Coding Clinic: 2008, Q2, P9-10

996.72 Due to other cardiac device, implant, and graft

Cardiac pacemaker or defibrillator:
  electrode(s), lead(s)
  subcutaneous pocket
Coronary artery bypass (graft)

> **Excludes** *occlusion due to atherosclerosis (414.00–414.07)*

Coding Clinic: 2008, Q3, P10-11; 2006, Q3, P8-9, 25; 2001, Q3, P20

996.73 Due to renal dialysis device, implant, and graft

Coding Clinic: 1991, Q2, P18

996.74 Due to vascular device, implant, and graft

> **Excludes** *occlusion of biological graft due to atherosclerosis (440.30–440.32)*

Coding Clinic: 2003, Q1, P16-18x2; 2000, Q1, P10

996.75 Due to nervous system device, implant, and graft

996.76 Due to genitourinary device, implant, and graft

Coding Clinic: 2009, Q1, P13; 2000, Q1, P15-16

996.77 Due to internal joint prosthesis

Use additional code to identify prosthetic joint (V43.60–V43.69)

996.78 Due to other internal orthopedic device, implant, and graft

Coding Clinic: 2003, Q2, P14

996.79 Due to other internal prosthetic device, implant, and graft

Coding Clinic: 2004, Q2, P7; 2001, Q1, P8-9; 1995, Q3, P14; 1992, Q3, P4-5

● **996.8 Complications of transplanted organ**

Transplant failure or rejection

Use additional code to identify nature of complication, such as:
  cytomegalovirus [CMV] infection (078.5)
  graft-versus-host disease (279.50–279.53)
  malignancy associated with organ transplant (199.2)
  post-transplant lymphoproliferative disorder (PTLD) (238.77)

Coding Clinic: 2003, Q1, P11; 2002, Q4, P53-54; 2001, Q3, P12-13; 1993, Q2, P11; Q1, P24

OGCR Section I.C.17.f.2.a

Transplant complications other than kidney: Codes under subcategory 996.8, Complications of transplanted organ, are for use for both complications and rejection of transplanted organs. A transplant complication code is only assigned if the complication affects the function of the transplanted organ. Two codes are required to fully describe a transplant complication, the appropriate code from subcategory 996.8 and a secondary code that identifies the complication. Pre-existing conditions or conditions that develop after the transplant are not coded as complications unless they affect the function of the transplanted organs.
See I.C.18.d.3 for transplant organ removal status
See I.C.2.i for malignant neoplasm associated with transplanted organ.

996.80 Transplanted organ, unspecified

996.81 Kidney

Coding Clinic: 2010, Q1, P15; 2008, Q4, P82-83; 2003, Q3, P16-17; 1998, Q3, P6x2&7; 1994, Q3, P8; Q2, P9; 1993, Q4, P32-33; Q1, P24-25

996.82 Liver

Coding Clinic: 2008, Q4, P82-83, 97-100; 2003, Q3, P16x2&17; 1998, Q3, P4

996.83 Heart

Coding Clinic: 2003, Q3, P16; 2002, Q4, P53-54; 2001, Q3, P13-14x2; 1998, Q3, P5; 1993, Q3, P13

996.84 Lung

Coding Clinic: 2003, Q2, P12; 1998, Q3, P5

996.85 Bone marrow

Coding Clinic: 2008, Q4, P90-91

996.86 Pancreas

996.87 Intestine

Coding Clinic: 2000, Q4, P47-48

996.89 Other specified transplanted organ

Coding Clinic: 1994, Q3, P5

● **996.9 Complications of reattached extremity or body part**

996.90 Unspecified extremity

996.91 Forearm

996.92 Hand

996.93 Finger(s)

996.94 Upper extremity, other and unspecified

996.95 Foot and toe(s)

996.96 Lower extremity, other and unspecified

996.99 Other specified body part

● **997 Complications affecting specified body systems, not elsewhere classified**

Use additional code to identify complication

> **Excludes** *the listed conditions when specified as:*
> *causing shock (998.0)*
> *complications of:*
> *anesthesia:*
> *adverse effect (001.0–799.9, 995.0–995.8)*
> *in labor or delivery (668.0–668.9)*
> *poisoning (968.0–969.9)*
> *implanted device or graft (996.0–996.9)*
> *obstetrical procedures (669.0–669.4)*
> *reattached extremity (996.90–996.96)*
> *transplanted organ (996.80–996.89)*

Coding Clinic: 1995, Q2, P7; 1993, Q2, P9-10; 1992, Q1, P13

● **997.0 Nervous system complications**

997.00 Nervous system complication, unspecified

997.01 Central nervous system complication

Anoxic brain damage
Cerebral hypoxia

> **Excludes** *Cerebrovascular hemorrhage or infarction (997.02)*

Coding Clinic: 2007, Q1, P22-23; 2006, Q1, P15-16

997.02 Iatrogenic cerebrovascular infarction or hemorrhage

Postoperative stroke

Coding Clinic: 2006, Q3, P6; 2004, Q2, P8-9

OGCR Section I.C.7.c

A cerebrovascular hemorrhage or infarction that occurs as a result of medical intervention is coded to 997.02. Documentation should clearly specify cause-and-effect relationship between the medical intervention and the cerebrovascular accident in order to assign this code. A secondary code from the code range 430-432 or from a code from subcategories 433 or 434 with a fifth digit of "1" should also be used to identify the type of hemorrhage or infarct.

997.09 Other nervous system complications

INJURY AND POISONING (800–999)

997.1 Cardiac complications
  Cardiac:
    arrest during or resulting from a procedure
    insufficiency during or resulting from a
      procedure
  Cardiorespiratory failure during or resulting from
    a procedure
  Heart failure during or resulting from a procedure

  | Excludes | *the listed conditions as long-term effects of cardiac surgery or due to the presence of cardiac prosthetic device (429.4)* |

  Coding Clinic: 2008, Q4, P177-180; 2000, Q2, P12; 1994, Q3, P9; Q1,
  P20; 1993, Q4, P37, 39-43; 5th Issue, P6-7

997.2 Peripheral vascular complications
  Phlebitis or thrombophlebitis during or resulting
    from a procedure

  | Excludes | *the listed conditions due to:*
    implant or catheter device (996.62)
    infusion, perfusion, or transfusion
      (999.2)
    complications affecting blood vessels
      (997.71–997.79) |

  Coding Clinic: 2003, Q1, P6-7; 2002, Q3, P24-27; 1993, Q1, P26

● **997.3 Respiratory complications**

  | Excludes | *iatrogenic [postoperative] pneumothorax (512.1)*
    iatrogenic pulmonary embolism (415.11)
    Mendelson's syndrome in labor and delivery (668.0)
      Aspiration into the lungs of gastric contents following vomiting or regurgitation
    specified complications classified elsewhere, such as:
      adult respiratory distress syndrome (518.5)
      pulmonary edema, postoperative (518.4)
      respiratory insufficiency, acute, postoperative (518.5)
      shock lung (518.5)
      tracheostomy complications (519.00–519.09)
      transfusion related acute lung injury (TRALI) (518.7) |

  Coding Clinic: 1997, Q1, P10; 1993, Q4, P43; Q2, P9-10; Q2, P3-4;
  1990, Q4, P25x2; 1989, Q1, P10

997.31 Ventilator associated pneumonia
  Ventilator associated pneumonitis

  | Use additional code to identify organism |

  Coding Clinic: 2008, Q4, P148-149; 2006, Q2, P25

997.39 Other respiratory complications
  Mendelson's syndrome resulting from a
    procedure
  Pneumonia (aspiration) resulting from a
    procedure

997.4 Digestive system complications
  Complications of:
    intestinal (internal) anastomosis and bypass, not
      elsewhere classified, except that involving
      urinary tract
  Hepatic failure specified as due to a procedure
  Hepatorenal syndrome specified as due to a
    procedure
    *Acute renal failure occurring along with cirrhosis or
      fulminant liver failure associated with portal
      hypertension*
  Intestinal obstruction NOS specified as due to a
    procedure

  | Excludes | *specified gastrointestinal complications classified elsewhere, such as:*
    blind loop syndrome (579.2)
    colostomy or enterostomy complications (569.60–569.69)
    complications of intestinal pouch (569.71–569.79)
    gastrojejunal ulcer (534.0–534.9)
    gastrostomy complications (536.40–536.49)
    infection of esophagostomy (530.86)
    infection of external stoma (569.61)
    mechanical complication of esophagostomy (530.87)
    pelvic peritoneal adhesions, female (614.6)
    peritoneal adhesions (568.0)
    peritoneal adhesions with obstruction (560.81)
    postcholecystectomy syndrome (576.0)
    postgastric surgery syndromes (564.2)
    pouchitis (569.71)
    vomiting following gastrointestinal surgery (564.3) |

  Coding Clinic: 2009, Q4, P129; 2003, Q1, P18; 2001, Q2, P4-6x2;
  1999, Q3, P4-5; Q2, P14; 1997, Q3, P7; Q1, P11; 1995, Q3,
  P7, 16; Q2, P7; 1993, Q1, P26; 1992, Q3, P15; 1989, Q2,
  P15; 1988, Q1, P14; 1987, Nov-Dec, P9; 1985, Sept-Oct, P11;
  Mar-April, P11

997.5 Urinary complications
  Complications of:
    external stoma of urinary tract
    internal anastomosis and bypass of urinary tract,
      including that involving intestinal tract
  Oliguria or anuria specified as due to procedure
  Renal (kidney):
    failure (acute) specified as due to procedure
    insufficiency (acute) specified as due to
      procedure
  Tubular necrosis (acute) specified as due to
    procedure

  | Excludes | *specified complications classified elsewhere, such as:*
    postoperative stricture of:
      ureter (593.3)
      urethra (598.2) |

  Coding Clinic: 2003, Q3, P13; 1996, Q3, P10-11,15; 1995, Q4,
  P72-73; 1994, Q1, P20; 1992, Q1, P13; 1989, Q2, P16

● **997.6 Amputation stump complication**

  | Excludes | *admission for treatment for a current traumatic amputation - code to complicated traumatic amputation*
    phantom limb (syndrome) (353.6) |

  Coding Clinic: 1996, Q4, P45-46

997.60 Unspecified complication

997.61 Neuroma of amputation stump

997.62 Infection (chronic)
Use additional code to identify the organism
Coding Clinic: 2005, Q1, P14-15; 2003, Q3, P14; 1996, Q4, P45-46

997.69 Other
Coding Clinic: 2005, Q1, P15

● **997.7 Vascular complications of other vessels**
Excludes *peripheral vascular complications (997.2)*

997.71 Vascular complications of mesenteric artery
Coding Clinic: 2001, Q4, P53

997.72 Vascular complications of renal artery

997.79 Vascular complications of other vessels

● **997.9 Complications affecting other specified body systems, not elsewhere classified**
Excludes *specified complications classified elsewhere, such as:*
broad ligament laceration syndrome (620.6)
postartificial menopause syndrome (627.4)
postoperative stricture of vagina (623.2)
Coding Clinic: 1994, Q1, P16; 1993, Q4, P41-42

997.91 Hypertension
Excludes *Essential hypertension (401.0–401.9)*

997.99 Other
Vitreous touch syndrome
Coding Clinic: 1994, Q2, P12; Q1, P17; Q1, P16-17

● **998 Other complications of procedures, NEC**
Excludes *fluid overload due to transfusion (blood) (276.61)* ◄
TACO (276.61) ◄
transfusion associated circulatory overload (276.61) ◄

998.0 Postoperative shock
Collapse NOS during or resulting from a surgical procedure
Shock (endotoxic) (hypovolemic) (septic) during or resulting from a surgical procedure
Excludes *shock:*
anaphylactic due to serum (999.4)
anesthetic (995.4)
electric (994.8)
following abortion (639.5)
obstetric (669.1)
traumatic (958.4)

● **998.1 Hemorrhage or hematoma or seroma complicating a procedure**
Excludes *hemorrhage, hematoma or seroma:*
complicating cesarean section or puerperal perineal wound (674.3)
due to implanted device or graft (996.70–996.79)
Coding Clinic: 2003, Q3, P13; 1993, Q1, P26; 1992, Q2, P15-16; 1987, Sept-Oct, P8

998.11 Hemorrhage complicating a procedure
Coding Clinic: 2003, Q3, P13; Q1, P4; 1997, Q4, P52; Q1, P10; 1994, Q1, P19-20

998.12 Hematoma complicating a procedure
Coding Clinic: 2006, Q3, P12; 2003, Q1, P6-7; 2002, Q3, P24-25; 1994, Q1, P20

998.13 Seroma complicating a procedure
Pocket of clear serous fluid that sometimes develops in the body after surgery
Coding Clinic: 1996, Q4, P46

998.2 Accidental puncture or laceration during a procedure
Accidental perforation by catheter or other instrument during a procedure on:
blood vessel
nerve
organ
Excludes *iatrogenic [postoperative] pneumothorax (512.1)*
puncture or laceration caused by implanted device intentionally left in operation wound (996.0–996.5)
specified complications classified elsewhere, such as:
broad ligament laceration syndrome (620.6)
dural tear (349.31)
incidental durotomy (349.31)
trauma from instruments during delivery (664.0–665.9)
Coding Clinic: 2010, Q1, P15; 2007, Q2, P11-12; 2006, Q1, P15; 2002, Q3, P24-27; 1994, Q3, P6; 1994, Q1, P17; 1990, Q3, P17-18; 1984, Nov-Dec, P12

● **998.3 Disruption of wound**
Dehiscence of operation wound
Splitting open
Disruption of any suture materials or other closure method
Rupture of operation wound
Excludes *disruption of:*
amputation of stump (997.69)
cesarean wound (674.1)
perineal wound, puerperal (674.2)
Coding Clinic: 2008, Q4, P149-152; 2002, Q4, P73; 1993, Q1, P19

998.30 Disruption of wound, unspecified
Disruption of wound NOS

998.31 Disruption of internal operation surgical wound
Disruption or dehiscence of closure of:
fascia, superficial or muscular
internal organ
muscle or muscle flap
ribs or rib cage
skull or craniotomy
sternum or sternotomy
tendon or ligament
Deep disruption or dehiscence of operation wound NOS
Excludes *complications of internal anastomosis of:*
gastrointestinal tract (997.4)
urinary tract (997.5)

998.32 Disruption of external operation (surgical) wound
Disruption or dehiscence of closure of:
cornea
mucosa
skin
subcutaneous tissue
Full-thickness skin disruption or dehiscence
Superficial disruption or dehiscence of operation wound
Coding Clinic: 2006, Q1, P8; 2005, Q1, P11; 2003, Q4, P104-107

998.33 Disruption of traumatic injury wound repair
Disruption or dehiscence of closure of traumatic laceration (external) (internal)

INJURY AND POISONING (800–999)

INJURY AND POISONING (800–999)

998.4 Foreign body accidentally left during a procedure
　　Adhesions due to foreign body accidentally left in operative wound or body cavity during a procedure
　　Obstruction due to foreign body accidentally left in operative wound or body cavity during a procedure
　　Perforation due to foreign body accidentally left in operative wound or body cavity during a procedure

　　Excludes *obstruction or perforation caused by implanted device intentionally left in body (996.0–996.5)*
　　Coding Clinic: 2009, Q1, P13; 1989, Q1, P9

● **998.5 Postoperative infection**

　　Excludes *bleb associated endophthalmitis (379.63)*
　　　　　infection due to:
　　　　　　implanted device (996.60–996.69)
　　　　　　infusion, perfusion, or transfusion (999.31–999.39)
　　　　　postoperative obstetrical wound infection (674.3)
　　Coding Clinic: 1996, Q4, P45-46; 1995, Q2, P7; 1994, Q3, P6; 1987, Jan-Feb, P13-14

　　998.51 Infected postoperative seroma
　　　　Use additional code to identify organism
　　　　Coding Clinic: 1996, Q4, P46

　　998.59 Other postoperative infection
　　　　Abscess: postoperative
　　　　　intra-abdominal postoperative
　　　　　stitch postoperative
　　　　　subphrenic postoperative
　　　　　wound postoperative
　　　　Septicemia postoperative

　　　　Use additional code to identify infection
　　　　Coding Clinic: 2006, Q2, P23-24; 2004, Q4, P75-76; 2003, Q4, P104-107; 1995, Q3, P5; Q2, P7, 11; 1993, Q1, P19

　　　　OGCR Section I.C.1.b.10.b
　　　　Sepsis due to postprocedural infection: In cases of postprocedural sepsis, the complication code, such as code 998.59, Other postoperative infection, or 674.3x, Other complications of obstetrical surgical wounds should be coded first followed by the appropriate sepsis codes (systemic infection code and either code 995.91 or 995.92). An additional code(s) for any acute organ dysfunction should also be assigned for cases of severe sepsis.

998.6 Persistent postoperative fistula
　　Coding Clinic: 1987, Jan-Feb, P14

998.7 Acute reaction to foreign substance accidentally left during a procedure
　　Peritonitis:
　　　aseptic
　　　chemical

● **998.8 Other specified complications of procedures, not elsewhere classified**
　　Coding Clinic: 1993, 5th Issue, P8, 15; 1989, Q1, P9; 1987, Jan-Feb, P13

　　998.81 Emphysema (subcutaneous) (surgical) resulting from a procedure

　　998.82 Cataract fragments in eye following cataract surgery

　　998.83 Non-healing surgical wound
　　　　Coding Clinic: 1996, Q4, P47

　　998.89 Other specified complications
　　　　Coding Clinic: 2009, Q2, P11; 2006, Q3, P9-10; 2005, Q3, P16-17; 1999, Q3, P13; 1998, Q2, P16

998.9 Unspecified complication of procedure, not elsewhere classified
　　Postoperative complication NOS

　　Excludes *complication NOS of obstetrical surgery or procedure (669.4)*
　　Coding Clinic: 1993, Q4, P41-42

● **999 Complications of medical care, not elsewhere classified**

　　Includes complications, not elsewhere classified, of:
　　　dialysis (hemodialysis) (peritoneal) (renal)
　　　extracorporeal circulation
　　　hyperalimentation therapy
　　　immunization
　　　infusion
　　　inhalation therapy
　　　injection
　　　inoculation
　　　perfusion
　　　transfusion
　　　vaccination
　　　ventilation therapy

　　Use additional code, where applicable, to identify specific complication

　　Excludes *specified complications classified elsewhere such as:*
　　　　complications of implanted device (996.0–996.9)
　　　　contact dermatitis due to drugs (692.3)
　　　　dementia dialysis (294.8)
　　　　　transient (293.9)
　　　　dialysis disequilibrium syndrome (276.0–276.9)
　　　　poisoning and toxic effects of drugs and chemicals (960.0–989.9)
　　　　postvaccinal encephalitis (323.51)
　　　　water and electrolyte imbalance (276.0–276.9)

999.0 Generalized vaccinia
　　Excludes *vaccinia not from vaccine (051.02)*

999.1 Air embolism
　　Air embolism to any site following infusion, perfusion, or transfusion
　　Excludes *embolism specified as:*
　　　　complicating:
　　　　　abortion (634–638 with .6, 639.6)
　　　　　ectopic or molar pregnancy (639.6)
　　　　　pregnancy, childbirth, or the puerperium (673.0)
　　　　due to implanted device (996.7)
　　　　traumatic (958.0)

999.2 Other vascular complications
　　Phlebitis following infusion, perfusion, or transfusion
　　Thromboembolism following infusion, perfusion, or transfusion
　　Thrombophlebitis following infusion, perfusion, or transfusion
　　Excludes *extravasation of vesicant drugs (999.81, 999.82)*
　　　　the listed conditions when specified as:
　　　　　due to implanted device (996.61–996.62, 996.72–996.74)
　　　　　postoperative NOS (997.2, 997.71–997.79)
　　Coding Clinic: 1997, Q2, P5

◀ New　◀┅ Revised　d̶e̶l̶e̶t̶e̶d̶ Deleted　Excludes　Includes　Use additional　Code first　Omit code
● Unacceptable Principal Diagnosis　● Use Additional Digit(s)　OGCR Official Guidelines　Coding Clinic

● **999.3 Other infection**

Infection following infusion, injection, transfusion, or vaccination

Sepsis following infusion, injection, transfusion, or vaccination

Septicemia following infusion, injection, transfusion, or vaccination

Use additional code to identify the specified infection, such as:
septicemia (038.0–038.9)

Excludes *the listed conditions when specified as:*
due to implanted device (996.60–996.69)
postoperative NOS (998.51–998.59)

Coding Clinic: 2001, Q2, P11-12; 1987, Jan-Feb, P14-15

999.31 Infection due to central venous catheter

Catheter-related bloodstream infection (CRBSI) NOS

Infection due to:
Hickman catheter
peripherally inserted central catheter (PICC)
portacath (port-a-cath)
triple lumen catheter
umbilical venous catheter

Excludes *infection due to:*
arterial catheter (996.62)
catheter NOS (996.69)
peripheral venous catheter (996.62)
urinary catheter (996.64)

Coding Clinic: 2008, Q4, P69-73, 192-193; 2007, Q4, P96-97

999.39 Infection following other infusion, injection, transfusion, or vaccination

999.4 Anaphylactic shock due to serum

Anaphylactic reaction due to serum

Excludes *shock:*
allergic NOS (995.0)
anaphylactic:
NOS (995.0)
due to drugs and chemicals (995.0)

999.5 Other serum reaction

Intoxication by serum	Serum sickness
Protein sickness	Urticaria due to serum
Serum rash	

Excludes *serum hepatitis (070.2–070.3)*

● **999.6 ABO incompatibility reaction due to transfusion of blood or blood products** ◀▥

~~Incompatible blood transfusion~~
~~Reaction to blood group incompatibility in infusion or transfusion~~

Excludes *minor blood group antigens reactions (Duffy) (E) (K(ell)) (Kidd) (Lewis) (M) (N) (P) (S) (999.89)*

999.60 ABO incompatibility reaction, unspecified ◀

ABO incompatible blood transfusion NOS ◀
Reaction to ABO incompatibility from transfusion NOS ◀

999.61 ABO incompatibility with hemolytic transfusion reaction not specified as acute or delayed ◀

ABO incompatibility with hemolytic transfusion reaction at unspecified time after transfusion ◀
Hemolytic transfusion reaction (HTR) due to ABO incompatibility ◀

999.62 ABO incompatibility with acute hemolytic transfusion reaction ◀

ABO incompatibility with hemolytic transfusion reaction less than 24 hours after transfusion ◀
Acute hemolytic transfusion reaction (AHTR) due to ABO incompatibility ◀

999.63 ABO incompatibility with delayed hemolytic transfusion reaction ◀

ABO incompatibility with hemolytic transfusion reaction 24 hours or more after transfusion ◀
Delayed hemolytic transfusion reaction (DHTR) due to ABO incompatibility ◀

999.69 Other ABO incompatibility reaction ◀

Delayed serologic transfusion reaction (DSTR) from ABO incompatibility ◀
Other ABO incompatible blood transfusion ◀
Other reaction to ABO incompatibility from transfusion ◀

● **999.7 Rh and other non-ABO incompatibility reaction due to transfusion of blood or blood products** ◀▥

~~Reactions due to Rh factor in infusion or transfusion~~

999.70 Rh incompatibility reaction, unspecified ◀

Reaction due to Rh factor in transfusion NOS ◀
Rh incompatible blood transfusion NOS ◀
Unspecified reaction due to incompatibility related to Rh antigens (C) (c) (D) (E) (e) ◀
Unspecified reaction to Rh incompatibility ◀

999.71 Rh incompatibility with hemolytic transfusion reaction not specified as acute or delayed ◀

Hemolytic transfusion reaction (HTR) due to Rh incompatibility ◀
HTR due to incompatibility related to Rh antigens (C) (c) (D) (E) (e), not specified as acute or delayed ◀
Rh incompatibility with hemolytic transfusion reaction at unspecified time after transfusion ◀

999.72 Rh incompatibility with acute hemolytic transfusion reaction ◀

Acute hemolytic transfusion reaction (AHTR) due to Rh incompatibility ◀
AHTR due to incompatibility related to Rh antigens (C) (c) (D) (E) (e) ◀
Rh incompatibility with hemolytic transfusion reaction less than 24 hours after transfusion ◀

999.73 Rh incompatibility with delayed hemolytic transfusion reaction ◀

Delayed hemolytic transfusion reaction (DHTR) due to Rh incompatibility ◀
DHTR due to incompatibility related to Rh antigens (C) (c) (D) (E) (e) ◀
Rh incompatibility with hemolytic transfusion reaction 24 hours or more after transfusion ◀

INJURY AND POISONING (800–999)

INJURY AND POISONING (800–999)

999.74 Other Rh incompatibility reaction ◀
     Delayed serologic transfusion reaction
         (DSTR) from Rh incompatibility ◀
     Other reaction due to incompatibility
         related to Rh antigens (C) (c) (D)
         (E) (e) ◀
     Other reaction to Rh incompatible blood
         transfusion ◀

**999.75 Non-ABO incompatibility reaction,
unspecified** ◀
     Non-ABO incompatible blood transfusion
         NOS ◀
     Reaction to non-ABO antigen
         incompatibility from transfusion
         NOS ◀
     Unspecified reaction due to incompatibility
         related to minor antigens (Duffy)
         (Kell) (Kidd) (Lewis) (M) (N) (P) (S) ◀

**999.76 Non-ABO incompatibility with hemolytic
transfusion reaction not specified as acute or
delayed** ◀
     Hemolytic transfusion reaction (HTR) due
         to non-ABO incompatibility ◀
     HTR from incompatibility related to minor
         antigens (Duffy) (Kell) (Kidd) (Lewis)
         (M) (N) (P) (S) ◀
     Non-ABO incompatibility with hemolytic
         transfusion reaction at unspecified
         time after transfusion ◀

**999.77 Non-ABO incompatibility with acute
hemolytic transfusion reaction** ◀
     Acute hemolytic transfusion reaction
         (AHTR) due to non-ABO
         incompatibility ◀
     AHTR from incompatibility related to
         minor antigens (Duffy) (Kell) (Kidd)
         (Lewis) (M) (N) (P) (S) ◀
     Non-ABO incompatibility with hemolytic
         transfusion reaction less than 24 hours
         after transfusion ◀

**999.78 Non-ABO incompatibility with delayed
hemolytic transfusion reaction** ◀
     Delayed hemolytic transfusion reaction
         (DHTR) due to non-ABO
         incompatibility ◀
     DHTR from incompatibility related to
         minor antigens (Duffy) (Kell) (Kidd)
         (Lewis) (M) (N) (P) (S) ◀
     Non-ABO incompatibility with hemolytic
         transfusion reaction 24 hours or more
         after transfusion ◀

**999.79 Other non-ABO incompatibility
reaction** ◀
     Delayed serologic transfusion reaction
         (DSTR) from non-ABO
         incompatibility ◀
     Other non-ABO incompatible blood
         transfusion ◀
     Other reaction due to incompatibility
         related to minor antigens (Duffy)
         (Kell) (Kidd) (Lewis) (M) (N) (P) (S) ◀
     Other reaction to non-ABO incompatibility
         from transfusion ◀

● **999.8 Other and unspecified infusion and transfusion
reaction** ◀⁃

> **Excludes**   *ABO incompatibility reactions
>   (999.60-999.69)* ◀
>   *febrile nonhemolytic transfusion reaction
>   (FNHTR) (780.66)* ◀
>   *hemochromatosis due to repeated red blood
>   cell transfusions (275.02)* ◀
>   *non-ABO incompatibility reactions
>   (999.70-999.79)* ◀
>   *postoperative shock (998.0)*
>   *posttransfusion purpura (287.41)* ◀
>   *Rh incompatibility reactions
>   (999.70-999.74)* ◀
>   *transfusion associated circulatory overload
>   (TACO) (276.61)* ◀
>   *transfusion related acute lung injury
>   (TRALI) (518.7)*

Coding Clinic: 2008, Q4, P152-155; 2000, Q3, P9

999.80 Transfusion reaction, unspecified ◀
     Incompatible blood transfusion NOS ◀
     Reaction to blood group incompatibility in
         infusion or transfusion NOS ◀

999.81 Extravasation of vesicant chemotherapy
     Infiltration of vesicant chemotherapy
     Coding Clinic: 2008, Q4, P152-155

999.82 Extravasation of other vesicant agent
     Infiltration of other vesicant agent

**999.83 Hemolytic transfusion reaction,
incompatibility unspecified** ◀
     Hemolytic transfusion reaction (HTR) with
         antigen incompatibility unspecified,
         not specified as acute or delayed ◀
     HTR with incompatibility unspecified at
         unspecified time after transfusion ◀

**999.84 Acute hemolytic transfusion reaction,
incompatibility unspecified** ◀
     Acute hemolytic transfusion reaction
         (AHTR) with antigen incompatibility
         unspecified ◀
     AHTR, incompatibility unspecified ◀

**999.85 Delayed hemolytic transfusion reaction,
incompatibility unspecified** ◀
     Delayed hemolytic transfusion reaction
         (DHTR) with antigen incompatibility
         unspecified ◀
     DHTR, incompatibility unspecified ◀

999.88 Other infusion reaction

999.89 Other transfusion reaction
     ~~Transfusion reaction NOS~~
     Delayed serologic transfusion reaction
         (DSTR), incompatibility unspecified ◀

> Use additional code to identify
>   graft-versus-host reaction (279.5)

**999.9 Other and unspecified complications of medical
care, not elsewhere classified**
     Complications, not elsewhere classified, of:
         electroshock therapy   ultrasound therapy
         inhalation therapy   ventilation therapy
     Unspecified misadventure of medical care

> **Excludes** *unspecified complication of:*
>   *phototherapy (990)*
>   *radiation therapy (990)*
>   *ventilator associated pneumonia (997.31)*

Coding Clinic: 2006, Q2, P25; 2003, Q1, P19; 1997, Q2, P5; 1994,
     Q3, P9

◀ New   ◀⁃ Revised   ~~deleted~~ Deleted   Excludes   Includes   Use additional   Code first   Omit code
● Unacceptable Principal Diagnosis   ● Use Additional Digit(s)   OGCR Official Guidelines   Coding Clinic

SUPPLEMENTARY CLASSIFICATION OF FACTORS INFLUENCING HEALTH STATUS AND CONTACT WITH HEALTH SERVICES (V01–V90) ◄◄◄

This classification is provided to deal with occasions when circumstances other than a disease or injury classifiable to categories 001–999 (the main part of ICD) are recorded as "diagnoses" or "problems." This can arise mainly in three ways:

a) When a person who is not currently sick encounters the health services for some specific purpose, such as to act as a donor of an organ or tissue, to receive prophylactic vaccination, or to discuss a problem which is in itself not a disease or injury. This will be a fairly rare occurrence among hospital inpatients, but will be relatively more common among hospital outpatients and patients of family practitioners, health clinics, etc.

b) When a person with a known disease or injury, whether it is current or resolving, encounters the health care system for a specific treatment of that disease or injury (e.g., dialysis for renal disease; chemotherapy for malignancy; cast change).

c) When some circumstance or problem is present which influences the person's health status but is not in itself a current illness or injury. Such factors may be elicited during population surveys, when the person may or may not be currently sick, or be recorded as an additional factor to be borne in mind when the person is receiving care for some current illness or injury classifiable to categories 001–999.

In the latter circumstances the V code should be used only as a supplementary code and should not be the one selected for use in primary, single cause tabulations. Examples of these circumstances are a personal history of certain diseases, or a person with an artificial heart valve in situ.

OGCR Section I.C.18.b
> **V codes use in any healthcare setting**
> V codes are for use in any healthcare setting. V codes may be used as either a first listed (principal diagnosis code in the inpatient setting) or secondary code, depending on the circumstances of the encounter. Certain V codes may only be used as first listed, others only as secondary codes.
> *See Section I.C.18.e,* **V Codes That May Only be Principal/ First-Listed Diagnosis.**

OGCR Section I.C.18.d.1
> Category V01 indicates contact with or exposure to communicable diseases. These codes are for patients who do not show any sign or symptom of a disease but have been exposed to it by close personal contact with an infected individual or are in an area where a disease is epidemic. These codes may be used as a first listed code to explain an encounter for testing, or, more commonly, as a secondary code to identify a potential risk.

PERSONS WITH POTENTIAL HEALTH HAZARDS RELATED TO COMMUNICABLE DISEASES (V01–V06)

> **Excludes** *family history of infectious and parasitic diseases (V18.8)*
> *personal history of infectious and parasitic diseases (V12.0)*

● **V01 Contact with or exposure to communicable diseases**
Coding Clinic: 2001, Q1, P10

  ● **V01.0 Cholera**
Conditions classifiable to 001

  ● **V01.1 Tuberculosis**
Conditions classifiable to 010–018

  ● **V01.2 Poliomyelitis**
Conditions classifiable to 045

  ● **V01.3 Smallpox**
Conditions classifiable to 050

  ● **V01.4 Rubella**
Conditions classifiable to 056

  ● **V01.5 Rabies**
Conditions classifiable to 071

  ● **V01.6 Venereal diseases**
Conditions classifiable to 090–099
Coding Clinic: 2007, Q4, P124-125x2

  ● **V01.7 Other viral diseases**
Conditions classifiable to 042–078, and V08, except as above

    V01.71 Varicella

    V01.79 Other viral diseases
Coding Clinic: 1992, Q2, P11

  ● **V01.8 Other communicable diseases**
Conditions classifiable to 001–136, except as above

    ● **V01.81 Anthrax**

    V01.82 Exposure to SARS-associated coronavirus
Coding Clinic: 2003, Q4, P46-48

    V01.83 Escherichia coli (E. coli)

    V01.84 Meningococcus

    ● **V01.89 Other communicable diseases**

  ● **V01.9 Unspecified communicable disease**

● **V02 Carrier or suspected carrier of infectious diseases**
> **Includes** Colonization status

  ● **V02.0 Cholera**

  ● **V02.1 Typhoid**

  ● **V02.2 Amebiasis**

  ● **V02.3 Other gastrointestinal pathogens**

  ● **V02.4 Diphtheria**

  ● **V02.5 Other specified bacterial diseases**

    ● **V02.51 Group B streptococcus**
Coding Clinic: 2006, Q3, P14; 2002, Q1, P14-15; 1998, Q4, P56; 1994, Q3, P4

    ● **V02.52 Other streptococcus**

    ● **V02.53 Methicillin susceptible Staphylococcus aureus**
MSSA colonization
Coding Clinic: 2008, Q4, P69-73

    ● **V02.54 Methicillin resistant Staphylococcus aureus**
MRSA colonization
Coding Clinic: 2008, Q4, P69-73

    ● **V02.59 Other specified bacterial diseases**
Meningococcal
Staphylococcal

  ● **V02.6 Viral hepatitis**

    ● **V02.60 Viral hepatitis carrier, unspecified**

    ● **V02.61 Hepatitis B carrier**

    ● **V02.62 Hepatitis C carrier**

    ● **V02.69 Other viral hepatitis carrier**

  ● **V02.7 Gonorrhea**

  ● **V02.8 Other venereal diseases**

  ● **V02.9 Other specified infectious organism**
Coding Clinic: 1994, Q4, P36; 1993, Q1, P22

V01-V91

◄ New   ◄◄◄ Revised   ~~deleted~~ Deleted   Excludes   Includes   Use additional   Code first
● Unacceptable Principal Diagnosis   ● Use Additional Digit(s)   OGCR Official Guidelines   Coding Clinic

1021

OGCR Section I.C.18.d.2

> Categories V03-V06 are for encounters for inoculations and vaccinations. They indicate that a patient is being seen to receive a prophylactic inoculation against a disease. The injection itself must be represented by the appropriate procedure code. A code from V03-V06 may be used as a secondary code if the inoculation is given as a routine part of preventive health care, such as a well-baby visit.

● **V03 Need for prophylactic vaccination and inoculation against bacterial diseases**

> **Excludes** *vaccination not carried out (V64.00–V64.09)*
> *vaccines against combinations of diseases (V06.0–V06.9)*

● **V03.0 Cholera alone**

● **V03.1 Typhoid-paratyphoid alone [TAB]**

● **V03.2 Tuberculosis [BCG]**

● **V03.3 Plague**

● **V03.4 Tularemia**

● **V03.5 Diphtheria alone**

● **V03.6 Pertussis alone**

● **V03.7 Tetanus toxoid alone**

● **V03.8 Other specified vaccinations against single bacterial diseases**

- ● **V03.81 Hemophilus influenza, type B [Hib]**

- ● **V03.82 Streptococcus pneumoniae [pneumococcus]**

- ● **V03.89 Other specified vaccination**
  Coding Clinic: 2000, Q2, P9

● **V03.9 Unspecified single bacterial disease**

● **V04 Need for prophylactic vaccination and inoculation against certain diseases**

> **Excludes** *vaccines against combinations of diseases (V06.0–V06.9)*

● **V04.0 Poliomyelitis**

● **V04.1 Smallpox**

● **V04.2 Measles alone**

● **V04.3 Rubella alone**

● **V04.4 Yellow fever**

● **V04.5 Rabies**

● **V04.6 Mumps alone**

● **V04.7 Common cold**

● **V04.8 Other viral diseases**

- ● **V04.81 Influenza**

- ● **V04.82 Respiratory syncytial virus (RSV)**
  Coding Clinic: 2009, Q1, P5; 2001, Q1, P4

- ● **V04.89 Other viral diseases**
  Coding Clinic: 2007, Q2, P11

● **V05 Need for prophylactic vaccination and inoculation against single diseases**

> **Excludes** *vaccines against combinations of diseases (V06.0–V06.9)*

● **V05.0 Arthropod-borne viral encephalitis**

● **V05.1 Other arthropod-borne viral diseases**

● **V05.2 Leishmaniasis**

● **V05.3 Viral hepatitis**

● **V05.4 Varicella**
  Chicken pox

● **V05.8 Other specified disease**
  Coding Clinic: 2001, Q1, P4; 1991, Q3, P20-21

● **V05.9 Unspecified single disease**

●**V06 Need for prophylactic vaccination and inoculation against combinations of diseases**

> **Note:** Use additional single vaccination codes from categories V03–V05 to identify any vaccinations not included in a combination code.

● **V06.0 Cholera with typhoid-paratyphoid [cholera TAB]**

● **V06.1 Diphtheria-tetanus-pertussis, combined [DTP] [DTaP]**
  Coding Clinic: 1998, Q3, P13-14

● **V06.2 Diphtheria-tetanus-pertussis with typhoid-paratyphoid [DTP TAB]**

● **V06.3 Diphtheria-tetanus-pertussis with poliomyelitis [DTP+polio]**

● **V06.4 Measles-mumps-rubella [MMR]**

● **V06.5 Tetanus-diphtheria [Td] [DT]**

● **V06.6 Streptococcus pneumoniae [pneumococcus] and influenza**

● **V06.8 Other combinations**

> **Excludes** *multiple single vaccination codes (V03.0–V05.9)*
> Coding Clinic: 1994, Q1, P19

● **V06.9 Unspecified combined vaccine**

PERSONS WITH NEED FOR ISOLATION, OTHER POTENTIAL HEALTH HAZARDS AND PROPHYLACTIC MEASURES (V07–V09)

● **V07 Need for isolation and other prophylactic or treatment measures ◀▥**

> **Excludes** *long-term (current) (prophylactic) use of certain specific drugs (V58.61-V58.69) ◀*
> *prophylactic organ removal (V50.41–V50.49)*

V07.0 Isolation
  Admission to protect the individual from his surroundings or for isolation of individual after contact with infectious diseases

● **V07.1 Desensitization to allergens**

● **V07.2 Prophylactic immunotherapy**
  Administration of:
  antivenin
  immune sera [gamma globulin]
  RhoGAM
  tetanus antitoxin

● **V07.3 Other prophylactic chemotherapy**

- ● **V07.31 Prophylactic fluoride administration**

- **V07.39 Other prophylactic chemotherapy**

> **Excludes** *maintenance chemotherapy following disease (V58.11)*

● **V07.4 Hormone replacement therapy (postmenopausal)**

V01-V91

◀ New ◀▥ Revised ~~deleted~~ Deleted Excludes Includes Use additional Code first
● Unacceptable Principal Diagnosis ● Use Additional Digit(s) **OGCR** Official Guidelines **Coding Clinic**

● **V07.5** ~~Prophylactic u~~Use of agents affecting estrogen receptors and estrogen levels ◄▭

    Code first, if applicable:
      malignant neoplasm of breast (174.0-174.9, 175.0-175.9)
      malignant neoplasm of prostate (185)

    Use additional code, if applicable, to identify:
      estrogen receptor positive status (V86.0)
      family history of breast cancer (V16.3)
      genetic susceptibility to cancer (V84.01-V84.09)
      personal history of breast cancer (V10.3)
      personal history of prostate cancer (V10.46)
      postmenopausal status (V49.81)

    | Excludes | *hormone replacement therapy (postmenopausal) (V07.4)* |

● **V07.51** ~~Prophylactic u~~Use of selective estrogen receptor modulators (SERMs) ◄▭
    ~~Prophylactic u~~Use of: ◄▭
      raloxifene (Evista)
      tamoxifen (Nolvadex)
      toremifene (Fareston)

● **V07.52** ~~Prophylactic u~~Use of aromatase inhibitors ◄▭
    ~~Prophylactic u~~Use of: ◄▭
      anastrozole (Arimidex)
      exemestane (Aromasin)
      letrozole (Femara)

● **V07.59** ~~Prophylactic u~~Use of other agents affecting estrogen receptors and estrogen levels ◄▭
    ~~Prophylactic u~~Use of: ◄▭
      estrogen receptor downregulators
      fulvestrant (Faslodex)
      gonadotropin-releasing hormone (GnRH) agonist
      goserelin acetate (Zoladex)
      leuprolide acetate (leuprorelin) (Lupron)
      megestrol acetate (Megace)

V07.8 Other specified prophylactic or treatment measure ◄▭
    Coding Clinic: 1992, Q1, P11

● **V07.9** Unspecified prophylactic or treatment measure ◄▭

OGCR Section I.C.1.d

  V08, Asymptomatic human immunodeficiency virus [HIV] infection, is to be applied when the patient without any documentation of symptoms is listed as being "HIV positive," "known HIV," "HIV test positive," or similar terminology. Do not use this code if the term "AIDS" is used or if the patient is treated for any HIV-related illness or is described as having any condition(s) resulting from HIV positive status; use 042 in these cases.

V08 Asymptomatic human immunodeficiency virus [HIV] infection status
    HIV positive NOS

    Note: This code is ONLY to be used when NO HIV infection symptoms or conditions are present. If any HIV infection symptoms or conditions are present, see code 042.

    | Excludes | *AIDS (042)* |
      human immunodeficiency virus [HIV] disease (042)
      exposure to HIV (V01.79)
      nonspecific serologic evidence of HIV (795.71)
      symptomatic human immunodeficiency virus [HIV] infection (042)

Coding Clinic: 2004, Q2, P11; 1999, Q2, P8

● **V09** Infection with drug-resistant microorganisms
    Note: This category is intended for use as an additional code for infectious conditions classified elsewhere to indicate the presence of drug-resistance of the infectious organism.
    Coding Clinic: 2008, Q4, P69-73

● **V09.0** Infection with microorganisms resistant to penicillins
    Coding Clinic: 2006, Q2, P16-17; 2003, Q4, P104-107; 1994, Q3, P4

● **V09.1** Infection with microorganisms resistant to cephalosporins and other B-lactam antibiotics

● **V09.2** Infection with microorganisms resistant to macrolides

● **V09.3** Infection with microorganisms resistant to tetracyclines

● **V09.4** Infection with microorganisms resistant to aminoglycosides

● **V09.5** Infection with microorganisms resistant to quinolones and fluoroquinolones
    ● **V09.50** Without mention of resistance to multiple quinolones and fluoroquinoles
    ● **V09.51** With resistance to multiple quinolones and fluoroquinoles

● **V09.6** Infection with microorganisms resistant to sulfonamides

● **V09.7** Infection with microorganisms resistant to other specified antimycobacterial agents
    | Excludes | *Amikacin (V09.4)* |
      Kanamycin (V09.4)
      Streptomycin [SM] (V09.4)

    ● **V09.70** Without mention of resistance to multiple antimycobacterial agents
    ● **V09.71** With resistance to multiple antimycobacterial agents

● **V09.8** Infection with microorganisms resistant to other specified drugs
    Vancomycin (glycopeptide) intermediate staphylococcus aureus (VISA/GISA)
    Vancomycin (glycopeptide) resistant enterococcus (VRE)
    Vancomycin (glycopeptide) resistant staphylococcus aureus (VRSA/GRSA)

    ● **V09.80** Without mention of resistance to multiple drugs
    ● **V09.81** With resistance to multiple drugs

● **V09.9** Infection with drug-resistant microorganisms, unspecified
    Drug resistance NOS

    ● **V09.90** Without mention of multiple drug resistance
    ● **V09.91** With multiple drug resistance
      Multiple drug resistance NOS

V01-V91

OGCR Section I.C.2.d

> When a primary malignancy has been previously excised or eradicated from its site and there is no further treatment directed to that site and there is no evidence of any existing primary malignancy, a code from category V10 should be used to indicate the former site of the malignancy. Any mention of extension, invasion, or metastasis to another site is coded as a secondary malignant neoplasm to that site. The secondary site may be the principal or first-listed with the V10 code used as a secondary code.

OGCR Section I.C.18.d.4

> Personal history codes explain a patient's past medical condition that no longer exists and is not receiving any treatment, but that has the potential for recurrence, and therefore may require continued monitoring. The exceptions to this general rule are category V14, Personal history of allergy to medicinal agents, and subcategory V15.0, Allergy, other than to medicinal agents. A person who has had an allergic episode to a substance or food in the past should always be considered allergic to the substance.

PERSONS WITH POTENTIAL HEALTH HAZARDS RELATED TO PERSONAL AND FAMILY HISTORY (V10–V19)

> **Excludes** *obstetric patients where the possibility that the fetus might be affected is the reason for observation or management during pregnancy (655.0–655.9)*

● **V10 Personal history of malignant neoplasm**
    Coding Clinic: 1994, Q2, P8

   ● **V10.0 Gastrointestinal tract**
        History of conditions classifiable to 140–159

    > **Excludes** *personal history of malignant carcinoid tumor (V10.91)*
    > *personal history of malignant neuroendocrine tumor (V10.91)*

      ● **V10.00 Gastrointestinal tract, unspecified**
      ● **V10.01 Tongue**
      ● **V10.02 Other and unspecified oral cavity and pharynx**
      ● **V10.03 Esophagus**
      ● **V10.04 Stomach**
      ● **V10.05 Large intestine**
            Coding Clinic: 1999, Q3, P7-8; 1995, Q1, P3-4
      ● **V10.06 Rectum, rectosigmoid junction, and anus**
      ● **V10.07 Liver**
      ● **V10.09 Other**
            Coding Clinic: 2003, Q4, P111

   ● **V10.1 Trachea, bronchus, and lung**
        History of conditions classifiable to 162

    > **Excludes** *personal history of malignant carcinoid tumor (V10.91)*
    > *personal history of malignant neuroendocrine tumor (V10.91)*

      ● **V10.11 Bronchus and lung**
      ● **V10.12 Trachea**

   ● **V10.2 Other respiratory and intrathoracic organs**
        History of conditions classifiable to 160, 161, 163–165

      ● **V10.20 Respiratory organ, unspecified**
      ● **V10.21 Larynx**
            Coding Clinic: 2003, Q4, P108,110
      ● **V10.22 Nasal cavities, middle ear, and accessory sinuses**
      ● **V10.29 Other**

   ● **V10.3 Breast**
        History of conditions classifiable to 174 and 175
        Coding Clinic: 2007, Q3, P4; Q1, P3-8; 2003, Q2, P3-5; 2001, Q4, P66; 1997, Q4, P50; 1995, Q4, P53; 1990, Q1, P21

   ● **V10.4 Genital organs**
        History of conditions classifiable to 179–187

      ● **V10.40 Female genital organ, unspecified**
      ● **V10.41 Cervix uteri**
            Coding Clinic: 2007, Q4, P99-101
      ● **V10.42 Other parts of uterus**
      ● **V10.43 Ovary**
      ● **V10.44 Other female genital organs**
      ● **V10.45 Male genital organ, unspecified**
      ● **V10.46 Prostate**
            Coding Clinic: 2009, Q1, P5; 1994, Q2, P12; 1984, May-June, P10
      ● **V10.47 Testis**
      ● **V10.48 Epididymis**
      ● **V10.49 Other male genital organs**

   ● **V10.5 Urinary organs**
        History of conditions classifiable to 188 and 189

    > **Excludes** *personal history of malignant carcinoid tumor (V10.91)* ◀
    > *personal history of malignant neuroendocrine tumor (V10.91)* ◀

        Coding Clinic: 1995, Q2, P8

      ● **V10.50 Urinary organ, unspecified**
      ● **V10.51 Bladder**
            Coding Clinic: 1995, Q2, P8;1985, July-Aug, P16
      ● **V10.52 Kidney**

        > **Excludes** *renal pelvis (V10.53)*

            Coding Clinic: 2004, Q2, P4
      ● **V10.53 Renal pelvis**
      ● **V10.59 Other**

   ● **V10.6 Leukemia**
        Conditions classifiable to 204–208

    > **Excludes** *leukemia in remission (204–208)*

        Coding Clinic: 1992, Q2, P13; 1985, May-June, P8-9

      ● **V10.60 Leukemia, unspecified**
      ● **V10.61 Lymphoid leukemia**
      ● **V10.62 Myeloid leukemia**
      ● **V10.63 Monocytic leukemia**
      ● **V10.69 Other**

   ● **V10.7 Other lymphatic and hematopoietic neoplasms**
        Conditions classifiable to 200–203

    > **Excludes** *listed conditions in 200–203 in remission*

        Coding Clinic: 1985, May-June, P8-9

      ● **V10.71 Lymphosarcoma and reticulosarcoma**
      ● **V10.72 Hodgkin's disease**
      ● **V10.79 Other**

   ● **V10.8 Personal history of malignant neoplasm of other sites**
        History of conditions classifiable to 170–173, 190–195

    > **Excludes** *personal history of malignant carcinoid tumor (V10.91)*
    > *personal history of malignant neuroendocrine tumor (V10.91)*

      ● **V10.81 Bone**
            Coding Clinic: 2003, Q2, P13
      ● **V10.82 Malignant melanoma of skin**
      ● **V10.83 Other malignant neoplasm of skin**

◀ New   ◀▥ Revised   ~~deleted~~ Deleted   Excludes   Includes   Use additional   Code first
● Unacceptable Principal Diagnosis   ● Use Additional Digit(s)   OGCR Official Guidelines   Coding Clinic

- ● V10.84 Eye
- ● V10.85 Brain
  Coding Clinic: 2001, Q1, P6-7
- ● V10.86 Other parts of nervous system
  > **Excludes** *peripheral, sympathetic, and parasympathetic nerves (V10.89)*
- ● V10.87 Thyroid
- ● V10.88 Other endocrine glands and related structures
- ● V10.89 Other
- ◐ V10.9 Other and unspecified personal history of malignant neoplasm
  - ● V10.90 Personal history of unspecified malignant neoplasm
    Personal history of malignant neoplasm NOS
    > **Excludes** *personal history of malignant carcinoid tumor (V10.91)*
    > *personal history of malignant neuroendocrine tumor (V10.91)*
    > *personal history of Merkel cell carcinoma (V10.91)*
  - ● V10.91 Personal history of malignant neuroendocrine tumor
    Personal history of malignant carcinoid tumor NOS
    Personal history of malignant neuroendocrine tumor NOS
    Personal history of Merkel cell carcinoma NOS
    Code first any continuing functional activity, such as:
    carcinoid syndrome (259.2)

- ◐ V11 Personal history of mental disorder
  - ● V11.0 Schizophrenia
    > **Excludes** *that in remission (295.0–295.9 with fifth-digit 5)*
    Coding Clinic: 1995, Q3, P6
  - ● V11.1 Affective disorders
    Personal history of manic-depressive psychosis
    > **Excludes** *that in remission (296.0–296.6 with fifth-digit 5, 6)*
  - ● V11.2 Neurosis
  - ● V11.3 Alcoholism
  - ● V11.4 Combat and operational stress reaction ◀
  - ● V11.8 Other mental disorders
  - ● V11.9 Unspecified mental disorder

- ◐ V12 Personal history of certain other diseases
  Coding Clinic: 2005, Q4, P94-100; 1992, Q3, P11
  - ◐ V12.0 Infectious and parasitic diseases
    > **Excludes** *personal history of infectious diseases specific to a body system*
    - ● V12.00 Unspecified infectious and parasitic disease
    - ● V12.01 Tuberculosis
    - ● V12.02 Poliomyelitis
    - ● V12.03 Malaria
    - ● V12.04 Methicillin resistant Staphylococcus aureus
      MRSA
      Coding Clinic: 2008, Q4, P69-73
    - ● V12.09 Other

- ● V12.1 Nutritional deficiency
- ● V12.2 Endocrine, metabolic, and immunity disorders
  > **Excludes** *history of allergy (V14.0–V14.9, V15.01–V15.09)*
  Coding Clinic: 2007, Q3, P5-6
- ● V12.3 Diseases of blood and blood-forming organs
- ◐ V12.4 Disorders of nervous system and sense organs
  - ● V12.40 Unspecified disorder of nervous system and sense organs
  - ● V12.41 Benign neoplasm of the brain
  - ● V12.42 Infections of the central nervous system
    Encephalitis
    Meningitis
  - ● V12.49 Other disorders of nervous system and sense organs
    Coding Clinic: 1998, Q4, P59-60
- ◐ V12.5 Diseases of circulatory system
  > **Excludes** *old myocardial infarction (412)*
  > *postmyocardial infarction syndrome (411.0)*
  - ● V12.50 Unspecified circulatory disease
  - ● V12.51 Venous thrombosis and embolism
    Pulmonary embolism
    Coding Clinic: 2006, Q3, P12; 2003, Q4, P108; 2002, Q1, P15-16
  - ● V12.52 Thrombophlebitis
  - ● V12.53 Sudden cardiac arrest
    Sudden cardiac death successfully resuscitated
    Coding Clinic: 2007, Q4, P99-101
  - ● V12.54 Transient ischemic attack (TIA), and cerebral infarction without residual deficits
    Prolonged reversible ischemic neurological deficit (PRIND)
    Reversible ischemic neurologic deficit (RIND)
    Stroke NOS without residual deficits
    > **Excludes** *history of traumatic brain injury (V15.52)*
    > *late effects of cerebrovascular disease (438.0–438.9)*
    Coding Clinic: 2007, Q4, P99-101; 2007, Q2, P3

    OGCR Section I.C.7.d.3
    Assign code V12.54, Transient ischemic attack (TIA), and cerebral infarction without residual deficits (and not a code from category 438) as an additional code for history of cerebrovascular disease when no neurologic deficits are present.
  - ● V12.59 Other
    Coding Clinic: 2007, Q2, P3; 1997, Q4, P35-37
- ◐ V12.6 Diseases of respiratory system
  > **Excludes** *tuberculosis (V12.01)*
  - ● V12.60 Unspecified disease of respiratory system
  - ● V12.61 Pneumonia (recurrent)
  - ● V12.69 Other diseases of respiratory system
- ◐ V12.7 Diseases of digestive system
  Coding Clinic: 1995, Q1, P3; 1992, Q3, P11; 1989, Q2, P16
  - ● V12.70 Unspecified digestive disease
  - ● V12.71 Peptic ulcer disease
  - ● V12.72 Colonic polyps
    Coding Clinic: 2002, Q3, P14-15
  - ● V12.79 Other

V01-V91

● **V13 Personal history of other diseases**
- ● **V13.0 Disorders of urinary system**
  - ● **V13.00 Unspecified urinary disorder**
  - ● **V13.01 Urinary calculi**
  - ● **V13.02 Urinary (tract) infection**
  - ● **V13.03 Nephrotic syndrome**
  - ● **V13.09 Other**
    - Coding Clinic: 1996, Q2, P7x2
- ● **V13.1 Trophoblastic disease**
  - Excludes   *supervision during a current pregnancy (V23.1)*
- ● **V13.2 Other genital system and obstetric disorders**
  - Excludes   *supervision during a current pregnancy of a woman with poor obstetric history (V23.0–V23.9)*
  - *habitual aborter recurrent pregnancy loss (646.3)* ◀▥
  - *without current pregnancy (629.81)*
  - ● **V13.21 Personal history of pre-term labor**
    - Excludes   *current pregnancy with history of pre-term labor (V23.41)*
  - ● **V13.22 Personal history of cervical dysplasia**
    - Personal history of conditions classifiable to 622.10–622.12
    - Excludes   *personal history of malignant neoplasm of cervix uteri (V10.41)*
    - Coding Clinic: 2007, Q4, P99-101
  - ● **V13.23 Personal history of vaginal dysplasia** ◀
    - Personal history of conditions classifiable to 623.0 ◀
    - Excludes   *personal history of malignant neoplasm of vagina (V10.44)* ◀
  - ● **V13.24 Personal history of vulvar dysplasia** ◀
    - Personal history of conditions classifiable to 624.01-624.02 ◀
    - Excludes   *personal history of malignant neoplasm of vulva (V10.44)* ◀
  - ● **V13.29 Other genital system and obstetric disorders**
- ● **V13.3 Diseases of skin and subcutaneous tissue**
- ● **V13.4 Arthritis**
- ● **V13.5 Other musculoskeletal disorders**
  - ● **V13.51 Pathologic fracture**
    - Healed pathologic fracture
    - Excludes   *personal history of traumatic fracture (V15.51)*
  - ● **V13.52 Stress fracture**
    - Healed stress fracture
    - Excludes   *personal history of traumatic fracture (V15.51)*
  - ● **V13.59 Other musculoskeletal disorders**
- ● **V13.6 Congenital (corrected) malformations** ◀▥
  - ● **V13.61 Personal history of (corrected) hHypospadias** ◀▥
  - ● **V13.62 Personal history of other (corrected) congenital malformations of genitourinary system** ◀
  - ● **V13.63 Personal history of (corrected) congenital malformations of nervous system** ◀
  - ● **V13.64 Personal history of (corrected) congenital malformations of eye, ear, face and neck** ◀
    - Corrected cleft lip and palate ◀

- ● **V13.65 Personal history of (corrected) congenital malformations of heart and circulatory system** ◀
- ● **V13.66 Personal history of (corrected) congenital malformations of respiratory system** ◀
- ● **V13.67 Personal history of (corrected) congenital malformations of digestive system** ◀
- ● **V13.68 Personal history of (corrected) congenital malformations of integument, limbs, and musculoskeletal systems** ◀
- ● **V13.69 Personal history of other (corrected) congenital malformations** ◀▥
  - Coding Clinic: 2004, Q1, P16-17
- ● **V13.7 Perinatal problems**
  - Excludes   *low birth weight status (V21.30–V21.35)*
- ● **V13.8 Other specified diseases**
- ● **V13.9 Unspecified disease**

● **V14 Personal history of allergy to medicinal agents**
- ● **V14.0 Penicillin**
- ● **V14.1 Other antibiotic agent**
- ● **V14.2 Sulfonamides**
- ● **V14.3 Other anti-infective agent**
- ● **V14.4 Anesthetic agent**
- ● **V14.5 Narcotic agent**
- ● **V14.6 Analgesic agent**
- ● **V14.7 Serum or vaccine**
- ● **V14.8 Other specified medicinal agents**
- ● **V14.9 Unspecified medicinal agent**

● **V15 Other personal history presenting hazards to health**
- Excludes   *personal history of drug therapy (V87.41–V87.49)*
- ● **V15.0 Allergy, other than to medicinal agents**
  - Excludes   *allergy to food substance used as base for medicinal agent (V14.0–V14.9)*
  - ● **V15.01 Allergy to peanuts**
  - ● **V15.02 Allergy to milk products**
    - Excludes   *lactose intolerance (271.3)*
    - Coding Clinic: 2003, Q1, P12
  - ● **V15.03 Allergy to eggs**
  - ● **V15.04 Allergy to seafood**
    - Seafood (octopus) (squid) ink
    - Shellfish
  - ● **V15.05 Allergy to other foods**
    - Food additives
    - Nuts other than peanuts
  - ● **V15.06 Allergy to insects and arachnids**
    - Bugs
    - Insect bites and stings
    - Spiders
  - ● **V15.07 Allergy to latex**
    - Latex sensitivity
  - ● **V15.08 Allergy to radiographic dye**
    - Contrast media used for diagnostic x-ray procedures
  - ● **V15.09 Other allergy, other than to medicinal agents**
- ● **V15.1 Surgery to heart and great vessels**
  - Excludes   *replacement by transplant or other means (V42.1–V42.2, V43.2–V43.4)*
  - Coding Clinic: 2004, Q1, P16-17
- ● **V15.2 Surgery to other organs**
  - Excludes   *replacement by transplant or other means (V42.0–V43.8)*

◀ New   ◀▥ Revised   ~~deleted~~ Deleted   Excludes   Includes   Use additional   Code first
● Unacceptable Principal Diagnosis   ● Use Additional Digit(s)   **OGCR** Official Guidelines   Coding Clinic

● **V15.21** **Personal history of undergoing in utero procedure during pregnancy**

● **V15.22** **Personal history of undergoing in utero procedure while a fetus**

● **V15.29** **Surgery to other organs**

● **V15.3** **Irradiation**
Previous exposure to therapeutic or other ionizing radiation

● **V15.4** **Psychological trauma**

> **Excludes** *history of condition classifiable to 290–316 (V11.0–V11.9)*

● **V15.41** **History of physical abuse**
Rape
Coding Clinic: 1999, Q3, P15

● **V15.42** **History of emotional abuse**
Neglect
Coding Clinic: 1999, Q3, P15

● **V15.49** **Other**
Coding Clinic: 1999, Q3, P15

● **V15.5** **Injury**

● **V15.51** **Traumatic fracture**
Healed traumatic fracture

> **Excludes** *personal history of pathologic and stress fracture (V13.51, V13.52)*

● **V15.52** **History of traumatic brain injury**

> **Excludes** *personal history of cerebrovascular accident (cerebral infarction) without residual deficits (V12.54)*

● **V15.53** **Personal history of retained foreign body fully removed** ◀

● **V15.59** **Other injury**

● **V15.6** **Poisoning**

● **V15.7** **Contraception**

> **Excludes** *current contraceptive management (V25.0–V25.4)*
> *presence of intrauterine contraceptive device as incidental finding (V45.5)*

● **V15.8** **Other specified personal history presenting hazards to health**

> **Excludes** *contact with and (suspected) exposure to:*
> *aromatic compounds and dyes (V87.11-V87.19)*
> *arsenic and other metals (V87.01-V87.09)*
> *molds (V87.31)*

● **V15.80** **History of failed moderate sedation**
History of failed conscious sedation

● **V15.81** **Noncompliance with medical treatment**

> **Excludes** *noncompliance with renal dialysis (V45.12)*

Coding Clinic: 2007, Q3, P11; 2006, Q4, P136; 2003, Q2, P7-8; 2001, Q2, P13; 1999, Q2, P17; Q1, P13-14; 1997, Q2, P11; 1996, Q3, P9

● **V15.82** **History of tobacco use**

> **Excludes** *tobacco dependence (305.1)*

Coding Clinic: 2009, Q1, P15

● **V15.83** **Underimmunization status**
Delinquent immunization status
Lapsed immunization schedule status

● **V15.84** **Contact with and (suspected) exposure to asbestos**

● **V15.85** **Contact with and (suspected) exposure to potentially hazardous body fluids**

● **V15.86** **Contact with and (suspected) exposure to lead**

● **V15.87** **History of extracorporeal membrane oxygenation [ECMO]**

● **V15.88** **History of fall**
At risk for falling
Coding Clinic: 2005, Q4, P94-100

● **V15.89** **Other**

> **Excludes** *contact with and (suspected) exposure to other potentially hazardous chemicals (V87.2)*
> *contact with and (suspected) exposure to other potentially hazardous substances (V87.39)* ◀▥

Coding Clinic: 2008, Q3, P6-7; 2007, Q3, P6; 1990, Q1, P21

● **V15.9** **Unspecified personal history presenting hazards to health**

OGCR Section I.C.18.d.3
Family history codes are for use when a patient has a family member(s) who has had a particular disease that causes the patient to be at higher risk of also contracting the disease.

● **V16** **Family history of malignant neoplasm**
Coding Clinic: 1985, Nov-Dec, P13

● **V16.0** **Gastrointestinal tract**
Family history of condition classifiable to 140–159
Coding Clinic: 1999, Q1, P4

● **V16.1** **Trachea, bronchus, and lung**
Family history of condition classifiable to 162

● **V16.2** **Other respiratory and intrathoracic organs**
Family history of condition classifiable to 160–161, 163–165

● **V16.3** **Breast**
Family history of condition classifiable to 174
Coding Clinic: 2004, Q4, P106-107; 2003, Q2, P3-5; 2000, Q2, P8-9; 1995, Q4, P61; 1992, Q1, P11; 1990, Q1, P21

● **V16.4** **Genital organs**
Family history of condition classifiable to 179–187

● **V16.40** **Genital organ, unspecified**

● **V16.41** **Ovary**
Coding Clinic: 2009, Q3, P21

● **V16.42** **Prostate**

● **V16.43** **Testis**

● **V16.49** **Other**
Coding Clinic: 2006, Q2, P3,4

● **V16.5** **Urinary organs**
Family history of condition classifiable to 188–189

● **V16.51** **Kidney**

● **V16.52** **Bladder**

● **V16.59** **Other**

● **V16.6** **Leukemia**
Family history of condition classifiable to 204–208

● **V16.7** **Other lymphatic and hematopoietic neoplasms**
Family history of condition classifiable to 200–203

● **V16.8** **Other specified malignant neoplasm**
Family history of other condition classifiable to 140–199

● **V16.9** **Unspecified malignant neoplasm**

V01-V91

◀ New   ◀▥ Revised   ~~deleted~~ Deleted   [Excludes]   [Includes]   [Use additional]   [Code first]
● Unacceptable Principal Diagnosis   ● Use Additional Digit(s)   **OGCR** Official Guidelines   Coding Clinic

V01-V91

● **V17**   **Family history of certain chronic disabling diseases**
     Coding Clinic: 1985, Nov-Dec, P13

   ● **V17.0**   **Psychiatric condition**

       | Excludes | *family history of mental retardation (V18.4)*

   ● **V17.1**   **Stroke (cerebrovascular)**

   ● **V17.2**   **Other neurological diseases**
       Epilepsy   Huntington's chorea

   ● **V17.3**   **Ischemic heart disease**

   ● **V17.4**   **Other cardiovascular diseases**
     Coding Clinic: 2004, Q1, P6-7

     ● **V17.41**   **Family history of sudden cardiac death (SCD)**

         | Excludes | *family history of ischemic heart disease (V17.3)*
            family history of myocardial infarction (V17.3)

     ● **V17.49**   **Family history of other cardiovascular diseases**
         Family history of cardiovascular disease NOS

   ● **V17.5**   **Asthma**

   ● **V17.6**   **Other chronic respiratory conditions**

   ● **V17.7**   **Arthritis**

   ● **V17.8**   **Other musculoskeletal diseases**

     ● **V17.81**   **Osteoporosis**

     ● **V17.89**   **Other musculoskeletal diseases**

● **V18**   **Family history of certain other specific conditions**
     Coding Clinic: 1985, Nov-Dec, P13

   ● **V18.0**   **Diabetes mellitus**
     Coding Clinic: 2005, Q2, P21; 2004, Q1, P8

   ● **V18.1**   **Other endocrine and metabolic diseases**

     ● **V18.11**   **Multiple endocrine neoplasia [MEN] syndrome**

     ● **V18.19**   **Other endocrine and metabolic diseases**

   ● **V18.2**   **Anemia**

   ● **V18.3**   **Other blood disorders**

   ● **V18.4**   **Mental retardation**

   ● **V18.5**   **Digestive disorders**

     ● **V18.51**   **Colonic polyps**

         | Excludes | *family history of malignant neoplasm of gastrointestinal tract (V16.0)*

     ● **V18.59**   **Other digestive disorders**

   ● **V18.6**   **Kidney diseases**

     ● **V18.61**   **Polycystic kidney**

     ● **V18.69**   **Other kidney diseases**

   ● **V18.7**   **Other genitourinary diseases**

   ● **V18.8**   **Infectious and parasitic diseases**

   ● **V18.9**   **Genetic disease carrier**

● **V19**   **Family history of other conditions**
     Coding Clinic: 1985, Nov-Dec, P13

   ● **V19.0**   **Blindness or visual loss**

   ● **V19.1**   **Other eye disorders**

   ● **V19.2**   **Deafness or hearing loss**

   ● **V19.3**   **Other ear disorders**

   ● **V19.4**   **Skin conditions**

   ● **V19.5**   **Congenital anomalies**

   ● **V19.6**   **Allergic disorders**

   ● **V19.7**   **Consanguinity**

   ● **V19.8**   **Other condition**

PERSONS ENCOUNTERING HEALTH SERVICES IN CIRCUMSTANCES RELATED TO REPRODUCTION AND DEVELOPMENT (V20–V29)

● **V20**   **Health supervision of infant or child**

   V20.0   **Foundling**

   ● **V20.1**   **Other healthy infant or child receiving care**
     Medical or nursing care supervision of healthy infant in cases of:
       maternal illness, physical or psychiatric
       socioeconomic adverse condition at home
       too many children at home preventing or interfering with normal care
     Coding Clinic: 2000, Q1, P25; 1993, Q4, P36; 1989, Q3, P14

   ● **V20.2**   **Routine infant or child health check**
     Developmental testing of infant or child
     Health check for child over 28 days old
     Immunizations appropriate for age
     Routine vision and hearing testing

     | Excludes | *health check for child under 29 days old (V20.31-V20.32)*
       newborn health supervision (V20.31-V20.32)
       special screening for developmental handicaps (V79.3)
     Use additional code(s) to identify:
       Special screening examination(s) performed (V73.0–V82.9)
     Coding Clinic: 2009, Q1, P15; 2004, Q1, P15-16x2

   ● **V20.3**   **Newborn health supervision**
     Health check for child under 29 days old

     | Excludes | *health check for child over 28 days old (V20.2)*

     ● **V20.31**   **Health supervision for newborn under 8 days old**
         Health check for newborn under 8 days old

     ● **V20.32**   **Health supervision for newborn 8 to 28 days old**
         Health check for newborn 8 to 28 days old
         Newborn weight check

● **V21**   **Constitutional states in development**

   ● **V21.0**   **Period of rapid growth in childhood**

   ● **V21.1**   **Puberty**

   ● **V21.2**   **Other adolescence**

   ● **V21.3**   **Low birth weight status**

     | Excludes | *history of perinatal problems (V13.7)*

     ● **V21.30**   **Low birth weight status, unspecified**

     ● **V21.31**   **Low birth weight status, less than 500 grams**

     ● **V21.32**   **Low birth weight status, 500–999 grams**
       Coding Clinic: 2009, Q4, P151

     ● **V21.33**   **Low birth weight status, 1000–1499 grams**

     ● **V21.34**   **Low birth weight status, 1500–1999 grams**

     ● **V21.35**   **Low birth weight status, 2000–2500 grams**

   ● **V21.8**   **Other specified constitutional states in development**

   ● **V21.9**   **Unspecified constitutional state in development**

◀ New   ◀▥ Revised   ~~deleted~~ Deleted | Excludes | Includes   Use additional   Code first
● Unacceptable Principal Diagnosis   ● Use Additional Digit(s)   OGCR Official Guidelines   Coding Clinic

● **V22 Normal pregnancy**

> | **Excludes** | *pregnancy examination or test, pregnancy unconfirmed (V72.40)*
> Coding Clinic: 2007, Q4, P124-125

> **OGCR** Section I.C.11.b.1
> For routine outpatient prenatal visits when no complications are present codes V22.0, Supervision of normal first pregnancy, and V22.1, Supervision of other normal pregnancy, should be used as the first-listed diagnoses. These codes should not be used in conjunction with chapter 11 codes.

● **V22.0 Supervision of normal first pregnancy**
> Coding Clinic: 1999, Q3, P16; 1990, Q1, P10; 1984, Nov-Dec, P18

● **V22.1 Supervision of other normal pregnancy**
> Coding Clinic: 1999, Q3, P16; 1990, Q1, P10

● **V22.2 Pregnant state, incidental**
> Pregnant state NOS
> Coding Clinic: 1998, Q2, P13-14; 1994, Q2, P14

> **OGCR** Section I.C.11.b.2
> For routine prenatal outpatient visits for patients with high-risk pregnancies, a code from category V23, Supervision of high-risk pregnancy, should be used as the first-listed diagnosis. Secondary chapter 11 codes may be used in conjunction with these codes if appropriate.

● **V23 Supervision of high-risk pregnancy**
> Coding Clinic: 1990, Q1, P10

● **V23.0 Pregnancy with history of infertility**

● **V23.1 Pregnancy with history of trophoblastic disease**
> Pregnancy with history of:
>   hydatidiform mole
>   vesicular mole
> | **Excludes** | *that without current pregnancy (V13.1)*

● **V23.2 Pregnancy with history of abortion**
> Pregnancy with history of conditions classifiable to 634–638
> | **Excludes** | ~~*habitual aborter*~~ *recurrent pregnancy loss:* ◀▥
>   *care during pregnancy (646.3)*
>   *that without current pregnancy (629.81)*

● **V23.3 Grand multiparity**
> | **Excludes** | *care in relation to labor and delivery (659.4)*
>   *that without current pregnancy (V61.5)*

● **V23.4 Pregnancy with other poor obstetric history**
> Pregnancy with history of other conditions classifiable to 630–676

  ● **V23.41 Pregnancy with history of pre-term labor**

  ● **V23.49 Pregnancy with other poor obstetric history**

● **V23.5 Pregnancy with other poor reproductive history**
> Pregnancy with history of stillbirth or neonatal death

● **V23.7 Insufficient prenatal care**
> History of little or no prenatal care

● **V23.8 Other high-risk pregnancy**
> Coding Clinic: 1998, Q4, P50-51

  ● **V23.81 Elderly primigravida**
> First pregnancy in a woman who will be 35 years of age or older at expected date of delivery
> | **Excludes** | *elderly primigravida complicating pregnancy (659.5)*
> Coding Clinic: 1998, Q4, P58

● **V23.82 Elderly multigravida**
> Second or more pregnancy in a woman who will be 35 years of age or older at expected date of delivery
> | **Excludes** | *elderly multigravida complicating pregnancy (659.6)*

● **V23.83 Young primigravida**
> First pregnancy in a female less than 16 years old at expected date of delivery
> | **Excludes** | *young primigravida complicating pregnancy (659.8)*

● **V23.84 Young multigravida**
> Second or more pregnancy in a female less than 16 years old at expected date of delivery
> | **Excludes** | *young multigravida complicating pregnancy (659.8)*

● **V23.85 Pregnancy resulting from assisted reproductive technology**
> Pregnancy resulting from in vitro fertilization

● **V23.86 Pregnancy with history of in utero procedure during previous pregnancy**
> | **Excludes** | *management of pregnancy affected by in utero procedure during current pregnancy (679.0–679.1)*

● **V23.89 Other high-risk pregnancy**
> Coding Clinic: 2006, Q3, P14

● **V23.9 Unspecified high-risk pregnancy**

> **OGCR** Section I.C.18.d.8
> The follow-up codes (V24, V67 and V89), are used to explain continuing surveillance following completed treatment of a disease, condition, or injury. They imply that the condition has been fully treated and no longer exists. They should not be confused with aftercare codes that explain current treatment for a healing condition or its sequelae. Follow-up codes may be used in conjunction with history codes to provide the full picture of the healed condition and its treatment. The follow-up code is sequenced first, followed by the history code. A follow-up code may be used to explain repeated visits. Should a condition be found to have recurred on the follow-up visit, then the diagnosis code should be used in place of the follow-up code.

● **V24 Postpartum care and examination**

V24.0 Immediately after delivery
> Care and observation in uncomplicated cases
> Coding Clinic: 2006, Q3, P11

> **OGCR** Section I.C.10.i.5
> When the mother delivers outside the hospital prior to admission and is admitted for routine postpartum care and no complications are noted, code V24.0, Postpartum care and examination immediately after delivery, should be assigned as the principal diagnosis.

● **V24.1 Lactating mother**
> Supervision of lactation

● **V24.2 Routine postpartum follow-up**

V01–V91

● **V25 Encounter for contraceptive management**
  ● **V25.0 General counseling and advice**
    ● **V25.01 Prescription of oral contraceptives**
    ● **V25.02 Initiation of other contraceptive measures**
        Fitting of diaphragm
        Prescription of foams, creams, or other agents
        Coding Clinic: 1997, Q3, P7
    ● **V25.03 Encounter for emergency contraceptive counseling and prescription**
        Encounter for postcoital contraceptive counseling and prescription
    ● **V25.04 Counseling and instruction in natural family planning to avoid pregnancy**
        Coding Clinic: 2007, Q4, P99-101
    ● **V25.09 Other**
        Family planning advice
  ● **V25.1 Encounter for insertion or removal of intrauterine contraceptive device** ◄▥
      Excludes *encounter for routine checking of intrauterine contraceptive device (V25.42)* ◄
    ● **V25.11 Encounter for insertion of intrauterine contraceptive device** ◄
    ● **V25.12 Encounter for removal of intrauterine contraceptive device** ◄
    ● **V25.13 Encounter for removal and reinsertion of intrauterine contraceptive device** ◄
        Encounter for replacement of intrauterine contraceptive device ◄
  V25.2 Sterilization
      Admission for interruption of fallopian tubes or vas deferens
  V25.3 Menstrual extraction
      Menstrual regulation
  ● **V25.4 Surveillance of previously prescribed contraceptive methods**
      Checking, reinsertion, or removal of contraceptive device
      Repeat prescription for contraceptive method
      Routine examination in connection with contraceptive maintenance
      Excludes *presence of intrauterine contraceptive device as incidental finding (V45.5)*
    ● **V25.40 Contraceptive surveillance, unspecified**
    ● **V25.41 Contraceptive pill**
    ● **V25.42 Intrauterine contraceptive device**
        Checking, reinsertion, or removal of intrauterine device ◄▥
        Excludes *insertion or removal of intrauterine contraceptive device (V25.11-V25.13)* ◄
        presence of intrauterine contraceptive device as incidental finding (V45.5) ◄
    ● **V25.43 Implantable subdermal contraceptive**
    ● **V25.49 Other contraceptive method**
        Coding Clinic: 1997, Q3, P7
  ● **V25.5 Insertion of implantable subdermal contraceptive**
  ● **V25.8 Other specified contraceptive management**
      Postvasectomy sperm count
      Excludes *sperm count following sterilization reversal (V26.22)*
      sperm count for fertility testing (V26.21)
      Coding Clinic: 1996, Q3, P9
  ● **V25.9 Unspecified contraceptive management**

● **V26 Procreative management**
  V26.0 Tuboplasty or vasoplasty after previous sterilization
      Coding Clinic: 1995, Q2, P10
  ● **V26.1 Artificial insemination**
  ● **V26.2 Investigation and testing**
      Excludes *postvasectomy sperm count (V25.8)*
      Coding Clinic: 1996, Q2, P9; 1985, Nov-Dec, P15
    ● **V26.21 Fertility testing**
        Fallopian insufflation
        Sperm count for fertility testing
        Excludes *genetic counseling and testing (V26.31–V26.39)*
    ● **V26.22 Aftercare following sterilization reversal**
        Fallopian insufflation following sterilization reversal
        Sperm count following sterilization reversal
    ● **V26.29 Other investigation and testing**
      OGCR Section I.C.18.d.3
        If the purpose of the encounter is genetic counseling associated with procreative management, a code from subcategory V26.3 should be assigned as the first-listed code, followed by a code from category V84, Genetic susceptibility to disease. Additional codes should be assigned for any applicable family or personal history.
  ● **V26.3 Genetic counseling and testing**
      Excludes *fertility testing (V26.21)*
      nonprocreative genetic screening (V82.71, V82.79)
      Coding Clinic: 2006, Q4, P117; 2005, Q4, P94-100
    ● **V26.31 Testing of female genetic disease carrier status**
    ● **V26.32 Other genetic testing of female**
        Use additional code to identify habitual aborter recurrent pregnancy loss (629.81, 646.3) ◄▥
    ● **V26.33 Genetic counseling**
    ● **V26.34 Testing of male for genetic disease carrier status**
    ● **V26.35 Encounter for testing of male partner of habitual aborter female with recurrent pregnancy loss** ◄▥
    ● **V26.39 Other genetic testing of male**
  ● **V26.4 General counseling and advice**
    ● **V26.41 Procreative counseling and advice using natural family planning**
        Coding Clinic: 2007, Q4, P99-101
    ● **V26.42 Encounter for fertility preservation counseling**
        Encounter for fertility preservation counseling prior to cancer therapy
        Encounter for fertility preservation counseling prior to surgical removal of gonads
    ● **V26.49 Other procreative management counseling and advice**
  ● **V26.5 Sterilization status**
    ● **V26.51 Tubal ligation status**
        Excludes *infertility not due to previous tubal ligation (628.0–628.9)*
    ● **V26.52 Vasectomy status**

◄ New   ◄▥ Revised   ~~deleted~~ Deleted   Excludes   Includes   Use additional   Code first
● Unacceptable Principal Diagnosis   ● Use Additional Digit(s)   OGCR Official Guidelines   Coding Clinic

● V26.8 **Other specified procreative management**

   ● V26.81 **Encounter for assisted reproductive fertility procedure cycle**
   Patient undergoing in vitro fertilization cycle
   Use additional code to identify the type of infertility
   Excludes *pre-cycle diagnosis and testing - code to reason for encounter*
   Coding Clinic: 2007, Q4, P99-101

   ● V26.82 **Encounter for fertility preservation procedure**
   Encounter for fertility preservation counseling prior to cancer therapy
   Encounter for fertility preservation procedure prior to surgical removal of gonads

   ● V26.89 **Other specified procreative management**

● V26.9 **Unspecified procreative management**

   OGCR Section I.C.11.h.3
   V27.0, Single liveborn, is the only outcome of delivery code appropriate for use with 650.

   OGCR Section I.C.11.k.4
   When an attempted termination of pregnancy results in a liveborn fetus assign code 644.21 with an appropriate code from category V27, Outcome of Delivery. The procedure code for the attempted termination of pregnancy should also be assigned.

   OGCR Section I.C.11.b.5
   An outcome of delivery code, V27.0-V27.9, should be included on every maternal record when a delivery has occurred. These codes are not to be used on subsequent records or on the newborn record.

● V27 **Outcome of delivery**
   Note: This category is intended for the coding of the outcome of delivery on the mother's record.
   Coding Clinic: 1991, Q2, P16

   ● V27.0 **Single liveborn**
   Coding Clinic: 2008, Q4, P192; 2005, Q4, P81; 2003, Q2, P9; 2002, Q2, P10; 2000, Q3, P5; 1998, Q4, P76-77

   ● V27.1 **Single stillborn**
   Coding Clinic: 2001, Q1, P11-12

   ● V27.2 **Twins, both liveborn**
   Coding Clinic: 1992, Q3, P10

   ● V27.3 **Twins, one liveborn and one stillborn**

   ● V27.4 **Twins, both stillborn**

   ● V27.5 **Other multiple birth, all liveborn**

   ● V27.6 **Other multiple birth, some liveborn**

   ● V27.7 **Other multiple birth, all stillborn**

   ● V27.9 **Unspecified outcome of delivery**
   routine prenatal care (V22.0–V23.9)

● V28 **Encounter for antenatal screening of mother**
   Excludes *abnormal findings on screening - code to findings suspected fetal conditions affecting management of pregnancy (655.00–655.93, 656.00–656.93, 657.00–657.03, 658.00–658.93) suspected fetal conditions not found (V89.01–V89.09)*

   OGCR Section I.C.18.d.5
   See V28, Antenatal screening; V73-V82 to report special screening examinations.

   ● V28.0 **Screening for chromosomal anomalies by amniocentesis**

● V28.1 **Screening for raised alpha-fetoprotein levels in amniotic fluid**

● V28.2 **Other screening based on amniocentesis**

● V28.3 **Encounter for routine screening for malformation using ultrasonics**
   Encounter for routine fetal ultrasound NOS
   Excludes *encounter for fetal anatomic survey (V28.81) genetic counseling and testing (V26.31–V26.39)*

● V28.4 **Screening for fetal growth retardation using ultrasonics**

● V28.5 **Screening for isoimmunization**

● V28.6 **Screening for Streptococcus B**

● V28.8 **Other specified antenatal screening**
   Coding Clinic: 1999, Q3, P16

   ● V28.81 **Encounter for fetal anatomic survey**

   ● V28.82 **Encounter for screening for risk of pre-term labor**

   ● V28.89 **Other specified antenatal screening**
   Chorionic villus sampling
   Genomic screening
   Nuchal translucency testing
   Proteomic screening

● V28.9 **Unspecified antenatal screening**

● V29 **Observation and evaluation of newborns for suspected condition not found**
   Note: This category is to be used for newborns, within the neonatal period (the first 28 days of life), who are suspected of having an abnormal condition resulting from exposure from the mother or the birth process, but without signs or symptoms, and which, after examination and observation, is found not to exist.
   Excludes *suspected fetal conditions not found (V89.01–V89.09)*
   Coding Clinic: 2000, Q1, P25-26

   V29.0 **Observation for suspected infectious condition**
   Coding Clinic: 2001, Q1, P10

   V29.1 **Observation for suspected neurological condition**

   V29.2 **Observation for suspected respiratory condition**

   ● V29.3 **Observation for suspected genetic or metabolic condition**
   Coding Clinic: 2005, Q2, P21; 2004, Q1, P8; 1998, Q4, P59

   V29.8 **Observation for other specified suspected condition**
   Coding Clinic: 2003, Q2, P15-16

   ● V29.9 **Observation for unspecified suspected condition**
   Coding Clinic: 2002, Q1, P6-7

OGCR Section I.C.15.d.1
Assign a code from category V29, Observation and evaluation of newborns and infants for suspected conditions not found, to identify those instances when a healthy newborn is evaluated for a suspected condition that is determined after study not to be present. Do not use a code from category V29 when the patient has identified signs or symptoms of a suspected problem; in such cases, code the sign or symptom. A code from category V29 may also be assigned as a principal code for readmissions or encounters when the V30 code no longer applies. Codes from category V29 are for use only for healthy newborns and infants for which no condition after study is found to be present.

V01-V91

OGCR Section I.C.15.d.2
A V29 code is to be used as a secondary code after the V30.

OGCR Section I.C.18.d.6
There are three observation V code categories. They are for use in very limited circumstances when a person is being observed for a suspected condition that is ruled out. The observation codes are not for use if an injury or illness or any signs or symptoms related to the suspected condition are present. In such cases the diagnosis/symptom code is used with the corresponding E code to identify any external cause. The observation codes are to be used as principal diagnosis only. The only exception to this is when the principal diagnosis is required to be a code from the V30, Live born infant, category. Then the V29 observation code is sequenced after the V30 code. Additional codes may be used in addition to the observation code but only if they are unrelated to the suspected condition being observed.

OGCR Section I.C.15.b
When coding the birth of an infant, assign a code from categories V30-V39, according to the type of birth. A code from this series is assigned as a principal diagnosis, and assigned only once to a newborn at the time of birth.

OGCR Section I.C.15.c
If the newborn is transferred to another institution, the V30 series is not used at the receiving hospital.

LIVEBORN INFANTS ACCORDING TO TYPE OF BIRTH (V30–V39)

Note: These categories are intended for the coding of liveborn infants who are consuming health care [e.g., crib or bassinet occupancy].

The following fourth-digit subdivisions are for use with categories V30–V39:

```
0   Born in hospital
1   Born before admission to hospital
●2  Born outside hospital and not hospitalized
```

The following two fifths-digits are for use with the fourth-digit .0, Born in hospital:

```
0   delivered without mention of cesarean delivery
1   delivered by cesarean delivery
```

● **V30 Single liveborn**
Coding Clinic: 2009, Q4, P151x2; 2006, Q3, P10-11; 2005, Q4, P83-89; Q2, P21; 2004, Q1, P8, 16; 2003, Q4, P67-68; Q2, P9; 2001, Q4, P50-51; 2000, Q1, P25-26; 1998, Q4, P46-47, 59; 1994, Q3, P4; 1993, Q4, P36

● **V31 Twin, mate liveborn**
Coding Clinic: 1992, Q3, P10

● **V32 Twin, mate stillborn**

● **V33 Twin, unspecified**

● **V34 Other multiple, mates all liveborn**

● **V35 Other multiple, mates all stillborn**

● **V36 Other multiple, mates live- and stillborn**

● **V37 Other multiple, unspecified**

● **V39 Unspecified**

PERSONS WITH A CONDITION INFLUENCING THEIR HEALTH STATUS (V40–V49)

Note: These categories are intended for use when these conditions are recorded as "diagnoses" or "problems."

● **V40 Mental and behavioral problems**
- ● **V40.0 Problems with learning**
- ● **V40.1 Problems with communication [including speech]**
- ● **V40.2 Other mental problems**
- ● **V40.3 Other behavioral problems**
- ● **V40.9 Unspecified mental or behavioral problem**

● **V41 Problems with special senses and other special functions**
- ● **V41.0 Problems with sight**
- ● **V41.1 Other eye problems**
- ● **V41.2 Problems with hearing**
- ● **V41.3 Other ear problems**
- ● **V41.4 Problems with voice production**
- ● **V41.5 Problems with smell and taste**
- ● **V41.6 Problems with swallowing and mastication**
- ● **V41.7 Problems with sexual function**

  Excludes *marital problems (V61.10)*
  psychosexual disorders (302.0–302.9)

- ● **V41.8 Other problems with special functions**
- ● **V41.9 Unspecified problem with special functions**

● **V42 Organ or tissue replaced by transplant**

  Includes homologous or heterologous (animal) (human) transplant organ status
  Coding Clinic: 1998, Q3, P5

  OGCR Section I.C.17.f.2.a
  Transplant complications other than kidney: Codes under subcategory 996.8, Complications of transplanted organ, are for use for both complications and rejection of transplanted organs. A transplant complication code is only assigned if the complication affects the function of the transplanted organ. Two codes are required to fully describe a transplant complication, the appropriate code from subcategory 996.8 and a secondary code that identifies the complication.
  Pre-existing conditions or conditions that develop after the transplant are not coded as complications unless they affect the function of the transplanted organs.
  See I.C.18.d.3) for transplant organ removal status.
  See I.C.2.i for malignant neoplasm associated with transplanted organ.

- ● **V42.0 Kidney**
  Coding Clinic: 2008, Q1, P10-13; 2003, Q1, P10-11; 2001, Q3, P12-13; 1994, Q2, P9x2
- ● **V42.1 Heart**
  Coding Clinic: 2003, Q3, P16; 2001, Q3, P13-14x2; 1994, Q2, P13
- ● **V42.2 Heart valve**
- ● **V42.3 Skin**
- ● **V42.4 Bone**
- ● **V42.5 Cornea**
- ● **V42.6 Lung**
- ● **V42.7 Liver**

◄ New   ◄ Revised   ~~deleted~~ Deleted   Excludes   Includes   Use additional   Code first
● Unacceptable Principal Diagnosis   ● Use Additional Digit(s)   OGCR Official Guidelines   Coding Clinic

V01-V91

OGCR Section I.C.17.f.2.b

Patients who have undergone kidney transplant may still have some form of chronic kidney disease (CKD) because the kidney transplant may not fully restore kidney function. Code 996.81 should be assigned for documented complications of a kidney transplant, such as transplant failure or rejection or other transplant complication. Code 996.81 should not be assigned for post kidney transplant patients who have chronic kidney (CKD) unless a transplant complication such as transplant failure or rejection is documented. If the documentation is unclear as to whether the patient has a complication of the transplant, query the provider. For patients with CKD following a kidney transplant, but who do not have a complication such as failure or rejection, *see section I.C.10.a.2, Chronic kidney disease and kidney transplant status.*

● **V42.8 Other specified organ or tissue**

    ● **V42.81 Bone marrow**

    ● **V42.82 Peripheral stem cells**

    ● **V42.83 Pancreas**
        Coding Clinic: 2003, Q1, P10-11; 2001, Q2, P16

    ● **V42.84 Intestines**
        Coding Clinic: 2000, Q4, P47-48

    ● **V42.89 Other**

● **V42.9 Unspecified organ or tissue**

● **V43 Organ or tissue replaced by other means**

    Includes organ or tissue assisted by other means
        replacement of organ by:
            artificial device
            mechanical device
            prosthesis

    Excludes *cardiac pacemaker in situ (V45.01)*
        fitting and adjustment of prosthetic device
          (V52.0–V52.9)
        renal dialysis status (V45.11)

● **V43.0 Eye globe**

● **V43.1 Lens**
    Pseudophakos

● **V43.2 Heart**

    ● **V43.21 Heart assist device**

    ● **V43.22 Fully implantable artificial heart**

● **V43.3 Heart valve**
    Coding Clinic: 2006, Q3, P7; 2002, Q3, P13-15

● **V43.4 Blood vessel**

● **V43.5 Bladder**

● **V43.6 Joint**
    Coding Clinic: 1991, Q1, P15

    ● **V43.60 Unspecified joint**

    ● **V43.61 Shoulder**

    ● **V43.62 Elbow**

    ● **V43.63 Wrist**

    ● **V43.64 Hip**
        Coding Clinic: 2009, Q1, P15; 2008, Q2, P3-5; 2006,
         Q3, P4-5; 2005, Q4, P83-89, 110-112; 2004,
         Q2, P15

    ● **V43.65 Knee**
        Coding Clinic: 2006, Q3, P5

    ● **V43.66 Ankle**

    ● **V43.69 Other**

● **V43.7 Limb**

● **V43.8 Other organ or tissue**

    ● **V43.81 Larynx**

    ● **V43.82 Breast**

    ● **V43.83 Artificial skin**

    ● **V43.89 Other**

● **V44 Artificial opening status**

    Excludes *artificial openings requiring attention or*
        management (V55.0–V55.9)

● **V44.0 Tracheostomy**
    Coding Clinic: 2003, Q4, P103-104, 107, 111; 2001, Q1, P6-7

● **V44.1 Gastrostomy**
    Coding Clinic: 2003, Q4, P103-104, 107-108, 110; 2001, Q1,
     P12; 1998, Q4, P42-44; 1997, Q3, P12-13; 1993, Q1,
     P26

● **V44.2 Ileostomy**
    Coding Clinic: 1988, Q2, P9-10

● **V44.3 Colostomy**
    Coding Clinic: 2003, Q4, P110

● **V44.4 Other artificial opening of gastrointestinal
    tract**

● **V44.5 Cystostomy**

    ● **V44.50 Cystostomy, unspecified**

    ● **V44.51 Cutaneous-vesicostomy**

    ● **V44.52 Appendico-vesicostomy**

    ● **V44.59 Other cystostomy**

● **V44.6 Other artificial opening of urinary tract**
    Nephrostomy
    Ureterostomy
    Urethrostomy

● **V44.7 Artificial vagina**

● **V44.8 Other artificial opening status**

● **V44.9 Unspecified artificial opening status**

● **V45 Other postprocedural states**

    Excludes *aftercare management (V51–V58.9)*
        malfunction or other complication-code to
         condition

● **V45.0 Cardiac device in situ**

    Excludes *artificial heart (V43.22)*
        heart assist device (V43.21)
    Coding Clinic: 1994, Q2, P10x2; 1993, 5th Issue, P12

    ● **V45.00 Unspecified cardiac device**

    ● **V45.01 Cardiac pacemaker**

        Excludes *cardiac defibrillator*
           with synchronous cardiac
           pacemaker (V45.02) ◄

    ● **V45.02 Automatic implantable cardiac
        defibrillator**
        With synchronous cardiac pacemaker ◄

    ● **V45.09 Other specified cardiac device**
        Carotid sinus pacemaker in situ

● **V45.1 Renal dialysis status**

    Excludes *admission for dialysis treatment or*
        session (V56.0)
    Coding Clinic: 2008, Q1, P7-8; 2007, Q4, P84-86; Q3, P11; 2006,
     Q4, P136; 2004, Q1, P22,23; 2001, Q2, P12-13; 1987,
     Sept-Oct, P8; Jan-Feb, P15

    ● **V45.11 Renal dialysis status**
        Hemodialysis status
        Patient requiring intermittent renal
          dialysis
        Peritoneal dialysis status
        Presence of arterial-venous shunt
          (for dialysis)
        Coding Clinic: 2008, Q4, P193; 2004, Q1, P23

    ● **V45.12 Noncompliance with renal dialysis**
        Coding Clinic: 2006, Q4, P136

V01-V91

V01-V91

● **V45.2 Presence of cerebrospinal fluid drainage device**
  Cerebral ventricle (communicating) shunt, valve, or device in situ

  | Excludes | *malfunction (996.2)* |

  Coding Clinic: 2003, Q4, P106-107

● **V45.3 Intestinal bypass or anastomosis status**

Excludes	*bariatric surgery status (V45.86)*
	gastric bypass status (V45.86)
	obesity surgery status (V45.86)

● **V45.4 Arthrodesis status**
  Coding Clinic: 1984, Nov-Dec, P18

● **V45.5 Presence of contraceptive device**

Excludes	~~*checking, reinsertion, or removal of*~~
	~~*device (V25.42)*~~
	~~*complication from device (996.32)*~~
	~~*insertion of device (V25.1)*~~

  ● **V45.51 Intrauterine contraceptive device**

Excludes	*checking of device (V25.42)* ◄
	complication from device (996.32) ◄
	insertion and removal of device (V25.11-V25.13) ◄

  ● **V45.52 Subdermal contraceptive implant**
    Coding Clinic: 1995, Q3, P14

  ● **V45.59 Other**

● **V45.6 States following surgery of eye and adnexa**

Excludes	*aphakia (379.31)*
	artificial:
	eye globe (V43.0)

  ● **V45.61 Cataract extraction status**
    Use additional code for associated artificial lens status (V43.1)

  ● **V45.69 Other states following surgery of eye and adnexa**
    Coding Clinic: 2001, Q2, P16-17

● **V45.7 Acquired absence of organ**

  V45.71 Acquired absence of breast and nipple

  | Excludes | *congenital absence of breast and nipple (757.6)* |

    Coding Clinic: 2001, Q4, P66; 1997, Q4, P50

  ● **V45.72 Acquired absence of intestine (large) (small)**

  ● **V45.73 Acquired absence of kidney**

  ● **V45.74 Other parts of urinary tract**
    Bladder

  ● **V45.75 Stomach**

  ● **V45.76 Lung**

  ● **V45.77 Genital organs**

  | Excludes | *acquired absence of cervix and uterus (V88.01–V88.03)* |
  | | *female genital mutilation status (629.20–629.29)* |

    Coding Clinic: 2003, Q1, P13-14x2

  ● **V45.78 Eye**

  ● **V45.79 Other acquired absence of organ**

  | Excludes | *acquired absence of pancreas (V88.11-V88.12)* ◄ |

● **V45.8 Other postprocedural status**

  ● **V45.81 Aortocoronary bypass status**
    Coding Clinic: 2003, Q4, P105-106; 2001, Q3, P15; 1997, Q3, P16

  ● **V45.82 Percutaneous transluminal coronary angioplasty status**
    Coding Clinic: 1995, Q2, P18

  ● **V45.83 Breast implant removal status**

  ● **V45.84 Dental restoration status**
    Dental crowns status
    Dental fillings status

  ● **V45.85 Insulin pump status**

  ● **V45.86 Bariatric surgery status**
    Gastric banding status
    Gastric bypass status for obesity
    Obesity surgery status

  | Excludes | *bariatric surgery status complicating pregnancy, childbirth or the puerperium (649.2)* |
  | | *intestinal bypass or anastomosis status (V45.3)* |

    Coding Clinic: 2009, Q2, P10

  ● **V45.87 Transplanted organ removal status**
    Transplanted organ previously removed due to complication, failure, rejection or infection

  | Excludes | *encounter for removal of transplanted organ – code to complication of transplanted organ (996.80–996.89)* |

  ● **V45.88 Status post administration of tPA (rtPA) in a different facility within the last 24 hours prior to admission to the current facility**

    Code first condition requiring tPA administration, such as:
    acute cerebral infarction (433.0–433.9 with fifth-digit 1, 434.0–434.9 with fifth digit 1)
    acute myocardial infarction (410.00–410.92)

  ● **V45.89 Other**
    Presence of neuropacemaker or other electronic device

  | Excludes | *artificial heart valve in situ (V43.3)* |
  | | *vascular prosthesis in situ (V43.4)* |

    Coding Clinic: 1995, Q1, P11

● **V46 Other dependence on machines and devices**

  ● **V46.0 Aspirator**

  ● **V46.1 Respirator [Ventilator]**
    Iron lung
    Coding Clinic: 2005, Q4, P94-100; 2004, Q4, P100-101

    V46.11 Dependence on respirator, status
      Coding Clinic: 2003, Q4, P104-105; 2001, Q1, P12

    V46.12 Encounter for respirator dependence during power failure

    V46.13 Encounter for weaning from respirator [ventilator]

    V46.14 Mechanical complication of respirator [ventilator]
      Mechanical failure of respirator [ventilator]

● **V46.2 Supplemental oxygen**
Long-term oxygen therapy

● **V46.3 Wheelchair dependence**
Wheelchair confinement status

Code first cause of dependence, such as:
muscular dystrophy (359.1)
obesity (278.00-278.03) ◀▥

● **V46.8 Other enabling machines**
Hyperbaric chamber
Possum [Patient-Operated-Selector-Mechanism]

Excludes *cardiac pacemaker (V45.0)*
kidney dialysis machine (V45.11)

● **V46.9 Unspecified machine dependence**

● **V47 Other problems with internal organs**

● **V47.0 Deficiencies of internal organs**

● **V47.1 Mechanical and motor problems with internal organs**

● **V47.2 Other cardiorespiratory problems**
Cardiovascular exercise intolerance with pain (with):
at rest
less than ordinary activity
ordinary activity

● **V47.3 Other digestive problems**

● **V47.4 Other urinary problems**

● **V47.5 Other genital problems**

● **V47.9 Unspecified**

● **V48 Problems with head, neck, and trunk**

● **V48.0 Deficiencies of head**

Excludes *deficiencies of ears, eyelids, and nose (V48.8)*

● **V48.1 Deficiencies of neck and trunk**

● **V48.2 Mechanical and motor problems with head**

● **V48.3 Mechanical and motor problems with neck and trunk**

● **V48.4 Sensory problem with head**

● **V48.5 Sensory problem with neck and trunk**

● **V48.6 Disfigurements of head**

● **V48.7 Disfigurements of neck and trunk**

● **V48.8 Other problems with head, neck, and trunk**

● **V48.9 Unspecified problem with head, neck, or trunk**

● **V49 Other conditions influencing health status**

● **V49.0 Deficiencies of limbs**

● **V49.1 Mechanical problems with limbs**

● **V49.2 Motor problems with limbs**

● **V49.3 Sensory problems with limbs**

● **V49.4 Disfigurements of limbs**

● **V49.5 Other problems of limbs**

● **V49.6 Upper limb amputation status**
Coding Clinic: 1998, Q4, P42-44

● **V49.60 Unspecified level**

● **V49.61 Thumb**

● **V49.62 Other finger(s)**
Coding Clinic: 2005, Q2, P7

● **V49.63 Hand**

● **V49.64 Wrist**
Disarticulation of wrist

● **V49.65 Below elbow**

● **V49.66 Above elbow**
Disarticulation of elbow

● **V49.67 Shoulder**
Disarticulation of shoulder

● **V49.7 Lower limb amputation status**
Coding Clinic: 2006, Q3, P5; 1998, Q4, P42-44

● **V49.70 Unspecified level**

● **V49.71 Great toe**

● **V49.72 Other toe(s)**

● **V49.73 Foot**

● **V49.74 Ankle**
Disarticulation of ankle

● **V49.75 Below knee**

● **V49.76 Above knee**
Disarticulation of knee
Coding Clinic: 2005, Q2, P14

● **V49.77 Hip**
Disarticulation of hip

● **V49.8 Other specified conditions influencing health status**

● **V49.81 Asymptomatic postmenopausal status (age-related) (natural)**

Excludes *menopausal and premenopausal disorders (627.0–627.9)*
postsurgical menopause (256.2)
premature menopause (256.31)
symptomatic menopause (627.0–627.9)
Coding Clinic: 2009, Q4, P151; 2000, Q4, P53-54

● **V49.82 Dental sealant status**

● **V49.83 Awaiting organ transplant status**
Coding Clinic: 2004, Q4, P101

● **V49.84 Bed confinement status**
Coding Clinic: 2005, Q4, P94-100

● **V49.85 Dual sensory impairment**
Blindness with deafness
Combined visual hearing impairment

Code first:
hearing impairment (389.00–389.9)
visual impairment (369.00–369.9)
Coding Clinic: 2007, Q4, P99-101

● **V49.86 Do not resuscitate status** ◀

● **V49.87 Physical restraints status** ◀

Excludes *restraint due to a procedure –
omit code* ◀

● **V49.89 Other specified conditions influencing health status**

● **V49.9 Unspecified**

PERSONS ENCOUNTERING HEALTH SERVICES FOR SPECIFIC PROCEDURES AND AFTERCARE (V50–V59)

Note: Categories V51–V58 are intended for use to indicate a reason for care in patients who may have already been treated for some disease or injury not now present, or who are receiving care to consolidate the treatment, to deal with residual states, or to prevent recurrence.

Excludes *follow-up examination for medical surveillance following treatment (V67.0–V67.9)*

● **V50 Elective surgery for purposes other than remedying health states**

V50.0 Hair transplant

V50.1 Other plastic surgery for unacceptable cosmetic appearance
Breast augmentation or reduction
Face-lift

Excludes *encounter for breast reduction (611.1)*
plastic surgery following healed injury or operation (V51.0–V51.8)

V01-V91

V01-V91

V50.2 Routine or ritual circumcision
Circumcision in the absence of significant
medical indication

● **V50.3 Ear piercing**

OGCR Section I.C.18.d.14

For encounters specifically for prophylactic
removal of breasts, ovaries, or another organ
due to a genetic susceptibility to cancer or a
family history of cancer, the principal or first
listed code should be a code from subcategory
V50.4, Prophylactic organ removal, followed by
the appropriate genetic susceptibility code and
the appropriate family history code.

● **V50.4 Prophylactic organ removal**

Excludes *organ donations (V59.0–V59.9)*
therapeutic organ removal-code to
condition
Coding Clinic: 2009, Q3, P21

V50.41 Breast
Coding Clinic: 2004, Q4, P106-107

V50.42 Ovary
Coding Clinic: 2009, Q3, P21x2

V50.49 Other
Coding Clinic: 2009, Q3, P21

● **V50.8 Other**

● **V50.9 Unspecified**

● **V51 Aftercare involving the use of plastic surgery**

Includes plastic surgery following healed injury or
operation

Excludes *cosmetic plastic surgery (V50.1)*
plastic surgery as treatment for current condition
or injury - code to condition or injury
repair of scar tissue - code to scar

**V51.0 Encounter for breast reconstruction following
mastectomy**

Excludes *deformity and disproportion of*
reconstructed breast (612.0–612.1)

**V51.8 Other aftercare involving the use of plastic
surgery**

● **V52 Fitting and adjustment of prosthetic device and implant**

Includes removal of device

Excludes *malfunction or complication of prosthetic device*
(996.0–996.7)
status only, without need for care
(V43.0–V43.8)

V52.0 Artificial arm (complete) (partial)

V52.1 Artificial leg (complete) (partial)

V52.2 Artificial eye

V52.3 Dental prosthetic device

V52.4 Breast prosthesis and implant
Elective implant exchange (different material)
(different size)
Removal of tissue expander without synchronous
insertion of permanent implant

Excludes *admission for initial breast implant*
insertion for breast augmentation
(V50.1)
complications of breast implant (996.54,
996.69, 996.79)
encounter for breast reconstruction
following mastectomy (V51.0)
Coding Clinic: 1995, Q4, P80.81

V52.8 Other specified prosthetic device
Coding Clinic: 2002, Q3, P12; Q2, P16-17

● **V52.9 Unspecified prosthetic device**

● **V53 Fitting and adjustment of other device**

Includes removal of device
replacement of device

Excludes *status only, without need for care (V45.0–V45.8)*

● **V53.0 Devices related to nervous system and special
senses**

**V53.01 Fitting and adjustment of cerebral
ventricle (communicating) shunt**
Coding Clinic: 1997, Q4, P51

**V53.02 Neuropacemaker (brain) (peripheral
nerve) (spinal cord)**

**V53.09 Fitting and adjustment of other devices
related to nervous system and special
senses**
Auditory substitution device
Visual substitution device
Coding Clinic: 1999, Q2, P3-4

● **V53.1 Spectacles and contact lenses**

● **V53.2 Hearing aid**

● **V53.3 Cardiac device**
Reprogramming
Coding Clinic: 1992, Q3, P3

V53.31 Cardiac pacemaker

Excludes *automatic implantable cardiac*
defibrillator with
synchronous cardiac
pacemaker (V53.32) ◀
mechanical complication
of cardiac pacemaker
(996.01)
Coding Clinic: 2002, Q1, P3; 1984, Nov-Dec, P18

**V53.32 Automatic implantable cardiac
defibrillator**
With synchronous cardiac pacemaker ◀
Coding Clinic: 2005, Q3, P3-9

V53.39 Other cardiac device
Coding Clinic: 2008, Q2, P9-10; 2007, Q1, P20

● **V53.4 Orthodontic devices**

● **V53.5 Other gastrointestinal appliance and device**

Excludes *colostomy (V55.3)*
ileostomy (V55.2)
other artifical opening of digestive tract
(V55.4)

● **V53.50 Fitting and adjustment of intestinal
appliance and device**

● **V53.51 Fitting and adjustment of gastric
lap band**

● **V53.59 Fitting and adjustment of other
gastrointestinal appliance and device**

● **V53.6 Urinary devices**
Urinary catheter

Excludes *cystostomy (V55.5)*
nephrostomy (V55.6)
ureterostomy (V55.6)
urethrostomy (V55.6)

● **V53.7 Orthopedic devices**
Orthopedic:
brace
cast
corset
shoes

Excludes *other orthopedic aftercare (V54)*

● **V53.8 Wheelchair**

◀ New   ◀▥ Revised   ~~deleted~~ Deleted | Excludes | | Includes | Use additional   Code first
● Unacceptable Principal Diagnosis   ● Use Additional Digit(s)   OGCR Official Guidelines   Coding Clinic

● **V53.9 Other and unspecified device**
Coding Clinic: 2003, Q2, P6-7

● **V53.90 Unspecified device**

● **V53.91 Fitting and adjustment of insulin pump**
Insulin pump titration

● **V53.99 Other device**
Coding Clinic: 2009, Q2, P10

● **V54 Other orthopedic aftercare**

| Excludes | fitting and adjustment of orthopedic devices (V53.7) |
malfunction of internal orthopedic device (996.40–996.49)
other complication of nonmechanical nature (996.60–996.79)

● **V54.0 Aftercare involving internal fixation device**

| Excludes | malfunction of internal orthopedic device (996.40–996.49) |
other complication of nonmechanical nature (996.60–996.79)
removal of external fixation device (V54.89)

V54.01 Encounter for removal of internal fixation device

V54.02 Encounter for lengthening/adjustment of growth rod

V54.09 Other aftercare involving internal fixation device
Coding Clinic: 2009, Q1, P15

● **V54.1 Aftercare for healing traumatic fracture**

| Excludes | aftercare following joint replacement (V54.81) |
aftercare for amputation stump (V54.89)

V54.10 Aftercare for healing traumatic fracture of arm, unspecified

V54.11 Aftercare for healing traumatic fracture of upper arm

V54.12 Aftercare for healing traumatic fracture of lower arm
Coding Clinic: 2007, Q1, P3-8

V54.13 Aftercare for healing traumatic fracture of hip
Coding Clinic: 2009, Q1, P15; 2007, Q1, P3-8; 2003, Q4, P103-105

V54.14 Aftercare for healing traumatic fracture of leg, unspecified

V54.15 Aftercare for healing traumatic fracture of upper leg

| Excludes | aftercare for healing traumatic fracture of hip (V54.13) |
Coding Clinic: 2006, Q3, P6

V54.16 Aftercare for healing traumatic fracture of lower leg
Coding Clinic: 2009, Q1, P14

V54.17 Aftercare for healing traumatic fracture of vertebrae

V54.19 Aftercare for healing traumatic fracture of other bone
Coding Clinic: 2005, Q1, P13

● **V54.2 Aftercare for healing pathologic fracture**

| Excludes | aftercare following joint replacement (V54.81) |

V54.20 Aftercare for healing pathologic fracture of arm, unspecified

V54.21 Aftercare for healing pathologic fracture of upper arm

V54.22 Aftercare for healing pathologic fracture of lower arm

V54.23 Aftercare for healing pathologic fracture of hip

V54.24 Aftercare for healing pathologic fracture of leg, unspecified

V54.25 Aftercare for healing pathologic fracture of upper leg

| Excludes | aftercare for healing pathologic fracture of hip (V54.23) |

V54.26 Aftercare for healing pathologic fracture of lower leg

V54.27 Aftercare for healing pathologic fracture of vertebrae
Coding Clinic: 2008, Q3, P4; 2003, Q4, P108-109

V54.29 Aftercare for healing pathologic fracture of other bone

● **V54.8 Other orthopedic aftercare**
Coding Clinic: 2001, Q3, P19; 1999, Q4, P5x2; 1990, Q1, P10, 20

V54.81 Aftercare following joint replacement

Use additional code to identify joint replacement site (V43.60–V43.69)
Coding Clinic: 2009, Q1, P14; 2006, Q3, P4; 2004, Q3, P12; Q2, P15

V54.89 Other orthopedic aftercare
Aftercare for healing fracture NOS
Coding Clinic: 2007, Q2, P8-9

● **V54.9 Unspecified orthopedic aftercare**

● **V55 Attention to artificial openings**

| Includes | adjustment or repositioning of catheter |
closure
passage of sounds or bougies
reforming
removal or replacement of catheter
toilet or cleansing

| Excludes | complications of external stoma (519.00–519.09, 569.60–569.69, ~~997.4~~, 997.5) ◀▥ |
status only, without need for care (V44.0–V44.9)

Coding Clinic: 1995, Q3, P13

V55.0 Tracheostomy

V55.1 Gastrostomy
Coding Clinic: 1999, Q4, P9; 1997, Q3, P7-8; 1996, Q1, P14; 1995, Q3, P13

V55.2 Ileostomy

V55.3 Colostomy
Coding Clinic: 2009, Q1, P14; 2005, Q2, P4-5; 1997, Q3, P9-10

V55.4 Other artificial opening of digestive tract
Coding Clinic: 2005, Q2, P14; 2003, Q1, P10

V55.5 Cystostomy

V55.6 Other artificial opening of urinary tract
Nephrostomy   Urethrostomy
Ureterostomy

V55.7 Artificial vagina

V55.8 Other specified artificial opening

● **V55.9 Unspecified artificial opening**

● **V56 Encounter for dialysis and dialysis catheter care**

Use additional code to identify the associated condition

| Excludes | dialysis preparation-code to condition |
Coding Clinic: 1993, Q1, P29

V56.0 Extracorporeal dialysis
Dialysis (renal) NOS

| Excludes | dialysis status (V45.11) |

Coding Clinic: 2005, Q4, P77-79; 2004, Q1, P23; 2000, Q4, P39-40; 1998, Q3, P6; Q2, P20-21; 1993, Q4, P34

◀ New   ◀▥ Revised   ~~deleted~~ Deleted | Excludes | Excludes   Includes Includes   Use additional Use additional   Code first Code first
● Unacceptable Principal Diagnosis   ● Use Additional Digit(s)   OGCR Official Guidelines   Coding Clinic

1037

V01-V91

V56.1 Fitting and adjustment of extracorporeal dialysis catheter
Removal or replacement of catheter
Toilet or cleansing

Use additional code for any concurrent extracorporeal dialysis (V56.0)
Coding Clinic: 1998, Q2, P20-21

● V56.2 Fitting and adjustment of peritoneal dialysis catheter

Use additional code for any concurrent peritoneal dialysis (V56.8)
Coding Clinic: 1998, Q4, P55

● V56.3 Encounter for adequacy testing for dialysis

● V56.31 Encounter for adequacy testing for hemodialysis

● V56.32 Encounter for adequacy testing for peritoneal dialysis
Peritoneal equilibration test

V56.8 Other dialysis
Peritoneal dialysis
Coding Clinic: 1998, Q4, P55

● V57 Care involving use of rehabilitation procedures
Use additional code to identify underlying condition
Coding Clinic: 2002, Q1, P18-19; 1997, Q3, P12

● V57.0 Breathing exercises

● V57.1 Other physical therapy
Therapeutic and remedial exercises, except breathing
Coding Clinic: 2006, Q3, P4; 2004, Q2, P15; 2002, Q4, P56; 1999, Q4, P5

● V57.2 Occupational therapy and vocational rehabilitation

● V57.21 Encounter for occupational therapy
Coding Clinic: 1999, Q4, P7

● V57.22 Encounter for vocational therapy

● V57.3 Speech-language therapy
Coding Clinic: 1997, Q4, P35-37

● V57.4 Orthoptic training

● V57.8 Other specified rehabilitation procedure

● V57.81 Orthotic training
Gait training in the use of artificial limbs

● V57.89 Other
Multiple training or therapy
Coding Clinic: 2007, Q4, P92-95; 2006, Q3, P6; 2003, Q4, P105-106, 108-109; Q2, P16; 2002, Q1, P16; 2001, Q3, P21; 1997, Q3, P11-13

● V57.9 Unspecified rehabilitation procedure

OGCR Section I.C.2.e.2

If a patient admission/encounter is solely for the administration of chemotherapy, immunotherapy or radiation therapy assign code V58.0, Encounter for radiation therapy, or V58.11, Encounter for antineoplastic chemotherapy, or V58.12, Encounter for antineoplastic immunotherapy as the first-listed or principal diagnosis. If a patient receives more than one of these therapies during the same admission more than one of these codes may be assigned, in any sequence.

The malignancy for which the therapy is being administered should be assigned as a secondary diagnosis.

● V58 Encounter for other and unspecified procedures and aftercare
Excludes convalescence and palliative care (V66.0–V66.9)

V58.0 Radiotherapy
Encounter or admission for radiotherapy
Excludes encounter for radioactive implant-code to condition
radioactive iodine therapy-code to condition
Coding Clinic: 1994, Q2, P10x2; 1993, Q4, P 36; 1987, Jan-Feb, P13

● V58.1 Encounter for chemotherapy and immunotherapy for neoplastic conditions
Encounter or admission for chemotherapy
Excludes chemotherapy and immunotherapy for nonneoplastic conditions-code to condition
Coding Clinic: 2005, Q4, P94-100; 2004, Q1, P13-14; 2003, Q2, P16-17; 2000, Q1, P23; 1993, Q4, P34, 36; Q3, P4x5; 1992, Q2, P16-17; 1991, Q2, P17; 1987, Sept-Oct, P8

V58.11 Encounter for antineoplastic chemotherapy
Coding Clinic: 2009, Q4, P152x2; 2008, Q4, P82-83, 152-155; 2007, Q4, P103-104; 2006, Q2, P20-22; 2004, Q1, P13-14

V58.12 Encounter for antineoplastic immunotherapy
Coding Clinic: 2004, Q1, P13-14

● V58.2 Blood transfusion, without reported diagnosis
Coding Clinic: 1994, Q1, P22

● V58.3 Attention to dressings and sutures
Change or removal of wound packing
Excludes attention to drains (V58.49)
planned postoperative wound closure (V58.41)
Coding Clinic: 2006, Q4, P117-118; 2005, Q2, P14

● V58.30 Encounter for change or removal of nonsurgical wound dressing
Encounter for change or removal of wound dressing NOS
Coding Clinic: 2009, Q4, P152x2

● V58.31 Encounter for change or removal of surgical wound dressing

● V58.32 Encounter for removal of sutures
Encounter for removal of staples

● V58.4 Other aftercare following surgery
Note: Codes from this subcategory should be used in conjunction with other aftercare codes to fully identify the reason for the aftercare encounter.
Excludes aftercare following sterilization reversal surgery (V26.22)
attention to artificial openings (V55.0–V55.9)
orthopedic aftercare (V54.0–V54.9)
Coding Clinic: 1999, Q4, P8-9

◄ New   ◄▥ Revised   ~~deleted~~ Deleted   Excludes   Includes   Use additional   Code first
● Unacceptable Principal Diagnosis   ● Use Additional Digit(s)   OGCR Official Guidelines   Coding Clinic

V58.41 Encounter for planned post-operative wound closure

> **Excludes** *disruption of operative wound (998.31–998.32)*
> *encounter for dressings and suture aftercare (V58.30–V58.32)*
>
> Coding Clinic: 1999, Q4, P15

V58.42 Aftercare following surgery for neoplasm
Conditions classifiable to 140–239

V58.43 Aftercare following surgery for injury and trauma
Conditions classifiable to 800–999

> **Excludes** *aftercare for healing traumatic fracture (V54.10–V54.19)*
>
> Coding Clinic: 2007, Q2, P8-9; 1987, Nov-Dec, P9

V58.44 Aftercare following organ transplant
Use additional code to identify the organ transplanted (V42.0–V42.9)
Coding Clinic: 2004, Q4, P101

V58.49 Other specified aftercare following surgery
Change or removal of drains
Coding Clinic: 1996, Q1, P8-9x2

V58.5 Orthodontics

> **Excludes** *fitting and adjustment of orthodontic device (V53.4)*

● **V58.6 Long-term (current) drug use**
Long-term (current) prophylactic drug use ◄

> **Excludes** *drug abuse (305.00–305.93)*
> *drug abuse and dependence complicating pregnancy (648.3–648.4)*
> *drug dependence (304.00–304.93)*
> *hormone replacement therapy (postmenopausal) (V07.4)*
> ~~*prophylactic*~~ *use of agents affecting estrogen receptors and estrogen levels (V07.51–V07.59)* ◄▥▥

V58.61 Long-term (current) use of anticoagulants

> **Excludes** *long-term (current) use of aspirin (V58.66)*
>
> Coding Clinic: 2008, Q4, P134-136; 2006, Q3, P13; 2004, Q3, P7; 2003, Q4, P108; 2003, Q1, P11-12; 2002, Q3, P13-16; Q1, P16

● **V58.62 Long-term (current) use of antibiotics**
Coding Clinic: 1998, Q4, P59-60

OGCR Section I.C.18.d.3

Codes from this subcategory (V58) indicate a patient's continuous use of a prescribed drug (including such things as aspirin therapy) for the long-term treatment of a condition or for prophylactic use. It is not for use for patients who have addictions to drugs. This subcategory is not for use of medications for detoxification or maintenance programs to prevent withdrawal symptoms in patients with drug dependence (e.g., methadone maintenance for opiate dependence). Assign the appropriate code for the drug dependence instead.

Assign a code from subcategory V58.6, Long-term (current) drug use, if the patient is receiving a medication for an extended period as a prophylactic measure (such as for the prevention of deep vein thrombosis) or as treatment of a chronic condition (such as arthritis) or a disease requiring a lengthy course of treatment (such as cancer). Do not assign a code from subcategory V58.6 for medication being administered for a brief period of time to treat an acute illness or injury (such as a course of antibiotics to treat acute bronchitis).

● **V58.63 Long-term (current) use of antiplatelets/ antithrombotics**

> **Excludes** *long-term (current) use of aspirin (V58.66)*

● **V58.64 Long-term (current) use of non-steroidal anti-inflammatories (NSAID)**

> **Excludes** *long-term (current) use of aspirin (V58.66)*

● **V58.65 Long-term (current) use of steroids**

V58.66 Long-term (current) use of aspirin
Coding Clinic: 2004, Q4, P102-103; 2003, Q1, P11-12

V58.67 Long-term (current) use of insulin
Coding Clinic: 2004, Q4, P53-56

V58.69 Long-term (current) use of other medications
Long term current use of methadone
Long term current use of opiate analgesic
Other high-risk medications
Coding Clinic: 2009, Q4, P152; Q3, P21; 2004, Q2, P10; Q1, P13-14; 2003, Q1, P11-12; 2000, Q2, P8-9; 1999, Q3, 13-14; 1996, Q3, P20; Q2, P7x2; 1995, Q4, P51, 61

● **V58.7 Aftercare following surgery to specified body systems, not elsewhere classified**

> Note: Codes from this subcategory should be used in conjunction with other aftercare codes to fully identify the reason for the aftercare encounter.
>
> **Excludes** *aftercare following organ transplant (V58.44)*
> *aftercare following surgery for neoplasm (V58.42)*
>
> Coding Clinic: 2003, Q4, P104-105

V58.71 Aftercare following surgery of the sense organs, NEC
Conditions classifiable to 360–379, 380–389

V58.72 Aftercare following surgery of the nervous system, NEC
Conditions classifiable to 320–359

> **Excludes** *aftercare following surgery of the sense organs, NEC (V58.71)*

V58.73 Aftercare following surgery of the circulatory system, NEC
Conditions classifiable to 390–459
Coding Clinic: 2009, Q2, P12

V58.74 Aftercare following surgery of the respiratory system, NEC
Conditions classifiable to 460–519

V58.75 Aftercare following surgery of the teeth, oral cavity and digestive system, NEC
Conditions classifiable to 520–579
Coding Clinic: 2005, Q2, P14

V58.76 Aftercare following surgery of the genitourinary system, NEC
Conditions classifiable to 580–629

> **Excludes** *aftercare following sterilization reversal (V26.22)*
>
> Coding Clinic: 2005, Q1, P11,12

V58.77 Aftercare following surgery of the skin and subcutaneous tissue, NEC
Conditions classifiable to 680–709

V58.78 Aftercare following surgery of the musculoskeletal system, NEC
Conditions classifiable to 710–739

> **Excludes** *orthopedic aftercare (V54.01–V54.9)*

◄ New   ◄▥▥ Revised   ~~deleted~~ Deleted   Excludes   Includes   Use additional   Code first
● Unacceptable Principal Diagnosis   ● Use Additional Digit(s)   **OGCR** Official Guidelines   Coding Clinic

1039

V01-V91

V01–V91

● **V58.8 Other specified procedures and aftercare**
Coding Clinic: 1994, Q2, P8x2

    V58.81 Fitting and adjustment of vascular catheter
        Removal or replacement of catheter
        Toilet or cleansing

        Excludes *complications of renal dialysis (996.73)*
            complications of vascular catheter (996.74)
            dialysis preparation—code to condition
            encounter for dialysis (V56.0–V56.8)
            fitting and adjustment of dialysis catheter (V56.1)

    V58.82 Fitting and adjustment of non-vascular catheter NEC
        Removal or replacement of catheter
        Toilet or cleansing

        Excludes *fitting and adjustment of peritoneal dialysis catheter (V56.2)*
            fitting and adjustment of urinary catheter (V53.6)

    V58.83 Encounter for therapeutic drug monitoring
        Use additional code for any associated long-term (current) drug use (V58.61–V58.69)

        Excludes *blood-drug testing for medicolegal reasons (V70.4)*
        Coding Clinic: 2004, Q2, P10-11; Q1, P13-14; 2002, Q3, P13-16

    V58.89 Other specified aftercare
        Coding Clinic: 2003, Q4, P106-107; 1998, Q4, P59-60

● **V58.9 Unspecified aftercare**

OGCR Section I.C.18.d.9
Category V59 is the donor codes. They are used for living individuals who are donating blood or other body tissue. These codes are only for individuals donating for others, not for self donations. They are not for use to identify cadaveric donations.

● **V59 Donors**
    Excludes *examination of potential donor (V70.8)*
        self-donation of organ or tissue--code to condition
    Coding Clinic: 2008, Q2, P8-9; 1995, Q4, P50x2

● **V59.0 Blood**
    Coding Clinic: 1990, Q1, P9-10

    ● **V59.01 Whole blood**

    ● **V59.02 Stem cells**
        Coding Clinic: 1995, Q4, P51

    ● **V59.09 Other**

    V59.1 Skin

    V59.2 Bone

    V59.3 Bone marrow
        Coding Clinic: 1985, Jan-Feb, P15

    V59.4 Kidney

    V59.5 Cornea

    V59.6 Liver

● **V59.7 Egg (oocyte) (ovum)**

    ● **V59.70 Egg (oocyte) (ovum) donor, unspecified**

    ● **V59.71 Egg (oocyte) (ovum) donor, under age 35, anonymous recipient**
        Egg donor, under age 35 NOS

    ● **V59.72 Egg (oocyte) (ovum) donor, under age 35, designated recipient**

    ● **V59.73 Egg (oocyte) (ovum) donor, age 35 and over, anonymous recipient**
        Egg donor, age 35 and over NOS

    ● **V59.74 Egg (oocyte) (ovum) donor, age 35 and over, designated recipient**

    V59.8 Other specified organ or tissue
        Coding Clinic: 2002, Q3, P20-21

    V59.9 Unspecified organ or tissue

PERSONS ENCOUNTERING HEALTH SERVICES IN OTHER CIRCUMSTANCES (V60–V69)

● **V60 Housing, household, and economic circumstances**

    ● **V60.0 Lack of housing**
        Hobos
        Social migrants
        Tramps
        Transients
        Vagabonds

    ● **V60.1 Inadequate housing**
        Lack of heating
        Restriction of space
        Technical defects in home preventing adequate care

    ● **V60.2 Inadequate material resources**
        Economic problem
        Poverty NOS

    ● **V60.3 Person living alone**

    ● **V60.4 No other household member able to render care**
        Person requiring care (has) (is):
            family member too handicapped, ill, or otherwise unsuited to render care
            partner temporarily away from home
            temporarily away from usual place of abode

        Excludes *holiday relief care (V60.5)*

    ● **V60.5 Holiday relief care**
        Provision of health care facilities to a person normally cared for at home, to enable relatives to take a vacation

    ● **V60.6 Person living in residential institution**
        Boarding school resident

    ● **V60.8 Other specified housing or economic circumstances**

        ● **V60.81 Foster care (status)**

        ● **V60.89 Other specified housing or economic circumstances**

    ● **V60.9 Unspecified housing or economic circumstance**

● **V61 Other family circumstances**
    Includes when these circumstances or fear of them, affecting the person directly involved or others, are mentioned as the reason, justified or not, for seeking or receiving medical advice or care

    ● **V61.0 Family disruption**

        ● **V61.01 Family disruption due to family member on military deployment**
        Individual or family affected by other family member being on deployment

        Excludes *family disruption due to family member on non-military extended absence from home (V61.08)*

◀ New   ◀⁞⁞⁞ Revised   ~~deleted~~ Deleted | Excludes | | Includes | Use additional   Code first
● Unacceptable Principal Diagnosis   ● Use Additional Digit(s)   **OGCR** Official Guidelines   Coding Clinic

● **V61.02 Family disruption due to return of family member from military deployment**
> Individual or family affected by other family member having returned from deployment (current or past conflict)

● **V61.03 Family disruption due to divorce or legal separation**

● **V61.04 Family disruption due to parent-child estrangement**
> | Excludes | other family estrangement (V61.09) |

● **V61.05 Family disruption due to child in welfare custody**

● **V61.06 Family disruption due to child in foster care or in care of non-parental family member**

● **V61.07 Family disruption due to death of family member**
> | Excludes | bereavement (V62.82) |

● **V61.08 Family disruption due to other extended absence of family member**
> | Excludes | family disruption due to family member on military deployment (V61.01) |

● **V61.09 Other family disruption**
> Family estrangement NOS

◐ **V61.1 Counseling for marital and partner problems**
> | Excludes | problems related to: psychosexual disorders (302.0–302.9) sexual function (V41.7) |

● **V61.10 Counseling for marital and partner problems, unspecified**
> Marital conflict
> Marital relationship problem
> Partner conflict
> Partner relationship problem

● **V61.11 Counseling for victim of spousal and partner abuse**
> | Excludes | encounter for treatment of current injuries due to abuse (995.80–995.85) |

● **V61.12 Counseling for perpetrator of spousal and partner abuse**

◐ **V61.2 Parent-child problems**

● **V61.20 Counseling for parent-child problem, unspecified**
> Concern about behavior of child
> Parent-child conflict
> Parent-child relationship problem

V61.21 Counseling for victim of child abuse
> Child battering
> Child neglect
> | Excludes | current injuries due to abuse (995.50–995.59) |

● **V61.22 Counseling for perpetrator of parental child abuse**
> | Excludes | counseling for non-parental abuser (V62.83) |

● **V61.23 Counseling for parent-biological child problem**
> Concern about behavior of biological child
> Parent-biological child conflict
> Parent-biological child relationship problem

● **V61.24 Counseling for parent-adopted child problem**
> Concern about behavior of adopted child
> Parent-adopted child conflict
> Parent-adopted child relationship problem

● **V61.25 Counseling for parent (guardian)-foster child problem**
> Concern about behavior of foster child
> Parent (guardian)-foster child conflict
> Parent (guardian)-foster child relationship problem

● **V61.29 Other parent-child problems**
> Coding Clinic: 1999, Q3, P16

● **V61.3 Problems with aged parents or in-laws**

◐ **V61.4 Health problems within family**

● **V61.41 Alcoholism in family**

● **V61.42 Substance abuse in family**

● **V61.49 Other**
> Care of sick or handicapped person in family or household
> Presence of sick or handicapped person in family or household

● **V61.5 Multiparity**

● **V61.6 Illegitimacy or illegitimate pregnancy**

● **V61.7 Other unwanted pregnancy**

● **V61.8 Other specified family circumstances**
> Problems with family members NEC
> Sibling relationship problem
> Coding Clinic: 1994, Q1, P21

● **V61.9 Unspecified family circumstance**

◐ **V62 Other psychosocial circumstances**
> | Includes | those circumstances or fear of them, affecting the person directly involved or others, mentioned as the reason, justified or not, for seeking or receiving medical advice or care |
>
> | Excludes | previous psychological trauma (V15.41–V15.49) |

● **V62.0 Unemployment**
> | Excludes | circumstances when main problem is economic inadequacy or poverty (V60.2) |

● **V62.1 Adverse effects of work environment**

◐ **V62.2 Other occupational circumstances or maladjustment**

● **V62.21 Personal current military deployment status**
> Individual (civilian or military) currently deployed in theater or in support of military war, peacekeeping and humanitarian operations

● **V62.22 Personal history of return from military deployment**
> Individual (civilian or military) with past history of military war, peacekeeping and humanitarian deployment (current or past conflict)

● **V62.29 Other occupational circumstances or maladjustment**
> Career choice problem
> Dissatisfaction with employment
> Occupational problem

● **V62.3 Educational circumstances**
> Academic problem
> Dissatisfaction with school environment
> Educational handicap

● **V62.4 Social maladjustment**
Acculturation problem
Cultural deprivation
Political, religious, or sex discrimination
Social:
  isolation
  persecution

● **V62.5 Legal circumstances**
Imprisonment   Litigation
Legal investigation   Prosecution

● **V62.6 Refusal of treatment for reasons of religion or conscience**

● **V62.8 Other psychological or physical stress, not elsewhere classified**

  ● **V62.81 Interpersonal problems, not elsewhere classified**
    Relational problem NOS

  ● **V62.82 Bereavement, uncomplicated**
    Excludes   *bereavement as adjustment reaction (309.0)*
    family disruption due to death of family member (V61.07)

  ● **V62.83 Counseling for perpetrator of physical/ sexual abuse**
    Excludes   *counseling for perpetrator of parental child abuse (V61.22)*
    counseling for perpetrator of spousal and partner abuse (V61.12)

  V62.84 Suicidal ideation
    Excludes   *suicidal tendencies (300.9)*
    Coding Clinic: 2005, Q4, P94-100

  V62.85 Homicidal ideation ◄

  ● **V62.89 Other**
    Borderline intellectual functioning
    Life circumstance problems
    Phase of life problems
    Religious or spiritual problem

● **V62.9 Unspecified psychosocial circumstance**

● **V63 Unavailability of other medical facilities for care**

  ● **V63.0 Residence remote from hospital or other health care facility**

  ● **V63.1 Medical services in home not available**
    Excludes   *no other household member able to render care (V60.4)*
    Coding Clinic: 2001, Q4, P67; Q1, P12

  ● **V63.2 Person awaiting admission to adequate facility elsewhere**
    Coding Clinic: 1994, Q1, P22-23

  ● **V63.8 Other specified reasons for unavailability of medical facilities**
    Person on waiting list undergoing social agency investigation

  ● **V63.9 Unspecified reason for unavailability of medical facilities**

● **V64 Persons encountering health services for specific procedures, not carried out**

  ● **V64.0 Vaccination not carried out**

    ● **V64.00 Vaccination not carried out, unspecified reason**

    ● **V64.01 Vaccination not carried out because of acute illness**

    ● **V64.02 Vaccination not carried out because of chronic illness or condition**

    ● **V64.03 Vaccination not carried out because of immune compromised state**

    ● **V64.04 Vaccination not carried out because of allergy to vaccine or component**

    ● **V64.05 Vaccination not carried out because of caregiver refusal**
    Guardian refusal   Parent refusal
    Excludes   *vaccination not carried out because of caregiver refusal for religious reasons (V64.07)*
    Coding Clinic: 2007, Q1, P12

    ● **V64.06 Vaccination not carried out because of patient refusal**

    ● **V64.07 Vaccination not carried out for religious reasons**

    ● **V64.08 Vaccination not carried out because patient had disease being vaccinated against**

    ● **V64.09 Vaccination not carried out for other reason**

  ● **V64.1 Surgical or other procedure not carried out because of contraindication**
    Coding Clinic: 1993, 5th Issue, P9-10; 1985, Mar-April, P13; 1984, May-June, P11

  ● **V64.2 Surgical or other procedure not carried out because of patient's decision**
    Coding Clinic: 2001, Q2, P8-9; 1999, Q1, P13-14; 1987, Jan-Feb, P13; 1985, July-Aug, P14

  ● **V64.3 Procedure not carried out for other reasons**

  ● **V64.4 Closed surgical procedure converted to open procedure**

    ● **V64.41 Laparoscopic surgical procedure converted to open procedure**
    Coding Clinic: 1997, Q4, P52

    ● **V64.42 Thoracoscopic surgical procedure converted to open procedure**

    ● **V64.43 Arthroscopic surgical procedure converted to open procedure**

● **V65 Other persons seeking consultation**

  V65.0 Healthy person accompanying sick person
    Boarder
    Coding Clinic: 1993, Q4, P36

  ● **V65.1 Person consulting on behalf of another person**
    Advice or treatment for nonattending third party
    Excludes   *concern (normal) about sick person in family (V61.41–V61.49)*

    ● **V65.11 Pediatric pre-birth visit for expectant parent(s)**
    Pre-adoption visit for adoptive parent(s)

    ● **V65.19 Other person consulting on behalf of another person**

  V65.2 Person feigning illness
    Malingerer
    Peregrinating patient
    Coding Clinic: 1999, Q3, P20

  ● **V65.3 Dietary surveillance and counseling**
    Dietary surveillance and counseling (in):
    NOS
    colitis
    diabetes mellitus
    food allergies or intolerance
    gastritis
    hypercholesterolemia
    hypoglycemia
    obesity
    Use additional code to identify Body Mass Index (BMI), if known (V85.0–V85.54)

V01-V91

● **V65.4 Other counseling, not elsewhere classified**
Health:
  advice
  education
  instruction

    | Excludes | counseling (for):
            contraception (V25.40–V25.49)
            genetic (V26.31–V26.39)
            on behalf of third party
              (V65.11–V65.19)
            procreative management
              (V26.41–V26.49)

  ● **V65.40 Counseling NOS**

  ● **V65.41 Exercise counseling**

  ● **V65.42 Counseling on substance use and abuse**

  ● **V65.43 Counseling on injury prevention**

  ● **V65.44 Human immunodeficiency virus [HIV] counseling**
      Coding Clinic: 1994, Q4, P35x3

      OGCR Section I.C.1.h
      When a patient returns to be informed of HIV test results use V65.44 if the results of the test are negative.

  ● **V65.45 Counseling on other sexually transmitted diseases**

  ● **V65.46 Encounter for insulin pump training**

  ● **V65.49 Other specified counseling**
      Coding Clinic: 2000, Q2, P8-9

● **V65.5 Person with feared complaint in whom no diagnosis was made**
  Feared condition not demonstrated
  Problem was normal state
  "Worried well"
  Coding Clinic: 1984, July-Aug, P20

● **V65.8 Other reasons for seeking consultation**
    | Excludes | *specified symptoms*
    Coding Clinic: 1992, Q3, P4

● **V65.9 Unspecified reason for consultation**

● **V66 Convalescence and palliative care**

  V66.0 Following surgery

  V66.1 Following radiotherapy

  V66.2 Following chemotherapy

  V66.3 Following psychotherapy and other treatment for mental disorder

  V66.4 Following treatment of fracture

● **V66.5 Following other treatment**

  V66.6 Following combined treatment

● **V66.7 Encounter for palliative care**
  End-of-life care
  Hospice care
  Terminal care

  Code first underlying disease
  Coding Clinic: 2008, Q3, P13-14; 2005, Q2, P9-10; 2003, Q4, P107; 1996, Q4, P47-48

● **V66.9 Unspecified convalescence**
  Coding Clinic: 1999, Q4, P8

OGCR Section I.C.18.d.8
The follow-up codes are used to explain continuing surveillance following completed treatment of a disease, condition, or injury. They imply that the condition has been fully treated and no longer exists. They should not be confused with aftercare codes that explain current treatment for a healing condition or its sequelae. Follow-up codes may be used in conjunction with history codes to provide the full picture of the healed condition and its treatment. The follow-up code is sequenced first, followed by the history code. A follow-up code may be used to explain repeated visits. Should a condition be found to have recurred on the follow-up visit, then the diagnosis code should be used in place of the follow-up code.

● **V67 Follow-up examination**

    | Includes | surveillance only following completed treatment

    | Excludes | *surveillance of contraception (V25.40–V25.49)*
    Coding Clinic: 2009, Q1, P14; 2003, Q2, P5

● **V67.0 Following surgery**
    Coding Clinic: 1997, Q4, P50; 1995, Q1, P4; 1992, Q3, P11; 1985, July-Aug, P16

  V67.00 Following surgery, unspecified

  V67.01 Follow-up vaginal pap smear
    Vaginal pap smear, status-post hysterectomy for malignant condition

    | Use additional | code to identify:
      acquired absence of uterus (V88.01–V88.03)
      personal history of malignant neoplasm (V10.40–V10.44)

    | Excludes | *vaginal pap smear status-post hysterectomy for non-malignant condition (V76.47)*

  V67.09 Following other surgery

    | Excludes | *sperm count following sterilization reversal (V26.22)*
      sperm count for fertility testing (V26.21)
    Coding Clinic: 2008, Q3, P6; 2003, Q3, P16; 2002, Q3, P14-15; 1995, Q4, P53; Q2, P8; 1993, Q4, P32; 1992, Q3, P11; 1984, May-June, P10

  V67.1 Following radiotherapy
    Coding Clinic: 1985, July-Aug, P16

  V67.2 Following chemotherapy
    Cancer chemotherapy follow-up
    Coding Clinic: 1985, July-Aug, P16

  V67.3 Following psychotherapy and other treatment for mental disorder

  V67.4 Following treatment of healed fracture
    | Excludes | *current (healing) fracture aftercare (V54.0–V54.9)*
    Coding Clinic: 2009, Q1, P14

● **V67.5 Following other treatment**

  V67.51 Following completed treatment with high-risk medication, not elsewhere classified

    | Excludes | *long-term (current) drug use (V58.61–V58.69)*
    Coding Clinic: 1999, Q1, P5-6x2; 1990, Q1, P18

  V67.59 Other

  V67.6 Following combined treatment

● **V67.9 Unspecified follow-up examination**

V01-V91

● **V68** **Encounters for administrative purposes**

  ● **V68.0** **Issue of medical certificates**

    | Excludes | *encounter for general medical examination (V70.0–V70.9)*

    ● **V68.01** **Disability examination**

      Use additional code(s) to identify: specific examination(s), screening and testing performed (V72.0–V82.9)

      Coding Clinic: 2007, Q4, P99-101

    ● **V68.09** **Other issue of medical certificates**

  ● **V68.1** **Issue of repeat prescriptions**

    Issue of repeat prescription for:
    appliance
    glasses
    medications

    | Excludes | *repeat prescription for contraceptives (V25.41–V25.49)*

  ● **V68.2** **Request for expert evidence**

  ● **V68.8** **Other specified administrative purpose**

    ● **V68.81** **Referral of patient without examination or treatment**

    ● **V68.89** **Other**

  ● **V68.9** **Unspecified administrative purpose**

● **V69** **Problems related to lifestyle**

  ● **V69.0** **Lack of physical exercise**

  ● **V69.1** **Inappropriate diet and eating habits**

    | Excludes | *anorexia nervosa (307.1)*
    bulimia (783.6)
    malnutrition and other nutritional deficiencies (260–269.9)
    other and unspecified eating disorders (307.50–307.59)

  ● **V69.2** **High-risk sexual behavior**

  ● **V69.3** **Gambling and betting**

    | Excludes | *pathological gambling (312.31)*

  V69.4 **Lack of adequate sleep**

    Sleep deprivation

    | Excludes | *insomnia (780.52)*

    Coding Clinic: 2004, Q4, P104

  ● **V69.5** **Behavioral insomnia of childhood**

  ● **V69.8** **Other problems related to lifestyle**

    Self-damaging behavior

  ● **V69.9** **Problem related to lifestyle, unspecified**

PERSONS WITHOUT REPORTED DIAGNOSIS ENCOUNTERED DURING EXAMINATION AND INVESTIGATION OF INDIVIDUALS AND POPULATIONS (V70–V82)

Note: Nonspecific abnormal findings disclosed at the time of these examinations are classifiable to categories 790–796.

● **V70** **General medical examination**

  Use additional code(s) to identify any special screening examination(s) performed (V73.0–V82.9)

  Coding Clinic: 1993, Q1, P28; 1985, Nov-Dec, P13

  ● **V70.0** **Routine general medical examination at a health care facility**

    Health checkup

    | Excludes | *health checkup of infant or child over 28 days old (V20.2)*
    health supervision of newborn 8 to 28 days old (V20.32)
    health supervision of newborn under 8 days old (V20.31)
    pre-procedural general physical examination (V72.83)

  ● **V70.1** **General psychiatric examination, requested by the authority**

  ● **V70.2** **General psychiatric examination, other and unspecified**

  ● **V70.3** **Other medical examination for administrative purposes**

    General medical examination for:
    admission to old age home
    adoption
    camp
    driving license
    immigration and naturalization
    insurance certification
    marriage
    prison
    school admission
    sports competition

    | Excludes | *attendance for issue of medical certificates (V68.0)*
    pre-employment screening (V70.5)

    Coding Clinic: 2008, Q3, P6

  V70.4 **Examination for medicolegal reasons**

    Blood-alcohol tests
    Blood-drug tests
    Paternity testing

    | Excludes | *examination and observation following:*
    accidents (V71.3, V71.4)
    assault (V71.6)
    rape (V71.5)

  V70.5 **Health examination of defined subpopulations**

    Armed forces personnel
    Inhabitants of institutions
    Occupational health examinations
    Pre-employment screening
    Preschool children
    Prisoners
    Prostitutes
    Refugees
    School children
    Students

  ● **V70.6** **Health examination in population surveys**

    | Excludes | *special screening (V73.0–V82.9)*

  V70.7 **Examination of participant in clinical trial**

    Examination of participant or control in clinical research

    Coding Clinic: 2006, Q2, P5-6

  ● **V70.8** **Other specified general medical examinations**

    Examination of potential donor of organ or tissue

  ● **V70.9** **Unspecified general medical examination**

OGCR Section I.C.18.d.6

There are three observation V code categories. They are for use in very limited circumstances when a person is being observed for a suspected condition that is ruled out. The observation codes are not for use if an injury or illness or any signs or symptoms related to the suspected condition are present. In such cases the diagnosis/symptom code is used with the corresponding E code to identify any external cause. The observation codes are to be used as principal diagnosis only. The only exception to this is when the principal diagnosis is required to be a code from the V30, Live born infant, category. Then the V29 observation code is sequenced after the V30 code. Additional codes may be used in addition to the observation code but only if they are unrelated to the suspected condition being observed.

◀ New   ◀▦ Revised   ~~deleted~~ Deleted | Excludes | Excludes   Includes Includes   Use additional Use additional   Code first Code first
● Unacceptable Principal Diagnosis   ● Use Additional Digit(s)   OGCR Official Guidelines   Coding Clinic Coding Clinic

● **V71 Observation and evaluation for suspected conditions not found**

> **Note:** This category is to be used when persons without a diagnosis are suspected of having an abnormal condition, without signs or symptoms, which requires study, but after examination and observation, is found not to exist. This category is also for use for administrative and legal observation status.
>
> **Excludes** *suspected maternal and fetal conditions not found (V89.01–V89.09)*
>
> Coding Clinic: 1990, Q1, P19; 1985, Nov-Dec, P10, 13

● **V71.0 Observation for suspected mental condition**

> **V71.01 Adult antisocial behavior**
> Dyssocial behavior or gang activity in adult without manifest psychiatric disorder
>
> **V71.02 Childhood or adolescent antisocial behavior**
> Dyssocial behavior or gang activity in child or adolescent without manifest psychiatric disorder
>
> **V71.09 Other suspected mental condition**

V71.1 Observation for suspected malignant neoplasm
> Coding Clinic: 1990, Q1, P21

V71.2 Observation for suspected tuberculosis

V71.3 Observation following accident at work

V71.4 Observation following other accident
> Examination of individual involved in motor vehicle traffic accident
> Coding Clinic: 2006, Q1, P9; 2004, Q1, P6-7

V71.5 Observation following alleged rape or seduction
> Examination of victim or culprit

V71.6 Observation following other inflicted injury
> Examination of victim or culprit

V71.7 Observation for suspected cardiovascular disease
> Coding Clinic: 2004, Q1, P6-7; 1993, 5th Issue, P17-24; 1990, Q1, P19; 1987, Sept-Oct, P10

● **V71.8 Observation and evaluation for other specified suspected conditions**

> **Excludes** *contact with and (suspected) exposure to (potentially) hazardous substances (V15.84–V15.86, V87.0–V87.31)*
>
> Coding Clinic: 1990, Q1, P19

> **V71.81 Abuse and neglect**
>
> > **Excludes** *adult abuse and neglect (995.80–995.85)*
> > *child abuse and neglect (995.50–995.59)*
> >
> > Coding Clinic: 2000, Q4, P54-55
>
> **V71.82 Observation and evaluation for suspected exposure to anthrax**
>
> **V71.83 Observation and evaluation for suspected exposure to other biological agent**
> > Coding Clinic: 2003, Q4, P46-48
>
> **V71.89 Other specified suspected conditions**
> > Coding Clinic: 2008, Q3, P6-7; 2003, Q2, P15-16

● **V71.9 Observation for unspecified suspected condition**
> Coding Clinic: 2002, Q1, P6-7

● **V72 Special investigations and examinations**

> **Includes** routine examination of specific system
>
> **Excludes** *general medical examination (V70.0–70.4)*
> *general screening examination of defined population groups (V70.5, V70.6, V70.7)*
> *health supervision of newborn 8 to 28 days old (V20.32)*
> *health supervision of newborn under 8 days old (V20.31)*
> *routine examination of infant or child over 28 days old (V20.2)*
>
> Use additional code(s) to identify any special screening examination(s) performed (V73.0–V82.9)
>
> Coding Clinic: 2004, Q1, P15-16; 1985, Nov-Dec, P13

V72.0 Examination of eyes and vision

● **V72.1 Examination of ears and hearing**
> Coding Clinic: 2004, Q1, P15-16

> ● **V72.11 Encounter for hearing examination following failed hearing screening**
> > Coding Clinic: 2006, Q4, P118
>
> ● **V72.12 Encounter for hearing conservation and treatment**
> > Coding Clinic: 2007, Q4, P99-101
>
> ● **V72.19 Other examination of ears and hearing**

● **V72.2 Dental examination**

● **V72.3 Gynecological examination**

> **Excludes** *cervical Papanicolaou smear without general gynecological examination (V76.2)*
> *routine examination in contraceptive management (V25.40–V25.49)*
>
> Coding Clinic: 2004, Q4, P104-105

> **V72.31 Routine gynecological examination**
> General gynecological examination with or without Papanicolaou cervical smear
> Pelvic examination (annual) (periodic)
>
> > Use additional code to identify:
> > human papillomavirus (HPV) screening (V73.81)
> > routine vaginal Papanicolaou smear (V76.47)
> >
> > Coding Clinic: 2006, Q2, P3,4
>
> **V72.32 Encounter for Papanicolaou cervical smear to confirm findings of recent normal smear following initial abnormal smear**
> > Coding Clinic: 2006, Q2, P3-4

● **V72.4 Pregnancy examination or test**
> Coding Clinic: 2005, Q4, P94-100; 2004, Q4, P105

> **V72.40 Pregnancy examination or test, pregnancy unconfirmed**
> Possible pregnancy, not (yet) confirmed
>
> **V72.41 Pregnancy examination or test, negative result**
>
> **V72.42 Pregnancy examination or test, positive result**

● **V72.5 Radiological examination, not elsewhere classified**
> Routine chest x-ray
>
> **Excludes** *radiologic examinations as part of pre-procedural testing (V72.81-V72.84)*
>
> Coding Clinic: 1990, Q1, P8, 10, 19-21; 1985, Nov-Dec, P13

◄ New ◄▦ Revised ~~deleted~~ Deleted Excludes Includes Use additional Code first
● Unacceptable Principal Diagnosis ● Use Additional Digit(s) OGCR Official Guidelines Coding Clinic

1045

V01-V91

Codes V72.5 and V72.62 may be used if the reason for the patient encounter is for routine laboratory/radiology testing in the absence of any signs, symptoms, or associated diagnosis. If routine testing is performed during the same encounter as a test to evaluate a sign, symptom, or diagnosis, it is appropriate to assign both the V code and the code describing the reason for the non-routine test.

● **V72.6 Laboratory examination**
Encounters for blood and urine testing
Coding Clinic: 2006, Q2, P4; 1994, Q4, P35; 1990, Q1, P22; 1985, Nov-Dec, P13

OGCR Section I.C.18.d.13 (outpatient)
V72.6 is not to be used if any sign or symptoms, or reason for a test is documented.

● **V72.60 Laboratory examination, unspecified**
● **V72.61 Antibody response examination**
Immunity status testing
Excludes encounter for allergy testing (V72.7)
● **V72.62 Laboratory examination ordered as part of a routine general medical examination**
Blood tests for routine general physical examination
● **V72.63 Pre-procedural laboratory examination**
Blood tests prior to treatment or procedure
Pre-operative laboratory examination
● **V72.69 Other laboratory examination**
● **V72.7 Diagnostic skin and sensitization tests**
Allergy tests
Skin tests for hypersensitivity
Excludes diagnostic skin tests for bacterial diseases (V74.0–V74.9)
Coding Clinic: 1985, Nov-Dec, P13
● **V72.8 Other specified examinations**
Excludes pre-procedural laboratory examinations (V72.63)
Coding Clinic: 1995, Q4, P51-52; 1990, Q1, P10; 1985, Nov-Dec, P13
V72.81 Preoperative cardiovascular examination
Pre-procedural cardiovascular examination
Coding Clinic: 1995, Q4, P51-52
V72.82 Preoperative respiratory examination
Pre-procedural respiratory examination
Coding Clinic: 1996, Q3, P14
V72.83 Other specified preoperative examination
Examination prior to chemotherapy
Other pre-procedural examination
Pre-procedural general physical examination
Excludes routine general medical examination (V70.0)
Coding Clinic: 1996, Q3, P14; 1995, Q4, P52
● **V72.84 Preoperative examination, unspecified**
Pre-procedural examination, unspecified
Coding Clinic: 1995, Q4, P52
● **V72.85 Other specified examination**
Coding Clinic: 2004, Q1, P12-13
● **V72.86 Encounter for blood typing**
● **V72.9 Unspecified examination**

● **V73 Special screening examination for viral and chlamydial diseases**
● **V73.0 Poliomyelitis**
● **V73.1 Smallpox**
● **V73.2 Measles**
● **V73.3 Rubella**
● **V73.4 Yellow fever**
● **V73.5 Other arthropod-borne viral diseases**
Dengue fever
Hemorrhagic fever
Viral encephalitis:
mosquito-borne
tick-borne
● **V73.6 Trachoma**
● **V73.8 Other specified viral and chlamydial diseases**
● **V73.81 Human papillomavirus (HPV)**
Coding Clinic: 2007, Q4, P99-101
● **V73.88 Other specified chlamydial diseases**
Coding Clinic: 2007, Q4, P124-125
● **V73.89 Other specified viral diseases**

OGCR Section I.C.1.h.
If a patient is being seen to determine his/her HIV status, use V73.89, Screening for other specified viral disease. Use V69.8, Other problems related to lifestyle, as a secondary code if an asymptomatic patient is in a known high risk group for HIV. Should a patient with signs or symptoms or illness, or a confirmed HIV related diagnosis be tested for HIV, code the signs and symptoms or the diagnosis. An additional counseling code V65.44 may be used if counseling is provided during the encounter for the test.

● **V73.9 Unspecified viral and chlamydial disease**
● **V73.98 Unspecified chlamydial disease**
● **V73.99 Unspecified viral disease**

● **V74 Special screening examination for bacterial and spirochetal diseases**
Includes diagnostic skin tests for these diseases
● **V74.0 Cholera**
● **V74.1 Pulmonary tuberculosis**
● **V74.2 Leprosy [Hansen's disease]**
● **V74.3 Diphtheria**
● **V74.4 Bacterial conjunctivitis**
● **V74.5 Venereal disease**
Screening for bacterial and spirochetal sexually transmitted diseases
Screening for sexually transmitted diseases NOS
Excludes special screening for nonbacterial sexually transmitted diseases (V73.81–V73.89, V75.4, V75.8)
Coding Clinic: 2007, Q4, P124-125
● **V74.6 Yaws**
● **V74.8 Other specified bacterial and spirochetal diseases**
Brucellosis
Leptospirosis
Plague
Tetanus
Whooping cough
● **V74.9 Unspecified bacterial and spirochetal disease**

◄ New   ◄ Revised   ~~deleted~~ Deleted   Excludes   Includes   Use additional   Code first
● Unacceptable Principal Diagnosis   ● Use Additional Digit(s)   OGCR Official Guidelines   Coding Clinic

● **V75　Special screening examination for other infectious diseases**

　● **V75.0　Rickettsial diseases**

　● **V75.1　Malaria**

　● **V75.2　Leishmaniasis**

　● **V75.3　Trypanosomiasis**
　　　　　Chagas' disease　　　Sleeping sickness

　● **V75.4　Mycotic infections**

　● **V75.5　Schistosomiasis**

　● **V75.6　Filariasis**

　● **V75.7　Intestinal helminthiasis**

　● **V75.8　Other specified parasitic infections**

　● **V75.9　Unspecified infectious disease**

● **V76　Special screening for malignant neoplasms**

　● **V76.0　Respiratory organs**

　● **V76.1　Breast**

　　● **V76.10　Breast screening, unspecified**

　　● **V76.11　Screening mammogram for high-risk patient**
　　　　　Coding Clinic: 2003, Q2, P3-5

　　● **V76.12　Other screening mammogram**
　　　　　Coding Clinic: 2009, Q4, P153; 2006, Q2, P10; Q2, P3-5

　　● **V76.19　Other screening breast examination**

　● **V76.2　Cervix**
　　　　Routine cervical Papanicolaou smear

　　　Excludes　*special screening for human papillomavirus (V73.81)*
　　　　　　that as part of a general gynecological examination (V72.31)

　● **V76.3　Bladder**

　● **V76.4　Other sites**

　　● **V76.41　Rectum**

　　● **V76.42　Oral cavity**

　　● **V76.43　Skin**

　　　V76.44　Prostate

　　● **V76.45　Testis**

　　● **V76.46　Ovary**

　　● **V76.47　Vagina**
　　　　Vaginal pap smear status-post hysterectomy for non-malignant condition

　　　Use additional code to identify acquired absence of uterus (V88.01–V88.03)

　　　Excludes　*vaginal pap smear status-post hysterectomy for malignant condition (V67.01)*

　　● **V76.49　Other sites**
　　　　　Coding Clinic: 1999, Q1, P4

　● **V76.5　Intestine**

　　● **V76.50　Intestine, unspecified**

　　● **V76.51　Colon**
　　　　Screening colonoscopy NOS ◄

　　　Excludes　*rectum (V76.41)*

　　　　Coding Clinic: 2004, Q1, P11-12; 2001, Q4, P55-56x2

　　● **V76.52　Small intestine**

　● **V76.8　Other neoplasm**

　　● **V76.81　Nervous system**

　　● **V76.89　Other neoplasm**

　● **V76.9　Unspecified**

● **V77　Special screening for endocrine, nutritional, metabolic, and immunity disorders**

　● **V77.0　Thyroid disorders**

　● **V77.1　Diabetes mellitus**

　● **V77.2　Malnutrition**

　● **V77.3　Phenylketonuria [PKU]**

　● **V77.4　Galactosemia**

　● **V77.5　Gout**

　● **V77.6　Cystic fibrosis**
　　　　Screening for mucoviscidosis

　● **V77.7　Other inborn errors of metabolism**

　● **V77.8　Obesity**

　● **V77.9　Other and unspecified endocrine, nutritional, metabolic, and immunity disorders**

　　● **V77.91　Screening for lipoid disorders**
　　　　Screening cholesterol level
　　　　Screening for hypercholesterolemia
　　　　Screening for hyperlipidemia

　　● **V77.99　Other and unspecified endocrine, nutritional, metabolic, and immunity disorders**

● **V78　Special screening for disorders of blood and blood-forming organs**

　● **V78.0　Iron deficiency anemia**

　● **V78.1　Other and unspecified deficiency anemia**

　● **V78.2　Sickle-cell disease or trait**

　● **V78.3　Other hemoglobinopathies**

　● **V78.8　Other disorders of blood and blood-forming organs**

　● **V78.9　Unspecified disorder of blood and blood-forming organs**

● **V79　Special screening for mental disorders and developmental handicaps**

　● **V79.0　Depression**

　● **V79.1　Alcoholism**

　● **V79.2　Mental retardation**

　● **V79.3　Developmental handicaps in early childhood**

　● **V79.8　Other specified mental disorders and developmental handicaps**

　● **V79.9　Unspecified mental disorder and developmental handicap**

● **V80　Special screening for neurological, eye, and ear diseases**

　● **V80.0　Neurological conditions**

　　● **V80.01　Traumatic brain injury**

　　● **V80.09　Other neurological conditions**

　● **V80.1　Glaucoma**

　● **V80.2　Other eye conditions**
　　　　Screening for:
　　　　　cataract
　　　　　congenital anomaly of eye
　　　　　senile macular lesions

　　　Excludes　*general vision examination (V72.0)*

　● **V80.3　Ear diseases**

　　　Excludes　*general hearing examination (V72.11–V72.19)*

● **V81　Special screening for cardiovascular, respiratory, and genitourinary diseases**

　● **V81.0　Ischemic heart disease**

　● **V81.1　Hypertension**

V01-V91

◄ New　◄▥ Revised　~~deleted~~ Deleted　[Excludes]　[Includes]　Use additional　Code first
● Unacceptable Principal Diagnosis　● Use Additional Digit(s)　OGCR Official Guidelines　Coding Clinic

1047

- V81.2 **Other and unspecified cardiovascular conditions**
- V81.3 **Chronic bronchitis and emphysema**
- V81.4 **Other and unspecified respiratory conditions**

Excludes	*screening for:*
	lung neoplasm (V76.0)
	pulmonary tuberculosis (V74.1)

- V81.5 **Nephropathy**
  Screening for asymptomatic bacteriuria
- V81.6 **Other and unspecified genitourinary conditions**

- V82 **Special screening for other conditions**
  - V82.0 **Skin conditions**
  - V82.1 **Rheumatoid arthritis**
  - V82.2 **Other rheumatic disorders**
  - V82.3 **Congenital dislocation of hip**
  - V82.4 **Maternal postnatal screening for chromosomal anomalies**

Excludes	*antenatal screening by amniocentesis (V28.0)*

  - V82.5 **Chemical poisoning and other contamination**
    Screening for:
    heavy metal poisoning
    ingestion of radioactive substance
    poisoning from contaminated water supply
    radiation exposure
  - V82.6 **Multiphasic screening**
  - V82.7 **Genetic screening**

Excludes	*genetic testing for procreative management (V26.31–V26.39)*

    Coding Clinic: 2006, Q4, P118
    - V82.71 **Screening for genetic disease carrier status**
    - V82.79 **Other genetic screening**
  - V82.8 **Other specified conditions**
    - V82.81 **Osteoporosis**

      Use additional code to identify:
      hormone replacement therapy
      (postmenopausal) status
      (V07.4)
      postmenopausal (natural) status
      (V49.81)
      Coding Clinic: 2000, Q4, P53-54
    - V82.89 **Other specified conditions**
  - V82.9 **Unspecified condition**

GENETICS (V83–V84)

OGCR Section I.C.18.d.3
Genetic carrier status indicates that a person carries a gene, associated with a particular disease, which may be passed to offspring who may develop that disease. The person does not have the disease and is not at risk of developing the disease.

- V83 **Genetic carrier status**
  - V83.0 **Hemophilia A carrier**
    - V83.01 **Asymptomatic hemophilia A carrier**
    - V83.02 **Symptomatic hemophilia A carrier**
  - V83.8 **Other genetic carrier status**
    - V83.81 **Cystic fibrosis gene carrier**
    - V83.89 **Other genetic carrier status**

OGCR Section I.C.18.d.3
Genetic susceptibility indicates that a person has a gene that increases the risk of that person developing the disease. Codes from category V84, Genetic susceptibility to disease, should not be used as principal or first-listed codes.

- V84 **Genetic susceptibility to disease**

Includes	Confirmed abnormal gene

  Use additional code, if applicable, for any associated family history of the disease (V16–V19)
  - V84.0 **Genetic susceptibility to malignant neoplasm**

    Code first, if applicable, any current malignant neoplasms (140.0–195.8, 200.0–208.9, 230.0–234.9)

    Use additional code, if applicable, for any personal history of malignant neoplasm (V10.0–V10.9)
    - V84.01 **Genetic susceptibility to malignant neoplasm of breast**
      Coding Clinic: 2004, Q4, P106-107
    - V84.02 **Genetic susceptibility to malignant neoplasm of ovary**
    - V84.03 **Genetic susceptibility to malignant neoplasm of prostate**
    - V84.04 **Genetic susceptibility to malignant neoplasm of endometrium**
    - V84.09 **Genetic susceptibility to other malignant neoplasm**
  - V84.8 **Genetic susceptibility to other disease**
    - V84.81 **Genetic susceptibility to multiple endocrine neoplasia [MEN]**
      Coding Clinic: 2007, Q4, P99-101
    - V84.89 **Genetic susceptibility to other disease**

BODY MASS INDEX (V85)

- V85 **Body mass index (BMI)**
  Kilograms per meters squared
  Note: BMI adult codes are for use for persons over 20 years old
  Coding Clinic: 2008, Q4, P191; 2005, Q4, P94-100
  - V85.0 **Body Mass Index less than 19, adult**
  - V85.1 **Body Mass Index between 19–24, adult**
  - V85.2 **Body Mass Index between 25–29, adult**
    - V85.21 **Body Mass Index 25.0–25.9, adult**
    - V85.22 **Body Mass Index 26.0–26.9, adult**
    - V85.23 **Body Mass Index 27.0–27.9, adult**
    - V85.24 **Body Mass Index 28.0–28.9, adult**
    - V85.25 **Body Mass Index 29.0–29.9, adult**
  - V85.3 **Body Mass Index between 30–39, adult**
    - V85.30 **Body Mass Index 30.0–30.9, adult**
    - V85.31 **Body Mass Index 31.0–31.9, adult**
    - V85.32 **Body Mass Index 32.0–32.9, adult**
    - V85.33 **Body Mass Index 33.0–33.9, adult**
    - V85.34 **Body Mass Index 34.0–34.9, adult**
    - V85.35 **Body Mass Index 35.0–35.9, adult**
    - V85.36 **Body Mass Index 36.0–36.9, adult**
    - V85.37 **Body Mass Index 37.0–37.9, adult**
    - V85.38 **Body Mass Index 38.0–38.9, adult**
    - V85.39 **Body Mass Index 39.0–39.9, adult**

V01-V91

● V85.4 **Body Mass Index 40 and over, adult** ◀═

   ● **V85.41 Body Mass Index 40.0-44.9, adult** ◀

   ● **V85.42 Body Mass Index 45.0-49.9, adult** ◀

   ● **V85.43 Body Mass Index 50.0-59.9, adult** ◀

   ● **V85.44 Body Mass Index 60.0-69.9, adult** ◀

   ● **V85.45 Body Mass Index 70 and over, adult** ◀

● V85.5 **Body Mass Index, pediatric**

   Note: BMI pediatric codes are for use for persons age 2–20 years old. These percentiles are based on the growth charts published by the Centers for Disease Control and Prevention (CDC)

   ● **V85.51 Body Mass Index, pediatric, less than 5th percentile for age**

   ● **V85.52 Body Mass Index, pediatric, 5th percentile to less than 85th percentile for age**

   ● **V85.53 Body Mass Index, pediatric, 85th percentile to less than 95th percentile for age**

   ● **V85.54 Body Mass Index, pediatric, greater than or equal to 95th percentile for age**

ESTROGEN RECEPTOR STATUS (V86)

● V86 **Estrogen receptor status**

   Code first malignant neoplasm of breast (174.0–174.9, 175.0–175.9)

   ● **V86.0 Estrogen receptor positive status [ER+]**

   ● **V86.1 Estrogen receptor negative status [ER-]**

OTHER SPECIFIED PERSONAL EXPOSURES AND HISTORY PRESENTING HAZARDS TO HEALTH (V87)

● V87 **Other specified personal exposures and history presenting hazards to health**

   ● **V87.0 Contact with and (suspected) exposure to hazardous metals**

      | Excludes | *exposure to lead (V15.86)* |
                    toxic effect of metals (984.0-985.9)

     ● **V87.01 Arsenic**

     ● **V87.09 Other hazardous metals**
         Chromium compounds
         Nickel dust

   ● **V87.1 Contact with and (suspected) exposure to hazardous aromatic compounds**

      | Excludes | *toxic effects of aromatic compounds (982.0, 983.0)* |

     ● **V87.11 Aromatic amines**

     ● **V87.12 Benzene**

     ● **V87.19 Other hazardous aromatic compounds**
         Aromatic dyes NOS
         Polycyclic aromatic hydrocarbons

   ● **V87.2 Contact with and (suspected) exposure to other potentially hazardous chemicals**
       Dyes NOS

      | Excludes | *exposure to asbestos (V15.84)* |
                    toxic effect of chemicals (980–989)

● **V87.3 Contact with and (suspected) exposure to other potentially hazardous substances**

    | Excludes | *contact with and (suspected) exposure to potentially hazardous body fluids (V15.85)* |
                   personal history of retained foreign body fully removed (V15.53) ◀
                   toxic effect of substances (980–989)

   ● **V87.31 Exposure to mold**

   ● **V87.32 Contact with and (suspected) exposure to algae bloom**

   ● **V87.39 Contact with and (suspected) exposure to other potentially hazardous substances**

● **V87.4 Personal history of drug therapy**

    | Excludes | *long-term (current) drug use (V58.61-V58.69)* |

   ● **V87.41 Personal history of antineoplastic chemotherapy**

   ● **V87.42 Personal history of monoclonal drug therapy**

   ● **V87.43 Personal history of estrogen therapy**

   ● **V87.44 Personal history of inhaled steroid therapy**

   ● **V87.45 Personal history of systemic steroid therapy**
         Personal history of steroid therapy NOS

   ● **V87.46 Personal history of immunosuppression therapy**

      | Excludes | *personal history of steroid therapy (V87.44, V87.45)* |

   ● **V87.49 Personal history of other drug therapy**

ACQUIRED ABSENCE OF OTHER ORGANS AND TISSUE (V88)

● V88 **Acquired absence of other organs and tissue**

   ● V88.0 **Acquired absence of cervix and uterus**

     ● **V88.01 Acquired absence of both cervix and uterus**
         Acquired absence of uterus NOS
         Status post total hysterectomy

     ● **V88.02 Acquired absence of uterus with remaining cervical stump**
         Status post partial hysterectomy with remaining cervical stump

     ● **V88.03 Acquired absence of cervix with remaining uterus**

   ● V88.1 **Acquired absence of pancreas** ◀

     Use additional code to identify any associated: ◀
     insulin use (V58.67) ◀
     secondary diabetes mellitus (249.00-249.91) ◀

     V88.11 Acquired total absence of pancreas ◀
        Acquired absence of pancreas NOS ◀

     V88.12 Acquired partial absence of pancreas ◀

V01-V91

◀ New   ◀═ Revised   ~~deleted~~ Deleted | Excludes | Includes   Use additional   Code first
● Unacceptable Principal Diagnosis   ● Use Additional Digit(s)   OGCR Official Guidelines   Coding Clinic

OTHER SUSPECTED CONDITIONS NOT FOUND (V89)

● **V89 Other suspected conditions not found**

  ● **V89.0 Suspected maternal and fetal conditions not found**

| Excludes | *known or suspected fetal anomalies affecting management of mother, not ruled out (655.00 655.93, 656.00–656.93, 657.00–657.03, 658.00–658.93) newborn and perinatal conditions – code to condition* |

    ● **V89.01 Suspected problem with amniotic cavity and membrane not found**
Suspected oligohydramnios not found
Suspected polyhydramnios not found

    ● **V89.02 Suspected placental problem not found**

    ● **V89.03 Suspected fetal anomaly not found**

    ● **V89.04 Suspected problem with fetal growth not found**

    ● **V89.05 Suspected cervical shortening not found**

    ● **V89.09 Other suspected maternal and fetal condition not found**

RETAINED FOREIGN BODY (V90) ◄

● **V90 Retained foreign body** ◄
Embedded fragment (status) ◄
Embedded splinter (status) ◄
Retained foreign body status ◄

| Excludes | *artificial joint prosthesis status (V43.60-V43.69) ◄ foreign body accidentally left during a procedure (998.4) ◄ foreign body entering through orifice (930.0-939.9) ◄ in situ cardiac devices (V45.00-V45.09) ◄ organ or tissue replaced by other means (V43.0-V43.89) ◄ organ or tissue replaced by transplant (V42.0-V42.9) ◄ personal history of retained foreign body removed (V15.53) ◄ superficial foreign body (splinter) (categories 910-917 and 919 with 4th character 6 or 7, 918.0) ◄* |

  ● **V90.0 Retained radioactive fragment** ◄

    V90.01 Retained depleted uranium fragments ◄

    V90.09 Other retained radioactive fragments ◄
Other retained depleted isotope fragments ◄
Retained nontherapeutic radioactive fragments ◄

  ● **V90.1 Retained metal fragments** ◄

| Excludes | *retained radioactive metal fragments (V90.01-V90.09) ◄* |

    V90.10 Retained metal fragments, unspecified ◄
Retained metal fragment NOS ◄

    V90.11 Retained magnetic metal fragments ◄

    V90.12 Retained nonmagnetic metal fragments ◄

  V90.2 Retained plastic fragments ◄
Acrylics fragments ◄
Diethylhexylphthalates fragments ◄
Isocyanate fragments ◄

● **V90.3 Retained organic fragments** ◄

  V90.31 Retained animal quills or spines ◄

  V90.32 Retained tooth ◄

  V90.33 Retained wood fragments ◄

  V90.39 Other retained organic fragments ◄

● **V90.8 Other specified retained foreign body** ◄

  V90.81 Retained glass fragments ◄

  V90.83 Retained stone or crystalline fragments ◄
Retained concrete or cement fragments ◄

  V90.89 Other specified retained foreign body ◄

  V90.9 Retained foreign body, unspecified material ◄

MULTIPLE GESTATION PLACENTA STATUS (V91) ◄

● **V91 Multiple gestation placenta status** ◄
Code first multiple gestation (651.0-651.9) ◄

  ● **V91.0 Twin gestation placenta status** ◄

    V91.00 Twin gestation, unspecified number of placenta, unspecified number of amniotic sacs ◄

    V91.01 Twin gestation, monochorionic/monoamniotic (one placenta, one amniotic sac) ◄

    V91.02 Twin gestation, monochorionic/diamniotic (one placenta, two amniotic sacs) ◄

    V91.03 Twin gestation, dichorionic/diamniotic (two placentae, two amniotic sacs) ◄

    V91.09 Twin gestation, unable to determine number of placenta and number of amniotic sacs ◄

  ● **V91.1 Triplet gestation placenta status** ◄

    V91.10 Triplet gestation, unspecified number of placenta and unspecified number of amniotic sacs ◄

    V91.11 Triplet gestation, with two or more monochorionic fetuses ◄

    V91.12 Triplet gestation, with two or more monoamniotic fetuses ◄

    V91.19 Triplet gestation, unable to determine number of placenta and number of amniotic sacs ◄

  ● **V91.2 Quadruplet gestation placenta status** ◄

    V91.20 Quadruplet gestation, unspecified number of placenta and unspecified number of amniotic sacs ◄

    V91.21 Quadruplet gestation, with two or more monochorionic fetuses ◄

    V91.22 Quadruplet gestation, with two or more monoamniotic fetuses ◄

    V91.29 Quadruplet gestation, unable to determine number of placenta and number of amniotic sacs ◄

  ● **V91.9 Other specified multiple gestation placenta status** ◄
Placenta status for multiple gestations greater than quadruplets ◄

    V91.90 Other specified multiple gestation, unspecified number of placenta and unspecified number of amniotic sacs ◄

    V91.91 Other specified multiple gestation, with two or more monochorionic fetuses ◄

    V91.92 Other specified multiple gestation, with two or more monoamniotic fetuses ◄

    V91.99 Other specified multiple gestation, unable to determine number of placenta and number of amniotic sacs ◄

◄ New   ◄▥ Revised   ~~deleted~~ Deleted   Excludes   Includes   Use additional   Code first
● Unacceptable Principal Diagnosis   ● Use Additional Digit(s)   OGCR Official Guidelines   Coding Clinic

Medicare Code Edit: E-codes are ICD-9-CM codes beginning with the letter E. They describe the circumstance causing an injury, not the nature of the injury, and therefore should not be used as a principal diagnosis.

SUPPLEMENTARY CLASSIFICATION OF EXTERNAL CAUSES OF INJURY AND POISONING (E000–E999)

This section is provided to permit the classification of environmental events, circumstances, and conditions as the cause of injury, poisoning, and other adverse effects. Where a code from this section is applicable, it is intended that it shall be used in addition to a code from one of the main chapters of ICD-9-CM, indicating the nature of the condition. Certain other conditions which may be stated to be due to external causes are classified in Chapters 1 to 16 of ICD-9-CM. For these, the "E" code classification should be used as an additional code for more detailed analysis.

Machinery accidents [other than those connected with transport] are classifiable to category E919, in which the fourth digit allows a broad classification of the type of machinery involved.

Categories for "late effects" of accidents and other external causes are to be found at E929, E959, E969, E977, E989, and E999.

(a) A transport accident (E800–E848) is any accident involving a device designed primarily for, or being used at the time primarily for, conveying persons or goods from one place to another.

Includes | accidents involving:
aircraft and spacecraft (E840–E845)
watercraft (E830–E838)
motor vehicle (E810–E825)
railway (E800–E807)
other road vehicles (E826–E829)

In classifying accidents which involve more than one kind of transport, the above order of precedence of transport accidents should be used.

Accidents involving agricultural and construction machines, such as tractors, cranes, and bulldozers, are regarded as transport accidents only when these vehicles are under their own power on a highway [otherwise the vehicles are regarded as machinery]. Vehicles which can travel on land or water, such as hovercraft and other amphibious vehicles, are regarded as watercraft when on the water, as motor vehicles when on the highway, and as off-road motor vehicles when on land, but off the highway.

Excludes | *accidents:*
in sports which involve the use of transport but where the transport vehicle itself was not involved in the accident
involving vehicles which are part of industrial equipment used entirely on industrial premises
occurring during transportation but unrelated to the hazards associated with the means of transportation [e.g., injuries received in a fight on board ship; transport vehicle involved in a cataclysm such as an earthquake]
to persons engaged in the maintenance or repair of transport equipment or vehicle not in motion, unless injured by another vehicle in motion

(b) A railway accident is a transport accident involving a railway train or other railway vehicle operated on rails, whether in motion or not.

Excludes | *accidents:*
in repair shops
in roundhouse or on turntable
on railway premises but not involving a train or other railway vehicle

(c) A railway train or railway vehicle is any device with or without cars coupled to it, designed for traffic on a railway.

Includes | interurban:
electric car (operated chiefly on its own right-of-way, not open to other traffic)
streetcar (operated chiefly on its own right-of-way, not open to other traffic)
railway train, any power [diesel] [electric] [steam]
funicular
monorail or two-rail
subterranean or elevated
other vehicle designed to run on a railway track

Excludes | *interurban electric cars [streetcars] specified to be operating on a right-of-way that forms part of the public street or highway [definition (n)]*

(d) A railway or railroad is a right-of-way designed for traffic on rails, which is used by carriages or wagons transporting passengers or freight, and by other rolling stock, and which is not open to other public vehicular traffic

(e) A motor vehicle accident is a transport accident involving a motor vehicle. It is defined as a motor vehicle traffic accident or as a motor vehicle nontraffic accident according to whether the accident occurs on a public highway or elsewhere.

Excludes | *injury or damage due to cataclysm*
injury or damage while a motor vehicle, not under its own power, is being loaded on, or unloaded from, another conveyance

(f) A motor vehicle traffic accident is any motor vehicle accident occurring on a public highway [i.e., originating, terminating, or involving a vehicle partially on the highway]. A motor vehicle accident is assumed to have occurred on the highway unless another place is specified, except in the case of accidents involving only off-road motor vehicles which are classified as nontraffic accidents unless the contrary is stated.

(g) A motor vehicle nontraffic accident is any motor vehicle accident which occurs entirely in any place other than a public highway.

(h) A public highway [trafficway] or street is the entire width between property lines [or other boundary lines] of every way or place, of which any part is open to the use of the public for purposes of vehicular traffic as a matter of right or custom. A roadway is that part of the public highway designed, improved, and ordinarily used, for vehicular travel.

Includes | approaches (public) to:
docks
public building
station

Excludes | *driveway (private)*
parking lot
ramp
roads in:
airfield
farm
industrial premises
mine
private grounds
quarry

E000–E999

(i) A motor vehicle is any mechanically or electrically powered device, not operated on rails, upon which any person or property may be transported or drawn upon a highway. Any object such as a trailer, coaster, sled, or wagon being towed by a motor vehicle is considered a part of the motor vehicle.

Includes
automobile [any type]
bus
construction machinery, farm and industrial machinery, steam roller, tractor, army tank, highway grader, or similar vehicle on wheels or treads, while in transport under own power
fire engine (motorized)
motorcycle
motorized bicycle [moped] or scooter
trolley bus not operating on rails
truck
van

Excludes
devices used solely to move persons or materials within the confines of a building and its premises, such as:
building elevator
coal car in mine
electric baggage or mail truck used solely within a railroad station
electric truck used solely within an industrial plant
moving overhead crane

(j) A motorcycle is a two-wheeled motor vehicle having one or two riding saddles and sometimes having a third wheel for the support of a sidecar. The sidecar is considered part of the motorcycle.

Includes
motorized:
bicycle [moped]
scooter
tricycle

(k) An off-road motor vehicle is a motor vehicle of special design, to enable it to negotiate rough or soft terrain or snow. Examples of special design are high construction, special wheels and tires, driven by treads, or support on a cushion of air.

Includes
all terrain vehicle [ATV]
army tank
hovercraft, on land or swamp
snowmobile

(l) A driver of a motor vehicle is the occupant of the motor vehicle operating it or intending to operate it. A motorcyclist is the driver of a motorcycle. Other authorized occupants of a motor vehicle are passengers.

(m) An other road vehicle is any device, except a motor vehicle, in, on, or by which any person or property may be transported on a highway.

Includes
animal carrying a person or goods
animal-drawn vehicle
animal harnessed to conveyance
bicycle [pedal cycle]
streetcar
tricycle (pedal)

Excludes *pedestrian conveyance [definition (q)]*

(n) A streetcar is a device designed and used primarily for transporting persons within a municipality, running on rails, usually subject to normal traffic control signals, and operated principally on a right-of-way that forms part of the traffic way. A trailer being towed by a streetcar is considered a part of the streetcar.

Includes
interurban or intraurban electric or streetcar, when specified to be operating on a street or public highway
tram (car)
trolley (car)

(o) A pedal cycle is any road transport vehicle operated solely by pedals.

Includes
bicycle
pedal cycle
tricycle

Excludes *motorized bicycle [definition (i)]*

(p) A pedal cyclist is any person riding on a pedal cycle or in a sidecar attached to such a vehicle.

(q) A pedestrian conveyance is any human powered device by which a pedestrian may move other than by walking or by which a walking person may move another pedestrian.

Includes
baby carriage
coaster wagon
heelies
ice skates
motorized mobility scooter ◀
perambulator
pushcart
pushchair
roller skates
scooter
skateboard
skis
sled
wheelchair (electric) ◀▥
wheelies

(r) A pedestrian is any person involved in an accident who was not at the time of the accident riding in or on a motor vehicle, railroad train, streetcar, animal-drawn or other vehicle, or on a bicycle or animal.

Includes
person:
changing tire of vehicle
in or operating a pedestrian conveyance
making adjustment to motor of vehicle
on foot

(s) A watercraft is any device for transporting passengers or goods on the water.

(t) A small boat is any watercraft propelled by paddle, oars, or small motor, with a passenger capacity of less than ten.

Includes
boat NOS
canoe
coble
dinghy
punt
raft
rowboat
rowing shell
scull
skiff
small motorboat

Excludes
barge
lifeboat (used after abandoning ship)
raft (anchored) being used as a diving platform
yacht

(u) An aircraft is any device for transporting passengers or goods in the air.

Includes
airplane [any type]
balloon
bomber
dirigible
glider (hang)
military aircraft
parachute

(v) A commercial transport aircraft is any device for collective passenger or freight transportation by air, whether run on commercial lines for profit or by government authorities, with the exception of military craft.

◀ New ◀▥ Revised ~~deleted~~ Deleted Excludes Includes Use additional Code first Omit code
● Unacceptable Principal Diagnosis ● Use Additional Digit(s) OGCR Official Guidelines Coding Clinic

E000-E999

EXTERNAL CAUSE STATUS (E000)

Note: A code from category E000 should be used in conjunction with the external cause code(s) assigned to a record to indicate the status of the person at the time the event occurred. A single code from category E000 should be assigned for an encounter.

● **E000 External cause status**

● **E000.0 Civilian activity done for income or pay**
Civilian activity done for financial or other compensation

> **Excludes** *military activity (E000.1)*

> Coding Clinic: 2009, Q4, P130

● **E000.1 Military activity**

> **Excludes** *activity of off duty military personnel (E000.8)*

E000.2 Volunteer activity ◄

> **Excludes** *activity of child or other family member assisting in compensated work of other family member (E000.8)* ◄

● **E000.8 Other external cause status**
Activity NEC
Activity of child or other family member assisting in compensated work of other family member ◄
Hobby not done for income
Leisure activity
Off-duty activity of military personnel
Recreation or sport not for income or while a student
Student activity
~~Volunteer activity~~

> **Excludes** *civilian activity done for income or compensation (E000.0)*
> *military activity (E000.1)*

> Coding Clinic: 2009, Q4, P130

● **E000.9 Unspecified external cause status**

ACTIVITY (E001-E030)

Note: Categories E001 to E030 are provided for use to indicate the activity of the person seeking healthcare for an injury or health condition, such as a heart attack while shoveling snow, which resulted from, or was contributed to, by the activity. These codes are appropriate for use for both acute injuries, such as those from chapter 17, and conditions that are due to the long-term, cumulative effects of an activity, such as those from chapter 13. They are also appropriate for use with external cause codes for cause and intent if identifying the activity provides additional information on the event.

These codes should be used in conjunction with other external cause codes for external cause status (E000) and place of occurrence (E849).

This section contains the following broad activity categories:

E001 Activities involving walking and running

E002 Activities involving water and water craft

E003 Activities involving ice and snow

E004 Activities involving climbing, rappelling, and jumping off

E005 Activities involving dancing and other rhythmic movement

E006 Activities involving other sports and athletics played individually

E007 Activities involving other sports and athletics played as a team or group

E008 Activities involving other specified sports and athletics

E009 Activity involving other cardiorespiratory exercise

E010 Activity involving other muscle strengthening exercises

E011 Activities involving computer technology and electronic devices

E012 Activities involving arts and handcrafts

E013 Activities involving personal hygiene and household maintenance

E014 Activities involving person providing caregiving

E015 Activities involving food preparation, cooking and grilling

E016 Activities involving property and land maintenance, building and construction

E017 Activities involving roller coasters and other types of external motion

E018 Activities involving playing musical instrument

E019 Activities involving animal care

E029 Other activity

E030 Unspecified activity

● **E001 Activities involving walking and running**

> **Excludes** *walking an animal (E019.0)*
> *walking or running on a treadmill (E009.0)*

● **E001.0 Walking, marching and hiking**
Walking, marching and hiking on level or elevated terrain

> **Excludes** *mountain climbing (E004.0)*

> Coding Clinic: 2009, Q4, P141

● **E001.1 Running**

● **E002 Activities involving water and water craft**

> **Excludes** *activities involving ice (E003.0-E003.9)*
> *boating and other watercraft transport accidents (E830-E838)*

● **E002.0 Swimming**

● **E002.1 Springboard and platform diving**

● **E002.2 Water polo**

● **E002.3 Water aerobics and water exercise**

● **E002.4 Underwater diving and snorkeling**
SCUBA diving

● **E002.5 Rowing, canoeing, kayaking, rafting and tubing**
Canoeing, kayaking, rafting and tubing in calm and turbulent water

● **E002.6 Water skiing and wake boarding**

● **E002.7 Surfing, windsurfing and boogie boarding**

● **E002.8 Water sliding**

● **E002.9 Other activity involving water and watercraft**
Activity involving water NOS
Parasailing
Water survival training and testing

E000-E999

● E003   **Activities involving ice and snow**
> **Excludes**   *shoveling ice and snow (E016.0)*

● E003.0   **Ice skating**
Figure skating (singles) (pairs)
Ice dancing
> **Excludes**   *ice hockey (E003.1)*

● E003.1   **Ice hockey**

● E003.2   **Snow (alpine) (downhill) skiing, snow boarding, sledding, tobogganing and snow tubing**
> **Excludes**   *cross country skiing (E003.3)*

● E003.3   **Cross country skiing**
Nordic skiing

● E003.9   **Other activity involving ice and snow**
Activity involving ice and snow NOS

● E004   **Activities involving climbing, rappelling and jumping off**
> **Excludes**   *hiking on level or elevated terrain (E001.0)*
> *jumping rope (E006.5)*
> *sky diving (E840-E844)*
> *trampoline jumping (E005.3)*

● E004.0   **Mountain climbing, rock climbing and wall climbing**

● E004.1   **Rappelling**

● E004.2   **BASE jumping**
Building, Antenna, Span, Earth jumping

● E004.3   **Bungee jumping**

● E004.4   **Hang gliding**

● E004.9   **Other activity involving climbing, rappelling and jumping off**

● E005   **Activities involving dancing and other rhythmic movement**
> **Excludes**   *martial arts (E008.4)*

● E005.0   **Dancing**

● E005.1   **Yoga**

● E005.2   **Gymnastics**
Rhythmic gymnastics
> **Excludes**   *trampoline (E005.3)*

● E005.3   **Trampoline**

● E005.4   **Cheerleading**

● E005.9   **Other activity involving dancing and other rhythmic movements**

● E006   **Activities involving other sports and athletics played individually**
> **Excludes**   *dancing (E005.0)*
> *gymnastics (E005.2)*
> *trampoline (E005.3)*
> *yoga (E005.1)*

● E006.0   **Roller skating (inline) and skateboarding**

● E006.1   **Horseback riding**

● E006.2   **Golf**

● E006.3   **Bowling**

● E006.4   **Bike riding**
> **Excludes**   *transport accident involving bike riding (E800-E829)*

● E006.5   **Jumping rope**

● E006.6   **Non-running track and field events**
> **Excludes**   *running (any form) (E001.1)*

● E006.9   **Other activity involving other sports and athletics played individually**
> **Excludes**   *activities involving climbing, rappelling, and jumping (E004.0-E004.9)*
> *activities involving ice and snow (E003.0-E003.9)*
> *activities involving walking and running (E001.0-E001.9)*
> *activities involving water and watercraft (E002.0-E002.9)*

● E007   **Activities involving other sports and athletics played as a team or group**
> **Excludes**   *ice hockey (E003.1)*
> *water polo (E002.2)*

● E007.0   **American tackle football**
Football NOS

● E007.1   **American flag or touch football**

● E007.2   **Rugby**

● E007.3   **Baseball**
Softball

● E007.4   **Lacrosse and field hockey**

● E007.5   **Soccer**

● E007.6   **Basketball**

● E007.7   **Volleyball (beach) (court)**

● E007.8   **Physical games generally associated with school recess, summer camp and children**
Capture the flag
Dodge ball
Four square
Kickball

● E007.9   **Other activity involving other sports and athletics played as a team or group**
Cricket

● E008   **Activities involving other specified sports and athletics**

● E008.0   **Boxing**

● E008.1   **Wrestling**

● E008.2   **Racquet and hand sports**
Handball
Racquetball
Squash
Tennis

● E008.3   **Frisbee**
Ultimate frisbee

● E008.4   **Martial arts**
Combatives

● E008.9   **Other specified sports and athletics activity**
> **Excludes**   *sports and athletics activities specified in categories E001-E007*

● E009   **Activity involving other cardiorespiratory exercise**
Activity involving physical training

● E009.0   **Exercise machines primarily for cardiorespiratory conditioning**
Elliptical and stepper machines
Stationary bike
Treadmill

● E009.1   **Calisthenics**
Jumping jacks
Warm up and cool down

● E009.2   **Aerobic and step exercise**

● E009.3   **Circuit training**

● E009.4   **Obstacle course**
Challenge course
Confidence course

● E009.5 **Grass drills**
    Guerilla drills

● E009.9 **Other activity involving other cardiorespiratory exercise**
    Excludes *activities involving cardiorespiratory exercise specified in categories E001-E008*

● E010 **Activity involving other muscle strengthening exercises**

  ● E010.0 **Exercise machines primarily for muscle strengthening**

  ● E010.1 **Push-ups, pull-ups, sit-ups**

  ● E010.2 **Free weights**
    Barbells
    Dumbbells

  ● E010.3 **Pilates**

  ● E010.9 **Other activity involving other muscle strengthening exercises**
    Excludes *activities involving muscle strengthening specified in categories E001-E009*

● E011 **Activities involving computer technology and electronic devices**
  Excludes *electronic musical keyboard or instruments (E018.0)*

  ● E011.0 **Computer keyboarding**
    Electronic game playing using keyboard or other stationary device

  ● E011.1 **Hand held interactive electronic device**
    Cellular telephone and communication device
    Electronic game playing using interactive device
    Excludes *electronic game playing using keyboard or other stationary device (E011.0)*

  ● E011.9 **Other activity involving computer technology and electronic devices**

● E012 **Activities involving arts and handcrafts**
  Excludes *activities involving playing musical instrument (E018.0-E018.3)*

  ● E012.0 **Knitting and crocheting**

  ● E012.1 **Sewing**

  ● E012.2 **Furniture building and finishing**
    Furniture repair

  ● E012.9 **Activity involving other arts and handcrafts**

● E013 **Activities involving personal hygiene and household maintenance**
  Excludes *activities involving cooking and grilling (E015.0-E015.9)*
    activities involving property and land maintenance, building and construction (E016.0-E016.9)
    activity involving persons providing caregiving (E014.0-E014.9)
    dishwashing (E015.0)
    food preparation (E015.0)
    gardening (E016.1)

  ● E013.0 **Personal bathing and showering**

  ● E013.1 **Laundry**

  ● E013.2 **Vacuuming**

  ● E013.3 **Ironing**

● E013.4 **Floor mopping and cleaning**

● E013.5 **Residential relocation**
    Packing up and unpacking involved in moving to a new residence

● E013.8 **Other personal hygiene activity**

● E013.9 **Other household maintenance**

● E014 **Activities involving person providing caregiving**

  ● E014.0 **Caregiving involving bathing**

  ● E014.1 **Caregiving involving lifting**

  ● E014.9 **Other activity involving person providing caregiving**

● E015 **Activities involving food preparation, cooking and grilling**

  ● E015.0 **Food preparation and clean up**
    Dishwashing

  ● E015.1 **Grilling and smoking food**

  ● E015.2 **Cooking and baking**
    Use of stove, oven and microwave oven

  ● E015.9 **Other activity involving cooking and grilling**

● E016 **Activities involving property and land maintenance, building and construction**

  ● E016.0 **Digging, shoveling and raking**
    Dirt digging
    Raking leaves
    Snow shoveling
    Coding Clinic: 2009, Q4, P141

  ● E016.1 **Gardening and landscaping**
    Pruning, trimming shrubs, weeding

  ● E016.2 **Building and construction**

  ● E016.9 **Other activity involving property and land maintenance, building and construction**

● E017 **Activities involving roller coasters and other types of external motion**

  ● E017.0 **Roller coaster riding** ◀◀

  ● E017.9 **Other activity involving external motion**

● E018 **Activities involving playing musical instrument**
  Activity involving playing electric musical instrument

  ● E018.0 **Piano playing**
    Musical keyboard (electronic) playing

  ● E018.1 **Drum and other percussion instrument playing**

  ● E018.2 **String instrument playing**

  ● E018.3 **Wind and brass instrument playing**

● E019 **Activities involving animal care**
  Excludes *horseback riding (E006.1)*

  ● E019.0 **Walking an animal**

  ● E019.1 **Milking an animal**

  ● E019.2 **Grooming and shearing an animal**

  ● E019.9 **Other activity involving animal care**

● E029 **Other activity**

  ● E029.0 **Refereeing a sports activity**

  ● E029.1 **Spectator at an event**

  ● E029.2 **Rough housing and horseplay**

  ● E029.9 **Other activity**

E030 **Unspecified activity**

E000-E999

◀ New   ◀◀ Revised   ~~deleted~~ Deleted   Excludes   Includes   Use additional   Code first   Omit code
● Unacceptable Principal Diagnosis   ● Use Additional Digit(s)   OGCR Official Guidelines   Coding Clinic

TRANSPORT ACCIDENTS (E800-E848)

Definitions and examples related to transport accidents

(a) A transport accident (E800-E848) is any accident involving a device designed primarily for, or being used at the time primarily for, conveying persons or goods from one place to another.

RAILWAY ACCIDENTS (E800-E807)

Note: For definitions of railway accident and related terms see definitions (a) to (d).

Excludes *accidents involving railway train and:*
aircraft (E840.0-E845.9)
motor vehicle (E810.0-E825.9)
watercraft (E830.0-E838.9)

The following fourth-digit subdivisions are for use with categories E800-E807 to identify the injured person:

> **0 Railway employee**
> Any person who by virtue of his employment in connection with a railway, whether by the railway company or not, is at increased risk of involvement in a railway accident, such as:
> catering staff of train
> driver
> guard
> porter
> postal staff on train
> railway fireman
> shunter
> sleeping car attendant
> **1 Passenger on railway**
> Any authorized person traveling on a train, except a railway employee.
>
> > **Excludes** *intending passenger waiting at station (8)*
> > *unauthorized rider on railway vehicle (8)*
>
> **2 Pedestrian**
> See definition (r)
> **3 Pedal cyclist**
> See definition (p)
> **8 Other specified person**
> Intending passenger or bystander waiting at station
> Unauthorized rider on railway vehicle
> **9 Unspecified person**

● ● **E800 Railway accident involving collision with rolling stock**

Requires fourth digit. See beginning of section E800-E845 for codes and definitions.

Includes collision between railway trains or railway vehicles, any kind
collision NOS on railway
derailment with antecedent collision with rolling stock or NOS

● ● **E801 Railway accident involving collision with other object**

Requires fourth digit. See beginning of section E800-E845 for codes and definitions.

Includes collision of railway train with:
buffers
fallen tree on railway
gates
platform
rock on railway
streetcar
other nonmotor vehicle
other object

Excludes *collision with:*
aircraft (E840.0-E842.9)
motor vehicle (E810.0-E810.9,
E820.0-E822.9)

● ● **E802 Railway accident involving derailment without antecedent collision**

Requires fourth digit. See beginning of section E800-E845 for codes and definitions.

● ● **E803 Railway accident involving explosion, fire, or burning**

Requires fourth digit. See beginning of section E800-E845 for codes and definitions.

Excludes *explosion or fire, with antecedent derailment (E802.0-E802.9)*
explosion or fire, with mention of antecedent collision (E800.0-E801.9)

● ● **E804 Fall in, on, or from railway train**

Requires fourth digit. See beginning of section E800-E845 for codes and definitions.

Includes fall while alighting from or boarding railway train

Excludes *fall related to collision, derailment, or explosion of railway train (E800.0-E803.9)*

● ● **E805 Hit by rolling stock**

Requires fourth digit. See beginning of section E800-E845 for codes and definitions.

Includes crushed by railway train or part
injured by railway train or part
killed by railway train or part
knocked down by railway train or part
run over by railway train or part

Excludes *pedestrian hit by object set in motion by railway train (E806.0-E806.9)*

● ● **E806 Other specified railway accident**

Requires fourth digit. See beginning of section E800-E845 for codes and definitions.

Includes hit by object falling in railway train
injured by door or window on railway train
nonmotor road vehicle or pedestrian hit by object set in motion by railway train
railway train hit by falling:
earth NOS
rock
tree
other object

Excludes *railway accident due to cataclysm (E908-E909)*

● ● **E807 Railway accident of unspecified nature**

Requires fourth digit. See beginning of section E800-E845 for codes and definitions.

Includes found dead on railway right-of-way NOS
injured on railway right-of-way NOS
railway accident NOS

◄ New   ◄▥ Revised   ~~deleted~~ Deleted   Excludes   Includes   Use additional   Code first   Omit code
● Unacceptable Principal Diagnosis   ● Use Additional Digit(s)   **OGCR** Official Guidelines   **Coding Clinic**

MOTOR VEHICLE TRAFFIC ACCIDENTS (E810-E819)

Note: For definitions of motor vehicle traffic accident, and related terms, see definitions (e) to (k).

| Excludes | *accidents involving motor vehicle and aircraft (E840.0-E845.9)* |

The following fourth-digit subdivisions are for use with categories E810-E819 to identify the injured person:

> 0 **Driver of motor vehicle other than motorcycle**
>   See definition (l)
> 1 **Passenger in motor vehicle other than motorcycle**
>   See definition (l)
> 2 **Motorcyclist**
>   See definition (l)
> 3 **Passenger on motorcycle**
>   See definition (l)
> 4 **Occupant of streetcar**
> 5 **Rider of animal; occupant of animal-drawn vehicle**
> 6 **Pedal cyclist**
>   See definition (p)
> 7 **Pedestrian**
>   See definition (r)
> 8 **Other specified person**
>   Occupant of vehicle other than above
>   Person in railway train involved in accident
>   Unauthorized rider of motor vehicle
> 9 **Unspecified person**

● ● **E810 Motor vehicle traffic accident involving collision with train**

Requires fourth digit. See beginning of section E800-E845 for codes and definitions.

| Excludes | *motor vehicle collision with object set in motion by railway train (E815.0-E815.9)*
railway train hit by object set in motion by motor vehicle (E818.0-E818.9) |

● ● **E811 Motor vehicle traffic accident involving re-entrant collision with another motor vehicle**

Requires fourth digit. See beginning of section E800-E845 for codes and definitions.

| Includes | collision between motor vehicle which accidentally leaves the roadway then re-enters the same roadway, or the opposite roadway on a divided highway, and another motor vehicle |

| Excludes | *collision on the same roadway when none of the motor vehicles involved have left and re-entered the roadway (E812.0-E812.9)* |

● ● **E812 Other motor vehicle traffic accident involving collision with motor vehicle**

Requires fourth digit. See beginning of section E800-E845 for codes and definitions.

| Includes | collision with another motor vehicle parked, stopped, stalled, disabled, or abandoned on the highway
motor vehicle collision NOS |

| Excludes | *collision with object set in motion by another motor vehicle (E815.0-E815.9)*
re-entrant collision with another motor vehicle (E811.0-E811.9) |

Coding Clinic: 2007, Q4, P105-107; 1996, Q4, P36.37

● ● **E813 Motor vehicle traffic accident involving collision with other vehicle**

Requires fourth digit. See beginning of section E800-E845 for codes and definitions.

| Includes | collision between motor vehicle, any kind, and:
other road (nonmotor transport) vehicle, such as:
animal carrying a person
animal-drawn vehicle
pedal cycle
streetcar |

| Excludes | *collision with:*
object set in motion by nonmotor road vehicle (E815.0-E815.9)
pedestrian (E814.0-E814.9)
nonmotor road vehicle hit by object set in motion by motor vehicle (E818.0-E818.9) |

● ● **E814 Motor vehicle traffic accident involving collision with pedestrian**

Requires fourth digit. See beginning of section E800-E845 for codes and definitions.

| Includes | collision between motor vehicle, any kind, and pedestrian
pedestrian dragged, hit, or run over by motor vehicle, any kind |

| Excludes | *pedestrian hit by object set in motion by motor vehicle (E818.0-E818.9)* |

Coding Clinic: 1996, Q4, P36.37

● ● **E815 Other motor vehicle traffic accident involving collision on the highway**

Requires fourth digit. See beginning of section E800-E845 for codes and definitions.

| Includes | collision (due to loss of control) (on highway) between motor vehicle, any kind, and:
abutment (bridge) (overpass)
animal (herded) (unattended)
fallen stone, traffic sign, tree, utility pole
guard rail or boundary fence
interhighway divider
landslide (not moving)
object set in motion by railway train or road vehicle (motor) (nonmotor)
object thrown in front of motor vehicle
safety island
temporary traffic sign or marker
wall of cut made for road
other object, fixed, movable, or moving |

| Excludes | *collision with:*
any object off the highway (resulting from loss of control) (E816.0-E816.9)
any object which normally would have been off the highway and is not stated to have been on it (E816.0-E816.9)
motor vehicle parked, stopped, stalled, disabled, or abandoned on highway (E812.0-E812.9)
moving landslide (E909.2)
motor vehicle hit by object:
set in motion by railway train or road vehicle (motor) (nonmotor) (E818.0-E818.9)
thrown into or on vehicle (E818.0-E818.9) |

● ● **E816 Motor vehicle traffic accident due to loss of control, without collision on the highway**

> Requires fourth digit. See beginning of section E800-E845 for codes and definitions.

> **Includes** motor vehicle:
>> failing to make curve and:
>>> colliding with object off the highway
>>> overturning
>>> stopping abruptly off the highway
>> going out of control (due to)
>>> blowout and:
>>>> colliding with object off the highway
>>>> overturning
>>>> stopping abruptly off the highway
>>> burst tire and:
>>>> colliding with object off the highway
>>>> overturning
>>>> stopping abruptly off the highway
>>> driver falling asleep and:
>>>> colliding with object off the highway
>>>> overturning
>>>> stopping abruptly off the highway
>>> driver inattention and:
>>>> colliding with object off the highway
>>>> overturning
>>>> stopping abruptly off the highway
>>> excessive speed and:
>>>> colliding with object off the highway
>>>> overturning
>>>> stopping abruptly off the highway
>>> failure of mechanical part and:
>>>> colliding with object off the highway
>>>> overturning
>>>> stopping abruptly off the highway

> **Excludes** *collision on highway following loss of control (E810.0-E815.9)*
>> *loss of control of motor vehicle following collision on the highway (E810.0-E815.9)*

● ● **E817 Noncollision motor vehicle traffic accident while boarding or alighting**

> Requires fourth digit. See beginning of section E800-E845 for codes and definitions.

> **Includes** fall down stairs of motor bus while boarding or alighting
>> fall from car in street while boarding or alighting
>> injured by moving part of the vehicle while boarding or alighting
>> trapped by door of motor bus boarding or alighting while boarding or alighting

● ● **E818 Other noncollision motor vehicle traffic accident**

> Requires fourth digit. See beginning of section E800-E845 for codes and definitions.

> **Includes** accidental poisoning from exhaust gas generated by motor vehicle while in motion
>> breakage of any part of motor vehicle while in motion
>> explosion of any part of motor vehicle while in motion
>> fall, jump, or being accidentally pushed from motor vehicle while in motion
>> fire starting in motor vehicle while in motion
>> hit by object thrown into or on motor vehicle while in motion
>> injured by being thrown against some part of, or object in motor vehicle while in motion
>> injury from moving part of motor vehicle while in motion
>> object falling in or on motor vehicle while in motion
>> object thrown on motor vehicle while in motion
>> collision of railway train or road vehicle except motor vehicle, with object set in motion by motor vehicle
>> motor vehicle hit by object set in motion by railway train or road vehicle (motor) (nonmotor)
>> pedestrian, railway train, or road vehicle (motor) (nonmotor) hit by object set in motion by motor vehicle

> **Excludes** *collision between motor vehicle and:*
>> *object set in motion by railway train or road vehicle (motor) (nonmotor) (E815.0-E815.9)*
>> *object thrown towards the motor vehicle (E815.0-E815.9)*
>> *person overcome by carbon monoxide generated by stationary motor vehicle off the roadway with motor running (E868.2)*

● ● **E819 Motor vehicle traffic accident of unspecified nature**

> Requires fourth digit. See beginning of section E800-E845 for codes and definitions.

> **Includes** motor vehicle traffic accident NOS
>> traffic accident NOS

> **Coding Clinic:** 2009, Q4, P141; 2008, Q4, P96-97; 2006, Q4, P100-102; 2003, Q1, P7; 1999, Q4, P11-12; Q1, P10; 1993, Q2, P4-5

◀ New   ◀▦ Revised   ~~deleted~~ Deleted   Excludes   Includes   Use additional   Code first   Omit code
● Unacceptable Principal Diagnosis   ● Use Additional Digit(s)   **OGCR** Official Guidelines   **Coding Clinic**

MOTOR VEHICLE NONTRAFFIC ACCIDENTS (E820-E825)

Note: For definitions of motor vehicle nontraffic accident and related terms see definition (a) to (k).

Includes accidents involving motor vehicles being used in recreational or sporting activities off the highway
collision and noncollision motor vehicle accidents occurring entirely off the highway

Excludes *accidents involving motor vehicle and:*
aircraft (E840.0-E845.9)
watercraft (E830.0-E838.9)
accidents, not on the public highway, involving agricultural and construction machinery but not involving another motor vehicle (E919.0, E919.2, E919.7)

The following fourth-digit subdivisions are for use with categories E820-E825 to identify the injured person:

> **0 Driver of motor vehicle other than motorcycle**
> See definition (l)
> **1 Passenger in motor vehicle other than motorcycle**
> See definition (l)
> **2 Motorcyclist**
> See definition (l)
> **3 Passenger on motorcycle**
> See definition (l)
> **4 Occupant of streetcar**
> **5 Rider of animal; occupant of animal-drawn vehicle**
> **6 Pedal cyclist**
> See definition (p)
> **7 Pedestrian**
> See definition (r)
> **8 Other specified person**
> Occupant of vehicle other than above
> Person on railway train involved in accident
> Unauthorized rider of motor vehicle
> **9 Unspecified person**

● ● **E820 Nontraffic accident involving motor-driven snow vehicle**

Requires fourth digit. See beginning of section E800-E845 for codes and definitions.

Includes breakage of part of motor-driven snow vehicle (not on public highway)
fall from motor-driven snow vehicle (not on public highway)
hit by motor-driven snow vehicle (not on public highway)
overturning of motor-driven snow vehicle (not on public highway)
run over or dragged by motor-driven snow vehicle (not on public highway)
collision of motor-driven snow vehicle with:
  animal (being ridden) (-drawn vehicle)
  another off-road motor vehicle
  other motor vehicle, not on public highway
  railway train
  other object, fixed or movable
injury caused by rough landing of motor-driven snow vehicle (after leaving ground on rough terrain)

Excludes *accident on the public highway involving motor driven snow vehicle (E810.0-E819.9)*

● ● **E821 Nontraffic accident involving other off-road motor vehicle**

Requires fourth digit. See beginning of section E800-E845 for codes and definitions.

Includes breakage of part of off-road motor vehicle, except snow vehicle (not on public highway)
fall from off-road motor vehicle, except snow vehicle (not on public highway)
hit by off-road motor vehicle, except snow vehicle (not on public highway)
overturning of off-road motor vehicle, except snow vehicle (not on public highway)
run over or dragged by off-road motor vehicle, except snow vehicle (not on public highway)
thrown against some part of or object in off-road motor vehicle, except snow vehicle (not on public highway)
collision with:
  animal (being ridden) (-drawn vehicle)
  another off-road motor vehicle, except snow vehicle
  other motor vehicle, not on public highway
  other object, fixed or movable

Excludes *accident on public highway involving off-road motor vehicle (E810.0-E819.9)*
collision between motor driven snow vehicle and other off-road motor vehicle (E820.0-E820.9)
hovercraft accident on water (E830.0-E838.9)

● ● **E822 Other motor vehicle nontraffic accident involving collision with moving object**

Requires fourth digit. See beginning of section E800-E845 for codes and definitions.

Includes collision, not on public highway, between motor vehicle, except off-road motor vehicle and:
  animal
  nonmotor vehicle
  other motor vehicle, except off-road motor vehicle
  pedestrian
  railway train
  other moving object

Excludes *collision with:*
motor-driven snow vehicle (E820.0-E820.9)
other off-road motor vehicle (E821.0-E821.9)

● ● **E823 Other motor vehicle nontraffic accident involving collision with stationary object**

Requires fourth digit. See beginning of section E800-E845 for codes and definitions.

Includes collision, not on public highway, between motor vehicle, except off-road motor vehicle, and any object, fixed or movable, but not in motion

E000-E999

● ● **E824 Other motor vehicle nontraffic accident while boarding and alighting**

    Requires fourth digit. See beginning of section E800–E845 for codes and definitions.

    Includes fall while boarding or alighting from motor vehicle except off-road motor vehicle, not on public highway

        injury from moving part of motor vehicle while boarding or alighting from motor vehicle except off-road motor vehicle, not on public highway

        trapped by door of motor vehicle while boarding or alighting from motor vehicle except off-road motor vehicle, not on public highway

● ● **E825 Other motor vehicle nontraffic accident of other and unspecified nature**

    Requires fourth digit. See beginning of section E800–E845 for codes and definitions.

    Includes accidental poisoning from carbon monoxide generated by motor vehicle while in motion, not on public highway

        breakage of any part of motor vehicle while in motion, not on public highway

        explosion of any part of motor vehicle while in motion, not on public highway

        fall, jump, or being accidentally pushed from motor vehicle while in motion, not on public highway

        fire starting in motor vehicle while in motion, not on public highway

        hit by object thrown into, towards, or on motor vehicle while in motion, not on public highway

        injured by being thrown against some part of, or object in motor vehicle while in motion, not on public highway

        injury from moving part of motor vehicle while in motion, not on public highway

        object falling in or on motor vehicle while in motion, not on public highway

        motor vehicle nontraffic accident NOS

    Excludes *fall from or in stationary motor vehicle (E884.9, E885.9)*

        overcome by carbon monoxide or exhaust gas generated by stationary motor vehicle off the roadway with motor running (E868.2)

        struck by falling object from or in stationary motor vehicle (E916)

OTHER ROAD VEHICLE ACCIDENTS (E826–E829)

    Note: Other road vehicle accidents are transport accidents involving road vehicles other than motor vehicles. For definitions of other road vehicle and related terms see definitions (m) to (o).

    Includes accidents involving other road vehicles being used in recreational or sporting activities

    Excludes *collision of other road vehicle [any] with:*
        aircraft (E840.0–E845.9)
        motor vehicle (E813.0–E813.9, E820.0–E822.9)
        railway train (E801.0–E801.9)

The following fourth-digit subdivisions are for use with categories E826–E829 to identify the injured person:

    0 Pedestrian
        See definition (r)
    1 Pedal cyclist
        See definition (p)
    2 Rider of animal
    3 Occupant of animal-drawn vehicle
    4 Occupant of streetcar
    8 Other specified person
    9 Unspecified person

● ● **E826 Pedal cycle accident**
    [0-9]

    Requires fourth digit. See beginning of section E800–E845 for codes and definitions.

    Includes breakage of any part of pedal cycle
        collision between pedal cycle and:
            animal (being ridden) (herded) (unattended)
            another pedal cycle
            nonmotor road vehicle, any
            pedestrian
            other object, fixed, movable, or moving, not set in motion by motor vehicle, railway train, or aircraft
        entanglement in wheel of pedal cycle
        fall from pedal cycle
        hit by object falling or thrown on the pedal cycle
        pedal cycle accident NOS
        pedal cycle overturned

● ● **E827 Animal-drawn vehicle accident**
    [0,2-4,8,9]

    Requires fourth digit. See beginning of section E800–E845 for codes and definitions.

    Includes breakage of any part of vehicle
        collision between animal-drawn vehicle and:
            animal (being ridden) (herded) (unattended)
            nonmotor road vehicle, except pedal cycle
            pedestrian, pedestrian conveyance, or pedestrian vehicle
            other object, fixed, movable, or moving, not set in motion by motor vehicle, railway train, or aircraft
        fall from animal-drawn vehicle
        knocked down by animal-drawn vehicle
        overturning of animal-drawn vehicle
        run over by animal-drawn vehicle
        thrown from animal-drawn vehicle

    Excludes *collision of animal-drawn vehicle with pedal cycle (E826.0–E826.9)*

◀ New   ◀▥▥ Revised   ~~deleted~~ Deleted   Excludes   Includes   Use additional   Code first   Omit code
● Unacceptable Principal Diagnosis   ● Use Additional Digit(s)   OGCR Official Guidelines   Coding Clinic

E000-E999

●● **E828 Accident involving animal being ridden**
[0,2,4,8,9]
Requires fourth digit. See beginning of section
E800-E845 for codes and definitions.

Includes collision between animal being ridden and:
another animal
nonmotor road vehicle, except pedal
cycle, and animal-drawn vehicle
pedestrian, pedestrian conveyance, or
pedestrian vehicle
other object, fixed, movable, or moving,
not set in motion by motor
vehicle, railway train, or aircraft
fall from animal being ridden
knocked down by animal being ridden
thrown from animal being ridden
trampled by animal being ridden
ridden animal stumbled and fell

Excludes *collision of animal being ridden with:*
animal-drawn vehicle (E827.0-E827.9)
pedal cycle (E826.0-E826.9)

●● **E829 Other road vehicle accidents**
[0,4,8,9]
Requires fourth digit. See beginning of section
E800-E845 for codes and definitions.

Includes accident while boarding or alighting from
streetcar
nonmotor road vehicle not classifiable
to E826-E828
blow from object in
streetcar
nonmotor road vehicle not classifiable
to E826-E828
breakage of any part of
streetcar
nonmotor road vehicle not classifiable
to E826-E828
caught in door of
streetcar
nonmotor road vehicle not classifiable
to E826-E828
derailment of
streetcar
nonmotor road vehicle not classifiable
to E826-E828
fall in, on, or from
streetcar
nonmotor road vehicle not classifiable
to E826-E828
fire in
streetcar
nonmotor road vehicle not classifiable
to E826-E828
collision between streetcar or nonmotor
road vehicle, except as in E826-E828,
and:
animal (not being ridden)
another nonmotor road vehicle not
classifiable to E826-E828
pedestrian
other object, fixed, movable, or moving,
not set in motion by motor
vehicle, railway train, or aircraft
nonmotor road vehicle accident NOS
streetcar accident NOS

Excludes *collision with:*
animal being ridden (E828.0-E828.9)
animal-drawn vehicle (E827.0-E827.9)
pedal cycle (E826.0-E826.9)

WATER TRANSPORT ACCIDENTS (E830-E838)

Note: For definitions of water transport accident and
related terms see definitions (a), (s), and (t).

Includes watercraft accidents in the course of
recreational activities

Excludes *accidents involving both aircraft, including*
objects set in motion by aircraft, and
watercraft (E840.0-E845.9)

The following fourth-digit subdivisions are for use with
categories E830-E838 to identify the injured person:

---

0 Occupant of small boat, unpowered
1 Occupant of small boat, powered
See definition (t)
Excludes *water skier (4)*

2 Occupant of other watercraft-crew
Persons:
engaged in operation of watercraft
providing passenger services [cabin attendants,
ship's physician, catering personnel]
working on ship during voyage in other
capacity [musician in band, operators of
shops and beauty parlors]
3 Occupant of other watercraft -- other than crew
Passenger
Occupant of lifeboat, other than crew, after
abandoning ship
4 Water skier
5 Swimmer
6 Dockers, stevedores
Longshoreman employed on the dock in loading
and unloading ships
7 Occupant of military watercraft, any type
8 Other specified person
Immigration and custom officials on board ship
Person:
accompanying passenger or member of crew
visiting boat
Pilot (guiding ship into port)
9 Unspecified person

●● **E830 Accident to watercraft causing submersion**
Requires fourth digit. See beginning of section
E800-E845 for codes and definitions.

Includes submersion and drowning due to:
boat overturning
boat submerging
falling or jumping from burning ship
falling or jumping from crushed
watercraft
ship sinking
other accident to watercraft

E000-E999

● ● **E831 Accident to watercraft causing other injury**

> Requires fourth digit. See beginning of section
> E800-E845 for codes and definitions.

> **Includes**   any injury, except submersion and
>   drowning, as a result of an accident
>   to watercraft
>   burned while ship on fire
>   crushed between ships in collision
>   crushed by lifeboat after abandoning ship
>   fall due to collision or other accident to
>   watercraft
>   hit by falling object due to accident to
>   watercraft
>   injured in watercraft accident involving
>   collision
>   struck by boat or part thereof after fall or
>   jump from damaged boat

> **Excludes**   *burns from localized fire or explosion on board
>   ship (E837.0-E837.9)*

● ● **E832 Other accidental submersion or drowning in water
transport accident**

> Requires fourth digit. See beginning of section
> E800-E845 for codes and definitions.

> **Includes**   submersion or drowning as a result of an
>   accident other than accident to the
>   watercraft, such as:
>   fall:
>   from gangplank
>   from ship
>   overboard
>   thrown overboard by motion of ship
>   washed overboard

> **Excludes**   *submersion or drowning of swimmer or diver
>   who voluntarily jumps from boat not
>   involved in an accident (E910.0-E910.9)*

● ● **E833 Fall on stairs or ladders in water transport**

> Requires fourth digit. See beginning of section
> E800-E845 for codes and definitions.

> **Excludes**   *fall due to accident to watercraft (E831.0-E831.9)*

● ● **E834 Other fall from one level to another in water
transport**

> Requires fourth digit. See beginning of section
> E800-E845 for codes and definitions.

> **Excludes**   *fall due to accident to watercraft
>   (E831.0-E831.9)*

● ● **E835 Other and unspecified fall in water transport**

> Requires fourth digit. See beginning of section
> E800-E845 for codes and definitions.

> **Excludes**   *fall due to accident to watercraft
>   (E831.0-E831.9)*

● ● **E836 Machinery accident in water transport**

> Requires fourth digit. See beginning of section
> E800-E845 for codes and definitions.

> **Includes**   injuries in water transport caused by:
>   deck machinery
>   engine room machinery
>   galley machinery
>   laundry machinery
>   loading machinery

● ● **E837 Explosion, fire, or burning in watercraft**

> Requires fourth digit. See beginning of section
> E800-E845 for codes and definitions.

> **Includes**   explosion of boiler on steamship
>   localized fire on ship

> **Excludes**   *burning ship (due to collision or explosion)
>   resulting in:
>   submersion or drowning (E830.0-E830.9)
>   other injury (E831.0-E831.9)*

● ● **E838 Other and unspecified water transport accident**

> Requires fourth digit. See beginning of section
> E800-E845 for codes and definitions.

> **Includes**   accidental poisoning by gases or fumes on
>   ship
>   atomic power plant malfunction in
>   watercraft
>   crushed between ship and stationary object
>   [wharf]
>   crushed between ships without accident to
>   watercraft
>   crushed by falling object on ship or while
>   loading or unloading
>   hit by boat while water skiing
>   struck by boat or part thereof (after fall
>   from boat)
>   watercraft accident NOS

AIR AND SPACE TRANSPORT ACCIDENTS (E840-E845)

Note: For definition of aircraft and related terms see definitions (u) and (v).

The following fourth-digit subdivisions are for use with categories E840-E845 to identify the injured person:

> **0 Occupant of spacecraft**
> **1 Occupant of military aircraft, any**
> Crew in military aircraft [air force] [army] [national guard] [navy]
> Passenger (civilian) (military) in military aircraft [air force] [army] [national guard] [navy]
> Troops in military aircraft [air force] [army] [national guard] [navy]
>
> > **Excludes** *occupants of aircraft operated under jurisdiction of police departments (5)*
> > *parachutist (7)*
>
> **2 Crew of commercial aircraft (powered) in surface-to-surface transport**
> **3 Other occupant of commercial aircraft (powered) in surface-to-surface transport**
> Flight personnel:
> not part of crew
> on familiarization flight
> Passenger on aircraft (powered) NOS
> **4 Occupant of commercial aircraft (powered) in surface-to-air transport**
> Occupant [crew] [passenger] of aircraft (powered) engaged in activities, such as:
> aerial spraying (crops) (fire retardants)
> air drops of emergency supplies
> air drops of parachutists, except from military craft
> crop dusting
> lowering of construction material [bridge or telephone pole]
> sky writing
> **5 Occupant of other powered aircraft**
> Occupant [crew] [passenger] of aircraft [powered] engaged in activities, such as:
> aerobatic flying
> aircraft racing
> rescue operation
> storm surveillance
> traffic surveillance
> Occupant of private plane NOS
> **6 Occupant of unpowered aircraft, except parachutist**
> Occupant of aircraft classifiable to E842
> **7 Parachutist (military) (other)**
> Person making voluntary descent
>
> > **Excludes** *person making descent after accident to aircraft (.1–.6)*
>
> **8 Ground crew, airline employee**
> Persons employed at airfields (civil) (military) or launching pads, not occupants of aircraft
> **9 Other person**

● ● **E840 Accident to powered aircraft at takeoff or landing**

Requires fourth digit. See beginning of section E800-E845 for codes and definitions.

> **Includes** collision of aircraft with any object, fixed, movable, or moving while taking off or landing
> crash while taking off or landing
> explosion on aircraft while taking off or landing
> fire on aircraft while taking off or landing
> forced landing

● ● **E841 Accident to powered aircraft, other and unspecified**

Requires fourth digit. See beginning of section E800-E845 for codes and definitions.

> **Includes** aircraft accident NOS
> aircraft crash or wreck NOS
> any accident to powered aircraft while in transit or when not specified whether in transit, taking off, or landing
> collision of aircraft with another aircraft, bird, or any object, while in transit
> explosion on aircraft while in transit
> fire on aircraft while in transit

● ● **E842 Accident to unpowered aircraft**
[6-9]

Requires fourth digit. See beginning of section E800-E845 for codes and definitions.

> **Includes** any accident, except collision with powered aircraft, to:
> balloon
> glider
> hang glider
> kite carrying a person
> hit by object falling from unpowered aircraft

● ● **E843 Fall in, on, or from aircraft**
[0-9]

Requires fourth digit. See beginning of section E800-E845 for codes and definitions.

> **Includes** accident in boarding or alighting from aircraft, any kind
> fall in, on, or from aircraft [any kind], while in transit, taking off, or landing, except when as a result of an accident to aircraft

● ● **E844 Other specified air transport accidents**
[0-9]

Requires fourth digit. See beginning of section E800-E845 for codes and definitions.

> **Includes** hit by aircraft without accident to aircraft
> hit by object falling from aircraft without accident to aircraft
> injury by or from machinery on aircraft without accident to aircraft
> injury by or from rotating propeller without accident to aircraft
> injury by or from voluntary parachute descent without accident to aircraft
> poisoning by carbon monoxide from aircraft while in transit without accident to aircraft
> sucked into jet without accident to aircraft
> any accident involving other transport vehicle (motor) (nonmotor) due to being hit by object set in motion by aircraft (powered)
>
> > **Excludes** *air sickness (E903)*
> > *effects of:*
> > *high altitude (E902.0-E902.1)*
> > *pressure change (E902.0-E902.1)*
> > *injury in parachute descent due to accident to aircraft (E840.0-E842.9)*

● ● **E845 Accident involving spacecraft**
[0,8,9]

Requires fourth digit. See beginning of section E800-E845 for codes and definitions.

> **Includes** launching pad accident
>
> > **Excludes** *effects of weightlessness in spacecraft (E928.0)*

VEHICLE ACCIDENTS NOT ELSEWHERE CLASSIFIABLE (E846–E848)

● **E846 Accidents involving powered vehicles used solely within the buildings and premises of industrial or commercial establishment**

Accident to, on, or   involving:
   battery-powered airport passenger vehicle
   battery-powered trucks (baggage) (mail)
   coal car in mine
   logging car
   self-propelled truck, industrial
   station baggage truck (powered)
   tram, truck, or tub (powered) in mine or quarry
Breakage of any part of vehicle
Collision with:
   pedestrian
   other vehicle or object within premises
Explosion of powered vehicle, industrial or commercial
Fall from powered vehicle, industrial or commercial
Overturning of powered vehicle, industrial or commercial
Struck by powered vehicle, industrial or commercial

Excludes *accidental poisoning by exhaust gas from vehicle not elsewhere classifiable (E868.2)*
injury by crane, lift (fork), or elevator (E919.2)

● **E847 Accidents involving cable cars not running on rails**

Accident to, on, or involving:
   cable car, not on rails
   ski chair-lift
   ski-lift with gondola
   teleferique
Breakage of cable
   caught or dragged by cable car, not on rails
   fall or jump from cable car, not on rails
   object thrown from or in cable car not on rails

● **E848 Accidents involving other vehicles, not elsewhere classifiable**

Accident to, on, or involving:
   ice yacht
   land yacht
   nonmotor, nonroad vehicle NOS

OGCR Section I.C.19.b

Use an additional code from category E849 to indicate the Place of Occurrence. The Place of Occurrence describes the place where the event occurred and not the patient's activity at the time of the event. Do not use E849.9 if the place of occurrence is not stated.

PLACE OF OCCURRENCE (E849) ◀▥

● **E849 Place of Occurrence**

Note: The following category is for use to denote the place where the injury or poisoning occurred.

● **E849.0 Home**
   Apartment
   Boarding house
   Farm house
   Home premises
   House (residential)
   Noninstitutional place of residence
   Private:
      driveway
      garage
      garden
      home
      walk
   Swimming pool in private house or garden
   Yard of home

Excludes *home under construction but not yet occupied (E849.3)*
institutional place of residence (E849.7)

● **E849.1 Farm**
   Buildings   Land under cultivation
Excludes *farm house and home premises of farm (E849.0)*

● **E849.2 Mine and quarry**
   Gravel pit   Tunnel under
   Sand pit   construction

● **E849.3 Industrial place and premises**
   Building under construction
   Dockyard
   Dry dock
   Factory
      building
      premises
   Garage (place of work)
   Industrial yard
   Loading platform (factory) (store)
   Plant, industrial
   Railway yard
   Shop (place of work)
   Warehouse
   Workhouse
   Coding Clinic: v 2003, Q4, P76-78

● **E849.4 Place for recreation and sport**
   Amusement park   Playground, including
   Baseball field   school playground
   Basketball court   Public park
   Beach resort   Racecourse
   Cricket ground   Resort NOS
   Fives court   Riding school
   Football field   Rifle range
   Golf course   Seashore resort
   Gymnasium   Skating rink
   Hockey field   Sports palace
   Holiday camp   Stadium
   Ice palace   Swimming pool, public
   Lake resort   Tennis court
   Mountain resort   Vacation resort

Excludes *that in private house or garden (E849.0)*

● **E849.5 Street and highway**
   Coding Clinic: 2009, Q4, P144; 1995, Q1, P10

● **E849.6 Public building**
   Building (including adjacent grounds) used
      by the general public or by a particular
      group of the public, such as:
   airport
   bank
   cafe
   casino
   church
   cinema
   clubhouse
   courthouse
   dance hall
   garage building (for car storage)
   hotel
   market (grocery or other commodity)
   movie house
   music hall
   nightclub
   office
   office building
   opera house
   post office
   public hall
   radio broadcasting station
   restaurant
   school (state) (public) (private)
   shop, commercial
   station (bus) (railway)
   store
   theater

Excludes *home garage (E849.0)*
industrial building or workplace (E849.3)

◀ New   ◀▥ Revised   ~~deleted~~ Deleted   **Excludes**   **Includes**   **Use additional**   **Code first**   **Omit code**
● Unacceptable Principal Diagnosis   ● Use Additional Digit(s)   **OGCR** Official Guidelines   **Coding Clinic**

● **E849.7 Residential institution**
　　Children's home
　　Dormitory
　　Hospital
　　Jail
　　Old people's home
　　Orphanage
　　Prison
　　Reform School

● **E849.8 Other specified places**
　　Beach NOS
　　Canal
　　Caravan site NOS
　　Derelict house
　　Desert
　　Dock
　　Forest
　　Harbor
　　Hill
　　Lake NOS
　　Mountain
　　Parking lot
　　Parking place
　　Pond or pool (natural)
　　Prairie
　　Public place NOS
　　Railway line
　　Reservoir
　　River
　　Sea
　　Seashore NOS
　　Stream
　　Swamp
　　Trailer court
　　Woods

● **E849.9 Unspecified place**

ACCIDENTAL POISONING BY DRUGS, MEDICINAL SUBSTANCES, AND BIOLOGICALS (E850-E858)

Includes　accidental overdose of drug, wrong drug given or taken in error, and drug taken inadvertently
　　accidents in the use of drugs and biologicals in medical and surgical procedures

Excludes　*administration with suicidal or homicidal intent or intent to harm, or in circumstances classifiable to E980-E989 (E950.0-E950.5, E962.0, E980.0-E980.5)*
　　correct drug properly administered in therapeutic or prophylactic dosage, as the cause of adverse effect (E930.0-E949.9)

Note:　See Alphabetic Index for more complete list of specific drugs to be classified under the fourth-digit subdivisions. The American Hospital Formulary numbers can be used to classify new drugs listed by the American Hospital Formulary Service (AHFS). See Appendix C.

● **E850 Accidental poisoning by analgesics, antipyretics, and antirheumatics**
　　Coding Clinic: 2008, Q3, P21

● **E850.0 Heroin**
　　Diacetylmorphine

● **E850.1 Methadone**

● **E850.2 Other opiates and related narcotics**
　　Codeine [methylmorphine]
　　Meperidine [pethidine]
　　Morphine
　　Opium (alkaloids)

● **E850.3 Salicylates**
　　Acetylsalicylic acid [aspirin]
　　Amino derivatives of salicylic acid
　　Salicylic acid salts

● **E850.4 Aromatic analgesics, not elsewhere classified**
　　Acetanilid
　　Paracetamol [acetaminophen]
　　Phenacetin [acetophenetidin]

● **E850.5 Pyrazole derivatives**
　　Aminophenazone [amidopyrine]
　　Phenylbutazone

● **E850.6 Antirheumatics [antiphlogistics]**
　　Gold salts
　　Indomethacin
　　Excludes　*salicylates (E850.3)*
　　　　steroids (E858.0)

● **E850.7 Other non-narcotic analgesics**
　　Pyrabital

● **E850.8 Other specified analgesics and antipyretics**
　　Pentazocine

● **E850.9 Unspecified analgesic or antipyretic**

● **E851 Accidental poisoning by barbiturates**
　　Amobarbital [amylobarbitone]
　　Barbital [barbitone]
　　Butabarbital [butabarbitone]
　　Pentobarbital [pentobarbitone]
　　Phenobarbital [phenobarbitone]
　　Secobarbital [quinalbarbitone]
　　Excludes　*thiobarbiturates (E855.1)*

● **E852 Accidental poisoning by other sedatives and hypnotics**

● **E852.0 Chloral hydrate group**

● **E852.1 Paraldehyde**

● **E852.2 Bromine compounds**
　　Bromides
　　Carbromal (derivatives)

● **E852.3 Methaqualone compounds**

● **E852.4 Glutethimide group**

● **E852.5 Mixed sedatives, not elsewhere classified**

● **E852.8 Other specified sedatives and hypnotics**

● **E852.9 Unspecified sedative or hypnotic**
　　Sleeping:
　　　drug NOS
　　　pill NOS
　　　tablet NOS

● **E853 Accidental poisoning by tranquilizers**

● **E853.0 Phenothiazine-based tranquilizers**
　　Chlorpromazine
　　Fluphenazine
　　Prochlorperazine
　　Promazine

● **E853.1 Butyrophenone-based tranquilizers**
　　Haloperidol
　　Spiperone
　　Trifluperidol

● **E853.2 Benzodiazepine-based tranquilizers**
　　Chlordiazepoxide　　Lorazepam
　　Diazepam　　　　　　Medazepam
　　Flurazepam　　　　　Nitrazepam
　　Coding Clinic: 2009, Q4, P150; 1991, Q3, P14

● **E853.8 Other specified tranquilizers**
　　Hydroxyzine
　　Meprobamate

● **E853.9 Unspecified tranquilizer**

E000-E999

E000-E999

● E854 Accidental poisoning by other psychotropic agents
  ● E854.0 Antidepressants
          Amitriptyline
          Imipramine
          Monoamine oxidase [MAO] inhibitors
          Coding Clinic: 2009, Q4, P150; 1991, Q3, P14

  ● E854.1 Psychodysleptics [hallucinogens]
          Cannabis derivatives
          Lysergide [LSD]
          Marihuana (derivatives)
          Mescaline
          Psilocin
          Psilocybin

  ● E854.2 Psychostimulants
          Amphetamine
          Caffeine
          Excludes central appetite depressants (E858.8)
          Coding Clinic: 2003, Q2, P11

  ● E854.3 Central nervous system stimulants
          Analeptics
          Opiate antagonists

  ● E854.8 Other psychotropic agents

● E855 Accidental poisoning by other drugs acting on central and autonomic nervous system
  ● E855.0 Anticonvulsant and anti-Parkinsonism drugs
          Amantadine
          Hydantoin derivatives
          Levodopa [L-dopa]
          Oxazolidine derivatives [paramethadione] [trimethadione]
          Succinimides

  ● E855.1 Other central nervous system depressants
          Ether
          Gaseous anesthetics
          Halogenated hydrocarbon derivatives
          Intravenous anesthetics
          Thiobarbiturates, such as thiopental sodium

  ● E855.2 Local anesthetics
          Cocaine
          Lidocaine [lignocaine]
          Procaine
          Tetracaine

  ● E855.3 Parasympathomimetics [cholinergics]
          Acetylcholine
          Anticholinesterase:
            organophosphorus
            reversible
          Pilocarpine

  ● E855.4 Parasympatholytics [anticholinergics and antimuscarinics] and spasmolytics
          Atropine
          Homatropine
          Hyoscine [scopolamine]
          Quaternary ammonium derivatives

  ● E855.5 Sympathomimetics [adrenergics]
          Epinephrine [adrenalin]
          Levarterenol [noradrenalin]

  ● E855.6 Sympatholytics [antiadrenergics]
          Phenoxybenzamine
          Tolazoline hydrochloride

  ● E855.8 Other specified drugs acting on central and autonomic nervous systems

  ● E855.9 Unspecified drug acting on central and autonomic nervous systems

● E856 Accidental poisoning by antibiotics

● E857 Accidental poisoning by other anti-infectives

● E858 Accidental poisoning by other drugs
          Coding Clinic: 2008, Q3, P21
  ● E858.0 Hormones and synthetic substitutes
  ● E858.1 Primarily systemic agents
  ● E858.2 Agents primarily affecting blood constituents
  ● E858.3 Agents primarily affecting cardiovascular system
  ● E858.4 Agents primarily affecting gastrointestinal system
  ● E858.5 Water, mineral, and uric acid metabolism drugs
  ● E858.6 Agents primarily acting on the smooth and skeletal muscles and respiratory system
  ● E858.7 Agents primarily affecting skin and mucous membrane, ophthalmological, otorhinolaryngological, and dental drugs
  ● E858.8 Other specified drugs
          Central appetite depressants
  ● E858.9 Unspecified drug

ACCIDENTAL POISONING BY OTHER SOLID AND LIQUID SUBSTANCES, GASES, AND VAPORS (E860-E869)

  Note: Categories in this section are intended primarily to indicate the external cause of poisoning states classifiable to 980–989. They may also be used to indicate external causes of localized effects classifiable to 001–799.

● E860 Accidental poisoning by alcohol, not elsewhere classified
  ● E860.0 Alcoholic beverages
          Alcohol in preparations intended for consumption
          Coding Clinic: 2009, Q4, P150; 1996, Q3, P161; 1991, Q3, P14

  ● E860.1 Other and unspecified ethyl alcohol and its products
          Denatured alcohol
          Ethanol NOS
          Grain alcohol NOS
          Methylated spirit

  ● E860.2 Methyl alcohol
          Methanol
          Wood alcohol

  ● E860.3 Isopropyl alcohol
          Dimethyl carbinol
          Isopropanol
          Rubbing alcohol substitute
          Secondary propyl alcohol

  ● E860.4 Fusel oil
          Alcohol:
            amyl
            butyl
            propyl

  ● E860.8 Other specified alcohols
  ● E860.9 Unspecified alcohol

● E861 Accidental poisoning by cleansing and polishing agents, disinfectants, paints, and varnishes
  ● E861.0 Synthetic detergents and shampoos
  ● E861.1 Soap products
  ● E861.2 Polishes
  ● E861.3 Other cleansing and polishing agents
          Scouring powders
  ● E861.4 Disinfectants
          Household and other disinfectants not ordinarily used on the person
          Excludes carbolic acid or phenol (E864.0)

◀ New   ◀◖▥ Revised   ~~deleted~~ Deleted   Excludes   Includes   Use additional   Code first   Omit code
● Unacceptable Principal Diagnosis   ● Use Additional Digit(s)   OGCR Official Guidelines   Coding Clinic

● **E861.5 Lead paints**

● **E861.6 Other paints and varnishes**
>   Lacquers
>   Oil colors
>   Paints, other than lead
>   Whitewashes

● **E861.9 Unspecified**

● **E862 Accidental poisoning by petroleum products, other solvents and their vapors, not elsewhere classified**

● **E862.0 Petroleum solvents**
>   Petroleum:
>   ether
>   benzine
>   naphtha

● **E862.1 Petroleum fuels and cleaners**
>   Antiknock additives to petroleum fuels
>   Gas oils
>   Gasoline or petrol
>   Kerosene
>   **Excludes**   *kerosene insecticides (E863.4)*

● **E862.2 Lubricating oils**

● **E862.3 Petroleum solids**
>   Paraffin wax

● **E862.4 Other specified solvents**
>   Benzene
>   **Coding Clinic: 2008, Q3, P6-7**

● **E862.9 Unspecified solvent**

● **E863 Accidental poisoning by agricultural and horticultural chemical and pharmaceutical preparations other than plant foods and fertilizers**
>   **Excludes**   *plant foods and fertilizers (E866.5)*

● **E863.0 Insecticides of organochlorine compounds**
>   Benzene hexachloride   Dieldrin
>   Chlordane   Endrine
>   DDT Toxaphene

● **E863.1 Insecticides of organophosphorus compounds**
>   Demeton   Parathion
>   Diazinon   Phenylsulphthion
>   Dichlorvos   Phorate
>   Malathion   Phosdrin
>   Methyl parathion

● **E863.2 Carbamates**
>   Aldicarb
>   Carbaryl
>   Propoxur

● **E863.3 Mixtures of insecticides**

● **E863.4 Other and unspecified insecticides**
>   Kerosene insecticides

● **E863.5 Herbicides**
>   2,4-Dichlorophenoxyacetic acid [2, 4-D]
>   2,4,5-Trichlorophenoxyacetic acid [2, 4, 5-T]
>   Chlorates
>   Diquat
>   Mixtures of plant foods and fertilizers with
>   herbicides
>   Paraquat

● **E863.6 Fungicides**
>   Organic mercurials (used in seed dressing)
>   Pentachlorophenols

● **E863.7 Rodenticides**
>   Fluoroacetates   Warfarin
>   Squill and derivatives Zinc phosphide
>   Thallium

● **E863.8 Fumigants**
>   Cyanides   Phosphine
>   Methyl bromide

● **E863.9 Other and unspecified**

● **E864 Accidental poisoning by corrosives and caustics, not elsewhere classified**
>   **Excludes**   *those as components of disinfectants (E861.4)*

● **E864.0 Corrosive aromatics**
>   Carbolic acid or phenol

● **E864.1 Acids**
>   Acid:
>   hydrochloric
>   nitric
>   sulfuric

● **E864.2 Caustic alkalis**
>   Lye

● **E864.3 Other specified corrosives and caustics**

● **E864.4 Unspecified corrosives and caustics**

● **E865 Accidental poisoning from poisonous foodstuffs and poisonous plants**
>   **Includes**   any meat, fish, or shellfish
>   plants, berries, and fungi eaten as, or in
>   mistake for food, or by a child
>   **Excludes**   *anaphylactic shock due to adverse food reaction*
>   *(995.60–995.69)* ◀▥
>   *food poisoning (bacterial) (005.0–005.9)*
>   *poisoning and toxic reactions to venomous*
>   *plants (E905.6–E905.7)*

● **E865.0 Meat**

● **E865.1 Shellfish**

● **E865.2 Other fish**

● **E865.3 Berries and seeds**

● **E865.4 Other specified plants**

● **E865.5 Mushrooms and other fungi**

● **E865.8 Other specified foods**

● **E865.9 Unspecified foodstuff or poisonous plant**

● **E866 Accidental poisoning by other and unspecified solid and liquid substances**
>   **Excludes**   *these substances as a component of:*
>   *medicines (E850.0-E858.9)*
>   *paints (E861.5-E861.6)*
>   *pesticides (E863.0-E863.9)*
>   *petroleum fuels (E862.1)*

● **E866.0 Lead and its compounds and fumes**

● **E866.1 Mercury and its compounds and fumes**

● **E866.2 Antimony and its compounds and fumes**

● **E866.3 Arsenic and its compounds and fumes**

● **E866.4 Other metals and their compounds and fumes**
>   Beryllium (compounds)
>   Brass fumes
>   Cadmium (compounds)
>   Copper salts
>   Iron (compounds)
>   Manganese (compounds)
>   Nickel (compounds)
>   Thallium (compounds)

● **E866.5 Plant foods and fertilizers**
>   **Excludes**   *mixtures with herbicides (E863.5)*

● **E866.6 Glues and adhesives**

● **E866.7 Cosmetics**

● **E866.8 Other specified solid or liquid substances**
>   **Coding Clinic: 1990, Q4, P25**

● **E866.9 Unspecified solid or liquid substance**

E000-E999

E000-E999

● **E867 Accidental poisoning by gas distributed by pipeline**
   Carbon monoxide from incomplete combustion of
      piped gas
   Coal gas NOS
   Liquefied petroleum gas distributed through pipes
      (pure or mixed with air)
   Piped gas (natural) (manufactured)

● **E868 Accidental poisoning by other utility gas and other
   carbon monoxide**

   ● **E868.0 Liquefied petroleum gas distributed in mobile
      containers**
         Butane or carbon monoxide from incomplete
            combustion of these gases
         Liquefied hydrocarbon gas NOS or carbon
            monoxide from incomplete combustion
            of these gases
         Propane or carbon monoxide from incomplete
            combustion of these gases

   ● **E868.1 Other and unspecified utility gas**
         Acetylene or carbon monoxide from
            incomplete combustion of these gases
         Gas NOS used for lighting, heating, or
            cooking or carbon monoxide from
            incomplete combustion of these gases
         Water gas or carbon monoxide from
            incomplete combustion of these gases

   ● **E868.2 Motor vehicle exhaust gas**
         Exhaust gas from:
            farm tractor, not in transit
            gas engine
            motor pump
            motor vehicle, not in transit
            any type of combustion engine not in
               watercraft
         | Excludes | *poisoning by carbon monoxide from:*
                        aircraft while in transit
                           (E844.0-E844.9)
                        motor vehicle while in transit
                           (E818.0-E818.9)
                        watercraft whether or not in transit
                           (E838.0-E838.9)

   ● **E868.3 Carbon monoxide from incomplete combustion
      of other domestic fuels**
         Carbon monoxide from incomplete
            combustion of:
            coal in domestic stove or fireplace
            coke in domestic stove or fireplace
            kerosene in domestic stove or fireplace
            wood in domestic stove or fireplace
         | Excludes | *carbon monoxide from smoke and*
                        fumes due to conflagration
                        (E890.0-E893.9)

   ● **E868.8 Carbon monoxide from other sources**
         Carbon monoxide from:
            blast furnace gas
            incomplete combustion of fuels in
               industrial use
            kiln vapor

   ● **E868.9 Unspecified carbon monoxide**

● **E869 Accidental poisoning by other gases and vapors**
   | Excludes | *effects of gases used as anesthetics (E855.1,*
                  E938.2)
               fumes from heavy metals (E866.0-E866.4)
               smoke and fumes due to conflagration or
                  explosion (E890.0-E899)

   ● **E869.0 Nitrogen oxides**

   ● **E869.1 Sulfur dioxide**

   ● **E869.2 Freon**

   ● **E869.3 Lacrimogenic gas [tear gas]**
         Bromobenzyl cyanide
         Chloroacetophenone
         Ethyliodoacetate

   ● **E869.4 Second-hand tobacco smoke**
         Coding Clinic: 1996, Q2, P10

   ● **E869.8 Other specified gases and vapors**
         Chlorine
         Hydrocyanic acid gas

   ● **E869.9 Unspecified gases and vapors**

MISADVENTURES TO PATIENTS DURING SURGICAL AND MEDICAL CARE
(E870-E876)

   | Excludes | *accidental overdose of drug and wrong drug*
                  given in error (E850.0-E858.9)
               surgical and medical procedures as the cause
                  of abnormal reaction by the patient,
                  without mention of misadventure at the
                  time of procedure (E878.0-E879.9)

   OGCR Section I.C.19.h.1
   Assign a code in the range of E870-E876 if
   misadventures are stated by the provider. **When
   applying the E code guidelines pertaining to
   sequencing, these E codes are considered causal
   codes.**

● **E870 Accidental cut, puncture, perforation, or hemorrhage
   during medical care**

   ● **E870.0 Surgical operation**
         Coding Clinic: 2010, Q1, P20-21

   ● **E870.1 Infusion or transfusion**

   ● **E870.2 Kidney dialysis or other perfusion**

   ● **E870.3 Injection or vaccination**

   ● **E870.4 Endoscopic examination**

   ● **E870.5 Aspiration of fluid or tissue, puncture, and
      catheterization**
         Abdominal paracentesis
         Aspirating needle biopsy
         Blood sampling
         Lumbar puncture
         Thoracentesis
         | Excludes | *heart catheterization (E870.6)*

   ● **E870.6 Heart catheterization**

   ● **E870.7 Administration of enema**

   ● **E870.8 Other specified medical care**

   ● **E870.9 Unspecified medical care**

● **E871 Foreign object left in body during procedure**

   ● **E871.0 Surgical operation**

   ● **E871.1 Infusion or transfusion**

   ● **E871.2 Kidney dialysis or other perfusion**

   ● **E871.3 Injection or vaccination**

   ● **E871.4 Endoscopic examination**

   ● **E871.5 Aspiration of fluid or tissue, puncture, and
      catheterization**
         Abdominal paracentesis
         Aspiration needle biopsy
         Blood sampling
         Lumbar puncture
         Thoracentesis
         | Excludes | *heart catheterization (E871.6)*

   ● **E871.6 Heart catheterization**

   ● **E871.7 Removal of catheter or packing**

   ● **E871.8 Other specified procedures**

   ● **E871.9 Unspecified procedure**

◄ New   ◄▮▮ Revised   ~~deleted~~ Deleted | Excludes | Includes   Use additional   Code first   Omit code
● Unacceptable Principal Diagnosis   ● Use Additional Digit(s)   **OGCR** Official Guidelines   **Coding Clinic**

● **E872 Failure of sterile precautions during procedure**

  ● **E872.0 Surgical operation**

  ● **E872.1 Infusion or transfusion**

  ● **E872.2 Kidney dialysis and other perfusion**

  ● **E872.3 Injection or vaccination**

  ● **E872.4 Endoscopic examination**

  ● **E872.5 Aspiration of fluid or tissue, puncture, and catheterization**
      Abdominal paracentesis
      Aspirating needle biopsy
      Blood sampling
      Lumbar puncture
      Thoracentesis
      Excludes *heart catheterization (E872.6)*

  ● **E872.6 Heart catheterization**

  ● **E872.8 Other specified procedures**

  ● **E872.9 Unspecified procedure**

● **E873 Failure in dosage**

      Excludes *accidental overdose of drug, medicinal or biological substance (E850.0-E858.9)*

  ● **E873.0 Excessive amount of blood or other fluid during transfusion or infusion**

  ● **E873.1 Incorrect dilution of fluid during infusion**

  ● **E873.2 Overdose of radiation in therapy**

  ● **E873.3 Inadvertent exposure of patient to radiation during medical care**

  ● **E873.4 Failure in dosage in electroshock or insulin-shock therapy**

  ● **E873.5 Inappropriate [too hot or too cold] temperature in local application and packing**

  ● **E873.6 Nonadministration of necessary drug or medicinal substance**

  ● **E873.8 Other specified failure in dosage**

  ● **E873.9 Unspecified failure in dosage**

● **E874 Mechanical failure of instrument or apparatus during procedure**

  ● **E874.0 Surgical operation**

  ● **E874.1 Infusion and transfusion**
      Air in system

  ● **E874.2 Kidney dialysis and other perfusion**

  ● **E874.3 Endoscopic examination**

  ● **E874.4 Aspiration of fluid or tissue, puncture, and catheterization**
      Abdominal paracentesis
      Aspirating needle biopsy
      Blood sampling
      Lumbar puncture
      Thoracentesis
      Excludes *heart catheterization (E874.5)*

  ● **E874.5 Heart catheterization**

  ● **E874.8 Other specified procedures**

  ● **E874.9 Unspecified procedure**

● **E875 Contaminated or infected blood, other fluid, drug, or biological substance**

      Includes presence of:
          bacterial pyrogens
          endotoxin-producing bacteria
          serum hepatitis-producing agent

  ● **E875.0 Contaminated substance transfused or infused**

  ● **E875.1 Contaminated substance injected or used for vaccination**

  ● **E875.2 Contaminated drug or biological substance administered by other means**

  ● **E875.8 Other**

  ● **E875.9 Unspecified**

● **E876 Other and unspecified misadventures during medical care**

  ● **E876.0 Mismatched blood in transfusion**

  ● **E876.1 Wrong fluid in infusion**

  ● **E876.2 Failure in suture and ligature during surgical operation**

  ● **E876.3 Endotracheal tube wrongly placed during anesthetic procedure**

  ● **E876.4 Failure to introduce or to remove other tube or instrument**
      Excludes *foreign object left in body during procedure (E871.0-E871.9)*

  ● **E876.5 Performance of wrong operation (procedure) on correct patient**
      Wrong device implanted into correct surgical site
      Excludes *correct operation (procedure) performed on wrong body part (E876.7)*
      Coding Clinic: 2006, Q3, P9-10

  ● **E876.6 Performance of operation (procedure) on patient not scheduled for surgery**
      Performance of operation (procedure) intended for another patient
      Performance of operation (procedure) on wrong patient

  ● **E876.7 Performance of correct operation (procedure) on wrong side/body part**
      Performance of correct operation (procedure) on wrong side
      Performance of correct operation (procedure) on wrong site
      Coding Clinic: 2009, Q4, P150-151

  ● **E876.8 Other specified misadventures during medical care**
      Performance of inappropriate treatment, NEC
      Coding Clinic: 2009, Q2, P11; 2008, Q4, P152-155

  ● **E876.9 Unspecified misadventure during medical care**

E000-E999

SURGICAL AND MEDICAL PROCEDURES AS THE CAUSE OF ABNORMAL REACTION OF PATIENT OR LATER COMPLICATION, WITHOUT MENTION OF MISADVENTURE AT THE TIME OF PROCEDURE (E878-E879)

Includes   procedures as the cause of abnormal
                reaction, such as:
                displacement or malfunction of
                    prosthetic device
                hepatorenal failure, postoperative
                malfunction of external stoma
                postoperative intestinal obstruction
                rejection of transplanted organ

Excludes   *anesthetic management properly carried
                out as the cause of adverse effect
                (E937.0-E938.9)*
                *infusion and transfusion, without mention
                of misadventure in the technique of
                procedure (E930.0-E949.9)*

OGCR Section I.C.19.h.2

Assign a code in the range of E878-E879 if the
provider attributes an abnormal reaction or later
complication to a surgical or medical procedure, but
does not mention misadventure at the time of the
procedure as the cause of the reaction.

- **E878** **Surgical operation and other surgical procedures as
  the cause of abnormal reaction of patient, or of later
  complication, without mention of misadventure at the
  time of operation**

  - **E878.0** **Surgical operation with transplant of whole
    organ**
    Transplantation of:
        heart
        kidney
        liver

  - **E878.1** **Surgical operation with implant of artificial
    internal device**
        Cardiac pacemaker
        Electrodes implanted in brain
        Heart valve prosthesis
        Internal orthopedic device

  - **E878.2** **Surgical operation with anastomosis, bypass,
    or graft, with natural or artificial tissues used as
    implant**
        Anastomosis:
            arteriovenous
            gastrojejunal
        Graft of blood vessel, tendon, or skin
        Excludes *external stoma (E878.3)*

  - **E878.3** **Surgical operation with formation of external
    stoma**
        Colostomy
        Cystostomy
        Duodenostomy
        Gastrostomy
        Ureterostomy

  - **E878.4** **Other restorative surgery**

  - **E878.5** **Amputation of limb(s)**

  - **E878.6** **Removal of other organ (partial) (total)**

  - **E878.8** **Other specified surgical operations and
    procedures**

  - **E878.9** **Unspecified surgical operations and procedures**

OGCR Section I.C.19.i.2

Assign a code in the range of E878-E879 if the provider attributes
an abnormal reaction or later complication to a surgical or
medical procedure, but does not mention misadventure at the
time of the procedure as the cause of the reaction.

- **E879** **Other procedures, without mention of misadventure
  at the time of procedure, as the cause of abnormal
  reaction of patient, or of later complication**

  - **E879.0** **Cardiac catheterization**

  - **E879.1** **Kidney dialysis**
    Coding Clinic: 2003, Q4, P60-61; 1994, Q3, P9

  - **E879.2** **Radiological procedure and radiotherapy**
        Excludes *radio-opaque dyes for diagnostic x-ray
                      procedures (E947.8)*
        Coding Clinic: 2006, Q4, P88-91

  - **E879.3** **Shock therapy**
        Electroshock therapy
        Insulin-shock therapy

  - **E879.4** **Aspiration of fluid**
        Lumbar puncture
        Thoracentesis

  - **E879.5** **Insertion of gastric or duodenal sound**

  - **E879.6** **Urinary catheterization**

  - **E879.7** **Blood sampling**

  - **E879.8** **Other specified procedures**
        Blood transfusion
        Coding Clinic: 1993, Q2, P3-4

  - **E879.9** **Unspecified procedure**

ACCIDENTAL FALLS (E880-E888)

Excludes *falls (in or from):*
            burning building (E890.8, E891.8)
            into fire (E890.0-E899)
            *into water (with submersion or drowning)
                (E910.0-E910.9)*
            machinery (in operation) (E919.0-E919.9)
            *on edged, pointed, or sharp object
                (E920.0-E920.9)*
            transport vehicle (E800.0-E845.9)
            *vehicle not elsewhere classifiable
                (E846-E848)*

- **E880** **Fall on or from stairs or steps**
  - **E880.0** **Escalator**
  - **E880.1** **Fall on or from sidewalk curb**
        Excludes *fall from moving sidewalk (E885.9)*
  - **E880.9** **Other stairs or steps**

- **E881** **Fall on or from ladders or scaffolding**
  - **E881.0** **Fall from ladder**
        Coding Clinic: 2007, Q1, P3-8
  - **E881.1** **Fall from scaffolding**
        Coding Clinic: 1999, Q4, P13

- **E882** **Fall from or out of building or other structure**
        Fall from:
            balcony
            bridge
            building
            flagpole
            tower
            turret
            viaduct
            wall
            window
        Fall through roof
        Excludes *collapse of a building or structure (E916)*
                      *fall or jump from burning building (E890.8,
                      E891.8)*

◀ New   ◀▥▥ Revised   ~~deleted~~ Deleted   Excludes   Includes   Use additional   Code first   Omit code
● Unacceptable Principal Diagnosis   ● Use Additional Digit(s)   **OGCR** Official Guidelines   **Coding Clinic**

E000-E999

● **E883 Fall into hole or other opening in surface**

    Includes   fall into:
                 cavity
                 dock
                 hole
                 pit
                 quarry
                 shaft
                 swimming pool
                 tank
                 well

    Excludes *fall into water NOS (E910.9)*
                  that resulting in drowning or submersion
                     without mention of injury
                     (E910.0-E910.9)

● **E883.0 Accident from diving or jumping into water [swimming pool]**
    Strike or hit:
       against bottom when jumping or diving
           into water
       wall or board of swimming pool
       water surface

    Excludes *diving with insufficient air supply (E913.2)*
                effects of air pressure from diving (E902.2)

● **E883.1 Accidental fall into well**

● **E883.2 Accidental fall into storm drain or manhole**

● **E883.9 Fall into other hole or other opening in surface**

● **E884 Other fall from one level to another**

● **E884.0 Fall from playground equipment**
    Excludes *recreational machinery (E919.8)*
    Coding Clinic: 2007, Q1, P3-8

● **E884.1 Fall from cliff**

● **E884.2 Fall from chair**

● **E884.3 Fall from wheelchair**
    Fall from motorized mobility scooter ◄
    Fall from motorized wheelchair ◄

● **E884.4 Fall from bed**

● **E884.5 Fall from other furniture**

● **E884.6 Fall from commode**
    Toilet

● **E884.9 Other fall from one level to another**
    Fall from:
       embankment
       haystack
       stationary vehicle
       tree

● **E885 Fall on same level from slipping, tripping, or stumbling**

● **E885.0 Fall from (nonmotorized) scooter**
    Excludes *fall from motorized mobility scooter (E884.3)* ◄
    Coding Clinic: 2002, Q4, P73

● **E885.1 Fall from roller skates**
    Heelies   Wheelies
    In-line skates

● **E885.2 Fall from skateboard**
    Coding Clinic: 2000, Q4, P61

● **E885.3 Fall from skis**
    Coding Clinic: 2007, Q2, P3-4

● **E885.4 Fall from snowboard**

● **E885.9 Fall from other slipping, tripping, or stumbling**
    Fall on moving sidewalk
    Coding Clinic: 2009, Q4, P150

● **E886 Fall on same level from collision, pushing, or shoving, by or with other person**
    Excludes *crushed or pushed by a crowd or human stampede (E917.1, E917.6)*

● **E886.0 In sports**
    Tackles in sports
    Excludes *kicked, stepped on, struck by object, in sports (E917.0, E917.5)*
    Coding Clinic: 2007, Q2, P3-4

● **E886.9 Other and unspecified**
    Fall from collision of pedestrian (conveyance) with another pedestrian (conveyance)

● **E887 Fracture, cause unspecified**

● **E888 Other and unspecified fall**
    Accidental fall NOS
    Fall on same level NOS
    Coding Clinic: 1993, Q4, P25-26

● **E888.0 Fall resulting in striking against sharp object**
    Use additional external cause code to identify object (E920)

● **E888.1 Fall resulting in striking against other object**

● **E888.8 Other fall**

● **E888.9 Unspecified fall**
    Fall NOS

ACCIDENTS CAUSED BY FIRE AND FLAMES (E890-E899)

    Includes asphyxia or poisoning due to conflagration or ignition
              burning by fire
              secondary fires resulting from explosion

    Excludes *arson (E968.0)*
              fire in or on:
                machinery (in operation) (E919.0-E919.9)
                transport vehicle other than stationary vehicle (E800.0-E845.9)
                vehicle not elsewhere classifiable (E846-E848)

● **E890 Conflagration in private dwelling**

    Includes conflagration in: conflagration in:
         apartment   lodging house
         boarding house   mobile home
         camping place   private garage
         caravan   rooming house
         farmhouse   tenement
         house
       conflagration originating from sources classifiable to E893-E898 in the above buildings

● **E890.0 Explosion caused by conflagration**

● **E890.1 Fumes from combustion of polyvinylchloride [PVC] and similar material in conflagration**

● **E890.2 Other smoke and fumes from conflagration**
    Carbon monoxide from conflagration in private building
    Fumes NOS from conflagration in private building
    Smoke NOS from conflagration in private building
    Coding Clinic: 2005, Q3, P10-11

● **E890.3 Burning caused by conflagration**

E000-E999

● **E890.8 Other accident resulting from conflagration**
　　　Collapse of burning private building
　　　Fall from burning private building
　　　Hit by object falling from burning private
　　　　building
　　　Jump from burning private building

● **E890.9 Unspecified accident resulting from
　　　conflagration in private dwelling**

● **E891 Conflagration in other and unspecified building or
　structure**
　　Conflagration in:
　　　barn
　　　church
　　　convalescent and other residential home
　　　dormitory of educational institution
　　　factory
　　　farm outbuildings
　　　hospital
　　　hotel
　　　school
　　　store
　　　theater
　　Conflagration originating from sources classifiable to
　　　E893-E898, in the above buildings

● **E891.0 Explosion caused by conflagration**

● **E891.1 Fumes from combustion of polyvinylchloride
　　　[PVC] and similar material in conflagration**

● **E891.2 Other smoke and fumes from conflagration**
　　　Carbon monoxide from conflagration in
　　　　building or structure
　　　Fumes NOS from conflagration in building or
　　　　structure
　　　Smoke NOS from conflagration in building or
　　　　structure

● **E891.3 Burning caused by conflagration**

● **E891.8 Other accident resulting from conflagration**
　　　Collapse of burning building or structure
　　　Fall from burning building or structure
　　　Hit by object falling from burning building or
　　　　structure
　　　Jump from burning building or structure

● **E891.9 Unspecified accident resulting from
　　　conflagration of other and unspecified building
　　　or structure**

● **E892 Conflagration not in building or structure**
　　Fire (uncontrolled) (in) (of):
　　　forest
　　　grass
　　　hay
　　　lumber
　　　mine
　　　prairie
　　　transport vehicle [any], except while in transit
　　　tunnel

● **E893 Accident caused by ignition of clothing**
　　Excludes *ignition of clothing:*
　　　　　from highly inflammable material (E894)
　　　　　with conflagration (E890.0-E892)

● **E893.0 From controlled fire in private dwelling**
　　　Ignition of clothing from:
　　　　normal fire (charcoal) (coal) (electric) (gas)
　　　　　(wood) in:
　　　　　brazier in private dwelling (as listed in
　　　　　　E890)
　　　　　fireplace in private dwelling (as listed
　　　　　　in E890)
　　　　　furnace in private dwelling (as listed in
　　　　　　E890)
　　　　　stove in private dwelling (as listed in
　　　　　　E890)

● **E893.1 From controlled fire in other building or
　　　structure**
　　　Ignition of clothing from:
　　　　normal fire (charcoal) (coal) (electric) (gas)
　　　　　(wood) in:
　　　　　brazier in other building or structure (as
　　　　　　listed in E891)
　　　　　fireplace in other building or structure
　　　　　　(as listed in E891)
　　　　　furnace in other building or structure (as
　　　　　　listed in E891)
　　　　　stove in other building or structure (as
　　　　　　listed in E891)

● **E893.2 From controlled fire not in building or
　　　structure**
　　　Ignition of clothing from:
　　　　bonfire (controlled)
　　　　brazier fire (controlled), not in building or
　　　　　structure
　　　　trash fire (controlled)
　　Excludes *conflagration not in building (E892)*
　　　　　trash fire out of control (E892)

● **E893.8 From other specified sources**
　　　Ignition of clothing from:
　　　　blowlamp
　　　　blowtorch
　　　　burning bedspread
　　　　candle
　　　　cigar
　　　　cigarette
　　　　lighter
　　　　matches
　　　　pipe
　　　　welding torch

● **E893.9 Unspecified source**
　　　Ignition of clothing (from controlled fire NOS)
　　　　(in building NOS) NOS

● **E894 Ignition of highly inflammable material**
　　Ignition of:
　　　benzine (with ignition of clothing)
　　　gasoline (with ignition of clothing)
　　　fat (with ignition of clothing)
　　　kerosene (with ignition of clothing)
　　　paraffin (with ignition of clothing)
　　　petrol (with ignition of clothing)
　　Excludes *ignition of highly inflammable material with:*
　　　　　conflagration (E890.0-E892)
　　　　　explosion (E923.0-E923.9)

● **E895 Accident caused by controlled fire in private
　dwelling**
　　Burning by (flame of) normal fire (charcoal) (coal)
　　　(electric) (gas) (wood) in:
　　　brazier in private dwelling (as listed in E890)
　　　fireplace in private dwelling (as listed in E890)
　　　furnace in private dwelling (as listed in E890)
　　　stove in private dwelling (as listed in E890)
　　Excludes *burning by hot objects not producing fire or
　　　　　flames (E924.0-E924.9)*
　　　　　ignition of clothing from these sources (E893.0)
　　　　　*poisoning by carbon monoxide from incomplete
　　　　　　combustion of fuel (E867-E868.9)*
　　　　　that with conflagration (E890.0-E890.9)

◀ New　　◀▥ Revised　　~~deleted~~ Deleted　　| Excludes |　　| Includes |　　Use additional　　Code first　　Omit code
　　　　● Unacceptable Principal Diagnosis　　● Use Additional Digit(s)　　OGCR Official Guidelines　　**Coding Clinic**

● **E896 Accident caused by controlled fire in other and unspecified building or structure**
> Burning by (flame of) normal fire (charcoal) (coal) (electric) (gas) (wood) in:
>> brazier in other building or structure (as listed in E891)
>> fireplace in other building or structure (as listed in E891)
>> furnace in other building or structure (as listed in E891)
>> stove in other building or structure (as listed in E891)

> | Excludes | *burning by hot objects not producing fire or flames (E924.0-E924.9)* |
> *ignition of clothing from these sources (E893.1)*
> *poisoning by carbon monoxide from incomplete combustion of fuel (E867-E868.9)*
> *that with conflagration (E891.0-E891.9)*

● **E897 Accident caused by controlled fire not in building or structure**
> Burns from flame of:
>> bonfire (controlled)
>> brazier fire (controlled), not in building or structure
>> trash fire (controlled)

> | Excludes | *ignition of clothing from these sources (E893.2)*
> *trash fire out of control (E892)*
> *that with conflagration (E892)*

● **E898 Accident caused by other specified fire and flames**

> | Excludes | *conflagration (E890.0-E892)*
> *that with ignition of:*
>> *clothing (E893.0-E893.9)*
>> *highly inflammable material (E894)*

● **E898.0 Burning bedclothes**
> Bed set on fire NOS

● **E898.1 Other**
> | Burning by: | Burning by: |
> | blowlamp | lamp |
> | blowtorch | lighter |
> | candle | matches |
> | cigar | pipe |
> | cigarette | welding torch |
> | fire in room NOS | |

● **E899 Accident caused by unspecified fire**
> Burning NOS

ACCIDENTS DUE TO NATURAL AND ENVIRONMENTAL FACTORS (E900-E909)

● **E900 Excessive heat**

● **E900.0 Due to weather conditions**
> Excessive heat as the external cause of:
>> ictus solaris
>> siriasis
>> sunstroke

● **E900.1 Of man-made origin**
> Heat (in):
>> boiler room
>> drying room
>> factory
>> furnace room
>> generated in transport vehicle
>> kitchen

● **E900.9 Of unspecified origin**

● **E901 Excessive cold**

● **E901.0 Due to weather conditions**
> Excessive cold as the cause of:
>> chilblains NOS
>> immersion foot

● **E901.1 Of man-made origin**
> Contact with or inhalation of:
>> dry ice
>> liquid air
>> liquid hydrogen
>> liquid nitrogen
> Prolonged exposure in:
>> deep freeze unit
>> refrigerator

● **E901.8 Other specified origin**

● **E901.9 Of unspecified origin**

● **E902 High and low air pressure and changes in air pressure**

● **E902.0 Residence or prolonged visit at high altitude**
> Residence or prolonged visit at high altitude as the cause of:
>> Acosta syndrome
>> Alpine sickness
>> altitude sickness
>> Andes disease
>> anoxia, hypoxia
>> barotitis, barodontalgia, barosinusitis, otitic barotrauma
>> hypobarism, hypobaropathy
>> mountain sickness
>> range disease

● **E902.1 In aircraft**
> Sudden change in air pressure in aircraft during ascent or descent as the cause of:
>> aeroneurosis
>> aviators' disease

● **E902.2 Due to diving**
> High air pressure from rapid descent in water as the cause of:
>> caisson disease
>> divers' disease
>> divers' palsy or paralysis
> Reduction in atmospheric pressure while surfacing from deep water diving as the cause of:
>> caisson disease
>> divers' disease
>> divers' palsy or paralysis

● **E902.8 Due to other specified causes**
> Reduction in atmospheric pressure while surfacing from under ground

● **E902.9 Unspecified cause**

● **E903 Travel and motion**

● **E904 Hunger, thirst, exposure, and neglect**

> | Excludes | *any condition resulting from homicidal intent (E968.0-E968.9)*
> *hunger, thirst, and exposure resulting from accidents connected with transport (E800.0-E848)*

● **E904.0 Abandonment or neglect of infants and helpless persons**
> Desertion of newborn
> Exposure to weather conditions resulting from abandonment or neglect
> Hunger or thirst resulting from abandonment or neglect
> Inattention at or after birth
> Lack of care (helpless person) (infant)

> | Excludes | *criminal [purposeful] neglect (E968.4)*

OGCR Section I.C.19.e.2

In cases of neglect when the intent is determined to be accidental E code E904.0 should be the first listed E code.

- ● **E904.1** **Lack of food**
  Lack of food as the cause of:
  inanition
  insufficient nourishment
  starvation
  | Excludes | *hunger resulting from abandonment or neglect (E904.0)*

- ● **E904.2** **Lack of water**
  Lack of water as the cause of:
  dehydration
  inanition
  | Excludes | *dehydration due to acute fluid loss (276.51)*

- ● **E904.3** **Exposure (to weather conditions), not elsewhere classifiable**
  Exposure NOS
  Humidity
  Struck by hailstones
  | Excludes | *struck by lightning (E907)*

- ● **E904.9** **Privation, unqualified**
  Destitution

- ● **E905** **Venomous animals and plants as the cause of poisoning and toxic reactions**
  | Includes | chemical released by animal
  insects
  release of venom through fangs, hairs, spines, tentacles, and other venom apparatus
  | Excludes | *eating of poisonous animals or plants (E865.0-E865.9)*

- ● **E905.0** **Venomous snakes and lizards**
  Cobra
  Copperhead snake
  Coral snake
  Fer de lance
  Gila monster
  Krait
  Mamba
  Rattlesnake
  Sea snake
  Snake (venomous)
  Viper
  Water moccasin
  | Excludes | *bites of snakes and lizards known to be nonvenomous (E906.2)*

- ● **E905.1** **Venomous spiders**
  Black widow spider
  Brown spider
  Tarantula (venomous)

- ● **E905.2** **Scorpion**

- ● **E905.3** **Hornets, wasps, and bees**
  Yellow jacket

- ● **E905.4** **Centipede and venomous millipede (tropical)**

- ● **E905.5** **Other venomous arthropods**
  Sting of:
  ant
  caterpillar

- ● **E905.6** **Venomous marine animals and plants**
  Puncture by sea urchin spine
  Sting of:
  coral
  jelly fish
  nematocysts
  sea anemone
  sea cucumber
  other marine animal or plant
  | Excludes | *bites and other injuries caused by nonvenomous marine animal (E906.2-E906.8)*
  bite of sea snake (venomous) (E905.0)

- ● **E905.7** **Poisoning and toxic reactions caused by other plants**
  Injection of poisons or toxins into or through skin by plant thorns, spines, or other mechanisms
  | Excludes | *puncture wound NOS by plant thorns or spines (E920.8)*

- ● **E905.8** **Other specified**

- ● **E905.9** **Unspecified**
  Sting NOS
  Venomous bite NOS

- ● **E906** **Other injury caused by animals**
  | Excludes | *poisoning and toxic reactions caused by venomous animals and insects (E905.0-E905.9)*
  road vehicle accident involving animals (E827.0-E828.9)
  tripping or falling over an animal (E885.9)

- ● **E906.0** **Dog bite**

- ● **E906.1** **Rat bite**

- ● **E906.2** **Bite of nonvenomous snakes and lizards**

- ● **E906.3** **Bite of other animal except arthropod**
  Cats
  Moray eel
  Rodents, except rats
  Shark

- ● **E906.4** **Bite of nonvenomous arthropod**
  Insect bite NOS

- ● **E906.5** **Bite by unspecified animal**
  Animal bite NOS

- ● **E906.8** **Other specified injury caused by animal**
  Butted by animal
  Fallen on by horse or other animal, not being ridden
  Gored by animal
  Implantation of quills of porcupine
  Pecked by bird
  Run over by animal, not being ridden
  Stepped on by animal, not being ridden
  | Excludes | *injury by animal being ridden (E828.0-E828.9)*

- ● **E906.9** **Unspecified injury caused by animal**

- ● **E907** **Lightning**
  | Excludes | *injury from:*
  fall of tree or other object caused by lightning (E916)
  fire caused by lightning (E890.0-E892)

- ● **E908** **Cataclysmic storms, and floods resulting from storms**
  | Excludes | *collapse of dam or man-made structure causing flood (E909.3)*

- ● **E908.0** **Hurricane**
  Storm surge
  "Tidal wave" caused by storm action
  Typhoon

- ● **E908.1** **Tornado**
  Cyclone   Twisters

- ● **E908.2** **Floods**
  Torrential rainfall   Flash flood
  | Excludes | *collapse of dam or man-made structure causing flood (E909.3)*

- ● **E908.3** **Blizzard (snow) (ice)**

- ● **E908.4** **Dust storm**

- ● **E908.8** **Other cataclysmic storms**

- ● **E908.9** **Unspecified cataclysmic storms, and floods resulting from storms**
  Storm NOS

◀ New   ◀░ Revised   ~~deleted~~ Deleted | Excludes | | Includes | Use additional   Code first   Omit code
● Unacceptable Principal Diagnosis   ● Use Additional Digit(s)   **OGCR** Official Guidelines   **Coding Clinic**

● **E909 Cataclysmic earth surface movements and eruptions**

  ● **E909.0 Earthquakes**

  ● **E909.1 Volcanic eruptions**
      Burns from lava   Ash inhalation

  ● **E909.2 Avalanche, landslide, or mudslide**

  ● **E909.3 Collapse of dam or man-made structure**

  ● **E909.4 Tidal wave caused by earthquake**
      Tidal wave NOS   Tsunami

Excludes	*tidal wave caused by tropical storm (E908.0)*

  ● **E909.8 Other cataclysmic earth surface movements and eruptions**

  ● **E909.9 Unspecified cataclysmic earth surface movements and eruptions**

ACCIDENTS CAUSED BY SUBMERSION, SUFFOCATION, AND FOREIGN BODIES (E910-E915)

● **E910 Accidental drowning and submersion**

Includes	immersion swimmers' cramp

Excludes	*diving accident (NOS) (resulting in injury except drowning) (E883.0)*
	diving with insufficient air supply (E913.2)
	drowning and submersion due to:
	  cataclysm (E908-E909)
	  machinery accident (E919.0-E919.9)
	  transport accident (E800.0-E845.9)
	effect of high and low air pressure (E902.2)
	injury from striking against objects while in running water (E917.2)

  ● **E910.0 While water-skiing**
      Fall from water skis with submersion or drowning

Excludes	*accident to water-skier involving a watercraft and resulting in submersion or other injury (E830.4, E831.4)*

  ● **E910.1 While engaged in other sport or recreational activity with diving equipment**
      Scuba diving NOS
      Skin diving NOS
      Underwater spear fishing NOS

  ● **E910.2 While engaged in other sport or recreational activity without diving equipment**
      Fishing or hunting, except from boat or with diving equipment
      Ice skating
      Playing in water
      Surfboarding
      Swimming NOS
      Voluntarily jumping from boat, not involved in accident, for swim NOS
      Wading in water

Excludes	*jumping into water to rescue another person (E910.3)*

  ● **E910.3 While swimming or diving for purposes other than recreation or sport**
      Marine salvage (with diving equipment)
      Pearl diving (with diving equipment)
      Placement of fishing nets (with diving equipment)
      Rescue (attempt) of another person (with diving equipment)
      Underwater construction or repairs (with diving equipment)

  ● **E910.4 In bathtub**

  ● **E910.8 Other accidental drowning or submersion**
      Drowning in:
        quenching tank
        swimming pool

  ● **E910.9 Unspecified accidental drowning or submersion**
      Accidental fall into water NOS
      Drowning NOS

● **E911 Inhalation and ingestion of food causing obstruction of respiratory tract or suffocation**
      Aspiration and inhalation of food [any] (into respiratory tract) NOS
      Asphyxia by food [including bone, seed in food, regurgitated food]
      Choked on food [including bone, seed in food, regurgitated food]
      Suffocation by food [including bone, seed in food, regurgitated food]
      Compression of trachea by food lodged in esophagus
      Interruption of respiration by food lodged in esophagus
      Obstruction of respiration by food lodged in esophagus
      Obstruction of pharynx by food (bolus)

Excludes	*injury, except asphyxia and obstruction of respiratory passage, caused by food (E915)* *obstruction of esophagus by food without mention of asphyxia or obstruction of respiratory passage (E915)*

● **E912 Inhalation and ingestion of other object causing obstruction of respiratory tract or suffocation**
      Aspiration and inhalation of foreign body except food (into respiratory tract) NOS
      Compression by foreign body in esophagus
      Foreign object [bean] [marble] in nose
      Interruption of respiration by foreign body in esophagus
      Obstruction of pharynx by foreign body
      Obstruction of respiration by foreign body in esophagus

Excludes	*injury, except asphyxia and obstruction of respiratory passage, caused by foreign body (E915)* *obstruction of esophagus by foreign body without mention of asphyxia or obstruction in respiratory passage (E915)*

● **E913 Accidental mechanical suffocation**

Excludes	*mechanical suffocation from or by:*
	  accidental inhalation or ingestion of:
	    food (E911)
	    foreign object (E912)
	  cataclysm (E908-E909)
	  explosion (E921.0-E921.9, E923.0-E923.9)
	  machinery accident (E919.0-E919.9)

  ● **E913.0 In bed or cradle**

Excludes	*suffocation by plastic bag (E913.1)*

  ● **E913.1 By plastic bag**

● **E913.2 Due to lack of air (in closed place)**
Accidentally closed up in refrigerator or other
airtight enclosed space
Diving with insufficient air supply

> **Excludes** | *suffocation by plastic bag (E913.1)*

● **E913.3 By falling earth or other substance**
Cave-in NOS

> **Excludes** | *cave-in caused by cataclysmic
earth surface movements and
eruptions (E909.8)
struck by cave-in without
asphyxiation or suffocation
(E916)*

● **E913.8 Other specified means**
Accidental hanging, except in bed or cradle

● **E913.9 Unspecified means**
Asphyxia, mechanical NOS
Strangulation NOS
Suffocation NOS

● **E914 Foreign body accidentally entering eye and adnexa**

> **Excludes** | *corrosive liquid (E924.1)*

● **E915 Foreign body accidentally entering other orifice**

> **Excludes** | *aspiration and inhalation of foreign body,
any, (into respiratory tract) NOS
(E911-E912)*

OTHER ACCIDENTS (E916-E928)

● **E916 Struck accidentally by falling object**
Collapse of building, except on fire
Falling:
    rock
    snowslide NOS
    stone
    tree
Object falling from:
    machine, not in operation
    stationary vehicle

> *Code first* collapse of building on fire (E890.0-E891.9)
    falling object in:
        cataclysm (E908-E909)
        machinery accidents (E919.0-E919.9)
        transport accidents (E800.0-E845.9)
        vehicle accidents not elsewhere classifiable
            (E846-E848)
    object set in motion by:
        explosion (E921.0-E921.9, E923.0-E923.9)
        firearm (E922.0-E922.9)
        projected object (E917.0-E917.9)

● **E917 Striking against or struck accidentally by objects or persons**

> **Includes** | bumping into or against
        object (moving) (projected) (stationary)
        pedestrian conveyance
        person
    colliding with
        object (moving) (projected) (stationary)
        pedestrian conveyance
        person
    kicking against
        object (moving) (projected) (stationary)
        pedestrian conveyance
        person
    stepping on
        object (moving) (projected) (stationary)
        pedestrian conveyance
        person
    struck by
        object (moving) (projected) (stationary)
        pedestrian conveyance
        person

> **Excludes** | *fall from:
        collision with another person, except when
            caused by a crowd (E886.0-E886.9)
        stumbling over object (E885.9)
        fall resulting in striking against object
            (E888.0-E888.1)
        injury caused by:
            assault (E960.0-E960.1, E967.0-E967.9)
            cutting or piercing instrument
                (E920.0-E920.9)
            explosion (E921.0-E921.9,
                E923.0-E923.9)
            firearm (E922.0-E922.9)
            machinery (E919.0-E919.9)
            transport vehicle (E800.0-E845.9)
            vehicle not elsewhere classifiable
                (E846-E848)*

● **E917.0 In sports without subsequent fall**
Kicked or stepped on during game (football)
    (rugby)
Struck by hit or thrown ball
Struck by hockey stick or puck
Coding Clinic: 2007, Q2, P3-4; 2006, Q1, P8; 2004, Q1, P9

● **E917.1 Caused by a crowd, by collective fear or panic
without subsequent fall**
Crushed by crowd or human stampede
Pushed by crowd or human stampede
Stepped on by crowd or human stampede

● **E917.2 In running water without subsequent fall**

> **Excludes** | *drowning or submersion
        (E910.0-E910.9) that in sports
        (E917.0, E917.5)*

● **E917.3 Furniture without subsequent fall**

> **Excludes** | *fall from furniture (E884.2,
        E884.4–E884.5)*

● **E917.4 Other stationary object without subsequent fall**
Bath tub
Fence
Lamp-post

● **E917.5 Object in sports with subsequent fall**
Knocked down while boxing
Coding Clinic: 2007, Q2, P3-4

● **E917.6 Caused by a crowd, by collective fear or panic
with subsequent fall**

● **E917.7 Furniture with subsequent fall**

> **Excludes** | *fall from furniture (E884.2,
        E884.4–E884.5)*

◀ New   ◀▥ Revised   ~~deleted~~ Deleted   Excludes   Includes   Use additional   Code first   Omit code
● Unacceptable Principal Diagnosis   ● Use Additional Digit(s)   OGCR Official Guidelines   Coding Clinic

● **E917.8 Other stationary object with subsequent fall**
    Bath tub
    Fence
    Lamp-post

● **E917.9 Other striking against with or without subsequent fall**

● **E918 Caught accidentally in or between objects**
    Caught, crushed, jammed, or pinched in or between
        moving or stationary objects, such as:
    escalator
    folding object
    hand tools, appliances, or implements
    sliding door and door frame
    under packing crate
    washing machine wringer

    | Excludes | *injury caused by:*
    cutting or piercing instrument (E920.0-
        E920.9)
    machinery (E919.0-E919.9)
    mechanism or component of firearm and
        air gun (E928.7)
    transport vehicle (E800.0-E845.9)
    vehicle not elsewhere classifiable
        (E846-E848)
    struck accidentally by:
        falling object (E916)
        object (moving) (projected) (E917.0-E917.9)

● **E919 Accidents caused by machinery**

    | Includes | burned by machinery (accident)
    caught between machinery and other
        object
    caught in (moving parts of) machinery
        (accident)
    collapse of machinery (accident)
    crushed by machinery (accident)
    cut or pierced by machinery (accident)
    drowning or submersion caused by
        machinery (accident)
    explosion of, on, in machinery (accident)
    fall from or into moving part of machinery
        (accident)
    fire starting in or on machinery (accident)
    mechanical suffocation caused by
        machinery (accident)
    object falling from, on, in motion by
        machinery (accident)
    overturning of machinery (accident)
    pinned under machinery (accident)
    run over by machinery (accident)
    struck by machinery (accident)
    thrown from machinery (accident)
    machinery accident NOS

    | Excludes | *accidents involving machinery, not in*
        operation (E884.9, E916-E918)
    injury caused by:
        electric current in connection with
            machinery (E925.0-E925.9)
        escalator (E880.0, E918)
        explosion of pressure vessel in connection
            with machinery (E921.0-E921.9)
        mechanism or component of firearm and
            air gun (E928.7)
        moving sidewalk (E885.9)
        powered hand tools, appliances,
            and implements (E916-E918,
            E920.0-E921.9, E923.0-E926.9)
        transport vehicle accidents involving
            machinery (E800.0-E848.9)
        poisoning by carbon monoxide generated by
            machine (E868.8)

● **E919.0 Agricultural machines**
    Animal-powered agricultural machine
    Combine
    Derrick, hay
    Farm machinery NOS
    Farm tractor
    Harvester
    Hay mower or rake
    Reaper
    Thresher

    | Excludes | *that being towed by another vehicle on*
        the highway (E810.0-E819.9,
        E827.0-E827.9, E829.0-E829.9)
    that in transport under own power on
        the highway (E810.0-E819.9)
    that involved in accident classifiable to
        E820-E829 (E820.0-E829.9)

● **E919.1 Mining and earth-drilling machinery**
    Bore or drill (land) (seabed)
    Shaft hoist
    Shaft lift
    Under-cutter

    | Excludes | *coal car, tram, truck, and tub in mine*
        (E846)

● **E919.2 Lifting machines and appliances**
    Chain hoist except in agricultural or mining
        operations
    Crane except in agricultural or mining
        operations
    Derrick except in agricultural or mining
        operations
    Elevator (building) (grain) except in
        agricultural or mining operations
    Forklift truck except in agricultural or mining
        operations
    Lift except in agricultural or mining
        operations
    Pulley block except in agricultural or mining
        operations
    Winch except in agricultural or mining
        operations

    | Excludes | *that being towed by another vehicle on*
        the highway (E810.0-E819.9,
        E827.0-E827.9, E829.0-E829.9)
    that in transport under own power on
        the highway (E810.0-E819.9)
    that involved in accident classifiable to
        E820-E829 (E820.0-E829.9)

● **E919.3 Metalworking machines**
    Abrasive wheel   Metal:
    Forging machine   milling machine
    Lathe   power press
    Mechanical shears   rolling-mill
    Metal: sawing machine
        drilling machine
    Coding Clinic: 2003, Q4, P76-78

● **E919.4 Woodworking and forming machines**
    Band saw   Overhead plane
    Bench saw   Powered saw
    Circular saw   Radial saw
    Molding machine   Sander

    | Excludes | *hand saw (E920.1)*

E000-E999

● **E919.5 Prime movers, except electrical motors**
  Gas turbine
  Internal combustion engine
  Steam engine
  Water driven turbine
  Excludes | *that being towed by other vehicle on*
  the highway (E810.0-E819.9,
  E827.0-E827.9, E829.0-E829.9)
  that in transport under own power on
  the highway (E810.0-E819.9)

● **E919.6 Transmission machinery**

Transmission:	Transmission:
belt	pinion
cable	pulley
chain	shaft
gear	

● **E919.7 Earth moving, scraping, and other excavating machines**

Bulldozer	Steam shovel
Road scraper	

  Excludes | *that being towed by other vehicle on*
  the highway (E810.0-E819.9)
  that in transport under own power on
  the highway (E810.0-E819.9)

● **E919.8 Other specified machinery**
  Machines for manufacture of:
    clothing
    foodstuffs and beverages
    paper
  Printing machine
  Recreational machinery
  Spinning, weaving, and textile machines

● **E919.9 Unspecified machinery**

● **E920 Accidents caused by cutting and piercing instruments or objects**
  Includes accidental injury (by) object:
    edged
    pointed
    sharp
  Excludes | *injury caused by mechanism or component of*
  firearm and air gun (E928.7)

● **E920.0 Powered lawn mower**

● **E920.1 Other powered hand tools**
  Any powered hand tool [compressed air]
    [electric] [explosive cartridge] [hydraulic
    power], such as:
    drill
    hand saw
    hedge clipper
    rivet gun
    snow blower
    staple gun
  Excludes | *band saw (E919.4)*
  bench saw (E919.4)

● **E920.2 Powered household appliances and implements**
  Blender
  Electric:
    beater or mixer
    can opener
    fan
    knife
    sewing machine
  Garbage disposal appliance

● **E920.3 Knives, swords, and daggers**

● **E920.4 Other hand tools and implements**
  Axe
  Can opener NOS
  Chisel
  Fork
  Hand saw
  Hoe
  Ice pick
  Needle (sewing)
  Paper cutter
  Pitchfork
  Rake
  Scissors
  Screwdriver
  Sewing machine, not powered
  Shovel

● **E920.5 Hypodermic needle**
  Contaminated needle
  Needle stick

● **E920.8 Other specified cutting and piercing instruments or objects**

Arrow	Nail
Broken glass	Plant thorn
Dart	Splinter
Edge of stiff paper	Tin can lid
Lathe turnings	

  Excludes | *animal spines or quills (E906.8)*
  flying glass due to explosion
  (E921.0-E923.9)
  Coding Clinic: 2001, Q3, P10

● **E920.9 Unspecified cutting and piercing instrument or object**

● **E921 Accident caused by explosion of pressure vessel**
  Includes accidental explosion of pressure vessels,
  whether or not part of machinery
  Excludes | *explosion of pressure vessel on transport*
  vehicle (E800.0-E845.9)

● **E921.0 Boilers**
  Coding Clinic: 2005, Q3, P10-11

● **E921.1 Gas cylinders**
  Air tank
  Pressure gas tank

● **E921.8 Other specified pressure vessels**
  Aerosol can
  Automobile tire
  Pressure cooker

  E921.9 Unspecified pressure vessel

● **E922 Accident caused by firearm and air gun missile**
  Excludes | *injury caused by mechanism or component*
  of firearm and air gun (E928.7)

● **E922.0 Handgun**
  Pistol
  Revolver
  Excludes | *Verey pistol (E922.8)*

● **E922.1 Shotgun (automatic)**

● **E922.2 Hunting rifle**

● **E922.3 Military firearms**
  Army rifle
  Machine gun

● **E922.4 Air gun**
  BB gun
  Pellet gun

● **E922.5 Paintball gun**
  Coding Clinic: 2002, Q4, P74

◀ New   ◀▥ Revised   ~~deleted~~ Deleted   Excludes   Includes   Use additional   Code first   Omit code
● Unacceptable Principal Diagnosis   ● Use Additional Digit(s)   OGCR Official Guidelines   Coding Clinic

● **E922.8 Other specified firearm missile**
Verey pistol [flare]

● **E922.9 Unspecified firearm missile**
Gunshot wound NOS
Shot NOS

● **E923 Accident caused by explosive material**

> **Includes** flash burns and other injuries resulting
> from explosion of explosive material
> ignition of highly explosive material with
> explosion

> **Excludes** *explosion:*
> *in or on machinery (E919.0-E919.9)*
> *on any transport vehicle, except stationary*
> *motor vehicle (E800.0-E848)*
> *with conflagration (E890.0, E891.0, E892)*
> *injury caused by mechanism or component*
> *of firearm and air gun (E928.7)*
> *secondary fires resulting from explosion*
> *(E890.0-E899)*

● **E923.0 Fireworks**

● **E923.1 Blasting materials**

Blasting cap	Explosive [any]
Detonator	used in blasting
Dynamite	operations

● **E923.2 Explosive gases**
Acetylene
Butane
Coal gas
Explosion in mine NOS
Fire damp
Gasoline fumes
Methane
Propane

● **E923.8 Other explosive materials**

Bomb	Torpedo
Explosive missile	Explosion in munitions:
Grenade	dump
Mine	factory
Shell	

● **E923.9 Unspecified explosive material**
Explosion NOS

● **E924 Accident caused by hot substance or object, caustic or corrosive material, and steam**

> **Excludes** *burning NOS (E899)*
> *chemical burn resulting from swallowing a*
> *corrosive substance (E860.0-E864.4)*
> *fire caused by these substances and objects*
> *(E890.0-E894)*
> *radiation burns (E926.0-E926.9)*
> *therapeutic misadventures (E870.0-E876.9)*

● **E924.0 Hot liquids and vapors, including steam**
Burning or scalding by:
boiling water
hot or boiling liquids not primarily caustic
or corrosive
liquid metal
other hot vapor
steam

> **Excludes** *hot (boiling) tap water (E924.2)*

● **E924.1 Caustic and corrosive substances**
Burning by:
acid [any kind]
ammonia
caustic oven cleaner or other substance
corrosive substance
lye
vitriol

● **E924.2 Hot (boiling) tap water**

● **E924.8 Other**
Burning by:
heat from electric heating appliance
hot object NOS
light bulb
steam pipe

● **E924.9 Unspecified**

● **E925 Accident caused by electric current**

> **Includes** electric current from exposed wire, faulty
> appliance, high voltage cable, live
> rail, or open electric socket as the
> cause of:
> burn
> cardiac fibrillation
> convulsion
> electric shock
> electrocution
> puncture wound
> respiratory paralysis

> **Excludes** *burn by heat from electrical appliance (E924.8)*
> *lightning (E907)*

● **E925.0 Domestic wiring and appliances**

● **E925.1 Electric power generating plants, distribution stations, transmission lines**
Broken power line

● **E925.2 Industrial wiring, appliances, and electrical machinery**
Conductors
Control apparatus
Electrical equipment and machinery
Transformers

● **E925.8 Other electric current**
Wiring and appliances in or on:
farm [not farmhouse]
outdoors
public building
residential institutions
schools

● **E925.9 Unspecified electric current**
Burns or other injury from electric current
NOS
Electric shock NOS
Electrocution NOS

E000-E999

● E926 **Exposure to radiation**

> Excludes | abnormal reaction to or complication
> of treatment without mention of
> misadventure (E879.2)
> atomic power plant malfunction in water
> transport (E838.0-E838.9)
> misadventure to patient in surgical and
> medical procedures (E873.2-E873.3)
> use of radiation in war operations
> (E996-E997.9)

● E926.0 **Radiofrequency radiation**
Overexposure to:
microwave radiation from:
high-powered radio and television
transmitters
industrial radiofrequency induction
heaters
radar installations
radar radiation from:
high-powered radio and television
transmitters
industrial radiofrequency induction
heaters
radar installations
radiofrequency from:
high-powered radio and television
transmitters
industrial radiofrequency induction
heaters
radar installations
radiofrequency radiation [any] from:
high-powered radio and television
transmitters
industrial radiofrequency induction
heaters
radar installations

● E926.1 **Infra-red heaters and lamps**
Exposure to infra-red radiation from heaters
and lamps as the cause of:
blistering   charring
burning   inflammatory change

> Excludes | physical contact with heater or lamp
> (E924.8)

● E926.2 **Visible and ultraviolet light sources**
Arc lamps
Black light sources
Electrical welding arc
Oxygas welding torch
Sun rays
Tanning bed

> Excludes | excessive heat from these sources
> (E900.1-E900.9)

Coding Clinic: 1996, Q3, P6

● E926.3 **X-rays and other electromagnetic ionizing
radiation**
Gamma rays
X-rays (hard) (soft)

● E926.4 **Lasers**

● E926.5 **Radioactive isotopes**
Radiobiologicals
Radiopharmaceuticals

● E926.8 **Other specified radiation**
Artificially accelerated beams of ionized
particles generated by:
betatrons
synchrotrons

● E926.9 **Unspecified radiation**
Radiation NOS

● E927 **Overexertion and strenuous and repetitive
movements or loads**

> Use additional code to identify activity (E001-E030)
> Coding Clinic: 2009, Q3, P18; 2008, Q3, P21

● E927.0 **Overexertion from sudden strenuous
movement**
Sudden trauma from strenuous movement

● E927.1 **Overexertion from prolonged static position**
Overexertion from maintaining prolonged
positions, such as:
holding
sitting
standing

● E927.2 **Excessive physical exertion from prolonged
activity**

● E927.3 **Cumulative trauma from repetitive motion**
Cumulative trauma from repetitive
movements
Coding Clinic: 2009, Q3, P20

● E927.4 **Cumulative trauma from repetitive impact**
Coding Clinic: 2009, Q3, P20x3, 21

● E927.8 **Other overexertion and strenuous and
repetitive movements or loads**

● E927.9 **Unspecified overexertion and strenuous and
repetitive movements or loads**

● E928 **Other and unspecified environmental and accidental
causes**

● E928.0 **Prolonged stay in weightless environment**
Weightlessness in spacecraft (simulator)

● E928.1 **Exposure to noise**
Noise (pollution)
Sound waves
Supersonic waves

● E928.2 **Vibration**

● E928.3 **Human bite**

● E928.4 **External constriction caused by hair**

● E928.5 **External constriction caused by other object**

● E928.6 **Environmental exposure to harmful algae
and toxins**
Algae bloom NOS
Blue-green algae bloom
Brown tide
Cyanobacteria bloom
Florida red tide
Harmful algae bloom
Pfiesteria piscicida
Red tide
Coding Clinic: 2007, Q4, P101-102

● E928.7 **Mechanism or component of firearm and
air gun**
Injury due to:
explosion of gun parts
recoil
Pierced, cut, crushed, or pinched by slide
trigger mechanism, scope or other gun
part
Powder burn from firearm or air gun

> Excludes | accident caused by firearm and air
> gun missile (E922.0-E922.9)

● E928.8 **Other**

◄ New   ◀▥ Revised   ~~deleted~~ Deleted   Excludes   Includes   Use additional   Code first   Omit code
● Unacceptable Principal Diagnosis   ● Use Additional Digit(s)   OGCR Official Guidelines   Coding Clinic

● **E928.9 Unspecified accident**
Accident NOS stated as accidentally inflicted
Blow NOS stated as accidentally inflicted
Casualty (not due to war) stated as accidentally inflicted
Decapitation stated as accidentally inflicted
Injury [any part of body, or unspecified] stated as accidentally inflicted, but not otherwise specified
Killed stated as accidentally inflicted, but not otherwise specified
Knocked down stated as accidentally inflicted, but not otherwise specified
Mangled stated as accidentally inflicted, but not otherwise specified
Wound stated as accidentally inflicted, but not otherwise specified

> **Excludes** *fracture, cause unspecified (E887)*
> *injuries undetermined whether accidentally or purposely inflicted (E980.0-E989)*
> Coding Clinic: 1996, Q3, P7; 1985, Nov-Dec, P15; 1984, Nov-Dec, P15

LATE EFFECTS OF ACCIDENTAL INJURY (E929)

Note: This category is to be used to indicate accidental injury as the cause of death or disability from late effects, which are themselves classifiable elsewhere. The "late effects" include conditions reported as such or as sequelae, which may occur at any time after the acute accidental injury.

● **E929 Late effects of accidental injury**

> **Excludes** *late effects of:*
> *surgical and medical procedures (E870.0-E879.9)*
> *therapeutic use of drugs and medicines (E930.0-E949.9)*

● **E929.0 Late effects of motor vehicle accident**
Late effects of accidents classifiable to E810-E825
Coding Clinic: 2008, Q4, P102-109; 1997, Q3, P12-13; 1995, Q1, P10; 1994, Q3, P4

● **E929.1 Late effects of other transport accident**
Late effects of accidents classifiable to E800-E807, E826-E838, E840-E848

● **E929.2 Late effects of accidental poisoning**
Late effects of accidents classifiable to E850-E858, E860-E869

● **E929.3 Late effects of accidental fall**
Late effects of accidents classifiable to E880-E888

● **E929.4 Late effects of accident caused by fire**
Late effects of accidents classifiable to E890-E899

● **E929.5 Late effects of accident due to natural and environmental factors**
Late effects of accidents classifiable to E900-E909

● **E929.8 Late effects of other accidents**
Late effects of accidents classifiable to E910-E928.8

● **E929.9 Late effects of unspecified accident**
Late effects of accidents classifiable to E928.9

OGCR Section I.C.17.e.1

Adverse Effect: When the drug was correctly prescribed and properly administered, code the reaction plus the appropriate code from the E930-E949 series. Codes from the E930-E949 series must be used to identify the causative substance for an adverse effect of drug, medicinal and biological substances, correctly prescribed and properly administered. The effect, such as tachycardia, delirium, gastrointestinal hemorrhaging, vomiting, hypokalemia, hepatitis, renal failure, or respiratory failure, is coded and followed by the appropriate code from the E930-E949 series.

DRUGS, MEDICINAL AND BIOLOGICAL SUBSTANCES CAUSING ADVERSE EFFECTS IN THERAPEUTIC USE (E930-E949)

> **Includes** correct drug properly administered in therapeutic or prophylactic dosage, as the cause of any adverse effect including allergic or hypersensitivity reactions

> **Excludes** *accidental overdose of drug and wrong drug given or taken in error (E850.0-E858.9)*
> *accidents in the technique of administration of drug or biological substance such as accidental puncture during injection, or contamination of drug (E870.0-E876.9)*
> *administration with suicidal or homicidal intent or intent to harm, or in circumstances classifiable to E950.0-E950.5, E962.0, E980.0-E980.5*

See Alphabetic Index for more complete list of specific drugs to be classified under the fourth-digit subdivisions. The American Hospital Formulary numbers can be used to classify new drugs listed by the American Hospital Formulary Service (AHFS). See appendix C.

● **E930 Antibiotics**

> **Excludes** *that used as eye, ear, nose, and throat [ENT], and local anti-infectives (E946.0-E946.9)*
> Coding Clinic: 2008, Q3, P21

● **E930.0 Penicillins**
Natural
Synthetic
Semisynthetic, such as:
ampicillin
cloxacillin
nafcillin
oxacillin
Coding Clinic: 2008, Q4, P128-131

● **E930.1 Antifungal antibiotics**
Amphotericin B
Griseofulvin
Hachimycin [trichomycin]
Nystatin

● **E930.2 Chloramphenicol group**
Chloramphenicol
Thiamphenicol

● **E930.3 Erythromycin and other macrolides**
Oleandomycin
Spiramycin

● **E930.4 Tetracycline group**
Doxycycline
Minocycline
Oxytetracycline
Coding Clinic: 1988, Q2, P9-10

● **E930.5 Cephalosporin group**
Cephalexin
Cephaloglycin
Cephaloridine
Cephalothin

E000-E999

◄ New　◄▬ Revised　~~deleted~~ Deleted　Excludes　Includes　Use additional　Code first　Omit code
● Unacceptable Principal Diagnosis　● Use Additional Digit(s)　OGCR Official Guidelines　Coding Clinic

1081

- **E930.6 Antimycobacterial antibiotics**
  - Cycloserine
  - Kanamycin
  - Rifampin
  - Streptomycin
- **E930.7 Antineoplastic antibiotics**
  - Actinomycins, such as:
    - bleomycin
    - cactinomycin
    - dactinomycin
    - daunorubicin
    - mitomycin
  - **Excludes** *other antineoplastic drugs (E933.1)*
  - Coding Clinic: 2007, Q2, P9-10
- **E930.8 Other specified antibiotics**
  - Coding Clinic: 1993, Q1, P29
- **E930.9 Unspecified antibiotic**

- **E931 Other anti-infectives**
  - **Excludes** *ENT, and local anti-infectives (E946.0-E946.9)*
  - **E931.0 Sulfonamides**
    - Sulfadiazine
    - Sulfafurazole
    - Sulfamethoxazole
  - **E931.1 Arsenical anti-infectives**
  - **E931.2 Heavy metal anti-infectives**
    - Compounds of:
      - antimony
      - bismuth
      - lead
      - mercury
    - **Excludes** *mercurial diuretics (E944.0)*
  - **E931.3 Quinoline and hydroxyquinoline derivatives**
    - Chiniofon
    - Diiodohydroxyquin
    - **Excludes** *antimalarial drugs (E931.4)*
  - **E931.4 Antimalarials and drugs acting on other blood protozoa**
    - Chloroquine phosphate
    - Cycloguanil
    - Primaquine
    - Proguanil [chloroguanide]
    - Pyrimethamine
    - Quinine (sulphate)
  - **E931.5 Other antiprotozoal drugs**
    - Emetine
  - **E931.6 Anthelmintics**
    - Hexylresorcinol
    - Male fern oleoresin
    - Piperazine
    - Thiabendazole
  - **E931.7 Antiviral drugs**
    - Methisazone
    - **Excludes** *amantadine (E936.4)*
      cytarabine (E933.1)
      idoxuridine (E946.5)
  - **E931.8 Other antimycobacterial drugs**
    - Ethambutol
    - Ethionamide
    - Isoniazid
    - Para-aminosalicylic acid derivatives
    - Sulfones
  - **E931.9 Other and unspecified anti-infectives**
    - Flucytosine
    - Nitrofuran derivatives

- **E932 Hormones and synthetic substitutes**
  - **E932.0 Adrenal cortical steroids**
    - Cortisone derivatives
    - Desoxycorticosterone derivatives
    - Fluorinated corticosteroids
    - Coding Clinic: 2008, Q4, P91-95; 2003, Q4, P108-109; 2000, Q3, P4-5
  - **E932.1 Androgens and anabolic congeners**
    - Nandrolone phenpropionate
    - Oxymetholone
    - Testosterone and preparations
    - Coding Clinic: 1985, July-Aug, P8
  - **E932.2 Ovarian hormones and synthetic substitutes**
    - Contraceptives, oral
    - Estrogens
    - Estrogens and progestogens combined
    - Progestogens
  - **E932.3 Insulins and antidiabetic agents**
    - Acetohexamide
    - Biguanide derivatives, oral
    - Chlorpropamide
    - Glucagon
    - Insulin
    - Phenformin
    - Sulfonylurea derivatives, oral
    - Tolbutamide
    - **Excludes** *adverse effect of insulin administered for shock therapy (E879.3)*
  - **E932.4 Anterior pituitary hormones**
    - Corticotropin
    - Gonadotropin
    - Somatotropin [growth hormone]
    - Coding Clinic: 1995, Q3, P15
  - **E932.5 Posterior pituitary hormones**
    - Vasopressin
    - **Excludes** *oxytocic agents (E945.0)*
  - **E932.6 Parathyroid and parathyroid derivatives**
  - **E932.7 Thyroid and thyroid derivatives**
    - Dextrothyroxine
    - Levothyroxine sodium
    - Liothyronine
    - Thyroglobulin
  - **E932.8 Antithyroid agents**
    - Iodides
    - Thiouracil
    - Thiourea
  - **E932.9 Other and unspecified hormones and synthetic substitutes**

- **E933 Primarily systemic agents**
  - **E933.0 Antiallergic and antiemetic drugs**
    - Antihistamines
    - Chlorpheniramine
    - Diphenhydramine
    - Diphenylpyraline
    - Thonzylamine
    - Tripelennamine
    - **Excludes** *phenothiazine-based tranquilizers (E939.1)*
    - Coding Clinic: 1997, Q2, P9-10

● **E933.1 Antineoplastic and immunosuppressive drugs**
   Azathioprine
   Busulfan
   Chlorambucil
   Cyclophosphamide
   Cytarabine
   Fluorouracil
   Mechlorethamine hydrochloride
   Mercaptopurine
   Triethylenethiophosphoramide [thio-TEPA]

   Excludes *antineoplastic antibiotics (E930.7)*

   Coding Clinic: 2009, Q4, P151; 2008, Q2, P6, 10-11; 2006, Q4,
      P69-73; Q2, P20; 2005, Q3, P11-12; 1999, Q3, P6-7;
      Q2, P9; 1996, Q2, P12; 1985, Mar-April, P14

● **E933.2 Acidifying agents**

● **E933.3 Alkalizing agents**

● **E933.4 Enzymes, not elsewhere classified**
   Penicillinase

● **E933.5 Vitamins, not elsewhere classified**
   Vitamin A
   Vitamin D

   Excludes *nicotinic acid (E942.2)*
                 vitamin K (E934.3)

● **E933.6 Oral bisphosphonates**
   Coding Clinic: 2007, Q4, P91-92, 102

● **E933.7 Intravenous bisphosphonates**
   Coding Clinic: 2007, Q4, P102

● **E933.8 Other systemic agents, not elsewhere classified**
   Heavy metal antagonists

● **E933.9 Unspecified systemic agent**

● **E934 Agents primarily affecting blood constituents**
   Coding Clinic: 1993, 5th Issue, P16

● **E934.0 Iron and its compounds**
   Ferric salts
   Ferrous sulphate and other ferrous salts

● **E934.1 Liver preparations and other antianemic agents**
   Folic acid

● **E934.2 Anticoagulants**
   Coumarin
   Heparin
   Phenindione
   Prothrombin synthesis inhibitor
   Warfarin sodium
   Coding Clinic: 2008, Q4, P134-136; 2006, Q3, P12-13; Q2,
      P17; 2004, Q3, P7; 1994, Q1, P22; 1990, Q3, P14

● **E934.3 Vitamin K [phytonadione]**

● **E934.4 Fibrinolysis-affecting drugs**
   Aminocaproic acid
   Streptodornase
   Streptokinase
   Urokinase

● **E934.5 Anticoagulant antagonists and other coagulants**
   Hexadimethrine bromide
   Protamine sulfate

● **E934.6 Gamma globulin**

● **E934.7 Natural blood and blood products**
   Blood plasma
   Human fibrinogen
   Packed red cells
   Whole blood
   Coding Clinic: 2006, Q4, P91-92; 2000, Q3, P9; 1997, Q2, P11

● **E934.8 Other agents affecting blood constituents**
   Macromolecular blood substitutes

● **E934.9 Unspecified agent affecting blood constituents**

● **E935 Analgesics, antipyretics, and antirheumatics**

● **E935.0 Heroin**
   Diacetylmorphine

● **E935.1 Methadone**

● **E935.2 Other opiates and related narcotics**
   Codeine [methylmorphine]
   Morphine
   Opium (alkaloids)
   Meperidine [pethidine]

● **E935.3 Salicylates**
   Acetylsalicylic acid [aspirin]
   Amino derivatives of salicylic acid
   Salicylic acid salts
   Coding Clinic: 1984, Nov-Dec, P15

● **E935.4 Aromatic analgesics, not elsewhere classified**
   Acetanilid
   Paracetamol [acetaminophen]
   Phenacetin [acetophenetidin]

● **E935.5 Pyrazole derivatives**
   Aminophenazone [aminopyrine]
   Phenylbutazone
   Coding Clinic: 1990, Q4, P26

● **E935.6 Antirheumatics [antiphlogistics]**
   Gold salts
   Indomethacin

   Excludes *salicylates (E935.3)*
                 steroids (E932.0)

● **E935.7 Other non-narcotic analgesics**
   Pyrabital

● **E935.8 Other specified analgesics and antipyretics**
   Pentazocine
   Coding Clinic: 1992, Q3, P16-17

● **E935.9 Unspecified analgesic and antipyretic**

● **E936 Anticonvulsants and anti-Parkinsonism drugs**

● **E936.0 Oxazolidine derivatives**
   Paramethadione
   Trimethadione

● **E936.1 Hydantoin derivatives**
   Phenytoin

● **E936.2 Succinimides**
   Ethosuximide
   Phensuximide

● **E936.3 Other and unspecified anticonvulsants**
   Beclamide
   Primidone

● **E936.4 Anti-Parkinsonism drugs**
   Amantadine
   Ethopropazine [profenamine]
   Levodopa [L-dopa]

● **E937 Sedatives and hypnotics**

● **E937.0 Barbiturates**
   Amobarbital [amylobarbitone]
   Barbital [barbitone]
   Butabarbital [butabarbitone]
   Pentobarbital [pentobarbitone]
   Phenobarbital [phenobarbitone]
   Secobarbital [quinalbarbitone]

   Excludes *thiobarbiturates (E938.3)*

● **E937.1 Chloral hydrate group**

● **E937.2 Paraldehyde**

● **E937.3 Bromine compounds**
   Bromide
   Carbromal (derivatives)

● **E937.4 Methaqualone compounds**

E000-E999

- E937.5 **Glutethimide group**
- E937.6 **Mixed sedatives, not elsewhere classified**
- E937.8 **Other sedatives and hypnotics**
- E937.9 **Unspecified**
    Sleeping:
        drug NOS
        pill NOS
        tablet NOS

● E938 **Other central nervous system depressants and anesthetics**

- E938.0 **Central nervous system muscle-tone depressants**
    Chlorphenesin (carbamate)
    Mephenesin
    Methocarbamol
- E938.1 **Halothane**
- E938.2 **Other gaseous anesthetics**
    Ether
    Halogenated hydrocarbon derivatives, except halothane
    Nitrous oxide
- E938.3 **Intravenous anesthetics**
    Ketamine
    Methohexital [methohexitone]
    Thiobarbiturates, such as thiopental sodium
- E938.4 **Other and unspecified general anesthetics**
- E938.5 **Surface and infiltration anesthetics**
    Cocaine
    Lidocaine [lignocaine]
    Procaine
    Tetracaine
- E938.6 **Peripheral nerve- and plexus-blocking anesthetics**
- E938.7 **Spinal anesthetics**
    Coding Clinic: 2004, Q2, P18; 2003, Q3, P12; 1987, Jan-Feb, P13-14
- E938.9 **Other and unspecified local anesthetics**

● E939 **Psychotropic agents**

- E939.0 **Antidepressants**
    Amitriptyline
    Imipramine
    Monoamine oxidase [MAO] inhibitors
    Coding Clinic: 2003, Q4, P75-76; 1992, Q3, P16
- E939.1 **Phenothiazine-based tranquilizers**
    Chlorpromazine   Prochlorperazine
    Fluphenazine   Promazine
    Phenothiazine
- E939.2 **Butyrophenone-based tranquilizers**
    Haloperidol
    Spiperone
    Trifluperidol
- E939.3 **Other antipsychotics, neuroleptics, and major tranquilizers**
    Coding Clinic: 2010, Q1, P20-21; 2006, Q4, P76-78
- E939.4 **Benzodiazepine-based tranquilizers**
    Chlordiazepoxide   Lorazepam
    Diazepam   Medazepam
    Flurazepam   Nitrazepam
- E939.5 **Other tranquilizers**
    Hydroxyzine
    Meprobamate
- E939.6 **Psychodysleptics [hallucinogens]**
    Cannabis (derivatives)
    Lysergide [LSD]
    Marihuana (derivatives)
    Mescaline
    Psilocin
    Psilocybin

- E939.7 **Psychostimulants**
    Amphetamine
    Caffeine
    Excludes *central appetite depressants (E947.0)*
- E939.8 **Other psychotropic agents**
- E939.9 **Unspecified psychotropic agent**

● E940 **Central nervous system stimulants**

- E940.0 **Analeptics**
    Lobeline
    Nikethamide
- E940.1 **Opiate antagonists**
    Levallorphan
    Nalorphine
    Naloxone
- E940.8 **Other specified central nervous system stimulants**
- E940.9 **Unspecified central nervous system stimulant**

● E941 **Drugs primarily affecting the autonomic nervous system**

- E941.0 **Parasympathomimetics [cholinergics]**
    Acetylcholine
    Anticholinesterase:
        organophosphorus
        reversible
    Pilocarpine
- E941.1 **Parasympatholytics [anticholinergics and antimuscarinics] and spasmolytics**
    Atropine
    Homatropine
    Hyoscine [scopolamine]
    Quaternary ammonium derivatives
    Excludes *papaverine (E942.5)*
- E941.2 **Sympathomimetics [adrenergics]**
    Epinephrine [adrenalin]
    Levarterenol [noradrenalin]
    Coding Clinic: 2002, Q3, P12
- E941.3 **Sympatholytics [antiadrenergics]**
    Phenoxybenzamine
    Tolazoline hydrochloride
    Coding Clinic: 2007, Q4, P77-79
- E941.9 **Unspecified drug primarily affecting the autonomic nervous system**

● E942 **Agents primarily affecting the cardiovascular system**

- E942.0 **Cardiac rhythm regulators**
    Practolol
    Procainamide
    Propranolol
    Quinidine
    Coding Clinic: 1986, Mar-April, P11-12
- E942.1 **Cardiotonic glycosides and drugs of similar action**
    Digitalis glycosides
    Digoxin
    Strophanthins
- E942.2 **Antilipemic and antiarteriosclerotic drugs**
    Cholestyramine
    Clofibrate
    Nicotinic acid derivatives
    Sitosterols
    Excludes *dextrothyroxine (E932.7)*
- E942.3 **Ganglion-blocking agents**
    Pentamethonium bromide

◀ New   ◀▥ Revised   ~~deleted~~ Deleted   Excludes   Includes   Use additional   Code first   Omit code
● Unacceptable Principal Diagnosis   ● Use Additional Digit(s)   OGCR Official Guidelines   Coding Clinic

E000-E999

● **E942.4 Coronary vasodilators**
    Dipyridamole
    Nitrates [nitroglycerin]
    Nitrites
    Prenylamine

● **E942.5 Other vasodilators**
    Cyclandelate
    Diazoxide
    Hydralazine
    Papaverine

● **E942.6 Other antihypertensive agents**
    Clonidine
    Guanethidine
    Rauwolfia alkaloids
    Reserpine

● **E942.7 Antivaricose drugs, including sclerosing agents**
    Monoethanolamine
    Zinc salts

● **E942.8 Capillary-active drugs**
    Adrenochrome derivatives
    Bioflavonoids
    Metaraminol

● **E942.9 Other and unspecified agents primarily affecting the cardiovascular system**

● **E943 Agents primarily affecting gastrointestinal system**

● **E943.0 Antacids and antigastric secretion drugs**
    Aluminum hydroxide
    Magnesium trisilicate

● **E943.1 Irritant cathartics**
    Bisacodyl
    Castor oil
    Phenolphthalein

● **E943.2 Emollient cathartics**
    Sodium dioctyl sulfosuccinate

● **E943.3 Other cathartics, including intestinal atonia drugs**
    Magnesium sulfate

● **E943.4 Digestants**
    Pancreatin
    Papain
    Pepsin

● **E943.5 Antidiarrheal drugs**
    Bismuth subcarbonate
    Kaolin
    Pectin
    Excludes *anti-infectives (E930.0-E931.9)*

● **E943.6 Emetics**

● **E943.8 Other specified agents primarily affecting the gastrointestinal system**

● **E943.9 Unspecified agent primarily affecting the gastrointestinal system**

● **E944 Water, mineral, and uric acid metabolism drugs**

● **E944.0 Mercurial diuretics**
    Chlormerodrin
    Mercaptomerin
    Mercurophylline
    Mersalyl

● **E944.1 Purine derivative diuretics**
    Theobromine
    Theophylline
    Excludes *aminophylline [theophylline ethylenediamine] (E945.7)*

● **E944.2 Carbonic acid anhydrase inhibitors**
    Acetazolamide

● **E944.3 Saluretics**
    Benzothiadiazides
    Chlorothiazide group

● **E944.4 Other diuretics**
    Ethacrynic acid
    Furosemide

● **E944.5 Electrolytic, caloric, and water-balance agents**

● **E944.6 Other mineral salts, not elsewhere classified**

● **E944.7 Uric acid metabolism drugs**
    Cinchophen and congeners
    Colchicine
    Phenoquin
    Probenecid

● **E945 Agents primarily acting on the smooth and skeletal muscles and respiratory system**

● **E945.0 Oxytocic agents**
    Ergot alkaloids
    Prostaglandins

● **E945.1 Smooth muscle relaxants**
    Adiphenine
    Metaproterenol [orciprenaline]
    Excludes *papaverine (E942.5)*

● **E945.2 Skeletal muscle relaxants**
    Alcuronium chloride
    Suxamethonium chloride

● **E945.3 Other and unspecified drugs acting on muscles**

● **E945.4 Antitussives**
    Dextromethorphan
    Pipazethate hydrochloride

● **E945.5 Expectorants**
    Acetylcysteine
    Cocillana
    Guaifenesin [glyceryl guaiacolate]
    Ipecacuanha
    Terpin hydrate

● **E945.6 Anti-common cold drugs**

● **E945.7 Antiasthmatics**
    Aminophylline [theophylline ethylenediamine]

● **E945.8 Other and unspecified respiratory drugs**

● **E946 Agents primarily affecting skin and mucous membrane, ophthalmological, otorhinolaryngological, and dental drugs**

● **E946.0 Local anti-infectives and anti-inflammatory drugs**

● **E946.1 Antipruritics**

● **E946.2 Local astringents and local detergents**

● **E946.3 Emollients, demulcents, and protectants**

● **E946.4 Keratolytics, keratoplastics, other hair treatment drugs and preparations**

● **E946.5 Eye anti-infectives and other eye drugs**
    Idoxuridine

● **E946.6 Anti-infectives and other drugs and preparations for ear, nose, and throat**

● **E946.7 Dental drugs topically applied**

● **E946.8 Other agents primarily affecting skin and mucous membrane**
    Spermicides

● **E946.9 Unspecified agent primarily affecting skin and mucous membrane**

E000-E999

● **E947 Other and unspecified drugs and medicinal substances**
- ● E947.0 Dietetics
- ● E947.1 Lipotropic drugs
- ● E947.2 Antidotes and chelating agents, not elsewhere classified
- ● E947.3 Alcohol deterrents
- ● E947.4 Pharmaceutical excipients
- ● E947.8 Other drugs and medicinal substances
  Contrast media used for diagnostic x-ray procedures
  Diagnostic agents and kits
- ● E947.9 Unspecified drug or medicinal substance

● **E948 Bacterial vaccines**
- ● E948.0 BCG vaccine
- ● E948.1 Typhoid and paratyphoid
- ● E948.2 Cholera
- ● E948.3 Plague
- ● E948.4 Tetanus
- ● E948.5 Diphtheria
- ● E948.6 Pertussis vaccine, including combinations with a pertussis component
- ● E948.8 Other and unspecified bacterial vaccines
- ● E948.9 Mixed bacterial vaccines, except combinations with a pertussis component

● **E949 Other vaccines and biological substances**

> **Excludes** *gamma globulin (E934.6)*
>
> Coding Clinic: 2008, Q3, P21

- ● E949.0 Smallpox vaccine
- ● E949.1 Rabies vaccine
- ● E949.2 Typhus vaccine
- ● E949.3 Yellow fever vaccine
- ● E949.4 Measles vaccine
- ● E949.5 Poliomyelitis vaccine
- ● E949.6 Other and unspecified viral and rickettsial vaccines
  Mumps vaccine
- ● E949.7 Mixed viral-rickettsial and bacterial vaccines, except combinations with a pertussis component

  > **Excludes** *combinations with a pertussis component (E948.6)*

- ● E949.9 Other and unspecified vaccines and biological substances

SUICIDE AND SELF-INFLICTED INJURY (E950-E959)

> **Includes** injuries in suicide and attempted suicide
> self-inflicted injuries specified as intentional

● **E950 Suicide and self-inflicted poisoning by solid or liquid substances**
- ● E950.0 Analgesics, antipyretics, and antirheumatics
  Coding Clinic: 1998, Q4, P50-51
- ● E950.1 Barbiturates
- ● E950.2 Other sedatives and hypnotics
- ● E950.3 Tranquilizers and other psychotropic agents
- ● E950.4 Other specified drugs and medicinal substances
- ● E950.5 Unspecified drug or medicinal substance
- ● E950.6 Agricultural and horticultural chemical and pharmaceutical preparations other than plant foods and fertilizers
- ● E950.7 Corrosive and caustic substances
  Suicide and self-inflicted poisoning by substances classifiable to E864
- ● E950.8 Arsenic and its compounds
- ● E950.9 Other and unspecified solid and liquid substances

● **E951 Suicide and self-inflicted poisoning by gases in domestic use**
- ● E951.0 Gas distributed by pipeline
- ● E951.1 Liquefied petroleum gas distributed in mobile containers
- ● E951.8 Other utility gas

● **E952 Suicide and self-inflicted poisoning by other gases and vapors**
- ● E952.0 Motor vehicle exhaust gas
- ● E952.1 Other carbon monoxide
- ● E952.8 Other specified gases and vapors
- ● E952.9 Unspecified gases and vapors

● **E953 Suicide and self-inflicted injury by hanging, strangulation, and suffocation**
- ● E953.0 Hanging
- ● E953.1 Suffocation by plastic bag
- ● E953.8 Other specified means
- ● E953.9 Unspecified means

● **E954 Suicide and self-inflicted injury by submersion [drowning]**

● **E955 Suicide and self-inflicted injury by firearms, air guns and explosives**
- ● E955.0 Handgun
- ● E955.1 Shotgun
- ● E955.2 Hunting rifle
- ● E955.3 Military firearms
- ● E955.4 Other and unspecified firearm
  Gunshot NOS
  Shot NOS
- ● E955.5 Explosives
- ● E955.6 Air gun
  BB gun
  Pellet gun
- ● E955.7 Paintball gun
- ● E955.9 Unspecified

● **E956 Suicide and self-inflicted injury by cutting and piercing instrument**

● **E957 Suicide and self-inflicted injuries by jumping from high place**
- ● E957.0 Residential premises
- ● E957.1 Other man-made structures
- ● E957.2 Natural sites
- ● E957.9 Unspecified

◄ New   ◀▥ Revised   ~~deleted~~ Deleted   Excludes   Includes   Use additional   Code first   Omit code
● Unacceptable Principal Diagnosis   ● Use Additional Digit(s)   OGCR Official Guidelines   Coding Clinic

E000-E999

- ● **E958 Suicide and self-inflicted injury by other and unspecified means**
  - ● **E958.0 Jumping or lying before moving object**
  - ● **E958.1 Burns, fire**
  - ● **E958.2 Scald**
  - ● **E958.3 Extremes of cold**
  - ● **E958.4 Electrocution**
  - ● **E958.5 Crashing of motor vehicle**
  - ● **E958.6 Crashing of aircraft**
  - ● **E958.7 Caustic substances, except poisoning**
    > **Excludes** *poisoning by caustic substance (E950.7)*
  - ● **E958.8 Other specified means**
  - ● **E958.9 Unspecified means**

- ● **E959 Late effects of self-inflicted injury**
  > **Note:** This category is to be used to indicate circumstances classifiable to E950-E958 as the cause of death or disability from late effects, which are themselves classifiable elsewhere. The "late effects" include conditions reported as such or as sequelae which may occur at any time after the attempted suicide or self-inflicted injury.

  OGCR Section I.C.19.d.1
  > When the cause of an injury or neglect is intentional child or adult abuse, the first listed E code should be assigned from categories E960-E968, Homicide and injury purposely inflicted by other persons, (except category E967). An E code from category E967, Child and adult battering and other maltreatment, should be added as an additional code to identify the perpetrator, if known.

HOMICIDE AND INJURY PURPOSELY INFLICTED BY OTHER PERSONS (E960-E969)

> **Includes** injuries inflicted by another person with intent to injure or kill, by any means

> **Excludes** *injuries due to:*
> *legal intervention (E970-E978)*
> *operations of war (E990-E999)*
> *terrorism (E979)*

- ● **E960 Fight, brawl, rape**
  - ● **E960.0 Unarmed fight or brawl**
    Beatings NOS
    Brawl or fight with hands, fists, feet
    Injured or killed in fight NOS
    > **Excludes** *homicidal:*
    > *injury by weapons (E965.0-E966, E969)*
    > *strangulation (E963)*
    > *submersion (E964)*
  - ● **E960.1 Rape**
    Coding Clinic: 1999, Q3, P15

- ● **E961 Assault by corrosive or caustic substance, except poisoning**
  Injury or death purposely caused by corrosive or caustic substance, such as:
  acid [any]
  corrosive substance
  vitriol
  > **Excludes** *burns from hot liquid (E968.3)*
  > *chemical burns from swallowing a corrosive substance (E962.0-E962.9)*

- ● **E962 Assault by poisoning**
  - ● **E962.0 Drugs and medicinal substances**
    Homicidal poisoning by any drug or medicinal substance
  - ● **E962.1 Other solid and liquid substances**
  - ● **E962.2 Other gases and vapors**
  - ● **E962.9 Unspecified poisoning**

- ● **E963 Assault by hanging and strangulation**
  Homicidal (attempt):
  garrotting or ligature
  hanging
  strangulation
  suffocation

- ● **E964 Assault by submersion [drowning]**

- ● **E965 Assault by firearms and explosives**
  - ● **E965.0 Handgun**
    Pistol
    Revolver
  - ● **E965.1 Shotgun**
  - ● **E965.2 Hunting rifle**
  - ● **E965.3 Military firearms**
  - ● **E965.4 Other and unspecified firearm**
  - ● **E965.5 Antipersonnel bomb**
  - ● **E965.6 Gasoline bomb**
  - ● **E965.7 Letter bomb**
  - ● **E965.8 Other specified explosive**
    Bomb NOS (placed in):
    car
    house
    Dynamite
  - ● **E965.9 Unspecified explosive**

- ● **E966 Assault by cutting and piercing instrument**
  Assassination (attempt), homicide (attempt) by any instrument classifiable under E920
  Homicidal:
  cut any part of body
  puncture any part of body
  stab any part of body
  Stabbed any part of body
  Coding Clinic: 1993, Q2, P4-5

- ● **E967 Perpetrator of child and adult abuse**
  > **Note:** Selection of the correct perpetrator code is based on the relationship between the perpetrator and the victim.
  - ● **E967.0 By father, stepfather, or boyfriend**
    Male partner of child's parent or guardian
  - ● **E967.1 By other specified person**
    Coding Clinic: 1999, Q3, P14-15
  - ● **E967.2 By mother, stepmother, or girlfriend**
    Female partner of child's parent or guardian
    Coding Clinic: 1996, Q4, P43-44
  - ● **E967.3 By spouse or partner**
    Abuse of spouse or partner by ex-spouse or ex-partner
    Coding Clinic: 1996, Q4, P43-44
  - ● **E967.4 By child**
  - ● **E967.5 By sibling**
  - ● **E967.6 By grandparent**
  - ● **E967.7 By other relative**
  - ● **E967.8 By non-related caregiver**
  - ● **E967.9 By unspecified person**

E000-E999

● **E968 Assault by other and unspecified means**

   ● **E968.0 Fire**
       Arson
       Homicidal burns NOS

        Excludes *burns from hot liquid (E968.3)*

   ● **E968.1 Pushing from a high place**

   ● **E968.2 Striking by blunt or thrown object**
       Coding Clinic: 1996, Q4, P43-44

   ● **E968.3 Hot liquid**
       Homicidal burns by scalding

   ● **E968.4 Criminal neglect**
       Abandonment of child, infant, or other
          helpless person with intent to injure or
          kill

   ● **E968.5 Transport vehicle**
       Being struck by other vehicle or run down
          with intent to injure
       Pushed in front of, thrown from, or dragged
          by moving vehicle with intent to injure

   ● **E968.6 Air gun**
       BB gun
       Pellet gun

   ● **E968.7 Human bite**

   ● **E968.8 Other specified means**
       Coding Clinic: 1999, Q3, P14-15x2

   ● **E968.9 Unspecified means**
       Assassination (attempt) NOS
       Homicidal (attempt):
         injury NOS
         wound NOS
       Manslaughter (nonaccidental)
       Murder (attempt) NOS
       Violence, non-accidental

E969 Late effects of injury purposely inflicted by other person

   Note: This category is to be used to indicate
      circumstances classifiable to E960-E968 as the
      cause of death or disability from late effects,
      which are themselves classifiable elsewhere.
      The "late effects" include conditions reported
      as such, or as sequelae which may occur at
      any time after the injury purposely inflicted by
      another person.

LEGAL INTERVENTION (E970-E978)

   Includes injuries inflicted by the police or other
      law-enforcing agents, including
      military on duty, in the course
      of arresting or attempting to
      arrest lawbreakers, suppressing
      disturbances, maintaining order, and
      other legal action
      legal execution

   Excludes *injuries caused by civil insurrections*
      (E990.0-E999)

● **E970 Injury due to legal intervention by firearms**
       Gunshot wound
       Injury by:
         machine gun
         revolver
         rifle pellet or rubber bullet
         shot NOS

● **E971 Injury due to legal intervention by explosives**
       Injury by:
         dynamite
         explosive shell
         grenade
         motor bomb

● **E972 Injury due to legal intervention by gas**
       Asphyxiation by gas
       Injury by tear gas
       Poisoning by gas

● **E973 Injury due to legal intervention by blunt object**
       Hit, struck by:
         baton (nightstick)
         blunt object
         stave

● **E974 Injury due to legal intervention by cutting and piercing instrument**
       Cut
       Incised wound
       Injured by bayonet
       Stab wound

● **E975 Injury due to legal intervention by other specified means**
       Blow
       Manhandling

● **E976 Injury due to legal intervention by unspecified means**

● **E977 Late effects of injuries due to legal intervention**
   Note: This category is to be used to indicate
      circumstances classifiable to E970-E976 as the
      cause of death or disability from late effects,
      which are themselves classifiable elsewhere.
      The "late effects" include conditions reported
      as such, or as sequelae which may occur at any
      time after the injury due to legal intervention.

● **E978 Legal execution**
       All executions performed at the behest of the judiciary
         or ruling authority [whether permanent or
         temporary] as:
       asphyxiation by gas
       beheading, decapitation (by guillotine)
       capital punishment
       electrocution
       hanging
       poisoning
       shooting
       other specified means

OGCR Section I.C.19.j.1-3

When the cause of an injury is identified by the Federal Government (FBI) as terrorism, the first-listed E-code should be a code from category E979, Terrorism. The definition of terrorism employed by the FBI is found at the inclusion note at E979. The terrorism E-code is the only E-code that should be assigned. Additional E codes from the assault categories should not be assigned.

When the cause of an injury is suspected to be the result of terrorism a code from category E979 should not be assigned. Assign a code in the range of E codes based circumstances on the documentation of intent and mechanism.

Assign code E979.9, Terrorism, secondary effects, for conditions occurring subsequent to the terrorist event. This code should not be assigned for conditions that are due to the initial terrorist act.

TERRORISM (E979)

● **E979 Terrorism**
Injuries resulting from the unlawful use of force or violence against persons or property to intimidate or coerce a Government, the civilian population, or any segment thereof, in furtherance of political or social objective
Coding Clinic: 2002, Q4, P74-77

● **E979.0 Terrorism involving explosion of marine weapons**
Depth-charge
Marine mine
Mine NOS, at sea or in harbour
Sea-based artillery shell
Torpedo
Underwater blast

● **E979.1 Terrorism involving destruction of aircraft**
Aircraft:
burned
exploded
shot down
Aircraft used as a weapon
Crushed by falling aircraft

● **E979.2 Terrorism involving other explosions and fragments**
Antipersonnel bomb (fragments)
Blast NOS
Explosion (of):
artillery shell
breech-block
cannon block
mortar bomb
munitions being used in terrorism
NOS
Fragments from:
artillery shell
bomb
grenade
guided missile
land-mine
rocket
shell
shrapnel
Mine NOS

● **E979.3 Terrorism involving fires, conflagration and hot substances**
Burning building or structure:
collapse of
fall from
hit by falling object in
jump from
Conflagration NOS
Fire (causing):
asphyxia
burns
NOS
other injury
Melting of fittings and furniture in burning
Petrol bomb
Smouldering building or structure

● **E979.4 Terrorism involving firearms**
Bullet:
carbine
machine gun
pistol
rifle
rubber (rifle)
Pellets (shotgun)

● **E979.5 Terrorism involving nuclear weapons**
Blast effects
Exposure to ionizing radiation from nuclear weapon
Fireball effects
Heat from nuclear weapon
Other direct and secondary effects of nuclear weapons

● **E979.6 Terrorism involving biological weapons**
Anthrax
Cholera
Smallpox

● **E979.7 Terrorism involving chemical weapons**
Gases, fumes, chemicals
Hydrogen cyanide
Phosgene
Sarin

● **E979.8 Terrorism involving other means**
Drowning and submersion
Lasers
Piercing or stabbing instruments
Terrorism NOS

● **E979.9 Terrorism secondary effects**
Note: This code is for use to identify conditions occurring subsequent to a terrorist attack not those that are due to the initial terrorist attack
Excludes late effect of terrorist attack (E999.1)

INJURY UNDETERMINED WHETHER ACCIDENTALLY OR PURPOSELY INFLICTED (E980-E989)

Note: Categories E980-E989 are for use when it is unspecified or it cannot be determined whether the injuries are accidental (unintentional), suicide (attempted), or assault.

● **E980 Poisoning by solid or liquid substances, undetermined whether accidentally or purposely inflicted**
● **E980.0 Analgesics, antipyretics, and antirheumatics**
● **E980.1 Barbiturates**
● **E980.2 Other sedatives and hypnotics**
● **E980.3 Tranquilizers and other psychotropic agents**
● **E980.4 Other specified drugs and medicinal substances**
● **E980.5 Unspecified drug or medicinal substance**
● **E980.6 Corrosive and caustic substances**
Poisoning, undetermined whether accidental or purposeful, by substances classifiable to E864
● **E980.7 Agricultural and horticultural chemical and pharmaceutical preparations other than plant foods and fertilizers**
● **E980.8 Arsenic and its compounds**
● **E980.9 Other and unspecified solid and liquid substances**

● **E981 Poisoning by gases in domestic use, undetermined whether accidentally or purposely inflicted**
● **E981.0 Gas distributed by pipeline**
● **E981.1 Liquefied petroleum gas distributed in mobile containers**
● **E981.8 Other utility gas**

E000-E999

● **E982 Poisoning by other gases, undetermined whether accidentally or purposely inflicted**
  ● E982.0 Motor vehicle exhaust gas
  ● E982.1 Other carbon monoxide
  ● E982.8 Other specified gases and vapors
  ● E982.9 Unspecified gases and vapors

● **E983 Hanging, strangulation, or suffocation, undetermined whether accidentally or purposely inflicted**
  ● E983.0 Hanging
  ● E983.1 Suffocation by plastic bag
  ● E983.8 Other specified means
  ● E983.9 Unspecified means

● **E984 Submersion [drowning], undetermined whether accidentally or purposely inflicted**

● **E985 Injury by firearms, air guns and explosives, undetermined whether accidentally or purposely inflicted**
  ● E985.0 Handgun
  ● E985.1 Shotgun
  ● E985.2 Hunting rifle
  ● E985.3 Military firearms
  ● E985.4 Other and unspecified firearm
  ● E985.5 Explosives
  ● E985.6 Air gun
    BB gun
    Pellet gun
  ● E985.7 Paintball gun

● **E986 Injury by cutting and piercing instruments, undetermined whether accidentally or purposely inflicted**

● **E987 Falling from high place, undetermined whether accidentally or purposely inflicted**
  ● E987.0 Residential premises
  ● E987.1 Other man-made structures
  ● E987.2 Natural sites
  ● E987.9 Unspecified site

● **E988 Injury by other and unspecified means, undetermined whether accidentally or purposely inflicted**
  ● E988.0 Jumping or lying before moving object
  ● E988.1 Burns, fire
  ● E988.2 Scald
  ● E988.3 Extremes of cold
  ● E988.4 Electrocution
  ● E988.5 Crashing of motor vehicle
  ● E988.6 Crashing of aircraft
  ● E988.7 Caustic substances, except poisoning
  ● E988.8 Other specified means
  ● E988.9 Unspecified means

● **E989 Late effects of injury, undetermined whether accidentally or purposely inflicted**
  Note: This category is to be used to indicate circumstances classifiable to E980-E988 as the cause of death or disability from late effects, which are themselves classifiable elsewhere. The "late effects" include conditions reported as such or as sequelae which may occur at any time after injury, undetermined whether accidentally or purposely inflicted.

INJURY RESULTING FROM OPERATIONS OF WAR (E990-E999)

Includes injuries to military personnel and civilians caused by war and civil insurrections and occurring during the time of war and insurrection, and peacekeeping missions

Excludes *accidents during training of military personnel, manufacture of war material and transport, unless attributable to enemy action*

● **E990 Injury due to war operations by fires and conflagrations**
  Includes asphyxia, burns, or other injury originating from fire caused by a fire-producing device or indirectly by any conventional weapon
  ● E990.0 From gasoline bomb
    Incendiary bomb
  ● E990.1 From flamethrower
  ● E990.2 From incendiary bullet
  ● E990.3 From fire caused indirectly from conventional weapon
    Excludes *fire aboard military aircraft (E994.3)*
  ● E990.9 From other and unspecified source

● **E991 Injury due to war operations by bullets and fragments**
  Excludes *injury due to bullets and fragments due to war operations, but occurring after cessation of hostilities (E998.0)*
    injury due to explosion of artillery shells and mortars (E993.2)
    injury due to explosion of improvised explosive device [IED] (E993.3-E993.5)
    injury due to sea-based artillery shell (E992.3)
  ● E991.0 Rubber bullets (rifle)
  ● E991.1 Pellets (rifle)
  ● E991.2 Other bullets
    Bullet [any, except rubber bullets and pellets]
    carbine
    machine gun
    pistol
    rifle
    shotgun
  ● E991.3 Antipersonnel bomb (fragments)
  ● E991.4 Fragments from munitions
    Fragments from:
    artillery shell
    bombs, except antipersonnel
    detonation of unexploded ordnance [UXO]
    grenade
    guided missile
    land mine
    rockets
    shell
  ● E991.5 Fragments from person-borne improvised explosive device [IED]
  ● E991.6 Fragments from vehicle-borne improvised explosive device [IED]
    IED borne by land, air, or water transport vehicle
  ● E991.7 Fragments from other improvised explosive device [IED]
    Roadside IED

◀ New ◀||| Revised ~~deleted~~ Deleted Excludes Includes Use additional Code first Omit code
● Unacceptable Principal Diagnosis ● Use Additional Digit(s) OGCR Official Guidelines Coding Clinic

● **E991.8 Fragments from weapons**
Fragments from:
   artillery
   autocannons
   automatic grenade launchers
   missile launchers
   mortars
   small arms

● **E991.9 Other and unspecified fragments**
Shrapnel NOS

● **E992 Injury due to war operations by explosion of marine weapons**

● **E992.0 Torpedo**

● **E992.1 Depth charge**

● **E992.2 Marine mines**
Marine mines at sea or in harbor

● **E992.3 Sea-based artillery shell**

● **E992.8 Other by other marine weapons**

● **E992.9 Unspecified marine weapon**
Underwater blast NOS

● **E993 Injury due to war operations by other explosion**
Injuries due to direct or indirect pressure or air
   blast of an explosion occurring during war
   operations

Excludes	*injury due to fragments resulting from an* *explosion (E991.0-E991.9)* *injury due to detonation of unexploded* *ordnance but occurring after cessation* *of hostilities (E998.0-E998.9)* *injury due to nuclear weapons* *(E996.0-E996.9)*

● **E993.0 Aerial bomb**

● **E993.1 Guided missile**

● **E993.2 Mortar**
Artillery shell

● **E993.3 Person-borne improvised explosive device [IED]**

● **E993.4 Vehicle-borne improvised explosive device [IED]**
IED borne by land, air, or water transport
   vehicle

● **E993.5 Other improvised explosive device [IED]**
Roadside IED

● **E993.6 Unintentional detonation of own munitions**
Unintentional detonation of own ammunition
   (artillery) (mortars)

● **E993.7 Unintentional discharge of own munitions launch device**
Unintentional explosion of own:
   autocannons
   automatic grenade launchers
   missile launchers
   small arms

● **E993.8 Other specified explosion**
Bomb
Grenade
Land mine

● **E993.9 Unspecified explosion**
Air blast NOS
Blast NOS
Blast wave NOS
Blast wind NOS
Explosion NOS

● **E994 Injury due to war operations by destruction of aircraft**

● **E994.0 Destruction of aircraft due to enemy fire or explosives**
Air to air missile
Explosive device placed on aircraft
Rocket propelled grenade [RPG]
Small arms fire
Surface to air missile

● **E994.1 Unintentional destruction of aircraft due to own onboard explosives**

● **E994.2 Destruction of aircraft due to collision with other aircraft**

● **E994.3 Destruction of aircraft due to onboard fire**

● **E994.8 Other destruction of aircraft**

● **E994.9 Unspecified destruction of aircraft**

● **E995 Injury due to war operations by other and unspecified forms of conventional warfare**

● **E995.0 Unarmed hand-to-hand combat**

Excludes	*intentional restriction of airway* *(E995.3)*

● **E995.1 Struck by blunt object**
Baton (nightstick)
Stave

● **E995.2 Piercing object**
Bayonet
Knife
Sword

● **E995.3 Intentional restriction of air and airway**
Intentional submersion
Strangulation
Suffocation

● **E995.4 Unintentional drowning due to inability to surface or obtain air**
Submersion

● **E995.8 Other forms of conventional warfare**

● **E995.9 Unspecified form of conventional warfare**

● **E996 Injury due to war operations by nuclear weapons**
Dirty bomb NOS

Excludes	*late effects of injury due to nuclear weapons* *(E999.1, E999.0)*

● **E996.0 Direct blast effect of nuclear weapon**
Injury to bodily organs due to blast
   pressure

● **E996.1 Indirect blast effect of nuclear weapon**
Injury due to being thrown by blast
Injury due to being struck or crushed
   by blast debris

● **E996.2 Thermal radiation effect of nuclear weapon**
Burns due to thermal radiation
Fireball effects
Flash burns
Heat effects

● **E996.3 Nuclear radiation effects**
Acute radiation exposure
Beta burns
Fallout exposure
Radiation sickness
Secondary effects of nuclear weapons

● **E996.8 Other effects of nuclear weapons**

● **E996.9 Unspecified effect of nuclear weapon**

E000-E999

● **E997 Injury due to war operations by other forms of unconventional warfare**

● **E997.0 Lasers**

● **E997.1 Biological warfare**

● **E997.2 Gases, fumes, and chemicals**

● **E997.3 Weapon of mass destruction [WMD], unspecified**

● **E997.8 Other specified forms of unconventional warfare**

● **E997.9 Unspecified form of unconventional warfare**

● **E998 Injury due to war operations but occurring after cessation of hostilities**

Injuries due to operations of war but occurring after cessation of hostilities by any means classifiable under E990-E997

Injuries by explosion of bombs or mines placed in the course of operations of war, if the explosion occurred after cessation of hostilities

● **E998.0 Explosion of mines**

● **E998.1 Explosion of bombs**

● **E998.8 Injury due to other war operations but occurring after cessation of hostilities**

● **E998.9 Injury due to unspecified war operations but occurring after cessation of hostilities**

● **E999 Late effect of injury due to war operations and terrorism**

Note: This category is to be used to indicate circumstances classifiable to E979, E990-E998 as the cause of death or disability from late effects, which are themselves classifiable elsewhere. The "late effects" include conditions reported as such or as sequelae which may occur at any time after injury resulting from operations of war or terrorism.

● **E999.0 Late effect of injury due to war operations**
Coding Clinic: 1998, Q1, P4; 1996, Q2, P12

● **E999.1 Late effect of injury due to terrorism**

◄ New ◄▥ Revised ~~deleted~~ Deleted Excludes Includes Use additional Code first Omit code
● Unacceptable Principal Diagnosis ● Use Additional Digit(s) OGCR Official Guidelines Coding Clinic

APPENDIX A
MORPHOLOGY OF NEOPLASMS

The World Health Organization has published an adaptation of the International Classification of Diseases for Oncology (ICD-O). It contains a coded nomenclature for the morphology of neoplasms, which is reproduced here for those who wish to use it in conjunction with Chapter 2 of the International Classification of Diseases, 9th Revision, Clinical Modification.

The morphology code numbers consist of five digits; the first four identify the histological type of the neoplasm and the fifth indicates its behavior. The one-digit behavior code is as follows:

/0 Benign
/1 Uncertain whether benign or malignant
      Borderline malignancy
/2 Carcinoma in situ
      Intraepithelial
      Noninfiltrating
      Noninvasive
/3 Malignant, primary site
/6 Malignant, metastatic site
      Secondary site
/9 Malignant, uncertain whether primary or metastatic site

In the nomenclature below, the morphology code numbers include the behavior code appropriate to the histological type of neoplasm, but this behavior code should be changed if other reported information makes this necessary. For example, "chordoma (M9370/3)" is assumed to be malignant; the term "benign chordoma" should be coded M9370/0. Similarly, "superficial spreading adenocarcinoma (M8143/3)" described as "noninvasive" should be coded M8143/2 and "melanoma (M8720/3)" described as "secondary" should be coded M8720/6.

The following table shows the correspondence between the morphology code and the different sections of Chapter 2:

Morphology Code Histology/Behavior			ICD-9-CM Chapter 2
Any	0	210-229	Benign neoplasms
M8000-M8004	1	239	Neoplasms of unspecified nature
M8010+	1	235-238	Neoplasms of uncertain behavior
Any	2	230-234	Carcinoma in situ
Any	3	140-195	Malignant neoplasms, stated or
		200-208	presumed to be primary
Any	6	196-198	Malignant neoplasms, stated or
			presumed to be secondary

The ICD-O behavior digit /9 is inapplicable in an ICD context, since all malignant neoplasms are presumed to be primary (/3) or secondary (/6) according to other information on the medical record.

Only the first-listed term of the full ICD-O morphology nomenclature appears against each code number in the list below. The ICD-9-CM Alphabetical Index (Volume 2), however, includes all the ICD-O synonyms as well as a number of other morphological names still likely to be encountered on medical records but omitted from ICD-O as outdated or otherwise undesirable.

A coding difficulty sometimes arises where a morphological diagnosis contains two qualifying adjectives that have different code numbers. An example is "transitional cell epidermoid carcinomas." "Transitional cell carcinoma NOS" is M8120/3 and "epidermoid carcinoma NOS" is M8070/3. In such circumstances, the higher number (M8120/3 in this example) should be used, as it is usually more specific.

CODED NOMENCLATURE FOR MORPHOLOGY OF NEOPLASMS

M800 Neoplasms NOS
M8000/0 *Neoplasm, benign*
M8000/1 *Neoplasm, uncertain whether benign or malignant*
M8000/3 *Neoplasm, malignant*
M8000/6 *Neoplasm, metastatic*

M8000/9 *Neoplasm, malignant, uncertain whether primary or metastatic*
M8001/0 *Tumor cells, benign*
M8001/1 *Tumor cells, uncertain whether benign or malignant*
M8001/3 *Tumor cells, malignant*
M8002/3 *Malignant tumor, small cell type*
M8003/3 *Malignant tumor, giant cell type*
M8004/3 *Malignant tumor, fusiform cell type*

M801-M804 Epithelial neoplasms NOS
M8010/0 *Epithelial tumor, benign*
M8010/2 *Carcinoma in situ NOS*
M8010/3 *Carcinoma NOS*
M8010/6 *Carcinoma, metastatic NOS*
M8010/9 *Carcinomatosis*
M8011/0 *Epithelioma, benign*
M8011/3 *Epithelioma, malignant*
M8012/3 *Large cell carcinoma NOS*
M8020/3 *Carcinoma, undifferentiated type NOS*
M8021/3 *Carcinoma, anaplastic type NOS*
M8022/3 *Pleomorphic carcinoma*
M8030/3 *Giant cell and spindle cell carcinoma*
M8031/3 *Giant cell carcinoma*
M8032/3 *Spindle cell carcinoma*
M8033/3 *Pseudosarcomatous carcinoma*
M8034/3 *Polygonal cell carcinoma*
M8035/3 *Spheroidal cell carcinoma*
M8040/1 *Tumorlet*
M8041/3 *Small cell carcinoma NOS*
M8042/3 *Oat cell carcinoma*
M8043/3 *Small cell carcinoma, fusiform cell type*

M805-M808 Papillary and squamous cell neoplasms
M8050/0 *Papilloma NOS (except Papilloma of urinary bladder M8120/1)*
M8050/2 *Papillary carcinoma in situ*
M8050/3 *Papillary carcinoma NOS*
M8051/0 *Verrucous papilloma*
M8051/3 *Verrucous carcinoma NOS*
M8052/0 *Squamous cell papilloma*
M8052/3 *Papillary squamous cell carcinoma*
M8053/0 *Inverted papilloma*
M8060/0 *Papillomatosis NOS*
M8070/2 *Squamous cell carcinoma in situ NOS*
M8070/3 *Squamous cell carcinoma NOS*
M8070/6 *Squamous cell carcinoma, metastatic NOS*
M8071/3 *Squamous cell carcinoma, keratinizing type NOS*
M8072/3 *Squamous cell carcinoma, large cell, nonkeratinizing type*
M8073/3 *Squamous cell carcinoma, small cell, nonkeratinizing type*
M8074/3 *Squamous cell carcinoma, spindle cell type*
M8075/3 *Adenoid squamous cell carcinoma*
M8076/2 *Squamous cell carcinoma in situ with questionable stromal invasion*
M8076/3 *Squamous cell carcinoma, microinvasive*
M8080/2 *Queyrat's erythroplasia*
M8081/2 *Bowen's disease*
M8082/2 *Lymphoepithelial carcinoma*

M809-M811 Basal cell neoplasms
M8090/1 *Basal cell tumor*
M8090/3 *Basal cell carcinoma NOS*
M8091/3 *Multicentric basal cell carcinoma*
M8092/3 *Basal cell carcinoma, morphea type*
M8093/3 *Basal cell carcinoma, fibroepithelial type*
M8094/3 *Basosquamous carcinoma*
M8095/3 *Metatypical carcinoma*
M8096/0 *Intraepidermal epithelioma of Jadassohn*
M8100/0 *Trichoepithelioma*
M8101/0 *Trichofolliculoma*
M8102/0 *Tricholemmoma*
M8110/0 *Pilomatrixoma*

M812-M813	**Transitional cell papillomas and carcinomas**
M8120/0	Transitional cell papilloma NOS
M8120/1	Urothelial papilloma
M8120/2	Transitional cell carcinoma in situ
M8120/3	Transitional cell carcinoma NOS
M8121/0	Schneiderian papilloma
M8121/1	Transitional cell papilloma, inverted type
M8121/3	Schneiderian carcinoma
M8122/3	Transitional cell carcinoma, spindle cell type
M8123/3	Basaloid carcinoma
M8124/3	Cloacogenic carcinoma
M8130/3	Papillary transitional cell carcinoma

M814-M838	**Adenomas and adenocarcinomas**
M8140/0	Adenoma NOS
M8140/1	Bronchial adenoma NOS
M8140/2	Adenocarcinoma in situ
M8140/3	Adenocarcinoma NOS
M8140/6	Adenocarcinoma, metastatic NOS
M8141/3	Scirrhous adenocarcinoma
M8142/3	Linitis plastica
M8143/3	Superficial spreading adenocarcinoma
M8144/3	Adenocarcinoma, intestinal type
M8145/3	Carcinoma, diffuse type
M8146/0	Monomorphic adenoma
M8147/0	Basal cell adenoma
M8150/0	Islet cell adenoma
M8150/3	Islet cell carcinoma
M8151/0	Insulinoma NOS
M8151/3	Insulinoma, malignant
M8152/0	Glucagonoma NOS
M8152/3	Glucagonoma, malignant
M8153/1	Gastrinoma NOS
M8153/3	Gastrinoma, malignant
M8154/3	Mixed islet cell and exocrine adenocarcinoma
M8160/0	Bile duct adenoma
M8160/3	Cholangiocarcinoma
M8161/0	Bile duct cystadenoma
M8161/3	Bile duct cystadenocarcinoma
M8170/0	Liver cell adenoma
M8170/3	Hepatocellular carcinoma NOS
M8180/0	Hepatocholangioma, benign
M8180/3	Combined hepatocellular carcinoma and cholangio-carcinoma
M8190/0	Trabecular adenoma
M8190/3	Trabecular adenocarcinoma
M8191/0	Embryonal adenoma
M8200/0	Eccrine dermal cylindroma
M8200/3	Adenoid cystic carcinoma
M8201/3	Cribriform carcinoma
M8210/0	Adenomatous polyp NOS
M8210/3	Adenocarcinoma in adenomatous polyp
M8211/0	Tubular adenoma NOS
M8211/3	Tubular adenocarcinoma
M8220/0	Adenomatous polyposis coli
M8220/3	Adenocarcinoma in adenomatous polyposis coli
M8221/0	Multiple adenomatous polyps
M8230/3	Solid carcinoma NOS
M8231/3	Carcinoma simplex
M8240/1	Carcinoid tumor NOS
M8240/3	Carcinoid tumor, malignant
M8241/1	Carcinoid tumor, argentaffin NOS
M8241/3	Carcinoid tumor, argentaffin, malignant
M8242/1	Carcinoid tumor, nonargentaffin NOS
M8242/3	Carcinoid tumor, nonargentaffin, malignant
M8243/3	Mucocarcinoid tumor, malignant
M8244/3	Composite carcinoid
M8250/1	Pulmonary adenomatosis
M8250/3	Bronchiolo-alveolar adenocarcinoma
M8251/0	Alveolar adenoma
M8251/3	Alveolar adenocarcinoma
M8260/0	Papillary adenoma NOS
M8260/3	Papillary adenocarcinoma NOS
M8261/1	Villous adenoma NOS
M8261/3	Adenocarcinoma in villous adenoma

M8262/3	Villous adenocarcinoma
M8263/0	Tubulovillous adenoma
M8270/0	Chromophobe adenoma
M8270/3	Chromophobe carcinoma
M8280/0	Acidophil adenoma
M8280/3	Acidophil carcinoma
M8281/0	Mixed acidophil-basophil adenoma
M8281/3	Mixed acidophil-basophil carcinoma
M8290/0	Oxyphilic adenoma
M8290/3	Oxyphilic adenocarcinoma
M8300/0	Basophil adenoma
M8300/3	Basophil carcinoma
M8310/0	Clear cell adenoma
M8310/3	Clear cell adenocarcinoma NOS
M8311/1	Hypernephroid tumor
M8312/3	Renal cell carcinoma
M8313/0	Clear cell adenofibroma
M8320/3	Granular cell carcinoma
M8321/0	Chief cell adenoma
M8322/0	Water-clear cell adenoma
M8322/3	Water-clear cell adenocarcinoma
M8323/0	Mixed cell adenoma
M8323/3	Mixed cell adenocarcinoma
M8324/0	Lipoadenoma
M8330/0	Follicular adenoma
M8330/3	Follicular adenocarcinoma NOS
M8331/3	Follicular adenocarcinoma, well differentiated type
M8332/3	Follicular adenocarcinoma, trabecular type
M8333/0	Microfollicular adenoma
M8334/0	Macrofollicular adenoma
M8340/3	Papillary and follicular adenocarcinoma
M8350/3	Nonencapsulated sclerosing carcinoma
M8360/1	Multiple endocrine adenomas
M8361/1	Juxtaglomerular tumor
M8370/0	Adrenal cortical adenoma NOS
M8370/3	Adrenal cortical carcinoma
M8371/0	Adrenal cortical adenoma, compact cell type
M8372/0	Adrenal cortical adenoma, heavily pigmented variant
M8373/0	Adrenal cortical adenoma, clear cell type
M8374/0	Adrenal cortical adenoma, glomerulosa cell type
M8375/0	Adrenal cortical adenoma, mixed cell type
M8380/0	Endometrioid adenoma NOS
M8380/1	Endometrioid adenoma, borderline malignancy
M8380/3	Endometrioid carcinoma
M8381/0	Endometrioid adenofibroma NOS
M8381/1	Endometrioid adenofibroma, borderline malignancy
M8381/3	Endometrioid adenofibroma, malignant

M839-M842	**Adnexal and skin appendage neoplasms**
M8390/0	Skin appendage adenoma
M8390/3	Skin appendage carcinoma
M8400/0	Sweat gland adenoma
M8400/1	Sweat gland tumor NOS
M8400/3	Sweat gland adenocarcinoma
M8401/0	Apocrine adenoma
M8401/3	Apocrine adenocarcinoma
M8402/0	Eccrine acrospiroma
M8403/0	Eccrine spiradenoma
M8404/0	Hidrocystoma
M8405/0	Papillary hydradenoma
M8406/0	Papillary syringadenoma
M8407/0	Syringoma NOS
M8410/0	Sebaceous adenoma
M8410/3	Sebaceous adenocarcinoma
M8420/0	Ceruminous adenoma
M8420/3	Ceruminous adenocarcinoma

M843	**Mucoepidermoid neoplasms**
M8430/1	Mucoepidermoid tumor
M8430/3	Mucoepidermoid carcinoma

M844-M849	**Cystic, mucinous, and serous neoplasms**
M8440/0	Cystadenoma NOS
M8440/3	Cystadenocarcinoma NOS
M8441/0	Serous cystadenoma NOS
M8441/1	Serous cystadenoma, borderline malignancy
M8441/3	Serous cystadenocarcinoma NOS

M8450/0	Papillary cystadenoma NOS
M8450/1	Papillary cystadenoma, borderline malignancy
M8450/3	Papillary cystadenocarcinoma NOS
M8460/0	Papillary serous cystadenoma NOS
M8460/1	Papillary serous cystadenoma, borderline malignancy
M8460/3	Papillary serous cystadenocarcinoma
M8461/0	Serous surface papilloma NOS
M8461/1	Serous surface papilloma, borderline malignancy
M8461/3	Serous surface papillary carcinoma
M8470/0	Mucinous cystadenoma NOS
M8470/1	Mucinous cystadenoma, borderline malignancy
M8470/3	Mucinous cystadenocarcinoma NOS
M8471/0	Papillary mucinous cystadenoma NOS
M8471/1	Papillary mucinous cystadenoma, borderline malignancy
M8471/3	Papillary mucinous cystadenocarcinoma
M8480/0	Mucinous adenoma
M8480/3	Mucinous adenocarcinoma
M8480/6	Pseudomyxoma peritonei
M8481/3	Mucin-producing adenocarcinoma
M8490/3	Signet ring cell carcinoma
M8490/6	Metastatic signet ring cell carcinoma

M850-M854 Ductal, lobular, and medullary neoplasms

M8500/2	Intraductal carcinoma, noninfiltrating NOS
M8500/3	Infiltrating duct carcinoma
M8501/2	Comedocarcinoma, noninfiltrating
M8501/3	Comedocarcinoma NOS
M8502/3	Juvenile carcinoma of the breast
M8503/0	Intraductal papilloma
M8503/2	Noninfiltrating intraductal papillary adenocarcinoma
M8504/0	Intracystic papillary adenoma
M8504/2	Noninfiltrating intracystic carcinoma
M8505/0	Intraductal papillomatosis NOS
M8506/0	Subareolar duct papillomatosis
M8510/3	Medullary carcinoma NOS
M8511/3	Medullary carcinoma with amyloid stroma
M8512/3	Medullary carcinoma with lymphoid stroma
M8520/2	Lobular carcinoma in situ
M8520/3	Lobular carcinoma NOS
M8521/3	Infiltrating ductular carcinoma
M8530/3	Inflammatory carcinoma
M8540/3	Paget's disease, mammary
M8541/3	Paget's disease and infiltrating duct carcinoma of breast
M8542/3	Paget's disease, extramammary (except Paget's disease of bone)

M855 Acinar cell neoplasms

M8550/0	Acinar cell adenoma
M8550/1	Acinar cell tumor
M8550/3	Acinar cell carcinoma

M856-M858 Complex epithelial neoplasms

M8560/3	Adenosquamous carcinoma
M8561/0	Adenolymphoma
M8570/3	Adenocarcinoma with squamous metaplasia
M8571/3	Adenocarcinoma with cartilaginous and osseous metaplasia
M8572/3	Adenocarcinoma with spindle cell metaplasia
M8573/3	Adenocarcinoma with apocrine metaplasia
M8580/0	Thymoma, benign
M8580/3	Thymoma, malignant

M859-M867 Specialized gonadal neoplasms

M8590/1	Sex cord-stromal tumor
M8600/0	Thecoma NOS
M8600/3	Theca cell carcinoma
M8610/0	Luteoma NOS
M8620/1	Granulosa cell tumor NOS
M8620/3	Granulosa cell tumor, malignant
M8621/1	Granulosa cell-theca cell tumor
M8630/0	Androblastoma, benign
M8630/1	Androblastoma NOS
M8630/3	Androblastoma, malignant
M8631/0	Sertoli-Leydig cell tumor
M8632/1	Gynandroblastoma
M8640/0	Tubular androblastoma NOS
M8640/3	Sertoli cell carcinoma

M8641/0	Tubular androblastoma with lipid storage
M8650/0	Leydig cell tumor, benign
M8650/1	Leydig cell tumor NOS
M8650/3	Leydig cell tumor, malignant
M8660/0	Hilar cell tumor
M8670/0	Lipid cell tumor of ovary
M8671/0	Adrenal rest tumor

M868-M871 Paragangliomas and glomus tumors

M8680/1	Paraganglioma NOS
M8680/3	Paraganglioma, malignant
M8681/1	Sympathetic paraganglioma
M8682/1	Parasympathetic paraganglioma
M8690/1	Glomus jugulare tumor
M8691/1	Aortic body tumor
M8692/1	Carotid body tumor
M8693/1	Extra-adrenal paraganglioma NOS
M8693/3	Extra-adrenal paraganglioma, malignant
M8700/0	Pheochromocytoma NOS
M8700/3	Pheochromocytoma, malignant
M8710/3	Glomangiosarcoma
M8711/0	Glomus tumor
M8712/0	Glomangioma

M872-M879 Nevi and melanomas

M8720/0	Pigmented nevus NOS
M8720/3	Malignant melanoma NOS
M8721/3	Nodular melanoma
M8722/0	Balloon cell nevus
M8722/3	Balloon cell melanoma
M8723/0	Halo nevus
M8724/0	Fibrous papule of the nose
M8725/0	Neuronevus
M8726/0	Magnocellular nevus
M8730/0	Nonpigmented nevus
M8730/3	Amelanotic melanoma
M8740/0	Junctional nevus
M8740/3	Malignant melanoma in junctional nevus
M8741/2	Precancerous melanosis NOS
M8741/3	Malignant melanoma in precancerous melanosis
M8742/2	Hutchinson's melanotic freckle
M8742/3	Malignant melanoma in Hutchinson's melanotic freckle
M8743/3	Superficial spreading melanoma
M8750/0	Intradermal nevus
M8760/0	Compound nevus
M8761/1	Giant pigmented nevus
M8761/3	Malignant melanoma in giant pigmented nevus
M8770/0	Epithelioid and spindle cell nevus
M8771/3	Epithelioid cell melanoma
M8772/3	Spindle cell melanoma NOS
M8773/3	Spindle cell melanoma, type A
M8774/3	Spindle cell melanoma, type B
M8775/3	Mixed epithelioid and spindle cell melanoma
M8780/0	Blue nevus NOS
M8780/3	Blue nevus, malignant
M8790/0	Cellular blue nevus

M880 Soft tissue tumors and sarcomas NOS

M8800/0	Soft tissue tumor, benign
M8800/3	Sarcoma NOS
M8800/9	Sarcomatosis NOS
M8801/3	Spindle cell sarcoma
M8802/3	Giant cell sarcoma (except of bone M9250/3)
M8803/3	Small cell sarcoma
M8804/3	Epithelioid cell sarcoma

M881-M883 Fibromatous neoplasms

M8810/0	Fibroma NOS
M8810/3	Fibrosarcoma NOS
M8811/0	Fibromyxoma
M8811/3	Fibromyxosarcoma
M8812/0	Periosteal fibroma
M8812/3	Periosteal fibrosarcoma
M8813/0	Fascial fibroma
M8813/3	Fascial fibrosarcoma
M8814/3	Infantile fibrosarcoma
M8820/0	Elastofibroma

M8821/1	*Aggressive fibromatosis*
M8822/1	*Abdominal fibromatosis*
M8823/1	*Desmoplastic fibroma*
M8830/0	*Fibrous histiocytoma NOS*
M8830/1	*Atypical fibrous histiocytoma*
M8830/3	*Fibrous histiocytoma, malignant*
M8831/0	*Fibroxanthoma NOS*
M8831/1	*Atypical fibroxanthoma*
M8831/3	*Fibroxanthoma, malignant*
M8832/0	*Dermatofibroma NOS*
M8832/1	*Dermatofibroma protuberans*
M8832/3	*Dermatofibrosarcoma NOS*

M884 **Myxomatous neoplasms**

M8840/0	*Myxoma NOS*
M8840/3	*Myxosarcoma*

M885-M888 **Lipomatous neoplasms**

M8850/0	*Lipoma NOS*
M8850/3	*Liposarcoma NOS*
M8851/0	*Fibrolipoma*
M8851/3	*Liposarcoma, well differentiated type*
M8852/0	*Fibromyxolipoma*
M8852/3	*Myxoid liposarcoma*
M8853/3	*Round cell liposarcoma*
M8854/3	*Pleomorphic liposarcoma*
M8855/3	*Mixed type liposarcoma*
M8856/0	*Intramuscular lipoma*
M8857/0	*Spindle cell lipoma*
M8860/0	*Angiomyolipoma*
M8860/3	*Angiomyoliposarcoma*
M8861/0	*Angiolipoma NOS*
M8861/1	*Angiolipoma, infiltrating*
M8870/0	*Myelolipoma*
M8880/0	*Hibernoma*
M8881/0	*Lipoblastomatosis*

M889-M892 **Myomatous neoplasms**

M8890/0	*Leiomyoma NOS*
M8890/1	*Intravascular leiomyomatosis*
M8890/3	*Leiomyosarcoma NOS*
M8891/1	*Epithelioid leiomyoma*
M8891/3	*Epithelioid leiomyosarcoma*
M8892/1	*Cellular leiomyoma*
M8893/0	*Bizarre leiomyoma*
M8894/0	*Angiomyoma*
M8894/3	*Angiomyosarcoma*
M8895/0	*Myoma*
M8895/3	*Myosarcoma*
M8900/0	*Rhabdomyoma NOS*
M8900/3	*Rhabdomyosarcoma NOS*
M8901/3	*Pleomorphic rhabdomyosarcoma*
M8902/3	*Mixed type rhabdomyosarcoma*
M8903/0	*Fetal rhabdomyoma*
M8904/0	*Adult rhabdomyoma*
M8910/3	*Embryonal rhabdomyosarcoma*
M8920/3	*Alveolar rhabdomyosarcoma*

M893-M899 **Complex mixed and stromal neoplasms**

M8930/3	*Endometrial stromal sarcoma*
M8931/1	*Endolymphatic stromal myosis*
M8932/0	*Adenomyoma*
M8940/0	*Pleomorphic adenoma*
M8940/3	*Mixed tumor, malignant NOS*
M8950/3	*Mullerian mixed tumor*
M8951/3	*Mesodermal mixed tumor*
M8960/1	*Mesoblastic nephroma*
M8960/3	*Nephroblastoma NOS*
M8961/3	*Epithelial nephroblastoma*
M8962/3	*Mesenchymal nephroblastoma*
M8970/3	*Hepatoblastoma*
M8980/3	*Carcinosarcoma NOS*
M8981/3	*Carcinosarcoma, embryonal type*
M8982/0	*Myoepithelioma*
M8990/0	*Mesenchymoma, benign*
M8990/1	*Mesenchymoma NOS*

M8990/3	*Mesenchymoma, malignant*
M8991/3	*Embryonal sarcoma*

M900-M903 **Fibroepithelial neoplasms**

M9000/0	*Brenner tumor NOS*
M9000/1	*Brenner tumor, borderline malignancy*
M9000/3	*Brenner tumor, malignant*
M9010/0	*Fibroadenoma NOS*
M9011/0	*Intracanalicular fibroadenoma NOS*
M9012/0	*Pericanalicular fibroadenoma*
M9013/0	*Adenofibroma NOS*
M9014/0	*Serous adenofibroma*
M9015/0	*Mucinous adenofibroma*
M9020/0	*Cellular intracanalicular fibroadenoma*
M9020/1	*Cystosarcoma phyllodes NOS*
M9020/3	*Cystosarcoma phyllodes, malignant*
M9030/0	*Juvenile fibroadenoma*

M904 **Synovial neoplasms**

M9040/0	*Synovioma, benign*
M9040/3	*Synovial sarcoma NOS*
M9041/3	*Synovial sarcoma, spindle cell type*
M9042/3	*Synovial sarcoma, epithelioid cell type*
M9043/3	*Synovial sarcoma, biphasic type*
M9044/3	*Clear cell sarcoma of tendons and aponeuroses*

M905 **Mesothelial neoplasms**

M9050/0	*Mesothelioma, benign*
M9050/3	*Mesothelioma, malignant*
M9051/0	*Fibrous mesothelioma, benign*
M9051/3	*Fibrous mesothelioma, malignant*
M9052/0	*Epithelioid mesothelioma, benign*
M9052/3	*Epithelioid mesothelioma, malignant*
M9053/0	*Mesothelioma, biphasic type, benign*
M9053/3	*Mesothelioma, biphasic type, malignant*
M9054/0	*Adenomatoid tumor NOS*

M906-M909 **Germ cell neoplasms**

M9060/3	*Dysgerminoma*
M9061/3	*Seminoma NOS*
M9062/3	*Seminoma, anaplastic type*
M9063/3	*Spermatocytic seminoma*
M9064/3	*Germinoma*
M9070/3	*Embryonal carcinoma NOS*
M9071/3	*Endodermal sinus tumor*
M9072/3	*Polyembryoma*
M9073/1	*Gonadoblastoma*
M9080/0	*Teratoma, benign*
M9080/1	*Teratoma NOS*
M9080/3	*Teratoma, malignant NOS*
M9081/3	*Teratocarcinoma*
M9082/3	*Malignant teratoma, undifferentiated type*
M9083/3	*Malignant teratoma, intermediate type*
M9084/0	*Dermoid cyst*
M9084/3	*Dermoid cyst with malignant transformation*
M9090/0	*Struma ovarii NOS*
M9090/3	*Struma ovarii, malignant*
M9091/1	*Strumal carcinoid*

M910 **Trophoblastic neoplasms**

M9100/0	*Hydatidiform mole NOS*
M9100/1	*Invasive hydatidiform mole*
M9100/3	*Choriocarcinoma*
M9101/3	*Choriocarcinoma combined with teratoma*
M9102/3	*Malignant teratoma, trophoblastic*

M911 **Mesonephromas**

M9110/0	*Mesonephroma, benign*
M9110/1	*Mesonephric tumor*
M9110/3	*Mesonephroma, malignant*
M9111/1	*Endosalpingioma*

M912-M916 **Blood vessel tumors**

M9120/0	*Hemangioma NOS*
M9120/3	*Hemangiosarcoma*
M9121/0	*Cavernous hemangioma*
M9122/0	*Venous hemangioma*
M9123/0	*Racemose hemangioma*
M9124/3	*Kupffer cell sarcoma*

M9130/0	*Hemangioendothelioma, benign*
M9130/1	*Hemangioendothelioma NOS*
M9130/3	*Hemangioendothelioma, malignant*
M9131/0	*Capillary hemangioma*
M9132/0	*Intramuscular hemangioma*
M9140/3	*Kaposi's sarcoma*
M9141/0	*Angiokeratoma*
M9142/0	*Verrucous keratotic hemangioma*
M9150/0	*Hemangiopericytoma, benign*
M9150/1	*Hemangiopericytoma NOS*
M9150/3	*Hemangiopericytoma, malignant*
M9160/0	*Angiofibroma NOS*
M9161/1	*Hemangioblastoma*

M917	**Lymphatic vessel tumors**
M9170/0	*Lymphangioma NOS*
M9170/3	*Lymphangiosarcoma*
M9171/0	*Capillary lymphangioma*
M9172/0	*Cavernous lymphangioma*
M9173/0	*Cystic lymphangioma*
M9174/0	*Lymphangiomyoma*
M9174/1	*Lymphangiomyomatosis*
M9175/0	*Hemolymphangioma*

M918-M920	**Osteomas and osteosarcomas**
M9180/0	*Osteoma NOS*
M9180/3	*Osteosarcoma NOS*
M9181/3	*Chondroblastic osteosarcoma*
M9182/3	*Fibroblastic osteosarcoma*
M9183/3	*Telangiectatic osteosarcoma*
M9184/3	*Osteosarcoma in Paget's disease of bone*
M9190/3	*Juxtacortical osteosarcoma*
M9191/0	*Osteoid osteoma NOS*
M9200/0	*Osteoblastoma*

M921-M924	**Chondromatous neoplasms**
M9210/0	*Osteochondroma*
M9210/1	*Osteochondromatosis NOS*
M9220/0	*Chondroma NOS*
M9220/1	*Chondromatosis NOS*
M9220/3	*Chondrosarcoma NOS*
M9221/0	*Juxtacortical chondroma*
M9221/3	*Juxtacortical chondrosarcoma*
M9230/0	*Chondroblastoma NOS*
M9230/3	*Chondroblastoma, malignant*
M9240/3	*Mesenchymal chondrosarcoma*
M9241/0	*Chondromyxoid fibroma*

M925	**Giant cell tumors**
M9250/1	*Giant cell tumor of bone NOS*
M9250/3	*Giant cell tumor of bone, malignant*
M9251/1	*Giant cell tumor of soft parts NOS*
M9251/3	*Malignant giant cell tumor of soft parts*

M926	**Miscellaneous bone tumors**
M9260/3	*Ewing's sarcoma*
M9261/3	*Adamantinoma of long bones*
M9262/0	*Ossifying fibroma*

M927-M934	**Odontogenic tumors**
M9270/0	*Odontogenic tumor, benign*
M9270/1	*Odontogenic tumor NOS*
M9270/3	*Odontogenic tumor, malignant*
M9271/0	*Dentinoma*
M9272/0	*Cementoma NOS*
M9273/0	*Cementoblastoma, benign*
M9274/0	*Cementifying fibroma*
M9275/0	*Gigantiform cementoma*
M9280/0	*Odontoma NOS*
M9281/0	*Compound odontoma*
M9282/0	*Complex odontoma*
M9290/0	*Ameloblastic fibro-odontoma*
M9290/3	*Ameloblastic odontosarcoma*
M9300/0	*Adenomatoid odontogenic tumor*
M9301/0	*Calcifying odontogenic cyst*
M9310/0	*Ameloblastoma NOS*
M9310/3	*Ameloblastoma, malignant*
M9311/0	*Odontoameloblastoma*
M9312/0	*Squamous odontogenic tumor*

M9320/0	*Odontogenic myxoma*
M9321/0	*Odontogenic fibroma NOS*
M9330/0	*Ameloblastic fibroma*
M9330/3	*Ameloblastic fibrosarcoma*
M9340/0	*Calcifying epithelial odontogenic tumor*

M935-M937	**Miscellaneous tumors**
M9350/1	*Craniopharyngioma*
M9360/1	*Pinealoma*
M9361/1	*Pineocytoma*
M9362/3	*Pineoblastoma*
M9363/0	*Melanotic neuroectodermal tumor*
M9370/3	*Chordoma*

M938-M948	**Gliomas**
M9380/3	*Glioma, malignant*
M9381/3	*Gliomatosis cerebri*
M9382/3	*Mixed glioma*
M9383/1	*Subependymal glioma*
M9384/1	*Subependymal giant cell astrocytoma*
M9390/0	*Choroid plexus papilloma NOS*
M9390/3	*Choroid plexus papilloma, malignant*
M9391/3	*Ependymoma NOS*
M9392/3	*Ependymoma, anaplastic type*
M9393/1	*Papillary ependymoma*
M9394/1	*Myxopapillary ependymoma*
M9400/3	*Astrocytoma NOS*
M9401/3	*Astrocytoma, anaplastic type*
M9410/3	*Protoplasmic astrocytoma*
M9411/3	*Gemistocytic astrocytoma*
M9420/3	*Fibrillary astrocytoma*
M9421/3	*Pilocytic astrocytoma*
M9422/3	*Spongioblastoma NOS*
M9423/3	*Spongioblastoma polare*
M9430/3	*Astroblastoma*
M9440/3	*Glioblastoma NOS*
M9441/3	*Giant cell glioblastoma*
M9442/3	*Glioblastoma with sarcomatous component*
M9443/3	*Primitive polar spongioblastoma*
M9450/3	*Oligodendroglioma NOS*
M9451/3	*Oligodendroglioma, anaplastic type*
M9460/3	*Oligodendroblastoma*
M9470/3	*Medulloblastoma NOS*
M9471/3	*Desmoplastic medulloblastoma*
M9472/3	*Medullomyoblastoma*
M9480/3	*Cerebellar sarcoma NOS*
M9481/3	*Monstrocellular sarcoma*

M949-M952	**Neuroepitheliomatous neoplasms**
M9490/0	*Ganglioneuroma*
M9490/3	*Ganglioneuroblastoma*
M9491/0	*Ganglioneuromatosis*
M9500/3	*Neuroblastoma NOS*
M9501/3	*Medulloepithelioma NOS*
M9502/3	*Teratoid medulloepithelioma*
M9503/3	*Neuroepithelioma NOS*
M9504/3	*Spongioneuroblastoma*
M9505/1	*Ganglioglioma*
M9506/0	*Neurocytoma*
M9507/0	*Pacinian tumor*
M9510/3	*Retinoblastoma NOS*
M9511/3	*Retinoblastoma, differentiated type*
M9512/3	*Retinoblastoma, undifferentiated type*
M9520/3	*Olfactory neurogenic tumor*
M9521/3	*Esthesioneurocytoma*
M9522/3	*Esthesioneuroblastoma*
M9523/3	*Esthesioneuroepithelioma*

M953	**Meningiomas**
M9530/0	*Meningioma NOS*
M9530/1	*Meningiomatosis NOS*
M9530/3	*Meningioma, malignant*
M9531/0	*Meningotheliomatous meningioma*
M9532/0	*Fibrous meningioma*
M9533/0	*Psammomatous meningioma*
M9534/0	*Angiomatous meningioma*

M9535/0	*Hemangioblastic meningioma*
M9536/0	*Hemangiopericytic meningioma*
M9537/0	*Transitional meningioma*
M9538/1	*Papillary meningioma*
M9539/3	*Meningeal sarcomatosis*

M954-M957   Nerve sheath tumor

M9540/0	*Neurofibroma NOS*
M9540/1	*Neurofibromatosis NOS*
M9540/3	*Neurofibrosarcoma*
M9541/0	*Melanotic neurofibroma*
M9550/0	*Plexiform neurofibroma*
M9560/0	*Neurilemmoma NOS*
M9560/1	*Neurinomatosis*
M9560/3	*Neurilemmoma, malignant*
M9570/0	*Neuroma NOS*

M958   Granular cell tumors and alveolar soft part sarcoma

M9580/0	*Granular cell tumor NOS*
M9580/3	*Granular cell tumor, malignant*
M9581/3	*Alveolar soft part sarcoma*

M959-M963   Lymphomas, NOS or diffuse

M9590/0	*Lymphomatous tumor, benign*
M9590/3	*Malignant lymphoma NOS*
M9591/3	*Malignant lymphoma, non Hodgkin's type*
M9600/3	*Malignant lymphoma, undifferentiated cell type NOS*
M9601/3	*Malignant lymphoma, stem cell type*
M9602/3	*Malignant lymphoma, convoluted cell type NOS*
M9610/3	*Lymphosarcoma NOS*
M9611/3	*Malignant lymphoma, lymphoplasmacytoid type*
M9612/3	*Malignant lymphoma, immunoblastic type*
M9613/3	*Malignant lymphoma, mixed lymphocytic-histiocytic NOS*
M9614/3	*Malignant lymphoma, centroblastic-centrocytic, diffuse*
M9615/3	*Malignant lymphoma, follicular center cell NOS*
M9620/3	*Malignant lymphoma, lymphocytic, well differentiated NOS*
M9621/3	*Malignant lymphoma, lymphocytic, intermediate differentiation NOS*
M9622/3	*Malignant lymphoma, centrocytic*
M9623/3	*Malignant lymphoma, follicular center cell, cleaved NOS*
M9630/3	*Malignant lymphoma, lymphocytic, poorly differentiated NOS*
M9631/3	*Prolymphocytic lymphosarcoma*
M9632/3	*Malignant lymphoma, centroblastic type NOS*
M9633/3	*Malignant lymphoma, follicular center cell, noncleaved NOS*

M964   Reticulosarcomas

M9640/3	*Reticulosarcoma NOS*
M9641/3	*Reticulosarcoma, pleomorphic cell type*
M9642/3	*Reticulosarcoma, nodular*

M965-M966   Hodgkin's disease

M9650/3	*Hodgkin's disease NOS*
M9651/3	*Hodgkin's disease, lymphocytic predominance*
M9652/3	*Hodgkin's disease, mixed cellularity*
M9653/3	*Hodgkin's disease, lymphocytic depletion NOS*
M9654/3	*Hodgkin's disease, lymphocytic depletion, diffuse fibrosis*
M9655/3	*Hodgkin's disease, lymphocytic depletion, reticular type*
M9656/3	*Hodgkin's disease, nodular sclerosis NOS*
M9657/3	*Hodgkin's disease, nodular sclerosis, cellular phase*
M9660/3	*Hodgkin's paragranuloma*
M9661/3	*Hodgkin's granuloma*
M9662/3	*Hodgkin's sarcoma*

M969   Lymphomas, nodular or follicular

M9690/3	*Malignant lymphoma, nodular NOS*
M9691/3	*Malignant lymphoma, mixed lymphocytic-histiocytic, nodular*
M9692/3	*Malignant lymphoma, centroblastic-centrocytic, follicular*
M9693/3	*Malignant lymphoma, lymphocytic, well differentiated, nodular*
M9694/3	*Malignant lymphoma, lymphocytic, intermediate differentiation, nodular*
M9695/3	*Malignant lymphoma, follicular center cell, cleaved, follicular*
M9696/3	*Malignant lymphoma, lymphocytic, poorly differentiated, nodular*
M9697/3	*Malignant lymphoma, centroblastic type, follicular*
M9698/3	*Malignant lymphoma, follicular center cell, noncleaved, follicular*

M970   Mycosis fungoides

M9700/3	*Mycosis fungoides*
M9701/3	*Sezary's disease*

M971-M972   Miscellaneous reticuloendothelial neoplasms

M9710/3	*Microglioma*
M9720/3	*Malignant histiocytosis*
M9721/3	*Histiocytic medullary reticulosis*
M9722/3	*Letterer-Siwe's disease*

M973   Plasma cell tumors

M9730/3	*Plasma cell myeloma*
M9731/0	*Plasma cell tumor, benign*
M9731/1	*Plasmacytoma NOS*
M9731/3	*Plasma cell tumor, malignant*

M974   Mast cell tumors

M9740/1	*Mastocytoma NOS*
M9740/3	*Mast cell sarcoma*
M9741/3	*Malignant mastocytosis*

M975   Burkitt's tumor

M9750/3	*Burkitt's tumor*

M980-M994   Leukemias

M980   Leukemias NOS

M9800/3	*Leukemia NOS*
M9801/3	*Acute leukemia NOS*
M9802/3	*Subacute leukemia NOS*
M9803/3	*Chronic leukemia NOS*
M9804/3	*Aleukemic leukemia NOS*

M981   Compound leukemias

M9810/3	*Compound leukemia*

M982   Lymphoid leukemias

M9820/3	*Lymphoid leukemia NOS*
M9821/3	*Acute lymphoid leukemia*
M9822/3	*Subacute lymphoid leukemia*
M9823/3	*Chronic lymphoid leukemia*
M9824/3	*Aleukemic lymphoid leukemia*
M9825/3	*Prolymphocytic leukemia*

M983   Plasma cell leukemias

M9830/3	*Plasma cell leukemia*

M984   Erythroleukemias

M9840/3	*Erythroleukemia*
M9841/3	*Acute erythremia*
M9842/3	*Chronic erythremia*

M985   Lymphosarcoma cell leukemias

M9850/3	*Lymphosarcoma cell leukemia*

M986   Myeloid leukemias

M9860/3	*Myeloid leukemia NOS*
M9861/3	*Acute myeloid leukemia*
M9862/3	*Subacute myeloid leukemia*
M9863/3	*Chronic myeloid leukemia*
M9864/3	*Aleukemic myeloid leukemia*
M9865/3	*Neutrophilic leukemia*
M9866/3	*Acute promyelocytic leukemia*

M987   Basophilic leukemias

M9870/3	*Basophilic leukemia*

M988   Eosinophilic leukemias

M9880/3	*Eosinophilic leukemia*

M989   Monocytic leukemias

M9890/3	*Monocytic leukemia NOS*
M9891/3	*Acute monocytic leukemia*
M9892/3	*Subacute monocytic leukemia*

M9893/3	*Chronic monocytic leukemia*		**M995-M997**	**Miscellaneous myeloproliferative and lymphoproliferative disorders**
M9894/3	*Aleukemic monocytic leukemia*		M9950/1	*Polycythemia vera*
M990-M994	**Miscellaneous leukemias**		M9951/1	*Acute panmyelosis*
M9900/3	*Mast cell leukemia*		M9960/1	*Chronic myeloproliferative disease*
M9910/3	*Megakaryocytic leukemia*		M9961/1	*Myelosclerosis with myeloid metaplasia*
M9920/3	*Megakaryocytic myelosis*		M9962/1	*Idiopathic thrombocythemia*
M9930/3	*Myeloid sarcoma*		M9970/1	*Chronic lymphoproliferative disease*
M9940/3	*Hairy cell leukemia*			

APPENDIX B

GLOSSARY OF MENTAL DISORDERS

Deleted as of October 1, 2004

APPENDIX C

CLASSIFICATION OF DRUGS BY AMERICAN HOSPITAL FORMULARY SERVICES LIST NUMBER AND THEIR ICD-9-CM EQUIVALENTS

The coding of adverse effects of drugs is keyed to the continually revised Hospital Formulary of the American Hospital Formulary Service (AHFS) published under the direction of the American Society of Hospital Pharmacists.

The following section gives the ICD-9-CM diagnosis code for each AHFS list.

AHFS List		ICD-9-CM Diagnosis Code
4:00	**ANTIHISTAMINE DRUGS**	**963.0**
8:00	**ANTI-INFECTIVE AGENTS**	
8:04	Amebicides	961.5
	hydroxyquinoline derivatives	961.3
	arsenical anti-infectives	961.1
8:08	Anthelmintics	961.6
	quinoline derivatives	961.3
8:12.04	Antifungal Antibiotics	960.1
	nonantibiotics	961.9
8:12.06	Cephalosporins	960.5
8:12.08	Chloramphenicol	960.2
8:12.12	The Erythromycins	960.3
8:12.16	The Penicillins	960.0
8:12.20	The Streptomycins	960.6
8:12.24	The Tetracyclines	960.4
8:12.28	Other Antibiotics	960.8
	antimycobacterial antibiotics	960.6
	macrolides	960.3
8:16	Antituberculars	961.8
	antibiotics	960.6
8:18	Antivirals	961.7
8:20	Plasmodicides (antimalarials)	961.4
8:24	Sulfonamides	961.0
8:26	The Sulfones	961.8
8:28	Treponemicides	961.2
8:32	Trichomonacides	961.5
	hydroxyquinoline derivatives	961.3
	nitrofuran derivatives	961.9
8:36	Urinary Germicides	961.9
	quinoline derivatives	961.3
8:40	Other Anti-Infectives	961.9
10:00	**ANTINEOPLASTIC AGENTS**	**963.1**
	antibiotics	960.7
	progestogens	962.2
12:00	**AUTONOMIC DRUGS**	
12:04	Parasympathomimetic (Cholinergic) Agents	971.0
12:08	Parasympatholytic (Cholinergic Blocking) Agents	971.1
12:12	Sympathomimetic (Adrenergic) Agents	971.2
12:16	Sympatholytic (Adrenergic Blocking) Agents	971.3
12:20	Skeletal Muscle Relaxants	975.2
	central nervous system muscle-tone depressants	968.0
16:00	**BLOOD DERIVATIVES**	**964.7**
20:00	**BLOOD FORMATION AND COAGULATION**	
20:04	Antianemia Drugs	964.1
20:04.04	Iron Preparations	964.0
20:04.08	Liver and Stomach Preparations	964.1
20:12.04	Anticoagulants	964.2
20:12.08	Antiheparin agents	964.5
20:12.12	Coagulants	964.5
20:12.16	Hemostatics	964.5
	capillary-active drugs	972.8
	fibrinolysis-affecting agents	964.4
	natural products	964.7

		ICD-9-CM Diagnosis Code
24:00	**CARDIOVASCULAR DRUGS**	
24:04	Cardiac Drugs	972.9
	cardiotonic agents	972.1
	rhythm regulators	972.0
24:06	Antilipemic Agents	972.2
	thyroid derivatives	962.7
24:08	Hypotensive Agents	972.6
	adrenergic blocking agents	971.3
	ganglion-blocking agents	972.3
	vasodilators	972.5
24:12	Vasodilating Agents	972.5
	coronary	972.4
	nicotinic acid derivatives	972.2
24:16	Sclerosing Agents	972.7
28:00	**CENTRAL NERVOUS SYSTEM DRUGS**	
28:04	General Anesthetics	968.4
	gaseous anesthetics	968.2
	halothane	968.1
	intravenous anesthetics	968.3
28:08	Analgesics and Antipyretics	965.9
	antirheumatics	965.6
	aromatic analgesics	965.4
	non-narcotics NEC	965.7
	opium alkaloids	965.00
	heroin	965.01
	methadone	965.02
	specified type NEC	965.09
	pyrazole derivatives	965.5
	salicylates	965.1
	specified type NEC	965.8
28:10	Narcotic Antagonists	970.1
28:12	Anticonvulsants	966.3
	barbiturates	967.0
	benzodiazepine-based tranquilizers	969.4
	bromides	967.3
	hydantoin derivatives	966.1
	oxazolidine derivative	966.0
	succinimides	966.2
28:16.04	Antidepressants	969.0
28:16.08	Tranquilizers	969.5
	benzodiazepine-based	969.4
	butyrophenone-based	969.2
	major NEC	969.3
	phenothiazine-based	969.1
28:16.12	Other Psychotherapeutic Agents	969.8
28:20	Respiratory and Cerebral Stimulants	970.9
	analeptics	970.0
	anorexigenic agents	977.0
	psychostimulants	969.7
	specified type NEC	970.8
28:24	Sedatives and Hypnotics	967.9
	barbiturates	967.0
	benzodiazepine-based tranquilizers	969.4
	chloral hydrate group	967.1
	glutethimide group	967.5
	intravenous anesthetics	968.3
	methaqualone	967.4
	paraldehyde	967.2
	phenothiazine-based tranquilizers	969.1
	specified type NEC	967.8
	thiobarbiturates	968.3
	tranquilizer NEC	969.5
36:00	**DIAGNOSTIC AGENTS**	**977.8**
40:00	**ELECTROLYTE, CALORIC, AND WATER BALANCE AGENTS NEC**	**974.5**
40:04	Acidifying Agents	963.2

ICD-9-CM, APPENDIX C

APPENDIX D

CLASSIFICATION OF INDUSTRIAL ACCIDENTS ACCORDING TO AGENCY

Annex B to the Resolution concerning Statistics of Employment Injuries adopted by the Tenth International Conference of Labor Statisticians on 12 October 1962

1 MACHINES

11   **Prime-Movers, except Electrical Motors**
111 *Steam engines*
112 *Internal combustion engines*
119 *Others*

12   **Transmission Machinery**
121 *Transmission shafts*
122 *Transmission belts, cables, pulleys, pinions, chains, gears*
129 *Others*

13   **Metalworking Machines**
131 *Power presses*
132 *Lathes*
133 *Milling machines*
134 *Abrasive wheels*
135 *Mechanical shears*
136 *Forging machines*
137 *Rolling-mills*
139 *Others*

14   **Wood and Assimilated Machines**
141 *Circular saws*
142 *Other saws*
143 *Molding machines*
144 *Overhand planes*
149 *Others*

15   **Agricultural Machines**
151 *Reapers (including combine reapers)*
152 *Threshers*
159 *Others*

16   **Mining Machinery**
161 *Under-cutters*
169 *Others*

19   **Other Machines Not Elsewhere Classified**
191 *Earth-moving machines, excavating and scraping machines, except means of transport*
192 *Spinning, weaving and other textile machines*
193 *Machines for the manufacture of foodstuffs and beverages*
194 *Machines for the manufacture of paper*
195 *Printing machines*
199 *Others*

2 MEANS OF TRANSPORT AND LIFTING EQUIPMENT

21   **Lifting Machines and Appliances**
211 *Cranes*
212 *Lifts and elevators*
213 *Winches*
214 *Pulley blocks*
219 *Others*

22   **Means of Rail Transport**
221 *Inter-urban railways*
222 *Rail transport in mines, tunnels, quarries, industrial establishments, docks, etc.*
229 *Others*

23   **Other Wheeled Means of Transport, Excluding Rail Transport**
231 *Tractors*
232 *Lorries*
233 *Trucks*
234 *Motor vehicles, not elsewhere classified*
235 *Animal-drawn vehicles*
236 *Hand-drawn vehicles*
239 *Others*

24   **Means of Air Transport**

25   **Means of Water Transport**
251 *Motorized means of water transport*
252 *Non-motorized means of water transport*

26   **Other Means of Transport**
261 *Cable-cars*
262 *Mechanical conveyors, except cable-cars*
269 *Others*

3 OTHER EQUIPMENT

31   **Pressure Vessels**
311 *Boilers*
312 *Pressurized containers*
313 *Pressurized piping and accessories*
314 *Gas cylinders*
315 *Caissons, diving equipment*
319 *Others*

32   **Furnaces, Ovens, Kilns**
321 *Blast furnaces*
322 *Refining furnaces*
323 *Other furnaces*
324 *Kilns*
325 *Ovens*

33   **Refrigerating Plants**

34   **Electrical Installations, Including Electric Motors, but Excluding Electric Hand Tools**
341 *Rotating machines*
342 *Conductors*
343 *Transformers*
344 *Control apparatus*
349 *Others*

35   **Electric Hand Tools**

36   **Tools, Implements, and Appliances, Except Electric Hand Tools**
361 *Power-driven hand tools, except electric hand tools*
362 *Hand tools, not power-driven*
369 *Others*

37   **Ladders, Mobile Ramps**

38   **Scaffolding**

39   **Other Equipment, Not Elsewhere Classified**

4 MATERIALS, SUBSTANCES, AND RADIATIONS

41   **Explosives**

42   **Dusts, Gases, Liquids and Chemicals, Excluding Explosives**
421 *Dusts*
422 *Gases, vapors, fumes*
423 *Liquids, not elsewhere classified*
424 *Chemicals, not elsewhere classified*

43   **Flying Fragments**

44   **Radiations**
441 *Ionizing radiations*
449 *Others*

49	**Other Materials and Substances Not Elsewhere Classified**		53	**Underground**

49   **Other Materials and Substances Not Elsewhere Classified**

ICD-9-CM, APPENDIX D

LIST OF THREE-DIGIT CATEGORIES

1. INFECTIOUS AND PARASITIC DISEASES

Intestinal infectious diseases (001–009)
001 Cholera
002 Typhoid and paratyphoid fevers
003 Other salmonella infections
004 Shigellosis
005 Other food poisoning (bacterial)
006 Amebiasis
007 Other protozoal intestinal diseases
008 Intestinal infections due to other organisms
009 Ill-defined intestinal infections

Tuberculosis (010–018)
010 Primary tuberculous infection
011 Pulmonary tuberculosis
012 Other respiratory tuberculosis
013 Tuberculosis of meninges and central nervous system
014 Tuberculosis of intestines, peritoneum, and mesenteric glands
015 Tuberculosis of bones and joints
016 Tuberculosis of genitourinary system
017 Tuberculosis of other organs
018 Miliary tuberculosis

Zoonotic bacterial diseases (020–027)
020 Plague
021 Tularemia
022 Anthrax
023 Brucellosis
024 Glanders
025 Melioidosis
026 Rat-bite fever
027 Other zoonotic bacterial diseases

Other bacterial diseases (030–041)
030 Leprosy
031 Diseases due to other mycobacteria
032 Diphtheria
033 Whooping cough
034 Streptococcal sore throat and scarlet fever
035 Erysipelas
036 Meningococcal infection
037 Tetanus
038 Septicemia
039 Actinomycotic infections
040 Other bacterial diseases
041 Bacterial infection in conditions classified elsewhere and of unspecified site

Human immunodeficiency virus (042)
042 Human immunodeficiency virus [HIV] disease

Poliomyelitis and other non-arthropod-borne viral diseases of central nervous system (045–049)
045 Acute poliomyelitis
046 Slow virus infection of central nervous system
047 Meningitis due to enterovirus
048 Other enterovirus diseases of central nervous system
049 Other non-arthropod-borne viral diseases of central nervous system

Viral diseases accompanied by exanthem (050–059)
050 Smallpox
051 Cowpox and paravaccinia
052 Chickenpox
053 Herpes zoster
054 Herpes simplex
055 Measles
056 Rubella
057 Other viral exanthemata
058 Other human herpesvirus
059 Other poxvirus infections

Arthropod-borne viral diseases (060–066)
060 Yellow fever
061 Dengue
062 Mosquito-borne viral encephalitis
063 Tick-borne viral encephalitis
064 Viral encephalitis transmitted by other and unspecified arthropods
065 Arthropod-borne hemorrhagic fever
066 Other arthropod-borne viral diseases

Other diseases due to viruses and Chlamydiae (070–079)
070 Viral hepatitis
071 Rabies
072 Mumps
073 Ornithosis
074 Specific diseases due to Coxsackie virus
075 Infectious mononucleosis
076 Trachoma
077 Other diseases of conjunctiva due to viruses and Chlamydiae
078 Other diseases due to viruses and Chlamydiae
079 Viral infection in conditions classified elsewhere and of unspecified site

Rickettsioses and other arthropod-borne diseases (080–088)
080 Louse-borne [epidemic] typhus
081 Other typhus
082 Tick-borne rickettsioses
083 Other rickettsioses
084 Malaria
085 Leishmaniasis
086 Trypanosomiasis
087 Relapsing fever
088 Other arthropod-borne diseases

Syphilis and other venereal diseases (090–099)
090 Congenital syphilis
091 Early syphilis, symptomatic
092 Early syphilis, latent
093 Cardiovascular syphilis
094 Neurosyphilis
095 Other forms of late syphilis, with symptoms
096 Late syphilis, latent
097 Other and unspecified syphilis
098 Gonococcal infections
099 Other venereal diseases

Other spirochetal diseases (100–104)
100 Leptospirosis
101 Vincent's angina
102 Yaws
103 Pinta
104 Other spirochetal infection

Mycoses (110–118)
110 Dermatophytosis
111 Dermatomycosis, other and unspecified
112 Candidiasis
114 Coccidioidomycosis
115 Histoplasmosis
116 Blastomycotic infection
117 Other mycoses
118 Opportunistic mycoses

Helminthiases (120–129)
120 Schistosomiasis [bilharziasis]
121 Other trematode infections
122 Echinococcosis
123 Other cestode infection
124 Trichinosis
125 Filarial infection and dracontiasis
126 Ancylostomiasis and necatoriasis
127 Other intestinal helminthiases

128 Other and unspecified helminthiases
129 Intestinal parasitism, unspecified

Other infectious and parasitic diseases (130–136)
130 Toxoplasmosis
131 Trichomoniasis
132 Pediculosis and phthirus infestation
133 Acariasis
134 Other infestation
135 Sarcoidosis
136 Other and unspecified infectious and parasitic diseases

Late effects of infectious and parasitic diseases (137–139)
137 Late effects of tuberculosis
138 Late effects of acute poliomyelitis
139 Late effects of other infectious and parasitic diseases

2. NEOPLASMS

Malignant neoplasm of lip, oral cavity, and pharynx (140–149)
140 Malignant neoplasm of lip
141 Malignant neoplasm of tongue
142 Malignant neoplasm of major salivary glands
143 Malignant neoplasm of gum
144 Malignant neoplasm of floor of mouth
145 Malignant neoplasm of other and unspecified parts of mouth
146 Malignant neoplasm of oropharynx
147 Malignant neoplasm of nasopharynx
148 Malignant neoplasm of hypopharynx
149 Malignant neoplasm of other and ill-defined sites within the lip, oral cavity, and pharynx

Malignant neoplasm of digestive organs and peritoneum (150–159)
150 Malignant neoplasm of esophagus
151 Malignant neoplasm of stomach
152 Malignant neoplasm of small intestine, including duodenum
153 Malignant neoplasm of colon
154 Malignant neoplasm of rectum, rectosigmoid junction, and anus
155 Malignant neoplasm of liver and intrahepatic bile ducts
156 Malignant neoplasm of gallbladder and extrahepatic bile ducts
157 Malignant neoplasm of pancreas
158 Malignant neoplasm of retroperitoneum and peritoneum
159 Malignant neoplasm of other and ill-defined sites within the digestive organs and peritoneum

Malignant neoplasm of respiratory and intrathoracic organs (160–165)
160 Malignant neoplasm of nasal cavities, middle ear, and accessory sinuses
161 Malignant neoplasm of larynx
162 Malignant neoplasm of trachea, bronchus, and lung
163 Malignant neoplasm of pleura
164 Malignant neoplasm of thymus, heart, and mediastinum
165 Malignant neoplasm of other and ill-defined sites within the respiratory system and intrathoracic organs

Malignant neoplasm of bone, connective tissue, skin, and breast (170–176)
170 Malignant neoplasm of bone and articular cartilage
171 Malignant neoplasm of connective and other soft tissue
172 Malignant melanoma of skin
173 Other malignant neoplasm of skin
174 Malignant neoplasm of female breast
175 Malignant neoplasm of male breast

Kaposi's sarcoma (176)
176 Kaposi's sarcoma

Malignant neoplasm of genitourinary organs (179–189)
179 Malignant neoplasm of uterus, part unspecified
180 Malignant neoplasm of cervix uteri
181 Malignant neoplasm of placenta

182 Malignant neoplasm of body of uterus
183 Malignant neoplasm of ovary and other uterine adnexa
184 Malignant neoplasm of other and unspecified female genital organs
185 Malignant neoplasm of prostate
186 Malignant neoplasm of testis
187 Malignant neoplasm of penis and other male genital organs
188 Malignant neoplasm of bladder
189 Malignant neoplasm of kidney and other and unspecified urinary organs

Malignant neoplasm of other and unspecified sites (190–199)
190 Malignant neoplasm of eye
191 Malignant neoplasm of brain
192 Malignant neoplasm of other and unspecified parts of nervous system
193 Malignant neoplasm of thyroid gland
194 Malignant neoplasm of other endocrine glands and related structures
195 Malignant neoplasm of other and ill-defined sites
196 Secondary and unspecified malignant neoplasm of lymph nodes
197 Secondary malignant neoplasm of respiratory and digestive systems
198 Secondary malignant neoplasm of other specified sites
199 Malignant neoplasm without specification of site

Malignant neoplasm of lymphatic and hematopoietic tissue (200–208)
200 Lymphosarcoma and reticulosarcoma
201 Hodgkin's disease
202 Other malignant neoplasm of lymphoid and histiocytic tissue
203 Multiple myeloma and immunoproliferative neoplasms
204 Lymphoid leukemia
205 Myeloid leukemia
206 Monocytic leukemia
207 Other specified leukemia
208 Leukemia of unspecified cell type

Neuroendocrine tumors (209)
209 Neuroendocrine tumors

Benign neoplasms (210–229)
210 Benign neoplasm of lip, oral cavity, and pharynx
211 Benign neoplasm of other parts of digestive system
212 Benign neoplasm of respiratory and intrathoracic organs
213 Benign neoplasm of bone and articular cartilage
214 Lipoma
215 Other benign neoplasm of connective and other soft tissue
216 Benign neoplasm of skin
217 Benign neoplasm of breast
218 Uterine leiomyoma
219 Other benign neoplasm of uterus
220 Benign neoplasm of ovary
221 Benign neoplasm of other female genital organs
222 Benign neoplasm of male genital organs
223 Benign neoplasm of kidney and other urinary organs
224 Benign neoplasm of eye
225 Benign neoplasm of brain and other parts of nervous system
226 Benign neoplasm of thyroid gland
227 Benign neoplasm of other endocrine glands and related structures
228 Hemangioma and lymphangioma, any site
229 Benign neoplasm of other and unspecified sites

Carcinoma in situ (230–234)
230 Carcinoma in situ of digestive organs
231 Carcinoma in situ of respiratory system
232 Carcinoma in situ of skin
233 Carcinoma in situ of breast and genitourinary system
234 Carcinoma in situ of other and unspecified sites

ICD-9-CM, APPENDIX E

Neoplasms of uncertain behavior (235–238)
235 Neoplasm of uncertain behavior of digestive and respiratory systems
236 Neoplasm of uncertain behavior of genitourinary organs
237 Neoplasm of uncertain behavior of endocrine glands and nervous system
238 Neoplasm of uncertain behavior of other and unspecified sites and tissues

Neoplasms of unspecified nature (239)
239 Neoplasm of unspecified nature

3. ENDOCRINE, NUTRITIONAL AND METABOLIC DISEASES, AND IMMUNITY DISORDERS

Disorders of thyroid gland (240–246)
240 Simple and unspecified goiter
241 Nontoxic nodular goiter
242 Thyrotoxicosis with or without goiter
243 Congenital hypothyroidism
244 Acquired hypothyroidism
245 Thyroiditis
246 Other disorders of thyroid

Diseases of other endocrine glands (249–259)
249 Secondary diabetes mellitus
250 Diabetes mellitus
251 Other disorders of pancreatic internal secretion
252 Disorders of parathyroid gland
253 Disorders of the pituitary gland and its hypothalamic control
254 Diseases of thymus gland
255 Disorders of adrenal glands
256 Ovarian dysfunction
257 Testicular dysfunction
258 Polyglandular dysfunction and related disorders
259 Other endocrine disorders

Nutritional deficiencies (260–269)
260 Kwashiorkor
261 Nutritional marasmus
262 Other severe protein-calorie malnutrition
263 Other and unspecified protein-calorie malnutrition
264 Vitamin A deficiency
265 Thiamine and niacin deficiency states
266 Deficiency of B-complex components
267 Ascorbic acid deficiency
268 Vitamin D deficiency
269 Other nutritional deficiencies

Other metabolic disorders and immunity disorders (270–279)
270 Disorders of amino-acid transport and metabolism
271 Disorders of carbohydrate transport and metabolism
272 Disorders of lipoid metabolism
273 Disorders of plasma protein metabolism
274 Gout
275 Disorders of mineral metabolism
276 Disorders of fluid, electrolyte, and acid-base balance
277 Other and unspecified disorders of metabolism
278 Obesity and other hyperalimentation
279 Disorders involving the immune mechanism

4. DISEASES OF BLOOD AND BLOOD-FORMING ORGANS

Diseases of the blood and blood-forming organs (280–289)
280 Iron deficiency anemias
281 Other deficiency anemias
282 Hereditary hemolytic anemias
283 Acquired hemolytic anemias
284 Aplastic anemia
285 Other and unspecified anemias
286 Coagulation defects
287 Purpura and other hemorrhagic conditions
288 Diseases of white blood cells
289 Other diseases of blood and blood-forming organs

5. MENTAL DISORDERS

Organic psychotic conditions (290–294)
290 Senile and presenile organic psychotic conditions
291 Alcoholic psychoses
292 Drug psychoses
293 Transient organic psychotic conditions
294 Other organic psychotic conditions (chronic)

Other psychoses (295–299)
295 Schizophrenic psychoses
296 Affective psychoses
297 Paranoid states
298 Other nonorganic psychoses
299 Psychoses with origin specific to childhood

Neurotic disorders, personality disorders, and other nonpsychotic mental disorders (300–316)
300 Neurotic disorders
301 Personality disorders
302 Sexual deviations and disorders
303 Alcohol dependence syndrome
304 Drug dependence
305 Nondependent abuse of drugs
306 Physiological malfunction arising from mental factors
307 Special symptoms or syndromes, not elsewhere classified
308 Acute reaction to stress
309 Adjustment reaction
310 Specific nonpsychotic mental disorders following organic brain damage
311 Depressive disorder, not elsewhere classified
312 Disturbance of conduct, not elsewhere classified
313 Disturbance of emotions specific to childhood and adolescence
314 Hyperkinetic syndrome of childhood
315 Specific delays in development
316 Psychic factors associated with diseases classified elsewhere

Mental retardation (317–319)
317 Mild mental retardation
318 Other specified mental retardation
319 Unspecified mental retardation

6. DISEASES OF THE NERVOUS SYSTEM AND SENSE ORGANS

Inflammatory diseases of the central nervous system (320–326)
320 Bacterial meningitis
321 Meningitis due to other organisms
322 Meningitis of unspecified cause
323 Encephalitis, myelitis, and encephalomyelitis
324 Intracranial and intraspinal abscess
325 Phlebitis and thrombophlebitis of intracranial venous sinuses
326 Late effects of intracranial abscess or pyogenic infection
327 Organic sleep disorders

Hereditary and degenerative diseases of the central nervous system (330–337)
330 Cerebral degenerations usually manifest in childhood
331 Other cerebral degenerations
332 Parkinson's disease
333 Other extrapyramidal disease and abnormal movement disorders
334 Spinocerebellar disease
335 Anterior horn cell disease
336 Other diseases of spinal cord
337 Disorders of the autonomic nervous system

Pain (338)
338 Pain, not elsewhere classified

Other headache syndromes (339)
339 Other headache syndromes

Other disorders of the central nervous system (340–349)
340   Multiple sclerosis
341   Other demyelinating diseases of central nervous system
342   Hemiplegia and hemiparesis
343   Infantile cerebral palsy
344   Other paralytic syndromes
345   Epilepsy
346   Migraine
347   Cataplexy and narcolepsy
348   Other conditions of brain
349   Other and unspecified disorders of the nervous system

Disorders of the peripheral nervous system (350–359)
350   Trigeminal nerve disorders
351   Facial nerve disorders
352   Disorders of other cranial nerves
353   Nerve root and plexus disorders
354   Mononeuritis of upper limb and mononeuritis multiplex
355   Mononeuritis of lower limb
356   Hereditary and idiopathic peripheral neuropathy
357   Inflammatory and toxic neuropathy
358   Myoneural disorders
359   Muscular dystrophies and other myopathies

Disorders of the eye and adnexa (360–379)
360   Disorders of the globe
361   Retinal detachments and defects
362   Other retinal disorders
363   Chorioretinal inflammations and scars and other disorders of choroid
364   Disorders of iris and ciliary body
365   Glaucoma
366   Cataract
367   Disorders of refraction and accommodation
368   Visual disturbances
369   Blindness and low vision
370   Keratitis
371   Corneal opacity and other disorders of cornea
372   Disorders of conjunctiva
373   Inflammation of eyelids
374   Other disorders of eyelids
375   Disorders of lacrimal system
376   Disorders of the orbit
377   Disorders of optic nerve and visual pathways
378   Strabismus and other disorders of binocular eye movements
379   Other disorders of eye

Diseases of the ear and mastoid process (380–389)
380   Disorders of external ear
381   Nonsuppurative otitis media and Eustachian tube disorders
382   Suppurative and unspecified otitis media
383   Mastoiditis and related conditions
384   Other disorders of tympanic membrane
385   Other disorders of middle ear and mastoid
386   Vertiginous syndromes and other disorders of vestibular system
387   Otosclerosis
388   Other disorders of ear
389   Hearing loss

7. DISEASES OF THE CIRCULATORY SYSTEM

Acute rheumatic fever (390–392)
390   Rheumatic fever without mention of heart involvement
391   Rheumatic fever with heart involvement
392   Rheumatic chorea

Chronic rheumatic heart disease (393–398)
393   Chronic rheumatic pericarditis
394   Diseases of mitral valve
395   Diseases of aortic valve
396   Diseases of mitral and aortic valves
397   Diseases of other endocardial structures
398   Other rheumatic heart disease

Hypertensive disease (401–405)
401   Essential hypertension
402   Hypertensive heart disease
403   Hypertensive renal disease
404   Hypertensive heart and renal disease
405   Secondary hypertension

Ischemic heart disease (410–414)
410   Acute myocardial infarction
411   Other acute and subacute form of ischemic heart disease
412   Old myocardial infarction
413   Angina pectoris
414   Other forms of chronic ischemic heart disease

Diseases of pulmonary circulation (415–417)
415   Acute pulmonary heart disease
416   Chronic pulmonary heart disease
417   Other diseases of pulmonary circulation

Other forms of heart disease (420–429)
420   Acute pericarditis
421   Acute and subacute endocarditis
422   Acute myocarditis
423   Other diseases of pericardium
424   Other diseases of endocardium
425   Cardiomyopathy
426   Conduction disorders
427   Cardiac dysrhythmias
428   Heart failure
429   Ill-defined descriptions and complications of heart disease

Cerebrovascular disease (430–438)
430   Subarachnoid hemorrhage
431   Intracerebral hemorrhage
432   Other and unspecified intracranial hemorrhage
433   Occlusion and stenosis of precerebral arteries
434   Occlusion of cerebral arteries
435   Transient cerebral ischemia
436   Acute but ill-defined cerebrovascular disease
437   Other and ill-defined cerebrovascular disease
438   Late effects of cerebrovascular disease

Diseases of arteries, arterioles, and capillaries (440–448)
440   Atherosclerosis
441   Aortic aneurysm and dissection
442   Other aneurysm
443   Other peripheral vascular disease
444   Arterial embolism and thrombosis
445   Atheroembolism
446   Polyarteritis nodosa and allied conditions
447   Other disorders of arteries and arterioles
448   Diseases of capillaries

Diseases of veins and lymphatics, and other diseases of circulatory system (451–459)
451   Phlebitis and thrombophlebitis
452   Portal vein thrombosis
453   Other venous embolism and thrombosis
454   Varicose veins of lower extremities
455   Hemorrhoids
456   Varicose veins of other sites
457   Noninfective disorders of lymphatic channels
458   Hypotension
459   Other disorders of circulatory system

8. DISEASES OF THE RESPIRATORY SYSTEM

Acute respiratory infections (460–466)
460   Acute nasopharyngitis [common cold]
461   Acute sinusitis
462   Acute pharyngitis
463   Acute tonsillitis
464   Acute laryngitis and tracheitis
465   Acute upper respiratory infections of multiple or unspecified sites
466   Acute bronchitis and bronchiolitis

ICD-9-CM, APPENDIX E

Other diseases of upper respiratory tract (470–478)

470 Deviated nasal septum
471 Nasal polyps
472 Chronic pharyngitis and nasopharyngitis
473 Chronic sinusitis
474 Chronic disease of tonsils and adenoids
475 Peritonsillar abscess
476 Chronic laryngitis and laryngotracheitis
477 Allergic rhinitis
478 Other diseases of upper respiratory tract

Pneumonia and influenza (480–488)

480 Viral pneumonia
481 Pneumococcal pneumonia [*Streptococcus pneumoniae* pneumonia]
482 Other bacterial pneumonia
483 Pneumonia due to other specified organism
484 Pneumonia in infectious diseases classified elsewhere
485 Bronchopneumonia, organism unspecified
486 Pneumonia, organism unspecified
487 Influenza
488 Influenza due to identified avian influenza virus

Chronic obstructive pulmonary disease and allied conditions (490–496)

490 Bronchitis, not specified as acute or chronic
491 Chronic bronchitis
492 Emphysema
493 Asthma
494 Bronchiectasis
495 Extrinsic allergic alveolitis
496 Chronic airways obstruction, not elsewhere classified

Pneumoconioses and other lung diseases due to external agents (500–508)

500 Coalworkers' pneumoconiosis
501 Asbestosis
502 Pneumoconiosis due to other silica or silicates
503 Pneumoconiosis due to other inorganic dust
504 Pneumopathy due to inhalation of other dust
505 Pneumoconiosis, unspecified
506 Respiratory conditions due to chemical fumes and vapors
507 Pneumonitis due to solids and liquids
508 Respiratory conditions due to other and unspecified external agents

Other diseases of respiratory system (510–519)

510 Empyema
511 Pleurisy
512 Pneumothorax
513 Abscess of lung and mediastinum
514 Pulmonary congestion and hypostasis
515 Postinflammatory pulmonary fibrosis
516 Other alveolar and parietoalveolar pneumopathy
517 Lung involvement in conditions classified elsewhere
518 Other diseases of lung
519 Other diseases of respiratory system

9. DISEASES OF THE DIGESTIVE SYSTEM

Diseases of oral cavity, salivary glands, and jaws (520–529)

520 Disorders of tooth development and eruption
521 Diseases of hard tissues of teeth
522 Diseases of pulp and periapical tissues
523 Gingival and periodontal diseases
524 Dentofacial anomalies, including malocclusion
525 Other diseases and conditions of the teeth and supporting structures
526 Diseases of the jaws
527 Diseases of the salivary glands
528 Diseases of the oral soft tissues, excluding lesions specific for gingiva and tongue
529 Diseases and other conditions of the tongue

Diseases of esophagus, stomach, and duodenum (530–538)

530 Diseases of esophagus
531 Gastric ulcer
532 Duodenal ulcer
533 Peptic ulcer, site unspecified
534 Gastrojejunal ulcer
535 Gastritis and duodenitis
536 Disorders of function of stomach
537 Other disorders of stomach and duodenum
538 Gastrointestinal mucositis (ulcerative)

Appendicitis (540–543)

540 Acute appendicitis
541 Appendicitis, unqualified
542 Other appendicitis
543 Other diseases of appendix

Hernia of abdominal cavity (550–553)

550 Inguinal hernia
551 Other hernia of abdominal cavity, with gangrene
552 Other hernia of abdominal cavity, with obstruction, but without mention of gangrene
553 Other hernia of abdominal cavity without mention of obstruction or gangrene

Noninfective enteritis and colitis (555–558)

555 Regional enteritis
556 Ulcerative colitis
557 Vascular insufficiency of intestine
558 Other noninfective gastroenteritis and colitis

Other diseases of intestines and peritoneum (560–569)

560 Intestinal obstruction without mention of hernia
562 Diverticula of intestine
564 Functional digestive disorders, not elsewhere classified
565 Anal fissure and fistula
566 Abscess of anal and rectal regions
567 Peritonitis
568 Other disorders of peritoneum
569 Other disorders of intestine

Other diseases of digestive system (570–579)

570 Acute and subacute necrosis of liver
571 Chronic liver disease and cirrhosis
572 Liver abscess and sequelae of chronic liver disease
573 Other disorders of liver
574 Cholelithiasis
575 Other disorders of gallbladder
576 Other disorders of biliary tract
577 Diseases of pancreas
578 Gastrointestinal hemorrhage
579 Intestinal malabsorption

10. DISEASES OF THE GENITOURINARY SYSTEM

Nephritis, nephrotic syndrome, and nephrosis (580–589)

580 Acute glomerulonephritis
581 Nephrotic syndrome
582 Chronic glomerulonephritis
583 Nephritis and nephropathy, not specified as acute or chronic
584 Acute renal failure
585 Chronic renal failure
586 Renal failure, unspecified
587 Renal sclerosis, unspecified
588 Disorders resulting from impaired renal function
589 Small kidney of unknown cause

Other diseases of urinary system (590–599)

590 Infections of kidney
591 Hydronephrosis
592 Calculus of kidney and ureter
593 Other disorders of kidney and ureter
594 Calculus of lower urinary tract
595 Cystitis

596 Other disorders of bladder
597 Urethritis, not sexually transmitted, and urethral syndrome
598 Urethral stricture
599 Other disorders of urethra and urinary tract

Diseases of male genital organs (600–608)
600 Hyperplasia of prostate
601 Inflammatory diseases of prostate
602 Other disorders of prostate
603 Hydrocele
604 Orchitis and epididymitis
605 Redundant prepuce and phimosis
606 Infertility, male
607 Disorders of penis
608 Other disorders of male genital organs

Disorders of breast (610–611)
610 Benign mammary dysplasias
611 Other disorders of breast
612 Deformity and disproportion of reconstructed breast

Inflammatory disease of female pelvic organs (614–616)
614 Inflammatory disease of ovary, fallopian tube, pelvic cellular tissue, and peritoneum
615 Inflammatory diseases of uterus, except cervix
616 Inflammatory disease of cervix, vagina, and vulva

Other disorders of female genital tract (617–629)
617 Endometriosis
618 Genital prolapse
619 Fistula involving female genital tract
620 Noninflammatory disorders of ovary, fallopian tube, and broad ligament
621 Disorders of uterus, not elsewhere classified
622 Noninflammatory disorders of cervix
623 Noninflammatory disorders of vagina
624 Noninflammatory disorders of vulva and perineum
625 Pain and other symptoms associated with female genital organs
626 Disorders of menstruation and other abnormal bleeding from female genital tract
627 Menopausal and postmenopausal disorders
628 Infertility, female
629 Other disorders of female genital organs

11. COMPLICATIONS OF PREGNANCY, CHILDBIRTH, AND THE PUERPERIUM

Ectopic and molar pregnancy and other pregnancy with abortive outcome (630–639)
630 Hydatidiform mole
631 Other abnormal product of conception
632 Missed abortion
633 Ectopic pregnancy
634 Spontaneous abortion
635 Legally induced abortion
636 Illegally induced abortion
637 Unspecified abortion
638 Failed attempted abortion
639 Complications following abortion and ectopic and molar pregnancies

Complications mainly related to pregnancy (640–649)
640 Hemorrhage in early pregnancy
641 Antepartum hemorrhage, abruptio placentae, and placenta previa
642 Hypertension complicating pregnancy, childbirth, and the puerperium
643 Excessive vomiting in pregnancy
644 Early or threatened labor
645 Prolonged pregnancy
646 Other complications of pregnancy, not elsewhere classified
647 Infective and parasitic conditions in the mother classifiable elsewhere but complicating pregnancy, childbirth, and the puerperium

648 Other current conditions in the mother classifiable elsewhere but complicating pregnancy, childbirth, and the puerperium
649 Other conditions or status of the mother complicating pregnancy, childbirth, or the puerperium

Normal delivery, and other indications for care in pregnancy, labor, and delivery (650–659)
650 Normal delivery
651 Multiple gestation
652 Malposition and malpresentation of fetus
653 Disproportion
654 Abnormality of organs and soft tissues of pelvis
655 Known or suspected fetal abnormality affecting management of mother
656 Other fetal and placental problems affecting management of mother
657 Polyhydramnios
658 Other problems associated with amniotic cavity and membranes
659 Other indications for care or intervention related to labor and delivery and not elsewhere classified

Complications occurring mainly in the course of labor and delivery (660–669)
660 Obstructed labor
661 Abnormality of forces of labor
662 Long labor
663 Umbilical cord complications
664 Trauma to perineum and vulva during delivery
665 Other obstetrical trauma
666 Postpartum hemorrhage
667 Retained placenta or membranes, without hemorrhage
668 Complications of the administration of anesthetic or other sedation in labor and delivery
669 Other complications of labor and delivery, not elsewhere classified

Complications of the puerperium (670–677)
670 Major puerperal infection
671 Venous complications in pregnancy and the puerperium
672 Pyrexia of unknown origin during the puerperium
673 Obstetrical pulmonary embolism
674 Other and unspecified complications of the puerperium, not elsewhere classified
675 Infections of the breast and nipple associated with childbirth
676 Other disorders of the breast associated with childbirth, and disorders of lactation
677 Late effect of complication of pregnancy, childbirth, and the puerperium

Other Maternal and Fetal Complications (678-679)
678 Other fetal conditions
679 Complications of in utero procedures

12. DISEASES OF THE SKIN AND SUBCUTANEOUS TISSUE

Infections of skin and subcutaneous tissue (680–686)
680 Carbuncle and furuncle
681 Cellulitis and abscess of finger and toe
682 Other cellulitis and abscess
683 Acute lymphadenitis
684 Impetigo
685 Pilonidal cyst
686 Other local infections of skin and subcutaneous tissue

Other inflammatory conditions of skin and subcutaneous tissue (690–698)
690 Erythematosquamous dermatosis
691 Atopic dermatitis and related conditions
692 Contact dermatitis and other eczema
693 Dermatitis due to substances taken internally
694 Bullous dermatoses

ICD-9-CM, APPENDIX E

695   Erythematous conditions
696   Psoriasis and similar disorders
697   Lichen
698   Pruritus and related conditions

Other diseases of skin and subcutaneous tissue (700–709)
700   Corns and callosities
701   Other hypertrophic and atrophic conditions of skin
702   Other dermatoses
703   Diseases of nail
704   Diseases of hair and hair follicles
705   Disorders of sweat glands
706   Diseases of sebaceous glands
707   Chronic ulcer of skin
708   Urticaria
709   Other disorders of skin and subcutaneous tissue

13. DISEASES OF THE MUSCULOSKELETAL SYSTEM AND CONNECTIVE TISSUE

Arthropathies and related disorders (710–719)
710   Diffuse diseases of connective tissue
711   Arthropathy associated with infections
712   Crystal arthropathies
713   Arthropathy associated with other disorders classified elsewhere
714   Rheumatoid arthritis and other inflammatory polyarthropathies
715   Osteoarthrosis and allied disorders
716   Other and unspecified arthropathies
717   Internal derangement of knee
718   Other derangement of joint
719   Other and unspecified disorder of joint

Dorsopathies (720–724)
720   Ankylosing spondylitis and other inflammatory spondylopathies
721   Spondylosis and allied disorders
722   Intervertebral disc disorders
723   Other disorders of cervical region
724   Other and unspecified disorders of back

Rheumatism, excluding the back (725–729)
725   Polymyalgia rheumatica
726   Peripheral enthesopathies and allied syndromes
727   Other disorders of synovium, tendon, and bursa
728   Disorders of muscle, ligament, and fascia
729   Other disorders of soft tissues

Osteopathies, chondropathies, and acquired musculoskeletal deformities (730–739)
730   Osteomyelitis, periostitis, and other infections involving bone
731   Osteitis deformans and osteopathies associated with other disorders classified elsewhere
732   Osteochondropathies
733   Other disorders of bone and cartilage
734   Flat foot
735   Acquired deformities of toe
736   Other acquired deformities of limbs
737   Curvature of spine
738   Other acquired deformity
739   Nonallopathic lesions, not elsewhere classified

14. CONGENITAL ANOMALIES

Congential anomalies (740–759)
740   Anencephalus and similar anomalies
741   Spina bifida
742   Other congenital anomalies of nervous system
743   Congenital anomalies of eye
744   Congenital anomalies of ear, face, and neck
745   Bulbus cordis anomalies and anomalies of cardiac septal closure

746   Other congenital anomalies of heart
747   Other congenital anomalies of circulatory system
748   Congenital anomalies of respiratory system
749   Cleft palate and cleft lip
750   Other congenital anomalies of upper alimentary tract
751   Other congenital anomalies of digestive system
752   Congenital anomalies of genital organs
753   Congenital anomalies of urinary system
754   Certain congenital musculoskeletal deformities
755   Other congenital anomalies of limbs
756   Other congenital musculoskeletal anomalies
757   Congenital anomalies of the integument
758   Chromosomal anomalies
759   Other and unspecified congenital anomalies

15. CERTAIN CONDITIONS ORIGINATING IN THE PERINATAL PERIOD

Maternal causes of perinatal morbidity and mortality (760–763)
760   Fetus or newborn affected by maternal conditions which may be unrelated to present pregnancy
761   Fetus or newborn affected by maternal complications of pregnancy
762   Fetus or newborn affected by complications of placenta, cord, and membranes
763   Fetus or newborn affected by other complications of labor and delivery

Other conditions originating in the perinatal period (764–779)
764   Slow fetal growth and fetal malnutrition
765   Disorders relating to short gestation and unspecified low birthweight
766   Disorders relating to long gestation and high birthweight
767   Birth trauma
768   Intrauterine hypoxia and birth asphyxia
769   Respiratory distress syndrome
770   Other respiratory conditions of fetus and newborn
771   Infections specific to the perinatal period
772   Fetal and neonatal hemorrhage
773   Hemolytic disease of fetus or newborn, due to isoimmunization
774   Other perinatal jaundice
775   Endocrine and metabolic disturbances specific to the fetus and newborn
776   Hematological disorders of fetus and newborn
777   Perinatal disorders of digestive system
778   Conditions involving the integument and temperature regulation of fetus and newborn
779   Other and ill-defined conditions originating in the perinatal period

16. SYMPTOMS, SIGNS, AND ILL-DEFINED CONDITIONS

Symptoms (780–789)
780   General symptoms
781   Symptoms involving nervous and musculoskeletal systems
782   Symptoms involving skin and other integumentary tissue
783   Symptoms concerning nutrition, metabolism, and development
784   Symptoms involving head and neck
785   Symptoms involving cardiovascular system
786   Symptoms involving respiratory system and other chest symptoms
787   Symptoms involving digestive system
788   Symptoms involving urinary system
789   Other symptoms involving abdomen and pelvis

Nonspecific abnormal findings (790–796)
790   Nonspecific findings on examination of blood
791   Nonspecific findings on examination of urine
792   Nonspecific abnormal findings in other body substances
793   Nonspecific abnormal findings on radiological and other examination of body structure
794   Nonspecific abnormal results of function studies

795 Nonspecific abnormal histological and immunological findings
796 Other nonspecific abnormal findings

Ill-defined and unknown causes of morbidity and mortality (797–799)
797 Senility without mention of psychosis
798 Sudden death, cause unknown
799 Other ill-defined and unknown causes of morbidity and mortality

17. INJURY AND POISONING

Fracture of skull (800–804)
800 Fracture of vault of skull
801 Fracture of base of skull
802 Fracture of face bones
803 Other and unqualified skull fractures
804 Multiple fractures involving skull or face with other bones

Fracture of spine and trunk (805–809)
805 Fracture of vertebral column without mention of spinal cord lesion
806 Fracture of vertebral column with spinal cord lesion
807 Fracture of rib(s), sternum, larynx, and trachea
808 Fracture of pelvis
809 Ill-defined fractures of bones of trunk

Fracture of upper limb (810–819)
810 Fracture of clavicle
811 Fracture of scapula
812 Fracture of humerus
813 Fracture of radius and ulna
814 Fracture of carpal bone(s)
815 Fracture of metacarpal bone(s)
816 Fracture of one or more phalanges of hand
817 Multiple fractures of hand bones
818 Ill-defined fractures of upper limb
819 Multiple fractures involving both upper limbs, and upper limb with rib(s) and sternum

Fracture of lower limb (820–829)
820 Fracture of neck of femur
821 Fracture of other and unspecified parts of femur
822 Fracture of patella
823 Fracture of tibia and fibula
824 Fracture of ankle
825 Fracture of one or more tarsal and metatarsal bones
826 Fracture of one or more phalanges of foot
827 Other, multiple, and ill-defined fractures of lower limb
828 Multiple fractures involving both lower limbs, lower with upper limb, and lower limb(s) with rib(s) and sternum
829 Fracture of unspecified bones

Dislocation (830–839)
830 Dislocation of jaw
831 Dislocation of shoulder
832 Dislocation of elbow
833 Dislocation of wrist
834 Dislocation of finger
835 Dislocation of hip
836 Dislocation of knee
837 Dislocation of ankle
838 Dislocation of foot
839 Other, multiple, and ill-defined dislocations

Sprains and strains of joints and adjacent muscles (840–848)
840 Sprains and strains of shoulder and upper arm
841 Sprains and strains of elbow and forearm
842 Sprains and strains of wrist and hand
843 Sprains and strains of hip and thigh
844 Sprains and strains of knee and leg
845 Sprains and strains of ankle and foot
846 Sprains and strains of sacroiliac region
847 Sprains and strains of other and unspecified parts of back
848 Other and ill-defined sprains and strains

Intracranial injury, excluding those with skull fracture (850–854)
850 Concussion
851 Cerebral laceration and contusion
852 Subarachnoid, subdural, and extradural hemorrhage, following injury
853 Other and unspecified intracranial hemorrhage following injury
854 Intracranial injury of other and unspecified nature

Internal injury of chest, abdomen, and pelvis (860–869)
860 Traumatic pneumothorax and hemothorax
861 Injury to heart and lung
862 Injury to other and unspecified intrathoracic organs
863 Injury to gastrointestinal tract
864 Injury to liver
865 Injury to spleen
866 Injury to kidney
867 Injury to pelvic organs
868 Injury to other intra-abdominal organs
869 Internal injury to unspecified or ill-defined organs

Open wound of head, neck, and trunk (870–879)
870 Open wound of ocular adnexa
871 Open wound of eyeball
872 Open wound of ear
873 Other open wound of head
874 Open wound of neck
875 Open wound of chest (wall)
876 Open wound of back
877 Open wound of buttock
878 Open wound of genital organs (external), including traumatic amputation
879 Open wound of other and unspecified sites, except limbs

Open wound of upper limb (880–887)
880 Open wound of shoulder and upper arm
881 Open wound of elbow, forearm, and wrist
882 Open wound of hand except finger(s) alone
883 Open wound of finger(s)
884 Multiple and unspecified open wound of upper limb
885 Traumatic amputation of thumb (complete) (partial)
886 Traumatic amputation of other finger(s) (complete) (partial)
887 Traumatic amputation of arm and hand (complete) (partial)

Open wound of lower limb (890–897)
890 Open wound of hip and thigh
891 Open wound of knee, leg [except thigh], and ankle
892 Open wound of foot except toe(s) alone
893 Open wound of toe(s)
894 Multiple and unspecified open wound of lower limb
895 Traumatic amputation of toe(s) (complete) (partial)
896 Traumatic amputation of foot (complete) (partial)
897 Traumatic amputation of leg(s) (complete) (partial)

Injury to blood vessels (900–904)
900 Injury to blood vessels of head and neck
901 Injury to blood vessels of thorax
902 Injury to blood vessels of abdomen and pelvis
903 Injury to blood vessels of upper extremity
904 Injury to blood vessels of lower extremity and unspecified sites

Late effects of injuries, poisonings, toxic effects, and other external causes (905–909)
905 Late effects of musculoskeletal and connective tissue injuries
906 Late effects of injuries to skin and subcutaneous tissues
907 Late effects of injuries to the nervous system
908 Late effects of other and unspecified injuries
909 Late effects of other and unspecified external causes

Superficial injury (910–919)
910 Superficial injury of face, neck, and scalp except eye
911 Superficial injury of trunk
912 Superficial injury of shoulder and upper arm

913 Superficial injury of elbow, forearm, and wrist
914 Superficial injury of hand(s) except finger(s) alone
915 Superficial injury of finger(s)
916 Superficial injury of hip, thigh, leg, and ankle
917 Superficial injury of foot and toe(s)
918 Superficial injury of eye and adnexa
919 Superficial injury of other, multiple, and unspecified sites

Contusion with intact skin surface (920–924)
920 Contusion of face, scalp, and neck except eye(s)
921 Contusion of eye and adnexa
922 Contusion of trunk
923 Contusion of upper limb
924 Contusion of lower limb and of other and unspecified sites

Crushing injury (925–929)
925 Crushing injury of face, scalp, and neck
926 Crushing injury of trunk
927 Crushing injury of upper limb
928 Crushing injury of lower limb
929 Crushing injury of multiple and unspecified sites

Effects of foreign body entering through orifice (930–939)
930 Foreign body on external eye
931 Foreign body in ear
932 Foreign body in nose
933 Foreign body in pharynx and larynx
934 Foreign body in trachea, bronchus, and lung
935 Foreign body in mouth, esophagus, and stomach
936 Foreign body in intestine and colon
937 Foreign body in anus and rectum
938 Foreign body in digestive system, unspecified
939 Foreign body in genitourinary tract

Burns (940–949)
940 Burn confined to eye and adnexa
941 Burn of face, head, and neck
942 Burn of trunk
943 Burn of upper limb, except wrist and hand
944 Burn of wrist(s) and hand(s)
945 Burn of lower limb(s)
946 Burns of multiple specified sites
947 Burn of internal organs
948 Burns classified according to extent of body surface involved
949 Burn, unspecified

Injury to nerves and spinal cord (950–957)
950 Injury to optic nerve and pathways
951 Injury to other cranial nerve(s)
952 Spinal cord injury without evidence of spinal bone injury
953 Injury to nerve roots and spinal plexus
954 Injury to other nerve(s) of trunk excluding shoulder and pelvic girdles
955 Injury to peripheral nerve(s) of shoulder girdle and upper limb
956 Injury to peripheral nerve(s) of pelvic girdle and lower limb
957 Injury to other and unspecified nerves

Certain traumatic complications and unspecified injuries (958–959)
958 Certain early complications of trauma
959 Injury, other and unspecified

Poisoning by drugs, medicinals and biological substances (960–979)
960 Poisoning by antibiotics
961 Poisoning by other anti-infectives
962 Poisoning by hormones and synthetic substitutes
963 Poisoning by primarily systemic agents
964 Poisoning by agents primarily affecting blood constituents
965 Poisoning by analgesics, antipyretics, and antirheumatics
966 Poisoning by anticonvulsants and anti-Parkinsonism drugs
967 Poisoning by sedatives and hypnotics
968 Poisoning by other central nervous system depressants and anesthetics

969 Poisoning by psychotropic agents
970 Poisoning by central nervous system stimulants
971 Poisoning by drugs primarily affecting the autonomic nervous system
972 Poisoning by agents primarily affecting the cardiovascular system
973 Poisoning by agents primarily affecting the gastrointestinal system
974 Poisoning by water, mineral, and uric acid metabolism drugs
975 Poisoning by agents primarily acting on the smooth and skeletal muscles and respiratory system
976 Poisoning by agents primarily affecting skin and mucous membrane, ophthalmological, otorhinolaryngological, and dental drugs
977 Poisoning by other and unspecified drugs and medicinals
978 Poisoning by bacterial vaccines
979 Poisoning by other vaccines and biological substances

Toxic effects of substances chiefly nonmedicinal as to source (980–989)
980 Toxic effect of alcohol
981 Toxic effect of petroleum products
982 Toxic effect of solvents other than petroleum-based
983 Toxic effect of corrosive aromatics, acids, and caustic alkalis
984 Toxic effect of lead and its compounds (including fumes)
985 Toxic effect of other metals
986 Toxic effect of carbon monoxide
987 Toxic effect of other gases, fumes, or vapors
988 Toxic effect of noxious substances eaten as food
989 Toxic effect of other substances, chiefly nonmedicinal as to source

Other and unspecified effects of external causes (990–995)
990 Effects of radiation, unspecified
991 Effects of reduced temperature
992 Effects of heat and light
993 Effects of air pressure
994 Effects of other external causes
995 Certain adverse effects, not elsewhere classified

Complications of surgical and medical care, not elsewhere classified (996–999)
996 Complications peculiar to certain specified procedures
997 Complications affecting specified body systems, not elsewhere classified
998 Other complications of procedures, not elsewhere classified
999 Complications of medical care, not elsewhere classified

SUPPLEMENTARY CLASSIFICATION OF FACTORS INFLUENCING HEALTH STATUS AND CONTACT WITH HEALTH SERVICES (V01–V86)

Persons with potential health hazards related to communicable diseases (V01–V09)
V01 Contact with or exposure to communicable diseases
V02 Carrier or suspected carrier of infectious diseases
V03 Need for prophylactic vaccination and inoculation against bacterial diseases
V04 Need for prophylactic vaccination and inoculation against certain viral diseases
V05 Need for other prophylactic vaccination and inoculation against single diseases
V06 Need for prophylactic vaccination and inoculation against combinations of diseases
V07 Need for isolation and other prophylactic measures
V08 Asymptomatic human immunodeficiency virus [HIV] infection status
V09 Infection with drug-resistant microorganisms

Persons with potential health hazards related to personal and family history (V10–V19)
V10 Personal history of malignant neoplasm
V11 Personal history of mental disorder
V12 Personal history of certain other diseases
V13 Personal history of other diseases

V14 Personal history of allergy to medicinal agents
V15 Other personal history presenting hazards to health
V16 Family history of malignant neoplasm
V17 Family history of certain chronic disabling diseases
V18 Family history of certain other specific conditions
V19 Family history of other conditions

Persons encountering health services in circumstances related to reproduction and development (V20–V29)
V20 Health supervision of infant or child
V21 Constitutional states in development
V22 Normal pregnancy
V23 Supervision of high-risk pregnancy
V24 Postpartum care and examination
V25 Encounter for contraceptive management
V26 Procreative management
V27 Outcome of delivery
V28 Antenatal screening
V29 Observation and evaluation of newborns and infants for suspected condition not found

Liveborn infants according to type of birth (V30–V39)
V30 Single liveborn
V31 Twin, mate liveborn
V32 Twin, mate stillborn
V33 Twin, unspecified
V34 Other multiple, mates all liveborn
V35 Other multiple, mates all stillborn
V36 Other multiple, mates live- and stillborn
V37 Other multiple, unspecified
V39 Unspecified

Persons with a condition influencing their health status (V40–V49)
V40 Mental and behavioral problems
V41 Problems with special senses and other special functions
V42 Organ or tissue replaced by transplant
V43 Organ or tissue replaced by other means
V44 Artificial opening status
V45 Other postsurgical states
V46 Other dependence on machines
V47 Other problems with internal organs
V48 Problems with head, neck, and trunk
V49 Problems with limbs and other problems

Persons encountering health services for specific procedures and aftercare (V50–V59)
V50 Elective surgery for purposes other than remedying health states
V51 Aftercare involving the use of plastic surgery
V52 Fitting and adjustment of prosthetic device
V53 Fitting and adjustment of other device
V54 Other orthopedic aftercare
V55 Attention to artificial openings
V56 Encounter for dialysis and dialysis catheter care
V57 Care involving use of rehabilitation procedures
V58 Other and unspecified aftercare
V59 Donors

Persons encountering health services in other circumstances (V60–V69)
V60 Housing, household, and economic circumstances
V61 Other family circumstances
V62 Other psychosocial circumstances
V63 Unavailability of other medical facilities for care
V64 Persons encountering health services for specific procedures, not carried out
V65 Other persons seeking consultation without complaint or sickness
V66 Convalescence and palliative care
V67 Follow-up examination
V68 Encounters for administrative purposes
V69 Problems related to lifestyle

Persons without reported diagnosis encountered during examination and investigation of individuals and populations (V70–V82)
V70 General medical examination
V71 Observation and evaluation for suspected conditions
V72 Special investigations and examinations
V73 Special screening examination for viral and chlamydial diseases
V74 Special screening examination for bacterial and spirochetal diseases
V75 Special screening examination for other infectious diseases
V76 Special screening for malignant neoplasms
V77 Special screening for endocrine, nutritional, metabolic, and immunity disorders
V78 Special screening for disorders of blood and blood-forming organs
V79 Special screening for mental disorders and developmental handicaps
V80 Special screening for neurological, eye, and ear diseases
V81 Special screening for cardiovascular, respiratory, and genitourinary diseases
V82 Special screening for other conditions

Genetics (V83–V84)
V83 Genetic carrier status
V84 Genetic susceptibility to malignant neoplasm

Body Mass Index (V85)
V85 Body mass index

Estrogen Receptor Status (V86)
V86 Estrogen receptor status

Other specified personal exposures and history presenting hazards to health (V87)
V87 Other specified personal exposures and history presenting hazards to health

Acquired absence of other organs and tissue (V88)
V88 Acquired absence of other organs and tissue

Other suspected conditions not found (V89)
V89 Other suspected conditions not found

SUPPLEMENTARY CLASSIFICATION OF EXTERNAL CAUSES OF INJURY AND POISONING (E800–E899)

Railway accidents (E800–E807)
E800 Railway accident involving collision with rolling stock
E801 Railway accident involving collision with other object
E802 Railway accident involving derailment without antecedent collision
E803 Railway accident involving explosion, fire, or burning
E804 Fall in, on, or from railway train
E805 Hit by rolling stock
E806 Other specified railway accident
E807 Railway accident of unspecified nature

Motor vehicle traffic accidents (E810–E819)
E810 Motor vehicle traffic accident involving collision with train
E811 Motor vehicle traffic accident involving re-entrant collision with another motor vehicle
E812 Other motor vehicle traffic accident involving collision with another motor vehicle
E813 Motor vehicle traffic accident involving collision with other vehicle
E814 Motor vehicle traffic accident involving collision with pedestrian
E815 Other motor vehicle traffic accident involving collision on the highway
E816 Motor vehicle traffic accident due to loss of control, without collision on the highway
E817 Noncollision motor vehicle traffic accident while boarding or alighting
E818 Other noncollision motor vehicle traffic accident
E819 Motor vehicle traffic accident of unspecified nature

ICD-9-CM, APPENDIX E

Motor vehicle nontraffic accidents (E820–E825)
E820 Nontraffic accident involving motor-driven snow vehicle
E821 Nontraffic accident involving other off-road motor vehicle
E822 Other motor vehicle nontraffic accident involving collision with moving object
E823 Other motor vehicle nontraffic accident involving collision with stationary object
E824 Other motor vehicle nontraffic accident while boarding and alighting
E825 Other motor vehicle nontraffic accident of other and unspecified nature

Other road vehicle accidents (E826–E829)
E826 Pedal cycle accident
E827 Animal-drawn vehicle accident
E828 Accident involving animal being ridden
E829 Other road vehicle accidents

Water transport accidents (E830–E838)
E830 Accident to watercraft causing submersion
E831 Accident to watercraft causing other injury
E832 Other accidental submersion or drowning in water transport accident
E833 Fall on stairs or ladders in water transport
E834 Other fall from one level to another in water transport
E835 Other and unspecified fall in water transport
E836 Machinery accident in water transport
E837 Explosion, fire, or burning in watercraft
E838 Other and unspecified water transport accident

Air and space transport accidents (E840–E845)
E840 Accident to powered aircraft at takeoff or landing
E841 Accident to powered aircraft, other and unspecified
E842 Accident to unpowered aircraft
E843 Fall in, on, or from aircraft
E844 Other specified air transport accidents
E845 Accident involving spacecraft

Vehicle accidents, not elsewhere classifiable (E846–E849)
E846 Accidents involving powered vehicles used solely within the buildings and premises of an industrial or commercial establishment
E847 Accidents involving cable cars not running on rails
E848 Accidents involving other vehicles, not elsewhere classifiable
E849 Place of occurrence

Accidental poisoning by drugs, medicinal substances, and biologicals (E850–E858)
E850 Accidental poisoning by analgesics, antipyretics, and antirheumatics
E851 Accidental poisoning by barbiturates
E852 Accidental poisoning by other sedatives and hypnotics
E853 Accidental poisoning by tranquilizers
E854 Accidental poisoning by other psychotropic agents
E855 Accidental poisoning by other drugs acting on central and autonomic nervous systems
E856 Accidental poisoning by antibiotics
E857 Accidental poisoning by anti-infectives
E858 Accidental poisoning by other drugs

Accidental poisoning by other solid and liquid substances, gases, and vapors (E860–E869)
E860 Accidental poisoning by alcohol, not elsewhere classified
E861 Accidental poisoning by cleansing and polishing agents, disinfectants, paints, and varnishes
E862 Accidental poisoning by petroleum products, other solvents and their vapors, not elsewhere classified
E863 Accidental poisoning by agricultural and horticultural chemical and pharmaceutical preparations other than plant foods and fertilizers
E864 Accidental poisoning by corrosives and caustics, not elsewhere classified
E865 Accidental poisoning from poisonous foodstuffs and poisonous plants

E866 Accidental poisoning by other and unspecified solid and liquid substances
E867 Accidental poisoning by gas distributed by pipeline
E868 Accidental poisoning by other utility gas and other carbon monoxide
E869 Accidental poisoning by other gases and vapors

Misadventures to patients during surgical and medical care (E870–E876)
E870 Accidental cut, puncture, perforation, or hemorrhage during medical care
E871 Foreign object left in body during procedure
E872 Failure of sterile precautions during procedure
E873 Failure in dosage
E874 Mechanical failure of instrument or apparatus during procedure
E875 Contaminated or infected blood, other fluid, drug, or biological substance
E876 Other and unspecified misadventures during medical care

Surgical and medical procedures as the cause of abnormal reaction of patient or later complication, without mention of misadventure at the time of procedure (E878–E879)
E878 Surgical operation and other surgical procedures as the cause of abnormal reaction of patient, or of later complication, without mention of misadventure at the time of operation
E879 Other procedures, without mention of misadventure at the time of procedure, as the cause of abnormal reaction of patient, or of later complication

Accidental falls (E880–E888)
E880 Fall on or from stairs or steps
E881 Fall on or from ladders or scaffolding
E882 Fall from or out of building or other structure
E883 Fall into hole or other opening in surface
E884 Other fall from one level to another
E885 Fall on same level from slipping, tripping, or stumbling
E886 Fall on same level from collision, pushing, or shoving, by or with other person
E887 Fracture, cause unspecified
E888 Other and unspecified fall

Accidents caused by fire and flames (E890–E899)
E890 Conflagration in private dwelling
E891 Conflagration in other and unspecified building or structure
E892 Conflagration not in building or structure
E893 Accident caused by ignition of clothing
E894 Ignition of highly inflammable material
E895 Accident caused by controlled fire in private dwelling
E896 Accident caused by controlled fire in other and unspecified building or structure
E897 Accident caused by controlled fire not in building or structure
E898 Accident caused by other specified fire and flames
E899 Accident caused by unspecified fire

Accidents due to natural and environmental factors (E900–E909)
E900 Excessive heat
E901 Excessive cold
E902 High and low air pressure and changes in air pressure
E903 Travel and motion
E904 Hunger, thirst, exposure, and neglect
E905 Venomous animals and plants as the cause of poisoning and toxic reactions
E906 Other injury caused by animals
E907 Lightning
E908 Cataclysmic storms, and floods resulting from storms
E909 Cataclysmic earth surface movements and eruptions

Accidents caused by submersion, suffocation, and foreign bodies (E910–E915)
E910 Accidental drowning and submersion
E911 Inhalation and ingestion of food causing obstruction of respiratory tract or suffocation
E912 Inhalation and ingestion of other object causing obstruction of respiratory tract or suffocation
E913 Accidental mechanical suffocation
E914 Foreign body accidentally entering eye and adnexa
E915 Foreign body accidentally entering other orifice

Other accidents (E916–E928)
E916 Struck accidentally by falling object
E917 Striking against or struck accidentally by objects or persons
E918 Caught accidentally in or between objects
E919 Accidents caused by machinery
E920 Accidents caused by cutting and piercing instruments or objects
E921 Accident caused by explosion of pressure vessel
E922 Accident caused by firearm missile
E923 Accident caused by explosive material
E924 Accident caused by hot substance or object, caustic or corrosive material, and steam
E925 Accident caused by electric current
E926 Exposure to radiation
E927 Overexertion and strenuous movements
E928 Other and unspecified environmental and accidental causes

Late effects of accidental injury (E929)
E929 Late effects of accidental injury

Drugs, medicinal and biological substances causing adverse effects in therapeutic use (E930–E949)
E930 Antibiotics
E931 Other anti-infectives
E932 Hormones and synthetic substitutes
E933 Primarily systemic agents
E934 Agents primarily affecting blood constituents
E935 Analgesics, antipyretics, and antirheumatics
E936 Anticonvulsants and anti-Parkinsonism drugs
E937 Sedatives and hypnotics
E938 Other central nervous system depressants and anesthetics
E939 Psychotropic agents
E940 Central nervous system stimulants
E941 Drugs primarily affecting the autonomic nervous system
E942 Agents primarily affecting the cardiovascular system
E943 Agents primarily affecting gastrointestinal system
E944 Water, mineral, and uric acid metabolism drugs
E945 Agents primarily acting on the smooth and skeletal muscles and respiratory system
E946 Agents primarily affecting skin and mucous membrane, ophthalmological, otorhinolaryngological, and dental drugs
E947 Other and unspecified drugs and medicinal substances
E948 Bacterial vaccines
E949 Other vaccines and biological substances

Suicide and self-inflicted injury (E950–E959)
E950 Suicide and self-inflicted poisoning by solid or liquid substances
E951 Suicide and self-inflicted poisoning by gases in domestic use
E952 Suicide and self-inflicted poisoning by other gases and vapors
E953 Suicide and self-inflicted injury by hanging, strangulation, and suffocation
E954 Suicide and self-inflicted injury by submersion [drowning]
E955 Suicide and self-inflicted injury by firearms and explosives
E956 Suicide and self-inflicted injury by cutting and piercing instruments
E957 Suicide and self-inflicted injuries by jumping from high place

E958 Suicide and self-inflicted injury by other and unspecified means
E959 Late effects of self-inflicted injury

Homicide and injury purposely inflicted by other persons (E960–E969)
E960 Fight, brawl, and rape
E961 Assault by corrosive or caustic substance, except poisoning
E962 Assault by poisoning
E963 Assault by hanging and strangulation
E964 Assault by submersion [drowning]
E965 Assault by firearms and explosives
E966 Assault by cutting and piercing instrument
E967 Child and adult battering and other maltreatment
E968 Assault by other and unspecified means
E969 Late effects of injury purposely inflicted by other person

Legal intervention (E970–E978)
E970 Injury due to legal intervention by firearms
E971 Injury due to legal intervention by explosives
E972 Injury due to legal intervention by gas
E973 Injury due to legal intervention by blunt object
E974 Injury due to legal intervention by cutting and piercing instruments
E975 Injury due to legal intervention by other specified means
E976 Injury due to legal intervention by unspecified means
E977 Late effects of injuries due to legal intervention
E978 Legal execution
E979 Terrorism

Injury undetermined whether accidentally or purposely inflicted (E980–E989)
E980 Poisoning by solid or liquid substances, undetermined whether accidentally or purposely inflicted
E981 Poisoning by gases in domestic use, undetermined whether accidentally or purposely inflicted
E982 Poisoning by other gases, undetermined whether accidentally or purposely inflicted
E983 Hanging, strangulation, or suffocation, undetermined whether accidentally or purposely inflicted
E984 Submersion [drowning], undetermined whether accidentally or purposely inflicted
E985 Injury by firearms and explosives, undetermined whether accidentally or purposely inflicted
E986 Injury by cutting and piercing instruments, undetermined whether accidentally or purposely inflicted
E987 Falling from high place, undetermined whether accidentally or purposely inflicted
E988 Injury by other and unspecified means, undetermined whether accidentally or purposely inflicted
E989 Late effects of injury, undetermined whether accidentally or purposely inflicted

Injury resulting from operations of war (E990–E999)
E990 Injury due to war operations by fires and conflagrations
E991 Injury due to war operations by bullets and fragments
E992 Injury due to war operations by explosion of marine weapons
E993 Injury due to war operations by other explosion
E994 Injury due to war operations by destruction of aircraft
E995 Injury due to war operations by other and unspecified forms of conventional warfare
E996 Injury due to war operations by nuclear weapons
E997 Injury due to war operations by other forms of unconventional warfare
E998 Injury due to war operations but occurring after cessation of hostilities
E999 Late effects of injury due to war operations

TABLE A

TABLE OF BACTERIAL FOOD POISONING

Bacteria Responsible	Description	Habitat	Types of Foods	Symptoms	Cause	Temperature Sensitivity
Staphylococcus aureus	Produces a heat-stable toxin.	Nose and throat of 30 to 50 percent of healthy population; also skin and superficial wounds.	Meat and seafood salads, sandwich spreads, and high salt foods.	Nausea, vomiting, and diarrhea within 4 to 6 hours. No fever.	Poor personal hygiene and subsequent temperature abuse.	No growth below 40° F. Bacteria are destroyed by normal cooking, but toxin is heat-stable.
Clostridium perfringens	Produces a spore and prefers low oxygen atmosphere. Live cells must be ingested.	Dust, soil, and gastrointestinal tracts of animals and man.	Meat and poultry dishes, sauces and gravies.	Cramps and diarrhea within 12 to 24 hours. No vomiting or fever.	Improper temperature control of hot foods and recontamination.	No growth below 40° F. Bacteria are killed by normal cooking, but a heat-stable spore can survive.
Clostridium botulinum	Produces a spore and requires a low oxygen atmosphere. Produces a heat-sensitive toxin.	Soils, plants, marine sediments, and fish.	Home-canned foods.	Blurred vision, respiratory distress, and possible DEATH.	Improper methods of home-processing foods.	Type E and Type B can grow at 38° F. Bacteria destroyed by cooking and the toxin is destroyed by boiling for 5 to 10 minutes. Heat-resistant spore can survive.
Vibrio parahaemolyticus	Requires salt for growth.	Fish and shellfish.	Raw and cooked seafood.	Diarrhea, cramps, vomiting, headache, and fever within 12 to 24 hours.	Recontamination of cooked foods or eating raw seafood.	No growth below 40° F. Bacteria killed by normal cooking.

PART IV

Procedures
Volume 3

A

Abbe operation
  construction of vagina 70.61
    with graft or prosthesis 70.63
  intestinal anastomosis - *see*
      Anastomosis, intestine
Abciximab, infusion 99.20
Abdominocentesis 54.91
Abdominohysterectomy 68.49
  laparoscopic 68.41
Abdominoplasty 86.83
Abdominoscopy 54.21
Abdominouterotomy 68.0
  obstetrical 74.99
Abduction, arytenoid 31.69
AbioCor® total replacement heart 37.52
Ablation
  biliary tract (lesion) by ERCP 51.64
  endometrial (hysteroscopic) 68.23
  inner ear (cryosurgery) (ultrasound)
      20.79
    by injection 20.72
  lesion
    esophagus 42.39
      endoscopic 42.33
    heart
      by peripherally inserted catheter
          37.34
      endovascular approach 37.34
      maze procedure (Cox-maze)
        endovascular approach 37.34
        open (trans-thoracic) approach
            37.33 ◄▥
        thoracoscopic approach 37.37 ◄
        trans-thoracic approach 37.33
      thoracoscopic approach 37.37 ◄
    intestine
      large 45.49
        endoscopic 45.43
      large intestine 45.49
        endoscopic 45.43
      liver 50.26
        laparoscopic 50.25
        open 50.23
        percutaneous 50.24
      lung 32.26
        bronchoscopic thermoplasty
            32.27 ◄
        open 32.23
        percutaneous 32.24
        thoracoscopic 32.25
      renal 55.35
        laparoscopic 55.34
        open 55.32
        percutaneous 55.33
    pituitary 07.69
      by
        Cobalt-60 92.32
        implantation (strontium-yttrium)
            (Y) NEC 07.68
          transfrontal approach 07.64
          transphenoidal approach 07.65
        proton beam (Bragg peak) 92.33
    prostate
      by
        cryoablation 60.62
        laser, transurethral 60.21
        radical cryosurgical ablation
            (RCSA) 60.62
        radiofrequency thermotherapy 60.97
        transurethral needle ablation
            (TUNA) 60.97

Ablation (*Continued*)
  tissue
    heart - *see* Ablation, lesion, heart
    liver – *see* Ablation, lesion, liver
    lung – *see* Ablation, lesion, lung
    renal – *see* Ablation, lesion, renal
Abortion, therapeutic 69.51
  by
    aspiration curettage 69.51
    dilation and curettage 69.01
    hysterectomy - *see* Hysterectomy
    hysterotomy 74.91
    insertion
      laminaria 69.93
      prostaglandin suppository 96.49
    intra-amniotic injection (saline)
        75.0
Abrasion
  corneal epithelium 11.41
    for smear or culture 11.21
  epicardial surface 36.39
  pleural 34.6
  skin 86.25
Abscission, cornea 11.49
Absorptiometry
  photon (dual) (single) 88.98
Aburel operation (intra-amniotic injection
    for abortion) 75.0
Accouchement forcé 73.99
Acetabulectomy 77.85
Acetabuloplasty NEC 81.40
  with prosthetic implant 81.52
Achillorrhaphy 83.64
  delayed 83.62
Achillotenotomy 83.11
  plastic 83.85
Achillotomy 83.11
  plastic 83.85
Acid peel, skin 86.24
Acromionectomy 77.81
Acromioplasty 81.83
  for recurrent dislocation of shoulder
      81.82
  partial replacement 81.81
  total replacement, NEC 81.80 ◄▥
    other 81.80 ◄
    reverse 81.88 ◄
Actinotherapy 99.82
Activities of daily living (ADL)
  therapy 93.83
  training for the blind 93.78
Acupuncture 99.92
  with smouldering moxa 93.35
  for anesthesia 99.91
Adams operation
  advancement of round ligament 69.22
  crushing of nasal septum 21.88
  excision of palmar fascia 82.35
Adenectomy - *see also* Excision, by site
  prostate NEC 60.69
  retropubic 60.4
Adenoidectomy (without tonsillectomy)
    28.6
  with tonsillectomy 28.3
Adhesiolysis - *see also* Lysis, adhesions
  for collapse of lung 33.39
  middle ear 20.23
Adipectomy 86.83
Adjustment
  cardiac pacemaker program
      (reprogramming) - *omit code*
  cochlear prosthetic device (external
      components) 95.49

Adjustment (*Continued*)
  dental 99.97
  gastric restrictive device (laparoscopic)
      44.98
  occlusal 24.8
  orthopedic device (noninvasive)
    external fixator - *omit code*
  spectacles 95.31
Administration (of) - *see also* Injection
  Activase® 99.10
  adhesion barrier substance 99.77
  Alteplase (tPA, generic) 99.10
  Anistreplase (tPA, generic) 99.10
  antitoxins NEC 99.58
    botulism 99.57
    diphtheria 99.58
    gas gangrene 99.58
    scarlet fever 99.58
    tetanus 99.56
  Bender Visual-Motor Gestalt test 94.02
  Benton Visual Retention test 94.02
  DrotAA 00.11
  Eminase® 99.10
  inhaled nitric oxide 00.12
  intelligence test or scale (Stanford-
      Binet) (Wechsler) (adult)
      (children) 94.01
    Minnesota Multiphasic Personality
        Inventory (MMPI) 94.02
    MMPI (Minnesota Multiphasic
        Personality Inventory) 94.02
  neuroprotective agent 99.75
  Proleukin® (low-dose) 99.28
    high-dose 00.15
  psychologic test 94.02
  Retavase® 99.10
  Reteplase (tPA, generic) 99.10
  Stanford-Binet test 94.01
  Streptase® 99.10
  Streptokinase (tPA, generic) 99.10
  Tenecteplase (tPA, generic) 99.10
  TNKase™ 99.10
  toxoid
    diphtheria 99.36
      with tetanus and pertussis,
          combined (DTP) 99.39
    tetanus 99.38
      with diphtheria and pertussis,
          combined (DTP) 99.39
  vaccine - *see also* Vaccination
    BCG 99.33
    measles-mumps-rubella (MMR)
        99.48
    poliomyelitis 99.41
    TAB 99.32
  Wechsler
    Intelligence Scale (adult) (children)
        94.01
    Memory Scale 94.02
  Xigris® 00.11
Adrenalectomy (unilateral) 07.22
  with partial removal of remaining
      gland 07.29
  bilateral 07.3
    partial 07.29
    subtotal 07.29
  complete 07.3
  partial NEC 07.29
  remaining gland 07.3
  subtotal NEC 07.29
  total 07.3
Adrenalorrhaphy 07.44
Adrenalotomy (with drainage) 07.41

◄ New ◀▥ Revised ~~deleted~~ Deleted ● Use Additional Digit(s) ▭ Omit code

Advancement
extraocular muscle 15.12
  multiple (with resection or recession) 15.3
eyelid muscle 08.59
eye muscle 15.12
  multiple (with resection or recession) 15.3
graft - *see* Graft
leaflet (heart) 35.10
pedicle (flap) 86.72
profundus tendon (Wagner) 82.51
round ligament 69.22
tendon 83.71
  hand 82.51
  profundus (Wagner) 82.51
  Wagner (profundus tendon) 82.51
AESOP® (Automated Endoscopic System for Optimal Positioning) - *see* category 17.4●
Albee operation
bone peg, femoral neck 78.05
graft for slipping patella 78.06
sliding inlay graft, tibia 78.07
Albert operation (arthrodesis of knee) 81.22
Aldridge (-Studdiford) **operation** (urethral sling) 59.5
Alexander operation
prostatectomy
  perineal 60.62
  suprapubic 60.3
shortening of round ligaments 69.22
Alexander-Adams operation (shortening of round ligaments) 69.22
Alimentation, parenteral 99.29
Allograft - *see* Graft
Almoor operation (extrapetrosal drainage) 20.22
Altemeier operation (perineal rectal pull-through) 48.49
Alveolectomy (interradicular) (intraseptal) (radical) (simple) (with graft) (with implant) 24.5
Alveoloplasty (with graft or implant) 24.5
Alveolotomy (apical) 24.0
Ambulatory cardiac monitoring (ACM) 89.50
Ammon operation (dacryocystotomy) 09.53
Amniocentesis (transuterine) (diagnostic) 75.1
with intra-amniotic injection of saline 75.0
Amniography 87.81
Amnioinfusion 75.37
Amnioscopy, internal 75.31
Amniotomy 73.09
to induce labor 73.01
Amputation (cineplastic) (closed flap) (guillotine) (kineplastic) (open) 84.91
abdominopelvic 84.19
above-elbow 84.07
above-knee (AK) 84.17
ankle (disarticulation) 84.13
  through malleoli of tibia and fibula 84.14
arm NEC 84.00
  through
    carpals 84.03
    elbow (disarticulation) 84.06
    forearm 84.05

Amputation (*Continued*)
arm NEC (*Continued*)
  through (*Continued*)
    humerus 84.07
    shoulder (disarticulation) 84.08
    wrist (disarticulation) 84.04
  upper 84.07
Batch-Spittler-McFaddin (knee disarticulation) 84.16
below-knee (BK) NEC 84.15
  conversion into above-knee amputation 84.17
Boyd (hip disarticulation) 84.18
Callander's (knee disarticulation) 84.16
carpals 84.03
cervix 67.4
Chopart's (midtarsal) 84.12
clitoris 71.4
Dieffenbach (hip disarticulation) 84.18
Dupuytren's (shoulder disarticulation) 84.08
ear, external 18.39
elbow (disarticulation) 84.06
finger, except thumb 84.01
  thumb 84.02
foot (middle) 84.12
forearm 84.05
forefoot 84.12
forequarter 84.09
Gordon-Taylor (hindquarter) 84.19
Gritti-Stokes (knee disarticulation) 84.16
Guyon (ankle) 84.13
hallux 84.11
hand 84.03
Hey's (foot) 84.12
hindquarter 84.19
hip (disarticulation) 84.18
humerus 84.07
interscapulothoracic 84.09
interthoracoscapular 84.09
King-Steelquist (hindquarter) 84.19
Kirk (thigh) 84.17
knee (disarticulation) 84.16
Kutler (revision of current traumatic amputation of finger) 84.01
Larry (shoulder disarticulation) 84.08
leg NEC 84.10
  above knee (AK) 84.17
  below knee (BK) 84.15
  through
    ankle (disarticulation) 84.13
    femur (AK) 84.17
    foot 84.12
    hip (disarticulation) 84.18
    tibia and fibula (BK) 84.15
Lisfranc
  foot 84.12
  shoulder (disarticulation) 84.08
Littlewood (forequarter) 84.09
lower limb NEC - *see also* Amputation, leg 84.10
Mazet (knee disarticulation) 84.16
metacarpal 84.03
metatarsal 84.11
  head (bunionectomy) 77.59
metatarsophalangeal (joint) 84.11
midtarsal 84.12
nose 21.4
penis (circle) (complete) (flap) (partial) (radical) 64.3
Pirogoff's (ankle amputation through malleoli of tibia and fibula) 84.14

Amputation (*Continued*)
ray
  finger 84.01
  foot 84.11
  toe (metatarsal head) 84.11
root (apex) (tooth) 23.73
  with root canal therapy 23.72
shoulder (disarticulation) 84.08
Sorondo-Ferre (hindquarter) 84.19
S. P. Rogers (knee disarticulation) 84.16
supracondylar, above-knee 84.17
supramalleolar, foot 84.14
Syme's (ankle amputation through malleoli of tibia and fibula) 84.14
thigh 84.17
thumb 84.02
toe (through metatarsophalangeal joint) 84.11
transcarpal 84.03
transmetatarsal 84.12
upper limb NEC - *see also* Amputation, arm 84.00
wrist (disarticulation) 84.04
Amygdalohippocampectomy 01.59 ◀
Amygdalohippocampotomy 01.39
Amygdalotomy 01.39
Analysis
cardiac rhythm device (AICD) (CRT-D) (CRT-P) (pacemaker) - *see* Interrogation
character 94.03
gastric 89.39
psychologic 94.31
transactional
  group 94.44
  individual 94.39
Anastomosis
abdominal artery to coronary artery 37.17
accessory-facial nerve 04.72
accessory-hypoglossal nerve 04.73
anus (with formation of endorectal ileal pouch) 45.95
aorta (descending)-pulmonary (artery) 39.0
aorta-renal artery 39.24
aorta-subclavian artery 39.22
aortoceliac 39.26
aorto(ilio)femoral 39.25
aortomesenteric 39.26
appendix 47.99
arteriovenous NEC 39.29
  for renal dialysis 39.27
artery (suture of distal to proximal end) 39.31
  with
    bypass graft 39.29
      extracranial-intracranial [EC-IC] 39.28
    excision or resection of vessel - *see* Arteriectomy, with anastomosis, by site
  revision 39.49
bile ducts 51.39
bladder NEC 57.88
  with
    isolated segment of intestine 57.87 [45.50]
      colon (sigmoid) 57.87 [45.52]
      ileum 57.87 [45.51]
      open loop of ileum 57.87 [45.51]
    to intestine 57.88
      ileum 57.87 [45.51]
bowel - *see also* Anastomosis, intestine 45.90

Anastomosis (Continued)
  bronchotracheal 33.48
  bronchus 33.48
  carotid-subclavian artery 39.22
  caval-mesenteric vein 39.1
  caval-pulmonary artery 39.21
  cervicoesophageal 42.59
  colohypopharyngeal (intrathoracic)
      42.55
    antesternal or antethoracic 42.65
  common bile duct 51.39
  common pulmonary trunk and left
      atrium (posterior wall) 35.82
  cystic bile duct 51.39
  cystocolic 57.88
  epididymis to vas deferens 63.83
  esophagocolic (intrathoracic) NEC
      42.56
    with interposition 42.55
    antesternal or antethoracic NEC
        42.66
      with interposition 42.65
  esophagocologastric (intrathoracic)
      42.55
    antesternal or antethoracic 42.65
  esophagoduodenal (intrathoracic) NEC
      42.54
    with interposition 42.53
  esophagoenteric (intrathoracic) NEC -
      see also Anastomosis, esophagus,
      to intestinal segment 42.54
    antesternal or antethoracic NEC - see
        also Anastomosis, esophagus,
        antesternal, to intestinal
        segment 42.64
  esophagoesophageal (intrathoracic)
      42.51
    antesternal or antethoracic 42.61
  esophagogastric (intrathoracic) 42.52
    antesternal or antethoracic 42.62
  esophagus (intrapleural) (intrathoracic)
      (retrosternal) NEC 42.59
    with
      gastrectomy (partial) 43.5
        complete or total 43.99
      interposition (of) NEC 42.58
        colon 42.55
        jejunum 42.53
        small bowel 42.53
    antesternal or antethoracic NEC
        42.69
      with
        interposition (of) NEC 42.68
          colon 42.65
          jejunal loop 42.63
          small bowel 42.63
        rubber tube 42.68
      to intestinal segment NEC 42.64
        with interposition 42.68
        colon NEC 42.66
          with interposition 42.65
        small bowel NEC 42.64
          with interposition 42.63
    to intestinal segment (intrathoracic)
        NEC 42.54
      with interposition 42.58
      antesternal or antethoracic NEC
          42.64
        with interposition 42.68
      colon (intrathoracic) NEC 42.56
        with interposition 42.55
        antesternal or antethoracic
            42.66
          with interposition 42.65

Anastomosis (Continued)
  esophagus NEC (Continued)
    to intestinal segment NEC
        (Continued)
      small bowel NEC 42.54
        with interposition 42.53
        antesternal or antethoracic
            42.64
          with interposition 42.63
  facial-accessory nerve 04.72
  facial-hypoglossal nerve 04.71
  fallopian tube 66.73
    by reanastomosis 66.79
  gallbladder 51.35
    to
      hepatic ducts 51.31
      intestine 51.32
      pancreas 51.33
      stomach 51.34
  gastroepiploic artery to coronary artery
      36.17
  hepatic duct 51.39
  hypoglossal-accessory nerve 04.73
  hypoglossal-facial nerve 04.71
  ileal loop to bladder 57.87 [45.51]
  ileoanal 45.95
  ileorectal 45.93
  inferior vena cava and portal vein
      39.1
  internal mammary artery (to)
    coronary artery (single vessel)
        36.15
      double vessel 36.16
    myocardium 36.2
  intestine 45.90
    large-to-anus 45.95
    large-to-large 45.94
    large-to-rectum 45.94
    large-to-small 45.93
    small-to-anus 45.95
    small-to-large 45.93
    small-to-rectal stump 45.92
    small-to-small 45.91
  intrahepatic 51.79
  intrathoracic vessel NEC 39.23
  kidney (pelvis) 55.86
  lacrimal sac to conjunctiva 09.82
  left-to-right (systemic-pulmonary
      artery) 39.0
  lymphatic (channel) (peripheral) 40.9
  mesenteric-caval 39.1
  mesocaval 39.1
  nasolacrimal 09.81
  nerve (cranial) (peripheral) NEC
      04.74
    accessory-facial 04.72
    accessory-hypoglossal 04.73
    hypoglossal-facial 04.71
  pancreas (duct) (to) 52.96
    bile duct 51.39
    gall bladder 51.33
    intestine 52.96
    jejunum 52.96
    stomach 52.96
  pleurothecal (with valve) 03.79
  portacaval 39.1
  portal vein to inferior vena cava 39.1
  pulmonary-aortic (Pott's) 39.0
  pulmonary artery and superior vena
      cava 39.21
  pulmonary-innominate artery (Blalock)
      39.0
  pulmonary-subclavian artery (Blalock-
      Taussig) 39.0

Anastomosis (Continued)
  pulmonary vein and azygos vein
      39.23
  pyeloileocutaneous 56.51
  pyeloureterovesical 55.86
  radial artery 36.19
  rectum, rectal NEC 48.74
    stump to small intestine 45.92
  renal (pelvis) 55.86
    vein and splenic vein 39.1
  renoportal 39.1
  salpingothecal (with valve) 03.79
  splenic to renal veins 39.1
  splenorenal (venous) 39.1
    arterial 39.26
  subarachnoid-peritoneal (with valve)
      03.71
  subarachnoid-ureteral (with valve)
      03.72
  subclavian-aortic 39.22
  superior vena cava to pulmonary
      artery 39.21
  systemic-pulmonary artery 39.0
  thoracic artery (to)
    coronary artery (single) 36.15
      double 36.16
    myocardium 36.2
  ureter (to) NEC 56.79
    bladder 56.74
    colon 56.71
    ileal pouch (bladder) 56.51
    ileum 56.71
    intestine 56.71
    skin 56.61
  ureterocalyceal 55.86
  ureterocolic 56.71
  ureterovesical 56.74
  urethra (end-to-end) 58.44
  vas deferens 63.82
  veins (suture of proximal to distal end)
      (with bypass graft) 39.29
    with excision or resection of vessel -
        see Phlebectomy, with
        anastomosis, by site
    mesenteric to vena cava 39.1
    portal to inferior vena cava 39.1
    revision 39.49
    splenic and renal 39.1
  ventricle, ventricular (intracerebral)
      (with valve) - see also Shunt,
      ventricular 02.2
  ventriculoatrial (with valve) 02.32
  ventriculocaval (with valve) 02.32
  ventriculomastoid (with valve) 02.31
  ventriculopleural (with valve) 02.33
  vesicle - see Anastomosis, bladder
Anderson operation (tibial lengthening)
    78.37
Anel operation (dilation of lacrimal duct)
    09.42
Anesthesia
  acupuncture for 99.91
  cryoanalgesia nerve (cranial)
      (peripheral) 04.2
  spinal - omit code
Aneurysmectomy 38.60
  with
    anastomosis 38.30
      abdominal
        artery 38.36
        vein 38.37
      aorta (arch) (ascending)
          (descending) 38.34
      head and neck NEC 38.32

◀ New   ⇐▥ Revised   ~~deleted~~ Deleted   ● Use Additional Digit(s)   ▭ Omit code

Aneurysmectomy *(Continued)*
  with *(Continued)*
    anastomosis *(Continued)*
      intracranial NEC 38.31
      lower limb
        artery 38.38
        vein 38.39
      thoracic NEC 38.35
      upper limb (artery) (vein) 38.33
    graft replacement (interposition)
        38.40
      abdominal
        aorta
          endovascular approach
              39.71
          open approach 38.44
          Zenith® Renu™ AAA graft
              39.71
        artery 38.46
        vein 38.47
      aorta (arch) (ascending)
          (descending thoracic)
        abdominal 38.44
        thoracic 38.45
        thoracoabdominal 38.45
            [38.44]
      head and neck NEC 38.42
      intracranial NEC 38.41
      lower limb
        artery 38.48
        vein 38.49
      thoracic NEC 38.45
      upper limb (artery) (vein)
          38.43
  abdominal
    artery 38.66
    vein 38.67
  aorta (arch) (ascending) (descending)
      38.64
  atrial, auricular 37.32
  head and neck NEC 38.62
  heart 37.32
  intracranial NEC 38.61
  lower limb
    artery 38.68
    vein 38.69
  sinus of Valsalva 35.39
  thoracic NEC 38.65
  upper limb (artery) (vein) 38.63
  ventricle (myocardium) 37.32
Aneurysmoplasty - *see*
    Aneurysmorrhaphy
Aneurysmorrhaphy NEC 39.52
  by or with
    anastomosis - *see* Aneurysmectomy,
        with anastomosis, by site
    clipping 39.51
    coagulation 39.52
    electrocoagulation 39.52
    endovascular graft
      abdominal aorta 39.71
      lower extremity artery(s) 39.79
      thoracic aorta 39.73
      upper extremity artery(s) 39.79
    excision or resection - *see also*
        Aneurysmectomy, by site
      with
        anastomosis - *see*
            Aneurysmectomy, with
            anastomosis, by site
        graft replacement - *see*
            Aneurysmectomy, with
            graft replacement, by
            site

Aneurysmorrhaphy NEC *(Continued)*
  by or with *(Continued)*
    filipuncture 39.52
    graft replacement - *see*
        Aneurysmectomy, with graft
        replacement, by site
    methyl methacrylate 39.52
    suture 39.52
    wiring 39.52
    wrapping 39.52
  Matas' 39.52
Aneurysmotomy - *see* Aneurysmectomy
Angiectomy
  with
    anastomosis 38.30
      abdominal
        artery 38.36
        vein 38.37
      aorta (arch) (ascending)
          (descending) 38.34
      head and neck NEC 38.32
      intracranial NEC 38.31
      lower limb
        artery 38.38
        vein 38.39
      thoracic vessel NEC 38.35
      upper limb (artery) (vein) 38.33
    graft replacement (interposition)
        38.40
      abdominal
        aorta 38.44
        artery 38.46
        vein 38.47
      aorta (arch) (ascending)
          (descending thoracic)
        abdominal 38.44
        thoracic 38.45
        thoracoabdominal 38.45 *[38.44]*
      head and neck NEC 38.42
      intracranial NEC 38.41
      lower limb
        artery 38.48
        vein 38.49
      thoracic vessel NEC 38.45
      upper limb (artery) (vein) 38.43
Angiocardiography (selective) 88.50
  carbon dioxide (negative contrast)
      88.58
  combined right and left heart 88.54
  intra-operative coronary fluorescence
      vascular 88.59 ◀▥
  left heart (aortic valve) (atrium)
      (ventricle) (ventricular outflow
      tract) 88.53
    combined with right heart 88.54
  right heart (atrium) (pulmonary valve)
      (ventricle) (ventricular outflow
      tract) 88.52
    combined with left heart 88.54
  SPY, coronary 88.59 ◀▥
  vena cava (inferior) (superior) 88.51
Angiography (arterial) - *see also*
    Arteriography 88.40
  by C.A.T. – *see* Scan, C.A.T., by site
  by computed tomography – *see* Scan,
      C.A.T., by site
  by magnetic resonance – *see* Imaging,
      magnetic resonance, by site ◀
  by radioisotope - *see* Scan, radioisotope,
      by site
  by ultrasound - *see* Ultrasonography,
      by site
  basilar 88.41
  brachial 88.49

Angiography *(Continued)*
  carotid (internal) 88.41
  celiac 88.47
  cerebral (posterior circulation) 88.41
  coronary NEC 88.57
    intra-operative fluorescence
        vascular 88.59
  eye (fluorescein) 95.12
  femoral 88.48
  heart 88.50
  intra-abdominal NEC 88.47
  intracranial 88.41
  intrathoracic vessels NEC 88.44
  lower extremity NEC 88.48
  neck 88.41
  non-coronary, intra-operative
      fluorescence 17.71 ◀
  placenta 88.46
  pulmonary 88.43
  renal 88.45
  specified artery NEC 88.49
  transfemoral 88.48
  upper extremity NEC 88.49
  veins - *see* Phlebography
  vertebral 88.41
Angioplasty (laser) - *see also* Repair, blood
    vessel

> Note: Also use 00.40, 00.41, 00.42, or
> 00.43 to show the total number of
> vessels treated. Use code 00.44 once to
> show procedure on a bifurcated vessel.
> In addition, use 00.45, 00.46, 00.47, or
> 00.48 to show the number of vascular
> stents inserted.

  balloon (percutaneous transluminal)
      NEC 39.50
    coronary artery 00.66
  coronary 36.09
    open chest approach 36.03
    percutaneous transluminal (balloon)
        00.66
  percutaneous transluminal (balloon)
      (single vessel)
    basilar 00.61
    carotid 00.61
    cerebral (intracranial) 00.62
    cerebrovascular
      cerebral (intracranial) 00.62
      precerebral (extracranial)
          00.61
        carotid 00.61
    coronary (balloon) 00.66
    femoropopliteal 39.50
    iliac 39.50
    lower extremity NOS 39.50
    mesenteric 39.50
    peripheral NEC 39.50
    precerebral (extracranial) 00.61
      carotid 00.61
    renal 39.50
    subclavian 39.50
    upper extremity NOS 39.50
    vertebral 00.61
  specified site NEC 39.50
    cerebrovascular
      cerebral (intracranial) 00.62
      precerebral (extracranial)
          00.61
    peripheral 39.50
Angiorrhaphy 39.30
  artery 39.31
  vein 39.32

Angioscopy, percutaneous 38.22
    eye (fluorescein) 95.12
Angiotomy 38.00
    abdominal
        artery 38.06
        vein 38.07
    aorta (arch) (ascending) (descending)
        38.04
    head and neck NEC 38.02
    intracranial NEC 38.01
    lower limb
        artery 38.08
        vein 38.09
    thoracic NEC 38.05
    upper limb (artery) (vein) 38.03
Angiotripsy 39.98
Ankylosis, production of - see
    Arthrodesis
Annuloplasty (heart) (posteromedial)
    35.33
Anoplasty 49.79
    with hemorrhoidectomy 49.46
Anoscopy 49.21
Antibiogram - see Examination,
    microscopic
Antiembolic filter, vena cava 38.7
Antiphobic treatment 94.39
Antrectomy
    mastoid 20.49
    maxillary 22.39
        radical 22.31
    pyloric 43.6
Antrostomy - see Antrotomy
Antrotomy (exploratory) (nasal sinus)
    22.2
    Caldwell-Luc (maxillary sinus)
        22.39
        with removal of membrane lining
            22.31
    intranasal 22.2
        with external approach (Caldwell-
            Luc) 22.39
        radical 22.31
    maxillary (simple) 22.2
        with Caldwell-Luc approach
            22.39
            with removal of membrane
                lining 22.31
        external (Caldwell-Luc approach)
            22.39
            with removal of membrane lining
                22.31
        radical (with removal of membrane
            lining) 22.31
Antrum window operation - see
    Antrotomy, maxillary
Aorticopulmonary window operation
    39.59
Aortogram, aortography (abdominal)
    (retrograde) (selective)
    (translumbar) 88.42
Aortoplasty (aortic valve) (gusset type)
    35.11
Aortotomy 38.04
Apexcardiogram (with ECG lead)
    89.57
Apheresis, therapeutic - see category
    99.7●
Apicectomy
    lung 32.39
        thoracoscopic 32.30
    petrous pyramid 20.59
    tooth (root) 23.73
        with root canal therapy 23.72

Apicoectomy 23.73
    with root canal therapy 23.72
Apicolysis (lung) 33.39
Apicostomy, alveolar 24.0
Aponeurectomy 83.42
    hand 82.33
Aponeurorrhaphy - see also Suture,
    tendon 83.64
    hand - see also Suture, tendon, hand
        82.45
Aponeurotomy 83.13
    hand 82.11
Appendectomy (with drainage) 47.09
    incidental 47.19
        laparoscopic 47.11
    laparoscopic 47.01
Appendicectomy (with drainage)
    47.09
    incidental 47.19
        laparoscopic 47.11
    laparoscopic 47.01
Appendicocecostomy 47.91
Appendicoenterostomy 47.91
Appendicolysis 54.59
    with appendectomy 47.09
        laparoscopic 47.01
        other 47.09
    laparoscopic 54.51
Appendicostomy 47.91
    closure 47.92
Appendicotomy 47.2
Application
    adhesion barrier substance 99.77
    anti-shock trousers 93.58
    arch bars (orthodontic) 24.7
        for immobilization (fracture)
            93.55
    barrier substance, adhesion 99.77
    Barton's tongs (skull) (with
        synchronous skeletal traction)
        02.94
    bone growth stimulator (surface)
        (transcutaneous) 99.86
    bone morphogenetic protein (Infuse™)
        (OP-1™) (recombinant) (rhBMP)
        84.52
    Bryant's traction 93.44
        with reduction of fracture or
            dislocation - see Reduction,
            fracture and Reduction,
            dislocation
    Buck's traction 93.46
    caliper tongs (skull) (with synchronous
        skeletal traction) 02.94
    cast (fiberglass) (plaster) (plastic) NEC
        93.53
        with reduction of fracture or
            dislocation - see Reduction,
            fracture and Reduction,
            dislocation
        spica 93.51
    cervical collar 93.52
        with reduction of fracture or
            dislocation - see Reduction,
            fracture and Reduction,
            dislocation
    clamp, cerebral aneurysm
        (Crutchfield) (Silverstone)
        39.51
    croupette, croup tent 93.94
    crown (artificial) 23.41
    Crutchfield tongs (skull) (with
        synchronous skeletal traction)
        02.94

Application (Continued)
    Dunlop's traction 93.44
        with reduction of fracture or
            dislocation - see Reduction,
            fracture and Reduction,
            dislocation
    elastic stockings 93.59
    electronic gaiter 93.59
    external fixator device (bone) 78.10
        carpal, metacarpal 78.14
        clavicle 78.11
        computer assisted (dependent) 84.73
        femur 78.15
        fibula 78.17
        humerus 78.12
        hybrid device or system 84.73
        Ilizarov type 84.72
        monoplanar system or device 84.71
        patella 78.16
        pelvic 78.19
        phalanges (foot) (hand) 78.19
        radius 78.13
        ring device or system 84.72
        scapula 78.11
        Sheffield type 84.72
        specified site NEC 78.19
        tarsal, metatarsal 78.18
        thorax (ribs) (sternum) 78.11
        tibia 78.17
        ulna 78.13
        vertebrae 78.19
    forceps, with delivery - see Delivery,
        forceps
    graft - see Graft
    gravity (G-) suit 93.59
    intermittent pressure device 93.59
    Jewett extension brace
        93.59
    Jobst pumping unit (reduction of
        edema) 93.59
    Lyman Smith traction 93.44
        with reduction of fracture or
            dislocation - see Reduction,
            fracture and Reduction,
            dislocation
    MAST (military anti-shock trousers)
        93.58
    Minerva jacket 93.52
    minifixator device (bone) - see category
        78.1●
    neck support (molded) 93.52
    obturator (orthodontic) 24.7
    orthodontic appliance (obturator)
        (wiring) 24.7
    pelvic sling 93.44
    with reduction of fracture or
        dislocation - see Reduction,
        fracture and Reduction,
        dislocation
    peridontal splint (orthodontic) 24.7
    plaster jacket 93.51
        Minerva 93.52
    pressure
        dressing (bandage) (Gibney)
            (Robert Jones') (Shanz)
            93.56
        trousers (anti-shock) (MAST)
            93.58
    prosthesis for missing ear 18.71
    Russell's traction 93.44
        with reduction of fracture or
            dislocation - see Reduction,
            fracture and Reduction,
            dislocation

◀ New   ⬅ Revised   ~~deleted~~ Deleted   ● Use Additional Digit(s)   ▨ Omit code

Application *(Continued)*
  splint, for immobilization (plaster)
      (pneumatic) (tray) 93.54
    with fracture reduction - *see*
        Reduction, fracture
  stereotactic head frame 93.59
  strapping (non-traction) 93.59
  substance, adhesion barrier 99.77
  Thomas collar 93.52
    with reduction of fracture or
        dislocation - *see* Reduction,
        fracture *and* Reduction,
        dislocation
  traction
    with reduction of fracture or
        dislocation - *see* Reduction,
        fracture *and* Reduction,
        dislocation
    adhesive tape (skin) 93.46
    boot 93.46
    Bryant's 93.44
    Buck's 93.46
    Cotrel's 93.42
    Dunlop's 93.44
    gallows 93.46
    Lyman Smith 93.44
    Russell's 93.44
    skeletal NEC 93.44
      intermittent 93.43
    skin, limbs NEC 93.46
    spinal NEC 93.42
      with skull device (caliper)
          (Crutchfield) (Gardner-
          Wells) (halo) (Vinke)
          (tongs) 93.41
        with synchronous insertion
            02.94
    Thomas' splint 93.45
  Unna's paste boot 93.53
  vasopneumatic device 93.58
  Velpeau dressing 93.59
  Vinke tongs (skull) (with synchronous
      skeletal traction) 02.94
  wound dressing NEC 93.57
Aquapheresis 99.78
Arc lamp - *see* Photocoagulation
Arcuplasty 81.66
Arrest
  bone growth (epiphyseal) 78.20
    by stapling - *see* Stapling,
        epiphyseal plate
    femur 78.25
    fibula 78.27
    humerus 78.22
    radius 78.23
    tibia 78.27
    ulna 78.23
  cardiac, induced (anoxic)
      (circulatory) 39.63
  circulatory, induced (anoxic)
      39.63
  hemorrhage - *see* Control,
      hemorrhage
Arslan operation (fenestration of inner
      ear) 20.61
Arteriectomy 38.60
  with
    anastomosis 38.30
      abdominal 38.36
      aorta (arch) (ascending)
          (descending) 38.34
      head and neck NEC 38.32
      intracranial NEC 38.31
      lower limb 38.38

Arteriectomy *(Continued)*
  with *(Continued)*
    anastomosis *(Continued)*
      thoracic NEC 38.35
      upper limb 38.33
    graft replacement (interposition)
        38.40
      abdominal
        aorta 38.44
      aorta (arch) (ascending)
          (descending thoracic)
          (thoracic)
        abdominal 38.44
        thoracic 38.45
        thoracoabdominal 38.45
            [38.44]
      head and neck NEC 38.42
      intracranial NEC 38.41
      lower limb 38.48
      thoracic NEC 38.45
      upper limb 38.43
  abdominal 38.66
  aorta (arch) (ascending) (descending)
      38.64
  head and neck NEC 38.62
  intracranial NEC 38.61
  lower-limb 38.68
  thoracic NEC 38.65
  upper limb 38.63
Arteriography (contrast) (fluoroscopic)
      (retrograde) 88.40
  by
    radioisotope - *see* Scan, radioisotope
    ultrasound (Doppler) - *see*
        Ultrasonography, by site
  aorta (arch) (ascending) (descending)
      88.42
  basilar 88.41
  brachial 88.49
  carotid (internal) 88.41
  cerebral (posterior circulation) 88.41
  coronary (direct) (selective) NEC
      88.57
    double catheter technique
        (Judkins) (Ricketts and
        Abrams) 88.56
    intra-operative fluorescence
        vascular 88.59
    single catheter technique (Sones)
        88.55
  Doppler (ultrasonic) - *see*
      Ultrasonography, by site
  femoral 88.48
  head and neck 88.41
  intra-abdominal NEC 88.47
  intrathoracic NEC 88.44
  lower extremity 88.48
  placenta 88.46
  pulmonary 88.43
  radioisotope - *see* Scan, radioisotope
  renal 88.45
  specified site NEC 88.49
  SPY, coronary 88.59 ◀▥
  superior mesenteric artery 88.47
  transfemoral 88.48
  ultrasound - *see* Ultrasonography, by
      site
  upper extremity 88.49
Arterioplasty - *see* Repair, artery
Arteriorrhaphy 39.31
Arteriotomy 38.00
  abdominal 38.06
  aorta (arch) (ascending) (descending)
      38.04

Arteriotomy *(Continued)*
  head and neck NEC 38.02
  intracranial NEC 38.01
  lower limb 38.08
  thoracic NEC 38.05
  upper limb 38.03
Arteriovenostomy 39.29
  for renal dialysis 39.27
Arthrectomy 80.90
  ankle 80.97
  elbow 80.92
  foot and toe 80.98
  hand and finger 80.94
  hip 80.95
  intervertebral disc - *see* category 80.5 ●
  knee 80.96
  semilunar cartilage 80.6
  shoulder 80.91
  specified site NEC 80.99
  spine NEC 80.99
  wrist 80.93
Arthrocentesis 81.91
  for arthrography - *see* Arthrogram
Arthrodesis (compression) (extra-
      articular) (intra-articular) (with bone
      graft) (with fixation device) 81.20
  ankle 81.11
  carporadial 81.25
  cricoarytenoid 31.69
  elbow 81.24
  finger 81.28
  foot NEC 81.17
  hip 81.21
  interphalangeal
    finger 81.28
    toe NEC 77.58
      claw toe repair 77.57
      hammer toe repair 77.56
  ischiofemoral 81.21
  knee 81.22
  lumbosacral, lumbar NEC 81.08
    ALIF (anterior lumbar interbody
        fusion) 81.06
    anterior column (interbody), ◀▥
        anterolateral (anterior) technique
            81.06 ◀▥
        posterior ~~(interbody), posterolateral~~
            technique 81.08 ◀▥
    axial lumber interbody fusion
        [AxiaLIF®] 81.08 ◀
    direct lateral interbody fusion
        [DLIF] 81.06 ◀
    extreme lateral interbody fusion
        [XLIF®] 81.06 ◀
    facet 81.07 ◀
    lateral transverse process technique
        81.07
    PLIF (posterior lumbar interbody
        fusion) 81.08
    TLIF (transforaminal lumbar
        interbody fusion) 81.08
  McKeever (metatarsophalangeal) 81.16
  metacarpocarpal 81.26
  metacarpophalangeal 81.27
  metatarsophalangeal 81.16
  midtarsal 81.14
  pantalar 81.11
  sacroiliac 81.08
  shoulder 81.23
  specified joint NEC 81.29
  spinal - *see also* Fusion, spinal 81.00
  subtalar 81.13
  tarsometatarsal 81.15
  tibiotalar 81.11

Arthrodesis (Continued)
   toe NEC 77.58
      claw toe repair 77.57
      hammer toe repair 77.56
   triple 81.12
   wrist 81.26
Arthroendoscopy - see Arthroscopy
Arthroereisis, subtalar joint 81.18
Arthrogram, arthrography 88.32
   temporomandibular 87.13
Arthrolysis 93.26
Arthroplasty (with fixation device) (with
      traction) 81.96
   ankle 81.49
   carpals 81.75
      with prosthetic implant 81.74
   carpocarpal, carpometacarpal 81.75
      with prosthetic implant 81.74
   Carroll and Taber (proximal
         interphalangeal joint) 81.72
   cup (partial hip) 81.52
   Curtis (interphalangeal joint) 81.72
   elbow 81.85
      with prosthetic replacement (partial)
         (total) 81.84
   femoral head NEC 81.40
      with prosthetic implant 81.52
   finger(s) 81.72
      with prosthetic implant 81.71
   foot (metatarsal) with joint replacement
      81.57
   Fowler (metacarpophalangeal joint)
      81.72
   hand (metacarpophalangeal)
         (interphalangeal) 81.72
      with prosthetic implant 81.71
   hip (with bone graft) 81.40
      cup (partial hip) 81.52
      femoral head NEC 81.40
         with prosthetic implant 81.52
            with total replacement 81.51
      partial replacement 81.52
      total replacement 81.51
   interphalangeal joint 81.72
      with prosthetic implant 81.71
   Kessler (carpometacarpal joint) 81.74
   knee - see also Repair, knee 81.47
      prosthetic replacement
            (bicompartmental) (hemijoint)
            (partial) (total)
            (tricompartmental)
            (unicompartmental) 81.54
      revision 81.55
   metacarpophalangeal joint 81.72
      with prosthetic implant 81.71
   shoulder 81.83
      prosthetic replacement (partial) 81.81
         total, NEC 81.80 ◀▥
            other 81.80 ◀
            reverse 81.88 ◀
      for recurrent dislocation 81.82
   temporomandibular 76.5
   toe NEC 77.58
      with prosthetic replacement 81.57
      for hallux valgus repair 77.59
   wrist 81.75
      with prosthetic implant 81.74
         total replacement 81.73
Arthroscopy 80.20
   ankle 80.27
   elbow 80.22
   finger 80.24
   foot 80.28
   hand 80.24
   hip 80.25

Arthroscopy (Continued)
   knee 80.26
   shoulder 80.21
   specified site NEC 80.29
   toe 80.28
   wrist 80.23
Arthrostomy - see also Arthrotomy
   80.10
Arthrotomy 80.10
   as operative approach - omit code
   with
      arthrography - see Arthrogram
      arthroscopy - see Arthroscopy
      injection of drug 81.92
      removal of prosthesis without
         replacement - see Removal,
         prosthesis, joint structures
   ankle 80.17
   elbow 80.12
   foot and toe 80.18
   hand and finger 80.14
   hip 80.15
   knee 80.16
   shoulder 80.11
   specified site NEC 80.19
   spine 80.19
   wrist 80.13
Artificial
   heart 37.52
      AbioCor® 37.52
      CardioWest™ (TAH-t) 37.52
   insemination 69.92
   kidney 39.95
   rupture of membranes 73.09
Arytenoidectomy 30.29
Arytenoidopexy 31.69
Asai operation (larynx) 31.75
Aspiration
   abscess - see Aspiration, by site
   anterior chamber, eye (therapeutic) 12.91
      diagnostic 12.21
   aqueous (eye) (humor) (therapeutic)
      12.91
      diagnostic 12.21
   ascites 54.91
   Bartholin's gland (cyst)
      (percutaneous) 71.21
   biopsy - see Biopsy, by site
   bladder (catheter) 57.0
      percutaneous (needle) 57.11
   bone marrow (for biopsy) 41.31
      from donor for transplant 41.91
      stem cell 99.79
   branchial cleft cyst 29.0
   breast 85.91
   bronchus 96.05
      with lavage 96.56
   bursa (percutaneous) 83.94
      hand 82.92
   calculus, bladder 57.0
   cataract 13.3
      with
         phacoemulsification 13.41
         phacofragmentation 13.43
            posterior route 13.42
   chest 34.91
   cisternal 01.01
   cranial (puncture) 01.09
   craniobuccal pouch 07.72
   craniopharyngioma 07.72
   cul-de-sac (abscess) 70.0
   curettage, uterus 69.59
      after abortion or delivery 69.52
      diagnostic 69.59
      to terminate pregnancy 69.51

Aspiration (Continued)
   cyst - see Aspiration, by site
   diverticulum, pharynx 29.0
   endotracheal 96.04
      with lavage 96.56
   extradural 01.09
   eye (anterior chamber) (therapeutic)
      12.91
      diagnostic 12.21
   fallopian tube 66.91
   fascia 83.95
      hand 82.93
   gallbladder (percutaneous) 51.01
   hematoma - see also Aspiration,
         by site
      obstetrical 75.92
         incisional 75.91
   hydrocele, tunica vaginalis 61.91
   hygroma - see Aspiration, by site
   hyphema 12.91
   hypophysis 07.72
   intracranial space (epidural)
         (extradural) (subarachnoid)
         (subdural) (ventricular) 01.09
   through previously implanted catheter
         or reservoir (Ommaya) (Rickham)
         01.02
   joint 81.91
      for arthrography - see Arthrogram
   kidney (cyst) (pelvis) (percutaneous)
         (therapeutic) 55.92
      diagnostic 55.23
   liver (percutaneous) 50.91
   lung (percutaneous) (puncture)
         (needle) (trocar) 33.93
      thoracoscopic 33.20
   middle ear 20.09
      with intubation 20.01
   muscle 83.95
      hand 82.93
   nail 86.01
   nasal sinus 22.00
      by puncture 22.01
      through natural ostium 22.02
   nasotracheal 96.04
      with lavage 96.56
   orbit, diagnostic 16.22
   ovary 65.91
   percutaneous - see Aspiration, by site
   pericardium (wound) 37.0
   pituitary gland 07.72
   pleural cavity 34.91
   prostate (percutaneous) 60.91
   Rathke's pouch 07.72
   seminal vesicles 60.71
   seroma - see Aspiration, by site
   skin 86.01
   soft tissue NEC 83.95
      hand 82.93
   spermatocele 63.91
   spinal (puncture) 03.31
   spleen (cyst) 41.1
   stem cell 99.79
   subarachnoid space (cerebral)
      01.09
   subcutaneous tissue 86.01
   subdural space (cerebral) 01.09
   tendon 83.95
      hand 82.93
   testis 62.91
   thymus 07.92
      thoracoscopic 07.95
   thyroid (field) (gland) 06.01
      postoperative 06.02

◀ New   ◀▥ Revised   ~~deleted~~ Deleted   ● Use Additional Digit(s)   ▨ Omit code

Aspiration *(Continued)*
  trachea 96.04
    with lavage 96.56
    percutaneous 31.99
  tunica vaginalis (hydrocele)
    (percutaneous) 61.91
  vitreous (and replacement) 14.72
    diagnostic 14.11
Assessment
  fitness to testify 94.11
  mental status 94.11
  nutritional status 89.39
  personality 94.03
  temperament 94.02
  vocational 93.85
Assistance
  cardiac - *see also* Resuscitation, cardiac
    extracorporeal circulation 39.61
  endotracheal respiratory - *see category*
    96.7●
  hepatic, extracorporeal 50.92
  respiratory (endotracheal)
    (mechanical) - *see* Ventilation,
    mechanical
Astragalectomy 77.98
Asymmetrogammagram - *see* Scan,
  radioisotope
Atherectomy
  cerebrovascular - *see* Angioplasty
  coronary - *see* Angioplasty
  peripheral 39.50
Atriocommissuropexy (mitral valve) 35.12
Atrioplasty NEC 37.99
  combined with repair of valvular and
    ventricular septal defects - *see*
    Repair, endocardial cushion defect
  septum (heart) NEC 35.71

Atrioseptopexy - *see also* Repair, atrial
  septal defect 35.71
Atrioseptoplasty - *see also* Repair, atrial
  septal defect 35.71
Atrioseptostomy (balloon) 35.41
Atriotomy 37.11
Atrioventriculostomy (cerebral-heart)
  02.32
Attachment
  abutment (screw) for prosthetic ear
    device
    percutaneous 20.99
  eye muscle
    orbicularis oculi to eyebrow
      08.36
    rectus to frontalis 15.9
  pedicle (flap) graft 86.74
    hand 86.73
    lip 27.57
    mouth 27.57
  pharyngeal flap (for cleft palate repair)
    27.62
    secondary or subsequent 27.63
  prosthetic ear device, abutment
    20.99
  retina - *see* Reattachment, retina
Atticoantrostomy (ear) 20.49
Atticoantrotomy (ear) 20.49
Atticotomy (ear) 20.23
Audiometry (Bekesy 5-tone) (impedance)
  (stapedial reflex response)
  (subjective) 95.41
Augmentation
  bladder 57.87
  breast - *see* Mammoplasty,
    augmentation
  buttock ("fanny-lift") 86.89

Augmentation *(Continued)*
  chin 76.68
  genioplasty 76.68
  mammoplasty - *see* Mammoplasty,
    augmentation
  outflow tract (pulmonary valve)
    (gusset type) 35.26
    in total repair of tetralogy of Fallot
      35.81
  vocal cord(s) 31.0
Auriculectomy 18.39
Autograft - *see* Graft
Autologous - *see* Blood, transfusion
Autopsy 89.8
Autotransfusion (whole blood) 99.02 - *see*
  Blood, transfusion
Autotransplant, autotransplantation - *see*
  also Reimplantation
  adrenal tissue (heterotopic)
    (orthotopic) 07.45
  kidney 55.61
  lung - *see* Transplant, transplantation,
    lung 33.5●
  ovary 65.72
    laparoscopic 65.75
  pancreatic tissue 52.81
  parathyroid tissue (heterotopic)
    (orthotopic) 06.95
  thyroid tissue (heterotopic) (orthotopic)
    06.94
  tooth 23.5
Avulsion, nerve (cranial) (peripheral)
  NEC 04.07
  acoustic 04.01
  phrenic 33.31
  sympathetic 05.29
Azygography 88.63

B

Bacterial smear - *see* Examination,
  microscopic
Baffes operation (interatrial transposition
  of venous return) 35.91
Baffle, atrial or interatrial 35.91
Balanoplasty 64.69
Baldy-Webster operation (uterine
  suspension) 69.22
Ballistocardiography 89.59
Balloon
  angioplasty - *see* Angioplasty, balloon
  pump, intra-aortic 37.61
  systostomy (atrial) 35.41
Ball operation
  herniorrhaphy - *see* Repair, hernia,
    inguinal
  undercutting 40.92
Bandage 93.37
  elastic 93.56
Banding
  gastric 44.68
    vertical 44.68
  pulmonary artery 38.85
Bankhart operation (capsular repair into
  glenoid, for shoulder dislocation) 81.82

Bardenheurer operation (ligation of
  innominate artery) 38.85
Barium swallow 87.61
Barkan operation (goniotomy) 12.52
  with goniopuncture 12.53
Barr operation (transfer of tibialis
  posterior tendon) 83.75
Barsky operation (closure of cleft hand)
  82.82
Basal metabolic rate 89.39
Basiotripsy 73.8
Bassett operation (vulvectomy with
  inguinal lymph node dissection)
  71.5 *[40.3]*
Bassini operation - *see* Repair, hernia,
  inguinal
Batch-Spittler-McFaddin operation (knee
  disarticulation) 84.16
Batista operation (partial ventriculectomy)
  (ventricular reduction) (ventricular
  remodeling) 37.35
Bearing surface, hip
  ceramic-on-ceramic 00.76
  ceramic-on-polyethylene
    00.77
  metal-on-metal 00.75
  metal-on-polyethylene 00.74

Beck operation
  aorta-coronary sinus shunt 36.39
  epicardial poudrage 36.39
Beck-Jianu operation (permanent
  gastrostomy) 43.19
Behavior modification 94.33
Bell-Beuttner operation (subtotal
  abdominal hysterectomy)
  68.39
  laparoscopic 68.31
Belsey operation (esophagogastric
  sphincter) 44.65
Benenenti operation (rotation of bulbous
  urethra) 58.49
Berke operation (levator resection of
  eyelid) 08.33
Bicuspidization of heart valve 35.10
  aortic 35.11
  mitral 35.12
Bicycle dynamometer 93.01
Biesenberger operation (size reduction of
  breast, bilateral) 85.32
  unilateral 85.31
Bifurcation, bone - *see also* Osteotomy
  77.30
Bigelow operation (litholapaxy) 57.0
Bililite therapy (ultraviolet) 99.82

B

Billroth I operation (partial gastrectomy with gastroduodenostomy) 43.6
Billroth II operation (partial gastrectomy with gastrojejunostomy) 43.7
Binnie operation (hepatopexy) 50.69
Biofeedback, psychotherapy 94.39
Biopsy
  abdominal wall 54.22
  adenoid 28.11
  adrenal gland NEC 07.11
    closed 07.11
    open 07.12
    percutaneous (aspiration) (needle) 07.11
  alveolus 24.12
  anus 49.23
  appendix 45.26
  artery (any site) 38.21
  aspiration - *see* Biopsy, by site
  bile ducts 51.14
    closed (endoscopic) 51.14
    open 51.13
    percutaneous (needle) 51.12
  bladder 57.33
    closed 57.33
    open 57.34
    transurethral 57.33
  blood vessel (any site) 38.21
  bone 77.40
    carpal, metacarpal 77.44
    clavicle 77.41
    facial 76.11
    femur 77.45
    fibula 77.47
    humerus 77.42
    marrow 41.31
    patella 77.46
    pelvic 77.49
    phalanges (foot) (hand) 77.49
    radius 77.43
    scapula 77.41
    specified site NEC 77.49
    tarsal, metatarsal 77.48
    thorax (ribs) (sternum) 77.41
    tibia 77.47
    ulna 77.43
    vertebrae 77.49
  bowel - *see* Biopsy, intestine
  brain NEC 01.13
    closed 01.13
    open 01.14
    percutaneous (needle) 01.13
  breast 85.11
    blind 85.11
    closed 85.11
    open 85.12
    percutaneous (needle) (Vimm-Silverman) 85.11
  bronchus NEC 33.24
    brush 33.24
    closed (endoscopic) 33.24
    open 33.25
    transbronchoscopic needle aspiration (TBNA) 33.24
    Wang needle (transbronchoscopic) 33.24
    washings 33.24
  bursa 83.21
  cardioesophageal (junction) 44.14
    closed (endoscopic) 44.14
    open 44.15
  cecum 45.25
    brush 45.25
    closed (endoscopic) 45.25
    open 45.26

Biopsy *(Continued)*
  cerebral meninges NEC 01.11
    closed 01.11
    open 01.12
    percutaneous (needle) 01.11
  cervix (punch) 67.12
    conization (sharp) 67.2
  chest wall 34.23
  clitoris 71.11
  colon 45.25
    brush 45.25
    closed (endoscopic) 45.25
    open 45.26
  conjunctiva 10.21
  cornea 11.22
  cul-de-sac 70.23
  diaphragm 34.27
  duodenum 45.14
    brush 45.14
    closed (endoscopic) 45.14
    open 45.15
  ear (external) 18.12
    middle or inner 20.32
  endocervix 67.11
  endometrium NEC 68.16
    by
      aspiration curettage 69.59
      dilation and curettage 69.09
    closed (endoscopic) 68.16
    open 68.13
  epididymis 63.01
  esophagus 42.24
    closed (endoscopic) 42.24
    open 42.25
  extraocular muscle or tendon 15.01
  eye 16.23
    muscle (oblique) (rectus) 15.01
  eyelid 08.11
  fallopian tube 66.11
  fascia 83.21
  fetus 75.33
  gallbladder 51.12
    closed (endoscopic) 51.14
    open 51.13
    percutaneous (needle) 51.12
  ganglion (cranial) (peripheral) NEC 04.11
    closed 04.11
    open 04.12
    percutaneous (needle) 04.11
    sympathetic nerve 05.11
  gum 24.11
  heart 37.25
  hypophysis - *see also* Biopsy, pituitary gland 07.15
  ileum 45.14
    brush 45.14
    closed (endoscopic) 45.14
    open 45.15
  intestine NEC 45.27
    large 45.25
      brush 45.25
      closed (endoscopic) 45.25
      open 45.26
    small 45.14
      brush 45.14
      closed (endoscopic) 45.14
      open 45.15
  intra-abdominal mass 54.24
    closed 54.24
    percutaneous (needle) 54.24
  iris 12.22

Biopsy *(Continued)*
  jejunum 45.14
    brush 45.14
    closed (endoscopic) 45.14
    open 45.15
  joint structure (aspiration) 80.30
    ankle 80.37
    elbow 80.32
    foot and toe 80.38
    hand and finger 80.34
    hip 80.35
    knee 80.36
    shoulder 80.31
    specified site NEC 80.39
    spine 80.39
    wrist 80.33
  kidney 55.23
    closed 55.23
    open 55.24
    percutaneous (aspiration) (needle) 55.23
  labia 71.11
  lacrimal
    gland 09.11
    sac 09.12
  larynx 31.43
    brush 31.43
    closed (endoscopic) 31.43
    open 31.45
  lip 27.23
  liver 50.11
    closed 50.11
    laparoscopic 50.14
    open 50.12
    percutaneous (aspiration) (needle) 50.11
    transjugular 50.13
    transvenous 50.13
  lung NEC 33.27
    brush 33.24
    closed (percutaneous) (needle) 33.26
      brush 33.24
      endoscopic 33.27
        brush 33.24
    endoscopic 33.27
      brush 33.24
    open 33.28
    thoracoscopic 33.20
    transbronchial 33.27
    transthoracic 33.26
  lymphatic structure (channel) (node) (vessel) 40.11
  mediastinum NEC 34.25
    closed 34.25
    open 34.26
    percutaneous (needle) 34.25
  meninges (cerebral) NEC 01.11
    closed 01.11
    open 01.12
    percutaneous (needle) 01.11
    spinal 03.32
  mesentery 54.23
  mouth NEC 27.24
  muscle 83.21
    extraocular 15.01
    ocular 15.01
  nasopharynx 29.12
  nerve (cranial) (peripheral) NEC 04.11
    closed 04.11
    open 04.12
    percutaneous (needle) 04.11
    sympathetic 05.11

◀ New   ◀|||| Revised   ~~deleted~~ Deleted   ● Use Additional Digit(s)   Omit code

Biopsy *(Continued)*
  nose, nasal 21.22
    sinus 22.11
      closed (endoscopic) (needle) 22.11
    open 22.12
  ocular muscle or tendon 15.01
  omentum
    closed 54.24
    open 54.23
    percutaneous (needle) 54.24
  orbit 16.23
    by aspiration 16.22
  ovary 65.12
    by aspiration 65.11
    laparoscopic 65.13
  palate (bony) 27.21
    soft 27.22
  pancreas 52.11
    closed (endoscopic) 52.11
    open 52.12
    percutaneous (aspiration) (needle)
      52.11
  pancreatic duct 52.14
    closed (endoscopic) 52.14
  parathyroid gland 06.13
  penis 64.11
  perianal tissue 49.22
  pericardium 37.24
  periprostatic 60.15
  perirectal tissue 48.26
  perirenal tissue 59.21
  peritoneal implant
    closed 54.24
    open 54.23
    percutaneous (needle) 54.24
  peritoneum
    closed 54.24
    open 54.23
    percutaneous (needle) 54.24
  periurethral tissue 58.24
  perivesical tissue 59.21
  pharynx, pharyngeal 29.12
  pineal gland 07.17
  pituitary gland 07.15
    transfrontal approach 07.13
    transsphenoidal approach 07.14
  pleura, pleural 34.24
    thoracoscopic 34.20
  prostate NEC 60.11
    closed (transurethral) 60.11
    open 60.12
    percutaneous (needle) 60.11
    transrectal 60.11
  rectum 48.24
    brush 48.24
    closed (endoscopic) 48.24
    open 48.25
  retroperitoneal tissue 54.24
  salivary gland or duct 26.11
    closed (needle) 26.11
    open 26.12
  scrotum 61.11
  seminal vesicle NEC 60.13
    closed 60.13
    open 60.14
    percutaneous (needle) 60.13
  sigmoid colon 45.25
    brush 45.25
    closed (endoscopic) 45.25
    open 45.26
  sinus, nasal 22.11
    closed (endoscopic) (needle) 22.11
    open 22.12
  skin (punch) 86.11

Biopsy *(Continued)*
  skull 01.15
  soft palate 27.22
  soft tissue NEC ~~83.21~~ 86.11 ◀▥
    closed (needle) (punch) 86.11 ◀
    open 83.21 ◀
  spermatic cord 63.01
  sphincter of Oddi 51.14
    closed (endoscopic) 51.14
    open 51.13
  spinal cord (meninges) 03.32
  spleen 41.32
    closed 41.32
    open 41.33
    percutaneous (aspiration) (needle)
      41.32
  stomach 44.14
    brush 44.14
    closed (endoscopic) 44.14
    open 44.15
  subcutaneous tissue (punch) 86.11
  supraglottic mass 29.12
  sympathetic nerve 05.11
  tendon 83.21
    extraocular 15.01
    ocular 15.01
  testis NEC 62.11
    closed 62.11
    open 62.12
    percutaneous (needle) 62.11
  thymus 07.16
  thyroid gland NEC 06.11
    closed 06.11
    open 06.12
    percutaneous (aspiration) (needle)
      06.11
      tongue 25.01
    closed (needle) 25.01
    open 25.02
  tonsil 28.11
  trachea 31.44
    brush 31.44
    closed (endoscopic) 31.44
    open 31.45
  tunica vaginalis 61.11
  umbilicus 54.22
  ureter 56.33
    closed (percutaneous) 56.32
      endoscopic 56.33
    open 56.34
    transurethral 56.33
  urethra 58.23
  uterus, uterine (endometrial) 68.16
    by
      aspiration curettage 69.59
      dilation and curettage 69.09
    closed (endoscopic) 68.16
    ligaments 68.15
      closed (endoscopic) 68.15
      open 68.14
    open 68.13
  uvula 27.22
  vagina 70.24
  vas deferens 63.01
  vein (any site) 38.21
  vulva 71.11
BiPAP 93.90
  delivered by
    endotracheal tube - *see* category 96.7 ●
    tracheostomy - *see* category 96.7 ●
BIS (bispectral index) monitoring 00.94
  [89.14]
Bischoff operation
  (ureteroneocystostomy) 56.74

Bisection - *see also* Excision
  hysterectomy 68.39
    laparoscopic 68.31
  ovary 65.29
    laparoscopic 65.25
  stapes foot plate 19.79
    with incus replacement 19.11
Bischoff operation (spinal myelotomy)
  03.29
Blalock operation (systemic-pulmonary
  anastomosis) 39.0
Blalock-Hanlon operation (creation of
  atrial septal defect) 35.42
Blalock-Taussig operation (subclavian-
  pulmonary anastomosis) 39.0
Blascovic operation (resection and
  advancement of levator palpebrae
  superioris) 08.33
Blepharectomy 08.20
Blepharoplasty - *see also* Reconstruction,
  eyelid 08.70
  extensive 08.44
Blepharorrhaphy 08.52
  division or severing 08.02
Blepharotomy 08.09
Blind rehabilitation therapy NEC 93.78
Block
  caudal - *see* Injection, spinal celiac
    ganglion or plexus 05.31
  dissection
    breast
      bilateral 85.46
      unilateral 85.45
    bronchus 32.6
    larynx 30.3
    lymph nodes 40.50
    neck 40.40
    vulva 71.5
  epidural, spinal - *see* Injection, spinal
  gasserian ganglion 04.81
  intercostal nerves 04.81
  intrathecal - *see* Injection, spinal
  nerve (cranial) (peripheral) NEC 04.81
  paravertebral stellate ganglion 05.31
  peripheral nerve 04.81
  spinal nerve root (intrathecal) - *see*
    Injection, spinal
  stellate (ganglion) 05.31
  subarachnoid, spinal - *see* Injection,
    spinal
  sympathetic nerve 05.31
  trigeminal nerve 04.81
Blood
  flow study, Doppler-type (ultrasound) -
    see Ultrasonography
  patch, spine (epidural) 03.95
  transfusion
    antihemophilic factor 99.06
    autologous
      collected prior to surgery 99.02
      intraoperative 99.00
      perioperative 99.00
      postoperative 99.00
      previously collected 99.02
      salvage 99.00
    blood expander 99.08
    blood surrogate 99.09
    coagulation factors 99.06
    exchange 99.01
    granulocytes 99.09
    hemodilution 99.03
    other substance 99.09
    packed cells 99.04
    plasma 99.07

Blood *(Continued)*
  transfusion *(Continued)*
    platelets 99.05
    serum, other 99.07
    thrombocytes 99.05
Blount operation
  femoral shortening (with blade plate) 78.25
    by epiphyseal stapling 78.25
Boari operation (bladder flap) 56.74
Bobb operation (cholelithotomy) 51.04
Bone
  age studies 88.33
  mineral density study 88.98
Bonney operation (abdominal hysterectomy) 68.49
  laparoscopic 68.41
Borthen operation (iridotasis) 12.63
Bost operation
  plantar dissection 80.48
  radiocarpal fusion 81.26
Bosworth operation
  arthroplasty for acromioclavicular separation 81.83
  fusion of posterior lumbar and lumbosacral spine 81.08
    for pseudarthrosis 81.38
  resection of radial head ligaments (for tennis elbow) 80.92
  shelf procedure, hip 81.40
Bottle repair of hydrocele, tunica-vaginalis 61.2
Boyd operation (hip disarticulation) 84.18
Brachytherapy
  intravascular 92.27
Brauer operation (cardiolysis) 37.10
Breech extraction - *see* Extraction, breech
Bricker operation (ileoureterostomy) 56.51
Brisement (forcé) 93.26
Bristow operation (repair of shoulder dislocation) 81.82
Brock operation (pulmonary valvotomy) 35.03
Brockman operation (soft tissue release for clubfoot) 83.84
Bronchogram, bronchography 87.32
  endotracheal 87.31
  transcricoid 87.32
Bronchoplasty 33.48
Bronchorrhaphy 33.41
Bronchoscopy NEC 33.23
  with biopsy 33.24
    lung 33.27
      brush 33.24
  fiberoptic 33.22
    with biopsy 33.24
      lung 33.27
        brush 33.24
  through tracheostomy 33.21
    with biopsy 33.24
      lung 33.27
        brush 33.24
Bronchospirometry 89.38
Bronchostomy 33.0
  closure 33.42
Bronchotomy 33.0
Browne (-Denis) operation (hypospadias repair) 58.45
Brunschwig operation (temporary gastrostomy) 43.19

Buckling, scleral 14.49
  with
    air tamponade 14.49
    implant (silicone) (vitreous) 14.41
    resection of sclera 14.49
    vitrectomy 14.49
    vitreous implant (silicone) 14.41
Bunionectomy (radical) 77.59
  with
    arthrodesis 77.52
    osteotomy of first metatarsal 77.51
    resection of joint with prosthetic implant 77.59
    soft tissue correction NEC 77.53
Bunnell operation (tendon transfer) 82.56
Burch procedure (retropubic urethral suspension for urinary stress incontinence) 59.5
Burgess operation (amputation of ankle) 84.14
Burn dressing 93.57
Burr holes 01.24
Bursectomy 83.5
  hand 82.31
Bursocentesis 83.94
  hand 82.92
Bursotomy 83.03
  hand 82.03
Burying of fimbriae in uterine wall 66.97
Bypass
  abdominal - coronary artery 36.17
  aortocoronary (catheter stent) (with prosthesis) (with saphenous vein graft) (with vein graft) 36.10
    one coronary vessel 36.11
    two coronary vessels 36.12
    three coronary vessels 36.13
    four coronary vessels 36.14
  arterial (graft) (mandril grown graft) (vein graft) NEC 39.29
    carotid-cerebral 39.28
    carotid-vertebral 39.28
    extracranial-intracranial [EC-IC] 39.28
    intra-abdominal NEC 39.26
    intrathoracic NEC 39.23
    peripheral NEC 39.29
  cardiopulmonary 39.61
    open 39.61
    percutaneous (closed) 39.66
  carotid-cerebral 39.28
  carotid-vertebral 39.28
  coronary - *see also* Bypass, aortocoronary 36.10
  extracranial-intracranial [EC-IC] 39.28
  gastric 44.39
    high 44.31
    laparoscopic 44.38
    Printen and Mason 44.31
  gastroduodenostomy (Jaboulay's) 44.39
    laparoscopic 44.38
    percutaneous [endoscopic] 44.32
  gastroenterostomy 44.39
    laparoscopic 44.38
  gastroepiploic - coronary artery 36.17
  gastrogastrostomy 44.39
    laparoscopic 44.38
  graft, pressurized treatment 00.16
  heart-lung (complete) (partial) 39.61
    open 39.61
    percutaneous (closed) 39.66
  high gastric 44.31
  ileo-jejunal 45.91
  internal mammary-coronary artery (single) 36.13
    double vessel 36.16

Bypass *(Continued)*
  jejunal-ileum 45.91
  pulmonary 39.61
    open 39.61
    percutaneous (closed) 39.66
  shunt
    intestine
      large-to-large 45.94
      small-to-large 45.93
      small-to-small 45.91
    stomach 44.39
      high gastric 44.31
      laparoscopic 44.38
  terminal ileum 45.93
  vascular (arterial) (graft) (mandril grown graft) (vein graft) NEC 39.29
    aorta-carotid-brachial 39.22
    aorta-iliac-femoral 39.25
    aorta-renal 39.24
    aorta-subclavian-carotid 39.22
    aortic-superior mesenteric 39.26
    aortocarotid 39.22
    aortoceliac 39.26
    aortocoronary - *see also* Bypass, aortocoronary 36.10
    aortofemoral 39.25
    aortofemoral-popliteal 39.25
    aortoiliac 39.25
      to popliteal 39.25
    aortoiliofemoral 39.25
    aortomesenteric 39.26
    aortopopliteal 39.25
    aortorenal 39.24
    aortosubclavian 39.22
    axillary-brachial 39.29
    axillary-femoral (superficial) 39.29
    axillofemoral (superficial) 39.29
    carotid-cerebral 39.28
    carotid-vertebral 39.28
    carotid to subclavian artery 39.22
    common hepatic-common iliac-renal 39.26
    coronary - *see also* Bypass, aortocoronary 36.10
    extracranial-intracranial [EC-IC] 39.28
    femoral-femoral 39.29
    femoroperoneal 39.29
    femoropopliteal (reversed saphenous vein) (saphenous) 39.29
    femorotibial (anterior) (posterior) 39.29
    iliofemoral 39.25
    ilioiliac 39.26
    internal mammary-coronary artery (single) 36.15
      double vessel 36.16
    intra-abdominal (arterial) NEC 39.26
      venous NEC 39.1
    intrathoracic NEC 39.23
    peripheral artery NEC 39.29
    popliteal-tibial 39.29
    renal artery 39.24
    splenorenal (venous) 39.1
      arterial 39.26
    subclavian-axillary 39.29
    subclavian-carotid 39.22
    subclavian-subclavian 39.22
    Y graft to renal arteries 39.24

◀ New   ◀▥ Revised   ~~deleted~~ Deleted   ● Use Additional Digit(s)   ▨ Omit code

C

Caldwell operation (sulcus extension) 24.91
Caldwell-Luc operation (maxillary sinusotomy) 22.39
  with removal of membrane lining 22.31
Calibration, urethra 89.29
Calicectomy (renal) 55.4
Callander operation (knee disarticulation) 84.16
Caloric test, vestibular function 95.44
Calycectomy (renal) 55.4
Calyco-ileoneocystostomy 55.86
Calycotomy (renal) 55.11
Campbell operation
  bone block, ankle 81.11
  fasciotomy (iliac crest) 83.14
  reconstruction of anterior cruciate ligament 81.45
Campimetry 95.05
Canaliculodacryocystorhinostomy 09.81
Canaliculoplasty 09.73
Canaliculorhinostomy 09.81
Canaloplasty, external auditory meatus 18.6
Cannulation - *see also* Insertion, catheter
  ampulla of Vater 51.99
  antrum 22.01
  arteriovenous 39.93
  artery 38.91
  caval-mesenteric vein 39.1
  cisterna chyli 40.61
  Eustachian tube 20.8
  lacrimal apparatus 09.42
  lymphatic duct, left (thoracic) 40.61
  nasal sinus (by puncture) 22.01
    through natural ostium 22.02
  pancreatic duct 52.92
    by retrograde endoscopy (ERP) 52.93
  renoportal 39.1
  sinus (nasal) (by puncture) 22.01
    through natural ostium 22.02
  splenorenal (venous) 39.1
    arterial 39.26
  thoracic duct (cervical approach) (thoracic approach) 40.61
Cannulization - *see* Cannulation
Canthocystostomy 09.82
Canthoplasty 08.59
Canthorrhaphy 08.52
  division or severing 08.02
Canthotomy 08.51
Capsulectomy
  joint - *see also* Arthrectomy 80.90
  kidney 55.91
  lens 13.65
    with extraction of lens 13.51
  ovary 65.29
    laparoscopic 65.25
Capsulo-iridectomy 13.65
Capsuloplasty - *see* Arthroplasty
Capsulorrhaphy 81.96
  with arthroplasty - *see* Arthroplasty
  ankle 81.94
  foot 81.94
  lower extremity NEC 81.95
  upper extremity 81.93
Capsulotomy
  joint - *see also* Division, joint capsule 80.40
    for claw toe repair 77.57

Capsulotomy (*Continued*)
  lens 13.64
    with
      discission of lens 13.2
      removal of foreign body 13.02
        by magnet extraction 13.01
Cardiac
  mapping 37.27
  massage (external) (closed chest) 99.63
    open chest 37.91
  retraining 93.36
Cardiac support device (CSD) 37.41
Cardiectomy (stomach) 43.5
Cardiocentesis 37.0
Cardiography - *see also* Angiocardiography 88.50
Cardiolysis 37.10
Cardiomyopexy 36.39
Cardiomyotomy 42.7
Cardio-omentopexy 36.39
Cardiopericardiopexy 36.39
Cardioplasty (stomach and esophagus) 44.65
  stomach alone 44.66
    laparoscopic 44.67
Cardioplegia 39.63
Cardiopneumopexy 36.39
Cardiorrhaphy 37.49
Cardioschisis 37.12
Cardiosplenopexy 36.39
Cardiotomy (exploratory) 37.11
Cardiovalvulotomy - *see* Valvulotomy, heart
Cardioversion (external) 99.62
  atrial 99.61
CardioWest™ Total Temporary Artificial Heart (TAH-t) 37.52
Carotid pulse tracing with ECG lead 89.56
Carpectomy (partial) 77.84
  total 77.94
Carroll and Taber arthroplasty (proximal interphalangeal joint) 81.72
Casting (for immobilization) NEC 93.53
  with fracture-reduction - *see* Reduction, fracture
Castration
  female (oophorectomy, bilateral) 65.51
    laparoscopic 65.53
  male 62.41
C.A.T. (computerized axial tomography) - *see also* Scan, C.A.T. 88.38
Catheterization - *see also* Insertion, catheter
  arteriovenous 39.93
  artery 38.91
  bladder, indwelling 57.94
    percutaneous (cystostomy) 57.17
    suprapubic NEC 57.18
  bronchus 96.05
    with lavage 96.56
  cardiac (right) 37.21
    combined left and right 37.23
    left 37.22
      combined with right heart 37.23
    right 37.21
      combined with left heart 37.23
  central venous NEC 38.93
    peripherally inserted central catheter (PICC) 38.93

Catheterization (*Continued*)
  chest 34.04
    revision (with lysis of adhesions) 34.04
      thoracoscopic 34.06
    thoracoscopic 34.06
  Eustachian tube 20.8
  heart (right) 37.21
    combined left and right 37.23
    left 37.22
      combined with right heart 37.23
    right 37.21
      combined with left heart 37.23
  hepatic vein 38.93
  inferior vena cava 38.93
  intercostal space (with water seal), for drainage 34.04
    revision (with lysis of adhesions) 34.04
      thoracoscopic 34.06
    thoracoscopic 34.06
  lacrimonasal duct 09.44
  laryngeal 96.05
  nasolacrimal duct 09.44
  pancreatic cyst 52.01
  renal vein 38.93
  Swan-Ganz (pulmonary) 89.64
  transtracheal for oxygenation 31.99
  umbilical vein 38.92
  ureter (to kidney) 59.8
    for retrograde pyelogram 87.74
  urethra, indwelling 57.94
  vein NEC 38.93
    for renal dialysis 38.95
Cattell operation (herniorrhaphy) 53.51
Cauterization - *see also* Destruction, lesion, by site
  anus NEC 49.39
    endoscopic 49.31
  Bartholin's gland 71.24
  broad ligament 69.19
  bronchus 32.09
    endoscopic 32.01
  canaliculi 09.73
  cervix 67.32
  chalazion 08.25
  choroid plexus 02.14
  conjunctiva 10.33
    lesion 10.32
  cornea (fistula) (ulcer) 11.42
  ear, external 18.29
  endometrial implant - *see* Excision, lesion, by site
  entropion 08.41
  esophagus 42.39
    endoscopic 42.33
  eyelid 08.25
    for entropion or ectropion 08.41
  fallopian tube 66.61
    by endoscopy (hysteroscopy) (laparoscopy) 66.29
  hemorrhoids 49.43
  iris 12.41
  lacrimal
    gland 09.21
    punctum 09.72
      for eversion 09.71
    sac 09.6
  larynx 30.09
  liver 50.29
  lung 32.29
    endoscopic 32.28
    thoracoscopic 32.20
  meibomian gland 08.25
  nose, for epistaxis (with packing) 21.03

Cauterization *(Continued)*
  ovary 65.29
    laparoscopic 65.25
  palate (bony) 27.31
  pannus (superficial) 11.42
  pharynx 29.39
  punctum, lacrimal 09.72
    for eversion 09.71
  rectum 48.32
    radical 48.31
  round ligament 69.19
  sclera 12.84
    with iridectomy 12.62
  skin 86.3
  subcutaneous tissue 86.3
  tonsillar fossa 28.7
  urethra 58.39
    endoscopic 58.31
  uterosacral ligament 69.19
  uterotubal ostia 66.61
  uterus 68.29
  vagina 70.33
  vocal cords 30.09
  vulva 71.3
Cavernoscopy 34.21
Cavernostomy 33.1
Cavernotomy, kidney 55.39
Cavography (inferior vena cava) 88.51
CCM (implantation of cardiac
    contractility modulation)
  rechargeable pulse generator only
    17.52
  total system 17.51
Cecectomy (with resection of terminal
    ileum)
  laparoscopic 17.32
  open and other 45.72
Cecil operation (urethral reconstruction)
    58.46
Cecocoloplicopexy 46.63
Cecocolostomy 45.94
Cecofixation 46.64
Ceco-ileostomy 45.93
Cecopexy 46.64
Cecoplication 46.62
Cecorrhaphy 46.75
Cecosigmoidostomy 45.94
Cecostomy (tube) - *see also* Colostomy 46.10
Cecotomy 45.03
Celiocentesis 54.91
Celioscopy 54.21
Celiotomy, exploratory 54.11
Cell block and Papanicolaou smear - *see*
    Examination, microscopic
CentriMag® acute circulatory support
    device 37.62
Cephalogram 87.17
  dental 87.12
  orthodontic 87.12
Cephalometry, cephalometrics 87.17
  echo 88.78
  orthodontic 87.12
  ultrasound (sonar) 88.78
  x-ray 87.81
Cephalotomy, fetus 73.8
Cerclage
  anus 49.72
  cervix 67.51
    transabdominal 67.51
    transvaginal 67.59
  isthmus uteri (cervix) 67.59
  retinal reattachment - *see also* Buckling,
    scleral 14.49
  sclera - *see also* Buckling, scleral 14.49

Cervicectomy (with synchronous
    colporrhaphy) 67.4
Cervicoplasty 67.69
Cesarean section 74.99
  classical 74.0
  corporeal 74.0
  extraperitoneal 74.2
  fundal 74.0
  laparotrachelotomy 74.1
  Latzko 74.2
  low cervical 74.1
  lower uterine segment 74.1
  peritoneal exclusion 74.4
  specified type NEC 74.4
  supravesical 74.2
  transperitoneal 74.4
    classical 74.0
    low cervical 74.1
  upper uterine segment 74.0
  vaginal 74.4
  Waters 74.2
Chamberlain procedure - *see*
    Mediastinotomy
Chandler operation (hip fusion) 81.21
Change - *see also* Replacement
  cast NEC 97.13
    lower limb 97.12
    upper limb 97.11
  cystostomy catheter or tube 59.94
  gastrostomy tube 97.02
  length
    bone - *see either category* 78.2●
      Shortening, bone *or category*
      78.3● Lengthening, bone
    muscle 83.85
      hand 82.55
    tendon 83.85
      hand 82.55
  nephrostomy catheter or tube 55.93
  pyelostomy catheter or tube 55.94
  splint 97.14
  tracheostomy tube 97.23
  ureterostomy catheter or tube 59.93
  urethral catheter, indwelling 57.95
Character analysis, psychologic 94.03
Charles operation (correction of
    lymphedema) 40.9
Charnley operation (compression
    arthrodesis)
  ankle 81.11
  hip 81.21
  knee 81.22
Cheatle-Henry operation - *see* Repair,
    hernia, femoral
Check
  automatic implantable cardioverter/
    defibrillator (AICD)
    (interrogation only) 89.49
  CRT-D (cardiac resynchronization
    defibrillator) (interrogation only)
    89.49
  CRT-P (cardiac resynchronization
    pacemaker) (interrogation only)
    89.45
  pacemaker, artificial (cardiac)
    (function) (interrogation only)
    (rate) 89.45
    amperage threshold 89.48
    artifact wave form 89.46
    electrode impedance 89.47
    voltage threshold 89.48
  vision NEC 95.09
Cheiloplasty 27.59
Cheilorrhaphy 27.51

Cheilostomatoplasty 27.59
Cheilotomy 27.0
Chemical peel, skin 86.24
Chemocauterization - *see also* Destruction,
    lesion, by site
  corneal epithelium 11.41
  palate 27.31
Chemodectomy 39.89 ◄▥
Chemoembolization 99.25
Chemolysis
  nerve (peripheral) 04.2
  spinal canal structure 03.8
Chemoneurolysis 04.2
Chemonucleolysis (nucleus pulposus)
    80.52
Chemopallidectomy 01.42
Chemopeel (skin) 86.24
Chemosurgery
  esophagus 42.39
    endoscopic 42.33
  Mohs' 86.24
  skin (superficial) 86.24
  stomach 43.49
    endoscopic 43.41
Chemothalamectomy 01.41
Chemotherapy - *see also* Immunotherapy
  Antabuse 94.25
  for cancer NEC 99.25
    brain wafer implantation 00.10
    CLO 17.70
    clofarabine 17.70
    CLOLAR® 17.70
    implantation of chemotherapeutic
      agent 00.10
    interstitial implantation 00.10
    intracavitary implantation 00.10
    wafer chemotherapy 00.10
  ithium 94.22
  methadone 94.25
  palate (bony) 27.31
Chevalier-Jackson operation (partial
    laryngectomy) 30.29
Child operation (radical subtotal
    pancreatectomy) 52.53
Cholangiocholangiostomy 51.39
Cholangiocholecystocholedochectomy
    51.22
Cholangio-enterostomy 51.39
Cholangiogastrostomy 51.39
Cholangiogram 87.54
  endoscopic retrograde (ERC) 51.11
  intraoperative 87.53
  intravenous 87.52
  percutaneous hepatic 87.51
  transhepatic 87.53
Cholangiography - *see also*
    Cholangiogram 87.54
Cholangiojejunostomy (intrahepatic) 51.39
Cholangiopancreatography, endoscopic
    retrograde (ERCP) 51.10
Cholangiostomy 51.59
Cholangiotomy 51.59
Cholecystectomy (total) 51.22
  partial 51.21
    laparoscopic 51.24
  total 51.22
    laparoscopic 51.23
Cholecystenterorrhaphy 51.91
Cholecystocecostomy 51.32
Cholecystocholangiogram 87.59
Cholecystocolostomy 51.32
Cholecystoduodenostomy 51.32
Cholecystoenterostomy (Winiwater) 51.32
Cholecystogastrostomy 51.34

◄ New   ◄▥ Revised   d̶e̶l̶e̶t̶e̶d̶ Deleted   ● Use Additional Digit(s)   ▭ Omit code

Cholecystogram 87.59
Cholecystoileostomy 51.32
Cholecystojejunostomy (Roux-en-Y)
    (with jejunojejunostomy) 51.32
Cholecystopancreatostomy 51.33
Cholecystopexy 51.99
Cholecystorrhaphy 51.91
Cholecystostomy NEC 51.03
    by trocar 51.02
Cholecystotomy 51.04
    percutaneous 51.01
Choledochectomy 51.63
Choledochoduodenostomy 51.36
Choledochoenterostomy 51.36
Choledochojejunostomy 51.36
Choledocholithotomy 51.41
    endoscopic 51.88
Choledocholithotripsy 51.41
    endoscopic 51.88
Choledochopancreatostomy 51.39
Choledochoplasty 51.72
Choledochorrhaphy 51.71
Choledochoscopy 51.11
Choledochostomy 51.51
Choledochotomy 51.51
Cholelithotomy 51.04
Chondrectomy 80.90
    ankle 80.97
    elbow 80.92
    foot and toe 80.98
    hand and finger 80.94
    hip 80.95
    intervertebral cartilage - see category
        80.5●
    knee (semilunar cartilage) 80.6
    nasal (submucous) 21.5
    semilunar cartilage (knee) 80.6
    shoulder 80.91
    specified site NEC 80.99
    spine - see category 80.5●
    wrist 80.93
Chondroplasty - see Arthroplasty
Chondrosternoplasty (for pectus
    excavatum repair) 34.74
Chondrotomy - see also Division, cartilage
    80.40
    nasal 21.1
Chopart operation (midtarsal
    amputation) 84.12
Chordectomy, vocal 30.22
Chordotomy (spinothalamic) (anterior)
    (posterior) NEC 03.29
    percutaneous 03.21
    stereotactic 03.21
Ciliarotomy 12.55
Ciliectomy (ciliary body) 12.44
    eyelid margin 08.20
Cinch, cinching
    for scleral buckling - see also Buckling,
        scleral 14.49
    ocular muscle (oblique) (rectus) 15.22
        multiple (two or more muscles) 15.4
Cineangiocardiography - see also
    Angiocardiography 88.50
Cineplasty, cineplastic prosthesis
    amputation - see Amputation
    arm 84.44
    biceps 84.44
    extremity 84.40
        lower 84.48
        upper 84.44
    leg 84.48
Cineradiograph - see Radiography
Cingulumotomy (brain) (percutaneous
    radiofrequency) 01.32

Circumcision (male) 64.0
    female 71.4
CISH [classic infrafascial SEMM
    hysterectomy] 68.31
Clagett operation (closure of chest wall
    following open flap drainage)
    34.72
Clamp and cautery, hemorrhoids 49.43
Clamping
    aneurysm (cerebral) 39.51
    blood vessel - see Ligation, blood vessel
    ventricular shunt 02.43
Clavicotomy 77.31
    fetal 73.8
Claviculectomy (partial) 77.81
    total 77.91
Clayton operation (resection of
    metatarsal heads and bases of
    phalanges) 77.88
Cleaning, wound 96.59
Clearance
    bladder (transurethral) 57.0
    pelvic
        female 68.8
        male 57.71
    prescalene fat pad 40.21
    renal pelvis (transurethral) 56.0
    ureter (transurethral) 56.0
Cleidotomy 77.31
    fetal 73.8
Clipping
    aneurysm (basilar) (carotid)
        (cerebellar) (cerebellopontine)
        (communicating artery)
        (vertebral) 39.51
    arteriovenous fistula 39.53
    frenulum, frenum
        labia (lips) 27.91
        lingual (tongue) 25.91
    left atrial appendage 37.36
    tip of uvula 27.72
Clitoridectomy 71.4
Clitoridotomy 71.4
Clivogram 87.02
Closure - see also Repair
    abdominal wall 54.63
        delayed (granulating wound) 54.62
        secondary 54.61
        tertiary 54.62
    amputation stump, secondary 84.3
    anular disc 80.54
        with graft or prosthesis 80.53
    anulus fibrosus 80.54
        with graft or prosthesis 80.53
    aorticopulmonary fenestration
        (fistula) 39.59
    appendicostomy 47.92
    artificial opening
        bile duct 51.79
        bladder 57.82
        bronchus 33.42
        common duct 51.72
        esophagus 42.83
        gallbladder 51.92
        hepatic duct 51.79
        intestine 46.50
            large 46.52
            small 46.51
        kidney 55.82
        larynx 31.62
        rectum 48.72
        stomach 44.62
        thorax 34.72
        trachea 31.72

Closure (Continued)
    artificial opening (Continued)
        ureter 56.83
        urethra 58.42
    atrial septal defect - see also Repair,
        atrial septal defect 35.71
        with umbrella device (King-Mills
            type) 35.52
        combined with repair of valvular
            and ventricular septal
            defects - see Repair,
            endocardial cushion
            defect
    bronchostomy 33.42
    cecostomy 46.52
    cholecystostomy 51.92
    cleft hand 82.82
    colostomy 46.52
    cystostomy 57.82
    diastema (alveolar) (dental) 24.8
    disrupted abdominal wall
        (postoperative) 54.61
    duodenostomy 46.51
    encephalocele 02.12
    endocardial cushion defect - see also
        Repair, endocardial cushion
        defect 35.73
    enterostomy 46.50
    esophagostomy 42.83
    fenestration
        aorticopulmonary 39.59
        septal, heart - see also Repair, heart,
            septum 35.70
    filtering bleb, corneoscleral
        (postglaucoma) 12.66
    fistula
        abdominothoracic 34.83
        anorectal 48.73
        anovaginal 70.73
        antrobuccal 22.71
        anus 49.73
        aorticopulmonary (fenestration) 39.59
        aortoduodenal 39.59
        appendix 47.92
        biliary tract 51.79
        bladder NEC 57.84
        branchial cleft 29.52
        bronchocutaneous 33.42
        bronchoesophageal 33.42
        bronchomediastinal 34.73
        bronchopleural 34.73
        bronchopleurocutaneous 34.73
        bronchopleuromediastinal 34.73
        bronchovisceral 33.42
        bronchus 33.42
        cecosigmoidal 46.76
        cerebrospinal fluid 02.12
        cervicoaural 18.79
        cervicosigmoidal 67.62
        cervicovesical 57.84
        cervix 67.62
        cholecystocolic 51.93
        cholecystoduodenal 51.93
        cholecystoenteric 51.93
        cholecystogastric 51.93
        cholecystojejunal 51.93
        cisterna chyli 40.63
        colon 46.76
        colovaginal 70.72
        common duct 51.72
        cornea 11.49
            with lamellar graft (homograft)
                11.62
            autograft 11.61

C

Closure *(Continued)*
  fistula *(Continued)*
    diaphragm 34.83
    duodenum 46.72
    ear, middle 19.9
    ear drum 19.4
    enterocolic 46.74
    enterocutaneous 46.74
    enterouterine 69.42
    enterovaginal 70.74
    enterovesical 57.83
    esophagobronchial 33.42
    esophagocutaneous 42.84
    esophagopleurocutaneous 34.73
    esophagotracheal 31.73
    esophagus NEC 42.84
    fecal 46.79
    gallbladder 51.93
    gastric NEC 44.63
    gastrocolic 44.63
    gastroenterocolic 44.63
    gastroesophageal 42.84
    gastrojejunal 44.63
    gastrojejunocolic 44.63
    heart valve - *see* Repair, heart, valve
    hepatic duct 51.79
    hepatopleural 34.73
    hepatopulmonary 34.73
    ileorectal 46.74
    ileosigmoidal 46.74
    ileovesical 57.83
    ileum 46.74
    in ano 49.73
    intestine 46.79
      large 46.76
      small NEC 46.74
    intestinocolonic 46.74
    intestinoureteral 56.84
    intestinouterine 69.42
    intestinovaginal 70.74
    intestinovesical 57.83
    jejunum 46.74
    kidney 55.83
    lacrimal 09.99
    laryngotracheal 31.62
    larynx 31.62
    lymphatic duct, left (thoracic) 40.63
    mastoid (antrum) 19.9
    mediastinobronchial 34.73
    mediastinocutaneous 34.73
    mouth (external) 27.53
    nasal 21.82
      sinus 22.71
    nasolabial 21.82
    nasopharyngeal 21.82
    oroantral 22.71
    oronasal 21.82
    oval window (ear) 20.93
    pancreaticoduodenal 52.95
    perilymph 20.93
    perineorectal 48.73
    perineosigmoidal 46.76
    perineourethroscrotal 58.43
    perineum 71.72
    perirectal 48.93
    pharyngoesophageal 29.53
    pharynx NEC 29.53
    pleura, pleural NEC 34.93
    pleurocutaneous 34.73
    pleuropericardial 37.49
    pleuroperitoneal 34.83
    pulmonoperitoneal 34.83
    rectolabial 48.73
    rectoureteral 56.84

Closure *(Continued)*
  fistula *(Continued)*
    rectourethral 58.43
    rectovaginal 70.73
    rectovesical 57.83
    rectovesicovaginal 57.83
    rectovulvar 48.73
    rectum NEC 48.73
    renal 55.83
    reno-intestinal 55.83
    round window 20.93
    salivary (gland) (duct) 26.42
    scrotum 61.42
    sigmoidovaginal 70.74
    sigmoidovesical 57.83
    splenocolic 41.95
    stomach NEC 44.63
    thoracic duct 40.63
    thoracoabdominal 34.83
    thoracogastric 34.83
    thoracointestinal 34.83
    thorax NEC 34.73
    trachea NEC 31.73
    tracheoesophageal 31.73
    tympanic membrane - *see also*
      Tympanoplasty 19.4
    umbilicourinary 57.51
    ureter 56.84
    ureterocervical 56.84
    ureterorectal 56.84
    ureterosigmoidal 56.84
    ureterovaginal 56.84
    ureterovesical 56.84
    urethra 58.43
    urethroperineal 58.43
    urethroperineovesical 57.84
    urethrorectal 58.43
    urethroscrotal 58.43
    urethrovaginal 58.43
    uteroenteric 69.42
    uterointestinal 69.42
    uterorectal 69.42
    uteroureteric 56.84
    uterovaginal 69.42
    uterovesical 57.84
    vagina 70.75
    vaginocutaneous 70.75
    vaginoenteric 70.74
    vaginoperineal 70.75
    vaginovesical 57.84
    vesicocervicovaginal 57.84
    vesicocolic 57.83
    vesicocutaneous 57.84
    vesicoenteric 57.83
    vesicometrorectal 57.83
    vesicoperineal 57.84
    vesicorectal 57.83
    vesicosigmoidal 57.83
    vesicosigmoidovaginal 57.83
    vesicoureteral 56.84
    vesicoureterovaginal 56.84
    vesicourethral 57.84
    vesicourethrorectal 57.83
    vesicouterine 57.84
    vesicovaginal 57.84
    vulva 71.72
    vulvorectal 48.73
  foramen ovale (patent) 35.71
    with
      prosthesis (open heart
        technique) 35.51
      closed heart technique
        35.52
      tissue graft 35.61

Closure *(Continued)*
  gastroduodenostomy 44.5
  gastrojejunostomy 44.5
  gastrostomy 44.62
  ileostomy 46.51
  jejunostomy 46.51
  laceration - *see also* Suture, by site
    liver 50.61
  laparotomy, delayed 54.62
  meningocele (spinal) 03.51
    cerebral 02.12
  myelomeningocele 03.52
  nephrostomy 55.82
  palmar cleft 82.82
  patent ductus arteriosus 38.85
  pelviostomy 55.82
  peptic ulcer (bleeding) (perforated)
    44.40
  perforation
    ear drum - *see also* Tympanoplasty
      19.4
    esophagus 42.82
    nasal septum 21.88
    tympanic membrane - *see also*
      Tympanoplasty 19.4
  proctostomy 48.72
  punctum, lacrimal (papilla) 09.91
  pyelostomy 55.82
  rectostomy 48.72
  septum defect (heart) - *see also* Repair,
    heart, septum 35.70
  sigmoidostomy 46.52
  skin (V-Y type) 86.59
  stoma
    bile duct 51.79
    bladder 57.82
    bronchus 33.42
    common duct 51.72
    esophagus 42.83
    gallbladder 51.92
    hepatic duct 51.79
    intestine 46.50
      large 46.52
      small 46.51
    kidney 55.82
    larynx 31.62
    rectum 48.72
    stomach 44.62
    thorax 34.72
    trachea 31.72
    ureter 56.83
    urethra 58.42
  thoracostomy 34.72
  tracheostomy 31.72
  ulcer (bleeding) (peptic) (perforated)
    44.40
    duodenum 44.42
    gastric 44.41
    intestine (perforated) 46.79
    skin 86.59
    stomach 44.41
  ureterostomy 56.83
  urethrostomy 58.42
  vagina 70.8
  vascular
    percutaneous puncture - *omit code*
  vesicostomy 57.22
  wound - *see also* Suture, by site
    with graft - *see* Graft
    with tissue adhesive 86.59
Coagulation, electrocoagulation - *see also*
  Destruction, lesion, by site
  aneurysm (cerebral) (peripheral vessel)
    39.52

◀ New   ◀≡ Revised   ~~deleted~~ Deleted   ● Use Additional Digit(s)   ▨ Omit code

Coagulation, electrocoagulation
(Continued)
arteriovenous fistula 39.53
brain tissue (incremental)
(radiofrequency) 01.59
broad ligament 69.19
cervix 67.32
ear
external 18.29
inner 20.79
middle 20.51
fallopian tube 66.61
gasserian ganglion 04.05
nose, for epistaxis (with packing)
21.03
ovary 65.29
laparoscopic 65.25
pharynx (by diathermy) 29.39
prostatic bed 60.94
rectum (polyp) 48.32
radical 48.31
retina (for)
destruction of lesion 14.21
reattachment 14.51
repair for tear 14.31
round ligament 69.19
semicircular canals 20.79
spinal cord (lesion) 03.4
urethrovesical junction, transurethral
57.49
uterosacral ligament 69.19
uterus 68.29
vagina 70.33
vulva 71.3
Coating, aneurysm of brain 39.52
Cobalt-60 therapy (treatment)
92.23
Coccygectomy (partial) 77.89
total 77.99
Coccygotomy 77.39
"Cocked hat" procedure (metacarpal
lengthening and transfer of local
flap) 82.69
Cockett operation (varicose vein)
lower limb 38.59
upper limb 38.53
Cody tack (perforation of footplate)
19.0
Coffey operation (uterine suspension)
(Meig's modification) 69.22
Cole operation (anterior tarsal wedge
osteotomy) 77.28
Colectomy (partial) (segmental)
(subtotal)
cecum (with terminal ileum)
laparoscopic 17.32
open and other 45.72
laparoscopic 17.39
left (Hartmann) (lower) (radical)
laparoscopic 17.35
open and other 45.75
multiple segmental
laparoscopic 17.31
open and other 45.71
open and other 45.79
right (radical)
laparoscopic 17.33
open and other 45.73
sigmoid
laparoscopic 17.36
open and other 45.76
terminal ileum with cecum
laparoscopic 17.32
open and other 45.72

Colectomy (Continued)
total
laparoscopic 45.81
open 45.82
other 45.83
unspecified 45.83
transverse
laparoscopic 17.34
open and other 45.74
Collapse, lung, surgical 33.39
by
destruction of phrenic nerve
33.31
pneumoperitoneum 33.33
pneumothorax, artificially-induced
33.32
thoracoplasty 33.34
Collection, sperm for artificial
insemination 99.96
Collis-Nissen operation (hiatal hernia
repair with esophagogastroplasty)
53.80
Colocentesis 45.03
Colocolostomy 45.94
proximal to distal segment 45.79
Colocystoplasty 57.87 [45.52]
Colofixation 46.64
Coloileotomy 45.00
Colonna operation
adductor tenotomy (first stage) 83.12
hip arthroplasty (second stage) 81.40
reconstruction of hip (second stage)
81.40
Colonoscopy 45.23
with
biopsy 45.25
rectum 48.24
stent - see Insertion, stent, colon
fiberoptic (flexible) 45.23
intraoperative 45.21
through stoma (artificial) 45.22
transabdominal 45.21
Colopexy 46.63
Coloplication 46.64
Coloproctostomy 45.94
Colorectosigmoidostomy 45.94
Colorectostomy 45.94
Colorrhaphy 46.75
Coloscopy - see Colonoscopy
Colosigmoidostomy 45.94
Colostomy (ileo-ascending)
(ileotransverse) (perineal)
(transverse) 46.10
with anterior rectal resection 48.62
delayed opening 46.14
loop 46.03
permanent (magnetic) 46.13
temporary 46.11
Colotomy 45.03
Colpectomy 70.4
Colpoceliocentesis 70.0
Colpocentesis 70.0
Colpocleisis (complete) (partial) 70.8
Colpohysterectomy 68.59
laparoscopically assisted (LAVH)
68.51
Colpoperineoplasty 70.79
with repair of urethrocele 70.51
with graft or prosthesis 70.53
Colpoperineorrhaphy 70.71
following delivery 75.69
Colpopexy 70.77
with graft or prosthesis 70.78
Colpoplasty 70.79

Colpopoiesis 70.61
vaginal construction 70.61
with graft or prosthesis 70.63
Colporrhaphy 70.71
anterior (cystocele repair) 70.51
with graft or prosthesis 70.54
for repair of
cystocele 70.51
with rectocele 70.50
with graft or prosthesis 70.53
enterocele 70.92
with graft or prosthesis 70.93
rectocele 70.52
with cystocele 70.50
with graft or prosthesis 70.53
urethrocele 70.51
with graft or prosthesis 70.54
posterior (rectocele repair) 70.52
with graft or prosthesis 70.55
Colposcopy 70.21
Colpotomy 70.14
for pelvic peritoneal drainage 70.12
Commando operation (radical
glossectomy) 25.4
Commissurotomy
closed heart technique - see
Valvulotomy, heart
open heart technique - see
Valvuloplasty, heart
Compression, trigeminal nerve 04.02
Conchectomy 21.69
Conchotomy 21.1
Conduction study, nerve 89.15
Conduitogram, ileum 87.78
Condylectomy - see category 77.8●
mandible 76.5
Condylotomy NEC - see also Division,
joint capsule 80.40
mandible (open) 76.62
closed 76.61
Conization
cervix (knife) (sharp) (biopsy) 67.2
by
cryosurgery 67.33
electroconization 67.32
Conjunctivocystorhinostomy 09.82
with insertion of tube or stent 09.83
Conjunctivodacryocystorhinostomy
(CDCR) 09.82
with insertion of tube or stent 09.83
Conjunctivodacryocystostomy 09.82
with insertion of tube or stent 09.83
Conjunctivoplasty 10.49
Conjunctivorhinostomy 09.82
with insertion of tube or stent 09.83
Constriction of globe, for scleral
buckling - see also Buckling, scleral
14.49
Construction
auricle, ear (with graft) (with implant)
18.71
ear
auricle (with graft) (with implant)
18.71
meatus (osseous) (skin-lined) 18.6
endorectal ileal pouch (H-pouch)
(J-pouch) (S-pouch) (with
anastomosis to anus) 45.95
esophagus, artificial - see Anastomosis,
esophagus
ileal bladder (open) 56.51
closed 57.87 [45.51]
ileal conduit 56.51
larynx, artificial 31.75

Construction (*Continued*)
patent meatus (ear) 18.6
penis (rib graft) (skin graft)
(myocutaneous flap) 64.43
pharyngeal valve, artificial 31.75
urethra 58.46
vagina, artificial 70.61
with graft or prosthesis 70.63
venous valves (peripheral) 39.59
Consultation 89.09
comprehensive 89.07
limited (single organ system) 89.06
specified type NEC 89.08
Continuous positive airway pressure
[CPAP] (non-invasive) 93.90
delivered by
endotracheal tube - *see* category
96.7●
tracheostomy – *see* category 96.7●
Control
atmospheric pressure and composition
NEC 93.98
antigen-free air conditioning 93.98
decompression chamber 93.97
mountain sanatorium 93.98
epistaxis 21.00
by
cauterization (and packing) 21.03
coagulation (with packing) 21.03
electrocoagulation (with packing)
21.03
excision of nasal mucosa with
grafting 21.07
ligation of artery 21.09
ethmoidal 21.04
external carotid 21.06
maxillary (transantral) 21.05
packing (nasal) (anterior) 21.01
posterior (and anterior) 21.02
specified means NEC 21.09
hemorrhage 39.98
abdominal cavity 54.19
adenoids (postoperative) 28.7
anus (postoperative) 49.95
bladder (postoperative) 57.93
chest 34.09
colon 45.49
endoscopic 45.43
duodenum (ulcer) 44.49
by
embolization (transcatheter)
44.44
suture (ligation) 44.42
endoscopic 44.43
esophagus 42.39
endoscopic 42.33
gastric (ulcer) 44.49
by
embolization (transcatheter)
44.44
suture (ligation) 44.41
endoscopic 44.43
intrapleural 34.09
postoperative (recurrent) 34.03
laparotomy site 54.12
nose - *see also* Control, epistaxis 21.00
peptic (ulcer) 44.49
by
embolization (transcatheter)
44.44
suture (ligation) 44.40
endoscopic 44.43
pleura, pleural cavity 34.09
postoperative (recurrent) 34.03

Control (*Continued*)
hemorrhage (*Continued*)
postoperative NEC 39.98
postvascular surgery 39.41
prostate 60.94
specified site NEC 39.98
stomach - *see* Control, hemorrhage,
gastric
thorax NEC 34.09
postoperative (recurrent)
34.03
thyroid (postoperative) 06.02
tonsils (postoperative) 28.7
Conversion
anastomosis - *see* Revision, anastomosis
atrial rhythm (to sinus rhythm)
99.61
cardiac rhythm NEC 99.69
to sinus rhythm 99.62
gastrostomy to jejunostomy
(endoscopic)
for feeding tube placement
46.32
obstetrical position - *see* Version
Cooling, gastric 96.31
CorCap™ 37.41
Cordectomy, vocal 30.22
Cordopexy, vocal 31.69
Cordotomy
spinal (bilateral) NEC 03.29
percutaneous 03.21
vocal 31.3
Corectomy 12.12
Corelysis 12.35
Coreoplasty 12.35
Corneoconjunctivoplasty 11.53
Corpectomy, (vertebral) 80.99
with diskectomy 80.99
Correction - *see also* Repair
atresia
esophageal 42.85
by magnetic forces 42.99
external meatus (ear) 18.6
nasopharynx, nasopharyngeal 29.4
rectum 48.0
tricuspid 35.94
atrial septal defect - *see also* Repair,
atrial septal defect 35.71
combined with repair of valvular and
ventricular septal defects - *see*
Repair, endocardial cushion
defect
blepharoptosis - *see also* Repair,
blepharoptosis 08.36
bunionette (with osteotomy) 77.54
chordee 64.42
claw toe 77.57
cleft
lip 27.54
palate 27.62
clubfoot NEC 83.84
coarctation of aorta
with
anastomosis 38.34
graft replacement 38.44
cornea NEC 11.59
refractive NEC 11.79
epikeratophakia 11.76
keratomileusis 11.71
keratophakia 11.72
radial keratotomy 11.75
esophageal atresia 42.85
by magnetic forces 42.99
everted lacrimal punctum 09.71

Correction (*Continued*)
eyelid
ptosis - *see also* Repair,
blepharoptosis 08.36
retraction 08.38
fetal defect 75.36
forcible, of musculoskeletal deformity
NEC 93.29
hammer toe 77.56
hydraulic pressure, open surgery
for penile inflatable prosthesis
64.99
urinary artificial sphincter 58.99
intestinal malrotation 46.80
large 46.82
small 46.81
inverted uterus - *see* Repair, inverted
uterus
lymphedema (of limb) 40.9
excision with graft 40.9
obliteration of lymphatics 40.9
transplantation of autogenous
lymphatics 40.9
nasopharyngeal atresia 29.4
overlapping toes 77.58
palate (cleft) 27.62
prognathism NEC 76.64
prominent ear 18.5
punctum (everted) 09.71
spinal pseudarthrosis - *see* Refusion,
spinal
syndactyly 86.85
tetralogy of Fallot
one-stage 35.81
partial - *see* specific procedure
total 35.81
total anomalous pulmonary venous
connection
one-stage 35.82
partial - *see* specific procedure
total 35.82
transposition, great arteries, total
35.84
tricuspid atresia 35.94
truncus arteriosus
one-stage 35.83
partial - *see* specific procedure
total 35.83
ureteropelvic junction 55.87
ventricular septal defect - *see also*
Repair, ventricular septal defect
35.72
combined with repair of valvular
and atrial septal defects - *see*
Repair, endocardial cushion
defect
Costectomy 77.91
with lung excision - *see* Excision, lung
associated with thoracic
operation - *omit code*
Costochondrectomy 77.91
associated with thoracic
operation - *omit code*
Costosternoplasty (pectus excavatum
repair) 34.74
Costotomy 77.31
Costotransversectomy 77.91
associated with thoracic
operation - *omit code*
Counseling (for) NEC 94.49
alcoholism 94.46
drug addiction 94.45
employers 94.49
family (medical) (social) 94.49

Counseling NEC (*Continued*)
  marriage 94.49
  ophthalmologic (with instruction)
      95.36
  pastoral 94.49
Countershock, cardiac NEC 99.62
Coventry operation (tibial wedge
      osteotomy) 77.27
CPAP (continuous positive airway
      pressure) 93.90
  delivered by
    endotracheal tube - *see* category
        96.7●
    tracheostomy – *see* category 96.7●
Craniectomy 01.25
  linear (opening of cranial suture) 02.01
  reopening of site 01.23
  strip (opening of cranial suture) 02.01
Cranioclasis, fetal 73.8
Cranioplasty 02.06
  with synchronous repair of
      encephalocele 02.12
Craniotomy 01.24
  as operative approach - *omit code*
  fetal 73.8
  for decompression of fracture 02.02
  reopening of site 01.23
Craterization, bone - *see also* Excision,
      lesion, bone 77.60
Crawford operation (tarso-frontalis sling
      of eyelid) 08.32
Creation - *see also* Formation
  cardiac device (defibrillator)
      (pacemaker) pocket
    with initial insertion of cardiac
        device - *omit code*
    new site (skin) (subcutaneous) 37.79
  conduit
    apical-aortic (AAC) 35.93 ◀
    ileal (urinary) 56.51
    left ventricle and aorta 35.93
    right atrium and pulmonary artery
        35.94
    right ventricle and pulmonary
        (distal) artery 35.92
      in repair of
        pulmonary artery atresia 35.92
        transposition of great vessels
            35.92
        truncus arteriosus 35.83
  endorectal ileal pouch (H-pouch) (J-
      pouch) (S-pouch) (with
      anastomosis to anus) 45.95
  esophagogastric sphincteric
      competence NEC 44.66
    laparoscopic 44.67
  Hartmann pouch - *see* Colectomy, by
      site
  interatrial fistula 35.42
  pericardial window 37.12
  pleural window, for drainage 34.09
  pocket
    cardiac device (defibrillator)
        (pacemaker)
      with initial insertion of cardiac
          device - *omit code*
      new site (skin) (subcutaneous)
          37.79
    loop recorder 37.79
    thalamic stimulator pulse generator
      with initial insertion of battery
          package - *omit code*
      new site (skin) (subcutaneous)
          86.09

Creation (*Continued*)
  shunt - *see also* Shunt
    arteriovenous fistula, for dialysis
        39.93
    left-to-right (systemic to pulmonary
        circulation) 39.0
  subcutaneous tunnel for esophageal
      anastomosis 42.86
    with anastomosis - *see* Anastomosis,
        esophagus, antesternal
  syndactyly (finger) (toe) 86.89
  thalamic stimulator pulse generator
    with initial insertion of battery
        package - *omit code*
    new site (skin) (subcutaneous) 86.09
  tracheoesophageal fistula 31.95
  window
    pericardial 37.12
    pleura, for drainage 34.09
Credé maneuver 73.59
Cricoidectomy 30.29
Cricothyreotomy (for assistance in
      breathing) 31.1
Cricothyroidectomy 30.29
Cricothyrostomy 31.1
Cricothyrotomy (for assistance in
      breathing) 31.1
Cricotomy (for assistance in breathing)
      31.1
Cricotracheotomy (for assistance in
      breathing) 31.1
Crisis intervention 94.35
Croupette, croup tent 93.94
Crown, dental (ceramic) (gold) 23.41
Crushing
  bone - *see* category 78.4●
  calculus
    bile (hepatic) passage 51.49
      endoscopic 51.88
    bladder (urinary) 57.0
    pancreatic duct 52.09
      endoscopic 52.94
  fallopian tube - *see also* Ligation,
      fallopian tube 66.39
  ganglion - *see* Crushing, nerve
  hemorrhoids 49.45
  nasal septum 21.88
  nerve (cranial) (peripheral) NEC
      04.03
    acoustic 04.01
    auditory 04.01
    phrenic 04.03
      for collapse of lung 33.31
    sympathetic 05.0
    trigeminal 04.02
    vestibular 04.01
  vas deferens 63.71
Cryoablation - *see* Ablation
Cryoanalgesia nerve (cranial) (peripheral)
      04.2
Cryoconization, cervix 67.33
Cryodestruction - *see* Destruction, lesion,
      by site
Cryoextraction, lens - *see also* Extraction,
      cataract, intracapsular 13.19
Cryohypophysectomy (complete) (total) -
      see also Hypophysectomy 07.69
Cryoleucotomy 01.32
Cryopexy, retinal - *see* Cryotherapy, retina
Cryoprostatectomy 60.62
Cryoretinopexy (for)
  reattachment 14.52
  repair of tear or defect 14.32
Cryosurgery - *see* Cryotherapy

Cryothalamectomy 01.41
Cryotherapy - *see also* Destruction, lesion,
      by site
  bladder 57.59
  brain 01.59
  cataract 13.19
  cervix 67.33
  choroid - *see* Cryotherapy, retina
  ciliary body 12.72
  corneal lesion (ulcer) 11.43
    to reshape cornea 11.79
  ear
    external 18.29
    inner 20.79
  esophagus 42.39
    endoscopic 42.33
  eyelid 08.25
  hemorrhoids 49.44
  iris 12.41
  nasal turbinates 21.61
  palate (bony) 27.31
  prostate 60.62
  retina (for)
    destruction of lesion 14.22
    reattachment 14.52
    repair of tear 14.32
  skin 86.3
  stomach 43.49
    endoscopic 43.41
  subcutaneous tissue 86.3
  turbinates (nasal) 21.61
  warts 86.3
    genital 71.3
Cryptectomy (anus) 49.39
  endoscopic 49.31
Cryptorchidectomy (unilateral) 62.3
  bilateral 62.41
Cryptotomy (anus) 49.39
  endoscopic 49.31
Cuirass 93.99
Culdocentesis 70.0
Culdoplasty 70.92
  with graft or prosthesis 70.93
Culdoscopy (exploration) (removal of
      foreign body or lesion) 70.22
Culdotomy 70.12
Culp-Deweerd operation (spiral flap
      pyeloplasty) 55.87
Culp-Scardino operation (ureteral flap
      pyeloplasty) 55.87
Culture (and sensitivity) - *see*
      Examination, microscopic
Curettage (with packing) (with secondary
      closure) - *see also* Dilation and
      curettage
  adenoids 28.6
  anus 49.39
    endoscopic 49.31
  bladder 57.59
    transurethral 57.49
  bone - *see also* Excision, lesion, bone
      77.60
  brain 01.59
  bursa 83.39
    hand 82.29
  cartilage - *see also* Excision, lesion, joint
      80.80
  cerebral meninges 01.51
  chalazion 08.25
  conjunctiva (trachoma follicles) 10.33
  corneal epithelium 11.41
    for smear or culture 11.21
  ear, external 18.29
  eyelid 08.25

Curettage (Continued)
joint - see also Excision, lesion, joint 80.80
meninges (cerebral) 01.51
spinal 03.4
muscle 83.32
hand 82.22
nerve (peripheral) 04.07
sympathetic 05.29
sclera 12.84
skin 86.3
spinal cord (meninges) 03.4
subgingival 24.31
tendon 83.39
sheath 83.31
hand 82.21
uterus (with dilation) 69.09
aspiration (diagnostic) NEC 69.59
after abortion or delivery 69.52
to terminate pregnancy 69.51
following delivery or abortion 69.02
Curette evacuation, lens 13.2
Curtis operation (interphalangeal joint arthroplasty) 81.72
Cutaneolipectomy 86.83
Cutdown, venous 38.94
Cutting
nerve (cranial) (peripheral) NEC 04.03
acoustic 04.01
auditory 04.01
root, spinal 03.1
sympathetic 05.0
trigeminal 04.02
vestibular 04.01
pedicle (flap) graft 86.71
pylorus (with wedge resection) 43.3

Cutting (Continued)
spinal nerve root 03.1
ureterovesical orifice 56.1
urethral sphincter 58.5
CVP (central venous pressure monitoring) 89.62
Cyclectomy (ciliary body) 12.44
eyelid margin 08.20
Cyclicotomy 12.55
Cycloanemization 12.74
Cyclocryotherapy 12.72
Cyclodialysis (initial) (subsequent) 12.55
Cyclodiathermy (penetrating) (surface) 12.71
Cycloelectrolysis 12.71
Cyclophotocoagulation 12.73
Cyclotomy 12.55
Cystectomy - see also Excision, lesion, by site
gallbladder - see Cholecystectomy
urinary (partial) (subtotal) 57.6
complete (with urethrectomy) 57.79
radical 57.71
with pelvic exenteration (female) 68.8
total (with urethrectomy) 57.79
Cystocolostomy 57.88
Cystogram, cystography NEC 87.77
Cystolitholapaxy 57.0
Cystolithotomy 57.19
Cystometrogram 89.22
Cystopexy NEC 57.89
Cystoplasty NEC 57.89

Cystoproctostomy 57.88
Cystoprostatectomy, radical 57.71
Cystopyelography 87.74
Cystorrhaphy 57.81
Cystoscopy (transurethral) 57.32
with biopsy 57.33
for
control of hemorrhage
bladder 57.93
prostate 60.94
retrograde pyelography 87.74
ileal conduit 56.35
through stoma (artificial) 57.31
Cystostomy
closed (suprapubic) (percutaneous) 57.17
open (suprapubic) 57.18
percutaneous (closed) (suprapubic) 57.17
suprapubic
closed 57.17
open 57.18
Cystotomy (open) (for removal of calculi) 57.19
Cystourethrogram (retrograde) (voiding) 87.76
Cystourethropexy (by) 59.79
levator muscle sling 59.71
retropubic suspension 59.5
suprapubic suspension 59.4
Cystourethroplasty 57.85
Cystourethroscopy 57.32
with biopsy
bladder 57.33
ureter 56.33
Cytology - see Examination, microscopic

D

Dacryoadenectomy 09.20
partial 09.22
total 09.23
Dacryoadenotomy 09.0
Dacryocystectomy (complete) (partial) 09.6
Dacryocystogram 87.05
Dacryocystorhinostomy (DCR) (by intubation) (external) (intranasal) 09.81
Dacryocystostomy 09.53
Dacryocystosyringotomy 09.53
Dacryocystotomy 09.53
Dahlman operation (excision of esophageal diverticulum) 42.31
Dana operation (posterior rhizotomy) 03.1
Danforth operation (fetal) 73.8
Darrach operation (ulnar resection) 77.83
da Vinci® (S HD) Surgical System – see category 17.4●
Davis operation (intubated ureterotomy) 56.2
Deaf training 95.49
Debridement
abdominal wall 54.3
bone - see also Excision, lesion, bone 77.60
fracture - see Debridement, open fracture

Debridement (Continued)
brain 01.59
burn (skin) 86.28
excisional 86.22
nonexcisional 86.28
bursa 83.5
cerebral meninges 01.51
dental 96.54
fascia 83.39
flap graft 86.75
graft (flap) (pedicle) 86.75
heart valve (calcified) - see Valvuloplasty, heart
infection (skin) 86.28
excisional 86.22
nail (bed) (fold) 86.27
nonexcisional 86.28
joint - see Excision, lesion, joint
meninges (cerebral) 01.51
spinal 03.4
muscle 83.45
hand 82.36
nail (bed) (fold) 86.27
nerve (peripheral) 04.07
open fracture (compound) 79.60
arm NEC 79.62
carpal, metacarpal 79.63
facial bone 76.2
femur 79.65
fibula 79.66
foot NEC 79.67

Debridement (Continued)
open fracture (Continued)
hand NEC 79.63
humerus 79.61
leg NEC 79.66
phalanges
foot 79.68
hand 79.64
radius 79.62
specified site NEC 79.69
tarsal, metatarsal 79.67
tibia 79.66
ulna 79.62
patella 77.66
pedicle graft 86.75
skin or subcutaneous tissue (burn) (infection) (wound) 86.28
cardioverter/defibrillator (automatic) pocket 37.79
excisional 86.22
graft 86.75
nail, nail bed, or nail fold 86.27
nonexcisional 86.28
pacemaker pocket 37.79
pocket
cardiac device NEC 37.79
cardiac pacemaker 37.79
cardioverter/defibrillator (automatic) 37.79
skull 01.25
compound fracture 02.02

C & D

Debridement (Continued)
spinal cord (meninges) 03.4
tendon 83.39
VersaJet™ 86.28
wound (skin) 86.28
excisional 86.22
nonexcisional 86.28
Decapitation, fetal 73.8
Decapsulation, kidney 55.91
Declotting - see also Removal, thrombus
arteriovenous cannula or shunt 39.49
Decompression
anus (imperforate) 48.0
biliary tract 51.49
by intubation 51.43
endoscopic 51.87
percutaneous 51.98
brain 01.24
carpal tunnel 04.43
cauda equina 03.09
chamber 93.97
colon 96.08
by incision 45.03
endoscopic (balloon) 46.85
common bile duct 51.42
by intubation 51.43
endoscopic 51.87
percutaneous 51.98
cranial 01.24
for skull fracture 02.02
endolymphatic sac 20.79
ganglion (peripheral) NEC 04.49
cranial NEC 04.42
gastric 96.07
heart 37.0
intestine 96.08
by incision 45.00
endoscopic (balloon) 46.85
intracranial 01.24
labyrinth 20.79
laminectomy 03.09
laminotomy 03.09
median nerve 04.43
muscle 83.02
hand 82.02
nerve (peripheral) NEC 04.49
auditory 04.42
cranial NEC 04.42
median 04.43
trigeminal (root) 04.41
orbit - see also Orbitotomy 16.09
pancreatic duct 52.92
endoscopic 52.93
pericardium 37.0
rectum 48.0
skull fracture 02.02
spinal cord (canal) 03.09
tarsal tunnel 04.44
tendon (sheath) 83.01
hand 82.01
thoracic outlet
by
myotomy (division of scalenus
anticus muscle) 83.19
tenotomy 83.13
trigeminal (nerve root) 04.41
Decortication
arterial 05.25
brain 01.51
cerebral meninges 01.51
heart 37.31
kidney 55.91
lung (partial) (total) 34.51
thoracoscopic 34.52

Decortication (Continued)
nasal turbinates - see Turbinectomy
nose 21.89
ovary 65.29
laparoscopic 65.25
periarterial 05.25
pericardium 37.31
ventricle, heart (complete)
37.31
Decoy, E2F 00.16
Deepening
alveolar ridge 24.5
buccolabial sulcus 24.91
lingual sulcus 24.91
Defatting, flap or pedicle graft
86.75
Defibrillation, electric (external)
(internal) 99.62
automatic cardioverter/defibrillator -
see category 37.9●
de Grandmont operation (tarsectomy)
08.35
Delaying of pedicle graft 86.71
Delivery (with)
assisted spontaneous 73.59
breech extraction (assisted) 72.52
partial 72.52
with forceps to aftercoming head
72.51
total 72.54
with forceps to aftercoming head
72.53
unassisted (spontaneous
delivery) - omit code
cesarean section - see Cesarean
section
Credé maneuver 73.59
De Lee maneuver 72.4
forceps 72.9
application to aftercoming head
(Piper) 72.6
with breech extraction
partial 72.51
total 72.53
Barton's 72.4
failed 73.3
high 72.39
with episiotomy 72.31
low (outlet) 72.0
with episiotomy 72.1
mid 72.29
with episiotomy 72.21
outlet (low) 72.0
with episiotomy 72.1
rotation of fetal head 72.4
trial 73.3
instrumental NEC 72.9
specified NEC 72.8
key-in-lock rotation 72.4
Kielland rotation 72.4
Malstrom's extraction 72.79
with episiotomy 72.71
manually assisted (spontaneous)
73.59
spontaneous (unassisted) 73.59
assisted 73.59
vacuum extraction 72.79
with episiotomy 72.71
Delorme operation
pericardiectomy 37.31
proctopexy 48.76
repair of prolapsed rectum
48.76
thoracoplasty 33.34

Denervation
aortic body 39.89 ◀▥
carotid body 39.89 ◀▥
facet, percutaneous (radiofrequency)
03.96
ovarian 65.94
paracervical uterine 69.3
uterosacral 69.3
Denker operation (radical maxillary
antrotomy) 22.31
Dennis-Barco operation - see Repair,
hernia, femoral
Denonvillier operation (limited
rhinoplasty) 21.86
Densitometry, bone (serial)
(radiographic) 88.98
Depilation, skin 86.92
Derlacki operation (tympanoplasty)
19.4
Dermabond 86.59
Dermabrasion (laser) 86.25
for wound debridement 86.28
Derotation - see Reduction, torsion
Desensitization
allergy 99.12
psychologic 94.33
Desmotomy - see also Division, ligament
80.40
Destruction
breast 85.20
chorioretinopathy - see also Destruction,
lesion, choroid 14.29
ciliary body 12.74
epithelial downgrowth, anterior
chamber 12.93
fallopian tube 66.39
with
crushing (and ligation) 66.31
by endoscopy (laparoscopy)
66.21
division (and ligation) 66.32
by endoscopy (culdoscopy)
(hysteroscopy)
(laparoscopy)
(peritoneoscopy)
66.22
ligation 66.39
with
crushing 66.31
by endoscopy
(laparoscopy)
66.21
division 66.32
by endoscopy
(culdoscopy)
(hysteroscopy)
(laparoscopy)
(peritoneoscopy)
66.22
fetus 73.8
hemorrhoids 49.49
by
cryotherapy 49.44
sclerotherapy 49.42
inner ear NEC 20.79
by injection 20.72
intervertebral disc (NOS) 80.50
by injection 80.52
by other specified method 80.59
herniated (nucleus pulposus)
80.51
LAA 37.36
lacrimal sac 09.6
left atrial appendage 37.36

Destruction (Continued)

lesion (local)
    anus 49.39
        endoscopic 49.31
    Bartholin's gland 71.24
        by
            aspiration 71.21
            excision 71.24
            incision 71.22
            marsupialization 71.23
    biliary ducts 51.69
        endoscopic 51.64
    bladder 57.59
        transurethral 57.49
    bone - see Excision, lesion, bone
    bowel - see Destruction, lesion,
        intestine
    brain (transtemporal approach)
        NEC 01.59
        by stereotactic radiosurgery
            92.30
            cobalt 60 92.32
            linear accelerator (LINAC)
                92.31
            multi-source 92.32
            particle beam 92.33
            particulate 92.33
            radiosurgery NEC 92.39
            single source photon 92.31
    breast NEC 85.20
    bronchus NEC 32.09
        endoscopic 32.01
    cerebral NEC 01.59
        meninges 01.51
    cervix 67.39
        by
            cauterization 67.32
            cryosurgery, cryoconization
                67.33
            electroconization 67.32
    choroid 14.29
        by
            cryotherapy 14.22
            diathermy 14.21
            implantation of radiation
                source 14.27
            photocoagulation 14.25
                laser 14.24
                xenon arc 14.23
            radiation therapy 14.26
    ciliary body (nonexcisional)
        12.43
        by excision 12.44
    conjunctiva 10.32
        by excision 10.31
    cornea NEC 11.49
        by
            cryotherapy 11.43
            electrocauterization 11.42
            thermocauterization 11.42
    cul-de-sac 70.32
    duodenum NEC 45.32
        by excision 45.31
            endoscopic 45.30
        endoscopic 45.30
    esophagus (chemosurgery)
        (cryosurgery)
        (electroresection)
        (fulguration) NEC 42.39
        by excision 42.32
            endoscopic 42.33
        endoscopic 42.33
    eye NEC 16.93
    eyebrow 08.25

Destruction (Continued)

lesion (Continued)
    eyelid 08.25
        excisional - see Excision, lesion,
            eyelid
    heart
        by catheter ablation 37.34
        by endovascular approach
            37.34
        by open approach 37.33
        by thoracoscopic approach
            37.37 ◄
        left atrial appendage 37.36
    intestine (large) 45.49
        by excision 45.41
            endoscopic 45.43
                polypectomy 45.42
        endoscopic 45.43
            polypectomy 45.42
        small 45.34
            by excision 45.33
    intranasal 21.31
    iris (nonexcisional) NEC 12.41
        by excision 12.42
    kidney 55.39
        by marsupialization 55.31
    lacrimal sac 09.6
    larynx 30.09
    liver 50.29
    lung 32.29
        endoscopic 32.28
        thoracoscopic 32.20
    meninges (cerebral) 01.51
        spinal 03.4
    nerve (peripheral) 04.07
        sympathetic 05.29
    nose 21.30
        intranasal 21.31
        specified NEC 21.32
    ovary
        by
            aspiration 65.91
            excision 65.29
                laparoscopic 65.25
        cyst by rupture (manual) 65.93
    palate (bony) (local) 27.31
        wide 27.32
    pancreas 52.22
        by marsupialization 52.3
        endoscopic 52.21
    pancreatic duct 52.22
        endoscopic 52.21
    penis 64.2
    pharynx (excisional) 29.39
    pituitary gland
        by stereotactic radiosurgery
            92.30
            cobalt 60 92.32
            linear accelerator (LINAC)
                92.31
            multi-source 92.32
            particle beam 92.33
            particulate 92.33
            radiosurgery NEC 92.39
            single source photon 92.31
    rectum (local) 48.32
        by
            cryosurgery 48.34
            electrocoagulation 48.32
            excision 48.35
            fulguration 48.32
            laser (Argon) 48.33
        polyp 48.36
        radical 48.31

Destruction (Continued)

lesion (Continued)
    retina 14.29
        by
            cryotherapy 14.22
            diathermy 14.21
            implantation of radiation
                source 14.27
            photocoagulation 14.25
                laser 14.24
                xenon arc 14.23
            radiation therapy 14.26
    salivary gland NEC 26.29
        by marsupialization 26.21
    sclera 12.84
    scrotum 61.3
    skin NEC 86.3
    sphincter of Oddi 51.69
        endoscopic 51.64
    spinal cord (meninges) 03.4
    spleen 41.42
        by marsupialization 41.41
    stomach NEC 43.49
        by excision 43.42
            endoscopic 43.41
        endoscopic 43.41
    subcutaneous tissue NEC 86.3
    testis 62.2
    tongue 25.1
    urethra (excisional) 58.39
        endoscopic 58.31
    uterus 68.29
nerve (cranial) (peripheral) (by
    cryoanalgesia) (by
    radiofrequency) 04.2
    sympathetic, by injection of
        neurolytic agent 05.32
neuroma
    acoustic 04.01
        by craniotomy 04.01
        by stereotactic radiosurgery 92.30
            cobalt 60 92.32
            linear accelerator (LINAC)
                92.31
            multi-source 92.32
            particle beam 92.33
            particulate 92.33
            radiosurgery NEC 92.39
            single source photon 92.31
    cranial 04.07
    Morton's 04.07
    peripheral
        Morton's 04.07
prostate (prostatic tissue)
    by
        cryotherapy 60.62
        microwave 60.96
        radiofrequency 60.97
    transurethral microwave
        thermotherapy (TUMT)
        60.96
    transurethral needle ablation
        (TUNA) 60.97
    TULIP (transurethral (ultrasound)
        guided laser induced
        prostatectomy) 60.21
    TUMT (transurethral microwave
        thermotherapy) 60.96
    TUNA (transurethral needle
        ablation) 60.97
semicircular canals, by injection
    20.72
tissue of heart - see Excision, lesion,
    heart ◄
vestibule, by injection 20.72

◄ New   ◄‖ Revised   ~~deleted~~ Deleted   ● Use Additional Digit(s)   ▨ Omit code

Detachment, uterosacral ligaments 69.3
Determination
    mental status (clinical) (medicolegal)
        (psychiatric) NEC 94.11
        psychologic NEC 94.09
    vital capacity (pulmonary) 89.37
Detorsion
    intestine (twisted) (volvulus) 46.80
        large 46.82
            endoscopic (balloon) 46.85
        small 46.81
    kidney 55.84
    ovary 65.95
    spermatic cord 63.52
        with orchiopexy 62.5
    testis 63.52
        with orchiopexy 62.5
    volvulus 46.80
        endoscopic (balloon) 46.85
Detoxification therapy 94.25
    alcohol 94.62
        with rehabilitation 94.63
        combined alcohol and drug 94.68
            with rehabilitation 94.69
    drug 94.65
        with rehabilitation 94.66
        combined alcohol and drug 94.68
            with rehabilitation 94.69
Devascularization, stomach 44.99
Device
    CorCap™ 37.41
    external fixator - see Fixator, external
Dewebbing
    esophagus 42.01
    syndactyly (fingers) (toes) 86.85
Dextrorotation - see Reduction, torsion
Dialysis
    hemodiafiltration, hemofiltration
        (extracorporeal) 39.95
    kidney (extracorporeal) 39.95
    liver 50.92
    peritoneal 54.98
    renal (extracorporeal) 39.95
Diaphanoscopy
    nasal sinuses 89.35
    skull (newborn) 89.16
Diaphysectomy - see category 77.8●
Diathermy 93.34
    choroid - see Diathermy, retina
    nasal turbinates 21.61
    retina
        for
            destruction of lesion 14.21
            reattachment 14.51
            repair of tear 14.31
    surgical - see Destruction, lesion,
        by site
    turbinates (nasal) 21.61
Dickson operation (fascial transplant)
    83.82
Dickson-Diveley operation (tendon
    transfer and arthrodesis to correct
    claw toe) 77.57
Dieffenbach operation (hip
    disarticulation) 84.18
Dilation
    achalasia 42.92
    ampulla of Vater 51.81
        endoscopic 51.84
    anus, anal (sphincter) 96.23
    biliary duct
        endoscopic 51.84
        pancreatic duct 52.99
            endoscopic 52.98

Dilation (Continued)
    biliary duct (Continued)
        percutaneous (endoscopy) 51.98
        sphincter
            of Oddi 51.81
                endoscopic 51.84
                pancreatic 51.82
                    endoscopic 51.85
    bladder 96.25
        neck 57.92
    bronchus 33.91
    cervix (canal) 67.0
        obstetrical 73.1
        to assist delivery 73.1
    choanae (nasopharynx) 29.91
    colon (endoscopic) (balloon) 46.85
        with insertion of colonic stent
            endoscopic 46.86
            other 46.87
    colostomy stoma 96.24
    duodenum (endoscopic) (balloon)
        46.85
        with insertion of colonic stent
            endoscopic 46.86
            other 46.87
    endoscopic - see Dilation, by site
    enterostomy stoma 96.24
    esophagus (by bougie) (by sound)
        42.92
    fallopian tube 66.96
    foreskin (newborn) 99.95
    frontonasal duct 96.21
    gastrojejunostomy site, endoscopic
        44.22
    heart valve - see Valvulotomy, heart
    ileostomy stoma 96.24
    ileum (endoscopic) (balloon) 46.85
        with insertion of colonic stent
            endoscopic 46.86
            other 46.87
    intestinal stoma (artificial) 96.24
    intestine (endoscopic) (balloon)
        46.85
        with insertion of colonic stent
            endoscopic 46.86
            other 46.87
    jejunum (endoscopic) (balloon) 46.85
        with insertion of colonic stent
            endoscopic 46.86
            other 46.87
    lacrimal
        duct 09.42
        punctum 09.41
    larynx 31.98
    lymphatic structure(s) (peripheral)
        40.9
    nares 21.99
    nasolacrimal duct (retrograde)
        09.43
        with insertion of tube or stent
            09.44
    nasopharynx 29.91
    pancreatic duct 52.99
        endoscopic 52.98
    pharynx 29.91
    prostatic urethra (transurethral)
        (balloon) 60.95
    punctum, lacrimal papilla 09.41
    pylorus
        by incision 44.21
        endoscopic 44.22
    rectum 96.22
    salivary duct 26.91
    sphenoid ostia 22.52

Dilation (Continued)
    sphincter
        anal 96.23
        cardiac 42.92
        of Oddi 51.81
            endoscopic 51.84
            pancreatic 51.82
                endoscopic 51.85
        pylorus, endoscopic 44.22
            by incision 44.21
    Stenson's duct 26.91
    trachea 31.99
    ureter 59.8
        meatus 56.91
    ureterovesical orifice 59.8
    urethra 58.6
        prostatic (transurethral) (balloon)
            60.95
    urethrovesical junction 58.6
    vagina (instrumental) (manual) NEC
        96.16
    vesical neck 57.92
    Wharton's duct 26.91
    Wirsung's duct 52.99
        endoscopic 52.98
Dilation and curettage, uterus
    (diagnostic) 69.09
    after
        abortion 69.02
        delivery 69.02
    to terminate pregnancy 69.01
Diminution, ciliary body 12.74
Disarticulation 84.91
    ankle 84.13
    elbow 84.06
    finger, except thumb 84.01
        thumb 84.02
    hip 84.18
    knee 84.16
    shoulder 84.08
    thumb 84.02
    toe 84.11
    wrist 84.04
Discectomy - see Diskectomy
Discission
    capsular membrane 13.64
    cataract (Wheeler knife) (Ziegler knife)
        13.2
        congenital 13.69
        secondary membrane 13.64
    iris 12.12
    lens (capsule) (Wheeler knife) (Ziegler
        knife) (with capsulotomy) 13.2
    orbitomaxillary, radical 16.51
    pupillary 13.2
    secondary membrane (after cataract)
        13.64
    vitreous strands (posterior approach)
        14.74
        anterior approach 14.73
Discogram, diskogram 87.21
Discolysis (by injection) 80.52
Diskectomy (discectomy), intervertebral
    80.51
    with corpectomy 80.99
    herniated (nucleus pulposus) 80.51
    percutaneous 80.59
Dispensing (with fitting)
    contact lens 95.32
    low vision aids NEC 95.33
    spectacles 95.31
Disruption
    blood brain barrier via infusion [BBBD]
        00.19

Dissection - *see also* Excision
  aneurysm 38.60
  artery-vein-nerve bundle 39.91
  branchial cleft fistula or sinus 29.52
  bronchus 32.1
  femoral hernia 53.29
  groin, radical 40.54
  larynx block (en bloc) 30.3
  mediastinum with pneumonectomy
      32.59
    thoracoscopic 32.50
  neck, radical 40.40
    with laryngectomy 30.4
    bilateral 40.42
    unilateral 40.41
  orbital fibrous bands 16.92
  pterygium (with reposition) 11.31
  radical neck - *see* Dissection, neck,
      radical
  retroperitoneal NEC 59.00
  thoracic structures (block) (en bloc)
      (radical) (brachial plexus,
      bronchus, lobe of lung, ribs, and
      sympathetic nerves) 32.6
  vascular bundle 39.91
Distention, bladder (therapeutic)
    (intermittent) 96.25
Diversion
  biliopancreatic (BPD) 43.7 *[45.51]*
      [45.91]
    with duodenal switch 43.89 *[45.51]*
        [45.91]
    urinary
      cutaneous 56.61
      ileal conduit 56.51
      internal NEC 56.71
      ureter to
          intestine 56.71
          skin 56.61
      uretero-ileostomy 56.51
Diversional therapy 93.81
Diverticulectomy
  bladder (suprapubic) 57.59
    transurethral approach 57.49
  duodenum 45.31
    endoscopic 45.30
  esophagus 42.31
    endoscopic 42.33
  esophagomyotomy 42.7
  hypopharyngeal (by cricopharyngeal
      myotomy) 29.32
  intestine
    large 45.41
      endoscopic 45.43
    small 45.33
  kidney 55.39
  Meckel's 45.33
  pharyngeal (by cricopharyngeal
      myotomy) 29.32
  pharyngoesophageal (by
      cricopharyngeal myotomy) 29.32
  stomach 43.42
    endoscopic 43.41
  urethra 58.39
    endoscopic 58.31
Division
  Achilles tendon 83.11
  adductor tendon (hip) 83.12
  adhesions - *see* Lysis, adhesions
  angle of mandible (open) 76.62
    closed 76.61
  anterior synechiae 12.32
  aponeurosis 83.13
  arcuate ligament (spine) - *omit code*

Division *(Continued)*
  arteriovenous fistula (with ligation)
      39.53
  artery (with ligation) 38.80
    abdominal 38.86
    aorta (arch) (ascending)
        (descending) 38.84
    head and neck NEC 38.82
    intracranial NEC 38.81
    lower limb 38.88
    thoracic NEC 38.85
    upper limb 38.83
  bladder neck 57.91
  blepharorrhaphy 08.02
  blood vessels, cornea 10.1
  bone - *see also* Osteotomy 77.30
  brain tissue 01.32
    cortical adhesions 02.91
  canaliculus 09.52
  canthorrhaphy 08.02
  cartilage 80.40
    ankle 80.47
    elbow 80.42
    foot and toe 80.48
    hand and finger 80.44
    hip 80.45
    knee 80.46
    shoulder 80.41
    specified site NEC 80.49
    spine 80.49
    wrist 80.43
  cerebral tracts 01.32
  chordae tendineae 35.32
  common wall between posterior left
      atrium and coronary sinus (with
      roofing of resultant defect with
      patch graft) 35.82
  congenital web
    larynx 31.98
    pharynx 29.54
  endometrial synechiae 68.21
  fallopian tube - *see* Ligation, fallopian
      tube
  fascia 83.14
    hand 82.12
  frenulum, frenum
    labial 27.91
    lingual 25.91
    tongue 25.91
  ganglion, sympathetic 05.0
  glossopharyngeal nerve 29.92
  goniosynechiae 12.31
  hypophyseal stalk - *see also*
      Hypophysectomy, partial 07.63
  iliotibial band 83.14
  isthmus
    horseshoe kidney 55.85
    thyroid 06.91
  joint capsule 80.40
    ankle 80.47
    elbow 80.42
    foot and toe 80.48
    hand and finger 80.44
    hip 80.45
    knee 80.46
    shoulder 80.41
    specified site NEC 80.49
    wrist 80.43
  labial frenum 27.91
  lacrimal ductules 09.0
  laryngeal nerve (external) (recurrent)
      (superior) 31.91
  ligament 80.40
    ankle 80.47

Division *(Continued)*
  ligament *(Continued)*
    arcuate (spine) - *omit code*
    canthal 08.36
    elbow 80.42
    foot and toe 80.48
    hand and finger 80.44
    hip 80.45
    knee 80.46
    palpebrae 08.36
    shoulder 80.41
    specified site NEC 80.49
    spine 80.49
      arcuate - *omit code*
      flavum - *omit code*
    uterosacral 69.3
    wrist 80.43
  ligamentum flavum (spine) - *omit code*
  meninges (cerebral) 01.31
  muscle 83.19
      hand 82.19
  nasolacrimal duct stricture (with
      drainage) 09.59
  nerve (cranial) (peripheral) NEC 04.03
    acoustic 04.01
    adrenal gland 07.42
    auditory 04.01
    glossopharyngeal 29.92
    lacrimal branch 05.0
    laryngeal (external) (recurrent)
        (superior) 31.91
    phrenic 04.03
      for collapse of lung 33.31
    root, spinal or intraspinal 03.1
    sympathetic 05.0
    tracts
      cerebral 01.32
      spinal cord 03.29
          percutaneous 03.21
    trigeminal 04.02
    vagus - *see also* Vagotomy 44.00
    vestibular 04.01
  otosclerotic process or material, middle
      ear 19.0
  papillary muscle (heart) 35.31
  patent ductus arteriosus 38.85
  penile adhesions 64.93
  posterior synechiae 12.33
  pylorus (with wedge resection) 43.3
  rectum (stricture) 48.91
  scalenus anticus muscle 83.19
  Skene's gland 71.3
  soft tissue NEC 83.19
      hand 82.19
  sphincter
    anal (external) (internal) 49.59
      left lateral 49.51
      posterior 49.52
    cardiac 42.7
    of Oddi 51.82
      endoscopic 51.85
    pancreatic 51.82
      endoscopic 51.85
  spinal
    cord tracts 03.29
      percutaneous 03.21
    nerve root 03.1
  symblepharon (with insertion of
      conformer) 10.5
  synechiae
    endometrial 68.21
    iris (posterior) 12.33
      anterior 12.32
  tarsorrhaphy 08.02

Division *(Continued)*
tendon 83.13
Achilles 83.11
adductor (hip) 83.12
hand 82.11
trabeculae carneae cordis (heart) 35.35
tympanum 20.23
uterosacral ligaments 69.3
vaginal septum 70.14
vas deferens 63.71
vein (with ligation) 38.80
abdominal 38.87
head and neck NEC 38.82
intracranial NEC 38.81
lower limb 38.89
varicose 38.59
thoracic NEC 38.85
upper limb 38.83
varicose 38.50
abdominal 38.57
head and neck NEC 38.52
intracranial NEC 38.51
lower limb 38.59
thoracic NEC 38.55
upper limb 38.53
vitreous, cicatricial bands (posterior
approach) 14.74
anterior approach 14.73
Doleris operation (shortening of round
ligaments) 69.22
D'Ombrain operation (excision of
pterygium with corneal graft) 11.32
Domestic tasks therapy 93.83
Dopplergram, Doppler flow mapping -
see also Ultrasonography
aortic arch 88.73
head and neck 88.71
heart 88.72
thorax NEC 88.73
Dorrance operation (push-back
operation for cleft palate) 27.62
Dotter operation (transluminal
angioplasty) 39.59
Douche, vagina 96.44
Douglas' operation (suture of tongue to
lip for micrognathia) 25.59
Downstream® System (AO therapy)
(aqueous oxygen) 00.49
Doyle operation (paracervical uterine
denervation) 69.3
Drainage
by
anastomosis - *see* Anastomosis
aspiration - *see* Aspiration
incision - *see* Incision
abdomen 54.19
percutaneous 54.91
abscess - *see also* Drainage, by site and
Incision, by site
appendix 47.2
with appendectomy 47.09
laparoscopic 47.01
parapharyngeal (oral) (transcervical)
28.0
peritonsillar (oral) (transcervical)
28.0
retropharyngeal (oral)
(transcervical) 28.0
thyroid (field) (gland) 06.09
percutaneous (needle) 06.01
postoperative 06.02
tonsil, tonsillar (oral) (transcervical)
28.0
antecubital fossa 86.04

Drainage *(Continued)*
appendix 47.91
with appendectomy 47.09
laparoscopic 47.01
abscess 47.2
with appendectomy 47.09
laparoscopic 47.01
axilla 86.04
bladder (without incision) 57.0
by indwelling catheter 57.94
percutaneous suprapubic (closed)
57.17
suprapubic NEC 57.18
buccal space 27.0
bursa 83.03
by aspiration 83.94
hand 82.92
hand 82.03
by aspiration 82.92
radial 82.03
ulnar 82.03
cerebrum, cerebral (meninges)
(ventricle) (incision)
(trephination) 01.39
by
anastomosis - *see* Shunt,
ventricular
aspiration 01.09
through previously implanted
catheter 01.02
chest (closed) 34.04
open (by incision) 34.09
thoracoscopic 34.06
cranial sinus (incision) (trephination)
01.21
by aspiration 01.09
cul-de-sac 70.12
by aspiration 70.0
cyst - *see also* Drainage, by site and
Incision, by site
pancreas (by catheter) 52.01
by marsupialization 52.3
internal (anastomosis) 52.4
pilonidal 86.03
spleen, splenic (by marsupialization)
41.41
duodenum (tube) 46.39
by incision 45.01
ear
external 18.09
inner 20.79
middle (by myringotomy) 20.09
with intubation 20.01
epidural space, cerebral (incision)
(trephination) 01.24
by aspiration 01.09
extradural space, cerebral (incision)
(trephination) 01.24
by aspiration 01.09
extraperitoneal 54.0
facial region 27.0
fascial compartments, head and neck
27.0
fetal hydrocephalic head (needling)
(trocar) 73.8
gallbladder 51.04
by
anastomosis 51.35
aspiration 51.01
incision 51.04
groin region (abdominal wall)
(inguinal) 54.0
skin 86.04
subcutaneous tissue 86.04

Drainage *(Continued)*
hematoma - *see* Drainage, by site and
Incision, by site
hydrocephalic head (needling) (trocar)
73.8
hypochondrium 54.0
intra-abdominal 54.19
iliac fossa 54.0
infratemporal fossa 27.0
intracranial space (epidural)
(extradural) (incision)
(trephination) 01.24
by aspiration 01.09
subarachnoid or subdural
(incision) (trephination)
01.31
by aspiration 01.09
intraperitoneal 54.19
percutaneous 54.91
kidney (by incision) 55.01
by
anastomosis 55.86
catheter 59.8
pelvis (by incision) 55.11
liver 50.0
by aspiration 50.91
Ludwig's angina 27.0
lung (by incision) 33.1
by punch (needle) (trocar)
33.93
midpalmar space 82.04
mouth floor 27.0
mucocele, nasal sinus 22.00
by puncture 22.01
through natural ostium 22.02
omentum 54.19
percutaneous 54.91
ovary (aspiration) 65.91
by incision 65.09
laparoscopic 65.01
palmar space (middle) 82.04
pancreas (by catheter) 52.01
by anastomosis 52.96
parapharyngeal 28.0
paronychia 86.04
parotid space 27.0
pelvic peritoneum (female) 70.12
male 54.19
pericardium 37.0
perigastric 54.19
percutaneous 54.91
perineum
female 71.09
male 86.04
perisplenic tissue 54.19
percutaneous 54.91
peritoneum 54.19
pelvic (female) 70.12
percutaneous 54.91
peritonsillar 28.0
pharyngeal space, lateral 27.0
pilonidal cyst or sinus 86.03
pleura (closed) 34.04
open (by incision) 34.09
thoracoscopic 34.06
popliteal space 86.04
postural 93.99
postzygomatic space 27.0
pseudocyst, pancreas 52.3
by anastomosis 52.4
pterygopalatine fossa 27.0
retropharyngeal 28.0
scrotum 61.0
skin 86.04

Drainage *(Continued)*
  spinal (canal) (cord) 03.09
    by anastomosis - *see* Shunt, spinal
    diagnostic 03.31
  spleen 41.2
    cyst (by marsupialization) 41.41
  subarachnoid space, cerebral (incision) (trephination) 01.31
    by aspiration 01.09
  subcutaneous tissue 86.04
  subdiaphragmatic 54.19
    percutaneous 54.91
  subdural space, cerebral (incision) (trephination) 01.31
    by aspiration 01.09
  subhepatic space 54.19
    percutaneous 54.91
  sublingual space 27.0
  submental space 27.0
  subphrenic space 54.19
    percutaneous 54.91
  supraclavicular fossa 86.04
  temporal pouches 27.0
  tendon (sheath) 83.01
    hand 82.01
  thenar space 82.04
  thorax (closed) 34.04
    open (by incision) 34.09
    thoracoscopic 34.06
  thyroglossal tract (by incision) 06.09
    by aspiration 06.01
  thyroid (field) (gland) (by incision) 06.09
    by aspiration 06.01
    postoperative 06.02

Drainage *(Continued)*
  tonsil 28.0
  tunica vaginalis 61.0
  ureter (by catheter) 59.8
    by
      anastomosis NEC - *see also* Anastomosis, ureter 56.79
      incision 56.2
  ventricle (cerebral) (incision) NEC 02.39
    by
      anastomosis - *see* Shunt, ventricular
      aspiration 01.09
        through previously implanted catheter 01.02
  vertebral column 03.09
Drawing test 94.08
Dressing
  burn 93.57
  ulcer 93.56
  wound 93.57
Drilling
  bone - *see also* Incision, bone 77.10
  ovary 65.99
Drotrecogin alfa (activated), infusion 00.11
Ductogram, mammary 87.35
Duhamel operation (abdominoperineal pull-through) 48.65
Duhrssen's
  incisions (cervix, to assist delivery) 73.93
  operation (vaginofixation of uterus) 69.22
Dunn operation (triple arthrodesis) 81.12

Duodenectomy 45.62
  with
    gastrectomy - *see* Gastrectomy
    pancreatectomy - *see* Pancreatectomy
Duodenocholedochotomy 51.51
Duodenoduodenostomy 45.91
  proximal to distal segment 45.62
Duodenoileostomy 45.91
Duodenojejunostomy 45.91
Duodenoplasty 46.79
Duodenorrhaphy 46.71
Duodenoscopy 45.13
  through stoma (artificial) 45.12
  transabdominal (operative) 45.11
Duodenostomy 46.39
Duodenotomy 45.01
Dupuytren operation
  fasciectomy 82.35
  fasciotomy 82.12
    with excision 82.35
  shoulder disarticulation 84.08
Durabond 86.59
Duraplasty 02.12
Durham (-Caldwell) operation (transfer of biceps femoris tendon) 83.75
DuToit and Roux operation (staple capsulorrhaphy of shoulder) 81.82
DuVries operation (tenoplasty) 83.88
Dwyer operation
  fasciotomy 83.14
  soft tissue release NEC 83.84
  wedge osteotomy, calcaneus 77.28

E

E2F decoy 00.16
Eagleton operation (extrapetrosal drainage) 20.22
ECG - *see* Electrocardiogram
Echocardiography 88.72
  intracardiac (heart chambers) (ICE) 37.28
  intravascular (coronary vessels) 00.24
  transesophageal 88.72
    monitoring (Doppler) (ultrasound) 89.68
Echoencephalography 88.71
Echography - *see* Ultrasonography
Echogynography 88.79
Echoplacentogram 88.78
ECMO (extracorporeal membrane oxygenation) 39.65
Eden-Hybinette operation (glenoid bone block) 78.01
Educational therapy (bed-bound children) (handicapped) 93.82
EEG (electroencephalogram) 89.14
  monitoring (radiographic) (video) 89.19
Effler operation (heart) 36.2
Effleurage 93.39
EGD (esophagogastroduodenoscopy) 45.13
  with closed biopsy 45.16

Eggers operation
  tendon release (patellar retinacula) 83.13
  tendon transfer (biceps femoris tendon) (hamstring tendon) 83.75
EKG - *see also* Electrocardiogram 89.52
Elastic hosiery 93.59
Electrocardiogram (with 12 or more leads) 89.52
  with vectorcardiogram 89.53
  fetal (scalp), intrauterine 75.32
  rhythm (with one to three leads) 89.51
Electrocautery - *see also* Cauterization
  cervix 67.32
  corneal lesion (ulcer) 11.42
  esophagus 42.39
    endoscopic 42.33
Electrocoagulation - *see also* Destruction, lesion, by site
  aneurysm (cerebral) (peripheral vessels) 39.52
  cervix 67.32
  cystoscopic 57.49
  ear
    external 18.29
    inner 20.79
    middle 20.51
  fallopian tube (lesion) 66.61
    for tubal ligation - *see* Ligation, fallopian tube

Electrocoagulation *(Continued)*
  gasserian ganglion 04.02
  nasal turbinates 21.61
  nose, for epistaxis (with packing) 21.03
  ovary 65.29
    laparoscopic 65.25
  prostatic bed 60.94
  rectum (polyp) 48.32
    radical 48.31
  retina (for)
    destruction of lesion 14.21
    reattachment 14.51
    repair of tear 14.31
  round ligament 69.19
  semicircular canals 20.79
  urethrovesical junction, transurethral 57.49
  uterine ligament 69.19
  uterosacral ligament 69.19
  uterus 68.29
  vagina 70.33
  vulva 71.3
Electrocochleography 20.31
Electroconization, cervix 67.32
Electroconvulsive therapy (ECT) 94.27
Electroencephalogram (EEG) 89.14
  monitoring (radiographic) (video) 89.19
Electrogastrogram 44.19
Electrokeratotomy 11.49

◀ New ◀◀ Revised ~~deleted~~ Deleted ● Use Additional Digit(s) ▨ Omit code

D & E

Note: Also use 00.40, 00.41, 00.42, or 00.43 to show the total number of vessels treated. Use code 00.44 once to show procedure on a bifurcated vessel. In addition, use 00.45, 00.46, 00.47, or 00.48 to show the number of vascular stents inserted.

Note: Also use 00.40, 00.41, 00.42, or 00.43 to show the total number of vessels treated. Use code 00.44 once to show procedure on a bifurcated vessel. In addition, use 00.45, 00.46, 00.47, or 00.48 to show the number of vascular stents inserted.

    percutaneous approach, intracranial
        vessel(s) 00.62

Endoscopy *(Continued)*
  intestine NEC *(Continued)*
    small 45.13
      esophagogastroduodenoscopy
          (EGD) 45.13
        with closed biopsy 45.16
      through stoma (artificial)
          45.12
      transabdominal (operative)
          45.11
    jejunum 45.13
      through stoma (artificial) 45.12
      transabdominal (operative) 45.11
    kidney 55.21
    larynx 31.42
      through stoma (artificial) 31.41
    lung - *see* Bronchoscopy
    mediastinum (transpleural) 34.22
    nasal sinus 22.19
    nose 21.21
    pancreatic duct 52.13
    pelvis 55.22
    peritoneum 54.21
    pharynx 29.11
    rectum 48.23
      through stoma (artificial) 48.22
      transabdominal (operative) 48.21
    sinus, nasal 22.19
    stomach NEC 44.13
      through stoma (artificial) 44.12
      transabdominal (operative) 44.11
    thorax (transpleural) 34.21
    trachea NEC 31.42
      through stoma (artificial) 31.41
    transpleural
      mediastinum 34.22
      thorax 34.21
    ureter 56.31
    urethra 58.22
    uterus 68.12
    vagina 70.21
Enema (transanal) NEC 96.39
  for removal of impacted feces 96.38
ENG (electronystagmogram) 95.24
Enlargement
  aortic lumen, thoracic 38.14
  atrial septal defect (pre-existing)
      35.41
    in repair of total anomalous
        pulmonary venous connection
        35.82
  eye socket 16.64
  foramen ovale (pre-existing) 35.41
    in repair of total anomalous
        pulmonary venous connection
        35.82
  intestinal stoma 46.40
    large intestine 46.43
    small intestine 46.41
  introitus 96.16
  orbit (eye) 16.64
  palpebral fissure 08.51
  punctum 09.41
  sinus tract (skin) 86.89
Enterectomy NEC 45.63
Enteroanastomosis
  large-to-large intestine 45.94
  small-to-large intestine 45.93
  small-to-small intestine 45.91
Enterocelectomy 53.9
  female 70.92
    with graft or prosthesis 70.93
  vaginal 70.92
    with graft or prosthesis 70.93

Enterocentesis 45.00
  duodenum 45.01
  large intestine 45.03
  small intestine NEC 45.02
Enterocholecystostomy 51.32
Enteroclysis (small bowel) 96.43
Enterocolectomy NEC 45.79
Enterocolostomy 45.93
Enteroentectropy 46.99
Enteroenterostomy 45.90
  small-to-large intestine 45.93
  small-to-small intestine 45.91
Enterogastrostomy 44.39
  laparoscopic 44.38
Enterolithotomy 45.00
Enterolysis 54.59
  laparoscopic 54.51
Enteropancreatostomy 52.96
Enterorrhaphy 46.79
  large intestine 46.75
  small intestine 46.73
Enterostomy NEC 46.39
  cecum - *see also* Colostomy 46.10
  colon (transverse) - *see also* Colostomy
      46.10
    loop 46.03
  delayed opening 46.31
  duodenum 46.39
    loop 46.01
  feeding NEC 46.39
    percutaneous (endoscopic) 46.32
  ileum (Brooke) (Dragstedt) 46.20
    loop 46.01
  jejunum (feeding) 46.39
    loop 46.01
    percutaneous (endoscopic) 46.32
  sigmoid colon - *see also* Colostomy
      46.10
    loop 46.03
  transverse colon - *see also* Colostomy
      46.10
    loop 46.03
Enterotomy 45.00
  large intestine 45.03
  small intestine 45.02
Enucleation - *see also* Excision, lesion, by
    site
  cyst
    broad ligament 69.19
    dental 24.4
    liver 50.29
    ovarian 65.29
      laparoscopic 65.25
    parotid gland 26.29
    salivary gland 26.29
    skin 86.3
    subcutaneous tissue 86.3
  eyeball 16.49
    with implant (into Tenon's
        capsule) 16.42
    with attachment of muscles
        16.41
EOG (electro-oculogram) 95.22
Epicardiectomy 36.39
Epididymectomy 63.4
  with orchidectomy (unilateral) 62.3
    bilateral 62.41
Epididymogram 87.93
Epididymoplasty 63.59
Epididymorrhaphy 63.81
Epididymotomy 63.92
Epididymovasostomy 63.83
Epiglottidectomy 30.21
Epikeratophakia 11.76

Epilation
  eyebrow (forceps) 08.93
    cryosurgical 08.92
    electrosurgical 08.91
  eyelid (forceps) NEC 08.93
    cryosurgical 08.92
    electrosurgical 08.91
  skin 86.92
Epiphysiodesis - *see also* Arrest, bone
    growth - *see* category 78.2●
Epiphysiolysis - *see also* Arrest, bone
    growth - *see* category 78.2●
Epiploectomy 54.4
Epiplopexy 54.74
Epiplorrhaphy 54.74
Episioperineoplasty 71.79
Episioperineorrhaphy 71.71
  obstetrical 75.69
Episioplasty 71.79
Episioproctotomy 73.6
Episiorrhaphy 71.71
  following episiotomy - *see*
      Episiotomy
  for obstetrical laceration 75.69
Episiotomy (with subsequent
    episiorrhaphy) 73.6
  high forceps 72.31
  low forceps 72.1
  mid forceps 72.21
  nonobstetrical 71.09
  outlet forceps 72.1
EPS (electrophysiologic stimulation)
  as part of intraoperative testing - *omit*
      code
  catheter based invasive
      electrophysiologic testing
      37.26
  device interrogation only without
      arrhythmia induction (bedside
      check) 89.45-89.49
  noninvasive programmed electrical
      stimulation (NIPS) 37.20
Eptifibatide, infusion 99.20
Equalization, leg
  lengthening - *see* category 78.3●
  shortening - *see* category 78.2●
Equilibration (occlusal) 24.8
Equiloudness balance 95.43
ERC (endoscopic retrograde
    cholangiography) 51.11
ERCP (endoscopic retrograde
    cholangiopancreatography)
    51.10
  cannulation of pancreatic duct
      52.93
ERG (electroretinogram) 95.21
ERP (endoscopic retrograde
    pancreatography) 52.13
Eruption, tooth, surgical 24.6
Erythrocytapheresis, therapeutic
    99.73
Escharectomy 86.22
Escharotomy 86.09
Esophageal voice training
    (postlaryngectomy) 93.73
Esophagectomy 42.40
  abdominothoracocervical (combined)
      (synchronous) 42.42
  partial or subtotal 42.41
  total 42.42
Esophagocologastrostomy (intrathoracic)
    42.55
  antesternal or antethoracic 42.65

Esophagocolostomy (intrathoracic) NEC 42.56
  with interposition of colon 42.55
  antesternal or antethoracic NEC 42.66
    with interposition of colon 42.65
Esophagoduodenostomy (intrathoracic) NEC 42.54
  with
    complete gastrectomy 43.99
    interposition of small bowel 42.53
Esophagoenterostomy (intrathoracic) NEC - see also Anastomosis, esophagus, to intestinal segment 42.54
  antesternal or antethoracic - see also Anastomosis, esophagus, antesternal, to intestinal segment 42.64
Esophagoesophagostomy (intrathoracic) 42.51
  antesternal or antethoracic 42.61
Esophagogastrectomy 43.99
Esophagogastroduodenoscopy (EGD) 45.13
  with closed biopsy 45.16
  through stoma (artificial) 45.12
  transabdominal (operative) 45.11
Esophagogastromyotomy 42.7
Esophagogastropexy 44.65
Esophagogastroplasty 44.65
Esophagogastroscopy NEC 44.13
  through stoma (artificial) 44.12
  transabdominal (operative) 44.11
Esophagogastrostomy (intrathoracic) 42.52
  with partial gastrectomy 43.5
  antesternal or antethoracic 42.62
Esophagoileostomy (intrathoracic) NEC 42.54
  with interposition of small bowel 42.53
  antesternal or antethoracic NEC 42.64
    with interposition of small bowel 42.63
Esophagojejunostomy (intrathoracic) NEC 42.54
  with
    complete gastrectomy 43.99
    interposition of small bowel 42.53
  antesternal or antethoracic NEC 42.64
    with interposition of small bowel 42.63
Esophagomyotomy 42.7
Esophagoplasty NEC 42.89
Esophagorrhaphy 42.82
Esophagoscopy NEC 42.23
  by incision (operative) 42.21
  with closed biopsy 42.24
  through stoma (artificial) 42.22
  transabdominal (operative) 42.21
Esophagostomy 42.10
  cervical 42.11
  thoracic 42.19
Esophagotomy NEC 42.09
Estes operation (ovary) 65.72
  laparoscopic 65.75
Estlander operation (thoracoplasty) 33.34
ESWL (extracorporeal shockwave lithotripsy) NEC 98.59
  bile duct 98.52
  bladder 98.51
  gallbladder 98.52

ESWL NEC (Continued)
  kidney 98.51
  Kock pouch (urinary diversion) 98.51
  renal pelvis 98.51
  specified site NEC 98.59
  ureter 98.51
Ethmoidectomy 22.63
Ethmoidotomy 22.51
Evacuation
  abscess - see Drainage, by site
  anterior chamber (eye) (aqueous) (hyphema) 12.91
  cyst - see also Excision, lesion, by site
    breast 85.91
    kidney 55.01
    liver 50.29
  hematoma - see also Incision, hematoma
    obstetrical 75.92
      incisional 75.91
  hemorrhoids (thrombosed) 49.47
  pelvic blood clot (by incision) 54.19
    by
      culdocentesis 70.0
      culdoscopy 70.22
  retained placenta
    with curettage 69.02
    manual 75.4
  streptothrix from lacrimal duct 09.42
Evaluation (of)
  audiological 95.43
  cardiac rhythm device (CRT-D) (CRT-P) (AICD) (pacemaker) - see Interrogation
  criminal responsibility, psychiatric 94.11
  functional (physical therapy) 93.01
  hearing NEC 95.49
  orthotic (for brace fitting) 93.02
  prosthetic (for artificial limb fitting) 93.03
  psychiatric NEC 94.19
    commitment 94.13
  psychologic NEC 94.08
  testimentary capacity, psychiatric 94.11
Evans operation (release of clubfoot) 83.84
Evisceration
  eyeball 16.39
    with implant (into scleral shell) 16.31
  ocular contents 16.39
    with implant (into scleral shell) 16.31
  orbit - see also Exenteration, orbit 16.59
  pelvic (anterior) (posterior) (partial) (total) (female) 68.8
    male 57.71
Evulsion
  nail (bed) (fold) 86.23
  skin 86.3
  subcutaneous tissue 86.3
Examination (for)
  breast
    manual 89.36
    radiographic NEC 87.37
    thermographic 88.85
    ultrasonic 88.73
  cervical rib (by x-ray) 87.43
  colostomy stoma (digital) 89.33
  dental (oral mucosa) (peridontal) 89.31
    radiographic NEC 87.12
  enterostomy stoma (digital) 89.33

Examination (Continued)
  eye 95.09
    color vision 95.06
    comprehensive 95.02
    dark adaptation 95.07
    limited (with prescription of spectacles) 95.01
    under anesthesia 95.04
  fetus, intrauterine 75.35
  general physical 89.7
  glaucoma 95.03
  gynecological 89.26
  hearing 95.47
  microscopic (specimen) (of) 91.9●

Note: Use the following fourth-digit subclassification with categories 90-91 to identify type of examination:
1 bacterial smear
2 culture
3 culture and sensitivity
4 parasitology
5 toxicology
6 cell block and Papanicolaou smear
9 other microscopic examination

  adenoid 90.3●
  adrenal gland 90.1●
  amnion 91.4●
  anus 90.9●
  appendix 90.9●
  bile ducts 91.0●
  bladder 91.3●
  blood 90.5●
  bone 91.5●
    marrow 90.6●
  brain 90.0●
  breast 91.6●
  bronchus 90.4●
  bursa 91.5●
  cartilage 91.5●
  cervix 91.4●
  chest wall 90.4●
  chorion 91.4●
  colon 90.9●
  cul-de-sac 91.1●
  dental 90.8●
  diaphragm 90.4●
  duodenum 90.8●
  ear 90.3●
  endocrine gland NEC 90.1●
  esophagus 90.8●
  eye 90.2●
  fallopian tube 91.4●
  fascia 91.5●
  female genital tract 91.4●
  fetus 91.4●
  gallbladder 91.0●
  hair 91.6●
  ileum 90.9●
  jejunum 90.9●
  joint fluid 91.5●
  kidney 91.2●
  large intestine 90.9●
  larynx 90.3●
  ligament 91.5●
  liver 91.0●
  lung 90.4●
  lymph (node) 90.7●
  meninges 90.0●
  mesentery 91.1●
  mouth 90.8●
  muscle 91.5●

Examination (*Continued*)
  microscopic (*Continued*)
    musculoskeletal system 91.5●
    nails 91.6●
    nerve 90.0●
    nervous system 90.0●
    nose 90.3●
    omentum 91.1●
    operative wound 91.7●
    ovary 91.4●
    pancreas 91.0●
    parathyroid gland 90.1●
    penis 91.3●
    perirenal tissue 91.2●
    peritoneum (fluid) 91.1●
    periureteral tissue 91.2●
    perivesical (tissue) 91.3●
    pharynx 90.3●
    pineal gland 90.1●
    pituitary gland 90.1●
    placenta 91.4●
    pleura (fluid) 90.4●
    prostate 91.3●
    rectum 90.9●
    retroperitoneum 91.1●
    semen 91.3●
    seminal vesicle 91.3●
    sigmoid 90.9●
    skin 91.6●
    small intestine 90.9●
    specified site NEC 91.8●
    spinal fluid 90.0●
    spleen 90.6●
    sputum 90.4●
    stomach 90.8●
    stool 90.9●
    synovial membrane 91.5●
    tendon 91.5●
    thorax NEC 90.4●
    throat 90.3●
    thymus 90.1●
    thyroid gland 90.1●
    tonsil 90.3●
    trachea 90.4●
    ureter 91.2●
    urethra 91.3●
    urine 91.3●
    uterus 91.4●
    vagina 91.4●
    vas deferens 91.3●
    vomitus 90.8●
    vulva 91.4●
  neurologic 89.13
  neuro-ophthalmology 95.03
  ophthalmoscopic 16.21
  panorex, mandible 87.12
  pelvic (manual) 89.26
    instrumental (by pelvimeter)
      88.25
    pelvimetric 88.25
  physical, general 89.7
  postmortem 89.8
  rectum (digital) 89.34
    endoscopic 48.23
      through stoma (artificial) 48.22
      transabdominal 48.21
  retinal disease 95.03
  specified type (manual) NEC 89.39
  thyroid field, postoperative 06.02
  uterus (digital) 68.11
    endoscopic 68.12
  vagina 89.26
    endoscopic 70.21
  visual field 95.05

Exchange transfusion 99.01
  intrauterine 75.2
Excision
  aberrant tissue - *see* Excision, lesion, by
    site of tissue origin
  abscess - *see* Excision, lesion, by site
  accessory tissue - *see also* Excision,
    lesion, by site of tissue origin
    lung 32.29
      endoscopic 32.28
      thoracoscopic 32.20
    spleen 41.93
  adenoids (tag) 28.6
    with tonsillectomy 28.3
  adenoma - *see* Excision, lesion, by site
  adrenal gland - *see also* Adrenalectomy
    07.22
  ampulla of Vater (with reimplantation
    of common duct) 51.62
  anal papilla 49.39
    endoscopic 49.31
  aneurysm (arteriovenous) - *see also*
    Aneurysmectomy 38.60
    coronary artery 36.91
    heart 37.32
    myocardium 37.32
    sinus of Valsalva 35.39
    ventricle (heart) 37.32
  anus (complete) (partial) 49.6
  aortic subvalvular ring 35.35
  apocrine gland 86.3
  aponeurosis 83.42
    hand 82.33
  appendage, left atrial 37.36
  appendiceal stump 47.09
    laparoscopic 47.01
  appendices epiploicae 54.4
  appendix - *see also* Appendectomy
    epididymis 63.3
    testis 62.2
  arcuate ligament (spine) - *omit code*
  arteriovenous fistula - *see also*
    Aneurysmectomy 38.60
  artery - *see also* Arteriectomy
    38.60
  Baker's cyst, knee 83.39
  Bartholin's gland 71.24
  basal ganglion 01.59
  bile duct 51.69
    endoscopic 51.64
  bladder - *see also* Cystectomy
  bleb (emphysematous), lung 32.29
    endoscopic 32.28
    thoracoscopic 32.20
  blood vessel - *see also* Angiectomy
    38.60
  bone (ends) (partial), except facial - *see*
    category 77.8●
    facial NEC 76.39
      total 76.45
        with reconstruction 76.44
    for graft (autograft) (homograft) -
      see category 77.7●
    fragments (chips) - *see also* Incision,
      bone 77.10
    joint - *see also* Arthrotomy 80.10
    necrotic - *see also* Sequestrectomy,
      bone 77.00
    heterotopic, from
      muscle 83.32
        hand 82.22
      skin 86.3
      tendon 83.31
        hand 82.21

Excision (*Continued*)
  bone, except facial (*Continued*)
    mandible 76.31
      with arthrodesis - *see* Arthrodesis
      total 76.42
        with reconstruction 76.41
    spur - *see* Excision, lesion, bone
    total, except facial - *see* category
      77.9●
      facial NEC 76.45
        with reconstruction 76.44
      mandible 76.42
        with reconstruction 76.41
  brain 01.59
    hemisphere 01.52
    lobe 01.53
  branchial cleft cyst or vestige 29.2
  breast - *see also* Mastectomy 85.41
    aberrant tissue 85.24
    accessory 85.24
    ectopic 85.24
    nipple 85.25
      accessory 85.24
    segmental 85.23
    supernumerary 85.24
    wedge 85.21
  broad ligament 69.19
  bronchogenic cyst 32.09
    endoscopic 32.01
  bronchus (wide sleeve) NEC 32.1
  buccal mucosa 27.49
  bulbourethral gland 58.92
  bulbous tuberosities (mandible)
    (maxilla) (fibrous) (osseous)
    24.31
  bunion - *see also* Bunionectomy 77.59
  bunionette (with osteotomy) 77.54
  bursa 83.5
    hand 82.31
  canal of Nuck 69.19
  cardioma 37.33
  carotid body (lesion) (partial) (total)
    39.89 ◄▥
  cartilage - *see also* Chondrectomy
    80.90
    intervertebral - *see* category
      80.5●
    knee (semilunar) 80.6
    larynx 30.29
    nasal (submucous) 21.5
  caruncle, urethra 58.39
    endoscopic 58.31
  cataract - *see also* Extraction, cataract
    13.19
    secondary membrane (after cataract)
      13.65
  cervical
    rib 77.91
    stump 67.4
  cervix (stump) NEC 67.4
    cold (knife) 67.2
    conization 67.2
    cryoconization 67.33
    electroconization 67.32
  chalazion (multiple) (single) 08.21
  cholesteatoma - *see* Excision, lesion, by
    site
  choroid plexus 02.14
  cicatrix (skin) 86.3
  cilia base 08.20
  ciliary body, prolapsed 12.98
  clavicle (head) (partial) 77.81
    total (complete) 77.91
  clitoris 71.4

Excision (Continued)

coarctation of aorta (end-to-end anastomosis) 38.64
  with
    graft replacement (interposition)
      abdominal 38.44
      thoracic 38.45
      thoracoabdominal 38.45
        [38.44]
common
  duct 51.63
  wall between posterior and coronary sinus (with roofing or resultant defect with patch graft) 35.82
condyle - see category 77.8 ●
  mandible 76.5
conjunctival ring 10.31
cornea 11.49
  epithelium (with chemocauterization) 11.41
    for smear or culture 11.21
costal cartilage 80.99
cul-de-sac (Douglas') 70.92
  with graft or prosthesis 70.93
cusp, heart valve 35.10
  aortic 35.11
  mitral 35.12
  tricuspid 35.14
cyst - see also Excision, lesion, by site
  apical (tooth) 23.73
    with root canal therapy 23.72
  Baker's (popliteal) 83.39
  breast 85.21
  broad ligament 69.19
  bronchogenic 32.09
    endoscopic 32.01
  cervix 67.39
  dental 24.4
  dentigerous 24.4
  epididymis 63.2
  fallopian tube 66.61
  Gartner's duct 70.33
  hand 82.29
  labia 71.3
  lung 32.29
    endoscopic 32.28
    thoracoscopic 32.20
  mesonephric duct 69.19
  Morgagni
    female 66.61
    male 62.2
  mullerian duct 60.73
  nasolabial 27.49
  nasopalatine 27.31
    by wide excision 27.32
  ovary 65.29
    laparoscopic 65.25
  parovarian 69.19
  pericardium 37.31
  periodontal (apical) (lateral) 24.4
  popliteal (Baker's), knee 83.39
  radicular 24.4
  spleen 41.42
  synovial (membrane) 83.39
  thyroglossal (with resection of hyoid bone) 06.7
  urachal (bladder) 57.51
    abdominal wall 54.3
  vagina (Gartner's duct) 70.33
cystic
  duct remnant 51.61
  hygroma 40.29
dentinoma 24.4
diaphragm 34.81

Excision (Continued)

disc, intervertebral NOS 80.50
  herniated (nucleus pulposus) 80.51
  other specified (diskectomy) 80.51
diverticulum
  ampulla of Vater 51.62
  anus 49.39
    endoscopic 49.31
  bladder 57.59
    transurethral 57.49
  duodenum 45.31
    endoscopic 45.30
  esophagus (local) 42.31
    endoscopic 42.33
  hypopharyngeal (by cricopharyngeal myotomy) 29.32
  intestine
    large 45.41
      endoscopic 45.43
    small NEC 45.33
  Meckel's 45.33
  pharyngeal (by cricopharyngeal myotomy) 29.32
  pharyngoesophageal (by cricopharyngeal myotomy) 29.32
  stomach 43.42
    endoscopic 43.41
  urethra 58.39
    endoscopic 58.31
  ventricle, heart 37.33
duct
  mullerian 69.19
  paramesonephric 69.19
  thyroglossal (with resection of hyoid bone) 06.7
ear, external (complete) NEC 18.39
  partial 18.29
    radical 18.31
ectopic
  abdominal fetus 74.3
  tissue - see also Excision, lesion, by site of tissue origin
    bone, from muscle 83.32
    breast 85.24
    lung 32.29
      endoscopic 32.28
      thoracoscopic 32.20
    spleen 41.93
empyema pocket, lung 34.09
epididymis 63.4
epiglottis 30.21
epithelial downgrowth, anterior chamber (eye) 12.93
epulis (gingiva) 24.31
esophagus - see also Esophagectomy 42.40
exostosis - see also Excision, lesion, bone 77.60
  auditory canal, external 18.29
  facial bone 76.2
  first metatarsal (hallux valgus repair) - see Bunionectomy
eye 16.49
  with implant (into Tenon's capsule) 16.42
    with attachment of muscles 16.41
eyelid 08.20
  redundant skin 08.86
falciform ligament 54.4

Excision (Continued)

fallopian tube - see Salpingectomy
fascia 83.44
  for graft 83.43
    hand 82.34
  hand 82.35
    for graft 82.34
fat pad NEC 86.3
  knee (infrapatellar) (prepatellar) 86.3
  scalene 40.21
fibroadenoma, breast 85.21
fissure, anus 49.39
  endoscopic 49.31
fistula - see also Fistulectomy
  anal 49.12
  arteriovenous - see also Aneurysmectomy 38.60
  ileorectal 46.74
  lacrimal
    gland 09.21
    sac 09.6
  rectal 48.73
  vesicovaginal 57.84
frenulum, frenum
  labial (lip) 27.41
  lingual (tongue) 25.92
ganglion (hand) (tendon sheath) (wrist) 82.21
  gasserian 04.05
  site other than hand or nerve 83.31
  sympathetic nerve 05.29
  trigeminal nerve 04.05
gastrocolic ligament 54.4
gingiva 24.31
glomus jugulare tumor 20.51
goiter - see Thyroidectomy
gum 24.31
hallux valgus - see also Bunionectomy
  with prosthetic implant 77.59
hamartoma, mammary 85.21
heart assist system - see Removal
hematocele, tunica vaginalis 61.92
hematoma - see Drainage, by site
hemorrhoids (external) (internal) (tag) 49.46
heterotopic bone, from
  muscle 83.32
    hand 82.22
  skin 86.3
  tendon 83.31
    hand 82.21
hydatid of Morgagni
  female 66.61
  male 62.2
hydatid cyst, liver 50.29
hydrocele
  canal of Nuck (female) 69.19
  male 63.1
  round ligament 69.19
  spermatic cord 63.1
  tunica vaginalis 61.2
hygroma, cystic 40.29
hymen (tag) 70.31
hymeno-urethral fusion 70.31
intervertebral disc - see Excision, disc, intervertebral (NOS) 80.50
intestine - see also Resection, intestine
  for interposition 45.50
    large 45.52
    small 45.51

Excision (Continued)

intestine (Continued)

  large (total)

    for interposition 45.52

    laparoscopic 45.81

    local 45.41

      endoscopic 45.43

    open 45.82

    other 45.83

    segmental

      laparoscopic 17.39

      multiple

        laparoscopic 17.31

        open and other 45.71

      open and other 45.79

    unspecified 45.83

  small (total) 45.63

    for interposition 45.51

    local 45.33

    partial 45.62

    segmental 45.62

      multiple 45.61

intraductal papilloma 85.21

iris prolapse 12.13

joint - see also Arthrectomy 80.90

keloid (scar), skin 86.3

LAA 37.36

labia - see Vulvectomy

lacrimal

  gland 09.20

    partial 09.22

    total 09.23

  passage 09.6

  sac 09.6

left atrial appendage 37.36

lesion (local)

  abdominal wall 54.3

  accessory sinus - see Excision, lesion, nasal sinus

  adenoids 28.92

  adrenal gland(s) 07.21

  alveolus 24.4

  ampulla of Vater 51.62

  anterior chamber (eye) NEC 12.40

  anus 49.39

    endoscopic 49.31

  apocrine gland 86.3

  artery 38.60

    abdominal 38.66

    aorta (arch) (ascending) (descending thoracic) 38.64

      with end-to-end anastomosis 38.45

        abdominal 38.44

        thoracic 38.45

        thoracoabdominal 38.45 [38.44]

      with graft interposition graft replacement 38.45

        abdominal 38.44

        thoracic 38.45

        thoracoabdominal 38.45 [38.44]

    head and neck NEC 38.62

    intracranial NEC 38.61

    lower limb 38.68

    thoracic NEC 38.65

    upper limb 38.63

  atrium 37.33

  auditory canal or meatus, external 18.29

    radical 18.31

  auricle, ear 18.29

    radical 18.31

Excision (Continued)

lesion (Continued)

  biliary ducts 51.69

    endoscopic 51.64

  bladder (transurethral) 57.49

    open 57.59

    suprapubic 57.59

  blood vessel 38.60

    abdominal

      artery 38.66

      vein 38.67

    aorta (arch) (ascending) (descending) 38.64

    head and neck NEC 38.62

    intracranial NEC 38.61

    lower limb

      artery 38.68

      vein 38.69

    thoracic NEC 38.65

    upper limb (artery) (vein) 38.63

  bone 77.60

    carpal, metacarpal 77.64

    clavicle 77.61

    facial 76.2

    femur 77.65

    fibula 77.67

    humerus 77.62

    jaw 76.2

      dental 24.4

    patella 77.66

    pelvic 77.69

    phalanges (foot) (hand) 77.69

    radius 77.63

    scapula 77.61

    skull 01.6

    specified site NEC 77.69

    tarsal, metatarsal 77.68

    thorax (ribs) (sternum) 77.61

    tibia 77.67

    ulna 77.63

    vertebrae 77.69

  brain (transtemporal approach) NEC 01.59

    by stereotactic radiosurgery 92.30

      cobalt 60 92.32

      linear accelerator (LINAC) 92.31

      multi-source 92.32

      particle beam 92.33

      particulate 92.33

      radiosurgery NEC 92.39

      single source photon 92.31

  breast (segmental) (wedge) 85.21

  broad ligament 69.19

  bronchus NEC 32.09

    endoscopic 32.01

  cerebral (cortex) NEC 01.59

    meninges 01.51

  cervix (myoma) 67.39

  chest wall 34.4

  choroid plexus 02.14

  ciliary body 12.44

  colon 45.41

    endoscopic NEC 45.43

      polypectomy 45.42

  conjunctiva 10.31

  cornea 11.49

  cranium 01.6

  cul-de-sac (Douglas') 70.32

  dental (jaw) 24.4

  diaphragm 34.81

  duodenum (local) 45.31

    endoscopic 45.30

Excision (Continued)

lesion (Continued)

  ear, external 18.29

    radical 18.31

  endometrium 68.29

  epicardium 37.31

  epididymis 63.3

  epiglottis 30.09

  esophagus NEC 42.32

    endoscopic 42.33

  eye, eyeball 16.93

    anterior segment NEC 12.40

  eyebrow (skin) 08.20

  eyelid 08.20

    by

      halving procedure 08.24

      wedge resection 08.24

    major

      full-thickness 08.24

      partial-thickness 08.23

    minor 08.22

  fallopian tube 66.61

  fascia 83.39

    hand 82.29

  groin region (abdominal wall) (inguinal) 54.3

    skin 86.3

    subcutaneous tissue 86.3

  gum 24.31

  heart ~~37.33~~ 37.34 ◄▦

    Cox-maze, open 37.33 ◄

    maze, modified, endovascular 37.34 ◄

    maze, modified, open 37.33 ◄

    open 37.33 ◄

    other approach, closed 37.34 ◄

  hepatic duct 51.69

  inguinal canal 54.3

  intestine

    large 45.41

      endoscopic NEC 45.43

        polypectomy 45.42

    small NEC 45.33

  intracranial NEC 01.59

  intranasal 21.31

  intraspinal 03.4

  iris 12.42

  jaw 76.2

    dental 24.4

  joint 80.80

    ankle 80.87

    elbow 80.82

    foot and toe 80.88

    hand and finger 80.84

    hip 80.85

    knee 80.86

    shoulder 80.81

    specified site NEC 80.89

    spine 80.89

    wrist 80.83

  kidney 55.39

    with partial nephrectomy 55.4

  labia 71.3

  lacrimal

    gland (frontal approach) 09.21

    passage 09.6

    sac 09.6

  larynx 30.09

  ligament (joint) - see also Excision, lesion, joint 80.80

    broad 69.19

    round 69.19

    uterosacral 69.19

◄ New   ◄▦ Revised   ~~deleted~~ Deleted   ● Use Additional Digit(s)   ▨ Omit code

Excision *(Continued)*
　lesion *(Continued)*
　　lip 27.43
　　　by wide excision
　　　　27.42
　　liver 50.29
　　lung NEC 32.29
　　　by lung volume reduction
　　　　surgery 32.22
　　　by wide excision 32.39
　　　　thoracoscopic 32.30
　　　endoscopic 32.28
　　　thoracoscopic 32.20
　　lymph structure(s) (channel) (vessel)
　　　NEC 40.29
　　　node - *see* Excision, lymph, node
　　mammary duct 85.21
　　mastoid (bone) 20.49
　　mediastinum 34.3
　　meninges (cerebral) 01.51
　　　spinal 03.4
　　mesentery 54.4
　　middle ear 20.51
　　mouth NEC 27.49
　　muscle 83.32
　　　hand 82.22
　　　ocular 15.13
　　myocardium 37.33
　　nail 86.23
　　nasal sinus 22.60
　　　antrum 22.62
　　　　with Caldwell-Luc approach
　　　　　22.61
　　　　specified approach NEC
　　　　　22.62
　　　ethmoid 22.63
　　　frontal 22.42
　　　maxillary 22.62
　　　　with Caldwell-Luc approach
　　　　　22.61
　　　　specified approach NEC
　　　　　22.62
　　　sphenoid 22.64
　　nasopharynx 29.3●
　　nerve (cranial) (peripheral)
　　　04.07
　　　sympathetic 05.29
　　nonodontogenic 24.31
　　nose 21.30
　　　intranasal 21.31
　　　polyp 21.31
　　　skin 21.32
　　　specified site NEC 21.32
　　odontogenic 24.4
　　omentum 54.4
　　orbit 16.92
　　ovary 65.29
　　　by wedge resection 65.22
　　　　laparoscopic 65.24
　　　that by laparoscope 65.25
　　palate (bony) 27.31
　　　by wide excision 27.32
　　　soft 27.49
　　pancreas (local) 52.22
　　　endoscopic 52.21
　　parathyroid 06.89
　　parotid gland or duct NEC
　　　26.29
　　pelvic wall 54.3
　　pelvirectal tissue 48.82
　　penis 64.2
　　pericardium 37.31
　　perineum (female) 71.3
　　　male 86.3

Excision *(Continued)*
　lesion *(Continued)*
　　periprostatic tissue 60.82
　　perirectal tissue 48.82
　　perirenal tissue 59.91
　　peritoneum 54.4
　　perivesical tissue 59.91
　　pharynx 29.39
　　　diverticulum 29.32
　　pineal gland 07.53
　　pinna 18.29
　　　radical 18.31
　　pituitary (gland) - *see also*
　　　Hypophysectomy, partial
　　　07.63
　　　by stereotactic radiosurgery
　　　　92.30
　　　　cobalt 60 92.32
　　　　linear accelerator (LINAC)
　　　　　92.31
　　　　multi-source 92.32
　　　　particle beam 92.33
　　　　particulate 92.33
　　　　radiosurgery NEC 92.39
　　　　single source photon
　　　　　92.31
　　pleura 34.59
　　pouch of Douglas 70.32
　　preauricular (ear) 18.21
　　presacral 54.4
　　prostate (transurethral) 60.61
　　pulmonary (fibrosis) 32.29
　　　endoscopic 32.28
　　　thoracoscopic 32.20
　　rectovaginal septum 48.82
　　rectum 48.35
　　　polyp (endoscopic) 48.36
　　retroperitoneum 54.4
　　salivary gland or duct NEC 26.29
　　　en bloc 26.32
　　sclera 12.84
　　scrotum 61.3
　　sinus (nasal) - *see* Excision, lesion,
　　　nasal sinus
　　Skene's gland 71.3
　　skin 86.3
　　　breast 85.21
　　　nose 21.32
　　　radical (wide) (involving
　　　　underlying or adjacent
　　　　structure) (with flap
　　　　closure) 86.4
　　　scrotum 61.3
　　skull 01.6
　　soft tissue NEC 83.39
　　　hand 82.29
　　spermatic cord 63.3
　　sphincter of Oddi 51.62
　　　endoscopic 51.64
　　spinal cord (meninges) 03.4
　　spleen (cyst) 41.42
　　stomach NEC 43.42
　　　endoscopic 43.41
　　　　polyp 43.41
　　　polyp (endoscopic) 43.41
　　subcutaneous tissue 86.3
　　　breast 85.21
　　subgingival 24.31
　　sweat gland 86.3
　　tendon 83.39
　　　hand 82.29
　　　ocular 15.13
　　　sheath 83.31
　　　　hand 82.21

Excision *(Continued)*
　lesion *(Continued)*
　　testis 62.2
　　thorax 34.4
　　thymus
　　　partial (open) (other) 07.81
　　　　thoracoscopic 07.83
　　　total (open) (other) 07.82
　　　　thoracoscopic 07.84
　　thyroid 06.31
　　　substernal or transsternal route
　　　　06.51
　　tongue 25.1
　　tonsil 28.92
　　trachea 31.5
　　tunica vaginalis 61.92
　　ureter 56.41
　　urethra 58.39
　　　endoscopic 58.31
　　uterine ligament 69.19
　　uterosacral ligament 69.19
　　uterus 68.29
　　vagina 70.33
　　vein 38.60
　　　abdominal 38.67
　　　head and neck NEC 38.62
　　　intracranial NEC 38.61
　　　lower limb 38.69
　　　thoracic NEC 38.65
　　　upper limb 38.63
　　ventricle (heart) 37.33
　　vocal cords 30.09
　　vulva 71.3
　ligament - *see also* Arthrectomy
　　80.90
　　broad 69.19
　　round 69.19
　　uterine 69.19
　　uterosacral 69.19
　ligamentum flavum (spine) -
　　omit code
　lingual tonsil 28.5
　lip 27.43
　liver (partial) 50.22
　loose body
　　bone - *see* Sequestrectomy, bone
　　joint 80.10
　lung (with mediastinal dissection)
　　32.59
　　accessory or ectopic tissue
　　　32.29
　　　endoscopic 32.28
　　　thoracoscopic 32.20
　　segmental 32.39
　　　thoracoscopic 32.30
　　specified type NEC 32.29
　　　endoscopic 32.28
　　　thoracoscopic 32.20
　　thoracoscopic 32.50
　　volume reduction surgery
　　　32.22
　　　biologic lung volume reduction
　　　　(BLVR) - *see category*
　　　　33.7●
　　wedge 32.29
　　　thoracoscopic 32.20
　lymph, lymphatic
　　drainage area 40.29
　　　radical - *see* Excision, lymph,
　　　　node, radical
　　　regional (with lymph node,
　　　　skin, subcutaneous tissue,
　　　　and fat) 40.3

Excision (Continued)
  lymph, lymphatic (Continued)
    node (simple) NEC 40.29
      with
        lymphatic drainage area
          (including skin,
          subcutaneous tissue, and
          fat) 40.3
        mastectomy - see Mastectomy,
          radical
        muscle and deep fascia - see
          Excision, lymph, node,
          radical
      axillary 40.23
        radical 40.51
        regional (extended) 40.3
      cervical (deep) (with excision of
        scalene fat pad) 40.21
        with laryngectomy 30.4
        radical (including muscle and
          deep fascia) 40.40
          bilateral 40.42
          unilateral 40.41
        regional (extended) 40.3
        superficial 40.29
      groin 40.24
        radical 40.54
        regional (extended) 40.3
      iliac 40.29
        radical 40.53
        regional (extended) 40.3
      inguinal (deep) (superficial)
        40.24
        radical 40.54
        regional (extended) 40.3
      jugular - see Excision, lymph,
        node, cervical
      mammary (internal) 40.22
        external 40.29
          radical 40.59
            regional (extended) 40.3
        radical 40.59
          regional (extended) 40.3
      paratracheal - see Excision,
        lymph, node, cervical
      periaortic 40.29
        radical 40.52
        regional (extended) 40.3
      radical 40.50
        with mastectomy - see
          Mastectomy, radical
        specified site NEC 40.59
      regional (extended) 40.3
      sternal - see Excision, lymph,
        node, mammary
    structure(s) (simple) NEC 40.29
      radical 40.59
      regional (extended) 40.3
  lymphangioma (simple) - see also
    Excision, lymph, lymphatic,
    node, 40.29
  lymphocele 40.29
  mastoid - see also Mastoidectomy
    20.49
  median bar, transurethral approach
    60.29
  meibomian gland 08.20
  meniscus (knee) 80.6
    acromioclavicular 80.91
    jaw 76.5
    sternoclavicular 80.91
    temporomandibular (joint) 76.5
    wrist 80.93
  mullerian duct cyst 60.73

Excision (Continued)
  muscle 83.45
    for graft 83.43
      hand 82.34
    hand 82.36
      for graft 82.34
  myositis ossificans 83.32
    hand 82.22
  nail (bed) (fold) 86.23
  nasolabial cyst 27.49
  nasopalatine cyst 27.31
    by wide excision 27.32
  neoplasm - see Excision, lesion, by site
  nerve (cranial) (peripheral) NEC
    04.07
    sympathetic 05.29
  neuroma (Morton's) (peripheral nerve)
    04.07
    acoustic
      by craniotomy 04.01
      by stereotactic radiosurgery
        92.30
        cobalt 60 92.32
        linear accelerator (LINAC)
          92.31
        multi-source 92.32
        particle beam 92.33
        particulate 92.33
        radiosurgery NEC 92.39
        single source photon 92.31
    sympathetic nerve 05.29
  nipple 85.25
    accessory 85.24
  odontoma 24.4
  orbital contents - see also Exenteration,
    orbit 16.59
  osteochondritis dissecans - see also
    Excision, lesion, joint 80.80
  ovary - see also Oophorectomy
    partial 65.29
      by wedge resection 65.22
        laparoscopic 65.24
      that by laparoscope 65.25
  Pancoast tumor (lung) 32.6
  pancreas (total) (with synchronous
    duodenectomy) 52.6
    partial NEC 52.59
      distal (tail) (with part of body)
        52.52
      proximal (head) (with part of
        body) (with synchronous
        duodenectomy) 52.51
      radical subtotal 52.53
    radical (one-stage) (two-stage)
      52.7
    subtotal 52.53
  paramesonephric duct 69.19
  parathyroid gland (partial) (subtotal)
    NEC - see also Parathyroidectomy
    06.89
  parotid gland - see also Excision,
    salivary gland 26.30
  parovarian cyst 69.19
  patella (complete) 77.96
    partial 77.86
  pelvirectal tissue 48.82
  perianal tissue 49.04
    skin tags 49.03
  pericardial adhesions 37.31
  periprostatic tissue 60.82
  perirectal tissue 48.82
  perirenal tissue 59.91
  periurethral tissue 58.92
  perivesical tissue 59.91

Excision (Continued)
  petrous apex cells 20.59
  pharyngeal bands 29.54
  pharynx (partial) 29.33
  pilonidal cyst or sinus (open) (with
    partial closure) 86.21
  pineal gland (complete) (total) 07.54
    partial 07.53
  pituitary gland (complete) (total) - see
    also Hypophysectomy 07.69
  pleura NEC 34.59
  polyp - see also Excision, lesion, by site
    esophagus 42.32
      endoscopic 42.33
    large intestine 45.41
      endoscopic 45.42
    nose 21.31
    rectum (endoscopic) 48.36
    stomach (endoscopic) 43.41
  preauricular
    appendage (remnant) 18.29
    cyst, fistula, or sinus (congenital)
      18.21
    remnant 18.29
  prolapsed iris (in wound) 12.13
  prostate - see Prostatectomy
  pterygium (simple) 11.39
    with corneal graft 11.32
  radius (head) (partial) 77.83
    total 77.93
  ranula, salivary gland NEC 26.29
  rectal mucosa 48.35
  rectum - see Resection, rectum
  redundant mucosa
    colostomy 45.41
      endoscopic 45.43
    duodenostomy 45.31
      endoscopic 45.30
    ileostomy 45.33
    jejunostomy 45.33
    perineum 71.3
    rectum 48.35
    vulva 71.3
  renal vessel, aberrant 38.66
  rib (cervical) 77.91
  ring of conjunctiva around cornea 10.31
  round ligament 69.19
  salivary gland 26.30
    complete 26.32
    partial 26.31
    radical 26.32
  scalene fat pad 40.21
  scar - see also Excision, lesion, by site
    epicardium 37.31
    mastoid 20.92
    pericardium 37.31
    pleura 34.59
    skin 86.3
    thorax 34.4
  secondary membrane, lens 13.65
  seminal vesicle 60.73
    with radical prostatectomy 60.5
  septum - see also Excision, by site
    uterus (congenital) 68.22
    vagina 70.33
  sinus - see also Excision, lesion, by site
    nasal - see Sinusectomy
    pilonidal 86.21
    preauricular (ear) (radical) 18.21
    tarsi 80.88
    thyroglossal (with resection of hyoid
      bone) 06.7
    urachal (bladder) 57.51
      abdominal wall 54.3

◀ New   ◀|||| Revised   ~~deleted~~ Deleted   ● Use Additional Digit(s)   ▨ Omit code

Excision (*Continued*)
Skene's gland 71.3
skin (local) 86.3
for graft (with closure of donor site) 86.91
radical (wide) (involving underlying or adjacent structure) (with flap closure) 86.4
tags
perianal 49.03
periauricular 18.29
soft tissue NEC 83.49
hand 82.39
spermatocele 63.2
spinous process 77.89
spleen (total) 41.5
accessory 41.93
partial 41.43
stomach - *see* Gastrectomy
sublingual gland (salivary) - *see also* Excision, salivary gland 26.30
submaxillary gland - *see also* Excision, salivary gland 26.30
supernumerary
breast 85.24
digits 86.26
sweat gland 86.3
synechiae - *see also* Lysis, synechiae
endometrial 68.21
tarsal plate (eyelid) 08.20
by wedge resection 08.24
tattoo 86.3
by dermabrasion 86.25
tendon (sheath) 83.42
for graft 83.41
hand 82.32
hand 82.33
for graft 82.32
thymus - *see also* Thymectomy 07.80
thyroglossal duct or tract (with resection of hyoid bone) 06.7
thyroid NEC - *see also* Thyroidectomy 06.39
tongue (complete) (total) 25.3
partial or subtotal 25.2
radical 25.4
tonsil 28.2
with adenoidectomy 28.3
lingual 28.5
tag 28.4
tooth NEC - *see also* Removal, tooth, surgical 23.19
from nasal sinus 22.60
torus
lingual 76.2
mandible, mandibularis 76.2
palate, palatinus 27.31
by wide excision 27.32
trabeculae carneae cordis (heart) 35.35
trochanteric lipomatosis 86.83
tumor - *see* Excision, lesion, by site
ulcer - *see also* Excision, lesion, by site
duodenum 45.31
endoscopic 45.30
stomach 43.42
endoscopic 43.41
umbilicus 54.3
urachus, urachal (cyst) (bladder) 57.51
abdominal wall 54.3

Excision (*Continued*)
ureter, ureteral 56.40
with nephrectomy - *see* Nephrectomy
partial 56.41
stricture 56.41
total 56.42
ureterocele 56.41
urethra, urethral 58.39
with complete cystectomy 57.79
endoscopic 58.31
septum 58.0
stricture 58.39
endoscopic 58.31
valve (congenital) 58.39
endoscopic (transurethral) (transvesical) 58.31
urethrovaginal septum 70.33
uterus (corpus) - *see also* Hysterectomy 68.9
cervix 67.4
lesion 67.39
lesion 68.29
septum 68.22
uvula 27.72
vagina (total) 70.4
varicocele, spermatic cord 63.1
vein - *see also* Phlebectomy 38.60
varicose 38.50
abdominal 38.57
head and neck NEC 38.52
intracranial NEC 38.51
lower limb 38.59
ovarian 38.67
thoracic NEC 38.55
upper limb 38.53
verucca - *see also* Excision, lesion, by site
eyelid 08.22
vesicovaginal septum 70.33
vitreous opacity 14.74
anterior approach 14.73
vocal cord(s) (submucous) 30.22
vulva (bilateral) (simple) - *see also* Vulvectomy 71.62
wart - *see also* Excision, lesion, by site
eyelid 08.22
wolffian duct 69.19
xanthoma (tendon sheath, hand) 82.21
site other than hand 83.31
Excisional biopsy - *see* Biopsy
Exclusion
left atrial appendage 37.36
pyloric
laparoscopic 44.38
open 44.39
Exenteration
ethmoid air cells 22.63
orbit 16.59
with
removal of adjacent structures 16.51
temporalis muscle transplant 16.59
therapeutic removal of bone 16.52
pelvic (organs) (female) 68.8
male 57.71
petrous pyramid air cells 20.59
Exercise (physical therapy) NEC 93.19
active musculoskeletal NEC 93.12
assisting 93.11
in pool 93.31

Exercise (*Continued*)
breathing 93.18
musculoskeletal
active NEC 93.12
passive NEC 93.17
neurologic 89.13
passive musculoskeletal NEC 93.17
resistive 93.13
Exfoliation, skin, by chemical 86.24
Exostectomy - *see also* Excision, lesion, bone 77.60
first metatarsal (hallux valgus repair) - *see* Bunionectomy
hallux valgus repair (with wedge osteotomy) - *see* Bunionectomy
Expiratory flow rate 89.38
Explant, explanation - *see* Removal
Exploration - *see also* Incision
abdomen 54.11
abdominal wall 54.0
adrenal (gland) 07.41
field 07.00
bilateral 07.02
unilateral 07.01
artery 38.00
abdominal 38.06
aorta (arch) (ascending) (descending) 38.04
head and neck NEC 38.02
intracranial NEC 38.01
lower limb 38.08
thoracic NEC 38.05
upper limb 38.03
auditory canal, external 18.02
axilla 86.09
bile duct(s) 51.59
common duct 51.51
endoscopic 51.11
for
relief of obstruction 51.42
endoscopic 51.84
removal of calculus 51.41
endoscopic 51.88
laparoscopic 51.11
for relief of obstruction 51.49
endoscopic 51.84
bladder (by incision) 57.19
endoscopic 57.32
through stoma (artificial) 57.31
bone - *see also* Incision, bone 77.10
brain (tissue) 01.39
breast 85.0
bronchus 33.0
endoscopic - *see* Bronchoscopy
bursa 83.03
hand 82.03
carotid body 39.89 ◀▥
carpal tunnel 04.43
choroid 14.9
ciliary body 12.44
colon 45.03
common bile duct 51.51
endoscopic 51.11
for
relief of obstruction 51.42
endoscopic 51.84
removal of calculus 51.41
endoscopic 51.88
coronary artery 36.99
cranium 01.24
cul-de-sac 70.12
endoscopic 70.22
disc space 03.09

◀ New   ◀ Revised   ~~deleted~~ Deleted   ● Use Additional Digit(s)   Omit code

Extraction *(Continued)*
cataract 13.19
after cataract (by)
capsulectomy 13.65
capsulotomy 13.64
discission 13.64
excision 13.65
iridocapsulectomy 13.65
mechanical fragmentation 13.66
needling 13.64
phacofragmentation (mechanical) 13.66
aspiration (simple) (with irrigation) 13.3
cryoextraction (intracapsular approach) 13.19
temporal inferior route (in presence of fistulization bleb) 13.11
curette evacuation (extracapsular approach) 13.2
emulsification (and aspiration) 13.41
erysiphake (intracapsular approach) 13.19
temporal inferior route (in presence of fistulization bleb) 13.11
extracapsular approach (with iridectomy) NEC 13.59
by temporal inferior route (in presence of fistulization bleb) 13.51
aspiration (simple) (with irrigation) 13.3
curette evacuation 13.2
emulsification (and aspiration) 13.41
linear extraction 13.2

Extraction *(Continued)*
cataract *(Continued)*
extracapsular approach NEC *(Continued)*
mechanical fragmentation with aspiration by
posterior route 13.42
specified route NEC 13.43
phacoemulsification (ultrasonic) (with aspiration) 13.41
phacofragmentation (mechanical) with aspiration by
posterior route 13.42
specified route NEC 13.43
ultrasonic (with aspiration) 13.41
rotoextraction (mechanical) with aspiration by
posterior route 13.42
specified route NEC 13.43
intracapsular (combined) (simple) (with iridectomy) (with suction) (with zonulolysis) 13.19
by temporal inferior route (in presence of fistulization bleb) 13.11
linear extraction (extracapsular approach) 13.2
phacoemulsification (and aspiration) 13.41
phacofragmentation (mechanical) with aspiration by
posterior route 13.42
specified route NEC 13.43
ultrasonic 13.41
rotoextraction (mechanical) with aspiration by
posterior route 13.42
specified route NEC 13.43

Extraction *(Continued)*
cataract *(Continued)*
secondary membranous (after cataract) (by)
capsulectomy 13.65
capsulotomy 13.64
discission 13.64
excision 13.65
iridocapsulectomy 13.65
mechanical fragmentation 13.66
needling 13.64
phacofragmentation (mechanical) 13.66
common duct stones (percutaneous) (through sinus tract) (with basket) 51.96
fat for graft or banking 86.90 ◄
foreign body - *see* Removal, foreign body
kidney stone(s), percutaneous 55.03
with fragmentation procedure 55.04
lens (eye) - *see also* Extraction, cataract 13.19
Malstrom's 72.79
with episiotomy 72.71
menstrual, menses 69.6
milk from lactating breast (manual) (pump) 99.98
tooth (by forceps) (multiple) (single) NEC 23.09
with mucoperiosteal flap elevation 23.19
deciduous 23.01
surgical NEC - *see also* Removal, tooth, surgical 23.19
vacuum, fetus 72.79
with episiotomy 72.71
vitreous - *see also* Removal, vitreous 14.72

E & F

F

Face lift 86.82
Facetectomy 77.89
Facilitation, intraocular circulation NEC 12.59
Failed (trial) forceps 73.3
Family
counselling (medical) (social) 94.49
therapy 94.42
Farabeuf operation (ischiopubiotomy) 77.39
Fasanella-Servatt operation (blepharoptosis repair) 08.35
Fasciaplasty - *see* Fascioplasty
Fascia sling operation - *see* Operation, sling
Fasciectomy 83.44
for graft 83.43
hand 82.34
hand 82.35
for graft 82.34
palmar (release of Dupuytren's contracture) 82.35
Fasciodesis 83.89
hand 82.89

Fascioplasty - *see also* Repair, fascia 83.89
hand - *see also* Repair, fascia, hand 82.89
Fasciorrhaphy - *see* Suture, fascia
Fasciotomy 83.14
Dupuytren's 82.12
with excision 82.35
Dwyer 83.14
hand 82.12
Ober-Yount 83.14
orbital - *see also* Orbitotomy 16.09
palmar (release of Dupuytren's contracture) 82.12
with excision 82.35
Fenestration
aneurysm (dissecting), thoracic aorta 39.54
aortic aneurysm 39.54
cardiac valve 35.10
chest wall 34.01
ear
inner (with graft) 20.61
revision 20.62
tympanic 19.55
labyrinth (with graft) 20.61
Lempert's (endaural) 19.9
operation (aorta) 39.54

Fenestration *(Continued)*
oval window, ear canal 19.55
palate 27.1
pericardium 37.12
semicircular canals (with graft) 20.61
stapes foot plate (with vein graft) 19.19
with incus replacement 19.11
tympanic membrane 19.55
vestibule (with graft) 20.61
Ferguson operation (hernia repair) 53.00
Fetography 87.81
Fetoscopy 75.31
Fiberoscopy - *see* Endoscopy, by site
Fibroidectomy, uterine 68.29
Fick operation (perforation of foot plate) 19.0
Filipuncture (aneurysm) (cerebral) 39.52
Filleting
hammer toe 77.56
pancreas 52.3
Filling, tooth (amalgam) (plastic) (silicate) 23.2
root canal - *see also* Therapy, root canal 23.70

Fimbriectomy - *see also* Salpingectomy,
    partial 66.69
  Uchida (with tubal ligation) 66.32
Finney operation (pyloroplasty) 44.29
Fissurectomy, anal 49.39
  endoscopic 49.31
  skin (subcutaneous tissue) 49.04
Fistulectomy - *see also* Closure, fistula, by
    site
  abdominothoracic 34.83
  abdominouterine 69.42
  anus 49.12
  appendix 47.92
  bile duct 51.79
  biliary tract NEC 51.79
  bladder (transurethral approach)
    57.84
  bone - *see also* Excision, lesion, bone
    77.60
  branchial cleft 29.52
  bronchocutaneous 33.42
  bronchoesophageal 33.42
  bronchomediastinal 34.73
  bronchopleural 34.73
  bronchopleurocutaneous 34.73
  bronchopleuromediastinal 34.73
  bronchovisceral 33.42
  cervicosigmoidal 67.62
  cholecystogastroenteric 51.93
  cornea 11.49
  diaphragm 34.83
  enterouterine 69.42
  esophagopleurocutaneous 34.73
  esophagus NEC 42.84
  fallopian tube 66.73
  gallbladder 51.93
  gastric NEC 44.63
  hepatic duct 51.79
  hepatopleural 34.73
  hepatopulmonary 34.73
  intestine
    large 46.76
    small 46.74
  intestinouterine 69.42
  joint - *see also* Excision, lesion, joint 80.80
  lacrimal
    gland 09.21
    sac 09.6
  laryngotracheal 31.62
  larynx 31.62
  mediastinocutaneous 34.73
  mouth NEC 27.53
  nasal 21.82
    sinus 22.71
  nasolabial 21.82
  nasopharyngeal 21.82
  oroantral 22.71
  oronasal 21.82
  pancreas 52.95
  perineorectal 71.72
  perineosigmoidal 71.72
  perirectal, not opening into rectum
    48.93
  pharyngoesophageal 29.53
  pharynx NEC 29.53
  pleura 34.73
  rectolabial 71.72
  rectourethral 58.43
  rectouterine 69.42
  rectovaginal 70.73
  rectovesical 57.83
  rectovulvar 71.72
  rectum 48.73
  salivary (duct) (gland) 26.42

Fistulectomy *(Continued)*
  scrotum 61.42
  skin 86.3
  stomach NEC 44.63
  subcutaneous tissue 86.3
  thoracoabdominal 34.83
  thoracogastric 34.83
  thoracointestinal 34.83
  thorax NEC 34.73
  trachea NEC 31.73
  tracheoesophageal 31.73
  ureter 56.84
  urethra 58.43
  uteroenteric 69.42
  uterointestinal 69.42
  uterorectal 69.42
  uterovaginal 69.42
  vagina 70.75
  vesicosigmoidovaginal 57.83
  vocal cords 31.62
  vulvorectal 71.72
Fistulization
  appendix 47.91
  arteriovenous 39.27
  cisterna chyli 40.62
  endolymphatic sac (for decompression)
    20.79
  esophagus, external 42.10
    cervical 42.11
    specified technique NEC 42.19
  interatrial 35.41
  labyrinth (for decompression) 20.79
  lacrimal sac into nasal cavity 09.81
  larynx 31.29
  lymphatic duct, left (thoracic) 40.62
  orbit 16.09
  peritoneal 54.93
  salivary gland 26.49
  sclera 12.69
    by trephination 12.61
    with iridectomy 12.65
  sinus, nasal NEC 22.9
  subarachnoid space 02.2
  thoracic duct 40.62
  trachea 31.29
  tracheoesophageal 31.95
  urethrovaginal 58.0
  ventricle, cerebral - *see also* Shunt,
    ventricular 02.2
Fistulogram
  abdominal wall 88.03
  chest wall 87.38
  retroperitoneum 88.14
  specified site NEC 88.49
Fistulotomy, anal 49.11
Fitting
  arch bars (orthodontic) 24.7
    for immobilization (fracture)
      93.55
  artificial limb 84.40
  contact lens 95.32
  denture (total) 99.97
    bridge (fixed) 23.42
      removable 23.43
    partial (fixed) 23.42
      removable 23.43
  hearing aid 95.48
  obturator (orthodontic) 24.7
  ocular prosthetics 95.34
  orthodontic
    appliance 24.7
    obturator 24.7
    wiring 24.7
  orthotic device 93.23

Fitting *(Continued)*
  periodontal splint (orthodontic) 24.7
  prosthesis, prosthetic device
    above knee 84.45
    arm 84.43
      lower (and hand) 84.42
      upper (and shoulder) 84.41
    below knee 84.46
    hand (and lower arm) 84.42
    leg 84.47
      above knee 84.45
      below knee 84.46
    limb NEC 84.40
    ocular 95.34
    penis (external) 64.94
    shoulder (and upper arm) 84.41
  spectacles 95.31
Five-in-one repair, knee 81.42
Fixation
  bone
    external, without reduction 93.59
      with fracture reduction - *see*
        Reduction, fracture
      cast immobilization NEC 93.53
      external fixator - *see* Fixator,
        external
      splint 93.54
      traction (skeletal) NEC 93.44
        intermittent 93.43
    internal (without fracture
      reduction) 78.50
      with fracture reduction - *see*
        Reduction, fracture
      carpal, metacarpal 78.54
      clavicle 78.51
      femur 78.55
      fibula 78.57
      humerus 78.52
      patella 78.56
      pelvic 78.59
      phalanges (foot) (hand) 78.59
      radius 78.53
      scapula 78.51
      specified site NEC 78.59
      tarsal, metatarsal 78.58
      thorax (ribs) (sternum) 78.51
        sternal fixation device with
          rigid plates 84.94 ◀
      tibia 78.57
      ulna 78.53
      vertebrae 78.59
  breast (pendulous) 85.6
  cardinal ligaments 69.22
  cervical collar 93.52
  duodenum 46.62
    to abdominal wall 46.61
  external (without manipulation for
    reduction) 93.59
    with fracture reduction - *see*
      Reduction, fracture
    cast immobilization NEC 93.53
    pressure dressing 93.56
    splint 93.54
    strapping (non-traction) 93.59
    traction (skeletal) NEC 93.44
      intermittent 93.43
  hip 81.40
  ileum 46.62
    to abdominal wall 46.61
  internal
    with fracture reduction - *see*
      Reduction, fracture
    without fracture reduction - *see*
      Fixation, bone, internal

Fixation (*Continued*)
intestine 46.60
  large 46.64
    to abdominal wall 46.63
  small 46.62
    to abdominal wall 46.61
    to abdominal wall 46.60
iris (bombé) 12.11
jejunum 46.62
  to abdominal wall 46.61
joint - *see* Arthroplasty
kidney 55.7
ligament
  cardinal 69.22
  palpebrae 08.36
omentum 54.74
parametrial 69.22
plaster jacket 93.51
  other cast 93.53
rectum (sling) 48.76
spine, with fusion - *see also* Fusion,
  spinal 81.00
spleen 41.95
splint 93.54
tendon 83.88
  hand 82.85
testis in scrotum 62.5
tongue 25.59
urethrovaginal (to Cooper's ligament)
  70.77
  with graft or prosthesis 70.78
uterus (abdominal) (vaginal)
  (ventrofixation) 69.22
vagina 70.77
  with graft or prosthesis 70.78
Fixator, external
computer assisted (dependent) 84.73
hybrid device or system 84.73
Ilizarov type 84.72
monoplanar system 84.71
ring device or system 84.72
Sheffield type 84.72
Flooding (psychologic desensitization)
  94.33
Flowmetry, Doppler (ultrasonic) - *see also*
  Ultrasonography
aortic arch 88.73
head and neck 88.71
heart 88.72
thorax NEC 88.73
Fluoroscopy - *see* Radiography
Fog therapy (respiratory) 93.94
Folding, eye muscle 15.22
multiple (two or more muscles) 15.4
Foley operation (pyeloplasty) 55.87
Fontan operation (creation of conduit
  between right atrium and
  pulmonary artery) 35.94
Foraminotomy 03.09
Forced extension, limb 93.25
Forceps delivery - *see* Delivery, forceps
Formation
adhesions
  pericardium 36.39
  pleura 34.6
anus, artificial - *see* Colostomy
duodenostomy 46.39
ileostomy - *see* Ileostomy
jejunostomy 46.39
  percutaneous (endoscopic) (PEJ)
    46.32
arteriovenous fistula (for kidney
  dialysis) (peripheral) (shunt) 39.27
  external cannula 39.93

Formation (*Continued*)
bone flap, cranial 02.03
cardiac device (defibrillator)
  (pacemaker) pocket
  with initial insertion of cardiac
    device - *omit code*
  new site (skin) (subcutaneous) 37.79
colostomy - *see* Colostomy
conduit
  apical-aortic (AAC) 35.93 ◄
  ileal (urinary) 56.51
  left ventricle and aorta 35.93
  right atrium and pulmonary artery
    35.94
  right ventricle and pulmonary
    (distal) artery 35.92
    in repair of
      pulmonary artery atresia
        35.92
      transposition of great vessels
        35.92
      truncus arteriosus 35.83
endorectal ileal pouch (H-pouch)
  (J-pouch) (S-pouch) (with
  anastomosis to anus) 45.95
fistula
  arteriovenous (for kidney dialysis)
    (peripheral shunt) 39.27
    external cannula 39.93
  bladder to skin NEC 57.18
    with bladder flap 57.21
    percutaneous 57.17
  cutaneoperitoneal 54.93
  gastric 43.19
    percutaneous (endoscopic)
      (transabdominal) 43.11
  mucous - *see* Colostomy
  rectovaginal 48.99
  tracheoesophageal 31.95
  tubulovalvular (Beck-Jianu)
    (Frank's) (Janeway) (Spivack's)
    (Ssabanejew-Frank) 43.19
  urethrovaginal 58.0
ileal
  bladder
    closed 57.87 [45.51]
    open 56.51
  conduit 56.51
interatrial fistula 35.42
mucous fistula - *see* Colostomy
pericardial
  baffle, interatrial 35.91
  window 37.12
pleural window (for drainage) 34.09
pocket
  cardiac device (defibrillator)
    (pacemaker)
    with initial insertion of cardiac
      device - *omit code*
    new site (skin) (subcutaneous)
      37.79
  loop recorder 37.79
  thalamic stimulator pulse generator
    with initial insertion of battery
      package - *omit code*
    new site (skin) (subcutaneous)
      86.09
pupil 12.39
  by iridectomy 12.14
rectovaginal fistula 48.99
reversed gastric tube (intrathoracic)
  (retrosternal) 42.58
  antesternal or antethoracic 42.68
septal defect, interatrial 35.42

Formation (*Continued*)
shunt
  abdominovenous 54.94
  arteriovenous 39.93
  peritoneojugular 54.94
  peritoneo-vascular 54.94
  pleuroperitoneal 34.05
  transjugular intrahepatic
    portosystemic (TIPS) 39.1
subcutaneous tunnel
  esophageal 42.86
    with anastomosis - *see*
      Anastomosis, esophagus,
      antesternal
  pulse generator lead wire 86.99
    with initial procedure - *omit code*
  thalamic stimulator pulse generator
    pocket
    with initial insertion of battery
      package - *omit code*
    new site (skin) (subcutaneous)
      86.09
syndactyly (finger) (toe) 86.89
tracheoesophageal 31.95
tubulovalvular fistula (Beck-Jianu)
  (Frank's) (Janeway) (Spivak's)
  (Ssabanejew-Frank) 43.19
uretero-ileostomy, cutaneous 56.51
ureterostomy, cutaneous 56.61
  ileal 56.51
urethrovaginal fistula 58.0
window
  pericardial 37.12
  pleural (for drainage) 34.09
  thoracoscopic 34.06
Fothergill (-Donald) operation (uterine
  suspension) 69.22
Fowler operation
arthroplasty of metacarpophalangeal
  joint 81.72
release (mallet finger repair) 82.84
tenodesis (hand) 82.85
thoracoplasty 33.34
Fox operation (entropion repair with
  wedge resection) 08.43
Fracture, surgical - *see also* Osteoclasis
  78.70
turbinates (nasal) 21.62
Fragmentation
lithotriptor - *see* Lithotripsy
mechanical
  cataract (with aspiration) 13.43
    posterior route 13.42
    secondary membrane 13.66
  secondary membrane (after cataract)
    13.66
ultrasonic
  cataract (with aspiration) 13.41
  stones, urinary (Kock pouch) 59.95
  urinary stones 59.95
    percutaneous nephrostomy 55.04
Franco operation (suprapubic cystotomy)
  57.18
Frank operation (permanent gastrostomy)
  43.19
Frazier (-Spiller) operation (subtemporal
  trigeminal rhizotomy) 04.02
Fredet-Ramstedt operation
  (pyloromyotomy) (with wedge
  resection) 43.3
Freeing
adhesions - *see* Lysis, adhesions
anterior synechiae (with injection of air
  or liquid) 12.32

Freeing (Continued)
  artery-vein-nerve bundle 39.91
  extraocular muscle, entrapped 15.7
  goniosynechiae (with injection of air or
      liquid) 12.31
  intestinal segment for interposition
      45.50
    large 45.52
    small 45.51
  posterior synechiae 12.33
  synechiae (posterior) 12.33
    anterior (with injection of air or
        liquid) 12.32
  vascular bundle 39.91
  vessel 39.91
Freezing
  gastric 96.32
  prostate 60.62
Frenckner operation (intrapetrosal
    drainage) 20.22
Frenectomy
  labial 27.41
  lingual 25.92
  lip 27.41
  maxillary 27.41
  tongue 25.92
Frenotomy
  labial 27.91
  lingual 25.91
Frenulumectomy - see Frenectomy
Frickman operation (abdominal
    proctopexy) 48.75
Frommel operation (shortening of
    uterosacral ligaments) 69.22
Fulguration - see also Electrocoagulation
    and Destruction, lesion, by site
  adenoid fossa 28.7
  anus 49.39
    endoscopic 49.31
  bladder (transurethral) 57.49
    suprapubic 57.59
  choroid 14.21
  duodenum 45.32
    endoscopic 45.30
  esophagus 42.39
    endoscopic 42.33
  large intestine 45.49
    endoscopic 45.43
      polypectomy 45.42
  penis 64.2
  perineum, female 71.3
  prostate, transurethral 60.29
  rectum 48.32
    radical 48.31
  retina 14.21
  scrotum 61.3
  Skene's gland 71.3
  skin 86.3
  small intestine NEC 45.34
    duodenum 45.32
      endoscopic 45.30
  stomach 43.49
    endoscopic 43.41
  subcutaneous tissue 86.3
  tonsillar fossa 28.7
  urethra 58.39
    endoscopic 58.31
  vulva 71.3

Function
  study - see also Scan, radioisotope
    gastric 89.39
    muscle 93.08
      ocular 95.25
    nasal 89.12
    pulmonary - see categories
        89.37-89.38
    renal 92.03
    thyroid 92.01
    urethral sphincter 89.23
Fundectomy, uterine 68.39
Fundoplication (esophageal) (Nissen's)
    44.66
  laparoscopic 44.67
Fundusectomy, gastric 43.89
Fusion
  atlas-axis (spine) - see Fusion, spinal,
      atlas-axis
  bone - see also Osteoplasty 78.40
  cervical (spine) (C2 level or below) - see
      Fusion, spinal, cervical
  claw toe 77.57
  craniocervical - see Fusion, spinal,
      craniocervical
  dorsal, dorsolumbar - see Fusion,
      spinal, dorsal, dorsolumbar
  epiphyseal-diaphyseal - see also Arrest,
      bone growth 78.20
  epiphysiodesis - see also Arrest, bone
      growth 78.20
  hammer toe 77.56
  joint (with bone graft) - see also
      Arthrodesis 81.20
    ankle 81.11
    claw toe 77.57
    foot NEC 81.17
    hammer toe 77.56
    hip 81.21
    interphalangeal, finger 81.28
    ischiofemoral 81.21
    metatarsophalangeal 81.16
    midtarsal 81.14
    overlapping toe(s) 77.58
    pantalar 81.11
    spinal - see also Fusion, spinal
        81.00
    subtalar 81.13
    tarsal joints NEC 81.17
    tarsometatarsal 81.15
    tibiotalar 81.11
    toe NEC 77.58
      claw toe 77.57
      hammer toe 77.56
      overlapping toe(s) 77.58
  lip to tongue 25.59
  lumbar, lumbosacral - see Fusion,
      spinal, lumbar, lumbosacral
  occiput-C2 (spinal) - see Fusion, spinal,
      occiput
  spinal, NOS (with graft) (with internal
      fixation) (with instrumentation)
      81.00 ◄▥
    anterior lumbar interbody fusion
        (ALIF) 81.06
    atlas-axis (anterior transoral)
        (posterior) 81.01
      for pseudarthrosis 81.31

Fusion (Continued)
  spinal, NOS (Continued)
    axial lumber interbody fusion
        [AxiaLIF®] 81.08 ◄
    cervical (C2 level or below) NEC
        81.02
      anterior column (interbody),
          anterolateral (anterior)
          technique 81.02 ◄▥
        for pseudarthrosis 81.32
      C1-C2 level (anterior) (posterior)
          81.01
        for pseudarthrosis 81.31
      for pseudarthrosis 81.32
      posterior column (interbody),
          posterolateral (posterior)
          technique 81.03 ◄▥
        for pseudarthrosis 81.33
    craniocervical (anterior transoral)
        (posterior) 81.01
      for pseudarthrosis 81.31
    direct lateral interbody fusion
        [DLIF] 81.06 ◄
    dorsal, dorsolumbar NEC 81.05
      anterior column (interbody),
          anterolateral (anterior)
          (extracavitary) technique
          81.04 ◄▥
        for pseudarthrosis 81.34
      for pseudarthrosis 81.35
      posterior column (interbody),
          posterolateral (posterior)
          technique 81.05 ◄▥
        for pseudarthrosis 81.35
    extreme lateral interbody fusion
        [XLIF®] 81.06 ◄
    facet 81.07 ◄
    lumbar, lumbosacral NEC 81.08
      anterior column (interbody), ◄▥
          anterolateral (anterior)
          technique 81.06 ◄▥
        for pseudarthrosis 81.36
      posterior (interbody),
          posterolateral technique
          81.08 ◄▥
        for pseudarthrosis 81.38 ◄
      lateral transverse process
          technique 81.07
        for pseudarthrosis 81.37
      posterior column, posterior
          (posterolateral) (transverse
          process) technique 81.07 ◄
    number of vertebrae - see codes
        81.62-81.64
    occiput-C2 (anterior transoral)
        (posterior) 81.01
      for pseudarthrosis 81.31
    posterior lumbar interbody fusion
        (PLIF) 81.08
    transforaminal lumbar interbody
        fusion (TLIF) 81.08

  Note: Also use either 81.62, 81.63, or
  81.64 as an additional code to show the
  total number of vertebrae fused.

  tongue (to lip) 25.59

◄ New   ◄▥ Revised   ~~deleted~~ Deleted   ● Use Additional Digit(s)   ▦ Omit code

G

Gait training 93.22
Galeaplasty 86.89
Galvanoionization 99.27
Games
    competitive 94.39
    organized 93.89
Gamma irradiation, stereotactic 92.32
Ganglionectomy
    gasserian 04.05
    lumbar sympathetic 05.23
    nerve (cranial) (peripheral) NEC 04.06
        sympathetic 05.29
    sphenopalatine (Meckel's) 05.21
    tendon sheath (wrist) 82.21
        site other than hand 83.31
    trigeminal 04.05
Ganglionotomy, trigeminal
    (radiofrequency) 04.02
Gant operation (wedge osteotomy of
    trochanter) 77.25
Garceau operation (tibial tendon transfer)
    83.75
Gardner operation (spinal meningocele
    repair) 03.51
Gas endarterectomy 38.10
    abdominal 38.16
    aorta (arch) (ascending) (descending)
        38.14
    coronary artery 36.09
    head and neck NEC 38.12
    intracranial NEC 38.11
    lower limb 38.18
    thoracic NEC 38.15
    upper limb 38.13
Gastrectomy (partial) (subtotal) NEC
    43.89
    with
        anastomosis (to) NEC 43.89
            duodenum 43.6
            esophagus 43.5
            gastrogastric 43.89
            jejunum 43.7
        esophagogastrostomy 43.5
        gastroduodenostomy (bypass) 43.6
        gastroenterostomy (bypass) 43.7
        gastrogastrostomy (bypass) 43.89
        gastrojejunostomy (bypass) 43.7
        jejunal transposition 43.81
    complete NEC 43.99
        with intestinal interposition 43.91
    distal 43.6
    Hofmeister 43.7
    Polya 43.7
    proximal 43.5
    radical NEC 43.99
        with intestinal interposition 43.91
    total NEC 43.99
        with intestinal interposition 43.91
Gastrocamera 44.19
Gastroduodenectomy - see Gastrectomy
Gastroduodenoscopy 45.13
    through stoma (artificial) 45.12
    transabdominal (operative) 45.11
Gastroduodenostomy (bypass)
    (Jaboulay's) 44.39
    with partial gastrectomy 43.6
Gastroenterostomy (bypass) NEC 44.39
    with partial gastrectomy 43.7
    laparoscopic 44.38
Gastrogastrostomy (bypass) 44.39
    with partial gastrectomy 43.89
    laparoscopic 44.38

Gastrojejunostomy (bypass) 44.39
    with partial gastrectomy 43.7
    laparoscopic 44.38
    percutaneous (endoscopic)
        for bypass 44.32
        for feeding tube placement 46.32
Gastrolysis 54.59
    laparoscopic 54.51
Gastropexy 44.64
Gastroplasty NEC 44.69
    laparoscopic 44.68
    vertical banded gastroplasty (VBG)
        44.68
Gastroplication 44.69
    laparoscopic 44.68
Gastropylorectomy 43.6
Gastrorrhaphy 44.61
Gastroscopy NEC 44.13
    through stoma (artificial) 44.12
    transabdominal (operative) 44.11
Gastrostomy (Brunschwig's)
    (decompression) (fine caliber tube)
    (Kader) (permanent) (Stamm)
    (Stamm-Kader) (temporary) (tube)
    (Witzel) 43.19
    Beck-Jianu 43.19
    Frank's 43.19
    Janeway 43.19
    percutaneous (endoscopic) (PEG)
        43.11
    Spivack's 43.19
    Ssabanejew-Frank 43.19
Gastrotomy 43.0
    for control of hemorrhage 44.49
Gavage, gastric 96.35
Gelman operation (release of clubfoot)
    83.84
Genioplasty (augmentation) (with graft)
    (with implant) 76.68
    reduction 76.67
Ghormley operation (hip fusion) 81.21
Gifford operation
    destruction of lacrimal sac 09.6
    keratotomy (delimiting) 11.1
        radial (refractive) 11.75
Gill operation
    arthrodesis of shoulder 81.23
    laminectomy 03.09
Gill-Stein operation (carporadial
    arthrodesis) 81.25
Gilliam operation (uterine suspension)
    69.22
Gingivectomy 24.31
Gingivoplasty (with bone graft) (with
    soft tissue graft) 24.2
Girdlestone operation
    laminectomy with spinal fusion
        81.00
    muscle transfer for claw toe repair
        77.57
    resection of femoral head and neck
        (without insertion of joint
        prosthesis) 77.85
        with replacement prosthesis - see
            Implant, joint, hip
    resection of hip prosthesis 80.05
        with replacement prosthesis - see
            Implant, joint, hip
Girdlestone-Taylor operation (muscle
    transfer for claw toe repair)
    77.57
Glenn operation (anastomosis of superior
    vena cava to right pulmonary
    artery) 39.21

Glenoplasty, shoulder 81.83
    with
        partial replacement 81.81
        total replacement, NEC 81.80
            other 81.80
            reverse 81.88
    for recurrent dislocation 81.82
Glomectomy
    carotid 39.89
    jugulare 20.51
Glossectomy (complete) (total) 25.3
    partial or subtotal 25.2
    radical 25.4
Glossopexy 25.59
Glossoplasty NEC 25.59
Glossorrhaphy 25.51
Glossotomy NEC 25.94
    for tongue tie 25.91
Glycoprotein IIB/IIIa inhibitor 99.20
Goebel-Frangenheim-Stoeckel
    operation (urethrovesical
    suspension) 59.4
Goldner operation (clubfoot release) 80.48
Goldthwaite operation
    ankle stabilization 81.11
    patellar stabilization 81.44
    tendon transfer for stabilization of
        patella 81.44
Gonadectomy
    ovary
        bilateral 65.51
            laparoscopic 65.53
        unilateral 65.39
            laparoscopic 65.31
    testis
        bilateral 62.41
        unilateral 62.3
Goniopuncture 12.51
    with goniotomy 12.53
Gonioscopy 12.29
Goniospasis 12.59
Goniotomy (Barkan's) 12.52
    with goniopuncture 12.53
Goodal-Power operation (vagina) 70.8
Gordon-Taylor operation (hindquarter
    amputation) 84.19
GP IIB/IIIa inhibitor, infusion 99.20
Graber-Duvernay operation (drilling of
    femoral head) 77.15
Graft, grafting
    aneurysm 39.52
        endovascular
            abdominal aorta 39.71
            lower extremity artery(s) 39.79
            thoracic aorta 39.73
            upper extremity artery(s) 39.79
    artery, arterial (patch) 39.58
        with
            excision or resection of vessel - see
                Arteriectomy, with graft
                replacement
            synthetic patch (Dacron) (Teflon)
                39.57
            tissue patch (vein) (autogenous)
                (homograft) 39.56
    blood vessel (patch) 39.58
        with
            excision or resection of vessel - see
                Angiectomy, with graft
                replacement
            synthetic patch (Dacron) (Teflon)
                39.57
            tissue patch (vein) (autogenous)
                (homograft) 39.56

Graft, grafting *(Continued)*
  bone (autogenous) (bone bank) (dual
      onlay) (heterogeneous) (inlay)
      (massive onlay) (multiple)
      (osteoperiosteal) (peg)
      (subperiosteal) (with metallic
      fixation) 78.00
    with
      arthrodesis - *see* Arthrodesis
      arthroplasty - *see* Arthroplasty
      gingivoplasty 24.2
      lengthening - *see* Lengthening,
          bone
    carpals, metacarpals 78.04
    clavicle 78.01
    facial NEC 76.91
      with total ostectomy 76.44
    femur 78.05
    fibula 78.07
    humerus 78.02
    joint - *see* Arthroplasty
    mandible 76.91
      with total mandibulectomy 76.41
    marrow - *see* Transplant, bone,
        marrow
    nose - *see* Graft, nose
    patella 78.06
    pelvic 78.09
    pericranial 02.04
    phalanges (foot) (hand) 78.09
    radius 78.03
    scapula 78.01
    skull 02.04
    specified site NEC 78.09
    spine 78.09
      with fusion - *see* Fusion, spinal
    tarsal, metatarsal 78.08
    thorax (ribs) (sternum) 78.01
    thumb (with transfer of skin flap)
        82.69
    tibia 78.07
    ulna 78.03
    vertebrae 78.09
      with fusion - *see* Fusion, spinal
  breast (*see also* Mammoplasty) 85.89
    fat graft 85.55 ◄
  buccal sulcus 27.99
  cartilage (joint) - *see also* Arthroplasty
    nose - *see* Graft, nose
  chest wall (mesh) (silastic) 34.79
  conjunctiva (free) (mucosa) 10.44
    for symblepharon repair 10.41
  cornea - *see also* Keratoplasty 11.60
  dermal-fat 86.69
  dermal regenerative 86.67
  dura 02.12
  ear
    auricle 18.79
    external auditory meatus 18.6
    inner 20.61
    pedicle preparation 86.71
  esophagus NEC 42.87
    with interposition (intrathoracic)
        NEC 42.58
      antesternal or antethoracic NEC
          42.68
      colon (intrathoracic) 42.55
        antesternal or antethoracic
            42.65
      small bowel (intrathoracic) 42.53
        antesternal or antethoracic
            42.63
  eyebrow - *see also* Reconstruction,
      eyelid, with graft 08.69

Graft, grafting *(Continued)*
  eyelid - *see also* Reconstruction, eyelid,
      with graft 08.69
    free mucous membrane 08.62
  eye socket (skin) (cartilage) (bone)
      16.63
  fallopian tube 66.79
  fascia 83.82
    with hernia repair - *see* Repair,
        hernia
    eyelid 08.32
    hand 82.72
    tarsal cartilage 08.69
  fat pad NEC 86.89
    with skin graft - *see* Graft, skin, full-
        thickness
  flap (advanced) (rotating) (sliding) - *see
      also* Graft, skin, pedicle
    tarsoconjunctival 08.64
  hair-bearing skin 86.64
  hand
    fascia 82.72
    free skin 86.62
    muscle 82.72
    pedicle (flap) 86.73
    tendon 82.79
  heart, for revascularization - *see*
      category 36.3●
  joint - *see* Arthroplasty
  larynx 31.69
  lip 27.56
    full-thickness 27.55
  lymphatic structure(s) (channel) (node)
      (vessel) 40.9
  mediastinal fat to myocardium 36.39
  meninges (cerebral) 02.12
  mouth, except palate 27.56
    full-thickness 27.55
  muscle 83.82
    hand 82.72
  myocardium, for revascularization 36.39
  nasolabial flaps 21.86
  nerve (cranial) (peripheral) 04.5
  nipple 85.86
  nose 21.89
    with
      augmentation 21.85
      rhinoplasty - *see* Rhinoplasty
      total reconstruction 21.83
    septum 21.88
    tip 21.86
  omentum 54.74
    to myocardium 36.39
  orbit (bone) (cartilage) (skin) 16.63
  outflow tract (patch) (pulmonary
      valve) 35.26
    in total repair of tetralogy of Fallot
        35.81
  ovary 65.92
  palate 27.69
    for cleft palate repair 27.62
  pedicle - *see* Graft, skin, pedicle
  penis (rib) (skin) 64.49
  pigskin 86.65
  pinch - *see* Graft, skin, free
  pocket - *see* Graft, skin, pedicle
  porcine 86.65
  postauricular (Wolff) 18.79
  razor - *see* Graft, skin, free
  rope - *see* Graft, skin, pedicle
  saphenous vein in aortocoronary
      bypass - *see* Bypass, aorto-
      coronary
  scrotum 61.49

Graft, grafting *(Continued)*
  skin (partial-thickness) (split-thickness)
      86.69
    amnionic membrane 86.66
    auditory meatus (ear) 18.6
    dermal-fat 86.69
      for breast augmentation 85.50
    dermal regenerative 86.67
    ear
      auditory meatus 18.6
      postauricular 18.79
    eyelid 08.61
    fat 86.87 ◄
    flap - *see* Graft, skin, pedicle
    free (autogenous) NEC 86.60
      breast
        deep inferior epigastric artery
            perforator (DIEP) flap,
            free 85.74
        gluteal artery perforator
            [GAP] flap, free 85.76
        superficial inferior epigastric
            artery (SIEA) flap, free
            85.75
        transverse rectus abdominis
            musculocutaneous
            (TRAM) flap, free 85.73
      lip 27.56
        thumb 86.62
          for
          pollicization 82.61
          reconstruction 82.69
    full-thickness 86.63
      breast 85.83
      hand 86.61
    hair-bearing 86.64
      eyelid or eyebrow 08.63
    hand 86.62
      full-thickness 86.61
    heterograft 86.65
    homograft 86.66
    island flap 86.70
    mucous membrane 86.69
      eyelid 08.62
    nose - *see* Graft, nose
    pedicle (flap) (tube) 86.70
      advancement 86.72
      attachment to site (advanced)
          (double) (rotating) (sliding)
          86.74
        hand (cross finger) (pocket)
            86.73
        lip 27.57
        mouth 27.57
        thumb 86.73
          for
          pollicization 82.61
          reconstruction NEC 82.69
      breast 85.84
        deep inferior epigastric artery
            perforator (DIEP) flap,
            free 85.74
        gluteal artery perforator (GAP)
            flap, free 85.76
        latissimus dorsi myocutaneous
            flap 85.71
        superficial inferior epigastric
            artery (SIEA) flap, free
            85.75
        transverse rectus abdominis
            musculocutaneous
            (TRAM) flap, free 85.73
        transverse rectus abdominis
            myocutaneous (TRAM)
            flap, pedicled 85.72

◄ New   ◄▥ Revised   ~~deleted~~ Deleted   ● Use Additional Digit(s)   ▨ Omit code

Graft, grafting (Continued)
  skin (Continued)
    pedicle (Continued)
      defatting 86.75
      delayed 86.71
      design and raising 86.71
      elevation 86.71
      preparation of (cutting) 86.71
      revision 86.75
      sculpturing 86.71
      transection 86.71
      transfer 86.74
      trimming 86.71
    postauricular 18.79
    rotation flap 86.70
    specified site NEC 86.69
      full-thickness 86.63
  tarsal cartilage 08.69
  temporalis muscle to orbit 16.63
    with exenteration of orbit 16.59
  tendon 83.81
    for joint repair - see Arthroplasty
    hand 82.79

Graft, grafting (Continued)
  testicle 62.69
  thumb (for reconstruction) NEC 82.69
  tongue (mucosal) (skin) 25.59
  trachea 31.79
  tubular (tube) - see Graft, skin, pedicle
  tunnel - see Graft, skin, pedicle
  tympanum - see also Tympanoplasty 19.4
  ureter 56.89
  vagina
    biological 70.94
    synthetic 70.95
  vein (patch) 39.58
    with
      excision or resection of vessel - see
        Phlebectomy, with graft
        replacement
      synthetic patch (Dacron) (Teflon)
        39.57
      tissue patch (vein)
        (autogenous)
        (homograft) 39.56
  vermilion border (lip) 27.56

Grattage, conjunctiva 10.31
Green operation (scapulopexy) 78.41
Grice operation (subtalar arthrodesis)
  81.13
Grip, strength 93.04
Gritti-Stokes operation (knee
  disarticulation) 84.16
Gross operation (herniorrhaphy)
  laparoscopic 53.43
    with graft or prosthesis 53.42
  other and open with graft or prosthesis
    53.41
  other open 53.49
Group therapy 94.44
Guttering, bone - see also Excision, lesion,
  bone 77.60
Guyon operation (amputation of ankle)
  84.13

H

Hagner operation (epididymotomy)
  63.92
Halsted operation - see Repair, hernia,
  inguinal
Hampton operation (anastomosis small
  intestine to rectal stump) 45.92
Hanging hip operation (muscle release)
  83.19
Harelip operation 27.54
Harrison-Richardson operation (vaginal
  suspension) 70.77
  with graft or prosthesis 70.78
Hartmann resection (of intestine) (with
  pouch) - see Colectomy, by site
Harvesting
  bone marrow 41.91
  fat for grafting or banking 86.90 ◄
  stem cells 99.79
Hauser operation
  achillotenotomy 83.11
  bunionectomy with adductor tendon
    transfer 77.53
  stabilization of patella 81.44
Heaney operation (vaginal hysterectomy)
  68.59
  laparoscopically assisted (LAVH)
    68.51
Hearing aid (with battery replacement)
  95.49
Hearing test 95.47
HeartMate® implantable heart assist
  system 37.66
HeartMate® II left ventricular assist
  system [LVAS] 37.66
Hegar operation (perineorrhaphy)
  71.79
Heine operation (cyclodialysis) 12.55
Heineke-Mikulicz operation
  (pyloroplasty) 44.29
Heller operation (esophagomyotomy)
  42.7

Hellström operation (transplantation of
  aberrant renal vessel) 39.55
Hemicolectomy
  left
    laparoscopic 17.35
    open and other 45.75
  right (extended)
    laparoscopic 17.33
    open and other 45.73
Hemicystectomy 57.6
Hemigastrectomy - see Gastrectomy
Hemiglossectomy 25.2
Hemilaminectomy (decompression)
  (exploration) 03.09
Hemilaryngectomy (anterior) (lateral)
  (vertical) 30.1
Hemimandibulectomy 76.31
Hemimastectomy (radical) 85.23
Hemimaxillectomy (with bone graft)
  (with prosthesis) 76.39
Heminephrectomy 55.4
Hemipelvectomy 84.19
Hemispherectomy (cerebral) 01.52
Hemithyroidectomy (with removal of
  isthmus) (with removal of portion of
  remaining lobe) 06.2
Hemodiafiltration (extracorporeal)
  39.95
Hemodialysis (extracorporeal) 39.95
Hemodilution 99.03
Hemofiltration (extracorporeal)
  39.95
Hemorrhage control - see Control,
  hemorrhage
Hemorrhoidectomy 49.46
  by
    cautery, cauterization 49.43
    crushing 49.45
    cryotherapy, cryosurgery 49.44
    excision 49.46
    injection 49.42
    ligation 49.45
Hemostasis - see Control, hemorrhage

Henley operation (jejunal transposition)
  43.81
Hepatectomy (complete) (total) 50.4
  partial or subtotal 50.22
Hepatic assistance, extracorporeal
  50.92
Hepaticocholangiojejunostomy 51.37
Hepaticocystoduodenostomy 51.37
Hepaticodochotomy 51.59
Hepaticoduodenostomy 51.37
Hepaticojejunostomy 51.37
Hepaticolithectomy 51.49
  endoscopic 51.88
Hepaticolithotomy 51.49
  endoscopic 51.88
Hepaticostomy 51.59
Hepaticotomy 51.59
Hepatocholangiocystoduodenostomy
  51.37
Hepatocholedochostomy 51.43
  endoscopic 51.87
Hepatoduodenostomy 50.69
Hepatogastrostomy 50.69
Hepatojejunostomy 50.69
Hepatolithotomy
  hepatic duct 51.49
  liver 50.0
Hepatopexy 50.69
Hepatorrhaphy 50.61
Hepatostomy (external) (internal)
  50.69
Hepatotomy (with packing) 50.0
Hernioplasty - see Repair, hernia
Herniorrhaphy - see Repair, hernia
Herniotomy - see Repair, hernia
Heterograft - see Graft
Heterotransplant, heterotransplantation -
  see Transplant
Hey operation (amputation of foot)
  84.12
Hey-Groves operation (reconstruction
  of anterior cruciate ligament)
  81.45

G & H

Heyman operation (soft tissue release for clubfoot) 83.84

Heyman-Herndon (-Strong) operation (correction of metatarsus varus) 80.48

Hibbs operation (lumbar spinal fusion) - *see* Fusion, lumbar

Higgins operation - *see* Repair, hernia, femoral

High forceps delivery 72.39
   with episiotomy 72.31

Hill-Allison operation (hiatal hernia repair, transpleural approach) 53.80

Hinging, mitral valve 35.12

His bundle recording 37.29

Hitchcock operation (anchoring tendon of biceps) 83.88

Hofmeister operation (gastrectomy) 43.7

Hoke operation
   midtarsal fusion 81.14
   triple arthrodesis 81.12

Holth operation
   iridencleisis 12.63
   sclerectomy 12.65

Homans operation (correction of lymph-edema) 40.9

Homograft - *see* Graft

Homotransplant, homotransplantation - *see* Transplant

Hosiery, elastic 93.59

Hutch operation (ureteroneocystostomy) 56.74

Hybinette-Eden operation (glenoid bone block) 78.01

Hydrocelectomy
   canal of Nuck (female) 69.19
     male 63.1
   round ligament 69.19
   spermatic cord 63.1
   tunica vaginalis 61.2

Hydrotherapy 93.33
   assisted exercise in pool 93.31
   whirlpool 93.32

Hymenectomy 70.31

Hymenoplasty 70.76

Hymenorrhaphy 70.76

Hymenotomy 70.11

Hyperalimentation (parenteral) 99.15

Hyperbaric oxygenation 93.95
   wound 93.59

Hyperextension, joint 93.25

Hyperthermia NEC 93.35
   for cancer treatment (interstitial) (local) (radiofrequency) (regional) (ultrasound) (whole-body) 99.85

Hypnodrama, psychiatric 94.32

Hypnosis (psychotherapeutic) 94.32
   for anesthesia - *omit code*

Hypnotherapy 94.32

Hypophysectomy (complete) (total) 07.69
   partial or subtotal 07.63
     transfrontal approach 07.61
     transsphenoidal approach 07.62
   specified approach NEC 07.68
   transfrontal approach (complete) (total) 07.64
     partial 07.61
   transsphenoidal approach (complete) (total) 07.65
     partial 07.62

Hypothermia (central) (local) 99.81
   gastric (cooling) 96.31
   freezing 96.32
   systemic (in open heart surgery) 39.62

Hypotympanotomy 20.23

Hysterectomy 68.9
   abdominal 68.49
     laparoscopic (total) [TLH] 68.41
     partial or subtotal (supracervical) (supravaginal) 68.39
     radical (modified) (Wertheim's) 68.69
       laparoscopic (total) [TLRH] 68.61

Hysterectomy (Continued)
   abdominal (Continued)
     supracervical 68.39
       classic infrafasical SEMM hysterectomy [CISH] 68.31
       laparoscopically assisted [LASH] 68.31
   vaginal (complete) (partial) (subtotal) (total) 68.59
     laparoscopically assisted (LAVH) 68.51
     radical (Schauta) 68.79
       laparoscopic [LRVH] 68.71

Hysterocolpectomy (radical) (vaginal) 68.79
   abdominal 68.69
     laparoscopic 68.61
   laparoscopic 68.71

Hysterogram NEC 87.85
   percutaneous 87.84

Hysterolysis 54.59
   laparoscopic 54.51

Hysteromyomectomy 68.29

Hysteropexy 69.22

Hysteroplasty 69.49

Hysterorrhaphy 69.41

Hysterosalpingography gas (contrast) 87.82
   opaque dye (contrast) 87.83

Hysterosalpingostomy 66.74

Hysteroscopy 68.12
   with
     ablation
       endometrial 68.23
     biopsy 68.16

Hysterotomy (with removal of foreign body) (with removal of hydatidiform mole) 68.0
   for intrauterine transfusion 75.2
   obstetrical 74.99
     for termination of pregnancy 74.91

Hysterotrachelectomy 67.4

Hysterotracheloplasty 69.49

Hysterotrachelorrhaphy 69.41

Hysterotrachelotomy 69.95

I

IAEMT (intraoperative anesthetic effect monitoring and titration) 00.94 [89.14]

ICCE (intracapsular cataract extraction) 13.19

Ileal
   bladder
     closed 57.87 [45.51]
     open (ileoureterostomy) 56.51
   conduit (ileoureterostomy) 56.51

Ileocecostomy 45.93

Ileocolectomy
   laparoscopic 17.33
   open and other 45.73

Ileocolostomy 45.93

Ileocolotomy 45.00

Ileocystoplasty (isolated segment anastomosis) (open loop) 57.87 [45.51]

Ileoduodenotomy 45.01

Ileoectomy (partial) 45.62
   with cecectomy
     laparoscopic 17.32
     open and other 45.72

Ileoentectropy 46.99

Ileoesophagostomy 42.54

Ileoileostomy 45.91
   proximal to distal segment 45.62

Ileoloopogram 87.78

Ileopancreatostomy 52.96

Ileopexy 46.61

Ileoproctostomy 45.95

Ileorectostomy 45.93

Ileorrhaphy 46.73

Ileoscopy 45.13
   through stoma (artificial) 45.12
   transabdominal (operative) 45.11

Ileosigmoidostomy 45.93

Ileostomy 46.20
   continent (permanent) 46.22
     for urinary diversion 56.51

Ileostomy (Continued)
   delayed opening 46.24
   Hendon (temporary) 46.21
   loop 46.01
   Paul (temporary) 46.21
   permanent 46.23
     continent 46.22
   repair 46.41
   revision 46.41
   tangential (temporary) 46.21
   temporary 46.21
   transplantation to new site 46.23
   tube (temporary) 46.21
   ureteral
     external 56.51
     internal 56.71

Ileotomy 45.02

Ileotransversostomy 45.93

Ileoureterostomy (Bricker's) (ileal bladder) 56.51

◀ New   ◀||| Revised   ~~deleted~~ Deleted   ● Use Additional Digit(s)   Omit code

H & I

Imaging (diagnostic)
   by
      optical coherence tomography
         (OCT) - *see* OCT and
         Tomography, optical
         coherence
   diagnostic, not elsewhere classified 88.90
   endovascular ultrasound - *see* Imaging,
      intravascular ultrasound
   intraoperative
      iMRI - *see* Imaging, magnetic
         resonance
      intravascular - *see* Imaging,
         intravascular ultrasound
   intravascular ultrasound (IVUS) 00.29
      aorta 00.22
      aortic arch 00.22
      carotid vessel 00.21
      cerebral vessel, extracranial 00.21
      coronary vessel 00.24
      intrathoracic vessel 00.22
      other specified vessel 00.28
      peripheral vessel 00.23
      renal vessel 00.25
      vena cava (inferior) (superior)
         00.22
   magnetic resonance (nuclear) (proton)
      NEC 88.97
      abdomen 88.97
      bladder (urinary) 88.95
      bone marrow blood supply 88.94
      brain (brain stem) 88.91
         intraoperative (iMRI) 88.96
         real-time 88.96
      chest (hilar) (mediastinal) 88.92
      computer assisted surgery (CAS)
         with MR/MRA 00.32
      extremity (lower) (upper) 88.94
      eye orbit 88.97
      face 88.97
      head NEC 88.97
      musculoskeletal 88.94
      myocardium 88.92
      neck 88.97
      orbit of eye 88.97
      prostate 88.95
      specified site NEC 88.97
      spinal canal (cord) (spine) 88.93
   VH™ - IVUS - *see* Imaging (diagnostic),
      intravascular ultrasound (IVUS),
      by site
   virtual histology intravascular
      ultrasound - *see* Imaging
      (diagnostic), intravascular
      ultrasound (IVUS), by site
Immobilization (by)
   with fracture-reduction - *see* Reduction,
      fracture
   bandage 93.59
   bone 93.53
   cast NEC 93.53
      with reduction of fracture or
         dislocation - *see* Reduction,
         fracture, *and* Reduction,
         dislocation
   device NEC 93.59
   pressure dressing 93.56
   splint (plaster) (tray) 93.54
      with reduction of fracture or
         dislocation - *see* Reduction,
         fracture, *and* Reduction,
         dislocation
   stereotactic head frame 93.59
   strapping (non-traction) 93.59

Immunoadsorption
   extracorporeal (ECI) 99.76
Immunization - *see also* Vaccination
   allergy 99.12
   autoimmune disease 99.13
   BCG 99.33
   brucellosis 99.55
   cholera 99.31
   diphtheria 99.36
   DPT 99.39
   epidemic parotitis 99.46
   German measles 99.47
   Hemophilus influenzae 99.52
   influenza 99.52
   measles 99.45
   meningococcus 99.55
   mumps 99.46
   pertussis 99.37
   plague 99.34
   poliomyelitis 99.41
   rabies 99.44
   rubella 99.47
   salmonella 99.55
   smallpox 99.42
   staphylococcus 99.55
   TAB 99.32
   tetanus 99.38
   triple vaccine 99.48
   tuberculosis 99.33
   tularemia 99.35
   typhoid-paratyphoid 99.32
   typhus 99.55
   viral NEC 99.55
   whooping cough 99.37
   yellow fever 99.43
Immunotherapy, antineoplastic
   99.28
   C-Parvum 99.28
   Interferon 99.28
   Interleukin-2 (low-dose) 99.28
      high-dose 00.15
   Levamisole 99.28
   Proleukin (low-dose) 99.28
      high-dose 00.15
   Thymosin 99.28
Impella® percutaneous external heart
   assist device 37.68
Implant, implantation
   abdominal artery to coronary artery
      36.17
   artery
      aortic branches to heart muscle
         36.2
      mammary to ventricular wall
         (Vineberg) 36.2
   baffle, atrial or interatrial 35.91
   biliary fistulous tract into stomach or
      intestine 51.39
   bipolar endoprosthesis (femoral head)
      81.52
   bladder sphincter, artificial (inflatable)
      58.93
   blood vessels to myocardium 36.2
   bone growth stimulator (invasive)
      (percutaneous) (semi-invasive) -
      see category 78.9●
   bone morphogenetic protein (Infuse™
      (OP-1™) (recombinant) (rhBMP)
      84.52
   bone void filler 84.55
      that with percutaneous vertebral
         augmentation 81.66
      that with percutaneous
         vertebroplasty 81.65

Implant, implantation *(Continued)*
   breast (for augmentation) (bilateral)
      85.54
      unilateral 85.53
   cardiac contractility modulation (CCM)
      rechargeable pulse generator only
         17.52
      total system 17.51
   cardiac resynchronization device
      defibrillator (biventricular) (BiV
         ICD) (BiV pacemaker with
         defibrillator) (BiV pacing with
         defibrillator) (CRT-D) (device
         and one or more leads) (total
         system) 00.51
         left ventricular coronary venous
            lead only 00.52
         pulse generator only 00.54
      pacemaker (BiV) (biventricular)
         (CRT-P) (device and one or
         more leads) (total system)
         00.50
         left ventricular coronary venous
            lead only 00.52
         pulse generator only 00.53
   cardiac support device (CSD) 37.41
   cardiomyostimulation system 37.67
   cardioverter/defibrillator (automatic)
      37.94
      leads only (patch electrode) (pacing)
         (sensing) 37.95
      pulse generator only 37.96
      total system 37.94
   CCM (cardiac contractility modulation)
      rechargeable pulse generator
         only 17.52
      total system 17.51
   chemotherapeutic agent
      00.10 ◀
   chest wall (mesh) (silastic) 34.79
   chin (polyethylene) (silastic)
      76.68
   cochlear (electrode) 20.96
      prosthetic device (electrode and
         receiver) 20.96
         channel (single) 20.97
            multiple 20.98
         electrode only 20.99
         internal coil only 20.99
   coil(s), endovascular 39.79
      head or neck vessels
         bare metal 39.75
         bioactive 39.76
   CorCap™ 37.41
   cornea 11.73
   CRT-D (biventricular defibrillator)
      (BiV ICD) (BiV pacemaker with
      defibrillator) (BiV pacing with
      defibrillator) (cardiac
      resynchronization defibrillator)
      (device and one or more leads)
      00.51
      left ventricular coronary venous
         lead only 00.52
      pulse generator only 00.54
   CRT-P (biventricular pacemaker)
      (BiV pacemaker) (cardiac
      resynchronization pacemaker)
      (device and one or more leads)
      00.50
      left ventricular coronary venous
         lead only 00.52
      pulse generator only 00.53
   custodis eye 14.41

Implant, implantation (Continued)
  dental (endosseous) (prosthetic)
      23.6
  device
      adjustable gastric band and port
          44.95
      bronchial device NOS 33.79
      bronchial substance NOS 33.79
      bronchial valve
          multiple lobes 33.73
          single lobe 33.71
      cardiac support device (CSD)
          37.41
      CorCap™ 37.41
      epicardial support device 37.41
      Lap-Band™ 44.95
      left atrial appendage 37.36
      left atrial filter 37.36
      left atrial occluder 37.36
      MitraClip® percutaneous mitral
          valve leaflet clip 35.97 ◄
      prosthetic cardiac support device
          37.41
      sternal fixation device with rigid
          plates 84.94 ◄
      subcutaneous for intracardiac or
          great vessel hemodynamic
          monitoring 00.57
      vascular access 86.07
      ventricular support device 37.41
  diaphragmatic pacemaker 34.85
  Dynesys® 84.82
  electrode(s)
      brain 02.93
          depth 02.93
          foramen ovale 02.93
          sphenoidal 02.96
      cardiac (initial) (transvenous)
          37.70
          atrium (initial) 37.73
              replacement 37.76
          atrium and ventricle (initial)
              37.72
              replacement 37.76
          epicardium (sternotomy or
              thoracotomy approach)
              37.74
          left ventricular coronary venous
              system 00.52
          temporary transvenous
              pacemaker system
              37.78
              during and immediately
                  following cardiac
                  surgery 39.64
          ventricle (initial) 37.71
              replacement 37.76
      carotid sinus 39.82 ◄▥
          with synchronous pulse
              generator implantation
              (total system) 39.81 ◄
      depth 02.93
      foramen ovale 02.93
      gastric 04.92
      heart - see also Implant, electrode(s),
          cardiac 37.70
      intracranial 02.93
      osteogenic (invasive) for bone
          growth stimulation - see
          category 78.9●
      peripheral nerve 04.92
      sacral nerve 04.92
      sphenoidal 02.96
      spine 03.93

Implant, implantation (Continued)
  electroencephalographic receiver
      brain 02.93
      intracranial 02.93
  electronic stimulator
      anus (subcutaneous) 49.92
      bladder 57.96
      bone growth (invasive)
          (percutaneous) (semi-invasive)
          78.9●
      brain - see Implant, neurostimulator,
          brain
      carotid sinus 39.83 ◄▥
          with synchronous lead(s)
              implantation (total system)
              39.81 ◄
      cochlear 20.96
          channel (single) 20.97
              multiple 20.98
      gastric 04.92
      intracranial - see Implant,
          neurostimulator,
          intracranial
      peripheral nerve - see Implant,
          neurostimulator, peripheral
          nerve
      phrenic nerve 34.85
      skeletal muscle 83.92
      spine - see Implant, neurostimulator,
          spine
      ureter 56.92
  electrostimulator - see Implant,
      electronic stimulator, by site
  endoprosthesis
      bile duct 51.87
      femoral head (bipolar) 81.52
      pancreatic duct 52.93
  endosseous (dental) 23.6
  epidural pegs 02.93
  epikeratoprosthesis 11.73
  estradiol (pellet) 99.23
  eye (Iowa type) 16.61
      integrated 16.41
  facial bone, synthetic (alloplastic) 76.92
  fallopian tube (Mulligan hood)
      (silastic tube) (stent) 66.93
      into uterus 66.74
  gastroepiploic artery to coronary
      artery 36.17
  hearing device, electromagnetic 20.95
  heart
      artificial 37.52
          total internal biventricular
              replacement system 37.52
              AbioCor® 37.52
              CardioWest™ (TAH-t) 37.52
      assist system
          CentriMag® – see Insertion,
              circulatory support device
          external heart assist device,
              percutaneous – see
              Insertion, circulatory
              support device
          external heart assist system, open
              approach 37.65
          extrinsic 37.68
          HeartMate® implantable heart
              assist system 37.66
          HeartMate® II left ventricular
              assist system [LVAS] 37.66
          Impella® percutaneous external
              circulatory assist device -
              see Insertion, circulatory
              support device

Implant, implantation (Continued)
  heart (Continued)
      assist system (Continued)
          implantable 37.66
          non-implantable – see Insertion,
              circulatory support device
          percutaneous external
              circulatory assist device –
              see Insertion, circulatory
              support device
          pulsation balloon 37.61
          pVAD (percutaneous VAD) – see
              Insertion, circulatory
              support device
          TandemHeart® - see Insertion,
              circulatory support
              device
          temporary non-implantable
              circulatory assist device -
              see Insertion, circulatory
              support device
          that for destination therapy (DT)
              37.66
      auxiliary ventricle 37.62
      cardiac support device (CSD)
          37.41
      circulatory assist system - see
          Implant, heart, assist system
      CorCap™ 37.41
      epicardial support device 37.41
      pacemaker - see also Implant,
          pacemaker, cardiac 37.80
      prosthetic cardiac support device
          37.41
      total internal biventricular
          replacement system 37.52
      valve(s)
          prosthesis or synthetic device
              (partial) (synthetic) (total)
              35.20
              aortic 35.22
              mitral 35.24
              pulmonary 35.26
              tricuspid 35.28
          tissue graft 35.20
              aortic 35.21
              mitral 35.23
              pulmonary 35.25
              tricuspid 35.27
      ventricular support device 37.41
  inert material
      breast (for augmentation) (bilateral)
          85.54
          unilateral 85.53
      larynx 31.0
      nose 21.85
      orbit (eye socket) 16.69
          reinsertion 16.62
      scleral shell (cup) (with evisceration
          of eyeball) 16.31
          reinsertion 16.62
      Tenon's capsule (with enucleation of
          eyeball) 16.42
          with attachment of muscles
              16.41
          reinsertion 16.62
      urethra 59.79
      vocal cord(s) 31.0
  infusion pump 86.06
  interbody spinal fusion device
      84.51
  intracardiac or great vessel
      hemodynamic monitor,
      subcutaneous 00.57

◄ New   ◄▥ Revised   ~~deleted~~ Deleted   ● Use Additional Digit(s)   ▨ Omit code

Implant, implantation *(Continued)*
  joint (prosthesis) (silastic) (Swanson
    type) NEC 81.96
    ankle (total) 81.56
      revision 81.59
    carpocarpal, carpometacarpal 81.74
    elbow (total) 81.84
      revision 81.97
    extremity (bioelectric) (cineplastic)
      (kineplastic) 84.40
      lower 84.48
        revision 81.59
      upper 84.44
        revision 81.97
    femoral (bipolar endoprosthesis)
      81.52
      revision NOS 81.53
        acetabular and femoral
          components (total) 00.70
        acetabular component only
          00.71
        acetabular liner and/or
          femoral head only 00.73
        femoral component only 00.72
        femoral head only and/or
          acetabular liner 00.73
        total (acetabular and femoral
          components) 00.70
    finger 81.71
    hand (metacarpophalangeal)
      (interphalangeal) 81.71
      revision 81.97
    hip (partial) 81.52
      revision NOS 81.53
        acetabular and femoral
          components (total) 00.70
        acetabular component only
          00.71
        acetabular liner and/or
          femoral head only 00.73
        femoral component only 00.72
        femoral head only and/or
          acetabular liner 00.73
        partial
          acetabular component only
            00.71
          acetabular liner and/or
            femoral head only
            00.73
          femoral component only
            00.72
          femoral head only and/or
            acetabular liner 00.73
        total (acetabular and femoral
          components) 00.70
      total 81.51
        revision (acetabular and
          femoral components)
    interphalangeal 81.71
      revision 81.97
    knee (partial) (total) 81.54
      revision NOS 81.55
        femoral component 00.82
        partial
          femoral component 00.82
          patellar component 00.83
          tibial component 00.81
          tibial insert 00.84
        patellar component 00.83
        tibial component 00.81
        tibial insert 00.84
        total (all components) 00.80
    metacarpophalangeal 81.71
      revision 81.97

Implant, implantation *(Continued)*
  joint NEC *(Continued)*
    shoulder (partial) 81.81
      revision 81.97
      total replacement, NEC 81.80 ◀▦
        other 81.80 ◀
        reverse 81.88 ◀
    toe 81.57
      for hallux valgus repair 77.59
      revision 81.59
    wrist (partial) 81.74
      revision 81.97
      total replacement 81.73
  kidney, mechanical 55.97
  Lap-Band™ 44.95
  larynx 31.0
  leads (cardiac) - *see* Implant,
    electrode(s), cardiac
  limb lengthening device, internal
    (NOS) 84.54
    with kinetic distraction 84.53
  mammary artery
    in ventricle (Vineberg) 36.2
    to coronary artery (single vessel)
      36.15
      double vessel 36.16
  M-Brace™ 84.82
  Mulligan hood, fallopian tube
    66.93
  nerve (peripheral) 04.79
  neuropacemaker - *see* Implant,
    neurostimulator, by site
  neurostimulator
    electrodes
      brain 02.93
      ~~carotid sinus 39.8~~
      gastric 04.92
      intracranial 02.93
      peripheral nerve 04.92
      sacral nerve 04.92
      spine 03.93
    pulse generator (subcutaneous)
      86.96 ◀▦
      cranial 01.20 ◀
      dual array 86.95
        rechargeable 86.98
      single array 86.94
        rechargeable 86.97
  nose 21.85
  Ommaya reservoir 02.2
  orbit 16.69
    reinsertion 16.62
  outflow tract prosthesis (heart) (gusset
    type)
    in
      pulmonary valvuloplasty
        35.26
      total repair of tetralogy of
        Fallot 35.81
  ovary into uterine cavity 65.72
    laparoscopic 65.75
  pacemaker
    brain - *see* Implant,
      neurostimulator, brain
    cardiac (device) (initial) (permanent)
      (replacement) 37.80
      dual-chamber device (initial)
        37.83
        replacement 37.87
      resynchronization device
        (biventricular pacemaker)
        (BiV pacemaker) (CRT-P)
        device only (initial)
          (replacement) 00.53

Implant, implantation *(Continued)*
  pacemaker *(Continued)*
    cardiac *(Continued)*
      resynchronization device
        (Continued)
        total system (device and one
          or more leads) 00.50
        transvenous lead into left
          ventricular coronary
          venous system 00.52
      single-chamber device (initial)
        37.81
        rate responsive 37.82
        replacement 37.85
          rate responsive 37.86
      temporary transvenous
        pacemaker system
        37.78
        during and immediately
          following cardiac
          surgery 39.64
    carotid sinus 39.89 ◀▦
    diaphragm 34.85
    gastric 04.92
    intracranial - *see* Implant,
      neurostimulator, intracranial
    neural - *see* Implant,
      neurostimulator, by site
    peripheral nerve - *see* Implant,
      neurostimulator, peripheral
      nerve
    spine - *see* Implant, neurostimulator,
      spine
  pancreas (duct) 52.96
  penis, prosthesis (internal)
    inflatable 64.97
    non-inflatable 64.95
  port, vascular access device 86.07
  premaxilla 76.68
  progesterone (subdermal) 99.23
  prosthesis, prosthetic device
    acetabulum (Aufranc-Turner) 81.52
    ankle (total) 81.56
    arm (bioelectric) (cineplastic)
      (kineplastic) 84.44
    breast (bilateral) (Cronin) (Dow-
      Corning) (Perras-Pappillon)
      85.54
      unilateral 85.53
    cardiac support device (CSD)
      (CorCap™) 37.41
    cochlear 20.96
      channel (single) 20.97
        multiple 20.98
    extremity (bioelectric) (cineplastic)
      (kineplastic) 84.40
      lower 84.48
      upper 84.44
    fallopian tube (Mulligan hood)
      (stent) 66.93
    femoral head (Austin-Moore)
      (bipolar) (Eicher) (Thompson)
      81.52
    revision NOS 81.53
      acetabular and femoral
        components (total)
        00.70
      acetabular component only
        00.71
      acetabular liner and/or
        femoral head only
        00.73
      femoral component only
        00.72

Implant, implantation (Continued)
  prosthesis, prosthetic device (Continued)
    femoral head (Continued)
      revision NOS (Continued)
        femoral head only and/or
          acetabular liner 00.73
        partial
          acetabular component only
            00.71
          acetabular liner and/or
            femoral head only
            00.73
          femoral component only
            00.72
          femoral head only and/or
            acetabular liner 00.73
        total (acetabular and
          femoral components
          00.70
    joint (Swanson type) NEC 81.96
      ankle (total) 81.56
      carpocarpal, carpometacarpal
        81.74
      elbow (total) 81.84
      finger 81.71
      hand (metacarpophalangeal)
        (interphalangeal) 81.71
      hip (partial) 81.52
        revision NOS 81.53
          acetabular and femoral
            components (total)
            00.70
          acetabular component only
            00.71
          acetabular liner and/or
            femoral head only
            00.73
          femoral component only
            00.72
          femoral head only and/or
            acetabular liner 00.73
          partial
            acetabular component
              only 00.71
            acetabular liner and/or
              femoral head only
              00.73
            femoral component only
              00.72
            femoral head only and/
              or acetabular liner
              00.73
          total (acetabular and
            femoral components)
            00.70
        total 81.51
          revision (acetabular and
            femoral components)
            00.70
      interphalangeal 81.71
      knee (partial) (total) 81.54
        revision NOS 81.55
          femoral component 00.82
          partial
            femoral component 00.82
            patellar component 00.83
            tibial component 00.81
            tibial insert 00.84
          patellar component 00.83
          tibial component 00.81
          tibial insert 00.84
          total (all components)
            00.80
      metacarpophalangeal 81.71

Implant, implantation (Continued)
  prosthesis, prosthetic device (Continued)
    joint NEC (Continued)
      shoulder (partial) 81.81
        total, NEC 81.80 ◀▥
          other 81.80 ◀
          reverse 81.88 ◀
      toe 81.57
        for hallux valgus repair 77.59
      wrist (partial) 81.74
        total 81.73
    leg (bioelectric) (cineplastic)
      (kineplastic) 84.48
    lens 13.91
    outflow tract (heart) (gusset type)
      in
        pulmonary valvuloplasty 35.26
        total repair of tetralogy of
          Fallot 35.81
    penis (internal) (non-inflatable)
      64.95
      inflatable (internal) 64.97
    skin (dermal regenerative) (matrix)
      86.67
    testicular (bilateral) (unilateral) 62.7
  pulsation balloon (phase-shift) 37.61
  pump, infusion 86.06
  radial artery 36.19
  radioactive isotope 92.27
  radium (radon) 92.27
  retinal attachment 14.41
    with buckling 14.41
  Rheos™ carotid sinus baroreflex
    activation device 39.81 ◀▥
  Rickham reservoir 02.2
  silicone
    breast (bilateral) 85.54
      unilateral 85.53
    skin (for filling of defect) 86.02
      for augmentation NEC 86.89
  spine NEC 84.59
    facet replacement device(s) 84.84
    interspinous process decompression
      device 84.80
    pedicle-based dynamic stabilization
      device(s) 84.82
    posterior motion preservation
      device(s) - see category 84.8●
  stimoceiver - see Implant,
    neurostimulator, by site
  stimulator
    electrodes ◀
      carotid sinus (baroreflex
        activation device) 39.8
        39.82 ◀▥
        with synchronous pulse
          generator implantation
          (total system) 39.81 ◀
    pulse generator ◀
      carotid sinus (baroreflex
        activation device) 39.83 ◀
        with synchronous electrode(s)
          implantation (total
          system) 39.81 ◀
  sudural
    grids 02.93
    strips 02.93
  Swanson prosthesis (joint) (silastic)
    NEC 81.96
    carpocarpal, carpometacarpal 81.74
    finger 81.71
    hand (interphalangeal)
      (metacarpophalangeal) 81.71
    interphalangeal 81.71

Implant, implantation (Continued)
  Swanson prosthesis NEC (Continued)
    knee (partial) (total) 81.54
      revision 81.55
    metacarpophalangeal 81.71
    toe 81.57
      for hallux valgus repair 77.59
    wrist (partial) 81.74
      total 81.73
  systemic arteries into myocardium
    (Vineberg type operation) 36.2
  Tandem™ heart 37.68
  telescope (IMT) (miniature) 13.91
  testicular prosthesis (bilateral)
    (unilateral) 62.7
  tissue expander (skin) NEC 86.93
    breast 85.95
  tissue mandril (for vascular graft)
    39.99
    with
      blood vessel repair 39.56
      vascular bypass or shunt - see
        Bypass, vascular
  tooth (bud) (germ) 23.5
    prosthetic 23.6
  umbrella, vena cava 38.7
  ureters into
    bladder 56.74
    intestine 56.71
      external diversion 56.51
    skin 56.61
  urethra
    for repair of urinary stress
      incontinence
      collagen 59.72
      fat 59.72
      polytef 59.72
  urethral sphincter, artificial (inflatable)
    58.93
  urinary sphincter, artificial (inflatable)
    58.93
  vascular access device 86.07
  vitreous (silicone) 14.75
    for retinal reattachment 14.41
      with buckling 14.41
  vocal cord(s) (paraglottic) 31.98
  X Stop™ 84.80
Implosion (psychologic desensitization)
  94.33
Incision (and drainage)
  with
    exploration - see Exploration
    removal of foreign body - see
      Removal, foreign body
  abdominal wall 54.0
    as operative approach - omit code
  abscess - see also Incision, by site
    antecubital fossa 86.04
    appendix 47.2
      with appendectomy 47.09
        laparoscopic 47.01
    axilla 86.04
    cheek 86.04
    extraperitoneal 54.0
    face 86.04
    gluteal 86.04
    groin region (abdominal wall)
      (inguinal) 54.0
      skin 86.04
      subcutaneous tissue 86.04
    hair follicle 86.04
    ischiorectal 49.01
    lip 27.0
    nailbed or nailfold 86.04

Incision (Continued)

abscess (Continued)
neck 86.04
omental 54.19
paronychia 86.04
perianal 49.01
perigastric 54.19
perineum (female) 71.09
male 86.04
perisplenic 54.19
peritoneal NEC 54.19
pelvic (female) 70.12
popliteal space 86.04
retroperitoneal 54.0
sclera 12.89
skin 86.04
subcutaneous tissue 86.04
subdiaphragmatic 54.19
subhepatic 54.19
submaxillary 86.04
subphrenic 54.19
supraclavicular fossa 86.04
vas deferens 63.6
adrenal gland 07.41
alveolus, alveolar bone 24.0
antecubital fossa 86.09
anus NEC 49.93
fistula 49.11
septum 49.91
appendix 47.2
artery 38.00
abdominal 38.06
aorta (arch) (ascending)
(descending) 38.04
head and neck NEC 38.02
intracranial NEC 38.01
lower limb 38.08
thoracic NEC 38.05
upper limb 38.03
atrium (heart) 37.11
auditory canal or meatus, external
18.02
auricle 18.09
axilla 86.09
Bartholin's gland or cyst 71.22
bile duct (with T or Y tube insertion)
NEC 51.59
common (exploratory) 51.51
for
relief of obstruction NEC 51.42
removal of calculus 51.41
for
exploration 51.59
relief of obstruction 51.49
bladder 57.19
neck (transurethral) 57.91
percutaneous suprapubic (closed)
57.17
suprapubic NEC 57.18
blood vessel - see also Angiotomy 38.00
bone 77.10
alveolus, alveolar 24.0
carpals, metacarpals 77.14
clavicle 77.11
facial 76.09
femur 77.15
fibula 77.17
humerus 77.12
patella 77.16
pelvic 77.19
phalanges (foot) (hand) 77.19
radius 77.13
scapula 77.11
skull 01.24

Incision (Continued)

bone (Continued)
specified site NEC 77.19
tarsals, metatarsals 77.18
thorax (ribs) (sternum) 77.11
tibia 77.17
ulna 77.13
vertebrae 77.19
brain 01.39
cortical adhesions 02.91
breast (skin) 85.0
with removal of tissue expander
85.96
bronchus 33.0
buccal space 27.0
bulbourethral gland 58.91
bursa 83.03
hand 82.03
pharynx 29.0
carotid body 39.89 ◀▥
cerebral (meninges) 01.39
epidural or extradural space
01.24
subarachnoid or subdural space
01.31
cerebrum 01.39
cervix 69.95
to
assist delivery 73.93
replace inverted uterus 75.93
chalazion 08.09
with removal of capsule 08.21
cheek 86.09
chest wall (for extrapleural drainage)
(for removal of foreign body)
34.01
as operative approach - omit code
common bile duct (for exploration)
51.51
for
relief of obstruction 51.42
removal of calculus 51.41
common wall between posterior left
atrium and coronary sinus (with
roofing of resultant defect with
patch graft) 35.82
conjunctiva 10.1
cornea 11.1
radial (refractive) 11.75
cranial sinus 01.21
craniobuccal pouch 07.72
cul-de-sac 70.12
cyst
dentigerous 24.0
radicular (apical) (periapical) 24.0
Duhrssen's (cervix, to assist delivery)
73.93
duodenum 45.01
ear
external 18.09
inner 20.79
middle 20.23
endocardium 37.11
endolymphatic sac 20.79
epididymis 63.92
epidural space, cerebral 01.24
epigastric region 54.0
intra-abdominal 54.19
esophagus, esophageal NEC 42.09
web 42.01
exploratory - see Exploration
extradural space (cerebral) 01.24
extrapleural 34.01
eyebrow 08.09

Incision (Continued)

eyelid 08.09
margin (trichiasis) 08.01
face 86.09
fallopian tube 66.01
fascia 83.09
with division 83.14
hand 82.12
hand 82.09
with division 82.12
fascial compartments, head and neck 27.0
fistula, anal 49.11
flank 54.0
furuncle - see Incision, by site
gallbladder 51.04
gingiva 24.0
gluteal 86.09
groin region (abdominal wall)
(inguinal) 54.0
skin 86.09
subcutaneous tissue 86.09
gum 24.0
hair follicles 86.09
heart 37.10
valve - see Valvulotomy
hematoma - see also Incision, by site
axilla 86.04
broad ligament 69.98
ear 18.09
episiotomy site 75.91
fossa (superficial) NEC 86.04
groin region (abdominal wall)
(inguinal) 54.0
skin 86.04
subcutaneous tissue 86.04
laparotomy site 54.12
mediastinum 34.1
perineum (female) 71.09
male 86.04
popliteal space 86.04
scrotum 61.0
skin 86.04
space of Retzius 59.19
subcutaneous tissue 86.04
vagina (cuff) 70.14
episiotomy site 75.91
obstetrical NEC 75.92
hepatic ducts 51.59
hordeolum 08.09
hygroma - see also Incision, by site
cystic 40.0
hymen 70.11
hypochondrium 54.0
intra-abdominal 54.19
hypophysis 07.72
iliac fossa 54.0
infratemporal fossa 27.0
ingrown nail 86.09
intestine 45.00
large 45.03
small 45.02
intracerebral 01.39
intracranial (epidural space)
(extradural space) 01.24
subarachnoid or subdural space
01.31
intraperitoneal 54.19
ischiorectal tissue 49.02
abscess 49.01
joint structures - see also Arthrotomy
80.10
kidney 55.01
pelvis 55.11
labia 71.09

Incision (*Continued*)
  lacrimal
    canaliculus 09.52
    gland 09.0
    passage NEC 09.59
    punctum 09.51
    sac 09.53
  larynx NEC 31.3
  ligamentum flavum (spine) - *omit code*
  liver 50.0
  lung 33.1
  lymphangioma 40.0
  lymphatic structure (channel) (node)
      (vessel) 40.0
  mastoid 20.21
  mediastinum 34.1
  meibomian gland 08.09
  meninges (cerebral) 01.31
    spinal 03.09
  midpalmar space 82.04
  mouth NEC 27.92
    floor 27.0
  muscle 83.02
    with division 83.19
      hand 82.19
    hand 82.02
      with division 82.19
  myocardium 37.11
  nailbed or nailfold 86.09
  nasolacrimal duct (stricture) 09.59
  neck 86.09
  nerve (cranial) (peripheral) NEC 04.04
    root (spinal) 03.1
  nose 21.1
  omentum 54.19
  orbit - *see also* Orbitotomy 16.09
  ovary 65.09
    laparoscopic 65.01
  palate 27.1
  palmar space (middle) 82.04
  pancreas 52.09
  pancreatic sphincter 51.82
    endoscopic 51.85
  parapharyngeal (oral) (transcervical)
      28.0
  paronychia 86.09
  parotid
    gland or duct 26.0
    space 27.0
  pelvirectal tissue 48.81
  penis 64.92
  perianal (skin) (tissue) 49.02
    abscess 49.01
  perigastric 54.19
  perineum (female) 71.09
    male 86.09
  peripheral vessels
    lower limb
      artery 38.08
      vein 38.09
    upper limb (artery) (vein) 38.03
  periprostatic tissue 60.81
  perirectal tissue 48.81
  perirenal tissue 59.09
  perisplenic 54.19
  peritoneum 54.95
    by laparotomy 54.19
    pelvic (female) 70.12
      male 54.19
  periureteral tissue 59.09
  periurethral tissue 58.91
  perivesical tissue 59.19
  petrous pyramid (air cells) (apex)
      (mastoid) 20.22

Incision (*Continued*)
  pharynx, pharyngeal (bursa) 29.0
    space, lateral 27.0
  pilonidal sinus (cyst) 86.03
  pineal gland 07.52
  pituitary (gland) 07.72
  pleura NEC 34.09
  popliteal space 86.09
  postzygomatic space 27.0
  pouch of Douglas 70.12
  prostate (perineal approach)
      (transurethral approach) 60.0
  pterygopalatine fossa 27.0
  pulp canal (tooth) 24.0
  Rathke's pouch 07.72
  rectovaginal septum 48.81
  rectum 48.0
    stricture 48.91
  renal pelvis 55.11
  retroperitoneum 54.0
  retropharyngeal (oral) (transcervical)
      28.0
  salivary gland or duct 26.0
  sclera 12.89
  scrotum 61.0
  sebaceous cyst 86.04
  seminal vesicle 60.72
  sinus - *see* Sinusotomy
  Skene's duct or gland 71.09
  skin 86.09
    with drainage 86.04
    breast 85.0
    cardiac pacemaker pocket, new site
        37.79
    ear 18.09
    nose 21.1
    subcutaneous tunnel for pulse
        generator lead wire 86.99
      with initial procedure - *omit code*
    thalamic stimulator pulse generator
        pocket, new site 86.09
      with initial insertion of battery
          package - *omit code*
    tunnel, subcutaneous for pulse
        generator lead wire 86.99
      with initial procedure - *omit code*
  skull (bone) 01.24
  soft tissue NEC 83.09
    with division 83.19
      hand 82.19
    hand 82.09
      with division 82.19
  space of Retzius 59.19
  spermatic cord 63.93
  sphincter of Oddi 51.82
    endoscopic 51.85
  spinal
    cord 03.09
    nerve root 03.1
  spleen 41.2
  stomach 43.0
  stye 08.09
  subarachnoid space, cerebral 01.31
  subcutaneous tissue 86.09
    with drainage 86.04
    tunnel
      esophageal 42.86
        with anastomosis - *see*
            Anastomosis, esophagus,
            antesternal
      pulse generator lead wire
          86.99
        with initial procedure - *omit
            code*

Incision (*Continued*)
  subdiaphragmatic space 54.19
  subdural space, cerebral 01.31
  sublingual space 27.0
  submandibular space 27.0
  submaxillary 86.09
    with drainage 86.04
  submental space 27.0
  subphrenic space 54.19
  supraclavicular fossa 86.09
    with drainage 86.04
  sweat glands, skin 86.04
  temporal pouches 27.0
  tendon (sheath) 83.01
    with division 83.13
      hand 82.11
    hand 82.01
      with division 82.11
  testis 62.0
  thenar space 82.04
  thymus (open) (other) 07.92
    thoracoscopic 07.95
  thyroid (field) (gland) NEC 06.09
    postoperative 06.02
  tongue NEC 25.94
    for tongue tie 25.91
  tonsil 28.0
  trachea NEC 31.3
  tunica vaginalis 61.0
  umbilicus 54.0
  urachal cyst 54.0
  ureter 56.2
  urethra 58.0
  uterus (corpus) 68.0
    cervix 69.96
    for termination of pregnancy
        74.91
    septum (congenital) 68.22
  uvula 27.71
  vagina (cuff) (septum) (stenosis)
      70.14
    for
      incisional hematoma
          (episiotomy) 75.91
      obstetrical hematoma NEC
          75.92
      pelvic abscess 70.12
  vas deferens 63.6
  vein 38.00
    abdominal 38.07
    head and neck NEC 38.02
    intracranial NEC 38.01
    lower limb 38.09
    thoracic NEC 38.05
    upper limb 38.03
  vertebral column 03.09
  vulva 71.09
    obstetrical 75.92
  web, esophageal 42.01
Incudectomy NEC 19.3
  with
    stapedectomy - *see also*
        Stapedectomy 19.19
    tympanoplasty - *see*
        Tympanoplasty
Incudopexy 19.19
Incudostapediopexy 19.19
  with incus replacement 19.11
Indentation, sclera, for buckling -
    see also Buckling, scleral
    14.49
Indicator dilution flow measurement
    89.68

◀ New   ◀▥ Revised   ~~deleted~~ Deleted   ● Use Additional Digit(s)   ▨ Omit code

Induction
abortion
by
D and C 69.01
insertion of prostaglandin
suppository 96.49
intra-amniotic injection
(prostaglandin) (saline)
75.0
labor
medical 73.4
surgical 73.01
intra- and extra-amniotic
injection 73.1
stripping of membranes
73.1
Inflation
belt wrap 93.99
Eustachian tube 20.8
fallopian tube 66.8
with injection of therapeutic agent
66.95
Infolding, sclera, for buckling - *see also*
Buckling, scleral 14.49
Infraction, turbinates (nasal) 21.62
Infundibulectomy
hypophyseal - *see also* Hypophysectomy,
partial 07.63
ventricle (heart) (right) 35.34
in total repair of tetralogy of Fallot
35.81
Infusion (intra-arterial) (intravenous)
with
disruption of blood brain barrier
[BBBD] 00.19
Abciximab 99.20
antibiotic
oxazolidinone class 00.14
antineoplastic agent
(chemotherapeutic) 99.25
biological response modifier [BRM]
99.28
cintredekin besudotox 99.28
CLO 17.70
clofarabine 17.70
CLOLAR® 17.70
high-dose interleukin-2 00.15
low-dose interleukin-2 99.28
biological response modifier [BRM],
antineoplastic agent 99.28
cintredekin besudotox 99.28
high-dose interleukin-2 00.15
low-dose interleukin-2 99.28
cancer chemotherapy agent NEC 99.25
cintredekin besudotox 99.28
CLO 17.70
clofarabine 17.70
CLOLAR® 17.70
drotrecogin alfa (activated) 00.11
electrolytes 99.18
enzymes, thrombolytic (streptokinase)
(tissue plasminogen activator)
(TPA) (urokinase)
direct coronary artery 36.04
intravenous 99.10
Eptifibatide 99.20
gamma globulin 99.14
GP IIB/IIIa inhibitor 99.20
hormone substance NEC 99.24
human B-type natriuretic peptide
(hBNP) 00.13
IgG (immunoglobulin) 99.14 ◀
immunoglobulin (IgG) (IVIG) (IVIg)
99.14 ◀

Infusion *(Continued)*
immunosuppressive antibody therapy
00.18
interleukin-2
high-dose 00.15
low-dose 99.28
IVIG (immunoglobulin) (IVIg)
99.14 ◀
nesiritide 00.13
neuroprotective agent 99.75
nimodipine 99.75
nutritional substance - *see* Nutrition
platelet inhibitor
direct coronary artery 36.04
intravenous 99.20
Proleukin (low-dose) 99.28
high-dose 00.15
prophylactic substance NEC 99.29
radioimmunoconjugate 92.28
radioimmunotherapy 92.28
radioisotope (liquid brachytherapy)
(liquid I-125) 92.20
recombinant protein 00.11
reteplase 99.10
therapeutic substance NEC
99.29
thrombolytic agent (enzyme)
(streptokinase) 99.10
with percutaneous transluminal
angioplasty

Note: Also use 00.40, 00.41, 00.42, or
00.43 to show the total number of
vessels treated.

coronary 00.66
non-coronary vessel(s)
39.50
specified site NEC 39.50
direct intracoronary artery 36.04
tirofiban (HCL) 99.20
vaccine
tumor 99.28
vasopressor 00.17
Injection (into) (hypodermically)
(intramuscularly) (intravenously)
(acting locally or systemically)
Actinomycin D, for cancer
chemotherapy 99.25
adhesion barrier substance 99.77
alcohol
nerve - *see* Injection, nerve
spinal 03.8
anterior chamber, eye (air) (liquid)
(medication) 12.92
antibiotic 99.21
oxazolidinone class 00.14
anticoagulant 99.19
anti-D (Rhesus) globulin 99.11
antidote NEC 99.16
anti-infective NEC 99.22
antineoplastic agent
(chemotherapeutic) NEC
99.25
biological response modifier
[BRM] 99.28
cintredekin besudotox 99.28
high-dose interleukin-2 00.15
low-dose interleukin-2 99.28
antivenin 99.16
barrier substance, adhesion 99.77
BCG
for chemotherapy 99.25
vaccine 99.33

Injection *(Continued)*
biological response modifier [BRM],
antineoplastic agent 99.28
cintredekin besudotox 99.28
high-dose interleukin-2 00.15
low-dose interleukin-2 99.28
bone marrow 41.92
transplant - *see* Transplant, bone,
marrow
breast (therapeutic agent) 85.92
inert material (silicone) (bilateral)
85.52
unilateral 85.51
bursa (therapeutic agent) 83.96
hand 82.94
cancer chemotherapeutic agent 99.25
caudal - *see* Injection, spinal
cintredekin besudotox 99.28
cortisone 99.23
costochondral junction 81.92
dinoprost-tromethine, intra-amniotic
75.0
disc, intervertebral (herniated) 80.52
ear, with alcohol 20.72
electrolytes 99.18
enzymes, thrombolytic (streptokinase)
(tissue plasminogen activator)
(TPA) (urokinase)
direct coronary artery 36.04
intravenous 99.10
epidural, spinal - *see* Injection, spinal
esophageal varices or blood vessel
(endoscopic) (sclerosing agent)
42.33
Eustachian tube (inert material) 20.8
eye (orbit) (retrobulbar) 16.91
anterior chamber 12.92
subconjunctival 10.91
fascia 83.98
hand 82.96
gamma globulin 99.14
ganglion, sympathetic 05.39
ciliary 12.79
paravertebral stellate 05.39
gel, adhesion barrier - *see* Injection,
adhesion barrier substance
globulin
anti-D (Rhesus) 99.11
gamma 99.14
Rh immune 99.11
heart 37.92
heavy metal antagonist 99.16
hemorrhoids (sclerosing agent) 49.42
hormone NEC 99.24
human B-type natriuretic peptide
(hBNP) 00.13
IgG (immunoglobulin) 99.14 ◀
immune sera 99.14
immunoglobulin (IgG) (IVIG) (IVIg)
99.14 ◀
inert material - *see* Implant, inert
material
inner ear, for destruction 20.72
insulin 99.17
intervertebral space for herniated disc
80.52
intra-amniotic
for induction of
abortion 75.0
labor 73.1
intrathecal - *see* Injection, spinal
IVIG (immunoglobulin) (IVIg) 99.14 ◀
joint (therapeutic agent) 81.92
temporomandibular 76.96

Injection *(Continued)*
  kidney (cyst) (therapeutic substance) NEC 55.96
  larynx 31.0
  ligament (joint) (therapeutic substance) 81.92
  liver 50.94
  lung, for surgical collapse 33.32
  Methotrexate, for cancer chemotherapy 99.25
  nerve (cranial) (peripheral) 04.80
    agent NEC 04.89
      alcohol 04.2
      anesthetic for analgesia 04.81
        for operative anesthesia - *omit code*
      neurolytic 04.2
      phenol 04.2
    laryngeal (external) (recurrent) (superior) 31.91
    optic 16.91
    sympathetic 05.39
      alcohol 05.32
      anesthetic for analgesia 05.31
      neurolytic agent 05.32
      phenol 05.32
  nesiritide 00.13
  neuroprotective agent 99.75
  nimodipine 99.75
  orbit 16.91
  pericardium 37.93
  peritoneal cavity
    air 54.96
    locally-acting therapeutic substance 54.97
  platelet inhibitor
    direct coronary artery 36.04
    intravenous 99.20
  prophylactic substance NEC 99.29
  prostate 60.92
  radioimmunoconjugate 92.28
  radioimmunotherapy 92.28
  radioisotopes (intracavitary) (intravenous) 92.28
  renal pelvis (cyst) 55.96
  retrobulbar (therapeutic substance) 16.91
    for anesthesia - *omit code*
  Rh immune globulin 99.11
  RhoGAM 99.11
  sclerosing agent NEC 99.29
    esophageal varices (endoscopic) 42.33
    hemorrhoids 49.42
    pleura 34.92
      treatment of malignancy (cytotoxic agent) 34.92 [99.25]
        with tetracycline 34.92 [99.21]
    varicose vein 39.92
    vein NEC 39.92
  semicircular canals, for destruction 20.72
  silicone - *see* Implant, inert material
  skin (sclerosing agent) (filling material) 86.02
  soft tissue 83.98
    hand 82.96
  spinal (canal) NEC 03.92
    alcohol 03.8
    anesthetic agent for analgesia 03.91
      for operative anesthesia - *omit code*
    contrast material (for myelogram) 87.21
    destructive agent NEC 03.8
    neurolytic agent NEC 03.8
    phenol 03.8

Injection *(Continued)*
  spinal NEC *(Continued)*
    proteolytic enzyme (chymodiactin) (chymopapain) 80.52
    saline (hypothermic) 03.92
    steroid NEC 03.92
  spinal nerve root (intrathecal) - *see* Injection, spinal
  steroid NEC 99.23
  subarachnoid, spinal - *see* Injection, spinal
  subconjunctival 10.91
  tendon 83.97
    hand 82.95
  testis 62.92
  therapeutic agent NEC 99.29
  thoracic cavity 34.92
  thrombolytic agent (enzyme) (streptokinase) 99.10
    with percutaneous transluminal angioplasty

> Note: Also use 00.40, 00.41, 00.42, or 00.43 to show the total number of vessels treated.

      coronary 00.66
      noncoronary vessels 39.50
      specified site NEC 39.50
    direct intracoronary artery 36.04
  trachea 31.94
  tranquilizer 99.26
  tunica vaginalis (with aspiration) 61.91
  tympanum 20.94
  urethra (inert material)
    for repair of urinary stress incontinence
      collagen implant 59.72
      endoscopic injection of implant 59.72
      fat implant 59.72
      polytef implant 59.72
  vaccine
    tumor 99.28
  varices, esophagus (endoscopic) (sclerosing agent) 42.33
  varicose vein (sclerosing agent) 39.92
    esophagus (endoscopic) 42.33
  vestibule, for destruction 20.72
  vitreous substitute (silicone) 14.75
    for reattachment of retina 14.59
  vocal cords 31.0
Inlay, tooth 23.3
Inoculation
  antitoxins - *see* Administration, antitoxins
  toxoids - *see* Administration, toxoids
  vaccine - *see* Administration, vaccine
Insemination, artificial 69.92
Insertion
  airway
    esophageal obturator 96.03
    nasopharynx 96.01
    oropharynx 96.02
  Allen-Brown cannula 39.93
  arch bars (orthodontic) 24.7
    for immobilization (fracture) 93.55
  atrial septal umbrella 35.52
  Austin-Moore prosthesis 81.52
  baffle, heart (atrial) (interatrial) (intra-atrial) 35.91
  bag, cervix (nonobstetrical) 67.0
    after delivery or abortion 75.8
    to assist delivery or induce labor 73.1

Insertion *(Continued)*
  Baker's (tube) (for stenting) 46.85
  balloon
    gastric 44.93
    heart (pulsation-type) (Kantrowitz) 37.61
    intestine (for decompression) (for dilation) 46.85
      with insertion of colonic stent
        endoscopic 46.86
        other 46.87
  band (adjustable)
    gastric, laparoscopic 44.95
    Lap-Band™ 44.95
  Barton's tongs (skull) (with synchronous skeletal traction) 02.94
  bipolar endoprosthesis (femoral head) 81.52
  Blakemore-Sengstaken tube 96.06
  bone growth stimulator (invasive) (percutaneous) (semi-invasive) - *see* category 78.9 ●
  bone morphogenetic protein (Infuse™) (OP-1™) (recombinant) (rhBMP) 84.52
  bone void filler 84.55
    that with percutaneous vertebral augmentation 81.66
    that with percutaneous vertebroplasty 81.65
  bougie, cervix, nonobstetrical 67.0
    to assist delivery or induce labor 73.1
  breast implant (for augmentation) (bilateral) 85.54
    unilateral 85.53
  bridge (dental) (fixed) 23.42
    removable 23.43
  bubble (balloon), stomach 44.93
  caliper tongs (skull) (with synchronous skeletal traction) 02.94
  cannula
    Allen-Brown 39.93
    for extracorporeal membrane oxygenation (ECMO) - *omit code*
    nasal sinus (by puncture) 22.01
      through natural ostium 22.02
    pancreatic duct 52.92
      endoscopic 52.93
    vessel to vessel 39.93
  cardiac resynchronization device
    defibrillator (biventricular defibrillator) (BiV ICD) (BiV pacemaker with defibrillator) (BiV pacing with defibrillator) (CRT- D) (device and one or more leads) (total system) 00.51
      left ventricular coronary venous lead only 00.52
      pulse generator only 00.54
    pacemaker (biventricular pacemaker) (BiV pacemaker) (CRT-P) (device and one or more leads) (total system) 00.50
      left ventricular coronary venous lead only 00.52
      pulse generator only 00.53

◀ New   ◀▥ Revised   ~~deleted~~ Deleted   ● Use Additional Digit(s)   ▨ Omit code

Insertion (*Continued*)
cardiac support device (CSD)
  (CorCap™) 37.41
carotid artery stent(s) (stent graft)
  00.63

> Note: Also use 00.40, 00.41, 00.42, or
> 00.43 to show the total number of
> vessels treated. Use code 00.44 once to
> show procedure on a bifurcated vessel.
> In addition, use 00.45, 00.46, 00.47, or
> 00.48 to show the number of vascular
> stents inserted.

catheter
  abdomen of fetus, for intrauterine
    transfusion 75.2
  anterior chamber (eye), for
    permanent drainage
    (glaucoma) 12.79
  artery 38.91
  bile duct(s) 51.59
    common 51.51
      endoscopic 51.87
    endoscopic 51.87
  bladder, indwelling 57.94
    suprapubic 57.18
      percutaneous (closed)
        57.17
  bronchus 96.05
    with lavage 96.56
  central venous NEC 38.93
    with guidance 38.97 ◄
    for
      hemodialysis 38.95
      pressure monitoring 89.62
    peripherally inserted central
      catheter (PICC) 38.93
  chest 34.04
    revision (with lysis of adhesions)
      34.04
      thoracoscopic 34.06
    thoracoscopic 34.06
  cranial cavity 01.26
    placement via burr hole(s) 01.28
  esophagus (nonoperative) 96.06
    permanent tube 42.81
  intercostal (with water seal), for
    drainage 34.04
    revision (with lysis of adhesions)
      34.04
      thoracoscopic 34.06
    thoracoscopic 34.06
  intracerebral 01.26
    placement via burr hole(s) 01.28
  spinal canal space (epidural)
    (subarachnoid) (subdural) for
    infusion of therapeutic or
    palliative substances 03.90
  Swan-Ganz (pulmonary) 89.64
  transtracheal for oxygenation 31.99
  vein NEC 38.93
    for renal dialysis 38.95
chest tube 34.04
  thoracoscopic 34.06
choledochohepatic tube (for
  decompression) 51.43
  endoscopic 51.87
circulatory support device
  CentriMag® 37.62
  external heart assist device
    biventricular 37.60
    Impella® 37.68
    percutaneous 37.68
    temporary 37.62

Insertion (*Continued*)
circulatory support device (*Continued*)
  non-implantable 37.62
  pVAD (percutaneous VAD) 37.68
  TandemHeart® 37.68
  temporary non-implantable
    circulatory assist device 37.62
cochlear prosthetic device - *see* Implant,
  cochlear prosthetic device
contraceptive device (intrauterine)
  69.7
CorCap™ 37.41
cordis cannula 54.98
coronary (artery)

> Note: Also use 00.40, 00.41, 00.42, or
> 00.43 to show the total number of
> vessels treated. Use code 00.44 once to
> show procedure on a bifurcated vessel.
> In addition, use 00.45, 00.46, 00.47, or
> 00.48 to show the number of vascular
> stents inserted.

  stent, drug-eluting 36.07
  stent, non-drug-eluting 36.06
Crosby-Cooney button 54.98
CRT-D (biventricular defibrillator) (BiV
  ICD) (BiV pacemaker with
  defibrillator) (BiV pacing with
  defibrillator) (cardiac
  resynchronization defibrillator)
  (device and one or more leads)
  00.51
  left ventricular coronary venous
    lead only 00.52
  pulse generator only 00.54
CRT-P (biventricular pacemaker) (BiV
  pacemaker) (cardiac
  resynchronization pacemaker)
  (device and one or more leads)
  00.50
  left ventricular coronary venous
    lead only 00.52
  pulse generator only 00.53
Crutchfield tongs (skull) (with
  synchronous skeletal traction)
  02.94
Davidson button 54.98
denture (total) 99.97
device
  adjustable gastric band and port
    44.95
  bronchial device NOS 33.79
  bronchial substance NOS 33.79
  bronchial valve(s)
    multiple lobes 33.73
    single lobe 33.71
  cardiac resynchronization - *see*
    Insertion, cardiac
    resynchronization device
  cardiac support device (CSD) 37.41
  CorCap™ 37.41
  epicardial support device 37.41
  Lap-Band™ 44.95
  left atrial appendage 37.90
  left atrial filter 37.90
  left atrial occluder 37.90
  MitraClip® mitral leaflet clip 35.97 ◄
  prosthetic cardiac support device
    37.41
  sternal fixation device with rigid
    plates 84.94 ◄
  vascular access 86.07
  ventricular support device 37.41
diaphragm, vagina 96.17

Insertion (*Continued*)
drainage tube
  kidney 55.02
    pelvis 55.12
  renal pelvis 55.12
Dynesys® 84.82
elbow prosthesis (total) 81.84
  revision 81.97
electrode(s)
  bone growth stimulator (invasive)
    (percutaneous) (semi-
    invasive) - *see* category 78.9●
  brain 02.93
    depth 02.93
    foramen ovale 02.93
    sphenoidal 02.96
  depth 02.93
  foramen ovale 02.93
  gastric 04.92
  heart (initial) (transvenous) 37.70
    atrium (initial) 37.73
      replacement 37.76
    atrium and ventricle (initial)
      37.72
      replacement 37.76
    epicardium (sternotomy or
      thoracotomy approach)
      37.74
    left ventricular coronary venous
      system 00.52
    temporary transvenous
      pacemaker system 37.78
      during and immediately
        following cardiac
        surgery 39.64
    ventricle (initial) 37.71
      replacement 37.76
  intracranial 02.93
  osteogenic (for bone growth
    stimulation) - *see* category
    78.9●
  peripheral nerve 04.92
  sacral nerve 04.92
  sphenoidal 02.96
  spine 03.93
electroencephalographic receiver - *see*
  Implant, electroencephalographic
  receiver, by site
electronic stimulator - *see* Implant,
  electronic stimulator, by site
electrostimulator - *see* Implant,
  electronic stimulator, by site
endograft(s), endovascular graft(s)
  endovascular, abdominal aorta
    39.71
  endovascular, head and neck vessels
    39.72
  endovascular, other vessels (for
    aneurysm) 39.79
  endovascular, thoracic aorta 39.73
endoprosthesis
  bile duct 51.87
  femoral head (bipolar) 81.52
  pancreatic duct 52.93
epidural pegs 02.93
external fixation device (bone) - *see*
  category 78.1●
facial bone implant (alloplastic)
  (synthetic) 76.92
filling material, skin (filling of defect)
  86.02
filter
  vena cava (inferior) (superior)
    (transvenous) 38.7

Insertion (*Continued*)
- fixator, mini device (bone) - *see* category 78.1●
- frame (stereotactic)
  - for radiosurgery 93.59
- Gardner Wells tongs (skull) (with synchronous skeletal traction) 02.94
- gastric bubble (balloon) 44.93
- globe, into eye socket 16.69
- Greenfield filter 38.7
- halo device (skull) (with synchronous skeletal traction) 02.94
- Harrington rod - *see also* Fusion, spinal, by level
  - with dorsal, dorsolumbar fusion 81.05
- Harris pin 79.15
- heart
  - assist system - *see* Implant, heart assist system
  - cardiac support device (CSD) 37.41
  - circulatory assist system - *see* Implant, heart assist system
  - CorCap™ 37.41
  - epicardial support device 37.41
  - Impella® 37.68
  - pacemaker - *see* Insertion, pacemaker, cardiac
  - prosthetic cardiac support device 37.41
  - pump (Kantrowitz) 37.62
  - valve - *see* Replacement, heart valve
  - ventricular support device 37.41
- hip prosthesis (partial) 81.52
  - revision NOS 81.53
    - acetabular and femoral components (total) 00.70
    - acetabular component only 00.71
    - acetabular liner and/or femoral head only 00.73
    - femoral component only 00.72
    - femoral head only and/or acetabular liner 00.73
    - partial
      - acetabular component only 00.71
      - acetabular liner and/or femoral head only 00.73
      - femoral component only 00.72
      - femoral head only and/or acetabular liner 00.73
    - total (acetabular and femoral components) 00.70
  - total 81.51
    - revision
      - acetabular and femoral components (total) 00.70
      - total (acetabular and femoral components) 00.70
- Holter valve 02.2
- Hufnagel valve - *see* Replacement, heart valve
- implant - *see* Insertion, prosthesis
- infusion pump 86.06
- interbody spinal fusion device 84.51
- intercostal catheter (with water seal) for drainage 34.04
  - revision (with lysis of adhesions) 34.04
    - thoracoscopic 34.06

Insertion (*Continued*)
- intra-arterial blood gas monitoring system 89.60
- intrauterine
  - contraceptive device 69.7
  - radium (intracavitary) 69.91
  - tamponade (nonobstetric) 69.91
- Kantrowitz
  - heart pump 37.62
  - pulsation balloon (phase-shift) 37.61
- keratoprosthesis 11.73
- King-Mills umbrella device (heart) 35.52
- Kirschner wire 93.44
  - with reduction of fracture or dislocation - *see* Reduction, fracture *and* Reduction, dislocation
- knee prosthesis (partial (total) 81.54
  - revision NOS 81.55
    - femoral component 00.82
    - partial
      - femoral component 00.82
      - patellar component 00.83
      - tibial component 00.81
      - tibial insert 00.84
    - patellar component 00.83
    - tibial component 00.81
    - tibial insert 00.84
    - total (all components) 00.80
- laminaria, cervix 69.93
- Lap-Band™ 44.95
- larynx, valved tube 31.75
- leads - *see* Insertion, electrode(s)
- lens, prosthetic (intraocular) 13.70
  - with cataract extraction, one-stage 13.71
  - secondary (subsequent to cataract extraction) 13.72
- limb lengthening device, internal, NOS 84.54
  - with kinetic distraction 84.53
- loop recorder 37.79
- metal staples into epiphyseal plate - *see also* Stapling, epiphyseal plate 78.20
- minifixator device (bone) - *see* category 78.1●
- M-Brace™ 84.82
- Mobitz-Uddin umbrella, vena cava 38.7
- mold, vagina 96.15
- Moore (cup) 81.52
- myringotomy device (button) (tube) 20.01
  - with intubation 20.01
- nasobiliary drainage tube (endoscopic) 51.86
- nasogastric tube
  - for
    - decompression, intestinal 96.07
    - feeding 96.6
- naso-intestinal tube 96.08
- nasolacrimal tube or stent 09.44
- nasopancreatic drainage tube (endoscopic) 52.97
- neuropacemaker - *see* Implant, neurostimulator, by site
- neurostimulator - *see* Implant, neurostimulator, by site

Insertion (*Continued*)
- non-coronary vessel stent(s) (stent graft)

> Note: Also use 00.40, 00.41, 00.42, or 00.43 to show the total number of vessels treated. Use code 00.44 once to show procedure on a bifurcated vessel. In addition, use 00.45, 00.46, 00.47, or 00.48 to show the number of vascular stents inserted.

- with angioplasty or atherectomy 39.50
- with bypass - *omit code*
- basilar 00.64
- carotid 00.63
- extracranial 00.64
- intracranial 00.65
- peripheral 39.90
  - bare, drug-coated 39.90
  - drug-eluting 00.55
- vertebral 00.64
- non-invasive (surface) (transcutaneous) stimulator 99.86
- obturator (orthodontic) 24.7
- ocular implant
  - with synchronous
    - enucleation 16.42
      - with muscle attachment to implant 16.41
    - evisceration 16.31
  - following or secondary to
    - enucleation 16.61
    - evisceration 16.61
- Ommaya reservoir 02.2
- orbital implant (stent) (outside muscle cone) 16.69
  - with orbitotomy 16.02
- orthodontic appliance (obturator) (wiring) 24.7
- outflow tract prosthesis (gusset type) (heart)
  - in
    - pulmonary valvuloplasty 35.26
    - total repair of tetralogy of Fallot 35.81
- pacemaker
  - brain - *see* Implant, neurostimulator, brain
  - cardiac (device) (initial) (permanent) (replacement) 37.80
    - dual-chamber device (initial) 37.83
      - replacement 37.87
    - during and immediately following cardiac surgery 39.64
    - resynchronization (biventricular pacemaker) (BiV pacemaker) (CRT-P) (device)
      - device only (initial) (replacement) 00.53
      - total system (device and one or more leads) 00.50
      - transvenous lead into left ventricular coronary venous system 00.52
    - single-chamber device (initial) 37.81
      - rate responsive 37.82
      - replacement 37.85
        - rate responsive 37.86

Insertion *(Continued)*
pacemaker *(Continued)*
cardiac *(Continued)*
temporary transvenous
pacemaker system 37.78
during and immediately
following cardiac
surgery 39.64
carotid 39.89 ◀▥
gastric 04.92
heart - *see* Insertion, pacemaker,
cardiac
intracranial - *see* Implant,
neurostimulator, intracranial
neural - *see* Implant,
neurostimulator, by site
peripheral nerve - *see* Implant,
neurostimulator, peripheral
nerve
spine - *see* Implant, neurostimulator,
spine
pacing catheter - *see* Insertion,
pacemaker, cardiac
pack
auditory canal, external 96.11
cervix (nonobstetrical) 67.0
after delivery or abortion 75.8
to assist delivery or induce labor
73.1
rectum 96.19
sella turcica 07.79
vagina (nonobstetrical) 96.14
after delivery or abortion 75.8
palatal implant 27.64
penile prosthesis (internal) (non-
inflatable) 64.95
inflatable (internal) 64.97
periodontal splint (orthodontic) 24.7
peripheral blood vessel - *see* non-
coronary
pessary
cervix 96.18
to assist delivery or induce labor
73.1
vagina 96.18
pharyngeal valve, artificial 31.75
port, vascular access 86.07
prostaglandin suppository (for
abortion) 96.49
prosthesis, prosthetic device
acetabulum (partial) 81.52
hip 81.52
revision NOS 81.53
acetabular and femoral
components (total)
00.70
acetabular component only
00.71
acetabular liner and/or
femoral head only
00.73
femoral component only
00.72
femoral head only and/or
acetabular liner 00.73
partial
acetabular component
only 00.71
acetabular liner and/or
femoral head only
00.73
femoral component only
00.72
femoral head only and/
or acetabular liner
00.73

Insertion *(Continued)*
prosthesis, prosthetic device *(Continued)*
acetabulum (partial) *(Continued)*
hip *(Continued)*
revision NOS *(Continued)*
total (acetabular and
femoral components)
00.70
revision 81.53
ankle (total) 81.56
arm (bioelectric) (cineplastic)
(kineplastic) 84.44
biliary tract 51.99
breast (bilateral) 85.54
unilateral 85.53
cardiac support device (CSD)
(CorCap™) 37.41
chin (polyethylene) (silastic) 76.68
elbow (total) 81.84
revision 81.97
extremity (bioelectric) (cineplastic)
(kineplastic) 84.40
lower 84.48
upper 84.44
fallopian tube 66.93
femoral head (Austin-Moore)
(bipolar) (Eicher) (Thompson)
81.52
hip (partial) 81.52
revision NOS 81.53
acetabular and femoral
components (total) 00.70
acetabular component only
00.71
acetabular liner and/or
femoral head only 00.73
femoral component only 00.72
femoral head only and/or
acetabular liner 00.73
partial
acetabular component only
00.71
acetabular liner and/or
femoral head only
00.73
femoral component only
00.72
femoral head only and/or
acetabular liner 00.73
total (acetabular and femoral
components) 00.70
total 81.51
revision
acetabular and femoral
components (total)
00.70
total (acetabular and
femoral components)
00.70
joint - *see* Arthroplasty
knee (partial) (total) 81.54
revision NOS 81.55
femoral component 00.82
partial
femoral component 00.82
patellar component 00.83
tibial component 00.81
tibial insert 00.84
patellar component 00.83
tibial component 00.81
tibial insert 00.84
total (all components) 00.80
leg (bioelectric) (cineplastic)
(kineplastic) 84.48

Insertion *(Continued)*
prosthesis, prosthetic device *(Continued)*
lens 13.91
ocular (secondary) 16.61
with orbital exenteration 16.42
outflow tract (gusset type) (heart)
in
pulmonary valvuloplasty 35.26
total repair of tetralogy of
Fallot 35.81
penis (internal) (noninflatable) 64.95
with
construction 64.43
reconstruction 64.44
inflatable (internal) 64.97
Rosen (for urinary incontinence) 59.79
shoulder
partial 81.81
revision 81.97
total, NEC 81.80 ◀▥
other 81.80 ◀
reverse 81.88 ◀
spine
artificial disc, NOS 84.60
cervical 84.62
nucleus 84.61
partial 84.61
total 84.62
lumbar, lumbosacral 84.65
nucleus 84.64
partial 84.64
total 84.65
thoracic (partial) (total) 84.63
other device 84.59
testicular (bilateral) (unilateral)
62.7
toe 81.57
hallux valgus repair 77.59
vagina
synthetic 70.95
pseudophakos - *see also* Insertion, lens
13.70
pump, infusion 86.06
radioactive isotope 92.27
radium 92.27
radon seeds 92.27,
Reuter bobbin (with intubation) 20.01
Rickham reservoir 02.2
Rosen prosthesis (for urinary
incontinence) 59.79
Scribner shunt 39.93
Sengstaken-Blakemore tube 96.06
sensor (lead)
intra-aneurysm sac pressure
monitoring device 00.58
intra-arterial, for continuous blood
gas monitoring 89.60
intracardiac or great vessel
hemodynamic monitoring
00.56
shunt - *see* Shunt
sieve, vena cava 38.7
skeletal muscle stimulator 83.92
skull
plate 02.05
stereotactic frame 93.59
tongs (Barton) (caliper) (Garder
Wells) (Vinke) (with
synchronous skeletal traction)
02.94
spacer (cement) (joint)
(methylmethacrylate) 84.56
spine 84.51
sphenoidal electrodes 02.96

◀ New ◀▥ Revised ~~deleted~~ Deleted ● Use Additional Digit(s) ▬ Omit code 1173

Insertion (*Continued*)
spine
bone void filler
that with percutaneous vertebral augmentation 81.66
that with percutaneous vertebroplasty 81.65
cage (BAK) 84.51
facet replacement device(s) 84.84
interbody spinal fusion device 84.51
interspinous process decompression device 84.80
non-fusion stabilization device - *see* category 84.8●
pedicle-based dynamic stabilization device(s) 84.82
posterior motion preservation device(s) - *see* category 84.8●
spacer 84.51
Spitz-Holter valve 02.2
Steinmann pin 93.44
with reduction of fracture or dislocation - *see* Reduction, fracture *and* Reduction, dislocation
stent(s) (stent graft)
artery (bare) (bonded) (drug coated) (non-drug-eluting)

Note: Also use 00.40, 00.41, 00.42, or 00.43 to show the total number of vessels treated. Use code 00.44 once to show procedure on a bifurcated vessel. In addition, use 00.45, 00.46, 00.47, or 00.48 to show the number of vascular stents inserted.

basilar 00.64
carotid 00.63
cerebrovascular
cerebral (intracranial) 00.65
precerebral (extracranial) 00.64
carotid 00.63
coronary (bare) (bonded) (drug coated) (non-drug-eluting) 36.06
drug-eluting 36.07
extracranial 00.64
carotid 00.63
femoral artery, superficial 39.90 ◀
drug-eluting 00.60 ◀
non-drug-eluting 39.90 ◀
intracranial 00.65
non-coronary vessel
basilar 00.64
carotid 00.63
extracranial 00.64
intracranial 00.65
peripheral 39.90
bare, drug-coated 39.90
drug-eluting 00.55
vertebral 00.64
bile duct 51.43
endoscopic 51.87
percutaneous transhepatic 51.98
colon
endoscopic (fluoroscopic guidance) 46.86
other 46.87

Insertion (*Continued*)
stent(s) (*Continued*)
coronary (artery) (bare) (bonded) (drug coated) (non-drug-eluting) 36.06

Note: Also use 00.40, 00.41, 00.42, or 00.43 to show the total number of vessels treated. Use code 00.44 once to show procedure on a bifurcated vessel. In addition, use 00.45, 00.46, 00.47, or 00.48 to show the number of vascular stents inserted.

drug-eluting 36.07
esophagus (endoscopic) (fluoroscopic) 42.81
mesenteric 39.90
bare, drug-coated 39.90
drug-eluting 00.55
non-coronary vessel

Note: Also use 00.40, 00.41, 00.42, or 00.43 to show the total number of vessels treated. Use code 00.44 once to show procedure on a bifurcated vessel. In addition, use 00.45, 00.46, 00.47, or 00.48 to show the number of vascular stents inserted.

with angioplasty or atherectomy 39.50
with bypass - *omit code*
basilar 00.64
carotid 00.63
extracranial 00.64
femoral artery, superficial 39.90 ◀
drug-eluting 00.60 ◀
non-drug-eluting 39.90 ◀
intracranial 00.65
mesenteric 39.90
bare, drug-coated 39.90
drug-eluting 00.55
peripheral 39.90
bare, drug-coated 39.90
drug-eluting 00.55
renal 39.90
bare, drug-coated 39.90
drug-eluting 00.55
vertebral 00.64
pancreatic duct 52.92
endoscopic 52.93
peripheral 39.90

Note: Also use 00.40, 00.41, 00.42, or 00.43 to show the total number of vessels treated. Use code 00.44 once to show procedure on a bifurcated vessel. In addition, use 00.45, 00.46, 00.47, or 00.48 to show the number of vascular stents inserted.

bare, drug-coated 39.90
drug-eluting 00.55
femoral artery, superficial, drug-eluting 00.60 ◀
precerebral 00.64

Note: Also use 00.40, 00.41, 00.42 or 00.43 to show the total number of vessels treated. Use code 00.44 once to show procedure on a bifurcated vessel. In addition, use 00.45, 00.46, 00.47, or 00.48 to show the number of vascular stents inserted.

Insertion (*Continued*)
stent(s) (*Continued*)
renal 39.90
bare, drug-coated 39.90
drug-eluting 00.55
sternal fixation device with rigid plates 84.94 ◀
subclavian 39.90

Note: Also use 00.40, 00.41, 00.42, or 00.43 to show the total number of vessels treated. Use code 00.44 once to show procedure on a bifurcated vessel. In addition, use 00.45, 00.46, 00.47, or 00.48 to show the number of vascular stents inserted.

bare, drug-coated 39.90
drug-eluting 00.55
tracheobronchial 96.05
vertebral 00.64

Note: Also use 00.40, 00.41, 00.42, or 00.43 to show the total number of vessels treated. Use code 00.44 once to show procedure on a bifurcated vessel. In addition, use 00.45, 00.46, 00.47, or 00.48 to show the number of vascular stents inserted.

stimoceiver - *see* Implant, neurostimulator, by site
stimulator for bone growth - *see* category 78.9●
subdural
grids 02.93
strips 02.93
suppository
prostaglandin (for abortion) 96.49
vagina 96.49
Swan-Ganz catheter (pulmonary) 89.64
tampon
esophagus 96.06
uterus 69.91
vagina 96.14
after delivery or abortion 75.8
Tandem™ heart 37.68
telescope (IMT) (miniature) 13.91
testicular prosthesis (bilateral) (unilateral) 62.7
tissue expander (skin) NEC 86.93
breast 85.95
tissue mandril (peripheral vessel) (Dacron) (Spark's type) 39.99
with
blood vessel repair 39.56
vascular bypass or shunt - *see* Bypass, vascular
tongs, skull (with synchronous skeletal traction) 02.94
totally implanted device for bone growth (invasive) - *see* category 78.9●
tube - *see also* Catheterization and Intubation
bile duct 51.43
endoscopic 51.87
chest 34.04
revision (with lysis of adhesions) 34.04
thoracoscopic 34.06
thoracoscopic 34.06
endotracheal 96.04
esophagus (nonoperative) (Sengstaken) 96.06
permanent (silicone) (Souttar) 42.81

Insertion *(Continued)*
  tube *(Continued)*
    feeding
      esophageal 42.81
      gastric 96.6
      nasogastric 96.6
    gastric
      by gastrostomy - *see* category
        43.1●
      for
        decompression, intestinal
          96.07
        feeding 96.6
    intercostal (with water seal), for
      drainage 34.04
      revision (with lysis of adhesions)
        34.04
      thoracoscopic 34.06
    Miller-Abbott (for intestinal
      decompression) 96.08
    nasobiliary (drainage) 51.86
    nasogastric (for intestinal
      decompression) NEC 96.07
    naso-intestinal 96.08
    nasopancreatic drainage
      (endoscopic) 52.97
    pancreatic duct 52.92
      endoscopic 52.93
    rectum 96.09
    stomach (nasogastric) (for intestinal
      decompression) NEC 96.07
      for feeding 96.6
    tracheobronchial 96.05
  umbrella device
    atrial septum (King-Mills) 35.52
    vena cava (Mobitz-Uddin) 38.7
  ureteral stent (transurethral) 59.8
    with ureterotomy 59.8 *[56.2]*
  urinary sphincter, artificial (AUS)
    (inflatable) 58.93
  vaginal mold 96.15
  valve(s)
    bronchus
      multiple lobes 33.73
      single lobe 33.71
    Holter 02.2
    Hufnagel - *see* Replacement, heart
      valve
    pharyngeal (artificial) 31.75
    Spitz-Holter 02.2
    vas deferens 63.95
  vascular access device, totally
    implantable 86.07
  vena cava sieve or umbrella 38.7
  Vinke tongs (skull) (with synchronous
    skeletal traction) 02.94
  X Stop™ 84.80
Instillation
  bladder 96.49
  digestive tract, except gastric gavage
    96.43
  genitourinary NEC 96.49
  radioisotope (intracavitary)
    (intravenous) 92.28
  thoracic cavity 34.92
Insufflation
  Eustachian tube 20.8
  fallopian tube (air) (dye) (gas) (saline)
    66.8
    for radiography - *see*
      Hysterosalpingography
    therapeutic substance 66.95
  lumbar retroperitoneal, bilateral
    88.15

Intercricothyroidotomy (for assistance
  in breathing) 31.1
Interleukin-2, infusion
  high-dose 00.15
  low-dose 99.28
Intermittent positive pressure breathing
  (IPPB) 93.91
Interposition operation
  esophageal reconstruction
    (intrathoracic) (retrosternal) NEC -
    see also Anastomosis, esophagus,
    with, interposition 42.58
  antesternal or antethoracic NEC - *see*
    also Anastomosis, esophagus,
    antesternal, with, interposition
    42.68
  uterine suspension 69.21
Interrogation
  cardioverter-defibrillator, automatic
    (AICD)
    with catheter based invasive
      electrophysiologic testing
      37.26
    with NIPS (arrhythmia induction)
      37.20
    interrogation only (bedside device
      check) 89.49
  CRT-D (cardiac resynchronization
    defibrillator)
    with catheter based invasive
      electrophysiologic testing
      37.26
    with NIPS (arrhythmia induction)
      37.20
    interrogation only (bedside device
      check) 89.49
  CRT-P (cardiac resynchronization
    pacemaker)
    with catheter based invasive
      electrophysiologic testing
      37.26
    with NIPS (arrhythmia induction)
      37.20
    interrogation only (bedside device
      check) 89.45
  pacemaker
    with catheter based invasive
      electrophysiologic testing
      37.26
    with NIPS (arrhythmia induction)
      37.20
    interrogation only (bedside device
      check) 89.45
Interruption
  vena cava (inferior) (superior) 38.7
Interview (evaluation) (diagnostic)
  medical, except psychiatric 89.05
    brief (abbreviated history) 89.01
    comprehensive (history and
      evaluation of new problem)
      89.03
    limited (interval history) 89.02
    specified type NEC 89.04
  psychiatric NEC 94.19
    follow-up 94.19
    initial 94.19
    pre-commitment 94.13
Intimectomy 38.10
  abdominal 38.16
  aorta (arch) (ascending) (descending)
    38.14
  head and neck NEC 38.12
  intracranial NEC 38.11
  lower limb 38.18

Intimectomy *(Continued)*
  thoracic NEC 38.15
  upper limb 38.13
Intraoperative anesthetic effect
  monitoring and titration (IAEMT)
  00.94 *[89.14]*
Introduction
  orthodontic appliance 24.7
  therapeutic substance (acting locally or
    systemically) NEC 99.29
    bursa 83.96
      hand 82.94
    fascia 83.98
      hand 82.96
    heart 37.92
    joint 81.92
      temporomandibular 76.96
    ligament (joint) 81.92
    pericardium 37.93
    soft tissue NEC 83.98
      hand 82.96
    tendon 83.97
      hand 82.95
    vein 39.92
Intubation - *see also* Catheterization and
  Insertion
  bile duct(s) 51.59
    common 51.51
      endoscopic 51.87
    endoscopic 51.87
  esophagus (nonoperative) (Sengstaken)
    96.06
    permanent tube (silicone) (Souttar)
      42.81
  Eustachian tube 20.8
  intestine (for decompression) 96.08
  lacrimal for
    dilation 09.42
    tear drainage, intranasal 09.81
  larynx 96.05
  nasobiliary (drainage) 51.86
  nasogastric
    for
      decompression, intestinal 96.07
      feeding 96.6
  naso-intestinal 96.08
  nasolacrimal (duct) (with irrigation)
    09.44
  nasopancreatic drainage (endoscopic)
    52.97
  respiratory tract NEC 96.05
  small intestine (Miller-Abbott)
    96.08
  stomach (nasogastric) (for
    intestinal decompression)
    NEC 96.07
    for feeding 96.6
  trachea 96.04
  ventriculocisternal 02.2
Invagination, diverticulum
  gastric 44.69
    laparoscopic 44.68
  pharynx 29.59
  stomach 44.69
    laparoscopic 44.68
Inversion
  appendix 47.99
  diverticulum
    gastric 44.69
      laparoscopic 44.68
    intestine
      large 45.49
        endoscopic 45.43
      small 45.34

Inversion *(Continued)*
  diverticulum *(Continued)*
    stomach 44.69
      laparoscopic 44.68
    tunica vaginalis 61.49
IOERT (intra-operative electron radiation therapy) 92.41
IOM (intra-operative neurophysiologic monitoring) 00.94
Ionization, medical 99.27
Iontherapy 99.27
Iontophoresis 99.27
Iridectomy (basal) (buttonhole) (optical) (peripheral) (total) 12.14
  with
    capsulectomy 13.65
    cataract extraction - *see* Extraction, cataract
    filtering operation (for glaucoma) NEC 12.65
    scleral
      fistulization 12.65
      thermocauterization 12.62
      trephination 12.61
Iridencleisis 12.63
Iridesis 12.63
Irido-capsulectomy 13.65
Iridocyclectomy 12.44
Iridocystectomy 12.42
Iridodesis 12.63
Iridoplasty NEC 12.39
Iridosclerectomy 12.65
Iridosclerotomy 12.69
Iridotasis 12.63

Iridotomy 12.12
  by photocoagulation 12.12
  with transfixion 12.11
  for iris bombé 12.11
  specified type NEC 12.12
Iron lung 93.99
Irradiation
  gamma, stereotactic 92.32
Irrigation
  anterior chamber (eye) 12.91
  bronchus NEC 96.56
  canaliculus 09.42
  catheter
    ureter 96.46
    urinary, indwelling NEC 96.48
    vascular 96.57
    ventricular 02.41
    wound 96.58
  cholecystostomy 96.41
  cornea 96.51
    with removal of foreign body 98.21
  corpus cavernosum 64.98
  cystostomy 96.47
  ear (removal of cerumen) 96.52
  enterostomy 96.36
  eye 96.51
    with removal of foreign body 98.21
  gastrostomy 96.36
  lacrimal
    canaliculi 09.42
    punctum 09.41
  muscle 83.02
    hand 82.02
  nasal
    passages 96.53
    sinus 22.00

Irrigation *(Continued)*
  nasolacrimal duct 09.43
    with insertion of tube or stent 09.44
  nephrostomy 96.45
  peritoneal 54.25
  pyelostomy 96.45
  rectal 96.39
  stomach 96.33
  tendon (sheath) 83.01
    hand 82.01
  trachea NEC 96.56
  traumatic cataract 13.3
  tube
    biliary NEC 96.41
    nasogastric NEC 96.34
    pancreatic 96.42
  ureterostomy 96.46
  ventricular shunt 02.41
  wound (cleaning) NEC 96.59
Irving operation (tubal ligation) 66.32
Irwin operation - *see also* Osteotomy 77.30
Ischiectomy (partial) 77.89
  total 77.99
Ischiopubiotomy 77.39
Isolation
  after contact with infectious disease 99.84
  ileal loop 45.51
  intestinal segment or pedicle flap
    large 45.52
    small 45.51
Isthmectomy, thyroid - *see also* Thyroidectomy, partial 06.39
IVUS - *see* Ultrasound, intravascular, by site

J

Jaboulay operation (gastroduodenostomy) 44.39
  laparoscopic 44.38
Janeway operation (permanent gastrostomy) 43.19
Jatene operation (arterial switch) 35.84
Jejunectomy 45.62
Jejunocecostomy 45.93
Jejunocholecystostomy 51.32
Jejunocolostomy 45.93

Jejunoileostomy 45.91
Jejunojejunostomy 45.91
Jejunopexy 46.61
Jejunorrhaphy 46.73
Jejunostomy (feeding) 46.39
  delayed opening 46.31
  loop 46.01
  percutaneous (endoscopic) (PEJ) 46.32
  revision 46.41
Jejunotomy 45.02
Johanson operation (urethral reconstruction) 58.46

Jones operation
  claw toe (transfer of extensor hallucis longus tendon) 77.57
    modified (with arthrodesis) 77.57
  dacryocystorhinostomy 09.81
  hammer toe (interphalangeal fusion) 77.56
    modified (tendon transfer with arthrodesis) 77.57
  repair of peroneal tendon 83.88
Joplin operation (exostectomy with tendon transfer) 77.53

K

Kader operation (temporary gastrostomy) 43.19
Kasai portoenterostomy 51.37
Kaufman operation (for urinary stress incontinence) 59.79
Kazanjiian operation (buccal vestibular sulcus extension) 24.91
Kehr operation (hepatopexy) 50.69
Keller operation (bunionectomy) 77.59

Kelly (-Kennedy) operation (urethrovesical plication) 59.3
Kelly-Stoeckel operation (urethrovesical plication) 59.3
Kelotomy 53.9
Keratectomy (complete) (partial) (superficial) 11.49
  for pterygium 11.39
    with corneal graft 11.32
Keratocentesis (for hyphema) 12.91
Keratomileusis 11.71

Keratophakia 11.72
Keratoplasty (tectonic) (with autograft) (with homograft) 11.60
  lamellar (nonpenetrating) (with homograft) 11.62
    with autograft 11.61
  penetrating (full-thickness) (with homograft) 11.64
    with autograft 11.63
  perforating - *see* Keratoplasty, penetrating

I, J, & K

Keratoplasty (Continued)
  refractive 11.71
  specified type NEC 11.69
Keratoprosthesis 11.73
Keratotomy (delimiting) (posterior) 11.1
  radial (refractive) 11.75
Kerr operation (low cervical cesarean
  section) 74.1
Kessler operation (arthroplasty,
  carpometacarpal joint) 81.74
Kidner operation (excision of accessory
  navicular bone) (with tendon
  transfer) 77.98
Killian operation (frontal sinusotomy)
  22.41
Kineplasty - see Cineplasty

King-Steelquist operation (hind-quarter
  amputation) 84.19
Kirk operation (amputation through
  thigh) 84.17
Kock pouch
  bowel anastomosis - omit code
  continent ileostomy 46.22
  cutaneous uretero-ileostomy 56.51
  ESWL (electrocorporeal shockwave
    lithotripsy) 98.51
  removal, calculus 57.19
  revision, cutaneous uretero-ileostomy
    56.52
  urinary diversion procedure 56.51
Kockogram (ileal conduitogram) 87.78
Kockoscopy 45.12

Kondoleon operation (correction of
  lymph-edema) 40.9
Krause operation (sympathetic
  denervation) 05.29
Kroener operation (partial
  salpingectomy) 66.69
Kroenlein operation (lateral orbitotomy)
  16.01
Kronig operation (low cervical cesarean
  section) 74.1
Krunkenberg operation (reconstruction
  of below-elbow amputation) 82.89
Kuhnt-Szymanowski operation
  (ectropion repair with lid
  reconstruction) 08.44
Kyphoplasty 81.66

L

Labbe operation (gastrotomy) 43.0
Labiectomy (bilateral) 71.62
  unilateral 71.61
Labyrinthectomy (transtympanic) 20.79
Labyrinthotomy (transtympanic) 20.79
Ladd operation (mobilization of intestine)
  54.95
Lagrange operation (iridosclerectomy)
  12.65
Lambrinudi operation (triple arthrodesis)
  81.12
Laminectomy (decompression) (for
  exploration) 03.09
  as operative approach - omit code
  with
    excision of herniated intervertebral
      disc (nucleus pulposus) 80.51
    excision of other intraspinal lesion
      (tumor) 03.4
    reopening of site 03.02
Laminography - see Radiography
Laminoplasty, expansile 03.09
Laminotomy (decompression) (for
  exploration) 03.09
  as operative approach - omit code
  reopening of site 03.02
Langenbeck operation (cleft palate
  repair) 27.62
Laparoamnioscopy 75.31
Laparorrhaphy 54.63
Laparoscopy 54.21
  with
    biopsy (intra-abdominal) 54.24
      uterine ligaments 68.15
      uterus 68.16
    destruction of fallopian tubes - see
      Destruction, fallopian tube
Laparotomy NEC 54.19
  as operative approach - omit code
  exploratory (pelvic) 54.11
  reopening of recent operative site (for
    control of hemorrhage) (for
    exploration) (for incision of
    hematoma) 54.12
Laparotrachelotomy 74.1
Lapidus operation (bunionectomy with
  metatarsal osteotomy) 77.51
Larry operation (shoulder disarticulation)
  84.08

Laryngectomy
  with radical neck dissection (with
    synchronous thyroidectomy)
    (with synchronous tracheostomy)
    30.4
  complete (with partial laryngectomy)
    (with synchronous tracheostomy)
    30.3
    with radical neck dissection (with
      synchronous thyroidectomy)
      (with synchronous
      tracheostomy) 30.4
  frontolateral partial (extended) 30.29
  glottosupraglottic partial 30.29
  lateral partial 30.29
  partial (frontolateral)
    (glottosupraglottic) (lateral)
    (submucous) (supraglottic)
    (vertical) 30.29
  radical (with synchronous
    thyroidectomy) (with
    synchronous tracheostomy)
    30.4
  submucous (partial) 30.29
  supraglottic partial 30.29
  total (with partial pharyngectomy) (with
    synchronous tracheostomy) 30.3
    with radical neck dissection (with
      synchronous thyroidectomy)
      (with synchronous
      tracheostomy) 30.4
  vertical partial 30.29
  wide field 30.3
Laryngocentesis 31.3
Laryngoesophagectomy 30.4
Laryngofissure 30.29
Laryngogram 87.09
  contrast 87.07
Laryngopharyngectomy (with
  synchronous tracheostomy) 30.3
  radical (with synchronous
    thyroidectomy) 30.4
Laryngopharyngoesophagectomy (with
  synchronous tracheostomy) 30.3
  with radical neck dissection (with
    synchronous thyroidectomy)
    30.4
Laryngoplasty 31.69
Laryngorrhaphy 31.61
Laryngoscopy (suspension) (through
  artificial stoma) 31.42

Laryngostomy (permanent) 31.29
  revision 31.63
  temporary (emergency) 31.1
Laryngotomy 31.3
Laryngotracheobronchoscopy 33.23
  with biopsy 33.24
Laryngotracheoscopy 31.42
Laryngotracheostomy (permanent) 31.29
  temporary (emergency) 31.1
Laryngotracheotomy (temporary) 31.1
  permanent 31.29
Laser - see also Coagulation, Destruction,
  and Photocoagulation by site
  angioplasty, percutaneous transluminal
    39.59
  coronary - see Angioplasty, coronary
Laser interstitial thermal therapy (LITT)
  under guidance
  lesion
    brain 17.61
    breast 17.69
    head and neck 17.62
    liver 17.63
    lung 17.69
    prostate 17.69
    thyroid 17.62
Lash operation
  internal cervical os repair 67.59
  laparoscopic supracervical
    hysterectomy 68.31
LASIK (Laser-assisted in situ
  keratomileusis) 11.71
Latzko operation
  cesarean section 74.2
  colpocleisis 70.8
Lavage
  antral 22.00
  bronchus NEC 96.56
    diagnostic (endoscopic)
      bronchoalveolar lavage (BAL)
      33.24
      bronchoalveolar lavage (BAL)
        33.24 ◀
      mini-bronchoalveolar lavage
        (mini-BAL) 33.29 ◀
  endotracheal 96.56
  gastric 96.33
  lung (total) (whole) 33.99
    diagnostic (endoscopic)
      bronchoalveolar lavage (BAL)
      33.24

Lavage *(Continued)*
  nasal sinus(es) 22.00
    by puncture 22.01
    through natural ostium 22.02
  peritoneal (diagnostic) 54.25
  trachea NEC 96.56
Leadbetter operation (urethral
  reconstruction) 58.46
Leadbetter-Politano operation
  (ureteroneocystostomy) 56.74
LEEP (loop electrosurgical excision
  procedure) of cervix 67.32
Le Fort operation (colpocleisis) 70.8
LeMesurier operation (cleft lip repair) 27.54
Lengthening
  bone (with bone graft) 78.30
    femur 78.35
    for reconstruction of thumb 82.69
    specified site NEC 78.39 - *see also*
      category 78.3●
    tibia 78.37
    ulna 78.33
  extraocular muscle NEC 15.21
    multiple (two or more muscles) 15.4
  fascia 83.89
    hand 82.89
  hamstring NEC 83.85
  heel cord 83.85
  leg
    femur 78.35
    tibia 78.37
  levator palpebrae muscle 08.38
  muscle 83.85
    extraocular 15.21
      multiple (two or more muscles)
        15.4
    hand 82.55
  palate 27.62
    secondary or subsequent 27.63
  tendon 83.85
    for claw toe repair 77.57
    hand 82.55
Leriche operation (periarterial
  sympathectomy) 05.25
Leucotomy, leukotomy 01.32
Leukopheresis, therapeutic 99.72
Lid suture operation (blepharoptosis) 08.31
Ligation
  adrenal vessel (artery) (vein) 07.43
  aneurysm 39.52
  appendages, dermal 86.26
  arteriovenous fistula 39.53
    coronary artery 36.99
  artery 38.80
    abdominal 38.86
    adrenal 07.43
    aorta (arch) (ascending)
      (descending) 38.84
    coronary (anomalous) 36.99
    ethmoidal 21.04
    external carotid 21.06
    for control of epistaxis - *see* Control,
      epistaxis
    head and neck NEC 38.82
    intracranial NEC 38.81
    lower limb 38.88
    maxillary (transantral) 21.05
    middle meningeal 02.13
    thoracic NEC 38.85
    thyroid 06.92
    upper limb 38.83
  atrium, heart 37.99
  auricle, heart 37.99
  bleeding vessel - *see* Control,
    hemorrhage

Ligation *(Continued)*
  blood vessel 38.80
    abdominal
      artery 38.86
      vein 38.87
    adrenal 07.43
    aorta (arch) (ascending)
      (descending) 38.84
    esophagus 42.91
      endoscopic 42.33
    head and neck 38.82
    intracranial NEC 38.81
    lower limb
      artery 38.88
      vein 38.89
    meningeal (artery) (longitudinal
      sinus) 02.13
    thoracic NEC 38.85
    thyroid 06.92
    upper limb (artery) (vein) 38.83
  bronchus 33.92
  cisterna chyli 40.64
  coronary
    artery (anomalous) 36.99
    sinus 36.39
  dermal appendage 86.26
  ductus arteriosus, patent 38.85
  esophageal vessel 42.91
    endoscopic 42.33
  ethmoidal artery 21.04
  external carotid artery 21.06
  fallopian tube (bilateral) (remaining)
    (solitary) 66.39
    by endoscopy (culdoscopy)
      (hysteroscopy) (laparoscopy)
      (peritoneoscopy) 66.29
    with
      crushing 66.31
        by endoscopy (laparoscopy)
          66.21
      division 66.32
        by endoscopy (culdoscopy)
          (laparoscopy)
          (peritoneoscopy) 66.22
      Falope ring 66.39
        by endoscopy (laparoscopy)
          66.29
    unilateral 66.92
  fistula, arteriovenous 39.53
    coronary artery 36.99
  gastric
    artery 38.86
    varices 44.91
      endoscopic 43.41
  hemorrhoids 49.45
  longitudinal sinus (superior) 02.13
  lymphatic (channel) (peripheral)
    40.9
    thoracic duct 40.64
  maxillary artery 21.05
  meningeal vessel 02.13
  spermatic
    cord 63.72
      varicocele 63.1
    vein (high) 63.1
  splenic vessels 38.86
  subclavian artery 38.85
  superior longitudinal sinus 02.13
  supernumerary digit 86.26
  thoracic duct 40.64
  thyroid vessel (artery) (vein) 06.92
  toes (supernumerary) 86.26
  tooth 93.55
    impacted 24.6

Ligation *(Continued)*
  ulcer (peptic) (base) (bed) (bleeding
    vessel) 44.40
    duodenal 44.42
    gastric 44.41
  ureter 56.95
  varices
    esophageal 42.91
      endoscopic 42.33
    gastric 44.91
      endoscopic 43.41
    peripheral vein (lower limb)
      38.59
      upper limb 38.53
  varicocele 63.1
  vas deferens 63.71
  vein 38.80
    abdominal 38.87
    adrenal 07.43
    head and neck NEC 38.82
    intracranial NEC 38.81
    lower limb 38.89
    spermatic, high 63.1
    thoracic NEC 38.85
    thyroid 06.92
    upper limb 38.83
    varicose 38.50
      abdominal 38.57
      esophagus 42.91
        endoscopic 42.33
      gastric 44.91
        endoscopic 43.41
      head and neck 38.52
      intracranial NEC 38.51
      lower limb 38.59
      stomach 44.91
      thoracic NEC 38.55
      upper limb 38.53
  vena cava, inferior 38.7
  venous connection between anomalous
    vein to
    left innominate vein 35.82
    superior vena cava 35.82
  wart 86.26
Light coagulation - *see* Photocoagulation
Lindholm operation (repair of ruptured
  tendon) 83.88
Lingulectomy, lung 32.39
Linton operation (varicose vein) 38.59
Lipectomy (subcutaneous tissue)
  (abdominal) (submental) 86.83
Liposuction 86.83
Lip reading training 95.49
Lip shave 27.43
Lisfranc operation
  foot amputation 84.12
  shoulder disarticulation
    84.08
Litholapaxy, bladder 57.0
  by incision 57.19
Lithotomy
  bile passage 51.49
  bladder (urinary) 57.19
  common duct 51.41
    percutaneous 51.96
  gallbladder 51.04
  hepatic duct 51.49
  kidney 55.01
    percutaneous 55.03
  ureter 56.2
Lithotripsy
  bile duct NEC 51.49
    extracorporeal shockwave (ESWL)
      98.52

◀ New   ◀◀ Revised   ~~deleted~~ Deleted   ● Use Additional Digit(s)   ▨ Omit code

Lithotripsy (Continued)
  bladder 57.0
    with ultrasonic fragmentation 57.0
      [59.95]
    extracorporeal shockwave (ESWL)
      98.51
  extracorporeal shockwave (ESWL)
    NEC 98.59
    bile duct 98.52
    bladder (urinary) 98.51
    gallbladder 98.52
    kidney 98.51
    Kock pouch 98.51
    renal pelvis 98.51
    specified site NEC 98.59
    ureter 98.51
  gallbladder NEC 51.04
    endoscopic 51.88
    extracorporeal shockwave (ESWL)
      98.52
  kidney 56.0
    extracorporeal shockwave (ESWL)
      98.51
    percutaneous nephrostomy with
      fragmentation (laser)
      (ultrasound) 55.04
  renal pelvis 56.0
    extracorporeal shockwave (ESWL)
      98.51
    percutaneous nephrostomy with
      fragmentation (laser)
      (ultrasound) 55.04
  ureter 56.0
    extracorporeal shock wave (ESWL)
      98.51
LITT (laser interstitial thermal therapy)
  under guidance
  lesion
    brain 17.61
    breast 17.69
    head and neck 17.62
    liver 17.63
    lung 17.69
    prostate 17.69
    thyroid 17.62
Littlewood operation (forequarter
  amputation) 84.09
LLETZ (large loop excision of the
  transformation zone) of cervix
  67.32
Lloyd-Davies operation
  (abdominoperineal resection), NOS
  48.50
  laparoscopic 48.51
  open 48.52
  other 48.59
Lobectomy
  brain 01.53
    partial 01.59
  liver (with partial excision of adjacent
    lobes) 50.3
  lung (complete) 32.49
    partial 32.39
      thoracoscopic 32.30
    segmental (with resection of
      adjacent lobes) 32.49
      thoracoscopic 32.41
    thoracoscopic 32.41
  thyroid (total) (unilateral) (with
    removal of isthmus) (with
    removal of portion of remaining
    lobe) 06.2
    partial - *see also* Thyroidectomy,
      partial 06.39

Lobectomy (Continued)
  thyroid (Continued)
    substernal 06.51
    subtotal - *see also* Thyroidectomy,
      partial 06.39
Lobotomy, brain 01.32
Localization, placenta 88.78
  by RISA injection 92.17
Longmire operation (bile duct
  anastomosis) 51.39
Loop ileal stoma (*see also* Ileostomy)
  46.01
Loopogram 87.78
Looposcopy (ileal conduit) 56.35
Lord operation
  dilation of anal canal for hemorrhoids
    49.49
  hemorrhoidectomy 49.49
  orchidopexy 62.5
Lower GI series (x-ray) 87.64
Lucas and Murray operation (knee
  arthrodesis with plate) 81.22
Lumpectomy
  breast 85.21
  specified site - *see* Excision, lesion, by
    site
Lymphadenectomy (simple) - *see also*
  Excision, lymph, node 40.29
Lymphadenotomy 40.0
Lymphangiectomy (radical) - *see also*
  Excision, lymph, node, by site,
  radical 40.50
Lymphangiogram
  abdominal 88.04
  cervical 87.08
  intrathoracic 87.34
  lower limb 88.36
  pelvic 88.04
  upper limb 88.34
Lymphangioplasty 40.9
Lymphangiorrhaphy 40.9
Lymphangiotomy 40.0
Lymphaticostomy 40.9
  thoracic duct 40.62
Lysis
  adhesions

> Note: blunt - *omit code*
>   digital - *omit code*
>   manual - *omit code*
>   mechanical - *omit code*
>   without instrumentation - *omit*
>   *code*

    abdominal 54.59
      laparoscopic 54.51
    appendiceal 54.59
      laparoscopic 54.51
    artery-vein-nerve bundle 39.91
    biliary tract 54.59
      laparoscopic 54.51
    bladder (neck) (intraluminal) 57.12
      external 59.11
        laparoscopic 59.12
      transurethral 57.41
    blood vessels 39.91
    bone - *see* category 78.4●
    bursa 83.91
      by stretching or manipulation
        93.28
      hand 82.91
    cartilage of joint 93.26
    chest wall 33.99

Lysis (Continued)
  adhesions (Continued)
    choanae (nasopharynx) 29.54
    conjunctiva 10.5
    corneovitreal 12.34
    cortical (brain) 02.91
    ear, middle 20.23
    Eustachian tube 20.8
    extraocular muscle 15.7
    extrauterine 54.59
      laparoscopic 54.51
    eyelid 08.09
      and conjunctiva 10.5
    eye muscle 15.7
    fallopian tube 65.89
      laparoscopic 65.81
    fascia 83.91
      hand 82.91
        by stretching or manipulation
          93.26
    gallbladder 54.59
      laparoscopic 54.51
    ganglion (peripheral) NEC 04.49
      cranial NEC 04.42
    hand 82.91
      by stretching or manipulation
        93.26
    heart 37.10
    intestines 54.59
      laparoscopic 54.51
    iris (posterior) 12.33
      anterior 12.32
    joint (capsule) (structure) - *see also*
      Division, joint capsule 80.40
    kidney 59.02
      laparoscopic 59.03
    labia (vulva) 71.01
    larynx 31.92
    liver 54.59
      laparoscopic 54.51
    lung (for collapse of lung) 33.39
    mediastinum 34.99
    meninges (spinal) 03.6
      cortical 02.91
    middle ear 20.23
    muscle 83.91
      by stretching or manipulation
        93.27
      extraocular 15.7
      hand 82.91
        by stretching or manipulation
          93.26
    nasopharynx 29.54
    nerve (peripheral) NEC 04.49
      cranial NEC 04.42
      roots, spinal 03.6
      trigeminal 04.41
    nose, nasal 21.91
    ocular muscle 15.7
    ovary 65.89
      laparoscopic 65.81
    pelvic 54.59
      laparoscopic 54.51
    penile 64.93
    pericardium 37.12
    perineal (female) 71.01
    peripheral vessels 39.91
    perirectal 48.81
    perirenal 59.02
      laparoscopic 59.03
    peritoneum (pelvic) 54.59
      laparoscopic 54.51
    periureteral 59.02
      laparoscopic 59.03

Lysis *(Continued)*
  adhesions *(Continued)*
    perivesical 59.11
      laparoscopic 59.12
    pharynx 29.54
    pleura (for collapse of lung) 33.39
    spermatic cord 63.94
    spinal (cord) (meninges) (nerve
      roots) 03.6
    spleen 54.59
      laparoscopic 54.51
    tendon 83.91
      by stretching or manipulation
        93.27
      hand 82.91
        by stretching or manipulation
          93.26

Lysis *(Continued)*
  adhesions *(Continued)*
    thorax 34.99
    tongue 25.93
    trachea 31.92
    tubo-ovarian 65.89
      laparoscopic 65.81
    ureter 59.02
      with freeing or repositioning of
        ureter 59.02
      intraluminal 56.81
      laparoscopic 59.03
    urethra (intraluminal) 58.5
    uterus 54.59
      intraluminal 68.21
      laparoscopic 54.51

Lysis *(Continued)*
  adhesions *(Continued)*
    uterus *(Continued)*
      peritoneal 54.59
        laparoscopic 54.51
      vagina (intraluminal) 70.13
      vitreous (posterior approach) 14.74
        anterior approach 14.73
      vulva 71.01
    goniosynechiae (with injection of air or
      liquid) 12.31
    synechiae (posterior) 12.33
      anterior (with injection of air or
        liquid) 12.32

M

Madlener operation (tubal ligation)
  66.31
Magnet extraction
  foreign body
    anterior chamber, eye 12.01
    choroid 14.01
    ciliary body 12.01
    conjunctiva 98.22
    cornea 11.0
    eye, eyeball NEC 98.21
      anterior segment 12.01
      posterior segment 14.01
    intraocular (anterior segment)
      12.01
    iris 12.01
    lens 13.01
    orbit 98.21
    retina 14.01
    sclera 12.01
    vitreous 14.01
Magnetic resonance imaging (nuclear) -
  see Imaging, magnetic resonance
Magnuson (-Stack) operation
  (arthroplasty for recurrent shoulder
  dislocation) 81.82
Mako Tactile Guidance System™ [TGS] -
  see category 17.4●
Malleostapediopexy 19.19
  with incus replacement 19.11
Malström's vacuum extraction 72.79
  with episiotomy 72.71
Mammaplasty - *see* Mammoplasty
Mammectomy - *see also* Mastectomy
  subcutaneous (unilateral) 85.34
    with synchronous implant 85.33
    bilateral 85.36
      with synchronous implant
        85.35
Mammilliplasty 85.87
Mammography NEC 87.37
Mammoplasty 85.89
  with
    full-thickness graft 85.83
    muscle flap 85.85
    pedicle graft 85.84
    split-thickness graft 85.82
  amputative (reduction) (bilateral)
    85.32
    unilateral 85.31

Mammoplasty *(Continued)*
  augmentation 85.50
    with
      breast implant (bilateral) 85.54
        unilateral 85.53
      injection into breast (bilateral)
        85.52
        unilateral 85.51
  reduction (bilateral) 85.32
    unilateral 85.31
  revision 85.89
  size reduction (gynecomastia)
    (bilateral) 85.32
    unilateral 85.31
Mammotomy 85.0
Manchester (-Donald) (-Fothergill)
  operation (uterine suspension)
  69.22
Mandibulectomy (partial) 76.31
  total 76.42
    with reconstruction 76.41
Maneuver (method)
  Bracht 72.52
  Credé 73.59
  De Lee (key-in-lock) 72.4
  Kristeller 72.54
  Loveset's (extraction of arms in breech
    birth) 72.52
  Mauriceau (-Smellie-Veit) 72.52
  Pinard (total breech extraction) 72.54
  Prague 72.52
  Ritgen 73.59
  Scanzoni (rotation) 72.4
  Van Hoorn 72.52
  Wigand-Martin 72.52
Manipulation
  with reduction of fracture or
    dislocation - *see* Reduction,
    fracture *and* Reduction,
    dislocation
  enterostomy stoma (with dilation)
    96.24
  intestine (intra-abdominal) 46.80
    large 46.82
    small 46.81
  joint
    adhesions 93.26
      temporomandibular 76.95
    dislocation - *see* Reduction,
      dislocation
  lacrimal passage (tract) NEC 09.49

Manipulation *(Continued)*
  muscle structures 93.27
  musculoskeletal (physical therapy)
    NEC 93.29
  nasal septum, displaced 21.88
  osteopathic NEC 93.67
    for general mobilization (general
      articulation) 93.61
    high-velocity, low-amplitude forces
      (thrusting) 93.62
    indirect forces 93.65
    isotonic, isometric forces 93.64
    low-velocity, high-amplitude forces
      (springing) 93.63
    to move tissue fluids 93.66
  rectum 96.22
  salivary duct 26.91
  stomach, intraoperative 44.92
  temporomandibular joint NEC 76.95
  ureteral calculus by catheter
    with removal 56.0
    without removal 59.8
  uterus NEC 69.98
    gravid 75.99
    inverted
      manual replacement (following
        delivery) 75.94
      surgical - *see* Repair, inverted
        uterus
Manometry
  esophageal 89.32
  spinal fluid 89.15
  urinary 89.21
Manual arts therapy 93.81
Mapping
  cardiac (electrophysiologic) 37.27
    doppler (flow) 88.72
  electrocardiogram only 89.52
Marckwald operation (cervical os repair)
  67.59
Marshall-Marchetti (-Krantz) operation
  (retropubic urethral suspension)
  59.5
Marsupialization - *see also* Destruction,
  lesion, by site
  cyst
    Bartholin's 71.23
    brain 01.59
    cervical (nabothian) 67.31
    dental 24.4
    dentigerous 24.4

◀ New   ◀||||| Revised   ~~deleted~~ Deleted   ● Use Additional Digit(s)   ▨ Omit code

Marsupialization (Continued)
   cyst (Continued)
      kidney 55.31
      larynx 30.01
      liver 50.21
      ovary 65.21
         laparoscopic 65.23
      pancreas 52.3
      pilonidal (open excision) (with
         partial closure) 86.21
      salivary gland 26.21
      spinal (intraspinal) (meninges)
         03.4
      spleen, splenic 41.41
   lesion
      brain 01.59
      cerebral 01.59
      liver 50.21
   pilonidal cyst or sinus (open excision)
      (with partial closure) 86.21
   pseudocyst, pancreas 52.3
   ranula, salivary gland 26.21
Massage
   cardiac (external) (manual) (closed)
      99.63
      open 37.91
   prostatic 99.94
   rectal (for levator spasm) 99.93
MAST (military anti-shock trousers)
   93.58
Mastectomy (complete) (prophylactic)
   (simple) (unilateral) 85.41
   with
      excision of regional lymph nodes
         85.43
         bilateral 85.44
      preservation of skin and nipple
         85.34
         with synchronous implant 85.33
         bilateral 85.36
            with synchronous implant
              85.35
   bilateral 85.42
   extended
      radical (Urban) (unilateral) 85.47
         bilateral 85.48
      simple (with regional
         lymphadenectomy)
         (unilateral) 85.43
         bilateral 85.44
   modified radical (unilateral) 85.43
      bilateral 85.44
   partial 85.23
   radical (Halsted) (Meyer) (unilateral)
      85.45
      bilateral 85.46
      extended (Urban) (unilateral) 85.47
         bilateral 85.48
      modified (unilateral) 85.43
         bilateral 85.44
   subcutaneous 85.34
      with synchronous implant 85.33
      bilateral 85.36
         with synchronous implant
            85.35
   subtotal 85.23
Masters' stress test (two-step) 89.42
Mastoidectomy (cortical) (conservative)
   20.49
   complete (simple) 20.41
   modified radical 20.49
   radical 20.42
      modified 20.49
   simple (complete) 20.41

Mastoidotomy 20.21
Mastoidotympanectomy 20.42
Mastopexy 85.6
Mastoplasty - see Mammoplasty
Mastorrhaphy 85.81
Mastotomy 85.0
Matas operation (aneurysmorrhaphy)
   39.52
Mayo operation
   bunionectomy 77.59
   herniorrhaphy
      laparoscopic 53.43
         with graft or prosthesis 53.42
      other and open with graft or
         prosthesis 53.41
      other open 53.49
   vaginal hysterectomy 68.59
      laparoscopically assisted (LAVH)
         68.51
Maze procedure ◄
   Cox-maze, open 37.33 ◄
   maze, modified, endovascular 37.34 ◄
   maze, modified, open 37.33 ◄
Mazet operation (knee disarticulation)
   84.16
McBride operation (bunionectomy with
   soft tissue correction) 77.53
McBurney operation - see Repair, hernia,
   inguinal
McCall operation (enterocele repair) 70.92
McCauley operation (release of clubfoot)
   83.84
McDonald operation (encirclement
   suture, cervix) 67.59
McIndoe operation (vaginal construction)
   70.61
   with graft or prosthesis 70.63
McKeever operation (fusion of first
   metatarsophalangeal joint for hallux
   valgus repair) 77.52
McKissock operation (breast reduction)
   85.33
McReynolds operation (transposition of
   pterygium) 11.31
McVay operation
   femoral hernia - see Repair, hernia,
      femoral
   inguinal hernia - see Repair, hernia,
      inguinal
Measurement
   airway resistance 89.38
   anatomic NEC 89.39
   arterial blood gases 89.65
      basal metabolic rate (BMR) 89.39
      blood gases
         arterial 89.65
            continuous intra-arterial
              89.60
         venous 89.66
   body 93.07
   cardiac output (by)
      Fick method 89.67
      indicator dilution technique 89.68
      oxygen consumption technique
         89.67
      thermodilution indicator 89.68
   cardiovascular NEC 89.59
   central venous pressure 89.62
   coronary blood flow 89.69
      fractional flow reserve (FFR)
         00.59
      intravascular pressure
         measurement 00.59
   gastric function NEC 89.39

Measurement (Continued)
   girth 93.07
   intelligence 94.01
   intracranial pressure 01.10
   intraocular tension or pressure 89.11
      as part of extended ophthalmologic
         work-up 95.03
   intrauterine pressure 75.35
   intravascular pressure 00.69
      coronary 00.59
      iliac 00.69
      intra-abdominal 00.69
      intrathoracic 00.67
         aorta 00.67
         aortic arch 00.67
         carotid 00.67
      mesenteric 00.69
      peripheral 00.68
      renal 00.69
   limb length 93.06
   lung volume 89.37
   mixed venous blood gases 89.66
   physiologic NEC 89.39
   portovenous pressure 89.62
   pulmonary airway flow, endoscopic
      33.72
   range of motion 93.05
   renal clearance 89.29
   respiratory NEC 89.38
   skin fold thickness 93.07
   skull circumference 93.07
   sphincter of Oddi pressure 51.15
   systemic arterial
      blood gases 89.65
         continuous intra-arterial 89.60
      pressure 89.61
   urine (bioassay) (chemistry) 89.29
   vascular 89.59
   venous blood gases 89.66
   vital capacity (pulmonary) 89.37
Meatoplasty
   ear 18.6
   urethra 58.47
Meatotomy
   ureter 56.1
   urethra 58.1
      internal 58.5
Mechanical ventilation - see Ventilation
Mediastinectomy 34.3
Mediastinoscopy 34.22
Mediastinotomy (Chamberlain
   procedure) 34.1
   with pneumonectomy 32.59
      thoracoscopic 32.50
Meloplasty, facial 86.82
Meningeorrhaphy (cerebral) 02.12
   spinal NEC 03.59
      for
         meningocele 03.51
         myelomeningocele 03.52
Meniscectomy (knee) NEC 80.6
   acromioclavicular 80.91
   sternoclavicular 80.91
   temporomandibular (joint) 76.5
   wrist 80.93
Menstrual extraction or regulation
   69.6
Mentoplasty (augmentation) (with graft)
   (with implant) 76.68
   reduction 76.67
Mesenterectomy 54.4
Mesenteriopexy 54.75
Mesenteriplication 54.75
Mesocoloplication 54.75

Mesopexy 54.75
Metatarsectomy 77.98
Metroplasty 69.49
Mid forceps delivery 72.29
Mikulicz operation (exteriorization of
    intestine) (first stage) 46.03
    second stage 46.04
Miles operation (proctectomy), NOS 48.50
    laparoscopic 48.51
    open 48.52
    other 48.59
Military anti-shock trousers (MAST) 93.58
Millard operation (cheiloplasty) 27.54
Miller operation
    midtarsal arthrodesis 81.14
    urethrovesical suspension 59.4
Millin-Read operation (urethrovesical
    suspension) 59.4
Mist therapy 93.94
Mitchell operation (hallux valgus repair)
    77.51
MitraClip® mitral valve leaflet clip
    35.97 ◀
Mobilization
    joint NEC 93.16
    mandible 76.95
    neostrophingic (mitral valve) 35.12
    spine 93.15
    stapes (transcrural) 19.0
    testis in scrotum 62.5
Mohs operation (chemosurgical excision
    of skin) 86.24
Molegraphy 87.81
Monitoring
    BIS (bispectral index) monitoring 00.94
        [89.14]
    brain temperature 01.17
    cardiac output (by)
        ambulatory (ACM) 89.50
        electrographic 89.54
            during surgery - omit code
        Fick method 89.67
        Holter-type device 89.50
        indicator dilution technique 89.68
        intracardiac or great vessel
            hemodynamic
            sensor (lead) 00.56
            subcutaneous device 00.57
        oxygen consumption technique 89.67
        specified technique NEC 89.68
        telemetry (cardiac) 89.54
        thermodilution indicator 89.68
        transesophageal (Doppler)
            (ultrasound) 89.68
    central venous pressure 89.62
    circulatory NEC 89.69
    continuous intra-arterial blood gas 89.60
    coronary blood flow (coincidence
        counting technique) 89.69
        fractional flow reserve (FFR) 00.59
        intravascular pressure measurement
            00.59
    electroencephalographic 89.19
        radio-telemetered 89.19
        video 89.19
    fetus (fetal heart)
        antepartum
            nonstress (fetal activity
                acceleration
                determinations) 75.34
            oxytocin challenge (contraction
                stress test) 75.35
            ultrasonography (early
                pregnancy) (Doppler) 88.78

Monitoring (Continued)
    fetus (Continued)
        intrapartum (during labor)
            (extrauterine) (external) 75.34
            auscultatory (stethoscopy) - omit
                code
            internal (with contraction
                measurements) (ECG) 75.32
            intrauterine (direct) (ECG) 75.32
            phonocardiographic
                (extrauterine) 75.34
            pulsed ultrasound (Doppler) 88.78
            transcervical fetal oxygen
                saturation monitoring
                75.38
            transcervical fetal SpO₂
                monitoring 75.38
    Holter-type device (cardiac) 89.50
    IAEMT (intraoperative anesthetic effect
        monitoring and titration) 00.94
        [89.14]
    intra-aneursym sac pressure 00.58
    intracranial oxygen 01.16
    intracranial pressure 01.10
    intraoperative anesthetic effect
        monitoring and titration
        (IAEMT) 00.94 [89.14]
    intravascular pressure 00.69
        coronary 00.59
        iliac 00.69
        intra-abdominal 00.69
        intrathoracic 00.67
            aorta 00.67
            aortic arch 00.67
            carotid 00.67
        mesenteric 00.69
        peripheral 00.68
        renal 00.69
    neurophysiologic
        intra-operative 00.94
    partial pressure of brain oxygen
        (PbtO₂) 01.16
    pulmonary artery
        pressure 89.63
        wedge 89.64
    sleep (recording) - see categories 89.17–
        89.18
    systemic arterial pressure 89.61
        intra-aneursym sac pressure 00.58
    telemetry (cardiac) 89.54
    transesophageal cardiac output
        (Doppler) 89.68
    ventricular pressure (cardiac) 89.62
Moore operation (arthroplasty) 81.52
Moschowitz
    enterocele repair 70.92
        with graft or prosthesis 70.93
    herniorrhaphy - see Repair, hernia,
        femoral
    sigmoidopexy 46.63
Mountain resort sanitarium 93.98
Mouth-to-mouth resuscitation 93.93
Moxibustion 93.35
MRI - see Imaging, magnetic resonance
Muller operation (banding of pulmonary
    artery) 38.85
Multiple sleep latency test (MSLT)
    89.18
Mumford operation (partial
    claviculectomy) 77.81
Musculoplasty - see also Repair, muscle
    83.87
    hand - see also Repair, muscle, hand
        82.89

Music therapy 93.84
Mustard operation (interatrial
    transposition of venous return)
    35.91
Myectomy 83.45
    anorectal 48.92
    eye muscle 15.13
        multiple 15.3
    for graft 83.43
        hand 82.34
    hand 82.36
        for graft 82.34
    levator palpebrae 08.33
    rectal 48.92
Myelogram, myelography (air) (gas)
    87.21
    posterior fossa 87.02
Myelotomy
    spine, spinal (cord) (tract) (one-stage)
        (two-stage) 03.29
        percutaneous 03.21
Myocardiectomy (infarcted area) 37.33
Myocardiotomy 37.11
Myoclasis 83.99
    hand 82.99
Myomectomy (uterine) 68.29
    broad ligament 69.19
Myoplasty - see also Repair, muscle 83.87
    hand - see also Repair, muscle, hand
        82.89
    mastoid 19.9
Myorrhaphy 83.65
    hand 82.46
Myosuture 83.65
    hand 82.46
Myotasis 93.27
Myotenontoplasty - see also Repair,
    tendon 83.88
    hand 82.86
Myotenoplasty - see also Repair, tendon
    83.88
    hand 82.86
Myotenotomy 83.13
    hand 82.11
Myotomy 83.02
    with division 83.19
        hand 82.19
    colon NEC 46.92
        sigmoid 46.91
    cricopharyngeal 29.31
        that for pharyngeal
            (pharyngoesophageal)
            diverticulectomy 29.32
    esophagus 42.7
    eye (oblique) (rectus) 15.21
        multiple (two or more muscles) 15.4
    hand 82.02
        with division 82.19
    levator palpebrae 08.38
    sigmoid (colon) 46.91
Myringectomy 20.59
Myringodectomy 20.59
Myringomalleolabyrinthopexy
    19.52
Myringoplasty (epitympanic, type I)
    (by cauterization) (by graft) 19.4
    revision 19.6
Myringostapediopexy 19.53
Myringostomy 20.01
Myringotomy (with aspiration) (with
    drainage) 20.09
    with insertion of tube or drainage
        device (button) (grommet)
        20.01

N

Nailing, intramedullary
with fracture reduction - *see*
Reduction, fracture with
internal fixation
internal (without fracture
reduction) 78.50
Narcoanalysis 94.21
Narcosynthesis 94.21
Narrowing, palpebral fissure 08.51
Nasopharyngogram 87.09
contrast 87.06
Necropsy 89.8
Needleoscopy (fetus) 75.31
Needling
Bartholin's gland (cyst) 71.21
cataract (secondary) 13.64
fallopian tube 66.91
hydrocephalic head 73.8
lens (capsule) 13.2
pupillary membrane (iris) 12.35
Nephrectomy (complete) (total)
(unilateral) 55.51
bilateral 55.54
partial (wedge) 55.4
remaining or solitary kidney 55.52
removal transplanted kidney 55.53
Nephrocolopexy 55.7
Nephrocystanastomosis NEC 56.73
Nephrolithotomy 55.01
Nephrolysis 59.02
laparoscopic 59.03
Nephropexy 55.7
Nephroplasty 55.89
Nephropyeloplasty 55.87
Nephropyeloureterostomy 55.86
Nephrorrhaphy 55.81
Nephroscopy 55.21
Nephrostolithotomy, percutaneous 55.03

Nephrostomy (with drainage tube) 55.02
closure 55.82
percutaneous 55.03
with fragmentation (ultrasound)
55.04
Nephrotomogram, nephrotomography
NEC 87.72
Nephrotomy 55.01
Nephroureterectomy (with bladder cuff)
55.51
Nephroureterocystectomy 55.51 [57.79]
Nerve block (cranial) (peripheral) NEC -
see also Block, by site 04.81
Neurectasis (cranial) (peripheral) 04.91
Neurectomy (cranial) (infraorbital)
(occipital) (peripheral) (spinal) NEC
04.07
gastric (vagus) - *see also* Vagotomy
44.00
opticociliary 12.79
paracervical 05.22
presacral 05.24
retrogasserian 04.07
sympathetic - *see* Sympathectomy
trigeminal 04.07
tympanic 20.91
Neurexeresis NEC 04.07
Neuroablation
radiofrequency 04.2
Neuroanastomosis (cranial) (peripheral)
NEC 04.74
accessory-facial 04.72
accessory-hypoglossal 04.73
hypoglossal-facial 04.71
Neurolysis (peripheral nerve) NEC 04.49
carpal tunnel 04.43
cranial nerve NEC 04.42
spinal (cord) (nerve roots) 03.6
tarsal tunnel 04.44
trigeminal nerve 04.41

Neuromonitoring
intra-operative 00.94
Neuroplasty (cranial) (peripheral) NEC
04.79
of old injury (delayed repair) 04.76
revision 04.75
Neurorrhaphy (cranial) (peripheral)
04.3
Neurotomy (cranial) (peripheral) (spinal)
NEC 04.04
acoustic 04.01
glossopharyngeal 29.92
lacrimal branch 05.0
retrogasserian 04.02
sympathetic 05.0
vestibular 04.01
Neurotripsy (peripheral) NEC 04.03
trigeminal 04.02
Nicola operation (tenodesis for
recurrent dislocation of shoulder)
81.82
Nimodipine, infusion 99.75
NIPS (non-invasive programmed
electrical stimulation) 37.20
Nissen operation (fundoplication of
stomach) 44.66
laparoscopic 44.67
Noble operation (plication of small
intestine) 46.62
Norman Miller operation (vaginopexy)
70.77
with graft or prosthesis 70.78
Norton operation (extraperitoneal
cesarean section) 74.2
Nuclear magnetic resonance imaging -
see Imaging, magnetic resonance
Nutrition, concentrated substances
enteral infusion (of) 96.6
parenteral, (total) 99.15
peripheral parenteral 99.15

O

Ober (-Yount) operation (gluteal-iliotibial
fasciotomy) 83.14
Obliteration
bone cavity - *see also* Osteoplasty 78.40
calyceal diverticulum 55.39
canaliculi 09.6
cerebrospinal fistula 02.12
cul-de-sac 70.92
with graft or prosthesis 70.93
frontal sinus (with fat) 22.42
lacrimal punctum 09.91
lumbar pseudomeningocele 03.51
lymphatic structure(s) (peripheral)
40.9
maxillary sinus 22.31
meningocele (sacral) 03.51
pelvic 68.8
pleural cavity 34.6
sacral meningocele 03.51
Skene's gland 71.3
tympanomastoid cavity 19.9
vagina, vaginal (partial) (total) 70.4
vault 70.8

Occlusal molds (dental) 89.31
Occlusion
artery
by embolization - *see* Embolization,
artery
by endovascular approach - *see*
Embolization, artery
by ligation - *see* Ligation, artery
fallopian tube - *see* Ligation, fallopian
tube
patent ductus arteriosus (PDA) 38.85
vein
by embolization - *see* Embolization,
vein
by endovascular approach - *see*
Embolization, vein
by ligation - *see* Ligation, vein
vena cava (surgical) 38.7
Occupational therapy 93.83
OCT (optical coherence tomography)
(intavascular imaging)
coronary vessel(s) 38.24
non-coronary vessel(s) 38.25
O'Donoghue operation (triad knee
repair) 81.43

Odontectomy NEC - *see also* Removal,
tooth, surgical 23.19
Oleothorax 33.39
Olshausen operation (uterine suspension)
69.22
Omentectomy 54.4
Omentofixation 54.74
Omentopexy 54.74
Omentoplasty 54.74
Omentorrhaphy 54.74
Omentotomy 54.19
Omphalectomy 54.3
Onychectomy 86.23
Onychoplasty 86.86
Onychotomy 86.09
with drainage 86.04
Oophorectomy (unilateral) 65.39
with salpingectomy 65.49
laparoscopic 65.41
bilateral (same operative episode)
65.51
laparoscopic 65.53
with salpingectomy 65.61
laparoscopic 65.63
laparoscopic 65.31

Oophorectomy (Continued)
  partial 65.29
    laparoscopic 65.25
    wedge 65.22
      that by laparoscope 65.24
  remaining ovary 65.52
    laparoscopic 65.54
    with tube 65.62
      laparoscopic 65.64
Oophorocystectomy 65.29
  laparoscopic 65.25
Oophoropexy 65.79
Oophoroplasty 65.79
Oophororrhaphy 65.71
  laparoscopic 65.74
Oophorostomy 65.09
  laparoscopic 65.01
Oophorotomy 65.09
  laparoscopic 65.01
Opening
  bony labyrinth (ear) 20.79
  cranial suture 02.01
  heart valve
    closed heart technique - see
      Valvulotomy, by site
    open heart technique - see
      Valvuloplasty, by site
  spinal dura 03.09
Operation
  Abbe
    construction of vagina 70.61
      with graft or prosthesis 70.63
    intestinal anastomosis - see
      Anastomosis, intestine
  abdominal (region) NEC 54.99
  abdominoperineal, NOS 48.50
    laparoscopic 48.51
    open 48.52
    other 48.59
  Aburel (intra-amniotic injection for
    abortion) 75.0
  Adams
    advancement of round ligament
      69.22
    crushing of nasal septum 21.88
    excision of palmar fascia 82.35
  adenoids NEC 28.99
  adrenal (gland) (nerve) (vessel) NEC
    07.49
  Albee
    bone peg, femoral neck 78.05
    graft for slipping patella 78.06
    sliding inlay graft, tibia 78.07
  Albert (arthrodesis, knee) 81.22
  Aldridge (-Studdiford) (urethral sling)
    59.5
  Alexander
    prostatectomy
      perineal 60.62
      suprapubic 60.3
    shortening of round ligaments of
      uterus 69.22
  Alexander-Adams (shortening of
    round ligaments of uterus) 69.22
  Almoor (extrapetrosal drainage) 20.22
  Altemeier (perineal rectal pull-
    through) 48.49
  Ammon (dacryocystotomy) 09.53
  Anderson (tibial lengthening) 78.37
  Anel (dilation of lacrimal duct) 09.42
  anterior chamber (eye) NEC 12.99
  anti-incontinence NEC 59.79
  antrum window (nasal sinus) 22.2
    with Caldwell-Luc approach 22.39

Operation (Continued)
  anus NEC 49.99
  aortic body NEC 39.89 ◀▥
  aorticopulmonary window 39.59
  appendix NEC 47.99
  Arslan (fenestration of inner ear) 20.61
  artery NEC 39.99
  Asai (larynx) 31.75
  Baffes (interatrial transposition of
    venous return) 35.91
  Baldy-Webster (uterine suspension)
    69.22
  Ball
    herniorrhaphy - see Repair, hernia,
      inguinal
    undercutting 49.02
  Bankhart (capsular repair into glenoid,
    for shoulder dislocation) 81.82
  Bardenheurer (ligation of innominate
    artery) 38.85
  Barkan (goniotomy) 12.52
    with goniopuncture 12.53
  Barr (transfer of tibialis posterior
    tendon) 83.75
  Barsky (closure of cleft hand) 82.82
  Bassett (vulvectomy with inguinal
    lymph node dissection) 71.5
    [40.3]
  Bassini (herniorrhaphy) - see Repair,
    hernia, inguinal
  Batch-Spittler-McFaddin (knee
    disarticulation) 84.16
  Batista (partial ventriculectomy)
    (ventricular reduction)
    (ventricular remodeling) 37.35
  Beck I (epicardial poudrage) 36.39
  Beck II (aorta-coronary sinus shunt)
    36.39
  Beck-Jianu (permanent gastrostomy)
    43.19
  Bell-Beuttner (subtotal abdominal
    hysterectomy) 68.39
  Belsey (esophagogastric sphincter)
    44.65
  Benenenti (rotation of bulbous
    urethra) 58.49
  Berke (levator resection eyelid) 08.33
  Biesenberger (size reduction of
    breast, bilateral) 85.32
    unilateral 85.31
  Bigelow (litholapaxy) 57.0
  biliary (duct) (tract) NEC 51.99
  Billroth I (partial gastrectomy with
    gastroduodenostomy) 43.6
  Billroth II (partial gastrectomy with
    gastrojejunostomy) 43.7
  Binnie (hepatopexy) 50.69
  Bischoff (ureteroneocystostomy)
    56.74
  bisection hysterectomy 68.39
    laparoscopic 68.31
  Bishoff (spinal myelotomy) 03.29
  bladder NEC 57.99
    flap 56.74
  Blalock (systemic-pulmonary
    anastomosis) 39.0
  Blalock-Hanlon (creation of atrial
    septal defect) 35.42
  Blalock-Taussig (subclavian-pulmonary
    anastomosis) 39.0
  Blascovic (resection and advancement
    of levator palpebrae superioris)
    08.33
  blood vessel NEC 39.99

Operation (Continued)
  Blount
    femoral shortening (with blade
      plate) 78.25
      by epiphyseal stapling 78.25
  Boari (bladder flap) 56.74
  Bobb (cholelithotomy) 51.04
  bone NEC - see category 78.4●
    facial 76.99
    injury NEC - see category 79.9●
    marrow NEC 41.98
    skull NEC 02.99
  Bonney (abdominal hysterectomy)
    68.49
    laparoscopic 68.41
  Borthen (iridotasis) 12.63
  Bost
    plantar dissection 80.48
    radiocarpal fusion 81.26
  Bosworth
    arthroplasty for acromioclavicular
      separation 81.83
    fusion of posterior lumbar spine
      81.08
      for pseudarthrosis 81.38
    resection of radial head ligaments
      (for tennis elbow) 80.92
    shelf procedure, hip 81.40
  Bottle (repair of hydrocele of tunica
    vaginalis) 61.2
  Boyd (hip disarticulation) 84.18
  brain NEC 02.99
  Brauer (cardiolysis) 37.10
  breast NEC 85.99
  Bricker (ileoureterostomy) 56.51
  Bristow (repair of shoulder dislocation)
    81.82
  Brock (pulmonary valvulotomy)
    35.03
  Brockman (soft tissue release for
    clubfoot) 83.84
  bronchus NEC 33.98
  Browne (-Denis) (hypospadias repair)
    58.45
  Brunschwig (temporary gastrostomy)
    43.19
  buccal cavity NEC 27.99
  Bunnell (tendon transfer) 82.56
  Burch procedure (retropubic urethral
    suspension for urinary stress
    incontinence) 59.5
  Burgess (amputation of ankle) 84.14
  bursa NEC 83.99
    hand 82.99
  bypass - see Bypass
  Caldwell (sulcus extension) 24.91
  Caldwell-Luc (maxillary sinusotomy)
    22.39
    with removal of membrane lining
      22.31
  Callander (knee disarticulation) 84.16
  Campbell
    bone block, ankle 81.11
    fasciotomy (iliac crest) 83.14
    reconstruction of anterior cruciate
      ligaments 81.45
  canthus NEC 08.99
  cardiac NEC 37.99
    septum NEC 35.98
    valve NEC 35.99
  carotid body or gland NEC 39.89 ◀▥
  Carroll and Taber (arthroplasty
    proximal interphalangeal joint)
    81.72

Operation (*Continued*)
Cattell (herniorrhaphy) 53.51
Cecil (urethral reconstruction) 58.46
cecum NEC 46.99
cerebral (meninges) NEC 02.99
cervix NEC 69.99
Chandler (hip fusion) 81.21
Charles (correction of lymphedema) 40.9
Charnley (compression arthrodesis)
    ankle 81.11
    hip 81.21
    knee 81.22
Cheatle-Henry - *see* Repair, hernia, femoral
chest cavity NEC 34.99
Chevalier-Jackson (partial laryngectomy) 30.29
Child (radical subtotal pancreatectomy) 52.53
Chopart (midtarsal amputation) 84.12
chordae tendineae NEC 35.32
choroid NEC 14.9
ciliary body NEC 12.98
cisterna chyli NEC 40.69
Clagett (closure of chest wall following open flap drainage) 34.72
Clayton (resection of metatarsal heads and bases of phalanges) 77.88
clitoris NEC 71.4
cocked hat (metacarpal lengthening and transfer of local flap) 82.69
Cockett (varicose vein)
    lower limb 38.59
    upper limb 38.53
Cody tack (perforation of footplate) 19.0
Coffey (uterine suspension) (Meigs' modification) 69.22
Cole (anterior tarsal wedge osteotomy) 77.28
Collis-Nissen (hiatal hernia repair) 53.80
colon NEC 46.99
Colonna
    adductor tenotomy (first stage) 83.12
    hip arthroplasty (second stage) 81.40
    reconstruction of hip (second stage) 81.40
commando (radical glossectomy) 25.4
conjunctiva NEC 10.99
    destructive NEC 10.33
cornea NEC 11.99
Coventry (tibial wedge osteotomy) 77.27
Cox-maze procedure (ablation or destruction of heart tissue) - *see* maze procedure
Crawford (tarso-frontalis sling of eyelid) 08.32
cul-de-sac NEC 70.92
Culp-Deweerd (spiral flap pyeloplasty) 55.87
Culp-Scardino (ureteral flap pyeloplasty) 55.87
Curtis (interphalangeal joint arthroplasty) 81.72
cystocele NEC 70.51
Dahlman (excision of esophageal diverticulum) 42.31
Dana (posterior rhizotomy) 03.1
Danforth (fetal) 73.8

Operation (*Continued*)
Darrach (ulnar resection) 77.83
Davis (intubated ureterotomy) 56.2
de Grandmont (tarsectomy) 08.35
Delorme
    pericardiectomy 37.31
    proctopexy 48.76
    repair of prolapsed rectum 48.76
    thoracoplasty 33.34
Denker (radical maxillary antrotomy) 22.31
Dennis-Varco (herniorrhaphy) - *see* Repair, hernia, femoral
Denonvillier (limited rhinoplasty) 21.86
dental NEC 24.99
    orthodontic NEC 24.8
Derlacki (tympanoplasty) 19.4
diaphragm NEC 34.89
Dickson (fascial transplant) 83.82
Dickson-Diveley (tendon transfer and arthrodesis to correct claw toe) 77.57
Dieffenbach (hip disarticulation) 84.18
digestive tract NEC 46.99
Doleris (shortening of round ligaments) 69.22
D'Ombrain (excision of pterygium with corneal graft) 11.32
Dorrance (push-back operation for cleft palate) 27.62
Dotter (transluminal angioplasty) 39.59
Douglas (suture of tongue to lip for micrognathia) 25.59
Doyle (paracervical uterine denervation) 69.3
Dühamel (abdominoperineal pull-through) 48.65
Duhrssen (vaginofixation of uterus) 69.22
Dunn (triple arthrodesis) 81.12
duodenum NEC 46.99
Dupuytren
    fasciectomy 82.35
    fasciotomy 82.12
        with excision 82.35
    shoulder disarticulation 84.08
Durham (-Caldwell) (transfer of biceps femoris tendon) 83.75
DuToit and Roux (staple capsulorrhaphy of shoulder) 81.82
DuVries (tenoplasty) 83.88
Dwyer
    fasciotomy 83.14
    soft tissue release NEC 83.84
    wedge osteotomy, calcaneus 77.28
Eagleton (extrapetrosal drainage) 20.22
ear (external) NEC 18.9
    middle or inner NEC 20.99
Eden-Hybinette (glenoid bone block) 78.01
Effler (heart) 36.2
Eggers
    tendon release (patellar retinacula) 83.13
    tendon transfer (biceps femoris tendon) (hamstring tendon) 83.75
Elliot (scleral trephination with iridectomy) 12.61

Operation (*Continued*)
Ellis Jones (repair of peroneal tendon) 83.88
Ellison (reinforcement of collateral ligament) 81.44
Elmslie-Cholmeley (tarsal wedge osteotomy) 77.28
Eloesser
    thoracoplasty 33.34
    thoracostomy 34.09
Emmet (cervix) 67.61
endorectal pull-through 48.41
epididymis NEC 63.99
esophagus NEC 42.99
Estes (ovary) 65.72
    laparoscopic 65.75
Estlander (thoracoplasty) 33.34
Evans (release of clubfoot) 83.84
extraocular muscle NEC 15.9
    multiple (two or more muscles) 15.4
        with temporary detachment from globe 15.3
    revision 15.6
    single 15.29
        with temporary detachment from globe 15.19
eyeball NEC 16.99
eyelid(s) NEC 08.99
face NEC 27.99
facial bone or joint NEC 76.99
fallopian tube NEC 66.99
Farabeuf (ischiopubiotomy) 77.39
Fasanella-Servatt (blepharoptosis repair) 08.35
fascia NEC 83.99
    hand 82.99
female (genital organs) NEC 71.9
    hysterectomy NEC 68.9
fenestration (aorta) 39.54
Ferguson (hernia repair) 53.00
Fick (perforation of footplate) 19.0
filtering (for glaucoma) 12.79
    with iridectomy 12.65
Finney (pyloroplasty) 44.29
fistulizing, sclera NEC 12.69
Foley (pyeloplasty) 55.87
Fontan (creation of conduit between right atrium and pulmonary artery) 35.94
Fothergill (-Donald) (uterine suspension) 69.22
Fowler
    arthroplasty of metacarpophalangeal joint 81.72
    release (mallet finger repair) 82.84
    tenodesis (hand) 82.85
    thoracoplasty 33.34
Fox (entropion repair with wedge resection) 08.43
Franco (suprapubic cystotomy) 57.19
Frank (permanent gastrostomy) 43.19
Frazier (-Spiller) (subtemporal trigeminal rhizotomy) 04.02
Fredet-Ramstedt (pyloromyotomy) (with wedge resection) 43.3
Frenckner (intrapetrosal drainage) 20.22
Frickman (abdominal proctopexy) 48.75
Frommel (shortening of uterosacral ligaments) 69.22

Operation (Continued)

Gabriel (abdominoperineal resection of rectum), NOS 48.50
  laparoscopic 48.51
  open 48.52
  other 48.59
gallbladder NEC 51.99
ganglia NEC 04.99
  sympathetic 05.89
Gant (wedge osteotomy of trochanter) 77.25
Garceau (tibial tendon transfer) 83.75
Gardner (spinal meningocele repair) 03.51
gastric NEC 44.99
Gelman (release of clubfoot) 83.84
genital organ NEC
  female 71.9
  male 64.99
Ghormley (hip fusion) 81.21
Giffod
  destruction of lacrimal sac 09.6
  keratotomy (delimiting) 11.1
Gill
  arthrodesis of shoulder 81.23
  laminectomy 03.09
Gill-Stein (carporadial arthrodesis) 81.25
Gilliam (uterine suspension) 69.22
Girdlestone
  laminectomy with spinal fusion 81.00
  muscle transfer for claw toe 77.57
  resection of femoral head and neck (without insertion of joint prosthesis) 77.85
    with replacement prosthesis - see Implant, joint, hip
  resection of hip prosthesis 80.05
    with replacement prosthesis - see Implant, joint, hip
Girdlestone-Taylor (muscle transfer for claw toe repair) 77.57
glaucoma NEC 12.79
Glenn (anastomosis of superior vena cava to right pulmonary artery) 39.21
globus pallidus NEC 01.42
Goebel-Frangenheim-Stoeckel (urethrovesical suspension) 59.4
Goldner (clubfoot release) 80.48
Goldthwaite
  ankle stabilization 81.11
  patella stabilization 81.44
  tendon transfer for patella dislocation 81.44
Goodall-Power (vagina) 70.4
Gordon-Taylor (hindquarter amputation) 84.19
Graber-Duvernay (drilling femoral head) 77.15
Green (scapulopexy) 78.41
Grice (subtalar arthrodesis) 81.13
Gritti-Stokes (knee disarticulation) 84.16
Gross (herniorrhaphy)
  laparoscopic 53.43
    with graft or prosthesis 53.42
  other and open with graft or prosthesis 53.41
  other open 53.49
gum NEC 24.39
Guyon (amputation of ankle) 84.13

Operation (Continued)

Hagner (epididymotomy) 63.92
Halsted - see Repair, hernia, inguinal
Halsted mastectomy 85.45
Hampton (anastomosis small intestine to rectal stump) 45.92
hanging hip (muscle release) 83.19
harelip 27.54
Harrison-Richardson (vaginal suspension) 70.77
  with graft or prosthesis 70.78
Hartmann - see Colectomy, by site
Hauser
  achillotenotomy 83.11
  bunionectomy with adductor tendon transfer 77.53
  stabilization of patella 81.44
Heaney (vaginal hysterectomy) 68.59
  laparoscopically assisted (LAVH) 68.51
heart NEC 37.99
  valve NEC 35.99
    adjacent structure NEC 35.39
Hegar (perineorrhaphy) 71.79
Heine (cyclodialysis) 12.55
Heineke-Mikulicz (pyloroplasty) - see category 44.2●
Heller (esophagomyotomy) 42.7
Hellström (transplantation of aberrant renal vessel) 39.55
hemorrhoids NEC 49.49
Henley (jejunal transposition) 43.81
hepatic NEC 50.99
hernia - see Repair, hernia
Hey (amputation of foot) 84.12
Hey-Groves (reconstruction of anterior cruciate ligament) 81.45
Heyman (soft tissue release for clubfoot) 83.84
Heyman-Herndon (-Strong) (correction of metatarsus varus) 80.48
Hibbs (lumbar spinal fusion) - see Fusion, lumbar
Higgins - see Repair, hernia, femoral
Hill-Allison (hiatal hernia repair, transpleural approach) 53.80
Hitchcock (anchoring tendon of biceps) 83.88
Hofmeister (gastrectomy) 43.7
Hoke
  midtarsal fusion 81.14
  triple arthrodesis 81.12
Holth
  iridencleisis 12.63
  sclerectomy 12.65
Homan (correction of lymphedema) 40.9
Hutch (ureteroneocystostomy) 56.74
Hybinette-Eden (glenoid bone block) 78.01
hymen NEC 70.91
hypopharynx NEC 29.99
hypophysis NEC 07.79
ileal loop 56.51
ileum NEC 46.99
intestine NEC 46.99
iris NEC 12.97
  inclusion 12.63
Irving (tubal ligation) 66.32
Irwin - see also Osteotomy 77.30
Jaboulay (gastroduodenostomy) 44.39
  laparoscopic 44.38

Operation (Continued)

Janeway (permanent gastrostomy) 43.19
Jatene (arterial switch) 35.84
jejunum NEC 46.99
Johanson (urethral reconstruction) 58.46
joint (capsule) (ligament) (structure) NEC 81.99
  facial NEC 76.99
Jones
  claw toe (transfer of extensor hallucis longus tendon) 77.57
    modified (with arthrodesis) 77.57
  dacryocystorhinostomy 09.81
  hammer toe (interphalangeal fusion) 77.56
  modified (tendon transfer with arthrodesis) 77.57
  repair of peroneal tendon 83.88
Joplin (exostectomy with tendon transfer) 77.53
Kader (temporary gastrostomy) 43.19
Kaufman (for urinary stress incontinence) 59.79
Kazanjiian (buccal vestibular sulcus extension) 24.91
Kehr (hepatopexy) 50.69
Keller (bunionectomy) 77.59
Kelly (-Kennedy) (urethrovesical plication) 59.3
Kelly-Stoeckel (urethrovesical plication) 59.3
Kerr (cesarean section) 74.1
Kessler (arthroplasty, carpometacarpal joint) 81.74
Kidner (excision of accessory navicular bone) (with tendon transfer) 77.98
kidney NEC 55.99
Killian (frontal sinusotomy) 22.41
King-Steelquist (hindquarter amputation) 84.19
Kirk (amputation through thigh) 84.17
Kock pouch
  bowel anastomosis - omit code
  continent ileostomy 46.22
  cutaneous uretero-ileostomy 56.51
  ESWL (electrocorporeal shock wave lithotripsy) 98.51
  removal, calculus 57.19
  revision, cutaneous uretero-ileostomy 56.52
  urinary diversion procedure 56.51
Kondoleon (correction of lymphedema) 40.9
Krause (sympathetic denervation) 05.29
Kroener (partial salpingectomy) 66.69
Kroenlein (lateral orbitotomy) 16.01
Kronig (low cervical cesarean section) 74.1
Krukenberg (reconstruction of below-elbow amputation) 82.89
Kuhnt-Szymanowski (ectropion repair with lid reconstruction) 08.44
Labbe (gastrotomy) 43.0
labia NEC 71.8
lacrimal
  gland 09.3
  system NEC 09.99
Ladd (mobilization of intestine) 54.95

◀ New   ◀▬ Revised   ~~deleted~~ Deleted   ● Use Additional Digit(s)   ▭ Omit code

Operation (*Continued*)
Lagrange (iridosclerectomy) 12.65
Lambrinudi (triple arthrodesis) 81.12
Langenbeck (cleft palate repair) 27.62
Lapidus (bunionectomy with metatarsal osteotomy) 77.51
Larry (shoulder disarticulation) 84.08
larynx NEC 31.98
Lash
 internal cervical os repair 67.59
 laparoscopic supracervical hysterectomy 68.31
Latzko
 cesarean section, extraperitoneal 74.2
 colpocleisis 70.8
Leadbetter (urethral reconstruction) 58.46
Leadbetter-Politano (ureteroneocystostomy) 56.74
Le Fort (colpocleisis) 70.8
LeMesurier (cleft lip repair) 27.54
lens NEC 13.90
Leriche (periarterial sympathectomy) 05.25
levator muscle sling
 eyelid ptosis repair 08.33
 urethrovesical suspension 59.71
 urinary stress incontinence 59.71
lid suture (blepharoptosis) 08.31
ligament NEC 81.99
 broad NEC 69.98
 round NEC 69.98
 uterine NEC 69.98
Lindholm (repair of ruptured tendon) 83.88
Linton (varicose vein) 38.59
lip NEC 27.99
Lisfranc
 foot amputation 84.12
 shoulder disarticulation 84.08
Littlewood (forequarter amputation) 84.09
liver NEC 50.99
Lloyd-Davies (abdominoperineal resection), NOS 48.50
 laparoscopic 48.51
 open 48.52
 other 48.59
Longmire (bile duct anastomosis) 51.39
Lord
 dilation of anal canal for hemorrhoids 49.49
 hemorrhoidectomy 49.49
 orchidopexy 62.5
Lucas and Murray (knee arthrodesis with plate) 81.22
lung NEC 33.99
lung volume reduction 32.22
 biologic lung volume reduction (BLVR) - *see* category 33.7●
lymphatic structure(s) NEC 40.9
 duct, left (thoracic) NEC 40.69
Madlener (tubal ligation) 66.31
Magnuson (-Stack) (arthroplasty for recurrent shoulder dislocation) 81.82
male genital organs NEC 64.99
Manchester (-Donald) (-Fothergill) (uterine suspension) 69.22
mandible NEC 76.99
 orthognathic 76.64

Operation (*Continued*)
Marckwald (cervical os repair) 67.59
Marshall-Marchetti (-Krantz) (retropubic urethral suspension) 59.5
Matas (aneurysmorrhaphy) 39.52
Mayo
 bunionectomy 77.59
 herniorrhaphy
  laparoscopic 53.43
   with graft or prosthesis 53.42
  other and open with graft or prosthesis 53.41
  other open 53.49
 vaginal hysterectomy 68.59
  laparoscopically assisted (LAVH) 68.51
maze procedure (ablation or destruction of heart tissue)
 by incision (open) 37.33
 by median sternotomy 37.33 ◄
 by peripherally inserted catheter 37.34
 by thoracotomy without thoracoscope 37.33 ◄
 endovascular approach 37.34
 trans-thoracic approach 37.33
Mazet (knee disarticulation) 84.16
McBride (bunionectomy with soft tissue correction) 77.53
McBurney - *see* Repair, hernia, inguinal
McCall (enterocele repair) 70.92
 with graft or prosthesis 70.93
McCauley (release of clubfoot) 83.84
McDonald (encirclement suture, cervix) 67.59
McIndoe (vaginal construction) 70.61
 with graft or prosthesis 70.63
McKeever (fusion of first metatarsophalangeal joint for hallux valgus repair) 77.52
McKissock (breast reduction) 85.33
McReynolds (transposition of pterygium) 11.31
McVay
 femoral hernia - *see* Repair, hernia, femoral
 inguinal hernia - *see* Repair, hernia, inguinal
meninges (spinal) NEC 03.99
 cerebral NEC 02.99
mesentery NEC 54.99
Mikulicz (exteriorization of intestine) (first stage) 46.03
 second stage 46.04
Miles (complete proctectomy), NOS 48.50
 laparoscopic 48.51
 open 48.52
 other 48.59
Millard (cheiloplasty) 27.54
Miller
 midtarsal arthrodesis 81.14
 urethrovesical suspension 59.4
Millin-Read (urethrovesical suspension) 59.4
Mitchell (hallux valgus repair) 77.51
Mohs (chemosurgical excision of skin) 86.24
Moore (arthroplasty) 81.52

Operation (*Continued*)
Moschowitz
 enterocele repair 70.92
  with graft or prosthesis 70.93
 herniorrhaphy - *see* Repair, hernia, femoral
 sigmoidopexy 46.63
mouth NEC 27.99
Muller (banding of pulmonary artery) 38.85
Mumford (partial claviculectomy) 77.81
muscle NEC 83.99
 extraocular - *see* Operation, extraocular
 hand NEC 82.99
 papillary heart NEC 35.31
musculoskeletal system NEC 84.99
Mustard (interatrial transposition of venous return) 35.91
nail (finger) (toe) NEC 86.99
nasal sinus NEC 22.9
nasopharynx NEC 29.99
nerve (cranial) (peripheral) NEC 04.99
 adrenal NEC 07.49
 sympathetic NEC 05.89
nervous system NEC 05.9
Nicola (tenodesis for recurrent dislocation of shoulder) 81.82
nipple NEC 85.99
Nissen (fundoplication of stomach) 44.66
 laparoscopic 44.67
Noble (plication of small intestine) 46.62
node (lymph) NEC 40.9
Norman Miller (vaginopexy) 70.77
 with graft or prosthesis 70.78
Norton (extraperitoneal cesarean operation) 74.2
nose, nasal NEC 21.99
 sinus NEC 22.9
Ober (-Yount) (gluteal-iliotibial fasciotomy) 83.14
obstetric NEC 75.99
ocular NEC 16.99
 muscle - *see* Operation, extraocular muscle
O'Donoghue (triad knee repair) 81.43
Olshausen (uterine suspension) 69.22
omentum NEC 54.99
ophthalmologic NEC 16.99
oral cavity NEC 27.99
orbicularis muscle sling 08.36
orbit NEC 16.98
oropharynx NEC 29.99
orthodontic NEC 24.8
orthognathic NEC 76.69
Oscar Miller (midtarsal arthrodesis) 81.14
Osmond-Clark (soft tissue release with peroneus brevis tendon transfer) 83.75
ovary NEC 65.99
Oxford (for urinary incontinence) 59.4
palate NEC 27.99
palpebral ligament sling 08.36
Panas (linear proctotomy) 48.0
Pancoast (division of trigeminal nerve at foramen ovale) 04.02

Operation (Continued)

pancreas NEC 52.99

pantaloon (revision of gastric anastomosis) 44.5

papillary muscle (heart) NEC 35.31

Paquin (ureteroneocystostomy) 56.74

parathyroid gland(s) NEC 06.99

parotid gland or duct NEC 26.99

Partsch (marsupialization of dental cyst) 24.4

Pattee (auditory canal) 18.6

Peet (splanchnic resection) 05.29

Pemberton

osteotomy of ilium 77.39

rectum (mobilization and fixation for prolapse repair) 48.76

penis NEC 64.98

Pereyra (paraurethral suspension) 59.6

pericardium NEC 37.99

perineum (female) NEC 71.8

male NEC 86.99

perirectal tissue NEC 48.99

perirenal tissue NEC 59.92

peritoneum NEC 54.99

periurethral tissue NEC 58.99

perivesical tissue NEC 59.92

pharyngeal flap (cleft palate repair) 27.62

secondary or subsequent 27.63

pharynx, pharyngeal (pouch) NEC 29.99

pineal gland NEC 07.59

Pinsker (obliteration of nasoseptal telangiectasia) 21.07

Piper (forceps) 72.6

Pirogoff (ankle amputation through malleoli of tibia and fibula) 84.14

pituitary gland NEC 07.79

plastic - see Repair, by site

pleural cavity NEC 34.99

Politano-Leadbetter (ureteroneocystostomy) 56.74

pollicization (with nerves and blood supply) 82.61

Polya (gastrectomy) 43.7

Pomeroy (ligation and division of fallopian tubes) 66.32

Poncet

lengthening of Achilles tendon 83.85

urethrostomy, perineal 58.0

Porro (cesarean section) 74.99

posterior chamber (eye) NEC 14.9

Potts-Smith (descending aorta-left pulmonary artery anastomosis) 39.0

Printen and Mason (high gastric bypass) 44.31

prostate NEC - see also Prostatectomy 60.69

specified type 60.99

pterygium 11.39

with corneal graft 11.32

Puestow (pancreaticojejunostomy) 52.96

pull-through NEC 48.49

pulmonary NEC 33.99

push-back (cleft palate repair) 27.62

Putti-Platt (capsulorrhaphy of shoulder for recurrent dislocation) 81.82

Operation (Continued)

pyloric exclusion 44.39

laparoscopic 44.38

pyriform sinus NEC 29.99

"rabbit ear" (anterior urethropexy) (Tudor) 59.79

Ramadier (intrapetrosal drainage) 20.22

Ramstedt (pyloromyotomy) (with wedge resection) 43.3

Rankin

exteriorization of intestine 46.03

proctectomy (complete), NOS 48.50

laparoscopic 48.51

open 48.52

other 48.59

Rashkind (balloon septostomy) 35.41

Rastelli (creation of conduit between right ventricle and pulmonary artery) 35.92

in repair of

pulmonary artery atresia 35.92

transposition of great vessels 35.92

truncus arteriosus 35.83

Raz-Pereyra procedure (bladder neck suspension) 59.79

rectal NEC 48.99

rectocele NEC 70.52

re-entry (aorta) 39.54

renal NEC 55.99

respiratory (tract) NEC 33.99

retina NEC 14.9

Ripstein (repair of rectal prolapse) 48.75

Rodney Smith (radical subtotal pancreatectomy) 52.53

Roux-en-Y

bile duct 51.36

cholecystojejunostomy 51.32

esophagus (intrathoracic) 42.54

gastroenterostomy 44.39

laparoscopic 44.38

gastrojejunostomy 44.39

laparoscopic 44.38

pancreaticojejunostomy 52.96

Roux-Goldthwait (repair of patellar dislocation) 81.44

Roux-Herzen-Judine (jejunal loop interposition) 42.63

Ruiz-Mora (proximal phalangectomy for hammer toe) 77.99

Russe (bone graft of scaphoid) 78.04

Saemisch (corneal section) 11.1

salivary gland or duct NEC 26.99

Salter (innominate osteotomy) 77.39

Sauer-Bacon (abdominoperineal resection), NOS 48.50

laparoscopic 48.51

open 48.52

other 48.59

Schanz (femoral osteotomy) 77.35

Schauta (-Amreich) (radical vaginal hysterectomy) 68.79

laparoscopic 68.71

Schede (thoracoplasty) 33.34

Scheie

cautery of sclera 12.62

sclerostomy 12.62

Schlatter (total gastrectomy) 43.99

Schroeder (endocervical excision) 67.39

Operation (Continued)

Schuchardt (nonobstetrical episiotomy) 71.09

Schwartze (simple mastoidectomy) 20.41

sclera NEC 12.89

Scott

intestinal bypass for obesity 45.93

jejunocolostomy (bypass) 45.93

scrotum NEC 61.99

Seddon-Brooks (transfer of pectoralis major tendon) 83.75

Semb (apicolysis of lung) 33.39

seminal vesicle NEC 60.79

Senning (correction of transposition of great vessels) 35.91

Sever (division of soft tissue of arm) 83.19

Sewell (heart) 36.2

sex transformation NEC 64.5

Sharrard (iliopsoas muscle transfer) 83.77

shelf (hip arthroplasty) 81.40

Shirodkar (encirclement suture, cervix) 67.59

sigmoid NEC 46.99

Silver (bunionectomy) 77.59

Sistrunk (excision of thyroglossal cyst) 06.7

Skene's gland NEC 71.8

skin NEC 86.99

skull NEC 02.99

sling

eyelid

fascia lata, palpebral 08.36

frontalis fascial 08.32

levator muscle 08.33

orbicularis muscle 08.36

palpebrae ligament, fascia lata 08.36

tarsus muscle 08.35

fascial (fascia lata)

eye 08.32

for facial weakness (trigeminal nerve paralysis) 86.81

palpebral ligament 08.36

tongue 25.59

tongue (fascial) 25.59

urethra (suprapubic) 59.4

retropubic 59.5

urethrovesical 59.5

Slocum (pes anserinus transfer) 81.47

Sluder (tonsillectomy) 28.2

Smith (open osteotomy of mandible) 76.62

Smith-Peterson (radiocarpal arthrodesis) 81.25

Smithwick (sympathectomy) 05.29

Soave (endorectal pull-through) 48.41

soft tissue NEC 83.99

hand 82.99

Sonneberg (inferior maxillary neurectomy) 04.07

Sorondo-Ferré (hindquarter amputation) 84.19

Soutter (iliac crest fasciotomy) 83.14

Spalding-Richardson (uterine suspension) 69.22

spermatic cord NEC 63.99

sphincter of Oddi NEC 51.89

spinal (canal) (cord) (structures) NEC 03.99

◀ New   ◀||| Revised   ~~deleted~~ Deleted   ● Use Additional Digit(s)   ▮ Omit code

Operation (*Continued*)

Spinelli (correction of inverted uterus) 75.93

Spivack (permanent gastrostomy) 43.19

spleen NEC 41.99

S.P. Rogers (knee disarticulation) 84.16

Ssabanejew-Frank (permanent gastrostomy) 43.19

Stacke (simple mastoidectomy) 20.41

Stallard (conjunctivocystorhinostomy) 09.82
  with insertion of tube or stent 09.83

Stamm (-Kader) (temporary gastrostomy) 43.19

Steinberg 44.5

Steindler
  fascia stripping (for cavus deformity) 83.14
  flexorplasty (elbow) 83.77
  muscle transfer 83.77

sterilization NEC
  female - *see also* specific operation 66.39
  male - *see also* Ligation, vas deferens 63.70

Stewart (renal plication with pyeloplasty) 55.87

stomach NEC 44.99

Stone (anoplasty) 49.79

Strassman (metroplasty) 69.49
  metroplasty (Jones modification) 69.49
  uterus 68.22

Strayer (gastrocnemius recession) 83.72

stress incontinence - *see* Repair, stress incontinence

Stromeyer-Little (hepatotomy) 50.0

Strong (unbridling of celiac artery axis) 39.91

Sturmdorf (conization of cervix) 67.2

subcutaneous tissue NEC 86.99

sublingual gland or duct NEC 26.99

submaxillary gland or duct NEC 26.99

Summerskill (dacryocystorhinostomy by intubation) 09.81

Surmay (jejunostomy) 46.39

Swenson
  bladder reconstruction 57.87
  proctectomy 48.49

Swinney (urethral reconstruction) 58.46

Syme
  ankle amputation through malleoli of tibia and fibula 84.14
  urethrotomy, external 58.0

sympathetic nerve NEC 05.89

Taarnhoj (trigeminal nerve root decompression) 04.41

Tack (sacculotomy) 20.79

Talma-Morison (omentopexy) 54.74

Tanner (devascularization of stomach) 44.99

TAPVC NEC 35.82

tarsus NEC 08.99
  muscle sling 08.35

tendon NEC 83.99
  extraocular NEC 15.9
  hand NEC 82.99

testis NEC 62.99

tetralogy of Fallot
  partial repair - *see* specific procedure
  total (one-stage) 35.81

Operation (*Continued*)

Thal (repair of esophageal stricture) 42.85

thalamus 01.41
  by stereotactic radiosurgery 92.32
    cobalt 60 92.32
    linear accelerator (LINAC) 92.31
    multi-source 92.32
    particle beam 92.33
    particulate 92.33
    radiosurgery NEC 92.39
    single source photon 92.31

Thiersch
  anus 49.79
  skin graft 86.69
    hand 86.62

Thompson
  cleft lip repair 27.54
  correction of lymphedema 40.9
  quadricepsplasty 83.86
  thumb apposition with bone graft 82.69

thoracic duct NEC 40.69

thorax NEC 34.99

Thorek (partial cholecystectomy) 51.21

three-snip, punctum 09.51

thymus NEC 07.99
  thoracoscopic, NEC 07.98

thyroid gland NEC 06.98

TKP (thermokeratoplasty) 11.74

Tomkins (metroplasty) 69.49

tongue NEC 25.99
  flap, palate 27.62
  tie 25.91

tonsil NEC 28.99

Torek (-Bevan) (orchidopexy) (first stage) (second stage) 62.5

Torkildsen (ventriculocisternal shunt) 02.2

Torpin (cul-de-sac resection) 70.92

Toti (dacryocystorhinostomy) 09.81

Touchas 86.83

Touroff (ligation of subclavian artery) 38.85

trabeculae corneae cordis (heart) NEC 35.35

trachea NEC 31.99

Trauner (lingual sulcus extension) 24.91

truncus arteriosus NEC 35.83

Tsuge (macrodactyly repair) 82.83

Tudor "rabbit ear" (anterior urethropexy) 59.79

Tuffier
  apicolysis of lung 33.39
  vaginal hysterectomy 68.59
    laparoscopically assisted (LAVH) 68.51

tunica vaginalis NEC 61.99

Turco (release of joint capsules in clubfoot) 80.48

Uchida (tubal ligation with or without fimbriectomy) 66.32

umbilicus NEC 54.99

urachus NEC 57.51

Urban (mastectomy) (unilateral) 85.47
  bilateral 85.48

ureter NEC 56.99

urethra NEC 58.99

urinary system NEC 59.99

uterus NEC 69.99
  supporting structures NEC 69.98

Operation (*Continued*)

uvula NEC 27.79

vagina NEC 70.91

vascular NEC 39.99

vas deferens NEC 63.99
  ligation NEC 63.71

vein NEC 39.99

vena cava sieve 38.7

vertebra NEC 78.49

vesical (bladder) NEC 57.99

vessel NEC 39.99
  cardiac NEC 36.99

Vicq d'Azyr (larynx) 31.1

Vidal (varicocele ligation) 63.1

Vineberg (implantation of mammary artery into ventricle) 36.2

vitreous NEC 14.79

vocal cord NEC 31.98

von Kraske (proctectomy) 48.64

Voss (hanging hip operation) 83.19

Vulpius (-Compere) (lengthening of gastrocnemius muscle) 83.85

vulva NEC 71.8

Ward-Mayo (vaginal hysterectomy) 68.59
  laparoscopically assisted (LAVH) 68.51

Wardill (cleft palate) 27.62

Waters (extraperitoneal cesarean section) 74.2

Waterston (aorta-right pulmonary artery anastomosis) 39.0

Watkins (-Wertheim) (uterus interposition) 69.21

Watson-Jones
  hip arthrodesis 81.21
  reconstruction of lateral ligaments, ankle 81.49
  shoulder arthrodesis (extra-articular) 81.23
  tenoplasty 83.88

Weir
  appendicostomy 47.91
  correction of nostrils 21.86

Wertheim (radical hysterectomy) 68.69
  laparoscopic 68.61

West (dacryocystorhinostomy) 09.81

Wheeler
  entropion repair 08.44
  halving procedure (eyelid) 08.24

Whipple (radical pancreaticoduodenectomy) 52.7
  Child modification (radical subtotal pancreatectomy) 52.53
  Rodney Smith modification (radical subtotal pancreatectomy) 52.53

White (lengthening of tendo calcaneus by incomplete tenotomy) 83.11

Whitehead
  glossectomy, radical 25.4
  hemorrhoidectomy 49.46

Whitman
  foot stabilization (talectomy) 77.98
  hip reconstruction 81.40
  repair of serratus anterior muscle 83.87
  talectomy 77.98
  trochanter wedge osteotomy 77.25

Wier (entropion repair) 08.44

Operation *(Continued)*
  Williams-Richardson (vaginal construction) 70.61
    with graft or prosthesis 70.63
  Wilms (thoracoplasty) 33.34
  Wilson (angulation osteotomy for hallux valgus) 77.51
  window
    antrum (nasal sinus) - *see* Antrotomy, maxillary
    aorticopulmonary 39.59
    bone cortex - *see also* Incision, bone 77.10
    facial 76.09
    nasoantral - *see* Antrotomy, maxillary
    pericardium 37.12
    pleural 34.09
  Winiwarter (cholecystoenterostomy) 51.32
  Witzel (temporary gastrostomy) 43.19
  Woodward (release of high riding scapula) 81.83
  Young
    epispadias repair 58.45
    tendon transfer (anterior tibialis) (repair of flat foot) 83.75
  Yount (division of iliotibial band) 83.14
  Zancolli
    capsuloplasty 81.72
    tendon transfer (biceps) 82.56
  Ziegler (iridectomy) 12.14
Operculectomy 24.6
Ophthalmectomy 16.49
  with implant (into Tenon's capsule) 16.42
    with attachment of muscles 16.41
Ophthalmoscopy 16.21
Opponensplasty (hand) 82.56
Optical coherence tomography (OCT) (intravascular imaging)
  coronary vessel(s) 38.24
  non-coronary vessel(s) 38.25
Orbitomaxillectomy, radical 16.51
Orbitotomy (anterior) (frontal) (temporofrontal) (transfrontal) NEC 16.09
  with
    bone flap 16.01
    insertion of implant 16.02
  Kroenlein (lateral) 16.01
  lateral 16.01
Orchidectomy (with epididymectomy) (unilateral) 62.3
  bilateral (radical) 62.41
  remaining or solitary testis 62.42
Orchidopexy 62.5
Orchidoplasty 62.69
Orchidorrhaphy 62.61
Orchidotomy 62.0
Orchiectomy (with epididymectomy) (unilateral) 62.3
  bilateral (radical) 62.41
  remaining or solitary testis 62.42
Orchiopexy 62.5
Orchioplasty 62.69
Orthoroentgenography - *see* Radiography
Oscar Miller operation (midtarsal arthrodesis) 81.14
Osmond-Clark operation (soft tissue release with peroneus brevis tendon transfer) 83.75

Ossiculectomy NEC 19.3
  with
    stapedectomy - *see also* Stapedectomy 19.19
    stapes mobilization 19.0
    tympanoplasty 19.53
      revision 19.6
Ossiculotomy NEC 19.3
Ostectomy (partial), except facial - *see also* category 77.8●
  facial NEC 76.39
    total 76.45
      with reconstruction 76.44
    first metatarsal head - *see* Bunionectomy
    for graft (autograft) (homograft) - *see also* category 77.7●
      mandible 76.31
        total 76.42
          with reconstruction 76.41
    total, except facial - *see also* category 77.9●
      facial NEC 76.45
        with reconstruction 76.44
      mandible 76.42
        with reconstruction 76.41
Osteoarthrotomy - *see also* Osteotomy 77.30
Osteoclasis 78.70
  carpal, metacarpal 78.74
  clavicle 78.71
  ear 20.79
  femur 78.75
  fibula 78.77
  humerus 78.72
  patella 78.76
  pelvic 78.79
  phalanges (foot) (hand) 78.79
  radius 78.73
  scapula 78.71
  specified site NEC 78.79
  tarsal, metatarsal 78.78
  thorax (ribs) (sternum) 78.71
  tibia 78.77
  ulna 78.73
  vertebrae 78.79
Osteolysis - *see* category 78.4●
Osteopathic manipulation - *see also* Manipulation, osteopathic 93.67
Osteoplasty NEC - *see* category 78.4●
  with bone graft - *see* Graft, bone
  for
    bone lengthening - *see* Lengthening, bone
    bone shortening - *see* Shortening, bone
    repair of malunion or nonunion of fracture - *see* Repair, fracture, malunion or nonunion
  carpal, metacarpal 78.44
  clavicle 78.41
  cranium NEC 02.06
    with
      flap (bone) 02.03
      graft (bone) 02.04
  facial bone NEC 76.69
  femur 78.45
  fibula 78.47
  humerus 78.42
  mandible, mandibular NEC 76.64
    body 76.63
    ramus (open) 76.62
      closed 76.61

Osteoplasty NEC *(Continued)*
  maxilla (segmental) 76.65
    total 76.66
  nasal bones 21.89
  patella 78.46
  pelvic 78.49
  phalanges (foot) (hand) 78.49
  radius 78.43
  scapula 78.41
  skull NEC 02.06
    with
      flap (bone) 02.03
      graft (bone) 02.04
  specified site NEC 78.49
  tarsal, metatarsal 78.48
  thorax (ribs) (sternum) 78.41
  tibia 78.47
  ulna 78.43
  vertebrae 78.49
Osteorrhaphy - *see also* Osteoplasty 78.40
Osteosynthesis (fracture) - *see* Reduction, fracture
Osteotomy (adduction) (angulation) (block) (derotational) (displacement) (partial) (rotational) 77.30
  carpals, metacarpals 77.34
    wedge 77.24
  clavicle 77.31
    wedge 77.21
  facial bone NEC 76.69
  femur 77.35
    wedge 77.25
  fibula 77.37
    wedge 77.27
  humerus 77.32
    wedge 77.22
  mandible (segmental) (subapical) 76.64
    angle (open) 76.62
      closed 76.61
    body 76.63
    Gigli saw 76.61
    ramus (open) 76.62
      closed 76.61
  maxilla (segmental) 76.65
    total 76.66
  metatarsal 77.38
    wedge 77.28
      for hallux valgus repair 77.51
  patella 77.36
    wedge 77.26
  pelvic 77.39
    wedge 77.29
  phalanges (foot) (hand) 77.39
    for repair of
      bunion - *see* Bunionectomy
      bunionette 77.54
      hallux valgus - *see* Bunionectomy
    wedge 77.29
      for repair of
        bunion - *see* Bunionectomy
        bunionette 77.54
        hallux valgus - *see* Bunionectomy
  radius 77.33
    wedge 77.23
  scapula 77.31
    wedge 77.21
  specified site NEC 77.39
    wedge 77.29
  tarsal 77.38
    wedge 77.28

Osteotomy *(Continued)*
  thorax (ribs) (sternum) 77.31
    wedge 77.21
  tibia 77.37
    wedge 77.27
  toe 77.39
    for repair of
      bunion - *see* Bunionectomy
      bunionette 77.54
      hallux valgus - *see*
        Bunionectomy
    wedge 77.29
      for repair of
        bunion - *see* Bunionectomy
        bunionette 77.54
        hallux valgus - *see*
          Bunionectomy
  ulna 77.33
    wedge 77.23

Osteotomy *(Continued)*
  vertebrae 77.39
    wedge 77.29
Otonecrectomy (inner ear) 20.79
Otoplasty (external) 18.79
  auditory canal or meatus 18.6
  auricle 18.79
  cartilage 18.79
    reconstruction 18.71
  prominent or protruding 18.5
Otoscopy 18.11
Outfolding, sclera, for buckling - *see also*
  Buckling, scleral 14.49
Outfracture, turbinates (nasal) 21.62
Output and clearance, circulatory 92.05
Overdistension, bladder (therapeutic)
  96.25
Overlapping, sclera, for buckling - *see*
  also Buckling, scleral 14.49

Oversewing
  left atrial appendage (LAA) 37.36
  pleural bleb 32.21
  ulcer crater (peptic) 44.40
    duodenum 44.42
    stomach 44.41
Oxford operation (for urinary
  incontinence) 59.4
Oximetry
  fetal pulse 75.38
Oxygenation 93.96
  extracorporeal membrane (ECMO) 39.65
  hyperbaric 93.95
    wound 93.59
  infusion therapy, Super 00.49
Oxygen therapy (catalytic) (pump) 93.96
  hyperbaric 93.95
  SuperSaturated 00.49

P

Pacemaker
  cardiac - *see also* Insertion, pacemaker,
    cardiac
    intraoperative (temporary) 39.64
    temporary (during and immediately
      following cardiac surgery)
      39.64
Packing - *see also* Insertion, pack
  auditory canal 96.11
  nose, for epistaxis (anterior) 21.01
    posterior (and anterior) 21.02
  rectal 96.19
  sella turcica 07.79
  vaginal 96.14
Palatoplasty 27.69
  for cleft palate 27.62
    secondary or subsequent 27.63
Palatorrhaphy 27.61
  for cleft palate 27.62
Pallidectomy 01.42
Pallidoansotomy 01.42
Pallidotomy 01.42
  by stereotactic radiosurgery 92.32
    cobalt 60 92.32
    linear accelerator (LINAC) 92.31
    multi-source 92.32
    particle beam 92.33
    particulate 92.33
    radiosurgery NEC 92.39
    single source photon 92.31
Panas operation (linear proctotomy)
  48.0
Pancoast operation (division of
  trigeminal nerve at foramen
  ovale) 04.02
Pancreatectomy (total) (with synchronous
  duodenectomy) 52.6
  partial NEC 52.59
    distal (tail) (with part of body) 52.52
    proximal (head) (with part of
      body) (with synchronous
      duodenectomy) 52.51
      radical 52.53
        subtotal 52.53
    radical 52.7
      subtotal 52.53

Pancreaticocystoduodenostomy 52.4
Pancreaticocystoenterostomy 52.4
Pancreaticocystogastrostomy 52.4
Pancreaticocystojejunostomy 52.4
Pancreaticoduodenectomy (total) 52.6
  partial NEC 52.59
    proximal 52.51
    radical subtotal
      52.53
  radical (one-stage) (two-stage) 52.7
  subtotal 52.53
Pancreaticoduodenostomy 52.96
Pancreaticoenterostomy 52.96
Pancreaticogastrostomy 52.96
Pancreaticoileostomy 52.96
Pancreaticojejunostomy 52.96
Pancreatoduodenectomy (total) 52.6
  partial NEC 52.59
  radical (one-stage) (two-stage)
    52.7
  subtotal 52.53
Pancreatogram 87.66
  endoscopic retrograde (ERP)
    52.13
Pancreatolithotomy 52.09
  endoscopic 52.94
Pancreatotomy 52.09
Pancreolithotomy 52.09
  endoscopic 52.94
Panendoscopy 57.32
  specified site, other than bladder - *see*
    Endoscopy, by site
  through artificial stoma 57.31
Panhysterectomy (abdominal) 68.49
  laparoscopic 68.41
  vaginal 68.59
    laparoscopically assisted (LAVH)
      68.51
Panniculectomy 86.83
Panniculotomy 86.83
Pantaloon operation (revision of gastric
  anastomosis) 44.5
Papillectomy, anal 49.39
  endoscopic 49.31
Papillotomy (pancreas) 51.82
  endoscopic 51.85
Paquin operation (ureteroneocystostomy)
  56.74

Paracentesis
  abdominal (percutaneous) 54.91
  anterior chamber, eye 12.91
  bladder 57.11
  cornea 12.91
  eye (anterior chamber) 12.91
  thoracic, thoracis 34.91
  tympanum 20.09
    with intubation 20.01
Parasitology - *see* Examination,
  microscopic
Parathyroidectomy (partial) (subtotal)
  NEC 06.89
  complete 06.81
  ectopic 06.89
  global removal 06.81
  mediastinal 06.89
  total 06.81
Parenteral nutrition, total 99.15
  peripheral 99.15
Parotidectomy 26.30
  complete 26.32
  partial 26.31
  radical 26.32
Partsch operation (marsupialization of
  dental cyst) 24.4
Passage - *see* Insertion and Intubation
Passage of sounds, urethra 58.6
Patch
  blood, spinal (epidural) 03.95
  graft - *see* Graft
  spinal, blood (epidural) 03.95
  subdural, brain 02.12
Patellapexy 78.46
Patellaplasty NEC 78.46
Patellectomy 77.96
  partial 77.86
Pattee operation (auditory canal) 18.6
Pectenotomy - *see also* Sphincterotomy,
  anal 49.59
PDT (percutaneous dilatational
  tracheostomy) – *see* Tracheostomy
Pedicle flap - *see* Graft, skin, pedicle
Peet operation (splanchnic resection) 05.29
PEG (percutaneous endoscopic
  gastrostomy) 43.11
PEGJJ (percutaneous [endoscopic]
  gastrojejunostomy) 44.32

O & P

PEJ (percutaneous endoscopic jejunostomy) 46.32
Pelvectomy, kidney (partial) 55.4
Pelvimetry 88.25
  gynecological 89.26
Pelviolithotomy 55.11
Pelvioplasty, kidney 55.87
Pelviostomy 55.12
  closure 55.82
Pelviotomy 77.39
  to assist delivery 73.94
Pelvi-ureteroplasty 55.87
Pemberton operation
  osteotomy of ilium 77.39
  rectum (mobilization and fixation for prolapse repair) 48.76
Penectomy 64.3
Pereyra operation (paraurethral suspension) 59.6
Perforation
  stapes footplate 19.0
Perfusion NEC 39.97
  carotid artery 39.97
  coronary artery 39.97
  for
    chemotherapy NEC 99.25
    hormone therapy NEC 99.24
  head 39.97
  hyperthermic (lymphatic), localized region or site 93.35
  intestine (large) (local) 46.96
    small 46.95
  kidney, local 55.95
  limb (lower) (upper) 39.97
  liver, localized 50.93
  neck 39.97
  subarachnoid (spinal cord) (refrigerated saline) 03.92
  total body 39.96
Pericardiectomy 37.31
Pericardiocentesis 37.0
Pericardiolysis 37.12
Pericardioplasty 37.49
Pericardiorrhaphy 37.49
Pericardiostomy (tube) 37.12
Pericardiotomy 37.12
Peridectomy 10.31
Perilimbal suction 89.11
Perimetry 95.05
Perineoplasty 71.79
Perineorrhaphy 71.71
  obstetrical laceration (current) 75.69
Perineotomy (nonobstetrical) 71.09
  to assist delivery - see Episiotomy
Periosteotomy - see also Incision, bone 77.10
  facial bone 76.09
Perirectofistulectomy 48.93
Peritectomy 10.31
Peritomy 10.1
Peritoneocentesis 54.91
Peritoneoscopy 54.21
Peritoneotomy 54.19
Peritoneumectomy 54.4
Phacoemulsification (ultrasonic) (with aspiration) 13.41
Phacofragmentation (mechanical) (with aspiration) 13.43
  posterior route 13.42
  ultrasonic 13.41
Phalangectomy (partial) 77.89
  claw toe 77.57
  cockup toe 77.58
  hammer toe 77.56

Phalangectomy (Continued)
  overlapping toe 77.58
  total 77.99
Phalangization (fifth metacarpal) 82.81
Pharyngeal flap operation (cleft palate repair) 27.62
  secondary or subsequent 27.63
Pharyngectomy (partial) 29.33
  with laryngectomy 30.3
Pharyngogram 87.09
  contrast 87.06
Pharyngolaryngectomy 30.3
Pharyngoplasty (with silastic implant) 29.4
  for cleft palate 27.62
    secondary or subsequent 27.63
Pharyngorrhaphy 29.51
  for cleft palate 27.62
Pharyngoscopy 29.11
Pharyngotomy 29.0
Phenopeel (skin) 86.24
Phlebectomy 38.60
  with
    anastomosis 38.30
      abdominal 38.37
      head and neck NEC 38.32
      intracranial NEC 38.31
      lower limb 38.39
      thoracic NEC 38.35
      upper limb 38.33
    graft replacement 38.40
      abdominal 38.47
      head and neck NEC 38.42
      intracranial NEC 38.41
      lower limb 38.49
      thoracic NEC 38.45
      upper limb 38.43
  abdominal 38.67
  head and neck NEC 38.62
  intracranial NEC 38.61
  lower limb 38.69
  thoracic NEC 38.65
  upper limb 38.63
  varicose 38.50
    abdominal 38.57
    head and neck NEC 38.52
    intracranial NEC 38.51
    lower limb 38.59
    thoracic NEC 38.55
    upper limb 38.53
Phlebogoniostomy 12.52
Phlebography (contrast) (retrograde) 88.60
  by radioisotope - see Scan, radioisotope, by site
  adrenal 88.65
  femoral 88.66
  head 88.61
  hepatic 88.64
  impedance 88.68
  intra-abdominal NEC 88.65
  intrathoracic NEC 88.63
  lower extremity NEC 88.66
  neck 88.61
  portal system 88.64
  pulmonary 88.62
  specified site NEC 88.67
  vena cava (inferior) (superior) 88.51
Phleborrhaphy 39.32
Phlebotomy 38.99
Phonocardiogram, with ECG lead 89.55
Photochemotherapy NEC 99.83
  extracorporeal 99.88

Photocoagulation
  ciliary body 12.73
  eye, eyeball 16.99
  iris 12.41
  macular hole - see Photocoagulation, retina
  orbital lesion 16.92
  retina
    for
      destruction of lesion 14.25
      reattachment 14.55
      repair of tear or defect 14.35
    laser (beam)
      for
        destruction of lesion 14.24
        reattachment 14.54
        repair of tear or defect 14.34
    xenon arc
      for
        destruction of lesion 14.23
        reattachment 14.53
        repair of tear or defect 14.33
Photography 89.39
  fundus 95.11
Photopheresis, therapeutic 99.88
Phototherapy NEC 99.83
  newborn 99.83
  ultraviolet 99.82
Phrenemphraxis 04.03
  for collapse of lung 33.31
Phrenicectomy 04.03
  for collapse of lung 33.31
Phrenicoexeresis 04.03
  for collapse of lung 33.31
Phrenicotomy 04.03
  for collapse of lung 33.31
Phrenicotripsy 04.03
  for collapse of lung 33.31
Phrenoplasty 34.84
Physical medicine - see Therapy, physical
Physical therapy - see Therapy, physical
Physiotherapy, chest 93.99
PICC (peripherally inserted central catheter) 38.93
Piercing ear, external (pinna) 18.01
Pigmenting, skin 86.02
Pilojection (aneurysm) (Gallagher) 39.52
Pinealectomy (complete) (total) 07.54
  partial 07.53
Pinealotomy (with drainage) 07.52
Pinning
  bone - see Fixation, bone, internal
  ear 18.5
Pinsker operation (obliteration of nasoseptal telangiectasia) 21.07
Piper operation (forceps) 72.6
Pirogoff operation (ankle amputation through malleoli of tibia and fibula) 84.14
Pituitectomy (complete) (total) - see also Hypophysectomy 07.69
Placentogram, placentography 88.46
  with radioisotope (RISA) 92.17
Planing, skin 86.25
Plantation, tooth (bud) (germ) 23.5
  prosthetic 23.6
Plasma exchange 99.07
Plasmapheresis, therapeutic 99.71
Plastic repair - see Repair, by site

◀ New   ◀⫤ Revised   ~~deleted~~ Deleted   ● Use Additional Digit(s)   Omit code

P

Procedure *(Continued)*
  diagnostic NEC *(Continued)*
    buccal 27.24
    bursa 83.29
    canthus 08.19
    cecum 45.28
    cerebral meninges 01.18
    cervix 67.19
    chest wall 34.28
    choroid 14.19
    ciliary body 12.29
    clitoris 71.19
    colon 45.28
    conjunctiva 10.29
    cornea 11.29
    cul-de-sac 70.29
    dental 24.19
    diaphragm 34.28
    duodenum 45.19
    ear
        external 18.19
        inner and middle 20.39
    epididymis 63.09
    esophagus 42.29
    Eustachian tube 20.39
    extraocular muscle or tendon
        15.09
    eye 16.29
        anterior chamber 12.29
        posterior chamber 14.19
    eyeball 16.29
    eyelid 08.19
    fallopian tube 66.19
    fascia (any site) 83.29
    fetus 75.35
    gallbladder 51.19
    ganglion (cranial) (peripheral)
        04.19
        sympathetic 05.19
    gastric 44.19
    globus pallidus 01.18
    gum 24.19
    heart 37.29
    hepatic 50.19
    hypophysis 07.19
    ileum 45.19
    intestine 45.29
        large 45.28
        small 45.19
    iris 12.29
    jejunum 45.19
    joint (capsule) (ligament) (structure)
        NEC 81.98
        facial 76.19
    kidney 55.29
    labia 71.19
    lacrimal (system) 09.19
    large intestine 45.28
    larynx 31.48
    ligament 81.98
        uterine 68.19
    liver 50.19
    lung 33.29
    lymphatic structure (channel)
        (gland) (node) (vessel) 40.19
    mediastinum 34.29
    meninges (cerebral) 01.18
        spinal 03.39
    mouth 27.29
    muscle 83.29
        extraocular (oblique) (rectus)
            15.09
        papillary (heart) 37.29
    nail 86.19

Procedure *(Continued)*
  diagnostic NEC *(Continued)*
    nasopharynx 29.19
    nerve (cranial) (peripheral) NEC
        04.19
        sympathetic 05.19
    nipple 85.19
    nose, nasal 21.29
        sinus 22.19
    ocular 16.29
        muscle 15.09
    omentum 54.29
    ophthalmologic 16.29
    oral (cavity) 27.29
    orbit 16.29
    orthodontic 24.19
    ovary 65.19
        laparoscopic 65.14
    palate 27.29
    pancreas 52.19
    papillary muscle (heart) 37.29
    parathyroid gland 06.19
    penis 64.19
    perianal tissue 49.29
    pericardium 37.29
    periprostatic tissue 60.18
    perirectal tissue 48.29
    perirenal tissue 59.29
    peritoneum 54.29
    periurethral tissue 58.29
    perivesical tissue 59.29
    pharynx 29.19
    pineal gland 07.19
    pituitary gland 07.19
    pleura 34.28
    posterior chamber, eye 14.19
    prostate 60.18
    pulmonary 33.29
    rectosigmoid 48.29
    rectum 48.29
    renal 55.29
    respiratory 33.29
    retina 14.19
    retroperitoneum 59.29
    salivary gland or duct 26.19
    sclera 12.29
    scrotum 61.19
    seminal vesicle 60.19
    sigmoid 45.28
    sinus, nasal 22.19
    skin 86.19
    skull 01.19
    soft tissue 83.29
    spermatic cord 63.09
    sphincter of Oddi 51.19
    spine, spinal (canal) (cord)
        (meninges) (structure)
        03.39
    spleen 41.39
    stomach 44.19
    subcutaneous tissue 86.19
    sympathetic nerve 05.19
    tarsus 09.19
    tendon NEC 83.29
        extraocular 15.09
    testicle 62.19
    thalamus 01.18
    thoracic duct 40.19
    thorax 34.28
    thymus 07.19
    thyroid gland 06.19
    tongue 25.09
    tonsils 28.19
    tooth 24.19

Procedure *(Continued)*
  diagnostic NEC *(Continued)*
    trachea 31.49
    tunica vaginalis 61.19
    ureter 56.39
    urethra 58.29
    uterus and supporting structures
        68.19
    uvula 27.29
    vagina 70.29
    vas deferens 63.09
    vesical 57.39
    vessel (blood) (any site) 38.29
    vitreous 14.19
    vulva 71.19
  fistulizing, sclera NEC 12.69
  miscellaneous (nonoperative) NEC
      99.99
  respiratory (nonoperative) NEC 93.99
  surgical - *see* Operation
Proctectasis 96.22
Proctectomy (partial) - *see also* Resection,
    rectum 48.69
  abdominoperineal, NOS 48.50
    laparoscopic 48.51
    open 48.52
    other 48.59
  complete (Miles) (Rankin), NOS
      48.50
    laparoscopic 48.51
    open 48.52
    other 48.59
  pull-through
    laparoscopic 48.42
    not otherwise specified 48.40
    open 48.43
    other 48.49
Proctoclysis 96.37
Proctolysis 48.99
Proctopexy (Delorme) 48.76
  abdominal (Ripstein) 48.75
Proctoplasty 48.79
Proctorrhaphy 48.71
Proctoscopy 48.23
  with biopsy 48.24
  through stoma (artificial) 48.22
  transabdominal approach 48.21
Proctosigmoidectomy - *see also* Resection,
    rectum 48.69
Proctosigmoidopexy 48.76
Proctosigmoidoscopy (rigid) 48.23
  with biopsy 48.24
  flexible 45.24
  through stoma (artificial) 48.22
  transabdominal approach 48.21
Proctostomy 48.1
Proctotomy (decompression) (linear)
    48.0
Production - *see also* Formation *and*
    Creation
  atrial septal defect 35.42
  subcutaneous tunnel for esophageal
      anastomosis 42.86
      with anastomosis - *see* Anastomosis,
          esophagus, antesternal
Prognathic recession 76.64
Prophylaxis, dental (scaling) (polishing)
    96.54
Prostatectomy (complete) (partial) NEC
    60.69
  loop 60.29
  perineal 60.62
  radical (any approach) 60.5
  retropubic (punch) (transcapsular) 60.4

◀ New   ◀▥ Revised   ~~deleted~~ Deleted   ● Use Additional Digit(s)   ▨ Omit code

Prostatectomy (Continued)
  suprapubic (punch) (transvesical) 60.3
  transcapsular NEC 60.69
    retropubic 60.4
  transperineal 60.62
  transurethral 60.29
    ablation (contact) (noncontact) by
      laser 60.21
    electrovaporization 60.29
    enucleative 60.29
    resection of prostate (TURP) 60.29
    ultrasound guided laser induced
      (TULIP) 60.21
  transvesical punch (suprapubic) 60.3
Prostatocystotomy 60.0
Prostatolithotomy 60.0
Prostatotomy (perineal) 60.0
Prostatovesiculectomy 60.5
Protection (of)
  individual from his surroundings
    99.84
  surroundings from individual 99.84
Psychoanalysis 94.31
Psychodrama 94.43
Psychotherapy NEC 94.39
  biofeedback 94.39
  exploratory verbal 94.37
  group 94.44
    for psychosexual dysfunctions
      94.41
  play 94.36
  psychosexual dysfunctions 94.34
  supportive verbal 94.38
PTCA (percutaneous transluminal
  coronary angioplasty) - see
  Angioplasty, balloon, coronary
Ptyalectasis 26.91
Ptyalithotomy 26.0
Ptyalolithotomy 26.0
Pubiotomy 77.39
  assisting delivery 73.94
Pubococcygeoplasty 59.71
Puestow operation
    (pancreaticojejunostomy) 52.96
Pull-through
  abdomino-anal 48.49
  abdominoperineal 48.49
    Duhamel type 48.65
  endorectal 48.41
Pulmowrap 93.99

Pulpectomy - see also Therapy, root canal
  23.70
Pulpotomy - see also Therapy, root canal
  23.70
Pump-oxygenator, for extracorporeal
  circulation 39.61
  percutaneous 39.66
Punch
  operation
    bladder neck, transurethral 57.49
    prostate - see Prostatectomy
  resection, vocal cords 30.22
Puncture
  antrum (nasal) (bilateral) (unilateral)
    22.01
  artery NEC 38.98
    for
      arteriography - see also
        Arteriography 88.40
    for
      coronary arteriography - see also
        Arteriography, coronary
        88.57
    percutaneous vascular closure - *omit
      code*
  bladder, suprapubic (for drainage)
    NEC 57.18
    needle 57.11
    percutaneous (suprapubic) 57.17
  bursa 83.94
    hand 82.92
  cisternal 01.01
    with contrast media 87.02
  cranial 01.09
    with contrast media 87.02
  craniobuccal pouch 07.72
  craniopharyngioma 07.72
  fallopian tube 66.91
  fontanel, anterior 01.09
  heart 37.0
    for intracardiac injection 37.92
  hypophysis 07.72
  iris 12.12
  joint 81.91
  kidney (percutaneous) 55.92
  larynx 31.98
  lumbar (diagnostic) (removal of dye)
    03.31
  lung (for aspiration) 33.93
  nasal sinus 22.01

Puncture (Continued)
  pericardium 37.0
  pituitary gland 07.72
  pleural cavity 34.91
  Rathke's pouch 07.72
  spinal 03.31
  spleen 41.1
    for biopsy 41.32
  sternal (for bone marrow biopsy) 41.31
    donor for bone marrow transplant
      41.91
  vein NEC 38.99
    for
      phlebography - see also
        Phlebography 88.60
      transfusion - see Transfusion
  ventricular shunt tubing 01.02
Pupillotomy 12.35
Push-back operation (cleft palate repair)
  27.62
Putti-Platt operation (capsulorrhaphy of
  shoulder for recurrent dislocation)
  81.82
pVAD (percutaneous ventricular assist
  device) 37.68
Pyelogram (intravenous) 87.73
  infusion (continuous) (diuretic) 87.73
  percutaneous 87.75
  retrograde 87.74
Pyeloileostomy 56.71
Pyelolithotomy 55.11
Pyeloplasty 55.87
Pyelorrhaphy 55.81
Pyeloscopy 55.22
Pyelostolithotomy, percutaneous 55.03
Pyelostomy 55.12
  closure 55.82
Pyelotomy 55.11
Pyeloureteroplasty 55.87
Pylorectomy 43.6
Pyloroduodenotomy - see category 44.2●
Pyloromyotomy (Ramstedt) (with wedge
  resection) 43.3
Pyloroplasty (Finney) (Heineke-Mikulicz)
  44.29
  dilation, endoscopic 44.22
    by incision 44.21
  not elsewhere classified 44.29
  revision 44.29
Pylorostomy - see Gastrostomy

Q

Quadrant resection of breast 85.22
Quadricepsplasty (Thompson) 83.86
Quarantine 99.84
Quenuthoracoplasty 77.31
Quotient, respiratory 89.38

R

Rachicentesis 03.31
Rachitomy 03.09
Radiation therapy - *see also* Therapy,
    radiation
    teleradiotherapy - *see*
        Teleradiotherapy
Radical neck dissection - *see*
    Dissection, neck
Radicotomy 03.1
Radiculectomy 03.1
Radiculotomy 03.1
Radiography (diagnostic) NEC 88.39
    abdomen, abdominal (flat plate) NEC
        88.19
        wall (soft tissue) NEC 88.09
    adenoid 87.09
    ankle (skeletal) 88.28
        soft tissue 88.37
    bone survey 88.31
    bronchus 87.49
    chest (routine) 87.44
        wall NEC 87.39
    clavicle 87.43
    computer assisted surgery (CAS) with
        fluoroscopy 00.33
    contrast (air) (gas) (radio-opaque
        substance) NEC
        abdominal wall 88.03
        arteries (by fluoroscopy) - *see*
            Arteriography
        bile ducts NEC 87.54
        bladder NEC 87.77
        brain 87.02
        breast 87.35
        bronchus NEC (transcricoid)
            87.32
            endotracheal 87.31
        epididymis 87.93
        esophagus 87.61
        fallopian tubes
            gas 87.82
            opaque dye 87.83
        fistula (sinus tract) - *see also*
            Radiography, contrast, by site
            abdominal wall 88.03
            chest wall 87.38
        gallbladder NEC 87.59
        intervertebral disc(s) 87.21
        joints 88.32
        larynx 87.07
        lymph - *see* Lymphangiogram
        mammary ducts 87.35
        mediastinum 87.33
        nasal sinuses 87.15
        nasolacrimal ducts 87.05
        nasopharynx 87.06
        orbit 87.14
        pancreas 87.66
        pelvis
            gas 88.12
            opaque dye 88.11
        peritoneum NEC 88.13
        retroperitoneum NEC 88.15
        seminal vesicles 87.91
        sinus tract - *see also* Radiography,
            contrast, by site
            abdominal wall 88.03
            chest wall 87.38
            nose 87.15
        skull 87.02

Radiography NEC (*Continued*)
    contrast (*Continued*)
        spinal disc(s) 87.21
        trachea 87.32
        uterus
            gas 87.82
            opaque dye 87.83
        vas deferens 87.94
        veins (by fluoroscopy) - *see*
            Phlebography
        vena cava (inferior) (superior)
            88.51
    dental NEC 87.12
    diaphragm 87.49
    digestive tract NEC 87.69
        barium swallow 87.61
        lower GI series 87.64
        small bowel series 87.63
        upper GI series 87.62
    elbow (skeletal) 88.22
        soft tissue 88.35
    epididymis NEC 87.95
    esophagus 87.69
        barium-swallow 87.61
    eye 95.14
    face, head, and neck 87.09
    facial bones 87.16
    fallopian tubes 87.85
    foot 88.28
    forearm (skeletal) 88.22
        soft tissue 88.35
    frontal area, facial 87.16
    genital organs
        female NEC 87.89
        male NEC 87.99
    hand (skeletal) 88.23
        soft tissue 88.35
    head NEC 87.09
    heart 87.49
    hip (skeletal) 88.26
        soft tissue 88.37
    intestine NEC 87.65
    kidney-ureter-bladder (KUB) 87.79
    knee (skeletal) 88.27
        soft tissue 88.37
    KUB (kidney-ureter-bladder) 87.79
    larynx 87.09
    lower leg (skeletal) 88.27
        soft tissue 88.37
    lower limb (skeletal) NEC 88.29
        soft tissue NEC 88.37
    lung 87.49
    mandible 87.16
    maxilla 87.16
    mediastinum 87.49
    nasal sinuses 87.16
    nasolacrimal duct 87.09
    nasopharynx 87.09
    neck NEC 87.09
    nose 87.16
    orbit 87.16
    pelvis (skeletal) 88.26
        pelvimetry 88.25
        soft tissue 88.19
    prostate NEC 87.92
    retroperitoneum NEC 88.16
    ribs 87.43
    root canal 87.12
    salivary gland 87.09
    seminal vesicles NEC 87.92
    shoulder (skeletal) 88.21
        soft tissue 88.35

Radiography NEC (*Continued*)
    skeletal NEC 88.33
        series (whole or complete) 88.31
    skull (lateral, sagittal or tangential
        projection) NEC 87.17
    spine NEC 87.29
        cervical 87.22
        lumbosacral 87.24
        sacrococcygeal 87.24
        thoracic 87.23
    sternum 87.43
    supraorbital area 87.16
    symphysis menti 87.16
    teeth NEC 87.12
        full-mouth 87.11
    thigh (skeletal) 88.27
        soft tissue 88.37
    thyroid region 87.09
    tonsils and adenoids 87.09
    trachea 87.49
    ultrasonic - *see* Ultrasonography
    upper arm (skeletal) 88.21
        soft tissue 88.35
    upper limb (skeletal) NEC 88.24
        soft tissue NEC 88.35
    urinary system NEC 87.79
    uterus NEC 87.85
        gravid 87.81
    uvula 87.09
    vas deferens NEC 87.95
    wrist 88.23
    zygomaticomaxillary complex
        87.16
Radioimmunotherapy 92.28
Radioisotope
    scanning - *see* Scan, radioisotope
    therapy - *see* Therapy, radioisotope
Radiology
    diagnostic - *see* Radiography
    therapeutic - *see* Therapy, radiation
Radiosurgery, stereotactic 92.30
    cobalt 60 92.32
    linear accelerator (LINAC) 92.31
    multi-source 92.32
    particle beam 92.33
    particulate 92.33
    radiosurgery NEC 92.39
    single source photon 92.31
Raising, pedicle graft 86.71
Ramadier operation (intrapetrosal
    drainage) 20.22
Ramisection (sympathetic) 05.0
Ramstedt operation (pyloromyotomy)
    (with wedge resection) 43.3
Range of motion testing 93.05
Rankin operation
    exteriorization of intestine 46.03
    proctectomy (complete), NOS
        48.50
        laparoscopic 48.51
        open 48.52
        other 48.59
Rashkind operation (balloon septostomy)
    35.41
Rastelli operation (creation of conduit
    between right ventricle and
    pulmonary artery) 35.92
    in repair of
        pulmonary artery atresia 35.92
        transposition of great vessels
            35.92
        truncus arteriosus 35.83

◀ New   ◀▥ Revised   ~~deleted~~ Deleted   ● Use Additional Digit(s)   ▨ Omit code

Raz-Pereyra procedure (bladder neck suspension) 59.79
RCSA (radical cryosurgical ablation) of prostate 60.62
Readjustment - *see* Adjustment
Reamputation, stump 84.3
Reanastomosis - *see* Anastomosis
Reattachment
    amputated ear 18.72
    ankle 84.27
    arm (upper) NEC 84.24
    choroid and retina NEC 14.59
        by
            cryotherapy 14.52
            diathermy 14.51
            electrocoagulation 14.51
            photocoagulation 14.55
                laser 14.54
                xenon arc 14.53
    ear (amputated) 18.72
    extremity 84.29
        ankle 84.27
        arm (upper) NEC 84.24
        fingers, except thumb 84.22
            thumb 84.21
        foot 84.26
        forearm 84.23
        hand 84.23
        leg (lower) NEC 84.27
        thigh 84.28
        thumb 84.21
        toe 84.25
        wrist 84.23
    finger 84.22
        thumb 84.21
    foot 84.26
    forearm 84.23
    hand 84.23
    joint capsule - *see also* Arthroplasty 81.96
    leg (lower) NEC 84.27
    ligament - *see also* Arthroplasty
        uterosacral 69.22
    muscle 83.74
        hand 82.54
        papillary (heart) 35.31
    nerve (peripheral) 04.79
    nose (amputated) 21.89
    papillary muscle (heart) 35.31
    penis (amputated) 64.45
    retina (and choroid) NEC 14.59
        by
            cryotherapy 14.52
            diathermy 14.51
            electrocoagulation 14.51
            photocoagulation 14.55
                laser 14.54
                xenon arc 14.53
    tendon (to tendon) 83.73
        hand 82.53
        to skeletal attachment 83.88
            hand 82.85
    thigh 84.28
    thumb 84.21
    toe 84.25
    tooth 23.5
    uterosacral ligament(s) 69.22
    vessels (peripheral) 39.59
        renal, aberrant 39.55
    wrist 84.23

Recession
    extraocular muscle 15.11
        multiple (two or more muscles) (with advancement or resection) 15.3
    gastrocnemius tendon (Strayer operation) 83.72
    levator palpebrae (superioris) muscle 08.38
    prognathic jaw 76.64
    tendon 83.72
        hand 82.52
Reclosure - *see also* Closure
    disrupted abdominal wall (postoperative) 54.61
Reconstruction (plastic) - *see also* Construction and Repair, by site
    alveolus, alveolar (process) (ridge) (with graft or implant) 24.5
    artery (graft) - *see* Graft, artery
    artificial stoma, intestine 46.40
    auditory canal (external) 18.6
    auricle (ear) 18.71
    bladder 57.87
        with
            ileum 57.87 [45.51]
            sigmoid 57.87 [45.52]
    bone, except facial - *see also* Osteoplasty 78.40
        facial NEC 76.46
            with total ostectomy 76.44
        mandible 76.43
            with total mandibulectomy 76.41
    breast, total, NOS 85.70
        deep inferior epigastric artery perforator (DIEP) flap, free 85.74
        gluteal artery perforator (GAP) flap, free 85.76
        latissimus dorsi myocutaneous flap 85.71
        other 85.79
        superficial inferior epigastric artery (SIEA) flap, free 85.75
        transverse rectus abdominis musculocutaneous (TRAM) flap, free 85.73
        transverse rectus abdominis myocutaneous (TRAM) flap, pedicled 85.72
    bronchus 33.48
    canthus (lateral) 08.59
    cardiac annulus 35.33
    chest wall (mesh) (silastic) 34.79
    cleft lip 27.54
    conjunctival cul-de-sac 10.43
        with graft (buccal mucous membrane) (free) 10.42
    cornea NEC 11.79
    diaphragm 34.84
    ear (external) (auricle) 18.71
        external auditory canal 18.6
        meatus (new) (osseous skin-lined) 18.6
        ossicles 19.3
        prominent or protruding 18.5
    eyebrow 08.70
    eyelid 08.70
        with graft or flap 08.69
            hair follicle 08.63
            mucous membrane 08.62
            skin 08.61

Reconstruction (*Continued*)
    eyelid (*Continued*)
        with graft or flap (*Continued*)
            tarsoconjunctival (one-stage) (two-stage) 08.64
            full-thickness 08.74
                involving lid margin 08.73
            partial-thickness 08.72
                involving lid margin 08.71
    eye socket 16.64
        with graft 16.63
    fallopian tube 66.79
    foot and toes (with fixation device) 81.57
        with prosthetic implant 81.57
    frontonasal duct 22.79
    hip (total) (with prosthesis) 81.51
    intraoral 27.59
    joint - *see* Arthroplasty
    lymphatic (by transplantation) 40.9
    mandible 76.43
        with total mandibulectomy 76.41
    mastoid cavity 19.9
    mouth 27.59
    nipple NEC 85.87
    nose (total) (with arm flap) (with forehead flap) 21.83
    ossicles (graft) (prosthesis) NEC 19.3
        with
            stapedectomy 19.19
            tympanoplasty 19.53
    pelvic floor 71.79
    penis (rib graft) (skin graft) (myocutaneous flap) 64.44
    pharynx 29.4
    scrotum (with pedicle flap) (with rotational flap) 61.49
    skin (plastic) (without graft) NEC 86.89
        with graft - *see* Graft, skin
    subcutaneous tissue (plastic) (without skin graft) NEC 86.89
        with graft - *see* Graft, skin
    tendon pulley (with graft) (with local tissue) 83.83
        for opponensplasty 82.71
        hand 82.71
    thumb (osteoplastic) (with bone graft) (with skin graft) 82.69
    trachea (with graft) 31.75
    umbilicus
        laparoscopic 53.43
            with graft or prosthesis 53.42
        other and open with graft or prosthesis 53.41
        other open 53.49
    ureteropelvic junction 55.87
    urethra 58.46
    vagina 70.62
        with graft or prosthesis 70.64
    vas deferens, surgically divided 63.82
Recontour, gingiva 24.2
Recreational therapy 93.81
Rectectomy - *see also* Resection, rectum 48.69
Rectopexy (Delorme) 48.76
    abdominal (Ripstein) 48.75
Rectoplasty 48.79
Rectorectostomy 48.74
Rectorrhaphy 48.71

Rectosigmoidectomy - *see also* Resection,
    rectum 48.69
    transsacral 48.61
Rectosigmoidostomy 45.94
Rectostomy 48.1
    closure 48.72
Red cell survival studies 92.05
Reduction - *see also* Excision, by site
    adipose tissue 86.83
    batwing arms 86.83
    breast (bilateral) 85.32
      unilateral 85.31
    bulbous tuberosities (mandible)
        (maxilla) (fibrous) (osseous)
        24.31
    buttocks 86.83
    diastasis, ankle mortise (closed) 79.77
      open 79.87
    dislocation (of joint) (manipulation)
        (with cast) (with splint) (with
        traction device) (closed) 79.70
      with fracture - *see* Reduction,
        fracture, by site
      ankle (closed) 79.77
        open 79.87
      elbow (closed) 79.72
        open 79.82
      finger (closed) 79.74
        open 79.84
      foot (closed) 79.78
        open 79.88
      hand (closed) 79.74
        open 79.84
      hip (closed) 79.75
        open 79.85
      knee (closed) 79.76
        open 79.86
      open (with external fixation)
        (with internal fixation)
        79.80
      specified site NEC 79.89
      shoulder (closed) 79.71
        open 79.81
      specified site (closed) NEC
        79.79
        open 79.89
      temporomandibular (closed)
        76.93
        open 76.94
      toe (closed) 79.78
        open 79.88
      wrist (closed) 79.73
        open 79.83
    elephantiasis, scrotum 61.3
    epistaxis - *see also* Control, epistaxis
      21.00
    fracture (bone) (with cast) (with splint)
        (with traction device) (closed)
        79.00
      with internal fixation 79.10
      alveolar process (with stabilization
        of teeth)
        mandible (closed) 76.75
          open 76.77
        maxilla (closed) 76.73
          open 76.77
        open 76.77
      ankle - *see* Reduction, fracture, leg
      arm (closed) NEC 79.02
        with internal fixation 79.12
        open 79.22
          with internal fixation 79.32
      blow-out - *see* Reduction, fracture,
        orbit

Reduction (*Continued*)
  fracture (*Continued*)
    carpal, metacarpal (closed) 79.03
      with internal fixation 79.13
      open 79.23
        with internal fixation 79.33
    epiphysis - *see* Reduction, separation
    facial (bone) NEC 76.70
      closed 76.78
      open 76.79
    femur (closed) 79.05
      with internal fixation 79.15
      open 79.25
        with internal fixation 79.35
    fibula (closed) 79.06
      with internal fixation 79.16
      open 79.26
        with internal fixation 79.36
    foot (closed) NEC 79.07
      with internal fixation 79.17
      open 79.27
        with internal fixation 79.37
    hand (closed) NEC 79.03
      with internal fixation 79.13
      open 79.23
        with internal fixation 79.33
    humerus (closed) 79.01
      with internal fixation 79.11
      open 79.21
        with internal fixation 79.31
    jaw (lower) - *see also* Reduction,
      fracture, mandible
      upper - *see* Reduction, fracture,
        maxilla
    larynx 31.64
    leg (closed) NEC 79.06
      with internal fixation 79.16
      open 79.26
        with internal fixation 79.36
    malar (closed) 76.71
      open 76.72
    mandible (with dental wiring)
      (closed) 76.75
      open 76.76
    maxilla (with dental wiring) (closed)
      76.73
      open 76.74
    nasal (closed) 21.71
      open 21.72
    open 79.20
      with internal fixation 79.30
      specified site NEC 79.29
        with internal fixation 79.39
    orbit (rim) (wall) (closed) 76.78
      open 76.79
    patella (open) (with internal
      fixation) 79.36
    phalanges
      foot (closed) 79.08
        with internal fixation 79.18
        open 79.28
          with internal fixation
            79.38
      hand (closed) 79.04
        with internal fixation
          79.14
        open 79.24
          with internal fixation
            79.34
    radius (closed) 79.02
      with internal fixation 79.12
      open 79.22
        with internal fixation 79.32
    skull 02.02

Reduction (*Continued*)
  fracture (*Continued*)
    specified site (closed) NEC 79.09
      with internal fixation 79.19
      open 79.29
        with internal fixation 79.39
    spine 03.53
    tarsal, metatarsal (closed) 79.07
      with internal fixation 79.17
      open 79.27
        with internal fixation 79.37
    tibia (closed) 79.06
      with internal fixation 79.16
      open 79.26
        with internal fixation 79.36
    ulna (closed) 79.02
      with internal fixation 79.12
      open 79.22
        with internal fixation 79.32
    vertebra 03.53
    zygoma, zygomatic arch (closed) 76.71
      open 76.72
  fracture dislocation - *see* Reduction,
    fracture
  heart volume 37.35
  hemorrhoids (manual) 49.41
  hernia - *see also* Repair, hernia
    manual 96.27
  intussusception (open) 46.80
    with
      fluoroscopy 96.29
      ionizing radiation enema 96.29
      ultrasonography guidance 96.29
    hydrostatic 96.29
    large intestine 46.82
      endoscopic (balloon) 46.85
    pneumatic 96.29
    small intestine 46.81
  lung volume 32.22
    biologic lung volume reduction
      (BLVR) - *see* category 33.7 ●
  malrotation, intestine (manual)
    (surgical) 46.80
    large 46.82
      endoscopic (balloon) 46.85
    small 46.81
  mammoplasty (bilateral) 85.32
    unilateral 85.31
  prolapse
    anus (operative) 49.94
    colostomy (manual) 96.28
    enterostomy (manual) 96.28
    ileostomy (manual) 96.28
    rectum (manual) 96.26
    uterus
      by pessary 96.18
      surgical 69.22
  ptosis overcorrection 08.37
  retroversion, uterus by pessary
    96.18
  separation, epiphysis (with internal
    fixation) (closed) 79.40
    femur (closed) 79.45
      open 79.55
    fibula (closed) 79.46
      open 79.56
    humerus (closed) 79.41
      open 79.51
    open 79.50
    specified site (closed) NEC - *see also*
      category 79.4 ●
      open - *see* category 79.5 ●
    tibia (closed) 79.46
      open 79.56

Reduction *(Continued)*
  size
    abdominal wall (adipose)
      (pendulous) 86.83
    arms (adipose) (batwing) 86.83
    breast (bilateral) 85.32
      unilateral 85.31
    buttocks (adipose) 86.83
    finger (macrodactyly repair)
      82.83
    skin 86.83
    subcutaneous tissue 86.83
    thighs (adipose) 86.83
  torsion
    intestine (manual) (surgical)
      46.80
      large 46.82
        endoscopic (balloon)
          46.85
      small 46.81
    kidney pedicle 55.84
    omentum 54.74
    spermatic cord 63.52
      with orchiopexy 62.5
    testis 63.52
      with orchiopexy 62.5
    uterus NEC 69.98
      gravid 75.99
  ventricular 37.35
  volvulus
    intestine 46.80
      large 46.82
        endoscopic (balloon) 46.85
      small 46.81
    stomach 44.92
Reefing, joint capsule - *see also*
  Arthroplasty 81.96
Re-entry operation (aorta) 39.54
Re-establishment, continuity - *see also*
  Anastomosis
  bowel 46.50
  fallopian tube 66.79
  vas deferens 63.82
Referral (for)
  psychiatric aftercare (halfway house)
    (outpatient clinic) 94.52
  psychotherapy 94.51
  rehabilitation
    alcoholism 94.53
    drug addiction 94.54
    psychologic NEC 94.59
    vocational 94.55
Reformation
  cardiac pacemaker pocket, new site
    (skin) (subcutaneous) 37.79
  cardioverter/defibrillator (automatic)
    pocket, new site (skin)
    (subcutaneous) 37.79
  chamber of eye 12.99
Refracture
  bone (for faulty union) - *see also*
    Osteoclasis 78.70
  nasal bones 21.88
Refusion
  spinal, NOS 81.30
    atlas-axis (anterior) (transoral)
      (posterior) 81.31
    axial lumber interbody fusion
      [AxiaLIF®] 81.38 ◀
    cervical (C2 level or below) NEC
      81.32
      anterior column (interbody),
        anterolateral (anterior)
        technique 81.32 ⬅||||

Reduction *(Continued)*
  spinal, NOS *(Continued)*
    cervical NEC *(Continued)*
      C1-C2 level (anterior) (posterior)
        81.31
        posterior column (interbody),
          posterolateral (posterior)
          technique 81.33 ⬅||||
      craniocervical (anterior) (transoral)
        (posterior) 81.31
      direct lateral interbody fusion
        [DLIF] 81.36 ◀
      dorsal, dorsolumbar NEC 81.35
        anterior column (interbody),
          anterolateral (anterior)
          (extracavitary) technique
          81.34 ⬅||||
        posterior column (interbody),
          posterolateral (posterior)
          technique 81.35 ⬅||||
      extreme lateral interbody fusion
        [XLIF®] 81.36 ◀
      facet 81.37 ◀
      lumbar, lumbosacral NEC 81.38
        anterior column (interbody), ⬅||||
          anterolateral (anterior)
            technique 81.36 ⬅||||
          posterior (interbody),
            posterolateral technique
            81.38 ⬅||||
        anterior lumbar interbody fusion
          (ALIF) 81.36
        lateral transverse process
          technique 81.37
        posterior column, posterior
          (posterolateral) (transverse
          process) technique 81.37 ◀
        posterior lumbar interbody
          fusion (PLIF) 81.38
        transforaminal lumbar interbody
          fusion (TLIF) 81.38
      number of vertebrae - *see codes*
        81.62–81.64
      occiput–C2 (anterior) (transoral)
        (posterior) 81.31
      refusion NEC 81.39

> Note: Also use either 81.62, 81.63, or
> 81.64 as an additional code to show the
> total number of vertebrae fused

Regional blood flow study 92.05
Regulation, menstrual 69.6
Rehabilitation programs NEC 93.89
  alcohol 94.61
    with detoxification 94.63
    combined alcohol and drug 94.67
      with detoxification 94.69
  drug 94.64
    with detoxification 94.66
    combined drug and alcohol
      94.67
      with detoxification 94.69
  sheltered employment 93.85
  vocational 93.85
Reimplantation
  adrenal tissue (heterotopic)
    (orthotopic) 07.45
  artery 39.59
    renal, aberrant 39.55
  bile ducts following excision of
    ampulla of Vater 51.62
  extremity - *see* Reattachment,
    extremity

Reimplantation *(Continued)*
  fallopian tube into uterus 66.74
  kidney 55.61
  lung 33.5 ●
  ovary 65.72
    laparoscopic 65.75
  pancreatic tissue 52.81
  parathyroid tissue (heterotopic)
    (orthotopic) 06.95
  pulmonary artery for hemitruncus
    repair 35.83
  renal vessel, aberrant 39.55
  testis in scrotum 62.5
  thyroid tissue (heterotopic) (orthotopic)
    06.94
  tooth 23.5
  ureter into bladder 56.74
Reinforcement - *see also* Repair, by site
  sclera NEC 12.88
    with graft 12.87
Reinsertion - *see also* Insertion or
  Revision
  cystostomy tube 59.94
  fixation device (internal) - *see also*
    Fixation, bone, internal 78.50
  heart valve (prosthetic) 35.95
  Holter (-Spitz) valve 02.42
  implant (expelled) (extruded)
    eyeball (with conjunctival graft)
      16.62
    orbital 16.62
  nephrostomy tube 55.93
  pyelostomy tube 55.94
  ureteral stent (transurethral) 59.8
    with ureterotomy 59.8 *[56.2]*
  ureterostomy tube 59.93
  valve
    heart (prosthetic) 35.95
    ventricular (cerebral) 02.42
Relaxation - *see also* Release training
  94.33
Release
  carpal tunnel (for nerve
    decompression) 04.43
  celiac artery axis 39.91
  central slip, extensor tendon hand
    (mallet finger repair) 82.84
  chordee 64.42
  clubfoot NEC 83.84
  de Quervain's tenosynovitis 82.01
  Dupuytren's contracture (by palmar
    fasciectomy) 82.35
    by fasciotomy (subcutaneous)
      82.12
    with excision 82.35
  Fowler (mallet finger repair) 82.84
  joint (capsule) (adherent)
    (constrictive) - *see also* Division,
    joint capsule 80.40
  laryngeal 31.92
  ligament - *see also* Division, ligament
    80.40
    median arcuate 39.91
    median arcuate ligament 39.91
  muscle (division) 83.19
    hand 82.19
  nerve (peripheral) NEC 04.49
    cranial NEC 04.42
    trigeminal 04.41
  pressure, intraocular 12.79
  scar tissue
    skin 86.84
    stoma - *see* Revision, stoma
  tarsal tunnel 04.44

Release (Continued)
  tendon 83.13
    hand 82.11
      extensor, central slip (repair
        mallet finger) 82.84
    sheath 83.01
      hand 82.01
    tenosynovitis 83.01
      abductor pollicis longus 82.01
      de Quervain's 82.01
      external pollicis brevis 82.01
      hand 82.01
  torsion
    intestine 46.80
      large 46.82
        endoscopic (balloon) 46.85
      small 46.81
    kidney pedicle 55.84
    ovary 65.95
    testes 63.52
  transverse carpal ligament (for nerve
    decompression) 04.43
  trigger finger or thumb 82.01
  urethral stricture 58.5
  Volkmann's contracture
    excision of scar, muscle 83.32
    fasciotomy 83.14
    muscle transplantation 83.77
  web contracture (skin) 86.84
Relief - *see* Release
Relocation - *see also* Revision
  cardiac device (CRT-D) (CRT-P)
    (defibrillator) (pacemaker)
    pocket, new site (skin)
    (subcutaneous) 37.79
  CRT-D pocket 37.79
  CRT-P pocket 37.79
  subcutaneous device pocket NEC
    86.09
Remobilization
  joint 93.16
  stapes 19.0
Remodel
  ventricle 37.35
Removal - *see also* Excision
  Abrams bar (chest wall) 34.01
  abscess - *see* Incision, by site
  adenoid tag(s) 28.6
  anal sphincter
    with revision 49.75
    without revision 49.76
  arch bars (orthodontic) 24.8
    immobilization device 97.33
  arterial graft or prosthesis 39.49
  arteriovenous shunt (device) 39.43
    with creation of new shunt 39.42
  artificial heart
    internal biventricular replacement
      system 37.55
  Barton's tongs (skull) 02.95
    with synchronous replacement
      02.94
  bladder sphincter, artificial 58.99
    with replacement 58.93
  blood clot - *see also* Incision, by site
    bladder (by incision) 57.19
      without incision 57.0
    kidney (without incision) 56.0
      by incision 55.01
    ureter
      by incision 56.2
  bone fragment (chip) - *see also* Incision,
    bone 77.10
    joint - *see also* Arthrotomy 80.10

Removal (Continued)
  bone fragment (Continued)
    necrotic - *see also* Sequestrectomy,
      bone 77.00
      joint - *see also* Arthrotomy 80.10
    skull 01.25
      with debridement of compound
        fracture 02.02
  bone growth stimulator - *see* category
    78.6●
  bony spicules, spinal canal 03.53
  brace 97.88
  breast implant 85.94
    tissue expander 85.96
  bronchial device or substance
    endoscopic 33.78
  calcareous deposit
    bursa 83.03
      hand 82.03
    tendon, intratendinous 83.39
      hand 82.29
  calcification, heart valve leaflets - *see*
    Valvuloplasty, heart
  calculus
    bile duct (by incision) 51.49
      endoscopic 51.88
      laparoscopic 51.88
      percutaneous 51.98
    bladder (by incision) 57.19
      without incision 57.0
    common duct (by incision) 51.41
      endoscopic 51.88
      laparoscopic 51.88
      percutaneous 51.96
    gallbladder 51.04
      endoscopic 51.88
      laparoscopic 51.88
    kidney (by incision) 55.01
      without incision (transurethral)
        56.0
      percutaneous 55.03
        with fragmentation
          (ultrasound) 55.04
      renal pelvis (by incision)
        55.11
        percutaneous nephostomy
          55.03
          with fragmentation
            55.04
      transurethral 56.0
    lacrimal
      canaliculi 09.42
        by incision 09.52
      gland 09.3
        by incision 09.0
      passage(s) 09.49
        by incision 09.59
      punctum 09.41
        by incision 09.51
      sac 09.49
        by incision 09.53
    pancreatic duct (by incision)
      52.09
      endoscopic 52.94
    perirenal tissue 59.09
    pharynx 29.39
    prostate 60.0
    salivary gland (by incision) 26.0
      by probe 26.91
    ureter (by incision) 56.2
      without incision 56.0
    urethra (by incision) 58.0
      without incision 58.6
  caliper tongs (skull) 02.95

Removal (Continued)
  cannula
    for extracorporeal membrane
      oxygenation (ECMO) - *omit*
      code
  cardiac pacemaker (device) (initial)
    (permanent) (cardiac
    resynchronization device,
    CRT-P) 37.89
    with replacement (by)
      cardiac resynchronization
        pacemaker (CRT-P)
        device only 00.53
        total system 00.50
      dual chamber device 37.87
      single-chamber device 37.85
      rate responsive 37.86
  cardioverter/defibrillator pulse
    generator
    without replacement (cardiac
      resynchronization
      defibrillator device
      (CRT-D)) 37.79
  cast 97.88
    with reapplication 97.13
      lower limb 97.12
      upper limb 97.11
  catheter (indwelling) - *see also*
    Removal, tube
    bladder 97.64
    cranial cavity 01.27
    middle ear (tympanum) 20.1
    ureter 97.62
    urinary 97.64
    ventricular (cerebral) 02.43
      with synchronous replacement
        02.42
  CCM (cardiac contractility modulation)
    without replacement
      (rechargeable pulse generator)
      (total system) 37.79
  cerclage material, cervix 69.96
  cerumen, ear 96.52
  corneal epithelium 11.41
    for smear or culture 11.21
  coronary artery obstruction (thrombus)
    36.09
    direct intracoronary artery infusion
      36.04
    open chest approach 36.03
    percutaneous transluminal (balloon)

> Note: Also use 00.40, 00.41, 00.42, or 00.43 to show the total number of vessels treated. Use code 00.44 once to show procedure on a bifurcated vessel. In addition, use 00.45, 00.46, 00.47, or 00.48 to show the number of vascular stents inserted.

  Crutchfield tongs (skull) 02.95
    with synchronous replacement
      02.94
  cyst - *see also* Excision, lesion, by site
    dental 24.4
    lung 32.29
      endoscopic 32.28
      thoracoscopic 32.20
  cystic duct remnant 51.61
  decidua (by)
    aspiration curettage 69.52
    curettage (D and C) 69.02
    manual 75.4

Removal (Continued)

dental wiring (immobilization device) 97.33
  orthodontic 24.8
device (therapeutic) NEC 97.89
  abdomen NEC 97.86
  bronchus 33.78
    valve 33.78
  digestive system NEC 97.59
  drainage - see Removal, tube
  external fixation device 97.88
    mandibular NEC 97.36
    minifixator (bone) - see category 78.6●
  for musculoskeletal immobilization NEC 97.88
  genital tract NEC 97.79
  head and neck NEC 97.39
  intrauterine contraceptive 97.71
  spine 80.09
  thorax NEC 97.49
  trunk NEC 97.87
  urinary system NEC 97.69
diaphragm, vagina 97.73
drainage device - see Removal, tube
dye, spinal canal 03.31
ectopic fetus (from) 66.02
  abdominal cavity 74.3
  extraperitoneal (intraligamentous) 74.3
  fallopian tube (by salpingostomy) 66.02
    by salpingotomy 66.01
    with salpingectomy 66.62
  intraligamentous 74.3
  ovarian 74.3
  peritoneal (following uterine or tubal rupture) 74.3
  site NEC 74.3
  tubal (by salpingostomy) 66.02
    by salpingotomy 66.01
    with salpingectomy 66.62
electrodes
  bone growth stimulator - see category 78.6●
  brain 01.22
    depth 01.22
      with synchronous replacement 02.93
    foramen ovale 01.22
      with synchronous replacement 02.93
    sphenoidal - omit code
      with synchronous replacement 02.96
  cardiac pacemaker (atrial) (transvenous) (ventricular) 37.77
    with replacement 37.76
  carotid sinus 04.93 39.87 ◄▥
    with synchronous pulse generator removal (total system) 39.86 ◄
    with synchronous replacement 04.92 39.82 ◄▥
  depth 01.22
    with synchronous replacement 02.93
  epicardial (myocardial) 37.77
    with replacement (by)
      atrial and/or ventricular lead(s) (electrode) 37.76
      epicardial lead 37.74

Removal (Continued)

electrodes (Continued)
  epidural pegs 01.22
    with synchronous replacement 02.93
  foramen ovale 01.22
    with synchronous replacement 02.93
  gastric 04.93
    with synchronous replacement 04.92
  intracranial 01.22
    with synchronous replacement 02.93
  peripheral nerve 04.93
    with synchronous replacement 04.92
  sacral nerve 04.93
  sphenoidal - omit code
    with synchronous replacement 02.96
  spinal 03.94
    with synchronous replacement 03.93
  temporary transvenous pacemaker system - omit code
electroencephalographic receiver (brain) (intracranial) 01.22
  with synchronous replacement 02.93
electronic
  stimulator - see Removal, neurostimulator, by site
    bladder 57.98
    bone 78.6●
    skeletal muscle 83.93
      with synchronous replacement 83.92
    ureter 56.94
electrostimulator - see Removal, electronic, stimulator, by site
embolus 38.00
  with endarterectomy - see Endarterectomy
  abdominal
    artery 38.06
    vein 38.07
  aorta (arch) (ascending) (descending) 38.04
  arteriovenous shunt or cannula 39.49
  bovine graft 39.49
  head and neck vessel
    endovascular approach 39.74
    open approach, intracranial vessels 38.01
    open approach, other vessels of head and neck 38.02
  intracranial vessel
    endovascular approach 39.74
    open approach, intracranial vessels 38.01
    open approach, other vessels of head and neck 38.02
  lower limb
    artery 38.08
    vein 38.09
  pulmonary (artery) (vein) 38.05
  thoracic vessel NEC 38.05
  upper limb (artery) (vein) 38.03
embryo - see Removal, ectopic fetus
encircling tube, eye (episcleral) 14.6
epithelial downgrowth, anterior chamber 12.93

Removal (Continued)

external fixation device 97.88
  mandibular NEC 97.36
  minifixator (bone) - see category 78.6●
extrauterine embryo - see Removal, ectopic fetus
eyeball 16.49
  with implant 16.42
    with attachment of muscles 16.41
fallopian tube - see Salpingectomy
feces (impacted) (by flushing) (manual) 96.38
fetus, ectopic - see Removal, ectopic fetus
fingers, supernumerary 86.26
fixation device
  external 97.88
    mandibular NEC 97.36
    minifixator (bone) - see category 78.6●
  internal 78.60
    carpal, metacarpal 78.64
    clavicle 78.61
    facial (bone) 76.97
    femur 78.65
    fibula 78.67
    humerus 78.62
    patella 78.66
    pelvic 78.69
    phalanges (foot) (hand) 78.69
    radius 78.63
    scapula 78.61
    specified site NEC 78.69
    tarsal, metatarsal 78.68
    thorax (ribs) (sternum) 78.61
    tibia 78.67
    ulna 78.63
    vertebrae 78.69
foreign body NEC - see also Incision, by site 98.20
  abdominal (cavity) 54.92
    wall 54.0
  adenoid 98.13
    by incision 28.91
  alveolus, alveolar bone 98.22
    by incision 24.0
  antecubital fossa 98.27
    by incision 86.05
  anterior chamber 12.00
    by incision 12.02
      with use of magnet 12.01
  anus (intraluminal) 98.05
    by incision 49.93
  artificial stoma (intraluminal) 98.18
  auditory canal, external 18.02
  axilla 98.27
    by incision 86.05
  bladder (without incision) 57.0
    by incision 57.19
  bone, except fixation device - see also Incision, bone 77.10
    alveolus, alveolar 98.22
      by incision 24.0
  brain 01.39
    without incision into brain 01.24
  breast 85.0
  bronchus (intraluminal) 98.15
    by incision 33.0
  bursa 83.03
    hand 82.03
  canthus 98.22
    by incision 08.51
  cerebral meninges 01.31

Removal *(Continued)*
  foreign body NEC *(Continued)*
    cervix (intraluminal) NEC 98.16
      penetrating 69.97
    choroid (by incision) 14.00
      with use of magnet 14.01
      without use of magnet 14.02
    ciliary body (by incision) 12.00
      with use of magnet 12.01
      without use of magnet 12.02
    conjunctiva (by magnet) 98.22
      by incision 10.0
    cornea 98.21
      by
        incision 11.1
        magnet 11.0
    duodenum 98.03
      by incision 45.01
    ear (intraluminal) 98.11
      with incision 18.09
    epididymis 63.92
    esophagus (intraluminal) 98.02
      by incision 42.09
    extrapleural (by incision) 34.01
    eye, eyeball (by magnet) 98.21
      anterior segment (by incision)
        12.00
        with use of magnet 12.01
        without use of magnet 12.02
      posterior segment (by incision)
        14.00
        with use of magnet 14.01
        without use of magnet
          14.02
      superficial 98.21
    eyelid 98.22
      by incision 08.09
    fallopian tube
      by salpingostomy 66.02
      by salpingotomy 66.01
    fascia 83.09
      hand 82.09
    foot 98.28
    gallbladder 51.04
    groin region (abdominal wall)
      (inguinal) 54.0
    gum 98.22
      by incision 24.0
    hand 98.26
    head and neck NEC 98.22
    heart 37.11
    internal fixation device - *see* Removal,
      fixation device, internal
    intestine
      by incision 45.00
      large (intraluminal) 98.04
        by incision 45.03
      small (intraluminal) 98.03
        by incision 45.02
    intraocular (by incision) 12.00
      with use of magnet 12.01
      without use of magnet 12.02
    iris (by incision) 12.00
      with use of magnet 12.01
      without use of magnet 12.02
    joint structures - *see also*
      Arthrotomy 80.10
    kidney (transurethral) (by
      endoscopy) 56.0
      by incision 55.01
      pelvis (transurethral) 56.0
        by incision 55.11
    labia 98.23
      by incision 71.09

Removal *(Continued)*
  foreign body NEC *(Continued)*
    lacrimal
      canaliculi 09.42
        by incision 09.52
      gland 09.3
        by incision 09.0
      passage(s) 09.49
        by incision 09.59
      punctum 09.41
        by incision 09.51
      sac 09.49
        by incision 09.53
    large intestine (intraluminal)
      98.04
      by incision 45.03
    larynx (intraluminal) 98.14
      by incision 31.3
    lens 13.00
      by incision 13.02
        with use of magnet 13.01
    liver 50.0
    lower limb, except foot 98.29
      foot 98.28
    lung 33.1
    mediastinum 34.1
    meninges (cerebral) 01.31
      spinal 03.01
    mouth (intraluminal) 98.01
      by incision 27.92
    muscle 83.02
      hand 82.02
    nasal sinus 22.50
      antrum 22.2
        with Caldwell-Luc approach
          22.39
      ethmoid 22.51
      frontal 22.41
      maxillary 22.2
        with Caldwell-Luc approach
          22.39
      sphenoid 22.52
    nerve (cranial) (peripheral) NEC
      04.04
      root 03.01
    nose (intraluminal) 98.12
      by incision 21.1
    oral cavity (intraluminal)
      98.01
      by incision 27.92
    orbit (by magnet) 98.21
      by incision 16.1
    palate (penetrating) 98.22
      by incision 27.1
    pancreas 52.09
    penis 98.24
      by incision 64.92
    pericardium 37.12
    perineum (female) 98.23
      by incision 71.09
      male 98.25
        by incision 86.05
    perirenal tissue 59.09
    peritoneal cavity 54.92
    perivesical tissue 59.19
    pharynx (intraluminal) 98.13
      by pharyngotomy 29.0
    pleura (by incision) 34.09
    popliteal space 98.29
      by incision 86.05
    rectum (intraluminal) 98.05
      by incision 48.0
    renal pelvis (transurethral) 56.0
      by incision 56.1

Removal *(Continued)*
  foreign body NEC *(Continued)*
    retina (by incision) 14.00
      with use of magnet 14.01
      without use of magnet 14.02
    retroperitoneum 54.92
    sclera (by incision) 12.00
      with use of magnet 12.01
      without use of magnet 12.02
    scrotum 98.24
      by incision 61.0
    sinus (nasal) 22.50
      antrum 22.2
        with Caldwell-Luc approach
          22.39
      ethmoid 22.51
      frontal 22.41
      maxillary 22.2
        with Caldwell-Luc approach
          22.39
      sphenoid 22.52
    skin NEC 98.20
      by incision 86.05
    skull 01.24
      with incision into brain 01.39
    small intestine (intraluminal) 98.03
      by incision 45.02
    soft tissue NEC 83.09
      hand 82.09
    spermatic cord 63.93
    spinal (canal) (cord) (meninges) 03.01
    stomach (intraluminal) 98.03
      bubble (balloon) 44.94
      by incision 43.0
    subconjunctival (by magnet) 98.22
      by incision 10.0
    subcutaneous tissue NEC 98.20
      by incision 86.05
    supraclavicular fossa 98.27
      by incision 86.05
    tendon (sheath) 83.01
      hand 82.01
    testis 62.0
    thorax (by incision) 34.09
    thyroid (field) (gland) (by incision)
      06.09
    tonsil 98.13
      by incision 28.91
    trachea (intraluminal) 98.15
      by incision 31.3
    trunk NEC 98.25
    tunica vaginalis 98.24
    upper limb, except hand 98.27
      hand 98.26
    ureter (transurethral) 56.0
      by incision 56.2
    urethra (intraluminal) 98.19
      by incision 58.0
    uterus (intraluminal) 98.16
    vagina (intraluminal) 98.17
      by incision 70.14
    vas deferens 63.6
    vitreous (by incision) 14.00
      with use of magnet 14.01
      without use of magnet 14.02
    vulva 98.23
      by incision 71.09
  gallstones
    bile duct (by incision) NEC 51.49
      endoscopic 51.88
    common duct (by incision) 51.41
      endoscopic 51.88
      percutaneous 51.96
    duodenum 45.01

◀ New   ◀‖ Revised   ~~deleted~~ Deleted   ● Use Additional Digit(s)   ▬ Omit code

Removal *(Continued)*
 gallstones *(Continued)*
  gallbladder 51.04
   endoscopic 51.88
   laparoscopic 51.88
  hepatic ducts 51.49
   endoscopic 51.88
  intestine 45.00
   large 45.03
   small NEC 45.02
  liver 50.0
 Gardner Wells tongs (skull) 02.95
  with synchronous replacement
   02.94
 gastric band (adjustable), laparoscopic
  44.97
 gastric bubble (balloon) 44.94
 granulation tissue - *see also* Excision,
   lesion, by site
  with repair - *see* Repair, by site
  cranial 01.6
  skull 01.6
 halo traction device (skull) 02.95
  with synchronous replacement
   02.94
 heart assist system
  with replacement 37.63
  intra-aortic balloon pump (IABP)
   97.44
  nonoperative 97.44
  open removal 37.64
  percutaneous external device
   97.44
 heart replacement system
  internal biventricular 37.55
 hematoma - *see* Drainage, by site
 Hoffman minifixator device (bone) - *see*
   category 78.6●
 hydatidiform mole 68.0
 impacted
  feces (rectum) (by flushing)
   (manual) 96.38
  tooth 23.19
  from nasal sinus (maxillary) 22.61
 implant
  breast 85.94
  cochlear prosthetic device 20.99
  cornea 11.92
  lens (prosthetic) 13.8
  middle ear NEC 20.99
  ocular 16.71
   posterior segment 14.6
  orbit 16.72
  retina 14.6
  tympanum 20.1
 implantable hemodynamic sensor
   (lead) and monitor device 37.79
 internal biventricular heart
   replacement system 37.55
 internal fixation device - *see* Removal,
   fixation device, internal
 intra-aortic balloon pump (IABP) 97.44
 intrauterine contraceptive device (IUD)
   97.71
 joint (structure) NOS 80.90
  ankle 80.97
  elbow 80.92
  foot and toe 80.98
  hand and finger 80.94
  hip 80.95
  knee 80.96
  other specified sites 80.99
  shoulder 80.91
  spine 80.99

Removal *(Continued)*
 joint NOS *(Continued)*
  toe 80.98
  wrist 80.93
 Kantrowitz heart pump 37.64
  nonoperative 97.44
 keel (tantalum plate), larynx 31.98
 kidney - *see also* Nephrectomy
  mechanical 55.98
  transplanted or rejected 55.53
 laminaria (tent), uterus 97.79
 leads (cardiac) - *see* Removal,
   electrodes, cardiac pacemaker
 lesion - *see* Excision, lesion, by site
 ligamentum flavum (spine) - *omit code*
 ligature
  fallopian tube 66.79
  ureter 56.86
  vas deferens 63.84
 limb lengthening device, internal - *see*
   category 78.6●
 loop recorder 86.05
 loose body
  bone - *see* Sequestrectomy, bone
  joint 80.10
  mesh (surgical) - *see* Removal,
   foreign body, by site
 lymph node - *see* Excision, lymph, node
 minifixator device (bone) - *see* category
   78.6●
  external fixation device 97.88
 Mulligan hood, fallopian tube 66.94
  with synchronous replacement 66.93
 muscle stimulator (skeletal) 83.93
  with replacement 83.92
 myringotomy device or tube 20.1
 nail (bed) (fold) 86.23
  internal fixation device - *see*
   Removal, fixation device,
   internal
 necrosis
  skin 86.28
   excisional 86.22
 neuropacemaker - *see* Removal,
   neurostimulator, by site
 neurostimulator
  electrodes
   brain 01.22
    with synchronous replacement
     02.93
   ~~carotid sinus 04.93~~
    ~~with synchronous replacement
     04.92~~
   gastric 04.93
   intracranial 01.22
    with synchronous replacement
     02.93
   peripheral nerve 04.93
    with synchronous replacement
     04.92
   sacral nerve 04.93
    with synchronous replacement
     04.92
   spinal 03.94
    with synchronous replacement
     03.93
  pulse generator (subcutaneous single
    array, dual array) 86.05 ◄▥
   with synchronous replacement
    86.96
   dual array 86.95
    rechargeable 86.98
   single array 86.94
    rechargeable 86.97

Removal *(Continued)*
 neurostimulator *(Continued)*
  pulse generator *(Continued)*
   cranial 01.29 ◄
    with synchronous replacement
     01.20 ◄
  nonabsorbable surgical material NEC -
    see Removal, foreign body,
    by site
  odontoma (tooth) 24.4
  orbital implant 16.72
  osteocartilagenous loose body, joint
    structures - *see also* Arthrotomy
    80.10
  outer attic wall (middle ear)
    20.59
  ovo-testis (unilateral) 62.3
   bilateral 62.41
  pacemaker
   brain (intracranial) - *see* Removal,
    neurostimulator
   cardiac (device) (initial) (permanent)
    37.89
    with replacement
     dual-chamber device 37.87
     single-chamber device 37.85
      rate responsive 37.86
    electrodes (atrial) (transvenous)
      (ventricular) 37.77
     with replacement 37.76
    epicardium (myocardium)
      37.77
     with replacement (by)
      atrial and/or ventricular
       lead(s) (electrode)
       37.76
      epicardial lead 37.74
    temporary transvenous
      pacemaker system - *omit
      code*
   intracranial - *see* Removal,
    neurostimulator
   neural - *see* Removal,
    neurostimulator
   peripheral nerve - *see* Removal,
    neurostimulator
   spinal - *see* Removal,
    neurostimulator
  pack, packing
   dental 97.34
   intrauterine 97.72
   nasal 97.32
   rectum 97.59
   trunk NEC 97.85
   vagina 97.75
   vulva 97.75
  pantopaque dye, spinal canal
    03.31
  patella (complete) 77.96
   partial 77.86
  pectus deformity implant device 34.01
  pelvic viscera, en masse (female) 68.8
   male 57.71
  pessary, vagina NEC 97.74
  pharynx (partial) 29.33
  phlebolith - *see* Removal, embolus
  placenta (by)
   aspiration curettage 69.52
   D and C 69.02
   manual 75.4
  plaque, dental 96.54
  plate, skull 02.07
   with synchronous replacement
    02.05

Removal *(Continued)*
  polyp - *see also* Excision, lesion, by site
    esophageal 42.32
      endoscopic 42.33
    gastric (endoscopic) 43.41
    intestine 45.41
      endoscopic 45.42
    nasal 21.31
  prosthesis
    bile duct 51.95
      nonoperative 97.55
    cochlear prosthetic device 20.99
    dental 97.35
    eye 97.31
    facial bone 76.99
    fallopian tube 66.94
      with synchronous replacement 66.93
    joint structures
      with replacement – *see* Revision, joint replacement by site
      without replacement
        ankle 80.07
        elbow 80.02
        foot and toe 80.08
        hand and finger 80.04
        hip 80.05
        knee 80.06
        shoulder 80.01
        specified site NEC 80.09
        spine 80.09
        unspecified site 80.00
        wrist 80.03
    lens 13.8
    penis (internal) without replacement 64.96
    Rheos™ carotid sinus baroreflex activation device 86.05
    Rosen (urethra) 59.99
    testicular, by incision 62.0
    urinary sphincter, artificial 58.99
      with replacement 58.93
  pseudophakos 13.8
  pterygium 11.39
    with corneal graft 11.32
  pulse generator
    cardiac pacemaker 37.86
    cardioverter/defibrillator 37.79
    carotid sinus 39.88 ◄
      with synchronous electrode removal (total system) 39.86 ◄
      with synchronous replacement 39.83 ◄
    neurostimulator - *see* Removal, neurostimulator, pulse generator
  pump assist device, heart 37.64
    with replacement 37.63
    nonoperative 97.44
  radioactive material - *see* Removal, foreign body, by site
  redundant skin, eyelid 08.86
  rejected organ
    kidney 55.53
    testis 62.42
  reservoir, ventricular (Ommaya) (Rickham) 02.43
    with synchronous replacement 02.42
  retained placenta (by)
    aspiration curettage 69.52
    D and C 69.02
    manual 75.4

Removal *(Continued)*
  retinal implant 14.6
  Rheos™ carotid sinus baroreflex activation device 86.05
  rhinolith 21.31
  rice bodies, tendon sheaths 83.01
    hand 82.01
  Roger-Anderson minifixator device (bone) - *see* category 78.6●
  root, residual (tooth) (buried) (retained) 23.11
  Rosen prosthesis (urethra) 59.99
  scleral buckle or implant 14.6
  Scribner shunt 39.43
  secondary membranous cataract (with iridectomy) 13.65
  secundines (by)
    aspiration curettage 69.52
    D and C 69.02
    manual 75.4
  sequestrum - *see* Sequestrectomy
  seton, anus 49.93
  Shepard's tube (ear) 20.1
  Shirodkar suture, cervix 69.96
  shunt
    arteriovenous 39.43
      with creation of new shunt 39.42
    lumbar-subarachnoid NEC 03.98
    pleurothecal 03.98
    salpingothecal 03.98
    spinal (thecal) NEC 03.98
    subarachnoid-peritoneal 03.98
    subarachnoid-ureteral 03.98
  silastic tubes
    ear 20.1
    fallopian tubes 66.94
      with synchronous replacement 66.93
  skin
    necrosis or slough 86.28
      excisional 86.22
        superficial layer (by dermabrasion) 86.25
  skull tongs 02.95
    with synchronous replacement 02.94
  spacer (cement) (joint) (methylmethacrylate) 84.57
  splint 97.88
  stent
    bile duct 97.55
    larynx 31.98
    ureteral 97.62
    urethral 97.65
  stimoceiver - *see* Removal, neurostimulator
  subdural
    grids 01.22
    strips 01.22
  supernumerary digit(s) 86.26
  suture(s) NEC 97.89
    abdominal wall 97.83
    by incision - *see* Incision, by site
    genital tract 97.79
    head and neck 97.38
    thorax 97.43
    trunk NEC 97.84
  symblepharon - *see* Repair, symblepharon
  temporary transvenous pacemaker system - *omit code*
  testis (unilateral) 62.3
    bilateral 62.41
    remaining or solitary 62.42

Removal *(Continued)*
  thrombus 38.00
    with endarterectomy - *see* Endarterectomy
    abdominal
      artery 38.06
      vein 38.07
    aorta (arch) (ascending) (descending) 38.04
    arteriovenous shunt or cannula 39.49
    bovine graft 39.49
    coronary artery 36.09
    head and neck vessel NEC 38.02
    intracranial vessel NEC 38.01
    lower limb
      artery 38.08
      vein 38.09
    pulmonary (artery) (vein) 38.05
    thoracic vessel NEC 38.05
    upper limb (artery) (vein) 38.03
  tissue expander (skin) NEC 86.05
    breast 85.96
  toes, supernumerary 86.26
  tongs, skull 02.95
    with synchronous replacement 02.94
  tonsil tag 28.4
  tooth (by forceps) (multiple) (single) NEC 23.09
    deciduous 23.01
    surgical NEC 23.19
      impacted 23.19
      residual root 23.11
      root apex 23.73
        with root canal therapy 23.72
  trachoma follicles 10.33
  T-tube (bile duct) 97.55
  tube
    appendix 97.53
    bile duct (T-tube) NEC 97.55
    cholecystostomy 97.54
    cranial cavity 01.27
    cystostomy 97.63
    ear (button) 20.1
    gastrostomy 97.51
    large intestine 97.53
    liver 97.55
    mediastinum 97.42
    nephrostomy 97.61
    pancreas 97.56
    peritoneum 97.82
    pleural cavity 97.41
    pyelostomy 97.61
    retroperitoneum 97.81
    small intestine 97.52
    thoracotomy 97.41
    tracheostomy 97.37
    tympanostomy 20.1
    tympanum 20.1
    ureterostomy 97.62
  ureteral splint (stent) 97.62
  urethral sphincter, artificial 58.99
    with replacement 58.93
  urinary sphincter, artificial 58.99
    with replacement 58.93
  utricle 20.79
  valve
    vas deferens 63.85
    ventricular (cerebral) 02.43
  vascular graft or prosthesis 39.49
  ventricular shunt or reservoir 02.43
    with synchronous replacement 02.42

◄ New   ◄▥ Revised   ~~deleted~~ Deleted   ● Use Additional Digit(s)   ▨ Omit code

Removal *(Continued)*
Vinke tongs (skull) 02.95
with synchronous replacement 02.94
vitreous (with replacement) 14.72
anterior approach (partial) 14.71
open sky technique 14.71
Wagner-Brooker minifixator device
(bone) - *see* category 78.6●
wiring, dental (immobilization device)
97.33
orthodontic 24.8
Renipuncture (percutaneous) 55.92
Renogram 92.03
Renotransplantation NEC 55.69

> Note: To report donor source:
> cadaver 00.93
> live non-related donor 00.92
> live related donor 00.91
> live unrelated donor 00.92

Reopening - *see also* Incision, by site
blepharorrhaphy 08.02
canthorrhaphy 08.02
cilia base 08.71
craniotomy or craniectomy site 01.23
fallopian tube (divided) 66.79
iris in anterior chambers 12.97
laminectomy or laminotomy site 03.02
laparotomy site 54.12
osteotomy site - *see also* Incision, bone
77.10
facial bone 76.09
tarsorrhaphy 08.02
thoracotomy site (for control of
hemorrhage) (for examination)
(for exploration) 34.03
thyroid field wound (for control of
hemorrhage) (for examination)
(for exploration) (for removal of
hematoma) 06.02
Repacking - *see* Replacement, pack, by
site
Repair
abdominal wall 54.72
adrenal gland 07.44
alveolus, alveolar (process) (ridge)
(with graft) (with implant)
24.5
anal sphincter 49.79
artificial sphincter
implantation 49.75
revision 49.75
laceration (by suture) 49.71
obstetric (current) 75.62
old 49.79
aneurysm (false) (true) 39.52
by or with
clipping 39.51
coagulation 39.52
coil, NEC (endovascular
approach) 39.79
head and neck
bare coils 39.75
bioactive coils 39.76
electrocoagulation 39.52
excision or resection of vessel -
see also Aneurysmectomy,
by site
with
anastomosis - *see*
Aneurysmectomy,
with anastomosis, by
site

Repair *(Continued)*
aneurysm *(Continued)*
by or with *(Continued)*
electrocoagulation *(Continued)*
with *(Continued)*
graft replacement - *see*
Aneurysmectomy,
with graft
replacement, by site
endovascular graft 39.79
abdominal aorta 39.71
head and neck 39.72
lower extremity artery(s) 39.79
thoracic aorta 39.73
upper extremity artery(s) 39.79
filipuncture 39.52
graft replacement - *see*
Aneurysmectomy, with
graft
replacement, by site
ligation 39.52
liquid tissue adhesive (glue)
39.79
endovascular approach 39.79
head and neck 39.72
methyl methacrylate 39.52
endovascular approach 39.79
head and neck 39.72
occlusion 39.52
endovascular approach 39.79
head and neck 39.72
suture 39.52
trapping 39.52
wiring 39.52
wrapping (gauze) (methyl
methacrylate) (plastic)
39.52
coronary artery 36.91
heart 37.32
sinus of Valsalva 35.39
thoracic aorta (dissecting), by
fenestration 39.54
anomalous pulmonary venous
connection (total)
one-stage 35.82
partial - *see* specific procedure
total 35.82
anular disc 80.54
with graft or prosthesis 80.53
anulus fibrosus 80.54
with graft or prosthesis 80.53
anus 49.79
laceration (by suture) 49.71
obstetric (current) 75.62
old 49.79
aorta 39.31
aorticopulmonary window 39.59
arteriovenous fistula 39.53
by or with
clipping 39.53
coagulation 39.53
coil, NEC (endovascular
approach) 39.79
head and neck vessels
bare coils 39.75
bioactive coils 39.76
division 39.53
excision or resection - *see also*
Aneurysmectomy, by site
with
anastomosis - *see*
Aneurysmectomy,
with anastomosis, by
site

Repair *(Continued)*
arteriovenous fistula *(Continued)*
by or with *(Continued)*
excision or resection *(Continued)*
with *(Continued)*
graft replacement - *see*
Aneurysmectomy,
with graft
replacement, by site
ligation 39.53
coronary artery 36.99
occlusion 39.53
endovascular approach
39.79
head and neck 39.72
suture 39.53
artery NEC 39.59
by
endovascular approach
abdominal aorta 39.71
head and neck (embolization
or occlusion) 39.72
other repair (of aneurysm)
39.79
percutaneous repair of
intracranial vessel(s)
(for stent insertion)
00.62

> Note: Also use 00.40, 00.41, 00.42, or
> 00.43 to show the total number of
> vessels treated. Use code 00.44 once to
> show procedure on a bifurcated vessel.
> In addition, use 00.45, 00.46, 00.47, or
> 00.48 to show the number of vascular
> stents inserted.

percutaneous repair of
precerebral (extracranial)
vessel(s) (for stent
insertion) 00.61

> Note: Also use 00.40, 00.41, 00.42, or
> 00.43 to show the total number of
> vessels treated. Use code 00.44 once to
> show procedure on a bifurcated vessel.
> In addition, use 00.45, 00.46, 00.47, or
> 00.48 to show the number of vascular
> stents inserted.

non-coronary percutaneous
transluminal angioplasty or
atherectomy

> Note: Also use 00.40, 00.41, 00.42, or
> 00.43 to show the total number of
> vessels treated. Use code 00.44 once to
> show procedure on a bifurcated vessel.
> In addition, use 00.45, 00.46, 00.47, or
> 00.48 to show the number of vascular
> stents inserted.

basilar 00.61
carotid 00.61
femoropopliteal 39.50
iliac 39.50
lower extremity NOS
39.50
mesenteric 39.50
renal 39.50
upper extremity NOS
39.50
vertebral 00.61

Repair *(Continued)*
  artery NEC *(Continued)*
    with
      patch graft 39.58
        with excision or resection of
          vessel - *see* Arteriectomy,
          with graft replacement,
          by site
        synthetic (Dacron) (Teflon)
          39.57
        tissue (vein) (autogenous)
          (homograft) 39.56
      suture 39.31
    coronary NEC 36.99
      by angioplasty - *see* Angioplasty,
        coronary
      by atherectomy - *see* Angioplasty,
        coronary
  artificial opening - *see* Repair, stoma
  atrial septal defect 35.71
    with
      prosthesis (open heart technique)
        35.51
        closed heart technique 35.52
      tissue graft 35.61
    combined with repair of valvular
      and ventricular septal defects -
      see Repair, endocardial cushion
      defect
    in total repair of total anomalous
      pulmonary venous connection
      35.82
  atrioventricular canal defect (any type)
    35.73
    with
      prosthesis 35.54
      tissue graft 35.63
  bifid digit (finger) 82.89
  bile duct NEC 51.79
    laceration (by suture) NEC
      51.79
      common bile duct 51.71
  bladder NEC 57.89
    exstrophy 57.86
    for stress incontinence - *see* Repair,
      stress incontinence
    laceration (by suture) 57.81
      obstetric (current) 75.61
      old 57.89
    neck 57.85
  blepharophimosis 08.59
  blepharoptosis 08.36
    by
      frontalis muscle technique (with)
        fascial sling 08.32
        suture 08.31
      levator muscle technique 08.34
        with resection or advancement
          08.33
      orbicularis oculi muscle sling 08.36
      tarsal technique 08.35
  blood vessel NEC 39.59
    with
      patch graft 39.58
        with excision or resection - *see*
          Angiectomy, with graft
          replacement
        synthetic (Dacron) (Teflon)
          39.57
        tissue (vein) (autogenous)
          (homograft) 39.56
      resection - *see* Angiectomy
      suture 39.30

Repair *(Continued)*
  blood vessel NEC *(Continued)*
    coronary artery NEC 36.99
      by angioplasty - *see* Angioplasty,
        coronary
      by atherectomy - *see* Angioplasty,
        coronary
    peripheral vessel NEC 39.59
      by angioplasty 39.50

  > Note: Also use 00.40, 00.41, 00.42, or
  > 00.43 to show the total number of
  > vessels treated. Use code 00.44 once to
  > show procedure on a bifurcated vessel.
  > In addition, use 00.45, 00.46, 00.47, or
  > 00.48 to show the number of vascular
  > stents inserted.

      by atherectomy 39.50

  > Note: Also use 00.40, 00.41, 00.42, or
  > 00.43 to show the total number of
  > vessels treated. Use code 00.44 once to
  > show procedure on a bifurcated vessel.
  > In addition, use 00.45, 00.46, 00.47, or
  > 00.48 to show the number of vascular
  > stents inserted.

      by endovascular approach
        39.79
  bone NEC - *see also* Osteoplasty - *see*
    category 78.4●
    by synostosis technique - *see*
      Arthrodesis
    accessory sinus 22.79
    cranium NEC 02.06
      with
        flap (bone) 02.03
        graft (bone) 02.04
    for malunion, nonunion, or delayed
      union of fracture - *see* Repair,
      fracture, malunion or
      nonunion
    nasal 21.89
    skull NEC 02.06
      with
        flap (bone) 02.03
        graft (bone) 02.04
  bottle, hydrocele of tunica vaginalis
    61.2
  brain (trauma) NEC 02.92
  breast (plastic) - *see also* Mammoplasty
    85.89
  broad ligament 69.29
  bronchus NEC 33.48
    laceration (by suture) 33.41
  bunionette (with osteotomy) 77.54
  canaliculus, lacrimal 09.73
  canthus (lateral) 08.59
  cardiac pacemaker NEC 37.89
    electrode(s) (lead) NEC 37.75
  cardioverter/defibrillator (automatic)
    pocket, (skin) (subcutaneous)
    37.99
  cerebral meninges 02.12
  cervix 67.69
    internal os 67.59
      transabdominal 67.51
      transvaginal 67.59
    aceration (by suture) 67.61
      obstetric (current) 75.51
      old 67.69
  chest wall (mesh) (silastic) NEC 34.79
  chordae tendineae 35.32

Repair *(Continued)*
  choroid NEC 14.9
    with retinal repair - *see* Repair, retina
  cisterna chyli 40.69
  claw toe 77.57
  cleft
    hand 82.82
    laryngotracheal 31.69
    lip 27.54
    palate 27.62
      secondary or subsequent 27.63
  coarctation of aorta - *see* Excision,
    coarctation of aorta
  cochlear prosthetic device 20.99
    external components only 95.49
  cockup toe 77.58
  colostomy 46.43
  conjunctiva NEC 10.49
    with scleral repair 12.81
    laceration 10.6
      with repair of sclera 12.81
    late effect of trachoma 10.49
  cornea NEC 11.59
    with
      conjunctival flap 11.53
      transplant - *see* Keratoplasty
    postoperative dehiscence 11.52
  coronary artery NEC 36.99
    by angioplasty - *see* Angioplasty,
      coronary
    by atherectomy - *see* Angioplasty,
      coronary
  cranium NEC 02.06
    with
      flap (bone) 02.03
      graft (bone) 02.04
  cusp, valve - *see* Repair, heart, valve
  cystocele 70.51
    with graft or prosthesis 70.54
    and rectocele 70.50
      with graft or prosthesis 70.53
  dental arch 24.8
  diaphragm NEC 34.84
  diastasis recti 83.65
  diastematomyelia 03.59
  ear (external) 18.79
    auditory canal or meatus 18.6
    auricle NEC 18.79
    cartilage NEC 18.79
    laceration (by suture) 18.4
    lop ear 18.79
    middle NEC 19.9
    prominent or protruding 18.5
  ectropion 08.49
    by or with
      lid reconstruction 08.44
      suture (technique) 08.42
      thermocauterization 08.41
      wedge resection 08.43
  encephalocele (cerebral) 02.12
  endocardial cushion defect 35.73
    with
      prosthesis (grafted to septa) 35.54
      tissue graft 35.63
  enterocele (female) 70.92
    with graft or prosthesis 70.93
    male 53.9
  enterostomy 46.40
  entropion 08.49
    by or with
      lid reconstruction 08.44
      suture (technique) 08.42
      thermocauterization 08.41
      wedge resection 08.43

◀ New   ◀‖‖‖ Revised   ~~deleted~~ Deleted   ● Use Additional Digit(s)   ▨ Omit code

Repair *(Continued)*
  epicanthus (fold) 08.59
  epididymis (and spermatic cord) NEC 63.59
    with vas deferens 63.89
  epiglottis 31.69
  episiotomy
    routine following delivery - *see* Episiotomy
    secondary 75.69
  epispadias 58.45
  esophagus, esophageal NEC 42.89
    fistula NEC 42.84
    stricture 42.85
  exstrophy of bladder 57.86
  eye, eyeball 16.89
    multiple structures 16.82
    rupture 16.82
    socket 16.64
      with graft 16.63
  eyebrow 08.89
    linear 08.81
  eyelid 08.89
    full-thickness 08.85
      involving lid margin 08.84
    laceration 08.81
      full-thickness 08.85
        involving lid margin 08.84
      partial-thickness 08.83
        involving lid margin 08.82
    linear 08.81
    partial-thickness 08.83
      involving lid margin 08.82
    retraction 08.38
  fallopian tube (with prosthesis) 66.79
    by
      reanastomosis 66.79
      reimplantation into
        ovary 66.72
        uterus 66.74
      suture 66.71
  false aneurysm - *see* Repair, aneurysm
  fascia 83.89
    by or with
      arthroplasty - *see* Arthroplasty
      graft (fascial) (muscle) 83.82
        hand 82.72
        tendon 83.81
          hand 82.79
      suture (direct) 83.65
        hand 82.46
    hand 82.89
      by
        graft NEC 82.79
          fascial 82.72
          muscle 82.72
        suture (direct) 82.46
    joint - *see* Arthroplasty
  filtering bleb (corneal) (scleral) (by excision) 12.82
    by
      corneal graft - *see also* Keratoplasty 11.60
      scleroplasty 12.82
      suture 11.51
        with conjunctival flap 11.53
  fistula - *see also* Closure, fistula
    anovaginal 70.73
    arteriovenous 39.53
      clipping 39.53
      coagulation 39.53
        endovascular approach 39.79
          head and neck 39.72

Repair *(Continued)*
  fistula *(Continued)*
    arteriovenous *(Continued)*
      division 39.53
      excision or resection - *see also* Aneurysmectomy, by site
        with
          anastomosis - *see* Aneurysmectomy, with anastomosis, by site
          graft replacement - *see* Aneurysmectomy, with graft replacement, by site
      ligation 39.53
        coronary artery 36.99
      occlusion 39.53
        endovascular approach 39.79
          head and neck 39.72
      suture 39.53
    cervicovesical 57.84
    cervix 67.62
    choledochoduodenal 51.72
    colovaginal 70.72
    enterovaginal 70.74
    enterovesical 57.83
    esophagocutaneous 42.84
    ileovesical 57.83
    intestinovaginal 70.74
    intestinovesical 57.83
    oroantral 22.71
    perirectal 48.93
    pleuropericardial 37.49
    rectovaginal 70.73
    rectovesical 57.83
    rectovesicovaginal 57.83
    scrotum 61.42
    sigmoidovaginal 70.74
    sinus
      nasal 22.71
      of Valsalva 35.39
    splenocolic 41.95
    urethroperineovesical 57.84
    urethrovesical 57.84
    urethrovesicovaginal 57.84
    uterovesical 57.84
    vagina NEC 70.75
    vaginocutaneous 70.75
    vaginoenteric NEC 70.74
    vaginoileal 70.74
    vaginoperineal 70.75
    vaginovesical 57.84
    vesicocervicovaginal 57.84
    vesicocolic 57.83
    vesicocutaneous 57.84
    vesicoenteric 57.83
    vesicointestinal 57.83
    vesicometrorectal 57.83
    vesicoperineal 57.84
    vesicorectal 57.83
    vesicosigmoidal 57.83
    vesicosigmoidovaginal 57.83
    vesicourethral 57.84
    vesicourethrorectal 57.83
    vesicouterine 57.84
    vesicovaginal 57.84
    vulva 71.72
    vulvorectal 48.73
  foramen ovale (patent) 35.71
    with
      prosthesis (open heart technique) 35.51
        closed heart technique 35.52
      tissue graft 35.61

Repair *(Continued)*
  fracture - *see also* Reduction, fracture
    larynx 31.64
    malunion or nonunion (delayed) NEC - *see* category 78.4●
      with
        graft - *see* Graft, bone
        insertion (of)
          bone growth stimulator (invasive) - *see* category 78.9●
          internal fixation device 78.5●
        manipulation for realignment - *see* Reduction, fracture, by site, closed
        osteotomy
          with
            correction of alignment - *see* category 77.3●
            with internal fixation device - *see* categories 77.3● [78.5]●
            with intramedullary rod - *see* categories 77.3● [78.5]●
        replacement arthroplasty - *see* Arthroplasty
        sequestrectomy - *see* category 77.0●
        Sofield type procedure - *see* categories 77.3● [78.5]●
        synostosis technique - *see* Arthrodesis
    vertebra 03.53
  funnel chest (with implant) 34.74
  gallbladder 51.91
  gastroschisis 54.71
  great vessels NEC 39.59
    laceration (by suture) 39.30
      artery 39.31
      vein 39.32
  hallux valgus NEC 77.59
    resection of joint with prosthetic implant 77.59
  hammer toe 77.56
  hand 82.89
    with graft or implant 82.79
      fascia 82.72
      muscle 82.72
      tendon 82.79
  heart 37.49
    assist system 37.63
    septum 35.70
      with
        prosthesis 35.50
        tissue graft 35.60
      atrial 35.71
        with
          prosthesis (open heart technique) 35.51
            closed heart technique 35.52
          tissue graft 35.61
      combined with repair of valvular and ventricular septal defects - *see* Repair, endocardial cushion defect
    in total repair of
      tetralogy of Fallot 35.81
      total anomalous pulmonary venous connection 35.82
      truncus arteriosus 35.83

R

Repair *(Continued)*
  heart *(Continued)*
    septum *(Continued)*
      combined with repair of
        valvular defect - *see*
        Repair,
        endocardial cushion
        defect
      ventricular 35.72
        with
          prosthesis (open heart
            technique) 35.53
            closed heart technique
              35.55
          tissue graft 35.62
        combined with repair of
          valvular and atrial septal
          defects - *see* Repair,
          endocardial cushion
          defect
        in total repair of
          tetralogy of Fallot 35.81
          total anomalous pulmonary
            venous connection
            35.82
          truncus arteriosus 35.83
    total internal biventricular
      replacement system 37.52
      implantable battery 37.54
      implantable controller 37.54
      thoracic unit 37.53
      transcutaneous energy transfer
        [TET] device 37.54
    valve (cusps) (open heart technique)
      35.10
      with prosthesis or tissue graft
        35.20
      aortic (without replacement)
        35.11
        with
          prosthesis 35.22
          tissue graft 35.21
        combined with repair of atrial
          and ventricular septal
          defects - *see* Repair,
          endocardial cushion
          defect
      mitral (without replacement)
        35.12
        with
          leaflet clip implant 35.97 ◀
          MitraClip® 35.97 ◀
          prosthesis 35.24
          tissue graft 35.23
        balloon, percutaneous
          35.96 ◀
        endovascular repair with
          implant 35.97 ◀
        percutaneous with leaflet clip
          implant 35.97 ◀
      pulmonary (without
        replacement) 35.13
        with
          prosthesis 35.26
            in total repair of
              tetralogy of Fallot
              35.81
          tissue graft 35.25
      tricuspid (without replacement)
        35.14
        with
          prosthesis 35.28
          tissue graft 35.27
  hepatic duct 51.79

Repair *(Continued)*
  hernia NEC 53.9
    anterior abdominal wall NEC
      (laparoscopic without graft or
      prosthesis) 53.59 ◀▥
      with prosthesis or graft
        laparoscopic 53.63
        other and open 53.69
    colostomy 46.42
    crural 53.29
    cul-de-sac (Douglas') 70.92
    diaphragmatic
      abdominal approach
        laparoscopic 53.71
        other and open 53.72
        unspecified 53.75
      thoracic, thoracoabdominal
        approach 53.80
        laparoscopic 53.83
        other and open 53.84
    epigastric 53.59
      with prosthesis or graft 53.69
    esophageal hiatus
      abdominal approach
        laparoscopic 53.71
        other and open 53.72
        unspecified 53.75
      thoracic, thoracoabdominal
        approach 53.80
    fascia 83.89
      hand 82.89
    femoral (unilateral) 53.29
      with prosthesis or graft 53.21
      bilateral 53.39
        with prosthesis or graft
          53.31
    Ferguson 53.00
    Halsted 53.00
    Hill-Allison (hiatal hernia repair,
      transpleural approach)
      53.80
    hypogastric 53.59
      with prosthesis or graft
        53.69
    incisional 53.51
      laparoscopic with prosthesis or
        graft 53.62
      other open with prosthesis or
        graft 53.61
    inguinal (unilateral) 53.00
      with prosthesis or graft
        53.05
      bilateral 53.10
        with prosthesis or graft
          53.17
          laparoscopic 17.24
        direct
          laparoscopic with graft or
            prosthesis 17.21
          other and open
            (laparoscopic without
            graft or prosthesis)
            53.11 ◀▥
            with prosthesis or graft
              53.14
        direct and indirect
          laparoscopic with graft or
            prosthesis 17.23
          other and open
            (laparoscopic without
            graft or prosthesis)
            53.13 ◀▥
            with prosthesis or graft
              53.16

Repair *(Continued)*
  hernia NEC *(Continued)*
    inguinal *(Continued)*
      bilateral *(Continued)*
        indirect
          laparoscopic with graft or
            prosthesis 17.22
          other and open
            (laparoscopic without
            graft or prosthesis)
            53.12 ◀▥
            with prosthesis or graft
              53.15
      direct (unilateral)
        with prosthesis or graft
          53.03
        and indirect (unilateral)
          laparoscopic with graft or
            prosthesis 17.11
          other and open
            (laparoscopic without
            graft or prosthesis)
            53.01 ◀▥
            with prosthesis or graft
              53.03
        laparoscopic with graft or
          prosthesis 17.11
        other and open (laparoscopic
          without graft or
          prosthesis) 53.01 ◀▥
          with prosthesis or graft
            53.03
      indirect (unilateral)
        laparoscopic with graft or
          prosthesis 17.12
        other and open (laparoscopic
          without graft or
          prosthesis) 53.02 ◀▥
          with prosthesis or graft
            53.04
      internal 53.9
      ischiatic 53.9
      ischiorectal 53.9
      laparoscopic with graft or
        prosthesis, NOS 17.13
      lumbar 53.9
      manual 96.27
      obturator 53.9
      omental 53.9
      paraesophageal
        laparoscopic 53.71
        other and open 53.72
        unspecified 53.75
      parahiatal
        laparoscopic 53.71
        other and open 53.72
        unspecified 53.75
      paraileostomy 46.41
      parasternal 53.82
      paraumbilical
        laparoscopic 53.43
          with graft or prosthesis
            53.42
        other and open with graft or
          prosthesis 53.41
        other open 53.49
      pericolostomy 46.42
      perineal (enterocele) 53.9
      preperitoneal 53.29
      pudendal 53.9
      retroperitoneal 53.9
      sciatic 53.9
      scrotal - *see* Repair, hernia,
        inguinal

◀ New   ◀▥ Revised   ~~deleted~~ Deleted   ● Use Additional Digit(s)   ▨ Omit code

Repair *(Continued)*
 hernia NEC *(Continued)*
  spigelian 53.59
   with prosthesis or graft 53.69
  umbilical
   laparoscopic 53.43
    with graft or prosthesis
     53.42
    other and open with graft or
     prosthesis 53.41
    other open 53.49
  uveal 12.39
  ventral (laparoscopic without graft
   or prosthesis) 53.59 ⬅▥
   with prosthesis or graft
    laparoscopic 53.63
    other and open 53.69
   incisional 53.51
    laparoscopic without graft or
     prosthesis 53.59 ◀
    other open with prosthesis or
     graft 53.61
 hydrocele
  round ligament 69.19
  spermatic cord 63.1
  tunica vaginalis 61.2
 hymen 70.76
 hypospadias 58.45
 ileostomy 46.41
 ingrown toenail 86.23
 intestine, intestinal NEC 46.79
  fistula - *see* Closure, fistula,
   intestine
  laceration
   large intestine 46.75
   small intestine NEC 46.73
  stoma - *see* Repair, stoma
 inverted uterus NEC 69.29
  manual
   nonobstetric 69.94
   obstetric 75.94
  obstetrical
   manual 75.94
   surgical 75.93
  vaginal approach 69.23
 iris (rupture) NEC 12.39
 jejunostomy 46.41
 joint (capsule) (cartilage) NEC - *see also*
  Arthroplasty 81.96
 kidney NEC 55.89
 knee (joint) NEC 81.47
  collateral ligaments 81.46
  cruciate ligaments 81.45
  five-in-one 81.42
  triad 81.43
 labia - *see* Repair, vulva
 laceration - *see* Suture, by site
 lacrimal system NEC 09.99
  canaliculus 09.73
  punctum 09.72
   for eversion 09.71
 laryngostomy 31.62
 laryngotracheal cleft 31.69
 larynx 31.69
  fracture 31.64
  laceration 31.61
 leads (cardiac) NEC 37.75
 ligament - *see also* Arthroplasty
  81.96
  broad 69.29
  collateral, knee NEC 81.46
  cruciate, knee NEC 81.45
  round 69.29
  uterine 69.29

Repair *(Continued)*
 lip NEC 27.59
  cleft 27.54
  laceration (by suture) 27.51
 liver NEC 50.69
  laceration 50.61
 lop ear 18.79
 lung NEC 33.49
 lymphatic (channel) (peripheral) NEC
  40.9
  duct, left (thoracic) NEC 40.69
 macrodactyly 82.83
 mallet finger 82.84
 mandibular ridge 76.64
 mastoid (antrum) (cavity) 19.9
 meninges (cerebral) NEC 02.12
  spinal NEC 03.59
   meningocele 03.51
   myelomeningocele 03.52
 meningocele (spinal) 03.51
  cranial 02.12
 mesentery 54.75
 mouth NEC 27.59
  laceration NEC 27.52
 muscle NEC 83.87
  by
   graft or implant (fascia) (muscle)
    83.82
    hand 82.72
   tendon 83.81
    hand 82.79
   suture (direct) 83.65
    hand 82.46
   transfer or transplantation
    (muscle) 83.77
    hand 82.58
  hand 82.89
   by
    graft or implant NEC
     82.79
     fascia 82.72
    suture (direct) 82.46
    transfer or transplantation
     (muscle) 82.58
 musculotendinous cuff, shoulder
  83.63
 myelomeningocele 03.52
 nasal
  septum (perforation) NEC 21.88
  sinus NEC 22.79
   fistula 22.71
 nasolabial flaps (plastic) 21.86
 nasopharyngeal atresia 29.4
 nerve (cranial) (peripheral) NEC
  04.79
  old injury 04.76
  revision 04.75
  sympathetic 05.81
 nipple NEC 85.87
 nose (external) (internal) (plastic)
  NEC - *see also* Rhinoplasty
  21.89
  laceration (by suture) 21.81
 notched lip 27.59
 omentum 54.74
 omphalocele
  laparoscopic 53.43
   with graft or prosthesis
    53.42
  other and open with graft or
   prosthesis 53.41
  other open 53.49
 orbit 16.89
  wound 16.81

Repair *(Continued)*
 ostium
  primum defect 35.73
   with
    prosthesis 35.54
    tissue graft 35.63
  secundum defect 35.71
   with
    prosthesis (open heart
     technique) 35.51
     closed heart technique 35.52
    tissue graft 35.61
 ovary 65.79
  with tube 65.73
   laparoscopic 65.76
 overlapping toe 77.58
 pacemaker
  cardiac
   device (permanent) 37.89
   electrodes (leads) NEC 37.75
   pocket (skin) (subcutaneous)
    37.79
 palate NEC 27.69
  cleft 27.62
   secondary or subsequent 27.63
  laceration (by suture) 27.61
 pancreas NEC 52.95
  Wirsung's duct 52.99
 papillary muscle (heart) 35.31
 patent ductus arteriosus 38.85
 pectus deformity (chest) (carinatum)
  (excavatum) 34.74
 pelvic floor NEC 70.79
  obstetric laceration (current) 75.69
  old 70.79
 penis NEC 64.49
  for epispadias or hypospadias 58.45
  inflatable prosthesis 64.99
  laceration 64.41
 pericardium 37.49
 perineum (female) 71.79
  laceration (by suture) 71.71
   obstetric (current) 75.69
   old 71.79
  male NEC 86.89
   laceration (by suture) 86.59
 peritoneum NEC 54.73
  by suture 54.64
 pharynx NEC 29.59
  laceration (by suture) 29.51
  plastic 29.4
 pleura NEC 34.93
 postcataract wound dehiscence 11.52
  with conjunctival flap 11.53
 pouch of Douglas 70.52
 primum ostium defect 35.73
  with
   prosthesis 35.54
   tissue graft 35.63
 prostate 60.93
 ptosis, eyelid - *see* Repair, blepharoptosis
 punctum, lacrimal NEC 09.72
  for correction of eversion 09.71
 quadriceps (mechanism) 83.86
 rectocele (posterior colporrhaphy)
  70.52
  with graft or prosthesis 70.55
  and cystocele 70.50
   with graft or prosthesis 70.53
 rectum NEC 48.79
  laceration (by suture) 48.71
  prolapse NEC 48.76
   abdominal approach 48.75
   STARR procedure 48.74

Repair *(Continued)*
  retina, retinal
    detachment 14.59
      by
        cryotherapy 14.52
        diathermy 14.51
        photocoagulation 14.55
          laser 14.54
          xenon arc 14.53
        scleral buckling - *see also*
          Buckling, scleral
          14.49
    tear or defect 14.39
      by
        cryotherapy 14.32
        diathermy 14.31
        photocoagulation 14.35
          laser 14.34
          xenon arc 14.33
  retroperitoneal tissue 54.73
  rotator cuff (graft) (suture) 83.63
  round ligament 69.29
  ruptured tendon NEC 83.88
    hand 82.86
  salivary gland or duct NEC 26.49
  sclera, scleral 12.89
    fistula 12.82
    staphyloma NEC 12.86
      with graft 12.85
  scrotum 61.49
  sinus
    nasal NEC 22.79
    of Valsalva (aneurysm) 35.39
  skin (plastic) (without graft) 86.89
    laceration (by suture) 86.59
  skull NEC 02.06
    with
      flap (bone) 02.03
      graft (bone) 02.04
  spermatic cord NEC 63.59
    laceration (by suture) 63.51
  sphincter ani 49.79
    laceration (by suture) 49.71
      obstetric (current) 75.62
        old 49.79
  spina bifida NEC 03.59
    meningocele 03.51
    myelomeningocele 03.52
  spinal (cord) (meninges) (structures)
    NEC 03.59
    meningocele 03.51
    myelomeningocele 03.52
  spleen 41.95
  sternal defect 78.41
  stoma
    bile duct 51.79
    bladder 57.22
    bronchus 33.42
    common duct 51.72
    esophagus 42.89
    gallbladder 51.99
    hepatic duct 51.79
    intestine 46.40
      large 46.43
      small 46.41
    kidney 55.89
    larynx 31.63
    rectum 48.79
    stomach 44.69
      laparoscopic 44.68
    thorax 34.79
    trachea 31.74
    ureter 56.62
    urethra 58.49

Repair *(Continued)*
  stomach NEC 44.69
    laceration (by suture) 44.61
      laparoscopic 44.68
  stress incontinence (urinary) NEC 59.79
    by
      anterior urethropexy 59.79
      Burch 59.5
      cystourethropexy (with levator
        muscle sling) 59.71
      injection of implant (fat)
        (collagen) (polytef) 59.72
      paraurethral suspension
        (Pereyra) 59.6
      periurethral suspension 59.6
      plication of urethrovesical
        junction 59.3
      pubococcygeal sling 59.71
      retropubic urethral suspension
        59.5
      suprapubic sling 59.4
      tension free vaginal tape 59.79
      urethrovesical suspension 59.4
        gracilis muscle transplant
          59.71
        levator muscle sling 59.71
  subcutaneous tissue (plastic)
    (without skin graft) 86.89
    laceration (by suture) 86.59
  supracristal defect (heart) 35.72
    with
      prosthesis (open heart technique)
        35.53
        closed heart technique 35.55
      tissue graft 35.62
  symblepharon NEC 10.49
    by division (with insertion of
      conformer) 10.5
    with free graft 10.41
  syndactyly 86.85
  synovial membrane, joint - *see*
    Arthroplasty
  telecanthus 08.59
  tendon 83.88
    by or with
      arthroplasty - *see* Arthroplasty
      graft or implant (tendon) 83.81
        fascia 83.82
          hand 82.72
        hand 82.79
        muscle 83.82
          hand 82.72
      suture (direct) (immediate)
        (primary) - *see also* Suture,
        tendon 83.64
        hand 82.45
      transfer for transplantation
        (tendon) 83.75
        hand 82.56
    hand 82.86
      by
        graft or implant (tendon)
          82.79
        suture (direct) (immediate)
          (primary) - *see also* Suture,
          tendon, hand) 82.45
        transfer or transplantation
          (tendon) 82.56
    rotator cuff (direct suture) 83.63
    ruptured NEC 83.88
      hand 82.86
    sheath (direct suture) 83.61
      hand 82.41
  testis NEC 62.69

Repair *(Continued)*
  tetralogy of Fallot
    partial - *see* specific procedure
    total (one-stage) 35.81
  thoracic duct NEC 40.69
  thoracostomy 34.72
  thymus (gland) 07.93
  tongue NEC 25.59
  tooth NEC 23.2
    by
      crown (artificial) 23.41
      filling (amalgam) (plastic)
        (silicate) 23.2
      inlay 23.3
  total anomalous pulmonary venous
    connection
    partial - *see* specific procedure
    total (one-stage) 35.82
  trachea NEC 31.79
    laceration (by suture) 31.71
  tricuspid atresia 35.94
  truncus arteriosus
    partial - *see* specific procedure
    total (one-stage) 35.83
  tunica vaginalis 61.49
    laceration (by suture) 61.41
  tympanum - *see* Tympanoplasty
  ureter NEC 56.89
    laceration (by suture) 56.82
  ureterocele 56.89
  urethra NEC 58.49
    laceration (by suture) 58.41
      obstetric (current) 75.61
        old 58.49
    meatus 58.47
  urethrocele (anterior colporrhaphy)
    (female) 70.51
    with graft or prosthesis 70.54
    and rectocele 70.50
      with graft or prosthesis 70.53
  urinary sphincter, artificial
    (component) 58.99
  urinary stress incontinence - *see* Repair,
    stress incontinence
  uterus, uterine 69.49
    inversion - *see* Repair, inverted
      uterus
    laceration (by suture) 69.41
      obstetric (current) 75.50
        old 69.49
    ligaments 69.29
      by
        interposition 69.21
        plication 69.22
  uvula 27.73
    with synchronous cleft palate repair
      27.62
  vagina, vaginal (cuff) (wall) NEC
    70.79
    anterior 70.51
      with graft or prosthesis 70.54
      with posterior repair 70.50
        with graft or prosthesis
          70.53
    cystocele 70.51
      with graft or prosthesis 70.54
      and rectocele 70.50
        with graft or prosthesis
          70.53
    enterocele 70.92
      with graft or prosthesis 70.93
    laceration (by suture) 70.71
      obstetric (current) 75.69
        old 70.79

◄ New   ◄▮ Revised   ~~deleted~~ Deleted   ● Use Additional Digit(s)   ▮ Omit code

Replacement *(Continued)*
  heart
    artificial
      total internal biventricular
        replacement system 37.52
        implantable battery 37.54
        implantable controller 37.54
        thoracic unit 37.53
        transcutaneous energy transfer
          [TET] device 37.54
      total internal biventricular
        replacement system 37.52
        implantable battery 37.54
        implantable controller 37.54
        thoracic unit 37.53
        transcutaneous energy transfer
          [TET] device 37.54
      valve (with prosthesis) (with tissue
        graft) 35.20
        aortic (with prosthesis) 35.22
          with tissue graft 35.21
        mitral (with prosthesis) 35.24
          with tissue graft 35.23
        poppet (prosthetic) 35.95
        pulmonary (with prosthesis)
          35.26
          with tissue graft 35.25
          in total repair of tetralogy of
            Fallot 35.81
        tricuspid (with prosthesis) 35.28
          with tissue graft 35.27
  hip (partial) (with fixation device)
    (with prosthesis) (with traction)
    81.52
    acetabulum 81.52
      revision 81.53
    femoral head 81.52
      revision 81.53
    total 81.51
      revision 81.53
  intervertebral disc
    artificial, NOS 84.60
      cervical 84.62
        nucleus 84.61
        partial 84.61
        total 84.62
      lumbar, lumbosacral 84.65
        nucleus 84.64
        partial 84.64
        total 84.65
      thoracic (partial) (total) 84.63
  inverted uterus - *see* Repair, inverted
    uterus
  iris NEC 12.39
  kidney, mechanical 55.97
  knee (bicompartmental) (hemijoint)
    (partial) (total)
    (tricompartmental)
    (unicompartmental) 81.54
    revision 81.55
  laryngeal stent 31.93
  leads (electrode)(s) - *see* Replacement,
    electrode(s)
  mechanical kidney 55.97
  mitral valve (with prosthesis) 35.24
    with tissue graft 35.23
  Mulligan hood, fallopian tube 66.93
  muscle stimulator (skeletal) 83.92
  nephrostomy tube 55.93
  neuropacemaker - *see* Implant,
    neurostimulator, by site
  neurostimulator - *see also* Implant,
    neurostimulator, by site
    skeletal muscle 83.92

Replacement *(Continued)*
  pacemaker
    brain - *see* Implant, neurostimulator,
      brain
    cardiac device (initial) (permanent)
      dual-chamber device 37.87
      resynchronization - *see*
        Replacement, CRT-P
      single-chamber device 37.85
        rate responsive 37.86
    electrode(s), cardiac (atrial)
      (transvenous) (ventricular)
      37.76
      epicardium (myocardium)
        37.74
      left ventricular coronary venous
        system 00.52
    gastric - *see* Implant,
      neurostimulator, gastric
    intracranial - *see* Implant,
      neurostimulator, intracranial
    neural - *see* Implant,
      neurostimulator, by site
    peripheral nerve - *see* Implant,
      neurostimulator, peripheral
      nerve
    sacral nerve - *see* Implant,
      neurostimulator, sacral
      nerve
    spine - *see* Implant, neurostimulator,
      spine
    temporary transvenous pacemaker
      system 37.78
  pack or bag
    nose 97.21
    teeth, tooth 97.22
    vagina 97.26
    vulva 97.26
    wound 97.16
  pessary, vagina NEC 97.25
  prosthesis
    acetabulum 81.53
    arm (bioelectric) (cineplastic)
      (kineplastic) 84.44
    biliary tract 51.99
    cochlear 20.96
    channel (single) 20.97
      multiple 20.98
    elbow 81.97
    extremity (bioelectric) (cineplastic)
      (kineplastic) 84.40
      lower 84.48
      upper 84.44
    fallopian tube (Mulligan hood)
      (stent) 66.93
    femur 81.53
    leg (bioelectric) (cineplastic)
      (kineplastic) 84.48
    penis (internal) (non-inflatable)
      64.95
      inflatable (internal) 64.97
    pulmonary valve (with prosthesis)
      35.26
      with tissue graft 35.25
      in total repair of tetralogy of Fallot
        35.81
  pyelostomy tube 55.94
  rectal tube 96.09
  Rheos™ carotid sinus baroreflex
    activation device 39.81 ◀▥
  sensor (lead)
    intracardiac or great vessel
      hemodynamic monitoring
      00.56

Replacement *(Continued)*
  shoulder NEC 81.83
    partial 81.81
    total, NEC 81.80 ◀▥
      other 81.80 ◀
      reverse 81.88 ◀
  skull
    plate 02.05
    tongs 02.94
  spacer (cement) (joint)
    (methylmethacrylate) 84.56
  specified appliance or device NEC 97.29
  spinal motion preservation device
    facet replacement device(s) 84.84
    interspinous process device(s) 84.80
    pedicle-based dynamic stabilization
      device(s) 84.82
  splint 97.14
  stent
    bile duct 97.05
    fallopian tube 66.93
    larynx 31.93
    pancreatic duct 97.05
    trachea 31.93
  stimoceiver - *see* Implant, stimoceiver,
    by site
  stimulator
    electrode(s) ◀
      carotid sinus 39.82 ◀▥
        with synchronous pulse
          generator replacement
          (total system) 39.81 ◀
    pulse generator ◀
      carotid sinus 39.83 ◀
        with synchronous electrode(s)
          replacement (total
          system) 39.81 ◀
  subdural
    grids 02.93
    strips 02.93
  testis in scrotum 62.5
  tongs, skull 02.94
  tracheal stent 31.93
  tricuspid valve (with prosthesis)
    35.28
    with tissue graft 35.27
  tube
    bile duct 97.05
    bladder 57.95
    cystostomy 59.94
    esophagostomy 97.01
    gastrostomy 97.02
    large intestine 97.04
    nasogastric 97.01
    nephrostomy 55.93
    pancreatic duct 97.05
    pyelostomy 55.94
    rectal 96.09
    small intestine 97.03
    tracheostomy 97.23
    ureterostomy 59.93
    ventricular (cerebral) 02.42
  umbilical cord, prolapsed 73.92
  ureter (with)
    bladder flap 56.74
    ileal segment implanted into
      bladder 56.89 *[45.51]*
  ureterostomy tube 59.93
  urethral sphincter, artificial 58.93
  urinary sphincter, artificial 58.93
  valve
    heart - *see also* Replacement, heart
      valve poppet (prosthetic) 35.95
    ventricular (cerebral) 02.42

◀ New   ◀▥ Revised   ~~deleted~~ Deleted   ● Use Additional Digit(s)   ▒ Omit code

Replacement *(Continued)*
  ventricular shunt (catheter) (valve)
      02.42
  Vinke tongs (skull) 02.94
  vitreous (silicone) 14.75
      for retinal reattachment 14.59
Replant, replantation - *see also*
      Reattachment
  extremity - *see* Reattachment, extremity
  penis 64.45
  scalp 86.51
  tooth 23.5
Reposition
  cardiac pacemaker
      electrode(s) (atrial) (transvenous)
          (ventricular) 37.75
      pocket 37.79
  cardiac resynchronization defibrillator
      (CRT-D) - *see* Revision, cardiac
      resynchronization defibrillator
  cardiac resynchronization pacemaker
      (CRT-P) - *see* Revision, cardiac
      resynchronization pacemaker
  cardioverter/defibrillator (automatic)
      lead(s) (epicardial patch) (pacing)
          (sensing) 37.75
      pocket 37.79
      pulse generator 37.79
  cilia base 08.71
  implantable hemodynamic sensor
      (lead) and monitor device 37.79
  iris 12.39
  neurostimulator
      leads
          subcutaneous, without device
              replacement 86.09
          within brain 02.93
          within or over gastric nerve
              04.92
          within or over peripheral nerve
              04.92
          within or over sacral nerve
              04.92
          within spine 03.93
      pulse generator
          subcutaneous, without device
              replacement 86.09
  renal vessel, aberrant 39.55
  subcutaneous device pocket NEC
      86.09
  thyroid tissue 06.94
  tricuspid valve (with plication)
      35.14
Resection - *see also* Excision, by site
  abdominoendorectal (combined),
      NOS 48.50
      laparoscopic 48.51
      open 48.52
      other 48.59
  abdominoperineal (rectum), NOS 48.50
      pull-through (Altemeier) (Swenson)
          NEC 48.49
          Duhamel type 48.65
          laparoscopic 48.42
          not otherwise specified 48.40
          open 48.43
  alveolar process and palate (en bloc)
      27.32
  aneurysm - *see* Aneurysmectomy
  aortic valve (for subvalvular stenosis)
      35.11
  artery - *see* Arteriectomy
  bile duct NEC 51.69
      common duct NEC 51.63

Resection *(Continued)*
  bladder (partial) (segmental)
      (transvesical) (wedge) 57.6
      complete or total 57.79
      lesion NEC 57.59
          transurethral approach 57.49
      neck 57.59
          transurethral approach 57.49
  blood vessel - *see* Angiectomy
  brain 01.59
      by
          stereotactic radiosurgery 92.30
              cobalt 60 92.32
              linear accelerator (LINAC)
                  92.31
              multi-source 92.32
              particle beam 92.33
              particulate 92.33
              radiosurgery NEC 92.39
              single source photon 92.31
      hemisphere 01.52
      lobe 01.53
  breast - *see also* Mastectomy
      quadrant 85.22
      segmental 85.23
  broad ligament 69.19
  bronchus (sleeve) (wide sleeve) 32.1
      block (en bloc) (with radical
          dissection of brachial plexus,
          bronchus, lobe of lung, ribs,
          and sympathetic nerves) 32.6
  bursa 83.5
      hand 82.31
  cecum (and terminal ileum)
      laparoscopic 17.32
      open and other 45.72
  cerebral meninges 01.51
  chest wall 34.4
  clavicle 77.81
  clitoris 71.4
  colon (partial) (segmental)
      ascending (cecum and terminal
          ileum)
          laparoscopic 17.32
          open and other 45.72
      cecum (and terminal ileum)
          laparoscopic 17.32
          open and other 45.72
      complete
          laparoscopic 45.81
          open 45.82
          other 45.83
          unspecified 45.83
      descending (sigmoid)
          laparoscopic 17.36
          open and other 45.76
      for interposition 45.52
      Hartmann
          laparoscopic 17.35
          open and other 45.75
      hepatic flexure
          laparoscopic 17.33
          open and other 45.73
      laparoscopic 17.39
      left radical (hemicolon)
          laparoscopic 17.35
          open and other 45.75
      multiple segmental
          laparoscopic 17.31
          open and other 45.71
      open and other 45.79
      right radical (hemicolon)
          (ileocolectomy)
          laparoscopic 17.33
          open and other 45.73

Resection *(Continued)*
  colon *(Continued)*
      segmental NEC
          laparoscopic 17.39
          multiple
              laparoscopic 17.31
              open and other 45.71
          open and other 45.79
      sigmoid
          laparoscopic 17.36
          open and other 45.76
      splenic flexure
          laparoscopic 17.35
          open and other 45.75
      total
          laparoscopic 45.81
          open 45.82
          other 45.83
          unspecified 45.83
      transverse
          laparoscopic 17.34
          open and other 45.74
  conjunctiva, for pterygium 11.39
  corneal graft 11.32
  cornual (fallopian tube) (unilateral)
      66.69
      bilateral 66.63
  diaphragm 34.81
  endaural 20.79
  endorectal (pull-through) (Soave)
      48.41
      combined abdominal, NOS 48.50
          laparoscopic 48.51
          open 48.52
          other 48.59
  esophagus (partial) (subtotal) - *see also*
      Esophagectomy 42.41
      total 42.42
  exteriorized intestine - *see* Resection,
      intestine, exteriorized
  fascia 83.44
      for graft 83.43
          hand 82.34
      hand 82.35
          for graft 82.34
  gallbladder (total) 51.22
  gastric (partial) (sleeve) (subtotal)
      NEC - *see also* Gastrectomy 43.89
      with anastomosis NEC 43.89
          esophagogastric 43.5
          gastroduodenal 43.6
          gastrogastric 43.89
          gastrojejunal 43.7
      complete or total NEC 43.99
          with intestinal interposition 43.91
      radical NEC 43.99
          with intestinal interposition 43.91
      wedge 43.42
          endoscopic 43.41
  hallux valgus (joint) - *see also*
      Bunionectomy with prosthetic
      implant 77.59
  hepatic
      duct 51.69
      flexure (colon)
          laparoscopic 17.33
          open and other 45.73
  infundibula, heart (right) 35.34
  intestine (partial) NEC
      cecum (with terminal ileum)
          laparoscopic 17.32
          open and other 45.72
      exteriorized (large intestine) 46.04
          small intestine 46.02

Resection *(Continued)*
  intestine NEC *(Continued)*
    for interposition 45.50
      large intestine 45.52
      small intestine 45.51
    hepatic flexure
      laparoscopic 17.33
      open and other 45.73
    ileum 45.62
      with cecum
        laparoscopic 17.32
        open and other 45.72
      laparoscopic 17.39
    large (partial) (segmental) NEC
      for interposition 45.52
      laparoscopic 17.39
      multiple segmental
        laparoscopic 17.31
        open and other 45.71
      other 45.79
      total
        laparoscopic 45.81
        open 45.82
        other 45.83
        unspecified 45.83
      unspecified 45.79
    left hemicolon
      laparoscopic 17.35
      open and other 45.75
    multiple segmental (large
        intestine)
      laparoscopic 17.31
      open and other 45.71
      small intestine 45.61
    open and other 45.79
    right hemicolon
      laparoscopic 17.33
      open and other 45.73
    segmental (large intestine)
      laparoscopic 17.39
      multiple
        laparoscopic 17.31
        open and other 45.71
      open and other 45.79
      small intestine 45.62
        multiple 45.61
    sigmoid
      laparoscopic 17.36
      open and other 45.76
    small (partial) (segmental) NEC
        45.62
      for interposition 45.51
      multiple segmental 45.61
      total 45.63
    total
      large intestine
        laparoscopic 45.81
        open 45.82
        other 45.83
        unspecified 45.83
      small intestine 45.63
  joint structure NEC - *see also*
      Arthrectomy 80.90
  kidney (segmental) (wedge) 55.4
  larynx - *see also* Laryngectomy
    submucous 30.29
  lesion - *see* Excision, lesion, by site
  levator palpebrae muscle 08.33
  ligament - *see also* Arthrectomy
      80.90
    broad 69.19
    round 69.19
    uterine 69.19
  lip (wedge) 27.43

Resection *(Continued)*
  liver (partial) (wedge) 50.22
    lobe (total) 50.3
    total 50.4
  lung (wedge) NEC 32.29
    endoscopic 32.28
    segmental (any part) 32.39
      thoracoscopic 32.30
    thoracoscopic 32.20
    volume reduction 32.22
      biologic lung volume reduction
          (BLVR) - *see* category 33.7●
  meninges (cerebral) 01.51
    spinal 03.4
  mesentery 54.4
  muscle 83.45
    extraocular 15.13
      with
        advancement or recession of
            other eye muscle 15.3
        suture of original insertion
            15.13
      levator palpebrae 08.33
      Muller's, for blepharoptosis 08.35
      orbicularis oculi 08.20
      tarsal, for blepharoptosis 08.35
    for graft 83.43
      hand 82.34
    hand 82.36
      for graft 82.34
    ocular - *see* Resection, muscle,
        extraocular
  myocardium 37.33
  nasal septum (submucous) 21.5
  nerve (cranial) (peripheral) NEC 04.07
    phrenic 04.03
      for collapse of lung 33.31
    sympathetic 05.29
    vagus - *see* Vagotomy
  nose (complete) (extended) (partial)
      (radical) 21.4
  omentum 54.4
  orbitomaxillary, radical 16.51
  ovary - *see also* Oophorectomy
    wedge 65.22
      laparoscopic 65.24
  palate (bony) (local) 27.31
    by wide excision 27.32
    soft 27.49
  pancreas (total) (with synchronous
      duodenectomy) 52.6
    partial NEC 52.59
      distal (tail) (with part of body)
          52.52
      proximal (head) (with part of
          body) (with synchronous
          duodenectomy) 52.51
      radical subtotal 52.53
    radical (one-stage) (two-stage) 52.7
    subtotal 52.53
  pancreaticoduodenal - *see also*
      Pancreatectomy 52.6
  pelvic viscera (en masse) (female) 68.8
    male 57.71
  penis 64.3
  pericardium (partial) (for)
    chronic constrictive pericarditis
        37.31
    drainage 37.12
    removal of adhesions 37.31
  peritoneum 54.4
  pharynx (partial) 29.33
  phrenic nerve 04.03
    for collapse of lung 33.31

Resection *(Continued)*
  prostate - *see also* Prostatectomy
    transurethral (punch) 60.29
  pterygium 11.39
  radial head 77.83
  rectosigmoid - *see also* Resection,
      rectum 48.69
  rectum (partial) NEC 48.69
    with
      pelvic exenteration 68.8
      transsacral sigmoidectomy
          48.61
    abdominoendorectal (combined),
        NOS 48.50
      laparoscopic 48.51
      open 48.52
      other 48.59
    abdominoperineal, NOS 48.50
      laparoscopic 48.51
      open 48.52
      other 48.59
      pull-through NEC 48.49
        Duhamel type 48.65
        laparoscopic 48.42
        not otherwise specified
            48.40
        open 48.43
    anterior 48.63
      with colostomy (synchronous)
          48.62
    Duhamel 48.65
    endorectal 48.41
      combined abdominal, NOS
          48.50
      laparoscopic 48.51
      open 48.52
      other 48.59
    posterior 48.64
    pull-through NEC 48.49
      endorectal 48.41
      laparoscopic 48.42
      not otherwise specified 48.40
      open 48.43
    STARR procedure 48.74
    submucosal (Soave) 48.41
      combined abdominal, NOS
          48.50
      laparoscopic 48.51
      open 48.52
      other 48.59
  rib (transaxillary) 77.91
    as operative approach - *omit code*
    incidental to thoracic
        operation - *omit code*
  right ventricle (heart), for infundibular
      stenosis 35.34
  root (tooth) (apex) 23.73
    with root canal therapy 23.72
    residual or retained 23.11
  round ligament 69.19
  sclera 12.65
    with scleral buckling - *see also*
        Buckling, scleral 14.49
    lamellar (for retinal reattachment)
        14.49
      with implant 14.41
  scrotum 61.3
  soft tissue NEC 83.49
    hand 82.39
  sphincter of Oddi 51.89
  spinal cord (meninges) 03.4
  splanchnic 05.29
  splenic flexure (colon) 45.75
  sternum 77.81

◀ New   ◀▥ Revised   ~~deleted~~ Deleted   ● Use Additional Digit(s)   ▨ Omit code

Resection *(Continued)*
  stomach (partial) (sleeve) (subtotal)
      NEC - *see also* Gastrectomy 43.89
    with anastomosis NEC 43.89
      esophagogastric 43.5
      gastroduodenal 43.6
      gastrogastric 43.89
      gastrojejunal 43.7
    complete or total NEC 43.99
      with intestinal interposition
          43.91
    fundus 43.89
    radical NEC 43.99
      with intestinal interposition
          43.91
    wedge 43.42
      endoscopic 43.41
  submucous
    larynx 30.29
    nasal septum 21.5
    vocal cords 30.22
  synovial membrane (complete)
      (partial) - *see also* Synovectomy
      80.70
  tarsolevator 08.33
  tendon 83.42
    hand 82.33
  thoracic structures (block) (en bloc)
      (radical) (brachial plexus,
      bronchus, lobes of lung, ribs, and
      sympathetic nerves) 32.6
  thorax 34.4
  tongue 25.2
    wedge 25.1
  tooth root 23.73
    with root canal therapy 23.72
    apex (abscess) 23.73
      with root canal therapy 23.72
    residual or retained 23.11
  trachea 31.5
  transurethral
    bladder NEC 57.49
    prostate 60.29
  transverse colon
    laparoscopic 17.34
    open and other 45.74
  turbinates - *see* Turbinectomy
  ureter (partial) 56.41
    total 56.42
  uterus - *see* Hysterectomy
  vein - *see* Phlebectomy
  ventricle (heart) 37.35
    infundibula 35.34
  vesical neck 57.59
    transurethral 57.49
  vocal cords (punch) 30.22
Respirator, volume-controlled (Bennett)
    (Byrd) - *see* Ventilation
Restoration
  cardioesophageal angle 44.66
    laparoscopic 44.67
  dental NEC 23.49
    by
      application of crown (artificial)
          23.41
      insertion of bridge (fixed)
          23.42
        removable 23.43
  extremity - *see* Reattachment,
      extremity
  eyebrow 08.70
    with graft 08.63
  eye socket 16.64
    with graft 16.63

Restoration *(Continued)*
  tooth NEC 23.2
    by
      crown (artificial) 23.41
      filling (amalgam) (plastic)
          (silicate) 23.2
      inlay 23.3
Restrictive
  gastric band, laparoscopic 44.95
Resurfacing, hip 00.86
  acetabulum 00.87
    with femoral head 00.85
  femoral head 00.86
    with acetabulum 00.85
  partial NOS 00.85
    acetabulum 00.87
    femoral head 00.86
  total (acetabulum and femoral head)
      00.85
Resuscitation
  artificial respiration 93.93
  cardiac 99.60
    cardioversion 99.62
      atrial 99.61
    defibrillation 99.62
    external massage 99.63
      open chest 37.91
    intracardiac injection 37.92
  cardiopulmonary 99.60
  endotracheal intubation 96.04
  manual 93.93
  mouth-to-mouth 93.93
  pulmonary 93.93
Resuture
  abdominal wall 54.61
  cardiac septum prosthesis 35.95
  chest wall 34.71
  heart valve prosthesis (poppet) 35.95
  wound (skin and subcutaneous tissue)
      (without graft) NEC 86.59
Retavase, infusion 99.10
Reteplase, infusion 99.10
Retightening (noninvasive)
  external fixator device - *omit code*
Retinaculotomy NEC - *see also* Division,
    ligament 80.40
  carpal tunnel (flexor) 04.43
Retraining
  cardiac 93.36
  vocational 93.85
Retrogasserian neurotomy 04.02
Revascularization
  cardiac (heart muscle) (myocardium)
      (direct) 36.10
    with
      bypass anastomosis
        abdominal artery to coronary
            artery 36.17
        aortocoronary (catheter stent)
            (homograft) (prosthesis)
            (saphenous vein graft)
            36.10
          one coronary vessel 36.11
          two coronary vessels 36.12
          three coronary vessels
              36.13
          four coronary vessels
              36.14
        gastroepiploic artery to
            coronary artery 36.17
        internal mammary-coronary
            artery (single vessel)
            36.15
          double vessel 36.16

Revascularization *(Continued)*
  cardiac *(Continued)*
    with *(Continued)*
      bypass anastomosis *(Continued)*
        specified type NEC 36.19
        thoracic artery-coronary artery
            (single vessel) 36.15
          double vessel 36.16
      implantation of artery into heart
          (muscle) (myocardium)
          (ventricle) 36.2
    indirect 36.2
    specified type NEC 36.39
    transmyocardial
      endoscopic 36.33
      endovascular 36.34
      open chest 36.31
      percutaneous 36.34
      specified type NEC 36.32
      thoracoscopic 36.33
Reversal, intestinal segment 45.50
  large 45.52
  small 45.51
Revision
  amputation stump 84.3
    current traumatic - *see* Amputation
  anastomosis
    biliary tract 51.94
    blood vessel 39.49
    gastric, gastrointestinal (with jejunal
        interposition) 44.5
    intestine (large) 46.94
      small 46.93
    pleurothecal 03.97
    pyelointestinal 56.72
    salpingothecal 03.97
    subarachnoid-peritoneal 03.97
    subarachnoid-ureteral 03.97
    ureterointestinal 56.72
  ankle replacement (prosthesis) 81.59
  anterior segment (eye) wound
      (operative) NEC 12.83
  arteriovenous shunt (cannula) (for
      dialysis) 39.42
  arthroplasty - *see* Arthroplasty
  bone flap, skull 02.06
  breast implant 85.93
  bronchostomy 33.42
  bypass graft (vascular) 39.49
    abdominal - coronary artery
        36.17
    aortocoronary (catheter stent)
        (with prosthesis) (with
        saphenous vein graft) (with
        vein graft) 36.10
      one coronary vessel 36.11
      two coronary vessels 36.12
      three coronary vessels 36.13
      four coronary vessels 36.14
    CABG - *see* Revision, aortocoronary
        bypass graft
    chest tube - *see* intercostal catheter
    coronary artery bypass graft (CABG)
        - *see* Revision, aortocoronary
        bypass graft, abdominal -
        coronary artery bypass, and
        internal mammary - coronary
        artery bypass
    intercostal catheter (with lysis of
        adhesions) 34.04
      thoracoscopic 34.06
    internal mammary - coronary artery
        (single) 36.15
      double vessel 36.16

Revision *(Continued)*
  cannula, vessel-to-vessel
    (arteriovenous) 39.94
  canthus, lateral 08.59
  cardiac pacemaker
    device (permanent) 37.89
    electrode(s) (atrial) (transvenous)
      (ventricular) 37.75
    pocket 37.79
  cardiac resynchronization defibrillator
    (CRT-D)
    device 37.79
    electrode(s) 37.75
    pocket 37.79
  cardiac resynchronization pacemaker
    (CRT-P)
    device (permanent) 37.89
    electrode(s) (atrial) (transvenous)
      (ventricular) 37.75
    pocket 37.79
  cardioverter/defibrillator (automatic)
    pocket 37.79
  cholecystostomy 51.99
  cleft palate repair 27.63
  colostomy 46.43
  conduit, urinary 56.52
  cystostomy (stoma) 57.22
  disc - *see* Revision, intervertebral disc
  elbow replacement (prosthesis) 81.97
  enterostomy (stoma) 46.40
    large intestine 46.43
    small intestine 46.41
  enucleation socket 16.64
    with graft 16.63
  esophagostomy 42.83
  exenteration cavity 16.66
    with secondary graft 16.65
  extraocular muscle surgery 15.6
  fenestration, inner ear 20.62
  filtering bleb 12.66
  fixation device (broken) (displaced) -
    see also Fixation, bone, internal
    78.50
  flap or pedicle graft (skin) 86.75
  foot replacement (prosthesis) 81.59
  gastric anastomosis (with jejunal
    interposition) 44.5
  gastric band, laparoscopic 44.96
  gastric port device
    laparoscopic 44.96
  gastroduodenostomy (with jejunal
    interposition) 44.5
  gastrointestinal anastomosis (with
    jejunal interposition) 44.5
  gastrojejunostomy 44.5
  gastrostomy 44.69
    laparoscopic 44.68
  hand replacement (prosthesis) 81.97
  heart procedure NEC 35.95
  hip replacement NOS 81.53
    acetabular and femoral components
      (total) 00.70
    acetabular component only
      00.71
    acetabular liner and/or femoral
      head only 00.73
    femoral component only 00.72
    femoral head only and/or
      acetabular liner 00.73
    partial
      acetabular component only
        00.71
      acetabular liner and/or femoral
        head only 00.73

Revision *(Continued)*
  hip replacement NOS *(Continued)*
    partial *(Continued)*
      femoral component only 00.72
      femoral head only and/or
        acetabular liner 00.73
      total (acetabular and femoral
        components) 00.70
  Holter (-Spitz) valve 02.42
  ileal conduit 56.52
  ileostomy 46.41
  intervertebral disc, artificial (partial)
    (total) NOS 84.69
    cervical 84.66
    lumbar, lumbosacral 84.68
    thoracic 84.67
  Jejunoileal bypass 46.93
  jejunostomy 46.41
  joint replacement
    acetabular and femoral components
      (total) 00.70
    acetabular component only 00.71
    acetabular liner and/or femoral
      head only 00.73
    ankle 81.59
    elbow 81.97
    femoral component only 00.72
    femoral head only and/or
      acetabular liner 00.73
    foot 81.59
    hand 81.97
    hip 81.53
      acetabular and femoral
        components (total) 00.70
      acetabular component only 00.71
      acetabular liner and/or femoral
        head only 00.73
      femoral component only 00.72
      femoral head only and/or
        acetabular liner 00.73
      partial
        acetabular component only
          00.71
        acetabular liner and/or
          femoral head only 00.73
        femoral component only
          00.72
        femoral head only and/or
          acetabular liner 00.73
      total (acetabular and femoral
        components) 00.70
    knee 81.55
    knee replacement NOS 81.55
      femoral component 00.82
      partial
        femoral component 00.82
        patellar component 00.83
        tibial component 00.81
        tibial insert 00.84
      patellar component 00.83
      tibial component 00.81
      tibial insert 00.84
      total (all components) 00.80
    lower extremity NEC 81.59
    toe 81.59
    upper extremity 81.97
    wrist 81.97
  knee replacement (prosthesis) NOS 81.55
    femoral component 00.82
    partial
      femoral component 00.82
      patellar component 00.83
      tibial component 00.81
      tibial insert 00.84

Revision *(Continued)*
  knee replacement NOS *(Continued)*
    patellar component 00.83
    tibial component 00.81
    tibial insert 00.84
    total (all components) 00.80
  laryngostomy 31.63
  lateral canthus 08.59
  mallet finger 82.84
  mastoid antrum 19.9
  mastoidectomy 20.92
  nephrostomy 55.89
  neuroplasty 04.75
  ocular implant 16.62
  orbital implant 16.62
  pocket
    cardiac device (defibrillator)
      (pacemaker)
      with initial insertion of cardiac
        device - *omit code*
      new site (cardiac device pocket)
        (skin) (subcutaneous) 37.79
    carotid sinus stimulation pulse
      generator 39.85 ◄
      with initial insertion of pulse
        generator - *omit code* ◄
    intracardiac hemodynamic
      monitoring 37.79
    subcutaneous device pocket NEC
      with initial insertion of generator
        or device - *omit code*
      new site 86.09
    thalamic stimulator pulse generator
      with initial insertion of battery
        package - *omit code*
      new site (skin) (subcutaneous)
        86.09
  previous mastectomy site - *see*
    categories 85.0–85.99
  proctostomy 48.79
  prosthesis
    acetabular and femoral components
      (total) 00.70
    acetabular component only 00.71
    acetabular liner and/or femoral
      head only 00.73
    ankle 81.59
    breast 85.93
    elbow 81.97
    femoral component only 00.72
    femoral head only and/or
      acetabular liner 00.73
    foot 81.59
    hand 81.97
    heart valve (poppet) 35.95
    hip 81.53
      acetabular component only 00.71
      acetabular liner and/or femoral
        head only 00.73
      femoral component only 00.72
      femoral head only and/or
        acetabular liner 00.73
      partial
        acetabular component only
          00.71
        acetabular liner and/or
          femoral head only 00.73
        femoral component only 00.72
        femoral head only and/or
          acetabular liner 00.73
      acetabular and femoral
        components (total) 00.70
      total (acetabular and femoral
        components) 00.70

S

Salpingo-oophorectomy (unilateral)
65.49
   that by laparoscope 65.41
   bilateral (same operative episode)
      65.61
      laparoscopic 65.63
   remaining or solitary tube and ovary
      65.62
      laparoscopic 65.64
Salpingo-oophoroplasty 65.73
   laparoscopic 65.76
Salpingo-oophororrhaphy 65.79
Salpingo-oophorostomy 66.72
Salpingo-oophorotomy 65.09
   laparoscopic 65.01
Salpingoplasty 66.79
Salpingorrhaphy 66.71
Salpingosalpingostomy 66.73
Salpingostomy (for removal of non-
   ruptured ectopic pregnancy)
   66.02
Salpingotomy 66.01
Salpingo-uterostomy 66.74
Salter operation (innominate osteotomy)
   77.39
Salvage (autologous blood)
   (intraoperative) (perioperative)
   (postoperative) 99.00
Sampling, blood for genetic
   determination of fetus 75.33
Sandpapering (skin) 86.25
Saucerization
   bone - see also Excision, lesion, bone
      77.60
   rectum 48.99
Sauer-Bacon operation (abdominoperineal
   resection), NOS 48.50
   laparoscopic 48.51
   open 48.52
   other 48.59
Scalenectomy 83.45
Scalenotomy 83.19
Scaling and polishing, dental 96.54
Scan, scanning
   C.A.T. (computerized axial
      tomography) 88.38
      with computer assisted surgery
         (CAS) 00.31
      abdomen 88.01
      bone 88.38
         mineral density 88.98
      brain 87.03
      cardiac 87.41
      coronary 87.41
      head 87.03
      kidney 87.71
      skeletal 88.38
         mineral density 88.98
      thorax 87.41
   computerized axial tomography
      (C.A.T.) - see also Scan, C.A.T.
      88.38
   C.T. - see Scan, C.A.T.
   gallium - see Scan, radioisotope
   liver 92.02
   MUGA (multiple gated acquisition) -
      see Scan, radioisotope
   positron emission tomography (PET) -
      see Scan, radioisotope
   radioisotope
      adrenal 92.09
      bone 92.14
         marrow 92.05
      bowel 92.04

Scan, scanning (Continued)
   radioisotope (Continued)
      cardiac output 92.05
      cardiovascular 92.05
      cerebral 92.11
      circulation time 92.05
      eye 95.16
      gastrointestinal 92.04
      head NEC 92.12
      hematopoietic 92.05
      intestine 92.04
      iodine-131 92.01
      kidney 92.03
      liver 92.02
      lung 92.15
      lymphatic system 92.16
      myocardial infarction 92.05
      pancreatic 92.04
      parathyroid 92.13
      pituitary 92.11
      placenta 92.17
      protein-bound iodine 92.01
      pulmonary 92.15
      radio-iodine uptake 92.01
      renal 92.03
      specified site NEC 92.19
      spleen 92.05
      thyroid 92.01
      total body 92.18
      uterus 92.19
   renal 92.03
   thermal - see Thermography
Scapulectomy (partial) 77.81
   total 77.91
Scapulopexy 78.41
Scarification
   conjunctiva 10.33
   nasal veins (with packing) 21.03
   pericardium 36.39
   pleura 34.6
      chemical 34.92
         with cancer chemotherapy
            substance 34.92
            [99.25]
         tetracycline 34.92 [99.21]
Schanz operation (femoral osteotomy)
   77.35
Schauta (-Amreich) operation (radical
   vaginal hysterectomy) 68.79
   laparoscopic 68.71
Schede operation (thoracoplasty)
   33.34
Scheie operation
   cautery of sclera 12.62
   sclerostomy 12.62
Schlatter operation (total gastrectomy)
   43.99
Schroeder operation (endocervical
   excision) 67.39
Schuchardt operation (nonobstetrical
   episiotomy) 71.09
Schwartze operation (simple
   mastoidectomy) 20.41
Scintiphotography - see Scan,
   radioisotope
Scintiscan - see Scan, radioisotope
Sclerectomy (punch) (scissors) 12.65
   for retinal reattachment 14.49
   Holth's 12.65
   trephine 12.61
      with implant 14.41
Scleroplasty 12.89
Sclerosis - see Sclerotherapy
Sclerostomy (Scheie's) 12.62

Sclerotherapy
   esophageal varices (endoscopic) 42.33
   hemorrhoids 49.42
   pleura 34.92
      treatment of malignancy (cytotoxic
         agent) 34.92 [99.25]
      with tetracycline 34.92 [99.21]
   varicose vein 39.92
   vein NEC 39.92
Sclerotomy (exploratory) 12.89
   anterior 12.89
      with
         iridectomy 12.65
         removal of vitreous 14.71
   posterior 12.89
      with
         iridectomy 12.65
         removal of vitreous 14.72
Scott operation
   intestinal bypass for obesity 45.93
   jejunocolostomy (bypass) 45.93
Scraping
   corneal epithelium 11.41
      for smear or culture 11.21
   trachoma follicles 10.33
Scrotectomy (partial) 61.3
Scrotoplasty 61.49
Scrotorrhaphy 61.41
Scrototomy 61.0
Scrub, posterior nasal (adhesions)
   21.91
Sculpturing, heart valve - see
   Valvuloplasty, heart
Section - see also Division and Incision
   cesarean - see Cesarean section
   ganglion, sympathetic 05.0
   hypophyseal stalk - see also
      Hypophysectomy, partial 07.63
   ligamentum flavum (spine) -
      omit code
   nerve (cranial) (peripheral) NEC
      04.03
      acoustic 04.01
      spinal root (posterior) 03.1
      sympathetic 05.0
      trigeminal tract 04.02
   Saemisch (corneal) 11.1
   spinal ligament 80.49
      arcuate - omit code
      flavum - omit code
   tooth (impacted) 23.19
Seddon-Brooks operation (transfer of
   pectoralis major tendon) 83.75
Semb operation (apicolysis of lung)
   33.39
Senning operation (correction of
   transposition of great vessels) 35.91
Separation
   twins (attached) (conjoined) (Siamese)
      84.93
   asymmetrical (unequal) 84.93
   symmetrical (equal) 84.92
Septectomy
   atrial (closed) 35.41
      open 35.42
      transvenous method (balloon)
         35.41
   submucous (nasal) 21.5
Septoplasty NEC 21.88
   with submucous resection of septum
      21.5
Septorhinoplasty 21.84
Septostomy (atrial) (balloon) 35.41
Septotomy, nasal 21.1

Sequestrectomy
bone 77.00
  carpals, metacarpals 77.04
  clavicle 77.01
  facial 76.01
  femur 77.05
  fibula 77.07
  humerus 77.02
  nose 21.32
  patella 77.06
  pelvic 77.09
  phalanges (foot) (hand) 77.09
  radius 77.03
  scapula 77.01
  skull 01.25
  specified site NEC 77.09
  tarsals, metatarsals 77.08
  thorax (ribs) (sternum) 77.01
  tibia 77.07
  ulna 77.03
  vertebrae 77.09
nose 21.32
skull 01.25
Sesamoidectomy 77.98
Setback, ear 18.5
Sever operation (division of soft tissue of arm) 83.19
Severing of blepharorrhaphy 08.02
Sewell operation (heart) 36.2
Sharrard operation (iliopsoas muscle transfer) 83.77
Shaving
bone - *see also* Excision, lesion, bone 77.60
cornea (epithelium) 11.41
  for smear or culture 11.21
patella 77.66
Shelf operation (hip arthroplasty) 81.40
Shirodkar operation (encirclement suture, cervix) 67.59
Shock therapy
chemical 94.24
electroconvulsive 94.27
electrotonic 94.27
insulin 94.24
subconvulsive 94.26
Shortening
bone (fusion) 78.20
  femur 78.25
  specified site NEC - *see* category 78.2●
  tibia 78.27
  ulna 78.23
endopelvic fascia 69.22
extraocular muscle NEC 15.22
  multiple (two or more muscles) 15.4
eyelid margin 08.71
eye muscle NEC 15.22
  multiple (two or more muscles) (with lengthening) 15.4
finger (macrodactyly repair) 82.83
heel cord 83.85
levator palpebrae muscle 08.33
ligament - *see also* Arthroplasty
  round 69.22
  uterosacral 69.22
muscle 83.85
  extraocular 15.22
    multiple (two or more muscles) 15.4
  hand 82.55
sclera (for repair of retinal detachment) 14.59
  by scleral buckling - *see also* Buckling, scleral 14.49

Shortening *(Continued)*
tendon 83.85
  hand 82.55
ureter (with reimplantation) 56.41
Shunt - *see also* Anastomosis and Bypass, vascular
abdominovenous 54.94
aorta-coronary sinus 36.39
aorta (descending)-pulmonary (artery) 39.0
aortocarotid 39.22
aortoceliac 39.26
aortofemoral 39.25
aortoiliac 39.25
aortoiliofemoral 39.25
aortomesenteric 39.26
aorto-myocardial (graft) 36.2
aortorenal 39.24
aortosubclavian 39.22
apicoaortic 35.93
arteriovenous NEC 39.29
  for renal dialysis (by)
    anastomosis 39.27
    external cannula 39.93
ascending aorta to pulmonary artery (Waterston) 39.0
axillary-femoral 39.29
carotid-carotid 39.22
carotid-subclavian 39.22
caval-mesenteric 39.1
corpora cavernosa-corpus spongiosum 64.98
corpora-saphenous 64.98
descending aorta to pulmonary artery (Potts-Smith) 39.0
endolymphatic (-subarachnoid) 20.71
endolymph-perilymph 20.71
extracranial-intracranial (EC-IC) 39.28
femoroperoneal 39.29
femoropopliteal 39.29
iliofemoral 39.25
ilioiliac 39.25
intestinal
  large-to-large 45.94
  small-to-large 45.93
  small-to-small 45.91
left subclavian to descending aorta (Blalock-Park) 39.0
left-to-right (systemic-pulmonary artery) 39.0
left ventricle (heart) (apex) and aorta 35.93
lienorenal 39.1
lumbar-subarachnoid (with valve) NEC 03.79
mesocaval 39.1
peritoneal-jugular 54.94
peritoneo-vascular 54.94
peritoneovenous 54.94
pleuroperitoneal 34.05
pleurothecal (with valve) 03.79
portacaval (double) 39.1
portal-systemic 39.1
portal vein to vena cava 39.1
pulmonary-innominate 39.0
pulmonary vein to atrium 35.82
renoportal 39.1
right atrium and pulmonary artery 35.94
right ventricle and pulmonary artery (distal) 35.92
  in repair of
    pulmonary artery atresia 35.92
    transposition of great vessels 35.92
    truncus arteriosus 35.83

Shunt *(Continued)*
salpingothecal (with valve) 03.79
semicircular subarachnoid 20.71
spinal (thecal) (with valve) NEC 03.79
  subarachnoid-peritoneal 03.71
  subarachnoid-ureteral 03.72
splenorenal (venous) 39.1
  arterial 39.26
subarachnoid-peritoneal (with valve) 03.71
subarachnoid-ureteral (with valve) 03.72
subclavian-pulmonary 39.0
subdural-peritoneal (with valve) 02.34
superior mesenteric-caval 39.1
systemic-pulmonary artery 39.0
transjugular intrahepatic portosystemic [TIPS] 39.1
vena cava to pulmonary artery (Green) 39.21
ventricular (cerebral) (with valve) 02.2
  to
    abdominal cavity or organ 02.34
    bone marrow 02.39
    cervical subarachnoid space 02.2
    circulatory system 02.32
    cisterna magna 02.2
    extracranial site NEC 02.39
    gallbladder 02.34
    head or neck structure 02.31
    intracerebral site NEC 02.2
    lumbar site 02.39
    mastoid 02.31
    nasopharynx 02.31
    peritoneal 02.34
    thoracic cavity 02.33
    ureter 02.35
    urinary system 02.35
    venous system 02.32
ventriculoatrial (with valve) 02.32
ventriculocaval (with valve) 02.32
ventriculocisternal (with valve) 02.2
ventriculolumbar (with valve) 02.39
ventriculomastoid (with valve) 02.31
ventriculonasopharyngeal 02.31
ventriculopleural (with valve) 02.33
Sialoadenectomy (parotid) (sublingual) (submaxillary) 26.30
complete 26.32
partial 26.31
radical 26.32
Sialoadenolithotomy 26.0
Sialoadenotomy 26.0
Sialodochoplasty NEC 26.49
Sialogram 87.09
Sialolithotomy 26.0
Sieve, vena cava 38.7
Sigmoid bladder 57.87 [45.52]
Sigmoidectomy
laparoscopic 17.36
open and other 45.76
Sigmoidomyotomy 46.91
Sigmoidopexy (Moschowitz) 46.63
Sigmoidoproctectomy - *see also* Resection, rectum 48.69
Sigmoidoproctostomy 45.94
Sigmoidorectostomy 45.94
Sigmoidorrhaphy 46.75
Sigmoidoscopy (rigid) 48.23
with biopsy 45.25
flexible 45.24
through stoma (artificial) 45.22
transabdominal 45.21

Sigmoidosigmoidostomy 45.94
  proximal to distal segment
    laparoscopic 17.36
    open and other 45.76
Sigmoidostomy - see also Colostomy
    46.10
Sigmoidotomy 45.03
Sign language 93.75
Silver operation (bunionectomy) 77.59
Sinogram
  abdominal wall 88.03
  chest wall 87.38
  retroperitoneum 88.14
Sinusectomy (nasal) (complete) (partial)
    (with turbinectomy) 22.60
  antrum 22.62
    with Caldwell-Luc approach
        22.61
  ethmoid 22.63
  frontal 22.42
  maxillary 22.62
    with Caldwell-Luc approach 22.61
  sphenoid 22.64
Sinusotomy (nasal) 22.50
  antrum (intranasal) 22.2
    with external approach (Caldwell-
        Luc) 22.39
      radical (with removal of
          membrane lining) 22.31
  ethmoid 22.51
  frontal 22.41
  maxillary (intranasal) 22.2
    external approach (Caldwell-Luc)
        22.39
      radical (with removal of
          membrane lining) 22.31
  multiple 22.53
  perinasal 22.50
  sphenoid 22.52
Sistrunk operation (excision of
    thyroglossal cyst) 06.7
Size reduction
  abdominal wall (adipose) (pendulous)
      86.83
  arms (adipose) (batwing) 86.83
  breast (bilateral) 85.32
    unilateral 85.31
  buttocks (adipose) 86.83
  skin 86.83
  subcutaneous tissue 86.83
  thighs (adipose) 86.83
Skeletal series (x-ray) 88.31
SKyphoplasty 81.66
Sling - see also Operation, sling
  fascial (fascia lata)
    for facial weakness (trigeminal
        nerve paralysis) 86.81
      mouth 86.81
    orbicularis (mouth) 86.81
    tongue 25.59
  levator muscle (urethrocystopexy)
      59.71
  pubococcygeal 59.71
  rectum (puborectalis) 48.76
  tongue (fascial) 25.59
Slitting
  canaliculus for
    passage of tube 09.42
    removal of streptothrix 09.42
  lens 13.2
  prepuce (dorsal) (lateral) 64.91
Slocum operation (pes anserinus transfer)
    81.47
Sluder operation (tonsillectomy) 28.2

Small bowel series (x-ray) 87.63
Smith operation (open osteotomy of
    mandible) 76.62
Smith-Peterson operation (radiocarpal
    arthrodesis) 81.25
Smithwick operation (sympathectomy)
    05.29
Snaring, polyp, colon (endoscopic) 45.42
Snip, punctum (with dilation) 09.51
Soave operation (endorectal pull-
    through) 48.41
Somatotherapy, psychiatric NEC 94.29
Sonneberg operation (inferior maxillary
    neurectomy) 04.07
Sorondo-Ferré operation (hindquarter
    amputation) 84.19
Soutter operation (iliac crest fasciotomy)
    83.14
Spaulding-Richardson operation (uterine
    suspension) 69.22
Spectrophotometry NEC 89.39
  blood 89.39
  placenta 89.29
  urine 89.29
Spectroscopy
  intravascular 38.23
  near infrared (NIR) 38.23
Speech therapy NEC 93.75
Spermatocelectomy 63.2
Spermatocystectomy 60.73
Spermatocystotomy 60.72
Sphenoidectomy 22.64
Sphenoidotomy 22.52
Sphincterectomy, anal 49.6
Sphincteroplasty
  anal 49.79
    obstetrical laceration (current) 75.62
      old 49.79
  bladder neck 57.85
  pancreas 51.83
  sphincter of Oddi 51.83
Sphincterorrhaphy, anal 49.71
  obstetrical laceration (current)
      75.62
    old 49.79
Sphincterotomy
  anal (external) (internal) 49.59
    left lateral 49.51
    posterior 49.52
  bladder (neck) (transurethral) 57.91
  choledochal 51.82
    endoscopic 51.85
  iris 12.12
  pancreatic 51.82
    endoscopic 51.85
  sphincter of Oddi 51.82
    endoscopic 51.85
  transduodenal ampullary 51.82
    endoscopic 51.85
Spinal anesthesia - *omit code*
Spinelli operation (correction of inverted
    uterus) 75.93
Spineoplasty 81.66
Spirometry (incentive) (respiratory) 89.37
Spivack operation (permanent
    gastrostomy) 43.19
Splanchnicectomy 05.29
Splanchnicotomy 05.0
Splenectomy (complete) (total) 41.5
  partial 41.43
Splenogram 88.64
  radioisotope 92.05
Splenolysis 54.59
  laparoscopic 54.51

Splenopexy 41.95
Splenoplasty 41.95
Splenoportogram (by splenic
    arteriography) 88.64
Splenorrhaphy 41.95
Splenotomy 41.2
Splinting
  dental (for immobilization) 93.55
    orthodontic 24.7
  musculoskeletal 93.54
  ureteral 56.2
Splitting - see also Division
  canaliculus 09.52
  lacrimal papilla 09.51
  spinal cord tracts 03.29
    percutaneous 03.21
  tendon sheath 83.01
    hand 82.01
Spondylosyndesis - see also Fusion, spinal
    81.00
S.P. Rogers operation (knee
    disarticulation) 84.16
Ssabanejew-Frank operation (permanent
    gastrostomy) 43.19
Stab, intercostal 34.09
Stabilization, joint - see also Arthrodesis
  patella (for recurrent dislocation)
      81.44
Stacke operation (simple mastoidectomy)
    20.41
Stallard operation
    (conjunctivocystorhinostomy)
    09.82
  with insertion of tube or stent 09.83
Stamm (-Kader) operation (temporary
    gastrostomy) 43.19
Stapedectomy 19.19
  with incus replacement (homograft)
      (prosthesis) 19.11
  revision 19.29
    with incus replacement 19.21
Stapediolysis 19.0
Stapling
  artery 39.31
  blebs, lung (emphysematous) 32.21
  diaphysis - see also Stapling, epiphyseal
      plate 78.20
  epiphyseal plate 78.20
    femur 78.25
    fibula 78.27
    humerus 78.22
    radius 78.23
    specified site NEC 78.29
    tibia 78.27
    ulna 78.23
  gastric varices 44.91
  graft - see Graft
  left atrial appendage 37.36
  vein 39.32
STARR (stapled transanal rectal resection)
    48.74
StaXx® FX Structural Kyphoplasty
    System 81.66
Steinberg operation 44.5
Steindler operation
  fascia stripping (for cavus deformity)
      83.14
  flexorplasty (elbow) 83.77
  muscle transfer 83.77
Stereotactic radiosurgery 92.30
  cobalt 60 92.32
  linear accelerator (LINAC) 92.31
  multi-source 92.32
  particle beam 92.33

◀ New   ◀◀ Revised   ~~deleted~~ Deleted   ● Use Additional Digit(s)   Omit code

Stereotactic radiosurgery (*Continued*)
  particulate 92.33
  radiosurgery NEC 92.39
  single source photon 92.31
Stereotactic head frame application
  93.59
Sterilization
  female - *see also* specific operation
    66.39
  male NEC - *see also* Ligation, vas
    deferens 63.70
Sternotomy 77.31
  as operative approach - *omit code*
  for bone marrow biopsy 41.31
Stewart operation (renal plication with
  pyeloplasty) 55.87
Stimulation (electronic) - *see also* Implant,
  electronic stimulator
  bone growth (percutaneous) - *see*
    category 78.9●
    transcutaneous (surface) 99.86
  cardiac (external) 99.62
    internal 37.91
  carotid sinus 99.64
  CaverMap™ 89.58
  defibrillator
    as part of intraoperative testing
     - *omit code*
    catheter based invasive
     electrophysiologic testing
     37.26
    device interrogation only without
     arrhythmia induction (bedside
     check) 89.45–89.49
    non-invasive programmed electrical
     stimulation (NIPS) 37.20
  electrophysiologic, cardiac
    as part of intraoperative testing
     - *omit code*
    catheter based invasive
     electrophysiologic testing
     37.26
    device interrogation only without
     arrhythmia induction (bedside
     check) 89.45–89.49
    noninvasive programmed electrical
     stimulation (NIPS) 37.20
  nerve
    CaverMap™ 89.58
    penile 89.58
    peripheral or spinal cord,
     transcutaneous 93.39
Stitch, Kelly-Stoeckel (urethra) 59.3
Stomatoplasty 27.59
Stomatorrhaphy 27.52
Stone operation (anoplasty) 49.79
Strapping (non-traction) 93.59
Strassman operation (metroplasty) 69.49
Strayer operation (gastrocnemius
  recession) 83.72
Stretching
  eyelid (with elongation) 08.71
  fascia 93.28
  foreskin 99.95
  iris 12.63
  muscle 93.27
  nerve (cranial) (peripheral) 04.91
  tendon 93.27
Stripping
  bone - *see also* Incision, bone 77.10
  carotid sinus 39.89 ⬅||||
  cranial suture 02.01
  fascia 83.14
    hand 82.12

Stripping (*Continued*)
  membranes for surgical induction of
    labor 73.1
  meninges (cerebral) 01.51
    spinal 03.4
  saphenous vein, varicose 38.59
  subdural membrane (cerebral) 01.51
    spinal 03.4
  varicose veins (lower limb) 38.59
    upper limb 38.53
  vocal cords 30.09
Stromeyer-Little operation (hepatotomy)
  50.0
Strong operation (unbridling of celiac
  artery axis) 39.91
Stryker frame 93.59
Study
  bone mineral density 88.98
  bundle of His 37.29
  color vision 95.06
  conduction, nerve (median) 89.15
  dark adaptation, eye 95.07
  electrophysiologic stimulation and
    recording, cardiac
    as part of intraoperative testing
     - *omit code*
    catheter based invasive
     electrophysiologic testing
     37.26
    device interrogation only without
     arrhythmia induction (bedside
     check) 89.45–89.49
    noninvasive programmed electrical
     stimulation (NIPS) 37.20
  function - *see also* Function, study
    radioisotope - *see* Scan,
     radioisotope
  lacrimal flow (radiographic) 87.05
  ocular motility 95.15
  pulmonary
    airway flow measurement,
     endoscopic 33.72
    function - *see* categories 89.37-89.38
  radiographic - *see* Radiography
  radio-iodinated triolein 92.04
  renal clearance 92.03
  spirometer 89.37
  tracer - *see also* Scan, radioisotope eye
    (P32) 95.16
  ultrasonic - *see* Ultrasonography
  visual field 95.05
  xenon flow NEC 92.19
    cardiovascular 92.05
    pulmonary 92.15
Sturmdorf operation (conization of
  cervix) 67.2
Submucous resection
  larynx 30.29
  nasal septum 21.5
Summerskill operation
  (dacryocystorhinostomy by
  intubation) 09.81
Surgery
  computer assisted (CAS) 00.39
    with robotics – *see* category 17.4●
    CAS with CT/CTA 00.31
    CAS with fluoroscopy 00.33
    CAS with MR/MRA 00.32
    CAS with multiple datasets 00.35
     imageless 00.34
     other CAS 00.39
    IGS - *see* Surgery, computer assisted
    image guided - *see* Surgery,
     computer assisted

Surgery (*Continued*)
  computer assisted (*Continued*)
    navigation (CT-free, IGN image
     guided, imageless) - *see*
     Surgery, computer assisted
  robotic assisted – *see* category 17.4●
Surmay operation (jejunostomy) 46.39
Suspension
  balanced, for traction 93.45
  bladder NEC 57.89
  diverticulum, pharynx 29.59
  kidney 55.7
  Olshausen (uterus) 69.22
  ovary 65.79
  paraurethral (Pereyra) 59.6
  periurethral 59.6
  urethra (retropubic) (sling) 59.5
  urethrovesical
    Goebel-Frangenheim-Stoeckel 59.4
    gracilis muscle transplant 59.71
    levator muscle sling 59.71
    Marshall-Marchetti (-Krantz) 59.5
    Millin-Read 59.4
    suprapubic 59.4
  uterus (abdominal or vaginal
    approach) 69.22
  vagina 70.77
    with graft or prosthesis 70.78
Suture (laceration)
  abdominal wall 54.63
    secondary 54.61
  adenoid fossa 28.7
  adrenal (gland) 07.44
  aneurysm (cerebral) (peripheral) 39.52
  anus 49.71
    obstetric laceration (current) 75.62
    old 49.79
  aorta 39.31
  aponeurosis - *see also* Suture, tendon
    83.64
  arteriovenous fistula 39.53
  artery 39.31
    percutaneous puncture
     closure - *omit code*
  bile duct 51.79
  bladder 57.81
    obstetric laceration (current) 75.61
  blood vessel NEC 39.30
    artery 39.31
     percutaneous puncture
      closure - *omit code*
    vein 39.32
  breast (skin) 85.81
  bronchus 33.41
  bursa 83.99
    hand 82.99
  canaliculus 09.73
  cecum 46.75
  cerebral meninges 02.11
  cervix (traumatic laceration) 67.61
    internal os, encirclement 67.59
    obstetric laceration (current) 75.51
    old 67.69
  chest wall 34.71
  cleft palate 27.62
  clitoris 71.4
  colon 46.75
  common duct 51.71
  conjunctiva 10.6
  cornea 11.51
    with conjunctival flap 11.53
  corneoscleral 11.51
    with conjunctival flap 11.53
  diaphragm 34.82

S

Suture (Continued)
  duodenum 46.71
    ulcer (bleeding) (perforated)
      44.42
      endoscopic 44.43
  dura mater (cerebral) 02.11
    spinal 03.59
  ear, external 18.4
  enterocele 70.92
    with graft or prosthesis 70.93
  entropion 08.42
  epididymis (and)
    spermatic cord 63.51
    vas deferens 63.81
  episiotomy - see Episiotomy
  esophagus 42.82
  eyeball 16.89
  eyebrow 08.81
  eyelid 08.81
    with entropion or ectropion repair
      08.42
  fallopian tube 66.71
  fascia 83.65
    hand 82.46
    to skeletal attachment 83.89
      hand 82.89
  gallbladder 51.91
  ganglion, sympathetic 05.81
  gingiva 24.32
  great vessel 39.30
    artery 39.31
    vein 39.32
  gum 24.32
  heart 37.49
  hepatic duct 51.79
  hymen 70.76
  ileum 46.73
  intestine 46.79
    large 46.75
    small 46.73
  jejunum 46.73
  joint capsule 81.96
    with arthroplasty - see Arthroplasty
    ankle 81.94
    foot 81.94
    lower extremity NEC 81.95
    upper extremity 81.93
  kidney 55.81
  labia 71.71
  laceration - see Suture, by site
  larynx 31.61
  ligament 81.96
    with arthroplasty - see Arthroplasty
    ankle 81.94
    broad 69.29
    Cooper's 54.64
    foot and toes 81.94
    gastrocolic 54.73
    knee 81.95
    lower extremity NEC 81.95
    sacrouterine 69.29
    upper extremity 81.93
    uterine 69.29
  ligation - see Ligation
  lip 27.51
  liver 50.61
  lung 33.43
  meninges (cerebral) 02.11
    spinal 03.59
  mesentery 54.75
  mouth 27.52
  muscle 83.65
    hand 82.46
    ocular (oblique) (rectus) 15.7

Suture (Continued)
  nerve (cranial) (peripheral) 04.3
    sympathetic 05.81
  nose (external) (internal) 21.81
    for epistaxis 21.09
  obstetric laceration NEC 75.69
    bladder 75.61
    cervix 75.51
    corpus uteri 75.52
    pelvic floor 75.69
    perineum 75.69
    periurethral 75.69
    rectum 75.62
    sphincter ani 75.62
    urethra 75.61
    uterus 75.50
    vagina 75.69
    vulva 75.69
  omentum 54.64
  ovary 65.71
    laparoscopic 65.74
  palate 27.61
    cleft 27.62
  palpebral fissure 08.59
  pancreas 52.95
  pelvic floor 71.71
    obstetric laceration (current) 75.69
  penis 64.41
  peptic ulcer (bleeding) (perforated)
    44.40
  pericardium 37.49
  perineum (female) 71.71
    after delivery 75.69
      episiotomy repair - see
        Episiotomy
    male 86.59
  periosteum 78.20
    carpal, metacarpal 78.24
    femur 78.25
    fibula 78.27
    humerus 78.22
    pelvic 78.29
    phalanges (foot) (hand) 78.29
    radius 78.23
    specified site NEC 78.29
    tarsal, metatarsal 78.28
    tibia 78.27
    ulna 78.23
    vertebrae 78.29
  peritoneum 54.64
  periurethral tissue to symphysis pubis
    59.5
  pharynx 29.51
  pleura 34.93
  rectum 48.71
    obstetric laceration (current) 75.62
  retina (for reattachment) 14.59
  sacrouterine ligament 69.29
  salivary gland 26.41
  scalp 86.59
    replantation 86.51
  sclera (with repair of conjunctiva)
    12.81
  scrotum (skin) 61.41
  secondary
    abdominal wall 54.61
    episiotomy 75.69
    peritoneum 54.64
  sigmoid 46.75
  skin (mucous membrane) (without
    graft) 86.59
    with graft - see Graft, skin
    breast 85.81
    ear 18.4

Suture (Continued)
  skin (Continued)
    eyebrow 08.81
    eyelid 08.81
    nose 21.81
    penis 64.41
    scalp 86.59
      replantation 86.51
    scrotum 61.41
    vulva 71.71
  specified site NEC - see Repair, by site
  spermatic cord 63.51
  sphincter ani 49.71
    obstetric laceration (current) 75.62
      old 49.79
  spinal meninges 03.59
  spleen 41.95
  stomach 44.61
    ulcer (bleeding) (perforated) 44.41
      endoscopic 44.43
  subcutaneous tissue (without skin
    graft) 86.59
    with graft - see Graft, skin
  tendon (direct) (immediate) (primary)
    83.64
    delayed (secondary) 83.62
      hand NEC 82.43
        flexors 82.42
    hand NEC 82.45
      delayed (secondary) 82.43
      flexors 82.44
        delayed (secondary) 82.42
    ocular 15.7
    rotator cuff 83.63
    sheath 83.61
      hand 82.41
    supraspinatus (rotator cuff repair)
      83.63
    to skeletal attachment 83.88
      hand 82.85
  Tenon's capsule 15.7
  testis 62.61
  thymus 07.93
  thyroid gland 06.93
  tongue 25.51
  tonsillar fossa 28.7
  trachea 31.71
  tunica vaginalis 61.41
  ulcer (bleeding) (perforated) (peptic)
    44.40
    duodenum 44.42
      endoscopic 44.43
    gastric 44.41
      endoscopic 44.43
    intestine 46.79
    skin 86.59
    stomach 44.41
      endoscopic 44.43
  ureter 56.82
  urethra 58.41
    obstetric laceration (current) 75.61
  uterosacral ligament 69.29
  uterus 69.41
    obstetric laceration (current) 75.50
      old 69.49
  uvula 27.73
  vagina 70.71
    obstetric laceration (current) 75.69
      old 70.79
  vas deferens 63.81
  vein 39.32
  vulva 71.71
    obstetric laceration (current) 75.69
      old 71.79

◀ New   ⬅ Revised   ~~deleted~~ Deleted   ● Use Additional Digit(s)   ▨ Omit code

Suture-ligation - *see also* Ligation
   blood vessel - *see* Ligation, blood vessel
Sweep, anterior iris 12.97
Swenson operation
   bladder reconstruction 57.87
   proctectomy 48.49
Swinney operation (urethral
   reconstruction) 58.46
Switch, switching
   coronary arteries 35.84
   great arteries, total 35.84
Syme operation
   ankle amputation through malleoli of
     tibia and fibula 84.14
   urethrotomy, external 58.0
Sympathectomy NEC 05.29
   cervical 05.22
   cervicothoracic 05.22
   lumbar 05.23
   periarterial 05.25

Sympathectomy NEC *(Continued)*
   presacral 05.24
   renal 05.29
   thoracolumbar 05.23
   tympanum 20.91
Sympatheticotripsy 05.0
Symphysiotomy 77.39
   assisting delivery (obstetrical)
     73.94
   kidney (horseshoe) 55.85
Symphysis, pleural 34.6
Synchondrotomy - *see also* Division,
   cartilage 80.40
Syndactylization 86.89
Syndesmotomy - *see also* Division,
   ligament 80.40
Synechiotomy
   endometrium 68.21
   iris (posterior) 12.33
     anterior 12.32

Synovectomy (joint) (complete) (partial)
   80.70
   ankle 80.77
   elbow 80.72
   foot and toe 80.78
   hand and finger 80.74
   hip 80.75
   knee 80.76
   shoulder 80.71
   specified site NEC 80.79
   spine 80.79
   tendon sheath 83.42
     hand 82.33
   wrist 80.73
Syringing
   lacrimal duct or sac 09.43
   nasolacrimal duct 09.43
     with
       dilation 09.43
       insertion of tube or stent 09.44

T

Taarnhoj operation (trigeminal nerve root
   decompression) 04.41
Tack operation (sacculotomy) 20.79
Tactile Guidance System™ [TGS] – *see*
   category 17.4●
Take-down
   anastomosis
     arterial 39.49
     blood vessel 39.49
     gastric, gastrointestinal 44.5
     intestine 46.93
     stomach 44.5
     vascular 39.49
     ventricular 02.43
   arterial bypass 39.49
   arteriovenous shunt 39.43
     with creation of new shunt 39.42
   cecostomy 46.52
   colostomy 46.52
   duodenostomy 46.51
   enterostomy 46.50
   esophagostomy 42.83
   gastroduodenostomy 44.5
   gastrojejunostomy 44.5
   ileostomy 46.51
   intestinal stoma 46.50
     large 46.52
     small 46.51
   jejunoileal bypass 46.93
   jejunostomy 46.51
   laryngostomy 31.62
   sigmoidostomy 46.52
   stoma
     bile duct 51.79
     bladder 57.82
     bronchus 33.42
     common duct 51.72
     esophagus 42.83
     gallbladder 51.92
     hepatic duct 51.79
     intestine 46.50
       large 46.52
       small 46.51
     kidney 55.82
     larynx 31.62
     rectum 48.72
     stomach 44.62

Take-down *(Continued)*
   stoma *(Continued)*
     thorax 34.72
     trachea 31.72
     ureter 56.83
     urethra 58.42
   systemic-pulmonary artery
       anastomosis 39.49
     in total repair of tetralogy of Fallot
       35.81
   tracheostomy 31.72
   vascular anastomosis or bypass 39.49
   ventricular shunt (cerebral) 02.43
Talectomy 77.98
Talma-Morison operation (omentopexy)
   54.74
Tamponade
   esophageal 96.06
   intrauterine (nonobstetric) 69.91
     after delivery or abortion 75.8
     antepartum 73.1
   vagina 96.14
     after delivery or abortion 75.8
     antepartum 73.1
Tanner operation (devascularization of
   stomach) 44.99
Tap
   abdomen 54.91
   chest 34.91
   cisternal 01.01
   cranial 01.09
   joint 81.91
   lumbar (diagnostic) (removal of dye)
     03.31
   perilymphatic 20.79
   spinal (diagnostic) 03.31
   subdural (through fontanel) 01.09
   thorax 34.91
Tarsectomy 08.20
   de Grandmont 08.35
Tarsoplasty - *see also* Reconstruction,
   eyelid 08.70
Tarsorrhaphy (lateral) 08.52
   division or severing 08.02
Tattooing
   cornea 11.91
   skin 86.02
Tautening, eyelid for entropion 08.42
Telemetry (cardiac) 89.54

Teleradiotherapy
   beta particles 92.25
     intra-operative 92.41
   Betatron 92.24
   cobalt-60 92.23
   electrons 92.25
     intra-operative 92.41
   iodine-125 92.23
   linear accelerator 92.24
   neutrons 92.26
   particulate radiation NEC 92.26
   photons 92.24
   protons 92.26
   radioactive cesium 92.23
   radioisotopes NEC 92.23
Temperament assessment 94.02
Temperature gradient study - *see also*
   Thermography 88.89
Tendinoplasty - *see* Repair, tendon
Tendinosuture (immediate) (primary) -
   see also Suture, tendon 83.64
   hand - *see also* Suture, tendon, hand
     82.45
Tendolysis 83.91
   hand 82.91
Tendoplasty - *see* Repair, tendon
Tenectomy 83.39
   eye 15.13
     levator palpebrae 08.33
     multiple (two or more tendons) 15.3
   hand 82.29
   levator palpebrae 08.33
   tendon sheath 83.31
     hand 82.21
Tenodesis (tendon fixation to skeletal
   attachment) 83.88
   Fowler 82.85
   hand 82.85
Tenolysis 83.91
   hand 82.91
Tenomyoplasty - *see also* Repair, tendon
   83.88
   hand - *see also* Repair, tendon, hand 82.86
Tenomyotomy - *see* Tenonectomy
Tenonectomy 83.42
   for graft 83.41
     hand 82.32
   hand 82.33
     for graft 82.32

S & T

Tenontomyoplasty - *see* Repair, tendon
Tenontoplasty - *see* Repair, tendon
Tenoplasty - *see also* Repair, tendon 83.88
  hand - *see also* Repair, tendon, hand
    82.86
Tenorrhaphy - *see also* Suture, tendon
  83.64
  hand - *see also* Suture, tendon, hand
    82.45
  to skeletal attachment 83.88
    hand 82.85
Tenosuspension 83.88
  hand 82.86
Tenosuture - *see also* Suture, tendon
  83.64
  hand - *see also* Suture, tendon, hand
    82.45
  to skeletal attachment 83.88
    hand 82.85
Tenosynovectomy 83.42
  hand 82.33
Tenotomy 83.13
  Achilles tendon 83.11
  adductor (hip) (subcutaneous) 83.12
  eye 15.12
    levator palpebrae 08.38
    multiple (two or more tendons)
      15.4
  hand 82.11
  levator palpebrae 08.38
  pectoralis minor tendon
    (decompression thoracic outlet)
    83.13
  stapedius 19.0
  tensor tympani 19.0
Tenovaginotomy - *see* Tenotomy
Tensing, orbicularis oculi 08.59
Termination of pregnancy
  by
    aspiration curettage 69.51
    dilation and curettage 69.01
    hysterectomy - *see* Hysterectomy
    hysterotomy 74.91
    intra-amniotic injection (saline)
      75.0
Test, testing (for)
  14 C-Urea breath 89.39
  auditory function NEC 95.46
  Bender Visual-Motor Gestalt 94.02
  Benton Visual Retention 94.02
  cardiac (vascular)
    function NEC 89.59
    stress 89.44
      bicycle ergometer 89.43
      Masters' two-step 89.42
      treadmill 89.41
  Denver developmental (screening)
    94.02
  fetus, fetal
    nonstress (fetal activity acceleration
      determinations) 75.34
    oxytocin challenge (contraction
      stress) 75.35
    sensitivity (to oxytocin) - *omit code*
  function
    cardiac NEC 89.59
    hearing NEC 95.46
    muscle (by)
      electromyography 93.08
      manual 93.04
    neurologic NEC 89.15
    vestibular 95.46
      clinical 95.44
  glaucoma NEC 95.26

Test, testing (Continued)
  hearing 95.47
    clinical NEC 95.42
  intelligence 94.01
  internal jugular-subclavian venous
    reflux 89.62
  intracarotid amobarbital (Wada) 89.10
  Masters' two-step stress (cardiac) 89.42
  muscle function (by)
    electromyography 93.08
    manual 93.04
  neurologic function NEC 89.15
  neurophysiologic monitoring
    intra-operative 00.94
  nocturnal penile tumescence 89.29
  provocative, for glaucoma 95.26
  psychologic NEC 94.08
  psychometric 94.01
  radio-cobalt B12 Schilling 92.04
  range of motion 93.05
  rotation (Bárány chair) (hearing) 95.45
  sleep disorder function - *see* categories
    89.17–89.18
  Stanford-Binet 94.01
  Thallium stress (transesophageal
    pacing) 89.44
  tuning fork (hearing) 95.42
  Urea breath, (14 C) 89.39
  vestibular function NEC 95.46
    thermal 95.44
  Wada (hemispheric function) 89.10
  whispered speech (hearing) 95.42
TEVAP (transurethral electrovaporization
  of prostate) 60.29
Thalamectomy 01.41
Thalamotomy 01.41
  by stereotactic radiosurgery 92.32
    cobalt 60 92.32
    linear accelerator (LINAC) 92.31
    multi-source 92.32
    particle beam 92.33
    particulate 92.33
    radiosurgery NEC 92.39
    single source photon 92.31
Thal operation (repair of esophageal
  stricture) 42.85
Theleplasty 85.87
Therapy
  Antabuse 94.25
  aqueous oxygen (AO) 00.49
  art 93.89
  aversion 94.33
  behavior 94.33
  Bennett respirator - *see* category
    96.7●
  blind rehabilitation NEC 93.78
  Byrd respirator - *see* category 96.7●
  carbon dioxide 94.25
  cobalt-60 92.23
  conditioning, psychiatric 94.33
  continuous positive airway pressure
    (CPAP) 93.90
    delivered by
      endotracheal tube - *see* category
        96.7●
      tracheostomy – *see* category
        96.7●
  croupette, croup tent 93.94
  daily living activities 93.83
    for the blind 93.78
  dance 93.89
  desensitization 94.33
  detoxification 94.25
  diversional 93.81

Therapy (Continued)
  domestic tasks 93.83
    for the blind 93.78
  Downstream® system 00.49
  educational (bed-bound children)
    (handicapped) 93.82
  electroconvulsive (ECT) 94.27
  electroshock (EST) 94.27
    subconvulsive 94.26
  electrotonic (ETT) 94.27
  encounter group 94.44
  extinction 94.33
  family 94.42
  fog (inhalation) 93.94
  gamma ray 92.23
  group NEC 94.44
    for psychosexual dysfunctions 94.41
  hearing NEC 95.49
  heat NEC 93.35
    for cancer treatment 99.85
  helium 93.98
  hot pack(s) 93.35
  hyperbaric oxygen 93.95
    wound 93.59
  hyperthermia NEC 93.35
    for cancer treatment 99.85
  individual, psychiatric NEC 94.39
    for psychosexual dysfunction
      94.34
  industrial 93.89
  infrared irradiation 93.35
  inhalation NEC 93.96
    nitric oxide 00.12
  insulin shock 94.24
  intermittent positive pressure
    breathing (IPPB) 93.91
  IPPB (intermittent positive pressure
    breathing) 93.91
  leech 99.99
  lithium 94.22
  LITT (laser interstitial thermal therapy)
    under guidance
    lesion
      brain 17.61
      breast 17.69
      head and neck 17.62
      liver 17.63
      lung 17.69
      prostate 17.69
      thyroid 17.62
  maggot 86.28
  manipulative, osteopathic - *see also*
    Manipulation, osteopathic
    93.67
  manual arts 93.81
  methadone 94.25
  mist (inhalation) 93.94
  music 93.84
  nebulizer 93.94
  neuroleptic 94.23
  nitric oxide 00.12
  occupational 93.83
  oxygen 93.96
    aqueous 00.49
    catalytic 93.96
    hyperbaric 93.95
      wound 93.59
    SuperSaturated 00.49
    wound (hyperbaric) 93.59
  paraffin bath 93.35
  physical NEC 93.39
    combined (without mention of
      components) 93.38
    diagnostic NEC 93.09

Therapy *(Continued)*
  play 93.81
    psychotherapeutic 94.36
  positive and expiratory pressure - *see*
    category 96.7●
  psychiatric NEC 94.39
    drug NEC 94.25
      lithium 94.22
  radiation 92.29
    contact (150 KVP or less) 92.21
    deep (200-300 KVP) 92.22
    electron, intra-operative 92.41
    high voltage (200-300 KVP) 92.22
    low voltage (150 KVP or less) 92.21
    megavoltage 92.24
    orthovoltage 92.22
    particle source NEC 92.26
    photon 92.24
    radioisotope (teleradiotherapy)
      92.23
    retinal lesion 14.26
    superficial (150 KVP or less) 92.21
    supervoltage 92.24
  radioisotope, radioisotopic NEC 92.29
    implantation or insertion 92.27
    injection or instillation 92.28
    teleradiotherapy 92.23
  radium (radon) 92.23
  recreational 93.81
  rehabilitation NEC 93.89
  respiratory NEC 93.99
    bi-level positive airway pressure
      [BiPAP] 93.90
      delivered by
        endotracheal tube - *see*
          category 96.7●
        tracheostomy – *see* category
          96.7●
    continuous positive airway pressure
      [CPAP] 93.90
      delivered by
        endotracheal tube - *see*
          category 96.7●
        tracheostomy – *see* category
          96.7●
    endotracheal respiratory assistance -
      see category 96.7●
    intermittent positive pressure
      breathing [IPPB] 93.91
    negative pressure (continuous)
      [CNP] 93.99
    nitric oxide 00.12
    non-invasive positive pressure
      (NIPPV) 93.90
    other continuous invasive
      (unspecified duration)
        96.70
      for less than 96 consecutive hours
        96.71
      for 96 consecutive hours or more
        96.72
    positive end expiratory pressure
      [PEEP]
      invasive - *see* category 96.7●
      non-invasive 93.90
  root canal 23.70
    with
      apicoectomy 23.72
      irrigation 23.71
  shock
    chemical 94.24
    electric 94.27
      subconvulsive 94.26
    insulin 94.24

Therapy *(Continued)*
  speech 93.75
    for correction of defect 93.74
  SuperOxygenation (SSO₂) 00.49
  SuperSaturated oxygen 00.49
  ultrasound
    heat therapy 93.35
    hyperthermia for cancer treatment
      99.85
    physical therapy 93.35
    therapeutic - *see* Ultrasound
  ultraviolet light 99.82
Thermocautery - *see* Cauterization
Thermography 88.89
  blood vessel 88.86
  bone 88.83
  breast 88.85
  cerebral 88.81
  eye 88.82
  lymph gland 88.89
  muscle 88.84
  ocular 88.82
  osteoarticular 88.83
  specified site NEC 88.89
  vein, deep 88.86
Thermokeratoplasty 11.74
Thermoplasty ◀
  bronchoscopic, bronchial (lung)
    32.27 ◀
Thermosclerectomy 12.62
Thermotherapy (hot packs) (paraffin
  bath) NEC 93.35
  prostate
    by
      microwave 60.96
      radiofrequency 60.97
    transurethral microwave
      thermotherapy (TUMT) 60.96
    transurethral needle ablation
      (TUNA) 60.97
    TUMT (transurethral microwave
      thermotherapy) 60.96
    TUNA (transurethral needle
      ablation) 60.97
Thiersch operation
  anus 49.79
  skin graft 86.69
    hand 86.62
Thompson operation
  cleft lip repair 27.54
  correction of lymphedema 40.9
  quadricepsplasty 83.86
  thumb apposition with bone graft
    82.69
Thoracectomy 34.09
  for lung collapse 33.34
Thoracentesis 34.91
Thoracocentesis 34.91
Thoracolysis (for collapse of lung) 33.39
Thoracoplasty (anterior) (extrapleural)
  (paravertebral) (posterolateral)
  (complete) partial) 33.34
Thoracoscopy, transpleural (for
  exploration) 34.21
Thoracostomy 34.09
  for lung collapse 33.32
Thoracotomy (with drainage) 34.09
  as operative approach - *omit code*
  exploratory 34.02
Thoratec® implantable ventricular assist
  device (IVAD™) 37.66
Thoratec® ventricular assist device
  (VAD) system 37.66

Three-snip operation, punctum 09.51
Thrombectomy 38.00
  with endarterectomy - *see*
    Endarterectomy
  abdominal
    artery 38.06
    vein 38.07
  aorta (arch) (ascending) (descending)
    38.04
  arteriovenous shunt or cannula 39.49
  bovine graft 39.49
  coronary artery 36.09
  head and neck vessel NEC 38.02
  intracranial vessel NEC 38.01
  lower limb
    artery 38.08
    vein 38.09
  mechanical
    endovascular
      head and neck 39.74
  pulmonary vessel 38.05
  thoracic vessel NEC 38.05
  upper limb (artery) (vein) 38.03
Thromboendarterectomy 38.10
  abdominal 38.16
  aorta (arch) (ascending) (descending)
    38.14
  coronary artery 36.09
    open chest approach 36.03
  head and neck NEC 38.12
  intracranial NEC 38.11
  lower limb 38.18
  thoracic NEC 38.15
  upper limb 38.13
Thymectomy 07.80
  partial (open) (other) 07.81
    thoracoscopic 07.83
  total (open) (other) 07.82
    thoracoscopic 07.84
  transcervical 07.99
Thyrochondrotomy 31.3
Thyrocricoidectomy 30.29
Thyrocricotomy (for assistance in
  breathing) 31.1
Thyroidectomy NEC 06.39
  by mediastinotomy - *see also*
    Thyroidectomy, substernal
      06.50
  with laryngectomy - *see* Laryngectomy
  complete or total 06.4
    substernal (by mediastinotomy)
      (transsternal route) 06.52
    transoral route (lingual) 06.6
  lingual (complete) (partial) (subtotal)
    (total) 06.6
  partial or subtotal NEC 06.39
    with complete removal of remaining
      lobe 06.2
    submental route (lingual) 06.6
    substernal (by mediastinotomy)
      (transsternal route) 06.51
  remaining tissue 06.4
  submental route (lingual) 06.6
  substernal (by mediastinotomy)
    (transsternal route) 06.50
    complete or total 06.52
    partial or subtotal 06.51
  transoral route (lingual) 06.6
  transsternal route - *see also*
    Thyroidectomy, substernal
      06.50
  unilateral (with removal of isthmus)
    (with removal of portion of other
    lobe) 06.2

◀ New   ◀▥ Revised   ~~deleted~~ Deleted   ● Use Additional Digit(s)   ▓ Omit code   **1225**

Thyroidorrhaphy 06.93
Thyroidotomy (field) (gland) NEC 06.09
   postoperative 06.02
Thyrotomy 31.3
   with tantalum plate 31.69
Tirofiban (HCL), infusion 99.20
Toilette
   skin - *see* Debridement, skin or
      subcutaneous tissue
   tracheostomy 96.55
Token economy (behavior therapy)
   94.33
Tomkins operation (metroplasty) 69.49
Tomography - *see also* Radiography
   abdomen NEC 88.02
   cardiac 87.42
   computerized axial NEC 88.38
      abdomen 88.01
      bone 88.38
         quantitative 88.98
      brain 87.03
      cardiac 87.41
      coronary 87.41
      head 87.03
      kidney 87.71
      skeletal 88.38
         quantitative 88.98
      thorax 87.41
   head NEC 87.04
   kidney NEC 87.72
   lung 87.42
   optical coherence (intravascular
      imaging)
      coronary vessel(s) 38.24
      non-coronary vessel(s) 38.25
   thorax NEC 87.42
Tongue tie operation 25.91
Tonography 95.26
Tonometry 89.11
Tonsillectomy 28.2
   with adenoidectomy 28.3
Tonsillotomy 28.0
Topectomy 01.32
Torek (-Bevan) operation (orchidopexy)
   (first stage) (second stage) 62.5
Torkildsen operation (ventriculocisternal
   shunt) 02.2
Torpin operation (cul-de-sac resection)
   70.92
Toti operation (dacryocystorhinostomy)
   09.81
Touchas operation 86.83
Touroff operation (ligation of subclavian
   artery) 38.85
Toxicology - *see* Examination, microscopic
TPN (total parenteral nutrition) 99.15
Trabeculectomy ab externo 12.64
Trabeculodialysis 12.59
Trabeculotomy ab externo 12.54
Trachelectomy 67.4
Trachelopexy 69.22
Tracheloplasty 67.69
Trachelorrhaphy (Emmet) (suture) 67.61
   obstetrical 75.51
Trachelotomy 69.95
   obstetrical 73.93
Tracheocricotomy (for assistance in
   breathing) 31.1
Tracheofissure 31.1
Tracheography 87.32
Tracheolaryngotomy (emergency) 31.1
   permanent opening 31.29
Tracheoplasty 31.79
   with artificial larynx 31.75

Tracheorrhaphy 31.71
Tracheoscopy NEC 31.42
   through tracheotomy (stoma) 31.41
Tracheostomy (emergency) (temporary)
   (for assistance in breathing) 31.1
   mediastinal 31.21
   percutaneous dilatational
      other permanent 31.29
      temporary 31.1
   permanent NEC 31.29
   revision 31.74
Tracheotomy (emergency) (temporary)
   (for assistance in breathing) 31.1
   percutaneous dilatational
      other permanent 31.29
      temporary 31.1
   permanent 31.29
Tracing, carotid pulse with ECG lead
   89.56
Traction
   with reduction of fracture or
      dislocation - *see* Reduction,
      fracture *and* Reduction,
      dislocation
   adhesive tape (skin) 93.46
   boot 93.46
   Bryant's (skeletal) 93.44
   Buck's 93.46
   caliper tongs 93.41
      with synchronous insertion of
         device 02.94
   Cortel's (spinal) 93.42
   Crutchfield tongs 93.41
      with synchronous insertion of
         device 02.94
   Dunlop's (skeletal) 93.44
   gallows 93.46
   Gardner Wells 93.41
      with synchronous insertion of
         device 02.94
   halo device, skull 93.41
      with synchronous insertion of
         device 02.94
   Lyman Smith (skeletal) 93.44
   manual, intermittent 93.21
   mechanical, intermittent 93.21
   Russell's (skeletal) 93.44
   skeletal NEC 93.44
      intermittent 93.43
   skin, limbs NEC 93.46
   spinal NEC 93.42
      with skull device (halo) (caliper)
         (Crutchfield) (Gardner Wells)
         (Vinke) (tongs) 93.41
      with synchronous insertion of
         device 02.94
   Thomas' splint 93.45
   Vinke tongs 93.41
      with synchronous insertion of
         device 02.94
Tractotomy
   brain 01.32
   medulla oblongata 01.32
   mesencephalon 01.32
   percutaneous 03.21
   spinal cord (one-stage) (two-stage) 03.29
   trigeminal (percutaneous)
      (radiofrequency) 04.02
Training (for) (in)
   ADL (activities of daily living) 93.83
      for the blind 93.78
   ambulation 93.22
   braille 93.77
   crutch walking 93.24

Training (*Continued*)
   dyslexia 93.71
   dysphasia 93.72
   esophageal speech (postlaryngectomy)
      93.73
   gait 93.22
   joint movements 93.14
   lip reading 93.75
   Moon (blind reading) 93.77
   orthoptic 95.35
   prenatal (natural childbirth) 93.37
   prosthetic or orthotic device usage 93.24
   relaxation 94.33
   speech NEC 93.75
      esophageal type 93.73
      for correction of defect 93.74
   use of lead dog for the blind 93.76
   vocational 93.85
TRAM (transverse rectus abdominis
   musculocutaneous) flap of breast
   free 85.73
   pedicled 85.72
Transactional analysis
   group 94.44
   individual 94.39
Transection - *see also* Division
   artery (with ligation) - *see also* Division,
      artery 38.80
      renal, aberrant (with reimplantation)
         39.55
   bone - *see also* Osteotomy 77.30
   fallopian tube (bilateral) (remaining)
      (solitary) 66.39
      by endoscopy 66.22
      unilateral 66.92
   isthmus, thyroid 06.91
   muscle 83.19
      eye 15.13
         multiple (two or more muscles)
          15.3
      hand 82.19
   nerve (cranial) (peripheral) NEC 04.03
      acoustic 04.01
      root (spinal) 03.1
      sympathetic 05.0
      tracts in spinal cord 03.29
      trigeminal 04.02
      vagus (transabdominal) - *see also*
         Vagotomy 44.00
   pylorus (with wedge resection) 43.3
   renal vessel, aberrant (with
      reimplantation) 39.55
   spinal
      cord tracts 03.29
      nerve root 03.1
   tendon 83.13
      hand 82.11
   uvula 27.71
   vas deferens 63.71
   vein (with ligation) - *see also* Division,
      vein 38.80
      renal, aberrant (with reimplantation)
         39.55
   varicose (lower limb) 38.59
Transfer, transference
   bone shaft, fibula into tibia 78.47
   digital (to replace absent thumb)
      82.69
   finger (to thumb) (same hand) 82.61
      to
         finger, except thumb 82.81
         opposite hand (with
          amputation) 82.69
          [84.01]

◀ New   ◀▥ Revised   ~~deleted~~ Deleted   ● Use Additional Digit(s)   ▭ Omit code

Transfer, transference (Continued)
    digital (Continued)
        toe (to thumb) (with amputation) 82.69 [84.11]
            to finger, except thumb 82.81 [84.11]
    fat pad NEC 86.89
        with skin graft - see Graft, skin, full-thickness
    finger (to replace absent thumb) (same hand) 82.61
        to
            finger, except thumb 82.81
            opposite hand (with amputation) 82.69 [84.01]
    muscle origin 83.77
        hand 82.58
    nerve (cranial) (peripheral) (radial anterior) (ulnar) 04.6
    pedicle graft 86.74
    pes anserinus (tendon) (repair of knee) 81.47
    tarsoconjunctival flap, from opposing lid 08.64
    tendon 83.75
        hand 82.56
        pes anserinus (repair of knee) 81.47
    toe-to-thumb (free) (pedicle) (with amputation) 82.69 [84.11]
Transfixion - see also Fixation
    iris (bombé) 12.11
Transfusion (of) 99.03
    antihemophilic factor 99.06
    antivenin 99.16
    autologous blood
        collected prior to surgery 99.02
        intraoperative 99.00
        perioperative 99.00
        postoperative 99.00
        previously collected 99.02
        salvage 99.00
    blood (whole) NOS 99.03
        expander 99.08
        surrogate 99.09
    bone marrow 41.00
        allogeneic 41.03
            with purging 41.02
        allograft 41.03
            with purging 41.02
        autograft 41.01
            with purging 41.09
        autologous 41.01
            with purging 41.09
    coagulation factors 99.06
    Dextran 99.08
    exchange 99.01
        intraperitoneal 75.2
        in utero (with hysterotomy) 75.2
    exsanguination 99.01
    gamma globulin 99.14
    granulocytes 99.09
    hemodilution 99.03
    intrauterine 75.2
    packed cells 99.04
    plasma 99.07
    platelets 99.05
    replacement, total 99.01
    serum NEC 99.07
    substitution 99.01
    thrombocytes 99.05
Transillumination
    nasal sinuses 89.35
    skull (newborn) 89.16

Translumbar aortogram 88.42
Transplant, transplantation

    Note: To report donor source:
                cadaver 00.93
                live non-related donor 00.92
                live related donor 00.91
                live unrelated donor 00.92

    artery 39.59
        renal, aberrant 39.55
    autotransplant - see Reimplantation
    blood vessel 39.59
        renal, aberrant 39.55
    bone - see also Graft, bone 78.00
        marrow 41.00
            allogeneic 41.03
                with purging 41.02
            allograft 41.03
                with purging 41.02
            autograft 41.01
                with purging 41.09
            autologous 41.01
                with purging 41.09
            stem cell
                allogeneic (hematopoietic) 41.05
                    with purging 41.08
                autologous (hematopoietic) 41.04
                    with purging 41.07
                cord blood 41.06
        stem cell
            allogeneic (hematopoietic) 41.05
                with purging 41.08
            autologous (hematopoietic) 41.04
                with purging 41.07
            cord blood 41.06
    combined heart-lung 33.6
    conjunctiva, for pterygium 11.39
    corneal - see also Keratoplasty 11.60
    dura 02.12
    fascia 83.82
        hand 82.72
    finger (replacing absent thumb) (same hand) 82.61
        to
            finger, except thumb 82.81
            opposite hand (with amputation) 82.69 [84.01]
    gracilis muscle (for) 83.77
        anal incontinence 49.74
        urethrovesical suspension 59.71
    hair follicles
        eyebrow 08.63
        eyelid 08.63
        scalp 86.64
    heart (orthotopic) 37.51
        combined with lung 33.6
    ileal stoma to new site 46.23
    intestine 46.97
    Islets of Langerhans (cells) 52.86
        allotransplantation of cells 52.85
        autotransplantation of cells 52.84
        heterotransplantation 52.85
        homotransplantation 52.84
    kidney NEC 55.69
    liver 50.59
        auxiliary (permanent) (temporary) (recipient's liver in situ) 50.51
        cells into spleen via percutaneous catheterization 38.91

Transplant, transplantation (Continued)
    lung 33.50
        bilateral 33.50
        combined with heart 33.6
        double 33.52
        single 33.51
        unilateral 33.51
    lymphatic structure(s) (peripheral) 40.9
    mammary artery to myocardium or ventricular wall 36.2
    muscle 83.77
        gracilis (for) 83.77
            anal incontinence 49.74
            urethrovesical suspension 59.71
        hand 82.58
        temporalis 83.77
            with orbital exenteration 16.59
    nerve (cranial) (peripheral) 04.6
    ovary 65.92
    pancreas 52.80
        heterotransplant 52.83
        homotransplant 52.82
        Islets of Langerhans (cells) 52.86
            allotransplantation of cells 52.85
            autotransplantation of cells 52.84
            heterotransplantation 52.85
            homotransplantation 52.84
        reimplantation 52.81
    pes anserinus (tendon) (repair of knee) 81.47
    renal NEC 55.69
        vessel, aberrant 39.55
    salivary duct opening 26.49
    skin - see Graft, skin
    spermatic cord 63.53
    spleen 41.94
    stem cells
        allogeneic (hematopoietic) 41.05
            with purging 41.08
        autologous (hematopoietic) 41.04
            with purging 41.07
        cord blood 41.06
    tendon 83.75
        hand 82.56
        pes anserinus (repair of knee) 81.47
        superior rectus (blepharoptosis) 08.36
    testis to scrotum 62.5
    thymus 07.94
    thyroid tissue 06.94
    toe (replacing absent thumb) (with amputation) 82.69 [84.11]
        to finger, except thumb 82.81 [84.11]
    tooth 23.5
    ureter to
        bladder 56.74
        ileum (external diversion) 56.51
            internal diversion only 56.71
        intestine 56.71
        skin 56.61
    vein (peripheral) 39.59
        renal, aberrant 39.55
    vitreous 14.72
        anterior approach 14.71
Transposition
    extraocular muscles 15.5
    eyelash flaps 08.63
    eye muscle (oblique) (rectus) 15.5

Transposition *(Continued)*
  finger (replacing absent thumb) (same hand) 82.61
    to
      finger, except thumb 82.81
      opposite hand (with amputation) 82.69 *[84.01]*
  interatrial venous return 35.91
  jejunal (Henley) 43.81
  joint capsule - *see also* Arthroplasty 81.96
  muscle NEC 83.79
    extraocular 15.5
    hand 82.59
  nerve (cranial) (peripheral) (radial anterior) (ulnar) 04.6
  nipple 85.86
  pterygium 11.31
  tendon NEC 83.76
    hand 82.57
  vocal cords 31.69
Transureteroureterostomy 56.75
Transversostomy - *see also* Colostomy 46.10
Trapping, aneurysm (cerebral) 39.52
Trauner operation (lingual sulcus extension) 24.91
Trephination, trephining
  accessory sinus - *see* Sinusotomy
  corneoscleral 12.89
  cranium 01.24
  nasal sinus - *see* Sinusotomy
  sclera (with iridectomy) 12.61
Trial (failed) forceps 73.3
Trigonectomy 57.6
Trimming, amputation stump 84.3

Triple arthrodesis 81.12
Trochanterplasty 81.40
Tsuge operation (macrodactyly repair) 82.83
Tuck, tucking - *see also* Plication
  eye muscle 15.22
    multiple (two or more muscles) 15.4
  levator palpebrae, for blepharoptosis 08.34
Tudor "rabbit ear" operation (anterior urethropexy) 59.79
Tuffier operation
  apicolysis of lung 33.39
  vaginal hysterectomy 68.59
    laparoscopically assisted (LAVH) 68.51
TULIP (transurethral ultrasound guided laser induced prostectomy) 60.21
TUMT (transurethral microwave thermotherapy) of prostate 60.96
TUNA (transurethral needle ablation) of prostate 60.97
Tunnel, subcutaneous (antethoracic) 42.86
  esophageal 42.68
    with anastomosis - *see* Anastomosis, esophagus, antesternal 42.68
  pulse generator lead wire 86.99
    with initial procedure - *omit code*
Turbinectomy (complete) (partial) NEC 21.69
  by
    cryosurgery 21.61
    diathermy 21.61
  with sinusectomy - *see* Sinusectomy

Turco operation (release of joint capsules in clubfoot) 80.48
TURP (transurethral resection of prostate) 60.29
Tylectomy (breast) (partial) 85.21
Tympanectomy 20.59
  with tympanoplasty - *see* Tympanoplasty
Tympanogram 95.41
Tympanomastoidectomy 20.42
Tympanoplasty (type I) (with graft) 19.4
  with
    air pocket over round window 19.54
    fenestra in semicircular canal 19.55
    graft against
      incus or malleus 19.52
      mobile and intact stapes 19.53
    incudostapediopexy 19.52
  epitympanic, type I 19.4
  revision 19.6
  type
    II (graft against incus or malleus) 19.52
    III (graft against mobile and intact stapes) 19.53
    IV (air pocket over round window) 19.54
    V (fenestra in semicircular canal) 19.55
Tympanosympathectomy 20.91
Tympanotomy 20.09
  with intubation 20.01

U

Uchida operation (tubal ligation with or without fimbriectomy) 66.32
UFR (uroflowmetry) 89.24
Ultrafiltration 99.78
  hemodiafiltration 39.95
  hemodialysis (kidney) 39.95
  removal, plasma water 99.78
  therapeutic plasmapheresis 99.71
Ultrasonography
  abdomen 88.76
  aortic arch 88.73
  biliary tract 88.74
  breast 88.73
  deep vein thrombosis 88.77
  digestive system 88.74
  eye 95.13
  head and neck 88.71
  heart 88.72
  intestine 88.74
  intravascular - *see* Ultrasound, intravascular (IVUS)
  lung 88.73
  midline shift, brain 88.71
  multiple sites 88.79
  peripheral vascular system 88.77
  retroperitoneum 88.76
  therapeutic - *see* Ultrasound
  thorax NEC 88.73
  total body 88.79
  urinary system 88.75
  uterus 88.79
    gravid 88.78

Ultrasound
  diagnostic - *see* Ultrasonography
  fragmentation (of)
    cataract (with aspiration) 13.41
    urinary calculus, stones (Kock pouch) 59.95
  heart
    intracardiac (heart chambers) (ICE) 37.28
    intravascular (coronary vessels) (IVUS) 00.24
    non-invasive 88.72
  inner ear 20.79
  intravascular (IVUS) (VH™-IVUS) 00.29
    aorta 00.22
    aortic arch 00.22
    cerebral vessel, extracranial 00.21
    coronary vessel 00.24
    intrathoracic vessel 00.22
    other specified vessel 00.28
    peripheral vessel 00.23
    renal vessel 00.25
    vena cava (inferior) (superior) 00.22
    VH™-IVUS - *see* Ultrasound, intravascular, by site
    virtual histology intravascular ultrasound - *see* Ultrasound, intravascular, by site
  therapeutic
    head 00.01
    heart 00.02
    neck 00.01
    other therapeutic ultrasound 00.09

Ultrasound *(Continued)*
  therapeutic *(Continued)*
    peripheral vascular vessels 00.03
    vessels of head and neck 00.01
    therapy 93.35
Umbilectomy 54.3
Unbridling
  blood vessel, peripheral 39.91
  celiac artery axis 39.91
Uncovering - *see* Incision, by site
Undercutting
  hair follicle 86.09
  perianal tissue 49.02
Unroofing - *see also* Incision, by site
  external
    auditory canal 18.02
    ear NEC 18.09
  kidney cyst 55.39
UPP (urethral pressure profile) 89.25
Upper GI series (x-ray) 87.62
UPPP (uvulopalatopharyngoplasty) 27.69 *[29.4]*
Uranoplasty (for cleft palate repair) 27.62
Uranorrhaphy (for cleft palate repair) 27.62
Uranostaphylorrhaphy 27.62
Urban operation (mastectomy) (unilateral) 85.47
  bilateral 85.48
Ureterectomy 56.40
  with nephrectomy 55.51
  partial 56.41
  total 56.42

T & U

◀ New   ◀ Revised   ~~deleted~~ Deleted   ● Use Additional Digit(s)   ▨ Omit code

V

V & W

Varicotomy, peripheral vessels (lower limb) 38.59
   upper limb 38.53
Vascular access device, totally implantable 86.07
Vascular closure, percutaneous puncture - *omit code*
Vascularization - *see* Revascularization
Vasectomy (complete) (partial) 63.73
Vasogram 87.94
Vasoligation 63.71
   gastric 38.86
Vasorrhaphy 63.81
Vasostomy 63.6
Vasotomy 63.6
Vasotripsy 63.71
Vasovasostomy 63.82
Vectorcardiogram (VCG) (with ECG) 89.53
Vectra® vascular access graft 86.07
Venectomy - *see* Phlebectomy
Venipuncture NEC 38.99
   for injection of contrast material - *see* Phlebography
Venography - *see* Phlebography
Venorrhaphy 39.32
Venotomy 38.00
   abdominal 38.07
   head and neck NEC 38.02
   intracranial NEC 38.01
   lower limb 38.09
   thoracic NEC 38.05
   upper limb 38.03
Venotripsy 39.98
Venovenostomy 39.29
Ventilation
   bi-level positive airway pressure [BiPAP] 93.90
      delivered by
         endotracheal tube - *see* category 96.7●
         tracheostomy – *see* category 96.7●
   continuous positive airway pressure [CPAP] 93.90
      delivered by
         endotracheal tube - *see* category 96.7●
         tracheostomy – *see* category 96.7●
   endotracheal respiratory assistance - *see* category 96.7●
   intermittent positive pressure breathing [IPPB] 93.91
   mechanical, NOS 93.90
      by endotracheal tube - *see* category 96.7●
      by tracheostomy - *see* category 96.7●
      endotracheal respiratory assistance - *see* category 96.7●

Ventilation (*Continued*)
   mechanical, NOS (*Continued*)
      invasive - *see* category 96.7●
      non-invasive [NIPPV] 93.90
      other continuous invasive (unspecified duration) 96.70
         for less than 96 consecutive hours 96.71
         for 96 consecutive hours or more 96.72
      negative pressure (continuous) [CNP] 93.99
      non-invasive positive pressure (NIPPV) 93.90
      positive end expiratory pressure [PEEP]
         invasive - *see* category 96.7●
         non-invasive 93.90
Ventriculectomy, heart
   partial 37.35
Ventriculocholecystostomy 02.34
Ventriculocisternostomy 02.2
Ventriculocordectomy 30.29
Ventriculogram, ventriculography (cerebral) 87.02
   cardiac
      left ventricle (outflow tract) 88.53
         combined with right heart 88.54
      right ventricle (outflow tract) 88.52
         combined with left heart 88.54
   radionuclide cardiac 92.05
Ventriculomyocardiotomy 37.11
Ventriculoperitoneostomy 02.34
Ventriculopuncture 01.09
   through previously implanted catheter or reservoir (Ommaya) (Rickham) 01.02
Ventriculoseptopexy - *see also* Repair, ventricular septal defect 35.72
Ventriculoseptoplasty - *see also* Repair, ventricular septal defect 35.72
Ventriculostomy 02.2
Ventriculotomy
   cerebral 02.2
   heart 37.11
Ventriculoureterostomy 02.35
Ventriculovenostomy 02.32
Ventrofixation, uterus 69.22
Ventrohysteropexy 69.22
Ventrosuspension, uterus 69.22
VEP (visual evoked potential) 95.23
Version, obstetrical (bimanual) (cephalic) (combined) (internal) (podalic) 73.21
   with extraction 73.22
   Braxton Hicks 73.21
      with extraction 73.22
   external (bipolar) 73.91

Version, obstetrical (*Continued*)
   Potter's (podalic) 73.21
      with extraction 73.22
   Wigand's (external) 73.91
   Wright's (cephalic) 73.21
      with extraction 73.22
Vertebroplasty, percutaneous 81.65
Vesicolithotomy (suprapubic) 57.19
Vesicostomy 57.21
Vesicourethroplasty 57.85
Vesiculectomy 60.73
   with radical prostatectomy 60.5
Vesiculogram, seminal 87.92
   contrast 87.91
Vesiculotomy 60.72
Vestibuloplasty (buccolabial) (lingual) 24.91
Vestibulotomy 20.79
VH™-IVUS - *see* Ultrasound, intravascular, by site
Vicq D'azyr operation (larynx) 31.1
Vidal operation (varicocele ligation) 63.1
Vidianectomy 05.21
Villusectomy - *see also* Synovectomy 80.70
Vision check 95.09
Visual evoked potential (VEP) 95.23
Vitrectomy (mechanical) (posterior approach) 14.74
   with scleral buckling 14.49
   anterior approach 14.73
Vocational
   assessment 93.85
   retraining 93.85
   schooling 93.82
Voice training (postlaryngectomy) 93.73
von Kraske operation (proctectomy) 48.64
Voss operation (hanging hip operation) 83.19
Vulpius (-Compere) operation (lengthening of gastrocnemius muscle) 83.85
Vulvectomy (bilateral) (simple) 71.62
   partial (unilateral) 71.61
   radical (complete) 71.5
   unilateral 71.61
V-Y operation (repair)
   bladder 57.89
      neck 57.85
   ectropion 08.44
   lip 27.59
   skin (without graft) 86.89
   subcutaneous tissue (without skin graft) 86.89
   tongue 25.59

W

Wada test (hemispheric function) 89.10
Wang needle aspiration biopsy
   bronchus 33.24
   lung 33.27 ◄
Ward-Mayo operation (vaginal hysterectomy) 68.59
   laparoscopically assisted (LAVH) 68.51

Washing - *see* Lavage and Irrigation
Waterston operation (aorta-right pulmonary artery anastomosis) 39.0
Watkins (-Wertheim) operation (uterus interposition) 69.21
Watson-Jones operation
   hip arthrodesis 81.21
   reconstruction of lateral ligaments, ankle 81.49

Watson-Jones operation (*Continued*)
   shoulder arthrodesis (extra-articular) 81.23
   tenoplasty 83.88
Webbing (syndactylization) 86.89
Weir operation
   appendicostomy 47.91
   correction of nostrils 21.86

◄ New   ◄▥ Revised   ~~deleted~~ Deleted   ● Use Additional Digit(s)   ▨ Omit code

Wertheim operation (radical
   hysterectomy) 68.69
   laparoscopic 68.61
West operation (dacryocystorhinostomy)
   09.81
Wheeler operation
   entropion repair 08.44
   halving procedure (eyelid) 08.24
Whipple operation (radical
   pancreaticoduodenectomy) 52.7
   Child modification (radical subtotal
      pancreatectomy) 52.53
   Rodney Smith modification (radical
      subtotal pancreatectomy) 52.53
White operation (lengthening of tendo
   calcaneus by incomplete tenotomy)
   83.11
Whitehead operation
   glossectomy, radical 25.4
   hemorrhoidectomy 49.46

Whitman operation
   foot stabilization (talectomy) 77.98
   hip reconstruction 81.40
   repair of serratus anterior muscle 83.87
   talectomy 77.98
   trochanter wedge osteotomy 77.25
Wier operation (entropion repair) 08.44
Williams-Richardson operation (vaginal
      construction) 70.61
   with graft or prosthesis 70.63
Wilms operation (thoracoplasty) 33.34
Wilson operation (angulation osteotomy
      for hallux valgus) 77.51
Window operation
   antrum (nasal sinus) - see Antrotomy,
      maxillary
   aorticopulmonary 39.59
   bone cortex - see also Incision, bone
      77.10
      facial 76.09

Window operation (Continued)
   nasoantral - see Antrotomy, maxillary
   pericardium 37.12
   pleura 34.09
Winiwarter operation
      (cholecystoenterostomy) 51.32
Wiring
   aneurysm 39.52
   dental (for immobilization) 93.55
      with fracture-reduction - see
         Reduction, fracture
   orthodontic 24.7
Wirsungojejunostomy 52.96
Witzel operation (temporary
      gastrostomy) 43.19
Woodward operation (release of high
      riding scapula) 81.83
Wrapping, aneurysm (gauze) (methyl
      methacrylate) (plastic) 39.52

X

Xenograft 86.65
Xerography, breast 87.36
Xeromammography 87.36
Xiphoidectomy 77.81

X-ray
   chest (routine) 87.44
      wall NEC 87.39
   contrast - see Radiography, contrast
   diagnostic - see Radiography

X-ray (Continued)
   injection of radio-opaque substance -
      see Radiography, contrast
   skeletal series, whole or complete 88.31
   therapeutic - see Therapy, radiation

Y

Young operation
   epispadias repair 58.45
   tendon transfer (anterior tibialis)
      (repair of flat foot) 83.75
Yount operation (division of iliotibial
      band) 83.14

Z

Zancolli operation
   capsuloplasty 81.72
   tendon transfer (biceps) 82.56
Zeus® Robotic Surgical System – see
   category 17.4●
Ziegler operation (iridectomy) 12.14
Zonulolysis (with lens extraction) - see
   also Extraction, cataract,
   intracapsular 13.19

Z-plasty
   epicanthus 08.59
   eyelid - see also Reconstruction, eyelid
      08.70
   hypopharynx 29.4
   skin (scar) (web contracture)
      86.84
      with excision of lesion 86.3

Code also note: This instruction is
   used in the Tabular List for two
   purposes:
1) To code components of a
   procedure that are performed
   at the same time, and
2) To code the use of special
   adjunctive procedures or
   equipment.

Includes note: This note appears
   immediately under a two- or
   three-digit code title. The
   information further defines, or
   gives examples of, the contents
   of the category.

Excludes note: Terms following
   the word "Excludes" are to be
   coded elsewhere as indicated
   in each case.

W, X, Y & Z

CLASSIFICATION OF PROCEDURES

PROCEDURES AND INTERVENTIONS, NEC (00)

0. PROCEDURES AND INTERVENTIONS, NOT ELSEWHERE CLASSIFIED (00)

00 Procedures and interventions, Not Elsewhere Classified

● **00.0 Therapeutic ultrasound**

| **Excludes** | *diagnostic ultrasound (non-invasive) (88.71–88.79)*
intracardiac echocardiography [ICE] (heart chamber(s)) (37.28)
intravascular imaging (adjunctive) (00.21–00.29) |

Coding Clinic: 2002, Q4, P90-92

00.01 Therapeutic ultrasound of vessels of head and neck
Anti-restenotic ultrasound
Intravascular non-ablative ultrasound

| **Excludes** | *diagnostic ultrasound of:*
eye (95.13)
head and neck (88.71)
that of inner ear (20.79)
ultrasonic:
angioplasty of non-coronary vessel (39.50)
embolectomy (38.01, 38.02)
endarterectomy (38.11, 38.12)
thrombectomy (38.01, 38.02) |

00.02 Therapeutic ultrasound of heart
Anti-restenotic ultrasound
Intravascular non-ablative ultrasound

| **Excludes** | *diagnostic ultrasound of heart (88.72)*
ultrasonic ablation of heart lesion (37.34)
ultrasonic angioplasty of coronary vessels (00.66, 36.09) |

00.03 Therapeutic ultrasound of peripheral vascular vessels
Anti-restenotic ultrasound
Intravascular non-ablative ultrasound

| **Excludes** | *diagnostic ultrasound of peripheral vascular system (88.77)*
ultrasonic angioplasty of:
non-coronary vessel (39.50) |

00.09 Other therapeutic ultrasound

| **Excludes** | *ultrasonic:*
fragmentation of urinary stones (59.95)
percutaneous nephrostomy with fragmentation (55.04)
physical therapy (93.35)
transurethral guided laser induced prostatectomy (TULIP) (60.21) |

● **00.1 Pharmaceuticals**

00.10 Implantation of chemotherapeutic agent
Brain wafer chemotherapy
Interstitial/intracavitary

| **Excludes** | *injection or infusion of cancer chemotherapeutic substance (99.25)* |

Coding Clinic: 2002, Q4, P93

00.11 Infusion of drotrecogin alfa (activated)
Infusion of recombinant protein
Coding Clinic: 2002, Q4, P93-94

00.12 Administration of inhaled nitric oxide
Nitric oxide therapy
Coding Clinic: 2002, Q4, P94

00.13 Injection or infusion of nesiritide
Human B-type natriuretic peptide (hBNP)
Coding Clinic: 2002, Q4, P94

00.14 Injection or infusion of oxazolidinone class of antibiotics
Linezolid injection
Coding Clinic: 2002, Q4, P95

00.15 High-dose infusion interleukin-2 [IL-2]
Infusion (IV bolus, CIV) interleukin
Injection of aldesleukin

| **Excludes** | *low-dose infusion interleukin-2 (99.28)* |

Coding Clinic: 2003, Q4, P92

00.16 Pressurized treatment of venous bypass graft [conduit] with pharmaceutical substance
Ex-vivo treatment of vessel
Hyperbaric pressurized graft [conduit]
Coding Clinic: 2004, Q4, P108

00.17 Infusion of vasopressor agent
Coding Clinic: 2004, Q4, P108-109

00.18 Infusion of immunosuppressive antibody therapy

| **Includes** | during induction phase of solid organ transplantation
monoclonal antibody therapy
polyclonal antibody therapy |

Coding Clinic: 2005, Q4, P101

00.19 Disruption of blood brain barrier via infusion [BBBD]
Infusion of substance to disrupt blood brain barrier

| Code also | chemotherapy (99.25) |

| **Excludes** | *other perfusion (39.97)* |

Coding Clinic: 2007, Q4, P103-104

● **00.2 Intravascular imaging of blood vessels**
Endovascular ultrasonography
Intravascular [ultrasound] imaging of blood vessels
Intravascular ultrasound (IVUS)
Virtual histology intravascular ultrasound (VH-IVUS)
Note: Real-time imaging of lumen of blood vessel(s) using sound waves

| Code also | any synchronous diagnostic or therapeutic procedures |

| **Excludes** | *adjunct vascular system procedures, number of vessels treated (00.40–00.43)*
diagnostic procedures on blood vessels (38.21–38.29)
diagnostic ultrasound of peripheral vascular system (88.77)
intravascular imaging of vessel(s) by OCT (38.24-38.25)
magnetic resonance imaging (MRI) (88.91–88.97)
therapeutic ultrasound (00.01–00.09) |

Coding Clinic: 2004, Q4, P109-111

00.21 Intravascular imaging of extracranial cerebral vessels
Common carotid vessels and branches
Intravascular ultrasound (IVUS), extracranial cerebral vessels

| **Excludes** | *diagnostic ultrasound (non-invasive) of head and neck (88.71)* |

◀ New   ◀ Revised   ~~deleted~~ Deleted   ● Use Additional Digit(s)   OGCR Official Guidelines   Coding Clinic

00.22   Intravascular imaging of intrathoracic vessels
Aorta and aortic arch
Intravascular ultrasound (IVUS), intrathoracic
   vessels
Vena cava (superior) (inferior)

> **Excludes** *diagnostic ultrasound (non-invasive) of
>   other sites of thorax (88.73)*

00.23   Intravascular imaging of peripheral vessels
Imaging of:
   vessels of arm(s)
   vessels of leg(s)
Intravascular ultrasound (IVUS), peripheral
   vessels

> **Excludes** *diagnostic ultrasound (non-invasive)
>   of peripheral vascular system
>   (88.77)*

00.24   Intravascular imaging of coronary vessels
Intravascular ultrasound (IVUS), coronary
   vessels

> **Excludes** *diagnostic ultrasound (non-invasive) of
>   heart (88.72)
>   intracardiac echocardiography [ICE]
>   (ultrasound of heart chamber(s))
>   (37.28)*

Coding Clinic: 2006, Q3, P8-9

00.25   Intravascular imaging of renal vessels
Intravascular ultrasound (IVUS), renal vessels
Renal artery

> **Excludes** *diagnostic ultrasound (non-invasive) of
>   urinary system (88.75)*

00.28   Intravascular imaging, other specified vessel(s)

00.29   Intravascular imaging, unspecified vessel(s)

● **00.3   Computer assisted surgery [CAS]**
CT-free navigation
Image guided navigation (IGN)
Image guided surgery (IGS)
Imageless navigation
That without the use of robotic(s) technology

> Code also diagnostic or therapeutic procedure

> **Excludes** *robotic assisted procedures (17.41–17.49)
>   stereotactic frame application only (93.59)*

00.31   Computer assisted surgery with CT/CTA

00.32   Computer assisted surgery with MR/MRA
Coding Clinic: 2004, Q4, P111-113

00.33   Computer assisted surgery with fluoroscopy

00.34   Imageless computer assisted surgery

00.35   Computer assisted surgery with multiple datasets

00.39   Other computer assisted surgery
Computer assisted surgery NOS

● **00.4   Adjunct vascular system procedures**
Note: These codes can apply to both coronary and
         peripheral vessels. These codes are to be
         used in conjunction with other therapeutic
         procedure codes to provide additional
         information on the number of vessels upon
         which a procedure was performed and/or
         the number of stents inserted. As appropriate,
         code both the number of vessels operated
         on (00.40–00.43), and the number of stents
         inserted (00.45–00.48).

> Code also any:
>   angioplasty or atherectomy (00.61–00.62, 00.66,
>   39.50)
>   endarterectomy (38.10–38.18)
>   insertion of vascular stent(s) (00.55, 00.63–00.65,
>   36.06–36.07, 39.90)
>   other removal of coronary artery obstruction (36.09)

00.40   Procedure on single vessel
Number of vessels, unspecified

> **Excludes** *(aorto)coronary bypass (36.10–36.19)
>   intravascular imaging of blood vessels
>   (00.21–00.29)*

Coding Clinic: 2009, Q3, P13; Q2, P12; 2007, Q1, P17; 2006,
Q3, P8-9; 2005, Q4, P69-72, 103-106

00.41   Procedure on two vessels

> **Excludes** *(aorto)coronary bypass (36.10–36.19)
>   intravascular imaging of blood vessels
>   (00.21–00.29)*

Coding Clinic: 2006, Q4, P119; 2005, Q4, P101-106

00.42   Procedure on three vessels

> **Excludes** *(aorto)coronary bypass (36.10–36.19)
>   intravascular imaging of blood vessels
>   (00.21–00.29)*

00.43   Procedure on four or more vessels

> **Excludes** *(aorto)coronary bypass (36.10–36.19)
>   intravascular imaging of blood vessels
>   (00.21–00.29)*

00.44   Procedure on vessel bifurcation
Note: This code is to be used to identify the
         presence of a vessel bifurcation; it does
         not describe a specific bifurcation stent.
         Use this code only once per operative
         episode, irrespective of the number of
         bifurcations in vessels.
Coding Clinic: 2006, Q4, P119

00.45   Insertion of one vascular stent
Number of stents, unspecified
Coding Clinic: 2009, Q3, P13; 2005, Q4, P69-72

00.46   Insertion of two vascular stents
Coding Clinic: 2009, Q2, P12; 2005, Q4, P103-106

00.47   Insertion of three vascular stents
Coding Clinic: 2006, Q4, P119

00.48   Insertion of four or more vascular stents

00.49   SuperSaturated oxygen therapy
Aqueous oxygen (AO) therapy
SSO$_2$
SuperOxygenation infusion therapy

> Code also any:
>   injection or infusion of thrombolytic agent
>   (99.10)
>   insertion of coronary artery stent(s)
>   (36.06-36.07)
>   intracoronary artery thrombolytic infusion
>   (36.04)
>   number of vascular stents inserted
>   (00.45-00.48)
>   number of vessels treated (00.40-00.43)
>   open chest coronary artery angioplasty
>   (36.03)
>   other removal of coronary obstruction
>   (36.09)
>   percutaneous transluminal coronary
>   angioplasty [PTCA] (00.66)
>   procedure on vessel bifurcation (00.44)

> **Excludes** *other oxygen enrichment (93.96)
>   other perfusion (39.97)*

Coding Clinic: 2008, Q4, P162-163

PROCEDURES AND INTERVENTIONS, NEC (00)

Excludes   **Includes**   Use additional   Code also   Omit code

PROCEDURES AND INTERVENTIONS, NEC (00)

● **00.5 Other cardiovascular procedures**
Coding Clinic: 2008, Q3, P18; 2002, Q4, P95-101

00.50 Implantation of cardiac resynchronization pacemaker without mention of defibrillation, total system [CRT-P]
BiV pacemaker
Biventricular pacemaker
Biventricular pacing without internal cardiac defibrillator
Implantation of cardiac resynchronization (biventricular) pulse generator pacing device, formation of pocket, transvenous leads including placement of lead into left ventricular coronary venous system, and intraoperative procedures for evaluation of lead signals.
That with CRT-P generator and one or more leads
Note: Device testing during procedure – *omit code*

Excludes *implantation of cardiac resynchronization defibrillator, total system [CRT-D] (00.51)*
insertion or replacement of any type pacemaker device (37.80–37.87)
replacement of cardiac resynchronization defibrillator pulse generator only [CRT-D] (00.54)
replacement of cardiac resynchronization pacemaker pulse generator only [CRT-P] (00.53)
Coding Clinic: 2008, Q3, P18; 2005, Q3, P3-9

00.51 Implantation of cardiac resynchronization defibrillator, total system [CRT-D]
BiV defibrillator
BiV ICD
BiV pacemaker with defibrillator
BiV pacing with defibrillator
Biventricular defibrillator
Biventricular pacing with internal cardiac defibrillator
Implantation of a cardiac resynchronization (biventricular) pulse generator with defibrillator [AICD], formation of pocket, transvenous leads, including placement of lead into left ventricular coronary venous system, intraoperative procedures for evaluation of lead signals, and obtaining defibrillator threshold measurements.
That with CRT-D generator and one or more leads
Note: Device testing during procedure – *omit code*

Excludes *implantation of cardiac resynchronization pacemaker, total system [CRT-P] (00.50)*
implantation or replacement of automatic cardioverter/ defibrillator, total system [AICD] (37.94)
replacement of cardiac resynchronization defibrillator pulse generator, only [CRT-D] (00.54)
Coding Clinic: 2008, Q3, P18; 2007, Q1, P16-17x2; 2005, Q3, P3-9; 2002, Q4, P99-100

00.52 Implantation or replacement of transvenous lead [electrode] into left ventricular coronary venous system

Excludes *implantation of cardiac resynchronization defibrillator, total system [CRT-D] (00.51)*
implantation of cardiac resynchronization pacemaker, total system [CRT-P] (00.50)
initial insertion of transvenous lead [electrode] (37.70–37.72)
replacement of transvenous atrial and/ or ventricular lead(s) [electrodes] (37.76)
Coding Clinic: 2008, Q3, P18; 2005, Q3, P3-9

00.53 Implantation or replacement of cardiac resynchronization pacemaker pulse generator only [CRT-P]
Implantation of CRT-P device with removal of any existing CRT-P or other pacemaker device
Note: Device testing during procedure – *omit code*

Excludes *implantation of cardiac resynchronization pacemaker, total system [CRT-P] (00.50)*
implantation or replacement of cardiac resynchronization defibrillator pulse generator only [CRT-D] (00.54)
insertion or replacement of any type pacemaker device (37.80–37.87)
Coding Clinic: 2005, Q3, P3-9

00.54 Implantation or replacement of cardiac resynchronization defibrillator pulse generator device only [CRT-D]
Implantation of CRT-D device with removal of any existing CRT-D, CRT-P, pacemaker, or defibrillator device
Note: Device testing during procedure – *omit code*

Excludes *implantation of automatic cardioverter/ defibrillator pulse generator only (37.96)*
implantation of cardiac resynchronization defibrillator, total system [CRT-D] (00.51)
implantation or replacement of cardiac resynchronization pacemaker pulse generator only [CRT-P] (00.53)
Coding Clinic: 2005, Q3, P3-9; 2002, Q4, P100

◄ New   ◄▌▌ Revised   ~~deleted~~ Deleted   ● Use Additional Digit(s)   OGCR Official Guidelines   Coding Clinic

00.55 **Insertion of drug-eluting** ~~peripheral vessel~~ **stent(s) of other peripheral vessel(s)** ◀▥

    Endograft(s)
    Endovascular graft(s)
    Stent grafts

    Code also any:
        angioplasty or atherectomy of other
           non-coronary vessel(s) (39.50)
        number of vascular stents inserted
           (00.45–00.48)
        number of vessels treated (00.40–00.43)
        procedure on vessel bifurcation (00.44)

    Excludes *drug-coated peripheral stents, e.g.,*
               heparin coated (39.90)
          insertion of cerebrovascular stent(s)
               (00.63–00.65)
          insertion of drug-eluting coronary
               artery stent (36.07)
          insertion of drug-eluting stent(s) of
               superficial femoral artery
               (00.60) ◀
          insertion of non-drug-eluting stent(s):
               coronary artery (36.06)
               peripheral vessel (39.90)
          ~~*that for aneurysm repair*~~ *that for*
               other endovascular procedure
               (39.71-39.79) ◀▥

    Coding Clinic: 2002, Q4, P101-103

00.56 **Insertion or replacement of implantable pressure sensor (lead) for intracardiac or great vessel hemodynamic monitoring**

    Code also any associated implantation or
        replacement of monitor (00.57)

    Excludes *circulatory monitoring (blood gas,*
            arterial or venous pressure,
            cardiac output and coronary
            blood flow) (89.60–89.69)
    Coding Clinic: 2006, Q4, P119-120

00.57 **Implantation or replacement of subcutaneous device for intracardiac or great vessel hemodynamic monitoring**

    Implantation of monitoring device with
        formation of subcutaneous pocket and
        connection to intracardiac pressure
        sensor (lead)

    Code also any associated insertion or
        replacement of implanted pressure sensor
        (lead) (00.56)
    Coding Clinic: 2006, Q4, P119-120

00.58 **Insertion of intra-aneurysm sac pressure monitoring device (intraoperative)**

    Insertion of pressure sensor during
        endovascular repair of abdominal or
        thoracic aortic aneurysm(s)
    Coding Clinic: 2008, Q4, P163-165

00.59 **Intravascular pressure measurement of coronary arteries**

    Includes fractional flow reserve (FFR)

    Code also any synchronous diagnostic or
        therapeutic procedures

    Excludes *intravascular pressure measurement of*
            intrathoracic arteries (00.67)
    Coding Clinic: 2008, Q4, P163-165

● **00.6** **Procedures on blood vessels**
    Coding Clinic: 2004, Q4, P114-116

00.60 **Insertion of drug-eluting stent(s) of superficial femoral artery** ◀

    Code also any: ◀
        angioplasty or atherectomy of other non-
           coronary vessel(s) (39.50) ◀
        non-drug-eluting peripheral stents (39.90) ◀
        number of vascular stents inserted
           (00.45-00.48) ◀
        number of vessels treated (00.40-00.43) ◀
        procedure on vessel bifurcation (00.44) ◀

    Excludes *insertion of drug-eluting stent(s) of*
            other peripheral vessel (00.55) ◀
          that for other endovascular procedure
            (39.71-39.79) ◀

00.61 **Percutaneous angioplasty or atherectomy of precerebral (extracranial) vessel(s)**
    Basilar   Vertebral
    Carotid

    Code also any:
        injection or infusion of thrombolytic agent
           (99.10)
        number of vascular stents inserted
           (00.45–00.48)
        number of vessels treated (00.40–00.43)
        percutaneous insertion of carotid artery
           stent(s) (00.63)
        percutaneous insertion of other precerebral
           artery stent(s) (00.64)
        procedure on vessel bifurcation (00.44)

    Excludes *angioplasty or atherectomy of other*
            non-coronary vessel(s) (39.50)
          removal of cerebrovascular obstruction
            of vessel(s) by open approach
            (38.01–38.02, 38.11–38.12,
            38.31–38.32, 38.41–38.42)

00.62 **Percutaneous angioplasty or atherectomy of intracranial vessel(s)**

    Code also any:
        injection or infusion of thrombolytic agent
           (99.10)
        number of vascular stents inserted
           (00.45–00.48)
        number of vessels treated (00.40–00.43)
        percutaneous insertion of intracranial
           stent(s) (00.65)
        procedure on vessel bifurcation (00.44)

    Excludes *angioplasty or atherectomy of other*
            non-coronary vessel(s) (39.50)
          removal of cerebrovascular obstruction
            of vessel(s) by open approach
            (38.01–38.02, 38.11–38.12,
            38.31–38.32, 38.41–38.42)

00.63 **Percutaneous insertion of carotid artery stent(s)**
    Includes the use of any embolic protection
        device, distal protection device, filter
        device, or stent delivery system
    Non-drug-eluting stent

    Code also any:
        number of vascular stents inserted
           (00.45–00.48)
        number of vessels treated (00.40–00.43)
        percutaneous angioplasty or atherectomy of
           precerebral vessel(s) (00.61)
        procedure on vessel bifurcation (00.44)

    Excludes *angioplasty or atherectomy of other*
            non-coronary vessel(s) (39.50)
          insertion of drug-eluting peripheral
            vessel stent(s) (00.55)

PROCEDURES AND INTERVENTIONS, NEC (00)

00.64 Percutaneous insertion of other precerebral (extracranial) artery stent(s)

Includes the use of any embolic protection device, distal protection device, filter device, or stent delivery system

Basilar stent

Vertebral stent

Code also any:

number of vascular stents inserted (00.45–00.48)

number of vessels treated (00.40–00.43)

percutaneous angioplasty or atherectomy of precerebral vessel(s) (00.61)

procedure on vessel bifurcation (00.44)

Excludes   *angioplasty or atherectomy of other non-coronary vessel(s) (39.50)*

insertion of drug-eluting peripheral vessel stent(s) (00.55)

00.65 Percutaneous insertion of intracranial vascular stent(s)

Includes the use of any embolic protection device, distal protection device, filter device, or stent delivery system

Code also any:

number of vascular stents inserted (00.45–00.48)

number of vessels treated (00.40–00.43)

percutaneous angioplasty or atherectomy of intracranial vessel(s) (00.62)

procedure on vessel bifurcation (00.44)

Excludes   *angioplasty or atherectomy of other non-coronary vessel(s) (39.50)*

insertion of drug-eluting peripheral vessel stent(s) (00.55)

00.66 Percutaneous transluminal coronary angioplasty [PTCA] or coronary atherectomy

Balloon angioplasty of coronary artery

Coronary atherectomy

Percutaneous coronary angioplasty NOS

PTCA NOS

Code also any:

injection or infusion of thrombolytic agent (99.10)

insertion of coronary artery stent(s) (36.06–36.07)

intracoronary artery thrombolytic infusion (36.04)

number of vascular stents inserted (00.45–00.48)

number of vessels treated (00.40–00.43)

procedure on vessel bifurcation (00.44)

SuperSaturated oxygen therapy (00.49)

Coding Clinic: 2009, Q2, P12; 2007, Q1, P17; 2006, Q3, P8-9; 2005, Q4, 69-72, P101-103; 2004, Q1, P10; Q2, P3

00.67 Intravascular pressure measurement of intrathoracic arteries

Assessment of:

aorta and aortic arch

carotid

Code also any synchronous diagnostic or therapeutic procedures

Coding Clinic: 2008, Q4, P163-165

00.68 Intravascular pressure measurement of peripheral arteries

Other peripheral vessels

Vessels of arm(s)

Vessels of leg(s)

Code also any synchronous diagnostic or therapeutic procedures

Coding Clinic: 2008, Q4, P163-165

00.69 Intravascular pressure measurement, other specified and unspecified vessels

Iliac vessels

Intra-abdominal vessels

Mesenteric vessels

Renal vessels

Code also any synchronous diagnostic or therapeutic procedures

Excludes   *intravascular pressure measurement of:*

coronary arteries (00.59)

intrathoracic arteries (00.67)

peripheral arteries (00.68)

Coding Clinic: 2008, Q4, P163-165

● **00.7 Other hip procedures**

Coding Clinic: 2005, Q4, P106-113

00.70 Revision of hip replacement, both acetabular and femoral components

Total hip revision

Code also any:

removal of (cement) (joint) spacer (84.57)

type of bearing surface, if known (00.74–00.77)

Excludes   *revision of hip replacement, acetabular component only (00.71)*

revision of hip replacement, femoral component only (00.72)

revision of hip replacement, Not Otherwise Specified (81.53)

revision with replacement of acetabular liner and/or femoral head only (00.73)

Coding Clinic: 2008, Q2, P3-4; 2008, Q1, P6; 2005, Q4, P110-112

00.71 Revision of hip replacement, acetabular component

Partial, acetabular component only

That with:

exchange of acetabular cup and liner

exchange of femoral head

Code also any type of bearing surface, if known (00.74–00.77)

Excludes   *revision of hip replacement, both acetabular and femoral components (00.70)*

revision of hip replacement, femoral component (00.72)

revision of hip replacement, Not Otherwise Specified (81.53)

revision with replacement of acetabular liner and/or femoral head only (00.73)

Coding Clinic: 2005, Q4, P110-112

00.72 Revision of hip replacement, femoral component
Partial, femoral component only
That with:
    exchange of acetabular liner
    exchange of femoral stem and head
  Code also any type of bearing surface, if
    known (00.74–00.77)
  Excludes *revision of hip replacement, acetabular*
    component (00.71)
    revision of hip replacement, both
    acetabular and femoral
    components (00.70)
    revision of hip replacement, not
    otherwise specified (81.53)
    revision with replacement of acetabular
    liner and/or femoral head only
    (00.73)

00.73 Revision of hip replacement, acetabular liner and/or femoral head only
  Code also any type of bearing surface, if
    known (00.74–00.77)

00.74 Hip bearing surface, metal on polyethylene

00.75 Hip bearing surface, metal-on-metal
Coding Clinic: 2006, Q4, P120-121

00.76 Hip bearing surface, ceramic-on-ceramic
Coding Clinic: 2005, Q4, P110-112

00.77 Hip bearing surface, ceramic-on-polyethylene

● **00.8 Other knee and hip procedures**
Note: Report up to two components using
00.81–00.83 to describe revision of knee
replacements. If all three components are
revised, report 00.80.
Coding Clinic: 2005, Q4, P113-117

00.80 Revision of knee replacement, total (all components)
Replacement of femoral, tibial, and patellar
components (all components)
  Code also any removal of (cement) (joint)
    spacer (84.57)
  Excludes *revision of only one or two components*
    (tibial, femoral or patellar
    component) (00.81–00.84)
Coding Clinic: 2008, Q1, P6

00.81 Revision of knee replacement, tibial component
Replacement of tibial baseplate and tibial insert
(liner)
  Excludes *revision of knee replacement, total (all*
    components) (00.80)
Coding Clinic: 2006, Q4, P103-104; 2005, Q4, P113-117

00.82 Revision of knee replacement, femoral component
That with replacement of tibial insert (liner)
  Excludes *revision of knee replacement, total (all*
    components) (00.80)
Coding Clinic: 2006, Q3, P9-10; 2005, Q4, P113-117

00.83 Revision of knee replacement, patellar component
  Excludes *revision of knee replacement, total (all*
    components) (00.80)

00.84 Revision of total knee replacement, tibial insert (liner)
Replacement of tibial insert (liner)
  Excludes *that with replacement of tibial*
    component (tibial baseplate and
    liner) (00.81)

00.85 Resurfacing hip, total, acetabulum and femoral head
Hip resurfacing arthroplasty, total
Coding Clinic: 2006, Q4, P121-122

00.86 Resurfacing hip, partial, femoral head
Hip resurfacing arthroplasty, NOS
Hip resurfacing arthroplasty, partial, femoral
head
  Excludes *that with resurfacing of acetabulum*
    (00.85)

00.87 Resurfacing hip, partial, acetabulum
Hip resurfacing arthroplasty, partial,
acetabulum
  Excludes *that with resurfacing of femoral head*
    (00.85)

● **00.9 Other procedures and interventions**

00.91 Transplant from live related donor
  Code also organ transplant procedure

00.92 Transplant from live non-related donor
  Code also organ transplant procedure
Coding Clinic: 2008, Q2, P8-9; 2004, Q4, P116-117

00.93 Transplant from cadaver
  Code also organ transplant procedure

00.94 Intra-operative neurophysiologic monitoring
Intra-operative neurophysiologic testing
IOM
Nerve monitoring
Neuromonitoring
  Includes Cranial nerve, peripheral nerve and
    spinal cord testing performed
    intra-operatively
  Excludes *brain temperature monitoring (01.17)*
    intracranial oxygen monitoring (01.16)
    intracranial pressure monitoring
    (01.10)
    plethysmogram (89.58)
Coding Clinic: 2009, Q2, P3; 2007, Q4, P104-105

PROCEDURES AND INTERVENTIONS, NEC (00)

(See Plates 86, 118, 472, 473, 500, 501, 502, 544, and 545 on pages NAP-6–NAP-14.)

1. OPERATIONS ON THE NERVOUS SYSTEM (01–05)

● **01 Incision and excision of skull, brain, and cerebral meninges**

● **01.0 Cranial puncture**

01.01 Cisternal puncture
Cisternal tap

> **Excludes** *pneumocisternogram (87.02)*

01.02 Ventriculopuncture through previously implanted catheter
Puncture of ventricular shunt tubing

01.09 Other cranial puncture
Aspiration of:
subarachnoid space
subdural space
Cranial aspiration NOS
Puncture of anterior fontanel
Subdural tap (through fontanel)
Coding Clinic: 2009, Q3, P15-16; 2007, Q4, P105-107

● **01.1 Diagnostic procedures on skull, brain, and cerebral meninges**

01.10 Intracranial pressure monitoring

> **Includes** insertion of catheter or probe for monitoring
Coding Clinic: 2009, Q3, P15-16; 2007, Q4, P105-107

01.11 Closed [percutaneous] [needle] biopsy of cerebral meninges
Burr hole approach

01.12 Open biopsy of cerebral meninges

01.13 Closed [percutaneous] [needle] biopsy of brain
Burr hole approach
Stereotactic method
Coding Clinic: 1987, Mar-April, P9

01.14 Open biopsy of brain

01.15 Biopsy of skull

01.16 Intracranial oxygen monitoring
Partial pressure of brain oxygen (PbtO$_2$)

> **Includes** insertion of catheter or probe for monitoring
Coding Clinic: 2007, Q4, P105-107

01.17 Brain temperature monitoring

> **Includes** insertion of catheter or probe for monitoring
Coding Clinic: 2007, Q4, P105-107

01.18 Other diagnostic procedures on brain and cerebral meninges

> **Excludes** *brain temperature monitoring (01.17)*
> *cerebral:*
> *arteriography (88.41)*
> *thermography (88.81)*
> *contrast radiogram of brain (87.01–87.02)*
> *echoencephalogram (88.71)*
> *electroencephalogram (89.14)*
> *intracranial oxygen monitoring (01.16)*
> *intracranial pressure monitoring (01.10)*
> *microscopic examination of specimen from nervous system and of spinal fluid (90.01–90.09)*
> *neurologic examination (89.13)*
> *phlebography of head and neck (88.61)*
> *pneumoencephalogram (87.01)*
> *radioisotope scan:*
> *cerebral (92.11)*
> *head NEC (92.12)*
> *tomography of head:*
> *C.A.T. scan (87.03)*
> *other (87.04)*
Coding Clinic: 1998, Q3, P12-13

01.19 Other diagnostic procedures on skull

> **Excludes** *transillumination of skull (89.16)*
> *x-ray of skull (87.17)*

● **01.2 Craniotomy and craniectomy**

> **Excludes** *decompression of skull fracture (02.02)*
> *exploration of orbit (16.01–16.09)*
> *that as operative approach –* omit code

01.20 Cranial implantation or replacement of neurostimulator pulse generator ◄

> Code also any associated lead implantation (02.93) ◄

> **Excludes** *implantation or replacement of subcutaneous neurostimulator pulse generator (86.94-86.98)* ◄

01.21 Incision and drainage of cranial sinus

01.22 Removal of intracranial neurostimulator lead(s)

> Code also any removal of neurostimulator pulse generator (86.05)

> **Excludes** *removal with synchronous replacement (02.93)*

01.23 Reopening of craniotomy site

01.24 Other craniotomy
Cranial:
decompression
exploration
trephination
Craniotomy NOS
Craniotomy with removal of:
epidural abscess
extradural hematoma
foreign body of skull

> **Excludes** *removal of foreign body with incision into brain (01.39)*
Coding Clinic: 1991, Q1, P14; 1984, July-Aug, P20

01.25 Other craniectomy
Debridement of skull NOS
Sequestrectomy of skull

> **Excludes** *debridement of compound fracture of skull (02.02)*
> *strip craniectomy (02.01)*
Coding Clinic: 2006, Q1, P6

01.26 Insertion of catheter(s) into cranial cavity or tissue

Code also any concomitant procedure (e.g. resection (01.59))

Excludes *placement of intracerebral catheter(s) via burr hole(s) (01.28)*
Coding Clinic: 2009, Q3, P16x2; 2005, Q4, P117-119

01.27 Removal of catheter(s) from cranial cavity or tissue
Coding Clinic: 2005, Q4, P117-119

01.28 Placement of intracerebral catheter(s) via burr hole(s)
Convection enhanced delivery
Stereotactic placement of intracerebral catheter(s)

Code also infusion of medication

Excludes *insertion of catheter(s) into cranial cavity or tissue(s) (01.26)*
Coding Clinic: 2009, Q3, P6; 2006, Q4, P122-123

01.29 Removal of cranial neurostimulator pulse generator ◄

● **01.3 Incision of brain and cerebral meninges**

01.31 Incision of cerebral meninges
Drainage of:
intracranial hygroma
subarachnoid abscess (cerebral)
subdural empyema

01.32 Lobotomy and tractotomy
Division of:
brain tissue
cerebral tracts
Percutaneous (radiofrequency) cingulotomy

01.39 Other incision of brain
Amygdalohippocampotomy
Drainage of intracerebral hematoma
Incision of brain NOS

Excludes *division of cortical adhesions (02.91)*
Coding Clinic: 2009, Q4, P84

● **01.4 Operations on thalamus and globus pallidus**

01.41 Operations on thalamus
Chemothalamectomy
Thalamotomy

Excludes *that by stereotactic radiosurgery (92.30–92.39)*

01.42 Operations on globus pallidus
Pallidoansectomy
Pallidotomy

Excludes *that by stereotactic radiosurgery (92.30–92.39)*

● **01.5 Other excision or destruction of brain and meninges**

01.51 Excision of lesion or tissue of cerebral meninges
Decortication of (cerebral) meninges
Resection of (cerebral) meninges
Stripping of subdural membrane of (cerebral) meninges

Excludes *biopsy of cerebral meninges (01.11–01.12)*

01.52 Hemispherectomy

01.53 Lobectomy of brain

01.59 Other excision or destruction of lesion or tissue of brain
Amygdalohippocampectomy ◄
Curettage of brain
Debridement of brain
Marsupialization of brain cyst
Transtemporal (mastoid) excision of brain tumor

Excludes *biopsy of brain (01.13–01.14)*
laser interstitial thermal therapy [LITT] of lesion or tissue of brain under guidance (17.61)
that by stereotactic radiosurgery (92.30–92.39)
Coding Clinic: 2005, Q4, P117-119; 1999, Q3, P7-8; Q1, P9-10; 1998, Q3, P12-13; Q1, P6-7; 1993, Q4, P33

01.6 Excision of lesion of skull
Removal of granulation tissue of cranium

Excludes *biopsy of skull (01.15)*
sequestrectomy (01.25)

● **02 Other operations on skull, brain, and cerebral meninges**

● **02.0 Cranioplasty**

Excludes *that with synchronous repair of encephalocele (02.12)*

02.01 Opening of cranial suture
Linear craniectomy
Strip craniectomy

02.02 Elevation of skull fracture fragments
Debridement of compound fracture of skull
Decompression of skull fracture
Reduction of skull fracture

Code also any synchronous debridement of brain (01.59)

Excludes *debridement of skull NOS (01.25)*
removal of granulation tissue of cranium (01.6)

02.03 Formation of cranial bone flap
Repair of skull with flap

02.04 Bone graft to skull
Pericranial graft (autogenous) (heterogenous)

02.05 Insertion of skull plate
Replacement of skull plate

02.06 Other cranial osteoplasty
Repair of skull NOS
Revision of bone flap of skull
Coding Clinic: 2006, Q1, P6-7; 2005, Q1, P11; 1998, Q3, P9-10

02.07 Removal of skull plate

Excludes *removal with synchronous replacement (02.05)*

● **02.1 Repair of cerebral meninges**

Excludes *marsupialization of cerebral lesion (01.59)*

02.11 Simple suture of dura mater of brain

02.12 Other repair of cerebral meninges
Closure of fistula of cerebrospinal fluid
Dural graft
Repair of encephalocele including synchronous cranioplasty
Repair of meninges NOS
Subdural patch

02.13 Ligation of meningeal vessel
Ligation of:
longitudinal sinus
middle meningeal artery

02.14 Choroid plexectomy
Cauterization of choroid plexus

OPERATIONS ON THE NERVOUS SYSTEM (01–05)

02.2 Ventriculostomy
Anastomosis of ventricle to:
   cervical subarachnoid space
   cisterna magna
Insertion of Holter valve
Ventriculocisternal intubation

● **02.3 Extracranial ventricular shunt**

   Includes   that with insertion of valve

   Coding Clinic: 1985, Sept-Oct, P12

02.31 Ventricular shunt to structure in head and neck
Ventricle to nasopharynx shunt
Ventriculomastoid anastomosis
Coding Clinic: 2004, Q4, P111-113

02.32 Ventricular shunt to circulatory system
Ventriculoatrial anastomosis
Ventriculocaval shunt

02.33 Ventricular shunt to thoracic cavity
Ventriculopleural anastomosis

02.34 Ventricular shunt to abdominal cavity and organs
Ventriculocholecystostomy
Ventriculoperitoneostomy

02.35 Ventricular shunt to urinary system
Ventricle to ureter shunt

02.39 Other operations to establish drainage of ventricle
Ventricle to bone marrow shunt
Ventricular shunt to extracranial site NEC

● **02.4 Revision, removal, and irrigation of ventricular shunt**

   Excludes *revision of distal catheter of ventricular shunt (54.95)*

02.41 Irrigation and exploration of ventricular shunt
Exploration of ventriculoperitoneal shunt at ventricular site
Re-programming of ventriculoperitoneal shunt

02.42 Replacement of ventricular shunt
Reinsertion of Holter valve
Replacement of ventricular catheter
Revision of ventriculoperitoneal shunt at ventricular site

02.43 Removal of ventricular shunt

● **02.9 Other operations on skull, brain, and cerebral meninges**

   Excludes *operations on:*
     pineal gland (07.17, 07.51–07.59)
     pituitary gland [hypophysis] (07.13–07.15, 07.61–07.79)

02.91 Lysis of cortical adhesions

02.92 Repair of brain

02.93 Implantation or replacement of intracranial neurostimulator lead(s)
Implantation, insertion, placement, or replacement of intracranial:
   brain pacemaker [neuropacemaker]
   depth electrodes
   epidural pegs
   electroencephalographic receiver
   foramen ovale electrodes
   intracranial electrostimulator
   subdural grids
   subdural strips

   Code also any: ◀▥
     insertion of cranial implantation or replacement of neurostimulator pulse generator (01.20) ◀
     insertion of subcutaneous neurostimulator pulse generator (86.94-86.98) ◀▥

02.94 Insertion or replacement of skull tongs or halo traction device
Coding Clinic: 2001, Q3, P8; 1996, Q3, P14

02.95 Removal of skull tongs or halo traction device

02.96 Insertion of sphenoidal electrodes

02.99 Other

   Excludes *chemical shock therapy (94.24)*
     electroshock therapy:
       subconvulsive (94.26)
       other (94.27)

● **03 Operations on spinal cord and spinal canal structures**

   Code also any application or administration of an adhesion barrier substance (99.77)

● **03.0 Exploration and decompression of spinal canal structures**

03.01 Removal of foreign body from spinal canal

03.02 Reopening of laminectomy site

03.09 Other exploration and decompression of spinal canal
Decompression:
   laminectomy
   laminotomy
Expansile laminoplasty
Exploration of spinal nerve root
Foraminotomy

   Code also any synchronous insertion, replacement and revision of posterior spinal motion preservation device(s), if performed (84.80–84.85)

   Excludes *drainage of spinal fluid by anastomosis (03.71–03.79)*
     laminectomy with excision of intervertebral disc (80.51)
     spinal tap (03.31)
     that as operative approach – omit code
   Coding Clinic: 2008, Q4, P109-110; Q2, P12; 2007, Q4, P116-120; Q1, P10; 2004, Q3, P6-7; 2002, Q4, P109-110; 2002, Q2, P15; 1999, Q4, P13-14; 1995, Q2, P9-10; 1990, 1997, Q2, P6; Q2, P23

03.1 Division of intraspinal nerve root
Rhizotomy

● **03.2 Chordotomy**

03.21 Percutaneous chordotomy
Stereotactic chordotomy

03.29 Other chordotomy
Chordotomy NOS
Tractotomy (one-stage) (two-stage) of spinal cord
Transection of spinal cord tracts

● **03.3 Diagnostic procedures on spinal cord and spinal canal structures**

03.31 Spinal tap
Lumbar puncture for removal of dye

   Excludes *lumbar puncture for injection of dye [myelogram] (87.21)*
   Coding Clinic: 1990, Q2, P23

03.32 Biopsy of spinal cord or spinal meninges

03.39 Other diagnostic procedures on spinal cord and spinal canal structures

   Excludes *microscopic examination of specimen from nervous system or of spinal fluid (90.01–90.09)*
     x-ray of spine (87.21–87.29)

03.4 Excision or destruction of lesion of spinal cord or spinal meninges
Curettage of spinal cord or spinal meninges
Debridement of spinal cord or spinal meninges
Marsupialization of cyst of spinal cord or spinal meninges
Resection of spinal cord or spinal meninges

   Excludes *biopsy of spinal cord or meninges (03.32)*
   Coding Clinic: 2008, Q2, P10; 1995, Q3, P5-6

● **03.5 Plastic operations on spinal cord structures**

03.51 Repair of spinal meningocele
Repair of meningocele NOS

03.52 Repair of spinal myelomeningocele

03.53 Repair of vertebral fracture
Elevation of spinal bone fragments
Reduction of fracture of vertebrae
Removal of bony spicules from spinal canal

> **Excludes** *percutaneous vertebral augmentation (81.66)*
> *percutaneous vertebroplasty (81.65)*

Coding Clinic: 2007, Q1, P20-21; 2004, Q4, P125-126; 2003, Q2, P22; 2002, Q2, P14; 1999, Q4, P12-13; 1996, Q3, P14

03.59 Other repair and plastic operations on spinal cord structures
Repair of:
diastematomyelia
spina bifida NOS
spinal cord NOS
spinal meninges NOS
vertebral arch defect
Coding Clinic: 2008, Q4, P109-110

03.6 Lysis of adhesions of spinal cord and nerve roots
Coding Clinic: 1998, Q2, P18

● **03.7 Shunt of spinal theca**

> **Includes** that with valve

03.71 Spinal subarachnoid-peritoneal shunt

03.72 Spinal subarachnoid-ureteral shunt

03.79 Other shunt of spinal theca
Lumbar-subarachnoid shunt NOS
Pleurothecal anastomosis
Salpingothecal anastomosis
Coding Clinic: 1997, Q1, P7

03.8 Injection of destructive agent into spinal canal
Coding Clinic: 2003, Q2, P6

● **03.9 Other operations on spinal cord and spinal canal structures**

03.90 Insertion of catheter into spinal canal for infusion of therapeutic or palliative substances
Insertion of catheter into epidural, subarachnoid, or subdural space of spine with intermittent or continuous infusion of drug (with creation of any reservoir)

> **Code also** any implantation of infusion pump (86.06)

03.91 Injection of anesthetic into spinal canal for analgesia

> **Excludes** *that for operative anesthesia — omit code*

Coding Clinic: 2000, Q3, P15; 1999, Q1, P7-8; 1998, Q2, P18; 1985, Mar-April, P15; 1984, May-June, P14; 1984, July-Aug, P20

03.92 Injection of other agent into spinal canal
Intrathecal injection of steroid
Subarachnoid perfusion of refrigerated saline

> **Excludes** *injection of:*
> *contrast material for myelogram (87.21)*
> *destructive agent into spinal canal (03.8)*

Coding Clinic: 2003, Q2, P6; 2000, Q3, P15; 1998, Q2, P18

03.93 Implantation or replacement of spinal neurostimulator lead(s)

> **Code also** any insertion of neurostimulator pulse generator (86.94-86.98)

Coding Clinic: 2000, Q1, P19-20

03.94 Removal of spinal neurostimulator lead(s)

> **Code also** any removal of neurostimulator pulse generator (86.05)

03.95 Spinal blood patch

03.96 Percutaneous denervation of facet

03.97 Revision of spinal thecal shunt
Coding Clinic: 1999, Q2, P4

03.98 Removal of spinal thecal shunt

03.99 Other
Coding Clinic: 1985, Mar-April, P15; 1984, May-June, P14; 1984, July-Aug, P20

● **04 Operations on cranial and peripheral nerves**

● **04.0 Incision, division, and excision of cranial and peripheral nerves**

> **Excludes** *opticociliary neurectomy (12.79)*
> *sympathetic ganglionectomy (05.21–05.29)*

04.01 Excision of acoustic neuroma
That by craniotomy

> **Excludes** *that by stereotactic radiosurgery (92.30–92.39)*

Coding Clinic: 1998, Q2, P20; 1995, Q2, P8

04.02 Division of trigeminal nerve
Retrogasserian neurotomy

04.03 Division or crushing of other cranial and peripheral nerves

> **Excludes** *that of:*
> *glossopharyngeal nerve (29.92)*
> *laryngeal nerve (31.91)*
> *nerves to adrenal glands (07.42)*
> *phrenic nerve for collapse of lung (33.31)*
> *vagus nerve (44.00–44.03)*

Coding Clinic: 1998, Q2, P20

04.04 Other incision of cranial and peripheral nerves

04.05 Gasserian ganglionectomy

04.06 Other cranial or peripheral ganglionectomy

> **Excludes** *sympathetic ganglionectomy (05.21–05.29)*

04.07 Other excision or avulsion of cranial and peripheral nerves
Curettage of peripheral nerve
Debridement of peripheral nerve
Resection of peripheral nerve
Excision of peripheral neuroma [Morton's]

> **Excludes** *biopsy of cranial or peripheral nerve (04.11–04.12)*

Coding Clinic: 1995, Q2, P8

● **04.1 Diagnostic procedures on peripheral nervous system**

04.11 Closed [percutaneous] [needle] biopsy of cranial or peripheral nerve or ganglion

04.12 Open biopsy of cranial or peripheral nerve or ganglion

04.19 Other diagnostic procedures on cranial and peripheral nerves and ganglia

> **Excludes** *microscopic examination of specimen from nervous system (90.01–90.09)*
> *neurologic examination (89.13)*

04.2 Destruction of cranial and peripheral nerves
Destruction of cranial or peripheral nerves by:
cryoanalgesia
injection of neurolytic agent
radiofrequency
Radiofrequency ablation
Coding Clinic: 2002, Q3, P10-11

04.3 Suture of cranial and peripheral nerves

● **04.4 Lysis of adhesions and decompression of cranial and peripheral nerves**

04.41 Decompression of trigeminal nerve root

04.42 Other cranial nerve decompression
Coding Clinic: 2002, Q3, P11-13; 1987, Mar-April, P8

OPERATIONS ON THE NERVOUS SYSTEM (01–05)

Excludes | Includes | Use additional | Code also | Omit code

04.43 Release of carpal tunnel
Coding Clinic: 1985, Nov-Dec, P11

04.44 Release of tarsal tunnel

04.49 Other peripheral nerve or ganglion decompression or lysis of adhesions
Peripheral nerve neurolysis NOS
Coding Clinic: 1993, Q2, P8

04.5 Cranial or peripheral nerve graft

04.6 Transposition of cranial and peripheral nerves
Nerve transplantation

● **04.7 Other cranial or peripheral neuroplasty**

04.71 Hypoglossal-facial anastomosis

04.72 Accessory-facial anastomosis

04.73 Accessory-hypoglossal anastomosis

04.74 Other anastomosis of cranial or peripheral nerve

04.75 Revision of previous repair of cranial and peripheral nerves

04.76 Repair of old traumatic injury of cranial and peripheral nerves

04.79 Other neuroplasty
Coding Clinic: 2006, Q1, P11

● **04.8 Injection into peripheral nerve**
| Excludes | *destruction of nerve (by injection of neurolytic agent) (04.2)*

04.80 Peripheral nerve injection, not otherwise specified

04.81 Injection of anesthetic into peripheral nerve for analgesia
| Excludes | *that for operative anesthesia –* omit code
Coding Clinic: 2000, Q1, P7-8

04.89 Injection of other agent, except neurolytic
| Excludes | *injection of neurolytic agent (04.2)*

● **04.9 Other operations on cranial and peripheral nerves**

04.91 Neurectasis

04.92 Implantation or replacement of peripheral neurostimulator lead(s)
Code also any insertion of neurostimulator pulse generator (86.94–86.98)
| Excludes | *implantation or replacement of carotid sinus stimulation lead(s) (39.82)* ◀
Coding Clinic: 2007, Q2, P10-11; 2006, Q2, P5-6; 2004, Q2, P7; 2001, Q3, P16-17; 1996, Q3, P12

04.93 Removal of peripheral neurostimulator lead(s)
Code also any removal of neurostimulator pulse generator (86.05)
Coding Clinic: 2001, Q3, P16-17

04.99 Other

● **05 Operations on sympathetic nerves or ganglia**
| Excludes | *paracervical uterine denervation (69.3)*

05.0 Division of sympathetic nerve or ganglion
| Excludes | *that of nerves to adrenal glands (07.42)*

● **05.1 Diagnostic procedures on sympathetic nerves or ganglia**
Coding Clinic: 2006, Q2, P7

05.11 Biopsy of sympathetic nerve or ganglion

05.19 Other diagnostic procedures on sympathetic nerves or ganglia

● **05.2 Sympathectomy**

05.21 Sphenopalatine ganglionectomy

05.22 Cervical sympathectomy

05.23 Lumbar sympathectomy

05.24 Presacral sympathectomy

05.25 Periarterial sympathectomy

05.29 Other sympathectomy and ganglionectomy
Excision or avulsion of sympathetic nerve NOS
Sympathetic ganglionectomy NOS
| Excludes | *biopsy of sympathetic nerve or ganglion (05.11)*
opticociliary neurectomy (12.79)
periarterial sympathectomy (05.25)
tympanosympathectomy (20.91)

● **05.3 Injection into sympathetic nerve or ganglion**
| Excludes | *injection of ciliary sympathetic ganglion (12.79)*

05.31 Injection of anesthetic into sympathetic nerve for analgesia

05.32 Injection of neurolytic agent into sympathetic nerve

05.39 Other injection into sympathetic nerve or ganglion

● **05.8 Other operations on sympathetic nerves or ganglia**

05.81 Repair of sympathetic nerve or ganglion

05.89 Other

05.9 Other operations on nervous system

---

2. OPERATIONS ON THE ENDOCRINE SYSTEM (06–07)

● **06 Operations on thyroid and parathyroid glands**
| Includes | incidental resection of hyoid bone

● **06.0 Incision of thyroid field**
| Excludes | *division of isthmus (06.91)*

06.01 Aspiration of thyroid field
Percutaneous or needle drainage of thyroid field
| Excludes | *aspiration biopsy of thyroid (06.11)*
drainage by incision (06.09)
postoperative aspiration of field (06.02)

06.02 Reopening of wound of thyroid field
Reopening of wound of thyroid field for:
control of (postoperative) hemorrhage
examination
exploration
removal of hematoma

06.09 Other incision of thyroid field
Drainage of hematoma by incision
Drainage of thyroglossal tract by incision
Exploration:
neck by incision
thyroid (field) by incision
Removal of foreign body by incision
Thyroidotomy NOS by incision
| Excludes | *postoperative exploration (06.02)*
removal of hematoma by aspiration (06.01)

● **06.1 Diagnostic procedures on thyroid and parathyroid glands**

    06.11 Closed [percutaneous] [needle] biopsy of thyroid gland
        Aspiration biopsy of thyroid

    06.12 Open biopsy of thyroid gland

    06.13 Biopsy of parathyroid gland

    06.19 Other diagnostic procedures on thyroid and parathyroid glands

        Excludes *radioisotope scan of:*
            parathyroid (92.13)
            thyroid (92.01)
            soft tissue x-ray of thyroid field (87.09)

● **06.2 Unilateral thyroid lobectomy**
    Complete removal of one lobe of thyroid (with removal of isthmus or portion of other lobe)
    Hemithyroidectomy

    Excludes *partial substernal thyroidectomy (06.51)*

● **06.3 Other partial thyroidectomy**

    06.31 Excision of lesion of thyroid

        Excludes *biopsy of thyroid (06.11–06.12)*
            laser interstitial thermal therapy [LITT] of lesion or tissue of neck under guidance (17.62)

    06.39 Other
        Isthmectomy
        Partial thyroidectomy NOS

        Excludes *partial substernal thyroidectomy (06.51)*

● **06.4 Complete thyroidectomy**

    Excludes *complete substernal thyroidectomy (06.52)*
        that with laryngectomy (30.3–30.4)

● **06.5 Substernal thyroidectomy**

    06.50 Substernal thyroidectomy, not otherwise specified

    06.51 Partial substernal thyroidectomy

    06.52 Complete substernal thyroidectomy

● **06.6 Excision of lingual thyroid**
    Excision of thyroid by:
        submental route
        transoral route

● **06.7 Excision of thyroglossal duct or tract**

● **06.8 Parathyroidectomy**

    06.81 Complete parathyroidectomy

    06.89 Other parathyroidectomy
        Parathyroidectomy NOS
        Partial parathyroidectomy

        Excludes *biopsy of parathyroid (06.13)*

● **06.9 Other operations on thyroid (region) and parathyroid**

    06.91 Division of thyroid isthmus
        Transection of thyroid isthmus

    06.92 Ligation of thyroid vessels

    06.93 Suture of thyroid gland

    06.94 Thyroid tissue reimplantation
        Autotransplantation of thyroid tissue

    06.95 Parathyroid tissue reimplantation
        Autotransplantation of parathyroid tissue
        Coding Clinic: 1995, Q1, P9

    06.98 Other operations on thyroid glands

    06.99 Other operations on parathyroid glands

● **07 Operations on other endocrine glands**

    Includes operations on:
        adrenal glands
        pineal gland
        pituitary gland
        thymus

    Excludes *operations on:*
        aortic and carotid bodies (39.81-39.89) ◀▥
        ovaries (65.0–65.99)
        pancreas (52.01–52.99)
        testes (62.0–62.99)

● **07.0 Exploration of adrenal field**

    Excludes *incision of adrenal (gland) (07.41)*

    07.00 Exploration of adrenal field, not otherwise specified

    07.01 Unilateral exploration of adrenal field

    07.02 Bilateral exploration of adrenal field

● **07.1 Diagnostic procedures on adrenal glands, pituitary gland, pineal gland, and thymus**

    07.11 Closed [percutaneous] [needle] biopsy of adrenal gland

    07.12 Open biopsy of adrenal gland

    07.13 Biopsy of pituitary gland, transfrontal approach

    07.14 Biopsy of pituitary gland, transsphenoidal approach

    07.15 Biopsy of pituitary gland, unspecified approach

    07.16 Biopsy of thymus

    07.17 Biopsy of pineal gland

    07.19 Other diagnostic procedures on adrenal glands, pituitary gland, pineal gland, and thymus

        Excludes *microscopic examination of specimen from endocrine gland (90.11–90.19)*
            radioisotope scan of pituitary gland (92.11)

● **07.2 Partial adrenalectomy**

    07.21 Excision of lesion of adrenal gland

        Excludes *biopsy of adrenal gland (07.11–07.12)*

    07.22 Unilateral adrenalectomy
        Adrenalectomy NOS

        Excludes *excision of remaining adrenal gland (07.3)*

    07.29 Other partial adrenalectomy
        Partial adrenalectomy NOS
        Coding Clinic: 2005, Q2, P4-5

● **07.3 Bilateral adrenalectomy**
    Excision of remaining adrenal gland

    Excludes *bilateral partial adrenalectomy (07.29)*

● **07.4 Other operations on adrenal glands, nerves, and vessels**

    07.41 Incision of adrenal gland
        Adrenalotomy (with drainage)

    07.42 Division of nerves to adrenal glands

    07.43 Ligation of adrenal vessels

    07.44 Repair of adrenal gland

    07.45 Reimplantation of adrenal tissue
        Autotransplantation of adrenal tissue

    07.49 Other

● **07.5 Operations on pineal gland**

    07.51 Exploration of pineal field

        Excludes *that with incision of pineal gland (07.52)*

OPERATIONS ON THE ENDOCRINE SYSTEM (06—07)

07.52　Incision of pineal gland

07.53　Partial excision of pineal gland

> **Excludes** *biopsy of pineal gland (07.17)*

07.54　Total excision of pineal gland
　　　　Pinealectomy (complete) (total)

07.59　Other operations on pineal gland

● 07.6　Hypophysectomy

07.61　Partial excision of pituitary gland, transfrontal approach
　　　　Cryohypophysectomy, partial transfrontal approach
　　　　Division of hypophyseal stalk transfrontal approach
　　　　Excision of lesion of pituitary [hypophysis] transfrontal approach
　　　　Hypophysectomy, subtotal transfrontal approach
　　　　Infundibulectomy, hypophyseal transfrontal approach

> **Excludes** *biopsy of pituitary gland, transfrontal approach (07.13)*

07.62　Partial excision of pituitary gland, transsphenoidal approach

> **Excludes** *biopsy of pituitary gland, transsphenoidal approach (07.14)*

Coding Clinic: 1992, Q3, P13

07.63　Partial excision of pituitary gland, unspecified approach

> **Excludes** *biopsy of pituitary gland NOS (07.15)*

07.64　Total excision of pituitary gland, transfrontal approach
　　　　Ablation of pituitary by implantation (strontium-yttrium) (Y) transfrontal approach
　　　　Cryohypophysectomy, complete transfrontal approach

07.65　Total excision of pituitary gland, transsphenoidal approach

07.68　Total excision of pituitary gland, other specified approach

07.69　Total excision of pituitary gland, unspecified approach
　　　　Hypophysectomy NOS
　　　　Pituitectomy NOS

● 07.7　Other operations on hypophysis

07.71　Exploration of pituitary fossa

> **Excludes** *exploration with incision of pituitary gland (07.72)*

07.72　Incision of pituitary gland
　　　　Aspiration of:
　　　　　　craniobuccal pouch
　　　　　　craniopharyngioma
　　　　　　hypophysis
　　　　　　pituitary gland
　　　　　　Rathke's pouch

07.79　Other
　　　　Insertion of pack into sella turcica

● 07.8　Thymectomy

07.80　Thymectomy, not otherwise specified

07.81　Other partial excision of thymus
　　　　Open partial excision of thymus

> **Excludes** *biopsy of thymus (07.16)*
> *thoracoscopic partial excision of thymus (07.83)*

07.82　Other total excision of thymus
　　　　Open total excision of thymus

> **Excludes** *thoracoscopic total excision of thymus (07.84)*

07.83　Thoracoscopic partial excision of thymus

> **Excludes** *other partial excision of thymus (07.81)*

Coding Clinic: 2007, Q4, P108-109

07.84　Thoracoscopic total excision of thymus

> **Excludes** *other total excision of thymus (07.82)*

Coding Clinic: 2007, Q4, P108-109

● 07.9　Other operations on thymus

07.91　Exploration of thymus field

> **Excludes** *exploration with incision of thymus (07.92)*

07.92　Other incision of thymus
　　　　Open incision of thymus

> **Excludes** *thoracoscopic incision of thymus (07.95)*

07.93　Repair of thymus

07.94　Transplantation of thymus

07.95　Thoracoscopic incision of thymus

> **Excludes** *other incision of thymus (07.92)*

Coding Clinic: 2007, Q4, P108-109

07.98　Other and unspecified thoracoscopic operations on thymus

07.99　Other and unspecified operations on thymus
　　　　Transcervical thymectomy

> **Excludes** *other thoracoscopic operations on thymus (07.98)*

(See Plates 81, 82, 87, and 90 on pages NAP-15–NAP-19.)

03.　OPERATIONS ON THE EYE (08–16)

● 08　Operations on eyelids

> **Includes** operations on the eyebrow

● 08.0　Incision of eyelid

08.01　Incision of lid margin

08.02　Severing of blepharorrhaphy

08.09　Other incision of eyelid

● 08.1　Diagnostic procedures on eyelid

08.11　Biopsy of eyelid

08.19　Other diagnostic procedures on eyelid

● 08.2 **Excision or destruction of lesion or tissue of eyelid**
> Code also any synchronous reconstruction (08.61–08.74)
>
> **Excludes** *biopsy of eyelid (08.11)*

08.20 **Removal of lesion of eyelid, not otherwise specified**
> Removal of meibomian gland NOS

08.21 **Excision of chalazion**

08.22 **Excision of other minor lesion of eyelid**
> Excision of:
>   verucca
>   wart

08.23 **Excision of major lesion of eyelid, partial-thickness**
> Excision involving one-fourth or more of lid margin, partial-thickness

08.24 **Excision of major lesion of eyelid, full-thickness**
> Excision involving one-fourth or more of lid margin, full-thickness
> Wedge resection of eyelid

08.25 **Destruction of lesion of eyelid**

● 08.3 **Repair of blepharoptosis and lid retraction**

08.31 **Repair of blepharoptosis by frontalis muscle technique with suture**

08.32 **Repair of blepharoptosis by frontalis muscle technique with fascial sling**

08.33 **Repair of blepharoptosis by resection or advancement of levator muscle or aponeurosis**

08.34 **Repair of blepharoptosis by other levator muscle techniques**

08.35 **Repair of blepharoptosis by tarsal technique**

08.36 **Repair of blepharoptosis by other techniques**
> Correction of eyelid ptosis NOS
> Orbicularis oculi muscle sling for correction of blepharoptosis

08.37 **Reduction of overcorrection of ptosis**

08.38 **Correction of lid retraction**

● 08.4 **Repair of entropion or ectropion**

08.41 **Repair of entropion or ectropion by thermocauterization**

08.42 **Repair of entropion or ectropion by suture technique**

08.43 **Repair of entropion or ectropion with wedge resection**

08.44 **Repair of entropion or ectropion with lid reconstruction**

08.49 **Other repair of entropion or ectropion**

● 08.5 **Other adjustment of lid position**

08.51 **Canthotomy**
> Enlargement of palpebral fissure

08.52 **Blepharorrhaphy**
> Canthorrhaphy
> Tarsorrhaphy

08.59 **Other**
> Canthoplasty NOS
> Repair of epicanthal fold

● 08.6 **Reconstruction of eyelid with flaps or grafts**
> **Excludes** *that associated with repair of entropion and ectropion (08.44)*

08.61 **Reconstruction of eyelid with skin flap or graft**

08.62 **Reconstruction of eyelid with mucous membrane flap or graft**

08.63 **Reconstruction of eyelid with hair follicle graft**

08.64 **Reconstruction of eyelid with tarsoconjunctival flap**
> Transfer of tarsoconjunctival flap from opposing lid

08.69 **Other reconstruction of eyelid with flaps or grafts**

● 08.7 **Other reconstruction of eyelid**
> **Excludes** *that associated with repair of entropion and ectropion (08.44)*
> Coding Clinic: 1996, Q2, P11

08.70 **Reconstruction of eyelid, not otherwise specified**

08.71 **Reconstruction of eyelid involving lid margin, partial-thickness**

08.72 **Other reconstruction of eyelid, partial-thickness**

08.73 **Reconstruction of eyelid involving lid margin, full-thickness**

08.74 **Other reconstruction of eyelid, full-thickness**

● 08.8 **Other repair of eyelid**

08.81 **Linear repair of laceration of eyelid or eyebrow**

08.82 **Repair of laceration involving lid margin, partial-thickness**

08.83 **Other repair of laceration of eyelid, partial-thickness**

08.84 **Repair of laceration involving lid margin, full-thickness**

08.85 **Other repair of laceration of eyelid, full-thickness**

08.86 **Lower eyelid rhytidectomy**

08.87 **Upper eyelid rhytidectomy**
> Coding Clinic: 1996, Q2, P11

08.89 **Other eyelid repair**
> Coding Clinic: 2000, Q1, P22-23

● 08.9 **Other operations on eyelids**

08.91 **Electrosurgical epilation of eyelid**

08.92 **Cryosurgical epilation of eyelid**

08.93 **Other epilation of eyelid**

08.99 **Other**

● 09 **Operations on lacrimal system**

09.0 **Incision of lacrimal gland**
> Incision of lacrimal cyst (with drainage)

● 09.1 **Diagnostic procedures on lacrimal system**

09.11 **Biopsy of lacrimal gland**

09.12 **Biopsy of lacrimal sac**

09.19 **Other diagnostic procedures on lacrimal system**
> **Excludes** *contrast dacryocystogram (87.05)*
> *soft tissue x-ray of nasolacrimal duct (87.09)*

● 09.2 **Excision of lesion or tissue of lacrimal gland**

09.20 **Excision of lacrimal gland, not otherwise specified**

09.21 **Excision of lesion of lacrimal gland**
> **Excludes** *biopsy of lacrimal gland (09.11)*

09.22 **Other partial dacryoadenectomy**
> **Excludes** *biopsy of lacrimal gland (09.11)*

09.23 **Total dacryoadenectomy**

09.3 **Other operations on lacrimal gland**

OPERATIONS ON THE EYE (08–16)

● **09.4 Manipulation of lacrimal passage**

> **Includes** removal of calculus
> that with dilation
>
> **Excludes** contrast dacryocystogram (87.05)

09.41 Probing of lacrimal punctum

09.42 Probing of lacrimal canaliculi

09.43 Probing of nasolacrimal duct

> **Excludes** that with insertion of tube or stent (09.44)

09.44 Intubation of nasolacrimal duct
Insertion of stent into nasolacrimal duct
Coding Clinic: 1994, Q2, P11

09.49 Other manipulation of lacrimal passage

● **09.5 Incision of lacrimal sac and passages**

09.51 Incision of lacrimal punctum

09.52 Incision of lacrimal canaliculi

09.53 Incision of lacrimal sac

09.59 Other incision of lacrimal passages
Incision (and drainage) of nasolacrimal duct NOS

● **09.6 Excision of lacrimal sac and passage**

> **Excludes** biopsy of lacrimal sac (09.12)

● **09.7 Repair of canaliculus and punctum**

> **Excludes** repair of eyelid (08.81–08.89)

09.71 Correction of everted punctum

09.72 Other repair of punctum

09.73 Repair of canaliculus

● **09.8 Fistulization of lacrimal tract to nasal cavity**

09.81 Dacryocystorhinostomy [DCR]

09.82 Conjunctivocystorhinostomy
Conjunctivodacryocystorhinostomy [CDCR]

> **Excludes** that with insertion of tube or stent (09.83)

09.83 Conjunctivorhinostomy with insertion of tube or stent

● **09.9 Other operations on lacrimal system**

09.91 Obliteration of lacrimal punctum

09.99 Other
Coding Clinic: 1994, Q2, P11

● **10 Operations on conjunctiva**

10.0 Removal of embedded foreign body from conjunctiva by incision

> **Excludes** removal of:
> embedded foreign body without incision (98.22)
> superficial foreign body (98.21)

10.1 Other incision of conjunctiva

● **10.2 Diagnostic procedures on conjunctiva**

10.21 Biopsy of conjunctiva

10.29 Other diagnostic procedures on conjunctiva

● **10.3 Excision or destruction of lesion or tissue of conjunctiva**

10.31 Excision of lesion or tissue of conjunctiva
Excision of ring of conjunctiva around cornea

> **Excludes** biopsy of conjunctiva (10.21)

Coding Clinic: 2000, Q4, P41; 1996, Q3, P7

10.32 Destruction of lesion of conjunctiva

> **Excludes** excision of lesion (10.31)
> thermocauterization for entropion (08.41)

10.33 Other destructive procedures on conjunctiva
Removal of trachoma follicles

● **10.4 Conjunctivoplasty**

10.41 Repair of symblepharon with free graft
Coding Clinic: 1996, Q3, P7

10.42 Reconstruction of conjunctival cul-de-sac with free graft

> **Excludes** revision of enucleation socket with graft (16.63)

10.43 Other reconstruction of conjunctival cul-de-sac

> **Excludes** revision of enucleation socket (16.64)

10.44 Other free graft to conjunctiva

10.49 Other conjunctivoplasty

> **Excludes** repair of cornea with conjunctival flap (11.53)

10.5 Lysis of adhesions of conjunctiva and eyelid
Division of symblepharon (with insertion of conformer)

10.6 Repair of laceration of conjunctiva

> **Excludes** that with repair of sclera (12.81)

● **10.9 Other operations on conjunctiva**

10.91 Subconjunctival injection
Coding Clinic: 1996, Q3, P7

10.99 Other

● **11 Operations on cornea**

11.0 Magnetic removal of embedded foreign body from cornea

> **Excludes** that with incision (11.1)

11.1 Incision of cornea
Incision of cornea for removal of foreign body

● **11.2 Diagnostic procedures on cornea**

11.21 Scraping of cornea for smear or culture

11.22 Biopsy of cornea

11.29 Other diagnostic procedures on cornea

● **11.3 Excision of pterygium**

11.31 Transposition of pterygium

11.32 Excision of pterygium with corneal graft

11.39 Other excision of pterygium

● **11.4 Excision or destruction of tissue or other lesion of cornea**

11.41 Mechanical removal of corneal epithelium
That by chemocauterization

> **Excludes** that for smear or culture (11.21)

Coding Clinic: 2002, Q3, P20-21

11.42 Thermocauterization of corneal lesion

11.43 Cryotherapy of corneal lesion

11.49 Other removal or destruction of corneal lesion
Excision of cornea NOS

> **Excludes** biopsy of cornea (11.22)

● **11.5 Repair of cornea**

11.51 Suture of corneal laceration
Coding Clinic: 1996, Q3, P7

11.52 Repair of postoperative wound dehiscence of cornea

11.53 Repair of corneal laceration or wound with conjunctival flap

11.59 Other repair of cornea

● **11.6 Corneal transplant**

> **Excludes** *excision of pterygium with corneal graft (11.32)*

    11.60 Corneal transplant, not otherwise specified
Keratoplasty NOS
Note: To report donor source - *see* codes 00.91–00.93

    11.61 Lamellar keratoplasty with autograft

    11.62 Other lamellar keratoplasty

    11.63 Penetrating keratoplasty with autograft
Perforating keratoplasty with autograft

    11.64 Other penetrating keratoplasty
Perforating keratoplasty (with homograft)

    11.69 Other corneal transplant

● **11.7 Other reconstructive and refractive surgery on cornea**

    11.71 Keratomileusis

    11.72 Keratophakia

    11.73 Keratoprosthesis

    11.74 Thermokeratoplasty

    11.75 Radial keratotomy

    11.76 Epikeratophakia

    11.79 Other

● **11.9 Other operations on cornea**

    11.91 Tattooing of cornea

    11.92 Removal of artificial implant from cornea

    11.99 Other
Coding Clinic: 2002, Q3, P20-21

● **12 Operations on iris, ciliary body, sclera, and anterior chamber**

> **Excludes** *operations on cornea (11.0–11.99)*

● **12.0 Removal of intraocular foreign body from anterior segment of eye**

    12.00 Removal of intraocular foreign body from anterior segment of eye, not otherwise specified

    12.01 Removal of intraocular foreign body from anterior segment of eye with use of magnet

    12.02 Removal of intraocular foreign body from anterior segment of eye without use of magnet

● **12.1 Iridotomy and simple iridectomy**

> **Excludes** *iridectomy associated with:*
> *cataract extraction (13.11–13.69)*
> *removal of lesion (12.41–12.42)*
> *scleral fistulization (12.61–12.69)*

    12.11 Iridotomy with transfixion

    12.12 Other iridotomy
Corectomy
Discission of iris
Iridotomy NOS

    12.13 Excision of prolapsed iris

    12.14 Other iridectomy
Iridectomy (basal) (peripheral) (total)

● **12.2 Diagnostic procedures on iris, ciliary body, sclera, and anterior chamber**

    12.21 Diagnostic aspiration of anterior chamber of eye

    12.22 Biopsy of iris

    12.29 Other diagnostic procedures on iris, ciliary body, sclera, and anterior chamber

● **12.3 Iridoplasty and coreoplasty**

    12.31 Lysis of goniosynechiae
Lysis of goniosynechiae by injection of air or liquid

    12.32 Lysis of other anterior synechiae
Lysis of anterior synechiae:
NOS
by injection of air or liquid

    12.33 Lysis of posterior synechiae
Lysis of iris adhesions NOS

    12.34 Lysis of corneovitreal adhesions

    12.35 Coreoplasty
Needling of pupillary membrane

    12.39 Other iridoplasty

● **12.4 Excision or destruction of lesion of iris and ciliary body**

    12.40 Removal of lesion of anterior segment of eye, not otherwise specified

    12.41 Destruction of lesion of iris, nonexcisional
Destruction of lesion of iris by:
cauterization
cryotherapy
photocoagulation

    12.42 Excision of lesion of iris

> **Excludes** *biopsy of iris (12.22)*

    12.43 Destruction of lesion of ciliary body, nonexcisional

    12.44 Excision of lesion of ciliary body

● **12.5 Facilitation of intraocular circulation**

    12.51 Goniopuncture without goniotomy

    12.52 Goniotomy without goniopuncture

    12.53 Goniotomy with goniopuncture

    12.54 Trabeculotomy ab externo

    12.55 Cyclodialysis

    12.59 Other facilitation of intraocular circulation
Coding Clinic: 1999, Q4, P13-14

● **12.6 Scleral fistulization**

> **Excludes** *exploratory sclerotomy (12.89)*

    12.61 Trephination of sclera with iridectomy

    12.62 Thermocauterization of sclera with iridectomy

    12.63 Iridencleisis and iridotasis

    12.64 Trabeculectomy ab externo

    12.65 Other scleral fistulization with iridectomy

    12.66 Postoperative revision of scleral fistulization procedure
Revision of filtering bleb

> **Excludes** *repair of fistula (12.82)*

Coding Clinic: 2001, Q2, P16-17

    12.69 Other fistulizing procedure
Coding Clinic: 1996, Q3, P4

● **12.7 Other procedures for relief of elevated intraocular pressure**

    12.71 Cyclodiathermy

    12.72 Cyclocryotherapy

    12.73 Cyclophotocoagulation

    12.74 Diminution of ciliary body, not otherwise specified

    12.79 Other glaucoma procedures
Coding Clinic: 1998, Q2, P16

OPERATIONS ON THE EYE (08–16)

● **12.8 Operations on sclera**

Excludes *those associated with:*
retinal reattachment (14.41–14.59)
scleral fistulization (12.61–12.69)

12.81 Suture of laceration of sclera
Suture of sclera with synchronous repair of conjunctiva

12.82 Repair of scleral fistula

Excludes *postoperative revision of scleral fistulization procedure (12.66)*

12.83 Revision of operative wound of anterior segment, not elsewhere classified

Excludes *postoperative revision of scleral fistulization procedure (12.66)*

12.84 Excision or destruction of lesion of sclera

12.85 Repair of scleral staphyloma with graft

12.86 Other repair of scleral staphyloma

12.87 Scleral reinforcement with graft

12.88 Other scleral reinforcement

12.89 Other operations on sclera
Exploratory sclerotomy

● **12.9 Other operations on iris, ciliary body, and anterior chamber**

12.91 Therapeutic evacuation of anterior chamber
Paracentesis of anterior chamber

Excludes *diagnostic aspiration (12.21)*

12.92 Injection into anterior chamber
Injection of:
air into anterior chamber
liquid into anterior chamber
medication into anterior chamber

12.93 Removal or destruction of epithelial downgrowth from anterior chamber

Excludes *that with iridectomy (12.41–12.42)*

12.97 Other operations on iris

12.98 Other operations on ciliary body

12.99 Other operations on anterior chamber

● **13 Operations on lens**

● **13.0 Removal of foreign body from lens**

Excludes *removal of pseudophakos (13.8)*

13.00 Removal of foreign body from lens, not otherwise specified

13.01 Removal of foreign body from lens with use of magnet

13.02 Removal of foreign body from lens without use of magnet

● **13.1 Intracapsular extraction of lens**

Code also any synchronous insertion of pseudophakos (13.71)

13.11 Intracapsular extraction of lens by temporal inferior route

13.19 Other intracapsular extraction of lens
Cataract extraction NOS
Cryoextraction of lens
Erysiphake extraction of cataract
Extraction of lens NOS

13.2 Extracapsular extraction of lens by linear extraction technique

Code also any synchronous insertion of pseudophakos (13.71)

13.3 Extracapsular extraction of lens by simple aspiration (and irrigation) technique
Irrigation of traumatic cataract

Code also any synchronous insertion of pseudophakos (13.71)

● **13.4 Extracapsular extraction of lens by fragmentation and aspiration technique**

Code also any synchronous insertion of pseudophakos (13.71)

13.41 Phacoemulsification and aspiration of cataract
Coding Clinic: 1996, Q3, P4; 1994, Q1, P16

13.42 Mechanical phacofragmentation and aspiration of cataract by posterior route
Code also any synchronous vitrectomy (14.74)

13.43 Mechanical phacofragmentation and other aspiration of cataract

● **13.5 Other extracapsular extraction of lens**

Code also any synchronous insertion of pseudophakos (13.71)

13.51 Extracapsular extraction of lens by temporal inferior route

13.59 Other extracapsular extraction of lens

● **13.6 Other cataract extraction**

Code also any synchronous insertion of pseudophakos (13.71)

13.64 Discission of secondary membrane [after cataract]

13.65 Excision of secondary membrane [after cataract]
Capsulectomy

13.66 Mechanical fragmentation of secondary membrane [after cataract]

13.69 Other cataract extraction

● **13.7 Insertion of prosthetic lens [pseudophakos]**

Excludes *implantation of intraocular telescope prosthesis (13.91)*

13.70 Insertion of pseudophakos, not otherwise specified

13.71 Insertion of intraocular lens prosthesis at time of cataract extraction, one-stage
Code also synchronous extraction of cataract (13.11–13.69)
Coding Clinic: 1996, Q3, P4

13.72 Secondary insertion of intraocular lens prosthesis

13.8 Removal of implanted lens
Removal of pseudophakos

● **13.9 Other operations on lens**
Coding Clinic: 2000, Q1, P9-10

13.90 Operation on lens, Not Elsewhere Classified

13.91 Implantation of intraocular telescope prosthesis
Implantable miniature telescope

Includes removal of lens, any method

Excludes *secondary insertion of ocular implant (16.61)*
Coding Clinic: 2006, Q4, P123-124

● **14 Operations on retina, choroid, vitreous, and posterior chamber**

● **14.0 Removal of foreign body from posterior segment of eye**

Excludes *removal of surgically implanted material (14.6)*

14.00 Removal of foreign body from posterior segment of eye, not otherwise specified

14.01 Removal of foreign body from posterior segment of eye with use of magnet

14.02 Removal of foreign body from posterior segment of eye without use of magnet

● 14.1 Diagnostic procedures on retina, choroid, vitreous, and posterior chamber

    14.11 Diagnostic aspiration of vitreous

    14.19 Other diagnostic procedures on retina, choroid, vitreous, and posterior chamber

● 14.2 Destruction of lesion of retina and choroid

    Includes   destruction of chorioretinopathy or isolated chorioretinal lesion

    Excludes   *that for repair of retina (14.31–14.59)*

    14.21 Destruction of chorioretinal lesion by diathermy

    14.22 Destruction of chorioretinal lesion by cryotherapy

    14.23 Destruction of chorioretinal lesion by xenon arc photocoagulation

    14.24 Destruction of chorioretinal lesion by laser photocoagulation

    14.25 Destruction of chorioretinal lesion by photocoagulation of unspecified type

    14.26 Destruction of chorioretinal lesion by radiation therapy

    14.27 Destruction of chorioretinal lesion by implantation of radiation source

    14.29 Other destruction of chorioretinal lesion
        Destruction of lesion of retina and choroid NOS

● 14.3 Repair of retinal tear

    Includes   repair of retinal defect

    Excludes   *repair of retinal detachment (14.41–14.59)*

    14.31 Repair of retinal tear by diathermy

    14.32 Repair of retinal tear by cryotherapy

    14.33 Repair of retinal tear by xenon arc photocoagulation

    14.34 Repair of retinal tear by laser photocoagulation
        Coding Clinic: 1994, Q1, P17

    14.35 Repair of retinal tear by photocoagulation of unspecified type

    14.39 Other repair of retinal tear

● 14.4 Repair of retinal detachment with scleral buckling and implant

    14.41 Scleral buckling with implant
        Coding Clinic: 1996, Q3, P6

    14.49 Other scleral buckling
        Scleral buckling with:
          air tamponade
          resection of sclera
          vitrectomy
        Coding Clinic: 1994, Q1, P16-17

● 14.5 Other repair of retinal detachment

    Includes   that with drainage

    14.51 Repair of retinal detachment with diathermy

    14.52 Repair of retinal detachment with cryotherapy

    14.53 Repair of retinal detachment with xenon arc photocoagulation

    14.54 Repair of retinal detachment with laser photocoagulation
        Coding Clinic: 1987, Nov-Dec, P10

    14.55 Repair of retinal detachment with photocoagulation of unspecified type

    14.59 Other

● 14.6 Removal of surgically implanted material from posterior segment of eye

● 14.7 Operations on vitreous

    14.71 Removal of vitreous, anterior approach
        Open sky technique
        Removal of vitreous, anterior approach (with replacement)

    14.72 Other removal of vitreous
        Aspiration of vitreous by posterior sclerotomy

    14.73 Mechanical vitrectomy by anterior approach
        Coding Clinic: 1996, Q3, P4-5

    14.74 Other mechanical vitrectomy
        Posterior approach
        Coding Clinic: 1996, Q3, P5

    14.75 Injection of vitreous substitute
        Excludes   *that associated with removal (14.71–14.72)*
        Coding Clinic: 1998, Q1, P6; 1996, Q3, P5; 1994, Q1, P17

    14.79 Other operations on vitreous
        Coding Clinic: 1999, Q3, P12; 1999, Q1, P11; 1998, Q1, P6

  14.9 Other operations on retina, choroid, and posterior chamber
    Coding Clinic: 1996, Q3, P5; 1993, 5th Issue, P13-14

● 15 Operations on extraocular muscles

● 15.0 Diagnostic procedures on extraocular muscles or tendons

    15.01 Biopsy of extraocular muscle or tendon

    15.09 Other diagnostic procedures on extraocular muscles and tendons

● 15.1 Operations on one extraocular muscle involving temporary detachment from globe

    15.11 Recession of one extraocular muscle
        Coding Clinic: 1996, Q3, P3-4

    15.12 Advancement of one extraocular muscle

    15.13 Resection of one extraocular muscle
        Coding Clinic: 1996, Q3, P4

    15.19 Other operations on one extraocular muscle involving temporary detachment from globe
        Excludes   *transposition of muscle (15.5)*

● 15.2 Other operations on one extraocular muscle

    15.21 Lengthening procedure on one extraocular muscle

    15.22 Shortening procedure on one extraocular muscle

    15.29 Other

  15.3 Operations on two or more extraocular muscles involving temporary detachment from globe, one or both eyes
    Coding Clinic: 1996, Q3, P3-4x2

  15.4 Other operations on two or more extraocular muscles, one or both eyes

  15.5 Transposition of extraocular muscles
    Excludes   *that for correction of ptosis (08.31–08.36)*

  15.6 Revision of extraocular muscle surgery

  15.7 Repair of injury of extraocular muscle
    Freeing of entrapped extraocular muscle
    Lysis of adhesions of extraocular muscle
    Repair of laceration of extraocular muscle, tendon, or Tenon's capsule

  15.9 Other operations on extraocular muscles and tendons

OPERATIONS ON THE EYE (08–16)

Excludes   Includes   Use additional   Code also   Omit code

● 16 **Operations on orbit and eyeball**

   Excludes *reduction of fracture of orbit (76.78–76.79)*

   ● 16.0 **Orbitotomy**

   16.01 **Orbitotomy with bone flap**
   Orbitotomy with lateral approach

   16.02 **Orbitotomy with insertion of orbital implant**
   Excludes *that with bone flap (16.01)*

   16.09 **Other orbitotomy**

   16.1 **Removal of penetrating foreign body from eye, not otherwise specified**
   Excludes *removal of nonpenetrating foreign body (98.21)*

   ● 16.2 **Diagnostic procedures on orbit and eyeball**

   16.21 **Ophthalmoscopy**

   16.22 **Diagnostic aspiration of orbit**

   16.23 **Biopsy of eyeball and orbit**

   16.29 **Other diagnostic procedures on orbit and eyeball**
   Excludes *examination of form and structure of eye (95.11–95.16)*
   general and subjective eye examination (95.01–95.09)
   microscopic examination of specimen from eye (90.21–90.29)
   objective functional tests of eye (95.21–95.26)
   ocular thermography (88.82)
   tonometry (89.11)
   x-ray of orbit (87.14, 87.16)

   ● 16.3 **Evisceration of eyeball**

   16.31 **Removal of ocular contents with synchronous implant into scleral shell**

   16.39 **Other evisceration of eyeball**

   ● 16.4 **Enucleation of eyeball**

   16.41 **Enucleation of eyeball with synchronous implant into Tenon's capsule with attachment of muscles**
   Integrated implant of eyeball

   16.42 **Enucleation of eyeball with other synchronous implant**

   16.49 **Other enucleation of eyeball**
   Removal of eyeball NOS

   ● 16.5 **Exenteration of orbital contents**

   16.51 **Exenteration of orbit with removal of adjacent structures**
   Radical orbitomaxillectomy

   16.52 **Exenteration of orbit with therapeutic removal of orbital bone**

   16.59 **Other exenteration of orbit**
   Evisceration of orbit NOS
   Exenteration of orbit with temporalis muscle transplant

● 16.6 **Secondary procedures after removal of eyeball**

   Excludes *that with synchronous:*
   enucleation of eyeball (16.41–16.42)
   evisceration of eyeball (16.31)

   16.61 **Secondary insertion of ocular implant**

   16.62 **Revision and reinsertion of ocular implant**

   16.63 **Revision of enucleation socket with graft**

   16.64 **Other revision of enucleation socket**

   16.65 **Secondary graft to exenteration cavity**

   16.66 **Other revision of exenteration cavity**

   16.69 **Other secondary procedures after removal of eyeball**

● 16.7 **Removal of ocular or orbital implant**

   16.71 **Removal of ocular implant**

   16.72 **Removal of orbital implant**

● 16.8 **Repair of injury of eyeball and orbit**

   16.81 **Repair of wound of orbit**
   Excludes *reduction of orbital fracture (76.78–76.79)*
   repair of extraocular muscles (15.7)

   16.82 **Repair of rupture of eyeball**
   Repair of multiple structures of eye
   Excludes *repair of laceration of:*
   cornea (11.51–11.59)
   sclera (12.81)

   16.89 **Other repair of injury of eyeball or orbit**

● 16.9 **Other operations on orbit and eyeball**

   Excludes *irrigation of eye (96.51)*
   prescription and fitting of low vision aids (95.31–95.33)
   removal of:
   eye prosthesis NEC (97.31)
   nonpenetrating foreign body from eye without incision (98.21)

   16.91 **Retrobulbar injection of therapeutic agent**
   Excludes *injection of radiographic contrast material (87.14)*
   opticociliary injection (12.79)

   16.92 **Excision of lesion of orbit**
   Excludes *biopsy of orbit (16.23)*

   16.93 **Excision of lesion of eye, unspecified structure**
   Excludes *biopsy of eye NOS (16.23)*

   16.98 **Other operations on orbit**

   16.99 **Other operations on eyeball**

3A. OTHER MISCELLANEOUS DIAGNOSTIC AND THERAPEUTIC PROCEDURES (17)

● 17 **Other miscellaneous procedures**

   ● 17.1 **Laparoscopic unilateral repair of inguinal hernia**
   Excludes *other and open unilateral repair of hernia (53.00 – 53.05)*
   Coding Clinic: 2008, Q4, P165-169

   17.11 **Laparoscopic repair of direct inguinal hernia with graft or prosthesis**
   Laparoscopic repair of direct and indirect inguinal hernia with graft or prosthesis

   17.12 **Laparoscopic repair of indirect inguinal hernia with graft or prosthesis**

   17.13 **Laparoscopic repair of inguinal hernia with graft or prosthesis, not otherwise specified**

● **17.2 Laparoscopic bilateral repair of inguinal hernia**

> **Excludes** *other and open bilateral repair of hernia (53.10 – 53.17)*
> Coding Clinic: 2008, Q4, P165-169

17.21 Laparoscopic bilateral repair of direct inguinal hernia with graft or prosthesis

17.22 Laparoscopic bilateral repair of indirect inguinal hernia with graft or prosthesis

17.23 Laparoscopic bilateral repair of inguinal hernia, one direct and one indirect, with graft or prosthesis

17.24 Laparoscopic bilateral repair of inguinal hernia with graft or prosthesis, not otherwise specified

● **17.3 Laparoscopic partial excision of large intestine**

> **Excludes** *other and open partial excision of large intestine (45.71- 45.79)*
> Coding Clinic: 2008, Q4, P169-172

17.31 Laparoscopic multiple segmental resection of large intestine

17.32 Laparoscopic cecectomy

17.33 Laparoscopic right hemicolectomy

17.34 Laparoscopic resection of transverse colon

17.35 Laparoscopic left hemicolectomy

17.36 Laparoscopic sigmoidectomy

17.39 Other laparoscopic partial excision of large intestine

● **17.4 Robotic assisted procedures**
Computer assisted robotic surgery
Computer-enhanced robotic surgery
Robotic procedure with computer assistance
Surgeon-controlled robotic surgery

Code first primary procedure

> **Excludes** *computer assisted surgery (00.31-00.35, 00.39)*

Note: This category includes use of a computer console with (3-D) imaging, software, camera(s), visualization and instrumentation *combined* with the use of robotic arms, device(s), or system(s) at the time of the procedure.
Coding Clinic: 2008, Q4, P172-174

17.41 Open robotic assisted procedure
Robotic assistance in open procedure

17.42 Laparoscopic robotic assisted procedure
Robotic assistance in laparoscopic procedure
Coding Clinic: 2009, Q3, P6

17.43 Percutaneous robotic assisted procedure
Robotic assistance in percutaneous procedure

17.44 Endoscopic robotic assisted procedure
Robotic assistance in endoscopic procedure

17.45 Thoracoscopic robotic assisted procedure
Robotic assistance in thoracoscopic procedure

17.49 Other and unspecified robotic assisted procedure
Robotic assistance in other and unspecified procedure

> **Excludes** *endoscopic robotic assisted procedure (17.44)*
> *laparoscopic robotic assisted procedure (17.42)*
> *open robotic assisted procedure (17.41)*
> *percutaneous robotic assisted procedure (17.43)*
> *thoracoscopic robotic assisted procedure (17.45)*

● **17.5 Additional cardiovascular procedures**

17.51 Implantation of rechargeable cardiac contractility modulation [CCM], total system
Note: Device testing during procedure – *omit code*
Implantation of CCM system includes formation of pocket, transvenous leads, including placement of leads, placement of catheter into left ventricle, intraoperative procedures for evaluation of lead signals, obtaining sensing threshold measurements, obtaining defibrillator threshold measurements.

> **Includes** implantation of device with removal of existing device

> **Code also** any concomitant:
> coronary bypass (36.10 – 36.19)
> extracorporeal circulation (39.61)
> insertion or replacement of automatic cardioverter/defibrillator, total system [AICD] (37.94)

> **Excludes** *implantation of CCM pulse generator only (17.52)*
> Coding Clinic: 2009, Q4, P141

17.52 Implantation or replacement of cardiac contractility modulation [CCM] rechargeable pulse generator only
Implantation of CCM device with removal of any existing CCM device
Note: Device testing during procedure – *omit code*

> **Code also** any concomitant:
> revision of device pocket (37.79)
> revision of lead [electrode] (37.75)

● **17.6 Laser interstitial thermal therapy [LITT] under guidance**
Focused laser interstitial thermal therapy [f-LITT] under MRI guidance
MRI-guided LITT

17.61 Laser interstitial thermal therapy [LITT] of lesion or tissue of brain under guidance
Focused laser interstitial thermal therapy [f-LITT] under MRI guidance
MRI-guided LITT of lesion or tissue of brain

> **Excludes** *laser interstitial thermal therapy [LITT] of lesion or tissue of head under guidance (17.62)*
> Coding Clinic: 2009, Q4, P144

17.62 Laser interstitial thermal therapy [LITT] of lesion or tissue of head and neck under guidance
Focused laser interstitial thermal therapy [f-LITT] under MRI guidance
MRI-guided LITT of lesion or tissue of head and neck

> **Excludes** *laser interstitial thermal therapy [LITT] of lesion or tissue of brain under guidance (17.61)*

17.63 Laser interstitial thermal therapy [LITT] of lesion or tissue of liver under guidance
Focused laser interstitial thermal therapy [f-LITT] under MRI guidance
MRI-guided LITT of lesion or tissue of liver

17.69 Laser interstitial thermal therapy [LITT] of lesion or tissue of other and unspecified site under guidance
Focused laser interstitial thermal therapy [f-LITT] under MRI guidance
MRI-guided LITT of lesion or tissue of breast
MRI-guided LITT of lesion or tissue of lung
MRI-guided LITT of lesion or tissue of prostate

> **Excludes** *laser interstitial thermal therapy [LITT] of lesion or tissue of brain under guidance (17.61)*
> *laser interstitial thermal therapy [LITT] of lesion or tissue of head and neck under guidance (17.62)*
> *laser interstitial thermal therapy [LITT] of lesion or tissue of liver under guidance (17.63)*

● **17.7 Other diagnostic and therapeutic procedures**

17.70 Intravenous infusion of clofarabine

> **Excludes** *injection or infusion of cancer chemotherapeutic substance (99.25)*

17.71 Non-coronary intra-operative fluorescence vascular angiography [IFVA] ◀
Intraoperative laser arteriogram ◀
SPY arteriogram ◀
SPY arteriography ◀

> **Excludes** *intra-operative coronary fluorescence vascular angiography (88.59)* ◀

(See Plates 92 and 93 on pages NAP-20–NAP-21.)

4. OPERATIONS ON THE EAR (18–20)

● **18 Operations on external ear**

> **Includes** operations on:
> external auditory canal
> skin and cartilage of:
> auricle
> meatus

● **18.0 Incision of external ear**

> **Excludes** *removal of intraluminal foreign body (98.11)*

18.01 Piercing of ear lobe
Piercing of pinna

18.02 Incision of external auditory canal

18.09 Other incision of external ear

● **18.1 Diagnostic procedures on external ear**

18.11 Otoscopy

18.12 Biopsy of external ear

18.19 Other diagnostic procedures on external ear

> **Excludes** *microscopic examination of specimen from ear (90.31–90.39)*

● **18.2 Excision or destruction of lesion of external ear**

18.21 Excision of preauricular sinus
Radical excision of preauricular sinus or cyst

> **Excludes** *excision of preauricular remnant [appendage] (18.29)*

18.29 Excision or destruction of other lesion of external ear
Cauterization of external ear
Coagulation of external ear
Cryosurgery of external ear
Curettage of external ear
Electrocoagulation of external ear
Enucleation of external ear
Excision of:
exostosis of external auditory canal
preauricular remnant [appendage]
Partial excision of ear

> **Excludes** *biopsy of external ear (18.12)*
> *radical excision of lesion (18.31)*
> *removal of cerumen (96.52)*

● **18.3 Other excision of external ear**

> **Excludes** *biopsy of external ear (18.12)*

18.31 Radical excision of lesion of external ear

> **Excludes** *radical excision of preauricular sinus (18.21)*

18.39 Other
Amputation of external ear

> **Excludes** *excision of lesion (18.21–18.29, 18.31)*

18.4 Suture of laceration of external ear

18.5 Surgical correction of prominent ear
Ear:
pinning
setback

18.6 Reconstruction of external auditory canal
Canaloplasty of external auditory meatus
Construction [reconstruction] of external meatus of ear:
osseous portion
skin-lined portion (with skin graft)

● **18.7 Other plastic repair of external ear**

18.71 Construction of auricle of ear
Prosthetic appliance for absent ear
Reconstruction:
auricle
ear

18.72 Reattachment of amputated ear

18.79 Other plastic repair of external ear
Otoplasty NOS
Postauricular skin graft
Repair of lop ear
Coding Clinic: 2003, Q3, P12-13

18.9 Other operations on external ear

> **Excludes** *irrigation of ear (96.52)*
> *packing of external auditory canal (96.11)*
> *removal of:*
> *cerumen (96.52)*
> *foreign body (without incision) (98.11)*

● **19 Reconstructive operations on middle ear**

19.0 Stapes mobilization
Division, otosclerotic:
material
process
Remobilization of stapes
Stapediolysis
Transcrural stapes mobilization

> **Excludes** *that with synchronous stapedectomy (19.11–19.19)*

● **19.1   Stapedectomy**

> **Excludes**   *revision of previous stapedectomy (19.21–19.29)*
> *stapes mobilization only (19.0)*

19.11   Stapedectomy with incus replacement
Stapedectomy with incus:
homograft
prosthesis

19.19   Other stapedectomy

● **19.2   Revision of stapedectomy**

19.21   Revision of stapedectomy with incus replacement

19.29   Other revision of stapedectomy

19.3   Other operations on ossicular chain
Incudectomy NOS
Ossiculectomy NOS
Reconstruction of ossicles, second stage

19.4   Myringoplasty
Epitympanic, type I
Myringoplasty by:
cauterization
graft
Tympanoplasty (type I)

● **19.5   Other tympanoplasty**

19.52   Type II tympanoplasty
Closure of perforation with graft against incus or malleus

19.53   Type III tympanoplasty
Graft placed in contact with mobile and intact stapes
Coding Clinic: 1985, Mar-April, P15

19.54   Type IV tympanoplasty
Mobile footplate left exposed with air pocket between round window and graft

19.55   Type V tympanoplasty
Fenestra in horizontal semicircular canal covered by graft

19.6   Revision of tympanoplasty

19.9   Other repair of middle ear
Closure of mastoid fistula
Mastoid myoplasty
Obliteration of tympanomastoid cavity

● **20   Other operations on middle and inner ear**

● **20.0   Myringotomy**

20.01   Myringotomy with insertion of tube
Myringostomy

20.09   Other myringotomy
Aspiration of middle ear NOS

20.1   Removal of tympanostomy tube
Coding Clinic: 1994, Q3, P7; 1987, Nov-Dec, P9

● **20.2   Incision of mastoid and middle ear**

20.21   Incision of mastoid

20.22   Incision of petrous pyramid air cells

20.23   Incision of middle ear
Atticotomy
Division of tympanum
Lysis of adhesions of middle ear

> **Excludes**   *division of otosclerotic process (19.0)*
> *stapediolysis (19.0)*
> *that with stapedectomy (19.11–19.19)*

● **20.3   Diagnostic procedures on middle and inner ear**

20.31   Electrocochleography

20.32   Biopsy of middle and inner ear

20.39   Other diagnostic procedures on middle and inner ear

> **Excludes**   *auditory and vestibular function tests (89.13, 95.41–95.49)*
> *microscopic examination of specimen from ear (90.31–90.39)*

● **20.4   Mastoidectomy**

Code also any:
skin graft (18.79)
tympanoplasty (19.4–19.55)

> **Excludes**   *that with implantation of cochlear prosthetic device (20.96–20.98)*

20.41   Simple mastoidectomy

20.42   Radical mastoidectomy

20.49   Other mastoidectomy
Atticoantrostomy
Mastoidectomy:
NOS
modified radical

● **20.5   Other excision of middle ear**

> **Excludes**   *that with synchronous mastoidectomy (20.41–20.49)*

20.51   Excision of lesion of middle ear

> **Excludes**   *biopsy of middle ear (20.32)*

20.59   Other
Apicectomy of petrous pyramid
Tympanectomy

● **20.6   Fenestration of inner ear**

20.61   Fenestration of inner ear (initial)
Fenestration of:
labyrinth with graft (skin) (vein)
semicircular canals with graft (skin) (vein)
vestibule with graft (skin) (vein)

> **Excludes**   *that with tympanoplasty, type V (19.55)*

20.62   Revision of fenestration of inner ear

● **20.7   Incision, excision, and destruction of inner ear**

20.71   Endolymphatic shunt

20.72   Injection into inner ear
Destruction by injection (alcohol):
inner ear
semicircular canals
vestibule

20.79   Other incision, excision, and destruction of inner ear
Decompression of labyrinth
Drainage of inner ear
Fistulization:
endolymphatic sac
labyrinth
Incision of endolymphatic sac
Labyrinthectomy (transtympanic)
Opening of bony labyrinth
Perilymphatic tap

> **Excludes**   *biopsy of inner ear (20.32)*

OPERATIONS ON THE EAR (18–20)

OPERATIONS ON THE EAR (18–20)

20.8 Operations on Eustachian tube
Catheterization of Eustachian tube
Inflation of Eustachian tube
Injection (Teflon paste) of Eustachian tube
Insufflation (boric acid-salicylic acid)
Intubation of Eustachian tube
Politzerization of Eustachian tube

● **20.9 Other operations on inner and middle ear**

20.91 Tympanosympathectomy

20.92 Revision of mastoidectomy
Coding Clinic: 1998, Q2, P20

20.93 Repair of oval and round windows
Closure of fistula:
oval window
perilymph
round window

20.94 Injection of tympanum

20.95 Implantation of electromagnetic hearing device
Bone conduction hearing device
| **Excludes** | *cochlear prosthetic device (20.96–20.98)* |
Coding Clinic: 2007, Q3, P5

20.96 Implantation or replacement of cochlear prosthetic device, not otherwise specified
Implantation of receiver (within skull) and
insertion of electrode(s) in the cochlea
| **Includes** | mastoidectomy |
| **Excludes** | *electromagnetic hearing device (20.95)* |

20.97 Implantation or replacement of cochlear prosthetic device, single channel
Implantation of receiver (within skull) and
insertion of electrode in the cochlea
| **Includes** | mastoidectomy |
| **Excludes** | *electromagnetic hearing device (20.95)* |

20.98 Implantation or replacement of cochlear prosthetic device, multiple channel
Implantation of receiver (within skull) and
insertion of electrodes in the cochlea
| **Includes** | mastoidectomy |
| **Excludes** | *electromagnetic hearing device (20.95)* |

20.99 Other operations on middle and inner ear
Attachment of percutaneous abutment (screw)
for prosthetic device
Repair or removal of cochlear prosthetic device
(receiver) (electrode)
| **Excludes** | *adjustment (external components) of cochlear prosthetic device (95.49) fitting of hearing aid (95.48)* |
Coding Clinic: 2007, Q3, P5

(See Plates 49, 57, 58, and 61 on pages NAP-22–NAP-25.)

5. **OPERATIONS ON THE NOSE, MOUTH, AND PHARYNX (21–29)**

● **21 Operations on nose**
| **Includes** | operations on: bone of nose skin of nose |

● **21.0 Control of epistaxis**

21.00 Control of epistaxis, not otherwise specified

21.01 Control of epistaxis by anterior nasal packing

21.02 Control of epistaxis by posterior (and anterior) packing
Coding Clinic: 1995, Q1, P5

21.03 Control of epistaxis by cauterization (and packing)

21.04 Control of epistaxis by ligation of ethmoidal arteries

21.05 Control of epistaxis by (transantral) ligation of the maxillary artery

21.06 Control of epistaxis by ligation of the external carotid artery

21.07 Control of epistaxis by excision of nasal mucosa and skin grafting of septum and lateral nasal wall

21.09 Control of epistaxis by other means
Coding Clinic: 1995, Q1, P5

21.1 Incision of nose
Chondrotomy
Incision of skin of nose
Nasal septotomy

● **21.2 Diagnostic procedures on nose**

21.21 Rhinoscopy

21.22 Biopsy of nose

21.29 Other diagnostic procedures on nose
| **Excludes** | *microscopic examination of specimen from nose (90.31–90.39) nasal: function study (89.12) x-ray (87.16) rhinomanometry (89.12)* |

● **21.3 Local excision or destruction of lesion of nose**
| **Excludes** | *biopsy of nose (21.22) nasal fistulectomy (21.82)* |

21.30 Excision or destruction of lesion of nose, not otherwise specified

21.31 Local excision or destruction of intranasal lesion
Nasal polypectomy

21.32 Local excision or destruction of other lesion of nose
Coding Clinic: 1989, Q2, P16

21.4 Resection of nose
Amputation of nose

21.5 Submucous resection of nasal septum

● **21.6 Turbinectomy**

21.61 Turbinectomy by diathermy or cryosurgery

21.62 Fracture of the turbinates

21.69 Other turbinectomy
| **Excludes** | *turbinectomy associated with sinusectomy (22.31–22.39, 22.42, 22.60–22.64)* |

● **21.7 Reduction of nasal fracture**

21.71 Closed reduction of nasal fracture

21.72 Open reduction of nasal fracture

◀ New   ◀|||| Revised   ~~deleted~~ Deleted   ● Use Additional Digit(s)   OGCR Official Guidelines   Coding Clinic

● **21.8 Repair and plastic operations on the nose**

  21.81 Suture of laceration of nose

  21.82 Closure of nasal fistula
       Nasolabial fistulectomy
       Nasopharyngeal fistulectomy
       Oronasal fistulectomy

  21.83 Total nasal reconstruction
       Reconstruction of nose with:
          arm flap
          forehead flap

  21.84 Revision rhinoplasty
       Rhinoseptoplasty
       Twisted nose rhinoplasty

  21.85 Augmentation rhinoplasty
       Augmentation rhinoplasty with:
          graft
          synthetic implant

  21.86 Limited rhinoplasty
       Plastic repair of nasolabial flaps
       Tip rhinoplasty

  21.87 Other rhinoplasty
       Rhinoplasty NOS

  21.88 Other septoplasty
       Crushing of nasal septum
       Repair of septal perforation
       Excludes   *septoplasty associated with submucous*
           resection of septum (21.5)

  21.89 Other repair and plastic operations on nose
       Reattachment of amputated nose

● **21.9 Other operations on nose**

  21.91 Lysis of adhesions of nose
       Posterior nasal scrub

  21.99 Other
       Excludes   *dilation of frontonasal duct (96.21)*
           irrigation of nasal passages (96.53)
           removal of:
              intraluminal foreign body without
                 incision (98.12)
              nasal packing (97.32)
           replacement of nasal packing (97.21)

● **22 Operations on nasal sinuses**

● **22.0 Aspiration and lavage of nasal sinus**

  22.00 Aspiration and lavage of nasal sinus, not otherwise specified

  22.01 Puncture of nasal sinus for aspiration or lavage

  22.02 Aspiration or lavage of nasal sinus through natural ostium

● **22.1 Diagnostic procedures on nasal sinus**

  22.11 Closed [endoscopic] [needle] biopsy of nasal sinus

  22.12 Open biopsy of nasal sinus

  22.19 Other diagnostic procedures on nasal sinuses
       Endoscopy without biopsy
       Excludes   *transillumination of sinus (89.35)*
           x-ray of sinus (87.15–87.16)

  22.2 Intranasal antrotomy
       Excludes   *antrotomy with external approach*
           (22.31–22.39)

● **22.3 External maxillary antrotomy**

  22.31 Radical maxillary antrotomy
       Removal of lining membrane of maxillary
          sinus using Caldwell-Luc approach

  22.39 Other external maxillary antrotomy
       Exploration of maxillary antrum with
          Caldwell-Luc approach

● **22.4 Frontal sinusotomy and sinusectomy**

  22.41 Frontal sinusotomy

  22.42 Frontal sinusectomy
       Excision of lesion of frontal sinus
       Obliteration of frontal sinus (with fat)
       Excludes   *biopsy of nasal sinus (22.11–22.12)*

● **22.5 Other nasal sinusotomy**

  22.50 Sinusotomy, not otherwise specified

  22.51 Ethmoidotomy

  22.52 Sphenoidotomy

  22.53 Incision of multiple nasal sinuses

● **22.6 Other nasal sinusectomy**
       Includes   that with incidental turbinectomy
       Excludes   *biopsy of nasal sinus (22.11–22.12)*

  22.60 Sinusectomy, not otherwise specified

  22.61 Excision of lesion of maxillary sinus with Caldwell-Luc approach

  22.62 Excision of lesion of maxillary sinus with other approach

  22.63 Ethmoidectomy

  22.64 Sphenoidectomy

● **22.7 Repair of nasal sinus**

  22.71 Closure of nasal sinus fistula
       Repair of oro-antral fistula

  22.79 Other repair of nasal sinus
       Reconstruction of frontonasal duct
       Repair of bone of accessory sinus

  22.9 Other operations on nasal sinuses
       Exteriorization of maxillary sinus
       Fistulization of sinus
       Excludes   *dilation of frontonasal duct (96.21)*

● **23 Removal and restoration of teeth**

● **23.0 Forceps extraction of tooth**

  23.01 Extraction of deciduous tooth

  23.09 Extraction of other tooth
       Extraction of tooth NOS

● **23.1 Surgical removal of tooth**

  23.11 Removal of residual root

  23.19 Other surgical extraction of tooth
       Odontectomy NOS
       Removal of impacted tooth
       Tooth extraction with elevation of
          mucoperiosteal flap

  23.2 Restoration of tooth by filling

  23.3 Restoration of tooth by inlay

● **23.4 Other dental restoration**

  23.41 Application of crown

  23.42 Insertion of fixed bridge

  23.43 Insertion of removable bridge

  23.49 Other

  23.5 Implantation of tooth

  23.6 Prosthetic dental implant
       Endosseous dental implant

● **23.7 Apicoectomy and root canal therapy**

  23.70 Root canal, not otherwise specified

  23.71 Root canal therapy with irrigation

  23.72 Root canal therapy with apicoectomy

  23.73 Apicoectomy

OPERATIONS ON THE NOSE, MOUTH, AND PHARYNX (21–29)

     Excludes   Includes   Use additional   Code also   Omit code

● **24 Other operations on teeth, gums, and alveoli**

24.0 Incision of gum or alveolar bone
Apical alveolotomy

● **24.1 Diagnostic procedures on teeth, gums, and alveoli**

24.11 Biopsy of gum

24.12 Biopsy of alveolus

24.19 Other diagnostic procedures on teeth, gums, and alveoli
Excludes dental:
examination (89.31)
x-ray:
full-mouth (87.11)
other (87.12)
microscopic examination of dental
specimen (90.81–90.89)

24.2 Gingivoplasty
Gingivoplasty with bone or soft tissue graft

● **24.3 Other operations on gum**

24.31 Excision of lesion or tissue of gum
Excludes biopsy of gum (24.11)
excision of odontogenic lesion (24.4)

24.32 Suture of laceration of gum

24.39 Other

24.4 Excision of dental lesion of jaw
Excision of odontogenic lesion

24.5 Alveoloplasty
Alveolectomy (interradicular) (intraseptal) (radical)
(simple) (with graft or implant)
Excludes biopsy of alveolus (24.12)
en bloc resection of alveolar process and palate
(27.32)

24.6 Exposure of tooth

24.7 Application of orthodontic appliance
Application, insertion, or fitting of:
arch bars
orthodontic obturator
orthodontic wiring
periodontal splint
Excludes nonorthodontic dental wiring (93.55)

24.8 Other orthodontic operation
Closure of diastema (alveolar) (dental)
Occlusal adjustment
Removal of arch bars
Repair of dental arch
Excludes removal of nonorthodontic wiring (97.33)

● **24.9 Other dental operations**

24.91 Extension or deepening of buccolabial or lingual sulcus

24.99 Other
Excludes dental:
debridement (96.54)
examination (89.31)
prophylaxis (96.54)
scaling and polishing (96.54)
wiring (93.55)
fitting of dental appliance [denture]
(99.97)
microscopic examination of dental
specimen (90.81–90.89)
removal of dental:
packing (97.34)
prosthesis (97.35)
wiring (97.33)
replacement of dental packing (97.22)

● **25 Operations on tongue**

● **25.0 Diagnostic procedures on tongue**

25.01 Closed [needle] biopsy of tongue

25.02 Open biopsy of tongue
Wedge biopsy

25.09 Other diagnostic procedures on tongue

25.1 Excision or destruction of lesion or tissue of tongue
Excludes biopsy of tongue (25.01–25.02)
frenumectomy:
labial (27.41)
lingual (25.92)
Coding Clinic: 2002, Q2, P5-6

25.2 Partial glossectomy

25.3 Complete glossectomy
Glossectomy NOS
Code also any neck dissection (40.40–40.42)

25.4 Radical glossectomy
Code also any:
neck dissection (40.40–40.42)
tracheostomy (31.1–31.29)

● **25.5 Repair of tongue and glossoplasty**

25.51 Suture of laceration of tongue

25.59 Other repair and plastic operations on tongue
Fascial sling of tongue
Fusion of tongue (to lip)
Graft of mucosa or skin to tongue
Excludes lysis of adhesions of tongue (25.93)
Coding Clinic: 1997, Q1, P5

● **25.9 Other operations on tongue**

25.91 Lingual frenotomy
Excludes labial frenotomy (27.91)

25.92 Lingual frenectomy
Excludes labial frenectomy (27.41)

25.93 Lysis of adhesions of tongue

25.94 Other glossotomy

25.99 Other

● **26 Operations on salivary glands and ducts**
Includes operations on:
lesser salivary gland and duct
parotid gland and duct
sublingual gland and duct
submaxillary gland and duct
Code also any neck dissection (40.40–40.42)

26.0 Incision of salivary gland or duct

● **26.1 Diagnostic procedures on salivary glands and ducts**

26.11 Closed [needle] biopsy of salivary gland or duct

26.12 Open biopsy of salivary gland or duct

26.19 Other diagnostic procedures on salivary glands and ducts
Excludes x-ray of salivary gland (87.09)

● **26.2 Excision of lesion of salivary gland**

26.21 Marsupialization of salivary gland cyst

26.29 Other excision of salivary gland lesion
Excludes biopsy of salivary gland (26.11–26.12)
salivary fistulectomy (26.42)

● **26.3 Sialoadenectomy**

26.30 Sialoadenectomy, not otherwise specified

26.31 Partial sialoadenectomy

26.32 Complete sialoadenectomy
En bloc excision of salivary gland lesion
Radical sialoadenectomy

● **26.4   Repair of salivary gland or duct**

26.41   Suture of laceration of salivary gland

26.42   Closure of salivary fistula

26.49   Other repair and plastic operations on salivary gland or duct
Fistulization of salivary gland
Plastic repair of salivary gland or duct NOS
Transplantation of salivary duct opening

● **26.9   Other operations on salivary gland or duct**

26.91   Probing of salivary duct

26.99   Other

● **27   Other operations on mouth and face**

Includes	operations on:

lips
palate
soft tissue of face and mouth, except tongue
and gingiva

Excludes	operations on:

gingiva (24.0–24.99)
tongue (25.01–25.99)

27.0   Drainage of face and floor of mouth
Drainage of:
facial region (abscess)
fascial compartment of face
Ludwig's angina

Excludes	*drainage of thyroglossal tract (06.09)*

27.1   Incision of palate

● **27.2   Diagnostic procedures on oral cavity**

27.21   Biopsy of bony palate

27.22   Biopsy of uvula and soft palate

27.23   Biopsy of lip

27.24   Biopsy of mouth, unspecified structure

27.29   Other diagnostic procedures on oral cavity

Excludes	*soft tissue x-ray (87.09)*

● **27.3   Excision of lesion or tissue of bony palate**

27.31   Local excision or destruction of lesion or tissue of bony palate
Local excision or destruction of palate by:
cautery
chemotherapy
cryotherapy

Excludes	*biopsy of bony palate (27.21)*

27.32   Wide excision or destruction of lesion or tissue of bony palate
En bloc resection of alveolar process and palate

● **27.4   Excision of other parts of mouth**

27.41   Labial frenectomy

Excludes	*division of labial frenum (27.91)*

27.42   Wide excision of lesion of lip

27.43   Other excision of lesion or tissue of lip

27.49   Other excision of mouth

Excludes	*biopsy of mouth NOS (27.24)*

excision of lesion of:
palate (27.31–27.32)
tongue (25.1)
uvula (27.72)
fistulectomy of mouth (27.53)
frenectomy of:
lip (27.41)
tongue (25.92)

Coding Clinic: 2005, Q2, P8-9

● **27.5   Plastic repair of lip and mouth**

Excludes	*palatoplasty (27.61–27.69)*

27.51   Suture of laceration of lip

27.52   Suture of laceration of other part of mouth

27.53   Closure of fistula of mouth

Excludes	*fistulectomy:*

nasolabial (21.82)
oro-antral (22.71)
oronasal (21.82)

27.54   Repair of cleft lip

27.55   Full-thickness skin graft to lip and mouth

27.56   Other skin graft to lip and mouth

27.57   Attachment of pedicle or flap graft to lip and mouth

27.59   Other plastic repair of mouth

● **27.6   Palatoplasty**

27.61   Suture of laceration of palate

27.62   Correction of cleft palate
Correction of cleft palate by push-back operation

Excludes	*revision of cleft palate repair (27.63)*

27.63   Revision of cleft palate repair
Secondary:
attachment of pharyngeal flap
lengthening of palate
Coding Clinic: 1996, Q1, P14

27.64   Insertion of palatal implant
Coding Clinic: 2004, Q4, P117-118

27.69   Other plastic repair of palate

Code also any insertion of palatal implant (27.64)

Excludes	*fistulectomy of mouth (27.53)*

Coding Clinic: 1999, Q3, P22; 1997, Q1, P5;
1985, Mar-April, P12

● **27.7   Operations on uvula**

27.71   Incision of uvula

27.72   Excision of uvula

Excludes	*biopsy of uvula (27.22)*

27.73   Repair of uvula

Excludes	*that with synchronous cleft palate repair (27.62)*

uranostaphylorrhaphy (27.62)

27.79   Other operations on uvula
Coding Clinic: 1992, Q3, P18; 1985, Mar-April, P12

● **27.9   Other operations on mouth and face**

27.91   Labial frenotomy
Division of labial frenum

Excludes	*lingual frenotomy (25.91)*

27.92   Incision of mouth, unspecified structure

Excludes	*incision of:*

gum (24.0)
palate (27.1)
salivary gland or duct (26.0)
tongue (25.94)
uvula (27.71)

27.99   Other operations on oral cavity
Graft of buccal sulcus

Excludes	*removal of:*

intraluminal foreign body (98.01)
penetrating foreign body from mouth without incision (98.22)

● **28   Operations on tonsils and adenoids**

28.0   Incision and drainage of tonsil and peritonsillar structures
Drainage (oral) (transcervical) of:
parapharyngeal abscess
peritonsillar abscess
retropharyngeal abscess
tonsillar abscess

Excludes	Includes	Use additional	Code also	Omit code

● 28.1 **Diagnostic procedures on tonsils and adenoids**

    28.11 **Biopsy of tonsils and adenoids**

    28.19 **Other diagnostic procedures on tonsils and adenoids**

        Excludes *soft tissue x-ray (87.09)*

28.2 **Tonsillectomy without adenoidectomy**
Coding Clinic: 1997, Q1, P5; 1990, Q2, P23

28.3 **Tonsillectomy with adenoidectomy**
Coding Clinic: 2005, Q2, P16

28.4 **Excision of tonsil tag**

28.5 **Excision of lingual tonsil**

28.6 **Adenoidectomy without tonsillectomy**
    Excision of adenoid tag

28.7 **Control of hemorrhage after tonsillectomy and adenoidectomy**
Coding Clinic: 2005, Q2, P16

● 28.9 **Other operations on tonsils and adenoids**

    28.91 **Removal of foreign body from tonsil and adenoid by incision**

        Excludes *that without incision (98.13)*

    28.92 **Excision of lesion of tonsil and adenoid**

        Excludes *biopsy of tonsil and adenoid (28.11)*

    28.99 **Other**
        Coding Clinic: 1990, Q2, P23

● 29 **Operations on pharynx**

    Includes operations on:
        hypopharynx
        nasopharynx
        oropharynx
        pharyngeal pouch
        pyriform sinus

29.0 **Pharyngotomy**
    Drainage of pharyngeal bursa

    Excludes *incision and drainage of retropharyngeal abscess (28.0)*
        removal of foreign body (without incision) (98.13)

● 29.1 **Diagnostic procedures on pharynx**

    29.11 **Pharyngoscopy**

    29.12 **Pharyngeal biopsy**
        Biopsy of supraglottic mass

29.19 **Other diagnostic procedures on pharynx**

    Excludes *x-ray of nasopharynx:*
        contrast (87.06)
        other (87.09)

29.2 **Excision of branchial cleft cyst or vestige**

    Excludes *branchial cleft fistulectomy (29.52)*

● 29.3 **Excision or destruction of lesion or tissue of pharynx**

    29.31 **Cricopharyngeal myotomy**

        Excludes *that with pharyngeal diverticulectomy (29.32)*

    29.32 **Pharyngeal diverticulectomy**

    29.33 **Pharyngectomy (partial)**

        Excludes *laryngopharyngectomy (30.3)*

    29.39 **Other excision or destruction of lesion or tissue of pharynx**

29.4 **Plastic operation on pharynx**
    Correction of nasopharyngeal atresia

    Excludes *pharyngoplasty associated with cleft palate repair (27.62–27.63)*
    Coding Clinic: 1999, Q3, P22; 1997, Q1, P5; 1992, Q3, P18; 1985, Mar-April, P12

● 29.5 **Other repair of pharynx**

    29.51 **Suture of laceration of pharynx**

    29.52 **Closure of branchial cleft fistula**

    29.53 **Closure of other fistula of pharynx**
        Pharyngoesophageal fistulectomy

    29.54 **Lysis of pharyngeal adhesions**

    29.59 **Other**

● 29.9 **Other operations on pharynx**

    29.91 **Dilation of pharynx**
        Dilation of nasopharynx

    29.92 **Division of glossopharyngeal nerve**

    29.99 **Other**

        Excludes *insertion of radium into pharynx and nasopharynx (92.27)*
        removal of intraluminal foreign body (98.13)

---

6.   OPERATIONS ON THE RESPIRATORY SYSTEM (30–34)

● 30 **Excision of larynx**

● 30.0 **Excision or destruction of lesion or tissue of larynx**

    30.01 **Marsupialization of laryngeal cyst**

    30.09 **Other excision or destruction of lesion or tissue of larynx**
        Stripping of vocal cords

        Excludes *biopsy of larynx (31.43)*
        laryngeal fistulectomy (31.62)
        laryngotracheal fistulectomy (31.62)

30.1 **Hemilaryngectomy**

● 30.2 **Other partial laryngectomy**

    30.21 **Epiglottidectomy**

    30.22 **Vocal cordectomy**
        Excision of vocal cords

    30.29 **Other partial laryngectomy**
        Excision of laryngeal cartilage

30.3 **Complete laryngectomy**
    Block dissection of larynx (with thyroidectomy) (with synchronous tracheostomy)
    Laryngopharyngectomy

    Excludes *that with radical neck dissection (30.4)*

30.4 **Radical laryngectomy**
    Complete [total] laryngectomy with radical neck dissection (with thyroidectomy) (with synchronous tracheostomy)

◄ New   ◄▥ Revised   ~~deleted~~ Deleted   ● Use Additional Digit(s)   OGCR Official Guidelines   Coding Clinic

● **31 Other operations on larynx and trachea**

31.0 Injection of larynx
Injection of inert material into larynx or vocal cords

31.1 Temporary tracheostomy
Temporary percutaneous dilatational tracheostomy [PDT]
Tracheotomy for assistance in breathing

Code also any synchronous bronchoscopy, if performed (33.21–33.24, 33.27)
Coding Clinic: 1997, Q1, P6

● **31.2 Permanent tracheostomy**

31.21 Mediastinal tracheostomy

31.29 Other permanent tracheostomy
Permanent percutaneous dilatational tracheostomy [PDT]

Excludes *that with laryngectomy (30.3–30.4)*

Code also any synchronous bronchoscopy, if performed (33.21–33.24, 33.27)
Coding Clinic: 2005, Q2, P8-9; 2002, Q2, P6

31.3 Other incision of larynx or trachea

Excludes *that for assistance in breathing (31.1–31.29)*

● **31.4 Diagnostic procedures on larynx and trachea**

31.41 Tracheoscopy through artificial stoma

Excludes *that with biopsy (31.43–31.44)*

31.42 Laryngoscopy and other tracheoscopy

Excludes *that with biopsy (31.43–31.44)*

31.43 Closed [endoscopic] biopsy of larynx

31.44 Closed [endoscopic] biopsy of trachea

31.45 Open biopsy of larynx or trachea

31.48 Other diagnostic procedures on larynx

Excludes *contrast laryngogram (87.07)*
microscopic examination of specimen from larynx (90.31–90.39)
soft tissue x-ray of larynx NEC (87.09)

31.49 Other diagnostic procedures on trachea

Excludes *microscopic examination of specimen from trachea (90.41–90.49)*
x-ray of trachea (87.49)

31.5 Local excision or destruction of lesion or tissue of trachea

Excludes *biopsy of trachea (31.44–31.45)*
laryngotracheal fistulectomy (31.62)
tracheoesophageal fistulectomy (31.73)

● **31.6 Repair of larynx**

31.61 Suture of laceration of larynx

31.62 Closure of fistula of larynx
Laryngotracheal fistulectomy
Take-down of laryngostomy

31.63 Revision of laryngostomy

31.64 Repair of laryngeal fracture

31.69 Other repair of larynx
Arytenoidopexy
Graft of larynx
Transposition of vocal cords

Excludes *construction of artificial larynx (31.75)*

● **31.7 Repair and plastic operations on trachea**

31.71 Suture of laceration of trachea

31.72 Closure of external fistula of trachea
Closure of tracheotomy

31.73 Closure of other fistula of trachea
Tracheoesophageal fistulectomy

Excludes *laryngotracheal fistulectomy (31.62)*

31.74 Revision of tracheostomy

31.75 Reconstruction of trachea and construction of artificial larynx
Tracheoplasty with artificial larynx

31.79 Other repair and plastic operations on trachea

● **31.9 Other operations on larynx and trachea**

31.91 Division of laryngeal nerve

31.92 Lysis of adhesions of trachea or larynx

31.93 Replacement of laryngeal or tracheal stent

31.94 Injection of locally-acting therapeutic substance into trachea

31.95 Tracheoesophageal fistulization

31.98 Other operations on larynx
Dilation of larynx
Division of congenital web of larynx
Removal of keel or stent of larynx

Excludes *removal of intraluminal foreign body from larynx without incision (98.14)*

31.99 Other operations on trachea

Excludes *removal of:*
intraluminal foreign body from trachea without incision (98.15)
tracheostomy tube (97.37)
replacement of tracheostomy tube (97.23)
tracheostomy toilette (96.55)

● **32 Excision of lung and bronchus**

Includes rib resection as operative approach
sternotomy as operative approach
sternum-splitting incision as operative approach
thoracotomy as operative approach

Code also any synchronous bronchoplasty (33.48)

Coding Clinic: 1988, Q4, P11

● **32.0 Local excision or destruction of lesion or tissue of bronchus**

Excludes *biopsy of bronchus (33.24–33.25)*
bronchial fistulectomy (33.42)

32.01 Endoscopic excision or destruction of lesion or tissue of bronchus

32.09 Other local excision or destruction of lesion or tissue of bronchus

Excludes *that by endoscopic approach (32.01)*

32.1 Other excision of bronchus
Resection (wide sleeve) of bronchus

Excludes *radical dissection [excision] of bronchus (32.6)*

● **32.2 Local excision or destruction of lesion or tissue of lung**
Coding Clinic: 2006, Q4, P124-126

32.20 Thoracoscopic excision of lesion or tissue of lung
Thoracoscopic wedge resection
Coding Clinic: 2007, Q4, P109-113

32.21 Plication of emphysematous bleb

32.22 Lung volume reduction surgery
Coding Clinic: 1997, Q1, P6; 1995, Q4, P64

32.23 Open ablation of lung lesion or tissue

Excludes   Includes   Use additional   Code also   Omit code

32.24 Percutaneous ablation of lung lesion or tissue

32.25 Thoracoscopic ablation of lung lesion or tissue
> Excludes | thoracoscopic excision of lesion or tissue of lung (32.20)

32.26 Other and unspecified ablation of lung lesion or tissue
> Excludes | bronchoscopic bronchial thermoplasty, ablation of smooth airway muscle (32.27) ◄

32.27 Bronchoscopic bronchial thermoplasty, ablation of airway smooth muscle ◄

32.28 Endoscopic excision or destruction of lesion or tissue of lung
> Excludes | ablation of lung lesion or tissue:
> open (32.23)
> other (32.26)
> percutaneous (32.24)
> thoracoscopic (32.25)
> biopsy of lung (33.26–33.27)

32.29 Other local excision or destruction of lesion or tissue of lung
Resection of lung:
NOS
wedge
> Excludes | ablation of lung lesion or tissue:
> open (32.23)
> other (32.26)
> percutaneous (32.24)
> thoracoscopic (32.25)
> biopsy of lung (33.26–33.27)
> laser interstitial thermal therapy [LITT] of lesion or tissue of lung under guidance (17.69)
> that by endoscopic approach (32.28)
> thoracoscopic excision of lesion or tissue of lung (32.20)
> wide excision of lesion of lung (32.3)
> Coding Clinic: 1999, Q3, P3-4

● 32.3 Segmental resection of lung
Partial lobectomy

32.30 Thoracoscopic segmental resection of lung
> Coding Clinic: 2007, Q4, P109-113

32.39 Other and unspecified segmental resection of lung
> Excludes | thoracoscopic segmental resection of lung (32.30)

● 32.4 Lobectomy of lung
Lobectomy with segmental resection of adjacent lobes of lung
> Excludes | that with radical dissection [excision] of thoracic structures (32.6)

32.41 Thoracoscopic lobectomy of lung
> Coding Clinic: 2007, Q4, P109-113

32.49 Other lobectomy of lung
> Excludes | thoracoscopic lobectomy of lung (32.41)

● 32.5 Pneumonectomy
Excision of lung NOS
Pneumonectomy (with mediastinal dissection)
> Coding Clinic: 1999, Q1, P6

32.50 Thoracoscopic pneumonectomy
> Coding Clinic: 2007, Q4, P109-113

32.59 Other and unspecified pneumonectomy
> Excludes | thoracoscopic pneumonectomy (32.50)

32.6 Radical dissection of thoracic structures
Block [en bloc] dissection of bronchus, lobe of lung, brachial plexus, intercostal structure, ribs (transverse process), and sympathetic nerves

32.9 Other excision of lung
> Excludes | biopsy of lung and bronchus (33.24–33.27)
> pulmonary decortication (34.51)

● 33 Other operations on lung and bronchus
> Includes | rib resection as operative approach
> sternotomy as operative approach
> sternum-splitting incision as operative approach
> thoracotomy as operative approach

33.0 Incision of bronchus

33.1 Incision of lung
> Excludes | puncture of lung (33.93)

● 33.2 Diagnostic procedures on lung and bronchus

33.20 Thoracoscopic lung biopsy
> Excludes | closed endoscopic biopsy of lung (33.27)
> closed [percutaneous] [needle] biopsy of lung (33.26)
> open biopsy of lung (33.28)
> Coding Clinic: 2007, Q4, P109-113

33.21 Bronchoscopy through artificial stoma
> Excludes | that with biopsy (33.24, 33.27)

33.22 Fiber-optic bronchoscopy
> Excludes | that with biopsy (33.24, 33.27)
> Coding Clinic: 2004, Q1, P4-5; 1986, Sept-Oct, P11

33.23 Other bronchoscopy
> Excludes | that for:
> aspiration (96.05)
> biopsy (33.24, 33.27)
> Coding Clinic: 2002, Q3, P18; 1999, Q1, P6

33.24 Closed [endoscopic] biopsy of bronchus
Bronchoscopy (fiberoptic) (rigid) with:
brush biopsy of "lung"
brushing or washing for specimen collection
excision (bite) biopsy
Diagnostic bronchoalveolar lavage (BAL)
Transbronchoscopic needle aspiration [TBNA] of bronchus ◄
> Excludes | closed biopsy of lung, other than brush biopsy of "lung" (33.26, 33.27)
> mini-bronchoalveolar lavage [mini-BAL] (33.29) ◄
> whole lung lavage (33.99)
> Coding Clinic: 2009, Q2, P8, 16; 2006, Q2, P20; 2004, Q3, P9; 2002, Q3, P16-17; 1991, Q3, P15; Q2, P15

33.25 Open biopsy of bronchus
> Excludes | open biopsy of lung (33.28)

33.26 Closed [percutaneous] [needle] biopsy of lung
Fine needle aspiration (FNA) of lung
Transthoracic needle biopsy of lung (TTNB)
> Excludes | endoscopic biopsy of lung (33.27)
> thoracoscopic lung biopsy (33.20)
> Coding Clinic: 1992, Q3, P12-13

33.27 Closed endoscopic biopsy of lung
Fiber-optic (flexible) bronchoscopy with fluoroscopic guidance with biopsy
Transbronchial lung biopsy
Transbronchoscopic needle aspiration [TBNA] of lung ◄
> Excludes | brush biopsy of "lung" (33.24)
> percutaneous biopsy of lung (33.26)
> thoracoscopic lung biopsy (33.20)
> Coding Clinic: 2009, Q2, P8, 16; 2004, Q3, P9; 2002, Q3, P16-17; 1991, Q3, P15; 1986, Sept-Oct, P11

33.28 Open biopsy of lung
> Coding Clinic: 1999, Q3, P3-4; 1992, Q3, P12-13

33.29 Other diagnostic procedures on lung and bronchus

> **Excludes** *bronchoalveolar lavage [BAL] (33.24)* ◄
> *contrast bronchogram:*
>   *endotracheal (87.31)*
>   *other (87.32)*
> *endoscopic pulmonary airway flow*
>   *measurement (33.72)*
> *lung scan (92.15)*
> *magnetic resonance imaging (88.92)*
> *microscopic examination of specimen*
>   *from bronchus or lung*
>   *(90.41–90.49)*
> *routine chest x-ray (87.44)*
> *ultrasonography of lung (88.73)*
> *vital capacity determination (89.37)*
> *x-ray of bronchus or lung NOS (87.49)*

● **33.3 Surgical collapse of lung**

33.31 Destruction of phrenic nerve for collapse of lung

33.32 Artificial pneumothorax for collapse of lung
   Thoracotomy for collapse of lung

33.33 Pneumoperitoneum for collapse of lung

33.34 Thoracoplasty

33.39 Other surgical collapse of lung
   Collapse of lung NOS

● **33.4 Repair and plastic operation on lung and bronchus**

33.41 Suture of laceration of bronchus

33.42 Closure of bronchial fistula
   Closure of bronchostomy
   Fistulectomy:
     bronchocutaneous
     bronchoesophageal
     bronchovisceral

> **Excludes** *closure of fistula:*
>   *bronchomediastinal (34.73)*
>   *bronchopleural (34.73)*
>   *bronchopleuromediastinal (34.73)*

33.43 Closure of laceration of lung

33.48 Other repair and plastic operations on bronchus

33.49 Other repair and plastic operations on lung

> **Excludes** *closure of pleural fistula (34.73)*

● **33.5 Lung transplant**
   Note: To report donor source - *see* codes 00.91–00.93

> **Excludes** *combined heart-lung transplantation (33.6)*

   Code also cardiopulmonary bypass [extracorporeal circulation] [heart-lung machine] (39.61)

33.50 Lung transplantation, not otherwise specified

33.51 Unilateral lung transplantation

33.52 Bilateral lung transplantation
   Double-lung transplantation
   En bloc transplantation

   Code also cardiopulmonary bypass [extracorporeal circulation] [heart-lung machine] (39.61)

33.6 Combined heart-lung transplantation
   Note: To report donor source - *see* codes 00.91–00.93

   Code also cardiopulmonary bypass [extracorporeal circulation] [heart-lung machine] (39.61)

● **33.7 Other endoscopic procedures in bronchus or lung**

> **Excludes** *insertion of tracheobronchial stent (96.05)*
> Coding Clinic: 2006, Q4, P126-127

33.71 Endoscopic insertion or replacement of bronchial valve(s), single lobe
   Endobronchial airflow redirection valve
   Intrabronchial airflow redirection valve

> **Excludes** *endoscopic insertion or replacement of bronchial valve(s), multiple lobes (33.73)*
> Coding Clinic: 2008, Q4, P174-175

33.72 Endoscopic pulmonary airway flow measurement
   Assessment of pulmonary airway flow

   Code also any diagnostic or therapeutic procedure if performed
   Coding Clinic: 2008, Q4, P174-175

33.73 Endoscopic insertion or replacement of bronchial valve(s), multiple lobes
   Endobronchial airflow redirection valve ◄
   Intrabronchial airflow redirection valve ◄

> **Excludes** *endoscopic insertion or replacement of bronchial valve(s), single lobe (33.71)*

33.78 Endoscopic removal of bronchial device(s) or substances

33.79 Endoscopic insertion of other bronchial device or substances
   Biologic Lung Volume Reduction NOS (BLVR)

● **33.9 Other operations on lung and bronchus**

33.91 Bronchial dilation
   Coding Clinic: 1997, Q1, P14

33.92 Ligation of bronchus

33.93 Puncture of lung

> **Excludes** *needle biopsy (33.26)*

33.98 Other operations on bronchus

> **Excludes** *bronchial lavage (96.56)*
> *removal of intraluminal foreign body from bronchus without incision (98.15)*

33.99 Other operations on lung
   Whole lung lavage

> **Excludes** *other continuous mechanical ventilation (96.70–96.72)*
> *respiratory therapy (93.90–93.99)*
> Coding Clinic: 2002, Q3, P17

● **34 Operations on chest wall, pleura, mediastinum, and diaphragm**

> **Excludes** *operations on breast (85.0–85.99)*

● **34.0 Incision of chest wall and pleura**

> **Excludes** *that as operative approach — omit code*

34.01 Incision of chest wall
   Extrapleural drainage

> **Excludes** *incision of pleura (34.09)*
> Coding Clinic: 2000, Q3, P12; 1992, Q1, P13

34.02 Exploratory thoracotomy

34.03 Reopening of recent thoracotomy site

34.04 Insertion of intercostal catheter for drainage
   Chest tube
   Closed chest drainage
   Revision of intercostal catheter (chest tube) (with lysis of adhesions)

> **Excludes** *thoracoscopic drainage of pleural cavity (34.06)*
> Coding Clinic: 2007, Q1, P14; 2003, Q2, P7-8; 1999, Q2, P12-13; Q1, P10; 1995, Q1, P5-6; 1992, Q1, P12

Excludes   Includes   Use additional   Code also   Omit code

34.05 Creation of pleuroperitoneal shunt

34.06 Thoracoscopic drainage of pleural cavity
Evacuation of empyema
Coding Clinic: 2007, Q4, P109-113

34.09 Other incision of pleura
Creation of pleural window for drainage
Intercostal stab
Open chest drainage

> Excludes   thoracoscopy (34.21)
> thoracotomy for collapse of lung
> (33.32)

Coding Clinic: 2002, Q3, P22-23x2; 1994, Q1, P8

34.1 Incision of mediastinum

> Excludes   mediastinoscopy (34.22)
> mediastinotomy associated with
> pneumonectomy (32.5)

Code also any biopsy, if performed

● **34.2 Diagnostic procedures on chest wall, pleura, mediastinum, and diaphragm**

34.20 Thoracoscopic pleural biopsy
Coding Clinic: 2007, Q4, P109-113

34.21 Transpleural thoracoscopy
Coding Clinic: 2002, Q3, P27

34.22 Mediastinoscopy
Code also any biopsy, if performed

34.23 Biopsy of chest wall

34.24 Other pleural biopsy

> Excludes   thoracoscopic pleural biopsy (34.20)

Coding Clinic: 2002, Q3, P22-23, 27

34.25 Closed [percutaneous] [needle] biopsy of mediastinum

34.26 Open mediastinal biopsy

34.27 Biopsy of diaphragm

34.28 Other diagnostic procedures on chest wall, pleura, and diaphragm

> Excludes   angiocardiography (88.50–88.58)
> aortography (88.42)
> arteriography of:
>   intrathoracic vessels NEC (88.44)
>   pulmonary arteries (88.43)
> microscopic examination of specimen
>   from chest wall, pleura, and
>   diaphragm (90.41–90.49)
> phlebography of:
>   intrathoracic vessels NEC (88.63)
>   pulmonary veins (88.62)
> radiological examinations of thorax:
>   C.A.T. scan (87.41)
>   diaphragmatic x-ray (87.49)
>   intrathoracic lymphangiogram
>   (87.34)
>   routine chest x-ray (87.44)
>   sinogram of chest wall (87.38)
>   soft tissue x-ray of chest wall NEC
>   (87.39)
>   tomogram of thorax NEC (87.42)
>   ultrasonography of thorax 88.73)

34.29 Other diagnostic procedures on mediastinum

> Excludes   mediastinal:
> pneumogram (87.33)
> x-ray NEC (87.49)

34.3 Excision or destruction of lesion or tissue of mediastinum

> Excludes   biopsy of mediastinum (34.25–34.26)
> mediastinal fistulectomy (34.73)

34.4 Excision or destruction of lesion of chest wall
Excision of lesion of chest wall NOS (with excision of ribs)

> Excludes   biopsy of chest wall (34.23)
> costectomy not incidental to thoracic
>   procedure (77.91)
> excision of lesion of:
>   breast (85.20–85.25)
>   cartilage (80.89)
>   skin (86.2–86.3)
> fistulectomy (34.73)

● **34.5 Pleurectomy**

34.51 Decortication of lung

> Excludes   thoracoscopic decortication of lung
> (34.52)

34.52 Thoracoscopic decortication of lung
Coding Clinic: 2007, Q4, P109-113

34.59 Other excision of pleura
Excision of pleural lesion

> Excludes   biopsy of pleura (34.24)
> pleural fistulectomy (34.73)

34.6 Scarification of pleura
Pleurosclerosis

> Excludes   injection of sclerosing agent (34.92)

Coding Clinic: 1992, Q1, P12

● **34.7 Repair of chest wall**

34.71 Suture of laceration of chest wall

> Excludes   suture of skin and subcutaneous tissue
> alone (86.59)

34.72 Closure of thoracostomy

34.73 Closure of other fistula of thorax
Closure of:
bronchopleural fistula
bronchopleurocutaneous fistula
bronchopleuromediastinal fistula

34.74 Repair of pectus deformity
Repair of:
pectus carinatum (with implant)
pectus excavatum (with implant)
Coding Clinic: 2004, Q2, P6-7

34.79 Other repair of chest wall
Repair of chest wall NOS
Coding Clinic: 2004, Q2, P6; 1987, Jan-Feb, P13

● **34.8 Operations on diaphragm**

34.81 Excision of lesion or tissue of diaphragm

> Excludes   biopsy of diaphragm (34.27)

34.82 Suture of laceration of diaphragm

34.83 Closure of fistula of diaphragm
Thoracicoabdominal fistulectomy
Thoracicogastric fistulectomy
Thoracicointestinal fistulectomy

34.84 Other repair of diaphragm

> Excludes   repair of diaphragmatic hernia
> (53.7–53.82)

34.85 Implantation of diaphragmatic pacemaker

34.89 Other operations on diaphragm

◀ New   ◀▥ Revised   ~~deleted~~ Deleted   ● Use Additional Digit(s)   OGCR Official Guidelines   Coding Clinic

● **34.9 Other operations on thorax**

34.91 Thoracentesis

34.92 Injection into thoracic cavity
    Chemical pleurodesis
    Injection of cytotoxic agent or tetracycline
    Instillation into thoracic cavity
    Requires additional code for any cancer
      chemotherapeutic substance (99.25)

    | **Excludes** | *that for collapse of lung (33.32)* |

    Coding Clinic: 2007, Q4, P109-113; Q1, P14; 1992, Q1, P12;
    1989, Q2, P17

34.93 Repair of pleura

(See Plates 141, 218, 219, 473, 500, 501, 502, 544, and 545 on pages NAP-9–NAP-14 and NAP-26–NAP-28.)

7. OPERATIONS ON THE CARDIOVASCULAR SYSTEM (35–39)

● **35 Operations on valves and septa of heart**

  | **Includes** | sternotomy (median) (transverse) as operative approach |
    thoracotomy as operative approach

  | Code also | cardiopulmonary bypass [extracorporeal circulation] [heart-lung machine] (39.61) |

● **35.0 Closed heart valvotomy**

  | **Excludes** | *percutaneous (balloon) valvuloplasty (35.96)* |

35.00 Closed heart valvotomy, unspecified valve

35.01 Closed heart valvotomy, aortic valve

35.02 Closed heart valvotomy, mitral valve

35.03 Closed heart valvotomy, pulmonary valve

35.04 Closed heart valvotomy, tricuspid valve

● **35.1 Open heart valvuloplasty without replacement**

  | **Includes** | open heart valvotomy |

  | **Excludes** | *that associated with repair of:* |
    endocardial cushion defect (35.54, 35.63, 35.73)
    percutaneous (balloon) valvuloplasty (35.96)
    valvular defect associated with atrial and ventricular septal defects (35.54, 35.63, 35.73)

  | Code also | cardiopulmonary bypass if performed [extracorporeal circulation] [heart-lung machine] (39.61) |
  Coding Clinic: 2008, Q2, P13

35.10 Open heart valvuloplasty without replacement, unspecified valve

35.11 Open heart valvuloplasty of aortic valve without replacement

35.12 Open heart valvuloplasty of mitral valve without replacement
    Coding Clinic: 2010, Q1, P7; 1997, Q1, P13; 1988, Q1, P10

35.13 Open heart valvuloplasty of pulmonary valve without replacement

35.14 Open heart valvuloplasty of tricuspid valve without replacement

34.99 Other

  | **Excludes** | *removal of:* |
    mediastinal drain (97.42)
    sutures (97.43)
    thoracotomy tube (97.41)
  Coding Clinic: 2000, Q1, P17; 1988, Q1, P9

● **35.2 Replacement of heart valve**

  | **Includes** | excision of heart valve with replacement |

  | Code also | cardiopulmonary bypass [extracorporeal circulation] [heart-lung machine] (39.61) |

  | **Excludes** | *that associated with repair of:* |
    endocardial cushion defect (35.54, 35.63, 35.73)
    valvular defect associated with atrial and ventricular septal defects (35.54, 35.63, 35.73)

35.20 Replacement of unspecified heart valve
    Repair of unspecified heart valve with tissue graft or prosthetic implant

35.21 Replacement of aortic valve with tissue graft
    Repair of aortic valve with tissue graft (autograft) (heterograft) (homograft)
    Coding Clinic: 1997, Q2, P8

35.22 Other replacement of aortic valve
    Repair of aortic valve with replacement:
    NOS
    prosthetic (partial) (synthetic) (total)
    Coding Clinic: 2008, Q4, P177-180; 1996, Q1, P11

35.23 Replacement of mitral valve with tissue graft
    Repair of mitral valve with tissue graft (autograft) (heterograft) (homograft)

35.24 Other replacement of mitral valve
    Repair of mitral valve with replacement:
    NOS
    prosthetic (partial) (synthetic) (total)

    | **Excludes** | *percutaneous repair with implant or leaflet clip (35.97)* ◄ |
    Coding Clinic: 2009, Q3, P19; 1997, Q4, P54-55

35.25 Replacement of pulmonary valve with tissue graft
    Repair of pulmonary valve with tissue graft (autograft) (heterograft) (homograft)
    Coding Clinic: 2007, Q1, P14-15; 2004, Q1, P16-17; 1997, Q2, P8

35.26 Other replacement of pulmonary valve
    Repair of pulmonary valve with replacement:
    NOS
    prosthetic (partial) (synthetic) (total)

35.27 Replacement of tricuspid valve with tissue graft
    Repair of tricuspid valve with tissue graft (autograft) (heterograft) (homograft)

35.28 Other replacement of tricuspid valve
    Repair of tricuspid valve with replacement:
    NOS
    prosthetic (partial) (synthetic) (total)

| Excludes | Includes | Use additional | Code also | Omit code |

OPERATIONS ON THE CARDIOVASCULAR SYSTEM (35–39)

● **35.3　Operations on structures adjacent to heart valves**

　　Code also cardiopulmonary bypass [extracorporeal circulation] [heart-lung machine] (39.61)

　35.31　Operations on papillary muscle
　　　Division of papillary muscle
　　　Reattachment of papillary muscle
　　　Repair of papillary muscle

　35.32　Operations on chordae tendineae
　　　Division of chordae tendineae
　　　Repair of chordae tendineae

　35.33　Annuloplasty
　　　Plication of annulus
　　　Coding Clinic: 1997, Q1, P13; 1988, Q1, P10

　35.34　Infundibulectomy
　　　Right ventricular infundibulectomy

　35.35　Operations on trabeculae carneae cordis
　　　Division of trabeculae carneae cordis
　　　Excision of trabeculae carneae cordis
　　　Excision of aortic subvalvular ring

　35.39　Operations on other structures adjacent to valves of heart
　　　Repair of sinus of Valsalva (aneurysm)

● **35.4　Production of septal defect in heart**

　35.41　Enlargement of existing atrial septal defect
　　　Rashkind procedure
　　　Septostomy (atrial) (balloon)

　35.42　Creation of septal defect in heart
　　　Blalock-Hanlon operation

● **35.5　Repair of atrial and ventricular septa with prosthesis**

　　Includes repair of septa with synthetic implant or patch

　　Code also cardiopulmonary bypass [extracorporeal circulation] [heart-lung machine] (39.61)

　35.50　Repair of unspecified septal defect of heart with prosthesis

　　　Excludes *that associated with repair of:*
　　　　endocardial cushion defect (35.54)
　　　　septal defect associated with
　　　　　valvular defect (35.54)

　35.51　Repair of atrial septal defect with prosthesis, open technique
　　　Atrioseptoplasty with prosthesis
　　　Correction of atrial septal defect with prosthesis
　　　Repair:
　　　　foramen ovale (patent)
　　　　with prosthesis ostium secundum defect with prosthesis

　　　Excludes *that associated with repair of:*
　　　　atrial septal defect associated with
　　　　　valvular and ventricular
　　　　　septal defects (35.54)
　　　　endocardial cushion defect (35.54)

　35.52　Repair of atrial septal defect with prosthesis, closed technique
　　　Insertion of atrial septal umbrella [King-Mills]
　　　Coding Clinic: 2005, Q2, 17-18; 1998, Q3, P11

　35.53　Repair of ventricular septal defect with prosthesis, open technique
　　　Correction of ventricular septal defect with prosthesis
　　　Repair of supracristal defect with prosthesis

　　　Excludes *that associated with repair of:*
　　　　endocardial cushion defect (35.54)
　　　　ventricular defect associated with
　　　　　valvular and atrial septal
　　　　　defects (35.54)
　　　Coding Clinic: 2007, Q1, P14-15

　35.54　Repair of endocardial cushion defect with prosthesis
　　　Repair:
　　　　atrioventricular canal with prosthesis
　　　　　(grafted to septa)
　　　　ostium primum defect with prosthesis
　　　　　(grafted to septa)
　　　　valvular defect associated with atrial
　　　　　and ventricular septal defects with
　　　　　prosthesis (grafted to septa)

　　　Excludes *repair of isolated:*
　　　　atrial septal defect (35.51–35.52)
　　　　valvular defect (35.20, 35.22, 35.24,
　　　　　35.26, 35.28)
　　　　ventricular septal defect (35.53)

　35.55　Repair of ventricular septal defect with prosthesis, closed technique

● **35.6　Repair of atrial and ventricular septa with tissue graft**

　　Code also cardiopulmonary bypass [extracorporeal circulation] [heart-lung machine] (39.61)

　35.60　Repair of unspecified septal defect of heart with tissue graft

　　　Excludes *that associated with repair of:*
　　　　endocardial cushion defect (35.63)
　　　　septal defect associated with
　　　　　valvular defect (35.63)

　35.61　Repair of atrial septal defect with tissue graft
　　　Atrioseptoplasty with tissue graft
　　　Correction of atrial septal defect with tissue graft
　　　Repair:
　　　　foramen ovale (patent) with tissue graft
　　　　ostium secundum defect with tissue graft

　　　Excludes *that associated with repair of:*
　　　　atrial septal defect associated with
　　　　　valvular and ventricular
　　　　　septal defects (35.63)
　　　　endocardial cushion defect (35.63)

　35.62　Repair of ventricular septal defect with tissue graft
　　　Correction of ventricular septal defect with tissue graft
　　　Repair of supracristal defect with tissue graft

　　　Excludes *that associated with repair of:*
　　　　endocardial cushion defect (35.63)
　　　　ventricular defect associate with
　　　　　valvular and atrial septal
　　　　　defects (35.63)

　35.63　Repair of endocardial cushion defect with tissue graft
　　　Repair of:
　　　　atrioventricular canal with tissue graft
　　　　ostium primum defect with tissue graft
　　　　valvular defect associated with atrial and
　　　　　ventricular septal defects with tissue
　　　　　graft

　　　Excludes *repair of isolated:*
　　　　atrial septal defect (35.61)
　　　　valvular defect (35.20–35.21, 35.23,
　　　　　35.25, 35.27)
　　　　ventricular septal defect (35.62)

● **35.7　Other and unspecified repair of atrial and ventricular septa**

　　Code also cardiopulmonary bypass [extracorporeal circulation] [heart-lung machine] (39.61)

　35.70　Other and unspecified repair of unspecified septal defect of heart
　　　Repair of septal defect NOS

　　　Excludes *that associated with repair of:*
　　　　endocardial cushion defect (35.73)
　　　　septal defect associated with
　　　　　valvular defect (35.73)

◀ New　◀▥ Revised　~~deleted~~ Deleted　● Use Additional Digit(s)　**OGCR** Official Guidelines　**Coding Clinic**

35.71 Other and unspecified repair of atrial septal defect
Repair NOS:
    atrial septum
    foramen ovale (patent)
    ostium secundum defect

> **Excludes** *that associated with repair of:*
>   *atrial septal defect associated with*
>   *valvular ventricular septal*
>   *defects (35.73)*
>   *endocardial cushion defect (35.73)*

35.72 Other and unspecified repair of ventricular septal defect
Repair NOS:
    supracristal defect
    ventricular septum

> **Excludes** *that associated with repair of:*
>   *endocardial cushion defect (35.73)*
>   *ventricular septal defect associated*
>   *with valvular and atrial septal*
>   *defects (35.73)*

35.73 Other and unspecified repair of endocardial cushion defect
Repair NOS:
    atrioventricular canal
    ostium primum defect
    valvular defect associated with atrial and
      ventricular septal defects

> **Excludes** *repair of isolated:*
>   *atrial septal defect (35.71)*
>   *valvular defect (35.20, 35.22, 35.24,*
>   *35.26, 35.28)*
>   *ventricular septal defect (35.72)*

● **35.8 Total repair of certain congenital cardiac anomalies**
    Note: For partial repair of defect [e.g. repair of atrial
    septal defect in tetralogy of Fallot] — *code to*
    specific procedure

35.81 Total repair of tetralogy of Fallot
One-stage total correction of tetralogy of Fallot
    with or without:
    commissurotomy of pulmonary valve
    infundibulectomy
    outflow tract prosthesis
    patch graft of outflow tract
    prosthetic tube for pulmonary artery
    repair of ventricular septal defect (with
      prosthesis)
    take-down of previous systemic-pulmonary
      artery anastomosis

35.82 Total repair of total anomalous pulmonary venous connection
One-stage total correction of total anomalous
    pulmonary venous connection with or
    without:
    anastomosis between (horizontal) common
      pulmonary trunk and posterior wall of
      left atrium (side-to-side)
    enlargement of foramen ovale
    incision [excision] of common wall between
      posterior left atrium and coronary
      sinus and roofing of resultant defect
      with patch graft (synthetic)
    ligation of venous connection (descending
      anomalous vein) (to left innominate
      vein) (to superior vena cava)
    repair of atrial septal defect (with prosthesis)

35.83 Total repair of truncus arteriosus
One-stage total correction of truncus arteriosus
    with or without:
    construction (with aortic homograft) (with
      prosthesis) of a pulmonary artery
      placed from right ventricle to arteries
      supplying the lung
    ligation of connections between aorta and
      pulmonary artery
    repair of ventricular septal defect (with
      prosthesis)

35.84 Total correction of transposition of great vessels, not elsewhere classified
Arterial switch operation [Jatene]
Total correction of transposition of great
    arteries at the arterial level by switching
    the great arteries, including the left or
    both coronary arteries, implanted in the
    wall of the pulmonary artery

> **Excludes** *baffle operation [Mustard] [Senning]*
>   *(35.91)*
>   *creation of shunt between right*
>   *ventricle and pulmonary artery*
>   *[Rastelli] (35.92)*

● **35.9 Other operations on valves and septa of heart**
    Code also cardiopulmonary bypass, if performed
    [extracorporeal circulation] [heart-lung
    machine] (39.61)

35.91 Interatrial transposition of venous return
Baffle:
    atrial
    interatrial
Mustard's operation
Resection of atrial septum and insertion of
    patch to direct systemic venous return to
    tricuspid valve and pulmonary venous
    return to mitral valve

35.92 Creation of conduit between right ventricle and pulmonary artery
Creation of shunt between right ventricle and
    (distal) pulmonary artery

> **Excludes** *that associated with total repair of*
>   *truncus arteriosus (35.83)*

    Coding Clinic: 2007, Q1, P14-15

35.93 Creation of conduit between left ventricle and aorta
Creation of apicoaortic shunt
Shunt between apex of left ventricle and aorta
    Coding Clinic: 2009, Q2, P8

35.94 Creation of conduit between atrium and pulmonary artery
Fontan procedure

35.95 Revision of corrective procedure on heart
Replacement of prosthetic heart valve poppet
Resuture of prosthesis of:
    septum
    valve

> **Excludes** *complete revision — code to specific*
>   *procedure*
>   *replacement of prosthesis or graft of:*
>   *septum (35.50–35.63)*
>   *valve (35.20–35.28)*

35.96 Percutaneous balloon valvuloplasty ◀
~~Percutaneous balloon valvuloplasty~~
Balloon dilation of valve ◀

> **Excludes** *mitral valve repair with implant*
>   *(35.97)* ◀

    Coding Clinic: 2009, Q3, P19x3; 2004, Q3, P10

35.97 Percutaneous mitral valve repair with implant ◀
Endovascular mitral valve repair ◀
Implantation of mitral valve leaflet clip ◀
Transcatheter mitral valve repair ◀

    Code also any transesophageal
      echocardiography [TEE] (88.72) ◀

> **Excludes** *percutaneous balloon valvuloplasty*
>   *(35.96)* ◀

35.98 Other operations on septa of heart
    Coding Clinic: 2007, Q1, P11-12

35.99 Other operations on valves of heart
    Coding Clinic: 2009, Q3, P19

OPERATIONS ON THE CARDIOVASCULAR SYSTEM (35–39)

OPERATIONS ON THE CARDIOVASCULAR SYSTEM (35–39)

● **36 Operations on vessels of heart**

Includes sternotomy (median) (transverse) as operative approach
thoracotomy as operative approach

Code also any:
cardiopulmonary bypass, if performed [extracorporeal circulation] [heart-lung machine] (39.61)
injection or infusion of platelet inhibitor (99.20)
injection or infusion of thrombolytic agent (99.10)
Coding Clinic: 1990, Q2, P23-24; 1985, July-Aug, P8-9

● **36.0 Removal of coronary artery obstruction and insertion of stent(s)**
Coding Clinic: 1994, Q2, P14; 1993, 5th Issue, P3

36.03 Open chest coronary artery angioplasty
Coronary (artery):
endarterectomy (with patch graft)
thromboendarterectomy (with patch graft)
Open surgery for direct relief of coronary artery obstruction

Excludes that with coronary artery bypass graft (36.10–36.19)

Code also any:
insertion of drug-eluting coronary stent(s) (36.07)
insertion of non-drug-eluting coronary stent(s) (36.06)
number of vascular stents inserted (00.45–00.48)
number of vessels treated (00.40–00.43)
procedure on vessel bifurcation (00.44)
Coding Clinic: 1994, Q1, P6; 1993, Q3, P7-8

36.04 Intracoronary artery thrombolytic infusion
That by direct coronary artery injection, infusion, or catheterization
Enzyme infusion
Platelet inhibitor

Excludes infusion of platelet inhibitor (99.20)
infusion of thrombolytic agent (99.10)
that associated with any procedure in 36.03
Coding Clinic: 2002, Q3, P20

36.06 Insertion of non-drug-eluting coronary artery stent(s)
Bare stent(s)
Bonded stent(s)
Drug-coated stent(s), i.e. heparin coated
Endograft(s)
Endovascular graft(s)
Stent grafts

Code also any:
number of vascular stents inserted (00.45–00.48)
number of vessels treated (00.40–00.43)
open chest coronary artery angioplasty (36.03)
percutaneous transluminal coronary angioplasty [PTCA] or coronary atherectomy (00.66)
procedure on vessel bifurcation (00.44)

Excludes insertion of drug-eluting coronary artery stent(s) (36.07)
Coding Clinic: 2009, Q2, P12; 2005, Q4, P69-72; 2001, Q2, P24; 2001, Q1, P9-10; 2000, Q1, P11-12; 1999, Q1, P17-18

36.07 Insertion of drug-eluting coronary artery stent(s)
Endograft(s)
Endovascular graft(s)
Stent graft(s)

Code also any:
number of vascular stents inserted (00.45–00.48)
number of vessels treated (00.40–00.43)
open chest coronary artery angioplasty (36.03)
percutaneous transluminal coronary angioplasty [PTCA] or coronary atherectomy (00.66)
procedure on vessel bifurcation (00.44)

Excludes drug-coated stents, e.g., heparin coated (36.06)
insertion of non-drug-eluting coronary artery stent(s) (36.06)
Coding Clinic: 2005, Q4, P103-106; 2002, Q4, P101-103

36.09 Other removal of coronary artery obstruction
Coronary angioplasty NOS

Code also any:
number of vascular stents inserted (00.45–00.48)
number of vessels treated (00.40–00.43)
procedure on vessel bifurcation (00.44)

Excludes that by open angioplasty (36.03)
that by percutaneous transluminal coronary angioplasty [PTCA] or coronary atherectomy (00.66)
Coding Clinic: 1990, Q2, P23

● **36.1 Bypass anastomosis for heart revascularization**
Note: Do not assign codes from series 00.40–00.43 with codes from series 36.10–36.19

Code also
cardiopulmonary bypass [extracorporeal circulation] [heart-lung machine] (39.61)
pressurized treatment of venous bypass graft [conduit] with pharmaceutical substance, if performed (00.16)
Coding Clinic: 2002, Q3, P3-91; 1993, Q3, P7-8; 1990, Q2, P24

36.10 Aortocoronary bypass for heart revascularization, not otherwise specified
Direct revascularization:
cardiac with catheter stent, prosthesis, or vein graft
coronary with catheter stent, prosthesis, or vein graft
heart muscle with catheter stent, prosthesis, or vein graft
myocardial with catheter stent, prosthesis, or vein graft
Heart revascularization NOS

36.11 (Aorto)coronary bypass of one coronary artery
Coding Clinic: 2002, Q3, P4-5,9; 1996, Q2, P7-8

36.12 (Aorto)coronary bypass of two coronary arteries
Coding Clinic: 2007, Q4, P121-122; 2002, Q3, P8; 1999, Q4, P15-16; 1996, Q2, P7-8; 1993, 5th Issue, P17-24

36.13 (Aorto)coronary bypass of three coronary arteries
Coding Clinic: 2002, Q3, P6-9; 1996, Q2, P7-8; 1993, 5th Issue, P17-24

36.14 (Aorto)coronary bypass of four or more coronary arteries
Coding Clinic: 2002, Q3, P5; 1996, Q2, P7-8

◀ New   ◀═ Revised   ~~deleted~~ Deleted   ● Use Additional Digit(s)   OGCR Official Guidelines   Coding Clinic

36.15 Single internal mammary-coronary artery bypass
Anastomosis (single):
    mammary artery to coronary artery
    thoracic artery to coronary artery
Coding Clinic: 2002, Q3, P4-9; 1999, Q4, P15-16; 1996, Q2, P7-8

36.16 Double internal mammary-coronary artery bypass
Anastomosis, double:
    mammary artery to coronary artery
    thoracic artery to coronary artery
Coding Clinic: 2002, Q3, P6,8-9; 1996, Q2, P7-8

36.17 Abdominal - coronary artery bypass
Anastomosis:
    gastroepiploic - coronary artery

36.19 Other bypass anastomosis for heart revascularization
Coding Clinic: 1996, Q2, P7-8

36.2 Heart revascularization by arterial implant
Implantation of:
    aortic branches [ascending aortic branches] into
        heart muscle
    blood vessels into myocardium
    internal mammary artery [internal thoracic artery]
        into:
        heart muscle
        myocardium
        ventricle
        ventricular wall
Indirect heart revascularization NOS

36.3 Other heart revascularization

36.31 Open chest transmyocardial revascularization

36.32 Other transmyocardial revascularization
Coding Clinic: 1998, Q4, P73-75

36.33 Endoscopic transmyocardial revascularization
Thoracoscopic transmyocardial revascularization
Coding Clinic: 2006, Q4, P127-128

36.34 Percutaneous transmyocardial revascularization
Endovascular transmyocardial revascularization
Coding Clinic: 2006, Q4, P127-128

36.39 Other heart revascularization
Abrasion of epicardium
Cardio-omentopexy
Intrapericardial poudrage
Myocardial graft:
    mediastinal fat
    omentum
    pectoral muscles

36.9 Other operations on vessels of heart
Code also cardiopulmonary bypass [extracorporeal circulation] [heart-lung machine] (39.61)

36.91 Repair of aneurysm of coronary vessel
Coding Clinic: 2008, Q2, P13

36.99 Other operations on vessels of heart
Exploration of coronary artery
Incision of coronary artery
Ligation of coronary artery
Repair of arteriovenous fistula
Coding Clinic: 2003, Q3, P18; 1999, Q4, P15-16

37 Other operations on heart and pericardium
Code also any injection or infusion of platelet inhibitor (99.20)
Coding Clinic: 2007, Q1, P11-12

37.0 Pericardiocentesis

37.1 Cardiotomy and pericardiotomy
Code also cardiopulmonary bypass [extracorporeal circulation] [heart-lung machine] (39.61)

37.10 Incision of heart, not otherwise specified
Cardiolysis NOS

37.11 Cardiotomy
Incision of:
    atrium
    endocardium
    myocardium
    ventricle

37.12 Pericardiotomy
Pericardial window operation
Pericardiolysis
Pericardiotomy
Coding Clinic: 1995, Q3, P7

37.2 Diagnostic procedures on heart and pericardium

37.20 Noninvasive programmed electrical stimulation (NIPS)
Excludes *that as part of intraoperative testing – omit code*
    catheter based invasive electrophysiologic testing (37.26)
    device interrogation only without arrhythmia induction (bedside check) (89.45–89.49)
Coding Clinic: 2006, Q4, P128-129

37.21 Right heart cardiac catheterization
Cardiac catheterization NOS
Excludes *that with catheterization of left heart (37.23)*
Coding Clinic: 2004, Q3, P10; 2003, Q3, P9-10; 1984, Nov-Dec, P12, 19; 1984, July-Aug, P19x2

37.22 Left heart cardiac catheterization
Excludes *that with catheterization of right heart (37.23)*
Coding Clinic: 2006, Q1, P69-72; 2005, Q4, P69-72; Q2, P10-11, 17-18; Q3, P14; 2004, Q3, P10; Q2, P3; 2000, Q1, P21; 1993, 5th Issue, P17-24

37.23 Combined right and left heart cardiac catheterization
Coding Clinic: 2007, Q1, P11-12; 2005, Q2, P17-18; 2004, Q3, P10; 2001, Q2, P8-9; 2000, Q1, P20-21; 1998, Q3, P11; 1996, Q1, P8; 1993, 5th Issue, P17-24; 1984, Nov-Dec, P19; 1984, July-Aug, P19

37.24 Biopsy of pericardium

37.25 Biopsy of heart
Coding Clinic: 2003, Q3, P16; 1994, Q3, P7-8

OPERATIONS ON THE CARDIOVASCULAR SYSTEM (35—39)

37.26　Catheter based invasive electrophysiologic testing
Electrophysiologic studies [EPS]

Code also any concomitant procedure

Excludes　*that as part of intraoperative testing – omit code*
device interrogation only without arrhythmia induction (bedside check) (89.45–89.49)
His bundle recording (37.29)
noninvasive programmed electrical stimulation (NIPS) (37.20)

Coding Clinic: 2003, Q3, P23; Q2, P19; 2002, Q1, P8-9; 1999, Q1, P3x21; 997, Q2, P10

37.27　Cardiac mapping

Code also any concomitant procedure

Excludes　*electrocardiogram (89.52)*
His bundle recording (37.29)

37.28　Intracardiac echocardiography
Echocardiography of heart chambers
ICE

Code also any synchronous Doppler flow mapping (88.72)

Excludes　*intravascular imaging of coronary vessels (intravascular ultrasound) (IVUS) (00.24)*

37.29　Other diagnostic procedures on heart and pericardium

Excludes　*angiocardiography (88.50–88.58)*
cardiac function tests (89.41–89.69)
cardiovascular radioisotopic scan and function study (92.05)
coronary arteriography (88.55–88.57)
diagnostic pericardiocentesis (37.0)
diagnostic ultrasound of heart (88.72)
x-ray of heart (87.49)

● **37.3　Pericardiectomy and excision of lesion of heart**

Code also cardiopulmonary bypass [extracorporeal circulation] [heart-lung machine], if performed (39.61) ◄▥

37.31　Pericardiectomy
Excision of:
　adhesions of pericardium
　constricting scar of:
　　epicardium
　　pericardium

37.32　Excision of aneurysm of heart
Repair of aneurysm of heart

37.33　Excision or destruction of other lesion or tissue of heart, open approach
Ablation or incision of heart tissue (cryoablation) (electrocautery) (laser) (microwave) (radiofrequency) (resection) (ultrasound), open chest approach ◄▥
Cox-maze procedure
Maze procedure
Modified maze procedure, trans-thoracic approach
That by median sternotomy ◄
That by thoracotomy without use of thoracoscope ◄

Excludes　*ablation, excision, or destruction of lesion or tissue of heart: ◄▥*
endovascular approach (37.34)
thoracoscopic approach (37.37) ◄
excision or destruction of left atrial appendate (LAA) (37.36)

Coding Clinic: 2006, Q3, P13-14; 2003, Q4, P93-95; 1994, Q2, P12

37.34　Excision or destruction of other lesion or tissue of heart, ~~other~~ endovascular approach ◄▥
Ablation of heart tissue (cryoablation) (electrocautery) (laser) (microwave) (radiofrequency) ~~(resection)~~ (ultrasound), via peripherally inserted catheter ◄▥
Modified maze procedure, ~~endovascular~~ percutaneous approach ◄▥

Excludes　*ablation, excision or destruction of lesion of tissue of heart: ◄*
open approach (37.33) ◄
thoracoscopic approach (37.37) ◄

Coding Clinic: 2003, Q4, P93-95; 2000, Q1, P20-21

37.35　Partial ventriculectomy
Ventricular reduction surgery
Ventricular remodeling

Code also any synchronous:
　mitral valve repair (35.02, 35.12)
　mitral valve replacement (35.23–35.24)
Coding Clinic: 2008, Q3, P9-10; 1997, Q4, P54-55

37.36　Excision or destruction of left atrial appendage (LAA)

Includes　Thoracoscopic approach, minithoracotomy approach
Clipping of left atrial appendage
Exclusion of left atrial appendage
Oversewing of left atrial appendage
Stapling of left atrial appendage

Code also any concomitant procedure performed

Excludes　*ablation, excision or destruction of lesion or tissue of heart, endovascular approach (37.34)*

Coding Clinic: 2008, Q4, P176; 2006, Q3, P13-14

37.37　Excision or destruction of other lesion or tissue of heart, thoracoscopic approach ◄
Ablation or incision of heart tissue (cryoablation) (electrocautery) (laser) (microwave) (radiofrequency) (resection) (ultrasound), via thoracoscope ◄
Modified maze procedure, thoracoscopic approach ◄
That via thoracoscopically-assisted approach (without thoracotomy) (with port access) (with sub-xiphoid incision) ◄

Excludes　*ablation, excision or destruction of lesion or tissue of heart: ◄*
open approach (37.33) ◄
endovascular approach (37.34) ◄
thoracoscopic excision or destruction of left atrial appendage [LAA] (37.36) ◄

● **37.4　Repair of heart and pericardium**
Coding Clinic: 1990, Q2, P24

37.41　Implantation of prosthetic cardiac support device around the heart
Cardiac support device (CSD)
Epicardial support device
Fabric (textile) (mesh) device
Ventricular support device on surface of heart

Code also any:
　cardiopulmonary bypass [extracorporeal circulation] [heart-lung machine] if performed (39.61)
　mitral valve repair (35.02, 35.12)
　mitral valve replacement (35.23–35.24)
　transesophageal echocardiography (88.72)

Excludes　*circulatory assist systems (37.61–37.68)*

Coding Clinic: 2005, Q4, P119-120

37.49　Other repair of heart and pericardium
Coding Clinic: 2008, Q3, P9-10

◄ New　◄▥ Revised　~~deleted~~ Deleted　● Use Additional Digit(s)　OGCR Official Guidelines　Coding Clinic

● **37.5   Heart replacement procedures**
     Coding Clinic: 2003, Q4, P96-98

    37.51   Heart transplantation

       Excludes   *combined heart-lung transplantation (33.6)*

       Coding Clinic: 2008, Q4, P180-182; 2005, Q2, P14-15

    37.52   Implantation of total internal biventricular heart replacement system
       Artificial heart

       Excludes   *implantation of heart assist system [VAD] (37.62, 37.65, 37.66, 37.68)*

       Note: This procedure includes substantial removal of part or all of the biological heart. Both ventricles are resected, and the native heart is no longer intact. Ventriculectomy is included in this procedure; do not code separately.

    37.53   Replacement or repair of thoracic unit of (total) replacement heart system

       Excludes   *replacement and repair of heart assist system [VAD] (37.63)*

    37.54   Replacement or repair of other implantable component of (total) replacement heart system
       Implantable battery
       Implantable controller
       Transcutaneous energy transfer [TET] device

       Excludes   *replacement and repair of heart assist system [VAD] (37.63)*
           replacement or repair of thoracic unit of (total) replacement heart system (37.53)

    37.55   Removal of internal biventricular heart replacement system
       Explantation of artificial heart

       Code also any concomitant procedure, such as:
           combined heart-lung transplantation (33.6)
           heart transplantation (37.51)
           implantation of internal biventricular heart replacement system (37.52)

       Excludes   *explantation [removal] of external heart assist system (37.64)*
           explantation [removal] of percutaneous external heart assist device (97.44)
           nonoperative removal of heart assist system (97.44)
           that with replacement or repair of heart replacement system (37.53, 37.54)

       Coding Clinic: 2008, Q4, P180-182

● **37.6   Implantation of heart and circulatory assist system(s)**

       Excludes   *implantation of prosthetic cardiac support system (37.41)*

       Coding Clinic: 2008, Q4, P177-180; 2004, Q4, P118-120

    37.60   Implantation or insertion of biventricular external heart assist system
       Temporary cardiac support for both left and right ventricles, inserted in the same operative episode

       Includes   open chest (sternotomy) procedure for cannulae attachments

       Note: Device (outside the body but connected to heart) with external circulation pump. Ventriculotomy is included; do not code separately.

       Excludes   *implantation of internal biventricular heart replacement system (artificial heart) (37.52)*
           implant of pulsation balloon (37.61)
           insertion of percutaneous external heart assist device (37.68)
           insertion of temporary non-implantable extracorporeal circulatory assist device (37.62)

    37.61   Implant of pulsation balloon
       Coding Clinic: 2005, Q3, P14

    37.62   Insertion of temporary non-implantable extracorporeal circulatory assist device
       ~~Acute circulatory support device~~
       Insertion of heart assist system, NOS
       Insertion of heart pump
       ~~Short-term circulatory support (up to six hours)~~

       Excludes   *implantation of total internal biventricular heart replacement system [artificial heart] (37.52)*
           implant of external heart assist system (37.65)
           insertion of implantable extracorporeal heart assist system (37.66)
           insertion of percutaneous external heart assist device (37.68)
           removal of heart assist system (37.64)

       Note: Includes explantation of this device; do not code separately.
       Coding Clinic: 2003, Q4, P116-117; 1990, Q2, P23

    37.63   Repair of heart assist system
       Replacement of parts of an existing ventricular assist device (VAD)

       Excludes   *replacement or repair of other implantable component of (total) replacement heart system [artificial heart] (37.54)*
           replacement or repair of thoracic unit of (total) replacement heart system [artificial heart] (37.53)

OPERATIONS ON THE CARDIOVASCULAR SYSTEM (35–39)

37.64 Removal of external heart assist system(s) or device(s)
Explantation of external device(s) providing left and right ventricular support
Explantation of single external device and cannulae

Excludes explantation [removal] of percutaneous external heart assist device (97.44)
nonoperative removal of heart assist system (97.44)
temporary non-implantable extracorporeal circulatory assist device (37.62)
that with replacement of implant (37.63)

Coding Clinic: 2008, Q4, P177-180

37.65 Implant of single ventricular (extracorporeal) external heart assist system
Insertion of one device into one ventricle

Includes open chest (sternotomy) procedure for cannulae attachments

Excludes implant of pulsation balloon (37.61)
implantation of total internal biventricular heart replacement system (37.52)
insertion of implantable heart assist system (37.66)
insertion of implantation of two external VADs for simultaneous right and left heart support (37.60)
insertion of percutaneous external heart assist device (37.68)
that without sternotomy (37.62)

Note: Insertion or implantation of one external VAD for left or right heart support.
Note: Device (outside the body but connected to heart) with external circulation and pump.

37.66 Insertion of implantable heart assist system
Axial flow heart assist system
Diagonal pump heart assist system
Left ventricular assist device (LVAD)
Pulsatile heart assist system
Right ventricular assist device (RVAD)
Rotary pump heart assist system
Transportable, implantable heart assist system
Ventricular assist device (VAD) not otherwise specified

Note: Device directly connected to the heart and implanted in the upper left quadrant of peritoneal cavity.
Note: This device can be used for either destination therapy (DT) or bridge-to-transplant (BTT)

Excludes implant of pulsation balloon (37.61)
implantation of total internal biventricular heart replacement system [artificial heart] (37.52)
insertion of percutaneous external heart assist device (37.68)

Coding Clinic: 2003, Q4, P116-117; 1998, Q1, P8

37.67 Implantation of cardiomyostimulation system
Note: Two-step open procedure consisting of transfer of one end of the latissimus dorsi muscle; wrapping it around the heart; rib resection; implantation of epicardial cardiac pacing leads into the right ventricle; tunneling and pocket creation for the cardiomyostimulator.

Coding Clinic: 1998, Q43, P75-76

37.68 Insertion of percutaneous external heart assist device
Includes percutaneous [femoral] insertion of cannulae attachments
Circulatory assist device
Extrinsic heart assist device
pVAD
Percutaneous heart assist device

Coding Clinic: 2009, Q3, P12; 2008, Q2, P12

● **37.7 Insertion, revision, replacement, and removal of leads; insertion of temporary pacemaker system; or revision of cardiac device pocket**

Code also any insertion and replacement of pacemaker device (37.80–37.87)

Excludes implantation or replacement of transvenous lead [electrode] into left ventricular cardiac venous system (00.52)

37.70 Initial insertion of lead [electrode], not otherwise specified

Excludes insertion of temporary transvenous pacemaker system (37.78)
replacement of atrial and/or ventricular lead(s) (37.76)

37.71 Initial insertion of transvenous lead [electrode] into ventricle

Excludes insertion of temporary transvenous pacemaker system (37.78)
replacement of atrial and/or ventricular lead(s) (37.76)

37.72 Initial insertion of transvenous leads [electrodes] into atrium and ventricle

Excludes insertion of temporary transvenous pacemaker system (37.78)
replacement of atrial and/or ventricular lead(s) (37.76)

Coding Clinic: 2008, Q4, P101-102; 1997, Q2, P4

37.73 Initial insertion of transvenous lead [electrode] into atrium

Excludes insertion of temporary transvenous pacemaker system (37.78)
replacement of atrial and/or ventricular lead(s) (37.76)

37.74 Insertion or replacement of epicardial lead [electrode] into epicardium
Insertion or replacement of epicardial by:
sternotomy
thoracotomy

Excludes replacement of atrial and/or ventricular lead(s) (37.76)

Coding Clinic: 2007, Q1, P20; 2005, Q3, P3-9

37.75 Revision of lead [electrode]
　　Repair of electrode [removal with re-insertion]
　　Repositioning of lead(s) (AICD) (cardiac
　　　device) (CRT-D) (CRT-P) (defibrillator)
　　　(pacemaker) (pacing) (sensing)
　　　[electrode]
　　Revision of lead NOS

> **Excludes** *repositioning of temporary transvenous
> pacemaker system — omit code*
> Coding Clinic: 2005, Q3, P3-9; 1999, Q2, P11-12

**37.76 Replacement of transvenous atrial and/or
ventricular lead(s) [electrode]**
　　Removal or abandonment of existing
　　　transvenous or epicardial lead(s) with
　　　transvenous lead(s) replacement

> **Excludes** *replacement of epicardial lead
> [electrode] (37.74)*
> Coding Clinic: 2005, Q3, P3-9

**37.77 Removal of lead(s) [electrode] without
replacement**
　　Removal:
　　　epicardial lead (transthoracic approach)
　　　transvenous lead(s)

> **Excludes** *removal of temporary transvenous
> pacemaker system — omit code
> that with replacement of:
> atrial and/or ventricular lead(s)
> [electrode] (37.76)
> epicardial lead [electrode] (37.74)*

**37.78 Insertion of temporary transvenous pacemaker
system**

> **Excludes** *intraoperative cardiac pacemaker
> (39.64)*
> Coding Clinic: 2005, Q3, P3-9; 1993, Q3, P12

**37.79 Revision or relocation of cardiac device
pocket**
　　Debridement and reforming pocket (skin and
　　　subcutaneous tissue)
　　Insertion of loop recorder
　　Relocation of pocket [creation of new pocket]
　　　pacemaker or CRT-P
　　Removal of cardiac device/pulse generator
　　　without replacement
　　Removal of the implantable hemodynamic
　　　pressure sensor (lead) and monitor device
　　Removal without replacement of cardiac
　　　resynchronization defibrillator device
　　Repositioning of implantable hemodynamic
　　　pressure sensor (lead) and monitor
　　　device
　　Repositioning of pulse generator
　　Revision of cardioverter/defibrillator
　　　(automatic) pocket
　　Revision of pocket for intracardiac
　　　hemodynamic monitoring
　　Revision or relocation of CRT-D pocket
　　Revision or relocation of pacemaker,
　　　defibrillator, or other implanted cardiac
　　　device pocket

> **Excludes** *removal of loop recorder (86.05)*
> Coding Clinic: 2005, Q3, P3-9; 1994, Q2, P10x2

● **37.8 Insertion, replacement, removal, and revision of
pacemaker device**
　　Note: Device testing during procedure – *omit code*

　　Code also any lead insertion, lead replacement, lead
　　　removal and/or lead revision (37.70–37.77)

> **Excludes** *implantation of cardiac resynchronization
> pacemaker [CRT-P] (00.50)
> implantation or replacement of cardiac
> resynchronization pacemaker pulse
> generator only [CRT-P] (00.53)*

**37.80 Insertion of permanent pacemaker, initial or
replacement, type of device not specified**

**37.81 Initial insertion of single-chamber device, not
specified as rate responsive**

> **Excludes** *replacement of existing pacemaker
> device (37.85–37.87)*

**37.82 Initial insertion of single-chamber device, rate
responsive**
　　Rate responsive to physiologic stimuli other
　　　than atrial rate

> **Excludes** *replacement of existing pacemaker
> device (37.85–37.87)*

37.83 Initial insertion of dual-chamber device
　　Atrial ventricular sequential device

> **Excludes** *replacement of existing pacemaker
> device (37.85–37.87)*
> Coding Clinic: 2008, Q4, P101-102; 1997, Q2, P4; 1997, Q2, P4

**37.85 Replacement of any type pacemaker device with
single-chamber device, not specified as rate
responsive**

**37.86 Replacement of any type of pacemaker device
with single-chamber device, rate responsive**
　　Rate responsive to physiologic stimuli other
　　　than atrial rate

**37.87 Replacement of any type pacemaker device with
dual-chamber device**
　　Atrial ventricular sequential device

37.89 Revision or removal of pacemaker device
　　Removal without replacement of cardiac
　　　resynchronization pacemaker device
　　　[CRT-P]
　　Repair of pacemaker device

> **Excludes** *removal of temporary transvenous
> pacemaker system — omit code
> replacement of existing pacemaker
> device (37.85–37.87)
> replacement of existing pacemaker
> device with CRT-P pacemaker
> device (00.53)*

● **37.9 Other operations on heart and pericardium**

37.90 Insertion of left atrial appendage device
　　Left atrial filter
　　Left atrial occluder
　　Transseptal catheter technique
　　Coding Clinic: 2004, Q4, P121-122

37.91 Open chest cardiac massage

> **Excludes** *closed chest cardiac massage (99.63)*
> Coding Clinic: 1988, Q4, P12

37.92 Injection of therapeutic substance into heart

**37.93 Injection of therapeutic substance into
pericardium**

37.94 Implantation or replacement of automatic cardioverter/defibrillator, total system [AICD]
> Implantation of defibrillator with leads
> (epicardial patches), formation of pocket
> (abdominal fascia) (subcutaneous),
> any transvenous leads, intraoperative
> procedures for evaluation of lead signals,
> and obtaining defibrillator threshold
> measurements
> Techniques:
> > lateral thoracotomy
> > medial sternotomy
> > subxiphoid procedure
>
> **Note:** Device testing during procedure –
> *omit code*
>
> Code also
> > extracorporeal circulation, if performed
> > (39.61)
> > any concomitant procedure [e.g., coronary
> > bypass (36.10–36.19) or CCM, total
> > system (17.51)]
>
> **Excludes** *implantation of cardiac
> resynchronization defibrillator,
> total system [CRT-D] (00.51)*
>
> Coding Clinic: 2009, Q4, P141; 2003, Q2, P19; 2001, Q3, P5-7;
> 1999, Q3, P12-13; Q1, P3; 1994, Q2, P12

37.95 Implantation of automatic cardioverter/defibrillator lead(s) only

37.96 Implantation of automatic cardioverter/defibrillator pulse generator only
> **Note:** Device testing during procedure –
> *omit code*
>
> **Excludes** *implantation or replacement of cardiac
> resynchronization defibrillator,
> pulse generator device only
> [CRT-D] (00.54)*

37.97 Replacement of automatic cardioverter/defibrillator lead(s) only
> **Excludes** *replacement of epicardial lead [electrode]
> into epicardium (37.74)
> replacement of transvenous lead
> [electrode] into left ventricular
> coronary venous system (00.52*
>
> Coding Clinic: 2005, Q3, P3-9

37.98 Replacement of automatic cardioverter/defibrillator pulse generator only
> **Note:** Device testing during procedure –
> *omit code*
>
> **Excludes** *replacement of cardiac resynchronization
> defibrillator, pulse generator
> device only [CRT-D] (00.54)*
>
> Coding Clinic: 1999, Q1, P3

37.99 Other
> **Excludes** *cardiac retraining (93.36)
> conversion of cardiac rhythm
> (99.60–99.69)
> implantation of prosthetic cardiac
> support device (37.41)
> insertion of left atrial appendage device
> (37.90)
> maze procedure (Cox-maze), open
> (37.33)
> maze procedure, endovascular approach
> (37.34)
> repositioning of pulse generator (37.79)
> revision of lead(s) (37.75)
> revision or relocation of pacemaker,
> defibrillator, or other implanted
> cardiac device pocket (37.79)*
>
> Coding Clinic: 2005, Q3, P3-9; Q2, P14-15; 1997, Q1, P12;
> 1994, Q1, P19; 1993, Q3, P12; 1989, Q1, P11

● **38 Incision, excision, and occlusion of vessels**
> Code also
> > any application or administration of an adhesion barrier
> > substance (99.77)
> > cardiopulmonary bypass [extracorporeal circulation]
> > [heart-lung machine] (39.61)
>
> **Excludes** *that of coronary vessels (00.66, 36.03, 36.04, 36.09,
> 36.10–36.99)*
>
> Coding Clinic: 1988, Q1, P11

The following fourth-digit subclassification is for use with
appropriate categories in section 38.0, 38.1, 38.3, 38.5, 38.6,
38.8, and 38.9 according to site. Valid fourth-digits are in
[brackets] at the end of each code/description.

> **0 unspecified site**
> **1 intracranial vessels**
> > Cerebral (anterior) (middle)
> > Circle of Willis
> > Posterior communicating artery
> **2 other vessels of head and neck**
> > Carotid artery (common) (external) (internal)
> > Jugular vein (external) (internal)
> **3 upper limb vessels**
> > Axillary
> > Brachial
> > Radial
> > Ulnar
> **4 aorta**
> **5 other thoracic vessels**
> > Innominate
> > Pulmonary (artery) (vein)
> > Subclavian
> > Vena cava, superior
> **6 abdominal arteries**
> > Celiac
> > Gastric
> > Hepatic
> > Iliac
> > Mesenteric
> > Renal
> > Splenic
> > Umbilical
> > **Excludes** *abdominal aorta (4)*
> **7 abdominal veins**
> > Iliac
> > Portal
> > Renal
> > Splenic
> > Vena cava (inferior)
> **8 lower limb arteries**
> > Femoral (common) (superficial)
> > Popliteal
> > Tibial
> **9 lower limb veins**
> > Femoral
> > Popliteal
> > Saphenous
> > Tibial

● **38.0 Incision of vessel**
[0-9]
> Embolectomy
> Thrombectomy
>
> **Excludes** *endovascular removal of obstruction from head
> and neck vessel(s) (39.74)
> puncture or catheterization of any:
> artery (38.91, 38.98)
> vein (38.92–38.95, 38.99)*
>
> Coding Clinic: 2003, Q1, P17-18; 1998, Q2, P23

◀ New   ◀▥ Revised   ~~deleted~~ Deleted   ● Use Additional Digit(s)   OGCR Official Guidelines   Coding Clinic

● **38.1 Endarterectomy**
[0-6, 8]   Endarterectomy with:
embolectomy
patch graft
temporary bypass during procedure
thrombectomy

Code also any:
number of vascular stents inserted (00.45–00.48)
number of vessels treated (00.40–00.43)
procedure on vessel bifurcation (00.44)
Coding Clinic: 2006, Q3, P20; 2002, Q1, P10-11; 2000, Q1, P16; 1999, Q2, P5; 1995, Q2, P16; 1985, Mar-April, P15

● **38.2 Diagnostic procedures on blood vessels**

Excludes *adjunct vascular system procedures (00.40–00.43)*

38.21 Biopsy of blood vessel

38.22 Percutaneous angioscopy

Excludes *angioscopy of eye (95.12)*

38.23 Intravascular spectroscopy
Intravascular chemography
Near infrared (NIR) spectroscopy

Includes spectroscopy of both coronary and peripheral vessels

Excludes *intravascular imaging of:*
coronary vessels (00.24, 38.24)
peripheral vessels (00.23, 38.25)
Coding Clinic: 2008, Q4, P182-183

38.24 Intravascular imaging of coronary vessel(s) by optical coherence tomography [OCT]

38.25 Intravascular imaging of non-coronary vessel(s) by optical coherence tomograpy [OCT]

Excludes *intravascular imaging of coronary vessel(s) by OCT (38.24)*

38.29 Other diagnostic procedures on blood vessels

Excludes *blood vessel thermography (88.86)*
circulatory monitoring (89.61–89.69)
contrast:
angiocardiography (88.50–88.58)
arteriography (88.40–88.49)
phlebography (88.60–88.67)
impedance phlebography (88.68)
peripheral vascular ultrasonography (88.77)
plethysmogram (89.58)
Coding Clinic: 2000, Q3, P16; 1999, Q1, P7

● **38.3 Resection of vessel with anastomosis**
[0-9]   Angiectomy
Excision of:
aneurysm (arteriovenous) with anastomosis
blood vessel (lesion) with anastomosis
Coding Clinic: 1985, Mar-April, P15; 1984, Nov-Dec, P10

● **38.4 Resection of vessel with replacement**
[0-9]   Angiectomy
Excision of:
aneurysm (arteriovenous) or blood vessel (lesion) with replacement
Partial resection with replacement

Excludes *endovascular repair of aneurysm (39.71–39.79)*
Coding Clinic: 2008, Q2, P13; 2006, Q3, P15-16; 1999, Q2, P5-6; Q1, P15; 1992, Q3, P10-11; 1985, Mar-April, P15; 1984, Nov-Dec, P10
Requires the use of one of the following fourth-digit subclassifications to identify site:

0 **unspecified site**
1 **intracranial vessels**
Cerebral (anterior) (middle)
Circle of Willis
Posterior communicating artery
2 **other vessels of head and neck**
Carotid artery (common) (external) (internal)
Jugular vein (external) (internal)
3 **upper limb vessels**
Axillary
Brachial
Radial
Ulnar
4 **aorta, abdominal**
Code also any thoracic vessel involvement (thoracoabdominal procedure) (38.45)
5 **thoracic vessels**
Aorta (thoracic)
Innominate
Pulmonary (artery) (vein)
Subclavian
Vena cava, superior
Code also any abdominal aorta involvement (thoracoabdominal procedure) (38.44)
6 **abdominal arteries**
Celiac
Gastric
Hepatic
Iliac
Mesenteric
Renal
Splenic
Umbilical

Excludes *abdominal aorta (4)*

7 **abdominal veins**
Iliac
Portal
Renal
Splenic
Vena cava (inferior)
8 **lower limb arteries**
Femoral (common) (superficial)
Popliteal
Tibial
9 **lower limb veins**
Femoral
Popliteal
Saphenous
Tibial

● **38.5 Ligation and stripping of varicose veins**
[0-3, 5, 7, 9]   Excludes *ligation of varices:*
esophageal (42.91)
gastric (44.91)
Coding Clinic: 1997, Q2, P7

OPERATIONS ON THE CARDIOVASCULAR SYSTEM (35–39)

● **38.6   Other excision of vessel**
[0-9]   Excision of blood vessel (lesion) NOS

> **Excludes** *excision of vessel for aortocoronary bypass (36.10–36.14)*
> *excision with:*
> *anastomosis (38.30–38.39)*
> *graft replacement (38.40–38.49)*
> *implant (38.40–38.49)*

Coding Clinic: 1995, Q3, P5-6; 1990, Q3, P17

38.7   Interruption of the vena cava
Insertion of implant or sieve in vena cava
Ligation of vena cava (inferior) (superior)
Plication of vena cava

Coding Clinic: 2007, Q2, P5; 1994, Q2, P9

● **38.8   Other surgical occlusion of vessels**
[0-9]   Clamping of blood vessel
Division of blood vessel
Ligation of blood vessel
Occlusion of blood vessel

> **Excludes** *adrenal vessels (07.43)*
> *esophageal varices (42.91)*
> *gastric or duodenal vessel for ulcer (44.40–44.49)*
> *gastric varices (44.91)*
> *meningeal vessel (02.13)*
> *percutaneous transcatheter infusion embolization (99.29)*
> *spermatic vein for varicocele (63.1)*
> *surgical occlusion of vena cava (38.7)*
> *that for chemoembolization (99.25)*
> *that for control of (postoperative) hemorrhage:*
> *anus (49.95)*
> *bladder (57.93)*
> *following vascular procedure (39.41)*
> *nose (21.00–21.09)*
> *prostate (60.94)*
> *tonsil (28.7)*
> *thyroid vessel (06.92)*
> *transcatheter (infusion) (99.29)*

Coding Clinic: 2005, Q1, P14; 2003, Q1, P15-16; 2000, Q3, P16; 2005, Q1, P14; 1999, Q1, P17-18; 1996, Q2, P7-8; 1996, Q1, P8; 1987, Mar-April, P9

● **38.9   Puncture of vessel**

> **Excludes** *that for circulatory monitoring (89.60–89.69)*

38.91   Arterial catheterization
Coding Clinic: 2005, Q1, P14; 1998, Q2, P24; 1995, Q1, P3; 1990, Q2, P23; 1988, Q1, P8; 1984, May-June, P11

38.92   Umbilical vein catheterization

38.93   Venous catheterization, not elsewhere classified

> **Excludes** *that for cardiac catheterization (37.21–37.23)*
> *that for renal dialysis (38.95)*
> *that with guidance (electrocardiogram) (fluoroscopy) (ultrasound) (38.97)* ◄

Coding Clinic: 2000, Q3, P9; 1998, Q2, P24; 1996, Q1, P5-6; 1992, Q2, P15-16; 1990, Q2, P24; 1985, July-Aug, P11

38.94   Venous cutdown

38.95   Venous catheterization for renal dialysis

> **Excludes** *insertion of totally implantable vascular access device [VAD] (86.07)*

Coding Clinic: 2008, Q4, P193; 1998, Q3, P13; 1994, Q2, P11

38.97   Central venous catheter placement with guidance ◄

> **Includes** guidance by: ◄
> electrocardiogram ◄
> fluoroscopy ◄
> ultrasound ◄

38.98   Other puncture of artery

> **Excludes** *that for:*
> *arteriography (88.40–88.49)*
> *coronary arteriography (88.55–88.57)*

38.99   Other puncture of vein
Phlebotomy

> **Excludes** *that for:*
> *angiography of veins (88.60–88.68)*
> *extracorporeal circulation (39.61, 50.92)*
> *injection or infusion of:*
> *sclerosing solution (39.92)*
> *therapeutic or prophylactic substance (99.11–99.29)*
> *perfusion (39.96–39.97)*
> *phlebography (88.60–88.68)*
> *transfusion (99.01–99.09)*

Coding Clinic: 1988, Q1, P11

● **39   Other operations on vessels**

> **Excludes** *those on coronary vessels (36.03–36.99)*

39.0   Systemic to pulmonary artery shunt
Descending aorta-pulmonary artery anastomosis (graft)
Left to right anastomosis (graft)
Subclavian-pulmonary anastomosis (graft)

> Code also cardiopulmonary bypass [extracorporeal circulation] [heart-lung machine] (39.61)

39.1   Intra-abdominal venous shunt
Anastomosis:
mesocaval
portacaval
portal vein to inferior vena cava
splenic and renal veins
transjugular intrahepatic portosystemic shunt (TIPS)

> **Excludes** *peritoneovenous shunt (54.94)*

Coding Clinic: 2002, Q2, P4; 1993, Q4, P31; Q2, P8

● **39.2   Other shunt or vascular bypass**

> Code also pressurized treatment of venous bypass graft [conduit] with pharmaceutical substance, if performed (00.16)

39.21   Caval-pulmonary artery anastomosis

> Code also cardiopulmonary bypass (39.61)

39.22   Aorta-subclavian-carotid bypass
Bypass (arterial):
aorta to carotid and brachial
aorta to subclavian and carotid
carotid to subclavian

39.23   Other intrathoracic vascular shunt or bypass
Intrathoracic (arterial) bypass graft NOS

> **Excludes** *coronary artery bypass (36.10–36.19)*

39.24   Aorta-renal bypass

39.25   Aorta-iliac-femoral bypass
Bypass:
aortofemoral
aortoiliac
aortoiliac to popliteal
aortopopliteal
iliofemoral [iliac-femoral]

Coding Clinic: 2003, Q1, P16-17; 1988, Q1, P10

39.26   Other intra-abdominal vascular shunt or bypass
Bypass:
aortoceliac
aortic-superior mesenteric
common hepatic-common iliac-renal
Intra-abdominal arterial bypass graft NOS

> **Excludes** *peritoneovenous shunt (54.94)*

39.27 Arteriovenostomy for renal dialysis
Anastomosis for renal dialysis
Formation of (peripheral) arteriovenous
fistula for renal [kidney] dialysis
Code also any renal dialysis (39.95)
Coding Clinic: 2007, Q1, P18; 2006, Q1, P10-11; 1985,
Sept-Oct, P12

39.28 Extracranial-intracranial (EC-IC) vascular bypass
Coding Clinic: 1992, Q2, P7

39.29 Other (peripheral) vascular shunt or bypass
Bypass (graft):
axillary-brachial
axillary-femoral [axillofemoral] (superficial)
brachial
femoral-femoral
femoroperoneal
femoropopliteal (arteries)
femorotibial (anterior) (posterior)
popliteal
vascular NOS

Excludes peritoneovenous shunt (54.94)
Coding Clinic: 2003, Q1, P17-18; 2002, Q2, P8; Q1, P13; 1985,
Sept-Oct, P13; 1984, July-Aug, P20

● **39.3 Suture of vessel**
Repair of laceration of blood vessel

Excludes any other vascular puncture closure device ––
omit code
suture of aneurysm (39.52)
that for control of hemorrhage (postoperative):
anus (49.95)
bladder (57.93)
following vascular procedure (39.41)
nose (21.00–21.09)
prostate (60.94)
tonsil (28.7)

39.30 Suture of unspecified blood vessel

39.31 Suture of artery
Coding Clinic: 2006, Q3, P9; 1998, Q2, P22

39.32 Suture of vein

● **39.4 Revision of vascular procedure**

39.41 Control of hemorrhage following vascular surgery

Excludes that for control of hemorrhage (post
operative):
anus (49.95)
bladder (57.93)
nose (21.00–21.09)
prostate (60.94)
tonsil (28.7)

39.42 Revision of arteriovenous shunt for renal dialysis
Conversion of renal dialysis:
end-to-end anastomosis to end-to-side
end-to-side anastomosis to end-to-end
vessel-to-vessel cannula to arteriovenous
shunt
Removal of old arteriovenous shunt and
creation of new shunt

Excludes replacement of vessel-to-vessel cannula
(39.94)
Coding Clinic: 1994, Q2, P15; 1993, Q4, P33

39.43 Removal of arteriovenous shunt for renal dialysis

Excludes that with replacement [revision] of
shunt (39.42)

39.49 Other revision of vascular procedure
Declotting (graft)
Revision of:
anastomosis of blood vessel
vascular procedure (previous)
Coding Clinic: 1999, Q2, P5; 1998, Q2, P17; 1994, Q2, P13,
P15; 1993, Q4, P33

● **39.5 Other repair of vessels**
Coding Clinic: 2002, Q1, P13; 2000, Q4, P63-64; 1998, Q2, P17; 1996,
Q4, P63

**39.50 Angioplasty or atherectomy of other
non-coronary vessel(s)**
Percutaneous transluminal angioplasty (PTA)
of non-coronary vessels:
Lower extremity vessels
Mesenteric artery
Renal artery
Upper extremity vessels

Code also any:
injection or infusion of thrombolytic agent
(99.10)
insertion of drug-eluting peripheral vessel
stent (00.55)
insertion of non-drug-eluting peripheral
vessel stent(s) or stent grafts(s)
(39.90)
number of vascular stents inserted
(00.45–00.48)
number of vessels treated (00.40–00.43)
procedure on vessel bifurcation (00.44)

Excludes percutaneous angioplasty or
atherectomy of precerebral or
cerebral vessel(s) (00.61–00.62)
Coding Clinic: 2009, Q3, P13; 2006, Q4, P119; 2003, Q3, P10;
2001, Q2, P23x2, 24; 2000, Q2, P10-11; Q1, P12;
1993, 5th Issue, P11

39.51 Clipping of aneurysm

Excludes clipping of arteriovenous fistula (39.53)

39.52 Other repair of aneurysm
Repair of aneurysm by:
coagulation
electrocoagulation
filipuncture
methyl methacrylate
suture
wiring
wrapping

Excludes endovascular repair of aneurysm
(39.71–39.79)
re-entry operation (aorta) (39.54)
that with:
graft replacement (38.40–38.49)
resection (38.30–38.49,
38.60–38.69)
Coding Clinic: 2002, Q3, P25-27x2; 1999, Q1, P15-17 x2; 1988,
Q1, P10

OPERATIONS ON THE CARDIOVASCULAR SYSTEM (35–39)

39.53 Repair of arteriovenous fistula
Embolization of carotid cavernous fistula
Repair of arteriovenous fistula by:
  clipping
  coagulation
  ligation and division

  | Excludes | *repair of:*
  arteriovenous shunt for renal
  dialysis (39.42)
  head and neck vessels, endovascular
  approach (39.72)
  that with:
  graft replacement (38.40–38.49)
  resection (38.30–38.49,
  38.60–38.69)

  Coding Clinic: 2006, Q3, P15-16; 2000, Q1, P8-9

39.54 Re-entry operation (aorta)
Fenestration of dissecting aneurysm of thoracic
  aorta

  Code also cardiopulmonary bypass
  [extracorporeal circulation] [heart-lung
  machine] (39.61)

39.55 Reimplantation of aberrant renal vessel

39.56 Repair of blood vessel with tissue patch graft

  | Excludes | *that with resection (38.40–38.49)*

  Coding Clinic: 2004, Q1, P16-17

39.57 Repair of blood vessel with synthetic patch graft

  | Excludes | *that with resection (38.40–38.49)*

**39.58 Repair of blood vessel with unspecified type of
patch graft**

  | Excludes | *that with resection (38.40–38.49)*

39.59 Other repair of vessel
Aorticopulmonary window operation
Arterioplasty NOS
Construction of venous valves (peripheral)
Plication of vein (peripheral)
Reimplantation of artery

  Code also cardiopulmonary bypass
  [extracorporeal circulation] [heart-lung
  machine] (39.61)

  | Excludes | *interruption of the vena cava (38.7)*
  reimplantation of renal artery (39.55)
  that with:
  graft (39.56–39.58)
  resection (38.30–38.49,
  38.60–38.69)

  Coding Clinic: 1993, Q4, P31-32; 5th Issue, P5; 1989, Q2, P17;
  1985, July-Aug, P8-9; Mar-April, P15

● **39.6 Extracorporeal circulation and procedures auxiliary to
heart surgery**

**39.61 Extracorporeal circulation auxiliary to open
heart surgery**
Artificial heart and lung
Cardiopulmonary bypass
Pump oxygenator

  | Excludes | *extracorporeal hepatic assistance*
  (50.92)
  extracorporeal membrane oxygenation
  [ECMO] (39.65)
  hemodialysis (39.95)
  percutaneous cardiopulmonary bypass
  (39.66)

  Coding Clinic: 2010, Q1, P14; 2009, Q2, P8; 2008, Q3, P9-10;
  2006, Q2, P13; 2004, Q1, P16-17; 2002, Q3, P5; 1997,
  Q4, P54-55; 1997, Q2, P8; 1995, Q1, P5-6; 1993, 5th
  Issue, P17-24; 1990, Q2, P24; 1985, July-Aug, P8-9

**39.62 Hypothermia (systemic) incidental to open heart
surgery**
  Coding Clinic: 1995, Q1, P5-6

39.63 Cardioplegia
Arrest:
  anoxic
  circulatory
  Coding Clinic: 1995, Q1, P5-6

39.64 Intraoperative cardiac pacemaker
Temporary pacemaker used during and
  immediately following cardiac surgery
  Coding Clinic: 1995, Q1, P5-6

39.65 Extracorporeal membrane oxygenation [ECMO]

  | Excludes | *extracorporeal circulation auxiliary to*
  open heart surgery (39.61)
  percutaneous cardiopulmonary bypass
  (39.66)

  Coding Clinic: 1990, Q2, P23; 1989, Q2, P17

39.66 Percutaneous cardiopulmonary bypass
Closed chest

  | Excludes | *extracorporeal circulation auxiliary to*
  open heart surgery (39.61)
  extracorporeal hepatic assistance
  (50.92)
  extracorporeal membrane oxygenation
  [ECMO] (39.65)
  hemodialysis (39.95)

  Coding Clinic: 1996, Q3, P11-12

● **39.7 Endovascular procedures on vessel(s)**
    Embolization
    Endoluminal repair
    Implantation
    Occlusion
    Removal
    Repair

    | Excludes | *angioplasty or atherectomy of other non-coronary vessel(s) (39.50)*
    insertion of non-drug-eluting peripheral vessel stent(s) (39.90)
    other repair of aneurysm (39.52)
    percutaneous insertion of carotid artery stent(s) (00.63)
    percutaneous insertion of intracranial stent(s) (00.65)
    percutaneous insertion of other precerebral artery stent(s) (00.64)
    resection of abdominal aorta with replacement (38.44)
    resection of lower limb arteries with replacement (38.48)
    resection of thoracic aorta with replacement (38.45)
    resection of upper limb vessels with replacement (38.43)

    Coding Clinic: 2000, Q4, P63-64

39.71 Endovascular implantation of graft in abdominal aorta
    Endovascular repair of abdominal aortic aneurysm with graft
    Stent graft(s)

    Code also intra-aneurysm sac pressure monitoring (intraoperative) (00.58)
    Coding Clinic: 2002, Q1, P13; 2000, Q4, P63-64

39.72 Endovascular embolization or occlusion of head and neck vessels
    Endograft(s)
    Endovascular graft(s)
    Liquid tissue adhesive (glue) embolization or occlusion
    Other implant or substance for repair, embolization or occlusion
    That for repair of aneurysm, arteriovenous malformation [AVM], or fistula

    | Excludes | *embolization of head or neck vessels using bare coils (39.75)*
    embolization of head or neck vessels using bioactive coils (39.76)
    mechanical thrombectomy of pre-cerebral and cerebral vessels (39.74)

    Coding Clinic: 2002, Q4, P103-105

39.73 Endovascular implantation of graft in thoracic aorta
    Endograft(s)
    Endovascular graft(s)
    Endovascular repair of defect of thoracic aorta with graft(s) or device(s)
    Stent graft(s) or device(s)
    That for repair of aneurysm, dissection, or injury

    | Excludes | *fenestration of dissecting aneurysm of thoracic aorta (39.54)*

    Code also intra-aneurysm sac pressure monitoring (intraoperative) (00.58)
    Coding Clinic: 2005, Q4, P120-121

39.74 Endovascular removal of obstruction from head and neck vessel(s)
    Endovascular embolectomy
    Endovascular thrombectomy of pre-cerebral and cerebral vessels
    Mechanical embolectomy or thrombectomy

    Code also :
      any injection or infusion of thrombolytic agent (99.10)
      number of vessels treated (00.40–00.43)
      procedure on vessel bifurcation (00.44)

    | Excludes | *endarterectomy of intracranial vessels and other vessels of head and neck (38.11–38.12)*
    occlusive endovascular embolization of head or neck vessel(s) using bare coils (39.75)
    occlusive endovascular embolization of head or neck vessel(s) using bioactive coils (39.76)
    open embolectomy or thrombectomy (38.01– 38.02)

    Coding Clinic: 2006, Q4, P129-130

39.75 Endovascular embolization or occlusion of vessel(s) of head or neck using bare coils
    Bare metal coils
    Bare platinum coils [BPC]
    That for treatment of aneurysm, arteriovenous malformation [AVM] or fistula

39.76 Endovascular embolization or occlusion of vessel(s) of head or neck using bioactive coils
    Biodegradable inner luminal polymer coils
    Coil embolization or occlusion utilizing bioactive coils
    Coils containing polyglycolic acid [PGA]
    That for treatment of aneurysm, arteriovenous malformation [AVM] or fistula
    Coding Clinic: 2009, Q4, P146

OPERATIONS ON THE CARDIOVASCULAR SYSTEM (35—39)

| Excludes | | Includes | | Use additional | | Code also | | Omit code |

39.79 Other endovascular procedures on other vessels
Endograft(s)
Endovascular graft(s)
Liquid tissue adhesive (glue) embolization or
  occlusion
Other coil embolization or occlusion
Other implant or substance for repair,
  embolization or occlusion
Repair of aneurysm

| Excludes | *abdominal aortic aneurysm resection*
[AAA] (38.44)
endovascular implantation of graft in
  abdominal aorta (39.71)
endovascular implantation of graft in
  thoracic aorta (39.73)
endovascular embolization or occlusion
  of head and neck vessels, bare
  metal coils (39.75)
endovascular embolization or occlusion
  of head and neck vessels,
  bioactive coils (39.76)
insertion of drug-eluting peripheral
  vessel stent(s) (00.55)
insertion of non-drug-eluting
  peripheral vessel(s) (for other
  than aneurysm repair) (39.90)
non-endovascular repair of
  arteriovenous fistula (39.53)
other surgical occlusion of vessels - see
  category 38.8
percutaneous transcatheter infusion
  (99.29)
thoracic aortic aneurysm resection
  (38.45)
transcatheter embolization for gastric
  or duodenal bleeding (44.44) |

Coding Clinic: 2010, Q1, P21; 2009, Q2, P7; 2006, Q2, P22,
23x2; 2002, Q4, P103-105; 2001, Q3, P17-18

● **39.8 Operations on carotid body, carotid sinus and other
vascular bodies**
~~Chemodectomy~~
~~Denervation of:~~
  ~~aortic body~~
  ~~carotid body~~
~~Electronic stimulator~~
~~Glomectomy, carotid~~
~~Implantation or replacement of carotid sinus~~
  ~~baroreflex activation device~~

| Excludes | excision of glomus jugulare (20.51)
~~replacement of carotid sinus lead(s) only (04.92)~~ |

Coding Clinic: 2007, Q2, P10-11

**39.81 Implantation or replacement of carotid sinus
stimulation device, total system** ◀
Carotid sinus baroreflex activation device ◀
Implantation of carotid sinus stimulator and
  lead(s) ◀

| Includes | carotid explorations ◀ |

| Excludes | *implantation or replacement of carotid*
sinus stimulation lead(s) only
(39.82) ◀
implantation or replacement of carotid
sinus stimulation pulse generator
only (39.83) ◀ |

**39.82 Implantation or replacement of carotid sinus
stimulation lead(s) only** ◀

| Excludes | *implantation or replacement of carotid*
sinus stimulation device, total
system (39.81) ◀ |

**39.83 Implantation or replacement of carotid sinus
stimulation pulse generator only** ◀

| Excludes | *implantation or replacement of carotid*
sinus stimulation device, total
system (39.81) ◀ |

**39.84 Revision of carotid sinus stimulation lead(s)
only** ◀
Repair of electrode [removal with
  re-insertion] ◀
Repositioning of lead(s) [electrode] ◀

**39.85 Revision of carotid sinus stimulation pulse
generator** ◀
Debridement and reforming pocket (skin and
  subcutaneous tissue) ◀
Relocation of pocket [creation of new pocket] ◀
Repositioning of pulse generator ◀
Revision of carotid sinus stimulation pulse
  generator pocket ◀

**39.86 Removal of carotid sinus stimulation device,
total system** ◀

**39.87 Removal of carotid sinus stimulation lead(s)
only** ◀

**39.88 Removal of carotid sinus stimulation pulse
generator only** ◀

**39.89 Other operations on carotid body, carotid sinus
and other vascular bodies** ◀
Chemodectomy ◀
Denervation of: ◀
  aortic body ◀
  carotid body ◀
Glomectomy, carotid ◀

| Excludes | *excision of glomus jugulare (20.51)* ◀ |

● **39.9 Other operations on vessels**
Coding Clinic: 1996, Q4, P63

**39.90 Insertion of non-drug-eluting, peripheral
(non-coronary) vessel stent(s)**
Bare stent(s)
Bonded stent(s)
Drug-coated stent(s), i.e., heparin coated
Endograft(s)
Endovascular graft(s)
Endovascular recanalization techniques
Stent graft(s)

Code also any:
  non-coronary angioplasty or atherectomy
    (39.50)
  number of vascular stents inserted
    (00.45–00.48)
  number of vessels treated (00.40–00.43)
  procedure on vessel bifurcation (00.44)

| Excludes | *insertion of drug-eluting peripheral*
vessel stent(s) (00.55)
percutaneous insertion of carotid artery
  stent(s) (00.63)
percutaneous insertion of intracranial
  stent(s) (00.65)
percutaneous insertion of other
  precerebral artery stent(s) (00.64)
that for aneurysm repair (39.71–39.79) |

Coding Clinic: 2009, Q3, P13; 2006, Q4, P119; 2001, Q2,
P23-24; 2000, Q1, P12

39.91 Freeing of vessel
Dissection and freeing of adherent tissue:
  artery-vein-nerve bundle
  vascular bundle
Coding Clinic: 2002, Q3, P12-13

39.92 Injection of sclerosing agent into vein

| Excludes | *injection:*
  esophageal varices (42.33)
  hemorrhoids (49.42) |

Coding Clinic: 1992, Q2, P17-18

39.93 Insertion of vessel-to-vessel cannula
Formation of:
  arteriovenous:
    fistula by external cannula
    shunt by external cannula

Code also any renal dialysis (39.95)

Coding Clinic: 1985, Sept-Oct, P12

39.94 Replacement of vessel-to-vessel cannula
Revision of vessel-to-vessel cannula

39.95 Hemodialysis
Artificial kidney   Hemofiltration
Hemodiafiltration   Renal dialysis

> Excludes *peritoneal dialysis (54.98)*

Coding Clinic: 2008, Q4, P193; 2007, Q3, P11; 2004, Q1, P22; 2003, Q4, P111-112; 2001, Q2, P4-6, 13; 2000, Q4, P39-40; 1998, Q2, P20-21; 1986, Sept-Oct, P10-11

39.96 Total body perfusion

> Code also substance perfused (99.21–99.29)

39.97 Other perfusion
Perfusion NOS
Perfusion, local [regional] of:
    carotid artery
    coronary artery
    head
    lower limb
    neck
    upper limb

> Code also substance perfused (99.21–99.29)

> Excludes *perfusion of:*
> *kidney (55.95)*
> *large intestine (46.96)*
> *liver (50.93)*
> *small intestine (46.95)*
> *SuperSaturated oxygen therapy (00.49)*

Coding Clinic: 2007, Q4, P103-104; 1996, Q3, P11-12

39.98 Control of hemorrhage, not otherwise specified
Angiotripsy
Control of postoperative hemorrhage NOS
Venotripsy

> Excludes *control of hemorrhage (postoperative):*
> *anus (49.95)*
> *bladder (57.93)*
> *following vascular procedure (39.41)*
> *nose (21.00–21.09)*
> *prostate (60.94)*
> *tonsil (28.7)*
> *that by:*
> *ligation (38.80–38.89)*
> *suture (39.30–39.32)*

39.99 Other operations on vessels

> Excludes *injection or infusion of therapeutic*
> *or prophylactic substance*
> *(99.11–99.29)*
> *transfusion of blood and blood*
> *components (99.01–99.09)*

Coding Clinic: 1989, Q1, P11

---

8. OPERATIONS ON THE HEMIC AND LYMPHATIC SYSTEM (40–41)

● **40 Operations on lymphatic system**
Coding Clinic: 1993, Q3, P12

40.0 Incision of lymphatic structures

● **40.1 Diagnostic procedures on lymphatic structures**

40.11 Biopsy of lymphatic structure
Transbronchoscopic needle aspiration [TBNA] of lymph node ◀
Coding Clinic: 2008, Q4, P90-91; 1984, Nov-Dec, P12

40.19 Other diagnostic procedures on lymphatic structures

> Excludes *lymphangiogram:*
> *abdominal (88.04)*
> *cervical (87.08)*
> *intrathoracic (87.34)*
> *lower limb (88.36)*
> *upper limb (88.34)*
> *microscopic examination of specimen*
> *(90.71–90.79)*
> *radioisotope scan (92.16)*
> *thermography (88.89)*

● **40.2 Simple excision of lymphatic structure**

> Excludes *biopsy of lymphatic structure (40.11)*

40.21 Excision of deep cervical lymph node

40.22 Excision of internal mammary lymph node

40.23 Excision of axillary lymph node
Coding Clinic: 2002, Q2, P7

40.24 Excision of inguinal lymph node

40.29 Simple excision of other lymphatic structure
Excision of:
    cystic hygroma
    lymphangioma
Simple lymphadenectomy
Coding Clinic: 1999, Q1, P6

40.3 Regional lymph node excision
Extended regional lymph node excision
Regional lymph node excision with excision of lymphatic drainage area including skin, subcutaneous tissue, and fat
Coding Clinic: 1992, Q2, P7

● **40.4 Radical excision of cervical lymph nodes**
Resection of cervical lymph nodes down to muscle and deep fascia

> Excludes *that associated with radical laryngectomy (30.4)*

40.40 Radical neck dissection, not otherwise specified

40.41 Radical neck dissection, unilateral
Coding Clinic: 2005, Q2, P8-9; 1999, Q2, P6-7

40.42 Radical neck dissection, bilateral

● **40.5 Radical excision of other lymph nodes**

> Excludes *that associated with radical mastectomy (85.45–85.48)*

40.50 Radical excision of lymph nodes, not otherwise specified
Radical (lymph) node dissection NOS

40.51 Radical excision of axillary lymph nodes

40.52 Radical excision of periaortic lymph nodes

40.53 Radical excision of iliac lymph nodes

40.54 Radical groin dissection

40.59 Radical excision of other lymph nodes

> Excludes *radical neck dissection (40.40–40.42)*

● **40.6 Operations on thoracic duct**

40.61 Cannulation of thoracic duct

40.62 Fistulization of thoracic duct

40.63 Closure of fistula of thoracic duct

40.64 Ligation of thoracic duct

40.69 Other operations on thoracic duct

Excludes   Includes   Use additional   Code also   Omit code

OPERATIONS ON THE HEMIC AND LYMPHATIC SYSTEM (40–41)

40.9 Other operations on lymphatic structures
Anastomosis of peripheral lymphatics
Dilation of peripheral lymphatics
Ligation of peripheral lymphatics
Obliteration of peripheral lymphatics
Reconstruction of peripheral lymphatics
Repair of peripheral lymphatics
Transplantation of peripheral lymphatics
Correction of lymphedema of limb, NOS

> **Excludes**   *reduction of elephantiasis of scrotum (61.3)*

● **41 Operations on bone marrow and spleen**
Coding Clinic: 1985, May-June, P18-19

● **41.0 Bone marrow or hematopoietic stem cell transplant**
Note: To report donor source - *see* codes 00.91–00.93

> **Excludes**   *aspiration of bone marrow from donor (41.91)*

41.00 Bone marrow transplant, not otherwise specified

41.01 Autologous bone marrow transplant without purging

> **Excludes**   *that with purging (41.09)*

41.02 Allogeneic bone marrow transplant with purging
Allograft of bone marrow with in vitro removal (purging) of T-cells

41.03 Allogeneic bone marrow transplant without purging
Allograft of bone marrow NOS

41.04 Autologous hematopoietic stem cell transplant without purging

> **Excludes**   *that with purging (41.07)*

41.05 Allogeneic hematopoietic stem cell transplant without purging

> **Excludes**   *that with purging (41.08)*

Coding Clinic: 2009, Q1, P9

41.06 Cord blood stem cell transplant

41.07 Autologous hematopoietic stem cell transplant with purging
Cell depletion
Coding Clinic: 2006, Q2, P20-22

41.08 Allogeneic hematopoietic stem cell transplant
Cell depletion

41.09 Autologous bone marrow transplant with purging
With extracorporeal purging of malignant cells from marrow
Cell depletion

41.1 Puncture of spleen

> **Excludes**   *aspiration biopsy of spleen (41.32)*

41.2 Splenotomy

● **41.3 Diagnostic procedures on bone marrow and spleen**

41.31 Biopsy of bone marrow
Coding Clinic: 1985, Jan-Feb, P15

41.32 Closed [aspiration] [percutaneous] biopsy of spleen

41.33 Open biopsy of spleen

41.38 Other diagnostic procedures on bone marrow

> **Excludes**   *microscopic examination of specimen from bone marrow (90.61–90.69)*
> *radioisotope scan (92.05)*

41.39 Other diagnostic procedures on spleen

> **Excludes**   *microscopic examination of specimen from spleen (90.61–90.69)*
> *radioisotope scan (92.05)*

● **41.4 Excision or destruction of lesion or tissue of spleen**
Code also any application or administration of an adhesion barrier substance (99.77)

> **Excludes**   *excision of accessory spleen (41.93)*

41.41 Marsupialization of splenic cyst

41.42 Excision of lesion or tissue of spleen

> **Excludes**   *biopsy of spleen (41.32–41.33)*

41.43 Partial splenectomy

41.5 Total splenectomy
Splenectomy NOS
Code also any application or administration of an adhesion barrier substance (99.77)

● **41.9 Other operations on spleen and bone marrow**
Code also any application or administration of an adhesion barrier substance (99.77)

41.91 Aspiration of bone marrow from donor for transplant

> **Excludes**   *biopsy of bone marrow (41.31)*

Coding Clinic: 1985, Jan-Feb, P15

41.92 Injection into bone marrow

> **Excludes**   *bone marrow transplant (41.00–41.03)*

Coding Clinic: 1996, Q3, P17

41.93 Excision of accessory spleen

41.94 Transplantation of spleen

41.95 Repair and plastic operations on spleen

41.98 Other operations on bone marrow
Coding Clinic: 2008, Q3, P19; 1994, Q3, P10

41.99 Other operations on spleen

◀ New   ⬅ Revised   ~~deleted~~ Deleted   ● Use Additional Digit(s)   OGCR Official Guidelines   Coding Clinic

(See Plate 284 on page NAP-29.)
9.   OPERATIONS ON THE DIGESTIVE SYSTEM (42–54)

● **42   Operations on esophagus**

●   **42.0   Esophagotomy**

   42.01   Incision of esophageal web

   42.09   Other incision of esophagus
        Esophagotomy NOS
        | Excludes | *esophagomyotomy (42.7)*
                    esophagostomy (42.10–42.19)

●   **42.1   Esophagostomy**

   42.10   Esophagostomy, not otherwise specified

   42.11   Cervical esophagostomy

   42.12   Exteriorization of esophageal pouch

   42.19   Other external fistulization of esophagus
        Thoracic esophagostomy
        Code also any resection (42.40–42.42)

●   **42.2   Diagnostic procedures on esophagus**

   42.21   Operative esophagoscopy by incision

   42.22   Esophagoscopy through artificial stoma
        | Excludes | *that with biopsy (42.24)*

   42.23   Other esophagoscopy
        | Excludes | *that with biopsy (42.24)*
        Coding Clinic: 2000, Q1, P20-21; 1998, Q3, P11

   42.24   Closed [endoscopic] biopsy of esophagus
        Brushing or washing for specimen collection
        Esophagoscopy with biopsy
        Suction biopsy of the esophagus
        | Excludes | *esophagogastroduodenoscopy [EGD]*
                    with closed biopsy (45.16)

   42.25   Open biopsy of esophagus

   42.29   Other diagnostic procedures on esophagus
        | Excludes | *barium swallow (87.61)*
                    esophageal manometry (89.32)
                    microscopic examination of specimen
                    from esophagus (90.81–90.89)
        Coding Clinic: 1996, Q3, P12-13

●   **42.3   Local excision or destruction of lesion or tissue of esophagus**

   42.31   Local excision of esophageal diverticulum

   42.32   Local excision of other lesion or tissue of esophagus
        | Excludes | *biopsy of esophagus (42.24–42.25)*
                    esophageal fistulectomy (42.84)

   42.33   Endoscopic excision or destruction of lesion or tissue of esophagus
        Ablation of esophageal neoplasm by
            endoscopic approach
        Control of esophageal bleeding by endoscopic
            approach
        Esophageal polypectomy by endoscopic
            approach
        Esophageal varices by endoscopic approach
        Injection of esophageal varices by endoscopic
            approach
        | Excludes | *biopsy of esophagus (42.24–42.25)*
                    fistulectomy (42.84)
                    open ligation of esophageal varices
                    (42.91)

   42.39   Other destruction of lesion or tissue of esophagus
        | Excludes | *that by endoscopic approach (42.33)*

●   **42.4   Excision of esophagus**
        | Excludes | *esophagogastrectomy NOS (43.99)*

   42.40   Esophagectomy, not otherwise specified

   42.41   Partial esophagectomy
        Code also any synchronous:
            anastomosis other than end-to-end
                (42.51–42.69)
            esophagostomy (42.10–42.19)
            gastrostomy (43.11–43.19)

   42.42   Total esophagectomy
        Code also any synchronous:
            gastrostomy (43.11–43.19)
            interposition or anastomosis other than
                end-to-end (42.51–42.69)
        | Excludes | *esophagogastrectomy (43.99)*
        Coding Clinic: 1988, Q4, P11

●   **42.5   Intrathoracic anastomosis of esophagus**
        Code also any synchronous:
            esophagectomy (42.40–42.42)
            gastrostomy (43.1)

   42.51   Intrathoracic esophagoesophagostomy

   42.52   Intrathoracic esophagogastrostomy

   42.53   Intrathoracic esophageal anastomosis with interposition of small bowel

   42.54   Other intrathoracic esophagoenterostomy
        Anastomosis of esophagus to intestinal
            segment NOS

   42.55   Intrathoracic esophageal anastomosis with interposition of colon

   42.56   Other intrathoracic esophagocolostomy
        Esophagocolostomy NOS

   42.58   Intrathoracic esophageal anastomosis with other interposition
        Construction of artificial esophagus
        Retrosternal formation of reversed gastric tube

   42.59   Other intrathoracic anastomosis of esophagus
        Coding Clinic: 1988, Q4, P11

●   **42.6   Antesternal anastomosis of esophagus**
        Code also any synchronous:
            esophagectomy (42.40–42.42)
            gastrostomy (43.1)

   42.61   Antesternal esophagoesophagostomy

   42.62   Antesternal esophagogastrostomy

   42.63   Antesternal esophageal anastomosis with interposition of small bowel

   42.64   Other antesternal esophagoenterostomy
        Antethoracic:
            esophagoenterostomy
            esophagoileostomy
            esophagojejunostomy

   42.65   Antesternal esophageal anastomosis with interposition of colon

   42.66   Other antesternal esophagocolostomy
        Antethoracic esophagocolostomy

   42.68   Other antesternal esophageal anastomosis with interposition

   42.69   Other antesternal anastomosis of esophagus

   42.7   Esophagomyotomy

●   **42.8   Other repair of esophagus**

   42.81   Insertion of permanent tube into esophagus
        Coding Clinic: 1997, Q1, P15

   42.82   Suture of laceration of esophagus

   42.83   Closure of esophagostomy

OPERATIONS ON THE DIGESTIVE SYSTEM (42–54)

42.84 Repair of esophageal fistula, not elsewhere classified

> **Excludes**   *repair of fistula:*
> *bronchoesophageal (33.42)*
> *esophagopleurocutaneous (34.73)*
> *pharyngoesophageal (29.53)*
> *tracheoesophageal (31.73)*

42.85 Repair of esophageal stricture

42.86 Production of subcutaneous tunnel without esophageal anastomosis

42.87 Other graft of esophagus

> **Excludes**   *antesternal esophageal anastomosis*
> *with interposition of:*
> *colon (42.65)*
> *small bowel (42.63)*
> *antesternal esophageal anastomosis*
> *with other interposition (42.68)*
> *intrathoracic esophageal anastomosis*
> *with interposition of:*
> *colon (42.55)*
> *small bowel (42.53)*
> *intrathoracic esophageal anastomosis*
> *with other interposition (42.58)*

42.89 Other repair of esophagus

● **42.9 Other operations on esophagus**

42.91 Ligation of esophageal varices

> **Excludes**   *that by endoscopic approach (42.33)*

42.92 Dilation of esophagus
Dilation of cardiac sphincter

> **Excludes**   *intubation of esophagus (96.03,*
> *96.06–96.08)*

42.99 Other

> **Excludes**   *insertion of Sengstaken tube (96.06)*
> *intubation of esophagus (96.03,*
> *96.06–96.08)*
> *removal of intraluminal foreign body*
> *from esophagus without incision*
> *(98.02)*
> *tamponade of esophagus (96.06)*

● **43 Incision and excision of stomach**

> Code also any application or administration of an
> adhesion barrier substance (99.77)
> Coding Clinic: 1989, Q3, P14

43.0 Gastrotomy

> **Excludes**   *gastrostomy (43.11–43.19)*
> *that for control of hemorrhage (44.49)*

● **43.1 Gastrostomy**

43.11 Percutaneous [endoscopic] gastrostomy [PEG]
Percutaneous transabdominal gastrostomy
Coding Clinic: 1994, Q2, P10-11

43.19 Other gastrostomy

> **Excludes**   *percutaneous [endoscopic] gastrostomy*
> *[PEG] (43.11)*
> Coding Clinic: 1992, Q1, P13-14; 1989, Q3, P14

43.3 Pyloromyotomy

● **43.4 Local excision or destruction of lesion or tissue of stomach**

43.41 Endoscopic excision or destruction of lesion or tissue of stomach
Gastric polypectomy by endoscopic approach
Gastric varices by endoscopic approach

> **Excludes**   *biopsy of stomach (44.14–44.15)*
> *control of hemorrhage (44.43)*
> *open ligation of gastric varices (44.91)*
> Coding Clinic: 1996, Q3, P10

43.42 Local excision of other lesion or tissue of stomach

> **Excludes**   *biopsy of stomach (44.14–44.15)*
> *gastric fistulectomy (44.62–44.63)*
> *partial gastrectomy (43.5–43.89)*

43.49 Other destruction of lesion or tissue of stomach

> **Excludes**   *that by endoscopic approach (43.41)*

43.5 Partial gastrectomy with anastomosis to esophagus
Proximal gastrectomy

43.6 Partial gastrectomy with anastomosis to duodenum
Billroth I operation
Distal gastrectomy
Gastropylorectomy

43.7 Partial gastrectomy with anastomosis to jejunum
Billroth II operation
Coding Clinic: 2003, Q3, P3-8

● **43.8 Other partial gastrectomy**

43.81 Partial gastrectomy with jejunal transposition
Henley jejunal transposition operation

> Code also any synchronous intestinal
> resection (45.51)

43.89 Other
Partial gastrectomy with bypass
gastrogastrostomy
Sleeve resection of stomach
Coding Clinic: 2003, Q3, P3-8

● **43.9 Total gastrectomy**

43.91 Total gastrectomy with intestinal interposition

43.99 Other total gastrectomy
Complete gastroduodenectomy
Esophagoduodenostomy with complete
gastrectomy
Esophagogastrectomy NOS
Esophagojejunostomy with complete
gastrectomy
Radical gastrectomy

● **44 Other operations on stomach**

> Code also any application or administration of an
> adhesion barrier substance (99.77)

● **44.0 Vagotomy**

44.00 Vagotomy, not otherwise specified
Division of vagus nerve NOS

44.01 Truncal vagotomy

44.02 Highly selective vagotomy
Parietal cell vagotomy
Selective proximal vagotomy

44.03 Other selective vagotomy

● **44.1 Diagnostic procedures on stomach**

44.11 Transabdominal gastroscopy
Intraoperative gastroscopy

> **Excludes**   *that with biopsy (44.14)*

44.12 Gastroscopy through artificial stoma

> **Excludes**   *that with biopsy (44.14)*

44.13 Other gastroscopy

> **Excludes**   *that with biopsy (44.14)*

44.14 Closed [endoscopic] biopsy of stomach
Brushing or washing for specimen collection

> **Excludes**   *esophagogastroduodenoscopy [EGD]*
> *with closed biopsy (45.16)*

44.15 Open biopsy of stomach

44.19 Other diagnostic procedures on stomach

> Excludes | gastric lavage (96.33)
> microscopic examination of specimen
> from stomach (90.81–90.89)
> upper GI series (87.62)

● **44.2 Pyloroplasty**

44.21 Dilation of pylorus by incision

44.22 Endoscopic dilation of pylorus
Dilation with balloon endoscope
Endoscopic dilation of gastrojejunostomy site
Coding Clinic: 2001, Q2, P17-18

44.29 Other pyloroplasty
Pyloroplasty NOS
Revision of pylorus
Coding Clinic: 1999, Q3, P3

● **44.3 Gastroenterostomy without gastrectomy**

44.31 High gastric bypass
Printen and Mason gastric bypass

44.32 Percutaneous [endoscopic] gastrojejunostomy
Bypass:
gastroduodenostomy
PEGJJ

> Excludes | percutaneous (endoscopic) feeding
> jejunostomy (46.32)

44.38 Laparoscopic gastroenterostomy
Bypass:
gastroduodenostomy
gastroenterostomy
gastrogastrostomy
Laparoscopic gastrojejunostomy without
gastrectomy NEC

> Excludes | gastroenterostomy, open approach
> (44.39)

Coding Clinic: 2004, Q4, P122

44.39 Other gastroenterostomy
Bypass:
gastroduodenostomy
gastroenterostomy
gastrogastrostomy
Gastrojejunostomy without gastrectomy NOS
Coding Clinic: 2003, Q3, P3-8; 2001, Q1, P16-17x2

● **44.4 Control of hemorrhage and suture of ulcer of stomach
or duodenum**

44.40 Suture of peptic ulcer, not otherwise specified

44.41 Suture of gastric ulcer site

> Excludes | ligation of gastric varices (44.91)

44.42 Suture of duodenal ulcer site
Coding Clinic: 1987, Jan-Feb, P11

**44.43 Endoscopic control of gastric or duodenal
bleeding**
Coding Clinic: 2004, Q2, P12-13; 1992, Q2, P17-18

**44.44 Transcatheter embolization for gastric or
duodenal bleeding**

> Excludes | surgical occlusion of abdominal vessels
> (38.86–38.87)

**44.49 Other control of hemorrhage of stomach or
duodenum**
That with gastrotomy

44.5 Revision of gastric anastomosis
Closure of:
gastric anastomosis
gastroduodenostomy
gastrojejunostomy
Pantaloon operation

● **44.6 Other repair of stomach**

44.61 Suture of laceration of stomach

> Excludes | that of ulcer site (44.41)

44.62 Closure of gastrostomy

44.63 Closure of other gastric fistula
Closure of:
gastrocolic fistula
gastrojejunocolic fistula

44.64 Gastropexy

44.65 Esophagogastroplasty
Belsey operation
Esophagus and stomach cardioplasty

**44.66 Other procedures for creation of esophagogastric
sphincteric competence**
Fundoplication
Gastric cardioplasty
Nissen's fundoplication
Restoration of cardio-esophageal angle

> Excludes | that by laparoscopy (44.67)

Coding Clinic: 2003, Q2, P12; 2001, Q2, P4, 5x2, 6x3; 1998,
Q3, P10

**44.67 Laparoscopic procedures for creation of
esophagogastric sphincteric competence**
Fundoplication
Gastric cardioplasty
Nissen's fundoplication
Restoration of cardio-esophageal angle
Coding Clinic: 2004, Q4, P122

44.68 Laparoscopic gastroplasty
Banding
Silastic vertical banding
Vertical banded gastroplasty (VBG)

> Code also any synchronous laparoscopic
> gastroenterostomy (44.38)

> Excludes | insertion, laparoscopic adjustable
> gastric band (restrictive
> procedure) (44.95)
> other repair of stomach, open approach
> (44.61–44.65, 44.69)

Coding Clinic: 2004, Q4, P123-124

44.69 Other
Inversion of gastric diverticulum
Repair of stomach NOS
Coding Clinic: 2003, Q3, P3-8; 1999, Q3, P3;
1984, Nov-Dec, P13

● **44.9 Other operations on stomach**

44.91 Ligation of gastric varices

> Excludes | that by endoscopic approach (43.41)

44.92 Intraoperative manipulation of stomach
Reduction of gastric volvulus

44.93 Insertion of gastric bubble (balloon)

44.94 Removal of gastric bubble (balloon)

44.95 Laparoscopic gastric restrictive procedure
Adjustable gastric band and port insertion

> Excludes | laparoscopic gastroplasty (44.68)
> other repair of stomach (44.69)

Coding Clinic: 2004, Q4, P123-124

**44.96 Laparoscopic revision of gastric restrictive
procedure**
Revision or replacement of:
adjustable gastric band
subcutaneous gastric port device
Coding Clinic: 2004, Q4, P123-124

OPERATIONS ON THE DIGESTIVE SYSTEM (42–54)

OPERATIONS ON THE DIGESTIVE SYSTEM (42–54)

44.97   Laparoscopic removal of gastric restrictive device(s)
Removal of either or both:
     adjustable gastric band
     subcutaneous port device

| Excludes | *nonoperative removal of gastric restrictive device(s) (97.86)*
open removal of gastric restrictive device(s) (44.99) |

Coding Clinic: 2004, Q4, P123-124

44.98   (Laparoscopic) adjustment of size of adjustable gastric restrictive device
Infusion of saline for device tightening
Withdrawal of saline for device loosening

Code also any:
     abdominal ultrasound (88.76)
     abdominal wall fluoroscopy (88.09)
     barium swallow (87.61)

Coding Clinic: 2004, Q4, P123-124

44.99   Other

| Excludes | *change of gastrostomy tube (97.02)*
dilation of cardiac sphincter (42.92)
gastric:
     cooling (96.31)
     freezing (96.32)
     gavage (96.35)
     hypothermia (96.31)
     lavage (96.33)
insertion of nasogastric tube (96.07)
irrigation of gastrostomy (96.36)
irrigation of nasogastric tube (96.34)
removal of:
     gastrostomy tube (97.51)
     intraluminal foreign body from stomach without incision (98.03)
replacement of:
     gastrostomy tube (97.02)
     (naso-)gastric tube (97.01) |

Coding Clinic: 2004, Q3, P5; 1985, Jan-Feb, P14-15

● **45   Incision, excision, and anastomosis of intestine**

Code also any application or administration of an adhesion barrier substance (99.77)

● **45.0   Enterotomy**

| Excludes | *duodenocholedochotomy (51.41–51.42, 51.51)*
that for destruction of lesion (45.30–45.34)
that of exteriorized intestine (46.14, 46.24, 46.31) |

45.00   Incision of intestine, not otherwise specified

45.01   Incision of duodenum

45.02   Other incision of small intestine

45.03   Incision of large intestine

| Excludes | *proctotomy (48.0)* |

● **45.1   Diagnostic procedures on small intestine**

Code also any laparotomy (54.11–54.19)

45.11   Transabdominal endoscopy of small intestine
Intraoperative endoscopy of small intestine

| Excludes | *that with biopsy (45.14)* |

45.12   Endoscopy of small intestine through artificial stoma

| Excludes | *that with biopsy (45.14)* |

45.13   Other endoscopy of small intestine
Esophagogastroduodenoscopy [EGD]

| Excludes | *that with biopsy (45.14, 45.16)* |

Coding Clinic: 2004, Q3, P5

45.14   Closed [endoscopic] biopsy of small intestine
Brushing or washing for specimen collection

| Excludes | *esophagogastroduodenoscopy [EGD] with closed biopsy (45.16)* |

45.15   Open biopsy of small intestine
Coding Clinic: 2005, Q2, P12; 2001, Q2, P9-11

45.16   Esophagogastroduodenoscopy [EGD] with closed biopsy
Biopsy of one or more sites involving esophagus, stomach, and/or duodenum
Coding Clinic: 2005, Q3, P17-18

45.19   Other diagnostic procedures on small intestine

| Excludes | *microscopic examination of specimen from small intestine (90.91–90.99)*
radioisotope scan (92.04)
ultrasonography (88.74)
x-ray (87.61–87.69) |

● **45.2   Diagnostic procedures on large intestine**

Code also any laparotomy (54.11–54.19)

45.21   Transabdominal endoscopy of large intestine
Intraoperative endoscopy of large intestine

| Excludes | *that with biopsy (45.25)* |

45.22   Endoscopy of large intestine through artificial stoma

| Excludes | *that with biopsy (45.25)* |

45.23   Colonoscopy
Flexible fiberoptic colonoscopy

| Excludes | *endoscopy of large intestine through artificial stoma (45.22)*
flexible sigmoidoscopy (45.24)
rigid proctosigmoidoscopy (48.23)
transabdominal endoscopy of large intestine (45.21) |

Coding Clinic: 2005, Q3, P17-18; 1995, Q1, P3-4

45.24   Flexible sigmoidoscopy
Endoscopy of descending colon

| Excludes | *rigid proctosigmoidoscopy (48.23)* |

45.25   Closed [endoscopic] biopsy of large intestine
Biopsy, closed, of unspecified intestinal site
Brushing or washing for specimen collection
Colonoscopy with biopsy

| Excludes | *proctosigmoidoscopy with biopsy (48.24)* |

Coding Clinic: 2003, Q1, P10-11

45.26   Open biopsy of large intestine

45.27   Intestinal biopsy, site unspecified

45.28   Other diagnostic procedures on large intestine

45.29   Other diagnostic procedures on intestine, site unspecified

| Excludes | *microscopic examination of specimen (90.91–90.99)*
scan and radioisotope function study (92.04)
ultrasonography (88.74)
x-ray (87.61–87.69) |

◀ New   ◀▥ Revised   ~~deleted~~ Deleted   ● Use Additional Digit(s)   OGCR Official Guidelines   Coding Clinic

● **45.3 Local excision or destruction of lesion or tissue of small intestine**

   45.30 Endoscopic excision or destruction of lesion of duodenum

       Excludes *biopsy of duodenum (45.14–45.15)*
                    control of hemorrhage (44.43)
                    fistulectomy (46.72)

   45.31 Other local excision of lesion of duodenum

       Excludes *biopsy of duodenum (45.14–45.15)*
                    fistulectomy (46.72)
                    multiple segmental resection (45.61)
                    that by endoscopic approach (45.30)

   45.32 Other destruction of lesion of duodenum

       Excludes *that by endoscopic approach (45.30)*

   45.33 Local excision of lesion or tissue of small intestine, except duodenum
       Excision of redundant mucosa of ileostomy

       Excludes *biopsy of small intestine (45.14–45.15)*
                    fistulectomy (46.74)
                    multiple segmental resection (45.61)

   45.34 Other destruction of lesion of small intestine, except duodenum

● **45.4 Local excision or destruction of lesion or tissue of large intestine**

   45.41 Excision of lesion or tissue of large intestine
       Excision of redundant mucosa of colostomy

       Excludes *biopsy of large intestine (45.25–45.27)*
                    endoscopic polypectomy of large intestine (45.42)
                    fistulectomy (46.76)
                    multiple segmental resection (17.31, 45.71)
                    that by endoscopic approach (45.42–45.43)
       Coding Clinic: 1987, Nov-Dec, P11

   45.42 Endoscopic polypectomy of large intestine

       Excludes *that by open approach (45.41)*
       Coding Clinic: 2005, Q2, P16-17; 1990, Q2, P25

   45.43 Endoscopic destruction of other lesion or tissue of large intestine
       Endoscopic ablation of tumor of large intestine
       Endoscopic control of colonic bleeding

       Excludes *endoscopic polypectomy of large intestine (45.42)*
       Coding Clinic: 2002, Q4, P61

   45.49 Other destruction of lesion of large intestine

       Excludes *that by endoscopic approach (45.43)*
       Coding Clinic: 1987, Nov-Dec, P11

● **45.5 Isolation of intestinal segment**

    Code also any synchronous:
       anastomosis other than end-to-end (45.90–45.94)
       enterostomy (46.10–46.39)

   45.50 Isolation of intestinal segment, not otherwise specified
       Isolation of intestinal pedicle flap
       Reversal of intestinal segment

   45.51 Isolation of segment of small intestine
       Isolation of ileal loop
       Resection of small intestine for interposition
       Coding Clinic: 2005, Q2, P12-13x2; 2003, Q3, P3-8; Q2, P11-12; 2000, Q3, P7-8

   45.52 Isolation of segment of large intestine
       Resection of colon for interposition

● **45.6 Other excision of small intestine**

    Code also any synchronous:
       anastomosis other than end-to-end (45.90–45.93, 45.95)
       colostomy (46.10–46.13)
       enterostomy (46.10–46.39)

       Excludes *cecectomy (17.32, 45.72)*
                    enterocolectomy (17.39, 45.79)
                    gastroduodenectomy (43.6–43.99)
                    ileocolectomy (17.33, 45.73)
                    pancreatoduodenectomy (52.51–52.7)

   45.61 Multiple segmental resection of small intestine
       Segmental resection for multiple traumatic lesions of small intestine

   45.62 Other partial resection of small intestine
       Duodenectomy
       Ileectomy
       Jejunectomy

       Excludes *duodenectomy with synchronous pancreatectomy (52.51–52.7)*
                    resection of cecum and terminal ileum (17.32, 45.72)
       Coding Clinic: 2010, Q1, P12; 2004, Q1, P10-11; 2003, Q1, P18

   45.63 Total removal of small intestine

● **45.7 Open and other partial excision of large intestine**

    Code also any synchronous:
       anastomosis other than end-to-end (45.92–45.94)
       enterostomy (46.10–46.39)

       Excludes *laparoscopic partial excision of large intestine (17.31–17.39)*
       Coding Clinic: 2009, Q1, P10x2

   45.71 Open and other multiple segmental resection of large intestine
       Segmental resection for multiple traumatic lesions of large intestine

   45.72 Open and other cecectomy
       Resection of cecum and terminal ileum

   45.73 Open and other right hemicolectomy
       Ileocolectomy
       Right radical colectomy
       Coding Clinic: 1999, Q3, P10-11

   45.74 Open and other resection of transverse colon

   45.75 Open and other left hemicolectomy

       Excludes *proctosigmoidectomy (48.41–48.69)*
                    second stage Mikulicz operation (46.04)
       Coding Clinic: 2002, Q4, P105-106

   45.76 Open and other sigmoidectomy
       Coding Clinic: 1996, Q1, P9; 1989, Q3, P15; 2002, Q4, P105-106

   45.79 Other and unspecified partial excision of large intestine
       Enterocolectomy NEC
       Coding Clinic: 2009, Q1, P11; 2003, Q1, P18; 1997, Q3, P9-10; 1991, Q1, P11

● **45.8 Total intra-abdominal colectomy**
    Excision of cecum, colon, and sigmoid

       Excludes *coloproctectomy (48.41–48.69)*
       Coding Clinic: 2008, Q4, P169-172

   45.81 Laparoscopic total intra-abdominal colectomy

   45.82 Open total intra-abdominal colectomy

   45.83 Other and unspecified total intra-abdominal colectomy

Excludes   Includes   Use additional   Code also   Omit code

OPERATIONS ON THE DIGESTIVE SYSTEM (42–54)

● **45.9　Intestinal anastomosis**

　　Code also any synchronous resection (45.31–45.8, 48.41–48.69)

　　Excludes　*end-to-end anastomosis — omit code*

　　Coding Clinic: 1999, Q3, P10-11

　45.90　Intestinal anastomosis, not otherwise specified

　45.91　Small-to-small intestinal anastomosis
　　Coding Clinic: 2010, Q1, P12; 2003, Q3, P3-8

　45.92　Anastomosis of small intestine to rectal stump
　　Hampton procedure
　　Coding Clinic: 2009, Q1, P5

　45.93　Other small-to-large intestinal anastomosis
　　Coding Clinic: 2009, Q1, P5; 2003, Q1, P18; 1986, Nov-Dec, P11

　45.94　Large-to-large intestinal anastomosis

　　Excludes　*rectorectostomy (48.74)*

　　Coding Clinic: 2009, Q1, P5; 1989, Q3, P15

　45.95　Anastomosis to anus
　　Formation of endorectal ileal pouch (H-pouch) (J-pouch) (S-pouch) with anastomosis of small intestine to anus
　　Coding Clinic: 2005, Q2, P13-14

● **46　Other operations on intestine**

　　Code also any application or administration of an adhesion barrier substance (99.77)

● **46.0　Exteriorization of intestine**

　　Includes　loop enterostomy
　　　　　　　multiple stage resection of intestine

　46.01　Exteriorization of small intestine
　　Loop ileostomy

　46.02　Resection of exteriorized segment of small intestine

　46.03　Exteriorization of large intestine
　　Exteriorization of intestine NOS
　　First stage Mikulicz exteriorization of intestine
　　Loop colostomy

　46.04　Resection of exteriorized segment of large intestine
　　Resection of exteriorized segment of intestine NOS
　　Second stage Mikulicz operation

● **46.1　Colostomy**

　　Code also any synchronous resection (45.49, 45.71–45.79, 45.8)

　　Excludes　*loop colostomy (46.03)*
　　　　　　　that with abdominoperineal resection of rectum (48.5)
　　　　　　　that with synchronous anterior rectal resection (48.62)

　46.10　Colostomy, not otherwise specified

　46.11　Temporary colostomy

　46.13　Permanent colostomy

　46.14　Delayed opening of colostomy

● **46.2　Ileostomy**

　　Code also any synchronous resection (45.34, 45.61–45.63)

　　Excludes　*loop ileostomy (46.01)*

　46.20　Ileostomy, not otherwise specified

　46.21　Temporary ileostomy

　46.22　Continent ileostomy

　46.23　Other permanent ileostomy

　46.24　Delayed opening of ileostomy

● **46.3　Other enterostomy**

　　Code also any synchronous resection (45.61–45.8)

　46.31　Delayed opening of other enterostomy

　46.32　Percutaneous (endoscopic) jejunostomy [PEJ]
　　Endoscopic conversion of gastrostomy to jejunostomy
　　Percutaneous (endoscopic) feeding enterostomy

　　Excludes　*percutaneous [endoscopic] gastrojejunostomy (bypass) (44.32)*

　46.39　Other
　　Duodenostomy
　　Feeding enterostomy
　　Coding Clinic: 1989, Q3, P15

● **46.4　Revision of intestinal stoma**

　46.40　Revision of intestinal stoma, not otherwise specified
　　Plastic enlargement of intestinal stoma
　　Reconstruction of stoma of intestine
　　Release of scar tissue of intestinal stoma

　　Excludes　*excision of redundant mucosa (45.41)*

　46.41　Revision of stoma of small intestine

　　Excludes　*excision of redundant mucosa (45.33)*

　　Coding Clinic: 2005, Q2, P11-12

　46.42　Repair of pericolostomy hernia

　46.43　Other revision of stoma of large intestine

　　Excludes　*excision of redundant mucosa (45.41)*

　　Coding Clinic: 2002, Q2, P9-10

● **46.5　Closure of intestinal stoma**

　　Code also any synchronous resection (45.34, 45.49, 45.61–45.8)

　46.50　Closure of intestinal stoma, not otherwise specified

　46.51　Closure of stoma of small intestine

　46.52　Closure of stoma of large intestine
　　Closure or take-down of:
　　　cecostomy
　　　colostomy
　　　sigmoidostomy
　　Coding Clinic: 2009, Q1, P5; 2005, Q2, P4-5; 1997, Q3, P9-10; 1987, Nov-Dec, P8

● **46.6　Fixation of intestine**

　46.60　Fixation of intestine, not otherwise specified
　　Fixation of intestine to abdominal wall

　46.61　Fixation of small intestine to abdominal wall
　　Ileopexy

　46.62　Other fixation of small intestine
　　Noble plication of small intestine
　　Plication of jejunum

　46.63　Fixation of large intestine to abdominal wall
　　Cecocoloplicopexy
　　Sigmoidopexy (Moschowitz)

　46.64　Other fixation of large intestine
　　Cecofixation
　　Colofixation

● **46.7　Other repair of intestine**

　　Excludes　*closure of:*
　　　　　　　ulcer of duodenum (44.42)
　　　　　　　vesicoenteric fistula (57.83)

　46.71　Suture of laceration of duodenum

　46.72　Closure of fistula of duodenum

　46.73　Suture of laceration of small intestine, except duodenum
　　Coding Clinic: 2010, Q1, P12

◀ New　　◀▦ Revised　　~~deleted~~ Deleted　　● Use Additional Digit(s)　　OGCR Official Guidelines　　Coding Clinic

46.74 Closure of fistula of small intestine, except duodenum

> **Excludes** closure of:
> artificial stoma (46.51)
> vaginal fistula (70.74)
> repair of gastrojejunocolic fistula (44.63)

46.75 Suture of laceration of large intestine

46.76 Closure of fistula of large intestine

> **Excludes** closure of:
> gastrocolic fistula (44.63)
> rectal fistula (48.73)
> sigmoidovesical fistula (57.83)
> stoma (46.52)
> vaginal fistula (70.72–70.73)
> vesicocolic fistula (57.83)
> vesicosigmoidovaginal fistula (57.83)

Coding Clinic: 1999, Q3, P8

46.79 Other repair of intestine
Duodenoplasty

● **46.8 Dilation and manipulation of intestine**
Coding Clinic: 2003, Q1, P14-15; 1998, Q43, P82-83

46.80 Intra-abdominal manipulation of intestine, not otherwise specified
Correction of intestinal malrotation
Reduction of:
intestinal torsion
intestinal volvulus
intussusception

> **Excludes** reduction of intussusception with:
> fluoroscopy (96.29)
> ionizing radiation enema (96.29)
> ultrasonography guidance (96.29)

46.81 Intra-abdominal manipulation of small intestine

46.82 Intra-abdominal manipulation of large intestine

46.85 Dilation of intestine
Dilation (balloon) of duodenum
Dilation (balloon) of jejunum
Endoscopic dilation (balloon) of large intestine
That through rectum or colostomy

> **Excludes** with insertion of colonic stent (46.86–46.87)

Coding Clinic: 2007, Q3, P6-7; 1989, Q3, P15

46.86 Endoscopic insertion of colonic stent(s)
Colonoscopy (flexible) (through stoma) with transendoscopic stent placement
Combined with fluoroscopic-guided insertion
Stent endoprosthesis of colon
Through the scope [TTS] technique

> **Excludes** other non-endoscopic insertion of colonic stent (46.87)

Coding Clinic: 2009, Q4, P148

46.87 Other insertion of colonic stent(s)

> **Includes** that by:
> fluoroscopic guidance only
> rectal guiding tube
> Non-endoscopic insertion

Code also any synchronous diagnostic procedure(s)

> **Excludes** endoscopic insertion of colonic stent (46.86)

● **46.9 Other operations on intestines**
46.91 Myotomy of sigmoid colon
46.92 Myotomy of other parts of colon
46.93 Revision of anastomosis of small intestine
46.94 Revision of anastomosis of large intestine
46.95 Local perfusion of small intestine
Code also substance perfused (99.21–99.29)
46.96 Local perfusion of large intestine
Code also substance perfused (99.21–99.29)
46.97 Transplant of intestine
Note: To report donor source - see codes 00.91–00.93
46.99 Other
Ileoentectropy

> **Excludes** diagnostic procedures on intestine (45.11–45.29)
> dilation of enterostomy stoma (96.24)
> intestinal intubation (96.08)
> removal of:
> intraluminal foreign body from large intestine without incision (98.04)
> intraluminal foreign body from small intestine without incision (98.03)
> tube from large intestine (97.53)
> tube from small intestine (97.52)
> replacement of:
> large intestine tube or enterostomy device (97.04)
> small intestine tube or enterostomy device (97.03)

Coding Clinic: 1999, Q3, P11; 1989, Q1, P11

● **47 Operations on appendix**

> **Includes** appendiceal stump

Code also any application or administration of an adhesion barrier substance (99.77)

● **47.0 Appendectomy**

> **Excludes** incidental appendectomy, so described
> laparoscopic (47.11)
> other (47.19)

Coding Clinic: 1992, Q3, P12

47.01 Laparoscopic appendectomy
Coding Clinic: 2001, Q1, P15-16; 1996, Q4, P64-65

47.09 Other appendectomy
Coding Clinic: 1997, Q4, P52

● **47.1 Incidental appendectomy**
Coding Clinic: 1987, Jan-Feb, P11-12

47.11 Laparoscopic incidental appendectomy
47.19 Other incidental appendectomy
Coding Clinic: 1996, Q4, P64-65; 1984, Nov-Dec, P12

47.2 Drainage of appendiceal abscess

> **Excludes** that with appendectomy (47.0)

● **47.9 Other operations on appendix**
47.91 Appendicostomy
47.92 Closure of appendiceal fistula
47.99 Other
Anastomosis of appendix

> **Excludes** diagnostic procedures on appendix (45.21–45.29)

Coding Clinic: 2001, Q3, P16

OPERATIONS ON THE DIGESTIVE SYSTEM (42–54)

Excludes   Includes   Use additional   Code also   Omit code

● 48 **Operations on rectum, rectosigmoid and perirectal tissue**

Code also any application or administration of an adhesion barrier substance (99.77)
Coding Clinic: 1999, Q3, P8-9

48.0 **Proctotomy**
Decompression of imperforate anus
Panas' operation [linear proctotomy]
| Excludes | incision of perirectal tissue (48.81)

48.1 **Proctostomy**

● 48.2 **Diagnostic procedures on rectum, rectosigmoid and perirectal tissue**

48.21 **Transabdominal proctosigmoidoscopy**
Intraoperative proctosigmoidoscopy
| Excludes | that with biopsy (48.24)

48.22 **Proctosigmoidoscopy through artificial stoma**
| Excludes | that with biopsy (48.24)

48.23 **Rigid proctosigmoidoscopy**
| Excludes | flexible sigmoidoscopy (45.24)
Coding Clinic: 2001, Q1, P8

48.24 **Closed [endoscopic] biopsy of rectum**
Brushing or washing for specimen collection
Proctosigmoidoscopy with biopsy
Coding Clinic: 2003, Q1, P12

48.25 **Open biopsy of rectum**

48.26 **Biopsy of perirectal tissue**

48.29 **Other diagnostic procedures on rectum, rectosigmoid and perirectal tissue**
| Excludes | digital examination of rectum (89.34)
lower GI series (87.64)
microscopic examination of specimen from rectum (90.91–90.99)

● 48.3 **Local excision or destruction of lesion or tissue of rectum**

48.31 **Radical electrocoagulation of rectal lesion or tissue**

48.32 **Other electrocoagulation of rectal lesion or tissue**
Coding Clinic: 1998, Q2, P18; 1987, Nov-Dec, P11

48.33 **Destruction of rectal lesion or tissue by laser**

48.34 **Destruction of rectal lesion or tissue by cryosurgery**

48.35 **Local excision of rectal lesion or tissue**
| Excludes | biopsy of rectum (48.24–48.25)
excision of perirectal tissue (48.82)
hemorrhoidectomy (49.46)
[endoscopic] polypectomy of rectum (48.36)
rectal fistulectomy (48.73)

48.36 **[Endoscopic] polypectomy of rectum**

● 48.4 **Pull-through resection of rectum**
Code also any synchronous anastomosis other than end-to-end (45.90, 45.92–45.95)
Coding Clinic: 2008, Q4, P169-172

48.40 **Pull-through resection of rectum, not otherwise specified**
Pull-through resection NOS
| Excludes | abdominoperineal pull-through NOS (48.50)

48.41 **Soave submucosal resection of rectum**
Endorectal pull-through operation

48.42 **Laparoscopic pull-through resection of rectum**

48.43 **Open pull-through resection of rectum**

48.49 **Other pull-through resection of rectum**
Abdominoperineal pull-through
Altemeier operation
Swenson proctectomy
| Excludes | Duhamel abdominoperineal pull-through (48.65)
laparoscopic pull-through resection of rectum (48.42)
open pull-through resection of rectum (48.43)
pull-through resection of rectum, not otherwise specified (48.40)
Coding Clinic: 2001, Q3, P8-9; 1999, Q2, P13

● 48.5 **Abdominoperineal resection of rectum**
Combined abdominoendorectal resection
Complete proctectomy
| Includes | with synchronous colostomy
Code also any synchronous anastomosis other than end-to-end (45.90, 45.92–45.95)
| Excludes | Duhamel abdominoperineal pull-through (48.65)
that as part of pelvic exenteration (68.8)
Coding Clinic: 1997, Q2, P5

48.50 **Abdominoperineal resection of the rectum, not otherwise specified**

48.51 **Laparoscopic abdominoperineal resection of the rectum**

48.52 **Open abdominoperineal resection of the rectum**

48.59 **Other abdominoperineal resection of the rectum**
| Excludes | abdominoperineal resection of the rectum, NOS (48.50)
laparoscopic abdominoperineal resection of the rectum (48.51)
open abdominoperineal resection of the rectum (48.52)

● 48.6 **Other resection of rectum**
Code also any synchronous anastomosis other than end-to-end (45.90, 45.92–45.95)

48.61 **Transsacral rectosigmoidectomy**

48.62 **Anterior resection of rectum with synchronous colostomy**
Coding Clinic: 1997, Q2, P5

48.63 **Other anterior resection of rectum**
| Excludes | that with synchronous colostomy (48.62)
Coding Clinic: 1996, Q1, P9

48.64 **Posterior resection of rectum**

48.65 **Duhamel resection of rectum**
Duhamel abdominoperineal pull-through

48.69 **Other**
Partial proctectomy
Rectal resection NOS
Coding Clinic: 2005, Q2, P13-14; 1987, Jan-Feb, P11; 1986, Nov-Dec, P11

● 48.7 **Repair of rectum**
| Excludes | repair of:
current obstetric laceration (75.62)
vaginal rectocele (70.50, 70.52, 70.53, 70.55)

48.71 **Suture of laceration of rectum**

48.72 **Closure of proctostomy**

48.73 Closure of other rectal fistula
Excludes fistulectomy:
perirectal (48.93)
rectourethral (58.43)
rectovaginal (70.73)
rectovesical (57.83)
rectovesicovaginal (57.83)

48.74 Rectorectostomy
Rectal anastomosis NOS
Stapled transanal rectal resection (STARR)

48.75 Abdominal proctopexy
Frickman procedure
Ripstein repair of rectal prolapse

48.76 Other proctopexy
Delorme repair of prolapsed rectum
Proctosigmoidopexy
Puborectalis sling operation
Excludes manual reduction of rectal prolapse (96.26)

48.79 Other repair of rectum
Repair of old obstetric laceration of rectum
Excludes anastomosis to:
large intestine (45.94)
small intestine (45.92–45.93)
repair of:
current obstetrica laceration (75.62)
vaginal rectocele (70.50, 70.52)

● **48.8 Incision or excision of perirectal tissue or lesion**
Includes pelvirectal tissue
rectovaginal septum

48.81 Incision of perirectal tissue
Incision of rectovaginal septum

48.82 Excision of perirectal tissue
Excludes perirectal biopsy (48.26)
perirectofistulectomy (48.93)
rectal fistulectomy (48.73)

● **48.9 Other operations on rectum and perirectal tissue**
48.91 Incision of rectal stricture
48.92 Anorectal myectomy
48.93 Repair of perirectal fistula
Excludes that opening into rectum (48.73)
Coding Clinic: 2007, Q1, P13

48.99 Other
Excludes digital examination of rectum (89.34)
dilation of rectum (96.22)
insertion of rectal tube (96.09)
irrigation of rectum (96.38–96.39)
manual reduction of rectal prolapse (96.26)
proctoclysis (96.37)
rectal massage (99.93)
rectal packing (96.19)
removal of:
impacted feces (96.38)
intraluminal foreign body from rectum without incision (98.05)
rectal packing (97.59)
transanal enema (96.39)

● **49 Operations on anus**
Code also any application or administration of an adhesion barrier substance (99.77)

● **49.0 Incision or excision of perianal tissue**
49.01 Incision of perianal abscess
Coding Clinic: 2005, Q2, P10

49.02 Other incision of perianal tissue
Undercutting of perianal tissue
Excludes anal fistulotomy (49.11)

49.03 Excision of perianal skin tags
49.04 Other excision of perianal tissue
Excludes anal fistulectomy (49.12)
biopsy of perianal tissue (49.22)
Coding Clinic: 2001, Q1, P8

● **49.1 Incision or excision of anal fistula**
Excludes closure of anal fistula (49.73)
49.11 Anal fistulotomy
49.12 Anal fistulectomy

● **49.2 Diagnostic procedures on anus and perianal tissue**
49.21 Anoscopy
49.22 Biopsy of perianal tissue
49.23 Biopsy of anus
49.29 Other diagnostic procedures on anus and perianal tissue
Excludes microscopic examination of specimen from anus (90.91–90.99)

● **49.3 Local excision or destruction of other lesion or tissue of anus**
Anal cryptotomy
Cauterization of lesion of anus
Excludes biopsy of anus (49.23)
control of (postoperative) hemorrhage of anus (49.95)
hemorrhoidectomy (49.46)
49.31 Endoscopic excision or destruction of lesion or tissue of anus
49.39 Other local excision or destruction of lesion or tissue of anus
Excludes that by endoscopic approach (49.31)
Coding Clinic: 2001, Q1, P8

● **49.4 Procedures on hemorrhoids**
49.41 Reduction of hemorrhoids
49.42 Injection of hemorrhoids
49.43 Cauterization of hemorrhoids
Clamp and cautery of hemorrhoids
49.44 Destruction of hemorrhoids by cryotherapy
49.45 Ligation of hemorrhoids
49.46 Excision of hemorrhoids
Hemorrhoidectomy NOS
Coding Clinic: 2007, Q1, P13
49.47 Evacuation of thrombosed hemorrhoids
49.49 Other procedures on hemorrhoids
Lord procedure

● **49.5 Division of anal sphincter**
49.51 Left lateral anal sphincterotomy
49.52 Posterior anal sphincterotomy
49.59 Other anal sphincterotomy
Division of sphincter NOS

49.6 Excision of anus
● **49.7 Repair of anus**
Excludes repair of current obstetric laceration (75.62)
49.71 Suture of laceration of anus
49.72 Anal cerclage
49.73 Closure of anal fistula
Excludes excision of anal fistula (49.12)
49.74 Gracilis muscle transplant for anal incontinence

OPERATIONS ON THE DIGESTIVE SYSTEM (42–54)

49.75 Implantation or revision of artificial anal sphincter
Removal with subsequent replacement
Replacement during same or subsequent operative episode

49.76 Removal of artificial anal sphincter
Explantation or removal without replacement
> **Excludes** *revision with implantation during same operative episode (49.75)*

49.79 Other repair of anal sphincter
Repair of old obstetric laceration of anus
> **Excludes** *anoplasty with synchronous hemorrhoidectomy (49.46)*
> *repair of current obstetric laceration (75.62)*
Coding Clinic: 1998, Q2, P16-17; 1997, Q1, P9-10

● **49.9 Other operations on anus**
> **Excludes** *dilation of anus (sphincter) (96.23)*

49.91 Incision of anal septum

49.92 Insertion of subcutaneous electrical anal stimulator

49.93 Other incision of anus
Removal of:
  foreign body from anus with incision
  seton from anus
> **Excludes** *anal fistulotomy (49.11)*
> *removal of intraluminal foreign body without incision (98.05)*

49.94 Reduction of anal prolapse
> **Excludes** *manual reduction of rectal prolapse (96.26)*

49.95 Control of (postoperative) hemorrhage of anus

49.99 Other

● **50 Operations on liver**
Code also any application or administration of an adhesion barrier substance (99.77)

50.0 Hepatotomy
Incision of abscess of liver
Removal of gallstones from liver
Stromeyer-Little operation

● **50.1 Diagnostic procedures on liver**

50.11 Closed (percutaneous) [needle] biopsy of liver
Diagnostic aspiration of liver
Coding Clinic: 2005, Q3, P24; 1994, Q3, P11; 1988, Q4, P12

50.12 Open biopsy of liver
Wedge biopsy
Coding Clinic: 2005, Q2, P13-14; 1984, Nov-Dec, P12

50.13 Transjugular liver biopsy
Transvenous liver biopsy
> **Excludes** *closed (percutaneous) [needle] biopsy of liver (50.11)*
> *laparoscopic liver biopsy (50.14)*
Coding Clinic: 2007, Q4, P113-114

50.14 Laparoscopic liver biopsy
> **Excludes** *closed (percutaneous) [needle] biopsy of liver (50.11)*
> *open biopsy of liver (50.12)*
> *transjugular liver biopsy (50.13)*
Coding Clinic: 2007, Q4, P113-114

50.19 Other diagnostic procedures on liver
> **Excludes** *laparoscopic liver biopsy (50.14)*
> *liver scan and radioisotope function study (92.02)*
> *microscopic examination of specimen from liver (91.01–91.09)*
> *transjugular liver biopsy (50.13)*

● **50.2 Local excision or destruction of liver tissue or lesion**
Coding Clinic: 2006, Q4, P124-126

50.21 Marsupialization of lesion of liver

50.22 Partial hepatectomy
Wedge resection of liver
> **Excludes** *biopsy of liver (50.11–50.12)*
> *hepatic lobectomy (50.3)*

50.23 Open ablation of liver lesion or tissue

50.24 Percutaneous ablation of liver lesion or tissue

50.25 Laparoscopic ablation of liver lesion or tissue

50.26 Other and unspecified ablation of liver lesion or tissue

50.29 Other destruction of lesion of liver
Cauterization of hepatic lesion
Enucleation of hepatic lesion
Evacuation of hepatic lesion
> **Excludes** *ablation of liver lesion or tissue:*
> *laparoscopic (50.25)*
> *open (50.23)*
> *other (50.26)*
> *percutaneous (50.24)*
> *laser interstitial thermal therapy [LITT] of lesion or tissue of liver under guidance (17.63)*
> *percutaneous aspiration of lesion (50.91)*
Coding Clinic: 2003, Q2, P9

50.3 Lobectomy of liver
Total hepatic lobectomy with partial excision of other lobe

50.4 Total hepatectomy
Coding Clinic: 2008, Q2, P8-9

● **50.5 Liver transplant**
Note: To report donor source - *see* codes 00.91–00.93

50.51 Auxiliary liver transplant
Auxiliary hepatic transplantation leaving patient's own liver in situ

50.59 Other transplant of liver
Coding Clinic: 2008, Q4, P120; Q2, P8-9

● **50.6 Repair of liver**

50.61 Closure of laceration of liver

50.69 Other repair of liver
Hepatopexy

● **50.9 Other operations on liver**
> **Excludes** *lysis of adhesions (54.5)*

50.91 Percutaneous aspiration of liver
> **Excludes** *percutaneous biopsy (50.11)*

50.92 Extracorporeal hepatic assistance
Liver dialysis
Coding Clinic: 2001, Q2, P21-22

50.93 Localized perfusion of liver

50.94 Other injection of therapeutic substance into liver

50.99 Other

◀ New   ◀|||| Revised   ~~deleted~~ Deleted   ● Use Additional Digit(s)   OGCR Official Guidelines   Coding Clinic

● **51 Operations on gallbladder and biliary tract**

Includes operations on:
    ampulla of Vater
    common bile duct
    cystic duct
    hepatic duct
    intrahepatic bile duct
    sphincter of Oddi

Code also any application or administration of an adhesion barrier substance (99.77)

● **51.0 Cholecystotomy and cholecystostomy**

51.01 Percutaneous aspiration of gallbladder
Percutaneous cholecystotomy for drainage
That by: needle or catheter
    Excludes *needle biopsy (51.12)*

51.02 Trocar cholecystostomy

51.03 Other cholecystostomy

51.04 Other cholecystotomy
Cholelithotomy NOS

● **51.1 Diagnostic procedures on biliary tract**

    Excludes *that for endoscopic procedures classifiable to 51.64, 51.84–51.88, 52.14, 52.21, 52.93–52.94, 52.97–52.98*

Coding Clinic: 1997, Q2, P7

51.10 Endoscopic retrograde cholangiopancreatography [ERCP]

    Excludes *endoscopic retrograde:*
        cholangiography [ERC] (51.11)
        pancreatography [ERP] (52.13)

Coding Clinic: 2003, Q3, P17-18; 2001, Q1, P8-9; 1999, Q2, P13-14; 1993, 5th Issue, P12

51.11 Endoscopic retrograde cholangiography [ERC]
Laparoscopic exploration of common bile duct

    Excludes *endoscopic retrograde:*
        cholangiopancreatography [ERCP]
        (51.10)
        pancreatography [ERP] (52.13)

Coding Clinic: 1996, Q1, P12-13; 1993, 5th Issue, P12; 1988, Q4, P7

51.12 Percutaneous biopsy of gallbladder or bile ducts
Needle biopsy of gallbladder

51.13 Open biopsy of gallbladder or bile ducts

51.14 Other closed [endoscopic] biopsy of biliary duct or sphincter of Oddi
Brushing or washing for specimen collection
Closed biopsy of biliary duct or sphincter of Oddi by procedures classifiable to 51.10–51.11, 52.13

51.15 Pressure measurement of sphincter of Oddi
Pressure measurement of sphincter by procedures classifiable to 51.10–51.11, 52.13

51.19 Other diagnostic procedures on biliary tract

    Excludes *biliary tract x-ray (87.51–87.59)*
    microscopic examination of specimen from biliary tract (91.01–91.09)

● **51.2 Cholecystectomy**

51.21 Other partial cholecystectomy
Revision of prior cholecystectomy
    Excludes *that by laparoscope (51.24)*

51.22 Cholecystectomy
    Excludes *laparoscopic cholecystectomy (51.23)*

Coding Clinic: 1997, Q4, P52; 1995, Q2, P11; 1993, 5th Issue, P11; 1992, Q2, P16; 1988, Q4, P7

51.23 Laparoscopic cholecystectomy
That by laser
Coding Clinic: 2008, Q4, P172-174; 1998, Q3, P10; 1997, Q4, P52; 1996, Q1, P12-13; 1995, Q2, P11; 1994, Q3, P11

51.24 Laparoscopic partial cholecystectomy
Coding Clinic: 1996, Q4, P69

● **51.3 Anastomosis of gallbladder or bile duct**

    Excludes *resection with end-to-end anastomosis (51.61–51.69)*

51.31 Anastomosis of gallbladder to hepatic ducts

51.32 Anastomosis of gallbladder to intestine

51.33 Anastomosis of gallbladder to pancreas

51.34 Anastomosis of gallbladder to stomach

51.35 Other gallbladder anastomosis
Gallbladder anastomosis NOS

51.36 Choledochoenterostomy

51.37 Anastomosis of hepatic duct to gastrointestinal tract
Kasai portoenterostomy
Coding Clinic: 2002, Q2, P12

51.39 Other bile duct anastomosis
Anastomosis of bile duct NOS
Anastomosis of unspecified bile duct to:
    intestine   pancreas
    liver   stomach

● **51.4 Incision of bile duct for relief of obstruction**

51.41 Common duct exploration for removal of calculus
    Excludes *percutaneous extraction (51.96)*
Coding Clinic: 1996, Q1, P12-13; 1988, Q4, P7

51.42 Common duct exploration for relief of other obstruction

51.43 Insertion of choledochohepatic tube for decompression
Hepatocholedochostomy
Coding Clinic: 1988, Q4, P7

51.49 Incision of other bile ducts for relief of obstruction

● **51.5 Other incision of bile duct**

    Excludes *that for relief of obstruction (51.41–51.49)*

51.51 Exploration of common duct
Incision of common bile duct
Coding Clinic: 1996, Q1, P12

51.59 Incision of other bile duct

● **51.6 Local excision or destruction of lesion or tissue of biliary ducts and sphincter of Oddi**

Code also anastomosis other than end-to-end (51.31, 51.36–51.39)

    Excludes *biopsy of bile duct (51.12–51.13)*

51.61 Excision of cystic duct remnant

51.62 Excision of ampulla of Vater (with reimplantation of common duct)

51.63 Other excision of common duct
Choledochectomy
    Excludes *fistulectomy (51.72)*

51.64 Endoscopic excision or destruction of lesion of biliary ducts or sphincter of Oddi
Excision or destruction of lesion of biliary duct by procedures classifiable to 51.10–51.11, 52.13
Coding Clinic: 1993, 5th Issue, P14

51.69 Excision of other bile duct
Excision of lesion of bile duct NOS
    Excludes *fistulectomy (51.79)*

OPERATIONS ON THE DIGESTIVE SYSTEM (42–54)

● **51.7 Repair of bile ducts**

51.71 Simple suture of common bile duct

51.72 Choledochoplasty
Repair of fistula of common bile duct

51.79 Repair of other bile ducts
Closure of artificial opening of bile duct NOS
Suture of bile duct NOS
> Excludes | *operative removal of prosthetic device (51.95)*

● **51.8 Other operations on biliary ducts and sphincter of Oddi**

51.81 Dilation of sphincter of Oddi
Dilation of ampulla of Vater
> Excludes | *that by endoscopic approach (51.84)*

51.82 Pancreatic sphincterotomy
Incision of pancreatic sphincter
Transduodenal ampullary sphincterotomy
> Excludes | *that by endoscopic approach (51.85)*

51.83 Pancreatic sphincteroplasty

51.84 Endoscopic dilation of ampulla and biliary duct
Dilation of ampulla and biliary duct by procedures classifiable to 51.10–51.11, 52.13

51.85 Endoscopic sphincterotomy and papillotomy
Sphincterotomy and papillotomy by procedures classifiable to 51.10–51.11, 52.13
Coding Clinic: 2003, Q3, P17.18; 1993, 5th Issue, P14

51.86 Endoscopic insertion of nasobiliary drainage tube
Insertion of nasobiliary tube by procedures classifiable to 51.10–51.11, 52.13

51.87 Endoscopic insertion of stent (tube) into bile duct
Endoprosthesis of bile duct
Insertion of stent into bile duct by procedures classifiable to 51.10–51.11, 52.13
> Excludes | *nasobiliary drainage tube (51.86)*
> *replacement of stent (tube) (97.05)*
Coding Clinic: 2003, Q3, P17

51.88 Endoscopic removal of stone(s) from biliary tract
Laparoscopic removal of stone(s) from biliary tract
Removal of biliary tract stone(s) by procedures classifiable to 51.10–51.11, 52.13
> Excludes | *percutaneous extraction of common duct stones (51.96)*
Coding Clinic: 2000, Q2, P11; 1997, Q2, P7; 1993, 5th Issue, P12

51.89 Other operations on sphincter of Oddi

● **51.9 Other operations on biliary tract**

51.91 Repair of laceration of gallbladder

51.92 Closure of cholecystostomy

51.93 Closure of other biliary fistula
Cholecystogastroenteric fistulectomy

51.94 Revision of anastomosis of biliary tract

51.95 Removal of prosthetic device from bile duct
> Excludes | *nonoperative removal (97.55)*

51.96 Percutaneous extraction of common duct stones
Coding Clinic: 1988, Q4, P7

51.98 Other percutaneous procedures on biliary tract
Percutaneous biliary endoscopy via existing T-tube or other tract for:
dilation of biliary duct stricture
removal of stone(s) except common duct stone
exploration (postoperative)
Percutaneous transhepatic biliary drainage
> Excludes | *percutaneous aspiration of gallbladder (51.01)*
> *percutaneous biopsy and/or collection of specimen by brushing or washing (51.12)*
> *percutaneous removal of common duct stone(s) (51.96)*
Coding Clinic: 1997, Q1, P14

51.99 Other
Insertion or replacement of biliary tract prosthesis
> Excludes | *biopsy of gallbladder (51.12–51.13)*
> *irrigation of cholecystostomy and other biliary tube (96.41)*
> *lysis of peritoneal adhesions (54.5)*
> *nonoperative removal of:*
> *cholecystostomy tube (97.54)*
> *tube from biliary tract or liver (97.55)*

● **52 Operations on pancreas**
> Includes   operations on pancreatic duct
> Code also   any application or administration of an adhesion barrier substance (99.77)

● **52.0 Pancreatotomy**

52.01 Drainage of pancreatic cyst by catheter

52.09 Other pancreatotomy
Pancreatolithotomy
> Excludes | *drainage by anastomosis (52.4, 52.96)*
> *incision of pancreatic sphincter (51.82)*
> *marsupialization of cyst (52.3)*

● **52.1 Diagnostic procedures on pancreas**

52.11 Closed [aspiration] [needle] [percutaneous] biopsy of pancreas

52.12 Open biopsy of pancreas

52.13 Endoscopic retrograde pancreatography [ERP]
> Excludes | *endoscopic retrograde:*
> *cholangiography [ERC] (51.11)*
> *cholangiopancreatography [ERCP] (51.10)*
> *that for procedures classifiable to 51.14–51.15, 51.64, 51.84–51.88, 52.14, 52.21, 52.92–52.94, 52.97–52.98*
Coding Clinic: 1993, 5th Issue, P12

52.14 Closed [endoscopic] biopsy of pancreatic duct
Closed biopsy of pancreatic duct by procedures classifiable to 51.10–51.11, 52.13

52.19 Other diagnostic procedures on pancreas
> Excludes | *contrast pancreatogram (87.66)*
> *endoscopic retrograde pancreatography [ERP] (52.13)*
> *microscopic examination of specimen from pancreas (91.01–91.09)*

● **52.2 Local excision or destruction of pancreas and pancreatic duct**

> **Excludes** *biopsy of pancreas (52.11–52.12, 52.14)*
> *pancreatic fistulectomy (52.95)*

52.21 Endoscopic excision or destruction of lesion or tissue of pancreatic duct
Excision or destruction of lesion or tissue of pancreatic duct by procedures classifiable to 51.10–51.11, 52.13

52.22 Other excision or destruction of lesion or tissue of pancreas or pancreatic duct

52.3 Marsupialization of pancreatic cyst

> **Excludes** *drainage of cyst by catheter (52.01)*

52.4 Internal drainage of pancreatic cyst
Pancreaticocystoduodenostomy
Pancreaticocystogastrostomy
Pancreaticocystojejunostomy

● **52.5 Partial pancreatectomy**

> **Excludes** *pancreatic fistulectomy (52.95)*

52.51 Proximal pancreatectomy
Excision of head of pancreas (with part of body)
Proximal pancreatectomy with synchronous duodenectomy

52.52 Distal pancreatectomy
Excision of tail of pancreas (with part of body)

52.53 Radical subtotal pancreatectomy
Coding Clinic: 2001, Q1, P13

52.59 Other partial pancreatectomy

52.6 Total pancreatectomy
Pancreatectomy with synchronous duodenectomy
Coding Clinic: 1996, Q4, P70-71

52.7 Radical pancreaticoduodenectomy
One-stage pancreaticoduodenal resection with choledochojejunal anastomosis, pancreaticojejunal anastomosis, and gastrojejunostomy
Two-stage pancreaticoduodenal resection (first stage) (second stage)
Radical resection of the pancreas
Whipple procedure

> **Excludes** *radical subtotal pancreatectomy (52.53)*

Coding Clinic: 2001, Q1, P13

● **52.8 Transplant of pancreas**
Note: To report donor source - *see* codes 00.91–00.93

52.80 Pancreatic transplant, not otherwise specified

52.81 Reimplantation of pancreatic tissue

52.82 Homotransplant of pancreas

52.83 Heterotransplant of pancreas

52.84 Autotransplantation of cells of Islets of Langerhans
Homotransplantation of islet cells of pancreas
Coding Clinic: 1996, Q4, P70-71

52.85 Allotransplantation of cells of Islets of Langerhans
Heterotransplantation of islet cells of pancreas
Coding Clinic: 1996, Q4, P70-71

52.86 Transplantation of cells of Islets of Langerhans, not otherwise specified

● **52.9 Other operations on pancreas**

52.92 Cannulation of pancreatic duct

> **Excludes** *that by endoscopic approach (52.93)*

52.93 Endoscopic insertion of stent (tube) into pancreatic duct
Insertion of cannula or stent into pancreatic duct by procedures classifiable to 51.10–51.11, 52.13

> **Excludes** *endoscopic insertion of nasopancreatic drainage tube (52.97)*
> *replacement of stent (tube) (97.05)*

Coding Clinic: 1997, Q2, P7

52.94 Endoscopic removal of stone(s) from pancreatic duct
Removal of stone(s) from pancreatic duct by procedures classifiable to 51.10–51.11, 52.13

52.95 Other repair of pancreas
Fistulectomy of pancreas
Simple suture of pancreas

52.96 Anastomosis of pancreas
Anastomosis of pancreas (duct) to:
intestine
jejunum
stomach

> **Excludes** *anastomosis to:*
> *bile duct (51.39)*
> *gallbladder (51.33)*

52.97 Endoscopic insertion of nasopancreatic drainage tube
Insertion of nasopancreatic drainage tube by procedures classifiable to 51.10–51.11, 52.13

> **Excludes** *drainage of pancreatic cyst by catheter (52.01)*
> *replacement of stent (tube) (97.05)*

52.98 Endoscopic dilation of pancreatic duct
Dilation of Wirsung's duct by procedures classifiable to 51.10–51.11, 52.13

52.99 Other
Dilation of pancreatic [Wirsung's] duct by open approach
Repair of pancreatic [Wirsung's] duct by open approach

> **Excludes** *irrigation of pancreatic tube (96.42)*
> *removal of pancreatic tube (97.56)*

OPERATIONS ON THE DIGESTIVE SYSTEM (42–54)

● **53 Repair of hernia**

Includes hernioplasty
herniorrhaphy

Code also any application or administration of an adhesion barrier substance (99.77)

Excludes manual reduction of hernia (96.27)

● **53.0 Other unilateral repair of inguinal hernia**

Excludes laparoscopic unilateral repair of inguinal hernia (17.11–17.13)
Coding Clinic: 1994, Q3, P8

53.00 Unilateral repair of inguinal hernia, not otherwise specified
Inguinal herniorrhaphy NOS
Coding Clinic: 2008, Q4, P165-169; 2003, Q3, P10-11

53.01 Other and open repair of direct inguinal hernia
Direct and indirect inguinal hernia
Coding Clinic: 1996, Q4, P65-66

53.02 Other and open repair of indirect inguinal hernia

53.03 Other and open repair of direct inguinal hernia with graft or prosthesis

53.04 Other and open repair of indirect inguinal hernia with graft or prosthesis

53.05 Repair of inguinal hernia with graft or prosthesis, not otherwise specified

● **53.1 Other bilateral repair of inguinal hernia**

Excludes laparoscopic bilateral repair of inguinal hernia (17.21–17.24)

53.10 Bilateral repair of inguinal hernia, not otherwise specified

53.11 Other and open bilateral repair of direct inguinal hernia
Coding Clinic: 1988, Q1, P9

53.12 Other and open bilateral repair of indirect inguinal hernia

53.13 Other and open bilateral repair of inguinal hernia, one direct and one indirect

53.14 Other and open bilateral repair of direct inguinal hernia with graft or prosthesis

53.15 Other and open bilateral repair of indirect inguinal hernia with graft or prosthesis

53.16 Other and open bilateral repair of inguinal hernia, one direct and one indirect, with graft or prosthesis

53.17 Bilateral inguinal hernia repair with graft or prosthesis, not otherwise specified

● **53.2 Unilateral repair of femoral hernia**

53.21 Unilateral repair of femoral hernia with graft or prosthesis

53.29 Other unilateral femoral herniorrhaphy

● **53.3 Bilateral repair of femoral hernia**

53.31 Bilateral repair of femoral hernia with graft or prosthesis

53.39 Other bilateral femoral herniorrhaphy

● **53.4 Repair of umbilical hernia**

Excludes repair of gastroschisis (54.71)

53.41 Other and open repair of umbilical hernia with graft or prosthesis

53.42 Laparoscopic repair of umbilical hernia with graft or prosthesis

53.43 Other laparoscopic umbilical herniorrhaphy

53.49 Other open umbilical herniorrhaphy

Excludes other laparoscopic umbilical herniorrhaphy (53.43)
repair of umbilical hernia with graft or prosthesis (53.41, 53.42)

● **53.5 Repair of other hernia of anterior abdominal wall (without graft or prosthesis)**

53.51 Incisional hernia repair
Coding Clinic: 2003, Q3, P6

53.59 Repair of other hernia of anterior abdominal wall
Repair of hernia:
epigastric
hypogastric
spigelian
ventral
That by laparoscopic approach ◄
Coding Clinic: 1996, Q3, P15

● **53.6 Repair of other hernia of anterior abdominal wall with graft or prosthesis**

53.61 Other open incisional hernia repair with graft or prosthesis

Excludes laparoscopic incisional hernia repair with graft or prosthesis (53.62)
Coding Clinic: 2006, Q2, P10-11

53.62 Laparoscopic incisional hernia repair with graft or prosthesis
Coding Clinic: 2003, Q3, P11

53.63 Other laparoscopic repair of other hernia of anterior abdominal wall with graft or prosthesis

53.69 Other and open repair of other hernia of anterior abdominal wall with graft or prosthesis

Excludes other laparoscopic repair of other hernia of anterior abdominal wall with graft or prothesis (53.63)

● **53.7 Repair of diaphragmatic hernia, abdominal approach**

53.71 Laparoscopic repair of diaphragmatic hernia, abdominal approach

53.72 Other and open repair of diaphragmatic hernia, abdominal approach

53.75 Repair of diaphragmatic hernia, abdominal approach, not otherwise specified

Excludes laparoscopic repair of diaphragmatic hernia (53.71)
other and open repair of diaphragmatic hernia (53.72)

● **53.8 Repair of diaphragmatic hernia, thoracic approach**

53.80 Repair of diaphragmatic hernia with thoracic approach, not otherwise specified
Thoracoabdominal repair of diaphragmatic hernia

53.81 Plication of the diaphragm

53.82 Repair of parasternal hernia

53.83 Laparoscopic repair of diaphragmatic hernia, with thoracic approach

53.84 Other and open repair of diaphragmatic hernia, with thoracic approach

Excludes repair of diaphragmatic hernia with thoracic approach, NOS (53.80)

53.9 Other hernia repair

Repair of hernia:
- ischiatic
- ischiorectal
- lumbar
- obturator

Repair of hernia:
- omental
- retroperitoneal
- sciatic

Excludes | relief of strangulated hernia with
exteriorization of intestine (46.01, 46.03)
repair of pericolostomy hernia (46.42)
repair of vaginal enterocele (70.92)

● 54 Other operations on abdominal region

Includes | operations on:
- epigastric region
- flank
- groin region
- hypochondrium
- inguinal region
- loin region
- pelvic cavity
- mesentery
- omentum
- peritoneum
- retroperitoneal tissue space

Code also any application or administration of an
adhesion barrier substance (99.77)

Excludes | hernia repair (53.00–53.9)
obliteration of cul-de-sac (70.92)
retroperitoneal tissue dissection (59.00–59.09)
skin and subcutaneous tissue of abdominal wall
(86.01–86.99)

Coding Clinic: 1997, Q1, P11; 1987, Nov-Dec, P12

54.0 Incision of abdominal wall

Drainage of:
- abdominal wall
- extraperitoneal abscess
- retroperitoneal abscess

Excludes | incision of peritoneum (54.95)
laparotomy (54.11–54.19)

Coding Clinic: 2006, Q2, P23-24; 2005, Q4, P74-77; 1993, 5th Issue, P9-10

● 54.1 Laparotomy

54.11 Exploratory laparotomy

Excludes | exploration incidental to intra-abdominal
surgery — omit code

Coding Clinic: 1989, Q3, P14; 1988, Q4, P12; 1987, Jan-Feb,
P11-12; 1984, Nov-Dec, P12

54.12 Reopening of recent laparotomy site

Reopening of recent laparotomy site for:
- control of hemorrhage
- exploration
- incision of hematoma

54.19 Other laparotomy

Drainage of intraperitoneal abscess or
hematoma

Excludes | culdocentesis (70.0)
drainage of appendiceal abscess (47.2)
exploration incidental to intra
abdominal surgery — omit code
Ladd operation (54.95)
percutaneous drainage of abdomen
(54.91)
removal of foreign body (54.92)

Coding Clinic: 2003, Q3, P16-17; 1992, Q1, P14

● 54.2 Diagnostic procedures of abdominal region

54.21 Laparoscopy

Peritoneoscopy

Excludes | laparoscopic cholecystectomy (51.23)
that incidental to destruction of
fallopian tubes (66.21–66.29)

Coding Clinic: 1996, Q4, P64-66

54.22 Biopsy of abdominal wall or umbilicus

54.23 Biopsy of peritoneum

Biopsy of:
- mesentery
- omentum
- peritoneal implant

Excludes | closed biopsy of:
omentum (54.24)
peritoneum (54.24)

54.24 Closed [percutaneous] [needle] biopsy of intra-abdominal mass

Closed biopsy of:
- omentum
- peritoneal implant
- peritoneum

Excludes | that of:
fallopian tube (66.11)
ovary (65.11)
uterine ligaments (68.15)
uterus (68.16)

Coding Clinic: 1997, Q4, P57

54.25 Peritoneal lavage

Diagnostic peritoneal lavage

Excludes | peritoneal dialysis (54.98)

Coding Clinic: 1998, Q2, P19-20; 1993, Q4, P31

54.29 Other diagnostic procedures on abdominal region

Excludes | abdominal lymphangiogram (88.04)
abdominal x-ray NEC (88.19)
angiocardiography of venae cava
(88.51)
C.A.T. scan of abdomen (88.01)
contrast x-ray of abdominal cavity
(88.11–88.15)
intra-abdominal arteriography NEC
(88.47)
microscopic examination of peritoneal
and retroperitoneal specimen
(91.11–91.19)
phlebography of:
intra-abdominal vessels NEC (88.65)
portal venous system (88.64)
sinogram of abdominal wall (88.03)
soft tissue x-ray of abdominal wall
NEC (88.09)
tomography of abdomen NEC (88.02)
ultrasonography of abdomen and
retroperitoneum (88.76)

54.3 Excision or destruction of lesion or tissue of abdominal wall or umbilicus

Debridement of abdominal wall
Omphalectomy

Excludes | biopsy of abdominal wall or umbilicus (54.22)
size reduction operation (86.83)
that of skin of abdominal wall (86.22, 86.26,
86.3)

Coding Clinic: 1989, Q1, P11

OPERATIONS ON THE DIGESTIVE SYSTEM (42–54)

OPERATIONS ON THE DIGESTIVE SYSTEM (42–54)

54.4 Excision or destruction of peritoneal tissue
Excision of:
  appendices epiploicae
  falciform ligament
  gastrocolic ligament
  lesion of:
    mesentery
    omentum
    peritoneum
  presacral lesion NOS
  retroperitoneal lesion NOS

Excludes | *biopsy of peritoneum (54.23)*
endometrectomy of cul-de-sac (70.32)

● **54.5 Lysis of peritoneal adhesions**
Freeing of adhesions of:
  biliary tract
  intestines
  liver
  pelvic peritoneum
  peritoneum
  spleen
  uterus

Excludes | *lysis of adhesions of:*
bladder (59.11)
fallopian tube and ovary
laparoscopic (65.81)
other (65.89)
kidney (59.02)
ureter (59.02)

54.51 Laparoscopic lysis of peritoneal adhesions
Coding Clinic: 2006, Q4, P130-134; 2003, Q3, P6-7; 1996, Q4, P65-66

54.59 Other lysis of peritoneal adhesions
Coding Clinic: 2010, Q1, P12; 2006, Q3, P15-16; 2003, Q3, P11; Q1, P14-15; 1996, Q4, P65-66; 1994, Q3, P8

● **54.6 Suture of abdominal wall and peritoneum**

54.61 Reclosure of postoperative disruption of abdominal wall

54.62 Delayed closure of granulating abdominal wound
Tertiary subcutaneous wound closure

54.63 Other suture of abdominal wall
Suture of laceration of abdominal wall

Excludes | *closure of operative wound — omit code*

54.64 Suture of peritoneum
Secondary suture of peritoneum

Excludes | *closure of operative wound — omit code*

● **54.7 Other repair of abdominal wall and peritoneum**

54.71 Repair of gastroschisis
Coding Clinic: 2002, Q2, P9

54.72 Other repair of abdominal wall

54.73 Other repair of peritoneum
Suture of gastrocolic ligament

54.74 Other repair of omentum
Epiplorrhaphy
Graft of omentum
Omentopexy
Reduction of torsion of omentum

Excludes | *cardio-omentopexy (36.39)*

Coding Clinic: 1987, Jan-Feb, P11

54.75 Other repair of mesentery
Mesenteric plication
Mesenteropexy

● **54.9 Other operations of abdominal region**

Excludes | *removal of ectopic pregnancy (74.3)*

54.91 Percutaneous abdominal drainage
Paracentesis

Excludes | *creation of cutaneoperitoneal fistula (54.93)*

Coding Clinic: 2007, Q4, P95-96; 1999, Q3, P9; 1999, Q2, P14; 1998, Q3, P12; 1990, Q2, P25

54.92 Removal of foreign body from peritoneal cavity
Coding Clinic: 1989, Q1, P11

54.93 Creation of cutaneoperitoneal fistula
Coding Clinic: 1995, Q2, P10

54.94 Creation of peritoneovascular shunt
Peritoneovenous shunt
Coding Clinic: 1988, Q1, P9

54.95 Incision of peritoneum
Exploration of ventriculoperitoneal shunt at peritoneal site
Ladd operation
Revision of distal catheter of ventricular shunt
Revision of ventriculoperitoneal shunt at peritoneal site

Excludes | *that incidental to laparotomy (54.11–54.19)*

54.96 Injection of air into peritoneal cavity
Pneumoperitoneum

Excludes | *that for:*
collapse of lung (33.33)
radiography (88.12–88.13, 88.15)

54.97 Injection of locally-acting therapeutic substance into peritoneal cavity

Excludes | *peritoneal dialysis (54.98)*

54.98 Peritoneal dialysis

Excludes | *peritoneal lavage (diagnostic) (54.25)*

Coding Clinic: 1993, Q4, P31

54.99 Other

Excludes | *removal of:*
abdominal wall suture (97.83)
peritoneal drainage device (97.82)
retroperitoneal drainage device (97.81)

Coding Clinic: 1999, Q1, P4

◄ New   ◄▭ Revised   ~~deleted~~ Deleted   ● Use Additional Digit(s)   **OGCR** Official Guidelines   **Coding Clinic**

10. OPERATIONS ON THE URINARY SYSTEM (55–59)

● **55 Operations on kidney**

  Includes operations on renal pelvis

  Code also any application or administration of an adhesion barrier substance (99.77)

  Excludes perirenal tissue (59.00–59.09, 59.21–59.29, 59.91–59.92)

● **55.0 Nephrotomy and nephrostomy**

  Excludes drainage by:
    anastomosis (55.86)
    aspiration (55.92)
    incision of kidney pelvis (55.11–55.12)

  55.01 Nephrotomy
    Evacuation of renal cyst
    Exploration of kidney
    Nephrolithotomy

  55.02 Nephrostomy
    Coding Clinic: 1997, Q2, P4; 1986, Sept-Oct, P11-12

  55.03 Percutaneous nephrostomy without fragmentation
    Nephrostolithotomy, percutaneous (nephroscopic)
    Percutaneous removal of kidney stone(s) by:
      basket extraction
      forceps extraction (nephroscopic)
    Pyelostolithotomy, percutaneous (nephroscopic)
    With placement of catheter down ureter

    Excludes percutaneous removal by fragmentation (55.04)
      repeat nephroscopic removal during current episode (55.92)
    Coding Clinic: 1996, Q2, P5

  55.04 Percutaneous nephrostomy with fragmentation
    Percutaneous nephrostomy with disruption of kidney stone by ultrasonic energy and extraction (suction) through endoscope
    With placement of catheter down ureter
    With fluoroscopic guidance

    Excludes repeat fragmentation during current episode (59.95)
    Coding Clinic: 1986, Sept-Oct, P11-12

● **55.1 Pyelotomy and pyelostomy**

  Excludes drainage by anastomosis (55.86)
    percutaneous pyelostolithotomy (55.03)
    removal of calculus without incision (56.0)

  55.11 Pyelotomy
    Exploration of renal pelvis
    Pyelolithotomy

  55.12 Pyelostomy
    Insertion of drainage tube into renal pelvis

● **55.2 Diagnostic procedures on kidney**

  55.21 Nephroscopy

  55.22 Pyeloscopy

  55.23 Closed [percutaneous] [needle] biopsy of kidney
    Endoscopic biopsy via existing nephrostomy, nephrotomy, pyelostomy, or pyelotomy

  55.24 Open biopsy of kidney

  55.29 Other diagnostic procedures on kidney

    Excludes microscopic examination of specimen from kidney (91.21–91.29)
      pyelogram:
        intravenous (87.73)
        percutaneous (87.75)
        retrograde (87.74)
      radioisotope scan (92.03)
      renal arteriography (88.45)
      tomography:
        C.A.T. scan (87.71)
        other (87.72)

● **55.3 Local excision or destruction of lesion or tissue of kidney**
    Coding Clinic: 2006, Q4, P124-126

  55.31 Marsupialization of kidney lesion

  55.32 Open ablation of renal lesion or tissue

  55.33 Percutaneous ablation of renal lesion or tissue

  55.34 Laparoscopic ablation of renal lesion or tissue

  55.35 Other and unspecified ablation of renal lesion or tissue

  55.39 Other local destruction or excision of renal lesion or tissue
    Obliteration of calyceal diverticulum

    Excludes ablation of renal lesion or tissue:
      laparoscopic (55.34)
      open (55.32)
      other (55.35)
      percutaneous (55.33)
      biopsy of kidney (55.23–55.24)
      partial nephrectomy (55.4)
      percutaneous aspiration of kidney (55.92)
      wedge resection of kidney (55.4)
    Coding Clinic: 1996, Q1, P10-11

  55.4 Partial nephrectomy
    Calycectomy
    Wedge resection of kidney

    Code also any synchronous resection of ureter (56.40–56.42)

● **55.5 Complete nephrectomy**

    Code also any synchronous excision of:
      adrenal gland (07.21–07.3)
      bladder segment (57.6)
      lymph nodes (40.3, 40.52–40.59)

  55.51 Nephroureterectomy
    Nephroureterectomy with bladder cuff
    Total nephrectomy (unilateral)

    Excludes removal of transplanted kidney (55.53)
    Coding Clinic: 2005, Q2, P4-5

  55.52 Nephrectomy of remaining kidney
    Removal of solitary kidney

    Excludes removal of transplanted kidney (55.53)

  55.53 Removal of transplanted or rejected kidney
    Coding Clinic: 2008, Q4, P82-83

  55.54 Bilateral nephrectomy

    Excludes complete nephrectomy NOS (55.51)

● **55.6 Transplant of kidney**
    Note: To report donor source - see codes 00.91–00.93

  55.61 Renal autotransplantation

  55.69 Other kidney transplantation
    Coding Clinic: 2004, Q4, P116-117; 1996, Q4, P70-71

55.7 **Nephropexy**
Fixation or suspension of movable [floating] kidney

● 55.8 **Other repair of kidney**

55.81 **Suture of laceration of kidney**

55.82 **Closure of nephrostomy and pyelostomy**

55.83 **Closure of other fistula of kidney**

55.84 **Reduction of torsion of renal pedicle**

55.85 **Symphysiotomy for horseshoe kidney**

55.86 **Anastomosis of kidney**
Nephropyeloureterostomy
Pyeloureterovesical anastomosis
Ureterocalyceal anastomosis
| **Excludes** | *nephrocystanastomosis NOS (56.73)* |

55.87 **Correction of ureteropelvic junction**

55.89 **Other**

● 55.9 **Other operations on kidney**
| **Excludes** | *lysis of perirenal adhesions (59.02)* |

55.91 **Decapsulation of kidney**
Capsulectomy of kidney
Decortication of kidney

55.92 **Percutaneous aspiration of kidney (pelvis)**
Aspiration of renal cyst
Renipuncture
| **Excludes** | *percutaneous biopsy of kidney (55.23)* |
Coding Clinic: 1984, Nov-Dec, P20

55.93 **Replacement of nephrostomy tube**

55.94 **Replacement of pyelostomy tube**

55.95 **Local perfusion of kidney**

55.96 **Other injection of therapeutic substance into kidney**
Injection into renal cyst

55.97 **Implantation or replacement of mechanical kidney**

55.98 **Removal of mechanical kidney**

55.99 **Other**
| **Excludes** | *removal of pyelostomy or nephrostomy tube (97.61)* |

● 56 **Operations on ureter**
Code also any application or administration of an adhesion barrier substance (99.77)
Coding Clinic: 1986, Sept-Oct, P11-12

56.0 **Transurethral removal of obstruction from ureter and renal pelvis**
Removal of:
blood clot from ureter or renal pelvis without incision
calculus from ureter or renal pelvis without incision
foreign body from ureter or renal pelvis without incision
Excludes	*manipulation without removal of obstruction (59.8)*
	that by incision (55.11, 56.2)
	transurethral insertion of ureteral stent for passage of calculus (59.8)

56.1 **Ureteral meatotomy**

56.2 **Ureterotomy**
Incision of ureter for:
drainage
exploration
removal of calculus
Excludes	*cutting of ureterovesical orifice (56.1)*
	removal of calculus without incision (56.0)
	transurethral insertion of ureteral stent for passage of calculus (59.8)
	urinary diversion (56.51–56.79)
Coding Clinic: 1986, Sept-Oct, P10

● 56.3 **Diagnostic procedures on ureter**

56.31 **Ureteroscopy**

56.32 **Closed percutaneous biopsy of ureter**
| **Excludes** | *endoscopic biopsy of ureter (56.33)* |

56.33 **Closed endoscopic biopsy of ureter**
Cystourethroscopy with ureteral biopsy
Transurethral biopsy of ureter
Ureteral endoscopy with biopsy through ureterotomy
Ureteroscopy with biopsy
| **Excludes** | *percutaneous biopsy of ureter (56.32)* |

56.34 **Open biopsy of ureter**

56.35 **Endoscopy (cystoscopy) (looposcopy) of ileal conduit**

56.39 **Other diagnostic procedures on ureter**
| **Excludes** | *microscopic examination of specimen from ureter (91.21–91.29)* |

● 56.4 **Ureterectomy**
Code also anastomosis other than end-to-end (56.51–56.79)
| **Excludes** | *fistulectomy (56.84)* |
| | *nephroureterectomy (55.51–55.54)* |

56.40 **Ureterectomy, not otherwise specified**

56.41 **Partial ureterectomy**
Excision of lesion of ureter
Shortening of ureter with reimplantation
| **Excludes** | *biopsy of ureter (56.32–56.34)* |

56.42 **Total ureterectomy**

● 56.5 **Cutaneous uretero-ileostomy**

56.51 **Formation of cutaneous uretero-ileostomy**
Construction of ileal conduit
External ureteral ileostomy
Formation of open ileal bladder
Ileal loop operation
Ileoureterostomy (Bricker's) (ileal bladder)
Transplantation of ureter into ileum with external diversion
| **Excludes** | *closed ileal bladder (57.87)* |
| | *replacement of ureteral defect by ileal segment (56.89)* |

56.52 **Revision of cutaneous uretero-ileostomy**
Coding Clinic: 1996, Q3, P15; 1988, Q4, P7

● 56.6 **Other external urinary diversion**

56.61 **Formation of other cutaneous ureterostomy**
Anastomosis of ureter to skin
Ureterostomy NOS

56.62 **Revision of other cutaneous ureterostomy**
Revision of ureterostomy stoma
| **Excludes** | *nonoperative removal of ureterostomy tube (97.62)* |

● **56.7 Other anastomosis or bypass of ureter**

> **Excludes** *ureteropyelostomy (55.86)*

56.71 Urinary diversion to intestine
Anastomosis of ureter to intestine
Internal urinary diversion NOS

> **Code also** any synchronous colostomy (46.10–46.13)

> **Excludes** *external ureteral ileostomy (56.51)*

56.72 Revision of ureterointestinal anastomosis

> **Excludes** *revision of external ureteral ileostomy (56.52)*

56.73 Nephrocystanastomosis, not otherwise specified

56.74 Ureteroneocystostomy
Replacement of ureter with bladder flap
Ureterovesical anastomosis

56.75 Transureteroureterostomy

> **Excludes** *ureteroureterostomy associated with partial resection (56.41)*

56.79 Other

● **56.8 Repair of ureter**

56.81 Lysis of intraluminal adhesions of ureter

> **Excludes** *lysis of periureteral adhesions (59.02–59.03)*
> *ureterolysis (59.02–59.03)*

56.82 Suture of laceration of ureter

56.83 Closure of ureterostomy

56.84 Closure of other fistula of ureter

56.85 Ureteropexy

56.86 Removal of ligature from ureter

56.89 Other repair of ureter
Graft of ureter
Replacement of ureter with ileal segment implanted into bladder
Ureteroplication

● **56.9 Other operations on ureter**

56.91 Dilation of ureteral meatus

56.92 Implantation of electronic ureteral stimulator

56.93 Replacement of electronic ureteral stimulator

56.94 Removal of electronic ureteral stimulator

> **Excludes** *that with synchronous replacement (56.93)*

56.95 Ligation of ureter

56.99 Other

> **Excludes** *removal of ureterostomy tube and ureteral catheter (97.62)*
> *ureteral catheterization (59.8)*

● **57 Operations on urinary bladder**

> **Code also** any application or administration of an adhesion barrier substance (99.77)

> **Excludes** *perivesical tissue (59.11–59.29, 59.91–59.92)*
> *ureterovesical orifice (56.0–56.99)*

Coding Clinic: 1986, Sept-Oct, P11-12

57.0 Transurethral clearance of bladder
Drainage of bladder without incision
Removal of:
blood clots from bladder without incision
calculus from bladder without incision
foreign body from bladder without incision

> **Excludes** *that by incision (57.19)*

● **57.1 Cystotomy and cystostomy**

> **Excludes** *cystotomy and cystostomy as operative approach — omit code*

57.11 Percutaneous aspiration of bladder

57.12 Lysis of intraluminal adhesions with incision into bladder

> **Excludes** *transurethral lysis of intraluminal adhesions (57.41)*

57.17 Percutaneous cystostomy
Closed cystostomy
Percutaneous suprapubic cystostomy

> **Excludes** *removal of cystostomy tube (97.63)*
> *replacement of cystostomy tube (59.94)*

57.18 Other suprapubic cystostomy

> **Excludes** *percutaneous cystostomy (57.17)*
> *removal of cystostomy tube (97.63)*
> *replacement of cystostomy tube (59.94)*

57.19 Other cystotomy
Cystolithotomy

> **Excludes** *percutaneous cystostomy (57.17)*
> *suprapubic cystostomy (57.18)*

Coding Clinic: 1986, Sept-Oct, P11-12

● **57.2 Vesicostomy**

> **Excludes** *percutaneous cystostomy (57.17)*
> *suprapubic cystostomy (57.18)*

57.21 Vesicostomy
Creation of permanent opening from bladder to skin using a bladder flap

57.22 Revision or closure of vesicostomy

> **Excludes** *closure of cystostomy (57.82)*

● **57.3 Diagnostic procedures on bladder**

57.31 Cystoscopy through artificial stoma

57.32 Other cystoscopy
Transurethral cystoscopy

> **Excludes** *cystourethroscopy with ureteral biopsy (56.33)*
> *retrograde pyelogram (87.74)*
> *that for control of hemorrhage (postoperative):*
> *bladder (57.93)*
> *prostate (60.94)*

Coding Clinic: 2001, Q1, P14; 1984, May-June, P10

57.33 Closed [transurethral] biopsy of bladder

57.34 Open biopsy of bladder
Coding Clinic: 2005, Q2, P12

57.39 Other diagnostic procedures on bladder

> **Excludes** *cystogram NEC (87.77)*
> *microscopic examination of specimen from bladder (91.31–91.39)*
> *retrograde cystourethrogram (87.76)*
> *therapeutic distention of bladder (96.25)*

● **57.4 Transurethral excision or destruction of bladder tissue**

57.41 Transurethral lysis of intraluminal adhesions

57.49 Other transurethral excision or destruction of lesion or tissue of bladder
Endoscopic resection of bladder lesion

> **Excludes** *transurethral biopsy of bladder (57.33)*
> *transurethral fistulectomy (57.83–57.84)*

Coding Clinic: 1996, Q1, P10-11

OPERATIONS ON THE URINARY SYSTEM (55–59)

● **57.5 Other excision or destruction of bladder tissue**

Excludes | *that with transurethral approach (57.41–57.49)*

57.51 Excision of urachus
Excision of urachal sinus of bladder

Excludes | *excision of urachal cyst of abdominal wall (54.3)*

57.59 Open excision or destruction of other lesion or tissue of bladder
Endometrectomy of bladder
Suprapubic excision of bladder lesion

Excludes | *biopsy of bladder (57.33–57.34)*
fistulectomy of bladder (57.83–57.84)

57.6 Partial cystectomy
Excision of bladder dome
Trigonectomy
Wedge resection of bladder

● **57.7 Total cystectomy**

Includes | total cystectomy with urethrectomy

57.71 Radical cystectomy
Pelvic exenteration in male
Removal of bladder, prostate, seminal vesicles, and fat
Removal of bladder, urethra, and fat in a female

Code also any:
lymph node dissection (40.3, 40.5)
urinary diversion (56.51–56.79)

Excludes | *that as part of pelvic exenteration in female (68.8)*

57.79 Other total cystectomy

● **57.8 Other repair of urinary bladder**

Excludes | *repair of:*
current obstetric laceration (75.61)
cystocele (70.50–70.51)
that for stress incontinence (59.3–59.79)

57.81 Suture of laceration of bladder

57.82 Closure of cystostomy

57.83 Repair of fistula involving bladder and intestine
Rectovesicovaginal fistulectomy
Vesicosigmoidovaginal fistulectomy

57.84 Repair of other fistula of bladder
Cervicovesical fistulectomy
Urethroperineovesical fistulectomy
Uterovesical fistulectomy
Vaginovesical fistulectomy

Excludes | *vesicoureterovaginal fistulectomy (56.84)*

57.85 Cystourethroplasty and plastic repair of bladder neck
Plication of sphincter of urinary bladder
V-Y plasty of bladder neck

57.86 Repair of bladder exstrophy

57.87 Reconstruction of urinary bladder
Anastomosis of bladder with isolated segment of ileum
Augmentation of bladder
Replacement of bladder with ileum or sigmoid [closed ileal bladder]

Code also resection of intestine (45.50–45.52)

Coding Clinic: 2005, Q2, P12-13x2; 2003, Q2, P11-12; 2000, Q3, P7-8

57.88 Other anastomosis of bladder
Anastomosis of bladder to intestine NOS
Cystocolic anastomosis

Excludes | *formation of closed ileal bladder (57.87)*

57.89 Other repair of bladder
Bladder suspension, not elsewhere classified
Cystopexy NOS
Repair of old obstetric laceration of bladder

Excludes | *repair of current obstetric laceration (75.61)*

● **57.9 Other operations on bladder**

57.91 Sphincterotomy of bladder
Division of bladder neck
Coding Clinic: 1994, Q3, P12; 1990, Q2, P23

57.92 Dilation of bladder neck

57.93 Control of (postoperative) hemorrhage of bladder

57.94 Insertion of indwelling urinary catheter

57.95 Replacement of indwelling urinary catheter

57.96 Implantation of electronic bladder stimulator

57.97 Replacement of electronic bladder stimulator

57.98 Removal of electronic bladder stimulator

Excludes | *that with synchronous replacement (57.97)*

57.99 Other

Excludes | *irrigation of:*
cystostomy (96.47)
other indwelling urinary catheter (96.48)
lysis of external adhesions (59.11)
removal of:
cystostomy tube (97.63)
other urinary drainage device (97.64)
therapeutic distention of bladder (96.25)

● **58 Operations on urethra**

Includes | operations on:
bulbourethral gland [Cowper's gland]
periurethral tissue

Code also any application or administration of an adhesion barrier substance (99.77)

58.0 Urethrotomy
Excision of urethral septum
Formation of urethrovaginal fistula
Perineal urethrostomy
Removal of calculus from urethra by incision

Excludes | *drainage of bulbourethral gland or periurethral tissue (58.91)*
internal urethral meatotomy (58.5)
removal of urethral calculus without incision (58.6)

58.1 Urethral meatotomy

Excludes | *internal urethral meatotomy (58.5)*

● **58.2 Diagnostic procedures on urethra**

58.21 Perineal urethroscopy

58.22 Other urethroscopy

58.23 Biopsy of urethra

58.24 Biopsy of periurethral tissue

58.29 Other diagnostic procedures on urethra and periurethral tissue

Excludes | *microscopic examination of specimen from urethra (91.31–91.39)*
retrograde cystourethrogram (87.76)
urethral pressure profile (89.25)
urethral sphincter electromyogram (89.23)

● **58.3 Excision or destruction of lesion or tissue of urethra**

> | Excludes | biopsy of urethra (58.23)
> excision of bulbourethral gland (58.92)
> fistulectomy (58.43)
> urethrectomy as part of:
>   complete cystectomy (57.79)
>   pelvic evisceration (68.8)
>   radical cystectomy (57.71)

58.31 Endoscopic excision or destruction of lesion or tissue of urethra
Fulguration of urethral lesion

58.39 Other local excision or destruction of lesion or tissue of urethra
Excision of:
    congenital valve of urethra
    lesion of urethra
    stricture of urethra
Urethrectomy

> | Excludes | that by endoscopic approach (58.31)

● **58.4 Repair of urethra**

> | Excludes | repair of current obstetric laceration (75.61)

58.41 Suture of laceration of urethra

58.42 Closure of urethrostomy

58.43 Closure of other fistula of urethra

> | Excludes | repair of urethroperineovesical fistula (57.84)

58.44 Reanastomosis of urethra
Anastomosis of urethra

58.45 Repair of hypospadias or epispadias
Coding Clinic: 1997, Q3, P6; 1996, Q4, P34-35

58.46 Other reconstruction of urethra
Urethral construction

58.47 Urethral meatoplasty

58.49 Other repair of urethra
Benenenti rotation of bulbous urethra
Repair of old obstetric laceration of urethra
Urethral plication

> | Excludes | repair of:
>   current obstetric laceration (75.61)
>   urethrocele (70.50–70.51)

Coding Clinic: 2009, Q1, P5

58.5 Release of urethral stricture
Cutting of urethral sphincter
Internal urethral meatotomy
Urethrolysis
Coding Clinic: 1997, Q1, P13-14

58.6 Dilation of urethra
Dilation of urethrovesical junction
Passage of sounds through urethra
Removal of calculus from urethra without incision

> | Excludes | urethral calibration (89.29)

Coding Clinic: 2001, Q1, P14; 1997, Q1, P13-14

● **58.9 Other operations on urethra and periurethral tissue**

58.91 Incision of periurethral tissue
Drainage of bulbourethral gland

58.92 Excision of periurethral tissue

> | Excludes | biopsy of periurethral tissue (58.24)
> lysis of periurethral adhesions
>   laparoscopic (59.12)
>   other (59.11)

58.93 Implantation of artificial urinary sphincter [AUS]
Placement of inflatable:
    bladder sphincter
    urethral sphincter
Removal with replacement of sphincter device [AUS]
With pump and/or reservoir

58.99 Other
Removal of inflatable urinary sphincter without replacement
Repair of inflatable sphincter pump and/or reservoir
Surgical correction of hydraulic pressure of inflatable sphincter device

> | Excludes | removal of:
>   intraluminal foreign body from urethra without incision (98.19)
>   urethral stent (97.65)

Coding Clinic: 2009, Q1, P5; 1995, Q4, P72-73

● **59 Other operations on urinary tract**

Code also any application or administration of an adhesion barrier substance (99.77)

● **59.0 Dissection of retroperitoneal tissue**

59.00 Retroperitoneal dissection, not otherwise specified

59.02 Other lysis of perirenal or periureteral adhesions

> | Excludes | that by laparoscope (59.03)

59.03 Laparoscopic lysis of perirenal or periureteral adhesions
Coding Clinic: 2006, Q4, P130-134

59.09 Other incision of perirenal or periureteral tissue
Exploration of perinephric area
Incision of perirenal abscess

● **59.1 Incision of perivesical tissue**

59.11 Other lysis of perivesical adhesions

59.12 Laparoscopic lysis of perivesical adhesions

59.19 Other incision of perivesical tissue
Exploration of perivesical tissue
Incision of hematoma of space of Retzius
Retropubic exploration

● **59.2 Diagnostic procedures on perirenal and perivesical tissue**

59.21 Biopsy of perirenal or perivesical tissue

59.29 Other diagnostic procedures on perirenal tissue, perivesical tissue, and retroperitoneum

> | Excludes | microscopic examination of specimen from:
>   perirenal tissue (91.21–91.29)
>   perivesical tissue (91.31–91.39)
>   retroperitoneum NEC (91.11–91.19)
>   retroperitoneal x-ray (88.14–88.16)

59.3 Plication of urethrovesical junction
Kelly-Kennedy operation on urethra
Kelly-Stoeckel urethral plication

59.4 Suprapubic sling operation
Goebel-Frangenheim-Stoeckel urethrovesical suspension
Millin-Read urethrovesical suspension
Oxford operation for urinary incontinence
Urethrocystopexy by suprapubic suspension

59.5 Retropubic urethral suspension
Burch procedure
Marshall-Marchetti-Krantz operation
Suture of periurethral tissue to symphysis pubis
Urethral suspension NOS
Coding Clinic: 1997, Q1, P11-12

59.6 Paraurethral suspension
Pereyra paraurethral suspension
Periurethral suspension

Excludes   Includes   Use additional   Code also   Omit code

● **59.7　Other repair of urinary stress incontinence**

59.71　Levator muscle operation for urethrovesical suspension
Cystourethropexy with levator muscle sling
Gracilis muscle transplant for urethrovesical suspension
Pubococcygeal sling

59.72　Injection of implant into urethra and/or bladder neck
Collagen implant
Endoscopic injection of implant
Fat implant
Polytef implant
Coding Clinic: 1995, Q4, P72-73

59.79　Other
Anterior urethropexy
Repair of stress incontinence NOS
Tudor "rabbit ear" urethropexy
Coding Clinic: 2001, Q2, P20; 2000, Q1, P14-15, 19-20; 1995, Q4, P72-73

59.8　Ureteral catheterization
Drainage of kidney by catheter
Insertion of ureteral stent
Ureterovesical orifice dilation

Code also any ureterotomy (56.2)

Excludes　that for:
retrograde pyelogram (87.74)
transurethral removal of calculus or clot from ureter and renal pelvis (56.0)
Coding Clinic: 2005, Q2, P12-13; 2003, Q2, P11-12; 2000, Q3, P7-8; 1994, Q3, P8

● **59.9　Other operations on urinary system**
Excludes　nonoperative removal of therapeutic device (97.61–97.69)

59.91　Excision of perirenal or perivesical tissue
Excludes　biopsy of perirenal or perivesical tissue (59.21)

59.92　Other operations on perirenal or perivesical tissue

59.93　Replacement of ureterostomy tube
Change of ureterostomy tube
Reinsertion of ureterostomy tube
Excludes　nonoperative removal of ureterostomy tube (97.62)

59.94　Replacement of cystostomy tube
Excludes　nonoperative removal of cystostomy tube (97.63)

59.95　Ultrasonic fragmentation of urinary stones
Shattered urinary stones
Excludes　percutaneous nephrostomy with fragmentation (55.04)
shock-wave disintegration (98.51)
Coding Clinic: 1986, Sept-Oct, P11-12; 1984, Nov-Dec, P20

59.99　Other
Excludes　instillation of medication into urinary tract (96.49)
irrigation of urinary tract (96.45–96.48)
Coding Clinic: 2008, Q2, P14

11.　OPERATIONS ON THE MALE GENITAL ORGANS (60–64)

● **60　Operations on prostate and seminal vesicles**
Includes　operations on periprostatic tissue
Code also any application or administration of an adhesion barrier substance (99.77)
Excludes　that associated with radical cystectomy (57.71)

60.0　Incision of prostate
Drainage of prostatic abscess
Prostatolithotomy
Excludes　drainage of periprostatic tissue only (60.81)

● **60.1　Diagnostic procedures on prostate and seminal vesicles**

60.11　Closed [percutaneous] [needle] biopsy of prostate
Approach:
transrectal
transurethral
Punch biopsy

60.12　Open biopsy of prostate

60.13　Closed [percutaneous] biopsy of seminal vesicles
Needle biopsy of seminal vesicles

60.14　Open biopsy of seminal vesicles

60.15　Biopsy of periprostatic tissue

60.18　Other diagnostic procedures on prostate and periprostatic tissue
Excludes　microscopic examination of specimen from prostate (91.31–91.39)
x-ray of prostate (87.92)

60.19　Other diagnostic procedures on seminal vesicles
Excludes　microscopic examination of specimen from seminal vesicles (91.31–91.39)
x-ray:
contrast seminal vesiculogram (87.91)
other (87.92)

- **60.2   Transurethral prostatectomy**

  Excludes *local excision of lesion of prostate (60.61)*

  Coding Clinic: 1993, 5th Issue, P9; 1985, Sept-Oct, P10

  - **60.21   Transurethral (ultrasound) guided laser induced prostatectomy (TULIP)**

    Ablation (contact) (noncontact) by laser
    Coding Clinic: 1995, Q4, P71; 1994, Q2, P9; 1992, Q3, P13

  - **60.29   Other transurethral prostatectomy**

    Excision of median bar by transurethral approach
    Transurethral electrovaporization of prostrate (TEVAP)
    Transurethral enucleative procedure
    Transurethral prostatectomy NOS
    Transurethral resection of prostate (TURP)
    Coding Clinic: 1997, Q3, P3; 1994, Q3, P12

- **60.3   Suprapubic prostatectomy**

  Transvesical prostatectomy

  Excludes *local excision of lesion of prostate (60.61)*
  radical prostatectomy (60.5)

- **60.4   Retropubic prostatectomy**

  Excludes *local excision of lesion of prostate (60.61)*
  radical prostatectomy (60.5)

- **60.5   Radical prostatectomy**

  Prostatovesiculectomy
  Radical prostatectomy by any approach

  Excludes *cystoprostatectomy (57.71)*

  Coding Clinic: 1993, Q3, P12

- **60.6   Other prostatectomy**

  - **60.61   Local excision of lesion of prostate**

    Excludes *biopsy of prostate (60.11–60.12)*
    laser interstitial thermal therapy [LITT] of lesion or tissue of prostate under guidance (17.69)

  - **60.62   Perineal prostatectomy**

    Cryoablation of prostate
    Cryoprostatectomy
    Cryosurgery of prostate
    Radical cryosurgical ablation of prostate (RCSA)

    Excludes *local excision of lesion of prostate (60.61)*

  - **60.69   Other**

- **60.7   Operations on seminal vesicles**

  - **60.71   Percutaneous aspiration of seminal vesicle**

    Excludes *needle biopsy of seminal vesicle (60.13)*

  - **60.72   Incision of seminal vesicle**

  - **60.73   Excision of seminal vesicle**

    Excision of Müllerian duct cyst
    Spermatocystectomy

    Excludes *biopsy of seminal vesicle (60.13–60.14)*
    prostatovesiculectomy (60.5)

  - **60.79   Other operations on seminal vesicles**

- **60.8   Incision or excision of periprostatic tissue**

  - **60.81   Incision of periprostatic tissue**

    Drainage of periprostatic abscess

  - **60.82   Excision of periprostatic tissue**

    Excision of lesion of periprostatic tissue

    Excludes *biopsy of periprostatic tissue (60.15)*

- **60.9   Other operations on prostate**

  - **60.91   Percutaneous aspiration of prostate**

    Excludes *needle biopsy of prostate (60.11)*

  - **60.92   Injection into prostate test link**

- **60.93   Repair of prostate**

- **60.94   Control of (postoperative) hemorrhage of prostate**

  Coagulation of prostatic bed
  Cystoscopy for control of prostatic hemorrhage

- **60.95   Transurethral balloon dilation of the prostatic urethra**

- **60.96   Transurethral destruction of prostate tissue by microwave thermotherapy**

  Transurethral microwave thermotherapy (TUMT) of prostate

  Excludes *prostatectomy:*
  other (60.61–60.69)
  radical (60.5)
  retropubic (60.4)
  suprapubic (60.3)
  transurethral (60.21–60.29)

- **60.97   Other transurethral destruction of prostate tissue by other thermotherapy**

  Radiofrequency thermotherapy
  Transurethral needle ablation (TUNA) of prostate

  Excludes *prostatectomy:*
  other (60.61–60.69)
  radical (60.5)
  retropubic (60.4)
  suprapubic (60.3)
  transurethral (60.21–60.29)

- **60.99   Other**

  Excludes *prostatic massage (99.94)*

  Coding Clinic: 1990, Q3, P13

- **61   Operations on scrotum and tunica vaginalis**

  - **61.0   Incision and drainage of scrotum and tunica vaginalis**

    Excludes *percutaneous aspiration of hydrocele (61.91)*

  - **61.1   Diagnostic procedures on scrotum and tunica vaginalis**

    - **61.11   Biopsy of scrotum or tunica vaginalis**

    - **61.19   Other diagnostic procedures on scrotum and tunica vaginalis**

  - **61.2   Excision of hydrocele (of tunica vaginalis)**

    Bottle repair of hydrocele of tunica vaginalis

    Excludes *percutaneous aspiration of hydrocele (61.91)*

  - **61.3   Excision or destruction of lesion or tissue of scrotum**

    Fulguration of lesion of scrotum
    Reduction of elephantiasis of scrotum
    Partial scrotectomy of scrotum

    Excludes *biopsy of scrotum (61.11)*
    scrotal fistulectomy (61.42)

  - **61.4   Repair of scrotum and tunica vaginalis**

    - **61.41   Suture of laceration of scrotum and tunica vaginalis**

    - **61.42   Repair of scrotal fistula**

    - **61.49   Other repair of scrotum and tunica vaginalis**

      Reconstruction with rotational or pedicle flaps

  - **61.9   Other operations on scrotum and tunica vaginalis**

    - **61.91   Percutaneous aspiration of tunica vaginalis**

      Aspiration of hydrocele of tunica vaginalis

    - **61.92   Excision of lesion of tunica vaginalis other than hydrocele**

      Excision of hematocele of tunica vaginalis

    - **61.99   Other**

      Excludes *removal of foreign body from scrotum without incision (98.24)*

OPERATIONS ON THE MALE GENITAL ORGANS (60–64)

Excludes   Includes   Use additional   Code also   Omit code

● **62 Operations on testes**

62.0 Incision of testis

● **62.1 Diagnostic procedures on testes**

62.11 Closed [percutaneous] [needle] biopsy of testis

62.12 Open biopsy of testis

62.19 Other diagnostic procedures on testes

62.2 Excision or destruction of testicular lesion
Excision of appendix testis
Excision of cyst of Morgagni in the male
Excludes *biopsy of testis (62.11–62.12)*

62.3 Unilateral orchiectomy
Orchidectomy (with epididymectomy) NOS

● **62.4 Bilateral orchiectomy**
Male castration
Radical bilateral orchiectomy (with epididymectomy)
Code also any synchronous lymph node dissection (40.3, 40.5)

62.41 Removal of both testes at same operative episode
Bilateral orchidectomy NOS

62.42 Removal of remaining testis
Removal of solitary testis

62.5 Orchiopexy
Mobilization and replacement of testis in scrotum
Orchiopexy with detorsion of testis
Torek (-Bevan) operation (orchidopexy) (first stage) (second stage)
Transplantation to and fixation of testis in scrotum

● **62.6 Repair of testes**
Excludes *reduction of torsion (63.52)*

62.61 Suture of laceration of testis

62.69 Other repair of testis
Testicular graft

62.7 Insertion of testicular prosthesis

● **62.9 Other operations on testes**

62.91 Aspiration of testis
Excludes *percutaneous biopsy of testis (62.11)*

62.92 Injection of therapeutic substance into testis

62.99 Other

● **63 Operations on spermatic cord, epididymis, and vas deferens**

● **63.0 Diagnostic procedures on spermatic cord, epididymis, and vas deferens**

63.01 Biopsy of spermatic cord, epididymis, or vas deferens

63.09 Other diagnostic procedures on spermatic cord, epididymis, and vas deferens
Excludes *contrast epididymogram (87.93)*
contrast vasogram (87.94)
other x-ray of epididymis and vas deferens (87.95)

63.1 Excision of varicocele and hydrocele of spermatic cord
High ligation of spermatic vein
Hydrocelectomy of canal of Nuck

63.2 Excision of cyst of epididymis
Spermatocelectomy

63.3 Excision of other lesion or tissue of spermatic cord and epididymis
Excision of appendix epididymis
Excludes *biopsy of spermatic cord or epididymis (63.01)*

63.4 Epididymectomy
Excludes *that synchronous with orchiectomy (62.3–62.42)*

● **63.5 Repair of spermatic cord and epididymis**

63.51 Suture of laceration of spermatic cord and epididymis

63.52 Reduction of torsion of testis or spermatic cord
Excludes *that associated with orchiopexy (62.5)*

63.53 Transplantation of spermatic cord

63.59 Other repair of spermatic cord and epididymis

63.6 Vasotomy
Vasostomy

● **63.7 Vasectomy and ligation of vas deferens**

63.70 Male sterilization procedure, not otherwise specified

63.71 Ligation of vas deferens
Crushing of vas deferens
Division of vas deferens

63.72 Ligation of spermatic cord

63.73 Vasectomy
Coding Clinic: 1998, Q2, P13

● **63.8 Repair of vas deferens and epididymis**

63.81 Suture of laceration of vas deferens and epididymis

63.82 Reconstruction of surgically divided vas deferens

63.83 Epididymovasostomy

63.84 Removal of ligature from vas deferens

63.85 Removal of valve from vas deferens

63.89 Other repair of vas deferens and epididymis

● **63.9 Other operations on spermatic cord, epididymis, and vas deferens**

63.91 Aspiration of spermatocele

63.92 Epididymotomy

63.93 Incision of spermatic cord

63.94 Lysis of adhesions of spermatic cord

63.95 Insertion of valve in vas deferens

63.99 Other

● **64 Operations on penis**
Includes operations on:
corpora cavernosa
glans penis
prepuce

64.0 Circumcision

● **64.1 Diagnostic procedures on the penis**

64.11 Biopsy of penis

64.19 Other diagnostic procedures on penis

64.2 Local excision or destruction of lesion of penis
Excludes *biopsy of penis (64.11)*

64.3 Amputation of penis

● **64.4 Repair and plastic operation on penis**

64.41 Suture of laceration of penis

64.42 Release of chordee
Coding Clinic: 1996, Q4, P34-35

64.43 Construction of penis

64.44 Reconstruction of penis

64.45 Replantation of penis
Reattachment of amputated penis

64.49 Other repair of penis

Excludes | repair of epispadias and hypospadias (58.45)

64.5 Operations for sex transformation, not elsewhere classified

● **64.9 Other operations on male genital organs**

64.91 Dorsal or lateral slit of prepuce

64.92 Incision of penis

64.93 Division of penile adhesions

64.94 Fitting of external prosthesis of penis
Penile prosthesis NOS

64.95 Insertion or replacement of non-inflatable penile prosthesis
Insertion of semi-rigid rod prosthesis into shaft of penis

Excludes | external penile prosthesis (64.94)
inflatable penile prosthesis (64.97)
plastic repair, penis (64.43–64.49)
that associated with:
construction (64.43)
reconstruction (64.44)

64.96 Removal of internal prosthesis of penis
Removal without replacement of non-inflatable or inflatable penile prosthesis

64.97 Insertion or replacement of inflatable penile prosthesis
Insertion of cylinders into shaft of penis and placement of pump and reservoir

Excludes | external penile prosthesis (64.94)
non-inflatable penile prosthesis (64.95)
plastic repair, penis (64.43–64.49)
Coding Clinic: 1990, Q2, P26

64.98 Other operations on penis
Corpora cavernosa-corpus spongiosum shunt
Corpora-saphenous shunt
Irrigation of corpus cavernosum

Excludes | removal of foreign body:
intraluminal (98.19)
without incision (98.24)
stretching of foreskin (99.95)
Coding Clinic: 1992, Q3, P9-10

64.99 Other

Excludes | collection of sperm for artificial insemination (99.96)

---

12. OPERATIONS ON THE FEMALE GENITAL ORGANS (65–71)

● **65 Operations on ovary**

Code also any application or administration of an adhesion barrier substance (99.77)

● **65.0 Oophorotomy**
Salpingo-oophorotomy

65.01 Laparoscopic oophorotomy

65.09 Other oophorotomy

● **65.1 Diagnostic procedures on ovaries**

65.11 Aspiration biopsy of ovary

65.12 Other biopsy of ovary

65.13 Laparoscopic biopsy of ovary
Coding Clinic: 1996, Q4, P66-67

65.14 Other laparoscopic diagnostic procedures on ovaries

65.19 Other diagnostic procedures on ovaries

Excludes | microscopic examination of specimen from ovary (91.41–91.49)

● **65.2 Local excision or destruction of ovarian lesion or tissue**

65.21 Marsupialization of ovarian cyst

Excludes | that by laparoscope (65.23)

65.22 Wedge resection of ovary

Excludes | that by laparoscope (65.24)

65.23 Laparoscopic marsupialization of ovarian cyst

65.24 Laparoscopic wedge resection of ovary

65.25 Other laparoscopic local excision or destruction of ovary

65.29 Other local excision or destruction of ovary
Bisection of ovary
Cauterization of ovary
Partial excision of ovary

Excludes | biopsy of ovary (65.11–65.13)
that by laparoscope (65.25)

● **65.3 Unilateral oophorectomy**
Coding Clinic: 1995, Q3, P15

65.31 Laparoscopic unilateral oophorectomy

65.39 Other unilateral oophorectomy

Excludes | that by laparoscope (65.31)

● **65.4 Unilateral salpingo-oophorectomy**

65.41 Laparoscopic unilateral salpingo-oophorectomy
Coding Clinic: 1996, Q4, P66-67

65.49 Other unilateral salpingo-oophorectomy

● **65.5 Bilateral oophorectomy**

65.51 Other removal of both ovaries at same operative episode
Female castration

Excludes | that by laparoscope (65.53)

65.52 Other removal of remaining ovary
Removal of solitary ovary

Excludes | that by laparoscope (65.54)

65.53 Laparoscopic removal of both ovaries at same operative episode

65.54 Laparoscopic removal of remaining ovary

● **65.6 Bilateral salpingo-oophorectomy**

65.61 Other removal of both ovaries and tubes at same operative episode

> **Excludes** *that by laparoscope (65.63)*
> Coding Clinic: 1996, Q4, P64-65

65.62 Other removal of remaining ovary and tube
Removal of solitary ovary and tube

> **Excludes** *that by laparoscope (65.64)*

65.63 Laparoscopic removal of both ovaries and tubes at same operative episode
> Coding Clinic: 2009, Q3, P6; 2006, Q4, P130-134; 1996, Q4, P68

65.64 Laparoscopic removal of remaining ovary and tube

● **65.7 Repair of ovary**

> **Excludes** *salpingo-oophorostomy (66.72)*

65.71 Other simple suture of ovary

> **Excludes** *that by laparoscope (65.74)*

65.72 Other reimplantation of ovary

> **Excludes** *that by laparoscope (65.75)*

65.73 Other salpingo-oophoroplasty

> **Excludes** *that by laparoscope (65.76)*

65.74 Laparoscopic simple suture of ovary

65.75 Laparoscopic reimplantation of ovary

65.76 Laparoscopic salpingo-oophoroplasty

65.79 Other repair of ovary
Oophoropexy

● **65.8 Lysis of adhesions of ovary and fallopian tube**

65.81 Laparoscopic lysis of adhesions of ovary and fallopian tube
> Coding Clinic: 1996, Q4, P66-67

65.89 Other lysis of adhesions of ovary and fallopian tube

> **Excludes** *that by laparoscope (65.81)*

● **65.9 Other operations on ovary**

65.91 Aspiration of ovary

> **Excludes** *aspiration biopsy of ovary (65.11)*

65.92 Transplantation of ovary

> **Excludes** *reimplantation of ovary*
> *laparoscopic (65.75)*
> *other (65.72)*

65.93 Manual rupture of ovarian cyst

65.94 Ovarian denervation

65.95 Release of torsion of ovary

65.99 Other
Ovarian drilling
> Coding Clinic: 1986, Nov-Dec, P9

● **66 Operations on fallopian tubes**

> Code also any application or administration of an adhesion barrier substance (99.77)

● **66.0 Salpingotomy and salpingostomy**

66.01 Salpingotomy

66.02 Salpingostomy

● **66.1 Diagnostic procedures on fallopian tubes**

66.11 Biopsy of fallopian tube

66.19 Other diagnostic procedures on fallopian tubes

> **Excludes** *microscopic examination of*
> *specimen from fallopian tubes*
> *(91.41–91.49)*
> *radiography of fallopian tubes*
> *(87.82–87.83, 87.85)*
> *Rubin's test (66.8)*

● **66.2 Bilateral endoscopic destruction or occlusion of fallopian tubes**

> **Includes** bilateral endoscopic destruction or
> occlusion of fallopian tubes by:
> culdoscopy
> endoscopy
> hysteroscopy
> laparoscopy
> peritoneoscopy
> endoscopic destruction of solitary
> fallopian tube

66.21 Bilateral endoscopic ligation and crushing of fallopian tubes

66.22 Bilateral endoscopic ligation and division of fallopian tubes

66.29 Other bilateral endoscopic destruction or occlusion of fallopian tubes

● **66.3 Other bilateral destruction or occlusion of fallopian tubes**

> **Includes** destruction of solitary fallopian tube

> **Excludes** *endoscopic destruction or occlusion of*
> *fallopian tubes (66.21–66.29)*

66.31 Other bilateral ligation and crushing of fallopian tubes

66.32 Other bilateral ligation and division of fallopian tubes
Pomeroy operation

66.39 Other bilateral destruction or occlusion of fallopian tubes
Female sterilization operation NOS

66.4 Total unilateral salpingectomy

● **66.5 Total bilateral salpingectomy**

> **Excludes** *bilateral partial salpingectomy for sterilization*
> *(66.39)*
> *that with oophorectomy (65.61–65.64)*

66.51 Removal of both fallopian tubes at same operative episode

66.52 Removal of remaining fallopian tube
Removal of solitary fallopian tube

● **66.6 Other salpingectomy**

> **Includes** salpingectomy by:
> cauterization
> coagulation
> electrocoagulation
> excision

> **Excludes** *fistulectomy (66.73)*

66.61 Excision or destruction of lesion of fallopian tube

> **Excludes** *biopsy of fallopian tube (66.11)*

66.62 Salpingectomy with removal of tubal pregnancy

> Code also any synchronous oophorectomy
> (65.31, 65.39)
> Coding Clinic: 1995, Q3, P15; 1985, Sept-Oct, P14

66.63 Bilateral partial salpingectomy, not otherwise specified

66.69 Other partial salpingectomy

● **66.7 Repair of fallopian tube**

66.71 Simple suture of fallopian tube

66.72 Salpingo-oophorostomy

66.73 Salpingo-salpingostomy

66.74 Salpingo-uterostomy

66.79 Other repair of fallopian tube
Graft of fallopian tube
Reopening of divided fallopian tube
Salpingoplasty
Coding Clinic: 1995, Q2, P10

66.8 Insufflation of fallopian tube
Insufflation of fallopian tube with:
air
dye
gas
saline
Rubin's test
| Excludes | *insufflation of therapeutic agent (66.95)*
that for hysterosalpingography (87.82–87.83)
Coding Clinic: 1990, Q2, P26

● **66.9 Other operations on fallopian tubes**

66.91 Aspiration of fallopian tube

66.92 Unilateral destruction or occlusion of fallopian tube
| Excludes | *that of solitary tube (66.21–66.39)*

66.93 Implantation or replacement of prosthesis of fallopian tube

66.94 Removal of prosthesis of fallopian tube

66.95 Insufflation of therapeutic agent into fallopian tubes

66.96 Dilation of fallopian tube

66.97 Burying of fimbriae in uterine wall

66.99 Other
| Excludes | *lysis of adhesions of ovary and tube*
laparoscopic (65.81)
other (65.89)
Coding Clinic: 1994, Q2, P11

● **67 Operations on cervix**
Code also any application or administration of an adhesion barrier substance (99.77)

67.0 Dilation of cervical canal
| Excludes | *dilation and curettage (69.01–69.09)*
that for induction of labor (73.1)

● **67.1 Diagnostic procedures on cervix**

67.11 Endocervical biopsy
| Excludes | *conization of cervix (67.2)*

67.12 Other cervical biopsy
Punch biopsy of cervix NOS
| Excludes | *conization of cervix (67.2)*

67.19 Other diagnostic procedures on cervix
| Excludes | *microscopic examination of specimen from cervix (91.41–91.49)*

67.2 Conization of cervix
| Excludes | *that by:*
cryosurgery (67.33)
electrosurgery (67.32)

● **67.3 Other excision or destruction of lesion or tissue of cervix**

67.31 Marsupialization of cervical cyst

67.32 Destruction of lesion of cervix by cauterization
Electroconization of cervix
LEEP (loop electrosurgical excision procedure)
LLETZ (large loop excision of the transformation zone)
Coding Clinic: 1998, Q1, P3

67.33 Destruction of lesion of cervix by cryosurgery
Cryoconization of cervix

67.39 Other excision or destruction of lesion or tissue of cervix
| Excludes | *biopsy of cervix (67.11–67.12)*
cervical fistulectomy (67.62)
conization of cervix (67.2)

67.4 Amputation of cervix
Cervicectomy with synchronous colporrhaphy

● **67.5 Repair of internal cervical os**
Coding Clinic: 2000, Q3, P11-12

67.51 Transabdominal cerclage of cervix

67.59 Other repair of internal cervical os
Cerclage of isthmus uteri
McDonald operation
Shirodkar operation
Transvaginal cerclage
| Excludes | *laparoscopically assisted supracervical hysterectomy [LASH] (68.31)*
transabdominal cerclage of cervix (67.51)
Coding Clinic: 2008, Q4, P124-125

● **67.6 Other repair of cervix**
| Excludes | *repair of current obstetric laceration (75.51)*

67.61 Suture of laceration of cervix

67.62 Repair of fistula of cervix
Cervicosigmoidal fistulectomy
| Excludes | *fistulectomy:*
cervicovesical (57.84)
ureterocervical (56.84)
vesicocervicovaginal (57.84)

67.69 Other repair of cervix
Repair of old obstetric laceration of cervix

● **68 Other incision and excision of uterus**
Code also any application or administration of an adhesion barrier substance (99.77)

68.0 Hysterotomy
Hysterotomy with removal of hydatidiform mole
| Excludes | *hysterotomy for termination of pregnancy (74.91)*

● **68.1 Diagnostic procedures on uterus and supporting structures**

68.11 Digital examination of uterus
| Excludes | *pelvic examination, so described (89.26)*
postpartal manual exploration of uterine cavity (75.7)

68.12 Hysteroscopy
| Excludes | *that with biopsy (68.16)*
Coding Clinic: 1990, Q2, P26

| Excludes | | Includes | | Use additional | | Code also | | Omit code |

68.13 Open biopsy of uterus

Excludes *closed biopsy of uterus (68.16)*

68.14 Open biopsy of uterine ligaments

Excludes *closed biopsy of uterine ligaments (68.15)*

68.15 Closed biopsy of uterine ligaments

Endoscopic (laparoscopy) biopsy of uterine adnexa, except ovary and fallopian tube

68.16 Closed biopsy of uterus

Endoscopic (laparoscopy) (hysteroscopy) biopsy of uterus

Excludes *open biopsy of uterus (68.13)*

68.19 Other diagnostic procedures on uterus and supporting structures

Excludes *diagnostic:*
aspiration curettage (69.59)
dilation and curettage (69.09)
microscopic examination of specimen from uterus (91.41–91.49)
pelvic examination (89.26)
radioisotope scan of:
placenta (92.17)
uterus (92.19)
ultrasonography of uterus (88.78–88.79)
x-ray of uterus (87.81–87.89)

● **68.2 Excision or destruction of lesion or tissue of uterus**

68.21 Division of endometrial synechiae

Lysis of intraluminal uterine adhesions

68.22 Incision or excision of congenital septum of uterus

68.23 Endometrial ablation

Dilation and curettage
Hysteroscopic endometrial ablation

68.29 Other excision or destruction of lesion of uterus

Uterine myomectomy

Excludes *biopsy of uterus (68.13, 68.16)*
uterine fistulectomy (69.42)

Coding Clinic: 2006, Q3, P18-19; 1996, Q1, P15

● **68.3 Subtotal abdominal hysterectomy**

68.31 Laparoscopic supracervical hysterectomy [LSH]

Classic infrafascial SEMM hysterectomy [CISH]
Laparoscopically assisted supracervical hysterectomy [LASH]

Coding Clinic: 2003, Q4, P98-99

68.39 Other and unspecified subtotal abdominal hysterectomy

Supracervical hysterectomy

Excludes *classic infrafascial SEMM hysterectomy [CISH] (68.31)*
laparoscopic supracervical hysterectomy [LSH] (68.31)

● **68.4 Total abdominal hysterectomy**

Code also any synchronous removal of tubes and ovaries (65.31–65.64)

Excludes *laparoscopic total abdominal hysterectomy (68.41)*
radical abdominal hysterectomy, any approach (68.61–68.69)

Coding Clinic: 1996, Q4, P64-65

68.41 Laparoscopic total abdominal hysterectomy

Total laparoscopic hysterectomy [TLH]

Coding Clinic: 2009, Q3, P6; 2006, Q4, P130-134

68.49 Other and unspecified total abdominal hysterectomy

Hysterectomy:
extended

● **68.5 Vaginal hysterectomy**

Code also any synchronous:
removal of tubes and ovaries (65.31–65.64)
repair of cystocele or rectocele (70.50–70.52)
repair of pelvic floor (70.79)

68.51 Laparoscopically assisted vaginal hysterectomy (LAVH)

Coding Clinic: 1996, Q4, P68

68.59 Other and unspecified vaginal hysterectomy

Excludes *laparoscopically assisted vaginal hysterectomy (LAVH) (68.51)*
radical vaginal hysterectomy (68.7)

● **68.6 Radical abdominal hysterectomy**

Code also any synchronous:
lymph gland dissection (40.3, 40.5)
removal of tubes and ovaries (65.31–65.64)

Excludes *pelvic evisceration (68.8)*

68.61 Laparoscopic radical abdominal hysterectomy

Laparoscopic modified radical hysterectomy
Total laparoscopic radical hysterectomy [TLRH]

Coding Clinic: 2006, Q4, P130-134

68.69 Other and unspecified radical abdominal hysterectomy

Modified radical hysterectomy
Wertheim's operation

Excludes *laparoscopic total abdominal hysterectomy (68.41)*
laparoscopic radical abdominal hysterectomy (68.61)

● **68.7 Radical vaginal hysterectomy**

Code also any synchronous:
lymph gland dissection (40.3, 40.5)
removal of tubes and ovaries (65.31–65.64)

Excludes *abdominal hysterectomy, any approach (68.31–68.39, 68.41–68.49, 68.61–68.69, 68.9)*

68.71 Laparoscopic radical vaginal hysterectomy [LRVH]

Coding Clinic: 2006, Q4, P130-134

68.79 Other and unspecified radical vaginal hysterectomy

Hysterocolpectomy
Schauta operation

68.8 Pelvic evisceration

Removal of ovaries, tubes, uterus, vagina, bladder, and urethra (with removal of sigmoid colon and rectum)

Code also any synchronous:
colostomy (46.12–46.13)
lymph gland dissection (40.3, 40.5)
urinary diversion (56.51–56.79)

68.9 Other and unspecified hysterectomy
Hysterectomy, NOS

> **Excludes** *abdominal hysterectomy, any approach (68.31–68.39, 68.41–68.49, 68.61–68.69)*
> *vaginal hysterectomy, any approach (68.51–68.59, 68.71–68.79)*

● **69 Other operations on uterus and supporting structures**
Code also any application or administration of an adhesion barrier substance (99.77)

● **69.0 Dilation and curettage of uterus**

> **Excludes** *aspiration curettage of uterus (69.51–69.59)*

69.01 Dilation and curettage for termination of pregnancy
Coding Clinic: 1993, Q3, P6

69.02 Dilation and curettage following delivery or abortion
Coding Clinic: 1993, Q3, P6

69.09 Other dilation and curettage
Diagnostic D and C
Coding Clinic: 1998, Q1, P4

● **69.1 Excision or destruction of lesion or tissue of uterus and supporting structures**

69.19 Other excision or destruction of uterus and supporting structures

> **Excludes** *biopsy of uterine ligament (68.14)*

● **69.2 Repair of uterine supporting structures**

69.21 Interposition operation
Watkins procedure

69.22 Other uterine suspension
Hysteropexy
Manchester operation
Plication of uterine ligament

69.23 Vaginal repair of chronic inversion of uterus

69.29 Other repair of uterus and supporting structures

69.3 Paracervical uterine denervation

● **69.4 Uterine repair**

> **Excludes** *repair of current obstetric laceration (75.50–75.52)*

69.41 Suture of laceration of uterus

69.42 Closure of fistula of uterus

> **Excludes** *uterovesical fistulectomy (57.84)*

69.49 Other repair of uterus
Repair of old obstetric laceration of uterus

● **69.5 Aspiration curettage of uterus**

> **Excludes** *menstrual extraction (69.6)*

69.51 Aspiration curettage of uterus for termination of pregnancy
Therapeutic abortion NOS

69.52 Aspiration curettage following delivery or abortion

69.59 Other aspiration curettage of uterus
Coding Clinic: 1998, Q1, P7

69.6 Menstrual extraction or regulation

69.7 Insertion of intrauterine contraceptive device

● **69.9 Other operations on uterus, cervix, and supporting structures**

> **Excludes** *obstetric dilation or incision of cervix (73.1, 73.93)*

69.91 Insertion of therapeutic device into uterus

> **Excludes** *insertion of:*
> *intrauterine contraceptive device (69.7)*
> *laminaria (69.93)*
> *obstetric insertion of bag, bougie, or pack (73.1)*

69.92 Artificial insemination

69.93 Insertion of laminaria

69.94 Manual replacement of inverted uterus

> **Excludes** *that in immediate postpartal period (75.94)*

69.95 Incision of cervix

> **Excludes** *that to assist delivery (73.93)*

69.96 Removal of cerclage material from cervix

69.97 Removal of other penetrating foreign body from cervix

> **Excludes** *removal of intraluminal foreign body from cervix (98.16)*

69.98 Other operations on supporting structures of uterus

> **Excludes** *biopsy of uterine ligament (68.14)*

69.99 Other operations on cervix and uterus

> **Excludes** *removal of:*
> *foreign body (98.16)*
> *intrauterine contraceptive device (97.71)*
> *obstetric bag, bougie, or pack (97.72)*
> *packing (97.72)*

● **70 Operations on vagina and cul-de-sac**
Code also any application or administration of an adhesion barrier substance (99.77)
Coding Clinic: 1990, Q2, P26

70.0 Culdocentesis

● **70.1 Incision of vagina and cul-de-sac**

70.11 Hymenotomy

70.12 Culdotomy

70.13 Lysis of intraluminal adhesions of vagina

70.14 Other vaginotomy
Division of vaginal septum
Drainage of hematoma of vaginal cuff

● **70.2 Diagnostic procedures on vagina and cul-de-sac**

70.21 Vaginoscopy

70.22 Culdoscopy

70.23 Biopsy of cul-de-sac

70.24 Vaginal biopsy

70.29 Other diagnostic procedures on vagina and cul-de-sac

● **70.3 Local excision or destruction of vagina and cul-de-sac**

70.31 Hymenectomy

70.32 Excision or destruction of lesion of cul-de-sac
Endometrectomy of cul-de-sac

> **Excludes** *biopsy of cul-de-sac (70.23)*

70.33 Excision or destruction of lesion of vagina

> **Excludes** *biopsy of vagina (70.24)*
> *vaginal fistulectomy (70.72–70.75)*

OPERATIONS ON THE FEMALE GENITAL ORGANS (65–71)

70.4 Obliteration and total excision of vagina
Vaginectomy
> **Excludes** *obliteration of vaginal vault (70.8)*

● **70.5 Repair of cystocele and rectocele**

70.50 Repair of cystocele and rectocele
> **Excludes** *repair of cystocele and rectocele with graft or prosthesis (70.53)*

70.51 Repair of cystocele
Anterior colporrhaphy (with urethrocele repair)
> **Excludes** *repair of cystocele and rectocele with graft or prosthesis (70.53)*
> *repair of cystocele with graft or prosthesis (70.54)*

Coding Clinic: 1984, Nov-Dec, P20

70.52 Repair of rectocele
Posterior colporrhaphy
> **Excludes** *repair of cystocele and rectocele with graft or prosthesis (70.53)*
> *repair of rectocele with graft or prosthesis (70.55)*
> *STARR procedure (48.74)*

Coding Clinic: 2006, Q1, P12

70.53 Repair of cystocele and rectocele with graft or prosthesis
Use additional code for biological substance (70.94) or synthetic substance (70.95), if known

70.54 Repair of cystocele with graft or prosthesis
Anterior colporrhaphy (with urethrocele repair)
Use additional code for biological substance (70.94) or synthetic substance (70.95), if known

70.55 Repair of rectocele with graft or prosthesis
Posterior colporrhaphy
Use additional code for biological substance (70.94) or synthetic substance (70.95), if known

● **70.6 Vaginal construction and reconstruction**

70.61 Vaginal construction
Coding Clinic: 2006, Q3, P18-19

70.62 Vaginal reconstruction
Coding Clinic: 1984, Nov-Dec, P20

70.63 Vaginal construction with graft or prosthesis
Use additional code for biological substance (70.94) or synthetic substance (70.95), if known
> **Excludes** *vaginal construction (70.61)*

70.64 Vaginal reconstruction with graft or prosthesis
Use additional code for biological substance (70.94) or synthetic substance (70.95), if known
> **Excludes** *vaginal reconstruction (70.62)*

● **70.7 Other repair of vagina**
> **Excludes** *lysis of intraluminal adhesions (70.13)*
> *repair of current obstetric laceration (75.69)*
> *that associated with cervical amputation (67.4)*

70.71 Suture of laceration of vagina
Coding Clinic: 1984, Nov-Dec, P20

70.72 Repair of colovaginal fistula

70.73 Repair of rectovaginal fistula

70.74 Repair of other vaginoenteric fistula

70.75 Repair of other fistula of vagina
> **Excludes** *repair of fistula:*
> *rectovesicovaginal (57.83)*
> *ureterovaginal (56.84)*
> *urethrovaginal (58.43)*
> *uterovaginal (69.42)*
> *vesicocervicovaginal (57.84)*
> *vesicosigmoidovaginal (57.83)*
> *vesicoureterovaginal (56.84)*
> *vesicovaginal (57.84)*

70.76 Hymenorrhaphy

70.77 Vaginal suspension and fixation

70.78 Vaginal suspension and fixation with graft or prosthesis
Use additional code for biological substance (70.94) or synthetic substance (70.95), if known

70.79 Other repair of vagina
Colpoperineoplasty
Repair of old obstetric laceration of vagina

70.8 Obliteration of vaginal vault
LeFort operation

● **70.9 Other operations on vagina and cul-de-sac**

70.91 Other operations on vagina
> **Excludes** *insertion of:*
> *diaphragm (96.17)*
> *mold (96.15)*
> *pack (96.14)*
> *pessary (96.18)*
> *suppository (96.49)*
> *removal of:*
> *diaphragm (97.73)*
> *foreign body (98.17)*
> *pack (97.75)*
> *pessary (97.74)*
> *replacement of:*
> *diaphragm (97.24)*
> *pack (97.26)*
> *pessary (97.25)*
> *vaginal dilation (96.16)*
> *vaginal douche (96.44)*

70.92 Other operations on cul-de-sac
Obliteration of cul-de-sac
Repair of vaginal enterocele

70.93 Other operations on cul-de-sac with graft or prosthesis
Repair of vaginal enterocele with graft or prosthesis
Use additional code for biological substance (70.94) or synthetic substance (70.95), if known

70.94 Insertion of biological graft
Allogenic material or substance
Allograft
Autograft
Autologous material or substance
Heterograft
Xenogenic material or substance

Code first these procedures when done with graft or prosthesis:
Other operations on cul-de-sac (70.93)
Repair of cystocele (70.54)
Repair of cystocele and rectocele (70.53)
Repair of rectocele (70.55)
Vaginal construction (70.63)
Vaginal reconstruction (70.64)
Vaginal suspension and fixation (70.78)

70.95 Insertion of synthetic graft or prosthesis
Artificial tissue

Code first these procedures when done
with graft or prosthesis:
Other operations on cul-de-sac (70.93)
Repair of cystocele (70.54)
Repair of cystocele and rectocele (70.53)
Repair of rectocele (70.55)
Vaginal construction (70.63)
Vaginal reconstruction (70.64)
Vaginal suspension and fixation (70.78)

● **71 Operations on vulva and perineum**

Code also any application or administration of an
adhesion barrier substance (99.77)

● **71.0 Incision of vulva and perineum**

71.01 Lysis of vulvar adhesions

71.09 Other incision of vulva and perineum
Enlargement of introitus NOS

Excludes | *removal of foreign body without
incision (98.23)*

● **71.1 Diagnostic procedures on vulva**

71.11 Biopsy of vulva

71.19 Other diagnostic procedures on vulva

● **71.2 Operations on Bartholin's gland**

71.21 Percutaneous aspiration of Bartholin's gland (cyst)

71.22 Incision of Bartholin's gland (cyst)

71.23 Marsupialization of Bartholin's gland (cyst)

71.24 Excision or other destruction of Bartholin's gland (cyst)

71.29 Other operations on Bartholin's gland

71.3 Other local excision or destruction of vulva and perineum
Division of Skene's gland

Excludes | *biopsy of vulva (71.11)*
vulvar fistulectomy (71.72)

Coding Clinic: 2007, Q4, P90-91

71.4 Operations on clitoris
Amputation of clitoris
Clitoridotomy
Female circumcision

71.5 Radical vulvectomy

Code also any synchronous lymph gland dissection
(40.3, 40.5)

● **71.6 Other vulvectomy**

71.61 Unilateral vulvectomy
Coding Clinic: 2006, Q2, P19

71.62 Bilateral vulvectomy
Vulvectomy NOS

● **71.7 Repair of vulva and perineum**

Excludes | *repair of current obstetric laceration (75.69)*

71.71 Suture of laceration of vulva or perineum

71.72 Repair of fistula of vulva or perineum

Excludes | *repair of fistula:*
urethroperineal (58.43)
urethroperineovesical (57.84)
vaginoperineal (70.75)

71.79 Other repair of vulva and perineum
Repair of old obstetric laceration of vulva or
perineum
Coding Clinic: 1997, Q1, P9-10

71.8 Other operations on vulva

Excludes | *removal of:*
foreign body without incision (98.23)
packing (97.75)
replacement of packing (97.26)

71.9 Other operations on female genital organs
Coding Clinic: 2004, Q4, P88-90; 2003, Q1, P13-14

---

13. OBSTETRICAL PROCEDURES (72–75)

● **72 Forceps, vacuum, and breech delivery**

72.0 Low forceps operation
Outlet forceps operation

72.1 Low forceps operation with episiotomy
Outlet forceps operation with episiotomy

● **72.2 Mid forceps operation**

72.21 Mid forceps operation with episiotomy

72.29 Other mid forceps operation

● **72.3 High forceps operation**

72.31 High forceps operation with episiotomy

72.39 Other high forceps operation

72.4 Forceps rotation of fetal head
DeLee maneuver
Key-in-lock rotation
Kielland rotation
Scanzoni's maneuver

Code also any associated forceps extraction
(72.0–72.39)

● **72.5 Breech extraction**

72.51 Partial breech extraction with forceps to aftercoming head

72.52 Other partial breech extraction

72.53 Total breech extraction with forceps to aftercoming head

72.54 Other total breech extraction

OPERATIONS ON THE FEMALE GENITAL ORGANS (65–71)

OBSTETRICAL PROCEDURES (72–75)

72.6 Forceps application to aftercoming head
Piper forceps operation

> **Excludes** *partial breech extraction with forceps to aftercoming head (72.51)*
> *total breech extraction with forceps to aftercoming head (72.53)*

● **72.7 Vacuum extraction**

> **Includes** Malström's extraction

72.71 Vacuum extraction with episiotomy

72.79 Other vacuum extraction
Coding Clinic: 2006, Q2, P5

72.8 Other specified instrumental delivery

72.9 Unspecified instrumental delivery

● **73 Other procedures inducing or assisting delivery**

● **73.0 Artificial rupture of membranes**

73.01 Induction of labor by artificial rupture of membranes
Surgical induction NOS

> **Excludes** *artificial rupture of membranes after onset of labor (73.09)*

Coding Clinic: 2000, Q3, P5

73.09 Other artificial rupture of membranes
Artificial rupture of membranes at time of delivery

73.1 Other surgical induction of labor
Induction by cervical dilation

> **Excludes** *injection for abortion (75.0)*
> *insertion of suppository for abortion (96.49)*

● **73.2 Internal and combined version and extraction**

73.21 Internal and combined version without extraction
Version NOS

73.22 Internal and combined version with extraction

73.3 Failed forceps
Application of forceps without delivery
Trial forceps

73.4 Medical induction of labor

> **Excludes** *medication to augment active labor —* omit code

● **73.5 Manually assisted delivery**

73.51 Manual rotation of fetal head

73.59 Other manually assisted delivery
Assisted spontaneous delivery
Crede maneuver
Coding Clinic: 1998, Q4, P76-77

73.6 Episiotomy
Episioproctotomy
Episiotomy with subsequent episiorrhaphy

> **Excludes** *that with:*
> *high forceps (72.31)*
> *low forceps (72.1)*
> *mid forceps (72.21)*
> *outlet forceps (72.1)*
> *vacuum extraction (72.71)*

Coding Clinic: 2008, Q4, P192; 2006, Q2, P5; 1992, Q1, P10-11

73.8 Operations on fetus to facilitate delivery
Clavicotomy on fetus
Destruction of fetus
Needling of hydrocephalic head

● **73.9 Other operations assisting delivery**

73.91 External version

73.92 Replacement of prolapsed umbilical cord

73.93 Incision of cervix to assist delivery
Dührssen's incisions

73.94 Pubiotomy to assist delivery
Obstetrical symphysiotomy

73.99 Other

> **Excludes** *dilation of cervix, obstetrical to induce labor (73.1)*
> *insertion of bag or bougie to induce labor (73.1)*
> *removal of cerclage material (69.96)*

● **74 Cesarean section and removal of fetus**

Code also any synchronous:
hysterectomy (68.3–68.4, 68.6, 68.8)
myomectomy (68.29)
sterilization (66.31–66.39, 66.63)

74.0 Classical cesarean section
Transperitoneal classical cesarean section

74.1 Low cervical cesarean section
Lower uterine segment cesarean section
Coding Clinic: 2001, Q1, P11-12

74.2 Extraperitoneal cesarean section
Supravesical cesarean section

74.3 Removal of extratubal ectopic pregnancy
Removal of:
ectopic abdominal pregnancy
fetus from peritoneal or extraperitoneal cavity following uterine or tubal rupture

> **Excludes** *that by salpingostomy (66.02)*
> *that by salpingotomy (66.01)*
> *that with synchronous salpingectomy (66.62)*

Coding Clinic: 1990, Q2, P25, 27; 1989, Q1, P11; 1985, Sept-Oct, P14

74.4 Cesarean section of other specified type
Peritoneal exclusion cesarean section
Transperitoneal cesarean section NOS
Vaginal cesarean section

● **74.9 Cesarean section of unspecified type**

74.91 Hysterotomy to terminate pregnancy
Therapeutic abortion by hysterotomy

74.99 Other cesarean section of unspecified type
Cesarean section NOS
Obstetrical abdominouterotomy
Obstetrical hysterotomy

● **75 Other obstetric operations**

75.0 Intra-amniotic injection for abortion
Injection of:
prostaglandin for induction of abortion
saline for induction of abortion
Termination of pregnancy by intrauterine injection

> **Excludes** *insertion of prostaglandin suppository for abortion (96.49)*

75.1 Diagnostic amniocentesis

75.2 Intrauterine transfusion
Exchange transfusion in utero
Insertion of catheter into abdomen of fetus for transfusion

Code also any hysterotomy approach (68.0)

● **75.3 Other intrauterine operations on fetus and amnion**

Code also any hysterotomy approach (68.0)

75.31 Amnioscopy
Fetoscopy
Laparoamnioscopy
Coding Clinic: 2006, Q3, P16-18

75.32 Fetal EKG (scalp)

75.33 Fetal blood sampling and biopsy

75.34 Other fetal monitoring
    Antepartum fetal nonstress test
    Fetal monitoring, not otherwise specified
    Excludes *fetal pulse oximetry (75.38)*

75.35 Other diagnostic procedures on fetus and amnion
    Intrauterine pressure determination
    Excludes *amniocentesis (75.1)*
        diagnostic procedures on gravid uterus and placenta (87.81, 88.46, 88.78, 92.17)
    Coding Clinic: 2006, Q3, P16-18

75.36 Correction of fetal defect
    OGCR Section I.C.10.a.2
    In cases when in utero surgery is performed on the fetus, a code from category 655 should be assigned identifying the fetal condition. Procedure code 75.36, Correction of fetal defect, should be assigned on the hospital inpatient record. No code from Chapter 15, the perinatal codes, should be used on the mother's record to identify fetal conditions. Surgery performed in utero on a fetus is still to be coded as an obstetric encounter.

75.37 Amnioinfusion
    Code also injection of antibiotic (99.21)
    Coding Clinic: 1998, Q4, P76-77

75.38 Fetal pulse oximetry
    Transcervical fetal oxygen saturation monitoring
    Transcervical fetal SpO$_2$ monitoring

75.4 Manual removal of retained placenta
    Excludes *aspiration curettage (69.52)*
        dilation and curettage (69.02)
    Coding Clinic: 2006, Q3, P11

● **75.5 Repair of current obstetric laceration of uterus**

    75.50 Repair of current obstetric laceration of uterus, not otherwise specified

    75.51 Repair of current obstetric laceration of cervix

    75.52 Repair of current obstetric laceration of corpus uteri
        Coding Clinic: 2008, Q2, P7-8

● **75.6 Repair of other current obstetric laceration**
    Code also episiotomy, if performed (73.6)
    Coding Clinic: 2008, Q4, P192; 1992, Q1, P10-11

    75.61 Repair of current obstetric laceration of bladder and urethra

    75.62 Repair of current obstetric laceration of rectum and sphincter ani

    75.69 Repair of other current obstetric laceration
        Episioperineorrhaphy
        Repair of:
            pelvic floor
            perineum
            vagina
            vulva
        Secondary repair of episiotomy
        Coding Clinic: 2008, Q4, P192; 2007, Q4, P125

75.7 Manual exploration of uterine cavity, postpartum

75.8 Obstetric tamponade of uterus or vagina
    Excludes *antepartum tamponade (73.1)*

● **75.9 Other obstetric operations**

    75.91 Evacuation of obstetrical incisional hematoma of perineum
        Evacuation of hematoma of:
            episiotomy
            perineorrhaphy

    75.92 Evacuation of other hematoma of vulva or vagina

    75.93 Surgical correction of inverted uterus
        Spintelli operation
        Excludes *vaginal repair of chronic inversion of uterus (69.23)*

    75.94 Manual replacement of inverted uterus

    75.99 Other
        Coding Clinic: 2006, Q3, P16-18

OBSTETRICAL PROCEDURES (72–75)

(See Plates 244 and 509 on pages NAP-30–NAP-31.)

14. OPERATIONS ON THE MUSCULOSKELETAL SYSTEM (76–84)

● **76 Operations on facial bones and joints**
    Excludes *accessory sinuses (22.00–22.9)*
        nasal bones (21.00–21.99)
        skull (01.01–02.99)

● **76.0 Incision of facial bone without division**

    76.01 Sequestrectomy of facial bone
        Removal of necrotic bone chip from facial bone

    76.09 Other incision of facial bone
        Reopening of osteotomy site of facial bone
        Excludes *osteotomy associated with orthognathic surgery (76.61–76.69)*
            removal of internal fixation device (76.97)

● **76.1 Diagnostic procedures on facial bones and joints**

    76.11 Biopsy of facial bone

    76.19 Other diagnostic procedures on facial bones and joints
        Excludes *contrast arthrogram of temporomandibular joint (87.13)*
            other x-ray (87.11–87.12, 87.14–87.16)
        Coding Clinic: 1987, Nov-Dec, P12

76.2 Local excision or destruction of lesion of facial bone
    Excludes *biopsy of facial bone (76.11)*
        excision of odontogenic lesion (24.4)

● **76.3 Partial ostectomy of facial bone**

    76.31 Partial mandibulectomy
        Hemimandibulectomy
        Excludes *that associated with temporomandibular arthroplasty (76.5)*
        Coding Clinic: 2005, Q2, P8-9

    Excludes   **Includes**   Use additional   Code also   Omit code

76.39 Partial ostectomy of other facial bone
Hemimaxillectomy (with bone graft or prosthesis)
Coding Clinic: 1987, Jan-Feb, P14

● **76.4 Excision and reconstruction of facial bones**

76.41 Total mandibulectomy with synchronous reconstruction

76.42 Other total mandibulectomy

76.43 Other reconstruction of mandible
Excludes genioplasty (76.67–76.68)
that with synchronous total mandibulectomy (76.41)
Coding Clinic: 2003, Q2, P13

76.44 Total ostectomy of other facial bone with synchronous reconstruction
Coding Clinic: 1993, Q3, P6

76.45 Other total ostectomy of other facial bone

76.46 Other reconstruction of other facial bone
Excludes that with synchronous total ostectomy (76.44)

76.5 Temporomandibular arthroplasty

● **76.6 Other facial bone repair and orthognathic surgery**
Code also any synchronous:
bone graft (76.91)
synthetic implant (76.92)
Excludes reconstruction of facial bones (76.41–76.46)

76.61 Closed osteoplasty [osteotomy] of mandibular ramus
Gigli saw osteotomy

76.62 Open osteoplasty [osteotomy] of mandibular ramus

76.63 Osteoplasty [osteotomy] of body of mandible

76.64 Other orthognathic surgery on mandible
Mandibular osteoplasty NOS
Segmental or subapical osteotomy
Coding Clinic: 2004, Q2, P9,10

76.65 Segmental osteoplasty [osteotomy] of maxilla
Maxillary osteoplasty NOS

76.66 Total osteoplasty [osteotomy] of maxilla

76.67 Reduction genioplasty
Reduction mentoplasty

76.68 Augmentation genioplasty
Mentoplasty:
NOS
with graft or implant

76.69 Other facial bone repair
Osteoplasty of facial bone NOS

● **76.7 Reduction of facial fracture**
Includes internal fixation
Code also any synchronous:
bone graft (76.91)
synthetic implant (76.92)
Excludes that of nasal bones (21.71–21.72)

76.70 Reduction of facial fracture, not otherwise specified

76.71 Closed reduction of malar and zygomatic fracture

76.72 Open reduction of malar and zygomatic fracture

76.73 Closed reduction of maxillary fracture

76.74 Open reduction of maxillary fracture

76.75 Closed reduction of mandibular fracture

76.76 Open reduction of mandibular fracture

76.77 Open reduction of alveolar fracture
Reduction of alveolar fracture with stabilization of teeth

76.78 Other closed reduction of facial fracture
Closed reduction of orbital fracture
Excludes nasal bone (21.71)

76.79 Other open reduction of facial fracture
Open reduction of orbit rim or wall
Excludes nasal bone (21.72)

● **76.9 Other operations on facial bones and joints**

76.91 Bone graft to facial bone
Autogenous graft to facial bone
Bone bank graft to facial bone
Heterogenous graft to facial bone

76.92 Insertion of synthetic implant in facial bone
Alloplastic implant to facial bone

76.93 Closed reduction of temporomandibular dislocation

76.94 Open reduction of temporomandibular dislocation

76.95 Other manipulation of temporomandibular joint

76.96 Injection of therapeutic substance into temporomandibular joint

76.97 Removal of internal fixation device from facial bone
Excludes removal of:
dental wiring (97.33)
external mandibular fixation device NEC (97.36)

76.99 Other

● **77 Incision, excision, and division of other bones**
Excludes laminectomy for decompression (03.09)
operations on:
accessory sinuses (22.00–22.9)
ear ossicles (19.0–19.55)
facial bones (76.01–76.99)
joint structures (80.00–81.99)
mastoid (19.9–20.99)
nasal bones (21.00–21.99)
skull (01.01–02.99)

The following fourth-digit subclassification is for use with appropriate categories in section 77 to identify the site. Valid fourth-digit categories are in brackets under each code.

0　unspecified site
1　scapula, clavicle, and thorax [ribs and sternum]
2　humerus
3　radius and ulna
4　carpals and metacarpals
5　femur
6　patella
7　tibia and fibula
8　tarsals and metatarsals
9　other
　　Pelvic bones
　　Phalanges (of foot) (of hand)
　　Vertebrae

● **77.0 Sequestrectomy**
[0-9]

● **77.1 Other incision of bone without division**
[0-9]　　Reopening of osteotomy site
Excludes aspiration of bone marrow (41.31, 41.91)
removal of internal fixation device (78.60–78.69)
Coding Clinic: 2002, Q1, P3-4

◀ New　　◀|||| Revised　　deleted Deleted　　● Use Additional Digit(s)　　OGCR Official Guidelines　　Coding Clinic

● **77.2 Wedge osteotomy**
[0-9]   Excludes   *that for hallux valgus (77.51)*

● **77.3 Other division of bone**
[0-9]   Osteoarthrotomy
     Excludes   *clavicotomy of fetus (73.8)*
         laminotomy or incision of vertebra
           (03.01–03.09)
         pubiotomy to assist delivery (73.94)
         sternotomy incidental to thoracic operation —
           omit code

● **77.4 Biopsy of bone**
[0-9]   Coding Clinic: 2006, Q3, P13; 1998, Q2, P12

● **77.5 Excision and repair of bunion and other toe deformities**

   77.51 Bunionectomy with soft tissue correction and osteotomy of the first metatarsal

   77.52 Bunionectomy with soft tissue correction and arthrodesis

   77.53 Other bunionectomy with soft tissue correction

   77.54 Excision or correction of bunionette
       That with osteotomy

   77.56 Repair of hammer toe
       Filleting of hammer toe
       Fusion of hammer toe
       Phalangectomy (partial) of hammer toe

   77.57 Repair of claw toe
       Capsulotomy of claw toe
       Fusion of claw toe
       Phalangectomy (partial) of claw toe
       Tendon lengthening of claw toe

   77.58 Other excision, fusion, and repair of toes
       Cockup toe repair
       Overlapping toe repair
       That with use of prosthetic materials

   77.59 Other bunionectomy
       Resection of hallux valgus joint with insertion of prosthesis

● **77.6 Local excision of lesion or tissue of bone**
[0-9]   Excludes   *biopsy of bone (77.40–77.49)*
         debridement of compound fracture
           (79.60–79.69)
   Coding Clinic: 2008, Q1, P3-4; 2004, Q4, P128-129; 2002, Q1, P3-49;
         2001, Q3, P9; 2000, Q2, P18-19; 1999, Q1, P8-9

● **77.7 Excision of bone for graft**
[0-9]   Coding Clinic: 2008, Q1, P5-6; 2007, Q2, P6; 2003, Q3, P19; 2003, Q2,
         P13; 2002, Q4, P107-110; 2002, Q2, P16; 2000, Q2, P12-13;
         1999, Q4, P12-13; 1995, Q2, P9;1994, Q2, P7

● **77.8 Other partial ostectomy**
[0-9]   Condylectomy
     Excludes   *amputation (84.00–84.19, 84.91)*
         arthrectomy (80.90–80.99)
         excision of bone ends associated with:
           arthrodesis (81.00–81.39, 81.62–81.66)
           arthroplasty (81.40–81.59, 81.71–81.85)
         excision of cartilage (80.5–80.6, 80.80–80.99)
         excision of head of femur with synchronous
           replacement (00.70–00.73, 81.51–81.53)
         hemilaminectomy (03.01–03.09)
         laminectomy (03.01–03.09)
         ostectomy for hallux valgus (77.51–77.59)
         partial amputation:
           finger (84.01)
           thumb (84.02)
           toe (84.11)
         resection of ribs incidental to thoracic
           operation — omit code
         that incidental to other operation —
           omit code
   Coding Clinic: 2002, Q2, P8

● **77.9 Total ostectomy**
[0-9]   Excludes   *amputation of limb (84.00–84.19, 84.91)*
         that incidental to other operation —
           omit code

● **78 Other operations on bones, except facial bones**
     Excludes   *operations on:*
         accessory sinuses (22.00–22.9)
         facial bones (76.01–76.99)
         joint structures (80.00–81.99)
         nasal bones (21.00–21.99)
         skull (01.01–02.99)
   Coding Clinic: 2002, Q2, P11

The following fourth-digit subclassification is for use with categories in section 78 to identify the site. Valid fourth-digit categories are in [brackets] under each code.

> 0 unspecified site
> 1 scapula, clavicle, and thorax [ribs and sternum]
> 2 humerus
> 3 radius and ulna
> 4 carpals and metacarpals
> 5 femur
> 6 patella
> 7 tibia and fibula
> 8 tarsals and metatarsals
> 9 other
>   Pelvic bones
>   Phalanges (of foot) (of hand)
>   Vertebrae

● **78.0 Bone graft**
[0-9]   Bone:
       bank graft
       graft (autogenous) (heterogenous)
   That with debridement of bone graft site (removal of
       sclerosed, fibrous, or necrotic bone or tissue)
   Transplantation of bone
     Code also   any excision of bone for graft (77.70–77.79)
     Excludes   *that for bone lengthening (78.30–78.39)*
   Coding Clinic: 2006, Q4, P103-104; 1998, Q2, P12; 1994, Q3, P10;
         1994, Q2, P7

● **78.1 Application of external fixator device**
[0-9]   Fixator with insertion of pins/wires/screws into bone
     Code also   any type of fixator device, if known
         (84.71–84.73)
     Excludes   *other immobilization, pressure, and attention*
         to wound (93.51–93.59)
   Coding Clinic: 2005, Q4, P127-129; 1994, Q2, P5

● **78.2 Limb shortening procedures**
[0, 2-5, 7-9]   Epiphyseal stapling
       Open epiphysiodesis
       Percutaneous epiphysiodesis
       Resection/osteotomy

● **78.3 Limb lengthening procedures**
[0, 2-5, 7-9]   Bone graft with or without internal fixation devices or
       osteotomy
   Distraction technique with or without corticotomy/
       osteotomy
     Code also   any application of an external fixation
       device (78.10–78.19)

Excludes   Includes   Use additional   Code also   Omit code

● **78.4　Other repair or plastic operations on bone**
[0-9]　　　Other operation on bone NEC
　　　　　Repair of malunion or nonunion fracture NEC

> **Excludes**　*application of external fixation device*
> *(78.10–78.19)*
> *limb lengthening procedures (78.30–78.39)*
> *limb shortening procedures (78.20–78.29)*
> *osteotomy (77.3)*
> *reconstruction of thumb (82.61–82.69)*
> *repair of pectus deformity (34.74)*
> *repair with bone graft (78.00–78.09)*

Coding Clinic: 2004, Q3, P9-10; 2002, Q3, P12; Q2, P14-16; 1999, Q4, P22; 1997, Q1, P5; 1991, Q3, P20; Q2, P20

● **78.5　Internal fixation of bone without fracture reduction**
[0-9]　　　Internal fixation of bone (prophylactic)
　　　　　Reinsertion of internal fixation device
　　　　　Revision of displaced or broken fixation device

> **Excludes**　*arthroplasty and arthrodesis (81.00–81.85)*
> *bone graft (78.00–78.09)*
> *insertion of sternal fixation device with rigid*
> *plates (84.94)* ◄
> *limb shortening procedures (78.20–78.29)*
> *that for fracture reduction (79.10–79.19,*
> *79.30–79.59)*

Coding Clinic: 2004, Q3, P6-7; 2003, Q2, P15; 1999, Q4, P13-14; 1995, Q3, P12

● **78.6　Removal of implanted devices from bone**
[0-9]　　　External fixator device (invasive)
　　　　　Internal fixation device
　　　　　Removal of bone growth stimulator (invasive)
　　　　　Removal of internal limb lengthening device
　　　　　Removal of pedicle screw(s) used in spinal fusion

> **Excludes**　*removal of cast, splint, and traction device*
> *(Kirschner wire) (Steinmann pin)*
> *(97.88)*
> *removal of posterior spinal motion*
> *preservation (facet replacement,*
> *pedicle-based dynamic stabilization,*
> *interspinous process) device(s) (80.09)*
> *removal of skull tongs or halo traction device*
> *(02.95)*

Coding Clinic: 2003, Q2, P14; 2002, Q4, P110; 2000, Q2, P18-19; Q1, P15-16; 1995, Q1, P10

● **78.7　Osteoclasis**
[0-9]

● **78.8　Diagnostic procedures on bone, not elsewhere**
[0-9]　　　**classified**

> **Excludes**　*biopsy of bone (77.40–77.49)*
> *magnetic resonance imaging (88.94)*
> *microscopic examination of specimen from*
> *bone (91.51–91.59)*
> *radioisotope scan (92.14)*
> *skeletal x-ray (87.21–87.29, 87.43,*
> *88.21–88.33)*
> *thermography (88.83)*

● **78.9　Insertion of bone growth stimulator**
[0-9]　　　Insertion of:
　　　　　bone stimulator (electrical) to aid bone healing
　　　　　osteogenic electrodes for bone growth stimulation
　　　　　totally implanted device (invasive)

> **Excludes**　*non-invasive (transcutaneous) (surface)*
> *stimulator (99.86)*

● **79　Reduction of fracture and dislocation**

> **Includes**　application of cast or splint reduction with
> insertion of traction device (Kirschner
> wire) (Steinmann pin)

Code also any:
　　　application of external fixator device (78.10–78.19)
　　　type of fixator device, if known (84.71–84.73)

> **Excludes**　*external fixation alone for immobilization of fracture*
> *(93.51–93.56, 93.59)*
> *internal fixation without reduction of fracture*
> *(78.50–78.59)*
> *operations on:*
> *facial bones (76.70–76.79)*
> *nasal bones (21.71–21.72)*
> *orbit (76.78–76.79)*
> *skull (02.02)*
> *vertebrae (03.53)*
> *removal of cast or splint (97.88)*
> *replacement of cast or splint (97.11–97.14)*
> *traction alone for reduction of fracture*
> *(93.41–93.46)*

The following fourth-digit subclassification is for use with
appropriate categories in section 79 to identify the site. Valid
fourth-digit categories are in [brackets] under each code.

0	unspecified site
1	humerus
2	radius and ulna
	Arm NOS
3	carpals and metacarpals
	Hand NOS
4	phalanges of hand
5	femur
6	tibia and fibula
	Leg NOS
7	tarsals and metatarsals
	Foot NOS
8	phalanges of foot
9	other specified bone

● **79.0　Closed reduction of fracture without internal fixation**
[0-9]　　> **Excludes**　*that for separation of epiphysis (79.40–79.49)*

Coding Clinic: 2005, Q4, P127-129; 1989, Q3, P16; 1988, Q4, P11

● **79.1　Closed reduction of fracture with internal fixation**
[0-9]　　> **Excludes**　*that for separation of epiphysis (79.40–79.49)*

Coding Clinic: 1994, Q2, P6-7; 1993, Q4, P35; 1993, Q1, P27; 1984, May-June, P11

● **79.2　Open reduction of fracture without internal fixation**
[0-9]　　> **Excludes**　*that for separation of epiphysis (79.50–79.59)*

● **79.3　Open reduction of fracture with internal fixation**
[0-9]　　> **Excludes**　*that for separation of epiphysis (79.50–79.59)*

Coding Clinic: 2007, Q1, P3-8; 2004, Q1, P9; 1998, Q2, P12; 1994, Q3, P10; Q2, P5, 7

● **79.4　Closed reduction of separated epiphysis**
[0-2, 5, 6, 9]　　Reduction with or without internal fixation

● **79.5　Open reduction of separated epiphysis**
[0-2, 5, 6, 9]　　Reduction with or without internal fixation

● **79.6　Debridement of open fracture site**
[0-9]　　　Debridement of compound fracture
Coding Clinic: 1995, Q3, P12

　　　◄ New　　◄■ Revised　　~~deleted~~ Deleted　　● Use Additional Digit(s)　　**OGCR** Official Guidelines　　**Coding Clinic**

● **79.7 Closed reduction of dislocation**

> **Includes** closed reduction (with external traction device)

> **Excludes** *closed reduction of dislocation of temporomandibular joint (76.93)*

79.70 **Closed reduction of dislocation of unspecified site**

79.71 **Closed reduction of dislocation of shoulder**

79.72 **Closed reduction of dislocation of elbow**

79.73 **Closed reduction of dislocation of wrist**

79.74 **Closed reduction of dislocation of hand and finger**

79.75 **Closed reduction of dislocation of hip**

79.76 **Closed reduction of dislocation of knee**

79.77 **Closed reduction of dislocation of ankle**

79.78 **Closed reduction of dislocation of foot and toe**

79.79 **Closed reduction of dislocation of other specified sites**

● **79.8 Open reduction of dislocation**

> **Includes** open reduction (with internal and external fixation devices)

> **Excludes** *open reduction of dislocation of temporomandibular joint (76.94)*

79.80 **Open reduction of dislocation of unspecified site**

79.81 **Open reduction of dislocation of shoulder**

79.82 **Open reduction of dislocation of elbow**

79.83 **Open reduction of dislocation of wrist**

79.84 **Open reduction of dislocation of hand and finger**

79.85 **Open reduction of dislocation of hip**

79.86 **Open reduction of dislocation of knee**

79.87 **Open reduction of dislocation of ankle**
> Coding Clinic: 2004, Q1, P9

79.88 **Open reduction of dislocation of foot and toe**

79.89 **Open reduction of dislocation of other specified sites**

● **79.9 Unspecified operation on bone injury**
[0-9]

● **80 Incision and excision of joint structures**

> **Includes** operations on:
> capsule of joint
> cartilage
> condyle
> ligament
> meniscus
> synovial membrane

> **Excludes** *cartilage of:*
> *ear (18.01–18.9)*
> *nose (21.00–21.99)*
> *temporomandibular joint (76.01–76.99)*

The following fourth-digit subclassification is for use with appropriate categories in section 80 to identify the site:

> 0 **unspecified site**
> 1 **shoulder**
> 2 **elbow**
> 3 **wrist**
> 4 **hand and finger**
> 5 **hip**
> 6 **knee**
> 7 **ankle**
> 8 **foot and toe**
> 9 **other specified sites**
>   Spine

● **80.0 Arthrotomy for removal of prosthesis without**
[0-9] **replacement**

> **Includes** removal of posterior spinal motion preservation (dynamic stabilization, facet replacement, interspinous process) device(s)

> Code also any:
> insertion of (cement) (joint) (methylmethacrylate) spacer (84.56)
> removal of (cement) (joint) (methylmethacrylate) spacer (84.57)

> **Excludes** *removal of pedicle screws used in spinal fusion (78.69)*
> Coding Clinic: 2008, Q2, P3-5; 1997, Q2, P10; 1992, Q2, P18; 1990, Q2, P27

● **80.1 Other arthrotomy**
[0-9] Arthrostomy

> **Excludes** *that for:*
> *arthrography (88.32)*
> *arthroscopy (80.20–80.29)*
> *injection of drug (81.92)*
> *operative approach —* omit code
> Coding Clinic: 2006, Q3, P22-23

● **80.2 Arthroscopy**
[0-9]

● **80.3 Biopsy of joint structure**
[0-9] Aspiration biopsy
> Coding Clinic: 2005, Q3, P13-14x2

● **80.4 Division of joint capsule, ligament, or cartilage**
[0-9] Goldner clubfoot release
Heyman-Herndon(-Strong) correction of metatarsus varus
Release of:
adherent or constrictive joint capsule
joint
ligament

> **Excludes** *symphysiotomy to assist delivery (73.94)*
> *that for:*
> *carpal tunnel syndrome (04.43)*
> *tarsal tunnel syndrome (04.44)*
> Coding Clinic: 2002, Q2, P16

● **80.5 Excision, destruction and other repair of intervertebral disc**
> Coding Clinic: 1986, Sept-Oct, P11-12

80.50 **Excision or destruction of intervertebral disc, unspecified**
Unspecified as to excision or destruction

80.51 **Excision of intervertebral disc**
Diskectomy
Removal of herniated nucleus pulposus
Level:
cervical
thoracic
lumbar (lumbosacral)
That by laminotomy or hemilaminectomy
That with decompression of spinal nerve root at same level
Requires additional code for any concomitant decompression of spinal nerve root at different level from excision site

> Code also any
> concurrent spinal fusion (81.00–81.09)
> repair of the anulus fibrosus (80.53–80.54)

> **Excludes** *intervertebral chemonucleolysis (80.52)*
> *laminectomy for exploration of intraspinal canal (03.09)*
> *laminotomy for decompression of spinal nerve root only (03.09)*
> *that for insertion of (non-fusion) spinal disc replacement device (84.60–84.69)*
> *that with corpectomy, (vertebral) (80.99)*
> Coding Clinic: 2009, Q2, P3; 2008, Q4, P183-184; Q4, P14-15; 2008, Q1, P5-6; 2008, Q1, P3-5; 2007, Q1, P9; 2006, Q1, P12-13; 2004, Q4, P129-133; 2003, Q3, P12; 1996, Q1, P7 x2; 1995, Q2, P9

OPERATIONS ON THE MUSCULOSKELETAL SYSTEM (76–84)

80.52 Intervertebral chemonucleolysis
With aspiration of disc fragments
With diskography
Injection of proteolytic enzyme into
intervertebral space (chymopapain)

Excludes	injection of anesthetic substance (03.91)
	injection of other substances (03.92)

80.53 Repair of the anulus fibrosus with graft or prosthesis
Anular disc repair
Closure (sealing) of the anulus fibrosus defect

Includes	microsurgical suture repair with fascial autograft
	soft tissue re-approximation repair with tension bands
	surgical mesh repair

Code also any:
application or administration of adhesion
barrier substance, if performed
(99.77)
intervertebral discectomy, if performed
(80.51)
locally harvested fascia for graft (83.43)
Coding Clinic: 2008, Q4, P183-184

80.54 Other and unspecified repair of the anulus fibrosus
Anular disc repair
Closure (sealing) of the anulus fibrosus
defect
Microsurgical suture repair without fascial
autograft
Percutaneous repair of the anulus fibrosus

Code also any:
application or administration of adhesion
barrier substance, if performed
(99.77)
intervertebral discectomy, if performed
(80.51)
Coding Clinic: 2008, Q4, P183-184

80.59 Other destruction of intervertebral disc
Destruction NEC
That by laser
Coding Clinic: 2002, Q3, P10; 1989, Q1, P11; 1988, Q4, P11

80.6 Excision of semilunar cartilage of knee
Excision of meniscus of knee
Coding Clinic: 2003, Q2, P18; 2000, Q3, P4; 1996, Q2, P4; 1993, Q1, P23

●**80.7 Synovectomy**
[0-9]   Complete or partial resection of synovial membrane

Excludes	excision of Baker's cyst (83.39)

Coding Clinic: 1984, Nov-Dec, P9

●**80.8 Other local excision or destruction of lesion of joint**
[0-9]   Coding Clinic: 2008, Q1, P7

●**80.9 Other excision of joint**
[0-9]
Excludes	cheilectomy of joint (77.80–77.89)
	excision of bone ends (77.80–77.89)

Coding Clinic: 2007, Q1, P20-21

●**81 Repair and plastic operations on joint structures**
●**81.0 Spinal fusion**

Includes	arthrodesis of spine with:
	bone graft
	internal fixation

Code also:
any insertion of interbody spinal fusion device
(84.51)
any insertion of recombinant bone morphogenetic
protein (84.52)
any synchronous excision of (locally) harvested
bone for graft (77.70–77.79)
the total number of vertebrae fused (81.62–81.64)

Note: Spinal fusion is classified by the anatomic
portion (column) fused and the technique
(approach) used to perform the fusion. ◀

For the anterior column, the body (corpus) of
adjacent vertebrae are fused (interbody fusion).
The anterior column can be fused using an
anterior, lateral, or posterior technique. ◀

For the posterior column, posterior structures
of adjacent vertebrae are fused (pedicle,
lamina, facet, transverse process, or "gutter"
fusion). A posterior column fusion can be
performed using a posterior, posterolateral, or
lateral transverse technique. ◀

Excludes	correction of pseudarthrosis of spine (81.30–81.39)
	refusion of spine (81.30–81.39)

Coding Clinic: 2009, Q2, P3

81.00 Spinal fusion, not otherwise specified

81.01 Atlas-axis spinal fusion
Craniocervical fusion by anterior, transoral, or
posterior technique
C1-C2 fusion by anterior, transoral, or posterior
technique
Occiput C2 fusion by anterior, transoral, or
posterior technique

81.02 Other cervical fusion of the, anterior column, anterior technique ◀▬
Arthrodesis of C2 level or below:
anterior (interbody technique) fusion ◀▬
anterolateral technique
Coding Clinic: 2003, Q4, P99-101; 2001, Q1, P6; 1996, Q1, P7x2

81.03 Other cervical fusion of the, posterior column, posterior technique ◀▬
Arthrodesis of C2 level or below:,
posterolateral technique ◀▬
posterior (interbody) technique
posterolateral technique

81.04 Dorsal and dorsolumbar fusion of the, anterior column, anterior technique ◀▬
Arthrodesis of thoracic or thoracolumbar
region:
anterior (interbody technique) fusion ◀▬
anterolateral technique
Extracavitary technique ◀
Coding Clinic: 2003, Q3, P19

81.05 Dorsal and dorsolumbar fusion of the, posterior column, posterior technique ◀▥

Arthrodesis of thoracic or thoracolumbar region:, posterolateral technique ◀▥
~~posterior (interbody) technique~~
~~posterolateral technique~~

81.06 Lumbar and lumbosacral fusion of the, anterior column, anterior technique ◀▥

Anterior lumbar interbody fusion (ALIF)
Arthrodesis of lumbar or lumbosacral region:
anterior (interbody ~~technique~~) fusion ◀▥
anterolateral technique
retroperitoneal ◀
transperitoneal ◀
Direct lateral interbody fusion [DLIF] ◀
Extreme lateral interbody fusion [XLIF] ◀
Coding Clinic: 2008, Q2, P14-15; 2007, Q1, P9-10,20-21; 2002, Q4, P107-108

81.07 Lumbar and lumbosacral fusion of the, posterior column, posterior ~~or lateral transverse process~~ technique ◀▥

Facet fusion ◀
Posterolateral technique ◀
Transverse process technique ◀
Coding Clinic: 2009, Q2, P3; 2002, Q4, P108

81.08 Lumbar and lumbosacral fusion of the, anterior column, posterior technique ◀▥

Arthrodesis of lumbar or lumbosacral region:, posterior (interbody) ~~technique~~ fusion ~~posterolateral technique~~ ◀▥
Axial lumbar interbody fusion [AxiaLIF] ◀
Posterior lumbar interbody fusion (PLIF)
Transforaminal lumbar interbody fusion (TLIF)
Coding Clinic: 2009, Q2, P3, 5; 2008, Q1, P5-6; 2006, Q1, P12-14x2; 2005, Q4, P122-123; 2002, Q4, P107-110; 2000, Q2, P12-13; 1999, Q4, P12-13; 1995, Q2, P9

● **81.1 Arthrodesis and arthroereisis of foot and ankle**

Includes arthrodesis of foot and ankle with:
bone graft
external fixation device

81.11 Ankle fusion
Tibiotalar fusion

81.12 Triple arthrodesis
Talus to calcaneus and calcaneus to cuboid and navicular

81.13 Subtalar fusion
Excludes arthroereisis (81.18)

81.14 Midtarsal fusion

81.15 Tarsometatarsal fusion

81.16 Metatarsophalangeal fusion

81.17 Other fusion of foot

81.18 Subtalar joint arthroereisis
Coding Clinic: 2005, Q4, P124

● **81.2 Arthrodesis of other joint**

Includes arthrodesis with:
bone graft
external fixation device
excision of bone ends and compression

81.20 Arthrodesis of unspecified joint

81.21 Arthrodesis of hip

81.22 Arthrodesis of knee

81.23 Arthrodesis of shoulder

81.24 Arthrodesis of elbow

81.25 Carporadial fusion

81.26 Metacarpocarpal fusion

81.27 Metacarpophalangeal fusion

81.28 Interphalangeal fusion

81.29 Arthrodesis of other specified joints

● **81.3 Refusion of spine**

Includes arthrodesis of spine with:
bone graft
internal fixation
correction of pseudarthrosis of spine

Code also:
any insertion of interbody spinal fusion device (84.51)
any insertion of recombinant bone morphogenetic protein (84.52)
any synchronous excision of (locally) harvested bone for graft (77.70–77.79)
the total number of vertebrae fused (81.62–81.64)

Note: Spine fusion is classified by the anatomic portion (column) fused and the technique (approach) used to perform the fusion. ◀

For the anterior column, the body (corpus) of adjacent vertebrae are fused (interbody fusion). The anterior column can be fused using an anterior, lateral, or posterior technique. ◀

For the posterior column, posterior structures of adjacent vertebrae are fused (pedicle, lamina, facet, transverse process, or "gutter" fusion). A posterior column fusion can be performed using a posterior, posterolateral, or lateral transverse technique. ◀
Coding Clinic: 2005, Q4, P122-123

81.30 Refusion of spine, not otherwise specified

81.31 Refusion of atlas-axis spine
Craniocervical fusion by anterior, transoral, or posterior technique
C1-C2 fusion by anterior, transoral, or posterior technique
Occiput C2 fusion by anterior, transoral, or posterior technique

81.32 Refusion of other cervical spine, anterior column, anterior technique ◀▥
Arthrodesis of C2 level or below:
anterior (interbody ~~technique~~) fusion ◀▥
anterolateral technique

81.33 Refusion of other cervical spine, posterior column, posterior technique ◀▥
Arthrodesis of C2 level or below:, posterolateral technique ◀▥
~~posterior (interbody) technique~~
~~posterolateral technique~~

81.34 Refusion of dorsal and dorsolumbar spine, anterior column, anterior technique ◀▥
Arthrodesis of thoracic or thoracolumbar region:
anterior (interbody ~~technique~~) fusion ◀▥
anterolateral technique
Extracavitary technique ◀

OPERATIONS ON THE MUSCULOSKELETAL SYSTEM (76–84)

81.35   Refusion of dorsal and dorsolumbar spine, posterior column, posterior technique ◀▥
        Arthrodesis of thoracic or thoracolumbar region:, posterolateral technique ◀▥
        ~~posterior (interbody) technique~~
        ~~posterolateral technique~~

81.36   Refusion of lumbar and lumbosacral spine, anterior column, anterior technique ◀▥
        Anterior lumbar interbody fusion (ALIF)
        Arthrodesis of lumbar or lumbosacral region:
        anterior (interbody ~~technique~~) fusion ◀▥
        anterolateral technique
        retroperitoneal ◀
        transperitoneal ◀
        Direct lateral interbody fusion [DLIF] ◀
        Extreme lateral interbody fusion [XLIF] ◀

81.37   Refusion of lumbar and lumbosacral spine, posterior column, posterior ~~or lateral transverse process~~ technique ◀▥
        Facet fusion ◀
        Posterolateral technique ◀
        Transverse process technique ◀

81.38   Refusion of lumbar and lumbosacral spine, anterior column, posterior technique ◀▥
        Arthrodesis of lumbar or lumbosacral region:, posterior (interbody~~) technique~~ fusion ~~posterolateral technique~~ ◀▥
        Axial lumbar interbody fusion [AxiaLIF] ◀
        Posterior lumbar interbody fusion (PLIF)
        Transforaminal lumbar interbody fusion (TLIF)

81.39   Refusion of spine, not elsewhere classified

● **81.4   Other repair of joint of lower extremity**
        Includes   arthroplasty of lower extremity with:
                external traction or fixation
                graft of bone (chips) or cartilage
                internal fixation device

81.40   Repair of hip, not elsewhere classified

81.42   Five-in-one repair of knee
        Medial meniscectomy, medial collateral ligament repair, vastus medialis advancement, semitendinosus advancement, and pes anserinus transfer

81.43   Triad knee repair
        Medial meniscectomy with repair of the anterior cruciate ligament and the medial collateral ligament
        O'Donoghue procedure

81.44   Patellar stabilization
        Roux-Goldthwait operation for recurrent dislocation of patella

81.45   Other repair of the cruciate ligaments

81.46   Other repair of the collateral ligaments
        Coding Clinic: 1995, Q1, P8

81.47   Other repair of knee
        Coding Clinic: 2006, Q2, P13-14; 2003, Q2, P18; 2000, Q1, P12-13; 1996, Q2, P4; 1995, Q1, P8; 1993, Q3, P5

81.49   Other repair of ankle
        Coding Clinic: 2001, Q2, P14-15; 2000, Q3, P4

● **81.5   Joint replacement of lower extremity**
        Note: Removal of prior prosthesis — *omit code*
        Includes   arthroplasty of lower extremity with:
                external traction or fixation
                graft of bone (chips) or cartilage
                internal fixation device or prosthesis

81.51   Total hip replacement
        Replacement of both femoral head and acetabulum by prosthesis
        Total reconstruction of hip
        Code also any type of bearing surface, if known (00.74–00.77)
        Coding Clinic: 2009, Q2, P3; 2004, Q4, P111-113; 1992, Q2, P18

81.52   Partial hip replacement
        Bipolar endoprosthesis
        Code also any type of bearing surface, if known (00.74–00.77)
        Coding Clinic: 1992, Q2, P18

81.53   Revision of hip replacement, not otherwise specified
        Revision of hip replacement, not specified as to components(s) replaced (acetabular, femoral, or both)
        Code also any:
                removal of (cement) (joint) spacer (84.57)
                type of bearing surface, if known (00.74–00.77)
        Excludes   *revision of hip replacement, components specified (00.70–00.73)*
        Coding Clinic: 2005, Q4, P106-113; 1997, Q3, P13

81.54   Total knee replacement
        Bicompartmental
        Partial knee replacement
        Tricompartmental
        Unicompartmental (hemijoint)
        Coding Clinic: 1985, Nov-Dec, P11

81.55   Revision of knee replacement, not otherwise specified
        Code also any removal of (cement) spacer (84.57)
        Excludes   *arthrodesis of knee (81.22)*
                revision of knee replacement, components specified (00.80–00.84)
        Coding Clinic: 2005, Q4, P113-117; 1997, Q2, P10

81.56   Total ankle replacement

81.57   Replacement of joint of foot and toe

81.59   Revision of joint replacement of lower extremity, not elsewhere classified
        Coding Clinic: 1988, Q1, P9

◀ New   ◀▥ Revised   ~~deleted~~ Deleted   ● Use Additional Digit(s)   OGCR Official Guidelines   Coding Clinic

● **81.6　Other procedures on spine**
　　Note: Number of vertebrae
　　The vertebral spine consists of 25 vertebrae in the
　　　　following order and number:
　　　　Cervical: C1 (atlas), C2 (axis), C3, C4, C5, C6, C7
　　　　Thoracic or Dorsal: T1, T2, T3, T4, T5, T6, T7, T8,
　　　　　　T9, T10, T11, T12
　　　　Lumbar and Sacral: L1, L2, L3, L4, L5, S1
　　Coders should report only one code from the series
　　　　81.62 or 81.63 or 81.64 to show the total number
　　　　of vertebrae fused on the patient.
　　Code also the level and approach of the fusion or
　　　　refusion (81.00–81.08, 81.30–81.39)

　81.62　Fusion or refusion of 2–3 vertebrae
　　　　Coding Clinic: 2009, Q2, P4; 2008, Q2, P14-15; 2008, Q1, P5-6;
　　　　　2006, Q1, P12-14x2; 2005, Q4, P122-123

　81.63　Fusion or refusion of 4–8 vertebrae
　　　　Coding Clinic: 2007, Q1, P20-21; 2003, Q4, P99-101

　81.64　Fusion or refusion of 9 or more vertebrae

　81.65　Percutaneous vertebroplasty
　　　　Injection of bone void filler (cement)
　　　　　(polymethylmethacrylate) (PMMA) into
　　　　　the diseased or fractured vertebral body
　　　　Excludes　*percutaneous vertebral augmentation*
　　　　　　(81.66)
　　　　Coding Clinic: 2008, Q2, P14-15; 2004, Q4, P125-126; 2002,
　　　　　Q2, P14-15

　81.66　Percutaneous vertebral augmentation
　　　　Insertion of inflatable balloon, bone tamp,
　　　　　or other device displacing (removing)
　　　　　(compacting) bone to create a space (cavity)
　　　　　(void) prior to the injection of bone void
　　　　　filler (cement) (polymethylmethacrylate)
　　　　　(PMMA) or other substance
　　　　Arcuplasty　　　　　　　Skyphoplasty
　　　　Kyphoplasty　　　　　　Spineoplasty
　　　　Excludes　*percutaneous vertebroplasty (81.65)*
　　　　Coding Clinic: 2008, Q2, P15; 2007, Q1, P3-8x2; 2006, Q3, P13;
　　　　　2004, Q4, P125-126; 2002, Q2, P14

● **81.7　Arthroplasty and repair of hand, fingers and wrist**
　　　　Includes　arthroplasty of hand and finger with:
　　　　　　external traction or fixation
　　　　　　graft of bone (chips) or cartilage
　　　　　　internal fixation device or prosthesis
　　　　Excludes　*operations on muscle, tendon and fascia of*
　　　　　　hand (82.01–82.99)

　81.71　Arthroplasty of metacarpophalangeal and
　　　　interphalangeal joint with implant

　81.72　Arthroplasty of metacarpophalangeal and
　　　　interphalangeal joint without implant
　　　　Coding Clinic: 1993, Q1, P28

　81.73　Total wrist replacement

　81.74　Arthroplasty of carpocarpal or carpometacarpal
　　　　joint with implant

　81.75　Arthroplasty of carpocarpal or carpometacarpal
　　　　joint without implant
　　　　Coding Clinic: 1993, Q3, P8

　81.79　Other repair of hand, fingers and wrist

● **81.8　Arthroplasty and repair of shoulder and elbow**
　　　　Includes　arthroplasty of upper limb NEC with:
　　　　　　external traction or fixation
　　　　　　graft of bone (chips) or cartilage
　　　　　　internal fixation device or prosthesis

　81.80　Other ̶Ttotal shoulder replacement ◀▥
　　　　Excludes　*reverse total shoulder replacement*
　　　　　　(81.88) ◀
　　　　Coding Clinic: 2008, Q2, P5-6

　81.81　Partial shoulder replacement

　81.82　Repair of recurrent dislocation of shoulder
　　　　Coding Clinic: 1995, Q3, P15

　81.83　Other repair of shoulder
　　　　~~Revision of arthroplasty of shoulder~~
　　　　Coding Clinic: 2004, Q1, P12; 2002, Q4, P110; Q1, P9-10;
　　　　　2001, Q4, P52; 2000, Q2, P14-15; 1993, Q3, P5

　81.84　Total elbow replacement
　　　　Partial elbow replacement

　81.85　Other repair of elbow

　81.88　Reverse total shoulder replacement ◀
　　　　Reverse ball-and-socket of the shoulder ◀
　　　　Excludes　*conversion of prior (failed) total*
　　　　　　shoulder ◀
　　　　　replacement (arthroplasty) to reverse
　　　　　　total shoulder replacement
　　　　　　(81.97) ◀

● **81.9　Other operations on joint structures**

　81.91　Arthrocentesis
　　　　Joint aspiration
　　　　Excludes　*that for:*
　　　　　　arthrography (88.32)
　　　　　　biopsy of joint structure
　　　　　　　(80.30–80.39)
　　　　　　injection of drug (81.92)

　81.92　Injection of therapeutic substance into joint or
　　　　ligament
　　　　Coding Clinic: 2000, Q2, P14-15; 1989, Q3, P16

　81.93　Suture of capsule or ligament of upper extremity
　　　　Excludes　*that associated with arthroplasty*
　　　　　　(81.71–81.75, 81.80–81.81, 81.84)

　81.94　Suture of capsule or ligament of ankle and foot
　　　　Excludes　*that associated with arthroplasty*
　　　　　　(81.56–81.59)

　81.95　Suture of capsule or ligament of other lower
　　　　extremity
　　　　Excludes　*that associated with arthroplasty*
　　　　　　(81.51–81.55, 81.59)

　81.96　Other repair of joint

　81.97　Revision of joint replacement of upper extremity
　　　　Partial
　　　　Removal of cement spacer
　　　　Revision of arthroplasty of shoulder ◀
　　　　Total
　　　　Coding Clinic: 2004, Q1, P12

　81.98　Other diagnostic procedures on joint structures
　　　　Excludes　*arthroscopy (80.20–80.29)*
　　　　　　biopsy of joint structure (80.30–80.39)
　　　　　　microscopic examination of specimen
　　　　　　　from joint (91.51–91.59)
　　　　　　thermography (88.83)
　　　　　　x-ray (87.21–87.29, 88.21–88.33)

　81.99　Other

● **82　Operations on muscle, tendon, and fascia of hand**
　　　　Includes　operations on:
　　　　　　aponeurosis
　　　　　　synovial membrane (tendon sheath)
　　　　　　tendon sheath

● **82.0　Incision of muscle, tendon, fascia, and bursa of hand**

　82.01　Exploration of tendon sheath of hand
　　　　Incision of tendon sheath of hand
　　　　Removal of rice bodies in tendon sheath of hand
　　　　Excludes　*division of tendon (82.11)*

OPERATIONS ON THE MUSCULOSKELETAL SYSTEM (76–84)

Excludes　　Includes　　Use additional　　Code also　　Omit code

82.02　Myotomy of hand
　　Excludes　myotomy for division (82.19)

82.03　Bursotomy of hand

82.04　Incision and drainage of palmar or thenar space

82.09　Other incision of soft tissue of hand
　　Excludes　incision of skin and subcutaneous tissue alone (86.01–86.09)
　　Coding Clinic: 1987, Nov-Dec, P10

● 82.1　Division of muscle, tendon, and fascia of hand

82.11　Tenotomy of hand
　　Division of tendon of hand

82.12　Fasciotomy of hand
　　Division of fascia of hand

82.19　Other division of soft tissue of hand
　　Division of muscle of hand

● 82.2　Excision of lesion of muscle, tendon, and fascia of hand

82.21　Excision of lesion of tendon sheath of hand
　　Ganglionectomy of tendon sheath (wrist)

82.22　Excision of lesion of muscle of hand

82.29　Excision of other lesion of soft tissue of hand
　　Excludes　excision of lesion of skin and subcutaneous tissue (86.21–86.3)

● 82.3　Other excision of soft tissue of hand
　　Code also　any skin graft (86.61–86.62, 86.73)
　　Excludes　excision of skin and subcutaneous tissue (86.21–86.3)

82.31　Bursectomy of hand

82.32　Excision of tendon of hand for graft

82.33　Other tenonectomy of hand
　　Tenosynovectomy of hand
　　Excludes　excision of lesion of:
　　　　tendon (82.29)
　　　　sheath (82.21)

82.34　Excision of muscle or fascia of hand for graft

82.35　Other fasciectomy of hand
　　Release of Dupuytren's contracture
　　Excludes　excision of lesion of fascia (82.29)

82.36　Other myectomy of hand
　　Excludes　excision of lesion of muscle (82.22)

82.39　Other excision of soft tissue of hand
　　Excludes　excision of skin (86.21–86.3)
　　　　excision of soft tissue lesion (82.29)

● 82.4　Suture of muscle, tendon, and fascia of hand

82.41　Suture of tendon sheath of hand

82.42　Delayed suture of flexor tendon of hand

82.43　Delayed suture of other tendon of hand

82.44　Other suture of flexor tendon of hand
　　Excludes　delayed suture of flexor tendon of hand (82.42)

82.45　Other suture of other tendon of hand
　　Excludes　delayed suture of other tendon of hand (82.43)

82.46　Suture of muscle or fascia of hand

● 82.5　Transplantation of muscle and tendon of hand

82.51　Advancement of tendon of hand

82.52　Recession of tendon of hand

82.53　Reattachment of tendon of hand

82.54　Reattachment of muscle of hand

82.55　Other change in hand muscle or tendon length

82.56　Other hand tendon transfer or transplantation
　　Excludes　pollicization of thumb (82.61)
　　　　transfer of finger, except thumb (82.81)
　　Coding Clinic: 1999, Q2, P10; 1998, Q43, P39-40

82.57　Other hand tendon transposition
　　Coding Clinic: 1993, Q3, P8; Q1, P28

82.58　Other hand muscle transfer or transplantation

82.59　Other hand muscle transposition

● 82.6　Reconstruction of thumb
　　Includes　digital transfer to act as thumb
　　Code also　any amputation for digital transfer (84.01, 84.11)

82.61　Pollicization operation carrying over nerves and blood supply

82.69　Other reconstruction of thumb
　　"Cocked-hat" procedure [skin flap and bone]
　　Grafts:
　　　　bone to thumb skin (pedicle) to thumb

● 82.7　Plastic operation on hand with graft or implant

82.71　Tendon pulley reconstruction
　　Reconstruction for opponensplasty

82.72　Plastic operation on hand with graft of muscle or fascia

82.79　Plastic operation on hand with other graft or implant
　　Tendon graft to hand

● 82.8　Other plastic operations on hand

82.81　Transfer of finger, except thumb
　　Excludes　pollicization of thumb (82.61)
　　Coding Clinic: 2005, Q2, P7

82.82　Repair of cleft hand

82.83　Repair of macrodactyly

82.84　Repair of mallet finger

82.85　Other tenodesis of hand
　　Tendon fixation of hand NOS

82.86　Other tenoplasty of hand
　　Myotenoplasty of hand

82.89　Other plastic operations on hand
　　Plication of fascia
　　Repair of fascial hernia
　　Excludes　that with graft or implant (82.71–82.79)

● 82.9　Other operations on muscle, tendon, and fascia of hand
　　Excludes　diagnostic procedures on soft tissue of hand (83.21–83.29)

82.91　Lysis of adhesions of hand
　　Freeing of adhesions of fascia, muscle, and tendon of hand
　　Excludes　decompression of carpal tunnel (04.43)
　　　　that by stretching or manipulation only (93.26)

82.92　Aspiration of bursa of hand

82.93　Aspiration of other soft tissue of hand
　　Excludes　skin and subcutaneous tissue (86.01)

82.94　Injection of therapeutic substance into bursa of hand

82.95　Injection of therapeutic substance into tendon of hand

82.96　Other injection of locally-acting therapeutic substance into soft tissue of hand
　　Excludes　subcutaneous or intramuscular injection (99.11–99.29)

82.99　Other operations on muscle, tendon, and fascia of hand

● **83 Operations on muscle, tendon, fascia, and bursa, except hand**

> **Includes**   operations on:
>> aponeurosis
>> synovial membrane of bursa and tendon
>>> sheaths
>> tendon sheaths

> **Excludes**   *diaphragm (34.81–34.89)*
>> *hand (82.01–82.99)*
>> *muscles of eye (15.01–15.9)*

● **83.0 Incision of muscle, tendon, fascia, and bursa**

83.01 Exploration of tendon sheath
> Incision of tendon sheath
> Removal of rice bodies from tendon sheath

83.02 Myotomy
> **Excludes**   *cricopharyngeal myotomy (29.31)*
> **Coding Clinic: 2008, Q4, P134-136**

83.03 Bursotomy
> Removal of calcareous deposit of bursa
> **Excludes**   *aspiration of bursa (percutaneous)*
>> *(83.94)*

83.09 Other incision of soft tissue
> Incision of fascia
> **Excludes**   *incision of skin and subcutaneous*
>> *tissue alone (86.01–86.09)*
> **Coding Clinic: 2009, Q1, P15**

● **83.1 Division of muscle, tendon, and fascia**

83.11 Achillotenotomy

83.12 Adductor tenotomy of hip

83.13 Other tenotomy
> Aponeurotomy
> Division of tendon
> Tendon release
> Tendon transection
> Tenotomy for thoracic outlet decompression

83.14 Fasciotomy
> Division of fascia
> Division of iliotibial band
> Fascia stripping
> Release of Volkmann's contracture by
>> fasciotomy
> **Coding Clinic: 2006, Q4, P100-102**

83.19 Other division of soft tissue
> Division of muscle
> Muscle release
> Myotomy for thoracic outlet decompression
> Myotomy with division
> Scalenotomy
> Transection of muscle

● **83.2 Diagnostic procedures on muscle, tendon, fascia, and bursa, including that of hand**

83.21 Open ~~B~~biopsy of soft tissue ◀▥
> **Excludes**   *biopsy of chest wall (34.23)*
>> *closed biopsy of skin and subcutaneous*
>>> *tissue (86.11)* ◀▥

83.29 Other diagnostic procedures on muscle, tendon, fascia, and bursa, including that of hand
> **Excludes**   *microscopic examination of specimen*
>> *(91.51–91.59)*
>> *soft tissue x-ray (87.09, 87.38–87.39,*
>>> *88.09, 88.35, 88.37)*
>> *thermography of muscle (88.84)*

● **83.3 Excision of lesion of muscle, tendon, fascia, and bursa**

> **Excludes**   *biopsy of soft tissue (83.21)*

83.31 Excision of lesion of tendon sheath
> Excision of ganglion of tendon sheath, except
>> of hand

83.32 Excision of lesion of muscle
> Excision of:
>> heterotopic bone
>> muscle scar for release of Volkmann's
>>> contracture
>> myositis ossificans

83.39 Excision of lesion of other soft tissue
> Excision of Baker's cyst
> **Excludes**   *bursectomy (83.5)*
>> *excision of lesion of skin and*
>>> *subcutaneous tissue (86.3)*
>> *synovectomy (80.70–80.79)*
> **Coding Clinic: 2005, Q2, P3-4; 1997, Q2, P6**

● **83.4 Other excision of muscle, tendon, and fascia**

83.41 Excision of tendon for graft

83.42 Other tenonectomy
> Excision of:
>> aponeurosis
>> tendon sheath
> Tenosynovectomy

83.43 Excision of muscle or fascia for graft

83.44 Other fasciectomy

83.45 Other myectomy
> Debridement of muscle NOS
> Scalenectomy
> **Coding Clinic: 1999, Q1, P8-9**

83.49 Other excision of soft tissue

● **83.5 Bursectomy**
> **Coding Clinic: 2006, Q2, P15x2; 1999, Q2, P10-11**

● **83.6 Suture of muscle, tendon, and fascia**

83.61 Suture of tendon sheath

83.62 Delayed suture of tendon

83.63 Rotator cuff repair
> **Coding Clinic: 2006, Q1, P6; 1993, Q2, P8**

83.64 Other suture of tendon
> Achillorrhaphy
> Aponeurorrhaphy
> **Excludes**   *delayed suture of tendon (83.62)*

83.65 Other suture of muscle or fascia
> Repair of diastasis recti

● **83.7 Reconstruction of muscle and tendon**
> **Excludes**   *reconstruction of muscle and tendon associated*
>> *with arthroplasty*

83.71 Advancement of tendon

83.72 Recession of tendon

83.73 Reattachment of tendon

83.74 Reattachment of muscle

83.75 Tendon transfer or transplantation

83.76 Other tendon transposition

83.77 Muscle transfer or transplantation
> Release of Volkmann's contracture by muscle
>> transplantation

83.79 Other muscle transposition

OPERATIONS ON THE MUSCULOSKELETAL SYSTEM (76-84)

● **83.8 Other plastic operations on muscle, tendon, and fascia**

> **Excludes** | *plastic operations on muscle, tendon, and fascia associated with arthroplasty*

83.81 Tendon graft

83.82 Graft of muscle or fascia
Coding Clinic: 2010, Q1, P14; 2001, Q3, P9

83.83 Tendon pulley reconstruction

83.84 Release of clubfoot, not elsewhere classified
Evans operation on clubfoot

83.85 Other change in muscle or tendon length
Hamstring lengthening
Heel cord shortening
Plastic achillotenotomy
Tendon plication

83.86 Quadricepsplasty

83.87 Other plastic operations on muscle
Musculoplasty
Myoplasty
Coding Clinic: 1997, Q1, P9-10

83.88 Other plastic operations on tendon
Myotenoplasty
Tendon fixation
Tenodesis
Tenoplasty

83.89 Other plastic operations on fascia
Fascia lengthening
Fascioplasty
Plication of fascia

● **83.9 Other operations on muscle, tendon, fascia, and bursa**

> **Excludes** | *nonoperative:*
> *manipulation (93.25–93.29)*
> *stretching (93.27–93.29)*

83.91 Lysis of adhesions of muscle, tendon, fascia, and bursa

> **Excludes** | *that for tarsal tunnel syndrome (04.44)*

83.92 Insertion or replacement of skeletal muscle stimulator
Implantation, insertion, placement, or replacement of skeletal muscle:
electrodes
stimulator
Coding Clinic: 1999, Q2, P10

83.93 Removal of skeletal muscle stimulator

83.94 Aspiration of bursa

83.95 Aspiration of other soft tissue

> **Excludes** | *that of skin and subcutaneous tissue (86.01)*

83.96 Injection of therapeutic substance into bursa

83.97 Injection of therapeutic substance into tendon

83.98 Injection of locally-acting therapeutic substance into other soft tissue

> **Excludes** | *subcutaneous or intramuscular injection (99.11–99.29)*

Coding Clinic: 2006, Q2, P11

83.99 Other operations on muscle, tendon, fascia, and bursa
Suture of bursa

● **84 Other procedures on musculoskeletal system**

● **84.0 Amputation of upper limb**

> **Excludes** | *revision of amputation stump (84.3)*

84.00 Upper limb amputation, not otherwise specified
Closed flap amputation of upper limb NOS
Kineplastic amputation of upper limb NOS
Open or guillotine amputation of upper limb NOS
Revision of current traumatic amputation of upper limb NOS

84.01 Amputation and disarticulation of finger

> **Excludes** | *ligation of supernumerary finger (86.26)*

84.02 Amputation and disarticulation of thumb

84.03 Amputation through hand
Amputation through carpals

84.04 Disarticulation of wrist

84.05 Amputation through forearm
Forearm amputation

84.06 Disarticulation of elbow

84.07 Amputation through humerus
Upper arm amputation

84.08 Disarticulation of shoulder

84.09 Interthoracoscapular amputation
Forequarter amputation

● **84.1 Amputation of lower limb**

> **Excludes** | *revision of amputation stump (84.3)*

84.10 Lower limb amputation, not otherwise specified
Closed flap amputation of lower limb NOS
Kineplastic amputation of lower limb NOS
Open or guillotine amputation of lower limb NOS
Revision of current traumatic amputation of lower limb NOS

84.11 Amputation of toe
Amputation through metatarsophalangeal joint
Disarticulation of toe
Metatarsal head amputation
Ray amputation of foot (disarticulation of the metatarsal head of the toe extending across the forefoot just proximal to the metatarsophalangeal crease)

> **Excludes** | *ligation of supernumerary toe (86.26)*

Coding Clinic: 2005, Q2, P7

84.12 Amputation through foot
Amputation of forefoot
Amputation through middle of foot
Chopart's amputation
Midtarsal amputation
Transmetatarsal amputation (amputation of the forefoot, including all the toes)

> **Excludes** | *ray amputation of foot (84.11)*

84.13 Disarticulation of ankle

84.14 Amputation of ankle through malleoli of tibia and fibula

84.15 Other amputation below knee
Amputation of leg through tibia and fibula NOS

84.16 Disarticulation of knee
Batch, Spitler, and McFaddin amputation
Mazet amputation
S.P. Roger's amputation

84.17 **Amputation above knee**
Amputation of leg through femur
Amputation of thigh
Conversion of below-knee amputation into
above-knee amputation
Supracondylar above-knee amputation
Coding Clinic: 2005, Q1, P16; 2003, Q3, P14-15; 1995, Q1, P10;
1988, Q4, P12

84.18 **Disarticulation of hip**

84.19 **Abdominopelvic amputation**
Hemipelvectomy
Hindquarter amputation

● 84.2 **Reattachment of extremity**

84.21 **Thumb reattachment**

84.22 **Finger reattachment**

84.23 **Forearm, wrist, or hand reattachment**

84.24 **Upper arm reattachment**
Reattachment of arm NOS

84.25 **Toe reattachment**

84.26 **Foot reattachment**

84.27 **Lower leg or ankle reattachment**
Reattachment of leg NOS
Coding Clinic: 1995, Q1, P8

84.28 **Thigh reattachment**

84.29 **Other reattachment**

84.3 **Revision of amputation stump**
Reamputation of stump
Secondary closure of stump
Trimming of stump

| **Excludes** | *revision of current traumatic amputation [revision by further amputation of current injury] (84.00–84.19, 84.91)* |

Coding Clinic: 2005, Q1, P14,16; 1999, Q4, P15; 1998, Q4, P12; Q2, P15

● 84.4 **Implantation or fitting of prosthetic limb device**

84.40 **Implantation or fitting of prosthetic limb device, not otherwise specified**

84.41 **Fitting of prosthesis of upper arm and shoulder**

84.42 **Fitting of prosthesis of lower arm and hand**

84.43 **Fitting of prosthesis of arm, not otherwise specified**

84.44 **Implantation of prosthetic device of arm**

84.45 **Fitting of prosthesis above knee**

84.46 **Fitting of prosthesis below knee**

84.47 **Fitting of prosthesis of leg, not otherwise specified**

84.48 **Implantation of prosthetic device of leg**

● 84.5 **Implantation of other musculoskeletal devices and substances**

| **Excludes** | *insertion of (non-fusion) spinal disc replacement device (84.60–84.69)* |

84.51 **Insertion of interbody spinal fusion device**
Insertion of: cages (carbon, ceramic, metal, plastic or titanium)
interbody fusion cage
synthetic cages or spacers
threaded bone dowels

Code also refusion of spine (81.30–81.39)

Code also spinal fusion (81.00–81.08)
Coding Clinic: 2008, Q2, P14-15; 2007, Q1, P20-21; 2005, Q4, P122-123; 2004, Q1, P21-22; 2003, Q2, P20; 2002, Q4, P108-110

84.52 **Insertion of recombinant bone morphogenetic protein rhBMP**
That via collagen sponge, coral, ceramic and other carriers

Code also primary procedure performed:
fracture repair (79.00–79.99)
spinal fusion (81.00–81.08)
spinal refusion (81.30–81.39)
Coding Clinic: 2009, Q2, P3; 2006, Q1, P13-14; 2002, Q4, P110-111

84.53 **Implantation of internal limb lengthening device with kinetic distraction**

Code also limb lengthening procedure (78.30–78.39)
Coding Clinic: 2004, Q4, P127

84.54 **Implantation of other internal limb lengthening device**
Implantation of internal limb lengthening device, Not Otherwise Specified (NOS)

Code also limb lengthening procedure (78.30–78.39)
Coding Clinic: 2004, Q4, P127

84.55 **Insertion of bone void filler**
Insertion of:
acrylic cement (PMMA)
bone void cement
calcium based bone void filler
polymethylmethacrylate (PMMA)

| **Excludes** | *that with percutaneous vertebral augmentation (81.66)*
that with percutaneous vertebroplasty (81.65) |

Coding Clinic: 2004, Q4, P128-129

84.56 **Insertion or replacement of (cement) spacer**
Insertion or replacement of joint (methylmethacrylate) spacer
Coding Clinic: 2008, Q2, P3-4; 2005, Q4, P124-125

84.57 **Removal of (cement) spacer**
Removal of joint (methylmethacrylate) spacer
Coding Clinic: 2008, Q2, P3-6; 2005, Q4, P124-125

84.59 **Insertion of other spinal devices**

| **Excludes** | *initial insertion of pedicle screws with spinal fusion—* omit code
insertion of facet replacement device(s) (84.84)
insertion of interspinous process device(s) (84.80)
insertion of pedicle-based dynamic stabilization device(s) (84.82) |

Coding Clinic: 2007, Q1, P9-10

● 84.6 **Replacement of spinal disc**

| **Includes** | non-fusion arthroplasty of the spine with insertion of artificial disc prosthesis |

84.60 **Insertion of spinal disc prosthesis, not otherwise specified**
Replacement of spinal disc, NOS

| **Includes** | diskectomy (discectomy) |

84.61 **Insertion of partial spinal disc prosthesis, cervical**
Nuclear replacement device, cervical
Partial artificial disc prosthesis (flexible), cervical
Replacement of nuclear disc (nucleus pulposus), cervical

| **Includes** | diskectomy (discectomy) |

| Excludes | **Includes** | Use additional | Code also | Omit code |

OPERATIONS ON THE MUSCULOSKELETAL SYSTEM (76–84)

84.62 Insertion of total spinal disc prosthesis, cervical
Replacement of cervical spinal disc, NOS
Replacement of total spinal disc, cervical
Total artificial disc prosthesis (flexible), cervical
Includes diskectomy (discectomy)

84.63 Insertion of spinal disc prosthesis, thoracic
Artificial disc prosthesis (flexible), thoracic
Replacement of thoracic spinal disc, partial or total
Includes diskectomy (discectomy)

84.64 Insertion of partial spinal disc prosthesis, lumbosacral
Nuclear replacement device, lumbar
Partial artificial disc prosthesis (flexible), lumbar
Replacement of nuclear disc (nucleus pulposus), lumbar
Includes diskectomy (discectomy)

84.65 Insertion of total spinal disc prosthesis, lumbosacral
Replacement of lumbar spinal disc, NOS
Replacement of total spinal disc, lumbar
Total artificial disc prosthesis (flexible), lumbar
Includes diskectomy (discectomy)
Coding Clinic: 2004, Q4, P129-133

84.66 Revision or replacement of artificial spinal disc prosthesis, cervical
Removal of (partial) (total) spinal disc prosthesis with synchronous insertion of new (partial) (total) spinal disc prosthesis, cervical
Repair of previously inserted spinal disc prosthesis, cervical

84.67 Revision or replacement of artificial spinal disc prosthesis, thoracic
Removal of (partial) (total) spinal disc prosthesis with synchronous insertion of new (partial) (total) spinal disc prosthesis, thoracic
Repair of previously inserted spinal disc prosthesis, thoracic

84.68 Revision or replacement of artificial spinal disc prosthesis, lumbosacral
Removal of (partial) (total) spinal disc prosthesis with synchronous insertion of new (partial) (total) spinal disc prosthesis, lumbosacral
Repair of previously inserted spinal disc prosthesis, lumbosacral

84.69 Revision or replacement of artificial spinal disc prosthesis, not otherwise specified
Removal of (partial) (total) spinal disc prosthesis with synchronous insertion of new (partial) (total) spinal disc prosthesis
Repair of previously inserted spinal disc prosthesis

● **84.7 Adjunct codes for external fixator devices**
Code also any primary procedure performed:
application of external fixator device (78.10, 78.12–78.13, 78.15, 78.17–78.19)
reduction of fracture and dislocation (79.00–79.89)

84.71 Application of external fixator device, monoplanar system
Excludes other hybrid device or system (84.73)
ring device or system (84.72)
Coding Clinic: 2005, Q4, P127-129

84.72 Application of external fixator device, ring system
Ilizarov type
Sheffield type
Excludes monoplanar device or system (84.71)
other hybrid device or system (84.73)

84.73 Application of hybrid external fixator device
Computer (assisted) (dependent) external fixator device
Hybrid system using both ring and monoplanar devices
Excludes monoplanar device or system, when used alone (84.71)
ring device or system, when used alone (84.72)

● **84.8 Insertion, replacement and revision of posterior spinal motion preservation device(s)**
Dynamic spinal stabilization device(s)
Includes any synchronous facetectomy (partial, total) performed at the same level
Code also any synchronous surgical decompression (foraminotomy, laminectomy, laminotomy), if performed (03.09)
Excludes fusion of spine (81.00–81.08, 81.30–81.39)
insertion of artificial disc prosthesis (84.60–84.69)
insertion of interbody spinal fusion device (84.51)
Coding Clinic: 2007, Q1, P9

84.80 Insertion or replacement of interspinous process device(s)
Interspinous process decompression device(s)
Interspinous process distraction device(s)
Excludes insertion or replacement of facet replacement device (84.84)
insertion or replacement of pedicle-based dynamic stabilization device (84.82)
Coding Clinic: 2007, Q4, P116-120

84.81 Revision of interspinous process device(s)
Repair of previously inserted interspinous process device(s)
Excludes revision of facet replacement device(s) (84.85)
revision of pedicle-based dynamic stabilization device (84.83)

84.82 Insertion or replacement of pedicle-based dynamic stabilization device(s)
Excludes initial insertion of pedicle screws with spinal fusion — omit code
insertion or replacement of facet replacement device(s) (84.84)
insertion or replacement of interspinous process device(s) (84.80)
replacement of pedicle screws used in spinal fusion (78.59)
Coding Clinic: 2007, Q4, P116-120

◀ New   ◀═ Revised   ~~deleted~~ Deleted   ● Use Additional Digit(s)   **OGCR** Official Guidelines   **Coding Clinic**

84.83 Revision of pedicle-based dynamic stabilization device(s)
Repair of previously inserted pedicle-based dynamic stabilization device(s)

> **Excludes** *removal of pedicle screws used in spinal fusion (78.69)*
> *replacement of pedicle screws used in spinal fusion (78.59)*
> *revision of facet replacement device(s) (84.85)*
> *revision of interspinous process device(s) (84.81)*

84.84 Insertion or replacement of facet replacement device(s)
Facet arthroplasty

> **Excludes** *initial insertion of pedicle screws with spinal fusion — omit code*
> *insertion or replacement of interspinous process device(s) (84.80)*
> *insertion or replacement of pedicle-based dynamic stabilization device(s) (84.82)*
> *replacement of pedicle screws used in spinal fusion (78.59)*

Coding Clinic: 2007, Q4, P116-120

84.85 Revision of facet replacement device(s)
Repair of previously inserted facet replacement device(s)

> **Excludes** *removal of pedicle screws used in spinal fusion (78.69)*
> *replacement of pedicle screws used in spinal fusion (78.59)*
> *revision of interspinous process device(s) (84.81)*
> *revision of pedicle-based dynamic stabilization device(s) (84.83)*

● **84.9 Other operations on musculoskeletal system**

> **Excludes** *nonoperative manipulation (93.25–93.29)*

84.91 Amputation, not otherwise specified

84.92 Separation of equal conjoined twins

84.93 Separation of unequal conjoined twins
Separation of conjoined twins NOS

84.94 Insertion of sternal fixation device with rigid plates ◄

> **Excludes** *insertion of sternal fixation device for internal fixation of fracture (79.39) ◄*
> *internal fixation of bone without fracture reduction (78.59) ◄*

84.99 Other

---

15. OPERATIONS ON THE INTEGUMENTARY SYSTEM (85–86)

● **85 Operations on the breast**

> **Includes** operations on the skin and subcutaneous tissue of:
> breast female or male
> previous mastectomy site female or male
> revision of previous mastectomy site

85.0 Mastotomy
Incision of breast (skin)
Mammotomy

> **Excludes** *aspiration of breast (85.91)*
> *removal of implant (85.94)*

Coding Clinic: 2004, Q1, P3-4; 1990, Q2, P27

● **85.1 Diagnostic procedures on breast**

85.11 Closed [percutaneous] [needle] biopsy of breast
Coding Clinic: 2000, Q2, P10; 1989, Q3, P17

85.12 Open biopsy of breast
Coding Clinic: 1989, Q3, P17; 1986, Mar-April, P11

85.19 Other diagnostic procedures on breast

> **Excludes** *mammary ductogram (87.35)*
> *mammography NEC (87.37)*
> *manual examination (89.36)*
> *microscopic examination of specimen (91.61–91.69)*
> *thermography (88.85)*
> *ultrasonography (88.73)*
> *xerography (87.36)*

● **85.2 Excision or destruction of breast tissue**

> **Excludes** *mastectomy (85.41–85.48)*
> *reduction mammoplasty (85.31–85.32)*

85.20 Excision or destruction of breast tissue, not otherwise specified

> **Excludes** *laser interstitial thermal therapy [LITT] of lesion or tissue of breast under guidance (17.69)*

85.21 Local excision of lesion of breast
Lumpectomy
Removal of area of fibrosis from breast

> **Excludes** *biopsy of breast (85.11–85.12)*

Coding Clinic: 1990, Q2, P27; 1989, Q3, P17; 1985, Sept-Oct, P12

85.22 Resection of quadrant of breast
Coding Clinic: 1985, Sept-Oct, P12

85.23 Subtotal mastectomy

> **Excludes** *quadrant resection (85.22)*

Coding Clinic: 1992, Q2, P7; 1985, Sept-Oct, P12

85.24 Excision of ectopic breast tissue
Excision of accessory nipple

85.25 Excision of nipple

> **Excludes** *excision of accessory nipple (85.24)*

● **85.3 Reduction mammoplasty and subcutaneous mammectomy**
Coding Clinic: 1995, Q4, P79-80

85.31 Unilateral reduction mammoplasty
Unilateral:
amputative mammoplasty
size reduction mammoplasty

85.32 Bilateral reduction mammoplasty
Amputative mammoplasty
Reduction mammoplasty (for gynecomastia)

85.33 Unilateral subcutaneous mammectomy with synchronous implant

> **Excludes** *that without synchronous implant (85.34)*

85.34 Other unilateral subcutaneous mammectomy
Removal of breast tissue with preservation of skin and nipple
Subcutaneous mammectomy NOS

85.35 Bilateral subcutaneous mammectomy with synchronous implant

> **Excludes** *that without synchronous implant (85.36)*

85.36 Other bilateral subcutaneous mammectomy

OPERATIONS ON THE INTEGUMENTARY SYSTEM (85–86)

● **85.4 Mastectomy**

85.41 Unilateral simple mastectomy
Mastectomy:
NOS
complete

85.42 Bilateral simple mastectomy
Bilateral complete mastectomy

85.43 Unilateral extended simple mastectomy
Extended simple mastectomy NOS
Modified radical mastectomy
Simple mastectomy with excision of regional
lymph nodes
Coding Clinic: 1984, May-June, P11

85.44 Bilateral extended simple mastectomy

85.45 Unilateral radical mastectomy
Excision of breast, pectoral muscles, and
regional lymph nodes [axillary, clavicular,
supraclavicular]
Radical mastectomy NOS

85.46 Bilateral radical mastectomy

85.47 Unilateral extended radical mastectomy
Excision of breast, muscles, and lymph nodes
[axillary, clavicular, supraclavicular,
internal mammary, and mediastinal]
Extended radical mastectomy NOS

85.48 Bilateral extended radical mastectomy

● **85.5 Augmentation mammoplasty**
Excludes *that associated with subcutaneous
mammectomy (85.33, 85.35)*
Coding Clinic: 1995, Q4, P80

**85.50 Augmentation mammoplasty, not otherwise
specified**

85.51 Unilateral injection into breast for augmentation
Excludes *injection of fat graft of breast (85.55) ◄*
Coding Clinic: 1997, Q3, P13

85.52 Bilateral injection into breast for augmentation
Injection into breast for augmentation NOS
Excludes *injection of fat graft of breast (85.55) ◄*

85.53 Unilateral breast implant
Coding Clinic: 2000, Q2, P18; 1998, Q2, P14

85.54 Bilateral breast implant
Breast implant NOS

85.55 Fat graft to breast ◄
Autologous fat transplantation or transfer ◄
Fat graft to breast NOS ◄
Fat graft to breast with or without use of
enriched graft ◄
Micro-fat grafting ◄
Includes extraction of fat for autologous
graft ◄
Excludes *that with reconstruction of breast
(85.70–85.79) ◄*

85.6 Mastopexy

● **85.7 Total reconstruction of breast**
Coding Clinic: 2008, Q4, P185-187; 1993, Q1, P27-28

**85.70 Total reconstruction of breast, not otherwise
specified**
Perforator flap, free

85.71 Latissimus dorsi myocutaneous flap

**85.72 Transverse rectus abdominis myocutaneous
(TRAM) flap, pedicled**
Excludes *transverse rectus abdominis
myocutaneous (TRAM) flap,
free (85.73)*

**85.73 Transverse rectus abdominis myocutaneous
(TRAM) flap, free**
Excludes *transverse rectus abdominis
myocutaneous (TRAM) flap,
pedicled (85.72)*

**85.74 Deep inferior epigastric artery perforator (DIEP)
flap, free**

**85.75 Superficial inferior epigastric artery (SIEA) flap,
free**

85.76 Gluteal artery perforator (GAP) flap, free

85.79 Other total reconstruction of breast
Excludes *deep inferior epigastric artery
perforator (DIEP) flap, free
(85.74)*
*gluteal artery perforator (GAP) flap,
free (85.76)*
*latissimus dorsi myocutaneous flap
(85.71)*
perforator flap, free (85.70)
*superficial inferior epigastric artery
(SIEA) flap, free (85.75)*
*total reconstruction of breast, not
otherwise specified (85.70)*
*transverse rectus abdominis
myocutaneous (TRAM) flap, free
(85.73)*
*transverse rectus abdominis
myocutaneous (TRAM) flap,
pedicled (85.72)*

● **85.8 Other repair and plastic operations on breast**
Excludes *that for:*
augmentation (85.50–85.54)
reconstruction (85.70–85.76, 85.79)
reduction (85.31–85.32)

85.81 Suture of laceration of breast

85.82 Split-thickness graft to breast

85.83 Full-thickness graft to breast

85.84 Pedicle graft to breast

85.85 Muscle flap graft to breast

85.86 Transposition of nipple
Coding Clinic: 1995, Q4, P79-80

85.87 Other repair or reconstruction of nipple

85.89 Other mammoplasty

● **85.9 Other operations on the breast**

85.91 Aspiration of breast
Excludes *percutaneous biopsy of breast (85.11)*

85.92 Injection of therapeutic agent into breast
Excludes *that for augmentation of breast
(85.51–85.52, 85.55) ◄*

85.93 Revision of implant of breast
Coding Clinic: 1998, Q2, P14

85.94 Removal of implant of breast
Coding Clinic: 1998, Q2, P14; 1992, Q3, P4-5

85.95 Insertion of breast tissue expander
Insertion (soft tissue) of tissue expander (one
or more) under muscle or platysma to
develop skin flaps for donor use

85.96 Removal of breast tissue expander
Coding Clinic: 2000, Q2, P18

85.99 Other
Coding Clinic: 1986, Nov-Dec, P9

◄ New　◄▦ Revised　~~deleted~~ Deleted　● Use Additional Digit(s)　OGCR Official Guidelines　Coding Clinic

● **86**   **Operations on skin and subcutaneous tissue**

   Includes   operations on:
       hair follicles
       male perineum
       nails
       sebaceous glands
       subcutaneous fat pads
       sudoriferous glands
       superficial fossae

   Excludes   *those on skin of:*
       anus (49.01–49.99)
       breast (mastectomy site) (85.0–85.99)
       ear (18.01–18.9)
       eyebrow (08.01–08.99)
       eyelid (08.01–08.99)
       female perineum (71.01–71.9)
       lips (27.0–27.99)
       nose (21.00–21.99)
       penis (64.0–64.99)
       scrotum (61.0–61.99)
       vulva (71.01–71.9)

● **86.0**   **Incision of skin and subcutaneous tissue**

   86.01   **Aspiration of skin and subcutaneous tissue**
     Aspiration of:
       abscess of nail, skin, or subcutaneous tissue
       hematoma of nail, skin, or subcutaneous tissue
       seroma of nail, skin, or subcutaneous tissue
     Coding Clinic: 1989, Q3, P16

   86.02   **Injection or tattooing of skin lesion or defect**
     Injection of filling material
     Insertion of filling material
     Pigmenting of skin of filling material

   86.03   **Incision of pilonidal sinus or cyst**
     Excludes   *marsupialization (86.21)*

   86.04   **Other incision with drainage of skin and subcutaneous tissue**
     Excludes   *drainage of:*
       fascial compartments of face and mouth (27.0)
       palmar or thenar space (82.04)
       pilonidal sinus or cyst (86.03)
     Coding Clinic: 2009, Q1, P15; 2008, Q3, P8-9; 2004, Q4, P75-76

   86.05   **Incision with removal of foreign body or device from skin and subcutaneous tissue**
     Removal of carotid sinus baroreflex activation device
     Removal of loop recorder
     Removal of neurostimulator pulse generator (single array, dual array)
     Removal of tissue expander(s) from skin or soft tissue other than breast tissue
     Excludes   *removal of foreign body without incision (98.20–98.29)*
     Coding Clinic: 1992, Q3, P9; 1986, Nov-Dec, P9

   86.06   **Insertion of totally implantable infusion pump**
     Code also any associated catheterization
     Excludes   *insertion of totally implantable vascular access device (86.07)*
     Coding Clinic: 1999, Q2, P4; 1993, 5th Issue, P11; 1988, Q1, P8

   86.07   **Insertion of totally implantable vascular access device [VAD]**
     Totally implanted port
     Excludes   *insertion of totally implantable infusion pump (86.06)*
     Coding Clinic: 2001, Q1, P13-14; 1996, Q1, P5-6x2; 1994, Q2, P11; 1993, 5th Issue, P11

   86.09   **Other incision of skin and subcutaneous tissue**
     Creation of thalamic stimulator pulse generator pocket, new site
     Escharotomy
     Exploration:
       sinus tract, skin
       superficial fossa
     Relocation of subcutaneous device pocket NEC
     Reopening subcutaneous pocket for device revision without replacement
     Undercutting of hair follicle
     Excludes   *creation of loop recorder pocket, new site, and insertion/relocation of device (37.79)*
       creation of pocket for implantable, patient-activated cardiac event recorder and insertion/relocation of device (37.79)
       removal of catheter from cranial cavity (01.27)
       that for drainage (86.04)
       that of:
         cardiac pacemaker pocket, new site (37.79)
         fascial compartments of face and mouth (27.0)
     Coding Clinic: 2005, Q1, P17; 2004, Q2, P3, 7-8x2; 1999, Q4, P21; 1995, Q3, P14; 1993, 5th Issue, P11; 1989, Q3, P17; 1985, July-Aug, P11; 1985, Mar-April, P15; 1984, May-June, P11, 14

● **86.1**   **Diagnostic procedures on skin and subcutaneous tissue**

   86.11   **Closed ~~B~~biopsy of skin and subcutaneous tissue** ◄▥
     Coding Clinic: 2008, Q4, P97-100

   86.19   **Other diagnostic procedures on skin and subcutaneous tissue**
     Excludes   *microscopic examination of specimen from skin and subcutaneous tissue (91.61–91.79)*

● **86.2**   **Excision or destruction of lesion or tissue of skin and subcutaneous tissue**

   86.21   **Excision of pilonidal cyst or sinus**
     Marsupialization of cyst
     Excludes   *incision of pilonidal cyst or sinus (86.03)*

   86.22   **Excisional debridement of wound, infection, or burn**
     Removal by excision of:
       devitalized tissue
       necrosis
       slough
     Excludes   *debridement of:*
       abdominal wall (wound) (54.3)
       bone (77.60–77.69)
       muscle (83.45)
         of hand (82.36)
       nail (bed) (fold) (86.27)
       nonexcisional debridement of wound, infection, or burn (86.28)
       open fracture site (79.60–79.69)
       pedicle or flap graft (86.75)
     Coding Clinic: 2008, Q3, P8-9; Q1, P3-4; 2006, Q3, P19-20; Q2, P11; 2005, Q2, P3-4; 2004, Q4, P138-139; Q2, P5; 2002, Q3, P23; Q1, P14-15; 2000, Q2, P9; 1999, Q1, P8-9; 1998, Q2, P15; 1995, Q3, P12; 1992, Q2, P17; 1991, Q3, P18-19; Q2, P18-19; 1989, Q3, P16

   Excludes   **Includes**   Use additional   Code also   Omit code

OGCR Section I.C.17.d

Excisional debridement involves surgical removal or cutting away, as opposed to a mechanical (brushing, scrubbing, washing) debridement. For coding purposes, excisional debridement is assigned to code 86.22. Nonexcisional debridement is assigned to code 86.28.

86.23　Removal of nail, nail bed, or nail fold

86.24　Chemosurgery of skin
Chemical peel of skin

86.25　Dermabrasion
That with laser

> Excludes | *dermabrasion of wound to remove embedded debris (86.28)*

86.26　Ligation of dermal appendage

> Excludes | *excision of preauricular appendage (18.29)*

86.27　Debridement of nail, nail bed, or nail fold
Removal of:
　necrosis
　slough

> Excludes | *removal of nail, nail bed, or nail fold (86.23)*

86.28　Nonexcisional debridement of wound, infection or burn
Debridement NOS
Maggot therapy
Removal of devitalized tissue, necrosis, and slough by such methods as:
　brushing
　irrigation (under pressure)
　scrubbing
　washing
Water scalpel (jet)
Coding Clinic: 2009, Q3, P13x3; 2007, Q1, P10-11; 2005, Q1, P14-15; 2004, Q2, P5,6; 2003, Q2, P15; 2002, Q3, P23; 2001, Q2, P18; 1991, Q3, P18-19; Q2, P18-19

OGCR Section I.C.17.d

Excisional debridement involves surgical removal or cutting away, as opposed to a mechanical (brushing, scrubbing, washing) debridement. For coding purposes, excisional debridement is assigned to code 86.22. Nonexcisional debridement is assigned to code 86.28.

86.3　Other local excision or destruction of lesion or tissue of skin and subcutaneous tissue
Destruction of skin by:
　cauterization cryosurgery
　fulguration
　laser beam
That with Z-plasty

> Excludes | *adipectomy (86.83)*
> *biopsy of skin (86.11)*
> *wide or radical excision of skin (86.4)*
> *Z-plasty without excision (86.84)*

Coding Clinic: 1996, Q1, P9; 1995, Q3, P14; 1990, Q2, P27; 1989, Q1, P12

86.4　Radical excision of skin lesion
Wide excision of skin lesion involving underlying or adjacent structure

> Code also any lymph node dissection (40.3–40.5)

●**86.5　Suture or other closure of skin and subcutaneous tissue**

86.51　Replantation of scalp

86.59　Closure of skin and subcutaneous tissue of other sites
Adhesives (surgical) (tissue)
Staples
Sutures

> Excludes | *application of adhesive strips (butterfly) — omit code*

●**86.6　Free skin graft**

> Includes | excision of skin for autogenous graft
> Excludes | *construction or reconstruction of:*
> *penis (64.43–64.44)*
> *trachea (31.75)*
> *vagina (70.61–70.64)*

86.60　Free skin graft, not otherwise specified

86.61　Full-thickness skin graft to hand

> Excludes | *heterograft (86.65)*
> *homograft (86.66)*

86.62　Other skin graft to hand

> Excludes | *heterograft (86.65)*
> *homograft (86.66)*

86.63　Full-thickness skin graft to other sites

> Excludes | *heterograft (86.65)*
> *homograft (86.66)*

86.64　Hair transplant

> Excludes | *hair follicle transplant to eyebrow or eyelash (08.63)*

86.65　Heterograft to skin
Pigskin graft
Porcine graft

> Excludes | *application of dressing only (93.57)*

Coding Clinic: 2002, Q3, P23

86.66　Homograft to skin
Graft to skin of:
　amnionic membrane from donor skin from donor

86.67　Dermal regenerative graft
Artificial skin, NOS
Creation of "neodermis"
Decellularized allodermis
Integumentary matrix implants
Prosthetic implant of dermal layer of skin
Regenerate dermal layer of skin

> Excludes | *heterograft to skin (86.65)*
> *homograft to skin (86.66)*

Coding Clinic: 2006, Q3, P19-20; 1998, Q43, P77-79

86.69　Other skin graft to other sites

> Excludes | *heterograft (86.65)*
> *homograft (86.66)*

Coding Clinic: 2010, Q1, P14; 1999, Q4, P15; 1998, Q43, P77-79

●**86.7　Pedicle grafts or flaps**

> Excludes | *construction or reconstruction of:*
> *penis (64.43–64.44)*
> *trachea (31.75)*
> *vagina (70.61–70.64)*

86.70　Pedicle or flap graft, not otherwise specified

86.71　Cutting and preparation of pedicle grafts or flaps
Elevation of pedicle from its bed
Flap design and raising
Partial cutting of pedicle or tube
Pedicle delay

> Excludes | *pollicization or digital transfer (82.61, 82.81)*
> *revision of pedicle (86.75)*

Coding Clinic: 2001, Q4, P66

86.72　Advancement of pedicle graft
Coding Clinic: 1999, Q3, P9-10

86.73　Attachment of pedicle or flap graft to hand

> Excludes | *pollicization or digital transfer (82.61, 82.81)*

86.74 Attachment of pedicle or flap graft to other sites
Attachment by:
advanced flap
double pedicled flap
pedicle graft
rotating flap
sliding flap
tube graft
Coding Clinic: 1999, Q3, P10; 1996, Q1, P15; 1993, Q2, P11

86.75 Revision of pedicle or flap graft
Debridement of pedicle or flap graft
Defatting of pedicle or flap graft

● **86.8 Other repair and reconstruction of skin and subcutaneous tissue**

86.81 Repair for facial weakness

86.82 Facial rhytidectomy
Face lift
> Excludes | *rhytidectomy of eyelid (08.86–08.87)*

86.83 Size reduction plastic operation
Liposuction
Reduction of adipose tissue of:
abdominal wall (pendulous)
arms (batwing)
buttock
thighs (trochanteric lipomatosis)
> Excludes | *breast (85.31–85.32)*
> *liposuction to harvest fat graft (86.90)* ◄
Coding Clinic: 2006, Q2, P10-11

86.84 Relaxation of scar or web contracture of skin
Z-plasty of skin
> Excludes | *Z-plasty with excision of lesion (86.3)*

86.85 Correction of syndactyly

86.86 Onychoplasty

86.87 Fat graft of skin and subcutaneous tissue ◄
Autologous fat transplantation or transfer ◄
Fat graft NOS ◄
Fat graft of skin and subcutaneous tissue with or without use of enriched graft ◄
Micro-fat grafting ◄
> Includes | extraction of fat for autologous graft ◄
> Excludes | *fat graft to breast (85.55)* ◄

86.89 Other repair and reconstruction of skin and subcutaneous tissue
> Excludes | *mentoplasty (76.67–76.68)*
Coding Clinic: 2002, Q4, P107-108; 2000, Q1, P26; 1998, Q2, P20; 1993, Q2, P11; 1992, Q2, P17

● **86.9 Other operations on skin and subcutaneous tissue**

86.90 Extraction of fat for graft or banking ◄
Harvest of fat for extraction of cells for future use ◄
Liposuction to harvest fat graft ◄
> Excludes | *that with graft at same operative episode (85.55, 86.87)* ◄

86.91 Excision of skin for graft
Excision of skin with closure of donor site
> Excludes | *that with graft at same operative episode (86.60- 86.69)*

86.92 Electrolysis and other epilation of skin
> Excludes | *epilation of eyelid (08.91–08.93)*

86.93 Insertion of tissue expander
Insertion (subcutaneous) (soft tissue) of expander (one or more) in scalp (subgaleal space), face, neck, trunk except breast, and upper and lower extremities for development of skin flaps for donor use
> Excludes | *flap graft preparation (86.71)*
> *tissue expander, breast (85.95)*

86.94 Insertion or replacement of single array neurostimulator pulse generator, not specified as rechargeable
Pulse generator (single array, single channel) for intracranial, spinal, and peripheral neurostimulator
> Code also any associated lead implantation (02.93, 03.93, 04.92)
> Excludes | *cranial implantation or replacement of neurostimulator pulse generator (01.20)* ◄
> *insertion or replacement of single array rechargeable neurostimulator pulse generator (86.97)*
Coding Clinic: 2004, Q4, P133-135

86.95 Insertion or replacement of dual array neurostimulator pulse generator, not specified as rechargeable
Pulse generator (dual array, dual channel) for intracranial, spinal, and peripheral neurostimulator
> Code also any associated lead implantation (02.93, 03.93, 04.92)
> Excludes | *cranial implantation or replacement of neurostimulator pulse generator (01.20)* ◄
> *insertion or replacement of dual array rechargeable neurostimulator pulse generator (86.98)*
Coding Clinic: 2004, Q4, P133-135

86.96 Insertion or replacement of other neurostimulator pulse generator
> Code also any associated lead implantation (02.93, 03.93, 04.92)
> Excludes | *cranial implantation or replacement of neurostimulator pulse generator (01.20)* ◄
> *insertion of dual array neurostimulator pulse generator (86.95, 86.98)*
> *insertion of single array neurostimulator pulse generator (86.94, 86.97)*
Coding Clinic: 2007, Q2, P10-11; 2006, Q2, P5-6; 2004, Q4, P133-135

86.97 Insertion or replacement of single array rechargeable neurostimulator pulse generator
Rechargeable pulse generator (single array, single channel) for intracranial, spinal, and peripheral neurostimulator
> Code also any associated lead implantation (02.93, 03.93, 04.92)
> Excludes | *cranial implantation or replacement of neurostimulator pulse generator (01.20)* ◄
Coding Clinic: 2005, Q4, P130-131

OPERATIONS ON THE INTEGUMENTARY SYSTEM (85–86)

86.98 Insertion or replacement of dual array rechargeable neurostimulator pulse generator
Rechargeable pulse generator (dual array, dual channel) for intracranial, spinal, and peripheral neurostimulator

Code also any associated lead implantation (02.93, 03.93, 04.92)

Excludes cranial implantation or replacement of neurostimulator pulse generator (01.20) ◄
Coding Clinic: 2005, Q4, P130-131

86.99 Other
Excludes removal of sutures from:
abdomen (97.83)
head and neck (97.38)
thorax (97.43)
trunk NEC (97.84)
wound catheter:
irrigation (96.58)
replacement (97.15)

16. MISCELLANEOUS DIAGNOSTIC AND THERAPEUTIC PROCEDURES (87–99)

● **87 Diagnostic Radiology**

● **87.0 Soft tissue x-ray of face, head, and neck**
Excludes angiography (88.40–88.68)

87.01 Pneumoencephalogram

87.02 Other contrast radiogram of brain and skull
Pneumocisternogram
Pneumoventriculogram
Posterior fossa myelogram

87.03 Computerized axial tomography of head
C.A.T. scan of head
Coding Clinic: 2005, Q3, P12-13; 1999, Q3, P7-8

87.04 Other tomography of head

87.05 Contrast dacryocystogram

87.06 Contrast radiogram of nasopharynx

87.07 Contrast laryngogram

87.08 Cervical lymphangiogram

87.09 Other soft tissue x-ray of face, head, and neck
Noncontrast x-ray of:
adenoid
larynx
nasolacrimal duct
nasopharynx
salivary gland
thyroid region
uvula
Excludes x-ray study of eye (95.14)

● **87.1 Other x-ray of face, head, and neck**
Excludes angiography (88.40–88.68)

87.11 Full-mouth x-ray of teeth

87.12 Other dental x-ray
Orthodontic cephalogram or cephalometrics
Panorex examination of mandible
Root canal x-ray

87.13 Temporomandibular contrast arthrogram

87.14 Contrast radiogram of orbit

87.15 Contrast radiogram of sinus

87.16 Other x-ray of facial bones
X-ray of:
frontal area
mandible
maxilla
nasal sinuses
nose
orbit
supraorbital area
symphysis menti
zygomaticomaxillary complex

87.17 Other x-ray of skull
Lateral projection of skull
Sagittal projection
Tangential projection

● **87.2 X-ray of spine**

87.21 Contrast myelogram

87.22 Other x-ray of cervical spine

87.23 Other x-ray of thoracic spine

87.24 Other x-ray of lumbosacral spine
Sacrococcygeal x-ray

87.29 Other x-ray of spine
Spinal x-ray NOS

● **87.3 Soft tissue x-ray of thorax**
Excludes angiocardiography (88.50–88.58)
angiography (88.40–88.68)

87.31 Endotracheal bronchogram

87.32 Other contrast bronchogram
Transcricoid bronchogram

87.33 Mediastinal pneumogram

87.34 Intrathoracic lymphangiogram

87.35 Contrast radiogram of mammary ducts

87.36 Xerography of breast

87.37 Other mammography
Coding Clinic: 1989, Q3, P17

87.38 Sinogram of chest wall
Fistulogram of chest wall

87.39 Other soft tissue x-ray of chest wall

● **87.4 Other x-ray of thorax**
Excludes angiocardiography (88.50–88.58)
angiography (88.40–88.68)

87.41 Computerized axial tomography of thorax
C.A.T. scan of
heart
thorax
Crystal linear scan of x-ray beam of thorax
Electronic subtraction of thorax
Photoelectric response of thorax
Tomography with use of computer, x-rays, and camera of thorax

87.42 Other tomography of thorax
Cardiac tomogram
Excludes C.A.T. scan of heart (87.41)

87.43 X-ray of ribs, sternum, and clavicle
Examination for:
cervical rib
fracture

87.44 Routine chest x-ray, so described
X-ray of chest NOS

OPERATIONS ON THE INTEGUMENTARY SYSTEM (85–86)

◄ New　◄▥ Revised　deleted Deleted　● Use Additional Digit(s)　OGCR Official Guidelines　**Coding Clinic**

87.49 Other chest x-ray
      X-ray of:
         bronchus NOS
         diaphragm NOS
         heart NOS
         lung NOS
         mediastinum NOS
         trachea NOS

● **87.5 Biliary tract x-ray**

   87.51 Percutaneous hepatic cholangiogram
         Coding Clinic: 1990, Q2, P28

   87.52 Intravenous cholangiogram

   87.53 Intraoperative cholangiogram
         Coding Clinic: 1996, Q1, P12-13; Q1, P12-13; 1990, Q2, P28

   87.54 Other cholangiogram
         Coding Clinic: 1988, Q4, P7

   87.59 Other biliary tract x-ray
         Cholecystogram

● **87.6 Other x-ray of digestive system**

   87.61 Barium swallow

   87.62 Upper GI series

   87.63 Small bowel series

   87.64 Lower GI series

   87.65 Other x-ray of intestine

   87.66 Contrast pancreatogram

   87.69 Other digestive tract x-ray

● **87.7 X-ray of urinary system**

   Excludes *angiography of renal vessels (88.45, 88.65)*

   87.71 Computerized axial tomography of kidney
         C.A.T. scan of kidney

   87.72 Other nephrotomogram

   87.73 Intravenous pyelogram
         Diuretic infusion pyelogram

   87.74 Retrograde pyelogram

   87.75 Percutaneous pyelogram

   87.76 Retrograde cystourethrogram

   87.77 Other cystogram

   87.78 Ileal conduitogram

   87.79 Other x-ray of the urinary system
         KUB x-ray

● **87.8 X-ray of female genital organs**

   87.81 X-ray of gravid uterus
         Intrauterine cephalometry by x-ray

   87.82 Gas contrast hysterosalpingogram

   87.83 Opaque dye contrast hysterosalpingogram

   87.84 Percutaneous hysterogram

   87.85 Other x-ray of fallopian tubes and uterus

   87.89 Other x-ray of female genital organs

● **87.9 X-ray of male genital organs**

   87.91 Contrast seminal vesiculogram

   87.92 Other x-ray of prostate and seminal vesicles

   87.93 Contrast epididymogram

   87.94 Contrast vasogram

   87.95 Other x-ray of epididymis and vas deferens

   87.99 Other x-ray of male genital organs

● **88 Other diagnostic radiology and related techniques**

● **88.0 Soft tissue x-ray of abdomen**

   Excludes *angiography (88.40–88.68)*

   88.01 Computerized axial tomography of abdomen
         C.A.T. scan of abdomen

      Excludes *C.A.T. scan of kidney (87.71)*

         Coding Clinic: 1998, Q2, P13

   88.02 Other abdomen tomography

      Excludes *nephrotomogram (87.72)*

   88.03 Sinogram of abdominal wall
         Fistulogram of abdominal wall

   88.04 Abdominal lymphangiogram

   88.09 Other soft tissue x-ray of abdominal wall

● **88.1 Other x-ray of abdomen**

   88.11 Pelvic opaque dye contrast radiography

   88.12 Pelvic gas contrast radiography
         Pelvic pneumoperitoneum

   88.13 Other peritoneal pneumogram

   88.14 Retroperitoneal fistulogram
         Coding Clinic: 1998, Q3, P8-9

   88.15 Retroperitoneal pneumogram

   88.16 Other retroperitoneal x-ray

   88.19 Other x-ray of abdomen
         Flat plate of abdomen
         Coding Clinic: 1999, Q3, P9

● **88.2 Skeletal x-ray of extremities and pelvis**

   Excludes *contrast radiogram of joint (88.32)*

   88.21 Skeletal x-ray of shoulder and upper arm

   88.22 Skeletal x-ray of elbow and forearm

   88.23 Skeletal x-ray of wrist and hand

   88.24 Skeletal x-ray of upper limb, not otherwise specified

   88.25 Pelvimetry

   88.26 Other skeletal x-ray of pelvis and hip

   88.27 Skeletal x-ray of thigh, knee, and lower leg

   88.28 Skeletal x-ray of ankle and foot
         Coding Clinic: 2003, Q4, P110

   88.29 Skeletal x-ray of lower limb, not otherwise specified

● **88.3 Other x-ray**

   88.31 Skeletal series
         X-ray of whole skeleton

   88.32 Contrast arthrogram

      Excludes *that of temporomandibular joint (87.13)*

   88.33 Other skeletal x-ray

      Excludes *skeletal x-ray of:*
            extremities and pelvis (88.21–88.29)
            face, head, and neck (87.11–87.17)
            spine (87.21–87.29)
            thorax (87.43)

   88.34 Lymphangiogram of upper limb

   88.35 Other soft tissue x-ray of upper limb

   88.36 Lymphangiogram of lower limb

   88.37 Other soft tissue x-ray of lower limb

      Excludes *femoral angiography (88.48, 88.66)*

MISCELLANEOUS DIAGNOSTIC AND THERAPEUTIC PROCEDURES (87–99)

88.38 Other computerized axial tomography
C.A.T. scan NOS

> **Excludes** *C.A.T. scan of:*
> *abdomen (88.01)*
> *head (87.03)*
> *heart (87.41)*
> *kidney (87.71)*
> *thorax (87.41)*

Coding Clinic: 2005, Q3, P13-14

88.39 X-ray, other and unspecified

● **88.4 Arteriography using contrast material**

> **Includes** angiography of arteries
> arterial puncture for injection of
> contrast material
> radiography of arteries (by
> fluoroscopy)
> retrograde arteriography

Note: The fourth-digit subclassification identifies the
site to be viewed, not the site of injection.

> **Excludes** *arteriography using:*
> *radioisotopes or radionuclides*
> *(92.01–92.19)*
> *ultrasound (88.71–88.79)*
> *fluorescein angiography of eye (95.12)*

Coding Clinic: 1985, Nov-Dec, P14

**88.40 Arteriography using contrast material,
unspecified site**

88.41 Arteriography of cerebral arteries
Angiography of:
basilar artery
carotid (internal)
posterior cerebral circulation
vertebral artery
Coding Clinic: 2000, Q1, P16; 1999, Q1, P7; 1995, Q2, P12

88.42 Aortography
Arteriography of aorta and aortic arch
Coding Clinic: 1999, Q1, P17

88.43 Arteriography of pulmonary arteries

88.44 Arteriography of other intrathoracic vessels

> **Excludes** *angiocardiography (88.50–88.58)*
> *arteriography of coronary arteries*
> *(88.55–88.57)*

88.45 Arteriography of renal arteries

88.46 Arteriography of placenta
Placentogram using contrast material

88.47 Arteriography of other intra-abdominal arteries
Coding Clinic: 2009, Q2, P7; 2000, Q1, P18-19

**88.48 Arteriography of femoral and other lower
extremity arteries**
Coding Clinic: 2006, Q2, P22-23; 2003, Q3, P10x2; Q1, P17-18;
1996, Q2, P7-8; 1989, Q2, P17

88.49 Arteriography of other specified sites

● **88.5 Angiocardiography using contrast material**

> **Includes** arterial puncture and insertion of arterial
> catheter for injection of contrast
> material
> cineangiocardiography
> selective angiocardiography

> **Code also** synchronous cardiac catheterization
> (37.21–37.23)

> **Excludes** *angiography of pulmonary vessels (88.43,*
> *88.62)*

Coding Clinic: 2008, Q3, P18; 2002, Q3, P20

88.50 Angiocardiography, not otherwise specified

88.51 Angiocardiography of venae cavae
Inferior vena cavography
Phlebography of vena cava (inferior) (superior)

88.52 Angiocardiography of right heart structures
Angiocardiography of:
pulmonary valve
right atrium
right ventricle (outflow tract)

> **Excludes** *intra-operative fluorescence vascular*
> *angiography (88.59)*
> *that combined with left heart*
> *angiocardiography (88.54)*

Coding Clinic: 2008, Q3, P18; 2007, Q1, P16-17

88.53 Angiocardiography of left heart structures
Angiocardiography of:
aortic valve
left atrium
left ventricle (outflow tract)

> **Excludes** *intra-operative fluorescence vascular*
> *angiography (88.59)*
> *that combined with right heart*
> *angiocardiography (88.54)*

Coding Clinic: 2007, Q1, P11-12, 17; 2005, Q4, P69-72; Q3,
P14; 2000, Q1, P20-21

**88.54 Combined right and left heart
angiocardiography**

> **Excludes** *intra-operative fluorescence vascular*
> *angiography (88.59)*

88.55 Coronary arteriography using a single catheter
Coronary arteriography by Sones technique
Direct selective coronary arteriography using a
single catheter

> **Excludes** *intra-operative fluorescence vascular*
> *angiography (88.59)*

Coding Clinic: 2006, Q2, P25-26; 2002, Q3, P20; 1992, Q3,
P10, 17-18

88.56 Coronary arteriography using two catheters
Coronary arteriography by:
Judkins technique
Ricketts and Abrams technique
Direct selective coronary arteriography using
two catheters

> **Excludes** *intra-operative fluorescence vascular*
> *angiography (88.59)*

Coding Clinic: 2006, Q3, P8-9; 2000, Q1, P20-21; 1992, Q3,
P17-18; Q3, P10

88.57 Other and unspecified coronary arteriography
Coronary arteriography NOS

> **Excludes** *intra-operative fluorescence vascular*
> *angiography (88.59)*

Coding Clinic: 2007, Q1, P15-16; 2006, Q2, P25-26; 2005, Q4,
P69-72; Q2, P10; Q3, P14; 2000, Q1, P21; 1992, Q3,
P10, 17-18

88.58 Negative-contrast cardiac roentgenography
Cardiac roentgenography with injection of
carbon dioxide

**88.59 Intra-operative coronary fluorescence vascular
angiography** ◀▥
Intraoperative laser arteriogram (SPY)
SPY arteriogram
SPY arteriography
Coding Clinic: 2007, Q4, P121-122; 2006, Q2, P25-26

● **88.6 Phlebography**

Includes   angiography of veins
             radiography of veins (by fluoroscopy)
             retrograde phlebography
             venipuncture for injection of contrast
                 material
             venography using contrast material

Note: The fourth-digit subclassification (88.60–88.67) identifies the site to be viewed, not the site of injection.

Excludes   *angiography using:*
           radioisotopes or radionuclides (92.01–92.19)
           ultrasound (88.71–88.79)
        fluorescein angiography of eye (95.12)

88.60 Phlebography using contrast material, unspecified site

88.61 Phlebography of veins of head and neck using contrast material

88.62 Phlebography of pulmonary veins using contrast material

88.63 Phlebography of other intrathoracic veins using contrast material
     Coding Clinic: 2008, Q3, P18

88.64 Phlebography of the portal venous system using contrast material
     Splenoportogram (by splenic arteriography)

88.65 Phlebography of other intra-abdominal veins using contrast material
     Coding Clinic: 2000, Q3, P9

88.66 Phlebography of femoral and other lower extremity veins using contrast material
     Coding Clinic: 2006, Q2, P22-23

88.67 Phlebography of other specified sites using contrast material

88.68 Impedance phlebography

● **88.7 Diagnostic ultrasound**

Includes   Echography
            Non-invasive ultrasound
            Ultrasonic angiography
            Ultrasonography

Excludes   *intravascular imaging (adjunctive) (IVUS)*
           (00.21–00.29)
        therapeutic ultrasound (00.01–00.09)

88.71 Diagnostic ultrasound of head and neck
     Determination of midline shift of brain
     Echoencephalography

Excludes   *eye (95.13)*

     Coding Clinic: 2002, Q1, P10-11; 1992, Q1, P11x2

88.72 Diagnostic ultrasound of heart
     Echocardiography
     Transesophageal echocardiography

Excludes   *echocardiography of heart chambers (37.28)*
        intracardiac echocardiography (ICE) (37.28)
        intravascular (IVUS) imaging of coronary vessels (00.24)

     Coding Clinic: 2007, Q1, P11-12; 2005, Q2, P17-18; Q3, P14; 2004, Q4, P121-122; Q1, P16-17; 2000, Q1, P20-21; 1999, Q1, P6; 1998, Q3, P11

88.73 Diagnostic ultrasound of other sites of thorax
     Aortic arch ultrasonography
     Breast ultrasonography
     Lung ultrasonography

88.74 Diagnostic ultrasound of digestive system

88.75 Diagnostic ultrasound of urinary system

88.76 Diagnostic ultrasound of abdomen and retroperitoneum
     Coding Clinic: 1999, Q2, P14

88.77 Diagnostic ultrasound of peripheral vascular system
     Deep vein thrombosis ultrasonic scanning

Excludes   *adjunct vascular system procedures (00.40–00.43)*

     Coding Clinic: 1999, Q4, P17-18; Q1, P13; Q1, P12-13; 1993, 5th Issue, P5; 1992, Q1, P11

88.78 Diagnostic ultrasound of gravid uterus
     Intrauterine cephalometry:
         echo
         ultrasonic
     Placental localization by ultrasound
     Coding Clinic: 2008, Q4, P124-125

88.79 Other diagnostic ultrasound
     Ultrasonography of:
         multiple sites
         nongravid uterus
         total body

● **88.8 Thermography**

88.81 Cerebral thermography

88.82 Ocular thermography

88.83 Bone thermography
     Osteoarticular thermography

88.84 Muscle thermography

88.85 Breast thermography

88.86 Blood vessel thermography
     Deep vein thermography

88.89 Thermography of other sites
     Lymph gland thermography
     Thermography NOS

● **88.9 Other diagnostic imaging**
     Coding Clinic: 2006, Q2, P25-26

88.90 Diagnostic imaging, not elsewhere classified

88.91 Magnetic resonance imaging of brain and brain stem

Excludes   *intraoperative magnetic resonance imaging (88.96)*
        laser interstitial thermal therapy [LITT] of lesion or tissue of brain under guidance (17.61)
        real-time magnetic resonance imaging (88.96)

88.92 Magnetic resonance imaging of chest and myocardium
     For evaluation of hilar and mediastinal lymphadenopathy

Excludes   *laser interstitial thermal therapy [LITT] of lesion or tissue of breast under guidance (17.69)*
        laser interstitial thermal therapy [LITT] of lesion or tissue of lung under guidance (17.69)

MISCELLANEOUS DIAGNOSTIC AND THERAPEUTIC PROCEDURES (87–99)

88.93 Magnetic resonance imaging of spinal canal
Spinal cord levels:
  cervical
  thoracic
  lumbar (lumbosacral)
Spinal cord
Spine

88.94 Magnetic resonance imaging of musculoskeletal
Bone marrow blood supply
Extremities (upper) (lower)

88.95 Magnetic resonance imaging of pelvis, prostate, and bladder

Excludes *laser interstitial thermal therapy [LITT] of lesion or tissue of prostate under guidance (17.69)*

88.96 Other intraoperative magnetic resonance imaging
iMRI
Real-time magnetic resonance imaging
Coding Clinic: 2002, Q4, P111

88.97 Magnetic resonance imaging of other and unspecified sites
Abdomen
Eye orbit
Face
Neck

Excludes *laser interstitial thermal therapy [LITT] of lesion or tissue of other and unspecified site under guidance (17.69)*

88.98 Bone mineral density studies
Dual photon absorptiometry
Quantitative computed tomography (CT) studies
Radiographic densitometry
Single photon absorptiometry

● **89 Interview, evaluation, consultation, and examination**

● **89.0 Diagnostic interview, consultation, and evaluation**

Excludes *psychiatric diagnostic interview (94.11–94.19)*

89.01 Interview and evaluation, described as brief
Abbreviated history and evaluation

89.02 Interview and evaluation, described as limited
Interval history and evaluation

89.03 Interview and evaluation, described as comprehensive
History and evaluation of new problem

89.04 Other interview and evaluation

89.05 Diagnostic interview and evaluation, not otherwise specified

89.06 Consultation, described as limited
Consultation on a single organ system

89.07 Consultation, described as comprehensive

89.08 Other consultation

89.09 Consultation, not otherwise specified

● **89.1 Anatomic and physiologic measurements and manual examinations — nervous system and sense organs**

Excludes *ear examination (95.41–95.49)*
eye examination (95.01–95.26)
the listed procedures when done as part of a general physical examination (89.7)

89.10 Intracarotid amobarbital test
Wada test

89.11 Tonometry

89.12 Nasal function study
Rhinomanometry

89.13 Neurologic examination

89.14 Electroencephalogram

Excludes *that with polysomnogram (89.17)*
Coding Clinic: 2005, Q3, P12-13

89.15 Other nonoperative neurologic function tests
Coding Clinic: 1995, Q3, P5-6; 1991, Q1, P14; 1987, Jan-Feb, P15-16

89.16 Transillumination of newborn skull

89.17 Polysomnogram
Sleep recording

89.18 Other sleep disorder function tests
Multiple sleep latency test [MSLT]

89.19 Video and radio-telemetered electroencephalographic monitoring
Radiographic EEG monitoring
Video EEG monitoring
Coding Clinic: 1992, Q1, P17; 1991, Q1, P14

● **89.2 Anatomic and physiologic measurements and manual examinations — genitourinary system**

Excludes *the listed procedures when done as part of a general physical examination (89.7)*

89.21 Urinary manometry
Manometry through:
  indwelling ureteral catheter
  nephrostomy
  pyelostomy
  ureterostomy

89.22 Cystometrogram
Coding Clinic: 1990, Q2, P27

89.23 Urethral sphincter electromyogram
Coding Clinic: 1990, Q2, P27

89.24 Uroflowmetry [UFR]
Coding Clinic: 1990, Q2, P27

89.25 Urethral pressure profile [UPP]
Coding Clinic: 1990, Q2, P27

89.26 Gynecological examination
Pelvic examination

89.29 Other nonoperative genitourinary system measurements
Bioassay of urine
Renal clearance
Urine chemistry

● **89.3 Other anatomic and physiologic measurements and manual examinations**

Excludes *the listed procedures when done as part of a general physical examination (89.7)*

89.31 Dental examination
Oral mucosal survey
Periodontal survey

89.32 Esophageal manometry
Coding Clinic: 1996, Q3, P13

89.33 Digital examination of enterostomy stoma
Digital examination of colostomy stoma

MISCELLANEOUS DIAGNOSTIC AND THERAPEUTIC PROCEDURES (87–99)

89.34 Digital examination of rectum

89.35 Transillumination of nasal sinuses

89.36 Manual examination of breast

89.37 Vital capacity determination

> Excludes | *endoscopic pulmonary airway flow measurement (33.72)*

89.38 Other nonoperative respiratory measurements
Plethysmography for measurement of respiratory function
Thoracic impedance plethysmography

> Excludes | *endoscopic pulmonary airway flow measurement (33.72)*

89.39 Other nonoperative measurements and examinations
14 C-Urea breath test
Basal metabolic rate [BMR]
Gastric:
  analysis
  function NEC

> Excludes | *body measurement (93.07)*
> *cardiac tests (89.41–89.69)*
> *fundus photography (95.11)*
> *limb length measurement (93.06)*
Coding Clinic: 2001, Q2, P9-11; 2000, Q3, P9; 1996, Q3, P12-13; 1994, Q1, P18

● **89.4 Cardiac stress tests, pacemaker and defibrillator checks**

89.41 Cardiovascular stress test using treadmill
Coding Clinic: 1988, Q1, P11

89.42 Masters' two-step stress test
Coding Clinic: 1988, Q1, P11

89.43 Cardiovascular stress test using bicycle ergometer
Coding Clinic: 1988, Q1, P11

89.44 Other cardiovascular stress test
Thallium stress test with or without transesophageal pacing

89.45 Artificial pacemaker rate check
Artificial pacemaker function check NOS
Bedside device check of pacemaker or cardiac resynchronization pacemaker [CRT-P]
Interrogation only without arrhythmia induction

> Excludes | *catheter based invasive electrophysiologic testing (37.26)*
> *noninvasive programmed electrical stimulation [NIPS] (arrhythmia induction) (37.20)*
Coding Clinic: 2002, Q1, P3

89.46 Artificial pacemaker artifact wave form check

89.47 Artificial pacemaker electrode impedance check

89.48 Artificial pacemaker voltage or amperage threshold check

89.49 Automatic implantable cardioverter/defibrillator (AICD) check
Bedside check of an AICD or cardiac resynchronization defibrillator [CRT-D]
Checking pacing thresholds of device
Interrogation only without arrhythmia induction

> Excludes | *catheter based invasive electrophysiologic testing (37.26)*
> *noninvasive programmed electrical stimulation [NIPS] (arrhythmia induction) (37.20)*
Coding Clinic: 2004, Q4, P135-136; 2002, Q1, P9

● **89.5 Other nonoperative cardiac and vascular diagnostic procedures**

> Excludes | *fetal EKG (75.32)*
Coding Clinic: 1984, July-Aug, P19

89.50 Ambulatory cardiac monitoring
Analog devices [Holter-type]
Coding Clinic: 1999, Q4, P21

89.51 Rhythm electrocardiogram
Rhythm EKG (with one to three leads)

89.52 Electrocardiogram
ECG NOS
EKG (with 12 or more leads)
Coding Clinic: 1988, Q1, P11

89.53 Vectorcardiogram (with ECG)

89.54 Electrographic monitoring
Telemetry

> Excludes | *ambulatory cardiac monitoring (89.50)*
> *electrographic monitoring during surgery — omit code*
Coding Clinic: 1988, Q1, P11; 1984, Nov-Dec, P12

89.55 Phonocardiogram with ECG lead

89.56 Carotid pulse tracing with ECG lead

> Excludes | *oculoplethysmography (89.58)*

89.57 Apexcardiogram (with ECG lead)
Coding Clinic: 1987, Jan-Feb, P15-16

89.58 Plethysmogram
Penile plethysmography with nerve stimulation

> Excludes | *plethysmography (for):*
> *measurement of respiratory function (89.38)*
> *thoracic impedance (89.38)*

89.59 Other nonoperative cardiac and vascular measurements
Coding Clinic: 2005, Q3, P21; 2004, Q4, P135-136; 2003, Q3, P23; 1992, Q2, P12

● **89.6 Circulatory monitoring**

> Excludes | *electrocardiographic monitoring during surgery — omit code*
> *implantation or replacement of subcutaneous device for intracardiac hemodynamic monitoring (00.57)*
> *insertion or replacement of implantable pressure sensor (lead) for intracardiac hemodynamic monitoring (00.56)*
Coding Clinic: 1984, July-Aug, P19

89.60 Continuous intra-arterial blood gas monitoring
Insertion of blood gas monitoring system and continuous monitoring of blood gases through an intra-arterial sensor
Coding Clinic: 2002, Q4, P111-112

89.61 Systemic arterial pressure monitoring

> Excludes | *intra-aneurysm sac pressure monitoring (intraoperative) (00.58)*
> *intravascular pressure measurement of intrathoracic arteries (00.67)*
> *intravascular pressure measurement of peripheral arteries (00.68)*

89.62 Central venous pressure monitoring

> Excludes | *intravascular pressure measurement, other specified and unspecified vessels (00.69)*

89.63 Pulmonary artery pressure monitoring

> Excludes | *pulmonary artery wedge monitoring (89.64)*
Coding Clinic: 1984, Nov-Dec, P19

MISCELLANEOUS DIAGNOSTIC AND THERAPEUTIC PROCEDURES (87–99)

89.64 Pulmonary artery wedge monitoring
Pulmonary capillary wedge [PCW] monitoring
Swan-Ganz catheterization
Coding Clinic: 1984, Nov-Dec, P19; July-Aug, P19

89.65 Measurement of systemic arterial blood gases
Excludes *continuous intra-arterial blood gas monitoring (89.60)*

89.66 Measurement of mixed venous blood gases

89.67 Monitoring of cardiac output by oxygen consumption technique
Fick method

89.68 Monitoring of cardiac output by other technique
Cardiac output monitor by thermodilution indicator

89.69 Monitoring of coronary blood flow
Coronary blood flow monitoring by coincidence counting technique
Excludes *intravascular pressure measurement of coronary arteries (00.59)*

89.7 General physical examination

89.8 Autopsy

● **90 Microscopic examination-I**
The following fourth-digit subclassification is for use with categories in section 90 to identify type of examination:

1 bacterial smear
2 culture
3 culture and sensitivity
4 parasitology
5 toxicology
6 cell block and Papanicolaou smear
9 other microscopic examination

● **90.0 Microscopic examination of specimen from nervous system and of spinal fluid**

● **90.1 Microscopic examination of specimen from endocrine gland, not elsewhere classified**

● **90.2 Microscopic examination of specimen from eye**

● **90.3 Microscopic examination of specimen from ear, nose, throat, and larynx**

● **90.4 Microscopic examination of specimen from trachea, bronchus, pleura, lung, and other thoracic specimen, and of sputum**

● **90.5 Microscopic examination of blood**

● **90.6 Microscopic examination of specimen from spleen and of bone marrow**

● **90.7 Microscopic examination of specimen from lymph node and of lymph**

● **90.8 Microscopic examination of specimen from upper gastrointestinal tract and of vomitus**

● **90.9 Microscopic examination of specimen from lower gastrointestinal tract and of stool**

● **91 Microscopic examination-II**
The following fourth-digit subclassification is for use with categories in section 91 to identify type of examination

1 bacterial smear
2 culture
3 culture and sensitivity
4 parasitology
5 toxicology
6 cell block and Papanicolaou smear
9 other microscopic examination

● **91.0 Microscopic examination of specimen from liver, biliary tract, and pancreas**

● **91.1 Microscopic examination of peritoneal and retroperitoneal specimen**

● **91.2 Microscopic examination of specimen from kidney, ureter, perirenal, and periureteral tissue**

● **91.3 Microscopic examination of specimen from bladder, urethra, prostate, seminal vesicle, perivesical tissue, and of urine and semen**

● **91.4 Microscopic examination of specimen from female genital tract**
Amnionic sac
Fetus

● **91.5 Microscopic examination of specimen from musculoskeletal system and of joint fluid**
Microscopic examination of:

bone	ligament
bursa	muscle
cartilage	synovial membrane
fascia	tendon

● **91.6 Microscopic examination of specimen from skin and other integument**
Microscopic examination of:

hair	skin
nails	

Excludes *mucous membrane — code to organ site that of operative wound (91.71–91.79)*

● **91.7 Microscopic examination of specimen from operative wound**

● **91.8 Microscopic examination of specimen from other site**

● **91.9 Microscopic examination of specimen from unspecified site**

● **92 Nuclear medicine**

● **92.0 Radioisotope scan and function study**

92.01 Thyroid scan and radioisotope function studies
Iodine-131 uptake
Protein-bound iodine
Radio-iodine uptake

92.02 Liver scan and radioisotope function study

92.03 Renal scan and radioisotope function study
Renal clearance study

92.04 Gastrointestinal scan and radioisotope function study
Radio-cobalt B12 Schilling test
Radio-iodinated triolein study

92.05 Cardiovascular and hematopoietic scan and radioisotope function study
Bone marrow scan or function study
Cardiac output scan or function study
Circulation time scan or function study
Radionuclide cardiac ventriculogram scan or function study
Spleen scan or function study
Coding Clinic: 1992, Q2, P7-8; 1988, Q1, P11

92.09 Other radioisotope function studies

● **92.1 Other radioisotope scan**

92.11 Cerebral scan
Pituitary

92.12 Scan of other sites of head
Excludes *eye (95.16)*

92.13 Parathyroid scan

92.14 Bone scan

92.15 Pulmonary scan

92.16 Scan of lymphatic system

92.17 Placental scan

92.18 Total body scan

92.19 Scan of other sites

◀ New ◀▥ Revised ~~deleted~~ Deleted ● Use Additional Digit(s) **OGCR** Official Guidelines **Coding Clinic**

● **92.2 Therapeutic radiology and nuclear medicine**

| Excludes | *that for:* |

    ablation of pituitary gland (07.64–07.69)
    destruction of chorioretinal lesion
      (14.26–14.27)

92.20 Infusion of liquid brachytherapy radioisotope
    I-125 radioisotope
    Intracavitary brachytherapy

| Includes | removal of radioisotope |

    Coding Clinic: 2005, Q4, P117-119; 2004, Q1, P3-5x2; 2000,
      Q1, P11-12; 1994, Q3, P11; 1994, Q2, P10

92.21 Superficial radiation
    Contact radiation [up to 150 KVP]

92.22 Orthovoltage radiation
    Deep radiation [200–300 KVP]

92.23 Radioisotopic teleradiotherapy
    Teleradiotherapy using:
      cobalt-60
      iodine-125
      radioactive cesium

92.24 Teleradiotherapy using photons
    Megavoltage NOS
    Supervoltage NOS
    Use of:
      Betatron
      linear accelerator

92.25 Teleradiotherapy using electrons
    Beta particles

| Excludes | *intra-operative electron radiation therapy (92.41)* |

92.26 Teleradiotherapy of other particulate radiation
    Neutrons
    Protons NOS

92.27 Implantation or insertion of radioactive elements
    Intravascular brachytherapy

| Code also | incision of site |

| Excludes | *infusion of liquid brachytherapy radioisotope (92.20)* |

    Coding Clinic: 2004, Q1, P3-5

92.28 Injection or instillation of radioisotopes
    Injection or infusion of
      radioimmunoconjugate
    Intracavitary injection or instillation
    Intravenous injection or instillation
    Iodine-131 [I-131] tositumomab
    Radioimmunotherapy
    Ytrium-90 [Y-90] ibritumomab tiuxetan

| Excludes | *infusion of liquid brachytherapy radioisotope (92.20)* |

92.29 Other radiotherapeutic procedure
    Coding Clinic: 2006, Q3, P14-15

● **92.3 Stereotactic radiosurgery**

| Code also | stereotactic head frame application (93.59) |

| Excludes | *stereotactic biopsy* |

92.30 Stereotactic radiosurgery, not otherwise specified

92.31 Single source photon radiosurgery
    High energy x-rays
    Linear accelerator (LINAC)

92.32 Multi-source photon radiosurgery
    Cobalt 60 radiation
    Gamma irradiation

92.33 Particulate radiosurgery
    Particle beam radiation (cyclotron)
    Proton accelerator

92.39 Stereotactic radiosurgery, not elsewhere classified

● **92.4 Intra-operative radiation procedures**

92.41 Intra-operative electron radiation therapy
    IOERT
    That using a mobile linear accelerator
    Coding Clinic: 2007, Q4, P122

● **93 Physical therapy, respiratory therapy, rehabilitation, and related procedures**

● **93.0 Diagnostic physical therapy**

93.01 Functional evaluation

93.02 Orthotic evaluation

93.03 Prosthetic evaluation

93.04 Manual testing of muscle function
    Coding Clinic: 1987, Jan-Feb, P15-16

93.05 Range of motion testing
    Coding Clinic: 1987, Jan-Feb, P15-16

93.06 Measurement of limb length

93.07 Body measurement
    Girth measurement
    Measurement of skull circumference

93.08 Electromyography

Excludes	*eye EMG (95.25)*
	that with polysomnogram (89.17)
	urethral sphincter EMG (89.23)

    Coding Clinic: 1987, Jan-Feb, P15-16

93.09 Other diagnostic physical therapy procedure

● **93.1 Physical therapy exercises**
    Coding Clinic: 1987, Jan-Feb, P15-16

93.11 Assisting exercise

| Excludes | *assisted exercise in pool (93.31)* |

93.12 Other active musculoskeletal exercise

93.13 Resistive exercise

93.14 Training in joint movements

93.15 Mobilization of spine

93.16 Mobilization of other joints

| Excludes | *manipulation of temporomandibular joint (76.95)* |

93.17 Other passive musculoskeletal exercise

93.18 Breathing exercise

93.19 Exercise, not elsewhere classified

● **93.2 Other physical therapy musculoskeletal manipulation**

93.21 Manual and mechanical traction

Excludes	*skeletal traction (93.43–93.44)*
	skin traction (93.45–93.46)
	spinal traction (93.41–93.42)

93.22 Ambulation and gait training

93.23 Fitting of orthotic device

93.24 Training in use of prosthetic or orthotic device
    Training in crutch walking

93.25 Forced extension of limb

93.26 Manual rupture of joint adhesions

93.27 Stretching of muscle or tendon

93.28 Stretching of fascia

93.29 Other forcible correction of deformity
    Coding Clinic: 1985, Nov-Dec, P11

MISCELLANEOUS DIAGNOSTIC AND THERAPEUTIC PROCEDURES (87–99)

● 93.3 **Other physical therapy therapeutic procedures**

93.31 **Assisted exercise in pool**

93.32 **Whirlpool treatment**

93.33 **Other hydrotherapy**

93.34 **Diathermy**

93.35 **Other heat therapy**
Acupuncture with smouldering moxa
Hot packs
Hyperthermia NEC
Infrared irradiation
Moxibustion
Paraffin bath
Excludes *hyperthermia for treatment of cancer (99.85)*

93.36 **Cardiac retraining**

93.37 **Prenatal training**
Training for natural childbirth

93.38 **Combined physical therapy without mention of the components**

93.39 **Other physical therapy**
Coding Clinic: 2005, Q2, P6-7; 2003, Q4, P105-106, 108-110; 1997, Q3, P12-13; 1991, Q3, P15; Q2, P15

● 93.4 **Skeletal traction and other traction**

93.41 **Spinal traction using skull device**
Traction using:
caliper tongs
Crutchfield tongs
halo device
Vinke tongs
Excludes *insertion of tongs or halo traction device (02.94)*
Coding Clinic: 2001, Q3, P8; 1996, Q3, P14

93.42 **Other spinal traction**
Cotrel's traction
Excludes *cervical collar (93.52)*

93.43 **Intermittent skeletal traction**

93.44 **Other skeletal traction**
Bryant's traction
Dunlop's traction
Lyman Smith traction
Russell's traction
Coding Clinic: 1989, Q3, P16

93.45 **Thomas' splint traction**

93.46 **Other skin traction of limbs**
Adhesive tape traction
Boot traction
Buck's traction
Gallows traction

● 93.5 **Other immobilization, pressure, and attention to wound**
Excludes *external fixator device (84.71–84.73)*
wound cleansing (96.58–96.59)

93.51 **Application of plaster jacket**
Excludes *Minerva jacket (93.52)*

93.52 **Application of neck support**
Application of:
cervical collar
Minerva jacket
molded neck support

93.53 **Application of other cast**

93.54 **Application of splint**
Plaster splint
Tray splint
Excludes *periodontal splint (24.7)*

93.55 **Dental wiring**
Excludes *that for orthodontia (24.7)*

93.56 **Application of pressure dressing**
Application of:
Gibney bandage
Robert Jones' bandage
Shanz dressing

93.57 **Application of other wound dressing**
Porcine wound dressing
Coding Clinic: 2002, Q3, P23

93.58 **Application of pressure trousers**
Application of:
anti-shock trousers
MAST trousers
vasopneumatic device
Coding Clinic: 1996, Q3, P13-14

93.59 **Other immobilization, pressure, and attention to wound**
Elastic stockings
Electronic gaiter
Intermittent pressure device
Oxygenation of wound (hyperbaric)
Stereotactic head frame application
Strapping (non-traction)
Velpeau dressing
Coding Clinic: 1999, Q3, P7-8; Q1, P12-13; 1991, Q1, P3-4; 1989, Q1, P12; 1988, Q4, P11

● 93.6 **Osteopathic manipulative treatment**

93.61 **Osteopathic manipulative treatment for general mobilization**
General articulatory treatment

93.62 **Osteopathic manipulative treatment using high-velocity, low-amplitude forces**
Thrusting forces

93.63 **Osteopathic manipulative treatment using low-velocity, high-amplitude forces**
Springing forces

93.64 **Osteopathic manipulative treatment using isotonic, isometric forces**

93.65 **Osteopathic manipulative treatment using indirect forces**

93.66 **Osteopathic manipulative treatment to move tissue fluids**
Lymphatic pump

93.67 **Other specified osteopathic manipulative treatment**

● 93.7 **Speech and reading rehabilitation and rehabilitation of the blind**

93.71 **Dyslexia training**

93.72 **Dysphasia training**

93.73 **Esophageal speech training**

93.74 **Speech defect training**

93.75 **Other speech training and therapy**
Coding Clinic: 2003, Q4, P105-106, 109-110; 1997, Q4, P35-37; Q3, P12-13

93.76 **Training in use of lead dog for the blind**

93.77 **Training in braille or Moon**

93.78 **Other rehabilitation for the blind**

● **93.8 Other rehabilitation therapy**

  93.81 Recreation therapy
    Diversional therapy
    Play therapy
    Excludes   *play psychotherapy (94.36)*

  93.82 Educational therapy
    Education of bed-bound children
    Special schooling for the handicapped

  93.83 Occupational therapy
    Daily living activities therapy
    Excludes   *training in activities of daily living for*
          the blind (93.78)
    Coding Clinic: 2005, Q2, P6-7; 2003, Q4, P105-106, 108; 1997,
    Q3, P12-13

  93.84 Music therapy

  93.85 Vocational rehabilitation
    Sheltered employment
    Vocational:
      assessment
      retraining
      training

  93.89 Rehabilitation, not elsewhere classified
    Coding Clinic: 2005, Q2, P6-7

● **93.9 Respiratory therapy**
    Excludes   *insertion of airway (96.01–96.05)*
          other continuous invasive (through
          endotracheal tube or tracheostomy)
          mechanical ventilation (96.70–96.72)
    Coding Clinic: 2004, Q3, P3; 2002, Q1, P12-13; 1998, Q3, P14

  93.90 Non-invasive mechanical ventilation
    Bi-level airway pressure
    BiPAP without (delivery through) endotracheal
      tube or tracheostomy
    CPAP without (delivery through) endotracheal
      tube or tracheostomy
    Mechanical ventilation NOS
    Non-invasive positive pressure (NIPPV)
    Non-invasive PPV
    NPPV
    That delivered by non-invasive interface:
      face mask
      nasal mask
      nasal pillow
      oral mouthpiece
      oronasal mask
    Excludes   *invasive (through endotracheal tube*
          or tracheostomy) continuous
          mechanical ventilation
          (96.70–96.72)
    Note: Patients admitted on *non-invasive*
      mechanical ventilation that
      subsequently require *invasive*
      mechanical ventilation; code both types
      of mechanical ventilation.
    Coding Clinic: 2008, Q4, P187-190; Q1, P8-9; 2004, Q3, P3

  93.91 Intermittent positive pressure breathing [IPPB]

  93.93 Nonmechanical methods of resuscitation
    Artificial respiration
    Manual resuscitation
    Mouth-to-mouth resuscitation
    Coding Clinic: 2003, Q2, P17

  93.94 Respiratory medication administered by
    nebulizer
    Mist therapy

  93.95 Hyperbaric oxygenation
    Excludes   *oxygenation of wound (93.59)*

  93.96 Other oxygen enrichment
    Catalytic oxygen therapy
    Cytoreductive effect
    Oxygenators
    Oxygen therapy
    Excludes   *oxygenation of wound (93.59)*
          SuperSaturated oxygen therapy
          (00.49)

  93.97 Decompression chamber

  93.98 Other control of atmospheric pressure and
    composition
    Antigen-free air conditioning
    Helium therapy
    Excludes   *inhaled nitric oxide therapy (INO)*
          (00.12)
    Coding Clinic: 2002, Q1, P14

  93.99 Other respiratory procedures
    Continuous negative pressure ventilation [CNP]
    Postural drainage
    Coding Clinic: 2003, Q4, P108-109; 1999, Q3, P11-12

● **94 Procedures related to the psyche**

  ● **94.0 Psychologic evaluation and testing**

    94.01 Administration of intelligence test
      Administration of:
        Stanford-Binet
        Wechsler Adult Intelligence Scale
        Wechsler Intelligence Scale for Children

    94.02 Administration of psychologic test
      Administration of:
        Bender Visual-Motor Gestalt Test
        Benton Visual Retention Test
        Minnesota Multiphasic Personality Inventory
        Wechsler Memory Scale

    94.03 Character analysis

    94.08 Other psychologic evaluation and testing

    94.09 Psychologic mental status determination, not
      otherwise specified

  ● **94.1 Psychiatric interviews, consultations, and evaluations**

    94.11 Psychiatric mental status determination
      Clinical psychiatric mental status
        determination
      Evaluation for criminal responsibility
      Evaluation for testimentary capacity
      Medicolegal mental status determination
      Mental status determination NOS

    94.12 Routine psychiatric visit, not otherwise specified

    94.13 Psychiatric commitment evaluation
      Pre-commitment interview

    94.19 Other psychiatric interview and evaluation
      Follow-up psychiatric interview NOS

MISCELLANEOUS DIAGNOSTIC AND THERAPEUTIC PROCEDURES (87–99)

MISCELLANEOUS DIAGNOSTIC AND THERAPEUTIC PROCEDURES (87–99)

● **94.2 Psychiatric somatotherapy**

94.21 Narcoanalysis
Narcosynthesis

94.22 Lithium therapy

94.23 Neuroleptic therapy

94.24 Chemical shock therapy

94.25 Other psychiatric drug therapy

94.26 Subconvulsive electroshock therapy

94.27 Other electroshock therapy
Electroconvulsive therapy (ECT)
EST

94.29 Other psychiatric somatotherapy

● **94.3 Individual psychotherapy**

94.31 Psychoanalysis

94.32 Hypnotherapy
Hypnodrome
Hypnosis

94.33 Behavior therapy
Aversion therapy
Behavior modification
Desensitization therapy
Extinction therapy
Relaxation training
Token economy

94.34 Individual therapy for psychosexual dysfunction

Excludes *that performed in group setting (94.41)*

94.35 Crisis intervention

94.36 Play psychotherapy

94.37 Exploratory verbal psychotherapy

94.38 Supportive verbal psychotherapy

94.39 Other individual psychotherapy
Biofeedback

● **94.4 Other psychotherapy and counseling**

94.41 Group therapy for psychosexual dysfunction

94.42 Family therapy

94.43 Psychodrama

94.44 Other group therapy

94.45 Drug addiction counseling

94.46 Alcoholism counseling

94.49 Other counseling

● **94.5 Referral for psychologic rehabilitation**

94.51 Referral for psychotherapy

94.52 Referral for psychiatric aftercare:
That in:
halfway house
outpatient (clinic) facility

94.53 Referral for alcoholism rehabilitation

94.54 Referral for drug addiction rehabilitation

94.55 Referral for vocational rehabilitation

94.59 Referral for other psychologic rehabilitation

● **94.6 Alcohol and drug rehabilitation and detoxification**

94.61 Alcohol rehabilitation

94.62 Alcohol detoxification

94.63 Alcohol rehabilitation and detoxification

94.64 Drug rehabilitation

94.65 Drug detoxification

94.66 Drug rehabilitation and detoxification

94.67 Combined alcohol and drug rehabilitation

94.68 Combined alcohol and drug detoxification

94.69 Combined alcohol and drug rehabilitation and detoxification

● **95 Ophthalmologic and otologic diagnosis and treatment**

● **95.0 General and subjective eye examination**

95.01 Limited eye examination
Eye examination with prescription of spectacles

95.02 Comprehensive eye examination
Eye examination covering all aspects of the visual system

95.03 Extended ophthalmologic work-up
Examination (for):
glaucoma
neuro-ophthalmology
retinal disease

95.04 Eye examination under anesthesia
Code also type of examination

95.05 Visual field study

95.06 Color vision study

95.07 Dark adaptation study

95.09 Eye examination, not otherwise specified
Vision check NOS

● **95.1 Examinations of form and structure of eye**

95.11 Fundus photography

95.12 Fluorescein angiography or angioscopy of eye

95.13 Ultrasound study of eye

95.14 X-ray study of eye

95.15 Ocular motility study

95.16 P32 and other tracer studies of eye

● **95.2 Objective functional tests of eye**

Excludes *that with polysomnogram (89.17)*

95.21 Electroretinogram [ERG]

95.22 Electro-oculogram [EOG]

95.23 Visual evoked potential [VEP]

95.24 Electronystagmogram [ENG]

95.25 Electromyogram of eye [EMG]

95.26 Tonography, provocative tests, and other glaucoma testing

● **95.3 Special vision services**

95.31 Fitting and dispensing of spectacles

95.32 Prescription, fitting, and dispensing of contact lens

95.33 Dispensing of other low vision aids

95.34 Ocular prosthetics

95.35 Orthoptic training

95.36 Ophthalmologic counseling and instruction
Counseling in:
adaptation to visual loss
use of low vision aids

◀ New   ◀▥ Revised   ~~deleted~~ Deleted   ● Use Additional Digit(s)   OGCR Official Guidelines   Coding Clinic

- **95.4 Nonoperative procedures related to hearing**
  - **95.41 Audiometry**
    - Békésy 5-tone audiometry
    - Impedance audiometry
    - Stapedial reflex response
    - Subjective audiometry
    - Tympanogram
  - **95.42 Clinical test of hearing**
    - Tuning fork test
    - Whispered speech test
  - **95.43 Audiological evaluation**
    - Audiological evaluation by:
      - Bárány noise machine
      - blindfold test
      - delayed feedback
      - masking
      - Weber lateralization
  - **95.44 Clinical vestibular function tests**
    - Thermal test of vestibular function
  - **95.45 Rotation tests**
    - Bárány chair
  - **95.46 Other auditory and vestibular function tests**
  - **95.47 Hearing examination, not otherwise specified**
  - **95.48 Fitting of hearing aid**

    > **Excludes** *implantation of electromagnetic hearing device (20.95)*

  - **95.49 Other nonoperative procedures related to hearing**
    - Adjustment (external components) of cochlear prosthetic device

- **96 Nonoperative intubation and irrigation**
  - **96.0 Nonoperative intubation of gastrointestinal and respiratory tracts**
    - **96.01 Insertion of nasopharyngeal airway**
    - **96.02 Insertion of oropharyngeal airway**
    - **96.03 Insertion of esophageal obturator airway**
    - **96.04 Insertion of endotracheal tube**
      - Coding Clinic: 2009, Q2, P11; 2007, Q1, P11; 2006, Q2, P8-9; 2005, Q4, P83-89; Q3, P10-11; Q2, P19-20; 2003, Q2, P17; 1993, 5th Issue, P11
    - **96.05 Other intubation of respiratory tract**

      > **Excludes** *endoscopic insertion or replacement of bronchial device or substance (33.71, 33.79)*

      - Coding Clinic: 1997, Q1, P14
    - **96.06 Insertion of Sengstaken tube**
      - Esophageal tamponade
    - **96.07 Insertion of other (naso-)gastric tube**
      - Intubation for decompression

      > **Excludes** *that for enteral infusion of nutritional substance (96.6)*

      - Coding Clinic: 2008, Q4, P138-140
    - **96.08 Insertion of (naso-)intestinal tube**
      - Miller-Abbott tube (for decompression)
    - **96.09 Insertion of rectal tube**
      - Replacement of rectal tube
  - **96.1 Other nonoperative insertion**

    > **Excludes** *nasolacrimal intubation (09.44)*

    - **96.11 Packing of external auditory canal**
    - **96.14 Vaginal packing**
    - **96.15 Insertion of vaginal mold**
    - **96.16 Other vaginal dilation**
    - **96.17 Insertion of vaginal diaphragm**
    - **96.18 Insertion of other vaginal pessary**
    - **96.19 Rectal packing**

- **96.2 Nonoperative dilation and manipulation**
  - **96.21 Dilation of frontonasal duct**
  - **96.22 Dilation of rectum**
  - **96.23 Dilation of anal sphincter**
  - **96.24 Dilation and manipulation of enterostomy stoma**
  - **96.25 Therapeutic distention of bladder**
    - Intermittent distention of bladder
  - **96.26 Manual reduction of rectal prolapse**
  - **96.27 Manual reduction of hernia**
  - **96.28 Manual reduction of enterostomy prolapse**
    - Coding Clinic: 1987, Nov-Dec, P11
  - **96.29 Reduction of intussusception of alimentary tract**
    - With:
      - fluoroscopy
      - ionizing radiation enema
      - ultrasonography guidance
    - Hydrostatic reduction
    - Pneumatic reduction

    > **Excludes** *intra-abdominal manipulation of intestine, not otherwise specified (46.80)*

    - Coding Clinic: 1998, Q43, P82-83
- **96.3 Nonoperative alimentary tract irrigation, cleaning, and local instillation**
  - **96.31 Gastric cooling**
    - Gastric hypothermia
  - **96.32 Gastric freezing**
  - **96.33 Gastric lavage**
  - **96.34 Other irrigation of (naso-)gastric tube**
  - **96.35 Gastric gavage**
  - **96.36 Irrigation of gastrostomy or enterostomy**
  - **96.37 Proctoclysis**
  - **96.38 Removal of impacted feces**
    - Removal of impaction:
      - by flushing
      - manually
  - **96.39 Other transanal enema**
    - Rectal irrigation

    > **Excludes** *reduction of intussusception of alimentary tract by ionizing radiation enema (96.29)*

- **96.4 Nonoperative irrigation, cleaning, and local instillation of other digestive and genitourinary organs**
  - **96.41 Irrigation of cholecystostomy and other biliary tube**
  - **96.42 Irrigation of pancreatic tube**
  - **96.43 Digestive tract instillation, except gastric gavage**
  - **96.44 Vaginal douche**
  - **96.45 Irrigation of nephrostomy and pyelostomy**
  - **96.46 Irrigation of ureterostomy and ureteral catheter**
    - Coding Clinic: 1985, July-Aug, P15
  - **96.47 Irrigation of cystostomy**
  - **96.48 Irrigation of other indwelling urinary catheter**
  - **96.49 Other genitourinary instillation**
    - Insertion of prostaglandin suppository
    - Coding Clinic: 2001, Q1, P5
- **96.5 Other nonoperative irrigation and cleaning**
  - **96.51 Irrigation of eye**
    - Irrigation of cornea

    > **Excludes** *irrigation with removal of foreign body (98.21)*

Excludes   Includes   Use additional   Code also   Omit code

96.52   **Irrigation of ear**
Irrigation with removal of cerumen

96.53   **Irrigation of nasal passages**

96.54   **Dental scaling, polishing, and debridement**
Dental prophylaxis
Plaque removal

96.55   **Tracheostomy toilette**

96.56   **Other lavage of bronchus and trachea**

| Excludes | *diagnostic bronchoalveolar lavage (BAL) (33.24)* |
| | *whole lung lavage (33.99)* |

Coding Clinic: 2002, Q3, P18

96.57   **Irrigation of vascular catheter**
Coding Clinic: 1993, Q3, P5

96.58   **Irrigation of wound catheter**

96.59   **Other irrigation of wound**
Wound cleaning NOS

| Excludes | *debridement (86.22, 86.27–86.28)* |

96.6   **Enteral infusion of concentrated nutritional substances**

● 96.7   **Other continuous invasive mechanical ventilation**

Includes	BiPAP delivered through endotracheal tube or tracheostomy (invasive interface)
	CPAP delivered through endotracheal tube or tracheostomy (invasive interface)
	Endotracheal respiratory assistance
	Invasive positive pressure ventilation [IPPV]
	Mechanical ventilation through invasive interface
	That by tracheostomy
	Weaning of an intubated (endotracheal tube) patient

Excludes	*continuous negative pressure ventilation [CNP] (iron lung) (cuirass) (93.99)*
	intermittent positive pressure breathing [IPPB] (93.91)
	non-invasive bi-level positive airway pressure [BiPAP] (93.90)
	non-invasive continuous positive airway pressure [CPAP] (93.90)
	non-invasive positive pressure (NIPPV) (93.90)
	that by face mask (93.90–93.99)
	that by nasal cannula (93.90–93.99)
	that by nasal catheter (93.90–93.99)

Code also any associated:
endotracheal tube insertion (96.04)
tracheostomy (31.1–31.29)

Note: Endotracheal Intubation

To calculate the number of hours (duration) of continuous mechanical ventilation during a hospitalization, begin the count from the start of the (endotracheal) intubation. The duration ends with (endotracheal) extubation.

If a patient is intubated prior to admission, begin counting the duration from the time of the admission. If a patient is transferred (discharged) while intubated, the duration would end at the time of transfer (discharge).

For patients who begin on (endotracheal) intubation and subsequently have a tracheostomy performed for mechanical ventilation, the duration begins with the (endotracheal) intubation and ends when the mechanical ventilation is turned off (after the weaning period).

Tracheostomy

To calculate the number of hours of continuous mechanical ventilation during a hospitalization, begin counting the duration when mechanical ventilation is started. The duration ends when the mechanical ventilator is turned off (after the weaning period).

If a patient has received a tracheostomy prior to admission and is on mechanical ventilation at the time of admission, begin counting the duration from the time of admission. If a patient is transferred (discharged) while still on mechanical ventilation via tracheostomy, the duration would end at the time of the transfer (discharge).

Coding Clinic: 2008, Q4, P187-190; 2004, Q3, P3, 11; 2003, Q2, P17; 2002, Q2, P19; 1998, Q3, P14

96.70   **Continuous invasive mechanical ventilation of unspecified duration**
Invasive mechanical ventilation NOS
Coding Clinic: 1992, Q2, P13-14x3

96.71   **Continuous invasive mechanical ventilation for less than 96 consecutive hours**
Coding Clinic: 2009, Q2, P11; 2007, Q3, P7-8; 2006, Q2, P8-9x2; 2005, Q3, P10-11; 2004, Q3, P3, 11; 2003, Q2, P17; 2002, Q1, P12-13; 2001, Q1, P6-7; 1993, 5th Issue, P11; 1992, Q2, P13-14x3

96.72   **Continuous invasive mechanical ventilation for 96 consecutive hours or more**
Coding Clinic: 2005, Q2, P19-20; 1992, Q2, P13-14x3

● 97   **Replacement and removal of therapeutic appliances**

● 97.0   **Nonoperative replacement of gastrointestinal appliance**

97.01   **Replacement of (naso-)gastric or esophagostomy tube**

97.02   **Replacement of gastrostomy tube**
Coding Clinic: 1997, Q1, P11

97.03   **Replacement of tube or enterostomy device of small intestine**
Coding Clinic: 2003, Q1, P10

97.04   **Replacement of tube or enterostomy device of large intestine**

97.05   **Replacement of stent (tube) in biliary or pancreatic duct**
Coding Clinic: 1999, Q2, P13-14

● 97.1   **Nonoperative replacement of musculoskeletal and integumentary system appliance**

97.11   **Replacement of cast on upper limb**

97.12   **Replacement of cast on lower limb**

97.13   **Replacement of other cast**

97.14   **Replacement of other device for musculoskeletal immobilization**
Splinting
Strapping

97.15   **Replacement of wound catheter**

97.16   **Replacement of wound packing or drain**

Excludes	*repacking of:*
	dental wound (97.22)
	vulvar wound (97.26)

● **97.2 Other nonoperative replacement**

  97.21 Replacement of nasal packing

  97.22 Replacement of dental packing

  97.23 Replacement of tracheostomy tube
         Coding Clinic: 1987, Nov-Dec, P11

  97.24 Replacement and refitting of vaginal diaphragm

  97.25 Replacement of other vaginal pessary

  97.26 Replacement of vaginal or vulvar packing or drain

  97.29 Other nonoperative replacements
         Coding Clinic: 1999, Q3, P9; 1998, Q3, P12; 1985, Mar-April, P11

● **97.3 Nonoperative removal of therapeutic device from head and neck**

  97.31 Removal of eye prosthesis
         Excludes *removal of ocular implant (16.71)*
                     removal of orbital implant (16.72)

  97.32 Removal of nasal packing

  97.33 Removal of dental wiring

  97.34 Removal of dental packing

  97.35 Removal of dental prosthesis

  97.36 Removal of other external mandibular fixation device

  97.37 Removal of tracheostomy tube

  97.38 Removal of sutures from head and neck

  97.39 Removal of other therapeutic device from head and neck
         Excludes *removal of skull tongs (02.94)*

● **97.4 Nonoperative removal of therapeutic device from thorax**

  97.41 Removal of thoracotomy tube or pleural cavity drain
         Coding Clinic: 1999, Q1, P10

  97.42 Removal of mediastinal drain

  97.43 Removal of sutures from thorax

  97.44 Nonoperative removal of heart assist system
         Explantation [removal] of circulatory assist device
         Explantation [removal] of percutaneous external heart assist device
         Intra-aortic balloon pump [IABP]
         Removal of extrinsic heart assist device
         Removal of pVAD
         Removal of percutaneous heart assist device
         Coding Clinic: 2001, Q4, P65

  97.49 Removal of other device from thorax
         Excludes *endoscopic removal of bronchial device(s) or substances (33.78)*
         Coding Clinic: 1986, Nov-Dec, P9

● **97.5 Nonoperative removal of therapeutic device from digestive system**

  97.51 Removal of gastrostomy tube

  97.52 Removal of tube from small intestine

  97.53 Removal of tube from large intestine or appendix

  97.54 Removal of cholecystostomy tube

  97.55 Removal of T-tube, other bile duct tube, or liver tube
         Removal of bile duct stent
         Coding Clinic: 2001, Q1, P8-9

  97.56 Removal of pancreatic tube or drain

  97.59 Removal of other device from digestive system
         Removal of rectal packing

● **97.6 Nonoperative removal of therapeutic device from urinary system**

  97.61 Removal of pyelostomy and nephrostomy tube

  97.62 Removal of ureterostomy tube and ureteral catheter

  97.63 Removal of cystostomy tube

  97.64 Removal of other urinary drainage device
         Removal of indwelling urinary catheter

  97.65 Removal of urethral stent

  97.69 Removal of other device from urinary system

● **97.7 Nonoperative removal of therapeutic device from genital system**

  97.71 Removal of intrauterine contraceptive device

  97.72 Removal of intrauterine pack

  97.73 Removal of vaginal diaphragm

  97.74 Removal of other vaginal pessary

  97.75 Removal of vaginal or vulvar packing

  97.79 Removal of other device from genital tract
         Removal of sutures

● **97.8 Other nonoperative removal of therapeutic device**

  97.81 Removal of retroperitoneal drainage device

  97.82 Removal of peritoneal drainage device
         Coding Clinic: 1993, 5th Issue, P8-9; 1990, Q2, P28; 1986, Sept-Oct, P12

  97.83 Removal of abdominal wall sutures

  97.84 Removal of sutures from trunk, not elsewhere classified

  97.85 Removal of packing from trunk, not elsewhere classified

  97.86 Removal of other device from abdomen

  97.87 Removal of other device from trunk

  97.88 Removal of external immobilization device
         Removal of:
           brace
           cast
           splint

  97.89 Removal of other therapeutic device

● **98 Nonoperative removal of foreign body or calculus**

● **98.0 Removal of intraluminal foreign body from digestive system without incision**
         Excludes *removal of therapeutic device (97.51–97.59)*

  98.01 Removal of intraluminal foreign body from mouth without incision

  98.02 Removal of intraluminal foreign body from esophagus without incision

  98.03 Removal of intraluminal foreign body from stomach and small intestine without incision
         Coding Clinic: 1985, Jan-Feb, P14-15

  98.04 Removal of intraluminal foreign body from large intestine without incision

  98.05 Removal of intraluminal foreign body from rectum and anus without incision

● **98.1 Removal of intraluminal foreign body from other sites without incision**
         Excludes *removal of therapeutic device (97.31–97.49, 97.61–97.89)*

  98.11 Removal of intraluminal foreign body from ear without incision

  98.12 Removal of intraluminal foreign body from nose without incision

  98.13 Removal of intraluminal foreign body from pharynx without incision

MISCELLANEOUS DIAGNOSTIC AND THERAPEUTIC PROCEDURES (87–99)

Excludes   Includes   Use additional   Code also   Omit code

98.14   Removal of intraluminal foreign body from larynx without incision

98.15   Removal of intraluminal foreign body from trachea and bronchus without incision

> **Excludes**   *endoscopic removal of bronchial device(s) or substances (33.78)*

98.16   Removal of intraluminal foreign body from uterus without incision

> **Excludes**   *removal of intrauterine contraceptive device (97.71)*

98.17   Removal of intraluminal foreign body from vagina without incision

98.18   Removal of intraluminal foreign body from artificial stoma without incision

98.19   Removal of intraluminal foreign body from urethra without incision

● **98.2**   Removal of other foreign body without incision

> **Excludes**   *removal of intraluminal foreign body (98.01–98.19)*

98.20   Removal of foreign body, not otherwise specified

98.21   Removal of superficial foreign body from eye without incision

98.22   Removal of other foreign body without incision from head and neck
> Removal of embedded foreign body from eyelid or conjunctiva without incision

98.23   Removal of foreign body from vulva without incision

98.24   Removal of foreign body from scrotum or penis without incision

98.25   Removal of other foreign body without incision from trunk except scrotum, penis, or vulva

98.26   Removal of foreign body from hand without incision
> Coding Clinic: 1987, Nov-Dec, P10

98.27   Removal of foreign body without incision from upper limb, except hand

98.28   Removal of foreign body from foot without incision

98.29   Removal of foreign body without incision from lower limb, except foot

● **98.5**   Extracorporeal shockwave lithotripsy [ESWL]
> Lithotriptor tank procedure
> Disintegration of stones by extracorporeal induced shockwaves
> That with insertion of stent

98.51   Extracorporeal shockwave lithotripsy [ESWL] of the kidney, ureter, and/or bladder

98.52   Extracorporeal shockwave lithotripsy [ESWL] of the gallbladder and/or bile duct

98.59   Extracorporeal shockwave lithotripsy of other sites

● **99**   Other nonoperative procedures

● **99.0**   Transfusion of blood and blood components
> Use additional code for that done via catheter or cutdown (38.92–38.94)

99.00   Perioperative autologous transfusion of whole blood or blood components
> Intraoperative blood collection
> Postoperative blood collection
> Salvage

99.01   Exchange transfusion
> Transfusion:
> exsanguination
> replacement
> Coding Clinic: 1989, Q2, P15

99.02   Transfusion of previously collected autologous blood
> Blood component
> Coding Clinic: 1990, Q1, P10; 1985, July-Aug, P16

99.03   Other transfusion of whole blood
> Transfusion:
> blood NOS
> hemodilution
> NOS

99.04   Transfusion of packed cells
> Coding Clinic: 2006, Q4, P91-92

99.05   Transfusion of platelets
> Transfusion of thrombocytes

99.06   Transfusion of coagulation factors
> Transfusion of antihemophilic factor

99.07   Transfusion of other serum
> Transfusion of plasma
> **Excludes**   *injection [transfusion] of: antivenin (99.16) gamma globulin (99.14)*
> Coding Clinic: 1985, Nov-Dec, P14

99.08   Transfusion of blood expander
> Transfusion of Dextran

99.09   Transfusion of other substance
> Transfusion of:
> blood surrogate
> granulocytes
> **Excludes**   *transplantation [transfusion] of bone marrow (41.0)*

● **99.1**   Injection or infusion of therapeutic or prophylactic substance
> **Includes**   injection or infusion given:
> hypodermically acting locally or systemically
> intramuscularly acting locally or systemically
> intravenously acting locally or systemically
> Coding Clinic: 2005, Q4, P101-103

99.10   Injection or infusion of thrombolytic agent
> Alteplase
> Anistreplase
> Reteplase
> Streptokinase
> Tenecteplase
> Tissue plasminogen activator (TPA)
> Urokinase
> **Excludes**   *aspirin — omit code*
> *GP IIB/IIIa platelet inhibitors (99.20)*
> *heparin (99.19)*
> *SuperSaturated oxygen therapy (00.49)*
> *warfarin — omit code*
> Coding Clinic: 2006, Q2, P22; 2001, Q2, P8-9; Q2, P7-8, 23

99.11 Injection of Rh immune globulin
  Injection of:
    Anti-D (Rhesus) globulin
    RhoGAM

99.12 Immunization for allergy
  Desensitization

99.13 Immunization for autoimmune disease

99.14 Injection or infusion of ~~gamma globulin~~ immunoglobulin ◄▥
  Injection of immune sera
  Injection or infusion of gamma globulin ◄

99.15 Parenteral infusion of concentrated nutritional substances
  Hyperalimentation
  Total parenteral nutrition [TPN]
  Peripheral parenteral nutrition [PPN]
  Coding Clinic: 2003, Q4, P104-105

99.16 Injection of antidote
  Injection of:
    antivenin
    heavy metal antagonist

99.17 Injection of insulin

99.18 Injection or infusion of electrolytes

99.19 Injection of anticoagulant
  | Excludes | infusion of drotrecogin alfa (activated) (00.11) |

● **99.2 Injection or infusion of other therapeutic or prophylactic substance**
  | Includes | injection or infusion given: |
    hypodermically acting locally or systemically
    intramuscularly acting locally or systemically
    intravenously acting locally or systemically
  | Excludes | SuperSaturated oxygen therapy (00.49) |
  Use additional code for:
  injection (into):
    breast (85.92)
    bursa (82.94, 83.96)
    intraperitoneal (cavity) (54.97)
    intrathecal (03.92)
    joint (76.96, 81.92)
    kidney (55.96)
    liver (50.94)
    orbit (16.91)
    other sites — see Alphabetic Index
  perfusion:
    NOS (39.97)
    intestine (46.95, 46.96)
    kidney (55.95)
    liver (50.93)
    total body (39.96)
  Coding Clinic: 2004, Q4, P138; 2002, Q3, P20; 1998, Q43, P85-86

99.20 Injection or infusion of platelet inhibitor
  Glycoprotein IIB/IIIa inhibitor
  GP IIB/IIIa inhibitor
  GP IIB-IIIa inhibitor
  | Excludes | infusion of heparin (99.19) |
  | | injection or infusion of thrombolytic agent (99.10) |
  Coding Clinic: 2006, Q3, P8-9; 2004, Q2, P3

99.21 Injection of antibiotic
  | Excludes | injection or infusion of oxazolidinone class of antibiotics (00.14) |
  Coding Clinic: 1998, Q43, P76-77; 1990, Q2, P24; 1989, Q3, P16; 1987, Mar-April, P9

99.22 Injection of other anti-infective
  | Excludes | injection or infusion of oxazolidinone class of antibiotics (00.14) |

99.23 Injection of steroid
  Injection of cortisone
  Subdermal implantation of progesterone
  Coding Clinic: 2000, Q3, P15; 1999, Q1, P7-8; 1996, Q3, P7; 1992, Q3, P9

99.24 Injection of other hormone
  Coding Clinic: 2006, Q1, P9-10

99.25 Injection or infusion of cancer chemotherapeutic substance
  Chemoembolization
  Injection or infusion of antineoplastic agent
  Use additional code for disruption of blood brain barrier, if performed [BBBD] (00.19)
Excludes	immunotherapy, antineoplastic (00.15, 99.28)
	implantation of chemotherapeutic agent (00.10)
	injection of radioisotope (92.28)
	injection or infusion of biological response modifier [BRM] as an antineoplastic agent (99.28)
	intravenous infusion of clofarabine (17.70)
  Coding Clinic: 2009, Q4, P79; 2008, Q4, P82-83; 2007, Q4, P103-104; 2003, Q2, P6, 16-17; 2000, Q1, P23-24; 1999, Q1, P4; 1998, Q1, P6-7; 1996, Q3, P11-12; 1992, Q2, P6-7; Q1, P12; 1988, Q1, P8; 1986, Nov-Dec, P11; 1985, July-Aug, P11; 1984, May-June, P11

99.26 Injection of tranquilizer

99.27 Iontophoresis

99.28 Injection or infusion of biological response modifier [BRM] as an antineoplastic agent
  Immunotherapy, antineoplastic
  Infusion of cintredekin besudotox
  Interleukin therapy
  Low-dose interleukin-2 (IL-2) therapy
  Tumor vaccine
  | Excludes | high-dose infusion interleukin-2 [IL-2] (00.15) |
  Coding Clinic: 2006, Q4, P122-123; 1999, Q2, P8; 1998, Q2, P10-11

99.29 Injection or infusion of other therapeutic or prophylactic substance
Excludes	administration of neuroprotective agent (99.75)
	immunization (99.31–99.59)
	infusion of blood brain barrier disruption substance (00.19)
	injection of sclerosing agent into: esophageal varices (42.33) hemorrhoids (49.42) veins (39.92)
	injection or infusion of human B-type natriuretic peptide (hBNP) (00.13)
	injection or infusion of nesiritide (00.13)
	injection or infusion of platelet inhibitor (99.20)
	injection or infusion of thrombolytic agent (99.10)
  Coding Clinic: 2010, Q1, P21-22; 2007, Q1, P11; 2004, Q4, P138; 2003, Q2, P10; 2002, Q3, P24-25; 2001, Q1, P15, 19-20; 2000, Q2, P14-15; Q1, P8-9, 18-19, 23-24; 1999, Q4, P17-18; 1998, Q2, P17-18, 23-24; Q1, P6; 1997, Q2, P11; 1996, Q3, P21; 1995, Q2, P12; 1990, Q2, P23-24; 1989, Q2, P17; 1988, Q1, P9; 1987, Sept-Oct, P11; 1984, Nov-Dec, P12

MISCELLANEOUS DIAGNOSTIC AND THERAPEUTIC PROCEDURES (87–99)

● **99.3   Prophylactic vaccination and inoculation against certain bacterial diseases**

  99.31   Vaccination against cholera

  99.32   Vaccination against typhoid and paratyphoid fever
      Administration of TAB vaccine

  99.33   Vaccination against tuberculosis
      Administration of BCG vaccine
      Coding Clinic: 1988, Q1, P8

  99.34   Vaccination against plague

  99.35   Vaccination against tularemia

  99.36   Administration of diphtheria toxoid
      | Excludes | *administration of:*
      diphtheria antitoxin (99.58)
      diphtheria-tetanus-pertussis, combined (99.39)

  99.37   Vaccination against pertussis
      | Excludes | *administration of diphtheria-tetanus-pertussis, combined (99.39)*

  99.38   Administration of tetanus toxoid
      | Excludes | *administration of:*
      diphtheria-tetanus-pertussis, combined (99.39)
      tetanus antitoxin (99.56)

  99.39   Administration of diphtheria-tetanus-pertussis, combined

● **99.4   Prophylactic vaccination and inoculation against certain viral diseases**

  99.41   Administration of poliomyelitis vaccine

  99.42   Vaccination against smallpox

  99.43   Vaccination against yellow fever

  99.44   Vaccination against rabies

  99.45   Vaccination against measles
      | Excludes | *administration of measles-mumps rubella vaccine (99.48)*

  99.46   Vaccination against mumps
      | Excludes | *administration of measles-mumps rubella vaccine (99.48)*

  99.47   Vaccination against rubella
      | Excludes | *administration of measles-mumps rubella vaccine (99.48)*

  99.48   Administration of measles-mumps-rubella vaccine

● **99.5   Other vaccination and inoculation**

  99.51   Prophylactic vaccination against the common cold

  99.52   Prophylactic vaccination against influenza

  99.53   Prophylactic vaccination against arthropod-borne viral encephalitis

  99.54   Prophylactic vaccination against other arthropod-borne viral diseases

  99.55   Prophylactic administration of vaccine against other diseases
      Vaccination against:
        anthrax
        brucellosis
        Rocky Mountain spotted fever
        Staphylococcus
        Streptococcus
        typhus
      Coding Clinic: 1994, Q1, P19

  99.56   Administration of tetanus antitoxin

  99.57   Administration of botulism antitoxin

  99.58   Administration of other antitoxins
      Administration of:
        diphtheria antitoxin
        gas gangrene antitoxin
        scarlet fever antitoxin

  99.59   Other vaccination and inoculation
      Vaccination NOS
      | Excludes | *injection of:*
      gamma globulin (99.14)
      Rh immune globulin (99.11)
      immunization for:
      allergy (99.12)
      autoimmune disease (99.13)

● **99.6   Conversion of cardiac rhythm**
      | Excludes | *open chest cardiac:*
      electric stimulation (37.91)
      massage (37.91)

  99.60   Cardiopulmonary resuscitation, not otherwise specified
      Coding Clinic: 1994, Q1, P16

  99.61   Atrial cardioversion
      Coding Clinic: 1993, Q3, P12

  99.62   Other electric countershock of heart
      Cardioversion:
        NOS
        external
      Conversion to sinus rhythm
      Defibrillation
      External electrode stimulation
      Coding Clinic: 2007, Q1, P17-18

  99.63   Closed chest cardiac massage
      Cardiac massage NOS
      Manual external cardiac massage

  99.64   Carotid sinus stimulation

  99.69   Other conversion of cardiac rhythm
      Coding Clinic: 1988, Q4, P11

● **99.7   Therapeutic apheresis or other injection, administration, or infusion of other therapeutic or prophylactic substance**

  99.71   Therapeutic plasmapheresis
      | Excludes | *extracorporeal immunoadsorption [ECI] (99.76)*

  99.72   Therapeutic leukopheresis
      Therapeutic leukocytapheresis

  99.73   Therapeutic erythrocytapheresis
      Therapeutic erythropheresis
      Coding Clinic: 1994, Q1, P20-21

  99.74   Therapeutic plateletpheresis

  99.75   Administration of neuroprotective agent

  99.76   Extracorporeal immunoadsorption
      Removal of antibodies from plasma with protein A columns
      Coding Clinic: 2002, Q4, P112-113

  99.77   Application or administration of adhesion barrier substance
      Coding Clinic: 2010, Q1, P21; 2002, Q4, P113

  99.78   Aquapheresis
      Plasma water removal
      Ultrafiltration [for water removal]
      | Excludes | *hemodiafiltration (39.95)*
      hemodialysis (39.95)
      therapeutic plasmapheresis (99.71)

  99.79   Other
      Apheresis (harvest) of stem cells
      Coding Clinic: 2008, Q3, P19; 2006, Q1, P12-14x2; 2005, Q1, P16-17; 1997, Q4, P55

● **99.8 Miscellaneous physical procedures**

99.81 Hypothermia (central) (local)

> | Excludes | *gastric cooling (96.31)*
> *gastric freezing (96.32)*
> *that incidental to open heart surgery
> (39.62)*

99.82 Ultraviolet light therapy
Actinotherapy

99.83 Other phototherapy
Phototherapy of the newborn

> | Excludes | *extracorporeal photochemotherapy
> (99.88)*
> *photocoagulation of retinal lesion
> (14.23–14.25, 14.33–14.35,
> 14.53–14.55)*

Coding Clinic: 1989, Q2, P15

99.84 Isolation
Isolation after contact with infectious
disease
Protection of individual from his
surroundings
Protection of surroundings from individual

99.85 Hyperthermia for treatment of cancer
Hyperthermia (adjunct therapy) induced by
microwave, ultrasound, low energy radio
frequency, probes (interstitial), or other
means in the treatment of cancer

> | Code also | any concurrent chemotherapy or
> radiation therapy

Coding Clinic: 1996, Q3, P11-12; 1989, Q3, P17

**99.86 Non-invasive placement of bone growth
stimulator**
Transcutaneous (surface) placement of pads
or patches for stimulation to aid bone
healing

> | Excludes | *insertion of invasive or semi-invasive
> bone growth stimulators (device)
> (percutaneous electrodes)
> (78.90–78.99)*

99.88 Therapeutic photopheresis
Extracorporeal photochemotherapy
Extracorporeal photopheresis

> | Excludes | *other phototherapy (99.83)*
> *ultraviolet light therapy (99.82)*

Coding Clinic: 1999, Q2, P7-8

● **99.9 Other miscellaneous procedures**

99.91 Acupuncture for anesthesia

99.92 Other acupuncture

> | Excludes | *that with smouldering mox (93.35)*

99.93 Rectal massage (for levator spasm)

99.94 Prostatic massage

99.95 Stretching of foreskin

99.96 Collection of sperm for artificial insemination

99.97 Fitting of denture

99.98 Extraction of milk from lactating breast

99.99 Other
Leech therapy

MISCELLANEOUS DIAGNOSTIC AND THERAPEUTIC PROCEDURES (87–99)

PART V

2011 Proposed
Inpatient Procedures

2011 PROPOSED INPATIENT PROCEDURES

The following list is part of the proposed changes to the Hospital Outpatient Prospective Payment System for Calendar Year 2011. Specifically, the file is Addendum E that lists the codes that are only payable as inpatient procedures as displayed at http://www.cms.hhs.gov/HospitalOutpatientPPS/HORD/list.asp#TopOfPage

For the 2011 final updates, see the companion website in December 2010 at: http://codingupdates.com

00176	01636	21155	22224	23332	27178	27536	32036	32851
00192	01638	21159	22226	23472	27181	27540	32095	32852
00211	01652	21160	22318	23900	27185	27556	32100	32853
00214	01654	21179	22319	23920	27187	27557	32110	32854
00215	01656	21180	22325	24900	27222	27558	32120	32855
00452	01756	21182	22326	24920	27226	27580	32124	32856
00474	01990	21183	22327	24930	27227	27590	32140	32900
00524	11004	21184	22328	24931	27228	27591	32141	32905
00540	11005	21188	22532	24940	27232	27592	32150	32906
00542	11006	21194	22533	25900	27236	27596	32151	32940
00546	11008	21196	22534	25905	27240	27598	32160	32997
00560	15756	21247	22548	25915	27244	27645	32200	33015
00561	15757	21255	22554	25920	27245	27646	32215	33020
00562	15758	21268	22556	25924	27248	27702	32220	33025
00567	16036	21343	22558	25927	27253	27703	32225	33030
00580	19271	21344	22585	26551	27254	27712	32310	33031
00604	19272	21346	22590	26553	27258	27715	32320	33050
00622	19305	21347	22595	26554	27259	27724	32402	33120
00632	19306	21348	22600	26556	27268	27725	32440	33130
00670	19361	21366	22610	26992	27269	27727	32442	33140
00792	19364	21422	22630	27005	27280	27880	32445	33141
00794	19367	21423	22632	27025	27282	27881	32480	33202
00796	19368	21431	22800	27030	27284	27882	32482	33203
00802	19369	21432	22802	27036	27286	27886	32484	33236
00844	20661	21433	22804	27054	27290	27888	32486	33237
00846	20664	21435	22808	27070	27295	28800	32488	33238
00848	20802	21436	22810	27071	27303	31225	32491	33243
00864	20805	21510	22812	27075	27365	31230	32500	33250
00865	20808	21615	22818	27076	27445	31290	32501	33251
00866	20816	21616	22819	27077	27447	31291	32503	33254
00868	20824	21620	22830	27078	27448	31360	32504	33255
00882	20827	21627	22840	27090	27450	31365	32540	33256
00904	20838	21630	22841	27091	27454	31367	32650	33257
00908	20930	21632	22842	27120	27455	31368	32651	33258
00932	20931	21705	22843	27122	27457	31370	32652	33259
00934	20936	21740	22844	27125	27465	31375	32653	33261
00936	20937	21750	22845	27130	27466	31380	32654	33265
00944	20938	21810	22846	27132	27468	31382	32655	33266
01140	20955	21825	22847	27134	27470	31390	32656	33300
01150	20956	22010	22848	27137	27472	31395	32657	33305
01212	20957	22015	22849	27138	27477	31584	32658	33310
01214	20962	22110	22850	27140	27485	31587	32659	33315
01232	20969	22112	22852	27146	27486	31725	32660	33320
01234	20970	22114	22855	27147	27487	31760	32661	33321
01272	21045	22116	22856	27151	27488	31766	32662	33322
01274	21141	22206	22857	27156	27495	31770	32663	33330
01402	21142	22207	22861	27158	27506	31775	32664	33332
01404	21143	22208	22862	27161	27507	31780	32665	33335
01442	21145	22210	22864	27165	27511	31781	32800	33400
01444	21146	22212	22865	27170	27513	31786	32810	33401
01486	21147	22214	23200	27175	27514	31800	32815	33403
01502	21151	22216	23210	27176	27519	31805	32820	33404
01634	21154	22220	23220	27177	27535	32035	32850	33405

33406	33610	33824	34804	35363	35634	38747	43326	44005
33410	33611	33840	34805	35371	35636	38765	43330	44010
33411	33612	33845	34806	35372	35637	38770	43331	44015
33412	33615	33851	34808	35390	35638	38780	43340	44020
33413	33617	33852	34812	35400	35642	39000	43341	44021
33414	33619	33853	34813	35450	35645	39010	43350	44025
33415	33641	33860	34820	35452	35646	39200	43351	44050
33416	33645	33861	34825	35454	35647	39220	43352	44055
33417	33647	33863	34826	35456	35650	39499	43360	44110
33420	33660	33864	34830	35480	35651	39501	43361	44111
33422	33665	33870	34831	35481	35654	39502	43400	44120
33425	33670	33875	34832	35482	35656	39503	43401	44121
33426	33675	33877	34833	35483	35661	39520	43405	44125
33427	33676	33880	34834	35501	35663	39530	43410	44126
33430	33677	33881	34900	35506	35665	39531	43415	44127
33460	33681	33883	35001	35508	35666	39540	43425	44128
33463	33684	33884	35002	35509	35671	39541	43460	44130
33464	33688	33886	35005	35510	35681	39545	43496	44132
33465	33690	33889	35013	35511	35682	39560	43500	44133
33468	33692	33891	35021	35512	35683	39561	43501	44135
33470	33694	33910	35022	35515	35691	39599	43502	44136
33471	33697	33915	35045	35516	35693	41130	43520	44137
33472	33702	33916	35081	35518	35694	41135	43605	44139
33474	33710	33917	35082	35521	35695	41140	43610	44140
33475	33720	33920	35091	35522	35697	41145	43611	44141
33476	33722	33922	35092	35523	35700	41150	43620	44143
33478	33724	33924	35102	35525	35701	41153	43621	44144
33496	33726	33925	35103	35526	35721	41155	43622	44145
33500	33730	33926	35111	35531	35741	42426	43631	44146
33501	33732	33930	35112	35533	35800	42845	43632	44147
33502	33735	33933	35121	35535	35820	42894	43633	44150
33503	33736	33935	35122	35536	35840	42953	43634	44151
33504	33737	33940	35131	35537	35870	42961	43635	44155
33505	33750	33944	35132	35538	35901	42971	43640	44156
33506	33755	33945	35141	35539	35905	43045	43641	44157
33507	33762	33960	35142	35540	35907	43100	43644	44158
33510	33764	33961	35151	35548	36660	43101	43645	44160
33511	33766	33967	35152	35549	36822	43107	43770	44187
33512	33767	33968	35182	35551	36823	43108	43771	44188
33513	33768	33970	35189	35556	37140	43112	43772	44202
33514	33770	33971	35211	35558	37145	43113	43773	44203
33516	33771	33973	35216	35560	37160	43116	43774	44204
33517	33774	33974	35221	35563	37180	43117	43775	44205
33518	33775	33975	35241	35565	37181	43118	43800	44210
33519	33776	33976	35246	35566	37182	43121	43810	44211
33521	33777	33977	35251	35570	37616	43122	43820	44212
33522	33778	33978	35271	35571	37617	43123	43825	44227
33523	33779	33979	35276	35583	37618	43124	43832	44300
33530	33780	33980	35281	35585	37660	43135	43840	44310
33533	33781	33981	35301	35587	37788	43279	43843	44314
33534	33782	33982	35302	35600	38100	43281	43845	44316
33535	33783	33983	35303	35601	38101	43282	43846	44320
33536	33786	34001	35304	35606	38102	43300	43847	44322
33542	33788	34051	35305	35612	38115	43305	43848	44345
33545	33800	34151	35306	35616	38380	43310	43850	44346
33548	33802	34401	35311	35621	38381	43312	43855	44602
33572	33803	34451	35331	35623	38382	43313	43860	44603
33600	33813	34502	35341	35626	38562	43314	43865	44604
33602	33814	34800	35351	35631	38564	43320	43880	44605
33606	33820	34802	35355	35632	38724	43324	43881	44615
33608	33822	34803	35361	35633	38746	43325	43882	44620

44625	47125	48153	50320	51575	57545	60521	61536	61686
44626	47130	48154	50323	51580	58140	60522	61537	61690
44640	47133	48155	50325	51585	58146	60540	61538	61692
44650	47135	48400	50327	51590	58150	60545	61539	61697
44660	47136	48500	50328	51595	58152	60600	61540	61698
44661	47140	48510	50329	51596	58180	60605	61541	61700
44680	47141	48520	50340	51597	58200	60650	61542	61702
44700	47142	48540	50360	51800	58210	61105	61543	61703
44715	47143	48545	50365	51820	58240	61107	61544	61705
44720	47144	48547	50370	51840	58267	61108	61545	61708
44721	47145	48548	50380	51841	58275	61120	61546	61710
44800	47146	48551	50400	51865	58280	61140	61548	61711
44820	47147	48552	50405	51900	58285	61150	61550	61735
44850	47300	48554	50500	51920	58293	61151	61552	61750
44899	47350	48556	50520	51925	58400	61154	61556	61751
44900	47360	49000	50525	51940	58410	61156	61557	61760
44960	47361	49002	50526	51960	58520	61210	61558	61850
45110	47362	49010	50540	51980	58540	61250	61559	61860
45111	47380	49020	50545	53415	58548	61253	61563	61863
45112	47381	49040	50546	53448	58605	61304	61564	61864
45113	47400	49060	50547	54125	58611	61305	61566	61867
45114	47420	49062	50548	54130	58700	61312	61567	61868
45116	47425	49203	50600	54135	58720	61313	61570	61870
45119	47460	49204	50605	54390	58740	61314	61571	61875
45120	47480	49205	50610	54411	58750	61315	61575	62005
45121	47550	49215	50620	54417	58752	61316	61576	62010
45123	47570	49220	50630	54430	58760	61320	61580	62100
45126	47600	49255	50650	54650	58822	61321	61581	62115
45130	47605	49425	50660	55605	58825	61322	61582	62116
45135	47610	49428	50700	55650	58940	61323	61583	62117
45136	47612	49605	50715	55801	58943	61332	61584	62120
45395	47620	49606	50722	55810	58950	61333	61585	62121
45397	47700	49610	50725	55812	58951	61340	61586	62140
45400	47701	49611	50728	55815	58952	61343	61590	62141
45402	47711	49900	50740	55821	58953	61345	61591	62142
45540	47712	49904	50750	55831	58954	61440	61592	62143
45550	47715	49905	50760	55840	58956	61450	61595	62145
45562	47720	49906	50770	55842	58957	61458	61596	62146
45563	47721	50010	50780	55845	58958	61460	61597	62147
45800	47740	50040	50782	55862	58960	61470	61598	62148
45805	47741	50045	50783	55865	59120	61480	61600	62161
45820	47760	50060	50785	55866	59121	61490	61601	62162
45825	47765	50065	50800	56630	59130	61500	61605	62163
46705	47780	50070	50810	56631	59135	61501	61606	62164
46710	47785	50075	50815	56632	59136	61510	61607	62165
46712	47800	50100	50820	56633	59140	61512	61608	62180
46715	47801	50120	50825	56634	59325	61514	61609	62190
46716	47802	50125	50830	56637	59350	61516	61610	62192
46730	47900	50130	50840	56640	59514	61517	61611	62200
46735	48000	50135	50845	57110	59525	61518	61612	62201
46740	48001	50205	50860	57111	59620	61519	61613	62220
46742	48020	50220	50900	57112	59830	61520	61615	62223
46744	48100	50225	50920	57270	59850	61521	61616	62256
46746	48105	50230	50930	57280	59851	61522	61618	62258
46748	48120	50234	50940	57296	59852	61524	61619	63043
46751	48140	50236	51525	57305	59855	61526	61624	63044
47010	48145	50240	51530	57307	59856	61530	61630	63050
47015	48146	50250	51550	57308	59857	61531	61635	63051
47100	48148	50280	51555	57311	60254	61533	61680	63077
47120	48150	50290	51565	57531	60270	61534	61682	63078
47122	48152	50300	51570	57540	60505	61535	61684	63081

63082	63191	63272	63302	64760	75959	99476	0095T	G0342
63085	63194	63273	63303	64809	92970	99477	0098T	G0343
63086	63195	63275	63304	64818	92971	99478	0157T	G0406
63087	63196	63276	63305	64866	92975	99479	0158T	G0407
63088	63197	63277	63306	64868	92992	99480	0163T	G0408
63090	63198	63278	63307	65273	92993	0048T	0164T	G0412
63091	63199	63280	63308	69155	99190	0050T	0165T	G0414
63101	63200	63281	63700	69535	99191	0051T	0166T	G0415
63102	63250	63282	63702	69554	99192	0052T	0167T	G0425
63103	63251	63283	63704	69950	99356	0053T	0169T	G0426
63170	63252	63285	63706	75900	99357	0075T	0184T	G0427
63172	63265	63286	63707	75952	99462	0076T	0195T	
63173	63266	63287	63709	75953	99468	0078T	0196T	
63180	63267	63290	63710	75954	99469	0079T	0202T	
63182	63268	63295	63740	75956	99471	0080T	0219T	
63185	63270	63300	64752	75957	99472	0081T	0220T	
63190	63271	63301	64755	75958	99475	0092T	G0341	